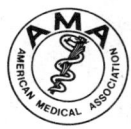

DRUG EVALUATIONS
6th edition

**Prepared by the
American Medical Association
Department of Drugs,
Division of Drugs
and Technology**

In cooperation with the
American Society for
Clinical Pharmacology
and Therapeutics

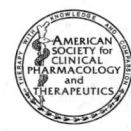

American Medical Association
Chicago, Illinois

First Edition—January 1971
Second Edition—September 1973
Third Edition—March 1977
    Second Printing—August 1977
Fourth Edition—February 1980
    Second Printing—October 1980
    Third Printing—September 1981
    Fourth Printing—February 1982
Fifth Edition—April 1983
    Second Printing—January 1984
    Third Printing—August 1984
    Fourth Printing—February 1985
Sixth Edition—September 1986

Printed in the United States of America

Additional copies may be purchased from:

Book & Pamphlet Fulfillment: OP-255/6
American Medical Association
P.O. Box 10946
Chicago, IL 60610

International Standard Book Number: 0-89970-200-7
Library of Congress Catalog Card Number: 76-9254

HBD: 85-359:60M: 9/86

Preface

Drug Evaluations (DE) is now in its second decade of use, and its original goal is unaltered: To provide physicians and other health care professionals with up-to-date, unbiased information on the *clinical* use of drugs. *DE* is intended to serve as a reference source for practical, comparative, evaluative information on drug therapy.

Evaluative Process for Drug Evaluations (DE): After chapters are prepared by the professional staff of the AMA Department of Drugs on the basis of the current scientific literature, they are reviewed by consultants and the medical staffs of the appropriate pharmaceutical manufacturers. Following consensus revision, the chapters are then reviewed by designees or members of the American Society for Clinical Pharmacology and Therapeutics (ASCPT). For this edition, 512 distinguished consultants contributed their comments to the drafts of the chapters. Thus, this publication is a joint scientific contribution to the field of applied therapeutics by the AMA, a large consultant body, and the ASCPT. The principles of therapeutics and comparative information contained in the introductions to the chapters and the individual drug evaluations that follow thus represent a distillation of the current scientific literature plus the combined wisdom of many experienced clinicians.

Drug evaluations are based upon the most recent information available. Every effort has been made to include information on newly introduced drugs and dosage forms and on significant investigational drugs. In a project of this scope, however, the inadvertent omission of some products and the inclusion of others no longer marketed are inevitable.

The inclusion of a particular drug in *DE* does not imply endorsement by the American Medical Association, nor should it be a criterion for approving use of that drug in any institution. An *evaluation* may be favorable, unfavorable, or both and represents a statement of the general merits of the preparation, not its specific usefulness in a given patient. The limitations of use, adverse reactions, contraindications, precautions, or dosage should be considered for each patient.

The opinions expressed in this book, particularly on controversial matters, may disagree with those from other sources. Statements are based on information from the scientific literature, unpublished data, the advice of consultants, and the opinions of reviewers representing the ASCPT. For other information, for basic data, and even for varying points of view, the physician is encouraged to consult other sources of information on drugs.

Scope and Organization of Drug Evaluations (DE): Like previous editions of *DE*, the sixth edition has been organized into sections and chapters that are based, insofar as possible, on therapeutic classifications. The three initial chapters contain *general information* on therapeutic principles or prescribing practices (ie, prescription practices and regulatory agencies, drug response variation and dosing information, drug interactions and adverse drug reactions).

In most of the remaining chapters, the introductions contain a discussion on the basic pharmacologic information, principles of therapeutics, pathogenesis of disease to the extent deemed necessary to facilitate the use of drugs in patients, and *comparative drug evaluations* within a pharmacologic or therapeutic category. Drug selection is based principally on the severity of the disease or disorder, the pharmacologic profile of each drug, and individual patient considerations. When possible, drugs of choice are recommended within the therapeutic or pharmacologic class. Discussions on the comparative merits of drugs have been expanded considerably for many of the chapters, and the utilization of tables for ready reference continues to increase.

The introductory section of each chapter is followed by *individual drug evaluations*, including selected mixtures. Information on investigational drugs and uses usually appears in the introductory section of the chapter; however, if an investigational drug's approval is deemed likely in the near future, an individual evaluation of the agent may appear. Evaluations on 76 new drugs marketed since the fifth edition and 103 investigational agents and uses have been added to the sixth edition. Listings of these newly marketed and investigational drugs follow the Acknowledgment Section.

Generally, titled headings in the evaluations include *Actions, Uses, Adverse Reactions and Precautions, Pharmacokinetics,* and *Dosage and Preparations.*

Discussion of drug *action* is limited to that deemed necessary to facilitate clinical drug use.

FDA-approved labeling limits the *use* of a drug for purposes of marketing and advertising, but does not constrain a physician's use of the drug in individual patients; therefore, because indications approved for labeling by the FDA may lag behind both the world literature and good medical practice, *DE* describes recognized uses of drugs regardless of their status in approved labeling.

Information on *adverse reactions* and *precautions* usually represents that most essential for use of the drugs. Accordingly, rare, minor, or unconfirmed reactions or precautions that relate to obvious or remote situations are sometimes omitted.

Pharmacokinetic information, especially that in the evaluations, continues to expand. Therapeutic drug blood concentrations are included when relevant.

The *dosage* information cited in *DE* falls within the ranges suggested by manufacturers and the FDA or that considered appropriate by other authorities. For many drugs, however, the correct dosage depends upon the size, age, and condition of the patient; response to treatment; sensitivity or tolerance; and the possible synergistic or antagonistic effect of concomitant medication. If the clinical situation permits, establishment of the dose should be cautious and exploratory unless a wide margin of safety prevails. However, if immediate disaster threatens because of therapeutic failure, treatment should be aggressive. In either situation, the physician should remember that improper dosage of the proper drug is probably as common a cause of inadequate response or therapeutic failure as the use of an improper drug. Accordingly, many doses are stated as ranges, but even the limits of these ranges are not inviolable. The upper limits given for most ranges, however, do suggest that larger amounts either may increase the risks of toxicity beyond what is ordinarily acceptable or may fail to provide a significant degree of additional therapeutic effect. Similarly, the lower limits often indicate that smaller doses will not provide therapeutic effects for most patients. For some drugs, no dosage is suggested.

The *preparations* listed for each drug, including those available generically, appear at the end of each evaluation. However, clinical experience often is limited to products of one or only a few manufacturers. Adequate clinical comparisons of all brands of the same drug are rarely available. For this reason, a valid comparison of brands has rarely been possible or attempted. Although most drugs described in this volume are dispensed exclusively or principally by prescription, many, of course, *can* be sold without prescription and these are so indicated.

The number of *cited* and/or *selected* references at the end of each chapter has increased considerably in the sixth edition. Specific statements in the evaluations often are cited, but general references also may be included for additional information.

The single comprehensive index that includes drug names (both generic and trademark), indications, and adverse reactions has been expanded to improve access to the information in this text.

An important addition to the sixth edition is Chapter 65, Antimicrobial Therapy and Chemoprophylaxis of Infectious Diseases. This initial chapter in the section on Anti-Infective Agents presents an overview of antimicrobial drug therapy and guidelines for drug selection for many common infectious diseases, including specific information on the treatment of sexually transmitted diseases and antimicrobial chemoprophylaxis for ambulatory and surgical patients. Another significant addition is Chapter 57, which furnishes background information and an update on the immune system to aid the physician in the selection and use of immunoreactive substances. These and the many other extensively revised chapters enhance the usefulness of the sixth edition for the practicing physician. The larger size and the new type face also increase the book's readability.

We hope that *DE* will continue to be a valuable reference for the medical profession and others who provide medical care. Suggestions for improving the usefulness of future editions are welcome.

JAMES H. SAMMONS, M.D.
Executive Vice President
American Medical Association

Contents

Acknowledgments

Appreciation is expressed to the following members of the staff of the AMA Department of Drugs, Division of Drugs and Technology, for their assistance in the preparation of this text:

SENIOR SCIENTISTS:

Donald R. Bennett, M.D., Ph.D.
Joseph W. Cranston, Jr., Ph.D.
R. Mark Evans, Ph.D.
Mary Ellen Kosman, Ph.D.
Kenneth F. Lampe, Ph.D.
William T. McGivney, Ph.D.
Barbara F. Murphy, M.S.
Carol M. Proudfit, Ph.D.
Norbert P. Rapoza, Ph.D.
Steven J. Smith, Ph.D.
Ross H. Weaver, Pharm.D.

SPECIAL CONTRIBUTORS:

John C. Ballin, Ph.D.
Steve Rosen, M.D.

EDITORIAL AND TECHNICAL STAFF:

Editor-in-Chief:

Kenneth F. Lampe, Ph.D.

Editors:

Sandra McVeigh
Beverly J. Rodgers

Research Associates:

Daniel R. Lee
Marsha Meyer

Technical Consultants:

Louis G. Schaaf
Donald O. Schiffman, Ph.D.

Technical Associates:

Joaquin Chang
Marilyn A. Krause
Mary Ann McCann
Betty J. Schiller

Technical Assistants:

Hermese J. Bryant
Patti Fitzgerald
Gayle Gregg
Diane Reuter
Beryl Schneiderman

DONALD R. BENNETT, M.D., Ph.D.
Acting Director
Division of Drugs and Technology

Consultants and Reviewers

The AMA Department of Drugs expresses its appreciation to the following individuals for their cooperation and assistance in reviewing the content of this edition of *Drug Evaluations*.

George N. Aagaard, M.D.
Jonathan Abrams, M.D.*
Elias Abrutyn, M.D.*
Louis M. Aledort, M.D.
Joseph S. Alpert, M.D.
Barbara Alving, Major, M.C.
Richard D. Amelar, M.D.
Arthur J. Ammann, M.D.
Douglas R. Anderson, M.D.
Jeffrey L. Anderson, M.D.
Richard L. Anderson, M.D.
Thomas Andrews, M.D.
William C. Andrews, M.D.
Vincent T. Andriole, M.D.*
David F. Archer, M.D.
Alan Askenase, M.D.
Richard H. Aster, M.D.
Arthur J. Atkinson, Jr., M.D.
Robert Austrian, M.D.
Louis V. Avioli, M.D.
Ross J. Baldessarini, M.D.
Robert Allen Barbee, M.D.*
Rachel Barcia-Morse, Ed.M., R.D.
Steven L. Barriere, Pharm.D.*
John G. Bartlett, M.D.*
Doris G. Bartuska, M.D.
Daniel C. Batlle, M.D.
John Baum, M.D.
Jules Baum, M.D.*
Tom Bell, M.D.*
John E. Bennett, M.D.*
William M. Bennett, M.D.
Al B. Benson III, M.D.
Kenneth G. Berge, M.D.
Tomas Berl, M.D.
Cheston M. Berlin, M.D.*
Frederic A. Berry, M.D.
Robert F. Betts, M.D.
Joseph Biederman, M.D.
Jerry G. Blaivas, M.D.*
Abby S. Bloch, M.S., R.D.
Robert E. Bolinger, M.D.
Robert O. Bonow, M.D.
Gerry R. Boss, M.D.
Talmadge A. Bowden, M.D.
George R. Braen, M.D.
George A. Bray, M.D.*
Paul F. Brenner, M.D.
Rubin Bressler, M.D.
Phillip O. Bridenbaugh, M.D.
Mark D. Brown, M.D., Ph.D.
Rex O. Brown, Pharm.D.
Howard A. Buechner, M.D.

Maurice B. Burg, M.D.
W. Arthur Burke, Pharm.D.
Robert P. Burns, M.D.
Maria Bustillo, M.D.
Andrei Calin, M.D.
Donald B. Calne, M.D.
Bruce M. Camitta, M.D.
Mario I. Canedo, M.D.
Paul J. Cannon, M.D.
Steve N. Caritis, M.D.*
Harold E. Carlson, M.D.
William T. Carpenter, Jr., M.D.
Vincent G. Caruso, M.D.
Donald O. Castell, M.D.
Frank B. Cerra, M.D.
Yung-Chi Cheng, Ph.D.
Richard Cheung, Pharm.D.
Ronald A. Chez, M.D.
Anthony W. Chow, M.D.
Robert E. Christensen, M.D.
James C. Cloyd, Pharm.D.
William E. Cobb, M.D.
Richard K. Cochran, M.D.
Jay D. Coffman, M.D.*
David J. Cohen, M.D.
Harry Cohen, M.D.*
Sidney Cohen, M.D.
Jay N. Cohn, M.D.
Ann C. Collier, M.D.
William S. Colucci, M.D.
John P. Conomy, M.D.
Marcel E. Conrad, M.D.
Lawrence Corey, M.D.
James E. Cottrell, M.D.
Benjamin G. Covino, M.D., Ph.D.*
Dr. Denis Craddock
Roy Cronnelly, M.D.
William H. Crosby, Jr., Col, M.C.*
Edward Crum, M.D.
Burke Cunha, M.D.*
Thomas R. Cupps, M.D.*
Donald J. Dalessio, M.D.*
Daniel T. Danahy, M.D.
Mayer B. Davidson, M.D.
Kenneth L. Davis, M.D.
Robert H. Demling, M.D.
Daniel Deykin, M.D.
Seymour Diamond, M.D.
Charles H. Dicken, M.D.
E. Rolland Dickson, M.D.
Joseph T. DiPiro, Pharm.D.*
Robert G. Dluhy, M.D.
W. Edwin Dodson, M.D.

James E. Doherty, M.D.
Daniel B. Drachman, M.D.
Leonard S. Dreifus, M.D.
F. E. Dreifuss, M.B.
Thomas D. Du Bose, Jr., M.D.*
Herbert L. DuPont, M.D.*
Carlos A. Dujovne, M.D.
A.K. Dutt, M.D.
Mervyn J. Eadie, M.D., Ph.D.
Paul Edelson, M.D.
John Edmeads, M.D.
Edmond I. Eger II, M.D.*
George M. Eliopoulos, M.D.
Michael D. Ellis, M.S., R.Ph.
Philip P. Ellis, M.D.*
Mary Allen Engle, M.D.*
Stephen E. Epstein, M.D.
James Ertle, M.D.
David S. Ettinger, M.D.
William E. Evans, Pharm.D.
Gerald A. Faich, M.D.
Constantine J. Falliers, M.D.
Eugene M. Farber, M.D.
Howard S. Farmer, M.D.*
Robert J. Fass, M.D.
Ralph D. Feigin, M.D.
F. Robert Fekety, Jr., M.D.
Robert L. Feldman, M.D.
Mark J. Finch, M.D.
Sydney M. Finegold, M.D.*
Alex E. Finkbeiner, M.D.
Brian G. Firth, M.D.
Thomas J. Fischer, M.D.*
Delbert A. Fisher, M.D.
Nicholas J. Fiumara, M.D.
Walter B. Forman, M.D.
Irving H. Fox, M.D.
Joseph A. Franciosa, M.D.*
S. Douglas Frasier, M.D.*
F.T. Fraunfelder, M.D.
Michael D. Freed, M.D.
Norbert Freinkel, M.D.
Edward D. Freis, M.D.
Arnold P. Friedman, M.D.
Edward D. Frohlich, M.D.
Lawrence A. Frohman, M.D.
Gerhard H. Fromm, M.D.
Koppel I. Furman, M.B.B.Ch.
Daniel Furst, M.D.
J. Lester Gabrilove, M.D.
R. Don Gambrell, Jr., M.D.
S. Samuel Gelbart, M.D.
Alan J. Gelenberg, M.D.
F. John Gennari, M.D.
Marvin C. Gershengorn, M.D.
Samuel Gershon, M.D.
Welton M. Gersony, M.D.*
Milo Gibaldi, Ph.D.*
Ray W. Gifford, Jr., M.D.*

William M. Glazer, M.D.
Charles J. Glueck, M.D.
Neil Goldberg, M.D.
Lewis Goldfrank, M.D.
Richard E. Goldsmith, M.D.
Robert A. Goldstein, M.D., Ph.D.
John F. Goodwin, M.D.
David Y. Graham, M.D.*
W. Morton Grant, M.D.
Robert G. Graw, M.D.
John R. Graybill, M.D.
Paul A. Greenberger, M.D.
David J. Greenblatt, M.D., Ph.D.
Harry L. Greene, M.D.
Tibor J. Greenwalt, M.D.
Roland Griffiths, Ph.D.
Alfred Grindon, M.D.*
Rolf M. Gunnar, M.D.
Theodore Hahn, M.D.
Robert N. Hamburger, M.D.
Lyle H. Hamilton, Ph.D.
Charles B. Hammond, M.D.
Stephen B. Hanauer, M.D.*
H. Hunter Handsfield, M.D.
Philip D. Hansten, Pharm.D.*
Donald C. Harrison, M.D.
Barry Hartman, M.D.
William H. Havener, M.D.
Robert H. Hayashi, M.D.*
Richard H. Helfant, M.D.
Paul Henkind, M.D., Ph.D.
Catherine G. Henry, M.D.
Victor Herbert, M.D., J.D.
William N.P. Herbert, M.D.
Mindy G. Hermann-Zaidins, R.D.
Paul E. Hermans, M.D.
John Hetherington, Jr., M.D.
Michael A. Heymann, M.D.
Margaret W. Hilgartner, M.D.
Alan R. Hinman, M.D.
Martin S. Hirsch, M.D.
Basil I. Hirschowitz, M.D.*
Alan F. Hofmann, M.D.*
William W. Hofmann, M.D.
William J. Holloway, M.D.
Edward W. Holmes, Jr., M.D.
King K. Holmes, M.D., Ph.D.
Jean E. Holt, M.D.
Leonard Horowitz, M.D.
David L. Horwitz, M.D.
H. Dunbar Hoskins, Jr., M.D.*
Walter T. Hughes, M.D.*
Sherwin J. Isenberg, M.D.
George G. Jackson, M.D.
Robert R. Jacobson, M.D., Ph.D.
Henry I. Jacoby, Ph.D.
R.L. Jamison, M.D.
Joseph Jankovic, M.D.
Joseph Jarabak, M.D., Ph.D.

Lissy F. Jarvik, M.D., Ph.D.
Murray E. Jarvik, M.D., Ph.D.
Manucher J. Javid, M.D.
K.N. Jeejeebhoy, M.B.B.S., Ph.D.*
Michael S. Jellinek, M.D.
John W. Jenne, M.D.*
Laverne C. Johnson, Ph.D.
William S. Jordan, Jr., M.D.
Franklyn N. Judson, M.D.
Thomas Kahn, M.D.
Allen B. Kaiser, M.D.*
Mitchell V. Kaminski, M.D.
John M. Kane, M.D.
William B. Kannel, M.D.
George W. Kaplan, M.D.
Harold I. Kaplan, M.D.
Norman M. Kaplan, M.D.
Solomon A. Kaplan, M.D.
Adolf W. Karchmer, M.D.*
John E. Kasik, M.D., Ph.D.*
Michael A. Kass, M.D.
Robert Katzman, M.D.
Ralph E. Kauffman, M.D.*
Herbert E. Kaufman, M.D.
Vincent C. Kelley, M.D.
James P. Kemp, M.D.
Thomas M. Kerkering, M.D.
William R. Keye, Jr., M.D.
Jay S. Keystone, M.D.
Charles Kilo, M.D.
Joseph B. Kirsner, M.D., Ph.D.*
Harold L. Klawans, M.D.
Donald F. Klein, M.D.
Stuart A. Kleit, M.D.
W. Peter Klinke, M.D.
Mark Knepper, M.D.
William Koller, M.D.
Anthony L. Komaroff, M.D.*
Burton I. Korelitz, M.D.
Stephen Kraus, M.D.*
Edward Krenzelok, Pharm.D.
Leslie A. Kuhn, M.D.
Howard E. Kulin, M.D.
Calvin M. Kunin, M.D.*
Peter G. Lacouture, M.S.
James W. Lance, M.D.
Ian R. Lange, M.B., Ch.B.
John Laszlo, M.D.*
Jack L. LeFrock, M.D.
William J. Ledger, M.D.*
Carl V. Leier, M.D.
Ilo E. Leppik, M.D.
Simmons Lessell, M.D.
Donald P. Levine, M.D.*
Joel S. Levine, M.D.*
Norman G. Levinsky, M.D.
Robert I. Levy, M.D.*
Edgar Lichstein, M.D.
Abraham N. Lieberman, M.D.

Theodore W. Lieberman, M.D.
Robert D. Lindeman, M.D.
Robert Lindsay, M.D.
Mortimer B. Lipsett, M.D.
Larry I. Lipshultz, M.D.
R. Bruce Logue, M.D.
Frederick J. Lovejoy, Jr., M.D.
Nicholas J. Lowe, M.D.
A. Harold Lubin, M.D.*
Nicolaos E. Madias, M.D.
Howard I. Maibach, M.D.*
Gerald L. Mandell, M.D.*
Theo C. Manschreck, M.D.
Edward Marut, M.D.
Lois Matsuoka, M.D.
John A. McCulloch, M.D.*
Jon E. McDermed, Pharm.D.
Dale E. McFarlin, M.D.
Marilynne McKay, M.D.
Edwin M. Meares, Jr., M.D.
Wallace B. Mendelson, M.D.
John L. Merritt, M.D.
Walter Mertz, M.D.
John Stirling Meyer, M.D.
Burt R. Meyers, M.D.*
Claude J. Migeon, M.D.
Larry Miller, M.D.
Myron Miller, M.D.*
Richard K. Miller, Ph.D.
John Mills, M.D.
Joel S. Mindel, M.D.
Daniel R. Mishell, Jr., M.D.
John A. Moore, M.D.
Mark Moran, M.D.
Neil C. Moran, M.D.
Edward A. Mortimer, M.D.
Marvin Moser, M.D.
Arnold M. Moses, M.D.
Harry Most, M.D.
Gilbert H. Mudge, M.D.
Hiltrud S. Mueller, M.D.
John F. Mueller, M.D.
Salim K. Mujais, M.D.
Ferid Murad, M.D., Ph.D.
Robert M. Naclerio, M.D.
Donald J. Nalebuff, D.M.D., M.D.
Theodore E. Nash, M.D.*
John D. Nelson, M.D.*
Harold C. Neu, M.D.*
Timothy E. Neufeld, M.D.
Franklin A. Neva, M.D.*
Ronald Lee Nichols, M.D.*
Stuart L. Nightingale, M.D.
Morris Notelovitz, M.D.
Thaddeus S. Nowinski, M.D.
E.J. O'Connell, M.D.
Robert A. O'Reilly, M.D.
Jack Orloff, M.D.
Steven J. Ory, M.D.

John A. Owen, Jr., M.D.
Charles Pak, M.D.
Mark G.A. Palazzo, M.B. Ch.B.
Susan K. Palmer, M.D.
A. Michael Parfitt, M.D.
William W. Parmley, M.D.
Madhu A. Pathak, Ph.D.*
Oglesby Paul, M.D.
David F. Paulson, M.D.
Harold E. Paulus, M.D.
Ronald G. Pearl, M.D.
Kay C. Pearson, R.Ph.
J. Kiffin Penry, M.D.
Mark A. Peppercorn, M.D.*
Robert H. Peter, M.D.
Thomas L. Petty, M.D.
Jeffrey P. Phelan, M.D.
William Edward Pierson, M.D.*
Gayle D. Pinchocofsky-Devin, R.D.
Stanley A. Plotkin, M.D.
Hiram C. Polk, Jr., M.D.
John M. Porter, M.D.
Roger J. Porter, M.D.
William B. Pratt, M.D.*
Irving Pruce, P.D.
Albert W. Pruitt, M.D.
Richard J. Ptachcinski, Pharm.D.
Richard Quintiliani, M.D.
James J. Rahal, M.D.*
Neil H. Raskin, M.D.
James E. Rasmussen, M.D.*
Geoffrey P. Redmond, M.D.
Samuel Refetoff, M.D.
Theobald Reich, M.D.
Marcus M. Reidenberg, M.D.
Michael F. Rein, M.D.*
L. Barth Reller, M.D.
Martin I. Resnick, M.D.*
Stuart Rich, M.D.*
Charles T. Richardson, M.D.*
Karl Rickels, M.D.
B. Lawrence Riggs, M.D.
Jacob Robbins, M.D.*
R.J. Roberts, M.D.
Rose Marie Robertson, M.D.
Henry J. Roenigk, M.D.
Allan R. Ronald, M.D.
Franz W. Rosa, M.D.
Ron G. Rosenfeld, M.D.
Robert L. Rosenfield, M.D.
Lawrence S. Ross, M.D.
Sanford Roth, M.D.
Richard B. Rothenberg, M.D.*
Lewis J. Rubin, M.D.
Lester B. Salans, M.D.
Jeff M. Sands, M.D.
Jay P. Sanford, M.D.
Joel R. Saper, M.D.*
Frank Sasinowski, J.D.

John J. Savarese, M.D.
Michael A. Savin, M.D.
Lawrence Schachner, M.D.*
Julius Schachter, Ph.D.
Anthony J. Schaeffer, M.D.
Irwin J. Schatz, M.D.
Isaac Schiff, M.D.
Stephen C. Schimpff, M.D.
Richard T.F. Schmidt, M.D.
Harold Schulman, M.D.
Alan B. Schwartz, M.D.
Franklin D. Schwartz, M.D.
Gwendolyn Scott, M.D.
Jack E. Sebben, M.D.
Edward M. Sellers, M.D., Ph.D.
Nasrollah T. Shahidi, M.D.
Mona M. Shangold, M.D.
David V. Sheehan, M.D.
Albert L. Sheffer, M.D.
Charles C. Shepard, M.D.
Dean Sheppard, M.D.
Maurice E. Shils, M.D., D.Sc.
Richard L. Shilsky, M.D.
David Shoch, M.D.
Ira Shoulson, M.D.*
Stanford T. Shulman, M.D.*
Joseph A. Sinkule, Pharm.D.
Boris Skurkovich, M.D.
Laurie J. Smith, M.D.
Leon G. Smith, M.D.
Lyman W. Smith, M.D.
Lynwood H. Smith, M.D.
N. Ty Smith, M.D.
R. Brian Smith, M.D.*
Thomas W. Smith, M.D.
Dixie E. Snider, M.D.
James B. Snow, Jr., M.D.
Rebecca Z. Sokol, M.D.
Yung Jai Sohn, M.D.*
Lawrence Solomon, M.D.
L. Paul Sonda, M.D.
Edmund H. Sonnenblick, M.D.
Sheldon L. Spector, M.D.*
Herta Spencer, M.D.
Leon Speroff, M.D.
Bruce V. Stadel, M.D.
Walter E. Stamm, M.D.*
Theodore H. Stanley, M.D.
Walter J. Stark, M.D.
William W. Stead, M.D.
Myron Stein, M.D.
Emanuel M. Steindler, M.S.
Robert K. Stoelting, M.D.
John B. Stokes, M.D.
H. Harlan Stone, M.D.
D. Eugene Strandness, M.D.
Arthur Straughn, Pharm.D.
Stephen E. Strauss, M.D.
Stephen B. Strum, M.D.

New Drugs and Uses Evaluated for Sixth Edition

Drug	Indication/Classification
Acebutolol Hydrochloride [Sectral]	Hypertension/Arrhythmias
Acetohydroxamic Acid [Lithostat]	Urinary calculus inhibitor
Acyclovir [Zovirax]	Antiviral agent, oral
Amdinocillin [Coactin]	Penicillin
Amiodarone Hydrochloride [Cordarone]	Arrhythmias
Ammonium Lactate [Lac-Hydrin]	Dermatologic agent
Amoxicillin/Clavulanate Potassium [Augmentin]	Antibacterial preparation
Amrinone Lactate [Inocor]	Inotropic agent
Atracurium Besylate [Tracrium]	Neuromuscular blocking agent
Auranofin [Ridaura]	Arthritis
Betaxolol Hydrochloride [Betoptic]	Glaucoma
Bitolterol Mesylate [Tornalate]	Bronchodilator
Bromocriptine Mesylate [Parlodel]	Acromegaly
Bumetanide [Bumex]	Diuretic
Buprenorphine Hydrochloride [Buprenex]	Analgesic
Butoconazole Nitrate [Femstat]	Antifungal agent
Cefonicid Sodium [Monocid]	Cephalosporin
Cefotetan Disodium [Cefotan]	Cephalosporin
Ceftazidime [Fortaz, Tazicef, Tazidime]	Cephalosporin
Ceftizoxime Sodium [Cefizox]	Cephalosporin
Ceftriaxone Sodium [Rocephin]	Cephalosporin
Ceforanide [Precef]	Cephalosporin
Cefuroxime Sodium [Zinacef]	Cephalosporin
Cellulose Sodium Phosphate [Calcibind]	Urinary calculus inhibitor
Chenodiol [Chenix]	Gallstone dissolution
Chymopapain [Chymodiactin, Discase]	Herniated lumbar disc
Ciclopirox Olamine [Loprox]	Antifungal agent
Clobetasol Propionate [Temovate]	Corticosteroid, topical
Cromolyn Sodium [Nasalcrom, Intal]	Allergy prophylaxis
Cromolyn Sodium [Opticrom]	Allergy, ocular
Cyclosporine [Sandimmune]	Immunomodulator
Diflorasone Diacetate [Florone, Maxiflor]	Corticosteroid, topical
Digoxin Immune Fab [Digibind]	Allergic rhinitis/Asthma
Dronabinol [Marinol]	Antiemetic
Econazole Nitrate [Spectazole]	Antifungal agent
Enalapril Maleate [Vasotec]	Hypertension/Congestive heart failure
Etomidate [Amidate]	Intravenous anesthetic
Etoposide [VePesid]	Antineoplastic agent
Flecainide Acetate [Tambocor]	Arrhythmias
Glipizide [Glucotrol]	Oral hypoglycemic agent
Glyburide [DiaBeta, Micronase]	Oral hypoglycemic agent
Gonadorelin Hydrochloride [Factrel]	Releasing hormone
Haemophilus B Polysaccharide Vaccine [b CAPSA I, Hib-Immune, HibVax]	Immunologic agent
Hemin for Injection [Panhematin]	Porphyrias
Imipenem/Cilastatin [Primaxin]	Antibacterial preparation
Indapamide [Lozol]	Hypertension/Diuretic
Indomethacin Sodium Trihydrate [Indocin IV]	Patent ductus arteriosus
Interferon, alfa A	Antineoplastic agent

Ketoprofen [Orudis]	Arthritis
Labetalol Hydrochloride [Trandate, Normodyne]	Hypertension
Levobunolol Hydrochloride [Betagan]	Glaucoma
Leuprolide Acetate [Lupron]	Antineoplastic agent
Mexiletine Hydrochloride [Mexitil]	Arrhythmias
Midazolam Hydrochloride [Versed]	Anesthetic induction agent
Monooctanoin [Moctanin]	Gallstone dissolution
Nabilone [Cesamet]	Antiemetic
Naltrexone Hydrochloride [Trexan]	Opioid abuse deterrent
Netilmicin Sulfate [Netromycin]	Aminoglycoside
Nicotine Polacrilex [Nicorette]	Smoking deterrent
Pentamidine Isethionate [Pentam 300]	Antiprotozoal agent
Pentoxifylline [Trental]	Intermittent claudication
Pimozide [Orap]	Tourette's syndrome
Polyethylene Glycol Electrolyte Preparation [Colyte, GoLYTELY]	Laxative preparation
Praziquantel [Biltricide]	Anthelmintic
Quazepam [Dormalin]	Sedative/Hypnotic
Ranitidine Hydrochloride [Zantac]	Peptic ulcer therapy
Ribavirin [Virazole]	Antiviral agent
Somatrem [Protropin]	Human growth hormone
Suprofen [Suprol]	Analgesic
Sufentanil Citrate [Sufenta]	Adjunct to anesthesia
Terfenadine [Seldane]	Antihistamine
Ticarcillin Disodium/Clavulanate Potassium [Timentin]	Antibacterial preparation
Tocainide Hydrochloride [Tonocard]	Arrhythmias
Trientine Hydrochloride [Cuprid]	Chelating agent
Trilostane [Modrastane]	Cushing's syndrome
Vecuronium Bromide [Norcuron]	Neuromuscular blocking agent

Investigational Drugs and Uses Evaluated in Sixth Edition

Drug	Indication/Classification
Acecainide Hydrochloride [NAPA]	Arrhythmias
Aclarubicin	Antineoplastic agent
Acrivastine	Antihistamine
Altretamine (Hexamethylmelamine)	Antineoplastic agent
Aminothiadiazole (A-TDA)	Antineoplastic agent
Amsacrine (m-AMSA) [Amsidyl]	Antineoplastic agent
Astemizole [Hismanal]	Antihistamine
Azacitidine [Mylosar]	Antineoplastic agent
Aziridinylbenzoquinone (A2Q)	Antineoplastic agent
Aztreonam [Azactam]	Antibacterial agent
BCG Vaccine	Immunostimulant
Budesonide [Rhinocort]	Rhinitis/Asthma
Buspirone Hydrochloride [Buspar]	Anxiety
Carboplatin (CBDCA)	Antineoplastic agent
CHIP	Antineoplastic agent
Cholestyramine Resin [Questran]	Hyperoxaluria
Clofazimine [Lamprene]	Leprosy
Compactin (Mevastatin)	Hyperlipidemia
Corynebacterium Parvum (CP)	Immunostimulant
Cyproheptadine Hydrochloride [Periactin]	Cushing's disease
Cytomegalovirus Immune Globulin	Immunologic agent
4-Deoxydoxorubicin (DxDx)	Antineoplastic agent
Dexamethasone, Dexamethasone Sodium Phosphate	Antiemetic (with cancer chemotherapy)
Dialyzable Transfer Factor	Immunostimulant
Difluoromethylornithine (DFMO)	Antineoplastic agent
Domperidone [Motilium]	Antiemetic
Encainide [Enkaid]	Antiarrhythmic agent
Enviroxime	Antiviral agent
Epoprostenol Sodium [Cyclo-Prostin]	Vasodilator/Antithrombotic agent
Ethionamide [Trecator-SC]	Leprosy
Etretinate [Tegison]	Psoriasis
Fenoterol Hydrobromide [Berotec]	Asthma
Fludarabine Phosphate	Antineoplastic agent
Fluocortin Butyl	Rhinitis
Flunitrazepam [Rohypnol]	Anesthetic premedication
Foscarnet Sodium	Antiviral agent
Guanfacine	Hypertension
Haemophilus Influenzae Type b Polysaccharide-Diphtheria Toxoid Conjugate Vaccine (PRP-D)	Immunologic agent
Homoharringtonine	Antineoplastic agent
Ifosamide [Ifex]	Antineoplastic agent
Indoramin Hydrochloride [Baratol]	Hypertension
Inosiplex [Isoprinosine]	Immunostimulant/Antiviral agent
Interferons	Antiviral agent
Interleukin-2	Antineoplastic agent
Ipratropium Bromide [Atrovent]	Asthma/Chronic bronchitis
Isotretinoin [Accutane]	Keratinization disorders/Antineoplastic agent

Ketanserin	Hypertension
Levamisole [Ergamisol]	Immunostimulant
Lidoflazine [Angex]	Angina
Lorazepam [Ativan]	Antiemetic (with cancer chemotherapy)
Lorcainide	Arrhythmias
Menogaril (7-Omen)	Antineoplastic agent
Meptazinol	Analgesic
Methyl-glyoxalbis-guanylhydrazone (MGBG)	Antineoplastic agent
Methylprednisolone Sodium Succinate [Solu-Medrol]	Antiemetic (with cancer chemotherapy)
Metrifonate	Schistosomiasis
Metyrapone Tartrate [Metopirone]	Cushing's syndrome
Mevinolin	Hyperlipidemia
Milrinone	Inotropic drug
Minoxidil [Regaine]	Alopecia
Misoprostol [Cytotec]	Peptic ulcer
Mitolactol (Dibromodulcitol)	Antineoplastic agent
Mitoxantrone Hydrochloride	Antineoplastic agent
Moricizine (Ethmozin) [Ethmozine]	Arrhythmias
Muramyl Dipeptide	Immunostimulant
Muromonab CD3 (Murine Monoclonal Antibody, Anti-CD3) [Orthoclone OKT3]	Immunosuppressant
N-Methylformamide (N-MF)	Antineoplastic agent
Niridazole [Ambilhar]	Schistosomiasis
Norfloxacin [Noroxin]	Antibacterial agent
Oxandrolone [Anavar]	Hyperlipidemia
Oxymetazoline [Oxylin]	Ocular decongestant
PCNU	Antineoplastic agent
Pentostatin [Potentiator]	Antineoplastic agent
Pergolide Mesylate	Parkinson's disease
Pirmenol	Arrhythmias
Potassium Citrate [Urocit-K]	Hyperoxaluria
Praziquantel [Biltricide]	Cestodiasis
Procaterol [Beta-Air]	Asthma
Propafenone [Rytmonorm]	Arrhythmias
Quinidine Gluconate	Malaria
Razoxane	Antineoplastic agent
Recombinant Human Tissue-Type Plasminogen Activator (tPA) [TPA]	Thrombolytic agent
Recombinant Yeast DNA Hepatitis B Vaccine	Immunologic agent
Rifampin [Rifadin, Rimactane]	Leprosy
Rotavirus Vaccine Live Oral Attenuated	Immunologic agent
Selegiline (Deprenyl) [Eldepryl]	Parkinson's disease
Semustine (Methyl CCNU)	Antineoplastic agent
Spirogermanium (NSC) [Spiro 32]	Antineoplastic agent
Suramin Sodium	Onchocerciasis
Tegafur (Ftorafur)	Antineoplastic agent
Teniposide (VM-26)	Antineoplastic agent
Terazosin Hydrochloride [Vasocard]	Hypertension
Tetrabenazine [Nitoman]	Extrapyramidal movement disorders
Thymic Hormones	Immunostimulants
Thymoxamine Hydrochloride	Alpha blocker, ophthalmic
Tiopronin [Thiola]	Cystinuria
Trimazosin [Cardovar]	Hypertension
Typhoid Vaccine Live Oral	Immunologic agent
Ursodeoxycholic Acid	Gallstone dissolving agent
Varicella-Zoster Vaccine Live Attenuated	Immunologic agent
Verapamil Hydrochloride [Calan, Isoptin]	Migraine headache
Vindesine Sulfate [Eldisine]	Antineoplastic agent
Zoladex	Antineoplastic agent

Prescription Practices and Regulatory Agencies

PRESCRIPTION PRACTICES

The prescription of a drug represents the culmination of a deliberative process between physician and patient aimed at the prevention, amelioration, or elimination of a disease or disorder. This deliberation requires that the physician understand a broad spectrum of scientific and psychosocial issues germane to the success of treatment. Following is a discussion of ways in which good prescription practices enhance a drug's efficacy and minimize misuse and abuse.

PATIENT MEDICATION INSTRUCTIONS. The American Medical Association-Patient Medication Instruction (AMA-PMI) program, initiated in 1982, provides physicians with easy to understand written information about widely used prescription drugs for distribution to their patients. These supplementary instructions present a balanced summary of the anticipated benefits and possible risks of the prescribed drug. The information is intended to augment, but not replace, the oral communication that should take place between the physician and the patient.

The Patient Medication Instruction sheet describes the uses of the prescribed drug or drug class. It includes background information that the patient should make known to the physician to facilitate selection of the optimal treatment regimen. Instructions for the proper use of the drug, as well as precau-

tions that the patient should be aware of are also specified. Finally, common documented side effects that may be anticipated are listed, as are more serious reactions that require notification of the physician and possibly discontinuation of the drug.

The Patient Medication Instruction program is intended to reinforce the importance of informing patients about their medications and instructing them in proper use. These supplementary written instructions enhance the physician's capacity to accomplish these two goals, thereby improving the effectiveness of drug therapy, reducing the risk of adverse reactions or improper use of the drugs, and reinforcing the physician-patient relationship. Patient Medication Instruction sheets can be obtained from the American Medical Association, 535 N Dearborn St, Chicago, IL 60610.

PATIENT CONTAINER LABEL. The American Medical Association encourages physicians to include the direction, "label as such," "l.a.s.," or merely "label" on the prescription. Exceptions should be made only when such disclosures are inadvisable for psychological reasons or detrimental to the welfare of the patient.

Numerous reasons exist for including the name and strength of a prescription drug on the container label. Container label information (1) helps to fulfill the right of the patient to be informed about the medications prescribed; (2) minimizes mistaken ingestion and may be lifesaving in accidental poisoning or overdose by providing immediate identification of the drug; (3) is of value when the patient has multiple attending physicians or moves to another locality; (4) identifies the drug for patients who have allergies or for those who develop an allergic reaction while taking the medication; and (5) alerts those given a prescription for a product on which a warning is subsequently issued.

COMPLIANCE. Strict adherence to a prescribed treatment plan is defined as compliance. Once the proper diagnosis, selection of drug therapy, dosage, and schedule and duration of administration have been determined, much of the responsibility for success of treatment falls upon the patient. The physician can influence the extent of compliance, however. Compliance is reported to be approximately 75% for short-term therapy but only 50% for long-term treatment (Sackett, 1980). Thus, the physician often overestimates the degree to which a patient is following the prescribed regimen (Roth and Caron, 1978). Recognition of the probability of noncompliance, especially during prolonged treatment, is a significant step toward improving compliance. Objective evidence of inadequate intake (eg, pill counts, blood drug concentration) is the only conclusive proof of noncompliance; lack of response to treatment and/or lack of side effects are only suggestive (Peck, 1980). Equally critical to compliance is a good physician-patient relationship. The patient's perception of the severity of the disorder and the efficacy of the prescribed treatment may be derived primarily from interaction with the physician (Solomon, 1980).

Studies have not determined the characteristics that identify patients unlikely to comply. Simplification of the drug regimen, patient education (eg, American Medical Association-Patient Medication Instruction program), parenteral therapy administered by medical personnel, and hospitalization improve compliance. Telephone calls to patients, home visits by nursing personnel, convenient packaging of medication, and monitoring of serum drug levels with positive feedback (eg, praise) also are beneficial (Peck, 1980).

Rapidly metabolized or excreted drugs whose effects must be maintained steadily for prolonged periods must be administered repeatedly at short intervals. Therefore, their use in timed-release form can simplify a drug regimen and thus improve compliance—*provided the medication is actually delivered in the even, measured manner that is intended.* On the other hand, the use of timed-release preparations of drugs with inherently long half-lives generally is not warranted. However, for patients who eliminate these drugs rapidly, a timed-release preparation may be useful if an effective plasma concentration can be maintained.

Mixtures (combination drugs) also can simplify a drug regimen by decreasing the number of medications that must be ingested. Thus, mixtures, like timed-release preparations, would be expected to improve compliance.

Finally, cost is a significant factor in compliance for some patients.

PRESCRIPTION COST. The physician's primary concern in prescribing a drug is the most expedient resolution of the patient's problem. Concern for expediency, however, should not preclude consideration of cost.

Generic Substitution: A generic drug is one that is no longer the exclusive property of the pharmaceutical company that developed it. The company that developed the drug may have marketed it exclusively for the life of the patent and/or cross-licensed other companies to manufacture and market the drug under the same or a different trademark. Following expiration of the patent, the drug can be marketed generically by a firm that fulfills the Food and Drug Administration's requirements for the proper manufacture and interstate marketing of a prescription drug product.

Every state has enacted legislation that permits, encourages, or even requires the substitution of a less costly generic equivalent for a more expensive drug that may have been prescribed. However, even in states with mandatory substitution laws, the physician can prohibit substitution. Many states also have compiled lists of acceptable (positive formulary) and unacceptable (negative formulary) drug product substitutions.

Concern about substitution of a generic for a trademark drug involves two basic questions: (1) Is the bioavailability of the generic drug equal to that of its trademark counterpart? (2) If so, will the patient benefit financially from use of the generic drug?

Nonequivalent bioavailability is a concern only when drug efficacy is altered. Altered efficacy may be manifested as therapeutic failure, diminished or enhanced therapeutic effect, or toxicity, although it is difficult to establish causality. Failure to recognize the reason for the altered patient response may result in improper diagnosis following patient re-evaluation. The problem may be further compounded if the pharmacist refills the prescription with the pioneer (trademark) product of known action or with a generic product that differs from both the original generic product dispensed and the pioneer product (Chodos, 1980). Many physicians assume that the company most experienced in producing a drug provides the preparation with the most consistent bioavailability. However, bioavailability for each drug product can be resolved only in controlled clinical studies. This information is often unavailable or may not be relevant for an individual patient.

The intent of state legislatures in enacting drug substitution laws was to pass on to the patient any savings that might accrue to the pharmacist as a result of competitive pricing, less complex inventories, and price reduction on bulk purchasing. Although patients can benefit financially from the prescription of a generic drug, the amount of money saved has varied from nothing to substantial sums (Horvitz, 1980).

In the final analysis, the drug that consistently provides the optimal therapeutic effect should be selected. An alternative to a proven drug, whether trademark or generic, should be prescribed only after careful consideration of the potential risks and benefits of substitution.

The sixth edition of FDA's *Approved Drug Products With Therapeutic Equivalency Evaluations*, published in October, 1985, lists currently marketed drug products that have been approved for safety and effectiveness. The list includes both prescription and OTC products with approved New Drug Applications, as well as approved blood and blood products. The annual publication is updated monthly by cumulative supplements. Therapeutic equivalence evaluations are provided for multisource products. Prepared as a cost containment aid to large purchasers of pharmaceuticals, the list is of value to community and hospital pharmacists seeking to determine whether a given drug product has been approved by the FDA. It enables prescribers and dispensers to determine if a generic drug is therapeutically equivalent to the reference drug.

Approved Drug Products With Therapeutic Equivalence Evaluations (ed 6) and cumulative supplements through January, 1987, can be obtained from the Superintendent of Documents, U.S. Government Printing Office, Washington, DC 20402 at a cost of $103.00 ($128.75 for foreign subscriptions).

Mixtures: Another suggestion for reducing the cost of drug therapy is the prescription of combination drug products, ie, a single preparation containing two or more active ingredients in a fixed ratio in which each ingredient contributes to overall therapeutic effectiveness. As with generic substitution, the selection of a mixture in preference to individual drugs is often controversial.

The purported advantages of a mixture are enhanced therapeutic effect, decreased potential for adverse reactions, and reduced cost (Weintraub, 1981). The therapeutic effect may be enhanced by synergism (eg, trimethoprim/sulfamethoxazole [Bactrim, Septra]), by improved efficacy of the primary ingredient (eg, levodopa/carbidopa [Sinemet]), or by improved patient compliance (ie, smaller number of medications). Adverse effects may be diminished by inclusion of a drug that antagonizes the undesirable effects of the primary agent (eg, isoniazid/pyridoxine). Cost should be reduced all along the producer-to-consumer chain, since only one medication must be handled (*Drug Ther Bull*, 1980).

Criticisms of selected mixtures include inflexibility of dosage ratio, inclusion of a low-potency drug(s) that contributes only marginally if at all to the therapeutic effect, or inclusion of an ingredient(s) that actually impairs the effectiveness of the primary ingredient (MacCannell and Giraud, 1980). In its Combination Drug Policy, the Food and Drug Administration requires that each component of a mixture contribute to the claimed therapeutic effects or, alternatively, that the added component enhance the safety or efficacy of the principal component or minimize its potential for abuse.

It is critical that the physician be aware of all active ingredients in a mixture, their indications, and their concentrations. Mixtures should be prescribed only if all of the active ingredients contribute significantly to the desired therapeutic effect and thus reduce patient discomfort, cost, and noncompliance.

Other Cost Factors: The amount and form cited on the prescription, the choice of pharmacy, and the judicious use of drugs for symptomatic relief are factors that can be manipulated to minimize the cost of drug therapy (Chilton, 1981). If a drug must be taken for a prolonged period, the correct dosage has been established, and the patient can be trusted to follow instructions properly, a prescription for a large quantity is often more economical than repeated prescriptions or refills for small quantities.

Physicians are urged to become informed about the quality and purity of drug products available from multiple sources and to supplement medical considerations with cost considerations when selecting the drug of choice for an individual patient.

The price of a particular drug can vary greatly from pharma-

cy to pharmacy. If an expensive product or prolonged therapy is required, the physician might suggest a pharmacy that dispenses the drug at a more reasonable price while maintaining the quality of its service. The relative cost to consumers charged by pharmacies can be determined by comparing their prices for one or more commonly used drugs (Chilton, 1981). Pharmacy and Therapeutics committees of local hospitals—which often base their review of products for inclusion in the hospital's formulary on reports in the literature, experiences of local physicians, availability, and cost in their region—also are valuable sources of information and guidance.

Finally, careful prescribing practices, including utilization of measures other than drug therapy to achieve symptomatic relief, can reduce the overall cost of treatment. Nondrug therapy is not always easily accomplished, however, because some patients consider the prescription of a drug to be the most tangible evidence of a meaningful interaction with the physician.

REFILLS. Refills for certain drugs are regulated by federal and state controlled substances acts (see the section on Controlled Substances). Prescriptions for all other drugs remain valid indefinitely if marked "refill prn," unless state law directs otherwise. However, an open-ended authorization for refills is usually not advisable. Limiting the number of refills allows the physician to monitor the patient's course of illness periodically, which is particularly important during long-term therapy to detect intolerance, tolerance, and drug interactions. After individual response variation and appropriate dosage have been determined, the number of refills may be increased for the patient's convenience.

ACCIDENTAL POISONING. An additional matter pertaining to almost any drug prescribed for administration at home is the possibility of accidental poisoning. The physician's control over this hazard is limited, but patients can at least be cautioned against having drugs accessible to young children.

The Poison Prevention Packaging Act (PPPA) requires that prescription drugs be dispensed in containers that meet child protection packaging standards. The purpose of this law is to protect against accidental poisoning of children because of easy access to unattended drug products. The PPPA applies to drugs dispensed both by the pharmacist and physician. The law does allow conventional packaging at the consumer's request or direction of the prescribing physician. This does not, however, exempt drugs dispensed by the physician from the provisions of the law, but rather allows the physician to determine whether childproof packaging is necessary for a particular patient.

Improper Prescription Practices

Societal concern with undermedication (underprescribing), overmedication (overprescribing), and drug abuse often is a significant factor in drug selection. When these concerns are pertinent, the physician must adopt the most effective therapeutic regimen, adapt it to the needs of the patient, and assure the treatment's conformity with the best interest of society as a whole.

The following discussion addresses ways in which good

prescription practices minimize the occurrence and thus the negative impact of these three issues. Ironically, these concerns have become prominent because of the large number of highly specific and effective therapeutic agents developed during the past three decades. The availability of these drugs has instilled high expectations in the general public. Improvements in diagnostic capability have expanded the array and increased the complexity of disease states that are presented to the physician for successful resolution.

Undermedication occurs when the patient fails to receive adequate drug therapy (Morgan, 1980). *Overmedication* is the unjustified or inappropriate use of a drug. The prescription of a drug is deemed unjustified when there is no proper indication for its use or when administration continues despite proven ineffectiveness or the achievement of the therapeutic goal. The use of a drug may be considered inappropriate when more effective or less hazardous drugs are available, when the dosage or duration of administration is excessive, or when a mixture is used and only one of the components is indicated. *Drug abuse* is the use of a drug, usually by self-administration, in a manner that deviates from the approved medical, legal, and social standards (Jaffe, 1980).

The prescription of psychotropic drugs is subject to federal and state regulation of controlled substances and is usually the focal point for discussion of good prescribing practices and appropriate drug therapy. The symptomatology of a disease state characterized by pain and/or psychic dysfunction is among the most difficult to categorize, quantify, establish causation for, and treat. The genuine mental suffering communicated by the patient is often totally subjective and provides few or no objective criteria to determine a rational treatment plan. The availability of a vast arsenal of psychotropic drugs to relieve such symptoms has been invaluable but also has resulted in many instances of undermedication, overmedication, and, especially, drug abuse.

Undermedication: Concern about the potential abuse of psychotropic agents traditionally has centered on the potent opioid analgesics, such as morphine. However, the negative impact of excessive concern about psychological and/or physical dependence is revealed by reports that the severe chronic pain accompanying terminal cancer is often inadequately treated. Potent analgesics, particularly opioids, are indicated for the sometimes excruciating pain of terminal cancer, and physicians should not hesitate to use them in these patients.

Inadequate pain relief with opioid analgesics is not limited to patients with terminal cancer. One study of opioid use in two New York teaching hospitals reported that, of 37 patients interviewed, 32% remained in severe distress and 41% in moderate distress despite administration of an opioid analgesic, usually meperidine (Marks and Sachar, 1973). The dosages prescribed were lower than those usually recommended and all patients received smaller amounts than were ordered.

Relief of suffering is a legitimate goal of medical practice. Failure to provide such relief may result from timidity ("pharmacophobia") (Symmers, 1973), incorrect or downgraded diagnosis, or lack of knowledge or faith in the value of a controversial drug, even when its administration is indicated. Patients may fail to comply or to convey the severity of their symptoms to the physician (Weintraub, 1981). Thus, the factors contributing to undermedication are diverse and disparate and span the fields of medicine, psychology, economics, and sociology. Society's genuine concern for the medical well being of the general population notwithstanding, drug therapy most effectively satisfies the emotional and physical needs of the individual patient when it evolves from close interaction and thorough discussion between physician and patient.

Overmedication: The enormous increase in the therapeutic use of psychotropic drugs should be viewed as generally positive. The development of benzodiazepines, such as diazepam and chlordiazepoxide, has provided more effective, less toxic alternatives to phenobarbital and meprobamate for the treatment of anxiety. However, criticism of the widespread use of these agents is sometimes justified. Drug therapy was never intended to be a panacea for the normal trials and tribulations of human existence. In most cases, the resolution of temporary difficulties without the use of drugs encourages the future successful and rewarding fulfillment of an individual's role in society. Treatment with benzodiazepines in such instances is of little or no benefit and constitutes overmedication. In contrast, when anxiety disorders impair normal function, a benzodiazepine may be warranted to achieve symptomatic relief. However, this therapeutic strategy should be selected only after consideration of (1) the most likely diagnosis to ensure the proper choice among antianxiety, antidepressant, antipsychotic, and hypnotic drugs; (2) the concomitant use of nonpharmacologic techniques to augment symptomatic relief and optimize drug requirements; and (3) the characteristics of the anxiety state to be treated (eg, chronic and persistent or infrequent and transient) to determine the optimum duration of therapy (Rosenbaum, 1982).

It can be concluded from extensive studies that irresponsible overprescription of benzodiazepines is infrequent and that these agents are exceptionally effective and safe for a broad spectrum of debilitating conditions ranging from anxiety to seizure disorders (Mellinger et al, 1978). Nevertheless, even the infrequent instance of irresponsible or unwitting misprescription of these drugs warrants increased sensitization and education in this area.

Drug Abuse: The issues of drug abuse and overmedication are often inextricably related. Acquisition of prescription drugs for purposes of abuse can occur by either illicit or licit means. The illicit mode has many variations, including prescription "kiting" (eg, alteration of written prescriptions), theft and forgery of prescription blanks, and thefts of drugs from manufacturers, wholesalers, pharmacies, and physicians' offices. The smuggling of drugs into the United States and the clandestine manufacture of drugs within this country are important illegal sources of otherwise legal medication, but federal officials estimate that more than 90% of diverted drugs are obtained at the retail level (ie, from individual pharmacies and physicians). In such cases, prescription drug abuse is synonymous with overmedication and may take any of the following forms (Council on Scientific Affairs, American Medical Association, 1982):

1. The willful and conscious misprescribing of controlled substances by physicians for abuse purposes, usually for

profit. These are the "script" doctors. Physicians responsible for this type of prescribing should be prosecuted to the full extent of the law.

2. Inappropriate prescribing by physicians who unwittingly acquiesce to insistent demands by patients for medication. These are "duped doctors." Drugs usually are prescribed in excessive amounts or for longer periods than necessary, which may initiate or perpetuate drug abuse or dependence or divert the drug to other persons for abuse purposes.

3. Uninformed prescribing by physicians who have not kept abreast of new developments in pharmacology and drug therapy. These are the "dated doctors." In addition to prescribing drugs in excessive quantities or for excessive periods, these physicians prescribe drugs for conditions that do not warrant such therapy or that might be better treated by other drugs.

4. Self-prescribing and administration by physicians who abuse or are dependent on drugs. These are "impaired doctors" who need treatment. Rehabilitation and disciplinary programs already exist in most states through medical societies and boards of medical examiners.

Iatrogenic drug abuse and dependence are adverse reactions every physician should seek to avoid (Lewis, 1974). To do so, the physician must guard against injudicious prescribing practices and avoid acquiescing to the demands of patients for instant chemical solutions to their problems. The physician should convey to patients through attitude and manner that drugs, no matter how helpful, are only one part of an overall plan of treatment and management. In essence, a preventive role can be played by the physician who exercises good judgment in administering and prescribing psychotropic drugs so that diversion to illicit use is averted and drug dependence is minimized or prevented.

Psychotropic drugs likely to be abused are subject to the Controlled Substances Act (Title II of the Federal Comprehensive Drug Abuse Prevention and Control Act of 1970) and include the drug classes outlined below.

Prescribing Controlled Psychotropic Drugs

ABUSE POTENTIAL AND DEPENDENCE LIABILITY. The major risk associated with a psychotropic drug is that a patient may feel compelled to continue experiencing the drug's reinforcing effects after the medical indications for its use have disappeared. Such compulsive use constitutes psychological dependence upon the drug. Tolerance characteristically develops and larger doses are necessary to achieve the same desired effects. Chronic self-administration of increasing doses often alters the normal physiologic state to such an extent that the abuser has become physically dependent upon the continuous use of the drug to prevent withdrawal symptoms, which range in severity from unpleasant (eg, insomnia) to life-threatening (eg, seizures).

The following is a brief discussion of the proper indications, abuse potential, and dependence liability of the major classes of controlled narcotic and psychotropic drugs. Included are the opioids, the antianxiety and hypnotic agents, and the central nervous system stimulants. More detailed information on the

benefits and risks associated with these drugs is presented in Chapters 4, 5, and 8 of this volume and in the AMA's handbook, *Drug Abuse: A Guide for the Primary Care Physician* (Wilford, 1981).

Opioids: Morphine and morphine-like drugs, such as codeine, have legitimate clinical usefulness, and the physician should not hesitate to prescribe them when indicated for patients who require analgesia or symptomatic relief not provided by nonopioid analgesics. The administration of these drugs is warranted to relieve moderate to severe pain (both acute and chronic) and, more specifically, the pain of terminal cancer; postoperative pain; severe pain associated with biliary, renal, or ureteral colic; pain of acute myocardial infarction; preoperative medication in anesthesia; certain forms of dyspnea; diarrhea; and insomnia due to pain or cough.

Ordinarily, opioids should be given in the smallest effective dose as infrequently as possible to minimize *tolerance and physical dependence*. This is particularly true when treating chronic diseases or conditions that might lead to drug abuse. The development of tolerance with prolonged use of opioids varies from patient to patient; some patients appear to develop little tolerance to the effects of these drugs, whereas others require increasing doses. An expressed need by the patient for an increased amount, therefore, should be evaluated in relation to the clinical situation to determine if the request is caused by worsening of pain, development of tolerance, or by anxiety.

The fact that these drugs have actions other than analgesia (eg, euphoria, relief of anxiety, sedation) also may lead to abuse. Such responses should be recognized and use of the drug monitored. Most patients given a morphine-like drug to relieve pain for longer than just a brief period are able to discontinue it without difficulty, even though they have developed mild physical dependence. A careful history aids in determining which patients must be followed closely.

Special attention should be given to patients with morphine-type drug dependence or a history of such dependence who also have other medical or surgical problems. If there is a genuine symptomatic need confirmed by adequate diagnostic evaluation and if other analgesics or nondrug therapy for pain are ineffective or impractical, it is the physician's responsibility to prescribe opioid analgesics as he would for any other patient. The physician must, however, remain constantly alert to certain considerations: (1) the patient may be simulating a disease in order to obtain a dependence-producing drug; (2) the effective dose level will vary, depending upon the degree of tolerance; and (3) abrupt discontinuation can precipitate a withdrawal syndrome increasing morbidity or causing death if the patient with an established dependence on a morphine-like drug undergoes major medical or surgical trauma. Drug dependence can be maintained until the patient begins to recover from the other illness. A regimen of gradual withdrawal should then be considered.

Antianxiety and Hypnotic Agents: The benzodiazepines, barbiturates, and other antianxiety and hypnotic agents depress the central nervous system to varying degrees. Although the specific indications for the benzodiazepines and barbiturates vary, their principal use is to relieve anxiety and/or insomnia. Other indications for some drugs in these categories include preanesthetic medication and seizure disorders. Drugs that are neither benzodiazepines nor barbiturates but that possess hypnotic activity as well as abuse potential and dependence liability include chloral hydrate, ethchlorvynol, ethinamate, glutethimide, and methyprylon. Meprobamate is a nonbenzodiazepine, nonbarbiturate drug with antianxiety action, abuse potential, and dependence liability. All of the above drugs are classified under the Controlled Substances Act.

The benzodiazepines are usually the drugs of choice when antianxiety and hypnotic activities are required because of their superior benefit/risk ratio. However, even the benzodiazepines are not recommended for trivial or minor distress or discomfort. Counseling is a more satisfactory therapeutic strategy in these instances. Even in moderate to severe disorders of this type, the physician initially should attempt to diagnose and treat the underlying disorders rather than rely on these drugs for symptomatic relief.

Prolonged use of the barbiturates may produce tolerance and psychological and/or physical dependence. The shorter acting barbiturates (secobarbital, amobarbital, and pentobarbital) have a greater abuse potential because of their rapid onset of action and the comparatively high intensity of their psychoactive effects. The longer acting barbiturates, phenobarbital and butabarbital, are absorbed slowly and do not penetrate the brain as readily, which probably account for their failure to produce the "high" sought by those who take drugs for recreational purposes. The shorter acting barbiturates are classified in Schedule II of the Controlled Substances Act, and the longer acting barbiturates are listed under Schedules III and IV. Because nonbarbiturate-nonbenzodiazepine hypnotics also have a high abuse potential, substituting one of these drugs for a barbiturate does not necessarily reduce the risk of drug dependence.

Abrupt withdrawal in a person with established physical dependence of the barbiturate type is followed in two or three days by an abstinence syndrome that usually is more severe than that produced by opioids. Convulsions, delirium, fever, and even coma and death may result. When physical dependence on a nonbenzodiazepine hypnotic is suspected, substitution of phenobarbital with gradual reduction of dosage is preferred to the benzodiazepines for withdrawal.

Long-term administration of benzodiazepines or meprobamate also may cause physical dependence. Symptoms are similar to those produced by chronic intoxication with barbiturates or alcohol. Withdrawal reactions may develop if the drug is discontinued abruptly. These reactions are similar to those produced by barbiturate withdrawal and may appear within 36 hours to one week, depending upon the drug's half-life and whether or not it is converted to an active metabolite. To avoid withdrawal reactions, the dosage of these drugs should be reduced gradually. Because dependence occurs, although relatively infrequently, these drugs are classified in Schedule IV.

Amphetamines and Other Stimulants: Amphetamines and several chemically related drugs are central nervous system stimulants. Small doses give the user a feeling of increased mental alertness and a sense of well being. As doses are increased, apprehension, decreased appetite, volubility, tremor, and excitement occur. Because tolerance and psychological dependence can develop rather quickly with large doses, the physician should prescribe amphetamines and other stimulants only for a limited time for a specific purpose.

The major medical uses of central nervous system stimulants, such as amphetamines and methylphenidate, are attention deficit disorder and narcolepsy. Amphetamines also have been widely used as anorexiants; however, because their efficacy over a long period has not been demonstrated and because of their high abuse potential, this use is not advocated. Also, the use of amphetamines to allay fatigue is unjustifiable except under extraordinary circumstances, for they serve only to impel the user to a greater expenditure of his own resources, sometimes to a hazardous point of fatigue of which he is not aware.

The administration of stimulants to alcohol- and barbiturate-dependent individuals is not appropriate, because such use can induce the patient to take increasing amounts of depressant drugs. Amphetamine-type drugs also are contraindicated in other dependence-prone individuals.

Polydrug abuse is common. "Uppers" in the morning with "downers" at bedtime is one abuse pattern of the polydrug type, as is the concurrent use of amphetamines with heroin or cocaine. In fact, problems associated with the depressant drug may bring the patient to the physician's attention and mask stimulant abuse.

The combined stimulant and euphoric effects of cocaine makes it the fastest growing form of drug abuse today, but its medical use is limited to topical anesthesia of the eye, nose, and oropharynx. There is considerable evidence that tolerance, profound psychological dependence, and perhaps physical dependence develop.

Amphetamine-type drugs were in widespread use before their dependence liability was recognized; as a result, several countries experienced epidemics of stimulant abuse. The drug of choice for abusers often is an amphetamine, but methylphenidate or another stimulant is often substituted when the preferred drug is not readily available. The chosen route of administration may be oral or intravenous. Under the Controlled Substances Act of 1970, amphetamines, phenmetrazine, and methylphenidate are included in Schedule II; other stimulant-anorexiants are classed as Schedule III or IV drugs. In addition, numerous states have adopted legislation or regulations restricting the prescribing of amphetamines to very narrow indications—usually only narcolepsy and attention deficit disorder.

The physician who prescribes stimulants for any indication must always be alert to their dependence liability and recognize that some patients may seek other sources of supply, either illegally or from another physician. There also is the danger that the efficacy of a stimulant in helping a person achieve a time-limited goal may predispose that person to regard amphetamine-type drugs as being desirable rather than potentially dangerous substances and thus may encourage future abuse. Dependence-prone persons who have been introduced to stimulants as anorexiants or to combat fatigue or depression can become chronic abusers.

Stimulant abuse can cause three types of medical problems: (1) medical complications associated with drug effects (eg, exacerbation of hypertension, arrhythmias, stroke, retinal damage due to intense vasospasm) or with drug administration (eg, septicemia and endocarditis from unclean needles); (2) emergency conditions, such as acute amphetamine psychosis, or hyperthermia and convulsions arising from use of toxic doses; and (3) signs and symptoms during the abstinence period following regular use that indicate drug dependence.

CONTROLLED SUBSTANCES ACT. The Controlled Substances Act (Title II of the Federal Comprehensive Drug Abuse Prevention and Control Act· of 1970) is designed to improve regulation of the manufacturing, distribution, and dispensing of controlled substances by providing a "closed" system for legitimate handlers of these drugs. If not specifically exempted, every person who manufactures, distributes, prescribes, administers, or dispenses any controlled substance must register annually with the Attorney General. Accurate records of drugs purchased, distributed, and dispensed must be maintained and kept on file for two years by all persons who regularly dispense and charge for controlled substances in the course of their practice.

Each drug or substance subject to control is assigned to one of five schedules depending upon the potential for abuse, medical usefulness, and degree of dependence if abused. The five schedules and the drugs included in them follow:

Schedule I: Drugs and other substances having a high potential for abuse and no current accepted medical usefulness. Included are certain opium derivatives (eg, heroin), some synthetic opioids (eg, alpha-methylfentanyl), and hallucinogens (eg, LSD).

Schedule II: Drugs having a high potential for abuse and accepted medical usefulness; abuse leads to severe psychological or physical dependence. In general, drugs in this schedule were previously controlled under the Narcotic Acts (eg, opium and derivatives, other opioids, cocaine). Stimulants, such as amphetamine and related compounds, and the short-acting barbiturates also are in this schedule.

Schedule III: Drugs having less abuse potential and accepted medical usefulness; abuse leads to moderate dependence. Included in this schedule are certain stimulants and depressants (eg, barbiturates not included in other schedules), as well as preparations containing limited quantities of certain opioid drugs.

Schedule IV: Drugs having a low abuse potential, accepted medical usefulness, and limited dependence. Included in this schedule are certain depressants not in another schedule (eg, chloral hydrate, phenobarbital, the benzodiazepines).

Schedule V: Drugs, including a few over-the-counter preparations, having a low abuse potential, accepted medical usefulness, and limited dependence. Mixtures containing limited quantities of opioids with nonopioid drugs are included in this schedule.

The Act also provides that no prescription order for drugs in Schedule II can be renewed. Emergency telephone prescriptions for drugs in this schedule may be dispensed if the practitioner furnishes a written, signed prescription order to the pharmacy within 72 hours and limits the amount to that needed during the emergency period. Prescription orders for drugs in Schedules III and IV may be redispensed up to five times within six months after the date of issue if authorized by the prescriber. Prescription orders for Schedule V drugs may be redispensed only as expressly authorized by the practitioner on the prescription.

Many states have controlled substances acts patterned after the federal law. Because there may be differences in the scheduling of drugs (some states are more restrictive, but none are less restrictive), physicians are urged to acquaint themselves with the provisions of the statutes and regulations in their local jurisdictions.

Precautions: The physician should take the following precautions to minimize the chances of controlled substances being procured illegally:

Keep prescription blanks where they cannot be stolen easily. Never sign them in advance and do not use them for writing notes. The prescriber's name, address, and DEA registration number and the full name and address of the patient must be given when controlled substances are prescribed.

The written prescription order should be precise and legible to enhance communication between physician and pharmacist.

The prescription order should indicate whether or not the prescription may be refilled and, if so, the number of times or duration of time a refill is authorized.

When prescribing a controlled substance, write out the actual amount in addition to giving an arabic number or roman numeral in order to discourage alterations in written prescription orders.

Use a separate prescription blank for each controlled substance prescribed. Avoid the use of prescription blanks that are preprinted with the name of a proprietary preparation.

Avoid writing prescription orders for large quantities of controlled drugs unless such amounts are absolutely necessary.

Maintain an accurate record of controlled drugs dispensed, as required by the Controlled Substances Act amendments of 1984 and state law.

Store office supplies of controlled drugs under lock and key.

Maintain only a minimum stock of controlled drugs in the medical bag, which should not be left unattended.

Assist any pharmacist who telephones to verify information about a written prescription order.

Institutions should discourage the use of institutional prescription blanks for prescribing controlled substances; if institutional prescription blanks are used, the physician should print his/her name, address, and DEA registration number on each blank.

OFFICIAL AND REGULATORY AGENCIES

There are several official governmental and quasi-official voluntary bodies concerned with standards for the manufacturing, distribution, labeling, and advertising of drug products. To acquaint the reader with the functions of these agencies and their spheres of influence as they pertain to medicinal agents, brief descriptions of their organization and duties follow.

FOOD AND DRUG ADMINISTRATION. The Food and Drug Administration (FDA) is charged by the federal Food, Drug and Cosmetic Act of 1938 and by the 1962 Kefauver-Harris Amendment to that Act with assuring the safety and efficacy of prescription drugs, including biologic products, marketed in interstate commerce. The FDA's regulatory jurisdiction over such drugs encompasses the standardization of nomenclature, the approval process for new drugs or new claims, official labeling and advertising, and methods of manufacture and distribution. The developmental history of this regulatory power has been summarized recently (Hayes, 1981).

Nomenclature: The Secretary of Health and Human Services is given the authority to designate an established name for any drug if he determines that such action is necessary or desirable in the interest of usefulness and simplicity. This name is to be used in any subsequent issue of any official compendium as the only official title for that drug. In practice, the official name will probably be one that has been recommended by the USAN Council (see the following discussion). Such an official established name is the only nonproprietary (generic) name, other than the chemical name or formula, that may appear on the manufacturer's label. This label, more commonly referred to as the official label, for a prescription drug must state the established drug name(s) and quantities of all active ingredients. This official name must appear in conjunction with the trademark name in other labeling (eg, package insert, patient information). The official label for an over-the-counter drug also must disclose the active ingredients but unfortunately is not required to reveal the quantities or ratios of these ingredients.

New Drug Approval: To market a new drug for human use in interstate commerce, a manufacturer must have an approved *New Drug Application* (NDA) from the FDA. Before an investigation of a new drug entity in humans can be initiated, the sponsor must submit to the FDA information specified as a *Notice of Claimed Investigational Exemption for a New Drug,* more commonly referred to as an "IND." The IND includes information about the chemical composition of the drug, results of all preclinical investigations (including animal safety studies), a protocol for the proposed clinical investigation, information on the experience of clinical investigators, agreements protecting the rights and safety of human subjects developed in accordance with the requirements of Human Subjects Protection Committees (Institutional Review Boards), and an agreement to submit annual progress reports. At least two to three years are often necessary to amass the required preclinical data for an IND for a new chemical entity. After the IND has been submitted to the FDA, the Agency has 30 days to review the proposed clinical study; the sponsor of the IND may proceed with the planned studies in humans after notification of approval or absence of comment from the FDA within the 30-day review period.

The FDA has formulated regulations for the clinical study of a new drug's safety and efficacy and has divided this evaluation into three phases. Phase I is intended to prove the safety of the new drug in normal subjects and to identify the tolerable dosage range. Pharmacokinetic data are also obtained in this usually small group of healthy volunteers. In phase II trials, controlled studies are performed in limited numbers of patients with the target disease or disorder to establish efficacy and appropriate dosage. Additional pharmacokinetic data are obtained and compared with the data from normal subjects. If phases I and II demonstrate that the drug is safe and potentially efficacious or may have benefits that outweigh any observed risks, more extensive clinical trials are initiated in phase III.

Phase III trials verify that the acceptable benefit/risk ratio determined in phase II studies persists under conditions of anticipated usage and in groups of patients large enough to identify statistically and clinically significant responses. Conferences between the sponsor and FDA, sometimes including outside medical experts, are held before and during phase III studies.

When the IND sponsor feels that data are sufficient to fulfill the requirements for approval of the drug by the FDA, an application for a New Drug Approval is filed. Four to six years are often required in the IND phase to complete the adequate and well-controlled trials necessary to support the claimed indications for an acceptable FDA application. By statute, the FDA must review the NDA application within 180 days. Usually, additional information and/or clarification is requested by the FDA and one to two years is required for NDA review and approval (Commission on the Federal Drug Approval Process, 1982).

Clinical experience with a new drug at the time of approval typically includes no more than 1,000 or 2,000 patients and often no more than a few hundred. The detection of adverse reactions occurring at frequencies of 1:1,000 or less is not reliable until hundreds of thousands of people are exposed. "Phase IV" postmarket surveillance studies may be conducted after NDA approval to obtain additional data to support safety and efficacy claims. The manufacturer or the FDA (through a contract organization) may initiate such a study. Thus, postmarketing surveillance is designed to improve detection of adverse reactions. Orderly postmarketing surveillance also permits better estimation of the incidence and severity of known adverse drug reactions, which in turn permits physicians to make more informed judgments in drug use and patient counseling.

Abbreviated New Drug Application (ANDA): On September 24, 1984, the President signed into law the Drug Price Competition and Patent Term Restoration Act of 1984 (Public Law 98-417). The new law provides the opportunity to extend patents on drug products to encourage the development of new drugs, as well as amends the Federal Food, Drug and Cosmetic Act to expand the universe of drugs for which the FDA may accept ANDAs. Before enactment of this new law, ANDAs were permitted only for duplicates, ie, generic versions of drug products first approved between 1938 and 1962. The new law provides for the submission of ANDAs for duplicates of any previously approved drug product, including post-1962 drug products. Additionally, this new law permits generic drug products to become available more quickly. Since the New Drug Approval process has already been satisfactorily completed (either by the same or a different manufacturer), the clinical investigations need not be repeated. However, the manufacturer must demonstrate that the proposed formulation meets FDA standards for identity, strength, quality, and purity. Bioavailability (at least 80% of the rate and extent of the innovator's product) testing may be required. Expanded use of the ANDA is advocated by the increasing number of pharmaceutical companies desiring to market generic versions of post-1962 drugs.

New Claims Approval: After a new drug has been marketed, the FDA requires further clinical proof of safety and efficacy if labeling claims or statements not included at the time of the original application are to be made.

As a general rule, whether new claims are added to the official label depends upon whether the pharmaceutical company has sufficient interest in the matter to initiate and follow the necessary procedures to obtain approval. Even if the manufacturer promptly responds to an obvious new opportunity for the marketed drug, the process of approval (although less demanding than the conventional NDA) still requires considerable time before the new claim can appear in the official label.

Postmarketing Surveillance: Manufacturers are required to submit to the FDA all reports of adverse effects, additional clinical experience, and other relevant data on marketed drugs. The following types of adverse drug reactions (ADRs) must be reported to the FDA by the manufacturer within 15 days: Reports of ADRs (domestic, foreign, literature, or study) (1) that are serious and not already listed on the label or (2) that are already labeled serious ADRs but that increase significantly in frequency. The agency can require label updating to keep precautionary information current. It also can take steps to have claims deleted that it considers no longer warranted, or even to revoke an NDA and remove the drug from the market if there is evidence that the drug is not safe and effective as originally believed. Legal remedies are available by which manufacturers may contest such actions if they disagree.

Official Labeling: The legal (Humphrey-Durham Act of 1951) distinction between a prescription drug and an over-the-counter drug is not founded upon relative safety per se, but rather involves a regulatory decision as to whether adequate directions for the proper (effective and safe) use of a particular drug can be written for the layman. If the FDA determines that adequate directions can be written, the manufacturer is not allowed to identify the drug with a prescription legend. Conversely, for a prescription drug, the manufacturer's directions or FDA-approved labeling (package insert) are intended for the physician and provide a summary of information about the chemical and physical nature of the product, pharmacology, indications and contraindications, means of administration, appropriate dosages, side effects and adverse reactions, how the drug is supplied, and any other information pertinent to its safe and effective use. This summary, or official label, is developed by discussions between the FDA and the sponsor. Drug product information published in the *Physicians' Desk Reference* is a verbatim presentation of the required label.

The FDA's jurisdiction over the uses of marketed drugs, dosage, and related matters extends only to what the manufacturer may recommend and must disclose in its labeling. It

was not the intent of the Congress (under the 1962 amendment of the Food, Drug and Cosmetic Act) to charge the FDA with dictating how a physician should practice medicine (Erickson et al, 1980; Roth, 1982). Rather, the FDA's concerns rest with sanctioning the marketing and assuring the availability of drugs that have demonstrated substantial safety and efficacy. The proper and successful therapeutic use of these drugs is the responsibility of the physician and requires a critical awareness and understanding of the present medical literature and careful monitoring of the patient's response.

The prescription of a drug for an unlabeled indication is entirely proper if based on rational scientific theory, reliable medical opinion, or controlled clinical studies. The FDA has made eminently clear that it neither has nor wants the authority to compel prescribers to adhere to officially labeled uses, because experience demonstrates that new uses for drugs already on the market are often first discovered through the serendipitous observations and therapeutic innovations of physicians (Hayes, 1981; *FDA Drug Bull*, 1982).

The physician is well advised to be *aware* of the content of a package insert and to give it due weight, especially the information on precautions, contraindications, and warnings. However, a decision on how to use a drug must be based on what is good medicine and best for the patient. This statement applies whether the physician's use of a drug conforms to official labeling or departs from it. In a professional liability suit, such drug labeling *may* have evidentiary weight for or against a physician, but drug labeling *per se* does not set the standard for what is good medical practice.

The FDA does not have jurisdiction over drug formulations that the physician may devise for use in the normal course of his practice, provided the physician does not introduce these products into interstate commerce. Such drugs include those compounded from separate ingredients, certain readily available chemicals, or other nonpharmaceutical products that have therapeutic uses.

Advertising: The Federal Food, Drug and Cosmetic Act provides that the advertising of prescription drugs must conform to the labeling in specified ways. Any advertisement that describes or alludes to a drug's use in patients must contain the generic name of the active ingredient(s), the name and address of the manufacturer, and a brief summary of prescribing information, including contraindications, warnings, and other pertinent information. A prescription drug advertisement that implies incorrectly that a drug is the treatment of choice or is useful for an unlabeled indication is unlawful. Manufacturers voluntarily may submit anticipated advertising to the FDA to ensure that the information conforms to legal requirements.

Regulation of advertising of nonprescription (over-the-counter) drugs is the responsibility of the Federal Trade Commission.

Manufacturing and Distribution: Detailed manufacturing information to assure uniform purity and potency of drugs is an important part of the NDA and continuing FDA inspection program. The method of preparing the drug must be outlined, along with a complete description of how quality, purity, and strength are maintained. The manufacturing facilities, production methods, and quality control measures of a pharmaceutical company are subject to FDA inspection and review. In addition, certification procedures conducted by the FDA are applied to insulin. Finally, the FDA is responsible for ensuring the safe distribution of drugs used in interstate commerce.

FEDERAL TRADE COMMISSION. The Federal Trade Commission (FTC) is an independent agency of the federal government with five commissioners appointed by the President. The Commission administers several laws, the principal one being the Federal Trade Commission Act, which deals with the regulation of commercial trade practices.

The principal power of the FTC with respect to drugs is contained in Title 15 of the Federal Trade Commission Act: This Act gives the Commission broad power to prevent the dissemination of false or misleading advertising of foods, drugs, and cosmetics to the general public. This power is circumscribed with respect to advertisements directed to the medical profession. Regulation of prescription drug advertising is the responsibility of the FDA. For nonprescription (OTC) drugs, the FTC relies upon FDA determinations and has taken action against advertising claims that are inconsistent with these.

DEPARTMENT OF JUSTICE. Responsibility for administration of the Controlled Substances Act is assigned to the Drug Enforcement Administration (DEA) in the Department of Justice. The DEA is charged with enforcing the provisions of the Act, which regulates the manufacture, purchase, prescribing, and dispensing of controlled substances and includes: (1) registration of physicians, pharmacists, and other handlers; (2) record-keeping requirements; (3) quotas on manufacturing; (4) restrictions on distribution; (5) restrictions on dispensing; (6) limitations on imports and exports; (7) conditions for storage of drugs; (8) reports of transactions to the government; and (9) criminal, civil, and administrative penalties for illegal acts. As a convenience, the *United States Pharmacopeia* (USP) includes the latest DEA regulations that affect practicing physicians and pharmacists.

CONSUMER PRODUCT SAFETY COMMISSION. The Consumer Product Safety Commission is responsible for administration of the Poison Prevention Packaging Act (PPPA). The Commission sets standards for childproof packaging, grants exemptions from these standards for certain products, and enforces the Act.

UNITED STATES PHARMACOPEIAL CONVENTION, INC. Under the General Committee of Revision, the United States Pharmacopeial Convention, Inc, issues the combined *United States Pharmacopeia (USP)* and the *National Formulary (NF)* at five-year intervals with cumulative annual *Supplements* and *Interim Revisions* as needed. This is a private body incorporated in the District of Columbia and composed of representatives from medical and pharmacy schools, state medical and pharmaceutical associations, the American Medical Association, the American Pharmaceutical Association, the American Chemical Society, many other scientific and trade associations, and various interested federal agencies.

Under authority of the Federal Food, Drug and Cosmetic Act, the standards for products described in *USP* and *NF* are official. Articles are admitted by the Committee of Revision on the basis of demonstrated therapeutic value, extent of use, or pharmaceutic necessity.

The Pharmacopeial Convention also publishes separately the annual, *USP Dispensing Information (USP-DI),* which includes (1) drug information for the pharmacist and other health professionals (an expansion of such information formerly included in the official compendia), as well as (2) information designed expressly for the patient in a section entitled, *Advice for the Patient* (also available separately).

USAN and the USP Dictionary of Drug Names, a cumulation of United States Adopted Names and other names for drugs, both current and retrospective, also is published by the United States Pharmacopeial Convention, Inc, annually.

USAN COUNCIL. The United States Adopted Names (USAN) Council, an agency formed to adopt appropriate nonproprietary names for all new drugs, was organized in January, 1964. It is sponsored by the American Medical Association, the American Pharmaceutical Association, and the United States Pharmacopeial Convention, Inc. The Council has five members: one member appointed by each sponsor, one member-at-large who must be approved by all three sponsors, and one member from the Food and Drug Administration.

The primary functions of the USAN Council are: (1) to negotiate with pharmaceutical manufacturers in the selection of meaningful and distinctive nonproprietary names for new drug entities; (2) to publicize the adopted names, the guiding principles used in devising these names, and the procedures involved in their adoption; and (3) to cooperate with other national and international agencies, particularly the World Health Organization, in standardizing, as much as possible, the nonproprietary nomenclature for drugs.

New USAN are published in *Clinical Pharmacology and Therapeutics* promptly after adoption and are cumulated annually. The current version of The Guiding Principles for Coining United States Adopted Names for Drugs appears in the annual cumulative publication, *USAN and the USP Dictionary of Drug Names.*

Cited References

Use of approved drugs for unlabeled indications. *FDA Drug Bull* 12:4-5, (April) 1982.

When are drug combinations justified? *Drug Ther Bull* 18:37-40, 1980.

Chilton L: Strategies for reducing prescription costs. *Pediatrics* 68:713-716, 1981.

Chodos DJ: Generic substitution: Form of pharmaceutical Russian roulette? in Lasagna L (ed): *Controversies in Therapeutics.* Philadelphia, WB Saunders, 1980, 72-81.

Commission on Federal Drug Approval Process: Final report. (March 31) 1982.

Council on Scientific Affairs, American Medical Association: Drug abuse related to prescribing practices. *JAMA* 247:862-866, 1982.

Erickson SH, et al: Use of drugs for unlabeled indications. *JAMA* 243:1543-1546, 1980.

Hayes AH Jr: Food and drug regulation after 75 years. *JAMA* 246:1223-1226, 1981.

Horvitz R: Generic substitution: A way to cut medical costs, in Lasagna L (ed): *Controversies in Therapeutics.* Philadelphia, WB Saunders, 1980, 63-71.

Jaffe JH: Drug addiction and drug abuse, in Gilman AG, et al (eds): *The Pharmacological Basis of Therapeutics,* ed 6. New York, Macmillan, 1980, 535-584.

Lewis JR: Misprescribing analgesics. *JAMA* 228:1155-1156, 1974.

MacCannell KL, Giraud G: Fixed ratio drug combinations: Sense and nonsense, in Lasagna L (ed): *Controversies in Therapeutics.* Philadelphia, WB Saunders, 1980, 172-179.

Marks RM, Sachar EJ: Undertreatment of medical inpatients with narcotic analgesics. *Ann Intern Med* 78:173-181, 1973.

Mellinger GD, et al: Psychic distress, life crisis, and use of psychotherapeutic medications: National household survey data. *Arch Gen Psychiatry* 35:1045-1052, 1978.

Morgan JP: Politics of medication, in Lasagna L (ed): *Controversies in Therapeutics.* Philadelphia, WB Saunders, 1980, 16-22.

Peck CC: Should we improve patient compliance with therapeutic regimens and if so how? in Lasagna L (ed): *Controversies in Therapeutics.* Philadelphia, WB Saunders, 1980, 559-566.

Rosenbaum JF: Drug treatment of anxiety. *N Engl J Med* 306:401-404, 1982.

Roth SH: Drug use, package insert, and practice of medicine, (editorial). *Arch Intern Med* 142:871-872, 1982.

Roth HP, Caron HS: Accuracy of doctors' estimates and patients' statements on adherence to drug regimen. *Clin Pharm Ther* 23:361-370, 1978.

Solomon HS: How to improve patient compliance, in Lasagna L (ed): *Controversies in Therapeutics.* Philadelphia, WB Saunders, 1980, 567-571.

Symmers WSC: Amphotericin pharmacophobia. *Br Med J* 4:460-463, 1973.

Weintraub M: Undertreatment: Who is to blame? *Drug Ther (Hosp)* 11:58-63, (Dec) 1981.

Wilford BB: *Drug Abuse: A Guide for the Primary Care Physician.* Chicago, American Medical Association, 1981, 263-283.

Drug Response Variation and Dosing Information

Administering a given dose of a drug to different patients yields a wide variety of responses. One subset may exhibit an inadequate or subtherapeutic response, a second subset may experience the desired therapeutic response, and a third subset may show signs of toxicity. Such variation in response to a drug generally is due, at least in part, to the large interpatient variability in pharmacokinetics and is often a major obstacle to optimal drug therapy. Individual variation may result from endogenous or exogenous factors. *Endogenous* factors include age, body weight, hormonal and nutritional status, sex, pregnancy, genetic differences, and diseases. *Exogenous* factors include diet and exposure to other drugs and various environmental chemicals.

The variation in response occurs most frequently to drugs with narrow therapeutic indexes. The therapeutic index (TI) can be defined as the ratio of the minimal drug concentration associated with a high probability of toxicity to the maximal drug concentration associated with a high probability of response and a low probability of toxicity. The TI is an average value and may differ in an individual patient. When the TI is small, ie, less than 2 or 3, pharmacokinetic variability can result in subtherapeutic, therapeutic, or toxic responses to identical doses.

Variations in response may be related to the drug, including its physiochemical properties (ie, ionization, molecular size, chemical reactivity, solubility), or the patient, including his physiologic status, which affects the biochemical kinetic processes (ie, binding, transport, enzyme-regulating activity) and drug receptor activity. These factors underlie the main elements of both the pharmacokinetic and pharmacodynamic properties of a drug.

APPLIED PHARMACOKINETICS

Applied pharmacokinetics provide relatively simple mathematical models that allow the clinician to individualize dosage regimens, thereby minimizing the potential for toxicity and enhancing the likelihood of obtaining the desired therapeutic response. Commonly used pharmacokinetic parameters are drug clearance, distribution volume, half-life, and bioavailability. These data permit computation of the dose and dosing interval most appropriate for an individual patient, but they do not take the place of careful clinical evaluation of the response to therapy. Awareness of such data can, however, raise a suspicion or confirm a clinical impression of inappropriate dosage.

The incidence of therapeutic failures and adverse drug reactions may be reduced if the physician is cognizant of factors that can alter this pharmacokinetic profile. However, it is important to note that many of the pharmacokinetic properties reported for drugs have been derived primarily from mean values obtained in healthy young adults, and this must be borne in mind before the information is applied to an individual patient.

Absorption

A drug is considered to be completely absorbed, ie, the total administered dose reaches the systemic circulation, when it is administered intravenously. Administration by any other route may result in less than complete absorption, and the fraction absorbed (F) may be less than 1.

The oral route of administration is used most commonly. Tablets and capsules must undergo a number of processes before reaching the systemic circulation (see Figure 1). Once ingested, they must disintegrate, deaggregate, and dissolve in the gastrointestinal fluids before they can be absorbed. A poorly designed pharmaceutical preparation may disintegrate or deaggregate too slowly, causing a drug to be lost in the stool. Absorption also may be incomplete because of the physicochemical properties of the drug (eg, solubility, molecular size, crystal form), presence of food or other substances in the intestine, gastric emptying and intestinal transit times, pH of the gastrointestinal tract, and biliary flow. Once in solution, a drug is susceptible to enzymatic degradation within the gastrointestinal lumen. The remaining drug, in general, passively diffuses through the wall of the small intestine (the most common site of absorption for weak acids and weak bases) into the portal circulation, through the liver, and into the systemic circulation. However, the intestinal wall and the liver are major sites of biotransformation, and a large fraction of a dose may diffuse into the intestinal wall and yet not reach the systemic circulation. Biotransformation that takes place before the drug reaches the systemic circulation is called the first-pass metabolism.

Other routes of administration tend to bypass the first-pass metabolism. Sublingual, buccal, and nasal administration can result in greater absorption of drugs degraded in the gastrointestinal tract or extensively metabolized by the liver. Rectally administered drugs may or may not bypass the liver, depending upon their site of absorption in the rectum (DeBoer et al, 1984). If absorbed in the upper rectum, a drug enters the portal circulation and must go through the liver before reaching the systemic circulation. On the other hand, if a drug is absorbed in the lower rectum, it enters directly into the systemic circulation and bypasses the liver.

The intramuscular and subcutaneous routes are commonly used to produce more rapid and complete absorption than with oral administration while minimizing the hazards of intravascular injection. The rate of absorption with these routes depends on drug solubility, concentration of the injected solution, site of administration, area blood flow, and activity of the patient. Absorption is most rapid after intramuscular injection into the deltoid, followed by injection into the vastus lateralis, and is slowest after injection into gluteal muscle (Niazi, 1979).

Bioavailability is defined as the rate and extent of absorption following nonvascular administration. It is determined by comparing the area under a serum drug concentration-time curve (AUC) following nonvascular administration with the AUC following intravenous administration, after correcting for any difference between doses.

Although a drug may be absorbed completely, the rate of absorption also may be important if it is too slow to achieve a therapeutic blood level or so rapid that high concentrations cause adverse effects.

Differences in the bioavailabilities of various pharmaceutical formulations of a given drug (ie, lack of bioequivalence) may have clinical significance, for therapeutic or toxic effects often depend upon serum drug concentrations. Differences in bioavailability between individuals and even in the same individual at different times make the determination of equivalent dosage difficult.

Problems are encountered most frequently during long-term therapy when a patient who is stabilized on one pharmaceutical formulation receives a nonequivalent substitute. Either inadequate therapy or toxicity due to bioinequivalence has been observed with phenytoin, digoxin, theophylline, triamterene, thyroid, aspirin, warfarin, prednisone, chloramphenicol, levodopa, and tolbutamide. Generic substitution should be restricted to drug formulations with demonstrated bioavailability, especially when treating a seriously ill patient or prescribing a drug with a low TI. (See Chapter 1, Prescription Practices and Regulatory Agencies, for a discussion on generic substitution.)

Timed-release preparations are formulated to release a drug slowly to increase its duration of action. These products deserve special consideration because of their potential variability in action. The general term, "timed-release," used to describe oral preparations in this text, is synonymous with the term, "controlled-release," used by the Food and Drug Administration, and includes formulations variously known as "delayed-action," "extended-release," "prolonged-action," "sustained-action," or "repeat-action."

Data on which to base an evaluation of effectiveness are

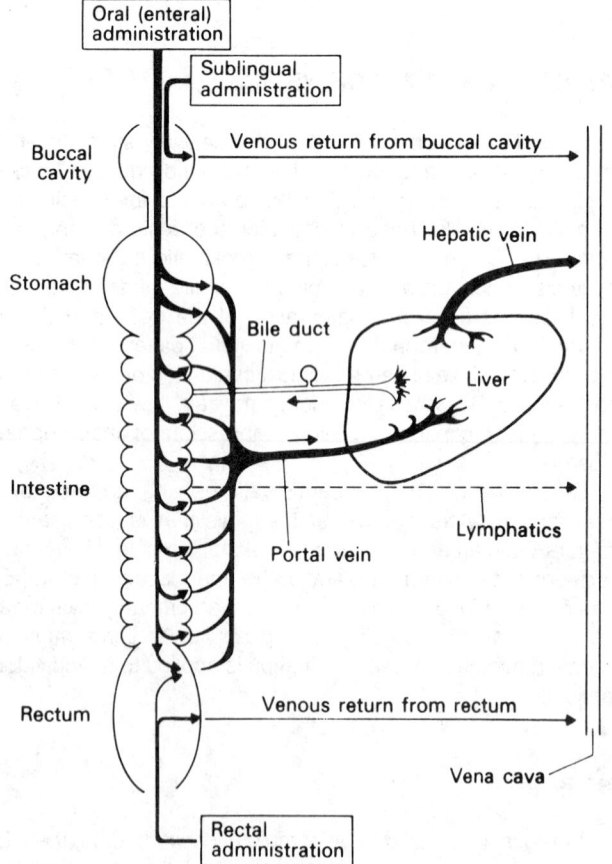

Figure 1. Absorptive processes following oral, sublingual, and rectal administration.
From Bowman WC, Rand MJ: Textbook of Pharmacology, ed 2. St. Louis, Blackwell Mosby, 1980. Reprinted with permission.

inadequate or unavailable for the timed-release forms of many drugs; however, specific drugs have been tested for effectiveness, and these are indicated in the individual evaluations. No precise product specifications have been established by the official compendia for timed-release preparations.

A number of factors stimulate interest in developing and marketing timed-release preparations. For a physician, these dosage forms increase patient compliance and minimize fluctuations in serum drug concentrations. For a pharmaceutical manufacturer, they may permit extension and/or retention of a competitive position in the marketplace (Gibaldi, 1984). The objective of timed-release preparations is to have the rate of release control the duration of drug effect. A number of pharmaceutical techniques are used to produce oral timed-release preparations; these include ion-exchange resins that bind the drug, semipermeable membranes with small laser-drilled holes, slowly eroding coatings or matrixes, and slowly dissolving physical or chemical forms.

In *parenteral* preparations, sustained release is achieved by using relatively insoluble salts or esters of the active drug or a special vehicle. It is doubtful whether such techniques can deliver a dose that is as precisely controlled as with intravenous infusion. Nevertheless, when some latitude in the range of safe and effective blood levels is permissible, substitution of slowly released preparations for intermittent injections may provide a more uniform blood concentration, and this type of preparation is certainly more convenient. The depot preparation of benzathine penicillin G is an example of a useful sustained-release formulation, but continuous intravenous infusion is still needed in some serious infections. Fluphenazine decanoate, a phenothiazine available in a sustained-release form, is useful in outpatients with a history of poor compliance, inadequate absorption of oral medication, or frequent relapses. Insulin also is available in sustained-release preparations, which have simplified the management of diabetes. Other satisfactory parenteral formulations are available for various corticosteroids, androgens, and estrogens.

Distribution

After entering the systemic circulation, a drug distributes throughout the body in a characteristic fashion that depends on its physicochemical characteristics (molecular size, solubility, degree of ionization) and the degree of binding to plasma and tissue proteins. For a few drugs, an equilibrium between tissue and plasma (or serum) drug concentrations is reached almost immediately. However, for most drugs, there is a measurable time lag before equilibrium can be obtained.

In general, factors affecting the rate of distribution are the diffusion rate, tissue perfusion rate, and the extent of binding to plasma and tissue proteins. Diffusion-rate limitation occurs when the rate of distribution is controlled by drug diffusion through a lipoid barrier and is a function of the partition coefficient, molecular weight, and degree of ionization. The rate of distribution of a drug that is highly water soluble, ionized, or has a large molecular weight is likely to be controlled by the rate of diffusion.

A perfusion-rate limitation predominates when the rate of

drug presentation, defined as the product of the rate of blood flow to the tissue and the arterial drug concentration, is the limiting factor. Such a limitation occurs with highly lipophilic drugs of low molecular weight (Rowland and Tozer, 1980).

The third major factor affecting drug distribution is the binding of drugs to plasma and tissue proteins. Drugs that are weak acids (eg, warfarin, phenytoin, aspirin) generally bind to albumin, while drugs that are weak bases (eg, propranolol, imipramine, quinidine) generally bind to lipoproteins and alpha-1-acid glycoprotein. Plasma protein binding is a reversible process, and the drug molecules constantly shift between the drug-protein complex and the free drug form but remain in overall equilibrium. With the exception of a few drugs (eg, disopyramide, valproic acid), the proportion of protein-bound drug in plasma remains constant throughout the therapeutic range. The total amount of drug in plasma changes constantly. Either the plasma concentration increases because another dose is administered, or the plasma concentration decreases because of elimination by metabolism or excretion. However, the equilibrium between bound and unbound drug maintains the two forms in the same proportions.

The fraction of drug bound to plasma proteins is affected by drugs and other substances that compete for protein binding sites, plasma protein concentration, and plasma pH. Because the free drug is the active form, increasing the unbound fraction may enhance pharmacologic activity acutely and lead to toxicity. However, usually the concentration of unbound drug returns to the preinsult level but the concentration of bound drug decreases resulting in a lower total (but not active) plasma drug concentration.

Most clinical laboratories measure total plasma concentration, which may be classified as subtherapeutic, therapeutic, or toxic even though only the unbound portion is clinically active. Patients have inadvertently received excessive doses because it was not recognized that the fraction of unbound drug in plasma was increased, and the dose was based on the total plasma drug concentration.

The *volume of distribution* is probably an even more important concept than the rate of distribution. A volume of distribution (Vd) is a hypothetical volume of fluid into which a drug distributes. It can be thought of as the volume required for a specific amount of drug in the body to produce a specific plasma or serum concentration. For example, if a patient weighing 67 kg is known to have 300 mg of theophylline in the body and the serum theophylline concentration is equal to 10 mg/L, the apparent Vd for theophylline is 30 L (0.45 L/kg).

Vd is a hypothetical volume with no physiologic basis. It is calculated as the total amount of drug in the body divided by the plasma drug concentration. For many drugs, the Vd is constant over a wide dosage range. For some drugs, it greatly exceeds total body weight. Digoxin, for example, has an average apparent Vd equal to 7.2 L/kg of body weight, due to extensive binding to cardiac and other tissue. Distribution volumes vary greatly, ranging from 0.06 L/kg for heparin to over 20 L/kg for nortriptyline.

Factors affecting the volume of distribution include lipid solubility, degree of ionization, molecular size, and the degree of binding to plasma and tissue proteins. The volume of distribution can be altered significantly by major illness. For example, severe renal failure markedly increases the Vd for phenytoin, probably because of decreased plasma protein binding (Tozer and Winter, 1980).

Clearance

Clearance often is considered to be the most important parameter for individualizing a dosage regimen. Clearance is not, as is commonly thought, the amount of drug eliminated over time; rather, it is the volume of biological fluid (eg, plasma, serum) from which a drug is removed over a period of time. Clearance is commonly adjusted for body weight or body surface area and is expressed as ml/minute, ml/kg/minute, L/kg/hour, ml/M²/minute, or L/M²/hour. It is analogous to the concept of renal clearance that was developed many years ago.

The total body clearance is a summation of clearances from the various drug metabolizing and drug eliminating organs. This is expressed as:

$$Cl_{total} = Cl_{hepatic} + Cl_{renal} + Cl_{pulmonary} + Cl_{other}$$

(Eq. 1)

Hepatic Metabolism: The liver may clear a drug from the body by excreting it unchanged in the biliary tract or, more commonly, by biotransformation. Biotransformation involves chemical alteration of a drug and can produce inactive metabolites that are readily excreted in the urine or pharmacologically active metabolites with unique physicochemical, pharmacokinetic, and pharmacodynamic properties.

Biotransformation consists of two types of chemical reactions, both of which tend to increase the drug's water solubility. In type I (or nonsynthetic) hepatic metabolic reactions, polar groups are added by oxidation, reduction, or hydrolysis. Oxidative-type reactions are by far the most important and most studied nonsynthetic reactions. One group of oxidative enzymes are the mixed-function oxidases, of which the cytochrome P-450 system is a component. The cytochrome P-450 enzymes can be induced by a number of exogenous factors, including cigarette smoking, environmental pollutants, dietary contents, and certain drugs (eg, phenytoin, phenobarbital, rifampin, carbamazepine). Cimetidine and possibly influenza vaccine inhibit their activity. Altered activity of the cytochrome P-450 enzymes causes many clinically important drug-drug interactions (see Chapter 3, Drug Interactions and Adverse Drug Reactions).

Type II (or synthetic) hepatic metabolic reactions involve conjugation with glucuronic acid, sulfate, or other groups. Conjugation reactions generally are not affected by liver disease or exogenous factors. The synthetic metabolites often are water soluble and, therefore, are rapidly excreted unchanged in the urine.

Hepatic Clearance: The rate of drug removal from the blood by the liver is a function of the hepatic blood flow (Q) and the efficiency of the organ to remove a drug as it perfuses through the liver.

$$Hepatic\ Clearance = Q \cdot E$$

(Eq. 2)

E is the fraction of drug removed from portal circulation as it leaves the liver; at least five factors affect the extraction ratio (E): the degree of binding to erythrocytes, the degree of binding to blood proteins, the diffusion rate between unbound drug in the blood and unbound drug within the hepatocyte, the rate of secretion of drug from the hepatocyte into the biliary tract, and the rate of hepatic biotransformation (Rowland and Tozer, 1980). The maximal ability of the liver to remove a drug by all pathways in the absence of blood flow limitations is designated by total intrinsic clearance (Cl_{int}) (Wilkinson and Shand, 1975). Accordingly,

$$Cl_{HEP} = Q \left[\frac{Cl_{int}}{Q + Cl_{int}} \right]$$

(Eq. 3)

When the hepatic intrinsic clearance is efficient (very high), the rate-limiting step is delivery of drug to the liver, that is, hepatic blood flow. Drugs in this category are classified as blood flow dependent and are referred to as high extraction ratio drugs.

Conversely, when the hepatic intrinsic clearance is very inefficient (very low), the rate-limiting step is the rate of removal from the blood, that is, the extraction rate. Drugs that meet this criteria are classified as blood flow independent and are referred to as low extraction drugs (Benet and Massoud, 1984).

These concepts help to explain why the clearance of certain metabolized drugs is affected greatly by changes in hepatic metabolic enzyme activity while the clearance of others is not. Drugs with a low extraction ratio, such as diazepam, phenylbutazone, phenytoin, procainamide, theophylline, salicylic acid, tolbutamide, and warfarin, are susceptible to hepatic enzyme induction and inhibition. However, their metabolic clearance is essentially unchanged by variations in hepatic blood flow. Conversely, drugs with a high extraction ratio, such as lidocaine, propoxyphene, meperidine, pentazocine, propranolol, and morphine, are resistant to changes in hepatic enzyme activity. They are, however, susceptible to changes in hepatic blood flow.

Drugs such as quinidine, desipramine, and nortriptyline have an intermediate extraction ratio and are affected by changes in intrinsic clearance and hepatic blood flow.

Renal Excretion: The elimination of drugs by the kidneys may involve glomerular filtration, tubular reabsorption, and tubular secretion. The kidneys receive about one-fourth of the total cardiac output, of which 10% is filtered by the glomerulus. The resulting glomerular filtration rate is approximately 125 ml/minute for the average adult. Blood cells, proteins, and drug molecules bound to them remain in the blood and are not filtered into the renal tubular lumen. Only the unbound fraction of drug in the blood is cleared by renal filtration. The maximal rate of drug clearance by renal filtration is equal to the product of the glomerular filtration rate and the fraction of drug unbound in the blood.

Renal tubular reabsorption usually is a passive process that decreases drug clearance. Reabsorption ranges from nearly absent to virtually complete. It occurs all along the nephron and tends to follow the movement of free water. The rate of reabsorption primarily depends upon the physicochemical properties of the drug, with nonionic lipophilic drugs being extensively reabsorbed. Altering the urinary pH markedly alters the rate of reabsorption; for example, the reabsorption of weak acids (eg, salicylic acid) can be decreased manyfold by increasing the urinary pH, which ionizes the drug.

Renal tubular secretion is an active process occurring primarily in the proximal tubule. Two separate systems actively secrete acids and bases, respectively, into the renal tubular lumen. Secretion is indicated when the rate of renal clearance of a drug exceeds the glomerular filtration rate.

Renal Elimination: Renal elimination is related to the fraction of drug removed by the kidneys per unit of time. It is affected by the fraction of drug excreted unchanged in the urine and renal function.

Changes in renal function are assessed by monitoring endogenous creatinine clearance. If creatinine clearance cannot be determined precisely, it can be estimated from a serum creatinine value if age, sex, and body weight are known and renal function is stable. Nomograms to facilitate the determination of this conversion have been published (eg, Siersbaek-Nielsen et al, 1971); an estimation for males may be calculated from the following equation (Cockcroft and Gault, 1976):

$$\text{Creatinine Clearance (men)} = \frac{(140 - \text{age}) \cdot (\text{body weight in kg})}{72 \cdot \text{serum creatinine}}$$

(Eq. 4)

For women, the creatinine clearance is 85% of the value calculated by this equation. The estimated creatinine clearance calculated from equation 4 may be higher than the actual creatinine clearance in certain patients (eg, pregnant women, patients with markedly reduced renal function [less than 10 ml/minute]). For individuals from 6 months to 20 years of age, the creatinine clearance can be calculated from the following equation (Schwartz et al, 1976):

$$\text{Creatinine Clearance (children)} = \frac{0.55 \cdot \text{length(cm)}}{\text{serum creatinine}}$$

(Eq. 5)

A dosage adjustment factor (equation 6) provides a method to design regimens for patients with impaired renal function empirically based on the creatinine clearance (Clcr) and the fraction of drug excreted unchanged in the urine of individuals with normal renal function (Fe).

$$\text{Dosage Adjustment Factor} = \frac{1}{\text{Fe}\left(\dfrac{\text{Cl}_{cr}}{120 \text{ ml/min}} - 1\right) + 1}$$

(Eq. 6)

The dosage adjustment factor can be used to prolong the dosing interval or reduce the dose in patients with impaired renal function. To adjust the interval in patients with renal impairment, the usual dosing interval for patients with normal renal function is multiplied by the dosage adjustment factor. Prolonging the interval may enhance patient compliance, but results in greater fluctuation in serum drug concentrations. If it is preferable to adjust the dose, the usual dose should be divided by the dosage adjustment factor.

Guidelines for specific drugs have been published (Bennett et al, 1983), and some are included in the evaluations.

PHARMACOKINETIC MODELS

Various pharmacokinetic models are used in which the body is divided into artificial compartments. For some drugs, the body may be viewed as a single homogeneous unit; for other drugs (eg, thiopental, lidocaine, vancomycin), multicompartment models are employed. However, for clinical purposes, the properties of many drugs can be assessed by utilizing a two-compartment open model in which there is a central (plasma) and a peripheral (tissue) compartment. It is assumed that absorption and elimination of the drug take place only to and from the central compartment.

First-Order Elimination

Drug elimination usually proceeds by *first-order kinetics*. The rate of elimination is proportional to the amount of drug in the body. Following intravenous administration and using the single-compartment model, the logarithm of the drug's plasma concentration plotted against time shows a linear decline (see

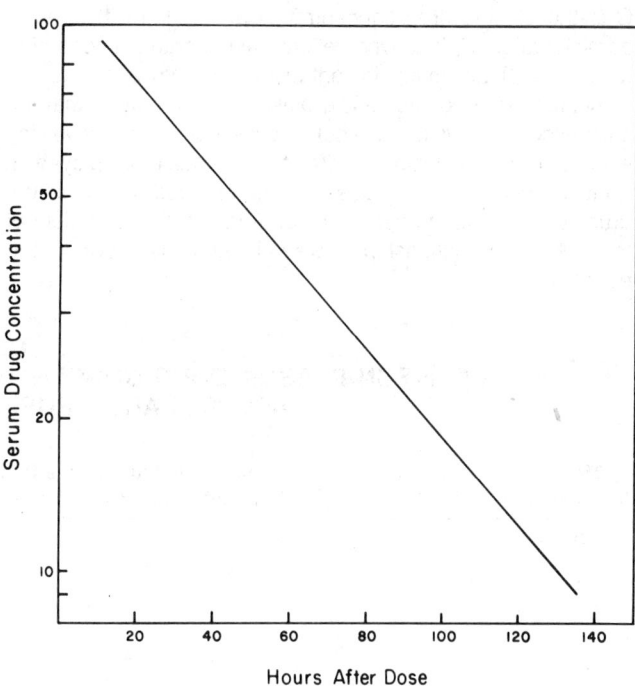

Figure 2. Semilogarithmic plot of the serum concentration versus time for a drug following one-compartment first-order model pharmacokinetic principles.

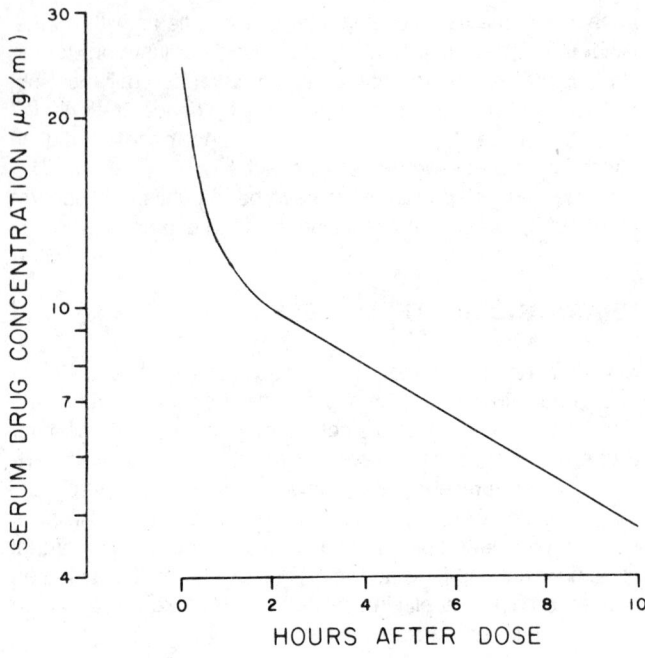

Figure 3. Semilogarithmic plot of the serum concentration versus time for a drug following two-compartment first-order model pharmacokinetic principles.

Figure 2). The slope of this line is the *elimination rate constant* (k). This process can be expressed mathematically as

$$C = C_0 \cdot e^{-kt}$$

(Eq. 7)

C is the plasma drug concentration at any time (t) after its administration, C_0 is a hypothetical plasma drug concentration at time = 0 assuming instantaneous mixing, and k is the elimination rate constant. The plasma concentration may be calculated from this formula but, to avoid calculations involving exponentials, the drug *half-life* ($t_{1/2}$) is usually employed in clinical practice. A half-life is the time required for the serum drug concentration to decline by one-half. It is independent of the dose. The relationship between $t_{1/2}$ and k is shown by the equation:

$$t_{1/2} = \frac{0.693}{k}$$

(Eq. 8)

A similar plot (logarithm of the plasma concentration of intravenous drug against time) may demonstrate a curve in the initial portion followed by a slower decline (Figure 3). This reflects a drug fitting the two-compartment open model. The first segment (α phase) primarily reflects the drug's distribution in the body; the second (β phase) primarily reflects its elimination. The elimination rate constant and the biologic half-life are determined from the β phase.

For practical purposes, a drug is usually considered to be eliminated in about four half-lives (over 90% eliminated) as shown in Table 1. If a drug is given repeatedly at fixed intervals, accumulation occurs until a plateau is reached. This *mean steady-state concentration* (C_{ssav}) is attained in about four half-lives. Thus, the longer the half-life of a drug, the longer it will take to reach a plateau level.

Nonlinear Elimination

Almost all drugs administered within their therapeutic dose range are removed from the plasma at a rate proportional to the amount of drug present, that is, by first-order kinetics. However, even at therapeutic concentrations, a few drugs will exceed the metabolic and/or excretory capacity of the body to behave in this manner. In the extreme of this situation, only a constant amount of the drug is cleared per unit of time, regardless of the concentration in the body. This capacity-limited process is generally described in the clinical literature as *nonlinear kinetics*. Of particular significance is the fact that increases in dose (or frequency of administration) will result in disproportionate increases in the plasma drug concentration and in the time required for elimination; these increases cannot be calculated by the same mathematical formulas employed for drugs that follow first-order kinetics. Dosage modifications for these drugs, notably phenytoin, dicumarol, probenecid, methotrexate, oral propranolol, salicylates, phenylbutazone,

TABLE 1.
DECLINE IN PLASMA DRUG CONCENTRATION FOLLOWING BOLUS INJECTION AND ACCUMULATION DURING CONTINUOUS INFUSION

Time (half-lives)	Single Bolus Intravenous Dose (% of initial plasma concentration)	Continuous Intravenous Infusion (% of steady-state plasma concentration)
0	100	0
1	50	50
2	25	75
3	12.5	87.5
4	6.25	93.75
5	3.12	96.88
6	1.56	98.44

alcohol, and, in some patients, theophylline are best determined by monitoring the clinical response or by measuring plasma levels. Nonlinear kinetics also are observed for drugs that bind to saturable sites in tissues or on plasma proteins and for drugs that alter their own distribution and clearance.

CLINICAL APPLICATIONS OF PHARMACOKINETIC PRINCIPLES

If the values for systemic clearance (Cl) and bioavailability (F) are known, it is possible to select a dosage regimen that will produce an average steady-state serum concentration (C_{ss}) by employing the following equation:

$$Dose = \frac{C_{ss} \cdot Cl \cdot \tau}{F}$$

(Eq. 9)

(τ is the dosing interval.) Equation 9 demonstrates that the dose must be modified if clearance is altered (eg, in patients with renal dysfunction, very young or very old patients).

If a therapeutic concentration must be achieved before approximately four half-lives elapse, a loading dose may be administered, followed by the maintenance dose at the desired dosing interval. A loading dose may be calculated by:

$$LD = \frac{C \cdot V}{F}$$

(Eq. 10)

C is a desired serum concentration.

If a drug having first-order elimination is administered by continuous intravenous infusion, the plateau level may be determined by:

$$C_{ss} = \frac{R_o}{Cl}$$

(Eq. 11)

R_0 is the rate of infusion in amount per unit of time. Doubling the rate of infusion doubles the plateau concentration; halving it halves the concentration. The time to reach plateau concentration by continuous intravenous infusion is about four times the half-life of the drug. Consequently, drugs with long half-lives reach plateau (C_{ssav}) slowly when given at a constant infusion rate. Therefore, a loading dose often is administered to achieve therapeutic drug concentrations rapidly.

Therapeutic Drug Monitoring

The blood, plasma, or serum concentration of a drug usually need not be monitored in uncomplicated cases or when the drug's toxic potential is not great, especially when information on well-defined clinical endpoints is available (eg, blood pressure, blood glucose, prothrombin time, urine output, ventilatory function).

Plasma drug concentrations may be helpful (Gugler and Azarnoff, 1976; Sjöqvist, 1977) (1) to confirm suspicions of under- or overdosage, particularly when the adverse effects of the drug are similar to disease symptoms (eg, nausea in congestive heart failure, muscle weakness in myasthenia gravis); (2) when initiating long-term therapy in patients with chronic diseases (eg, epilepsy, congestive heart failure, asthma); (3) to achieve therapeutic serum drug concentrations rapidly in patients with acute and serious disorders; (4) to establish optimum dosage schedules for drugs that either have a normal TI or do not follow first-order kinetics (eg, phenytoin); (5) when multiple drug therapy is planned and clinically relevant interactions are likely; (6) to identify selected cases of noncompliance, errors of medication, development of tolerance, lack of bioavailability, or an unusual pharmacogenetic reaction; and (7) to monitor the results of treatment in selected patients experiencing toxic reactions.

Nonlinear kinetics often is evident after overdosage, which can be detected with multiple sampling; this establishes the severity of the toxicity and provides an index to monitor the efficacy of management and to estimate the duration of the excessive plasma level of the drug.

Sampling Time: One of the most frequent errors in therapeutic drug monitoring is obtaining blood samples at inappropriate (or unrecorded) times. At best, measuring a serum drug concentration without regard to the timing provides useless information at a relatively high expense; at worst, it misleads a physician into altering a dosage regimen based on faulty data, thus exposing a patient to the risk of subtherapeutic response or toxicity.

When interpreting a serum drug concentration, the drug, route of administration, and condition of the patient must be considered. The serum concentrations of a drug with a short half-life fluctuate markedly between doses; thus, the timing of the sample is critical. If, however, a drug is administered by continuous intravenous infusion, a sample may be obtained anytime after steady state is reached.

The time at which a blood sample is drawn for measuring the serum concentration of a drug with a very long half-life or a timed-release preparation is less critical; once steady state is reached, the specimen usually can be obtained at any time between the completion of the distribution phase and the next dose.

For orally administered drugs, the most common time to draw a blood sample for determining drug concentrations is immediately before the next dose (trough concentration). Sampling at this time minimizes the effects of absorption and distribution.

An acutely ill patient requires more aggressive monitoring than a stabilized one. A serum drug concentration may be determined within a few minutes after a loading dose to ensure that the concentration is within the therapeutic range. On occasion, samples are drawn before steady state in order to forecast whether the concentrations are likely to be subtherapeutic, therapeutic, or toxic at steady state.

Protein Binding and Active Metabolites: Routine determinations of drug serum concentration usually reflect both protein bound and free drug. However, pharmacologic actions generally correlate better with the amount of free drug in the plasma. Only rarely is a change in dosage required because of

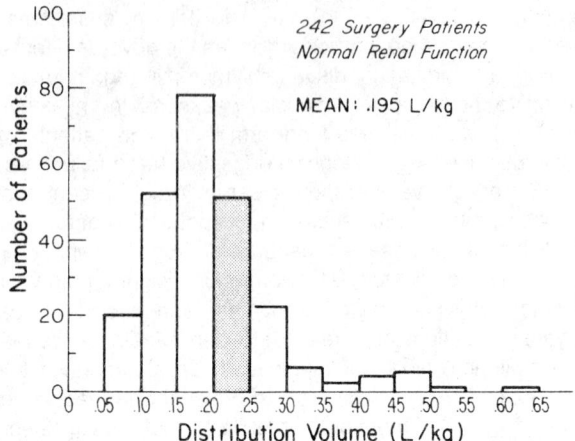

Figure 4. Example of idiopathic interpatient variability. This histogram displays the wide range of distribution volumes for gentamicin in 242 surgery patients with normal measured serum creatinines. From Zaske et al, 1980. Reprinted with permission.

altered binding. A problem can arise if the total serum concentration is employed as a guide to dosage and the binding in the patient differs from that of the general population.

A number of drugs have active metabolites. The metabolites should be considered when monitoring serum concentrations because, unless specifically requested by a physician, their serum concentration is not determined by most clinical laboratories. Active metabolites occasionally have pharmacokinetic and pharmacodynamic characteristics that are quite different from those of the parent compound and may accumulate to toxic levels, especially in patients with impaired renal function.

FACTORS AFFECTING PATIENT RESPONSE TO DRUGS

Probably the most important and least understood factor affecting patient response to a drug is the idiopathic variation

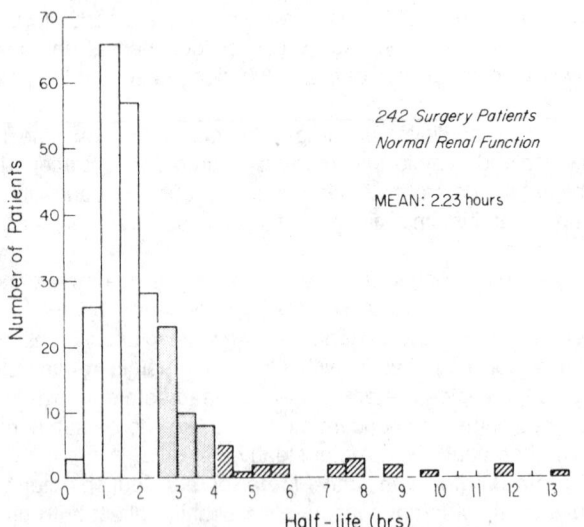

Figure 5. An example of idiopathic interpatient variability. This histogram displays the wide range of gentamicin halflives in 242 surgery patients with measured serum creatinines less than 1.5 mg/dl. From Zaske et al, 1980. Reprinted with permission.

in pharmacokinetic parameters among apparently similar patients (see Figures 4 and 5). There is a large variation in the distribution and clearance of many drugs that cannot be explained by factors such as patient age, gender, or renal and hepatic function. The interpatient variability in pharmacokinetics seems to be as important as the interpatient variability in intrinsic sensitivity to the drug.

Influence of Diet and Environmental Chemicals

Chemical determinants of the response to drugs include food, other drugs, and other xenobiotics (chemicals associated with household products, incidental environmental exposure, occupation, and social activities).

Drug interaction is a term used broadly by some authors to describe alterations of drug effects caused by other drugs, food, or an environmental chemical (Alvares, 1978; Alvares et al, 1979; Dollery et al, 1979). More information on interactions, especially drug-drug interactions encountered in clinical practice, is presented in Chapter 3, Drug Interactions and Adverse Drug Reactions.

Food: The diet may affect the absorption, distribution, metabolism, and elimination of drugs. Serious vitamin and protein deficiencies can affect drug binding, biotransformation, or patient response. Dietary fat can alter the absorption of lipid-soluble drugs (eg, griseofulvin).

Most food-drug interactions decrease the rate or extent of drug absorption (Welling, 1984). Some are clinically relevant (eg, tetracycline and milk) but most are not. Variation in absorption can be minimized by taking drugs on an empty stomach with an adequate volume (150 to 200 ml) of fluid. In a few instances, however, giving certain drugs with food may avoid gastrointestinal irritation (eg, iron preparations, metronidazole, nitrofurantoin, potassium salts, nonsteroidal anti-inflammatory agents) or even enhance absorption (eg, griseofulvin, isotretinoin). When applicable, this information is included in the drug evaluations.

Adverse food-drug interactions also may occur. For example, headache and occasional hypertensive crisis may follow the ingestion of tyramine-rich foods (eg, cheddar cheese, chicken liver, aged or tenderized meats, Chianti or sherry wine, broad beans) by patients receiving monoamine oxidase inhibitors (isocarboxazid, tranylcypromine, phenelzine).

Nondrug Chemicals: The average individual in the United States is exposed to numerous nondrug chemicals in the form of food additives and contaminants. In addition, occupational or household chemical exposures orally, dermally, or by inhalation must be taken into account. The clinical relevance of this chemical burden is unknown, but the physician should be aware that he is giving drugs to patients who are exposed to nondrug chemicals. Since most nondrug chemicals do not appear in patient histories or drug profiles, the suspicion and identification of an occupational or household chemical exposure may help explain therapeutic failure or an adverse drug reaction (eg, the disulfiram-like response to alcohol-containing preparations by workers exposed to cyanamide or tetramethylthiuram disulfide).

Cigarette smoke contains polycyclic hydrocarbons that induce mixed-function hepatic oxidases, particularly in the young (Vestal and Wood, 1980). This enhancement of metabolism increases the dosage requirement for theophylline. The plasma levels of imipramine and antipyrine also are decreased in smokers. Other hydrocarbons (eg, chlorinated hydrocarbons in pesticides such as DDT and lindane; the flame retardant polychlorinated biphenyls; polycyclic hydrocarbons in charcoal broiled meat) also can increase the biotransformation of antipyrine and theophylline.

Alcohol has numerous actions that can alter the response to many drugs. Because of its widespread use, alcohol has the most clinically significant drug interaction capacity of any single nondietary nondrug chemical. Its actions are variable and depend upon the degree and duration of intake. Acute alcohol ingestion may inhibit the biotransformation of drugs. Conversely, chronic alcohol use (more than 200 g/day) induces microsomal oxidation enzymes that metabolize many drugs (Iber, 1977). In the absence of acute intoxication, the chronic alcoholic metabolizes some substances (eg, barbiturates) more rapidly and thus shows considerable tolerance to these agents. Conversely, in the later stages of hepatic cirrhosis, the chronic alcoholic may become sensitive to drugs that depend upon hepatic metabolism for elimination.

Influence of Pharmacogenetics

Variability among individuals in their response to drugs is due, in part, to genetic differences (Weinshilboum, 1984; Vesell, 1985). Individuals with genetic variants may fail to respond to or may experience adverse effects with usual therapeutic doses.

Genetic Differences in Drug Biotransformation: Because most drugs are biotransformed rather than excreted unchanged, genetic variations in metabolic pathways or rate of biotransformation may have important clinical implications. Some drugs have multiple pathways of biotransformation; the resulting metabolites may be inactive, have activity similar to that of the parent drug, or show an entirely different activity.

Drug oxidation appears to be controlled by two alleles at a single gene locus (genetic polymorphism) (Eichelbaum, 1984). The disposition of phenformin, tricyclic antidepressants, phenytoin, metoprolol, alprenolol, perhexilene, tolbutamide, and phenylbutazone has been studied in twins and in families, and a major contributor to the variability in response to these drugs is genetically controlled.

Several drugs are biotransformed by acetylation; the metabolite may be inactive (eg, N-acetylisoniazid) or active (eg, N-acetylprocainamide). The general population can be divided into slow or fast acetylators. Because of this genetic distinction, individualization of therapy based on acetylator phenotype may avoid therapeutic failure or toxic reactions. Rapid inactivators are homozygous or heterozygous for a gene controlling an "acetylating" enzyme, while slow inactivation is a homozygous recessive trait. Approximately one-half of American whites and blacks are slow inactivators of isoniazid, but this trait is uncommon among Japanese and rare in Eskimos. Liver damage is more common in rapid acetylators, apparently because a metabolite of isoniazid, acetylhydrazine, accumulates in these individuals; acetylhydrazine is converted to an acylating agent that causes hepatocellular necrosis. In slow acetylators, the maintenance of higher plasma levels of isoniazid may predispose to dose-related neuropathies and may interfere with the biotransformation of other drugs (eg, phenytoin).

Slow acetylators of hydralazine and sulfasalazine, but probably not phenelzine, experience adverse effects more frequently than fast acetylators in whom usual doses may be less effective. Hydralazine-induced lupus erythematosus occurs almost exclusively in slow acetylators and may be related to an altered ratio of the two principal metabolites.

Hereditary Diseases That Alter Drug Response: Hereditary diseases in which symptoms of the disease and/or other adverse effects are precipitated by specific drugs are good examples of the influence of genetic factors on drug response. In other genetic disorders, the response to certain drugs is enhanced, diminished, or abnormal, and these agents may be useful to detect heterozygotes.

A number of drugs produce *hemolytic anemia* in individuals with an inherited deficiency of glucose-6-phosphate dehydrogenase (G6PD). Enzyme-deficient cells cannot protect themselves as efficiently as normal erythrocytes against oxidant drugs or metabolites; in the presence of these agents, essential cell components are oxidized and hemolysis occurs. This inborn error of metabolism is frequently called "primaquine sensitivity," because it was originally observed in patients receiving antimalarial drugs (primaquine, pamaquine, pentaquine). Hemolytic anemia also has developed in susceptible individuals after administration of some sulfonamides, nitrofurans, sulfones, antipyretic-analgesics (acetanilid, phenacetin, and, in some extreme variants, aspirin), chloramphenicol, aminosalicylic acid, quinidine, methylene blue, and vitamin K. It also has occurred after contact with naphthalene or ingestion of fava beans. Most individuals with G6PD deficiency do not experience hematologic symptoms unless they are exposed to these agents.

The geographical distribution of G6PD deficiency closely follows the distribution of *Plasmodium falciparum* malaria, which suggests that the trait provides some selective advantage against this disease. It appears most frequently in populations of African and Mediterranean descent and occurs in about 10% to 13% of black American males. Oxidant drugs or metabolites often cause more severe symptoms in whites with G6PD deficiency than in affected blacks. Also, hemolysis may be induced in whites by agents that have no hemolytic effect on enzyme-deficient blacks (eg, chloramphenicol, aminosalicylic acid, fava beans).

Influence of Biological Rhythms

The pharmacologic activity of a drug is affected by inherent biological rhythms in physiologic sensitivity (chronesthesy) and drug disposition (chronopharmacokinetics) (Reinberg and Smolensky, 1982). *Chronopharmacology* is the study of drug effects in relation to biological rhythms. Biological rhythms recur at daily (circadian), weekly (circasesten), monthly (circatrigintan), and yearly (circannual) intervals (known as periods) and are defined by the peak time in relation to the period (acrophase), the within-period variability (amplitude), and the mean for the period (mesor).

Chronopharmacology has significant clinical implications, and the chronopharmacokinetics of aspirin, theophylline, nortriptyline, alcohol, cisplatin, phenytoin, and corticosteroids have been studied in man. It has been noted that doses of corticosteroid given at 7 AM and at 11 PM are more likely to produce the desired effects in Addison's disease than three doses administered with meals (Reinberg, 1978). The nephrotoxicity of cisplatin may be minimized when this drug is administered from 5 PM to 6 PM (Hrushesky and Rushing, 1984), and the toxicity of doxorubicin may be minimized when it is administered at 6 AM (Hrushesky, 1985). The role of chronopharmacology in other drug therapy remains to be determined.

Influence of Disease

RENAL IMPAIRMENT. Renal dysfunction can alter the absorption, distribution, metabolism, and excretion of drugs.

Absorption: The effect of renal function on the absorption of oral drugs has not been fully explored. Many patients in renal failure are given aluminum-containing antacids to bind and prevent phosphate absorption, but the absorption of other drugs also may be impaired.

The absorption of a number of drugs was thought to be decreased in patients with renal failure, but studies now show that changes in serum concentrations may be due to altered drug distribution and clearance rather than absorption (Gambertoglio, 1984).

Distribution: Drug distribution may be affected by (1) changes in systemic pH, such as the acidosis of uremia or the alkalosis following severe potassium depletion; (2) alterations in protein binding that result from hypoalbuminemia produced by the nephrotic syndrome, by displacement of drugs by endogenous acids that accumulate in those with uremia, or by the altered configuration of albumin in that condition; and (3) other factors that are imperfectly understood. These changes in drug distribution have been placed into two categories (Brater, 1980): effects that change the total plasma concentration of the drug (eg, phenytoin, warfarin, digoxin) and effects that leave the total plasma concentration unchanged but modify the free fraction (diazoxide, salicylates, phenobarbital, thiopental).

In endstage renal disease, digoxin's volume of distribution is reduced and a smaller than usual loading dose will produce the normal therapeutic range of plasma drug concentrations. In uremia or hypoalbuminemia, protein binding of a number of drugs (eg, phenytoin, warfarin, diazepam, triamterene, sulfonamides, penicillin) is decreased. The resulting increase in unbound drug would be expected to intensify the pharmacologic action or cause toxicity, but there is usually a compensatory increase in clearance. The therapeutic dose of phenytoin, for example, usually remains the same, but the total plasma concentration may be one-half to one-third that of patients with normal renal function.

Systemic acidosis increases the permeability of the central nervous system to salicylates and phenobarbital but does not affect the plasma concentration of these agents. Similarly, decreased protein binding intensifies the activity of diazoxide and thiopental. Whether increased sensitivity to other drugs is due to similar alterations in distribution has not been established (eg, encephalopathy produced by large parenteral doses of penicillin in uremic patients, obtunded cardioaccelerator response to atropine in those with chronic renal failure).

Metabolism: The clinical significance of drug metabolism within the kidneys, which may be considerable (Anders, 1980), has not been evaluated and, historically, has been ignored. Renal disease sometimes affects hepatic metabolism. The mechanism is clear when changes in protein binding and volume of distribution are involved, but is as yet obscure and unpredictable when enzymatic processes are concerned.

Excretion: Drugs that are excreted mostly unchanged by the kidney (eg, aminoglycosides, cephalosporins, some sulfonamides, digoxin, lithium, ethambutol, methotrexate) or those with pharmacologically active metabolites that are eliminated by renal excretion (eg, allopurinol, clofibrate, procainamide, meperidine, amobarbital, some oral sulfonylureas) may produce adverse effects in patients with impaired renal function if usual doses are administered.

To prevent accumulation and toxic effects caused by increased plasma concentrations of the drug or metabolite, the rate of administration must be reduced. This can be accomplished by reducing the size of the dose while maintaining the usual dosing interval or by increasing the interval while using the standard dose. For the aminoglycosides, it generally is preferable to give standard doses at increased intervals to prevent toxic or subtherapeutic peak levels or toxic trough levels.

Dosage adjustment may be important if renal function is less than 50% of normal, if the percentage of drug excreted unchanged is greater than 50%, or if active metabolites are extensively excreted by the kidney. As the percentage of drug excreted by the kidney decreases with reduction in renal function, there is a corresponding increase in the importance of extrarenal routes (biliary and metabolic) of elimination. If extrarenal elimination also is compromised, compensation must be considered *in addition* to the dosage adjustment made for the loss in renal function.

HEPATIC IMPAIRMENT. The importance of hepatic dysfunction as a determinant of pharmacokinetics depends, for the most part, on the extent that the liver contributes to the drug's elimination. The extraction ratio (see the discussion on Hepatic Clearance for definition) may be modified by changes in protein binding (cirrhosis, ascites, renal disease). Changes in hepatic blood flow also may alter hepatic clearance. The metabolizing capacity is reduced following hepatic necrosis, is enhanced by microsomal enzyme induction by some drugs or environmental chemicals, or is variably modified by alcohol. Disorders of biliary excretion affect the clearance of drugs excreted primarily in the bile, which are mostly agents of high molecular weight (eg, rifampin).

Dosage guidelines for patients with cirrhosis and hepatitis are being developed (Sjöqvist et al, 1980). Unfortunately, in contrast to renal disease, there is no quantitative method for adjusting dosage in patients with liver disease because of the variability of involvement and lack of ability to measure hepatic clearance (Bennett, 1981).

OTHER DISEASE STATES. Diseases that reduce cardiac output or hepatic blood flow decrease the elimination of drugs whose clearance is limited by perfusion. In *congestive heart failure*, the clearance of lidocaine may be reduced by 50%. Edema can alter transport processes at many sites. Gastrointestinal mucosal edema in patients with congestive heart failure significantly decreases the absorption of quinidine, furosemide, procainamide, and hydrochlorothiazide.

Pulmonary disease (cor pulmonale, acute hypoxia) may produce hemodynamic disturbances that decrease renal and hepatic blood flow, which reduces the clearance of drugs with flow-dependent elimination. The half-life of aminoglycosides is prolonged significantly in preterm neonates with hypoxia, and the clearance of theophylline is reduced up to 75% in patients with severe respiratory insufficiency. Hypoxia may affect a drug's metabolic pathways and extent of metabolism (eg, increased liberation of the nephrotoxic fluoride ion from halothane).

For the effect of *gastrointestinal disease* on drug absorption, see the section on Absorption and Bank et al, 1980.

Hypo- and hyperthyroidism can influence bioavailability (riboflavin), biotransformation (propylthiouracil), and renal excretion (digoxin) of drugs.

Pregnancy may significantly decrease the protein binding of drugs (Dean et al, 1980), increase their renal excretion (Krauer and Krauer, 1977), and variably affects their metabolism. The binding of phenytoin to serum proteins, for example, is reduced markedly during the last trimester of pregnancy (Ruprah et al, 1980), thus accelerating clearance, decreasing drug plasma concentrations, and adversely affecting seizure control. The disposition of most drugs during pregnancy has not been studied.

In *obesity,* the dosage of water-soluble drugs with a narrow margin of safety (eg, digoxin, aminoglycosides) should be calculated on the basis of ideal weight rather than on actual body weight. Little information is available to establish dosage guidelines for fat-soluble drugs in these patients. For theophylline, it has been suggested that the loading dose be based on actual weight, but that the maintenance dosage be calculated on the basis of ideal weight. Ideal body weight can be calculated by the following equations:

$$IBW \text{ (male)} = 50 \text{ kg} + 2.3 \text{ kg/inch over 5 feet}$$
$$IBW \text{ (female)} = 45 \text{ kg} + 2.3 \text{ kg/inch over 5 feet}$$

Modification of receptor sensitivity, destruction of acetylcholine receptor sites (in myasthenia gravis), and loss of dopaminergic receptors (in parkinsonism) illustrate the considerable range of effects that diseases have on the pharmacodynamic response to a drug. Receptor activity also may be increased. Thus, one to two weeks after acute denervation (soft tissue trauma, major burns, cord transection), succinylcholine may liberate sufficient potassium from the affected muscle to induce cardiac arrest.

Influence of Age

The patient's age may be responsible for variations in drug response. Particular problems in dosage selection occur in the very young and the very old; the former are undergoing nonuniform organ maturation while the latter are experiencing nonuniform organ deterioration. Both of these extreme age groups differ from young adults in the kinetics of absorption and elimination, volume of distribution, and receptor sensitivity.

PEDIATRIC PATIENTS. There are many difficulties in choosing the most appropriate drugs and determining the dosage in pediatric patients, who are usually divided into three age groups: newborn, 0 to 4 weeks (perinatal, 26 weeks gestation to end of first postnatal month); infant, 5 to 52 weeks; child, 1 to 16 years (adolescent, 12 to 16 years). Whether children and infants will respond to a particular drug in the same manner as adults can be determined only through research and experience. Indeed, their responses to many drugs are known to be different. The age and size of the individual, as well as the disease state, affect dosage in these patients.

The pharmacokinetics of many drugs change with the continuing development of several physiologic functions. Many metabolic mechanisms in premature and newborn infants are not fully developed, and drugs may accumulate to toxic concentrations if dosage is based upon traditional criteria. In fact, the infant's response to drugs during the first weeks of life probably varies more, overall, from that of a 1-year-old than the response of a 1-year-old varies from that of an adult.

Although an increasing number of studies are being conducted on the pharmacokinetics of drugs in pediatric patients, data on which to base dosage recommendations for specific drugs are limited. Consequently, most drugs do not have established doses for infants and children. Nevertheless, some generalizations can be made on the basis of the information available.

The basic pharmacokinetic functions (absorption, distribution, metabolism, and excretion) affect a drug's concentration at receptor sites and hence its actions, and these should be considered when treating pediatric patients.

Absorption: Differences in gastrointestinal function that may affect the absorption of drugs occur primarily in the newborn and infant. (In general, there are no important differences between the healthy child and adult.) Peristalsis is irregular during the first several weeks, gastric emptying is prolonged until about 6 to 12 months of age, and gastric pH is neutral and does not reach adult values until about 3 years of age. The oral absorption of nalidixic acid, phenytoin, and acetaminophen is delayed in neonates, and the absorption of phenobarbital is delayed and reduced during the first two weeks of life. Because gastric acidity is decreased during the neonatal period, there is increased absorption of acid-labile penicillins in infants and children up to 3 years. In older infants and children, the rate of absorption of several anticonvulsants (phenobarbital, ethosuximide, valproic acid, clonazepam, diazepam) and imipramine is increased; thus, their frequency of administration may require reduction. It should be kept in mind that diseases of the gastrointestinal tract may alter the absorption rate of orally administered drugs.

Intramuscular absorption in infants may be decreased and erratic, but percutaneous absorption is more rapid and extensive in infants than in adults because of differences in skin thickness.

Distribution: The distribution of drugs in neonates and infants may differ from that in older children and adults because body composition varies markedly with age. The proportion of body water (total and extracellular) is greater in the newborn but gradually decreases to adult values by about 12 months. The relative mass of subcutaneous tissue also varies; it is greatest at 9 months, decreases until about 6 years, and increases again in adolescence. These changes affect the distribution of lipid-soluble drugs.

Plasma protein binding also affects drug disposition. For some drugs, this is decreased in the newborn, but adult values are reached in about 10 to 12 months. Protein binding of salicylates, penicillins, sulfonamides, phenytoin, phenylbutazone, phenobarbital, and imipramine is decreased in infants. The protein binding of diazepam and digoxin is similar in infants and adults. In neonates with hyperbilirubinemia, drugs that are highly bound to plasma proteins (eg, sulfonamides, salicylates, phenytoin) may displace bilirubin and cause kernicterus.

Since cardiac output and blood flow are related to body surface rather than to body weight, drug distribution and equilibration rates are faster in children than in adults.

Metabolism: In general, the capacity of the infant's liver to metabolize drugs is low and develops rapidly in the first months after birth. It varies for different drugs depending upon the enzymes involved, since not all enzyme systems are affected to the same degree and do not attain adult values at the same rate.

Drugs that depend upon hepatic metabolism for elimination may have longer apparent plasma half-lives in infants; for those drugs, the interval between doses should be increased and the daily dose decreased. Certain drugs administered to the mother during pregnancy may affect metabolism in the newborn through induction of hepatic enzymes. For example, phenytoin and carbamazepine have shorter half-lives in neonates who were exposed to these drugs prenatally. In addition, an inducing agent given to the mother may affect its own plasma half-life and that of certain other drugs given to the infant. Therefore, the possibility of previous exposure to an inducing agent might be considered when administering drugs to a newborn infant, although the clinical significance of prenatal enzyme induction has not been assessed.

Data on specific drugs are limited; the plasma half-life of diazepam, digoxin, indomethacin, nalidixic acid, nortriptyline, acetaminophen, phenylbutazone, phenobarbital, phenytoin, salicylates, and tolbutamide appears to be longer in infants. Conversely, theophylline, phenylbutazone, and most anticonvulsants are metabolized faster in older children than in adults. It should be kept in mind that hepatic disease may affect the metabolizing ability in children as well as in adults.

Excretion: Renal function in relation to body surface area is greatly reduced in neonates and infants but approaches adult values in about 6 to 12 months. Drugs that depend upon renal excretion for elimination are disposed of slowly in infants and have longer apparent half-lives. Therefore, the dosage of these drugs must be adjusted to avoid accumulation and toxic reactions.

Dosage schedules for several antibiotics (eg, penicillins, gentamicin, kanamycin) that are eliminated by the kidney have been developed (see the appropriate chapters in Section XI). Other drugs that are excreted at reduced rates include indomethacin, salicylic acid, acetaminophen, and sulfonamides. The renal clearance of digoxin, as a function of body surface area, is low at 1 month of age but increases to within the adult range at about 6 months. (See the section on Renal Impairment.)

Calculation of Doses for Children: It must be emphasized that any method devised to calculate drug dosage for both children and adults provides an estimate only, to be verified or corrected by clinical experience and/or measurement of drug concentrations. Usually, the dose for children is given in terms of mg/kg of body weight, mg/M^2 of body surface area, or as a fraction proportionate to the weight of the child in comparison with that of an average adult. However, the dose of many drugs is not a simple linear function of body weight, and to calculate the dose as so much per kilogram of body weight is often inaccurate. Another common practice in determining a child's dose has been to give some fraction of an adult dose, using the age of the patient as a rough guide. Because of the great variation in size among children of the same age, this method is satisfactory only for drugs with a wide margin of safety.

Experience has shown that the dose of many drugs is more nearly proportionate to weight to the 0.7 power (Wt$^{0.7}$). The surface area of the body (in square meters) also may be approximated by Wt (lb)$^{0.7}$ X 0.055. Although the validity of this method has been criticized because body surface area may not be related directly to physiologic and metabolic function, it does provide a practical and useful basis for the estimation of drug dosage in children. Thus, dosage expressed as grams or milligrams per square meter of surface area rather than per unit of body weight may provide a more accurate method of adjusting the dose to the age or size of the patient for some drugs. Surface area, however, is not a satisfactory basis for dosage calculations in premature infants or neonates.

Statements of pediatric dosage for individual drugs in this book follow the method of conversion developed for the particular drug. Thus, some conversions are based upon age, some upon weight, and some upon body surface area. If adequate dosage information based on actual pediatric use is either nonexistent or not readily available, suggested guidelines sometimes are furnished even when it is recognized that more data would be desirable; for some drugs, lack of information has been specifically acknowledged. When the dosage for children has been established, it is given in the text and should be used in preference to any calculated dose. When information is inadequate, it is suggested that the body surface area be taken as the criterion—*provided* there is no evidence that a child will react to the drug differently from an adult. Calculation of a fractional exponential function of weight is too forbidding for practical use, but the task may be simplified by employing a table (see Table 2).

GERIATRIC PATIENTS. Elderly patients also should receive special consideration when determining the dosage of certain drugs. Two-thirds of all Americans over the age of 65 take at least one prescription drug. Of those who take prescription drugs, at least one-third take three or more (American Association of Retired Persons, 1984). Because they use relatively

TABLE 2.
DETERMINATION OF CHILDREN'S DOSES
FROM ADULT DOSES ON THE BASIS OF BODY SURFACE AREA

Age	Weight*		Surface area*	
	(kg.)	(lb.)	(Sq. M.)	Fraction of adult dose†
	2.0	4.4	0.15	0.09
Birth	3.4	7.4	0.21	0.12
3 Weeks	4.0	8.8	0.25	0.14
3 months	5.7	12.5	0.29	0.17
6 months	7.4	16	0.36	0.21
9 months	9.1	20	0.44	0.25
1 year	10	22	0.46	0.27
1½ years	11	25	0.50	0.29
2 years	12	27	0.54	0.31
3 years	14	31	0.60	0.35
4 years	16	36	0.68	0.39
5 years	19	41	0.73	0.42
6 years	21	47	0.82	0.47
7 years	24	53	0.90	0.52
8 years	27	59	0.97	0.56
9 years	29	65	1.05	0.61
10 years	32	71	1.12	0.65
11 years	36	78	1.20	0.70
12 years	39	86	1.28	0.74

*Approximate average for age.
†Based on adult surface area of 1.73 sq. M.
From Done AK, 1972.

more drugs than other age groups, the appropriate choice of drugs and dosage is of primary importance in their health care.

Although a specific age cannot be applied to define this group, patients over 60 or 65 are usually included. However, it should be kept in mind that chronological age does not correspond well to physiologic age in the elderly. There is a gradual deterioration of all systems, but some organs may be affected more than others in a given individual. The differences between individuals of the same age is therefore so great that increased biological variation is characteristic of this age group. Each patient must be evaluated individually.

When prescribing drugs for the elderly, special attention should be given to the following general principles:

(1) The physician should ascertain what other medications, including OTC products, the patient is taking. Elderly people often take many drugs, some of which may not be needed and should be discontinued. The patient should receive as few drugs as possible.

(2) The dosage schedule should be as simple as possible, and the dosage form should be easily self-administered. Directions for taking the medication should be understood by the patient; over one-half of Americans over 65 desire written instructions (American Association of Retired Persons, 1984).

Patient medication instructions for a number of drugs are available from the American Medical Association, Department of Drugs, 535 N Dearborn, Chicago, IL 60610.

(3) Patients should be followed closely to determine compliance, drug efficacy, and adverse effects.

(4) Any physiologic or pathologic changes that may affect the dosage and response to the drug must be considered. However, these factors are often difficult to identify and studies on the pharmacokinetics of drugs in the elderly have been limited. Nevertheless, available evidence indicates that changes in several physiologic functions occur with aging and these may affect the actions of certain drugs.

Absorption: There is little evidence that the extent of absorption of passively absorbed drugs is diminished in the elderly. Other factors are usually responsible for altered drug effects in the elderly. However, conditions such as decreased gastric acidity and gastrointestinal motility, which reduce gastric emptying, and possibly decreased trypsin production may delay or impair drug absorption. Drugs that affect these functions (eg, antacids, anticholinergics) may affect the absorption of other agents. The active absorption of nutrients, vitamins, and minerals also may be impaired in the elderly. For example, it has been reported that iron, calcium, thiamine, galactose, vitamin B_{12}, and 3-methylglucose absorption is decreased and, thus, larger doses may be necessary (Massoud, 1984).

Distribution: Alterations in circulation and changes in body composition may affect the distribution and equilibration rate of drugs. Total body weight may decrease, especially in the very elderly, but the ratio of fat to lean is usually greater. Adipose tissue increases from an average of 18% to 30% in men and from 35% to 48% in women (Greenblatt et al, 1982). The enlarged fat compartment may increase the distribution volume of lipid-soluble drugs (eg, diazepam, lidocaine) and decrease the volume of water-soluble drugs (eg, acetaminophen, alcohol). In addition, the plasma albumin concentration may decrease, which elevates the free (active) fraction of drugs that are highly protein bound (eg, warfarin). Because the effects of warfarin or other anticoagulants may be enhanced in geriatric patients, therapy should be monitored carefully. Furthermore, since displacement of one drug by another from protein-binding sites is one mechanism of drug-drug interaction (eg, phenylbutazone, salicylate, sulfadiazine) (see Chapter 3), it is particularly important to consider this possibility in the elderly.

Metabolism: The relationship between aging and hepatic enzyme metabolic capacity is complex and depends on the type of metabolic reaction (oxidative versus conjugation reactions) and the patient's gender. Oxidative capacity declines with age, but the decline is greater in elderly men than in elderly women (Greenblatt et al, 1984) and there is considerable intersubject variability (Vestal et al, 1975). Environmental factors such as cigarette smoking may have a greater influence than age per se. The effect on oxidative metabolism is consistent for most drugs with low hepatic extraction ratios. The data are less clear regarding drugs with high extraction ratios, because their rate of metabolism depends on hepatic blood flow in addition to hepatic metabolic enzyme activity. The rate of hepatic conjugation appears to be unaffected by age.

Excretion: Between the ages of 20 and 90, there is an almost linear decline in glomerular filtration rate and tubular secretion by 35% to 50%. This is accompanied by decreased renal blood flow. In addition, most patients over age 60 have some renal pathology, which further reduces renal function. Therefore, it is important to consider the geriatric patient's renal function when determining the dose of certain drugs. Doses may need to be reduced or dosage intervals lengthened to prevent accumulation. Some elderly patients have relatively normal renal function, and care must be taken to avoid underdosing as well as overdosing. The patient should be monitored carefully; determination of serum drug concentrations may be useful.

Drugs excreted by the kidney that are used commonly in elderly patients and that may require reduction of the maintenance dose include digoxin, quinidine, aminoglycosides, colistin, ethambutol, tetracyclines (except doxycycline), amantadine, cimetidine, and lithium. Loading doses usually are the same in the elderly as in other patients. The evaluations on these drugs should be consulted for dosages in patients with decreased renal function. See also the section on Renal Impairment.

The clearance of drugs that are eliminated by active tubular secretion (eg, organic bases [procainamide]) also is decreased with age independently of the glomerular filtration rate (creatinine clearance). Thus, the elderly require smaller doses than middle-aged adults, just as the young may require larger doses.

Pharmacodynamics: Elderly patients appear to be more sensitive to some drug effects, but the mechanisms involved are not known. Increased receptor sensitivity is difficult to determine and explain pharmacologically. Changes in hormone, adrenergic, and biogenic amine receptors occur with aging, but their influence on drug action has not yet been determined.

In general, the elderly are more sensitive to narcotics: Morphine produces increased pain relief but more variable serum concentrations, and meperidine has a longer half-life and causes more adverse reactions. Barbiturates produce erratic and paradoxical effects, possibly due to diminished sensory input in a patient with an already limited global orientation; drug half-lives are prolonged but the mechanism is unknown. The tricyclic antidepressants cause confusion and disorientation, which may result from increased sensitivity to their anticholinergic effects. The incidence of phenothiazine-induced extrapyramidal reactions and orthostatic hypotension may be increased. The thiazides also produce orthostatic hypotension more often, which may result from impaired compensatory action. Thiazides cause hypokalemia more frequently in elderly patients, which potentiates the effects of digitalis. The incidence of hyperkalemia is higher in older patients taking potassium-sparing diuretics, possibly because renal function is impaired in these individuals. The elderly may be more susceptible to hypoglycemia with use of sulfonylureas. With aspirin, the incidence of occult blood loss may be higher and may lead to iron deficiency anemia; larger than usual doses of supplemental iron may be required because of decreased absorption.

Additional factors that affect drug response in the elderly are various disease states, the simultaneous use of a number of drugs, a marginal diet, drug-induced nutritional deficits, and, very importantly, *uneven compliance* with the medication schedule. As a general rule, both the effective dose and the toxic dose decline with advancing age.

Selected References

Bioavailability

DeBoer AG, et al: Drug absorption by sublingual and rectal routes. *Br J Anaesth* 56:69-82, 1984.

Gibaldi M: Prolonged-release medication. *Perspect Clin Pharmacol* 2:17-20, 25-27, 33-35, 41-43, 49-53, 1984.

Diet and Environmental Chemicals

Alvares AP: Interactions between environmental chemicals and drug biotransformation in man. *Clin Pharmacokinet* 3:462-477, 1978.

Alvares AP, et al: Regulation of drug metabolism in man by environmental factors. *Drug Metab Rev* 9:185-205, 1979.

Dollery CT, et al: Contribution of environmental factors to variability in human drug metabolism. *Drug Metab Rev* 9:207-220, 1979.

George CF: Food, drugs, and bioavailability. *Br Med J* 289:1093-1094, 1984.

Iber FL: Drug metabolism in heavy consumers of ethyl alcohol. *Clin Pharmacol Ther* 22:735-742, 1977.

Vestal RE, Wood AJJ: Influence of age and smoking on drug kinetics in man: Studies using model compounds. *Clin Pharmacokinet* 5:309-319, 1980.

Welling PG: Interactions affecting drug absorption. *Clin Pharmacokinet* 9:404-434, 1984.

Geriatric Patients

American Association of Retired Persons: *Prescription Drugs: A Survey of Consumer Uses, Attitudes, and Behavior*. Washington, DC, AARP, 1984.

Goldberg PB, Roberts J: Pharmacologic basis for developing rational drug regimens for elderly patients. *Med Clin North Am* 67:315-331, 1983.

Greenblatt DJ, et al: Drug disposition in old age. *N Engl J Med* 306:1081-1088, 1982.

Greenblatt DJ, et al: Pharmacokinetic risk factors in the elderly, in Moore SR, Teal TW (eds): *Geriatric Drug Use: Clinical and Social Perspectives*. New York, Pergamon Press, 1984, 153-159.

Massoud N: Pharmacokinetic considerations in geriatric patients, in Benet LZ, et al (eds): *Pharmacokinetic Basis for Drug Treatment*. New York, Raven Press, 1984, 283-310.

Mayersohn M: "Xylose test" to assess gastrointestinal absorption in the elderly: Pharmacokinetic evaluation of literature. *J Gerontol* 37:300-305, 1982.

Vestal RE, Dawson GW: Pharmacology and aging, in Finch CE, Schneider EL (eds): *Handbook of the Biology of Aging*, ed 2. New York, Van Nostrand, 1985, 744-819.

Vestal RE, et al: Antipyrine metabolism in man: Influence of age, alcohol, caffeine, and smoking. *Clin Pharmacol Ther* 18:425-432, 1975.

Hepatic, Cardiovascular, and Other Disease States

Bank S, et al: Gastrointestinal and hepatic diseases, in Avery GS (ed): *Drug Treatment: Principles and Practice of Clinical Pharmacology and Therapeutics*, ed 2. Sydney, ADIS Press, 1980, 683-759.

Bennett WM: Altering drug dose in patients with diseases of the kidney and liver, in Anderson RJ, Schrier RW (eds): *Clinical Use of Drugs in Patients with Kidney and Liver Disease*. Philadelphia, WB Saunders, 1981, 16-29.

Dean M, et al: Serum protein binding of drugs during and after pregnancy in humans. *Clin Pharmacol Ther* 28:253-261, 1980.

Krauer B, Krauer F: Drug kinetics in pregnancy. *Clin Pharmacokinet* 2:167-181, 1977.

Ruprah M, et al: Decreased serum protein binding of phenytoin in late pregnancy. *Lancet* 2:316-317, 1980.

Sjöqvist F, et al: Fundamentals of clinical pharmacology, in Avery GS (ed): *Drug Treatment: Principles and Practice of Clinical Pharmacology and Therapeutics,* ed 2. Sydney, ADIS Press, 1980, 1-61.

Wilkinson GR, Shand DG: Physiological approach to hepatic drug clearance. *Clin Pharmacol Ther* 18:377-390, 1975.

Williams RL, Benet LZ: Drug pharmacokinetics in cardiac and hepatic disease. *Annu Rev Pharmacol Toxicol* 20:389-413, 1980.

Pediatric Patients

Done AK: Drugs for children, in Modell W (ed): *Drugs of Choice 1972-1973*, St Louis, CV Mosby, 1982.

George SL, Gehan EA: Methods for measurement of body surface area. *J Pediatr* 94:342, 1979.

Green TP, Mirkin BL: Clinical pharmacokinetics: Pediatric considerations, in Benet LZ, et al (eds): *Pharmacokinetic Basis for Drug Treatment*. New York, Raven Press, 1984, 269-282.

Haycock GB, et al: Geometric method for measuring body surface area: Height-weight formula validated in infants, children, and adults. *J Pediatr* 93:62-66, 1978.

Morselli PL, et al: Clinical pharmacokinetics in newborns and infants: Age-related differences and therapeutic implications. *Clin Pharmacokinet* 5:485-527, 1980.

Nation RL: Drug kinetics in childbirth. *Clin Pharmacokinet* 5:340-364, 1980.

Roberts RJ: Pharmacologic principles in therapeutics in infants, in: *Drug Therapy in Infants: Pharmacologic Principles and Clinical Experience*. Philadelphia, WB Saunders, 1984, 3-24.

Triggs EJ, et al: Influence of age on drug metabolism. *Med J Aust* 141:823-827, 1984.

Pharmacogenetics and Chronopharmacology

Eichelbaum M: Polymorphic drug oxidation in humans. *Federation Proc* 43:2298-2302, 1984.

Hrushesky WMJ: Circadian timing of cancer chemotherapy. *Science* 228:73-75, 1985.

Hrushesky WJM, Rushing D: Circadian chronopharmacokinetics and chronotoxicology of doxorubicin and cisplatin in human beings with cancer. *Proceedings of the First International Montreaux Conference of Chronopharmacology*. Montreux, Switzerland, March 26-30, 1984, 305.

Reinberg A: Clinical chronopharmacology, an experimental basis for chronotherapy. *Arzneim Forsch* 28:1861-1867, 1978.

Reinberg A, Smolensky MH: Circadian changes of drug disposition in man. *Clin Pharmacokinet* 7:401-420, 1982.

Vesell ES: Genetic host factors: Determinants of drug response, (editorial). *N Engl J Med* 313:261-262, 1985.

Weinshilboum RM: Human pharmacogenetics. *Federation Proc* 43:2295-2297, 1984.

Pharmacokinetics

Benet LZ, Massoud N: Pharmacokinetics, in Benet LZ, et al (eds): *Pharmacokinetic Basis for Drug Treatment*. New York, Raven Press, 1984, 1-28.

Bowman WC, Rand MJ: *Textbook of Pharmacology*, ed 2. London, Blackwell Scientific, 1980, 40.1-40.58.

Committee for Pharmacokinetic Nomenclature: *Manual of Symbols, Equations & Definitions in Pharmacokinetics*. Philadelphia, Committee for Pharmacokinetic Nomenclature, 1982.

Niazi S: *Textbook of Biopharmaceutics and Clinical Pharmacokinetics*. New York, Appleton-Century-Crofts, 1979, 86.

Riegelman S, Collier P: Application of statistical moment theory to evaluation of in vivo dissolution time and absorption time. *J Pharmacokinet Biopharm* 8:509-534, 1980.

Rowland M, Tozer TN: *Clinical Pharmacokinetics: Concepts and Applications*. Philadelphia, Lea & Febiger, 1980.

Tozer TN, Winter ME: Phenytoin, in Evans WE, et al (eds): *Applied Pharmacokinetics*. San Francisco, Applied Therapeutics, 1980, 275-314.

Renal Disease

Anders MW: Metabolism of drugs by the kidney. *Kidney Int* 18:636-647, 1980.

Bennett WM, et al: Drug prescribing in renal failure: Dosing guidelines for adults. *Am J Kidney Dis* 3:155-193, 1983.

Brater DC: Pharmacological role of the kidney. *Drugs* 19:31-48, 1980.

Cockcroft DW, Gault MH: Prediction of creatinine clearance from serum creatinine. *Nephron* 16:31-41, 1976.

Dettli L: Drug dosage in renal disease. *Clin Pharmacokinet* 1:126-134, 1976.

Gambertoglio JG: Effects of renal disease: Altered pharmacokinetics, in Benet LZ, et al (eds): *Pharmacokinetic Basis for Drug Treatment*. New York, Raven Press, 1984, 149-171.

Reidenberg MM, Drayer DE: Drug therapy in renal failure. *Annu Rev Pharmacol Toxicol* 20:45-54, 1980.

Schwartz GJ, et al: Simple estimate of glomerular filtration rate in children derived from body length and plasma creatinine. *Pediatrics* 58:259-263, 1976.

Siersbaek-Nielsen K, et al: Rapid evaluation of creatinine clearance. *Lancet* 1:1133-1134, 1971.

Therapeutic Drug Monitoring

Evans WE, et al (eds): *Applied Therapeutics: Principles of Therapeutic Drug Monitoring*, ed 2. San Francisco, Applied Therapeutics, 1986.

Gugler R, Azarnoff DL: Clinical use of plasma drug concentrations. *Ration Drug Ther* 10:1-7, (Nov) 1976.

Kauffman RE: Clinical interpretation and application of drug concentration data. *Pediatr Clin North Am* 28:35-45, 1981.

Koch-Weser J: Serum level approach to individualization of drug dosage. *Eur J Clin Pharmacol* 9:1-8, 1975.

McCoy HG, Cipolle RJ: Toward optimal drug therapy: Benefits of therapeutic drug monitoring. *Postgrad Med* 74:121-134, (Oct) 1983.

Sjöqvist F: Clinical use of drug plasma level determinations, in Azarnoff DL, et al (eds): *Year Book of Drug Therapy*. Chicago, Year Book Medical Publishers, 1977, 13-20.

Zaske DE, et al: Gentamicin dosage requirements: Wide interpatient variations in 242 surgery patients with normal renal function. *Surgery* 87:164-169, 1980.

Drug Interactions and Adverse Drug Reactions

DRUG INTERACTIONS

Drugs may interact with food, environmental chemicals, or other drugs. The influence of diet and environmental chemicals on the response to drugs is discussed in Chapter 2, Drug Response Variation and Dosing Information. *Drug-drug interaction* refers specifically to interactions between drugs (prescription or nonprescription); the broader term, drug interaction, often is substituted. Physicians must be aware of the varied type of interaction that may occur.

Many drug interactions cause undesirable effects and account for a significant number of adverse reactions. They also can limit bioavailability or block desired effects. However, many drug interactions are clinically valuable. For example, probenecid prolongs the activity and thereby increases the effectiveness of penicillin, diuretics enhance the action of other antihypertensive drugs, and certain drugs are used as antidotes to overdosage of other agents (eg, chelating agents for metals, leucovorin for methotrexate, protamine for heparin).

Mechanisms

Drug interactions are chemically based (ie, one drug is physically or chemically incompatible with another drug), pharmacokinetically based (ie, one drug affects the absorption, distribution, biotransformation, or excretion of a second drug), physiologically based (ie, one drug alters the overt activity of a second drug at a separate site of action), or pharmacodynamically based (ie, one drug alters the activity of a second drug at or near the receptor site). Most drug interactions are classified according to the mechanism of the interaction.

Inactivation: This includes the direct physical or chemical inactivation of drugs: the degradation of sodium nitroprusside by light, the adsorption of insulin onto glass, the binding of nitroglycerin by intravenous tubing, and the neutralization or precipitation of drugs that are mixed in the same intravenous bottle (eg, tobramycin and carbenicillin). Inactivation or incompatibility reduces bioavailability by decreasing the amount of active drug. Most hospital pharmacies have reference sources, such as the *Handbook on Injectable Drugs* (Trissel, 1985), on the inactivation of parenteral drugs.

Absorption: A drug may affect the rate and/or extent of absorption (ie, bioavailability) of another drug through physical or chemical binding in the gastrointestinal tract, slowing or accelerating gastrointestinal motility, altering bacterial flora, or elevating gastric pH. Generally, interactions due to drug binding decrease bioavailability. For example, cholestyramine resin adsorbs a number of drugs, including digoxin and thyroid hormone, thus decreasing their bioavailability. This type of interaction can be minimized by separating the time of administration by at least four hours. Drug binding in the gastrointestinal tract also can be used for therapeutic purposes. Activated charcoal is commonly administered to counteract an acute drug overdose by binding the toxic agent in the gastrointestinal tract, thereby decreasing the amount of toxin absorbed. This type of drug interaction has been termed "gastrointestinal dialysis" (Levy, 1982).

Drugs that alter gastrointestinal motility modify the bioavailability of agents that are absorbed poorly, slowly, or by saturable carrier proteins. Fortunately, this type of interaction rarely is clinically relevant.

Drugs also can modify the bioavailability of other drugs by altering the bacterial flora or elevating gastric pH. Oral neomycin changes the bacterial flora and, in most patients, decreases the rate and extent of absorption of concomitantly administered digoxin. However, the natural bacterial flora of a small subsection of the population (less than 10%) degrade digoxin to inactive metabolites, and neomycin increases the bioavailability of digoxin in these individuals. Elevating the gastric pH by administering sodium bicarbonate decreases the absorption of some forms of tetracycline.

Distribution: For most drugs, the plasma concentration of free drug, rather than the total plasma concentration, correlates with the clinical response. Drugs that are bound to plasma proteins may be displaced by chemicals or other drugs, but clinically relevant interactions are unlikely unless the original drug is at least 85% bound. With this high degree of binding, small changes in the bound fraction can temporarily double or triple the free drug concentration and increase pharmacologic activity until compensation takes place. The rate and extent of compensation depend upon biotransformation and/or elimination of the drug. For example, adequate compensation occurs quickly if excess free drug is eliminated rapidly or distributed widely (ie, has a large volume of distribution). These compensatory mechanisms probably explain why most protein-binding displacement interactions are not very serious clinically. Conversely, a serious interaction may occur when a highly bound drug that is not widely distributed and that requires biotransformation for inactivation is displaced in a patient with impaired hepatic or renal function. For example, phenylbutazone not only displaces warfarin, which is highly plasma protein bound, but also inhibits its hepatic metabolism; therefore, severe bleeding may result from impaired elimination of the increased concentration of free warfarin.

Biotransformation: Biotransformation of drugs is usually a process of detoxification, but toxicity may result when the metabolite is more toxic than the parent molecule. The quinone formed by oxidation of acetaminophen is hepatotoxic, especially when the amount of glutathione available is limited.

Biotransformation of drugs (most of which are fat soluble) is performed by two different enzyme systems. Oxygen or other chemical entities are inserted into the parent molecule to produce one or more water-soluble groups (eg, hydroxyl) during phase I biotransformation. Some products of phase I metabolism are sufficiently water soluble to be excreted readily from the body; others undergo additional biotransformation (phase II), which consists largely of conjugation reactions (eg, glucuronidation, acetylation, sulfation) that further enhance water solubility and promote excretion. Most phase I oxidations are performed by a family of isoenzymes known as P-450 cytochrome enzymes or hepatic microsomal mixed-function oxidases. The type and degree of biotransformation of any given drug vary among individuals due principally to genetic differences that control the availability and activity of metabolizing enzymes, particularly the phase I type.

Many environmental chemicals and drugs administered to animals chronically or subchronically increase the synthesis or activity of drug metabolizing enzymes, ie, *enzyme induction* (Park and Breckenridge, 1981). Since multiple mechanisms are operating simultaneously, interactions predicted from animal studies may not be observed clinically, however. For example, phenylbutazone induces drug metabolizing enzymes in animals but, in man, it also inhibits enzyme activity.

Because enzyme activity is determined genetically, the degree of enzyme induction varies considerably. Many drugs are not given for sufficient periods in large enough doses to produce clinically significant enzyme induction. Nevertheless, those that are potent enzyme inducers (ie, barbiturates, especially phenobarbital; phenytoin; rifampin) markedly alter the response to a second drug, especially when they are used for prolonged periods. Carbamazepine, alcohol, glutethimide, phenylbutazone, tobacco smoking, and some constituents of the diet also induce enzymes. Studies suggest that the inducibility of hepatic enzymes is related to the patient's age: The systemic clearance of antipyrine in elderly smokers is not significantly different from that in elderly nonsmokers (Vestal and Wood, 1980).

Drug metabolizing processes (ie, oxidation, reduction, hydrolysis, conjugation) are also susceptible to *enzyme inhibition* (Park and Breckenridge, 1981). Compensatory mechanisms, such as increased enzyme synthesis, may diminish the effects of enzyme inhibition but are not inevitable (eg, no compensation occurs with the inhibition of tolbutamide oxidation by sulfaphenazole).

A number of these mechanisms are useful therapeutically. The therapeutic use of disulfiram is based on its ability to block the oxidation of acetaldehyde. Allopurinol blocks the metabolism of purines to uric acid by xanthine oxidase and increases blood levels of mercaptopurine by the same mechanism. Azathioprine reacts similarly with allopurinol, and serious toxicity has been observed with combined use of allopurinol and azathioprine.

Chloramphenicol, dicumarol, disulfiram, cimetidine, phenylbutazone, and propoxyphene may cause serious adverse drug interactions clinically by inhibiting hepatic microsomal mixed-function oxidases, especially if the second drug exhibits zero-order (dose-dependent) biotransformation kinetics (eg, alcohol, phenytoin, aspirin, dicumarol). The monoamine oxidase inhibitors do not affect the hepatic mixed-function oxidases but do inhibit the monoamine oxidase enzymes that terminate the action of some sympathomimetic amines, thus enhancing the magnitude of their effects.

The principal function of the liver in drug disposition is biotransformation. Mild or moderate liver dysfunction generally does not affect drug biotransformation; thus, a clinically significant effect occurs only in individuals with severe liver impairment (as determined by routine laboratory tests). Other determinants of hepatic function (age, genetic profile, nutritional status, disease, hepatic blood flow) may predispose to interactions when one drug is a hepatotoxin and the second drug is biotransformed in the liver. Unfortunately, there is no good correlation between any of the routine laboratory liver function tests and a change in the rate of hepatic drug biotransformation. Therefore, monitoring of the patient, determination of plasma drug concentrations (if indicated), and individualization of dosage are especially important to avoid such interactions.

Excretion: Drug-induced alterations in renal blood flow, glomerular filtration, tubular reabsorption, or tubular secretion can result in drug interaction. The nephrotoxic aminoglycoside antibiotics can produce additive impairment of renal function when administered with other potentially nephrotoxic drugs (eg, cephalothin, polymyxin B, ethacrynic acid, furosemide). Tubular reabsorption can be especially sensitive to tubular fluid pH, and both reabsorption and secretion are affected by competing normal metabolites (eg, uric acid) or exogenous chemicals. Tubular secretory mechanisms are either anionic or cationic; the cationic transport system has greater specificity. Many anionic metabolites or drugs (eg, uric acid, salicylates, sulfonamides, sulfates, glycine and glucuronide conjugates, penicillin, probenecid, thiazides) are eliminated by the same transport system and thus can competitively block each other's excretion.

Receptor Action: Certain drug responses are mediated by the activation of specific receptors. When two drugs are given concurrently, activation of one drug's receptor may enhance or decrease the response of the second drug's receptor. This type of interaction may involve the same or different receptors. Although these receptors are sometimes considered a specialized compartment of distribution, this interaction is usually categorized as pharmacodynamic rather than pharmacokinetic. There are many examples of pharmacodynamic drug interactions. Additive pharmacologic or toxicologic effects are generally considered to be more common than antagonistic effects. However, a less than anticipated therapeutic response resulting from drug interaction-induced antagonism is often subtle and difficult to detect; therefore, many antagonistic drug interactions are missed. The anticholinergic effects of tricyclic antidepressants, quinidine, antihistamines, and certain phenothiazines operate through the same muscarinic cholinergic receptor, while the potentiation of central nervous system depression with combined administration of a narcotic and a barbiturate operates through different receptors. Naloxone's ability to antagonize opiate-induced respiratory depression is a beneficial drug interaction in which the same receptor is affected by the antagonist and agonist.

Potentially Serious Undesirable Drug Interactions

Drug-drug interactions can cause therapeutic failure by decreasing bioavailability, inducing enzymes, increasing clearance, or antagonizing the desired effect. Interactions caused by alteration of drug absorption in the gastrointestinal tract and drug incompatibilities most commonly decrease bioavailability. Generally, absorption interactions may be avoided by staggering the times of oral administration of two interacting drugs, and incompatibilities can be avoided by appropriate preparation and administration of parenteral drugs.

The concomitant administration of two drugs that act on the same physiologic system to produce an additive effect (or, less often, an antagonistic effect) often leads to an adverse drug reaction. Additive central nervous system depression, anticholinergic activity, nephrotoxicity, ototoxicity, hypotension, gastric irritation, and neuromuscular depression are well documented examples. Less common but often more serious reactions result from potentiation of toxicity. One drug's interference with the biotransformation and/or elimination of a second drug may potentiate the latter's toxicity, especially when liver or kidney function is compromised by age or disease. Adverse drug reactions resulting from these types of interactions can be avoided or minimized by selecting an alternative drug, altering the dose or dosage schedule initially, and/or periodic clinical or laboratory monitoring.

Specific information on clinically relevant drug interactions is included in the introductions to the chapters and the drug evaluations. In addition, Table 1 cites examples of potentially serious drug interactions in which (1) a time interval is recommended between the administration of two drugs when both are given orally, (2) alternative drug therapy should be considered if possible, (3) it is highly desirable to alter initial doses, and/or (4) a symptom, laboratory test, or physical sign should be monitored periodically (especially quantitatively) to assure a good therapeutic response without drug toxicity.

ADVERSE DRUG REACTIONS

The World Health Organization's broad definition of an adverse drug reaction is "any response to a drug that is noxious and unintended and that occurs at doses used in man for prophylaxis, diagnosis or therapy of disease, or for the modification of physiological function." Effects of errors in medication are not included in this definition since the routine, appropriate use of the drug is implied. Inadequate doses, problems of bioavailability that result in therapeutic failure, drug abuse, noncompliance, and accidental or suicidal poisoning are not usually classified as adverse drug reactions, although they are considered in the broader context of the overall risk associated with a drug. Drug interactions can be classified as adverse reactions when the circumstances and clinical outcome meet the criteria specified in the WHO definition.

Definite adverse drug reactions are not always caused by the primary active ingredient of a product; impurities formed during manufacture, preservatives, vehicles, degradation products, and excipients may be responsible. Patients have had adverse reactions to tincture of orange, metabisulfite, polyethylene glycol, benzyl alcohol, propylene glycol, and azo dyes (including tartrazine) (Napke and Stevens, 1984).

Adverse drug reactions result from known and as yet unknown actions that produce predictable minor and major toxicity, as well as unpredictable idiosyncrasy and hypersensitivity. Information on adverse reactions is always incomplete when a drug is first introduced into clinical use. Premarketing exposure to an investigational drug is limited usually to 1,000 to 3,000 persons. Therefore, the probability of identifying adverse drug reactions with a frequency of less than 1:1,000 is remote. The full range of adverse reactions may not be known until a drug has been used (1) in patients with a wide variety of diseases, disorders, or conditions, (2) in hundreds of thou-

TABLE 1.
CLINICALLY IMPORTANT AND WELL DOCUMENTED UNDESIRABLE DRUG INTERACTIONS

Drug/Class	Interacts With	Producing	Comments

ALCOHOL	Clonidine
	Methyldopa
	Reserpine
	
	Analgesics, opioid
	Antianxiety drugs
	Anticholinergics, centrally
	  acting
	Anticonvulsants
	Antihistamines
	Antipsychotics
	Central skeletal muscle
	  relaxants
	Hypnotics
	Magnesium salts
	  (parenteral)
	Tricyclic antidepressants
		additive sedation	Patient should avoid or limit alcohol intake and be warned of the danger of driving or operating machinery. Patients receiving any combination of drugs with the potential for producing CNS depression should be observed more frequently, especially during the initiation of therapy.

	Aspirin and other salicylates	additive gastric irritation	Concurrent use should be avoided, especially in patients with a history of gastric irritation or bleeding. Acetaminophen is a useful alternative for analgesia or antipyresis.
	Cefamandole Cefoperazone Chlorpropamide Metronidazole Moxalactam	disulfiram-like reaction (facial flushing, sweating, nausea, tachycardia)	Patients should avoid or limit alcohol intake.
AMINOGLYCOSIDES	Cephalothin Ethacrynic acid	additive ototoxicity	Avoid combination if possible, especially in patients with renal damage. If combination is required, periodic monitoring of hearing is recommended.
	Azlocillin Carbenicillin Mezlocillin Piperacillin Ticarcillin	diminished aminoglycoside activity in patients with impaired renal function	The extended spectrum penicillins accumulate in the blood and the aminoglycoside is inactivated.
ANTICOAGULANTS, ORAL	Amiodarone Aspirin Chloral hydrate Cimetidine Clofibrate Glucagon Metronidazole Phenylbutazone Sulfinpyrazone Anabolic steroids Salicylates Sulfonamides Thyroid hormones	enhanced anticoagulant activity	Severe hemorrhage may occur when anticoagulants are given with aspirin or phenylbutazone; thus, their concurrent use is not recommended. Bleeding and/or prolonged prothrombin times have been reported with concomitant administration of an anticoagulant and one of the other drugs listed; however, their combined use is not contraindicated when periodic examination for bleeding and monitoring of prothrombin times are done and appropriate adjustment in dosage made.

(Continued on next page)

Drug/Class	Interacts With	Producing	Comments
	Carbamazepine Cholestyramine Ethchlorvynol Glutethimide Griseofulvin Phytonadione Rifampin Barbiturates	diminished anticoagulant activity	Oral anticoagulants should be taken one hour before or no less than four hours after cholestyramine to reduce effects on their absorption. Concurrent administration of the vitamin K preparation, phytonadione, should be avoided unless it is needed to antagonize the anticoagulant effect. The remaining drugs listed are enzyme inducers and, when they are discontinued, severe bleeding may occur if they have been administered with an oral anticoagulant; therefore, monitoring is recommended.
BETA BLOCKERS	Indomethacin	reduced antihypertensive response	Indomethacin impairs the hypotensive effects of beta blockers by a pharmacodynamic rather than pharmacokinetic mechanism. Concurrent use should be avoided when possible. Other nonsteroidal anti-inflammatory agents may produce a similar effect.
CAPTOPRIL	Indomethacin	diminished or abolished antihypertensive effect	Concurrent use should be avoided. Other prostaglandin synthetase inhibitors may produce a similar effect.
CARBAMAZEPINE	Erythromycin Isoniazid Propoxyphene Troleandomycin	enhanced carbamazepine activity	The listed drugs inhibit the hepatic metabolism of carbamazepine. Toxicity (ie, diplopia, nausea, vomiting, nystagmus, ataxia, drowsiness) may occur. Adjustment of the dose is usually necessary.
CARMUSTINE	Cimetidine	additive bone marrow suppression	Concurrent use should be avoided if possible.
CLONIDINE	Propranolol	rebound hypertension	Termination of clonidine therapy in a patient also receiving a nonselective beta-blocking drug has resulted in hypertension. Gradual withdrawal of clonidine and appropriate monitoring of blood pressure are recommended.
CYCLOSPORINE	Ketoconazole	enhanced cyclosporine activity	Concurrent use should be avoided if possible. If ketoconazole is necessary, the serum cyclosporine concentration should be monitored and the dose adjusted accordingly.
DIGITOXIN	Rifampin	diminished digitoxin activity	Rifampin stimulates the hepatic metabolism of digitoxin. Underdigitalization may result. Adjustment of the dose is usually necessary.
DIGOXIN AND OTHER DIGITALIS GLYCOSIDES	Cholestyramine resin Colestipol Kaolin Antacids	decreased bioavailability of digoxin and related compounds	Following oral administrations of digoxin, a one- to two-hour interval is recommended before the drugs listed are given.

(Continued on next page)

Drug/Class	Interacts With	Producing	Comments
	Neomycin (oral) Penicillamine	decreased serum digitalis concentration	Patients should be monitored closely and doses adjusted accordingly.
	Amphotericin B Corticosteroids Thiazide and loop diuretics	potassium depletion and enhanced potential for cardiotoxicity	Potassium supplementation is recommended for patients receiving digoxin and potassium-depleting drugs but only if determination of a baseline serum potassium concentration followed by periodic monitoring to avoid hyperkalemia is part of the management program. A potassium-sparing diuretic (amiloride, spironolactone, triamterene) may be a better alternative than a thiazide or loop diuretic in selected patients.
	Amiodarone Erythromycin base Quinidine Tetracycline Verapamil	enhanced potential for cardiotoxicity	Serum digitalis concentration may increase during concurrent therapy. Patients should be monitored closely and dosage adjusted accordingly.
DISULFIRAM	Metronidazole	acute psychoses	Concurrent use should be avoided. Mechanism of this interaction is unknown.
DOXYCYCLINE	Carbamazepine Phenobarbital Phenytoin	diminished doxycycline activity	The listed drugs may stimulate the hepatic metabolism of doxycycline. Another tetracycline should be substituted or the doxycycline dosage doubled.
EPINEPHRINE	Halothane	enhanced potential for cardiotoxicity	Arrhythmias induced by the rapid intravenous administration of epinephrine in the presence of halothane can be life-threatening. The dosage of epinephrine should be reduced if it must be used. Indirect-acting sympathomimetic agents are less likely to be potentiated.
GUANETHIDINE	Chlorpromazine Dextroamphetamine Sympathomimetic amines, indirect-acting Tricyclic antidepressants	diminished antihypertensive activity	Another antihypertensive drug should be selected or the concurrent use of guanethidine and listed drugs should be avoided.
HEPARIN	Aspirin	enhanced anticoagulant activity	Aspirin inhibits platelet function and should be used with caution in patients receiving heparin. Acetaminophen, sodium salicylate, or other analgesics are suggested substitutes.
INSULIN	Fenfluramine Propranolol Monoamine oxidase inhibitors	enhanced hypoglycemic activity	The insulin dose may require reduction during concurrent fenfluramine therapy. The potential of propranolol to interfere with carbohydrate metabolism also may necessitate adjustment of insulin dose. The concurrent use of insulin and monoamine oxidase inhibitors should be avoided if possible.

(Continued on next page)

Drug/Class	Interacts With	Producing	Comments
KETAMINE			
	Halothane	decreased cardiac output, stroke volume, and blood pressure and increased arteriolar resistance	When halothane anesthesia is used, ketamine should be administered cautiously and cardiac function monitored closely.
LIDOCAINE			
	Cimetidine Propranolol	increased serum lidocaine concentration	Cimetidine and propranolol reduce the hepatic clearance of lidocaine. It may be necessary to reduce the dose of lidocaine to avoid toxicity.
LINCOMYCIN			
	Kaolin	decreased lincomycin bioavailability	Concurrent use should be avoided.
LITHIUM			
	Nonsteroidal anti-inflammatory agents Thiazide-type diuretics	increased serum lithium concentration	Indomethacin and thiazide-type diuretics decrease the renal clearance of lithium. Serum lithium concentration and patient response should be monitored and the dose adjusted accordingly.
	Probenecid	decreased renal excretion of lithium	Serum concentration and patient response should be monitored and the dosage adjusted accordingly.
	Theophylline	decreased serum lithium concentration	Theophylline increases the renal clearance of lithium. The dose of lithium may need to be increased.
MEPERIDINE			
	Monoamine oxidase inhibitors	enhanced central nervous system toxicity (excitement, convulsions, hyperpyrexia, severe respiratory depression)	The combination has caused fatalities and avoidance is recommended even though the interaction does not always occur. The cautious use of small doses of morphine is recommended if a narcotic analgesic is required.
MERCAPTOPURINE AZATHIOPRINE	Allopurinol	enhanced toxicity of mercaptopurine and azathioprine	The dose of mercaptopurine or azathioprine should be reduced by one-third to one-fourth if allopurinol is administered concurrently. Maintenance doses are adjusted on the basis of clinical response.
METHOTREXATE			
	Aspirin and other salicylates Probenecid	increased serum methotrexate concentration	The concurrent use of aspirin, other salicylates, and propranolol with methotrexate should be avoided. Acetaminophen (for analgesia and antipyresis) and indomethacin (for anti-inflammatory action) appear to be acceptable alternatives to salicylates.
METHOXYFLURANE			
	Tetracycline Barbiturates	increased risk of nephrotoxicity	Concurrent use should be avoided when possible.
METOPROLOL PROPRANOLOL	Chlorpromazine Cimetidine Oral contraceptives	enhanced beta-blocking activity	The drugs listed inhibit the hepatic metabolism of metoprolol and propranolol. Dosage of beta blocker may need to be reduced.

(Continued on next page)

Drug/Class	Interacts With	Producing	Comments
	Rifampin Barbiturates	diminished beta-blocking activity	Rifampin and barbiturates induce hepatic metabolism of metoprolol and propranolol. Dosage of beta blockers may need to be increased.
MEXILETINE	Phenytoin Rifampin	diminished mexiletine activity	Hepatic enzyme inducers, such as phenytoin and rifampin, may decrease serum mexiletine concentration. Patient response should be monitored and the dose adjusted accordingly.
MONOAMINE OXIDASE INHIBITORS	Sympathomimetic amines, indirect-acting	hypertension	Anorexiants, amphetamines, ephedrine, phenylephrine, phenylpropanolamine, pseudoephedrine, methylphenidate, tyramine-containing foods, and nonprescription drugs containing such sympathomimetic amines have been reported to be responsible for this interaction. Avoidance of these drugs, a diet low in tyramine, and, if needed, cautious substitution of direct-acting sympathomimetic agents are recommended.
NONDEPOLARIZING MUSCLE RELAXANTS	Ketamine Quinidine Aminoglycosides Polymyxins	enhanced neuromuscular blockade	To avoid respiratory depression, extreme caution is necessary if listed drugs are given with neuromuscular blocking agents during surgery or the postoperative period. Concurrent use may make weaning from a respirator more difficult.
ORAL CONTRACEPTIVES	Phenytoin Primidone Rifampin Barbiturates	diminished contraceptive activity	Because all of these drugs are enzyme inducers, they can enhance estrogen metabolism, resulting in breakthrough bleeding, reduced oral contraceptive efficacy, and unplanned pregnancy. Although the degree of enzyme induction is variable among patients, other contraceptive methods are recommended if pregnancy must be avoided.
	Ampicillin Tetracycline	diminished contraceptive activity	Ampicillin and tetracycline may interfere with the enterohepatic circulation of estrogens by reducing bacterial hydrolysis of conjugated estrogen in the intestine.
PHENOBARBITAL	Valproic acid	increased serum phenobarbital concentration	Valproic acid inhibits hepatic metabolism of phenobarbital. The phenobarbital dosage should be decreased when valproic acid therapy is initiated.
PHENYTOIN	Chloramphenicol Cimetidine Dicumarol Disulfiram Isoniazid Phenylbutazone Trimethoprim Sulfonamides	increased serum phenytoin concentration	Concurrent use of the listed drugs may produce phenytoin toxicity. Patients should be monitored and the dose adjusted accordingly.

(Continued on next page)

Drug/Class	Interacts With	Producing	Comments
	Diazoxide Folic acid	decreased serum phenytoin concentration	Diazoxide appears to enhance the hepatic metabolism of phenytoin. Phenytoin dosage may need to be increased. Folic acid and phenytoin may reduce each other's serum concentrations. Patients should be monitored for evidence of folic acid deficiency and/or subtherapeutic response to phenytoin.
POTASSIUM SPARING DIURETICS	Potassium supplements	hyperkalemia	Concurrent use is one of the most common causes of hyperkalemia.
PRAZOSIN	Beta-adrenergic blockers	enhanced orthostatic hypotension associated with the first dose of prazosin	
PRIMIDONE	Phenytoin	enhanced primidone activity	Reduction of primidone dosage may be required to avoid phenobarbital (a primidone metabolite) toxicity.
PROBENECID	Aspirin and other salicylates	antagonism of uricosuric activity	Another analgesic is recommended.
PROPRANOLOL (See also METOPROLOL and BETA BLOCKERS)	Epinephrine	marked increase in systolic and diastolic blood pressure and decrease in heart rate	Epinephrine should be avoided in patients receiving propranolol. When epinephrine is administered, the beta-adrenergic activity is inhibited while the alpha-adrenergic activity is unopposed. Also, patients taking propranolol tend to be very resistant to the favorable effects of epinephrine in acute anaphylaxis.
QUINIDINE	Amiodarone Cimetidine	enhanced quinidine activity	Amiodarone increases serum quinidine concentration by an unknown mechanism. Serum quinidine concentrations and patient response should be monitored and the dose adjusted accordingly. Cimetidine increases serum quinidine levels by reducing quinidine metabolism.
	Phenytoin Rifampin Barbiturates	diminished quinidine activity	The drugs listed induce the hepatic enzymes, decreasing the serum quinidine concentration. Serum quinidine concentrations and patient response should be monitored and the dose adjusted accordingly.
SUCCINYLCHOLINE	Cyclophosphamide Lidocaine Trimethaphan	enhanced neuromuscular blockade	Cyclophosphamide, trimethaphan, and possibly lidocaine decrease plasma cholinesterase enzyme activity. Concurrent use should be avoided if possible.
SULFINPYRAZONE	Aspirin and other salicylates	diminished uricosuric activity	Concurrent use should be avoided.

(Continued on next page)

Drug/Class	Interacts With	Producing	Comments
SULFONYLUREAS	Chloramphenicol Dicumarol Phenylbutazone Sulfonamides	enhanced hypoglycemic activity	Chloramphenicol, dicumarol, sulfonamides, and phenylbutazone inhibit the hepatic metabolism of certain sulfonylureas. A lower dose of the sulfonylurea may be required.
	Clofibrate	enhanced hypoglycemic activity	Clofibrate may impair the renal excretion of chlorpropamide; however, clofibrate also appears to have intrinsic hypoglycemic activity.
	Salicylates	enhanced hypoglycemic activity	Salicylates alter glucose tolerance and glucose metabolism and may enhance insulin secretion. Further, salicylates compete with sulfonylureas for protein binding sites.
SYMPATHOMIMETIC AMINES, DIRECT-ACTING (epinephrine, methenamine, norepinephrine, phenylephrine)	Tricyclic antidepressants	enhanced cardiovascular action (arrhythmias, hypertension, tachycardia) of direct-acting sympathomimetic drugs	Monitoring of cardiovascular status is recommended if concurrent administration is necessary.
SYMPATHOMIMETIC AMINES, INDIRECT-ACTING (ephedrine, mephentermine)	Tricyclic antidepressants	diminished cardiovascular activity	
TETRACYCLINES	Antacids Calcium compounds Iron compounds Magnesium compounds	decreased bioavailability of tetracyclines	Antacids, calcium compounds, and magnesium compounds chelate with all tetracyclines except doxycycline and perhaps minocycline. Iron compounds decrease the bioavailability of all tetracyclines. If concurrent use is necessary, oral administration should be separated by an interval of at least three hours.
THEOPHYLLINE	Cimetidine Erythromycin Troleandomycin	enhanced theophylline activity	Cimetidine, erythromycin, and troleandomycin inhibit the hepatic metabolism of theophylline and aminophylline. Serum theophylline concentration and patient response should be monitored and the dose adjusted accordingly.
	Nadolol Pindolol Propranolol Timolol	diminished effect of theophylline on the bronchial muscles	The use of these noncardioselective beta blockers should be avoided in patients receiving theophylline.
	Phenytoin	diminished theophylline activity	Phenytoin induces enzyme activity and increases the clearance of theophylline. The dose of both drugs may need to be increased.

sands of patients, especially for adverse events with an incidence of less than 1 to 10:10,000, and (3) for a prolonged period or only long after exposure to the drug (eg, diethylstilbestrol and vaginal cancer).

Assessment of Causality

Proving that a specific drug is responsible for an adverse event in an individual may be extremely difficult (Karch and Lasagna, 1975) because of multiple drug exposures and underlying illnesses. The physician should report a suspected, new, serious, adverse drug reaction even if considerable uncertainty exists (see the section on Reporting Adverse Drug Reactions).

Criteria have been developed by the Reports Evaluation Branch of the FDA's Division of Drug and Biological Product Experience in the form of an algorithm (see the Figure) that is

ALGORITHM FOR ESTABLISHING CAUSAL RELATIONSHIP BETWEEN DRUG AND EVENT

START HERE*

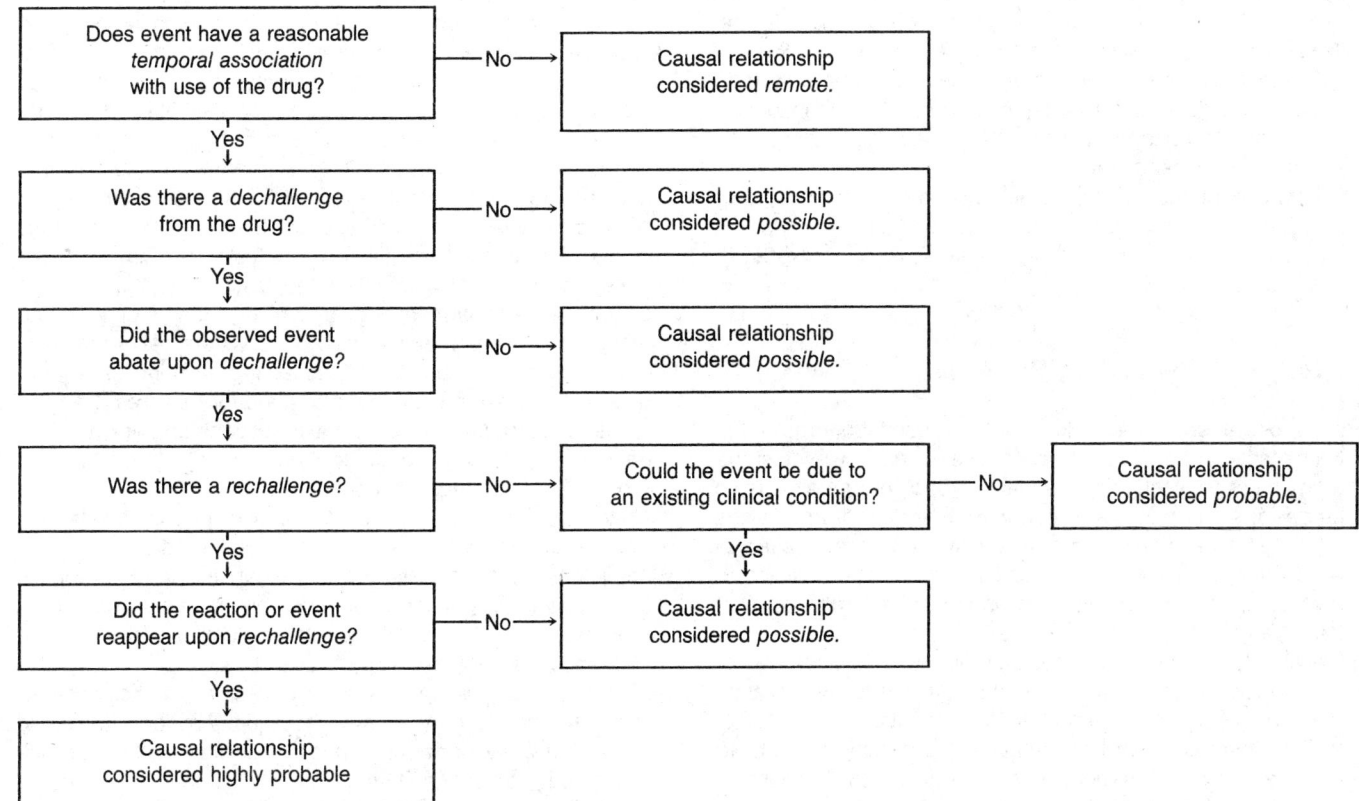

* Each drug is carried through independently; if more than one drug was dechallenged or rechallenged simultaneously, causality for all is considered to be remote or possible.

QUESTIONS:
1. Did the reaction follow a reasonable temporal sequence?
2. Did the patient improve after stopping the drug?
3. Did the reaction appear on repeated exposure (rechallenge)?
4. Could the reaction be reasonably explained by the known characteristics of the patient's *clinical state?*

From Jones, 1982.

used to evaluate causality (Jones, 1982). Other algorithms have been developed to improve the reliability of adverse drug reaction information (Kramer et al, 1979; Hutchinson et al, 1979; Busto et al, 1982). All of these algorithms include the following criteria: (1) a *temporal* relationship between the suspected drug and the adverse reaction; (2) the presence of a positive *dechallenge,* ie, improvement after removal of the drug; (3) the presence of a positive *rechallenge,* ie, recurrence of the adverse reaction when administration of the drug is resumed; and (4) the lack of a confounding effect (eg, concomitant disease is not likely to cause the same type of disorder). The adverse reaction can then be classified as follows:

Highly Probable: A reaction that follows a reasonable temporal sequence from administration of the drug or in which the drug level has been established in body fluids or tissues; that follows a known response pattern to the suspected drug; and that is confirmed by improvement on stopping or reducing the dose of the drug (dechallenge), and reappearance of the reaction on repeated exposure (rechallenge).

Probable: A reaction that follows a reasonable temporal sequence from administration of the drug; that follows a known response pattern to the suspected drug; that is confirmed by dechallenge; and that could not be reasonably explained by the known characteristics of the patient's clinical state.

Possible: A reaction that follows a reasonable temporal sequence from administration of the drug and follows a known response pattern to the suspected drug but that could have been produced by the patient's clinical state or other modes of therapy administered to the patient.

Remote: Any reaction that does not meet the criteria above, especially if the event has no reasonable temporal association with use of the drug.

The true causality of any new adverse reaction cannot usually be established on the basis of a single case. Thus, the FDA uses these criteria more to establish a range of relative likelihood of association in the context of multiple reports. These issues are discussed in a review (Venulet, 1982).

The potential for adverse drug reactions is relatively high among the elderly and newborn (see the section on Influence of Age on Response to Drugs in Chapter 2, Drug Response Variation and Dosing Information).

Because of the additional determinants of adverse drug reactions during pregnancy and breast feeding, reactions that may occur in the mother and infant are discussed separately in this chapter.

Avoiding Adverse Drug Reactions

Almost all drugs cause known and reasonably predictable toxic reactions when given in excessive doses; however, some drugs must be given in doses that approach or reach the toxic range for some patients. When more than one drug must be administered and an interaction is likely, appropriate observation is needed to detect the approach or onset of toxicity, to reverse it, and to avoid its progression to intolerable proportions. Drugs often have not been tested in seriously ill patients, the elderly, pregnant women, and infants before marketing. When prescribing newly released drugs, particular attention must be given to dosage and adverse effects.

The most important information that a physician can have about adverse drug reactions is knowing which reactions to anticipate with each drug prescribed. When a drug is known to cause severe organ damage relatively frequently, relevant baseline studies and periodic surveillance for specific toxic endpoints are recommended. Serious toxicity often can be avoided by teaching patients to be alert for its early signs. In this book, the usual custom has been to warn of reactions but not to attempt detailed advice on monitoring them. Suggestions for periodic evaluation of symptoms, signs, and laboratory tests are ordinarily reserved for situations in which these are of definite value. More commonly, reliance is placed upon the physician's judgment to determine the details of monitoring. Even when laboratory tests are recommended, it seldom has been practical to specify frequency, for it is impossible to devise a precise routine that is ideal for all patients.

When toxic reactions occur gradually or their overt manifestations appear slowly, abnormal laboratory test results may precede the appearance of symptoms and warn of toxicity. For example, drugs that cause megaloblastic anemia with prolonged use, such as some anticonvulsants and folic acid antagonists, warrant the periodic performance of blood studies. On the other hand, much routine laboratory testing done in the absence of symptoms or signs is wasteful and may lead to a false sense of security, as when efforts are made to anticipate reactions that occur precipitously. For example, warning the patient to alert the physician to any significant untoward event (eg, infection) is more important in preventing agranulocytosis than prodigious numbers of hemograms. If

such an event occurs, immediate laboratory evaluation is indicated, even when a recent hemogram was normal.

Drug-induced liver disease of an allergic or hypersensitivity type presents the greatest problem in early detection. Many drugs produce liver damage (without apparent relation to dosage) in hypersensitive patients, and serious hypersensitivity reactions tend to develop precipitously. A number of cofactors increase the likelihood or severity of drug-induced liver damage, including continued use of the causative drug after the development of hepatitis and administration to elderly and female patients (Feinberg, 1981). Unfortunately, there is little evidence that such reactions can be diagnosed routinely by performing frequent liver function tests before symptoms develop. Minor abnormalities in these tests are often difficult to assess in terms of cause or importance, and striking ones seldom precede symptoms by a significant length of time. The most important precaution is to observe the patient for malaise, abdominal discomfort, anorexia, dark urine, and jaundice and to perform appropriate laboratory studies if any of these reactions occur. Cholestatic reactions are typically less dangerous than the hepatocellular type, but both must be regarded as potentially serious.

Occasionally, drug-induced nephrotoxicity occurs with dramatic suddenness. Usually, however, kidney damage develops subtly well before symptoms appear. When a nephrotoxic drug is given for prolonged periods, routine urinalyses, measurements of serum creatinine, and an occasional creatinine clearance test may be useful.

The following suggestions may lessen the incidence or minimize the severity of adverse drug reactions, including those that arise from interactions. (See the sections on Adverse Drug Reactions During Pregnancy and Breast Feeding for similar recommendations for these special situations.)

Individualize drug therapy by assessing the endogenous and exogenous determinants that alter drug responsiveness. An adequate history and physical examination identify hereditary diseases and health status. Identifying important exogenous factors requires determination of occupational or environmental chemical exposures, dietary intake, and the use of alcohol, tobacco, and other drugs (prescription and nonprescription).

Refer to the literature for information on potentially serious drug interactions (Table 1 in this chapter; American Pharmaceutical Association, 1976, 1978; Avery, 1977; Davies, 1981; *Medical Letter Handbook of Drug Interactions*, 1983; Dukes, 1984; Lerman and Weibert, 1982; Hansten, 1985), particularly if the drug(s) intended for use has not been prescribed recently. Avoid compilations that make no attempt to establish the clinical relevance of the drug interactions listed. The clinical relevance of drug interactions requires perspective. A considerable number of reported interactions are of no clinical relevance because they are based on (1) animal studies not confirmed in humans, (2) limited studies (eg, case reports) not substantiated by well controlled studies, (3) hypothetical situations, or (4) clinically insignificant changes. Even when drug interactions are confirmed and clinically relevant, the benefit/risk ratio must be evaluated in each individual case rather than avoiding a combination altogether.

Anticipate that patients requiring prolonged drug therapy

(eg, those with heart disease, hypertension, diabetes, epilepsy, or psychoses) are most likely to react adversely when new therapy is initiated or terminated. Adverse reactions occurring at termination of part or all of a therapeutic program are often overlooked (eg, loss of metabolic enzyme induction or enzyme inhibition, withdrawal from drug dependence). During such periods, it may be important to schedule more frequent visits, offer additional patient education, and monitor symptoms, signs, and laboratory tests.

Teach patients to identify early signs and symptoms associated with potentially serious adverse reactions, and to contact the physician as soon as possible when these are noted. Serious toxicity often can be avoided when the patient knows what to anticipate.

Optimize drug therapy by giving the least number of drugs that achieves the desired effect; the risk of an adverse drug reaction is proportional to the number of drugs prescribed.

Suspect drug-induced disease. It is not always possible to prevent every adverse drug reaction, but early detection will minimize morbidity and mortality. A high index of suspicion is required to detect and distinguish adverse drug reactions from other clinical events. Suspicion of drug-induced disease coupled with an understanding of the major criteria for assessing drug association (eg, selective monitored dechallenge and, in selected cases, rechallenge) can sometimes resolve this question promptly (Jones, 1982).

Adverse Drug Reactions During Pregnancy and FDA Pregnancy Categories

Administration of a drug to pregnant women presents a unique problem to the physician (*Obstet Gynecol,* 1981). Not only must adverse drug reactions in the mother be considered, but the fetus also must be regarded as a potential target.

The type of reaction produced in the fetus depends upon the stage of development in which drug exposure occurs (Beeley, 1981 A and B; Miller, 1981). Although not strictly a part of gestation, ova lie dormant for decades and are exposed to drugs and other environmental chemicals before conception. Four major stages of human gestation are recognized: (1) Preimplantation lasts about 12 days from conception to implantation. (2) Organogenesis occurs during days 13 to 56. Preimplantation and organogenesis comprise that period of embryonic development referred to as the first trimester of pregnancy. (3) The second and third trimesters are the periods of fetal development during which considerable growth and functional development occur in the teeth and central nervous, endocrine, genital, and immune systems. (4) The relatively short labor-delivery stage completes the time during pregnancy when maternal drug administration may influence the fetus.

TERATOGENS. Teratology is the study of congenital malformations that are grossly visible at birth and are induced by exogenous agents (teratogens) in the first trimester, especially during organogenesis. This definition may be extended to include any birth defect (ie, morphologic, biochemical, behavioral) induced at any stage of gestation and detected at birth or later in life. The incidence of congenital malformations does not appear to have increased during the last 30 years despite the dramatic increase in the number of new chemical entities available. Congenital abnormalities are increasing as a proportion of infant mortality, but this reflects a greater salvage rate for infants who previously died from other causes.

The incidence of major birth defects in the United States is 2% to 4% or about 90,000 births per year. The causes of 65% to 70% of these birth defects are unknown; 25% are ascribed to genetic factors, 3% to chromosomal aberrations, and 3% (range, 1% to 5%) to environmental factors (ie, maternal infection, radiation, drug administration).

The presence and severity of a drug-induced congenital malformation depend upon many factors: the drug's nature (ie, whether it is a potent, weak, or nonteratogen), its accessibility in unbound form to the embryo or fetus, the period of gestation during which it is administered, the dose and duration of action, the synergistic or antagonistic effects of concomitantly administered drugs, and the genetic constitution and susceptibility of the fetus, which, in turn, is dependent upon the age, nutritional status, and health of the mother (Iams and Rayburn, 1982).

Teratogen Testing: The identification of a teratogen in man is exceedingly difficult, and selected principles of teratology and epidemiology are often used to illustrate this (Howard and Hill, 1979). Consequently, teratogen identification in man has been limited to unique defects or patterns of defects caused by specific drugs (eg, thalidomide, warfarin, isotretinoin, phenytoin, lithium, trimethadione, alcohol, penicillamine, diethylstilbestrol and other sex hormones, antineoplastic drugs).

The doses used in experimental teratology are usually much greater than those used clinically. Furthermore, species susceptibility varies. This makes it very difficult to predict clinical effects on the basis of animal studies. Despite this inability to extrapolate, the medical community is conservative about using drugs that are teratogenic in animals, even when no such effect has been documented in man after prolonged use.

Individual case reports and epidemiologic surveys are used to identify teratogens retrospectively. Although individual case reports have limitations (ie, dependence on voluntary reporting, incompleteness of data, unreliability of recall), most of the drugs that are known to be teratogenic in humans have been identified by astute observations of practicing physicians. Thus, case reports are the primary mechanism for alerting the medical community to potent teratogens. Epidemiologic studies are desirable for confirmation; however, an almost impractically large number of pregnant women must be monitored to distinguish between congenital malformations induced by a weak teratogen and those due to other mechanisms. An association between a congenital malformation and a drug does not necessarily imply causality; the disorder may be produced by the condition for which the drug is used or some other confounding factor.

FDA PREGNANCY CATEGORIES. Five categories of prescription drugs for use in pregnant women have been established by the FDA for inclusion in the precautions section of the package insert (Millstein, 1980). All prescription drugs absorbed systemically or those known to have a potential for harm to the fetus are categorized according to the level of risk as follows:

FDA Pregnancy Category A: Controlled studies in women

fail to demonstrate a risk to the fetus in the first trimester (and there is no evidence of a risk in later trimesters), and the possibility of fetal harm appears remote.

FDA Pregnancy Category B: Either animal reproduction studies have not demonstrated a fetal risk but there are no controlled studies in pregnant women, or animal reproduction studies have shown an adverse effect (other than decreased fertility) that was not confirmed in controlled studies on women in the first trimester (and there is no evidence of a risk in later trimesters).

FDA Pregnancy Category C: Either studies in animals have revealed adverse effects on the fetus (teratogenic, embryocidal, or other effects) and there are no controlled studies in women, or studies in women and animals are not available. Drugs in this category should be given only if the potential benefit justifies the risk to the fetus.

FDA Pregnancy Category D: There is positive evidence of human fetal risk, but the benefits for pregnant women may be acceptable despite the risk, as in life-threatening or serious diseases for which safer drugs cannot be used or are ineffective. An appropriate statement must appear in the "warnings" section of the labeling of drugs in this category.

FDA Pregnancy Category X: Studies in animals or humans have demonstrated fetal abnormalities, there is evidence of fetal risk based on human experience, or both, and the risk of using the drug in pregnant women clearly outweighs any possible benefit. The drug is contraindicated in women who are or may become pregnant. An appropriate statement must appear in the "contraindications" section of the labeling of drugs in this category.

ADVERSE DRUG REACTIONS DURING LATER STAGES OF PREGNANCY. Not all adverse drug reactions that occur during the last two trimesters are of the teratogenic type. Genetic constitution and individual susceptibility generally are considered to be less significant than the nature, dose, and duration of some drugs given during the second and third trimesters. For example, the excessive and prolonged maternal use of opiates and barbiturates during pregnancy and up to the time of delivery causes withdrawal symptoms (eg, hyperirritability, vomiting, shrill cry) in many exposed infants at delivery. Similarly, administration of large doses of most central nervous system depressants during labor will impair respiration in many infants at birth (Committee on Drugs, American Academy of Pediatrics, 1978).

The labeling described above for teratogens also includes available information on maternal and fetal effects of drugs that have a recognized use during labor or delivery, whether or not the use is stated in the indications section of the labeling.

AVOIDING ADVERSE DRUG REACTIONS DURING PREGNANCY. It is desirable for the physician to have information on a drug's potential risk to the fetus so that the risk can be weighed against the potential benefit to the mother. Unfortunately, this information is seldom complete; however, review articles are available on drugs that might be used in pregnancy (Berkowitz et al, 1981; Hays, 1981; Miller, 1981; Rayburn and Zuspan, 1982) or agents that are of greatest concern (Hill and Stern, 1979; Howard and Hill, 1979; Golbus, 1980; Wood and Beeley, 1981).

Absolute safety for the fetus cannot be guaranteed even by

practicing therapeutic nihilism for all women between the ages of 14 and 45. Furthermore, this would deny women the medications necessary to treat many serious disorders. Failure to treat a serious maternal condition may be more hazardous to the fetus than the drug. An appreciation by the physician of the scope of potential effects of drugs upon the embryo and fetus, together with curtailment in drug prescribing, appears to be a more sensible approach. To that end, Table 2 illustrates the scope and types of adverse drug reactions that may occur when certain drugs are used during various stages of pregnancy. The list is not inclusive but cites the major adverse reactions observed.

In this book, an effort has been made to include information on known or reasonably assumed hazards of drugs given during pregnancy. For many drugs, particularly new ones, little or no information is available on use during pregnancy. Accordingly, it often is necessary to warn that a drug should be given only if the expected benefits exceed the risks to mother and fetus, even when inadequate data exist to specify what risks, if any, are present. Such a warning serves as a reminder that, unless a systemically absorbed drug has been studied extensively in pregnant women, it should be given only if an appropriate need exists, and the possibility of fetal toxicity should be borne in mind.

PHYSICIANS' RESPONSIBILITIES IN DRUG EXPOSURE DURING PREGNANCY. The physician's four responsibilities concerning drug exposures during pregnancy are (1) to avoid unnecessary drug use and choose the drug with the least hazardous risk/benefit ratio; (2) to inform patients about the implications of drug exposures during pregnancy; (3) with necessary or inadvertent drug exposures, to advise patients on the priority for birth avoidance measures; and (4) when birth defects are observed, to determine unusual exposures and report these.

The physician is often faced with the need to advise patients on inadvertent or necessary drug exposures in early pregnancy. Concerns are magnified by widespread publicity regarding teratogenic controversies, uncertainty of risks, and legal and moral issues. From the preceding discussion, it is apparent that *unnecessary* drug exposures should be avoided. However, this should not be misconstrued to indicate that necessary treatment should be avoided or that necessary or inadvertent drug exposure is a reason for interrupting a pregnancy, except possibly for the few instances in which the maternal risk is high and well established (see following discussion).

Mothers will be exposed to numerous environmental chemicals in every pregnancy, and little risk can be attributed to most of these. On the other hand, every pregnancy, regardless of such exposures, carries a substantial fetal risk that cannot be avoided. When reassuring pregnant patients regarding drug exposures, the inherent risk should always be conveyed and the physician should never advise that an adverse outcome is not possible in the absence of drug exposure. Relative to this presently unavoidable risk, the risk associated with exposure to a drug not known to be a human teratogen is probably small.

The causal association between cigarette smoking and fetal growth retardation is unequivocal and these avoidable risks should be emphasized.

TABLE 2.
ADVERSE DRUG REACTIONS DURING PREGNANCY

The following noninclusive list illustrates the scope and type of adverse drug reactions that may occur when certain drugs are used during the various stages of pregnancy. The data very considerably regarding completeness of animal and clinical studies, years of therapeutic use and follow-up, and the number and validity of literature reports available. For that reason, the reliability of the findings is scaled as follows:

X: Known effects in man that are well documented and conclusive. The risk of use of the drug clearly outweighs any possible benefit.

K: Known effects in man that are generally well documented but not necessarily demonstrated conclusively in every case listed.

S: Suspected effects in man that are based on a number of clinical studies and/or case reports.

Q: Questionable effects in man that are based on sporadic case reports.

U: Unknown effects in man that are based on no known effects on the conceptus or a lack of reported studies.

A: Animal documented effects only.

D: Disease-related effects, which implies that the drug is used for treatment of a disease in pregnancy and that the disease itself produces abnormalities in the conceptus occasionally even in the absence of the drug.

Extrapolation of an adverse reaction for any agent listed to other members of the same therapeutic class is not warranted; for reference to specific information on the use of a drug during pregnancy, see the index.

Category/Agent	1st Trimester (Embryonic Development)	2nd and 3rd Trimesters (Fetal Development)	Labor-Delivery
ADRENERGIC DRUGS			
Beta Antagonist			
Propranolol	U/A general malformations	K intrauterine growth retardation K decreased fetal cardiac output	K decreased cardiac output, fetal hypoglycemia K neonatal hypoglycemia
Beta Agonists			
Ritodrine	U	K inhibition of uterine contractions	K inhibition of labor[2]
Terbutaline	U	K fetal tachycardia	K fetal tachycardia
Albuterol (Salbutamol)	U		
ANALGESICS			
Opioids			
Meperidine	U/A		K neonatal respiratory depression K decreased fetal heart rate
Morphine	U/A		K neonatal respiratory depression K neonatal withdrawal after prolonged maternal administration
Heroin	U/A	K intrauterine growth retardation K increased neonatal mortality K premature labor	K decreased fetal heart rate
Propoxyphene	U/A	U	U
Nonsteroidal Anti-inflammatory Analgesics			
Aspirin	U/A	U	K closure of ductus arteriosus K fetal bleeding K prolonged gestation

(Continued on next page)

Category/Agent	1st Trimester (Embryonic Development)	2nd and 3rd Trimesters (Fetal Development)	Labor-Delivery
Indomethacin	U	U	K closure of ductus arteriosus K fetal bleeding K prolonged gestation
ANESTHETICS, LOCAL			
Mepivacaine	U	U	S fetal bradycardia
Chloroprocaine	U	U	S fetal bradycardia
Lidocaine	U	U	K fetal acidosis, depression, bradycardia
ANTIBIOTICS			
Chloramphenicol	U	K neonatal-gray baby	K neonatal-gray baby
Streptomycin	K 8th nerve damage, multiple defects, micromelia	K 8th nerve damage	U
Gentamicin	S 8th nerve damage	S 8th nerve damage	U
Kanamycin	S 8th nerve damage	S 8th nerve damage	U
Nitrofurantoin	U	K hyperbilirubinemia K hemolytic anemia	K hyperbilirubinemia K hemolytic anemia
Sulfonamides	U	K hyperbilirubinemia	K hyperbilirubinemia
Tetracycline	K inhibition of bone growth S micromelia S syndactyly	K staining of deciduous teeth K inhibition of bone growth S enamel hypoplasia	K staining of deciduous teeth
Sulfamethoxazole/ Trimethoprim	Q/A malformations	U	U
Metronidazole	U/A tumors	U	U
ANTICHOLINERGICS	Q	K fetal bradycardia	K fetal bradycardia
ANTICOAGULANTS			
Warfarin	D/K syndrome: stippled cartilage, midline facial depression, blindness	K intrauterine growth retardation, mental retardation, hemorrhage	K neonatal hemorrhage
Heparin	U	U	U
Dicumarol	K syndrome: (see Warfarin)	K intrauterine growth retardation, mental retardation, hemorrhage	K neonatal hemorrhage

(Continued on next page)

Category/Agent	1st Trimester (Embryonic Development)	2nd and 3rd Trimesters (Fetal Development)	Labor-Delivery
ANTICONVULSANTS			
Phenytoin	D cardiac abnormalities K syndrome: midline hypoplasia, ptosis, wide mouth, inner epicanthal folds, short neck, mild webbing, hypoplastic nails, short phalanges	S intrauterine growth retardation S mental retardation	S neonatal hemorrhage
Trimethadione	D cardiac abnormalities K syndrome: abnormal facies, V-shaped eyebrows, cardiac abnormalities, cleft palate	S mental retardation	U
Paramethadione	D cardiac abnormalities K syndrome: abnormal facies, V-shaped eyebrows, cardiac abnormalities, cleft palate	S mental retardation	U
Phenobarbital	D cardiac abnormalities S general malformations	U/A enzyme induction	K neonatal respiratory depression K neonatal withdrawal after prolonged maternal administration
Diazepam	D cardiac abnormalities S cleft lip, palate		K neonatal hypotonia, apnea (floppy infant syndrome) K neonatal respiratory depression Q neonatal withdrawal after prolonged maternal administration
Valproate	K neural tube defects		
ANTIDIABETIC DRUGS			
Insulin	D skeletal malformations	U	U
Chlorpropamide	U/A CNS effects		K neonatal hypoglycemia
Tolbutamide	U/A CNS effects		K neonatal hypoglycemia

(Continued on next page)

Category/Agent	1st Trimester (Embryonic Development)	2nd and 3rd Trimesters (Fetal Development)	Labor-Delivery
ANTIHISTAMINES			
Brompheniramine	Q malformations	U	U
Meclizine	U/A	U	U
Cyclizine	U/A	U	U
ANTIHYPERTENSIVE DRUGS			
Methyldopa	U	D stillbirths	D stillbirths, neonatal death
Hydralazine	U/A skeletal malformations	U	U
Diazoxide	U/A	Q hyperbilirubinemia, thrombocytopenia, hypoglycemia (intrauterine growth retardation)	Q hyperbilirubinemia, thrombocytopenia, hypoglycemia (intrauterine growth retardation)
ANTIMALARIAL DRUGS			
Quinine	K general malformations, abortion, 8th nerve damage	S deafness, thrombocytopenia	U
Chloroquine	S 8th nerve damage	S 8th nerve damage	U
ANTIMYCOBACTERIAL DRUGS			
Rifampin	U/A CNS effects	U	U
Streptomycin	See Antibiotics		
Isoniazid	Q CNS effects	U	U
Ethionamide	U/A	U	U
ANTITHYROID DRUGS			
Iodide 125, 131	K goiter, thyroid ablation >10 weeks	K goiter, thyroid ablation	U
Propylthiouracil	Q mental status K goiter	Q mental status K goiter	U
Methimazole	K goiter	K goiter	U
CENTRAL NERVOUS SYSTEM DRUGS			
Lysergic Acid	Q CNS effects, limb abnormalities	U	U
Phenothiazines	Q general malformations	U	U
Lithium	S cardiac malformations	U	U
Thalidomide	X general malformations, phocomelia	U	U
Haloperidol	Q general malformations	U	U

(Continued on next page)

Category/Agent	1st Trimester (Embryonic Development)	2nd and 3rd Trimesters (Fetal Development)	Labor-Delivery
Imipramine	Q general malformations	U	U
Reserpine	U/A	U/A	K neonatal nasal congestion K neonatal depression K neonatal galactosemia
Antianxiety Drugs Meprobamate	Q general malformations	U	U
Chlordiazepoxide	Q general malformations	U	U
Diazepam	S cleft palate		K neonatal respiratory depression K apnea, hypotonia (floppy infant syndrome) Q neonatal withdrawal after prolonged maternal administration
CORTICOSTEROIDS Hydrocortisone	U/A	U	U promotes lung maturity[2]
Prednisone	U/A	Q intrauterine growth retardation	U promotes lung maturity[2]
CYTOTOXIC DRUGS Busulfan Cyclophosphamide	S multiple anomalies	S intrauterine growth retardation	
Mercaptopurine	S intrauterine growth retardation	S abortion	
Idoxuridine Fluorouracil	S abortion		
Folic Acid Antagonists Aminopterin	X multiple anomalies X craniofacial anomalies X abortion X intrauterine growth retardation	K intrauterine growth retardation K mental retardation K abortion	K intrauterine growth retardation K mental retardation
Pyrimethamine	U/A/D high risk	U	U
Methotrexate	K multiple anomalies K craniofacial anomalies K intrauterine growth retardation	K intrauterine growth retardation	U

(Continued on next page)

Category/Agent	1st Trimester (Embryonic Development)	2nd and 3rd Trimesters (Fetal Development)	Labor-Delivery
DIURETICS			
Acetazolamide	U/A general malformations	U	U
Thiazides	S maternal potassium and water imbalance	S fetal jaundice, thrombocytopenia S ion imbalances	S neonatal jaundice, thrombocytopenia S ion imbalances
IMMUNOSUPPRESSANTS			
Corticosteroids	See Corticosteroids		
Azathioprine	Q adrenal hypoplasia	Q adrenal hypoplasia	U
DRUGS ACTING ON THE REPRODUCTIVE SYSTEM			
Clomiphene	Q/D neural tube defect, assorted anomalies, Down's syndrome	U	U
Diethylstilbestrol	X vaginal tumors X uterine and cervical malformations X adenosis X male genital malformations	K/A vaginal tumors K/A uterine malformations K/A adenosis K/A male genital malformations Q behavioral effects	U
Oral Contraceptives	Q	U	U
Synthetic Progestins	S limb reduction K masculinization of female fetus	Q behavioral effects U	U U
Androgens	X masculinization of female fetus	U	U
MISCELLANEOUS			
Acetohydroxamic Acid	U/A general malformations, clubbed limbs in rats	U/A	U
Ergot Alkaloids	K oxytocic properties	K oxytocic properties	K
Isotretinoin	X spontaneous abortions, malformed ears, cardiac defects, CNS malformations	X	X
X Irradiation Diagnostic	Q leukemia	Q leukemia	Q leukemia

(Continued on next page)

Category/Agent	1st Trimester (Embryonic Development)	2nd and 3rd Trimesters (Fetal Development)	Labor-Delivery
High dose	K general malformations K abortion	K intrauterine growth retardation CNS effects, gonadal effects Q leukemia	
Microwaves	U/A skeletal malformations	U/A abortion	U
Ethanol (chronic, binge)	K/A syndrome: midline hypoplasia, microcephaly, low set ears, cardiac abnormalities, female genital malformations	K intrauterine growth retardation, mental retardation, neonatal withdrawal, decreased fetal breathing	K neonatal depression
Hyperthermia	Q/A general malformations, abortion	U/A intrauterine growth retardation, abortion	U
Methylmercury	X mental retardation	X mental retardation	
Tobacco smoking	K intrauterine growth retardation	K intrauterine growth retardation K increased perinatal mortality K decreased fetal breathing	K increased perinatal mortality K decreased fetal breathing
Mebendazole	U/A	U	U
Caffeine (at least 7 cups of coffee/day)	Q increased reproductive loss A general malformations	Q increased reproductive loss	K fetal tachycardia

¹Adapted from Miller RK, 1981.
²Action may be useful therapeutically.

Questions regarding preconception drug exposures to the father are also raised. Birth defects resulting from preconception drug exposure have not been confirmed in the limited number of epidemiologic studies available and are unlikely unless effects persist into the period of embryogenesis. This question needs further study.

There are only a few drugs or drug classes for which teratogenic risks have been established sufficiently to justify terminating pregnancy. These include the following:

Isotretinoin [Accutane] is *contraindicated* in all women of childbearing age unless effective contraception is insured. Isotretinoin is a proven teratogen in animals and in humans. The risk of spontaneous abortions or congenital malformations is very high when the drug is taken in the second month of gestation. Clinical findings include malformed or absent ears, severe congenital heart defects, and central nervous system malformations, including hydrocephalus and microcephaly. Similar findings are reported in animal studies. The drug appears to disrupt the migration of neural tissue in the early stages of development. Pregnancy therefore must be ruled out before a woman of childbearing age can be given isotretinoin. If pregnancy does occur while a woman is receiving the drug, she should be advised about the serious risks to her fetus.

Antineoplastic agents, especially aminopterin, carry a high risk of teratogenesis and avoidance of pregnancy is usually recommended. Nevertheless, with the exception of aminopterin, normal infants have been delivered in most of the small number of pregnancies that have been allowed to proceed to term. Expert detailed information is necessary for the occasional mother who may wish to consider continuing pregnancy while receiving antineoplastic therapy. The limited data available for various types of antineoplastics have been reviewed (Nicholson, 1968; Shepard, 1979; Gililland and Weinstein, 1983).

The range of reported frequencies of birth defects after use of *anticonvulsants* illustrates the difficulties in extrapolating from epidemiologic studies; estimates of the proportion of children affected range from 0% to more than 30%. Even expert reviewers differ widely in their conclusions (Shepard, 1979; Committee on Drugs, American Academy of Pediatrics, 1979). A syndrome similar to the fetal alcohol syndrome has been observed with hydantoins and other anticonvulsants, but frequency estimates have been subjective and appear to be influenced by knowledge of exposure. Selected defects (especially neurologic, cleft, and heart defects) appear to occur about twice as frequently in offspring of treated epileptic mothers compared to those of untreated epileptic women. Valproic acid exposure has recently been associated with neural tube defects, particularly spina bifida, and may warrant prenatal testing (Committee on Drugs, American Academy of Pediatrics, 1983 A).

Authorities agree that anticonvulsants should be continued as needed, despite the apparent risk of malformations. The data are probably insufficient to justify substituting one anticonvulsant for another after selecting the agent(s) that appears to have the best risk/benefit ratio for the patient and type of seizure. The mother should be advised that increased risks have been observed but that the chances are favorable for delivering a normal infant, although interruption of pregnancy is justified in a few patients. For pregnancies carried to term, vitamin K should be given to the infant postpartum because hemorrhage has been induced by anticonvulsants (including barbiturates).

Estrogens, particularly potent *nonsteroidal* agents such as diethylstilbestrol (DES), are associated with a rare vaginal cancer (incidence, approximately 1 in 1,000 exposures) and more often with other changes in the genitourinary tract of both male and female offspring (DES Task Force, 1978). Despite precautions, inadvertent exposures still occur. Effects are related to the type of agent, the potency, and the time of exposure.

Inadvertent exposure to *oral contraceptives* has been reported to be hazardous in some studies, but the risk has not been confirmed in other studies (Wilson and Brent, 1981). The risk does not appear to justify interruption of pregnancy. *Danazol*, an impeded estrogen used to treat endometriosis and fibrocystic breast disease, has been associated with masculinization of female fetuses when taken by the mother in early pregnancy.

Masculinization of the fetal external genitalia is a basic biological phenomenon with administration of *testosterone*. Significant maternal exposure (rare) poses sufficient hazard to the female embryo to consider termination of pregnancy. The incidence with testosterone-derived progestins (usually found in oral contraceptives) is low and that with other progestational agents apparently is negligible.

Antiandrogenic effects (hypospadias, cryptorchidism, microphallus, and possible effects on fertility and behavior) on the male fetus from exposure to extrinsic sex hormones have been suggested by several epidemiologic studies and have been supported by observations in animals, including primates. The number of exposures is too small to establish clear-cut risks relative to specific types of sex hormones, but the hazard is best established for DES (Gill et al, 1979). Although the dimensions of the risks, especially those influencing behavior and fertility, are not defined, the observed overt relative risks are low.

Antithyroid drugs cross the placenta and can produce fetal hypothyroidism and goiter; therefore, pregnancy should be avoided when using these drugs. However, hyperthyroidism may develop initially during pregnancy (incidence, 0.2%) and, if untreated, can result in premature birth. The goitrogenic effects of thiouracil derivatives and iodine are generally reversible. Therefore, if hyperthyroidism must be treated during pregnancy, the lowest effective dose of propylthiouracil (which crosses the placenta less readily than methimazole) is recommended. Thyroid hormone given with propylthiouracil cannot be recommended (Cooper, 1984). Radioactive iodine preparations also should not be used because of the possibility of thyroid ablation after eight weeks of pregnancy.

Lithium appears to be associated with characteristic right sided heart damage, although well controlled data are unavailable to establish the level of risk. Lithium is also goitrogenic. Although exposure during pregnancy is a concern, many normal infants have been delivered; thus, when lithium is deemed essential, the lowest possible dose should be given. Lithium is the only psychotropic drug for which there is sufficient evidence of teratogenesis to consider termination of pregnancy (Committee on Drugs, American Academy of Pediatrics, 1983 B).

Coumarin anticoagulants (eg, warfarin) cause nasal hypoplasia, stippling of secondary epiphyses, and growth retardation; blindness and hydrocephalus also have been observed. Although the incidence of long-term effects is not established, only a small proportion of infants have been affected (Pauli et al, 1980). Warfarin therapy is usually temporary and termination of a pregnancy that has occurred during such therapy may be considered. However, most infants have been normal. Heparin is generally considered the drug of choice when anticoagulation is required, especially during the first trimester, because it does not cross the placenta and is not teratogenic. However, heparin may cause major problems and the rate of fetal loss is high when it is given in the third trimester.

Penicillamine, a drug used to treat Wilson's disease, heavy metal poisoning, cystinuria, rheumatoid arthritis, and other conditions, is associated with a characteristic collagen defect. However, authorities recommend continuation of penicillamine in pregnant women with Wilson's disease, since the risk/benefit ratio with moderate doses (1 g/day or less) is low. The drug should be withheld from pregnant women with cystinuria if possible. If stones continue to form, the dose should be limited to 1 g/day. Alternative management of rheumatoid arthritis is recommended during pregnancy.

Administration of *tetracyclines* during the third trimester of pregnancy is associated with interference of calcification in the fetus; this effect results in abnormal osteogenesis and hypoplasia of dental enamel. The most obvious effect is permanent yellow-brown discoloration of the teeth. Therefore, tetracyclines should not be prescribed during the latter half of pregnancy unless there are compelling reasons.

Malaria prophylaxis has been widely used during pregnancy and has not been observed to be injurious, whereas malaria during pregnancy is hazardous. However, it may be desirable to avoid high-dose chloroquine therapy for rheumatoid conditions during pregnancy.

Adverse Drug Reactions During Breast Feeding

The number of mothers who breast-feed has increased from 28% in 1975 to more than 50% at present. This has led to increased questioning of the physician concerning the potential toxicity of drugs taken by lactating women that may appear in breast milk. Unfortunately, data on the short- and long-term effects and safety of many maternally ingested drugs upon the suckling infant are incomplete.

The mechanisms that determine the concentration of a drug in breast milk are similar to those existing elsewhere within the organism. Drugs generally traverse membranes by passive diffusion, and the ultimate concentration achieved depends upon the existing concentration gradient, molecular weight, degree of ionization, lipid solubility, and extent of drug-maternal plasma protein binding (Berlin, 1981; Welch and Findlay, 1981). Breast milk (pH, 7.0 to 7.6; mean pH, 7.2) is more acid than plasma (pH, 7.4), and weak bases become more ionized as the pH decreases; thus, these drugs generally have higher concentrations in milk than in plasma as the relatively membrane-impermeable ionized form is retained or "trapped" within breast milk. The opposite occurs with weak acids. However, the influence of molecular weight (eg, sulfasalazine, heparin), lipid solubility, and protein binding (eg, warfarin) may be more significant than the coefficient of ionization (pKa).

Milk/plasma ratios signify only that the drug is present in milk. They indicate nothing about the total amount absorbed by the infant or the possibility of adverse effects, which are of concern to the individual patient. It is now quite clear that, with very few exceptions, all drugs present in the maternal circulation are transferred into milk; however, the maximum amount secreted into milk seldom exceeds 1% to 2% of the maternal dose. Thus, the decision to breast-feed is based primarily on the incidence and types of adverse reactions reported rather than the presence of the drug in breast milk.

Drugs that are received by nursing infants in milk are most often placed in one of four general categories throughout this book. The information is located in the Precautions or Adverse Reactions and Precautions section for individual drugs or drug classes when appropriate. These categories include situations when breast-feeding is contraindicated, when periodic monitoring of the nursing infant is recommended, when no significant adverse reactions in the nursing infant have been reported, or when available data are insufficient to evaluate and recommend the safety of the drug during breast-feeding.

A number of authors (*Med Lett Drugs Ther*, 1979; Beeley, 1981 B; Berlin, 1981; Committee on Drugs, American Academy of Pediatrics, 1983 B) agree that antimetabolites, chloramphenicol, radioactive pharmaceuticals, and phenindione should be contraindicated during breast-feeding. Lithium is considered to be contraindicated by most authorities, because high concentrations can occur in the plasma of nursing infants. Isotretinoin also is contraindicated during breast feeding. Although the amount excreted in milk is unknown, the drug is a known teratogen, and exposure in infants should be minimized. Some authorities also express concern about the use of isoniazid because of the possible hepatotoxic action of its acetylated metabolite in the infant. Other drugs that are relatively contraindicated include sulfonamides; dapsone and nitrofurantoin, which may produce hemolytic anemia, especially in G6PD-deficient infants; and antithyroid drugs (especially methimazole) and iodides, which may inhibit thyroid function. However, propylthiouracil does not appear to be present in clinically significant concentrations in human milk (Kampmann et al, 1980).

The use of low-dose combination or progestin only-minipill oral contraceptives is generally considered safe. The amount of estrogen ingested by a suckling infant is similar whether the estrogen is exogenous from a combination oral contraceptive or endogenous produced by a lactating mother. The progestin component of combination oral contraceptives is also found in breast milk, whereas endogenous progesterone is not (Committee on Drugs, American Academy of Pediatrics, 1981).

Physical signs in the infant should be monitored to identify serious adverse reactions when certain agents or drugs are used by the nursing mother, eg, drowsiness with alcohol, barbiturates, benzodiazepines, certain antihistamines, and other agents with a sedative action; diarrhea and candidiasis with ampicillin; dependence with prolonged use of large doses of opiates and opioids.

Evidence supports the contention that milk is produced continuously rather than stored and that the maternal plasma concentration reflects the milk concentration. Thus, if the nursing mother waits for one half-life of the drug to elapse before nursing, the amount of drug in breast milk decreases by about 50%.

Atropine, oral contraceptives, and diuretics are reported to impair milk production in nursing mothers, although this has never been documented.

The major decision to be considered is whether medication is necessary in nursing mothers rather than whether the medicated mother should nurse. Drugs should not be prescribed for the nursing mother to relieve trivial symptoms.

REPORTING ADVERSE DRUG REACTIONS

An Adverse Drug Reaction Reporting Program has been established by the Division of Drug and Biologic Product Experience of the Food and Drug Administration, Parklawn Building, Rockville, MD, 20857. This Division is especially interested in receiving *new* adverse drug reactions not currently included in the drug's labeling, especially those associated with suspected drug interactions, carcinogenicity, congenital anomalies, and deaths. Previously reported reactions also are of interest if they are more severe or occur in clusters within a hospital or clinic. These reported reactions are one of the most important components of overall postmarketing drug surveillance, and the information is used to update the labeling and occasionally to modify the drug's indications for use or precautions. Studies have documented that new adverse reactions are discovered more efficiently from spontaneous reporting than from other methods, including large postmarketing studies (Rossi et al, 1983; Venning, 1983). Confidentiality with regard to the patients' and doctors' names is assured.

A report form, FDA-1639 (periodically attached to the *Food and Drug Bulletin* sent to most health care professionals), is distributed by the Food and Drug Administration, Department of Health and Human Services, Washington, DC, 20204. A mailer copy of the FDA-1639 form with accompanying instructions appears at the end of this book for convenience in order to promote this important activity. The hospital pharmacist can serve as an important resource to coordinate the information requested in the report. Attachment of other relevant data is encouraged. Practicing physicians, hospital pharmacists, and selected nursing personnel are in key positions to contribute to the success of this monitoring program. Health professionals submit over 30,000 reports yearly, either to the drug manufacturer (who must notify the FDA) or directly to the FDA.

Cited References

Drug therapy and pregnancy: Maternal, fetal and neonatal considerations, (symposium). *Obstet Gynecol* 58(suppl):1-105, (Nov) 1981.

The Medical Letter Handbook of Drug Interactions. New Rochelle, NY, The Medical Letter, 1983.

Update: Drugs in breast milk. *Med Lett Drugs Ther* 21:21-24, 1979.

American Pharmaceutical Association: *Evaluations of Drug Interactions,* ed 2. Washington, DC, American Pharmaceutical Association, 1976.

American Pharmaceutical Association: *Evaluations of Drug Interactions,* ed 2 (supplement). Washington, DC, American Pharmaceutical Association, 1978.

Avery GS: Drug interactions that really matter: Guide to major important drug interactions. *Drugs* 14:132-146, 1977.

Beeley L: Adverse effects of drugs in later pregnancy. *Clin Obstet Gynaecol* 8:275-289, 1981 A.

Beeley L: Drugs and breast feeding. *Clin Obstet Gynaecol* 8:291-295, 1981 B.

Berkowitz RL, et al (eds): *Handbook for Prescribing Medications During Pregnancy.* Boston, Little, Brown and Company, 1981.

Berlin CM Jr: Pharmacologic considerations of drug use in lactating mother. *Obstet Gynecol* 58(suppl):17-23, (Nov) 1981.

Busto U, et al: Comparison of two recently published algorithms for assessing probability of adverse drug reactions. *Br J Clin Pharmacol* 13:223-227, 1982.

Committee on Drugs, American Academy of Pediatrics: Effect of medication during labor and delivery on infant outcome. *Pediatrics* 62:402-403, 1978.

Committee on Drugs, American Academy of Pediatrics: Anticonvulsants and pregnancy. *Pediatrics* 63:331-333, 1979.

Committee on Drugs, American Academy of Pediatrics: Breast-feeding and contraception. *Pediatrics* 68:138-140, 1981.

Committee on Drugs, American Academy of Pediatrics: Valproate teratogenicity. *Pediatrics* 71:980, 1983 A.

Committee on Drugs, American Academy of Pediatrics: Transfer of drugs and other chemicals into human breast milk. *Pediatrics* 72:375-383, 1983 B.

Cooper DS: Antithyroid drugs. *N Engl J Med* 311:1353-1362, 1984.

Davies DM: *Textbook of Adverse Drug Reactions,* ed 2. New York, Oxford University Press, 1981.

DES Task Force, Summary Report 1978. NIH Publication no. 81-1688. Bethesda, Md, National Institutes of Health, 1978.

Dukes MNG: *Side Effects of Drugs,* ed 8. Princeton, Excerpta Medica, 1984.

Feinberg LE: Drug-induced hepatitis, in Anderson RJ, Schrier RW (eds): *Clinical Use of Drugs in Patients with Kidney and Liver Disease.* Philadelphia, WB Saunders, 1981, 136-152.

Gililland J, Weinstein L: Effects of cancer chemotherapy agents on developing fetus. *Obstet Gynecol Surv* 38:6-13, 1983.

Gill WB, et al: Association of diethylstilbestrol exposure in utero with cryptorchidism, testicular hypoplasia, and semen abnormalities. *J Urol* 122:36-39, 1979.

Golbus MS: Teratology for obstetrician: Current status. *Obstet Gynecol* 55:269-277, 1980.

Hansten PD: *Drug Interactions,* ed 5. Philadelphia, Lea & Febiger, 1985.

Hays DP: Teratogenesis: Review of basic principles with discussion of selected agents, parts I and II. *Drug Intell Clin Pharm* 15:444-450, 542-561, 1981.

Hill RM, Stern L: Drugs in pregnancy: Effects on fetus and newborn. *Drugs* 17:182-197, 1979.

Howard FM, Hill JM: Drugs in pregnancy. *Obstet Gynecol Surv* 34:643-653, 1979.

Hutchinson TA, et al: Algorithm for operational assessment of adverse drug reactions. II. Demonstration of reproducibility and validity. *JAMA* 242:633-638, 1979.

Iams JD, Rayburn WF: Drug effects on fetus, in Rayburn WF, Zuspan FP (eds): *Drug Therapy in Obstetrics and Gynecology.* Norwalk, CT, Appleton-Century-Crofts, 1982, 9-17.

Jones JK: Adverse drug reactions in community health setting: Approaches to recognizing, counseling, and reporting. *Fam Commun Health* 5:58-67, 1982.

Kampmann JP, et al: Propylthiouracil in human milk: Revision of dogma. *Lancet* 1:736-738, 1980.

Karch FE, Lasagna L: Adverse drug reactions: Critical review. *JAMA* 234:1236-1241, 1975.

Kramer MS, et al: Algorithm for operational assessment of adverse drug reactions. I. Background, description, and instructions for use. *JAMA* 242:623-632, 1979.

Lerman F, Weibert RT: *Drug Interactions Index.* Oradell, NJ, Medical Economics, 1982.

Levy G: Gastrointestinal clearance of drugs with activated charcoal, (editorial). *N Engl J Med* 307:676-678, 1982.

Miller RK: Drugs during pregnancy: Therapeutic dilemma. *Ration Drug Ther* 15:1-9, (July) 1981.

Millstein LG: FDA's "pregnancy categories," (letter). *N Engl J Med* 303:706, 1980.

Napke E, Stevens DGH: Excipients and additives: Hidden hazards in drug products and in product substitution. *Can Med Assoc J* 131:1449-1452, 1984.

Nicholson HO: Cytotoxic drugs in pregnancy: Review of reported cases. *J Obstet Gynaecol Br Comm* 75:307-312, 1968.

Park BK, Breckenridge AM: Clinical implications of enzyme induction and enzyme inhibition. *Clin Pharmacokinet* 6:1-24, 1981.

Pauli RM, et al: Risks of anticoagulation in pregnancy. *Am Heart J* 100:761-762, 1980.

Rayburn WF, Zuspan FP: *Drug Therapy in Obstetrics and Gynecology.* Norwalk, CT, Appleton-Century-Crofts, 1982.

Rossi AC, et al: Discovery of adverse drug reactions: Comparison of selected phase IV studies with spontaneous reporting methods. *JAMA* 249:2226-2228, 1983.

Shepard TH: Teratogenicity of therapeutic agents. *Curr Probl Pediatr* 10:1-42, 1979.

Trissel LA: *Handbook on Injectable Drugs,* ed 4. Bethesda, MD, American Society of Hospital Pharmacists, 1985.

Venning GR: Identification of adverse reactions to new drugs, I-IV. *Br Med J* 286:199-202; 289-292; 365-368; 458-460; 544-547, 1983.

Venulet J: *Assessing Causes of Adverse Drug Reactions with Special Reference to Standardized Methods.* London, Academic Press, 1982.

Vestal RE, Wood AJJ: Influence of age and smoking on drug kinetics in man: Studies using model compounds. *Clin Pharmacokinet* 5:309-319, 1980.

Welch RM, Findlay JWA: Excretion of drugs in human breast milk. *Drug Metab Rev* 12:261-277, 1981.

Wilson JG, Brent RL: Are female sex hormones teratogenic? *Am J Obstet Gynecol* 141:567-580, 1981.

Wood SM, Beeley L (eds): Prescribing in pregnancy. *Clin Obstet Gynaecol* 8:248-528, 1981.

General Analgesics

The analgesics discussed in this chapter are divided into two groups: (1) the opioids, which bind to opioid receptors, and (2) the nonopioids (analgesic-antipyretics), which have no affinity for these receptors. Although drugs in both groups have analgesic properties, their other pharmacologic actions differ and they are discussed separately. Mixtures containing drugs from each group are discussed in a third section.

OPIOIDS

The opioids can be classified as agonists, which resemble morphine in most of their actions, or as mixed agonist-antagonists, which act as agonists at one type of opioid receptor and as competitive antagonists at another or as weak or partial agonists. The agonists include the natural opium alkaloids (morphine, codeine, a mixture of opium alkaloids [Pantopon]), their analogues (hydrocodone in mixtures), hydromorphone [Dilaudid], oxycodone (in mixtures), oxymorphone [Numorphan], and the following synthetic compounds: phenylpiperidine derivatives (meperidine [Demerol], alphaprodine [Nisentil]), a morphinan derivative (levorphanol [Levo-Dromoran]), and diphenylheptane derivatives (methadone [Dolophine], propoxyphene [Darvon]). The mixed agonist-antagonists include a morphinan derivative, butorphanol [Stadol]; a phenanthrene derivative, nalbuphine [Nubain]; a benzomorphan derivative, pentazocine [Talwin]; an oripavine derivative, buprenorphine [Buprenex]; and an azepine, meptazinol (investigational drug).

Pharmacodynamics

The concept of analgesic receptors that interact with various compounds to produce analgesia was proposed many years ago, but only recently have specific opioid binding sites been identified as receptors and their anatomical distribution determined. The density of opioid binding sites varies markedly in different regions of the central nervous system. Densities are high in anatomical areas associated with physiologic functions affected by opioids; this suggests a correlation between site of action and effect.

Neurochemical evidence has indicated that the receptors are associated with synapses of the brain, and they appear to function as sites for a natural neurotransmitter. Endogenous polypeptides that bind to opioid binding sites and mimic some of the actions of opioids have been found in brain tissue; they have been identified as a mixture of two pentapeptides, met (methionine)-enkephalin and leu (leucine)-enkephalin. A larger peptide with similar activity, beta-endorphin, has been found in the pituitary. Beta-endorphin is comprised of the amino acid sequence 61-91 of the pituitary peptide, beta-lipotropin, and met-enkephalin is comprised of the amino acid sequence 61-65 of beta-lipotropin. Another pituitary peptide, designated dynorphin, was identified later and is more potent than beta-endorphin and leu-enkephalin. It contains leu-enkephalin, which may be a cleavage product of dynorphin, and appears to be a selective κ (kappa) agonist. Several possible functions, including neurotransmission, have been suggested for the endorphins and enkephalins, but their mechanism of analgesic action is not clear.

Although the opioids have various chemical structures, they all interact with opioid receptors. Relative analgesic efficacy appears to be related to their affinity for specific binding sites, as determined by in vitro studies. For example, morphine has a greater affinity for opioid binding sites than codeine.

Different types or subclasses of opioid receptors have been postulated to explain the various actions of the opioids. On the basis of studies in dogs, three types of receptors were proposed and now are established firmly: The μ (mu) receptor mediates morphine-like analgesia and euphoria; the κ (kappa) receptor probably mediates pentazocine-like analgesia, sedation, and miosis; and the σ (sigma) receptor mediates dysphoria and psychotomimetic effects produced by pentazocine and other drugs with antagonist activity. Subsequently, at least two other types of receptors, designated δ (delta) and ϵ (epsilon), have been proposed to explain the actions of the opioids and endorphins on the mouse and rat vas deferens and guinea pig ileum. The δ receptor also has been found in the central nervous system and is selective for enkephalins, while the ϵ receptor has high selectivity for beta-endorphin but lacks affinity for enkephalins. There is considerable evidence that the δ receptor plays a role in opioid-induced respiratory depression. Studies in rats support the view that the μ receptor is associated with reduced tidal volume and the δ receptor with reduced respiratory rate. The μ receptor may exist as two subtypes, μ_1 and μ_2. The μ_1 receptor is present only in the central nervous system and is associated with supraspinal analgesia, prolactin release, hypothermia, and catalepsy. The μ_2 receptor is associated with bradycardia and reduced tidal volume. The investigational drug, meptazinol, is an agonist that acts primarily at the putative μ_1 receptor. Although these studies suggest that different receptors mediate different effects, more research is needed to determine their exact nature and role.

Indications

Morphine is the prototype of many opioids, all of which have qualitatively similar actions on the central nervous system. The relative usefulness of the morphine-like opioid analgesics is determined by the type and severity of pain, the onset and duration of action by different routes of administration, and the severity of adverse reactions. The availability of several analgesics in each category, including those with "strong or potent" or "weak or mild" activity, as well as those with mixed agonist-antagonist properties, permits considerable latitude in the selection of an agent for a specific situation. Thus, the physician may meet the needs of most patients by becoming familiar with the properties of representative drugs.

Acute Pain: Opioids are most effective for relieving moderate to severe acute pain from various causes. They alter the psychological response to pain as well as its perception, partially at a spinal level, and suppress anxiety and apprehension. They act on higher centers of the central nervous system to produce analgesia without loss of consciousness, although, at least initially, fully effective doses usually cause sedation. Small to moderate doses relieve constant dull pain, and moderate to large parenteral doses are usually required to alleviate intermittent sharp pain caused by trauma or of visceral origin. Agents that are weaker than morphine are useful for mild or moderate pain but not for severe pain. The stronger analgesics generally should not be used for pain that can be relieved by weaker drugs or nonopioid analgesics. However, the more potent drugs should not be withheld for short-term therapy but should be administered in sufficient doses when indicated (eg, for pain occurring postoperatively or after injuries).

Chronic Pain: The treatment of chronic pain depends upon its cause. When analgesics are indicated, adequate relief usually can be attained initially with a nonopioid (eg, acetaminophen, aspirin, diflunisal, ibuprofen, naproxen sodium). If pain is not controlled by one of these drugs, concurrent use of an opioid or an agonist-antagonist with low dependence liability may be tried. Strong analgesics should be reserved until necessary. Their prolonged administration in chronic pain of nonmalignant etiology produces tolerance and may lead to complications more debilitating than the pain itself (ie, drug dependence), or may result in conditioned pain behavior.

Withdrawal of strong analgesics and re-evaluation of therapy may be necessary in some patients with chronic pain not associated with malignant disease. Other treatment, such as nerve blocks, should be considered. Drugs of other classes, particularly small doses of antidepressants, also are frequently useful. For this purpose, all antidepressants appear to be equivalent in effectiveness. It may be necessary to refer certain patients to a pain clinic where multidisciplinary attention is available and neurosurgical interruption of the pain pathway may be considered. Additional discussions of management are included in several reviews (Foley, 1985).

Neoplastic Disease: The management of patients with chronic pain associated with neoplastic disease, especially in its terminal phase, requires special consideration. A primary concern is maintenance of the patient's comfort; nonmedical aspects (eg, physical, social, mental, spiritual) also must be taken into account in the total care program. The choice of analgesic depends upon the status of the disease and the response. It may be necessary to try several compounds, and the drug regimen should be changed as required to obtain relief. A nonopioid (acetaminophen, aspirin, diflunisal, ibuprofen, naproxen sodium, suprofen, or other nonsteroidal anti-inflammatory drugs) should be tried initially. Usual doses of weak opioids often are no more effective than nonopioids, but both types of drugs may be given concomitantly, since their effects are additive. If this combined therapy does not relieve the pain, an oral agonist-antagonist with or without a nonopiate may be tried before a strong analgesic is prescribed. Because agonist-antagonists may precipitate withdrawal symptoms in opioid-dependent patients, a "wash-out" period may be necessary before they can be used.

The oral route is preferred and is usually adequate unless pain is very severe. Although the oral/parenteral effectiveness ratio of morphine and some closely related drugs is not as favorable as that of other strong analgesics (eg, codeine, methadone, levorphanol, oxycodone, oxymorphone), morphine may be effective orally if the dosage is adjusted appropriately (see the evaluation). The concomitant administration of aspirin, acetaminophen, or other nonopioid and a strong opioid given orally often provides additional relief. If oral administration is inadequate or cannot be tolerated, a parenteral route must be used. However, it is generally advisable to continue concomitant therapy with an oral nonopioid.

Many authorities believe that strong analgesics should be administered on a fixed schedule rather than as needed when treating chronic pain. The dose, route, and schedule *must be individualized* according to the efficacy and duration of action of the analgesic and the response of the patient. A drug with a long duration of action is preferred to reduce the frequency of administration. Results of trials utilizing self-administration indicate that many patients take less medication under these conditions.

Although tolerance may develop to the strong analgesics, it seldom is a practical problem. Dosage requirements also may increase because of progression of the disease. In any case, cross-tolerance is not absolute, and patients who become tolerant to one opioid can be given another. Iatrogenic dependence should not be considered a primary problem when treating the severe pain of neoplastic disease and must never be a reason to withhold strong analgesics from patients who may benefit from them (McGivney and Crooks, 1984; Foley, 1985).

Myocardial Infarction: The aim in treating the severe pain of acute myocardial infarction is to provide adequate relief without excessive untoward effects, especially those affecting the respiratory and cardiovascular systems. Morphine is generally considered the drug of choice for this use. When prompt relief is required, a dilute solution may be given slowly intravenously in divided doses. Hemodynamic effects are slight and may be beneficial (eg, reduction of left ventricular work index). Although morphine may produce adverse reactions (eg, nausea, vomiting, respiratory depression), it relieves pain and reduces anxiety. If excessive bradycardia, hypotension, or respiratory depression occurs, naloxone [Narcan] may be given.

Meperidine also is used in myocardial infarction, particularly that associated with bradycardia; in comparable doses, its effects are similar to those of morphine. The hemodynamic effects of nalbuphine appear to resemble those of morphine, but blood pressure is not reduced and no deleterious hemodynamic effects have been observed. Thus, nalbuphine may be useful in myocardial infarction, but greater experience is needed to determine whether it has advantages over conventional drugs. Pentazocine and butorphanol increase left ventricular workload and myocardial oxygen demands, and are not as desirable as morphine.

Obstetric Analgesia: Use of a strong analgesic in obstetric patients requires considerable experience and judgment to provide adequate analgesia for the mother while avoiding interference with the progress of labor and preventing respiratory depression in the newborn infant. Meperidine is widely used for this purpose; however, like all strong analgesics, it crosses the placenta and may depress fetal respiration (see the evaluation). If opioid-induced respiratory depression is suspected in the neonate, naloxone should be given as an adjunct to mechanical ventilatory support. Administration of an antagonist to the mother before delivery to counteract fetal depression is not recommended.

Preanesthetic Medication and Anesthesia: Strong analgesics are useful for preanesthetic medication because their sedative, antianxiety, and analgesic properties afford smoother induction and maintenance of anesthesia and reduce excitement during emergence. However, in the absence of preoperative pain, antianxiety agents (eg, diazepam [Valium], triazolam [Halcion]) may be preferred to reduce postoperative nausea and vomiting and avoid postoperative respiratory depression (see Chapter 17, Adjuncts to Anesthesia). Certain strong analgesics (meperidine, morphine, fentanyl, and hydromorphone) are used to supplement the hypnotic and analgesic effects of nitrous oxide. Large doses of morphine, fentanyl, and some other strong analgesics are administered intravenously in balanced anesthesia, primarily in those undergoing cardiac surgery and in other poor-risk patients. See Chapter 16, General Anesthetics.

Pulmonary Edema: Patients with dyspnea of pulmonary edema secondary to acute left ventricular failure may benefit from administration of morphine if ventilation is adequately controlled or equipment for artificial ventilation is readily available. Morphine allays the anxiety caused by hypoxemia and produces peripheral pooling of blood, which reduces the workload on the heart. Other measures (eg, rotating tourniquets, oxygen and IPPB combined with etiologic management) also are essential. Although acute left ventricular failure is the most common cause of pulmonary edema, the specific etiology should be determined and treatment instituted accordingly. Morphine generally should not be given when pulmonary edema is caused by a chemical respiratory irritant. It should be used very cautiously in patients with bronchial asthma and should not be given during an asthmatic attack.

Cough: The cough reflex is depressed or abolished by opioids, but use of strong analgesics for this purpose should be restricted to patients with painful cough that cannot be controlled by codeine or non-narcotic agents (see Chapter 21, Decongestant, Cough, and Cold Preparations) or when cough suppression is required during certain procedures. When an active cough reflex is desired along with analgesia, meperidine may be preferred because it lacks an antitussive effect.

Gastrointestinal and Urinary Tract Disorders: Although morphine and related strong analgesics produce adverse gastrointestinal effects (eg, nausea, vomiting, constipation), their antiperistaltic action is useful in the symptomatic treatment of diarrhea (see Chapter 53, Agents Used in Disorders of the Lower Intestinal Tract). However, prolonged use may cause severe constipation even after therapy is discontinued. Although acute severe pain associated with biliary, renal, or ureteral colic can be relieved by a strong analgesic, antispasmodic therapy also should be considered, since morphine and related agents may increase smooth muscle tone. Strong analgesics should not be administered if the presence and site of pain are necessary for diagnosis.

Adverse Reactions and Precautions

Opioids cause adverse reactions that limit their usefulness: respiratory depression, nausea, vomiting, constipation, cardiovascular effects (hypotension, bradycardia), and increased intracranial pressure. Constipation may be a problem, particularly with prolonged use, but may be prevented by concomitant administration of a senna derivative or other stimulant laxative. Other reactions include miosis, spasm of the biliary and urinary tracts, and, rarely, hypersensitivity phenomena (urticaria, rash, and anaphylactoid reactions with intravenous administration).

Respiratory depression is the most dangerous acute reaction produced by the morphine-like analgesics, although it is rarely severe with usual doses. Severe hypoventilation or apnea is most likely to develop in elderly debilitated patients and in those with respiratory disorders characterized by chronic hypoxia. If severe respiratory depression occurs or appears to be imminent, intravenous naloxone should be given (see Chapter 80, Drugs Used in the Treatment of Poisoning) or mechanical support of respiration should be provided.

Opioids should be used cautiously in patients with excessive respiratory secretions (eg, in chronic obstructive lung disease), because they decrease ciliary activity, reduce the cough reflex, and increase bronchomotor tone.

Opioids should be given in reduced doses or withheld from patients in shock or those with decreased blood volume, for severe hypotension may develop. Because these analgesics may cause hypoventilation and hypercapnia, resulting in cerebrovascular dilatation and increased intracranial pressure, they must be used with extreme caution (unless mechanical ventilation is provided) in patients with head injuries, intracranial lesions or tumors, or other conditions in which increased intracranial pressure should be avoided. Morphine and other strong analgesics may produce miosis and their use in patients with suspected head injuries or in those undergoing intracranial surgery may mask the dilation of one or both pupils that is an important sign of increased intracranial pressure.

Drowsiness and clouding of the sensorium and mental processes are the most prominent central effects of opioids. Although these effects are often desirable, impairment of the ability to concentrate limits the usefulness of these agents in some ambulatory patients.

Since opioid analgesics are metabolized by the liver, they should be used with caution in patients with hepatic insufficiency, for their duration of action may be prolonged.

Strong analgesics are not necessarily contraindicated in patients with impaired renal function, but individualization of dosage may be required since prolonged respiratory depression and narcosis have been reported after morphine was given to patients with uremia or various other disorders of renal function (Sear et al, 1985). Opioids decrease urine production directly by acting on the kidney and indirectly by stimulating the release of antidiuretic hormone. Their spasmogenic effect on the sphincter of the urinary bladder may cause acute urinary retention in patients with prostatic hypertrophy or urethral stricture.

The dose of analgesic should be reduced in patients with myxedema, hypothyroidism, or hypoadrenalism.

Drug Interactions: The dose of opioids should be reduced in patients receiving other drugs that depress the central nervous system (eg, antipsychotic agents, barbiturates, antianxiety agents), or the dose of the latter agents should be adjusted. Severe adverse reactions have occurred following the administration of meperidine [Demerol] to patients receiving monoamine oxidase inhibitors; these have not been observed with morphine.

Tolerance and Dependence: Tolerance may develop after prolonged use of morphine-like drugs. Therefore, any increase in the dosage requirement should be evaluated to determine if it is caused by worsening of pain due to progression of the pathologic process or by the development of tolerance. In chronic pain associated with terminal cancer, tolerance is seldom a problem; pain often can be controlled by around-the-clock maintenance doses of oral morphine, which can be administered for prolonged periods without any need for further increments.

The opioid analgesics have effects on the central nervous system other than analgesia, which may lead to abuse by some patients. The dependence occurring with use of these drugs is referred to generally as morphine-type dependence to distinguish it from that produced by alcohol, barbiturates, and other central nervous system depressants. The dependence may be qualitatively and quantitatively different among drugs in the group. Results of studies designed to determine dependence liability indicated that butorphanol [Stadol], nalbuphine [Nubain], pentazocine [Talwin], propoxyphene [Darvon], and codeine have less abuse potential than morphine.

The physician should not assume that patients with pathologic pain will experience the same effects from morphine-like drugs as the "street addict" or that iatrogenic dependence will develop consistently. In fact, dependence is extremely unlikely following the short-term use of even large doses of strong parenteral analgesics in patients with acute pain. Anxiety about dependence should not be permitted to result in undermedication for acute pain that causes unnecessary suffering. Most patients given an opioid for analgesia are able to discontinue its use without difficulty. However, it should be kept in mind that physical dependence without psychological dependence may develop after prolonged use (eg, multiple daily doses for at least 20 days) of a strong analgesic; therefore the dose should be decreased gradually after the drug is no longer needed to avoid the discomfort of a withdrawal syndrome.

Although it often is difficult to identify dependence-prone patients, physicians should make every effort to do so. Patients who are emotionally unstable, those with a history of dependence or abuse of other psychotropic agents (including alcohol), and patients with affective disorders may be predisposed to analgesic abuse. Opioid use should be monitored very carefully in these patients, but they should not be deprived of necessary analgesics.

Ordinarily, morphine or its congeners should be given in the smallest effective dose to minimize tolerance and physical dependence. This is particularly important for patients with chronic diseases or conditions that may lead to drug abuse. (See also the section on Prescribing Controlled Psychotropic Drugs in Chapter 1.) The use of methadone for the management of opioid abusers is discussed later in this chapter; the use of naltrexone [Trexan] for this purpose is described in Chapter 80, Drugs Used in the Treatment of Poisoning.

Intrathecal and Epidural Opioid Analgesia

The epidural or intrathecal administration of opioids is being investigated to avoid the side effects of large systemic doses. The epidural route is used most commonly. Various opioids have been employed, but a preservative-free solution of morphine is used most frequently. The primary differences among opioids are rate of onset of action, segmental spread, and duration. Both spread and duration are increased as the hydrophilic property of the opioid is increased. An epidural dose of morphine 5 mg, one of the most hydrophilic opioids, may provide good to excellent pain relief for 24 to 36 hours. Single-dose, intermittent, and continuous epidural administration have been used for chronic pain, postoperative pain, the first stage of labor, and following cesarean section. Implanted infusion pumps with intrathecal catheters and reservoirs that can be refilled percutaneously have been utilized for chronic pain.

The advantages of this technique are the long duration of action and, unlike spinal or epidural local anesthesia, there is no sympathetic blockade (permitting ambulation), loss of motor tone, or loss of sensitivity to temperature or pinprick.

The most serious adverse effect is respiratory depression; because the onset of the respiratory effect may be delayed, adequate patient monitoring is required. This adverse reaction occurs much less frequently with epidural than intrathecal administration. It probably is more pronounced with lipophilic opioids, eg, morphine. When this procedure is utilized for the relief of postoperative pain, respiratory depression may be minimized by avoiding the concomitant use of systemic opioids and by maintaining the patient in a 30° head-up position.

Other side effects include pruritus, nausea and vomiting, and urinary retention. Both the pruritus and the nausea and vomiting respond to doses of naloxone too small to affect analgesia. Urinary retention generally is associated only with the initial use of opioids by these routes. Partial agonist or agonist-antagonist opioids should not be used epidurally or intrathecally in patients who have received pure agonist opioids systemically for a prolonged period because severe opioid withdrawal with shock may develop.

Drug selection and comparison of the epidural and intrathecal routes are discussed in greater detail in Cousins and Mather, 1984; Hughes et al, 1984; Kotelko et al, 1984; and Stenseth et al, 1985. Limitations of the technique in patients with chronic cancer pain, particularly the development of tolerance, are described by Max et al, 1985.

Dosage and Routes of Administration

Dosage of the strong analgesics should be individualized and based on the severity of pain. For rapid onset of effect, these agents must be given parenterally; however, oral administration can produce analgesia equivalent to that achieved after intramuscular injection if the dose is increased in accordance with the oral/parenteral potency ratio for the particular drug. Some analgesics (eg, codeine, levorphanol [Levo-Dromoran], methadone) have a more favorable oral/parenteral potency ratio than morphine.

Intravenous administration produces a more rapid onset of action with greater dosage control. Since rapid intravenous injection produces sudden, profound respiratory depression and possibly hypotension, a dilute solution should be injected over several minutes; a narcotic antagonist and equipment for mechanical ventilation must be available. In patients confined to bed, the incidence of hypotension, dizziness, nausea, and vomiting is minimized.

Drug Evaluations

AGONISTS

Opium Alkaloids and Derivatives

MORPHINE SULFATE

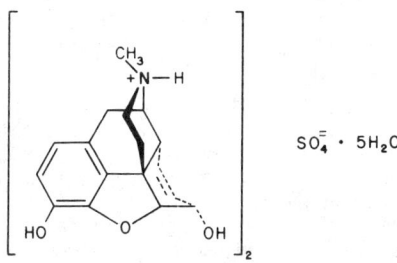

Morphine is the prototype of the strong analgesics (see the Introduction for actions, uses, adverse reactions, and precautions). It is classified as a Schedule II drug under the Controlled Substances Act.

This agent is usually given parenterally to assure rapid and complete relief of pain. It is considerably less potent orally because of rapid metabolism in the intestinal wall and liver; thus, only a small percentage of an oral dose reaches the systemic circulation. However, this does not preclude use of the oral route in cancer patients in whom sufficient relief can be obtained by using an adequate dose.

Maximal analgesic action usually occurs within one hour after parenteral administration; analgesia persists for approximately four hours (range, two and one-half to seven hours). The peak effect occurs later and the duration of action is longer after oral use than after intramuscular injection.

For use of morphine by the epidural and intrathecal routes, see the section on Intrathecal and Epidural Opioid Analgesia in the Introduction.

Morphine is classified in FDA Pregnancy Category C.

PHARMACOKINETICS. The volume of distribution is 3.2 ± 0.3 L/kg, the elimination half-life is 2.9 ± 0.5 hours, and the clearance rate is 14.7 ± 0.9 ml/min/kg (Stanski et al, 1978). Elderly patients may be more sensitive to morphine and have higher, more variable serum levels than younger patients; thus, age should be considered when determining the dosing interval (Kaiko, 1980).

There are only minor differences in the kinetic patterns of morphine in pediatric patients (1 month to 15 years) and no differences in their sensitivity to morphine (Dahlström et al, 1979). However, in infants under 1 week, the elimination half-life is prolonged to 6.8 hours (range, 4.6 to 8.9) and the clearance is less than 50% that of older infants (6.3 ml/min/kg; range, 3.6 to 7.6) (Lynn and Slattery, 1985).

The response to morphine may be enhanced in patients with uremia, various renal disorders, and renal ischemia (Sear et al, 1985). However, the mean elimination half-life and clearance were similar in patients with renal failure and in normal subjects (Aitkenhead et al, 1983).

DOSAGE AND PREPARATIONS.
Intramuscular, Subcutaneous: Adults, 10 mg/70 kg (range, 5 to 20 mg), depending upon the cause of the pain and the response of the patient; *children* (subcutaneous), 0.1 to 0.2 mg/kg (maximal dose, 15 mg).

Intravenous: Except in general anesthesia and during acute pulmonary edema or myocardial infarction, this route of administration is employed only rarely. It may be useful when prompt analgesia is important. *Adults,* 2.5 to 15 mg in 4 to 5 ml of water for injection, administered over four to five minutes.

Epidural (Lumbar): Adults, 5 mg. Smaller doses may be effective in the elderly.

Intrathecal: Adults, 0.2 to 1 mg.
> *Generic.* Solution 2, 4, 5, 8, 10, and 15 mg/ml in 1 ml and half-filled 2 ml containers; tablets (soluble) 10, 15, and 30 mg.
> *Duramorph PF* (Elkins-Sinn). Solution (sterile) 0.5 and 1 mg/ml in 10 ml containers (preservative-free).
> NOTE: *Only preservative-free morphine sulfate should be employed for epidural or intrathecal administration.*

Oral: Oral morphine is one-third to one-sixth as potent as intramuscular morphine in total effect. The dose must be individualized because of variation in bioavailability; 20 to 25 mg may be sufficient for some patients, but others may require 75 mg or more every four hours. The timed-release preparation is administered at 8- to 12-hour intervals.
> *Generic.* Tablets 15 and 30 mg; solution 10 and 20 mg/5 ml (alcohol 10%).
> *M S Contin* (Purdue Frederick). Tablets (timed-release) 30 mg.

Rectal: The dose must be individualized. *Adults,* 10 to 20 mg every four hours.
> *Generic.* Suppositories 5, 10, and 20 mg.

Buccal, Sublingual: These routes provide good absorption and avoid first-pass metabolism. The dosage is the same as for intramuscular administration (Bell et al, 1985).

CODEINE PHOSPHATE

CODEINE SULFATE

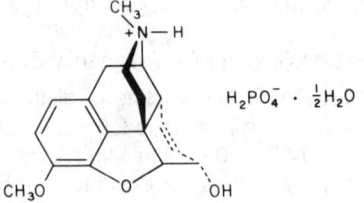

$$H_2PO_4^- \cdot \tfrac{1}{2}H_2O$$

ACTIONS AND USES. Codeine relieves mild to moderate pain and is usually administered orally with nonopioid analgesics (see the section on Mixtures).

Results of controlled studies have shown that oral codeine 65 mg is approximately equivalent to aspirin 650 mg or acetaminophen 650 mg; doses lower than 15 mg usually are ineffective. Codeine has been reported to be less effective than aspirin in postpartum, uterine, or dental pain; it has been suggested that inhibition of prostaglandin synthesis and an anti-inflammatory action may play a role in aspirin's superiority.

When administered intramuscularly, codeine 120 to 130 mg is approximately equivalent to morphine sulfate 10 mg but causes more adverse reactions.

For the use of codeine as an antitussive, see Chapter 21, Decongestant, Cough, and Cold Preparations.

ADVERSE REACTIONS AND PRECAUTIONS. The adverse reactions of codeine resemble those of other morphine-like drugs. Constipation is noted occasionally, but nausea, vomiting, and drowsiness are minimal after usual oral doses. Dizziness may occur in ambulatory patients. The larger doses necessary to relieve more severe pain cause most of the adverse effects observed with morphine, including respiratory depression. Naloxone antagonizes the respiratory depression caused by overdosage.

Significant quantities of histamine may be released after large doses of codeine are administered and may produce hypotension, cutaneous vasodilation, urticaria, and, more rarely, bronchoconstriction. This histamine-releasing action appears to be stronger than that of morphine in equianalgesic doses; therefore, codeine should not be administered intravenously.

Codeine is classified in FDA Pregnancy Category C.

DEPENDENCE LIABILITY. The dependence liability of codeine is somewhat less than that of morphine, and physical dependence occurs only rarely after oral analgesic use. However, abuse of the drug, particularly in the form of cough syrup, is not uncommon. Codeine (except in mixtures) is classified as a Schedule II drug under the Controlled Substances Act.

PHARMACOKINETICS. Codeine is absorbed rapidly following oral administration. Peak plasma levels occur in about one hour and the plasma half-life is about 3.5 hours. After intramuscular injection, peak plasma levels occur in about 30 minutes and the half-life is about three hours. The bioavailability of codeine is greater than that of morphine after oral administration; its oral:parenteral analgesic potency ratio is 1:1.5.

Codeine is metabolized primarily in the liver and is excreted in the urine as conjugated products; however, a portion is demethylated to form morphine, which has been postulated to contribute to the analgesic effect. The plasma concentration does not correlate with the brain concentration or relief of pain, however.

DOSAGE AND PREPARATIONS.
Oral, Subcutaneous, Intramuscular: For analgesia, *adults,* 30 to 60 mg four to six times daily as needed; *children,* 0.5 mg/kg four to six times daily.

For antitussive use, see Chapter 21.

CODEINE PHOSPHATE:
Generic. Solution 30 mg/ml in 1, 2, and 20 ml containers and 60 mg/ml in 1 and 2 ml containers; tablets (soluble) 15, 30, and 60 mg; powder.
CODEINE SULFATE:
Generic. Tablets (soluble, oral) 15, 30, and 60 mg.

HYDROCHLORIDES OF OPIUM ALKALOIDS
[Pantopon]

This preparation is a mixture of purified opium alkaloids in solution as the hydrochloride salts (20 mg of the mixture contains the equivalent of 15 mg of morphine sulfate). The indications are the same as for morphine and it is used most commonly for postoperative pain. Claims that the analgesic and sedative effects of morphine are enhanced, while adverse effects are minimized by other constituents in the preparation, have not been substantiated by controlled clinical studies; thus, it has no proven advantage over an equivalent amount of morphine.

This product is classified as a Schedule II drug under the Controlled Substances Act and in FDA Pregnancy Category C.

DOSAGE AND PREPARATIONS.
Intramuscular, Subcutaneous: The manufacturer's suggested dosage is: *Adults,* 5 to 20 mg.
Pantopon (Roche). Solution 20 mg/ml in 1 ml containers (alcohol 6%).

HYDROMORPHONE HYDROCHLORIDE
[Dilaudid]

Hydromorphone, a derivative of morphine, has the same actions and uses (see the Introduction); however, it is about eight times more potent on a milligram basis and has a slightly shorter duration. This analgesic is about one-fifth as potent orally as intramuscularly; the peak effect occurs later and the duration of action is longer with oral administration. The elimination half-life is about 2.5 hours after intravenous or oral administration.

Hydromorphone is more soluble than morphine; thus, higher concentrations may be injected if necessary. The greater solubility permits smaller intramuscular or subcutaneous injection volume. This is an advantage if multiple daily administration is required in patients with diminished tissue mass due to terminal illness.

Adverse reactions are the same as those produced by morphine in equianalgesic doses (see the Introduction).

Hydromorphone is classified as a Schedule II drug under the Controlled Substances Act.

DOSAGE AND PREPARATIONS.
Intramuscular, Intravenous (slow), Subcutaneous: Adults, 1 to 1.5 mg every four to six hours as required; the dose may be increased for severe pain. Concentrated solutions of hydromorphone [Dilaudid-HP] are intended only for administration to opioid-tolerant patients. In cancer patients with chronic pain, subcutaneous or intramuscular doses of 1 to 14 mg are usually satisfactory, but this range may be exceeded as required. There is little experience with the intravenous use of the concentrate; if necessary, it should be given slowly over a period of two to three minutes.
Generic. Solution 1, 2, 3, and 4 mg/ml in half-filled 2 ml containers.
Dilaudid (Knoll). Solution 1 and 4 mg/ml in 1 ml containers and 2 mg/ml in 1 and 20 ml containers; powder in 900 mg containers (for compounding).
Dilaudid-HP (Knoll). Solution 10 mg/ml in 1 ml containers.
Oral: Adults, 2 to 4 mg every four hours as required; the dose may be increased if necessary.
Dilaudid (Knoll). Tablets 1, 2, 3, and 4 mg.
Rectal: Adults, 3 mg every six to eight hours.
Dilaudid (Knoll). Suppositories 3 mg.

OXYMORPHONE HYDROCHLORIDE
[Numorphan]

Oxymorphone is a derivative of morphine and is closely related chemically to hydromorphone. This analgesic is about ten times as potent as morphine on a weight basis. Its actions, uses, and duration of effect are similar to those of hydromorphone and morphine, except that oxymorphone appears to possess little antitussive activity. When administered by rectal suppository, it is about one-tenth as potent as when injected intramuscularly.

Adverse reactions are similar to those produced by morphine and other narcotic analgesics in equianalgesic doses. See the Introduction for indications and adverse reactions.

Oxymorphone is classified as a Schedule II drug under the Controlled Substances Act and in FDA Pregnancy Category C.

DOSAGE AND PREPARATIONS.
Intramuscular, Subcutaneous: Adults, 1 to 1.5 mg every four to six hours. For obstetric analgesia, 0.5 to 1 mg intramuscularly.
Intravenous: Adults, 0.5 mg initially.
Numorphan (DuPont). Solution 1 mg/ml in 1 ml containers and 1.5 mg/ml in 1 and 10 ml containers.
Rectal: Adults, 5 mg every four to six hours.
Numorphan (DuPont). Suppositories 5 mg.

Synthetic Compounds

MEPERIDINE HYDROCHLORIDE
[Demerol]

ACTIONS AND USES. Meperidine, a phenylpiperidine derivative, is a synthetic opioid analgesic. Many of its pharmacologic properties and indications are similar to those of morphine, but meperidine has no effect on cough and is much less constipating. It is one-eighth as potent as morphine on a weight basis when administered parenterally. Meperidine is about one-third to one-fourth as potent orally as parenterally.

This analgesic is widely used in anesthetic premedication, in balanced anesthesia, and in obstetric analgesia. It is preferred to morphine for obstetric use because the incidence of vomiting is lower and it may not penetrate the blood-brain barrier of the fetus as easily. Nevertheless, it can produce significant respiratory depression in the newborn infant proportional to the fetal blood concentration. This can be minimized by giving small incremental doses of 25 mg intravenously during labor.

The maximal analgesic effect occurs 30 to 50 minutes after intramuscular injection. The duration of action (two to four hours) is shorter than that of morphine. Results of studies on the relationship between blood concentration of meperidine and analgesic response have indicated that 0.7 mcg/ml would relieve severe pain in 95% of patients. Because absorption varies among individuals following intramuscular administration, blood concentrations adequate to produce analgesia may not be achieved with usual doses in about 5% of patients. It has been suggested that intravenous infusion with blood concentration determinations may be more effective for pain relief (Austin et al, 1980; Hug, 1980).

ADVERSE REACTIONS, PRECAUTIONS, AND INTERACTIONS. The most commonly observed adverse reactions include dizziness, nausea, and vomiting (especially in ambulatory patients). Meperidine is less constipating than morphine, but its sedative effect is comparable. Extreme asthenia, hyperhidrosis, syncope, dysphoria, and nightmares also have been observed. Equianalgesic doses of meperidine and morphine produce similar respiratory depression, which can be reversed by a narcotic antagonist. With prolonged administration, large amounts of normeperidine may accumulate, particularly in patients with decreased renal function. Both meperidine and normeperidine cause excitatory phenomena, including convulsions. However, a definite relationship between blood concentration of the metabolite and toxic reactions has not been established (Austin et al, 1981). Pain, induration, and abscess may occur at the injection site after repeated subcutaneous administration.

Contraindications to the use of meperidine are similar to those for morphine and other opioid analgesics. They include elevated cerebrospinal fluid pressure and hypersensitivity.

Because changes in drug disposition have been reported in patients with liver disease and the elderly, dosage must be reduced in these individuals (Mather and Meffin, 1978).

The dose of meperidine should be reduced when antipsychotic agents, sedative-hypnotics, or other drugs that depress the central nervous system are given concurrently. Severe toxic reactions (eg, restlessness, excitement, fever) have followed the use of meperidine in patients receiving monoamine oxidase inhibitors.

Meperidine is classified as a Schedule II drug under the Controlled Substances Act.

PHARMACOKINETICS. Following intravenous administration of meperidine in healthy individuals, the volume of distribution at steady state was 269 L (range, 198 to 333 L); plasma clearance was 1.06 L/min (range, 0.71 to 1.32), and the elimination half-life was 3.6 hours (range, 3.1 to 4.1). There is evidence that the disposition of meperidine varies between day and night, with the elimination half-life being shorter and the plasma clearance greater at night. This suggests that larger doses might be required at night (Ritschel et al, 1983). Bioavailability after oral administration is about 50% due to first-pass metabolism in the liver.

The drug is excreted in the urine, primarily as normeperidine, meperidinic acid and its conjugates, and normeperidinic acid and its conjugates; about 5% of the dose is excreted as unchanged drug. Normeperidine is the only metabolite that has been detected in the blood. It is about one-half as active as an analgesic but more active as a convulsant than the parent drug.

DOSAGE AND PREPARATIONS.
Intramuscular, Intravenous (slow), Oral, Subcutaneous: Adults, 100 mg (range, 50 to 150 mg), repeated at intervals of three to four hours if required. The intramuscular route is preferred to subcutaneous injection if repeated administration is anticipated. For obstetric analgesia, 50 to 100 mg intramuscularly or subcutaneously, repeated three or four times at one- to three-hour intervals if necessary. *Children,* 1 to 1.5 mg/kg (maximal dose, 100 mg) intramuscularly, orally, or subcutaneously, repeated at intervals of three to four hours if necessary.

> *Generic.* Solution 10 mg/ml in 30 ml containers, 25 and 75 mg/ml in 1 and half-filled 2 ml containers, 50 mg/ml in 1, 2, and 30 ml containers, and 100 mg/ml in 1 and 20 ml containers; syrup 50 mg/5 ml; tablets 50 and 100 mg.
> *Demerol* (Winthrop-Breon). Solution 25 mg/ml in 0.5 and 1 ml containers, 50 mg/ml in 1 and 30 ml containers, 75 mg/ml in 1 and 1.5 ml containers, and 100 mg/ml in 1, 2, and 20 ml containers; syrup 50 mg/5 ml; tablets 50 and 100 mg.

ALPHAPRODINE HYDROCHLORIDE
[Nisentil]

This drug is related chemically and pharmacologically to meperidine, but it is more potent on a weight basis and has a more rapid onset and shorter duration of action. Alphaprodine is useful when rapid analgesia of short duration is desirable (eg, in obstetrics; in urologic examinations and procedures [cystoscopy]; preoperatively in major surgery; in minor surgery, especially orthopedic, ophthalmologic, rhinologic, and laryngologic procedures; in children requiring analgesia during dental procedures).

Adverse reactions and precautions are similar to those described for meperidine (see that evaluation and the Introduction). Alphaprodine is classified as a Schedule II drug under the Controlled Substances Act.

PHARMACOKINETICS. Following intravenous administration, the onset of action occurs in one to two minutes and the duration is 30 to 90 minutes. The onset after subcutaneous administration is about ten minutes with a duration of one to two hours. The elimination half-life of alphaprodine following intravenous administration was reported to be 131 ± 9 minutes; its apparent volume of distribution was 1.90 ± 0.16 L/kg. The drug is metabolized by the liver and is excreted primarily in the urine; trace amounts are excreted in human milk.

DOSAGE AND PREPARATIONS.
Intravenous: Adults, 0.4 to 0.6 mg/kg injected slowly over three or four minutes. For cystoscopy, initially, 20 to 30 mg. For major surgery, 10 to 20 mg; for minor surgery, 20 mg. The initial dose should not exceed 30 mg and the total dose should not exceed 240 mg in 24 hours. Respiratory depression may develop when the drug is given intravenously. The patient should be lying down and naloxone and resuscitative facilities should be immediately available.
Subcutaneous: Adults, initially, 0.4 to 1.2 mg/kg (maximum, 60 mg). For obstetric analgesia, initially, 40 to 60 mg after cervical dilation has begun, repeated at two-hour intervals if necessary. For major surgery, 20 to 40 mg; for minor surgery, 40 mg. The total amount should not exceed 240 mg in 24 hours.
Submucosal: Children, 0.3 to 0.6 mg/kg. Alphaprodine should be used with great caution and in reduced dosage in pediatric dental patients who are receiving other central nervous system depressants. Pediatric use for other indications is not recommended.
Intramuscular: The drug should not be given by this route because its absorption is unpredictable.
    Nisentil (Roche). Solution 40 mg/ml in 1 ml containers and 60 mg/ml in 10 ml containers.

LEVORPHANOL TARTRATE
[Levo-Dromoran]

This synthetic analgesic is a morphinan derivative related chemically and pharmacologically to morphine, and it has the same indications (see the Introduction). Levorphanol is four to eight times more potent than morphine after intramuscular injection, has a similar duration of action, and is relatively more effective orally. It is about one-half as potent orally as intramuscularly.

The adverse reactions and precautions of levorphanol are similar to those of morphine. Although some reports suggest that levorphanol is less likely to cause nausea, vomiting, and constipation, any difference in the incidence of adverse reactions is slight. (See the Introduction.) Levorphanol is classified as a Schedule II drug under the Controlled Substances Act.

DOSAGE AND PREPARATIONS.
Oral, Subcutaneous: Adults, 2 to 3 mg.
    Levo-Dromoran (Roche). Solution 2 mg/ml in 1 and 10 ml containers; tablets 2 mg.

METHADONE HYDROCHLORIDE
[Dolophine Hydrochloride]

ACTIONS. Methadone is a synthetic analgesic that differs chemically from morphine, although its actions and analgesic potency are similar. Following a single intramuscular injection, the duration of analgesia and subjective effects are the same as for morphine. It is approximately one-half as potent orally as intramuscularly and has a longer duration of action. The half-life of methadone averages 25 hours; this comparatively long period may be related to its extensive binding to plasma proteins. The drug accumulates upon repeated administration.

USES. Since methadone can prevent or relieve acute withdrawal symptoms produced by morphine-like drugs, it is useful orally in the detoxification of patients dependent upon these agents. The withdrawal of methadone itself produces symptoms that are less intense but more prolonged than those of heroin or morphine withdrawal, and the syndrome develops more slowly. Methadone also is useful orally in maintenance programs for individuals dependent on heroin or other morphine-like drugs.

The Food and Drug Administration has promulgated regulations providing for strict control over the distribution, use, and dispensing of methadone to reduce abuse and diversion. Under the conditions established by these regulations, methadone may be used to treat severe pain in hospitalized patients and outpatients, for the detoxification and temporary maintenance treatment of hospitalized narcotic addicts, and for maintenance treatment under approved methadone programs. Although methadone depresses the cough reflex, labeling for use as an antitussive is no longer permitted.

Methadone is classified as a Schedule II drug under the Controlled Substances Act.

ADVERSE REACTIONS AND PRECAUTIONS. Nausea, vomiting, constipation, dizziness, dryness of the mouth, and mental depression occur more frequently in ambulatory patients. Contraindications are the same as for morphine. Because it accumulates with repeated administration, methadone should be used cautiously, particularly in the elderly and debilitated, for conditions requiring prolonged parenteral medication. Subcutaneous injection may be irritating.

DOSAGE AND PREPARATIONS.

Intramuscular, Subcutaneous: Adults, for relief of pain, 2.5 to 10 mg, repeated when necessary. Dosage should be individualized to prevent accumulation.

   Dolophine Hydrochloride (Lilly). Solution 10 mg/ml in 1 and 20 ml containers.

Oral: Adults, for relief of pain, dosage should be individualized according to the severity of pain and response of the patient: (tablets) 2.5 to 10 mg every six to eight hours; (solution) 5 to 20 mg every six to eight hours. After initial pain relief is maintained for three to five days, the dose should be adjusted to prevent accumulation and toxic effects; administration every 8 to 12 hours may be adequate (Hansen et al, 1982).

   Dolophine Hydrochloride (Lilly), *Methadone Hydrochloride* (Roxane). Tablets 5 and 10 mg.
   Methadone Hydrochloride (Lilly). Tablets (dispersible) 40 mg (for detoxification and maintenance treatment only).
   Methadone Hydrochloride (Roxane). Solution (oral) 1 mg/ml (alcohol-free) and 2 mg/ml (alcohol 8%).

PROPOXYPHENE HYDROCHLORIDE
   [Darvon]

PROPOXYPHENE NAPSYLATE
   [Darvon-N]

ACTIONS AND USES. Propoxyphene is related chemically to methadone and is used orally to relieve mild to moderate pain. Although this drug is an opioid, analgesic efficacy is less than that of other opioids. It is estimated that the milligram potency of propoxyphene hydrochloride is one-half to two-thirds that of codeine, and 65 mg is no more effective, and usually less so, than 650 mg of aspirin or acetaminophen. Studies comparing the two salts of propoxyphene show that equianalgesic effects are produced by equimolar amounts of the salts (100 mg of napsylate is equivalent to 65 mg of hydrochloride).

Propoxyphene does not possess anti-inflammatory or antipyretic actions and has little or no antitussive activity, although the nonanalgesic levorotatory isomer has been used for this purpose.

ADVERSE REACTIONS AND PRECAUTIONS. The most common adverse reactions are dizziness, drowsiness, nausea, and vomiting, which are more prominent in ambulatory patients. Some reactions may be alleviated if the patient is recumbent. Less common untoward effects include constipation, abdominal pain, rash, and headache. Asthenia, euphoria, dysphoria, and minor visual disturbances have been reported rarely. Concomitant ingestion of alcohol or other central nervous system depressants produces additive effects.

Propoxyphene should not be prescribed for pregnant women since adverse effects on fetal development have not been ruled out. Furthermore, withdrawal symptoms have occurred in the neonate when the drug was used by the mother near term.

The *dependence liability* of propoxyphene, as determined in controlled studies, is less than that of codeine. However, abuse with development of morphine-type dependence has been reported. Propoxyphene preparations are classified as Schedule IV drugs under the Controlled Substances Act.

POISONING. Propoxyphene, alone and in combination with alcohol and other central nervous system depressants, has caused a number of deaths from drug overdose. Most of these fatalities were associated with suicidal or frank abuse, but some apparently resulted from accidental overdose. Because propoxyphene may be abused and overdosage may be fatal, physicians should use caution in prescribing this drug (only the number of doses required for a specific condition should be prescribed and the number of refills, if any, should be limited).

Overdosage is manifested by respiratory depression; extreme somnolence, which may be followed by coma; pupillary constriction; and acute circulatory failure. In addition to these symptoms characteristic of narcotic poisoning, focal and generalized convulsions usually are prominent. Arrhythmias and pulmonary edema have been reported occasionally; apnea, cardiac arrest, and death have occurred. The narcotic antagonist, naloxone, overcomes severe respiratory depression and should be given following airway management and initiation of respiratory support.

PHARMACOKINETICS. Propoxyphene is completely absorbed after oral administration, but systemic availability is reduced because of the first-pass elimination of 30% to 70% of a dose. The major metabolite is norpropoxyphene, which is largely eliminated in the urine. The oral clearance is 1.3 to 3.6 L/min and systemic clearance is 0.6 to 1.2 L/min. The apparent volume of distribution is 700 to 1,800 L. The half-life of propoxyphene is 14.6 hours (range, 8 to 24) and that of norpropoxyphene is 22.9 hours (range, 18 to 29) (Gram et al, 1979).

DOSAGE AND PREPARATIONS.

Oral: Adults, 65 mg (hydrochloride) every three to four hours or 100 mg (napsylate) every four hours as needed.

   PROPOXYPHENE HYDROCHLORIDE:
   Darvon (Lilly), *Generic.* Capsules 32 and 65 mg.
   Additional Trademarks.
   Dolene (Lederle), *SK-65* (Smith Kline & French).
   PROPOXYPHENE NAPSYLATE:
   Darvon-N (Lilly). Suspension 50 mg/5 ml; tablets 100 mg.

MIXED AGONIST-ANTAGONISTS

PENTAZOCINE HYDROCHLORIDE
[Talwin NX]

PENTAZOCINE LACTATE
[Talwin]

ACTIONS. Pentazocine was the first mixed agonist-antagonist analgesic to be marketed. It is an agonist at the kappa and sigma opioid receptors and has a weak antagonist action at the mu receptor. Results of controlled clinical studies have shown that parenteral pentazocine is one-fourth to one-sixth as potent as morphine on a weight basis, and it is about one-third as potent orally as parenterally.

Pentazocine has a more rapid onset and a shorter duration of action than morphine; thus, its time-effect curve resembles that of meperidine. Following intramuscular injection, maximal analgesia usually occurs within 30 to 60 minutes and lasts two to three hours. After oral ingestion, the peak effect occurs in one to three hours and lasts somewhat longer than after intramuscular injection.

USES. Pentazocine relieves moderate pain but may be less effective than morphine in severe pain. It is useful in chronic pain when given before appreciable physical dependence on opiates has developed. This drug also is administered for preoperative medication. When used for obstetric analgesia, pentazocine causes fetal respiratory depression comparable to that produced by meperidine.

Pentazocine has been used to relieve the pain of myocardial infarction. However, the cardiac workload tends to increase because of increased pulmonary arterial and central venous pressure. For this reason, morphine is preferred to pentazocine for this use, except in hypotensive patients who would benefit from increased aortic pressure.

ADVERSE REACTIONS AND PRECAUTIONS. Adverse reactions are generally similar to those produced by other strong analgesics, except as indicated below. Nausea, vomiting, and dizziness occur most frequently. Other effects observed occasionally include euphoria, diaphoresis, constipation, urinary retention, and transient hypertension. The degree of drowsiness and sedation produced by pentazocine is approximately the same or greater than that produced by equianalgesic doses of morphine or meperidine.

As with other strong analgesics, pentazocine produces respiratory depression. The severity of respiratory depression following parenteral administration of 20 mg of pentazocine is equivalent to that produced by 10 mg of morphine. However, increasing the dose of pentazocine above 30 mg does not cause a proportionate increase in respiratory depression as with morphine.

Psychotomimetic effects (dysphoria, nightmares, feelings of depersonalization, and most commonly, visual hallucinations) may occur with usual doses but are more common following larger doses. Epileptiform electroencephalographic abnormalities and grand mal convulsions have been observed rarely after large intravenous doses.

Pentazocine is contraindicated if increased intracranial pressure, head injury, or other intracranial lesions are present unless mechanical support of respiration is being employed. The drug is partially metabolized in the liver and partially excreted by the kidney unchanged; therefore, it should be used with caution in patients with impaired renal or hepatic function. Care should be exercised in patients with myocardial infarction when nausea and vomiting are present, in those with respiratory depression, and in those undergoing surgery of the biliary tract. Ambulatory patients should be warned not to operate machinery or drive cars while taking the drug.

Repeated injection into a single area can produce sterile abscess, ulceration, and scarring of the subcutaneous tissue and muscle. If long-term administration is required and oral pentazocine cannot be utilized, the injection site should be rotated and the intramuscular route employed.

This drug is classified in FDA Pregnancy Category C.

DEPENDENCE LIABILITY. Because of its mixed agonist-antagonist properties, pentazocine has less dependence liability than conventional narcotics; nevertheless, psychic and physical dependence have been reported, primarily after parenteral administration. Abuse of pentazocine in combination with pyribenzamine also has been reported. In most of these individuals, prior dependence or abuse of other drugs had been established. Thus, pentazocine should be used with caution and carefully monitored in dependence-prone or emotionally unstable individuals.

Abrupt withdrawal following prolonged parenteral use has caused abdominal cramps, fever, lacrimation, rhinorrhea, anxiety, and restlessness in some patients. These symptoms rarely require treatment; if they are severe, pentazocine can be readministered and the dose reduced gradually. A benzodiazepine controls withdrawal symptoms in some patients. Methadone or other opiates should not be substituted for pentazocine to treat these symptoms because of their greater potential for dependence.

Pentazocine, like other narcotic antagonists, can precipitate an acute withdrawal syndrome in patients physically dependent on opiates; the severity of the reaction is related to the extent of the patient's prior narcotic experience and the dose of pentazocine. In addition, pentazocine can antagonize the analgesic effect of an agonist (eg, meperidine) in nontolerant patients.

Pentazocine is classified as a Schedule IV drug under the Controlled Substances Act. In some states, it is included in Schedule II.

POISONING. The most common toxic effects of pentazocine

are dysphoria, delusions, and hallucinations. Naloxone is effective in the treatment of overdosage. Oxygen, mechanical support of ventilation, and supportive measures should be used as needed.

PHARMACOKINETICS. Pentazocine is well absorbed by all routes of administration, but there is considerable individual variation. Bioavailability after oral administration is 18.4% ± 7.8%; the reduction is due to first-pass metabolism. The elimination half-life is 203 ± 71 minutes following intravenous administration and 177 ± 34 minutes following oral administration. The volume of distribution at steady state is 396 ± 136 L. In cirrhotic patients, the elimination half-life is doubled and the rate of clearance halved. Oral bioavailability in these patients is increased from about 20% to approximately 70% (Bullingham et al, 1983). Pentazocine is metabolized extensively and excreted in urine as conjugated and unchanged drug (Ehrnebo et al, 1977).

DOSAGE AND PREPARATIONS.
(Strengths are expressed in terms of the base.)
Oral: Adults, 50 mg every three or four hours as needed, increased to 100 mg if necessary (maximum, 600 mg daily). These tablets contain naloxone, an opioid antagonist, to diminish the abuse potential. *Children under 12 years,* dosage not established.

PENTAZOCINE HYDROCHLORIDE:
Talwin NX (Winthrop-Breon). Tablets 50 mg with naloxone hydrochloride 0.5 mg.

Intramuscular, Intravenous, Subcutaneous: Adults, 30 mg every three to four hours as necessary; single doses in excess of 30 mg intravenously or 60 mg intramuscularly or subcutaneously are not advisable, and the total daily dose should not exceed 360 mg. The subcutaneous route should not be used unless necessary because of possible tissue damage. (Pentazocine should not be mixed in the same syringe with soluble barbiturates because precipitation will occur.) *Children under 12 years,* dosage not established.

For obstetric analgesia, 20 or 30 mg as a single intramuscular dose. When contractions become regular, 20 mg may be given intravenously and repeated two or three times at two- to three-hour intervals as needed.

PENTAZOCINE LACTATE:
Talwin (Winthrop-Breon). Solution 30 mg/ml in 1, 1.5, 2, and 10 ml containers.

BUPRENORPHINE HYDROCHLORIDE
[Buprenex]

ACTIONS AND USES. Buprenorphine is a derivative of the opium alkaloid, thebaine. This potent opioid analgesic possesses both agonist and antagonist properties, which ac-

counts for some of its unique actions. In numerous clinical trials, as well as in clinical use, buprenorphine has relieved moderate to severe pain associated with surgical procedures (eg, abdominal, thoracic, orthopedic, hysterectomy), cancer, neuralgias, labor, renal colic, and myocardial infarction. When this drug was used to treat chronic pain for several months, efficacy varied with the nature of the pain, but tolerance to the analgesic effect did not develop.

Buprenorphine can be given parenterally, (intravenous, intramuscular, subcutaneous), orally, and sublingually. It also has been given extradurally but should not be used by this route in patients who have received systemic opioids for prolonged periods because serious hypotension may occur (Christensen and Anderson, 1982).

In clinical studies, buprenorphine was found to be 20 to 30 times more potent than morphine on a weight basis. It has a longer duration of action (up to six hours) than morphine, pentazocine, and meperidine. Onset of analgesia occurs within 15 minutes after intramuscular injection and sooner after intravenous administration.

When used with nitrous oxide and flunitrazepam in balanced anesthesia, buprenorphine produced satisfactory analgesia for minor surgery but was usually inadequate when used alone. When it was given intravenously or intramuscularly after induction of anesthesia with nitrous oxide and fentanyl, the anesthetic and respiratory depressant effects of fentanyl were reversed but the analgesic effects were prolonged. Buprenorphine apparently acted as an opioid antagonist, but its agonist effect extended the duration of analgesia. Additional studies are necessary to determine the usefulness of buprenorphine in balanced anesthesia.

The drug's cardiovascular effects are similar to those produced by morphine in equianalgesic doses. Slight reductions in heart rate and systolic blood pressure with little or no change in diastolic pressure were observed. Myocardial contractility was not affected. Buprenorphine has been used to relieve the pain of myocardial infarction in a limited number of patients and no clinically significant hemodynamic effects have been observed; however, additional studies are needed to establish the efficacy of buprenorphine in this condition.

ADVERSE REACTIONS AND PRECAUTIONS. In general, the adverse reactions of buprenorphine resemble those of other opioid analgesics. Drowsiness occurs most frequently (50% to 85%) and is most pronounced during the first hour after administration. The incidence of nausea and vomiting is 10% to 20%. Other reactions include constipation, diaphoresis, dizziness, dryness of the mouth, miosis, bradycardia, and hypotension. Psychotomimetic effects were rarely observed.

Like other opioid analgesics, buprenorphine can produce respiratory depression resembling that caused by morphine at equianalgesic doses, but the onset is delayed and the duration is longer. However, severe respiratory depression has not been reported clinically. Unlike morphine, large doses of naloxone only partially reverse the depression produced by buprenorphine. Doxapram, a respiratory stimulant, has been reported to reverse the decreased respiration. As with other strong analgesics, buprenorphine should be used with caution in patients with head injuries or respiratory disorders unless mechanical support of respiration is provided and in those receiving other central nervous system depressants.

This drug is classified in FDA Pregnancy Category C.

DEPENDENCE LIABILITY. Results of studies in animals and man to determine the dependence liability of buprenorphine indicate that its abuse potential is low and may be less than that of codeine or propoxyphene. In studies in former addicts, buprenorphine produced typical morphine-like effects following single doses or long-term administration. The intensity of abstinence symptoms after prolonged administration was less than with morphine and similar to codeine, propoxyphene, nalorphine, pentazocine, and butorphanol. Symptoms develop gradually and do not reach maximum intensity for 14 to 15 days.

Naloxone does not precipitate withdrawal symptoms when given during prolonged administration of buprenorphine as it does with other opioid analgesics. Buprenorphine blocks the effects of large doses of morphine for about 30 hours. On the basis of these findings, it was suggested that this analgesic could be used for maintenance therapy in the treatment of narcotic addiction (Jasinski et al, 1978). In one study, buprenorphine suppressed the self-administration of heroin in addicts, and its withdrawal did not produce opiate abstinence symptoms, but further studies are needed to determine whether buprenorphine is useful for maintenance therapy of heroin dependence (Mello and Mendelson, 1980). Dependence on or abuse of buprenorphine was not reported in a postmarketing surveillance study (Harcus et al, 1979). Its abuse potential can be better assessed after wider clinical use. Buprenorphine should be prescribed with the same care as other opioids.

Buprenorphine is classified as a Schedule V drug under the Controlled Substances Act.

PHARMACOKINETICS. Buprenorphine is absorbed rapidly after intramuscular injection. Peak plasma concentrations occur in two to five minutes; after five minutes, concentrations are equal to those achieved with intravenous injection. After intramuscular administration, buprenorphine is excreted unchanged, mainly in the feces (68%), with smaller amounts (27%) excreted in the urine as conjugates of the unchanged drug and the dealkylated derivative.

Absorption is variable and delayed following sublingual administration; the peak blood level occurs in about three hours (range, 90 to 360 minutes) and absorption is essentially complete within five hours. Analgesia is attained in 15 to 45 minutes. There appears to be no direct relationship between plasma concentration and pharmacologic effect. Bioavailability after sublingual administration was about 50%. The drug is highly protein bound (about 96%).

Following intravenous administration, buprenorphine has a volume of distribution of 187.8 ± 35.3 L at steady state, a plasma clearance of 1275 ± 88.9 ml/min, and an elimination half-life of approximately five hours (Bullingham et al, 1983).

DOSAGE AND PREPARATIONS.
Intramuscular, Intravenous (slow): *Adults,* 0.3 to 0.6 mg, repeated every six to eight hours as required. Dosage has not been established for *children under 13 years.*

Buprenex (Norwich Eaton). Solution 0.3 mg/ml in 1 ml containers.

BUTORPHANOL TARTRATE
[Stadol]

ACTIONS AND USES. Although butorphanol is related chemically to levorphanol, its actions resemble those of pentazocine. The antagonist potency of butorphanol on a weight basis is about 10 to 30 times that of pentazocine and about one-tenth to one-fortieth that of naloxone, as determined by animal studies.

In controlled clinical studies, butorphanol relieved moderate to severe pain; its effectiveness in acute postoperative pain was comparable to that of morphine, meperidine, or pentazocine, but it was 3.5 to 7 times as potent on a weight basis as morphine, 30 to 40 times as potent as meperidine, and 20 times as potent as pentazocine. The peak analgesic effect occurs in about 30 minutes and the duration of effect after intramuscular injection is about three to four hours.

When given in increments of 1 mg to women in active labor, butorphanol resembles meperidine with respect to pain relief and effects on the neonate.

Butorphanol also appears to be comparable to meperidine when used for preanesthetic medication, except that it produces more sedation. It was as effective as morphine and meperidine as a supplement to balanced anesthesia.

The hemodynamic effects of butorphanol, as determined in a relatively small number of patients, appear to resemble those of pentazocine more than those of morphine. Butorphanol appears to increase pulmonary arterial pressure and pulmonary vascular resistance, left ventricular end-diastolic pressure, systemic arterial pressure, and possibly, the workload of the heart, which limits its usefulness in myocardial infarction. The administration of butorphanol for this condition should be restricted to patients who cannot tolerate morphine or meperidine.

Results of animal studies have demonstrated that butorphanol has antitussive activity, but this property has not been studied in man.

ADVERSE REACTIONS AND PRECAUTIONS. Adverse reactions are similar to those produced by other strong analgesics; those reported most frequently are sedation, nausea, and sweating. Other reactions with an incidence of more than 1% include headache, vertigo, feeling of floating, dizziness, lethargy, confusion, and lightheadedness. Psychotomimetic effects (eg, hallucinations, unusual dreams, depersonalization) reported with other antagonists have occurred only rarely with butorphanol. Cardiovascular (eg, palpitation) and dermatologic (eg, rash) effects also have been observed only rarely.

The respiratory depressant effects of butorphanol are similar to those of morphine in equianalgesic doses. Depression does not increase proportionally with larger doses as with morphine but lasts longer. Naloxone antagonizes respiratory depression.

Butorphanol does not induce withdrawal reactions in patients who are dependent on opioids. It should be used cautiously in patients with respiratory depression or in conjunction with other drugs that cause respiratory depression. It also should be administered cautiously in reduced doses to patients with hepatic or renal impairment, for these conditions may affect its metabolism and elimination.

DEPENDENCE LIABILITY. Studies in animals and a small number of human volunteers designed to determine dependence liability indicated that butorphanol has a low potential for dependence. Symptoms resembling those of opioid withdrawal were observed when the drug was discontinued or an antagonist was administered to individuals who received large doses for several weeks; however, drug-seeking behavior was not exhibited. Subjective effects were similar to those produced by morphine, but euphoria did not occur and the overall pharmacologic profile resembled that of central nervous system depressants such as barbiturates more closely than that of morphine. To minimize abuse, butorphanol should be prescribed with the same precautions used for opioids.

Butorphanol is not classified under the Controlled Substances Act.

PHARMACOKINETICS. Butorphanol is absorbed rapidly and essentially completely after intramuscular injection. Peak plasma levels occur in 30 to 60 minutes, and the elimination half-life is 2.5 to 4 hours. The volume of distribution at steady state is 350 L and the plasma clearance has been reported to be 2,700 to 4,065 ml/min (Bullingham et al, 1983). This agent is metabolized primarily to the inactive hydroxybutorphanol, which is excreted mainly in the urine; some is eliminated in the bile. When butorphanol was administered to women in labor, unchanged drug and glucuronide were found in the serum of the neonate. It is not known whether the drug is excreted in human milk.

DOSAGE AND PREPARATIONS.
Intramuscular: Adults, 2 mg, repeated every three to four hours as necessary (range, 1 to 4 mg), depending upon the severity of the pain.
Intravenous: Adults, 1 mg, repeated every three to four hours as necessary (range, 0.5 to 2 mg), depending upon the severity of the pain. *Children,* dosage has not been established.
   Stadol (Bristol). Solution 1 mg/ml in 1 ml containers and 2 mg/ml in 1, 2, and 10 ml containers.

MEPTAZINOL

ACTIONS AND USES. Meptazinol is an investigational drug (marketed in the United Kingdom) thought to act as a partial agonist with relative selectivity at the μ_1 receptor (Hoffbrand and Turner, 1983; Pasternak and Turner, 1985). This is presumed to confer the advantage of producing minimal respiratory depression. Parenteral meptazinol 100 mg is approximately equivalent in analgesic effect to meperidine 100 mg or morphine 8 mg. Oral meptazinol 200 mg is equivalent to pentazocine 50 mg. Meptazinol-induced analgesia is reversed by naloxone. Meptazinol reverses acute morphine overdosage in animals and precipitates an abstinence syndrome in opioid-dependent animals.

Meptazinol does not produce constipation. Miosis is slight and does not mask neurologic signs. Mood is rarely affected. This drug could not be differentiated from placebo and was not recognized to be similar to any drug of abuse by opioid addicts. Meptazinol cannot be substituted for an opioid in patients physically dependent on opioids.

Parenteral meptazinol has a rapid onset but short duration of action. It has been effective in obstetric analgesia, postoperative pain, dental pain, and acute pain produced by gallbladder and kidney stones. Because tolerance to its analgesic action and physical dependence do not develop, oral meptazinol may be useful in chronic pain.

ADVERSE REACTIONS AND PRECAUTIONS. In usual analgesic doses (30 or 60 mg intramuscularly), meptazinol did not significantly affect arterial pressure, heart rate, or the arterial PaO_2 and $PaCO_2$. The drug does not decrease the ventilatory response to hypercapnia. In a study employing doses up to 4 mg/kg in anesthetized patients, systemic and pulmonary vascular resistance was unchanged but cardiac output, mean arterial pressure, and heart rate decreased significantly. This dose did not induce myocardial depression.

The most common side effects are nausea and vomiting, which occur significantly more often than with morphine; the incidence is similar to that experienced with meperidine. If meptazinol is employed in anesthetic premedication or for postoperative pain, nausea and vomiting can be reduced or prevented by the coadministration of scopolamine. The frequency and severity of dizziness, sweating, and peripheral vasodilation also is much greater than with morphine. Sedation is uncommon. All side effects are dose dependent and less severe following oral administration. Meptazinol does not appear to enhance central nervous system depression produced by other drugs, such as alcohol, thiopental, benzodiazepines, or general anesthetics.

There is little information on overdosage. In one case report, the patient ingested the equivalent of 14 200-mg capsules without developing symptoms and demonstrated a normal pupillary response to light. After gastric lavage, the patient remained asymptomatic. Unfortunately, the blood concentration of the drug was not reported.

PHARMACOKINETICS. Intramuscular administration of meptazinol relieves pain within 30 minutes but the duration of action is brief, diminishing rapidly after two hours. Less than 5% of a dose is excreted unchanged. Metabolites have no significant activity. The principal metabolite, a glucuronide conjugate, is eliminated by the kidney. Protein binding is 20% to 25%. The elimination half-life is about two hours in adults and approximately three hours in neonates following administration to the mother during labor.

The mean oral bioavailability is 8.7%. Since approximately 70% of an oral dose is excreted as metabolites by the kidney, this suggests extensive first-pass metabolism by the liver.

Although the half-life is prolonged in the elderly (about 3.4 hours), no accumulation occurred when 200 mg was administered at six-hour intervals.

Meptazinol (Wyeth).
(Investigational drug)

NALBUPHINE HYDROCHLORIDE
[Nubain]

ACTIONS. Nalbuphine is related chemically to oxymorphone and the opioid antagonist, naloxone. It has both agonist and antagonist properties, thus resembling pentazocine pharmacologically (Errick and Heel, 1983).

The analgesic potency of parenteral nalbuphine on a milligram basis is approximately the same as that of morphine and about three to four times greater than that of pentazocine; its antagonistic potency is about ten times greater than that of pentazocine. The onset of action is two to three minutes after intravenous administration and 15 minutes after intramuscular or subcutaneous administration; the duration of effect is three to six hours.

USES. In clinical studies, nalbuphine relieved moderate to severe pain from a variety of causes (eg, postoperative, trauma, cancer, renal or biliary colic). Nalbuphine 10 to 15 mg was compared to meperidine 75 to 100 mg as an obstetric analgesic during labor and was found to have similar effects on the mother and the neonate. When used for preanesthetic medication, nalbuphine's analgesic and sedative effects were comparable to those of morphine.

Use of this analgesic in patients with chronic pain has been limited, but satisfactory relief was reported and less tolerance developed than with morphine.

Results of comparative studies on the hemodynamic effects of nalbuphine and morphine in patients with acute myocardial infarction indicated that nalbuphine may have advantages over morphine, since it relieved pain and reduced myocardial oxygen demands without decreasing blood pressure.

ADVERSE REACTIONS AND PRECAUTIONS. In general, the adverse reactions of nalbuphine are the same as those of morphine and other strong analgesics. The most common reaction is sedation, which occurs in about one-third of patients. This effect may be desirable, but ambulatory patients should be advised to avoid driving a car or operating machinery while taking the drug.

Less frequent reactions include a sweaty clammy feeling, nausea and vomiting, dizziness and vertigo, dryness of the mouth, and headache. Other central nervous system effects (incidence 1% or less) include nervousness, depression, crying, confusion, hallucinations, and dysphoria. The incidence of psychotomimetic effects is lower than with pentazocine.

Respiratory depression may occur with usual doses of nalbuphine and is comparable to that produced by an equianalgesic dose of morphine. However, unlike the latter, depression is not increased by larger doses (greater than 30 mg) of nalbuphine. Naloxone reverses respiratory depression.

Cardiovascular reactions (hypertension, hypotension, bradycardia, tachycardia), gastrointestinal effects (dyspepsia, cramps), and dermatologic reactions (pruritus, burning, urticaria) have been reported infrequently.

Because of its antagonist property, nalbuphine may precipitate withdrawal symptoms in opioid-dependent patients. Other precautions for the use of nalbuphine are the same as for other strong analgesics (see the Introduction).

DEPENDENCE LIABILITY. The abrupt withdrawal of nalbuphine following prolonged administration causes opiate-like abstinence symptoms, which are milder than those of morphine but more intense than those of pentazocine. Although the abuse potential is low and may be similar to that of pentazocine, this drug should be prescribed with the same caution as other strong analgesics.

Nalbuphine is not classified under the Controlled Substances Act.

PHARMACOKINETICS. There are no published studies. In the manufacturer's literature, the elimination half-life is reported to be approximately five hours. About 7% of unchanged drug and two metabolites are excreted in the urine. The oral potency (not a utilized route of administration) is about 20% of intramuscular potency. A summary of reported plasma concentrations as a function of time following administration is given by Bullingham et al, 1983.

DOSAGE AND PREPARATIONS.
Subcutaneous, Intramuscular, Intravenous: *Adults,* 10 mg, repeated every three to six hours as necessary, depending on the severity of the pain (maximum, 20 mg single dose and 160 mg total daily dose). *Children,* dosage has not been established.

Nubain (DuPont). Solution 10 mg/ml in 1, 2, and 10 ml containers and 20 mg/ml in 1 and 10 ml containers.

NONOPIOID ANALGESICS

The drugs discussed in this section do not bind to opioid receptors and are not classified under the Controlled Substances Act. They have principally analgesic, antipyretic, and anti-inflammatory actions.

Pharmacodynamics: The exact mechanism of action of these agents is not known. Evidence from animal studies has shown that the analgesic effect of aspirin and acetaminophen on induced pain is principally peripheral (blockade of pain impulse generation). Their primary clinical effects appear to be related to inhibition of prostaglandin synthesis, since the actions of the prostaglandins have been reported to include hyperalgesia (pain), fever, edema, and erythema. The precise mechanism of the various inhibitors cannot be stated definitely (Zipser and Laffi, 1985).

Although the therapeutic actions of this group of drugs may result from inhibition of prostaglandin synthesis, this property also may produce many of their adverse reactions. Effects of long-term, continuous use include inhibition of platelet aggregation with prolonged bleeding time; exacerbation of gastroesophageal reflux; gastrointestinal irritation and ulceration; decreased renal function with increased BUN and creatinine levels, which may progress to renal failure or result in the nephrotic syndrome; and less common renal disturbances including interstitial nephritis, papillary necrosis, and hyperkalemia (Khokhar, 1984; Allen et al, 1986; Bailie, 1986; Epstein, 1986). Nonimmunologic syndromes with bronchospasm, rhinitis, angioedema, and urticaria may follow a single dose or occur in patients who previously received these drugs without untoward incident (Settipane, 1981; Zeitz and Jarmoszuk, 1985).

Indications: In general, nonopioid analgesics alleviate headache, myalgia, arthralgia, and other pain arising from integumental structures. Mild to moderate postoperative and postpartum pain, pain from neoplasms, and some other types of visceral pain also may respond to these drugs. They are generally not useful in severe pain, but some newer nonsteroidal analgesic agents with anti-inflammatory actions have been effective in moderate to severe postoperative pain and these agents, as well as aspirin, have been somewhat effective in moderate to severe bone pain. The antipyretic action of the nonopioid analgesics presumably results from inhibition of production of prostaglandin E_2 within the preoptic division of the anterior hypothalamus. All of the nonsteroidal anti-inflammatory drugs are equipotent in this regard. Interestingly, acetaminophen, which has only weak peripheral anti-inflammatory activity, is as potent an antipyretic as aspirin or ibuprofen. Although antipyretics generally are used to reduce fever, certain conditions have been identified in which reduction of elevated body temperature (more than 102 F) is indicated (Gray and Blaschke, 1985). These include young children with a history of febrile seizures, fever secondary to head trauma or central nervous system disease, fever-induced hallucinations in psychotic patients, fever associated with coronary artery and other cardiovascular disease, and fever during early pregnancy. Because of the epidemiologic association of an increased incidence of Reye's syndrome with the use of aspirin during the prodromal phase of influenza B or A or varicella (chickenpox) infections, only acetaminophen is recommended as an antipyretic for fever of unknown etiology in children and adolescents. Either drug may be employed in adults and both are preferred to other nonopioid analgesics for this purpose.

Dysmenorrhea may be caused by increased endometrial production of prostaglandin. Several drugs that inhibit prostaglandin synthesis have been tested for their effectiveness in this condition. Ibuprofen [Advil, Motrin, Nuprin, Rufen], indomethacin [Indocin], mefenamic acid [Ponstel], naproxen [Naprosyn], naproxen sodium [Anaprox], and suprofen [Suprol] are among those found to be effective. Aspirin is a weak inhibitor of prostaglandin synthesis in the uterus and is less effective in dysmenorrhea.

Drug Selection: The choice of analgesic depends upon the effectiveness and adverse reactions of a particular preparation in the individual patient. The most widely used agents of this group are aspirin and acetaminophen. They have equivalent analgesic and antipyretic properties, but their pharmacologic actions and adverse effects differ. Of the newer analgesic/anti-inflammatory drugs, diflunisal [Dolobid], fenoprofen [Nalfon], ibuprofen, naproxen, naproxen sodium, and suprofen are as or more effective than aspirin, acetaminophen, or codeine (see the evaluations). Evidence supporting the analgesic efficacy of mefenamic acid [Ponstel] is limited. It has not been shown to be more effective than aspirin or similar mild analgesics and has caused a number of serious adverse reactions. With the exception of aspirin and acetoaminophen, acute poisoning from the nonsteroidal anti-inflammatory agents employed as mild analgesics is rare and the associated clinical manifestations are usually mild (Vale and Meredith, 1986).

Other drugs possessing analgesic and antipyretic properties include indomethacin and phenylbutazone [Azolid, Butazolidin], but they are not used as general purpose mild analgesics because of their potential to cause serious adverse reactions; they are discussed in Chapter 59, Antiarthritic Drugs, and Chapter 60, Agents Used in Gout and Hyperuricemia.

Drug Evaluations

SALICYLIC ACID DERIVATIVES

ASPIRIN

USES. This prototype of the nonopioid analgesics is a drug of choice when a mild analgesic is indicated. Aspirin is more useful in the treatment of headache, neuralgia, myalgia, arthralgia, and other pain arising from integumental structures than in acute severe pain of visceral origin. However, it may relieve moderate postoperative, postpartum, or other visceral pain, such as that secondary to trauma or cancer. In the latter, aspirin may provide adequate relief and should be tried prior to use of strong analgesics. Aspirin can be given with an opioid to increase the analgesic effect.

Large doses have an anti-inflammatory action, which may contribute to relief of pain when inflammation is a factor. This drug is the primary agent in the management of some rheumatic diseases (see Chapter 59, Antiarthritic Drugs). Aspirin is less effective than the newer nonsteroidal anti-inflammatory agents in dysmenorrhea.

When therapy is indicated to reduce fever, aspirin is one of the most effective drugs. Epidemiologic evidence suggests the possible association between the use of aspirin to treat fever in children during the prodromal phase of varicella (chickenpox) or influenza B or A infections and the subsequent development of Reye's syndrome. At present, the data are fragmentary and more studies are necessary to define the nature of the relationship, if any, between the use of aspirin or other salicylates in such illnesses and the occurrence of Reye's syndrome. In balancing the risk of Reye's syndrome with the benefits of aspirin therapy, the current opinion of the Committee on Infectious Diseases of the American Academy of Pediatrics is that "aspirin should not be prescribed under usual circumstances for children with varicella or those suspected of having influenza on the basis of clinical or epidemiologic evidence" (Committee on Infectious Diseases, 1982). If control of fever is necessary, acetaminophin may be employed.

In rheumatic fever, the amount of aspirin required to relieve pain and joint swelling exceeds usual analgesic doses. The inflammatory process is suppressed but progression of the disease is not affected. Penicillin and other appropriate therapy should be administered concomitantly.

Because aspirin inhibits platelet function, it has been tried in various thromboembolic diseases. Results of clinical trials indicate that aspirin reduces recurrent transient ischemic attacks in patients of both sexes who have experienced transient ischemia of the brain due to fibrin platelet emboli, but it may prevent stroke in men only. Stroke was not prevented in women and there is no evidence that aspirin is beneficial in completed stroke in men or women. Additional evidence is needed to determine whether aspirin is beneficial in other thromboembolic diseases, eg, myocardial infarction (see Chapter 33, Agents Used for Anticoagulant Therapy), or for the prevention of hypertension and pre-eclampsia in angiotensin II-sensitive primigravid women (Wallenburg et al, 1986).

ADVERSE REACTIONS AND PRECAUTIONS. Serious adverse reactions occur infrequently with usual analgesic doses. Gastrointestinal symptoms (gastric distress, heartburn, or nausea) are most common. Gastric distress may be diminished by taking aspirin with food or a full glass of water. Occult gastrointestinal bleeding occurs in many patients but apparently is not correlated with gastric distress. The amount of blood lost is usually insignificant clinically but, with prolonged administration, iron deficiency anemia may result. Massive gastrointestinal hemorrhage occurs rarely in relation to the frequency of aspirin use but may be life-threatening. This effect may be due to the action of aspirin on the stomach mucosa, platelet dysfunction, or both in susceptible individuals (ie, those with ulcer, bleeding problems). Aspirin may cause gastric ulcers after long-term use. There is no evidence that it produces duodenal ulcers. Aspirin should not be used in patients with a recent history of peptic ulcer or gastrointestinal bleeding. Patients should be advised that alcohol may increase gastrointestinal bleeding when ingested with aspirin.

Large doses taken for several days can cause hypoprothrombinemia, which may be reversed by phytonadione (vitamin K_1). This effect usually is not significant except in susceptible patients (eg, those receiving anticoagulants, patients with severe liver disease). Even usual analgesic doses of aspirin inhibit platelet aggregation and increase bleeding time. Because of the role of platelets in hemostasis, this effect may be an important factor in gastrointestinal and other bleeding. Aspirin is contraindicated in patients with bleeding disorders (eg, hemophilia). The drug should be discontinued one week prior to surgery to prevent or minimize postoperative bleeding.

Reversible hepatotoxicity has been associated with the large doses given to children with rheumatic disease and adults with lupus erythematosus or rheumatoid arthritis. The effect is dependent upon salicylate blood concentrations (a level exceeding 25 mg/dl is likely to cause hepatic injury), the disease state (eg, rheumatic or collagen disease), and pre-existing liver disease. Liver function tests should be performed periodically in patients with these conditions.

An acute intolerance to aspirin occurs in about 0.3% of the population, usually adults, many of whom have taken the drug without incident for many years. In a typical reaction, which occurs between 15 minutes and three hours after ingestion, there is a profuse and inappropriate rhinorrhea; macular erythema, nausea, vomiting, intestinal cramps, and diarrhea also may occur. Shortly after rhinorrhea begins, an acute asthmatic attack occurs. The reaction may be severe and there are many reports in the older medical literature of death following administration of one or two aspirin tablets. Epinephrine or theophylline may be required to counteract bronchospasm. The acute reaction normally terminates after about two hours (Zeitz and Jarmoszuk, 1985).

The reaction is nonimmunologic, but its mechanism is not known. Some authors distinguish two subgroups in the intolerant population: one that demonstrates primarily a bronchospastic response and another that demonstrates primarily urticaria and angioedema (Settipane, 1981).

The intolerance to aspirin is specific and does not extend to sodium salicylate, salicylic acid esters, choline salicylate, or thiosalicylate. Many patients who cannot tolerate aspirin also cannot tolerate other nonsteroidal anti-inflammatory drugs; cross-intolerance has been reported to mefenamic acid, flufenamic acid, ibuprofen, and naproxen. Indomethacin is particularly reactive, but phenylbutazone usually elicits reactions only at higher doses. Cross-intolerance also extends to tartrazine (FD&C Yellow No. 5), a dye often used in foods and pharmaceuticals.

Aspirin does not appear to have any teratogenic effects in man. Prolonged pregnancy and labor with increased bleeding before and after delivery may be correlated with chronic ingestion of aspirin producing high blood salicylate concentrations during the week preceding parturition.

POISONING. The most common signs of chronic aspirin overdosage is tinnitus, a sensation of fullness in the ears, and muffled hearing. These effects may be abolished within 24 hours by reducing the dose. Reversible deafness also occurs with large, acute doses. It is advisable to determine if tinnitus is present in patients receiving large doses for prolonged periods. Otic symptoms will not occur in patients with pre-existing hearing loss or in infants and young children. The most common sign of overdosage in the latter is hyperventilation.

Acute intoxication from accidental overdosage of aspirin is a common cause of fatal drug poisoning in children, although the number of deaths has been declining in recent years as a result of safety closures on bottles, public education, and increased substitution of acetaminophen. Toxic doses disturb the acid-base balance, which is manifested as metabolic acidosis in infants and young children and as compensated respiratory alkalosis in older children and adults. Salicylates uncouple oxidative phosphorylation, which is manifested as hypoglycemia and hyperpyrexia, particularly in infants and young children. Marked hyperpnea and tachypnea, tachycardia, nausea, and vomiting occur; stupor and coma may develop.

The severity of intoxication can be determined by measuring the blood salicylate concentration six hours or more after acute ingestion or any time that chronic intoxication is suspected. A serum salicylate concentration of 50 mg/dl indicates mild toxicity; amounts above 75 mg/dl are potentially fatal. Plasma salicylate measurements may be unreliable when enteric-coated preparations have been ingested and are misleading in chronic overdosage or severe acidosis. As a general rule, the acute oral dose causing serious intoxication is 100 mg/kg in a child and 10 g in an adult.

The sequence of management in salicylate overdosage depends on the severity of intoxication. Primary resuscitation is begun if needed. Dehydration, acidosis, and hypoglycemia should be corrected. Hyperthermia is managed by external cooling. Salicylate may be retained in the stomach for up to 24 hours as the result of prostaglandin inhibition and should be removed by induced emesis or lavage as indicated. This is followed by gastric instillation of activated charcoal, which binds salicylate, thus preventing further absorption. Thereafter, management is directed toward reducing the body burden of salicylate. This is most readily accomplished by increasing the pH of the urine with bicarbonate. If the urine remains very acidic but the flow is adequate, potassium chloride should be added to the intravenous fluids. If urine flow is markedly diminished in the presence of adequate hydration, pulmonary edema, or progressive deterioration of the patient's status, hemodialysis may be required. Following massive overdosage, the prophylactic administration of phytonadione (vitamin K_1) may be appropriate.

DRUG INTERACTIONS. Because aspirin is widely used, its interactions with other drugs must be considered, although relatively few are clinically important. Large doses of aspirin taken for several days decrease prothrombin production, thus increasing the prothrombin time; even smaller doses may increase bleeding time by inhibiting platelet aggregation. Because of this, aspirin should not be used by patients taking oral anticoagulants.

Large doses of salicylates decrease blood glucose concentration and may enhance the effect of the oral hypoglycemics. These drugs should not be given concomitantly unless the dosage of the hypoglycemic agent is reduced to the extent indicated by determinations of blood glucose.

Although large doses of a salicylate have a uricosuric effect, usual analgesic doses cause uric acid retention, which produces hyperuricemia in some patients. Salicylates antagonize the activity of uricosuric agents, and patients with gout must be advised to avoid their use.

The incidence of gastric ulceration may be increased if aspirin is given with other ulcerogenic agents, such as corticosteroids or any of the NSAIDs. Concurrent use of these agents should be avoided.

Aspirin has been reported to displace methotrexate from protein binding sites, thereby increasing the latter drug's plasma concentration to toxic levels; however, the therapeutic effect is also increased. If the two drugs are used together, the patient must be monitored closely.

PHARMACOKINETICS. Aspirin is absorbed primarily from the small intestine and secondarily from the stomach. Absorption is rapid following oral administration of conventional tablets or capsules, but the rate is affected by gastric emptying time and the release characteristics of the dosage form. Absorption is most rapid when aspirin is given in solution.

Aspirin is rapidly hydrolyzed, partly by esterases during absorption and partly by the liver, to salicylic acid before entering the systemic circulation. Both aspirin and salicylic acid enter the central nervous system. Hydrolysis by plasma esterases is rapid. Salicylic acid is cleared by renal excretion and by metabolism. It is conjugated with glycine (forming salicyluric acid) and glucuronic acid (forming salicylphenolic glucuronide and salicylacyl glucuronide). A small fraction of salicylic acid is oxidized to gentisic acid.

The enzymes forming salicyluric acid and salicylphenolic glucuronide are saturable and follow Michaelis-Menten kinetics. Therefore, the pharmacokinetics of salicylate elimination are complex, since both the ratio of metabolites and clearance are dose dependent. Approximately 70% to 90% of salicylic acid is bound to serum albumin, and the apparent volume of distribution ranges from 0.1 to 0.35 L/kg, depending on drug concentration. The half-life of salicylate increases with the dose: 3.1 to 3.2 hours with 300 to 650 mg, 5 hours with 1 g, and 9 hours with 2 g. As the half-life increases, urinary excretion decreases. Thus, increasing the dose without increasing the dosage interval may result in accumulation with toxic effects. However, there is marked variation in the rate of elimination among individuals, possibly because of differences in salicyluric acid-forming capacity. Therefore, the dosage must be individualized when large amounts are required (Levy, 1981; Netter et al, 1985; Needs and Brooks, 1985).

FORMULATIONS. The rate of absorption or bioavailability of aspirin depend upon its rate of dissolution from the dosage form, the most common of which is plain (unbuffered) tablets. Several studies have shown that differences among various formulations affect the rate of dissolution and absorption, and thus the levels achieved in the blood. However, the relationship of blood levels to the onset and intensity of analgesic effect is uncertain.

Antacids or buffering ingredients are combined with aspirin (buffered aspirin) to reduce gastric irritation. The relatively small amount of antacid present in most products does not increase the gastric pH significantly but increases the dissolution rate of aspirin, resulting in more rapid absorption. Although some individuals claim that they tolerate buffered preparations better than plain aspirin, results of controlled clinical studies have been contradictory. As with plain tablets, buffered aspirin products have variable dissolution rates and certain preparations may be less bioavailable than some unbuffered tablets. Furthermore, it has not been demonstrated conclusively that buffered aspirin has a faster onset of action, greater peak intensity, or longer analgesic effect.

Aspirin is also available in highly buffered effervescent preparations; when dissolved, the aspirin is present as sodium acetylsalicylate. Results of studies have shown that this form has a more rapid rate of absorption and produces a higher blood salicylate level than tablet formulations. In addition, highly buffered sodium acetylsalicylate solution causes less gastric irritation and gastrointestinal bleeding, although the effect on platelets is unchanged. Because effervescent preparations contain more absorbable antacid, repeated use of large doses alkalizes the urine, resulting in faster excretion and decreased salicylate blood concentration. Nevertheless, because of the rapid absorption of aspirin from effervescent preparations, they are an effective form for occasional use. These preparations should not be used by patients who must restrict sodium intake.

Enteric-coated preparations may be used to avoid gastric reactions. The incidence of gastrointestinal mucosal lesions is reduced with these preparations, but absorption of aspirin is delayed and varies among different products. Although this type of preparation may be useful when administered repeatedly to treat rheumatoid arthritis, it does not relieve pain promptly. Timed-release preparations offer no advantage over standard tablets.

Rectal suppositories are used in patients unable to take oral medication. However, the rectal absorption of aspirin is variable; it may be slow and incomplete or rapid and cause adverse reactions. Also, aspirin may cause rectal irritation. For these reasons, suppositories are of questionable usefulness.

DOSAGE AND PREPARATIONS.
Oral: For analgesia and antipyresis, *adults and children over 12 years,* 650 mg every four hours as necessary or 500 mg to 1 g initially, followed by 500 mg every three hours or 1 g every six hours as necessary (maximum, 4 g daily).

Children under 12 years, 1.5 g/M^2 daily in divided doses. For convenience, the following dosage schedule may be used: *2 to 3 years,* 160 mg; *4 to 5 years,* 240 mg; *6 to 8 years,* 320 mg; *9 to 10 years,* 400 mg; *11 years,* 480 mg. Doses may be repeated every four hours as necessary.

For prophylaxis of stroke (males) and transient ischemic attacks, see Chapter 33, Agents Used For Anticoagulant Therapy.

For acute rheumatic fever, *adults,* 6 to 8 g daily; *children,* 3 g daily (optimum salicylate level, 25 to 30 mg/dl).

NOTE: Because most manufacturers express dosage sizes of aspirin in grains rather than milligrams, the grain sizes with *approximate* milligram equivalents are given.
Generic. Tablets 5, 7 1/2, and 10 gr (325, 500, and 650 mg); tablets (buffered) 5 gr (325 mg); tablets (enteric-coated) 5 and 10 gr (325 and 650 mg); suppositories 1, 2, 3, 5, 10. and 20 gr (60, 130, 195, 325, and 650 mg and 1.2 g) (all forms nonprescription).
Available Trademarks.
(Examples of various formulations; all nonprescription)
Alka-Seltzer (Miles). Tablets (highly buffered, effervescent) 324 mg with sodium bicarbonate 1.9 g and citric acid 1 g (sodium 55 mg/tablet).
Ascriptin (Rorer). Tablets (buffered) 325 mg with magnesium and aluminum hydroxide 150 or 300 mg (*Ascriptin A/D*).
Bufferin (Bristol-Myers). Tablets (buffered) 325 mg with aluminum glycinate 48.6 mg and magnesium carbonate 97.2 mg.
Cama (Dorsey). Tablets (buffered) 600 mg with magnesium hydroxide 150 mg and aluminum hydroxide 150 mg.
Ecotrin (Menley & James). Tablets (enteric-coated) 325 mg.
Measurin (Winthrop-Breon). Tablets (timed-release) 650 mg.

SODIUM SALICYLATE

Sodium salicylate is less effective than equal doses of aspirin in relieving pain and reducing fever. However, individuals who are hypersensitive to aspirin may tolerate sodium salicylate.

In general, this salicylate produces the same adverse reactions as aspirin (see that evaluation), but there is less occult gastrointestinal bleeding. Platelet function is not affected but, as with aspirin, prothrombin time is increased. Patients on a low-sodium diet should not receive this drug.

DOSAGE AND PREPARATIONS.
Oral: 650 mg every four hours as necessary (range, 325 mg to 4 g daily).
Generic. Tablets (plain, enteric-coated) 325 and 650 mg (nonprescription).

DIFLUNISAL
[Dolobid]

ACTIONS AND USES. Diflunisal differs chemically from aspirin and other salicylates but, like them, has analgesic, antiinflammatory, and antipyretic properties and also inhibits prostaglandin synthetase.

Diflunisal is useful for the acute or long-term symptomatic treatment of mild to moderate pain. In controlled clinical studies, this drug relieved postoperative pain of meniscectomy, episiotomy, and dental, orthopedic, and various other procedures. It also controlled the pain of musculoskeletal conditions, such as sprains and strains, trauma, and low back disorders, and of cancer (Brogden et al, 1980).

In various comparative studies, single doses of diflunisal 500 mg were comparable in analgesic efficacy to aspirin 650 mg, acetaminophen 600 or 650 mg, and propoxyphene napsylate 100 mg with acetaminophen 650 mg. A single dose of diflunisal 1 g was as effective as the combination of codeine 60 mg and acetaminophen 600 mg. When administered repeatedly, diflunisal 500 mg twice daily was comparable in analgesic effect to codeine 25 mg four times daily, pentazocine 50 mg four times daily, propoxyphene 65 mg and acetaminophen 650 mg three times daily, or propoxyphene napsylate 100 mg and aspirin 650 mg four times daily. In most patients, the duration of analgesic action of diflunisal (up to 12 hours) was notably longer than that of other drugs in these studies. The onset of analgesia usually occurs within one hour and the maximum effect within two to three hours.

Diflunisal also is effective in arthritis (see Chapter 59). Although it has antipyretic activity, this drug has not been effective in febrile patients.

Diflunisal also has a uricosuric effect. Analgesic doses increased renal clearance of uric acid and decreased serum uric acid (Dresse et al, 1979; van Loenhout et al, 1981). It is not known whether diflunisal interferes with the activity of other uricosuric agents or has a useful uricosuric action in the treatment of gout.

ADVERSE REACTIONS AND PRECAUTIONS. Diflunisal is generally well tolerated. The most frequent adverse reactions are nausea, dyspepsia, gastrointestinal pain, and diarrhea. Rash and headache are observed in 3% to 9% of patients. Other reactions with an incidence of 1% to 3% include vomiting, constipation, flatulence, dizziness, tinnitus, fatigue, somnolence, and insomnia.

In comparative studies, the incidence of gastrointestinal reactions, as well as dizziness, edema, and tinnitus, was lower than with aspirin. In addition, comparative studies in normal volunteers showed that fecal blood loss with diflunisal 1 g twice daily was about one-half that with aspirin 1.3 g twice daily (no significant differences in fecal blood loss were observed with diflunisal 500 mg twice daily and placebo). However, gastrointestinal bleeding and peptic ulceration (incidence, less than 1 in 100) have been reported, and patients with a history of upper gastrointestinal tract disease should be monitored carefully during therapy. In those with active peptic ulcer or gastrointestinal bleeding, the benefit/risk ratio should be considered and appropriate ulcer therapy instituted if diflunisal is administered.

The effect of diflunisal on platelet function and bleeding time is dose related but reversible, even when large doses (1 g twice daily) are used. However, patients at risk should be observed carefully.

Acute interstitial nephritis and acute renal failure have been reported with diflunisal therapy (Wharton et al, 1982). These reactions and nephrotic syndrome also have been observed with other nonsteroidal anti-inflammatory drugs and may be associated with inhibition of prostaglandin synthesis (Bailie, 1986). Because diflunisal is eliminated primarily by the kidney and its half-life is increased in the presence of renal insufficiency, patients with significantly impaired renal function should be monitored carefully and lower doses should be used.

Since peripheral edema has been observed, the drug should be used with caution in patients with compromised cardiac function, hypertension, or other conditions predisposing to fluid retention.

Borderline elevations of one or more liver function tests may occur in up to 15% of those receiving diflunisal, as with other nonsteroidal anti-inflammatory drugs. In controlled clinical trials, significant elevations (three times the upper limit of normal) of SGPT (ALT) or SGOT (AST) occurred in less than 1% of patients. Although severe hepatic reactions are rare, jaundice and fatal hepatitis have been reported with other nonsteroidal anti-inflammatory drugs. If signs or symptoms suggesting liver dysfunction develop or liver function tests are abnormal, the patient should be evaluated for evidence of more severe hepatic reactions; if abnormalities persist or worsen, the drug should be discontinued.

Because cross-sensitivity may occur, diflunisal should not be given to patients who experienced rhinitis, acute asthmatic attacks, urticaria, or angioedema with aspirin or other nonsteroidal anti-inflammatory drugs.

Since no adequate, well-controlled studies have been conducted in pregnant women, diflunisal should not be used during the first two trimesters unless it is clearly indicated (FDA Pregnancy Category C). It should not be administered during the third trimester because of the potential effects of prostaglandin inhibitors on the fetal cardiovascular system (premature closure of ductus arteriosus). See Chapter 26, Agents Used in Miscellaneous Cardiovascular Disorders.

DRUG INTERACTIONS. When diflunisal and indomethacin were given to normal volunteers, the renal clearance of indomethacin was decreased and the plasma levels were increased. Since fatal gastrointestinal hemorrhage has been associated with the concomitant use of these drugs, they should not be administered concurrently.

Clinical data on the concomitant use of diflunisal and other nonsteroidal anti-inflammatory drugs are not available; thus, their combined administration cannot be recommended. However, studies on some of these drugs have been carried out in normal volunteers with the following results: When diflunisal was administered with acetaminophen, the plasma concentrations of the latter drug were significantly increased but those of diflunisal were not affected. When multiple doses of aspirin and diflunisal were administered together, the plasma concentrations of diflunisal were decreased slightly. Concomitant administration of diflunisal and naproxen did not affect plasma concentrations of either drug, but significantly decreased the urinary excretion of naproxen and its glucuronide metabolite. The administration of sulindac with diflunisal did not significantly affect plasma concentrations of the active sulfide metabolite of sulindac.

Concomitant administration of antacids and diflunisal may reduce the bioavailability of the latter drug; the effect is slight with occasional doses of antacids, but may be clinically significant during repeated administration.

The dosage of oral anticoagulants may need adjustment when diflunisal is given concomitantly, for prothrombin time was prolonged in normal volunteers when both drugs were administered.

When hydrochlorothiazide and diflunisal were given to normal volunteers, the plasma levels of the thiazide were increased and its hyperuricemic effect was decreased. A similar decrease in hyperuricemic effect but not diuretic activity was observed when furosemide and diflunisal were given together.

In diabetic patients receiving diflunisal and tolbutamide, tolbutamide plasma levels or fasting blood glucose were not significantly affected.

POISONING. Drowsiness, disorientation, and stupor were the most common symptoms of overdosage. Most patients recover without permanent sequelae, but fatalities have been reported. Treatment should include emptying the stomach, symptomatic and supportive measures, and careful observation of the patient. Because of extensive protein binding, hemodialysis may not be effective.

PHARMACOKINETICS. Diflunisal is well absorbed following

oral administration; peak plasma levels are reached within two to three hours. When given with food, absorption of the drug is delayed slightly but not decreased.

Like salicylic acid, diflunisal exhibits dose-dependent nonlinear pharmacokinetics, ie, doubling the dose more than doubles drug plasma concentrations. The time required to reach steady state and the plasma half-life increase with larger doses. The plasma half-life of diflunisal is three to four times longer than that of salicylic acid. Its elimination half-life ranged from 8 hours with doses of 125 mg twice daily to 15 hours with doses of 500 mg twice daily. The volume of distribution is 0.1 L/kg. Clearance of a single 500-mg dose is 8 ml/min. Steady-state plasma levels were attained in three to four days with 125 mg twice daily and in seven to nine days with 500 mg twice daily. The half-life is increased as the creatinine clearance is reduced.

Diflunisal is converted to two soluble glucuronide conjugates and about 90% is excreted in the urine. Little or none is excreted in the feces. Approximately 2% to 7% of the concentration in plasma appears in the milk of lactating mothers. The drug is more than 99% bound to plasma proteins (Steelman et al, 1978; Verbeeck et al, 1983).

DOSAGE AND PREPARATIONS.
Oral: The dosage should be individualized depending upon the severity of pain, the presence of other disorders, and the patient's weight, age, and renal function. *Adults,* for mild to moderate pain, an initial loading dose of 1 g, followed by 500 mg every 8 to 12 hours. Doses of 500 mg initially, followed by 250 mg every 8 to 12 hours, may be appropriate for some patients. *Children,* dosage has not been established.
Dolobid (Merck Sharp & Dohme). Tablets 250 and 500 mg.

PARA-AMINOPHENOL DERIVATIVE

ACETAMINOPHEN

USES. Acetaminophen, an analgesic and antipyretic, is as effective as aspirin. It is used to treat headache, mild to moderate myalgia, arthralgia, chronic pain of cancer, postpartum pain, postoperative pain, and fever. It is the preferred alternative to aspirin for patients who cannot tolerate the latter, those with a coagulation disorder (eg, hemophilia), or individuals with a history of peptic ulcer. In children requiring only analgesia or antipyresis, acetaminophen may be preferred to aspirin because it is less toxic if an accidental overdose occurs. (Interestingly, acetaminophen overdosage in children under 6 is rarely, if ever, associated with hepatotoxicity, but such protection is lost by adolescence.) Further, no relationship has been demonstrated between acetaminophen and the incidence of Reye's syndrome in children or adolescents with influenza B or A or varicella (chickenpox). Acetaminophen is unsatisfactory for conditions requiring potent anti-inflammatory activity (rheumatic disease, juvenile arthritis, dysmenorrhea, sunburn). Unlike aspirin, acetaminophen does not antagonize the effects of uricosuric agents and may be used in patients with gouty arthritis who are taking a uricosuric.

ADVERSE REACTIONS. Adverse reactions occur infrequently and hypersensitivity only rarely. Acetaminophen is a metabolite of phenacetin and acetanilid but, unlike these drugs, produces little or no methemoglobinemia and reports of hemolytic anemia have been rare. It does not cause gastrointestinal bleeding. Although large doses have been reported to potentiate the action of oral anticoagulants, small doses have no effect on prothrombin time. It is not known whether prolonged use of acetaminophen can cause the type of renal injury associated with abuse of analgesic mixtures containing phenacetin.

POISONING. Large doses (15 g as a single dose or 5 to 8 g/day for several weeks) of acetaminophen may cause severe hepatic damage and death. The first signs of toxicity occur about 12 to 24 hours after acute overdose and include nausea, vomiting, diarrhea, diaphoresis, pallor, and abdominal pain. Hepatic injury is manifested about 24 to 48 hours after overdose by increased serum transaminases, lactic dehydrogenase, prothrombin time, and serum bilirubin concentrations. Severe hepatic damage may progress to hepatic failure, encephalopathy, coma, and death. In addition to appropriate supportive therapy, liver injury may be minimized by administering acetylcysteine. For details of treatment, see Chapter 80, Drugs Used in the Treatment of Poisoning.

PHARMACOKINETICS. Acetaminophen is rapidly and almost completely absorbed from the gastrointestinal tract following oral administration. Peak plasma concentrations of 5 to 20 mcg/ml occur in 30 to 60 minutes with usual analgesic doses, but there is no correlation between serum concentration and analgesic effect. Significant serum protein binding does not occur with therapeutic doses. The apparent volume of distribution is about 1 L/kg. The plasma half-life in healthy subjects ranges from 1 to 2.5 hours (Forrest et al, 1982).

Acetaminophen is metabolized in the liver, largely to glucuronide and sulfate conjugates, and eliminated in the urine. In patients with impaired renal function, the conjugated metabolites accumulate in the blood but the unchanged drug does not. A minor fraction is metabolized to hydroxylates and deacetylated derivatives. It has been suggested that the hydroxylated metabolite is responsible for hepatotoxicity with overdosage (Levy, 1981). There is evidence that some forms of liver disease decrease the conjugation of acetaminophen and increase its half-life. It is not known if this increases the incidence or severity of hepatotoxicity, but the possibility should be considered in patients with pre-existing liver disorders.

DOSAGE AND PREPARATIONS.
Oral: Adults and children over 12 years, 325 to 650 mg at four-hour intervals, if needed, or 500 mg to 1 g initially, followed by 500 mg every three hours or 1 g every six hours as needed (maximum, 4 g daily).

Children under 12 years, 1.5 g/M^2 daily in divided doses. For convenience, the following dosage schedule may be used: *2 to 3 years,* 160 mg; *4 to 5 years,* 240 mg; *6 to 8 years,* 320 mg; *9 to 10 years,* 400 mg; *11 years,* 480 mg. Doses may be repeated every four hours as necessary.

74

Rectal: The relative potency of the suppository formulation is about one-half that of the oral tablet; however, as with other drugs, the bioavailability of acetaminophen may vary, depending upon the composition of the suppository base. Since comparative data are not available, no dosage is suggested.

Generic. Capsules 300 and 500 mg; capsules (timed-release) 500 mg; drops 60 mg/0.6 ml; elixir 120 mg/5 ml; tablets 325, 500, and 650 mg; suppositories 120, 325, and 650 mg (all forms nonprescription).

Available Trademarks.
Anacin-3 (Whitehall), *Liquiprin* (Norcliff Thayer), *Phenaphen* (Robins), *Tempra* (Mead Johnson), *Tylenol* (McNeil), *Valadol* (Squibb) (all nonprescription).

ANTHRANILIC ACID DERIVATIVE

MEFENAMIC ACID
[Ponstel]

ACTIONS AND USES. Mefenamic acid is related chemically to meclofenamate, an antiarthritic drug. It has analgesic, antipyretic, and anti-inflammatory actions and is claimed to relieve mild to moderate pain, but therapy should not exceed one week. Results of comparative studies have shown that mefenamic acid is no more effective than aspirin and other mild analgesics. Because it has been associated with a number of serious adverse reactions, other mild analgesics are preferred.

Results of several studies have indicated that mefenamic acid relieves the pain of primary dysmenorrhea and that associated with intrauterine devices. Comparative studies with other prostaglandin inhibitors (eg, ibuprofen, naproxen) have not been performed but, since the latter agents are better tolerated, they are preferable for this use.

ADVERSE REACTIONS AND PRECAUTIONS. Gastrointestinal symptoms are the most common adverse effects. Diarrhea occurs in a significant number of patients and usually recurs when mefenamic acid is given a second time. Occult gastrointestinal bleeding is noted less frequently than with aspirin. Dyspepsia, constipation, nausea, abdominal pain, vomiting, headache, drowsiness, vertigo, and dizziness have been observed. Elevated blood urea nitrogen levels were reported in one study. Hemolytic anemia, agranulocytosis, thrombocytopenic purpura, and megaloblastic anemia also have been reported.

If diarrhea or rash occurs, the drug should be discontinued and not used thereafter. Mefenamic acid is contraindicated in patients with gastrointestinal inflammation or ulceration and in those with impaired renal function and should be used with caution in asthmatics because it may exacerbate this condition.

The safety of mefenamic acid during pregnancy or in children under 14 years has not been established (FDA Pregnancy Category C).

PHARMACOKINETICS. Mefenamic acid is metabolized to 3'-hydroxymethyl and 3'-carboxylate derivatives. These metabolites are excreted in the urine as their acyl glucuronides with unchanged drug. About 20% of the dose is eliminated as the unconjugated 3'-carboxyl derivative in the feces. The elimination half-life is three to four hours. The volume of distribution and clearance have not been published. The drug is extensively bound to plasma protein (Verbeeck et al, 1983).

DOSAGE AND PREPARATIONS.
Oral: *Adults and children over 14 years,* 500 mg initially, followed by 250 mg every six hours as needed for no longer than one week. The drug should be taken with food.

Ponstel (Parke-Davis). Capsules 250 mg.

PHENYLPROPIONIC ACID DERIVATIVES AND RELATED DRUGS

FENOPROFEN CALCIUM
[Nalfon]

ACTIONS AND USES. Fenoprofen is chemically and pharmacologically similar to ibuprofen. Like aspirin, it has anti-inflammatory, analgesic, and antipyretic properties. Results of several controlled studies indicated that fenoprofen 200 mg was similar in effectiveness to aspirin 650 mg, codeine 60 mg, or propoxyphene napsylate 100 mg in patients with various painful conditions (eg, trauma, episiotomy, postpartum and postoperative pain). Single or repeated doses of fenoprofen 400 mg reduced fever associated with acute and chronic respiratory disease, but additional studies are needed to establish the optimum dose for this use.

ADVERSE REACTIONS. The most common adverse reactions are drowsiness, dizziness, sweating, and asthenia. Gastrointestinal effects (eg, dyspepsia, constipation, nausea, vomiting) also have occurred. Gastrointestinal bleeding is less than with aspirin. However, since a few cases of ulceration have been observed, the drug should be used with caution in patients with a history of peptic ulcer. (For other adverse reactions, see Chapter 59, Antiarthritic Drugs.)

PHARMACOKINETICS. Fenoprofen is well absorbed after oral administration. It is extensively bound (more than 99%) to plasma protein and thus does not appear in breast milk, amniotic fluid, cord blood, or saliva. The volume of distribution is 0.08 to 0.10 L/kg. The drug is metabolized almost completely (98%) to fenoprofen glucuronide (45%), 4'-

dihydroxyfenoprofen glucuronide (45%), and 4'-hydroxyprofen. These metabolites are excreted by the kidney. Small amounts of unchanged drug are recovered in the feces (even after intravenous administration). The elimination half-life is two to three hours (Verbeeck et al, 1983).

DOSAGE AND PREPARATIONS.
Oral: Adults, 200 mg every four to six hours as needed. *Children,* dosage has not been established.
    Nalfon (Dista). Capsules 200 and 300 mg; tablets 600 mg (strengths expressed in terms of the base).

IBUPROFEN
    [Advil, Medipren, Motrin, Nuprin, Rufen]

$$CH_3CHCH_2 \underset{CH_3}{\;} \text{—} \quad \text{—} \overset{O}{\underset{CH_3}{CHCOH}}$$

ACTIONS AND USES. Ibuprofen has analgesic, anti-inflammatory, and antipyretic actions. It relieves mild to moderate postoperative pain (eg, dental, episiotomy), dysmenorrhea, and headache. In a limited number of studies, its effectiveness was comparable to or greater than that of aspirin, codeine, or propoxyphene (Miller, 1981).

ADVERSE REACTIONS AND PRECAUTIONS. The overall incidence of adverse reactions is low, and this agent appears to be better tolerated than aspirin. The most common reactions are nausea and vomiting; diarrhea, constipation, heartburn, and epigastric pain occur less frequently. Patients receiving ibuprofen experienced less gastrointestinal bleeding than those receiving aspirin. However, since ulcer occurred in a few patients, it is advisable to use this agent with caution in those with peptic ulcer or a history of such ulcers. (For other adverse reactions, see Chapter 59.)

PHARMACOKINETICS. About 80% of an oral dose is absorbed. Peak plasma concentrations are attained within 0.5 to 1.5 hours if the drug is taken on an empty stomach. Ibuprofen is eliminated by metabolism; only 1% is excreted in the urine unchanged. The urinary metabolites include: 2-(2-carboxypropyl)-phenylpropionic acid (37%), 2-(p-2-hydroxy-2-methyl propyl)-phenylpropionic acid (25%), and conjugated ibuprofen (14%). The drug is tightly bound to plasma protein (99%). It is not excreted in breast milk. The elimination half-life is 2 to 2.5 hours (Verbeeck et al, 1983).

DOSAGE AND PREPARATIONS. This drug may be taken with meals or milk to reduce gastrointestinal distress.
Oral: Adults, 200 to 400 mg every four to six hours as necessary. For primary dysmenorrhea, 400 mg every four to six hours. For fever, 200 mg every four to six hours. *Children,* dosage has not been established.
    Generic. Tablets 400 and 600 mg.
    Advil (Whitehall), **Medipren** (McNeil), **Nuprin** (Bristol-Myers). Tablets 200 mg (nonprescription).
    Motrin (Upjohn). Tablets 300, 400, and 600 mg.
    Rufen (Boots). Tablets 400 mg and 600 mg.

NAPROXEN
    [Naprosyn]

NAPROXEN SODIUM
    [Anaprox]

$$CH_3O \text{—} \quad \text{—} \overset{O}{\underset{CH_3}{CHCOH}}$$

ACTIONS AND USES. Like aspirin, naproxen has analgesic, anti-inflammatory, and antipyretic actions. The sodium salt is absorbed more rapidly and produces a higher peak plasma level than the acid. Otherwise, the properties and actions of the two forms are the same.

The analgesic activity of naproxen has been demonstrated in various conditions, such as postoperative pain, including orthopedic and dental, as well as postpartum uterine cramps, acute or chronic musculoskeletal and soft tissue inflammation, headache, and primary dysmenorrhea. Results of several comparative studies showed that the analgesic effect of naproxen is comparable to or greater than that of aspirin, aspirin with codeine, acetaminophen, or pentazocine, and is of longer duration. Naproxen was as effective as indomethacin in relieving pain of musculoskeletal disorders and trauma.

In animal studies, naproxen was found to be a more potent antipyretic than aspirin. In children, naproxen 7.5 mg/kg was as effective as aspirin 15 mg/kg and had a much longer duration of action.

ADVERSE REACTIONS AND PRECAUTIONS. The most common adverse reactions are nausea, dizziness, heartburn, headache, abdominal discomfort, and drowsiness. Less gastrointestinal bleeding has been observed than with aspirin; however, this reaction occasionally may be severe and ulceration has been reported. Therefore, naproxen should be used with caution in patients with a history of peptic ulcer. It should not be given to patients who are sensitive to aspirin or other prostaglandin inhibitors. (For other adverse reactions, see Chapter 59, Antiarthritic Drugs.)

This drug is classified in FDA Pregnancy Category B.

PHARMACOKINETICS. Naproxen is rapidly and completely absorbed following oral or rectal administration. Binding to plasma protein is concentration dependent: 99.6% at 23 to 40 mcg/ml and 97.4% at 473 mcg/ml. The apparent volume of distribution is approximately 0.1 L/kg.

About 60% of the drug is eliminated by the kidney, primarily as glucuronide. An additional 28% is excreted as the glucuronide of the 6-demethylated metabolite. Less than 10% is excreted in the urine unchanged. Less than 3% of naproxen and its metabolites is eliminated in the feces. The elimination half-life is not dose dependent and ranges from 12 to 15 hours (Verbeeck et al, 1983).

DOSAGE AND PREPARATIONS.
Oral: Adults, for mild to moderate pain and primary dysmenorrhea, (naproxen sodium) 550 mg initially, followed by 275 mg

every six to eight hours as needed, or (naproxen) 500 mg initially, followed by 250 mg every six to eight hours as required. The daily dose should not exceed 1.25 g.

For mild to moderately severe acute or chronic musculoskeletal and soft tissue inflammation, (naproxen sodium) 275 mg twice daily or 275 mg in the morning and 550 mg in the evening, or (naproxen) 250 or 375 mg twice daily. During long-term administration, the dose should be adjusted in accordance with the patient's response.

NAPROXEN:
Naprosyn (Syntex). Tablets 250, 375, and 500 mg.
NAPROXEN SODIUM:
Anaprox (Syntex). Tablets 275 mg equivalent to 250 mg naproxen base (sodium 1 mEq/tablet).

SUPROFEN
[Suprol]

ACTIONS AND USES. Suprofen, a new nonsteroidal anti-inflammatory and antipyretic drug (*Pharmacology*, 1983; Todd and Heel, 1985) is related to ibuprofen and naproxen. Like other drugs of this class, it acts by inhibiting prostaglandin synthesis. There is some evidence that it also reduces pain induced by bradykinin and uterine contractions induced by bradykinin, arachidonic acid, and prostaglandins. Little information is available on its anti-inflammatory action. It exerts a uricosuric effect in analgesic doses.

Oral suprofen was shown to be more effective in relieving acute pain than acetaminophen, aspirin, codeine, oxycodone, propoxyphene, and combinations of the latter three with aspirin. Its antipyretic potency is exceeded only by that of indomethacin, and suprofen is more potent in dysmenorrhea. Its value in the management of chronic pain remains to be assessed.

ADVERSE REACTIONS AND PRECAUTIONS. The most frequent complaint is gastrointestinal distress. Although suprofen causes less bleeding than aspirin in equipotent doses, peptic ulceration has been reported. Other side effects include headache, somnolence, dizziness, and skin rash, but their incidence and significance have not been determined.

Analgesic doses of suprofen do not displace warfarin or phenytoin from serum protein. Other drug interactions have not been reported.

A single case of overdosage of suprofen has been reported (Freestone and Critchley, 1984). A heroin addict with abnormal liver function ingested forty 200-mg capsules six hours prior to admission. She was conscious and recovery was uncomplicat-

ed. The plasma concentration on admission was 66.2 mg/dl, fortyfold higher than peak concentrations after a 200-mg dose in healthy subjects. In 12 hours, the concentration decreased to 4.6 mg/dl, showing nondose-dependent (linear) elimination kinetics with a half-life of 3.1 hours.

PHARMACOKINETICS. Analgesia occurs within 30 to 60 minutes and lasts four to six hours. The absolute bioavailability after a 200-mg dose is 92.2%, indicating little first-pass metabolism. Accumulation has not occurred with repeated doses. Plasma concentrations and elimination kinetics are the same in elderly and younger subjects.

The pharmacokinetics of suprofen are not dose dependent. The volume of distribution at steady state is 12.2 L and the plasma clearance is 114.7 ml/min. The elimination half-life is approximately 76 minutes (Zulliger and Fassolt, 1983, 1985).

About 90% of oral suprofen is eliminated in the urine, chiefly as an acyl glucuronide, but a small concentration of hydroxylated metabolites also is present.

DOSAGE AND PREPARATIONS.
Oral: *Adults,* for analgesia and relief of dysmenorrhea, 200 mg every four to six hours or 400 mg twice daily. *Children,* no dosage has been established.

For its antipyretic effect (investigational indication), *adults and children,* 5 mg/kg. Larger doses do not produce an additional effect (Todd and Heel, 1985).
Suprol (McNeil, Ortho). Capsules 200 mg.

MIXTURES

Mixtures of analgesic agents or an analgesic with drugs of another class are among the most widely used pharmaceutical products. Most are formulated on the theoretical basis that they will produce a greater analgesic effect, provide broader therapeutic uses, or cause fewer or less severe untoward effects than a single ingredient.

The various analgesic mixtures are divided into three groups on the basis of composition: (1) mixtures of nonopioid (analgesic-antipyretic) drugs, (2) mixtures of a nonopioid with an opioid, and (3) mixtures of analgesics with nonanalgesics. Despite the widespread use of these products, relatively few well-controlled studies have been performed to determine their comparative effectiveness (Beaver, 1975, 1981).

Mixtures of Nonopioid (Analgesic-Antipyretic) Drugs

Many products contain two or more analgesic-antipyretic drugs, eg, aspirin and acetaminophen. The analgesic effect of such a combination is theoretically no greater than the sum of effects of the individual drugs, and no advantage has been demonstrated by combining them. Since the common adverse reactions of these agents are not dose related within the therapeutic range, the smaller amount of each agent in the mixture does not necessarily produce fewer or less severe adverse reactions.

Although results of some studies have suggested that

caffeine may increase the analgesic effect of aspirin or acetaminophen, others have not substantiated such enhancement. Thus, mixtures of analgesic-antipyretic drugs with or without caffeine have not been proved to be superior to optimal doses of the individual components.

Mixtures of a Nonopioid with an Opioid

The combination of an opioid with a nonopioid (analgesic-antipyretic) appears to be rational because the mechanism of action of each drug differs and the analgesic effects of the individual drugs are additive. Since the nonopioids have a ceiling analgesic effect and the dosage of opioids should be limited to prevent adverse effects, a combination of this type may provide greater pain relief with a minimum of adverse effects in a convenient form for the patient.

Codeine and propoxyphene are the most common opioid ingredients in such mixtures; however, few comparative studies have been performed to determine the relative efficacies of the various combinations. Since propoxyphene is usually less effective than codeine in comparable doses, combinations containing propoxyphene may be less effective than similar combinations containing codeine.

Preparations containing acetaminophen lack the anti-inflammatory action produced by those containing aspirin, although each combination has an antipyretic action. Since the mixture of aspirin and caffeine has not been shown to be more effective than either aspirin or acetaminophen alone, combinations containing this mixture with an opioid have no advantage over the simpler mixtures.

Hydrocodone, a semisynthetic analogue of codeine, also is an ingredient in some mixtures and has the same action as other opioids. It is more potent on a milligram basis than codeine and its dependence liability is similar to that of other potent oral analgesics.

Combinations of meperidine with acetaminophen are available for use as oral analgesics. However, meperidine is less effective orally than parenterally, and no well-controlled studies have been performed to demonstrate the contribution of each ingredient.

Oxycodone, a codeine analogue, has pharmacologic properties similar to those of the morphine-like drugs. It is effective orally and, on a milligram basis, its analgesic potency and dependence liability are similar to those of morphine. In the United States, it is available only as an ingredient of mixtures with acetaminophen or aspirin. Dependence on products containing oxycodone has been reported; thus, these mixtures should be prescribed with the same caution as other opioids.

The combination of pentazocine with aspirin is indicated to relieve moderate pain. In one controlled study, this combination provided greater relief of pain in patients with cancer than aspirin alone; effectiveness was comparable to that of combinations of codeine and aspirin or oxycodone and aspirin.

The adverse reactions and precautions of these combinations are those of the individual ingredients. More serious untoward effects are usually caused by the more potent opioid component.

These analgesic mixtures are divided into groups on the basis of their opioid component. The quantitative formula of the most widely used products in each group is listed for information; this does not imply that such products have merit over similar products not listed.

Mixtures Containing Codeine

These mixtures are classified in Schedule III of the Controlled Substances Act.

> ***Acetaminophen with Codeine*** (Generic). Each tablet contains acetaminophen 300 mg and codeine 15, 30, or 60 mg; each 5 ml of elixir contains acetaminophen 120 mg and codeine 12 mg.
>
> ***Ascriptin with Codeine*** (Rorer). Each tablet contains aspirin 325 mg, codeine phosphate 15 (No. 2) or 30 (No. 3) mg, and magnesium-aluminum hydroxide 150 mg.
>
> ***Aspirin with Codeine*** (Generic). Each tablet contains aspirin 325 mg and codeine phosphate 15, 30, or 60 mg.
>
> ***Empirin with Codeine*** (Burroughs Wellcome). Each tablet contains aspirin 325 mg and codeine phosphate 15 mg (No. 2), 30 mg (No. 3), or 60 mg (No. 4).
>
> ***Empracet with Codeine Phosphate*** (Burroughs Wellcome). Each tablet contains acetaminophen 300 mg and codeine phosphate 30 mg (No. 3) or 60 mg (No. 4).
>
> ***Phenaphen with Codeine*** (Robins). Each capsule contains acetaminophen 325 mg and codeine phosphate 15 mg (No. 2), 30 mg (No. 3), or 60 mg (No. 4).
>
> ***Phenaphen-650 with Codeine*** (Robins). Each tablet contains acetaminophen 650 mg and codeine 30 mg.
>
> ***Tylenol with Codeine*** (McNeil). Each capsule contains acetaminophen 300 mg and codeine phosphate 30 mg (No. 3) or 60 mg (No. 4); each tablet contains acetaminophen 300 mg and codeine phosphate 7.5 mg (No. 1), 15 mg (No. 2), 30 mg (No. 3), or 60 mg (No. 4); each 5 ml of elixir contains acetaminophen 120 mg and codeine phosphate 12 mg (alcohol 7%).

Mixtures Containing Hydrocodone

These mixtures are classified as Schedule III drugs under the Controlled Substances Act.

> ***Generic.*** Tablets containing hydrocodone bitartrate 5 or 7 mg and acetaminophen 500 mg or hydrocodone bitartrate 7.5 mg and acetaminophen 650 mg or 1 g.
>
> ***Lortab*** (Russ). Each 5 ml of liquid contains hydrocodone bitartrate 25 mg and acetaminophen 120 mg; each tablet contains hydrocodone bitartrate 5 or 7 mg and acetaminophen 500 mg.
>
> ***Vicodin*** (Knoll). Each tablet contains hydrocodone bitartrate 5 mg and acetaminophen 500 mg.

Mixture Containing Meperidine

This mixture is classified in Schedule II of the Controlled Substances Act.

> ***Demerol APAP*** (Breon). Each tablet contains meperidine hydrochloride 50 mg and acetaminophen 300 mg.

Mixtures Containing Oxycodone

These mixtures are classified in Schedule II of the Controlled Substances Act.

> ***Percodan*** (DuPont). Each tablet contains oxycodone hydrochlor-

ide 4.5 mg, oxycodone terephthalate 0.38 mg, and aspirin 325 mg; each **Percodan-Demi** tablet contains oxycodone hydrochloride 2.25 mg, oxycodone terephthalate 0.19 mg, and aspirin 325 mg.

Percocet-5 (DuPont). Each tablet contains oxycodone hydrochloride 5 mg and acetaminophen 325 mg.

Tylox (McNeil). Each capsule contains oxycodone hydrochloride 4.5 mg, oxycodone terephthalate 0.38 mg, and acetaminophen 500 mg.

Mixtures Containing Pentazocine

Talacen (Winthrop-Breon). Each tablet contains pentazocine hydrochloride equivalent to 25 mg of the base and acetaminophen 650 mg.

Talwin Compound (Winthrop). Each tablet contains pentazocine hydrochloride equivalent to 12.5 mg of the base and aspirin 325 mg (Schedule IV).

Mixtures Containing Propoxyphene

These mixtures are classified as Schedule IV substances under the Controlled Substances Act.

Darvon Compound (Lilly). Each capsule contains aspirin 389 mg, caffeine 32.4 mg, and propoxyphene hydrochloride 32 mg.

Darvon Compound-65 (Lilly). Each capsule contains aspirin 389 mg, caffeine 32.4 mg, and propoxyphene hydrochloride 65 mg.

Darvon-N with A.S.A. (Lilly), **Generic**. Each tablet contains propoxyphene napsylate 100 mg and aspirin 325 mg.

Darvocet-N 50, -100 (Lilly). Each tablet contains propoxyphene napsylate 50 or 100 mg and acetaminophen 325 or 650 mg.

Wygesic (Wyeth). Each tablet contains propoxyphene hydrochloride 65 mg and acetaminophen 650 mg.

Mixtures Containing Analgesics With Nonanalgesics

Drugs with a sedative action (sedative-hypnotics, antianxiety agents, centrally acting skeletal muscle relaxants, antihistamines) are components of several widely used analgesic mixtures. They allegedly enhance analgesic effectiveness and relieve muscle spasm or anxiety accompanying pain.

On theoretical grounds, a sedative might be expected to alter a patient's reaction to pain, and a muscle relaxant might be useful in patients with certain musculoskeletal problems. It has not been definitely shown that the skeletal muscle relaxants have a selective muscle relaxant action or that antihistamines have activity separate from their sedative effect. (See Chapter 12, Drugs Used in Disorders Affecting Skeletal Muscle.) Results of some studies have suggested that a combination of a muscle relaxant and an analgesic provides greater benefit in patients with acute musculoskeletal problems than similar doses of analgesic alone. However, since few properly controlled studies have been designed to determine the relative efficacy of the various products, it cannot be concluded that one is superior to another.

There is some evidence that a combination containing a barbiturate is more effective in tension headache than the analgesic component alone (see Chapter 13, Drugs Used to Treat Migraine and Other Headaches). It should be kept in mind that the duration of action of the sedative may differ from that of the mild analgesic, that the actions of the drugs with repeated use might not coincide, and that abuse of a preparation containing a barbiturate may occur. It has been reported that meprobamate augments pain but, when given with aspirin, the latter drug antagonizes this effect.

Cited References

Suprofen. *Pharmacology* 27(suppl 1):1-96, 1983.

Aitkenhead AR, et al: Pharmacokinetics of single dose I.V. morphine in normal volunteers and patients with end stage renal failure. *Br J Anaesth* 55:905P, 1983.

Allen RC, et al: Renal papillary necrosis in children with chronic arthritis. *Am J Dis Child* 140:20-22, 1986.

Austin KL, et al: Relationship between blood meperidine concentrations and analgesic response: Preliminary report. *Anesthesiology* 53:460-466, 1980.

Austin KL, et al: Rate of formation of norpethidine from pethidine. *Br J Anaesth* 53:255-257, 1981.

Bailie MD: Renal papillary necrosis in children with chronic arthritis. *Am J Dis Child* 140:16-17, 1986.

Beaver WT: Analgesic combinations, in Lasagna L (ed): *Combination Drugs: Their Use and Regulation.* New York, Stratton Intercontinental, 1975.

Beaver WT: Aspirin and acetaminophen as constituents of analgesic combinations. *Arch Intern Med* 141:293-300, 1981.

Bell MDD, et al: Buccal morphine: New route for analgesia? *Lancet* 1:71-73, 1985.

Brogden RN, et al: Diflunisal: Review of its pharmacological properties and therapeutic use in pain and musculoskeletal strain and sprains and pain in osteoarthritis. *Drugs* 19:84-106, 1980.

Bullingham RES, et al: Clinical pharmacokinetics of narcotic agonist-antagonistic drugs. *Clin Pharmacokinet* 8:332-343, 1983.

Christensen FR, Andersen LW: Adverse reaction to extradural buprenorphine, (letter). *Br J Anaesth* 54:476, 1982.

Committee on Infectious Diseases: Special report. *Pediatrics* 69:810-812, 1982.

Cousins MJ, Mather LE: Intrathecal and epidural administration of opioids. *Anesthesiology* 61:276-310, 1984.

Dahlström B, et al: Morphine kinetics in children. *Clin Pharmacol Ther* 26:354-365, 1979.

Dresse A, et al: Uricosuric properties of diflunisal in man. *Br J Clin Pharm* 7:267-272, 1979.

Ehrnebo M, et al: Bioavailability and first-pass metabolism of oral pentazocine in man. *Clin Pharmacol Ther* 22:888-892, 1977.

Epstein M (ed): Prostaglandins and the kidney. *Am J Med* 80(suppl 1A):1-84, 1986.

Errick JK, Heel RC: Nalbuphine: Preliminary review of its pharmacological properties and therapeutic efficacy. *Drugs* 26:191-211, 1983.

Foley KM: Treatment of cancer pain. *N Engl J Med* 313:84-95, 1985.

Forrest JAH, et al: Clinical pharmacokinetics of paracetamol. *Clin Pharmacokinet* 7:93-107, 1982.

Freestone S, Critchley JAJH: Self poisoning with sutoprofen. *Br Med J* 289:470, 1984.

Gram LF, et al: d-Propoxyphene kinetics after single oral and intravenous doses in man. *Clin Pharmacol Ther* 26:473-482, 1979.

Gray JD, Blaschke TF: Fever: To treat or not to treat. *Ration Drug Ther* 19:1-6, (Dec) 1985.

Hansen J, et al: Clinical evaluation of oral methadone in treatment of cancer pain. *Acta Anaesth Scand* Suppl 74:124-127, 1982.

Harcus AW, et al: Methodology of monitored release of new preparation: Buprenorphine. *Br Med J* 2:163-165, 1979.

Hoffbrand BI, Turner P: Clinical experience with injectable meptazinol: New strong analgesic. *Postgrad Med J* 59(suppl 1):1-94, 1983.

Hug CC Jr: Improving analgesic therapy. *Anesthesiology* 53:441-443, 1980.

Hughes SC, et al: Maternal and neonatal effects of epidural morphine for labor and delivery. *Anesth Analg* 63:319-324, 1984.

Jasinski DR, et al: Human pharmacology and abuse potential of analgesic buprenorphine: Potential agent for treating narcotic addiction. *Arch Gen Psychiatry* 35:501-516, 1978.

Kaiko RF: Age and morphine analgesia in cancer patients with postoperative pain. *Clin Pharmacol Ther* 28:823-826, 1980.

Khokhar N: Nephrotoxicity of nonsteroidal anti-inflammatory drugs. *Am Fam Physician* 30:123-128, (July) 1984.

Kotelko DM, et al: Epidural morphine analgesia after cesarean delivery. *Obstet Gynecol* 63:409-413, 1984.

Levy G: Comparative pharmacokinetics of aspirin and acetaminophen. *Arch Intern Med* 141:279-281, 1981.

Lynn AM, Slattery JT: Pharmacokinetics of morphine sulfate in early infancy. *Anesthesiology* 63:A349, 1985.

Mather LE, Meffin PJ: Clinical pharmacokinetics of pethidine. *Clin Pharmacokinet* 3:352-368, 1978.

Max MB, et al: Epidural and intrathecal opiates: Cerebrospinal fluid and plasma profiles in patients with chronic cancer pain. *Clin Pharmacol Ther* 38:631-641, 1985.

McGivney WT, Crooks GM (eds): Care of patients with severe chronic pain in terminal illness. *JAMA* 251:1182-1188, 1984.

Mello NK, Mendelson JH: Buprenorphine suppresses heroin use by heroin addicts. *Science* 207:657-659, 1980.

Miller RR: Evaluation of analgesic efficacy of ibuprofen. *Pharmacotherapy* 1:21-27, (July-Aug) 1981.

Needs CJ, Brooks PM: Clinical pharmacokinetics of salicylates. *Clin Pharmacokinet* 10:164-177, 1985.

Netter P, et al: Salicylate kinetics in old age. *Clin Pharmacol Ther* 38:6-11, 1985.

Pasternak GW, Turner P (eds): Meptazinol: Novel analgesic. *Postgrad Med J* 61(suppl 2):1-34, 1985.

Ritschel WA, et al: Pilot study on disposition and pain relief after intramuscular administration of meperidine during day or night. *Int J Clin Pharmacol Ther Toxicol* 21:218-223, 1983.

Sear J, et al: Morphine kinetics and kidney transplantation: Morphine removal is influenced by renal ischemia. *Anesth Analg* 64:1065-1070, 1985.

Settipane GA: Adverse reactions to aspirin and related drugs. *Arch Intern Med* 141:328-332, 1981.

Stanski DR, et al: Kinetics of intravenous and intramuscular morphine. *Clin Pharmacol Ther* 24:52-59, 1978.

Steelman SL, et al: Chemistry, pharmacology and clinical pharmacology of diflunisal. *Curr Med Res Opin* 5:506, 1978.

Stenseth R, et al: Epidural morphine for postoperative pain: Experience with 1085 patients. *Acta Anaesthesiol Scand* 29:148-156, 1985.

Todd PA, Heel RC: Suprofen: Review of its pharmacodynamic and pharmacokinetic properties and analgesic efficacy. *Drugs* 30:514-538, 1985.

Vale JA, Meredith TJ: Acute poisoning due to non-steroidal anti-inflammatory drugs. Clinical features and management. *Med Toxicol* 1:12-31, 1986.

van Loenhout JWA, et al: Persistent hypouricemic effect of long term diflunisal administration. *J Rheumatol* 8:639-642, 1981.

Verbeeck RK, et al: Clinical pharmacokinetics of non-steroidal anti-inflammatory drugs. *Clin Pharmacokinet* 8:297-331, 1983.

Wallenburg HCS, et al: Low-dose aspirin prevents pregnancy-induced hypertension and pre-eclampsia in angiotensin-sensitive primigravidae. *Lancet* 1:1-3, 1986.

Wharton JG, et al: Acute renal failure associated with diflunisal. *Postgrad Med J* 58:104-105, 1982.

Zeitz JK, Jarmoszuk I: Nasal polyps, bronchial asthma, and aspirin sensitivity: Samter syndrome. *Compr Ther* 11:21-26, (June) 1985.

Zipser RD, Laffi G: Prostaglandins, thromboxanes and leukotrienes in clinical medicine. *West J Med* 143:485-497, 1985.

Zulliger HW, Fassolt A: Suprofen kinetics in healthy male volunteers after intramuscular injection of increasing dosages. *Arzneim-Forsch* 33:1322-1326, 1983.

Zulliger HW, Fassolt A: Pharmacokinetics and bioavailability of suprofen injection solution after intravenous application versus capsules on six healthy male volunteers. *Arzneim-Forsch* 35:976-980, 1985.

Drugs Used for Anxiety and Sleep Disorders 5

ANXIETY

Description and Classification

Anxiety is apprehension, tension, or uneasiness that stems from the anticipation of danger that may be internal or external (American Psychiatric Association, 1980). Anxiety may be a response to stress associated with environmental stimuli or it may be devoid of any apparent precipitating stimulus.

Anxiety usually is a normal response in that an individual's past experience justifies the magnitude of the anxiety. When anxiety is disproportionate to the presenting or anticipated situation or when it occurs without an identifiable stimulus, it can disrupt normal function. It is at this point that treatment generally becomes necessary, although the point on the continuum of anxiety where treatment is indicated is not clearly demarcated. Rather, the decision to treat results from deliberations of the patient and physician based upon a careful exposition, if possible, of the situation by the patient and/or family and a circumspect consideration of this history by the physician.

The following summarizes the classification of anxiety disorders and the pharmacologic approaches available for treatment.

A diagnosis of primary anxiety disorder can be made only when the disorder is not situational (ie, secondary to another condition or situation). Primary anxiety disorder must be differentiated from situational anxiety, which can be caused by medical disorders (eg, hyperthyroidism, pheochromocytoma), substance abuse (intoxication or withdrawal), or psychiatric disorders (schizophrenia, affective disorder, or organic mental disorder). Situational anxiety also can be precipitated by psychosocial stressors (eg, unpleasant social interactions, bereavement, business losses, marital conflict, stage fright).

The anxiety disorders, as categorized in the third edition of the *Diagnostic and Statistical Manual of Mental Disorders (DSM III)* (American Psychiatric Association, 1980), include the anxiety states (anxiety neuroses) and the phobic disorders (phobic neuroses). Disorders classified as anxiety states are panic disorder, generalized anxiety disorder, obsessive-compulsive disorder, post-traumatic stress disorder (acute or chronic), and atypical anxiety disorder. Phobic disorders include agoraphobia, social phobia, and simple phobia.

Anxiety States: *Panic disorder* is characterized by spontaneous, unexplained, recurrent, acute attacks of anxiety (panic) accompanied by feelings of terror and autonomic manifestations of anxiety. For diagnosis, at least three panic attacks must occur within a three-week period and a minimum of four of the following signs and symptoms must be present: dyspnea, palpitations, chest pain or discomfort; choking or smothering sensation; dizziness, vertigo, or unsteady feeling; a sense of unreality; paresthesias (tingling in the hands or feet); hot and cold flashes; sweating; faintness; trembling or shaking; fear of dying, going crazy, or doing something uncontrollable during an attack.

Generalized anxiety disorder is diagnosed when generalized anxiety persists for at least one month in a patient older than 18 years and at least three of the following general manifestations of anxiety are present: motor tension, autonomic hyperactivity, apprehensive expectation, and vigilance and scanning. The manifestations of vigilance and scanning are reflected in the patient's complaints of feeling "on edge" or irritable or in difficulties with attention span and sleeping. If anxiety is pronounced and denial is present, the patient's complaints may be largely somatic (eg, headache, gastrointestinal dysfunction, cervical or back pain) rather than psychological. Mild depressive symptoms also are common.

Obsessive-compulsive disorder is characterized by anxiety arising from either (1) recurrent obsessive ideas, thoughts, images, or impulses that are perceived by the patient as invasions of consciousness and considered senseless or repugnant, or (2) compulsions that appear to be purposeful (eg, handwashing) performed in a repetitive and stereotyped manner. The actions are motivated by a desire to ward off some future event or situation, but the compulsive activity is either totally unconnected in reality with the feared event or is grossly excessive. It is initially resisted, pleasureless, and distressful and interferes with function but is subjectively compelling and provides some relief from tension.

Post-traumatic stress disorder follows the occurrence of a recognizable stressor that would evoke significant symptoms of distress in almost anyone (eg, rape, assault, airplane accident, natural disasters). Responsiveness to the environment generally begins to decline soon after the event. The individual frequently feels detached or estranged from others, is commonly depressed, and often is unable to experience the same level of involvement with others that he had prior to the event. The patient subsequently may relive the event in dreams. Intrusive thoughts, sudden actions, nightmares, and insomnia are common. At least two of the following symptoms must be present for diagnosis and must not have existed prior to the traumatic event: hyperalertness or exaggerated startle response, sleep disturbance, guilt about surviving when others have not or about behavior required for survival, impaired memory or concentration, avoidance of activities that arouse recollection of the traumatic event, intensification of symptoms by exposure to events that symbolize or resemble the traumatic event.

The fifth anxiety state, *atypical anxiety disorder*, represents a residual category for patients who do not meet the criteria for the other four anxiety states, but who have significant anxiety.

Phobic Disorders: Phobic disorders are characterized by irrational fear of objects, activities, or situations and by the compelling desire to avoid them, notwithstanding the individual's understanding that the fear is grossly disproportionate to any real threat.

Three major phobic disorders are recognized (American Psychiatric Association, 1980).

Agoraphobia is the most common of the three phobic disorders treated (American Psychiatric Association, 1980). It is characterized by a marked fear of being alone or in public places, especially those from which escape might be difficult or help not available in case of sudden incapacitation (eg, crowds, tunnels, bridges, public transportation). Normal activities become increasingly constricted, and avoidance behavior dominates the individual's life.

Social phobia consists of a persistent and irrational fear of being scrutinized by others or of behaving in a humiliating or embarrassing way. The individual (often an adolescent) recognizes that the fear is excessive or unreasonable. Usually, social phobia is limited to one activity (eg, fear of speaking, eating, or using lavatories in public places). The disorder often is chronic and, unlike agoraphobia, is usually distressing rather than incapacitating.

Simple phobia is a persistent and irrational fear of any object or focus of concern not described as objects or situations of agoraphobia or social phobia (eg, spiders, snakes, heights). Thus, simple phobia represents a residual category for the phobic disorders. A simple phobia seldom is incapacitating.

Management

Panic and Phobic Disorders: Therapy is based principally upon the type and degree of anxiety. The severe, disabling anxiety that accompanies panic disorder, social phobia, or agoraphobia should be treated with tricyclic antidepressants or monoamine oxidase inhibitors. Imipramine, a tricyclic agent, is the most thoroughly studied of these agents and should be considered the drug of choice. Phenelzine [Nardil], a monoamine oxidase inhibitor, has been especially effective in those resistant to other treatment modalities; however, this drug can cause serious adverse reactions (Sheehan, 1982 A) (see Chapter 7, Drugs Used in Affective Disorders). Alprazolam [Xanax], a triazolo-substituted benzodiazepine, also has been effective in panic disorders and agoraphobia (Sheehan, 1982 B; Chouinard et al, 1982). It has a rapid onset of action, and adverse reactions are not severe and their incidence is low. However, it should be noted that many patients experience marked difficulty during withdrawal of the medication. Evidence is accumulating that many other benzodiazepines may be effective in panic disorder and agoraphobia (Noyes et al, 1984).

Selection of the appropriate dosage is more important than the choice of a particular drug. The dose should be increased gradually until side effects become a problem. In two studies in agoraphobia and mixed phobias (Zitrin et al, 1983) and panic disorder (Garakani et al, 1984), imipramine 25 mg was given before bedtime and the amount was increased every second night by 25 mg up to 150 mg. If panic attacks did not cease, the dosage was increased to 225 mg/day and then to a maximum of 300 mg/day. Mean effective daily doses were 204 mg for agoraphobia and mixed phobias and 160 mg for panic disorder. The initial dose of alprazolam generally should be 0.5 mg three times daily, increased by 0.5 mg/day every two days until significant improvement or excessive sedation becomes evident; 3 to 6 mg/day usually is effective, although doses up to 9 mg/day have been suggested (Sheehan, 1982 A). For phenelzine, the average effective daily dose is between 45 and 60 mg (range, 45 to 90 mg). Amounts exceeding 90 mg can be administered if side effects do not develop and beneficial actions are evident after one week at this dosage level. Because of phenelzine's potential for serious interactions with some foods and drugs, the patient or the person supervising drug administration should receive written instructions regarding appropriate dietary and drug restrictions.

Once substantial improvement has occurred, maintenance doses should be given for six months and possibly up to 12 months, although this requires further study. The maintenance amount probably can be reduced without affecting the therapeutic response. After this 6- to 12-month interval, a drug-free period should be tried. Recurrence of a dysfunctional anxiety state indicates the need for indefinite drug therapy.

An incomplete resolution of agoraphobia or social phobia by drug therapy suggests that addition of behavioral techniques may be beneficial as adjunctive therapy. The most successful techniques utilize exposure to the feared stimulus to eliminate the anxious response (Marks, 1976). Behavioral therapy is the treatment of choice for simple phobia. Exposure to the feared object or situation often eliminates the tendency to avoid, which then extinguishes anticipatory anxiety.

Generalized Anxiety Disorder: Generalized anxiety disorder is best treated by one or more of the following: supportive psychotherapy, relaxation therapy, meditation, pharmacotherapy. Antianxiety agents may play an important role in controlling anxious feelings and allow the patient to participate more fully in supportive treatment (Nemiah, 1980). The benzodiazepines are the drugs of choice. A small but significant subgroup of patients with persistent chronic anxiety of this type may require continuous therapy for six months or more. Recent studies have focused on the long-term efficacy of the benzodiazepines (Rickels et al, 1983 A) and indicate that prolonged drug therapy is of value.

Obsessive-Compulsive Disorder: This anxiety disorder, which occurs infrequently in the general population, is relatively easy to diagnose but difficult to treat. The three most beneficial treatment modalities are behavioral therapy; drug therapy; and, for severe, recalcitrant cases, neurosurgery (Jenike, 1983). The tricyclic antidepressants, especially the investigational drug, clomipramine, have been reported to be effective (Thorén et al, 1980; Asberg et al, 1982) and are drugs of choice (Jenike, 1983). The monoamine oxidase inhibitors may be useful when phobic anxiety or panic attacks also are present (Jenike et al, 1983).

Situational Anxiety: Acute anxiety in response to an obvious environmental stimulus (eg, job stress, marital discord) is termed situational anxiety. In situational anxiety, counseling may be all that is needed. Antianxiety drugs may be prescribed briefly when there is genuine suffering and interference with normal functioning. When an anxiety disorder follows a traumatic event, antianxiety agents may be beneficial initially, but long-term administration rarely is indicated.

Anxiety Secondary to Medical Disease: Anxiety may be a response to a catastrophic illness or chronic disease or may be symptomatic of a physical disorder. In such cases, initial therapy should be directed to the cure or improvement of the physical disorder. In patients with chronic illness (eg, cardiac disease) or terminal illness, educational efforts, supportive psychotherapy (especially in group settings), and behavioral therapy are beneficial. These forms of treatment may be augmented by judicious use of antianxiety agents, especially the benzodiazepines (Schuckit, 1983), in times of particular distress.

SLEEP DISORDERS

The essential function of sleep is still unknown, although it is generally recognized to have a restorative quality, diminishing fatigue and dysphoria. The occurrence of sleep is correlated with circadian body temperature rhythms, but the length of prior wakefulness is a factor in sleep duration. There is no recommended daily optimum amount of sleep for any individual or age group; however, it is possible to determine the optimum quantity required by an individual. A shortened (common in the elderly) or lengthened total sleep time is not considered pathologic in the absence of complaints. However, extremes of sleep correlate with increased mortality, although no causal relationship has been demonstrated (Kripke et al, 1979).

Disorders of sleep and arousal have been separated into four categories to improve diagnosis (Sleep Disorders Classification Committee, 1979) and treatment: (1) disorders of initiating and maintaining sleep (insomnias); (2) disorders of excessive somnolence (hypersomnias); (3) dysfunctions associated with sleep, sleep stages, or partial arousals (parasomnias); and (4) disorders of the sleep wake schedule.

Disorders of Initiating and Maintaining Sleep (Insomnias)

Description and Classification: Insomnia encompasses a broad spectrum of disorders with diverse underlying causes. Insomnia may be associated with a psychiatric disorder, the use of drugs or alcohol, respiratory impairment, myoclonus or "restless legs," or other medical, toxic, or environmental conditions.

The insomnias are by far the most common sleep problem. Inability to fall asleep and/or maintain the sleep state at night are frequent complaints. One-third of the U.S. population complains of poor sleep and one-third of this group believes it to be a major problem (Mendelson, 1980). Common subjective daytime complaints that correlate with nighttime sleeplessness include drowsiness, fatigue, lack of energy, dysphoria, and lack of alertness. Daytime sleepiness in the absence of nighttime sleep complaints is less common, and objective data on daytime performance are not available. Thus, the urgency of a patient-presumed greater sleep need in this latter group must be evaluated on the basis of genuine unpleasantness and/or on interference with daytime function.

The temporal classification of insomnias as transient, short-term, or long-term is most useful (National Institutes of Health, 1983). In transient insomnia, an acute stressor or situation adversely affects sleep and this most commonly lasts only a few days. Short-term insomnia usually is associated with situational stress and can last up to three weeks. Sleep difficulty may be caused by the loss of a loved one; job pressures; concerns regarding examinations; anticipation or reaction to life changes, such as marriage or divorce; environmental factors, such as overcrowding, excessive noise, and poor bedding or housing conditions; physical restrictions or lack of physical activity; nightshift work and travel across time zones (jet lag), which upset internal biological rhythms; certain drugs (eg, amphetamines, caffeine); or withdrawal of some drugs (eg, alcohol, nicotine).

Long-term insomnia persists for more than three weeks and, in one-third to one-half of patients, it is due to an underlying psychiatric disorder. Chronic drug abuse (eg, alcohol) and/or dependence causes long-term insomnia in a second major group of patients. Other causes include medical conditions, such as arthritis, neurogenic pain, and various types of headache. The daytime pain experienced by the latter patients may be magnified greatly at night when sleep is attempted, environmental stimuli are decreased, and more attention is focused internally. In patients with malignancies, pain can be severe and fear and anxiety over the ultimate consequences of the illness often are overwhelming. Patients with angina pectoris and/or arrhythmias often are afraid to sleep because of fear that an attack may occur during the night when they feel most vulnerable and helpless. Other causes of long-term insomnia include sleep apnea, nocturnal myoclonus, restless legs syndrome, 24-hour rhythm disturbances (eg, advanced and delayed sleep phase), or undefined psychological or physiologic stressors (National Institutes of Health, 1983).

Management: A sleep complaint, whether it is nighttime sleeplessness, daytime sleepiness, decreased daytime performance, or excessive daytime sleep, requires careful diagnostic evaluation prior to therapy (Coleman et al, 1982). An accurate diagnosis requires that the underlying cause of insomnia be determined. The awake-state symptomatology that usually accompanies nighttime insomnia is not diagnostic, for it is often present in other sleep disorders (ie, hypersomnias, parasomnias, sleep-wake schedule disorders). A medical history, including a detailed sleep, drug, and psychiatric history; physical examination; and appropriate laboratory procedures also may be needed for differential diagnosis.

The treatment of an insomnia depends on the underlying cause and the duration of the complaint. Both pharmacologic and nonpharmacologic treatment modalities can be tailored to meet the needs of the individual patient.

Transient insomnia most often is related directly to a minor situational stress (eg, hospitalization for elective surgery, jet travel) and drug treatment may or may not be needed. When a drug is prescribed, a small dose of a rapidly eliminated hypnotic may be adequate unless sustained sedation is desired or daytime anxiety is a problem. Treatment may be needed for one to three nights.

Short-term insomnia also often results from situational stress. Removal from the stressful situation or improvement in coping skills may be all that is needed. Counseling, brief training in relaxation techniques, and education in sleep hygiene (eg, desirable sleep routines; avoiding naps, caffeine-containing beverages, and strenuous exercise three to four hours before bedtime; regular waking time) are beneficial. If, despite good sleep hygiene, a hypnotic is needed, the smallest effective dose should be given for not more than three weeks. Intermittent use is advisable during this period: After administration for one or two nights results in good sleep, the next day's dose can be skipped followed by resumption of use for one or two days (National Institutes of Health, 1983).

The causes of long-term insomnia are more numerous and require special medical, physiologic, and psychiatric evaluations. If a major psychiatric disorder is present, it should be treated appropriately. In drug abusers, the offending agent(s) must be identified and detoxification and rehabilitation started. When pain causes loss of sleep, analgesics should be administered. Nocturnal myoclonus, a disorder characterized by rhythmic myoclonic jerks that occur during sleep, may be relieved by clonazepam [Klonopin]. Insomnia due to certain other conditions may respond to concomitant behavioral treatment.

In many of these conditions, counseling, psychotherapy, and behavior modification may obviate the need for drugs. Exercise, decreased caffeine intake, elimination of drugs, and a trial of biofeedback (relaxation) and other stress reduction techniques should be tried initially. A concomitant short trial (less than one month) of sleep-promoting medication also may be indicated (National Institutes of Health, 1983). However, it must be kept in mind that a hypnotic is only an adjunct to achieving the main therapeutic goal of breaking the vicious cycle of insomnia, fear of sleeplessness, more emotional and physiologic arousal, and insomnia (Kales et al, 1983). The presence of sleep apnea, daytime sleepiness, or heavy snoring may be contraindications to sleep-promoting medications for long-term insomnia.

Although hypnotics often alleviate insomnia, they do not induce normal sleep as defined by objective sleep parameters. Sleep laboratory studies have demonstrated that hypnotic doses of most of these agents reduce the amount of REM (rapid eye movement) sleep. The benzodiazepines, the usual drugs of choice, are least active in this respect; however, they reduce stage 3 and 4 sleep, but the clinical significance of this alteration is unknown. The nonbenzodiazepine-nonbarbiturate hypnotics and the barbiturates have similar effects on objective sleep parameters, except for chloral hydrate, which has only a minimal effect (Kales et al, 1977).

When hypnotics are indicated for patients with sleep disorders, appropriate guidelines should be followed: (1) Special caution is required for patients with respiratory difficulties, suicidal tendencies, or a history of alcoholism, drug dependence, or substance abuse. (2) The potential for impairment of daytime performance should be discussed with the patient. It should be stressed that the patient may be unaware of his impairment. (3) Because of individual response variation, conservative use is especially necessary to avoid drug interactions in the elderly, in patients with associated illnesses, in those who drink alcohol, or in those taking other medication, especially antihistamines. (4) The minimum effective amount should be administered, and dose escalation should be avoided. (5) Hypnotics should not be prescribed beyond the period of effectiveness demonstrated in well-controlled studies. (6) Periodic monitoring is necessary to reassess drug effectiveness, minimize nightly reliance on medication, and determine toxic or other factors that would alter the risk of continuing hypnotic use. (7) Drug therapy should be discontinued when goals have been met. Gradual dosage reduction is essential after long-term administration to minimize insomnia and possible withdrawal signs.

Disorders of Excessive Somnolence (Hypersomnias)

The hypersomnias are a diverse group of functional and organic conditions with the primary symptoms of inappropriate and undesirable sleepiness during waking hours, decreased cognitive and motor performance, excessive tendency to sleep, unavoidable napping, increase in total 24-hour sleep, and difficulty in achieving full arousal on awakening (Sleep Disorders Classification Committee, 1979). Most people who complain about hypersomnia and are seen in sleep disorder centers have narcolepsy or sleep apnea. Hypersomnias, like the insomnias, also may be associated with other medical or psychiatric disorders, eg, depression (particularly bipolar), substance abuse (tolerance to or withdrawal from central nervous system stimulants, prolonged use of central nervous system depressants).

Narcolepsy: The classical diagnostic tetrad of the primary symptoms of narcolepsy (Parkes, 1977; Ferriss, 1982) is (1) excessive daytime sleepiness with a history of falling asleep episodically, rapidly, and often inappropriately while performing a daily task; (2) episodic cataplectic attacks of muscular weakness precipitated by emotional stimulation (ie, humor, anger, fear, surprise); (3) hypnagogic hallucinations, which may be visual, auditory, or tactile, occurring during the transition from wakefulness to sleep; and (4) sleep paralysis characterized by consciousness and inability to move or cry out during the transition from wakefulness to sleep but more often upon awakening. All narcoleptics have sleep attacks and 60% to 70% experience cataplexy; less than one-fourth of patients have all four symptoms (Browman et al, 1983). Common secondary signs and symptoms include automatic behavior with complete retrograde amnesia, as well as disturbed nocturnal sleep characterized by frequent awakenings. A polysomnograph showing a transition from wakefulness directly into REM rather than NREM sleep helps to confirm the diagnosis. Narcoleptics usually fall asleep extremely rapidly.

Narcolepsy usually develops between ages 15 and 25; it rarely appears after age 40. The disorder generally persists for life, although some adaptation occurs. A small proportion of patients with mild narcolepsy prefer to take no medications. However, for most narcoleptics, treatment with central nervous system stimulants and/or antidepressants is necessary. Such treatment must meet the specific needs of the individual patient (eg, only during work periods).

Methylphenidate, dextroamphetamine, and pemoline are the central nervous system stimulants most often indicated. These drugs control the excessive daytime sleepiness characteristic of the disorder. The tricyclic antidepressants, protriptyline and imipramine, also may diminish daytime sleepiness, but the consistency of this effect is controversial. There is general agreement that the antidepressants control other symptoms of the disorder, such as cataplexy, hypnagogic hallucinations, or sleep paralysis, and thus decrease the required dose of central nervous system stimulant.

Methylphenidate and dextroamphetamine have a duration of action of two to five hours, whereas pemoline's therapeutic effects persist for eight to ten hours. For the patient whose narcolepsy is almost controlled by regularization of nocturnal sleep schedule plus a convenient schedule of napping, an average daily dose of 20 mg of methylphenidate (10 mg twice daily) may be sufficient (Regestein et al, 1983). If cataplexy is severe, protriptyline or imipramine can be added in small doses initially and the amount increased gradually over two to four weeks while the maintenance dose that maximizes therapeutic effect and minimizes adverse effects is determined. The therapeutic actions of protriptyline and imipramine in narcolepsy are immediate, unlike their antidepressant activities.

In severe narcolepsy, it is difficult to control daytime sleepiness with doses of central nervous system stimulants that do not interfere with nighttime sleep. The dose and schedule of administration should be adjusted to provide the minimal effective amount during periods demanding concentrated effort and sustained activity.

Tolerance often develops both to the central nervous system stimulants and to the antidepressants. This tolerance may be minimized by instituting drug holidays one day a week. Another approach is gradual withdrawal, followed by resumption of therapy at a lower dose. The patient should be cautioned not to drive or engage in other potentially hazardous activities during withdrawal.

Sleep Apnea: This disorder is characterized by cessation of breathing that is centrally induced or caused by upper airway obstruction, or it is a mixed type with both components (Chokroverty and Sharp, 1981). Episodes may occur hundreds of times each night. Severe bradycardia, hypoxemia, and hypercapnia occur during the apneic episodes. Life-threatening arrhythmias may result if apnea persists; however, it usually stops before serious arrhythmias occur.

The apneic patient has no memory of these difficulties and consequently complains only of daytime fatigue and sleepiness. The obstructive disorder is most common in elderly obese men who snore; however, infants and children can be affected quite severely (Brouillette et al, 1982) and increased awareness is necessary to provide earlier treatment and reduce morbidity in this age group. Questioning the patient's bed partner or examining the sleeping infant or child may be necessary for a presumptive diagnosis when all of the classical features of the disorder are not present. The diagnosis of sleep apnea can be confirmed only by polysomnographic recordings.

Therapy for obstructive sleep apnea includes weight loss, removal of obstructing tissue, and avoidance of sedatives. In children, particular attention should be paid to the possibilities of anatomic obstruction of the upper airways, such as tonsillar or adenoid hypertrophy and deviated nasal septum, which can be corrected surgically. In adults, tracheostomy is the definitive treatment for severe obstructive sleep apnea, although more conservative approaches can be tried first.

Protriptyline, imipramine, and medroxyprogesterone have been effective in some cases of obstructive sleep apnea. Protriptyline 30 mg/day decreased daytime sleepiness in one study with a limited number of subjects (Brownell et al, 1982). Medroxyprogesterone 20 mg three times daily reduced heart failure, peripheral edema, and daytime somnolence (Orr et al,

1979). Results with other treatments, such as mechanical interventions and oxygen therapy, have been inconsistent.

Effective therapy for central apneas has not been established. Respiratory stimulants, theophylline, and progestational agents have not been very effective (Hudgel, 1981). Acetazolamide 250 mg four times daily reduced daytime somnolence in five of six patients in one study (White et al, 1982), but supporting data have not been reported.

Parasomnias

Drug therapy is seldom indicated for parasomnias (eg, childhood enuresis, childhood night terrors, sleepwalking at any age). Behavioral modification, reassurance, and injury prevention techniques, respectively, are the modalities of choice. Rarely, an antidepressant may be appropriate for unresponsive childhood enuresis (see Chapter 31, Agents Used to Treat Urologic Disorders) or a benzodiazepine may be effective for severe, persistent night terrors (clinical data are available only for diazepam).

ANTIANXIETY AND HYPNOTIC DRUGS

Antianxiety and hypnotic drugs are listed in Table 1. Principles of use and drug selection follow.

Benzodiazepines

Indications: The benzodiazepines are usually the drugs of choice when an antianxiety, sedative, or hypnotic action is needed. Other indications for selected benzodiazepines include preanesthetic medication, alcohol withdrawal, seizure disorders, spasticity, localized skeletal muscle spasm, and nocturnal myoclonus. The benzodiazepines have distinct advantages over other drugs when their respective adverse reactions, abuse or dependence liability, drug interactions, and lethality are compared. The pharmacokinetics of these drugs greatly affect their efficacy and adverse reactions and thus influence drug selection.

In agoraphobia and panic disorder, alprazolam [Xanax] appears to be the most effective benzodiazepine. However, further examination of the efficacy of large doses of benzodiazepines in these disorders is necessary to clearly establish the superiority of one benzodiazepine over another.

All benzodiazepines alleviate the uncomplicated anxiety of generalized anxiety disorder and improve situational anxiety.

Some patients with chronic anxiety benefit from the long-term administration of these drugs. If discontinuation of prolonged benzodiazepine administration has resulted in a return to previous poor levels of function or is otherwise inadvisable, long-term therapy with these drugs may be necessary and is entirely appropriate (Greenblatt et al, 1983).

Flurazepam, triazolam, and temazepam are used most commonly to treat insomnia. Quazepam has recently been approved and is effective in the treatment of insomnia. Diazepam, oxazepam, and lorazepam are also effective hypnotic agents. When drug therapy is indicated to alleviate problems of initiating sleep, triazolam is most effective because of its rapid onset of action and ability to decrease sleep latency. Flurazepam and temazepam are most effective in preventing repeated awakenings during sleep because of the longer duration of their hypnotic effect. When impairment of daytime skills (eg, alertness, manual dexterity) should be minimized or is especially undesirable, triazolam and temazepam are preferred. However, rebound insomnia upon abrupt discontinuation of therapy has been reported with these two benzodiazepines (Kales et al, 1983), especially with triazolam (Bixler et al, 1985).

As with all drugs, there is a need for clear directions and warnings to the patient about the use of benzodiazepines; frequent clinical reappraisal of treatment efficacy and vigilant monitoring for toxic effects or risk factors that would make continued use of the drug hazardous (eg, renal or hepatic disease, alcoholism, depression) are also essential.

Actions: The site and mechanism of action mediating the antianxiety, sedative, hypnotic, and anticonvulsant effects of the benzodiazepines remain speculative. Facilitation of inhibitory gamma-aminobutyric acid (GABA) neurotransmission presently is the most satisfactory hypothesis: Interaction of the benzodiazepines with a benzodiazepine-specific receptor amplifies or facilitates the inhibitory presynaptic and/or postsynaptic actions of GABA through an allosteric mechanism on the GABA receptor complex.

Recent evidence suggests that there are two types of benzodiazepine receptors: Postsynaptic benzodiazepine receptors (Type I) are found in the hippocampus, and high concentrations of presynaptic benzodiazepine receptors (Type II) are found in the cerebellum. These two receptor types can be differentiated further because Type I receptor function does not appear to be regulated by chloride ion fluxes. Differences in localization, binding affinity, and control mechanisms for these receptors suggest that further elucidation of the way molecular events translate into an organism's function will make possible more specific and effective drug therapy (Snyder, 1984).

Pharmacokinetics: The pharmacokinetic properties of the benzodiazepines often provide the rationale for the proper selection of these compounds. Absorption, volume of distribution, and metabolic route are prime determinants of onset of action, duration of effect, and the need for special caution in debilitated patients (eg, the elderly, those with hepatic disease), respectively.

As previously discussed, onset of action has significant implications for the pharmacologic management of insomnia (disorders of initiating sleep) and, to a lesser extent, the short-term treatment of anxiety. After oral administration, a drug's onset of action is determined mainly by the rapidity of absorption from the gastrointestinal tract (see Table 2). Clorazepate, diazepam, and flurazepam are absorbed most rapidly, while halazepam, oxazepam, prazepam, and temazepam are absorbed slowly.

Chlordiazepoxide, diazepam, and lorazepam also are available for parenteral use. Since chlordiazepoxide is absorbed erratically after intramuscular injection, intravenous use is preferred when parenteral therapy is required. Lorazepam is

and reliably after intramuscular administra-
injection also may affect the absorption rate.
...e probability of rapid and complete absorption
...ar diazepam is enhanced by injection into the
...cle area (Greenblatt et al, 1983).

Du... ...n of action is related largely to the drug's lipophilicity.
The more lipophilic a benzodiazepine is, the more rapid its
onset and the shorter its duration of action. Highly lipophilic
drugs, such as diazepam, enter brain tissue rapidly but also
redistribute rapidly to other regions of the body. The effect of a
drug's volume of distribution becomes less apparent when
multiple doses are given over a one- or two-week period.

The direct relationship between lipophilicity and duration of
action is confounded somewhat by the biotransformation of
certain benzodiazepines to active metabolites. Clorazepate,
chlordiazepoxide, diazepam, halazepam, flurazepam, and
prazepam are transformed to active metabolites, primarily by
oxidation to N-dealkylated products with half-lives longer than
those of the parent drugs. Alprazolam and triazolam undergo
hydroxylation to weak or inactive metabolites. These metabolic characteristics are particularly significant in elderly and
newborn patients, individuals with liver disease, or those
taking other drugs that undergo hepatic metabolism, for the
hepatic oxidation process tends to be impaired when any one
of these conditions is present.

The elimination half-life of a benzodiazepine is prolonged in
elderly patients because of the following age-related changes
(Ochs et al, 1981): (1) The enzyme systems necessary for
metabolism of the long-acting benzodiazepines (ie, hepatic
N-demethylation, aliphatic hydroxylation) become less active
with age. (2) The proportion of fat to total body weight
increases with age, which increases the volume of distribution
of lipid-soluble drugs, including benzodiazepines. The effect
on volume of distribution also explains in part the more rapid
elimination half-life of some benzodiazepines in men, because
men have a lower proportion of fat to total body weight than
women.

Since monitoring the drug concentration in blood is not
established as helpful, dosage adjustments and multiple daily
doses may be necessary initially until the desired response
and acceptable level of untoward effects are established. After
the optimum total daily dosage is determined, single daily
doses may be given to some patients; other patients require
multiple daily doses, even when benzodiazepines with long
half-lives are prescribed.

For specific pharmacokinetic data, see Table 2.

Adverse Reactions: Daytime sedation and hangover are
the most common initial untoward effects of the benzodiazepines, but they appear to occur less frequently than with the
barbiturates. Other common adverse effects with oral use are
dizziness and ataxia, which are dose related.

Untoward reactions noted occasionally are blurred vision,
diplopia, hypotension, amnesia, slurred speech, tremor, urinary incontinence, constipation, and leukopenia.

Fatigue, dysarthria, muscle weakness, dryness of the
mouth, and gastrointestinal discomfort (nausea and vomiting)
also have been reported, but a causal relationship has not
been established definitely. The gastrointestinal disturbances
may be reduced by administering the drug with or immediately

after meals. Rash, chills, fever, and, rarely, blood dyscrasias
have been noted.

Paradoxical aggression (increased irritability, insomnia, hyperactivity, and even violent hostile rage reactions) has been
reported rarely. An increased frequency of vivid dreams also
has been associated with benzodiazepine use or withdrawal.
Depression may represent an undiagnosed, concomitant, previously masked condition. Suicidal impulses have been reported in several patients taking diazepam 40 to 60 mg daily.

Respiratory depression, apnea, and cardiac arrest have
occurred rarely, usually following intravenous administration.
These reactions are most common in elderly or severely ill
patients, in those receiving other central nervous system
depressants, or in those with limited ventilatory reserve.
Intravenous injection of diazepam may cause local pain and
thrombophlebitis. There also is tentative evidence that benzodiazepines may further suppress respiration in patients with
undiagnosed sleep apnea or chronic lung disease.

Precautions: Sedation may be lessened by prescribing
relatively small doses initially and increasing the amount
gradually to produce the desired antianxiety effect without
oversedation; however, if tolerance develops, the dosage and
continued use of the drug should be reassessed. Patients
should be cautioned to avoid undertaking activities that require
mental alertness, judgment, and physical coordination (eg,
driving a car, operating dangerous machinery) during initial
therapy when sedation may be pronounced. The concomitant
use of alcohol may be hazardous.

Ataxia, dizziness, and headache often are observed during
the early period of dosage adjustment. Elderly and debilitated
patients develop drowsiness and ataxia more often than
younger patients. In addition, symptoms of organic brain
disease in the elderly may be aggravated if they receive the
larger doses appropriate for younger patients.

Caution is required when prescribing benzodiazepines for
patients with severely impaired hepatic function, especially
agents with long-acting active metabolites.

Many benzodiazepines accumulate until steady-state concentrations are reached (several days to two weeks). Drugs
with long elimination half-lives (chlordiazepoxide, clorazepate,
diazepam, flurazepam, halazepam, quazepam, prazepam) are
most likely to accumulate excessively. Cumulative clinical
effects do not always result, possibly because of tolerance or
the poor correlation of plasma concentrations with clinical
effects. However, some patients, particularly the elderly, may
be subjectively unaware of sedation or impairment of performance, although they function less effectively after a week or
two of benzodiazepine therapy.

Pregnancy and Breast Feeding: The association between
the use of benzodiazepines during the first trimester of pregnancy and the development of cleft lip with or without cleft
palate has been reported; however, the most recent data
suggest that such exposure to diazepam does not materially
affect the risk of cleft lip with or without cleft palate or of cleft
palate alone (Rosenberg et al, 1983). Dysmorphogenic changes in rib formation were observed in two animal species given
50 to 100 times the human dose. Overall, data are not
adequate to assess the safety of the benzodiazepines during
pregnancy. Therefore, unless a pressing need exists, it is

TABLE 1.
ANTIANXIETY AND HYPNOTIC DRUGS:
PRINCIPAL USES AND GENERAL PRESCRIBING INFORMATION

DRUG	Anxiety	Insomnia	Preanesthetic Medication	IV Anesthetic Induction	Alcohol Withdrawal
BENZODIAZEPINES					
Compounds with Active Metabolites					
Chlordiazepoxide [Libritabs, Librium]	+		+		+
Clorazepate [Tranxene]	+				+
Diazepam [Valium, Valrelease]	+		+	+	+
Flurazepam [Dalmane]		+			
Halazepam [Paxipam]	+				
Prazepam [Centrax]	+				
Compounds with Weakly Active, Short-lived, or Inactive Metabolites					
Alprazolam [Xanax]	+				
Clonazepam [Klonopin]					
Flunitrazepam* [Rohypnol]				+	
Lorazepam [Ativan]	+	+	+		+*
Midazolam [Versed]				+	
Oxazepam [Serax]	+				+
Quazepam [Dormalin]		+			
Temazepam [Restoril]		+			
Triazolam [Halcion]		+	+		
BARBITURATES					
Phenobarbital	+	+			
Mephobarbital [Mebaral]					
Amobarbital [Amytal]		+	+		
Pentobarbital [Nembutal]		+	+		
Secobarbital [Seconal]		+	+		
NONBENZODIAZEPINE-NONBARBITURATES					
Antianxiety Agents					
Buspirone* [Buspar]	+				
Hydroxyzine [Atarax, Orgatrax, Vistaril]	+		+		+
Meprobamate [Equanil, Meprospan, Miltown]	+				
Propranolol [Inderal] (Investigational use)	+				
Hypnotic Agents (prescription)					
Chloral Hydrate		+	+		

USES				GENERAL PRESCRIBING INFORMATION		
Barbiturate Withdrawal	Seizure Disorders	Skeletal Muscle Hyperactivity	Nocturnal Myoclonus	Parenteral Preparation Available	Generic Form Available	Controlled Substance Schedule
				YES	YES	IV
	+			NO	NO	IV
	+	+		YES	YES	IV
				NO	NO	IV
				NO	NO	IV
				NO	NO	IV
				NO	NO	IV
	+		+	NO	NO	IV
				YES	NO	**
	+*			YES	NO	IV
				YES	NO	IV
				NO	NO	IV
						IV
				NO	NO	IV
				NO	NO	**
+	+			YES	YES	IV
	+			NO	YES	IV
				YES	YES	II
				YES	YES	II
				YES	YES	II
				YES	YES	NONE
				NO	YES	IV
				YES	NO	NONE
				NO	YES	IV

(continued on next page)

TABLE 2 (continued)

DRUG					PRINCIPAL
	Anxiety	Insomnia	Preanesthetic Medication	IV Anesthetic Induction	Alcohol Withdrawal
Ethchlorvynol [Placidyl]		+			
Ethinamate [Valmid]		+			
Glutethimide [Doriden]		+			
Methyprylon [Noludar]		+			
Paraldehyde		+			+
Hypnotic Agents (antihistamines [nonprescription])					
Diphenhydramine [Nervine, Nytol, Sleep-Eze 3, Sominex 2]		+			
Doxylamine [Unisom]		+			
Pyrilamine [Dormarex]		+			

*Investigational   **Not determined

advisable to avoid the benzodiazepines during pregnancy, especially during the first trimester. Alprazolam, halazepam, and lorazepam (parenteral) are classified in FDA Pregnancy Category D. Temazepam and triazolam are classified in FDA Pregnancy Category X.

Diazepam and desmethyldiazepam cross the placenta during labor and fetal concentrations exceed those in the mother. Available evidence suggests that intramuscular or intravenous administration of more than 30 mg of diazepam during the final 15 hours of labor can produce low Apgar scores, apnea, hypothermia, and poor sucking in newborn infants (the floppy-infant syndrome). Hypothermia and delayed feeding, particularly in preterm infants, also were associated with large doses of intravenous lorazepam given before delivery. Full-term neonates whose mothers received oral lorazepam had no complications other than delayed feeding associated with relatively large doses in 7 of 29 cases (Whitelaw et al, 1981).

Withdrawal symptoms and signs can be expected in infants born to mothers who are physically dependent on benzodiazepines during the last trimester.

Although detectable amounts of diazepam appear in breast milk, effects in the nursing infant probably are insignificant. If it is essential to prescribe any benzodiazepine for a nursing mother, the infant should be monitored closely.

Poisoning: When alcohol or other central nervous system depressants are not used concomitantly, the benzodiazepines are the safest antianxiety and hypnotic agents and have a wide margin of safety in overdosage; in combination with alcohol, these agents become substantially more toxic. When overdose occurs, usual supportive measures often are adequate. However, in more severe cases (eg, acute circulatory failure and coma), treatment is similar to that for barbiturate overdose, except that dialysis is of limited value.

Tolerance: Tolerance to the sedation and ataxia produced by benzodiazepines develops with continued administration of the same dosage, but tolerance to the antianxiety effect develops much more slowly, if at all (Rickels et al, 1983 A; Greenblatt et al, 1983). A rapidly developing tolerance (tachyphylaxis) to the hypnotic, respiratory, and cardiovascular actions occurs with overdosage. The benzodiazepine blood concentration may remain well above the normal range associated with sleep or even anesthesia during recovery from overdose when the patient is awake and vital signs are stable. Metabolic tolerance (liver enzyme induction) does not appear to be of clinical significance.

Abuse and Dependence Liability: The potential for abuse of benzodiazepines is mild in comparison to drugs such as pentobarbital, hydromorphone, and cocaine. Long-term administration of larger than usual or, in some cases, even usual therapeutic doses of benzodiazepines can cause physical dependence (Rickels et al, 1983 A; Owen and Tyrer, 1983). The benzodiazepines are classified under Schedule IV of the Controlled Substances Act.

Dependence occurs relatively frequently in individuals with a history of alcohol and drug abuse, and the benzodiazepines should be avoided in these patients if possible. Withdrawal symptoms are similar to those produced by barbiturate or alcohol dependence and usually include anxiety, agitation, irritability, insomnia, tremor, headache, dizziness, muscle twitches and pain, anorexia, nausea and vomiting, diarrhea, hyperosmia, photophobia, diaphoresis, hyperacusis, incoordination, weakness, and appreciable weight loss. Depersonalization and depression are not uncommon. The onset of a withdrawal reaction may be delayed for 36 hours to one week following cessation of the drug, depending upon the specific compound's half-life and whether it is converted to an active metabolite.

If physical dependence is well established, withdrawal reactions may occur if the drugs are discontinued abruptly, espe-

USES				GENERAL PRESCRIBING INFORMATION		
Barbiturate Withdrawal	Seizure Disorders	Skeletal Muscle Hyperactivity	Nocturnal Myoclonus	Parenteral Preparation Available	Generic Form Available	Controlled Substance Schedule
				NO	NO	IV
				NO	NO	IV
				NO	YES	III
				NO	NO	III
				YES	YES	IV
				NO	YES	NONE
				NO	NO	NONE
				NO	YES	NONE

cially short-acting benzodiazepines, although seizures do not usually develop during withdrawal from these benzodiazepines. *Therefore, very gradual reduction of dosage is recommended* (5% to 10% per day or less for 10 to 14 days). A long-acting benzodiazepine may be substituted temporarily to control the signs and symptoms of withdrawal.

Long-acting benzodiazepines may be withdrawn abruptly from patients without a history of seizures if no other risk factors, such as alcohol, barbiturate, or opiate abuse, are present. However, tapering of dosage is still desirable if possible. Patients with a history of seizures who are dependent on large doses of long-acting benzodiazepines should be hospitalized and the dose reduced gradually to complete withdrawal over a 20-day period (Robinson and Sellers, 1982). Some authorities prefer to use phenobarbital (substitutive treatment) even when there is no history of seizures. Propranolol [Inderal] may be a useful supplement in some patients (Tyrer et al, 1981). The physician should closely supervise the dosage and duration of use of these drugs in all patients, especially those with a history of drug dependence.

Psychological dependence is more common than physical dependence and can occur with any dose. This type of drug reliance is difficult to distinguish from a recurrence of the original anxiety disorder. Consequently, good medical practice demands that these agents be prescribed initially only when a disorder known to respond to such therapy can be diagnosed with reasonable assurance, and their use should be continued only for the shortest time required.

Drug Interactions: Additive central nervous system depression may occur with concomitant use of a benzodiazepine and other central nervous system depressants (eg, other antianxiety and hypnotic drugs, alcohol, heterocyclic antidepressants, opioid analgesics, antipsychotics, antihistamines including nonprescription sleep aids and cold remedies). The combination of a benzodiazepine and another central nervous system

depressant is not necessarily contraindicated, although the dose of the benzodiazepine may require reduction, close follow-up of the patient may be necessary initially, and/or precautionary advice about activities that require alertness should be stressed.

Acute ingestion of alcohol impairs the metabolic disposition of diazepam, desmethyldiazepam, and chlordiazepoxide (Sellers and Busto, 1982). However, central nervous system function is only slightly more depressed than with either alcohol or the benzodiazepine alone. A psychodynamic interaction between these drugs is primarily responsible.

Cimetidine [Tagamet] inhibits the hepatic microsomal enzymes responsible for the N-dealkylation and hydroxylation of benzodiazepines metabolized by oxidation, but this interaction appears to be of minimal clinical importance (Greenblatt et al, 1984).

Isoniazid prolongs the elimination half-life of diazepam by approximately 30%, probably through inhibition of hepatic microsomal enzymes. (A reduced clearance would be expected for benzodiazepines affected similarly by cimetidine [see above].) However, if the patient also is receiving rifampin, the latter's enzyme-inducing action usually overwhelms the effect of isoniazid; as a result, clearance is increased and the elimination half-life of diazepam is shortened (Ochs et al, 1981). Dosage adjustment of diazepam may be necessary.

Low-dose estrogen-containing oral contraceptives prolong the elimination half-life of diazepam, presumably through inhibition of hepatic microsomal enzymes (Abernethy et al, 1982). Because a direct relationship between diazepam's plasma concentration and clinical effect has not been clearly established, the clinical significance of these interactions has not been established conclusively.

Issues in Prescribing Benzodiazepines: In recent years, the medical use of benzodiazepines has received much attention. There is concern that these drugs, when used as antianxi-

TABLE 2.
ANTIANXIETY AND HYPNOTIC DRUGS: PHARMACOKINETIC DATA

Drug	Oral Absorption: t max hours (Relative Rate)	Most Significant Biologically Active Compounds in Blood	Mean (Range) Elimination Half-life hours	Volume of Distribution L/kg	Clearance ml/min/kg
BENZODIAZEPINES					
Compounds With Active Metabolites					
Chlordiazepoxide	0.5-4	Chlordiazepoxide Desmethylchlor-diazepoxide	9.9 (8-24) (24-96)	0.3 ± 0.03	0.37 ± 0.06
Clorazepate	1-2	Desmethyldiazepam	(50-100)	0.93-1.27	
Diazepam	1.5-2	Diazepam Desmethyldiazepam	(20-50) (50-100)	0.95-2 0.93-1.27	0.38 ± 0.06
Flurazepam	0.5-2	Desalkylflurazepam	(74-160)*		
Halazepam	1-3	Halazepam Desmethyldiazepam	14 (50-100)		
Prazepam	6	Desmethyldiazepam	(50-100)		
Compounds With Weakly Active, Short-lived, or Inactive Metabolites					
Alprazolam	1-2	Alprazolam	12.1 (11.1-19)	1.1	
Clonazepam	1-2	Clonazepam	(18-50)		
Lorazepam	2	Lorazepam	15 (8-25)	1.0-1.3	0.7-1.2
Midazolam	IV USE	Midazolam	2.5 ± 2.17	1.72 ± 0.05	8.1
Oxazepam	1-4	Oxazepam	(5-15)	0.6-2	0.9-2
Quazepam	2	Quazepam	39		
Temazepam	2-3	Temazepam	14.7 (8-38)	1.4-1.5	1.1-1.4
Triazolam	1.3	Triazolam	2.6 (1.7-5.2)	0.8-1.3	3.7-10.6
BARBITURATES					
Phenobarbital	6-18	Phenobarbital	79 (53-118)		
Mephobarbital	6-18	Mephobarbital Phenobarbital	79 (53-118)		
Amobarbital	2	Amobarbital	25 (16-40)		
Pentobarbital	2	Pentobarbital	(15-50)		
Secobarbital	2	Secobarbital	28 (15-40)		

(continued on next page)

Drug	Oral Absorption: t max hours (Relative Rate)	Most Significant Biologically Active Compounds in Blood	Mean (Range) Elimination Half-life hours	Volume of Distribution L/kg	Clearance ml/min/kg
NONBENZODIAZEPINE-NONBARBITURATES					
Antianxiety Agents					
Hydroxyzine		Hydroxyzine	(2.5-3.4)		
Meprobamate	2-3	Meprobamate	(10-24)		
Propranolol (Investigational use)	1-3	Propranolol Hydroxypropranolol	3.9 ± 0.4	3.9 ± 0.6	12 ± 3
Hypnotic Agents (prescription)					
Chloral Hydrate		Trichloroethanol	(4-9.5)		
Ethchlorvynol		Ethchlorvynol	(10-25)		
Ethinamate		Ethinamate	2.5		
Glutethimide		Glutethimide	(5-22)		
Methyprylon		Methyprylon	4		
Paraldehyde	0.5-1	Paraldehyde	7.4 (3.4-9.8)	0.8-1.2	
Hypnotic Agents (antihistamines [nonprescription])					
Diphenhydramine		Diphenhydramine			
Doxylamine		Doxylamine	9.3 (4-12)		
Pyrilamine		Pyrilamine			

Mean half-life (hours): young males, 74; elderly males, 160; young females, 90; elderly females, 120

ety agents and hypnotics, are overprescribed both in terms of the absolute number of people receiving them and in the length of time that patients take them. Questions also have arisen about prescription practices in certain portions of the population, such as women and the elderly.

The charge that the benzodiazepines are overprescribed in this country has not been borne out by analyses of prescription practices (Mellinger and Balter, 1983), which have characterized the prescription of psychotherapeutic agents as moderate if not conservative. Short-term and infrequent use of antianxiety agents and hypnotics are more common than long-term daily use. A total of 1.6% of all adults between 18 and 79 years used these drugs daily for one year or longer. Further analysis of this figure indicated that the long-term use was associated with bona fide health problems being treated within the health care system (Mellinger et al, 1984).

These data raise the question about the long-term efficacy of benzodiazepines as antianxiety agents and hypnotics. More rigorously controlled studies must be carried out on this subject. Some studies suggest that tolerance to diazepam's anxiolytic effect does not develop for as long as 22 weeks (Rickels et al, 1983 A) and that the investigational benzodiazepines, lormetazepam and nitrazepam, retain significant efficacy as hypnotics over 24 weeks (Oswald et al, 1982). Confirmation and extension of these studies are necessary.

More women use antianxiety agents than men, but a study of indications for such use also has deemed such therapy appropriate. Gender differences may reflect a male's reluctance to admit to being sick and to seek medical care. Also, men are more likely to use alcohol to relieve anxiety. Men and women are equally likely to use benzodiazepines for long periods and the tendency for long-term use increases with age in association with the treatment of significant medical problems.

Summary: The benzodiazepines are effective antianxiety and hypnotic agents that should be reserved for patients with significant subjective distress whose ability to function normally has been compromised. The prescribing physician must monitor the patient carefully to assure the need for continuing drug therapy as well as the continuing efficacy and safety of the drug. Dosage and duration of therapy should be minimized. The manner in which the pharmacokinetics of the individual benzodiazepines can be manipulated to maximize the therapeutic effect also should be considered. The benzodiazepines should be used cautiously in a patient with a history of abuse or drug dependence or in a pregnant woman.

Barbiturates

Indications: Derivatives of barbituric acid possess hypnotic and anticonvulsant activity. Of the longer acting barbiturates, phenobarbital and mephobarbital are administered principally for seizure disorders; phenobarbital and butabarbital also are labeled for use as sedatives. The former is preferred during withdrawal after prolonged use of barbiturates and the nonbenzodiazepine-nonbarbiturate drugs (ie, chloral hydrate, ethchlorvynol, ethinamate, glutethimide, meprobamate, methyprylon, paraldehyde). (See also the discussion on Dependence in this section.)

Phenobarbital is prescribed in some cases of congenital hyperbilirubinemia because it enhances the metabolism of bilirubin by enzyme induction.

Amobarbital, pentobarbital, and secobarbital are shorter acting barbiturates labeled for use as hypnotics. However, they lack the specificity of action of the benzodiazepines and, thus, have a lower therapeutic index. These three drugs also are administered orally or parenterally as preanesthetic medication (see Chapter 17) and intravenously to provide regional anesthesia.

The ultrashort-acting barbiturates, thiopental, methohexital, and thiamylal, are used as intravenous general anesthetics. Barbiturate-induced anesthesia decreases brain oxygen utilization by approximately 50% and increases glycogen and high energy phosphate. Because of these actions, barbiturates may be of value for brain resuscitation in metabolic, toxic, or infectious encephalopathy (Frost, 1981; Safar, 1981; Michenfelder, 1982).

Actions: The barbiturates are believed to facilitate inhibitory neurotransmission in the central nervous system, presumably by interacting with proteins of the gamma-aminobutyric acid (GABA) chloride ionophore complex to open chloride ion channels and hyperpolarize neuronal membranes (Brunello and Cheney, 1981). The known actions of barbiturates on membrane lipids, protein synthesis, neurotransmitters other than GABA, and ion regulation have been reviewed (Ho and Harris, 1981).

Pharmacokinetics: All barbiturates are weak acids that are well absorbed orally and intramuscularly, especially their salts. Distribution, in turn, is related to lipid solubility and plasma and protein binding. Phenobarbital, which has the longest onset and duration of action clinically, also has the lowest degree of lipid solubility and protein binding.

All barbiturates are metabolized principally to inactive derivatives by the microsomal enzyme system of the liver. An exception is mephobarbital, which is metabolized in part to phenobarbital. The inactive metabolites are conjugated with glucuronic acid and excreted in the urine, but 25% to 50% of a dose of phenobarbital also is eliminated unchanged in the urine.

See also Table 2 and Breimer, 1977.

Adverse Reactions and Precautions: Drowsiness and lethargy are common in sensitive individuals (eg, the elderly, those with severe liver disease) or in patients taking large doses; residual sedation ("hangover") is common after hypnotic doses. For these reasons, ambulatory patients should be specifically warned to be cautious of or avoid activities that require mental alertness, judgment, and physical coordination (eg, driving a vehicle, operating dangerous machinery), especially if alcohol is ingested concomitantly.

Reactions noted infrequently include skin eruptions (eg, urticaria, angioedema, generalized morbilliform rash, Stevens-Johnson syndrome, discrete violaceous macules) and gastrointestinal disturbances, such as nausea and vomiting. Paradoxical restlessness or excitement and exacerbation of the symptoms of certain organic brain disorders may develop, especially in elderly patients and children.

Because barbiturates may aggravate acute intermittent porphyria by inducing the enzymes responsible for porphyrin synthesis, their use is contraindicated in patients with this disease (Smith and DeMatteis, 1980). Drug-induced hepatitis has been reported with phenobarbital (Lane and Peterson, 1984).

Since the liver is the major site of barbiturate degradation, caution should be observed when these drugs are given to patients with hepatic disease. Pulmonary insufficiency is a relative contraindication, for serious ventilatory depression may occur in these patients.

Great caution should be taken to avoid intra-arterial injection or extravasation of the highly alkaline sodium salts of barbiturates. Injection into an artery provokes intense, prolonged, spastic vasoconstriction and ischemia and has caused gangrene of the extremity. Acute excruciating pain, edema, erythema, inflammation, and obliteration of the distal pulse are rapidly evident in the affected limb. For treatment of this complication, see Chapter 16, General Anesthetics.

Physicians should assess a patient's susceptibility to drug abuse before prescribing a barbiturate. See also Chapter 1, Prescription Practices and Regulatory Agencies.

Pregnancy and Breast Feeding: Reproductive studies in animals reveal no evidence of impaired fertility or harm to the fetus; no adequate controlled studies are available in pregnant women. Results of retrospective, case-controlled studies in pregnant women have suggested that there is an association between maternal consumption of phenobarbital and a higher than expected incidence of fetal abnormalities, but this has not been established. Barbiturates are classified in FDA Pregnancy Category D.

Barbiturates readily cross the placenta and can depress the

neonate's respiration and central nervous system. Withdrawal symptoms and signs are likely to occur in infants born to mothers who are physically dependent on barbiturates during the last trimester.

Cautions concerning the special use of phenobarbital and mephobarbital in epileptics who become pregnant are discussed in Chapter 9.

Small amounts of most barbiturates appear in breast milk, and thus caution should be used when a barbiturate is administered to a nursing mother.

Poisoning: Barbiturates remain one of the leading causes of fatal drug poisoning. Acute poisoning is usually the result of ingestion for suicidal purposes. Some cases have been attributed to a state of drug-induced confusion (automatism) in which the patient forgets having taken the medication and takes more, but there is substantial doubt that this phenomenon exists. The direct or indirect effects of barbiturates and other central nervous system or cardiovascular depressants (eg, alcohol, heterocyclic antidepressants, antihistamines, opiates) taken concomitantly can be fatal. The usual safeguard is to prescribe small quantities of the drug, but some patients may accumulate a supply of medication until they have enough to attempt suicide.

Overdosage of the barbiturates can cause tachycardia, hypotension, profound shock, ventilatory depression, areflexia, coma, and death due to cardioventilatory failure secondary to depression of the vital medullary centers. Good nursing care is of primary importance in barbiturate poisoning, and this may be all that is required if the ventilatory and cardiovascular systems are functioning adequately and there is a positive response to painful stimuli.

If the patient is still conscious and less than four hours have elapsed since ingestion, vomiting may be induced by syrup of ipecac.

Gastric lavage and activated charcoal are used in comatose patients only after an open airway has been secured, if necessary by endotracheal intubation. An adequate airway should be maintained, arterial blood gases should be monitored, and sufficient oxygen should be given to prevent hypoxemia. Controlled ventilation must be instituted if ventilatory failure develops.

Osmotic diuretics and alkalization of the urine significantly increase the renal excretion of phenobarbital. In severe poisoning, hemodialysis or charcoal hemoperfusion may be lifesaving, especially if vigorous diuresis cannot be maintained.

Complications can be avoided by changing the patient's position hourly to prevent pressure sores and hypostatic pneumonia, maintaining adequate hydration and nutrition with parenteral administration of fluids, and providing all standard supportive therapy.

Tolerance: Two types of tolerance may be observed with the barbiturates. Metabolic tolerance may occur when a barbiturate or other drug accelerates the hepatic inactivation of the barbiturate. This type of tolerance is most common with barbiturates that have relatively short half-lives. Pharmacodynamic tolerance results when the depressant effect on the central nervous system decreases after repeated administration. This is noted most frequently with the long-acting barbiturate, phenobarbital, and with large doses of the shorter acting barbiturates. Cross tolerance develops among the barbiturates and between these drugs and alcohol. It is important to remember that, although tolerance develops to the hypnotic effects of barbiturates, the lethal dose does not increase significantly.

Dependence: Chronic intoxication occurs most commonly with use of the short-acting barbiturates, and symptoms are similar to those of alcohol intoxication (eg, disorientation, ataxia, euphoria). Prolonged, uninterrupted use of escalating doses of barbiturates, particularly the short-acting drugs, may result in physical and psychological dependence. Withdrawal reactions have been reported in neonates after maternal ingestion of these drugs.

If a barbiturate appears to have lost its effectiveness after long-term administration, it should be withdrawn slowly. The patient should be warned that unpleasant symptoms (eg, increased frequency and intensity of dreaming, nightmares) may occur. Abrupt withdrawal after several months of use (600 mg or more daily of pentobarbital or secobarbital) may be followed within 24 hours by a severe withdrawal syndrome that is more serious than that caused by opiates. The syndrome usually lasts approximately one week. Status epilepticus may occur with grand mal convulsions (which develop between 12 hours and 12 days after withdrawal), delirium, and, sometimes, progressive hyperpyrexia, coma, and death.

Gradual withdrawal of the offending agent (nonsubstitutive treatment) over ten days to three weeks, depending upon the severity of dependence, is necessary to minimize the signs and symptoms of withdrawal. Because of its long duration of action, phenobarbital is often used as an alternative treatment (substitutive). It is administered in place of the offending drug until signs and symptoms have stabilized (eg, approximately 30 mg of phenobarbital is substituted for each 100 mg of the shorter acting barbiturates). The dose of phenobarbital then is reduced gradually by 10% every 24 hours. Phenobarbital also can be used for substitutive treatment in patients withdrawing from chloral hydrate, ethchlorvynol, ethinamate, glutethimide, methaqualone, methyprylon, paraldehyde, and meprobamate.

An alternative procedure avoids subjective assessment of the degree of drug dependence to determine dose equivalents of phenobarbital (Robinson et al, 1981). With this technique, administration of phenobarbital is not begun until drug blood levels have fallen to twice the upper limit of the normal therapeutic range for the barbiturate or hypnotic abused; this avoids treating patients who are intoxicated on admission but clearly at risk from withdrawal. The loading dose of phenobarbital (120 mg/hour) is given orally until at least three of the following five signs or symptoms are present: nystagmus, drowsiness, ataxia, dysarthria, emotional lability. Major inclusion criteria include (1) a history of seizures or delirium during withdrawal; (2) barbiturate dosage at least 500 mg daily for longer than four weeks; (3) comparable dependence on other hypnotics that produce cross tolerance to barbiturates; and (4) toxic drug level on admission without clinical intoxication (ie, tolerance). The technique reduces the period of hospitalization and allows earlier rehabilitation and development of alternative coping mechanisms.

Amobarbital, pentobarbital, and secobarbital are classified

as Schedule II agents, and butabarbital and phenobarbital are classified as Schedule III and IV agents, respectively. (See Chapter 1, Prescription Practices and Regulatory Agencies, for additional information.)

Drug Interactions: The dosage of barbiturates must be reduced when they are given with other central nervous system depressants (eg, alcohol, other hypnotic and antianxiety agents, heterocyclic antidepressants, opiate analgesics, antipsychotics, antihistamines). Barbiturates must be used with caution in patients receiving monoamine oxidase inhibitors (isocarboxazid, phenelzine, tranylcypromine), since these drugs may potentiate the depressant effects of the barbiturates.

Phenobarbital increases the synthesis and activity of hepatic microsomal enzymes involved in the metabolism of warfarin and dicumarol; the shorter acting barbiturates are less likely to produce this effect. The benzodiazepines are preferred in patients who are also receiving anticoagulants.

Barbiturates may enhance the metabolism of heterocyclic antidepressants, phenytoin, griseofulvin, and adrenal corticosteroids. For example, the administration of phenobarbital to asthmatic patients dependent on corticosteroids has been reported to exacerbate asthma; this effect was reversed when phenobarbital was discontinued. It may be necessary to adjust the dosage schedule of these drugs to maintain control of the disorder.

Summary: The use of the barbiturates as antianxiety agents and sedative-hypnotics has been superseded by that of the benzodiazepines. The benzodiazepines exhibit less abuse and dependence liability and have a greater therapeutic index.

Nonbenzodiazepine-Nonbarbiturates

The benzodiazepines have largely replaced these compounds. Pharmacokinetic data on these agents are fragmentary (see Table 2). Adverse reactions, precautions, and poisoning are discussed in the evaluations. For information on dependence, see the evaluations and the discussion of Dependence in the section on Barbiturates.

Anxiety: Buspirone (investigational drug) is an azaspirodecanedione that has been shown in clinical studies to have an anxiolytic action comparable to that of diazepam (Goldberg and Finnerty, 1982; Rickels et al, 1982). In these studies, diazepam was more effective in reducing somatic symptoms and buspirone appeared to be more effective in reducing symptoms of cognitive and interpersonal problems (Gershon and Eison, 1983). Buspirone produced less sedation, lethargy, and depression and had less tendency to interact with common medications than diazepam. Also, studies in animals and man failed to demonstrate abuse potential. Further studies are necessary to define the exact role of this drug in the treatment of anxiety disorders.

Propranolol and other beta blockers generally are not as effective as benzodiazepines in the treatment of anxiety (Rickels et al, 1983 A). When somatic symptoms of anxiety (eg, tremor, palpitations, tachycardia) are more prominent than psychological symptoms, beta blockers may be useful alone or adjunctively (Frishman et al, 1981); this situation is most common in psychocardiac disorders causally related to anxiety rather than to cardiac ischemia. Controlled studies have suggested that, when psychological symptoms are primary and little somatization is present, beta blockers produce little improvement.

There is interest in the use of beta blockers for acute, situational, anticipatory anxiety (eg, public speaking, stage fright, competitive activities). When functional incapacitation arising from anticipatory anxiety cannot be managed by self-discipline, counseling, and behavioral modification, small doses of beta blockers may be useful. However, the effectiveness of beta blockers under these circumstances is not established conclusively because well-controlled clinical trials have not been performed.

Meprobamate and hydroxyzine are less effective than the benzodiazepines in the treatment of anxiety. Long-term use of larger than usual doses of meprobamate produces physical dependence and this further limits its use. Hydroxyzine, an antihistamine with antiemetic activity, has limited abuse potential and, thus, some usefulness in patients with anxiety who have a history of drug abuse.

Tricyclic antidepressants and monoamine oxidase inhibitors are effective in panic disorders and agoraphobia.

Insomnia: Chloral hydrate is an effective sedative and hypnotic. Because of its rapid onset of action and short half-life, it is especially useful when there is difficulty in falling asleep. Some tolerance to the hypnotic action generally develops within five weeks. Although the benefit/risk ratio is not as good as that of the benzodiazepines, this drug may be the preferred alternative among the nonbenzodiazepine hypnotics in selected patients.

Ethinamate, ethchlorvynol, glutethimide, and methyprylon have very limited or variable antianxiety action and are marketed only for treatment of insomnia. Ethinamate and ethchlorvynol have low potency and, like chloral hydrate, have a rapid onset and brief duration of action. In some studies, the hypnotic effect was reported to be less predictable than that of chloral hydrate, and their overall safety is judged to be comparable to that of the barbiturates.

The effect of the two piperidinedione derivatives, glutethimide and methyprylon, on electroencephalographic sleep patterns is similar to that of the barbiturates. Management of overdosage with these drugs can be very difficult, especially the cardiovascular manifestations. Glutethimide and methyprylon rarely, if ever, should be considered drugs of choice for insomnia.

Since serotonin plays a role in inducing and maintaining normal sleep, *l*-tryptophan has been administered orally to increase brain levels of serotonin. Although a dose of 1 g significantly decreased sleep latency and total time awake without altering sleep patterns, the hypnotic action is observed only during the early part of the sleep cycle, is unpredictable, and is not characterized by a satisfactory dose-response relationship (Hartmann, 1977). Because the hypnotic action has not been confirmed in other studies, this use of *l*-tryptophan must be considered investigational and the drug is not recommended in routine clinical practice.

An OTC Sedative, Sleep-Aid and Tranquilizer Panel appointed by the FDA concluded that short-term use of certain antihistamines as sleep aids may be acceptable, but the Panel urged that better controlled studies be conducted to establish their usefulness and safety. Subsequent studies (Rickels et al, 1983 B, 1984) demonstrated that diphenhydramine and doxylamine produced significantly more improvement in several sleep parameters, including sleep latency, the target symptom for OTC sleep aids, than did placebo. However, these effects were less pronounced than those of the benzodiazepines. Pyrilamine also is available as a single-entity OTC sleep-aid.

Drug Evaluations

BENZODIAZEPINES

ALPRAZOLAM
[Xanax]

USES. Alprazolam, a novel triazolobenzodiazepine compound with antianxiety and sedative-hypnotic actions, is effective in the treatment of panic disorder, agoraphobia, situational anxiety, and generalized anxiety disorder. Studies have indicated that alprazolam also may be useful in major depressive episodes (Feighner et al, 1983; Rickels et al, 1985), but further clinical study is necessary to define alprazolam's role in this disorder.

ADVERSE REACTIONS AND PRECAUTIONS. Drowsiness is the most common side effect reported but is generally less than that noted with diazepam at equieffective doses. Other reactions are similar to those of other benzodiazepines. Although these occasionally may be severe, most are mild and seldom require discontinuation of therapy. Caution should be observed when other drugs possessing sedative actions are given with alprazolam.

Physical or psychological dependence is likely when larger than usual doses are prescribed or therapy is prolonged. Withdrawal reactions, including seizures, have been reported in patients receiving long-term alprazolam therapy in whom the dose was decreased rapidly or the drug was discontinued abruptly. Thus, as with all benzodiazepines, treatment should be terminated by gradually reducing the dose.

See the Introduction for additional information on adverse reactions, precautions, interactions, use during pregnancy, poisoning, and dependence. This drug is classified in FDA Pregnancy Category D.

PHARMACOKINETICS. Alprazolam is rapidly and well absorbed orally. The time to peak blood level is one to two hours. Protein binding is about 70%, generally less than for other benzodiazepines. Although this benzodiazepine is biotransformed, the range of half-life in many patients overlaps the ranges for lorazepam, oxazepam, and temazepam. The elimination half-life is longer in elderly males (19 hours) than in young males (11.1 hours). The major metabolite, alpha-hydroxyalprazolam, is conjugated and excreted rapidly and is eliminated principally in the urine as the glucuronide conjugate. When given three times a day, steady-state levels of alprazolam are attained in two to five days.

DOSAGE AND PREPARATIONS.

Oral: For anxiety, *adults,* 0.25 to 0.5 mg three times a day (maximum daily dose, 4 mg); *elderly or debilitated patients,* 0.25 mg two or three times daily.

For panic disorder or agoraphobia, *adults,* 0.5 mg three times daily after meals for two days. The dose is increased by adding 0.5 mg to one of the existing doses every two days until 2 mg three times daily is given. The upward titration should be stopped when significant improvement or excessive sedation becomes evident. Doses of 3 to 6 mg/day usually are necessary for therapeutic effect.

Xanax (Upjohn). Tablets 0.25, 0.5, and 1 mg.

CHLORDIAZEPOXIDE
[Libritabs]

CHLORDIAZEPOXIDE HYDROCHLORIDE
[Librium]

USES. Chlordiazepoxide is effective in the management of situational anxiety and generalized anxiety disorder and also is used to ameliorate the symptoms of alcohol withdrawal and as a preanesthetic medication. It is slightly more useful in relieving anxiety than nonbenzodiazepines. Its anticonvulsant and muscle relaxant actions are less pronounced than those of diazepam.

ADVERSE REACTIONS AND PRECAUTIONS. Large doses have caused hypotension and syncope, and usual oral doses have exacerbated ventilatory failure in patients with chronic bronchitis. Increased or decreased libido, agranulocytosis, jaundice, and a lupus erythematosus-like syndrome have been reported rarely. In one patient, parkinsonism was exacerbated upon initiation of chlordiazepoxide treatment. This drug also may cause excitement, depression, confusion, and hallucinations.

Long-term use of larger than usual doses may produce psychological and physical dependence. Withdrawal symptoms were reported in twin neonates during the third week of life when the mother had taken 20 to 30 mg daily throughout pregnancy.

Chlordiazepoxide has a wide margin of safety unless taken with alcohol or other central nervous system depressants. Although coma has been reported after ingestion of 300 mg, it has not developed after ingestion of 1 g, and patients have recovered after taking as much as 2.5 g in a single dose.

See the Introduction for additional information on adverse reactions, precautions, interactions, use during pregnancy, poisoning, and dependence.

PHARMACOKINETICS. Chlordiazepoxide is absorbed more rapidly and predictably after oral than after intramuscular administration, but blood levels vary widely among individuals. The elimination half-life of the major active metabolite, desmethylchlordiazepoxide, ranges from one to four days; therefore, cumulative effects can occur with repeated daily administration.

DOSAGE AND PREPARATIONS.

Oral: Adults, for anxiety, 15 to 100 mg divided into three or four doses or once daily at bedtime; *elderly or debilitated patients,* 5 mg two to four times daily; *children over 6 years,* 5 mg two to four times daily. Information is inadequate to establish dosage for *children under 6 years.*

CHLORDIAZEPOXIDE:
Libritabs (Roche). Tablets 5, 10, and 25 mg.
CHLORDIAZEPOXIDE HYDROCHLORIDE:
Librium (Roche), **Generic.** Capsules 5, 10, and 25 mg.

Intravenous: For severe withdrawal symptoms in acute alcoholism, *adults,* 50 to 100 mg given cautiously over at least one minute, repeated, if necessary, in two to four hours. The dose may be reduced to 25 to 50 mg three or four times daily if necessary. The total daily dose should not exceed 300 mg. Oral administration should be substituted as soon as possible. The dose should be reduced by one-half in *elderly or debilitated patients.*

CHLORDIAZEPOXIDE HYDROCHLORIDE:
Librium (Roche). Powder 100 mg in 5 ml containers.

CLORAZEPATE DIPOTASSIUM
[Tranxene]

USES. Clorazepate is used in the treatment of situational and generalized anxiety disorders, seizure disorders, and alcohol withdrawal. Its anxiolytic efficacy is equal to that of diazepam and depends upon conversion of the parent compound to active metabolites.

ADVERSE REACTIONS AND PRECAUTIONS. The most common adverse effects are similar to those of the other benzodiazepines. In addition, blurred vision, confusion, and depression occur occasionally.

Long-term therapy with larger than usual doses may produce psychological and physical dependence. Clorazepate is contraindicated in patients with acute angle-closure glaucoma.

See the Introduction for additional information on adverse reactions, precautions, interactions, use during pregnancy, poisoning, and dependence.

PHARMACOKINETICS. Clorazepate undergoes decarboxylation to desmethyldiazepam in liquid, and the rate of conversion is accelerated at low pH. Therefore, the drug is almost totally converted to desmethyldiazepam in the stomach and is absorbed rapidly by the gastrointestinal tract, primarily in this form. Accumulation occurs with repeated administration until steady-state plasma concentrations of desmethyldiazepam are reached (one to two weeks).

DOSAGE AND PREPARATIONS.

Oral: Adults, for anxiety, 15 to 60 mg in two to four divided doses or a single dose at bedtime; *elderly or debilitated patients,* initially, 7.5 to 15 mg daily.

Tranxene (Abbott). Capsules and tablets 3.75, 7.5, and 15 mg; tablets 11.25 and 22.5 mg (*Tranxene-SD*).

DIAZEPAM
[Valium, Valrelease]

USES. Diazepam is effective in the management of situational anxiety and generalized anxiety disorder in appropriately selected patients. It is also used for skeletal muscle relaxation, for seizure disorders, for preanesthetic medication or intravenous anesthetic induction, and for alleviating abstinence symptoms during alcohol withdrawal. See the Introduction and Table 1 for additional information.

ADVERSE REACTIONS AND PRECAUTIONS. The most common adverse reactions are similar to those of other benzodiazepines (see the Introduction). Untoward effects noted occasionally are blurred vision, diplopia, hypotension, amnesia, slurred speech, tremor, urinary incontinence, and constipation; one case of transitory leukopenia has been reported. Diazepam causes paradoxical aggression and excitement rarely. Depression probably represents an undiagnosed, concomitant, previously masked condition. Suicidal impulses have been reported in several patients taking 40 to 60 mg daily. Apnea and cardiac arrest have occurred rarely, usually after intravenous administration, in elderly or severely ill patients, in those receiving other central nervous system depressant drugs, or in those with limited ventilatory reserve. Intravenous injection may cause local pain and thrombophlebitis. Gynecomastia has been reported with the long-term use or abuse of diazepam.

Diazepam is subject to abuse and may produce physical

dependence after prolonged administration. It is classified as a Schedule IV agent under the Controlled Substances Act.

PREGNANCY AND LACTATION. Cleft lip, with or without cleft palate, has been reported when diazepam was used during the first trimester of pregnancy. More recent data suggest that exposure to diazepam during the first trimester does not materially affect the risk of cleft lip with or without cleft palate or of cleft palate alone. Diazepam and desmethyldiazepam cross the placenta during labor, and fetal concentrations may exceed those in the mother. Available evidence suggests that intramuscular or intravenous administration of more than 30 mg during the final 15 hours of labor can produce low Apgar scores, apnea, hypothermia, and poor sucking in the newborn infant (floppy-infant syndrome).

Although detectable amounts of diazepam appear in breast milk, effects on the nursing infant are insignificant if doses do not exceed 10 mg daily.

PHARMACOKINETICS. Diazepam is absorbed rapidly and predictably after oral administration. Injection into the deltoid muscle area increases the likelihood of rapid and complete absorption after intramuscular administration (Divoll et al, 1983). Cumulative effects can occur with repeated administration until steady-state plasma concentrations are achieved (one to two weeks). The half-life ranges from 20 to 70 hours; however, the major active metabolite of diazepam, desmethyldiazepam, has a half-life ranging from 50 to 100 hours. Another active metabolite, temazepam, has a very short half-life and is clinically unimportant after usual therapeutic doses of diazepam are administered. The half-lives of diazepam and its major active metabolites are usually increased in neonates, the elderly, and those with severe hepatic disorders.

DOSAGE AND PREPARATIONS.
Oral: Adults, for anxiety, 4 to 40 mg daily in two to four divided doses or a single dose of 2.5 to 10 mg at bedtime; *elderly or debilitated patients and those taking other central nervous system depressants concomitantly,* initially, 2 to 2.5 mg once or twice daily, increased gradually as needed or tolerated. *Children,* 0.12 to 0.8 mg/kg daily in three or four divided doses. A timed-release preparation [Valrelease] is recommended only when it has been determined that the optimal dose of diazepam is at least 5 mg three times daily. The usual daily dose is one or two capsules depending on the severity of symptoms.

   Valium (Roche), ***Generic.*** Tablets 2, 5, and 10 mg.
   Valrelease (Roche). Capsules (timed-release) 15 mg.

Intravenous, Intramuscular (deep): When used intravenously, the solution should be injected slowly, taking at least one minute for each 5 mg (1 ml) given. Small veins, such as those on the dorsum of the hand or wrist, should not be used. Extreme care should be taken to avoid intra-arterial administration or extravasation. Diazepam should not be mixed with other solutions or drugs or added to intravenous fluids. If it is not feasible to administer diazepam directly, it may be injected slowly through the infusion tubing as close as possible to the vein insertion.

For severe anxiety or severe muscle spasm associated with local trauma, spasticity, akathisia, or tetanus, *adults,* initially, 5 to 10 mg, repeated in three to four hours if necessary; larger doses may be required for tetanus. *Children,* 0.04 to 0.2 mg/kg

initially, repeated in three to four hours if necessary (maximum, 0.6 mg/kg in an eight-hour period). Diazepam should not be used in spastic patients with respiratory difficulty unless equipment for assisted ventilation is available.

For acute alcohol withdrawal, *adults,* initially, 5 to 20 mg intravenously, then 5 to 10 mg in three to four hours if necessary, followed by oral therapy.

   Valium (Roche). Solution 5 mg/ml in 2 and 10 ml containers.

FLURAZEPAM HYDROCHLORIDE
[Dalmane]

USES. Flurazepam is chemically and pharmacologically similar to the other benzodiazepines. This drug is marketed exclusively for use in insomnia. Results of well-controlled clinical and sleep laboratory studies have shown that flurazepam significantly reduces sleep-induction time, number of awakenings, and time spent awake and increases the duration of sleep. Hypnotic effects begin an average of 17 minutes after oral administration and last seven to eight hours. In a small controlled sleep study, flurazepam was reported to maintain its effectiveness for up to four weeks.

Flurazepam produces, at least initially, residual daytime sedation in most patients due to the production of a long-acting metabolite. Therefore, the drug is most appropriate for the intermittent treatment of long-term insomnia and for short-term therapy when a benzodiazepine with a long elimination half-life and a resulting daytime anxiolytic effect is desirable (Mitler et al, 1984).

The percentage of REM sleep is reduced during therapy because total sleep time is increased significantly without a proportional increase in the amount of REM sleep, almost entirely due to an increase in Stage 2 sleep. Like other benzodiazepines, flurazepam reduces sleep in Stages 3 and 4. After discontinuing therapy, the sleep stage pattern returns to normal. The clinical significance of the alteration in sleep pattern has not been established.

Rebound insomnia is not as prominent, if it occurs at all, with flurazepam as it is with shorter acting benzodiazepines (Kales et al, 1979).

ADVERSE REACTIONS AND PRECAUTIONS. Ataxia and vertigo may occur, especially in elderly or debilitated patients. Paradoxical reactions (eg, excitement, nervousness, euphoria, irritability) also have been observed.

Flurazepam is contraindicated in pregnant women. Also, patients should be cautioned that an additive central nervous system depressant effect may occur if alcohol is consumed the day after flurazepam administration.

See the Introduction for additional information on adverse reactions, precautions, interactions, use during pregnancy, poisoning, and dependence.

PHARMACOKINETICS. The major metabolite of flurazepam, N-desalkylflurazepam, is active and has a long half-life. Mean half-lives (in hours) are: 74 for young males and 160 for elderly males; 90 for young females and 120 for elderly females (Greenblatt et al, 1981). Accumulation of this metabolite may be responsible for some degree of drowsiness or impairment of daytime skills, especially with doses of 30 mg. However, these effects do not consistently parallel the actual increase in plasma concentration of N-desalkylflurazepam, possibly because of adaptation. Slow elimination of this metabolite on termination of therapy probably accounts for minimal rebound insomnia.

DOSAGE AND PREPARATIONS.
Oral: For sleep induction, *adults,* 30 mg at bedtime (15 mg may be adequate in some patients); *elderly or debilitated patients,* 15 mg. Information is inadequate to establish a dosage in *children under 15 years.*

Dalmane (Roche). Capsules 15 and 30 mg.

HALAZEPAM
[Paxipam]

USES. Halazepam is indicated for situational anxiety and generalized anxiety disorder or for the short-term relief of symptoms when anxiety associated with other disorders is not controlled by more specific medication. Tolerance did not develop to the antianxiety action after four months. In animal studies, halazepam demonstrated hypnotic, anticonvulsant, and muscle relaxant properties.

See the Introduction for additional information on anxiety and its management.

ADVERSE REACTIONS, PRECAUTIONS, AND DRUG INTERACTIONS. The most common side effect is drowsiness (incidence, 29%). Other central nervous system effects (incidence, 9%) include headache, apathy, psychomotor retardation, disorientation, confusion, euphoria, dysarthria, depression, and syncope. Dizziness (8%), ataxia (5%), fatigue (4%), and paradoxical agitation or rage reaction (1%) also occurred. Gastrointestinal disturbances were observed in 9% of patients.

Like other benzodiazepines, halazepam has a low order of acute toxicity. One study (Jaffe et al, 1983) indicated that its abuse potential may be lower than that of diazepam. Overdosage is characterized by confusion, impaired coordination, respiratory depression, hypotension, and coma.

No adverse drug interactions peculiar to halazepam have been reported. Additive sedation with alcohol and other central nervous system depressant drugs occur (see the Introduction).

Precautions for the use of halazepam include those for the benzodiazepines in general: avoidance of alcohol and hazardous tasks, as well as use in suicidal patients or those with a history of drug abuse.

PREGNANCY AND LACTATION. Sufficient data are unavailable to evaluate the use of halazepam during pregnancy or lactation. Because benzodiazepines potentially cause fetal harm when administered to pregnant women and because of its chemical similarity to diazepam, halazepam is classified in FDA Pregnancy Category D. The drug crosses the placenta and appears in breast milk.

Until more data become available, it is assumed that the use of halazepam just prior to delivery is likely to depress the neonate (neonatal flaccidity or floppy-infant syndrome). Mothers dependent on halazepam during the third trimester are likely to deliver dependent infants who require additional management.

PHARMACOKINETICS. Oral bioavailability is good and the rate of absorption is rapid (time to peak effect, one to three hours). Protein binding is at least 90%. The elimination half-life of the parent compound is 14 hours, but that of desmethyldiazepam ranges from 50 to 100 hours. Accumulation can occur with repeated doses, especially in the elderly or those with significant hepatic (but not renal) impairment.

DOSAGE AND PREPARATIONS.
Oral: For anxiety, *adults,* 20 to 40 mg three or four times a day; *elderly or sensitive patients,* 20 mg once or twice a day. Information is inadequate to establish a dose in *children under 18 years.*

Paxipam (Schering). Tablets 20 and 40 mg.

LORAZEPAM
[Ativan]

USES. Lorazepam is an effective antianxiety and hypnotic agent (Ameer and Greenblatt, 1981). Because of its amnesic action when given parenterally, it is used as a preanesthetic medication. Lorazepam also may be useful in the treatment of status epilepticus (Walker et al, 1979; Leppik et al, 1983), the acute alcohol abstinence syndrome (Solomon et al, 1983; O'Brien et al, 1983), and neuroleptic-induced catatonia (Fricchione et al, 1983) (see Chapters 17, Adjuncts to Anesthesia; 9, Antiepileptic Drugs; and 8, Drugs Used in Other Mental Disorders).

ADVERSE REACTIONS AND PRECAUTIONS. The most common untoward effects of lorazepam are sedation (15.9%), dizziness (6.9%), weakness (4.2%), and ataxia (3.4%). These reactions abate in over 50% of patients during continued administration; the remainder usually respond to reduction of the dose. Other reactions are similar to those of benzodiazepines in general (see the Introduction). Only minimal effects on respiration and cardiovascular reflexes have been noted, even when large doses were given.

Some patients developed leukopenia and elevated lactic dehydrogenase levels; therefore, periodic monitoring during long-term therapy is suggested. Systematic clinical studies have not been performed to determine whether lorazepam is effective for more than four months. Longer therapy should be based on periodic reassessment of the drug's effectiveness.

Based on lorazepam's chemical structure and actions, dependence liability is expected to be similar to that with other benzodiazepines.

Until sufficient clinical experience is available, the drug should be avoided in pregnant and nursing women and in children younger than 12 years. The parenteral form of lorazepam is classified in FDA Pregnancy Category D.

See the Introduction for additional information on adverse reactions, precautions, interactions, use during pregnancy, poisoning, and dependence.

PHARMACOKINETICS. Like oxazepam, lorazepam is not metabolized to an active derivative. It is eliminated principally as the inactive glucuronide, and cumulative effects are not likely after daily administration. This drug has a relatively short half-life of 15 hours (range, 8 to 25 hours) (Greenblatt, 1981). Lorazepam also resembles oxazepam in that the half-life, volume of distribution, and systemic clearance are reported to be unaltered by age (up to the seventh decade) or alcoholic cirrhosis or acute viral hepatitis (Kraus et al, 1978). The drug should be used cautiously in elderly patients and in those with impaired renal function.

Although it is almost completely absorbed, absorption after oral administration is somewhat slow (the peak effect and peak plasma concentrations occur in about two hours). The parenteral formulation is reliably absorbed intramuscularly; however, pain at the injection site has been reported occasionally.

DOSAGE AND PREPARATIONS.
Oral: Adults, for anxiety, initially, 1 to 2 mg two or three times daily; the usual range is 2 to 6 mg daily in divided doses. The dose can be increased gradually if needed to a maximum of 10 mg daily in two or three divided doses. For insomnia associated with anxiety or transient situational stress, a single dose of 2 to 4 mg is given at bedtime. These doses should be reduced by one-half initially in *elderly or debilitated patients.*
  Ativan (Wyeth), *Generic.* Tablets 0.5, 1, and 2 mg.

OXAZEPAM
  [Serax]

ACTIONS AND USES. This drug is similar to the other benzodiazepines in its effectiveness in situational anxiety, generalized anxiety disorder, alcohol withdrawal, and insomnia.

ADVERSE REACTIONS AND PRECAUTIONS. The incidence of adverse reactions is low. Drowsiness is most common and may occur after a daily dose of 60 mg. Reactions noted occasionally include rash, nausea, dizziness, syncope, hypotension, tachycardia, edema, nightmares, lethargy, slurred speech, and such paradoxical reactions as excitement and confusion. The incidence of ataxia is less than with related drugs. Leukopenia, eosinophilia, and hepatic dysfunction have occurred rarely. The long-term use of larger than usual doses may result in psychological and physical dependence.

See the Introduction for additional information on adverse reactions, precautions, interactions, use during pregnancy, poisoning, and dependence.

PHARMACOKINETICS. Oxazepam has a short elimination half-life (5 to 15 hours), because it, like lorazepam and temazepam, is metabolized to inactive glucuronide metabolites; thus, accumulation is less likely. The inactive glucuronide is eliminated by the kidney. Since no metabolically active products are formed, the pharmacokinetic parameters of oxazepam are not altered significantly by liver disease (alcoholic cirrhosis, acute viral hepatitis). Nevertheless, until more data are available on possible receptor sensitivity to oxazepam in the elderly and those with hepatic and renal disorders, this drug should be used cautiously in these patients.

DOSAGE AND PREPARATIONS.
Oral: For anxiety, *adults,* 30 to 120 mg daily divided into three or four doses. *Elderly patients,* initially, 30 mg daily divided into three doses; if necessary, the dose may be increased cautiously to 45 to 60 mg daily divided into three or four doses. *Children 6 to 12 years,* information is inadequate to establish a dosage; this agent should not be used in *children under 6 years.*
  Serax (Wyeth). Capsules 10, 15, and 30 mg; tablets 15 mg.

PRAZEPAM
  [Centrax]

Prazepam is effective in the treatment of situational anxiety and generalized anxiety disorder (Greenblatt and Shader, 1978).

ADVERSE REACTIONS AND PRECAUTIONS. The untoward effects are similar to those of other benzodiazepines. Reactions observed most frequently are fatigue (11.6%), dizziness (8.7%), weakness (7.7%), drowsiness (6.8%), lightheadedness (6.8%), and ataxia (5%).

Prazepam is excreted in breast milk and should be avoided in nursing mothers. It is not recommended for use during pregnancy or in children and is contraindicated in patients with acute angle-closure glaucoma.

Based on prazepam's chemical structure, metabolism, and available data, tolerance, intoxication, dependence, and interactions are expected to resemble those of other benzodiazepines. (See the Introduction.)

PHARMACOKINETICS. Like diazepam, halazepam, and clorazepate, prazepam is converted primarily to desmethyldiazepam, which appears to be the principal active metabolite. This conversion occurs relatively slowly in the liver, and peak levels of desmethyldiazepam are observed approximately six hours after oral administration. A mean half-life of 60 hours (range, 50 to 100 hours) has been reported, which represents desmethyldiazepam.

DOSAGE AND PREPARATIONS.
Oral: For anxiety, *adults,* initially, 20 mg as a single dose; if necessary, the dose may be increased to 40 to 60 mg daily given in divided amounts or as a single dose, usually at bedtime. *Elderly or debilitated patients,* 10 to 15 mg.

Centrax (Parke-Davis). Capsules 5, 10, and 20 mg; tablets 10 mg.

QUAZEPAM
[Dormalin]

USES. Quazepam is useful in the treatment of insomnia characterized by difficulty in falling asleep, frequent nocturnal awakenings, and/or early morning awakenings. It has been shown to decrease sleep latency and total wake time and increase total sleep time.

ADVERSE REACTIONS AND PRECAUTIONS. The most frequent side effect associated with quazepam is daytime drowsiness. Headache, fatigue, dizziness, dry mouth, and dyspepsia also are common. Paradoxical reactions (eg, excitement, nervousness, agitation, hallucinations) have been observed.

Quazepam is contraindicated in patients with known hypersensitivity to it or other benzodiazepines. It is also contraindicated in patients with established or suspected sleep apnea. Quazepam is contraindicated during pregnancy because the potential risks outweigh the possible benefits. Patients taking quazepam should be cautioned about the potential for an additive central nervous system depressant effect if alcohol is consumed within several days of quazepam administration.

See the Introduction for additional information on adverse reactions, precautions, interactions, use during pregnancy, poisoning, and dependence.

PHARMACOKINETICS. This drug is rapidly absorbed after oral administration. Quazepam, the active parent compound, is metabolized in the liver to 2-oxoquazepam and N-desalkyl-2-oxoquazepam, which have exhibited central nervous system activity in animal models. Quazepam is approximately 95% bound to plasma protein. The mean elimination half-life of quazepam is 39 hours; its two active metabolites have half-lives of 39 and 73 hours, respectively.

DOSAGE AND PREPARATIONS.
Oral: Adults, initially, 15 mg until the response is determined. In some patients, the dose may be reduced to 7.5 mg. In *elderly and debilitated patients*, an attempt should be made to reduce the nightly dose. Information is inadequate to establish a dosage for *children under 18 years*.

Dormalin (Schering). Tablets 15 mg.

TEMAZEPAM
[Restoril]

USES. Temazepam, a hydroxylated minor metabolite of diazepam, is marketed only for the treatment of insomnia, although it also has been shown to have an antianxiety action in clinical studies. The drug decreases the total number of awakenings, increases total sleep time, and improves the subjective quality of sleep. Sleep latency (onset of sleep) was not affected in controlled studies, probably because temazepam is absorbed slowly. Thus, when taken at bedtime, this drug does not induce sleep (Kales et al, 1983). This problem may be circumvented by taking temazepam one to two hours before bedtime, but flurazepam and triazolam are generally preferred when trouble falling asleep is the presenting complaint.

Suggested adult doses of 30 mg (elderly, 15 mg) may impair daytime performance; hypnotic doses of 15 mg do not impair daytime skills, except in some elderly patients. Doses of 40 mg or more significantly reduce respiratory function and body temperature in some patients.

See the Introduction for additional information on insomnia and its management.

ADVERSE REACTIONS AND PRECAUTIONS. Side effects are usually mild and diminish with continued administration. Those reported most frequently are morning drowsiness (17%), dizziness (7%), lethargy (5%), confusion (2% to 3%), and gastrointestinal disturbances (anorexia, diarrhea) (1% to 2%). Reactions with an incidence of less than 1% include vertigo, dryness of the mouth, paresthesias, tachycardia, panic reaction, nystagmus, paradoxical excitement, and hallucinations.

Like other benzodiazepines, temazepam has a low order of acute toxicity. Overdosage is characterized principally by confusion, impaired coordination, respiratory depression, coma, and hypotension.

Precautions for the use of temazepam include those for benzodiazepines in general: avoidance of alcohol and hazardous tasks, as well as use in patients with a history of drug abuse or suicidal tendencies.

Tolerance or withdrawal reactions were not observed after nightly administration for one month. However, patients should be advised that sleep may be somewhat disturbed for a night or two following termination of therapy.

No adverse drug interactions peculiar to temazepam have been reported. Additive sedation with alcohol and other central nervous system depressant drugs would be anticipated, but not that reported with cimetidine (see the Introduction).

Dysmorphogenic changes in rib formation were observed in two animal species given 50 to 100 times the human dose. Use of temazepam during pregnancy should be avoided (FDA Pregnancy Category X).

PHARMACOKINETICS. Oral bioavailability is 100%, but the rate of absorption is relatively slow (mean time to peak concentration in young adults, 2.18 to 2.75 hours). Volume of distribution ranges from 1.4 to 1.53 L/kg and clearance from 1.10 to 1.36 ml/kg/min. The elimination half-life ranges from 8 to 38 hours (mean, 14.7 hours) (Divoll et al, 1981). In earlier studies, the reported elimination half-life was 15 to 30 hours in the elderly.

Temazepam is conjugated principally with glucuronic acid and excreted in the urine, but a small amount is N-demethylated prior to conjugation. As with lorazepam and oxazepam, hepatic dysfunction should have little effect on the elimination half-life of temazepam. Metabolic enzyme induction was not evident after five to seven days of administration. Accumulation after repeated use is generally not a problem, but further study in the elderly is required.

DOSAGE AND PREPARATIONS.
Oral: For sleep induction, *adults,* 30 mg at bedtime; in some patients, 15 mg may be sufficient. *Elderly or sensitive patients,* 15 mg. Information is inadequate to establish a dosage for *children under 18 years.*
   Restoril (Sandoz). Capsules 15 and 30 mg.

TRIAZOLAM
[Halcion]

USES. This triazolobenzodiazepine compound is effective in the treatment of insomnia. Triazolam is appropriate for use in transient insomnia and for intermittent administration in short-term or long-term insomnia when daytime sedation and an antianxiety action are not needed.

The sleep induced by triazolam is characterized by (1) shortened sleep-onset time, (2) delay in the onset but not the total percentage of REM sleep, (3) reduction of Stage 4 sleep but increased total sleep time, (4) decreased number of nocturnal awakenings, (5) a quality of sleep described as good in controlled studies, and (6) absence of REM rebound.

Rebound insomnia with use of triazolam has been reported in a number of studies.

Single doses of 0.125 to 0.25 mg at bedtime were more effective than placebo in controlled studies and were not associated with residual daytime impairment. In controlled studies, a single dose of 0.5 mg at bedtime was more effective than 0.25 mg and was equivalent to 30 mg of flurazepam; however, many individuals experienced daytime impairment with this dose. Recent evidence suggests that the initial dose should be limited to 0.25 mg or less.

Tolerance to the hypnotic effect does not appear to develop after one to two months of treatment.

See the Introduction for additional information on insomnia and its management.

ADVERSE REACTIONS AND PRECAUTIONS. The most common side effects are drowsiness, dizziness, and headache; however, in controlled studies, these symptoms occur as frequently with a placebo. Hallucinations have been reported (0.1%), as has moderate to marked confusion (frequency uncertain). Intrahepatic cholestasis has been associated with the use of triazolam, but a causal relationship has not been demonstrated conclusively.

Additive sedation with alcohol and other central nervous system depressant drugs would be anticipated. No adverse interactions were observed in a six-week study of 56 psychiatric inpatients who were receiving one to five additional psychoactive drugs.

Like other benzodiazepines, triazolam has a low order of acute toxicity. Overdosage is characterized principally by respiratory depression, coma, and hypotension.

Precautions for the use of triazolam include those for benzodiazepines in general: avoidance of alcohol and hazardous tasks, as well as in suicidal patients and in those with a history of drug abuse.

Data are inadequate to evaluate the use of this drug during pregnancy or lactation, but triazolam is classified in FDA Pregnancy Category X.

PHARMACOKINETICS. Triazolam is rapidly and well absorbed orally. Time to peak concentration is 1.25 hours. Protein binding is about 90%. Volume of distribution is 0.8 to 1.3 L/kg. Clearance is 3.7 to 10.6 ml/min/kg, and no significant difference is noted between sexes or with age. The elimination half-life is 2.6 hours (range, 1.7 to 5.2 hours). The two major metabolites of triazolam have little if any hypnotic activity, and their elimination half-lives are less than four hours. Following hydroxylation and subsequent glucuronide conjugation, metabolites of triazolam are eliminated in the urine (Eberts et al, 1981). Accumulation does not occur with daily use for at least three months.

DOSAGE AND PREPARATIONS.
Oral: For insomnia, *adults,* initially, 0.25 mg or less (range, 0.125 to 0.5 mg) but, as with all medications, the lowest effective dose should given. *Elderly or sensitive patients,* initially, 0.125 mg until individual response is determined; up to 0.25 mg may be given. Information is inadequate to establish a dose for *children under 18 years.*
   Halcion (Upjohn). Tablets 0.125 mg, 0.25 and 0.5 mg.

BARBITURATES

PHENOBARBITAL

PHENOBARBITAL SODIUM

ACTIONS AND USES. Phenobarbital differs from shorter acting analogues in that it is used in seizure disorders (see Chapter 9) and occasionally as a daytime sedative or for mild anxiety. This barbiturate is generally given orally but may be administered parenterally if necessary. Phenobarbital also is employed to treat barbiturate and other nonbenzodiazepine withdrawal syndromes (see the Introduction).

Since phenobarbital decreases serum bilirubin levels, it has been used in newborn infants to prevent physiologic jaundice and to treat hyperbilirubinemia, but a hemorrhagic diathesis has been observed occasionally. Phenobarbital also reduces elevated serum bilirubin levels in older children and adults with Gilbert's disease (familial nonhemolytic nonobstructive jaundice). This action may be mediated, at least in part, by the enhanced formation of bilirubin glucuronide. Phenobarbital is also given to control signs and symptoms of withdrawal in infants of mothers addicted to opioids and short-acting barbiturates. (See Chapter 8, Drugs Used in Other Mental Disorders.)

PRECAUTIONS. Long-term use of larger than usual doses may result in physical and psychological dependence. See the Introduction for adverse reactions, other precautions, and interactions.

The safety of this agent during pregnancy has not been established, but barbiturates are classified in FDA Pregnancy Category D. See also Chapter 9, Antiepileptic Drugs.

PHARMACOKINETICS. When phenobarbital is given orally, 80% of the dose is absorbed and peak blood levels occur after 6 to 18 hours; the half-life is three to four days. Ten to thirty percent of the maternal plasma concentration is present in breast milk, and fetal and maternal plasma concentrations are almost equal. Approximately 25% of a dose is eliminated unchanged in the urine; the remainder is converted to inactive hydroxylated products that are then conjugated.

Phenobarbital is a potent inducer of hepatic microsomal enzymes and thus can influence the hepatic biotransformation of drugs (eg, oral anticoagulants, chlorpromazine). Pharmacodynamic tolerance may develop in the central nervous system but the mechanism is unknown; this is observed primarily when large doses are taken. Death can occur after ingestion of several grams. The fatal blood level in nontolerant individuals is usually 8 to 12 mg/dl.

DOSAGE AND PREPARATIONS.
PHENOBARBITAL:
Oral: For anxiety, *adults,* 30 to 120 mg daily in two or three divided doses; *children,* 6 mg/kg daily in three divided doses. For sleep induction, *adults,* 100 to 320 mg. Because phenobarbital has a very long half-life, timed-release preparations do not offer any significant advantage over ordinary dosage forms.

Generic. Elixir 20 mg/5 ml; tablets 8, 16, 32, 65, and 100 mg.
PHENOBARBITAL SODIUM:
Intramuscular, Intravenous: These routes should be used only when oral administration is impossible or impractical. For sleep induction, *adults,* 100 to 320 mg; for sedation, same as oral dosage. Patients should be observed carefully during intravenous injection; the rate must not exceed 100 mg (2 ml of 5% solution)/min. Relaxation, drowsiness, yawning, and slowing of speech and motor activity usually indicate that only a small additional amount is necessary; 15 minutes or longer may be required before a peak concentration is attained in the brain.

Generic. Powder for injection in 120 mg containers; solution 30, 60, 65, and 130 mg/ml in 1 ml containers.

AMOBARBITAL
[Amytal]

AMOBARBITAL SODIUM
[Amytal Sodium]

Amobarbital is effective as a sedative and hypnotic (but not antianxiety) agent and is usually given orally. It is most commonly used to induce sleep. Its action is comparable to that of secobarbital or pentobarbital but, like similar agents, it may lose its effectiveness by the second week of continued administration. The parenteral routes should be used for insomnia only when oral administration is impossible or impractical.

The fatal blood level is usually 3 to 6 mg/dl. See the Introduction for information on adverse reactions, precautions, poisoning, dependence, and interactions.

DOSAGE AND PREPARATIONS.
AMOBARBITAL:
Oral: Same as oral dosage for sodium salt.
Amytal (Lilly). Tablets 15, 30, 50, and 100 mg.
AMOBARBITAL SODIUM:
Intramuscular: For sleep induction, *adults,* 65 to 500 mg. No more than 5 ml should be injected at any one site.
Intravenous (10% aqueous solution): For sleep induction, *adults and children over 6 years,* 65 to 500 mg; the injection rate should not exceed 1 ml/min. The final dosage is determined largely by the patient's response as the dose is adjusted.

Generic. Powder.
Amytal Sodium (Lilly). Powder (sterile) 250 and 500 mg.
Oral: For sedation, *adults and children over 12 years,* 50 to 300 mg daily in divided doses; *children under 12 years,* 6

mg/kg/day divided into three doses. For sleep induction, *adults and children over 12 years,* 65 to 200 mg at bedtime.
　　Generic. Capsules 200 mg.
　　Amytal Sodium (Lilly). Capsules 65 and 200 mg.

PENTOBARBITAL
[Nembutal]

PENTOBARBITAL SODIUM
[Nembutal Sodium]

This short-acting barbiturate is effective as a sedative and hypnotic (but not antianxiety) agent and is usually given orally. Parenteral routes should be used to induce sleep only when oral administration is impossible or impractical. It is prescribed more frequently for sleep induction than for sedation but, like similar agents, may lose its effectiveness by the second week of continued administration.

Pentobarbital is frequently abused by drug-dependent individuals. Death can occur after ingestion of more than 3 g; the fatal blood level usually is 1 to 2.5 mg/dl.

See the Introduction for information on adverse reactions, precautions, poisoning, dependence, and interactions.

DOSAGE AND PREPARATIONS.
PENTOBARBITAL:
Oral: Same as oral dosage for sodium salt.
　　Nembutal (Abbott). Elixir 20 mg/5 ml (strength expressed in terms of sodium salt) (alcohol 18%).
PENTOBARBITAL SODIUM:
Intramuscular: For sleep induction, *adults,* 150 to 200 mg. No more than 250 mg or 5 ml should be injected at any one site because of possible tissue irritation. Injection should be made only into a large muscle mass, preferably the upper outer quadrant of the gluteus maximus.
Intravenous: For sleep induction, *adults,* 100 mg initially; when the effect is determined (after at least one minute), additional small incremental doses to a total of 500 mg may be given slowly until the desired effect is obtained. *Children,* 50 mg initially.
　　Generic. Solution 50 mg/ml in 1 and 2 ml containers.
　　Nembutal Sodium (Abbott). Solution 50 mg/ml in 2, 20, and 50 ml containers.
Oral: For sedation, *adults,* 30 mg three or four times daily or 100 mg in the morning; *children,* 6 mg/kg daily in three divided doses. For sleep induction, *adults,* 100 mg.
　　Nembutal Sodium (Abbott), *Generic.* Capsules 50 and 100 mg.
Rectal: For sedation or sleep induction, *adults,* 120 or 200 mg; for sedation, *children,* 6 mg/kg daily in three divided doses.
　　Nembutal Sodium (Abbott). Suppositories 30, 60, 120, and 200 mg.

SECOBARBITAL SODIUM
[Seconal Sodium]

The hypnotic effectiveness of this barbiturate is comparable to that of pentobarbital sodium; secobarbital is not an antianxiety agent. It is usually given orally; parenteral routes should be used to induce sleep only when oral administration is impossible or impractical. Secobarbital is used more frequently for hypnosis than for sedation but, like similar drugs, may lose its effectiveness by the second week of continued administration. For injection, an aqueous solution is preferred to preparations containing polyethylene glycol, because the latter may be irritating to the kidney, especially in patients with renal insufficiency.

Secobarbital is commonly abused by drug-dependent individuals. The fatal blood level is usually 1 to 2.5 mg/dl.

See the Introduction for information on adverse reactions, precautions, poisoning, dependence, and interactions.

DOSAGE AND PREPARATIONS.
Intramuscular: For sleep induction, *adults,* 100 to 200 mg; *children,* 3 to 5 mg/kg (maximum, 100 mg).
Intravenous: For sleep induction, *adults,* 50 to 250 mg; the injection rate should not exceed 50 mg/15 seconds. Administration should be discontinued as soon as the desired effect is attained.
　　Generic. Solution 50 mg/ml in 1 and 2 ml containers.
　　Seconal Sodium (Lilly). Solution 50 mg/ml in 20 ml containers.
Oral: For sleep induction, *adults,* 100 mg at bedtime. For sedation, *children,* 6 mg/kg daily in three divided doses.
　　Generic. Capsules 50 and 100 mg; tablets 100 mg.
　　Seconal Sodium (Lilly), *Generic.* Capsules 50 and 100 mg.
Rectal: For sedation or sleep induction, *adults,* 120 to 200 mg; for sedation, *children,* 6 mg/kg daily in three divided doses.
　　Seconal Sodium (Lilly). Suppositories 120 and 200 mg.

NONBENZODIAZEPINE-NONBARBITURATES

BUSPIRONE HYDROCHLORIDE
[Buspar]

ACTIONS AND USES. In clinical trials, the efficacy of this investigational agent in relieving anxiety was comparable to that of diazepam. The mechanism of the antianxiety action is not known, but buspirone appears to interact only with the brain's dopaminergic system in a manner analogous to that of both dopamine agonists and antagonists (Riblet et al, 1982). Buspirone lacks the hypnotic, anticonvulsant, and muscle relaxant properties of diazepam and does not potentiate the depressant effects of alcohol. The abuse or dependence liability of buspirone appears to be negligible.

ADVERSE REACTIONS AND PRECAUTIONS. Nervousness, restlessness, headache, weakness, dizziness, depression, and nausea have been reported with use of buspirone. The incidence of depression and drowsiness was significantly lower than with diazepam and was comparable to placebo. Nervousness was more common in patients taking buspirone (Newton et al, 1982), but this drug produced less psychological impairment than diazepam and did not affect driving skills. Larger doses (eg, 40 mg) caused dysphoric effects (Cole et al, 1982). Concern that buspirone's interaction with the brain's dopamine systems might produce tardive dyskinesia has not been borne out by clinical observation.

Buspar (Mead Johnson).
(Investigational drug)

CHLORAL HYDRATE

$$Cl_3C-CH(OH)_2$$

USES. Chloral hydrate is a relatively safe, rapidly effective, reliable sedative and hypnotic agent for short-term use. It is especially useful in insomnia characterized by difficulty in falling asleep. The lethal to therapeutic dose ratio is much lower than with the benzodiazepines and barbiturates. Chloral hydrate may be the preferred alternative to benzodiazepines in selected patients, but some tolerance to the hypnotic action generally develops within five weeks. The antianxiety action of chloral hydrate is too limited and variable to be useful.

The unpleasant taste and odor of chloral hydrate can be minimized by the use of chilled vehicles, the capsule form, or rectal administration.

ADVERSE REACTIONS AND PRECAUTIONS. Gastric irritation occurs in some patients. Paradoxical excitement is observed rarely. The continued use of large doses causes peripheral vasodilation, hypotension, ventilatory depression, arrhythmias, and myocardial depression.

Overdosage may result in coma, and pinpoint pupils are observed occasionally. The narcotic antagonist, naloxone, does not overcome these symptoms.

Chloral hydrate may potentiate the action of oral anticoagulants because its major metabolite displaces the anticoagulants from their protein binding sites. A benzodiazepine might be a better choice in patients also receiving oral anticoagulants. Clinically relevant enzyme induction does not occur.

Long-term use of larger than usual doses may result in psychological and physical dependence. Chloral hydrate is contraindicated in patients with marked hepatic or renal impairment, severe cardiac disease, and gastritis. This drug is classified in FDA Pregnancy Category C.

See the Introduction and Tables 1 and 2 for more information on hypnotic drugs.

PHARMACOKINETICS. Trichloroethanol is the active metabolite of chloral hydrate; it is formed rapidly by a large first-pass hepatic effect and has a mean half-life of 8 (range, 4 to 9.5) hours. Chloral hydrate is excreted in the urine, in part as trichloroethanol glucuronide, which may give false-positive results of tests for glucose.

DOSAGE AND PREPARATIONS.
Oral, Rectal: For sedation, *adults,* 250 mg three times daily after meals; *children,* 25 mg/kg daily divided into three or four doses. For sleep induction, *adults,* 500 mg to 1 g 15 to 30 minutes before bedtime; *children,* 50 mg/kg. The daily dose for adults should not exceed 2 g, and no more than 1 g should be given as a single dose in children.

Generic. Capsules 250 and 500 mg; syrup 250 and 500 mg/5 ml; suppositories 500 mg.
Available Trademark.
Noctec (Squibb).

ETHCHLORVYNOL
[Placidyl]

$$CH_3CH_2C(OH)(C{\equiv}CH)CH{=}CHCl$$

USES. This drug is a tertiary acetylenic alcohol used as a hypnotic agent for short-term therapy. The hypnotic action of ethchlorvynol may be less predictable than that of the benzodiazepines, barbiturates, or chloral hydrate. The elimination half-life is 10 to 25 hours. Clinical situations that warrant selection of ethchlorvynol over a benzodiazepine are extremely rare.

ADVERSE REACTIONS AND PRECAUTIONS. Hypotension, nausea or vomiting, aftertaste, blurred vision, dizziness, facial numbness, urticaria, and toxic amblyopia have been reported occasionally. One case of fatal immune thrombocytopenia has been described.

Long-term use of larger than usual doses may result in psychological and physical dependence. A daily dose of 1.5 g may be sufficient to induce the latter. Withdrawal symptoms, including convulsions, may occur when ethchlorvynol is discontinued abruptly.

This drug is classified in FDA Pregnancy Category C.

POISONING. Overdose with ethchlorvynol can produce prolonged unconsciousness. Pancytopenia and hemolysis also have been reported. Because large amounts of ethchlorvynol are taken up by adipose tissue, the blood concentration does not accurately indicate the magnitude of overdose.

Intravenous overdosage of ethchlorvynol causes primarily noncardiac pulmonary edema in contrast to the central nervous system depression produced by large oral doses (Schottstaedt et al, 1981). Experimentally, the drug has been shown to exert a direct toxic action on the alveolar-capillary membrane.

Charcoal and/or amberlite hemoperfusion may be most effective for removing this drug.

See the Introduction and Tables 1 and 2 for further information on hypnotic drugs.

DOSAGE AND PREPARATIONS.
Oral: For sleep induction, *adults,* 500 mg to 1 g at bedtime. The 1-g dose is usually reserved for unusually severe insomnia. This drug should not be used in *children.*
   Placidyl (Abbott). Capsules 200, 500, and 750 mg.

ETHINAMATE
[Valmid]

ACTIONS AND USES. This carbamic acid ester of alcohol is a relatively weak hypnotic with a rapid onset and brief duration of action; therefore, it is used only in patients who have difficulty in falling asleep. Ethinamate is not effective for more than seven days. Clinical situations that warrant selection of ethinamate over a benzodiazepine are extremely rare.

   Minimal pharmacokinetic data are available, and the effects of this compound on REM sleep are unknown. Ethinamate undergoes hepatic hydroxylation and subsequent glucuronide conjugation. The elimination half-life is 2.5 hours.

   See the Introduction and Tables 1 and 2 for further information on hypnotic drugs.

ADVERSE REACTIONS AND PRECAUTIONS. Paradoxical excitement in children, mild gastrointestinal disturbances, and rash occur occasionally. Thrombocytopenic purpura and fever have been reported rarely. Death has occurred after ingestion of 15 g, but survival has been reported after ingestion of 28 g. Long-term use of larger than usual doses may result in psychological and physical dependence. Withdrawal symptoms, including convulsions, may occur when ethinamate is discontinued abruptly.

   This drug is classified in FDA Pregnancy Category C.

DOSAGE AND PREPARATIONS.
Oral: For sleep induction, *adults,* 500 mg or 1 g 20 minutes before bedtime; *elderly or debilitated patients,* 500 mg. The safety and effectiveness of ethinamate in *children less than 15 years* has not been established.
   Valmid (Dista). Capsules 500 mg.

GLUTETHIMIDE
[Doriden]

USES. Glutethimide is a hypnotic drug but, like similar agents, loses its effectiveness by the second week of continued administration. This agent has no therapeutic advantage over the benzodiazepines, barbiturates, or chloral hydrate and clinical situations that warrant selection of glutethimide over a

benzodiazepine are extremely rare. The elimination half-life ranges from 5 to 22 hours.

ADVERSE REACTIONS, PRECAUTIONS, AND DRUG INTERACTIONS. Generalized rash may occur but usually disappears within two or three days after withdrawal of the drug. Nausea, residual sedation, paradoxical excitement, blurred vision, acute hypersensitivity reactions, acute intermittent porphyria, thrombocytopenic purpura, aplastic anemia, urticaria, exfoliative dermatitis, and leukopenia have been reported rarely.

   If coumarin anticoagulants are used with glutethimide, their metabolism is increased and their dosage may require adjustment, because glutethimide induces hepatic microsomal enzymes. Concurrent ingestion of glutethimide and alcohol may increase blood levels of the latter by approximately 10%, resulting in greater central nervous system depression than when either agent is used alone.

   Long-term use of larger than usual doses may result in psychological and physical dependence. A daily dose of more than 2.5 g may be sufficient to cause the latter. Withdrawal symptoms, including convulsions, may occur when glutethimide is discontinued abruptly. The drug is contraindicated in patients with porphyria.

   Glutethimide is classified in FDA Pregnancy Category C.

POISONING. Overdosage (20 to 30 times the usual dose) has caused areflexia, fever, and prolonged coma, sometimes with unilateral clinical findings. Toxic doses produce less respiratory depression than the barbiturates but circulatory depression is more profound. The long duration and fluctuating depth of the coma are partly due to the production of a potent active metabolite. Although death has been reported after ingestion of 12 g, patients have recovered after doses as large as 15 g. The fatal blood level is usually 1.5 to 3 mg/dl.

   This agent is very insoluble in water and catharsis removes residual amounts from the intestines. Most authorities feel that peritoneal dialysis or hemodialysis is ineffective in treating overdosage but, because of the drug's low water solubility, lipid dialysis may be more effective. Intensive supportive therapy alone frequently is satisfactory.

   See the Introduction and Tables 1 and 2 for further information on hypnotic drugs.

DOSAGE AND PREPARATIONS.
Oral: For sleep induction, *adults,* 250 to 500 mg at bedtime; *children under 12 years,* information is inadequate to establish dosage.
   Generic. Capsules 500 mg; tablets 250 and 500 mg.
   Doriden (USV). Tablets 250 and 500 mg.

HYDROXYZINE HYDROCHLORIDE
[Atarax, Orgatrax, Vistaril]

HYDROXYZINE PAMOATE
[Vistaril]

ACTIONS AND USES. Hydroxyzine is a less potent antianxiety agent than the benzodiazepines, but it also possesses antiemetic and antihistaminic effects. Consequently, it is used for motion sickness, preanesthetic medication, alcohol withdrawal, and allergic dermatoses, especially when a mild antianxiety action is beneficial. The long-term effectiveness of hydroxyzine as an antianxiety agent (ie, more than four months) has not been assessed by systematic clinical studies. The elimination half-life is 2.5 to 3.4 hours.

See the Introduction and Tables 1 and 2 for additional information on antianxiety drugs.

ADVERSE REACTIONS, PRECAUTIONS, AND DRUG INTERACTIONS. The incidence of untoward effects appears to be low; drowsiness usually is transient. Fatal overdosage is uncommon and withdrawal reactions have not been observed.

Some teratogenic effects have been reported in animals when doses substantially above the human therapeutic range were administered, but these findings are difficult to evaluate and inconclusive with respect to human pregnancy. Therefore, until more data are available, hydroxyzine is contraindicated in early pregnancy (see the discussion on drugs used during pregnancy in Chapter 2, Drug Response Variation and Dosing Information).

The dose of opioids or barbiturates given with hydroxyzine must be reduced by 50%, because their central nervous system depressant action is potentiated. Hydroxyzine is an antihistamine and may interfere with responses to skin test antigens.

DOSAGE AND PREPARATIONS.
Oral: For anxiety, *adults,* 75 to 400 mg daily divided into four doses.

HYDROXYZINE HYDROCHLORIDE:
Atarax (Roerig), *Generic.* Syrup 10 mg/5 ml (alcohol 10.5%, *Atarax*); tablets 10, 25, 50, and 100 mg.
HYDROXYZINE PAMOATE:
Generic. Capsules 25, 50, and 100 mg.
Vistaril (Pfizer). Capsules 25, 50, and 100 mg; oral suspension 25 mg/5 ml (equivalent to hydrochloride).

Intramuscular: For severe anxiety, *adults,* 50 to 100 mg every four to six hours as needed.

HYDROXYZINE HYDROCHLORIDE:
Generic. Solution 25 and 50 mg/ml in 1, 1.5, 2, and 10 ml containers.
Orgatrax (Organon). Solution 50 mg/ml in 1, 2, and 10 ml containers.
Vistaril (Pfipharmecs). Solution 25 mg/ml in 1 and 10 ml containers and 50 mg/ml in 1, 1.5, 2, and 10 ml containers.

MEPROBAMATE
[Equanil, Meprospan, Miltown]

$$H_2NCOCH_2\underset{\underset{CH_2CH_2CH_3}{|}}{\overset{\overset{CH_3}{|}}{C}}CH_2OCNH_2$$

Meprobamate is useful in the treatment of anxiety, but it appears to be somewhat less effective than the benzodiazepines.

ADVERSE REACTIONS AND PRECAUTIONS. The most common untoward effect is drowsiness, which develops with doses larger than 1.2 g daily. Thrombocytopenia, leukopenia, dermatitis, urticaria, anaphylactic reactions, hypotension and syncope, blurred vision, weakness of the extremities, and paradoxical euphoria and anger occur rarely. Agranulocytosis and aplastic anemia have been reported, although no causal relationship has been established.

Meprobamate appears in breast milk in concentrations two to four times that in maternal plasma. Therefore, the risks to the nursing baby should be considered when treatment of anxiety in a nursing mother is being evaluated.

The use of meprobamate is contraindicated in patients with acute intermittent porphyria or a history of allergic or idiosyncratic reactions to drugs such as carisoprodol.

Long-term use of larger than usual doses may result in psychological and physical dependence. Withdrawal symptoms may occur when meprobamate is discontinued abruptly after the prolonged daily administration of 1.6 to 2.4 g, and convulsions may develop after a daily dose of approximately 6 g. Death has occurred during withdrawal of this drug. Death from poisoning has been reported after ingestion of 12 g, but patients have survived after ingestion of 40 g.

See the Introduction and Tables 1 and 2 for additional information on antianxiety drugs.

PHARMACOKINETICS. Efficacy coincides with the peak plasma concentration, which is attained two to three hours after ingestion. Induction of hepatic microsomal enzymes occurs but does not appear to be a problem with usual doses. Consistent bioavailability of the timed-release preparation has been demonstrated; however, because meprobamate has a mean half-life of 10 to 24 hours, timed-release preparations do not offer any significant advantage over ordinary dosage forms for most patients.

DOSAGE AND PREPARATIONS.
Oral: Adults, 1.2 to 1.6 g (maximum, 2.4 g) daily divided into three or four doses. *Children 6 to 12 years,* 100 to 200 mg two or three times daily; *children under 6 years,* not recommended.

Equanil (Wyeth). Tablets 200 and 400 mg; tablets (coated) 400 mg (*Wyseals*).
Meprospan (Wallace). Capsules (timed-release) 200 and 400 mg.
Miltown (Wallace), *Generic.* Tablets 200, 400, and 600 mg (*Miltown* only).

METHYPRYLON
[Noludar]

Methyprylon is used only as a hypnotic and is effective for at least seven consecutive nights. Clinical situations that warrant selection of methyprylon over a benzodiazepine are extremely rare. The elimination half-life is about four hours.

See the Introduction and Tables 1 and 2 for further information on hypnotic agents.

ADVERSE REACTIONS AND PRECAUTIONS. Dizziness, mild to moderate gastrointestinal upset, headache, paradoxical excitement, and rash have been reported occasionally. Although death has occurred after ingestion of 6 g, patients have recovered after doses as high as 37 g. Long-term use of larger than usual therapeutic doses may result in psychological and physical dependence. Withdrawal symptoms, including convulsions, may occur when methyprylon is discontinued abruptly.

This drug is classified in FDA Pregnancy Category B.

DOSAGE AND PREPARATIONS.

Oral: Adults, 200 to 400 mg at bedtime. *Children 12 years and older,* the effective dose varies greatly and, therefore, should be individualized; initially, 50 mg is suggested and the amount may be increased up to 200 mg if required. This drug should not be used in *children under 12 years.*

Noludar (Roche). Capsules 300 mg; tablets 50 and 200 mg.

MIXTURES

Mixtures containing one or more barbiturates, most commonly amobarbital, butabarbital, pentobarbital, phenobarbital, or secobarbital (eg, Tuinal), or other hypnotic and antianxiety agents have been used extensively for many years, but any alleged advantage of such combination products is hypothetical. The effects of these mixtures may only be additive, often without any compensating advantage to the patient. Furthermore, fixed-ratio combinations do not permit careful adjustment of the dosage of each drug, which may be important when administering two or more drugs with different durations of action. For these reasons, use of this type of mixture is not recommended.

For the same reasons, fixed-ratio combinations of two or more antianxiety agents or antianxiety agents with anorexiants, antihypertensive agents, estrogens, mild analgesics, antianginal agents, or antispasmodics are not recommended. Such mixtures are marketed for the treatment of anxiety, pain, menopausal symptoms, angina pectoris, obesity, hypertension, and musculoskeletal and gastrointestinal disorders.

Cited References

Abernethy DR, et al: Impairment of diazepam metabolism by low-dose estrogen-containing oral-contraceptive steroids. *N Engl J Med* 306:791-792, 1982.

Ameer B, Greenblatt DJ: Lorazepam: Review of its clinical pharmacological properties and therapeutic uses. *Drugs* 21:161-200, 1981.

American Psychiatric Association: *Diagnostic and Statistical Manual of Mental Disorders,* ed 3. Washington, DC, American Psychiatric Association, 1980.

Asberg M, et al: Psychopharmacologic treatment of obsessive-compulsive disorder: Clomipramine treatment of obsessive disorder; biochemical and clinical aspects. *Psychopharmacol Bull* 18:13-21, 1982.

Bixler EO, et al: Rebound insomnia and elimination half-life: Assessment of individual subject response. *J Clin Pharmacol* 25:115-124, 1985.

Breimer DD: Clinical pharmacokinetics of hypnotics. *Clin Pharmacokinet* 2:93-109, 1977.

Brouillette RT, et al: Obstructive sleep apnea in infants and children. *J Pediatr* 100:31-40, 1982.

Browman CP, et al: Hypersomnia: Diagnosis and management. *Compr Ther* 9:67-74, (June) 1983.

Brownell LG, et al: Protriptyline in obstructive sleep apnea: Double-blind trial. *N Engl J Med* 307:1037-1042, 1982.

Brunello N, Cheney DL: Septal-hippocampal cholinergic pathway: Role in antagonism of pentobarbital anesthesia and regulation by various afferents. *J Pharmacol Exp Ther* 219:489-495, 1981.

Chokroverty S, Sharp JT: Primary sleep apnoea syndrome. *J Neurol Neurosurg Psychiatry* 44:970-982, 1981.

Chouinard G, et al: Alprazolam in treatment of generalized anxiety and panic disorders: Double-blind placebo-controlled study. *Psychopharmacology* 77:229-233, 1982.

Cole JO, et al: Assessment of abuse liability of buspirone in recreational sedative users. *J Clin Psychiatry* 43(12, sec 2):69-74, 1982.

Coleman RM, et al: Sleep-wake disorders based on polysomnographic diagnosis: National cooperative study. *JAMA* 247:997-1003, 1982.

Divoll M, et al: Effect of age and gender on disposition of temazepam. *J Pharm Sci* 70:1104-1107, 1981.

Divoll M, et al: Absolute bioavailability of oral and intramuscular diazepam: Effects of age and sex. *Anesth Analg* 62:1-8, 1983.

Eberts FS Jr, et al: Triazolam disposition. *Clin Pharmacol Ther* 29:81-93, 1981.

Feighner JP, et al: Comparison of alprazolam, imipramine and placebo in treatment of depression. *JAMA* 249:3057-3064, 1983.

Ferriss GS: Narcolepsy. *Contin Educat* 16:41-48, (May) 1982.

Fricchione GL, et al: Intravenous lorazepam in neuroleptic-induced catatonia. *J Clin Psychopharmacol* 3:338-342, 1983.

Frishman WH, et al: Beta-adrenoceptor blockade in anxiety states: New approach to therapy? *Cardiovasc Rev Rep* 2:447-459, 1981.

Frost EAM: Brain preservation. *Anesth Analg* 60:821-832, 1981.

Garakani H, et al: Treatment of panic disorder with imipramine alone. *Am J Psychiatry* 141:446-448, 1984.

Gershon S, Eison AS: Anxiolytic profiles. *J Clin Psychiatry* 44(11, sec 2):45-56, 1983.

Goldberg HL, Finnerty R: Comparison of buspirone in two separate studies. *J Clin Psychiatry* 43(12, sec 2):87-91, 1982.

Greenblatt DJ: Clinical pharmacokinetics of oxazepam and lorazepam. *Clin Pharmacokinet* 6:89-105, 1981.

Greenblatt DJ, Shader RI: Prazepam and lorazepam: Two new benzodiazepines. *N Engl J Med* 299:1342-1344, 1978.

Greenblatt DJ, et al: Kinetics and clinical effects of flurazepam in young and elderly noninsomniacs. *Clin Pharmacol Ther* 30:475-486, 1981.

Greenblatt DJ, et al: Current status of benzodiazepines, parts 1 and 2. *N Engl J Med* 309:354-358, 410-415, 1983.

Greenblatt DJ, et al: Clinical importance of interaction of diazepam and cimetidine. *N Engl J Med* 310:1639-1643, 1984.

Hartmann E: L-tryptophan: Rational hypnotic with clinical potential. *Am J Psychiatry* 134:366-370, 1977.

Hudgel DW: Diagnosis and therapy of sleep apnea. *J Fam Pract* 12:1001-1007, 1981.

Ho IK, Harris RA: Mechanism of action of barbiturates. *Am Rev Pharmacol* 21:83-111, 1981.

Jaffe JH, et al: Abuse potential of halazepam and of diazepam in patients recently treated for acute alcohol withdrawal. *Clin Pharmacol Ther* 34:623-630, 1983.

Jenike MA: Obsessive compulsive disorder. *Compr Psychiatry* 24:99-115, (March/April) 1983.

Jenike MA, et al: Monoamine oxidase inhibitors in obsessive-compulsive disorder. *J Clin Psychiatry* 44:131-132, 1983.

Kales A, et al: Comparative effectiveness of nine hypnotic drugs: Sleep laboratory studies. *J Clin Pharmacol* 17:207-213, 1977.

Kales A, et al: Rebound insomnia: Potential hazard following withdrawal of certain benzodiazepines. *JAMA* 241:1692-1695, 1979.

Kales JD, et al: Treatment of sleep disorders: I. Insomnia. *Ration Drug Ther* 17:1-7, (Feb) 1983.

Kraus JW, et al: Effects of aging and liver disease on disposition of lorazepam. *Clin Pharmacol Ther* 24:411-419, 1978.

Kripke DF, et al: Short and long sleep and sleeping pills: Is increased mortality associated? *Arch Gen Psychiatry* 36:103-116, 1979.

Lane T, Peterson EA: Hepatitis as manifestation of phenobarbital hypersensitivity, (letter). *South Med J* 77:94, 1984.

Leppik IE, et al: Double-blind study of lorazepam and diazepam in status epilepticus. *JAMA* 249:1452-1454, 1983.

Marks IM: Current status of behavioral psychotherapy: Theory and practice. *Am J Psychiatry* 133:253-261, 1976.

Mellinger GD, Balter MB: Psychotherapeutic drugs: Current assessment of prevalence and patterns of use, in Morgan JP, Kagan DV (eds): *Society and Medication: Conflicting Signals for Prescribers and Patients.* Lexington, MA, Lexington Books, 1983, 137-154.

Mellinger GD, et al: Prevalence and correlates of long-term regular use of anxiolytics. *JAMA* 251:375-379, 1984.

Mendelson WB: Prevalence of sleep disturbance and hypnotic use, in Mendelson WB: *The Use and Misuse of Sleeping Pills: A Clinical Guide.* New York, Plenum Medical Book Company, 1980, 25-37.

Michenfelder JD: Barbiturates for brain resuscitation: Yes and no, (editorial). *Anesthesiology* 57:74-75, 1982.

Mitler MM, et al: Comparative hypnotic effects of flurazepam, triazolam, and placebo: Long-term simultaneous nighttime and daytime study. *J Clin Psychopharmacol* 4:2-16, 1984.

National Institutes of Health: *Drugs and Insomnia Consensus Development Conference Summary,* volume 4, number 10, 1983.

Nemiah JC: Anxiety state (anxiety neurosis), in Kaplan HI, et al (eds): *Comprehensive Textbook of Psychiatry/III,* ed 3. Baltimore, Williams & Wilkins, 1980, vol 2, 1483-1492.

Newton RE, et al: Side effect profile of buspirone in comparison to active controls and placebo. *J Clin Psychiatry* 43(12, sec 2):100-102, 1982.

Noyes R, et al: Diazepam and propranolol in panic disorder and agoraphobia. *Arch Gen Psychiatry* 41:287-292, 1984.

O'Brien JE, et al: Double-blind comparison of lorazepam and diazepam in treatment of acute alcohol abstinence syndrome. *Curr Ther Res* 34:825-831, 1983.

Ochs HR, et al: Diazepam kinetics in relation to age and sex. *Pharmacology* 23:24-30, 1981.

Orr WC, et al: Progesterone therapy in obese patients with sleep apnea. *Arch Intern Med* 139:109-111, 1979.

Oswald I, et al: Benzodiazepine hypnotics remain effective for 24 weeks. *Br Med J* 284:860-863, 1982.

Owen RT, Tyrer P: Benzodiazepine dependence: Review of the evidence. *Drugs* 25:385-398, 1983.

Parkes JD: The sleepy patient. *Lancet* 1:990-993, 1977.

Regestein QR, et al: Narcolepsy: Initial clinical approach. *J Clin Psychiatry* 44:166-172, 1983.

Riblet LA, et al: Pharmacology and neurochemistry of buspirone. *J Clin Psychiatry* 43(12, sec 2):11-16, 1982.

Rickels K, et al: Buspirone and diazepam in anxiety: Controlled study. *J Clin Psychiatry* 43(12, sec 2):81-86, 1982.

Rickels K, et al: Long-term diazepam therapy and clinical outcome. *JAMA* 250:767-771, 1983 A.

Rickels K, et al: Diphenhydramine in insomniac family practice patients: Double blind study. *J Clin Pharmacol* 23:235-242, 1983 B.

Rickels K, et al: Doxylamine succinate in insomniac family practice patients: Double-blind study. *Curr Ther Res* 35:532-540, 1984.

Rickels K, et al: Alprazolam, doxepin and placebo in treatment of depression. *Arch Gen Psychiatry* 42:134-141, 1985.

Robinson GM, Sellers EM: Diazepam withdrawal seizures. *Can Med Assoc J* 126:944-945, 1982.

Robinson GM, et al: Barbiturate and hypnosedative withdrawal by multiple oral phenobarbital loading dose technique. *Clin Pharmacol Ther* 30:71-76, 1981.

Rosenberg L, et al: Lack of relation of oral clefts to diazepam use during pregnancy. *N Engl J Med* 309:1282-1285, 1983.

Safar P: Cerebral resuscitation. *Mt Sinai J Med* 48:385-388, 1981.

Schottstaedt MW, et al: Placidyl abuse: Dimorphic picture. *Crit Care Med* 9:677-679, 1981.

Schuckit MA: Anxiety related to medical disease. *J Clin Psychiatry* 44(11, sec 2):31-36, 1983.

Sellers EM, Busto U: Benzodiazepines and ethanol: Assessment of effects and consequences of psychotropic drug interactions. *J Clin Psychopharmacol* 2:249-262, 1982.

Sheehan DV: Current views of treatment of panic and phobic disorders. *Drug Ther* 12:518-525, 1982 A.

Sheehan DV: Panic attacks and phobias. *N Engl J Med* 307:156-158, 1982 B.

Sleep Disorders Classification Committee: Diagnostic classification of sleep and arousal disorders. *Sleep* 2:17-18, 1979.

Smith AG, DeMatteis F: Drugs and hepatic porphyrias. *Clin Haematol* 9:399-424, 1980.

Snyder SH: Drug and neurotransmitter receptors in the brain. *Science* 224:22-31, 1984.

Solomon J, et al: Double-blind comparison of lorazepam and chlordiazepoxide in treatment of acute alcohol abstinence syndrome. *Clin Therapeut* 6:52-58, 1983.

Thorén P, et al: Clomipramine treatment of obsessive-compulsive disorder: Controlled clinical trial. *Arch Gen Psychiatry* 37:1281-1285, 1980.

Tyrer P, et al: Benzodiazepine withdrawal symptoms and propranolol. *Lancet* 1:520-522, 1981.

Walker JE, et al: Lorazepam in status epilepticus. *Ann Neurol* 6:207-213, 1979.

White DP, et al: Central sleep apnea: Improvement with acetazolamide therapy. *Arch Intern Med* 142:1816-1819, 1982.

Whitelaw AGL, et al: Effect of maternal lorazepam on neonate. *Br Med J* 282:1106-1108, 1981.

Zitrin CM, et al: Treatment of phobias: I. Comparison of imipramine hydrochloride and placebo. *Arch Gen Psychiatry* 40:125-138, 1983.

Antipsychotic Drugs

Active psychoses are characterized by one or more of the following: diminished and distorted capacity to process information and draw logical conclusions, impaired judgment, disordered perceptions, hallucinations, extreme excitement, violent aggression, and delusions (Anderson and Kuehnle, 1981). When the underlying disorder is an acute organic mental syndrome (delirium), fluctuating levels of consciousness, disorientation, and loss of recent memory also are observed.

Antipsychotic drugs ameliorate the symptoms of active psychoses. They are useful in mania, acute exacerbations of schizophrenia, schizoaffective disorder, paranoia, atypical psychotic disorders such as those that develop in critical care units following surgery or myocardial infarction, rage reactions, severe agitated major depression with psychotic features, and sensory deprivation syndromes, as well as in acute psychotic episodes associated with either delirium or complex partial seizures. Other conditions that respond to antipsychotic drugs are intractable hiccups, the chorea of Huntington's disease, ballismus, Tourette's syndrome, and agitated behavior associ-

ated with severe mental retardation. These drugs are of unproven value in borderline personality disorder and other severe personality disorders, such as schizotypal personality. Antipsychotic drugs are variably useful in chronic schizophrenia, in which they reduce the rate of exacerbations.

Classification: Antipsychotic drugs are also referred to as *neuroleptics,* because of their potential to induce neurologic side effects. The classes of drugs having antipsychotic activity include the phenothiazines, thioxanthenes, butyrophenones, dihydroindolones, dibenzoxazepines, dibenzodiazepines, and diphenylbutylpiperidines (see Table 1). Phenothiazines are classified on the basis of their chemistry (aliphatic, piperidine, or piperazine compounds), pharmacologic actions, and potency. The thioxanthene derivatives, chlorprothixene [Taractan] and thiothixene [Navane], are related chemically to the aliphatic and piperazine phenothiazines, respectively. Haloperidol [Haldol], a butyrophenone; molindone [Moban], a dihydroindolone; and loxapine [Loxitane], a dibenzoxazepine, are the only representatives of their respective chemical classes available in the United States that are commonly used to treat

TABLE 1.
ANTIPSYCHOTIC DRUGS

Drug	Chemical Classification	Therapeutically Equivalent Oral Dose (mg)	Effects		
			Sedation	Autonomic[1]	Extrapyramidal Reactions[2]
Fluphenazine Permitil (Schering) Prolixin (Squibb)	Phenothiazine: Piperazine Compound	2	+	+	+++
Haloperidol Haldol (McNeil)	Butyrophenone	2	+	+	+++
Thiothixene Navane (Roerig)	Thioxanthene	4	+	+	+++
Trifluoperazine[3] Stelazine (Smith Kline & French)	Phenothiazine: Piperazine Compound	5	++	+	+++
Perphenazine Trilafon (Schering)	Phenothiazine: Piperazine Compound	10	++	+	++/+++
Molindone Moban (DuPont)	Dihydroindolone	10	++	+	+
Loxapine Loxitane (Lederle)	Dibenzoxazepine	15	++	+/++	++/+++
Prochlorperazine[3, 4] Compazine (Smith Kline & French)	Phenothiazine: Piperazine Compound	15	++	+	+++
Acetophenazine Tindal (Schering)	Phenothiazine: Piperazine Compound	20	++	+	+++
Triflupromazine Vesprin (Squibb)	Phenothiazine: Aliphatic Compound	30	+++	++/+++	++
Mesoridazine Serentil (Boehringer Ingelheim)	Phenothiazine: Piperidine Compound	50	+++	++	+
Chlorpromazine[3] Thorazine (Smith Kline & French)	Phenothiazine: Aliphatic Compound	100	+++	+++	++
Chlorprothixene Taractan (Roche)	Thioxanthene	100	+++	+++	+/++
Thioridazine[3] Mellaril (Sandoz)	Phenothiazine: Piperidine Compound	100	+++	+++	+

[1]Alpha antiadrenergic and anticholinergic effects
[2]Excluding tardive dyskinesia which appears to be produced to the same degree and frequency by all agents with equieffective antipsychotic doses
[3]Available generically
[4]Used rarely, if ever, as an antipsychotic agent

psychiatric patients, although droperidol [Inapsine], a short-acting butyrophenone, has potent sedative and antipsychotic actions. A diphenylbutylpiperidine, pimozide [Orap], is used for the treatment of Tourette's syndrome, although it too is a potent antipsychotic agent. These compounds are pharmacologically, but not chemically, related to the piperazine phenothiazines.

An investigational drug, penfluridol, is a diphenylbutylpiperi-dine compound with potent antipsychotic properties. It is effective orally when given only once weekly, which may improve compliance. The decanoate and enanthate salts of fluphenazine [Prolixin Decanoate, Prolixin Enanthate] and a depot preparation of haloperidol (decanoate salt) are market-ed as long-acting depot preparations for intramuscular or subcutaneous administration (see Table 2).

Mechanism of Action: The etiology of schizophrenia and

TABLE 2.
LONG-ACTING ANTIPSYCHOTIC DRUGS

Drug	Chemical Classification	Route of Administration	Duration of Action	Status
Fluphenazine Decanoate Prolixin Decanoate (Squibb)	Phenothiazine Piperazine	Intramuscular Subcutaneous	2-3 weeks	Available
Fluphenazine Enanthate Prolixin Enanthate (Squibb)	Phenothiazine Piperazine	Intramuscular Subcutaneous	2 weeks	Available
Haloperidol Decanoate Haldol Decanoate (McNeil)	Butyrophenone	Intramuscular	3-4 weeks	Available
Penfluridol Semap (McNeil)	Diphenylbutylpiperidine	Oral	1 week	Investigational

most nontoxic nondelirious psychoses unrelated to coarse brain diseases is unknown and, thus, the specific mechanism by which antipsychotic drugs exert their therapeutic effects is not completely understood. It is known, however, that antipsychotic drugs bind strongly to and block dopaminergic receptors of the forebrain and basal ganglia (as well as other tissues). They have variable antagonistic interactions with muscarinic, alpha-adrenergic, histaminergic, and serotonergic receptors in the brain and peripheral tissues.

The dopaminergic receptor systems have been characterized as follows: (1) dopamine (D-1) receptors that are associated with stimulation of dopamine-sensitive adenylate cyclase and are blocked by most neuroleptics (roughly in proportion to their clinical efficacy) but only weakly by butyrophenone and diphenylbutylpiperidine compounds, and (2) dopamine (D-2) receptors that may inhibit dopamine-sensitive adenylate cyclase in some tissues and are blocked by nearly all types of neuroleptic agents including butyrophenones. The clinical potency of the antipsychotic drugs correlates best with their affinity for D-2 receptors. Antipsychotic drugs have weak and variable interactions at binding sites defined by dopamine agonists.

Because nearly all antipsychotic drugs block the action of dopamine centrally, a current hypothesis postulates that their clinical actions and characteristic neurologic side effects are mediated by antagonism of dopaminergic activity in the brain. However, there is no compelling evidence that this effect is necessary for antipsychotic activity or that psychosis is a hyperdopaminergic state.

Dopamine neurons and pathways are located principally in the mesolimbic, mesocortical, tuberoinfundibular, and nigrostriatal areas of the brain. The antagonism of dopamine in the mesolimbic and mesocortical areas probably contributes to the therapeutic actions of the antipsychotic drugs. Antagonism of dopamine's action in the striatum (caudate and putamen) probably accounts for many of the characteristic neurotoxic effects (eg, parkinsonism, dystonia, akathisia, dyskinesias) of neuroleptic agents. Antagonism of dopamine's neurohormonal action to prevent release of prolactin by the anterior pituitary accounts for the sustained hyperprolactinemia associated with neuroleptics and other antidopaminergic agents. The site of

the antiemetic action of the antipsychotics is probably the chemoreceptor trigger zone of the medulla.

The ciliary and vagal antimuscarinic antiparasympathetic activities of the antipsychotic drugs, especially the low-potency agents, probably produce blurred vision, dry mouth, and urinary retention and may contribute to excessive sedation or confusion. The alpha (α_1)-adrenergic actions may cause sedation, orthostatic hypotension, and lightheadedness, especially with low-potency neuroleptics. The antihistaminergic activities of these drugs probably contribute to drowsiness and sedation as well.

It is probable that some interplay of these actions is responsible for both therapeutic and adverse effects.

Schizophrenia (Schizophrenic Disorders)

Diagnosis: Psychotic symptoms are common, nonspecific, and may be present in such conditions as delirium, anticholinergic poisoning, hypoglycemia, Wernicke-Korsakoff's syndrome, mania, melancholia, dementia, and drug intoxication (eg, phencyclidine). Thus, an accurate diagnosis is required for appropriate treatment (Manschreck, 1983).

Schizophrenia represents a group of ill-defined, chronic, idiopathic, psychotic disorders characterized primarily by distinctive changes in concept formations and reality relationships. Symptoms typically become evident during adolescence or early adulthood. The schizophrenic disorders probably have some degree of genetic transmission but their etiology remains unknown. Exacerbations can be activated in susceptible individuals by psychosocial stressors (Manschreck, 1981; Strauss and Carpenter, 1981).

The third edition of the *Diagnostic and Statistical Manual of Mental Disorders (DSM III)* (American Psychiatric Association, 1980) defines schizophrenia (schizophrenic disorders) more precisely. Its criteria include:

(1) The presence of at least one of the following: (a) Bizarre delusions relating to thought content (such as broadcasting one's own thoughts, thought insertions, thought withdrawal, thought controlled by others). (b) Alterations in thought form (ie, loosening of thought associations to the point of incoher-

ence or impoverished speech and blunted, flat, or inappropriate affect; delusions or hallucinations; or catatonic or other grossly disorganized behavior). (c) Other grandiose, religious, nihilistic, or somatic delusions and persecutory or jealous delusions if accompanied by prominent hallucinations of any type and disorganized thinking (to distinguish schizophrenia from paranoia). (d) Auditory hallucinations, usually of a type in which a voice comments in more than a few words on the individual's thoughts or behavior.

(2) Deterioration of work, social relations, or self-care; goal-directed activities (volition) are especially affected, and a loss of ego boundaries (sense of self) occurs frequently.

(3) Persistence of the illness for at least six months (with or without a prodromal or residual phase) during which at least one of the above signs and symptoms was present.

(4) Onset of the prodromal or active phase before age 45 (usually before age 30).

(5) Any organic mental disorder, or mental retardation, or primary affective (mood) disorder, or personality disorder has been excluded. Although delusions, hallucinations, incoherence, and blunted affect are often present in organic mental disorders, impairment of intellect and memory, disorientation, and fluctuating levels of consciousness distinguish these disorders from schizophrenia.

(6) If there is a history of a major depressive or manic episode, it developed after the psychotic symptoms or was brief in duration relative to the symptoms described above.

A prodromal phase of schizophrenia is common and is characterized by subtle changes (eg, low levels of self-care and role or social functioning; oddities of behavior and ideation; diminished affect and reasoning; illogical thinking; social withdrawal; speech is vague, overelaborate, circumstantial, idiosyncratic, or metaphorical). In the active phase or during acute exacerbations, signs and symptoms are more flagrant; a residual phase usually follows in which only a few signs and symptoms (usually of diminished intensity) persist.

Although a schizophrenic disorder may go into partial remission, exacerbations are common and signify the presence of chronic schizophrenia. Patients with chronic schizophrenic disorder often experience progression of impairments of affect, volition, insight, and judgment. Chronic schizophrenia also is of particular concern because the antipsychotic drugs are less effective in sustained or progressive impairments. Some authorities believe that their principal or only benefit in a chronic schizophrenic disorder is to prevent acute exacerbations (Crow, 1980). Whether antipsychotic drugs play a therapeutic or prophylactic role, controlled studies demonstrate that they reduce the exacerbation rate in chronic schizophrenia by about two and one-half times in medication-responsive schizophrenic patients (Davis and Casper, 1977).

Management: The pharmacologic treatment of acute active schizophrenia usually is indicated when there is significant disruption of the patient's ability to perform important daily routines at work and at home. In more severe and critical cases, loss of behavioral control may threaten the well-being of the individual and those who come in contact with him.

Severe, acute, active schizophrenia often is managed by parenteral (usually intramuscular) administration of an antipsy-

chotic drug. Parenteral therapy may hasten the onset of sedative, if not antipsychotic, activity; for example, haloperidol's effect becomes apparent about three hours after oral administration and 20 to 30 minutes after intramuscular administration. Such rapidity of action may be important in agitated, combative patients. Additionally, parenteral administration assures bioavailability.

When intramuscular administration is indicated, 2 to 5 mg of fluphenazine hydrochloride [Prolixin], haloperidol, thiothixene, or the equivalent is given intramuscularly every four to eight hours; total daily doses of 10 to 20 mg are usually sufficient. Not all patients respond satisfactorily, however, perhaps because of the marked individual variation in absorption, metabolism, and elimination of antipsychotic drugs. Thus, careful monitoring of patient response and appropriate titration of dose are essential.

The value and safety of more rapid escalation of dosage in acute active psychosis are not proved (Ericksen et al, 1978; Kirkpatrick and Burnett, 1982; Donaldson et al, 1984). Several controlled studies concluded that control of severe psychosis is expedited by use of such regimens as intramuscular injection of 5 to 10 mg of haloperidol, thiothixene, or fluphenazine every 30 to 60 minutes (maximum, 60 mg) or the induction of gross sedation. Current strategies stress rapid initiation of therapy rather than rapid escalation of dosage. The incidence of acute dystonic reactions increases when larger doses of antipsychotics are given more frequently (especially in young men), and deaths rarely have been associated with such aggressive, rapid dosing. Some authorities recommend the prophylactic use of a centrally acting anticholinergic drug (eg, oral benztropine [Cogentin] 1 to 2 mg/day) beginning with the first dose of antipsychotic drug and continued during the initial weeks of treatment to minimize the risk of acute dystonic reactions commonly associated with large doses of potent neuroleptic agents. However, strong opposition to this practice also exists.

If symptoms of an acute active psychosis are less severe, initial daily oral doses of 200 to 600 mg chlorpromazine [Thorazine] or the equivalent are appropriate. The amount can be increased as the response improves or adverse reactions intervene. The rate of increase depends upon the patient's age and weight and the severity of symptoms. An effective daily dosage range after several days of treatment is generally 500 to 800 mg of chlorpromazine. Although the maximum recommended daily dose is 2 g, amounts exceeding 1 g rarely improve the response. Indeed, daily doses of 300 to 500 mg often are effective (Donaldson et al, 1984) and those below 300 mg are well tolerated and adequate in many acutely psychotic patients (Cohen et al, 1980 A). Patients under 40 years and those who are agitated or have severe psychoses generally require a larger daily dose. Although too gradual an increase in dosage and administration of inadequate amounts sometimes cause early treatment failure, excessive dosing and too rapid increase of dose during the first days and weeks of treatment are more common errors. The lowest dose that achieves the maximum therapeutic effect should be used.

The response to antipsychotic drugs in newly diagnosed patients should be evident within one to two days of adequate treatment. Many symptoms (eg, agitation, combativeness, hallucinations, paranoia) improve within six to eight weeks in about 95% of patients. No patient should be considered a treatment failure without an intensive course of carefully monitored therapy. If the desired therapeutic effect is not attained after an adequate trial of therapy (generally considered to be about six weeks at doses equivalent to up to 800 mg of chlorpromazine or 30 mg of a high-potency agent), substitution of a drug from a different chemical class may be justified. Substitution of a near equivalent dose of the new drug usually can be made gradually, but equivalent doses of high-potency and low-potency agents cannot be substituted rapidly because of side effects.

Sound practice requires individualization of dose rather than routine or generalized dosage regimens, as well as continuous and careful monitoring, especially during initial treatment. Larger than usual doses can be given rarely when required.

The oral route is preferred (Kessler and Waletzky, 1981) unless the severity of illness dictates otherwise. Liquid preparations are absorbed somewhat more readily but may be inconvenient; successively less reliable are tablets and capsules. The half-life of most antipsychotic drugs is 10 to 30 hours and thus timed-release oral preparations are not needed and may decrease drug absorption.

The relapse or exacerbation rate after successful medical treatment for acute schizophrenia is 5% to 10% of patients per month for at least one year. Maintenance drug therapy decreases the relapse rate by 50%, but also carries the risk of extrapyramidal side effects and tardive dyskinesia. However, in view of the success of prophylactic antipsychotic therapy, the use of these drugs generally is justified for at least 6 to 12 months.

As in acute active schizophrenia, the maintenance dose should be the least amount that maintains the therapeutic response, causes the fewest side effects, allows optimum function, and prevents relapse. In one study utilizing several maintenance protocols with chlorpromazine 150 mg to 2 g daily (Baldessarini and Davis, 1980), no correlation between dose and efficacy was found. Other evidence also suggests that large doses are not necessarily more effective than smaller amounts in preventing relapse (Aubree and Lader, 1980), and effective maintenance doses may be less than 100 mg/day (chlorpromazine or equivalent) in many patients (Baldessarini, 1984). Thus, a constant reduction of dose should be attempted when establishing the maintenance level, especially in outpatients in partial remission (Kane, 1984).

Both the intramuscular depot and oral routes are effective for maintenance therapy. With oral administration, the drug is given daily; depot intramuscular preparations are given at intervals of two weeks or longer.

When the oral route is selected, the daily dose can be given in divided amounts to minimize adverse reactions until a satisfactory maintenance dose has been established. Thereafter one, or occasionally two, doses daily are administered unless adverse reactions increase. A single dose at bedtime is preferred to take advantage of the sedation produced and, possibly, to decrease the incidence of orthostatic hypotension; additional sedation often is unnecessary and the patient is less likely to be drowsy during the day. Selected patients may benefit from the daytime sedation produced by divided doses, and daytime administration may permit use of lower total doses.

Administration of depot formulations circumvents variations in absorption and the more extensive first-pass hepatic metabolism characteristic of oral administration. These preparations are often preferred in noncompliant patients. A disadvantage of depot formulations is that elimination of the drug is gradual, which may prolong the duration of side effects. There is also growing evidence that large doses may produce excessive neurotoxicity and inferior antipsychotic responses (Teicher and Baldessarini, 1985), and "forced" compliance may have deleterious effects in some schizophrenic patients.

The patient's progress and drug regimen should be reviewed periodically. Maintenance therapy greatly increases the likelihood of retaining the improvement gained during initial treatment and is more effective if there is continued, supportive contact with the patient and his family. It has been suggested that medication be continued for at least six months after the first acute episode of schizophrenia and for one year or more after the second episode. The antipsychotic drugs may be required indefinitely or at least intermittently if three or more relapses occur. The severity of the episode should influence the duration of therapy for newly diagnosed schizophrenic patients.

Use of depot preparations or continuous daily oral administration may assure compliance, but periodic reduction or even cautious interruption of treatment is advisable to minimize drug accumulation, to unmask symptoms of tardive dyskinesia (Task Force on Late Neurologic Effects of Antipsychotic Drugs, 1980) and facilitate its early diagnosis (see also the discussion on Withdrawal Symptoms), and to assess the need for furthur treatment.

A therapeutic option presently under study is early intervention, time-limited, targeted pharmacotherapy (Carpenter and Heinrichs, 1984). In this regimen, patients do not receive drugs and are followed until prodromal signs of relapse appear. An antipsychotic agent is then administered to avert an impending acute psychotic episode and is discontinued gradually when the condition stabilizes. Close monitoring and extensive family and patient education are required. Preliminary results have shown this method to be effective, but further study is needed.

Traditional insight-oriented psychotherapy offers little benefit for schizophrenia, although counseling by the physician can help both patient and family understand the disorder and facilitate rehabilitation and cooperation. The therapeutic alliance between physician and patient is important to optimize compliance and appropriate dosage adjustment. Behavioral therapy may reduce stress and enhance coping skills (Falloon and Lieberman, 1983). Social support systems (family, social services, occupational therapy) help to develop skills and vocational training in a sheltered environment. Initial treatment in an institutional setting may be essential.

Drug Selection: Numerous controlled studies have determined that patterns of response to any antipsychotic drug are similar among patients with various types of schizophrenia (eg, disorganized, paranoid, catatonic, undifferentiated). Thus, despite differences in potency, all antipsychotic drugs are equally effective in equivalent doses (Davis, 1975; Davis and Casper, 1977). Selection of an antipsychotic drug is determined mainly by the potential adverse effects. The incidence and severity of untoward effects produced by each drug should be taken into account, for the potential adverse reactions that the patient accepts are essential considerations in compliance.

Other factors also influence drug selection. The history of a favorable response to a particular antipsychotic agent by the patient or close family members suggests its use initially. Conversely, a previously unfavorable response to adequate doses tends to militate against use of that drug. The patient's age and physical condition and the cost of the drug (Davis, 1976) are other significant factors. Since sensitivity varies among patients and in a given patient over time, individualization of dosage and treatment procedures is required.

Antipsychotic drugs are arranged in decreasing order of potency in Table 1. High-potency drugs have less sedative and autonomic blocking activity but are more likely to produce extrapyramidal reactions (dystonia, akathisia, parkinsonism); with minor exceptions, the reverse is noted as potency decreases. Allergic, systemic (hepatic and bone marrow), cutaneous, and ocular reactions are more prominent with low-potency drugs. There is no evidence that a given antipsychotic drug is more or less likely than another to produce tardive dyskinesia (Tarsy and Baldessarini, 1984). A rational approach is for the physician to become proficient in the use of at least one low-potency and one high-potency drug.

Antipsychotic drugs are equally efficacious when administered by intramuscular injection. Fluphenazine hydrochloride, trifluoperazine, thiothixene, loxapine, and haloperidol are often administered intramuscularly, although the latter is relatively costly. These high-potency antipsychotic drugs are preferred for injection because less discomfort and tissue damage are observed and the incidence of hypotensive reactions is considerably reduced compared to chlorpromazine and other low-potency antipsychotic drugs given by this route.

Monitoring Blood Drug Concentration: The phenothiazines, thioxanthenes, loxapine, and molindone are extensively metabolized and haloperidol is biotransformed via reduction to an active compound. Monitoring the blood drug concentration is not useful routinely, but may aid in assessing compliance and evaluating patients refractory to conventional therapy. Several analytical methods are available: gas chromatography (sometimes combined with mass spectroscopy [GC/MS] in research laboratories) and high pressure liquid chromatography are preferred techniques for measurement of the plasma concentration. Also a radio receptor assay is available to determine active forms of a drug and its metabolites (Cohen and Baldessarini, 1984). However, standardization of optimal therapeutic plasma levels remains poor.

Combination Therapy: Combinations of neuroleptics are no more effective than adequate doses of a single agent. The beneficial effects of some antipsychotic agents (eg, thioridazine, fluphenazine) may be increased when a benzodiazepine is added to the regimen, but schizophrenic symptoms may increase if a stimulant or antidepressant is added to overcome the sedation produced by an antipsychotic drug. The addition of lithium to antipsychotic drug treatment in refractory patients may enhance the therapeutic response, but this combination needs more study. A review of drugs other than antipsychotics in the treatment of schizophrenia is available (Donaldson et al, 1984).

Other Indications

Acute Mania: Lithium is a relatively selective agent for acute mania. However, because it has a longer latent period than the antipsychotic drugs, an antipsychotic agent often is administered alone or with lithium in initial treatment, especially for severe manifestations. Once behavior has been controlled and lithium has become effective, the antipsychotic drug may be discontinued or the dosage reduced (see also Chapter 7, Drugs Used in Affective Disorders).

Schizoaffective Disorder: This poorly defined disorder should be diagnosed only when schizophrenia and affective disorder cannot be differentiated (American Psychiatric Association, 1980). Antipsychotic drugs may be beneficial, although the specificity of the antidepressant effect is disputed. Lithium or a heterocyclic antidepressant may have to be added to the regimen for complete control. Lithium may be preferred for long-term prophylaxis. (See Chapter 7.)

Paranoia: This is a relatively rare disorder characterized by a well organized, persistent delusional system in an otherwise relatively normal personality without features of schizophrenia (Manschreck and Petri, 1978). Paranoia of this type is sometimes resistant to antipsychotic drugs, especially in elderly patients; however, some patients respond adequately and may require prolonged treatment.

Paranoid features (the paranoid syndrome) may be found in many psychiatric, neurologic, metabolic, and endocrine disorders, as well as in substance-induced psychoses (eg, alcohol, amphetamine, phencyclidine). The same antipsychotic drug regimen described for other acute psychoses is used for acute psychosis with predominant or extensive paranoid features.

Although the antipsychotic drugs are useful in amphetamine-induced toxic psychosis, they may increase symptoms in patients who have abused hallucinogens. Toxic delirium caused by drugs with considerable anticholinergic activity may be exacerbated and prolonged by antipsychotic agents, which also have anticholinergic properties.

Organic Mental Syndromes: Antipsychotic drugs are less useful in acute psychotic episodes associated with organic mental syndromes, including substance-induced syndromes (toxic psychoses or delirium), than in acute idiopathic psychoses. Establishment of the etiology is extremely important. Elimination of the toxic compound may be all that is necessary. Further, antipsychotic drugs may compound the toxicity. Nevertheless, the cautious administration of small doses may be justified and may reduce confusion, agitation, and hyperactivity in patients with delirium or dementia with psychotic features.

These drugs may be of benefit for short-term use in demented patients to control behavioral problems that impair their management or that place the patient at great risk of personal injury and in those who do not respond to behavior modification therapy and appropriate nursing care (see Chapter 8, Drugs Used in Other Mental Disorders).

Pervasive Developmental Disorder (Autism): The benefit of antipsychotic drug therapy as an adjunct to psychosocial and/or behavioral therapies in autistic children is controversial. The low-potency agents are probably less effective or less well tolerated than high-potency agents. In some studies, the high-potency antipsychotic, haloperidol, has been effective in children with prominent symptoms of withdrawal, hyperactivity, and aggressive and stereotyped behavior (Campbell et al, 1984). Haloperidol combined with behavioral therapy also improved the acquisition of language. Other clinical experience suggests that only the overt behavioral manifestations improve (Biederman and Jellinek, 1984).

Mental Retardation: Antipsychotic agents are sometimes used empirically in agitated patients with severe mental retardation. These drugs may alleviate irritability, disturbed sleep, agitation, hostility, and combativeness and may improve social behavior and concentration. However, they do not improve speech, communication, or the mental deficiency. Although haloperidol often is prescribed for this purpose, there is no evidence that it is superior to low doses of other high-potency antipsychotic agents; low-potency antipsychotics are not preferred due to excessive sedation and other side effects. Because of the danger of tardive dyskinesia, use of antipsychotic drugs in children and adolescents with behavior disorders other than schizophrenia or autism should be restricted and reviewed critically on a regular basis.

Huntington's Disease: Although antipsychotic drugs do not reverse or halt the progression of dementia or other neurologic deficits in Huntington's disease, they ameliorate and control chorea, especially in earlier stages. Dopamine-depleting drugs, such as tetrabenazine and reserpine, are also being investigated (see Chapter 11, Drugs Used in Extrapyramidal Movement Disorders).

Tourette's Syndrome: Antipsychotic agents, such as haloperidol, can be effective in Tourette's syndrome, an uncommon disorder manifested by severe motor tics, barking cries, grunts, and explosive outbursts of obscene expletives (Murray, 1978). Precise dosage adjustment is difficult in these patients. The development of a school avoidance syndrome in young patients or a social phobia in older patients is an unusual adverse reaction to haloperidol (Mikkelsen et al, 1981). If this reaction occurs or the response is poor, clonidine [Catapres] is an acceptable alternative in about two-thirds of patients. Chlorpromazine (Cohen et al, 1980 B) or pimozide [Orap] also may be tried. (See Chapter 11, Drugs Used in Extrapyramidal Movement Disorders.)

Ballismus (Ballism): This disorder is characterized by continual, usually unilateral (hemiballismus), purposeless, "flinging" movements of the extremities (particularly the arms). This extrapyramidal syndrome is almost always produced by acute vascular infarctions of the subthalamic nucleus. Control of the disorder, survival, and even disappearance of the syndrome have occurred in a number of patients within three to six months when haloperidol 3 to 12 mg was administered daily (Klawans et al, 1978). Individuals who cannot tolerate haloperidol may be controlled with chlorpromazine 100 to 200 mg daily or other neuroleptics.

Miscellaneous Uses: Chlorpromazine is indicated in the treatment of *intractable hiccups*, which is one of the rare conditions requiring intravenous administration of a phenothiazine (Wagner and Stapczynski, 1982).

Because they potentiate the effects of hypnotic, analgesic, and anesthetic agents, some antipsychotic drugs are occasionally used as *adjuncts to anesthesia* (see Chapter 17).

With the exception of mesoridazine and thioridazine, the antipsychotic drugs have a pronounced *antiemetic* action (see Chapter 14, Drugs Used in Vertigo and Vomiting).

Antipsychotic agents are of no value in uncomplicated acute or chronic alcoholism, but may be useful when hallucinations or psychosis complicate such disorders. They may precipitate seizures during acute alcohol withdrawal reactions, and fatalities have followed intravenous administration.

All antipsychotic drugs produce varying degrees of sedation and depression of mood. Accordingly, they have been inappropriately termed major tranquilizers and prescribed for patients with anxiety. Benzodiazepines are more effective, safer, and better tolerated by most anxious patients than even small doses of the antipsychotic drugs. An antidepressant is usually preferred when anxiety is associated with depression and in the panic-agoraphobia syndrome.

Adverse Reactions

Antipsychotic drugs are characterized by a high therapeutic index, although side effects occur routinely at therapeutic doses. Overdose is seldom fatal in adults and most adverse reactions are not life-threatening. However, the neurologic side effects of the antipsychotics are particularly troublesome, often limit the tolerated dose, and may interfere with therapeutic effects. Close clinical observation is essential to monitor the patient's progress and detect adverse reactions promptly. Although laboratory profiles are advisable to establish baseline values, frequent laboratory tests are unnecessary and have little predictive value.

BEHAVIORAL EFFECTS. Sedation is common after use of all antipsychotic drugs and is especially pronounced after large doses of the low-potency phenothiazines (chlorpromazine, triflupromazine [Vesprin], mesoridazine [Serentil], thioridazine [Mellaril], and chlorprothixene [Taractan]) (see Table 1). It can be minimized by reducing the dose or substituting a less sedating agent. However, sedation decreases during long-term treatment and many patients become tolerant to this effect. Daytime somnolence usually can be avoided by giving a single dose at bedtime.

Toxic psychosis may be difficult to differentiate from deterioration of the schizophrenic state. Reactions are characterized by exacerbation of psychotic symptomatology, confusion, insomnia, or marked sedation associated with bizarre dreams and general impairment of psychomotor activity. Dosage reduction usually ameliorates the condition, although nonspecific withdrawal symptoms may follow discontinuation of treatment, especially with low-potency agents. Substituting an antipsychotic drug with less anticholinergic activity also may be helpful, particularly if an anticholinergic drug is being prescribed simultaneously.

EXTRAPYRAMIDAL REACTIONS. Three of these common reactions, dystonia, akathisia, and parkinsonism, occur early during treatment (within hours to weeks) and are more characteristic of the high-potency antipsychotic drugs (see Table 1). The low-potency piperidine phenothiazines, mesoridazine and thioridazine, are least likely to produce extrapyramidal symptoms. The fourth reaction, tardive dyskinesia, usually is not observed for months to years after initiation of therapy but appears to occur with similar frequency with all antipsychotic drugs. (See the discussion on Tardive Dyskinesia and Chapter 11, Drugs Used in Extrapyramidal Movement Disorders.)

Dystonia: Dystonic reactions are noted most frequently following parenteral administration, especially in male patients under 25 years. Acute reactions often are bizarre and abrupt in onset; they may be confused with tetanus, hysteria, epilepsy, meningitis, encephalitis, stroke, or strychnine poisoning, and patients have been treated erroneously.

Acute torsion dystonia generally appears first (within hours or a few days). It is characterized primarily by abnormal, long-sustained, posturing movements of the neck, jaw, trunk, and eyes (ie, spastic torticollis, opisthotonus, grimacing, perioral spasms, dysphagia) often with protrusion of the tongue, masseter spasms, and oculogyric crisis. Hyperhidrosis, pallor, fever, marked anxiety or tremor, laryngeal and pharyngeal spasm with dysphagia or dyspnea, asphyxia, and cyanosis also have been reported and fatalities have occurred.

Dystonia rarely persists but should be treated by temporarily discontinuing antipsychotic therapy and administering a centrally acting anticholinergic agent (eg, benztropine [Cogentin] 1 to 2 mg intramuscularly or intravenously) or an antihistamine (eg, diphenhydramine [Benadryl] 25 to 50 mg intramuscularly) to alleviate symptoms during the adaptive phase. Parenteral administration of an anticholinergic or antihistaminic agent may be preferable to oral therapy for more rapid termination of abnormal movements, especially when life-threatening laryngospasm develops.

Akathisia: This disorder is characterized by a feeling of restlessness, and the resultant uncontrollable pacing and agitation may mimic dyskinesia. It can appear immediately but most commonly appears within a few weeks to a few months after initiation of therapy, and may persist. Because this condition is often mistaken for psychotic agitation, the dose of the antipsychotic agent may be increased unnecessarily, which exacerbates the akathisia. If a reduction in dose is not feasible, central anticholinergic drugs can be used and a sedating agent, such as diazepam [Valium], often may be added temporarily. However, the most promising treatment is propranolol [Inderal] 10 to 60 mg/day (Zubenko et al, 1984). After akathisia is controlled, the antipsychotic drug usually can be continued with the antiakathisic medication. If adaptation to this disorder occurs, the antipsychotic drug can be administered alone.

Parkinsonism: Parkinsonian symptoms consist of rigidity, bradykinesia, shuffling gait, postural abnormalities, mask-like facies, hypersalivation, and variable tremor occurring within a few weeks to a few months after initiating therapy. This syndrome is clinically indistinguishable from postencephalitic or idiopathic Parkinson's disease. Symptoms are most prominent after parenteral administration of usual doses; severe catatonic reactions, sometimes with malignant complications (infection, fever, myoglobinuria), may develop. It is important not to confuse the bradykinesia, mask-like facies, and apathy of parkinsonism with the diminished affect of major depression or the apathy of schizophrenia. Oral administration of a central anticholinergic drug or amantadine [Symmetrel] often controls this condition; the dose of antipsychotic drug may be reduced if psychotic symptoms do not worsen.

Although anticholinergic drugs reduce the severity of extrapyramidal effects, there is some concern regarding their routine prophylactic use with antipsychotic drugs. Those who oppose routine concomitant administration emphasize the risks, which include additive anticholinergic toxicity. Those who favor prophylactic use note that some extrapyramidal side effects are subtle and easy to miss. In addition, avoidance of side effects improves compliance and, in certain situations (eg, outpatients who reside at a considerable distance from a physician), prophylactic therapy might prove reasonable.

Initial treatment with antipsychotics alone (adding anticholinergics later if necessary) or with both classes of drugs is acceptable. When the latter regimen is selected, it is important to remember that dystonia, akathisia, and parkinsonism occur early in treatment. Therefore, if extrapyramidal side effects do not occur by the third or fourth month, the dose of the anticholinergic should be reduced gradually and discontinued if possible. If slow withdrawal precipitates extrapyramidal symptoms, the anticholinergic drug may be added again. These agents are often hard to withdraw. It is important to realize that their half-life is much shorter than that of antipsychotics; thus, when both are to be discontinued, the anticholinergic should be withdrawn more gradually and not simultaneously with the antipsychotic drug.

Tardive Dyskinesia: This condition is characterized principally by choreiform movements of the face, jaw, tongue, trunk, and extremities. Dystonic and ballistic movements also may be present. Each choreiform movement is a single muscle jerk (tic); however, a novel pattern of locomotion emerges because the patient attempts to mask the tics by carrying out semipurposeful movements. A to-and-fro pattern of trunk movement and sustained posturing movements (dystonia) can complicate the differentiation of this condition from parkinsonian tremor and acute dystonia, respectively. Tardive dyskinesia, like most dyskinesias, disappears during sleep and worsens with heightened arousal or anxiety. The disorder ranges in severity from isolated dyskinesias, usually of the choreiform type, to widespread disabling dystonias (rare) that interfere with walking and eating.

A Task Force of the American Psychiatric Association (Task Force on Late Neurologic Effects of Antipsychotic Drugs, 1980) reported that 10% to 20% of patients given antipsychotic drugs for one year or more develop clinically significant tardive dyskinesia (rates corrected for the 5% to 10% risk of spontaneous dyskinesias in similar populations not treated with neuroleptics). The elderly and perhaps women and young men may be at increased risk. Symptoms are characteristically unmasked or aggravated by the abrupt discontinuance of antipsychotic drugs and persist long after medication is withdrawn (as withdrawal-emergent dyskinesias). Many patients improve significantly within months, while some patients require one year or more (Glazer et al, 1984); rates of spontaneous remission are greater if the neuroleptic is withdrawn or the dose reduced. The elderly usually experience more prolonged and severe episodes of tardive dyskinesia that are less readily reversible (Tarsy and Baldessarini, 1984).

There is evidence that the mechanism of tardive dyskinesia involves supersensitivity of postsynaptic dopamine receptors along with subsensitivity of muscarinic receptors (Stahl et al, 1982; Friedman et al, 1983). Other mechanisms may contribute to this movement disorder.

Differential diagnosis of tardive dyskinesia is complex (Granacher, 1981) and criteria vary widely. For example, some observers include minor movements that are difficult to distinguish from habit spasms, mannerisms, or the spontaneous chewing movements seen in many normal elderly patients (senile chorea).

The Task Force also points out that the drugs available to treat tardive dyskinesia are not satisfactory in most patients (see Chapter 11, Drugs Used in Extrapyramidal Movement Disorders). Therefore, the prevention of the disorder is critical and the following guidelines have been recommended: (1) Antipsychotic drugs should be reserved for the short-term treatment of acute psychosis, including first attacks or exacerbations of schizophrenia, paranoia, mania, some cases of toxic or organic psychoses, childhood psychoses, and as adjuncts in psychotic depression. (2) Their use for over six months is indicated only in chronic psychotic disorders, primarily schizophrenia, and only when a continuing response can be shown. (3) Antipsychotic therapy should be evaluated at least once yearly by reducing the dose by about 10% every three to seven days until the drug has been stopped completely or the clinical condition worsens. This procedure indicates whether antipsychotic medication is still beneficial and also helps to detect early symptoms of dyskinesia upon withdrawal.

Because there are no alternative drugs to treat psychoses, the Task Force concludes that the clinician, in consultation with the patient and family, must balance the risks of continuing treatment in a patient who develops tardive dyskinesia against the benefits of antipsychotic therapy. They stress that tardive dyskinesia does not seem to be uniformly relentless and progressive and that continuing treatment, at least in the short term, is usually justifiable if the patient has an active psychosis.

Neuroleptic Malignant Syndrome: This syndrome is a relatively rare reaction associated with antipsychotics, especially the high-potency drugs. It is characterized by severe muscular hypertonicity and akinesia (rigidity, catatonia), dysarthria, and fluctuating levels of consciousness, including stupor and mutism, as well as fever and variable autonomic disturbances of heart rate and blood pressure. Physical exhaustion, dehydration, and pneumonia or emboli may be predisposing or complicating factors (Caroff, 1980). Neurolep-

tic malignant syndrome is twice as common in males as in females; 80% of cases occur in patients under 40 years of age. The prevalence is uncertain, but as many as 1% of patients treated with antipsychotic drugs may be at risk (Manschreck, 1983). The mortality rate is 20% (Weinberg and Twersky, 1983).

Specific treatment for the neuroleptic malignant syndrome is emerging. Initially, antipsychotic medication should be discontinued immediately, followed by supportive therapy (ie, control of hyperthermia with antipyretics and cooling blankets, intravenous fluids). Some success with drug therapy has been reported. Amantadine (McCarron et al, 1982; Amdurski et al, 1983), bromocriptine [Parlodel] (Mueller et al, 1983), dantrolene [Dantrium] (May et al, 1983), and a combination of dantrolene and bromocriptine (Granato et al, 1983) have been reported to produce remission in severe cases, but more extensive study is necessary (Birkhimer and DeVane, 1984). Bromocriptine 10 to 50 mg every 24 hours is especially promising and is well tolerated.

AUTONOMIC NERVOUS SYSTEM EFFECTS. Most antipsychotic agents have both alpha antiadrenergic and some anticholinergic actions, especially the low-potency drugs (see Table 1). These effects are common after oral administration but are most pronounced after parenteral administration. Autonomic reactions rarely necessitate drug withdrawal, but reduced doses may be advisable if effects are severe.

Orthostatic hypotension is the most troublesome antiadrenergic effect; it improves temporarily if the patient lies down, and patients should be advised to stand and/or begin walking slowly and carefully. Acute hypotensive crises may occur in elderly or debilitated patients and after large parenteral doses. If hypotension is severe, intravenous fluids should be administered cautiously to correct hypovolemia. Norepinephrine [Levophed] or phenylephrine [Neo-Synephrine] is required only rarely. Beta-adrenergic amines (eg, epinephrine, isoproterenol) are contraindicated, for they may cause a paradoxical worsening of hypotension. As with other drugs having antiadrenergic actions, the antipsychotic agents, especially thioridazine, may inhibit ejaculation.

Anticholinergic-autonomic effects include dryness of the mouth, tachycardia, blurred vision, urinary retention, and constipation. Death has resulted from adynamic ileus or fulminating infection of the bladder. Antipsychotic agents impair central thermoregulatory mechanisms, which may be a problem in hot temperatures. Anticholinergic drugs generally should not be used with antipsychotic drugs to avoid additive anticholinergic activity (see also discussion on Tardive Dyskinesia).

ALLERGIC AND IDIOSYNCRATIC EFFECTS. Cholestatic jaundice is noted most often with use of aliphatic phenothiazines, usually during the first few weeks of treatment. This may be a hypersensitivity reaction and is usually mild and self-limited; however, if hyperbilirubinemia or jaundice is detected, the drug should be withdrawn immediately and an agent from a different chemical group administered.

Cutaneous allergic reactions, manifested as urticarial, maculopapular, or petechial lesions, occur infrequently. Serious reactions (eg, exfoliative dermatitis) have been reported occasionally. If these effects are noted, the drug should be discontinued and therapy resumed later with a drug from a different chemical class.

Photosensitivity usually is manifested as an acute hypersensitivity reaction to sun with severe sunburn or rash. A chronic skin reaction manifested by dark purplish brown pigmentation also may develop. This idiosyncratic reaction is generally mild and seldom requires dosage adjustment. It occurs most often when the aliphatic phenothiazines, especially chlorpromazine, are given for prolonged periods in large doses (800 mg or more daily). The risk of photosensitivity may be minimized by using the lowest effective dose, avoiding exposure to ultraviolet light, and using sunscreen preparations.

See the section on Hematologic Effects for a discussion on agranulocytosis.

NEUROENDOCRINE EFFECTS. Delayed ovulation and menstruation, amenorrhea, and galactorrhea in women and gynecomastia, edema, and weight gain in men have been reported occasionally. These effects are generally transient. They are considered to be manifestations of neuroendocrine imbalance caused by altered hypothalamic and pituitary function. Thioridazine is especially risky in this regard (Brown et al, 1981).

Sexual dysfunction in both men and women has been reported with the use of antipsychotics (Mitchell and Popkin, 1982; Oyewumi, 1983). In women, these drugs can cause loss of libido and inability to achieve orgasm. In men, erectile and ejaculatory deficiencies, as well as loss of libido, have been reported. Most types of sexual dysfunction disappear when the drugs are discontinued. Priapism, although rare, may persist and eventually may require surgical intervention.

All neuroleptic drugs produce hyperprolactinemia by blocking the inhibitory action of dopamine on prolactin secretion (Gruen et al, 1978). Although prolactin increases the incidence and growth of some mammary tumors in mice and rats and some human metastatic breast carcinomas are prolactin-dependent, it also exerts a protective effect against some carcinogen-induced breast tumors in rodents. Results of limited studies have not shown an association between long-term administration of antipsychotic drugs and antidopaminergic antihypertensive agents (all of which induce sustained hyperprolactinemia) and the development of mammary tumors in humans. Epidemiologic studies are continuing. Until conclusive data are available, however, physicians should be aware of this potential problem, particularly in women with previously detected breast cancer or in those with a strong family history of this neoplasm.

CARDIAC EFFECTS. Thioridazine may produce electrocardiographic alterations resembling hypokalemia (ie, prolonged QT interval, appearance of U waves). Similar disturbances in ventricular repolarization have been reported in patients receiving large doses of low-potency drugs. Elderly patients may require high-potency neuroleptics to avoid these reactions.

RESPIRATORY EFFECTS. Respiratory dysfunction has been reported rarely and may be due to the sedative or extrapyramidal actions of these drugs. The sedative effects may exacerbate acute problems in patients with a history of chronic obstructive lung disease. Extrapyramidal actions may result in pharyngeal and laryngeal paralysis leading to dysphagia and aspiration. Respiratory distress also may be associated with tardive dyskinesia (Young and Patel, 1984).

OCULAR EFFECTS. Dose-related pigmentary keratopathy, conjunctival melanosis, and glaucoma have been observed when large doses of chlorpromazine were employed for long periods. Opacities of the cornea and lens due to deposition of fine particulate matter were detectable on slit-lamp examination. Generally, vision is not impaired and changes regress after withdrawal of therapy. However, chlorpromazine has been implicated in one case of optic atrophy.

Large doses of thioridazine have caused pigmentary retinopathy, and the patchy loss of visual acuity (scotoma) is sometimes irreversible. For this reason, the maximal recommended dose of thioridazine is 800 mg daily.

HEMATOLOGIC EFFECTS. Although these reactions appear to be most frequent with low-potency neuroleptics, they may be associated with any of these agents. Some depression of leukopoiesis is detectable in most patients, particularly with large doses of low-potency phenothiazines (eg, chlorpromazine, thioridazine), but rarely persists. Agranulocytosis is a potentially catastrophic idiosyncratic reaction that usually appears within the first three months of phenothiazine therapy. Although the incidence is extremely low (about 1 in 10,000), mortality is high. Therefore, appearance of fever, sore throat, or cellulitis is an indication for discontinuing the phenothiazine and performing white blood cell and differential counts immediately. After recovery, low doses of a high-potency neuroleptic can be substituted.

Precautions

Patient Reassurance: After discharge from the hospital, both patient and family should be advised that medication must be continued even though the patient feels well; reassurance about needless fears of addiction is important. The effects of drowsiness on such tasks as driving or operating machinery should be stressed, and dosage schedules that minimize interference with the patient's ability to perform these tasks should be employed. The patient should be further warned about the possible additive effects of other central nervous system depressants (eg, antianxiety agents, hypnotics, centrally acting anticholinergics, tricyclic antidepressants) and specifically about the additive depressant effects of alcoholic beverages.

Informed Consent: The principles of informed consent govern antipsychotic drug treatment as they do other therapies and procedures in medicine. Despite the presence of psychotic symptoms, patients are generally considered legally competent to participate in informed consent procedures. However, the physician may wish to inform relatives or other responsible members of the patient's household of the risks and benefits of treatment.

In the acute phases of illness, it is generally considered sufficient to give reasonable indication of the purposes, anticipated benefits, and short-term risks of antipsychotic drug therapy. The medical record should note that this information has been discussed. In long-term treatment, the risk of serious complications, such as tardive dyskinesia, is greater. When treatment lasts for more than 6 to 12 months, a formal discussion of the risks is indicated. The patient also should be advised of the risks associated with discontinuation of therapy (eg, exacerbation of symptoms). Alternative strategies for using antipsychotic drugs may be reviewed. The record should reflect that discussion of these issues has taken place and that the patient has consented to this treatment strategy. Some clinicians believe that written informed consent may provide better documentation that the patient has been advised of risks, benefits, and alternative treatment strategies. This seems particularly important when evidence of dyskinesia has been observed.

There is no evidence that engaging in informed consent decreases compliance or undermines a therapeutic strategy. On the contrary, there is evidence that this process enhances the therapeutic alliance.

Because lack of insight is a common feature of schizophrenia, doctor and patient will often disagree about the presence of illness and desirability of treatment. Overriding the patient's right to refuse treatment is indicated only in emergencies. Otherwise, a continued effort to gain the patient's cooperation is required. Guidelines for defining emergencies that permit forcible medication of the psychotic patient vary among states and federal jurisdictions. The physician faced with this dilemma must be familiar with local standards.

Children: Antipsychotic drugs are used in children only when normal functioning is significantly impaired and only as adjuncts to other forms of therapy (eg, behavioral, psychological, educational) (Oyewumi, 1983). Most clinicians prefer low doses of high-potency antipsychotic drugs. The lowest effective dose should be employed for an adequate period (eg, six weeks). There is no evidence that children are more vulnerable to adverse reactions, although further study is needed. It is important to note that tardive dyskinesia can occur in children.

Older Patients: The incidence of adverse effects, especially hypotension and neurologic reactions, is higher in patients over 55 years. To minimize these reactions, the dose should be reduced to the lowest effective level, the patient should be observed closely, and the maintenance regimen should be reviewed periodically.

Since sleep disturbances are more common in elderly patients, the administration of antipsychotic agents once daily at bedtime may be appropriate. However, when higher dosage levels are indicated, smaller amounts at more frequent intervals may be necessary, since the drug may not be eliminated quickly enough to avoid excessive plasma concentrations. Some clinicians prefer medium-potency drugs, such as perphenazine and piperacetazine, in geriatric patients.

Psychiatric syndromes in the elderly can be caused by drugs or organic (brain or systemic) disease. In these instances, withdrawal of the precipitating drug or treatment of the medical condition should supersede antipsychotic medication and may obviate the need for these agents. Because the elderly are particularly prone to develop adverse effects from antipsychotic drugs, these agents should not be used when other drugs are effective.

Coexisting Medical Problems: A history of liver disease is not an absolute contraindication to use of antipsychotic agents, but smaller doses may be required because metabolic clearance is decreased. The more potent antipsychotics (piperazine phenothiazines, thiothixene [Navane], or haloperidol [Haldol]) are preferred in these patients.

Although tolerance to the hypotensive effect develops with prolonged treatment, caution is required when antipsychotic drugs are given to patients in whom a sudden drop in blood pressure is undesirable.

Antipsychotic agents may be given to epileptics receiving adequate anticonvulsant therapy. The increased incidence of seizures that has been observed occasionally may be averted by increasing the dose of the anticonvulsant. Patients with a family history of seizures or febrile convulsions are more likely to develop seizures than those without such history. Thioridazine [Mellaril], mesoridazine [Serentil], fluphenazine [Permitil, Prolixin], and molindone [Moban] are least epileptogenic. Specific guidelines for antipsychotic drug selection and management of epileptic patients have been reviewed (Itil and Soldatos, 1980).

Drug Interactions: Antipsychotic drugs may enhance the action of other central nervous system depressants (eg, antianxiety agents, hypnotics, analgesics). The doses of preanesthetic drugs having sedative action and general anesthetics may need to be reduced with concomitant use. Antipsychotic agents should be discontinued temporarily in patients receiving spinal or epidural anesthesia to allow time for the remaining drug to be metabolized.

Concurrent use of heterocyclic antidepressants or anticholinergic agents may cause additive central nervous system depression and anticholinergic activity. Antipsychotic drugs may interfere with the neuronal uptake of guanethidine [Ismelin], which antagonizes its antihypertensive effect.

Tolerance, Dependence, and Withdrawal Symptoms: Some tolerance to the sedative, anticholinergic, and antiadrenergic (hypotensive) effects of antipsychotic drugs develops within weeks to months. Little tolerance to the antipsychotic action occurs in spite of the adaptive dopamine supersensitivity that develops and that is postulated to cause tardive dyskinesia. There are, however, recent reports of probable tolerance after three years of continuous treatment with parenteral fluphenazine in about 10% of patients with chronic schizophrenia.

Although drug dependence does not occur, some physiologic adaptation is evident, because abrupt withdrawal after prolonged therapy results in the following cluster of symptoms in about one-third of patients, especially with low-potency agents: nausea, vomiting, diaphoresis, headache, restlessness, and insomnia (Lacoursiere et al, 1976; Luchins et al, 1980). The mechanism may be related to altered sensitivity of cholinergic neurons following prolonged anticholinergic blockade, because the low-potency antipsychotic drugs with stronger anticholinergic effects are more likely to produce the phenomenon. However, these withdrawal symptoms are also produced by the concomitant withdrawal of high-potency antipsychotic and anticholinergic drugs given to alleviate extrapyramidal reactions.

Withdrawal signs and symptoms occur in two to three days and may persist for two weeks. A gradual (over one to two weeks) reduction in dosage is recommended when terminating antipsychotic drug therapy. An anticholinergic drug given concomitantly also should be withdrawn gradually, but not simultaneously with the antipsychotic drug. Drug holidays should be utilized cautiously for patients sensitive to withdrawal symptoms.

Withdrawal psychosis has been suggested to explain the rapid exacerbation of schizophrenic symptoms in some patients undergoing dosage reduction or discontinuation of therapy. However, these observations are also compatible with recurrence of symptoms following reduction of effective therapy and the withdrawal hypothesis has not yet been confirmed.

Teratogenicity: Data on the teratogenicity of antipsychotic drugs are fragmentary, contradictory, and mainly report on experience with the older antipsychotic drugs.

Antipsychotic drugs have been identified in maternal and fetal plasma, amniotic fluid, and the urine of newborn infants. Prolonged extrapyramidal effects may appear in the infant, and there is a possibility of behavioral teratogenesis (Coyle et al, 1974). Thus, the use of antipsychotic drugs should be avoided during the first trimester if possible, but the slightly increased risk of teratogenicity may be outweighed by the need for treatment (Edlund and Craig, 1984). Therapy should be discontinued one or two weeks before delivery to avoid neonatal distress (see discussion on the use of drugs during pregnancy in Chapter 3).

Lactation: Antipsychotic drugs are secreted in low concentrations into breast milk (Oyewumi, 1983). Breast feeding should be discouraged when a mother requires antipsychotic medication. If a mother who needs continuous therapy nurses her infant, close supervision of the infant is mandatory.

Drug Evaluations

The efficacy of most antipsychotic agents in current clinical use in the United States is similar and doses may be equated with 100 mg of of chlorpromazine (see Table 1). Differences among compounds are related to the presence of other pharmacologic properties, to the prevalence of particular adverse reactions, and to variation in individual response.

The pharmacologic properties and the prevalence of particular adverse reactions depend principally on the chemical class; therefore, the following evaluations are arranged by chemical class. Information on dosage is given for each member of a class, but information pertaining to the class is included in the first evaluation (ie, prototype drug) in each category.

PHENOTHIAZINE DERIVATIVES

Aliphatic Compounds

CHLORPROMAZINE HYDROCHLORIDE
[Thorazine]

ACTIONS AND USES. Chlorpromazine was the first antipsychotic agent marketed and is the prototype of the aliphatic phenothiazines. This agent is used primarily to treat schizophrenia and acute active psychoses and to control the manifestations of mania; it is used less commonly in schizoaffective disorder, paranoia, intractable hiccups, disturbed behavior associated with mental retardation, and nausea and vomiting.

Chlorpromazine is sometimes used to treat ballismus, Tourette's syndrome, and the chorea of Huntington's disease, although it is not labeled for these indications (see the Introduction).

Chlorpromazine has a relatively low potency. It is one of the most sedative antipsychotic drugs, but tolerance to this effect usually develops. Chlorpromazine probably is best tolerated by patients under 40 years. In older patients, the incidence of dizziness, hypotension, ocular changes, and dyskinesias increases, although the latter is more commonly associated with the more potent neuroleptics.

ADVERSE REACTIONS. Chlorpromazine is less likely to cause extrapyramidal symptoms (other than tardive dyskinesia) than some other phenothiazines; parkinsonism and akathisia occur more frequently than dystonia.

Because chlorpromazine has pronounced antiadrenergic and anticholinergic properties, orthostatic hypotension, dryness of the mouth, blurred vision, urinary retention, and constipation are common. These reactions tend to diminish after the first week of continual therapy. Chlorpromazine appears to have the greatest propensity among the phenothiazines to produce agranulocytosis and cholestatic jaundice, but both are rare. Allergic skin reactions are uncommon, but mild photosensitivity occurs relatively often and the patient should be so informed. A lupus-like illness with a lupus-like coagulation inhibitor has been reported (Alberti-Flor, 1983; Tollefson et al, 1984). Patients should be examined periodically for conjunctival melanosis, pigmentary opacities in the cornea and lens, and glaucoma. Menstrual irregularities, galactorrhea, gynecomastia, and impotence have been reported occasionally.

For further information on indications, adverse reactions, and precautions, see the Introduction.

PHARMACOKINETICS. Although intestinal absorption is complete, the oral bioavailability is 32% ± 19% because of variable metabolism in the intestinal wall and liver (marked first-pass effect). Time to peak plasma concentration is two to four hours. After intramuscular administration, plasma concentrations are four to ten times higher than after oral administration; onset of action occurs within 20 to 30 minutes, and the peak effect is noted in two to three hours. Volume of distribution (21 ± 9 L/kg) and plasma binding (95% to 98%) are extensive. The plasma half-life is 30 ± 7 hours; however, some metabolites are eliminated slowly (months) in the urine.

At least 100 metabolites of chlorpromazine appear in man. Several of these, norchlorpromazine, 11-hydroxychlorpromazine, and 7-hydroxychlorpromazine, are pharmacologically active.

Enzyme induction varies considerably among individuals. Clearance after intramuscular administration is 8.6 ± 2.9 ml/min/kg. Less than 1% of the drug is excreted unchanged by the kidney.

DOSAGE AND PREPARATIONS. This drug generally should not be used in children under 6 months.

Intramuscular: For acute active psychoses in hospitalized *adults,* 25 to 100 mg initially, repeated in one to four hours as necessary until control is achieved. Most patients respond to 0.5 to 1 g daily. *Elderly or debilitated patients,* doses in the lower range for adults generally control symptoms. *Children,* 0.5 mg/kg every six to eight hours, gradually increased until symptoms are controlled; the total daily dose should not exceed 40 mg in children under 5 years or 75 mg in older children. Oral administration should be substituted when symptoms are controlled.

Intravenous: This route is highly irritating and should be used only for intractable hiccups.

> *Thorazine* (Smith Kline & French), **Generic**. Solution (aqueous) 25 mg/ml in 1, 2, and 10 ml containers.

Oral: For severe psychosis, *adults,* initially, 200 to 600 mg daily in divided doses, increased if necessary until symptoms are controlled or adverse reactions intervene (maximum, 2 g daily). A dose of 500 to 800 mg/day is usually adequate after several days of treatment. Although the maximum recommended daily dose is 2 g, amounts exceeding 1 g rarely increase the response. *Elderly or debilitated patients,* one-third to one-half the usual adult dose, increased more gradually (20- to 25-mg increments). *Children,* 0.5 mg/kg every four to six hours.

For all patients, after two weeks at optimal dosage, the amount should be reduced gradually to the minimum effective level for maintenance. The average dose in patients under 40 years is 300 to 800 mg daily. The response of older patients seldom improves with doses exceeding 300 mg daily. Amounts greater than 1 g daily usually confer no additional advantage and may produce a higher incidence of adverse reactions.

> **Generic**. Concentrate 30 and 100 mg/ml; tablets 10, 25, 50, 100, and 200 mg.
> *Thorazine* (Smith Kline & French). Capsules (timed-release) 30, 75, 150, 200, and 300 mg; concentrate 30 and 100 mg/ml; syrup 10 mg/5 ml; tablets 10, 25, 50, 100, and 200 mg.

Rectal: *Children,* 1 mg/kg every six to eight hours.

> *Thorazine* (Smith Kline & French). Suppositories 25 and 100 mg (equivalent to base).

TRIFLUPROMAZINE HYDROCHLORIDE
[Vesprin]

Triflupromazine has the same actions and indications as chlorpromazine and is equally effective (see Table 1). For information on indications, adverse reactions, and precautions, see the Introduction and the evaluation on Chlorpromazine Hydrochloride.

DOSAGE AND PREPARATIONS.

Intramuscular: For acute active psychoses in hospitalized patients, *adults,* initially, 60 to 150 mg daily; *elderly or debili-* *tated patients,* 10 to 75 mg daily; *children over 2 1/2 years,* 0.2 to 0.25 mg/kg (maximum, 10 mg daily). Oral administration should be substituted when symptoms are controlled.

> *Vesprin* (Squibb). Solution 10 mg/ml in 10 ml containers and 20 mg/ml in 1 ml containers.

Oral: Initially, *adults,* 50 to 150 mg daily in divided doses; *children,* 2 mg/kg daily in divided doses. When symptoms are controlled, the dosage should be reduced gradually to the minimum effective level for maintenance.

> *Vesprin* (Squibb). Tablets 10, 25, and 50 mg.

Piperidine Compounds

THIORIDAZINE HYDROCHLORIDE
[Mellaril]

ACTIONS AND USES. This low-potency phenothiazine is widely used. Its efficacy is similar to that of chlorpromazine in equivalent doses (see Table 1). Thioridazine is generally considered to be the prototype of the piperidine compounds; however, its effectiveness may be due principally to the formation of the more active metabolite, mesoridazine, which is also widely used.

Thioridazine is administered primarily to treat schizophrenia and acute active psychoses. Thioridazine and mesoridazine also have been suggested to relieve anxiety, agitation, and depression associated with affective disorders (Gershon et al, 1981), and both drugs have been used extensively in schizo-affective disorders. See the Introduction for other indications.

ADVERSE REACTIONS. Sedation and orthostatic hypotension are similar to those observed with chlorpromazine. The pronounced anticholinergic activity of thioridazine (and its relatively weak antidopaminergic action) may explain the low incidence of extrapyramidal reactions, other than tardive dyskinesia. Large doses may inhibit ejaculation and have been associated with retrograde ejaculation. Electrocardiographic changes have been noted more frequently with thioridazine than with other phenothiazines and may occur after short-term therapy with daily doses of 300 mg or more. Agranulocytosis is rare. Agranulocytosis with hepatitis that progressed to hepatic encephalopathy was reported in one patient; jaundice was not previously associated with thioridazine. Photosensitivity has developed rarely.

Pigmentary retinopathy occurs frequently in patients receiving more than 800 mg/day; diminished visual acuity may be irreversible. Smaller daily doses have impaired vision without detectable retinal changes. Because of these ocular reactions, 800 mg/day is the maximum dose; the manufacturer recommends that doses exceeding 300 mg/day be used only in patients with severe psychoses. Thus, if large doses are required for long periods or if 800 mg/day is inadequate, another antipsychotic agent should be substituted.

The combination of thioridazine and lithium has been reported rarely to produce severe neurotoxicity manifested by seizures, delirium, encephalopathy, EEG abnormalities, and, in one patient, choreoathetoid movements. The risk of cardiac conduction problems is increased when thioridazine is given with a heterocyclic antidepressant.

For further information on indications, adverse reactions, and precautions, see the Introduction.

PHARMACOKINETICS. Bioavailability data are limited, but thioridazine produces peak plasma concentrations one to four hours after oral administration. The drug is sulfoxidized principally to mesoridazine and small amounts of sulforidazine, which are pharmacologically active, and thioridazine-5-sulfoxide, which is inactive. Both thioridazine and mesoridazine are widely distributed, and the ratio of bound to free drug is 3:1 and 2:1, respectively. Both drugs have equal receptor-binding affinity, but the concentration of free mesoridazine is relatively higher and this agent forms fewer inactive metabolites and is inactivated more slowly than thioridazine. These factors may account for its greater clinical potency and the response of thioridazine-refractory patients to mesoridazine (Gershon et al, 1981).

DOSAGE AND PREPARATIONS.
Oral: Adults, initially, 150 to 300 mg daily in divided doses; this may be increased gradually to a maximum of 800 mg daily in hospitalized patients. For maintenance therapy, the dose should be reduced gradually to the minimum effective level. *Elderly or debilitated patients,* one-third to one-half the usual adult dosage. *Children 2 years or older,* 1 mg/kg daily in divided doses; *under 2 years,* information is inadequate to establish a dosage.

   Generic. Concentrate 30 mg/ml; tablets 10, 25, 50, 100, 150, and 200 mg.
   Mellaril (Sandoz). Concentrate 30 mg/ml (alcohol 3%) and 100 mg/ml (alcohol 4.2%); suspension 25 and 100 mg/5 ml (equivalent to hydrochloride) (*Mellaril-S*); tablets 10, 15, 25, 50, 100, 150, and 200 mg.

MESORIDAZINE BESYLATE
[Serentil]

Mesoridazine, the major active metabolite of thioridazine, is an effective low-potency antipsychotic agent (see Table 1).

For information on indications, adverse reactions, and pharmacokinetics, see the Introduction and the evaluation on Thioridazine Hydrochloride.

DOSAGE AND PREPARATIONS.
Intramuscular: For acute psychoses, *adults and children over 12 years,* 25 to 175 mg daily in divided doses. Since

intramuscular injection is irritating, oral administration should be substituted when symptoms are controlled.
   Serentil (Boehringer Ingelheim). Solution 25 mg/ml in 1 ml containers.
Oral: Adults and children over 12 years, initially, 150 mg daily in divided doses, increased gradually in 50-mg increments until symptoms are controlled, then reduced gradually to the minimum effective amount for maintenance (range, 100 to 400 mg daily). *Elderly or debilitated patients,* one-third to one-half the usual adult dosage. *Children under 12 years,* information is inadequate to establish a dosage.
   Serentil (Boehringer Ingelheim). Concentrate 25 mg/ml (alcohol 0.61%); tablets 10, 25, 50, and 100 mg.

Piperazine Compounds

TRIFLUOPERAZINE HYDROCHLORIDE
[Stelazine]

ACTIONS AND USES. Trifluoperazine is a prototype of the piperazine phenothiazines, which are high-potency antipsychotic drugs (see Table 1). Trifluoperazine is used primarily to treat schizophrenia and acute active psychoses. It also is used in schizoaffective disorder, paranoid syndrome, and mental retardation with disturbed behavior (see the Introduction). The piperazine phenothiazines also have potent antiemetic activity. Trifluoperazine has been used investigationally to treat ballismus and Tourette's syndrome.

ADVERSE REACTIONS AND PRECAUTIONS. The piperazines have less sedative effect than other phenothiazines. The incidence of autonomic effects (eg, orthostatic hypotension) is also lower, but extrapyramidal reactions occur more frequently, particularly when large doses are used in patients over 40 years.

Piperazine compounds are less likely to produce blood dyscrasias or jaundice, although transient leukopenia has been reported occasionally. Ocular changes have developed rarely with trifluoperazine but have not yet been noted with other piperazine compounds.

Since no marked electrocardiographic changes have been observed, piperazine compounds may be preferred for patients with cardiovascular disease. However, a few patients with angina pectoris have reported increased pain during therapy with trifluoperazine. Therefore, patients with angina should be observed carefully and the drug withdrawn if an unfavorable response occurs.

For further information on indications, adverse reactions, and precautions, see the Introduction.

PHARMACOKINETICS. Pharmacokinetic data on trifluoperazine are limited but bioavailability, onset of action, time to peak effect, first-pass effect, metabolism, and elimination half-lives appear to resemble those of chlorpromazine.

DOSAGE AND PREPARATIONS.

Intramuscular: For acute psychoses, *adults,* 1 to 2 mg by deep intramuscular injection every four to six hours, as needed. Doses exceeding 6 mg/24 hours are rarely necessary. *Elderly and debilitated patients,* one-third to one-half of the usual adult dose given at longer intervals. *Children 6 years and older,* 1 mg once or twice daily; *under 6 years,* information is inadequate to establish a dosage. When symptoms are controlled, oral administration should be substituted.

   Stelazine (Smith Kline & French). Solution 2 mg/ml in 10 ml containers.

Oral: Initially, *adults (outpatients),* 2 to 4 mg daily in divided doses; *(hospitalized),* 4 to 10 mg daily in divided doses, increased gradually to the optimum amount. *Elderly or debilitated patients,* one-third to one-half the usual adult dose. *Children 6 years or older,* 1 to 2 mg daily, gradually increased to the optimum amount (rarely more than 15 mg daily).

   When symptoms are controlled, the dosage should be reduced gradually for all patients to the minimum effective amount for maintenance. The concentrate should be diluted in fruit juice or another suitable vehicle just prior to administration.

   Stelazine (Smith Kline & French), **Generic.** Concentrate 10 mg/ml; tablets 1, 2, 5, and 10 mg.

ACETOPHENAZINE MALEATE
   [Tindal]

   See the Introduction and the evaluation on Trifluoperazine Hydrochloride.

DOSAGE AND PREPARATIONS.

Oral: Adults, initially, 60 mg daily in divided doses, increased in 20-mg increments until the optimum level (usually 80 to 120 mg daily for hospitalized patients) is reached or adverse effects intervene. As much as 400 mg daily may be used. *Elderly or debilitated patients,* one-third to one-half the usual adult dosage. *Children,* information is inadequate to establish a dosage.

   In all patients, when symptoms have been controlled, the dosage should be reduced gradually to the minimum effective amount for maintenance.

   Tindal (Schering). Tablets 20 mg.

FLUPHENAZINE DECANOATE
   [Prolixin Decanoate]

FLUPHENAZINE ENANTHATE
   [Prolixin Enanthate]

FLUPHENAZINE HYDROCHLORIDE
   [Permitil, Prolixin]

ACTIONS AND USES. Fluphenazine has the highest milligram potency of the phenothiazines (see Table 1).

   The duration of action of the depot forms, fluphenazine decanoate and fluphenazine enanthate, is two to three weeks. An interval of four weeks or longer between injections may be adequate for maintenance therapy in selected patients. Depot forms are useful in outpatients with a history of poor compliance, inadequate absorption of oral medication, or frequent relapses (Groves and Mandel, 1975; Glazer, 1984).

   Close supervision and individualization of dosage are required. Hospitalization may be necessary initially and a short-acting oral form used to determine dosage (fluphenazine hydrochloride). Initial doses of a depot form and the intervals between doses then should be determined carefully, based on the patient's personal and family drug history. Although there is no precise formula for conversion from oral to depot preparations, one study suggested that for each 10 mg of fluphenazine hydrochloride required daily, fluphenazine decanoate 12.5 mg be given intramuscularly every three weeks (Schooler and Levine, 1976).

   If extrapyramidal reactions occurred previously (particularly following use of high-potency drugs or a chemical class that produces a lower incidence of these symptoms), it is advisable to use a test depot dose (usually, 12.5 mg) and increase the amount every 10 to 14 days during the first month until a therapeutic response has been attained. After the patient has been stabilized on the optimum dose, the amount should be adjusted to provide the minimum effective maintenance dose as infrequently as possible. Continued supervision and a flexible dosage regimen usually are necessary for optimum response. In physically healthy patients with refractory chronic schizophrenia, optimal doses of parenteral preparations have been used successfully for years without producing severe extrapyramidal reactions.

ADVERSE REACTIONS AND PRECAUTIONS. With the exception of tardive dyskinesia, extrapyramidal reactions usually appear during the first few weeks of therapy but they may occur even after the patient's condition is stabilized. Occasionally, usual doses of anticholinergic drugs do not adequately control extrapyramidal symptoms, and increased amounts may precipitate toxic psychosis. In such cases, smaller doses or less frequent administration of fluphenazine generally controls symptoms.

   Depending upon dosage and individual sensitivity, sedation, anticholinergic side effects, and hypotensive episodes have been observed. Usually these reactions are mild and subside spontaneously. Rarely, jaundice occurs with oral use of fluphenazine; the depot forms have not yet been reported to cause this reaction. Only the risk of extrapyramidal reactions appears to be increased by use of the depot form (Glazer, 1984).

PHARMACOKINETICS. Time to maximum blood concentration after intramuscular injection of fluphenazine enanthate was two to four days, and the plasma half-life was 3.6 and 3.7 days in two patients compared to 2 to 4 hours and about 12 hours, respectively, for fluphenazine hydrochloride. Time to maximum blood concentration after intramuscular injection of the decanoate salt was 12 to 24 hours, and plasma half-life was 6.8 and 9.6 days in two patients.

DOSAGE AND PREPARATIONS.

Intramuscular, Subcutaneous (depot preparations): For sustained effects, *adults,* initially, 12.5 mg, followed by 25 mg every two to three weeks to establish appropriate dosage. Dosage and intervals must be individualized, but the amount rarely should exceed 100 mg every two to six weeks; if the dose exceeds 50 mg, increases should be made in increments of. 12.5 mg. *Debilitated patients or those with a history of extrapyramidal reactions,* initially, 2.5 mg, followed by 2.5 to 5 mg every 10 to 14 days. *Children,* information is inadequate to establish a dosage.

> FLUPHENAZINE DECANOATE:
> *Prolixin Decanoate* (Squibb). Solution 25 mg/ml (in sesame oil) in 1 and 5 ml containers.
> FLUPHENAZINE ENANTHATE:
> *Prolixin Enanthate* (Squibb). Solution 25 mg/ml (in sesame oil) in 1 and 5 ml containers.

Intramuscular: For acute active psychosis, *adults,* initially, 1.25 to 2.5 mg every six to eight hours until symptoms are controlled; amounts exceeding 10 mg are seldom required. When symptoms are controlled, oral administration should be substituted. *Elderly or debilitated patients,* one-third to one-half the usual adult dose. *Children,* information is inadequate to establish a dosage.

> FLUPHENAZINE HYDROCHLORIDE:
> *Prolixin* (Squibb). Solution 2.5 mg/ml in 10 ml containers.

Oral: Adults, initially, 2.5 to 10 mg, reduced gradually to a usual maintenance dose of 1 to 5 mg daily (maintenance doses exceeding 3 mg are rarely necessary). *Elderly or debilitated patients,* 1 to 2.5 mg daily, depending upon response. *Children,* information is inadequate to establish a dosage, although 0.75 to 10 mg/day has been used in *children 5 to 12 years.* The concentrate should be diluted with water, fruit juice, or other suitable vehicle before administration.

> FLUPHENAZINE HYDROCHLORIDE:
> *Permitil* (Schering). Concentrate 5 mg/ml (alcohol 1%); tablets 2.5, 5, and 10 mg.
> *Prolixin* (Squibb). Elixir 2.5 mg/5 ml (alcohol 14%); tablets 1, 2.5, 5, and 10 mg.

PERPHENAZINE
[Trilafon]

See the Introduction and the evaluation on Trifluoperazine Hydrochloride.

DOSAGE AND PREPARATIONS.

Intramuscular: Adults, for acute active psychoses, initially, 5 to 10 mg; 5 mg may be given every six hours thereafter, but the total amount should not exceed 15 mg daily in ambulatory patients or 30 mg daily in hospitalized patients. *Elderly or debilitated patients,* one-third to one-half the usual adult dose. *Children under 12 years,* information is inadequate to establish a dosage; *over 12 years,* lowest limit of adult dose. When symptoms are controlled, oral administration should be substituted.

> *Trilafon* (Schering). Solution 5 mg/ml in 1 ml containers.

Oral: Adults, 8 to 32 mg daily in divided doses. Daily doses greater than 64 mg should be used very cautiously. When symptoms have been controlled, the dosage should be reduced gradually to the minimum effective level. *Elderly or debilitated patients,* one-third to one-half the usual adult dose. Pediatric dosage has not been established but the following amounts have been given in divided doses: *Children 1 to 6 years,* 4 to 6 mg daily; *6 to 12 years,* 6 mg daily; *over 12 years,* 6 to 12 mg daily. The concentrate should be diluted in fruit juice or another suitable liquid vehicle (tea is not recommended) prior to administration.

> *Trilafon* (Schering). Concentrate 16 mg/5 ml (alcohol <0.1%); tablets 2, 4, 8, and 16 mg; tablets (timed-release) 8 mg.

THIOXANTHENE DERIVATIVES

CHLORPROTHIXENE
[Taractan]

The pharmacologic actions of chlorprothixene, a low-potency xanthene compound, are very similar to those of chlorpromazine. For information on indications and adverse reactions, see the Introduction and the evaluation on Chlorpromazine Hydrochloride.

DOSAGE AND PREPARATIONS.

Intramuscular: For acute active psychoses, *adults and children over 12 years,* 75 to 200 mg daily in divided doses. *Elderly or debilitated patients,* 30 to 100 mg daily in divided doses. When symptoms are controlled, oral administration should be substituted. *Children under 12 years,* information is inadequate to establish a dosage.

> *Taractan* (Roche). Solution 12.5 mg/ml in 2 ml containers (as hydrochloride).

Oral: Adults, 75 to 200 mg daily in divided doses, increased gradually until symptoms are controlled or adverse reactions intervene. The optimum dose rarely exceeds 600 mg daily. *Elderly or debilitated patients and children over 6 years,* 30 to 100 mg daily in divided doses. When symptoms are controlled, the dosage should be reduced gradually to the minimum effective level. *Children under 6 years,* information is inadequate to establish a dosage.

> *Taractan* (Roche). Concentrate 100 mg/5 ml (as lactate and hydrochloride); tablets 10, 25, 50, and 100 mg.

THIOTHIXENE
[Navane]

THIOTHIXENE HYDROCHLORIDE
[Navane]

The chemical structure and pharmacologic actions of thiothixene, a high-potency compound, are very similar to those of the piperazine phenothiazines. For information on indications and adverse reactions, see the Introduction and the evaluation on Trifluoperazine Hydrochloride.

DOSAGE AND PREPARATIONS.
Intramuscular: For acute active psychoses, *adults and children 12 years or older,* initially, 4 mg two to four times daily, increased gradually until symptoms are controlled (maximum, 30 mg daily). *Elderly or debilitated patients*, one-third to one-half the usual adult dose. When symptoms are controlled, oral administration should be substituted. *Children under 12 years,* use not recommended because the drug's safety in pediatric patients has not been established.
    THIOTHIXENE HYDROCHLORIDE:
    Navane (Roerig). Solution 2 and 5 mg/ml (equivalent to base) in 2 ml containers.
Oral: Adults, 6 to 10 mg daily in divided doses, increased gradually if necessary. The usual optimal dose is 20 to 30 mg daily, and amounts in excess of 60 mg daily rarely enhance the response. When symptoms are controlled, the dose should be reduced gradually to the minimum effective level. *Elderly or debilitated patients,* initially, one-third to one-half the usual adult dosage. *Children under 12 years,* use not recommended because the drug's safety in pediatric patients has not been established.
    THIOTHIXENE:
    Navane (Roerig). Capsules 1, 2, 5, 10, and 20 mg.
    THIOTHIXENE HYDROCHLORIDE:
    Navane (Roerig). Concentrate 5 mg/ml (alcohol 7%) (equivalent to base).

BUTYROPHENONE DERIVATIVE

HALOPERIDOL
[Haldol]

HALOPERIDOL LACTATE
[Haldol]

HALOPERIDOL DECANOATE
[Haldol Decanoate]

ACTIONS AND USES. Haloperidol is pharmacologically, but not chemically, related to the high-potency piperazine phenothiazines (Ayd, 1978). This drug is used primarily to treat schizophrenia and acute active psychoses; it is also used in schizoaffective disorder, paranoid syndrome, ballismus, and Tourette's syndrome (drug of choice) and occasionally as adjunctive therapy in mental retardation and the chorea of Huntington's disease (see the Introduction). It also is a potent antiemetic.

Haloperidol decanoate is a long-acting injectable depot preparation for the prophylactic treatment of chronic schizophrenia (*Int Drug Ther Newslett*, 1980).

ADVERSE REACTIONS. Like the piperazine phenothiazines, haloperidol is relatively nonsedating and is likely to produce extrapyramidal reactions (see Table 1), especially if there is a history of such reactions to other antipsychotic agents. Akathisia and acute dystonias occasionally are severe. Persistent extrapyramidal symptoms usually are dose related but have also occurred following use of relatively small amounts.

Haloperidol causes fewer autonomic effects than the phenothiazines, although transient orthostatic hypotension has been reported occasionally. Also, it does not appear to produce any electrocardiographic changes.

Dermatologic reactions are rare and the risk of adverse hepatic effects is minimal. Mild, transient hematologic changes have occurred, but only one case of agranulocytosis has been reported.

Malformations occurred in two infants following maternal use of haloperidol and other medications. Epidemiologic studies have not confirmed a teratogenic effect of haloperidol, and a causal relationship was not established in either case.

For further information on indications, adverse reactions, and precautions, see the Introduction.

PHARMACOKINETICS. Haloperidol is well absorbed orally; however, a first-pass effect results in 60% (range, 44% to 74%) relative oral to intravenous bioavailability. Time to peak effect after intramuscular and oral administration is one and three hours, respectively. Volume of distribution is 20 L/kg. Haloperidol undergoes extensive hepatic degradation that includes N-dealkylation and glucuronidation; less than 1% of unchanged haloperidol is excreted in the urine. Plasma half-lives after oral administration vary from 12 to 38 hours.

The activity of haloperidol decanoate, a depot preparation, depends upon the enzymatic hydrolysis of the ester to haloperidol. Haloperidol decanoate, given once monthly (in amounts approximately 20 times the daily oral maintenance dose of haloperidol), has maintained patients with chronic schizophrenia for over one year. Steady-state plasma concentrations of 2 to 8 ng/ml are reached by the third monthly injection.

DOSAGE AND PREPARATIONS.
Intramuscular (regular preparation): For acute psychoses with marked agitation, *adults,* initially, 2 to 5 mg. Depending upon response, subsequent doses may be administered as often as every hour (although four- to eight-hour intervals are satisfactory in most patients) until symptoms are controlled. A dose of 10 mg daily usually is sufficient, and doses above 15 mg daily are seldom required. Oral administration should then

be substituted and the dosage individualized. *Elderly or debilitated patients and children under 12 years,* information is inadequate to establish a dosage.

HALOPERIDOL LACTATE:
Haldol (McNeil). Solution 5 mg/ml in 1 and 10 ml containers.

Intramuscular (depot formulation): The manufacturer suggests the following: For chronic psychoses, patients should be stabilized on antipsychotic medication before conversion to haloperidol decanoate. Furthermore, patients considered for haloperidol decanoate therapy should be given oral haloperidol first to exclude sensitivity to haloperidol. Close clinical supervision is required during initial dose adjustment to minimize overdosage or reappearance of psychotic symptoms before the next injection. During dose adjustment or exacerbations of psychosis, therapy can be supplemented with short-acting forms of haloperidol.

The initial dose of haloperidol decanoate should be based on the patient's clinical history, physical condition, and response to previous antipsychotic therapy. Small doses should be given initially and the amount increased as needed. The initial dose of haloperidol decanoate should be 10 to 15 times the previous daily dose in oral haloperidol equivalents, but no more than a maximum initial dose of 100 mg (2 ml). Haloperidol decanoate has been effective when administered at monthly intervals in several clinical studies. However, variation in patient response may dictate a need to adjust the interval as well as the dose.

Lower initial doses and more gradual adjustment are recommended for elderly or debilitated patients.

Clinical experience with haloperidol decanoate in doses greater than 300 mg (6 ml) per month has been limited.

HALOPERIDOL DECANOATE:
Haldol Decanoate (McNeil). Solution (in sesame oil) 70.5 mg (equivalent to 50 mg of base)/ml in 1 ml containers.

Oral: For acute active psychoses, *adults and children over 12 years,* initially, 0.5 to 2 mg for moderate symptoms and 3 to 5 mg for severe symptoms; this amount is given every 8 to 12 hours until psychotic symptoms are controlled. Doses of 10 mg daily are usually sufficient and doses above 15 mg daily are seldom required. When control has been obtained, the dose should be reduced gradually to the minimum effective maintenance level (usually, 2 to 8 mg daily). *Elderly or debilitated patients,* initially, 0.5 to 2 mg, gradually increased in increments of 0.5 mg.

For chronic schizophrenia, *adults and children over 12 years,* initially, 6 to 15 mg in divided doses, gradually increased until control is achieved (100 mg daily is required rarely for severely disturbed or resistant patients) and then gradually reduced to maintenance levels (usually, 15 to 20 mg daily). *Elderly or debilitated patients,* initially, 0.5 to 1.5 mg, increased gradually in small increments; the usual maintenance dose is 2 to 8 mg daily. *Children 3 to 12 years,* initially, 0.5 mg daily, increased by 0.5 mg at five- to seven-day intervals until the desired therapeutic effect is obtained. The total daily dose may be given in two or three divided amounts. Maintenance doses usually range from 0.05 to 0.15 mg/kg/day for psychotic disorders. *Children under 3 years,* information is inadequate to establish dosage.

HALOPERIDOL:

Haldol (McNeil). Tablets 0.5, 1, 2, 5, 10, and 20 mg.
HALOPERIDOL LACTATE:
Haldol (McNeil), *Generic.* Concentrate 2 mg/ml.

DIBENZOXAZEPINE DERIVATIVE

LOXAPINE HYDROCHLORIDE
[Loxitane C, Loxitane IM]

LOXAPINE SUCCINATE
[Loxitane]

ACTIONS AND USES. This dibenzoxazepine derivative represents a new class of tricyclic antipsychotic agents that is chemically distinct from the phenothiazines, butyrophenones, thioxanthenes, and dihydroindolone compounds. However, the major pharmacologic actions of loxapine do not differ appreciably from those of the older antipsychotic drugs. Loxapine has antiemetic, sedative, anticholinergic, and alpha-antiadrenergic actions.

This compound is effective in the treatment of schizophrenia and acute active psychoses. A closely related derivative, amoxapine [Asendin], is an antidepressant.

ADVERSE REACTIONS AND PRECAUTIONS. The incidence of extrapyramidal reactions, other than tardive dyskinesia, is intermediate between the aliphatic and piperazine phenothiazines (see Table 1). Lens opacities, pigmentary retinopathy, and skin pigmentation have not been reported. Loxapine, like other neuroleptics, decreases the seizure threshold and should be used with caution in patients with a history of convulsive disorders. Hepatitis has been associated rarely with use of loxapine.

For further information on indications, adverse reactions, and precautions, see the Introduction.

PHARMACOKINETICS. Loxapine is well absorbed orally. Times to peak serum levels after oral and intramuscular administration are two hours and one hour, respectively. Major metabolites are 8-hydroxyloxapine (antipsychotic activity) and 8-hydroxyamoxapine (antidepressant activity). Mean elimination half-lives of loxapine, 8-hydroxyloxapine, and 8-hydroxyamoxapine are 3.4, 9, and 30 hours, respectively.

DOSAGE AND PREPARATIONS.
Oral: Adults and adolescents 16 years or older, initially, 10 mg twice daily; a maximum of 50 mg daily may be given to severely psychotic patients. Dosage should be increased rapidly over the next week to ten days until control is achieved. For maintenance, dosage should be reduced gradually to the minimum effective level (usually, 60 to 100 mg daily) with a maximum dose of 250 mg daily. *Elderly and debilitated patients,* initially, one-third to one-half the usual adult dose. *Children under 16 years,* information is inadequate to estab-

lish a dosage. The concentrate should be diluted in fruit juice prior to administration.

LOXAPINE HYDROCHLORIDE:
Loxitane C (Lederle). Concentrate 25 mg/ml (equivalent to base).
LOXAPINE SUCCINATE:
Loxitane (Lederle). Capsules 5, 10, 25, and 50 mg (equivalent to base).

Intramuscular: 12.5 to 50 mg every four to six hours or at longer intervals, depending upon the response. Once symptoms are controlled, oral therapy should be substituted. This preparation should *not* be injected intravenously.

LOXAPINE HYDROCHLORIDE:
Loxitane IM (Lederle). Solution 50 mg/ml (equivalent to base) in 1 and 10 ml containers.

DIHYDROINDOLONE DERIVATIVE

MOLINDONE HYDROCHLORIDE
[Moban]

Molindone is chemically unrelated to the phenothiazines, butyrophenones, or thioxanthenes. It is effective in schizophrenia and acute active psychoses.

Pharmacokinetic data are fragmentary. The time to maximum plasma concentration is about 1.5 hours. The parent drug is metabolized rapidly and extensively, but the clinical effect persists for 24 to 36 hours.

ADVERSE REACTIONS AND PRECAUTIONS. The extrapyramidal and antiadrenergic effects of molindone generally are less severe than those of the other antipsychotics. The sedative effects are intermediate between the aliphatic and piperazine phenothiazines (see Table 1). Molindone decreases the convulsive threshold experimentally. Lens opacities and pigmentary retinopathy have not been reported.

For further information on adverse reactions and precautions, see the Introduction.

DOSAGE AND PREPARATIONS.
Oral: *Adults,* initially, 50 to 75 mg daily in divided doses, gradually increased if necessary until symptoms are controlled; as much as 225 mg daily has been used. When symptoms are controlled, the dose should be reduced gradually to the minimum effective level for maintenance. *Elderly or debilitated patients,* initially, one-third to one-half the usual adult dosage. *Children under 12 years,* information is inadequate to establish a dosage.
Moban (DuPont). Concentrate 20 mg/ml; tablets 5, 10, 25, 50, and 100 mg.

Cited References

Haloperidol decanoate: Latest depot neuroleptic. *Int Drug Ther Newslett* 15:5-8, (Feb) 1980.

Alberti-Flor JJ: Chlorpromazine-induced lupus-like illness. *Am Fam Physician* 27:151-152, (April) 1983.

Amdurski S, et al: Therapeutic trial of amantadine in haloperidol-induced malignant neuroleptic syndrome. *Curr Ther Res* 33:225-229, 1983.

American Psychiatric Association: *Diagnostic and Statistical Manual of Mental Disorders,* ed 3. Washington, DC, American Psychiatric Association, 1980, 181-193, 199-203.

Anderson WH, Kuehnle JC: Diagnosis and early management of acute psychosis. *N Engl J Med* 305:1128-1130, 1981.

Aubree JC, Lader MH: High and very high dosage antipsychotics: Critical review. *J Clin Psychiatry* 41:341-350, 1980.

Ayd FJ Jr: Haloperidol: Twenty years' clinical experience. *J Clin Psychiatry* 39:807-814, 1978.

Baldessarini RJ (ed): Antipsychotic drugs, in: *Psychiatric Treatment.* Washington, DC, American Pyschiatric Association, 1984.

Baldessarini RJ, Davis JM: What is best maintenance dose of neuroleptics for schizophrenia? *Psychiatry Res* 3:115-122, 1980.

Biederman J, Jellinek MS: Psychopharmacology in children. *N Engl J Med* 310:968-971, 1984.

Birkhimer LJ, DeVane CL: Neuroleptic malignant syndromes: Presentation and treatment. *Drug Intell Clin Pharm* 18:462-465, 1984.

Brown WA, et al: Differential effects of neuroleptic agents on pituitary-gonadal axis in men. *Arch Gen Psychiatry* 38:1270-1272, 1981.

Campbell M, et al: Psychopharmacological treatment of children with syndrome of autism. *Pediatr Ann* 13:309-316, 1984.

Caroff SN: Neuroleptic malignant syndrome. *J Clin Psychiatry* 41:79-83, 1980.

Carpenter WT Jr, Heinrichs DW: Early intervention, time-limited, targeted pharmacotherapy of schizophrenia, in: Carpenter WT Jr, Schooler NR (eds): *New Directions in Drug Treatment for Schizophrenia.* Rockville, MD, National Institute of Mental Health, 1984, 34-43.

Cohen BM, et al: Neuroleptic blood levels and therapeutic effect. *Psychopharmacology* 70:191-194, 1980 A.

Cohen DJ, et al: Clonidine ameliorates Gilles de la Tourette syndrome. *Arch Gen Psychiatry* 37:1350-1357, 1980 B.

Cohen BM, Baldessarini RJ: Blood neuroleptic levels as guide to clinical treatment. *Direct Psychiatry* 4:1-7, 1984.

Coyle J, et al: Teratogenesis: Critical evaluation. *Pharmacol Biochem Behav* 4:191-200, 1974.

Crow TJ: Molecular pathology of schizophrenia: More than one disease process? *Br Med J* 280:66-68, 1980.

Davis JM: Overview: Maintenance therapy in psychiatry: I. Schizophrenia. *Am J Psychiatry* 132:1237-1245, 1975.

Davis JM: Comparative doses and costs of antipsychotic medication. *Arch Gen Psychiatry* 33:858-861, 1976.

Davis JM, Casper R: Antipsychotic drugs: Clinical pharmacology and therapeutic use. *Drugs* 14:260-282, 1977.

Donaldson SR, et al: Pharmacologic treatment of schizophrenia: Progress report, in Carpenter WT Jr, Schooler NR (eds): *New Directions in Drug Treatment for Schizophrenia.* Rockville, MD, National Institute of Mental Health, 1984, 5-28.

Edlund MJ, Craig TJ: Antipsychotic drug use and birth defects: Epidemiologic reassessment. *Compr Psychiatry* 25:32-37, (Jan/Feb) 1984.

Ericksen SE, et al: Haloperidol dose, plasma levels, and clinical response: Double-blind study. *Psychopharmacol Bull* 14:15-16, 1978.

Falloon IRH, Lieberman RP: Interactions between drug and psychosocial therapy in schizophrenia. *Schizophren Bull* 9:543-554, 1983.

Friedman E, et al: Chronic fluphenazine and clozapine elicit opposite changes in brain muscarinic receptor binding: Implications for understanding tardive dyskinesia. *J Pharmacol Exp Ther* 226:7-12, 1983.

Gershon S, et al: Mesoridazine: Pharmacodynamic and pharmacokinetic profile. *J Clin Psychiatry* 42:463-469, 1981.

Glazer WM: Depot fluphenazine: Risk/benefit ratio. *J Clin Psychiatry* 45(5, sec 2):28-35, 1984.

Glazer WM, et al: Tardive dyskinesia. *Arch Gen Psychiatry* 41:623-627, 1984.

Granacher RP Jr: Differential diagnosis of tardive dyskinesia: Overview. *Am J Psychiatry* 138:1288-1297, 1981.

Granato JE, et al: Neuroleptic malignant syndrome: Successful treatment with dantrolene and bromocriptine. *Ann Neurol* 14:89-90, 1983.

Groves JE, Mandel MR: Long-acting phenothiazines. *Arch Gen Psychiatry* 32:893-900, 1975.

Gruen PH, et al: Prolactin responses to neuroleptics in normal and schizophrenic subjects. *Arch Gen Psychiatry* 35:108-116, 1978.

Itil TM, Soldatos C: Epileptogenic side effects of psychotropic drugs: Practical recommendations. *JAMA* 244:1460-1463, 1980.

Kane JM: Low dose medication strategies in maintenance treatment of schizophrenia, in Carpenter WT Jr, Schooler NR (eds): *New Directions in Drug Treatment for Schizophrenia.* Rockville, MD, National Institute of Mental Health, 1984, 29-33.

Kessler KA, Waletzky JP: Clinical use of antipsychotics. *Am J Psychiatry* 138:202-209, 1981.

Kirkpatrick B, Burnett GB: Observations on neuroleptic use in acute psychotic patients. *J Clin Psychopharmacol* 2:205-207, 1982.

Klawans HL, et al: Combating hemiballismus with neuroleptics. *Drug Ther (Hosp)* 3:65-68, (March) 1978.

Lacoursiere RB, et al: Medical effects of abrupt neuroleptic withdrawal. *Compr Psychiatry* 17:285-293, (March-April) 1976.

Luchins DJ, et al: Role of cholinergic supersensitivity in medical symptoms associated with withdrawal of antipsychotic drugs. *Am J Psychiatry* 137:1395-1398, 1980.

Manschreck TC: Schizophrenic disorders. *N Engl J Med* 305:1628-1632, 1981.

Manschreck TC: Drug treatment of schizophrenia: Principles and limitations. *Drug Ther* 13:185-204, (Sept) 1983.

Manschreck TC, Petri M: Paranoid syndrome. *Lancet* 2:251-253, 1978.

May DC, et al: Neuroleptic malignant syndrome: Response to dantrolene sodium. *Ann Intern Med* 98:183-184, 1983.

McCarron MM, et al: Case of neuroleptic malignant syndrome successfully treated with amantadine. *J Clin Psychiatry* 43:381-382, 1982.

Mikkelsen EJ, et al: School avoidance and social phobia triggered by haloperidol in patients with Tourette's syndrome. *Am J Psychiatry* 138:1572-1576, 1981.

Mitchell JE, Popkin MK: Antipsychotic drug therapy and sexual dysfunction in men. *Am J Psychiatry* 139:633-637, 1982.

Mueller PS, et al: Neuroleptic malignant syndrome: Successful treatment with bromocriptine. *JAMA* 249:386-388, 1983.

Murray TJ: Tourette's syndrome: Treatable tic. *Can Med Assoc J* 118:1407-1410, 1978.

Oyewumi LK: Neuroleptics under high risk conditions. *Can J Psychiatry* 28:398-403, 1983.

Schooler NR, Levine J: Initiation of long-term pharmacotherapy in schizophrenia: Dosage and side effect comparisons between oral and depot fluphenazine. *Pharmakopsychiatr Neuropsychopharmacakol* 9:159-169, 1976.

Stahl SM, et al: Neuropharmacology of tardive dyskinesia, spontaneous dyskinesia, and other dystonias. *J Clin Psychopharmacol* 2:321-328, 1982.

Strauss JS, Carpenter WT: Schizophrenia. *J Nerv Mental Dis* 169:113-119, 1981.

Tarsy D, Baldessarini RJ: Tardive dyskinesia. *Am Rev Med* 35:605-623, 1984.

Task Force on Late Neurologic Effects of Antipsychotic Drugs: Tardive dyskinesia: Summary of task force report of American Psychiatric Association. *Am J Psychiatry* 137:1163-1172, 1980.

Telcher MH, Baldessarini RJ: Selection of neuroleptic dosage. *Arch Gen Psychiatry* 42:636-637, 1985.

Tollefson G, et al: Circulating lupus-like coagulation inhibitor induced by chlorpromazine. *J Clin Psychopharmacol* 4:49-51, 1984.

Wagner MS, Stapczynski JS: Persistent hiccups. *Ann Emerg Med* 11:24-26, 1982.

Weinberg S, Twersky RS: Neuroleptic malignant syndrome. *Anesth Analg* 62:848-850, 1983.

Young LK, Patel MM: Respiratory complications of antipsychotic drugs in medically ill patients. *Res Staff Physician* 30:73-80, (Nov) 1984.

Zubenko G, et al: Comparison of metoprolol and propranolol in treatment of akathisia. *Psychiatry Res* 11:143-149, 1984.

Drugs Used in Affective Disorders

7

Depression that occurs alone or accompanies a medical disorder usually is diagnosed and treated initially by a primary care physician and is the psychiatric disorder most frequently encountered by such physicians. Treatment by a psychiatrist usually is required if initial drug therapy has failed and/or the disorder has progressed considerably (Richardson and Richelson, 1984). Optimum drug therapy requires an understanding of the dynamics of depression, the clinical pharmacology of available drugs, and the individual needs of the patient.

AFFECTIVE DISORDERS

Clinically significant disturbances in mood define the major characteristic of the affective disorders. Such disturbances are manifested as full or partial depressive and/or manic episodes in the major affective disorders (major depression and the bipolar disorders) or as chronic, less severe aberrations in mood in other affective disorders, such as cyclothymic disorder, dysthymic disorder, and atypical depression. The following is a discussion of the criteria for diagnosis and pharmacologic treatment of the affective disorders.

A depressive episode, as defined in the third edition of the *Diagnostic and Statistical Manual of Mental Disorders (DSM III)* (American Psychiatric Association, 1980), is characterized by dysphoric mood or loss of interest or pleasure in all or almost all usual activities and pastimes. The mood disturbance must be prominent and relatively persistent but is not necessarily the dominant symptom. Some or all of the following symptoms also may be present: (1) inability to experience joy or pleasure in usual activities or decreased sexual drive; (2) feelings of helplessness, worthlessness, self-reproach, or inappropriate guilt; (3) inability to concentrate, slowed thinking, and indecisiveness; (4) recurrent thoughts of death and hopelessness commonly linked to suicidal plans and acts; (5) psychomotor agitation or retardation, blunted affect, or tearfulness; (6) insomnia, usually in the early morning but occasionally on retiring (hypersomnia occurs more rarely); (7) anorexia with significant weight loss or, occasionally, hyperphagia; and (8) fatigue or loss of energy. Widely variable degrees of anxiety occur in almost all depressed patients, and when prominent, can lead to misdiagnosis with incorrect treatment. Uncommonly, psychotic morbid preoccupation with depressive symptoms (particularly somatic concerns) ensues that can result in total decompensation. Delusions may occur in more severe forms and further impair the ability to cope with normal social, personal, and work functions.

In a manic episode, the patient exhibits (1) emotional lability (euphoria to frustration) and distractibility by trivial events; (2) lack of need for sleep; (3) flight of ideas (racing thoughts); (4) pressure of speech; (5) overactivity at work, play, or sex or excessive sociability; (6) extreme self-confidence with delusions of importance and grandiose ideas; and (7) excessive involvement in activities with a high potential for unrecognized painful consequences (eg, inappropriate gambling, buying sprees, sexual indiscretions, foolish business investments, reckless driving). Milder forms (hypomania) are less easily recognized, and individuals may appear to be highly energetic and innovative and often are successful professionally. In hypomania, pathology may not become obvious until behavior exceeds rational limits.

Classification: The *DSM III* terminology for affective disorders supports the dichotomy traditionally recognized for the depressive illnesses, ie, bipolar for patients who experience episodes of both mania and depression, unipolar for patients who experience one or more major depressive episodes but who have never had a manic episode.

Bipolar disorder is subclassified as manic, depressed, or mixed, depending upon the signs and symptoms observed during typically recurring episodes. Diagnosis is based on the duration of episodes (depression for at least two weeks, mania for at least one week) and their severity (presence of at least four of the eight major signs and symptoms listed above for depression and/or three of the seven signs described for mania). Classification is complete when it can be recognized that the disorder is in remission or that associated psychotic features occur, ie, delusions and hallucinations that are either mood-congruent or mood-incongruent.

Major depression (unipolar depression) occurs at least ten times as frequently as bipolar disorder. In addition to the primary symptom of dysphoric mood or loss of interest or pleasure in all or almost all usual activities and pastimes, at least four of the eight signs and symptoms of depression described above must be present nearly every day for at least two weeks for diagnosis.

Endogenous depression has been replaced in *DSM III* by the term "major depression with melancholia" to designate a subtype of major depression characterized by a pervasive loss of pleasure in all activities, complete lack of reactivity to usually pleasurable stimuli, and at least three of the following: (1) depressed mood perceived as distinctly different from that associated with uncomplicated grief (loss); (2) depression worse in the morning; (3) early morning awakening; (4) marked psychomotor retardation or agitation; (5) significant anorexia and weight loss; or (6) excessive or inappropriate guilt.

Cyclothymic disorder is a chronic illness (at least two years' duration) with recurring episodes of hypomania and depression that are not of sufficient duration and severity for a diagnosis of bipolar disorder.

Dysthymic disorder must be of at least two years' duration in adults and one year in children. Some signs and symptoms resemble those of major depression but are less severe and of shorter duration. Unlike major depression, a personality disorder often coexists with dysthymic depression or some of the following symptoms appear: hypochondriacal concerns, dependency, poor interpersonal and social adjustment, obsessional tendencies, irritability and anger, manipulative suicidal threats, self-pity, substance abuse, negative pessimistic behavior, emotional lability, histrionic behavior, and severe anxiety. Dysthymic disorder is closely related to conditions once termed neurotic depression, reactive depression, or chronic characterological depression.

In *DSM III*, atypical depression is a residual category for depressive symptoms that are not classifiable as bipolar, major, cyclothymic, or dysthymic. However, the concept of atypical depression usually is applied to a disorder of mood with reversal of the classical vegetative (endogenous) features (eg, early age of onset; rarity of attempted suicide; increase in weight, appetite, libido, and sleep; diurnal variation in that the patient feels worse in the evening and has insomnia on retiring; mood lability and irritability; prominent anxiety) (Davidson et al, 1982). Atypical depressions represent a significant proportion of mood disorders encountered by primary care physicians. Diagnosis generally must be made by a psychiatrist.

It is important to distinguish among bipolar disorder, major depression, cyclothymic disorder, dysthymic disorder, and atypical depression, because their prognosis and management, especially responsiveness to drug therapy, differ. For the same reasons, primary disorders should be differentiated from any secondary form (reactive depression) that occurs during the course of some other primary psychiatric or medical disorder.

Alcoholism is a common cause of *substance-induced depression*; street drug abuse or adverse reactions to a number of prescription drugs also cause cause this type of depression.

Uncomplicated bereavement from a significant loss (eg, spouse, employment, friend, position) is not classified as a depressive disorder, but is considered a normal self-limited grief reaction. It is much more common than all of the primary and secondary depressive disorders.

Major depression in the elderly often mimics dementia. A definitive diagnosis is critical to ensure appropriate treatment, although a therapeutic trial with an antidepressant may be warranted when the diagnosis cannot be established. Such depression can be distinguished from dementia on the basis of the following characteristics: The onset of depression is quite abrupt, the progression is usually rapid, the patient is aware of deficits and complains of memory loss, impairment is not usually worse at night, the mood is depressed, and the patient has a history of psychiatric disturbance. In the demented patient, the onset of symptomatology is insidious, progression of the disorder is usually slow, the patient is less aware of and tries to hide memory loss, impairment usually is worse at night, the patient typically is happy, and a history of psychiatric disturbance is uncommon (Finlayson and Martin, 1982).

Etiology: Delineation of the underlying causes of the major affective disorders has been difficult. Psychoanalytical and behavioral explanations gradually are losing credibility to biological theories. Although neurochemical research has produced many promising leads, definitive characterization of the primary cause remains elusive.

Neurochemical hypotheses of the major affective disorders

and major depression, in particular, have focused attention on the neuroendocrine regulatory system and the central neurotransmitter systems. The view of major depression as a neuroendocrine disorder focuses primarily on aberrations in the hypothalamic-pituitary-adrenal axis and secondarily on irregularities in the hypothalamic-pituitary-thyroid axis. The former suggests that noradrenergic tonic inhibition of the hypothalamic release of corticotropin releasing factor (CRF) is deficient, which results in excessive serum concentrations of cortisol. Patients with depression have increased cortisol secretion, an increased number of secretory episodes, and markedly elevated plasma cortisol concentrations (Sachar, 1973). More recent evidence suggests that the endogenous opioid system also may be involved in the pathogenesis of major depression (Cohen et al, 1984).

Focus on neurotransmitter systems has become diffuse as studies implicate more transmitter systems in the etiology of major depression. Historically, the adrenergic amine-depleting activity of the antihypertensive drug, reserpine, was shown to induce severe depression, and this observation formed the basis for the biogenic amine hypothesis. This hypothesis proposes that affective disorders are due to genetically determined deficiencies in the functional activities of norepinephrine and/or serotonin. Studies examining the effects of antidepressants support this hypothesis, for they suggest that the major pharmacologic effects of these drugs involve alteration of adrenergic and serotonergic function in the central nervous system (van Praag, 1982).

Cholinergic mechanisms also may play a causative role in the development of affective disorders. Most heterocyclic antidepressants block muscarinic cholinergic receptors in the central nervous system at therapeutic concentrations (Snyder and Yamamura, 1977). Workers exposed for long periods to acetylcholinesterase inhibitors often become markedly depressed. Sleep disturbances frequently are associated with major depression and are characterized by short, shallow, and fragmented sleep. REM sleep is characteristically advanced toward sleep onset and is associated with increased cholinergic and decreased aminergic activity (Gillin, 1983).

In summary, many individuals with major affective disorders appear to be genetically vulnerable. At present, it is not known which neuromodulatory system(s) are most responsible. However, recent evidence suggests that an aberration in the complex interrelationship among many such systems may be causative.

Treatment Modalities: Drug therapy and psychotherapy have proven efficacy in the treatment of the major affective disorders and, thus, constitute the major treatment modalities in use today. Electroconvulsive therapy is particularly effective in the treatment of major depression, but generally is reserved for patients who exhibit considerable potential for suicide or those unresponsive to drug therapy (Crowe, 1984).

Drug therapy for the major affective disorders utilizes the heterocyclic antidepressants, the monoamine oxidase inhibitors, or lithium and other alternative drugs (eg, carbamazepine [Tegretol]). The heterocyclic antidepressants are most useful in both the acute treatment and prophylaxis of major depressive disorders; they also are effective in secondary forms.

Lithium alone or with an antidepressant is effective in the treatment of depressive episodes of bipolar disorders.

Although anxiety often accompanies depression, antidepressants, particularly the monoamine oxidase inhibitors, usually resolve the anxiety and insomnia along with the depressive symptoms. Therefore, adjunctive antianxiety drugs should not be prescribed routinely, substituted inappropriately for antidepressants, or given for longer than two to three weeks without re-evaluation of the disorder. If antianxiety therapy is warranted, the benzodiazepines usually are the drugs of choice; compared to the barbiturates, benzodiazepines have a wider margin of safety, cause fewer clinically significant drug interactions, and do not depress plasma levels of heterocyclic antidepressants (see Chapter 5, Drugs Used for Anxiety and Sleep Disorders).

Psychotherapy for the major affective disorders includes cognitive therapy, interpersonal psychotherapy, and behavioral therapy. Currently, the National Institute of Mental Health is in the late stages of a multi-institutional trial comparing the effectiveness of antidepressant drugs to psychotherapy. Regardless of the ultimate outcome of these studies, therapy must be tailored to meet the individual needs of the patient as defined by diagnosis, family history, medical and psychiatric history, and previous response to treatment. Evidence from controlled studies suggests that, in general, the combination of an antidepressant with psychotherapy may be the most effective treatment for depressed patients (Glass, 1981); counseling that embodies nonjudgmental listening, empathy, and reassurance is essential in all patients and may improve compliance with drug therapy.

Drug Therapy: The role of drugs in the treatment of specific affective disorders has been outlined above. Apart from an established diagnosis and a personal or family history of response to a particular antidepressant, secondary pharmacologic actions (eg, stimulation versus sedation) of the individual drugs have implications for both the therapeutic response and the occurrence of side effects and, thus, are additional factors for consideration in the selection process. Onset of action also has been promoted as an important determinant of drug selection, but there is no consistent clinical evidence to support distinctions among antidepressants on this basis.

In the *manic* form of bipolar disorder (manic-depressive illness), up to 85% of patients respond to lithium, especially when the classic symptoms recur without intermittent depressive episodes. Carbamazepine has been suggested as a useful alternative drug for recurring mania in patients who cannot tolerate or do not respond to an adequate course of lithium (Ballenger and Post, 1980; Post et al, 1984). An antipsychotic drug and lithium are indicated if mania is severe and psychotic symptoms are present. Their concomitant use should be discontinued when symptoms are controlled.

The signs and symptoms of the *depressed* phase of bipolar disorder are essentially the same as those of *major depression*. Both respond to heterocyclic antidepressants and electroconvulsive therapy. Major depression with melancholia responds especially well to the heterocyclic drugs. The sudden appearance of a manic episode following successful treatment

DRUGS USED IN AFFECTIVE DISORDERS

Classification	Drug	Aliphatic Amine Type	Sedative Activity	Anticholinergic Activity	Usual Adult (Outpatient) Daily Dose Range During Initial Treatment* (mg)
ANTIDEPRESSANTS					
HETEROCYCLIC COMPOUNDS					
Dibenzazepines	Desipramine Norpramin (Merrell Dow) Pertofrane (USV)	Secondary	Minimal	Minimal	75**-150
	Imipramine Janimine (Abbott) SK-Pramine (Smith Kline & French) Tofranil (Geigy)	Tertiary	Intermediate	Intermediate	75**-150
	Trimipramine Surmontil (Wyeth)	Tertiary	Maximal	Intermediate	75**-150
Dibenzocycloheptadienes	Protriptyline Vivactil (Merck Sharp & Dohme)	Secondary	Minimal	Intermediate	15**-40
	Nortriptyline Aventyl (Lilly) Pamelor (Sandoz)	Secondary	Intermediate	Minimal	20**-100
	Amitriptyline Elavil (Merck Sharp & Dohme) Endep (Roche)	Tertiary	Maximal	Maximal	75**-150
Dibenzoxepin	Doxepin Adapin (Pennwalt) Sinequan (Roerig)	Tertiary	Maximal	Maximal	75**-150
Dibenzoxazepine	Amoxapine Asendin (Lederle)	Not Applicable	Minimal	Minimal	75**-200
Tetracyclic Compound					
	Maprotiline Ludiomil (CIBA)	Secondary	Intermediate	Intermediate	75**-150
Triazolopyridine Compound					
	Trazodone Desyrel (Mead Johnson)	Not Applicable	Intermediate	Minimal	150**-300
MONOAMINE OXIDASE INHIBITORS					
Hydrazines	Isocarboxazid Marplan (Roche)				30-40
	Phenelzine Nardil (Parke-Davis)				45-90
Nonhydrazine	Tranylcypromine Parnate (Smith Kline & French)				20-40

(Continued on next page)

Classification	Drug	Aliphatic Amine Type	Sedative Activity	Anticholinergic Activity	Usual Adult (Outpatient) Daily Dose Range During Initial Treatment* (mg)
ANTIMANIC	Lithium Cibalith-S (CIBA) Eskalith (Smith Kline & French) Lithane (Miles) Lithobid (CIBA) Lithonate (Rowell) Lithotabs (Rowell)				600-1800 (Initial) 900-1200 (Maintenance)

Initial treatment (treatment of the initial phase) is regarded as the 4- to 8-week period until the patient becomes nearly symptom-free; treatment usually is instituted with the smaller dose of the range listed and gradually increased to the larger dose, if required (see the following footnote). Doses larger than those listed often are required in severely depressed inpatients or in drug-resistant patients (see the evaluations). Continuation treatment at the optimal daily dose (or somewhat less) determined during initial treatment usually is then instituted for a period of approximately 20 consecutive weeks. Controlled studies are in progress to determine if maintenance treatment is indicated beyond continuation treatment, usually at a lower daily dose than that utilized during continuation treatment.

**One useful schedule that lessens the intensity of undesirable sedative, hypotensive, and anticholinergic effects initially in outpatients and makes dosage adjustment easier follows: Imipramine (or an equivalent dose of the antidepressants other than the monoamine oxidase inhibitors and lithium) 25 mg twice daily for three days, 50 mg twice daily for three days, and 75 mg twice daily for the next ten days. A minimum of five days between dosage adjustments may be more appropriate in the elderly, the debilitated, or patients with cardiac disease and may be particularly desirable to avoid undue sedation and hypotension that may result in injury. (If insomnia is prominent, it may be preferable to give the initial daily amount as a single dose at bedtime to obtain the full benefit of sedation and minimize functional impairment and drowsiness during the day.) After two to three weeks of therapy, a single daily dose is commonly given at bedtime. If limited benefit is observed by the third week, the daily dose is increased, usually weekly, until satisfactory improvement, intolerable adverse reactions, or the recommended maximum dose is reached (see the evaluations).*

of a depressive episode may signify the presence of a previously undiagnosed bipolar disorder.

The *mixed* form of bipolar disorder may respond to lithium alone, although optimum management usually requires the cautious concomitant use of an antidepressant. Rarely, lithium alone is adequate for maintenance during the first year of stabilization.

The role of antidepressants is not established in *dysthymic disorder*. Although heterocyclic antidepressants are used most frequently, a monoamine oxidase inhibitor may be preferred in selected patients (Ravaris et al, 1980).

The response to drug treatment is also highly individualized in patients with *atypical depressions*. Certain subtypes, such as atypical depression with panic attacks and hysteroid dysphoria, seem to be more responsive to the monoamine oxidase inhibitors than to the heterocyclic antidepressants (Stern et al, 1980; Davidson et al, 1982; Liebowitz et al, 1984). Nevertheless, patients with dysthymic or atypical depressive disorders usually do not respond as completely to heterocyclic antidepressants or monoamine oxidase inhibitors as patients with major depression.

Simultaneous treatment with antipsychotic drugs and/or heterocyclic antidepressants and/or lithium occasionally is necessary for patients with *schizoaffective disorder* and *paranoid schizophrenia*. Monoamine oxidase inhibitors generally should not be used because they often stimulate patients with schizophrenia; heterocyclic compounds also have been re-

ported to possess this action. (See Chapter 6, Antipsychotic Drugs.)

Many therapeutic agents are known to cause *drug-induced depression*, but the antipsychotic agents, barbiturates, alcohol, oral contraceptives, and centrally acting antihypertensive agents (eg, reserpine, methyldopa [Aldomet]) are most commonly implicated (Whitlock and Evans, 1978). Reducing the dose or discontinuing therapy and counseling are indicated. Antidepressants are usually not necessary.

Uncomplicated bereavement requires drug therapy infrequently; counseling is usually adequate. A few patients may benefit from the temporary use of antianxiety agents to produce sedation and sleep without interfering with the normal grief reaction.

Class discussion of the antidepressants (heterocyclic compounds and monoamine oxidase inhibitors) and antimanic drugs (lithium and carbamazepine) follows. Drugs evaluated individually include the heterocyclic compounds, the monoamine oxidase inhibitors, lithium, and selected mixtures. For convenience, the Table summarizes pertinent information on marketed drugs used in affective disorders.

HETEROCYCLIC ANTIDEPRESSANTS

Uses: The available heterocyclic antidepressants (amitriptyline, amoxapine, desipramine, doxepin, imipramine, maprotiline, nortriptyline, protriptyline, trazodone, and trimipramine) elevate mood, increase physical activity and mental alertness, improve appetite and sleep patterns, and reduce morbid preoccupation in 60% to 70% of patients with major depression. In addition to their usefulness in treating acute depressive episodes, these drugs are effective to prevent relapse and as maintenance therapy to prevent recurrence of major depressive episodes. Additionally, some heterocyclic compounds are effective in the treatment of panic or phobic disorders and have been used in dysthymic and atypical depression.

Other indications for heterocyclic antidepressants that remain investigational, controversial, or incompletely established include hysteroid dysphoria, obsessive-compulsive disorder, school phobia, attention deficit disorder, narcolepsy, chronic pain, migraine, anorexia nervosa, bulimia, peptic ulcer, peripheral diabetic neuropathy, sleep apnea, and acute paranoid disorder.

Mechanism of Action: The mechanism of action of the heterocyclic antidepressants remains undefined despite the large body of knowledge that has accumulated (van Praag, 1982). Their pharmacologic effects are most apparent when evaluation is based on the time (acute versus chronic) and site (blockade of reuptake versus blockade of receptors) of their actions.

On an acute basis, the heterocyclic antidepressants block the reuptake of norepinephrine and serotonin into their respective nerve terminals within the central nervous system. They also block serotonergic, noradrenergic (alpha$_1$), histaminergic (H$_1$ more than H$_2$), and muscarinic receptors. These combined effects on reuptake and receptor occupation reduce the synthesis and turnover of norepinephrine and serotonin and reduce the firing rates of neurons of these two transmitters.

On a chronic basis, blockade of the neuronal reuptake of norepinephrine and serotonin continues with a gradual return to normal turnover and firing rates. A decrease in beta- and alpha$_2$-adrenergic receptor sensitivity is characteristic. There is probably no change or a slight increase in alpha$_1$-adrenergic receptor sensitivity, and the overall effects on the serotonergic receptor system are uncertain. There is no change or some increase in the number of muscarinic receptors.

Correlation of specific neurochemical actions of the heterocyclic antidepressants with their therapeutic effects must take into consideration the one to three weeks that elapse before such effects are apparent. Some chronic effects of these drugs have been established, but it is not known which of these account for therapeutic benefit.

Pharmacokinetics: All heterocyclic compounds are well absorbed orally, extensively metabolized, highly protein-bound in plasma and tissue, and slowly eliminated. Mean half-life and/or range (in hours) for the heterocyclic antidepressants are: desipramine 17.1 (12.5 to 24.7), nortriptyline 26.6 (12.8 to 48.2), imipramine 7.6 (4 to 17.6), amitriptyline 15.1 (10.3 to 25.3), doxepin 16.8 (8.2 to 24.5), protriptyline 78.4 (54.6 to 124), amoxapine 8, maprotiline 43 to 51, and trazodone 4 to 9. The half-lives of metabolites are: desipramine from imipramine 29.9 (13.5 to 61.5), nortriptyline from amitriptyline 26.6 (16.5 to 35.7), and 8-hydroxyamoxapine from

amoxapine 30 (Amsterdam et al, 1980). Because half-lives are prolonged in patients over 55 years, the initial dose for older patients may require modification. The antidepressant response is often slow (one to three weeks) and is not accelerated appreciably by parenteral administration. Electroconvulsive therapy may, therefore, be the treatment of choice in suicidal patients.

Although the correlations between plasma concentration of some heterocyclic compounds and therapeutic efficacy are statistically significant, drug concentrations often are too variable to have predictive value in the individual patient (Robinson et al, 1978, 1981; Hollister, 1981). The individual variation in metabolism of these drugs is between ten- and thirtyfold; therefore, signs and symptoms are used to adjust dosage. Plasma concentrations may aid in optimizing therapy in unresponsive patients, in detecting noncompliance, and possibly in managing overdosage (Amsterdam et al, 1980).

A curvilinear relationship in the form of an inverted U is proposed to exist between nortriptyline plasma concentrations and efficacy in responsive patients with major depression; maximal efficacy is attained at concentrations between 50 and 150 ng/ml. Limited evidence suggests that the relationship between imipramine (plus its active metabolite, desipramine) plasma concentrations and efficacy is linear in hospitalized patients with major depression; threshold concentrations for therapeutic response appear to exceed 95 ng/ml for imipramine and 225 to 240 ng/ml for combined imipramine and desipramine. Data are insufficient to define the relationship between plasma concentration and efficacy for amitriptyline, desipramine, doxepin, maprotiline, protriptyline, and trazodone.

Administration and Dosage: The *initial treatment* period is considered to be the four to eight weeks needed for the patient to become nearly symptom-free. Outpatient treatment usually is instituted with the smaller dose of the range listed in the Table and the amount is gradually increased to the larger dose if required. The initial two to three weeks of heterocyclic drug therapy are critical. A common cause of inadequate treatment in outpatients is oversedation during the first few days caused by an excessive initial dose, which results in noncompliance. Different schedules have been utilized to initiate therapy. For one useful schedule in outpatients that lessens the intensity of undesirable sedative, hypotensive, and anticholinergic side effects and makes dosage adjustment easier, see the footnote in the Table.

In hospitalized patients, closer monitoring is possible, the initial daily dose is generally larger, and the time needed to attain a maximum daily dose is usually shorter. Doses larger than those listed in the Table and evaluations often are required.

Following initial treatment, the duration of *continuation treatment* usually is approximately six months. The daily dose is reduced four to eight weeks after initial control of depression is achieved to lessen adverse effects and improve patient compliance. However, some psychiatrists concerned about relapse with this strategy prefer to administer 150 mg of imipramine or the equivalent daily or continue the initial dose for approximately six months unless side effects are intolerable.

For recurrent depressive episodes that necessitate *maintenance treatment*, the duration of therapy depends upon the type and severity of depression, the previous pattern of episodes, the adverse consequences of a new recurrence, and the patient's ability to tolerate the drug. Daily doses of 50 mg (in the elderly) to 150 mg of imipramine or another heterocyclic compound are reported to have prophylactic value. Studies of long-term preventive maintenance have not evaluated the effectiveness of doses exceeding 150 mg/day or the optimal duration of therapy. If a patient remains free of recurrence for a period equal to several previous cycle lengths, therapy may be discontinued provided a family member or friend is available to alert the physician to the signs of relapse. In general, the stronger the indications for instituting maintenance therapy, the longer its duration should be (National Institutes of Health Consensus Development Conference, 1984).

Since the rates of metabolism and, hence, plasma concentrations of these drugs vary widely, individualization of dose on the basis of clinical effect is more important than strict adherence to recommendations for initial, maintenance, and maximum doses. Some patients may require more than the usual maximum dose. If patients do not respond to an adequate trial with one heterocyclic antidepressant, a different drug of this class occasionally proves useful.

Drug therapy should be discontinued gradually over a few weeks. This avoids the withdrawal syndrome that may follow abrupt discontinuation of the heterocyclic antidepressant and allows minimum dosage alteration if symptoms and signs of relapse occur. The simultaneous administration of barbiturates may cause refractoriness to heterocyclic drugs. Conversely, the toxic effects of heterocyclic compounds may be potentiated by alcohol and the barbiturates; the mechanism of this interaction is not known.

Adverse Reactions: The most common adverse reactions of the heterocyclic compounds are due to their anticholinergic and alpha-adrenergic blocking activities: flushing, diaphoresis, dryness of the mouth, blurred vision, constipation, tachycardia, and hypotension. Tachycardia, orthostatic hypotension, aggravation of angle-closure glaucoma, urinary retention, adynamic ileus, and confusion as a component of toxic delirium may be especially hazardous in elderly patients with other diseases.

The anticholinergic activity of the heterocyclic antidepressants is variable. Tertiary amines, such as amitriptyline and doxepin, exhibit greater anticholinergic activity than secondary amines. The anticholinergic activity of trazodone is minimal.

Allergic skin reactions and photosensitivity are relatively uncommon, as are agranulocytosis, cholestatic jaundice, leukopenia, leukocytosis, Loeffler's syndrome, eosinophilia, and thrombocytopenia. Hypertension and convulsions have been reported following a course of imipramine in a patient with undiagnosed pheochromocytoma. Delayed, inhibited, or retrograde ejaculation can occur.

Central nervous system effects include sedation (see the Table), fine tremor, speech blockage, and anxiety or insomnia. Increased appetite with overeating occurs in some patients. These drugs may produce seizures, particularly in patients prone to such disorders, including those with a history of

severe alcoholism. Amoxapine, imipramine, and especially maprotiline lower the seizure threshold more than desipramine and the monoamine oxidase inhibitors. Thus, the latter drugs are preferred in patients with seizure disorders (Richardson and Richelson 1984).

Parkinsonism occurs occasionally, especially on abrupt withdrawal of the drug; antidepressants with minimal anticholinergic activity are implicated most commonly. Heterocyclic drugs are reported to produce tardive dyskinesia rarely after prolonged use of large doses, but there are no controlled studies to substantiate this finding. Amoxapine is a derivative of the antipsychotic, loxapine, and can produce tardive dyskinesia. Hyponatremia resulting from a syndrome of inappropriate secretion of antidiuretic hormone (SIADH) has been observed rarely.

Serious cardiac reactions are uncommon unless overdosage occurs or these drugs are used in patients with preexisting cardiac dysfunction. Effects include (1) direct cardiac action (increased rate caused by anticholinergic activity [vagal inhibition], delayed conduction and disturbance in rhythm because of quinidine-like bundle of His sensitivity, and impaired contractility), and (2) action on the peripheral vasculature (orthostatic hypotension caused by central or peripheral alpha-adrenergic receptor blockade) (Blackwell, 1981). Thus, a baseline ECG and periodic monitoring, especially determination of the width of the QRS complex, are recommended for elderly patients and those with prior or existing cardiac impairment, particularly those receiving quinidine, procainamide, or disopyramide. In addition, pretreatment and regular monitoring of supine and standing blood pressure should be undertaken to minimize consequences of orthostatic hypotension.

There is little evidence of substantial differences in cardiotoxicity among the heterocyclic antidepressants in therapeutic doses. Anecdotal evidence suggests that amoxapine may be less cardiotoxic than other heterocyclics, but atrial flutter and fibrillation has been reported with use of this drug (Cassem, 1982).

The triazolopyridine, trazodone, also has been reported to be cardiotoxic (Lippmann et al, 1983); in patients with preexisting myocardial irritability, increased frequency of beats and ventricular tachycardia have been associated with its use. Cardiotoxicity has been reported only after overdose of maprotiline, but studies have shown that significant changes in the ECG are produced by both maprotiline and imipramine (Mielke et al, 1979).

Precautions: The heterocyclic antidepressants should not be used in acutely agitated schizophrenic patients, and they should be used cautiously in those with mixed mania and depression, since they may unmask mania. Particular attention should be given to patients with suicidal tendencies when they start to respond to therapy, for the risk of suicide may be greatest when recovery begins and the patient becomes more active.

These compounds should be used with caution in elderly patients and in those with a history of a seizure disorder (especially maprotiline), renal failure, or severely impaired hepatic function. Close supervision is advised if treatment is considered in patients with angle-closure glaucoma, urinary retention or obstruction, or those at risk of developing ileus.

The risks should be weighed very carefully in patients with cardiac disease. It is also important to monitor the blood pressure, for hypotensive side effects are common and serious, especially in elderly patients with hypertension or orthostatic hypotension. Relative contraindications to the use of the heterocyclic antidepressants include bundle branch block, the postmyocardial infarction period, and tachycardia being treated with quinidine.

Routine precautions should be followed when these drugs are used during pregnancy and breast feeding (see the discussion in Chapter 3).

Because of reported withdrawal effects, the dose of these drugs should be reduced gradually in patients who have been receiving large amounts.

Poisoning: Overdosage of the heterocyclic antidepressants can produce symptoms of anticholinergic and cardiac toxicity (Marshall and Forker, 1982). Fatal overdose has been reported in enuretic children or their siblings and in children who have taken pills belonging to their parents. A single oral dose of 1 g of amitriptyline, imipramine, or doxepin produces severe toxic reactions in adults, and doses exceeding 2 g are sometimes fatal. All patients who have received such overdoses should be hospitalized to permit continuous cardiac monitoring. A widened QRS complex is a presumptive sign of overdosage. The first symptoms usually do not appear for one to four hours after ingestion, and patients who are alert when first seen may become comatose later.

Respiratory depression, shock, serious atrial and ventricular arrhythmias (ranging from marked bradycardia to supraventricular and ventricular tachycardia), hyperthermia, agitation, ataxia, delirium, and coma may be observed. Other neurologic effects include dilated pupils, nystagmus, hyperactive tendon reflexes, tremor, myoclonus, choreoathetosis, bladder and bowel paralysis, and convulsions. Severe poisoning is characterized by coma, seizures, and arrhythmias.

Treatment consists of general supportive measures, *including correction of acidosis* to enhance protein binding of the heterocyclic compounds, thus reducing the concentration of free drug in the blood. Gastric lavage with activated charcoal is recommended even as late as six to eight hours following ingestion. Continued instillation of activated charcoal via nasogastric tube (with appropriate endotracheal intubation) is indicated for comatose patients, because the parent drug and its active metabolites undergo enterohepatic recirculation. Forced diuresis, peritoneal dialysis, hemodialysis, and exchange transfusion are of no value, and hemoperfusion is of limited value. Hyperpyrexia is managed by physical cooling procedures, but hypothermia may occur instead.

Cardiovascular abnormalities must be monitored carefully and may be particularly difficult to manage. The antiarrhythmic drugs, disopyramide, procainamide, and quinidine, are contraindicated because of their additive depressant effect on cardiac conduction; lidocaine, propranolol, and phenytoin are the drugs of choice. Physostigmine [Antilirium] (1 to 3 mg intravenously in divided doses) may help control myoclonus, choreoathetosis, delirium, coma, and some cardiotoxic reactions, but this agent must be used with caution because it can cause potentially serious cholinergic effects, including excessive salivation requiring suction, bradycardia, bronchoconstriction, and convulsions. Repeated injections may be required because physostigmine has a short duration of action. (See Chapter 80, Drugs Used in the Treatment of Poisoning.) Cardioversion and/or electrical pacing may be necessary to control the arrhythmias, and diazepam [Valium] may be used to control convulsions. Drugs that further impair cardiac conduction and depress the central nervous system probably should be avoided.

Drug Interactions: Since drugs used to treat cardiovascular disease, hypertension, and depression have numerous effects on biogenic amines, there are many interactions between drugs in these classes. Guanethidine [Ismelin] should not be given to patients receiving the heterocyclic compounds (trazodone may be given) because the antidepressants interfere with the action of this antihypertensive agent. The effect of clonidine [Catapres] also may be antagonized by some heterocyclic antidepressants.

Direct-acting adrenergic drugs (eg, epinephrine, certain sympathomimetic amines) may be potentiated by heterocyclic antidepressants. Methylphenidate [Ritalin] may inhibit the metabolism of heterocyclic drugs and increase their blood concentrations. The noradrenergic anorexiant, fenfluramine [Pondimin], has sedative properties and markedly potentiates this effect of the heterocyclic antidepressants; therefore, the combination should be avoided.

The prominent anticholinergic effects of the heterocyclic drugs are additive with those produced by other drugs with a similar action (eg, centrally acting anticholinergic drugs used in parkinsonism, antihistamines, antipsychotic agents). A toxic confusional and delirious state may result, particularly in the elderly.

Gastric emptying may be delayed in some individuals, thus limiting the bioavailability of some concurrently administered drugs. Physicians are advised to administer other agents one to two hours before or after the heterocyclic drugs.

Extreme caution should be exercised if a heterocyclic compound is given with or soon after a monoamine oxidase inhibitor, for their concomitant use rarely may produce tremors, excitability, hyperpyrexia, muscle rigidity, generalized clonic convulsions, delirium, and death. Based on theoretical considerations, an interval of at least seven days is suggested after a heterocyclic compound is discontinued before the monoamine oxidase inhibitor is given, and a two-week interval after a monoamine oxidase inhibitor is discontinued before the heterocyclic compound is given.

Some specialists have concluded that concurrent administration of heterocyclic agents and monoamine oxidase inhibitors may not be dangerous if the dosage of each drug is titrated carefully and if the monoamine oxidase inhibitor is begun after the heterocyclic antidepressant is started, but not vice versa. Combined therapy should be undertaken only by those familiar with the procedure.

Heterocyclic drugs that cause significant sedation (ie, doxepin, amitriptyline, nortriptyline, imipramine, trimipramine, trazodone, maprotiline) interact additively with alcohol. Adynamic ileus and excessive hepatic lipids also have been reported after use of such combinations. Moderate to heavy alcohol consumption should be avoided, especially if the patient drives or works in a hazardous occupation.

Certain antipsychotic drugs impair the hepatic metabolism and clearance of heterocyclic antidepressants, which increases the serum concentrations of the latter. The dosage of the heterocyclic antidepressant may require adjustment when an antipsychotic drug is used concurrently.

The effectiveness of the heterocyclic drugs may be reduced by heavy smoking and by concurrent administration of barbiturates, which induce hepatic microsomal enzymes that hasten the metabolism of the heterocyclics.

The simultaneous administration of barbiturates may cause refractoriness to heterocyclic drugs. Conversely, the toxic effects of heterocyclic compounds may be potentiated by alcohol and the barbiturates; the mechanism of this interaction is not known.

Drug Selection: The therapeutic efficacy and the onset of action of the heterocyclic antidepressants are essentially equivalent. All other factors being equal, the more established heterocyclic antidepressants, such as amitriptyline and imipramine, might be considered first-line drugs in the treatment of major depression because they have a long record of proven effectiveness and tend to be less expensive.

When medical disorders coexist with depression, differences in side effects assume a greater significance (Richardson and Richelson, 1984). Maprotiline may be preferred in patients with congestive heart failure, ischemic heart disease, or conduction defects. In patients with hypertension being treated with guanethidine, trimipramine and trazodone are the most appropriate choices due to their minimal inhibition of norepinephrine uptake. Protriptyline and desipramine can be used safely in hypertensive patients being treated with either prazosin or clonidine.

In patients with parkinsonism, the anticholinergic activity of amitriptyline, protriptyline, trimipramine, doxepin, maprotiline, and imipramine may ameliorate the medical disorder as well as the depression. As mentioned above, desipramine or a monoamine oxidase inhibitor is preferred in patients with a history of seizure disorders.

The antihistaminic activity of doxepin, trimipramine, amitriptyline, and maprotiline can be utilized to alleviate symptoms of an allergic disorder while also treating depression. Conversely, the anticholinergic activity of heterocyclics may produce or exacerbate confusional episodes in the elderly or exacerbate constipation or glaucoma; antidepressants with minimal anticholinergic activity (trazodone, amoxapine, nortriptyline, and desipramine) should be tried first when anticholinergic activity is particularly undesirable.

MONOAMINE OXIDASE INHIBITORS

The monoamine oxidase (MAO) inhibitors (isocarboxazid, phenelzine, and tranylcypromine) have long been considered second-line drugs in the treatment of affective disorders; however, recognition of their usefulness has increased with refinement of the definition and classification of the affective disorders and with greater understanding of the need to titrate

doses carefully. Nevertheless it must be recognized that the risk of hypertensive crisis due to drug-food or drug-drug interaction is significant with MAO inhibitors and the necessity to avoid certain foods and drugs must receive due consideration when they are prescribed.

Isocarboxazid, phenelzine, and tranylcypromine are effective in patients with atypical depression (Liebowitz et al, 1984) and panic or phobic disorders (Sheehan, 1984). These drugs also may be preferred in selected patients with dysthymic disorder. The monoamine oxidase inhibitors are useful in major depression, particularly when psychomotor agitation or anxiety is a presenting symptom (Davidson, 1983) or when heterocyclic antidepressants have failed. However, the latter are generally more effective and are drugs of choice for major depression, especially with melancholia. Recent evidence suggests that the monoamine oxidase inhibitors also may be effective in the treatment of bulimia (Walsh et al, 1982; Pope et al, 1983 A).

Patients who cannot adhere to dietary restrictions; those who consume alcohol; those with severe cardiovascular, hepatic, or renal disease; and those with pheochromocytoma should not receive MAO inhibitors. Asthmatics and patients who require pressor agents should be given MAO inhibitors with great caution.

Mechanism of Action: The mechanism of action of the monoamine oxidase inhibitors remains undefined. However, as with the heterocyclic antidepressants, much is known about the acute and chronic pharmacologic actions of these drugs (Murphy et al, 1984).

The three monoamine oxidase inhibitors marketed in the United States irreversibly inhibit both monoamine oxidase A and B. Monoamine oxidase A preferentially deaminates norepinephrine and serotonin, while monoamine oxidase B selectively degrades benzylamine and phenethylamine. When administered on an acute basis, the MAO inhibitors transiently elevate the cytoplasmic and vesicular concentrations of norepinephrine and serotonin. This activates a feedback loop that reduces the synthesis of these monoamines. If administration continues, there is a reduction in the number and activity of beta-adrenergic receptors, as well as in the number of alpha$_2$-adrenergic and serotonergic receptor sites.

As with the heterocyclic antidepressants, the therapeutic response to the monoamine oxidase inhibitors is delayed. An association between the specific chronic pharmacologic actions of these drugs and the delayed therapeutic response has yet to be demonstrated.

Administration and Dosage: The monoamine oxidase inhibitors are well absorbed orally. These drugs are metabolized and excreted relatively rapidly; however, the inhibited enzyme requires several weeks for regeneration.

The principles of administration and dosage for the heterocyclic compounds also apply to the monoamine oxidase inhibitors. These drugs should be administered only to patients who can be observed closely. It may be prudent to monitor blood pressure in the elderly to detect significant orthostatic hypotension (Robinson et al, 1982). The dose that relieves symptoms without causing undesirable effects is given daily, usually in divided amounts. Because of tranylcypromine's mild stimulant effect, this drug should not be given in the evening.

The duration of therapy is based on response. Maintenance doses may be necessary for patients with recurrent depressive episodes. If the recurrences are part of a manic-depressive illness, concurrent administration of lithium should be considered. As with heterocyclic antidepressants, abrupt discontinuation of monoamine oxidase inhibitors may precipitate a withdrawal syndrome. The recommended drug and dietary restrictions should be enforced for two to three weeks after discontinuation of the drug.

Adverse Reactions: The most common reactions to the monoamine oxidase inhibitors are drowsiness, dryness of the mouth, orthostatic hypotension, blurred vision, dysuria, and constipation. Orthostatic hypotension (dizziness, vertigo) is seldom severe enough to require discontinuation of therapy. Sexual dysfunction (impotence or inability to ejaculate) is reported in about 10% of males. Weight gain, insomnia, and jerky movements during sleep are less common. Insomnia associated with euphoria, tremors, and hypomanic agitated behavior may reflect overdosage or sensitivity to the drugs.

If headache, tachycardia, palpitation, nausea, vomiting, and hypertension occur together, it may indicate a hypertensive crisis caused by a food- or drug-drug interaction. (See the section on Drug Interactions.) Leukopenia, skin eruptions, photosensitivity, hepatotoxicity, hallucinations, and polyneuropathy have been reported rarely. Bilateral edema of the extremities is infrequent and may not respond to thiazide or loop diuretics; if it does not, the dose of the monoamine oxidase inhibitor should be reduced or therapy discontinued.

Precautions: It is important to educate patients concerning the untoward effects produced by monoamine oxidase inhibitors, especially the potential for severe interactions with certain foods and drugs. Physicians also should be alert for signs of severe hypotension. The monoamine oxidase inhibitors may exacerbate agitation and schizophrenic conditions and, thus, should be avoided in patients with these conditions. Patients should be instructed to inform other physicians treating them and pharmacists that they are taking monoamine oxidase inhibitors. They should carry a card stating that they are taking these drugs; information on potential food and drug interactions also may be included on the card.

Poisoning: There is currently little data on the mean lethal dose of the monoamine oxidase inhibitors. Death has been reported with doses of 170 to 650 mg tranylcypromine and 375 to 1,500 mg phenelzine. Toxic effects may not appear for 12 hours or more after ingestion and are largely adrenergic in nature: agitation, increased ventilatory and cardiac rates, dilated pupils, hyperreflexia, tremors, ataxia, sweating, hyperthermia, heart block, hypotension, delirium, convulsions, and coma. Aggressive supportive therapy to maintain vital functions, physical cooling procedures, forced diuresis, and acidification of the urine are indicated. Because monoamine oxidase inhibitors decrease gut motility, gastric lavage should be performed up to several hours after ingestion. Rapid recovery has occurred following hemodialysis after tranylcypromine and phenelzine overdose (Tollefson, 1983).

Food and Drug Interactions: Hypertension has been associated with the concomitant use of monoamine oxidase inhibitors and foods or beverages containing a large amount of tyramine, a naturally occurring pressor amine. These hypertensive crises are characterized by headache, tachycardia, palpitation, hypertension, nausea, and vomiting. Occasionally, pulmonary edema or subarachnoid or intracranial hemorrhage manifested by stiffness of the neck, decreasing consciousness, and syncope results from severe hypertension. Therefore, patients should be warned to avoid foods and beverages with a high tyramine content (eg, cheese, red wines, kippered [dried, salted] and pickled herring, chicken livers, canned figs, broad beans [fava beans], large amounts of chocolate, beer, brewer's yeast, aged meats and meat extracts, nonpasteurized yogurt). Protein-rich food that may be spoiled, aged, fermented, smoked, or pickled should be avoided as these foods may be subject to protein breakdown. A complete list of such foods and beverages should be given to any patient receiving monoamine oxidase inhibitors (*Med Lett Drugs Ther,* 1980). The effects of other indirect-acting adrenergic drugs (eg, amphetamines, methylphenidate [Ritalin], ephedrine, cocaine, sympathomimetic amines including those in cold or asthma remedies) are markedly potentiated and these drugs also should be avoided. Phentolamine [Regitine] and parenteral chlorpromazine [Thorazine] have been used to counteract the hypertensive crises.

In life-threatening situations that require use of a sympathomimetic agent, it appears to be theoretically preferable to use a direct-acting drug (eg, norepinephrine [Levophed], dopamine [Dopastat, Intropin]) because, unlike the heterocyclic compounds, the monoamine oxidase inhibitors do not block catecholamine reuptake.

Levodopa [Dopar, Larodopa] should be withdrawn two to four weeks prior to institution of monoamine oxidase inhibitors. Methyldopa [Aldomet], tryptophan, and 5-hydroxytryptophan also are relatively contraindicated.

Severe toxic reactions characterized by excitation and hyperpyrexia may occur when dextromethorphan (a common ingredient of over-the-counter cough preparations) or meperidine [Demerol] and related analgesics are given to patients receiving monoamine oxidase inhibitors. If emergency surgery is necessary, meperidine should be avoided and the recommended dose of the narcotic chosen should be reduced by at least 25% to 50%. The central nervous system depressant action of anesthetics and alcohol is also markedly potentiated.

Furazolidone [Furoxone], an antimicrobial drug, and procarbazine [Matulane], an antineoplastic agent, act as monoamine oxidase inhibitors when given for more than five days; therefore, caution should be observed if these drugs are administered with other monoamine oxidase inhibitors.

Insulin-dependent patients should be monitored for hypoglycemia at the start of monoamine oxidase inhibitor therapy; the dosage of insulin may require adjustment.

Tranylcypromine should be administered with caution to patients receiving disulfiram [Antabuse], because severe toxicity, including convulsions and death, have been noted in animals.

When changing from one MAO inhibitor to another, a washout period may be advisable. Hypertensive crisis and stroke have been reported when substituting tranylcypromine for phenelzine.

For interactions between heterocyclic and monoamine oxidase inhibitor antidepressants, see the section on Heterocyclic Antidepressants.

Drug Selection: Phenelzine, isocarboxazid, and tranylcypromine have similar pharmacologic profiles. Phenelzine may be the most effective monoamine oxidase inhibitor for the treatment of panic and phobic disorders. Of these drugs, only tranylcypromine has a clinically detectable amphetamine-like psychostimulant effect, usually manifested only with larger doses. The incidence of intracranial hemorrhage (sometimes fatal) associated with severe occipital headache and paradoxical hypertension appears to be greater with tranylcypromine than with other monoamine oxidase inhibitors.

CENTRAL NERVOUS SYSTEM STIMULANTS

Recent anecdotal evidence has suggested that psychomotor stimulants (eg, dextroamphetamine [Dexedrine], methylphenidate [Ritalin]) may be helpful in selected patients with affective disorders. These drugs may be beneficial in elderly patients with medical problems. Also, these stimulants may be effective adjuncts to antidepressant therapy in resistant patients. Psychomotor stimulants should not be used routinely, however, in patients with affective disorders. The potential for tolerance and abuse is high, and these drugs may produce adverse cardiovascular effects, especially in the elderly. A few physicians employ dextroamphetamine (10 or 15 mg once or twice daily for one or two days) as a diagnostic tool to determine the probable efficacy of heterocyclic antidepressant therapy; however, this technique has not been beneficial in any controlled study and it is not recommended for routine use.

Additional information on these drugs is presented in Chapter 8, Drugs Used in Other Mental Disorders.

ANTIMANIC DRUGS

Lithium is effective in 60% to 80% of all acute hypomanic and manic episodes. The onset of the therapeutic effect is slow (five days to three weeks), but larger doses may shorten the time to clinical response. Alternatively, antipsychotic agents alone or with lithium usually are employed in the initial treatment of highly agitated, hyperactive manic patients. When the acute episode is controlled, the antipsychotic agent may be withdrawn gradually and lithium continued as the sole therapeutic agent. Careful dosage adjustment of both drugs is essential for optimum effectiveness and to lessen any additive central nervous system toxicity (Spring, 1979; Hansen, 1981).

Lithium decreases the intensity and frequency of successive episodes in cyclic mania and depression (Davis, 1976) and, thus, is clearly indicated in the prophylaxis of bipolar disorder. However, it is not effective in all patients and should be given indefinitely only when it reduces the frequency and/or intensity of recurrent manic and depressive episodes. An antidepressant drug also may be required in breakthrough depression. Likewise, if mania is observed during use of antidepressants in patients with recurring depressive episodes, combination therapy with lithium may be helpful. Although lithium alone is reported to be effective in some patients experiencing acute episodes of major depression, heterocyclic antidepressants are preferred.

The combined use of lithium and an antipsychotic agent may be helpful for schizoaffective disorders associated with manic signs and symptoms. Lithium has been proposed for use in a variety of other psychiatric disorders (eg, recurrent alcoholism, socially unacceptable aggressive behavior, organic brain syndromes, choreiform disorders, hyperkinesis and other behavior or character disorders in children). However, its efficacy in these conditions has not been established.

Open clinical studies support the efficacy of lithium in cluster headache (Ekbom, 1981), but exacerbation of migraine headaches has occurred (Peatfield, 1981). (See also Chapter 13, Drugs Used to Treat Migraine and Other Headaches.)

Lithium carbonate also is reported to control the diarrhea of pancreatic cholera syndrome that is presumably caused by vasoactive intestinal peptides or similar substances secreted from pancreatic nonbeta islet cell tumors (Pandol et al, 1980). Finally, lithium produces leukocytosis in most patients treated for up to two years and may be useful in the management of certain leukopenic conditions (Pi et al, 1983).

Carbamazepine [Tegretol], an anticonvulsant, is a useful adjunct when lithium is inadequate or not tolerated in patients requiring both acute treatment and prophylaxis of manic episodes (Ballenger and Post, 1980; Post, 1982; Post et al, 1984). More than one-half of patients who failed to respond to lithium derived significant benefit from the use of carbamazepine (*Int Drug Ther News*, 1982). It is more effective in mania than depression (Jann et al, 1984). Further study of carbamazepine in the treatment of bipolar affective disorders is necessary to define its role.

Drug Evaluations

HETEROCYCLIC COMPOUNDS

IMIPRAMINE HYDROCHLORIDE
[Janimine, SK-Pramine, Tofranil]

IMIPRAMINE PAMOATE
[Tofranil-PM]

USES. Imipramine is the prototype of the heterocyclic antidepressants and is effective in the treatment of the major depressive episodes of major depression, mixed bipolar disorder, and depressed bipolar disorder. Imipramine also is useful in dysthymic disorder, panic disorder, or the phobic disorders. This drug may be given to treat atypical depression, but the monoamine oxidase inhibitors generally are preferred.

Imipramine may improve eating behavior in patients with bulimia, but its role in this disorder awaits the results of further studies (Pope et al, 1983 B).

The pamoate form offers no advantage over the hydrochloride salt, which is inherently long acting.

ADVERSE REACTIONS AND PRECAUTIONS. The untoward effects of imipramine are characteristic of all heterocyclic antidepressants. Sedation and anticholinergic effects are most common. Allergic reactions, blood dyscrasias, endocrine effects, and jaundice are uncommon. A case of tremor (Kronfol et al, 1983) and a patient with intolerable vasospasm of the hands and feet (Appelbaum and Kapoor, 1983) have been reported. Cardiac and central nervous system toxicity may be prominent with overdosage.

Abrupt cessation of treatment after long-term therapy may produce withdrawal symptoms (eg, headache, malaise, anorexia, fatigue). An akathisia-like syndrome also has been reported when administration of large doses (300 mg or more daily) was stopped suddenly. Although most fatal cases of poisoning have occurred after ingestion of more than 1.5 g, individual sensitivity varies; death has been reported after as little as 500 to 750 mg and recovery has occurred after ingestion of 5.4 g.

See the Introduction for a more complete discussion on adverse reactions, precautions, and the use of imipramine with other drugs.

DOSAGE AND PREPARATIONS. Dosage should be individualized on the basis of clinical response.
Intramuscular: *Adults,* initially, up to 100 mg daily in divided doses. The oral route should be substituted as soon as possible.

IMIPRAMINE HYDROCHLORIDE:
Tofranil (Geigy). Solution 12.5 mg/ml in 2 ml containers.
Oral: *Adults (hospitalized),* initially, 100 mg daily in divided doses, increased gradually to 200 mg daily; 250 to 300 mg daily may be given if there is no response after two weeks. *Adults (outpatients),* initially, 75 mg increased to 150 mg daily in divided doses; a useful schedule to minimize sedation and anticholinergic effects is described in the footnote to the Table. A single daily dose or the major portion of the daily dose may be given at bedtime if insomnia is prominent or undue sedation occurs during the day. If little benefit is noted by the third week, the dose may be increased (eg, by 50 mg daily every week) until clinical improvement, intolerable side effects, or the maximum recommended daily dose is reached (ie, 200 mg). For maintenance, the lowest dose that will maintain remission is recommended. *Elderly patients and adolescents,* initially, 25 to 50 mg daily, increased to 100 mg daily in divided doses.

IMIPRAMINE HYDROCHLORIDE:
Janimine (Abbott), *SK-Pramine* (Smith Kline & French), *Tofranil* (Geigy), *Generic.* Tablets 10, 25, and 50 mg.
IMIPRAMINE PAMOATE:

Tofranil-PM (Geigy). Capsules equivalent to 75, 100, 125, and 150 mg of imipramine hydrochloride.

AMITRIPTYLINE HYDROCHLORIDE
[Elavil, Endep]

USES. Amitriptyline is as effective as imipramine in the treatment of the major depressive episodes of major depression, mixed bipolar disorder, and depressed bipolar disorder. This drug also may be useful in dysthymic disorder, panic disorder, phobic disorders, and atypical depression. Concomitant administration of amitriptyline with an antipsychotic can be beneficial in schizoaffective disorder.

Amitriptyline may control abnormal eating behavior in bulimic patients (Mitchell and Groat, 1984). This agent also is useful in the prophylaxis of migraine headache and in some patients with chronic muscle-contraction headache that is unresponsive to analgesic therapy (see Chapter 13, Drugs Used to Treat Migraine and Other Headaches).

ADVERSE REACTIONS AND PRECAUTIONS. Effective doses have a moderate to marked sedative action. Because anticholinergic activity may be pronounced with amitriptyline, confusional episodes may occur more frequently, especially in elderly patients. Leukopenia and an increased appetite for carbohydrates with resultant weight gain also have been reported.

Although most fatal cases of poisoning have resulted from ingestion of more than 1.3 g, death has been reported after ingestion of 500 mg and recovery after ingestion of almost 4 g.

See the Introduction for a more complete discussion on indications, adverse reactions, precautions, and the use of heterocyclic antidepressants with other drugs.

DOSAGE AND PREPARATIONS.
Intramuscular: *Adults,* initially, 20 to 30 mg four times a day. The oral route should be substituted as soon as possible.
Elavil (Merck Sharp & Dohme), *Generic.* Solution 10 mg/ml in 10 ml containers.
Oral: *Adults (hospitalized),* initially, 100 mg daily in divided doses, increased gradually to 200 mg daily if necessary; some patients may require as much as 300 mg daily. *Adults (outpatients),* initially, 75 mg increased to 150 mg daily in divided doses; a useful schedule to minimize sedation and anticholinergic effects is described in the footnote to the Table. A single daily dose or the major portion of the daily dose may be given at bedtime if insomnia is prominent or undue sedation occurs during the day. If little benefit is noted by the third week, the dose may be increased (eg, by 50 mg daily every week) until clinical improvement, intolerable side effects, or the maximum recommended daily dose is reached (ie, 300 mg). For maintenance, the lowest dose that will maintain remission is recommended. *Elderly patients and adolescents,* initially, 25 to 50 mg daily, increased to 100 mg daily in divided doses.

Elavil (Merck Sharp & Dohme), *Endep* (Roche), *Generic*. Tablets 10, 25, 50, 75, 100, and 150 mg.

AMOXAPINE
[Asendin]

Amoxapine is the only member of the dibenzoxazepine class of tricyclic compounds (Lydiard and Gelenberg, 1981; Smith and Ayd, 1981). Its chemical structure is similar to that of the antipsychotic drug, loxapine, and it has some dopamine receptor antagonist action.

USES. Results of controlled studies show that the antidepressant action of amoxapine is equivalent to that of imipramine and amitriptyline. Amoxapine is more effective in relieving anxiety and agitation than imipramine. As with other heterocyclic drugs, amoxapine generally is more effective in major depression than in dysthymic or atypical depression. It has relatively weak sedative and anticholinergic activities compared to imipramine or amitriptyline. The manufacturer claims that the onset of action is more rapid than with more traditional heterocyclic antidepressants and that more than 80% of patients who respond do so within two weeks; however, this finding has not been consistent (Prusoff et al, 1981; Rickels et al, 1981; Click and Zisook, 1982; Winsauer and O'Hair, 1984).

ADVERSE REACTIONS AND PRECAUTIONS. Although sedation and anticholinergic effects are minimal, caution is advised when prescribing this drug for patients who perform hazardous tasks that require alertness or for those with a history of urinary retention or angle-closure glaucoma. Sexual disturbances, constipation, and elevated serum prolactin levels with galactorrhea have been reported.

Extrapyramidal side effects have been observed infrequently and may be caused by the 7-hydroxyamoxapine metabolite, which is a dopamine antagonist. Dyskinesias have been reported, but it is not clear whether they are tardive or withdrawal dyskinesias. One case of neuroleptic malignant syndrome has developed (Hunt-Fugate et al, 1984).

Thus far, tachycardia and arrhythmias have been reported less frequently than anticipated on the basis of experience with more traditional heterocyclic compounds; nevertheless, caution is advised when amoxapine is used in individuals with cardiac abnormalities, and the drug is not recommended during the immediate period following myocardial infarction.

Seizures have been reported infrequently, most often after overdose or use of large therapeutic doses. Amoxapine should be used with caution in epileptic patients. Skin rashes occur infrequently. Agranulocytosis has occurred (Christenson, 1983).

DRUG INTERACTIONS. Drug interactions with amoxapine are similar to those observed with traditional heterocyclic drugs, ie, additive central nervous system depression with any drug that also has this effect (eg, antianxiety drugs, hypnotics, alcohol, antipsychotic agents, central anticholinergic agents, antihistamines). Long-term concurrent administration of barbiturates may reduce the effectiveness of any heterocyclic compound by inducing drug metabolizing enzymes.

The concurrent administration of monoamine oxidase inhibitors or administration of amoxapine within 10 to 14 days following such therapy can cause a severe syndrome of hypertension, hyperpyrexia, seizures, and even death.

PREGNANCY AND LACTATION. Embryotoxic and fetotoxic effects, as well as decreased postnatal survival (intrauterine death, stillbirth, decreased weight gain), occurred in animals given three to ten times the human dose, but no teratogenic effects were observed. Amoxapine should be used during pregnancy only if the benefit justifies the risk to the fetus (FDA Pregnancy Category C).

Amoxapine and 8-hydroxyamoxapine are detectable in human breast milk and this drug is not recommended for use in nursing women.

See the Introduction for a more complete discussion of indications, adverse reactions, interactions, and management of overdose.

PHARMACOKINETICS. Amoxapine is rapidly and well absorbed when given orally (time to peak effect is about 80 minutes). Protein binding is about 90%. The drug is metabolized to 7-hydroxyamoxapine and 8-hydroxyamoxapine. The latter has antidepressant activity and a longer half-life (30 hours) than the parent compound (eight hours). Although 7-hydroxyamoxapine (half-life, 6.5 hours) is not an antidepressant, it does have antipsychotic activity and may contribute to side effects. After conjugation with glucuronic acid, the metabolites are excreted in the urine.

DOSAGE AND PREPARATIONS.
Oral: Adults, initially, 75 mg, increased to 200 mg daily in divided doses; a useful schedule to minimize sedation and anticholinergic effects is described in the footnote to the Table. A single daily dose or the major portion of the daily dose may be given at bedtime if insomnia is prominent or undue sedation occurs during the day. If little benefit is noted by the third week, the dose may be increased (eg, by 50 mg daily every week) until clinical improvement, intolerable side effects, or the maximum recommended daily dose is reached (ie, *outpatients,* 400 mg; *inpatients,* 600 mg). For maintenance, the lowest dose that will maintain remission is recommended. *Elderly patients and adolescents,* initially, 25 to 50 mg daily, increased to 100 mg daily in divided doses.

Asendin (Lederle). Tablets 25, 50, 100, and 150 mg.

DESIPRAMINE HYDROCHLORIDE
[Norpramin, Pertofrane]

Desipramine, a metabolite of imipramine, has actions and uses similar to those of the parent compound and is as effective as imipramine in the treatment of depression.

Untoward effects are similar to those produced by imipramine, but its anticholinergic and sedative actions are less pronounced. Thus, desipramine may be especially useful in patients who are particularly sensitive to these effects.

See the Introduction for more complete information on indications, adverse reactions, precautions, and the use of heterocyclic antidepressants with other drugs.

DOSAGE AND PREPARATIONS.

Oral: *Adults (hospitalized),* initially, 75 mg daily in divided doses, increased gradually to 200 mg daily. If necessary, after two weeks, the dosage may be increased gradually to a maximum of 300 mg daily. *Adults (outpatients),* initially, 75 mg increased to 150 mg daily in divided doses; a useful schedule to minimize sedation and anticholinergic effects is described in the footnote to the Table. A single daily dose or the major portion of the daily dose may be given at bedtime if insomnia is prominent or undue sedation occurs during the day. If little benefit is noted by the third week, the dose may be increased (eg, by 50 mg daily every week) until clinical improvement, intolerable side effects, or the maximum recommended daily dose is reached (ie, 300 mg). For maintenance, the lowest dose that will maintain remission is recommended. *Elderly patients and adolescents,* initially, 25 to 50 mg daily, increased to 100 mg daily in divided doses.

    Norpramin (Merrell Dow). Tablets 10, 25, 50, 75, 100, and 150 mg.
    Pertofrane (USV). Capsules 25 and 50 mg.

DOXEPIN HYDROCHLORIDE
[Adapin, Sinequan]

Doxepin, a heterocyclic antidepressant, is as effective as imipramine in the treatment of the major depressive episodes of major depression, mixed bipolar disorder, and depressed bipolar disorder. It also may be effective in the depressive periods of dysthymic disorder and in atypical depression.

Therapeutic doses produce marked anticholinergic effects and pronounced sedation. Untoward effects are similar to those of other heterocyclic antidepressants. Most fatal cases of poisoning have resulted from ingestion of more than 1.5 g; however, recovery has occurred after ingestion of 5 g.

See the Introduction for additional information on indications, adverse reactions, precautions, and the use of heterocyclic antidepressants with other drugs.

DOSAGE AND PREPARATIONS.

Oral: *Adults (hospitalized),* initially, 75 mg daily in divided doses for patients with mild to moderate illness. Higher doses may be required in more severely ill patients. The usual optimum dosage is 75 to 150 mg daily. The dosage may be increased gradually after two weeks to a maximum of 300 mg daily. *Adults (outpatients),* initially, 75 mg daily in divided doses; the usual optimum dosage is 75 to 150 mg daily. A useful schedule to minimize sedation and anticholinergic effects is described in the footnote to the Table. A single daily dose or the major portion of the daily dose may be given at bedtime if insomnia is prominent or undue sedation occurs during the day. If little benefit is noted by the third week, the dose may be increased (eg, by 50 mg daily every week) until clinical improvement, intolerable side effects, or the maximum recommended daily dose is reached (ie, 300 mg). For maintenance, the lowest dose that will maintain remission is recommended. Doses as low as 25 to 50 mg/day have controlled patients with mild symptomatology or depression accompanying organic disease. *Elderly patients and adolescents,* initially, 25 to 50 mg daily, increased to 100 mg daily in divided doses.

    Adapin (Pennwalt). Capsules 10, 25, 50, 75, and 100 mg.
    Sinequan (Roerig). Capsules 10, 25, 50, 75, 100, and 150 mg; oral concentrate 10 mg/ml.

MAPROTILINE HYDROCHLORIDE
[Ludiomil]

ACTIONS AND USES. Maprotiline is the first tetracyclic antidepressant to be marketed in the United States (Wells and Gelenberg, 1981). Its pharmacologic and clinical profiles, as well as its efficacy, resemble those of imipramine. Maprotiline blocks the neuronal uptake of norepinephrine more than that of serotonin. Some patients respond within one week, but optimum effects usually are not observed for two to three weeks.

ADVERSE REACTIONS AND PRECAUTIONS. Drowsiness and anticholinergic effects are the most common reactions reported. They appear to be less severe than with doxepin or amitriptyline. Skin rashes occur no more frequently with maprotiline than with imipramine or amitriptyline. Cardiotoxic effects are less severe than with imipramine or amitriptyline, but the incidence is similar for all three drugs. Therefore, maprotiline should be used cautiously in patients with a history of myocardial infarction or cardiac disorders.

Seizures are observed more often than with other heterocyclic compounds. They have occurred over a broad dose range, after even modest increases in the daily dosage, and during stabilized dosing regimens (Mendelis, 1983). Likewise, they have been reported to develop rapidly after initiation of therapy, as well as during prolonged treatment. Maprotiline has caused convulsions in 25% of patients who received overdoses. Therefore, the drug should not be used in patients with known or suspected seizure disorders. The risk may be diminished by starting therapy at a low dosage for two weeks before gradually increasing the amount to recommended levels.

DRUG INTERACTIONS. Drug interactions with maprotiline are similar to those of other heterocyclic drugs, ie, acute additive central nervous system depression with any drug that also has this effect (eg, antianxiety drugs, hypnotics, alcohol, antipsychotic drugs, central anticholinergic drugs, antihistamines). Severe adverse reactions (hypertension, hyperpyrexia, seizures, and death) may occur after concurrent administration of MAO inhibitors or administration of maprotiline within 10 to 14 days following their use.

See the Introduction for a more complete discussion of indications, adverse reactions, drug interactions, and management of overdose.

PREGNANCY AND LACTATION. No teratogenic, embryotoxic, or fetotoxic effects have been observed in animals. No adequate, well-controlled studies have been performed in pregnant women to assure the safety of the fetus; therefore, maprotiline should be administered during pregnancy only if the benefit justifies the risk to the fetus (FDA Pregnancy Category B).

Concentrations of maprotiline in breast milk are similar to those in the blood; therefore, its use should be discouraged in nursing women.

PHARMACOKINETICS. Although maprotiline is completely absorbed, peak plasma concentrations are not attained for 9 to 16 hours in normal individuals. Protein binding is about 90% and the volume of distribution is 23 L/kg. The elimination half-life of unchanged drug ranges from 43 to 51 hours. Maprotiline is extensively metabolized by a first-order process, and approximately 70% of the metabolites are excreted in the urine.

DOSAGE AND PREPARATIONS.
Oral: Adults (hospitalized), initially, 100 to 150 mg daily in divided doses, gradually increased as required and tolerated. Most hospitalized patients with moderate to severe depression respond to 150 mg daily, although as much as 225 mg (maximum) may be required.

Adults (outpatients), initially, 75 mg daily in single or divided doses for two weeks. If little benefit is noted by the third week, the dose may be increased gradually (eg, by 25 mg daily every week) until clinical improvement, intolerable side effects, or the maximum recommended daily dose is reached (ie, 225 mg). For maintenance, the lowest dose that will maintain remission is recommended. *Elderly patients,* initially, 25 to 50 mg daily; 50 to 75 mg daily is usually satisfactory for maintenance.
   Ludiomil (CIBA). Tablets 25, 50, and 75 mg.

NORTRIPTYLINE HYDROCHLORIDE
[Aventyl Hydrochloride, Pamelor]

Nortriptyline, the N-demethylated metabolite of amitriptyline, is as effective as imipramine in the treatment of the major depressive episodes of major depression, mixed bipolar disorder, and depressed bipolar disorder. It also may be useful in the depressive periods of dysthymic disorder and in atypical depression. Depression that follows stroke also may respond to nortriptyline (Lipsey et al, 1984).

Plasma concentrations below 50 ng/ml are generally ineffective and those exceeding 175 ng/ml are often associated with a suboptimal response; therefore, excessive dosage may diminish responsiveness. In addition, active metabolites of nortriptyline may accumulate in elderly patients and toxic side effects may develop despite plasma nortriptyline concentrations below 150 ng/ml.

See the Introduction for additional information on indications, adverse reactions, precautions, and the use of heterocyclic antidepressants with other drugs.

DOSAGE AND PREPARATIONS.
Oral: Adults (hospitalized), initially, 40 mg daily in three or four divided doses, increased to a maximum of 150 mg daily after two weeks, if necessary. After adjustment as needed, the total dose can be given once daily at bedtime.

Adults (outpatients), dosage should begin at a low level and be increased as required to 25 mg three or four times daily. A useful schedule to minimize sedation and anticholinergic effects is described in the footnote to the Table. Doses above 150 mg are not recommended. For maintenance, the lowest dose that maintains remission should be given. *Adolescents and elderly patients,* 30 to 50 mg daily in divided doses.
   Aventyl Hydrochloride (Lilly). Capsules 10 and 25 mg; liquid 10 mg/5 ml (alcohol 4%).
   Pamelor (Sandoz). Capsules 10, 25, and 75 mg; oral solution 10 mg/5 ml (alcohol 4%).

PROTRIPTYLINE HYDROCHLORIDE
[Vivactil]

Protriptyline, a heterocyclic antidepressant, is effective in the treatment of major depression, mixed bipolar disorder, and depressed bipolar disorder. It also may be useful in the treatment of the depressive periods of dysthymic disorder.

Unlike most of the other heterocyclic antidepressants, protriptyline causes little, if any, sedation. Because of this, it may be particularly useful in narcolepsy and depression associated with psychomotor retardation, apathy, and fatigue and is less beneficial when agitation and anxiety are prominent. This drug has a long elimination half-life (three to five days).

See the Introduction for additional information on indications, adverse reactions, precautions, and the use of heterocyclic antidepressants with other drugs.

DOSAGE AND PREPARATIONS.
Oral: Adults (hospitalized), 15 mg daily in one or two doses, increased to a maximum of 60 mg daily after two weeks, if necessary. After adjustment as needed, the total dose can be given once daily, usually in the morning. *Adults (outpatients),* initially, 15 to 40 mg daily in three or four doses. Doses should

begin at a low level and be increased gradually. A useful schedule to minimize sedation and anticholinergic effects is described in the footnote to the Table. Doses above 60 mg daily are not recommended. For maintenance, the lowest dose that maintains remission should be given. *Adolescents and elderly patients,* initially, 10 to 15 mg daily in one or two divided doses, increased gradually if necessary. In elderly patients, the cardiovascular system must be monitored closely if the daily dose exceeds 20 mg.

   Vivactil (Merck Sharp & Dohme). Tablets 5 and 10 mg.

TRAZODONE HYDROCHLORIDE
   [Desyrel]

ACTIONS. Trazodone is a phenylpiperazine propyl derivative of triazolopyridine and is chemically unrelated to tricyclic or tetracyclic antidepressants (Rickels et al, 1980; Brogden et al, 1981; Goldberg and Finnerty, 1980). It has no monoamine oxidase inhibiting or amphetamine-like properties. Trazodone is a serotonin antagonist in low doses in rodents, and therapeutic doses inhibit the neuronal uptake of serotonin in man. Prolonged administration decreases the number of serotonin receptors experimentally; norepinephrine uptake is essentially unaffected. After long-term administration, the number of presynaptic alpha$_2$-adrenergic receptors may be decreased.

USES. Controlled studies have demonstrated that trazodone is as effective as amitriptyline and imipramine in patients with major depressive disorders. It is as effective as amitriptyline in some patients with dysthymic disorder; however, the number of controlled studies are inadequate to define the role of trazodone in subsets of depressive disorders. Trazodone does not aggravate psychotic symptoms in patients with schizophrenia or schizoaffective disorders.

   Onset of action in initial studies was reported to be three to seven days in most patients, and an optimum effect was noted in two to six weeks.

ADVERSE REACTIONS AND PRECAUTIONS. Trazodone is well tolerated. Drowsiness is the most common side effect (incidence, 15% to 20%). Nausea and vomiting also are common. Anticholinergic effects (ie, dryness of the mouth, constipation, urinary retention) occur infrequently. Agitation is noted in less than 1% of patients. Seizures, extrapyramidal reactions, and hepatotoxicity are rare. Priapism has been associated with trazodone therapy (Lansky and Selzer, 1984) and may lead to permanent impotence.

   The cardiotoxicity, neurotoxicity, and respiratory depression commonly encountered after overdose of heterocyclic antidepressants are less severe with trazodone (Lesar et al, 1983). However, death has occurred in patients who ingested trazodone with another central nervous system depressant.

DRUG INTERACTIONS. Interaction with other drugs occurs infrequently; however, because trazodone causes drowsiness in some patients, caution is advised when this drug is used with other central nervous system depressants, including alcohol.

PREGNANCY AND LACTATION. Trazodone is classified in FDA Pregnancy Category C because it is associated with increased fetal resorption in rats and congenital anomalies in rabbits. There are no adequate well-controlled studies in man. Small amounts of trazodone and its metabolites are present in breast milk; therefore, caution is advised in nursing mothers.

PHARMACOKINETICS. When given orally, trazodone is absorbed rapidly, bioavailability is essentially complete, and the mean time to peak effect is about 1.5 (range, 0.5 to 2) hours in fasting and 2.5 hours in nonfasting patients. However, the manufacturer recommends that the drug be taken after a light meal or snack to improve total absorption and diminish the incidence of dizziness and lightheadedness. Data on distribution are fragmentary; protein binding is 96% (at 1 ng/ml).

   Trazodone is extensively metabolized by hepatic microsomal enzymes, but enzyme induction has not been observed. Major metabolites include m-chlorophenylpiperazine (possibly active) and oxotriazolopyridin propionic acid. Two-thirds of the drug and its metabolites are excreted in the urine and one-third appears in the feces. The mean plasma elimination half-life of parent drug ranges from 3.9 to 6.3 hours; however, the beta elimination half-life for total radioactivity ranges from 7 to 13 hours. Based on the limited data available at this time, it is not clear whether there is a direct relationship between trazodone plasma levels and its therapeutic effects.

DOSAGE AND PREPARATIONS.
Oral: Adults (hospitalized), initially, 150 mg daily in divided doses, increased by 50 mg daily every three to four days. Severely depressed inpatients may require 400 to 600 mg daily.

   Adults (outpatients), initially, 150 mg increased to 250 mg daily in divided doses; a useful schedule to minimize sedation and anticholinergic effects is described in the footnote to the Table. A single daily dose or the major portion of the daily dose may be given at bedtime if insomnia is prominent or undue sedation occurs during the day. If little benefit is noted by the third week, the dose may be increased (eg, by 50 mg daily every week) until clinical improvement, intolerable side effects, or the maximum recommended daily dose is reached (ie, 400 mg). For maintenance, the lowest dose that will maintain remission is recommended. *Elderly patients and adolescents,* initially, 25 to 50 mg daily, increased to 100 to 150 mg daily in divided doses, depending upon the response and tolerance.

   Desyrel (Mead Johnson). Tablets 50, 100, and 150 mg (Dividose).

TRIMIPRAMINE MALEATE
   [Surmontil]

Trimipramine is an effective antidepressant that resembles the other dibenzazepines (ie, desipramine, imipramine); however, unlike the latter compounds, the sedation produced is equivalent to that observed with amitriptyline and doxepin. Therapeutic doses have intermediate anticholinergic activity.

The indications, adverse reactions, and precautions of trimipramine are similar to those of the other heterocyclic compounds (see the Introduction). The potential risk to the fetus is unknown.

DOSAGE AND PREPARATIONS.

Oral: Adults (hospitalized), initially, 100 mg daily in divided doses, increased gradually to 200 mg daily; if improvement does not occur in two to three weeks, the dose may be increased to a maximum of 250 to 300 mg.

Adults (outpatients), initially, 75 mg increased to 150 mg daily in divided doses; a useful schedule to minimize sedation and anticholinergic effects is described in the footnote to the Table. A single daily dose or the major portion of the daily dose may be given at bedtime if insomnia is prominent or undue sedation occurs during the day. If little benefit is noted by the third week, the dose may be increased (eg, by 50 mg daily every week) until clinical improvement, intolerable side effects, or the maximum recommended daily dose is reached (ie, 200 mg). For maintenance, dosage should be adjusted to the lowest level required for symptomatic relief. *Elderly patients and adolescents,* initially, 25 to 50 mg daily, increased to 100 mg daily in divided doses.

Surmontil (Wyeth). Capsules 25, 50, and 100 mg.

MONOAMINE OXIDASE INHIBITORS

PHENELZINE SULFATE
[Nardil]

USES. Phenelzine is effective in the treatment of some depressed patients, particularly those with dysthymic disorder and atypical depression. It also is useful in the treatment of panic disorder and the phobic disorders. Like other monoamine oxidase inhibitors, however, phenelzine may be less effective than the heterocyclic drugs in major depressive episodes, such as major depression with melancholia. Some patients refractory to the heterocyclic drugs respond to phenelzine, especially those with severe anxiety. Studies have shown phenelzine and amitriptyline to be equieffective in outpatients with depression (Rowan et al, 1980; Ravaris et al, 1980).

Phenelzine has improved eating behavior in some patients with bulimia; however, phenelzine's role in this disorder awaits the results of controlled clinical trials.

PRECAUTIONS. Because all monoamine oxidase inhibitors have the potential to produce serious adverse reactions, patients should be reliable and supervised closely. Dietary restrictions and precautions regarding concomitant medication should be adhered to and vasoactive drugs avoided or used in reduced dosage.

Although several fatal cases of poisoning have occurred after ingestion of 375 mg to 1.5 g, recovery was reported after ingestion of doses within this range.

See the Introduction for a discussion on adverse reactions, precautions, and the use of monoamine oxidase inhibitors with other drugs.

PHARMACOKINETICS. Phenelzine is acetylated rapidly or slowly, depending upon the patient's genetic profile; however, there is evidence that acetylation is not a major metabolic pathway for phenelzine, and no relationship has been demonstrated between acetylator phenotype and therapeutic or adverse effects (Davidson et al, 1978; Robinson et al, 1978).

DOSAGE AND PREPARATIONS. The dose must be individualized to achieve adequate therapeutic results with minimal adverse effects.

Oral: Adults (outpatients), initially, 45 to 75 mg daily in two or three divided doses; alternatively, 1 mg/kg daily. The dose can be increased to 90 mg if there is no response after 21 days. Most patients require at least 60 mg to inhibit monoamine oxidase by about 80%, but the dose should be decreased if untoward effects develop. A few patients may require more than 90 mg. It is often useful to maintain patients on a therapeutic dose for at least six months after improvement is noted. If long-term maintenance therapy is indicated for recurrent illness, the total daily dose should be reduced to the lowest effective amount, usually 45 to 60 mg daily. Information is inadequate to establish a dosage for *children under 16 years.*

Nardil (Parke-Davis). Tablets 15 mg.

ISOCARBOXAZID
[Marplan]

USES. Isocarboxazid is effective in the treatment of some depressed patients, particularly those with dysthymic disorder and atypical depression. It also is useful in the treatment of panic disorder and the phobic disorders. Although isocarboxazid has been effective in major depression with melancholia (Giller et al, 1984), the heterocyclic antidepressants generally are the drugs of choice in this disorder. In depression without melancholia, a daily dose of 50 mg was more effective than 30 mg in alleviating depression and anxiety.

Because all monoamine oxidase inhibitors can produce serious adverse reactions, patients should be supervised closely. Recovery has been reported after ingestion of 300 to 500 mg of isocarboxazid.

See the Introduction for additional information on indications, adverse reactions, precautions, and the use of monoamine oxidase inhibitors with other drugs.

DOSAGE AND PREPARATIONS.

Oral: Adults (outpatients), initially, 30 mg daily in divided doses; the amount may be increased to 50 mg in refractory patients. The dosage should be reduced as soon as clinical improvement is observed; 10 to 20 mg daily or less is the usual amount given for maintenance. However, the actual maintenance dose has never been established in controlled trials, and a higher dose may be necessary. Information is inadequate to establish dosage for *children under 16 years.*

Marplan (Roche). Tablets 10 mg.

TRANYLCYPROMINE SULFATE
[Parnate]

Tranylcypromine differs structurally from the hydrazines, phenelzine and isocarboxazid, in that it is formed from cyclization of the side chain of amphetamine. This monoamine oxidase inhibitor is effective in the treatment of dysthymic disorder and atypical depression. It also is useful in panic and phobic disorders. Tranylcypromine is less effective than the heterocyclic antidepressants in the treatment of major depressive episodes.

Adverse reactions are generally comparable to those of other monoamine oxidase inhibitors. However, because of its amphetamine-like structure, tranylcypromine may cause psychomotor stimulation at doses higher than those used for depression. The incidence of intracranial hemorrhage (sometimes fatal) associated with paradoxical hypertension and severe occipital headache appears to be greater than with phenelzine or isocarboxazid. Dependence has been reported occasionally; therefore, the drug should be used with care in patients prone to drug abuse.

A small number of deaths resulted from ingestion of more than 350 mg; however, recovery also has occurred after ingestion of this amount.

See the Introduction for additional information on indications, adverse reactions, precautions, and the use of monoamine oxidase inhibitors with other drugs.

DOSAGE AND PREPARATIONS.
Oral: Adults (outpatients), initially, 20 to 40 mg daily in two equally divided doses in the morning and afternoon for two weeks. Subsequent doses should be adjusted according to the patient's response; the lowest effective dose should be given in divided amounts. Doses exceeding 30 mg daily are rarely necessary, although 50 mg has been used in hospitalized patients with severe depression. Information is inadequate to establish a dosage for *children under 16 years.*

Parnate (Smith Kline & French), *Generic.* Tablets 10 mg.

ANTIMANIC DRUG

LITHIUM CARBONATE
[Eskalith, Lithane, Lithobid, Lithonate, Lithotabs]

LITHIUM CITRATE
[Cibalith-S]

ACTIONS AND USES. Lithium counteracts mood changes and is considered to be the only specific antimanic drug for the prophylaxis and treatment of bipolar disorder. Acute hypomanic and manic episodes respond to lithium, but combined therapy with an antipsychotic agent may be preferred to control behavior initially. Lithium may be effective as maintenance therapy for major depression, although antidepressants are preferred. It is under investigation for use in a number of other psychiatric and medical conditions.

Lithium has little effect on otherwise healthy patients except for mild sedation and has no antiadrenergic or anticholinergic action. Its antimanic mechanism of action has not been fully elucidated.

ADVERSE REACTIONS. Patients receiving lithium require close clinical observation, careful dosage adjustment, and frequent monitoring of blood levels to avoid toxic effects. To prevent toxicity, the dosage should be maintained within a critical and narrow range, for adverse reactions may occur at doses that are close to therapeutic levels. Patients can tolerate larger doses of lithium during acute manic episodes. However, as the attack subsides, the dose should be reduced rapidly to prevent accumulation. *Serum lithium levels should not exceed 2.0 mEq/L (preferably 0.75 to 1.5 for most patients) during initial treatment and should be kept within a range of 0.4 to 1.0 mEq/L during maintenance.*

The following clinical manifestations are useful guidelines for evaluating most patients, and serum lithium levels alone should not be substituted for clinical observation:

Transient mild to moderate side effects occur in most patients at serum levels of 1.5 to 2 mEq/L but may be observed at lower levels, depending upon the patient's tolerance. The most common reactions include nausea, diarrhea, malaise, and fine hand tremor. Other common untoward effects are thirst, polyuria, polydipsia, and fatigue, which may persist throughout treatment but are reversible when the drug is discontinued. Hand tremor occasionally can be modified with propranolol if it is necessary to maintain the dosage for antimanic effectiveness.

Drowsiness, vomiting, muscle weakness, ataxia, dryness of the mouth, abdominal pain, lethargy, dizziness, slurred speech, and nystagmus are early symptoms of intoxication. These reactions may occur at concentrations above 1.5 mEq/L and are common at concentrations of 2 mEq/L.

Moderate to severe adverse reactions may occur at serum concentrations above 2 mEq/L. At levels of 2 to 2.5 mEq/L, symptoms include anorexia, persistent nausea and vomiting, blurred vision, fasciculations, clonic movements of whole limbs, hyperactive deep tendon reflexes, choreoathetoid movements, epileptiform convulsions, toxic psychosis, syncope, electroencephalographic changes, acute circulatory failure, stupor, and coma. At serum levels above 2.5 mEq/L, symptoms may progress rapidly to generalized convulsions, oliguria, and death.

When the serum lithium level exceeds 1.5 mEq/L or adverse

reactions become bothersome regardless of the serum lithium level, the drug generally should be discontinued for 24 hours and therapy resumed at a lower dose. The patient and those living in his household should be cautioned to notify the physician immediately if untoward symptoms or unexplained illnesses occur.

Prolonged administration of lithium has resulted in impaired renal function. Of greatest clinical significance is a reduction in urine concentrating ability that may present as nephrogenic diabetes insipidus. The impairment is usually reversed when lithium is withdrawn and cannot be corrected by vasopressin. Salt restriction or diuretic therapy should not be instituted, since these measures only enhance lithium toxicity (Waller and George, 1984). Diffuse thyroid enlargement with no change in thyroid function or, occasionally, hypothyroidism also may occur after long-term treatment. The administration of thyroid hormones controls the glandular enlargement, and thyroid function generally returns to normal when lithium is withdrawn. Thyroid function tests should be performed periodically in all patients receiving long-term therapy.

Persistent neurologic deficits rarely are associated with the use of lithium (Donaldson and Cuningham, 1983; Green, 1984). Manifestations include an akinetic hypertonic state with cogwheel rigidity, tremor, dysarthria, mask-like facies, and mutism. These manifestations of neurologic damage are similar to acute signs except cerebellar signs are more conspicuous and responsiveness is not decreased. Pseudotumor cerebri (increased intracranial pressure and papilledema) has been reported.

A wide range of cutaneous adverse effects has been associated with lithium therapy (Deandrea et al, 1982). Maculopapular, follicular, and acneiform eruptions occur. The first two reactions may clear despite continued lithium therapy, whereas the acneiform reaction may necessitate decreasing the dose or discontinuing therapy. Lithium also may induce or exacerbate psoriasis and, more rarely, may be associated with exfoliative dermatitis.

Mild leukocytosis (white blood count, 10,000 to 18,000) occurs frequently throughout therapy, but it is reversible when lithium is discontinued. Reversible electrocardiographic alterations (flattening and inversion of T waves, occasional bradycardia, rare disturbance in sinus node function, or sinoatrial block and widening of the QRS complex) that do not respond to potassium therapy also have been noted (Mitchell and MacKenzie, 1982). Transient hyperglycemia, headache, peripheral edema, weight gain, hair loss, metallic taste, and hypertension have been reported infrequently.

An acute brain syndrome occurs infrequently and is characterized by a toxic confusional state, convulsions, and changes in the electroencephalogram; there are no other signs of lithium toxicity and toxic serum levels are not present. This reaction is observed most commonly within three weeks after initiating therapy and responds rapidly to discontinuation of the drug or reduction of the dose. Patients with schizophrenia and organic brain disease may be hypersensitive to this action of lithium.

TREATMENT OF POISONING. No specific antidote for lithium poisoning is known. However, when frank symptoms of toxicity occur or serum levels exceed 2 mEq/L, lithium should be discontinued and fluid and electrolyte replacement therapy initiated. Excretion of lithium is facilitated by alkalization of urine and administration of osmotic diuretics (urea, mannitol), acetazolamide, and theophylline. Electrocardiograms and measurements of serum hematocrit should be performed periodically. Anticonvulsants may be necessary if seizures occur. Peritoneal dialysis is less effective than hemodialysis; the latter should be used routinely when lithium levels exceed 2.5 mEq/L or when renal function is impaired.

PRECAUTIONS. If the clinical situation permits, a complete physical examination and selected laboratory studies are useful before initiating therapy; this should include tests for cardiovascular, hepatic, thyroid, and renal function; total and differential white blood counts; hemoglobin levels; and complete urinalysis. Serum lithium levels should be determined monthly during the acute phase and quarterly after the maintenance dosage has been established. Blood samples should be drawn 8 to 12 hours after the last dose, and this time interval should remain fairly constant to keep results comparable.

The effects of lithium on renal function have been summarized (Waller and George, 1984). To avoid renal dysfunction, the following guidelines are recommended: (1) Long-term treatment with lithium should be reserved for established indications and continued only in responsive patients. (2) Baseline tests of renal function, including repetition of these tests at the first signs of polyuria or nocturia, may be helpful. (3) Lithium plasma levels should be monitored often enough to determine the lowest concentration compatible with optimal efficacy. (4) Toxicity and high tubular concentrations of lithium may be avoided by maintaining a fluid intake of at least 2 L of water evenly distributed throughout the day to minimize dehydration.

Since lithium is excreted mainly by the kidneys, its elimination depends upon normal renal function and adequate salt and fluid intake (at least 2 L daily). Lithium usually is relatively contraindicated in patients with renal or cardiac disease (eg, sick sinus syndrome) when interference with excretion is likely (eg, in those with decreased renal blood flow) or when electrolyte imbalance is present. In the presence of sodium deficiency, lithium ion is selectively reabsorbed in the renal tubules and may accumulate to toxic levels because of dehydration and sodium and potassium depletion. Therefore, lithium should be used cautiously in patients receiving diuretics or in those on a "crash" or low-salt diet. If lithium must be used with diuretics, the serum lithium and electrolyte levels should be monitored closely and the dosage of lithium reduced as indicated. Loop diuretics may be preferable to other diuretics (Jefferson and Kalin, 1979). If excessive and prolonged diarrhea, profuse perspiration, or vomiting occurs, lithium should be discontinued and supplemental salt and fluid administered. The drug should not be given to debilitated or dehydrated individuals or to those with severe infections.

Special precautions are necessary when lithium is used in the elderly, since the rate of renal excretion tends to decline with age. Use of small doses with very gradual increases and frequent determination of serum lithium levels generally are necessary. Optimal efficacy is usually obtainable in a range of 0.6 to 0.8 mEq/L or less in the elderly.

Although lithium is not contraindicated in diabetics, it has increased serum insulin levels. Blood sugar and electrolyte levels should be monitored periodically.

PREGNANCY AND LACTATION. An increase in the rate of congenital abnormalities, especially heart defects, has been reported in infants exposed to lithium during early pregnancy. Therefore, its use is relatively contraindicated during the first trimester. If lithium is considered for use after the third month of pregnancy to avoid postpartum psychosis, the risk to the fetus or infant should be weighed against the expected benefits (FDA Pregnancy Category D). Lithium crosses the placenta and is present in equivalent concentrations in the mother and fetus. Since the half-life of lithium is prolonged in newborn infants, the dose should be decreased or the drug discontinued seven to ten days prior to delivery.

The hemodynamic and metabolic alterations that occur during delivery may cause toxic accumulation of lithium in both mother and infant. During delivery, water deprivation, infusion of hypertonic sodium chloride, or injection of pituitary hormones should be avoided. Additionally, the concentration of lithium in breast milk is one-third to one-half that in maternal plasma; therefore, mothers taking lithium probably should not breast-feed their infants.

DRUG INTERACTIONS. The combined use of lithium and iodine should be avoided, for synergistic antithyroid effects have been reported; patients receiving lithium should be warned to avoid medications that contain iodides (eg, cough medicines, multivitamin preparations).

Two nonsteroidal anti-inflammatory prostaglandin synthetase inhibitors, indomethacin and phenylbutazone, have been shown to elevate serum lithium concentrations by reducing its renal clearance. Although ibuprofen did not produce this phenomenon, caution is advised when concurrent administration of lithium and this type of drug is necessary (Ragheb et al, 1980).

PHARMACOKINETICS. Lithium is completely absorbed six to eight hours after oral administration. Since the onset of action is slow (five to ten days), parenteral use is of no advantage. Plasma half-life varies among patients from 17 to 36 hours, and this drug is eliminated almost entirely by the kidneys. About 80% of filtered lithium is reabsorbed. The normal variations in urinary flow rate and dietary sodium intake do not appreciably affect the rate of excretion.

Lithium ion is not protein bound, is distributed in total body water, and is concentrated in various tissues to different degrees. After a steady state has been achieved, the lithium level in cerebrospinal fluid is about 40% of that in serum, and renal clearance for an individual remains relatively constant.

There is a good correlation between the serum concentration of lithium ion and therapeutic efficacy and toxicity. Therefore, noncompliance can be suspected in a patient with an adequate serum concentration who takes a few doses of lithium prior to testing if the lithium RBC/plasma ratio is well below the normal range.

DOSAGE AND PREPARATIONS. Dosage should be individualized on the basis of serum levels and response, and the drug should be discontinued if a satisfactory response is not obtained in a few weeks.

Oral: Adults, for acute mania, initially, 0.6 to 1.8 g daily in three divided doses, increased or decreased daily or every other day by 0.3 g (maximum, 2.4 g) to produce a serum level of 0.75 to 1.5 mEq/L. During acute manic episodes, some patients show increased tolerance to ordinarily toxic blood levels. When the acute attack subsides, the dose should be reduced rapidly to obtain a serum level of 0.4 to 1.0 mEq/L. Lithium therapy should be used cautiously in *debilitated or elderly patients. Children under 12,* information is inadequate to establish safety and efficacy in this age group.

LITHIUM CARBONATE:
Generic. Capsules, tablets 300 mg.
Eskalith (Smith Kline & French). Capsules, tablets 300 mg; tablets (timed-release) 450 mg (*Eskalith CR*).
Lithane (Miles), *Lithotabs* (Rowell). Tablets 300 mg.
Lithobid (CIBA). Tablets (timed-release) 300 mg.
Lithonate (Rowell). Capsules 300 mg.
LITHIUM CITRATE:
Cibalith-S (CIBA), *Generic.* Syrup 300 mg (8 mEq)/5 ml (equivalent to lithium carbonate).

MIXTURES

MIXTURES CONTAINING AN ANTIDEPRESSANT AND ANTIPSYCHOTIC DRUG

Combination products containing amitriptyline and perphenazine are available for use in patients with schizoaffective disorders. Some of these patients require only an antipsychotic drug, although amitriptyline occasionally is useful adjunctively to control symptoms of depression. However, the amounts supplied in fixed-ratio combinations are usually not suitable for such patients. Antipsychotic agents are contraindicated in the treatment of depressive disorders and other neurotic illnesses. Tardive dyskinesia has been reported with the antipsychotics, and their use should be restricted to patients with clear-cut indications for this combination.

DOSAGE AND PREPARATIONS. See the manufacturers' labeling for dosage.

Etrafon (Schering), *Triavil* (Merck Sharp & Dohme). Tablets containing perphenazine 2 mg and amitriptyline hydrochloride 10 mg (*Etrafon 2-10, Triavil 2-10*) or 25 mg (*Etrafon, Triavil 2-25*); tablets containing perphenazine 4 mg and amitriptyline hydrochloride 10 mg (*Etrafon-A, Triavil 4-10*), 25 mg (*Etrafon-Forte, Triavil 4-25*), or 50 mg (*Triavil 4-50*).

MIXTURE CONTAINING AN ANTIDEPRESSANT AND ANTIANXIETY DRUG

The combination product, Limbitrol, contains amitriptyline and chlordiazepoxide and is promoted for patients with moderate to severe depression associated with moderate to severe anxiety. Since most anxiety accompanying depression is ultimately relieved during the course of treatment with an antidepressant drug alone, antianxiety drugs are not required routinely. Thus, combined use for initial therapy is not recommended by most clinicians. Further, antidepressant drugs require individual titration of dose to obtain optimum response, and this is less easily accomplished with a fixed-dose combination. Safe use of Limbitrol during pregnancy and lactation has not been established.

See the section on Heterocyclic Antidepressants in this chapter and the evaluation on Chlordiazepoxide in Chapter 5, Drugs Used For Anxiety and Sleep Disorders, for additional information on adverse reactions and precautions.

DOSAGE AND PREPARATIONS. See the manufacturer's labeling for dosage.

    Limbitrol (Roche). Tablets containing amitriptyline hydrochloride 12.5 or 25 mg and chlordiazepoxide 5 or 10 mg.

Cited References

Carbamazepine's acute and prophylactic effects in manic and depressive illness: Update. *Int Drug Ther News* 17:5-10, (Feb/March) 1982.

Monoamine oxidase inhibitors for depression. *Med Lett Drugs Ther* 22:58-60, 1980.

American Psychiatric Association: *Diagnostic and Statistical Manual of Mental Disorders,* ed 3. Washington, DC, American Psychiatric Association, 1980.

Amsterdam J, et al: Clinical application of tricyclic antidepressant pharmacokinetics and plasma levels. *Am J Psychiatry* 137:653-662, 1980.

Appelbaum PS, Kapoor W: Imipramine-induced vasospasm: Case report. *Am J Psychiatry* 140:913-915, 1983.

Ballenger JC, Post RM: Carbamazepine in manic-depressive illness: New treatment. *Am J Psychiatry* 137:782-790, 1980.

Blackwell B: Adverse effects of antidepressant drugs. I. Monoamine oxidase inhibitors and tricyclics. II. 'Second generation' antidepressants and rational decision making in antidepressant therapy. *Drugs* 21:201-219, 273-282, 1981.

Brogden RN, et al: Trazodone: Review of pharmacological properties and therapeutic efficacy in depression and anxiety. *Drugs* 21:401-429, 1981.

Cassem N: Cardiovascular effects of antidepressants. *J Clin Psychiatry* 43(11, sec 2):22-28, 1982.

Christenson BC: Agranulocytosis associated with amoxapine. *Am J Psychiatry* 140:921-922, 1983.

Click MA Jr, Zisook S: Amoxapine and amitriptyline: Serum levels and clinical response in patients with primary unipolar depression. *J Clin Psychiatry* 43:369-371, 1982.

Cohen MR, et al: Plasma cortisol and β-endorphin immunoreactivity in nonmajor and major depression. *Am J Psychiatry* 141:628-632, 1984.

Crowe RR: Electroconvulsive therapy: Current perspective. *N Engl J Med* 311:163-166, 1984.

Davidson J: When and how to use MAO inhibitors. *Drug Ther* 13:197-202, (Jan) 1983.

Davidson J, Turnbull C: Importance of dose in isocarboxazid therapy. *J Clin Psychiatry* 45(7, sec 2):49-52, 1984.

Davidson J, et al: Acetylation phenotype, platelet monoamine oxidase inhibition, and effectiveness of phenelzine in depression. *Am J Psychiatry* 135:467-469, 1978.

Davidson JRT, et al: Atypical depression. *Arch Gen Psychiatry* 39:527-534, 1982.

Davis JM: Overview: Maintenance therapy in psychiatry. II. Affective disorders. *Am J Psychiatry* 133:1-13, 1976.

Deandrea D, et al: Dermatological reactions to lithium: Critical review of literature. *J Clin Psychopharmacol* 2:199-204, 1982.

Donaldson IM, Cuningham J: Persisting neurologic sequelae of lithium carbonate therapy. *Arch Neurol* 40:747-751, 1983.

Ekbom K: Lithium for cluster headache: Review of literature and preliminary results of long-term treatment. *Headache* 21:132-139, 1981.

Finlayson RE, Martin LM: Recognition and management of depression in the elderly. *Mayo Clin Proc* 57:115-120, 1982.

Giller E Jr, et al: Assessing treatment response to monoamine oxidase inhibitor isocarboxazid. *J Clin Psychiatry* 45(7, sec 2):44-48, 1984.

Gillin JC: Sleep studies in affective illness: Diagnostic, therapeutic, and pathophysiological implications. *Psychiatr Ann* 13:368-384, 1983.

Glass RM: Recent developments in psychotherapy of depression. *Psychosomatics* 22:110-113, 1981.

Goldberg HL, Finnerty RJ: Trazodone in treatment of neurotic depression. *J Clin Psychiatry* 41:430-434, 1980.

Green JB: Permanent neurological deficits resulting from lithium toxicity, (letter). *Ann Neurol* 15:111, 1984.

Hansen HE: Renal toxicity of lithium. *Drugs* 22:461-476, 1981.

Hollister LE: Current antidepressant drugs: Clinical use. *Drugs* 22:129-152, 1981.

Hunt-Fugate AK, et al: Adverse reactions due to dopamine blockade by amoxapine: Case report and review of literature. *Pharmacotherapy* 4:35-39, 1984.

Jann MW, et al: Alternative drug therapies for mania: Literature review. *Drug Intell Clin Pharm* 18:577-589, 1984.

Jefferson JW, Kalin NH: Serum lithium levels and long-term diuretic use. *JAMA* 241:1134-1136, 1979.

Kronfol Z, et al: Imipramine-induced tremor: Effects of beta-adrenergic blocking agent. *J Clin Psychiatry* 44:225-226, 1983.

Lansky MR, Selzer J: Priapism associated with trazodone therapy: Case report. *J Clin Psychiatry* 45:232-233, 1984.

Lesar T, et al: Trazodone overdose. *Ann Emerg Med* 12:221-223, 1983.

Liebowitz MR, et al: Phenelzine versus imipramine in atypical depression: Preliminary report. *Arch Gen Psychiatry* 41:669-677, 1984.

Lippmann S, et al: Trazodone cardiotoxicity, (letter). *Am J Psychiatry* 140:1383, 1983.

Lipsey JR, et al: Nortriptyline treatment of post-stroke depression: Double-blind study. *Lancet* 1:297-300, 1984.

Lydiard RB, Gelenberg AJ: Amoxapine: Antidepressant with some neuroleptic properties? Review of its chemistry, animal pharmacology and toxicology, human pharmacology, and clinical efficacy. *Pharmacotherapy* 1:163-178, 1981.

Marshall JB, Forker AD: Cardiovascular effects of tricyclic antidepressant drugs: Therapeutic usage, overdose, and management of complications. *Am Heart J* 103:401-414, 1982.

Mendelis PS: Maprotiline and convulsions. *ADR Highlights* 83:1-10, (Oct 11) 1983.

Mielke DH, et al: Controlled evaluation of tetracyclic (maprotiline) and tricyclic (imipramine) antidepressant and their effects on heart. *Curr Ther Res* 25:738-742, 1979.

Mitchell JE, Groat R: Placebo-controlled, double-blind trial of amitriptyline in bulimia. *J Clin Psychopharmacol* 4:186-193, 1984.

Mitchell JE, MacKenzie TB: Cardiac effects of lithium therapy in man: Review. *J Clin Psychiatry* 43:47-51, 1982.

Murphy DL, et al: New contributions from basic science to understanding effects of monoamine oxidase inhibiting antidepressants. *J Clin Psychiatry* 45(7, sec 2):37-43, 1984.

National Institutes of Health Consensus Development Conference: *Mood Disorders: Pharmacologic Prevention of Recurrences.* Bethesda, National Institutes of Health, vol 5, 1984.

Pandol SJ, et al: Beneficial effect of oral lithium carbonate in treatment of pancreatic cholera syndrome. *N Engl J Med* 302:1403-1404, 1980.

Peatfield RC: Lithium in migraine and cluster headache: Review. *J R Soc Med* 74:432-436, 1981.

Pi EH, et al: Effect of lithium on leukocytes: Two-year follow-up. *J Clin Psychiatry* 44:139-140, 1983.

Pope HG Jr, et al: Antidepressant treatment of bulimia: Preliminary experience and practical recommendations. *J Clin Psychopharmacol* 3:274-281, 1983 A.

Pope HG Jr, et al: Bulimia treated with imipramine: Placebo-controlled, double-blind study. *Am J Psychiatry* 140:554-558, 1983 B.

Post RM: Carbamazepine's acute and prophylactic effects in manic and depressive illness: Update. *Int Drug Ther Newslett* 17:5-9, 1982.

Post RM, et al: Selective response to anticonvulsant carbamazepine in manic-depressive illness: Case study. *J Clin Psychopharmacol* 4:178-185, 1984.

Prusoff BA, et al: Speed of symptom reduction in depressed outpatients treated with amoxapine and amitriptyline. *Curr Ther Res* 30:843-855, 1981.

Ragheb M, et al: Interaction of indomethacin and ibuprofen with lithium in manic patients under steady-state lithium level. *J Clin Psychiatry* 41:397-398, 1980.

Ravaris CL, et al: Phenelzine and amitriptyline in treatment of depression: Comparison of present and past studies. *Arch Gen Psychiatry* 37:1075-1080, 1980.

Richardson JW III, Richelson E: Antidepressants: Clinical update for medical practitioners. *Mayo Clin Proc* 59:330-337, 1984.

Rickels K, et al: Trazodone: New broad-spectrum antidepressant. Symposium, 11th Congress of Collegium Internationale Neuro-Psychopharmacologicum. Amsterdam, Excerpta Medica, 1980, 86-101.

Rickels K, et al: Amoxapine and imipramine in treatment of depressed outpatients: Controlled study. *Am J Psychiatry* 138:20-24, 1981.

Robinson DS, et al: Clinical pharmacology of phenelzine. *Arch Gen Psychiatry* 35:629-635, 1978.

Robinson DS, et al: Plasma levels of antidepressants and therapeutic effects. *Adv Biol Psychiatry* 7:198-207, 1981.

Robinson DS, et al: Cardiovascular effects of phenelzine and amitriptyline in depressed outpatients. *J Clin Psychiatry* 43:8-15, 1982.

Rowan P, et al: Comparative effects of phenelzine and amitriptyline: Placebo controlled trial. *Neuropharmacology* 19:1223-1225, 1980.

Sachar EJ, et al: Disrupted 24-hour patterns of cortisol secretion in psychotic depression. *Arch Gen Psychiatry* 28:19-23, 1973.

Sheehan DV: Delineation of anxiety and phobic disorders responsive to monoamine oxidase inhibitors: Implications for classification. *J Clin Psychiatry* 45(7, sec 2):29-36, 1984.

Smith RS Jr, Ayd FJ Jr: Critical appraisal of amoxapine. *J Clin Psychiatry* 42:238-242, 1981.

Snyder SH, Yamamura HI: Antidepressants and the muscarinic acetylcholine receptor. *Arch Gen Psychiatry* 34:236-239, 1977.

Spiegel K, et al: Analgesic activity of tricyclic antidepressants. *Ann Neurol* 13:462-465, 1983.

Spring GK: Neurotoxicity with combined use of lithium and thioridazine. *J Clin Psychiatry* 40:135-138, 1979.

Stern SL, et al: Toward rational pharmacotherapy of depression. *Am J Psychiatry* 137:545-552, 1980.

Tollefson GD: Monoamine oxidase inhibitors: Review. *J Clin Psychiatry* 44:280-288, 1983.

van Praag HM: Depression. *Lancet* 2:1259-1264, 1982.

Waller DG, George CF: Lithium and the kidney. *Adv Drug React Acc Pois Rev* 3:65-89, 1984.

Walsh BT, et al: Treatment of bulimia with monoamine oxidase inhibitors. *Am J Psychiatry* 139:1629-1630, 1982.

Wells BG, Gelenberg AJ: Chemistry, pharmacology, pharmacokinetics, adverse effects, and efficacy of antidepressant maprotiline hydrochloride. *Pharmacotherapy* 1:121-139, 1981.

Whitlock FA, Evans LEJ: Drugs and depression. *Drugs* 15:53-71, 1978.

Winsauer HJ, O'Hair DE: Rapid onset of action of amoxapine in depressive illness. *Curr Ther Res* 35:815-825, 1984.

Drugs Used in Other Mental Disorders

8

ALCOHOLISM AND CIGARETTE SMOKING

The abuse of psychoactive drugs has received widespread public attention. Such attention is warranted, for drug abuse exacts an enormous human and monetary toll from our society.

Alcoholism and cigarette smoking are two of the most insidious forms of drug abuse because they have the implicit, if not explicit, approval of society. Such approval persists despite widespread agreement that the excessive use of alcohol and any use of cigarettes cause hundreds of thousands of premature deaths, contribute billions of dollars to the total national health expenditure, and account for billions more in lost productivity. Alcoholism and cigarette smoking are recognized substance use disorders and, for most abusers of these drugs, constitute an addiction.

The treatment for these substance use disorders primarily involves counseling; behavior modification and/or psychological therapy often are included. Pharmacologic intervention is available to aid in withdrawal and, for alcoholism, to prevent relapse. The value of available drugs for this last indication is controversial.

Alcohol

PROPERTIES OF ALCOHOL. Alcohol readily affects body function. Because it is completely miscible in water, every cell in the body is subject to interaction with and harm from the drug. Alcohol is converted to acetaldehyde, an even more toxic water-soluble compound. Oxidation of alcohol increases the ratio of NADH:NAD, thus altering the metabolism of compounds that depend upon the NADH:NAD system. Alcohol has caloric but no nutritive value and, furthermore, prevents absorption of amino acids, vitamins, and other nutritive substances in the gastrointestinal tract. Although it is not a carcinogen, alcohol may enhance the carcinogenic activity of other such compounds.

Pharmacologic Activity: Alcohol has both central and peripheral pharmacologic activity. In the central nervous system, it is a nonspecific depressant. Such depression and disinhibition contribute to feelings of relaxation, confidence, and euphoria that often accompany the use of alcohol in a social setting. The mechanism by which this general depression occurs is uncertain, but evidence suggests that alcohol inhibits the release of a Ca^{2+}-dependent neurotransmitter. This inhibition may be due to reduced entry of Ca^{2+} into nerve terminals through voltage-dependent channels. Presumably, alcohol alters these channels by interacting with a site in the presynaptic membrane (Littleton, 1983).

Depression of central nervous system function becomes manifest as blood alcohol concentrations rise. Reasoning, memory, and coordination deteriorate. Loss of inhibitions and impaired judgment may lead to dangerous or violent behavior and disregard for social norms. Susceptibility to the effects of alcohol varies widely and is based partly on constitutional factors, nutritional status, and degree of tolerance. Thus, it is difficult to associate particular blood alcohol concentrations with specific degrees of impairment. However, if alcohol is not abused chronically, blood concentrations of 200 to 300 mg/dl generally are associated with slurred speech and ataxia, and concentrations of 300 to 400 mg/dl may produce stupor, coma, and anesthesia. Although some chronic alcoholics tolerate blood concentrations of 500 to 600 mg/dl without marked

153

impairment of consciousness, levels exceeding 500 mg/dl are potentially lethal if attained rapidly. Death is due to respiratory depression.

Moderate doses of alcohol produce vasodilation, especially of cutaneous vessels. Gastric and salivary secretions usually are stimulated. A diuretic effect occurs due to inhibition of the release of antidiuretic hormone and to decreased tubular reabsorption of water. Finally, alcohol mobilizes fat from peripheral tissues and enhances lipid anabolism in the liver, establishing conditions leading to the development of fatty liver.

Pharmacokinetics: In the fasting state, alcohol is absorbed from the stomach (20%) and small intestine (80%) and is widely distributed. Approximately 90% to 98% of a dose undergoes dose-dependent oxidation by hepatic cytosolic alcohol dehydrogenase and microsomal enzymes to carbon dioxide and water via the intermediate products, acetaldehyde and acetate. When alcohol is oxidized, some of the resulting changes (eg, increased production of lactate and fatty acid, hyperuricemia) appear to be caused by the increased ratio of NADH:NAD.

In nontolerant individuals, the liver can metabolize approximately 1 to 1.5 ounces of 80 to 100 proof whiskey, a 4-ounce glass of wine, or 12 ounces of beer per hour, although this also at least partially is a function of body size.

Ingestion in excess of the individual rate of metabolism will lead to accumulation. The rate of metabolism often is increased in alcoholics who have been drinking recently and in smokers, perhaps because of enzyme induction. The increase in metabolism and/or development of pharmacodynamic tolerance may be masked by hepatitis, advanced cirrhosis of the liver, or nutritional deficiencies. Hyperthyroid patients may metabolize alcohol twice as rapidly as normal individuals. In the elderly, serum alcohol concentrations may be 25% to 30% more than those in younger patients who have ingested identical amounts of alcohol.

Use of Alcohol During Pregnancy: Alcohol readily crosses the placenta, and its use during pregnancy can produce the fetal alcohol syndrome (Clarren and Smith, 1978; Iosub et al, 1981). Infants with this syndrome have poor motor development and growth and usually are mentally retarded. They exhibit a cluster of distinctive facial features (ie, short upturned nose with sunken nasal bridge, small and underdeveloped midface, short palpebral fissures and epicanthal folds, absent or minimal ridges between nose and mouth, hypoplastic maxilla and underdeveloped jaw). The incidence of various malformations of the cardiac, urogenital, and skeletal systems also is increased in these infants. The risk of fetal alcohol syndrome is increased if alcohol is consumed during the first trimester.

Even moderate alcohol consumption during pregnancy increases the risk of spontaneous abortion and low birth weight. A safe level of alcohol intake, if any, during pregnancy has not been established but is the subject of considerable debate and investigation.

Drug Interactions: Alcohol is ingested by most individuals in the United States, and numerous interactions between alcohol and other drugs occur (Linnoila et al, 1979; Lieber, 1980). The most important is enhanced central nervous system depression induced by the concomitant use of alcohol and other drug(s) with a similar action. These include general anesthetics, opioid analgesics, hypnotic and antianxiety drugs, antihistamines, antipsychotic agents, heterocyclic antidepressants, central skeletal muscle relaxants, centrally acting anticholinergic agents, anticonvulsants, and certain antihypertensive agents (reserpine, methyldopa, clonidine).

The mechanism may be pharmacodynamic and/or pharmacokinetic; the latter occurs because alcohol competes with many endogenous and exogenous chemicals that utilize a common biotransformation pathway, ie, oxidation by hepatic microsomal enzymes. Some adaptive tolerance occurs gradually to both alcohol and other central nervous system depressants (eg, general anesthetics, hypnotics, antianxiety agents) and diminishes the sedative effect. Nevertheless, patients should be cautioned to avoid any combination of the following: alcohol intake (even as little as a single drink), any other central nervous system depressant, and performing tasks requiring alertness (eg, operation of a motor vehicle or other machinery).

Additive orthostatic hypotension is less common but significant. This interaction results from concomitant use of alcohol and drugs with vasodilator activity (eg, reserpine, methyldopa, hydralazine, guanethidine, nitroglycerin).

Potentially severe interactions occur with ingestion of alcohol and the salicylates, including aspirin; antidiabetic drugs, including insulin; anticonvulsants; and anticoagulants. Alcohol should be avoided when aspirin is ingested, because the combination promotes gastrointestinal bleeding. Severe hypoglycemia may occur when alcohol is taken with insulin or oral hypoglycemic agents, because alcohol interferes with the metabolism of the latter and may rarely produce hypoglycemia when given alone. Alcohol also interferes with the metabolism of oral anticoagulants and anticonvulsants and higher than expected serum concentrations of these agents may be obtained. Conversely, chronic intake of alcohol can increase the metabolizing activity of microsomal enzymes and actually shorten the half-life of anticoagulants, oral hypoglycemic agents, and anticonvulsants, thus reducing their effectiveness. Such enzyme induction may account for therapeutic failures, but the clinical relevance of these interactions is unknown. The effect of enzyme induction can be offset by the liver damage induced by alcohol and/or nutritional deficiency, which may affect the capacity of the liver to detoxify drugs. Accordingly, the dosage of anticoagulants, oral hypoglycemic agents, and anticonvulsants may require adjustment upon initiation and termination of therapy in chronic alcoholics. Careful monitoring of the patient is essential.

The enhanced susceptibility of chronic alcoholics to hepatitis induced by acetaminophen, isoniazid, and carbon tetrachloride also is explained by enzyme induction, because the biotransformation to toxic metabolites is enhanced.

The hypertensive reaction that occurs when monoamine oxidase inhibitors are taken with alcoholic beverages appears to result from dihydroxyphenylalanine and/or tyramine rather than alcohol itself.

Chronic Excessive Alcohol Ingestion

Alcoholism is a term that lacks precise definition. For the purpose of this discussion, however, it can be defined as a behavior pattern maintained by psychological dependence on the behavior of drinking and/or physical dependence on the drug, alcohol. Such a behavior pattern generally disrupts normal functioning at all levels and is harmful to health. When one or both types of dependencies is well established, use of the drug becomes compulsive and constitutes an addiction.

MANIFESTATIONS. Chronic alcoholism is characterized by the episodic or habitual consumption of alcohol that may result in one or more of the following effects: (1) psychological problems (anxiety, depression, loss of control of drinking); (2) social deterioration (decreased performance at work, disrupted family life); and (3) physiologic derangement (eg, tremors, impaired memory and coordination, liver disease). Each alcoholic patient represents a different conglomerate of biological (genetic, physiologic), psychological (personality disorder, depression, psychosis), and social (peer pressure, cultural background, religion) factors that predispose to alcoholism (Kissin and Begleiter, 1977; Skinner, 1981).

Severe hypoglycemia is uncommon in chronic alcoholics but may occur during withdrawal from a prolonged bout of drinking (Kallas and Sellers, 1975). This reaction is caused by inadequate carbohydrate intake, low glycogen stores, and inhibition of gluconeogenesis that results from an increased NADH:NAD ratio, which diverts pyruvic acid to lactic acid. Lactic acidemia and ketoacidosis may occur as well.

Inadequate dietary intake and/or malabsorption are responsible for the malnutrition that may be present. Folic acid and protein deficiencies, pancreatic insufficiency, abnormal biliary secretions, and mucosal abnormalities are induced directly by alcohol and cause malabsorption of fat, protein, sodium, water, thiamine, folic acid, vitamin B_{12}, and D-xylose. A nutritious diet with little or no alcohol intake reverses many of these abnormalities (Green and Tall, 1979). Prolonged malnutrition, especially thiamine deficiency, and early cerebral atrophy, possibly due to the direct effects of alcohol and its metabolic products on the central nervous system, produce Wernicke's encephalopathy (confusion, nystagmus, abnormal ocular muscle movement) and the amnesic syndrome (Korsakoff's psychosis), which is characterized by confabulation, polyneuropathy, and selective amnesia (particularly short-term memory) for events after the onset of the illness.

Chronic excessive intake of alcohol may lead initially to fatty liver. Hepatic necrosis and, ultimately, cirrhosis are caused by the direct toxic effects of alcohol. Elevated gamma glutamyl transpeptidase and serum glutamic oxaloacetic transaminase levels may be indications of hepatic injury. An isolated elevation of the former without the latter probably represents enzyme induction, whereas an elevation of the latter usually signifies liver damage. However, there is no correlation between the magnitude of the elevations and the degree of functional impairment or histologic changes in the liver. Only liver biopsy accurately ascertains the type and extent of damage.

Hyperlipidemia, hyperuricemia, hypomagnesemia, pancrea-

titis, myopathy including cardiomyopathy, increased risk of cancer (tongue, mouth, oropharynx, hypopharynx, esophagus, larynx, and liver), sexual and reproductive dysfunction, depression and suicide, traffic and industrial accidents, and sociopathology (eg, family violence, child abuse, rape, assault) are additional complications of alcoholism (Lieber, 1976; West, 1984).

TOLERANCE AND PHYSICAL DEPENDENCE. Chronic use of alcohol results in the development of tolerance and physical dependence. Initially, tolerance appears to be related to both increased metabolism (drug-dispositional) and cellular adaptation (pharmacodynamic) to the pharmacologic activity of alcohol. Metabolic tolerance may decrease temporarily in the presence of hepatitis or permanently with severe cirrhosis.

Cellular adaptation in the central nervous system to the chronic influx of alcohol eventually establishes a state of physical dependence. Such dependence becomes apparent when abstention from alcohol causes subjective distress and objective signs of withdrawal. Upon abrupt withdrawal, the adaptive neurophysiologic and biochemical changes that occurred in the central nervous system to meet the constant challenge of alcohol manifest themselves physiologically as hypersensitivity of the sensory modalities. Depending upon the degree of physical dependence, any or all of the following signs and symptoms may be present: irritability; anxiety; insomnia; nightmares; tremulousness; nausea; vomiting; sweating and flushing; hyperreflexia; increased muscle tone and tremor; tactile, auditory, and visual disturbances; seizures; delirium (global confusion); hypertension; and arrhythmias.

TREATMENT. The management of alcoholism can be divided into three phases: acute intoxication, the withdrawal syndrome, and long-term rehabilitation.

Therapy for severe acute intoxication is only supportive and drugs usually are not required. The essential elements of management include mechanical ventilatory support; maintenance of body temperature; correction of dehydration, acid-base abnormalities, electrolyte imbalance, and/or hypoglycemia; and lavage (rarely indicated).

In 80% to 85% of alcoholic patients, withdrawal is expressed as a mild to moderate abstinence syndrome. Onset and peak of withdrawal symptoms usually occur 6 to 8 and 24 to 36 hours, respectively, after cessation of drinking. For the remaining 15% to 20% of alcoholics, symptoms are more severe and may even be life-threatening. These symptoms usually peak in 96 to 120 hours, then gradually subside over the next 72 hours. Delirium tremens occurs in less than 1% of patients.

Detoxification usually does not require the use of psychoactive drugs, but a well-organized and trained staff is essential (Whitfield et al, 1978; Naranjo et al, 1983). When drug therapy is needed, the benzodiazepines are preferred because they are as efficacious as and less toxic than alcohol, barbiturates, chloral hydrate, paraldehyde, hydroxyzine and other antihistamines, and antipsychotic drugs (Lewis and Femino, 1982).

Mild signs and symptoms of alcohol withdrawal may be managed with oral benzodiazepines. Diazepam [Valium] and chlordiazepoxide [Librium] have been used more extensively than clorazepate [Tranxene]. Because of pharmacokinetic considerations, benzodiazepines that are not metabolized to active derivatives and possess relatively shorter half-lives (eg, oxazepam [Serax], lorazepam [Ativan]) may be preferred in older patients or in those with severe liver disease (Sellers and Kalant, 1976); the use of lorazepam to treat alcohol withdrawal is investigational.

One regimen (Sellers et al, 1983) for moderate to severe alcohol withdrawal utilized an initial oral loading dose of diazepam 20 mg plus supportive care with subsequent 20-mg doses every one to two hours as needed to control symptoms. In this study, the median number of doses required was three given over 7.6 hours. All patients receiving diazepam were effectively treated.

Oral administration of the benzodiazepines usually is effective. Peak concentrations of diazepam and chlordiazepoxide occur about 45 minutes after oral ingestion. If needed, however, parenteral preparations are available. The intravenous route is preferred for chlordiazepoxide, because absorption from intramuscular sites may be erratic. Diazepam and lorazepam are well absorbed after intramuscular administration. Transition to oral use usually can be initiated within 12 hours. For the dosage employed in alcohol withdrawal, see the evaluations in Chapter 5, Drugs Used for Anxiety and Sleep Disorders.

A single oral or parenteral dose of thiamine 100 mg may be given routinely early during treatment of withdrawal.

Complicated cases or delirium tremens may require additional therapy. Hypokalemia, hypochloremic alkalosis, and volume deficit should be corrected. Since seizures usually are self-limited, intravenous diazepam generally is not indicated. However, in patients with a documented history of seizures unrelated to alcohol withdrawal, an oral or intravenous loading dose of phenytoin [Dilantin], with subsequent maintenance doses daily for five days, prevents recurrence (see Chapter 9, Antiepileptic Drugs, for dosage). Infrequently, seizures are associated with hypomagnesemia.

Lidocaine [Xylocaine] or procainamide [Procan, Pronestyl] may be needed to treat arrhythmias; propranolol [Inderal] also is useful and may be especially effective for uncontrolled, severe tremor. The potent piperazine phenothiazines (eg, fluphenazine [Permitil, Prolixin]) or the butyrophenone, haloperidol [Haldol], should be given for hallucinations or paranoid ideation.

In the long-term management of alcoholic patients, pharmacotherapy is much less important than counseling of the patient and family and a program of rehabilitation. Supportive care to facilitate the development of coping mechanisms is essential, especially in the early phases of treatment. Referral to support groups (eg, Alcoholics Anonymous) should take into account the presence of other psychiatric disorders, age, sex, socioeconomic status, religious orientation, and orientation toward group therapy.

Avoidance of increased anxiety during early treatment is important. The physician must accept relapses and encourage the patient to return to treatment. Active intervention and outreach are critical for the establishment of trust. Finally, disulfiram [Antabuse] may be an effective adjunct to behavior modification or psychotherapy. Some controlled clinical trials support the short-term effectiveness of disulfiram, but the long-term efficacy of the drug in decreasing or terminating

alcohol use and abuse has not been established (see the evaluation).

Alcohol-Sensitizing Drugs: The interaction between alcohol and disulfiram can be used therapeutically to control alcohol intake. The threatened or actual occurrence of a strong, unpleasant physiologic response to alcohol in combination with a prior dose of disulfiram constitutes an adverse event that conditions behavior to the avoidance of alcohol ingestion. However, the efficacy of this approach for improving behavioral or medical problems is questionable (Peachey and Naranjo, 1984).

Disulfiram or carbimide (not available in the United States) produce an aversive effect by inhibiting the conversion of acetaldehyde, a metabolite of alcohol, to acetic acid by aldehyde dehydrogenase. Elevation of blood acetaldehyde concentrations is believed to be responsible for the occurrence of the aversive effect. The enzymatic inhibition produced by disulfiram is irreversible and, thus, persists longer than the reversible inhibition produced by carbimide. Compared to disulfiram, carbimide's side effects appear to be less frequent and less severe. These alcohol-sensitizing drugs should be restricted to recovering alcoholics who clearly seek abstinence, who wish to take the drug, and who have no medical or psychosocial reasons to avoid their use (Peachey and Naranjo, 1984) (see evaluation on Disulfiram).

Metronidazole [Flagyl, Protostat], procarbazine [Matulane], monoamine oxidase inhibitors, chloramphenicol, quinacrine [Atabrine], furazolidone [Furoxone], and chlorpropamide [Diabinese] have been reported to produce mild disulfiram-like actions when alcohol is ingested. Controlled studies have not substantiated this finding for metronidazole. Further, acetaldehyde blood levels are not always significantly elevated following use of alcohol and chlorpropamide. Flushing as a result of a chlorpropamide-alcohol interaction may be a genetic marker for noninsulin-dependent diabetes even before the onset of glucose intolerance (Hansten, 1981). The disulfiram-like reactions produced by these drugs are considered to be of minor significance, since they are much less severe than disulfiram-alcohol and carbimide-alcohol reactions.

Drug Evaluation

DISULFIRAM
[Antabuse]

$$(C_2H_5)_2N\overset{\overset{S}{\|}}{C}-S-S-\overset{\overset{S}{\|}}{C}N(C_2H_5)_2$$

ACTIONS AND USES. Disulfiram, a thiuram derivative, interferes with the conversion of acetaldehyde to acetic acid by aldehyde dehydrogenase (Eneanya et al, 1981). When taken with alcohol, this drug increases the blood acetaldehyde concentration and produces several uncomfortable symptoms. The unpleasantness of this interaction is the basis for disulfiram's adjunctive use to decrease alcohol consumption.

Although some controlled clinical trials support the short-term effectiveness of disulfiram when employed with behavioral and psychological counseling, the drug's efficacy in the long-term treatment of chronic alcoholism has not been established (Sellers et al, 1981). Compliance with long-term therapy is a major problem. Disulfiram should never be used without supportive counseling or psychotherapy.

The alcohol-disulfiram reaction may be manifested by flushing, dyspnea, nausea, thirst, chest pain, palpitation, and vertigo; hyperventilation, tachycardia, vomiting, hyperhidrosis, hypotension, syncope, and confusion also may occur. Blood pressure may fall to shock level. The reaction usually lasts 30 minutes to several hours, and drowsiness and sleep follow. The intensity of the reaction varies among individuals but generally is proportional to the amount of alcohol ingested and the dose of disulfiram and time elapsed since its administration.

The true incidence of mild reactions is a subject of controversy (Gragg, 1982). Severe reactions, which include respiratory depression, acute circulatory failure, arrhythmias, myocardial infarction, acute congestive heart failure, syncope, and convulsions, may be fatal. During severe reactions, individuals should be treated as for shock (see Chapter 27). Inhalation of 95% oxygen with 5% carbon dioxide, as well as other symptomatic treatment, may be useful. The serum potassium level should be monitored and maintained, particularly in patients receiving digitalis, since hypokalemia has been reported. The resynthesis of aldehyde dehydrogenase to normal levels generally requires about a week (but may require two weeks or more) after termination of disulfiram therapy; patients should be warned not to ingest alcohol during this period.

ADVERSE REACTIONS. In the absence of alcohol, disulfiram may cause transient mild drowsiness, fatigue, impotence, headache, acneiform eruptions, allergic dermatitis, or a metallic- or garlic-like aftertaste, especially during the first two weeks of therapy. These effects usually disappear spontaneously with continued therapy, but sometimes dosage reduction is required.

Psychotic reactions have been noted rarely. These have included symptomatic configurations of severe depression, schizophrenia, mania, and organic encephalopathy. Polyneuropathy, peripheral neuritis, and, rarely, optic neuropathy also have occurred. It has been suggested that these reactions may be caused by carbon disulfide, a metabolite of disulfiram.

Disulfiram has been reported to be hepatotoxic in a few patients (Eneanya et al, 1981). A latent period of 3 to 25 weeks may elapse before symptoms of liver disease occur. Hepatotoxicity may be masked by the natural tendency to attribute any hepatic impairment to alcohol.

PRECAUTIONS. Disulfiram should be used cautiously in patients with diabetes mellitus, hypothyroidism, epilepsy, cerebral damage, chronic or acute nephritis, or severe hepatic cirrhosis or insufficiency, as well as during pregnancy. It is contraindicated in patients with symptomatic ischemic heart disease, coronary thrombosis, psychosis, depression, neuropathy, or hypersensitivity and in those recently treated with paraldehyde or who have a measurable blood alcohol concentration due to recent ingestion of alcohol or an alcohol-containing product (eg, foods, elixirs, cough syrups). Lotions with a high alcohol content that are liberally applied topically also should be used cautiously. Before treatment commences,

the patient should be fully informed of the purpose, procedure, and consequences of disulfiram administration.

Although disulfiram has the potential to produce severe adverse reactions in its own right, some patients experience only occasional drowsiness or skin rash. Nevertheless, it may be advisable for those undergoing treatment with disulfiram to carry identification cards describing the most common symptoms of the disulfiram-alcohol reaction and designating the attending physician. (Identification cards may be obtained from the manufacturer.)

DRUG INTERACTIONS. Disulfiram inhibits the metabolism of several drugs other than alcohol, and the consequences should be borne in mind. In particular, toxic levels of phenytoin, warfarin, isoniazid, rifampin, and benzodiazepines with active long-acting metabolites (eg, clorazepate, diazepam, flurazepam, chlordiazepoxide, halazepam, prazepam) may accumulate when disulfiram is given concomitantly. It may be necessary to adjust the dosage of such drugs during or upon discontinuation of disulfiram therapy.

PHARMACOKINETICS. With oral administration, 70% to 90% of a dose is absorbed rapidly, and the time to peak serum concentration is one to two hours. Disulfiram is first rapidly reduced to diethyldithiocarbamate, which is methylated, glucuronidated, or sulfated and undergoes oxidation to diethylamine and carbon disulfide. Half-life data are unavailable for most metabolites; however, the inhibition of aldehyde dehydrogenase by disulfiram develops slowly over 12 hours and is irreversible. The duration of action is the six days or more required for resynthesis of the enzyme.

DOSAGE AND PREPARATIONS. When initiating disulfiram therapy, the patient must not be acutely intoxicated, must not have significant withdrawal signs and symptoms, and should not have a blood alcohol content; the latter generally means that the patient should not have used alcohol for at least 12 hours before disulfiram treatment is begun.
Oral: Adults, initially, a maximum of 500 mg daily as a loading dose for one week. For maintenance, 250 mg daily (range, 125 to a maximum of 500 mg) is given for months to years, depending upon the individual. However, because of potential liver toxicity and unproved efficacy, administration for more than six months should be undertaken with caution. Liver enzymes should be monitored at suitable intervals during long-term therapy.

Antabuse (Ayerst), *Generic.* Tablets 250 and 500 mg.

Cigarette Smoking

Fifty-five million Americans smoke cigarettes. Three of every five smokers have tried to quit, and nine of ten smokers say they want to quit (Richmond, 1983). Most smokers are physically dependent upon nicotine and psychologically dependent upon the behavior of smoking. For most individuals, cigarette smoking is an addiction.

PROPERTIES OF NICOTINE. Nicotine is a central nervous system and ganglionic stimulant. Its actions are mediated by nicotine-specific receptors. Administration of the drug to animals and humans characteristically produces tremors and respiratory excitation; at higher doses, convulsions may occur. The central stimulant effect of nicotine is believed to contribute to fortification and maintenance of the behavior of cigarette smoking, although this is not entirely clear (Griffiths and Henningfield, 1982).

Nicotine can cause nausea and vomiting by a combination of central and peripheral actions. Peripheral vasoconstriction, tachycardia, and elevated blood pressure are produced by stimulation of the sympathetic ganglia, the adrenal medulla, and chemoreceptors of the aortic and carotid bodies. Nicotine initially stimulates salivary and bronchial secretions but later inhibits them (Taylor, 1980). Finally, nicotine is chemotactic for neutrophils and enhances neutrophil responsiveness to chemotactic peptides (Totti et al, 1984).

Pharmacokinetics: Nicotine is absorbed readily from the respiratory tract, buccal mucosa, and skin. After oral administration, it is absorbed largely from the intestine. Pulmonary absorption of nicotine after inhalation of cigarette smoke is extremely rapid.

Nicotine is metabolized in the lung and liver after inhalation and oral administration, respectively. The major metabolites are cotinine, which has one-fifth the pharmacologic activity of nicotine, and nicotine-1-N-oxide. Nicotine and these metabolites are rapidly eliminated by the kidneys; the rate of urinary excretion decreases as the urine becomes increasingly alkaline. The plasma half-life of nicotine after inhalation or parenteral administration is 30 to 60 minutes. Nicotine is excreted in breast milk (Taylor, 1980).

Cigarette Smoking During Pregnancy: Smoking during pregnancy tends to decrease birth weight and increase the risk of abortion and premature birth. The incidence of stillbirth also is increased. Fetal breathing time is decreased. At present, there is no definitive evidence that cigarette smoking during pregnancy produces congenital malformations. Hyperkinesia and hyperirritability are more evident in the infant.

Drug Interactions: Cigarette smoking can alter the pharmacokinetics and activity of many drugs. The mechanism of such interactions usually is induction of liver microsomal enzyme activity by the polycyclic hydrocarbons in cigarette smoke. This enzyme induction differs qualitatively and quantitatively from that produced by phenobarbital. Enzyme activity remains elevated up to six months after cessation of smoking.

Smokers tend to have decreased blood concentrations and/or effects with concomitant use of theophylline, pentazocine [Talwin], propranolol [Inderal], propoxyphene [Darvon], heparin, and, possibly, heterocyclic antidepressants, phenothiazines, caffeine, and benzodiazepines. The dosage of these drugs may need to be increased in smokers, especially in heavy smokers. Also, diabetics who smoke tend to require larger doses of insulin. Smoking increases the potential for serious adverse effects in women taking oral contraceptives.

In most cases, there is little evidence of a recognizable hazard from an interaction per se. Exceptions are limited to insulin, propoxyphene, propranolol, and theophylline (D'arcy, 1984).

Chronic Cigarette Smoking

Cigarette smoking is considered a substance use disorder under the criteria established in the third edition of the *Diagnostic and Statistical Manual of Mental Disorders (DSM-III)* (American Psychiatric Association, 1980). Dependence upon nicotine can be diagnosed if an individual has smoked continuously for at least one month and if at least one of the following is present: (1) serious attempts to stop or significantly reduce the amount of tobacco use on a permanent basis have been unsuccessful, (2) attempts to stop smoking have led to the occurrence of a withdrawal syndrome, and (3) the individual continues to smoke despite the presence of a serious physical disorder that is known to be exacerbated by smoking.

Chronic cigarette smoking is a major risk factor for coronary artery disease and arteriosclerotic peripheral vascular disease. It is a causative factor in cancer of the lung, mouth, larynx, and esophagus and is a contributory factor for cancer of the bladder, pancreas, and kidney. Chronic bronchitis and emphysema are more common in cigarette smokers (*Surgeon General's Report on Smoking and Health*, 1979).

TOLERANCE AND PHYSICAL DEPENDENCE. Tolerance develops to some of the effects of nicotine. The dizziness, nausea, and vomiting that often are reported by nonhabituated individuals do not occur in experienced smokers. Such tolerance probably is pharmacodynamic in nature.

Physical dependence upon nicotine is manifested by the rapid onset of a withdrawal syndrome after cessation of smoking. The most consistent signs and symptoms are nausea, headache, constipation, diarrhea, and increased appetite. Drowsiness, fatigue, insomnia, irritability, and inability to concentrate also are common. Heart rate and diastolic blood pressure decrease as soon as six hours after withdrawal and persist for up to three days. Weight gain and the craving for cigarettes are long-term manifestations of withdrawal. In one study, 21% of former smokers reported craving cigarettes at least intermittently five to nine years after cessation (Jarvik, 1979; Jaffe, 1980).

Both tolerance to the adverse effects of cigarette smoking and physical dependence upon nicotine contribute to maintenance of the smoking behavior. Physical dependence appears to be a significant obstacle to long-term abstinence after cessation of smoking.

TREATMENT. Long-term fulfillment of the desire to stop smoking requires mastery of both the short-term and residual effects of the psychological and physical dependence that contribute to preservation of the addiction. A variety of techniques, including counseling programs, educational campaigns, proprietary or public service clinics, hypnosis, sensory deprivation, behavior modification, and aversion therapy, have achieved modest success in producing long-term abstinence. These techniques have been reviewed elsewhere (*Surgeon General's Report on Smoking and Health*, 1979).

The results of clinical studies (Fagerström, 1982; Jarvis et al, 1982; Russell et al, 1983) have shown that nicotine chewing gum, nicotine polacrilex (nicotine resin complex) [Nicorette], is moderately beneficial as a temporary adjunct in helping individuals quit smoking. Initiation of use of the gum coincident with complete cessation of smoking aids in overcoming the psychological dependence independently of the physical dependence. The benefit derived correlates positively with the increasing physical dependence on nicotine and those who are highly motivated to quit derive the greatest benefit.

Use of nicotine polacrilex constitutes substitution of a less hazardous vehicle and route of administration (eg, chewing gum with buccal absorption) for a more dangerous one (eg, inhalation of cigarette smoke including chemical and particulate matter). This substitution has two objectives: First, the gum provides blood concentrations of nicotine comparable to those achieved by the smoking of cigarettes and, thus, sufficient to prevent withdrawal signs. Second, by alleviating the usual physical consequences of the cessation of smoking, the gum allows the patient to focus attention and energies on overcoming the psychological component of the addiction. Thus, environmental situations that normally elicit smoking behavior (eg, stress at work) can be worked through and mechanisms to cope with the desire to smoke can be developed and fortified. Nicotine polacrilex is most useful at the time of or within the first few months after cessation of smoking and in conjunction with behavioral or psychological therapy to provide intensive treatment. As coping mechanisms develop and the urge to smoke fades, patients gradually reduce the number of pieces of gum chewed each day. Initiation of this gradual withdrawal should be possible within two or three months. Use of the gum for longer than three months has not been demonstrated to be beneficial.

The physician plays a crucial role in the planning, implementation, and management of a therapeutic regimen that optimizes the patient's chances for abstaining from smoking permanently. Patients who are sufficiently motivated to stop smoking should be identified, and a detailed smoking history (eg, how long and how much the patient has smoked, when and how the patient has tried to quit) should be taken. The physician must assess the risks and benefits associated with nicotine polacrilex (eg, versus self-administration of nicotine via cigarette smoking).

It is important that the patient clearly understand the rationale, benefits, and risks of treatment. Counseling, behavioral or psychological therapy, or formal programs to be followed in conjunction with use of the gum must be outlined. The physician should take careful note of the patient's progress; offer encouragement; provide direct, unequivocal instructions and analysis of that progress; and monitor the gradual withdrawal from the gum. Finally, follow-up consultation to promote continued abstention from cigarette smoking should be provided.

Drug Evaluation

NICOTINE POLACRILEX (Nicotine Resin Complex)
[Nicorette]

Nicotine chewing gum is of moderate therapeutic value as a temporary adjunct to behavioral or psychological therapy for smokers who are physically dependent upon nicotine and wish to quit smoking. The success of this program correlates positively with the patient's motivation and the physician's acumen, enthusiasm, and encouragement. See previous discussion.

ADVERSE REACTIONS AND PRECAUTIONS. Adverse effects associated with use of nicotine polacrilex generally are mild and transient. Gastrointestinal and central nervous system disturbances and those related to the mechanics and process of chewing and absorption are most prevalent. Nonspecific gastrointestinal distress, eructation, and nausea and/or vomiting occur in approximately 10%, 6%, and 19% of patients, respectively. Lightheadedness, insomnia, irritability, and headache occur in 1% to 2% of patients. Mouth (including ulcers) and throat soreness have been reported in about 37% of patients, while muscle ache of the jaw has been noted in 18% of patients. The incidence of hiccups and excessive salivation is 15% and 2%, respectively.

Abuse potential is minimal. However, it should be kept in mind that use of the gum maintains the patient's physical dependence on nicotine, and it may be difficult to withdraw the gum. Withdrawal should be accomplished by gradually decreasing the daily dose.

In one short-term study conducted to assess the cardiovascular effects of one 4-mg piece of nicotine gum, changes in heart rhythm, blood pressure, finger skin temperature, and calf and hand blood flow were insignificant. A small increase (10% to 12%) in heart rate was observed (Nyberg et al, 1982).

Except for adverse effects from the mechanics of chewing, reactions are characteristic of those associated with smoking nicotine. Since only the vehicle and route of administration are different, it is not surprising that the adverse effects do not disrupt the therapeutic process or present a significant hazard.

The use of nicotine chewing gum is contraindicated in nonsmokers; during the immediate postmyocardial infarction period; in those with life-threatening arrhythmias; in patients with severe or worsening angina pectoris; in those with active temporomandibular joint disease; and during pregnancy (FDA Pregnancy Category X).

Special caution must be exercised when the gum is used by patients with certain cardiovascular, endocrine, and gastrointestinal diseases. Specific examples include coronary heart disease, serious arrhythmias, hypertension, vasospastic diseases, hyperthyroidism, pheochromocytoma, insulin-dependent diabetes, and peptic ulcer. The drug should be used cautiously in patients with oral or pharyngeal inflammation or dental problems that may be exacerbated by chewing gum. During lactation, consideration should be given to discontinuing either the nursing or the gum after evaluation of the risk to the child and the benefit derived by the mother.

POISONING. The minimal oral lethal dose of nicotine is approximately 40 to 60 mg (MacArthur and Williams, 1983; Taylor, 1980). However, the likelihood of overdose by accidental swallowing of the gum is small. Adult volunteers swallowed 10 pieces containing 4 mg of nicotine each, and the resulting blood concentrations were similar to those produced by smoking one cigarette.

Two factors prevent serious adverse sequelae following oral overdose: First, the nicotine in the gum is bound to an ion exchange resin and is released only during chewing. Second, nicotine released from the gum in the gastrointestinal tract and absorbed is largely inactivated by the microsomal enzyme system on first-pass through the liver. Notwithstanding this, the patient should be instructed to contact a physician or the local poison control center immediately in case of accidental overdose or if a child chews or swallows one or more pieces of the gum.

PHARMACOKINETICS. The nicotine in the chewing gum is bound to an ion exchange resin, and the gum must be chewed for release of nicotine. The blood concentration of nicotine depends upon the vigor and duration of chewing. One study showed that chewing one piece of gum containing 2 mg of nicotine hourly produced a mean steady-state plasma nicotine level of 11.8 ng/ml. This compared with a mean plasma nicotine trough concentration during usual smoking of 15.7 ng/ml.

The pattern of blood nicotine concentration differs after pulmonary and buccal absorption. Smoking cigarettes produces peak blood concentrations immediately, which decline thereafter. In contrast, the nicotine chewing gum produces a constant blood nicotine concentration sufficient to prevent signs of abstinence (McNabb et al, 1982).

DOSAGE AND PREPARATIONS. The patient must be motivated to give up smoking and should be instructed to stop smoking immediately prior to initiation of therapy.

Buccal: One piece of gum is chewed whenever the urge to smoke occurs and each piece should be chewed slowly and intermittently for 30 minutes. Most patients require approximately 10 pieces of gum per day during the first month of treatment. Patients should be instructed not to exceed 30 pieces of gum per day. The use of nicotine resin complex for more than six months is not recommended.

Nicorette (Merrell Dow). Chewing gum 2 mg per square (sugar free).

DEMENTIA

The treatment of dementia presents a significant challenge to the medical community. Optimal care for the patient requires that the physician and others providing such care understand a broad spectrum of medical, scientific, and psychosocial issues. The prevalence of severe dementia in those 65 years and older is about 4% to 5% and that of mild dementia is reported to be 2.6% to 15.4%. Thus, in this country, about 3 million individuals over age 65 are affected by dementia.

DIAGNOSIS. Dementia is a loss of memory and other cognitive functions that places an individual on a level significantly below that expected based on his/her previous performance, education, and achievements. The deterioration of these functions is determined by a history of decline in performance, by clinical examination, and by neuropsychological testing. In general, significant dementia interferes with a patient's ability to cope adequately with the environment, although the demands of each situation must be taken into account.

Dementia is one disorder of mental function in a larger set that includes confusion, delirium, lethargy, stupor, coma, mental retardation, mania, schizophrenia, thought disorder, depression, aphasia, amnesia, apraxia, and agnosia. It may be confused with any of the foregoing because of overlap. However, dementia can be distinguished by three central features: deterioration from a previously higher level of function; restriction of the defining features to memory and other cognitive functions; and the global nature of the impairment. Dementia cannot be diagnosed when the patient's consciousness is impaired or when other medical problems interfere with evaluation. Diagnosis is behavioral; dementia cannot be determined by CAT scan or EEG, although specific causes may be distinguished by these means.

Dementia includes numerous specific disorders that have been subclassified as described below. For successful management, dementia must be differentiated from delirium or the dementia syndrome of depression. The ability to distinguish between primary and secondary dementia also is crucial to therapeutic outcome.

Delirium is a global impairment of cognitive functioning that is of relatively brief duration (days to weeks) and is generally reversible. Cognitive function is difficult to evaluate because delirium is characterized by the acute onset (hours to days) of clouding of consciousness that fluctuates irregularly and unpredictably. It tends to be most severe at night. A primary part of the disturbance probably results from derangement of cerebral regions that subserve activation, arousal, and the sleep-wakefulness cycle, because inattentiveness, incoherent speech, insomnia, daytime sleepiness, irregular episodes of sleep and wakefulness, as well as increased or decreased psychomotor activity and difficulty in distinguishing perceptions and images from dreams and visual hallucinations may occur. Neurologic signs generally are limited to abnormal movements; tremor, bilateral asterixis, and/or multifocal myoclonus of facial and shoulder muscles are common late in the disease.

Individuals at risk for delirium include the elderly; those dependent on drugs or alcohol; patients with brain damage or chronic renal, hepatic, pulmonary, or cardiac failure; and those who are sensory or sleep deprived, immobilized, undergoing significant psychological stress, or receiving multiple drugs that can lead to drug intoxication (eg, drugs with anticholinergic or sedative activity).

Dementia also is a global impairment of cognitive functioning but is usually progressive and interferes with social or occupational activity. The core cognitive impairment in moderate to severe dementia includes deficits of memory and/or impaired directed or abstract thinking, judgment, and intellectual performance. Onset is gradual (months to years) and consciousness is not clouded, but orientation often is reduced. Depression, delusions, and/or hallucinations also may be present. Mild to moderate dementia is often difficult to distinguish from benign senescent forgetfulness, a nonprogressive decline in memory.

Depression is common in geriatric patients, often mimics

dementia, and may resemble organic brain syndrome or be superimposed upon it. The major clinical features used to distinguish the dementia syndrome of depression from dementia can be summarized as follows (Wells, 1979). The onset of the dementia syndrome of depression can be dated with some precision while the onset of dementia can be defined only within broad limits. The course of the dementia syndrome of depression is rapid, whereas dementia develops slowly. In the dementia syndrome of depression, a history of previous psychiatric dysfunction is common, whereas in dementia it is unusual. Patients with the dementia syndrome of depression often complain of cognitive loss, emphasize their disability, highlight their failures, and make little effort to perform even simple tasks. Conversely, demented patients complain little of cognitive loss, conceal their disability, delight in their accomplishments, and struggle to perform tasks. Finally, for patients with the dementia syndrome of depression, attention and concentration often are well preserved, "don't know" answers are typical, and memory loss for recent and remote events usually is equally severe. For demented patients, attention and concentration usually are faulty, "near miss" answers are frequent, and memory loss for recent events is more severe.

After dementia has been identified, a critical next step is to differentiate primary dementia from that secondary to other diseases or disorders. About 80% of all cases of dementia are considered primary and include primary degenerative dementia (often referred to as dementia of the Alzheimer type) and multi-infarct dementia. Primary degenerative dementia is associated in part with the insidious malignant deterioration of both cortical and subcortical neurons (DeBoni and McLachlan, 1980; Bondareff et al, 1982; Coyle et al, 1983), but the precise etiology remains to be defined. Multi-infarct dementia is more abrupt in onset than the Alzheimer type and progresses incrementally rather than gradually as new microinfarcts destroy cortical tissue. This form of primary dementia is common in patients with hypertension, vascular disease, and diabetes. The two types can be difficult to distinguish, and the Hachinsky Ischemic Scale may be helpful.

Dementia is classified as secondary (ie, due to progression of an underlying disorder, such as parkinsonism, infection, trauma, neoplasm, nutritional deficiency, or substance abuse) in approximately 20% of affected patients. Diagnosis is critical because secondary dementia usually is reversible with therapy.

The differential diagnosis of dementia has been reviewed (Task Force of National Institute on Aging, 1980; Small et al, 1981; Dahl, 1983).

MANAGEMENT. The long-term management of primary dementia differs in several respects from that of other terminal illnesses. The following will focus on devising a framework to optimize long-term care of patients with primary degenerative dementia, although much of this information also applies to patients with multi-infarct dementia. Several principles of these disorders and their sociology must be recognized:

1. No interventions are known that will alter the course of the disease.

2. The disease is of long duration and total disability occurs late in its course. For most of the duration, the patient is ambulatory and able to aid in daily living activities to some extent. Furthermore, the patient is able to express and, apparently, experience interpersonal emotions.

3. Most families choose to care for the patient at home for as long as possible rather than place the individual in an institution.

4. In most other disorders, the patient's response to the illness is the focus for psychological intervention. In dementia, significant grieving occurs also in the caretaker and other family members; thus, emotional support systems must be available.

5. The social milieu of demented patients should remain as fixed as possible. These patients are very sensitive to changes in residence and in caretakers. A demented patient is much more likely to retain functional effectiveness in a familiar environment.

Given these principles, management of the demented patient in a noninstitutional setting, most likely the home, will be the first line of long-term care. Before the decision for home management can be endorsed, however, the health, emotional state, and coping skills of the primary caretaker should be assessed. Those with severe deficiencies in one of these areas should be encouraged to consider alternatives to home management. Adequate support for the primary caretaker also is an important requirement if home care is to be undertaken.

When home management becomes impractical, institutionalization is the sole option. For the demented patient in a nursing home, requirements similar to those of home management must be met (eg, competent staff, optimization of physical environment, availability of physicians). The level of expertise must be higher, since the magnitude of the nursing problems will be greater.

The uncertain etiology of primary degenerative dementia has precluded the development of specific therapy to prevent the disease or impede progression. Thus, treatment regimens focus on amelioration of symptoms.

Nondrug Therapy: Nondrug therapy is most important in dementia of the Alzheimer type and includes environmental management, family counseling and support, and psychotherapy. These behavioral and psychological approaches seek both to maintain the patient's optimal awareness of the time, place, and composition of his/her environment and to enhance the family's understanding of the patient's needs and limitations and of their own as caretakers.

Awareness of the environment is best maintained by the constant and continuous presentation of cues to stimulate the patient. Management of that environment should include: (1) Prominent color-coded displays of calendars, clocks, and checklists to facilitate orientation; (2) access to nightlights, radio, and television to minimize sensory deprivation; (3) photographs and other objects to help create a familiar and, therefore, stable environment; (4) appraisal of the need for corrective glasses and hearing aids; (5) routine hygienic measures to minimize the effects of minor illnesses and prevent bedsores; (6) adequate nutrition and fluid intake to minimize constipation and prevent nutritional deficiencies that may aggravate the disorder; and (7) accident prevention techniques to minimize falls and burns.

Drug Therapy: Pharmacologic treatment of primary degenerative dementia is limited, particularly because of poor understanding of its etiology and pathogenesis. Until more specific information is available, drug therapy is investigational and is aimed at (1) facilitating function in neural elements that may be involved in memory and other cognitive processes, and (2) increasing cerebral metabolism in a nonspecific way.

The ability of drugs to alter central neurotransmitter function is receiving considerable attention because of the success of this type of treatment in functional psychoses and parkinsonism (Crook and Gershon, 1981). Cholinomimetic agents and neuropeptides are being investigated most intensively. Choline and lecithin, precursors of acetylcholine, are being studied because of the memory deficits produced by the centrally acting anticholinergic antagonist, scopolamine, and the short-term effect of the acetylcholinesterase inhibitor, physostigmine, in alleviating memory loss in patients with central nervous system trauma. Although these drugs have enhanced memory in some individuals, their efficacy in patients with primary degenerative dementia has not been encouraging (Davis, 1979; *Int Drug Ther Newslett*, 1981).

The mixture of ergoloid mesylates [Deapril-ST, Hydergine] is thought to enhance cerebral metabolism and, in some studies, has been reported to produce modest improvements in confusional states, depressed mood, dizziness, unsociability, and self-care; however, it is difficult to predict which patients will benefit. A therapeutic trial with this mixture may be indicated in patients with accurately diagnosed dementia who are receiving the best nondrug management possible but who continue to have clinically significant mental impairment.

Although specific drug therapy for the disease process is lacking, disruptive and debilitating symptoms—such as psychotic behavior, depression, anxiety, and insomnia—are amenable to treatment with drugs commonly used for these manifestations. However, serious consideration of the pharmacodynamic and pharmacokinetic alterations characteristic of the elderly is critical before drug therapy is initiated. Generally, drugs with short half-lives should be administered in doses lower than those given to younger patients. A drug's spectrum and potential for producing adverse effects, as well as its potential for interaction with other drugs the patient is taking, must be considered. Finally, the individual supervising administration of the drug must fully understand the appropriate dosing schedule, the expectation for improvement, and the potential for harm.

ATTENTION DEFICIT DISORDER

Attention deficit disorder occurs in approximately 3% of prepuberal children and is characterized by developmentally inappropriate inattentiveness and impulsiveness (Kinsbourne and Caplan, 1979; Biederman, 1982; Dubey, 1982). Hyperactivity may or may not be present. Accordingly, *DSM-III* (American Psychiatric Association, 1980) recommends that this disorder be subclassified as attention deficit disorder with hyperactivity, attention deficit disorder without hyperactivity, and attention deficit disorder, residual type (hyperactivity is no longer present, but attention deficit and impulsiveness persist).

DSM-III rejects the older terminology (minimal brain dysfunction, minimal brain damage, and hyperkinetic syndrome) because inattentiveness must be present for diagnosis, hyperactivity is an inconsistent finding, and organic lesions of the brain are not demonstrable.

DIAGNOSIS. The diagnosis of attention deficit disorder is based upon the major criteria of inattention, impulsivity, and hyperactivity. At least three of the following signs of inattention must be present: failure to complete projects started, easy distractibility, failure to listen, and difficulty in adhering to a play activity. At least three of the following signs of impulsivity must be present: the tendency to act before thinking, a sudden shift from one activity to another, difficulty in organizing work, the need for excessive supervision, and difficulty in waiting for one's turn at play or in a game. For a diagnosis of attention deficit disorder with hyperactivity, at least two of the following signs must be present: excessive running and/or climbing, difficulty in sitting still or excessive fidgeting, and motor restlessness during sleep. Onset of the disorder must occur before age 7, and the disorder must have persisted for at least six months (Laufer and Shetty, 1980).

Attention deficit disorder must be differentiated from age-appropriate overactivity, learning disability, severe and profound mental retardation, conduct disorder, schizophrenia, affective disorder with mania, and absence seizures (American Psychiatric Association, 1980; Laufer and Shetty, 1980). Children with age-appropriate overactivity may be especially active; however, their activity is much more organized and purposeful than that of children with attention deficit disorder. A learning disability is manifested by a more selective lag in development for a particular element of academic performance, while mental retardation is characterized by a more uniform and broad deficiency in academic performance than that usually seen with attention deficit disorder. Many patients with conduct disorder have signs of impulsivity, inattention, and hyperactivity, and the additional diagnosis of attention deficit disorder frequently is warranted. Some patients with mental retardation present with the characteristic symptoms of attention deficit disorder. In such cases, the additional diagnosis of attention deficit disorder is warranted. Schizophrenia and affective disorders with mania may be characterized by features of attention deficit disorder; however, these diagnoses pre-empt that of the latter. It should also be noted that many children with attention deficit disorder have an associated learning disorder. Finally, the child in school who experiences frequent absence seizures may react with hyperactivity out of sheer frustration, and an electroencephalogram may be necessary to establish the correct diagnosis.

MANAGEMENT. Attention deficit disorder has a profound impact on the child's emotional life and usually requires counseling for the affected child. Adjunctive therapy, such as remedial education, behavior modification, and counseling with the child's parents and teachers, also are indicated (Wolraich, 1977; Kinsbourne and Caplan, 1979). Parents and teachers must establish an environment of predictable structure with experiences of manageable intensity for the child (Laufer and Shetty, 1980); such an environment will diminish anxiety and facilitate normal maturation.

Drug Therapy: The goal of pharmacotherapy is to enhance

the child's capacity to exert control when desired rather than to control the child. Many controlled studies utilizing both subjective and objective criteria to judge outcome indicate that central nervous system stimulants decrease symptoms. They can improve short-term learning; prolong attention span; improve goal-directed activity, concentration, and classroom behavior; and reduce impulsiveness, hyperactivity, and aggressive behavior. These drugs are effective but are not a specific curative treatment (Biederman and Jellinek, 1984), and no data are available to demonstrate conclusively that they improve learning for long periods. Follow-up studies indicate that these children may continue to have difficulty in school, exhibit behavioral disorders, and have poor self-esteem into adolescence or even into adulthood (Milman, 1979; Weiss, 1981; Amado and Lustman, 1982). There is limited information on treatment of adolescents and adults with attention deficit disorder.

Dextroamphetamine [Dexedrine], methylphenidate [Ritalin], and pemoline [Cylert] appear to be useful. Some investigators feel that methylphenidate is the drug of choice, but others believe that dextroamphetamine is equally effective. Pemoline is less frequently the drug of choice, because improvement is more gradual with recommended initial doses than with methylphenidate or dextroamphetamine. However, its longer duration of action allows once daily dosing and is an advantage in many children.

Because amphetamine sulfate, the racemic form of amphetamine, has less central nervous system activity and a more pronounced effect on the cardiovascular system than the dextrorotatory isomer, dextroamphetamine, the latter is preferred. Another form, methamphetamine [Desoxyn], is essentially equivalent to dextroamphetamine in its central nervous system and cardiovascular effects but has been extensively abused; therefore, dextroamphetamine is preferred.

Although dextroamphetamine and methylphenidate are known to facilitate dopamine release, albeit by different mechanisms (Lawson-Wendling et al, 1981), their mechanism of action in attention deficit disorder remains speculative. Their proposed calming action is nonspecific and has been reported in normal children as well (Weingartner et al, 1980; Rapoport et al, 1978). The latter investigators conclude that, on this basis, the diagnostic use of these agents is unwarranted. Other investigators consider the comparison of drug action on children with attention deficit disorder to be inappropriate, because normal children do not have the same problems; thus, they recommend the diagnostic use of these drugs for a limited period (Kinsbourne and Caplan, 1979). Because dextroamphetamine and methylphenidate are short acting (two to four hours), they require frequent administration during the day and have been associated with behavioral deterioration in some cases. Drug administration should be interrupted occasionally to determine whether behavioral symptoms require continued therapy.

The prolonged use of dextroamphetamine, methylphenidate, and pemoline may limit linear growth and weight, presumably because of appetite suppression, decreased food intake, and altered secretion of growth hormone. Therefore, weight gain and linear growth must be monitored closely. One two-year study showed that methylphenidate depressed linear growth slightly in the first year of therapy, but this was offset by a greater than expected growth rate in the second year (Satterfield et al, 1979). It also was reported that total dosage and summer drug holidays may influence weight, but not height, deficits. The goal is to use doses that reduce hyperactivity without suppressing weight. Pemoline also was reported to depress longitudinal growth for up to 18 months; however, these children caught up to their normal peers in subsequent months (Friedmann et al, 1981).

Central nervous system stimulants have been alleged to precipitate Tourette's syndrome in susceptible children (Lowe et al, 1982), necessitating substitution of other psychotropic drugs, including haloperidol (see Chapter 6, Antipsychotic Drugs). Children with a history of tics or a diagnosis of Tourette's disorder should not receive these stimulants, and those with a family history of similar disorders should be given the drug only under careful supervision.

Heterocyclic antidepressants also are used to treat attention deficit disorder. Imipramine usually is preferred to amitriptyline because of the marked sedative action of the latter in children. Beneficial results have been not as great or as consistent as with the stimulant drugs (Winsberg et al, 1980; Garfinkel et al, 1983). Nevertheless, these antidepressants may be appropriate alternatives in some patients, particularly those who cannot tolerate or do not respond to dextroamphetamine and methylphenidate. Side effects and adverse reactions are potentially more serious than with the central nervous system stimulants, and children given heterocyclic drugs should be monitored closely. (See Chapter 7, Drugs Used in Affective Disorders.)

Antipsychotic drugs (eg, haloperidol [Haldol]) also have been utilized. Their potential for significant neurologic sequelae (extrapyramidal movement disorders) is still present in children. However, for those severely affected, antipsychotics may be very helpful.

Diet Therapy: Diet therapy has been advocated for children with attention deficit disorder. The Feingold diet is essentially free of artificial flavors and colors that are purported to be etiologic agents. Although synthetic food dyes adversely affect learning (Swanson and Kinsbourne, 1980) and behavior (Weiss et al, 1980) in some children with attention deficit disorder, the results achieved with this diet are not encouraging (Conners, 1980). A conference (National Institutes of Health Consensus Conference, 1982) agreed that additive-free diets are not effective for most children but did not object to their use on a trial basis, because they may be beneficial adjuncts to drugs and other therapies (Kolata, 1982).

Drug Evaluations

DEXTROAMPHETAMINE SULFATE
[Dexedrine]

USES. Dextroamphetamine is useful with remedial measures in the management of children with attention deficit disorder (see the Introduction) and as an alternative to methylphenidate in patients with narcolepsy (see Chapter 5, Drugs Used for Anxiety and Sleep Disorders). Dextroamphetamine generally is preferred to amphetamine because it has less effect on the cardiovascular system. All amphetamines are classified as Schedule II drugs under the Controlled Substances Act.

A summary of other uses for dextroamphetamine follows:

Obesity: Although amphetamines temporarily produce slightly more weight loss in users than in control subjects, their long-term benefit is insignificant because of the development of tolerance. Moreover, the potential for abuse is considerable. For these reasons, alternative management programs, preferably nondrug, are recommended and the use of amphetamines is strongly discouraged. (See Chapter 51, Agents Used in Obesity.)

Motion Sickness: Concomitant administration of scopolamine and dextroamphetamine is effective in severe motion sickness, but such use is not recommended routinely. (See Chapter 14, Drugs Used in Vertigo and Vomiting.)

Idiopathic Edema: This disorder occurs almost exclusively in women and is diagnosed by exclusion (Streeten, 1978). Most patients experience diurnal fluctuations in the severity of edema, which is aggravated by prolonged standing and sitting. Dextroamphetamine and methylphenidate have been used experimentally as part of a management program that also includes diuretic therapy (see Chapter 29), reduction of excessive salt intake, and avoidance of prolonged standing and sitting. Altered dopaminergic transmission may play a role in the pathogenesis, and a recent study suggests that bromocriptine (investigational use) may be helpful (Sowers et al, 1982). Many authorities feel that the use of these drugs for idiopathic edema is entirely inappropriate, because patients with idiopathic edema overuse diuretics for psychogenic reasons and may be potential amphetamine drug abusers (MacGregor et al, 1979).

Depression: Short-term use of a small dose of dextroamphetamine is recommended by a few physicians (1) for patients with reactive depressions who cannot tolerate other antidepressants (usually the elderly), and (2) in difficult diagnostic situations to determine the probable efficacy of heterocyclic drugs. Neither indication is supported by controlled studies. See Chapter 7, Drugs Used in Affective Disorders.

Fatigue: The use of amphetamines to allay fatigue is unjustifiable except under the most extraordinary circumstances. They are dangerous for drivers and those engaged in comparable activities, and they have no legitimate role in athletics. Indeed, their use may contribute to increased athletic injuries.

ADVERSE REACTIONS AND PRECAUTIONS. Untoward effects of the amphetamines, particularly their sympathomimetic effects, are related to their pharmacologic actions. These agents may cause nervousness, restlessness, tremors, insomnia, cardiovascular disturbances (eg, tachycardia, arrhythmias, hypertension), dizziness, mydriasis, dryness of the mouth, and gastrointestinal disturbances (eg, nausea, constipation, diarrhea). Anorexia and temporary growth retardation have been observed in children. Dosage should not be increased unnecessarily because larger amounts may produce marked restlessness, irritability, and aggressiveness.

More serious central nervous system reactions occur rarely and include psychic changes and dystonic movements of the head, neck, and extremities. Serious depressive reactions and toxic psychoses have followed prolonged use, especially of large doses.

Generally, the amphetamines should not be prescribed for patients with cardiovascular disease or hyperthyroidism because their sympathomimetic effect may aggravate these conditions. They also should not be given to those known to be susceptible to drug abuse. These drugs should be used with caution in patients who are sensitive to adrenergic agents.

Reproduction studies in mammals utilizing large multiples of the human dose have suggested that the amphetamines have both an embryotoxic and a teratogenic potential. Fetal malformations also have been reported clinically but have not been established conclusively (see Chapter 3). One retrospective study of offspring of women who took dextroamphetamine during pregnancy showed no effect on neonatal birthweight when the drug was taken before the third trimester and only a small effect when it was taken during the third trimester. Neither length nor head circumference was affected (Naeye, 1983) (FDA Pregnancy Category C).

POISONING. In general, acute overdosage accentuates the usual pharmacologic effects of excitement, agitation, hypertension, tachycardia, mydriasis, slurred speech, ataxia, tremor, chills, hyperreflexia, tachypnea, fever, headache, and toxic psychoses characterized by auditory and visual hallucinations and paranoid delusions. If these symptoms develop, lavage, sedatives, custodial care, and psychotherapy should be employed when indicated. Chlorpromazine may block the central nervous system effects but aggravates similar signs and symptoms produced by anticholinergic drugs if these have been taken concurrently. Excretion can be hastened by acidification of the urine.

In severe cases, overdosage may cause hyperpyrexia, chest pain, acute circulatory failure, convulsions, and coma. Fatalities have occurred in adults after doses of only 100 to 500 mg.

ABUSE. Susceptible patients may develop marked psychological dependence on amphetamines. Individuals who abuse these Schedule II drugs frequently inject as much as several grams daily (parenteral amphetamine preparations are not available commercially). In general, the toxic features of chronic abuse include a distinctive amphetamine psychosis that resembles schizophrenia and is characterized by paranoia, stereotyped behavior, picking at the skin, preoccupation with one's own thoughts, and auditory and visual hallucinations.

Abrupt termination of large doses of amphetamines may unmask symptoms of chronic fatigue, mental depression, paranoid psychosis, tremor, and gastrointestinal disturbances. Fatigue may be followed by drowsiness and prolonged sleep. Such reactions often are considered to be a type of abstinence syndrome.

DRUG INTERACTIONS. Amphetamines interfere with the hypotensive effect of guanethidine, and animal studies have indicated that amphetamines have a similar effect when they are given with methyldopa. Therefore, amphetamines should not be used with these drugs.

Amphetamines also are contraindicated in patients receiving monoamine oxidase inhibitors, because their use may precipitate a hypertensive crisis. Although the amphetamines are resistant to monoamine oxidase, their actions are potentiated by the monoamine oxidase inhibitors, presumably as a result of the release of biogenic amines. They may initiate arrhythmias through their catecholamine-releasing effect in patients receiving general anesthetics that sensitize the heart to epinephrine.

Amphetamines can increase blood levels of the heterocyclic antidepressants by interfering with their metabolism. Antipsychotic drugs antagonize most of the central nervous system actions of the amphetamines.

PHARMACOKINETICS. The amphetamines are well absorbed orally, are not highly bound to protein, and are excreted largely by the kidney. Their half-lives range from 7 to 14 hours (10 ± 1.7 hours) if the urine is acid; this may be extended to 30 hours if the urine is alkaline.

DOSAGE AND PREPARATIONS.
Oral: For attention deficit disorder, individualization of dosage is very important; optimal amounts for the morning, afternoon, and evening administration need not be the same. A few children may require only two doses per day, and a few may require an extra dose at bedtime, particularly those who often awaken during the night and in whom loss of sleep impairs learning in the classroom the following day. *Children 3 to 5 years,* 2.5 mg daily initially, increased by 2.5 mg at weekly intervals until an optimum response is obtained; *6 years and older,* 5 mg once or twice daily initially, increased by 5 mg at weekly intervals until an optimum response is obtained. The effective dosage range is 5 to 20 mg daily (maximum, 40 mg/day).

Since the effects of a single dose may not persist for more than four hours, the following alternative schedule utilizes administration three times daily during the waking hours. This often improves behavior and interpersonal relationships at home as well as in school (Kinsbourne and Caplan, 1979). *Children 6 years and older,* initially, 2.5 mg three times a day, usually 30 minutes before meals, increased by 2.5 mg/dose every three or four days until satisfactory improvement is reported, intolerable side effects occur, or signs and symptoms of overfocusing appear (ie, the child becomes withdrawn, tearful, suspicious, or dulled in interactions with others). The maximum recommended dosage is 40 mg/day.

For narcolepsy, *adults and children over 6 years,* 5 to 60 mg daily in divided doses, depending upon the patient's requirements. Tolerance is a major problem when large doses are administered daily for prolonged periods. An occasional drug holiday or withholding therapy during nonworking periods restores sensitivity to the drug and allows the dosage to be decreased when therapy is reinstituted.

Generic. Capsules (timed-release) 15 mg; tablets 5 and 10 mg.
Dexedrine (Smith Kline & French). Capsules (timed-release) 5, 10, and 15 mg; elixir 5 mg/5 ml (alcohol 10%); tablets 5 mg.

Similar Drug.
METHAMPHETAMINE HYDROCHLORIDE:

Desoxyn (Abbott). Tablets 5 mg; tablets (timed-release) 5, 10, and 15 mg.

METHYLPHENIDATE HYDROCHLORIDE
[Ritalin]

ACTIONS AND USES. This central nervous system stimulant is useful as an adjunct to remedial measures (psychological, educational, or social) in the management of children with attention deficit disorder. In comparative studies, methylphenidate was statistically superior to dextroamphetamine and pemoline in a few measurements of improvement. Behavioral improvement appeared to be sustained for at least two years as judged by subjective criteria.

Methylphenidate also may be useful in narcolepsy (see Chapter 5, Drugs Used for Anxiety and Sleep Disorders) and idiopathic edema (see the evaluation on Dextroamphetamine Sulfate).

ADVERSE REACTIONS AND PRECAUTIONS. The most common adverse reactions are nervousness and insomnia. Anorexia, weight loss, and growth retardation may occur during prolonged therapy. Occasional reactions include dizziness, dyskinesia, rash, nausea, abdominal pain, hypertension, hypotension, palpitation, changes in the pulse rate, tachycardia, arrhythmias, and headache. Toxic psychosis has been reported rarely.

Psychological dependence has occurred after long-term use of large doses but has not been reported during treatment of attention deficit disorder in children. Misuse of methylphenidate does not appear to be a problem in patients under adequate medical supervision when recommended dose levels are administered, but the drug should be given cautiously to patients with a history of substance abuse. Methylphenidate has been substituted for amphetamines by individuals who abuse drugs and is classified as a Schedule II drug under the Controlled Substances Act.

This drug is contraindicated in patients with marked anxiety, tension, agitation, or glaucoma, and it should be used cautiously in epileptic and hypertensive patients. Methylphenidate should be discontinued if seizures occur.

DRUG INTERACTIONS. Methylphenidate may increase the serum level of anticonvulsants (phenytoin, phenobarbital, and primidone), coumarin anticoagulants, phenylbutazone, and tricyclic antidepressants if these drugs are administered concurrently. The drug should be used cautiously with pressor agents and monoamine oxidase inhibitors. It may decrease the hypotensive effect of guanethidine. Therefore, the dosage of these agents should be adjusted when they are given with methylphenidate.

PHARMACOKINETICS. Methylphenidate is rapidly and well absorbed after oral administration. Peak plasma concentrations are attained in one to two hours. One study showed that oral administration of the drug with breakfast accelerated rather than impeded absorption compared to administration 30 minutes before breakfast, and no significant differences were noted in behavioral, cognitive, or electrophysiologic effects (Swanson et al, 1983; Chan et al, 1983). The plasma half-life is reported to be one to two hours.

The duration of action usually is no more than four to six hours, but there is considerable individual variation. Methylphenidate is principally (80%) hydrolyzed to ritalinic acid, which is excreted in the urine.

DOSAGE AND PREPARATIONS.

Oral: For attention deficit disorder, individualization of the dose is very important; optimal amounts for the morning, afternoon, and evening administration need not be the same. Some children may require only two doses per day, and a few may require an extra dose at bedtime, particularly those who often awaken during the night and in whom loss of sleep impairs learning in the classroom the following day. *Children 6 years and older,* initially, 5 mg twice daily (before breakfast and lunch); this dose may be gradually increased by 5 or 10 mg at weekly intervals. The usual effective dosage range is 0.3 to 0.5 mg/kg daily (10 to 20 mg daily for the average child). The maximum daily dose is 2 mg/kg or a total of 60 mg. If improvement is not observed after one month, the drug should be discontinued.

Since the effects of a single dose usually do not persist for more than four hours, the following alternative schedule utilizes administration three times daily during the waking hours. This often improves behavior and interpersonal relationships at home as well as in school (Kinsbourne and Caplan, 1979). *Children 6 years and older,* initially, 5 mg three times a day, usually 30 minutes before meals, increased by 5 mg/dose every three or four days until satisfactory improvement, intolerable side effects, or signs and symptoms of overfocusing occur (ie, the child becomes withdrawn, tearful, suspicious, or dulled in interactions with others). The maximum recommended dose is 60 mg/day.

For narcolepsy, *adults,* 10 mg two or three times daily (range, 10 to 60 mg daily). Tolerance is a major problem when large doses are administered daily for prolonged periods. An occasional drug holiday or withholding therapy during nonworking periods restores sensitivity to the drug and allows the dosage to be decreased when therapy is reinstituted.

Generic. Tablets 5, 10, and 20 mg.
Ritalin (CIBA). Tablets 5, 10, and 20 mg; tablets (timed-release) 20 mg *(Ritalin-SR).*

PEMOLINE
[Cylert]

ACTIONS AND USES. This central nervous system stimulant is an oxazolidine. It is indicated as an adjunct to remedial measures in the management of children with attention deficit disorder. In controlled clinical studies, it improved the condition of children with this disorder as judged by physicians, parents, and teachers and by the results of psychological test scores.

In comparative studies, results were similar with pemoline, dextroamphetamine, and methylphenidate, except that the latter drug was statistically superior in a few measurements of improvement. The beneficial effects occurred more rapidly with the other stimulants than with pemoline. However, pemoline was administered once daily while the other drugs were given twice daily. As with methylphenidate and dextroamphetamine, subjective improvement appeared to be sustained over a period of two years.

The activity of pemoline in combating depression and fatigue and enhancing performance has been studied, but its effectiveness in these conditions has not been demonstrated.

ADVERSE REACTIONS AND PRECAUTIONS. The most common adverse effects of pemoline are insomnia and anorexia. The insomnia may be transient or severe enough to necessitate adjustment of dosage. Anorexia may result in weight loss, particularly during the early weeks of therapy, but weight gain occurs after three to six months of continued administration and the weight curve approximates normal. A decrease in expected linear growth has been reported after long-term use, but the effect appears to be only temporary (see the Introduction). Onset of puberty was not delayed in the limited number of patients studied to determine this effect.

Other adverse reactions reported infrequently include dizziness, drowsiness, headache, depression, hallucinations, rash, nausea, and gastrointestinal distress. No clinically significant sympathomimetic effects (increased pulse rate or blood pressure) were observed with pemoline.

Elevated SGOT, SGPT, and LDH levels occurred in a few patients and jaundice has been reported. The hepatic dysfunction appears to be a delayed hypersensitivity reaction. These reactions generally developed after several months of therapy and usually were reversible upon withdrawal of the drug. The enzyme levels decreased within three to nine months after discontinuation of pemoline; however, in a few patients, liver enzyme levels continued to increase after discontinuation. Periodic monitoring of hepatic function during therapy is advisable; one case of fatal hepatic dysfunction has been reported. No significant hematologic effects or changes in blood urea nitrogen, uric acid, or bilirubin values were observed in long-term studies.

Although no potential for abuse was found in studies in primates, psychotic symptoms have been reported in adults who misused the drug. Because pemoline has properties similar to those of other central nervous system stimulants, it is classified as a Schedule IV drug, although its abuse potential is low.

PHARMACOKINETICS. Pemoline is well absorbed orally and has a half-life of approximately 12 hours. It is excreted principally by the kidney.

DOSAGE AND PREPARATIONS.

Oral: For attention deficit disorder, *children 6 years and over,* initially, 37.5 mg daily as a single dose in the morning, increased by 18.75 mg at one-week intervals until the desired response is observed. The usual effective range is 56.25 to 75 mg daily (maximum, 112.5 mg daily). Improvement is gradual and may not be observed for three to four weeks.

Cylert (Abbott). Tablets 18.75, 37.5, and 75 mg; tablets (chewable) 37.5 mg.

Cited References

Neurotransmitter treatment of senile dementia, Alzheimer's type. *Int Drug Ther Newslett* 16:5-8, (Feb) 1981.

Surgeon General's Report on Smoking and Health. Washington, DC, US Department of Health, Education and Welfare, 1979.

Amado H, Lustman PJ: Attention deficit disorders persisting in adulthood: Review. *Compr Psychiatry* 23:300-314, (July-Aug) 1982.

American Psychiatric Association: *Diagnostic and Statistical Manual of Mental Disorders,* ed 3. Washington, DC, American Psychiatric Association, 1980.

Biederman J: New directions in pediatric psychopharmacology. *Drug Ther* 12:147-168, (May) 1982.

Biederman J, Jellinek MS: Psychopharmacology in children. *N Engl J Med* 310:968-972, 1984.

Bondareff W, et al: Loss of neurons of origin of adrenergic projection to cerebral cortex (nucleus locus ceruleus) in senile dementia. *Neurology* 23:164-168, 1982.

Chan Y-PM, et al: Methylphenidate hydrochloride given with or before breakfast: II. Effects on plasma concentration of methylphenidate and ritalinic acid. *Pediatrics* 72:56-59, 1983.

Clarren SK, Smith DW: Fetal alcohol syndrome. *N Engl J Med* 298:1063-1067, 1978.

Conners CK: *Food Additives and Hyperactive Children.* New York, Plenum Press, 1980.

Coyle JT, et al: Alzheimer's disease: Disorder of cortical cholinergic innervation. *Science* 219:1184-1190, 1983.

Crook T, Gershon S (eds): *Strategies for the Development of an Effective Treatment for Senile Dementia.* New Canaan, CT, Mark Powley Associates, 1981.

Dahl DS: Diagnosis of Alzheimer's disease. *Postgrad Med* 73:217-221, (April) 1983.

D'arcy PF: Tobacco smoking and drugs: Clinically important interactions? *Drug Intell Clin Pharm* 18:302-307, 1984.

Davis KL: Cholinomimetic treatment of neuropsychiatric disorders: Review of recent developments. *Mt Sinai J Med* 46:455-459, 1979.

DeBoni U, McLachlan DRC: Senile dementia and Alzheimer's disease: Current view. *Life Sci* 27:1-14, 1980.

Dubey DR: Hyperkinetic child: Current status. *Compr Ther* 8:58-67, (May) 1982.

Eneanya DI, et al: Actions and metabolic fate of disulfiram. *Annu Rev Pharmacol Toxicol* 21:575-596, 1981.

Fagerström K-O: Comparison of psychological and pharmacological treatment in smoking cessation. *J Behav Med* 5:343-351, 1982.

Friedmann N, et al: Effect on growth in pemoline-treated children with attention deficit disorder. *Am J Dis Child* 135:329-332, 1981.

Garfinkel BD, et al: Tricyclic antidepressant and methylphenidate treatment of attention deficit disorder in children. *J Am Acad Child Psychiatry* 22:343-348, 1983.

Gragg DM: Drugs to decrease alcohol consumption, (letter). *N Engl J Med* 306:747, 1982.

Green PHR, Tall AR: Drugs, alcohol and malabsorption. *Am J Med* 67:1066-1076, 1979.

Griffiths RR, Henningfield JE: Pharmacology of cigarette smoking behavior. *Trends Pharmacol Sci* 3:260-263, (June) 1982.

Hansten PD: Chlorpropamide and alcohol. *Drug Interact Newslett* 1:39-40, (Oct) 1981.

Iosub S, et al: Fetal alcohol syndrome revisited. *Pediatrics* 68:475-479, 1981.

Jaffe JH: Drug addiction and drug abuse, in Gilman AG, et al (eds): *The Pharmacological Basis of Therapeutics,* ed 6. New York, Macmillan, 1980.

Jarvik ME: Biological influences on cigarette smoking, in: *The Behavioral Aspects of Smoking.* NIDA Monograph, vol 26, 1979.

Jarvis MJ, et al: Randomised controlled trial of nicotine chewing gum. *Br Med J* 285:537-540, 1982.

Kallas P, Sellers EM: Blood glucose in intoxicated chronic alcoholics. *Can Med Assoc J* 112:590-592, 1975.

Kinsbourne M, Caplan PJ: *Children's Learning and Attention Problems.* Boston, Little, Brown and Company, 1979.

Kissin B, Begleiter H (eds): *The Biology of Alcoholism, Vol 5: Treatment and Rehabilitation of the Chronic Alcoholic.* New York, Plenum Press, 1977.

Kolata G: Consensus on diets and hyperactivity. *Science* 215:958, 1982.

Laufer MW, Shetty T: Attention deficit disorders, in Kaplan HI, et al (eds): *Comprehensive Textbook of Psychiatry/III,* ed 3. Baltimore, Williams & Wilkins, 1980, 2538-2550.

Lawson-Wendling KL, et al: Differential effects of (+)-amphetamine, methylphenidate, and amfonelic acid on catecholamine synthesis in selected regions of rat brain. *J Pharm Pharmacol* 33:803-804, 1981.

Lewis DC, Femino J: Management of alcohol withdrawal. *Ration Drug Ther* 16:1-5, (Feb) 1982.

Lieber CS: Metabolism of alcohol. *Sci Am* 234:25-33, (March) 1976.

Lieber CS: Interaction of ethanol with drug toxicity. *Am J Gastroenterol* 74:313-320, 1980.

Linnoila M, et al: Drug interactions with alcohol. *Drugs* 18:299-311, 1979.

Littleton JM: Tolerance and physical dependence on alcohol at level of synaptic membranes: Review. *J R Soc Med* 76:593-601, 1983.

Lowe TL, et al: Stimulant medications precipitate Tourette's syndrome. *JAMA* 247:1168-1169, 1982.

MacArthur DR, Williams GW: Nicotine gum in smoking cessation. *Pharmaceut J* 230:45-46, (Jan 15) 1983.

MacGregor GA, et al: Is "idiopathic" oedema idiopathic? *Lancet* 1:397-400, 1979.

McNabb ME, et al: Plasma nicotine levels produced by chewing nicotine gum. *JAMA* 248:865-868, 1982.

Milman DH: Minimal brain dysfunction in childhood: Outcome in late adolescence and early adult years. *J Clin Psychiatry* 40:371-380, 1979.

Naeye RL: Maternal use of dextroamphetamine and growth of fetus. *Pharmacology* 26:117-120, 1983.

Naranjo CA, et al: Nonpharmacologic intervention in acute alcohol withdrawal. *Clin Pharmacol Ther* 34:214-219, 1983.

National Institutes of Health Consensus Conference: Defined diets and childhood hyperactivity. *JAMA* 248:290-292, 1982.

Nyberg G, et al: Cardiovascular effects of nicotine chewing gum in healthy non-smokers. *Eur J Clin Pharmacol* 23:303-307, 1982.

Peachey JE, Naranjo CA: Role of drugs in treatment of alcoholism. *Drugs* 27:171-182, 1984.

Rapoport J, et al: Dextroamphetamine: Cognitive and behavioral effects in normal prepubertal boys. *Science* 199:560-563, 1978.

Richmond JB: Ending the cigarette pandemic. *NY State J Med* 83:1259, 1983.

Russell MAH, et al: Effect of nicotine chewing gum as adjunct to general practitioners' advice against smoking. *Br Med J* 287:1782-1784, 1983.

Satterfield JH, et al: Growth of hyperactive children treated with methylphenidate. *Arch Gen Psychiatry* 36:212-217, 1979.

Sellers EM, Kalant H: Alcohol intoxication and withdrawal. *N Engl J Med* 294:757-762, 1976.

Sellers EM, et al: Drugs to decrease alcohol consumption. *N Engl J Med* 305:1255-1262, 1981.

Sellers EM, et al: Diazepam loading: Simplified treatment of alcohol withdrawal. *Clin Pharmacol Ther* 34:822-826, 1983.

168

Skinner HA: Primary syndromes of alcohol abuse: Their measurement and correlates. *Br J Addict* 76:63-76, 1981.

Small GW, et al: Diagnosis and treatment of dementia in the aged. *West J Med* 135:469-481, 1981.

Sowers J, et al: Effects of bromocriptine on renin, aldosterone, and prolactin responses to posture and metoclopramide in idiopathic edema: Possible therapeutic approach. *J Clin Endocrinol Metab* 54:510-516, 1982.

Streeten DHP: Idiopathic edema: Pathogenesis, clinical features, and treatment. *Metabolism* 27:353-383, 1978.

Swanson JM, et al: Methylphenidate hydrochloride given with or before breakfast: I. Behavioral, cognitive, and electrophysiologic effects. *Pediatrics* 72:49-55, 1983.

Swanson JM, Kinsbourne M: Artificial colors and hyperactive behavior, in Knights R, Bakker D (eds): *Treatment of Hyperactive and Learning Disabled Children: Current Research.* Baltimore, University Park Press, 1980, 131-150.

Task Force of National Institute on Aging: Senility reconsidered: Treatment possibilities for mental impairment in the elderly. *JAMA* 244:259-263, 1980.

Taylor P: Ganglionic stimulating and blocking agents, in Gilman AG, et al (eds): *The Pharmacological Basis of Therapeutics*, ed 6. New York, Macmillan, 1980, 211-219.

Totti N III, et al: Nicotine is chemotactic for neutrophils and enhances neutrophil responsiveness to chemotactic peptides. *Science* 223:169-171, 1984.

Weingartner H, et al: Cognitive processes in normal and hyperactive children and their response to amphetamine treatment. *J Abnorm Psychol* 89:25-37, 1980.

Weiss G: Controversial issues of pharmacotherapy of hyperactive child. *Can J Psychiatry* 26:385-392, 1981.

Weiss B, et al: Behavioral responses to artificial food colors. *Science* 107:1487-1488, 1980.

Wells CE: Pseudodementia. *Am J Psychiatry* 136:895-900, 1979.

West LJ (moderator): UCLA Conference, Alcoholism. *Ann Intern Med* 100:405-416, 1984.

Whitfield CL, et al: Detoxification of 1,024 alcoholic patients without psychoactive drugs. *JAMA* 239:1409-1410, 1978.

Winsberg BG, et al: Ineffectiveness of imipramine in children who fail to respond to methylphenidate. *J Autism Development Disord* 10:129-137, 1980.

Wolraich ML: Stimulant drug therapy in hyperactive children: Research and clinical implications. *Pediatrics* 60:512-518, 1977.

Antiepileptic Drugs

Seizures are manifestations of a focal or generalized disturbance of the brain. Epilepsies are chronic seizure disorders characterized by a tendency for recurrent seizures. Seizures (and some epilepsies) are caused by congenital or birth defects, degenerative disease, trauma of the central nervous system, anoxia, fever, metabolic disturbances, anaphylaxis, infection, neoplasm, cerebrovascular disease, poisoning, and withdrawal of alcohol and certain drugs. In some cases, seizures may occur in the absence of any diagnosable conditions. In most acute conditions, the seizures are temporary and treatment is directed primarily at the underlying cause.

Patients with epilepsy may experience sudden loss or disturbance of consciousness often associated with motor, sensory, autonomic, and/or inappropriate behavioral phenomena. The age-adjusted prevalence of epilepsy in this country is 6.25/1,000 population (Hauser and Kurland, 1975). Complex partial, simple partial, and generalized tonic-clonic seizures are the most prevalent types observed in epileptic syndromes. The overall incidence of epilepsy is greatest in the first year of life, declines over fivefold in the next ten years, reaches a minimum by age 30 to 40, and begins to increase again at 50 (Hauser and Kurland, 1975; Browne and Feldman, 1983).

Seizures have been classified into two broad groups: partial seizures and generalized seizures (convulsive and nonconvulsive) (Commission on Classification and Terminology of the International League Against Epilepsy, 1981) (see Table 1). Epilepsy also may be classified etiologically as symptomatic or idiopathic; the former category implies that a cause has been determined. The cause of seizures should be sought, since the underlying disorder may respond to definitive treatment. Most idiopathic epilepsies begin during childhood or adolescence. Epilepsy that occurs in infancy usually results from developmental defects, metabolic disease, or birth injury. Epilepsy that begins during adulthood is thought to be caused by trauma, stroke, tumors, or other recognizable brain disease, but in many cases the etiology cannot be determined.

Seizures are caused by hyperexcitable neurons. In experimental models, localized hypoxia or cooling, interference with utilization of substrate, alteration of ion permeability, or the topical application of certain chemicals to the brain (eg, cobalt, penicillin, alumina gel) may cause sudden focal hyperexcitability and electrical discharge. However, the etiology and self-perpetuating discharge of an idiopathic epileptogenic focus are less well understood. An area of abnormal electrical activity, as defined by electroencephalography, may be present in many epilepsies.

In recently developed experimental models, subconvulsive electrical stimuli delivered intermittently to a single area of the brain over a period of time results in the development of seizures that become longer and more intense following repeated stimulation. This process, known as kindling, produces enhanced neuronal sensitivity and provides a potentially informative model for epilepsy. In this model, the continued application of electrical stimuli leads to the development of a

TABLE 1.
EPILEPTIC SEIZURES: CLASSIFICATION AND CHARACTERISTICS

Seizure Classification	Clinical Characteristics
I. PARTIAL SEIZURES (FOCAL SEIZURES)	

A. Simple partial seizures
  1. with motor symptoms
  2. with somatosensory or special sensory symptoms
  3. with autonomic symptoms
  4. with psychic symptoms
	Most common in older children and adults. Consciousness usually not impaired. Paroxysmal attacks limited to functional disturbances of sensory, motor, and/or autonomic nerves and to anatomical regions of the brain, depending on the particular cortical area of involvement. Seizures with motor (Jacksonian seizure) and special sensory symptoms (odor, taste) are most common.

B. Complex partial seizures
  1. simple partial onset followed by impairment of consciousness
  2. with impairment of consciousness at the onset
	Most common in older children and adults. Often daily episodes of impaired consciousness (eg, amnesia, unresponsiveness), usually characterized by brief (1 to 2 minutes) loss of contact with environment. Clinical manifestations varied; most commonly consist of automatisms (eg, staring, chewing movements or smacking of lips, bizarre purposeless motor or psychic performances, mumbled speech or unintelligible sounds). Confusion may persist for 1 to 2 minutes after attack subsides. EEG is helpful for diagnosis, because unusual variants of this disorder may be extremely difficult to distinguish from purely functional psychiatric disorders.

C. Partial seizures evolving to secondarily generalized seizures
  1. simple partial seizures (A) evolving to generalized seizures
  2. complex partial seizures (B) evolving to generalized seizures
  3. simple partial seizures evolving to complex partial seizures evolving to generalized seizures
	On occasion, partial seizures may spread and become generalized tonic-clonic seizures.

II. GENERALIZED SEIZURES (CONVULSIVE OR NONCONVULSIVE)	
A. Absence seizures (petit mal seizures) 1. atypical absence seizures	Onset usually between 4 and 8 years; rarely occurs before age 3 or after age 15. An absence attack is an abrupt, brief loss of consciousness, amnesia, or unawareness characterized by staring and a 3/second spike and wave pattern in the EEG, which may be associated with mild clonic movements (eye blinking, jerking movements), automatisms, or changes in postural tone. No postictal or confused state follows attack. Duration of attack is 10 to 30 seconds, and attacks may occur as frequently as 50 to 100 times a day. Atypical seizures have more heterogeneous EEG pattern onset and/or cessation is not abrupt.
B. Myoclonic seizures	Single or multiple sudden, brief, "shock-like" contractions may be generalized or confined to the face and trunk or to one or more extremities. Many cases of myoclonic jerks and action myoclonus are not classified as epileptic seizures.
C. Clonic seizures	Clonic seizures are characterized by repetitive clonic jerks that lack a tonic component. Clonic jerks may be symmetrical, asymmetrical, rhythmic, or arrhythmic; these seizures are relatively rare, occurring primarily in early childhood.
D. Tonic seizures	Tonic contraction of certain muscle groups is accompanied by altered consciousness, but there is no progression to clonic phase. Duration of seizures is brief (10 seconds). Ocular phenomena are common and include fixation of the eyes, eyelid retraction, superior ocular deviation, nystagmus, and mydriasis. Autonomic signs also prominent: tachycardia, hypertension, respiratory distress, capillary restriction with cyanosis. Seizures usually activated by sleep.

(Continued on next page)

TABLE 1 (continued)
EPILEPTIC SEIZURES: CLASSIFICATION AND CHARACTERISTICS

Seizure Classification	Clinical Characteristics
E. Tonic-clonic seizures	These types of seizures are the most commonly encountered primary and secondary generalized seizures and can occur at any age. While some patients experience a vague aura, the majority lose consciousness without premonitory signs. Seizures begin with a sudden tonic contraction of muscles (if respiratory muscle is affected, there is stridor); the patient falls to the ground and remains rigid (10 to 30 seconds). The tonic phase gives way to the clonic phase (30 to 50 seconds) and muscle relaxation interrupts tonic contraction. Muscle tone returns in rhythmic flexor spasms, which become less frequent as the seizure subsides. Following this, the patient remains unconscious for variable periods. Seizures usually last two to five minutes. Urinary and fecal incontinence may occur in the clonic phase.
F. Atonic seizures	Sudden reduction of muscle tone may selectively affect muscle groups leading to head drop with slackening of the jaw, the dropping of a limb, or loss of all muscle tone leading to a slumping to the ground. When attacks are brief, they are called "drop attacks." Other conditions, such as narcolepsy cataplexy syndrome and brainstem ischemia, also cause "drop attacks."
III. UNCLASSIFIED EPILEPTIC SEIZURES	Inadequate data for classification. This category includes some neonatal seizures (eg, rhythmic eye movements, chewing and swimming movements)

Adapted from Commission on Classification and Terminology of the International League Against Epilepsy, 1981.

neuronal state of spontaneous recurrent generalized seizures that usually arise from sites remote but synaptically connected to the original site of stimulation. The neuronal reorganization underlying kindling is thought to involve both the kindled site and synaptically related secondary foci. Thus, epileptic propagation depends upon recruitment of normal neurons that ultimately results in a clinical seizure. An understanding of the reorganization that occurs with kindling (development of secondary foci and the nature of their spontaneous discharge) may explain the latency and repetitive discharge of an epileptogenic focus (Penry and Porter, 1979).

ANTIEPILEPTIC DRUGS

Mechanism of Action

The antiepileptic drugs are categorized in Table 2 according to seizure type and their usage in epilepsy. Even those in the same chemical class may have no common site or mechanism of action. Many antiepileptic drugs prevent the spread of neural excitation rather than suppressing the focus of discharge itself, and normal excitability is generally unaffected by doses that modify idiopathic and electrically or chemically induced local or systemic hyperexcitability. Therefore, the phrase, neuronal membrane stabilizing effect, often is used to describe the overall action of the antiepileptic drugs.

The molecular sites of antiepileptic action of these drugs are poorly understood; however, several drugs are known to affect gamma aminobutyric acid (GABA), an inhibitory neurotransmitter. Certain agents that produce seizures (eg, tetanus antitoxin, allyl glycine, picrotoxin, bicuculline, pentylenetetrazol) diminish the activity of GABA. Clonazepam, diazepam, phenobarbital, and valproic acid (Hammond et al, 1981) enhance the activity of the GABA-mediated inhibitory system. Postsynaptic receptors for the benzodiazepines have been discovered that facilitate the binding of GABA to its receptor, leading to greater chloride ion influx through chloride channels and thus greater inhibition of the postsynaptic neuron. Barbiturates and phenytoin also may increase GABA-mediated chloride conduction in postsynaptic membranes.

Based on the hypothesis that spontaneous electrical discharges result from GABA-neuron dysfunction, a new generation of antiepileptic agents (eg, progabide, gamma vinyl GABA) is being developed to enhance GABA-mediated inhibition (Meldrum, 1984): A number of GABA prodrugs have been synthesized that deliver GABA across the blood-brain barrier. One receptor-specific agonist, progabide, may be active against partial and generalized seizures; the incidence of adverse reactions was low in a limited number of patients (Martínez-Lage et al, 1984), but the drug is not free of hepatotoxicity.

Dysfunction in other neurotransmitters may also occur in epilepsy. Ethosuximide, valproic acid, and trimethadione, but not phenytoin or phenobarbital, block seizures induced by leucine enkephalin, which suggests that the enkephalinergic neurotransmitter system may be involved in the genesis of absence epilepsy (Snead and Bearden, 1980).

Phenytoin also may alter neurotransmitter inhibitory systems. Post-tetanic potentiation of synaptic transmission is reduced and post-tetanic hyperpolarization is abolished. These actions are ascribed to modifications of sodium, calcium, and potassium ion transport that result in membrane stabilization (Woodbury, 1980; Woodbury et al, 1982).

Drug Selection

Initial drug therapy is based principally on seizure pattern (see Table 1). Once the epileptic syndrome is diagnosed, drug selection is determined by the efficacy and adverse reactions of the principal antiepileptic drugs: phenytoin [Dilantin], pheno-

TABLE 2.
ANTIEPILEPTICS

Seizure Type	Commonly Used	Infrequently Used
PARTIAL SEIZURES (FOCAL SEIZURES) A. Simple Partial Seizures B. Complex Partial Seizures C. Partial seizures evolving to secondarily generalized seizures	Phenytoin [Dilantin] Carbamazepine [Tegretol] Phenobarbital Primidone [Mysoline]	Phenacemide [Phenurone] Ethotoin [Peganone] Mephenytoin [Mesantoin] Mephobarbital [Mebaral] Metharbital [Gemonil] Acetazolamide [Diamox] Valproic Acid [Depakene, Depakote]
GENERALIZED SEIZURES Absence	Ethosuximide [Zarontin] Valproic Acid [Depakene, Depakote] Clonazepam [Klonopin]	Acetazolamide [Diamox] Clorazepate [Tranxene] Diazepam [Valium] Methsuximide [Celontin] Phensuximide [Milontin] Paramethadione [Paradione] Trimethadione [Tridione]
Tonic-Clonic Seizures	Phenytoin [Dilantin] Carbamazepine [Tegretol] Phenobarbital Valproic Acid [Depakene, Depakote]	Primidone [Mysoline] Bromides, inorganic Ethotoin [Peganone] Mephenytoin [Mesantoin] Mephobarbital [Mebaral] Metharbital [Gemonil] Acetazolamide [Diamox]
Myoclonic Seizures Infantile Spasms, Lennox-Gastaut Syndrome	Corticotropin (ACTH) Corticosteroids Clonazepam [Klonopin]	Carbamazepine [Tegretol] Phenytoin [Dilantin] Phenobarbital Primidone [Mysoline]
Myoclonic Seizures (Including Postanoxic Myoclonus)	Valproic Acid [Depakene, Depakote] Clonazepam [Klonopin] L-5 hydroxytryptophan	Bromides, inorganic Carbamazepine [Tegretol] Phenytoin [Dilantin] Phenobarbital Diazepam [Valium] Metharbital [Gemonil]
Atonic Seizures	Valproic Acid [Depakene, Depakote] Clonazepam [Klonopin]	Ethosuximide [Zarontin] Trimethadione [Tridione]

barbital, carbamazepine [Tegretol], primidone [Mysoline], valproic acid [Depakene, Depakote], and ethosuximide [Zarontin]. A long-term, multicenter, randomized, double-blind trial has been conducted to compare the efficacy and adverse reactions of the major antiepileptic drugs in patients with partial and generalized tonic-clonic seizures (Mattson et al, 1985). The patient's age and response to previous drug therapy (Penry and Newmark, 1979; Wilder and Bruni, 1981), as well as the dosage form and frequency of administration also influence drug selection.

Epileptic Seizures: For the initial treatment of *generalized tonic-clonic* or *partial (focal) seizures,* monotherapy with phenytoin, phenobarbital, primidone, or carbamazepine is currently recommended. Although their antiepileptic activity is similar, the clinically important differences are determined by the adverse reactions they produce.

In adults, comparative clinical trial data indicate that the efficacy of the drugs is equivalent in secondarily generalized tonic-clonic seizures and that carbamazepine is the most effective antiepileptic drug in partial seizures (Mattson et al, 1985). However, the choice among these drugs is still debated. Phenytoin is preferred by many neurologists for initial treatment of adults and older children because of the long experience with its use and its effectiveness when used alone. Mephenytoin [Mesantoin] and ethotoin [Peganone] are less commonly used alternatives to phenytoin. Mephenytoin is effective but may be toxic to the bone marrow. Ethotoin is safer than phenytoin but is less effective, possibly because of its shorter elimination half-life (Korberly et al, 1981).

A growing number of neurologists choose carbamazepine, especially in women and children over 5 years, because it does not cause the coarsening of facial features, hirsutism, and gingival hyperplasia induced by phenytoin. In addition, carbamazepine is often effective alone, and its administration is less complicated than that of phenytoin, since it follows linear pharmacokinetics. Fears of its potentially serious hematologic toxicity have decreased in recent years and neuropsychological reactions may occur less frequently with carbamazepine than with phenytoin.

Phenobarbital is more often reserved for initial use in children under 5 years. However, there is growing evidence that barbiturates exert subtle effects on cognitive ability in both children and adults. Therefore, these drugs may be less desirable than carbamazepine or phenytoin, but this has not been definitely established. The actions of mephobarbital [Mebaral] and metharbital [Gemonil] resemble those of phenobarbital, but they are less potent and appear to have no advantages over the latter. The short-acting barbiturates are not useful prophylactically, for their hypnotic action tends to parallel their antiepileptic effect.

Primidone is associated with a higher failure rate than phenytoin, phenobarbital, or carbamazepine because of a greater incidence of side effects during initial therapy, even with low doses; however, in those patients who are able to tolerate the drug, seizure control is similar to that with carbamazepine or phenytoin.

Valproic acid was reported to be as effective as phenytoin (Covanis et al, 1982; Wilder et al, 1983 A; Turnbull et al, 1985) in primary generalized tonic-clonic seizures. However, its role in generalized tonic-clonic and partial seizures has not yet been established conclusively. Although there is concern over the possibility of hepatotoxicity, this effect is rare (see the evaluation).

Benzodiazepines are variably effective but sedation limits their use (Porter and Theodore, 1983). The succinimides and oxazolidinediones are ineffective in generalized tonic-clonic seizures and very rarely may precipitate them in susceptible patients. Phenacemide [Phenurone] occasionally is effective in complex partial seizures, but it often produces severe adverse reactions and is therefore rarely used. It is not recommended unless the benefit justifies the considerable risk. Inorganic bromides (eg, sodium or potassium bromide) have some antiepileptic activity in generalized tonic-clonic seizures. It is believed that toxicity is uncommon when the serum concentration of bromide remains within the therapeutic range, but there is little data on adverse reactions associated with prolonged therapy. Their use alone is obsolete, but some neurologists continue to regard them as useful adjuncts in selected patients. Dextroamphetamine is rarely used as an adjunct to the sedating antiepileptic drugs to reduce central nervous system depression. Most clinicians prefer a less sedating antiepileptic drug.

If seizures are not controlled by maximally tolerated doses of one of the four primary drugs, the initial drug may be replaced gradually by another drug of choice. If seizures continue, a second antiepileptic drug should be added to the regimen. Combination therapy is occasionally more effective than monotherapy (Mattson et al, 1985), but drug interactions make overall management more complex. The combination of phenytoin and carbamazepine has been recommended for maximum control of generalized tonic-clonic or partial seizures (Porter, 1984). Primidone is frequently used adjunctively with phenytoin or carbamazepine when the response to a single drug is not satisfactory. Acetazolamide is used only rarely as a temporary adjunct in generalized tonic-clonic or partial seizures because tolerance develops. Clorazepate [Tranxene] is used adjunctively in the management of partial seizures.

Drugs that are effective in *absence seizures* include ethosuximide, valproic acid, clonazepam [Klonopin], and trimethadione [Tridione]. Ethosuximide is the drug of choice when absence seizures are not associated with generalized tonic-clonic seizures. Some clinicians prefer valproic acid initially for absence seizures, but others reserve it for use when therapeutic failure or intolerance to ethosuximide occurs because of the possibility of serious idiosyncratic hepatotoxicity. If seizure control is not complete with either drug alone, they can be given together. Clonazepam represents a third alternative; it is very effective but tolerance develops and seizures may recur (Aird et al, 1984). The other succinimides, methsuximide [Celontin] and phensuximide [Milontin], also may be effective but are less commonly used. Of the oxazolidinediones, trimethadione is more effective than paramethadione [Paradione] but, because of toxicity, both should be reserved for patients refractory to safer drugs. Acetazolamide can be used as an adjunct to other drugs in selected patients.

About one-half of patients with absence seizures also develop generalized tonic-clonic seizures. Most neurologists prefer to treat such patients with valproic acid, which is usually effective in both types of primary generalized seizures. Some clinicians employ carbamazepine or phenytoin for the generalized tonic-clonic seizures, but phenytoin may increase the frequency of absence attacks. When these drugs are used and a therapeutic plasma concentration is attained, ethosuximide therapy is initiated. Phenobarbital and primidone are not usually employed because they increase the frequency of absence attacks.

Both typical and *atypical absence seizures* have been treated with the benzodiazepines, clonazepam, diazepam [Valium] (less preferred), or clorazepate, with variable success. These agents should be considered alternative therapy for absence seizures in patients who do not respond to ethosuximide or valproic acid.

Myoclonic seizures occur alone or with absence or generalized tonic-clonic seizures and often are refractory to drug therapy. Drug selection is based principally on the age of the patient at onset. Some myoclonic seizures respond well to valproic acid and some authorities consider it the drug of choice. Clonazepam also may be beneficial; although sedation and tolerance may limit its usefulness (Browne, 1978), these effects have not occurred consistently (Mikkelsen et al, 1981). Both drugs also have been given concomitantly (Iivanainen and Himberg, 1982).

Infantile myoclonic epilepsy (infantile spasm) occurs from age 3 months to 2 years and *Lennox-Gastaut syndrome* occurs from age 3 to 7 years. Corticotropin (ACTH) or an adrenal corticosteroid is sometimes effective. Some data suggest that ACTH is more effective than prednisone (Snead et al, 1983). Initially, ACTH 40 to 80 units is given daily for three months or for one month after spasms are controlled completely. The daily dose is then decreased by 20 units/ month until 20 units daily is given for one month, at which time an alternate-day schedule is established. After one month of alternate-day therapy, the dose is reduced by 10 and 5 units for the next two months, respectively, and then discontinued. Alternatively, 80 units is given on alternate days for about ten months, starting within one month of the diagnosis, to improve seizure control and halt mental deterioration (Singer et al, 1980). A smaller daily dose (20 units) given for a shorter period is effective in selected patients and may be necessary if hypertension develops with use of larger doses (Hrachovy et al, 1980). Clonazepam is the drug of second choice when steroids are not tolerated or ineffective. A controlled study comparing ACTH and nitrazepam is being conducted.

For older children, a ketogenic diet is recommended as adjunctive therapy when drug refractoriness is a problem (Livingston et al, 1979). The value of ketogenic diets remains to be assessed by controlled clinical trials.

Myoclonic seizures generally do not respond to phenytoin, phenobarbital, primidone, or carbamazepine.

Posthypoxic myoclonus is a subset of myoclonic seizures that has also been classified as a movement disorder. It may respond to the investigational drug, L-5-hydroxytryptophan (L-5HTP) (Van Woert and Hwang, 1978; Thal et al, 1980), which appears to be relatively specific for this disorder. A relative deficiency of serotonin (the decarboxylation product of L-5HTP) has been suggested as the cause of the myoclonus. Concomitant administration with the 5-HTP decarboxylase inhibitor, carbidopa, to minimize adverse reactions is being studied.

Valproic acid and clonazepam are given for *atonic seizures*. Ethosuximide and trimethadione are drugs of second choice or adjuncts, especially when the preferred agents are ineffective. Most patients respond poorly to all available medications.

Status Epilepticus: Status epilepticus has been defined as epileptic seizures that are repeated so frequently or are so prolonged that they create a fixed and continuous epileptic condition. Persistent tonic-clonic status epilepticus is an emergency requiring prompt and vigorous treatment. Most episodes in patients with prior epilepsy result from noncompliance, abrupt withdrawal of antiepileptic medication, withdrawal of alcohol and hypnotic drugs, and fever. Hypoglycemia, hypocalcemia, hyponatremia, stroke, meningitis, encephalitis, head injury, or drugs (amphetamines, phenothiazines, antianxiety agents, tricyclic antidepressants) are less common causes.

Establishment of an adequate airway and an intravenous line, as well as ventilatory support if needed, are required initially for management. After obtaining a blood sample for glucose determination, a 50-ml bolus of 50% dextrose (for adolescents or adults) is often administered immediately.

Drug selection often is based on the physician's familiarity with a particular drug and method of administration. Although some authorities employ intravenous phenytoin initially, intravenous diazepam is usually the drug of choice for initial control of generalized tonic-clonic status epilepticus because it has a more rapid onset of action and is equally effective (see Table 3). Intravenous lorazepam is longer acting and as effective as diazepam in status epilepticus but its superiority as a longer acting agent has not been demonstrated (Leppik et al, 1983). Since diazepam has a short duration of action, a loading dose of phenytoin should be administered simultaneously or immediately after control of seizures to establish a therapeutic

serum concentration rapidly (see Table 3). For discussion of the loading dose concept, see Chapter 2, Drug Response Variation and Dosing Information, and Cloyd et al, 1980.

Phenytoin is usually preferred to phenobarbital for status epilepticus because it causes less hypotension and depression of the respiratory and central nervous systems in patients who have received diazepam. However, if seizures are not controlled by diazepam and a loading dose of phenytoin, phenobarbital should be given intravenously to produce a therapeutic plasma concentration as rapidly as possible (Browne, 1982).

Phenobarbital is the preferred initial drug in very young children, during barbiturate or primidone withdrawal, and when phenytoin is relatively contraindicated (eg, in patients with cardiac conduction disturbances, such as sinus arrest and second- or third-degree A-V block; profound hypotension; or severe congestive heart failure).

If seizures do not respond to diazepam, phenobarbital, and phenytoin, parenteral administration of paraldehyde may be tried (see the evaluation). Although this agent has several disadvantages, it also can be given rectally. Alternatively, lidocaine [Xylocaine] has been given by slow intravenous infusion, although this drug itself may produce seizures (see the evaluation) and its use is discouraged by a number of specialists. For conservative treatment, a general anesthetic may be administered under the supervision of an anesthesiologist; resuscitative equipment should be immediately available.

When tonic-clonic seizures are not continuous but separated by prolonged periods of stupor, a loading dose of intravenous phenytoin initially may avoid the use of diazepam, which may further depress consciousness and respiration.

Treatment of partial and complex partial status epilepticus is generally the same as for the tonic-clonic type. For absence status epilepticus, intravenous diazepam is usually preferred initially. Oral ethosuximide or valproic acid then should be administered to establish an effective serum concentration as rapidly as possible.

Nonepileptic Seizures: A *febrile seizure* most often occurs in children between 3 months and 5 years of age; it is associated with fever but there is no evidence of intracranial infection or any other cause. A Consensus Development Conference of the National Institutes of Health (Freeman, 1980) concluded that two significant risks are associated with a febrile seizure: a 30% to 40% risk of recurrent febrile seizures and a very slightly increased risk of epilepsy.

Daily administration of antiepileptic drugs does not appear to prevent epilepsy but does reduce the likelihood of recurrence of febrile seizures from 1:3 to 1:10 when given for at least two years; therapy should be discontinued slowly over one to two months. Seizure prophylaxis should not be instituted routinely but may be considered (1) when neurologic development is abnormal (eg, cerebral palsy syndromes, mental retardation, microcephaly); (2) when a febrile seizure lasts longer than 15 minutes, is focal, or is followed by transient or persistent neurologic abnormalities; (3) when there is a history of nonfebrile seizures of genetic origin in a parent or sibling; or (4) in very young children who have the highest risk of recurrence.

Phenobarbital is the most commonly used agent and should

TABLE 3.
PARENTERAL THERAPY FOR STATUS EPILEPTICUS

Drug	Dosage/Route	Comments
Diazepam [Valium]	*Intravenous: Adults,* 5 to 10 mg given at a rate of 1 ml (5 mg)/min, repeated at 10- to 15-minute intervals (maximum, 30 mg). This dose may be repeated in two to four hours if necessary. For intravenous drip, diazepam 100 mg is diluted in 500 ml of 5% dextrose in water and given at a rate of 40 ml/hr to maintain a serum concentration of 0.2 to 0.8 mcg/ml. *Children 5 years or older,* 1 mg every two to five minutes (maximum, 10 mg), repeated in two to four hours if necessary. *Infants over 30 days and children under 5 years,* 0.2 to 0.5 mg every two to five minutes (maximum, 5 mg). Intravenous therapy is much preferred; however, if convulsions make slow intravenous injection impossible in children, intramuscular administration may be substituted.	Because of its rapid action, diazepam is considered by many epileptologists to be the drug of choice for initial control of continuous generalized tonic-clonic and absence status epilepticus. However, some authorities prefer to initiate therapy with intravenous phenytoin, particularly in patients with status epilepticus induced by head trauma, in those whose attacks have temporarily ceased, or in those who experience prolonged consciousness between attacks (Browne, 1982; Cloyd et al, 1980; Delgado Escueta et al, 1982; Porter, 1984). Since diazepam is rapidly redistributed, resulting in a lowered brain concentration, a parenteral loading dose of the longer acting phenytoin is usually administered concomitantly to provide long-term control. Sedation, hypotension, and respiratory depression are potential side effects of diazepam, especially in the young and elderly.
Lorazepam [Ativan]	*Intravenous: Adults,* although no dosage or rate of administration has been firmly established, 4 mg given at a rate of 1 ml (2 mg)/min has been effective (Leppik et al, 1983). This dose can be repeated at 10-minute intervals if needed. *Children,* experience is limited.	Lorazepam is as effective as diazepam in the initial control of generalized tonic-clonic status epilepticus. Controlled clinical studies have shown no difference in onset of action or incidence of respiratory depression between lorazepam and diazepam. However, further studies are needed to determine whether its duration of action is longer than with diazepam.
Phenytoin [Dilantin]	*Intravenous: Adults and children,* a loading dose of 15 mg/kg undiluted is administered at a rate not to exceed 50 mg/min. (Pediatric loading dose also may be calculated on the basis of 250 mg/M^2 given at a rate of 1 to 2 mg/kg/min.) An additional 5 mg/kg is given after 12 hours (Morris, 1981). Alternatively, 20 mg/kg diluted with 0.45% or 0.9% sodium chloride solution to produce 20 to 30 mg/ml phenytoin is administered at a rate not to exceed 50 mg/min. This is usually the only dose required in 24 hours (Cloyd et al, 1980). With either regimen, therapeutic serum concentrations are between 10 and 25 mcg/ml for 24 hours in most patients. Phenytoin should be administered in an intensive care unit so that heart rate, blood pressure, and electrocardiographic activity can be monitored.	Phenytoin has a slower onset of action than diazepam but is as effective in controlling generalized tonic-clonic status epilepticus. To prevent recurrence of seizures, phenytoin is administered with or immediately after diazepam. In epileptics, prior treatment with phenytoin does not lead to drug toxicity when it is used in status epilepticus. Phenytoin has been recommended as the initial drug in status epilepticus associated with head trauma or other neurosurgical disorders in which changes in the patient's consciousness are not desirable. Phenytoin is generally preferred to phenobarbital as a longer acting antiepileptic because it is more effective and causes less respiratory and central nervous system depression and hypotension in combination with diazepam.

(Continued on next page)

TABLE 3 (continued)

Drug	Dosage/Route	Comments
Phenobarbital	*Intravenous, Intramuscular: Adults,* the loading dose is 5 to 10 mg/kg. One-fifth of the total dose given intravenously undiluted at a rate of less than 50 mg/min every 5 to 10 minutes helps prevent respiratory depression. If the patient has previously been given phenytoin without success or an unknown serum level of phenobarbital is present, 2 mg/kg of phenobarbital should be administered intravenously every 15 minutes until adequate response is obtained, hypotension and/or respiratory depression develops, or a cumulative dose of 1 g/24 hours has been given. Intravenous administration is preferred, but intramuscular administration may be utilized if necessary; the initial dose is 3 to 5 mg/kg. *Children,* 10 to 15 mg/kg. One-fifth of total dose given intravenously undiluted at a rate of less than 50 mg/min every 5 to 10 minutes helps prevent respiratory depression. Dosage is adjusted to maintain serum concentration of 15 to 40 mcg/ml. If patient had previously been given phenytoin without success or an unknown serum level of phenobarbital is present, a dose of 2 mg/kg of phenobarbital should be administered intravenously every 15 minutes until an adequate response is obtained or hypotension and/or respiratory depression develops. Intravenous administration is preferred, but intramuscular administration may be utilized if necessary; the initial dose is 3 to 5 mg/kg. *Neonates,* the loading dose is 15 to 20 mg/kg.	Phenobarbital is often the preferred alternative to phenytoin in very young children, during withdrawal from barbiturates, in noncompliant patients, and when phenytoin is relatively contraindicated because of cardiac conduction and automaticity disorders.

be given in doses that produce a serum concentration of 15 mcg/ml (see the evaluation). Behavioral changes (ie, hyperactivity to extreme irritability, rarely somnolence) and sleep pattern disturbances (ie, prolonged nocturnal awakening) require discontinuation of phenobarbital in 25% of children. Because this drug may interfere with higher cortical or cognitive functions (eg, defects in short-term memory formation and general comprehension, attention deficit), many pediatricians advocate close monitoring during prolonged therapy (see Adverse Reactions). Diazepam and valproic acid are alternatives to phenobarbital. Their beneficial effects in this relatively benign condition must be weighed carefully against the risk of serious adverse reactions, especially with valproic acid.

Convulsive seizures are sometimes associated with the *drug withdrawal syndrome* in persons physically dependent on the barbiturates, alcohol, benzodiazepines, and other nonbarbiturate-nonbenzodiazepine antianxiety and hypnotic drugs. Phenobarbital or benzodiazepines are used most often to alleviate moderate to severe signs and symptoms, depending on the etiology of the syndrome (see Chapter 5, Drugs Used for Anxiety and Sleep Disorders). Since these drugs have an anticonvulsant action, additional antiepileptic drugs usually are not required. The addition of phenytoin is indicated only in high-risk patients (eg, those with a history of seizures, patients with extremely poor nutrition). Carbamazepine and valproic acid also have been used adjunctively. Carbamazepine's ability to attenuate mood swings in bipolar disorders

may be of value in selected patients. The potential for hepatotoxicity with barbiturates, phenytoin (rare), and valproic acid must be considered.

Antipsychotic drugs are inappropriate because most of these agents lower the seizure threshold; however, when psychotic signs and symptoms occur during withdrawal, haloperidol [Haldol] is efficacious and does not increase the frequency of seizures or cause extensive vasodilation with hypotension (Wilbur and Kulik, 1981).

The use of antiepileptic drugs in the prophylaxis of *post-traumatic epilepsy* is controversial. Phenytoin and/or phenobarbital may reduce the incidence of post-traumatic epilepsy in some patients but data are inconclusive. Patients who may benefit from therapy have been defined as having (1) penetrating head injuries; (2) closed brain injuries with neurologic symptoms of brain contusion or abnormal EEG; and (3) closed brain injuries without contusion when coma lasts more than three hours and epilepsy is present in family members or there is a history of abnormal delivery or febrile convulsions in childhood.

Drug Therapy

General Principles: The objective of drug therapy is to control seizures as completely as possible without causing intolerable adverse reactions. Antiepileptic therapy must be individualized; the appropriate dosage of a drug or combination of drugs depends upon the size, age, and condition of the patient; the response to treatment; and the interactions between concomitantly administered medication.

Initially, a single drug should be given in doses that produce serum concentrations known to be therapeutic in most individuals. Properly individualized monotherapy controls approximately 80% of the more common forms of epilepsy and avoids drug interactions. The dose is increased gradually until seizures are controlled or toxicity makes further increases inadvisable. The dose for children is usually 50% to 100% larger on a weight basis than that for adults.

A common error in the management of epilepsy is failure to allow time for the drug to reach steady state before evaluating its effectiveness. Based on pharmacokinetic principles, at least five drug half-lives must elapse before steady-state serum concentrations are achieved. Rapid-onset or rapidly recurring seizures may mandate a more immediate attainment of steady-state antiepileptic serum concentrations; this may be achieved by giving a loading dose at the onset of therapy or larger doses at any stage before the steady state is reached. Loading doses may be given intravenously, intramuscularly, or orally depending on the preparation.

Initially, antiepileptic drugs may cause central nervous system depression or gastrointestinal disturbances but the effects are transient and are not indications to discontinue treatment.

If untoward effects continue, the dose should be reduced to the tolerated level. Only when serious adverse reactions develop should another drug be substituted (Reynolds and Shorvon, 1981). When the initial drug is inadequate, another agent (preferably from a different chemical class) should be substituted or added to the regimen. Any alteration in therapy (substitution or addition) should be made gradually and effectiveness judged over a long period (with particular attention to the time required to reach a new steady state). When adding a second agent, the serum concentration of the initial drug should be held constant until the dosage of the second drug is optimized. Medication should not be stopped abruptly unless a serious adverse reaction occurs; in this event, another antiepileptic drug should be substituted promptly. Patients should be warned of the dangers of discontinuing any medication, informed of possible adverse reactions, and advised of the necessity of reporting any untoward effects to the physician.

Most treatment failures are caused by noncompliance. It is, therefore, important for the patient to understand and accept his disorder. It is also important for the physician to appreciate the social, psychological, and economic needs of the patient, which may require a multidisciplinary approach (Penry and Newmark, 1979; Boshes, 1980). Patient visits should be scheduled regularly to evaluate the efficacy and adverse reactions of the medication, to measure drug serum concentrations when indicated, and to adjust the dose if necessary. Other steps to improve compliance include simplification of dosage schedule, maintenance of medication calendar, individualized medicine containers, and patient education.

Uncontrolled epilepsy may lead to intractable epilepsy; data from kindling experiments support the view that seizures are self-perpetuating and repetitive brain stimulation leads to neuronal changes that cause spontaneous electrical discharge. If drugs do not reduce the frequency of seizures by approximately 85% within one year, the patient should be referred to a specialized epilepsy center.

Withdrawal of Medication: Unless a progressive underlying disease is involved, spontaneous remissions may occur, especially with idiopathic epilepsies that usually begin during childhood. (The great majority of absence seizures are limited to childhood.) Accordingly, the eventual discontinuation of an antiepileptic drug regimen should be considered.

Guidelines for discontinuation of therapy in children are being developed but some controversy persists. Two studies (Emerson et al, 1981; Thurston et al, 1982) support the view that 70% or more of children who originally experienced only a few seizures, who have remained seizure-free for four years with antiepileptic medication, and who have a normal or mildly abnormal EEG will remain seizure-free after withdrawal of antiepileptic medication. A recent study has shown that, in selected patients, a seizure-free interval of two years may permit discontinuation of medication (Shinnar et al, 1985). In addition, this study demonstrated that EEG improvement without slowing or spikes at the time of proposed discontinuation had the best prognosis for the patient remaining seizure free. There is general agreement that factors against discontinuation of therapy include epilepsy of long duration (eg, six years) prior to control and the presence of partial seizures, atypical febrile seizures, a combination of seizure types (mixed seizure disorders or Lennox-Gastaut syndrome), EEG with spikes and slowing (Shinnar et al, 1985), neurologic dysfunction, or mental retardation. Family history and age at proposed discontinuation of antiepileptic drug therapy are not significant. There is disagreement on whether the following are risk factors: onset of epilepsy prior to age 2 years, total number of seizures prior to control, and type and cause of seizure. It is generally believed that these risk factors may be minor (Berg, 1982; Gordon, 1982).

The dose of one drug at a time should be reduced very gradually while maintaining the serum concentration of the second drug in the therapeutic range, since sudden withdrawal may precipitate seizures and is one of the most common causes of status epilepticus. The optimal length of time for withdrawal of medication has not been established; a minimum of a few months and a maximum of six months have been advocated. Until these issues are resolved, the physician is urged to seek consultant opinion before discontinuing drug therapy.

Monitoring Therapeutic Drug Concentrations: Because there is a significant relationship between the serum concentration of an antiepileptic drug and its therapeutic effect, determination of drug serum concentrations may be helpful, particularly during initial dosage adjustment and to confirm compliance. The usual therapeutic ranges have been determined for most antiepileptic drugs. However, values vary among different clinics and laboratories, as well as among patients, and the therapeutic range should serve only as a guideline. For comparative purposes, it is recommended that blood samples be drawn before the first dose of the day (trough concentration).

Drug monitoring improves the overall management of epileptic patients by (1) identifying baseline concentrations of antiepileptic drugs associated with an optimal therapeutic regimen in an individual patient; (2) allowing adjustments in dose to compensate for changing physiologic states (eg, stress, pregnancy, puberty, old age) or disease states (eg, acute uremia, hepatic disease); (3) confirming compliance with the drug regimen; and (4) determining the effect of drug interactions on serum concentrations.

Because of the importance of drug serum concentrations in determining adequate therapy, considerable pharmacokinetic data are available for all commonly used antiepileptic drugs (see Table 4 and Hvidberg and Dam, 1976; Eadie and Tyrer, 1980; So and Penry, 1981). Two pharmacokinetic observations of special interest are: (1) Within the first few weeks of administration, carbamazepine induces hepatic enzymes that are responsible for its own biotransformation. The degree of autoinduction is variable, but an increase in dosage is usually required. Autoinduction and heteroinduction also contribute to drug interactions. (2) The biotransformation of phenytoin is characterized by dose-dependent kinetics; thus, as the metabolism of phenytoin approaches saturation, even small dosage increases may cause unexpected toxicity as a result of disproportionately large increases in the serum concentration and the apparent half-life of the drug. The enzymatic biotransformation of phenytoin also is inhibited by a number of drugs, resulting in unexpected toxicity. (See also Table 4.)

Adverse Reactions and Precautions: Most antiepileptic drugs produce gastrointestinal disturbances, especially during the early stages of treatment. The symptoms may be reduced by decreasing the dose or by administering the drugs after meals, although this may alter either the rate or the amount of drug absorbed. Patients should follow a consistent pattern when taking their medication.

All antiepileptic drugs depress the central nervous system to varying degrees at therapeutic concentrations. Usual doses of carbamazepine, phenytoin, ethosuximide, and valproic acid exert the least effect. Sedation is most noticeable during initial therapy but tolerance usually develops. Paradoxical excitement occurs rarely with the benzodiazepines (diazepam and clonazepam) but is common when phenobarbital is prescribed for young children and the elderly. Dose-related and idiopathic neurologic reactions, such as ataxia, seizures, pseudodementia, bradykinesia, and choreoathetosis, also have been observed. Phenacemide [Phenurone] often causes profound personality changes, including psychoses and suicidal depression.

All antiepileptic drugs, especially in combination, occasionally produce subacute cognitive or behavioral syndromes. They impair attention, concentration, memory, and mental or motor speed (Reynolds and Trimble, 1985). There is concern

TABLE 4
PHARMACOKINETIC DATA ON COMMONLY USED ANTIEPILEPTIC DRUGS

Drug	Usual Therapeutic Serum Concentration (Range, mcg/ml)	Steady State Requirement (Days)	Serum Half-Life Hours (Mean ± SD)	
			Adults	Children
Carbamazepine [Tegretol]	4-12	3-4	12±6 (initially the mean may be 30-35 hours; values listed are obtained at 3-4 weeks because of variable autoinduction)	8±4
Clonazepam [Klonopin]	0.02-0.08	6	23±5 to 34±8	23±10
Ethosuximide [Zarontin]	40-100	7-10	55±5	30±6
Phenobarbital	15-40 10-25	>21	120-144	72-96
Phenytoin [Dilantin]	10-20	variable (7-8)	24±12 (dose dependent, eg, 18.5 at 3.1 mg/kg/day, 35.5 at 6.5 mg/kg/day)	20±2
Primidone [Mysoline]	5-12	4-7	15 (monotherapy) 9 (combination therapy)	8±4.8
Valporic Acid [Depakene, Depakote]	50-100	1-4	15±7 (monotherapy) 10-12 (combination therapy)	11±4 (monotherapy) 7±4 (combination therapy)

that nonintoxicating serum concentrations of antiepileptic drugs also impair cognitive skills. Studies in normal volunteers and epileptics receiving monotherapy implicated barbiturates and hydantoins most often; these effects were less common with carbamazepine and valproic acid.

Based on these studies, the American Academy of Pediatrics (Committee on Drugs, 1985) recommends the following: (1) A thorough understanding of the natural history of the seizure disorder is required to decide whether to initiate or discontinue therapy (eg, in those with febrile seizures). (2) When selecting an antiepileptic drug, its specificity for the seizure type and its adverse reactions should be considered. (3) As follow-up to therapy, careful attention should be given to parental, teacher, and office observations of cognitive function, mood, and behavior. (4) If significant changes occur, consideration should be given to reducing the dose or substituting another antiepileptic drug. (5) Neuropsychological screening tests may detect subtle behavioral and intellectual effects. (6) Studies designed to evaluate and compare behavioral and cognitive effects of antiepileptic drugs in children should be performed.

Many antiepileptic drugs cause rash as a hypersensitivity reaction; the eruptions are usually morbilliform and require discontinuance of the drug. Drug sensitivity reactions cannot be predicted, but they usually become apparent after 10 to 14 days of therapy. A skin reaction rarely precedes the development of systemic lupus erythematosus, Stevens-Johnson syndrome, angioedema, serum sickness, or polyarteritis nodosa.

Anaphylaxis is extremely rare.

Megaloblastic anemias have been observed with several antiepileptic drugs, particularly the hydantoins, some barbiturates, and primidone. Usually therapy may be continued if the anemia responds to folic acid. Even in the absence of anemia, there is some evidence that reduction of folic acid concentrations by antiepileptic drugs may cause reversible symptoms of mental deterioration. Poor memory, inattentiveness, lethargy, and slow learning may result from other effects of antiepileptic drugs or may be evidence of brain damage. However, if such symptoms occur in the presence of low folate blood concentrations, treatment with folic acid may be warranted. It should be noted that folic acid may decrease phenytoin concentrations.

Among the most dangerous reactions to antiepileptic drugs are those that result from damage to the bone marrow, liver, and kidneys. Baseline and periodic blood studies should be performed in patients receiving these drugs. Although periodic blood studies detect leukopenias, they do not always predict the more serious reactions that occur precipitously (eg, agranulocytosis, thrombocytopenia, aplastic anemia). Since early recognition of the dyscrasia and discontinuance of the offending drug are essential, the patient should be advised to report promptly such symptoms as sore throat, fever, easy bruising, petechiae, epistaxis, or other signs of infection or bleeding tendency. Clinical and laboratory evaluations are necessary if such symptoms occur. Severe blood dyscrasias occur most commonly with phenacemide and mephenytoin and rarely with other antiepileptic drugs including paramethadione and tri-

Volume of Distribution (L/kg)	Plasma Protein Binding (Percent)	Clearance (ml/kg/min)	Biotransformation Site-Percent	Biologically Active Compounds in Blood
1.4±0.12	60-70	0.58±0.12	hepatic 98%	carbamazepine 10,11 epoxide of carbamazepine (shorter half-life than parent)
3.2±1.1	87	0.92±0.25	hepatic 98%	clonazepam 7-amino clonazepam (slight activity)
0.72±0.07	nil	0.26±0.05	hepatic 80%-90%	ethosuximide
0.8±0.33	40-60	0.09±0.04	hepatic 40%-60% renal 10%-40% unchanged	phenobarbital
0.64±0.04	90	VM=8.4±4.6 mg/kg/day (dose dependent)	hepatic 95%	phenytoin
0.8	20	0.78±0.62	hepatic 30%-90% renal 10%-70%	primidone (t½ about 8 hours) phenobarbital (t½ about 96 hours) phenylethyl malonamide (t½, about 30 hours)
0.13±0.04	80-94	0.12±0.04	hepatic 96%	valproic acid

methadione. Recent data suggest that the risk of severe blood dyscrasias is similar for phenytoin and carbamazepine. Although the risk of blood dyscrasias is diminished after the first year of treatment, the physician should be alert to their possible occurrence. The mortality from aplastic anemia is particularly high and recovery is slow in surviving patients.

Baseline liver function studies should be performed before antiepileptic drug treatment is initiated, and patients should be instructed to report promptly any symptoms of hepatotoxicity, such as jaundice, dark urine, anorexia, abdominal discomfort, or other gastrointestinal symptoms. Severe, sometimes fatal, hepatitis has occurred with phenacemide and more rarely with other antiepileptic drugs, including the hydantoins, carbamazepine, and valproic acid. Since this drug-induced hepatitis is probably idiosyncratic, the value of performing periodic laboratory studies in asymptomatic patients is doubtful. Patients receiving phenacemide and valproic acid (see the evaluation) may be exceptions, for abnormal results of liver function tests may herald the development of serious hepatic disease. As with most idiosyncratic reactions, the vulnerable period is the first three to six months of treatment.

Nephropathies have developed occasionally during antiepileptic therapy especially with trimethadione and paramethadione. These reactions usually develop insidiously. The appearance of any significant renal abnormality is an indication for discontinuing the drug.

Antiepileptic drugs can cause intermittent porphyria and lymphadenopathy.

A frequently cited paradoxical effect of antiepileptic drugs is the tendency of agents effective for one type of seizure to aggravate or precipitate seizures of another type. However, seizure types tend to be mixed in epileptic disorders, and the apparent aggravation of one type very often is a manifestation of the natural course of disease and reflects the ineffectiveness of the particular drug for that type of seizure. Alternatively, the aggravation may be due to multiple drug therapy. Carbamazepine has been reported to exacerbate atypical absence seizures in children with mixed partial and generalized epilepsy (Snead and Hosey, 1985). However, these children also were receiving other antiepileptic drugs and the increase in seizure frequency may have resulted from increased metabolism of the other antiepileptic drugs following enzyme induction by carbamazepine. Failure to maintain therapeutic serum concentrations of other antiepileptic drugs as carbamazepine is integrated into the regimen may increase seizure frequency. Some authorities believe that increasing doses of phenytoin may exacerbate seizures and that seizure control is obtained by reducing the dose. In general, precipitation of seizures by antiepileptic drugs probably is rare. There is no question, however, that their abrupt withdrawal can precipitate seizures. When a drug is to be discontinued, the dose should be reduced gradually unless rapid withdrawal and substitution of another drug is mandatory because of a serious adverse reaction.

Drug Interactions: The potential for antiepileptic drug interactions is considerable since a number of the most commonly used antiepileptic drugs share one or more of the following characteristics: (1) enzyme induction and/or inhibition of hepatic microsomal enzymes involved in biotransformation; (2) acidic pH and alteration of the protein binding of some drugs commonly used in combination for mixed epilepsies; and (3) administration for long periods.

Most drug interactions are pharmacokinetic, but some are pharmacodynamic (they produce additive central nervous system depression). The pharmacokinetically based drug interactions commonly increase (promote toxicity) or decrease (result in therapeutic failure) drug serum concentrations. Fortunately, two major approaches are available to evaluate drug interactions: (1) patient monitoring for signs and symptoms of toxicity, and (2) therapeutic drug monitoring (there is a reasonably good correlation between therapeutic failure or toxicity and the serum concentrations of most antiepileptic drugs).

Table 5 summarizes the average daily maintenance doses and therapeutic serum concentrations of commonly used antiepileptic drugs, signs and symptoms of acute toxicity, and drug interactions that affect drug serum concentrations (Eadie and Tyrer, 1980; So and Penry, 1981; Perucca, 1982). For interactions of antiepileptic drugs with other drugs, see the evaluations and Chapter 3, Drug Interactions and Adverse Drug Reactions.

Use in Pregnancy: Although the risk of congenital abnormalities with use of antiepileptic drugs during pregnancy is small, the benefit must be weighed carefully against the risk for each patient. Women of childbearing age who are receiving antiepileptic drugs should be informed that the chance of having a normal child is greater than 90%, but the risk of a congenital malformation may be about two to three times greater than in the general population because of the drug and/or the disease. It is not possible to determine whether malformations result from epilepsy in general, genetic predisposition to both epilepsy and these birth defects, antiepileptic drugs (either as a result of their direct action or pharmacokinetic distribution), or drug-induced deficiency states. The best evidence indicates that all these factors probably are contributory.

The most common major malformations are cleft lip and/or palate and congenital heart disease. The incidence of congenital heart disease in the general population is approximately 5/1,000 births, and the incidence of cleft lip/palate is approximately 2/1,000 births. In children born to epileptic women taking antiepileptic drugs, the incidence of both defects is approximately 18/1,000 (Committee on Maternal and Fetal Medicine, American College of Obstetricians and Gynecologists, 1984).

Most congenital malformations have been associated with use of phenytoin or phenobarbital, either alone or in combination, which may reflect their wider use. The pattern of some abnormalities caused by hydantoins and barbiturates has been referred to as the "fetal hydantoin syndrome" or "fetal barbiturate syndrome." However, the evidence is insufficient to firmly establish the existence of such syndromes.

Trimethadione is used less often than phenytoin and phenobarbital but is a very potent teratogen; birth defects or spontaneous abortions have occurred in 80% of conceptuses exposed to this agent in utero. Trimethadione should not be prescribed for females of childbearing age unless absolutely necessary; if pregnancy occurs during treatment, the patient should have the option of terminating it. Spina bifida recently has been associated with use of valproic acid; several case-control studies indicate that the incidence may be 1% to 2% in children of women taking this drug.

Presently, there is no reason to substitute other antiepileptic drugs for phenytoin, phenobarbital, or valproic acid in the pregnant patient. In women desiring to become pregnant, some authorities consider substituting carbamazepine for other antiepileptic drugs and evaluating its effectiveness prior to pregnancy. Withdrawal of effective antiepileptic medications may lead to seizures with serious consequences for mother and fetus.

See also the discussion on avoiding adverse drug reactions during pregnancy in Chapter 3.

Serum concentrations of antiepileptic drugs tend to decrease during pregnancy. The concentrations should be monitored frequently and the dosage adjusted accordingly. Monitoring should continue for six months postpartum. Fetal monitoring is recommended during labor because depression of clotting factors and hemorrhages may occur. The administration of vitamin K to the mother during labor and to the infant is recommended. Bleeding and coagulation studies should be performed periodically during the first 24 to 48 hours and additional vitamin K administered if required.

Nursing is not contraindicated in mothers receiving antiepileptic medications; however, drug concentrations in the nursing infant may require monitoring if problems develop (eg, sedation in the infant induced by phenobarbital, primidone, or the benzodiazepines).

Drug Evaluations

COMMONLY USED ANTICONVULSANTS

CARBAMAZEPINE
[Tegretol]

ACTIONS AND USES. This tricyclic (iminostilbene) compound is related chemically to the tricyclic antidepressant, imipramine. It has potent antiepileptic properties and is effective alone or with other antiepileptic drugs in partial seizures, especially complex partial seizures, generalized tonic-clonic seizures, and combinations of these seizure types. Carbamazepine is ineffective for and may exacerbate absence, myoclonic, and atonic seizures.

Comparative clinical trial data indicate that carbamazepine is more effective than other antiepileptic drugs in simple and complex partial seizures, but individual responses vary (Mattson et al, 1985). Many clinicians consider carbamazepine a drug of choice for initial therapy, especially in children and women. This drug is increasingly preferred to phenobarbital in

pediatric patients because it has less effect on alertness and behavior. It is reported to have psychotropic activity that may increase alertness and elevate mood in depressed epileptic patients, but not in otherwise normal patients.

ADVERSE REACTIONS AND PRECAUTIONS. Reactions that occur most commonly during early treatment are drowsiness, dizziness, lightheadedness, ataxia, nausea, and vomiting. These side effects usually subside spontaneously within a week or after a reduction in dose. They may be minimized by initiating therapy with a small dose and increasing it gradually. Less common neurologic reactions include confusion, headache, fatigue, blurred vision, transient diplopia and oculomotor disturbances, dysphasia, abnormal involuntary movements, peripheral neuritis and paresthesias, depression with agitation, talkativeness, nystagmus, and tinnitus. Rarely, certain childhood seizures increase when carbamazepine is administered (Snead and Hosey, 1985).

Gastrointestinal reactions include gastric distress and abdominal pain, diarrhea, constipation, and anorexia. Dryness of the mouth, glossitis, and stomatitis also occur.

Dermatologic reactions (pruritic and erythematous rashes, urticaria, Stevens-Johnson syndrome, photosensitivity, altered skin pigmentation, exfoliative dermatitis, alopecia, hyperhidrosis, erythema multiforme, erythema nodosum, and aggravation of systemic lupus erythematosus) occur in 6% of patients. They usually necessitate discontinuation of carbamazepine.

Hematopoietic reactions (leukopenia, agranulocytosis, eosinophilia, leukocytosis, purpura, aplastic anemia, and thrombocytopenia) are rare but may be serious; aplastic anemia and thrombocytopenia may be fatal. Leukopenia occurs only rarely in younger people. Since its onset is gradual and reversible upon dosage reduction, patients should be advised to notify their physician if fever, sore throat, aphthous stomatitis, easy bruising, petechial or purpuric hemorrhage, or other signs of hematologic toxicity appear. It should be noted that a modest depression of the neutrophil count is common and does not necessitate discontinuation of the drug.

Cardiovascular, genitourinary, metabolic, hepatic, and other reactions have been reported rarely. These include aggravation of hypertension or ischemic heart disease, arrhythmias, hypotension, syncope, edema, hyponatremia, congestive heart failure, recurrence of thrombophlebitis, urinary frequency, acute urinary retention, albuminuria, glycosuria, elevated blood urea nitrogen levels, microscopic deposits in the urine, impotence, cholestatic and hepatocellular jaundice, fever and chills, lymphadenopathy, myalgia and arthralgia, leg cramps, and conjunctivitis.

Water intoxication caused by inappropriate secretion of antidiuretic hormone occurs occasionally and may be related to high serum concentrations of carbamazepine. Clinical signs of severe water retention are lethargy, weakness, nausea, vomiting, confusion or hostility, neurologic abnormalities, stupor, and convulsions.

Baseline blood and platelet counts, urinalysis, and hepatic and renal function studies should be performed before initiating treatment and at regular intervals during treatment. However, excessively frequent and specialized monitoring is unwarranted and costly (Hart and Easton, 1982). Complete

TABLE 5.
SERUM CONCENTRATIONS AND RELATED DRUG INTERACTIONS
OF COMMONLY USED ANTIEPILEPTIC DRUGS

Drug	Average Daily Maintenance Dose		Usual Therapeutic Serum Concentration Range (mcg/ml)	Signs and Symptoms Usually Associated with Elevated Serum Concentrations or Toxicity of Cited Drugs
	Adults (mg/kg)	Children (mg/kg)		
Carbamazepine [Tegretol]	10-20	20-30	4-12	Vertigo, lethargy, nystagmus, blurred vision, diplopia, confusion, ataxia, stupor
Clonazepam [Klonopin]	0.05-0.2	0.1-0.2	0.02-0.08	Sedation, confusion, slurred speech, somnolence, respiratory depression, coma, hypotension
Ethosuximide [Zarontin]	20-40	20-30	40-100	Nausea, vomiting, gastric distress, drowsiness, ataxia
Phenobarbital	2-3	3-5	15-40 10-25	Sedation, drowsiness, slurred speech, nystagmus, confusion, somnolence, ataxia, respiratory depression, coma, hypotension
Primidone [Mysoline]	10-25	10-25	5-21	Same as phenobarbital
Phenytoin [Dilantin]	3-5	4-7	10-20	Vertigo, ataxia, slurred speech, nystagmus, diplopia, somnolence, coma (arrhythmias with rapid intravenous administration)

Pharmacodynamic and/or Pharmacokinetic Interactions with Other Antiepileptics by Cited Antiepileptic Drug	Antiepileptic Drugs that Alter Serum Concentration of Cited Drug		Nonantiepileptic Drugs that Alter Serum Concentration of Cited Drug	
	Increase	Decrease	Increase	Decrease
Carbamazepine decreases serum concentration of clonazepam, diazepam, ethosuximide, phenytoin, phenobarbital, primidone, and valproic acid by enzyme induction, but extent and incidence vary greatly among patients for all of these drug interactions.		Carbamazepine (autoinduction) Phenobarbital (infrequent in man) Phenytoin	Erythromycin Isoniazid Propoxyphene Troleandomycin	
Clonazepam does not appear to produce any consistent change in serum concentration of carbamazepine, phenobarbital, phenytoin, or primidone. Pharmacodynamically, it may exhibit additive central nervous system depression with any other agent that also has this action.		Carbamazepine Phenytoin Phenobarbital Primidone		
Ethosuximide does not produce any significant consistent change in serum concentration of other antipileptic drugs.		Carbamazepine Phenobarbital Phenytoin Primidone		
Phenobarbital infrequently increases biotransformation of phenytoin by enzyme induction, thus reducing the serum concentration. However, these effects may be partially or completely offset by phenobarbital's inhibition of phenytoin metabolism. The net effect on phenytoin concentrations is variable. Pharmacodynamically, phenobarbital may produce additive central nervous system depression with any other antiepileptic drug that has a sedative action.	Phenytoin Valproic Acid	Carbamazepine Phenytoin (sometimes)		Folic Acid
Same as phenobarbital	Same as phenobarbital		Isoniazid	
Phenytoin may reduce serum concentration of carbamazepine, valproic acid, ethosuximide, and primidone by enzyme induction. The effect on serum concentration of phenobarbital is variable.	Valproic Acid (note also decrease—see Valproic Acid for Mechanism)	Carbamazepine Phenobarbital (infrequent in man) Valproic Acid	Chloramphenicol Cimetidine Dicumarol Disulfiram Isoniazid Phenylbutazone Sulfonamides Trimethoprim	Folic Acid Alcohol (chronic ingestion) Diazoxide

(Continued on next page)

TABLE 5 (continued)

Drug	Average Daily Maintenance Dose		Usual Therapeutic Serum Concentration Range (mcg/ml)	Signs and Symptoms Usually Associated with Elevated Serum Concentrations or Toxicity of Cited Drugs
	Adults (mg/kg)	Children (mg/kg)		
Valproic Acid [Depakene, Depakote]	15-30 (monotherapy) 30-45 (combination therapy)	20-30 (monotherapy) 40-60 (combination therapy)	50-100	Sedation, gastric disturbance, diarrhea, ataxia, somnolence, coma

blood counts should be performed every two weeks for the first two months and quarterly thereafter if no abnormalities appear. Patients should be instructed to contact their physician immediately if petechiae, pallor, weakness, fever, or infection occurs.

PREGNANCY. Assessing the teratogenic potential of carbamazepine is difficult because of its use with other agents and because the epileptic disorder also contributes to this effect. Although more data are required, birth defects may be increased when carbamazepine is used with other antiepileptic drugs (Rosa, 1983), and the risks and benefits of drug therapy should be weighed. This drug is classified in FDA Pregnancy Category C.

DRUG INTERACTIONS. Since carbamazepine is chemically related to the tricyclic compounds, it should not be administered to patients who are sensitive to these drugs. The possibility of activating latent psychosis or inducing confusion or agitation in elderly patients also exists.

Approximately 60% to 70% of carbamazepine is bound to plasma albumin, but it is not displaced by acidic drugs as phenytoin is and it does not displace the latter. Carbamazepine decreases the serum concentration of clonazepam, diazepam, ethosuximide, phenytoin, phenobarbital, primidone, and valproic acid, as a result of enzyme induction, and phenytoin decreases the serum concentration of carbamazepine. Erythromycin, isoniazid, propoxyphene, and troleandomycin increase the serum concentration of carbamazepine. Carbamazepine is a potent enzyme inducer and, like phenytoin, it may be expected to decrease the effectiveness of oral anticoagulants, certain antibiotics (tetracycline, rifampin, and chloramphenicol), oral contraceptives, and quinidine.

PHARMACOKINETICS. The oral absorption of carbamazepine is variable; peak serum concentrations after use of solid dosage forms occur 6 to 12 hours after initiation of therapy (Bertilsson, 1978) and as early as two to three hours after chronic administration. Absorption is about 70% when the drug is taken with meals. With monotherapy, the usual therapeutic serum concentration is 4 to 12 mcg/ml, but concentrations as high as 17 mcg/ml may be required to control seizures without producing unacceptable adverse reactions or toxicity. With concomitant use of other antiepileptic drugs, concentrations as low as 4 mcg/ml may be associated with toxicity.

Carbamazepine is metabolized in the liver to an active 10,11-epoxide derivative, which has a shorter half-life than the parent compound. Carbamazepine induces its own metabolism; as a result, the usual initial mean half-life of 35 hours is reduced to 12 ± 6 hours (adults) or 8 ± 4 hours (children) after three or four weeks of administration. Pregnancy does not appear to alter plasma steady-state concentrations (Battino et al, 1985).

For other pharmacokinetic data, see Table 4.

DOSAGE AND PREPARATIONS.
Oral: Children under 6 years, 100 mg daily; *6 to 12 years,* 100 mg twice daily on the first day. The amount is increased by 100 mg daily at appropriate intervals (usually one to two weeks) and given in three or four divided doses until the desired response is obtained (usual maximum dose, 1 g). The usual maintenance dose is 400 to 800 mg (20 to 30 mg/kg) daily; the frequency of administration must be individualized. *Adults and adolescents,* initially, 400 mg divided into two doses on the first day, increased by 200 mg daily at appropriate intervals (usually one to two weeks) and administered in three or four

Pharmacodynamic and/or Pharmacokinetic Interactions with Other Antiepileptics by Cited Antiepileptic Drug	Antiepileptic Drugs that Alter Serum Concentration of Cited Drug		Nonantiepileptic Drugs that Alter Serum Concentration of Cited Drug	
	Increase	Decrease	Increase	Decrease
In patients already receiving phenobarbital, addition of valproic acid increases serum phenobarbital by 25% to 68%. This interaction can lead to marked sedation and is therefore potentially serious.		Carbamazepine Phenobarbital Primidone Phenytoin		
Valproic acid initially may increase the free phenytoin concentration within a few days usually followed by a fall in the total phenytoin concentration within several weeks; in turn, this is followed by a gradual return to normal within one to four months. (See the drug interaction section of the evaluation on Valproic Acid for an explanation of the mechanism of this complex interaction.)				
Valproic acid displaces diazepam from protein binding sites and may augment sedative action of diazepam, especially early in therapy.				
Valproic acid inhibits parahydroxylation of phenobarbital, thus increasing its serum concentration.				

divided doses. The usual maintenance dose is 800 mg to 1.2 g (10 to 20 mg/kg) daily. The usual maximum dose is 1 g daily in *children 12 to 15 years* and 1.2 g in patients *over 15 years*. Up to 2 g daily has been given to *adults* when necessary.

Tegretol (Geigy). Tablets 200 mg; tablets (chewable) 100 mg.

CLONAZEPAM
[Klonopin]

ACTIONS AND USES. Clonazepam may be useful alone or with other drugs to control myoclonic or atonic seizures and photosensitive epilepsy (Browne, 1978). Although this drug also is effective in absence seizures, tolerance develops and breakthrough seizures usually occur after one or two months. Increasing the dose may re-establish partial control in some patients. For this reason, ethosuximide or valproic acid is preferred. In addition, the incidence of drowsiness and ataxia is higher with prolonged use of clonazepam than with ethosuximide. Although sedation and tolerance may limit its usefulness, these effects have not occurred consistently (Mikkelsen et al, 1981).

Clonazepam may be helpful in status epilepticus, but parenteral forms are not available.

Clonazepam is seldom effective in generalized tonic-clonic or partial seizures and actually increased the number of generalized tonic-clonic seizures in some patients.

In sleep-related nocturnal myoclonus, a nonepileptic condition affecting adults, consciousness or awareness is not altered but episodic repetitive leg jerks occur during the night and cause insomnia and daytime sleepiness; uncontrollable movements of the legs without myoclonic jerks is a variant (restless legs syndrome). Anecdotal and open studies support the use of clonazepam in these conditions (Boghen, 1980). Attacks are suppressed or eliminated by doses of 0.5 mg taken at bedtime or three times a day.

ADVERSE REACTIONS AND PRECAUTIONS. The most common adverse reactions of clonazepam affect the central nervous system. Approximately one-half of patients experience drowsiness, about one-third ataxia, and up to one-quarter personality changes. These effects appear to be dose related, occur early in the course of therapy, and may partially subside with long-term administration. The sedation may be minimized by initiating therapy with a small dose and increasing the amount gradually. Other neurologic effects include abnormal eye movements, slurred speech, tremor, vertigo, and confusion.

Minor, but sometimes troublesome, reactions involving the cardiovascular, gastrointestinal, and genitourinary systems have been observed. Skin rashes, anemia, leukopenia, thrombocytopenia, and eosinophilia also have occurred. Clonazepam causes respiratory depression and hypersecretion in the upper respiratory passages; therefore, it should be used with caution in individuals with respiratory tract disease. This drug is contraindicated in those with a history of sensitivity to the benzodiazepines, significant liver disease, or acute angle-closure glaucoma.

Both psychological and physical dependence have been reported; withdrawal symptoms similar to those observed for the barbiturates have occurred following sudden withdrawal of clonazepam. Rapid withdrawal may precipitate status epilepticus. This drug is classified as a Schedule IV substance under the Controlled Substances Act.

The effects of clonazepam on the fetus and nursing infant are not known; therefore, this drug should be used during pregnancy only if the expected benefits outweigh the potential hazards (see the Introduction). Nursing infants should be monitored for excessive sedation.

DRUG INTERACTIONS. Interactions between clonazepam and other antiepileptic drugs usually are not significant. Clonazepam does not consistently alter the serum concentrations of carbamazepine, phenobarbital, phenytoin, or primidone, but carbamazepine, phenytoin, phenobarbital, and primidone may decrease the serum concentration of clonazepam. Additive central nervous system depression may occur when clonazepam is given with another drug that has this action, especially barbiturates. The combination of clonazepam and valproic acid has been associated with nonconvulsive spike wave stupor in a few patients.

PHARMACOKINETICS. Peak serum concentrations occur one to three hours after oral administration. The mean plasma half-life in adults ranges from 23 ± 5 hours to 34 ± 8 hours; the half-life in children is 23 ± 10 hours. Seizure control is usually achieved with serum concentrations of 0.02 to 0.08 mcg/ml. It should be noted that clonazepam serum concentrations are affected by enzyme induction of other drugs given concomitantly. For other pharmacokinetic data, see Table 4.

DOSAGE AND PREPARATIONS.
Oral: Adults, initially, 1.5 mg daily in three divided doses, increased by 0.5 to 1 mg every third day until seizures are adequately controlled or adverse effects intervene (maximum, 20 mg daily). The daily maintenance dose is usually 0.05 to 0.2 mg/kg. *Infants and children up to 10 years or 30 kg,* 0.01 to 0.03 (maximum, 0.05) mg/kg daily in two or three divided doses, increased by 0.25 to 0.5 mg every third day until a maintenance dose of 0.1 to 0.2 mg/kg/day has been reached.
   Klonopin (Roche). Tablets 0.5, 1, and 2 mg.

DIAZEPAM
[Valium, Valrelease]

ACTIONS AND USES. Intravenous diazepam is potentially life-saving in continuous tonic-clonic status epilepticus and is a drug of choice for initial control of seizures because of its almost immediate onset of action. Therapeutic serum concentrations are achieved in two to six minutes (Woodbury et al, 1982). Its duration of action is short due to rapid redistribution from the brain, and a loading dose of intravenous phenytoin sodium should be given concomitantly or immediately after control of seizures to maintain antiepileptic activity. Intravenous diazepam also may be useful with or as an alternative to magnesium sulfate to control the seizures of eclampsia. A rectal solution (not available in the United States) appears to be useful for status epilepticus in children.

Oral diazepam is sometimes helpful as an adjunct to other antiepileptic drugs in myoclonic spasms and atonic seizures, which often do not respond to other drugs.

ADVERSE REACTIONS AND PRECAUTIONS. When diazepam is given parenterally for status epilepticus, the patient must be observed for signs of respiratory and central nervous system depression and hypotension, especially when it is administered with other antiepileptic agents. Young and elderly patients are most vulnerable. However, the overall safety of the drug appears to compare favorably with that of other agents used for this emergency. The injectable form contains sodium benzoate and benzoic acid as buffers, which have been shown to displace bilirubin from albumin in vitro; thus, the possibility of kernicterus in newborn infants must be considered.

The most common adverse effects after oral use are drowsiness, dizziness, fatigue, and ataxia, which are dose related. Paradoxical excitement or stimulation occurs infrequently.

For further information on adverse reactions, precautions, drug interactions, and other uses, see Chapters 5, Drugs Used for Anxiety and Sleep Disorders; 12, Drugs Used in Disorders Affecting Skeletal Muscle; and 17, Adjuncts to Anesthesia. Diazepam is classified as a Schedule IV substance under the Controlled Substances Act.

PHARMACOKINETICS. Onset of action is almost immediate after intravenous administration. The volume of distribution is reported to be 0.95 to 2 L/kg. The half-lives of diazepam and its active derivative, desmethyldiazepam, are 27 to 37 and 50 to 100 hours, respectively; however, rapid redistribution out of the brain occurs within 30 minutes after injection, which reduces its effectiveness.

Effective plasma concentrations of diazepam and desmethyldiazepam have not been determined definitively, but minimal concentrations of 0.3 to 0.7 mcg/ml are required to terminate status epilepticus. The plasma concentration of diazepam exceeds 0.5 mcg/ml immediately after intravenous injection. Concentrations between 0.1 and 1 mcg/ml have been reported after long-term oral therapy.

For complete pharmacokinetic data, see Chapter 5, Drugs Used for Anxiety and Sleep Disorders.

DOSAGE AND PREPARATIONS.
Intravenous (slow): For status epilepticus, see Table 3.
   Valium (Roche). Solution 5 mg/ml in 2 and 10 ml containers.
Oral: Adults, 2 to 10 mg two to four times daily, beginning with a small dose and increasing the amount gradually. *Elderly or debilitated patients,* initially, 2 mg. *Children,* initially, 2 to 4 mg daily in divided doses; subsequent doses are lower than those

used for adults. A timed-release form (capsules, 15 mg) should be used only when it has been determined that 5 mg three times daily is the optimal daily dose.

   Valium (Roche), *Generic.* Tablets 2, 5, and 10 mg.
   Valrelease (Roche). Capsules (timed-release) 15 mg.

ETHOSUXIMIDE
[Zarontin]

ACTIONS AND USES. Ethosuximide is the drug of choice for absence seizures unaccompanied by other types of seizures. It abolishes seizures in 50% of patients and reduces seizure frequency by one-half in another 25%; some reports indicate that it controls absence seizures in 90% of newly diagnosed patients. Ethosuximide is preferred to other succinimides because it is more effective and less likely to produce drowsiness and gastrointestinal upset. Although valproic acid is equally effective, the rare but serious hepatotoxicity caused by this drug favors the initial use of ethosuximide.

   Ethosuximide also may be effective in myoclonic seizures and akinetic epilepsy but is generally ineffective in complex partial or generalized tonic-clonic seizures.

ADVERSE REACTIONS AND PRECAUTIONS. The most common adverse reactions are gastrointestinal disturbances (eg, nausea, vomiting, anorexia). Drowsiness, ataxia, headache, dizziness, euphoria, hiccup, rash, urticaria, and behavioral changes have been observed occasionally. Psychotic reactions with hallucinations may occur at high serum concentrations, but they seldom occur in young children with typical absence seizures who have no previous history of psychiatric disturbances. Serious untoward effects occur less frequently than with trimethadione and paramethadione. Systemic lupus erythematosus, aplastic anemia, thrombocytopenia, leukopenia, pancytopenia, and eosinophilia have been reported rarely. (See also the Introduction.)

   Psychometric studies on the effect of ethosuximide in children of normal intelligence who had absence seizures and minimal or no evidence of nervous system abnormalities have shown that the drug had a positive effect on test results in approximately one-half of the children (Browne and Feldman, 1983).

   Ethosuximide does not consistently alter the serum concentration of other antiepileptic drugs; however, carbamazepine, phenytoin, phenobarbital, and primidone may decrease the serum concentration of ethosuximide.

PHARMACOKINETICS. Ethosuximide is well absorbed orally and peak serum concentration occurs in one to four hours. The plasma half-life averages 30 ± 6 hours in children and 55 ± 5 hours in adults. Maximum control of absence seizures usually is achieved with serum concentrations of 40 to 100 mcg/ml. Concentrations up to 160 mcg/ml are sometimes tolerated. For other pharmacokinetic data, see Table 4.

DOSAGE AND PREPARATIONS.
Oral: Adults and children over 6 years, initially, 500 mg daily, increased, if necessary, by 250 mg every four to seven days until seizures are controlled or untoward effects develop. The daily maintenance dose is usually 20 to 40 mg/kg. Doses exceeding 1 g daily are seldom more effective than smaller amounts. *Children 3 to 6 years,* initially, 250 mg daily with incremental increases in dosage as for older patients. The daily maintenance dose is usually 20 to 30 mg/kg.

   Zarontin (Parke-Davis). Capsules 250 mg; syrup 250 mg/5 ml.

PHENOBARBITAL

PHENOBARBITAL SODIUM

ACTIONS AND USES. Phenobarbital, a long-acting barbiturate, is one of the most widely employed antiepileptic drugs. It is effective in generalized tonic-clonic and simple partial (with motor or somatosensory symptoms) seizures. Complex partial seizures do not respond as well, and absence seizures are not relieved and may be exacerbated. Phenobarbital is useful in seizures caused by barbiturate withdrawal in dependent individuals.

   This barbiturate often is used as the initial drug in young children. However, because of increasing concern about adverse neuropsychologic reactions to sedative/hypnotic antiepileptic drugs, some neurologists prefer less sedating drugs, such as carbamazepine, phenytoin, or valproic acid (Porter and Theodore, 1983).

   Phenobarbital sodium is used parenterally to treat status epilepticus, although diazepam or lorazepam is the initial drug of choice (see Table 3). A full antiepileptic dose should be given initially to prevent recurrence of seizures.

ADVERSE REACTIONS AND PRECAUTIONS. With the exception of significant cognitive and behavioral effects, phenobarbital may cause the least systemic toxicity of all antiepileptic drugs. Neurotoxicity is its major adverse effect. Drowsiness is the most common adverse reaction and, although tolerance usually develops, a significant percentage of patients continue to be bothered by sedation. A substantial number of adults develop depression. An occasional patient may become excitable; children and the elderly are most susceptible. In children, disturbances in cognitive function may be subtle and result in a decline in school performance (see the Introduction). Ataxia sometimes occurs; if it persists, a reduction in dosage is required.

   Barbiturates are contraindicated in patients with acute intermittent porphyria. Abrupt termination of therapy may exacerbate seizures, but drug dependence is unlikely with usual antiepileptic doses. (See also the Introduction.)

Skin eruptions are uncommon but rarely progress to exfoliative dermatitis. Megaloblastic anemia also is uncommon.

When phenobarbital is given during pregnancy, the possibility of congenital malformations or a coagulation defect and hemorrhage in the newborn must be considered (FDA Pregnancy Category D). Nursing infants whose mothers are receiving phenobarbital should be monitored for excessive sedation, since phenobarbital concentrations in milk may exceed those in maternal plasma (Nau et al, 1982).

DRUG INTERACTIONS. Phenobarbital infrequently increases the biotransformation of phenytoin by enzyme induction, thus reducing the latter's serum concentration. However, these effects may be partially or completely offset by the inhibition of phenytoin metabolism by phenobarbital. The net effect is unpredictable for a given patient. Phenobarbital may either increase or decrease the serum concentration of phenytoin. Conversely, phenytoin's effect on phenobarbital concentrations is variable.

Valproic acid increases and folic acid and carbamazepine decrease the serum concentration of phenobarbital.

Phenobarbital is a potent enzyme inducer and may decrease the effectiveness of oral anticoagulants, oral contraceptives, griseofulvin, quinidine, and certain antibiotics (chloramphenicol, rifampin, and tetracycline). Phenobarbital may produce additive central nervous system depression when used with another drug having a sedative action.

PHARMACOKINETICS. Phenobarbital is almost completely absorbed orally, but one to six hours may be necessary to achieve peak serum concentrations. Because of its long half-life, timed-release preparations are unnecessary. The drug also is well absorbed after intramuscular injection. The average plasma half-life is three to four days in children and five to six days in adults; consequently, three or more weeks are required to attain steady-state plasma concentrations. Doubling the dose for the first four days of therapy provides effective plasma concentrations more promptly, but sedation is prominent.

Serum concentrations of 15 to 40 mcg/ml are usually optimal for the control of epilepsy; concentrations greater than 40 mcg/ml are often accompanied by symptoms of toxicity, but higher concentrations may be tolerated by some patients. For other pharmacokinetic data, see Table 4.

DOSAGE AND PREPARATIONS.

PHENOBARBITAL:

Oral: Adults, 50 to 100 mg two times daily; alternatively, 2 to 3 mg/kg daily in two divided doses. *Children,* 15 to 50 mg two times daily; alternatively, 3 to 5 mg/kg daily in two divided doses. Administration once daily should be adequate in children and adults after the daily maintenance dose is determined. Due to phenobarbital's long half-life (120 to 144 hours in adults and 72 to 96 hours in children), the use of timed-release dosage forms is unnecessary.

Generic. Elixir 20 mg/5 ml; tablets 8, 16, 32, 65, and 100 mg.

PHENOBARBITAL SODIUM:

Intramuscular, Intravenous (slow): For status epilepticus, see Table 3.

Generic. Powder in 120 mg containers; solution 30, 60, 65, and 130 mg/ml in 1 ml containers.

PHENYTOIN
[Dilantin]

PHENYTOIN SODIUM
[Dilantin Sodium]

USES. Phenytoin is useful in generalized tonic-clonic, complex partial, and simple partial seizures and frequently is chosen for initial therapy, particularly in adults. Because of phenytoin's adverse reactions (hirsutism, gingival hyperplasia, coarsening of facial features), phenobarbital is often prescribed for infants and young children. Many authorities consider carbamazepine to be the major alternative to phenytoin when cosmetic adverse reactions are a concern. Phenytoin is commonly given with phenobarbital, primidone, carbamazepine, or valproic acid when monotherapy fails. It is ineffective in absence, myoclonic, and atonic seizures.

Intravenous phenytoin sodium is effective for status epilepticus (see Table 3) and can be used as the initial drug to terminate seizures, but its onset of action is much slower than that of diazepam. Therefore, it usually is given in addition to intravenous diazepam.

This drug also may prevent seizures in high-risk patients being treated for the alcohol withdrawal syndrome and in certain cases of head trauma (see the Introduction).

Phenytoin has been advocated for many other disorders, but conclusive evidence of effectiveness is inadequate for most proposed indications. However, the effectiveness of intravenous phenytoin in certain arrhythmias has been established (see Chapter 24, Antiarrhythmic Agents). Trigeminal neuralgia is sometimes relieved by phenytoin, but carbamazepine and baclofen are preferred (see Chapter 10, Drugs Used to Treat Neuralgias).

ADVERSE REACTIONS AND PRECAUTIONS. Phenytoin produces little or no sedation in usual amounts. Ataxia is a common effect of all hydantoins and requires dosage reduction. Although the evidence is conflicting, these drugs probably cause permanent cerebellar damage if toxic concentrations are maintained for prolonged periods. In very young patients, drug-induced ataxia may be confused with the natural unsteadiness of the toddler.

Ocular signs and symptoms, such as nystagmus and diplopia, may necessitate reduction of dosage. Peripheral neuropathy may develop after years of use. Skin eruptions occur frequently but are only rarely serious and are unrelated to the dose.

Gingival hyperplasia is common and often severe in children. Scrupulous oral hygiene may prevent secondary inflammation but has little or no effect on the incidence or severity of this complication. Repeated gingivectomies may be required if use of the drug is continued. (In children, gingival hyperplasia seldom occurs with mephenytoin and has not been reported with ethotoin.) Hypertrichosis and hirsutism are less common but do occur, especially in children.

Rare but serious idiosyncratic reactions include hepatitis, bone marrow depression, systemic lupus erythematosus, Stevens-Johnson syndrome, and lymphadenopathy resembling malignant lymphomas. Usually lymphadenopathy begins to disappear one to two weeks after therapy is discontinued. A few cases of true lymphoma and Hodgkin's disease have been reported and a causal relationship to hydantoin therapy seems possible.

Folic acid depletion may occur and sometimes causes megaloblastic anemia. Folic acid replacement, however, may increase the rate of phenytoin's metabolism and excretion, thus decreasing the antiepileptic action; thus, folic acid should not be administered routinely to patients without anemia.

Interference with vitamin D metabolism may cause osteomalacia but this has not occurred in noninstitutionalized, intellectually normal, ambulatory patients who receive adequate sunshine.

When phenytoin is given during pregnancy, the possibility of congenital malformations and coagulation defect with hemorrhage in the newborn infant must be considered. Low concentrations of phenytoin appear in breast milk. See the section on Adverse Reactions in the Introduction.

DRUG INTERACTIONS. Phenytoin may reduce the serum concentration of carbamazepine, valproic acid, ethosuximide, and primidone by enzyme induction. Phenytoin's effect on phenobarbital concentrations is variable. Phenytoin-carbamazepine combinations are becoming a more common regimen for partial and generalized seizures. Serum concentrations of both drugs should be monitored to assure that adequate serum concentrations of both agents are maintained.

Drugs that significantly increase the serum concentration of phenytoin include chloramphenicol, cimetidine, dicumarol, disulfiram, isoniazid, phenylbutazone, sulfonamides, and trimethoprim. Folic acid, prolonged ingestion of alcohol, carbamazepine, and possibly phenobarbital decrease the phenytoin serum concentration. The interaction of valproic acid with phenytoin is complex; serum concentrations of phenytoin may be increased or decreased (see Table 5 and the evaluation on Valproic Acid).

Phenytoin is a relatively potent enzyme inducer and decreases the effectiveness of oral anticoagulants, certain antibiotics (tetracycline, rifampin, and chloramphenicol), oral contraceptives, and quinidine.

PHARMACOKINETICS. Oral absorption is variable (30% to 97%) among patients but, except for alterations in gastrointestinal physiology, tends to remain constant in a given patient. Time to peak serum concentration ranges from 1.5 to 3 and 4 to 12 hours for prompt and timed-release phenytoin sodium capsules, respectively.

Plasma protein binding is 90%. The plasma half-life depends on the concentration and increases with higher serum concentrations; it is approximately 24 hours at concentrations less than 10 mcg/ml and 24 to 48 hours at concentrations of 10 to 20 mcg/ml.

Serum concentrations are not related linearly to the daily dose (dose-dependent or saturation kinetics), and small increases in dose greatly increase the serum concentration throughout the therapeutic range as saturation of drug metabolizing enzymes is approached. Serum concentrations of 10 to 20 mcg/ml are usually optimal. In general, concentrations above 20 mcg/ml are progressively associated with the following symptoms of toxicity: 20 mcg/ml, nystagmus; 30 mcg/ml, ataxia; and 40 mcg/ml, lethargy. However, doses producing these adverse reactions occasionally are tolerated when a therapeutic effect is otherwise unobtainable. The serum concentration of free phenytoin can be increased by hyperbilirubinemia (eg, in neonates, in those with liver disease), hypoalbuminemia (eg, in the elderly, in those with liver disease), and uremia. Salivary monitoring using appropriate precautions is a reproducible and consistent reflection of the serum concentration of free phenytoin (Knott et al, 1982).

Phenytoin's saturable kinetics accentuates the variations in the rate of dissolution and absorption among the various dosage forms and products. Thus, phenytoin serum concentrations may differ significantly from one product to another. If it is necessary to change products, serum concentrations should be determined and adjustments in dosage made to maintain optimum serum concentrations.

For other pharmacokinetic data, see Table 4.

DOSAGE AND PREPARATIONS.
Oral: The dosage must be individualized according to the patient's response and the drug serum concentrations. Initially, phenytoin may be administered in divided doses (usually twice daily). Once-daily administration usually is sufficient to maintain serum concentrations in the therapeutic range once steady state has been achieved and improves compliance. However, once-daily dosage may not be practical in patients who are bothered by adverse reactions at peak serum concentrations, in patients in whom good seizure control is not achieved, and in children because they metabolize phenytoin more rapidly.

Adults, initially, 300 mg daily in two divided doses; the maintenance dose is usually 300 to 400 mg or 3 to 5 mg/kg daily (maximum, usually 600 mg). Incremental increases can be made using chewable 50-mg tablets or 30-mg capsules. The tablets can be broken in half to provide further refinement of the dosage increment. There are formulation differences between tablet and capsules that may cause problems due to nonlinear kinetics. When mixing the two forms, the tablets (free acid phenytoin) contain 8% more phenytoin than the phenytoin sodium capsules. Many physicians avoid these difficulties by using only 100-mg and 30-mg capsules (Porter, 1984). *Children,* initially, 5 mg/kg daily in two divided doses with the maintenance dose individualized. A suggested initial maintenance dose is 4 to 7 mg/kg daily (maximum, 300 mg daily). *Children over 6 years* may require the minimum adult dose (300 mg daily).

PHENYTOIN:
Dilantin (Parke-Davis). Suspension 30 (pediatric) and 125 mg/5 ml (alcohol <0.6%); tablets (pediatric, chewable) 50 mg.
PHENYTOIN SODIUM:
Generic. Capsules (plain, timed-release) 100 mg.

Dilantin (Parke-Davis). Capsules (timed-release) 30 and 100 mg.
Additional Trademark.
Diphenylan (Lannett).
Intravenous: For status epilepticus, see Table 3.
   PHENYTOIN SODIUM:
   Dilantin (Parke-Davis), **Generic**. Solution 50 mg/ml in 2 and 5 ml containers.
Intramuscular: Intramuscular injection is not recommended, because it is painful, crystals are precipitated at the site of injection, and absorption is very erratic.

PRIMIDONE
[Mysoline]

ACTIONS AND USES. This deoxybarbiturate is closely related chemically to the barbiturates. It is converted to two active metabolites, phenobarbital and phenylethylmalonamide (PEMA). Primidone is used principally in generalized tonic-clonic and complex and simple partial seizures; some clinicians believe that the drug has specific usefulness for complex partial seizures. Recent data show that the failure rate with primidone is higher than with carbamazepine and phenytoin in the treatment of partial seizures (Mattson et al, 1985). This was attributed to a greater incidence of adverse reactions during initial therapy with primidone. In those patients able to tolerate this drug, antiepileptic effectiveness was equal to that of carbamazepine or phenytoin. Primidone is commonly given with phenytoin but monotherapy is often preferred. It is not effective in absence seizures.

ADVERSE REACTIONS AND PRECAUTIONS. Sedation is common but often diminishes with continued administration. As with phenobarbital, if the dose is increased gradually, incapacitating drowsiness may be avoided. Ataxia and some of the minor reactions caused by barbiturates also have been observed with primidone. Skin eruptions, such as maculopapular or morbilliform rash, are noted occasionally. Megaloblastic anemia, which responds to folic acid, has been reported.

In general, drug interactions are similar to those described for phenobarbital (see the evaluation). When the drug is given during pregnancy, the same precautions should be observed as with use of barbiturates (see the Introduction). Primidone, like the barbiturates, is contraindicated in patients with acute intermittent porphyria.

PHARMACOKINETICS. Primidone is rapidly and completely absorbed after oral administration; peak serum concentrations are attained in 30 minutes to 9 hours. Serum concentrations vary widely during long-term therapy but average approximately 1 mcg/ml per mg/kg of daily dose; 5 to 10 mcg/ml is the usual therapeutic range. Serum concentrations of phenobarbital produced by biotransformation of primidone average 2 mcg/ml per mg/kg of the daily dose of primidone; concentrations of PEMA are between the two. Because of the considerable interdosage fluctuation in steady-state primidone concen-

trations, it is often more convenient to adjust the dosage according to the serum concentrations of phenobarbital and the patient's response. Significant ataxia and lethargy usually occur when primidone concentrations acutely exceed 12 mcg/ml. It should be noted that much of the toxicity is related to PEMA and phenobarbital. Concentrations of primidone in excess of 20 mcg/ml may be well tolerated if phenobarbital concentrations are low. Primidone concentrations are sensitive to enzyme induction produced by other antiepileptic drugs.

For other pharmacokinetic data, see Table 4.

DOSAGE AND PREPARATIONS.
Oral: *Adults and older children,* 250 mg daily at bedtime to 2 g daily in divided doses; alternatively, 10 to 25 mg/kg daily in two or three divided doses. *Children under 8 years,* one-half the adult dosage; alternatively, 10 to 25 mg/kg daily in two or three divided doses. Adverse reactions may necessitate smaller doses with more gradual increase.
   Generic. Tablets 250 mg.
   Mysoline (Ayerst). Suspension 250 mg/5 ml; tablets 50 and 250 mg.

VALPROIC ACID
[Depakene, Depakote]

ACTIONS AND USES. Results of clinical trials with valproic acid (as sodium valproate) (Lewis, 1978; Bruni and Wilder, 1979; Browne, 1980) have shown that this drug reduced the frequency of several types of seizures, but was more effective in generalized than in partial seizures. It may be as effective as phenytoin in newly diagnosed cases of partial seizures.

Valproic acid is most useful in typical absence seizures and photosensitive seizures. Results were also promising in atypical absence seizures (variant of petit mal). It is as effective as ethosuximide in patients with absence seizures alone; although some clinicians prefer valproic acid, the American Academy of Pediatrics (Committee on Drugs, 1982) recommended that it be reserved for use when therapeutic failure or intolerance to ethosuximide occurs because valproic acid causes rare but potentially fatal hepatotoxicity. Valproic acid is considered the drug of choice by many neurologists for patients with both absence and generalized tonic-clonic seizures. Its efficacy is about the same as in patients with the latter type alone.

In the majority of patients studied with tonic-clonic seizures, valproic acid was added to the regimen when other antiepileptic drugs failed to maintain control. The frequency of seizures was reduced by 75% or more in about 50% of these patients. The dose of other antiepileptic drugs could be reduced in many patients, and it was possible to discontinue other drugs in a few. About 30% of patients failed to respond.

In a study evaluating the treatment of tonic-clonic or partial seizures, valproic acid and phenytoin were equally effective with respect to two-year remission time or time to first seizure following initiation of drug treatment (Turnbull et al, 1985). This drug may be preferred in many stimulus sensitive (reflex) epilepsies.

Valproic acid is the drug of choice in some adolescents and adults with juvenile myoclonic epilepsy. It is not effective for infantile spasms and may be dangerous in children receiving polytherapy.

In general, atonic and akinetic seizures in patients with Lennox-Gastaut syndrome are less responsive.

Since this drug has been useful in some patients refractory to all other antiepileptic drugs, it may warrant a trial in unresponsive patients regardless of seizure type.

ADVERSE REACTIONS AND PRECAUTIONS. Adverse reactions generally appear early in the course of therapy and are mild and transient. Hematologic and gastrointestinal reactions, sedation, elevated liver enzyme levels, and hyperammonemia usually are not major concerns when considering the benefit of valproic acid therapy. However, fatal hepatotoxicity has developed rarely.

The incidence of gastrointestinal disturbances (nausea, vomiting, anorexia, heartburn) ranges from 6% to 45% (Turnbull, 1983). Symptoms are transient and require drug withdrawal in only 0.9% of adults and 2.9% of children (Schmidt, 1984). The frequency of such reactions has been reduced by administering the enteric-coated preparation [Depakote] (Wilder et al, 1983 B). Diarrhea, abdominal cramps, and constipation were reported occasionally. Increased appetite with weight gain is common and can be controlled by diet; however, in some cases excessive weight gain may require drug withdrawal (Turnbull, 1983).

Sedation and drowsiness developed in about 5% of patients but in only 0.2% of those receiving valproic acid alone. These effects usually disappeared when the dose of concurrently administered antiepileptic drugs was reduced. Central nervous system stimulation and excitement have been observed when valproic acid was given alone, and aggressiveness and hyperactivity were noted in some children. Hand tremor, resembling benign essential tremor, is the most common neurologic adverse reaction with chronic therapy and occasionally is severe enough to interfere with writing. Tremor occurs more frequently with doses greater than 750 mg/day and may improve with dosage reduction (Turnbull, 1983). Other central nervous system effects reported rarely include ataxia and headache. In normal volunteers, cognitive impairment was less with valproic acid than with phenytoin.

Alopecia was reported in 2.6% to 12% of patients, was usually temporary, and did not necessitate withdrawal of the drug. Regrown hair may differ from the original in color and texture. Rash was observed rarely.

Valproic acid inhibits the secondary phase of platelet aggregation, but this is unlikely to be of clinical significance unless patients are receiving other drugs that affect coagulation. Prolonged bleeding times have been reported. Thrombocytopenia has been observed occasionally, but the incidence of this reaction is not known.

The benefit of determining bleeding time before initiating therapy is unproven. Platelet function should be monitored before surgery. Caution is recommended when administering drugs that affect coagulation to patients receiving valproic acid, and dosage adjustments should be made when necessary.

Rarely, severe or fatal pancreatitis has been reported and the physician should be prepared to treat this complication if severe abdominal pain and vomiting occur (Wyllie et al, 1984).

Transient elevations of liver transaminases (eg, serum glutamic oxaloacetic transaminase [SGOT]) are common. Liver enzyme levels often return to normal with or without dosage adjustment and usually are not related to serious liver dysfunction, but severe hepatotoxicity has occurred rarely when valproic acid was used as monotherapy (1/37,000 patients) and was relatively more common when this drug was used in polytherapy (1/6,500 patients) (Dreifuss and Santilli, 1986). Between 1978 and 1984, 37 fatalities related to valproic acid were reported, mostly in children. The risk of fatal hepatotoxicity was lowest in those over 2 years, especially if they received monotherapy, and was greatest in children from birth to 2 years receiving multiple antiepileptic drugs (1/500) and in patients with mental retardation, congenital abnormalities, and other neurologic diseases. Prodromal illness characterized by muscular weakness, lethargy, anorexia, and vomiting often was present. The reactions usually developed after an average of two months (range, three days to six months) of therapy.

Guidelines recommended by the American Academy of Pediatrics (Committee on Drugs, 1982) include: (1) Current standard therapy should be utilized initially whenever possible, eg, in absence and febrile seizures, although valproic acid is effective in many of these and other types of seizures. (2) Valproic acid should not be given to patients with hepatic disease or dysfunction, critically ill children, and children receiving other medication that affects coagulation. (3) Liver function should be assessed prior to therapy, three to five weeks after initiation of treatment, approximately monthly during the first six months of use, and periodically thereafter. (4) Patients and their parents should be instructed to report symptoms, such as malaise, lethargy, gastrointestinal distress, jaundice, easy bruising, and loss of seizure control, since laboratory assays alone are inadequate to diagnose valproic acid-induced hepatotoxicity. However, if laboratory tests indicate clinically important hepatic dysfunction, consideration should be given to discontinuing this drug. (5) Dosage should be maintained at the lowest amount that produces optimal seizure control. Routine monitoring of liver function does not always detect hepatotoxicity of rapid onset, since it may not be preceded by elevation of SGOT (Turnbull, 1983; Powell-Jackson et al, 1984; Green, 1984; Isom, 1984).

Valproic acid therapy commonly produces reversible hyperammonemia, but the clinical significance of this reaction in the absence of liver dysfunction is unknown. Although most pediatric patients were asymptomatic, the relationship between this reaction and acute confusional and stuporous states must be determined (Turnbull, 1983).

If other antiepileptic drugs, particularly barbiturates, are given concomitantly, serum levels should be determined periodically and the dosage adjusted to obtain optimum therapeutic concentrations.

Since valproic acid is partly eliminated as a ketone-containing metabolite, the urine ketone test may show false-positive results.

TERATOGENICITY. Valproic acid has teratogenic effects in mice, rats, and rabbits, usually manifested as increased resorption, retarded fetal growth, and major developmental abnormalities, including skeletal defects. The incidence was about the same as with phenytoin at similar dose levels. Neural tube abnormalities occurred in about 1% of infants whose mothers received valproic acid alone or with other antiepileptic drugs during pregnancy (Turnbull, 1983; Jeavons, 1984). Although an accurate estimate of risks cannot be determined precisely, physicians should carefully weigh the risks and benefits when prescribing valproic acid to women of childbearing age (FDA Pregnancy Category D). Low concentrations (3% of maternal serum concentration) of valproic acid appear in breast milk. (See the Introduction.)

OVERDOSAGE. One case of overdosage of valproic acid (36 g) taken with phenobarbital (1 g) and phenytoin (300 mg) has been reported. The patient became comatose about four hours after ingesting the drugs but gradually recovered and was discharged from the hospital the following day. On the other hand, overdosage of three times the daily recommended initial amount of valproic acid daily for five days was reported to cause profound lethargy and to be at least partially responsible for the death of one patient (Tift, 1980). The treatment of overdosage consists of general supportive measures, including maintenance of adequate urinary output to facilitate elimination of the drug. Intravenous naloxone 0.01 mg/kg reversed coma caused by valproic acid ingestion in one patient (Steiman et al, 1979).

DRUG INTERACTIONS. When valproic acid is given with phenobarbital, the serum phenobarbital concentration is increased by 25% to 68% (Rimmer and Richens, 1985); this can cause marked sedation or intoxication. Therefore, a 30% to 75% reduction in phenobarbital dosage is required when valproic acid is added to the regimen, and two to three weeks must elapse before a new steady-state level is achieved.

The interaction between valproic acid and phenytoin is complex (Hansten, 1981). Valproic acid displaces phenytoin from serum albumin, which temporarily increases the ratio of free/bound drug; toxicity may result if phenytoin concentrations were high prior to administration of valproic acid. The increased availability of free phenytoin decreases the total serum concentration by about 30% during the first several weeks of therapy but usually does not result in recurrence of seizures because the free phenytoin concentration does not change. However, valproic acid may also inhibit the biotransformation of phenytoin, which, over the next 4 to 16 weeks, produces a gradual return of phenytoin serum concentrations to previous values. Most patients do not require dosage adjustment, but phenytoin toxicity may develop or seizures may recur. Careful patient monitoring rather than aggressive therapeutic drug monitoring is recommended. (See also Table 5.) Free phenytoin measurements may be useful to explain the onset of central nervous system toxicity when the total serum phenytoin concentration is in the therapeutic range.

Valproic acid displaces diazepam from protein binding sites and may augment its sedative action.

Other interactions between valproic acid and phenobarbital, primidone, phenytoin, and carbamazepine result from the enzyme-inducing effects of the latter drugs, which reduce the half-life of valproic acid. The half-life was not affected by ethosuximide or the benzodiazepines. Valproic acid does not induce liver enzymes.

PHARMACOKINETICS. Valproic acid is absorbed rapidly and completely following oral administration; peak serum concentrations occur 1.5 to 2 hours after ingestion of liquid preparations and 1.5 to 4 hours after enteric-coated preparations. If taken with food, absorption is delayed but the bioavailability is unaffected. The plasma half-life is 11 ± 4 hours in children and 15 ± 7 hours in adults. The concomitant use of enzyme-inducing drugs decreases the half-life in children to 7 ± 4 hours and in adults to 10 to 12 hours. Therapeutic serum concentrations range from 50 to 100 mcg/ml. Active and toxic metabolites are formed during biotransformation but are present only in very low concentrations. Their importance has not been determined. For other pharmacokinetic data, see Table 4.

DOSAGE AND PREPARATIONS.
Oral: Adults, initially, 5 to 10 mg/kg daily; maintenance dose, 15 to 20 mg/kg/day. When used with other antiepileptic drugs, the initial dose is 10 mg/kg/day and the maintenance dose is 30 to 45 mg/kg/day. *Children*, initially, 10 to 15 mg/kg/day; maintenance dose, 20 to 30 mg/kg/day. When used with other antiepileptic drugs, the initial dose is 15 to 20 mg/kg/day and the maintenance dose is 40 to 60 mg/kg/day.
Depakene (Abbott). Capsules 250 mg; syrup 250 mg/5 ml (as sodium valproate).
Depakote (Abbott). Tablets (enteric-coated) 125, 250, and 500 mg (as divalproex sodium).

INFREQUENTLY USED ANTICONVULSANTS

ACETAZOLAMIDE
[Diamox]

This carbonic anhydrase inhibitor has been used in absence, generalized tonic-clonic, and partial seizures. It is most often administered as an adjunct to other drugs, but its usefulness is limited by the rapid development of tolerance in some patients. Acetazolamide is often helpful when intermittent administration is required (eg, in women whose seizure frequency increases with menstruation).

For adverse reactions and other uses, see Chapter 18, Agents Used to Treat Glaucoma, and Chapter 29, Diuretics.

DOSAGE AND PREPARATIONS.
Oral: Adults and children, 8 to 30 mg/kg daily in divided doses (range, 375 mg to 1 g daily).
Generic. Tablets 250 mg.
Diamox (Lederle). Tablets 125 and 250 mg.

LIDOCAINE HYDROCHLORIDE
[Xylocaine Hydrochloride]

As an alternative to general anesthesia, this local anesthetic is sometimes infused intravenously as a last resort in status epilepticus after the drugs of choice have failed. However, many epileptologists recommend that general anesthesia be used instead for prolonged status epilepticus. Overdosage of lidocaine causes convulsions and great care is required with its use. (See also Chapter 15, Local Anesthetics, and Chapter 24, Antiarrhythmic Agents.)

Caution should be exercised in patients receiving tocainide as an antiarrhythmic agent when lidocaine is given intravenously because of their additive effects.

DOSAGE AND PREPARATIONS.

Intravenous: Adults, initially, 100 mg, followed by 50 mg in 20 minutes; an appropriate maintenance dose then is administered by continuous infusion at a rate of 1 to 3 mg/min, using a pump if possible. Dosage should be reduced in patients with severe liver disease and heart failure. Control of seizures usually is achieved with the patient maintaining consciousness. Early symptoms and signs of overdose include hypotension, confusion, and tremors. The rate of infusion is reduced periodically until the drug can be discontinued; this may require several days. *Children,* 1.5 mg/kg initially, followed by 0.75 mg/kg in 20 minutes; the maintenance dose is 30 mcg/kg/min.

Generic. Solution (without preservatives) 1% and 2% in 2 to 50 ml containers.

Xylocaine Hydrochloride (Astra). Solution for bolus injection 2% in 5 ml containers; solution for preparation of infusion solutions only (without sodium chloride or preservatives) 4% in 25 and 50 ml containers; solution 20% in 5 and 10 ml containers.

MEPHOBARBITAL
[Mebaral]

Mephobarbital is metabolized to phenobarbital and thus has similar properties and uses, but larger doses must be given. There is no evidence that it has any advantage over phenobarbital. (See the Introduction and the evaluation on Phenobarbital.) This drug is classified in FDA Pregnancy Category D.

DOSAGE AND PREPARATIONS. The serum concentrations given for phenobarbital may be used as a guide to adjust the dosage of mephobarbital (see the evaluation).

Oral: Adults, 400 to 600 mg daily in divided doses. *Children* *under 5 years,* 16 to 32 mg three or four times daily; *over 5 years,* 32 to 64 mg three or four times daily.

Mebaral (Winthrop-Breon). Tablets 32, 50, 100, and 200 mg.

PARALDEHYDE

This drug may be used in status epilepticus when other agents are not effective. Intravenous administration must be slow or severe coughing ensues that may add to the difficulty of administration and may even cause pulmonary hemorrhage. Intramuscular injection can cause tissue necrosis and sterile abscess but is relatively safe if care is taken to avoid peripheral nerves. Rectal administration also is employed, most commonly in children; however, the dose is more difficult to control by this route and the absorption is very slow.

Fatalities have occurred with use of paraldehyde. Bronchopulmonary disease is a relative contraindication, since a significant amount is excreted by the lungs. The sedative effect may be intensified and prolonged in patients with liver disease. Thrombophlebitis is a frequent complication of intravenous administration. Coughing, possibly related to pulmonary edema, and hypotension have been reported.

DOSAGE AND PREPARATIONS. Outdated drug may be toxic. Plastic devices must be avoided; only glass syringes and containers and rubber tubing are advised.

Intramuscular, Intravenous: Intramuscular injection should be deep and no more than 5 ml should be given at a single site. Intravenous injection must be slow, preferably by drip, and the drug should be diluted to 8% or less in sodium chloride or 5% dextrose injection. Care should be taken to avoid extravasation.

Adults and children, for status epilepticus, doses vary but frequently exceed those for more benign conditions. The usual dose is 0.15 to 0.3 ml/kg; a moderate additional dose (0.05 ml/kg) may be needed, especially for smaller children. The dose may be repeated in two to six hours.

Generic. Liquid in 5 and 30 ml containers.

Rectal: Children, 0.3 ml/kg dissolved in an equal quantity of olive oil. Dilution in milk also has been suggested to improve tolerance.

Generic. Liquid in 30 ml containers.

TRIMETHADIONE
[Tridione]

USES. This drug is effective in absence seizures but should be reserved for refractory cases because of toxicity.

ADVERSE REACTIONS AND PRECAUTIONS. Serious reactions, some of which were fatal, include rash that may progress to exfoliative dermatitis or erythema multiforme, nephropathy, hepatitis, and bone marrow depression with aplastic anemia, neutropenia, or agranulocytosis. Pseudolymphomas, systemic lupus erythematosus, and a myasthenia gravis-like syndrome also have been reported. Drowsiness, alopecia, and hiccup may occur during early treatment. Reversible visual disturbances, particularly hemeralopia (defective vision in bright light), have been reported.

A high incidence of congenital abnormalities has been associated with the use of trimethadione during pregnancy. Accordingly, this drug should be avoided in females of child-bearing age. (See the Introduction.)

PHARMACOKINETICS. Trimethadione is rapidly and well absorbed orally; time to peak serum concentration is 0.5 to 2 hours. Protein binding is insignificant, and the volume of distribution is 60% of body weight. Trimethadione is demethylated by hepatic microsomal enzymes to the active metabolite, dimethadione, which has a half-life of 6 to 13 days. Serum concentrations of trimethadione average 0.6 mcg/ml per mg/kg of daily dose. The serum concentration of dimethadione averages 12 mcg/ml per mg/kg of daily dose and is used to guide dosage adjustment. Adequate seizure control is usually obtained with dimethadione concentrations above 700 mcg/ml.

DOSAGE AND PREPARATIONS.

Oral: Adults, initially, 900 mg daily in three or four divided doses, increased by 300 mg daily at weekly intervals to a maximum of 2.4 g daily. *Children,* initially, 40 mg/kg (300 to 900 mg) daily in three or four divided doses.

    Tridione (Abbott). Capsules 300 mg; solution 40 mg/ml; tablets (chewable) 150 mg.

PHENYTOIN SODIUM AND PHENOBARBITAL

Use of this fixed-dose combination of antiepileptic drugs is not advisable for initial therapy, since the dosage of each drug should be established *individually* in accordance with the clinical response and drug serum concentrations. Additionally, monotherapy should first be attempted to control seizures. If this has been done and the concentrations present in the mixture correspond to the ratio and quantities required, it may be used for convenience to improve compliance until a subsequent dosage adjustment is necessary.

    Dilantin with Phenobarbital (Parke-Davis). Each capsule contains phenytoin sodium 100 mg and phenobarbital 16 or 32 mg.

Cited References

Aird RB, et al: *The Epilepsies: A Critical Review.* New York, Raven Press, 1984.

Battino D, et al: Plasma concentrations of carbamazepine and carbamazepine-10,11-epoxide during pregnancy and after delivery. *Clin Pharmacokinet* 10:279-284, 1985.

Berg BO: Prognosis of childhood epilepsy: Another look. *N Engl J Med* 306:861-862, 1982.

Bertilsson L: Clinical pharmacokinetics of carbamazepine. *Clin Pharmacokinet* 3:128-143, 1978.

Boghen D: Successful treatment of restless legs with clonazepam, (letter). *Ann Neurol* 8:341, 1980.

Boshes LD: Rights of epileptic patient. *Chicago Med* 83:1109-1112, 1980.

Browne TR: Clonazepam. *N Engl J Med* 299:812-816, 1978.

Browne TR: Valproic acid. *N Engl J Med* 302:661-666, 1980.

Browne TR: Therapy of status epilepticus. *Compr Ther* 8:28-36, (May) 1982.

Browne TR, Feldman RG (eds): *Epilepsy: Diagnosis and Management.* Boston, Little, Brown and Company, 1983.

Bruni J, Wilder BJ: Valproic acid: Review of new antiepileptic drug. *Arch Neurol* 36:393-398, 1979.

Cloyd JC, et al: Status epilepticus: Role of intravenous phenytoin. *JAMA* 244:1479-1481, 1980.

Commission on Classification and Terminology of the International League Against Epilepsy: Proposal for revised clinical and electroencephalographic classification of epileptic seizures. *Epilepsia* 22:489-501, 1981.

Committee on Drugs, American Academy of Pediatrics: Valproic acid: Benefits and risks. *Pediatrics* 70:316-319, 1982.

Committee on Drugs, American Academy of Pediatrics: Behavioral and cognitive effects of anticonvulsants. *Pediatrics* 76:644-647, 1985.

Committee on Maternal and Fetal Medicine, American College of Obstetricians and Gynecologists: Anticonvulsants and pregnancy. *ACOG Committee Statement.* Washington, DC, ACOG, 1984.

Covanis A, et al: Sodium valproate: Monotherapy vs polytherapy. *Epilepsia* 23:693-720, 1982.

Delgado-Escueta AV, et al: Management of status epilepticus. *N Engl J Med* 306:1337-1340, 1982.

Dreifuss FE, Santilli N: Valproic acid hepatic fatalities: Analysis of United States cases. *Neurology* 36(suppl):175, 1986.

Eadie MJ, Tyrer JH: *Anticonvulsant Therapy: Pharmacological Basis and Practice,* ed 2. New York, Churchill Livingstone, 1980.

Emerson R, et al: Stopping medication in children with epilepsy: Predictors of outcome. *N Engl J Med* 304:1125-1129, 1981.

Freeman JM: Febrile seizures: Consensus of significance, evaluation, and treatment. *Pediatrics* 66:1009-1012, 1980.

Gordon N: Duration of treatment for childhood epilepsy. *Dev Med Child Neurol* 24:84-88, 1982.

Green SH: Sodium valproate and routine liver function tests. *Arch Dis Child* 59:813-814, 1984.

Hammond EJ, et al: Central actions of valproic acid in man and experimental models of epilepsy. *Life Sci* 29:2561-2574, 1981.

Hansten PD: Interactions of valproic acid with other anticonvulsants. *Drug Interact Newslett* 1:27-30, (July) 1981.

Hart RG, Easton JD: Carbamazepine and hematological monitoring. *Ann Neurol* 11:309-312, 1982.

Hauser WA, Kurland LT: Epidemiology of epilepsy in Rochester, Minnesota, 1935 through 1967. *Epilepsia* 16:1-66, 1975.

Hrachovy RA, et al: Controlled study of ACTH therapy in infantile spasms. *Epilepsia* 21:631-636, 1980.

Hvidberg EF, Dam M: Clinical pharmacokinetics of anticonvulsants. *Clin Pharmacokinet* 1:161-188, 1976.

Iivanainen M, Himberg J-J: Valproate and clonazepam in treatment of severe progressive myoclonus epilepsy. *Arch Neurol* 39:236-238, 1982.

Isom JB: On toxicity of valproic acid, (editorial). *Am J Dis Child* 138:901-903, 1984.

Jeavons PM: Non-dose-related side effects of valproate. *Epilepsia* 25(suppl 1):S50-S55, 1984.

Knott C, et al: Phenytoin-valproate interaction: Importance of saliva monitoring in epilepsy. *Br Med J* 284:13-16, 1982.

Korberly BH, et al: Ethotoin use in pediatric seizure patients. *Am J Dis Child* 135:1139-1140, 1981.

Leppik IE, et al: Double-blind study of lorazepam and diazepam in status epilepticus. *JAMA* 249:1452-1454, 1983.

Lewis JR: Valproic acid (Depakene): New anticonvulsant agent. *JAMA* 240:2190-2192, 1978.

Livingston S, et al: Medical treatment of epilepsy: Introduction. *Pediatr Ann* 8:210-274, 1979.

Martínez-Lage JM, et al: Progabide treatment in severe epilepsy: Double-blind cross-over trial versus placebo. *Epilepsia* 25:586-593, 1984.

Mattson RH, et al: Comparison of carbamazepine, phenobarbital, phenytoin, and primidone in partial and secondarily generalized tonic-clonic seizures. *N Engl J Med* 313:145-151, 1985.

Meldrum B: Amino acid neurotransmitters and new approaches to anticonvulsant drug action. *Epilepsia* 25(suppl 2):S140-S149, 1984.

Mikkelsen B, et al: Clonazepam (Rivotril) and carbamazepine (Tegretol) in psychomotor epilepsy: Randomized multicenter trial. *Epilepsia* 22:415-420, 1981.

Morris HH III: Current treatment of status epilepticus. *J Fam Pract* 13:987-991, 1981.

Nau H, et al: Anticonvulsants during pregnancy and lactation: Transplacental, maternal, and neonatal pharmacokinetics. *Clin Pharmacokinet* 7:508-543, 1982.

Penry JK, Newmark ME: Use of antiepileptic drugs. *Ann Intern Med* 90:207-218, 1979.

Penry JK, Porter RJ: Epilepsy: Mechanisms and therapy. *Med Clin North Am* 63:801-812, 1979.

Perucca E: Pharmacokinetic interactions with antiepileptic drugs. *Clin Pharmacokinet* 7:57-84, 1982.

Porter RJ: *Epilepsy: 100 Elementary Principles. Major Problems in Neurology.* Philadelphia, WB Saunders, vol 12, 1984.

Porter RJ, Theodore WH: Nonsedative regimens in treatment of epilepsy. *Arch Intern Med* 143:945-947, 1983.

Powell-Jackson PR, et al: Hepatotoxicity to sodium valproate: Review. *Gut* 25:673-681, 1984.

Reynolds EH, Shorvon SD: Single drug or combination therapy for epilepsy? *Drugs* 21:374-382, 1981.

Reynoids EH, Trimble MR: Adverse neuropsychiatric effects of anticonvulsants. *Drugs* 29:570-581, 1985.

Rimmer EM, Richens A: Update on sodium valproate. *Pharmacotherapy* 5:171-184, 1985.

Rosa FW: Pregnancy outcomes with maternal carbamazepine exposure. *ADR Highlights* 1-10, (Oct 13) 1983.

Schmidt D: Adverse effects of valproate. *Epilepsia* 25(suppl 1):S44-S49, 1984.

Shinnar S, et al: Discontinuing antiepileptic medication in children with epilepsy after two years without seizures: Prospective study. *N Engl J Med* 313:976-980, 1985.

Singer WD, et al: Effect of ACTH therapy upon infantile spasms. *J Pediatr* 96:485-489, 1980.

Snead OC III, Bearden LJ: Anticonvulsants specific for petit mal antagonist epileptogenic effect of leucine enkephalin. *Science* 210:1031-1033, 1980.

Snead OC III, Hosey LC: Exacerbation of seizures in children by carbamazepine. *N Engl J Med* 313:916-921, 1985.

Snead OC, et al: ACTH and prednisone in childhood seizure disorders. *Neurology* 33:966-970, 1983.

So EL, Penry JK: Epilepsy in adults. *Ann Neurol* 9:3-16, 1981.

Steiman GS, et al: Treatment of accidental sodium valproate overdose with opiate antagonist, (letter). *Ann Neurol* 6:274, 1979.

Thal LJ, et al: Treatment of myoclonus with L-5-hydroxytryptophan and carbidopa: Clinical, electrophysiological, and biochemical observations. *Ann Neurol* 7:570-576, 1980.

Thurston JH, et al: Prognosis in childhood epilepsy: Additional follow-up of 148 children 15 to 23 years after withdrawal of anticonvulsant therapy. *N Engl J Med* 306:831-836, 1982.

Tift JP: Valproic acid, (letter). *N Engl J Med* 303:394, 1980.

Turnbull DM: Adverse effects of valproate. *Adv Drug React Acc Pois Rev* 2:191-216, 1983.

Turnbull DM, et al: Which drug for adult epileptic patient: Phenytoin or valproate? *Br Med J* 290:815-819, 1985.

Van Woert MH, Hwang EC: Biochemistry and pharmacology of myoclonus, in Klawans HL (ed): *Clinical Neuropharmacology.* New York, Raven Press, vol 3, 1978, 167-184.

Wilbur R, Kulik FA: Anticonvulsant drugs in alcohol withdrawal: Use of phenytoin, primidone, carbamazepine, valproic acid, and sedative anticonvulsants. *Am J Hosp Pharm* 38:1138-1143, 1981.

Wilder BJ, Bruni J: *Seizure Disorders: A Pharmacological Approach to Treatment.* New York, Raven Press, 1981.

Wilder BJ, et al: Comparison of valproic acid and phenytoin in newly diagnosed tonic-clonic seizures. *Neurology* 33:1474-1476, 1983 A.

Wilder BJ, et al: Gastrointestinal tolerance of divalproex sodium. *Neurology* 33:808-811, 1983 B.

Woodbury DM: Convulsant drugs: Mechanisms of action, in Glaser GH, et al (eds): *Antiepileptic Drugs: Mechanisms of Action.* New York, Raven Press, 1980, 249-303.

Woodbury DM, et al (eds): *Antiepileptic Drugs,* ed 2. New York, Raven Press, 1982.

Wyllie E, et al: Pancreatitis associated with valproic acid therapy. *Am J Dis Child* 138:912-914, 1984.

Drugs Used to Treat Neuralgias

10

TRIGEMINAL AND GLOSSOPHARYNGEAL
NEURALGIAS

    Drug Evaluations

POSTHERPETIC NEURALGIA

DIABETIC NEUROPATHY

CHEMONUCLEOLYSIS FOR SCIATICA CAUSED BY
HERNIATED LUMBAR DISC

    Drug Evaluation

A variety of drugs with anticonvulsant, antispastic, antidepressant, or enzymatic activity are used to manage neuralgias. These compounds are often more useful than agents with general analgesic properties, but the mechanisms by which they alleviate pain are not well understood. Some of these agents may exert their analgesic activity by inhibiting polysynaptic pain transmission.

The causes of neuralgic pain are diverse and the pain may be episodic or chronic. For example, disease or injuries affecting different portions of the nervous system cause the chronic pain associated with tabes dorsalis, postherpetic neuralgia, and diabetic peripheral neuropathy. Sciatica due to herniated lumbar disc results from nerve compression by the disc material. The causes of trigeminal neuralgia include nerve compression by arterial loop(s), multiple sclerosis, small tumors, and bony defects; in some patients, the cause is idiopathic.

Evaluating the efficacy of agents used to manage the pain of neuralgias is difficult because of the spontaneous remissions that occur, inadequate follow-up of drug therapy, the subjective nature of the pain, and the substantial number of patients who exhibit a placebo response. The discussion of therapy for neuralgias in this chapter is limited to conditions in which drug treatment may be beneficial.

TRIGEMINAL AND GLOSSOPHARYNGEAL NEURALGIAS

Trigeminal neuralgia, an episodic facial pain syndrome, occurs most often in elderly patients. Unilateral paroxysms of severe shooting pain within one or more divisions of the trigeminal nerve are followed by a period of relief and then by another episode of severe pain. This pain is characteristically triggered by tactile stimuli on the face.

Carbamazepine [Tegretol] is the drug of choice and should be used initially. If attacks are not controlled completely by carbamazepine or the patient cannot tolerate this agent, the addition of baclofen [Lioresal] has been effective (Fromm et al, 1980, 1984). Phenytoin [Dilantin] may be added as a third drug when results are suboptimal. It also may be given alone or with carbamazepine, but its effectiveness is less than that of baclofen.

Clonazepam [Klonopin], a benzodiazepine anticonvulsant, and chlorphenesin [Maolate], a muscle relaxant, have been reported to be effective in a limited number of patients, but studies comparing these drugs with carbamazepine and baclofen are needed to determine their place in pharmacotherapy.

Remissions are not unusual in trigeminal neuralgia and a drug holiday should be tried by gradually reducing the dose of carbamazepine and other drugs over one to two weeks following a pain-free period of several months. If pain recurs, drug treatment can be reinstituted.

Between 25% and 50% of patients receiving drug therapy for trigeminal neuralgia relapse (Dalessio, 1982). When drug therapy fails to control pain or produces unacceptable side effects, surgery should be recommended. Although a permanent sensory deficit and anesthesia dolorosa may result, surgical treatment is invariably effective.

Glossopharyngeal neuralgia is much less common than trigeminal neuralgia and is characterized by similar paroxysms of lancinating pain in the pharynx, tonsils, and ear. Pain is often triggered by swallowing and accompanied by syncope that is thought to be due to increased vagal activity. Carbamazepine is the drug of choice. If pain persists, cocainization of the pharynx may provide temporary relief. When glossopharyngeal neuralgia is refractory to carbamazepine, surgical section of the ninth cranial nerve root is recommended (Bruyn, 1983).

Drug Evaluations

BACLOFEN
[Lioresal]

$$H_2NCH_2CHCH_2COOH$$

ACTIONS. Baclofen is an analogue of gamma aminobutyric acid (GABA) and acts presynaptically at a bicuculline-insensitive GABA receptor. This drug acts by antagonizing excitatory neurotransmission, possibly by blocking the release of the putative excitatory transmitters, glutamic and aspartic acids, from primary afferent fibers and Substance P from cutaneous nociceptive afferent nerve endings. In experimental animals, baclofen has been shown to depress excitatory transmission and enhance segmental inhibition in the spinal trigeminal nucleus (Fromm et al, 1980).

USES. This drug sometimes is effective alone for long-term control in newly diagnosed patients who cannot tolerate carbamazepine. However, because it appears to have a synergistic action with carbamazepine and phenytoin, baclofen is more commonly used with these drugs in previously uncontrolled patients. Baclofen alone appears to be less effective than carbamazepine but more effective than phenytoin (Fromm et al, 1984).

ADVERSE REACTIONS. Baclofen appears to be well tolerated in responsive patients treated for trigeminal neuralgia (Fromm et al, 1984). Drowsiness, nausea, and vomiting are the most common adverse effects and occur more frequently when baclofen is administered with carbamazepine. Hallucinations, seizures, or both may develop after abrupt dosage reduction or discontinuation of treatment after more than two months.

See Chapter 12, Drugs Used in Disorders Affecting Skeletal Muscle, for a more detailed discussion of adverse reactions.

DOSAGE AND PREPARATIONS.
Oral: Adults, initially, 10 mg three times daily; the amount is increased by 10 mg/day every other day to 60 to 80 mg/day in three or four divided doses by the end of the second week. The average maintenance dose is 50 to 60 mg/day for patients receiving baclofen alone and 30 to 40 mg/day when baclofen is given with carbamazepine or phenytoin (Fromm et al, 1984). A lower initial dose (5 mg three times daily) that is increased more gradually should be given to elderly patients and those taking other central nervous system depressants.

Lioresal (Geigy). Tablets 10 and 20 mg.

CARBAMAZEPINE
[Tegretol]

ACTIONS AND USES. Carbamazepine, a primary antiepileptic drug, is related chemically to the tricyclic compounds. Its antineuralgic action may result from reduction of excitatory synaptic transmission in the spinal trigeminal nucleus by increasing the latency of trigeminal neuronal response and decreasing the number of neuronal discharges (Fromm et al, 1981). A similar action has been reported for phenytoin and baclofen. Carbamazepine-10,11-epoxide, a major metabolite of carbamazepine, also has considerable antineuralgic activity (Tomson and Bertilsson, 1984).

Carbamazepine is the drug of choice for trigeminal and glossopharyngeal neuralgia. Satisfactory relief of pain is obtained in 70% to 90% of patients within 24 to 72 hours and effectiveness may persist for many years; however, in one study, 19% of patients developed resistance (Taylor et al, 1981). When a relapse occurs during therapy, the dose may be increased; if this is ineffective or not tolerated, the concomitant administration of baclofen and/or phenytoin may be helpful. Patients who do not respond to drug therapy may require surgery.

Carbamazepine also is effective in the lightning pains of tabes dorsalis, although clinical experience with this use of the drug is more limited than in trigeminal neuralgia. It has been used to relieve pain in multiple sclerosis, acute idiopathic polyneuritis (Guillain-Barré syndrome), peripheral diabetic neuropathy, phantom limb, post-traumatic paresthesia, bilateral superior laryngeal neuralgia, and painful hemifacial spasms. It should be kept in mind that carbamazepine is not a general analgesic but is specific for certain types of pain; thus, it should not be used to treat trivial facial pain or minor pain at other sites.

ADVERSE REACTIONS AND PRECAUTIONS. The reactions that occur most commonly during early treatment are drowsiness, dizziness, lightheadedness, ataxia, nausea, and vomiting; they usually subside spontaneously within a week or after a reduction in dose. Their incidence may be minimized by utilizing a small dose initially and increasing the amount gradually.

Dermatologic reactions occur occasionally and include pruritic and erythematous rashes, urticaria, Stevens-Johnson syndrome, exfoliative dermatitis, erythema multiforme, erythema nodosum, and aggravation of systemic lupus erythematosus. These effects may be severe enough to necessitate discontinuation of therapy.

Hematopoietic reactions (leukopenia, agranulocytosis, eosinophilia, leukocytosis, purpura, aplastic anemia, and thrombocytopenia) develop rarely but may be serious. Aplastic anemia and thrombocytopenia may be fatal. Therefore, patients should be advised to notify their physician if signs of hematologic toxicity appear (eg, fever, sore throat, aphthous stomatitis, easy bruising, petechial or purpuric hemorrhage).

Cardiovascular, genitourinary, metabolic, hepatic, and other reactions have been reported rarely. Although the antidiuretic action of carbamazepine rarely causes water intoxication and hyponatremia, caution should be used when treating elderly patients with cardiovascular disease. If symptoms of water intoxication occur, the plasma sodium level and osmolality should be measured. If hyponatremia develops, carbamazepine should be discontinued or the dosage reduced.

It is advisable to perform blood and platelet counts, liver function tests, urinalysis, and blood urea nitrogen determinations prior to treatment and to repeat these tests at regular intervals during treatment.

Since carbamazepine is related chemically to the tricyclic antidepressants, it should not be administered to patients sensitive to these compounds. The possibility of activating latent psychosis or, in elderly patients, of precipitating confusion or agitation also exists.

This drug is classified in FDA Pregnancy Category C.

For other adverse reactions, see Chapter 9, Antiepileptic Drugs.

PHARMACOKINETICS. The absorption of carbamazepine from the gastrointestinal tract is slow and variable; peak serum concentrations occur in 6 to 12 hours (Bertilsson, 1978). Because carbamazepine induces its own metabolism, the plasma half-life varies. Initially, the usual mean half-life is 35 hours, but is reduced to 17 ± 8 hours after three to four weeks. With a half-life of 35 hours, approximately one week is required to attain a steady-state plasma concentration. After induction of hepatic metabolism, the established steady-state concentration may be subtherapeutic and attacks of pain may recur. A positive correlation between drug plasma levels and pain relief has been demonstrated; levels between 5.7 and 10.1 mcg/ml were most effective. Side effects were not observed with plasma levels below 7.9 mcg/ml (Tomson et al, 1980).

Carbamazepine is metabolized in the liver to an epoxide and several other metabolites, which are excreted in the bile and urine. This drug is highly bound to plasma albumin but, unlike phenytoin, it is not displaced by acidic drugs and does not displace the latter.

DRUG INTERACTIONS. Carbamazepine enhances the metabolism of phenytoin through enzyme induction, and plasma levels of phenytoin may be reduced when these drugs are given concomitantly. Conversely, carbamazepine serum concentrations may be reduced by phenytoin.

There is evidence that erythromycin, isoniazid, and propoxyphene inhibit carbamazepine metabolism and thus may cause toxic effects (dizziness, drowsiness, nausea). Patients receiving carbamazepine should be monitored for signs of toxicity when these drugs are administered. The dosage of carbamazepine may have to be reduced.

If carbamazepine is given with warfarin, the half-life of the latter is reduced and the dose must be increased to maintain the anticoagulant effect. See also Chapter 9, Antiepileptic Drugs.

DOSAGE AND PREPARATIONS.

Oral: Adults, 200 mg to a maximum of 1.2 g daily; small doses should be used initially and the amount increased gradually (eg, 100 mg twice on the first day, increased by 100 mg every 12 hours until freedom from pain is achieved or toxicity occurs). A pain-free state usually can be maintained with 400 to 800 mg daily.

Carbamazepine should be administered in the minimal effective dose with meals. Since many individuals experience spontaneous prolonged remissions every few months, an attempt should be made to discontinue therapy occasionally. If pain recurs when the drug is withdrawn, reinstitution of therapy is effective.

Tegretol (Geigy). Tablets (chewable) 100 mg; tablets 200 mg.

PHENYTOIN
[Dilantin]

PHENYTOIN SODIUM
[Dilantin]

Phenytoin is sometimes used in trigeminal neuralgia, although it is less effective than carbamazepine and baclofen. Like these drugs, phenytoin depresses the excitatory synaptic transmission in the spinal trigeminal nucleus. It may be tried in patients who do not respond to carbamazepine or baclofen or it may be given with these drugs.

Phenytoin has been reported to be effective in several other pain syndromes (eg, peripheral neuralgia, phantom limb pain, Fabry's disease, thalamic pain, dysesthesia, postherpetic neuralgia), but adequate controlled studies to establish its usefulness are lacking (Walson et al, 1975). In one double-blind crossover study, phenytoin did not significantly improve symptoms of diabetic symmetric polyneuropathy (Saudek et al, 1977).

The most common adverse reactions include nausea, dizziness, ataxia, dyspepsia, and nystagmus. See Chapter 9, Antiepileptic Drugs for a more detailed discussion of adverse reactions.

DOSAGE AND PREPARATIONS.

Oral: For trigeminal neuralgia, *adults,* 300 to 400 mg daily. Since relief of pain does not correlate with drug blood levels, dosage may be increased until pain is relieved or toxic effects occur (Loeser, 1977).

PHENYTOIN:
Dilantin (Parke-Davis). Suspension 125 mg/5 ml.
PHENYTOIN SODIUM:
Dilantin (Parke-Davis), *Generic.* Capsules (plain, timed-release) 100 mg.

POSTHERPETIC NEURALGIA

Postherpetic neuralgia is a complication of acute herpes zoster and occurs almost exclusively in those over 60 years. Chronic pain characterized as severe and sharp or sometimes as a burning sensation is often associated with hyperesthesia. Unlike the episodic pain of trigeminal neuralgia, the constant pain of postherpetic neuralgia usually is not alleviated by carbamazepine or phenytoin, although their trial may be justified. Intralesional and subcutaneous injection of long-acting corticosteroids in conjunction with tricyclic antidepressants has been useful (Stein and Warfield, 1982).

Results of clinical trials have shown amitriptyline [Elavil, Endep, SK-Amitriptyline] to be effective in the management of postherpetic neuralgia (Watson et al, 1982). The analgesic action of amitriptyline appears to be independent of its antidepressant action, because analgesia occurs rapidly at doses below those needed to treat depression. The drug was given initially in a single dose of 12.5 to 25 mg at bedtime and the amount was increased by 12.5 mg every two to five days to a mean daily dose of 75 mg (range, 25 to 138 mg) (Watson et al, 1982). It has been suggested that a "therapeutic window effect" occurs in some patients treated with amitriptyline. This concept implies that a dosage range may exist below which and above which pain relief is not achieved and within which analgesia occurs. Since this effect may occur at a lower dosage range than for depression, amitriptyline should be administered in small amounts with reassessment and gradual incremental increases until analgesia is achieved (Watson, 1984). Additional controlled studies to confirm the usefulness of antidepressants in postherpetic neuralgia are needed.

DIABETIC NEUROPATHY

Peripheral nerve disorders are late complications of diabetes mellitus. Disabling spontaneous pains, dysesthesias, and paresthesias are common in sensory polyneuropathy. The pain of diabetic neuropathy often does not respond to drug therapy.

The management of diabetic neuropathy should include control of blood glucose concentrations and the administration of nonopiate analgesics, although their effect on pain of this nature is limited. Shooting or stabbing pains can be multifocal and may respond to carbamazepine or phenytoin (Brown and Asbury, 1984). The deep, constant, aching pain may be relieved by tricyclic antidepressants. Results of a small controlled clinical trial with imipramine [Janimine, SK-Pramine, Tofranil] demonstrated its effectiveness in 7 of 12 patients with pain, paresthesia, dysesthesia, and numbness (Kvinesdal et al, 1984). Patients received 50 mg/day the first week and 100 mg/day for the remaining four weeks. Amitriptyline 25 to 150 mg taken orally at bedtime also may be beneficial (Brown and Asbury, 1984). The use of phenothiazines, such as fluphenazine [Permitil, Prolixin], in combination with tricyclic antidepressants is based on anecdotal reports. Some physicians do not recommend the prolonged use of phenothiazines because of the risks of extrapyramidal and cardiovascular side effects and

tardive dyskinesia, which may develop after drug withdrawal. The aldose reductase inhibitor, sorbinil, is being evaluated for diabetic neuropathy but further clinical trials are needed (Jaspan et al, 1983).

CHEMONUCLEOLYSIS FOR SCIATICA CAUSED BY HERNIATED LUMBAR DISC

Lumbar nerve root compression caused by a ruptured intervertebral disc is characterized primarily by leg (including buttock) pain and back pain, with the former being the dominant complaint. The pain is usually felt in one leg and follows a typical sciatic nerve distribution.

Enzymatic digestion of the disc material (ie, chemonucleolysis, discolysis) offers a practical alternative to surgery in properly selected patients. The objective of chemonucleolysis is to deliver a hydrolytic enzyme to the intradiscal space, and thus the ruptured disc material, by transcutaneous injection without injuring adjacent structures. Chymopapain, which hydrolyzes the noncollagenous proteoglycan portion of the disc material, is effective for chemonucleolysis.

Disc prolapse causes symptoms in less than 10% of patients with back pain and sciatica (Fraser, 1985). Intradiscal injection of chymopapain should be administered only to patients with documented herniated lumbar intervertebral discs who have not responded to an adequate period of conservative therapy.

Intradiscal injection of collagenase [Nucleolysin] (investigational) hydrolyzes the Type I and II collagen matrix of the nucleus pulposus and may be effective in the treatment of ruptured lumbar discs, but there is less experience with this agent than with chymopapain. Collagenase may offer an alternative to surgery in patients previously treated with chymopapain who may be sensitized to this enzyme. The rate of anaphylaxis with collagenase has not yet been determined.

Drug Evaluation

CHYMOPAPAIN
[Chymodiactin, Discase]

ACTIONS. Chymopapain, a proteolytic enzyme, hydrolyzes the noncollagenous proteoglycan portion of the nucleus pulposus of the intervertebral disc. Disruption of the proteoglycan complex significantly decreases the water-binding capacity, which reduces the volume and intradiscal pressure of the nucleus pulposus. It is hypothesized that pain relief and improvements in neurologic deficits result from the reduction of the mass of herniated material pressing on the nerve roots.

Some controversy exists as to whether chymopapain relieves the tension on the nerve root by altering the disc protrusion or by narrowing the disc space (Spencer and Miller, 1983). The specificity of chymopapain for the nucleus pulposus may be explained by the electrostatic attraction between the enzyme, which has a net positive charge at physiologic pH, and proteoglycan, which bears a negative charge under the same conditions. Significant proteolytic activity outside the disc appears to be limited by the inhibitory activity of plasma α_2-macroglobulin.

USES. Intradiscal chymopapain is effective in sciatica caused by documented compression of a lumbar nerve root by protrusion of an intervertebral disc. An adequate period of conservative therapy is recommended before chymopapain (and other methods of intervention) is considered. Radiculopathy of nondiscogenic origin, such as impingement of the nerve root by hypertrophic bony spurs, spondylolisthesis or spinal stenosis, intraspinal tumor, spinal arteriovenous malformation, and arachnoiditis, does not respond to chymopapain (Ramirez and Javid, 1984).

Success rates in controlled and uncontrolled studies have varied from 59% to 80% (McCulloch, 1981; Fraser, 1982; Javid et al, 1983; Simmons et al, 1984). Optimal effectiveness with chymopapain depends upon careful patient selection, and detailed criteria have been published (McCulloch and MacNab, 1983; Brown, 1983). In general, patients who benefit from intradiscal chymopapain should have the following signs: radicular pain and paresthesias localized to specific dermatomal distribution and affecting one leg or rarely both legs; positive straight leg raising of less than 50 degrees with pain below the knee that is increased by dorsiflexion of the foot; two of the following neurologic signs: sensory alteration, depressed reflex activity, muscle weakness, and muscle wasting; and diagnosis of herniated disc confirmed by a myelogram and/or computer-assisted tomography (CAT scan).

ADVERSE REACTIONS. Serious but rare adverse reactions caused by chymopapain are anaphylaxis and neurologic complications due to subarachnoid injection. Mild to severe anaphylaxis develops in approximately 0.5% of patients not known to be previously sensitized; data indicate that the overall incidence is higher in women than in men and with general anesthesia than with local anesthesia (Smith Laboratories, 1984).

Almost all anaphylactic reactions occur immediately but may be observed up to two hours after injection. Since the intervertebral disc is avascular, release of chymopapain into the bloodstream is delayed. Thus, the patient should be observed closely for 30 minutes after injection and for an additional 90 minutes in the recovery room. The signs and symptoms of anaphylaxis include almost immediate hypotension and/or bronchospasm, which may proceed to laryngeal edema, tachycardia, arrhythmia, cardiac arrest, coma, and death.

Chymopapain is extremely toxic if injected into the subarachnoid space. The enzyme hydrolyzes the basement membranes of the small vessels in the pia-arachnoid, and the resulting subarachnoid hemorrhage may cause immediate unconsciousness, convulsions, or delayed fibrosis of the cauda equina, which may interfere with bowel and bladder control and lower extremity function; death may result.

Serious neurologic complications, such as paraplegia and cerebral hemorrhage, have been reported in a small number of patients soon after chymopapain injection.

Transverse myelitis occurs in about 1 in 18,000 patients injected with chymopapain and is characterized by the development of paraplegia and paraparesis after two to three weeks without prior signs or symptoms. This adverse reaction may result from leakage of dye and enzyme into the subarachnoid space. Patients undergoing discography immediately preceding chemonucleolysis may be at greatest risk (Smith Laboratories, 1984). Therefore, discography before chemonucleolysis should be avoided when possible.

Back pain, stiffness, and soreness are observed in 50% of patients. Muscle spasm occurs in 20% to 30% of patients immediately following injection. Back pain from muscle spasm may be incapacitating, but rarely lasts more than one day and does not appear to affect the outcome of chymopapain treatment.

Rash, urticaria, or pruritus may occur as late as two weeks after chymopapain injection. The incidence is less than 1%. Rash may occur alone or as part of the anaphylactic reaction and is associated with pruritus, which may be managed with intravenous diphenhydramine (Ramirez and Javid, 1984). Urticaria with pruritus may develop suddenly seven to ten days after injection and is twice as common as anaphylaxis.

PRECAUTIONS. Safe and effective use of chymopapain requires specialized training in chemonucleolysis. Since nerve root compression may result from conditions other than herniated disc, extensive training and experience in the diagnosis and management of all spinal disorders are required for proper patient selection. Additionally, physicians and support personnel should be aware of the potential complications from the use of chymopapain, including anaphylaxis, in order to take immediate and appropriate action.

A history of allergy to papaya or its extracts precludes the use of chymopapain. This enzyme may be self-sensitizing, and a repeat injection is contraindicated due to the lack of a reliable immunologic screening test for potential anaphylaxis. The determination of chymopapain-specific IgE plasma levels and skin sensitivity testing using inactivated chymopapain may aid in identifying high-risk patients (Tsay et al, 1984; McCulloch et al, in press; Bernstein et al, 1985). Further studies are needed to refine the accuracy and reliability of these tests. Although still under clinical investigation, chemonucleolysis with collagenase may offer an alternative to surgery in patients with prior exposure to chymopapain (Brown, 1983).

Because of the possibility of an anaphylactic reaction to chymopapain, some surgeons advocate that corticosteroids and antihistamines be given preoperatively (Brown, 1983); other authorities feel that routine premedication has not been proven to be beneficial (McCulloch and MacNab, 1983). Whether or not patients are pretreated with antihistamines and steroids, when anaphylaxis occurs, the physician must be prepared to make an immediate diagnosis and administer epinephrine and large amounts of fluids.

Some authorities prefer local anesthesia during chemonucleolysis, because it allows early detection of anaphylactic reactions and does not interfere with subsequent treatment. It should be noted that halothane and epinephrine may interact to cause cardiac arrhythmias. There are currently some differences in opinion among surgeons regarding the choice of anesthesia (general versus local) for chemonucleolysis (Brown, 1983; *F-D-C Reports,* 1985; McCulloch, 1984).

Nerve root scarification from previous operations may increase the possibility of neurologic complications (eg, transverse myelitis) and should be considered before chemonucleolysis is chosen.

Studies to determine the safety of chymopapain in children are in progress, and preliminary information indicates that this enzyme can be used safely in this group.

Because its safety during any phase of pregnancy also remains to be determined, chemonucleolysis with chymopapain is contraindicated during pregnancy or suspected pregnancy (FDA Pregnancy Category C).

PHARMACOKINETICS. Fragments of chymopapain immunoreactive protein have been detected in the plasma as early as 30 minutes after intradiscal injection. The inhibitory activity of α_2-macroglobulin prevents significant chymopapain activity outside the disc.

DOSAGE AND PREPARATIONS. Some protocols for chemonucleolysis recommend the administration of a test dose of chymopapain to assess the potential for anaphylaxis, but the predictive value has been questioned (Bernstein, 1984).

CHYMODIACTIN:

Intradiscal Injection: Adults, 2,000 to 4,000 picoKatal units/ disc in a solution of sterile water containing 2,000 units/ml. The preferred dose is 3,000 units or 1.5 ml/disc. The maximal dose for a patient with multiple disc herniation is 8,000 units.

   Chymodiactin (Smith). Lyophilized powder 4,000 and 10,000 picoKatal units/vial.

DISCASE:

Intradiscal Injection: Adults, 5 nanoKatal units (1 nanoKatal unit = 1,000 picoKatal units)/disc or 2 ml/disc. The maximal dose in a patient with multiple disc herniation is 10 nanoKatal units.

   Discase (Travenol). Lyophilized powder 12.5 nanoKatal units/vial.

Cited References

General anesthesia should remain option for chemonucleolysis. *F-D-C Reports*. April 15, 1985.

Bernstein IL: Anaphylaxis from chymopapain, (letter reply). *JAMA* 251:1953-1954, 1984.

Bernstein DI, et al: Prospective evaluation of chymopapain sensitivity in patients undergoing chemonucleolysis. *J Allergy Clin Immunol* 76:458-465, 1985.

Bertilsson L: Clinical pharmacokinetics of carbamazepine. *Clin Pharmacokinet* 3:128-143, 1978.

Brown MD: *Intradiscal Therapy: Chymopapain or Collagenase*. Chicago, Year Book Medical Publishers, 1983.

Brown MJ, Asbury, AK: Diabetic neuropathy. *Ann Neurol* 15:2-12, 1984.

Bruyn GW: Glossopharyngeal neuralgia. *Cephalalgia* 3:143-157, 1983.

Dalessio DJ: Trigeminal neuralgia: Practical approach to treatment. *Drugs* 24:248-255, 1982.

Fraser RD: Chymopapain for treatment of intervertebral disc herniation: Preliminary report of double-blind study. *Spine* 7:608-612, 1982.

Fraser RD: Treatment of intervertebral disc prolapse by intradiscal injection of chymopapain. *Med J Aust* 142:431-434, 1985.

Fromm GH, et al: Baclofen in trigeminal neuralgia: Effect on spinal trigeminal nucleus: Pilot study. *Arch Neurol* 37:768-771, 1980.

Fromm GH, et al: Role of inhibitory mechanisms in trigeminal neuralgia. *Neurology* 31:683-687, 1981.

Fromm GH, et al: Baclofen in treatment of trigeminal neuralgia: Double blind study and long-term follow-up. *Ann Neurol* 15:240-244, 1984.

Jaspan J, et al: Treatment of severely painful diabetic neuropathy with an aldolase reductase inhibitor: Relief of pain and improved somatic and autonomic nerve function. *Lancet* 2:758-762, 1983.

Javid MJ, et al: Safety and efficacy of chymopapain (Chymodiactin) in herniated nucleus pulposus with sciatica: Results of randomized double-blind study. *JAMA* 249:2489-2494, 1983.

Kvinesdal B, et al: Imipramine treatment of painful diabetic neuropathy. *JAMA* 251:1727-1730, 1984.

Loeser JD: Management of tic douloureux. *Pain* 3:155-162, 1977.

McCulloch JA: Chemonucleolysis for relief of sciatica due to herniated intervertebral disc. *Can Med Assoc J* 124:879-882, 1981.

McCulloch JA: Chemonucleolysis: State of the art, in Genant HK (ed): *Spine Update 1984: Perspectives in Radiology, Orthopaedic Surgery, and Neurosurgery*. San Francisco, University of California, 1984, 127-130.

McCulloch JA, MacNab I: *Sciatica and Chymopapain*. Baltimore, Williams & Wilkins, 1983.

McCulloch J, et al: Skin testing for chymopapain allergy: Preliminary report (in press).

Ramirez LF, Javid MJ: Chymopapain: New alternative for herniated discs. *Drug Ther (Hosp)* 9:80-90, (March) 1984.

Saudek CD, et al: Phenytoin in treatment of diabetic symmetrical polyneuropathy. *Clin Pharmacol Ther* 22:196-199, 1977.

Simmons JW, et al: Update and review of chemonucleolysis. *Clin Orthopaed Relat Res* 183:51-60, 1984.

Smith Laboratories: *Post-Marketing Surveillance Reports*, 1984.

Spencer DL, Miller JAA: Mechanism of sciatic pain relief by chemonucleolysis. *Orthopedics* 6:1600-1603, 1983.

Stein JM, Warfield CA: Herpes zoster and postherpetic neuralgia. *Hosp Pract* 17:96A-960, (Sept) 1982.

Taylor JC, et al: Long-term treatment of trigeminal neuralgia with carbamazepine. *Postgrad Med J* 57:16-18, 1981.

Tomson T, Bertilsson L: Potent therapeutic effect of carbamazepine-10,11-epoxide in trigeminal neuralgia. *Arch Neurol* 41:598-601, 1984.

Tomson T, et al: Carbamazepine therapy in trigeminal neuralgia: Clinical effects in relation to plasma concentration. *Arch Neurol* 37:699-703, 1980.

Tsay Y-G, et al: Preoperative chymopapain sensitivity test for chemonucleolysis candidates. *Spine* 9:764-768, 1984.

Walson P, et al: New uses for phenytoin. *JAMA* 233:1385-1389, 1975.

Watson CPN: Therapeutic window for amitriptyline analgesia. *Can Med Assoc J* 130:105-106, 1984.

Watson CP, et al: Amitriptyline versus placebo in postherpetic neuralgia. *Neurology* 32:671-673, 1982.

Other Selected References

Management of trigeminal neuralgia. *Drug Ther Bull* 21:97-99, 1983.

Anthony M: Relief of facial pain. *Drugs* 18:122-129, 1979.

Crill WE: Carbamazepine. *Ann Intern Med* 79:844-847, 1973.

Penovich PE, Morgan JP: Carbamazepine: Review. *Drug Ther* 6:187-193, (Feb) 1976.

Drugs Used in Extrapyramidal Movement Disorders

11

The extrapyramidal nervous system consists of multisynaptic neurons located in the basal ganglia, thalamic and subthalamic nuclei, red nucleus, substantia nigra, and parts of the reticular formation, cerebellum, and cerebrum. These neurons modulate and integrate motor, as well as cognitive, emotional, and language impulses arising in the pyramidal system. Normal extrapyramidal-coordinated movement depends in part on the maintenance of physiologic levels of dopamine and acetylcholine within the striatum neural pathways. Dopamine is believed to act principally as an inhibitory neurotransmitter and acetylcholine as an excitatory neurotransmitter. Although the dopaminergic pathway is the most important, alterations in many other neurotransmitters can produce either hypokinetic (eg, parkinsonism) or hyperkinetic syndromes (eg, chorea).

Extrapyramidal movement disorders are characterized by abnormal involuntary movements or dyskinesias (eg, myoclonus, tremors, tics, chorea, athetosis, ballismus), bradykinesia, changes in muscle tone (ie, dystonia, rigidity), and impaired postural reflexes. Paralysis, spasticity, and increased reflexes (stretch, Babinski sign) are less prominent than in conditions associated more exclusively with impairment of the pyramidal system. The primary extrapyramidal symptoms occuring in classic Parkinson's disease are tremor, bradykinesia, rigidity, and impaired postural reflexes. Many other diseases exhibit one or two of these features (eg, olivopontocerebellar degeneration, Creutzfeldt-Jakob disease).

PARKINSONISM

Parkinson's disease (primary parkinsonism) is a nonhereditary progressive neurologic disorder of the extrapyramidal system. Its etiology is still unknown, although there is some evidence to support environmental causes (eg, the appearance of parkinsonism in drug addicts who used meperidine analogues contaminated with 1-methyl-4 phenyl-tetrahydropyridine [MPTP]).

The extrapyramidal manifestations result largely from a deficiency of dopamine in the striatum (ie, caudate nucleus and putamen), which may be part of a more generalized structural or regulatory defect. Degeneration of the large pigmented neurons in the substantia nigra occurs in both idiopathic and postencephalitic parkinsonism, and the dopamine deficiency is proportional to cell loss.

In addition to the classic features (resting tremor, lead-pipe rigidity, bradykinesia, loss of normal postural reflexes, and impaired gait), cognitive, perceptual, and memory deficits and even global dementia occur in approximately one-third of patients (Lieberman, 1979). Data on the incidence of dementia in Parkinson's disease are controversial, however. Alzheimer's disease is six times more common in patients with Parkinson's disease than in age-matched controls (Boller et al, 1980). Depression occurs in approximately one-half of patients. Impaired speech, sialorrhea, dysphagia, and seborrheic dermatitis are also present in many patients.

Parkinsonian symptoms may be associated with more extensive central nervous system dysfunction, such as that seen in progressive supranuclear palsy, Shy-Drager syndrome, olivopontocerebellar degeneration, Wilson's disease, and the Westphal (rigid) variant of Huntington's disease.

Drug-induced parkinsonism may result from blockade of dopamine receptors by antipsychotic drugs or metoclopramide or depletion of brain dopamine by rauwolfia alkaloids. Signs and symptoms also may be produced by midbrain tumors or central nervous system injury from chronic manganese, MPTP, carbon monoxide, carbon tetrachloride, or carbon disulfide poisoning.

The discovery that the parkinsonian symptoms observed in some drug addicts were caused by MPTP, a neurotoxic byproduct of the synthesis of some meperidine analogues, has led to expanded research on the underlying mechanism of Parkinson's disease. MPTP is converted by monoamine oxidase B to a metabolite that appears to selectively destroy dopamine-producing neurons in the substantia nigra (Langston et al, 1983; Markey et al, 1984).

The goals in the treatment of parkinsonism are to provide maximum symptomatic relief and to maintain maximum independence of movement for as long as possible. Therapy is symptomatic, not curative, and it is directed toward replenishing striatal dopamine and, to a lesser extent, blocking central cholinergic receptors. Bradykinesia, rigidity, tremor, and disorders of posture and gait are alleviated by drug therapy.

Although pharmacotherapy is the basis for the management of Parkinson's disease, nondrug measures also are important. Exercise, speech therapy, physical therapy, and psychotherapy are beneficial. Family support and involvement are critical for effective care. Their familiarity with dosage schedules can be helpful in planning activities and in maintaining the patient on regular medication.

Drug Selection

The choice of drugs (see Table 1) is related principally to the severity of the disease and may change as a result of the disease's progression or the patient's ability to tolerate adverse reactions (Perlik et al, 1980; Pearce, 1984).

Mild Involvement: In the early stages of Parkinson's disease, asymmetrical tremor and bradykinesia may predominate, and medication is usually not required if patients function relatively well. As the disease begins to impair activities, one or more drugs with central anticholinergic activity may be considered, or amantadine [Symmetrel] may be preferred (Pearce, 1984).

Anticholinergic drugs are usually selected for younger patients who will require long-term therapy and for patients who are particularly troubled by tremor. Tremor and rigidity respond well to anticholinergic drugs, but bradykinesia and loss of postural reflexes are less affected. These drugs produce significant central nervous system side effects, particularly in older patients.

Unless tremor is predominant, many neurologists consider amantadine the initial drug of choice. This drug usually relieves all signs and symptoms for extended periods. Because amantadine is excreted primarily unchanged by the kidney, the renal function of older patients should be monitored to prevent toxicity. The combination of amantadine and an anticholinergic drug may have additive therapeutic and adverse effects.

Fully Developed Disease: Patients who do not respond to anticholinergic drugs or amantadine or those who are only partially responsive are usually given levodopa, most often combined with carbidopa, a peripheral decarboxylase inhibitor [Sinemet]; the combination minimizes the peripheral adverse reactions, especially nausea and vomiting, of levodopa alone [Dopar, Larodopa]. Sinemet contains carbidopa and levodopa in a ratio of 1:4 or 1:10 (see the evaluation). Another combination, Madopa, which contains benserazide and levodopa in a ratio of 1:4, is available only for investigational use in the United States, but it has been compared extensively with Sinemet. Although a few patients may respond better to one of these mixtures than the other, their efficacy and safety are similar (Diamond et al, 1978; Lieberman et al, 1978).

There is controversy over when to use levodopa and the dose to employ. Some neurologists believe that the progression of Parkinson's disease and the development of adverse reactions correlate with the duration of levodopa treatment (Fahn and Bressman, 1984) and recommend that this drug be reserved for use in later stages of the disease. Those opposing this view believe that late management problems with levodopa result from progression of the disease (Muenter, 1984; Markham and Diamond, 1981) and that therapy thus should begin at the earliest onset of disabling symptoms. In general, most clinicians initiate levodopa therapy on the basis of degree of disability and the social and occupational needs of the patient (Calne, 1984; Legg, 1983; Pearce, 1984). If symptoms preclude a normal work or social life, it is generally agreed that levodopa therapy is indicated (Calne, 1984).

Although re-establishment of normal motor function is desirable, many neurologists conservatively administer levodopa in the smallest dose that permits performance of daily activities (Lang and Blair, 1984; Calne, 1984). Amantadine, anticholinergic drugs, and/or bromocriptine may be given concomitantly to enhance control.

Advanced Disease: The response to levodopa gradually diminishes after two to five years and fluctuations in motor performance or adverse mental changes often occur at this time. Three types of problems develop during prolonged levodopa therapy. The first consists of dose-related and thus dose-limiting reactions. These include various psychiatric problems (eg, disruption of sleep cycle, vivid dreams or nightmares, hallucinations) and involuntary movements or dyskinesias. The severity of these reactions frequently require reduction of dose with subsequent loss of efficacy. The addition of amantadine or bromocriptine [Parlodel] to the regimen may allow dosage reduction.

Problems in the second category are usually difficult to modulate by manipulating the dose of levodopa. Most common is end-of-dose akinesia or "wearing-off," which may occur one to four hours after the last dose and require more frequent administration of levodopa/carbidopa. The addition of amantadine to the regimen is believed to be helpful, but its benefit is

TABLE 1.
DRUGS USED IN THE MANAGEMENT OF PARKINSON'S DISEASE

Drugs	Comment
EARLY STAGES OF DISEASE	
Anticholinergic Agents Benztropine [Cogentin] Biperiden [Akineton] Diphenhydramine [Benadryl] Ethopropazine [Parsidol] Orphenadrine [Disipal] Procyclidine [Kemadrin] Trihexyphenidyl [Artane]	If symptoms are mild, drug therapy may not be necessary. When treatment is required, either anticholinergics or amantadine is usually effective. Because of age-related central nervous system adverse reactions, an anticholinergic may be most appropriate in younger patients and in those in whom tremor is the major complaint.
Amantadine [Symmetrel]	When tremor is not the major symptom, many neurologists consider amantadine to be a good initial drug. All signs and symptoms may improve in many patients.
FULLY DEVELOPED DISEASE	
Levodopa and Carbidopa [Sinemet] Levodopa [Dopar, Larodopa]	Levodopa therapy is usually begun when anticholinergics and/or amantadine do not provide sufficient improvement and disability threatens employment or a reasonable lifestyle. The combination of levodopa-carbidopa is preferred by most neurologists. The combination reduces gastrointestinal side effects. Dosage should be individualized so that the minimal amount is administered. The aim of this dosage is to provide sufficient improvement so that daily activities can be performed, usually with some parkinsonian signs. Amantadine, bromocriptine, and/or anticholinergics may be given concomitantly.
LATE STAGES OF DISEASE	
Levodopa [Dopar, Larodopa] Levodopa and Carbidopa [Sinemet]	After one to five years of levodopa therapy, late-stage management problems with levodopa often occur and include dyskinesia and hallucinations, "wearing-off" of drug effect, "on-off" oscillations, and overall loss of drug effectiveness. Dyskinesia and hallucinations may require dosage reduction. The common problem of "wearing-off" may be treated by more frequent administration of levodopa. Rapid and unpredictable motor fluctuations usually are unresponsive to dosage changes. A levodopa holiday has been utilized to combat manifestations of levodopa toxicity.
Bromocriptine [Parlodel] Pergolide (investigational) Lisuride (investigational)	Use of the direct-acting dopamine agonist, bromocriptine, is initially effective but its efficacy in combination with levodopa is usually not sustained. Other investigational dopamine agonists, such as pergolide and lisuride, may also show waning effectiveness.
Amantadine [Symmetrel] Selegiline (deprenyl) (investigational)	Amantadine also may be helpful in combination with levodopa. Its effectiveness may be prolonged by a temporary withdrawal, which seems to restore activity. Addition of selegiline also has provided modest improvement in function.

often temporary. With the recurrence of "wearing-off," some neurologists withdraw amantadine for one month to restore the effectiveness of this agent.

Another problem in this category, rapid and unpredictable fluctuations between mobility and immobility ("on-off" effects), is a serious obstacle in the drug management of late stage Parkinson's disease. These fluctuations can occur rapidly and may not appear to be linked to the dosing schedule. The fluctuation may be partially explained by interference with the absorption of levodopa by food and by competition between large neutral amino acids and levodopa for transport to the brain (Nutt et al, 1984). Attention to the timing of protein intake

and the separation of drug administration and meals may be helpful. Bromocriptine may be added to the regimen of these individuals; best results are obtained by reducing the dose of levodopa (by 50% in some cases) while increasing that of bromocriptine (Calne, 1982). Amantadine is an alternative to bromocriptine. Although these drugs are often helpful, especially bromocriptine, neither consistently stabilizes the response for long.

There is evidence that substitution of other dopaminergic agonists may improve the response (Goetz et al, 1984). The investigational dopaminergic agonists, pergolide and lisuride, have an action resembling that of bromocriptine and may be useful in managing "wearing-off" and "on-off" phenomena (Goetz et al, 1983; LeWitt et al, 1983). As with bromocriptine, the effectiveness of pergolide decreases with time (Lieberman et al, 1984).

The relatively specific type B monoamine oxidase inhibitor, selegiline (deprenyl), may prolong the action of dopamine. Clinical evaluation (primarily European) of its effectiveness as an adjunct to levodopa/carbidopa has indicated that selegiline is useful in managing "on-off" fluctuations in some patients. It has a levodopa-sparing effect and reduction of levodopa dosage by 30% is usually possible. There is some suggestion that the addition of selegiline to levodopa and a decarboxylase inhibitor may slow the progression of illness (Birkmayer, 1983), but the usefulness of this regimen must be validated in appropriately controlled studies.

The final type of problem encountered with levodopa therapy in advanced Parkinson's disease is loss of drug effectiveness. It is not clear whether this effect is secondary to progression of the underlying disease or overstimulation (leading to down-regulation) of dopamine receptors. Total re-evaluation of diagnosis, redetermination of concomitant medications (eg, antipsychotic agents, reserpine, metoclopramide [Reglan]), and rescreening for metabolic disorders such as hypothyroidism are recommended to rule out underlying causes. The addition of bromocriptine or amantadine to levodopa/carbidopa therapy may improve the response temporarily. Alternatively, although potentially hazardous and controversial (Friedman, 1985), some authorities recommend temporary withdrawal of levodopa (Direnfeld et al, 1980; Weiner et al, 1980). Because parkinsonism may become more severe during drug withdrawal, hospitalization is generally recommended. There are two goals of initiating a drug holiday from levodopa. The first is to eliminate or reduce adverse drug effects (eg, hallucinations) and the second is to reverse down-regulation of dopamine receptors, thus restoring the effectiveness of levodopa. Recent results do not support the efficacy of this form of therapy (Mayeux et al, 1985).

Drug Evaluations

DRUGS WITH CENTRAL ANTICHOLINERGIC ACTIVITY

ACTIONS AND USES. The efficacy of these drugs appears to be related to their central cholinergic blocking action. Inhibition of dopamine reuptake into presynaptic nerve terminals also may be involved. The belladonna alkaloids, atropine and scopolamine, were the first of these agents used in parkinsonism. They have now been replaced by synthetic drugs that are equally effective but produce fewer peripheral side effects. The synthetic drugs include the piperidyl compounds (trihexyphenidyl [Artane]), their analogues (biperiden [Akineton], procyclidine [Kemadrin]), and the tropanol derivative, benztropine [Cogentin]. The antihistamines (diphenhydramine [Benadryl], orphenadrine [Disipal]) and the phenothiazine derivative, ethopropazine [Parsidol], also have some antiparkinson activity attributable to their anticholinergic properties.

In most patients not receiving levodopa, the maximal tolerated dose of a single anticholinergic drug often is not adequate. In such instances, a second and, if needed, a third drug from another class may be added; the dose of each drug should be individualized. The durations of action of these anticholinergic drugs differ, and patients may tolerate one drug better than another. Otherwise, none has any advantages over the others.

Trihexyphenidyl, biperiden, benztropine, or ethopropazine is usually preferred for initiating therapy. Ethopropazine is thought to be especially effective in reducing tremor. Antihistamines, particularly diphenhydramine, are used primarily as adjuncts. However, they may be used alone for initial therapy in mild parkinsonism and for maintenance therapy in elderly patients who cannot tolerate the more potent anticholinergic drugs.

After long-term administration of anticholinergic agents, patients frequently become refractory to their effects. This often is caused by progression of the disease, but extraneous factors, such as trauma, unrelated illness, or emotional stress, may exacerbate symptoms. Increasing the dose or substituting a drug from another class sometimes restores responsiveness. Levodopa or amantadine may be added later if needed. When therapy is initiated with levodopa, a central anticholinergic agent may be added later to achieve maximal improvement.

The anticholinergic and antihistaminic drugs also are used to control some acute extrapyramidal reactions (dystonias, akathisia, and parkinsonism induced by antipsychotic drugs). Although diphenhydramine commonly causes excessive sedation, it often is preferred because of its low toxicity.

ADVERSE REACTIONS AND PRECAUTIONS. Most untoward effects are related to the peripheral or central cholinergic blocking activity of these drugs. Adverse effects occur least often with the antihistamines and ethopropazine, for their anticholinergic activity is milder. However, some undesirable effects can be expected when therapeutic doses of any of these agents are administered.

The most common adverse reactions are dryness of the mouth, mydriasis, cycloplegia, tachycardia, constipation, urinary retention, and psychic disturbances. Patients with prostatic hypertrophy should be observed carefully for signs of urinary retention, and those with hypomotile gastrointestinal disorders should be monitored for signs of constipation or intestinal obstruction. Fatal adynamic ileus has occurred in patients receiving combinations of drugs with anticholinergic properties. Patients with a tendency to develop tachycardia should receive the smallest effective dose. Large doses of anticholinergic drugs can markedly elevate body temperature.

Because of their mydriatic effect, anticholinergic drugs can precipitate an attack of acute glaucoma in patients predisposed to angle closure. This has occurred occasionally after parenteral administration but only rarely after oral use. As a rule, anticholinergic drugs can be given safely to patients with open-angle glaucoma who are receiving miotics.

Confusion and excitement may occur with large doses or in susceptible patients (eg, the elderly, patients with pre-existing mental disorders, those taking tricyclic antidepressants with anticholinergic activity to overcome the depression often seen in patients with Parkinson's disease). More serious mental disturbances (agitation, disorientation, delirium, paranoid reaction, and hallucinations) are usually drug induced and do not represent an intensification of the existing symptoms of parkinsonism.

Great care must be taken when administering anticholinergic agents to elderly patients, especially those with any degree of dementia. Anticholinergic drug-induced impairment of memory is very common in this group. Susceptible patients should be observed carefully, because the adverse effects may be subtle, may develop only with prolonged use, and often are not detectable until drugs are discontinued or the dose is reduced.

The antihistamines also have adverse effects unrelated to their anticholinergic action. Drowsiness and dizziness are common with therapeutic doses. Anorexia, nausea, and vomiting may occur. Other reactions reported occasionally include euphoria, hypotension, headache, weakness, tingling, and heaviness of the hands.

Drowsiness, dizziness, inability to concentrate, and confusion are the most common adverse effects of ethopropazine. Mild anticholinergic side effects also have been reported. Muscle cramps, epigastric discomfort, paresthesia, heaviness of the limbs, hypotension, and rash occur occasionally.

DOSAGE AND PREPARATIONS. Therapy with anticholinergic drugs should be initiated with a small amount that is increased gradually until optimal benefits are attained or unacceptable untoward effects occur. Younger patients and those with postencephalitic parkinsonism may tolerate larger doses than older patients with the idiopathic form. If the anticholinergic drugs must be discontinued, a stepwise reduction of dose should be employed (unless acute toxicity occurs) to lessen exacerbating parkinsonian symptoms.

See Table 2 for dosage and preparations.

TABLE 2.
CENTRALLY ACTIVE ANTICHOLINERGIC DRUGS

Drug and Chemical Structure	Usual Dosage	Preparations
PIPERIDYL COMPOUNDS		
Biperiden Hydrochloride Biperiden Lactate	*Oral:* For idiopathic and postencephalitic parkinsonism, *adults,* initially, 2 mg three times daily. The dose may be gradually increased up to 20 mg daily if required and tolerated. For drug-induced extrapyramidal reactions, *adults,* 2 mg one to three times daily.	*Akineton* (Knoll). Tablets 2 mg [hydrochloride].
	Intramuscular: For drug-induced extrapyramidal reactions, except tardive dyskinesia, *adults,* 2 mg, *children,* 0.04 mg/kg. This dose may be repeated every one-half hour if required, but no more than four consecutive doses should be given within a 24-hour period.	Solution (for injection) 5 mg in 1 ml containers [lactate].
Procyclidine Hydrochloride	*Oral:* For idiopathic and postencephalitic parkinsonism, *adults,* initially, 5 mg twice daily. The dose may be increased gradually to 20 to 30 mg daily if required and tolerated. For drug-induced extrapyramidal reactions, except tardive dyskinesia, *adults,* initially, 2 to 2.5 mg three times daily. The dose may then be increased by 2 to 2.5 mg daily until symptoms are controlled. Generally, symptomatic relief is obtained with 10 to 20 mg daily.	*Kemadrin* (Burroughs Wellcome). Tablets 5 mg.
Trihexyphenidyl Hydrochloride	*Oral:* (Tablets or elixir is preferred, as the efficacy of timed-release capsules has not been established.) For idiopathic and postencephalitic parkinsonism, *adults,* initially, 2 mg two or three times daily. The dose is gradually increased until the desired therapeutic effect is obtained or until severe adverse reactions preclude a further increase. Doses larger than 15 to 20 mg daily are rarely required or tolerated, but some patients with postencephalitic parkinsonism may tolerate 40 to 50 mg daily.	*Generic.* Tablets 2 and 5 mg. *Artane* (Lederle). Capsules (timed-release) 5 mg; elixir 2 mg/5 ml; tablets 2 and 5 mg.
	For drug-induced extrapyramidal reactions, except tardive dyskinesia, *adults,* initially, 1 mg. If symptoms are not controlled within a few hours, subsequent doses are increased until symptoms subside. The usual total daily dose is 5 to 15 mg.	

TROPANOL DERIVATIVES
Benztropine Mesylate

CH₃SO₃⁻

Oral: For idiopathic and postencephalitic parkinsonism, *adults,* initially, 0.5 to 1 mg at bedtime. Patients with postencephalitic parkinsonism often tolerate an initial dose of 2 mg. The dosage may be gradually increased to 4 to 6 mg daily if required and tolerated.

Oral, Intramuscular, Intravenous: For drug-induced extrapyramidal reactions, except tardive dyskinesia, *adults,* 1 to 4 mg once or twice daily. In acute dystonic reactions, initially, 1 to 2 mg intramuscularly or intravenously; to prevent recurrence, 1 to 2 mg orally twice daily.

Cogentin
(Merck Sharp & Dohme).
Tablets 0.5, 1, and 2 mg; solution (for injection) 1 mg/ml in 2 ml containers.

ANTIHISTAMINES
Diphenhydramine Hydrochloride

Cl⁻

Oral: For idiopathic and postencephalitic parkinsonism, *adults,* initially, 25 mg three times daily. The dosage may be gradually increased to 50 mg four times daily if required. For extrapyramidal reactions, *children,* 5 mg/kg daily in divided doses at six-hour intervals.

Intramuscular (deep), Intravenous: For drug-induced extrapyramidal reactions, except tardive dyskinesia, *adults,* 10 to 50 mg. The maximal single dose is 100 mg and the total daily dose should not exceed 400 mg. *Children* (intramuscular), 5 mg/kg daily. The maximal daily dose should not exceed 300 mg in 24 hours.

Benadryl
(Parke-Davis).
Capsules 25 and 50 mg; elixir 12.5 mg/5 ml (alcohol 14%).
Solution (for injection) 10 mg/ml in 10 and 30 ml containers and 50 mg/ml in 1 and 10 ml containers.

Orphenadrine Hydrochloride

Cl⁻

Oral: For idiopathic and postencephalitic parkinsonism, *adults,* initially, 50 mg three times daily. The dosage may be gradually increased up to 250 mg daily if required and tolerated.

Disipal
(Riker).
Tablets 50 mg.

PHENOTHIAZINE
Ethopropazine Hydrochloride

Cl⁻

Oral: For idiopathic and postencephalitic parkinsonism, *adults,* initially, 50 mg once or twice daily. The dosage may be gradually increased, if required, to a total daily dose of 100 to 400 mg in mild or moderate cases. Patients with severe impairment may require 500 to 600 mg.

Parsidol
(Parke-Davis).
Tablets 10 and 50 mg.

DRUGS AFFECTING BRAIN DOPAMINE

Dopamine-releasing Drug

AMANTADINE HYDROCHLORIDE
[Symmetrel]

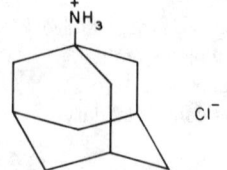

Cl⁻

ACTIONS AND USES. This antiviral agent reduces signs and symptoms and improves functional capacity in some patients with parkinsonism. It is believed to act by augmenting the release of dopamine and other catecholamines from neuronal storage sites, by delaying the reuptake of these neurotransmitters into synaptic vesicles, and by exerting anticholinergic effects. Amantadine is less effective than levodopa, but it generally produces a more rapid response (two to five days) and fewer untoward reactions, and the dosage is easier to adjust. Initial clinical improvement may not be sustained, however, and performance may deteriorate after three to six months (Timberlake and Vance, 1978).

Amantadine may be most effective when used alone for initial therapy but is also useful when given with anticholinergic drugs or levodopa. This agent is particularly beneficial in patients who cannot tolerate maximally effective doses of levodopa or in whom the response to levodopa fluctuates.

ADVERSE REACTIONS AND PRECAUTIONS. Amantadine is usually well tolerated. Some adverse effects are similar to those produced by anticholinergic agents: changes in mood, dizziness, nervousness, inability to concentrate, ataxia, slurred speech, insomnia, lethargy, blurred vision, urinary retention, dryness of the mouth, gastrointestinal hypomotility, and rash.

Approximately 25% of patients develop difficulty in thinking, confusion, lightheadedness, hallucinations, and anxiety. These symptoms are usually mild, occur shortly after therapy is initiated, are reversible following withdrawal of the drug, and often cease even when administration is continued. Activities requiring mental alertness (eg, driving) should be avoided until it is reasonable to assume that this cluster of symptoms will not recur.

Livedo reticularis (mottling of the skin) is relatively common in patients (particularly women) receiving amantadine for one month or longer. This reaction may subside during continued administration but can persist throughout therapy. It disappears gradually within days or weeks after amantadine is discontinued. There is no association between livedo reticularis and any underlying systemic disorder.

Edema of the feet, ankles, and legs (usually associated with livedo reticularis) has been noted in some patients.

Large doses of amantadine are embryotoxic and teratogenic in certain laboratory animals; therefore, the drug should not be used during pregnancy unless the benefits to the mother outweigh the risks to the fetus (FDA Pregnancy Category C). Amantadine is excreted in milk and should not be given to nursing mothers.

DRUG INTERACTIONS. Both the peripheral and central adverse effects of anticholinergic drugs are increased by amantadine. Combined therapy has induced acute psychotic reactions identical to those caused by atropine poisoning. If signs of central toxicity occur during combined therapy, the dose of the anticholinergic drug should be reduced. Psychotic reactions are not uncommon in patients receiving amantadine with levodopa.

PHARMACOKINETICS. Amantadine is well absorbed orally; the elimination half-life ranges from 9.7 to 14.5 hours (mean, 11.8 ± 2.1 hours) in normal subjects. Since more than 90% of this drug is excreted unchanged in the urine, the dose must be adjusted in patients with renal impairment (Horadam et al, 1981). Hemodialysis is relatively ineffective in removing amantadine.

DOSAGE AND PREPARATIONS.
Oral: For idiopathic or postencephalitic parkinsonism, initially, 25 to 50 mg daily of amantadine syrup increased gradually to 200 mg/day. The syrup preparation allows smaller initial dosage and helps lessen the risk of early side effects. Amounts exceeding 200 mg daily generally provide little

additional relief and may be associated with increasing toxicity.

Symmetrel (DuPont). Capsules 100 mg; syrup 50 mg/5 ml.

Drugs That Increase Brain Levels of Dopamine

LEVODOPA
[Dopar, Larodopa]

ACTIONS. Although dopamine does not enter the brain in sufficient quantities to be of value in the treatment of parkinsonism, levodopa, its immediate precursor, penetrates the blood-brain barrier and is then converted to dopamine by the enzyme, L-aromatic amino acid decarboxylase. The amount of this enzyme in peripheral tissues is far in excess of that in the brain and, therefore, large doses of levodopa are required to achieve therapeutic levels of dopamine in the central nervous system.

USES. Most neurologists administer levodopa in combination with the decarboxylase inhibitor, carbidopa, which minimizes peripheral adverse reactions (eg, nausea and vomiting) and allows reduction of the dose of levodopa. However, in patients not bothered by these adverse reactions, levodopa alone may be appropriate.

When administered in gradually increasing doses for an adequate period of time, levodopa relieves symptoms and improves functional capacity in about 75% of patients with parkinsonism. In one-half of patients, the quality of life is improved markedly for many years. Levodopa is so specific and effective in Parkinson's disease that an initial lack of response is cause to question the accuracy of diagnosis; some unresponsive patients have multisystem degenerative diseases involving brain sites in addition to the dopaminergic nigrostriatal pathway.

Levodopa does not halt progression of the underlying disease, but symptoms improve substantially and life expectancy is prolonged an average of more than three years over that observed with previously available therapy. This may be attributed partially to better medical care, more frequent visits that identify complications early, and better control of complications, such as infections (Shaw et al, 1980).

Levodopa is useful in both idiopathic and postencephalitic parkinsonism; patients with the postencephalitic form may require smaller doses. All major parkinsonian symptoms may be ameliorated, particularly bradykinesia, rigidity, and, to a lesser extent, tremor. Balance, posture, gait, and handwriting improve promptly; mood may be elevated; and seborrhea and drooling may diminish. Although intellectual function improves initially, this effect often is transient; mental deterioration and dementia may develop during long-term therapy. It has not been established whether mental changes reflect progression of degenerative disease or a direct effect of levodopa (Fahn and Bressman, 1984; Lang and Blair, 1984; Markham and Diamond, 1981).

Although levodopa is more effective than the central anticholinergic drugs and amantadine, it is usually reserved for patients with more marked functional impairment. When initiating therapy in patients already receiving anticholinergic drugs or amantadine, some neurologists decrease the doses of these drugs and observe the effect of levodopa. If treatment is initiated with levodopa/carbidopa, anticholinergic drugs, amantadine, and/or bromocriptine may be added later to achieve optimal effects. It is best to avoid combining an anticholinergic agent and levodopa if there is a history of psychosis.

This drug also is effective in parkinsonism due to neural damage resulting from chronic manganese exposure, carbon monoxide poisoning, or MPTP intoxication.

More studies are necessary to determine whether levodopa can reverse parkinsonian symptoms produced by antipsychotic drugs. Because this syndrome results from dopamine receptor blockade, it is presumed that the quantity of dopamine available from levodopa is inadequate to overcome the blockade.

ADVERSE REACTIONS AND PRECAUTIONS.

Gastrointestinal: Nausea, vomiting, and anorexia occur in most patients if the initial daily dose is large or increased too rapidly. To avoid nausea and vomiting, the dose should be titrated slowly. Symptoms usually are diminished by temporarily reducing the daily dose, by administering smaller doses more frequently, or by giving the drug with food. However, in chronic therapy, the tentative relationship between high-protein meals and "on-off" symptoms may require separation of dosing and meals (Nutt et al, 1984). Antiemetics (eg, phenothiazines, thioxanthenes, butyrophenones, metoclopramide) should be avoided because they may counteract levodopa's therapeutic effect. An exception may be the investigational dopamine antagonist, domperidone, which acts on the medullary chemoreceptor trigger zone outside the blood-brain barrier (see the evaluation in Chapter 14, Drugs Used in Vertigo and Vomiting).

Other gastrointestinal disturbances occasionally reported but questionably related to levodopa therapy include abdominal pain, diarrhea, constipation, and activation of peptic ulcer.

Neurologic: Abnormal involuntary movements often occur just before or soon after the optimal therapeutic response is obtained and are the major dose-limiting factors in levodopa therapy. Mild, intermittent dyskinesias (usually choreiform movements) involving the mouth, tongue, face, and neck are common after a few months of therapy. Dyskinesias of the limbs, particularly the hands, are even more common than facial dyskinesia but are not as well recognized. Some tolerance develops to these dyskinesias, and many patients are either unaware of them or willingly tolerate them in order to obtain the beneficial effects of levodopa. The incidence of peak-dose dyskinesias is as high as 80% in patients receiving prolonged levodopa therapy (Shaw et al, 1980).

Severe, generalized, drug-induced dyskinesias generally occur after prolonged administration of large doses. Choreiform, choreoathetoid, dystonic, myoclonic, or a combination of these movements may occur. They are usually associated with improved control of parkinsonism and may disappear when the dose is reduced, although parkinsonian symptoms then may increase. In some patients, abnormal involuntary movements recur at progressively lower doses.

Episodes of akinesia, tremor, and rigidity lasting a few minutes to several hours are often seen in patients after more than one year of levodopa therapy. At least two forms of these fluctuations have been described: (1) End-of-dose akinesia ("wearing off" effect), which occurs at increasingly shorter intervals between doses of levodopa and may initially be improved by reducing the interval between doses. Concomitant use of amantadine also may be helpful but its effect is often temporary. End-of-dose akinesia is associated with low plasma concentrations of levodopa. (2) The on-off phenomenon representing unpredictable and rapid motor fluctuations is less common than end-of-dose deterioration. It bears no relationship to the time of the last dose and may be alleviated by adding amantadine or bromocriptine to the regimen and adjusting the diet and timing of meals (see the Introduction). A third form, akinesia paradoxica (sometimes called "transient freezing"), often develops suddenly during a dyskinetic episode; no satisfactory treatment is available, and the mechanism of this phenomenon remains unexplained. All of these fluctuations may appear in the same patient, and some physicians regard all three forms as manifestations of on-off phenomena.

Headache, mydriasis, widening of the palpebral fissures, and activation of cluster headache (Horton's syndrome) occasionally have been associated with levodopa therapy. Exacerbation of oculogyric crisis by levodopa has been reported in patients with postencephalitic parkinsonism.

Respiratory: Respiratory abnormalities may develop independently, most commonly in patients with postencephalitic parkinsonism, but some respiratory dysfunction may develop during drug therapy. Symptoms include cough, hoarseness, postnasal drip, tachypnea, bradypnea, gasping, panting, sniffing, and feelings of pressure in the chest. These phenomena may represent dyskinesias of the diaphragm and intercostal muscles and are much more common in patients with parkinsonism and Shy-Drager syndrome.

Psychiatric: Psychic disturbances are common, particularly in elderly patients receiving other antiparkinson drugs, especially anticholinergic drugs, concomitantly. Euphoria, restlessness, anxiety, irritability, hyperactivity, insomnia, hallucinations, and vivid dreams are common. Agitation, hypomanic and paranoid reactions, delirium, and severe depression, including aggressive or suicidal behavior, have developed occasionally, most often in patients with pre-existing dementia or a history of mental illness. In some cases, levodopa may unmask a previously unrecognized dementia. The mental changes generally respond to a reduction in dose but occasionally require discontinuation of levodopa.

Cardiovascular: If the initial daily dose of levodopa is large or is increased too rapidly, the standing systolic and diastolic blood pressures may be reduced by 20 to 30 mm Hg. This effect usually is well tolerated, but significant orthostatic hypotension with syncope may occur, especially in patients taking diuretics and/or tricyclic antidepressants concomitantly. This reaction tends to diminish in time and often can be alleviated by wearing elastic bandages or stockings, temporarily reducing the dose of levodopa, increasing the intake of salt, and, in extreme cases (eg, Shy-Drager syndrome), administering a salt-retaining steroid. When the latter measures are employed, the patient should be monitored closely for symptoms of hypervolemia and congestive heart failure.

Both minor disturbances of cardiac rate and rhythm (tachycardia and premature ventricular contractions) and severe arrhythmias have developed occasionally. It is not clear whether levodopa was a causal factor or whether the arrhythmia was related to underlying heart disease. Cardiac rhythm should be monitored during dosage adjustment. Arrhythmias do not usually require antiarrhythmic drugs and it is seldom necessary to discontinue levodopa therapy. No significant difference in the severity of ventricular arrhythmias or in the incidence of orthostatic hypotension was noted in patients receiving levodopa/carbidopa compared to levodopa alone (Leibowitz and Lieberman, 1975).

Transient flushing of the skin is common during levodopa therapy. Palpitations may occur but often disappear with continued therapy.

Hypertension, myocardial infarction, and venous thrombosis have been reported occasionally, but there is no evidence that these complications are more common in patients receiving levodopa than in a comparable age group not receiving the drug. If myocardial infarction occurs during therapy, modification of the treatment program may be required.

LABORATORY FINDINGS. Results of laboratory studies have not revealed evidence of serious hematologic, renal, hepatic, or thyroid dysfunction due to levodopa. Large doses may cause hypokalemia associated with increased plasma levels of aldosterone; this effect is substantially reduced by adding carbidopa to the regimen. The white blood cell count decreased temporarily in a few patients. Positive Coombs' tests occur occasionally, and there have been a few reports of reduced hemoglobin and hematocrit levels unrelated to a hemolytic process.

Mild, transient elevations of blood urea nitrogen occur and usually can be controlled by increasing fluid intake. Elevation of the SGOT level has been noted in a few patients, but this usually returned to normal despite continued drug administration. Increased blood LDH, bilirubin, and alkaline phosphatase levels are rare. Elevations of uric acid have been noted using the colorimetric method of measurement but have not been reported in tests using the uricase method.

Levodopa increases plasma growth hormone levels and may produce mild carbohydrate intolerance, but signs of acromegaly or diabetes mellitus have not occurred during long-term therapy. Dark-colored sweat and changes in urine color (red-tinged when voiding, black when exposed to air) have been reported but are not indications for discontinuing the drug.

TERATOGENICITY. Levodopa (alone or with carbidopa) has caused visceral and skeletal malformations in rabbits; levodopa alone has depressed fetal and postnatal growth and viability in rodents. This drug is not recommended during pregnancy, in nursing mothers, or in children under 12 years.

DRUG INTERACTIONS. The therapeutic response to levodopa alone may be reduced or abolished by pyridoxine in doses as low as 5 mg daily, but not when levodopa is combined with sufficient amounts of carbidopa (approximately 100 mg/day). This has been attributed to the accelerated decarboxylation of levodopa in peripheral tissues. Patients receiving levodopa alone should avoid multiple vitamin preparations containing more than the minimal daily requirement of pyridoxine (see Chapter 47, Vitamins and Minerals).

The effectiveness of levodopa also may be reduced by phenothiazines, butyrophenones, thioxanthenes, rauwolfia alkaloids, phenytoin, papaverine, and metoclopramide.

Since a hypertensive crisis may occur if levodopa is given with a nonspecific monoamine oxidase inhibitor, these drugs always should be discontinued two weeks prior to initiation of levodopa therapy.

Methyldopa may decrease the antiparkinson effect of levodopa. Additive hypotensive effects also have been noted in patients receiving levodopa and other antihypertensive drugs.

If general anesthetics are required during therapy, it is recommended that levodopa be discontinued the night before anesthesia and reinstituted at the same dose as soon as possible after surgery. When therapy is interrupted for longer periods, the dosage should be adjusted gradually.

PHARMACOKINETICS. Levodopa is well absorbed by the amino acid transport system in the small bowel. Since the drug is substantially decarboxylated to dopamine by a first-pass hepatic effect, the concomitant administration of a decarboxylase inhibitor markedly increases the amount of levodopa available to enter the systemic circulation and brain. Levodopa has a relatively short plasma half-life (one to three hours). Dopamine is rapidly metabolized, principally to 3,4-dihydroxyphenylacetic acid and homovanillic acid, and many minor metabolites.

DOSAGE AND PREPARATIONS. Levodopa should be given under close medical supervision and the dosage must be individualized. When initiating therapy, patients in good general health who have only moderate neurologic impairment may be treated as outpatients if they are seen at regular intervals and good compliance is anticipated. Hospitalization should be reserved for patients with marked disability, those having coexisting systemic disorders that should be monitored daily, or those for whom drug administration cannot be properly supervised on an outpatient basis. All patients should be seen at regular intervals and the dosage modified as necessary for optimal results.

Oral: Levodopa is usually administered three or four times daily during the waking hours, but may be given much more frequently, depending upon the patient's response. It can be given with food to reduce gastrointestinal disturbances, but this may reduce absorption and therapeutic effect. The initial daily dose ranges from 500 mg to 1 g, depending upon the patient's tolerance, and may then be increased by 100 to 500 mg every two or three days, or less frequently in less tolerant patients (eg, 75 mg every three to seven days), until the desired therapeutic response is obtained or adverse reactions supervene. If adverse reactions are severe, the dose should be reduced or the drug discontinued temporarily. Optimal dosage generally is attained in six to eight weeks and usually ranges from 4 to 8 g daily. After several months to one year, a satisfactory clinical response often can be maintained with a lower dose.

Generic. Capsules 500 mg.
Dopar (Norwich Eaton). Capsules 100, 250, and 500 mg.
Larodopa (Roche). Capsules and tablets 100, 250, and 500 mg.

LEVODOPA AND CARBIDOPA
[Sinemet]

ACTIONS AND USES. The combination of levodopa/carbidopa is considered the preparation of choice by most neurologists when symptoms of Parkinson's disease significantly interfere with normal daily activities.

Approximately 95% of an oral dose of levodopa is decarboxylated in peripheral tissues, leaving only 5% for diffusion across the blood-brain barrier. Thus, large doses are required to achieve therapeutic levels of dopamine in the central nervous system. However, these amounts frequently cause nausea and vomiting, presumably because of an effect of dopamine on the chemoreceptor trigger zone, which is located outside the blood-brain barrier.

Carbidopa is a dopa decarboxylase inhibitor that does not cross the blood-brain barrier and therefore does not prevent the central conversion of levodopa to dopamine. By preventing the extracerebral metabolism of levodopa, carbidopa increases the amount available in the brain for decarboxylation to dopamine, thereby enhancing the therapeutic response and reducing side effects caused by peripheral actions of dopamine and other catecholamines.

Carbidopa alone [Lodosyn] is available to physicians only on request and is reserved primarily for investigational use. The combination product [Sinemet] is recommended for general use.

Sinemet contains carbidopa and levodopa in ratios of 1:4 or 1:10. The combination increases the plasma concentrations of levodopa, reduces dosage requirements for levodopa by approximately 75%, and decreases the incidence of nausea and vomiting significantly. Therefore, the dosage can be increased more rapidly and the response is somewhat smoother. Sinemet is preferred by most physicians for initial therapy, because higher brain concentrations of levodopa are attained with fewer peripheral side effects than with a comparable dose of levodopa alone.

Most adults require 70 to 200 mg daily of carbidopa for maximum inhibition of peripheral dopa decarboxylase, and the 1:10 ratio of Sinemet 10-100 may deliver less than the minimum requirement when only small doses of levodopa are desired. In such instances, it may be useful to prescribe the preparation containing a 1:4 ratio of carbidopa/levodopa [Sinemet 25-100] to permit saturation of peripheral dopa decarboxylase and deliver less than 700 mg daily of levodopa. Responsiveness increases and adverse reactions decrease (Hoehn, 1980).

ADVERSE REACTIONS. Approximately 2% to 5% of patients experience persistent nausea and vomiting; as with levodopa alone, these reactions can be minimized by giving the combination with food. Combined therapy does not significantly decrease the dyskinesias and psychiatric disturbances induced by levodopa alone. In fact, since the dose can be increased rapidly, these reactions may appear earlier and be more severe than with levodopa alone. In other respects, the adverse effects and interactions produced by this combination are similar to those seen with levodopa. No adverse reactions have been attributed to carbidopa alone.

DOSAGE AND PREPARATIONS. Like all fixed-dose combinations, Sinemet is not suitable for all patients. Dosage must be titrated carefully to obtain the desired therapeutic response with minimal adverse effects. The patient should be observed closely during dosage adjustment and, if adverse reactions are seen, the dose should be reduced or the compound temporarily discontinued.

Oral: Most authorities prefer to initiate therapy with a half-tablet of Sinemet 10-100 or of the 25-100 formulation two to four times daily; the dosage is then increased by one-half to one tablet/day every two to three days to minimize adverse effects. The manufacturer recommends using Sinemet 25-100 to provide adequate carbidopa. If a larger daily dose of levodopa is needed, one tablet of Sinemet 25-250 three or four times daily may be given. This may be increased by one-half to one tablet daily or every other day if necessary. The usual maintenance dose is three to a maximum of eight tablets of Sinemet 25-250 daily in divided amounts. If further adjustment is indicated, levodopa may be added to the regimen.

In patients being transferred from levodopa to levodopa/carbidopa, levodopa should be discontinued at least 12 hours before initiating therapy with Sinemet. The initial daily dose should provide approximately 25% of the previous amount of levodopa. The suggested initial dosage is one tablet of Sinemet 10-100 or Sinemet 25-100 three or four times daily for patients who have been maintained on less than 1.5 g of levodopa daily. Patients maintained on larger doses of levodopa may eventually require one tablet of Sinemet 25-250 three or four times daily.

Patients who require or tolerate only small doses of levodopa (ie, 0.75 to 1 g daily) may benefit from Sinemet 25-100 (1:4 ratio) rather than Sinemet 10-100 (1:10 ratio) to ensure an adequate daily intake of the decarboxylase inhibitor.

Sinemet (Merck Sharp & Dohme). Tablets containing carbidopa 10 mg and levodopa 100 mg [**Sinemet 10-100**] or carbidopa 25 mg and levodopa 100 mg [**Sinemet 25-100**] or 250 mg [**Sinemet 25-250**].

SELEGILINE (Deprenyl)

ACTIONS AND USES. Early clinical trials revealed that monoamine oxidase inhibitors potentiated the antiparkinson actions of levodopa, presumably by inhibiting the degradation of dopamine, but their concomitant use produced hypertension. Monoamine oxidase occurs in at least two forms, which differ in substrate specificity: Type A is associated principally with the oxidative deamination of noradrenalin and serotonin; type B has preferential activity for dopamine.

A double-blind crossover study was conducted in Europe to determine the role of selegiline, a relatively specific type B monoamine oxidase inhibitor, in extending the duration of action and effectiveness of levodopa (Lees et al, 1977). Total daily doses of 5 to 10 mg decreased the amount of levodopa required by an average of 200 mg daily (approximately 30%). Selegiline with levodopa alone or levodopa/carbidopa increased the duration of action of levodopa and was beneficial in overcoming early morning immobility and stiffness and mild on-off disabilities (Yahr et al, 1983). Results of studies in the United States evaluating the usefulness of selegiline as an adjunct in the management of on-off symptoms have been mixed (Eisler et al, 1981; Schachter et al, 1980).

Some European investigators suggest that the drug be considered prior to the addition or substitution of bromocriptine. Selegiline may play a limited but significant role as an adjunct in the management of parkinsonism.

Recent data indicating that the neurotoxin, MPTP, requires enzymatic activation by monoamine oxidase B have increased interest in selegiline in this country. Selegiline and other specific enzyme inhibitors prevent MPTP-induced parkinsonism in animals (Langston et al, 1984; Heikkila et al, 1984). In addition, there is a report that selegiline may prolong the lifespan of patients with idiopathic Parkinson's disease by slowing the disease process (Birkmayer, 1983).

Selegiline in doses up to 15 mg daily has no antiparkinson activity. It is metabolized extensively to methamphetamine and amphetamine (Reynolds et al, 1978). In one controlled study on a small group of patients, the conversion of selegiline to amphetamine was confirmed; this drug also counteracted the dose-related fluctuations in response to optimal levodopa therapy without causing serious side effects (Schachter et al, 1980).

It has not been established whether release of dopamine, blockade of dopamine reuptake by selegiline metabolites, and/or inhibition of monoamine oxidase type B is responsible for the improved efficacy of levodopa.

ADVERSE REACTIONS. Dyskinesia occurs in about one-third of patients, and this reaction is severe and disabling in one-third of those affected. The increase in its incidence may have resulted from failure to reduce the dose of levodopa upon initiation of selegiline. Mental changes also are very common (eg, depression, dementia, paranoid ideation, psychotic episodes). The incidence of nausea, dryness of the mouth, confusion, and dizziness is 10% to 20% and that of orthostatic hypotension, syncope, circumoral paresthesias, hallucinations, and unpleasant taste is 5% or less. Hypertension following ingestion of tyramine-containing foods and hepatotoxicity have not been observed; however, 1 patient in a group of 32 developed hypertension that resolved on cessation of selegiline therapy.

DOSAGE AND PREPARATIONS.
Oral: The recommended daily dose is 5 mg, increased to a maximum of 10 mg if no response occurs. Alternate-day administration can be considered if a good response is obtained.

Eldepryl (Britannia Pharmaceuticals Limited). Tablets 5 mg. (Investigational drug)

Dopamine Receptor Agonists

The gradual loss of responsiveness to levodopa that occurs over one to five years may be caused in part by the decreasing capacity of nigrostriatal neurons to synthesize and store dopamine. This assumption reinforced the search for specific agonists that act directly on striatal dopamine receptor sites. Natural and semisynthetic ergolines derived from ergot alkaloids are the primary sources of such agonists.

Bromocriptine is the only clinically useful direct-acting dopamine receptor agonist presently available for the treatment of parkinsonism (Vance et al, 1984; Lang and Blair, 1984; Parkes, 1979; Hoehn, 1980). Lisuride (a soluble ergoline derivative) and pergolide (a semisynthetic derivative of ergot) are dopamine receptor agonists that are considerably more potent on a milligram basis than bromocriptine and appear to be promising antiparkinson drugs. The short duration of action of lisuride may limit its usefulness in patients with diurnal fluctuations in performance (Parkes et al, 1981), but it has the advantage of intravenous administration. In contrast, pergolide has a longer duration of action and its efficacy is similar to that of bromocriptine (LeWitt et al, 1983).

A number of partial agonists, including the nonergot, ciladopa, is being investigated. The lower affinity of these agonists for dopamine receptors should increase selectivity of action for supersensitive postsynaptic striatal receptors over other central dopamine receptors and thus may decrease adverse reactions (Lieberman et al, 1985).

BROMOCRIPTINE MESYLATE
[Parlodel]

USES. Bromocriptine may be more effective than the anticholinergic drugs and amantadine in parkinsonism. However, levodopa alone or with carbidopa is still the therapy of choice.

The primary indications for bromocriptine in parkinsonism are (1) as an adjunct to levodopa or levodopa/carbidopa in patients experiencing significant fluctuations in therapeutic response, end-of-dose akinesia, and painful muscle cramps; the decrease in fluctuations may be related to bromocriptine's longer duration of action, which supports the view that bromocriptine and levodopa may affect different dopamine receptors and/or sites; (2) as an alternative to levodopa if that drug is contraindicated or not tolerated; and (3) in patients unresponsive to levodopa (not all of these patients respond to bromocriptine).

The dose of levodopa or levodopa/carbidopa should be reduced as the dose of bromocriptine is increased. This may reduce the incidence of dyskinesias and dystonias induced by levodopa, for bromocriptine appears to have less of a tendency than levodopa to produce these involuntary movements.

There is less experience with bromocriptine as the initial drug for long-term management of Parkinson's disease. The debate is similar to that on levodopa: when and in what dose to begin therapy (Calne, 1984).

Approximately 50% to 60% of previously untreated patients given maximum tolerated doses of bromocriptine respond favorably (ie, 25% reduction in disability score). The remainder show no response or experience adverse effects severe enough to necessitate drug withdrawal (Lees and Stern, 1981).

ADVERSE REACTIONS. There is considerable individual variation in response to bromocriptine. Careful titration of dose to determine the maximum benefit/risk ratio is required.

Transient dizziness and nausea often occur with total daily doses of 10 to 50 mg. Administering bromocriptine with food or antacids, reducing the dose, and increasing the daily dose more gradually may alleviate nausea in severe cases. Domperidone, a peripheral dopamine antagonist, has controlled marked nausea and vomiting (see Chapter 14, Drugs Used in Vertigo and Vomiting).

Hypotension occurs less frequently but can be severe, even with doses of 2.5 mg, especially when initiating therapy. Colicky abdominal pain, constipation, blurred vision with or without diplopia, and digital vasospasm on exposure to cold are observed occasionally. Hepatotoxicity is rare and resolves with discontinuation of the drug.

Asymptomatic elevations of serum transaminase and alkaline phosphatase levels have been reported. No other liver function or routine laboratory tests appear to be affected.

More serious adverse reactions generally occur with total daily doses of 50 to 100 mg (but can occur even at lower dosages) and include erythromelalgia, mental disturbances, and dyskinesias. Erythromelalgia is characterized by red, tender, warm, edematous lower extremities. Mental disturbances may be limited to confusion and vivid dreams or, less frequently, paranoid delusions and visual hallucinations. Dyskinesias resemble the choreiform movements induced by levodopa. Pulmonary infiltrates and thickening of the pleura have occurred in a few patients receiving doses in this range. All effects are reversible upon decreasing the dose or discontinuing the drug.

PHARMACOKINETICS. Following oral administration, 28% of a dose is absorbed from the gastrointestinal tract. Absorption is rapid and time to peak effect and peak concentration is about 1.2 hours. The drug is 90% to 96% bound to serum albumin.

The mean elimination half-life (including inactive polar metabolites) is about 50 hours. The mean half-life for the parent compound is 3 ± 0.5 hours and that for the nonpolar metabo-

lites formed as bromocriptine undergoes phase I-type metabolism is 7.5 hours (Schran et al, 1980).

Bromocriptine is extensively metabolized by first-order kinetics in the liver, and 98% of an oral dose is excreted in the feces; the remaining 2% is excreted in the urine (Vance et al, 1984). Active metabolites have not been identified.

DOSAGE AND PREPARATIONS.

Oral: It is important to initiate treatment with a small dose and increase the amount slowly until a maximum therapeutic response is achieved. Initially, 1.25 mg twice daily is suggested to lessen nausea and hypotensive effects. The dose is increased biweekly or monthly by 1.25 to 2.5 mg until beneficial effects or intolerable adverse reactions are noted. Most patients respond to 10 to 20 mg daily but a few with advanced disease may require up to 100 mg daily (maximum).

Parlodel (Sandoz). Capsules 5 mg; tablets 2.5 mg.

PERGOLIDE MESYLATE

ACTIONS AND USES. This investigational drug is a synthetic ergoline with direct dopaminergic activity. Unlike other dopamine agonists, pergolide has both D_1 and D_2 receptor activity. Pergolide is more potent than bromocriptine and has a longer half-life. However, its overall efficacy in combination with levodopa/carbidopa in advanced parkinsonism is similar to that of bromocriptine (LeWitt et al, 1983). When given with levodopa, this drug is effective in managing the on-off and wearing-off symptoms observed during long-term levodopa therapy (LeWitt et al, 1983; Lieberman et al, 1984; Goetz et al, 1983). Its efficacy declines after six months (Lieberman et al, 1984), perhaps because of desensitization of dopamine receptors, progression of the disease, or both.

Restoration of the effect of levodopa/carbidopa/dopamine agonist therapy has been reported following substitution of pergolide for bromocriptine (Goetz et al, 1984). Thus, failure of one dopaminergic agonist may not rule out response to a second.

ADVERSE REACTIONS. Adverse reactions are similar to those of bromocriptine. At optimal dosage, the most common reactions are mild nausea, loss of appetite, dry mouth, and lightheadedness (LeWitt et al, 1983). Asymptomatic hypotension has occurred. Sedation and hallucinations are less common. Initial reports of increased arrhythmias were not substantiated (Tanner et al, 1985). As with bromocriptine and methysergide, prolonged administration of pergolide may produce rare pleural fibrosis, which may resolve with cessation of the drug.

DOSAGE AND PREPARATIONS.

Oral: Initially, 0.1 mg daily, increased by 0.1 to 0.4 mg daily to a maximum daily dose of 5 mg (Lieberman et al, 1984).

Pergolide Mesylate (Lilly).
(Investigational drug)

OTHER DYSKINETIC DISORDERS

MYOCLONUS. This disorder is characterized by brief, lightning-like muscular contractions of sudden onset; a small group or several groups of muscles may be involved. The contractions may be repetitive and are typically arrhythmic and unpredictable. Myoclonic disorders are closely related to epileptic seizures and many result from structural central nervous system lesions. Drugs such as 5-hydroxytryptophan for postanoxic myoclonus and others used in the treatment of myoclonic seizures are discussed in Chapter 9, Antiepileptic Drugs.

TICS. Tics (habit spasms) resemble choreic movements in that they are isolated muscle twitches or jerks that are often repetitive and stereotyped; they are not strictly involuntary, because they can be temporarily suppressed or modified. They occasionally are induced by drugs and are commonly associated with anxiety. An antianxiety drug may be useful in some simple tic disorders; however, the complex multiple tic disorder, Tourette's syndrome, may require treatment with the antipsychotic drugs, haloperidol and pimozide [Orap] (see the evaluation), or clonidine [Catapres] (see Chapter 6, Antipsychotic Drugs).

DYSTONIAS. These are long-sustained, often bizarre, posturing movements of the neck, jaw, trunk, and extremities often associated with protrusion of the tongue, masseter spasms, blepharospasm, and oculogyric crisis. Idiopathic and hereditary dystonias and those caused by perinatal cerebral injury, head trauma, and encephalitis occur most frequently. However, acute dystonia also is a common adverse reaction to the initial administration of antipsychotic drugs and other antidopaminergic agents, such as the antiemetic, metoclopramide [Reglan]. Acute, drug-induced dystonias generally respond rapidly to parenteral administration of an antihistamine (eg, diphenhydramine [Benadryl]) or a centrally acting anticholinergic agent (eg, benztropine [Cogentin], biperiden [Akineton]); see the section on Adverse Reactions in Chapter 6, Antipsychotic Drugs.

BALLISMUS. Ballismus is characterized by continual, usually unilateral (hemiballismus), purposeless, flinging movements of the upper extremities. It is most often produced by acute vascular infarction of the subthalamic nucleus. Some authorities believe that this disorder represents a severe form of chorea. Ballismus is usually self-limiting but responds to antipsychotic drugs (see Chapter 6).

TREMOR. Tremor is a repetitive, rhythmic, oscillatory (to and fro) movement consisting of alternate contractions of opposing muscle groups. It may be static (present at rest), action or postural (present throughout the range of movement), or intention (accentuated towards the end of movement). The tremors associated with parkinsonism are static, those occurring with senility or thyrotoxicosis are action or postural, and those that develop with delirium tremens, multiple sclerosis, and cerebellar disease are intention.

Essential tremor, a common form of action or postural tremor, primarily involves the upper extremities and develops in adults with no other demonstrable neurologic abnormalities; it is often familial (benign hereditary tremor). The intensity is variable and may be aggravated by stress and fatigue. The frequency of this fine tremor ranges from 4 to 12 Hz. It is thought to represent an exaggeration of physiologic tremor and resembles that associated with anxiety, thyrotoxicosis, or senility or induced by epinephrine, amphetamines, tricyclic antidepressants, or lithium.

Although alcohol cannot be recommended for control of essential tremor due to its abuse potential, under certain circumstances it may be the most effective agent for some patients (Koller and Biary, 1984 A). Alcohol usually acts within a few minutes but efficacy decreases with continued use (Larsen and Calne, 1983).

Beta-adrenergic blocking drugs are the agents of choice for essential tremor. Although propranolol [Inderal] (see evaluation) has been used most extensively, metoprolol [Lopressor], timolol [Blocadren], atenolol [Tenormin], and sotalol (investigational) also are effective. Primidone [Mysoline] is being investigated as an antitremor agent (Koller, 1985).

Senile tremor also may respond to beta-adrenergic blocking agents.

CHOREA. This abnormal involuntary movement disorder involves brief contraction of small muscle groups in the face, trunk, or extremities. A novel pattern of movement often emerges when the patient attempts to mask these contractions by carrying out semipurposeful movements.

Chorea occurs as a component of Huntington's disease and spontaneous or drug-induced oral masticatory syndrome; it occurs rarely with hyperthyroidism, systemic lupus erythematosus, after rheumatic fever (Sydenham's chorea) or encephalitis, during pregnancy, or with use of contraceptive drugs (chorea gravidarum), levodopa, amphetamine, methylphenidate [Ritalin], and phenytoin [Dilantin]. Choreiform, and occasionally dystonic, movements are a component of antipsychotic drug-induced tardive (late onset) dyskinesia.

Athetosis consists of slow, writhing, involuntary movements of the limb muscles that often accompany chorea (choreoathetosis) as a sequel of birth injury (cerebral palsy).

Huntington's Disease: Huntington's disease is a progressive, autosomal dominant, genetic disorder characterized by choreiform movements and behavioral abnormalities (Folstein and Folstein, 1981). Widespread degenerative changes produce a relative excess of dopamine in nigrostriatal neurotransmission and striatal reductions in GABA, acetylcholine, substance P, and enkephalins. Symptoms usually develop in the third to fifth decade of life. Juvenile-onset (first or second decade) Huntington's disease (akinetic-rigid form) is characterized by bradykinesia and hypertonicity resembling parkinsonism more than chorea. Seizures and mental retardation are present in some juvenile patients.

Drug therapy is only a small part of the overall management of adults with Huntington's disease (Folstein and Folstein, 1981). Pharmacotherapy is limited to symptomatic treatment of the movement disorder and depression but provides only transient relief and does not alter the functional decline. It also is important to recognize and treat associated depression and schizophrenic-like psychoses in patients with this disease.

Levodopa may be of short-term palliative value in juvenile-onset Huntington's disease. However, this drug markedly increases choreiform activity in the adult-onset form and may aggravate behavioral abnormalities. Recent localization of the gene for Huntington's disease to the short arm of chromosome 4 offers promise of reliable presymptomatic detection.

Antichoreic therapy is usually reserved for patients with disabling features, but attempts to mask choreic movements completely are not recommended. Antichoreic drugs are usually administered in the minimum amount with frequent drug holidays. The goal of therapy is to reduce brain dopaminergic transmission or enhance cholinergic activity. Dopamine transmission can be reduced by agents that inhibit the presynaptic synthesis and storage of dopamine or that antagonize dopamine receptors postsynaptically. Antipsychotic agents antagonize dopamine and usually lessen the chorea temporarily in adult-onset Huntington's disease. No particular antipsychotic drug appears to be most effective. The use of larger doses may restore control, but prolonged administration may increase the incidence of tardive dyskinesia (Shoulson, 1979).

The dopamine-depleting drug, tetrabenazine [Nitoman], also reduces the chorea of Huntington's disease (Toglia et al, 1978; Bird, 1980; Shoulson and Goldblatt, 1981; Jankovic, 1982). However, tetrabenazine also has dopamine-blocking effects and rarely may cause dystonic reactions. It is available only on an investigational basis in the United States. Another investigational agent, alpha-methyl-paratyrosine (AMPT), a catecholamine synthesis inhibitor, has been shown to increase the antichoreic effect of tetrabenazine (Lang and Marsden, 1982).

Oral choline has been claimed to enhance cholinergic activity. Although choline exerted antichoreic effects in a limited number of patients (Davis et al, 1976), the overall benefit of antichoreic drugs with cholinergic activity has been questioned (Nutt, 1983).

Individuals with Huntington's disease have a regional and selective loss of GABA, acetylcholine, and a variety of neuropeptides in the brain paralleling neurodegenerative changes in the striatum and other basal ganglia structures. However, the administration of various agents to increase GABA or mimic its action (eg, muscimol, THIP, gama-vinyl GABA, baclofen [Lioresal], isoniazid [Nydrazid]) has been of little clinical value (Foster et al, 1983; Scigliano et al, 1984; Perry et al, 1982).

TARDIVE DYSKINESIA. Classic tardive dyskinesia is characterized by involuntary, repetitive, choreiform movements of the cheek, mouth, and tongue. Lip smacking, chewing, tongue thrusting or protruding, lateral jaw movements, and sucking maneuvers result and are frequently termed the buccolingual masticatory or oral masticatory syndrome. As with all involuntary movement disorders, the dyskinesia disappears during sleep and is aggravated by stress. Tardive dyskinesia may take other forms, including choreiform movements of the hands and feet, athetoid movements of the extremities, and dystonic posturing of the neck and trunk.

The prevalence of tardive dyskinesia has increased in the last two decades following the use of antipsychotic drugs (Jeste and Wyatt, 1981 A; Kane and Smith, 1982). In addition, there are subsets of this disorder that are either unrelated to drug therapy or can occur during or following such drug therapy, making differential diagnosis much more difficult (Burke, 1984).

The pathogenesis of drug-induced tardive dyskinesia has been attributed to the development of supersensitivity of postsynaptic dopamine receptors rather than to reduction of cholinergic activity as in Huntington's disease. Other mechanisms also may be involved in the etiology of tardive dyskinesia (Jeste and Wyatt, 1981 B). No one antipsychotic drug has a greater or lesser chance of producing tardive dyskinesia (Burke, 1984).

A Task Force of the American Psychiatric Association has reviewed the late neurologic effects of antipsychotic drugs (Task Force on Late Neurological Effects of Antipsychotic Drugs, 1980). A summary of their findings on the risk factors, pathogenesis, differential diagnosis, and prognosis appears in the section on Adverse Reactions in Chapter 6, Antipsychotic Drugs. That section also includes guidelines to reduce the incidence of this type of tardive dyskinesia, since the Task Force felt that prophylaxis was more beneficial than current therapy.

If tardive dyskinesia develops during antipsychotic drug therapy, the first step should be discontinuation of the antipsychotic drug or dosage reduction if the underlying psychotic disorder permits this approach. A drug-free period should follow to allow for spontaneous remission of symptoms.

In general, drug treatment of tardive dyskinesia is not recommended. However, when disabling tardive dyskinesia persists for years after antipsychotic drug withdrawal, treatment with a dopamine depletor may be attempted, although the success of such therapy is limited. Improvement has been reported with reserpine, and this drug may be helpful as initial therapy. Tetrabenazine has been useful, but its dopamine receptor antagonist action may aggravate tardive dyskinesia in some patients (Burke, 1984).

Bromocriptine and levodopa also have been given to modify dopaminergic action. Low doses of bromocriptine are postulated to act on dopamine presynaptic autoreceptors to inhibit dopamine synthesis and release. Approximately 20 mg daily improved symptoms in 20% of patients (Jeste and Wyatt, 1982). This use of bromocriptine is investigational. The use of levodopa is based on the hypothesis that a temporary increase in dopamine levels would reduce receptor supersensitivity. Results of studies have shown that improvement may be achieved, but patients with severe tardive dyskinesia may not tolerate this drug (Jeste and Wyatt, 1982; Burke, 1984).

Reinstitution of antipsychotic drug therapy may be tried as a last resort. Once control is established, the drug is withdrawn gradually over one year or more (Burke, 1984). Some authorities reinstitute antipsychotic drug therapy only if psychosis recurs.

Of the cholinergic agents used to obtain a more favorable acetylcholine/dopamine ratio in the brain, choline has been advocated most commonly (Davis et al, 1976). However, studies to date have not demonstrated its usefulness and role in tardive dyskinesia. Since lecithin also improves tardive dyskinesia and is better tolerated than choline, it may be more acceptable, but controlled studies are necessary to substantiate its value (Simpson et al, 1982; Jeste and Wyatt, 1982).

Anecdotal reports and open studies indicate that lithium, baclofen [Lioresal], methyldopa [Aldomet], valproic acid [Depakene], clonidine [Catapres], amantadine [Symmetrel], clozapine (investigational), and clonazepam [Klonopin] may be effective in tardive dyskinesia, but controlled studies are necessary (Simpson et al, 1982; Jeste and Wyatt, 1982; Meltzer and Luchins, 1984). One small controlled clinical trial has indicated that the investigational drug, sulpiride, may be useful in treating tardive dyskinesia (Quinn and Marsden, 1984). Larger studies are needed to determine its role in this disorder.

Drug Evaluations

TETRABENAZINE
[Nitoman]

ACTIONS AND USES. Results of a number of controlled studies suggest that use of this investigational dopamine-depleting agent may control the involuntary movements of Huntington's chorea and other hyperkinetic movement disorders (Toglia et al, 1978; Bird, 1980; Jankovic, 1982). It was originally introduced as an antipsychotic drug and has actions similar to those of reserpine, which it resembles pharmacologically. Tetrabenazine does not possess many of the peripheral actions of reserpine, but it depletes catecholamines in the central nervous system. It does exert dopamine blocking effects and has been implicated as the cause of dystonic reactions and tardive dyskinesia. More long-term controlled studies are required to evaluate the role of tetrabenazine in the treatment of chorea.

Since tetrabenazine is not available in the United States, reserpine 1 to 5 mg daily has been used as a substitute.

ADVERSE REACTIONS. The most frequent adverse reactions are drowsiness and depression. More serious, less common effects include orthostatic hypotension and dysphagia.

Drug interactions are essentially the same as those observed with reserpine (see Chapter 28, Antihypertensive Agents).

DOSAGE AND PREPARATIONS.
Oral: For disease- or drug-induced chorea, *adults,* initially, 25 mg four times daily, increased by 25 mg daily every three to four days until the desired response is obtained, intolerable adverse effects occur, or a maximal daily dose of 200 mg is given.
Nitoman (Roche [United Kingdom, Australia]).
(Investigational drug)

PIMOZIDE
[Orap]

ACTIONS AND USES. This diphenylbutylpiperidine derivative has neuroleptic activity and is marketed for the suppression of phonic and motor tics in patients with Tourette's syndrome. In short-term studies, the efficacy of pimozide in Tourette's syndrome was similar to that of haloperidol (Shapiro and Shapiro, 1984). Although the precise mechanism of action is unknown, blockade of postsynaptic dopamine receptors has been postulated. Because of the limited experience with

pimozide in young patients (2 to 15 years), the manufacturer suggests that this drug be used only when motor and phonic tics become disabling and treatment with haloperidol has failed.

ADVERSE REACTIONS. The incidence of adverse reactions is similar to that of other neuroleptics. Extrapyramidal reactions and tardive dyskinesia are a risk with long-term use. Ventricular arrhythmias are rare but may be serious. An electrocardiogram should be performed before initiation of therapy and again in one month. Prolongation of the Q-T interval may necessitate withdrawal of the drug. Sedation is the most common reaction and anticholinergic reactions, such as dry mouth, constipation, and blurred vision, may occur.

PHARMACOKINETICS. Pimozide is well absorbed orally and has a long plasma half-life. Peak serum concentrations occur within six to eight hours and the mean half-life is 55 hours.

Pimozide is metabolized primarily in the liver by oxidative N-dealkylation. The drug and its major metabolites are excreted primarily by the kidneys (McNeil Pharmaceuticals, 1984).

DOSAGE AND PREPARATIONS.
Oral: Initially, 1 to 2 mg daily in divided doses, increased gradually every other day to a maximum of 0.3 mg/kg or 20 mg daily. The dose should be individualized so that the suppression of motor and phonic tics is balanced against adverse reactions. The usual daily maintenance dose is less than 0.2 mg/kg or 10 mg daily, whichever is less. Periodic attempts to reduce the dose have been recommended by the manufacturer. The effective dosage for *children under 12 years* has not been determined.
Orap (McNeil). Tablets 2 mg.

PROPRANOLOL HYDROCHLORIDE
[Inderal]

ACTIONS AND USES. Propranolol is the drug of choice for the management of essential tremor in patients for whom it is not contraindicated. Therapy is usually initiated when tremor disrupts or limits occupational and social activities. Hand tremor responds best; head tremor also has been shown to respond (Koller, 1984). Voice tremor may be more resistant (Larsen and Calne, 1983). Response to therapy is variable among patients and no definite predictive factors have been identified to aid in selecting those who will receive satisfactory symptomatic relief. However, younger patients with tremor of short duration (Dupont et al, 1973), older patients, and those with slow tremor frequencies (Teravainen et al, 1976) appear to respond well. In general, those more severely affected are refractory to therapy. Tremor may be suppressed completely in some patients, but tremor intensity is reduced 60% to 80% in most patients (Sørensen et al, 1981).

In asthmatic patients who cannot tolerate propranolol, metoprolol has been an effective alternative (Koller and Biary, 1984 B). There appears to be very little therapeutic overlap among the beta blockers with antitremor activity (eg, nadolol, metoprolol, propranolol); patients who do not respond to propranolol are unlikely to respond to another beta blocker.

The mechanism of action of propranolol in this disorder is

unknown. Further studies are required to determine whether this drug acts on central beta$_2$ receptors or peripheral receptors in skeletal muscle.

For adverse reactions, precautions, and pharmacokinetics, see Chapter 25, Antianginal Agents.

DOSAGE AND PREPARATIONS.

Oral: Although propranolol blood concentrations do not appear to correlate with effectiveness, clinical improvement is related to dosage and is generally achieved when 120 to 240 mg is given daily in three divided doses. A few patients respond to as little as 60 mg daily (Sørensen et al, 1981).

    Generic. Tablets 10, 20, 40, and 80 mg.

    Inderal (Ayerst). Tablets 10, 20, 40, 60, 80, and 90 mg.

    Inderal LA (Ayerst). Capsules (timed-release) 80, 120, and 160 mg.

Cited References

Bird ED: Chemical pathology of Huntington's disease. *Annu Rev Pharmacol Toxicol* 20:533-551, 1980.

Birkmayer W: Deprenyl (selegiline) in treatment of Parkinson's disease. *Acta Neurol Scand* Suppl 95:103-106, 1983.

Boller F, et al: Parkinson disease, dementia, and Alzheimer disease: Clinicopathological correlations. *Ann Neurol* 7:329-335, 1980.

Burke RE: Tardive dyskinesia: Current clinical issues. *Neurology* 34:1348-1358, 1984.

Calne DB: Role of various forms of treatment in management of Parkinson's disease. *Clin Neuropharmacol* 5(suppl 1):S38-S43, 1982.

Calne DB: Progress in Parkinson's disease, (editorial). *N Engl J Med* 310:523-524, 1984.

Davis KL, et al: Choline in tardive dyskinesia and Huntington's disease. *Life Sci* 19:1507-1515, 1976.

Diamond SG, et al: Double-blind comparison of levodopa, Madopa, and Sinemet in Parkinson disease. *Ann Neurol* 3:267-272, 1978.

Direnfeld LK, et al: Is L-dopa drug holiday useful? *Neurology* 30:785-788, 1980.

Dupont E, et al: Treatment of benign essential tremor with propranolol. *Acta Neurol Scand* 49:75-84, 1973.

Eisler T, et al: Deprenyl in Parkinson's disease. *Neurology* 31:19-23, 1981.

Fahn S, Bressman SB: Should levodopa therapy for parkinsonism be started early or late? Evidence against early treatment. *Can J Neurol Sci* 11:200-206, 1984.

Folstein S, Folstein M: Diagnosis and treatment of Huntington's disease. *Compr Ther* 7:60-66, (April) 1981.

Foster NL, et al: THIP treatment of Huntington's disease. *Neurology* 33:637-639, 1983.

Friedman JH: 'Drug holidays' in treatment of Parkinson's disease: Brief review. *Arch Intern Med* 145:913-915, 1985.

Goetz CG, et al: Pergolide in Parkinson's disease. *Arch Neurol* 40:785-787, 1983.

Goetz CG, et al: Chronic agonist therapy for Parkinson's disease: 5-year study of bromocriptine and pergolide. *Neurology* 34(suppl 12):218, 1984.

Heikkila RE, et al: Protection against dopaminergic neurotoxicity of 1-methyl-4-phenyl-1, 2, 5, 6-tetrahydropyridine by monoamine oxidase inhibitors. *Nature* 311:467-469, 1984.

Hoehn MM: Increased dosage of carbidopa in patients with Parkinson's disease receiving low doses of levodopa: Pilot study. *Arch Neurol* 37:146-149, 1980.

Horadam VW, et al: Pharmacokinetics of amantadine hydrochloride in subjects with normal and impaired renal function. *Ann Intern Med* 94:454-458, 1981.

Jankovic J: Treatment of hyperkinetic movement disorders with tetrabenazine: Double-blind crossover study. *Ann Neurol* 11:41-47, 1982.

Jeste DV, Wyatt RJ: Changing epidemiology of tardive dyskinesia: Overview. *Am J Psychiatry* 138:297-309, 1981 A.

Jeste DV, Wyatt RJ: Dogma disputed: Is tardive dyskinesia due to postsynaptic dopamine receptor supersensitivity. *J Clin Psychiatry* 42:455-457, 1981 B.

Jeste DV, Wyatt RJ: Therapeutic strategies against tardive dyskinesia: Two decades of experience. *Arch Gen Psychiatry* 39:803-816, 1982.

Kane JM, Smith JM: Tardive dyskinesia: Prevalence and risk factors, 1959 to 1979. *Arch Gen Psychiatry* 39:473-481, 1982.

Koller WC: Propranolol therapy for essential tremor of the head. *Neurology* 34:1077-1079, 1984.

Koller W: Efficacy of primidone in essential tremor, (abstract P73). 110th Annual Meeting of the Neurological Association, Chicago, Oct 2-5, 1985.

Koller WC, Biary N: Effect of alcohol on tremors: Comparison with propranolol. *Neurology* 34:221-222, 1984 A.

Koller WC, Biary N: Metoprolol compared with propranolol in treatment of essential tremor. *Arch Neurol* 41:171-172, 1984 B.

Lang AE, Blair RDG: Parkinson's disease in 1984: Update. *Can Med Assoc J* 131:1031-1037, 1984.

Lang AE, Marsden CD: Alpha-methylparatyrosine and tetrabenazine in movement disorders. *Clin Neuropharmacol* 5:375-387, 1982.

Langston JW, et al: Chronic parkinsonism in humans due to product of meperidine-analog synthesis. *Science* 219:979-980, 1983.

Langston JW, et al: Pargyline prevents MPTP-induced parkinsonism in primates. *Science* 225:1480-1482, 1984.

Larsen TA, Calne DB: Essential tremor. *Clin Neuropharmacol* 6:185-206, 1983.

Lees AJ, Stern GM: Sustained bromocriptine therapy in previously untreated patients with Parkinson's disease. *J Neurol Neurosurg Psychiatry* 44:1020-1023, 1981.

Lees AJ, et al: Deprenyl in Parkinson's disease. *Lancet* 2:791-795, 1977.

Legg NJ: Parkinson's disease: Course and management. *Practitioner* 227:375-379, 1983.

Leibowitz M, Lieberman A: Comparison of dopa decarboxylase inhibitor (carbidopa) combined with levodopa and levodopa alone on cardiovascular system of patients with Parkinson's disease. *Neurology* 25:917-921, 1975.

LeWitt PA, et al: Comparison of pergolide and bromocriptine therapy in parkinsonism. *Neurology* 33:1009-1014, 1983.

Lieberman AN: Dementia in Parkinson disease. *Ann Neurol* 6:355-359, 1979.

Lieberman A, et al: Comparative effectiveness of two extracerebral DOPA decarboxylase inhibitors in Parkinson disease. *Neurology* 28:964-968, 1978.

Lieberman AN, et al: Long-term treatment with pergolide: Decreased efficacy with time. *Neurology* 34:223-226, 1984.

Lieberman AN, et al: Use of partial dopamine agonist ciladopa in advanced Parkinson disease, (abstract). *Neurology* 35(suppl 1):203, 1985.

Markey SP, et al: Intraneuronal generation of pyridinium metabolite may cause drug-induced parkinsonism. *Nature* 311:464-467, 1984.

Markham CH, Diamond SG: Evidence to support early levodopa therapy in Parkinson disease. *Neurology* 31:125-131, 1981.

Mayeux R, et al: Reappraisal of temporary levodopa withdrawal ("drug holiday") in Parkinson's disease. *N Engl J Med* 313:724-728, 1985.

McNeil Pharmaceuticals, 1984 (personal communication).

Meltzer HY, Luchins DJ: Effect of clozapine in severe tardive dyskinesia: Case report. *J Clin Psychopharmacol* 4:286-287, 1984.

Muenter MD: Should levodopa be started early or late? *Can J Neurol Surg* 11:195-199, 1984.

Nutt JG: Effect of cholinergic agents in Huntington's disease: Reappraisal. *Neurology* 33:932-935, 1983.

Nutt JG, et al: "On-off" phenomenon in Parkinson's disease: Relation to levodopa absorption and transport. *N Engl J Med* 310:483-488, 1984.

Parkes JD: Bromocriptine in treatment of parkinsonism. *Drugs* 17:365-382, 1979.

Parkes JD, et al: Lisuride in parkinsonism. *Ann Neurol* 9:48-52, 1981.

Pearce JMS: Drug treatment in Parkinson's disease. *Br Med J* 288:1777-1778, 1984.

Perlik SJ, et al: Parkinsonism: Is your treatment appropriate? *Geriatrics* 35:65-70, (Nov) 1980.

Perry TL, et al: Double-blind clinical trial of isoniazid in Huntington's disease. *Neurology* 32:354-358, 1982.

Quinn N, Marsden CD: Double blind trial of sulpiride in Huntington's disease and tardive dyskinesia. *J Neurol Neurosurg Psychiatry* 47:844-847, 1984.

Reynolds GP, et al: Deprenyl is metabolized to methamphetamine and amphetamine in man. *Br J Clin Pharmacol* 6:542-544, 1978.

Schachter M, et al: Deprenyl in management of response fluctuations in patients with Parkinson's disease on levodopa. *J Neurol Neurosurg Psychiatry* 43:1016-1021, 1980.

Schran HF, et al: Pharmacokinetics of bromocriptine in man, in Goldstein M, et al (eds): *Ergot Compounds and Brain Function: Neuroendocrine and Neuropsychiatric Aspects.* New York, Raven Press, 1980.

Scigliano G, et al: Gamma-vinyl GABA treatment of Huntington's disease. *Neurology* 34:94-96, 1984.

Shapiro AK, Shapiro E: Controlled study of pimozide vs placebo in Tourette's syndrome. *J Am Acad Child Psychiatry* 23:161-173, 1984.

Shaw KM, et al: Impact of treatment with levodopa on Parkinson's disease. *Q J Med* 49:283-293, 1980.

Shoulson I: Huntington's disease: Overview of experimental therapeutics, in Chase TN, et al: *Huntington's Disease.* New York, Raven Press, 1979.

Shoulson I, Goldbatt D: Huntington's disease: Effect of tetrabenazine and antipsychotic drugs on motor features, (abstract). *Neurology* 31:81, 1981.

Simpson GM, et al: Management of tardive dyskinesia: Current update. *Drugs* 23:381-393, 1982.

Sørensen PS, et al: Essential tremor treated with propranolol: Lack of correlation between clinical effect and plasma propranolol levels. *Ann Neurol* 9:53-57, 1981.

Tanner CM, et al: Pergolide mesylate: Lack of cardiac toxicity in patients with cardiac disease. *Neurology* 35:918-921, 1985.

Task Force on Late Neurological Effects of Antipsychotic Drugs: Tardive dyskinesia: Summary of task force report of American Psychiatric Association. *Am J Psychiatry* 137:1163-1172, 1980.

Teravainen H, et al: Effect of propranolol on essential tremor. *Neurology* 26:27-30, 1976.

Timberlake WH, Vance MA: Four-year treatment of patients with parkinsonism using amantadine alone or with levodopa. *Ann Neurol* 3:119-128, 1978.

Toglia JU, et al: Tetrabenazine in treatment of Huntington's chorea and other hyperkinetic movement disorders. *J Clin Psychiatry* 39:81-87, 1978.

Vance ML, et al: Bromocriptine. *Ann Intern Med* 100:78-91, 1984.

Weiner WJ, et al: Drug holiday and management of Parkinson disease. *Neurology* 30:1257-1261, 1980.

Yahr MD, et al: Treatment of Parkinson's disease in early and late phases: Use of pharmacological agents with special reference to deprenyl (selegiline). *Acta Neurol Scand* Suppl 95:95-102, 1983.

Drugs Used in Disorders Affecting Skeletal Muscle

Drugs discussed in this chapter are useful in managing myasthenia gravis and in treating the common symptoms of upper motor neuron lesions (spasticity), and involuntary muscle contractions (spasms). Drug therapy for inflammatory myopathies and multiple sclerosis is also reviewed.

MYASTHENIA GRAVIS

ETIOLOGY. Myasthenia gravis is an autoimmune disorder characterized by progressive weakness and rapid fatigability of skeletal muscle due to impaired neuromuscular transmission (Grob, 1981; Havard and Scadding, 1983; Penn et al, 1984; Scheife et al, 1981; Seybold, 1983). Episodes of muscle weakness of variable severity occur, sometimes in association with infection, stress, and loss of sleep. When involvement is limited, usually only those muscles innervated by the cranial nerves (ie, extraocular, facial, pharyngeal, laryngeal) are affected. With moderate to severe involvement, the ability of axial muscles and those in the extremities to sustain adequate contractile power may be affected.

Myasthenia is caused by a deficiency of the postsynaptic neuromuscular acetylcholine receptor complex. Receptor deficiency may result from postsynaptic membrane lysis or antigenic modulation. Lysis of the postsynaptic membrane is produced by antireceptor antibody and the C9 component of complement. With antigenic modulation, postsynaptic receptors are cross-linked, degraded, and cleared much faster than normal. A combination of these actions reduces the number of available acetylcholine receptors in the involved muscles by as much as 70% to 90%. Hence, the number of interactions between the acetylcholine released by nerve impulses and the receptors is decreased, which reduces muscle strength or causes progressive failure of contraction from repeated nerve stimulation.

A thymic abnormality is present in almost all patients with generalized myasthenia under the age of 45; thymic hyperplasia is present in 70% to 85% and malignant thymoma(s) in 10% to 15% of affected patients. Tomograms of the anterior mediastinum are generally included in the initial evaluation of all newly diagnosed patients to look for a thymoma.

Circulating antibodies to acetylcholine receptor have been demonstrated in 70% to 90% of those with myasthenia, although the severity of the disease does not correlate with antibody titer. Since myasthenic antibodies are polyclonal, this lack of correlation may reflect the differing capacities of monoclonal antibodies to produce lysis and antigenic modulation. Further, in some patients who lack circulating antibodies, cytochemical studies show that antibody and complement are localized at the motor endplate. However, the severity of clinical signs increases with the proportion of receptors bound by antibody. Decreased antibody titers have been reported after thymectomy and, since thymectomy benefits many myasthenic patients, clinical improvement may be associated with reduction of antireceptor antibody levels over a period of several years. However, thymectomy does not always reduce the antibody titer. The transient effectiveness of plasmapheresis is explained by the acute depletion of circulating antibody.

Other forms of myasthenia include pure ocular myasthenia (symptoms confined to extraocular muscles) and penicillamine-induced myasthenia (usually in patients with rheumatoid arthritis treated with penicillamine). Extremely high antibody titers in pregnant patients with myasthenia may cause neonatal myasthenia gravis (Donaldson et al, 1981), although these infants may develop myasthenia even when the maternal antibody titer is undetectable or not particularly high. Congenital myasthenia includes a diverse group of disorders that may be genetic and involve presynaptic changes (Havard and Scadding, 1983).

DIAGNOSIS. The diagnosis of myasthenia gravis usually can be made on the basis of the patient's history and symptoms and can be substantiated by a number of procedures. The presence of antiacetylcholine receptor antibody in plasma is usually determined routinely. Although antibody and complement can be cytochemically localized at the endplate (Engel et al, 1982), this procedure is rarely performed.

A typical myasthenic decremental response on electromyography (EMG) using repetitive, mixed nerve stimulation of proximal muscles is almost always present. In doubtful cases, myasthenia can be differentiated from other neuromuscular diseases by the parenteral administration of the short-acting anticholinesterase, edrophonium [Tensilon], or the longer acting agent, neostigmine methylsulfate [Prostigmin]. An appropriate focal deficit, such as ptosis, diplopia, or weakness of a specific muscle group, should be selected as an endpoint for evaluation and the effect of drug administration followed closely and quantitatively, if possible. Muscle strength usually improves in patients with myasthenia gravis, whereas those with other disorders experience either no increase or even a slight weakness and also may develop fasciculations, especially in the eyelids. Some physicians routinely administer saline initially as a placebo or atropine to improve interpretation of the test results. The Tensilon and neostigmine tests are not specific for autoimmune myasthenia gravis; they only indicate a decrease in neuromuscular transmission. In view of the accuracy and availability of these tests, the use of potentially dangerous systemic curare to determine weakness is obsolete.

MANAGEMENT. The primary goal in the management of myasthenia gravis is to reduce or eliminate antibody with drugs or other measures (eg, thymectomy, plasmapheresis). Management varies according to the severity of the disease, the age of the patient, and the type of myasthenia. Controversy exists as to the most effective sequence and combination of the main therapeutic modalities, which include anticholinesterase drugs, corticosteroids, immunosuppressants, thymectomy, and plasmapheresis (Havard and Scadding, 1983). Data

from well-controlled, comparative, clinical trials to guide management are lacking. Close supervision by the physician is required to assess the patient's symptoms and psychological status.

When myasthenic patients must be treated for other disorders or infection, it should be noted that certain drugs may exacerbate their condition, although this need not preclude their use when necessary. Drugs that depress neuromuscular transmission (eg, aminoglycoside, polymyxin, and tetracycline antibiotics), antiarrhythmic agents (eg, procainamide [Procan, Pronestyl], quinidine, propranolol [Inderal]), chlorpromazine [Thorazine], lithium, phenytoin [Dilantin], thyroid hormones, and methoxyflurane [Penthrane] aggravate or unmask myasthenia gravis (Adams et al, 1984; Argov and Mastaglia, 1979). Myasthenic patients are sensitive to central nervous system depressants, which should be used with caution because of their inhibitory effects on the respiratory drive.

Management of myasthenia usually begins with the early removal of thymoma, when present. When thymoma is absent, reversible anticholinesterase drugs are usually given initially to enhance the function of remaining normal acetylcholine receptors. Their use alone is limited to the treatment of mild myasthenia (before and after thymectomy). Since spontaneous remissions can occur during initial anticholinesterase therapy, it has been recommended that these drugs be given for 6 to 12 months before thymectomy is considered (Oosterhuis, 1984). If no remission occurs after this time, patients 10 to 40 years of age may be suitable candidates for thymectomy (irrespective of their response to anticholinesterase drugs). Thymectomy in patients over 40 years is more controversial unless a thymoma is present. For further information on patient selection, see Rowland, 1980; Snead et al, 1980; Craven et al, 1981; Grob, 1981; Havard and Scadding, 1983; Mulder et al, 1983; and Olanow et al, 1982.

Thymectomy improves the condition or induces remissions in 20% to 50% of patients, especially young adults and female adolescents. It has decreased the postoperative antibody titer by an average of -18.3% (range, -84% to +28%) (Tindall, 1980). The time to maximum response (clinical and antibody titer) may be a few weeks or as long as two to five years.

Thymectomy should not be performed in all patients, however, and should not be performed in emergency situations. Although the value of thymectomy is established, an adequate vigorous trial of anticholinesterase drugs to improve symptoms and corticosteroids to reduce antibodies may be equally effective in selected patients (Snead et al, 1980; Pascuzzi et al, 1984).

Corticosteroids are usually effective and relatively safe in patients of all ages with moderate to severe myasthenia, especially elderly males who also respond more promptly. Anticholinesterase agents are often given concomitantly.

The use of immunosuppressants is reserved for severe myasthenia in patients refractory to corticosteroids or to those who cannot tolerate these drugs. Azathioprine [Imuran] is most commonly used and may be combined with prednisone in many individuals with severe disease (Oosterhuis, 1984). Azathioprine has been used more extensively in Europe, where this use of immunosuppressants is more accepted. In one study, the remission rate with azathioprine was 40% (78 patients) with daily doses of 150 to 200 mg (Mertens et al, 1981). A similar remission rate (44%) was reported in a more recent study, but relapse occurred in all patients when the drug was withdrawn (Witte et al, 1984). Azathioprine is a weak immunosuppressant and the doses used to treat severe myasthenia are similar to those used to maintain allografts. The incidence of severe adverse reactions also is similar, and, since significant improvement usually takes months to appear, the risks with long-term administration should be considered carefully before initiating therapy.

Plasmapheresis is useful in refractory patients with severe myasthenia gravis. It should be employed only in conjunction with other treatment modalities, especially corticosteroids and immunosuppressive drugs (Dau, 1980). Although improvement is relatively transient, plasmapheresis in combination with prednisone has been recommended for emergencies, such as respiratory crisis, to avoid tracheostomy (Oosterhuis, 1984).

ANTICHOLINESTERASE AGENTS. The principal reversible anticholinesterases used to treat myasthenia gravis are pyridostigmine bromide [Mestinon, Regonol] and neostigmine bromide [Prostigmin]; ambenonium chloride [Mytelase] is used occasionally.

Actions and Uses: These drugs are used alone for mild symptoms and as adjuncts to corticosteroids for moderate to severe symptoms. They act by inhibiting acetylcholinesterase, the enzyme that hydrolyzes acetylcholine, thereby increasing the duration of action of acetylcholine released at the motor endplate. Thus, the number of interactions between the transmitter and receptors is increased and muscular strength and response to repetitive nerve stimulation improve.

Although the anticholinesterases may improve the condition of some patients, muscle strength remains below normal in others. In addition, in any given patient, strength may improve in some muscle groups, while no improvement or even deterioration may occur in others. A beneficial effect is dose dependent, but the improvement with larger doses must be weighed against the danger of overdosage. The potency of individual anticholinesterase agents varies but the maximal achievable muscle strength in any one patient is approximately the same. The optimal dose and timing of administration must be determined empirically for each patient, taking into account fluctuations in strength and variations in the patient's needs. When anticholinesterases are used alone, sacrificing the strength of some muscle groups may be necessary if respiration is compromised at the same dose.

The dose often must be increased in the presence of infection and, occasionally, premenstrually and during stress. Mild exacerbations of myasthenia are treated by increasing the dose of oral medication very gradually and carefully; dosage adjustment should continue as long as symptomatic improvement results. Although critically ill patients often are refractory to anticholinesterase medication, responsiveness to adjunctive anticholinesterase medication can sometimes be restored by reducing the dose temporarily or withdrawing medication completely for 72 hours in hospitalized patients (who usually will require respiratory support).

There are no adequately controlled studies that unequivocally document differences in efficacy among the available agents. However, many physicians regard pyridostigmine as the drug of choice for maintenance when the symptoms are mild to moderate because it produces fewer adverse effects than neostigmine or ambenonium.

Pharmacokinetics: These quaternary ammonium derivatives are poorly and variably absorbed orally, especially with regard to extent as compared to rate of absorption. The ratio of effectiveness of a parenteral to oral dose is about 30:1. The volume of distribution and plasma half-life of pyridostigmine are 1.1 ± 0.3 L/kg and 1.9 ± 0.2 hours, respectively. The compounds are extensively metabolized by plasma esterases and hepatic enzymes to inactive metabolites; unchanged drug and metabolites are excreted in the urine. Therapeutic drug monitoring is not useful; dosage alterations are based on clinical response.

Adverse Reactions: The most common adverse reactions of anticholinesterase agents are caused by excessive cholinergic stimulation and include both muscarinic and nicotinic effects. The former consist of abdominal cramps, nausea, vomiting, diarrhea, hypersalivation, increased bronchial secretions, lacrimation, miosis, and diaphoresis. Nicotinic effects include muscle cramps, fasciculations, and weakness. Only the muscarinic effects can be counteracted by atropine. However, atropine should not be administered routinely to control the anticholinesterase side effects, for these reactions are warning signs and masking them may inadvertently lead to cholinergic crisis. Further, many patients use the severity of anticholinesterase side effects as a guide to optimum dosage. Use of atropine also may result in drying and inspissation of bronchial secretions.

The anticholinesterase compounds are contraindicated in the presence of mechanical obstruction of the intestinal or urinary tract. They should be used with extreme caution in patients with bronchial asthma. Compounds containing the bromide ion (pyridostigmine bromide, neostigmine bromide) should not be used in patients with a history of sensitivity to this ion. These drugs are classified in FDA Pregnancy Category C.

Precautions: Myasthenic weakness may worsen suddenly, often without recognizable cause. Such exacerbations are characterized by decreased responsiveness to drug therapy that cannot be overcome by administration of larger doses and may progress to a *myasthenic crisis,* which is characterized by severe muscular weakness with dysphagia and ventilatory insufficiency. Ventilatory support, cautious intravenous or intramuscular administration of pyridostigmine bromide or neostigmine methylsulfate, corticosteroids, or plasmapheresis may be beneficial.

Overdosage may occur when patients in a refractory phase of myasthenia gravis receive increasing amounts of an anticholinesterase drug in an attempt to control symptoms. In these patients, the maximal obtainable strength is below normal and the administration of excessive doses may convert a myasthenic crisis into a *cholinergic crisis.* It has been suggested that these agents may produce depolarization-induced inactivation of the voltage-sensitive ion channels of the sarcolemma near the endplate. In any event, overdosage increases the amount of acetylcholine present but reduces the number of ion channels available for activation, thereby increasing muscle weakness. Fasciculations and cholinergic side effects, which are common symptoms of overdosage in normal individuals, may be mild or absent in myasthenic patients; instead, generalized weakness may be the principal sign.

The symptoms of myasthenic crisis may be difficult to distinguish from those of cholinergic crisis. The differential diagnosis cannot always be made on the basis of signs and symptoms. Since myasthenic crisis is much more common (Rowland, 1980), ventilation must be supported and the patient observed until a diagnosis is possible. Pharmacologic tests should be performed only after endotracheal intubation and controlled ventilation have been instituted. A small intravenous dose (1 to 2 mg) of edrophonium may improve strength temporarily if the patient has not received enough of the anticholinesterase agent but will aggravate the weakness if too much has been given.

Poisoning: If overdosage has occurred, establishment of an endotracheal tube is the first priority; 1 to 2 mg of atropine should be given intravenously to counteract the muscarinic effects. Controlled ventilation and suction also may be necessary. The cholinesterase reactivator, pralidoxime [Protopam], is much less effective against reversible than irreversible anticholinesterases and thus is seldom used.

ADRENAL CORTICOSTEROIDS. Adrenal corticosteroids are beneficial in patients with moderate to severe myasthenic muscle weakness. There is general agreement that their indications include (1) inadequate control with anticholinesterase drugs (ie, most patients with more than mild involvement, those with rapidly progressing disease); (2) older adults (usually over 40 years) with moderate to severe involvement, whether or not they have undergone thymectomy; (3) possibly for an interim period following thymectomy because of the delayed response often associated with this procedure; (4) patients who refuse or do not respond to thymectomy; (5) maintenance therapy after surgical removal of an invasive thymoma; and (6) possibly to prepare patients for thymectomy (Scheife et al, 1981), although the increased risk of infection and delay in postoperative healing often make this use of steroids inadvisable. The use of corticosteroids for ocular myasthenia gravis that cannot be managed with anticholinesterase drugs or lid-crutches, occlusion, or prism has been recommended (Oosterhuis, 1984; Havard and Scadding, 1983), but this use is controversial.

Steroids probably act by suppressing the immune system. Therapy is not curative, as evidenced by recurrence of symptoms within three months after steroids are discontinued. Therefore, their administration may be required indefinitely or reinstituted periodically when needed.

Employment of a high-dose, alternate-day, maintenance regimen has minimized adverse effects while improving muscular strength. This regimen may prevent lethal weakness and permanent damage to the neuromuscular system as long as it is continued. A short-acting steroid (eg, prednisone) is preferred for the alternate-day regimen because there is less interference with the normal ACTH-cortisol cycle and no accumulation of drug, thus reducing the likelihood of deleterious effects on the tissues.

When large doses of steroids are used initially, weakness is exacerbated in about 80% of patients. Therefore, treatment should be started with relatively small doses, which are then increased gradually, even though this may slow the rate of improvement. Maximum response is usually noted in about five months. Optimal doses of anticholinesterase medication should be continued, especially during initiation of steroid treatment. The need for anticholinesterase drugs may decrease as the patient improves. It has been suggested that patients on a steroid alternate-day regimen receive a high-protein, low-carbohydrate diet supplemented with potassium and possibly antacids.

Drug Evaluations

ANTICHOLINESTERASE AGENTS

PYRIDOSTIGMINE BROMIDE
[Mestinon, Regonol]

USES. Pyridostigmine, given orally, is the most widely used anticholinesterase agent for the treatment of myasthenia gravis. It is given alone for mild muscle weakness and is combined with corticosteroids for moderate to severe impairment. The drug also may be administered parenterally with great caution to treat neonatal myasthenia, exacerbations of myasthenia, and as an alternative to edrophonium for diagnosis. Because of marked fluctuations in drug serum concentrations after intramuscular administration, very slow intravenous infusion is preferable when parenteral medication is essential.

The therapeutic response is similar to that observed with neostigmine, but pyridostigmine has a slightly longer duration of action.

ADVERSE REACTIONS AND PRECAUTIONS. Adverse effects after therapeutic doses occur less frequently with pyridostigmine than with neostigmine. For a discussion of adverse reactions and precautions, see the Introduction to this section.

DOSAGE AND PREPARATIONS. Dosage requirements vary widely among patients because of differences in absorption, metabolism, and excretion of the drug; thus, the dose and timing of administration must be determined empirically. Careful record keeping by the patient is helpful in adjusting the dosage schedule. An early attempt should be made to reduce or eliminate doses during rest or sleep in order to maintain sensitivity to the drug and reduce direct endplate damage.

The syrup is useful for infants, young children, and patients who cannot swallow tablets or when the dose is in fractions of tablet size; it may be given by nasogastric tube if necessary. Some patients find that taking a timed-release tablet at night improves strength upon awakening in the morning.

Oral: Adults, initially, 60 to 120 mg every three to four hours; the intervals are altered as necessary on the basis of response. In severe myasthenia, 600 mg to 1.5 g daily has been recommended by the manufacturer. *Children,* 7 mg/kg daily in divided doses and timed as required.

If timed-release preparations are used, the usual dose is 180 to 540 mg once or twice daily. Because of the delayed onset of action, regular tablets or syrup may be needed supplementally. Use of timed-release preparations may increase the risk of cholinergic crises.

> *Mestinon* (Roche). Syrup 60 mg/5 ml (alcohol 5%); tablets 60 mg; tablets (timed-release) 180 mg.

Intramuscular, Intravenous (preferred): For exacerbations of myasthenia gravis or when oral administration is impractical, *adults,* approximately one-thirtieth of the oral dose. For *newborn infants* of myasthenic mothers, 0.05 to 0.15 mg/kg.

> *Mestinon* (Roche). Solution 5 mg/ml in 2 ml containers.
> *Regonol* (Organon). Solution 5 mg/ml in 2 and 5 ml containers.

NEOSTIGMINE BROMIDE
[Prostigmin]

NEOSTIGMINE METHYLSULFATE
[Prostigmin]

USES. Neostigmine bromide is used orally alone to treat mild myasthenia gravis and with corticosteroids for moderate to severe muscle weakness. The therapeutic response is similar to that obtained with pyridostigmine and ambenonium, but neostigmine has a shorter duration of action and is more potent than pyridostigmine; 15 mg of neostigmine is approximately equivalent to 60 mg of pyridostigmine. The methylsulfate salt is given parenterally to patients who are unable to swallow. It also is an alternative to edrophonium for diagnosis.

ADVERSE REACTIONS AND PRECAUTIONS. Adverse effects after therapeutic doses occur more frequently with neostigmine than with pyridostigmine or ambenonium. For adverse reactions and precautions, see the Introduction to this section.

DOSAGE AND PREPARATIONS.
NEOSTIGMINE BROMIDE:
Oral: The dose and frequency of administration must be individualized according to the response of the patient (see evaluation on Pyridostigmine Bromide). *Adults,* initially, 15 mg every three to four hours; the dose and frequency of administration are then adjusted in accordance with the patient's requirements. *Children,* 2 mg/kg daily in divided doses as required.

> *Generic.* Powder; tablets 15 mg.
> *Prostigmin* (Roche). Tablets 15 mg.

NEOSTIGMINE METHYLSULFATE:
Intramuscular, Subcutaneous: For treatment of exacerbations of myasthenia gravis when oral therapy is impractical, *adults,* 0.5 mg. Subsequent dosage should be adjusted according to the patient's response. *Infants and children,* 0.01 to 0.04 mg/kg every two to three hours.

Atropine (0.01 mg/kg intramuscularly or subcutaneously) should not be used routinely but can be given with each dose or with alternate doses to control adverse effects.

Intravenous: When the patient cannot take anticholinesterase agents orally (eg, following thymectomy), very slow intravenous infusion may be preferable. A suggested dose is 1 mg dissolved in 100 ml of saline and infused at a rate of 25 ml/hr.

> *Generic.* Solution 0.25 mg/ml in 1 ml containers, 0.5 mg/ml in 1 and 10 ml containers, and 1 mg/ml in 10 ml containers.
> *Prostigmin* (Roche). Solution 0.25 mg/ml in 1 ml containers, 0.5 mg/ml in 1 and 10 ml containers, and 1 mg/ml in 1 ml containers.

AMBENONIUM CHLORIDE
[Mytelase]

Ambenonium is given orally to treat mild myasthenia gravis. It produces fewer cholinergic side effects than neostigmine, but may have a longer duration of action and a greater tendency to accumulate. Ambenonium is used less commonly than pyridostigmine or neostigmine but may be preferred in patients who cannot tolerate these drugs because of sensitivity to the bromide ion.

For adverse reactions and precautions, see the Introduction to this section.

DOSAGE AND PREPARATIONS.
Oral: The dose and frequency of administration vary greatly and must be individualized according to the response of the patient (see the evaluation on Pyridostigmine Bromide). *Adults,* initially, 5 mg three or four times daily, increased as required; the dosage should be adjusted at intervals of one to two days to avoid accumulation. *Children,* initially, 0.3 mg/kg daily in divided doses, increased, if necessary, to 1.5 mg/kg daily in divided doses.

> *Mytelase* (Winthrop-Breon). Tablets l0 mg.

EDROPHONIUM CHLORIDE
[Tensilon]

USES. Edrophonium is used in the diagnosis of myasthenia gravis. It has a more rapid onset and shorter duration of action than pyridostigmine and neostigmine methylsulfate. Administration of atropine is usually unnecessary, but this agent should be readily available, especially for older patients. After intravenous administration, muscle strength increases in myasthenic patients within one to three minutes and lasts for five to ten minutes.

A smaller dose of edrophonium is used to differentiate a myasthenic crisis from a cholinergic crisis: An intravenous dose produces a brief remission of symptoms if these are caused by an exacerbation of the illness, but further weakens patients suffering from an overdose of medication.

For untoward effects, see the Introduction to this section.

DOSAGE AND PREPARATIONS.

Intravenous: For diagnosis, *adults,* 2 mg injected within 15 to 30 seconds; if no response occurs within 45 seconds, an additional 8 mg should be given. The test may be repeated after one to two hours (see manufacturer's labeling for details). Atropine should be readily available, although it is not administered routinely. *Children under 34 kg,* 1 mg; *over 34 kg,* 2 mg. If no response is observed after 45 seconds, an additional dose of up to 5 mg in children under 34 kg and up to 10 mg in children over 34 kg should be administered.

For differential diagnosis of myasthenic crisis and cholinergic crisis, *adults,* 1 to 2 mg. This test should be undertaken only if facilities for endotracheal intubation and controlled ventilation are immediately available.

Intramuscular: For diagnosis, *infants,* 0.5 mg as a single dose. *Children under 34 kg,* 2 mg; *over 34 kg,* 5 mg. There is a delay of two to ten minutes before a response is noted with this route of administration.

   Tensilon (Roche). Solution (sterile) 10 mg/ml in 1 and 10 ml containers.

ADRENAL CORTICOSTEROID

PREDNISONE

Oral treatment with a short-acting corticosteroid, such as prednisone, is beneficial in patients with moderate to severe myasthenia gravis. The success rate is high, but treatment may have to be continued indefinitely and the patient must be observed closely for adverse effects.

ADVERSE REACTIONS AND PRECAUTIONS. The adverse reactions usually associated with prolonged use of steroids may occur and must be treated appropriately. Alternate-day therapy minimizes these reactions. For a more detailed discussion, see the Introduction to this section and Chapter 61, Adrenal Corticosteroids in Nonendocrine Diseases.

DOSAGE AND PREPARATIONS. The following oral dosages should serve only as a guide. The patient's clinical status should be evaluated carefully before each dosage change. If there is an exacerbation of myasthenic weakness following an increase in the dose of prednisone, the amount should be reduced or maintained without further increases until the patient's condition stabilizes.

Oral: Initially, 25 mg daily for two days, increased by 5 mg every two days until an optimal response occurs (usually, 50 to 60 mg daily). An alternate-day program is gradually substituted by adding 10 mg to the first day's dose (60 mg) and subtracting 10 mg from the second day's dose (40 mg) each week until improvement reaches a plateau (ie, the patient experiences weakness on the "off" day) or until 100 mg is given every other day. The dosage then should be reduced very gradually over many months to establish a minimal maintenance dose to be given on alternate days (often as much as 30 to 60 mg). Patients with severe myasthenia gravis who do not respond to 100 mg every other day usually do not respond to dosage increases. In these patients, it may be preferable to add an immunosuppressive drug, such as azathioprine. The dosage of anticholinesterase drugs should be adjusted as necessary during steroid therapy.

For preparations, see Chapter 61.

MYOPATHIES

MUSCULAR DYSTROPHIES. These hereditary disorders include Duchenne's, facioscapulohumeral, limb-girdle muscular, distal muscular, ocular, oculopharyngeal, and myotonic dystrophies. They are characterized by progressive weakness and muscle wasting. There is no effective drug therapy.

METABOLIC MYOPATHIES. This group of genetic disorders, which are characterized by altered muscle metabolism, consists of glycogen storage diseases (including McArdle's disease), mitochondrial and lipid storage myopathies, and myoglobinuria. With few exceptions, no drugs are effective. Various diet therapies have been employed to circumvent metabolic deficiencies and increase muscle strength. Supplemental dextrose or fats have not been successful in McArdle's disease but one report indicated that a high-protein diet was beneficial (Slonim and Goans, 1985).

Hyperkalemic and *hypokalemic periodic paralysis* can be managed prophylactically with oral acetazolamide (investigational indication). This drug is postulated to act by altering muscle membrane function (increased uptake of glucose and decreased uptake of potassium). In hypokalemic paralysis, acetazolamide reduces the number of attacks as well as residual muscle weakness. The daily oral dose in familial hypokalemic periodic paralysis is 250 to 750 mg for adults and 125 mg for children; this amount is divided into two or three doses. Since periodic paralysis may be precipitated by hypokalemia due to renal or gastrointestinal loss, diuretic or steroid therapy, excessive licorice ingestion, or thyrotoxicosis, overall treatment should be directed toward correcting the causes if possible.

A serious complication of anesthesia, *malignant hyperthermia,* appears to result from a genetic disorder of muscle metabolism. Regulation of intracellular calcium is altered, and an abnormal increase in sarcoplasmic calcium concentration follows depolarization; this, in turn, markedly increases aerobic and anaerobic metabolism. Attacks are usually fatal. Intravenous dantrolene [Dantrium] is the drug of choice for this condition. It decreases the release of calcium from the sarcoplasmic reticulum and reduces muscle contraction. See the discussion on Agents Used in Malignant Hyperthermia in Chapter 17, Adjuncts to Anesthesia.

Alcoholic and drug-induced myopathies are treated by abstinence from alcohol and withdrawal of the myopathic agent, respectively.

INFLAMMATORY MYOPATHIES. These disorders constitute a large and heterogeneous group and are the most common acquired myopathies. Causative factors include infection (eg, viral, bacterial, fungal, parasitic), drugs (penicillamine), and immunologic abnormalities (Mastaglia and Ojeda, 1985). Treatment of the underlying disorder or discontinuation of the offending drugs usually corrects myopathies produced by infections or drugs.

Myopathies produced by immunologic abnormalities (idiopathic myopathies) are manifested by inflammatory muscle lesions that vary in severity, pattern of involvement, pathologic characteristics, and response to therapy. The myopathy may be isolated in muscle (polymyositis) or associated with cutaneous alterations in approximately one-third of patients (dermatomyositis). Muscle pain and tenderness usually do not occur acutely in polymyositis and, during the subacute and chronic stages, muscle weakness commonly affects the proximal limb muscle most severely. Dermatomyositis is additionally characterized by an erythematous rash in a butterfly distribution over the face. Rash also may occur over the forehead, neck, shoulders, chest, and limbs.

The main indication for treatment is muscle weakness severe enough to cause disability. Corticosteroids are the initial agents used to treat polymyositis or dermatomyositis. Only general guidelines are available for their use; the optimal initial dose or duration of therapy and the usefulness of alternate-day therapy remain to be determined. In one regimen, therapy is initiated with prednisone 1 to 2 mg/kg daily for two to three months. The dose can be decreased gradually after initial response. Improvement in muscle strength and serum creatine phosphokinase concentrations may be used as guides to determine the timing of dosage reduction (Henriksson and Sandstedt, 1982). Usually, the dose is reduced by 5 mg/day at weekly intervals until 30 mg/day is given; further reduction is carried out in weekly steps of 2.5 mg until serum enzyme concentrations become stable and control of symptoms is maintained (Mastaglia and Ojeda, 1985). More abrupt reduction of the dose may cause recurrence of weakness and an increase in serum creatine phosphokinase. Maintenance therapy may be required for years.

Patients who fail to respond to corticosteroids or who relapse during therapy have been managed with immunosuppressants (eg, azathioprine [Imuran], methotrexate [Folex, Mexate], cyclophosphamide [Cytoxan, Neosar], lymphocyte immune globulin). (See Chapter 61, Adrenal Corticosteroids in Nonendocrine Diseases, and Chapter 63, Immunomodulators.)

DEMYELINATING DISORDER

Multiple Sclerosis

Multiple sclerosis is characterized by motor, sensory, and visual dysfunction caused by scattered patches of demyelination or subsequent replacement of demyelinated patches with scar tissue localized to central but not peripheral nerve fibers.

Motor symptoms vary considerably. In mild cases, slight muscle weakness may occur during exercise; in rapidly progressive cases, slight lower extremity paralysis may progress to paraplegia in a matter of days. In progressive unremitting forms, chronic paraparesis or hemiparesis may progress slowly.

Currently, no therapeutic or prophylactic measure has been shown to alter the course of multiple sclerosis. Effective therapy is difficult to determine because of (1) lack of indicators of disease activity, (2) marked clinical variations in severity of the disease in any one patient, and (3) lack of specific diagnostic tests (McFarlin, 1983).

Symptomatic treatment of multiple sclerosis is directed toward relieving spasticity and bladder dysfunction, which is usually manifested by urinary incontinence. Results of controlled trials have shown that corticotropin provides slight but significant improvement in acute attacks, and baclofen, [Lioresal] and other antispastic drugs are employed to relieve spasticity (see the section on Spasticity). Hyperreflexic bladder usually is treated with the anticholinergic agent, propantheline [Pro-Banthine] (see Chapter 31, Agents Used to Treat Urologic Disorders). Immunosuppressive agents (eg, cyclophosphamide [Cytoxan, Neosar], chlorambucil [Leukeran], azathioprine [Imuran], cyclosporine [Sandimmune], interferon, copolymer I) have been used investigationally; the condition improved for at least one year with use of these drugs, but they were not effective in more prolonged management (Noseworthy et al, 1984). The results of treatment with hyperbaric oxygen therapy have been marginal (McFarlin, 1983).

SPASTICITY

Spasticity, a common symptom of upper motor neuron lesions characterized by altered muscle tone, affects six million people in the United States (Bishop, 1977; Young and Delwaide, 1981; Delisa and Little, 1982). The primary element of spasticity is a velocity-dependent increase in tonic stretch reflexes that causes hyperactive reflexes. Other symptoms include flexor or extensor spasms and loss of dexterity.

Closed head injuries and stroke are the most common causes of spasticity. Other etiologies include cerebral palsy, multiple sclerosis (two-thirds of patients experience moderate to severe spasticity), spinal cord trauma, and other neurologic disorders. The variable mixture of true spasticity and dystonia (persistently increased flexor or extensor tone) that occurs in spasticity of cerebral origin may determine the response to antispastic drug therapy, for dystonia is less responsive to these drugs.

Antispastic drugs are used in conjunction with physical therapy, including an exercise program that emphasizes daily stretching, reduction of nociceptive stimuli, and education to ensure confidence and full use of residual capabilities (Merritt, 1981).

Electromyography and clinical assessment of the musculoskeletal system are used to monitor drug therapy, but reduction in spasticity does not necessarily correlate with overall functional improvement, because paralysis and other motor deficits are often associated. Drug therapy may actually be detrimental if reduction of extensor tone in the legs unmasks severe muscle weakness that compromises the ability to stand and walk to an intolerable degree.

DRUG SELECTION. The three primary antispastic drugs are diazepam [Valium] and baclofen [Lioresal], which act centrally, and dantrolene [Dantrium], which acts peripherally (Davidoff, 1978).

Because the degree and type of spasticity vary considerably both in an individual patient and among patients and the placebo response is high, only carefully controlled studies are of value in determining the response to drugs. Results of such studies confirm that diazepam, baclofen, and dantrolene are superior to placebo in reducing spasticity and pain. The choice among the three drugs depends upon the condition being treated, its initial or presenting status, associated illness, and the drugs' other pharmacologic actions.

Response rates are higher in patients with traumatic spinal cord lesions (65% to 75%) or multiple sclerosis (30% to 65%) than in those with purely cerebral lesions. Baclofen appears to be most effective in relieving spasticity due to increased cutaneous or flexor reflexes in multiple sclerosis. Dantrolene appears to be most effective in spasticity of cerebral origin, but the incidence of dose-related hepatotoxicity limits its wider use (see the evaluation). In spasticity caused by stroke, dantrolene occasionally is beneficial; diazepam and baclofen are of limited usefulness because of their central nervous system side effects and the tolerance that may develop with prolonged administration. These drugs are not effective in rigidity associated with parkinsonism or Huntington's chorea.

Baclofen may be preferred to diazepam in patients who are already experiencing considerable sedation, poor coordination, and/or ataxia associated with marginal cerebellar function, and dantrolene tends to be less satisfactory than diazepam and baclofen in patients with borderline strength (Schmidt et al, 1976).

Diazepam has had the longest history of successful use, although baclofen is preferred by some physicians (Delisa and Little, 1982). The antispastic action of diazepam does not appear to differ from that of other benzodiazepines, although there are few controlled clinical studies using related benzodiazepines for spasticity.

Phenothiazines with alpha-adrenergic blocking activity (eg, aliphatic and piperidine compounds) also have been used to treat spasticity. Although chlorpromazine [Thorazine] has been effective in some patients, the response is unpredictable and sedation and lethargy have limited its use. In animal studies, phenytoin [Dilantin] was shown to enhance the antispastic action of chlorpromazine, but the mechanism is not well understood. One controlled clinical study confirmed that concomitant administration of chlorpromazine and phenytoin was more effective than either agent alone (Cohan et al, 1980). Further confirmation is required before these drugs can be considered definitive therapy for spasticity, and comparative studies are needed to establish the role of this combination in spastic disorders.

Local injection of dilute solutions of absolute alcohol or phenol into affected muscle "motor points" or intrathecal injection (chemical neurolysis) also has been tried. However, these techniques are difficult to perform, the effect often does not persist for more than several months, and irreversible destruction may occur.

Depolarizing or nondepolarizing neuromuscular blocking drugs and the central skeletal muscle relaxant drugs that are given for localized muscle spasm are of no value in spastic disorders.

Drug Evaluations

CENTRALLY ACTING DRUGS

BACLOFEN
[Lioresal]

$$H_2NCH_2CHCH_2COH$$

ACTIONS. Baclofen is a chemical analogue of the inhibitory neurotransmitter, gamma aminobutyric acid (GABA). It has no direct effect on the neuromuscular junction but diminishes the transmission of monosynaptic extensor and polysynaptic flexor reflexes in the spinal cord. This action may occur presynaptically at a bicuculline-insensitive GABA receptor (Bowery et al, 1980) by inhibiting the release of the putative excitatory transmitters, glutamic and aspartic acids, from primary afferent fibers. Interference with the release of substance P and other putative excitatory neurotransmitters from cutaneous nociceptive afferent nerve endings that produce flexor reflexes also may contribute to the effectiveness of baclofen. An analgesic action is also demonstrable in animals; however, it is not known whether this effect is responsible for the relief of painful flexor spasms observed clinically, since doses much larger than those used clinically were used in animals.

USES. Baclofen relieves some of the primary components of spinal spasticity: involuntary flexor and extensor spasms and resistance to passive movements. Spasticity induced by spinal lesions is more responsive than that of cerebral origin.

A controlled study comparing baclofen, dantrolene, and diazepam in patients with multiple sclerosis showed baclofen to be the most effective (response rate, up to 65%); in comparison, the placebo response rate was 10% to 30% (Hedley et al, 1975). Other controlled studies comparing placebo and baclofen confirm the latter's efficacy in multiple sclerosis (Duncan et al, 1976; Levine et al, 1977; Feldman et al, 1978). The degree of response is limited but clinically relevant in terms of improved comfort, progression to a more independent state of self-care, less disruption of sleep, and ability to participate in a more aggressive rehabilitation program. The efficacy of baclofen in spasticity caused by stroke is being investigated but this drug often is unsatisfactory in these patients.

Unlike dantrolene, baclofen has no peripheral muscle relaxant activity; consequently, this drug may theoretically be a more appropriate choice for patients with borderline strength.

One open-label study demonstrated that an investigational intravenous preparation of baclofen (but not oral tablets) relieved urethral sphincter spasticity associated with traumatic paraplegia (Hachen and Krucker, 1977).

Baclofen is reported to be effective in stiff-man syndrome (Miller and Korsvik, 1981), which is characterized by episodic tightening of the axial musculature. Simultaneous involvement of both agonist and antagonist muscle groups makes willed movements progressively difficult.

This drug is not effective in the rigidity of parkinsonism or Huntington's chorea.

ADVERSE REACTIONS. Baclofen is relatively well tolerated and severe adverse reactions are uncommon. Drowsiness, lassitude, and dizziness occur most frequently, especially when full therapeutic doses are administered initially. Ataxia may develop even at therapeutic dose levels. These effects are often transient and may disappear with continued treatment. Their incidence is reported to be less than with diazepam at equieffective doses and can be reduced appreciably by using a small initial dose and increasing it gradually. Patients over 40 years and those with cerebral lesions appear to be most susceptible.

Severe muscle weakness does not appear to be a direct effect of the drug and probably represents paresis that is unmasked when muscle tone is reduced. This phenomenon is a common reason for withdrawal from therapy.

Side effects with a reported incidence of 1% to 10% are nausea, mild gastrointestinal upset, constipation or diarrhea, insomnia, headache, confusion, symptomatic hypotension, and urinary frequency. Reduced bladder and bowel responses have been observed in patients with paraplegia. Allergic skin reactions and effects on renal, hepatic, cardiac, and bone marrow function are uncommon. Neuropsychiatric signs and symptoms (eg, euphoria, depression, paresthesias, muscle pain, impaired coordination, tremor, dystonia, nystagmus, accommodation disorders, hallucinations, seizures, dysuria, enuresis) occur rarely and often are difficult to differentiate from those of the underlying disease.

PRECAUTIONS. There are no absolute contraindications to baclofen therapy other than hypersensitivity. This drug should be used with caution when spasticity actually sustains upright posture and balance in locomotion or is utilized to sustain function. Dosage reduction should be considered in patients with impaired renal function and in those receiving other central nervous system depressants concurrently.

There have been reports that baclofen adversely affected seizure control in a few epileptic patients, but one study employing therapeutic doses showed no effect on seizures controlled by antiepileptic drugs (Terrence et al, 1983).

Rarely, asymptomatic elevations of the SGOT, alkaline phosphatase, and blood glucose levels have occurred; there-fore, appropriate laboratory tests should be performed periodically in patients with liver disease or diabetes.

Baclofen has not caused dependence or been abused. Gradual reduction of the dose over a one- to two-week period is recommended, for abrupt withdrawal causes a rebound increase in the number of flexor spasms. In addition, auditory and visual hallucinations, paranoid ideation, agitated behavior, and seizures (especially in patients with cerebral lesions) have been reported after abrupt termination of therapy that exceeded two months.

Baclofen crosses the placenta. Its safety during pregnancy and in children under 12 years has not been established. It is not known whether the drug is excreted in breast milk.

TOXICITY. With overdosage, signs of central nervous system depression are most prominent. Severe intoxication is characterized by seizures, coma, respiratory depression, and muscular hypotonia with absent limb reflexes. Bradycardia and hypotension also have been observed.

Emergency management of acute baclofen intoxication includes respiratory support followed by gastric lavage and diuresis (Haubenstock et al, 1983). No specific antidote is available. During the recovery phase, seizures and myoclonic tics have been reported in many patients. Seizures have been managed with diazepam or clonazepam (Haubenstock et al, 1983), although these drugs may prolong unconsciousness.

Patients with underlying cardiovascular disease should be observed carefully for one week to detect late onset tachycardia and/or hypertension.

PHARMACOKINETICS. Baclofen is rapidly and well absorbed orally. The peak serum concentration is attained in two to three hours (Brogden et al, 1974). Protein binding is about 30%. The plasma:brain distribution ratio is about 10, and the drug is cleared slowly from the brain.

About 70% to 85% of a dose is eliminated unchanged in the urine within one day and complete elimination takes three days. The mean half-life is three to four hours, but there is considerable individual variation.

DOSAGE AND PREPARATIONS. The initial daily dose should be low and increased gradually. Administration several times daily appears to control spasticity more evenly with fewer side effects.

Oral: Adults, some authorities prefer to initiate therapy with 5 or 10 mg daily for the first three days to minimize drowsiness, dizziness, and ataxia. However, the manufacturer recommends 5 mg three times daily for three days, increased by 5 mg three times daily every three days until the optimum effect has been achieved or a maximum of 80 mg daily has been reached; the usual optimal dose ranges from 40 to 80 mg daily. However, some patients may require up to 120 mg daily to achieve beneficial effects. When therapy is to be terminated, the dosage should be reduced gradually over one or two weeks. *Children,* 1 to 1.5 mg/kg daily has been reported to be effective. Treatment should begin with 5 mg/day and the amount increased gradually (Melnick and Shellenberger, 1982).

Lioresal (Geigy). Tablets 10 and 20 mg (**Lioresal DS**).

DIAZEPAM
[Valium, Valrelease]

ACTIONS. Diazepam has an antispastic action in addition to its antianxiety, hypnotic, and antiepileptic properties. The muscle relaxant action of diazepam is thought to result from its ability to enhance gamma aminobutyric acid (GABA)-mediated presynaptic inhibition in the central nervous system and to depress neurons in the descending lateral reticular system that facilitate the gamma motor neurons; however, neither the spinal nor supraspinal sites of action have been established conclusively. Unfortunately, diazepam also depresses neurons in the ascending reticular activating system that mediate wakefulness. The resulting sedation and lethargy generally detract from its antispastic effect and may be the most common reason for drug withdrawal. Diazepam does not alter the synthesis, release, reuptake, or enzymatic degradation of GABA.

USES. Diazepam may be useful in a variety of chronic upper motor neuron disorders in which spasticity is a component. It is superior to placebo in spasticity associated with spinal cord lesions, multiple sclerosis, and cerebral disorders, although improvement is less pronounced in the latter. Other benzodiazepines may have similar activity but few controlled, comparative clinical studies have been published.

The central side effects of diazepam may make this drug less useful in patients with pre-existing sedation and marginal cerebellar function. Unlike dantrolene, diazepam has no peripheral muscle relaxant activity; consequently, this drug may be appropriate for patients with borderline strength.

Diazepam is useful adjunctively in acute, localized, severe, traumatic disorders associated with painful muscle spasm (see the section on Spasm).

This drug alleviates the widespread tightness and pain of the stiff-man syndrome, but it often produces profound sedation at the doses required.

Diazepam may be useful in the motor restlessness of akathisia, although its antianxiety action is probably of greater significance than its antispastic action in this condition (see Chapter 11, Drugs Used in Extrapyramidal Movement Disorders).

When given intravenously, diazepam is a useful adjunct in muscle spasms caused by tetanus toxin (Alfery and Rauscher, 1979) or strychnine, although the anticonvulsant rather than antispastic action may play some role.

ADVERSE REACTIONS AND PRECAUTIONS. Drowsiness is the primary side effect of diazepam, although some adaptation occurs with long-term therapy. Alcohol enhances central sedation. Oversedation in elderly patients may be a problem, even at the lower limits of the dosage range. Impairment of coordination (hand coordination and speed, walking speed, station stability) also usually occurs. Prolonged uninterrupted use of diazepam may lead to physical and psychological dependence.

For a more complete discussion of the mechanism of action, pharmacokinetics, adverse reactions, precautions, and dosage of the benzodiazepines, see Chapter 5, Drugs Used for Anxiety and Sleep Disorders.

DOSAGE AND PREPARATIONS.
Oral: Adults, for spasticity or severe localized muscle spasms, 2 to 10 mg three or four times daily. *Children,* 0.12 to 0.8 mg/kg daily divided into three or four doses. A timed-release preparation [Valrelease] should be used only when it has been determined that the optimal daily dose of diazepam is 5 mg three times a day.

Valium (Roche), *Generic.* Tablets 2, 5, and 10 mg.
Valrelease (Roche). Capsules (timed-release) 15 mg.

Intravenous: The solution should be injected slowly, allowing at least one minute for each 5 mg (1 ml). Although the manufacturer recommends that diazepam not be added to intravenous fluids, intravenous infusion has been used. Since diazepam is significantly absorbed by plastic containers and intravenous administration sets, large-volume glass containers and careful dose titration are necessary. Diazepam should not be mixed with other drugs for intravenous use (Mason et al, 1981).

Adults, for spasticity or severe localized muscle spasm, 2 to 10 mg, repeated in three to four hours, if necessary. *Children,* initially, 0.04 to 0.2 mg/kg (maximum, 0.6 mg/kg in an eight-hour period).

Intravenous diazepam should not be used in spastic patients with respiratory difficulty.

Valium (Roche). Solution 5 mg/ml in 2 and 10 ml containers.

PERIPHERALLY ACTING DRUG

DANTROLENE SODIUM
[Dantrium]

ACTIONS. This unique skeletal muscle relaxant reduces muscle contractility. It acts at a site beyond the neuromuscular junction and interferes with the intramuscular release of calcium ions from the sarcoplasmic reticulum (Pinder et al, 1977) in extrafusal and intrafusal muscle fibers. Fast muscle units (rapid contraction with large increases in tension) are affected more than slow muscle units (slow, tonic contraction with limited increases in tension). Unlike the neuromuscular blocking agents, dantrolene cannot decrease contractile activity by more than 75% to 80%.

Therapeutic doses have little or no effect on cardiac and smooth muscles. The drug has no specific antispastic action on hyperactive neurons.

USES. Dantrolene is superior to placebo in spasticity induced by spinal cord and cerebral injuries or lesions associated with multiple sclerosis, cerebral palsy, and possibly stroke. It can be used in spastic patients, especially those with cerebral spasticity, who are in a stable neurologic state and in whom spasticity causes pain, discomfort, or distress or diminishes the ability to utilize residual motor function. It must be given cautiously to ambulatory patients, because relief of spasticity is due to weakness that may worsen the patient's overall functional capacity. The benefit of reducing muscle stiffness versus the possible disadvantage of reducing muscle strength must be weighed individually; however, dantrolene generally is less useful in patients with borderline strength.

Dantrolene is not indicated in fibrositis, rheumatoid spondylitis, bursitis, arthritis, or acute muscle spasm of local origin. The drug should not be given to patients with amyotrophic lateral sclerosis, for these individuals have a very low tolerance to the muscle weakness induced by dantrolene.

Intravenous dantrolene is indicated when a presumptive diagnosis of malignant hyperthermia has been made; it also is used prophylactically in patients with a history of this disorder (see Chapter 17, Adjuncts to Anesthesia). Dantrolene has been used investigationally to treat the symptoms of neuroleptic malignant syndrome and to relieve exercise-induced pain in Duchenne's muscular dystrophy.

ADVERSE REACTIONS AND PRECAUTIONS. Muscle weakness, drowsiness, and diarrhea are the most common reactions. Severe persistent diarrhea may require treatment, reduction in dose, or temporary cessation of therapy. Anorexia, nausea, vomiting, and an acne-like rash are also significant side effects. Less frequently, dizziness, headache, nervousness, insomnia, and depression have occurred. Pleuropericardial reactions and visual disturbances develop rarely.

The most serious adverse reaction is idiosyncratic or hypersensitivity-mediated hepatocellular injury, which occurs rarely and has been fatal. The risk appears to be greatest in patients over 35 years and in women, especially women receiving estrogen therapy. Hepatotoxicity occurs most frequently between 3 and 12 months after initiation of therapy. Therefore, routine baseline hepatic function studies should be performed prior to therapy, and SGOT or SGPT and alkaline phosphatase levels should be determined at appropriate intervals during therapy. The lowest effective dose (preferably no more than 400 mg daily) should be prescribed. Therapy should be continued for more than 60 days only if symptoms are relieved and there is no evidence of hepatic injury. Dantrolene is contraindicated in patients with active hepatic disease. Hepatotoxicity was not observed in children under 10 years in the largest retrospective study conducted to date (Utili et al, 1977).

Dantrolene should be given cautiously to patients with impaired respiratory function and frequent monitoring is essential.

The safety of dantrolene during pregnancy has not been established, although it does not cross the placenta.

No clinically significant drug interactions have been confirmed.

PHARMACOKINETICS. About one-third of a dose of dantrolene is absorbed orally and the absorption half-life is about 30 minutes. Dantrolene is metabolized to 5-hydroxydantrolene (major) and acetylamino dantrolene (minor), which are only weakly active. The blood concentrations of dantrolene and 5-hydroxydantrolene after 400 mg/day has been given for several weeks are not significantly different from those obtained after a single oral dose of 100 mg. This finding does not appear to be related to enzyme induction, but rather to capacity-limited absorption or protein binding (Meyler et al, 1981).

The plasma half-life is five to eight hours. After two weeks of therapy, a linear dose-concentration relationship is observed in the therapeutic dose range (daily doses of 50, 100, and 200 mg), but not with doses of 400 mg daily. There is no correlation between blood concentration and clinical improvement; oral doses exceeding 100 mg daily often do not increase the drug's effect.

Less than 1% of dantrolene and about 10% of its metabolites are recovered in the urine.

DOSAGE AND PREPARATIONS.

Oral: Dosage must be individualized. *Adults,* initially, 25 mg once or twice daily, increased to 25 mg three or four times daily, and then, by increments, to 50 to 100 mg four times daily. Each dosage level should be maintained for four to seven days to determine response. The dose should not be increased beyond the amount that produces maximal benefit with an acceptable level of adverse effects. (The manufacturer's literature specifies that most patients respond to 400 mg/day or less; 100 to 200 mg daily often is adequate.) *Children,* a similar schedule should be utilized, starting with 0.5 mg/kg once or twice daily (maximum, 100 mg four times daily or 3 mg/kg four times daily).

Dantrium (Norwich Eaton). Capsules 25, 50, and 100 mg.

Intravenous: For the treatment and prophylaxis of malignant hyperthermia, see Chapter 17, Adjuncts to Anesthesia.

Dantrium (Norwich Eaton). Powder (sterile, lyophilized) 20 mg. Concentration following reconstitution is approximately 0.32 mg/ml in 10 ml containers.

SPASM

Spasm is an involuntary contraction of a muscle or group of muscles, usually attended by pain and limited function. Reflex muscle spasm (splinting) often occurs as a protective response to local injury but may be exaggerated and require therapy. Drug therapy depends upon the etiology of the spasm (eg, antiepileptic drugs for epileptic myoclonic seizures, calcium for hypocalcemic muscle spasm, analgesics and/or central skeletal muscle relaxants for spasm associated with acute pain syndromes). Acetazolamide [Diamox] and phenytoin [Dilantin] have been reported to be useful in treating myotonia congenita.

Most muscle strains and minor injuries are self-limited and respond rapidly to rest and physical therapy. Initial immobilization of the affected part with casts, pressure bandages, neck collars, arm slings, or crutches; cold compresses; and whirlpool baths often obviate the need for drugs other than mild analgesics. Occasionally, an anti-inflammatory drug may be prescribed when there is considerable tissue damage and edema, although there is no evidence that these drugs reduce the healing time.

Cramps are a form of muscle spasm that are abrupt in onset and last for minutes at a time. Common precipitating factors include vigorous exercise, excessive sweating (resulting in water and sodium loss), vomiting, diarrhea, hypotension, hypokalemia, or drugs (eg, diuretics, corticosteroids). Cramps usually involve the calf or foot and are treated by rubbing and stretching the affected muscle. Night cramps are common in elderly patients, pregnant women, diabetics, and patients with peripheral vascular disease. For frequent nocturnal leg cramps, quinine [Quinamm] is most commonly used (see the evaluation). There is less experience with other agents for this condition.

More severe acute or chronic local spasms may be produced by strains and sprains, trauma, and cervical or lumbar radiculopathy resulting from degenerative osteoarthritis, herniated disc, spondylolysis, chemonucleolysis, or laminectomy. These spasms are characterized by local pain, tenderness on palpation, increased muscle consistency, and limitation of motion and daily activities. In an extensive randomized study (Wiesel et al, 1980), bedrest decreased absence from work by 50%, whereas analgesic and anti-inflammatory agents had no effect on work attendance, although they did provide adjunctive pain relief. The use of chymopapain for herniated disc is discussed in Chapter 10, Drugs Used to Treat Neuralgias.

Central Skeletal Muscle Relaxants and Quinine

These drugs include carisoprodol [Rela, Soma], chlorphenesin [Maolate], chlorzoxazone [Paraflex], methocarbamol [Delaxin, Robaxin], orphenadrine [Norflex], and cyclobenzaprine [Flexeril], which is chemically related to the tricyclic antidepressants. Diazepam is also used in muscle spasms associated with injury (see the evaluation in the section on Spasticity).

Actions: Experimentally, central skeletal muscle relaxants depress spinal polysynaptic reflexes preferentially over monosynaptic reflexes, as well as facilitative and inhibitory neuronal activity affecting muscle stretch reflexes, primarily in the lateral reticular area of the brainstem. Most of these drugs produce sedation, which may reflect depression of neuronal activity in the medial reticular ascending system that is essential for wakefulness. In man, the oral doses of all these drugs are well below the amount required experimentally to elicit muscle relaxant activity; thus, some investigators conclude that their muscle relaxant activity is related only to their sedative effect. However, relief of muscle spasm is not always associated with sedation, which may contribute to overall improvement in some patients but is considered a side effect in others.

Uses: All spasmolytic drugs are superior to placebo in alleviating the symptoms and signs of localized muscle spasm. However, none of these agents have been shown to be more effective than analgesic/anti-inflammatory drugs in relieving the pain of acute or chronic localized muscle spasm.

Methocarbamol and orphenadrine can be administered intravenously to relieve severe, acute muscle spasm of local origin caused by inflammation or trauma. Intravenous methocarbamol also reduces spasticity in selected patients being prepared for physical therapy.

Oral administration of skeletal muscle relaxant drugs is only slightly effective in spasticity induced by cerebrospinal trauma, cerebral palsy, or demyelinating disorders, such as multiple sclerosis. Thus, these agents are not recommended for oral therapy in spastic disorders. In general, skeletal muscle relaxants are not useful in rheumatoid arthritis, but they have been used with anti-inflammatory agents.

Drug Selection: Comparative, controlled, crossover studies to identify drugs of choice to treat spasm are difficult to conduct because of the subjective, variable, and self-limited nature of these illnesses. Extensive reviews of the literature support this view and further emphasize the numerous errors in design and interpretation of clinical studies (Elenbaas, 1980; Deyo, 1983). No one central skeletal muscle relaxant appears to be more effective than another in acute disorders and all have similar side effects. Available data support the use of cyclobenzaprine and diazepam in skeletal muscle spasms (Basmajian, 1978).

Some central skeletal muscle relaxants are available in combination with analgesics: carisoprodol with aspirin [Soma Compound], chlorzoxazone with acetaminophen [Blanex, Parafon Forte], methocarbamol with aspirin [Robaxisal], orphenadrine with aspirin and caffeine [Norgesic, Norgesic Forte]. The Drug Efficacy and Safety Implementation Program of the Food and Drug Administration has categorized all such combination products as possibly effective.

Adverse Reactions: The following adverse reactions and precautions occur with use of all skeletal muscle relaxants except cyclobenzaprine and diazepam. For specific adverse reactions and precautions, see the evaluations.

Drowsiness, lightheadedness, and dizziness are observed most frequently. Occasionally, nausea, vomiting, heartburn, abdominal distress, constipation, diarrhea, or ataxia may occur. Blurred vision, flushing, asthenia, lethargy, and lassitude are more common after intravenous administration than after oral use and are usually transient. With the exception of carisoprodol, areflexia, flaccid paralysis, respiratory depression, tachycardia, and hypotension occur occasionally after large oral doses. Acute poisoning is rarely fatal and is treated in the same manner as barbiturate or benzodiazepine intoxication (see Chapter 5, Drugs Used for Anxiety and Sleep Disorders). Dialysis is of limited value in overdosage of diazepam or cyclobenzaprine.

The centrally acting agents should be discontinued if rash, pruritus, or other evidence of hypersensitivity occurs. Serious allergic manifestations (eg, anaphylactic reactions, leukopenia) have been observed rarely.

Precautions: Patients receiving these drugs should not undertake activities that require mental alertness, judgment, and physical coordination (eg, driving a vehicle, operating dangerous machinery) until it is known that drowsiness or other incapacitating effects will not develop. Caution is necessary if skeletal muscle relaxants and other central nervous system depressants (eg, alcohol, hypnotics, antianxiety drugs, antipsychotic drugs, antidepressants) are used concomitantly, since their effects may be additive. Symptoms of organic brain disease in elderly patients may be aggravated.

Psychic or physical dependence may develop after long-term administration of large doses of some of these agents, especially in patients with a known tendency to abuse drugs. Abrupt discontinuance after prolonged use of large amounts may produce severe withdrawal symptoms, including seizures.

Routine precautions should be followed if these drugs are given during pregnancy (see the discussion on use of drugs during pregnancy in Chapter 3). Unless specifically stated in the evaluations, there is no information on the presence of these compounds in the milk of lactating women.

Drug Evaluations

CARISOPRODOL
[Rela, Soma]

ACTIONS AND USES. Carisoprodol, a congener of meprobamate, is useful as an adjunct to rest, physical therapy, and other appropriate measures to treat the pain of local muscle spasm. It is not effective in spastic or dyskinetic movement disorders.

ADVERSE REACTIONS AND PRECAUTIONS. The most common untoward effect is drowsiness (10%). Idiosyncratic reactions (eg, extreme asthenia, transient quadriplegia, dizziness, ataxia, diplopia, agitation, confusion, disorientation) have occurred rarely after initial administration. Carisoprodol is contraindicated in patients with acute intermittent porphyria. See the Introduction to this section for additional information on adverse reactions and precautions.

PHARMACOKINETICS. The onset of action is rapid and the duration is four to six hours. The elimination half-life is eight hours. (Manufacturers' unpublished data indicate the drug has a half-life of 1 to 1.5 hours.) The compound is metabolized in the liver and the products formed are eliminated in the urine. Carisoprodol is present in the milk of lactating women.

DOSAGE AND PREPARATIONS.
Oral: Adults, 350 mg four times daily; *children under 12 years,* information is inadequate to establish a dosage.
  Rela (Schering), *Soma* (Wallace), *Generic.* Tablets 350 mg.

CHLORPHENESIN CARBAMATE
[Maolate]

USES. This analogue of mephenesin is useful as an adjunct to rest, physiotherapy, and other appropriate measures to treat the pain of local muscle spasm. It is not effective in spastic or dyskinetic movement disorders.

ADVERSE REACTIONS. The most common untoward effects are drowsiness and dizziness. Adverse reactions noted occasionally include gastrointestinal disturbances, paradoxical stimulation, nervousness, insomnia, headache, and asthenia. Rash, pruritus, and blood dyscrasias occur rarely. See the Introduction to this section for additional information on adverse reactions and precautions.

PHARMACOKINETICS. The half-life of chlorphenesin is 3.5 ± 0.2 (2.3 to 5.1) hours. The compound is conjugated, principally with glucuronic acid, and eliminated in the urine.

DOSAGE AND PREPARATIONS.
Oral: Adults, initially, 800 mg three times daily until the desired effect is obtained; for maintenance, 400 mg four times daily or less frequently, as required. *Children,* information is inadequate to establish a dosage.
  Maolate (Upjohn). Tablets 400 mg.

CHLORZOXAZONE
[Paraflex]

USES. Chlorzoxazone, a benzoxalinone, is chemically distinct from all other muscle relaxants. It is useful as an adjunct to rest, physical therapy, and other appropriate measures to treat the pain of local muscle spasm. Chlorzoxazone is not effective in spastic or dyskinetic movement disorders.

ADVERSE REACTIONS AND PRECAUTIONS. The most common side effect is drowsiness (15%). Other reactions include headache, gastrointestinal irritation, and, rarely, gastrointestinal bleeding and hypersensitivity reactions.

Hepatic dysfunction and jaundice have been reported, but a causal relationship cannot be established. Nevertheless, chlorzoxazone should be used cautiously in patients with a history of liver disease. Patients should be monitored closely for signs of liver damage, and the drug should be discontinued if hepatic dysfunction develops.

See the Introduction to this section for additional information on adverse reactions and precautions.

PHARMACOKINETICS. Chlorzoxazone is absorbed rapidly after oral administration, and peak blood concentrations are attained in three to four hours. It is extensively metabolized in the liver, conjugated with glucuronic acid, and excreted by the kidney. The elimination half-life is 1.1 hours.

DOSAGE AND PREPARATIONS.
Oral: Adults, 250 to 750 mg three or four times daily; *children,* 125 to 500 mg three or four times daily.
  Paraflex (McNeil), *Generic.* Tablets 250 mg.

CYCLOBENZAPRINE HYDROCHLORIDE
[Flexeril]

ACTIONS AND USES. Cyclobenzaprine is structurally and pharmacologically related to the tricyclic antidepressants. It is useful as an adjunct to rest, physical therapy, and other appropriate measures in the short-term treatment of painful local muscle spasm. Only a few comparative controlled studies have been published. Results of these studies suggest that a total daily dose of 30 mg is necessary to distinguish this drug's effects from those of a placebo. Oral doses of 60 mg daily do not affect spasticity of spinal or cerebral origin.

ADVERSE REACTIONS AND PRECAUTIONS. The most common side effects are drowsiness (39%), dryness of the mouth (27%), and dizziness (11%). These reactions reflect the sedative and anticholinergic activities of most tricyclic compounds. Tachycardia, weakness, dyspepsia, paresthesia, blurred vision, unpleasant taste, nausea, and insomnia occur less frequently. Sweating, myalgia, dyspnea, abdominal pain, constipation, coated tongue, tremors, dysarthria, euphoria, nervousness, disorientation, confusion, headache, urinary retention, decreased bladder tonus, ataxia, and allergic reactions are rare. No unexpected adverse reactions have been identified in postmarketing surveillance studies, and the incidence of the most common adverse reactions (somnolence, dry mouth, dizziness) was significantly lower than in controlled trials (Nibbelink and Strickland, 1980).

Short-term studies to assess uses other than muscle spasm usually employed somewhat larger doses than those recommended for spasm, and some of the more serious central nervous system reactions noted with the tricyclic antidepressants occurred.

Because of its anticholinergic properties, caution is advised when administering cyclobenzaprine to patients with angle-closure glaucoma or prostatic hypertrophy. Its sedative effects may be additive with those of other central nervous system depressants.

Cyclobenzaprine is contraindicated during the acute recovery phase of myocardial infarction and in patients with arrhythmias, heart block, conduction disturbances, or congestive heart failure.

For general adverse reactions, precautions, and management of overdosage for tricyclic antidepressants, see Chapter 7, Drugs Used in Affective Disorders.

The safe use of cyclobenzaprine during pregnancy has not been established (FDA Pregnancy Category B). Its safety in nursing mothers and children younger than 15 years also remains to be determined.

DRUG INTERACTIONS. Cyclobenzaprine may interact with monoamine oxidase inhibitors when given concomitantly or within 14 days after their discontinuation. It may enhance the effects of alcohol, other central nervous system depressants, and drugs with anticholinergic actions. The antihypertensive action of guanethidine and related drugs may be antagonized.

PHARMACOKINETICS. Doses of 5 to 30 mg are absorbed rapidly, but absorption may be saturated with these amounts. A considerable first-pass effect occurs in the intestine and/or liver of some individuals.

Cyclobenzaprine is highly bound to plasma proteins (93%) and is extensively metabolized to derivatives that are excreted by the kidney, principally as glucuronide conjugates. These effects probably account, in part, for the large variation in plasma concentrations observed among patients.

An elimination half-life of one to three days and a duration of action of 12 to 24 hours have been reported; however, postmarketing surveillance suggests that administration three times daily is appropriate for most patients.

DOSAGE AND PREPARATIONS.
Oral: Adults, 10 mg three times daily (maximum, 60 mg daily). The manufacturer recommends that treatment be limited to two or three weeks.
Flexeril (Merck Sharp & Dohme). Tablets 10 mg.

METHOCARBAMOL
[Delaxin, Robaxin]

USES. This analogue of mephenesin is useful as an adjunct to rest and physical therapy to alleviate the pain of local muscle spasm. The drug can be given parenterally in severe cases or when oral administration is not feasible. Methocarbamol is not effective orally in spastic or dyskinetic movement disorders but it may be given intravenously to reduce spasticity in selected patients being prepared for physical therapy.

ADVERSE REACTIONS AND PRECAUTIONS. Dizziness, drowsiness, headache, anorexia, vertigo, and mild nausea occur occasionally after oral administration, and skin eruptions have been reported rarely. Flushing, metallic taste, nausea, nystagmus, diplopia, mild ataxia, hypotension, and bradycardia have been observed after parenteral administration. These untoward effects may be lessened by giving the injection at a rate not exceeding 3 ml/min. Parenteral administration is contraindicated in patients with impaired renal function, because the polyethylene glycol 300 vehicle may be nephrotoxic.

Safe use during pregnancy or lactation is not established (FDA Pregnancy Category C).

PHARMACOKINETICS. Data are limited, but time to peak blood concentration is 30 minutes. Methocarbamol is largely metabolized. The elimination half-life is 0.9 to 2.2 hours.

DOSAGE AND PREPARATIONS.
Oral: Adults, initially, 1.5 to 2 g four times daily for 48 to 72 hours; for maintenance, 1 g four times daily. The safety and effectiveness of this drug in *children under 12 years* are not established.

Delaxin (Ferndale). Tablets 500 mg.
Robaxin (Robins), *Generic.* Tablets 500 and 750 mg.

Intramuscular: *Adults,* 500 mg alternately in each gluteal region every eight hours.

Intravenous: *Adults,* 1 to 3 g daily at a rate not exceeding 3 ml/min; some physicians substitute oral administration after 1 or 2 g has been administered. The drug should not be given by this route for more than three days.

Generic. Solution 100 mg/ml in 10 ml containers.
Robaxin (Robins). Solution (aqueous) 100 mg/ml with polyethylene glycol 300 50% in 10 ml containers.

ORPHENADRINE CITRATE
[Norflex]

This analogue of the antihistamine, diphenhydramine, is useful as an adjunct to rest, physiotherapy, and other appropriate measures to relieve the pain of local muscle spasm. The drug can be given parenterally in severe cases or when oral administration is not feasible. Orphenadrine is not effective in spastic or dyskinetic movement disorders.

ADVERSE REACTIONS AND PRECAUTIONS. The most common side effects of orphenadrine reflect its anticholinergic activity and include blurred vision, dryness of the mouth and skin, and mild excitation. This agent is contraindicated in patients with angle-closure glaucoma or myasthenia gravis, and it should be used with caution in those with tachycardia, cardiac decompensation, or urinary retention. Dosage reduction may be required in the elderly to avoid intolerable side effects. Some patients experience transient dizziness, lightheadedness, or syncope, which may impair their ability to perform potentially hazardous activities. Hypersensitivity reactions are uncommon. Hypoglycemic reactions have developed rarely when propoxyphene or a phenothiazine was given concomitantly. This drug is classified in FDA Pregnancy Category C.

For a more complete discussion of the adverse reactions and precautions of centrally acting anticholinergic drugs, see Chapter 11, Drugs Used in Extrapyramidal Movement Disorders.

PHARMACOKINETICS. Data in man are limited; orphenadrine is largely metabolized and the elimination half-life is about 14 hours.

DOSAGE AND PREPARATIONS.

Oral: *Adults,* 100 mg twice daily.
Generic. Tablets 100 mg; tablets (timed-release) 100 mg.
Norflex (Riker). Tablets (timed-release) 100 mg.

Intramuscular, Intravenous: *Adults,* 60 mg twice daily.
Generic. Solution 30 mg/ml in 2, 10 and 30 ml containers.
Norflex (Riker). Solution (aqueous) 30 mg/ml in 2 ml containers.
Additional Trademark.
Banflex (Forest).

QUININE SULFATE
[Quinamm]

ACTIONS AND USES. This antimalarial drug is used to prevent nocturnal leg cramps. Its effectiveness has not been established by controlled clinical trial, but quinine has a long history of use for this indication and is widely believed to be effective. One small clinical trial with nine patients who were maintained on hemodialysis for chronic renal failure demonstrated that quinine was significantly more effective than placebo in reducing the number and severity of associated muscle cramps (Kaji et al, 1976).

The Food and Drug Administration has stated that until controlled clinical trials are conducted on quinine's use in nocturnal leg cramps, it should not be generally regarded as safe and effective for this indication (*Federal Register,* 1985).

A number of effects on skeletal muscle have been attributed to quinine: (1) increased refractory period, (2) decreased excitability of the motor endplate to acetylcholine (curare-like effect), and (3) redistribution of calcium in muscle fiber. However, the degree to which these effects occur with therapeutic doses of quinine has not been determined.

ADVERSE REACTIONS. The dose used for nocturnal leg cramps (about one-fourth that given for malaria) probably does not produce symptoms of cinchonism (eg, tinnitus, headache, altered auditory acuity, blurred vision, nausea, diarrhea). For adverse reactions, see the evaluation in Chapter 77, Antiprotozoal Agents.

PRECAUTIONS. Quinine should not be given to patients who are hypersensitive to this agent or to individuals with glucose-6-phosphate dehydrogenase deficiency. Thrombocytopenic purpura may follow its administration in highly sensitive individuals. Quinine should be avoided in patients with optic neuritis and tinnitus or a history of blackwater fever. It should be discontinued if the patient experiences ringing in the ears, deafness, skin rash, or visual disturbances or nausea and vomiting occur.

Because this drug readily crosses the placenta and has been associated with fetal malformations (eg, auditory nerve hypoplasia, limb anomalies, visceral defects), it should not be taken during pregnancy (FDA Pregnancy Category X) and the manufacturer advises caution when it is given to nursing mothers.

DRUG INTERACTIONS. Alkalization of the urine with acetazolamide or sodium bicarbonate may lead to toxic serum concentrations of quinine by decreasing the urinary excretion of the drug. Antacids containing aluminum may decrease quinine's effectiveness by delaying or decreasing absorption.

Quinine antagonizes the action of anticholinesterase drugs,

such as pyridostigmine, and should not be given to myasthenic patients.

Increased plasma concentrations of digoxin and digitoxin have been demonstrated after concomitant administration of quinine. Therefore, plasma digoxin and digitoxin concentrations should be determined periodically for individuals taking either of these glycosides and quinine.

Quinine has the potential to depress hepatic enzyme systems and thus vitamin K factors. The action of warfarin and other oral anticoagulants may be enhanced by the resulting hypoprothrombinemia.

PHARMACOKINETICS. This drug is well absorbed and peak plasma concentrations are attained one to three hours after ingestion of a single oral dose. The elimination half-life of quinine ranges from 5 to 16 hours. Approximately 70% of a dose is bound to plasma protein and degradation primarily occurs in the liver. Quinine and its metabolites are eliminated mainly by renal excretion; only 5% of the dose is excreted unaltered in the urine.

DOSAGE AND PREPARATIONS.
Oral: Adults, 200 to 300 mg once daily at bedtime (Webster, 1985) or twice daily after dinner and at bedtime if necessary. Treatment should be interrupted after several days to determine whether continued therapy is required.

> *Generic.* Capsules 130, 195, 200, 300, and 325 mg; tablets 260 and 325 mg.
> *Quinamm* (Merrell Dow). Tablets 260 mg.

Cited References

Internal analgesic, antipyretic, and antirheumatic drug products for over-the-counter human use; tentative final monograph for drug products for treatment and/or prevention of nocturnal leg cramps. *Federal Register* 50:46588-46954, 1985.

Adams SL, et al: Drugs that may exacerbate myasthenia gravis. *Ann Emerg Med* 13:532-538, 1984.

Alfery DD, Rauscher LA: Tetanus: Review. *Crit Care Med* 7:176-181, 1979.

Argov Z, Mastaglia FL: Disorders of neuromuscular transmission caused by drugs. *N Engl J Med* 301:409-413, 1979.

Basmajian JV: Cyclobenzaprine hydrochloride effect on skeletal muscle spasm in lumbar region and neck: Two double-blind controlled clinical and laboratory studies. *Arch Phys Med Rehabil* 59:58-63, 1978.

Bishop B: Spasticity: Its physiology and management. *Phys Ther* 57:371-401, 1977.

Bowery NG, et al: Baclofen decreases neurotransmitter release in mammalian CNS by action at novel GABA receptor. *Nature* 283:92-93, 1980.

Brogden RN, et al: Baclofen: Preliminary report of its pharmacological properties and therapeutic efficacy in spasticity. *Drugs* 8:1-14, 1974.

Cohan SL, et al: Phenytoin and chlorpromazine in treatment of spasticity. *Arch Neurol* 37:360-364, 1980.

Craven C, et al: Effect of corticosteroids on thymus in myasthenia gravis. *Muscle Nerve* 4:425-428, 1981.

Dau PC: Plasmapheresis therapy in myasthenia gravis. *Muscle Nerve* 3:468-482, 1980.

Davidoff RA: Pharmacology of spasticity. *Neurology* 28:46-51, 1978.

Delisa JA, Little J: Managing spasticity. *Am Fam Physician* 26:117-122, (Sept) 1982.

Deyo RA: Conservative therapy for low back pain: Distinguishing useful from useless therapy. *JAMA* 250:1057-1062, 1983.

Donaldson JO, et al: Antiacetylcholine receptor antibody in neonatal myasthenia gravis. *Am J Dis Child* 135:222-226, 1981.

Duncan GW, et al: Evaluation of baclofen treatment for certain symptoms in patients with spinal cord lesions. *Neurology* 26:441-446, 1976.

Elenbaas JK: Centrally acting oral skeletal muscle relaxants. *Am J Hosp Pharm* 37:1313-1323, 1980.

Engel AG, et al: Immunopathology of acquired myasthenia gravis. *Ann NY Acad Sci* 377:158-174, 1982.

Feldman RG, et al: Baclofen for spasticity in multiple sclerosis: Double-blind crossover and three-year study. *Neurology* 28:1094-1098, 1978.

Grob D (ed): Myasthenia gravis: Pathophysiology and management. *Ann NY Acad Sci* 377:1-902, 1981.

Hachen HJ, Krucker V: Clinical and laboratory assessment of efficacy of baclofen (Lioresal) on urethral sphincter spasticity in patients with traumatic paraplegia. *Eur Urol* 3:237-240, 1977.

Haubenstock A, et al: Baclofen (Lioresal) intoxication: Report of 4 cases and review of literature. *Clin Toxicol* 20:59-68, 1983.

Havard CWH, Scadding GK: Myasthenia gravis: Pathogenesis and current concepts in management. *Drugs* 26:174-184, 1983.

Hedley DW, et al: Evaluation of baclofen (Lioresal) for spasticity in multiple sclerosis. *Postgrad Med J* 51:615-618, 1975.

Henriksson KG, Sandstedt P: Polymyositis: Treatment and prognosis: Study of 107 patients. *Acta Neurol Scand* 65:280-300, 1982.

Kaji DM, et al: Prevention of muscle cramps in haemodialysis patients by quinine sulphate. *Lancet* 2:66-67, 1976.

Levine IM, et al: Lioresal, new muscle relaxant in treatment of spasticity: Double-blind quantitative evaluation. *Dis Nerv Syst* 38:1011-1015, 1977.

Mason NA, et al: Factors affecting diazepam infusion: Solubility, administration-set composition, and flow rate. *Am J Hosp Pharm* 38:1449-1454, 1981.

Mastaglia FL, Ojeda VJ: Inflammatory myopathies, part 2. *Ann Neurol* 17:317-323, 1985.

McFarlin DE: Treatment of multiple sclerosis, (editorial). *N Engl J Med* 308:215-217, 1983.

Melnick ME, Shellenberger MK: Management of pediatric spasticity. *Compr Ther* 8:20-26, (Oct) 1982.

Merritt JL: Management of spasticity in spinal cord injury. *Mayo Clin Proc* 56:614-622, 1981.

Mertens HG, et al: Effect of immunosuppressive drugs (azathioprine). *Ann NY Acad Sci* 377:691-698, 1981.

Meyler WJ, et al: Effect of dantrolene sodium in relation to blood levels in spastic patients after prolonged administration. *J Neurol Neurosurg Psychiatry* 44:334-339, 1981.

Miller F, Korsvik H: Baclofen in treatment of stiff-man syndrome. *Ann Neurol* 9:511-512, 1981.

Mulder DG, et al: Thymectomy for myasthenia gravis. *Am J Surg* 146:61-66, 1983.

Nibbelink DW, Strickland SC: Cyclobenzaprine (Flexeril): Report of postmarketing surveillance program. *Curr Ther Res* 28:894-903, 1980.

Noseworthy JH, et al: Therapeutic trials in multiple sclerosis. *Can J Neurol Sci* 11:355-362, 1984.

Olanow CW, et al: Prospective study of thymectomy and serum acetylcholine receptor antibodies in myasthenia gravis. *Ann Surg* 196:113-121, 1982.

Oosterhuis HJGH: Treating myasthenic patient, in: *Myasthenia Gravis: Clinical Neurology and Neurosurgery Monographs.* Edinburgh, Churchill Livingstone, 1984, vol 5, 175-261.

Pascuzzi RM, et al: Long-term corticosteroid treatment of myasthenia gravis: Report of 116 patients. *Ann Neurol* 15:291-298, 1984.

Penn AS, et al: Therapy of myasthenia gravis, in Serratrice G, et al (eds): *Neuromuscular Disease.* New York, Raven Press, 1984, 495-501.

Pinder RM, et al: Dantrolene sodium: Review of pharmacological properties and therapeutic efficacy in spasticity. *Drugs* 13:3-23, 1977.

Rowland LP: Controversies about treatment of myasthenia gravis. *J Neurol Neurosurg Psychiatry* 43:644-659, 1980.

Scheife RT, et al: Myasthenia gravis: Signs, symptoms, diagnosis, immunology, and current therapy. *Pharmacotherapy* 1:39-54, 1981.

Schmidt RT, et al: Comparison of dantrolene sodium and diazepam in treatment of spasticity. *J Neurol Neurosurg Psychiatry* 39:350-356, 1976.

Seybold ME: Myasthenia gravis: Clinical and basic science review. *JAMA* 250:2516-2521, 1983.

Slonim AE, Goans PJ: Myopathy in McArdle's syndrome: Improvement with high-protein diet. *N Engl J Med* 312:355-359, 1985.

Snead OC III, et al: Juvenile myasthenia gravis. *Neurology* 30:732-739, 1980.

Terrence CF, et al: Baclofen: Effect on seizure frequency. *Arch Neurol* 40:28-29, 1983.

Tindall RSA: Humoral immunity in myasthenia gravis: Effects of steroids and thymectomy. *Neurology* 30:554-557, 1980.

Utili R, et al: Dantrolene-associated hepatic injury: Incidence and character. *Gastroenterology* 72:610-616, 1977.

Webster LT: Drugs used in chemotherapy of protozoal infections: Malaria, in Gilman AG, et al (eds): *The Pharmacological Basis of Therapeutics*, ed 7. New York, Macmillan, 1985, 1044.

Wiesel SW, et al: Acute low-back pain: Objective analysis of conservative therapy. *Spine* 5:324-330, 1980.

Witte AS, et al: Azathioprine in treatment of myasthenia gravis. *Ann Neurol* 15:602-605, 1984.

Young RR, Delwaide PJ: Spasticity, parts I and II. *N Engl J Med* 304:28-33, 96-99, 1981.

Drugs Used to Treat Migraine and Other Headaches

13

INTRODUCTION

VASCULAR HEADACHE OF THE MIGRAINE TYPE

Migraine Headache

Cluster Headache

MUSCLE-CONTRACTION AND COMBINED HEADACHE

DRUG EVALUATIONS

Ergot Alkaloids

Beta-blocking Agents

Calcium Channel Blocking Agents

Antidepressants

Mixtures (Table)

Headache, one of the most common symptoms experienced by man, may be precipitated by a great variety of stimuli: emotional stress; fatigue; sensitivity to certain foods and beverages, including alcohol; medications; and acute illness. There may be no apparent underlying cause. In some individuals, headaches occur frequently but irregularly; however, they are usually acute and short lived and can be relieved by over-the-counter preparations containing aspirin or acetaminophen. This type of headache is usually not debilitating and does not require physician consultation.

In contrast, chronic recurrent headache, for which patients most often consult physicians, is associated with various medical, neurologic, or psychogenic disorders. Appropriate therapy depends upon an accurate diagnosis of the type of headache. For texts discussing diagnostic procedures, see the references at the end of this chapter.

The Ad Hoc Committee of the National Institute of Neurological and Communicative Disorders and Stroke has developed the most complete classification of headache (Ad Hoc Committee on Classification of Headache, 1962). This classification includes painful and nonpainful disorders of the entire head and is based on the underlying pain mechanisms proposed at that time. Although it still serves as a general framework for diagnosis, the established categories for certain headaches (eg, migraine, muscle-contraction headache) are currently being re-examined. Some authorities feel that vascular mechanisms underlying migraine and cluster headaches are secondary to a central neurogenic disorder (Blau 1984; Drummond and Lance 1984; Pearce 1984). A review of the clinical research on muscle-contraction headache has shown a poor correlation between pain and contraction of scalp muscle (see section on Muscle-Contraction and Combined Headache). Further, it has been proposed that muscle-contraction and migraine headache differ only in their relative position along a continuum of pain severity (Waters, 1973; Anderson and Franks, 1981; Featherstone, 1985). Further research may eventually necessitate reclassification of headache types. This chapter will follow the currently accepted classification.

A major type of headache that must be considered in differential diagnosis is that caused by underlying disease: intracranial disturbances (eg, vascular anomalies, tumors, trauma), systemic diseases (eg, allergies; hypertension; cervical osteoarthritis; diseases of eye, ear, nose, throat), and cranial (eg, trigeminal) neuralgia. These headaches usually can be relieved by specific therapy for the underlying disorder, eg, surgical correction of tumors, antibiotics for infections, antirheumatic drugs for osteoarthritis. Drug treatment for cranial neuralgias is discussed in Chapter 10, Drugs Used to Treat Neuralgias.

Considerations in the management of recurrent muscle-contraction, migraine, or cluster headaches are: (1) No single therapy is effective in all patients with the same type of headache, which serves to underscore the uncertainty about the pathophysiology of the disorder. Therefore, drug therapy must be individualized and trial of different therapies and drugs may be required to establish an effective regimen. (2) In addition to abortive therapy, some patients should receive prophylactic therapy; prophylaxis is valuable in chronic muscle-contraction, migraine, and cluster headaches. These patients should be monitored closely and adjustments made in choice of therapy or dosage when necessary. (3) Many patients with chronic headaches have received drugs that may cause drug dependence (eg, barbiturates, antianxiety agents, ergotamine, narcotics, analgesic and caffeine mixtures), and their withdrawal along with instruction regarding their proper use is necessary. This last consideration may be a primary obstacle in the long-term relief of headache (Medina and Diamond, 1977; Saper and Van Meter, 1980).

VASCULAR HEADACHE OF THE MIGRAINE TYPE

Migraine Headache

Migraine headaches can begin during childhood, but 60% to 70% of patients are women in their late teens, twenties, and thirties (Waters and O'Connor, 1975). Headache pain is usually characterized as steady or throbbing and is most severe in the temporal and frontal regions. The headache is often unilateral, frequently occurs at night or on awakening, and may be associated with nausea, vomiting, photophobia, irritability, and constipation or diarrhea. Local or generalized edema, pallor, dizziness, and sweating also may occur.

Migraine may be precipitated by tyramine-containing foods, alcohol, noise, glare, menses, anxiety, fatigue, or stress. Prodromal aura (visual, sensory, motor, or any combination) are sharply defined in "classic" migraine but are absent in "common" migraine; the vast majority of those with migraine have the common type. A patient may experience classic migraine headache at one time and that resembling the common type at others. Combined muscle-contraction/ migraine headache is not unusual. Severe forms of classic migraine, including hemiplegic, ophthalmoplegic, basilar-artery, and atypical migraine, are rare but should be considered in differential diagnosis.

The pathophysiology of migraine remains to be determined. Although biphasic intracerebral vasoconstriction followed by extracerebral arterial dilation is known to occur during classic migraine, there is some controversy as to whether the attack results from primary vascular instability or some underlying neuronal disturbance (Pearce, 1984; Blau, 1984). Many authorities now believe that the initial intracerebral vasoconstriction of classic migraine may be secondary to a wave of cortical excitation followed by depression of neuronal function spreading over both cerebral hemispheres. The headache phase is often associated with distention of extracranial vessels; sensitization of the vascular wall by serotonin, histamine, or bradykinin; and deficiencies in brain serotonin and endorphin levels that regulate pain control (Lance, 1982; Salmon et al, 1982). It has been suggested that hypothalamic disturbances may account for the periodicity of migraine attacks (Pearce, 1984). Much of the pharmacotherapy of migraine is directed at modifying cerebrovascular physiology.

A family history of migraine exists in 65% to 70% of affected patients and aids in diagnosis. Migraine patients may be genetically predisposed to headache by variant patterns of monoamine metabolism, which make them vulnerable to changes in monoamine transmitters in the central nervous system, as well as platelet-released serotonin (Lance, 1982).

The effective management of recurrent migraine may require combined medical and nonmedical therapy, including the control or elimination of underlying factors that precipitate an attack. Among the nonpharmacologic techniques, many headache specialists have found biofeedback to be effective. Its beneficial action may be mediated through generalized reduction of sympathetic tone, which decreases blood flow in supraorbital and superficial temporal arteries (Dalessio et al, 1979). A reduction in catecholamines and decreased monoamine oxidase activity also have been observed (Mathew et al, 1980). Biofeedback reduced the intensity and frequency of headaches in some patients, and some authorities consider it especially effective in children (Diamond, 1983). However, in a recent review of the data, the American College of Physicians concluded that there is insufficient evidence of the efficacy of biofeedback in mixed migraine and muscle-contraction headaches and that, while biofeedback may be useful adjunctively, this therapy is no more effective than relaxation techniques for migraine or muscle-contraction headaches (Health and Public Policy Committee, American College of Physicians, 1985).

Pharmacotherapy consists of symptomatic treatment of the acute attack (abortive) and prophylactic (interval) therapy to reduce the frequency and severity of headaches.

Drug Selection for Acute Migraine: The goal of drug therapy for acute migraine headache is to relieve pain and reduce or prevent accompanying nausea and vomiting. Drugs should be administered during the earliest stages of an attack to obtain the greatest therapeutic effect. The early stages of classic migraine are the easiest to identify; the aura serves as a signal to begin abortive measures. Once the headache has been established, oral drugs are generally poorly absorbed due to gastric stasis, nausea, or both.

Nonspecific symptomatic relief of mild attacks may be obtained with mild analgesics (aspirin, acetaminophen), sedatives (eg, barbiturates), or antianxiety drugs. Some mixtures containing sedatives and analgesics (eg, Fiorinal, Midrin) also may be helpful but may be habituating. If mild analgesics are ineffective, stronger analgesics (eg, aspirin with codeine, propoxyphene [Darvon]) may be employed, but their effectiveness is limited once the attack has begun because of gastric stasis. Metoclopramide [Reglan] 10 to 20 mg has been recommended to restore gastric motility, permit absorption of analgesics, and prevent nausea and vomiting (Selby, 1983; Kunkel, 1985). It should be given 10 to 20 minutes prior to analgesics. This drug probably should not be used in young children because it can cause extrapyramidal reactions in this age group (although adults also may develop dyskinesias with metoclopramide).

If symptoms of migraine headache cannot be managed with analgesics, subsequent attacks should be aborted with ergotamine tartrate, which is available as a sublingual [Ergomar, Ergostat] or inhalation [Medihaler Ergotamine] preparation or in combination with caffeine [Cafergot, Wigraine] in oral or rectal preparations. Caffeine has been reported to increase the absorption and effectiveness of ergotamine (Schmidt and Fanchamps, 1974). Of the available ergot alkaloids, ergotamine has the most prolonged effect and most consistently aborts migraine headaches when an adequate dose is administered as soon as possible after the onset of the migraine prodrome or attack. However, the major side effects and contraindications for the use of this drug should be borne in mind (see the evaluation).

Concomitant oral administration of metoclopramide may

prevent the severe nausea and vomiting caused by ergotamine (or the migraine attack) and enhance ergotamine's absorption (Tfelt-Hansen et al, 1980; Bradfield, 1976). Some physicians prefer phenothiazine antiemetics, such as prochlorperazine [Compazine] or promethazine [Phenergan], which can be administered either rectally or intramuscularly. The belladonna alkaloids present in mixtures containing ergotamine (eg, Cafergot P-B) also are claimed to allay nausea and vomiting. The sublingual or inhalation route may be more practical when nausea occurs. When used properly, the inhalation preparation provides rapid systemic availability of the drug.

In patients who cannot tolerate ergotamine, the mixture of isometheptene mucate, dichloralphenazone, and acetaminophen [Midrin] may be an effective alternative. Contraindications to the use of isometheptene are similar to those for ergotamine (see Table). Clinical data indicate that Midrin is superior to acetaminophen alone (Diamond, 1976).

The ergotamine derivative, dihydroergotamine [D.H.E. 45], may be a useful alternative to ergotamine when high serum drug concentrations are needed. This drug is administered intramuscularly or intravenously and is considered by some authorities to be the agent of choice in physicians' offices and hospital emergency rooms for patients with severe migraine headache (Diamond, 1983; Raskin and Raskin, 1984). Sublingual and inhalation forms of ergotamine may be considered second choices in these situations. Severe headaches that fail to respond to ergot preparations may be relieved by a strong analgesic (eg, meperidine [Demerol]). However, strong analgesics should be given cautiously, since there is potential for abuse; patients taking such drugs should be followed closely.

Rarely, migraine headache becomes intractable to both ergotamine therapy and strong analgesics and may persist for days or weeks (status migrainosus). Dexamethasone acetate 16 mg intramuscularly has been reported to produce dramatic improvement (Diamond and Medina, 1980 A). Alternatively, oral prednisone is effective when a large dose (60 to 80 mg) is given for the first two days with the amount reduced gradually over a few days. The combined intravenous administration of dihydroergotamine 0.5 mg and metoclopramide 10 mg every eight hours also has been reported to terminate attacks of status migrainosus (Raskin and Raskin, 1984).

Migraine in children is usually treated with biofeedback, cyproheptadine, or aspirin. Ergotamine is almost never used as the initial drug to treat migraine in young patients, but when the above therapy is inadequate, ergotamine can be used safely and effectively.

Drug Selection for Prophylactic Therapy: The decision to begin prophylactic therapy for migraine headaches is based on the frequency and severity of the attacks, the response to abortive therapy, and coexisting medical conditions. Usually, patients who experience one or two disabling attacks per week are candidates for prophylactic therapy. However, if the attacks respond well to abortive therapy with ergotamine and the dose does not exceed recommended safety limits, prophylactic therapy is not required. Conversely, if abortive therapy is inadequate or contraindicated, preventive therapy is the only alternative. For children, the use of continuous medication to prevent intermittent headaches (eg, three or four per month)

should be weighed carefully. Since spontaneous remissions occur, prolonged, uninterrupted prophylactic treatment without a drug-free interval is not advisable.

Ergotamine is generally not recommended for prophylaxis because its potent peripheral vasoconstrictor action may produce arterial insufficiency and dependence may result from prolonged daily use. In dependent patients, a self-sustaining headache-medication cycle is established in which drug withdrawal precipitates a rebound headache that necessitates readministration of ergotamine. Certain patients may be predisposed to this rebound syndrome. The headache that follows ergotamine withdrawal is debilitating and lasts longer than a typical migraine headache (Saper, 1983). Nevertheless, withdrawal must be attempted to re-establish headache control, since prophylactic agents are often ineffective in ergotamine-dependent patients. Some authorities still favor intermittent use of ergotamine to prevent predictable migraine attacks, such as those occurring on weekends, in association with menstruation, or resulting from a known stressful situation. Caution should be exercised when ergotamine is used in these circumstances.

Methysergide [Sansert] and beta blockers are the most effective agents for migraine prophylaxis. Many authorities prefer beta blocker therapy because of the potential occurrence of serious fibrotic adverse reactions with methysergide (Diamond and Medina, 1980 A). Most experience has been gained with propranolol, but other beta blockers (ie, atenolol [Tenormin], metoprolol [Lopressor], nadolol [Corgard], timolol [Blocadren]) were effective in controlled clinical trials (Steiner and Joseph, 1984; Turner, 1984). No significant difference in effectiveness between these beta blockers and propranolol has been demonstrated.

Prophylactic therapy with beta blockers may be particularly useful in patients who cannot take ergot preparations (eg, those with hypertension, cerebrovascular disease, angina pectoris, severe peripheral vascular disease, thyrotoxicosis). However, these drugs should not be used when beta blockade would be harmful (see the evaluation). If the patient fails to respond to beta blockers or these drugs are contraindicated, a number of alternative agents may be appropriate.

Methysergide is considered by some authorities to be the most effective prophylactic drug available but, because of its potential for serious adverse reactions, this drug must be used with caution and treatment should be interrupted after four to six months. Some authorities use methysergide only after tricyclic antidepressants, calcium channel blocking agents, and nonsteroidal anti-inflammatory agents (eg, naproxen [Naprosyn]) have failed. Methysergide is not effective in an acute migraine attack or muscle-contraction headache and should be restricted to short-term use in patients under age 50 who are not at risk for vascular disease.

Although the use of calcium channel blocking drugs, such as verapamil [Calan, Isoptin], nimodipine [Nimotop] (investigational drug), or nifedipine [Procardia], for migraine prophylaxis is investigational, these drugs reduced the frequency and duration of attacks of both common and classic migraine in controlled clinical trials (Holmes et al, 1984; Markley et al, 1984; Meyer, 1985; Solomon et al, 1983). Verapamil reduced the frequency of attacks in patients refractory to ergotamine, propranolol, and amitriptyline (Markley et al, 1984). The lower incidence and milder nature of side effects with verapamil and other calcium blockers may make these agents an alternative to methysergide or propranolol (see the evaluation on Verapamil Hydrochloride).

Cyproheptadine [Periactin], an antihistamine with antiserotonin and calcium antagonist activity, was considered to be effective for prophylaxis in some patients, but results of controlled studies have shown that it is only slightly better than placebo. Adverse effects include drowsiness and increased appetite with weight gain. Children appear to tolerate this drug better than adults, however, and some clinicians consider cyproheptadine to be a drug of choice for prophylactic therapy in pediatric patients (Diamond and Medina, 1980 B). A related compound, pizotyline (pizotifen), is not available in the United States, but it reduced the frequency and severity of migraine attacks in clinical trials (Louis and Spierings, 1982; Selby, 1983). This drug is widely used in Canada, Australia, and Europe; it has the same spectrum of adverse reactions as cyproheptadine, but is considered superior to the latter for migraine prophylaxis.

In a limited number of studies, amitriptyline, a tricyclic antidepressant, was effective prophylactically for some patients with migraine or muscle-contraction headache. This drug also may be useful in the prophylaxis of mixed migraine/muscle-contraction headache. In one controlled study, amitriptyline was more effective than placebo in preventing migraine, and its action did not appear to be related to the antidepressant effect (Couch and Hassanein, 1979). Thus, this drug may be an alternative to methysergide when propranolol is not tolerated or is ineffective.

Another antidepressant, the monoamine oxidase inhibitor, phenelzine [Nardil], was reported to be beneficial in some patients refractory to other prophylactic therapy. However, because the response is variable and the adverse effects are potentially severe, it should be reserved for patients with severe migraine or chronic mixed migraine/muscle-contraction headache that does not respond to prophylactic therapy with other drugs.

Antianxiety agents may be used for short-term prophylaxis to allay stress.

Clonidine [Catapres] has been recommended for patients sensitive to foods containing tyramine in whom the response rate was 30% (Diamond, 1983). However, this is no greater than the placebo response rate observed in most controlled clinical trials. If used for migraine prophylaxis, the manufacturer recommends 0.025 to 0.075 mg twice daily. Clonidine should be withdrawn gradually in order to avoid hypertensive crises but this is considered unlikely at these dosages and in normotensive patients.

There is some indirect evidence that prostaglandins play a role in the development of a migraine attack. Thus, several inhibitors of prostaglandin synthetase and platelet aggregation have been studied as prophylactic drugs. The results from a small number of studies with aspirin, indomethacin [Indocin], and dipyridamole [Persantine] have not been convincing (Masel et al, 1980; O'Neil and Mann, 1978; Diamond and Medina, 1980 A). However, a controlled double-blind trial with naproxen demonstrated that this drug moderately reduced the frequency and duration of migraine attacks (Ziegler and Ellis, 1985). Newer nonsteroidal anti-inflammatory drugs (eg, ibuprofen [Advil, Motrin, Nuprin, Rufen], fenoprofen [Nalfon]) that inhibit prostaglandin synthesis also may prevent migraine, but further studies are needed to determine their ultimate role for this use.

Other agents (eg, progestins, papaverine, bromocriptine [Parlodel], diuretics) and histamine desensitization have been suggested for prophylaxis of migraine, but there are minimal data to assess their efficacy.

Cluster Headache

Cluster headache (also known as Horton's syndrome, histaminic cephalalgia, migrainous neuralgia, and by many other names) is related to migraine but differs sufficiently to be considered a separate type of vascular headache. The typical form, classified as *episodic* or *periodic*, is characterized by brief (30 to 40 minutes), excruciating, nonthrobbing, unilateral, oculofrontal or oculotemporal pain occurring in a series or "cluster" of closely spaced attacks, often at night. Associated signs are conjunctival injection, lacrimation, nasal congestion, facial blanching or flushing, and, occasionally, ptosis and miosis on the side of the pain. Unlike migraine headaches, prodromata or aura do not precede the headache and nausea and vomiting are absent. Clusters generally last 4 to 12 weeks, with remissions of months or years.

In *chronic cluster headache*, the periods of remission are diminished. In one form (chronic paroxysmal hemicrania, CPH), attacks occur more than six times daily. Although cluster headaches are observed more frequently in men than in women (5:1), CPH is distinguished by its almost exclusive occurrence in women, the great frequency of attacks, and its response to indomethacin. There is usually no family history of cluster headache (Kudrow, 1979).

The pathogenesis of cluster headache is not known, but numerous studies indicate that certain changes in cephalic blood flow, as well as biochemical changes (eg, histamine, serotonin, and hormone levels) result from a neurogenic mechanism. Unilateral increases in blood flow usually follow the onset of pain and it has been postulated that vascular changes are initiated by a vasodilator pathway involving the trigeminal nerve and greater superficial petrosal nerve afferent-efferent arc (Drummond and Lance, 1984).

Drug Selection: Preventive therapy is the treatment of choice of most headache specialists, but abortive medication also may be required. The choice of therapy depends on the age and health of the patient, the frequency of attacks, duration of the cluster, and the response to previous therapy (Saper, 1983). The primary prophylactic medications are methysergide, lithium carbonate, and corticosteroids. Ergotamine tartrate also has been effective for short episodes that occur at predictable times (Lance, 1982; Raskin and Appenzeller, 1980; Speed, 1985). Methysergide is more effective in preventing episodic cluster headache than the chronic type and is especially beneficial in patients under 30 years.

Lithium is effective in the prophylactic management of chronic cluster headache refractory to methysergide (Ekbom, 1981; Manzoni et al, 1983; Mathew, 1984). Lithium also may be effective in episodic clusters; this drug is regarded by some authorities as a second-line drug and is preferred to corticosteroids when methysergide fails. Corticosteroids are very effective in terminating and preventing cluster headache. Because of the self-limited nature of cluster headache and the side effects of the corticosteroids, the recommended course of therapy is about three weeks. The dosage varies; in one regimen, oral prednisone 60 mg is given daily for four days followed by a six-day stepwise reduction of the dose to zero (Saper, 1983).

Individual cataclysmic attacks that break through preventive therapy or that occur before prophylactic therapy becomes effective may be terminated by an ergot preparation; unless contraindicated, parenteral dihydroergotamine is preferred by some clinicians for prompt relief but may not be practical for regular use. As an alternative, rectal administration of ergotamine/caffeine suppositories has been recommended. Because the attacks are brief, oral and sublingual preparations of ergotamine are usually ineffective. The inhalant form of ergotamine provides fast relief in selected patients, but variability in dosing and constriction of pulmonary arteries require patient education in its use (Raskin and Appenzeller, 1980). When a large number of attacks occur daily, overmedication may occur.

Cluster headache also may be aborted by inhaling 100% oxygen (8 to 10 L/minute for 5 to 10 minutes) through a tight-fitting mask. The mechanism of action is unknown, but this form of therapy has been reported to be useful in 57% to 93% of cases (Kudrow, 1981).

Initial studies with calcium channel blockers (eg, verapamil, nifedipine, nimodipine [investigational]) suggest that these drugs may have prophylactic activity; nimodipine was reported to be the most effective. However, more studies are required before the usefulness of calcium antagonists in cluster headache is established (Meyer and Hardenberg, 1983).

CPH usually responds completely to oral indomethacin 25 to 50 mg three times daily (Saper, 1983; Mathew, 1984).

MUSCLE-CONTRACTION AND COMBINED HEADACHE

Clinicians have defined muscle-contraction headaches as those characterized by mild to moderate nonthrobbing pain, tightness, or pressure around the head and neck unassociated with autonomic disturbances. This type of headache (also referred to as tension headache) represents the most common one for which a physician is consulted. Acute muscle-contraction headache often develops in response to stress, aggravation, frustration, eye strain, or positional effects.

The mechanism of muscular headache has been proposed to result from sustained contraction of the neck and scalp muscles, which constrict scalp arteries and produce ischemia (Friedman, 1979). However, electromyography of the frontalis muscle demonstrated that there is poor correlation between muscle contraction and pain (Bakal and Kaganov, 1977). This finding has led some headache specialists to question the existence of muscle-contraction headache as a separate entity and to propose a more central pain disorder as the basis. Migraine and muscle-contraction headaches also have been described as representing degrees of pain intensity existing along a headache severity continuum (Waters, 1973; Featherstone, 1985).

Muscular and migraine-like headaches often occur together (Cohen and McArthur et al, 1981; Anderson and Franks, 1981; Joffe et al, 1983; Saper, 1983) and a significant portion of patients with chronic headache have "mixed" headaches with migraine and muscular features (Ziegler, 1985).

Current physiologic, psychological, and clinical studies have blurred the traditional distinction between muscle-contraction and common migraine headaches. Several clinical patterns have been described for mixed headaches. One type consists predominantly of migraine symptoms with some symptoms of muscle-contraction headache. Another type is expressed as muscle-contraction headache (occurring for hours or days) with accompanying migraine-like features, such as photosensitivity, gastrointestinal distress, and vasomotor phenomena. Most difficult to treat is the chronic headache syndrome that begins in early years as migraine headache and evolves later in adult life into a relatively constant muscle-contraction-like headache. This type of mixed headache is most common in women and frequently is accompanied by depression, anxiety, and sleep disturbances. The chronic nature of this pain increases the potential for analgesic abuse.

Muscle-contraction headaches also have been referred to as psychogenic headaches. Although these headaches are frequently precipitated by emotional factors, especially anxiety, they must be differentiated from headaches accompanying severe psychological disorders. To avoid confusion, it is proposed that the class, psychogenic, be restricted to headaches that do not have known physiologic pain-producing mechanisms and in which the pain represents the primary expression of an underlying psychiatric disorder. The psychogenic class includes conversion, delusional, and hypochondriacal headaches (Packard, 1976; Weatherhead, 1980).

Muscle-contraction headaches also must be differentiated from those caused by certain disorders of muscles or joints (inflammation or infection of the muscles of the head and neck, cervical osteoarthritis, disorders of the temporal-mandibular joint). Treatment or correction of the underlying condition is important in the management of these headaches.

Drug Selection: Treatment of chronic combined headache represents a therapeutic challenge to the headache specialist. Many authorities recommend hospitalization and withdrawal of all analgesics taken daily. Chlorpromazine (or another phenothiazine) has been given during analgesic withdrawal; antianxiety agents may also be useful. A multidisciplinary approach is usually required including physical therapy, biofeedback, relaxation techniques, psychotherapy, and drug therapy (Ziegler,

1978; Martin, 1978; Nuechterlein and Holroyd, 1980). The combination of propranolol (or another appropriate beta blocker) and amitriptyline has been useful in prophylaxis (Mathew, 1981; Dexter et al, 1980). Monoamine oxidase inhibitors also are reported to be effective (Saper, 1983).

Antidepressants, such as amitriptyline, imipramine, and desipramine, are useful because of their analgesic activity and their effect on the depression commonly associated with chronic muscle-contraction and combined headaches.

An acute attack of mixed muscle-contraction/migraine headache is usually managed by treating the symptoms of the dominant headache type (eg, ergotamine for migraine, analgesics or antidepressants for muscle contraction). Combined administration of ergotamine and simple analgesics may be required.

Acute muscle-contraction headaches with mild to moderate pain may be treated with a nonopiate analgesic (eg, aspirin, acetaminophen, ibuprofen, other nonsteroidal anti-inflammatory analgesics); an antidepressant; or an antianxiety agent (eg, diazepam [Valium]), given alone or with an analgesic. Drugs with high dependence liability should be avoided. Certain combination products containing a barbiturate (eg, Fiorinal) or other sedative (eg, meprobamate [Micrainin]) with an analgesic are useful in this type of headache (see Table). However, because these mixtures have high abuse potential, they should be avoided in patients with chronic headaches (Medina and Diamond, 1977; Friedman, 1979).

Many patients with muscle-contraction headache have associated depressive symptoms. Pain is often worse in the morning than in the evening, is generalized rather than localized, is accompanied by scalp formication, and is associated with symptoms common in depression, such as sleep disturbances with early and frequent awakening. The tricyclic antidepressants may be more effective than analgesics if such symptoms are present. However, there is growing evidence to indicate that antidepressants reduce headache pain independent of the presence of depression. A nighttime dose may relieve both sleep disturbances and headache.

Drug Evaluations

ERGOT ALKALOIDS

ERGOTAMINE TARTRATE
[Medihaler Ergotamine, Ergomar, Ergostat]

ACTIONS AND USES. Ergotamine is the drug of choice in the treatment of acute attacks of migraine. It also may be used to alleviate or prevent acute attacks of cluster headache.

The long-term prophylactic use of ergotamine is generally inadvisable because of its potential adverse reactions, but short-term daily use may be appropriate in certain cases. For example, patients experiencing daily attacks of cluster headaches may receive the drug for 10 to 14 days to help terminate a bout.

Ergotamine causes peripheral vasoconstriction, especially in the dilated external carotid arterial bed. It acts as a vasoconstrictor if the tonus of the vessel is low and as a vasodilator if the tonus is high. Although this drug's peripheral vasoconstrictor action is important in relieving migraine attacks, its effect on central serotonergic neurons may also play a role. In therapeutic doses, ergotamine does not act as an adrenergic blocking agent but potentiates epinephrine and norepinephrine and inhibits the reuptake of these amines after nerve stimulation (Fozard, 1975).

To be most effective, adequate doses must be administered early in the migraine attack, ie, the drug should be taken immediately after the onset of any prodromal symptoms. The dosage should be individualized to determine an appropriate amount for subsequent attacks. Ergotamine is poorly absorbed when given orally (available only in combination products) or sublingually, and there is considerable variation among individuals; if these routes are ineffective, rectal suppositories (available only in combination products) should be tried since higher plasma levels have been reported after administration by this route than after oral use. The drug also may be given by inhalation, which produces a more rapid effect than the oral route.

ADVERSE REACTIONS AND PRECAUTIONS. Ergotamine may produce nausea, vomiting, epigastric discomfort, diarrhea, polydipsia, and drowsiness. More serious adverse reactions include paresthesias of the extremities, cramps and weakness of the legs, myalgia (eg, stiffness of thigh and neck muscles), angina-like precordial pain and distress, transient sinus tachycardia and bradycardia, and, in sensitive patients, localized edema, pruritus, and peripheral vasoconstriction.

Symptoms of chronic overdosage (eg, malaise, nausea, headache) have occurred when 7 to 10 mg per week was taken continuously (Hokkanen et al, 1978). These effects may be followed by severe vasoconstriction and endarteritis. Gangrene of the extremities is rare when usual doses are given to patients who do not have peripheral vascular disease or other contraindicating disorders. If ergotamine-induced peripheral ischemia occurs, it may be relieved by infusion of sodium nitroprusside or administration of prazosin; the latter may be preferred because it can be given orally (Cobaugh, 1980). Sympathetic ganglionic blockade also has been reported to be effective (Robb, 1975).

Patients taking ergotamine daily for prolonged periods may become dependent on the drug. This may cause rebound vasoconstriction, vasodilation, and headache (Saper and Van Meter, 1980); therefore, ergotamine should be discontinued gradually.

Ergotamine is contraindicated in patients with peripheral vascular disease (eg, Raynaud's disease, thromboangiitis obliterans, thrombophlebitis, marked arteriosclerosis), severe hypertension, ischemic heart disease or anginal pain after exertion, peptic ulcer, renal or hepatic disease, malnutrition, or hypersensitivity to ergot preparations. It should not be used in the presence of infections. Since ergotamine has oxytocic properties, it should not be given to pregnant women (FDA Pregnancy Category X). Ergotamine preparations should be used cautiously in children; a product without ergotamine, eg, Midrin, may be preferred.

DRUG INTERACTIONS. The abortive use of ergotamine for breakthrough migraine headaches in patients receiving propranolol for prophylaxis is usually well tolerated. There is the potential, however, for this combination to cause excessive vasoconstriction. This interaction is probably rare, but one patient receiving propranolol with intermittent use of ergotamine/caffeine suppositories developed severe peripheral ischemia (Baumrucker, 1973).

PHARMACOKINETICS. Following oral administration of 2 mg, the serum concentration is less than 0.1 ng/ml after 10 minutes and up to two days after ingestion. Rectal administration produces low variable serum concentrations with a mean level of 0.16 ng/ml (Ibraheem et al, 1983). Estimates of bioavailability are 2% for the oral route and 5% for the rectal route (Ibraheem et al, 1983). Sublingual absorption of ergotamine also is poor (Tfelt-Hansen et al, 1982). The low bioavailability of oral ergotamine is the result of a significant first-pass effect in which 97% of the absorbed drug is degraded. Good therapeutic response has been correlated with serum concentrations of ergotamine and metabolites that reached 0.2 ng/ml or higher in less than one hour (Ala-Hurula, 1982).

Ergotamine is distributed rapidly to the tissues and is metabolized in the liver; metabolites are excreted primarily (90%) in bile, with only traces (3% to 4%) found in the urine. The plasma half-life is 96 ± 24 minutes (Orton and Richardson, 1982), but ergotamine and metabolites have a slow elimination half-life of 21 to 34 hours (Meier and Schreier, 1976), which may account for the prolonged therapeutic effect and toxicity (Rall and Schleifer, 1980).

DOSAGE AND PREPARATIONS.
Inhalation: Adults, a single inhalation (0.36 mg) at the onset of an attack, repeated if necessary at intervals of no less than five minutes to a total of six inhalations in 24 hours (maximum, 15 inhalations in one week). Patients should be monitored for compliance, and excessive use should be avoided. The risk of provoking bronchospasm in asthmatic patients should be kept in mind when ergotamine is administered by this route.
   Medihaler Ergotamine (Riker). Solution 9 mg/ml in 2.5 ml containers. Each dose (a single inhalation) contains approximately 0.36 mg of ergotamine tartrate.
Sublingual: Adults, 2 mg at the onset of an attack, followed by 2 mg every 30 minutes if necessary (maximum, 6 mg in 24 hours and 10 mg in one week).
   Ergomar (Fisons), **Ergostat** (Parke-Davis). Tablets 2 mg.
AVAILABLE MIXTURES. See Table.

DIHYDROERGOTAMINE MESYLATE
[D.H.E. 45]

ACTIONS AND USES. Dihydroergotamine, given intramuscularly or intravenously, is considered by some authorities to be the drug of choice for terminating a migraine or cluster headache attack in the emergency room or office setting. These routes are inconvenient if repeated self-administration is required. Intravenous dihydroergotamine has terminated status migrainosus and repeated intravenous administration terminated the cycles of attacks (Raskin and Raskin, 1984). Although the incidence of gastrointestinal reactions appears to be less than with parenteral administration of ergotamine tartrate (investigational), the vasoconstrictor effect of dihydroergotamine is less pronounced and a smaller percentage of patients respond to this agent.

For adverse reactions and precautions, see the evaluation on Ergotamine Tartrate.

PHARMACOKINETICS. Peak plasma concentrations are reached in 2 to 11 minutes. The drug is quickly eliminated from the plasma; the mean alpha phase half-life is 1.35 minutes and beta phase half-life is 23 minutes (Kanto, 1983).

DOSAGE AND PREPARATIONS.
Intramuscular: Adults, 1 mg at the onset of an attack, repeated if necessary at hourly intervals to a total of 3 mg. This route is preferred.
Intravenous: For rapid effect, *adults,* 1 mg, repeated if necessary once after one hour. The total dose should not exceed 2 mg.

   D.H.E. 45 (Sandoz). Solution 1 mg/ml in 1 ml containers.

METHYSERGIDE MALEATE
[Sansert]

MIXTURES

Preparation	Ingredients	Comment
Cafergot (Sandoz), Wigraine (Organon), Generic	Each tablet contains ergotamine tartrate 1 mg and caffeine 100 mg	Clinical experience and comparative trials indicate that caffeine increases the effectiveness of ergotamine, probably by increasing its enteral absorption (Schmidt and Fanchamps, 1974). (FDA Pregnancy Category X)
Cafergot (Sandoz), Wigraine (Organon)	Each suppository contains ergotamine tartrate 2 mg and caffeine 100 mg	
Cafergot P-B (Sandoz)	Each tablet contains ergotamine tartrate 1 mg, caffeine 100 mg, levorotatory belladonna alkaloids as malates 0.125 mg, and pentobarbital sodium 30 mg	Belladonna alkaloids are claimed to allay the nausea and vomiting caused by the migraine attack or by ergotamine. Barbiturate may be helpful, but the sedative preferably should be prescribed separately to allow more flexibility in adjusting the dose and to reduce abuse potential. (FDA Pregnancy Category X)
	Each suppository contains ergotamine tartrate 2 mg, caffeine 100 mg, levorotatory belladonna alkaloids as malates 0.25 mg, and pentobarbital 60 mg	
Bellergal (Dorsey)	Each tablet contains ergotamine tartrate 0.3 mg, phenobarbital 20 mg, levorotatory belladonna alkaloids as malates 0.1 mg	Bellergal is claimed to be useful in migraine prophylaxis when attacks occur frequently. This preparation is not useful for aborting acute attacks since the amount of ergotamine is insufficient. Most authorities believe that prolonged administration of an ergot preparation is not advisable, because peripheral vasoconstriction and ergot habituation may occur. Also, the potential abuse of the barbiturate component may compound the problems. (FDA Pregnancy Category X)
Bellergal-S (Dorsey)	Each timed-release tablet contains ergotamine tartrate 0.6 mg, phenobarbital 40 mg, and levorotatory belladonna alkaloids as malates 0.2 mg	
Axotal (Adria)	Each tablet contains butalbital 50 mg and aspirin 650 mg	These mixtures may be indicated to relieve muscle-contraction (tension) headache and may be helpful as analgesics in migraine headache. Fixed-dose combinations do not permit adjustment of dose to suit the needs of individual patients. It may be preferable to prescribe the sedative separately; however, butalbital is not available as a single-entity agent. If a sedative is required for muscle-contraction or migraine headache, an agent other than butalbital must be prescribed. Use in chronic muscle-contraction headache may lead to abuse.
Esgic (Gilbert)	Each tablet contains butalbital 50 mg, acetaminophen 325 mg, and caffeine 40 mg	
Fiorinal (Sandoz)	Each capsule or tablet contains butalbital 50 mg, aspirin 325 mg, and caffeine 40 mg	For adverse reactions and precautions, see Chapter 4, General Analgesics, and Chapter 7, Drugs Used for Anxiety and Sleep Disorders. (FDA Pregnancy Category D)
Micrainin (Wallace)	Each tablet contains aspirin 325 mg and meprobamate 200 mg	
Phrenilin, Phrenilin Forte (Carnrick)	Each tablet or capsule contains butalbital 50 mg and acetaminophen 325 mg or 650 mg (Forte capsule)	

Usual Dosage

Oral: Adults, two tablets at onset of migraine attack, then if needed, one additional tablet every 30 minutes. Total dose should not exceed six tablets/attack or ten/week.
Children, one-half tablet initially, then if needed, one-half tablet every 30 minutes (maximum, three tablets).

Rectal: Adults, appropriate tolerated dose should be determined for each patient between headache attacks (usually one-half suppository at the beginning of an attack, but some patients require only 0.25 to 0.5 mg). If necessary, dose is repeated after one hour. Total amount should not exceed two suppositories/attack or five suppositories/week.

Oral: Same as Cafergot (see above).

Rectal: Same as Cafergot (see above).

Oral: Adults, four plain tablets daily (one in the morning, one at noon, and two at bedtime) or two timed-release tablets daily (one in the morning and one in the evening).

Oral: Adults, one or two tablets or capsules every four hours maximum, six tablets or capsules daily. (Phrenilin Forte, one capsule every four to six hours with maximum of three capsules daily.) No dosage has been established for *children under 12 years*.

(continued on next page)

USES. This agent is a semisynthetic ergot alkaloid that is related chemically to the oxytocic agent, methylergonovine. It is not useful in aborting acute migraine headaches or in preventing or treating muscle-contraction headache. Methysergide is an effective prophylactic agent for migraine and episodic cluster headaches. However, since rare but serious fibrotic reactions occur with prolonged therapy, methysergide is reserved for the management of severe disabling migraine headaches that do not respond to other prophylactic agents, such as propranolol. Careful supervision is required and a four-week drug holiday must be instituted after four to six months of therapy to reduce the incidence of serious adverse reactions.

Although methysergide is claimed to be more beneficial in severe classic migraine, there is no evidence to indicate that it is more effective in preventing classic than common migraine (Selby, 1983).

Methysergide may be used as the initial drug in the prophylaxis of episodic cluster headache, since the duration of treatment is usually brief (2 to 10 weeks). Younger patients with episodic cluster may respond best to therapy (Mathew, 1984).

ACTIONS. The exact mechanism of action of this agent in preventing migraine has not been established definitely. Although methysergide potentiates the vasoconstrictor effects of catecholamines, it has only mild vasoconstrictor properties, which may explain its failure to abort acute migraine or a cluster attack. The drug is a potent peripheral serotonin antagonist and acts centrally as a serotonin agonist. One hypothesis suggests that migraine headache results from disruption of the serotonin/endorphin control of the pain suppressor system during an attack; disruption of nociceptive function results from decreased serotonin in the midbrain (Salmon et al, 1982). Methysergide may mimic the actions of serotonin centrally in regulating pain. Additional actions include inhibition of histamine release and stabilization of platelets against spontaneous release of serotonin.

ADVERSE REACTIONS. Adverse reactions occur with moderate frequency. Many are mild and disappear with continued use of methysergide, but serious reactions necessitate discontinuance of therapy.

Among the serious but uncommon adverse reactions are fibrotic changes in retroperitoneal, pleuropulmonary, and cardiac tissues that may occur with long-term, uninterrupted administration. Retroperitoneal fibrosis may obstruct the urinary tract. Early clinical manifestations are flank pain and dysuria; typical deviation and obstruction of one or both ureters may be demonstrated by intravenous pyelography. Vascular insufficiency of the lower limbs with pain, edema, muscular atrophy, and thrombophlebitis caused by involvement of the aorta, vena cava, and common iliac vessels also may occur.

Usual signs of pleuropulmonary fibrosis are dyspnea, chest pain, and pleural friction rubs or effusion. Murmurs and dyspnea are signs of fibrosis of the aortic valve, mitral valve, and root of the aorta.

MIXTURES continued

Preparation	Ingredients	Comment
Midrin (Carnrick)	Each capsule contains isometheptene mucate 65 mg, dichloralphenazone 100 mg, and acetaminophen 325 mg	Midrin appears to be more effective for abortive than preventive treatment and may be useful in patients who cannot tolerate ergotamine. The results of a few controlled studies indicate that the combination is no more effective than isometheptene, the active ingredient, which is not available alone; Midrin is more effective than placebo (Diamond, 1976). Isometheptene is claimed to act as a cerebral vasoconstrictor, and results of studies show that Midrin reduces regional cerebral blood flow in migraine patients (Yamamoto and Meyer, 1980). Results of studies comparing Midrin and ergotamine have been inconsistent. Adverse reactions include drowsiness, dizziness, feeling of weakness, and palpitations. This mixture should not be used in patients with hypertension, heart disease, or peripheral vascular disease.

Administration of methysergide should be discontinued if signs of retroperitoneal, pleuropulmonary, or cardiac fibrosis are noted. Partial and even complete regression of the process may occur after the drug is discontinued, but surgery may be necessary. Incompetent valves may require replacement.

Although methysergide has only weak vasoconstrictor properties, vascular insufficiency may occur. Angina-like pain has been precipitated or increased. Symptoms of peripheral vascular insufficiency include cold, numb, painful extremities with or without paresthesias and diminished or absent pulse. If these symptoms occur, the drug should be discontinued to prevent severe tissue ischemia.

Central nervous system reactions include insomnia, nervousness, euphoria, dizziness, ataxia, rapid speech, difficulty in thinking, feeling of depersonalization, nightmares, and hallucinations. Drowsiness, lethargy, loss of initiative, and mental depression also have been reported.

Gastrointestinal reactions (eg, nausea, vomiting, diarrhea, abdominal pain) are common during early therapy. Administration of methysergide to patients with peptic ulcer has caused pronounced elevations in gastric hydrochloric acid levels. Other adverse reactions include dermatitis, alopecia, peripheral and localized edema, weight gain, arthralgia, and myalgia. Neutropenia and eosinophilia have occurred rarely.

PRECAUTIONS. Patients should be seen frequently during therapy with methysergide, and they should be instructed to report symptoms such as chest pain, leg cramps, edema of ankles or hands, change in skin color, or paresthesias in the extremities. These symptoms can be evaluated by repeated examination of the blood supply to the extremities to avoid dangerous sequelae. However, retroperitoneal fibrosis can develop without symptoms or positive results from laboratory studies. Some authorities advocate periodic urograms, while others believe that the risk of repeated injections of contrast medium exceeds the risk of ureteral compression from short-term methysergide therapy and advocate instead a careful clinical follow-up.

Contraindications are the same as for ergotamine (see the evaluation). In addition, methysergide should not be used in patients with pulmonary disease, valvular heart disease, rheumatoid arthritis or other collagen diseases, and conditions that may progress to fibrosis.

Methysergide should not be used continuously for more than six months without imposing a reasonable drug-free period (three to four weeks). However, the dosage should be reduced gradually during the two to three weeks preceding discontinuation of the drug to avoid rebound headache.

DOSAGE AND PREPARATIONS.
Oral: Adults, for prophylaxis of migraine, initially, 2 mg with meals on the first day, increased by 2 mg on days two and three until 6 mg daily is administered.

For prophylaxis of cluster headache, initially, 2 mg daily with meals, increased gradually to 8 mg daily (Mathew, 1984).
Sansert (Sandoz). Tablets 2 mg.

BETA-BLOCKING AGENTS

Clinical trials have demonstrated the efficacy of propranolol in the prevention of migraine headache. Other studies have shown that atenolol, timolol, metoprolol, and nadolol are equally effective for prophylaxis (Stellar et al, 1984; Olsson et al, 1984; Forssman et al, 1983; Ryan et al, 1983). However, oxprenolol, pindolol, practolol, and alprenolol were ineffective, which suggests that beta blockade does not account for the activity of these drugs in migraine prophylaxis. All of the active drugs lack intrinsic sympathomimetic activity and antagonize beta$_1$ receptors. They are generally well tolerated.

The initial doses of metoprolol, timolol, and atenolol used investigationally are similar to those given for the treatment of hypertension (Olsson et al, 1984; Stellar et al, 1984; Forssman et al, 1983) (see Chapter 28, Antihypertensive Agents). The initial dose of nadolol was 80 mg daily increased gradually to 160 mg (Ryan et al, 1983).

Usual Dosage

Oral: Adults, two capsules at the onset of attack, followed by one capsule every hour until pain is relieved (maximum, five capsules in 12-hour period).

PROPRANOLOL HYDROCHLORIDE
[Inderal]

ACTIONS AND USES. Many authorities consider propranolol the preferred drug for the prophylaxis of migraine in patients in whom it is not contraindicated. Although only a very small number of patients become headache-free, over 60% experience a reduction in the frequency and severity of attacks. The efficacy of propranolol in the treatment of an acute attack has not been established and this drug does not prevent cluster headache.

The mechanism by which propranolol prevents migraine attacks is not understood. This nonselective beta blocker prevents cephalic arterial dilation; the rationale for use of this drug is based on the hypothesis that the pain of migraine results from dilation of extracranial arteries. However, clinical trials with beta-blocking drugs of variable selectivity indicate that beta blockade does not entirely account for their effect in migraine. Propranolol also prevents platelet aggregation and lipolysis induced by catecholamines. The latter action decreases prostaglandin synthesis, which may be important in preventing migraine (Diamond and Medina, 1980 A).

ADVERSE REACTIONS AND PRECAUTIONS. Propranolol is generally well tolerated. Nausea, lightheadedness, fatigue, insomnia, and diarrhea have been reported occasionally. Cold extremities are common, and arterial insufficiency has been reported rarely with concomitant use of propranolol and ergotamine. Mild mental dulling also occurs rarely. Heart rate and blood pressure are reduced. The heart rate should be monitored; in general, when full beta-blocking doses are used, the pulse rate is less than 60 beats per minute.

Propranolol should not be used in patients with asthma, chronic obstructive lung disease, congestive heart failure, or atrioventricular conduction disturbances.

For other adverse reactions and precautions, see Chapter 25, Antianginal Agents.

DOSAGE AND PREPARATIONS.
Oral: Since doses vary widely (160 to 240 mg daily), the dosage must be individualized. *Adults,* initially, usually 20 to 40 mg two or three times per day, increased gradually by 20 to 40 mg every third or fourth day until a therapeutic effect is observed or adverse reactions occur. *Children,* dosage must be individualized, but approximates 0.6 to 1.5 mg/kg/day (Lai et al, 1982). Once the maintenance dose has been achieved, the timed-release formulation, Inderal LA, may be considered for convenience and compliance.

If the drug must be discontinued, the dose should be reduced gradually over two weeks, for abrupt withdrawal may precipitate headache or angina pectoris in patients with pre-existing coronary disease.

Generic. Tablets 10, 20, 40, and 80 mg.
Inderal (Ayerst). Tablets 10, 20, 40, 60, 80, and 90 mg.
Inderal LA (Ayerst). Capsules (timed-release) 80, 120, and 160 mg.

CALCIUM CHANNEL BLOCKING AGENTS

Calcium antagonists are used in the treatment of cardiovascular disorders such as hypertension, dysrhythmias, Raynaud's disease, and vasospastic angina. Their inhibitory action on vascular smooth muscle contraction has been postulated to be the basis for their prophylactic activity against migraine headaches (Peroutka, 1983), but they may act at sites within the central nervous system. These drugs block the entrance of calcium through the membrane channels regardless of the triggering agent (eg, serotonin, norepinephrine, prostaglandins, ethanol, thrombin). Since intracerebral vessels appear to depend exclusively on extracellular calcium for contraction, calcium channel blocking drugs should inhibit the initial vasoconstriction that occurs during the first phase of the migraine attack.

Many calcium blockers are being investigated for use in migraine prophylaxis. Verapamil has been effective in patients who did not respond to ergotamine, propranolol, or amitriptyline (Holmes et al, 1984; Markley et al, 1984; Solomon et al, 1983). In controlled clinical trials, flunarizine appeared to be equally effective in common and classic migraine and was more effective in younger patients (Holmes et al, 1984; Peroutka, 1983). The frequency and severity of migraine attacks were decreased by over one-half in most patients studied; progressive improvement was noted over a three-month period (Diamond and Schenbaum, 1983; Frenken and Nuijten, 1984). Flunarizine has a half-life of 17 days and long-term safety has not been established. A closely related calcium antagonist, cinnarizine, also has prophylactic activity (Holmes et al, 1984), as do nimodipine and nifedipine; nimodipine has greater selectivity for cerebral vessels (Meyer and Hardenberg, 1983). The frequency of attacks decreased within one month after beginning use of nimodipine, compared to two months with flunarizine. Nimodipine also may be active in cluster headache.

Some established migraine prophylactic drugs also act by antagonizing calcium channel influx. Cyproheptadine has significant nonspecific calcium channel blocking activity at doses used for migraine prophylaxis (Peroutka, 1983). Experimentally, amitriptyline inhibits basilar artery contraction induced by serotonin and norepinephrine.

The initial results of clinical trials with these drugs indicate that they may become useful alternatives to established prophylactic agents, providing more flexibility in the management of migraine headache. Additional controlled clinical studies are necessary to determine their place in the prophylaxis of vascular headaches.

VERAPAMIL HYDROCHLORIDE
[Calan, Isoptin]

ACTIONS. Verapamil is postulated to be effective through its ability to inhibit intracerebral arterial vasoconstriction by inhibiting calcium influx into vascular smooth muscle. Verapamil also produces vasodilation, blocks platelet serotonin release, and inhibits platelet aggregation.

USES. This drug has prevented migraine headaches that failed to respond to other prophylactic agents (Markley et al, 1984). Results of a limited number of studies report that verapamil completely prevented headaches in a small number of patients with intractable headache and reduced the frequency and duration (but not the severity) of the attack in over one-half of those treated (Markley et al, 1984; Solomon et al, 1983).

Verapamil may be considered in patients refractory to propranolol, methysergide, or amitriptyline; in those who cannot tolerate these drugs; or when these agents are contraindicated.

ADVERSE REACTIONS AND PRECAUTIONS. The incidence of side effects is low compared to that with methysergide. The most common reactions were constipation, lightheadedness, transient hypotension, and headache (Markley et al, 1984; Solomon et al, 1983). (See the evaluation in Chapter 25, Antianginal Agents, for other adverse reactions.)

Verapamil should not be used in patients with congestive heart failure, hypotension, sick sinus syndrome, cardiac conduction disease, and renal or hepatic failure or in combination with beta blockers.

DOSAGE AND PREPARATIONS.
Oral: Adults, for migraine prophylaxis, 80 mg three or four times daily (Markley et al, 1984; Solomon et al, 1983).
    Calan (Searle), *Isoptin* (Knoll). Tablets 80 and 120 mg.
    (Investigational indication)

ANTIDEPRESSANTS

AMITRIPTYLINE HYDROCHLORIDE
[Elavil, Endep, SK-Amitriptyline]

ACTIONS AND USES. This tricyclic compound is useful in the prophylaxis of migraine. Results of one controlled study indicated that amitriptyline was most effective in nondepressed patients with severe migraine and depressed patients with less severe migraine (Couch and Hassanein, 1979). In some studies, amitriptyline was as effective as methysergide but, in others, the drug was no better than placebo (Diamond and Medina, 1980 A). Thus, patient selection appears to be important for optimum results.

Amitriptyline inhibits the reuptake of norepinephrine and serotonin at nerve endings, but its exact mechanism of action in migraine is not known. Its effect is relatively independent of antidepressant action.

This drug also is effective in patients with chronic muscle-contraction headache that has not responded to analgesic therapy, as well as in patients with mixed vascular and muscle-contraction headache.

ADVERSE REACTIONS AND PRECAUTIONS. The usual adverse effects are dryness of the mouth, blurred vision, constipation, urinary retention, and tachycardia. Amitriptyline should be used with caution in patients with angle-closure glaucoma, urinary retention or obstruction, and cardiac disease.

For other uses and a more complete discussion of adverse reactions and precautions, see Chapter 7, Drugs Used in Affective Disorders.

DOSAGE AND PREPARATIONS.
Oral: For migraine prophylaxis, *adults*, initially, 25 mg daily at bedtime, increased by 25 mg every one to two weeks to a daily dose of 100 to 200 mg, if necessary (Diamond and Medina, 1980 A). Tolerance may be improved by giving three or four doses daily rather than one bedtime dose.

For muscle-contraction headaches, initially, 50 to 75 mg at bedtime, increased every two to three weeks to 200 to 250 mg daily (Diamond, 1983). The drug can be discontinued after the patient has been headache-free for one or two months. If headaches recur, the course may be repeated.
    Elavil (Merck Sharp & Dohme), *Endep* (Roche), *SK-Amitriptyline* (Smith Kline & French), *Generic*. Tablets 10, 25, 50, 75, 100, and 150 mg.

LITHIUM CARBONATE
[Eskalith, Lithobid, Lithane, Lithonate]

ACTIONS AND USES. The mechanism of action of lithium carbonate in chronic cluster headache is unknown. The use of this agent for cluster headache was based on its effectiveness in another cyclical neurologic disorder, manic depressive psychosis. Few agents prevent chronic cluster headache, and lithium is considered the drug of choice by many headache specialists (Ekbom, 1981; Mathew, 1984). Patients have reported dramatic relief in the first week of treatment, but approximately 60% of initial responders experienced breakthrough attacks, which were claimed to be less severe and of short duration. Lithium may be effective in episodic cluster headache and some specialists use it when methysergide is not effective or contraindicated. The apparent effectiveness of lithium decreases with long-term administration but can be re-established by providing a two-week drug holiday before readministering the drug (Saper, 1983).

Patients receiving lithium must be closely monitored for side effects and toxicity with repeated measurement of lithium blood levels (see the evaluation in Chapter 7, Drugs Used in Affective Disorders).

DOSAGE AND PREPARATIONS.

Oral: Adults, 300 mg two to four times daily (Mathew, 1984). Timed-release tablets are usually given twice daily at approximately 12-hour intervals.

   Generic. Capsules, tablets 300 mg.
   Eskalith (Smith Kline & French). Capsules, tablets 300 mg; tablets (timed-release) 450 mg (*Eskalith CR*).
   Lithane (Miles), *Lithotabs* (Rowell). Tablets 300 mg.
   Lithobid (CIBA). Tablets (timed-release) 300 mg.
   Lithonate (Rowell). Capsules 300 mg.

Cited References

Ad Hoc Committee on Classification of Headache: Classification of headache. *JAMA* 179:717-718, 1962.

Ala-Hurula V: Correlation between pharmacokinetics and clinical effects of ergotamine in patients suffering from migraine. *Eur J Clin Pharmacol* 21:397-402, 1982.

Anderson CD, Franks RD: Migraine and tension headache: Is there a physiologic difference? *Headache* 21:63-71, 1981.

Bakal DA, Kaganov JA: Muscle contraction and migraine headache: Psychophysiologic comparison. *Headache* 17:208-215, 1977.

Baumrucker JF: Drug interaction: Propranolol and cafergot, (letter). *N Engl J Med* 288:916-917, 1973.

Blau JN: Migraine pathogenesis: Neural hypothesis reexamined. *J Neurol Neurosurg Psychiatry* 47:437-442, 1984.

Bradfield JM: New look at use of ergotamine. *Drugs* 12:449-453, 1976.

Cobaugh DS: Prazosin treatment of ergotamine-induced peripheral ischemia. *JAMA* 244:1360, 1980.

Cohen MJ, McArthur DL: Classification of migraine and tension headache from survey of 10,000 headache diaries. *Headache* 21:25-29, 1981.

Couch JR, Hassanein RS: Amitriptyline in migraine prophylaxis. *Arch Neurol* 36:695-699, 1979.

Dalessio DJ, et al: Conditioned adaptation-relaxation reflex in migraine therapy. *JAMA* 242:2102-2104, 1979.

Dexter JD, et al: Concomitant use of amitriptyline and propranolol in intractable headache, (abstract). *Headache* 20:157, 1980.

Diamond S: Treatment of migraine with isometheptene, acetaminophen, and dichloralphenazone combination: Double-blind, crossover trial. *Headache* 15:282-287, 1976.

Diamond S: Rational approach to diagnosing and treating headache. Part III: Therapy. *Fam Med Rep* 1:39-44, (Sept 26) 1983.

Diamond S, Medina JL: Current thoughts on migraine. *Headache* 20:208-212, 1980 A.

Diamond S, Medina JL: Newer drug therapies for headache. *Postgrad Med* 68:125-140, 1980 B.

Diamond S, Schenbaum H: Flunarizine, a calcium channel blocker, in prophylactic treatment of migraine. *Headache* 23:39-42, 1983.

Drummond PD, Lance JW: Thermographic changes in cluster headache. *Neurology* 34:1292-1298, 1984.

Ekbom K: Lithium for cluster headache: Review of literature and preliminary results of long-term treatment. *Headache* 21:132-139, 1981.

Featherstone HJ: Migraine and muscle contraction headaches: Continuum. *Headache* 25:194-198, 1985.

Forssman B, et al: Atenolol for migraine prophylaxis. *Headache* 23:188-190, 1983.

Fozard JR: Animal pharmacology of drugs used in treatment of migraine. *J Pharm Pharmacol* 27:297-321, 1975.

Frenken CWCM, Nuijten STM: Flunarizine, new preventive approach to migraine: Double-blind comparison with placebo. *Clin Neurol Neurosurg* 86:17-20, 1984.

Friedman AP: Muscle contraction headache. *Am Fam Physician* 20:109-113, (Nov) 1979.

Health and Public Policy Committee, American College of Physicians: Position paper: Biofeedback for headaches. *Ann Intern Med* 102:128-131, 1985.

Hokkanen E, et al: Toxic effects of ergotamine used for migraine. *Headache* 18:95-98, 1978.

Holmes B, et al: Flunarizine: Review of its pharmacodynamic and pharmacokinetic properties and therapeutic use. *Drugs* 27:6-44, 1984.

Ibraheem JJ, et al: Low bioavailability of ergotamine tartrate after oral and rectal administration in migraine sufferers. *Br J Clin Pharmacol* 16:695-699, 1983.

Joffe R, et al: Self-observation study of headache symptoms in children. *Headache* 23:20-25, 1983.

Kanto J: Clinical pharmacokinetics of ergotamine, dihydroergotamine, ergotoxine, bromocriptine, methysergide and lergotrile. *Int J Clin Pharmacol Ther Toxicol* 21:135-142, 1983.

Kudrow L: Cluster headache: Diagnosis and management. *Headache* 19:142-150, 1979.

Kudrow L: Response of cluster headache attacks to oxygen inhalation. *Headache* 21:1-4, 1981.

Kunkel RS: Pharmacologic management of migraine—1985. *Cleve Clin Q* 52:95-101, (Spring) 1985.

Lai C-W, et al: Hemiplegic migraine in childhood: Diagnostic and therapeutic aspects. *J Pediatr* 100:696-699, 1982.

Lance JW: Pathogenesis of migraine, in: *Mechanism and Management of Headache*, ed 4. Boston, Butterworth Scientific, 1982, 152-177.

Louis P, Spierings ELH: Comparison of flunarizine (Sibelium) and pizotifen (Sandomigran) in migraine treatment: Double-blind study. *Cephalalgia* 2:197-203, 1982.

Manzoni GC, et al: Lithium carbonate in cluster headache: Assessment of its short- and long-term therapeutic efficacy. *Cephalalgia* 3:109-114, 1983.

Markley HG, et al: Verapamil in prophylactic therapy of migraine. *Neurology* 34:973-976, 1984.

Martin MJ: Psychogenic factors in headache. *Med Clin North Am* 62:559-570, 1978.

Masel BE, et al: Platelet antagonists in migraine prophylaxis: Clinical trial using aspirin and dipyridamole. *Headache* 20:13-18, 1980.

Mathew NT: Prophylaxis of migraine and mixed headache: Randomized controlled study. *Headache* 21:105-109, 1981.

Mathew NT: Prophylactic pharmacotherapy of cluster headache, in: *Cluster Headache*. New York, Spectrum Publications, 1984, 97-109.

Mathew RJ, et al: Catecholamines and migraine: Evidence based on biofeedback induced changes. *Headache* 20:247-252, 1980.

Medina JL, Diamond S: Drug dependency in patients with chronic headaches. *Headache* 17:12-14, 1977.

Meier J, Schreier E: Human plasma levels of some anti-migraine drugs. *Headache* 16:96-104, 1976.

Meyer JS: Calcium channel blockers in prophylactic treatment of vascular headache, (editorial). *Ann Intern Med* 102:395-397, 1985.

Meyer JS, Hardenberg J: Clinical effectiveness of calcium entry blockers in prophylactic treatment of migraine and cluster headache. *Headache* 23:266-277, 1983.

Nuechterlein KH, Holroyd JC: Biofeedback in treatment of tension headache: Current status. *Arch Gen Psychiatry* 37:866-873, 1980.

Olsson JE, et al: Metoprolol and propranolol in migraine prophylaxis: Double-blind multicentre study. *Acta Neurol Scand* 70:160-168, 1984.

O'Neil BP, Mann JD: Aspirin prophylaxis in migraine. *Lancet* 2:1179-1181, 1978.

Orton DA, Richardson RJ: Ergotamine absorption and toxicity. *Postgrad Med J* 58:6-11, 1982.

Packard RC: What is psychogenic headache? *Headache* 16:20-23, 1976.

Pearce JMS: Migraine: Cerebral disorder. *Lancet* 2:86-89, 1984.

Peroutka SJ: Pharmacology of calcium channel antagonists: Novel class of anti-migraine agents? *Headache* 23:273-283, 1983.

Rall TW, Schleifer LS: Oxytocin, prostaglandins, ergot alkaloids and other agents, in Gilman AG, et al (eds): *The Pharmacological Basis of Therapeutics*, ed 6. New York, Macmillan, 1980, 935-950.

Raskin NH, Appenzeller O: *Headache*. Philadelphia, WB Saunders, 1980.

Raskin NH, Raskin KE: Repetitive intravenous dihydroergotamine for treatment of intractable migraine, (abstract). *Neurology* 34:245, 1984.

Robb LG: Severe vasospasm following ergot administration. *West J Med* 123:231-235, 1975.

Ryan RE Sr, et al: Nadolol: Its use in prophylactic treatment of migraine. *Headache* 23:26-31, 1983.

Salmon S, et al: Putative S-HT central feedback in migraine and cluster headache attacks. *Adv Neurol* 33:265-274, 1982.

Saper JR (ed): *Headache Disorders: Current Concepts and Treatment Strategies*. Boston, John Wright, 1983.

Saper JR, Van Meter MJ: Ergotamine habituation: Analysis and profile. *Headache* 20:159, 1980.

Schmidt R, Fanchamps A: Effect of caffeine on intestinal absorption of ergotamine in man. *Eur J Clin Pharmacol* 7:213-216, 1974.

Selby G: Treatment, in: *Migraine and Its Variants*. Boston, ADIS Health Science Press, 1983, 107-149.

Solomon GD, et al: Verapamil prophylaxis of migraine: Double-blind, placebo-controlled study. *JAMA* 250:2500-2502, 1983.

Speed WG III: Cluster Rx: Variety of options. *Mod Med* 69-73, (Feb) 1985.

Steiner TJ, Joseph R: Practical experience of beta-blockade in migraine: Personal view. *Postgrad Med J* 60(suppl 2):56-60, 1984.

Stellar S, et al: Migraine prevention with timolol: Double-blind crossover study. *JAMA* 252:2576-2580, 1984.

Tfelt-Hansen P, et al: Double blind study of metoclopramide in treatment of migraine attacks. *J Neurol Neurosurg Psychiatry* 43:369-371, 1980.

Tfelt-Hansen P, et al: Bioavailability of sublingual ergotamine. *Br J Clin Pharmacol* 13:239-240, 1982.

Turner P: Beta-blocking drugs in migraine. *Postgrad Med J* 60(suppl 2):51-55, 1984.

Waters WE: Epidemiological enigma of migraine. *Int J Epidemiol* 2:189-194, 1973.

Waters WE, O'Connor TJ: Prevalence of migraine. *J Neurol Neurosurg Psychiatry* 30:613, 1975.

Weatherhead AD: Psychogenic headache. *Headache* 20:47-54, 1980.

Yamamota M, Meyer JS: Hemicranial disorders of vasomotor adrenoreceptors in migraine and cluster headache. *Headache* 20:321-335, 1980.

Ziegler DK: Tension headache. *Med Clin North Am* 62:495-505, 1978.

Ziegler DK: Headache symptom: How many entities? *Arch Neurol* 42:273-274, 1985.

Ziegler DK, Ellis DJ: Naproxen in prophylaxis of migraine. *Arch Neurol* 42:582-584, 1985.

Other Selected References

Critchley M, et al (eds): Headache: Physiopathological and clinical concepts, in: *Advances in Neurology*. New York, Raven Press, 1982, vol 33.

Dalessio DJ (ed): *Wolff's Headache and Other Head Pain*, ed 4. New York, Oxford University Press, 1980.

Diamond S, Dalessio DJ (eds): *The Practicing Physician's Approach to Headache*, ed 2. Baltimore, Williams & Wilkins, 1978.

Lance JW: *Mechanism and Management of Headache*, ed 4. London-Boston, Butterworths, 1982.

Ryan RE Sr, Ryan RE Jr (eds): *Headache and Head Pain: Diagnosis and Treatment*. St Louis, CV Mosby, 1978.

Drugs Used in Vertigo and Vomiting

Vertigo, nausea, and vomiting are only indications of altered function; they are not diseases. Rational therapy depends upon diagnosis of the underlying disorder and may or may not include drugs (Barbezat, 1981).

The drugs discussed in this chapter are effective in combating vertigo or the nausea and vomiting associated with motion sickness, pregnancy, the postoperative period, toxins (metabolic toxins [eg, uremia, hypercalcemia], microbial toxins), radiation therapy, and cancer chemotherapy drugs. Nausea and vomiting induced by other drugs (eg, opiates, digitalis, estrogens, aminophylline, levodopa, iron preparations) are obviated by reducing the dose, changing the preparation, altering the route or time of administration, or substituting another drug. Although reducing the dosage of an opiate alleviates drug-induced nausea and vomiting, use of an antiemetic may be preferred.

Nausea and vomiting related to pathology of the abdominal organs, increased intraluminal pressure in the intestine, food allergies, hypo- or hyperglycemia, increased intracranial pressure, and of psychogenic origin or vertigo related to central nervous system tumor, infection, multiple sclerosis, migraine, vascular insufficiency, diabetes, hypothyroidism, or orthostatic hypotension are reduced by correcting the underlying disorder.

The pharmacodynamic classification (see the Table) of drugs used to prevent and treat vertigo and vomiting is of more value in defining anticipated side effects than efficacy. Useful drugs include (1) the anticholinergic agent, scopolamine, which appears to act by reducing the excitability of labyrinth receptors, thus depressing conduction in vestibular cerebellar pathways or preventing recruitment of impulses at the chemoreceptor trigger zone; (2) H_1 antihistamines (buclizine [Bucladin-S], cyclizine [Marezine], dimenhydrinate [Dramamine], diphenhydramine [Benadryl], hydroxyzine [Atarax, Orgatrax, Vistaril], meclizine [Antivert, Bonine], promethazine [Phenergan]), which are assumed to affect neural pathways originating in the labyrinth (many of these agents also have anticholinergic activity that may contribute to their effectiveness in motion sickness); and (3) antidopaminergic drugs, which include metoclopramide [Reglan], domperidone [Motilium] (investigational), many phenothiazines, and the butyrophenones, droperidol [Inapsine] and haloperidol [Haldol]; these drugs act primarily upon the chemoreceptor trigger zone and, to a lesser degree, by inhibiting peripheral autonomic afferent impulses to the vomiting center via the vagus nerve. In addition to their antidopaminergic activity at the chemoreceptor trigger zone, metoclopramide and domperidone also appear to act by stimulating upper gastrointestinal motility (but not secretion), which enhances gastric emptying. Both increase lower esophageal sphincter pressure. The incidence of extrapyramidal side effects is lower with domperidone, and this drug may be particularly useful in children to lessen nausea and vomiting caused by gastroenteritis or cancer chemotherapy.

AVAILABLE PREPARATIONS AND PRINCIPAL USES
OF ANTIVERTIGO AND ANTIEMETIC DRUGS

Drug Classification	Available Preparations		
	Parenteral	Suppository	Oral
ANTICHOLINERGIC			
Scopolamine Hydrobromide	×		×
Scopolamine [Transderm-Scop]	× (dermal)		
ANTIHISTAMINIC			
Buclizine Hydrochloride [Bucladin-S]			×
Cyclizine Hydrochloride [Marezine]			×
Cyclizine Lactate [Marezine]	×		
Dimenhydrinate [Dramamine]	×		×
Diphenhydramine Hydrochloride [Benadryl]	×		×
Hydroxyzine Hydrochloride [Atarax, Orgatrax, Vistaril]	×		×
Hydroxyzine Pamoate [Vistaril]			×
Meclizine Hydrochloride [Antivert, Bonine]			×
Promethazine Hydrochloride [Phenergan]	×	×	×
ANTIDOPAMINERGIC			
Aliphatic Phenothiazines			
Chlorpromazine [Thorazine]		×	
Chlorpromazine Hydrochloride [Thorazine]	×		×
Promazine Hydrochloride [Sparine]	×		×
Triflupromazine Hydrochloride [Vesprin]	×		
Piperazine Phenothiazines			
Fluphenazine Hydrochloride [Permitil, Prolixin]	×		×
Perphenazine [Trilafon]	×		×
Prochlorperazine [Compazine]		×	
Prochlorperazine Edisylate [Compazine]	×		×
Prochlorperazine Maleate [Compazine]			×
Thiethylperazine Malate [Torecan]	×		
Thiethylperazine Maleate [Torecan]		×	×
Butyrophenones			
Droperidol [Inapsine]	×		
Haloperidol [Haldol]			×
Haloperidol Lactate [Haldol]	×		×
Miscellaneous Antidopaminergic Agents			
Domperidone[3] [Motilium]	(×)	(×)	(×)
Metoclopramide [Reglan]	×	(×)	×
MISCELLANEOUS			
Benzquinamide Hydrochloride [Emete-Con]	×		
Diphenidol Hydrochloride [Vontrol]			×

| | | Principal Uses | | | |
Vertigo	Motion Sickness	Pregnancy[1]	Postoperative Emesis	Cancer Chemotherapy	Toxins[2] Radiation Therapy
	++		+		
+	++				
±	+				
+	+	+	++		
+	+	+	++		
++	++	+			
+	+	+		+	
±	+		+		
±	+				
++	+	+			+
+	++	+	+	+	+
				+	±
				+	±
			+		±
			+	±	±
			+	±	+
			+	±	+
			+	+	+
			++	+	++
+			++	+	
			++		+
			++	+	+
			(+)	(+)	(++)
			(+)	++	(+)
			+	+	
+			+	+	+

(continued on next page)

AVAILABLE PREPARATIONS AND PRINCIPAL USES
OF ANTIVERTIGO AND ANTIEMETIC DRUGS (continued)

Drug Classification	Available Preparations		
	Parenteral	Suppository	Oral
Trimethobenzamide Hydrochloride [Tigan]	×	×	×
Benzodiazepines Diazepam [Valium, Valrelease]	×		×
Lorazepam [Ativan]	×		
Cannabinoids Dronabinol (delta-9-tetrahydrocannabinol) [Marinol]			×
Nabilone [Cesamet]			×
Corticosteroids Dexamethasone[3] [Decadron]	×		×
Methylprednisolone[3] [Solu-Medrol]	×		

[1] *Antiemetics generally are not recommended during pregnancy (see text).*
[2] *Toxins include metabolic toxins (eg, uremia, hypercalcemia) and other exogenous toxins (eg, microbial, chemicals).*

Phenothiazines used most commonly for their antiemetic effect include those in the aliphatic group (chlorpromazine [Thorazine], promazine [Sparine], and triflupromazine [Vesprin]) and the piperazine group (fluphenazine [Permitil, Prolixin], perphenazine [Trilafon], prochlorperazine [Compazine], and thiethylperazine [Torecan]). The piperidine phenothiazines (eg, thioridazine [Mellaril]) are *not* effective antiemetics. Although promethazine is an aliphatic phenothiazine, it is used as an antihistamine because it has only weak dopamine antagonist activity, possesses considerable antihistaminic activity, and, unlike other phenothiazines but like antihistamines, is effective in vertigo and motion sickness.

Three miscellaneous agents, diphenidol [Vontrol], trimethobenzamide [Tigan], and benzquinamide [Emete-Con], also are used as antiemetics. Diphenidol is thought to act upon the aural vestibular apparatus and the latter two drugs primarily upon the chemoreceptor trigger zone.

Clinical studies have demonstrated that dronabinol (delta-9-tetrahydrocannabinol) [Marinol], the active ingredient of marijuana, and nabilone [Cesamet] are useful in controlling vomiting caused by cancer chemotherapy (Carey et al, 1983; Laszlo, 1983). Their antiemetic action is not related to an antidopaminergic mechanism (Shannon et al, 1978). Other agents useful in chemotherapy-induced nausea and vomiting are corticosteroids (eg, dexamethasone) and benzodiazepines (eg, lorazepam [Ativan]) (Bowcock et al, 1984; Markman et al, 1984).

VERTIGO

True (objective) vertigo is associated with a hallucination of movement (commonly, but not exclusively, rotational). It can be produced by any lesion or process affecting the brain, the eighth cranial nerve, or the labyrinthine system. Common causes of chronic episodic or unremitting true vertigo include cerebral ischemia or atrophy, vestibular or labyrinthine neuronitis, benign positional vertigo, and Meniere's disease. It also may be associated with migraine headache or hearing loss. Nausea and vomiting are not always present, although they are more likely to be associated with true rather than subjective vertigo. The diagnosis (Turner, 1975) and management (Jackson et al, 1980) of true vertigo, including selection of appropriate drug therapy if indicated, depend upon the etiology, rapidity of onset, and character (episodic or unremitting) of the disorder.

The dizziness of *subjective vertigo* is characterized mainly by the presyncopal feeling of lightheadedness, fainting, or altered consciousness, sometimes associated with a vague sensation of motion described as being within the head. Subjective vertigo may be associated with disorders that result in inadequate blood supply to the cochlea and/or vestibular apparatus (eg, severe anemia, heart block, hypersensitive carotid sinus syndrome, sick sinus syndrome, transient ischemic attack, stroke, trauma). The latter three disorders also may cause true vertigo, depending upon the location of the impairment. In addition, subjective vertigo may be associated with psychiatric disturbances, especially when hyperventilation is present.

Drug-induced vertigo occurs most frequently after use of agents that damage the eighth nerve (eg, aminoglycoside antibiotics, ethacrynic acid [Edecrin], furosemide [Lasix]) or produce orthostatic hypotension (eg, antihypertensive agents, phenothiazines).

Drug Selection: Side effects markedly limit the use of scopolamine in vertigo, especially the chronic types. The antihistaminic drugs (dimenhydrinate, meclizine, and promethazine) are often beneficial in *true (objective) vertigo.* Diazepam [Valium] may suppress vestibular responses and reduce the anxiety that may accompany vertigo, but its

| | | | Principal Uses | | |
Vertigo	Motion Sickness	Pregnancy[1]	Postoperative Emesis	Cancer Chemotherapy	Toxins[2] Radiation Therapy
			+		+
+	±				
				(+)	
				+	
				+	
				(++)	+
				(++)	(+)

[3]*Investigational drug or indication*
+ = *relative effectiveness based on available data*

effectiveness is not dependent upon its sedative action. Although these drugs are generally satisfactory, severe vomiting associated with vertigo may require the use of antidopaminergic agents or diphenidol. Use of diphenidol generally is limited to hospitalized patients or closely supervised outpatients, because of the potential severity of its adverse effects.

If vertigo is severe enough to produce intolerable anxiety or severe depression, patients may benefit from the use of antianxiety agents or antidepressants (see Chapters 5 and 7, respectively).

In *Meniere's disease,* an attempt is made to suppress the vestibular symptoms and to modify the underlying pathologic feature of endolymphatic hydrops. The therapeutic efficacy of drugs used to manage vertigo associated with this disorder is difficult to evaluate because spontaneous remission occurs in 60% of patients (Brookes, 1983).

Oral diazepam controls symptoms in 60% to 70% of patients. In refractory cases, meclizine 25 to 100 mg orally, dimenhydrinate 50 mg orally or intramuscularly, scopolamine 0.6 mg orally or subcutaneously, droperidol 5 mg intravenously, or diazepam 5 to 20 mg *slowly* intravenously may be required. Prochlorperazine 5 to 10 mg orally and cinnarizine 15 to 30 mg orally every eight hours also were reported to be effective in vertigo resulting from Meniere's disease (Brookes, 1983). Dehydration and electrolyte imbalance caused by emesis should be corrected. Diuretics and salt restriction, in conjunction with diazepam or other antiemetics, are generally employed in the management of Meniere's disease, but evidence is not sufficiently definitive to support their efficacy.

The use of papaverine, histamine, betahistine, nylidrin, and other vasodilators to improve blood flow to the labyrinth and brainstem has produced some short-term improvement in patients with vertigo, tinnitus, and deafness, but their role in the symptomatic treatment and to arrest progression of Meniere's disease has not been defined.

Antivertigo drugs usually play less of a role in the treatment of *subjective vertigo* than management of the underlying disorder. In drug-induced vertigo, withdrawing the offending drug or reducing the dose is preferred to administering labyrinthine suppressants.

VOMITING

Emesis is a complex reflex that is coordinated by the vomiting center in the medulla. Stimuli are relayed to this center from peripheral areas (eg, gastric mucosa, peritoneum). Major sensory stimuli also arise within the central nervous system itself (ie, cerebral cortex, otic vestibular apparatus) and may be transmitted through the chemoreceptor trigger zone sensory nucleus (CTZ) in the medulla to the vomiting center. The vomiting center frequently is stimulated directly. The efferent arc is completed by excitatory impulses transmitted to the salivary glands and the muscles of the diaphragm, anterior abdominal wall, gastric antrum, and duodenum. Inhibitory impulses to the muscles of the gastric fundus, gastroesophageal sphincter, and esophagus arrive simultaneously.

Nausea and vomiting may be symptoms of serious organic disturbances of almost any of the viscera of the chest or abdomen or may be produced by infections, drugs, radiation, painful or noxious stimuli, metabolic and emotional disturbances, exposure to unfamiliar environmental forces, audiovisual-proprioceptive sensory mismatch phenomena (eg, air or ship travel, amusement park rides, prolonged car or train travel, exposure to large centrifugal forces), or vertigo. Whenever possible, the underlying cause should be corrected. The use of antiemetics is justified only when no alternative therapy exists and the benefits outweigh the risks of adverse reactions or of masking more serious underlying conditions.

In general, drug therapy is more effective for prophylaxis

than for treatment of vomiting, especially that caused by motion sickness, radiation, or chemotherapy. Oral dosage forms are most useful for prophylaxis; suppository and parenteral forms are preferred for treatment.

Vomiting Associated with Gastroenteritis: Because of the self-limited nausea and vomiting associated with acute gastroenteritis, antiemetics may be required only when intravenous hydration and nutrition, electrolyte replenishment, rest, and fasting do not improve the patient's condition.

Vomiting Associated with Motion Sickness: Motion sickness includes sea, air, car, and space sickness. The principal subjective components of the motion sickness syndrome are nausea, vomiting, pallor, and cold sweating, which occur on exposure to certain types of real or apparent motion. Tolerance develops in two or three days if the intensity of the stimulus does not increase. The prophylactic use of drugs (usually one to two hours before travel) is more effective than treatment.

An adhesive unit containing scopolamine [Transderm-Scōp] for placement behind the ear delivers a sufficient dose at a constant rate transdermally to prevent motion sickness in most patients. Transdermal delivery of scopolamine decreases the incidence of most side effects (primarily drowsiness, dryness of the mouth, and blurred vision) observed with oral and parenteral scopolamine and prolongs effectiveness for several days (Price et al, 1979). Although oral or parenteral scopolamine may be more effective than transdermal delivery, the use of these routes is limited because of the higher incidence of untoward effects. The oral or parenteral form of scopolamine may be especially useful for severe motion sickness of brief duration when only a few small doses are required. Repeated doses may have a cumulative effect.

The antihistamines are less effective than oral or parenteral scopolamine but produce fewer adverse effects. Buclizine, cyclizine, dimenhydrinate, meclizine, diphenhydramine, and hydroxyzine prevent mild to moderate motion sickness. Controlled studies comparing transdermal scopolamine to dimenhydrinate found them to be about equally effective, but neither was as effective as oral or parenteral scopolamine. Cinnarizine (not available in United States) has been reported to reduce vomiting in children known to be susceptible to car sickness (Macnair, 1983). The duration of action of antihistamines ranges from four to six hours; the action of meclizine is claimed to persist for 24 hours.

Promethazine is the most effective antihistamine for the prophylaxis of moderate to severe motion sickness and also is usually beneficial in the treatment of vomiting associated with this disorder. However, the considerable sedative action of promethazine and the other antihistamines, which may contribute to their effectiveness, may limit their use. Promethazine is especially useful when combined with ephedrine. A more potent phenothiazine may be required for intractable vomiting but phenothiazines are ineffective in the prophylaxis of motion sickness.

Vomiting During Pregnancy: Drugs should not be used to treat vomiting during pregnancy unless absolutely necessary. Although morning sickness may occur in 50% to 80% of pregnant patients during the sixth to fourteenth weeks of gestation, a very small percentage experience nausea and vomiting of sufficient severity to necessitate antiemetic drug therapy. Nondrug therapy (eg, alteration of diet and time of eating, rest) should always be tried before antiemetics are prescribed. Emetrol (a mixture of fructose, dextrose, and orthophosphoric acid) and cola syrup frequently are employed for morning sickness. However, cola syrup contains caffeine and its use during pregnancy is discouraged by the Food and Drug Administration. If a more potent antiemetic action is necessary, cyclizine or meclizine may be used initially. If persistent vomiting compromises maternal nutrition, promethazine or an antidopaminergic drug (see the Table) may be considered.

Postoperative Vomiting: Postoperative vomiting has many causes and thus may be particularly difficult to prevent. The *routine* postoperative use of antiemetics is unwarranted because less than 3% of individuals require such therapy. Their administration to prevent postoperative vomiting is indicated only in a few clinical situations: when vomiting would endanger the results of surgery (eg, intraocular, ear, or oral surgery [when the jaws have been wired together]), in debilitated patients at risk of dehydration or electrolyte imbalance, or when labyrinthine activity is increased, which occurs during almost all ear surgery.

Drugs useful for the treatment of postoperative vomiting are prochlorperazine, perphenazine, cyclizine, benzquinamide, haloperidol, and droperidol. In a study comparing intramuscular antiemetics, haloperidol 2 mg, droperidol 5 mg, and prochlorperazine 10 mg all provided significant antiemetic activity but differed in onset and duration of action. Haloperidol became effective in 0 to 30 minutes and the duration of activity was four hours, prochlorperazine became effective in 30 minutes and had a duration of four hours, and droperidol reached peak effectiveness in three to four hours and the antiemetic effect lasted 24 hours (Loeser et al, 1979).

Although droperidol is very effective, it probably should be reserved for preoperative prophylaxis because of the disturbing mental effects that sometimes occur during the recovery period when doses greater than 5 mg are used. Droperidol's longer duration of action and low incidence of adverse reactions compared to other antidopaminergic agents make it the agent of choice in certain cases (Palazzo and Strunin, 1984). Droperidol, promethazine, prochlorperazine, or benzquinamide usually is administered in patients having ear surgery. Some physicians use promethazine or hydroxyzine for premedication in patients with a history of nausea and vomiting after general anesthesia.

Vomiting Due to Cancer Chemotherapy: Nausea and vomiting are major adverse reactions in patients receiving cancer chemotherapy. The use of antiemetics is indicated to prevent medical complications (esophageal tearing [Mallory-Weiss syndrome], anorexia, malnutrition, dehydration), to alleviate patient discomfort, to prevent anticipatory nausea and vomiting, and to improve compliance with therapy. The effective management of vomiting induced by antineoplastic agents also should consider the patient's physiologic condition (eg, maintenance of hydration), provide emotional support and, possibly, employ behavioral relaxation techniques, especially for anticipatory nausea and vomiting (Stoudemire et al, 1984).

The primary agents for the management of nausea and vomiting are high-dose metoclopramide (intravenous), dexamethasone, phenothiazines (prochlorperazine), droperidol, lorazepam, and dronabinol. The mechanism(s) by which antineoplastic agents induce nausea and vomiting is not well understood. The emetic action of these agents is diffuse and is characterized by some degree of delayed (1 to 12 hours) onset of vomiting (with the exception of mechlorethamine) and multiphasic time courses (Borison and McCarthy, 1983). Delayed vomiting suggests that drug metabolites or cellular material released as a result of tissue toxicity may be partly responsible.

The complex nature of the sensory and stimulatory input underlying chemotherapy-induced nausea and vomiting may explain why single-agent antiemetic therapy is usually not completely effective. Combinations of antiemetics that simultaneously block cholinergic (scopolamine, promethazine), histaminergic H_1 (promethazine, other antihistamines), or dopaminergic D_2 (phenothiazines, butyrophenones) receptors have been suggested (Peroutka and Snyder, 1982). Such combinations are being studied and may prove to be useful.

The effectiveness of antiemetic therapy, for the most part, depends on the emetic potential of the antineoplastic agent and dose; the most effective anticancer agents, cisplatin [Platinol] and doxorubicin [Adriamycin], are the most potent emetics. The comparative efficacy of antiemetics used to relieve the nausea and vomiting associated with different chemotherapeutic agents has been reviewed (Laszlo, 1983).

Many authorities prefer to use repeated courses of intravenous metoclopramide (1 to 3 mg/kg) in combination with other antiemetics to prevent acute nausea and vomiting induced by cisplatin alone, cisplatin in combination with other drugs (Gralla, 1983; Strum et al, 1982; Eyre and Ward, 1984; Kris et al, 1985), and moderate to highly emetic regimens not containing cisplatin (Strum et al, 1984; Fortner et al, 1985; Strum et al, 1985). Controlled clinical trials have demonstrated that a large intravenous dose of metoclopramide alone provides significant antiemetic activity in patients receiving cisplatin 35 to 120 mg/M² (Gralla et al, 1984; Strum et al, 1982). Approximately one-third to one-half of treated patients may be protected completely from emesis. Although nausea and vomiting are substantially reduced in many of the remaining patients, a significant portion continue to experience unacceptable emesis.

The response may be improved by the concurrent administration of intravenous dexamethasone. In controlled trials, complete protection has been demonstrated in 66% to 81% of patients and most patients preferred this combination to metoclopramide alone (Kris et al, 1985; Strum et al, 1985). Diphenhydramine often is added to this antiemetic regimen to prevent metoclopramide-induced extrapyramidal reactions. Lorazepam also is regarded by a number of oncologists (and by more than 90% of treated patients) as a useful adjunct to the above agents (*Oncology Times*, 1985). This drug produces antegrade amnesia that lasts for four to six hours and this action apparently is the basis for patient acceptance. Lorazepam may be particularly useful in patients not receiving

complete antiemetic protection with high-dose metoclopramide, dexamethasone, and diphenhydramine.

Intravenous butyrophenones (haloperidol and droperidol) are less effective than metoclopramide for acute cisplatin-induced nausea and vomiting but can provide complete protection in some patients (30% with haloperidol) (Neidhart et al, 1981; Wilson et al, 1981; Citron et al, 1984). There is less experience with intravenous butyrophenone/dexamethasone combinations than with metoclopramide/dexamethasone regimens. Dronabinol has some activity against cisplatin-induced emesis but is less effective than high-dose metoclopramide.

Late-onset nausea and vomiting (appearing after 24 hours and lasting one week) are common with cisplatin chemotherapy. Antiemetics are used orally for prophylaxis. Combinations of metoclopramide/dexamethasone and prochlorperazine/dexamethasone have provided a high degree of protection in a limited number of patients (Strum et al, 1985).

For more immediate (2 to 12 hours) nausea and vomiting induced by mildly emetic agents, phenothiazines, butyrophenones, dronabinol, nabilone, and dexamethasone have been useful preventive agents. Phenothiazines (prochlorperazine, thiethylperazine) are most commonly used, but few patients prefer them to other effective agents (Markman et al, 1984) with the exception of dronabinol in the elderly (Wampler, 1983). Dronabinol and nabilone were shown to be as effective and possibly superior to prochlorperazine in a number of controlled studies. The antiemetic action of dronabinol closely parallels its psychoactive effects and, for this reason, it usually is reserved for patients refractory to phenothiazines (Vincent et al, 1983). Droperidol and nabilone are alternatives in patients who do not respond to phenothiazines. Combinations of dronabinol and a phenothiazine may be effective and allow use of smaller doses of both agents, but more studies are needed to demonstrate an additive effect. Intravenous dexamethasone followed by oral administration is more effective than prochlorperazine; more than two-thirds of patients were completely protected from nausea and vomiting (Markman et al, 1984).

In clinical trials, the antiemetic activity of the antihistamines, cyclizine and cinnarizine, was inadequate (Morran et al, 1979; Moertel et al, 1963). Although promazine, meclizine, and dimenhydrinate have not been thoroughly studied, most oncologists consider them ineffective regardless of the emetic potential of the chemotherapy. Some authorities believe diphenhydramine enhances the antiemetic effect of high-dose metoclopramide/dexamethasone, in addition to reducing the incidence of extrapyramidal reactions. Domperidone is under investigation for nausea and vomiting induced by a variety of chemotherapeutic combinations, including those containing cisplatin (Brogden et al, 1982).

Adverse Reactions and Precautions

Caution is required with use of all antiemetics because they may mask the symptoms of organic disease (eg, gastrointestinal or central nervous system disorders) or the toxic effects of other drugs. The drowsiness commonly produced by these drugs may account for some of the antiemetic action. Individuals whose activities require alertness, such as those operating vehicles or machinery, should not use antiemetics. The actions of other central nervous system depressants may be potentiated.

Anticholinergic and Antihistaminic Drugs: Drowsiness is the most common untoward effect; anticholinergic side effects also may be anticipated, even with the antihistamines. Promethazine [Phenergan, Remsed] is relatively free of the extrapyramidal reactions observed with the phenothiazines and the butyrophenone, haloperidol [Haldol].

Buclizine [Bucladin-S], cyclizine [Marezine], hydroxyzine [Orgatrax, Vistaril], and meclizine [Antivert, Bonine] are teratogenic in animals when given in very large doses. However, large drug surveillance programs have not demonstrated that birth defects occur in the dosage ranges employed clinically. After review of the existing epidemiologic data on pregnant women, the Food and Drug Administration concluded that these data do not support a restriction on the use of meclizine or cyclizine or a pregnancy warning (*Federal Register,* 1979). (See the discussion on adverse reactions during pregnancy in Chapter 3.)

Antidopaminergic Drugs: Phenothiazines in the piperazine group (fluphenazine [Prolixin], perphenazine [Trilafon], prochlorperazine [Compazine], and thiethylperazine [Torecan]) are less likely to cause drowsiness, orthostatic hypotension, dryness of the mouth, and nasal congestion than those in the aliphatic group (chlorpromazine [Thorazine], promazine [Sparine], and triflupromazine [Vesprin]). Cholestatic jaundice, granulocytopenia, urticaria, dermatitis, thrombocytopenia, leukopenia, agranulocytosis, purpura, pancytopenia, and gastroenteritis have occurred after use of all phenothiazines. Less common reactions include galactorrhea, photosensitivity, and edema of the extremities. The incidence of these reactions is quite low when phenothiazines are used as antiemetics, since the duration of administration is short and the dosage relatively small.

Extrapyramidal reactions, including akathisia, dystonia, parkinsonian syndrome, and dysarthria, have been associated with use of all phenothiazines, haloperidol, and metoclopramide, and they may occur after a single dose. The incidence of these reactions is higher with phenothiazines in the piperazine group than with those in the aliphatic group. Diphenhydramine rapidly reverses these reactions (see the evaluation).

The extrapyramidal symptoms and signs that may be produced, particularly after parenteral administration of large doses, may be confused with the central nervous system signs of an undiagnosed primary disease responsible for the vomiting (eg, Reye's syndrome, other encephalopathy). Thus, use of these drugs and other hepatotoxic agents should be avoided in children and adolescents with signs and symptoms suggesting Reye's syndrome.

Phenothiazines are contraindicated in patients with a history of hypersensitivity to any phenothiazine. Although they are usually contraindicated in patients with bone marrow depression, their intermittent use in preventing vomiting due to cancer chemotherapy should not be precluded on this basis, since bone marrow depression is a common consequence of chemotherapy. Phenothiazines should be used with caution in patients with a history of dyskinetic reactions and, since these drugs are detoxified primarily in the liver, in those with moderate to severe hepatic dysfunction.

The action of phenothiazines and butyrophenones may be potentiated if other central nervous system depressants are used concomitantly. Sedation may be desirable in some patients (eg, those with malignancies) but undesirable in others. Phenothiazines are contraindicated when marked central nervous system depression or hypotension is present. They also may augment the fall in blood pressure when given to patients receiving spinal or epidural anesthesia or adrenergic blocking agents. Caution should be used in pregnant women with pre-eclampsia, since some patients with this condition have labile blood pressure and may experience a significant fall in pressure. See also Chapter 6, Antipsychotic Drugs, and the evaluation on Haloperidol.

Miscellaneous Drugs: See the evaluations.

Drug Evaluations

ANTICHOLINERGIC DRUG

SCOPOLAMINE
[Transderm-Scōp]

SCOPOLAMINE HYDROBROMIDE
[Triptone]

ACTIONS AND USES. Scopolamine is the most effective single agent for motion sickness, especially when it is severe and of brief duration. This drug acts primarily by reducing the excitability of the labyrinthine receptors and by depressing conduction in the vestibular cerebellar pathway. Before the advent of transdermal delivery, scopolamine had been largely supplanted by the antihistaminic antiemetics, principally because of its untoward effects. The transdermal delivery system (an adhesive unit containing scopolamine) causes fewer anticholinergic side effects. When the adhesive unit is applied postauricularly, scopolamine is released at a uniform rate for 72 hours, which protects most individuals susceptible to motion sickness. However, there is some evidence to suggest that the therapeutic response to this system of delivery decreases before 72 hours and that pharmacokinetic differences between individuals may account for the variability in effectiveness (Clissold and Heel, 1985).

Results of controlled studies in individuals subjected to severe motion indicate that there is a synergistic effect when oral scopolamine 0.3 to 0.6 mg was given with dextroamphetamine 5 to 10 mg, respectively, or when scopolamine 0.6 mg was given with ephedrine or promethazine 25 mg (Wood and Graybiel, 1972). The combination of scopolamine and promethazine or ephedrine has the additional advantages of producing fewer untoward effects and having little abuse potential (Wood, 1979). These combinations are indicated only for intense conditions of motion (eg, storms at sea, aerobatics, severe rotary experimental circumstances) or for individuals who are highly susceptible to moderately rough conditions of motion when transdermal scopolamine does not afford adequate protection.

In adults, scopolamine hydrobromide 0.2 to 0.4 mg is useful when given with morphine prior to surgery and is more effective than either atropine or glycopyrrolate in preventing postoperative nausea and vomiting. Transdermal scopolamine is superior to placebo in reducing the number of vertigo attacks.

ADVERSE REACTIONS AND PRECAUTIONS. Anticholinergic side effects (blurred vision, mydriasis, dryness of the mouth, changes in pulse rate, drowsiness, amnesia, and fatigue) often occur with use of scopolamine, especially in large doses. Less frequent but more severe effects (urinary retention, constipation, disorientation) may develop, especially in children and elderly patients. A toxic psychosis consisting of excitement, restlessness, hallucinations, or delirium occurs infrequently. Scopolamine should not be used in patients with glaucoma and should be used cautiously in those with prostatic enlargement.

The incidence of anticholinergic side effects is reduced with the adhesive unit, although dryness of the mouth occurs in most patients (67%) and drowsiness is frequent (16%) (Clissold and Heel, 1985). The hands should be washed thoroughly following application of the adhesive unit to prevent mydriasis from finger-to-eye exposure to scopolamine. Transdermal scopolamine should be avoided in children because it is not known if the dose delivered by this system produces serious adverse reactions.

The benefit of this drug during pregnancy must be weighed against potential risks (FDA Pregnancy Category C).

DOSAGE AND PREPARATIONS.
SCOPOLAMINE HYDROBROMIDE:
Oral: Adults, for prophylaxis of motion sickness, initially, 0.25 mg one hour before anticipated travel, repeated in four hours if necessary.

Triptone (Commerce). Capsules 0.25 mg (nonprescription).

Subcutaneous: Adults, for prevention and treatment of motion sickness, initially, 0.6 mg, then 0.3 mg every six hours if required; *children,* 0.006 mg/kg.

Generic. Solution 0.4 mg/ml in 0.5 and 1 ml containers and 0.3 and 1 mg/ml in 1 ml containers.
SCOPOLAMINE:
Topical: Adults, one transdermal adhesive unit is applied to clean dry skin in the postauricular area four to six hours before antiemetic protection is required. The unit delivers 1.5 mg over a period of 72 hours. This system may not be suitable for use in *children.*

Transderm-Scōp (CIBA). Adhesive unit 2.5 cm² containing 1.5 mg scopolamine.

ANTIHISTAMINIC DRUGS

BUCLIZINE HYDROCHLORIDE
[Bucladin-S]

Buclizine, a piperazine antihistamine, is useful in preventing motion sickness, but controlled studies are insufficient to evaluate its effectiveness in vertigo. The duration of action is four to six hours.

Drowsiness, dryness of the mouth, headache, and agitation may occur. Buclizine is contraindicated during early pregnancy; see the Introduction for a discussion of the drug's teratogenic effects in animals.

DOSAGE AND PREPARATIONS.
Oral: For motion sickness, *adults,* 50 mg at least one-half hour before departure and four to six hours later, if necessary. For vertigo, the usual dosage is 50 mg twice daily.

Bucladin-S (Stuart). Tablets 50 mg.

CYCLIZINE HYDROCHLORIDE
[Marezine]

CYCLIZINE LACTATE
[Marezine]

USES. Cyclizine prevents and relieves motion sickness, vertigo, and symptoms of aural vestibular disorders. The duration of action is about four hours. Intramuscular cyclizine is a drug of choice in the treatment of postoperative nausea and vomiting (Palazzo and Strunin, 1984); the incidence of side effects is lower than with the phenothiazines. Cyclizine generally does not relieve vomiting due to cancer chemotherapeutic agents (Morran et al, 1979).

ADVERSE REACTIONS AND PRECAUTIONS. Large doses may cause drowsiness and dryness of the mouth. A large-scale study, including pregnant women receiving cyclizine during the first trimester, failed to demonstrate any teratogenic effect with the doses employed clinically (Milkovich and van den Berg, 1976). After review of the existing epidemiologic data on pregnant women, the Food and Drug Administration concluded that these data do not support a restriction on the use of cyclizine or a pregnancy warning (*Federal Register,* 1979).

DOSAGE AND PREPARATIONS.
Oral: For motion sickness, *adults,* 50 mg one-half hour before departure, then every four to six hours as necessary (maxi-

mum, 200 mg daily); *children 6 to 10 years,* 3 mg/kg divided into three doses during a 24-hour period.

CYCLIZINE HYDROCHLORIDE:
Marezine (Burroughs Wellcome). Tablets 50 mg.
Intramuscular: *Adults,* 50 mg every four to six hours as necessary.

CYCLIZINE LACTATE:
Marezine (Burroughs Wellcome). Solution 50 mg/ml in 1 ml containers.

DIMENHYDRINATE
[Dramamine]

This chlorotheophylline salt of diphenhydramine is especially useful in preventing and treating vertigo, including that associated with Meniere's disease, and motion sickness; it also is effective in nausea and vomiting during pregnancy. As with other antihistamines, dimenhydrinate generally is ineffective against nausea and vomiting induced by cancer chemotherapeutic agents. The duration of action is four to six hours. Mild drowsiness occurs.

DOSAGE AND PREPARATIONS.
Intramuscular: *Adults,* 50 mg every three to four hours as needed; *children,* 1 to 1.5 mg/kg every six hours (maximum, 300 mg/day).
Intravenous: *Adults,* 50 mg diluted in 10 ml of sodium chloride injection administered over a period of two minutes; *children,* no dosage has been established.
Generic. Solution 50 mg/ml in 1 and 10 ml containers.
Dramamine (Searle). Solution 50 mg/ml in 1 and 5 ml containers.
Oral: *Adults,* 50 to 100 mg every four hours; *children,* 1 to 1.5 mg/kg every six hours (maximum, 300 mg/day).
Dramamine (Searle), *Generic.* Liquid 12.5 mg/4 ml (alcohol 5% [*Dramamine*]) (nonprescription); tablets 50 mg (nonprescription).

DIPHENHYDRAMINE HYDROCHLORIDE
[Benadryl]

This antihistamine has actions similar to those of cyclizine. It is effective in the prevention and treatment of vertigo, motion sickness, and nausea and vomiting during pregnancy. When given intravenously, it is the drug of choice for the treatment of extrapyramidal reactions induced by the dopaminergic blocking agents because of its high degree of effectiveness. Primarily for this reason, it has become a component of antiemetic regimens containing metoclopramide. The duration of action is four to six hours.

The incidence of drowsiness is high. Individuals whose activities require alertness, such as those operating vehicles or machinery, should not use diphenhydramine.

DOSAGE AND PREPARATIONS.
Intramuscular (deep), Intravenous: *Adults,* 10 mg initially; if sedation is not severe, the subsequent dose may be increased to 20 to 50 mg every two or three hours (maximum, 400 mg/day). For extrapyramidal reactions (oculogyric crises, torticollis, and akathisia) produced by phenothiazines, butyrophenones, and metoclopramide, 50 mg is administered intravenously over two to three minutes. When used with metoclopramide and dexamethasone in conjunction with cisplatin, this dose is given 30 minutes prior to chemotherapy and is repeated in four hours.
Intramuscular (deep): *Children,* 1 to 1.5 mg/kg every six hours (maximum, 300 mg/day).
Generic. Solution 10 mg/ml in 10 and 30 ml containers and 50 mg/ml in 1, 5, and 10 ml containers.
Benadryl (Parke-Davis). Solution (sterile) 10 mg/ml in 10 and 30 ml containers and 50 mg/ml in 1 and 10 ml containers.
Oral: For motion sickness, *adults,* 50 mg one-half hour before departure and 50 mg before each meal; *children,* 1 to 1.5 mg/kg every six hours (maximum, 300 mg/day).
Generic. Capsules 25 and 50 mg; elixir and syrup 12.5 mg/5 ml.
Benadryl (Parke-Davis). Capsules 25 and 50 mg; elixir 12.5 mg/5 ml (alcohol 14%).

HYDROXYZINE HYDROCHLORIDE
[Atarax, Orgatrax, Vistaril]

HYDROXYZINE PAMOATE
[Vistaril]

Hydroxyzine, an antianxiety and antihistaminic agent, also possesses antiemetic properties. This drug was shown to reduce nausea and vomiting when given intramuscularly after induction of anesthesia (McKenzie et al, 1981). It also is useful for the treatment of motion sickness and, possibly, vertigo. The duration of action is four to six hours. The incidence of drowsiness is low.

Hydroxyzine potentiates the central nervous system depressant actions of narcotics and barbiturates; therefore, the dose of these drugs should be reduced by at least 50% when hydroxyzine is used concurrently. It was demonstrated in one study that hydroxyzine enhances opioid analgesia (Beaver and Feise, 1976), which allows reduction of the opioid dosage, but this effect is not universally accepted.

See the Introduction for a discussion on the drug's teratogenic effects in animals.

DOSAGE AND PREPARATIONS.
Intramuscular: For postoperative vomiting, *adults,* 25 to 100 mg; *children,* 1 mg/kg, repeated every six hours if necessary.

HYDROXYZINE HYDROCHLORIDE:
Generic. Solution 25 mg/ml in 1 and 10 ml containers; 50 mg/ml in 1, 2, and 10 ml containers; 75 mg/ml in 1.5 ml containers; and 100 mg/ml in 2 ml containers.
Orgatrax (Organon). Solution 50 mg/ml in 1, 2, and 10 ml containers.
Vistaril (Pfipharmecs). Solution 25 mg/ml in 1 and 10 ml containers and 50 mg/ml in 1, 1.5, 2, and 10 ml containers.

Oral: *Adults,* 25 to 100 mg three or four times daily; *children under 6 years,* 12.5 mg every six hours; *over 6 years,* 12.5 to 25 mg every six hours.

HYDROXYZINE HYDROCHLORIDE:
Atarax (Roerig), *Generic.* Syrup 10 mg/5 ml (alcohol 0.5% *[Atarax]*); tablets 10, 25, 50, and 100 mg.
HYDROXYZINE PAMOATE:
Generic. Capsules 25, 50, and 100 mg.
Vistaril (Pfizer). Capsules 25, 50, and 100 mg; suspension 25 mg/5 ml (strengths expressed in terms of the hydrochloride salt).

MECLIZINE HYDROCHLORIDE
[Antivert, Bonine]

Meclizine is effective in preventing and treating motion sickness. It has a slower onset and longer duration of action (24 hours) than most other antihistamines used for motion sickness. Meclizine also is one of the most useful antiemetics to prevent and treat nausea and vomiting associated with vertigo of vestibular origin (eg, labyrinthitis, Meniere's disease) and occasionally prevents vomiting associated with radiation sickness. It helps alleviate nausea and vomiting associated with pregnancy when conservative measures are ineffective (see the Introduction).

Drowsiness, blurred vision, dryness of the mouth, and fatigue have occurred following administration of meclizine. After review of the existing epidemiologic data on pregnant women, the Food and Drug Administration concluded that these data do not support a restriction on the use of meclizine or a pregnancy warning (*Federal Register,* 1979). (FDA Pregnancy Category B)

DOSAGE AND PREPARATIONS.
Oral: *Adults,* for motion sickness, 25 to 50 mg once daily; the initial dose should be taken at least one hour prior to departure. For vertigo and radiation sickness, 25 to 100 mg daily in divided doses, depending upon clinical response. *Children,* dosage has not been established.

Generic. Tablets 12.5 and 25 mg; tablets (chewable) 25 mg. (Generic preparations may be nonprescription depending upon manufacturers' labeling.)
Antivert (Roerig). Tablets 12.5, 25, and 50 mg; tablets (chewable) 25 mg.
Bonine (Pfipharmecs). Tablets (chewable) 25 mg (nonprescription).

PROMETHAZINE HYDROCHLORIDE
[Phenergan]

ACTIONS AND USES. Unlike other phenothiazines, promethazine has pronounced antihistaminic activity in addition to strong central cholinergic blocking activity, is effective in the prevention and treatment of vertigo and motion sickness, and has limited, if any, effect upon vomiting caused by stimulation of the chemoreceptor trigger zone. The central cholinergic blocking action may account for promethazine's effectiveness against motion sickness. It is useful in preventing postoperative nausea and vomiting, although it should not be used routinely for this purpose. Promethazine is less effective than the antidopaminergic agents in vomiting induced by toxins, radiation, and cancer chemotherapeutic agents. The duration of action is four to six hours.

Results of controlled studies in individuals subjected to severe motion indicate that a synergistic effect occurs when promethazine 25 mg is combined with ephedrine 12.5 mg (Wood, 1979).

ADVERSE REACTIONS AND PRECAUTIONS. The most frequent and prominent side effect of promethazine is sedation. Anticholinergic and antiadrenergic adverse reactions occur infrequently after oral administration (see the Introduction).

In the usual antiemetic dose, promethazine is relatively free of the extrapyramidal stimulation associated with some phenothiazine and butyrophenone derivatives. However, the drug should be avoided in children and adolescents whose symptoms and signs suggest Reye's syndrome (see the Introduction).

DOSAGE AND PREPARATIONS.
Intramuscular, Rectal: For treatment of nausea and vomiting, *adults,* initially, 25 mg, then 12.5 to 25 mg as needed every four to six hours. A dose of 12.5 mg (which is usually effective) should be tried initially in selected high-risk postoperative patients, because hypotension is observed more frequently when the 25-mg dose is given parenterally postoperatively. *Children under 12 years,* the dose should be adjusted on the basis of the age and weight of the patient and severity of the condition, and no more than one-half the suggested adult dose should be administered; if given as an adjunct to premedication, the suggested dose is 1.1 mg/kg.
Generic. Solution 25 and 50 mg/ml in 1 and 10 ml containers.
Phenergan (Wyeth). Solution 25 and 50 mg/ml in 1 ml containers; suppositories 12.5, 25, and 50 mg.

Oral, Rectal: For motion sickness, *adults,* 25 mg twice daily. Administration one-half to one hour before anticipated travel is most beneficial. *Children,* 12.5 to 25 mg twice daily. Tablets, syrup, or rectal suppositories may be used.
Phenergan (Wyeth), *Generic.* Syrup 6.25 and 25 mg/5 ml; tablets 12.5, 25, and 50 mg; suppositories (*Phenergan* only) 12.5, 25, and 50 mg.

ANTIDOPAMINERGIC DRUGS

CHLORPROMAZINE
[Thorazine]

CHLORPROMAZINE HYDROCHLORIDE
[Thorazine]

ACTIONS AND USES. Chlorpromazine is the prototype of the aliphatic phenothiazines. This drug's antiemetic activity is based on its antagonism of dopamine receptors in the chemoreceptor trigger zone, which reduces neural impulses to the vomiting center.

This phenothiazine is less potent as an antiemetic than prochlorperazine, thiethylperazine, and perphenazine; however, the incidence of dystonias is less with chlorpromazine than with the latter drugs, especially with intramuscular administration. Because of the greater degree of sedation and the higher incidence of orthostatic hypotension encountered with chlorpromazine than with prochlorperazine, most specialists prefer the latter or thiethylperazine to prevent chemotherapy-induced nausea and vomiting. As with other phenothiazines, chlorpromazine is useful with mildly emetic regimens but does not ameliorate nausea and vomiting due to strong emetic agents, such as cisplatin, doxorubicin, mechlorethamine, dacarbazine, or dactinomycin.

Chlorpromazine does not prevent vertigo or motion sickness, although it may be useful in treating severe vomiting produced by these disorders.

ADVERSE REACTIONS AND PRECAUTIONS. Unacceptable drowsiness may occur, although tolerance usually develops after continued use. Chlorpromazine prolongs postanesthesia sleeping time.

Serious untoward effects may occur after long-term use or administration of large doses and include extrapyramidal reactions, orthostatic hypotension, cholestatic jaundice, and leukopenia. Because of the severity of these adverse reactions, chlorpromazine should be considered only when vomiting cannot be controlled by less toxic antiemetics. Since all phenothiazines have the potential to produce extrapyramidal reactions, these drugs should be avoided in children and adolescents whose symptoms and signs suggest Reye's syndrome (see the Introduction and Chapter 6, Antipsychotic Drugs).

DOSAGE AND PREPARATIONS. This drug generally should not be used in *children under 6 months* except when it is potentially lifesaving. The manufacturers' suggested dosages are:
CHLORPROMAZINE:
Rectal: Adults, 50 to 100 mg every six to eight hours; *children,* 1 mg/kg every six to eight hours.

Thorazine (Smith Kline & French). Suppositories 25 and 100 mg.
CHLORPROMAZINE HYDROCHLORIDE:
Intramuscular: Adults, initially, 25 mg. If hypotension does not occur, 25 to 50 mg is given every three or four hours until vomiting stops; the drug is then given orally. *Children,* 0.5 mg/kg every six to eight hours; maximum daily doses, *up to 5 years* (22.5 kg), 40 mg; *5 to 12 years* (22.5 to 45 kg), 75 mg.
  Generic. Solution 25 mg/ml in 10 ml containers.
  Thorazine (Smith Kline & French). Solution (aqueous) 25 mg/ml in 1, 2, and 10 ml containers.
Oral: Adults, 10 to 25 mg every four to six hours; *children,* 0.5 mg/kg every four to six hours. Since all phenothiazines have prolonged half-lives (12 to 20 hours), the timed-release preparation has no significant advantage over the ordinary oral dosage forms for most patients.
  Generic. Concentrate 30 and 100 mg/ml; tablets 10, 25, 50, 100, and 200 mg.
  Thorazine (Smith Kline & French). Capsules (timed-release) 30, 75, 150, 200, and 300 mg; concentrate 30 and 100 mg/ml; syrup 10 mg/5 ml; tablets 10, 25, 50, 100, and 200 mg.

DOMPERIDONE
[Motilium]

ACTIONS AND USES. This investigational antidopaminergic drug has antiemetic activity similar to that of metoclopramide, although the incidence of extrapyramidal side effects is lower because domperidone does not readily cross the blood-brain barrier. Intravenous or oral administration increases lower esophageal sphincter pressure, the duration of antral and duodenal contractions, and the gastric emptying of liquids and semisolids.

In open and controlled studies in adults and children (Dhondt et al, 1978; Reyntjens, 1979), domperidone was more effective than placebo. This drug appears to be particularly effective in chronic postprandial dyspepsia, postprandial nausea and vomiting, and that associated with gastroenteritis. For the latter purpose, it may become the drug of choice in infants and children (Hoffbrand, 1979). Domperidone may prove to be useful for nausea and vomiting associated with dysmenorrhea, migraine, head injury, hemodialysis, and radiation therapy. It is of *no* value for nausea and vomiting induced by narcotics. In postoperative vomiting, this drug was effective when given after the first vomiting episode but not when given before induction or at the end of anesthesia. Intravenous domperidone may relieve nausea and vomiting due to cancer chemotherapeutic agents of moderate emetic potency (Brogden et al, 1982).

ADVERSE REACTIONS. When domperidone is administered as an intravenous bolus (more than 50 mg), cardiac dysrhythmias have been reported. An intravenous infusion avoids this risk and is advised for patients with hypokalemia or heart disease and those receiving concomitant cytotoxic chemotherapy. The lack of extrapyramidal reactions may be because the drug is poorly distributed to the central nervous system and does not block dopaminergic receptors in the basal ganglia. Because it rarely causes dystonias, domperidone may be especially useful in infants and children.

Domperidone, like metoclopramide, may increase serum prolactin concentrations. A few cases of galactorrhea have been reported after prolonged use (Cann et al, 1983).

PHARMACOKINETICS. Domperidone is well absorbed when given intramuscularly, orally, or rectally. Peak plasma concentrations are attained 10 to 30 minutes after intramuscular and oral administration and one to two hours after rectal administration. Systemic bioavailability of intramuscular domperidone is approximately 90%, whereas that of oral domperidone is 13% to 17% due to first-pass hepatic and gut wall metabolism. Bioavailability after oral administration is increased when domperidone is taken 90 minutes after a meal.

Domperidone undergoes extensive hepatic biotransformation and is excreted in the bile (60%). The half-life is approximately seven hours.

DOSAGE AND PREPARATIONS.
Intravenous, Intramuscular: *Adults,* 10 mg up to six times daily (maximum, 1 mg/kg daily). *Children,* 0.1 to 0.2 mg/kg three to six times daily (maximum, 1 mg/kg daily).
Oral: *Adults,* 20 to 40 mg three or four times daily; *children,* 0.6 mg/kg three or four times daily (Brogden et al, 1982).

For chronic postprandial dyspepsia, the usual *adult* dose is 10 mg three times a day 15 to 30 minutes before meals and at bedtime. *Children,* (1% solution) 0.3 mg/kg three times a day 15 to 30 minutes before meals and, if necessary, at bedtime. The daily dose for adults and children may be doubled if there is no significant improvement after two weeks of therapy.
Rectal: *Adults,* 60 mg two to four times daily. *Children 1 to 2 years,* 10 mg two to four times daily; *2 to 4 years,* 30 mg once or twice daily; *4 to 6 years,* 30 mg up to three times daily; *6 to 10 years,* 30 mg up to four times daily.
   Motilium (Janssen).
   (Investigational drug)

DROPERIDOL
[Inapsine]

Because extrapyramidal reactions, hypotension, and sedation occur less frequently and are less severe than with phenothiazines and because of its longer duration of action, droperidol may be preferred for prophylaxis of nausea and vomiting associated with anesthesia and surgery (Palazzo and Strunin, 1984). This drug is employed occasionally to alleviate nausea and vomiting in Meniere's syndrome. An intravenous loading dose of droperidol followed by either continuous infusion or repeated intravenous administration was effective in some cases of cisplatin-induced nausea and vomiting.

For a more detailed discussion on droperidol, see Chapter 16, General Anesthetics.
DOSAGE AND PREPARATIONS.
Intramuscular: For premedication, *adults,* 2.5 to 10 mg (1 to 4 ml). The dosage must be individualized according to the physical status of the patient and is reduced in the elderly or when other depressant drugs are used concomitantly. *Children 2 to 12 years,* 1 to 1.5 mg (0.4 to 0.6 ml)/9 to 11 kg.
Intravenous: For Meniere's syndrome, *adults,* 5 mg. To prevent postoperative nausea and vomiting, *adults,* 1.25 mg to 2.5 mg five minutes prior to termination of anesthesia, repeated intramuscularly during the first 24 hours after surgery if the patient complains of nausea, retches, or vomits; *children 1 to 15 years,* 0.05 mg/kg.

As an antiemetic in cancer chemotherapy, *adults,* 2.5 to 5 mg 30 to 60 minutes prior to treatment; the same or one-half the dose is given intramuscularly after therapy on request but no more than once every hour; *children,* 1.25 mg (0.5 ml)/20 kg repeated intramuscularly as necessary, but no more than once every hour.

For nausea and vomiting induced by cisplatin or other strong emetic agents, *adults,* a loading dose of 15 mg, followed by 7.5 mg every two hours for seven doses (Citron et al, 1984).
   Inapsine (Janssen). Solution 2.5 mg/ml in 2, 5, and 10 ml containers.

FLUPHENAZINE HYDROCHLORIDE
[Permitil, Prolixin]

USES. Fluphenazine, a piperazine phenothiazine, is effective in the management of postoperative nausea and vomiting and that caused by toxins and radiation. There is little evidence to support its use in cancer chemotherapy but fluphenazine probably can be used for nausea and vomiting induced by mildly emetic chemotherapy. This phenothiazine has little sedative effect and does not appreciably prolong postanesthesia sleeping time when given preoperatively.

Fluphenazine does not prevent vertigo or motion sickness.

ADVERSE REACTIONS AND PRECAUTIONS. The incidence of extrapyramidal reactions is higher with fluphenazine than with most other phenothiazines. The drug should be avoided in children and adolescents whose symptoms and signs suggest Reye's syndrome (see the Introduction). Fluphenazine has little tendency to produce orthostatic hypotension; however, other anticholinergic effects (blurred vision, dryness of the mouth, and urinary retention) have been reported. See also Chapter 6, Antipsychotic Drugs.

DOSAGE AND PREPARATIONS.
Intramuscular, Oral: *Adults,* 1.25 mg repeated at six- to eight-hour intervals if needed; *children,* dosage is reduced.

Permitil (Schering). Concentrate (oral) 5 mg/ml (alcohol 1%); tablets 0.25, 2.5, 5, and 10 mg.

Prolixin (Squibb). Elixir 2.5 mg/5 ml (alcohol 14%); tablets 1, 2.5, 5, and 10 mg; solution (for injection, aqueous, sterile) 2.5 mg/ml in 10 ml containers.

HALOPERIDOL
[Haldol]

HALOPERIDOL LACTATE
[Haldol]

ACTIONS AND USES. The antiemetic action of this antidopaminergic butyrophenone is achieved mainly through inhibition of stimuli at the chemoreceptor trigger zone. The duration of action of haloperidol is longer than that of droperidol.

Haloperidol has been administered to alleviate nausea and vomiting associated with narcotics, anesthesia and surgery, radiation therapy, cancer chemotherapy, and gastrointestinal disorders.

Haloperidol does not prevent vertigo or motion sickness and is not recommended for use during pregnancy until more clinical data are available.

ADVERSE REACTIONS AND PRECAUTIONS. The adverse reactions produced by haloperidol closely resemble those of the piperazine phenothiazines (see the Introduction and Chapter 6, Antipsychotic Drugs), but they occur only rarely with the small doses and short-term therapy employed to relieve nausea and vomiting.

As with other antiemetics, haloperidol must be given with great caution to patients with gastrointestinal disorders to avoid masking the development of life-threatening conditions that may be amenable to surgery. Because this drug has a marked potential to produce akathisia and other extrapyramidal reactions, it should be avoided in children and adolescents. Elderly or debilitated patients may be more sensitive to the drug.

DOSAGE AND PREPARATIONS.

Intramuscular: Adults, 1, 2, or 5 mg every 12 hours as needed.

HALOPERIDOL LACTATE:
Haldol (McNeil). Solution 5 mg/ml in 1 and 10 ml containers.

Oral: Adults, 1, 2, or 5 mg twice daily.

HALOPERIDOL:
Haldol (McNeil). Tablets 0.5, 1, 2, 5, 10, and 20 mg.

HALOPERIDOL LACTATE:
Haldol (McNeil). Concentrate 2 mg/ml.

METOCLOPRAMIDE
[Reglan]

ACTIONS AND USES. Like the phenothiazines, metoclopramide has an antidopaminergic effect at the chemoreceptor trigger zone, but it also increases gastrointestinal motility.

High-dose intravenous metoclopramide is regarded by many authorities as the initial drug of choice in preventing nausea and vomiting induced by cisplatin (especially at doses greater than 100 mg/M²) and other highly emetic antineoplastic agents, such as dacarbazine, dactinomycin, mechlorethamine, and doxorubicin (Kris et al, 1985; Strum et al, 1984; Strum et al, 1985). Optimal control of nausea and vomiting is obtained with a combination of intravenous metoclopramide, dexamethasone, and diphenhydramine (Strum et al, 1985). As with other antiemetics, its efficacy is reduced in the presence of anticipatory nausea and vomiting.

Gastric stasis induced by morphine is reversed by metoclopramide, and this antiemetic is effective for narcotic-induced nausea and vomiting (eg, opioid-induced postoperative vomiting). There is evidence that metoclopramide may be useful preoperatively to empty the stomach prior to emergency surgery. Additionally, it tightens the lower esophageal sphincter to prevent aspiration when emergency general anesthesia must be given. Metoclopramide also may alleviate nausea and vomiting induced by toxins and radiation. Like other antidopaminergic agents, it does *not* prevent motion sickness.

Metoclopramide is useful for diabetic gastroparesis (see Chapter 52, Agents Used in Disorders of the Upper Gastrointestinal Tract) and enhances the response to ergotamine and analgesics in migraine headache (see Chapter 13, Drugs Used to Treat Migraine and Other Headaches).

ADVERSE REACTIONS AND PRECAUTIONS. The principal adverse effects of metoclopramide are sedation and diarrhea, which develop in most patients given the larger doses needed to alleviate vomiting induced by antineoplastic agents.

Extrapyramidal reactions, including parkinsonian symptoms and tardive dyskinesia, have been noted when metoclopramide was used for many months or years (Kataria et al, 1978). Parkinsonian symptoms usually resolve in a few weeks following drug withdrawal, but may persist for several months. Dystonic reactions (oculogyric crises, trismus, torticollis, opisthotonos) and akathisia are more likely to occur within the first 72 hours of treatment. They are common in children, young adults, patients with renal impairment, and with the larger doses used in chemotherapy patients. Usually, extrapyramidal reactions are readily reversible by diphenhydramine.

Metoclopramide may increase the sedative actions of central nervous system depressants and may increase the severity and frequency of extrapyramidal reactions produced by medications given concurrently, particularly phenothiazines. It is contraindicated in the presence of gastrointestinal obstruction, hemorrhage, or perforation; convulsive disorders; and pheochromocytoma.

Occasional reactions include agitation, irritability, urticarial or maculopapular rash, dryness of the mouth, glossal or periorbital edema, and neck pain and rigidity. Methemoglobinemia has been reported in neonates who received excessive doses.

This drug is classified in FDA Pregnancy Category B.

PHARMACOKINETICS. With the exception of simple conjugation, this drug undergoes little hepatic metabolism. The half-life is five to six hours in patients with normal renal function and is not dose dependent. In one study, blood concentrations of metoclopramide (more than 850 ng/ml) correlated with antiemetic efficacy (Meyer et al, 1984), but this finding was not substantiated in a second study (Strum et al, 1985).

DOSAGE AND PREPARATIONS. Dosage should be reduced by approximately 60% in patients with severe renal impairment.

Intravenous: Adults, to alleviate nausea and vomiting induced by moderately emetic cancer chemotherapeutic agents, 0.5 to 0.75 mg/kg diluted in 50 ml of a large-volume parenteral solution and infused slowly over a 15-minute period 30 minutes prior to chemotherapy and at intervals of two, five, and eight hours after the first dose. When used with dexamethasone, 0.5 mg/kg given intravenously at the same intervals is effective.

For highly emetic regimens containing cisplatin, 2 to 3 mg/kg is administered one-half hour before chemotherapy and then at two- and four-hour intervals. Dexamethasone and diphenhydramine also are given intravenously 30 minutes prior to chemotherapy and the dose of diphenhydramine is repeated in four hours. For highly emetic noncisplatin-containing regimens, 1 mg/kg is given intravenously 30 minutes before chemotherapy and two hours later; subsequent doses are given orally.

Solutions may be diluted more than one hour prior to use but partially used material should not be stored for later administration. Dexamethasone and diphenhydramine are administered in the same dosage as for cisplatin-containing regimens (see above).

Children, the incidence of extrapyramidal reactions is unacceptably high with doses of 1 to 2 mg/kg (even with concomitant use of diphenhydramine). Further studies are needed to determine a safe and effective dosage.

Reglan (Robins). Solution 5 mg/ml (monohydrochloride) in 2, 10, and 30 ml containers.

Oral: Adults, for delayed-onset nausea and vomiting caused by cisplatin, 0.5 mg/kg four times a day for six days beginning 24 hours after chemotherapy. Concomitant use with oral dexamethasone is most effective (see the evaluation).

Reglan (Robins). Syrup 5 mg/ml (monohydrochloride); tablets (monohydrochloride) 10 mg.

PERPHENAZINE
[Trilafon]

This piperazine phenothiazine is effective in the management of postoperative nausea and vomiting and for that caused by narcotics, toxins, and radiation. It is not widely used as an antiemetic in cancer chemotherapy regimens but its effectiveness may be similar to that of other antidopaminergic agents. Perphenazine does *not* prevent vertigo or motion sickness.

Untoward effects include extrapyramidal reactions, blurred or double vision, nasal congestion, dryness of the mouth, salivation, headache, and, occasionally, drowsiness. The drug should be avoided in children and adolescents whose symptoms and signs suggest Reye's syndrome (see the Introduction and Chapter 6, Antipsychotic Drugs).

DOSAGE AND PREPARATIONS. No dosage has been established for *children under 12 years.*
Intramuscular: *Adults,* 5 or, rarely, 10 mg.
Trilafon (Schering). Solution 5 mg/ml in 1 ml containers.
Oral: Adults, 2 to 4 mg every four to six hours. Since all phenothiazines have prolonged half-lives (12 to 20 hours), the timed-release preparation has no significant advantage over ordinary oral dosage forms for most patients.
Trilafon (Schering). Concentrate 16 mg/5 ml (alcohol less than 0.1%); tablets 2, 4, 8, and 16 mg; tablets (timed-release) 8 mg.

PROCHLORPERAZINE
[Compazine]

PROCHLORPERAZINE EDISYLATE
[Compazine]

PROCHLORPERAZINE MALEATE
[Compazine]

Prochlorperazine is effective in the management of postoperative nausea and vomiting in adults and that caused by toxins, radiation, and mildly emetic cancer chemotherapeutic agents, especially when minimal sedation is desired. Prochlorperazine is less useful for vomiting caused by moderately to severely emetic cancer chemotherapy. This drug does *not* prevent vertigo or motion sickness.

ADVERSE REACTIONS AND PRECAUTIONS. This piperazine phenothiazine frequently causes extrapyramidal reactions. Although these effects are most likely to occur with large doses, signs may appear abruptly in patients taking only moderate doses. Consideration should be given to the increased potential for extrapyramidal side effects when prochlorperazine is used in repeated cycles of radiation therapy.

Drowsiness, dizziness, cutaneous reactions, and amenorrhea occur occasionally, and orthostatic hypotension, neutropenia, and cholestasis have been reported rarely.

Particular caution is necessary in patients who are sensitive to other phenothiazines, in those with hepatic disease, and in children. The drug should be avoided in children undergoing surgery and in children and adolescents whose symptoms and signs suggest Reye's syndrome (see the Introduction). Prochlorperazine also should not be used in children under 2 years or less than 9 kg unless it is potentially lifesaving. See also Chapter 6, Antipsychotic Drugs.

DOSAGE AND PREPARATIONS.

PROCHLORPERAZINE:

Rectal: *Adults,* 25 mg twice daily; *children 9 to 14 kg,* 2.5 mg every 12 to 24 hours; *14 to 18 kg,* 2.5 mg every 8 to 12 hours; *18 to 39 kg,* 2.5 mg every 8 hours or 5 mg every 12 hours.
   Compazine (Smith Kline & French). Suppositories 2.5, 5, and 25 mg.

PROCHLORPERAZINE EDISYLATE:

Intramuscular (deep): *Adults,* 5 to 10 mg every three or four hours (maximum, 40 mg daily); *children over 10 kg,* 0.13 mg/kg; intramuscular administration usually is not repeated in children.
   Generic. Solution 5 mg/ml in 2 ml containers.
   Compazine (Smith Kline & French). Solution (aqueous) 5 mg/ml in 2 and 10 ml containers.

Oral: *Adults,* 5 to 10 mg three or four times daily; *children 9 to 14 kg,* 2.5 mg every 12 to 24 hours; *14 to 18 kg,* 2.5 mg every 8 to 12 hours; *18 to 39 kg,* 2.5 mg every 8 hours or 5 mg every 12 hours.
   Compazine (Smith Kline & French). Syrup 5 mg/5 ml.

PROCHLORPERAZINE MALEATE:

Oral: Same as oral dosage for edisylate salt. Since all phenothiazines have prolonged half-lives (12 to 20 hours), the timed-release preparation has no significant advantage over ordinary oral dosage forms for most patients.
   Generic. Tablets 5, 10, and 25 mg.
   Compazine (Smith Kline & French). Capsules (timed-release) 10, 15, and 30 mg; tablets 5, 10, and 25 mg.

PROMAZINE HYDROCHLORIDE
[Sparine]

Promazine, an aliphatic phenothiazine, is effective in postoperative nausea and vomiting. It has not been studied extensively in emesis caused by cancer chemotherapeutic agents, radiation sickness, or toxins. However, as with other phenothiazine antiemetics, promazine is unlikely to prevent nausea and vomiting due to moderately or severely emetic chemotherapy.

ADVERSE REACTIONS AND PRECAUTIONS. The incidence of adverse reactions (eg, drowsiness, orthostatic hypotension) is similar to that of the other aliphatic phenothiazines, especially after parenteral administration. The hypotensive action may be detrimental in patients with cardiac or cerebrovascular insufficiency, and the anticholinergic actions may be detrimental in patients with ileus, angle-closure glaucoma, or urinary retention.

Extrapyramidal reactions are infrequent. Although relatively rare, agranulocytosis is reported to occur more frequently than with chlorpromazine or prochlorperazine. The drug should be avoided in children and adolescents whose symptoms and signs suggest Reye's syndrome (see the Introduction).

DOSAGE AND PREPARATIONS.

Oral: *Adults,* 25 to 50 mg every four to six hours.
   Sparine (Wyeth). Syrup 10 mg/5 ml; tablets 25, 50, and 100 mg.
Intramuscular: *Adults,* 50 mg.
   Generic. Solution 25 and 50 mg/ml in 10 ml containers.
   Sparine (Wyeth). Solution 25 mg/ml in 1 and 10 ml containers and 50 mg/ml in 1, 2, and 10 ml containers.

THIETHYLPERAZINE MALATE
[Torecan]

THIETHYLPERAZINE MALEATE
[Torecan]

USES. Thiethylperazine is particularly useful to treat nausea and vomiting associated with surgery; it also relieves nausea and vomiting caused by mildly emetic cancer chemotherapeutic agents, radiation therapy, and toxins. This piperazine phenothiazine does *not* prevent vertigo or motion sickness.

ADVERSE REACTIONS AND PRECAUTIONS. Untoward effects are infrequent, mild, and transitory with usual doses. Adverse reactions noted occasionally include drowsiness, dizziness, dryness of the mouth and nose, tachycardia, and anorexia. Moderate hypotension has occurred occasionally within 30 minutes after administration to patients recovering from general anesthesia.

Like other phenothiazines, thiethylperazine may produce extrapyramidal reactions. Symptoms may appear even after a single dose but abate if therapy is discontinued. For severe reactions, such as oculogyric crisis and torticollis, diphenhydramine 50 mg given intravenously abolishes symptoms within minutes. Thiethylperazine should be avoided in children and adolescents whose symptoms and signs suggest Reye's syndrome (see the Introduction and Chapter 6, Antipsychotic Drugs).

DOSAGE AND PREPARATIONS. No dosage has been established for *children.*

Intramuscular: Adults, 10 mg one to three times daily.
 THIETHYLPERAZINE MALATE:
 Torecan (Boehringer Ingelheim). Solution (aqueous) 5 mg/ml in 2 ml containers.
Oral, Rectal: Adults, 10 mg one to three times daily.
 THIETHYLPERAZINE MALEATE:
 Torecan (Boehringer Ingelheim). Tablets 10 mg; suppositories 10 mg.

TRIFLUPROMAZINE HYDROCHLORIDE
 [Vesprin]

USES. This aliphatic phenothiazine is effective in postoperative nausea and vomiting. Its effectiveness in preventing nausea and vomiting induced by cancer chemotherapeutic agents, radiation sickness, or toxins has not been well studied. Like other phenothiazine antiemetics, triflupromazine may be useful only against vomiting due to mildly emetic agents. It does *not* prevent vertigo or motion sickness.

ADVERSE REACTIONS AND PRECAUTIONS. Triflupromazine produces less sedation than some other phenothiazines (eg, promazine), but it prolongs the postanesthesia sleep time. Extrapyramidal reactions have been observed following even single doses of this compound. The drug should be avoided in children and adolescents whose symptoms and signs suggest Reye's syndrome (see the Introduction and Chapter 6, Antipsychotic Drugs) and should not be used in children less than 2 1/2 years.

DOSAGE AND PREPARATIONS.
Intramuscular: Adults, 5 to 15 mg, repeated every four hours if necessary (maximum, 60 mg daily); *elderly or debilitated patients,* 2.5 mg every four hours if necessary; *children over 2 1/2 years,* 0.07 mg/kg three times a day (maximum, 10 mg daily).
Intravenous: Adults, 1 to 3 mg.
 Vesprin (Squibb). Solution 10 mg/ml in 10 ml containers and 20 mg/ml in 1 ml containers.

MISCELLANEOUS DRUGS

BENZQUINAMIDE HYDROCHLORIDE
 [Emete-Con]

ACTIONS AND USES. Like the antidopaminergic drugs, this short-acting benzquinoline derivative apparently inhibits stimuli at the chemoreceptor trigger zone. Benzquinamide is used primarily to prevent and treat postoperative nausea and vomiting. It is more effective than the phenothiazines in preventing nausea and vomiting produced by cancer chemotherapy. Although only rarely effective against cisplatin- or mechlorethamine-induced emesis, benzquinamide eliminated vomiting in 20% of patients receiving doxorubicin (Neidhart et al, 1981). Data are not sufficient to justify the use of benzquinamide during pregnancy or in children.

ADVERSE REACTIONS AND PRECAUTIONS. Results of a few controlled studies suggest that benzquinamide produces fewer serious adverse reactions than the phenothiazines; however, there is less overall experience with this agent. Drowsiness is noted most frequently. Shivering, chills, and mild anticholinergic reactions also have been reported.

 Persistent tachycardia, transient hypotension, and increased cardiac output and respiratory rate have been noted. A sudden increase in blood pressure has occurred with rapid intravenous administration. Arrhythmias may develop in anesthetized patients regardless of the route of administration, even at doses below those required for antiemetic effect. Use of benzquinamide in patients with moderate to severe hypertension or severe cardiovascular disease is questionable, particularly if the drug is given intravenously during anesthesia.

DOSAGE AND PREPARATIONS.
Intramuscular (preferred route): *Adults,* 0.5 to 1 mg/kg at least 15 minutes prior to administration of antineoplastic drugs or emergence from anesthesia. (The plasma half-life is approximately 40 minutes.) This dose may be repeated in one hour and then every three to four hours as required.
Intravenous: When therapeutic concentrations are desired in less than 15 minutes, a single dose of 0.2 to 0.4 mg/kg is given to *adults;* the drug may be diluted in 5% dextrose in water, sodium chloride injection, or lactated Ringer's injection and administered over one to three minutes or given as an intravenous infusion. Subsequent doses should be given intramuscularly.
 Emete-Con (Roerig). Powder equivalent to benzquinamide 50 mg.

DIPHENIDOL HYDROCHLORIDE
 [Vontrol]

ACTIONS AND USES. Diphenidol acts upon the aural vestibular apparatus and is useful in nausea and vomiting associated with general anesthesia, toxins, radiation therapy, and cancer chemotherapeutic agents. In adults, this drug also is effective in vertigo following surgery of the middle and inner ear and in Meniere's disease.

Because of possible rare adverse effects, such as hallucinations, disorientation, or confusion, diphenidol should be used only when close supervision is possible. Its use in the treatment of vertigo in children has not been investigated.

ADVERSE REACTIONS AND PRECAUTIONS. Because of its central anticholinergic actions, diphenidol may induce visual or auditory hallucinations, disorientation, or confusion. These effects usually occur within a few days after initiation of therapy (incidence, about 1 in 350 patients) and subside spontaneously within three days after the drug is discontinued.

Diphenidol occasionally has produced drowsiness, dryness of the mouth, tachycardia, and dizziness. Untoward effects reported rarely include rash, heartburn, headache, nausea, indigestion, blurred vision, malaise, and mild, transient hypotension.

Since over 90% of diphenidol is eliminated by the kidney, the drug is contraindicated in patients with severe renal impairment.

DOSAGE AND PREPARATIONS.
This drug should not be used in *infants under 6 months of age or weighing less than 12 kg.*
Oral: *Adults,* 25 to 50 mg four times daily; *children over 6 months or more than 12 kg,* 0.9 mg/kg initially, repeated in one hour if necessary; thereafter, doses may be given every four hours as needed (maximum, 5.5 mg/kg daily).
  Vontrol (Smith Kline & French). Tablets 25 mg.

TRIMETHOBENZAMIDE HYDROCHLORIDE
[Tigan]

ACTIONS AND USES. This drug inhibits stimuli at the chemoreceptor trigger zone in animals and has been promoted for use in alleviating nausea and reducing the frequency of vomiting during the immediate postoperative period, in radiation sickness, and in gastroenteritis. It is not as effective as the phenothiazines postoperatively. Trimethobenzamide has little or no value in the prevention or treatment of vertigo, motion sickness, or nausea and vomiting due to cancer chemotherapy.

In general, the effectiveness of the oral form appears to be somewhat unpredictable, which may be related to problems of bioavailability; reformulations of oral and suppository forms are currently being explored.

ADVERSE REACTIONS AND PRECAUTIONS. With usual doses, the incidence of adverse effects is low; with larger doses, drowsiness, vertigo, diarrhea, and cutaneous hypersensitivity reactions may occur. Extrapyramidal reactions or convulsions also have been noted; the latter occur more often in children and the elderly.

Pain at the site of injection and local irritation after rectal administration have been noted. Although the association between Reye's syndrome and trimethobenzamide has not

been proved, this drug should be avoided in children with signs and symptoms suggesting Reye's syndrome.

DOSAGE AND PREPARATIONS.
Intramuscular: *Adults,* 200 mg three or four times daily. To prevent postoperative vomiting, a single dose of 200 mg may be given before or during surgery; this dose may be repeated three hours after termination of anesthesia if needed. This route should not be used in *children.*
  Tigan (Beecham), **Generic.** Solution 100 mg/ml in 2 and 20 ml containers.
Oral: *Adults,* 250 mg three or four times daily; *children,* 4 to 5 mg/kg every six to eight hours.
  Generic. Capsules 250 mg.
  Tigan (Beecham). Capsules 100 and 250 mg.
Rectal: *Adults,* 200 mg three or four times daily; *children,* 4 to 5 mg/kg every six to eight hours. This route should not be used in *premature or newborn infants.*
  Tigan (Beecham), **Generic.** Suppositories 100 (pediatric) and 200 mg with benzocaine 2% (*Tigan* only).

Cannabinoids

DRONABINOL (delta-nine-tetrahydrocannabinol, THC)
[Marinol]

USES. This agent is the principal psychoactive component of marijuana. Although its antiemetic efficacy when given orally during cancer chemotherapy has been confirmed in a number of controlled studies (Cocchetto et al, 1981), superiority over other antiemetics has not been proved (Carey et al, 1983).

Dronabinol may be indicated for patients who do not respond to metoclopramide, butyrophenones, or phenothiazines or who develop tolerance to their antiemetic effect. It may be used initially in those patients who are less likely to be troubled by the drug's central nervous system adverse reactions. Dronabinol is useful in selected patients receiving certain antineoplastic drugs, such as methotrexate. It has reduced nausea and vomiting caused by high-dose cisplatin; in one study, the number of vomiting episodes was reduced to less than two in approximately one-third of patients (Gralla et al, 1984). This drug is less effective during chemotherapy with other agents (eg, cyclophosphamide, doxorubicin, mechlorethamine) (Gralla et al, 1984).

There is little experience with the use of dronabinol for nausea and vomiting associated with anesthesia and surgery, radiation therapy, and toxins.

ADVERSE REACTIONS AND PRECAUTIONS. Psychoactive effects occur with the antiemetic use of dronabinol and the duration of these effects and the antiemetic action is similar (about two to three hours). These effects (eg, mood changes, distortions in visual and time sense, somnolence) may be unacceptable to some patients, especially the elderly. Occasional dysphoria or hallucinations limit the usefulness of this drug in patients with psychiatric disorders. Since dronabinol has been reported to enhance seizure activity, it should be administered with caution to epileptic patients.

Dronabinol may produce transient tachycardia and large doses may cause orthostatic hypotension; these effects should be considered before the drug is used in patients with angina, mitral stenosis, and similar cardiovascular disorders.

The safety of dronabinol during pregnancy has not been determined (FDA Pregnancy Category B).

PHARMACOKINETICS. Dronabinol is slowly and erratically absorbed from the intestine. The peak plasma concentration is attained in 60 to 90 minutes, but the latent period may be significantly more prolonged. The systemic bioavailability is 10% to 20%. Dronabinol is 97% to 99% protein bound. The initial apparent volume of distribution is 0.036 L/kg, but this increases one hundredfold with long-term use as THC partitions into body fat.

Following oral administration, dronabinol is converted to 11-hydroxy-dronabinol (Lemberger et al, 1973), which possesses equivalent activity. This, in turn, is converted into even more polar and acidic compounds. Metabolism is impaired in patients with severe hepatic dysfunction. The metabolites and their conjugates are eliminated in the feces and urine. Urinary excretion of unchanged dronabinol and 11-hydroxy-dronabinol is negligible. The rate-limiting step is the return of dronabinol to the plasma from tissue binding sites. The terminal elimination half-life of dronabinol is about 19 hours and that of its metabolites is about 48 hours (Anderson and McGuire, 1981).

Currently, dronabinol is not available for intravenous or inhalational use; however, the pharmacokinetics after these routes has been compared with those observed after oral administration (Ohlsson et al, 1980).

DOSAGE AND PREPARATIONS.
Oral: Initially, 5 to 7.5 mg/M² every three to four hours beginning 4 to 12 hours before chemotherapy and continuing for 8 to 24 hours after therapy. The second dose can be increased by 2.5 mg/M² if the desired results are not achieved and if adverse reactions are not unacceptable. The manufacturer recommends a maximum dose of 15 mg/M².
Marinol (Roxane). Capsules (liquid, in sesame seed oil) 2.5, 5, and 10 mg.

NABILONE
[Cesamet]

Nabilone is a synthetic derivative of dronabinol. Its antiemetic activity is similar to that of the parent drug, but it may be more effective against vomiting induced by certain cancer chemotherapy agents, such as cisplatin. Clinical trials have demonstrated that nabilone is more effective than prochlorperazine in alleviating nausea and vomiting induced by moderately emetic agents (Vincent et al, 1983). Nabilone reduces the severity and duration of vomiting in 50% to 70% of patients refractory to other agents (Ward and Holmes, 1985). It also may relieve nausea and vomiting associated with low-dose cisplatin therapy (45 to 70 mg/M²) (Steele et al, 1980) and may be effective for nausea and vomiting refractory to phenothiazine therapy.

ADVERSE REACTIONS. Therapeutic doses cause side effects similar to those of dronabinol (Vincent et al, 1983), except for a lower incidence of tachycardia. Drowsiness, dizziness, and vertigo occur in 60% to 70% of patients. Orthostatic hypotension, ataxia, visual disturbances, and toxic psychoses have been reported and may necessitate withdrawal of the drug (Ward and Holmes, 1985).

PHARMACOKINETICS. Nabilone has a half-life of approximately two hours, but its active metabolites have half-lives of approximately 35 hours (Rubin et al, 1977). Following oral administration, peak plasma concentrations are reached in 60 to 120 minutes. This drug is excreted primarily in the bile (67%) (Lemberger et al, 1982).

DOSAGE AND PREPARATIONS.
Oral: 1 to 2 mg every 6 to 12 hours (Vincent et al, 1983).
Cesamet (Lilly).

Benzodiazepines

DIAZEPAM
[Valium, Valrelease]

Diazepam acts as a vestibular depressant. It may be useful in vertigo (particularly when associated with anxiety), Meniere's disease, and nausea and vomiting of psychogenic origin. In addition, this drug may relieve the anxiety associated with cancer chemotherapy.

For adverse reactions and precautions, see Chapter 5, Drugs Used for Anxiety and Sleep Disorders.

PHARMACOKINETICS. About 85% to 100% of a dose is absorbed from the gastrointestinal tract; peak plasma levels are attained about one hour after oral administration. The volume of distribution is 1.1 L/kg (0.95 to 2 L/kg), and 98% is protein bound.

Diazepam is metabolized by demethylation and hydroxylation. All metabolites are active. The final metabolic products are excreted in the urine as inactive conjugates. The half-life of diazepam ranges from 21 to 46 hours. It is prolonged in premature infants, elderly patients, and those with hepatic disease, who require a reduction in dosage. Dosage adjustment is not required in patients with renal disease.

DOSAGE AND PREPARATIONS.

Oral: *Adults,* for Meniere's disease, 5 mg every three hours.
  Valium (Roche), **Generic.** Tablets 2, 5, and 10 mg.
  Valrelease (Roche). Capsules (timed-release) 15 mg.
Intravenous: *Adults,* for Meniere's disease, 5 mg initially (maximum dose, 20 mg).
  Valium (Roche). Solution 5 mg/ml in 2 and 10 ml containers.

LORAZEPAM
[Ativan]

Although the use of lorazepam in nausea and vomiting induced by cancer chemotherapy is investigational, this drug may be a useful adjunct to established prophylactic agents (metoclopramide/dexamethasone). Lorazepam alone has weak antiemetic activity. Its primary effect may be induction of antegrade amnesia for four to six hours in approximately 50% of patients receiving 2 mg and in almost 100% of those receiving 4 mg.

Lorazepam has a high degree of subjective acceptance even in patients whose vomiting is not relieved. Further clinical studies are needed to determine the optimal dose and use of this agent, however. Most authorities employ lorazepam as an adjunct to metoclopramide/dexamethasone when this combination does not achieve a satisfactory response.

Mild to marked sedation and urinary incontinence are the most common side effects (Bowcock et al, 1984; *Oncology Times,* 1985).

DOSAGE AND PREPARATIONS.

Intravenous, Intramuscular: *Adults,* a single dose of 0.025 to 0.05 mg/kg injected slowly intravenously or given intramuscularly 30 minutes before chemotherapy (*Oncology Times,* 1985). The maximum dose should not exceed 4 mg. The initial intravenous or intramuscular dose may be supplemented with sublingual lorazepam 1 to 2 mg hourly as needed to maintain mild to moderate sedation.
  Ativan (Wyeth). Solution 2 and 4 mg/ml in 1, 2, and 10 ml containers; tablets 0.5, 1, and 2 mg.
  (Investigational indication)

Corticosteroids

DEXAMETHASONE

DEXAMETHASONE SODIUM PHOSPHATE

USES. Studies have shown that dexamethasone is superior to prochlorperazine in reducing nausea and vomiting caused by moderately emetic cancer chemotherapeutic regimens (eg, cyclophosphamide/methotrexate/fluorouracil) (Cassileth et al, 1983; Markman et al, 1984). In one study, it relieved or significantly reduced nausea and vomiting induced by cisplatin (50 to 75 mg/M^2) in approximately 65% of patients undergoing repeated courses of chemotherapy (Aapro and Alberts, 1981). This effect has not been demonstrated universally, but subjective patient preference for this agent has been noted (Strum et al, 1985). Currently, dexamethasone is used with high-dose intravenous metoclopramide and diphenhydramine for cisplatin-containing regimens and for highly emetic noncisplatin-containing regimens (see the Introduction). Dexamethasone decreases the incidence of diarrhea caused by high-dose metoclopramide. It also may prevent radiation-induced emesis.

The intermittent, short-term use of glucocorticoids generally is not associated with toxicity (see Chapter 61, Adrenal Corticosteroids in Nonendocrine Diseases).

DOSAGE AND PREPARATIONS. The optimal dose and schedule for dexamethasone in the treatment of nausea and vomiting caused by cancer chemotherapeutic agents have not been determined.

Intravenous: *Adults,* for mild vomiting caused by chemotherapy (eg, methotrexate, fluorouracil, vinblastine, vincristine, etoposide), 10 mg administered over three to five minutes 30 minutes before chemotherapy, followed by oral administration (if needed) of 8 mg 6, 12, and 18 hours after therapy.

For moderately severe vomiting caused by chemotherapy (eg, cyclophosphamide 500 mg to 1.1 g/M^2, doxorubicin more than 50 mg/M^2, carmustine 100 to 200 mg/M^2, lomustine less than 60 mg/M^2), 10 to 20 mg (Markman et al, 1984) 30 minutes before chemotherapy plus metoclopramide 0.5 mg/kg (see the evaluation on Metoclopramide). Dexamethasone 8 mg is then given orally every six hours for three doses (Strum et al, 1985).

For severe vomiting caused by chemotherapy (eg, cisplatin, mechlorethamine, cyclophosphamide more than 1.2 g/M^2, dactinomycin, dacarbazine more than 300 mg/M^2, carmustine more than 300 mg/M^2, lomustine more than 60 mg/M^2), 20 mg 30 minutes before chemotherapy plus metoclopramide 1 to 3 mg/kg and diphenhydramine 50 mg given concomitantly (Strum et al, 1985; Kris et al, 1985). (See the evaluation on Metoclopramide.)

Oral: *Adults,* for delayed nausea and vomiting caused by cisplatin, 24 hours after chemotherapy, 4 mg every eight hours for three days, then 2 mg every eight hours for three days; oral metoclopramide 0.5 mg/kg is given concomitantly every six hours for six days. Alternatively, 8 mg every eight hours on day 1 and every 12 hours on day 2, then 4 mg every 12 hours for three days. Oral prochlorperazine is given concomitantly in the following dosage: 20 to 30 mg every eight hours on day 1, 30 mg twice on day 2, and 15 mg twice daily for three days (Strum et al, 1985).

   See Chapter 61 for preparations.
   (Investigational indication)

METHYLPREDNISOLONE SODIUM SUCCINATE
[Solu-Medrol]

Methylprednisolone has been used investigationally as an antiemetic in cancer chemotherapy. The mechanism of action is unknown, although it has been postulated that inhibition of prostaglandin formation may be responsible for the antiemetic effect of corticosteroids.

Intravenous administration of large doses of methylprednisolone in combination with droperidol and chlorpromazine has been reported to relieve vomiting induced by cisplatin 120 mg/M^2 (Mason et al, 1982).

The intermittent, short-term use of glucocorticoids generally is not associated with toxicity (see Chapter 61, Adrenal Corticosteroids in Nonendocrine Diseases).

DOSAGE AND PREPARATIONS.

Intravenous: The definitive dosage for this investigational use of methylprednisolone has not been determined. Bolus doses of 125 to 500 mg have been given before chemotherapy and once or twice at six-hour intervals after chemotherapy.

   Solu-Medrol (Upjohn), **Generic.** Powder 40, 125, and 500 mg and 1 g.
   (Investigational indication)

MIXTURES

No controlled studies exist to support the contention that fixed-ratio combinations are as effective as single-entity preparations.

   Emetrol (Rorer). Solution (oral) containing balanced amounts of fructose, dextrose, and orthophosphoric acid with controlled hydrogen ion concentration (nonprescription). The manufacturer's recommended dose is one to two tablespoonsful, repeated every 15 minutes as needed.
   WANS (Webcon). Each suppository contains pyrilamine maleate 25 mg and pentobarbital sodium 30 mg (pediatric) or pyrilamine maleate 50 mg and pentobarbital sodium 50 or 100 mg. (FDA Pregnancy Category D)

Cited References

Antiemetic drug products for over-the-counter human use; tentative final order. *Federal Register* 44:41064-41073, (July 13) 1979.

Proceedings of investigational review—June 10, 1983: Lorazepam as adjunct in cancer chemotherapy. *Oncology Times* 7(suppl):1-27, (Feb) 1985.

Aapro MS, Alberts DS: High-dose dexamethasone for prevention of *cis*-platin-induced vomiting. *Cancer Chemother Pharmacol* 7:11-14, 1981.

Anderson PO, McGuire GG: Delta-9-tetrahydrocannabinol as antiemetic. *Am J Hosp Pharm* 38:639-646, 1981.

Barbezat GO: The vomiting patient: Rational approach. *Drugs* 22:246-253, 1981.

Beaver WT, Feise G: Comparison of analgesic effects of morphine, hydroxyzine, and their combination in patients with postoperative pain. *Adv Pain Res Ther* 1:553-557, 1976.

Borison HL, McCarthy LE: Neuropharmacology of chemotherapy-induced emesis. *Drugs* 25(suppl 1):8-17, 1983.

Bowcock SJ, et al: Antiemetic prophylaxis with high dose metoclopramide or lorazepam in vomiting induced by chemotherapy. *Br Med J* 288:1879, 1984.

Brogden RN, et al: Domperidone: Review of pharmacological activity, pharmacokinetics and therapeutic efficacy in symptomatic treatment of chronic dyspepsia and as antiemetic. *Drugs* 24:360-400, 1982.

Brookes GB: Meniere's disease: Practical approach to management. *Drugs* 25:77-89, 1983.

Cann PA, et al: Galactorrhoea as side effect of domperidone. *Br Med J* 286:1395-1396, 1983.

Carey MP, et al: Delta-9-tetrahydrocannabinol in cancer chemotherapy: Research problems and issues. *Ann Intern Med* 99:106-114, 1983.

Cassileth PA, et al: Antiemetic efficacy of dexamethasone therapy in patients receiving cancer chemotherapy. *Arch Intern Med* 143:1347-1349, 1983.

Citron ML, et al: Droperidol: Optimal dose and time of initiation, (abstract). *Proc Am Assoc Cancer Res/Am Soc Clin Oncol* 25:106, 1984.

Clissold SP, Heel RC: Transdermal hyoscine (scopolamine): Preliminary review of its pharmacodynamic properties and therapeutic efficacy. *Drugs* 29:189-207, 1985.

Cocchetto DM, et al: Critical review of safety and antiemetic efficacy of delta-9-tetrahydrocannabinol. *Drug Intell Clin Pharm* 15:867-875, 1981.

Dhondt F, et al: Domperidone (R33 812) suppositories: Effective antiemetic agent in diverse pediatric conditions: Multicenter trial. *Curr Ther Res* 24:912-923, 1978.

Eyre HJ, Ward JH: Control of cancer chemotherapy-induced nausea and vomiting. *Cancer* 54:2642-2648, 1984.

Fortner CL, et al: Combination antiemetic therapy in control of chemotherapy-induced emesis. *Drug Intell Clin Pharm* 19:21-24, 1985.

Gralla RJ: Metoclopramide: Review of antiemetic trials. *Drugs* 25(suppl 1):63-73, 1983.

Gralla RJ, et al: Antiemetic therapy: Review of recent studies and report of random assignment trial comparing metoclopramide with delta-9-tetrahydrocannabinol. *Cancer Treat Rep* 68:163-172, 1984.

Hoffbrand BI (ed): Domperidone in treatment of upper gastro-intestinal symptoms, (symposium). *Postgrad Med J* 55(suppl):1-54, 1979.

Jackson RT, et al: Ear, nose and throat diseases, in Avery GS (ed): *Drug Treatment: Principles and Practice of Clinical Pharmacology and Therapeutics,* ed 2. Sydney, ADIS Press, 1980, 335-361.

Kataria M, et al: Extrapyramidal side-effects of metoclopramide. *Lancet* 2:1254-1255, 1978.

Kris MG, et al: Improved control of cisplatin-induced emesis with high-dose metoclopramide and with combinations of metoclopramide, dexamethasone, and diphenhydramine: Results of consecutive trials in 255 patients. *Cancer* 55:527-534, 1985.

Laszlo J (ed): *Antiemetics and Cancer Chemotherapy.* Baltimore, Williams & Wilkins, 1983.

Lemberger L, et al: Comparative pharmacology of Δ^9-tetrahydrocannabinol and its metabolite, 11-OH-Δ^9-tetrahydrocannabinol. *J Clin Invest* 52:2411-2417, 1973.

Lemberger L, et al: Pharmacokinetics, metabolism and drug abuse potential of nabilone. *Cancer Treat Rep* 9(suppl B):17-23, 1982.

Loeser EA, et al: Comparison of droperidol, haloperidol and prochlorperazine as postoperative antiemetics. *Can Anaesth Soc J* 26:125-127, 1979.

Macnair AL: Cinnarizine in prophylaxis of car sickness in children. *Curr Med Res Opinion* 8:451-455, 1983.

Markman M, et al: Antiemetic efficacy of dexamethasone: Randomized, double-blind, crossover study with prochlorperazine in patients receiving cancer chemotherapy. *N Engl J Med* 311:549-552, 1984.

Mason BA, et al: Effective control of cisplatin-induced nausea using high-dose steroids and droperidol. *Cancer Treat Rep* 66:243-245, 1982.

McKenzie R, et al: Antiemetic effectiveness of intramuscular hydroxyzine compared with intramuscular droperidol. *Anesth Analg* 60:783-788, 1981.

Meyer BR, et al: Optimizing metoclopramide control of cisplatin-induced emesis. *Ann Intern Med* 100:393-395, 1984.

Milkovich I, van den Berg BJ: Evaluation of teratogenicity of certain antinauseant drugs. *Am J Obstet Gynecol* 125:244-248, 1976.

Moertel CG, et al: Controlled clinical evaluation of antiemetic drugs. *JAMA* 186:116-118, 1963.

Morran C, et al: Incidence of nausea and vomiting with cytotoxic chemotherapy: Prospective randomised trial of antiemetics. *Br Med J* 1:1323-1324, 1979.

Neidhart JA, et al: Specific antiemetics for specific cancer chemotherapeutic agents: Haloperidol versus benzquinamide. *Cancer* 47:1439-1443, 1981.

Ohlsson A, et al: Plasma delta-9-tetrahydrocannabinol concentrations and clinical effects after oral and intravenous administration and smoking. *Clin Pharmacol Ther* 28:409-416, 1980.

Palazzo MGA, Strunin L: Anaesthesia and emesis II: Prevention and management. *Can Anaesth Soc J* 31:407-415, 1984.

Peroutka SJ, Snyder SH: Antiemetics: Neurotransmitter receptor binding predicts therapeutic actions. *Lancet* 1:658-659, 1982.

Price N, et al: Transdermal delivery of scopolamine for prevention of motion-induced nausea in rough seas. *Clin Ther* 2:258-262, 1979.

Reyntjens A: Domperidone as antiemetic: Summary of research reports. *Postgrad Med J* 55:50-54, 1979.

Rubin A, et al: Physiologic disposition of nabilone, cannabinol derivative, in man. *Clin Pharmacol Ther* 22:85-91, 1977.

Shannon HE, et al: Lack of antiemetic effects of delta-9-tetrahydrocannabinol in apomorphine-induced emesis in the dog. *Life Sci* 23:49-54, 1978.

Steele N, et al: Double-blind comparison of antiemetic effects of nabilone and prochlorperazine on chemotherapy-induced emesis. *Cancer Treat Rep* 64:219-224, 1980.

Stoudemire A, et al: Recent advances in pharmacologic and behavioral management of chemotherapy-induced emesis. *Arch Intern Med* 144:1029-1033, 1984.

Strum SB, et al: Intravenous metoclopramide: Effective antiemetic in cancer chemotherapy. *JAMA* 247:2683-2686, 1982.

Strum SB, et al: Intravenous metoclopramide: Prevention of chemotherapy-induced nausea and vomiting; preliminary evaluation. *Cancer* 53:1432-1439, 1984.

Strum SB, et al: Control of acute onset and delayed-onset chemotherapy-induced nausea and emesis with metoclopramide-based regimens. *IM* 6:104-117, 1985.

Turner JS Jr: Practical approach to patient with vertigo: Outline of diagnosis and management for nonspecialist. *South Med J* 68:241-245, 1975.

Vincent BJ, et al: Review of cannabinoids and their antiemetic effectiveness. *Drugs* 25(suppl 1):52-62, 1983.

Wampler G: Pharmacology and clinical effectiveness of phenothiazines and related drugs for managing chemotherapy-induced emesis. *Drugs* 25(suppl 1):35-51, 1983.

Ward A, Holmes B: Nabilone: Preliminary review of its pharmacological properties and therapeutic use. *Drugs* 30:127-144, 1985.

Wilson J, et al: Continuous infusion droperidol: Anti-emetic therapy for cis-platinum (DDP) toxicity, (abstract). *Proc Am Assoc Cancer Res/Am Soc Clin Oncol* 22:241, 1981.

Wood CD: Antimotion sickness and antiemetic drugs. *Drugs* 17:471-479, 1979.

Wood CD, Graybiel A: Theory of antimotion sickness drug mechanisms. *Aerospace Med* 43:249-252, 1972.

Local Anesthetics   15

INTRODUCTION

REGIONAL ANESTHETIC TECHNIQUES

Infiltration Anesthesia

Peripheral Nerve Block Anesthesia

Epidural Anesthesia

Spinal (Subarachnoid) Anesthesia

Topical (Surface) Anesthesia

ADJUNCTS TO REGIONAL ANESTHETICS

ADVERSE REACTIONS AND PRECAUTIONS

DRUG EVALUATIONS

Local anesthetics produce loss of sensation and prevent muscle activity in circumscribed areas of the body by reversibly blocking nerve conduction (regional anesthesia). Local anesthetics (other than benzocaine) are amines. They are classified as esters or amides depending upon whether they are derivatives of para-aminobenzoic acid (eg, procaine) or aniline (eg, lidocaine). This chemical classification is clinically significant in that it indicates the principal site of biotransformation and the potential for allergic sensitization. Certain antihistaminic, anticholinergic, and adrenergic agents having a similar configuration also exhibit local anesthetic activity. The intrathecal or epidural administration of opioids alone or in conjunction with local anesthetics to relieve pain is discussed in Chapter 4, General Analgesics.

Local anesthetic bases are relatively insoluble in water but are soluble in lipid vehicles (eg, ointments). Salts of local anesthetic bases are water soluble and stable. In tissue water, the ratio of the nonionized base to the cationic (ionized) form depends upon the pKa of the compound (range, 7.6 to 9.0) and tissue fluid pH (see Table 1). The nonionized base penetrates the nerve sheath and membrane more readily than the cation. After re-equilibration at the internal pH of the axon, the cation is quantitatively the principal form that blocks nerve conduction.

The cationic form attaches to the internal axoplasmic membrane, possibly a phospholipid receptor, to decrease ion flux, particularly sodium. The rate of increase and amplitude of the nerve action potential are depressed to the degree that depolarization is not sufficient for a propagated action potential. At least 1 cm of nerve should be exposed to the local anesthetic to ensure conduction blockade, because the impulse in myelinated fibers is capable of skipping over two or three nodes of Ranvier.

The nonionized base also blocks nerve conduction, but this action is less prominent. The site appears to be the lipophilic areas of the nerve membrane, and the mechanism is believed to be similar to that of the general anesthetics, which are thought to act through a physicochemical mechanism rather than through specific receptors. After the anesthetic occupies a critical volume fraction of the nerve membrane, the membrane expands; this interferes with the conformational changes of the protein necessary for ion flux and depolarization. Topical anesthetics that possess a very low pKa (eg, benzocaine: pKa 3.5) or certain non-nitrogenous local anesthetic alcohols (eg, benzyl alcohol) may produce nerve block almost exclusively through the physicochemical mechanism.

The onset of anesthesia (essentially the rate and degree of penetration into individual nerves) principally depends upon the lipid solubility, molecular size, and quantity of available nonionized form of the local anesthetic (see Table 1). Thus, those with a high lipid solubility and/or a low pKa have a more rapid onset. The anesthetic's vasoactive action, the blood flow and pH at the site of injection, and the total volume and concentration of the anesthetic solution also are important determinants of onset of action.

Although carefully controlled studies have identified many exceptions (eg, brachial plexus block), which may be related to neurovascularity, it is believed that nerves generally are blocked in sequence according to their size. Thus, small nonmyelinated autonomic C fibers, thinly myelinated sensory delta A fibers (carrying pain, pressure, fine touch, and temperature sensations), and myelinated autonomic preganglionic B fibers are blocked before larger myelinated A fibers that transmit visceral sensory proprioception and motor functions. The clinical appearance of sensory or motor loss may vary from this order in larger nerves because of the geographical

TABLE 1.
PHYSICOCHEMICAL PROPERTIES OF LOCAL ANESTHETIC AGENTS

	Local Anesthetic	Partition Coefficient[a]	Protein Binding %	pKa	% Free Base [b]				
					pH 6.8	7.0	7.2	7.4	7.6
ESTERS	Chloroprocaine	0.14	NA[c]	8.7	1.2	2.0	3.1	4.8	7.4
	Procaine	0.02	5.8[d]	8.9	0.8	1.2	2.0	3.1	4.8
	Tetracaine	4.1	75.6[e]	8.5	2.0	3.1	4.8	7.4	11
AMIDES	Bupivacaine	27.5	95.6[e]	8.1	4.8	7.4	11	17	24
	Etidocaine	141	94[e]	7.7	11	17	24	33	44
	Lidocaine	2.9	64.3[e]	7.9	7.4	11	17	24	33
	Mepivacaine	0.8	77.5[e]	7.6	14	20	28	39	50
	Prilocaine	0.9	55 approx.	7.9	7.4	11	17	24	33

[a]n-Heptane/Buffer, pH 7.4

$$b \begin{cases} pH = pKa - \log \dfrac{[BH^+]}{[B]} \\ \% \text{ Free Base} = \dfrac{100}{1 + \dfrac{[BH^+]}{[B]}} \end{cases}$$

[c]NA = Not Available
[d]nerve homogenate binding
[e]plasma protein binding

location of fibers (either near the surface or core of the nerve). The concentration of drug required to block large nerve trunks is greater than that needed for smaller peripheral nerves. The duration of the block depends upon all of the factors listed for onset of anesthesia, as well as upon the extent of protein binding and whether or not a vasoconstrictor is added to the solution.

Pharmacokinetics: After the local anesthetic is absorbed from its site of administration into the systemic circulation, it is redistributed to other tissues and cleared from the body by metabolism and excretion. The anesthetic is redistributed to the various body tissues in proportion to its tissue/blood partition coefficient and the mass and perfusion of the tissue. The partition coefficient is affected in vivo by the extent to which the agent is bound to tissue and erythrocyte proteins, by its nonspecific binding to albumin and specific binding to alpha$_1$-acid glycoproteins in the plasma, and by the pH gradient. These factors determine the amount of free drug available for crossing membranes and the extent of ion trapping.

Ester-type local anesthetics are partly or completely hydrolyzed by plasma cholinesterase and, to a much lesser extent, by hepatic cholinesterase; the metabolites are excreted in the urine. After regional blockade with usual doses, hydrolysis is so rapid that only small concentrations of the ester anesthetics may be detected in the plasma. An exception is cocaine, 10% to 12% of which is excreted unchanged. The elimination half-life (t$1/2\beta$) for chloroprocaine is less than four minutes (Zsigmond and Kothary, 1979) and that of procaine is 7.7 minutes (Seifen et al, 1979). The t$1/2\beta$ is not available for tetracaine. The half-life of cocaine is dose dependent and may be determined by using the equation, t$1/2\beta$ = 13.5 + 24.5 x dose (mg/kg) (Barnett et al, 1981). The amides are metabolized in the liver by microsomal enzymes; the small quantity of unchanged amide that is excreted in the urine is not usually relevant in patients with impaired renal function. In contrast to the esters, appreciable concentrations of the amide anesthetics may appear in the plasma and may accumulate after multiple administrations.

Pharmacokinetic data for the commonly employed amides are shown in Table 2. The metabolism of both the esters and amides may be reduced in patients with hepatic disease, and the metabolism of the ester anesthetics is decreased in patients with suppressed or genetically atypical esterases. Conditions that decrease the volume of distribution (eg, congestive heart failure) may increase the plasma level of the local anesthetic and thus increase the likelihood of side effects. Factors that diminish protein binding can significantly elevate the plasma levels of the pharmacologically active form of those agents that are usually bound in excess of 90% (see Table 1); in the neonate, there is a compensatory increase in the volume of distribution. The specific binding capacity of the alpha$_1$-acid glycoproteins is limited. Thus, the greater the vascular concentration of a local anesthetic, such as bupivacaine, the greater will be the unbound fraction.

For most local anesthetics, the perineural concentration necessary to produce block is several hundredfold greater than the plasma level associated with side effects; therefore, the drug should be injected precisely at the appropriate site to avoid systemic toxicity. In general, the greatest rate of absorption, and hence the highest plasma level, is achieved by use of large volumes or high concentrations. Plasma levels are relatively unaffected by the speed of injection (except with the intravenous route) or by the age (except the very young and very old) of the patient. Thus, the least volume of the most dilute solution that is effective should be administered. Injection into highly vascular sites (eg, head and neck region, intercostal and paracervical blocks) and topical application to respiratory mucous membranes must be conducted with care. Solutions containing epinephrine may be efficacious in vascular sites.

Solutions of local anesthetics are usually isotonic to avoid edema, local irritation, and inflammation at the site of injection.

TABLE 2.
MEAN PHARMACOKINETIC DATA FOR AMIDE LOCAL ANESTHETICS

	$t\frac{1}{2}\alpha$ minutes	$t\frac{1}{2}\beta$ minutes	Vdss liters	Cltot liters/minute	% Excreted Unchanged
Bupivacaine	2.7	210	72	0.47	5
Etidocaine	2.2	156	133	1.22	1
Lidocaine	1.0	96	91	0.95	10
Mepivacaine	0.7	114	84	0.78	16

Solutions for subarachnoid anesthesia can be prepared in varying baricity to obtain the desired level of anesthesia.

REGIONAL ANESTHETIC TECHNIQUES

Regional (conduction) anesthetic techniques are classified according to the site of application: (1) infiltration (local), including extravascular and intravascular (intravenous regional anesthesia, Bier block); (2) peripheral nerve block (nerve or field block); (3) central neural block, ie, epidural (peridural, extradural, caudal), subarachnoid (spinal, intrathecal); and (4) topical (surface). The agents most commonly employed for these applications are listed in Tables 3 and 4.

To prevent accidental intravascular injection, needle placement *always* must be verified by gentle aspiration with a syringe before injection and periodically during administration. An intravenous infusion *always* should be started prior to injecting a substantial dose of a local anesthetic. Apparatus for administering oxygen and artificial ventilation, diazepam [Valium], vasopressors, intravenous fluids, succinylcholine [Anectine, Quelicin, Sucostrin], thiopental [Pentothal], and any additional drugs and equipment that may be useful for resuscitation should be available (de Jong, 1978).

Infiltration Anesthesia: Extravascular anesthesia includes the conventional technique of injecting the anesthetic in the immediate area of surgery.

In *intravascular anesthesia,* which is synonymous with *intravenous regional anesthesia* or *Bier block,* usually the entire distal portion of an extremity is anesthetized. A needle is inserted into a distal peripheral vein and secured in place. The extremity then is exsanguinated by gravity or with an elastic wrap (eg, Esmarch). A pneumatic tourniquet is then applied to the upper arm or leg. For surgery on the hand, it is applied nearly always to the upper arm and, for the foot, it is applied below the knee. The cuff is inflated to a pressure that occludes arterial flow. This technique is not applicable to the entire leg because of the large quantity of anesthetic that would be required. Tourniquet discomfort is relieved by use of a double tourniquet or by administration of small intravenous doses of an analgesic. A dilute solution of local anesthetic without preservatives or epinephrine is then injected and diffuses from the veins and capillaries to produce an evenly distributed infiltration to all nerves in the occluded limb. Satisfactory anesthesia is obtained within several minutes and is maintained as long as the circulation is occluded.

Prilocaine [Citanest] 0.5% *without epinephrine* is preferred for this technique by some anesthesiologists (Holmes, 1980), but 0.25% to 0.5% lidocaine is employed most commonly.

TABLE 3.
LOCAL ANESTHETICS PRINCIPALLY EMPLOYED FOR INJECTION

	Infiltration	Nerve Block	Intravenous Regional	Epidural	Subarachnoid
AMIDES					
Bupivacaine [Marcaine, Sensorcaine]	0.25%	0.25–0.5%	NR	0.25–0.75%	—
Dibucaine [Nupercaine]	—	—	—	—	0.25% (†)
Etidocaine [Duranest]	0.5%	0.5–1%	—	0.5–1.5%	—
Lidocaine [Xylocaine]	0.5%	0.5–2%	0.5%*	1–2%	1.5–5%
Mepivacaine [Carbocaine]	0.5–1%	1–2%	—	1–2%	—
Prilocaine [Citanest]	1–2%	1–3%	0.5%*	1–3%	—
AMINOBENZOATE ESTERS					
Chloroprocaine [Nesacaine]	1%	—	NR	2–3%	NR
Procaine [Novocain]	0.25–0.5%	1–2%	—	NR	10%
Tetracaine [Pontocaine]	NR	NR	—	NR	1%

(†) = Infrequent application   — = Not in current use or ineffective   NR = Not recommended   * = Without epineprine

TABLE 4.
LOCAL ANESTHETICS EMPLOYED FOR TOPICAL (SURFACE) APPLICATION

	Eye	Ear	Nose	Throat	Urethra	Rectum	Skin
AMIDES							
Dibucaine [Nupercainal]	–	+	–	–	–	+	+
Lidocaine [Xylocaine]	–	–	–	–	–	–	+
Lidocaine Hydrochloride [Xylocaine]	–	+	+	+	+	–	–
ESTERS							
Benzoic Acid Esters							
Cocaine Hydrochloride	NR*	+	+	+	–	–	–
Hexylcaine Hydrochloride [Cyclaine]	NR	–	+	+	+	–	–
Proparacaine Hydrochloride [Alcaine, Ophthaine]	+	–	–	–	–	–	–
Aminobenzoate Esters							
Benzocaine [Americaine]	–	+	+	+	+	+	+
Butamben Picrate [Butesin Picrate]	–	–	–	–	–	–	+
Tetracaine Hydrochloride [Pontocaine]	+	+	+	+	–	+	+
MISCELLANEOUS							
Dyclonine Hydrochloride [Dyclone]	–	–	–	+	+	+	+
Pramoxine Hydrochloride [Tronolane, Tronothane]	–	–	–	+	–	+	+

+ = In current use   – = Not in current use or ineffective   NR = Not Recommended   *See text

Peripheral Nerve Block Anesthesia: In *field block anesthesia*, the solution is injected close to the nerves around the area to be anesthetized. In *nerve block anesthesia*, a localized perineural injection is made at an access point along the course of a nerve distant from the operative site. More concentrated solutions of drug often are required because these nerves have a sheath and a relatively large diameter.

The drugs most commonly used for infiltration and peripheral nerve block anesthesia include chloroprocaine [Nesacaine], lidocaine [Xylocaine], mepivacaine [Carbocaine], prilocaine [Citanest], and procaine [Novocain]. Bupivacaine [Marcaine, Sensorcaine] and etidocaine [Duranest] are indicated if a more prolonged block is desired.

Epidural Anesthesia: Epidural anesthesia is accomplished by injecting a local anesthetic into the epidural space (Bromage, 1978; Cousins and Bridenbaugh, 1980). In lumbar epidural anesthesia, the injection is usually made in an interspace between the second lumbar and first sacral vertebrae to avoid injury to the spinal cord, which ends at the first lumbar vertebra in 95% of individuals. In caudal anesthesia, the solution is introduced into the caudal canal (a continuation of the epidural space) through the sacral hiatus.

In general, the number of spinal segments blocked is determined by the site of injection (lumbar or caudal), the position of the patient (fewer segments with sitting), the quantity of drug injected (more segments with larger dose), possibly the age of the patient (more segments in children and the elderly), pregnancy (more segments at term), and extent of arteriosclerosis (more segments if occlusive arterial disease is present). Increasing the concentration of the anesthetic shortens the onset time and increases the degree of motor blockade. Cephalad spread of anesthetic occurs more readily than sacral spread following lumbar epidural injection; a significant delay or absence of anesthesia at the first and second sacral

segments frequently is observed (Concepcion and Covino, 1984).

Physiologic changes are slower in onset with epidural anesthesia than with subarachnoid anesthesia. Many physicians believe that a test dose should be administered at least five minutes before the main dose in an attempt to detect inadvertent intravenous or subarachnoid (spinal) injection. The addition of 1:200,000 epinephrine to the test dose aids in the recognition of an intravascular injection. The relatively large dose needed and the great vascularity of the epidural space increase the possibility of systemic reactions. Repeated fractional injections through an in situ catheter (continuous epidural anesthesia) may be used to prolong epidural anesthesia.

The drugs most commonly employed for epidural anesthesia are chloroprocaine, lidocaine, or mepivacaine for surgical procedures of one to two hours and bupivacaine or etidocaine for procedures lasting longer than two hours. Selection is based on the degree of motor blockade desired, if any, and the required duration of sensory blockade (see the evaluations). Prilocaine 3% without epinephrine in total doses of less than 600 mg is useful if a vasoconstrictor must be avoided. This drug should not be used, however, in obstetrics. The anesthetics differ in the degree of motor nerve blockade produced by anesthetic doses. This is most marked with bupivacaine, which in a concentration of 0.25% to 0.5% produces adequate analgesia for obstetrics or postoperative pain relief with minimal motor blockade (Concepcion and Covino, 1984).

To minimize the danger of injecting a solution contaminated by chemicals or bacteria, only single-dose containers should be used. Epinephrine reduces the peak blood concentration of most local anesthetics.

Spinal (Subarachnoid) Anesthesia: With this technique, the local anesthetic agent is injected into the subarachnoid space, usually in an interspace between the second and fifth lumbar vertebrae. The level of anesthesia is determined by the site of injection, density and volume of the solution, and position of the patient during and immediately after administration of the anesthetic. Pregnancy or abdominal tumors decrease spinal fluid volume, resulting in a significant reduction in the dosage requirement. Factors that do not affect the spread of spinal anesthetic solutions are the rate of injection, age or body weight (if the length and volume of the subarachnoid space are the same), sudden increases in cerebrospinal fluid pressure (eg, occurring during coughing, straining, or Valsalva maneuver), or the presence in the anesthetic solution of a vasoconstrictor (Greene, 1981).

In addition to isobaric solutions for use in spinal anesthesia, hyperbaric (with dextrose) solutions possessing a density greater than 1.007 or hypobaric (in distilled water) solutions with a density less than 1.005 are available to assure that the specific gravity is higher or lower than that of cerebrospinal fluid, respectively. The hypobaric (light) solutions gravitate caudad and the hyperbaric (heavy) solutions gravitate cephalad when the patient is in the head-down (Trendelenburg) position.

Consciousness is preserved at all times unless the reticular activating system is obtunded during high levels of spinal anesthesia or, more commonly, profound arterial hypotension develops secondary to the sympathetic blockade that is always produced. The degree of sympathetic blockade is determined by the level of anesthesia but extends further cephalad than either sensory or motor blockade. Hypotension is the most important complication commonly associated with spinal anesthesia. It is intensified by changes in position that promote diminished venous return and by pre-existing hypertension, hypovolemia, pregnancy, or old age. The patient is at greatest risk during the first 30 minutes after spinal anesthesia is induced. Individual tolerance for hypotension varies; as a general rule, a reduction of 25% of the preanesthetic pressure requires intervention (Greene, 1981). If practical, the patient should be placed in a head-down position with the legs raised to promote venous return. Oxygen should be administered. The cardiac output can be increased by the administration of ephedrine or mephentermine [Wyamine] and the judicious use of increased fluid administration.

The duration of anesthesia depends upon the rate at which the drug leaves the nerve tissue, primarily by vascular absorption. The local anesthetic diffuses within the cerebrospinal fluid and is removed primarily by the venous circulation; a small quantity is removed by lymphatic drainage. Enzymatic hydrolysis of the drugs in cerebrospinal fluid is insignificant. Duration may be increased 50% to 100% by adding epinephrine to the solution. Fractional injections of solutions without a vasoconstrictor through an in situ catheter (continuous spinal anesthesia) also may be used to prolong spinal anesthesia. The repeated injection of a local anesthetic is associated with diminished effectiveness and duration of action (tachyphylaxis), probably as the result of local pH changes. If the concentration of the anesthetic in solution is increased, the duration is increased, but not proportionally.

Tetracaine and lidocaine are most widely used for spinal anesthesia; procaine, dibucaine [Nupercaine], and bupivacaine also can be administered. To minimize the danger of injecting a contaminated solution, only single-dose containers should be employed, and only local anesthetics specifically prepared for subarachnoid anesthesia should be used.

The dose administered for spinal anesthesia generally is too small, even if injected intravascularly, to produce systemic toxicity or to exert any direct depressant effects upon the fetus when given during labor and delivery.

Topical (Surface) Anesthesia: Cationic forms of local anesthetics do not penetrate intact skin, but nonionized (base) forms do penetrate to a limited degree. As a result, only certain local anesthetics (see Table 4) are capable of relieving pruritus, burning, and surface pain on intact skin and the less sensitive mucous membranes (anus and rectum).

Both cationic and nonionized forms penetrate abraded skin. Wounds, ulcers, and burns are treated with preparations that are relatively insoluble in tissue fluids. This generally reduces the possibility of systemic toxicity if the area of application is not too extensive and administration is not repeated too frequently. Mucous membranes of the nose, mouth, pharynx, larynx, trachea, bronchi, vagina, and urethra are readily anesthetized by both cationic and nonionized forms. However, since absorption from certain of these areas may be quite rapid, the smallest dose required for adequate analgesia should be administered to minimize the possibility of systemic reactions. The addition of a vasoconstrictor generally does not lessen the incidence of these reactions.

The use of local anesthetics on conjunctival and corneal tissues represents a form of topical application. Because benoxinate and proparacaine [Ak-Taine, Alcaine, Ophthaine, Ophthetic] are used only topically on the eye, they are discussed in Chapter 20, Miscellaneous Ophthalmic Preparations. The ophthalmologic use of cocaine and tetracaine [Pontocaine] also is discussed in Chapter 20; however, in view of their more widespread local anesthetic use, their evaluations appear in this chapter as well.

ADJUNCTS TO REGIONAL ANESTHETICS

Vasoconstrictors may be added to local anesthetic solutions used for infiltration, peripheral nerve block, epidural, and subarachnoid anesthesia to decrease the rate of absorption. In general, this prolongs the anesthetic effect and reduces the risk of systemic reactions, as well as increases the frequency of complete conduction blocks at low anesthetic concentration. The addition of a vasoconstrictor is more appropriate than increasing the concentration to prolong the duration. Epinephrine is the vasoconstrictor most commonly used for infiltration, nerve block, epidural, and spinal anesthesia.

Local anesthetic solutions containing epinephrine should not be used for nerve blocks in areas supplied by end-arteries (eg, digits, ears, nose, penis) because they may cause ischemia, which could progress to necrosis. The total dosage of epinephrine should not exceed 0.2 mg, and concentrations exceeding 1:200,000 are not recommended. Solutions containing epinephrine for infiltration and nerve blocks should be used with caution in patients in labor because of the danger of producing vasoconstriction in uterine blood vessels, which may decrease placental circulation, diminish the intensity of uterine contractions, and prolong labor. It also is undesirable to use solutions containing epinephrine in patients with thyrotoxicosis. The risk of using vasoconstrictor-containing solutions in patients with severe cardiovascular disease must be assessed individually. The systemic effects of epinephrine may be potentiated in patients receiving tricyclic antidepressants or monoamine oxidase inhibitors. Epinephrine should not be injected into areas with diminished blood flow resulting from severe peripheral vascular disease.

Cocaine is the only local anesthetic that exhibits an inherent vasoconstrictor action, although there is some evidence that low concentrations of mepivacaine and lidocaine may also possess this effect (Blair, 1975). Moderate to high concentrations of all local anesthetics, except cocaine, have a vasodilator effect.

ADVERSE REACTIONS AND PRECAUTIONS

Hypersensitivity Reactions: Unpredictable adverse reactions (ie, hypersensitivity, including anaphylaxis) are extremely rare. If a patient is hypersensitive to a particular local anesthetic, a drug from a different chemical group should be substituted. Allergic reactions usually are associated with ester-type agents, which are derivatives of p-aminobenzoic acid, a potent sensitizer. Use of a test dose to determine hypersensitivity may not be reliable. If rash, urticaria, edema, or other manifestations of allergy develop during use of a topical anesthetic, the drug should be discontinued. To minimize the possibility of a serious allergic reaction, topical preparations should not be applied for prolonged periods except under continual supervision.

Systemic Reactions: The most common cause of toxic reactions to local anesthetics is inadvertent intravascular injection. Predictable central nervous system reactions occur when plasma concentrations reach a critical level and are qualitatively similar for all local anesthetics. However, when absorption is slow, peak plasma levels (and presumably the possibility of prolonged systemic reactions) may not be observed for 20 to 30 minutes after the drug is injected. Because of accumulation, systemic reactions are more likely to occur after repeated doses. The reactions primarily involve the central nervous system and, secondarily, the cardiovascular system.

Signs and symptoms of central nervous system toxicity are restlessness, lightheadedness and dizziness, circumoral paresthesias, tinnitus, difficulty in focusing, and tremors; convulsions may follow. Subconvulsive doses of lidocaine [Xylocaine] and procaine [Novocain] are often associated with sedation or sleep, which has not been reported with other local anesthetics (Covino and Vassallo, 1976). If the drug plasma level is high, ventilatory depression, progressing to respiratory arrest and coma, may develop as a result of generalized central nervous system depression.

The most important and initial treatment should be to ensure and maintain a patent airway and to support ventilation with oxygen and assisted or controlled respiration if required.

Persistent convulsions may be controlled by the intravenous administration of diazepam in 2.5-mg increments. Some authors suggest that adequate doses of short-acting barbiturates or succinylcholine be given to permit controlled ventilation. Usual preoperative doses of barbiturates have little or no value in averting central nervous system reactions. However, diazepam 0.1 to 0.15 mg/kg has been recommended for prophylaxis.

Cardiovascular toxicity is characterized by bradycardia, hypotension, and heart block that may ultimately progress to cardiac arrest. Cardiovascular symptoms usually begin after signs of central nervous system toxicity are established and may reflect hypoxia more than a direct action of the anesthetic. However, rapid inadvertent intravenous injection can cause an abrupt hypotensive episode. In animal studies, bupivacaine and etidocaine have been associated with nodal or ventricular arrhythmias before or at the onset of convulsions and in the absence of such predisposing factors as hypoxemia, acidemia, and hyperkalemia. It is recommended that injection of large doses of these agents be made in fractional increments of 30 mg given at two-minute intervals with monitoring for symptoms of overdosage (Marx, 1984).

Acute circulatory failure is treated with fluids and vasopressors (eg, ephedrine) administered intravenously. If respiratory arrest occurs or asystole is suspected, artificial ventilation and external cardiac massage must be instituted immediately.

Systemic effects (anxiety, restlessness, tremors, palpitations, tachycardia, anginal pain, dizziness, headache, and hypertension) may be produced by the epinephrine that is added to local anesthetics for parenteral use. These reactions are seen most frequently in office dentistry and are usually mild and transient when a 1:200,000 concentration is used.

Local Reactions: The most common local adverse reaction caused by local anesthetics is contact dermatitis characterized by erythema and pruritus that may progress to vesiculation and oozing. This occurs most commonly in individuals (eg, physicians, dentists) who are frequently exposed to ester-type local anesthetics or those receiving prolonged self-medication (eg, hemorrhoidal preparations). These reactions have become rare since the amides were introduced.

Repeated corneal application of topical anesthetics should be avoided since keratitis, which occasionally may lead to permanent reduction in visual acuity, can occur.

Effects on Infants: Local anesthetics diffuse readily through the placenta and reports have appeared of diminished muscle strength and tone and decreased rooting behavior in the newborn infant, although Apgar scores are normal. If used in excessive quantities, particularly in paracervical block, the increased absorption of these agents may cause fetal bradycardia and central nervous system depression after birth.

Bupivacaine [Marcaine, Sensorcaine] and etidocaine [Duranest] have much lower umbilical vein/maternal vein plasma concentration ratios than alternative agents. This may be related to their high degree of protein binding (94% to 96%) or it may reflect their greater uptake by fetal tissues. Both drugs have high lipid partition coefficients and are absorbed by fetal tissues in greater amounts than lidocaine. In neurobehavioral tests administered to infants a few hours after birth, epidural anesthesia with bupivacaine was reported to cause less depression than with lidocaine or mepivacaine.

Drug Evaluations

Selected uses of currently available local anesthetics appear in Tables 3 and 4. When allergic, pharmacokinetic, or individual factors necessitate use of a different agent, selection of an alternative drug will depend upon the factor or factors involved. Some topical preparations may contain a small quantity of antimicrobial agent as a preservative, but no claim is made for antimicrobial action.

Suggested maximum single doses appear in the evaluations for those local anesthetics recommended for injection; however, there is considerable evidence that these amounts may be excessive in some clinical situations (Covino, 1978). Therefore, suggested doses should be considered only as guidelines.

BENZOCAINE
[Americaine]

Benzocaine is used for surface anesthesia of the skin and mucous membranes. It is one of the most widely used agents for relief of sunburn, pruritus, and minor burns. Ointments containing less than 10% benzocaine or acidic preparations are ineffective on intact or mildly sunburned skin.

Since benzocaine is poorly soluble in water and poorly absorbed, the incidence of systemic toxic reactions is low. The possibility of sensitization should always be considered. Preparations containing benzocaine may cause methemoglobinemia in susceptible infants. For additional information on adverse reactions and precautions, see the Introduction.

DOSAGE AND PREPARATIONS.
Topical: The appropriate preparation is applied as required.
   Generic. Cream 5% (nonprescription); bulk (crystals, powder).
   Americaine Anesthetic (American Critical Care). Aerosol containing benzocaine 20% in a water-dispersible base in 20, 60, and 120 ml containers (nonprescription).
   Americaine Hemorrhoidal Ointment (American Critical Care). Ointment containing benzocaine 20% and benzethonium chloride 0.1% in a water-soluble polyethylene glycol base in 30 g containers (nonprescription).
   Americaine Anesthetic Lubricant (American Critical Care). Gel containing benzocaine 20% and benzethonium chloride 0.1% in a water-soluble base of polyethylene glycol 300 and 4,000 in 2.5 and 30 g containers.
   Americaine Otic (American Critical Care). Solution 20% in a water-soluble base (1% [w/w] glycerin and polyethylene glycol 300) with benzethonium chloride 0.1% in 15 ml containers.

BUPIVACAINE HYDROCHLORIDE
[Marcaine, Sensorcaine]

ACTIONS AND USES. This amide, related chemically to mepivacaine, is used for infiltration, nerve block, spinal, and epidural anesthesia. Its most important property is its long duration of action. Bupivacaine is particularly useful when administered by continuous epidural techniques to relieve pain during labor, since the need for supplemental doses is less than with mepivacaine or lidocaine. When the 0.5% solution is used in obstetrics, the interval between doses is usually two to three hours. Although bupivacaine may accumulate in the mother during continuous epidural anesthesia, few systemic toxic reactions have been reported, since delivery usually occurs before toxic plasma levels are attained. It is contraindicated for paracervical block and is not recommended for intravenous regional block. This anesthetic is classified in FDA Pregnancy Category C. Data on use of bupivacaine in children under 12 years is incomplete.

The potency of bupivacaine is similar to that of etidocaine (ie, four times greater than that of mepivacaine, lidocaine, and prilocaine). In general, the onset of action is slower and the interval to maximal anesthesia is longer with bupivacaine than with lidocaine. The duration of action is two to three times longer than with mepivacaine and lidocaine. Some peripheral nerve blocks may last more than 24 hours.

ADVERSE REACTIONS AND PRECAUTIONS. The systemic reactions produced by bupivacaine are qualitatively similar to those produced by other local anesthetics. However, ventricular arrhythmias have been observed following intravenous administration (Clarkson and Hondeghem, 1985). For additional information on adverse reactions and precautions, see the Introduction.

DOSAGE AND PREPARATIONS.
Injection: As a general guide, the maximal single dose in healthy *adults* should not exceed 175 mg without epinephrine and 225 mg with epinephrine 1:200,000. This dose should not be repeated at intervals of less than three hours. A maximal total dosage of 400 mg (8 mg/kg) in 24 hours generally should not be exceeded.

If the 0.5% solution without epinephrine is used for continuous epidural anesthesia in obstetric patients, the total dose probably should not exceed 320 mg over a 12-hour period. In epidural anesthesia in nonobstetric patients, the 0.5% concentration produces moderate motor blockade but analgesia may be inadequate in 5% to 10% of patients; the 0.75% solution produces good analgesia and motor blockade of long duration. Solutions of 0.75% are not recommended for obstetric anesthesia.
Infiltration: Without epinephrine, up to 70 ml of the 0.25% solution (approximate duration of analgesia, 200 minutes); with epinephrine, up to 90 ml of the 0.25% solution (approximate duration of analgesia, 400 minutes).
Intravenous regional: The use of bupivacaine for intravenous regional anesthesia is not recommended.
Nerve block: Without epinephrine, up to 70 ml of the 0.25% solution or 35 ml of the 0.5% solution; with epinephrine, up to 90 ml of the 0.25% solution or 45 ml of the 0.5% solution. The 0.5% solution is required to produce a consistent complete motor block of the larger nerves. Onset of anesthesia is slow

(approximately 10 to 20 minutes). The duration of analgesia with either concentration is about 400 minutes and is little affected by epinephrine. A concentration of 0.75% is employed for retrobulbar block, but this concentration is not recommended for other nerve blocks.

Caudal: With or without epinephrine, for obstetrical analgesia and perineal surgery, up to 30 ml of the 0.25% solution; for surgery of the lower extremities, up to 30 ml of the 0.5% solution. A single dose of either the 0.25% or 0.5% solution does not reliably produce motor block and, when used for a continuous technique, supplemental doses of the 0.25% or 0.5% solution are necessary. Only single-dose containers should be used.

Lumbar epidural: With epinephrine, for obstetrical analgesia and perineal surgery and for relief of postoperative pain, up to 20 ml of the 0.25% solution; for obstetrical analgesia and surgery of the lower extremities, up to 20 ml of the 0.5% solution with or without epinephrine. When used for a continuous technique, supplemental 5- to 10-ml doses of the 0.25% or 0.5% solution usually produce excellent sensory analgesia. Motor block, such as that required for abdominal surgery, usually can be obtained by use of up to 20 ml of the 0.75% solution. Repeated use of the 0.75% solution for continuous epidural anesthesia is inadvisable because of the possibility of accumulation. Only single-dose containers should be used.

Generic. Solution 0.25%, 0.5%, and 0.75%.

Marcaine (Winthrop-Breon). Solution 0.25% and 0.5% in 10, 30, and 50 ml containers; 0.75% in 10 and 30 ml containers; 0.25% and 0.5% with epinephrine 1:200,000 in 10, 30, and 50 ml containers; 0.75% with epinephrine 1:200,000 in 30 ml containers; 0.75% with 8.25% dextrose in 2 ml containers for spinal anesthesia. Solutions that do not contain epinephrine may be autoclaved. Solutions in multiple-dose (50 ml) containers also contain methylparaben.

Sensorcaine (Astra). Solution (sterile) 0.25% and 0.5% in 30 and 50 ml containers; 0.75% in 30 ml containers; 0.5% and 0.75% with epinephrine 1:200,000 in 30 ml containers.

BUTAMBEN PICRATE
[Butesin Picrate]

Butamben is used on the skin to relieve pruritus and burning. Since it is relatively insoluble in water and thus poorly absorbed, this drug may remain in contact with the skin for a prolonged period with a low incidence of systemic reactions.

Butamben picrate may cause a rash in sensitive individuals. For additional information on adverse reactions and precautions, see the Introduction.

DOSAGE AND PREPARATIONS.
Topical: The ointment is applied to affected areas as required.

Butesin Picrate (Abbott). Ointment 1% in 28.4 g containers (nonprescription).

CHLOROPROCAINE HYDROCHLORIDE
[Nesacaine, Nesacaine-CE]

Chloroprocaine, a chlorinated analogue of procaine, is used for infiltration, peripheral nerve block, caudal, and epidural anesthesia. The drug is not effective topically and has not been studied sufficiently to be used for subarachnoid anesthesia. Its anesthetic potency is slightly greater than that of procaine; its onset of action is more rapid and the duration is slightly shorter. Nerve blocks last an average of one hour. The addition of epinephrine 1:200,000 prolongs the duration to as much as one and one-half hours.

ADVERSE REACTIONS AND PRECAUTIONS. The systemic toxicity of chloroprocaine is less than that of all other local anesthetics because of its rapid hydrolysis by plasma cholinesterase (even in the presence of decreased maternal and fetal cholinesterase activity at term), which shortens the plasma half-life. This anesthetic is classified in FDA Pregnancy Category C.

Neural irritation may follow accidental subarachnoid administration of a large volume of chloroprocaine solution (Gissen et al, 1984; Wang et al, 1984).

For additional information on adverse reactions and precautions, see the Introduction.

DOSAGE AND PREPARATIONS.
Injection: As a general guide, the maximal single dose is 800 mg (20 mg/kg) without epinephrine and 1 g with epinephrine 1:200,000. Repeated doses of up to 300 mg without epinephrine and 600 mg with epinephrine 1:200,000 may be given at 50-minute intervals.

Infiltration: Without epinephrine, up to 80 ml of the 1% solution; with epinephrine 1:200,000, 100 ml of the 1% solution. Three ml of 1% chloroprocaine is injected at each of four sites for paracervical block; 3 to 4 ml of the 1% solution without epinephrine may be used for digital blocks.

Peripheral nerve block: The dose of the 1% or 2% solution, with or without epinephrine 1:200,000, depends upon the type of block and intensity and duration of effect needed: 10 ml of a 2% solution on each side for pudendal nerve block, 30 to 40 ml of a 2% solution for brachial plexus block, 2 to 3 ml of a 2% solution for mandibular block, and 0.5 to 1 ml of a 2% solution for infraorbital block.

Caudal: Initially, 15 to 25 ml (depending upon the size of the patient) of the 2% or 3% *Nesacaine-CE* solution. Repeated doses may be given at 40- to 60-minute intervals as required; epinephrine 1:200,000 may be used to prolong the action.

Lumbar and sacral epidural: The usual total initial dose, with or without epinephrine 1:200,000, is 15 to 25 ml of the 2% or 3% *Nesacaine-CE* solution. Supplemental doses of 10 to 20 ml may be given at 40- to 50-minute intervals.

Nesacaine (Astra). Solution 1% and 2% in 30 ml containers (2% not for caudal or epidural anesthesia).

Nesacaine-CE (Astra). Solution 2% and 3% in 30 ml containers (for caudal or epidural anesthesia; contains no preservative).

COCAINE HYDROCHLORIDE

ACTIONS AND USES. Cocaine is a naturally occurring alkaloid that produces excellent topical anesthesia and intense vasoconstriction when applied to mucous surfaces. It is used for anesthesia in the ear, nose, and throat and in bronchoscopy. The addition of epinephrine is not only unnecessary (it does not delay absorption), but it may increase the likelihood of cardiac arrhythmias. The moistening of dry cocaine powder with epinephrine solution to form so-called "cocaine mud" for use on the nasal mucosa is particularly dangerous and is not recommended. Cocaine is not used parenterally.

Onset of action is rapid (one minute) with a duration of approximately one hour, depending upon the dose and concentration applied.

ADVERSE REACTIONS AND PRECAUTIONS. Toxic symptoms occur frequently because cocaine is absorbed readily after topical application, in spite of its vasoconstrictor action, and dosage is difficult to monitor carefully. The toxic signs differ slightly from those observed with other local anesthetics in that pronounced central and peripheral sympathetic activity occur concurrently. The central nervous system effects include euphoria and cortical stimulation manifested by excitement, restlessness, and tremors followed by grand mal seizures. Tachycardia and elevated blood pressure also are observed initially.

Repeated use results in psychic dependence and tolerance; therefore, cocaine is classified as a Schedule II drug under the Controlled Substances Act.

Cocaine exerts an indirect adrenergic effect by interfering with the tissue uptake of circulating catecholamines. This effect potentiates the actions of endogenous and exogenous epinephrine and norepinephrine. Ventricular fibrillation caused by absorption of excessive amounts of cocaine may occur, particularly if a general anesthetic that sensitizes the myocardium to catecholamines also is being administered. For this reason, cocaine should be used with extreme caution, if at all, in patients with hypertension, severe cardiovascular disease, or thyrotoxicosis or in patients taking drugs that also potentiate catecholamines (eg, guanethidine, monoamine oxidase inhibitors). For additional information on adverse reactions and precautions, see the Introduction.

Solutions of cocaine are unstable and deteriorate on standing; boiling and autoclaving cause decomposition.

DOSAGE AND PREPARATIONS.
Topical: For the ear, nose, and throat and for bronchoscopy, concentrations of 4% are used. A 0.25% to 0.5% solution is satisfactory for corneal anesthesia, but cocaine has largely been replaced by other agents because of its tendency to produce transient irregularity of the corneal epithelium (see also Chapter 20, Miscellaneous Ophthalmic Preparations). As a general guide, the maximal dose is 150 to 200 mg. The lowest concentration and smallest volume possible should be applied. Concentrations greater than 4% may decrease time to onset of anesthesia slightly, but their use is not advisable because of the potential for increasing the incidence and severity of systemic toxic reactions.

Generic. Tablets (soluble) 135 mg; solution (topical) 40 and 100 mg/ml; bulk (crystals, powder).

DIBUCAINE
[Nupercainal]

DIBUCAINE HYDROCHLORIDE
[Nupercaine]

Dibucaine is one of the most potent and toxic of the long-acting anesthetics when used parenterally. It is 15 to 20 times more potent and 15 times more toxic than procaine when injected. The parenteral dosage form is indicated only for spinal anesthesia. Hyperbaric (heavy), hypobaric (light), and isobaric solutions are available for subarachnoid anesthesia. The onset of action is relatively slow (up to 15 minutes); the duration of spinal anesthesia is three to four hours but can be prolonged to six hours by the addition of epinephrine. Dibucaine is metabolized but a portion may be eliminated unchanged.

The topical dosage form is applied to the ear, skin, and rectal mucocutaneous junction for long-acting surface anesthesia.

For adverse reactions and precautions, see the Introduction. This anesthetic is classified in FDA Pregnancy Category C.

DOSAGE AND PREPARATIONS.
Topical:
Skin: The 0.5% cream or 1% ointment is applied as required.
Rectum: The ointment is used morning and night, preferably following bowel movements.

DIBUCAINE:
Generic. Ointment 1% (nonprescription).
Nupercainal (CIBA). Cream 0.5% in 45 g containers; ointment 1% in 30 and 60 g containers (both forms nonprescription).

Injection:
Subarachnoid: Saddle block (rectal, urologic, and obstetrical anesthesia not involving abdomen), 2.5 to 5 mg (1 to 2 ml of hyperbaric solution); lower extremities, 4 mg (6 ml of hypobaric solution); abdomen, 7.5 to 10 mg (11 to 15 ml of hypobaric solution). For dosage for isobaric subarachnoid anesthesia, see the manufacturers' literature.

DIBUCAINE HYDROCHLORIDE:
Generic. Bulk.
Nupercaine (CIBA). Solution (for spinal anesthesia only) 2.5 mg/ml (0.25%) with dextrose 100 mg (5%) in 2 ml containers (hyperbaric); 0.667 mg/ml (1:1,500) in 20 ml containers (hypobaric); and 5 mg/ml (0.5%) (1:200) in 2 ml containers (isobaric).

DYCLONINE HYDROCHLORIDE
[Dyclone]

Dyclonine is used topically to anesthetize mucous membranes prior to endoscopy, to suppress the gag reflex, to relieve the pain of minor burns, to relieve the discomfort of gynecologic or proctologic procedures, and in the management of pruritus ani or vulvae. This drug is not used in cystoscopic procedures following intravenous pyelography with contrast media containing iodine because of formation of a precipitate that interferes with visualization.

The potency of dyclonine is comparable to that of cocaine. Generally, up to ten minutes are required for onset of action and the duration is up to one hour.

The toxicity of dyclonine is presumed to be low. For additional information on adverse reactions and precautions, see the Introduction.

DOSAGE AND PREPARATIONS.

Either the 0.5% or the 1% solution may be used for most of the indications described below. When continuous or repetitive application is anticipated, as in some oral or anogenital uses, the 0.5% solution may be preferred to reduce transmucosal absorption and the attendant possibility of cumulative systemic toxicity.

Topical: As a general guide, the maximal single dose is 200 mg.

Skin: 0.5% or 1% solution is applied as required.

Mouth, esophagus, oral endoscopy: For relief of oral pain, 5 to 10 ml of the 0.5% or 1% solution is swabbed, gargled, or sprayed and then expectorated. For esophagoscopy after pharyngeal anesthesia, 10 to 15 ml of the 0.5% solution is swallowed. For relief of esophageal pain, 5 to 15 ml of the 0.5% solution is swallowed.

Bronchoscopy: The tongue is pulled forward and the larynx and trachea are sprayed with 2 ml of the 1% solution every five minutes until the laryngeal reflex is abolished. This usually requires two or three sprayings. Five minutes should be allowed before instrumentation.

Urologic endoscopy: 6 to 30 ml of the 0.5% to 1% solution (usually 10 to 15 ml) is instilled into the urethra and retained for five to ten minutes before instrumentation.

Gynecology: 0.5% or 1% solution is used as a wet compress or spray.

Proctology: A cotton pledget saturated with the 0.5% or 1% solution is applied for relief of pain and discomfort.

> **Dyclone** (Astra). Solution 0.5% and 1% with chlorobutanol in 30 ml containers.

ETIDOCAINE HYDROCHLORIDE
[Duranest]

ACTIONS AND USES. Etidocaine is currently employed for infiltration, peripheral nerve block, and epidural (but not subarachnoid) anesthesia. A 0.5% concentration, with or without epinephrine, is generally adequate for infiltration anesthesia. Solutions of 0.5%, with or without epinephrine, are used for peripheral nerve blocks. The addition of epinephrine does not prolong the duration of analgesia but maintains lower plasma concentrations of the anesthetic. A 1% or 1.5% concentration is suggested for epidural anesthesia; onset of sensory block is rapid (about five minutes) with complete block in 12 minutes.

This agent differs from other local anesthetics in that it produces a profound motor nerve blockade after epidural administration; this may be preferred for abdominal surgery but is less desirable for normal obstetric delivery. Regression of anesthesia following epidural administration is similar to that seen with spinal anesthesia, ie, the patient may experience pain at the operative site while motor block is still present.

The onset of action of this amide is more rapid than that of bupivacaine and, at equipotent levels of anesthesia, the duration is comparable to that of bupivacaine and usually at least twice as long as that of lidocaine.

Although etidocaine and bupivacaine elicit seizures at the same plasma concentration, the decreased rate of absorption, more rapid plasma decay, and increased volume of distribution are probably responsible for the fact that, experimentally, etidocaine is less toxic than bupivacaine after injection of the same dose.

Like other amides, etidocaine is metabolized primarily by the liver, and metabolic products are excreted in the urine; little unchanged drug is excreted.

ADVERSE REACTIONS AND PRECAUTIONS. See the Introduction. This anesthetic is classified in FDA Pregnancy Category B.

DOSAGE AND PREPARATIONS.

Injection: A 0.5% solution is recommended for infiltration and peripheral nerve block; however, this concentration is no longer available commercially. The 1% solution may be more appropriate for major peripheral nerve blocks and is recommended for epidural nerve blocks in various gynecologic and obstetric procedures. A total dose of the 0.5%, 1%, or 1.5% solution for infiltration and nerve blocks should not exceed 5.5 mg/kg (400 mg) for solutions with epinephrine and 4 mg/kg (300 mg) for solutions without epinephrine.

The 1.5% solution may be required in intra-abdominal procedures and cesarean sections. The usual dose is 100 to 300 mg for intra-abdominal or pelvic surgery, 150 to 300 mg for lower limb surgery and cesarean section, and 50 to 150 mg for vaginal obstetrics.

> **Duranest** (Astra). Solution (sterile) 1% with and without epinephrine 1:200,000 in 30 ml containers; 1.5% with epinephrine 1:200,000 in 20 ml containers. Single-dose (30 ml) containers without epinephrine may be autoclaved.

HEXYLCAINE HYDROCHLORIDE
[Cyclaine]

Hexylcaine is used for surface anesthesia of intact mucous membranes in endoscopy, intubations, and manipulations of the respiratory, upper gastrointestinal, and urinary tracts. Anesthesia is produced in five minutes and lasts approximately 30 minutes. The topical solution is not suitable for ophthalmologic use. Hexylcaine is not injected because of its local and systemic toxicity.

Tissue irritation, burning, swelling, and tissue necrosis with slough have been reported after topical or inadvertent parenteral administration. For additional information on adverse reactions and precautions, see the Introduction.

DOSAGE AND PREPARATIONS.

Topical: Adults, as a general guide, the maximal single dose is 500 mg. A 1% or 2% concentration usually gives adequate anesthesia.

Nose: The area is swabbed, packed, or sprayed with a 0.5% to 5% solution. A concentration of 1% or more may be required for antral puncture.

Bronchoscopy, endotracheal intubation: No more than 10 ml (500 mg) of a 5% solution should be used.

Gastroscopy: The patient should gargle four times with the 1% or 2% solution; the procedure is repeated twice at five-minute intervals. The excess should not be swallowed. The total amount of hexylcaine 5% to be diluted and used as a gargle should not exceed 5 ml.

Genitourinary: The dose ordinarily should not exceed 10 ml of the 5% solution.

Cyclaine (Merck Sharp & Dohme). Solution 5% with propylparaben 0.02% and methylparaben 0.15% in 60 ml containers.

LIDOCAINE
[Xylocaine]

LIDOCAINE HYDROCHLORIDE
[Xylocaine]

ACTIONS AND USES. This amide is one of the most widely used local anesthetics for infiltration, intravenous regional, nerve block, epidural, and subarachnoid anesthesia; it also is commonly used for topical anesthesia.

Compared to procaine, the action of lidocaine is more rapid in onset, more intense, and of longer duration; lidocaine also is more potent. This anesthetic has excellent powers of diffusion and penetration. It has a local vasodilator action but is usually administered with epinephrine. When used alone, anesthesia after perineural injection lasts 60 to 75 minutes; with epinephrine, anesthesia lasts up to two hours.

ADVERSE REACTIONS AND PRECAUTIONS. When administered by extravascular injection, lidocaine is approximately one and one-half times as toxic as procaine. When given intravenously, lidocaine is twice as toxic as procaine. Rapid absorption of large amounts generally causes convulsions, but central nervous system depression rather than stimulation

may occur in some patients. Even therapeutic doses may cause drowsiness, lassitude, and amnesia. Other systemic reactions are similar to those produced by local anesthetics in general.

Lidocaine is not irritating and produces relatively little sensitization when used topically.

This anesthetic is classified in FDA Pregnancy Category B. For additional information on adverse reactions and precautions, see the Introduction.

DOSAGE AND PREPARATIONS

As a general guide, in healthy *adults* with normal hepatic function and hepatic blood flow, the maximal single dose recommended by the manufacturer for topical use is 300 mg and for injection (excluding subarachnoid) is 300 mg (4.5 mg/kg) without epinephrine or 500 mg (7 mg/kg) with epinephrine. This dose should not be repeated at intervals of less than two hours. The vascularity of tissue at the site of injection also should be considered when estimating total dose. In normal *children,* the dose (preferably of the 0.5% or 1% solution) should be reduced according to the type of block and the age of the child (see Chapter 2).

Topical: The 2% solution is generally recommended for topical anesthesia, particularly in infants. The 4% solution is used principally for laryngotracheal anesthesia. The maximal recommended dose is 10 ml of the 2% or 5 ml of the 4% concentration.

Skin: The maximal dose is 35 g of the 2.5% or 5% ointment daily.

Nose and nasopharynx: 1 to 5 ml of a 1% to 4% solution is sprayed or used on cotton applicators, depending upon the procedure. *Mouth, pharynx, and upper digestive tract:* The 2% viscous solution is used. The preparation can be moved around the mouth and pharynx by the cheeks and tongue and then swallowed. The adult dose should not exceed 15 ml (300 mg) every three hours or 120 ml in 24 hours. This anesthetic may obtund the pharyngeal stage of swallowing. Therefore, the patient should not eat or drink for one hour after application to avoid the danger of aspiration.

Respiratory tract: 1 to 5 ml of the 4% solution is sprayed or used by applicator or pack to produce anesthesia of the pharynx, larynx, and trachea for laryngoscopy, endotracheal intubation, and bronchoscopy. In addition, 2 to 3 ml of the 4% solution may be injected through the cricothyroid membrane (transtracheal), but a total dose of 5 ml generally should not be exceeded. Endotracheal tubes may be lubricated with 2% lidocaine hydrochloride jelly or 5% lidocaine ointment.

Urology: A 2% aqueous solution or 2% jelly may be used. *Men,* prior to catheterization, 5 to 10 ml of the 2% jelly is instilled slowly into the urethra and retained by penile clamp for five to ten minutes. For sounding or cystoscopy, 10 to 15 ml is given initially; an additional 15 ml is instilled after the clamp is removed. The maximal dose is 30 ml in 12 hours. In *women,* the dose is 3 to 5 ml. Several minutes should be allowed prior to performing urologic procedures.

LIDOCAINE, LIDOCAINE HYDROCHLORIDE:
Generic. Ointment 5%.
Xylocaine (Astra). Ointment 2.5% in 35 g containers (nonprescription) and 5% in 3.5 and 35 g containers; jelly 2% (hydrochlor-

ide) with methylparaben and propylparaben in 30 ml containers; solution (viscous) 2% (hydrochloride) in 20, 100, and 450 ml containers; solution (sterile) 4% (hydrochloride) with methylparaben in 50 and 100 ml containers.

Injection:

Infiltration: Onset of anesthesia is almost immediate. Without epinephrine, for extensive procedures, 25 to 60 ml of a 0.5% solution (duration of analgesia, approximately 75 minutes) or 10 to 30 ml of a 1% solution (duration of analgesia, approximately 90 minutes); for minor surgery and relief of pain, 2 to 50 ml of a 0.5% solution. With epinephrine 1:200,000, the duration of analgesia is approximately 150 minutes for the 0.5% solution and 240 minutes for the 1% solution. For dentistry, a 2% solution with epinephrine 1:100,000 is employed; the approximate duration of analgesia or anesthesia is 150 minutes. The maximum single dose is 7 mg/kg.

Intravenous regional: 40 to 50 ml of a 0.5% solution without epinephrine is used for the arm and approximately 60 ml for the leg.

Nerve block: For minor nerve blocks (eg, ulnar, intercostal), a 0.5% solution is adequate. For major nerve blocks (eg, pudendal, brachial plexus), a 0.5% or 1% solution is used. The addition of epinephrine 1:200,000 is recommended if large volumes are required. The approximate duration is 60 minutes without and 120 minutes with epinephrine. The maximum recommended volumes are, without epinephrine, up to 30 ml of a 1% solution or 15 ml of a 2% solution; with epinephrine 1:200,000, up to 50 ml of a 1% or 25 ml of a 2% solution. The usual doses are 15 to 20 ml of a 1.5% solution for brachial plexus, 1 to 5 ml of a 2% solution for mandibular, 3 ml of a 1% solution for intercostal, 3 to 5 ml of a 1% solution for paravertebral, and 10 ml of a 1% solution on each side for pudendal nerve block; for cervical nerve (stellate ganglion) block, the dose is 5 ml of a 1% solution; for lumbar sympathetic block, 5 to 10 ml of a 1% solution. Retrobulbar block lasting 90 minutes can be accomplished with 4 ml of the 4% solution of lidocaine.

Caudal: Without epinephrine, for obstetrical analgesia, up to 30 ml of the 1% solution; for surgical anesthesia, up to 20 ml of the 1.5% solution. With epinephrine 1:200,000, for surgical anesthesia, up to 30 ml of the 1.5% solution or 25 ml of the 2% solution. Analgesia during labor may be obtained with 20 to 30 ml of a 0.5% solution. Only single-dose containers should be used.

Lumbar epidural: Without epinephrine, for obstetrical or postoperative analgesia, 8 to 15 ml of the 1% solution; for surgical anesthesia, 15 to 20 ml of the 1.5% or 10 to 15 ml of the 2% solution. The dose depends upon the level of analgesia required but cannot be predicted accurately. With epinephrine 1:200,000, up to 20 ml of the 1%, 1.5%, or 2% solution. Analgesia during labor may be obtained with 8 to 10 ml of a 0.5% solution of lidocaine. Only single-dose containers should be used.

Subarachnoid: The 1.5% and 5% solutions with 7.5% dextrose (hyperbaric) are used for subarachnoid anesthesia. For vaginal delivery, 0.8 or 1 ml (40 or 50 mg) of the 5% solution or 2 ml (30 mg) of the 1.5% solution will provide perineal anesthesia for about one hour; analgesia lasts an additional 40 minutes. For cesarean section, 1.5 ml (75 mg) of the 5% solution may be used.

LIDOCAINE HYDROCHLORIDE:

Generic. Solution 1% and 2% with and without epinephrine, 4% without epinephrine.

Xylocaine (Astra). Solution 0.5% in 50 ml containers and with epinephrine 1:200,000 in 50 ml containers; 1% in 2, 2.5, 5, 10, 20, 30, and 50 ml containers, with epinephrine 1:200,000 in 30 ml containers, and with epinephrine 1:100,000 in 20 and 50 ml containers; 1.5% in 20 ml containers, with dextrose 7.5% in 2 ml containers, and with epinephrine 1:200,000 in 30 ml containers; 2% in 2, 10, 20, and 50 ml containers and 1.8 ml dental cartridges, with epinephrine 1:200,000 in 20 ml containers, and with epinephrine 1:100,000 in 20 and 50 ml containers and 1.8 ml dental cartridges; 4% in 5 ml containers; 5% with dextrose 7.5% in 2 ml containers. Aqueous solutions without epinephrine can be autoclaved repeatedly if necessary; preparations containing dextrose should not be autoclaved more than once or twice. All multiple-dose (20 or 50 ml) containers contain methylparaben 1 mg/ml.

MEPIVACAINE HYDROCHLORIDE

[Carbocaine, Polocaine]

ACTIONS AND USES. This amide is chemically related to bupivacaine but pharmacologically related to lidocaine. It is indicated for infiltration, nerve block, and epidural anesthesia. Mepivacaine is effective topically only in large doses and therefore should not be used by this route.

The potency of mepivacaine is similar to that of lidocaine. Anesthesia develops in three to five minutes and lasts two to two and one-half hours. Conventional doses may be used without epinephrine for most purposes. Unless contraindicated, epinephrine should be added to reduce plasma levels of mepivacaine when larger doses must be given.

ADVERSE REACTIONS. The systemic reactions produced by mepivacaine are similar to those caused by other local anesthetics, but drowsiness, lassitude, and amnesia occur less frequently than with lidocaine. Therefore, mepivacaine may be desirable for outpatient surgery.

Because the potentially high maternal blood concentration and rapid placental transfer can produce a high blood level in the fetus, utilization of mepivacaine in pudendal or paracervical nerve blocks for obstetric analgesia is not recommended (FDA Pregnancy Category C).

For additional information on adverse reactions and precautions, see the Introduction.

DOSAGE AND PREPARATIONS.

Injection: Adults, as a general guide, the doses of mepivacaine are similar to those of lidocaine. The maximal single dose is 7 mg/kg or 400 mg, whichever is less. This dose should not be repeated at intervals of less than 90 minutes, and no more than 1 g should be administered during any 24-hour period. The dose should be reduced in elderly or debilitated patients. The *pediatric* dose should be carefully measured as a percentage of the total adult dose based on weight and should not exceed 5 to 6 mg/kg (2.5 to 3 mg/lb) in children, especially those weighing less than 30 lb. In children under 3 years or weighing less than 30 lb, concentrations less than 2% (eg, 0.5% to 1.5%) should be employed.

Infiltration: Up to 80 ml of a 0.5% or 40 ml of the 1% solution.

Nerve block: 5 to 40 ml of the 1% or 5 to 20 ml of the 1.5% solution.

Epidural: 15 to 25 ml of the 1% solution, 10 to 20 ml of the 1.5% solution, or 10 to 20 ml of the 2% solution. Only single-dose containers should be used.

   Carbocaine (Winthrop-Breon). Solution 1% and 2% with methylparaben 0.1% in 30 and 50 ml containers; 1.5% in 30 ml containers; and 2% in 20 and 50 ml containers.

   Polocaine (Astra). Solution 3% in 1.8 ml dental cartridges.

PRAMOXINE HYDROCHLORIDE
[Tronolane, Tronothane]

$$CH_3CH_2CH_2CH_2O—\bigcirc—OCH_2CH_2CH_2—\overset{H}{\underset{}{N^+}}\bigcirc O \quad Cl^-$$

Pramoxine is derived from morpholine and, since it is chemically different from ester- or amide-type compounds, may be useful in patients who are sensitive to these classes of drugs. The potency of pramoxine is comparable to that of benzocaine. Onset of action is within three to five minutes.

Pramoxine is applied topically to the skin or mucous membranes to relieve pain caused by minor burns and wounds and to relieve pruritus secondary to dermatoses or hemorrhoids. It also may be used to facilitate sigmoidoscopic examinations and to anesthetize laryngopharyngeal surfaces prior to endotracheal intubation. However, it does not abolish the gag reflex. This anesthetic should not be injected or applied to the nasal mucosa, for it may irritate the tissue, and it should not be used for bronchoscopy or gastroscopy.

For adverse reactions and precautions, see the Introduction.

DOSAGE AND PREPARATIONS.
Topical:

Skin, mucous membranes: The 1% cream or jelly is applied as required, usually every three or four hours. For severe discomfort, preparations may be applied every two or three hours for one or two days; applications should be decreased thereafter to every four hours.

Larynx, trachea: The 1% jelly is used on endotracheal and intragastric tubes.

   Tronolane (Abbott). Cream 1% in 30 and 90 g containers; suppositories 1% (both forms nonprescription).

   Tronothane (Abbott). Cream (water-miscible) 1% in 30 g containers; jelly (water-soluble) 1% in 30 g containers (both forms nonprescription).

PRILOCAINE HYDROCHLORIDE
[Citanest]

$$\bigcirc\overset{CH_3}{\underset{}{}}—NHCCHNH_2CH_2CH_2CH_3 \quad Cl^-$$

ACTIONS AND USES. Prilocaine is similar pharmacologically to lidocaine and is used for infiltration, intravenous regional (preferred agent), peripheral nerve block, and epidural anesthesia. It is not used topically or for subarachnoid anesthesia. The effectiveness of prilocaine and lidocaine in equivalent doses is comparable, but the action of prilocaine is slightly slower in onset and of slightly longer duration. Epinephrine prolongs its effect.

Since prilocaine is more rapidly metabolized and excreted and has a larger volume of distribution than lidocaine, it is approximately 40% less toxic. For the same reasons, prilocaine blood levels are lower, which probably accounts for the lack of psychomotor impairment compared to that with bupivacaine, etidocaine, and lidocaine at equianesthetic doses. Therefore, this anesthetic may be desirable for outpatient surgery.

ADVERSE REACTIONS AND PRECAUTIONS. Two metabolites of prilocaine, ortho-toluidine and nitroso-toluidine, form methemoglobin. Doses in excess of 600 mg may produce a grayish or slate-blue cyanosis of the lips, mucous membranes, and nail beds, but respiratory and circulatory distress apparently do not occur. Methemoglobinemia also has been observed in neonates whose mothers received prilocaine shortly before delivery. In one clinical study, there were no signs of inadequate oxygen transport in healthy individuals who received 1.2 g of prilocaine. Although methemoglobinemia is readily reversed by the intravenous administration of methylene blue (1 to 2 mg/kg of a 1% solution injected over a five-minute period), the therapeutic effect may be short-lived because methylene blue may be cleared before conversion of all the methemoglobin to hemoglobin. Prilocaine should not be administered to patients with idiopathic or congenital methemoglobinemia, anemia, or cardiac or ventilatory failure with hypoxia; it should be used with caution for continuous epidural anesthesia since the methemoglobinemic effect of individual doses is additive.

This anesthetic is classified in FDA Pregnancy Category B. For additional information on adverse reactions and precautions, see the Introduction.

DOSAGE AND PREPARATIONS.
Injection: As a general guide, in normal healthy *adults,* the maximal single dose is 600 mg or 8 mg/kg in a two-hour period or no more than 1.2 g in a four-hour period. A 0.5% to 1% concentration should be used in *children,* and the dose should be reduced appropriately according to the type of block and the age, weight, and height of the child.

Infiltration: Up to 30 ml of the 1% or 2% solution.

Intravenous regional (Bier Block): Investigational. *Adults,* 0.5%, arm 40 to 50 ml, hand 10 ml; *children,* arm 5 mg/kg.

Nerve block: Up to 30 ml of the 2% solution or 15 to 20 ml of the 3% solution.

Caudal: 20 to 30 ml of the 1% solution is adequate for most routine vaginal deliveries. For surgical procedures requiring more profound anesthesia, 20 to 30 ml of the 2% solution or 15 to 20 ml of the 3% solution.

Lumbar epidural: 15 to 25 ml of the 1% or 2% solution or 15 to 20 ml of the 3% solution.

   Citanest (Astra). Solution 1% and 2% with methylparaben 0.1% in 30 ml containers; 3% in 20 ml containers; 4% with and without epinephrine 1:200,000 in 1.8 ml dental cartridges.

PROCAINE HYDROCHLORIDE
[Novocain]

$$H_2N \ \text{—} \ \overset{O}{\underset{}{C}}OCH_2CH_2\overset{+}{N}H \ \begin{matrix} CH_2CH_3 \\ CH_2CH_3 \end{matrix} \quad Cl^-$$

Procaine was the preferred local anesthetic for injection for many years, but it has been largely supplanted by other local anesthetics. Procaine has a slower onset of action than lidocaine and prilocaine; its duration of action is about one hour. It is ineffective topically.

Procaine is metabolized rapidly, which accounts for its safety. Much of it is hydrolyzed by plasma cholinesterase; the remainder is metabolized in the liver. The adverse reactions produced by procaine are similar to those of other synthetic local anesthetics. This anesthetic is classified in FDA Pregnancy Category C.

For additional information on adverse reactions and precautions, see the Introduction.

DOSAGE AND PREPARATIONS.
Injection: As a general guide, the maximal single dose for *adults* (excluding subarachnoid anesthesia) is 500 or 600 mg with epinephrine 1:200,000.

Infiltration: With or without epinephrine 1:200,000, up to 100 ml of a 0.25% or 0.5% solution.

Nerve block: With or without epinephrine 1:200,000, up to 50 ml of the 1% or 25 ml of the 2% solution.

Caudal, lumbar epidural: Procaine is not indicated for caudal or epidural anesthesia.

Subarachnoid: The 10% solution diluted with 10% dextrose prepared for subarachnoid anesthesia (hyperbaric) is used. For saddle block (perineum), 0.5 ml of the 10% solution diluted with 0.5 ml of 10% dextrose injection; for lower extremities, 1 ml of the 10% solution diluted with 1 ml of 10% dextrose injection; for level to costal margin, 2 ml of the 10% solution diluted with 1 ml of 10% dextrose injection. Onset is rapid and the duration of analgesia is 30 to 45 minutes.

> **Generic.** Solution 1% and 2%.
> **Novocain** (Winthrop-Breon). Solution 1% (isotonic) in 2 and 6 ml containers and with chlorobutanol 0.25% in 30 ml containers; solution (isotonic) 2% with chlorobutanol 0.25% in 30 ml containers; solution 10% in 2 ml containers (for spinal anesthesia; autoclaving more than once is not recommended).

TETRACAINE HYDROCHLORIDE
[Pontocaine]

$$CH_3CH_2CH_2CH_2NH \ \text{—} \ \overset{O}{\underset{}{C}}OCH_2CH_2\overset{+}{N}H \ \begin{matrix} CH_3 \\ CH_3 \end{matrix} \quad Cl^-$$

Tetracaine is the drug most widely used for subarachnoid anesthesia. It is not recommended for infiltration, peripheral nerve, or lumbar epidural blocks. Tetracaine is approximately ten times more potent and toxic than procaine. The onset of action is slow (approximately five minutes) after injection, but the duration of anesthesia is more than twice as long as that of procaine (two to three hours). Onset of action also develops slowly following topical application, and the duration of anesthesia is approximately 45 minutes. Tetracaine is metabolized in the plasma and liver at a slower rate than procaine.

This anesthetic is classified in FDA Pregnancy Category C. For information on adverse reactions and precautions, see the Introduction.

DOSAGE AND PREPARATIONS.
Topical:

Skin, anus: The 0.5% ointment or 1% cream is used. No more than 30 g for *adults* or 7.5 g for *children* should be applied in a 24-hour period.

Nose, pharynx: Up to 2 ml of a 1% solution.

Esophageal and laryngeal reflexes: 2 ml of a 1% solution effectively abolishes reflexes in preparation for esophagoscopy, bronchoscopy, and bronchography. These doses should not be exceeded because of the risk of systemic toxicity caused by rapid absorption of the drug.

> **Pontocaine** (Winthrop-Breon). Cream 1% in 30 g containers (nonprescription); ointment 0.5% in 30 g containers (nonprescription); solution 2% in 30 and 118 ml containers (rhinolaryngology).

Injection:

Infiltration, peripheral nerve block, caudal: Tetracaine is not recommended for these procedures because of its slow onset of action and great systemic toxicity.

Subarachnoid: The 1% solution diluted with an equal volume of 10% dextrose prepared for spinal anesthesia (hyperbaric) is used. For obstetrical saddle block, 2 to 4 mg; for lower extremities and perineal operations, 3 to 6 mg; for most cesarean sections and lower abdominal surgery, 9 to 12 mg; for upper abdominal surgery, 12 to 15 mg. Doses exceeding 15 mg are rarely administered. Epinephrine 1:1,000 (0.1 to 0.2 mg) may be added to prolong the duration of anesthesia by 30% to 50% in the average adult.

> **Generic.** Powder.
> **Pontocaine** (Winthrop-Breon). Solution 0.2% with dextrose 6% in 2 ml containers, 0.3% with dextrose 6% in 5 ml containers (saddle block, perineal), 1% in 2 ml containers (subarachnoid), and 0.5% in 15 ml containers (topical, ophthalmology).

Cited References

Barnett G, et al: Cocaine pharmacokinetics in humans. *J Ethnopharmacol* 3:353-366, 1981.

Blair MA: Cardiovascular pharmacology of local anesthetics. *Br J Anaesth* 47:247-252, 1975.

Bromage PR: *Epidural Analgesia.* Philadelphia, WB Saunders, 1978.

Clarkson CW, Hondeghem LM: Mechanism for bupivacaine depression of cardiac conduction: Fast block of sodium channels during the action potential with slow recovery from block during diastole. *Anesthesiology* 62:396-405, 1985.

Concepcion M, Covino BG: Rational use of local anesthetics. *Drugs* 27:256-270, 1984.

Cousins MJ, Bridenbaugh PO (eds): *Neural Blockade in Clinical Anesthesia and Management of Pain.* Philadelphia, JB Lippincott, 1980.

Covino BG: Systemic toxicity of local anesthetic agents. *Anesth Analg* 57:387-388, 1978.

Covino BG, Vassallo HG: *Local Anesthetics: Mechanisms of Action and Clinical Use.* New York, Grune & Stratton, 1976.

de Jong RH: Toxic effects of local anesthetics. *JAMA* 239:1166-1168, 1978.

Gissen AJ, et al: Chloroprocaine controversy II. Is chloroprocaine neurotoxic? *Reg Anesth* 9:135-145, 1984.

Greene NM: *Physiology of Spinal Anesthesia*, ed 3. Baltimore, Williams & Wilkins, 1981.

Holmes CMcK: Intravenous regional neural blockade, in Cousins MJ, Bridenbaugh PO (eds): *Neural Blockade in Clinical Anesthesia and Management of Pain*. Philadelphia, JB Lippincott, 1980, 343-354.

Marx GF: Cardiotoxicity of local anesthetics: The plot thickens. *Anesthesiology* 60:3-5, 1984.

Seifen AB, et al: Pharmacokinetics of intravenous procaine infusion in humans. *Anesth Analg* 58:382-386, 1979.

Wang BC, et al: Chronic neurological deficits and Nesacaine-CE: Effect of the anesthetic, 2-chloroprocaine, or the antioxidant, sodium bisulfite? *Anesth Analg* 63:445-447, 1984.

Zsigmond EK, Kothary SP: *2-Chloroprocaine: Clinical pharmacology, pharmacokinetics and its safety in regional anesthesia*, (exhibit).

International Anesthesia Research Society, Hollywood, FL, March 11-15, 1979.

Other Selected References

Katz RL (ed): Regional anesthesia. *Semin Anesth* 2:1-80, 1983.

Local Anesthestic Human Prescription Drugs Class Labeling Guideline for Professional Labeling. *Federal Register Notice* 47 FR: 41636, September 21, 1982.

Ralston DH, Shnider SM: Fetal and neonatal effects of regional anesthesia in obstetrics. *Anesthesiology* 48:34-64, 1978.

Tucker GT, Mather LE: Pharmacokinetics of local anesthetic agents. *Br J Anaesth* 47:213-224, 1975.

Tucker GT, Mather LE: Clinical pharmacokinetics of local anesthetics. *Clin Pharmacokinet* 4:241-278, 1979.

General Anesthetics

16

ADVERSE REACTIONS AND PRECAUTIONS

DRUG EVALUATIONS

Gas

Volatile Liquids

Intravenous Anesthetics

Barbiturates

Benzodiazepines

Miscellaneous Agents

COMBINATION ANESTHESIA

Balanced Anesthesia

Neuroleptanalgesia and Neuroleptanesthesia

Drug Evaluations

General anesthetics induce various degrees of analgesia; depression of consciousness, circulation, and respiration; relaxation of skeletal muscle; reduction of reflex activity; and amnesia. There are two types of general anesthetics, inhalation and intravenous. The arterial concentration required to induce anesthesia with either type varies with the condition of the patient, the desired depth of anesthesia, and the concomitant use of other drugs.

A single agent is used only infrequently to produce anesthesia. Anesthesia almost always is induced by administration of an intravenous anesthetic and maintained with an inhalation or intravenous agent or a combination. A muscle relaxant also may be required for intubation or during the intraoperative period. Thus, for most general anesthetic procedures, a number of drugs are administered. The concomitant use of certain inhalation and intravenous anesthetics, often in conjunction with opioid analgesics, neuroleptic drugs, or muscle relaxants, is referred to as combination anesthesia. Special types of combination anesthesia (ie, balanced anesthesia, neuroleptanesthesia) are discussed later in this chapter.

Inhalation Anesthetics: These are gases or volatile liquids that vary greatly in the rate at which they induce anesthesia; potency; the degree of circulatory, respiratory, or neuromuscular depression they produce; and analgesic effects (see the Table). Inhalation anesthetics have advantages over intravenous agents in that the depth of anesthesia can be changed rapidly by altering the inhaled concentration. Because of their

rapid elimination, they do not contribute to postoperative respiratory depression.

The rate at which the partial pressure of an inhalation anesthetic in the arterial blood approaches that in the inspired gas depends largely upon the drug's solubility in blood (the blood gas partition coefficient at 37 C [Eger, 1974]). When solubility is low, equilibrium is approached rapidly and induction, changes in anesthetic depth, and recovery times are rapid.

The clinical potency of an inhalation anesthetic is often defined in terms of MAC: the minimum alveolar concentration necessary to prevent movement in 50% of individuals subjected to a painful stimulus, usually skin incision (Eger, 1974; Quasha et al, 1980). For clinical purposes, MAC is an additive function; thus, 0.5 MAC nitrous oxide plus 0.5 MAC halothane will suppress movement in 50% of patients subjected to a painful stimulus. The volatile anesthetics (volatility is expressed as vapor pressure [VP] in mm Hg at 20 C) usually are given with 40% to 70% nitrous oxide, which reduces the required dose of volatile anesthetic. Anesthetic requirements (MAC) are not affected by the sex of the patient, the duration of the procedure, the arterial pH, PaO_2 or $PaCO_2$ (14 to 95 torr), the basal metabolic rate, or the usual doses of atropine or scopolamine given preoperatively. MAC decreases with increasing age and also is reduced by hypothermia, pregnancy, hypotension (mean blood pressure, <40 to 50 mm Hg), and the concurrent administration of other central nervous system

PHYSICAL CONSTANTS OF INHALATIONAL ANESTHETIC AGENTS

	Anesthetic	Blood/Gas Partition Coefficient (37 C)	Minimum Alveolar Concentration (MAC) vols %	Vapor Pressure (20 C)	Percentage Recovered As Metabolites*
VOLATILE LIQUIDS					
Hydrocarbon	Halothane [Fluothane]	2.54**	0.8	243	15–20
Ethers	Enflurane [Ethrane]	2.11**	1.7	172	2.4
	Isoflurane [Forane]	1.46**	1.2	240	0.17
	Methoxyflurane [Penthrane]	15.44**	0.2	23	50
GAS					
Inorganic	Nitrous Oxide	0.5	100+	gas	0

*Eger, 1980
+Hornbein et al, 1982
**Eger and Eger, 1985

depressants (opioids, sedative-hypnotics, or neuroleptic agents).

The only commercially available anesthetic *gas* is nitrous oxide. The *volatile liquids*, halothane [Fluothane], methoxyflurane [Penthrane], enflurane [Ethrane], and isoflurane [Forane], are halogenated compounds. (Methoxyflurane no longer is employed as a general anesthetic, but may be used as an on-demand, intermittent analgesic, particularly in obstetrics.)

Intravenous Anesthetics: The ultrashort-acting barbiturates, thiopental [Pentothal], methohexital [Brevital], and thiamylal [Surital], are used for induction. Loss of consciousness is rapid and induction is pleasant, but there is little muscle relaxation and reflexes frequently are not reduced adequately. Repeated administration results in accumulation and prolongs the recovery time. Since these agents have little if any analgesic activity, they are seldom used alone except in brief minor procedures.

Ketamine [Ketalar], a short-acting nonbarbiturate anesthetic, may be given intravenously or intramuscularly. It induces a dissociative state in which the patient may appear to be awake but is unconscious and does not respond to pain. Ketamine has been used in various diagnostic procedures; in brief, minor surgical procedures that do not require substantial skeletal muscle relaxation; and for changing dressings in burn patients. It also may be used as an induction agent, especially when cardiovascular or sympathetic depression is undesirable. When combined with nitrous oxide, diazepam [Valium] or lorazepam [Ativan], and a muscle relaxant, ketamine may be employed for major surgical procedures. Ketamine is not widely used because it increases cerebral blood flow and postoperative hallucinations occur occasionally.

Diazepam and midazolam are benzodiazepines given intravenously for induction. Large doses produce anterograde amnesia that is useful in anesthesia. Diazepam is used alone to produce basal sedation for diagnostic procedures (eg, endoscopy).

Etomidate [Amidate] may be given intravenously to induce anesthesia or as a supplement to nitrous oxide or an analgesic in combination anesthesia. It can be used as a substitute for thiopental in patients with asthma, severe cardiovascular disease, or peripheral circulatory failure. Because etomidate is metabolized by hydrolysis, presumably it could be used in patients with acute intermittent porphyria. This agent may find specific applications in neurosurgery because cerebral vascular flow and intracranial pressure are decreased.

Opioids, particularly fentanyl [Sublimaze] or sufentanil [Sufenta], may be given with oxygen and muscle relaxants for induction and maintenance of anesthesia in selected high-risk patients (see the section on Combination Anesthesia).

Adverse Reactions and Precautions

Inhalation Anesthetics: Delirium may develop during induction and recovery, but drugs given for premedication, particularly scopolamine, may be responsible (see Chapter 17, Adjuncts to Anesthesia). Gastroesophageal reflux or vomiting with aspiration may occur during induction, and nausea and vomiting may develop postoperatively.

Enflurane and halothane produce dose-related myocardial depression when present in useful anesthetic concentrations. Myocardial depression is less when isoflurane and nitrous oxide are used. Enflurane, isoflurane, and nitrous oxide may increase the heart rate; halothane does not have this effect. Arrhythmias may develop during administration of any inhalation anesthetic. Supraventricular arrhythmias are common and usually benign except when cardiac output and arterial pressure are reduced. Loss of the P wave (junctional rhythm, nodal rhythm, isorhythmic A-V dissociation) is very common during inhalation anesthesia. If myocardial function is borderline from any cause, decreased arterial pressure and cardiac output are inevitable. Therefore, the blood pressure should be determined immediately if the P wave disappears; conversely, a rapid fall in blood pressure requires immediate assessment of the electrocardiogram. Ventricular arrhythmias occur only rarely unless hypoxia or hypercapnia is present but are more likely to occur with use of halothane than with enflurane, isoflurane, or methoxyflurane. Halothane sensitizes the heart to the actions of catecholamines. Therefore, use of epinephrine, norepinephrine [Levophed], or isoproterenol [Isuprel] during halothane anesthesia may increase the risk of ventricular arrhythmias. Administration of halothane may increase the risk of ventricular arrhythmias in patients with high levels of endogenous catecholamines (eg, pheochromocytoma, severe anxiety). Isoflurane and, to a lesser extent, enflurane reduce systemic vascular resistance; halothane has no effect. Isoflurane decreases coronary vascular resistance and may produce a steal of myocardial blood flow in patients with severe coronary artery disease. Whether this causes appreciable myocardial ischemia remains controversial.

Respiratory depression occurs at all levels of general anesthesia with inhalation anesthetics. At a given level, the most profound depression is produced by enflurane. Controlled ventilation is recommended if normocapnia must be guaranteed. The ventilatory response to hypoxia is depressed by subanesthetic concentrations and is lost at anesthetic concentrations of all inhalation agents. The ventilatory response to hypercapnia is depressed at anesthetizing concentrations and is lost at 1.5 to 3 times MAC.

The cause of transient, slight abnormalities in the results of liver function tests is uncertain, but such changes are relatively common after any general anesthetic technique; serious liver damage is rare. Although halothane apparently is associated with hepatitis, no cause-and-effect relationship has been established and the diagnosis remains one of exclusion under normal circumstances (Stock and Strunin, 1985).

Reversible oliguria results from reduced renal blood flow and glomerular filtration during general anesthesia. This may be minimized if the patient is hydrated adequately and deep levels of anesthesia are avoided. However, methoxyflurane can produce direct, dose-related tubular injury with high-output renal failure and is contraindicated in patients with impaired renal function and in those receiving other potentially nephrotoxic agents (eg, aminoglycosides, tetracyclines). Because this complication is dose related and caused by the free fluoride ion produced by metabolism of the drug, methoxyflurane must be administered in diminishing concentrations during prolonged procedures. In comparison to methoxyflurane, enflurane produces substantially less free fluoride ion, isoflurane minimal amounts, and halothane essentially none. Metabolism of enflurane may be increased appreciably in patients taking isoniazid.

Body temperature tends to fall during anesthesia because of exposure, vasodilation, and suppression of thermoregulation. Postoperative shivering is common after anesthesia with the potent inhalation agents.

Malignant hyperthermia is a rare, often fatal complication that may be triggered by the potent inhalation anesthetics in genetically susceptible individuals (see Chapter 17, Adjuncts to Anesthesia, for a more detailed discussion).

Nitrous oxide, enflurane, halothane, isoflurane, and methoxyflurane elevate intracranial pressure by increasing cerebral blood flow, but this appears to be significant only in patients with intracranial lesions. Halothane increases cerebral blood flow more than enflurane or isoflurane. Cerebral auto-regulation is lost during halothane anesthesia but not during isoflurane anesthesia. Hypocapnia induced by hyperventilation essentially eliminates the increase in intracranial pressure. Patients with intracranial lesions should not receive halothane until hyperventilation has been instituted; hyperventilation may be instituted concomitantly with the administration of isoflurane. Enflurane should be used with care in these patients, because it may produce seizures in the presence of hypocapnia; convulsions are less likely if concentrations are maintained below 1.5% to 2%. Thiopental constricts cerebral vessels and also may be used to attenuate the increase in intracranial pressure during the use of volatile anesthetics.

Although enflurane, halothane, isoflurane, and nitrous oxide were teratogenic in some animal studies, they are not known to affect the human fetus. However, it is inadvisable to administer these agents during the first trimester unless such use is unavoidable. General anesthesia per se is not teratogenic. Neonatal depression can be anticipated if high concentrations of potent inhalation agents are administered during a prolonged delivery. However, general anesthesia is not used routinely for vaginal deliveries because of the advantages of regional anesthesia in this situation. During cesarean section, fetal exposure to anesthesia is generally very short. Nitrous oxide does not relax uterine muscle or increase uterine bleeding. Anesthetizing concentrations of enflurane, halothane, and isoflurane relax the uterus and may increase postpartum bleeding. Equipotent doses of volatile anesthetics have the same effect. Concentrations ranging from 0.5 to 1.5 MAC produced no significant change in myometrial depression (Paull and Ziccone, 1980). The use of high concentrations of volatile anesthetics for uterine surgery during the first trimester of pregnancy (eg, dilation and curettage) also is associated with increased blood loss.

The dose of nondepolarizing neuromuscular blocking agents (tubocurarine, metocurine [Metubine], pancuronium [Pavulon], atracurium [Tracrium], vecuronium [Norcuron], and gallamine [Flaxedil]) should be reduced when used with the volatile anesthetics because the latter potentiate the muscle relaxant effects. Halothane is the least and enflurane and isoflurane are the most potent in this regard.

Intravenous Anesthetics: Yawning, coughing, and laryngeal spasm may occur during induction of anesthesia with barbiturates. Hypotension may develop, particularly in hypovolemic patients or in those with diminished cardiac contractility. Undesirably light anesthesia due to rapid redistribution from the central nervous system can occur, particularly in young patients. Pronounced respiratory depression and apnea may develop immediately after rapid injection or overdosage. Shivering or excitement and delirium in the presence of pain may be observed during recovery.

The barbiturates may exacerbate acute intermittent porphyria and are *contraindicated* in patients with this disease. Care should be taken to avoid extravasation or intra-arterial injection of these drugs, particularly thiopental, for tissue necrosis and gangrene may occur.

See the evaluations for adverse reactions and precautions to be observed with the nonbarbiturate anesthetics.

Drug Evaluations

INHALATION ANESTHETICS

Gas

NITROUS OXIDE

ACTIONS AND USES. Nitrous oxide (blood/gas solubility 0.5, MAC 104% of one atmosphere) (Hornbein et al, 1982) is nonexplosive, but combustible items will burn in nitrous oxide. It must always be administered with at least 25% to 30% oxygen during induction and maintenance. Induction with 70% nitrous oxide is facilitated by premedication with an opioid analgesic or barbiturate.

For surgical anesthesia, nitrous oxide must be supplemented with other agents (eg, thiopental, benzodiazepines, opioid analgesics, more potent inhalation agents). It reduces the requirement for other inhalation anesthetics, and thus is included as one of the inhalation agents in almost all patients undergoing general anesthesia. A neuromuscular blocking agent often is given concomitantly if muscle relaxation is necessary.

Nitrous oxide has good analgesic properties and thus is useful as the sole analgesic in brief procedures and in the second stage of labor. It is employed also as a sedative in regional anesthesia with local anesthetics.

ADVERSE REACTIONS AND PRECAUTIONS. Serious adverse effects on the cardiovascular or ventilatory systems, liver, kidneys, or metabolic function usually do not occur when the inhalation mixture contains an adequate concentration of oxygen and ventilation is maintained. Severe hypotension may occur when hypovolemia, shock, or significant heart disease exists.

Because nitrous oxide is 35 times more soluble in blood than nitrogen, more nitrous oxide diffuses into a closed air-containing cavity than nitrogen diffuses out. If the cavity has rigid walls, the pressure within it rises; if the cavity does not have rigid walls, the volume increases. Therefore, nitrous oxide should be used with extreme caution in the presence of conditions such as air embolism, pneumothorax, pulmonary air cysts, or acute intestinal obstruction and during or after recent pneumoencephalography. Because nitrous oxide also can diffuse into the cuff of the endotracheal tube, periodic deflation is recommended.

To avoid the diffusion hypoxia that may develop after discontinuing prolonged anesthesia with nitrous oxide, oxygen should be employed briefly during emergence. Recovery is rapid unless large doses of supplemental agents have been used. Postoperative nausea and vomiting occur in 30% to 60% of patients, and develop more frequently if nitrous oxide is used to supplement a more potent anesthetic.

Nitrous oxide should not be used to produce analgesia or light narcosis for longer than 48 hours (eg, in patients receiving artificial ventilation) because of its tendency to produce leuko-penia. Megaloblastic bone marrow changes occur after two to four hours.

Epidemiologic and experimental evidence indicates that long exposure to trace concentrations of nitrous oxide may produce abortion. Similar but less complete evidence suggests that prolonged exposure also may cause neurologic, hepatic, and renal injury and congenital anomalies.

Nitrous oxide inactivates vitamin B_{12}, which is an essential cofactor of methionine synthase; thus, the serum tetrahydrofolate and methionine concentrations are reduced during anesthesia. The reduction of tetrahydrofolate can cause leukopenia and megaloblastic anemia or neurologic injury and may be responsible for the teratogenic or fetotoxic action of nitrous oxide (Nunn, 1984).

DOSAGE AND PREPARATIONS.

Inhalation: There is considerable variability in the responses of patients to nitrous oxide. Generally, sedation is produced by nitrous oxide 25%. Analgesia requires 25% to 50%. Laryngeal incompetence may develop with use of the 50% concentration. For maintenance, 30% to 70% nitrous oxide may be used, depending upon the patient's condition and the type and amount of supplemental agents used. Because of its low potency, nitrous oxide cannot be used as the sole agent for induction without large doses of a narcotic for premedication.

Generic. Available in metal cylinders color-coded with blue paint.

Volatile Liquids

ENFLURANE
[Ethrane]

$$
\begin{array}{ccc}
\text{F} & & \text{F} \text{F} \\
| & & | | \\
\text{HCOCCH} \\
| & & | | \\
\text{F} & & \text{F} \text{Cl}
\end{array}
$$

ACTIONS, USES, AND INTERACTIONS. Enflurane (VP 172 torr, blood/gas solubility 2.11, MAC 1.7%) is a nonflammable, halogenated ether anesthetic that provides rapid induction with little or no excitement. The rapidity of induction, however, may be limited due to breath holding or coughing caused by the pungency of this agent. Although salivary and bronchiolar secretions are increased slightly, use of atropine-like drugs for premedication is not essential. To avoid the cardiovascular depression and central nervous system stimulation produced by high concentrations, this agent usually is given in a low concentration (1% to 2%) with nitrous oxide. Enflurane provides better muscle relaxation than halothane. Neuromuscular blocking agents may be used to enhance the muscle relaxation, but the usual dosage of nondepolarizing drugs must be reduced significantly (see Chapter 17, Adjuncts to Anesthesia).

With low concentrations, the cardiovascular system remains relatively stable, although blood pressure is often reduced and the pulse rate is increased; cardiac rhythm is only slightly affected. Results of some studies in man suggest that this anesthetic does not sensitize the heart to catecholamines, but other studies show that enflurane does sensitize the heart but less than halothane. The dose-response relationships are more variable and unpredictable than with halothane. A suggested maximum dose of subcutaneous or submucosal (not intravenous) epinephrine is 2 mcg/kg over a 10-minute period in at least a 1:100,000 dilution during enflurane anesthesia; the concomitant administration of lidocaine decreases any tendency to arrhythmogenicity. Enflurane has been used during resection of pheochromocytoma, and it appears to be useful when increased catecholamine concentrations are anticipated.

Enflurane 1% with nitrous oxide, oxygen, and controlled ventilation significantly decreases intraocular pressure and is useful for eye surgery.

Relaxation of the uterus is dose related, but concentrations below 3% do not prevent the uterine response to oxytocic agents. Analgesic concentrations (0.25% to 1.25%) do not interrupt spontaneous uterine activity or produce excessive bleeding.

Enflurane is suitable for both induction and maintenance of anesthesia in children, although most anesthesiologists find that its pungency makes this anesthetic less acceptable than halothane.

Recovery is usually very rapid and uneventful; shivering from hypothermia is relatively common, but restlessness, delirium, nausea, and vomiting are infrequent. The speed of recovery may necessitate earlier administration of analgesics to relieve postoperative pain.

ADVERSE REACTIONS AND PRECAUTIONS. Enflurane causes profound respiratory depression. The ventilatory rate remains essentially constant or slightly elevated, but the tidal volume is decreased with resulting depression of minute volume. In adults, spontaneous ventilation may be sufficient at light levels of anesthesia but, as the depth increases, controlled ventilation is required to avoid hypercapnia.

Transient, slight abnormalities in the results of liver function tests similar to those observed after use of other volatile anesthetics have been noted. There have been several reports of hepatic damage related to enflurane anesthesia, but analysis of these cases does not support a causal relationship.

The clinical implications of the biotransformation of enflurane to free fluoride ion require further study. Plasma concentrations of fluoride ion are considerably below the toxic threshold in normal individuals, but may approach toxic levels in patients receiving isoniazid. The renal excretion of fluoride ion is promoted by an alkaline urine.

Central nervous system stimulation, manifested by increased electrical activity and seizure-like electroencephalographic patterns, occurs as anesthesia deepens; these changes usually appear when inspired concentrations exceed 3%. Paroxysms of tonic-clonic or twitching movements of the facial muscles and extremities developed in a few patients, usually in association with deep anesthesia *and* hypocapnia. These can be terminated without sequelae by lightening anesthesia and reducing minute ventilation or by substituting another anesthetic agent. Children are more sensitive to this effect and may exhibit grand mal seizures at concentrations in excess of 4%. These seizures are not harmful if oxygenation is sustained. Seizure activity is not exacerbated in patients with

pre-existing convulsive disorders if normocapnia is maintained.

This anesthetic agent is classified in FDA Pregnancy Category B.

DOSAGE AND PREPARATIONS.
Inhalation: For induction, 2% to 4.5% vaporized by a flow of oxygen or a nitrous oxide-oxygen mixture. Generally, 0.5% to 3% is administered for maintenance.
  Ethrane (Anaquest). Liquid in 125 and 250 ml containers.

HALOTHANE
[Fluothane]

$$\begin{array}{ccc} Cl & & F \\ | & & | \\ HC & - & COCH_3 \\ | & & | \\ Cl & & F \end{array}$$

ACTIONS, USES, AND INTERACTIONS. Halothane (VP 243 torr, blood/gas solubility 2.54, MAC 0.8%) is a nonflammable, halogenated, hydrocarbon anesthetic that provides relatively rapid induction with little or no excitement. Analgesia may not be adequate. Nitrous oxide is generally given concomitantly. Because halothane may not produce sufficient muscle relaxation, neuromuscular blocking agents may be required.

Halothane is far less irritating to the respiratory tract than enflurane or isoflurane. It depresses pharyngeal and laryngeal reflexes, dilates the bronchioles, and reduces salivation and bronchial secretions. It depresses the depth of respiration, produces tachypnea, and increases the alveolar-arterial oxygen difference; ventilation may need to be controlled to avoid respiratory acidosis.

Halothane diminishes sympathetic activity, augments vagal tone, depresses the contractility of the heart, and induces venodilation. Cardiac output, arterial pressure, and pulse rate are reduced, usually in proportion to the depth of anesthesia. Severe hypotension and circulatory failure may occur with overdosage. Supraventricular arrhythmias or nodal rhythm may be observed during induction or deep anesthesia; ventricular arrhythmias may be increased over awake levels but are uncommon unless ventilation is inadequate. Small doses of epinephrine (1 to 1.5 mcg/kg) may be administered subcutaneously or submucosally with halothane when adequate ventilation is assured. Exceeding this dose is potentially hazardous, however, since this anesthetic sensitizes the heart to catecholamines. The concomitant administration of lidocaine and epinephrine decreases the risk of arrhythmias.

Transient, slight abnormalities in the results of liver function tests have been observed after a single administration. The changes are similar to those noted following administration of other anesthetics but occur more frequently than with enflurane or isoflurane. Although many cases of liver damage, ranging from mild hepatitis to massive hepatic necrosis, have been reported after such use, the incidence of unexplained cases of massive hepatic necrosis is about 1 in 35,000 anesthetic administrations. There is evidence suggesting that liver damage is more likely to develop if there is intraoperative or postoperative hypoxia. Halothane should not be given to patients who developed jaundice or acute liver damage after previous exposure to this drug unless other obvious causes for the hepatic damage have been demonstrated. It also may be unwise to give halothane to patients who developed a similar response after exposure to methoxyflurane and possibly to other halogenated anesthetics, although there is no evidence to substantiate this precaution.

Dose-dependent, reversible effects on the kidney (eg, decreased renal blood flow, glomerular filtration rate, and urine volume) have been observed during anesthesia, particularly in dehydrated patients or those with intraoperative hypotension. No significant metabolic disturbances have been noted. Renal oxygen consumption is reduced.

Controlled studies have indicated that low concentrations of halothane may increase uterine hemorrhage when this agent is used during early pregnancy (therapeutic abortion). Concentrations of halothane above 0.5% relax the uterus, thus inhibiting natural or induced uterine contractions and delaying delivery. Halothane in concentrations above 1% interferes with the action of the oxytocic drugs, oxytocin and ergonovine, and considerable uterine hemorrhage may occur.

Recovery from anesthesia is usually rapid and uneventful. Shivering is common. Restlessness, delirium, nausea, and vomiting are infrequent.

DOSAGE AND PREPARATIONS.
Inhalation: For induction, a 1% to 4% concentration vaporized by a flow of oxygen or a nitrous oxide-oxygen mixture. For maintenance, a 0.5% to 2% concentration.
  Generic. Liquid in 250 ml containers.
  Fluothane (Ayerst). Liquid in 125 and 250 ml containers.

ISOFLURANE
[Forane]

$$\begin{array}{c} \quad\ F \\ \quad\ | \\ HC-O-CHCF_3 \\ \ |\qquad\ | \\ \ F\qquad Cl \end{array}$$

ACTIONS AND USES. Isoflurane (VP 240 torr, blood/gas solubility 1.46, MAC 1.2%) is a nonflammable, halogenated ether anesthetic. Although it is a structural isomer of enflurane, there are many pharmacologic differences between the two agents.

This anesthetic has a pungent odor, which limits the rate of increase in the inspired concentration that is acceptable to the patient; coughing and breath holding may occur. Induction is smoother and excitement is decreased when premedication is given and when nitrous oxide and oxygen are administered concomitantly. However, induction is more often accomplished with intravenous agents. Relaxation of the jaw, although not as profound as with halothane, is satisfactory for endotracheal intubation. The effects of nondepolarizing neuromuscular blocking drugs are markedly potentiated in the presence of isoflurane; therefore, their dose must be reduced by one-third to two-thirds (see Chapter 17, Adjuncts to Anesthesia).

With concentrations of 1 to 2 MAC, little myocardial depression is observed in normal, normocapnic patients. Reduction of blood pressure is dose related and secondary to peripheral vasodilation rather than decreased cardiac output. There is little tendency to develop arrhythmias and the myocardium is not sensitized to catecholamines. The pulse rate may increase, and occasional patients experience tachycardia that is not suppressed by increasing the concentration of isoflurane. After ruling out hypoxia or malignant hyperthermia, the pulse rate usually can be decreased with small doses of opioid (eg, 0.1 mg fentanyl, 8 to 10 mg morphine), using care to compensate for the greater ventilatory depression, or propranolol 0.5 to 2 mg.

Depression of minute volume can be counteracted by adjusting the dose. Controlled ventilation may be required for normocapnia and is required for hypocapnia.

Isoflurane is metabolized minimally; the major metabolites are trifluoroacetic acid and fluoride ion in a ratio of about 2:1. In one study, serum fluoride ion concentrations were dose related (maximum, 5.5 micromoles [mcM]/L). In another study, serum fluoride ion concentrations at the end of anesthesia averaged 3.6 mcM/L (maximum, 12 mcM/L). In comparison, methoxyflurane produced serum fluoride ion concentrations as high as 200 mcM/L and enflurane as high as 80 mcM/L. Subtle laboratory evidence of defects in renal concentrating ability occurs at serum fluoride ion concentrations above 50 mcM/L, and overt damage is observed at concentrations greater than approximately 100 mcM/L. There is no evidence of renal dysfunction following use of isoflurane. Likewise, no alterations in hepatic function due to isoflurane itself have been observed.

Unlike enflurane, no central nervous system stimulation is evident with deep anesthesia. Isoflurane increases cerebral blood flow at concentrations exceeding 1.1 MAC and may increase intracranial pressure. However, hyperventilation may be used to decrease cerebral blood flow and pressure since hypocapnia does not induce seizure activity during isoflurane anesthesia. At 1 MAC, cerebral blood flow is significantly greater with halothane. Autoregulation of cerebral blood flow is maintained with isoflurane but not with halothane. Cerebral protrusion is less with isoflurane or enflurane than with halothane. Increases in blood pressure minimally increase protrusion during isoflurane or enflurane anesthesia, whereas increases in blood pressure may more than double protrusion during halothane anesthesia.

The safety of isoflurane during pregnancy and delivery has not been established. As with other inhaled anesthetics, isoflurane produces teratogenic changes in animals. Analgesic concentrations of 0.3% to 0.7% do not depress the frequency or force of uterine contractions or increase maternal blood loss.

Mental alertness is depressed for two to three hours after anesthesia; however, postoperative nausea, vomiting, and excitation are uncommon.

DOSAGE AND PREPARATIONS.
Inhalation: For induction, 3% to 3.5% vaporized in oxygen or in a nitrous oxide-oxygen mixture. Concentrations between 0.5% and 3% are satisfactory for maintenance. Rarely is more than 3% required when isoflurane is given with oxygen alone.
  Forane (Anaquest). Liquid containing no additives or chemical stabilizers in 100 ml containers.

METHOXYFLURANE
[Penthrane]

$$HC-COCH_3$$

with Cl, F substituents shown: CH bearing Cl (top) and Cl (bottom), adjacent C bearing F (top) and F (bottom), bonded to OCH_3

ACTIONS AND USES. Methoxyflurane (VP 23 torr, blood/gas solubility 15.44, MAC 0.2%) is a potent halogenated ether anesthetic with a fruity odor. Because of its low vapor pressure and high solubility in blood and certain components of the anesthesia delivery circle (rubber, soda lime), induction may be slow and recovery prolonged unless the carrier gas includes at least 50% nitrous oxide.

Methoxyflurane provides adequate analgesia and can be used alone in dentistry. At concentrations of 0.25% to 0.5%, methoxyflurane does not affect uterine contractions and may be used in obstetrical patients, particularly for intermittent analgesia during the first stage of labor.

Currently, methoxyflurane is rarely used for surgical anesthesia. If so employed, it should be administered with nitrous oxide to achieve a relatively light level of anesthesia, and a neuromuscular blocking agent should be given concurrently to obtain the desired degree of muscular relaxation. The upper MAC-hour limit described (see Precautions) should be observed. Since methoxyflurane augments the neuromuscular blocking effects of nondepolarizing muscle relaxants, the dose of the latter should be markedly reduced (see Chapter 17, Adjuncts to Anesthesia).

ADVERSE REACTIONS, PRECAUTIONS, AND INTERACTIONS. Methoxyflurane depresses the cardiovascular system to approximately the same degree as halothane. Cardiac contractility is reduced and cardiac output and arterial pressure are decreased in proportion to the concentration of inhaled vapor. The heart rate is relatively unchanged, although atropine-responsive sinus bradycardia may occur and nodal escape rhythm may develop during deep anesthesia. Arrhythmias are uncommon, even in the presence of hypercapnia. The drug only moderately sensitizes the heart to catecholamines and does not stimulate the sympathetic nervous system if adequate ventilation and depth of anesthesia are maintained.

Methoxyflurane does not irritate the respiratory tract or increase secretions, and premedication with belladonna drugs is not required. Ventilation is depressed only slightly at light levels of anesthesia, and this may be used as a guide to depth of anesthesia. Respiration may need to be assisted or controlled when deeper levels of anesthesia are attained, for minute volume is diminished markedly.

Transient, slight abnormalities in the results of liver function tests have been observed, and there are a number of anecdotal reports of hepatic damage, including massive hepatic necrosis. Methoxyflurane should not be administered to patients who developed acute unexplained liver damage after previous exposure to this drug. It also may be unwise to give methoxyflurane to patients who responded similarly to halothane.

Other anesthetics should be used in patients with renal damage, since impaired renal function has been associated with use of methoxyflurane, particularly after administration for long periods without time-dependent dosage reductions. The symptoms are usually those of vasopressin-resistant, high-output renal failure and include output of a large volume of dilute urine; dehydration; weight loss; increased serum osmolality; significantly increased blood sodium, urea nitrogen, and creatinine levels; elevated serum and urine concentrations of inorganic fluoride; and increased excretion of oxalic acid. Most patients recover completely, but some develop oliguric renal failure, a few develop chronic renal failure, and, rarely, a patient dies. High-output renal failure is dose related and is caused by the free fluoride ion produced by metabolism of the drug; fluoride ion interferes with sodium transport necessary for concentrating urine and also may render the appropriate renal tubules unresponsive to antidiuretic hormone.

The severity of nephrotoxicity depends primarily upon the dose (ie, concentration and time or MAC-hours) of methoxyflurane and secondarily upon the degree of metabolism, the presence of enzyme induction (eg, from barbiturates), and variations in sensitivity to fluoride ion. Subclinical nephropathy occurs after about 2.5 MAC-hours of methoxyflurane, which results in about 50 to 60 mcM/L serum fluoride. As much as 50% to 70% of methoxyflurane reaching the systemic circulation is metabolized by the liver. It is important that the presence of a normal arterial pressure not be assumed to indicate that a light level of anesthesia is being maintained, as this may result in administration of a nephrotoxic dose. Methoxyflurane should not be given to patients receiving other potentially nephrotoxic drugs (eg, aminoglycosides, tetracyclines), because concurrent use of these agents has been associated with irreversible renal failure.

Nausea and vomiting may occur postoperatively. Recovery from anesthesia is prolonged but there is a good analgesic effect in the immediate postoperative period.

This anesthetic is classified in FDA Pregnancy Category C.

DOSAGE AND PREPARATIONS.
Inhalation: For analgesia, 0.3% to 0.8% in air. A draw-over device is acceptable when the drug is inhaled only to produce analgesia. It may be wise to limit the amount of drug used for self-administration during labor to 15 ml.

An intravenous agent should be used for induction of anesthesia.

For maintenance, at least 50% nitrous oxide is employed and supplemental neuromuscular blocking agents are used, if required, so that the lowest effective total dose of methoxyflurane is given. See the manufacturer's literature for tables indicating stepwise dose reductions with exposure duration. Since subclinical nephrotoxicity has been detected after the administration of one MAC (0.16%) for 2 1/2 hours, *the total dose of methoxyflurane should not exceed this MAC-hour limit*. This effectively restricts this drug's usefulness to relatively few indications.

When methoxyflurane is administered to produce anesthesia, a vaporizer calibrated for methoxyflurane must be used, and it must be placed outside the anesthesia delivery circle.

Penthrane (Abbott). Liquid in 15 and 125 ml containers.
Also available for self-administered analgesia by inhaler (**Analgizer**).

INTRAVENOUS ANESTHETICS

Barbiturates

THIOPENTAL SODIUM
[Pentothal]

ACTIONS AND USES. This barbiturate is useful to induce general anesthesia, since loss of consciousness occurs within 30 to 60 seconds after intravenous administration. Thiopental usually is not employed for maintenance (even with nitrous oxide) for procedures lasting longer than 15 to 20 minutes, because the cumulative dose results in delayed awakening. It has poor analgesic properties. The use of nitrous oxide 67% decreases requirements for thiopental by two-thirds. Depending upon the type of surgery, narcotic analgesics and neuromuscular blocking agents also may be required. Usual doses have no significant effects at the myoneural junction. Uterine muscle tone is not affected.

Although this anesthetic may be administered rectally for basal sedation or anesthesia, absorption of a thiopental suspension from the rectum is unpredictable.

ADVERSE REACTIONS AND PRECAUTIONS. In some instances, the arterial pressure is only slightly affected by thiopental. Frequently, a reduction in cardiac output and arterial pressure caused by myocardial depression and peripheral vasodilation occurs immediately after rapid intravenous injection of enough thiopental to produce deep anesthesia. In hypovolemic patients and those with myocardial disease or untreated hypertension, the drug must be administered more slowly, in dilute solution, and incrementally, if at all.

Thiopental is a potent respiratory depressant, and apnea may occur immediately after intravenous injection, particularly in the presence of hypovolemia, cranial trauma, or preanesthetic medication with opioid drugs. Tidal volume is depressed to a greater extent than the respiratory rate. Respiratory depression may be prolonged in patients with myasthenia gravis.

Rapid redistribution of thiopental out of the brain can result in light anesthesia characterized in part by reflex hyperactivity of the airway to mechanical stimulation (eg, intubation, instrumentation, secretions, blood). Therefore, an adequate depth of anesthesia should be assured in patients sensitive to bronchospasm; in those with upper airway obstruction; when coughing, hiccupping, or straining is undesirable; and to avoid laryngospasm, which might otherwise occur at any time from direct or indirect stimulation (eg, rectal dilation). Introduction of an artificial airway or painful stimulus also may cause hypertension and tachycardia in lightly anesthetized patients. This may increase myocardial oxygen demand profoundly, which is undesirable in patients with coronary artery disease.

Transient, slight alterations in the results of liver function tests similar to those observed following administration of other anesthetics may occur after use of thiopental. Pre-existing liver disease is not a contraindication to the usual induction dose.

Thiopental decreases urine output by reducing perfusion pressure, constricting renal arteries, and releasing antidiuretic hormone, but it does not cause renal damage.

Thiopental is absolutely contraindicated in patients with acute intermittent porphyria or other hepatic porphyrias.

Anaphylaxis has been reported following injection of thiopental, but this response is *very* rare.

Care should be taken to avoid extravasation or intra-arterial injection, for neuritis and skin slough may occur with the former (especially with concentrations exceeding 25 mg/ml) and arteritis, followed by vasospasm, edema, thrombosis, and gangrene, with the latter. Damage is reduced when dilute solutions are administered; concentrations should not exceed 2.5%. Intra-arterial injection usually produces immediate intense pain prior to loss of consciousness. The injection must be discontinued immediately and a vasodilator (eg, nitroprusside) or a local anesthetic without epinephrine (eg, lidocaine) must be injected locally (preferably through the needle used for the thiopental). If the needle has been removed from the artery, the vasodilator should be injected into the subclavian artery, since the affected artery will be in spasm (Dundee and Wyant, 1974). Local injection of heparin may reduce thrombosis, and sympathetic block or general anesthesia with halothane may relieve pain and vascular spasm and assist in opening collateral circulation. Infiltration of the area with a local anesthetic without epinephrine (eg, 1% lidocaine) may ameliorate the consequences of extravasation.

Consciousness returns rapidly unless large doses have been given. Postoperative nausea and vomiting are uncommon, but shivering occurs often and excitement and delirium may develop during recovery in the presence of pain.

This drug is classified in FDA Pregnancy Category C.

PHARMACOKINETICS. The duration of unconsciousness after a single dose of thiopental is determined by the rate of redistribution from the central nervous system into muscle. Factors that diminish blood flow into muscle, eg, hypovolemia, delay awakening. Thiopental is almost completely metabolized (more than 99%) in the liver. The half-life is 11.5 hours, the apparent volume of distribution at steady state is 1.4 L/kg, and the clearance is 150 ml/min. These values are increased during pregnancy; at term, the half-life is 26.1 hours, the apparent volume of distribution is 4.1 L/kg, and the clearance rate is 286 ml/min (Morgan et al, 1981). The elimination half-life in pediatric patients is one-half that in adults; the clearance values are 6.6 ml/kg/min in children and 3.1 mg/ml/kg in adults (Sorbo et al, 1984). Morbid obesity markedly increases the volume of distribution to 7.9 L/kg and the half-life to 27.85 hours (Jung et al, 1982).

DOSAGE AND PREPARATIONS.

Intravenous: The dose required to induce and maintain anesthesia varies with premedication, concurrent nitrous oxide administration, physical status, pre-existing disease, and adequacy of the respiratory and circulatory systems. Age, sex, weight, and serum albumin levels have little effect on thiopental requirements. Adherence to a strict "usual" dose regimen is discouraged. Tolerance has been reported following repeated use, as in burn patients.

For induction, *adults,* after a 2-ml test dose of a freshly prepared 2.5% solution, 50 or 100 mg is injected intermittently every 30 to 40 seconds until the desired effect is obtained, or a single injection of 3 to 5 mg/kg is given. For maintenance, 50 to 100 mg of a 2.5% solution is injected as required. *Children 5 to 15 years,* a 2.5% solution is injected slowly and intermittently at 30-second intervals. The total dose recommended for induction is 4 to 5 mg/kg in relatively healthy, unpremedicated patients. For maintenance, the usual total dose for children weighing 30 to 50 kg is 25 to 50 mg injected intermittently.

  Pentothal (Abbott). Powder (for solution) 0.25, 0.4, 0.5, 1, 2.5, and 5 g.

Rectal: For basal anesthesia in *children,* 30 mg/kg in a 40% suspension.

  Pentothal (Abbott). Suspension 400 mg/g in 2 g containers.

METHOHEXITAL SODIUM
[Brevital Sodium]

Methohexital has a short duration of action. It may be used for induction or for procedures in which momentary loss of consciousness is desirable, eg, electroshock therapy. Adverse effects are similar to those noted with thiopental. Hiccups may occur after rapid intravenous injection. Involuntary muscle movements have been observed more frequently with methohexital than with thiopental.

PHARMACOKINETICS. The short duration of action of methohexital results largely from its rapid distribution out of the central nervous system. In addition, this barbiturate is cleared more rapidly (9.9 ± 2.9 ml/kg/min) than thiopental (3.4 ± 0.5 ml/kg/min). The elimination half-life of methohexital is 4 ± 2.5 hours and its apparent volume of distribution is 2.1 ± 0.7 L/kg (Hudson et al, 1982).

DOSAGE AND PREPARATIONS.

Intravenous: Adults, for induction, after a 2-ml test dose, 5 to 12 ml of a 1% solution is injected at the rate of 1 ml every five seconds. For maintenance, 2 to 4 ml of a 1% solution injected as required.

Rectal: Children, for basal anesthesia, 20 to 30 mg/kg in a 10% solution in lukewarm tap water.

  Brevital Sodium (Lilly). Powder (for solution) 0.5, 2.5, and 5 g.

THIAMYLAL SODIUM
[Surital]

The uses and adverse effects of this rapid-acting barbiturate are similar to those of thiopental sodium.

DOSAGE AND PREPARATIONS.

Intravenous: Adults, for induction, after a 2-ml test dose of a freshly prepared 2.5% solution, 2 or 4 ml is injected every 30 to 40 seconds until the desired effect is obtained, or a single injection of 3 to 5 mg/kg is given. For maintenance, 2 to 4 ml of a 2.5% solution is injected as required.

  Surital (Parke-Davis). Powder (for solution) 1, 5, and 10 g.

Benzodiazepines

DIAZEPAM
[Valium]

ACTIONS AND USES. Diazepam is administered intravenously to produce basal sedation during regional anesthesia, for cardioversion, and in endoscopic and dental procedures. It also is used occasionally as an induction agent, particularly in patients with cardiovascular disease. Otherwise, it is considered less satisfactory than the ultrashort-acting barbiturates for induction because of its slightly slower onset of action (at least one minute) and especially because the recovery period is more prolonged. Sleep and altered consciousness usually are preceded by nystagmus and slurred speech but not excitement. Diazepam also is used for premedication (see Chapter 17), as a component of neuroleptanalgesia, and to control convulsions caused by local anesthetics (see Chapter 15).

Since diazepam has no analgesic action, concurrent use of local or topical anesthetics improves anesthetic management in some patients (eg, prior to endoscopy). Diazepam has no analgesic effect and will not enhance the analgesic action of opioid drugs or potentiate the effects of neuromuscular blocking agents.

ADVERSE REACTIONS, PRECAUTIONS, AND INTERACTIONS. The intravenous administration of diazepam may cause mild tachycardia and slight respiratory depression, but acute circulatory failure has occurred in a healthy adult and respiratory arrest was observed in a healthy elderly patient after intravenous injections of 20 mg and 10 mg, respectively. Such effects may be anticipated if the drug is administered too rapidly. Respiratory arrest also has been noted after use of the drug during anesthesia, particularly if an opioid analgesic was included in the premedication. It is advisable to decrease the dose of opioid drugs used for premedication by at least one-third and to administer them in small increments. In high-dose opioid anesthesia, even small amounts (2.5 to 5 mg) of intravenous diazepam can decrease blood pressure and cardiac output profoundly. Smaller doses of diazepam (usually 2 to 5 mg) should be used for elderly or debilitated patients or when other sedative drugs are administered.

The half-life of diazepam is 20 or more hours; thus, outpatients must be accompanied home because of the slow recovery of psychomotor skills.

Superficial, painless venous thrombosis develops at the site of injection in 15% of patients; the incidence increases with age. A high incidence of phlebitis has been reported following the intravenous use of diazepam. Injection into small veins (such as on the back of the hand) frequently causes pain and is not recommended. Care should be taken to avoid intra-arterial injection, which can cause extensive tissue necrosis.

Although Apgar scores are little affected when diazepam is used for vaginal delivery, hypotonicity, hypoactivity, and hypothermia may occur in infants after doses of 20 to 50 mg are given to the mother. Therefore, diazepam is *not* recommended for obstetrical patients.

PHARMACOKINETICS. Diazepam is metabolized to an active derivative. Its half-life depends upon age, ranging from 20 hours at age 20 years to 90 hours at age 80 years, a relationship which parallels the age-related increase in the initial volume of distribution. However, the plasma clearance remains nearly constant (20 to 32 ml/minute) regardless of age. Therefore, when this drug is given for prolonged periods, dose corrections for age are unnecessary. The apparent volume of distribution at steady state is 1.1 L/kg.

DOSAGE AND PREPARATIONS.

Intravenous: Diazepam should not be mixed with solutions of other drugs. To prevent prolonged exposure of the vein to a high concentration of the solvent and to reduce venous thrombosis, diazepam is injected through the intravenous tubing as close as possible to the vein insertion with the intravenous fluid flowing rapidly.

For induction of anesthesia, 0.1 to 1.5 mg/kg is required. Although some healthy patients may fall asleep with doses of 0.4 mg/kg, or even 0.2 mg/kg if an opioid analgesic is used for premedication, 0.8 to 1.5 mg/kg is required if sleep is to be assured. This combination is dangerous in poor-risk patients because of the risk of cardiovascular depression. Diazepam should be injected slowly (no more than 5 mg [1 ml]/min in adults and no more than 0.25 mg/kg/3 min in children).

For basal sedation, increments of 2.5 mg are given at 30-second intervals until the patient falls into a light sleep or nystagmus, ptosis, or slurred speech develops. Ptosis covering half of the pupil is a reproducible endpoint. Generally, 5 to 30 mg is required.

Valium (Roche). Solution 5 mg/ml in 2 and 10 ml containers.

MIDAZOLAM HYDROCHLORIDE
[Versed]

ACTIONS AND USES. This induction agent differs from other benzodiazepines in that it is water soluble. Intravenous administration rarely causes pain or thrombophlebitis. Induction (approximately 80 seconds) is more rapid than with diazepam or flunitrazepam but slower than with thiopental (30 to 60 seconds).

The degree of respiratory depression produced by midazolam is similar to that observed with diazepam. A brief period of apnea may occur about two minutes after intravenous administration. The incidence and duration of apnea are less than with an equivalent dose of thiopental and its onset is later. Oxygen should be employed during spontaneous ventilation. As with diazepam, slightly increased airway resistance is noted occasionally.

The cardiovascular system remains stable during induction. There is a slight, dose-dependent reduction in blood pressure but the heart rate, cardiac output, and rhythm are not affected in normal subjects. The drug appears to be satisfactory for induction in patients with ischemic heart disease (Reves et al, 1978).

Midazolam has no effects on gastrointestinal smooth muscle. It does not affect the response to muscle relaxants. Intraocular pressure is reduced, but the increase in intraocular pressure produced by succinylcholine or intubation is not prevented. The cerebral blood flow in healthy volunteers was reduced by one-third, suggesting that midazolam might be appropriate for induction in neurosurgical patients with intracranial hypertension (Forster, et al, 1982).

Fetal transfer of midazolam is significantly less than that of diazepam, and it may be possible to employ this agent in obstetrical patients without producing fetal hypotonia or hypothermia.

No renal, hepatic, or other complications have been reported.

Midazolam produces anterograde but not retrograde amnesia. Since this effect may be related to the duration of the sedative action, midazolam is inferior to the other benzodiazepines if the latter effect is desired. It has no analgesic action and will not enhance the analgesic effect of opioids.

PHARMACOKINETICS. Midazolam is metabolized in the liver to two hydroxylated derivatives that are excreted by the kidney. Neither metabolite possesses a soporific action. The duration of hypnotic action is approximately 4.5 minutes (Brown et al, 1979). Midazolam is extensively protein bound (more than 95%). With an intravenous dose of 0.075 mg/kg, the half-life is 68 minutes, the apparent volume of distribution is 0.23 L/kg, and the clearance is 13 ml/min/kg (Kanto et al, 1984).

DOSAGE AND PREPARATIONS.

Intravenous: *Adults*, for sedation, 5 mg. For induction, 0.2 mg/kg if an opioid analgesic is used for premedication. There is considerable variation in the dose required for induction; some adults are resistant to 30 mg. Since these patients readily accept a mask after the administration of midazolam, induction may be completed with the planned maintenance agent.

No dosage has been established for *children* or for *obstetric procedures.*

Versed (Roche). Solution (buffered, aqueous) 5 mg/ml.

Miscellaneous Agents

ETOMIDATE
[Amidate]

ACTIONS AND USES. Etomidate is a new, nonbarbiturate anesthetic (Giese and Stanley, 1983) used primarily to induce surgical anesthesia. It does not produce analgesia, but can be employed in a totally intravenous technique in which continuous infusion is combined with intermittent or continuous administration of fentanyl.

The advantages of etomidate are its minimal effects on the cardiovascular system and respiration during induction. It does not cause the liberation of histamine. An induction dose reduces cardiac output, stroke volume, and arterial pressure and produces a compensatory increase in heart rate. All of these alterations are within acceptable limits. Arrhythmias are uncommon. No significant changes in pulmonary or vascular resistance are noted, although peripheral blood flow may be increased. The effects are similar in normal patients and in those with severe cardiovascular disease. Etomidate decreases cerebral blood flow (by 35% to 50%), cerebral metabolic rate, and intracranial pressure and thus may be useful in neurosurgery.

ADVERSE REACTIONS AND PRECAUTIONS. Pain is common during administration but can be reduced by rapid injection into a large vein or premedication with an analgesic (eg, meperidine). In marked contrast to the barbiturates, etomidate produces no adverse effects following inadvertent intra-arterial injection.

Spontaneous muscle movements occur during induction in about 60% of patients not given premedication. These movements are not epileptogenic and their severity is not dose related. They subside rapidly and may be ameliorated by premedication with an opioid.

Since etomidate lacks analgesic action, intubation following its use for induction may be accompanied by pronounced

tachycardia and hypertension. These effects usually can be prevented by analgesic premedication in patients at risk.

Transient apnea (15 to 20 seconds) may occur during induction, particularly in elderly patients, and this may be prolonged by analgesic or benzodiazepine premedication. Coughing and hiccupping also have been observed, but their incidence is not dose related. Laryngospasm is uncommon.

Postoperative nausea and vomiting are more common with etomidate than with thiopental and occur more frequently (in up to 50% of patients) following multiple doses. Hypersensitivity reactions apparently are infrequent. Rash has been reported occasionally, but anaphylactic responses (eg, hypotension, bronchospasm) have not been observed.

Etomidate reversibly suppresses adrenocortical function. Prolonged infusion may produce hypotension, oliguria, and electrolyte disturbances that respond to glucocorticoids. For this reason, etomidate should not be employed for long surgical procedures or for prolonged sedation in intensive care patients.

This drug is classified in FDA Pregnancy Category C.

PHARMACOKINETICS. After administration of the usual induction dose (0.3 mg/kg), unconsciousness occurs within one minute and responsiveness returns within two to three minutes. Recovery time is dose dependent. Etomidate is hydrolyzed rapidly in the plasma and liver to an inactive metabolite. The plasma elimination half-life has been fitted to a triexponential equation to give $t1/2\alpha$ 2.6 $\pm$ 1.3 minutes, $t1/2\beta$ 28.7 $\pm$ 14.0 minutes, and $t1/2\gamma$ 4.6 $\pm$ 2.6 hours. The volume of distribution is 0.31 $\pm$ 0.152 L/kg and clearance is 0.699 $\pm$ 0.177 L/kg/hr (Van Hamme et al, 1978). The drug is 78% bound to serum albumin.

DOSAGE AND PREPARATIONS.

Intravenous: *Adults and children over 10 years*, the usual dose is 0.3 mg/kg (0.2 to 0.6 mg/kg) injected over a period of 30 to 60 seconds. This drug is not recommended for use during pregnancy or lactation or for children under 10 years.

Amidate (Abbott). Solution 2 mg/ml in 10 and 20 ml containers.

KETAMINE HYDROCHLORIDE
[Ketalar]

ACTIONS AND USES. Ketamine is a nonbarbiturate anesthetic that can be administered intravenously or intramuscularly. It induces a state of sedation and amnesia during which the patient may appear to be awake but is dissociated from the environment, immobile, and unresponsive to pain. Induction of anesthesia is rapid, even after intramuscular injection. Like thiopental, ketamine's anesthetic action is terminated by redistribution out of the central nervous system in approximately 10 minutes. Recovery from the postanesthetic psychic effects is more prolonged and may depend on elimination.

Because this anesthetic is rapidly effective when administered intramuscularly, it is particularly useful for repeated anesthesia in burn patients, for diagnostic studies, for sedating uncontrollable patients (eg, the mentally retarded), and for minor surgical procedures in young children. A small dose (0.5 to 1 mg/kg intramuscularly) can be used to calm agitated children and facilitate insertion of an intravenous cannula. The analgesic properties of ketamine may contribute to its usefulness for these purposes.

Ketamine also may be of value to induce anesthesia, particularly when a barbiturate cannot be used or cardiovascular depression must be avoided (eg, shock, severe dehydration, severe anemia, constrictive pericarditis). It is particularly useful in the presence of bronchospasm. However, it is not satisfactory as the sole agent for abdominal or other major surgical procedures because skeletal muscle relaxation is inadequate and adverse effects occur.

An anticholinergic drug should be given for premedication to reduce secretions. The concomitant use of diazepam, hydroxyzine, or a barbiturate increases recovery time. Another general anesthetic and a neuromuscular blocking agent can be used with ketamine if required. Ketamine potentiates the neuromuscular blocking effects of tubocurarine but not of pancuronium or succinylcholine. Postoperative analgesia may be produced when ketamine is administered intraoperatively.

ADVERSE REACTIONS AND PRECAUTIONS. Muscular rigidity, athetoid motions of the mouth and tongue, swallowing, random movements of the extremities, vocalization, laryngeal spasm, fasciculations, tremors, and generalized extensor spasm have occurred occasionally. Frank convulsions are extremely rare.

Although arrhythmias are seldom observed, ketamine usually increases heart rate and cardiac output, and the arterial pressure may increase as much as 25%, principally from stimulation of the central sympathetic nervous system and inhibition of norepinephrine reuptake. There is little change in systemic vascular resistance. The drug should be used with care in patients with mild, uncomplicated hypertension and is contraindicated when a significant elevation of blood pressure would constitute a serious hazard (in patients with aneurysms, angina, heart failure, cerebral trauma, or thyrotoxicosis) and in those who are hypersensitive to the drug. The indirect cardiovascular stimulant properties of ketamine are blocked when halothane or enflurane is given concomitantly and the direct myocardial depressant action of ketamine then becomes evident. Hypotension also may be observed in severely ill patients (eg, septic shock) or in patients with depleted cardiovascular stores of catecholamines (eg, chronic congestive failure).

Transient respiratory depression may occur immediately after intravenous administration of anesthetic doses and respiratory arrest has occurred in neonates. Laryngeal reflexes are depressed but retained during anesthesia. Aspiration of stomach contents has been reported, and an endotracheal tube should be used when any doubt exists concerning gastric content. Upper airway infection may increase the incidence of laryngospasm after use of ketamine, but there are no controlled studies to substantiate this finding. Tracheobronchial secretions are increased. Pre-existing bronchospasm usually is abolished by the smooth muscle relaxant action of ketamine.

Ketamine increases cerebrospinal fluid pressure and intracranial blood flow and should be used with extreme caution in patients with evidence of increased intracranial pressure or a space-occupying lesion. It has been suggested that ketamine does not always produce satisfactory analgesia in patients with cerebral cortical disease; the mechanism is unknown.

Ketamine may increase intraocular pressure slightly; thus, its use for some intraocular surgical procedures is inappropriate. It may be wise to avoid this anesthetic in patients with pre-existing elevation of intraocular pressure.

Studies on ketamine's effects on the fetus when used during delivery indicate that doses greater than 2 mg/kg are likely to cause fetal depression. Although smaller doses (0.25 to 0.5 mg/kg) appear to be safe for analgesia, caution is advised.

Ketamine may cause vomiting, hypersalivation, lacrimation, shivering, and transient cutaneous reactions. There is some evidence that the drug interacts with thyroid medication to produce severe hypertension and tachycardia.

Recovery from ketamine anesthesia sometimes takes up to several hours. Psychic disturbances during emergence (unpleasant dreams, irrational behavior, excitement, disorientation, illusions, delirium, hallucinations) may occur more frequently in adults (particularly women) than in children. The reported incidence varies between 3% and 50%. Several techniques can reduce the incidence of such reactions: (1) Oral premedication with lorazepam 4 mg or diazepam 10 mg; (2) intravenous administration of diazepam 0.15 to 0.3 mg/kg at the end of anesthesia; (3) use of no more than 2 mg/kg as the induction dose and maintenance of anesthesia with doses of 0.5 to 1 mg/kg; (4) use of a low-dose microdrip intravenous infusion; (5) use of glycopyrrolate instead of atropine or scopolamine; and (6) maintenance of anesthesia with other agents. Of these, premedication with 4 mg of oral lorazepam 30 to 40 minutes prior to induction is the most effective in preventing the emergence phenomena but sedation is increased and recovery may be prolonged. Although there is no evidence that psychic disturbances have any residual effect, it may be advisable to avoid ketamine in patients with preoperative psychiatric problems.

PHARMACOKINETICS. Ketamine is metabolized in the liver. The half-life is 2.5 to 4 hours, the apparent volume of distribution is 3.3 L/kg, and the clearance rate is 1.3 L/min.

DOSAGE AND PREPARATIONS. Tachyphylaxis has been observed when ketamine is given for repeated operative, diagnostic, or therapeutic procedures.

Intravenous: For induction, single-dose method, 2 mg/kg (range, 1 to 4.5 mg/kg) administered over 60 seconds. Unconsciousness persists for 10 to 15 minutes and analgesia persists for an additional 30 minutes. For maintenance, one-half of the full induction dose, repeated as necessary.

Using the low-dose, microdrip technique, a 0.1% concentration is administered at a rate of 20 ml/min as needed for induction. The rate is adjusted according to the patient's blood pressure, pulse rate, and response to surgical stimulation. When this technique is employed for maintenance with nitrous oxide and a muscle relaxant, the total dose of ketamine required is only one-third to one-half of the amount employed for bolus administration.

An anesthetic technique that minimizes the adverse cardiovascular response to ketamine may be accomplished by premedication with diazepam 10 mg orally 30 to 120 minutes prior to induction and atropine sulfate 0.4 mg intravenously at induction. Induction is initiated by infusing ketamine 0.1% in a dose of 1.5 mg/kg in three minutes; at the beginning of each minute, 5 mg of diazepam is given for a total of 15 mg. During the second minute, 0.6 mg/kg of tubocurarine (pancuronium is not satisfactory) is given intravenously as a bolus. After intubation, ventilation is maintained with nitrous oxide and oxygen. Maintenance doses of ketamine during the first hour are 0.2 mg/kg/hr by infusion with intermittent boluses of diazepam 5 mg every 30 minutes. For the second and subsequent hours, the dose of ketamine is reduced to 0.1 mg/kg/hr and of diazepam to 2.5 mg every 30 minutes. Additional amounts of tubocurarine are given as needed (Aldrete and McDonald, 1980; Wilson et al, 1980).

Intramuscular: For induction, 6.5 to 13 mg/kg. For maintenance, one-half of the full induction dose, repeated as necessary. For analgesia (eg, burn patients), 2 mg/kg.

> **Ketalar** (Parke-Davis). Solution (equivalent to base) 10 mg/ml in 20 and 50 ml containers, 50 mg/ml in 10 ml containers, and 100 mg/ml in 5 ml containers.

COMBINATION ANESTHESIA

Balanced Anesthesia

Components: Because of its low potency, nitrous oxide must be supplemented with other agents to produce conditions suitable for surgery. The use of more potent inhalation or intravenous agents to achieve this goal has been discussed. The intravenous use of an ultrashort-acting barbiturate, an opioid analgesic, a neuromuscular blocking agent, and nitrous oxide to produce general anesthesia is termed "balanced anesthesia." Meperidine [Demerol], morphine, fentanyl [Sublimaze], and sufentanil [Sufenta] are the most widely employed analgesics and, in combination with a barbiturate, supplement the hypnotic and analgesic effects of nitrous oxide. Meperidine was the first opioid analgesic used in this manner but is not as satisfactory as fentanyl because of its tendency to produce myocardial depression when given in large doses.

An opioid analgesic often is included in the premedication and anesthesia is induced with a barbiturate and nitrous oxide. The opioid then is given intravenously in increments over five to ten minutes until adequate analgesia has been produced. Additional small amounts may be required during surgery if the patient reacts to painful stimuli (eg, increasing pulse rate and arterial pressure, pupillary dilation, sweating, muscle movement). If used judiciously in this manner and if avoided during the last one to two hours of *prolonged* surgery, adequate intraoperative analgesia usually can be achieved without the need for postoperative ventilatory support. If a neuromuscular blocking agent is used, controlled ventilation is mandatory during surgery. If a neuromuscular blocking agent is not used, spontaneous ventilation may be satisfactory during short

procedures; however, controlled ventilation generally is advisable.

The following combination is often used for short surgical procedures (15 to 20 minutes in adults): fentanyl 1 to 2 mcg/kg intravenously two minutes prior to induction, thiopental 4 mg/kg for induction, and 70% nitrous oxide-30% oxygen for maintenance, plus supplemental doses of thiopental 1 to 2 mg/kg and fentanyl 0.25 to 0.5 mcg/kg. This regimen permits rapid recovery and is useful for outpatient surgery in adults. Sufentanil 0.2 to 0.3 mcg/kg initially with thiopental 2 to 3 mg/kg for induction and 0.05 to 0.1 mcg/kg as needed for maintenance may be substituted for fentanyl.

Morphine became popular in balanced anesthesia for cardiac surgery and for poor-risk patients in general because it usually did not affect myocardial function or cardiovascular dynamics. Large intravenous doses (0.5 to 3 mg/kg) were administered with nitrous oxide or halothane. However, later studies indicated that the administration of nitrous oxide in concentrations greater than 60% or halothane 0.21% to 0.23% after use of morphine 1 mg/kg produced cardiovascular depression (eg, decreased arterial pressure and cardiac index).

When large doses of morphine are used alone with 100% oxygen, amnesia may not be achieved and a higher proportion of patients may require appropriate measures to combat hypertension. Anterograde amnesia is provided by the concurrent administration of diazepam 0.5 mg/kg. Controlled ventilation must be employed postoperatively, at least during the first 12 to 24 hours. The easy transition from intraoperative to postoperative analgesia and ventilatory support is one of the major advantages of this technique in these poor-risk patients.

Fentanyl or sufentanil can be substituted for morphine, but the rapid administration of these drugs may produce muscular rigidity that interferes with ventilation. This effect may be minimized by slow administration, pretreatment with or concomitant administration of a nondepolarizing muscle relaxant, or premedication with a benzodiazepine (Stanley, 1982). To avoid cardiovascular depression produced by nitrous oxide, sufentanil 8 mcg/kg or more or fentanyl 50 mcg/kg or more administered incrementally may be used with oxygen and a muscle relaxant for cardiovascular surgery or neurosurgical procedures requiring a sitting position.

The narcotic antagonist, naloxone [Narcan], may be administered to overcome the residual effects of the opioid analgesic at the end of surgery. However, this reduces or eliminates postoperative analgesia and sometimes increases sympathetic stimulation, which results in arrhythmias and increased myocardial work. It also can be hazardous if the effect of the narcotic antagonist ends before that of the analgesic. If a narcotic antagonist is used in this manner, the patient must be observed carefully and additional doses of the antagonist given as necessary. (See Chapter 80, Drugs Used in the Treatment of Poisoning.)

The dosage schedules discussed above represent only general guidelines. In practice, the technique of balanced anesthesia remains somewhat empirical: The choice of opioid analgesic, the dose used, and the frequency of administration differ and always must be individualized. The adequacy of spontaneous ventilation always must be evaluated carefully and objectively during the postoperative period.

Advantages and Disadvantages: Clinical experience and data from some controlled trials indicate that properly administered balanced anesthesia minimizes intraoperative cardiovascular depression and may increase peripheral resistance; there is an early return of consciousness, and the incidence of postoperative nausea, vomiting, excitement, and pain is low.

Balanced anesthesia is contraindicated when an FIO_2 of 0.25 to 0.4 cannot be tolerated or in patients with anemia that limits the oxygen-carrying capacity of the blood. Care must be taken not to "cover up" inadequate analgesia with muscle relaxants. Patient awareness during surgery has been reported.

Neuroleptanalgesia and Neuroleptanesthesia

Neuroleptanalgesia historically refers to administration of both an opioid analgesic and droperidol [Inapsine], a neuroleptic (antipsychotic) drug, to produce an altered state of consciousness and awareness. Alternative combinations used in clinical studies include diazepam [Valium], ketamine [Ketalar], or droperidol with meperidine [Demerol], morphine, fentanyl [Sublimaze], or sufentanil [Sufenta].

Consciousness is not lost during neuroleptanalgesia and the technique may be useful for diagnostic and therapeutic procedures performed under local anesthesia (eg, cardiac catheterization, repeated burn dressings).

When nitrous oxide is used to supplement these combinations, the term, neuroleptanesthesia, is employed. A muscle relaxant also may be included. This technique often provides satisfactory general anesthesia and may be particularly valuable when the patient's cooperation is required during the procedure, for consciousness returns soon after the flow of nitrous oxide is terminated.

The opioid analgesic, fentanyl, has been used most commonly with the butyrophenone, droperidol, in neuroleptanesthesia. Droperidol and fentanyl are available as single-entity products or in fixed-dose combination [Innovar].

Drug Evaluations

FENTANYL CITRATE
[Sublimaze]

ACTIONS. On a milligram basis, fentanyl is 50 to 100 times more potent than morphine, which is approximately eight to ten times more potent than meperidine. The analgesia produced by morphine lasts two to three times longer than that of fentanyl and approximately two times longer than that of meperidine. Fentanyl resembles thiopental in that moderate single doses are short acting due to redistribution. Multiple doses or large amounts accumulate and prolong recovery time.

USES. For balanced anesthesia with nitrous oxide or another inhalation agent and a muscle relaxant, repeated doses of 0.05 to 0.1 mg of fentanyl can be used instead of meperidine and total doses of 0.015 to 0.1 mg/kg can replace morphine in cardiac surgery and poor-risk patients. Fentanyl does not cause the moderate to marked vasodilation produced by morphine and meperidine. Fentanyl can be used for induction of surgical anesthesia and as the sole anesthetic agent with oxygen and a muscle relaxant for cardiovascular, neurologic, or orthopedic surgery in selected patients.

Fentanyl is used with the butyrophenone, droperidol, in neuroleptanalgesia and with both droperidol and nitrous oxide in neuroleptanesthesia (see the evaluation on Droperidol and Fentanyl).

ADVERSE REACTIONS AND PRECAUTIONS. If a therapeutic dose of fentanyl is administered rapidly intravenously, a generalized increase in muscle tone, including chest wall spasm, may develop; such rigidity also can occur with use of meperidine or morphine. The incidence of rigidity increases with age (Bailey et al, 1985) and is caused by a central action of fentanyl. Thoracic compliance decreases markedly, which impairs the ability to assist or control ventilation. The incidence and severity of rigidity can be decreased by premedication with a small dose of a nondepolarizing muscle relaxant (eg, pancuronium 0.022 mg/kg) (Stanley, 1982; Bailey et al, 1985). Rigidity also is exacerbated by nitrous oxide but can be relieved or prevented by general anesthesia with thiopental or halothane, or by use of a neuromuscular blocking agent and controlled ventilation.

Slowing of the heart rate, which is easily reversed by atropine, may occur when fentanyl is given.

PHARMACOKINETICS. Fentanyl 6.4 mcg/kg given intravenously has an elimination half-life of 3.6 hours, an apparent volume of distribution of 4 L/kg, and a clearance of 0.96 L/min. It is 81% protein bound (McClain and Hug, 1980). The pharmacokinetic data from several sources have been reviewed (Mather, 1983).

DOSAGE AND PREPARATIONS.
Intramuscular: Adults, for premedication, 0.05 to 0.1 mg (1 to 2 ml) 30 to 60 minutes prior to surgery. This dose should be decreased in the elderly or poor-risk patient.
Intravenous: Adults, for induction, 0.05 to 0.1 mg (1 to 2 ml) initially, repeated at two- to three-minute intervals until satisfactory induction is achieved. If attenuation of sympathetic activity is desired (eg, coronary artery disease), a total dose of 30 to 40 mcg/kg is required. The dose should be reduced to 0.025 to 0.05 mg (0.5 to 1 ml) in elderly or poor-risk patients. For maintenance, 0.025 mg to one-half the loading dose may be administered if lightening of anesthesia is manifested by movement or change in vital signs. *Children 2 to 12 years,* for

induction and maintenance, 2 to 3 mcg/kg. See also the evaluation on Droperidol and Fentanyl Citrate.

Sublimaze (Janssen). Solution 0.05 mg/ml in 2, 5, 10, and 20 ml containers.

SUFENTANIL CITRATE
[Sufenta]

ACTIONS. This opioid is a derivative of fentanyl and is pharmacologically similar. On a weight basis, sufentanil is 5 to 12 times more potent than fentanyl and 625 times more potent than morphine. When given to induce anesthesia, the onset of action of sufentanil is about 15% to 20% more rapid than that of fentanyl. At low dosage, recovery time is equivalent for the two agents. After induction of general anesthesia, recovery is significantly more rapid than with an equivalent anesthetic dose of fentanyl. The duration of action, like that of fentanyl, is determined by redistribution from the central nervous system. Because sufentanil is cleared more rapidly from tissue storage sites, there presumably is less tendency for accumulation.

USES. Sufentanil is used for balanced anesthesia in general surgery as an adjunct to nitrous oxide and oxygen. It also may be used for induction of surgical anesthesia and as the sole anesthetic agent with a muscle relaxant and oxygen for cardiovascular and neurosurgical procedures.

ADVERSE REACTIONS AND PRECAUTIONS. Like fentanyl, the rapid intravenous administration of sufentanil may produce a general increase in skeletal muscle tone, including chest wall spasm. The incidence of this response can be reduced by the prior or concomitant administration of a nondepolarizing muscle relaxant. Bradycardia occurs in about 3% of patients and responds to atropine. Both hypotension and hypertension have been reported.

PHARMACOKINETICS. Sufentanil 5 mcg/kg given intravenously is metabolized rapidly (elimination half-life, 2.4 hours). The apparent volume of distribution is 2.5 L/kg and the clearance is 0.8 L/min (Bovill et al, 1981). It is 92.5% protein bound (Meuldermans et al, 1982).

DOSAGE AND PREPARATIONS.
Intravenous: For general surgery requiring intubation and mechanical ventilation, *adults*, 1 to 2 mcg/kg with nitrous oxide/oxygen; for maintenance, 10 to 25 mcg (0.2 to 0.5 ml) as needed.

For major surgical procedures requiring some attenuation of sympathetic response to surgical stimuli, *adults*, 2 to 8 mcg/kg with nitrous oxide/oxygen; for maintenance, 25 to 50 mcg (0.5 to 1 ml) as needed.

For induction in patients undergoing cardiovascular or neurosurgical procedures in the sitting position, *adults*, 8 mcg/kg or more with oxygen and a nondepolarizing (curariform) muscle relaxant; for maintenance, 25 to 50 mcg (0.5 to 1 ml) as

needed. Postoperative mechanical ventilation will be required with these doses. *Children 2 to 12 years undergoing cardiovascular surgery*, 10 mcg/kg or more with oxygen only.

Children under 2 years, no dosage has been established because of insufficient data. However, the agent appears to be safe for cardiovascular procedures in this population.

Sufenta (Janssen). Solution 50 mcg/ml in 1, 2, and 5 ml containers (preservative free).

DROPERIDOL
[Inapsine]

ACTIONS AND USES. Droperidol, a butyrophenone, produces an altered state of awareness, sedation, and, in many patients, dysphoria. It causes little or no amnesia and has an antiemetic action. It is not an analgesic. Intravenous administration causes a slight, transient fall in arterial pressure secondary to peripheral vasodilation that may be due to block of alpha-adrenergic receptors, direct vasodilation, or both. There is little change in ventilation and the drug appears to have little effect on the respiratory depressant action of fentanyl. A dose of 10 mg reduces total body oxygen consumption by approximately 25%.

When droperidol was not used previously during the procedure, intravenous administration of 0.075 mg/kg at the termination of general anesthesia reduced the incidence of postoperative vomiting. However, because this drug may produce untoward effects and the incidence of severe, protracted postoperative vomiting is less than 3%, its prophylactic use for antiemetic effect should be reserved for procedures in which vomiting could interfere with the results of surgery (eg, intraocular surgery). (See also Chapter 14, Drugs Used in Vertigo and Vomiting.)

ADVERSE REACTIONS AND PRECAUTIONS. Droperidol occasionally produces extrapyramidal reactions (protrusion and uncontrolled movements of the tongue, dysphagia, lateral movements of the head, torticollis, twitching of limbs, restlessness, agitation, and parkinsonian crises) within 24 to 48 hours. Signs and symptoms can be relieved rapidly by diphenhydramine or benztropine (see Chapter 11, Drugs Used in Extrapyramidal Movement Disorders). Patients occasionally have reported dysphoric reactions when droperidol was given for premedication.

DRUG INTERACTIONS. Anecdotal evidence suggests that droperidol may antagonize the effects of levodopa resulting in reappearance of parkinsonian symptoms. Because of the drug's prolonged action (usually 12 to 24 hours), other central nervous system depressants should be given cautiously and in reduced doses during the early postoperative period.

PHARMACOKINETICS. Droperidol has an elimination half-life

of approximately 2.2 hours (Cressman et al, 1973). Other pharmacokinetic parameters have not been reported.

DOSAGE AND PREPARATIONS. See the evaluation on Droperidol and Fentanyl Citrate.

> *Inapsine* (Janssen). Solution 2.5 mg/ml in 2, 5, and 10 ml containers.

DROPERIDOL AND FENTANYL CITRATE
[Innovar]

ACTIONS AND USES. This fixed-dose combination contains the narcotic analgesic, fentanyl (0.05 mg/ml), and the neuroleptic butyrophenone, droperidol (2.5 mg/ml). These drugs usually provide satisfactory amnesia and analgesia, and the mixture has been used to produce neuroleptanalgesia and neuroleptanesthesia. As with all combinations, its use is appropriate only when both drugs are to be administered at the same time and in the dosage ratio present in the mixture; otherwise, the two drugs should be administered separately as necessary.

Droperidol and fentanyl can be administered safely to patients who have previously experienced malignant hyperpyrexia under general anesthesia.

ADVERSE REACTIONS AND PRECAUTIONS. Cardiac output is reduced and systemic vascular resistance is increased initially but return to normal as surgery continues. The arterial pressure and pulse rate tend to remain stable, but the heart rate may decrease. Ventricular arrhythmias are uncommon unless the sympathetic nervous system is stimulated by accumulation of carbon dioxide due to inadequate ventilation. Profound depression of the ventilatory rate and minute volume and apnea (caused by fentanyl) are to be expected. Apnea may result from central nervous system depression or peripheral muscle rigidity and can be treated by controlled ventilation. Muscle rigidity can be overcome by neuromuscular blocking agents.

Transient, slight abnormalities in the results of liver function tests similar to those observed after other anesthetic techniques have developed. Hyperglycemia occurs, but there is no evidence of metabolic acidosis. Pupils are constricted, intraocular tension is unchanged, and, if hypercapnia is avoided, cerebrospinal fluid pressure is reduced in patients with and without space-occupying lesions. In contrast, the volatile agents may increase pressure, even with normocapnia.

Consciousness and spontaneous respiration return rapidly when nitrous oxide and controlled ventilation are stopped if large doses have not been administered repeatedly. Postoperative nausea, vomiting, and shivering due to hypothermia may occur, but restlessness and delirium are uncommon. Extrapyramidal reactions may develop if a large dose of droperidol has been used (see the evaluation on Droperidol).

Evidence that the combination reduces laryngeal competence suggests that this mixture should be used only with great caution and in small quantities to facilitate "awake intubation" indicated for a full stomach.

See also the evaluations on Fentanyl Citrate and Droperidol.

DOSAGE AND PREPARATIONS.

Intravenous: Neuroleptanesthesia can be induced with 1 ml/9 to 12 kg (smaller doses may be adequate) administered slowly (1 ml every one to two minutes), followed by nitrous oxide and oxygen when drowsiness develops. Thiopental 100 mg also may be used to hasten induction. Anesthesia can be maintained with nitrous oxide or with fentanyl alone (usual dose, 0.05 to 0.1 mg every 30 to 60 minutes) when clinical signs indicate that anesthesia may be too light (voluntary movements, rapid or irregular ventilation, increasing pulse rate and arterial pressure, lacrimation). The mixture should not be used for maintenance unless the patient specifically requires the pharmacologic effects of both drugs.

Neuromuscular blocking agents and controlled ventilation should be utilized as indicated. If the former are not required, assisted ventilation may be adequate if the total dose of fentanyl does not exceed approximately 3 mcg/kg. A narcotic antagonist can be given to reverse severe respiratory depression but, unless carefully titrated to a satisfactory level of depression, it will antagonize the analgesic effect as well. The patient must be observed carefully after use of the narcotic antagonist in case the effect of the antagonist ends before that of fentanyl.

Because droperidol is long acting and has a relatively slow onset (10 to 15 minutes) and fentanyl has a relatively rapid onset (one to two minutes) but a short duration of action, an alternative technique that avoids the use of Innovar has been described: Induction is started with a single dose of droperidol 0.15 mg/kg; six to eight minutes later, fentanyl 0.002 to 0.003 mg/kg is given incrementally over six to eight minutes. Nitrous oxide is started when drowsiness develops and anesthesia is maintained as described above.

> *Innovar* (Janssen). Each milliliter of solution contains fentanyl citrate 0.05 mg and droperidol 2.5 mg in 2 and 5 ml containers.

Cited References

Aldrete JA, McDonald JS: Low-dose ketamine-diazepam prevents adverse reactions, in Aldrete JA, Stanley TH (eds): *Trends in Intravenous Anesthesia*. Chicago, Year Book Medical Publishers, 1980, 331-341.

Bailey PL, et al: Anesthetic induction with fentanyl. *Anesth Analg* 64:48-53, 1985.

Bovill JG, et al: Kinetics of alfentanil and sufentanil: Comparison. *Anesthesiology* 55:A174, 1981.

Brown CR, et al: Clinical, electroencephalographic, and pharmacokinetic studies of a water-soluble benzodiazepine, midazolam maleate. *Anesthesiology* 50:467-470, 1979.

Cressman WA, et al: Absorption, metabolism and excretion of droperidol by human subjects following intramuscular and intravenous administration. *Anesthesiology* 38:363-369, 1973.

Dundee JW, Wyant GM: *Intravenous Anesthesia*. Edinburgh, Churchill Livingstone, 1974.

Eger EI II: *Anesthetic Uptake and Action*. Baltimore, Williams & Wilkins, 1974.

Eger EI II: *American Society of Anesthesiology Annual Refresher Course*, 1980.

Eger RR, Eger EI II: Effect of temperature and age on solubility of enflurane, halothane, isoflurane, and methoxyflurane in human blood. *Anesth Analg* 64:640-642, 1985.

Forster A, et al: Effects of midazolam on cerebral blood flow in human volunteers. *Anesthesiology* 56:453-455, 1982.

Giese JL, Stanley TH: Etomidate: New intravenous anesthetic induction agent. *Pharmacotherapy* 3:251-258, 1983.

Hornbein TF, et al: Minimum alveolar concentration of nitrous oxide in man. *Anesth Analg* 61:553-556, 1982.

Hudson PJ, et al: Comparative pharmacokinetics of methohexital and thiopental. *Anesthesiology* 57:A240, 1982.

Jung D, et al: Thiopental disposition in lean and obese patients undergoing surgery. *Anesthesiology* 56:269-274, 1982.

Kanto J, et al: Pharmacokinetics and sedative effect of midazolam in connection with Caesarean section performed under epidural anesthesia. *Acta Anaesthiol Scand* 28:116-118, 1984.

Mather LE: Clinical pharmacokinetics of fentanyl and its newer derivatives. *Clin Pharmacokinet* 8:422-446, 1983.

McClain DA, Hug CC Jr: Intravenous fentanyl kinetics. *Clin Pharmacol Ther* 28:106-114, 1980.

Meuldermans WEG, et al: Plasma protein binding and distribution of fentanyl, sufentanil, alfentanil and lofentanil in blood. *Arch Int Pharmacodyn* 257:4-19, 1982.

Morgan DJ, et al: Pharmacokinetics and plasma binding of thiopental. I. Studies in surgical patients. II. Studies at cesarean section. *Anesthesiology* 54:468-473, 474-480, 1981.

Nunn JF: Interaction of nitrous oxide and vitamin B_{12}. *Trends Pharmacol Sci* 5:225-227, 1984.

Paull J, Ziccone S: Halothane, enflurane, methoxyflurane, and isolated human uterine muscle. *Anaesth Intens Care* 8:397-401, 1980.

Quasha AL, et al: Determination and applications of MAC. *Anesthesiology* 53:315-334, 1980.

Reves JG, et al: Comparison of two benzodiazepines for anesthesia induction: Midazolam and diazepam. *Can Anaesth Soc J* 25:211-214, 1978.

Sorbo S, et al: Pharmacokinetics of thiopental in pediatric surgical patients. *Anesthesiology* 61:666-670, 1984.

Stanley TH: High-dose narcotic anesthesia. *Semin Anesth* 1:21-32, 1982.

Stock JGL, Strunin L: Unexplained hepatitis following halothane. *Anesthesiology* 63:424-439, 1985.

Van Hamme MJ, et al: Pharmacokinetics of etomidate, new intravenous anesthetic. *Anesthesiology* 49:274-277, 1978.

Wilson RD, et al: Cardiovascular effects of ketamine infusion, in Aldrete JA, Stanley TH (eds): *Trends in Intravenous Therapy*. Chicago, Year Book Medical Publishers, 1980, 343-354.

Other Selected References

Adams AP: Enflurane in clinical practice. *Br J Anaesth* 53(suppl 1):27-41, 1981.

Clarke RSJ, Norman J (eds): Symposium on anesthetic pharmacology. *Br J Anaesth* 51:577-710, 1979.

Cohen EN: Toxicity of inhalation anesthetic agents. *Br J Anaesth* 50:665-675, 1978.

Davie IT: Specific drug interactions in anesthesia. *Anaesthesia* 32:1000-1008, 1977.

Duvaldestin P: Pharmacokinetics in intravenous anaesthetic practice. *Clin Pharmacokinet* 6:61-82, 1981.

Eger EI II: Isoflurane. *Semin Anesth* 1:1-13, 1982.

Eger EI II: *Nitrous Oxide/N_2O*. New York, Elsevier, 1985.

Estafanous FG (ed): *Opioids in Anesthesia*. Boston, Butterworth, 1984.

Farrell G, et al: Halothane hepatitis. Detection of a constitutional susceptibility factor. *N Engl J Med* 313:1310-1314, 1985.

Gray TC, et al (eds): *General Anesthesia*, ed 4. London, Butterworth, vols I and II, 1980.

Korttila K: Pharmacokinetics of intravenous non-narcotic anesthetics, in Aldrete JA, Stanley TH (eds): *Trends in Intravenous Therapy*. Chicago, Year Book Medical Publishers, 1980, 13-42.

Miller RD (ed): *Anesthesia*. New York, Churchill Livingstone, vols I and II, 1981.

Steen PA, Michenfelder JD: Neurotoxicity of anesthetics. *Anesthesiology* 50:437-453, 1979.

Whitwam JG: Adverse reactions to I.V. induction agents. *Br J Anaesth* 50:677-687, 1978.

Adjuncts to Anesthesia *17*

AGENTS USED FOR PREMEDICATION

   Analgesics

   Barbiturates

   Benzodiazepines

   Neuroleptic Drugs

   Anticholinergic Drugs

NEUROMUSCULAR BLOCKING DRUGS

   Nondepolarizing (Competitive) Blocking Drugs

   Depolarizing Blocking Drug

MISCELLANEOUS ADJUNCTIVE DRUGS

   Vasodilators

   Agents Used In Pheochromocytoma

   Agents Used In Malignant Hyperthermia

   Agent Used in Pre-eclampsia and Eclampsia

   Respiratory Stimulants (Analeptics)

A number of drugs commonly used as adjuncts to anesthesia have additional therapeutic indications and may be discussed in more detail in other chapters. Agents given to reduce the incidence of postoperative nausea and vomiting are discussed in Chapter 14, Drugs Used in Vertigo and Vomiting. Drugs used in the prevention and management of aspiration pneumonitis are discussed in Chapter 52, Agents Used in Disorders of the Upper Gastrointestinal Tract.

AGENTS USED FOR PREMEDICATION

Generally, a patient's usual medication need not be altered when surgery is indicated, but potential complications or drug interactions must be evaluated. Medications that must be continued (eg, antianginal drugs, anticonvulsants, antihypertensive agents) may necessitate modification of the anesthetic technique. The dose of insulin may require adjustment to avoid intraoperative hypoglycemia or hyperglycemia and ketosis. Glucocorticoids should be continued in patients who received high-dose therapy in the preceding six months (Knudsen et al, 1981) or in those with chronic asthma. Opioid analgesics frequently are required in patients with moderate to severe preoperative pain and in opioid-dependent individuals. Defects in hydration, electrolyte balance, hemoglobin levels, and nutritional status should be corrected before surgery if possible.

Historically, drugs were administered before the induction of anesthesia with diethyl ether to sedate the patient, reduce apprehension, facilitate induction, diminish the dose of anesthetic, inhibit salivary and airway secretions, and prevent bradycardia. Morphine was used to achieve the first four effects, and atropine or scopolamine was given to achieve the remaining two. During the last several decades, other analgesics, hypnotics, benzodiazepines, and neuroleptics have been used instead of morphine, but definitive comparative studies have not been conducted.

Analgesics: There are few important differences among the individual analgesics. Euphoria is not a characteristic of the preanesthetic use of opioids unless these agents are administered to relieve preoperative pain. Most opiates and opioids produce sedation but generally do not reduce apprehension or cause amnesia. All may increase the incidence of pre- and

TABLE 1.
AGENTS USED FOR PREMEDICATION

Drug	Route	Dosage
ANALGESICS		
Fentanyl Citrate [Sublimaze]	Intramuscular	*Adults,* 0.05 to 0.1 mg.
Morphine Sulfate	Subcutaneous Intramuscular	*Adults,* 10 mg (range, 5 to 12 mg); *children 1 year and over,* 0.1 mg/kg (maximum, 10 mg).
Meperidine Hydrochloride [Demerol Hydrochloride]	Subcutaneous Intramuscular	*Adults,* 100 mg (range, 50 to 150 mg); *children 1 year and over,* 1 mg/kg (maximum, 100 mg).
Pentazocine Lactate [Talwin Lactate]	Subcutaneous Intramuscular	*Adults,* 20 to 40 mg.
BARBITURATES		
Pentobarbital Sodium [Nembutal Sodium]	Intramuscular	*Adults,* 100 to 150 mg (range, 75 to 200 mg); *children 6 months and over,* 2 to 4 mg/kg (maximum, 100 mg).
Secobarbital Sodium [Seconal Sodium]	Intramuscular	*adults,* 100 to 150 mg (range, 75 to 200 mg); *children 6 months and over,* 2 to 4 mg/kg (maximum, 100 mg).
BENZODIAZEPINES		
Chlordiazepoxide Hydrochloride [Librium]	Oral Intramuscular	*Adults,* 50 to 100 mg.
Diazepam [Valium, Valrelease]	Oral Intravenous Rectal	*Adults,* 10 mg; *children 2 years and over,* 0.25 mg/kg. *Adults,* 10 to 20 mg. *children,* 0.4 to 0.5 mg/kg.
Flunitrazepam* [Rohypnol]	Oral Intramuscular	*Adults,* 1 to 2 mg. *Adults,* 2 mg.
Lorazepam [Ativan]	Oral Intramuscular Intravenous	*Adults,* 4 mg. *Adults,*** 0.05 mg/kg (maximum, 4 mg) two hours prior to surgery. *Adults,*** 0.044 mg/kg (maximum, 2 mg).
Midazolam [Versed]	Intravenous Intramuscular	*Adults,* 5 mg. *Adults,* 0.07 to 0.1 mg/kg.
Temazepam [Restoril]	Oral	*Adults,* 20 to 30 mg.
Triazolam [Halcion]	Oral	*Adults,* 0.125 to 0.25 mg (maximum, 0.5 mg).
NEUROLEPTIC DRUGS		
Droperidol [Inapsine]	Intramuscular	*Adults,* 2.5 to 5 mg.
Droperidol and Fentanyl Citrate [Innovar]	Intramuscular	*Adults,* 0.5 to 2 ml (fentanyl 0.05 mg/ml and droperidol 2.5 mg/ml).

(Continued on next page)

Drug	Route	Dosage
ANTICHOLINERGIC DRUGS		
Atropine Sulfate	Oral	*Adults,* 2 mg.
	Intramuscular	*Adults,* 0.6 mg; *newborn infants,* 0.1 mg; *4 to 12 months,* 0.2 mg; *1 to 3 years,* 0.3 mg; *3 to 14 years,* 0.4 mg.
Glycopyrrolate [Robinul Injectable]	Intramuscular	*Adults,* 0.0044 mg/kg; *children up to 12 years,* 0.0044 to 0.0088 mg/kg 60 minutes prior to induction.
Scopolamine Hydrobromide	Oral	*Adults,* 1 mg.
	Intramuscular	*Adults,* 0.4 to 0.6 mg; *infants 4 to 7 months,* 0.1 mg; *7 months to 3 years,* 0.15 mg; *3 to 8 years,* 0.2 mg; *8 to 12 years,* 0.3 mg.

Subcutaneous or intramuscular doses are administered 45 to 60 minutes before anesthesia and oral doses one to four hours before anesthesia. The amounts should be reduced in elderly or debilitated patients.

Drugs may also be given intravenously. They should be given slowly, with caution, ie, titrated to effect. The intravenous doses are generally smaller than those recommended for other parenteral routes.

*Investigational drug

**Not recommended for patients under 18 years.

postoperative nausea and vomiting. Other adverse effects include dizziness, tachycardia, sweating, and, less commonly, hypotension, restlessness or excitement, and respiratory depression with a marked reduction in the respiratory response to increases in PCO_2.

If scopolamine is given with morphine or meperidine [Demerol], the incidence of sedation and delayed awakening may be increased, while that of apprehension and pre- and postoperative nausea and vomiting may be reduced.

The effects of pentazocine [Talwin] are similar to those of morphine. Undesirable psychotomimetic effects occur in some adults, particularly the elderly, receiving more than 40 mg and marked emetic effects develop with doses of 60 mg.

Intramuscular fentanyl [Sublimaze] has an inappropriate onset and too short a duration of action for routine preanesthetic use. When administered intravenously just prior to induction of general or regional anesthesia, it produces good to profound sedation.

See also Table 1 for dosages and Chapter 4, General Analgesics.

Barbiturates: In an attempt to avoid the adverse effects of opiate and opioid analgesics, secobarbital [Seconal] and pentobarbital [Nembutal] were tried. However, preanesthetic doses of these drugs may depress respiration and do not provide analgesia; disorientation or delirium may develop in the presence of pain. Circulation is only slightly affected and nausea or vomiting is rare. Barbiturates must not be used in patients with hepatic porphyria.

Barbiturates now are being replaced by benzodiazepines, which produce more anterograde amnesia and less respiratory depression. See also Table 1 for dosages and Chapter 5, Drugs Used for Anxiety and Sleep Disorders.

Benzodiazepines: The benzodiazepines may be preferred to the opiate and opioid analgesics and the short-acting barbiturates for premedication. These drugs provide sedation and anterograde amnesia and reduce anxiety to varying degrees. At recommended doses, the incidence and intensity of sedation are least with chlordiazepoxide [Librium] and most with lorazepam [Ativan]. The antianxiety action is most pronounced with flunitrazepam [Rohypnol] (investigational drug) 2 mg orally and lorazepam 2.5 mg orally (Kanto, 1981). Anterograde amnesia is more marked and prolonged with lorazepam than with diazepam [Valium] (Ameer and Greenblatt, 1981). Triazolam [Halcion] has a potent sedative-hypnotic action. Newer benzodiazepines employed for premedication include flunitrazepam (Male et al, 1980; Mattila and Larni, 1980), midazolam [Versed] (Dundee et al, 1984; Reves et al, 1985), and temazepam [Restoril] (Beechey et al, 1981).

Excitement, dizziness, tachycardia, hypotension, and pre- or postoperative nausea and vomiting are uncommon, although the combined use of lorazepam and scopolamine may produce severe restlessness. Benzodiazepines slightly reduce lower esophageal sphincter pressure, which increases the possibility of reflux. Following premedication with intravenous diazepam 0.14 mg/kg, the minute ventilation, respiratory frequency, and mean inspiratory flow rate were reduced by 17%, 12%, and 19%, respectively (Clergue et al, 1981). The other benzodiazepines are presumed to cause equivalent respiratory depression.

Since benzodiazepines are absorbed reliably from the gastrointestinal tract, the oral route often is used. The onset of action is rapid after parenteral administration, but absorption following intramuscular injection of diazepam may be erratic because of this drug's low water solubility. Absorption is more rapid following injection into the upper thigh or deltoid rather than the buttock. Pain may persist at the injection site.

In children, benzodiazepines produce effective sedation, few nightmares, and, possibly, better acceptance of the anesthetic face mask; the incidence of postoperative vomiting also is lower than with opioids.

See also Table 1 for dosages and Chapters 5, Drugs Used for Anxiety and Sleep Disorders; 9, Antiepileptic Drugs; and 16, General Anesthetics.

Neuroleptic Drugs: When used as the sole preanesthetic medication in adults, intramuscular droperidol [Inapsine] 5 mg causes drowsiness significantly more often than 100 mg of secobarbital but less often than 10 mg of either morphine or diazepam. In addition, the incidence of extrapyramidal reactions (dystonia, akathisia, and oculogyric crises), dysphoria, tachycardia, and hypotension is higher than with a placebo.

Droperidol alone does not always lessen postoperative nausea and vomiting more than a placebo, and the severity of preoperative nausea and vomiting may be similar to that experienced with 10 mg of morphine. One controlled study demonstrated that droperidol had significant pre- and postoperative antiemetic action when given with meperidine (Tornetta, 1977). When droperidol 2.5 mg is given with fentanyl citrate 0.05 mg (available in this ratio as the fixed-dose combination, Innovar) for premedication, the quality of sedation may be better than that produced by 10 mg of morphine. The incidence of preoperative nausea and vomiting with the combination is low and that of postoperative nausea and vomiting is significantly less than with 10 mg of morphine. In general, droperidol alone is unsatisfactory for preanesthetic medication in adults unless an analgesic is given concomitantly to prevent dysphoria. See Table 1 for dosages and the section on Neuroleptanesthesia in Chapter 16, General Anesthetics.

Controlled studies comparing the phenothiazine derivatives, chlorpromazine [Thorazine] and promethazine [Phenergan], with meperidine plus atropine showed that, at doses inducing comparable sedation, apprehension was relieved to a greater degree by the phenothiazines; however, the incidence of preoperative tachycardia and/or hypotension and restlessness appeared to be greater with their use. Some phenothiazines also produce postoperative dyskinesia. The usefulness of most phenothiazines for premedication is severely curtailed by these adverse effects. See also Chapter 6, Antipsychotic Drugs.

Anticholinergic Drugs: Atropine, scopolamine, or glycopyrrolate [Robinul] is given to reduce excessive salivary and other airway secretions caused by some inhalation anesthetics and ketamine [Ketalar]. They are also used to protect against bradycardia, sinus arrest, and hypotension induced by succinylcholine [Anectine, Quelicin, Sucostrin] during tracheal intubation or certain surgical manipulations (eg, stimulation of the peritoneum, pressure on the eye, traction of ocular muscles).

Atropine is preferred to scopolamine for preventing reflex bradycardia because it has a more sustained accelerating effect on the heart rate. However, usual preanesthetic doses (0.4 or 0.5 mg intramuscularly) do not block the cardiac vagal nerves (this requires 1.5 to 2 mg), and the vagolytic action of an intramuscular or intravenous dose is usually brief (30 minutes). Small doses (up to 0.4 mg) of scopolamine may slow rather than accelerate the heart rate; therefore, this drug is preferred to atropine when tachycardia must be avoided (eg, in patients with mitral stenosis).

Scopolamine is a more potent antisialogogue than atropine. It has a significant sedative effect and may reduce the incidence of postoperative nausea and vomiting. However, scopolamine also may produce dizziness, delay awakening, and prolong postoperative confusion, especially in the elderly. Scopolamine alone does not produce anterograde amnesia as effectively as lorazepam, but it does cause significant additive amnesia when used with a benzodiazepine or opiate.

The quaternary ammonium anticholinergic, glycopyrrolate, is a more potent antisialogogue than atropine and often is used for preanesthetic medication because it lacks central anticholinergic activity. The duration of parasympathetic blockade is two to three hours, and secretions are reduced for up to seven hours.

Anticholinergic drugs inhibit heat loss, presumably by suppressing perspiration, and should be given cautiously to patients with fever, particularly children, to avoid hyperpyrexia. All anticholinergic drugs reduce the tone of the lower esophageal sphincter, which may increase gastric reflux.

If anticholinergic premedication is required in patients predisposed to increased intraocular pressure, the hazard of inducing acute glaucoma can be minimized by instilling one drop of 1% pilocarpine in each eye. Anticholinergic drugs can be given safely to patients with open-angle glaucoma (80% of glaucoma patients have the open-angle type), particularly if they are being treated with miotics, and to patients who have undergone peripheral iridectomy.

Atropine and scopolamine, but not glycopyrrolate, readily cross the blood-brain barrier and can cause confusion, particularly in children and the elderly. The intraoperative use of atropine or scopolamine may prolong postanesthetic somnolence or cause emergence delirium postoperatively (especially in elderly individuals or patients in pain).

Physostigmine salicylate [Antilirium] administered intravenously is the specific antidote for central anticholinergic intoxication; delirium is reduced with doses of 1 mg, and 2 mg may be required to lessen somnolence (see the discussion on Respiratory Stimulants in this chapter and Chapter 80, Drugs Used in the Treatment of Poisoning).

See Table 1 for dosages.

NEUROMUSCULAR BLOCKING DRUGS

Nondepolarizing (competitive) or depolarizing neuromuscular blocking agents are used to provide skeletal muscle relaxation during surgical procedures, particularly abdominal surgery. These drugs also are used to facilitate endotracheal intubation, relieve laryngospasm, provide adequate muscle relaxation during diagnostic procedures performed under general anesthesia, prevent dislocations and fractures during electroconvulsive shock therapy, produce apnea to facilitate controlled ventilation during thoracic surgery and neurosurgery, control muscle spasms in tetanus, and facilitate controlled ventilation by eliminating inadequate spontaneous efforts in patients with ventilatory failure. Because these drugs have no anesthetic or analgesic properties, they should not be used to compensate for inadequate anesthesia.

Ventilation must be controlled whenever neuromuscular blocking agents are used. An objective evaluation of residual muscular paralysis (ie, the ability of the patient to breathe adequately, maintain an open airway, take a deep breath and cough, lift his head holding the mouth closed, exhibit hand grip strength) must be conducted upon completion of surgery. In infants, the ability to keep the eyes open or hold up the legs indicates restoration of neuromuscular function. For patients who are not sufficiently awake to permit satisfactory evaluation of ventilatory recovery, a peripheral nerve stimulator can be used to determine residual paralysis more precisely. Nerve stimulators also are commonly used to assess the magnitude of neuromuscular blockade during surgery.

Nondepolarizing (Competitive) Blocking Drugs

The nondepolarizing blocking drugs (tubocurarine, meto-curine [Metubine], gallamine [Flaxedil], pancuronium [Pavulon], atracurium [Tracrium], and vecuronium [Norcuron]) compete with acetylcholine for cholinergic receptor sites on the postjunctional membrane but lack the transmitter action of acetylcholine. They also may have significant presynaptic depressant activities.

The nondepolarizing muscle relaxants display multicompartment pharmacokinetics (Lee and Katz, 1980). Schedules for loading doses, infusions, and use in various pathologic states and obstetrics have been designed (Ramzan et al, 1981). The pharmacokinetic properties of the nondepolarizing muscle relaxants are compared in Table 2.

Antagonists: The competitive block can be antagonized by anticholinesterases, such as neostigmine [Prostigmin] (adults, 2.5 to 5 mg; children, 0.08 mg/kg), pyridostigmine [Mestinon, Regonol] (adults, 10 to 20 mg; children, 0.4 mg/kg), or edrophonium [Enlon, Tensilon] (adults, 30 to 50 mg; children, 0.5 to 1 mg/kg).

TABLE 2.
PHARMACOKINETICS OF NEUROMUSCULAR BLOCKING AGENTS

Agent	t½β min	Vdss L/kg	Cl ml/min/kg	Reference
NORMOTHERMIC YOUNG ADULTS				
Atracurium	21	0.16	5.3	Ward and Neill, 1983
Gallamine	150	0.29	1.6	Ramzan et al, 1980
Metocurine	269	0.45	1.1	Matteo et al, 1985
Pancuronium	107	0.28	1.8	Duvaldestin et al, 1982
Tubocurarine	173	0.43	1.7	Matteo et al, 1985
Vecuronium	71	0.27	5.2	Cronnelly et al, 1983
ELDERLY PATIENTS				
Metocurine	530	0.28	0.4	Matteo et al, 1985
Pancuronium	201	0.32	1.2	Duvaldestin et al, 1982
Tubocurarine	268	0.28	0.8	Matteo et al, 1985
PATIENTS IN RENAL FAILURE				
Atracurium	18	0.17	6.3	de Bros et al, 1985
Metocurine	10.7 hrs	—	0.4	Brotherton and Matteo, 1980
Pancuronium	257	0.30	0.9	Somogyi et al, 1977 A
Tubocurarine	330	—	—	Miller et al, 1977
Vecuronium	97	0.24	2.5	Fahey et al, 1981 B
PATIENTS WITH HEPATIC CIRRHOSIS				
Vecuronium	84	0.25	2.7	Lebrault et al, 1985
Pancuronium	208	0.42	1.5	Duvaldestin et al, 1978
PATIENTS WITH HEPATIC AND RENAL FAILURE				
Atracurium	22	0.21	6.5	Ward and Neill, 1983
PATIENTS WITH BILIARY OBSTRUCTION				
Gallamine	220	0.26	0.9	Westra et al, 1981
Pancuronium	224	0.43	1.5	Westra et al, 1981
Vecuronium	270	0.31	0.97	Somogyi et al, 1977 B

TABLE 3.
PHARMACOKINETICS OF ANTICHOLINESTERASE AGENTS
EMPLOYED FOR REVERSAL OF NEUROMUSCULAR BLOCKADE

Agent	t½β min	Vdss L/kg	Cl ml/min/kg	Reference
Edrophonium	110	1.1	9.6	Morris et al, 1981 A
Neostigmine	104	1.0	9.4	Cronnelly and Morris, 1982
Pyridostigmine	112	1.1	8.6	Cronnelly et al, 1980
With Renal Failure				
Edrophonium	206	0.7	2.7	Morris et al, 1981 B
Neostigmine	183	0.78	3.4	Cronnelly and Morris, 1982
Pyridostigmine	379	1.0	2.1	Cronnelly et al, 1980

Pyridostigmine has a slower onset (13 minutes) than edrophonium (three minutes) or neostigmine (six to eight minutes), but a longer duration of action than either. The pharmacokinetic properties of anticholinesterase agents employed to reverse neuromuscular blockade appear in Table 3.

Anticholinesterase drugs have undesirable vagal and muscarinic properties; thus, atropine (adults and children, 0.015 to 0.02 mg/kg) or glycopyrrolate (adults and children, 0.2 mg for each 1 mg of neostigmine or 5 mg of pyridostigmine) must be administered prior to or with these cholinesterase inhibitors. Atropine 0.007 mg/kg must be given with edrophonium to prevent bradycardia. The anticholinesterase drugs must be used cautiously in patients with cardiac rhythm or conduction disturbances. Bronchial asthma does not present a problem.

The effectiveness of anticholinesterases in reversing skeletal muscle paralysis depends upon the dose of the nondepolarizing blocking agent used, and, more importantly, upon the extent of neuromuscular block (percentage of spontaneous recovery from block) at the time of reversal.

Depolarizing Blocking Drug

The depolarizing drug, succinylcholine [Anectine, Quelicin, Sucostrin], is believed to depolarize the postsynaptic membrane in a manner similar to the normal neurotransmitter, acetylcholine. Initially, muscle fasciculations occur that are usually visible. Continued occupation of the receptors by succinylcholine (which dissociates less readily from the receptor than acetylcholine) results in persistent (phase I) blockade and paralysis. Phase I block is not antagonized by anticholinesterase drugs; indeed, since anticholinesterase agents inhibit plasma cholinesterase (the enzyme responsible for the primary metabolism of succinylcholine), as well as acetylcholinesterase, these drugs may prolong the block.

Decreased receptor sensitivity may occur after a single large dose, repeated administration, or prolonged infusion of succinylcholine. This causes a desensitization block (dual, antidepolarizing, or phase II block), which is superficially similar to that produced by the nondepolarizing drugs. The safest treatment of phase II block is maintenance of controlled ventilation until the block reverses spontaneously. However, antagonism of phase II block with edrophonium 10 to 20 mg may be a reasonable alternative when succinylcholine is not in the circulation. Thus, succinylcholine can produce two types of block with different characteristics, durations, and responses to antagonists.

Drug Selection

The choice between the two classes of neuromuscular blocking drugs is determined by the expected duration of the operative procedure (succinylcholine has the shortest duration of action), the possibility of interactions between the blocking agent and the general anesthetic or other drugs, and the presence of pathologic conditions that may influence the patient's pharmacokinetic response (Wingard and Cook, 1977). Generally, a single dose of succinylcholine is used to produce brief relaxation or to facilitate endotracheal intubation. For longer surgical procedures and to facilitate controlled ventilation, repeated doses of nondepolarizing agents are used or, less commonly, succinylcholine is administered by continuous infusion for short periods.

Adverse Reactions and Precautions

Prolonged paralysis may occur with succinylcholine if the plasma cholinesterase level is low or atypical or if magnesium sulfate is being administered. The dose should be reduced when plasma cholinesterase levels are low (eg, in those with severe parenchymatous liver disease or malnutrition, after administration of anticholinesterase miotic drugs or exposure to organophosphate insecticides).

Succinylcholine is a powerful triggering agent for malignant hyperthermia in susceptible patients and is contraindicated when there is a history or suspicion of this syndrome. Succinylcholine should be avoided in recovering burn patients, paraplegic and quadriplegic patients, and others in whom muscle denervation may have occurred (eg, massive crush injury), because it may induce significant hyperkalemia.

Gallamine, pancuronium, metocurine, and tubocurarine depend on renal function for clearance (see Table 2), but succinylcholine, atracurium, and vecuronium do not. The latter two are the nondepolarizing muscle relaxants of choice in patients with renal failure.

The main hazard with use of all neuromuscular blocking agents is inadequate postoperative ventilation. Their actions are prolonged by overdose; interactions between the blocking agent and other drugs (including potent inhalation anesthetics, calcium channel blocking drugs, and certain antibiotics, such as aminoglycosides, tetracyclines, polymyxins, lincomycin [Lincocin], and clindamycin [Cleocin]); or certain pathologic conditions (eg, myasthenia gravis, Eaton-Lambert syndrome, amyotrophic lateral sclerosis) (Miller and Savarese, 1981). Respiratory acidosis, hypomagnesemia, hypocalcemia, and hypokalemia may enhance the action of nondepolarizing drugs and make the block resistant to reversal. Use of a peripheral nerve stimulator should prevent an absolute or relative overdose.

Tachycardia and a slight increase in arterial pressure due to a vagolytic action follow administration of gallamine and, to a lesser extent, pancuronium. In contrast, tubocurarine induces histamine release and ganglionic blockade, thus reducing arterial pressure and producing bradycardia. The muscarinic effects of succinylcholine can cause bradycardia, sinus arrest, and severe arrhythmias, particularly after repeated doses in children; atropine prevents or abolishes these effects.

Any nondepolarizing muscle relaxant is safe for use in patients with penetrating wounds of the eye, but succinylcholine generally is not recommended because intraocular pressure may increase from muscle fasciculations and sympathetic stimulation (see the evaluation).

Histamine release induced by tubocurarine, metocurine, and atracurium may cause or exacerbate bronchiolar spasm. This mechanism also may be responsible for increased intracranial pressure. Intracranial pressure also may be increased by the pressor action of succinylcholine.

Drug Evaluations

NONDEPOLARIZING (COMPETITIVE) BLOCKING DRUGS

ATRACURIUM BESYLATE
[Tracrium]

ACTIONS AND USES. This symmetrical bis-quaternary ester is approximately 2.5 times as potent as tubocurarine, but its duration of action is shorter. Atracurium is of particular value in patients with renal and/or hepatic impairment because neither condition alters the duration of block. Cardiovascular effects are minimal when recommended doses are given. The duration of action is similar in young adults and the elderly (Lowry et al, 1985). Paralysis is antagonized readily by neostigmine, edrophonium, or pyridostigmine.

ADVERSE REACTIONS AND PRECAUTIONS. Most adverse effects associated with atracurium appear to be caused by histamine release. Urticaria, rash, local erythema, wheezing, and hypotension occur occasionally. Atracurium is classified in FDA Pregnancy Category C.

PHARMACOKINETICS. Atracurium is presumed to be inactivated by two degradative pathways, hydrolysis of an ester group and Hofmann elimination, both of which lead to breaks in the chain between quaternary nitrogen atoms. The relative contributions of these pathways have not been determined. Metabolites have no muscle relaxant action. See Table 2 for the pharmacokinetic profile of atracurium.

DOSAGE AND PREPARATIONS. Dosage requirements vary and a peripheral nerve stimulator aids in determining the appropriate amount. Enflurane, isoflurane, and to a lesser extent halothane decrease the dosage requirement.
Intravenous: Initially, 0.4 to 0.5 mg/kg; subsequent doses, 0.08 to 0.1 mg/kg. If atracurium is given after succinylcholine-assisted intubation, 0.3 to 0.4 mg/kg is recommended initially.
   Tracrium (Burroughs Wellcome). Solution 10 mg/ml in 5 and 10 ml containers.

GALLAMINE TRIETHIODIDE
[Flaxedil]

ACTIONS AND USES. This synthetic agent has a longer duration of action than tubocurarine at equipotent doses; very large doses may have a prolonged effect. The actions of gallamine are similar to those of tubocurarine, but this agent blocks the cardiac vagus and may cause sinus tachycardia and, occasionally, hypertension and increased cardiac output; therefore, it should be used cautiously in patients at risk from increased heart rate but may be preferred for patients with bradycardia. In contrast to their effects on tubocurarine, respiratory acidosis diminishes and alkalosis enhances the blocking effect of gallamine. See also the evaluation on Tubocurarine Chloride.

Since gallamine is excreted unchanged solely by the kidneys, another agent should be used in patients with renal damage. A slightly larger dose of neostigmine may be required to reverse the effect of gallamine than of tubocurarine.

PHARMACOKINETICS. See Table 2.

DOSAGE AND PREPARATIONS. The required dose varies greatly and a peripheral nerve stimulator aids in determining the appropriate amount. The doses listed are for use with nitrous oxide as the only inhalation agent; they must be reduced if gallamine is used with more potent inhalation agents. The size of subsequent doses depends upon the anticipated duration of the procedure.
Intravenous: Adults and children, initially, 1 mg/kg; subsequent doses, 0.3 to 0.5 mg/kg. *Infants up to 1 month*, initially, 1 mg/kg; subsequent doses, 0.5 mg/kg.
   Flaxedil (Davis & Geck). Solution 20 mg/ml in 10 ml containers.

METOCURINE IODIDE (Dimethyl Tubocurarine Iodide)
[Metubine]

This semisynthetic derivative of tubocurarine is approximately twice as potent as the parent drug and, at equipotent dosage, has a similar or slightly longer duration of action. Since metocurine causes less histamine release and less ganglionic blockade, its effect on the circulatory system is not as prominent as that of tubocurarine. Differences in pharmacokinetic profile are shown in Table 2.

For uses and adverse reactions, see the evaluation on Tubocurarine Chloride. Metocurine is classified in FDA Pregnancy Category C.

DOSAGE AND PREPARATIONS. The required dose varies greatly and a peripheral nerve stimulator may aid in determining the appropriate amount. The doses listed are for use with nitrous oxide as the only inhalation agent; they must be reduced if metocurine is used with more potent inhalation agents. The size of subsequent doses depends upon the anticipated duration of the procedure.

Intravenous: Adults, initially, 0.1 to 0.3 mg/kg; subsequent doses, 0.02 to 0.05 mg/kg.

Metubine (Lilly). Solution 2 mg/ml in 20 ml containers.

PANCURONIUM BROMIDE
[Pavulon]

ACTIONS AND USES. The effects and indications for pancuronium appear to be similar to those of tubocurarine; however, there are some important differences in actions. Pancuronium is approximately five times more potent than tubocurarine. The onset of action of the two drugs is comparable. Endotracheal intubation is accomplished with ease in approximately three minutes. At equipotent dosage, pancuronium has a shorter duration of action than tubocurarine.

Unlike tubocurarine, pancuronium does not cause hypotension, presumably because it lacks ganglionic blocking action and rarely, if ever, causes release of histamine. It may increase heart rate, cardiac output, and arterial pressure, primarily because of its vagolytic action and secondarily because it blocks the neuronal reuptake of norepinephrine.

Atrioventricular conduction is accelerated, but cardiac contractility and total peripheral resistance are unaffected. Ventricular extrasystoles occur occasionally. In the elderly, neuromuscular block may be prolonged with delayed recovery of normal tone (Duvaldestin et al, 1982). For other adverse reactions, see the evaluation on Tubocurarine Chloride.

Only insignificant quantities of pancuronium enter the fetal blood stream, which suggests that the drug may be used safely in obstetrical anesthesia.

PHARMACOKINETICS. See Table 2.

DOSAGE AND PREPARATIONS. The required dose varies greatly and a peripheral nerve stimulator aids in determining the appropriate amount. The doses listed are for use with nitrous oxide as the only inhalation agent; they must be reduced if pancuronium is used with more potent inhalation agents. The size of subsequent doses depends upon the anticipated duration of the procedure.

Intravenous: Adults and children, initially, 0.04 to 0.1 mg/kg; for intubation, 0.1 mg/kg; subsequently, 0.01 to 0.02 mg/kg, repeated as required (generally every 20 to 40 minutes).

Pavulon (Organon). Solution 1 mg/ml in 10 ml containers and 2 mg/ml in 2 and 5 ml containers.

TUBOCURARINE CHLORIDE

ACTIONS AND USES. Tubocurarine (curare) is used to produce muscle relaxation during surgical procedures of moderate or long duration, to reduce the severity of muscle spasms in severe tetanus, to facilitate controlled ventilation, and, occasionally, in the diagnosis of myasthenia gravis (see Chapter 12, Drugs Used in Disorders Affecting Skeletal Muscle). Tubocurarine does not readily cross the placenta in significant quantities and does not affect the tone of the uterus; therefore, it may be used in obstetrical anesthesia. However, repeated use of large doses may result in fetal paralysis (FDA Pregnancy Category C).

Tubocurarine causes flaccid paralysis of all skeletal muscles. The muscles of the eyes are affected first, followed by those of the face, limbs, and trunk; then the intercostal muscles and, finally, the diaphragm become paralyzed. Paralysis of abdominal muscles cannot be achieved without substantial paralysis of the ventilatory muscles. The neuromuscular blocking effect can be reversed when there is a muscle response to peripheral nerve stimulation or when signs of returning muscle activity begin; administration of neostigmine, edrophonium, or pyridostigmine intravenously at this time is appropriate.

DRUG INTERACTIONS. Various drugs potentiate or prolong the action of tubocurarine at the neuromuscular junction. Of the volatile anesthetics, enflurane and isoflurane cause the greatest potentiation, methoxyflurane somewhat less, and halothane the least. When tubocurarine is given with enflurane or isoflurane, the dose of the blocking agent should be reduced to one-third to one-half of that used with nitrous oxide and one-half to two-thirds that used with halothane.

Many antibiotics (eg, streptomycin, neomycin, polymyxin B, colistin, kanamycin, bacitracin, gentamicin, amikacin, lincomycin, clindamycin) enhance the neuromuscular block produced by tubocurarine and other nondepolarizing agents. If extremely large doses of these drugs have been used recently, especially in patients with renal failure, controlled ventilation may be required postoperatively. Quinidine, magnesium sulfate, and trimethaphan (but not sodium nitroprusside) also have been reported to potentiate the neuromuscular blocking action of tubocurarine.

ADVERSE REACTIONS AND PRECAUTIONS. Tubocurarine may cause hypotension when large doses are given intravenously. This effect tends to be transient and is related directly to the depth of anesthesia and the volemic status; it is due to peripheral vasodilatation, which, in turn, is believed to be caused by release of histamine and ganglionic blockade. The hypotensive effect can be minimized by administering incremental doses.

Tubocurarine has been reported to cause bronchospasm due to the release of histamine. Although this effect is considered to be clinically unimportant in normal patients, pancuronium may be preferred in patients with asthma.

Respiratory acidosis and hypokalemia enhance and respiratory alkalosis diminishes the blocking effect of tubocurarine. Patients with myasthenia gravis are sensitive to the blocking effects of nondepolarizing agents; therefore, the dose of these drugs should be reduced considerably in these patients.

Tubocurarine does not readily penetrate the blood-brain barrier; therefore, it is devoid of central nervous system effects when administered in therapeutic doses. However, adequate ventilation must be assured, for hypoventilation may result in hypercarbia, cerebral vasodilation, and increased intracranial pressure. Intracranial pressure also may be increased as the result of histamine release, which causes cerebral vasodilation.

PHARMACOKINETICS. A single intravenous dose of tubocurarine produces maximum paralysis in three to five minutes, and the clinical effect may persist for more than 60 minutes. About 40% of the dose is excreted unchanged by the kidneys over 24 hours. When repeated doses are used, the amount of each succeeding fraction generally should be reduced. See Table 2 for this drug's pharmacokinetic profile.

DOSAGE AND PREPARATIONS. The required dose varies greatly and a peripheral nerve stimulator is of value in determining the appropriate amount. The doses that follow are for use with nitrous oxide as the only inhalation agent; they must be reduced if tubocurarine is used with more potent inhalation agents. The size of subsequent doses depends upon the anticipated duration of the procedure.

Intravenous: *Adults and children,* initially, 0.2 to 0.5 mg/kg; subsequent doses, 0.04 to 0.1 mg/kg. *Infants up to 1 month,* initially, 0.3 mg/kg; subsequent doses, 0.1 mg/kg.

Generic. Solution 3 mg/ml in 10 and 20 ml containers.

VECURONIUM BROMIDE
[Norcuron]

ACTIONS AND USES. This monoquaternary analogue of pancuronium has equivalent potency and a similar rate of onset, but the duration of vecuronium's effect is about one-third to one-half that of pancuronium (Krieg et al, 1980 A; Fahey et al, 1981 A). Vecuronium does not produce significant ganglionic or vagal blockade or interfere with the uptake of norepinephrine and it is essentially free of histamine-releasing action. Therefore, it does not affect the heart rate or blood pressure (Gregoretti et al, 1982). Intracranial pressure is unaffected.

Vecuronium is used during endotracheal intubation and surgery (Krieg et al, 1980 B). The duration of action is similar in young adults and the elderly (Lowry et al, 1985), but recovery time in infants is approximately twice as long (73 minutes) as in young children (35 minutes) (Fisher et al, 1985). The block produced by vecuronium is readily reversed by neostigmine, pyridostigmine, or edrophonium.

This drug is classified in FDA Pregnancy Category C.

PHARMACOKINETICS. About 10% to 25% of a dose is eliminated by the kidney; the major portion is excreted in the bile. In patients with chronic renal failure, clearance is reduced by 12% but neuromuscular block is prolonged by only 32% (Morris et al, 1980). In patients with impaired hepatic function, both the intensity and duration of neuromuscular blockade are increased (Durant et al, 1979; Lebrault et al, 1985). For further information on pharmacokinetics, see Table 2.

DOSAGE AND PREPARATIONS. The required dose varies greatly and a peripheral nerve stimulator may be of value in determining the appropriate amount. The doses that follow are for use with nitrous oxide and/or halothane as inhalation agents; they may be reduced 20% to 30% if vecuronium is used with enflurane or isoflurane.

Intravenous: *Adults,* for intubation, 0.08 to 0.1 mg/kg; subsequent intraoperative doses, 0.01 to 0.015 mg/kg, repeated as required. If vecuronium is given after succinylcholine-assisted intubation, 0.04 to 0.06 mg/kg is recommended as the initial dose.

Children 1 to 10 years may require a slightly larger initial dose and more frequent supplemental doses than adults; *infants under 1 year* are more sensitive to vecuronium than adults and recovery time may be more prolonged.

Norcuron (Organon). Powder (for solution) 2 mg/ml in 5 ml containers with diluent.

DEPOLARIZING BLOCKING DRUG

SUCCINYLCHOLINE CHLORIDE
[Anectine, Quelicin, Sucostrin]

$$\left[\begin{array}{l} \text{O} \\ \| \\ \text{COCH}_2\text{CH}_2\text{N}^+(\text{CH}_3)_3 \\ | \\ (\text{CH}_2)_2 \\ | \\ \text{COCH}_2\text{CH}_2\text{N}^+(\text{CH}_3)_3 \\ \| \\ \text{O} \end{array} \right] 2\text{Cl}^-$$

ACTIONS AND USES. Succinylcholine has a rapid onset (one minute) and short duration of action (five to ten minutes) after doses of 1 mg/kg. It undergoes rapid hydrolysis by plasma cholinesterase. A single dose usually causes transient, visible muscle fasciculations, followed by profound flaccid paralysis of all skeletal muscles.

Succinylcholine is used primarily during brief procedures, such as endotracheal intubation; to relieve laryngospasm; in endoscopy; in orthopedic manipulation; and in electroconvulsive therapy.

Since succinylcholine is almost completely hydrolyzed by plasma cholinesterase, prolonged postoperative apnea can occur in patients with abnormal plasma cholinesterase activity caused by a genetically determined variant of plasma cholinesterase or diminished hepatic synthesis of normal cholinesterase. The plasma cholinesterase level also can be reduced significantly after exposure to organophosphorus pesticides or topical use of long-acting anticholinesterase agents (eg, echothiophate) for open-angle glaucoma or accommodative esotropia. Complications can be avoided by using a small test dose and observing the response to a peripheral nerve stimulator.

Prolonged postoperative apnea caused by phase II block also can develop in normal patients receiving repeated or increasing doses. The dose-response curve is quite steep for succinylcholine (1 to 3 mg/kg for phase I block; 3 to 5 mg/kg for phase II block), and a peripheral nerve stimulator aids in monitoring the block when succinylcholine is used to provide continuous muscle relaxation. Prolonged postoperative apnea can be avoided if the infusions are interrupted frequently to evaluate the rate of return of neuromuscular function.

The response to succinylcholine may be prolonged in the presence of hypokalemia. Patients with myasthenia gravis may be resistant to depolarizing agents and have a predisposition to phase II block.

ADVERSE REACTIONS AND PRECAUTIONS. Succinylcholine has been reported to cause nodal and ventricular arrhythmias, decreased or increased heart rate, and increased arterial pressure. Nodal arrhythmias, bradycardia, and sinus arrest have occurred after intravenous injection (particularly in children) or after fractional doses were given intravenously at three- to ten-minute intervals to patients also receiving halothane. These effects usually can be avoided by administering atropine prior to the repeated doses or by using the intramuscular route in children. Intravenous administration following intramuscular injection can produce bradyarrhythmia. The complex cardiovascular effects of this blocking agent have been attributed in part to autonomic ganglionic stimulation.

Severe ventricular arrhythmias and cardiac arrest have followed administration of succinylcholine to patients with severe burns, major crush injuries, upper motor neuron lesions due to stroke or tumor, spinal cord injuries, multiple sclerosis of recent onset, tetanus, or diffuse lower motor neuron disease. These adverse effects have been attributed to a pronounced increase in plasma potassium levels following depolarization of the supersensitive denervated muscle. This sensitivity develops one to two weeks after the onset of motor paralysis and persists for several months, sometimes up to a year or more. Sensitivity may begin somewhat sooner in those with lower motor neuron disease and lasts until recovery of neuromuscular function or atrophy of the muscle occurs. The vulnerable period following burns is 5 to 120 days after injury. Succinylcholine should be avoided in these patients.

Succinylcholine increases intraocular pressure markedly within one minute. This effect is transient (five to ten minutes) and occurs during the stage of generalized muscle fasciculations. It can be attenuated by the prior administration of a nondepolarizing relaxant. Succinylcholine should not be used alone after the eye has been opened surgically or is already open at the beginning of anesthesia (eg, penetrating wounds, iris prolapse). Since the effect on intraocular pressure is brief, succinylcholine is not contraindicated in patients with open-angle glaucoma or those predisposed to angle closure. In these patients, one or two drops of pilocarpine may be instilled prior to surgery.

Succinylcholine does not cross the placenta in appreciable quantities and is safe for use in obstetrical anesthesia unless the patient has atypical or depressed plasma cholinesterase activity (FDA Pregnancy Category C).

Reduced maintenance doses may be required if the patient is receiving magnesium sulfate concurrently, for this agent has been reported to potentiate neuromuscular blockade.

Patients with myotonia congenita (Thomsen's disease) or myotonia dystrophica (Steinert's disease) respond to succinylcholine with contracture that ranges from clenched fists to a whole body response with legs drawn up, back arched, spasm of masseter muscles, laryngospasm, and contraction of the diaphragm. Contracture is also an immediate or early sign of succinylcholine-induced malignant hyperthermia, a rare complication of general anesthesia that may have a genetic basis. Its management is discussed later in this chapter.

Postoperative pain and stiffness in the neck, shoulder, subcostal, and back muscles are common after use of succinylcholine, particularly in patients aged 20 to 50; these effects apparently do not occur in children under 3 years. The incidence varies from 10% in patients maintained on bed rest for one day to 70% in ambulatory patients. Symptoms generally appear 12 to 24 hours after administration and last for several hours to a few days. The incidence of pain and stiffness may be reduced by giving tubocurarine 3 mg or gallamine 20 mg three minutes prior to succinylcholine; however, the dose of succinylcholine should be increased by approximately 50% to produce an equal degree of relaxation.

Diazepam 0.05 to 0.15 mg/kg also diminishes the incidence of postoperative muscle pain without necessitating an increase in the dose of succinylcholine.

When the angle of the cardioesophageal sphincter is normal, the increase in pressure required to open the sphincter is 28 cm/water. Succinylcholine-induced abdominal muscle fasciculations increase intragastric pressure: 1 mg/kg increases pressure to 40 cm/water and larger doses may increase pressure to 85 cm/water, which may result in regurgitation, particularly in young adults. Pretreatment with nondepolarizing relaxants may prevent this complication.

About 40% of prepuberal children exhibit myoglobinuria. This effect is not related to the apparent severity of the fasciculations. Myoglobinuria occurs only rarely in adults.

DOSAGE AND PREPARATIONS. The dose required varies greatly and a peripheral nerve stimulator aids in regulating the rate of infusion.

Intravenous: Adults, initially, 0.3 to 1.5 mg/kg; subsequent doses, 0.01 to 0.05 mg/kg. For continuous infusion, a 0.1% (1 mg/ml) or 0.2% (2 mg/ml) solution is administered at an average rate of 2.5 to 7.5 mg/min. The dose necessary to maintain paralysis is reduced in pregnant women. *Infants,* 2 mg/kg. *Children,* 1 mg/kg. Continuous infusion of succinylcholine is not recommended for neonates and young children.

Intramuscular: Infants, 4 mg/kg; *children,* 2 to 3 mg/kg (not to exceed a total dose of 150 mg).

  Generic. Solution 20 mg/ml in 10 ml containers.
  Anectine (Burroughs Wellcome). Powder (sterile) 500 mg and 1 g; solution 20 mg/ml in 10 ml containers.
  Quelicin (Abbott). Solution 20 and 50 mg/ml in 10 ml containers and 100 mg/ml in 5, 10, and 20 ml containers.
  Sucostrin (Squibb). Solution (aqueous) 20 and 100 mg/ml in 10 ml containers.

MISCELLANEOUS ADJUNCTIVE DRUGS

Vasodilators

Controlled Hypotension: Hypotensive drugs may be given during certain surgical procedures (eg, plastic, vessel, or neurosurgery) to reduce bleeding that would interfere with the technique. They may be used during intracerebral aneurysm ligation to decrease transmural pressure and reduce the risk of rupture during manipulation prior to clipping. Controlled hypotension may be appropriate to reduce large volume blood losses during hip replacement, Harrington rod insertion, prostatectomy, or radical neck or pelvic surgery and in threatened hemorrhage. In addition, hypotensive drugs can improve myocardial performance by decreasing cardiac preload and afterload.

In some instances, an adequate hypotensive effect can be accomplished by deepening general anesthesia. For example, a mean blood pressure of 60 to 70 torr can be maintained by isoflurane alone without untoward effects. This technique may be used during orthopedic, oral, and vascular surgery.

Peripheral vasodilation may be induced through blockade of sympathetic outflow of the spinal cord by epidural or spinal anesthesia. However, because the resulting hypotension is not readily reversed and controlled ventilation is usually required, this approach has had limited application.

Agents used to induce controlled hypotension are the ganglionic blocking drug, trimethaphan [Arfonad], and the direct-acting smooth muscle relaxant, sodium nitroprusside [Nipride, Nitropress]. Trimethaphan can produce tachycardia by blockade of vagal ganglia; it also depresses cardiac sympathetic tone, which reduces organ perfusion as the cardiac output is diminished at mean arterial pressures of 50 mm Hg. Sodium nitroprusside may not decrease perfusion at this pressure. There is evidence that trimethaphan may produce direct cerebral toxic effects at doses required to induce a mean arterial pressure of 50 mm Hg. Thus, trimethaphan is used less often than sodium nitroprusside, which lacks direct autonomic and cardiac effects and has a shorter duration of action. However, some patients are resistant to its effects and fatal cyanide poisoning may occur if the drug is not administered as indicated. Since sodium nitroprusside tends to increase cardiac output reflexly, it has been speculated that it may not produce as dry a surgical field as trimethaphan.

Hypotension should be induced gradually over five to ten minutes. The blood pressure (measured directly via an indwelling catheter attached to a pressure transducer), arterial blood gas levels, electrocardiogram, and urinary output must be monitored continuously. Scrupulous attention to respiration is essential. Hyperventilation must be avoided, since normocarbia is required for autoregulation of cerebral perfusion. Although positive fluid balance opposes induced hypotension, hypovolemia can produce irreversible shock. If inadequate circulatory volume is suspected, infusion of the hypotensive agent should be discontinued at intervals until the pressure rises in order to assess the reversibility of hypotension. Overdosage usually results in an undesirable fall in blood pressure before the effect on recovery time becomes significant. Diuretics, antihypertensive agents, and beta blockers enhance the action of the hypotensive agents. Consideration should be given to the risk/benefit ratio of this technique in patients with hypertension, anemia, coronary artery disease, renal insufficiency, Addison's disease, or deficient cerebral circulation. This technique is not recommended during pregnancy.

Induced hypotension should be performed only by anesthesiologists familiar with the interrelationships between blood volume, blood pressure, muscle relaxants, anesthetics, and end-expiratory pressure with the perfusion of the brain, heart, kidney, and liver.

Other Indications: In addition to inducing controlled hypotension, vasodilators are used to control pre- or intraoperative hypertension during surgery, to treat myocardial ischemia or ventricular failure, and to improve forward flow in patients with valvular insufficiency. These effects are achieved by reducing preload (venous dilation) or afterload (arteriolar dilation).

The selection of an appropriate agent permits a whole range of vasodilating activity from predominant dilation of the venous vascular bed to predominant arteriolar dilation according to the following sequence: morphine, nitroglycerin, spinal anesthesia, fentanyl, general anesthesia with enflurane or isoflurane, sodium nitroprusside, phentolamine. Nitroglycerin is a venodilator and sodium nitroprusside an arteriolar dilator, but these agents dilate both venous and arterial beds to some extent. The dominant vascular response may be matched to the clinical situation.

Drug Evaluations

NITROGLYCERIN
[Nitro-Bid IV, Nitrostat IV, Tridil]

ACTIONS AND USES. Nitroglycerin relaxes vascular, bronchial, gastrointestinal, ureteral, and uterine smooth muscle. Following rapid intravenous administration, transient arteriolar dilation occurs in association with increased stroke volume, cardiac output, and coronary flow. This is followed within one minute by reflex arteriolar constriction. Venous capacitance increases, left ventricular filling pressure declines markedly, and ventricular volume and cardiac work are reduced. With continuous infusion, preload is affected more than afterload, usually with little change in cardiac output. Discontinuation of the infusion is followed by restoration of baseline vascular parameters within nine minutes (Hill et al, 1981).

ADVERSE REACTIONS. Side effects of intravenous nitroglycerin occasionally include bradycardia (of vagal origin), hypoxemia (due to increased pulmonary ventilation-perfusion abnormalities), and, perhaps, methemoglobinemia. (This has not been reported during intraoperative use of nitroglycerin; see Chapter 25, Antianginal Agents, for management.) Hypotension and bradycardia are managed by discontinuing the infusion, assuring an adequate airway and oxygenation, and administering a vasoconstrictor if required.

DOSAGE AND PREPARATIONS.
Intravenous Infusion: (An infusion pump is preferred.) 0.1 to 1 mg/kg/min.
  Generic. Solution 5 mg/ml in 5 ml containers (alcohol 50%).
  Nitro-Bid IV (Marion). Solution 5 mg/ml in 1, 5, and 10 ml containers (alcohol 70%).
  Nitrostat IV (Parke-Davis). Solution 0.8 mg/ml in 10 ml containers with or without delivery set (alcohol 5%).
  Tridil (American Critical Care). Solution 5 mg/ml in 5 and 10 ml containers with or without delivery set (**Tridilset**) (alcohol 30%).

SODIUM NITROPRUSSIDE
[Nipride, Nitropress]

$$Na_2Fe(CN)_5NO \cdot 2H_2O$$

ACTIONS AND USES. Sodium nitroprusside acts directly to dilate resistance and, in larger doses, capacitance vessels. Peripheral resistance, central venous pressure, and pulmonary artery pressure are reduced. The drug has no direct action on the myocardium or on the central and autonomic nervous systems. The fall in blood pressure is dose dependent and, therefore, is related to the rate of infusion. There may be a reflex increase in heart rate and a variable increase in cardiac output, sometimes as great as 30%, depending upon the type

and depth of anesthesia. When the infusion is slowed or stopped, the blood pressure usually increases immediately and returns to pretreatment levels in one to ten minutes.

The dose response is extremely variable and the infusion rate requires individual titration; some patients are relatively resistant to the drug's action. Tachyphylaxis is rare. Increasing tolerance and metabolic acidosis are early indications of toxicity.

See also the discussion on Controlled Hypotension.

PHARMACOKINETICS AND ADVERSE REACTIONS. Nitroprusside is metabolized to cyanide. The major elimination pathway of cyanide is conversion to thiocyanate, which is excreted by the kidney. If the rate of conversion is adequate, no toxic effects are observed with short-term treatment. If the production of cyanide is excessive, a reaction with cellular cytochrome oxidase interferes with cellular respiration, resulting in decreased A-VO$_2$ difference and lactic acidosis. The infusion of nitroprusside should be stopped and a 25% solution of sodium thiosulfate in dextrose 5% in water should be injected over a 10- to 15-minute period to a total dose of 150 mg/kg. Sodium nitrite 3% then should be injected at a rate of 2.5 to 5 ml/min to a total dose of 5 mg/kg. (Sodium thiosulfate is a cofactor for the conversion of cyanide to thiocyanate, and sodium nitrite forms methemoglobin, which produces an inactive cyanide derivative.)

The concurrent administration of a 0.1% solution of hydroxocobalamin in 5% dextrose in water at a rate of 25 mg/hour during nitroprusside administration reduces the accumulation of cyanide ion (Cottrell et al, 1979) and significantly decreases the tendency toward lactic acidosis. Experimental work suggests that sodium thiosulfate 75 mg/kg is effective in preventing cyanide accumulation (Krapez et al, 1981). If prolonged exposure to maximum doses of sodium nitroprusside is anticipated, the prophylactic use of an antagonist should be considered.

The precautions for the use of nitroprusside are those common to the induction of hypotensive anesthesia (see the discussion on Controlled Hypotension).

DOSAGE AND PREPARATIONS.
Intravenous Infusion: (An infusion pump is preferred.) *Adults and children*, 0.5 to 10 mcg/kg/min. Infusion rates greater than 10 mcg/kg/min should not be employed.
  Nipride (Roche), **Nitropress** (Abbott), **Generic.** Powder equivalent to sodium nitroprusside dihydrate 50 mg in 5 ml containers for dilution in dextrose injection 5% in water to 1,000 ml (50 mcg/ml), 500 ml (100 mcg/ml), or 250 ml (200 mcg/ml).

TRIMETHAPHAN CAMSYLATE
[Arfonad]

ACTIONS AND USES. Trimethaphan reduces peripheral resistance, primarily by ganglionic blockade; it also has direct peripheral dilating activity. It is a weak histamine liberator. The usual rate of administration produces maximal hypotension in two to ten minutes. After discontinuation of the infusion, blood pressure increases in three to five minutes with return to a systolic pressure greater than 100 mm Hg within ten minutes. Occasionally, return to prehypotensive levels may be delayed for as long as 30 minutes, particularly when large doses are used for prolonged periods.

Some patients are resistant to the hypotensive effect of ganglionic blocking agents, and repeated administration of large doses is not recommended. In many patients, an appropriate hypotensive response occurs initially but tachyphylaxis then develops. The mechanism of this response has not been determined.

About one-third of the dose is excreted unchanged by the kidney. The fate of the remainder is unknown.

See also the discussion on Controlled Hypotension.

ADVERSE REACTIONS AND PRECAUTIONS. In elderly patients, the usual response to trimethaphan-induced hypotension is bradycardia. In contrast, children and young adults usually exhibit some degree of tachycardia. The resultant increase in cardiac output reduces the hypotensive effect, which may necessitate the administration of increased amounts of the drug or augmentation with halothane. If the patient's condition permits, treatment with small incremental intravenous doses of a beta-blocking agent (eg, propranolol 0.01 to 0.05 mg/kg) also may prevent the increased heart rate.

The precautions for the use of trimethaphan are those common to the induction of hypotensive anesthesia (see the discussion on Controlled Hypotension). Ganglionic blocking agents may conceal the signs of hypoglycemia in diabetics and interfere with sympathetically mediated gluconeogenesis.

DOSAGE AND PREPARATIONS.
Intravenous Infusion: Adults, a 0.1% solution (1 mg/ml) in dextrose injection 5% is infused at a rate of 3 to 4 mg/min initially; the amount is titrated to maintain the desired level of hypotension.

> **Arfonad** (Roche). Solution 50 mg/ml in 10 ml containers for dilution in dextrose 5% to 500 ml.

Agents Used in Pheochromocytoma

The alpha-adrenergic blocking agents, phenoxybenzamine [Dibenzyline] and phentolamine [Regitine]; the beta-adrenergic blocking agents, propranolol [Inderal] and metoprolol [Lopressor]; and sodium nitroprusside are used in the surgical management of patients with pheochromocytoma. Phenoxybenzamine and propranolol also are used preoperatively, the former to control hypertension and sometimes to estimate the intravascular volume for volume replacement, and the latter to control sinus tachycardia and frequent premature ventricular contractions. Since the beta-adrenergic blocking agents may increase peripheral vascular resistance significantly as a result of unopposed alpha-adrenergic activity, they should not be used alone.

Paroxysms of severe hypertension may be controlled during anesthesia by infusion of sodium nitroprusside, by intravenous injection of 1 to 5 mg of phentolamine, or by infusion of a 0.01% (0.1 mg/ml) solution of phentolamine. Serious ventricular arrhythmias may be controlled by the slow intravenous injection of propranolol in increments of 0.5 to 1 mg to a total of 3 to 5 mg in adults.

If severe hypotension develops after removal of the tumor, the infusion of norepinephrine may be indicated (see also Chapter 27, Agents Used to Treat Shock, and Chapter 28, Antihypertensive Agents).

Agents Used in Malignant Hyperthermia

This potentially fatal syndrome may develop in genetically susceptible individuals receiving general anesthesia (Steward, 1979). The syndrome may be induced by any volatile anesthetic, but the onset is usually more abrupt when succinylcholine is used, either alone or in conjunction with volatile agents. Premedication with a belladonna alkaloid may increase the incidence of this aberrant response.

Signs: The earliest sign of malignant hypertension in susceptible patients is usually unexplained tachycardia or tachyarrhythmia. Other early signs include tachypnea, labile blood pressure (usually a moderate increase), and flushing followed by cyanotic mottling. Blood pH falls quickly due to production of carbon dioxide and later to formation of lactic acid. Serum potassium levels become elevated. Muscle rigidity develops later and usually is noted first in the jaw muscles, but does not occur in about 25% of patients.

Hyperthermia is a late sign. Heat produced in the skeletal muscle elevates core temperature rapidly, which ultimately rises to more than 110° F (42° C). Disseminated intravascular coagulation and oozing of blood at the surgical site may develop. Acute pulmonary edema secondary to left ventricular failure often appears in the terminal stage. Creatine phosphokinase may increase during the crisis but reaches maximal levels (20,000 to 100,000 IU) 24 to 48 hours later. Levels of lactic dehydrogenase and hepatic transaminases are also elevated.

Treatment: An operating room protocol should be established to guide therapy (Ryan, 1979; Gronert, 1983). Appropriate steps are: (1) discontinue anesthesia immediately; (2) administer 100% oxygen with hyperventilation; (3) administer dantrolene [Dantrium] by continuous, rapid intravenous push, beginning with a minimum of 2 mg/kg and continuing until symptoms subside or a total dose of 10 mg/kg has been reached; (4) correct acidosis with sodium bicarbonate 1 to 2 mEq/kg immediately, thereafter guided by measurements of arterial pH and PCO_2; (5) control hyperkalemia by administering 10 units of regular insulin in 10 ml of dextrose injection 50%; (6) initiate cooling until the temperature is 38° to 39° C (surface cooling with ice in children; intravenous iced saline in adults, 1,000 ml every ten minutes to a maximum of 3,000 ml); and (7) maintain urinary output above 2 ml/kg/hour to protect against renal damage from myoglobinuria. The electrocardiogram, temperature, and urinary output should be monitored. In addition, an arterial line for measuring blood gases, electrolytes, and blood pressure should be inserted. If the physiologic and metabolic abnormalities reappear, the drug regimen should be repeated. It has been recommended that dantrolene be readministered 12 hours after termination of the acute episode. Frequent monitoring should be continued for 24 to 48 hours after the acute episode.

Anesthesia for the Susceptible Patient: No anesthetic technique is completely safe for patients susceptible to malignant hyperthermia, since even stress may trigger an attack. The incidence can be reduced by selecting techniques that are rarely associated with an unfavorable reaction, administering prophylactic doses of dantrolene preoperatively (see evaluation), monitoring the patient closely, and instituting remedial measures immediately if necessary (Relton, 1979).

Neuroleptanalgesia is the preferred technique (see Chapter 16, General Anesthetics). In addition to dantrolene, a barbiturate or benzodiazepine may be used for premedication with or without a narcotic. The belladonna alkaloids should be avoided. Nondepolarizing muscle relaxants may be used as needed, but succinylcholine and inhalation anesthetics should not be given.

DANTROLENE SODIUM
[Dantrium]

USES. See above discussion on malignant hyperthermia.

ADVERSE REACTIONS AND PRECAUTIONS. The use of dantrolene in acute hyperthermic emergencies or for the preoperative preparation of patients susceptible to malignant hyperthermia is not associated with the hepatotoxicity and pleural effusion that can occur during prolonged administration (see Chapter 12, Drugs Used in Disorders Affecting Skeletal Muscle). However, the large doses used for premedication may produce nausea, diarrhea, blurred vision, muscle weakness, and incoordination.

DOSAGE AND PREPARATIONS.
Intravenous: For malignant hyperthermia, the dose for *adults* and *children* is the same: Intravenous push, beginning with a minimum dose of 2 mg/kg and continuing until symptoms subside or a cumulative dose of 10 mg/kg has been reached. If the physiologic and metabolic abnormalities reappear, administration of dantrolene and the other drugs (oxygen, sodium bicarbonate) should be repeated.

For prophylaxis, 2 mg/kg approximately 15 minutes prior to induction of anesthesia, repeated in five to eight hours.
Dantrium Intravenous (Norwich Eaton). Powder (sterile, lyophilized) 20 mg for reconstitution to 70 ml.
Oral: For prophylaxis, 4 to 8 mg/kg/day in four divided doses for one to two days prior to surgery, with the last dose given three to five hours prior to surgery. The larger dose may cause considerable weakness.
Dantrium (Norwich Eaton). Capsules 25, 50, and 100 mg.

Agent Used in Pre-eclampsia and Eclampsia

MAGNESIUM SULFATE

ACTIONS AND USES. Magnesium sulfate is used to prevent or control convulsions in patients with pre-eclampsia and eclampsia. It acts at the myoneural junction to prevent the presynaptic release of acetylcholine and to decrease the amplitude of the motor endplate potential. Uterine contractions are inhibited and uterine blood flow is enhanced. Although magnesium sulfate causes some peripheral vasodilation, its antihypertensive action is slight and unpredictable; therefore, an antihypertensive drug (usually hydralazine) must be used concomitantly to reduce blood pressure (Pritchard, 1980).

Magnesium should be reserved for patients who experienced a significant increase in blood pressure with imminent or recent eclampsia (Lubbe, 1984). Less severe hypertensive change usually responds to combination therapy with alpha- and beta-adrenergic blocking agents.

ADVERSE REACTIONS AND PRECAUTIONS. Magnesium ion rapidly crosses the placenta but rarely causes hypermagnesemia in the neonate. Toxicity in the mother is indicated by loss of deep tendon reflexes, which occurs with magnesium plasma concentrations of 7 to 10 mEq/L. Plasma concentrations exceeding 10 mEq/L affect the respiratory muscles. This action can be antagonized by calcium gluconate or calcium chloride (10 ml of 10% solution infused over a three-minute period). High plasma levels of magnesium also produce heart block.

Magnesium sulfate potentiates the neuromuscular blocking effects of succinylcholine and the nondepolarizing muscle relaxants. It should be given cautiously to patients with impaired renal function.

DOSAGE AND PREPARATIONS.
Intravenous (by constant infusion pump): *Adults*, loading dose, 2 to 4 g (4 to 8 ml of a 50% solution) over a five-minute period; constant infusion, 1 to 2 g/hr (8 ml of 50% solution in 230 ml of dextrose injection 5% = 1 g magnesium sulfate/60 ml). Intravenous boluses are not recommended for maintenance. Magnesium is eliminated by renal excretion; if the urine output is below 30 ml/hr, the rate of administration must be reduced (Barford and Sokol, 1981).

Intramuscular administration no longer is recommended in patients with pre-eclampsia or eclampsia because absorption is unpredictable due to vasospasm and abnormal extracellular fluid distribution.
Generic. Solution 10% in 10 and 20 ml containers; 12.5% in 8 ml containers; 25% (concentrate) in 150 ml containers; and 50% in 2, 5, 10, 20, and 30 ml containers.

Respiratory Stimulants (Analeptics)

Analeptics are general central nervous system stimulants; they stimulate respiration, enhance the response to sensory stimulation, and hasten the return of normal reflexes. However, studies have demonstrated that analeptics are of limited usefulness in the supportive treatment of ventilatory insufficiency or arrest caused by anesthetics or other drugs with hypnotic activity. None of these drugs have the high specificity of action of the narcotic antagonists or anticholinesterase agents and should not be substituted for these agents when respiratory depression is caused by narcotics or neuromuscular blocking drugs. They are ineffective in ventilatory depression caused by cardiac arrest, airway obstruction, bronchospasm, or overdosage of other central nervous system depressants.

Analeptics act directly on nervous tissue. When ventilation is improved, their site of action is in the brain stem, particularly the medulla; certain analeptics (eg, doxapram [Dopram]) act on the carotid chemoreceptors as well. Reflex activity is improved when the spinal cord is stimulated in addition to the brain stem. Arousal occurs when higher centers are stimulated. Any improvement in cardiovascular reflexes results from improved central nervous system function rather than direct myocardial stimulation.

Convulsions may occur with increasing doses of any analeptic. Large doses given frequently may depress respiration. The margin between the analeptic and convulsant dose is narrow with the older analeptics (picrotoxin, nikethamide [Coramine], pentylenetetrazol [Cardiazol]). Doxapram is safer and has supplanted the older agents when analeptic therapy is elected to stimulate ventilation; its usefulness in hastening arousal is less established (Winnie, 1973; Sebel et al, 1980).

The xanthines, caffeine and theophylline, are not recommended for general analeptic use, but they are given to treat apnea in premature infants.

Analeptics, particularly caffeine sodium benzoate and the amphetamines, have been promoted to overcome the "hangover" effects of drug-induced coma. However, their administration for this purpose is neither logical nor advisable.

Physostigmine [Antilirium] reduces the arousal time in postoperative patients who received anticholinergic drugs, antihistamines, benzodiazepines, and droperidol and alleviates the disorientation and agitation occasionally caused by these agents, but its routine use is not recommended. Physostigmine also has been administered to arouse patients for brief periods during neuroleptanesthesia when their cooperation is required (eg, in certain neurosurgical procedures). Central depression produced by inhalation anesthetics, opiates and opioids, ketamine (Drummond et al, 1979), or barbiturates is not affected by physostigmine.

See the evaluation on Physostigmine Salicylate in Chapter 80, Drugs Used in the Treatment of Poisoning, for adverse reactions, precautions, and dosage.

Drug Evaluations

DOXAPRAM HYDROCHLORIDE
[Dopram]

ACTIONS AND USES. Animal studies have demonstrated that this analeptic causes arousal, stimulates ventilation, and increases arterial pressure. Studies in patients with normal central nervous and respiratory systems confirmed that doxapram increased the ventilatory response to carbon dioxide and the minute ventilation by increasing tidal volume and, to a lesser extent, the ventilatory rate. However, the drug also increased oxygen uptake, reduced carbon dioxide tension, and elevated pH, oxygen tension, and oxygen saturation. The adverse effects did not necessitate reducing the rate of administration.

Controlled double-blind studies reveal that doxapram hastens arousal when administered during the immediate postoperative period. It is not widely used, however, perhaps because the clinical usefulness and possible hazards remain unclear.

The availability of other simple tests (eg, evaluation of the ventilatory rate and pattern, measurement of inspiratory and expiratory airway pressures, ability of the patient to lift his head, response to peripheral nerve stimulation) renders the diagnostic use of doxapram in postanesthetic apnea or hypoventilation of minimal clinical value.

ADVERSE REACTIONS AND PRECAUTIONS. Generalized warmth, sweating, dyspnea, restlessness, hyperreflexia, laryngospasm, coughing, breathholding, retching, tachycardia, hypertension, nausea, lightheadedness, headache, and tremor may occur, particularly if large doses are given. Agitation and hallucinations are rare.

Doxapram is contraindicated in patients with convulsive disorders, hypertension, cerebral edema, hyperthyroidism, or pheochromocytoma and in those taking monoamine oxidase inhibitors or adrenergic agents. It is not recommended in patients with known or suspected pulmonary embolism, pneumothorax, or airway obstruction. Because controlled ventilation and standard supportive therapy are effective in ventilatory failure, doxapram *should not be used* in patients with drug-induced coma.

PHARMACOKINETICS. Doxapram is extensively metabolized; less than 5% of an intravenous dose is excreted unchanged in the urine. The mean half-life is 3.4 hours. The apparent volume of distribution is 1.5 L/kg, and the clearance is 370 ml/min (Robson and Prescott, 1978).

DOSAGE AND PREPARATIONS. The manufacturer's suggested dosages are:

Intravenous: Adults, for ventilatory depression following anesthesia, 0.5 to 1 mg/kg is injected as a single dose and repeated at five-minute intervals until a maximum of 2 mg/kg has been given. Alternatively, 1.5 to 2 mg/kg is infused. The calculated total dose is added to dextrose 5% or 10% or sodium chloride injection and administered at an initial rate of approximately 5 mg/min until a satisfactory response is observed; for maintenance, an infusion rate of 1 to 3 mg/min is suggested. The maximal dosage by infusion is 4 mg/kg or 300 mg for adults of average weight.

To hasten arousal during the recovery period, 1 to 1.5 mg/kg is injected. The total amount is given as a single dose or in divided doses at five-minute intervals.

Doxapram is not labeled for use in *children* or during pregnancy.

Dopram (Robins). Solution 20 mg/ml in 20 ml containers.

METHYLXANTHINES

ACTIONS AND USES. The methylxanthines, caffeine and theophylline, are effective in the treatment of primary apnea of prematurity (Higbee and Bosso, 1979; Aranda et al, 1981). This disorder has been defined as an absence of respiratory effort lasting more than 20 seconds; cyanosis and/or bradycardia also may be present.

The methylxanthines decrease the frequency of apneic episodes, probably through a central action. Regularization of breathing is associated with increased alveolar ventilation and increased sensitivity of the medullary respiratory center to carbon dioxide. Lung compliance, PaO_2, pH, respiratory rate, and blood pressure usually are not affected by methylxanthine therapy, although $PaCO_2$ often is decreased when apneic episodes are reduced (Davi et al, 1978).

ADVERSE REACTIONS AND PRECAUTIONS. The frequency and severity of adverse reactions to methylxanthines are minimal if care is taken to keep the serum concentration of the stimulant, particularly theophylline, within the recommended range (Howell et al, 1981). Both caffeine and theophylline increase central nervous system activity. Two times the recommended serum concentration of theophylline (more than 20 mcg/ml) has been associated with tachypnea, tachycardia, jitteriness, and vomiting while four times the recommended serum concentration (more than 40 to 60 mcg/ml) has produced seizures. Too rapid intravenous administration of either agent can induce hypotension. Caffeine has a much greater therapeutic index than theophylline and there are fewer reports of toxicity with its use in apnea of prematurity. Both caffeine and theophylline may increase serum glucose.

PHARMACOKINETICS. The plasma clearance of methylxanthines, especially caffeine, is markedly prolonged in premature infants and may change significantly during therapy as the infant matures. There also is wide variability in plasma clearance among infants, and dosage is best determined by monitoring the drug plasma concentration. This is especially important in premature infants.

Unlike adults, premature infants metabolize theophylline in part to caffeine (Tserng et al, 1983; Aranda et al, 1984). The fraction of the dose excreted as caffeine and other metabolites is a function of gestational age and birth weight and decreases with postnatal maturation. It has been recommended that the total plasma concentration of methylxanthines (caffeine plus theophylline) be determined in order to adjust the dose of theophylline.

A summary of pharmacokinetic studies in premature infants (Roberts, 1984) shows that theophylline has an approximate half-life of 28 hours (range, 12 to 58 hours) and a volume of distribution of 0.7 L/kg; clearance is about 17 ml/hr/kg in premature infants 6 to 11 days old and increases to about 31 ml/kg/hr by the ninth week. There have been fewer studies on caffeine pharmacokinetics in the premature infant. The values

reported in most available studies (Gorodischer and Karplus, 1982) are: half-life, 60 to 100 hours; volume of distribution, 0.8 to 0.9 L/kg; and clearance, 8 to 9 ml/kg/hr (Roberts, 1984).

DOSAGE AND PREPARATIONS. Theophylline is administered orally by nasogastric tube, preferably as a nonalcoholic syrup. Theophylline also may be given intravenously. Caffeine usually is administered orally as a solution of caffeine citrate; however, an intravenous solution of caffeine citrate can be prepared by the hospital pharmacy.

THEOPHYLLINE:

Doses are given as theophylline base.

Oral (nasogastric tube): A loading dose of 5 mg/kg is followed by a maintenance dose of 2 mg/kg every 12 hours. Plasma concentrations of total methylxanthines should be monitored, with the first determination made within 24 hours after starting the maintenance dose. Generally, 5 to 12 mcg/ml are effective theophylline plasma concentrations. The smallest effective dose should be used; many premature infants respond satisfactorily to plasma concentrations of 3 to 5 mcg/ml. Toxicity often occurs at methylxanthine concentrations greater than 20 mcg/ml. Smaller doses may be given more frequently to maintain a more constant, effective concentration without high, possibly toxic, peak concentrations. It may be necessary to increase the daily dose occasionally to maintain therapeutic blood concentrations, because the clearance of theophylline increases with age during the first month of life.

Intravenous: A loading dose of 2.5 to 5 mg/kg of theophylline (commercial preparations of aminophylline may contain 79% or 85% theophylline equivalent), followed by a constant intravenous infusion of 2 mg/kg every 12 hours, *with frequent monitoring of plasma concentrations,* until a plasma theophylline concentration of 2 to 12 mcg/ml is attained.

See Chapter 22, Drugs Used in Bronchial Disorders, for a list of available theophylline products.

CAFFEINE:

Preparations containing sodium benzoate should not be employed in the neonate.

Oral (nasogastric tube): A loading dose of caffeine 10 mg/kg (caffeine citrate contains 50% caffeine), followed by 2.5 mg/kg once daily. Serum levels should be monitored if possible; generally, 5 to 12 mcg/ml of caffeine is effective. Toxic signs may develop at plasma concentrations above 20 mcg/ml and are common with concentrations above 50 mcg/ml.

Intravenous: A loading dose of 10 mg/kg (as caffeine base) is followed by 2.5 mg/kg/day beginning 24 hours after the loading dose.

Generic. Powder.

Cited References

Ameer B, Greenblatt DJ: Lorazepam: Review of clinical pharmacological properties and therapeutic uses. *Drugs* 21:161-200, 1981.

Aranda JV, et al: Pharmacologic considerations in therapy of neonatal apnea. *Pediatr Clin North Am* 28:113-133, 1981.

Aranda JV, et al: Ontogeny of human caffeine and theophylline metabolism. *Dev Pharmacol Ther* 7(suppl 1):18-25, 1984.

Barford DAG, Sokol RJ: Modern approach to severe preeclampsia. *Drug Ther* 6:31-35, (Feb) 1981.

Beechey APG, et al: Temazepam as premedication in day surgery. *Anaesthesia* 36:10-15, 1981.

Brotherton WP, Matteo RS: Pharmacokinetics of metocurine in man with renal failure, (abstract). *Anesthesiology* 53(suppl):268, (Sept) 1980.

Clergue F, et al: Depression of respiratory drive by diazepam as premedication. *Br J Anaesth* 53:1059-1063, 1981.

Cottrell JE, et al: Prevention of nitroprusside-induced cyanide toxicity with hydroxocobalamin. *N Engl J Med* 298:809-811, 1979.

Cronnelly R, Morris RB: Antagonism of neuromuscular blockade. *Br J Anaesth* 54:183-194, 1982.

Cronnelly R, et al: Pyridostigmine kinetics with and without renal function. *Clin Pharmacol Ther* 28:78-81, 1980.

Cronnelly R, et al: Pharmacokinetics and pharmacodynamics of vecuronium (ORG NC45) and pancuronium in anesthetized humans. *Anesthesiology* 58:405-408, 1983.

Davi MJ, et al: Physiologic changes induced by theophylline in treatment of apnea in preterm infants. *J Pediatr* 92:91-95, 1978.

de Bros FM, et al: Pharmacokinetics and pharmacodynamics of atracurium under isoflurane anesthesia in normal and anephric patients, (abstract). *Anesth Analg* 64:207, 1985.

Drummond JC, et al: Randomized evaluation of reversal of ketamine by physostigmine. *Can Anaesth Soc J* 26:288-295, 1979.

Dundee JW, et al: Midazolam: Review of its pharmacological properties and therapeutic use. *Drugs* 28:519-543, 1984.

Durant NN, et al: Hepatic elimination of Org-NC45 and pancuronium, (abstract). *Anesthesiology* 51(suppl):267, (Sept) 1979.

Duvaldestin P, et al: Pancuronium pharmacokinetics in patients with liver cirrhosis. *Br J Anaesth* 50:1131-1136, 1978.

Duvaldestin P, et al: Pharmacokinetics, pharmacodynamics, and dose-response relationships of pancuronium in control and elderly subjects. *Anesthesiology* 56:36-40, 1982.

Fahey MR, et al: Clinical pharmacology of ORG NC45 (Norcuron): New nondepolarizing muscle relaxant. *Anesthesiology* 55:6-11, 1981 A.

Fahey MR, et al: Pharmacokinetics of ORG NC45 (Norcuron) in patients with and without renal failure. *Br J Anaesth* 53:1049-1053, 1981 B.

Fisher DM, et al: Pharmacokinetics and pharmacodynamics of vecuronium in anesthetized infants and children, (abstract). *Anesth Analg* 64:212, 1985.

Gorodischer R, Karplus M: Pharmacokinetic aspects of caffeine in premature infants with apnea. *Eur J Clin Pharmacol* 22:47-52, 1982.

Gregoretti SM, et al: Heart rate and blood pressure changes after ORG NC45 (vecuronium) and pancuronium during halothane and enflurance anesthesia. *Anesthesiology* 56:392-395, 1982.

Gronert GA: Malignant hyperthermia. *Semin Anesth* 2:197-204, 1983.

Higbee MD, Bosso JA: Apnea of prematurity. *Drug Intell Clin Pharm* 13:24-29, 1979.

Hill NS, et al: Intravenous nitroglycerin: Review of pharmacology, indications, therapeutic effects and complications. *Chest* 79:69-76, 1981.

Howell J, et al: Adverse effects of caffeine and theophylline in newborn infant. *Semin Perinatol* 5:359-369, 1981.

Kanto J: Benzodiazepines as oral premedicants. *Br J Anaesth* 53:1179-1188, 1981.

Knudsen L, et al: Hypotension during and after operation in glucocorticoid-treated patients. *Br J Anaesth* 53:295-301, 1981.

Krapez JR, et al: Effects of cyanide antidotes used with sodium nitroprusside infusions: Sodium thiosulphate and hydroxocobalamin given prophylactically to dogs. *Br J Anaesth* 53:793-804, 1981.

Krieg N, et al: Relative potency of Org NC45, pancuronium, alcuronium and tubocurarine in anaesthetized man. *Br J Anaesth* 52:783-787, 1980 A.

Krieg N, et al: Intubation conditions and reversibility of new nondepolarizing neuromuscular blocking agent, Org-NC45. *Acta Anaesthesiol Scand* 24:423-425, 1980 B.

Lebrault C, et al: Pharmacokinetics and pharmacodynamics of vecuronium (ORG NC45) in patients with cirrhosis. *Anesthesiology* 62:601-605, 1985.

Lee C, Katz RL: Neuromuscular pharmacology: Clinical update and commentary. *Br J Anaesth* 52:173-188, 1980.

Lowry KG, et al: Vecuronium and atracurium in the elderly: Clinical comparison with pancuronium. *Acta Anaesthesiol Scand* 29:405-408, 1985.

Lubbe WF: Hypertension in pregnancy: Pathophysiology and management. *Drugs* 28:170-188, 1984.

Male CG, et al: Comparison of three benzodiazepines for oral premedication in minor gynaecological surgery. *Br J Anaesth* 52:429-436, 1980.

Matteo RS, et al: Pharmacokinetics and pharmacodynamics of d-tubocurarine and metocurine in the elderly. *Anesth Analg* 64:23-29, 1985.

Mattila MAK, Larni HM: Flunitrazepam: Review of pharmacological properties and therapeutic use. *Drugs* 20:353-374, 1980.

Miller RD, et al: Pharmacokinetics of d-tubocurarine in man with and without renal failure. *J Pharmacol Exp Ther* 202:1-7, 1977.

Miller RD, Savarese JJ: Pharmacology of muscle relaxants, their antagonists, and monitoring of neuromuscular function, in Miller RD (ed): *Anesthesia*. New York, Churchill Livingstone, 1981, vol 1, 487-538.

Morris R, et al: Pharmacokinetics of Norcuron in patients with normal and impaired renal function. *Anesthesiology* 53(suppl):267, (Sept) 1980.

Morris RB, et al: Pharmacokinetics of edrophonium and neostigmine when antagonizing d-tubocurarine neuromuscular blockade in man. *Anesthesiology* 54:399-402, 1981 A.

Morris RB, et al: Pharmacokinetics of edrophonium in anephric and renal transplant patients. *Br J Anaesth* 53:1311-1314, 1981 B.

Pritchard JA: Management of preeclampsia and eclampsia. *Kidney Int* 18:259-266, 1980.

Ramzan MJ, et al: Pharmacokinetic studies in man with gallamine triethiodide. II. Single 4 and 6 mg/kg IV doses. *Eur J Clin Pharmacol* 17:145-152, 1980.

Ramzan MI, et al: Clinical pharmacokinetics of nondepolarizing muscle relaxants. *Clin Pharmacokinet* 6:25-60, 1981.

Relton JES: Anesthesia for elective surgery in patients susceptible to malignant hyperthermia. *Int Anesthesiol Clin* 17:141-151, (Winter) 1979.

Reves JG, et al: Midazolam: Pharmacology and uses. *Anesthesiology* 62:310-324, 1985.

Roberts RJ: *Drug Therapy in Infants: Pharmacologic Principles and Clinical Experience*. Philadelphia, WB Saunders, 1984, 119-137.

Robson RH, Prescott LF: Pharmacokinetic study of doxapram in patients and volunteers. *Br J Clin Pharmacol* 7:81-87, 1978.

Ryan JF: Treatment of acute hyperthermia crises. *Int Anesthesiol Clin* 17:153-168, (Winter) 1979.

Sebel PS, et al: Effects of doxapram on postoperative pulmonary complications following thoracotomy. *Br J Anaesth* 52:81-84, 1980.

Somogyi AA, et al: Effect of renal failure on disposition and neuromuscular blocking action of pancuronium bromide. *Eur J Clin Pharmacol* 12:23-29, 1977 A.

Somogyi AA, et al: Disposition kinetics of pancuronium bromide in patients with total biliary obstruction. *Br J Anaesth* 49:1103-1108, 1977 B.

Steward DJ: Malignant hyperthermia: Acute crisis. *Int Anesthesiol Clin* 17:1-9, (Winter) 1979.

Tornetta FJ: Comparison of droperidol, diazepam and hydroxyzine hydrochloride as premedication. *Anesth Analg* 56:496-500, 1977.

Tserng K-Y, et al: Developmental aspects of theophylline metabolism in premature infants. *Clin Pharm Ther* 33:522-528, 1983.

Ward S, Neill EAM: Pharmacokinetics of atracurium in acute hepatic failure (with acute renal failure). *Br J Anaesth* 55:1169-1172, 1983.

Westra P, et al: Hepatic and renal disposition of pancuronium and gallamine in patients with extrahepatic cholestasis. *Br J Anaesth* 53:331-338, 1981.

Wingard LB, Cook DR: Clinical pharmacokinetics of muscle relaxants. *Clin Pharmacokinet* 2:330-343, 1977.

Winnie AP: Chemical respirogenesis: Comparative study. *Acta Anaesthesiol Scand* Suppl 51:1-32, 1973.

Agents Used to Treat Glaucoma

18

The primary goal in the treatment of chronic open-angle glaucoma is to prevent damage to the optic nerve fibers and loss of visual field by reducing elevated intraocular pressure. Other goals may include the prevention of damage to aqueous humor outflow channels (in chronic angle closure), prevention of ocular enlargement (in infantile glaucomas), and relief of ocular symptoms.

The drugs used in glaucoma therapy reduce intraocular pressure by decreasing resistance to outflow of aqueous humor (miotics and epinephrine), by decreasing aqueous production (carbonic anhydrase inhibitors and beta-adrenergic blocking drugs), or by transiently reducing the volume of intraocular fluids (osmotic agents).

Aqueous humor is produced in the ciliary epithelium and transported into the posterior chamber from which it passes through the pupil into the anterior chamber. The aqueous humor leaves the eye by flowing through the trabecular meshwork in the anterior chamber angle, entering Schlemm's canal, and passing into the venous system. Another route is through uveoscleral pathways. Most forms of glaucoma result from interference with aqueous outflow within the trabecular meshwork or from closure of the angle by the iris.

TYPES OF GLAUCOMA

Primary Open-Angle (Chronic Simple) Glaucoma: In primary open-angle glaucoma, which is by far the most common form, outflow resistance is increased because of abnormalities in the trabecular meshwork-Schlemm's canal system. Histologic studies suggest that the changes in these structures may represent an exaggeration of the normal aging process (Fine et al, 1981).

Primary open-angle glaucoma is a chronic, slowly progressing, multifactorial disorder that usually is asymptomatic until extensive, irreversible loss of visual field has occurred. Drug therapy is the primary treatment; laser trabeculoplasty or filtering surgery is reserved for patients whose intraocular pressure has not been lowered sufficiently to prevent further optic nerve damage and visual field loss despite maximally tolerated therapy with a miotic, epinephrine and/or a beta-blocking drug, and a carbonic anhydrase inhibitor. When evaluating the results of treatment, the intraocular pressure should be measured at different times of day, since variations of as much as 10 mm Hg may occur over a 24-hour period and, if unrecognized, may lead to progressive ocular damage.

Special consideration should be given to treatment of open-angle glaucoma in patients with cataracts. Epinephrine or a beta blocker may be preferred for topical therapy because miotics may further impair vision, and the long-acting miotics may exacerbate cataracts and increase the risk of complications during or after cataract surgery. In addition, prolonged use of miotics (particularly the long-acting agents) may lead to permanent miosis and thus interfere with evaluation of the patient (Van Buskirk, 1982).

Ocular Hypertension: Patients with a mild or moderate elevation in intraocular pressure but no visual field loss or glaucomatous cupping of the optic disc may be observed closely without treatment unless the presence of significant risk factors suggest that the advantages of therapy outweigh potential risks. Risk factors with high prognostic significance are a particularly high intraocular pressure during the period of observation, the presence of small splinter hemorrhages on or adjacent to the optic disc, advanced age, the presence of systemic vascular disease, and a positive family history.

Normal-Tension ("Low-Tension") Glaucoma: When glaucomatous cupping and visual field loss occur in the presence of normal intraocular pressure, the possibility of intermittent increases in pressure should be ascertained by measuring pressure at different times of day. The effect of low ocular rigidity (which may give falsely low intraocular pressure readings on Schiøtz and other indentation tonometers) should be excluded by applanation tonometry. The possibility of a past pressure elevation (eg, from trauma or topical corticosteroid therapy) should be considered. Other causes of optic atrophy (eg, intracranial tumors, ischemic optic neuropathy) should also be ruled out. A history of severe hypotension or other cardiovascular crises should be determined, since these conditions may damage the optic nerve. After ruling out these other possible causes of optic nerve damage, treatment should be directed toward reducing the intraocular pressure to the lowest possible level as in open-angle glaucoma.

Primary Angle-Closure (Narrow-Angle) Glaucoma: This form of glaucoma occurs as an acute episode of severe pressure elevation. Aqueous humor outflow is blocked by contact between the peripheral iris and the trabecular meshwork, which usually occurs because iris-lens contact has partially blocked the flow of aqueous humor from the posterior to the anterior chamber (relative pupillary block), resulting in aqueous accumulation in the posterior chamber. Eyes with shallow anterior chambers and narrow angles are predisposed to angle-closure glaucoma. Dilation of the pupil by drugs, emotional stress, or darkness may precipitate an acute attack. Moderate dilation (5 to 6 mm) is more likely to induce an attack than wide dilation because, with wide mydriasis, pupillary block is relieved. Some cases of angle closure occur with gradual partial closure of the angle and present with an asymptomatic, chronic, low-grade pressure elevation that mimics chronic open-angle glaucoma.

Laser surgical iridotomy or standard surgical iridectomy is the definitive treatment for primary angle-closure glaucoma. Short-acting miotics, osmotic agents, carbonic anhydrase inhibitors, and a topical beta blocker are used in an acute attack to prepare the patient for surgery. To avoid a bilateral attack, the unaffected eye is often also treated with a miotic. Although usually protective, prophylactic therapy may rarely precipitate acute angle closure in the second eye, and it is prudent to confirm by gonioscopy that the miotic does indeed open the angle. For this reason, many ophthalmologists advise prophylactic laser iridotomy in the second eye.

Residual glaucoma that persists after surgery for angle closure is treated in the same manner as open-angle glaucoma.

Secondary Glaucomas: The secondary glaucomas are associated with various ocular or systemic diseases, trauma, or the use of certain drugs and may be of the open-angle or closed-angle (synechial) variety. The primary goal is to control the underlying disorder if possible. Drugs employed in primary open-angle glaucoma are useful in most cases of noninflammatory secondary glaucoma. In glaucoma associated with inflammation, miotics should be avoided because they may worsen the inflammation and increase synechia formation. Mydriatics and cycloplegics are useful to treat the iritis, and beta blockers, carbonic anhydrase inhibitors, and epinephrine are used to reduce the intraocular pressure.

Infantile Glaucoma: Primary congenital glaucoma is essentially a surgical problem. Surgery is also the first approach in other types of childhood glaucoma but is less often successful. Drugs may be used preoperatively to obtain optimum conditions for surgery and postoperatively to treat residual glaucoma.

MIOTICS

Actions and Uses

The miotics are cholinergic drugs that stimulate parasympathetic effector cells directly (parasympathomimetic agents) or indirectly by inhibiting cholinesterase, the enzyme that destroys acetylcholine (anticholinesterase agents). When applied topically to the eye, these drugs induce constriction of the pupil, contraction of the ciliary muscle, and a fall in intraocular pressure that is associated with decreased resistance to the outflow of aqueous humor.

In chronic open-angle glaucoma, a miotic has long been the principal and initial drug used, but beta-blocking drugs are now often employed as initial therapy. Miotics lower intraocular pressure in open-angle glaucoma by reducing outflow resistance. This probably occurs as a result of contraction of the ciliary muscle producing traction on the scleral spur and widening of spaces within the trabecular meshwork. The reduction in outflow resistance is the desired effect; miosis and spasm of accommodation are side effects that may interfere with vision and cause discomfort.

In contrast, the beneficial effect of miotics in angle-closure glaucoma results from constriction of the pupil, which pulls the peripheral iris away from the trabecular meshwork. In some instances, miotics (particularly strong miotics) may close rather than open the angle and worsen angle closure. This paradoxical effect results from increased pupillary block induced by miosis and/or forward movement of the lens associated with ciliary muscle contraction.

Although miotics are beneficial in many forms of noninflammatory secondary glaucoma, they are not useful when obstruction of the outflow channels is due to particulate matter (eg, lens cortex or macrophages with lens material in phacolytic glaucoma; zonular fragments in alpha-chymotrypsin-induced glaucoma; viscous material in sodium hyaluronate-induced glaucoma; inflammatory cells in iridocyclitis; tumor cells; red blood cells). Miotics should be avoided when iritis is present because they may aggravate the inflammatory process. Moreover, iridolenticular adhesions (posterior synechiae) may result from inflammation and are particularly undesirable in the presence of a small pupil.

Short-Acting Miotics: The parasympathomimetic agent, pilocarpine, has long been the preferred miotic for initial and maintenance therapy in primary open-angle glaucoma and many other chronic glaucomas. It often controls intraocular pressure when used alone. Pilocarpine should be given in a dosage adequate to maintain the intraocular pressure at the level required to prevent further damage to the optic disc and progressive loss of visual field. Variations in pressure at different times of day should be taken into consideration. Stronger concentrations may be required in patients with dark irides, because topical miotics are less effective in heavily pigmented eyes. In addition to the eyedrop preparation, pilocarpine is available in a long-acting gel formulation [Pilopine HS Gel] and a timed-release system [Ocusert].

In patients over age 50 who do not have cataracts, pilocarpine is relatively free of undesirable effects and is better tolerated than other miotics available in the United States. Carbachol may be substituted if resistance or intolerance develops to pilocarpine or if a slightly longer acting drug is needed. The short-acting anticholinesterase drug, physostigmine (eserine), is not well tolerated and is not commonly used today for prolonged therapy.

Pilocarpine is also the miotic usually given (in low concentrations) for emergency treatment of acute angle-closure glaucoma. It generally should not be administered for long periods to avoid or postpone surgery, especially if the pressure remains elevated, because 40% of patients experience a recurrence of acute angle closure despite miotic therapy and others may develop chronic angle closure with formation of peripheral anterior synechiae. In selected cases, especially in very elderly patients, pilocarpine has been used for long-term therapy if the pressure is controlled and the angle opens more widely. However, it is not commonly used for this purpose since the advent of laser iridotomy. Pilocarpine is also used for long-term therapy after laser or conventional surgery if the intraocular pressure remains elevated.

Long-Acting Miotics: Demecarium [Humorsol] and the organophosphorus compounds, isoflurophate [Floropryl] and echothiophate [Phospholine], are long-acting, potent cholinesterase inhibitors employed in the treatment of chronic open-angle glaucoma. Because of their cataractogenic properties and the rare precipitation of retinal detachment, these drugs should be reserved for patients refractory to short-acting miotics, epinephrine, beta-blocking drugs, and, possibly, carbonic anhydrase inhibitors. Some authorities now prefer filtering surgery or laser trabeculoplasty to long-acting miotics, especially if the lens is present. In the absence of the lens, some ophthalmologists are less hesitant to use strong miotics if there is no sign suggesting an imminent risk of retinal detachment, and these agents often are used to treat chronic glaucoma in aphakic patients. Strong miotics should not be administered for a few weeks prior to surgery in patients with narrow angles because they may aggravate pupillary block and angle closure. They also increase the frequency of hemorrhage during surgery. Long-acting miotics also should be avoided in other types of glaucoma caused by unrelieved pupillary block. These agents may be used after surgery if continued drug therapy is required and weaker miotics are inadequate.

Adverse Reactions and Precautions

Miotics, particularly the long-acting anticholinesterase agents, cause a variety of untoward reactions as a result of their local effects on ocular structures. Accommodative myopia can be troublesome in younger patients, and pupillary constriction may interfere with vision, particularly in patients with central lens opacities. An optical correction may be indicated for the induced myopia but is usually unsatisfactory because of the variability of this condition. Presbyopic patients may need a change in eyeglass prescription if a miotic is discontinued because the "pinhole" effect of a small pupil compensates for presbyopia.

Most patients taking miotics have poor vision in dim light, making night driving hazardous. Other common local effects include twitching of the eyelids, browache, headache, ocular pain, ciliary and conjunctival congestion, and lacrimation. Localized allergy, manifested by conjunctivitis and contact dermatitis, may develop. This complication was more prevalent when physostigmine solutions were used frequently. Long-term therapy with the strong miotics may cause conjunctival thickening and obstruction of the nasolacrimal canals.

Cataract development may be hastened by treatment with long-acting anticholinesterase agents, particularly in patients over 60 years of age. These cataracts are characterized by the appearance of anterior subcapsular vacuoles. Although pilocarpine has on occasion been suspected to be cataractogenic with long-term use, such an association is difficult to prove. Many patients have retained clear lenses after using pilocarpine for several decades.

When long-acting miotics are administered for prolonged periods, rounded nodules of the pigmentary epithelium may develop at the pupillary margin of the iris, especially in children. These nodules may enlarge sufficiently to interfere with vision and rarely may rupture or break free into the aqueous. The nodules generally disappear when the drug is discontinued, and their incidence may be reduced if one drop of phenylephrine 2.5% is used simultaneously.

Pupillary block, local vascular congestion, and occasional forward movement of the lens induced by the strong miotics may cause a sudden or, more often, an insidious closure of the angle and an increase in intraocular pressure even in eyes with only moderately narrow angles. Patients with swollen lenses due to advanced cataracts may be particularly at risk. Strong miotics are contraindicated prior to iridectomy in angle-closure glaucoma, in open-angle glaucoma with an excessively narrow angle (combined mechanism glaucoma), and in secondary glaucomas caused by unrelieved pupillary block. Occasionally, short-acting miotics have similarly aggravated angle closure in predisposed eyes. Rarely, if either short- or long-acting miotics are administered after surgery for angle closure, the anterior chamber may become very shallow and the intraocular pressure may rise due to development of malignant (ciliary block) glaucoma. Cycloplegics, carbonic anhydrase inhibitors, and osmotic agents are needed in these patients.

When there is an active inflammatory process (eg, in glaucoma secondary to anterior uveitis), miotics usually are of little therapeutic value and predispose to the development of posterior synechiae. Long-acting miotics may increase the frequency of hemorrhage during and after ocular surgery and promote formation of posterior synechiae. If possible, these agents should be discontinued several weeks prior to ocular surgery.

Following prolonged (months to years) use of miotics, particularly the cholinesterase inhibitors, miosis may persist when the drug is discontinued. This complication may be caused by fibrosis of the sphincter muscle, by loss of tone of the dilator muscle, or occasionally by the formation of dense posterior synechiae. Periodic pharmacologic mydriasis (at least twice a year) may prevent this complication.

Retinal detachment, an occasional complication of miotic therapy in predisposed individuals, may result from drug-induced spasm of accommodation, which causes the lens and vitreous to move forward and create a retinal tear. Retinal detachment may occur from one hour to several weeks after beginning miotic therapy (Beasley and Fraunfelder, 1979). Miotics should be used with caution in patients at high risk of retinal detachment (eg, aphakic or myopic patients, those with retinovitreal pathology or previous retinal detachment in the opposite eye), and the peripheral retina should be examined prior to administration. If retinal holes are present, consideration should be given to prophylactic cryoretinopexy before miotic therapy is started.

Topical miotics, particularly echothiophate and demecarium, occasionally cause systemic effects. Such reactions are very rare following routine administration of pilocarpine, carbachol, or the rapidly hydrolyzed anticholinesterase, isoflurophate, but have been seen with excessive treatment. Symptoms of systemic anticholinesterase toxicity include muscle weakness, hypersalivation, sweating, nausea, vomiting, abdominal pain, urinary incontinence, diarrhea, bradycardia, severe hypotension, and bronchospasm. These agents should be used cautiously in patients with bronchial asthma, bradycardia, or hypotension. An increase in blood pressure may occur occasionally due to a nicotinic effect on sympathetic ganglia.

Toxic doses of anticholinesterase drugs can cause central nervous system (CNS) effects (ataxia, confusion, convulsions, coma) and muscular paralysis. Death can result from respiratory failure. Patients who have undergone lacrimal surgery with placement of lacrimal drainage tubes are at increased risk because of enhanced drug absorption.

The most common symptoms of systemic toxicity in children are abdominal cramps and diarrhea; mild rhinorrhea, lacrimation, and upper respiratory congestion also may be observed (Apt and Gaffney, 1976). Children with Down's syndrome may be particularly likely to develop CNS disturbances from anticholinesterase miotics.

Systemic drug absorption can be reduced and corneal contact time prolonged by keeping the eyes gently closed for five minutes after application of eyedrops (which reduces the action of the nasolacrimal pump) and by occlusion of the lacrimal puncta by pressing the fingers over the inner canthal area (which minimizes drainage into the nose and throat). Severe toxic reactions are treated with intravenous atropine; pralidoxime [Protopam] may be used concomitantly when required.

Drug Interactions: Plasma cholinesterase levels are depressed significantly during topical therapy with long-acting anticholinesterase miotics, and prolonged apnea and cardiovascular collapse may develop if succinylcholine is given to patients using these drugs. Long-acting miotics should be discontinued, if possible, two to four weeks prior to administration of succinylcholine, and the anesthesiologist should be informed that the patient has been receiving an anticholinesterase drug. The hydrolysis of procaine also is decreased by topical anticholinesterase agents.

Because of possible adverse additive effects, anticholinesterase miotics should be administered cautiously to patients with myasthenia gravis who are receiving systemic anticholinesterase therapy. Conversely, caution should be exercised in the use of a systemic anticholinesterase drug for myasthenia gravis when the patient is already receiving topical therapy with a strong miotic. An adverse interaction between organophosphate miotics and organophosphate insecticides is possible, and these miotics are considered hazardous in farm workers exposed to insecticides. The cardiac and pulmonary side effects of these drugs may be additive with those of the beta blockers.

There is evidence from animal studies that chronic administration of a long-acting cholinesterase inhibitor may cause prolonged (up to several months) subsensitivity to pilocarpine.

Drug Evaluations

PARASYMPATHOMIMETIC AGENTS

PILOCARPINE HYDROCHLORIDE
[Adsorbocarpine, Akarpine, Isopto Carpine, Pilocar]

PILOCARPINE NITRATE
[P.V. Carpine]

ACTIONS AND USES. Pilocarpine is the miotic of choice for initial and maintenance therapy in primary open-angle glaucoma and many other chronic glaucomas and in the emergency treatment of acute angle-closure glaucoma. This agent penetrates the eye well. After topical instillation, miosis begins in 15 to 30 minutes and lasts four to eight hours. The maximal reduction of intraocular pressure occurs in two to four hours, which correlates with the maximal decrease in outflow resistance. Pilocarpine does not appear to have a clinically important effect on aqueous production.

A weak concentration of pilocarpine (0.125%) is useful to demonstrate denervation supersensitivity in patients with Adie's (tonic pupil) syndrome (Bourgon et al, 1978).

ADVERSE REACTIONS AND PRECAUTIONS. Pilocarpine generally is tolerated better than other miotics. Nevertheless, stinging and local irritation may occur and ciliary spasm and miosis may be troublesome initially. Allergic reactions and systemic effects are uncommon. (See also the section on Adverse Reactions and Precautions in the Introduction.)

DOSAGE AND PREPARATIONS.

Topical: In primary open-angle glaucoma and other chronic glaucomas, pilocarpine should be given in a dosage adequate to maintain intraocular pressure at the level necessary to prevent further damage to the optic nerve and progressive loss of visual field. Initially, one drop of a 1% or 2% solution is instilled in the conjunctival sac every four to eight hours. The concentration and frequency of administration may be adjusted later as needed. For maintenance, drops are usually instilled four times daily (range, three to six times daily). Concentrations of 4% may be necessary, especially in patients with heavily pigmented irides or advanced glaucoma. Concentrations of 6% to 8% may rarely provide still better control. Stronger concentrations may have a longer duration of action but cause side effects more frequently.

In primary angle-closure glaucoma prior to surgery, initially, drops (usually the 1% or 2% solution) are instilled frequently (eg, three or four times in a 30-minute period). Occasionally, pilocarpine is unsuccessful in opening the angle, particularly when the pressure is high enough to impede circulation to the sphincter muscle. The unaffected eye may be treated every six to eight hours to avoid a bilateral attack.

In congenital glaucoma, a constricted iris protects the lens during surgery; therefore, some surgeons apply one drop of a 2% solution to the affected eye every six hours for 24 hours before surgery.

All preparations are available as ophthalmic solutions.

PILOCARPINE HYDROCHLORIDE:
Generic. Solution 0.5%, 1%, 2%, 3%, 4%, 6%, and 8%.
Adsorbocarpine (Alcon). Solution (sterile) 1%, 2%, and 4% with benzalkonium chloride 0.004% and edetate disodium 0.1% in 15 ml containers.
Akarpine (Akorn). Solution (aqueous) 0.5%, 1%, 2%, 4%, and 6% with benzalkonium chloride 0.01% and edetate disodium 0.01% in 15 ml containers.
Isopto Carpine (Alcon). Solution (sterile) 0.25%, 0.5%, 1%, 2%, 3%, 4%, 5%, 6%, 8%, and 10% with benzalkonium chloride 0.01% in 15 ml (0.25%, 8%, and 10% concentrations only) and 30 ml containers.
Pilocar (CooperVision). Solution (sterile) 0.5%, 1%, 2%, 3%, 4%, and 6% with benzalkonium chloride and edetate disodium in 15 ml containers.

Pilocarpine Steri-Units (Alcon). Solution (sterile) 1%, 2%, 4%, and 8% in 2 ml presterilized containers (preservative free).
Additional Trademarks.
Almocarpine (Ayerst), **Ocu-Carpine** (Ocumed), **Pilocel** (Optopics), **Pilokair** (Pharmafair).
PILOCARPINE NITRATE:
P.V. Carpine Liquifilm (Allergan). Solution (sterile) 1%, 2%, and 4% with chlorobutanol 0.5% in 15 ml containers.

OCUSERT PILO-20/PILO-40 OCULAR THERAPEUTIC SYSTEM

ACTIONS AND USES. The Ocusert pilocarpine system is a drug delivery unit consisting of two outer membranes with a central reservoir of pilocarpine. It is designed for use in patients with chronic open-angle glaucoma. When placed in the upper or lower cul-de-sac, pilocarpine gradually diffuses across the two outer polymeric layers that serve as rate-controlling membranes. The unit is available in two strengths, Pilo-20 and -40, which correspond in effectiveness roughly to 0.5% or 1% and 2% or 3% pilocarpine. Patients who are inadequately controlled with the Pilo-40 unit may require concomitant use of other antiglaucoma drugs. The Ocusert System is more expensive than eyedrops, but it may provide better diurnal control of intraocular pressure and improve compliance in unreliable patients. In younger patients, miosis and spasm of accommodation are reduced but, because these symptoms can be troublesome during the first few hours after insertion of a new unit, the device should be inserted at bedtime or it may be soaked in a glass of water for one hour before placing it in the cul-de-sac.

Although the Ocusert System is labeled for replacement every seven days, the duration of action and rate of release of pilocarpine are variable.

ADVERSE REACTIONS AND PRECAUTIONS. Conjunctival irritation may be noted, particularly during initial use. Occasionally, sudden leakage of pilocarpine has produced marked miosis and decreased vision associated with a further fall in intraocular pressure. Rarely, the Ocusert may migrate onto the cornea, obstructing vision and causing pain. Some patients, particularly those with loose lids, have difficulty retaining the Ocusert and may lose it without noting the loss. Since the unit may fall out at night, the patient should be instructed to make sure that it is in place every morning.

DOSAGE AND PREPARATIONS.

Topical: The unit is placed in the upper or lower cul-de-sac at bedtime and should be replaced every seven days.

Ocusert Pilo-20 Ocular Therapeutic System (20 mcg/hour for one week), **Ocusert Pilo-40 Ocular Therapeutic System** (40 mcg/hour for one week) (Alza). Ophthalmic sustained-release systems (sterile) in packages of eight units.

PILOCARPINE GEL
[Pilopine HS Gel]

ACTIONS AND USES. This long-acting preparation contains pilocarpine hydrochloride in an aqueous gel. It is used to treat chronic open-angle glaucoma. After one application, intraocular pressure is lowered for 18 to 24 hours.

ADVERSE REACTIONS AND PRECAUTIONS. Pilocarpine gel often causes irritation, blurred vision, and transient superficial punctate keratitis. Some patients are bothered by their eyelids sticking together in the morning. During prolonged therapy, persistent superficial corneal haze develops in one-fifth of patients. The long-term effect of this corneal change is unknown (Johnson et al, 1984).

DOSAGE AND PREPARATIONS.
Topical: One-half inch is applied to the lower conjunctival cul-de-sac once daily at bedtime. More frequent application may be required in some patients.

> *Pilopine HS Gel* (Alcon). Gel (sterile) containing pilocarpine hydrochloride 4% with benzalkonium chloride 0.008% in 5 g containers.

CARBACHOL
[Isopto Carbachol]

$$H_2NCOCH_2CH_2\overset{+}{N}(CH_3)_3 \quad Cl^-$$

ACTIONS AND USES. Carbachol is used in primary open-angle glaucoma and other chronic glaucomas, usually to replace pilocarpine when resistance or intolerance to the latter has developed or when a slightly longer acting drug is needed. It has been used for emergency treatment of acute angle-closure glaucoma, but pilocarpine is preferred because it is less likely to aggravate pupillary block and its action is easier to reverse.

Carbachol does not penetrate the eye as well as pilocarpine and is usually prepared with a wetting agent to enhance corneal penetration.

ADVERSE REACTIONS AND PRECAUTIONS. Carbachol may cause more accommodative spasm and headache than pilocarpine and produces slight conjunctival hyperemia. Resistance has been reported to develop suddenly. Other local and systemic adverse reactions occur rarely (see the section on Adverse Reactions and Precautions in the Introduction).

DOSAGE AND PREPARATIONS.
Topical: In primary open-angle glaucoma and other chronic glaucomas, carbachol should be given in a dosage adequate to maintain the intraocular pressure at the level necessary to prevent further optic nerve damage and progressive visual field loss. Initially, one drop of a 0.75% to 3% solution is instilled in the conjunctival sac every eight hours.

> All preparations are available as ophthalmic solutions.
> *Isopto Carbachol* (Alcon). Solution (sterile) 0.75%, 1.5%, 2.25%, and 3% with benzalkonium chloride 0.005% in 15 and 30 ml containers.

SHORT-ACTING ANTICHOLINESTERASE AGENTS

PHYSOSTIGMINE SULFATE (Eserine Sulfate)

PHYSOSTIGMINE SALICYLATE
[0.5% Eserine]

ACTIONS AND USES. Although not currently popular for primary therapy, physostigmine has been used to treat open-angle glaucoma. It is also employed occasionally to treat accommodative esotropia (overconvergence caused by excessive accommodation). Miosis occurs in about 30 minutes and may last 12 to 36 hours.

ADVERSE REACTIONS AND PRECAUTIONS. Physostigmine often causes hyperemia of the conjunctiva and iris. It is rarely tolerated for prolonged periods because conjunctivitis and allergic reactions occur frequently. Long-term administration can produce follicles in the cul-de-sac. In blacks, prolonged treatment with physostigmine ointment may cause depigmentation of the lid margins. See also the section on Adverse Reactions and Precautions in the Introduction.

Solutions are sensitive to light and heat and should not be used if discolored. Ointments may cause blurred vision and usually are reserved for nighttime use.

DOSAGE AND PREPARATIONS.
Topical: In primary open-angle glaucoma and other chronic glaucomas, one drop of solution is applied every four to six hours or, more commonly, the ointment is used at night. The lowest effective concentration should be applied no more frequently than required to maintain the intraocular pressure at the level necessary to prevent further damage to the optic nerve and progressive loss of visual field.

> All preparations are available in ophthalmic form.
> PHYSOSTIGMINE SULFATE:
> Drug available under the name Eserine Sulfate: Ointment 0.25%.
> PHYSOSTIGMINE SALICYLATE:
> *0.5% Eserine Steri-Unit* (Alcon). Solution (sterile) 0.5% in 2 ml containers (preservative free).

PHYSOSTIGMINE SALICYLATE AND PILOCARPINE HYDROCHLORIDE

Combinations of miotics offer no advantages over adequate doses of a single-entity drug. A disadvantage of this combination is the difference in duration of action of the two components. It also has been suggested that their combined effect may be competitive rather than additive or synergistic and that resistance may develop to both components during long-term therapy.

Preparation is available as ophthalmic solution.

Isopto P-ES (Alcon). Solution (sterile) containing physostigmine salicylate 0.25% and pilocarpine hydrochloride 2% with chlorobutanol 0.15% in 15 ml containers.

LONG-ACTING ANTICHOLINESTERASE AGENTS

DEMECARIUM BROMIDE
[Humorsol]

ECHOTHIOPHATE IODIDE
[Phospholine Iodide]

ISOFLUROPHATE (DFP)
[Floropryl]

ACTIONS AND USES. These potent, long-acting miotics are used to treat primary open-angle glaucoma and other chronic glaucomas when short-acting miotics and other agents are inadequate. They are used most frequently to treat glaucoma in aphakic patients. Maximal reduction of intraocular pressure occurs within 24 hours after a single instillation, and residual effects may persist for days. When instilled once daily for a number of days, a cumulative effect occurs; the maximal reduction in pressure is attained after several days of therapy.

In addition to their use in glaucoma, the strong miotics have been employed to diagnose and treat accommodative esotropia. By inducing accommodation peripherally, they decrease accommodative effort and thereby reduce accommodative convergence. The lowest effective concentration should be employed.

ADVERSE REACTIONS AND PRECAUTIONS. The development of cataracts after long-term administration has limited the usefulness of these agents in glaucoma therapy. Although cataract formation has not been observed in children or young adults, the usefulness of these agents in young patients with strabismus must be balanced against the potential risk that these agents will hasten the development of cataracts later in life. (See also the section on Adverse Reactions and Precautions in the Introduction.)

DOSAGE AND PREPARATIONS. These strong miotics should be administered in the lowest effective dosage.

DEMECARIUM BROMIDE:

Topical: In primary open-angle glaucoma and other chronic glaucomas, initially, one drop of a 0.125% or 0.25% solution instilled in the conjunctival sac every 12 to 48 hours.

Humorsol (Merck Sharp & Dohme). Solution (sterile, aqueous) 0.125% and 0.25% with benzalkonium chloride 0.02% in 5 ml containers.

ECHOTHIOPHATE IODIDE:

Topical: In primary open-angle glaucoma and other chronic glaucomas, initially, one drop of a 0.03% to 0.06% solution instilled in the conjunctival sac every 12 to 48 hours. A stronger concentration (0.125% or 0.25%) is often required in highly pigmented eyes.

Phospholine Iodide (Ayerst). Powder (lyophilized) 1.5, 3, 6.25, and 12.5 mg with 5 ml of diluent containing mannitol 1.2%, boric acid 0.06%, exsiccated sodium phosphate 0.026%, and chlorobutanol 0.5% to make 0.03%, 0.06%, 0.125%, and 0.25% solution, respectively.

ISOFLUROPHATE:

Topical: In primary open-angle glaucoma and other chronic glaucomas, initially, a one-quarter inch strip of ointment is applied every 8 to 72 hours.

Floropryl (Merck Sharp & Dohme). Ointment (sterile) 0.025% in polyethylene-mineral oil gel in 3.5 g containers.

EPINEPHRINE

EPINEPHRINE BITARTRATE
[Epitrate]

EPINEPHRINE HYDROCHLORIDE
[Epifrin, Glaucon]

EPINEPHRYL BORATE
[Epinal, Eppy/N]

ACTIONS. The dilator muscle of the iris contains mainly alpha-adrenergic receptors, and activation of these receptors causes pupillary dilation. Although the sphincter and ciliary muscles are largely under parasympathetic control, adrenergic receptors have also been described in these tissues, primarily beta receptors in the ciliary muscle and both alpha and beta receptors in the sphincter muscle of the iris. The function of these receptors in the regulation of aqueous production and outflow facility is not clearly understood, since both adrenergic agonists and antagonists lower intraocular pressure. Current evidence suggests that aqueous formation is modulated primarily by beta-adrenergic mechanisms: stimulation of beta receptors in the ciliary processes increases aqueous production, while blockade of these receptors decreases production (Schenker et al, 1981). Activation of adrenergic receptors in the outflow channels increases outflow facility, but whether this effect is mediated by alpha or beta receptors is highly controversial. This action may involve stimulation of prostaglandin synthesis (Camras et al, 1985).

Epinephrine acts on both alpha- and beta-adrenergic receptors. When instilled in eyes with primary open-angle glaucoma, it reduces intraocular pressure for 12 to 24 hours or rarely longer. Brief constriction of the conjunctival vessels is followed by a more prolonged vasodilation. Brief mydriasis may occur in some patients. The mechanism by which epinephrine reduces intraocular pressure is independent of its mydriatic action and results primarily from an increase in outflow facility. Early studies suggested that epinephrine also decreases aqueous formation, but more recent data indicate that it actually increases aqueous production slightly.

USES. Epinephrine is used to treat primary open-angle glaucoma and other chronic glaucomas. It may be administered alone for initial treatment, especially in patients who cannot tolerate miotic therapy (ie, relatively young patients with active accommodation, older patients with cataracts whose vision is reduced by a small pupil). Epinephrine is also used to supplement miotics and/or carbonic anhydrase inhibitors.

The responsiveness of each individual should be determined before long-term epinephrine therapy is begun because of variability in responsiveness and because a paradoxical transient elevation of intraocular pressure may occur occasionally, even in eyes with open angles. Highly pigmented eyes require stronger concentrations.

ADVERSE REACTIONS AND PRECAUTIONS. Epinephrine produces browache, headache, blurred vision, ocular irritation, and lacrimation in some patients. Epinephryl borate may cause less local discomfort than the hydrochloride and especially the bitartrate salts. Repeated use of epinephrine may cause reactive hyperemia, allergic conjunctivitis, and contact dermatitis. About 20% or more of patients cannot tolerate prolonged use of this agent because of these reactions. Corneal edema has been reported very rarely after long-term administration.

Of particular importance in aphakic eyes is the possibility of inducing cystoid macular edema. This complication has been reported in 10% to 20% of aphakic patients during long-term therapy. Fortunately, the maculopathy is usually reversible if epinephrine is discontinued when visual acuity first begins to decrease. Many ophthalmologists prefer not to use epinephrine in aphakic eyes unless the glaucoma is sufficiently severe to justify the risk.

Topical epinephrine can cause pupillary dilation, even when used with miotics, and the mydriatic effect is enhanced by timolol. It is contraindicated preoperatively in angle-closure glaucoma because it may precipitate an acute attack. When instilled without miotics in patients with open-angle glaucoma, epinephrine rarely may cause a temporary elevation of intraocular pressure upon initial administration. This phenomenon may be associated with release of pigment particles from the iris into the aqueous humor (aqueous floaters). With long-term administration, melanin-like deposits may appear in the bulbar or palpebral conjunctiva, in roughened or edematous areas of the cornea, or in soft contact lenses.

Supersensitivity, manifested by mydriasis and lid retraction, has been reported after long-term topical therapy. Prolonged use rarely contributes to the development of benign ocular mucous membrane pemphigoid.

The ocular hypotensive effect of epinephrine is partially inhibited by oral indomethacin (Camras et al, 1985).

Systemic reactions to topical epinephrine include tachycardia, premature ventricular contractions, hypertension, headache, sweating, tremors, blanching, and disorientation. In several instances, systemic effects occurred when the drug was applied after conjunctival permeability was increased by tonometry or administration of local anesthetics.

As with any drug, the lowest effective concentration should be used. Occasionally, the 0.25% strength is effective and the 0.5% strength is frequently sufficient. Gentle eyelid closure for five minutes after administration and pressure at the inner canthus reduce the risk of systemic reactions and prolong ocular contact time.

Epinephrine should be used with care in patients with arrhythmias, hypertension, hyperthyroidism, recent myocardial infarction, or arteriosclerotic heart disease. It may cause ventricular premature contractions, tachycardia, and fibrillation in patients undergoing general anesthesia with halothane, cyclopropane, or other agents that sensitize the heart to catecholamines.

DOSAGE AND PREPARATIONS. Discoloration of solutions indicates that an oxidation product has been formed; these solutions should be discarded.

Topical: In primary open-angle glaucoma and other chronic glaucomas, one drop of a 0.25% to 2% solution is instilled in the conjunctival sac, usually once or twice daily. The stronger concentration may be required in patients with dark irides.

It should be noted that, with different salts, the same percentage may not contain the same amount of active base. The 2% bitartrate solution is equivalent to 1% epinephrine hydrochloride.

All preparations are available for ophthalmic use.

EPINEPHRINE BITARTRATE:
Epitrate (Ayerst). Solution (sterile, aqueous) 2% (equivalent to 1.1% base) with chlorobutanol 0.5% in 7.5 ml containers.

EPINEPHRINE HYDROCHLORIDE:
Generic. Solution 1:1,000.
Epifrin (Allergan). Solution (sterile) equivalent to 0.25%, 0.5%, 1%, and 2% free base with benzalkonium chloride in 5 ml (0.5%, 1%, and 2% concentrations) and 15 ml (all strengths) containers.
Glaucon (Alcon). Solution (sterile) equivalent to 0.5%, 1%, or 2% base with benzalkonium chloride 0.01% in 10 ml containers.

EPINEPHRYL BORATE:
Epinal (Alcon). Solution (sterile) equivalent to 0.5% or 1% base with benzalkonium chloride 0.01% in 7.5 ml containers.
Eppy/N (Barnes-Hind). Solution (sterile) equivalent to 0.5%, 1%, and 2% levo-epinephrine free base with benzalkonium chloride 0.01% in 7.5 ml containers.

DIPIVEFRIN HYDROCHLORIDE (Dipivalyl Epinephrine)
[Propine]

ACTIONS AND USES. The prodrug, dipivefrin, is a lipophilic analogue of epinephrine formed by the addition of two pivalic acid side chains to the parent compound. Prodrugs require biotransformation to the parent compound before they are therapeutically active. Dipivefrin is converted to epinephrine by esterases in the ocular tissues. Because of its lipophilic properties, dipivefrin penetrates the eye more readily than epinephrine and reduces intraocular pressure at a lower concentration. The onset of action occurs in 30 minutes and the maximal reduction in pressure is attained in one hour.

Dipivefrin is an effective ocular hypotensive agent in patients with open-angle glaucoma. Its effect on intraocular pressure is slightly less than that of 2% epinephrine hydrochloride, but its mydriatic effect is comparable (Kass et al, 1979; Kohn et al, 1979).

ADVERSE REACTIONS. Dipivefrin produces less burning and irritation than epinephrine and may cause fewer allergic reactions. Allergic or follicular conjunctivitis may occur during long-term therapy (Theodore and Leibowitz, 1979). As with epinephrine, cystoid macular edema has been reported. Because a lower concentration is required for corneal penetration, systemic side effects may be reduced.

For other potential adverse effects, see the previous evaluation.

DOSAGE AND PREPARATIONS.
Topical: In primary open-angle glaucoma and other chronic glaucomas, one drop is instilled in the conjunctival sac every 12 hours.
> *Propine* (Allergan). Solution (sterile) 0.1% with benzalkonium chloride 0.004% in 5, 10, and 15 ml containers.

EPINEPHRINE BITARTRATE AND PILOCARPINE HYDROCHLORIDE

Mixtures containing pilocarpine and epinephrine are convenient for treating open-angle glaucoma when both drugs are required and one of the available combinations is effective in controlling intraocular pressure. Many ophthalmologists are opposed to use of the combination products because more epinephrine than necessary is delivered if the medication is used four times daily.
> Preparations are available as ophthalmic solutions.
> *E-Pilo, E-Pilo-2, E-Pilo-3, E-Pilo-4,* and *E-Pilo-6* (CooperVision). Solution (sterile) containing epinephrine bitartrate 1% (equivalent to 0.55% base) and pilocarpine hydrochloride 1%, 2%, 3%, 4%, or 6% with benzalkonium chloride and edetate disodium in 10 ml containers.
> *P1E1, P2E1, P3E1, P4E1,* and *P6E1* (Alcon). Solution (sterile) containing epinephrine bitartrate 1% (equivalent to 0.5% base) and pilocarpine hydrochloride 1%, 2%, 3%, 4%, or 6% with benzalkonium chloride 0.01% in 15 ml containers.

BETA-ADRENERGIC BLOCKING DRUGS

Beta-adrenergic receptors are located primarily in the heart, the arteries and arterioles of skeletal muscle, and the bronchi, where they subserve cardiac excitation, vasodilation, and bronchial relaxation. Beta receptors also have been identified in ocular tissue, primarily in the ciliary body and, along with alpha receptors, in the sphincter muscle of the iris. Beta-blocking drugs combine reversibly with these receptors to block the response to sympathetic nerve stimulation or circulating catecholamines. The various beta-blocking drugs differ in their affinity for cardiac (beta$_1$) and noncardiac (beta$_2$) receptors, and some show local anesthetic and partial agonist activity.

Beta-blocking agents lower intraocular pressure by decreasing the production of aqueous humor. It is not known whether this effect is actually due to beta blockade because beta-receptor agonists, such as isoproterenol, also have an ocular hypotensive effect. The effect of beta-blocking drugs on intraocular pressure occurs after either topical or systemic administration of both cardioselective (beta$_1$) and nonselective (beta$_{1,2}$) agents. The topical route is usually preferred because of a lower incidence of systemic side effects. Oral therapy may be useful when there are additional indications for a beta-blocking drug (eg, systemic hypertension, angina pectoris).

TIMOLOL MALEATE
[Timoptic]

ACTIONS. Timolol is a long-acting nonselective beta-blocking agent. In animal studies, it lacked significant partial agonist or local anesthetic properties. Mild local anesthetic properties have been noted in some patients, however, after prolonged use (Van Buskirk, 1979). Following topical application of a single dose, intraocular pressure is reduced within 20 minutes and the effect is still evident after 24 hours. If timolol is withdrawn following long-term therapy, the ocular hypotensive effect does not disappear completely for at least two weeks.

When given alone, timolol does not alter pupillary diameter or reactivity to light, but it enhances the mydriatic effect of epinephrine. Because it does not cause spasm of accommodation or miosis, timolol is better tolerated than miotics in young adults and in older patients with cataracts.

USES. Timolol lowers the intraocular pressure of patients with primary open-angle glaucoma and some secondary glaucomas. It has been used successfully to treat chronic glaucoma in aphakia and to prevent or treat glaucoma induced by alpha chymotrypsin, sodium hyaluronate, or laser procedures. Timolol also may be useful in the emergency treatment of acute angle-closure glaucoma when given with systemic ocular hypotensive drugs and pilocarpine.

In patients with open-angle glaucoma who respond to timolol, the ocular hypotensive effect is maximal when treatment is begun but may diminish during the first few days, particularly when the baseline pressure is high. This "escape" phenomenon should be watched for in evaluating initial efficacy. The residual improvement is often maintained but, after several months, partial tolerance may develop and is not overcome by increasing the drug concentration (Boger, 1979).

In patients with open-angle glaucoma, timolol appears to be as effective as pilocarpine or epinephrine and is better tolerated by some patients (Boger et al, 1978 A; Moss et al, 1978; Radius et al, 1978). Although both timolol and acetazolamide lower intraocular pressure by reducing aqueous production, their combined effect on pressure and aqueous production is greater than that of either drug alone (Berson and Epstein, 1981; Dailey et al, 1982; Kass et al, 1982). The effect of this combination is not fully additive, however. Timolol also may further reduce intraocular pressure in patients receiving miotics or multiple drug therapy (Boger et al, 1978 B; Zimmerman et al, 1979).

Unlike the additive effects of timolol with miotics, the benefit of combining timolol with epinephrine is uncertain and currently in doubt. The initial effect appears to depend upon the sequence of administration, ie, additive effects occur only if timolol is added to the regimen of patients who are already receiving epinephrine (Schenker et al, 1981). This initial enhancement tends to disappear during long-term combined therapy (Korey et al, 1982; Thomas and Epstein, 1981), although a more sustained additive effect was reported when the two drugs were instilled hours, rather than minutes, apart (Cyrlin et al, 1982).

Timolol is a suitable alternative to pilocarpine for initial and maintenance therapy. It is of particular benefit in young individuals with active accommodation and in older patients with lens opacities, particularly when epinephrine is ineffective, not tolerated, or contraindicated. Timolol also may be given with a miotic and/or carbonic anhydrase inhibitor to patients requiring combined therapy, and it usually should be added before the carbonic anhydrase inhibitor. The combination of timolol, a miotic, and a carbonic anhydrase inhibitor should be used as tolerated before resorting to surgery.

ADVERSE REACTIONS, PRECAUTIONS, AND INTERACTIONS. Timolol may cause mild ocular irritation, conjunctival hyperemia, ocular pain, headache, corneal anesthesia, transitory dry-eye syndrome, local hypersensitivity reactions, superficial punctate keratitis, blepharoptosis, and blurring of central vision (sometimes associated with a reversible myopia). In one study, blurred vision was the reason most often cited for discontinuation of timolol therapy (Wilson et al, 1980).

An abrupt rise in intraocular pressure may occur when timolol replaces existing antiglaucoma medication, and the pressure should be checked shortly after the previous drug is discontinued. Since timolol enhances the mydriatic effect of epinephrine, combined therapy may be dangerous in patients with narrow filtration angles. Aqueous suppression therapy with timolol and/or acetazolamide has occasionally caused hypotony and ciliochoroidal detachment after filtering surgery.

Other ocular reactions for which a cause-and-effect relationship has not been proved include aphakic macular edema, retinal detachment, macular hemorrhage, uveitis, and cataracts (McMahon et al, 1979; Van Buskirk, 1980).

Timolol is absorbed into the systemic circulation and may produce side effects related to blockade of cardiac and noncardiac beta receptors. Its effects are additive with those of other beta-blocking drugs, and patients who are also receiving a systemically administered beta blocker should be observed carefully. Timolol also may have additive effects with calcium channel blocking agents. If the patient is being treated by another physician for a cardiac disorder, this physician should be consulted prior to instituting therapy. Gentle eyelid closure for five minutes reduces the likelihood of systemic reactions while increasing ocular contact time, and there may be added benefit from digital pressure at the inner canthus to block lacrimal drainage (Passo et al, 1984; Zimmerman et al, 1984).

Bradycardia is the most common systemic side effect of timolol and blood pressure also may be decreased; therefore, pulse rate and blood pressure should be monitored. A paradoxical increase in blood pressure has developed in some patients (Wilson et al, 1980; Van Buskirk, 1980). (The possibility of a drug interaction should be considered in these cases, because systemically administered beta blockers occasionally have caused hypertensive reactions in the presence of increased levels of exogenous or endogenous circulating catecholamines.) Congestive heart failure, syncope, heart block, atrial fibrillation with a slow ventricular rate, and myocardial infarction have been reported rarely. Timolol should be used cautiously in patients with uncontrolled congestive heart failure or A-V conduction disturbances. Sudden death has occurred occasionally shortly after timolol therapy was instituted, but a cause-and-effect relationship has not been established in all cases (Van Buskirk, 1980).

Timolol significantly reduces forced expiratory volume in patients with chronic obstructive airway disease and may precipitate bronchospasm (Schoene et al, 1981). A number of fatalities from status asthmaticus have been reported. Like other nonselective beta blockers, timolol should not be used in patients with a history of asthma or chronic bronchitis. Both the cardiac and the pulmonary side effects of timolol may be additive with those of the anticholinesterase miotics. Timolol occasionally has increased the frequency of hypoglycemic episodes and masked the symptoms of hypoglycemia in diabetics receiving insulin.

Central nervous system effects are similar to those reported with systemically administered beta blockers and include fatigue, lethargy, depression, anxiety, psychic dissociation, confusion, and hallucinations (McMahon et al, 1979; Van Buskirk, 1980). Timolol also may cause sexual dysfunction (impotence, decreased libido). It has occasionally aggravated symptoms of myasthenia gravis.

Anorexia, nausea, and dyspepsia have been reported. Reversible nail pigmentation has occurred rarely.

Very high blood levels of timolol occur in infants after ocular administration, and this may lead to episodes of apnea and other complications (Passo et al, 1984).

Timolol is excreted in breast milk and should be used cautiously in nursing mothers. Its safety in pregnancy has not been determined (FDA Pregnancy Category C).

DOSAGE AND PREPARATIONS.
Topical: In primary open-angle glaucoma and other chronic glaucomas, initially, one drop of the 0.25% solution is instilled in the conjunctival sac twice daily. If a satisfactory response is not obtained, dosage may be increased to one drop of the 0.5% solution twice daily. Occasionally, once-daily application of the 0.5% solution may be sufficient for maintenance. If a

patient with severe glaucoma is being transferred from another antiglaucoma drug, the previously used medication should not be discontinued for three weeks or longer and the pressure should then be checked to confirm that an abrupt rise has not occurred.

Timoptic (Merck Sharp & Dohme). Solution (sterile, aqueous) 0.25% and 0.5% with benzalkonium chloride 0.01% in 5, 10, and 15 ml containers.

BETAXOLOL HYDROCHLORIDE
[Betoptic]

Betaxolol is a topical beta-blocking drug that acts primarily on beta$_1$ receptors. It recently became available for treating chronic open-angle glaucoma. Betaxolol appears to be as effective as timolol (Berry et al, 1984) and may be safer in asthmatics (Schoene et al, 1984), but experience with its use is still limited.

For adverse effects produced by topical beta blockers, see the evaluation on Timolol Maleate.

DOSAGE AND PREPARATIONS.
Topical: Initially, in primary open-angle glaucoma and other chronic glaucomas, one drop is instilled twice daily.

Betoptic (Alcon). Solution (sterile, aqueous) 0.5% (as base) with benzalkonium chloride 0.01% in 5 and 10 ml containers.

LEVOBUNOLOL HYDROCHLORIDE
[Betagan]

Levobunolol, the stereoisomer of timolol, is a long-acting nonselective beta blocker for topical treatment of chronic open-angle glaucoma. It is as effective as timolol and has similar side effects (Berson et al, 1985, Long et al, 1985).

For adverse effects of topical beta blockers, see the evaluation on Timolol Maleate. This drug is classified in FDA Pregnancy Category C.

DOSAGE AND PREPARATIONS.
Topical: In primary open-angle glaucoma and other chronic glaucomas, initially, one drop is instilled once or twice daily.

Betagan (Allergan). Solution (sterile) 0.5% with benzalkonium chloride 0.004% and edetate disodium in 5 and 10 ml containers.

CARBONIC ANHYDRASE INHIBITORS

ACTIONS. Carbonic anhydrase inhibitors (acetazolamide, dichlorphenamide, methazolamide) are given systemically to reduce intraocular pressure. These drugs were originally introduced as diuretics, but their effect on intraocular pressure does not depend upon diuresis. They reduce aqueous production and thus lower pressure by blocking ocular carbonic anhydrase in the ciliary epithelium. Systemic acidosis adds to the ocular hypotensive effect. When maximal doses are given, carbonic anhydrase inhibitors reduce aqueous flow by about 50%.

USES. The major use of carbonic anhydrase inhibitors is for long-term treatment of primary open-angle glaucoma and other chronic glaucomas refractory to short-acting miotics, epinephrine, and timolol. (Most ophthalmologists prefer to use a carbonic anhydrase inhibitor before a strong miotic is substituted for a weak one in the phakic eye.)

Carbonic anhydrase inhibitors are used with osmotic agents, miotics, and topical beta blockers for the emergency treatment of acute angle-closure glaucoma. By reducing aqueous formation, carbonic anhydrase inhibitors decrease pressure behind the iris and thus assist in opening the angle. They should be used only for *short-term* treatment prior to surgery because the lowered pressure may mask the fact that the angle remains partly closed. Peripheral anterior synechiae may then develop and result in permanent closure of the angle.

Carbonic anhydrase inhibitors also are used in some secondary glaucomas (eg, glaucomatocyclitic crisis syndrome; glaucoma induced by alpha chymotrypsin, sodium hyaluronate, or laser procedures; glaucoma secondary to anterior uveitis or trauma) and in the preoperative treatment of congenital glaucoma.

ADVERSE REACTIONS, PRECAUTIONS, AND INTERACTIONS. Carbonic anhydrase inhibitors commonly cause malaise, anorexia, weight loss, fatigue, headache, weakness, nervousness, loss of libido, impotence, paresthesias, and, in infants, failure to thrive. Lethargy and depression are common and often unrecognized until the drug is discontinued and the patient notices a sudden improvement in emotional state. Many patients cannot tolerate the drugs for prolonged periods because of this malaise syndrome. Transient myopia has been reported and may result from changes in lens hydration or forward movement of the lens caused by ciliary body swelling. Confusion, ataxia, tremor, and tinnitus have been reported rarely. Carbonic anhydrase inhibitors are better tolerated by patients under 40 years of age than by older patients.

The frequency and intensity of side effects are dose related, and some are associated with systemic acidosis. An attempt should be made to relieve symptoms by adjusting dosage. In many patients, one-fourth of the previously recommended full dosage is as effective as larger doses and less likely to cause side effects. If dosage adjustment is unsuccessful, sodium bicarbonate 80 mEq daily may alleviate some symptoms, despite the fact that this treatment has little effect on the serum CO$_2$-combining power. Sodium bicarbonate has been employed primarily in patients with advanced glaucoma who are about to discontinue the carbonic anhydrase inhibitor because of the malaise syndrome (Epstein and Grant, 1978). Carbonic anhydrase inhibitor therapy alters the taste of carbonated drinks. Because of their effect on acid-base balance, carbonic anhydrase inhibitors increase the risk of salicylate intoxication in patients receiving large doses of aspirin.

Carbonic anhydrase inhibitors frequently cause gastric distress, nausea, vomiting, and diarrhea. Constipation has also been reported. These effects appear to be caused by a local irritant action and may respond to measures such as taking the drug with food or sodium bicarbonate or substituting a different preparation. Acetazolamide in timed-release capsules may be better tolerated than the tablet form.

Diuresis may be troublesome initially but often subsides during continued therapy. The serum potassium level may fall during the first few weeks of treatment but usually returns to a low normal level unless a potassium-wasting diuretic (thiazide, loop diuretic) is taken concurrently. The hypokalemia is not associated with a clinically significant reduction in total body potassium. Although theoretically possible, no serious problems (eg, enhanced digitalis toxicity) have been associated with the initial hypokalemia or with prolonged therapy unless a potassium-wasting diuretic is given concomitantly. Potassium supplements do not alleviate the symptomatic side effects of carbonic anhydrase inhibitors in normokalemic patients and are no longer given routinely. Serum potassium levels should be monitored in patients receiving concurrent therapy with another potassium-wasting diuretic.

Renal colic, hematuria, and oliguria or anuria may occur during prolonged therapy and are usually evidence of ureteral calculus formation. The renal stones may be precipitated by the reduced urinary excretion of citrate and/or magnesium, which decreases the solubility of calcium. Nephrolithiasis may occur more frequently with acetazolamide than with methazolamide (Grant, 1973; Epstein and Grant, 1978). Very rarely, renal symptoms have occurred early during therapy without evidence of urinary calculi. A sulfonamide-like nephropathy may be involved in these cases, and a few patients have died in acute renal failure.

The carbonic anhydrase inhibitors reduce uric acid excretion and increase the blood uric acid level. The hyperuricemia is usually asymptomatic but rarely has led to an exacerbation of gout. Other untoward effects reported with these drugs include rash (due to sulfonamide sensitivity) and, rarely, drug fever, hirsutism, thrombocytopenia, leukopenia, agranulocytosis, and aplastic anemia.

Since carbonic anhydrase inhibitors may have teratogenic effects, these drugs should be avoided during early pregnancy. Negligible amounts of acetazolamide are excreted in breast milk.

Carbonic anhydrase inhibitors should be used cautiously in patients with obstructive pulmonary disease because they may precipitate acute respiratory failure. Rarely, carbonic anhydrase inhibitors have caused severe hyperchloremic acidosis in diabetic patients.

Postoperative use of carbonic anhydrase inhibitors may adversely affect the outcome of filtering operations by reducing the size of the resultant drainage bleb and delaying reformation of the anterior chamber. Aqueous suppression therapy with timolol and/or acetazolamide has occasionally caused hypotony and ciliochoroidal detachment after filtration surgery.

PHARMACOKINETICS. Carbonic anhydrase inhibitors are widely distributed throughout the body, with the highest concentrations present in tissues containing high concentrations of carbonic anhydrase, especially erythrocytes and the renal cortex. The drugs also enter the aqueous humor.

Different brands of acetazolamide may vary in bioavailability, and significant lot-to-lot variation has been found in some products. For this reason, bioequivalence requirements have been proposed for all carbonic anhydrase inhibitors. Therapeutic plasma levels of acetazolamide range from 4 to 10 mcg/ml. Acetazolamide is 93% protein bound. It is not metabolized, and 70% of an administered dose is recovered in the urine within 24 hours. The half-life is five hours.

Methazolamide is well absorbed. It is only 55% protein bound and diffuses into tissues more readily than acetazolamide. Only 25% of a dose is excreted unchanged in the urine, but there is no information about metabolites.

Dichlorphenamide appears to be well absorbed, and maximal effects are observed two to four hours after administration. Its pharmacokinetic properties have not been studied extensively.

DOSAGE AND PREPARATIONS.
ACETAZOLAMIDE:
Oral: *Adults,* 62.5 to 250 mg (tablets) two to four times daily or 500 mg (capsules) once or twice daily. The timed-release preparation given once daily is better tolerated by some patients, but the magnitude of the ocular hypotensive effect is less than with larger doses. *Children,* 10 to 15 mg/kg daily in divided doses.
   Ak-Zol (Akorn), **Generic.** Tablets 250 mg.
   Diamox (Lederle). Capsules (timed-release) 500 mg; tablets 125 and 250 mg.
ACETAZOLAMIDE SODIUM:
Intravenous, Intramuscular: *Adults,* initially, 500 mg; the dose may be repeated, if necessary, in two to four hours. *Infants and children,* 5 to 10 mg/kg every six hours.
   Diamox [parenteral] (Lederle). Powder 500 mg (should be reconstituted with at least 5 ml of sterile water for injection).
DICHLORPHENAMIDE:
Oral: *Adults,* 50 to 200 mg every six to eight hours.
   Daranide (Merck Sharp & Dohme). Tablets 50 mg.
METHAZOLAMIDE:
Oral: *Adults,* 25 to 50 mg two or three times daily.
   Neptazane (Lederle). Tablets 50 mg.

OSMOTIC AGENTS

Hypertonic solutions of glycerin [Glyrol, Osmōglyn], isosorbide [Ismotic], urea [Ureaphil], or mannitol [Osmitrol] are used for the short-term reduction of intraocular pressure and vitreous volume. By increasing blood osmolarity, these agents induce the withdrawal of fluid from the eyeball by an osmotic effect. They cause an immediate, marked fall in intraocular pressure and reduction of vitreous volume and are generally effective even in patients who do not respond to miotics and carbonic anhydrase inhibitors.

In acute angle-closure glaucoma, osmotic agents are used to reduce intraocular pressure rapidly prior to surgery and to help clear corneal edema. When the pressure elevation is pronounced, the iris sphincter becomes ischemic and may not respond to miotics unless pressure is reduced initially with an osmotic agent. Osmotic agents also may aid in opening the angle by reducing the volume of the posterior segment of the eye and transiently reducing pressure behind the iris. If the miotic is then effective in opening the angle, the pressure may remain normal even after the osmotic effect has worn off.

In chronic glaucomas, osmotic agents are used only for pre- and postoperative treatment. They also are used pre- and postoperatively in congenital glaucoma, retinal detachment surgery, routine cataract extraction, and keratoplasty, and they may be of temporary benefit in some secondary glaucomas. Since their action is dependent upon an intact blood-aqueous barrier, osmotic agents are sometimes ineffective in inflammatory secondary glaucomas.

Mannitol and urea are given intravenously; they are equally effective in reducing intraocular pressure and vitreous volume, but mannitol is more convenient to administer and less toxic. Orally administered glycerin and isosorbide are not as rapidly effective as the intravenous agents, but often are preferred because of their safety and convenience. Ethanol also has an osmotic action and may be given orally to reduce intraocular pressure in an emergency.

See the evaluations for adverse reactions and precautions.

GLYCERIN
[Glyrol, Osmōglyn]

$$CH_2OH$$
$$|$$
$$CHOH$$
$$|$$
$$CH_2OH$$

USES. Oral glycerin is used to reduce intraocular pressure and vitreous volume prior to various ocular surgical procedures, such as cataract surgery and iridectomy, and for short-term treatment of some secondary glaucomas. Glycerin is probably safer than the intravenously administered agents, urea and mannitol, but it has a slower onset of action. A maximal reduction in intraocular pressure and vitreous volume occurs about one hour after administration, with a return to the pretreatment level in about five hours. Because it is rapidly metabolized, glycerin produces little diuresis, and routine urinary bladder catheterization for surgery is not required.

ADVERSE REACTIONS AND PRECAUTIONS. Headache, nausea, and vomiting are the most common untoward effects. Diarrhea occurs occasionally. Glycerin may cause hyperglycemia and glycosuria and should be used cautiously in diabetics. Confusion and amnesia may occur in older patients, but frank hyperosmolar nonketotic coma is a rare complication. The systemic effects of dehydration that occur with use of the intravenous osmotic agents are less likely with glycerin. Glycerin should not be given intravenously because it can cause hemolysis.

DOSAGE AND PREPARATIONS.
Oral: *Adults and children,* 1 to 1.5 g/kg, given as a 50% or 75% solution. The drug may be administered more than once daily, if necessary. Lemon juice or instant coffee may be added to unflavored preparations. Palatability is also enhanced by pouring the solution over crushed ice and drinking through a straw, but patients should not be permitted to drink additional water.
Available generically in bulk form (unflavored) and may be diluted.
Glyrol (CooperVision). Solution (oral) 75% (0.94 g/ml).
Osmōglyn (Alcon). Solution (oral) 50% (0.6 g/ml).

ISOSORBIDE
[Ismotic]

Isosorbide is an oral osmotic agent used to reduce intraocular pressure and vitreous volume prior to ocular surgical procedures and for short-term treatment of some secondary glaucomas. It apparently has the same onset and duration of action as glycerin.

Untoward effects also are similar, although isosorbide does not adversely affect blood glucose levels and is preferred in diabetics. It also may cause less nausea and vomiting. Isosorbide produces a more significant diuresis than glycerin and catheterization may be necessary. It also may cause diarrhea.

DOSAGE AND PREPARATIONS.
Oral: *Adults,* initially, 1.5 g/kg. The drug may be given up to four times daily, if indicated. It may be poured over cracked ice to increase palatability.
Note: Isosorbide should not be confused with isosorbide dinitrate, an antianginal drug.
Ismotic (Alcon). Solution (oral) 45% (0.45 g/ml).

MANNITOL
[Osmitrol]

$$CH_2OH$$
$$|$$
$$HOCH$$
$$|$$
$$HOCH$$
$$|$$
$$HCOH$$
$$|$$
$$HCOH$$
$$|$$
$$CH_2OH$$

ACTIONS AND USES. Mannitol is given intravenously to reduce intraocular pressure and vitreous volume prior to ocular surgical procedures and for short-term treatment of some secondary glaucomas. A maximal reduction in intraocular pressure occurs in 30 to 60 minutes and lasts six to eight hours.

If an intravenous osmotic agent is indicated, mannitol is generally preferred to urea because it is more convenient and less toxic. Impaired renal function is not a contraindication to its use, and it does not cause tissue necrosis if extravasation occurs. Mannitol may be less likely than urea to penetrate ocular fluids in the presence of inflammation and, in this situation, it would be more effective than urea.

ADVERSE REACTIONS AND PRECAUTIONS. Headache, nausea, vomiting, dehydration, and massive diuresis are common untoward effects of mannitol. Urinary bladder catheterization should be considered in patients who are undergoing surgery. Chills, dizziness, and chest pain also have been reported. The drug occasionally has caused agitation, disorientation, convulsions, and anaphylactoid reactions. Cardiovascular status should be evaluated before using mannitol. Because of the large fluid volumes required, an acute increase in intravascular volume with subsequent overload may result in pulmonary edema or intracranial hemorrhage. Fatalities have been reported.

DOSAGE AND PREPARATIONS.
Intravenous: *Adults and children,* 0.5 to 2 g/kg as a 20% solution is infused over a period of 30 to 60 minutes. Administration may be discontinued when the desired effect has been

obtained, even if the full dose has not been given. A total dose of 1 g/kg is usually sufficient, and smaller doses are sometimes effective.

Note: Mannitol should not be confused with mannitol hexanitrate, an antianginal drug.

Generic. Solution 5%, 10%, 15%, 20%, and 25%.

Osmitrol (Travenol). Solution 5% in 1,000 ml containers, 10% in 500 and 1,000 ml containers, 15% in 150 and 500 ml containers, and 20% in 250 and 500 ml containers.

UREA FOR INJECTION

[Ureaphil]

$$\begin{array}{c} NH_2 \\ | \\ C=O \\ | \\ NH_2 \end{array}$$

Urea is used less commonly than other osmotic agents. Because the eye is permeable to urea, a rebound elevation in intraocular pressure and vitreous volume may occur after the ocular hypotensive effect has terminated (about 8 to 12 hours after administration), but this is not usually a significant clinical problem.

The systemic toxicity of urea is similar to that of mannitol. Urea is irritating to the tissues; it causes pain at the site of infusion and necrosis may result if extravasation occurs. Superficial and deep thrombosis may develop if urea is infused into the veins of the lower extremities. This agent should not be used in patients with severely impaired renal or hepatic function. Cardiovascular status should be evaluated before administering urea.

Urea is often reconstituted with invert sugar solution. Invert sugar contains fructose, which can cause severe reactions (hypoglycemia, nausea, vomiting, tremors, coma, and convulsions) in patients with hereditary fructose intolerance (aldolase deficiency).

DOSAGE AND PREPARATIONS. The solution should be prepared just prior to use.

Intravenous: *Adults,* 0.5 to 2 g/kg of a 30% solution is administered at a rate of 60 drops/min. *Children,* 0.5 to 1.5 g/kg of a 30% solution is infused over a 30-minute period.

Ureaphil (Abbott). Powder (lyophilized, for injection) 40 g.

INVESTIGATIONAL AGENTS

Parasympathomimetic Agents

Aceclidine, a miotic not yet available in the United States, has an ocular hypotensive effect similar to that of pilocarpine. It causes less shallowing of the anterior chamber and less accommodative spasm than pilocarpine (Drance, 1978).

Carbachol does not readily penetrate the cornea. A lipid-soluble compound, N-demethylated carbachol hydrochloride, is under investigation.

Adrenergic Agonist and Antagonists

Advances in knowledge concerning the role of adrenergic receptors in regulating aqueous production and outflow have stimulated a search for ocular hypotensive drugs that are better tolerated and more effective than epinephrine. Research has focused on the effects of related catecholamines, agents that enhance the effects of catecholamines, adrenergic blocking drugs, and agents with both central and peripheral actions (Ross and Drance, 1975; Sears, 1976; Leopold, 1978).

Catecholamines: The catecholamine, isoproterenol, stimulates beta₁ and beta₂ receptors. When applied topically, its ocular hypotensive effect is comparable to that of epinephrine. The usefulness of isoproterenol is limited, however, by the frequent occurrence of local discomfort and systemic side effects (tachycardia). The beta agonist, albuterol, which selectively stimulates beta₂ (noncardiac) receptors, also is effective when applied topically, but it often causes severe hyperemia and local irritation and tolerance may develop during prolonged therapy (Ross and Drance, 1975; Sears, 1976).

Norepinephrine may prove useful in patients who experience allergic reactions to epinephrine (Pollack and Rossi, 1975). Norepinephrine acts primarily on alpha receptors. A stable ophthalmic preparation (borate salt) is currently under investigation. The ocular hypotensive effect of norepinephrine borate 4% appears to be comparable to that of epinephryl borate 1%. Conjunctival hyperemia is the only significant side effect reported. A prodrug analogue, norepinephrine dipivalate, is also under study (Stewart et al, 1981).

Agents That Enhance the Effects of Catecholamines: Another approach has been to increase the ocular hypotensive effect of epinephrine or norepinephrine by administering agents that prevent the reuptake of catecholamines into sympathetic nerve terminals. Preliminary data suggest that the antihypertensive drug, labetalol [Normodyne, Trandate], may lower intraocular pressure by this mechanism when applied topically.

In other studies, an attempt has been made to induce a state of denervation supersensitivity to exogenous epinephrine by topical application of guanethidine, a drug that prevents reuptake and blocks release of catecholamines. In initial studies, the ocular hypotensive effect of epinephrine was enhanced by prior administration of 5% guanethidine, but some patients developed superficial punctate lesions in the corneal epithelium, severe hyperemia, and ptosis. More recently, a 1% concentration of guanethidine has been used in fixed-dose combination with 0.5 to 1% epinephrine. This combination is well tolerated and is more effective than epinephrine alone.

When administered by the subconjunctival route, 6-hydroxydopamine selectively destroys sympathetic nerve terminals in the anterior uvea, thereby increasing the response to catecholamines (denervation supersensitivity). A single injection (0.2 ml of a 2% solution) enhances the response to epinephrine eyedrops for periods ranging from a few weeks to six months. The subsequent loss of effectiveness is presumably due to nerve regeneration, and most patients require repeated injections. 6-hydroxydopamine may be useful in patients who do not respond to maximal medical therapy or in those who cannot tolerate miotics (Talusan et al, 1981). However, this treatment is not usually practical on a long-term basis because the duration of effect is limited, and repeated subconjunctival injections are uncomfortable.

Alpha-Adrenergic Blocking Agents: Alpha-blocking drugs constrict the pupil by blocking alpha receptors in the dilator muscle of the iris, thereby permitting parasympathetic dominance via the sphincter muscle. They have no significant effect on the ciliary muscle or aqueous outflow system. One such agent, thymoxamine hydrochloride, has been effective in the emergency treatment of acute angle-closure glaucoma and may be useful diagnostically to distinguish between angle-closure glaucoma and open-angle glaucoma with a narrow angle (Wand and Grant, 1976). It also has been used to reverse the mydriatic effect of phenylephrine (see Chapter 19, Mydriatics and Cycloplegics). Thymoxamine is not currently under active investigation in the United States, but some investigators have obtained supplies of the drug by filing an individual IND with the FDA.

Beta-Adrenergic Blocking Agents: Timolol, betaxolol, and levobunolol are the only beta-blocking drugs available in the United States in ophthalmic formulations. Topical preparations of propranolol and practolol were used abroad to treat open-angle glaucoma, but propranolol proved to be unsuitable for long-term therapy because of its local anesthetic effect, and practolol was withdrawn from the market because of systemic toxicity. Topical preparations of atenolol, metoprolol, and pindolol are under investigation abroad or in the United States. The diacetyl derivative of nadolol also is under study for ophthalmic use in this country.

Agents with Both Central and Peripheral Actions: Clonidine [Catapres], which is used to treat systemic hypertension, reduces intraocular pressure when given orally, intravenously, or topically. Clonidine stimulates alpha-adrenergic receptors in the central nervous system and, to a lesser extent, in the peripheral blood vessels. Both mechanisms have been suggested to explain its ocular hypotensive effect.

Marijuana and some of its derivatives reduce intraocular pressure when smoked, after oral or parenteral administration, and, in animals, when applied topically. Marijuana is believed to reduce sympathetic tone by a central action and also may have peripheral adrenergic and antiadrenergic actions. Frequent side effects limit its usefulness for systemic therapy, and topical application does not appear to be effective in humans.

Miscellaneous Agents: Forskolin represents a new class of antiglaucoma drugs in the early stages of investigation. Forskolin lowers intraocular pressure by decreasing aqueous humor formation. It is thought to act by stimulating a receptor enzyme complex in the ciliary epithelium to increase intracellular concentrations of cyclic adenosine monophosphate (cAMP). When applied topically as a 1% solution to the human eye, forskolin lowers intraocular pressure for at least five hours (Caprioli and Sears, 1983).

Topical carbonic anhydrase inhibitors are also being investigated in the hope of finding an effective compound that lacks the systemic side effects of the oral drugs. One agent under study is an analogue of ethoxzolamide (Lewis et al, 1984).

Cited References

Apt L, Gaffney WL: Toxicity of topical eye medications used in childhood strabismus, in Leopold IH, Burns RP (eds): *Symposium on Ocular Therapy.* New York, John Wiley & Sons, 1976, vol 8, 1-10.

Beasley H, Fraunfelder FT: Retinal detachments and topical ocular miotics. *Ophthalmology* 86:95-98, 1979.

Berry DP Jr, et al: Betaxolol and timolol: Comparison of efficacy and side effects. *Arch Ophthalmol* 102:42-45, 1984.

Berson FG, Epstein DL: Separate and combined effects of timolol maleate and acetazolamide in open-angle glaucoma. *Am J Ophthalmol* 92:788-791, 1981.

Berson FG, et al: Levobunolol compared with timolol for long-term control of elevated intraocular pressure. *Arch Ophthalmol* 103:379-382, 1985.

Boger WP III: Timolol: Short-term "escape" and long term "drift." *Ann Ophthalmol* 11:1239-1242, 1979.

Boger WP III, et al: Clinical trial comparing timolol ophthalmic solution to pilocarpine in open-angle glaucoma. *Am J Ophthalmol* 86:8-18, 1978 A.

Boger WP III, et al: Long-term experience with timolol ophthalmic solution in patients with open-angle glaucoma. *Ophthalmology* 85:259-267, 1978 B.

Bourgon P, et al: Cholinergic supersensitivity of iris sphincter in Adie's tonic pupil. *Am J Ophthalmol* 85:373-377, 1978.

Camras CB, et al: Inhibition of epinephrine-induced reduction of intraocular pressure by systemic indomethacin in humans. *Am J Ophthalmol* 100:169-175, 1985.

Caprioli J, Sears M: Forskolin lowers intraocular pressure in rabbits, monkeys, and man. *Lancet* 1:958-960, 1983.

Cyrlin MN, et al: Additive effect of epinephrine to timolol therapy in primary open angle glaucoma. *Arch Ophthalmol* 100:414-418, 1982.

Dailey RA, et al: Effects of timolol maleate and acetazolamide on rate of aqueous formation in normal human subjects. *Am J Ophthalmol* 93:232-237, 1982.

Drance SM: Use of miotics in management of intraocular pressure, in Leopold IH, Burns RP (eds): *Symposium on Ocular Therapy.* New York, John Wiley & Sons, 1978, vol 11, 1-9.

Epstein DL, Grant WM: Management of carbonic anhydrase inhibitor side effects, in Leopold IH, Burns RP (eds): *Symposium on Ocular Therapy.* New York, John Wiley & Sons, 1978, vol 11, 51-64.

Fine BS, et al: Clinicopathologic study of four cases of primary open-angle glaucoma compared to normal eyes. *Am J Ophthalmol* 91:88-105, 1981.

Grant WM: Antiglaucoma drugs: Problems with carbonic anhydrase inhibitors, in Leopold IH (ed): *Symposium on Ocular Therapy.* St Louis, CV Mosby, 1973, vol 6, 19-38.

Johnson DH, et al: One-year multicenter clinical trial of pilocarpine gel. *Am J Ophthalmol* 97:723-729, 1984.

Kass MA, et al: Dipivefrin and epinephrine treatment of elevated intraocular pressure: Comparative study. *Arch Ophthalmol* 97:1865-1866, 1979.

Kass MA, et al: Timolol and acetazolamide: Study of concurrent administration. *Arch Ophthalmol* 100:941-942, 1982.

Kohn AN, et al: Clinical comparison of dipivalyl epinephrine and epinephrine in treatment of glaucoma. *Am J Ophthalmol* 87:196-201, 1979.

Korey JS, et al: Timolol and epinephrine: Long-term evaluation of concurrent administration. *Arch Ophthalmol* 100:742-745, 1982.

Leopold IH: Changing scene in drug therapy of glaucoma, in Leopold IH, Burns RP (eds): *Symposium on Ocular Therapy.* New York, John Wiley & Sons, 1978, vol 11, 11-28.

Lewis RA, et al: Ethoxzolamide analogue gel: Topical carbonic anhydrase inhibitor. *Arch Ophthalmol* 102:1821-1824, 1984.

Long D, et al: Minimum concentration of levobunolol required to control intraocular pressure in patients with primary open-angle glaucoma or ocular hypertension. *Am J Ophthalmol* 99:18-22, 1985.

McMahon CD, et al: Adverse effects experienced by patients taking timolol. *Am J Ophthalmol* 88:736-738, 1979.

Moss AP, et al: Comparison of effects of timolol and epinephrine on intraocular pressure. *Am J Ophthalmol* 86:489-495, 1978.

Passo MS, et al: Plasma timolol in glaucoma patients. *Ophthalmology* 91:1361-1363, 1984.

Pollack IP, Rossi H: Norepinephrine in treatment of ocular hypertension and glaucoma. *Arch Ophthalmol* 93:173-177, 1975.

Radius RL, et al: Timolol: New drug for management of chronic simple glaucoma. *Arch Ophthalmol* 96:1003-1008, 1978.

Ross RA, Drance SM: Effects of catecholamines and related drugs on intraocular pressure. *Can J Ophthalmol* 10:162-167, 1975.

Schenker HI, et al: Fluorophotometric study of epinephrine and timolol in human subjects. *Arch Ophthalmol* 99:1212-1216, 1981.

Schoene RB, et al: Timolol-induced bronchospasm in asthmatic bronchitis. *JAMA* 245:1400-1461, 1981.

Schoene RB, et al: Effects of topical betaxolol, timolol, and placebo on pulmonary function in asthmatic bronchitis. *Am J Ophthalmol* 97:86-92, 1984.

Sears ML: Adrenergic therapy of open angle glaucoma, in Leopold IH, Burns RP (eds): *Symposium on Ocular Therapy.* New York, John Wiley & Sons, 1976, vol 8, 67-78.

Stewart RH, et al: Norepinephrine dipivalylate dose-response in ocular hypertensive subjects. *Ann Ophthalmol* 13:1279-1283, 1981.

Talusan E, et al: 6-hydroxydopamine in treatment of open-angle glaucoma. *Am J Ophthalmol* 92:792-798, 1981.

Theodore J, Leibowitz HM: External ocular toxicity of dipivalyl epinephrine. *Am J Ophthalmol* 88:1013-1016, 1979.

Thomas JV, Epstein DL: Timolol and epinephrine in primary open angle glaucoma: Transient additive effect. *Arch Ophthalmol* 99:91-95, 1981.

Van Buskirk EM: Corneal anesthesia after timolol maleate therapy. *Am J Ophthalmol* 88:739-743, 1979.

Van Buskirk EM: Adverse reactions from timolol administration. *Ophthalmology* 87:447-450, 1980.

Van Buskirk EM: Hazards of medical glaucoma therapy in cataract patient. *Ophthalmology* 89:238-241, 1982.

Wand M, Grant WM: Thymoxamine hydrochloride: Effects on facility of outflow and intraocular pressure. *Invest Ophthalmol* 15:400-403, 1976.

Wilson RP, et al: Place of timolol in practice of ophthalmology. *Ophthalmology* 87:451-454, 1980.

Zimmerman TJ, et al: Timolol plus maximum-tolerated antiglaucoma therapy. *Arch Ophthalmol* 97:278-279, 1979.

Zimmerman TJ, et al: Improving therapeutic index of topically applied ocular drugs. *Arch Ophthalmol* 102:551-553, 1984.

Other Selected References

Chandler PA, Grant WM: *Glaucoma,* ed 2. Philadelphia, Lea & Febiger, 1979.

Ellis PP: *Ocular Therapeutics and Pharmacology,* ed 7. St Louis, CV Mosby, 1985.

Fraunfelder FT: *Drug-induced Ocular Side Effects and Drug Interactions,* ed 2. Philadelphia, Lea & Febiger, 1982.

Kolker AE, Hetherington J: *Becker-Shaffer's Diagnosis and Therapy of the Glaucomas,* ed 5. St Louis, CV Mosby, 1983.

Mydriatics and Cycloplegics   *19*

USES

Anticholinergic drugs are applied topically to the eye to produce paralysis of accommodation (cycloplegia) and pupillary dilation (mydriasis). These muscarinic antagonists paralyze the ciliary and iris sphincter muscles, which are innervated by the parasympathetic nervous system. They are used primarily as an aid in refraction, internal examination of the eye, and other diagnostic procedures; to produce mydriasis and cycloplegia before, during, and after intraocular surgery; and to treat anterior uveitis and some secondary glaucomas. The anticholinergic drugs available commercially as ophthalmic preparations include atropine, scopolamine (hyoscine), homatropine, cyclopentolate [Ak-Pentolate, Cyclogyl], and tropicamide [Mydriacyl].

Alpha-adrenergic agonists produce mydriasis without cycloplegia by contracting the dilator muscle of the iris. Phenylephrine and epinephrine act directly on receptors, whereas hydroxyamphetamine [Paredrine] and cocaine have an indirect action. Hydroxyamphetamine releases intraneuronal stores of norepinephrine and cocaine prevents neuronal reuptake of the neurotransmitter, thereby increasing its concentration at the neuronal synapse.

Phenylephrine, the most commonly administered topical adrenergic drug, is useful for diagnostic purposes, ocular surgery, and as an adjunct in the treatment of anterior uveitis to prevent formation of synechiae (adhesions). Epinephrine dilates the pupil when a dilute solution is instilled into the anterior chamber during ophthalmic surgery. It does not produce significant mydriasis when applied topically unless the corneal epithelium is disturbed or the patient is also receiving a beta blocker such as timolol [Timoptic]. Since adrenergic and anticholinergic drugs act by different mechanisms, wider mydriasis can be obtained by using both.

Diagnosis

Refraction: Both the cycloplegic and mydriatic actions of anticholinergic drugs are useful in estimating errors of refraction. Cycloplegia prevents accommodation during refraction and reveals latent refractive errors in hyperopia; dilation of the pupil facilitates retinoscopic estimation of the refractive error. The presence of mydriasis does not necessarily indicate adequate cycloplegia, for mydriasis generally occurs more rapidly than cycloplegia, persists longer, and can be obtained with a lower drug concentration. Highly pigmented eyes are relatively resistant to topical cycloplegics and more frequent instillation or use of a stronger solution may be required.

Atropine is the most potent mydriatic-cycloplegic drug in clinical use. It has a slow onset and a very long duration of action; in adults, residual cycloplegia may persist for six days or more and mydriasis for two or three weeks. Because of its prolonged action, atropine is not used for refraction in adults, but it is useful for children up to 5 or 6 years of age, especially when esotropia is present (Hiatt and Jerkins, 1983). Scopolamine has a cycloplegic effect almost equal to that of atropine. Although its duration of action is somewhat shorter (approximately three days), it is still too long for refraction in adults.

The shorter acting cycloplegics, homatropine, cyclopentolate, and tropicamide, are used for refraction in adults, older children, and sometimes in young children. Homatropine has the slowest onset and most prolonged action of these three drugs; residual cycloplegia may persist for 36 to 48 hours. Cyclopentolate induces maximal cycloplegia in 25 to 75 minutes with complete recovery in 6 to 24 hours. Cyclopentolate is preferred to atropine by some ophthalmologists for refraction in children over 2 to 3 years of age, including those with convergent strabismus. Tropicamide is a weaker cycloplegic, but its potency and duration of action are sufficient for refraction in adults. Examination must be performed within 20 to 35 minutes or it may be necessary to instill an additional drop. Complete recovery of accommodation occurs two to six hours after administration (Gettes and Belmont, 1961). Mydriasis, especially of blue irides, may persist for 24 to 36 hours with cyclopentolate and rarely with tropicamide.

Intraocular Examination: Adrenergic and short-acting anticholinergic drugs are used to dilate the pupil for examination of the intraocular structures (Gambill et al, 1967). Since phenylephrine and hydroxyamphetamine produce mydriasis without cycloplegia, the patient is spared the inconvenience of residual blurring of vision. This is an important consideration in patients who must drive home after the examination.

Light from an ophthalmoscope evokes iris sphincter contraction. If an anticholinergic agent is not used concomitantly with the adrenergic drug, much of the mydriasis produced by the latter may be counteracted by sphincter muscle contraction. Phenylephrine 2.5% may be combined with tropicamide or cyclopentolate (in a single solution or administered five minutes apart) to achieve wider mydriasis. Given in this manner, cyclopentolate (0.5%) and tropicamide (0.5% or 1%) have comparable mydriatic effects. The combination eliminates the need for multiple instillations and usually produces adequate mydriasis in patients with dark irides and in those receiving miotic therapy; the mydriatic effect is enhanced by prior instillation of a local anesthetic (Apt and Henrick, 1980; Sinclair et al, 1980).

Another short-acting anticholinergic, eucatropine, has a more delayed onset of action than tropicamide or cyclopentolate but has the advantage of producing little or no cycloplegia. An ophthalmic preparation of eucatropine is not commercially available, and this drug may be difficult to obtain in some areas.

If pupillary dilation is necessary for ophthalmoscopic examination of a patient with potential angle-closure glaucoma, a weak cycloplegic, such as tropicamide, may be safer than an adrenergic agonist. Cycloplegics tend to pull the lens posteriorly and flatten it, often reducing pupillary block and widening the chamber angle. They also paralyze the iris sphincter, reducing the pull of the iris against the lens. For examination of the posterior pole, a wick of cotton moistened with epinephrine 1:1,000 may be placed in the inferior cul-de-sac for three minutes to dilate only the inferior sector of the iris (Shaffer, 1967). Since mydriatic drugs can precipitate an attack of acute angle-closure glaucoma, patients at risk should be examined after the procedure to make certain that the pupil has returned to normal size, the angle is gonioscopically open, and the intraocular pressure is normal.

The alpha-adrenergic blocking agent, thymoxamine (investigational, available by individual IND only), is widely used abroad to reverse the mydriatic effect of phenylephrine. When used for this purpose, this drug is as effective as pilocarpine, is longer acting, and appears to be safer in eyes predisposed to angle closure (Mapstone, 1977; Saheb et al, 1982).

Provocative Test for Angle-closure Glaucoma: Not all patients with anatomically narrow filtration angles will develop acute angle-closure glaucoma. Provocative tests are sometimes performed to detect those who might. No available test is highly reliable and all entail some degree of risk. The safest and most physiologic procedures are the dark room test and the prone test, which may be performed simultaneously and do not require instillation of a mydriatic drug (Wand, 1974).

In mydriatic provocative testing, a short-acting agent, such as hydroxyamphetamine, eucatropine, tropicamide, or phenylephrine, is instilled and results are considered positive if the pressure increases by 8 mm Hg within one hour and the angle is gonioscopically closed at the time of the elevation. Gonioscopy is essential in interpreting the results because cycloplegia alone may increase intraocular pressure by reducing outflow facility. If results are positive, a mydriatic provocative test may be difficult to reverse unless phenylephrine is used and thymoxamine is available to reverse it. Only one eye should be tested at a time and the patient should be forewarned that iridectomy or iridotomy may be necessary if the angle remains closed.

Horner's Syndrome: Unilateral Horner's syndrome can be diagnosed with bilateral instillation of cocaine eyedrops. Results of this test are evaluated 30 minutes after instillation of a 10% solution or 60 minutes after instillation of a 5% solution. The test is positive if there is an increase in the difference of the diameters of the two pupils, the abnormal pupil being smaller. Once the presence of Horner's syndrome is confirmed, the lesion usually can be localized by instilling hydroxyamphetamine 1% in each eye. The denervated pupil should dilate if the lesion is preganglionic but not if it is postganglionic. The hydroxyamphetamine test is more accurate in confirming the presence of a postganglionic lesion than in predicting the site of the lesion when this is unknown (Maloney et al, 1980). The two tests should be separated by 48 hours.

Intraocular Surgery

Mydriatic eyedrops are instilled prior to some ocular surgical procedures, particularly to facilitate round pupil cataract extraction and to locate the retinal break during retinal detachment operations. Atropine or a shorter acting agent, such as phenylephrine or cyclopentolate, may be instilled preoperatively for this purpose. For wider mydriasis, an anticholinergic drug may be supplemented with an adrenergic agent (eg, cyclopentolate and phenylephrine [Cyclomydril]). Short-acting mydriatics are preferred if a posterior chamber intraocular lens is to be implanted.

Pupillary constriction induced by surgical trauma may be mediated by prostaglandins. Prostaglandin synthetase inhibitors (eg, indomethacin) have been given investigationally prior to surgery in an attempt to reduce the miosis. By the same action, inhibition of platelet aggregation could cause troublesome bleeding during surgery. Systemic therapy has not been consistently effective, but pretreatment with topical indomethacin or flurbiprofen (investigational preparations) may prevent or reduce surgically induced miosis (Keates and McGowan, 1984; Keulen-De Vos et al, 1983).

Epinephrine hydrochloride [Adrenalin Chloride] is used in very dilute solutions (1:10,000 to 1:100,000) intracamerally for mydriasis during surgery. It is best to use Adrenalin Chloride 1:1,000 without preservative (most preservatives are highly toxic to the corneal endothelium) and to dilute the preparation with a solution appropriate for intraocular use.

The pupil is dilated daily after some ocular surgical procedures to prevent formation of posterior synechiae. Atropine, scopolamine, or a shorter acting anticholinergic may be instilled one to several times daily until slit-lamp examination shows minimal iritis. An alpha-adrenergic agent, such as phenylephrine, may be used as well. It should be kept in mind that the duration of mydriatic action is reduced by inflammation. If postoperative inflammation is prolonged, continued mydriatic-cycloplegic therapy is advisable. In addition to their use for postoperative iritis, cycloplegics are useful to prevent or treat a flat anterior chamber after filtering surgery.

Mydriatics and cycloplegics are *not* used after extracapsular cataract surgery with placement of a posterior chamber intraocular lens, because mydriasis may cause the iris to become trapped behind the lens. Intraocular miotics, such as acetylcholine [Miochol], or carbachol [Miostat], are used at the end of this procedure.

Anterior Uveitis

Topical corticosteroids are the mainstay in the treatment of anterior uveitis (see Chapter 20, Miscellaneous Ophthalmic Preparations). Cycloplegics are used adjunctively, and local and systemic antibiotics are given when ocular infection is present.

Cycloplegics have three beneficial actions in anterior uveitis: They relax the intraocular muscles, thereby relieving pain and photophobia, and they reduce abnormal vascular permeability and dilate the pupil, which prevent complications. Atropine and scopolamine are often preferred for treating anterior uveitis because the duration of action of shorter acting agents is further reduced in the inflamed eye and because the latter drugs are more expensive. The cycloplegic may be supplemented with phenylephrine for maximal mydriasis. Shorter acting anticholinergics are used in mild inflammatory conditions and may be preferred when the intraocular pressure is elevated. Some ophthalmologists also employ the shorter acting agents in acute iritis to keep the iris in motion and prevent it from becoming sealed in a mydriatic position.

Secondary Glaucomas

Glaucoma Associated with Intraocular Inflammation: In acute anterior uveitis, increased permeability of the blood vessels of the ciliary body and iris leads to an outpouring of protein and inflammatory cells into the anterior chamber. The exudates may obstruct the trabecular meshwork and increase resistance to outflow of aqueous humor. If the inflammation persists, permanent obstruction may occur due to adhesions that seal the iris to the angle structures (peripheral anterior synechiae). These may occur with or without pupillary block.

Treatment of anterior uveitis with topical corticosteroids and cycloplegics may prevent these complications. Topical timolol [Timoptic] and/or epinephrine and systemic antiglaucoma drugs (a carbonic anhydrase inhibitor and, for short-term therapy, an osmotic agent) may be used to reduce elevated intraocular pressure. (See Chapter 18, Agents Used To Treat Glaucoma.) Miotics should be avoided in the presence of active inflammation, but may be helpful later if glaucoma persists after uveitis has subsided. It is important to rule out steroid therapy as a cause of the glaucoma.

Pupillary block is another potential complication of chronic or recurrent anterior uveitis. Contact between the inflamed iris and the anterior surface of the lens leads to the formation of adhesions that seal the iris to the lens. These posterior synechiae prevent passage of aqueous humor from the posterior to the anterior chamber through the pupil (pupillary block). As a result, the iris bulges forward (iris bombé) closing the filtration angle and causing the intraocular pressure to rise. Pupillary block also may occur in the absence of the lens (aphakia) when posterior synechiae seal the iris to the bulging vitreous face or lens capsule. Predisposing causes are an occluded iridectomy or iridotomy and wound leak.

Dilation of the pupil reduces contact between the iris and the lens or the vitreous face and may prevent formation of posterior synechiae or aid in breaking them once they have formed. Intensive mydriatic-cycloplegic therapy with atropine or scopolamine and phenylephrine may be required, along with topical corticosteroids (if inflammation is active) and antiglaucoma therapy as described above. By reducing vitreous volume, an osmotic agent may be particularly helpful to break pupillary block in the aphakic eye. Subconjunctival injection of 0.1 ml of a mixture containing equal proportions of cocaine 4%, atropine 1%, and epinephrine 1:1,000 has been used rarely to break resistant synechiae in aphakia; the blood pressure should be monitored when this combination is used because it will rise alarmingly in an occasional patient. If medical treatment fails to relieve pupillary block, surgery should be performed.

Malignant (Ciliary Block) Glaucoma: Mydriatic-cycloplegic therapy may be useful in malignant glaucoma, a rare complication of ocular surgery (usually for glaucoma). In this condition, forward displacement of the lens, ciliary processes, and iris flattens the anterior chamber and closes the filtration angle, and aqueous humor becomes trapped in the vitreous. Blockage of aqueous flow past the ciliary process (ciliary block), increased vitreous pressure, and an abnormal laxity in the zonules of the lens are believed to be causative factors.

Therapy with atropine (or scopolamine) and phenylephrine may promote re-formation of the anterior chamber and opening of the angle, presumably by increasing tension in the zonules and by relieving ciliary block. An osmotic agent and a carbonic anhydrase inhibitor are also administered to reduce pressure from within the vitreous. If drug therapy is successful, the systemic drugs and phenylephrine may be discontinued but, in many cases, the cycloplegic must be administered indefinitely (Chandler et al, 1968; Shaffer and Hoskins, 1978). Surgery may be necessary in unresponsive patients. Medical therapy is rarely effective in aphakic malignant (ciliovitreal block) glaucoma; laser disruption of the anterior hyaloid may be the treatment of choice.

Lens Subluxation: Although mydriatic-cycloplegic drugs have been used to treat acute glaucoma associated with anterior dislocation of the lens, pupillary dilation in the presence of a dislocated lens in the posterior chamber may promote anterior migration of the loose lens.

Miscellaneous Uses

Cycloplegic drugs have been used to discourage accommodation in other ocular disorders. In patients with severe functional spasm of accommodation, atropine is sometimes applied daily for three or four weeks to provide a period of accommodative rest.

Because of increasing evidence that close work may contribute to the progression of myopia, there has been a resurgence of interest in the use of atropine and bifocals to retard progression (Brodstein et al, 1984). The efficacy of chronic cycloplegia for treating myopia remains highly controversial and the potential adverse effects of long-term therapy are of concern.

In suppression amblyopia when occlusion therapy is unsuccessful or not feasible, atropine has been employed to blur vision in the normal eye, thus forcing fixation with the amblyopic eye. Atropine is most effective if the fixing eye is significantly hypermetropic because cycloplegia impairs both near and distance vision in hypermetropes, while it mainly blurs near vision in myopes and emmetropes.

Atropine has been used occasionally in accommodative esotropia to prevent convergence by paralyzing accommodation. This form of therapy is not consistently effective because the blurred vision induced by the cycloplegic may increase accommodative effort and thereby increase the degree of esotropia, especially initially or as the effect of the drug wears off.

Short-acting mydriatic agents have been employed with some success to reposition dislocated intraocular lens implants, especially the iris-clip type.

Adverse Reactions and Precautions

Local Reactions: Both anticholinergic and adrenergic mydriatics can precipitate an attack of acute angle-closure glaucoma in eyes with anatomically narrow angles. An abrupt elevation of intraocular pressure occurs when the pupil is mid-dilated because this position maximizes iris-lens contact and blocks the forward movement of aqueous through the pupil (pupillary block). The increased pressure behind the iris causes it to bow forward, obstructing outflow through the filtration angle. The attack of angle closure sometimes reverses spontaneously but often requires therapy to break the block. Long-acting mydriatics (atropine or scopolamine) should not be used preoperatively in eyes predisposed to angle closure, and shorter acting mydriatics should be used cautiously, if at all.

Topical anticholinergic drugs increase intraocular pressure to some degree in about one of four eyes with mild primary open-angle glaucoma and occasionally in normal eyes. The pressure rise is self-limited and is not caused by closure of the angle. It appears to be due to increased resistance to aqueous outflow associated with loss of ciliary muscle tone or to blocking of the trabecular meshwork by pigment liberated from the iris. Phenylephrine 2.5% is preferred to an anticholinergic drug for diagnostic purposes in patients with open-angle glaucoma.

When treating inflammation of the anterior segment, posterior synechiae may form if mydriatic drugs (particularly the long-acting agents) are applied for prolonged periods without moving the pupil. Posterior synechiae are especially likely to develop if there are inflammatory exudates in the angle. Gonioscopy is necessary to confirm their presence. Concurrent corticosteroid therapy minimizes this problem. If slit-lamp examination shows that synechiae are forming, the mydriatic may be discontinued briefly.

Anticholinergic drugs cause blurred vision, glare, and photophobia. Atropine may cause contact dermatitis of the lids and allergic conjunctivitis. Allergic reactions are less common with the other anticholinergic agents.

Atropine and scopolamine should be used with care in patients with keratoconus and Down's syndrome because they may induce permanent mydriasis.

Adrenergic drugs may cause browache, headache, blurred vision, hypersensitivity reactions, pain, and lacrimation. Pigment granules (aqueous floaters) may appear in the anterior chamber several minutes after instillation. They disappear within 12 to 24 hours and occur with decreasing frequency when the drug is administered repeatedly. These granules are apparently released from the iris and are derived from degenerated cells in the iris pigment epithelium that rupture when the dilator muscle contracts. They occur most commonly in older patients with dark irides and in those with exfoliation syndrome. Release of pigment is sometimes associated with a marked increase in intraocular pressure, which may be most pronounced in diabetics and patients with exfoliation syndrome. If the angle of the anterior chamber is open, the effect is transient and usually requires no treatment, unless the optic nerve is vulnerable.

Mydriatic solutions should be used with caution in eyes with intraocular lens implants, especially the iris-plane type, because of the risk of dislocation.

Systemic Reactions: Systemic reactions may occur after ocular application of anticholinergic or adrenergic drugs, particularly in children and elderly patients. These drugs should be instilled in the lowest effective concentration and no more often than needed to obtain the desired response. Systemic absorption can be reduced and corneal contact time prolonged by gentle eyelid closure for five minutes after instillation (which reduces the action of the nasolacrimal pump) and pressure at the inner canthus (which minimizes drainage into the nose and throat). Excess solution should be blotted with a tissue.

Children with fair complexions, Down's syndrome, or brain damage appear to be especially susceptible to anticholinergic toxicity. Anticholinergic toxicity also may explain some cases of delirium seen after cataract surgery (Summers and Reich, 1979). Symptoms include dryness of the mouth and skin, flushing, fever, rash, thirst, tachycardia, irritability, dizziness, depression, weeping, hyperactivity, ataxia, confusion, somnolence, hallucinations, delirium, and, rarely, convulsions, coma, and death. Systemic reactions are most common after instillation of atropine, scopolamine, or cyclopentolate 2% [Cyclogyl]. Cyclopentolate in particular has been associated with a transient, acute psychosis, especially in children and recently also documented in adults. Cyclopentolate 0.5% affects gastrointestinal function in preterm infants, while a 0.25% solution does not (Isenberg et al, 1985).

For ophthalmoscopy, one drop of a dilute solution of a combination of phenylephrine and tropicamide or cyclopentolate provides adequate mydriasis and reduces the risk of systemic toxicity from multiple applications and/or higher concentrations (Brown and Hanna, 1978; Apt and Henrick, 1980; Sinclair et al, 1980). Physostigmine salicylate is an effective antidote for anticholinergic toxicity (see Chapter 80, Drugs Used in the Treatment of Poisoning).

Tachycardia, hypertension, ventricular arrhythmias, anginal pain, myocardial infarction, cardiac arrest, subarachnoid hemorrhage, hyperhidrosis, blanching, tremors, agitation, and confusion may occur following ocular instillation of adrenergic drugs. These systemic reactions are most common when a strong concentration (phenylephrine 10%) is instilled repeatedly (Fraunfelder and Scafidi, 1978). Neonates, elderly patients, adults with orthostatic hypotension, and patients given systemic atropine are particularly at risk. For neonates, elderly patients, and those with known cardiovascular disease, the 2.5% solution is safer than the 10% solution but is still too concentrated for low-weight (less than 1,600 g) neonates. A solution containing cyclopentolate 0.2% and phenylephrine 1% [Cyclomydril] appears to be safe and effective for mydriasis in premature infants (Isenberg et al, 1984).

Drug Evaluations

ANTICHOLINERGIC AGENTS

ATROPINE SULFATE
[Atropine-Care, Atropisol, Isopto Atropine]

ACTIONS AND USES. Atropine is a potent, long-acting mydriatic and cycloplegic. Its effect on accommodation may last six days or longer and mydriasis may persist for two or three weeks. Atropine is used for pre- and postoperative mydriasis, in anterior uveitis, and in some secondary glaucomas. It may be used for refraction in children up to age 5 or 6 years and is the most potent cycloplegic for use in children with convergent strabismus (Hiatt and Jerkins, 1983). Because of its long duration of action, atropine is not useful for refraction in adults.

ADVERSE REACTIONS AND PRECAUTIONS. Acute angle-closure glaucoma may occur if atropine is instilled in eyes with anatomically narrow angles. This agent also may increase intraocular pressure in eyes with open-angle glaucoma and in some normal eyes. Systemic reactions may occur, particularly in children and elderly patients. Contact dermatitis and allergic conjunctivitis are not uncommon. See also the section on Adverse Reactions and Precautions in the Introduction.

DOSAGE AND PREPARATIONS.

Topical: For preoperative mydriasis, one drop of a 1% solution, often supplemented with one drop of phenylephrine, is instilled prior to surgery. Some surgeons prefer to instill drops for several days prior to surgery as well.

In anterior segment inflammation, the concentration and frequency of administration are determined by the severity of inflammation and the pupillary response. Atropine may be supplemented with phenylephrine for maximal mydriasis.

For anterior uveitis or postoperative mydriasis, one drop of a 1% to 2% solution instilled once daily is often adequate, but more frequent use may be required in the presence of severe inflammation. A 0.5% solution or ointment applied one to three times daily is often adequate in children. When slit-lamp examination reveals minimal inflammation, a less potent agent, such as homatropine, may be substituted.

To break posterior synechiae, drops may be instilled more frequently, eg, one drop of a 2% solution (alternately with phenylephrine 10%) every five to ten minutes for five applications of each. The risk of toxicity from each drug is increased with increasing dosage.

For malignant (ciliary block) glaucoma, initially, one drop of a 1% or 2% solution and one drop of phenylephrine 10% three or four times daily. For maintenance, one drop of a 1% or 2% solution daily or every other day.

For refraction in *children,* see Table 1.

All preparations available in topical ophthalmic forms.

Atropine-Care (Akorn). Solution (sterile) 1% with benzalkonium chloride 0.01% in 5 and 15 ml containers.

Atropine Sulfate (Allergan). Solution (sterile) 1% with chlorobutanol 0.5% in 15 ml containers; ointment (sterile) 0.5% and 1% with chlorobutanol 0.5% in 3.5 g containers.

Atropine Sulfate Steri-Unit (Alcon). Solution (sterile) 1% and 2% (preservative free) in 2 ml containers.

Atropisol (CooperVision). Solution (sterile) 0.5%, 1%, and 2% with benzalkonium chloride in 1 ml containers and 1% with benzalkonium chloride and edetate disodium in 5 and 15 ml containers.

Isopto Atropine (Alcon). Solution (sterile) 0.5%, 1%, and 3% with benzalkonium chloride 0.01% in 5 and 15 ml (1% concentration only) containers.

Ophthalmic forms also marketed by other manufacturers under generic name: Solution 1% and 2%; ointment 1%.

TABLE 1.
AGENTS USED FOR REFRACTION

Drug	Dosage (Topical)
Atropine Sulfate [Atropine-Care, Atropisol, Isopto Atropine]	*Children:* One drop of 0.125% solution (in infants less than 1 year), 0.25% solution (in children 1 to 5 years and in all children with blue irides), 0.5% solution or ointment (in children over 5 years), or 1% solution or ointment (in children with dark irides) is applied three times daily for three days prior to refraction and once on the morning of refraction.* Administration should be discontinued if systemic effects occur.
Cyclopentolate Hydrochloride [Ak-Pentolate, Cyclogyl]	*Adults:* One drop of 1% solution (or 2% in patients with dark irides) is instilled once, or one drop of 0.5% solution is instilled and repeated in five minutes. *Children:* One drop of 1% solution is instilled and repeated in ten minutes. *Infants under 1 year,* a 0.5% solution should be used.
Homatropine Hydrobromide [Isopto Homatropine]	*Adults and Children:* One drop of 2% or 5% solution is instilled and may be repeated if necessary in 5 to 10 minutes.
Scopolamine Hydrobromide [Isopto Hyoscine]	*Children:* One drop of 0.25% solution is applied twice daily for two days before the refraction.*
Tropicamide [Mydriacyl]	*Adults:* One drop of 1% solution. If the examination cannot be performed within 20 to 35 minutes, an additional drop may be instilled.

* If ointment is used, it should not be applied for several hours immediately prior to refraction because it will impair the transparency of the cornea and alter the regularity of its refraction.

CYCLOPENTOLATE HYDROCHLORIDE
[Ak-Pentolate, Cyclogyl]

ACTIONS AND USES. Cyclopentolate is an effective mydriatic and cycloplegic with a rapid onset and relatively short duration of action. Cycloplegia is maximal 25 to 75 minutes after instillation, and recovery of accommodation is complete in 6 to 24 hours. This drug is used as an aid in refraction, for ophthalmoscopy, and for preoperative mydriasis. The mydriatic effect may be greater than that of other cycloplegic drugs and is enhanced by phenylephrine. One drop of a solution containing 0.5% cyclopentolate and 2.5% phenylephrine is usually adequate for ophthalmoscopy; maximal effects occur 60 minutes after instillation.

ADVERSE REACTIONS AND PRECAUTIONS. Cyclopentolate has caused systemic reactions in both children and adults. Mild reactions of short duration are common. Severe central nervous system disturbances, manifested by ataxia, hallucinations, and grand mal seizures, have occurred rarely in children. Vomiting, abdominal distention, and adynamic ileus developed in a pair of premature twins following instillation of six drops of the 1% solution. One of the twins subsequently died from necrotizing enterocolitis. Even the 0.5% solution affects gastric function in premature infants (Isenberg et al, 1985) and

full-term neonates (Hermansen and Sullivan, 1985). Acute angle closure may occur if cyclopentolate is instilled in eyes with anatomically narrow angles. See also the section on Adverse Reactions and Precautions in the Introduction.

DOSAGE AND PREPARATIONS.
Topical: For refraction, see Table 1. For ophthalmoscopy, see Table 2.

Ak-Pentolate (Akorn). Solution (ophthalmic, sterile) 0.5% and 1% with edetate disodium 0.01% and benzalkonium chloride 0.01% in 15 ml containers.

Cyclogyl (Alcon). Solution (ophthalmic, sterile) 0.5%, 1%, and 2% with edetate disodium and benzalkonium chloride 0.01% in 2, 5, and 15 ml containers.

Ophthalmic forms also marketed by other manufacturers under generic name: Solution 0.1% and 1%.

CYCLOPENTOLATE HYDROCHLORIDE AND PHENYLEPHRINE HYDROCHLORIDE
[Cyclomydril]

This combination is used to produce wide mydriasis for ophthalmoscopy and for preoperative mydriasis. It may be the mydriatic of choice in premature neonates (Isenberg et al, 1984).

See the evaluations on Cyclopentolate Hydrochloride and Phenylephrine Hydrochloride and the section on Adverse Reactions and Precautions in the Introduction.

DOSAGE AND PREPARATIONS.
Topical: For ophthalmoscopy, see Table 2.

Cyclomydril (Alcon). Solution (ophthalmic, sterile) containing cyclopentolate hydrochloride 0.2% and phenylephrine hydro-

TABLE 2.
AGENTS USED FOR OPHTHALMOSCOPY

Drug	Dosage (Topical)
Cyclopentolate Hydrochloride [Ak-Pentolate, Cyclogyl]	One drop of 0.5% solution. For *preterm infants,* a 0.2% solution should be used. For wider mydriasis in *older children and adults,* one drop of a solution containing 0.5% cyclopentolate and 2.5% phenylephrine.
Cyclopentolate and Phenylephrine [Cyclomydril]	One drop of solution containing 0.2% cyclopentolate and 1% phenylephrine. (May be used safely in *preterm infants).*
Eucatropine Hydrochloride	One drop of 5% or 10% solution, repeated in 10 to 15 minutes if necessary.
Tropicamide [Mydriacyl]	One drop of 0.5% solution. For wider mydriasis, one drop of a solution containing 0.5% tropicamide and 2.5% phenylephrine. For examination of patients with primary open-angle glaucoma who are being treated with miotics, a solution containing equal parts of 0.5% tropicamide and 10% phenylephrine may be used.
Phenylephrine Hydrochloride [Ak-Dilate, Mydfrin, Neo-Synephrine Hydrochloride]	One drop of 2.5% solution.
Hydroxyamphetamine Hydrobromide [Paredrine]	One drop of 1% solution.

chloride 1% with edetate disodium and benzalkonium chloride 0.01% in 2 and 5 ml containers.

EUCATROPINE HYDROCHLORIDE

Eucatropine, a weak anticholinergic drug, produces mydriasis that lasts for two to four hours with little or no cycloplegia. It is occasionally used for ophthalmoscopy and provocative testing for angle-closure glaucoma.

Eucatropine may be difficult to obtain in some areas. Some pharmacies will prepare an ophthalmic solution upon special request but the solution is unstable.

For adverse effects, see the section on Adverse Reactions and Precautions in the Introduction.

DOSAGE AND PREPARATIONS.
Topical: For ophthalmoscopy, see Table 2. As a provocative test for angle-closure glaucoma, two drops of a 5% solution are instilled in one eye. (For details, see the discussion on provocative testing in the Introduction.) At the conclusion of the provocative test, the patient should be examined to make certain that the pupil has returned to normal size, the angle is gonioscopically open, and the intraocular pressure is normal.

No commercial ophthalmic preparation available. Compounding necessary for prescription.

HOMATROPINE HYDROBROMIDE
[Isopto Homatropine]

Homatropine is a mydriatic and cycloplegic used for refraction and for treatment of anterior uveitis. Repeated instillation of the 2% solution at ten-minute intervals produces maximal cycloplegia in 60 minutes. Effects may persist for 36 to 48 hours.

For adverse effects, see the section on Adverse Reactions and Precautions in the Introduction.

DOSAGE AND PREPARATIONS.
Topical: For refraction, see Table 1. For mild anterior uveitis, one drop of a 2% or 5% solution is instilled two or three times daily. When homatropine is used for continuing therapy after administration of atropine or scopolamine, the drops may be instilled initially one or more times daily, followed by twice weekly administration.

All preparations available as topical ophthalmic solutions.

Homatropine Hydrobromide (CooperVision). Solution (sterile) 2% and 5% with benzalkonium chloride in 1 ml containers and 2% and 5% with edetate disodium and benzalkonium chloride in 5 ml containers.

Isopto Homatropine (Alcon). Solution (sterile) 2% and 5% with benzalkonium chloride 0.01% (2% concentration) or benzethonium chloride 0.005% (5% concentration) in 5 and 15 ml containers.

Homatropine Hydrobromide Steri-Unit (Alcon). Solution 5% (preservative free) in 2 ml containers.
Drug also marketed by other manufacturers under generic name: Powder.

SCOPOLAMINE HYDROBROMIDE
[Isopto Hyoscine]

Br^- · $3H_2O$

ACTIONS AND USES. Scopolamine is a potent mydriatic and cycloplegic. In the concentrations used clinically, it has a shorter duration of action than atropine; cycloplegia may persist for three days. Scopolamine rarely causes local allergic reactions and is useful in patients who are allergic to atropine. It is administered occasionally for refraction in children but is employed most commonly for postoperative mydriasis, in anterior uveitis, and in some secondary glaucomas.

ADVERSE REACTIONS AND PRECAUTIONS. Scopolamine can cause acute angle-closure glaucoma if instilled in eyes with anatomically narrow angles. It also may increase intraocular pressure in eyes with open-angle glaucoma. Acute psychotic reactions with systemic effects may occur, particularly in children and elderly patients (see the section on Adverse Reactions and Precautions in the Introduction). Scopolamine may cause drowsiness.

DOSAGE AND PREPARATIONS.
Topical: In anterior segment inflammation, the concentration and frequency of administration are determined by the severity of inflammation and pupillary response. Scopolamine may be supplemented with phenylephrine for maximal mydriasis.

For postoperative mydriasis, one drop of a 0.25% solution instilled once daily is often adequate.

For anterior uveitis, one drop of a 0.25% solution is instilled once daily or more frequently in severe inflammation. When slit-lamp examination reveals minimal inflammation, a less potent agent, such as homatropine, may be substituted.

To break posterior synechiae, one drop of solution is instilled more frequently and may be alternated with phenylephrine 10% to enhance the mydriatic effect. The risk of toxicity from each drug is increased with increasing dosage.

For malignant (ciliary block) glaucoma, initially, one drop of a 0.25% solution and one drop of phenylephrine 10% three or four times daily or more often if required. For maintenance, one drop of a 0.25% or 0.3% solution once daily.

For refraction in children, see Table 1.
All preparations available in topical ophthalmic forms.
Isopto Hyoscine (Alcon). Solution (sterile) 0.25% with benzalkonium chloride 0.01% in 5 and 15 ml containers.
Available Mixture.
Murocoll-2 (Muro). Solution (sterile) containing scopolamine 0.3% and phenylephrine 10% with benzalkonium chloride 0.01% in 5 ml containers.

TROPICAMIDE
[Mydriacyl]

ACTIONS AND USES. Tropicamide is an effective mydriatic and cycloplegic with a rapid onset and short duration of action. It is used as an aid in refraction, for ophthalmoscopy and retinal photography, and occasionally in provocative testing for acute angle-closure glaucoma. Maximal cycloplegia occurs within 20 to 35 minutes after two drops of the 1% solution are instilled five minutes apart. The duration of action is very brief and complete recovery of accommodation occurs in two to six hours. Combination eyedrops containing 0.5% tropicamide and 2.5% phenylephrine produce maximal pupillary dilation within 45 minutes.

ADVERSE REACTIONS AND PRECAUTIONS. Because of its short duration of action, this drug rarely causes systemic reactions. For adverse effects of anticholinergic drugs, see the section on Adverse Reactions and Precautions in the Introduction.

DOSAGE AND PREPARATIONS.
Topical: For refraction, see Table 1. For ophthalmoscopy and retinal photography, see Table 2.
Mydriacyl (Alcon). Solution (sterile) 0.5% and 1% with benzalkonium chloride 0.01% in 15 ml containers.
Drug also marketed under generic name: Solution 0.5% and 1%.

ADRENERGIC AGENTS

PHENYLEPHRINE HYDROCHLORIDE
[Ak-Dilate, Mydfrin, Neo-Synephrine Hydrochloride]

ACTIONS AND USES. Phenylephrine is an alpha-adrenergic agonist. It is used to produce mydriasis without cycloplegia for examination of the intraocular structures; to facilitate ocular surgery; as an adjunct in the treatment of anterior uveitis, postoperative inflammation, and some secondary glaucomas; and occasionally for provocative testing for acute angle-closure glaucoma. It is often given with an anticholinergic drug to achieve wider mydriasis.

After ocular instillation of a 10% solution, maximal mydriasis is obtained in 60 to 90 minutes and recovery occurs in about six hours. For preoperative mydriasis, a 2.5% solution was as effective as a 10% solution when given every 15 minutes for 90 minutes (Smith et al, 1976), but the 10% solution was more effective (particularly in highly pigmented eyes) when three applications were given in conjunction with cyclopentolate (Duffin et al, 1983). A solution containing 2.5% phenylephrine and 0.5% tropicamide or cyclopentolate is useful for ophthalmoscopy (Apt and Henrick, 1980).

ADVERSE REACTIONS, PRECAUTIONS, AND INTERAC-
TIONS. Local adverse reactions include transient pain, release
of aqueous floaters with a transitory increase in intraocular
pressure, and occlusion of structurally narrow angles resulting
in angle-closure glaucoma. Because of the adrenergic effect
on Mueller's muscle, striking lid retraction may be observed;
therefore, patients should not be evaluated for ptosis surgery
or thyroid disease after instillation of phenylephrine eyedrops.
In patients over 50, rebound miosis has been noted 24 hours
after instillation, and the mydriatic response to subsequent
doses is diminished. Subconjunctival hemorrhage has occurred rarely. In animal studies, phenylephrine had a cytotoxic
effect on the endothelium when the corneal epithelium had
been removed; when the epithelium was intact, the damage
was limited to the epithelial cells.

Phenylephrine occasionally may cause systemic reactions
(eg, tachycardia, hypertension, anginal pain, ventricular arrhythmias, myocardial infarction, cardiac arrest, subarachnoid
hemorrhage), particularly when a strong concentration is
instilled repeatedly. Application in a cotton conjunctival pack
should be avoided because of the number of severe systemic
effects that have been reported. Although the incidence of
severe hypertensive responses to 10% phenylephrine eyedrops may be low (Brown et al, 1980), a pronounced increase
in blood pressure may occur in neonates and elderly patients.
Severe nausea and vomiting resulting in dehydration, hyperviscosity, venous thrombosis, and pulmonary embolism were
reported in a diabetic who received the 10% solution.

Adverse cardiovascular effects usually can be avoided by
use of the 2.5% solution (Fraunfelder and Scafidi, 1978; Meyer
and Fraunfelder, 1980). The 10% solution should be used
cautiously, if at all, in patients with hypertension and/or
coronary artery disease and should be avoided in neonates
and elderly patients. Even the 2.5% solution can increase the
blood pressure markedly in preterm infants and patients with
idiopathic orthostatic hypotension.

Monoamine oxidase inhibitors and tricyclic antidepressants
may increase the pressor response to phenylephrine. There is
one report of an adverse cardiovascular reaction to phenylephrine eyedrops that was attributed to an interaction with
propranolol; however, in a controlled study on hypertensive
patients, beta blockade did not enhance the pressor effect of
phenylephrine (Myers, 1984).

See also the section on Adverse Reactions and Precautions
in the Introduction.

DOSAGE AND PREPARATIONS. Phenylephrine solutions are
unstable and should not be exposed to light, heat, or air.
Topical: For ophthalmoscopy, see Table 2. For preoperative
mydriasis, one drop of a 2.5% solution every 15 minutes for
two to four doses.

For postoperative mydriasis after iridectomy, one drop of a
10% solution is instilled once or twice daily. Atropine should be
substituted if inflammation is severe. After cyclodialysis, one
drop of a 10% solution is instilled once daily for three days in
conjunction with miotics.

For use of phenylephrine to supplement atropine or scopolamine, see the evaluations on these drugs.

All preparations available as topical ophthalmic solutions.
Ak-Dilate (Akorn). Solution (sterile) 2.5% and 10% with edetate
disodium and benzalkonium chloride 0.01% in 5 and 15 ml
containers.
Mydfrin (Alcon). Solution (sterile) 2.5% with edetate disodium
and benzalkonium chloride 0.01% in 5 ml containers.
Neo-Synephrine Hydrochloride (Winthrop-Breon). Solution
(sterile) 2.5% with benzalkonium chloride 0.013% in 15 ml
containers; 10% (viscous, nonviscous) with benzalkonium chloride 0.01% in 5 ml containers.
Phenylephrine Hydrochloride (CooperVision). Solution (sterile)
10% with edetate disodium and benzalkonium chloride in 5 ml
containers or with thimerosal 0.01% in 1 ml containers.
Drug also marketed by other manufacturers under generic name:
Solution 10%.

HYDROXYAMPHETAMINE HYDROBROMIDE
[Paredrine]

Hydroxyamphetamine is used to produce mydriasis for
ophthalmoscopy, to localize the lesion in Horner's syndrome,
and occasionally in provocative testing for acute angle-closure
glaucoma. It is a weaker mydriatic than phenylephrine; maximal mydriasis is produced in 45 to 60 minutes and recovery
occurs in about six hours.

See also the section on Adverse Reactions and Precautions
in the Introduction.

DOSAGE AND PREPARATIONS.
Topical: For ophthalmoscopy, see Table 2. To localize the
lesion in Horner's syndrome after baseline pupillary measurements, one drop is instilled in each eye and administration is
repeated in five minutes. Pupillography is repeated 30 minutes
later. The denervated pupil will dilate if the lesion is preganglionic but not if it is postganglionic.
Paredrine (Smith Kline & French). Solution (ophthalmic) 1% with
thimerosal 0.002% in 15 ml containers.

ALPHA-ADRENERGIC BLOCKING AGENT

THYMOXAMINE HYDROCHLORIDE

ACTIONS. This alpha-adrenergic blocking agent (investigational by individual IND only) constricts the pupil by blocking
alpha receptors in the dilator muscle of the iris, thereby
permitting parasympathetic dominance via the sphincter muscle. Since thymoxamine has no effect on the ciliary muscle, it

induces miosis without causing shallowing of the anterior chamber as occurs with cholinergic drugs (Saheb et al, 1980; Susanna et al, 1978).

USES. When applied topically, thymoxamine induces a rapid and sustained reversal of phenylephrine-induced mydriasis and it appears to be safer than pilocarpine for this purpose in eyes with narrow angles (Mapstone, 1977; Saheb et al, 1982). Thymoxamine also may be useful in glaucoma therapy (see Chapter 18) and in the differential diagnosis and treatment of lid retraction (Dixon et al, 1979).

ADVERSE REACTIONS. The 0.5% concentration may cause ocular irritation. Marked chemosis and ptosis have occurred with stronger concentrations.

DOSAGE AND PREPARATIONS.
Topical: For reversing phenylephrine-induced mydriasis, one drop of a 0.5% solution induces significant miosis, which may persist for 24 hours.

Thymoxamine Hydrochloride (Warner Lambert). Solution (ophthalmic) 0.5%. (This drug is not in active clinical trial, but some investigators have received supplies after getting official permission from the FDA and obtaining an IND number.)
(Investigational drug)

Cited References

Apt L, Henrick A: Pupillary dilatation with single eyedrop mydriatic combinations. *Am J Ophthalmol* 89:553-559, 1980.

Brodstein RS, et al: Treatment of myopia with atropine and bifocals: Long-term prospective study. *Ophthalmology* 91:1373-1379, 1984.

Brown C, Hanna C: Use of dilute drug solutions for routine cycloplegia and mydriasis. *Am J Ophthalmol* 86:820-824, 1978.

Brown MM, et al: Lack of side effects from topically administered 10% phenylephrine eyedrops: Controlled study. *Arch Ophthalmol* 98:487-489, 1980.

Chandler PA, et al: Malignant glaucoma: Medical and surgical treatment. *Am J Ophthalmol* 66:495-502, 1968.

Dixon RS, et al: Use of thymoxamine in eyelid retraction. *Arch Ophthalmol* 97:2147-2150, 1979.

Duffin RM, et al: 2.5% v 10% phenylephrine in maintaining mydriasis during cataract surgery. *Arch Ophthalmol* 101:1903-1906, 1983.

Fraunfelder FT, Scafidi AF: Possible adverse effects from topical ocular 10% phenylephrine. *Am J Ophthalmol* 85:447-453, 1978.

Gambill HD, et al: Mydriatic effect of four drugs determined with pupillograph. *Arch Ophthalmol* 77:740-746, 1967.

Gettes BC, Belmont O: Tropicamide: Comparative cycloplegic effects. *Arch Ophthalmol* 66:336-340, 1961.

Hermansen MC, Sullivan LS: Feeding intolerance following ophthalmologic examination. *Am J Dis Child* 139:367-368, 1985.

Hiatt RL, Jerkins G: Comparison of atropine and tropicamide in esotropia. *Ann Ophthalmol* 15:341-343, 1983.

Isenberg S, et al: Comparison of mydriatic eyedrops in low-weight infants. *Ophthalmology* 91:278-279, 1984.

Isenberg SJ, et al: Effects of cyclopentolate eyedrops on gastric secretory function in preterm infants. *Ophthalmology* 92:698-700, 1985.

Keates RH, McGowan KA: Clinical trial of flurbiprofen to maintain pupillary dilation during cataract surgery. *Ann Ophthalmol* 16:919-921, 1984.

Keulen-De Vos HCJ, et al: Effect of indomethacin in preventing surgically induced miosis. *Br J Ophthalmol* 67:94-96, 1983.

Maloney WF, et al: Evaluation of causes and accuracy of pharmacologic localization in Horner's syndrome. *Am J Ophthalmol* 90:394-402, 1980.

Mapstone R: Dilating dangerous pupils. *Br J Ophthalmol* 61:517-524, 1977.

Meyer SM, Fraunfelder FT: Phenylephrine hydrochloride. *Ophthalmology* 87:1177-1180, 1980.

Myers MG: Beta adrenoceptor antagonism and pressor response to phenylephrine. *Clin Pharmacol Ther* 36:57-63, 1984.

Saheb NE, et al: Effect of thymoxamine and pilocarpine on depth of anterior chamber. *Can J Ophthalmol* 15:170-171, 1980.

Saheb NE, et al: Thymoxamine versus pilocarpine in reversal of phenylephrine-induced mydriasis. *Can J Ophthalmol* 17:266-267, 1982.

Shaffer RN: Problems in use of autonomic drugs in ophthalmology, in Leopold IH (ed): *Ocular Therapy: Complications and Management.* St Louis, CV Mosby, 1967, vol 2, 18-23.

Shaffer RN, Hoskins HD: Ciliary block (malignant) glaucoma. *Trans Am Acad Ophthalmol Otolaryngol* 85:215-221, 1978.

Sinclair SH, et al: Mydriatic solution for outpatient indirect ophthalmoscopy. *Arch Ophthalmol* 98:1572-1574, 1980.

Smith RB, et al: Mydriatic effect of phenylephrine. *Eye Ear Nose Throat Mon* 55:133-134, 1976.

Summers WK, Reich TC: Delirium after cataract surgery: Review and two cases. *Am J Psychiatry* 136(4A):386-391, 1979.

Susanna R, et al: Effects of thymoxamine on anterior chamber depth in human eyes. *Can J Ophthalmol* 13:250-251, 1978.

Wand M: Provocative tests in angle-closure glaucoma: Brief review with commentary. *Ophthalmic Surg* 5:32-37, 1974.

Other Selected References

Apt L, Gaffney WL: Toxicity of topical eye medications used in childhood strabismus, in Leopold IH, Burns RP (eds): *Symposium on Ocular Therapy.* New York, John Wiley & Sons, 1976, vol 8, 1-9.

Fraunfelder FT: *Drug-Induced Ocular Side Effects and Drug Interactions,* ed 2. Philadelphia, Lea & Febiger, 1982.

Grant WM: *Toxicology of the Eye,* ed 2. Springfield, Charles C Thomas, 1974.

Kolker AE, Hetherington J Jr: *Becker-Shaffer's Diagnosis and Therapy of the Glaucomas,* ed 5. St Louis, CV Mosby, 1983.

Miscellaneous Ophthalmic Preparations

20

ANTI-INFLAMMATORY AGENTS

LOCAL ANESTHETICS

DYES

ENZYMES

INTRAOCULAR MIOTICS

CHELATING AGENTS

CORNEAL DEHYDRATING AGENTS

IRRIGATING SOLUTIONS

DEMULCENTS

EMOLLIENTS

DECONGESTANTS

ANTIALLERGIC AGENTS

ASTRINGENTS

ANTI-INFLAMMATORY AGENTS

ADRENAL CORTICOSTEROIDS

ACTIONS AND USES. Adrenal corticosteroids are used to control ocular inflammation, reduce scarring, and prevent visual loss. Steroid therapy is useful in ocular allergic disorders (eg, vernal conjunctivitis, contact dermatitis of the lids and conjunctiva, allergic blepharitis), Thygeson's superficial punctate keratopathy, sterile uveal tract inflammation (iritis, iridocyclitis, posterior uveitis), episcleritis, scleritis, temporal arteritis, orbital inflammation associated with Graves' disease, chalazia, and congenital hemangiomas. The efficacy of corticosteroids in optic neuritis has not been clearly established.

Corticosteroids are useful in treating postoperative iridocyclitis, but the benefits of prophylactic use must be weighed against potential adverse effects, ie, delayed wound healing, increased susceptibility to or masking of postoperative infection. Steroids do not significantly reduce the incidence of uveitis or choroidal detachment following retinal detachment surgery, and they do not prevent the increase in intraocular pressure frequently associated with laser trabeculoplasty.

Use of steroids in ocular infections requires concomitant antimicrobial therapy aimed at the specific causative organism. Corticosteroids may weaken ocular defense mechanisms and worsen the course of infectious disease. Exceptions are the local use of corticosteroids in chronic herpes zoster ophthalmicus and epidemic keratoconjunctivitis. Herpes simplex stromal keratitis and uveitis may be treated cautiously with steroids, but an antiviral agent should be used concomitantly to prevent reactivation of the epithelial infection.

ROUTES OF ADMINISTRATION. Topical therapy usually controls inflammations of the lids, conjunctiva, cornea, and anterior sclera. Ophthalmologists also inject solutions or suspensions of corticosteroids by the subconjunctival route to supplement topical therapy in resistant inflammations. For a more prolonged action, the repository form of methylprednisolone or triamcinolone acetonide is used. Intralesional injection of these long-acting steroids has been effective in resolving chalazia and congenital hemangiomas of the lids.

Anterior uveitis sometimes is controlled by steroids applied topically or injected subconjunctivally, but systemic therapy also may be needed. Inflammatory disorders of the posterior segment of the globe (eg, posterior uveitis, scleritis) may require both systemic and periocular (posterior subconjunctival or retrobulbar) administration.

Hydrocortisone, hydrocortisone acetate, dexamethasone, dexamethasone sodium phosphate, fluorometholone, medrysone, prednisolone acetate, and prednisolone sodium phosphate are available as drops or ointment for topical application. Medrysone, hydrocortisone, and low concentrations of prednisolone (0.125%) have mild anti-inflammatory activity, and are useful for treating superficial inflammatory conditions (eg, allergic conjunctivitis). Dexamethasone and its esters and stronger concentrations of prednisolone and its esters readily penetrate the cornea and are preferred for treatment of corneal inflammatory disorders and anterior uveitis. Fluorometholone and fluorometholone acetate (investigational) also may be useful in anterior segment inflammation, but their anti-inflammatory activity in vivo appears to be less than that of dexamethasone or prednisolone.

Many steroid preparations are available only as suspensions, which may be packaged in opaque bottles. Their liquid phases contain corticosteroid at saturation concentrations, but their particulate phases tend to settle with gravity. Therefore, unequal doses may be administered if the patient does not shake the bottle sufficiently (Apt et al, 1979).

Information on corticosteroids used for topical ophthalmic therapy appears in Table 1, and a list of commercially available preparations will be found at the end of this section.

TABLE 1.
TOPICAL OPHTHALMIC CORTICOSTEROIDS

Agent	Concentration[1]
Hydrocortisone	0.5% (ointment)
Hydrocortisone Acetate	0.5% (ointment)
Dexamethasone	0.1% (suspension)
Dexamethasone Sodium Phosphate	0.1% (solution) 0.05% (ointment)
Fluorometholone	0.1% (suspension)
Fluorometholone Acetate[2]	0.1% (suspension)
Medrysone	1% (suspension)
Prednisolone Acetate	0.12% and 1% (suspension)
Prednisolone Sodium Phosphate	0.125%, 0.5%, and 1% (solution) 0.125% and 1% (suspension)

[1]In severe inflammatory conditions, drops are applied every one or two hours until a response is obtained; the frequency is then reduced. Ointments are applied three or four times daily or as night-time medication. The patient should be instructed to shake suspensions vigorously.

[2]Investigational

ADVERSE REACTIONS AND PRECAUTIONS. Topically applied corticosteroids may cause stinging and burning and, occasionally, mydriasis and ptosis. Although the severe adverse reactions associated with systemic therapy occur only rarely, corticosteroid eyedrops are absorbed in amounts sufficient to cause partial adrenal suppression in adults and occasionally Cushing's syndrome in young children.

Corticosteroids should not be used without prior slit-lamp examination of the cornea for evidence of herpes simplex involvement, and long-term use requires periodic re-examination for this purpose. Corticosteroids should be given in the lowest effective concentration, and long-term use should be avoided when possible. Exacerbation of active but controlled inflammation may occur if the corticosteroid is discontinued abruptly; therefore, the interval between applications should be lengthened gradually.

Corticosteroids lower resistance to fungal, bacterial, and some viral infections and, by reducing inflammation, they can mask the warning symptoms of pain and hyperemia. The concomitant use of an antibiotic and the presence of a corneal abrasion may increase susceptibility to fungal infections. If steroids are used to treat stromal herpes simplex of the cornea or herpetic uveitis, an antiviral drug should be given concomitantly to prevent reactivation of the epithelial infection.

Repeated local administration of corticosteroids may increase intraocular pressure. This response has been attributed to a reduction in the facility of outflow of aqueous humor through the trabecular meshwork. The elevation in pressure is not accompanied by pain and is reversible upon discontinuation of the drug; if undetected, it may damage the optic nerve.

The ocular hypertensive response to prolonged administration of corticosteroids is variable and may be genetically determined. In the general population, an insignificant pressure elevation occurs in about 65% of individuals. Marked elevations occur frequently in patients with primary open-angle glaucoma and their relatives, myopes, diabetics, and males with connective tissue disorders. The magnitude of the pressure elevation also depends upon the drug used, the concentration, frequency of administration, and duration of treatment. Dexamethasone and its esters and prednisolone and its esters produce the greatest pressure elevations (Mindel et al, 1979). The pressure elevation produced by fluorometholone 0.1% is one-half that caused by dexamethasone 0.1% but is four times that caused by medrysone 1% (Mindel et al, 1980). A clinically important increase in pressure is rare with medrysone, hydrocortisone 0.5%, or dilute concentrations of more potent steroids, eg, 0.01% dexamethasone (Podos and Becker, 1972).

Intraocular pressure should be measured before initiation of long-term topical therapy and then every two months or more frequently in patients predisposed to a steroid-induced pressure elevation. Particular caution should be observed when using repository corticosteroids in predisposed individuals. Increased intraocular pressure is less common with systemic therapy.

Posterior subcapsular cataracts have developed during long-term corticosteroid therapy. This complication was first noted in patients receiving large systemic doses but also has been associated with topical use. Early lens changes may regress when steroids are discontinued but, if the opacities are more distinct, regression is uncommon and the cataracts may progress. Intraocular inflammation also may cause cataracts, and it is difficult to distinguish those caused by disease from those promoted by therapy.

Corticosteroids may delay wound healing. After cataract surgery, this may result in wound dehiscence and the development of a filtering bleb.

An association has been reported between topical corticosteroid therapy and the development of acute anterior uveitis in individuals (primarily blacks) with no history of pre-existing ocular inflammation or infection. In most cases, the uveitis developed after the steroid was discontinued. No permanent ocular damage was observed.

Topical corticosteroid preparations should be used sparingly in any conditions that cause thinning of the cornea, as perforation may occur.

Retrobulbar injection of repository steroids has rarely caused atrophy of orbital rim fat and delayed hypersensitivity reactions.

PREPARATIONS.
DEXAMETHASONE:
Maxidex Suspension (Alcon). Suspension (sterile) 0.1% with benzalkonium chloride 0.01% in 5 and 15 ml containers.
DEXAMETHASONE SODIUM PHOSPHATE:
Generic. Ointment 0.05% in 3.8 g containers; solution 0.1% in 5 ml containers.
Decadron Phosphate (Merck Sharp & Dohme). Ointment (sterile) 0.05% in 3.5 g containers; solution (sterile) 0.1% with sodium bisulfite 0.1%, phenylethanol 0.25%, and benzalkonium chloride 0.02% in 5 ml containers.
Maxidex Ointment (Alcon). Ointment (sterile) 0.05% (dexamethasone phosphate equivalent) in 3.5 g containers.
FLUOROMETHOLONE:
FML (Allergan). Suspension (sterile) 0.1% with polyvinyl alcohol 1.4%, benzalkonium chloride, and edetate disodium in 5, 10, and 15 ml containers.
HYDROCORTISONE:
Generic. Ointment 0.5% in 3.5 g containers.
HYDROCORTISONE ACETATE:
Generic. Ointment 0.5% in 3.5 g containers.
MEDRYSONE:
HMS (Allergan). Suspension (sterile) 1% with polyvinyl alcohol 1.4%, benzalkonium chloride, and edetate disodium in 5 and 10 ml containers.
PREDNISOLONE ACETATE:
Ak-Tate (Akorn). Suspension (aqueous, sterile) 1% with benzalkonium chloride and edetate disodium in 5, 10, and 15 ml containers.
Econopred, Econopred Plus (Alcon). Suspension (sterile) 0.125% (**Econopred**) or 1% (**Econopred Plus**) with benzalkonium chloride 0.01% in 5 and 10 ml containers.
Pred Mild, Pred Forte (Allergan). Suspension (sterile) 0.12% (**Mild**) or 1% (**Forte**) with benzalkonium chloride in 5 and 10 ml (**Mild**) and 5, 10, and 15 ml (**Forte**) containers.
Predate (Muro). Suspension (sterile) 1% with benzalkonium chloride 0.01% in 5 ml containers.
PREDNISOLONE SODIUM PHOSPHATE:
Ak-Pred (Akorn). Suspension (aqueous, sterile) 0.125% or 1% (equivalent to 0.1% or 0.8% base) with benzalkonium chloride 0.01% in 5 and 15 ml containers.
Inflamase (CooperVision). Solution (sterile) 0.125% (**Mild**) and 1% (**Forte**) (equivalent to 0.1% or 0.8% base) with benzalkonium chloride 0.01% in 5 and 10 ml containers.

Metreton (Schering). Solution (sterile) 0.5% (prednisolone phosphate equivalent) with edetate disodium and benzalkonium chloride 0.02% in 5 ml containers.

STEROID-ANTIBACTERIAL MIXTURES

Mixtures containing a fixed-dose combination of a corticosteroid and one or more antibacterial agents are used by some ophthalmologists to treat conditions in which both may be required, eg, marginal keratitis secondary to staphylococcal infection, allergic conjunctivitis with chronic bacterial conjunctivitis, blepharoconjunctivitis, phlyctenular keratoconjunctivitis, selected cases of postoperative inflammation. These mixtures should not be used to treat conjunctivitis or blepharitis of unknown origin. Corticosteroids reduce resistance to infection and may have an adverse effect if the invading organism is resistant to the antibiotic. See Chapter 73, Topical Antiinfective Agents: Otic and Ophthalmic Preparations.

PREPARATIONS.
CHLORAMPHENICOL AND STEROID:
Chloromycetin Ophthalmic (Parke-Davis). Powder (sterile) containing chloramphenicol 12.5 mg and hydrocortisone acetate 25 mg (preservative free) with 15 ml sterile water for suspension.
CHLORAMPHENICOL, POLYMYXIN B, AND STEROID:
Ophthocort (Parke-Davis). Ointment (sterile) containing chloramphenicol 1%, polymyxin B sulfate 10,000 units/g, and hydrocortisone acetate 0.5% (preservative free) in 3.5 g containers.
NEOMYCIN AND STEROID:
Ak-Neo-Cort (Akorn), **Cor-Oticin** (Maurry). Suspension (aqueous, sterile) containing neomycin sulfate 0.5% (equivalent to 0.35% base) and hydrocortisone acetate 1.5% with chlorobutanol 0.5% in 5 ml containers.
Neo-Cortef Ophthalmic (Upjohn). Ointment (sterile) containing neomycin sulfate 0.5% (equivalent to 0.35% base) and hydrocortisone acetate 0.5% or 1.5% with chlorobutanol 0.65% in 3.5 g containers; suspension (sterile) containing neomycin sulfate 0.5% (equivalent to 0.35% base) and hydrocortisone acetate 0.5% or 1.5% in 2.5 ml (1.5% hydrocortisone acetate only) and 5 ml containers.
NeoDecadron Ophthalmic (Merck Sharp & Dohme). Ointment (sterile) containing neomycin sulfate 0.5% (equivalent to 0.35% base) and dexamethasone sodium phosphate 0.05% (equivalent to dexamethasone phosphate 0.05%) in 3.5 g containers; solution (sterile) containing neomycin sulfate 0.5% (equivalent to 0.35% base) and dexamethasone sodium phosphate (equivalent to dexamethasone phosphate 0.1%) with benzalkonium chloride 0.02% and sodium bisulfite 0.1% in 5 ml containers.
Neo-Delta-Cortef Ophthalmic (Upjohn). Ointment (sterile) containing neomycin sulfate 0.5% (equivalent to 0.35% base) and prednisolone acetate 0.25% or 0.5% with chlorobutanol 0.65% in 3.5 g containers; suspension (sterile) containing neomycin sulfate 0.5% (equivalent to 0.35% base) and prednisolone acetate 0.25% in 5 ml containers.
NEOMYCIN, POLYMYXIN B, BACITRACIN, AND STEROID:
Cortisporin Ophthalmic (Burroughs Wellcome). Ointment (sterile) containing neomycin sulfate 0.5% (equivalent to 0.35% base), polymyxin B sulfate 10,000 units/g, bacitracin zinc 400 units/g, and hydrocortisone 1% in 3.5 g containers; suspension (sterile) containing neomycin sulfate 0.5% (equivalent to 0.35% base), polymyxin B sulfate 10,000 units/ml, and hydrocortisone 1% with thimerosal 0.001% in 7.5 ml containers.
NEOMYCIN, POLYMYXIN B, AND STEROID:
Maxitrol (Alcon). Ointment (sterile) containing neomycin sulfate 0.5% (equivalent to 0.35% base), polymyxin B sulfate 10,000

units/g, and dexamethasone 0.1% with methylparaben 0.05% and propylparaben 0.01% in 3.5 g containers; suspension (sterile) containing neomycin sulfate 0.5% (equivalent to 0.35% base), polymyxin B sulfate 10,000 units/ml, and dexamethasone 0.1% with benzalkonium chloride 0.004% in 5 ml containers.

Poly-Pred Ophthalmic (Allergan). Suspension (sterile) containing neomycin sulfate 0.5% (equivalent to 0.35% base), polymyxin B sulfate 10,000 units/ml, and prednisolone acetate 0.5% with thimerosal 0.001% in 5 ml containers.

SULFACETAMIDE SODIUM AND STEROID:

Ak-Cide (Akorn). Ointment (sterile) containing sulfacetamide sodium 10% and prednisolone acetate 0.05% in 3.5 g containers; suspension (sterile) containing sulfacetamide sodium 10% and prednisolone acetate 0.5% with benzalkonium chloride 0.01% in 5 and 15 ml containers.

Blephamide (Allergan). Suspension (sterile) containing sulfacetamide sodium 10% and prednisolone acetate 0.2% with benzalkonium chloride in 5 and 10 ml containers.

Blephamide S.O.P. (Allergan). Ointment (sterile) containing sulfacetamide sodium 10% and prednisolone acetate 0.2% with phenylmercuric acetate 0.0008% in 3.5 g containers.

Cetapred (Alcon). Ointment (sterile) containing sulfacetamide sodium 10% and prednisolone acetate 0.25% with methylparaben 0.05% and propylparaben 0.01% in 3.5 g containers.

Isopto Cetapred (Alcon). Suspension (sterile) containing sulfacetamide sodium 10% and prednisolone acetate 0.25% with methylparaben 0.05%, propylparaben 0.01%, and benzalkonium chloride 0.025% in 5 and 15 ml containers.

Metimyd (Schering). Ointment (sterile) containing sulfacetamide sodium 10% and prednisolone acetate 0.5% with methylparaben 0.05% and propylparaben 0.01% in 3.5 g containers; suspension (sterile) containing sulfacetamide sodium 10% and prednisolone acetate 0.5% with phenylethyl alcohol 0.5% and benzalkonium chloride 0.025% in 5 ml containers.

Optimyd (Schering). Solution (sterile) containing sulfacetamide sodium 10% and prednisolone sodium phosphate 0.55% (equivalent to prednisolone phosphate 0.5%) with benzalkonium chloride 0.025% and phenylethyl alcohol 0.5% in 5 ml containers.

Sulphrin (Muro). Suspension (sterile) containing sulfacetamide sodium 10% and prednisolone acetate 0.5% with methylparaben 0.05% and propylparaben 0.01% in 5 ml containers.

Vasocidin (CooperVision). Solution (sterile) containing sulfacetamide sodium 10%, prednisolone sodium phosphate 0.25% (equivalent to prednisolone 0.2%), and phenylephrine hydrochloride 0.125% with methylparaben and propylparaben in 5, 10, and 15 ml containers.

NONSTEROIDAL ANTI-INFLAMMATORY DRUGS

Nonsteroidal anti-inflammatory agents are used occasionally to treat ocular inflammatory disorders (Leopold and Murray, 1979; Podos and Sugar, 1980). There has been particular interest in the role of prostaglandins in ocular inflammation and the effect of agents that inhibit their synthesis or release. Aspirin and indomethacin [Indocin], which inhibit prostaglandin synthesis, has been given systemically to treat uveitis, episcleritis, and postsurgical cystoid macular edema, but there are conflicting reports on their efficacy. A recent report suggests that aspirin may be useful as an adjunct in the treatment of vernal conjunctivitis. Systemically administered phenylbutazone [Azolid, Butazolidin] has been reported to be useful in patients with scleritis, episcleritis, and mild anterior uveitis.

Pre- and postoperative administration of indomethacin eyedrops (not available commercially) prevents surgically induced miosis. Topically applied indomethacin also may reduce the short-term risk of cystoid macular edema associated with cataract or retinal detachment surgery, but does not appear to improve long-term prognosis (Jampol, 1982; Kraff et al, 1982; Miyake et al, 1980, 1983; Yannuzzi et al, 1981). Oxyphenbutazone eyedrops have been used abroad in the management of postoperative ocular inflammation, superficial eye injuries, and episcleritis. Newer agents, such as ibuprofen, fenoprofen, and flurbiprofen, have been studied for their effects on ocular inflammation in laboratory animals and limited data suggest that they may be useful clinically.

IMMUNOSUPPRESSIVE AGENTS

Immunosuppressive and antineoplastic agents have been effective in some patients with severe inflammatory disorders refractory to corticosteroids, but toxicity often limits their usefulness (Burns et al, 1976). Results of recent studies suggest that cyclosporine may reduce inflammation and improve visual acuity in some patients with refractory posterior uveitis (Nussenblatt et al, 1983).

LOCAL ANESTHETICS

Agents Used for Surface Anesthesia

COCAINE HYDROCHLORIDE

PROPARACAINE HYDROCHLORIDE
[Ak-Taine, Alcaine, Ophthaine, Ophthetic]

TETRACAINE HYDROCHLORIDE
[Pontocaine]

ACTIONS AND USES. These agents are applied topically to the eye to anesthetize the conjunctiva and cornea. Surface anesthesia alone provides sufficient analgesia for superficial procedures, such as tonometry, gonioscopy, removal of superficial foreign bodies and sutures, conjunctival and corneal scrapings, and lacrimal canalicular manipulation. Topical anesthetics also may be used as adjuncts to locally injected anesthetics for operations on deeper structures.

Topical anesthetics produce adequate corneal anesthesia within one minute after instillation. The duration of anesthesia (which may be increased by repeated application) is approximately 15 minutes with 0.5% proparacaine or 0.5% tetracaine. Cocaine 4% may have a slightly shorter duration of action (Jordan and Baum, 1980), but its vasoconstrictor effect is useful in conjunctival operations. It also may loosen the corneal epithelium more readily than other anesthetics, thus facilitating debridement or total removal of the surface epithelium.

ADVERSE REACTIONS AND PRECAUTIONS. Topical anesthetics cause transient irregularities in the surface of the corneal epithelium that may interfere with visualization of the intraocular structures. Because protective eyelid reflexes are suppressed, the corneal epithelium may become dry. Repeated administration may retard healing and cause pitting and sloughing of the corneal epithelium with formation of a yellow-white ring in the corneal stroma around the original area of disease (Burns et al, 1977). Cocaine may be more toxic in this respect than other topical anesthetics, but all of these agents may damage the cornea.

The patient should be warned not to rub the eye after instillation. Topical anesthetics should not be used repeatedly except under close medical supervision, and they should not be given to the patient for self-medication. Long-term unsupervised use has caused corneal scarring and permanent loss of vision.

Proparacaine causes less local discomfort than the other topical anesthetics, although this varies with the proprietary product. Allergic reactions have been reported most frequently with tetracaine, which may reflect its more widespread use. Allergy to the preservative also may occur occasionally. Single-dose sterile containers without preservative are sometimes preferred (Smith and Everett, 1973) but are expensive.

Cocaine dilates the pupil and has precipitated acute angle closure in predisposed eyes.

The amount of anesthetic absorbed after topical application to the eye is usually not sufficient to cause systemic reactions, but excessive doses can cause central nervous system disturbances.

DOSAGE AND PREPARATIONS.
See Table 2.

Agents Used For Local Injection

BUPIVACAINE HYDROCHLORIDE
[Marcaine]

ETIDOCAINE HYDROCHLORIDE
[Duranest]

LIDOCAINE HYDROCHLORIDE
[Xylocaine]

MEPIVACAINE HYDROCHLORIDE
[Carbocaine]

PROCAINE HYDROCHLORIDE
[Novocain]

ACTIONS AND USES. These agents are injected locally inside the muscle cone (retrobulbar injection) or in the region of the facial nerve (facial nerve akinesia) to reduce pain and to prevent eye and lid movements during surgery. Epinephrine may be added to the solution to reduce systemic absorption and thereby prolong the action and decrease the toxicity of the anesthetic, but it is usually not required when slowly absorbed

TABLE 2.
AGENTS USED FOR SURFACE ANESTHESIA

Drug	Dosage (Topical)	Ophthalmic Preparation
Cocaine Hydrochloride, U.S.P.	One or two drops of 0.5% to 2% solution instilled before procedure.	No pharmaceutical dosage form available; compounding necessary for prescription.
Proparacaine Hydrochloride	One or two drops of 0.5% solution instilled before procedure. For deeper anesthesia, more frequent instillation required.	*Ak-Taine* (Akorn). Solution (sterile) 0.5% with benzalkonium chloride and chlorobutanol in 15 ml containers. *Alcaine* (Alcon). Solution (sterile) 0.5% with glycerin, sodium hydroxide and/or hydrochloric acid, and benzalkonium chloride in 15 ml containers. *Ophthaine* (Squibb). Solution (sterile) 0.5% with glycerin, sodium hydroxide or hydrochloric acid, chlorobutanol, and benzalkonium chloride in 15 ml containers. *Ophthetic* (Allergan). Solution (sterile) 0.5% with glycerin, sodium chloride, and benzalkonium chloride in 15 ml containers.
Tetracaine Hydrochloride	One or two drops of 0.5% solution instilled before the procedure. For deeper anesthesia, two to four instillations required.	*Generic.* Solution 0.5% in 1, 2, and 15 ml containers. *Pontocaine* (Winthrop-Breon). Solution 0.5% with chlorobutanol 0.4% in 15 and 60 ml containers. *Tetracaine Steri-Units* (Alcon). Solution (sterile) 0.5% in 2 ml containers (preservative free).

TABLE 3.
AGENTS USED FOR LOCAL INJECTION

| Drug | Dosage[1] | | | Preparations[4] |
	Facial Nerve Akinesia[2]	Retrobulbar Block[3]	Infiltration Anesthesia	

Procaine Hydrochloride	4 to 10 ml of 1% to 2% solution	2 to 4 ml of 1% to 2% solution	0.25% to 0.5% solution	*Generic.*
				   Solution 1% and 2% (with and without epinephrine).
				Novocain (Winthrop-Breon).
				   Solution 1% and 2%.

Lidocaine Hydrochloride	4 to 10 ml of 1% to 2% solution	2 to 4 ml of 2% or 4% solution	0.5% solution	*Generic.*
				   Solution 1% and 2% (with and without epinephrine).
				Xylocaine Hydrochloride (Astra).
				   Solution 0.5%, 1%, 1.5%, and 2% (with and without epinephrine 1:200,000) and 4% (without epinephrine)

Mepivacaine Hydrochloride	4 to 10 ml of 2% solution	2 to 4 ml of 2% solution	1% to 2% solution	*Carbocaine.* (Winthrop-Breon). Solution 1%, 1.5%, and 2%.
Bupivacaine Hydrochloride	5 to 10 ml of 0.5% solution or 5 to 7 ml of 0.75% solution	2 to 4 ml of 0.75% solution	—	*Marcaine* (Winthrop-Breon). Solution 0.25%, 0.5%, and 0.75% (all with and without epinephrine bitartrate 1:200,000). Solutions without epinephrine may be reautoclaved.
Etidocaine Hydrochloride	5 ml of 1% solution	2 to 4 ml of 1% solution	—	*Duranest* (Astra). Solution 1% (with and without epinephrine); 1.5% (with epinephrine). Solutions without epinephrine may be reautoclaved.

[1]*Epinephrine (1:200,000) may be added to prolong the action of the anesthetic. Hyaluronidase may be added to increase diffusion of the anesthetic.*

[2]*Solution is injected in region of terminal branches of facial nerve or around the proximal trunk of the nerve.*

[3]*Solution is injected inside the muscle cone behind the globe. Low pressure may be applied to the eye intermittently for three to five minutes after the injection. Some ophthalmologists combine two different anesthetics for retrobulbar block (eg, 2 ml lidocaine and 2 ml bupivacaine).*

[4]*For complete product information, see Chapter 15, Local Anesthetics.*

agents, such as mepivacaine and bupivacaine, are employed. Hyaluronidase [Wydase] enhances diffusion of the anesthetic into the tissues (see the evaluation).

Procaine, lidocaine, and mepivacaine also are used to block nerve endings in the immediate area of surgery (infiltration anesthesia) for procedures such as minor lid surgery. Subconjunctival infiltration anesthesia is sometimes employed prior to intraocular surgery or some operations on the surface of the eye (eg, pterygium).

Because it is metabolized rapidly, procaine has a short duration of action and is relatively safe. Lidocaine diffuses more readily than procaine and is more potent, longer acting, and more toxic on a milligram-for-milligram basis. In a comparative study, the duration of near maximal akinesia of the extraocular muscles was measured following retrobulbar block with procaine 4% or lidocaine 4%, each administered with epinephrine (Russell and Guyton, 1954). The mean duration of action of procaine was 40 minutes and of lidocaine, 90 minutes. The duration of akinesia was reduced, however, when hyaluronidase was added to the solution (procaine, 30 minutes; lidocaine, 60 minutes).

Mepivacaine is similar to lidocaine in potency and toxicity, but it may have a longer action. Bupivacaine, which is related structurally to mepivacaine, has the longest duration of action but time to onset of action is variable. When compared to 2% lidocaine, bupivacaine (0.75% solution with epinephrine and/or hyaluronidase) had a slower onset of action but the duration of akinesia was considerably longer (11 hours versus 4 hours) and analgesia was also more prolonged (Chin and Almquist, 1983). Etidocaine also has a long duration of action (Ellingsson and Aasved, 1979). Etidocaine exhibits frequency dependency, ie, motor neurons, which fire more frequently than sensory neurons, tend to take up the anesthetic more rapidly. For this reason, the duration of akinesia is often longer than the duration of anesthesia.

ADVERSE REACTIONS AND PRECAUTIONS. Allergic reactions are less common with the amide group of local anesthetics (lidocaine, mepivacaine, bupivacaine, etidocaine) than with the ester group (procaine). Transient pain may follow the injection of bupivacaine. Occlusion of the central retinal artery has occurred following retrobulbar injection of anesthetics.

Locally injected anesthetics can cause convulsions, respiratory and cardiac arrest, and other severe systemic reactions if excessive amounts are absorbed or if the anesthetic is given intravenously (see Chapter 15, Local Anesthetics). Respiratory arrest, without accompanying convulsions or cardiovascular collapse, occurred following retrobulbar injection of bupivacaine (Smith, 1981). This reaction was attributed to brain stem anesthesia caused by local anesthetic gaining access to the subarachnoid space (Chang et al, 1984). Systemic reactions (eg, tachycardia, hypertension) also may occur if sufficient quantities of epinephrine are absorbed. The blood catecholamine levels produced by fear or pain can exceed those produced by the anesthetic solution.

See also Ellis, 1976, and Smith and Everett, 1973.

DOSAGE AND PREPARATIONS.
See Table 3.

DYES

FLUORESCEIN SODIUM

ACTIONS AND USES. Fluorescein is an indicator dye that appears yellow-green in normal tear film and bright green in a more alkaline medium, such as the aqueous humor. Fluorescence is activated by blue and ultraviolet light.

Fluorescein is applied topically to detect corneal epithelial defects. Because it makes the tear fluid visible, this dye is used to fit hard contact lenses and to delineate the margins of the applanated area in applanation tonometry. Since the intensity of green fluorescence increases when the dye is in contact with aqueous humor, fluorescein is useful for locating the site of a wound leak (eg, in patients with a persistent flat anterior chamber after cataract surgery). It also is instilled in the eye to test lacrimal patency; if drainage is normal, the dye will appear in the nasal secretions.

The usual fluorescein products should not be used to fit soft contact lenses, because the lens will absorb the dye. Fluorexon [Fluorosoft] is available for use with soft contact lenses having less than 60% water content. This solution can be removed by repeated rinsing with physiologic saline.

A nondiagnostic use of topical fluorescein is for irrigation of the eye after injury by an indelible pencil. The aniline dyes in these pencils cause edema and necrosis of ocular tissue that may result in loss of vision unless detoxified.

Fluorescein is given intravenously as an aid in retinal angioscopy and angiography. It is used to evaluate diabetic retinopathy and to detect occlusion or obliteration of retinal vessels, vascular malformations, neovascularization, changes in vascular permeability, ocular tumors, defects in the retinal pigment epithelium, and abnormalities of the iris vasculature (iris angiography). Intravenous administration or multiple topical applications may be used to study aqueous humor flow rate. Measurement of the arm-to-retina circulation time is employed for diagnosis of carotid artery occlusion. Fluorescein may also be given orally to investigate retinal conditions in which the normal barriers to leakage of fluids are disrupted, such as cystoid macular edema (Kelley and Kincaid, 1979).

ADVERSE REACTIONS AND PRECAUTIONS. Preservatives with positive charges are inactivated by the negatively charged fluorescein molecule. Contaminated fluorescein solutions have been a source of ocular infections, particularly by *Pseudomonas* organisms. Sterile, single-dose containers and individually packaged filter-paper strips impregnated with fluorescein are safer than multiple-dose containers. Fluress, a fluorescein-benoxinate mixture for topical use, has rarely caused grand mal seizures.

Nausea and vomiting occur occasionally when fluorescein is given intravenously. Pruritus, urticaria, paresthesias, dizziness, and syncope also have been reported. Anaphylactic reactions have occurred only rarely, but facilities to treat these reactions should be available (Stein and Parker, 1971). Acute pulmonary edema, myocardial infarction, and cardiac arrest are also uncommon complications of intravenous fluorescein.

DOSAGE AND PREPARATIONS.
Topical: To detect epithelial defects, a fluorescein strip moistened with ophthalmic irrigating solution is used to touch the conjunctiva, or one drop of a 0.5% to 2% solution is placed in the conjunctival sac. To provide contrast between the lesion and surrounding areas, excess dye may be removed by use of an irrigating solution.

To fit hard contact lenses, with the contact lens in place, a fluorescein strip moistened with ophthalmic irrigating solution is lightly touched to the superior conjunctiva or one drop of a 2% solution is applied. The patient should be instructed to blink several times to circulate the dye. Under blue light, areas that lack fluorescein-stained tears appear black, indicating that the contact lens is touching the cornea at those points.

In applanation tonometry, following topical anesthesia, one drop of a 0.25% solution or a fluorescein strip moistened with ophthalmic irrigating solution is applied to the eye immediately before tonometry. Combination products containing benoxinate or proparacaine and fluorescein may be used for simultaneous staining and local anesthesia. Tetracaine generally should be avoided because it may reduce the intensity of fluorescence.

To test lacrimal patency, one drop of a 2% solution is instilled in the conjunctival sac. The patient should be instructed to blink at least four times after the dye is instilled. After six minutes, nasal secretions are examined under blue light; the presence of traces of the dye indicates that the nasolacrimal drainage system is open. In a modification of this procedure (Hecht, 1978), one drop of the 2% solution is instilled three times at 15-minute intervals. One minute after instillation of the third drop, the patient is instructed to place his head downward at a 45° angle to prevent posterior loss of the dye and to avoid sniffing back the fluid. The nasal secretions are then examined after 10 minutes.

To test for aqueous leak following ocular surgery, one drop

of a 2% solution is instilled in the affected eye. Gentle pressure on the globe may be necessary to determine the site of the leak.

As an antidote to poisoning by aniline dyes, following removal of the pencil point, the eye is irrigated with a 2% solution every 10 minutes until a visible precipitate no longer forms. Irrigation is then repeated every 30 minutes for 12 to 24 hours.

All preparations available in ophthalmic forms.

Generic. Solution 2% in 1 and 15 ml containers.

Ful-Glo (Barnes-Hind). Sterile applicators impregnated with fluorescein sodium 0.6 mg/strip in boxes containing 300 individual strips.

Fluor-I-Strip (Ayerst). Sterile applicators impregnated with fluorescein sodium 9 mg/strip (lint free) with chlorobutanol 0.5% in individual envelopes in boxes containing 200 envelopes.

Fluor-I-Strip A.T. (Ayerst). Sterile applicators impregnated with fluorescein sodium 1 mg/strip (lint free) with chlorobutanol 0.5% in boxes containing 100 envelopes (2 strips/envelope).

Fluorescein Sodium Steri-Units (Alcon). Solution (sterile) 2% with phenylmercuric nitrate 0.04% in 2 ml containers.

Available Mixtures.

Fluoracaine (Akorn). Solution (sterile) containing fluorescein sodium 0.25% and proparacaine hydrochloride 0.5% with thimerosal 0.01% in 5 ml containers.

Fluress (Barnes-Hind). Solution (sterile) containing fluorescein sodium 0.25% and benoxinate hydrochloride 0.4% with chlorobutanol 1% in 5 ml containers.

Product Used for Fitting Soft Contact Lenses With Water Content <60%:

FLUOREXON:

Fluoresoft (Holles Laboratories). Solution (sterile, without preservatives) 0.35% in 0.5 ml containers.

Intravenous: Adults, 500 mg (10 ml of a 5% solution or 5 ml of a 10% solution) is injected rapidly into an arm vein. Some investigators believe that better visualization can be attained with 3 ml of a 25% solution (750 mg). The dye should appear in the central retinal artery in 9 to 15 seconds.

Fluorescite (Alcon). Solution (sterile) 5% in 10 ml containers, 10% in 5 ml containers, 10% in 5 and 10 ml containers, and 25% in 2 ml containers.

Funduscein (CooperVision). Solution 10% in 5 ml containers and 25% in 3 ml containers.

ROSE BENGAL

Rose bengal is a vital stain that does not stain the precorneal tear film but has a particular affinity for devitalized or abraded corneal and conjunctival epithelium. When viewed under the slit-lamp, the stain consists of rose-colored dots; if inflammation or hemorrhage interferes with visibility, a green filter will give the stain a purplish blue cast. Rose bengal is used to determine the extent of epithelial damage in various conjunctival or corneal disorders. It is particularly useful for diagnosis of keratoconjunctivitis sicca (Laibson, 1980; Lamberts, 1983) and for the fine differentiation of the margin of corneal ulcers, especially those caused by herpes simplex virus.

Although rose bengal is more irritating to the eye than fluorescein, a local anesthetic is generally not necessary if small amounts are used. Rose bengal discolors the lids and surrounding facial area for several days when the undiluted 1% solution is applied in the form of eyedrops.

DOSAGE AND PREPARATIONS.

Topical: Ocular irritation and staining of the lids and surrounding facial area can be minimized by placing a drop of the 1% solution on the stick end of a cotton-tipped applicator, which permits application of about one-fourth of a normal drop. Alternatively, the 1% solution may be diluted and then instilled in drop form or ophthalmic strips impregnated with rose bengal may be used.

Rose Bengal (Akorn). Solution (ophthalmic, sterile) 1% with thimerosal 0.01% in 5 ml containers.

Rose Bengal Ophthalmic Strips (Barnes-Hind). Sterile strips impregnated with 1.3 mg in packages containing 100 strips.

ENZYMES

CHYMOTRYPSIN

[Alpha Chymar, Catarase, Zolyse]

ACTIONS AND USES. Chymotrypsin is a proteolytic enzyme used to dissolve the zonules of the lens (zonulysis) during intracapsular cataract extraction. It is introduced behind the iris into the posterior chamber where it dissolves the zonular fibers within two to four minutes.

ADVERSE REACTIONS AND PRECAUTIONS. A transient increase in intraocular pressure is a common untoward effect of chymotrypsin; if the pressure is very high, ocular pain and corneal edema may occur. Enzyme-induced glaucoma may persist for a week. The cause is unknown but may involve the accumulation of zonular fragments in the trabecular meshwork or a toxic effect on the trabecular meshwork and ciliary body. The use of chymotrypsin also has been associated with wound disruption and loss of the anterior chamber. These complications apparently result from the enzyme-induced glaucoma; the incidence can be reduced by use of multiple corneoscleral sutures and postoperative administration of a topical beta blocker and a systemic carbonic anhydrase inhibitor.

Chymotrypsin is extremely toxic to the retina and should not be allowed to penetrate into the vitreous. In patients with fluid vitreous, enzymatic zonulysis can result in loss of the lens posteriorly and, possibly, entry of chymotrypsin into the vitreous body. Uveitis also has been observed. Systemic reactions have not been reported.

DOSAGE AND PREPARATIONS. The anterior chamber should be free of unclotted blood, because blood rapidly inactivates the enzyme.

Intraocular: 0.2 to 0.5 ml of a freshly prepared 1:5,000 to 1:10,000 solution is injected slowly behind the iris into the posterior chamber. A second application of chymotrypsin may be required if the zonules are resistant.

> *Alpha Chymar* (Barnes-Hind). Powder (lyophilized, for solution) 750 units with 10 ml of diluent.
>
> *Catarase* (two strengths) (CooperVision). Two-compartment vial containing lyophilized chymotrypsin 150 or 300 units in the lower compartment and sodium chloride injection 2 ml in the upper compartment.
>
> *Zolyse* (Alcon). Powder (lyophilized, for solution) 750 units with 9 ml of diluent.

HYALURONIDASE
[Wydase]

ACTIONS AND USES. Hyaluronidase is an enzyme that hydrolyzes hyaluronic acid, a polysaccharide found in interstitial spaces of tissues where it blocks invasive substances. Hyaluronidase is used during ophthalmic surgical procedures to enhance diffusion of locally injected anesthetics by increasing tissue permeability. When hyaluronidase is added to the injection solution, the time required for induction of complete akinesia is reduced (Mindel, 1978) and anesthesia is enhanced. Hyaluronidase may increase the rate of absorption of the anesthetic and thus reduce its duration of action, but this problem can usually be avoided if epinephrine is added to the injection solution (Ellis, 1976).

ADVERSE REACTIONS AND PRECAUTIONS. Adverse reactions are rare. Local irritation and allergic reactions have been reported. Subconjunctival injection may cause transient myopia and astigmatism that resolves within a few weeks. An association between use of hyaluronidase and development of cystoid macular edema has been suggested.

DOSAGE AND PREPARATIONS.

Injection: 150 units are added to each 10 ml of anesthetic solution.

> *Wydase* (Wyeth). Powder (lyophilized) 150 and 1,500 units with lactose and thimerosal; solution (stabilized) 150 units/ml with edetate disodium and thimerosal in sterile sodium chloride injection in 1 and 10 ml containers.

SODIUM HYALURONATE
[Healon]

ACTIONS AND USES. Sodium hyaluronate is the sodium salt of hyaluronic acid. A highly purified fraction of this naturally occurring substance is available as a 1% transparent, noninflammatory, viscoelastic solution for use as an aid in ophthalmic surgery.

Cataract Surgery-Intraocular Lens Implant: When placed in the anterior chamber prior to lens extraction, sodium hyaluronate reduces endothelial cell loss and serves to maintain the anterior chamber (Pape and Balazs, 1980). During extracapsular cataract extraction, it may help prevent rupture of the posterior capsule. Sodium hyaluronate is particularly useful to protect the corneal endothelium during primary or secondary implantation of an intraocular lens (Miller and Stegmann, 1981, 1982; Polack et al, 1981).

Filtering Operations for Glaucoma: In conjunction with trabeculectomy, injection of sodium hyaluronate into the anterior chamber and subconjunctival space may deepen the anterior chamber and promote formation of a superior filtration bleb (Pape and Balazs, 1980).

Keratoplasty: When placed in the anterior chamber after removal of the corneal button, sodium hyaluronate facilitates graft suturing and protects the donor graft (Pape and Balazs, 1980; Polack et al, 1981).

Vitrectomy and Retinal Detachment Surgery: Sodium hyaluronate also has been injected into the vitreous cavity to flatten the retina and thus facilitate retinal detachment surgery (Stenkula et al, 1981).

ADVERSE REACTIONS AND PRECAUTIONS. The intraocular pressure should be carefully monitored during the first 24 hours after use of sodium hyaluronate in anterior segment surgery, because an increase in pressure may occur (Pape, 1980). If a significant elevation occurs, a carbonic anhydrase inhibitor and/or a topical beta blocker should be given until the intracameral sodium hyaluronate is diluted by newly formed aqueous (Pape and Balazs, 1980). Replacement of sodium hyaluronate by balanced salt solution or physiologic saline at the end of the operation may minimize the increase in pressure (Miller and Stegmann, 1981; Pape, 1980).

Increased intraocular pressure has also been reported after injection of large amounts of sodium hyaluronate for posterior segment surgery; this complication is most common in aphakic diabetics.

Rarely, iritis, hypopyon, corneal edema, and corneal decompensation have been reported postoperatively. Their relationship to sodium hyaluronate has not been established.

DOSAGE AND PREPARATIONS.

Intracameral: For cataract surgery-intraocular lens implant, a sufficient amount is introduced slowly and carefully into the anterior chamber (using a cannula or needle) before or after delivery of the lens. Injection prior to lens delivery is preferred to protect the corneal endothelium during surgery. Additional amounts may be added to replace any that is lost during surgery. Sodium hyaluronate also may be used to coat intraocular lenses and surgical instruments.

For glaucoma surgery, in conjunction with trabeculectomy, a sufficient amount of sodium hyaluronate is injected slowly and carefully through a corneal paracentesis to reconstitute the anterior chamber. Additional amounts may be injected to permit the preparation to extrude into the subconjunctival filtration site through and around the sutured outer scleral flap.

For corneal graft surgery, after removal of the corneal button, the anterior chamber is filled with sodium hyaluronate, the donor graft is then placed on top of the preparation and sutured in place. Additional amounts may be injected to replace any lost during the procedure.

> *Healon* (Pharmacia). Solution (sterile, ophthalmic) 10 mg/ml with sodium chloride 8.5 mg, disodium hydrogen phosphate dihydrate, 0.28 mg, and sodium dihydrogen phosphate 0.04 mg in 0.4, 0.75, and 2 ml containers.

INTRAOCULAR MIOTICS

ACETYLCHOLINE CHLORIDE
[Miochol]

$$CH_3COCH_2CH_2\overset{+}{N}-CH_3 \quad Cl^-$$

ACTIONS AND USES. Acetylcholine is the neurohumoral transmitter at numerous sites in the nervous system, including the neuroeffector junction of the iris sphincter muscle. When applied topically to the eye, acetylcholine is of no therapeutic value because of poor corneal penetration and rapid hydrolysis by acetylcholinesterase. However, it produces prompt, pronounced miosis when introduced into the anterior chamber and is useful during certain surgical procedures on the anterior segment of the eye.

Acetylcholine is commonly used to produce miosis during cataract surgery. By increasing the iris surface, it helps protect the vitreous face and facilitates placement of sutures. It also may prevent formation of peripheral anterior synechiae. Acetylcholine is particularly useful during implantation of an intraocular lens to prevent subluxation of the implant into the anterior chamber.

During peripheral iridectomy, acetylcholine may be introduced into the anterior chamber to permit excision of only peripheral iris tissue and to aid in repositing of the iris. It also is used during penetrating keratoplasty to facilitate suturing of the graft, to protect the lens, and to prevent incarceration of the iris (Rizzuti, 1967).

Acetylcholine has a shorter duration of action than other miotics, which is an advantage during ocular surgery, because prolonged miosis can cause severe postoperative pain or predispose to pupillary block. If miosis is desired postoperatively, a longer acting miotic (ie, carbachol, pilocarpine) must be instilled.

ADVERSE REACTIONS AND PRECAUTIONS. Because it is rapidly inactivated, acetylcholine seldom produces adverse effects. Systemic reactions (hypotension, bradycardia, flushing, sweating, and dyspnea) occur rarely. The bradycardia should be treated with intravenous atropine. Bronchospasm has been reported following intraocular administration of acetylcholine to a patient who was taking a beta blocker (Rasch et al, 1983).

No local toxic effects produced by acetylcholine itself have been reported; however, the hypertonic solution may cause transient lens opacities. Serious ocular complications (corneal edema, intraocular inflammation, opacity of the anterior lens capsule, retinal toxicity, and optic atrophy) have occurred when acetylcholine was gas sterilized, because the ethylene oxide used in the process enters through or around the rubber stopper of the two-compartment vial and reacts chemically with the water and/or chloride ion in the pharmaceutical product. Ethylene glycol and/or ethylene chlorhydrin may form, and both are highly toxic to the eye.

DOSAGE AND PREPARATIONS.
Intracameral: 0.5 to 2 ml of a freshly prepared 1:100 solution is instilled into the anterior chamber.
  Miochol (CooperVision). Two-compartment vial containing lyophilized acetylcholine chloride 20 mg and mannitol 60 mg in the lower compartment and sterile water 2 ml in the upper compartment.

CARBACHOL
[Miostat]

$$H_2NCOCH_2CH_2\overset{+}{N}-CH_3 \quad Cl^-$$

ACTIONS AND USES. This parasympathomimetic agent may be preferred to acetylcholine during ocular surgery when more prolonged miosis is desired. In contrast to the transient effect of acetylcholine, the miosis induced by carbachol is still evident 15 hours after intracameral injection. Carbachol has not been used as extensively as acetylcholine, but the two drugs are equally effective in producing prompt, complete miosis after cataract extraction (Beasley, 1971). An advantage of carbachol is its stability in solution; unlike acetylcholine, it need not be freshly prepared prior to instillation.

ADVERSE REACTIONS AND PRECAUTIONS. Corneal edema may occur if excessive amounts of carbachol are introduced into the anterior chamber or if the drug is used in patients with an already compromised endothelium, eg, Fuchs' dystrophy, corneal transplants, cataract surgery that requires more manipulation than usual (Fraunfelder, 1980).

DOSAGE AND PREPARATIONS.
Intracameral: 0.4 to 0.5 ml of a 0.01% solution is instilled into the anterior chamber.
  Miostat (Alcon). Solution (sterile, for intraocular use) 0.01% in 1.5 ml containers.

CHELATING AGENTS

DEFEROXAMINE MESYLATE
[Desferal]

$$\overset{+}{H_3N}(CH_2)_5\overset{O}{NC}(CH_2)_2CNH(CH_2)_5\overset{O}{NC}(CH_2)_2CNH(CH_2)_5\overset{O}{NCCH_3} \quad CH_3SO_3^-$$

ACTIONS AND USES. This chelating agent may be applied locally to the eye to treat ocular siderosis involving the cornea. It is given topically to remove superficial iron deposits and subconjunctivally for deposits in the stroma or iris.

ADVERSE REACTIONS AND PRECAUTIONS. Hyperemia and allergic reactions have been reported after local use.

DOSAGE AND PREPARATIONS.
Topical: A 10% solution of deferoxamine in 1% methylcellulose is applied four times daily for several weeks, or a 5% concentration in an ointment base is given.

Subconjunctival: 0.5 ml of a 10% solution is injected twice weekly for eight to ten weeks.

Desferal (CIBA). Powder (lyophilized, sterile) 500 mg.

EDETATE DISODIUM (EDTA)
[Chealamide, Endrate]

ACTIONS AND USES. This chelating agent is applied topically to remove corneal calcium deposits that impair vision or cause pain. It dissolves calcium deposits of endogenous origin (eg, band keratopathy and other calcific corneal deposits associated with chronic uveitis, advanced interstitial keratitis, hypercalcemia). Edetate disodium also is useful for emergency management and subsequent treatment of calcium hydroxide burns of the eye (Grant, 1952) and has been suggested for decontaminating the eye after injury by zinc chloride (Johnstone et al, 1973).

Edetate disodium extracts calcium from the conjunctiva, corneal epithelium, and anterior layers of the stroma but does not affect deposits in the deep stroma. The removal of superficial calcium deposits should improve vision unless scarring and vascularization have occurred; however, calcium deposits of endogenous origin tend to recur. Edetate disodium does not penetrate the corneal epithelium. Unless the deposit extends to the surface, the epithelium must be removed completely before application.

ADVERSE REACTIONS AND PRECAUTIONS. Edetate disodium is well tolerated when applied topically. Transient stinging and chemosis may occur. The stronger concentration (1.85%) may cause stromal edema.

DOSAGE AND PREPARATIONS.
Topical: For removal of exogenous or endogenous calcium deposits from the anterior layers of the stroma, a local anesthetic should be instilled before the procedure; cocaine is often preferred because it facilitates epithelial removal. The corneal epithelium is then completely removed and the denuded area is irrigated with edetate disodium (0.35% to 1.85% solution) for 15 to 20 minutes. The solution is applied as a corneal bath, by continuous irrigation, or by application of a pledget soaked in the solution to the cornea. After the procedure, the eye should be irrigated with sodium chloride injection or a balanced salt solution.

For emergency treatment of calcium hydroxide burns, the eye should first be flushed with water as quickly as possible and then irrigated with a 0.35% to 1.85% solution of edetate disodium for 15 minutes.

For emergency treatment of zinc chloride injury, after flushing with water, the eye may be irrigated with a 1.7% solution for 15 minutes. Treatment may be ineffective if not begun within two minutes after injury.

No ophthalmic preparation is available. The intravenous solution must be diluted to the desired concentration with isotonic sodium chloride injection.

Chealamide (Vortech), **Endrate** (Abbott), **Generic.** Solution (injection) 150 mg/ml in 20 ml containers.

CORNEAL DEHYDRATING AGENTS

ANHYDROUS GLYCERIN
[Ophthalgan]

HYPERTONIC SODIUM CHLORIDE
[Adsorbonac, Hypersal, Muro-128]

ACTIONS AND USES. These dehydrating agents are applied topically to reduce corneal edema. They act by rendering the precorneal tear film hypertonic, thereby extracting water from the corneal epithelium. Hypertonic agents are effective in the short- and long-term treatment of epithelial edema to clear the cornea and improve visual acuity. Topical osmotherapy extracts only a small volume of stromal fluid and does not reduce stromal edema. Hypertonic agents also do not improve visual acuity if scarring of the epithelium or stroma has occurred (Dohlman, 1983).

Glycerin is used prior to ophthalmoscopy or gonioscopy when the cornea is too edematous to permit diagnosis. It is very effective as a dehydrating agent, but instillation is painful and long-term therapy is not well tolerated.

Hypertonic sodium chloride is used for prolonged treatment of epithelial edema associated with cataract extraction, corneal transplantation, trauma, or recurrent corneal erosions. When treating bullous keratopathy in patients with corneal edema of long duration, best results may be obtained when the patient is also fitted with a hydrophilic soft contact lens (Gasset and Kaufman, 1971). The lens usually relieves pain, may improve corneal pathology, and occasionally improves visual acuity. The lens must be sterilized carefully to prevent infection, particularly when epithelial disease is present. See also *Federal Register*, 1980.

ADVERSE REACTIONS AND PRECAUTIONS. Topical osmotic agents may cause transient stinging and burning. Glycerin causes more local discomfort than sodium chloride.

DOSAGE AND PREPARATIONS.
ANHYDROUS GLYCERIN:
Topical: To facilitate diagnosis, one to three drops are instilled prior to the examination. A topical anesthetic should be instilled before glycerin is applied.

Ophthalgan (Ayerst). Solution (ophthalmic, sterile) with chlorobutanol 0.55% in 7.5 ml containers.
HYPERTONIC SODIUM CHLORIDE:
Topical: For treatment of corneal edema, one or two drops of the solution are instilled every three or four hours or as needed and the ointment may be applied at bedtime. In patients with bullous keratopathy, topical osmotherapy should be avoided if the eye is painful. After pain has subsided, one or two drops of the 5% solution are instilled as needed to control edema. (When used with a hydrophilic soft contact lens, the solution is

preferred to the ointment because the latter may become trapped in the lens-cornea interface and interfere with vision.) The frequency of administration may be reduced or the drug discontinued as edema subsides.

All preparations available in topical ophthalmic form.

Adsorbonac (Alcon). Solution (sterile) 2% and 5% with thimerosal 0.004% and edetate disodium 0.1% in 15 ml containers (nonprescription).

Hypersal (Barnes-Hind). Solution (sterile) 5% with benzalkonium chloride 0.005% and edetate disodium 0.02% in 15 ml containers.

Muro-128 (Muro). Ointment (sterile) 5% in 3.5 g containers; solution (sterile) 5% with methylparaben 0.023% and propylparaben 0.01% in 15 and 30 ml containers (nonprescription).

IRRIGATING SOLUTIONS

Internal Irrigating Solutions: These preparations are administered during ocular surgery to irrigate the anterior chamber, extraocular muscles, or lacrimal system; to wash out portions of the lens during cataract surgery; to irrigate the eye during vitrectomy; and to moisten the cornea. Irrigating solutions may differ in their ability to preserve corneal endothelial structure and function and to maintain lens clarity. In corneal perfusion studies, glutathione-bicarbonate-Ringer's solution [BSS Plus] was more effective than lactated Ringer's solution in maintaining corneal thickness and endothelial structure (Edelhauser et al, 1978). BSS Plus caused less corneal swelling than lactated Ringer's on the first day after pars plana vitrectomy in diabetic patients, but, by the seventh postoperative day, there was no significant difference between the two solutions (Benson et al, 1981).

BSS (Alcon). Solution (sterile) containing sodium chloride 0.49%, potassium chloride 0.075%, calcium chloride 0.048%, magnesium chloride 0.03%, sodium acetate 0.39%, sodium citrate 0.17%, and sodium hydroxide and/or hydrochloric acid in 15 ml containers and with sodium chloride 0.64% in 15, 250, and 500 ml containers.

BSS Plus (Alcon). Two-container preparation: (Part I) Solution (sterile) containing sodium chloride 7.44 mg, potassium chloride 0.395 mg, dried sodium phosphate 0.433 mg, sodium bicarbonate 2.19 mg/ml, and sodium hydroxide and/or hydrochloric acid to be reconstituted with (Part II) solution (sterile) containing calcium chloride dihydrate 3.85 mg, magnesium chloride hexahydrate 5 mg, dextrose 23 mg, and glutathione disulfide 4.6 mg/ml.

External Irrigating Solutions: These solutions are used for flushing the eye to remove foreign bodies, air pollutants, chemicals, and gases and for irrigation after diagnostic procedures. The boric acid present in some preparations may form an insoluble complex with the polyvinyl alcohol contained in some contact lens wetting solutions.

All preparations available in topical ophthalmic forms.

Ak-Rinse (Akorn). Solution (sterile) containing sodium chloride 0.49%, potassium chloride 0.075%, calcium chloride 0.048%, magnesium chloride 0.03%, sodium acetate 0.39%, sodium citrate 0.17%, and benzalkonium chloride 0.013% in 118 ml containers (nonprescription).

Collyrium (Wyeth). Solution containing boric acid, sodium borate, thimerosal 0.002%, and antipyrine 0.4% in 180 ml containers (nonprescription).

Dacriose (CooperVision). Solution (sterile) containing sodium chloride, potassium chloride, sodium phosphate, sodium hydroxide, benzalkonium chloride, and edetate disodium in 15, 30, and 120 ml containers (nonprescription).

Eye-Stream (Alcon). Each milliliter contains a balanced salt solution of sodium chloride 0.49%, potassium chloride 0.075%, calcium chloride 0.48%, magnesium chloride 0.03%, sodium acetate 0.39%, sodium citrate 0.17%, sodium hydroxide and/or hydrochloric acid, purified water, and benzalkonium chloride 0.013% (nonprescription).

Neo-Flo (American Optical). Solution (sterile) containing boric acid, sodium chloride, potassium chloride, sodium carbonate, and benzalkonium chloride 1:15,000 in 112 ml containers (nonprescription).

DEMULCENTS

ACTIONS AND USES. Ocular demulcents (artificial tears) are used to prevent corneal damage and alleviate symptoms in patients with keratoconjunctivitis sicca, neuroparalytic keratitis, exposure keratopathy, and other dry-eye syndromes. They also are used in normal eyes for temporary relief of discomfort and dryness caused by exposure to irritants, wind, or sun. These preparations contain water-soluble polymers (usually cellulose esters or polyvinyl alcohol) that act as a substitute for natural tears. They increase the thickness of the precorneal tear film, possibly by dragging water with them as they spread over the ocular surface with each blink (Benedetto et al, 1975).

The comfort of an artificial tear preparation is influenced by various factors, including pH, tonicity, and preservative, and the choice of the best preparation for an individual patient should be determined by trial and error (Laibson, 1980).

Formulations containing higher concentrations of cellulose esters are more viscous than those containing polyvinyl alcohol, but retention times are comparable. Preparations reported to be mucomimetic (eg, Adsorbotear, Tears Naturale) may be retained longer and have been suggested for use in mucus-deficient dry-eye conditions, such as ocular pemphigoid (Lemp et al, 1975). Some patients with keratoconjunctivitis sicca prefer a hypotonic solution [Hypotears], which may help to balance the hyperosmolarity of tears found in these patients (Gilbard et al, 1978). A dilute 0.1% solution of sodium hyaluronate also may be useful.

Patients who require frequent administration of artificial tear solutions may benefit from Lacrisert. This timed-release ocular insert consists of a water-soluble hydroxypropylcellulose pellet that is placed in the lower conjunctival cul-de-sac once or twice daily. The most common problems associated with Lacrisert have been blurred vision and inadvertent loss of the insert (Lamberts, 1983).

In addition to their use in artificial tear preparations, cellulose esters and polyvinyl alcohol are employed as vehicles for ophthalmic drugs and as lubricants to moisten hard contact lenses and to protect the cornea during gonioscopy. A product [Enuclene] containing the detergent, tyloxapol, is used to lubricate artificial eyes.

ADVERSE REACTIONS AND PRECAUTIONS. Ophthalmic demulcents are nonirritating to ocular tissue and can be used for prolonged periods without damaging the eye. Viscous preparations may cause discomfort if excess solution is allowed to dry on the upper lid (see also *Federal Register*, 1980).

DOSAGE AND PREPARATIONS.

Topical: Artificial tears must be used regularly and as often as necessary to keep the conjunctiva moist. In patients with dry-eye syndrome, it may be necessary to apply the drops as often as every 15 minutes during warm dry weather. Occlusion of the lacrimal puncta by cauterization or insertion of punctum plugs may help to preserve existing lacrimal secretion and to prolong the retention of artificial tears.

All preparations available in ophthalmic form.

ARTIFICIAL TEARS.
HYDROXYETHYLCELLULOSE:
Clērz (CooperVision). Solution (sterile) with thimerosal 0.001% in 25 ml containers (nonprescription).
Clērz 2 (CooperVision). Solution (sterile, preservative free) in 15 ml containers (nonprescription).
Lyteers (Barnes-Hind). Solution (sterile) with edetate disodium 0.05% and benzalkonium chloride 0.01% in 15 ml containers (nonprescription).
HYDROXYPROPYLCELLULOSE (Sterile Ocular Insert):
Lacrisert (Merck Sharp & Dohme). Water-soluble insert containing hydroxypropylcellulose 5 mg in packages containing 60 units.
HYDROXYPROPYLMETHYLCELLULOSE:
Isopto Alkaline (Alcon). Solution (sterile) 1% with benzalkonium chloride 0.01% in 15 ml containers (nonprescription).
Isopto Plain (Alcon). Solution 0.5% with benzalkonium chloride 0.01% in 15 ml containers (nonprescription).
Isopto Tears (Alcon). Solution (sterile) 0.5% with benzalkonium chloride 0.01% in 15 and 30 ml containers (nonprescription).
Lacril (Allergan). Solution 0.5% with gelatin A 0.01% and chlorobutanol 0.5% in 15 ml containers (nonprescription).
Muro Tears (Muro). Solution (sterile) 0.5% and dextran 40 with benzalkonium chloride 0.01% in 15 ml containers (nonprescription).
Tearisol (CooperVision). Solution (sterile) 0.5% with benzalkonium chloride 0.01% and edetate disodium 0.01% in 15 ml containers (nonprescription).
METHYLCELLULOSE:
Methulose (American Optical). Solution (sterile) 0.25% with benzalkonium chloride 0.004% in 15 and 30 ml containers (nonprescription).
Murocel (Muro). Solution (sterile) 1% with propylparaben 0.01% and methylparaben in 15 ml containers (nonprescription).
Visculose (American Optical). Solution (sterile) 0.5% or 1% with benzalkonium chloride 0.004% in 15 ml containers (nonprescription).
POLYVINYL ALCOHOL:
hy-FLOW (CooperVision). Solution (sterile, mildly hypertonic) with edetate disodium 0.025% and benzalkonium chloride 0.01% in 60 ml containers (nonprescription).
Liquifilm Tears (Allergan). Solution (sterile) 1.4% with chlorobutanol 0.5% in 15 and 30 ml containers (nonprescription).
Liquifilm Forte (Allergan). Solution (sterile) 3% with thimerosal 0.002% and edetate disodium in 15 and 30 ml containers (nonprescription).
Pre-Sert (Allergan). Solution (sterile) 3% with benzalkonium chloride 0.004% in 15 ml containers (nonprescription).
Tears Plus (Allergan). Solution 1.4% with chlorobutanol 0.5% in 15 and 30 ml containers.
Total (Allergan). Solution (sterile) with edetate disodium and benzalkonium chloride in 60 and 120 ml containers (nonprescription).
Wetting Solution (Barnes-Hind). Solution (sterile) with edetate disodium 0.02% and benzalkonium chloride 0.004% in 35 and 60 ml containers (nonprescription).
POLYVINYL ALCOHOL AND CELLULOSE ESTER:
Contique Wetting Solution (Alcon). Solution with hydroxypropylmethylcellulose, benzalkonium chloride 0.004%, and edetate disodium 0.025% in 60 ml containers (nonprescription).
Lensine 5 (CooperVision). Solution (sterile, mildly hypertonic) with hydroxyethylcellulose, edetate disodium 0.05%, and benzalkonium chloride 0.01% in 60 and 120 ml containers (nonprescription).

Lens-Mate (Alcon). Solution with hydroxypropylmethylcellulose, benzalkonium chloride 0.1%, and edetate disodium 0.1% in 59 ml containers (nonprescription).
Liquifilm Wetting Solution (Allergan). Solution with hydroxypropylmethylcellulose and benzalkonium chloride 0.004% in 20 and 60 ml containers (nonprescription).
Neo-Tears (Barnes-Hind). Solution (sterile) containing hydroxyethylcellulose with thimerosal not to exceed 0.004% and edetate disodium 0.02% in 15 ml containers (nonprescription).
Visalens Wetting Solution (Leeming). Solution (sterile) with hydroxypropylmethylcellulose, sodium chloride, edetate disodium 0.1%, and benzalkonium chloride 0.01% in 60 ml containers (nonprescription).
OTHER POLYMERIC SYSTEMS:
Adapettes (Alcon). Solution (sterile) containing water-soluble polymers, povidone, thimerosal 0.004%, and edetate disodium 0.1% in 15 ml containers (nonprescription).
Adsorbotear (Alcon). Solution (sterile) containing water-soluble polymers, povidone 1.67%, hydroxyethylcellulose 0.44%, thimerosal 0.004%, and edetate disodium 0.1% in 15 ml containers (nonprescription).
Comfort Drops (Barnes-Hind). Solution (sterile) with edetate disodium 0.02% and benzalkonium chloride 0.005% in 15 ml containers (nonprescription).
Contique Dual Wet (Alcon). Solution containing Duasorb water-soluble polymers, polyvinyl alcohol, benzalkonium chloride 0.01%, and edetate disodium 0.05% in 60 ml containers (nonprescription).
Hypotears (CooperVision). Solution (sterile, hypotonic) containing *Lipiden* polymeric system with benzalkonium chloride 0.01% and edetate disodium 0.03% (tonicity adjusted with nonionic agents) in 15 and 30 ml containers (nonprescription).
Tears Naturale (Alcon). Solution containing *Duasorb* water-soluble polymers, benzalkonium chloride 0.01%, and edetate disodium 0.05% in 15 and 30 ml containers (nonprescription).
ARTIFICIAL EYE LUBRICANT.
Enuclene (Alcon). Solution (sterile) containing tyloxapol 0.25% and benzalkonium chloride 0.02% in 15 ml containers (nonprescription).
GONIOSCOPY LUBRICANT.
Gonioscopic Prism Solution (Alcon). Solution (sterile) containing hydroxyethylcellulose with thimerosal 0.004% and edetate disodium 0.1% in 15 ml containers (nonprescription).
Goniosol (CooperVision). Solution (sterile) containing hydroxypropylmethylcellulose 2.5% with benzalkonium chloride 0.01% and edetate disodium in 15 ml containers (nonprescription).

EMOLLIENTS

ACTIONS AND USES. Emollients are sterile, bland ointments that usually contain petrolatum, mineral oil, and lanolin derivatives. They form an occlusive film on the surface of the eye and are used to lubricate and protect the eye from drying during and after surgery, exposure to wind or sun, or foreign body removal. Emollients are useful to protect the cornea of patients with dry-eye syndromes, particularly as nighttime medication. They also are used as vehicles for ophthalmic drugs.

ADVERSE REACTIONS AND PRECAUTIONS. Emollients cause temporary blurring of vision. Although oleaginous vehicles are toxic to the interior of the eye, no adverse effects have been reported when emollients were used immediately after ocular surgery or in the presence of corneal abrasions or corneal ulcers (*Federal Register*, 1980).

DOSAGE AND PREPARATIONS.
Topical: One-fourth inch of ointment is applied to the inside of the lower lid.

All preparations available in topical ophthalmic form.
Duolube (Muro). Ointment (sterile) containing white petrolatum and mineral oil in 3.5 g containers (nonprescription).
Duratears (Alcon). Ointment (sterile) with white petrolatum, anhydrous liquid lanolin, mineral oil, methylparaben 0.05%, and propylparaben 0.01% in 3.5 g containers (nonprescription).
Lacri-Lube S.O.P. (Allergan). Ointment (sterile) with white petrolatum 55%, mineral oil 42.5%, nonionic lanolin derivatives 2%, and chlorobutanol 0.5% in 3.5 and 7 g containers and 0.7 g unit dose (nonprescription).

DECONGESTANTS

NAPHAZOLINE HYDROCHLORIDE

PHENYLEPHRINE HYDROCHLORIDE

TETRAHYDROZOLINE HYDROCHLORIDE

OXYMETAZOLINE (Investigational)

ACTIONS AND USES. These topically applied adrenergic drugs constrict dilated conjunctival vessels and are widely used by the public to whiten the eye. The FDA Advisory Review Panel on OTC Ophthalmic Drug Products has found the following concentrations to be safe and effective for relief of redness of the eye due to minor irritations: phenylephrine 0.08% to 0.2%, naphazoline 0.01% to 0.03%, and tetrahydrozoline 0.01% to 0.05% (*Federal Register*, 1980).

ADVERSE REACTIONS AND PRECAUTIONS. In the concentrations present in decongestant products, adrenergic drugs rarely cause serious untoward effects. However, prolonged or indiscriminate use should be avoided, since this could lead to neglect of symptoms of serious eye disease.

Ocular stinging and burning and reactive hyperemia may occur with excessive use. Mydriasis develops occasionally, particularly in patients with light irides, in those who wear contact lenses, or in those with corneal abrasions. Mydriasis may precipitate an attack of acute angle-closure glaucoma in predisposed eyes.

For local and systemic adverse effects of stronger concentrations of adrenergic drugs, see Chapter 18, Agents Used to Treat Glaucoma, and Chapter 19, Mydriatics and Cycloplegics.

Naphazoline and tetrahydrozoline are more stable in solution than phenylephrine, as the activity of phenylephrine is greatly reduced by oxidation.

DOSAGE AND PREPARATIONS.
Topical: One or two drops instilled up to four times daily.
All preparations available in topical ophthalmic form.
NAPHAZOLINE HYDROCHLORIDE:
Ak-Con (Akorn). Solution (sterile) 0.1% with benzalkonium chloride 0.01% and edetate disodium 0.01% in 15 ml containers.
Albalon (Allergan). Solution (sterile) 0.1% with benzalkonium chloride and edetate disodium in 5 and 15 ml containers.
Clear Eyes (Abbott). Solution (sterile) 0.012% with edetate disodium 0.1% and benzalkonium chloride 0.01% in 15 and 45 ml containers (nonprescription).
Degest 2 (Barnes-Hind). Solution (sterile) 0.012% with benzalko-

nium chloride 0.0067% and edetate disodium 0.02% in 15 ml containers (nonprescription).
Muro's Opcon (Muro). Solution (sterile) 0.1% with benzalkonium chloride 0.01% in 15 ml containers.
Naphcon (Alcon). Solution 0.012% (nonprescription) or 0.1% (prescription) (*Naphcon Forte*) with benzalkonium chloride 0.01% in 15 ml containers.
VasoClear (CooperVision). Solution (sterile) 0.02% in **Lipiden** polymeric system with benzalkonium chloride 0.01% in 15 ml containers (nonprescription).
Vasocon Regular (CooperVision). Solution (sterile) 0.1% with benzalkonium chloride in 15 ml containers.
PHENYLEPHRINE HYDROCHLORIDE:
Ak-Nefrin (Akorn). Solution (sterile) 0.12% with benzalkonium chloride 0.01% in 15 ml containers (nonprescription).
Isopto Frin (Alcon). Solution (sterile) 0.12% with benzethonium chloride 0.01% in 15 ml containers (nonprescription).
Prefrin (Allergan). Solution (sterile) 0.12% with benzalkonium chloride 0.004% in 20 ml containers (nonprescription).
Tear-Efrin (CooperVision). Solution (sterile) 0.12% with benzalkonium chloride and edetate disodium in 15 ml containers (nonprescription).
TETRAHYDROZOLINE HYDROCHLORIDE:
Murine Plus (Abbott). Solution (sterile) 0.05% with edetate disodium 0.1% and benzalkonium chloride 0.01% in 18 and 45 ml containers (nonprescription).
Soothe (Alcon). Solution (sterile) 0.15% with benzalkonium chloride 0.004% and edetate disodium 0.1% in 15 ml containers (nonprescription).
Visine (Leeming). Solution (sterile) 0.05% with edetate disodium 0.1% and benzalkonium chloride 0.01% in 15, 22.5, and 30 ml containers (nonprescription).
OXYMETAZOLINE (Investigational):
Oxylin (Allergan). Solution 0.025%.

ANTIALLERGIC AGENTS

CROMOLYN
[Opticrom]

ACTIONS AND USES. Cromolyn inhibits the release of histamine and other mediators of immediate hypersensitivity reactions from mast cells, possibly by interfering with calcium transport across the mast cell membrane.

When applied topically, cromolyn may be useful in certain atopic diseases of the eye, particularly vernal keratoconjunctivitis, an uncommon seasonal disorder affecting young people. Vernal keratoconjunctivitis is characterized by pruritus, inflammation, photophobia, thick mucous discharge, formation of giant papillae on the conjunctival tarsus, superficial punctate keratitis, limbal edema and infiltration, white limbal spots consisting of eosinophils (Trantas' dots), and, in severe cases, corneal ulcers. Cromolyn relieves pruritus and inflammation, decreases mucus secretion, and may improve punctate keratitis (Foster and Duncan, 1980). Additional therapy with corticosteroid eyedrops may be required during acute exacerbations and in severe cases, and oral aspirin may be useful.

In patients with ragweed rhinitis and conjunctivitis, cromolyn eyedrops relieved both ocular and nasal symptoms in those with low preseasonal IgE antibody levels; in those with high antibody levels, only the nasal symptoms improved (Welsh et al, 1979).

ADVERSE REACTIONS AND PRECAUTIONS. Cromolyn eyedrops may cause transient stinging. Pruritus, erythema, and chemosis have occurred rarely.

DOSAGE AND PREPARATIONS.

Topical: *Adults and children*, one drop instilled four to six times daily. Efficacy depends upon regular prophylactic use and symptoms may not improve until the drops have been used for a number of days.

> **Opticrom** (Fisons). Solution (ophthalmic) 4% with phenylethyl alcohol 0.4%, benzalkonium chloride 0.01%, and edetate disodium 0.01% in 10 ml containers.

ANTIHISTAMINES WITH DECONGESTANTS

ACTIONS AND USES. Products containing an antihistamine and decongestant are promoted for the treatment of allergic conjunctivitis. In studies using a histamine model of ocular allergy, pretreatment with a topical antihistamine-decongestant combination prevented redness and pruritus induced by application of histamine to the eye. There is little evidence that these products prevent or relieve symptoms of allergic conjunctivitis clinically.

The antihistamines used in ophthalmic solutions are H_1 blockers. H_2 receptors are also present in ocular tissue and may play a role in ocular allergy (Abelson and Udell, 1981).

ADVERSE REACTIONS AND PRECAUTIONS. Antihistamines can cause eczematous contact dermatitis following topical use. Individuals sensitized to one antihistamine may show cross sensitivity to other antihistamines or related agents. These agents may dilate the pupil and, in patients predisposed to angle-closure glaucoma, could precipitate an acute attack.

All preparations available in topical ophthalmic form.

> **Albalon-A** (Allergan). Solution (sterile) containing antazoline phosphate 0.5% and naphazoline hydrochloride 0.05% with benzalkonium chloride 0.004% and edetate disodium in 5 and 15 ml containers.
>
> **Muro's Opcon-A** (Muro). Solution (sterile) containing pheniramine maleate 0.3% and naphazoline hydrochloride 0.025% with benzalkonium chloride 0.01% in 15 ml containers.
>
> **Naphcon-A** (Alcon). Solution (sterile) containing pheniramine maleate 0.3% and naphazoline hydrochloride 0.025% with benzalkonium chloride 0.01% in 15 ml containers.
>
> **Prefrin-A** (Allergan). Solution (sterile) containing pyrilamine maleate 0.1% and phenylephrine hydrochloride 0.12% with benzalkonium chloride 0.1% in 15 ml containers.
>
> **Vasocon-A** (CooperVision). Solution (sterile) containing antazoline phosphate 0.5% and naphazoline hydrochloride 0.05% with phenylmercuric acetate 0.002% in 15 ml containers.

ASTRINGENTS

ZINC SULFATE

Zinc sulfate has mild astringent properties when applied topically to the eye. In the concentration used in ophthalmic products, it may act by clearing mucus from the surface of the eye. The FDA Advisory Review Panel on OTC Ophthalmic Drug Products has found the 0.25% solution (which is usually marketed in combination with a decongestant) to be safe and effective for temporary relief of discomfort caused by minor eye irritation (*Federal Register*, 1980).

Zinc sulfate may cause transient stinging or burning. Other adverse effects have not been reported.

DOSAGE AND PREPARATIONS.

Topical: One or two drops of a 0.25% solution are instilled into the affected eye(s) up to four times daily.

> All preparations available in topical ophthalmic forms.
>
> **Neozin** (American Optical). Solution (sterile) 0.25% with phenylephrine hydrochloride 0.125% and benzalkonium chloride 0.004% in 15 ml containers (nonprescription).
>
> **Op-Thal-Zin** (Alcon). Solution (sterile) 0.25% with benzalkonium chloride 0.01% in 15 ml containers (nonprescription).
>
> **Visine-A.C.** (Leeming). Solution (sterile, isotonic) 0.25% with tetrahydrozoline hydrochloride 0.05% and benzalkonium chloride 0.01% in 15 and 30 ml containers (nonprescription).
>
> **Zincfrin** (Alcon). Solution (sterile) 0.25% with phenylephrine hydrochloride 0.12% and benzalkonium chloride 0.01% in 15 ml containers (nonprescription).

INFUSION OF ROSE PETALS
[Estivin]

This product contains an extract of *Rosa gallica* buds and has been used by the laity for many years to treat conjunctivitis caused by hay fever as well as other minor eye irritations. The FDA Advisory Panel on OTC Ophthalmic Drug Products concluded that this preparation is safe and effective in reducing ocular irritation encountered in those adapting to contact lenses. However, the Panel recommended that further studies be performed to determine the active ingredient(s) and the effective concentration.

> **Estivin** (Alcon). Solution (sterile) containing infusion of rose petals with thimerosal 0.01% in 7.5 ml containers (nonprescription).

Cited References

Ophthalmic drug products for over-the-counter human use; establishment of a monograph, proposed rulemaking. *Federal Register* 45:30002-30050, (May 6) 1980.

Abelson MB, Udell IJ: H_2-receptors in human ocular surface. *Arch Ophthalmol* 99:302-304, 1981.

Apt L, et al: Patient compliance with use of topical ophthalmic corticosteroid suspensions. *Am J Ophthalmol* 87:210-214, 1979.

Beasley H: Miotics in cataract surgery. *Trans Am Ophthal Soc* 69:237-244, 1971.

Benedetto DA, et al: Instilled fluid dynamics and surface chemistry of polymers in preocular tear film. *Invest Ophthalmol* 14: 887-902, 1975.

Benson WE, et al: Intraocular irrigating solutions for pars plana vitrectomy: Prospective, randomized, double-blind study. *Arch Ophthalmol* 99:1013-1015, 1981.

Burns RP, et al: Immunosuppressive therapy in ophthalmology, in Leopold IH, Burns RP (eds): *Symposium on Ocular Therapy.* New York, John Wiley & Sons, 1976, vol 8, 11-15.

Burns RP, et al: Chronic toxicity of local anesthetics on cornea, in Leopold IH, Burns RP (eds): *Symposium on Ocular Therapy.* New York, John Wiley & Sons, 1977, vol 10, 31-44.

Chang JL, et al: Brain stem anesthesia following retrobulbar block. *Anesthesiology* 61:789-790, 1984.

Chin GN, Almquist HT: Bupivacaine and lidocaine retrobulbar anesthesia: Double-blind clinical study. *Ophthalmology* 90:369-372, 1983.

Dohlman CH: Physiology of the cornea: Corneal edema, in Smolin G, Throft RA (eds): *The Cornea: Scientific Foundations and Clinical Practice*. Boston, Little, Brown and Company, 1983, 3-17.

Edelhauser HF, et al: Intraocular irrigating solutions: Comparative study of BSS Plus and lactated Ringer's solution. *Arch Ophthalmol* 96:516-520, 1978.

Ellingsson A, Aasved H: Etidocaine and lidocaine in ophthalmic surgery. *Acta Ophthalmol* 57:543-546, 1979.

Ellis PP: Local anesthetics, in Leopold IH, Burns RP (eds): *Symposium on Ocular Therapy*. New York, John Wiley & Sons, 1976, vol 8, 17-24.

Foster CS, Duncan J: Randomized clinical trial of topically administered cromolyn sodium for vernal keratoconjunctivitis. *Am J Ophthalmol* 90:175-181, 1980.

Fraunfelder FT: Recent advances in ocular toxicology, in Srinivasan BD (ed): *Ocular Therapeutics*. New York, Masson Publishing USA, Inc, 1980, 123-126.

Gasset AR, Kaufman HE: Bandage lenses in treatment of bullous keratopathy. *Am J Ophthalmol* 72:376-380, 1971.

Gilbard JP, et al: Osmolarity of tear microvolumes in keratoconjunctivitis sicca. *Arch Ophthalmol* 96:677-681, 1978.

Grant WM: New treatment for calcific corneal opacities. *Arch Ophthalmol* 48:681-685, 1952.

Hecht SD: Evaluation of the lacrimal drainage system. *Ophthalmology* 85:1250-1258, 1978.

Jampol LM: Pharmacologic therapy of aphakic cystoid macular edema. *Ophthalmology* 80:891-897, 1982.

Johnstone MA, et al: Experimental zinc chloride ocular injury and treatment with disodium edetate. *Am J Ophthalmol* 76:137-142, 1973.

Jordan A, Baum J: Basic tear flow: Does it exist? *Ophthalmology* 87:920-930, 1980.

Kelley JS, Kincaid M: Retinal fluorography using oral fluorescein. *Arch Ophthalmol* 97:2331-2332, 1979.

Kraff MC, et al: Prophylaxis of pseudophakic cystoid macular edema with topical indomethacin. *Ophthalmology* 89:885-890, 1982.

Laibson PR: Diagnosis and treatment of keratoconjunctivitis sicca, in: *Symposium on Medical and Surgical Disease of the Cornea*. St Louis, CV Mosby Co, 1980, 36-47.

Lamberts DW: Keratoconjunctivitis sicca, in Smolin G, Throft RA (eds): *The Cornea: Scientific Foundations and Clinical Practice*. Boston, Little, Brown and Company, 1983, 293-309.

Lemp MA, et al: Effect of tear substitutes on tear film break-up time. *Invest Ophthalmol* 14:255-258, 1975.

Leopold IH, Murray D: Noncorticosteroidal anti-inflammatory agents in ophthalmology. *Ophthalmology* 86:142-155, 1979.

Miller D, Stegmann R: Use of sodium hyaluronate in human IOL implantation. *Ann Ophthalmol* 13:811-815, 1981.

Miller D, Stegmann R: Secondary intraocular lens implantation using sodium hyaluronate. *Ann Ophthalmol* 14:621-623, 1982.

Mindel JS: Value of hyaluronidase in ocular surgical akinesia. *Am J Ophthalmol* 85:643-646, 1978.

Mindel JS, et al: Similarity of intraocular pressure response to different corticosteroid esters when compliance is controlled. *Ophthalmology* 86:99-107, 1979.

Mindel JS, et al: Comparative ocular pressure elevation by medrysone, fluorometholone, and dexamethasone phosphate. *Arch Ophthalmol* 98:1577-1578, 1980.

Miyake K, et al: Long-term follow-up study on prevention of aphakic cystoid macular oedema by topical indomethacin. *Br J Ophthalmol* 64:324-328, 1980.

Miyake K, et al: Incidence of cystoid macular edema after retinal detachment surgery and use of topical indomethacin. *Am J Ophthalmol* 95:451-456, 1983.

Nussenblatt RB, et al: Cyclosporin A therapy in treatment of intraocular inflammatory disease resistant to systemic corticosteroids and cytotoxic agents. *Am J Ophthal* 96:275-282, 1983.

Pape LG: Intracapsular and extracapsular technique of lens implantation with Healon. *Ann Intraoc Implant Soc J* 6:342-343, 1980.

Pape LG, Balazs EA: Use of sodium hyaluronate (Healon) in human anterior segment surgery. *Ophthalmology* 87:699-705, 1980.

Podos SM, Becker B: Intraocular pressure effects of diluted and new topical corticosteroids, in Leopold IH (ed): *Symposium on Ocular Therapy*. St Louis, CV Mosby Co, 1972, vol 5, 90-95.

Podos SM, Sugar A: Use of nonsteroidal anti-inflammatory drugs in ocular conditions, in Srinivasan BD (ed): *Ocular Therapeutics*. New York, Masson Publishing USA, Inc, 1980, 73-81.

Polack FM, et al: Sodium hyaluronate (Healon) in keratoplasty and IOL implantation. *Ophthalmology* 88:425-431, 1981.

Rasch D, et al: Bronchospasm following intraocular injection of acetylcholine in patient taking metropolol. *Anesthesiology* 59:583-585, 1983.

Rizzuti AB: Acetylcholine in surgery of lens, iris, and cornea. *Am J Ophthalmol* 63:484-487, 1967.

Russell DA, Guyton JS: Retrobulbar injection of lidocaine (Xylocaine) for anesthesia and akinesia. *Am J Ophthalmol* 38:78-84, 1954.

Smith JL: Retrobulbar Marcaine can cause respiratory arrest. *J Clin Neuroophthalmol* 1:171-172, 1981.

Smith RB, Everett WG: Physiology and pharmacology of local anesthetic agents. *Int Ophthalmol Clin* 13:35-60, 1973.

Stein MR, Parker CW: Reactions following intravenous fluorescein. *Am J Ophthalmol* 72:861-868, 1971.

Stenkula S, et al: Use of sodium-hyaluronate (Healon) in treatment of retinal detachment. *Ophthal Surg* 12:435-437, 1981.

Welsh PW, et al: Topical ocular administration of cromolyn sodium for treatment in seasonal ragweed conjunctivitis. *J Allergy Clin Immunol* 64:209-215, 1979.

Yannuzzi LA, et al: Incidence of aphakic cystoid macular edema with use of topical indomethacin. *Ophthalmology* 88:947-954, 1981.

Other Selected References

Ellis PP: *Ocular Therapeutics and Pharmacology*, ed 7. St. Louis, CV Mosby Co, 1985

Fraunfelder FT: *Drug-Induced Ocular Side Effects and Drug Interactions*, ed 2. Philadelphia, Lea & Febiger, 1982.

Fraunfelder FT, Roy FH (eds): *Current Ocular Therapy*, ed 2. Philadelphia, WB Saunders, 1985.

Havener WH: *Ocular Pharmacology*, ed 5. St Louis, CV Mosby Co, 1983.

Decongestant, Cough, and Cold Preparations

A large proportion of all days lost from work and school is caused by respiratory tract illnesses. Considerations of the pertinent anatomy and physiology of the respiratory tract can serve as a basis for rational management of respiratory disease.

Nasal Physiology: The main functions of the nose are to modify the temperature and humidity of inspired air for maximum suitability for the lungs and to filter a large portion of inhaled foreign material. The vasculature of the nose plays an important role in regulating the patency of the nasal airway. Neural control of the vascular smooth muscle allows for delicate adjustment of capillary and arterial blood flow, which are responsible for changes in the cross sectional diameter of the nasal airway.

The nose accounts for about one-half of total respiratory tract resistance to air flow. The resistance varies with the individual and is affected by the degree of nasal vascular congestion, anatomic variations, posture, exercise, air temperature, irritants, medications, time of day, and disease states. Normally, the greatest resistance to air flow occurs at the anterior nares, which have the smallest cross sectional diameter. When mucosal congestion over the turbinates becomes severe, air flow resistance increases markedly (Proctor and Anderson, 1982).

The development of nasal vascular congestion depends primarily on autonomic neural controls that respond reflexly to changes in the inspired air. Cold air increases resistance, as does change in posture when moving from a standing or sitting position to a recumbent one. In contrast, exercise initially decreases resistance. These normal variations in nasal congestion alter nasal air flow resistance, which often is confused with that associated with disease. There is a normal, reciprocal fluctuation in the patency of each side of the nose (the nasal cycle). Some disorders, such as the common cold, inflammation of the nose and sinuses, and hypothyroidism, increase nasal congestion. Certain drugs (eg, reserpine, estrogens), as well as the rebound after prolonged administration of topical vasoconstrictors (nasal sprays), also may increase nasal congestion.

Normal functioning of the nose is not always sufficient to protect the respiratory tract from illness, a fact attested to by the prevalence of the common cold. Colds are not only major nuisances but associated complications, including ear, throat, and sinus disorders, may predispose to more severe illnesses. Upper respiratory tract infections may be associated with bronchial hyperreactivity that exacerbates bronchial asthma or chronic bronchitis.

Pulmonary Physiology: Airway obstruction results from

bronchospasm, mucosal edema, increased secretions, and/or airway inflammation. During normal breathing, the airway widens during inspiration and closes slightly during expiration. Conditions such as asthma and viral infections increase bronchial muscle reactivity and/or airway inflammation and narrow the airways, especially during expiration. The diameter of the larger airways may be modified by drugs that regulate autonomic function.

RHINITIS

Signs and symptoms of noninfectious upper respiratory disorders caused by inflammatory conditions (eg, allergic and nonallergic rhinitis) often resemble those of infection (eg, the common cold).

Allergy frequently causes noninfectious acute rhinitis. It is estimated that seasonal allergic rhinitis (hay fever, pollinosis) affects more than 17 million Americans. Symptoms are caused by the release of histamine and other chemical mediators (see Chapter 58, Histamine and Antihistamines). Sneezing, nasal stuffiness, runny nose, nasal and ocular pruritus, increased lacrimation, and postnasal drip can predispose to chronic nasal or sinus infection or otitis media with effusion.

Chronic or nonseasonal rhinitis, often referred to as perennial rhinitis, is defined as inflammation of the nasal mucosa that results in daily episodes of rhinorrhea, nasal congestion, and sneezing for several weeks (Simons, 1984). Chronic rhinitis is caused by various allergic and nonallergic nasal disorders; nonallergic nasal disease is responsible for a high percentage of cases. Several types of chronic rhinitis can coexist in the same patient. Asthma may also be present.

Common types of chronic rhinitis include vasomotor rhinitis and nonallergic or allergic rhinitis with eosinophilia (Meltzer et al, 1983; Ballow, 1984). Vasomotor rhinitis results from a local autonomic imbalance with exaggerated parasympathetic stimulation of the nasal mucosa. This disorder is exacerbated by emotion, airway irritants such as tobacco smoke, changes in weather or ambient temperature, or an alteration in general health. Agents with adrenergic activity or those that block parasympathetic responses may be helpful for symptomatic treatment. Distinct from allergic rhinitis with eosinophilia is a relatively new entity, nonallergic rhinitis with eosinophilia, which resembles allergic rhinitis but lacks evidence of an IgE-mediated reaction; eosinophils are present in nasal secretions in both disorders. Symptoms of chronic rhinitis can be caused by drugs (eg, adrenergic blocking agents, cholinesterase inhibitors, estrogen preparations including contraceptives), pregnancy, and hypothyroidism. Other causes include septal deviation, foreign body, ciliary disorders, neoplasia, Wegener's granulomatosis, and cerebrospinal rhinorrhea. For a detailed discussion of etiologic, diagnostic, and therapeutic aspects of chronic rhinitis, see Meltzer et al, 1983.

NONDRUG THERAPY. Nondrug therapy for rhinitis and the common cold is similar. Exposure to cigarette smoke, pollutants, known allergens, and other irritants should be avoided. In patients with pharyngitis, saline gargles and warm mist therapy may be helpful, but the latter may be hazardous due to mold growth in the vaporizer. When nasal congestion is severe, nasal irrigation with warm (37° C) isotonic saline solution is often beneficial (see Adjunctive Therapy). Patients should drink plenty of liquids. Vigorous regular exercise may reduce nasal obstruction, especially in patients with vasomotor rhinitis. Immunotherapy can be successful in selected patients with chronic or recurrent allergic rhinitis.

DRUG THERAPY. Treatment of allergic rhinitis is directed at preventing the release of inflammatory mediators or blocking their effects after they are released. Antihistamines are the most widely used agents for this condition and are often chosen for initial therapy. They help relieve rhinorrhea, sneezing, nasal pruritus, and conjunctivitis but do not affect nasal congestion. If they are ineffective or produce excessive sedation, a nasal decongestant can be substituted. Nasal decongestants shrink swollen turbinates and are the most effective agents for nasal congestion but have little effect on sneezing and rhinorrhea. Since oral decongestants are much less likely to cause rebound congestion, they are more suitable than topical products for long-term use. However, tachyphylaxis is common with prolonged use of oral agents and they can increase blood pressure and exacerbate peripheral ischemic disease.

Cromolyn nasal spray [Nasalcrom] appears to be as effective as the antihistamines in patients with seasonal allergic rhinitis. This agent is more effective if used prior to the onset of symptoms, but it may also be of value in patients with mild symptoms to prevent marked nasal obstruction. Cromolyn may be less useful for chronic allergic rhinitis and has no effect in nonallergic nasal disorders. Minimal adverse effects have been observed with this agent.

Corticosteroids are the most effective drugs for allergic rhinitis. Intranasal administration can be utilized if symptoms are not controlled by the previously mentioned agents or when patients cannot tolerate these drugs. Discomfort is decreased in up to 90% of patients with allergic rhinitis after treatment with an intranasal steroid alone; some patients may require oral or parenteral steroids for optimal management of severe allergic rhinitis (eg, during the pollen season in ragweed areas). The safety of long-term treatment with intranasal corticosteroids has not been established but their use for periods beyond one year may not cause significant adverse effects.

Anticholinergic agents, which are often administered preoperatively to decrease respiratory tract secretions, are occasionally used in rhinitis. Some patients with severe rhinorrhea and congestion obtain more relief from propantheline [Pro-Banthīne] or belladonna alkaloids than from nasal decongestants. Atropine nasal spray can relieve rhinorrhea, but adverse effects, such as dry mouth and tachycardia, decrease acceptance of this agent. Ipratropium, an investigational atropine analogue, produces fewer adverse effects and is being studied in the treatment of rhinitis.

None of these drugs are likely to abolish symptoms completely. Severely affected patients may require concurrent administration of an antihistamine, a nasal decongestant, and an anticholinergic drug given separately or in a proprietary mixture. Cromolyn or a topical steroid also may be required to help control symptoms.

It is claimed that the sedative effect of the traditional

antihistamines is balanced by the stimulant effect of nasal decongestants, but this action is unpredictable. For maximal control and fewest side effects, separate administration is preferable so that the dose of each can be titrated (see also the section on Mixtures).

Antihistamine/decongestant combinations are widely used in the prophylaxis of otitis media with effusion, but their value is controversial. The results of double-blind studies demonstrate that such combinations are ineffective in childhood serous otitis media (Cantekin et al, 1983; Bhambhani et al, 1983). However, they may be of some benefit in children with associated symptoms such as allergy, nasal congestion, or upper respiratory infection (*Pediatr Alert*, 1983).

ADJUNCTIVE THERAPY. Nasal irrigation with warm isotonic saline solution may relieve severe nasal congestion and obstruction, although no controlled trials have been performed. This procedure may help liquify secretions, cleanse allergens, and decrease mucous crust formation (Wood, 1984). It is a safe alternative when used properly in young infants, in whom nasal decongestants are not recommended by some authorities. Irrigation before use of a topical nasal preparation enhances the efficacy of the latter. Some physicians advocate nasal irrigation with saline after rather than before the topical medication.

The saline solution can be prepared by dissolving one level teaspoonful each of table salt and baking soda in one pint (one quart in children) of warm (37° C) tap water. Patients must be instructed on appropriate technique. The head should be down with chin on chest. Using a small rubber bulb ear syringe, each nostril is irrigated with about one cup of saline solution until thick mucus is no longer flushed out. This procedure should be performed upon arising, at bedtime, and during the waking hours as necessary (Wood, 1984; Crawford and Cohen, 1985). If ear pain or discomfort occurs during irrigation, the procedure should be stopped.

Drug Selection

The rational selection of drugs requires that noninfectious rhinitis be distinguished from infectious rhinitis associated with the common cold because most agents useful for noninfectious rhinitis (antihistamines, cromolyn nasal spray, intranasal corticosteroids) have little value in patients with the common cold. Nasal decongestants are often beneficial in both conditions. Antibiotics should be reserved for patients with bacterial infections.

A broad variety of medicines is available over-the-counter for rhinitis and other minor respiratory illnesses. Because the components are often similar to those of prescription medicines, they are subject to the same advantages and problems.

ANTIHISTAMINES. Antihistamines are the most widely prescribed drugs for allergic rhinitis. They are effective alone when the disorder is mild to moderately severe and are particularly effective in seasonal allergic rhinitis when sneezing and rhinorrhea predominate and edema and congestion are minimal. Antihistamines are more effective if taken before symptoms occur. They should be taken regularly by sensitive patients during the allergen exposure period or season even when symptoms are absent. Their premature discontinuation can result in recurrence of symptoms. When nasal congestion and turbinate swelling are prominent symptoms, as in vasomotor rhinitis and nonallergic eosinophilic rhinitis, antihistamines are less useful than decongestants.

Drowsiness, the most common adverse effect of the traditional antihistamines, is better tolerated by many patients after a few days to weeks of therapy. A single daily dose of an antihistamine with a relatively long half-life taken at bedtime may be beneficial in adults. The availability of the nonsedating antihistamine, terfenadine [Seldane], and the expected approval of similar drugs will extend the usefulness of these drugs (see Chapter 58, Histamine and Antihistamines).

NASAL DECONGESTANTS. Alpha-adrenergic agonists constrict dilated blood vessels in the nasal mucosa, reducing blood flow to engorged, edematous tissue. These drugs promote drainage of the sinuses, relieve the stuffy feeling in the nose, and improve nasal ventilation. Nasal decongestants provide temporary, symptomatic relief in acute rhinitis associated with the common cold and other respiratory infections, as well as in hay fever, nonseasonal allergic rhinitis, and other forms of acute and chronic rhinitis and sinusitis. Decongestants are also used topically to facilitate visualization of nasal and nasopharyngeal membranes during diagnostic procedures and to reduce mucosal swelling prior to application of topical steroids or nasal surgery. Because of rebound congestion, topical decongestants should not be used to treat chronic rhinitis except for occasional relief of exacerbations.

Administration: Nasal decongestants can be administered topically or orally. Topical decongestants have the advantages of greater efficacy and more rapid onset of action. However, their topical use for more than five days can result in rebound nasal congestion, which leads to rhinitis medicamentosa (see Adverse Reactions and Precautions). Although this condition occasionally occurs after prolonged use of oral decongestants, the symptoms are less severe, and, therefore, oral forms are preferred for prolonged treatment. Oral decongestants also may reach areas inaccessible to topical application and have a longer duration of action. However, they may produce undesirable systemic effects.

Topical nasal decongestants are available as drops, sprays, and vapors. (Solutions applied by means of wet tampons and nasal packs injure nasal cilia and are no longer used except for diagnostic or surgical procedures in the office or hospital.)

Drops instilled onto the nasal mucosa have the advantage of working their way backward from the vestibule if a lateral, head-low position is used; if not, drops may trickle rapidly over the surface of the nasal mucosa and pass into the nasopharynx where they are swallowed. *Sprays* deliver a mist containing drops in finely divided form. When instilled properly, drops cover a larger area of nasal mucosa than can be reached by an equal volume of spray if obstruction does not impede distribution (Hardy et al, 1985). Improper use can result in repeated delivery to a localized area resulting in mucosal damage at that site. For short-term intermittent use, *vaporizers* containing a volatile base of certain nasal decongestants (eg, propylhexedrine [Benzedrex]) are among the most effective agents for reaching the desired areas of the nasal mucosa. Vaporizers are particularly useful when rapid decongestion of the nasal mucosa and possibly the eustachian orifices is required, as during airplane descent.

When treating barotitis by producing vasoconstriction in the mucosa near the orifices of the eustachian tubes, drops should be instilled as follows: The patient lies supine, but not hyperextended, with the head turned 15° toward the affected ear. Nose drops are instilled into the affected side and allowed to run along the floor of the nose and "puddle" at the eustachian orifice, which is positioned at the low point. The patient should remain in this position for about five minutes. If necessary, the procedure is repeated for the other side.

In children, maintaining the head in an upright position minimizes accumulation, since the spray and secretions drip anteriorly from the nostril and are not swallowed. For children under 6 years, drops are preferred to a spray because of the difficulty of controlling dosage with the latter, which may release enough medication to cause overdose in these patients. Accordingly, drops and sprays for children always should be administered by an adult. Because of the risks of systemic absorption, some physicians suggest that nasal decongestants should not be used in infants and small children.

Adverse Reactions and Precautions: The most common adverse effects of oral nasal decongestants are insomnia and irritability. Isolated reports have suggested that antihistamine/decongestant combinations containing pseudoephedrine cause hallucinations in children. However, most of these reports used larger doses than those usually recommended or patients had predisposing factors, such as febrile conditions.

Since the nasal vessels are not more sensitive to adrenergic drugs than other blood vessels, oral doses large enough to produce nasal decongestion constrict other vascular beds, thus redistributing blood flow and causing cardiac stimulation. In normal individuals, usual decongestant doses do not increase blood pressure; susceptible patients, however, can develop marked tachycardia, arrhythmias, and increased blood pressure.

Topical nasal decongestants sometimes cause temporary local discomfort, including stinging, burning, or dryness of the mucosa. Inhaled vapors of volatile bases (eg, propylhexedrine) may dry the mucosa rapidly and interfere with ciliary action, but these effects are usually clinically insignificant.

Use of topical decongestants can produce rebound congestion and chronic administration can lead to rhinitis medicamentosa, a disorder characterized by chronic swelling and a red, boggy, edematous appearance of the nasal mucosa. Rebound congestion probably results from tachyphylaxis and an irritant effect on the nasal mucosa. As the decongestant effect of each application wears off, congestion recurs with increasing severity, thereby encouraging repeated use at shorter intervals. Swelling of the mucosa that is often worse than the original congestion then occurs. Dryness, severe soreness, and a burning sensation also develop.

Discontinuation of the topical nasal decongestant relieves soreness and burning within 48 to 72 hours but nasal congestion and other symptoms of chronic rhinitis worsen. Some patients have great difficulty in discontinuing topical nasal decongestants. Those with severe congestion may require an oral decongestant or systemic steroid.

Topical decongestants also may produce systemic reactions, especially in infants and young children in whom decreased body temperature, central nervous system depression, and even coma can develop. Significant absorption from the nasal mucosa or gastrointestinal tract occurs if excess solution is swallowed. Proper use of nasal sprays may be the best way to avoid systemic absorption.

Overdosage of most adrenergic drugs causes transient hypertension, nervousness, nausea, dizziness, palpitations, arrhythmias, and, occasionally, central nervous system stimulation with seizures. There is no evidence that the appetite is suppressed by usual doses of these drugs.

Overdoses of two imidazolines, tetrahydrozoline [Tyzine] and naphazoline [Privine], have caused severe reactions characterized by hypertension, sweating, drowsiness, deep sleep, coma, and even hypotension and bradycardia. These effects are most common in children. The possibility that such reactions may occur with other adrenergic decongestants should be kept in mind. The topical nasal decongestants, especially the imidazolines, should be used sparingly, if at all, and with particular caution in infants, young children, and patients with cardiovascular disease.

All adrenergic agents should be given with caution to patients with thyroid disease, hypertension, diabetes mellitus, and heart disease and to those receiving tricyclic antidepressants (in whom additive pressor effects can occur). Nasal decongestants should not be used in patients receiving monoamine oxidase inhibitors or in individuals whose sensitivity to even small doses is manifested by insomnia, dizziness, weakness, tremor, and arrhythmias.

Topical solutions quickly become contaminated after use and can serve as reservoirs for bacteria and fungi. Patients should be cautioned not to place the dropper in the nostril or to allow more than one person to use the same dropper bottle. The bottle or spray pack should be discarded when the medication is no longer needed. Discoloration of the normally clear solutions indicates decomposition. Nasal solutions of many adrenergic agents, especially naphazoline and probably the other imidazolines, should not be used in atomizers having aluminum parts because they interact with this metal.

CROMOLYN. The nasal spray preparation of cromolyn is probably as effective as an oral antihistamine in preventing the symptoms of allergic rhinitis. Cromolyn is usually of limited value in relieving established symptoms, although it may prevent progression of mild symptoms. Patients with seasonal allergic rhinitis are more responsive than those with the chronic form. The greatest effect is observed in patients with positive skin tests to allergens, elevated IgE levels, or nasal eosinophilia. Nasal cromolyn is less effective than the intranasal corticosteroids for both seasonal and chronic allergic rhinitis. It is ineffective for nasal polyps, nonallergic eosinophilic rhinitis, vasomotor rhinitis, and other nonallergic conditions. Sneezing, nasal pruritus, rhinorrhea, and, in some patients, watery itchy eyes are relieved more than nasal congestion.

Cromolyn is an alternative to antihistamines in patients who cannot tolerate drowsiness. However, it is not likely to be effective in patients refractory to antihistamines. The therapeutic advantage of cromolyn over other medications used for allergic rhinitis is its lack of adverse effects.

TOPICAL CORTICOSTEROIDS. Topical steroid preparations exert a marked anti-inflammatory effect on the nasal mucosa by inhibiting the release of inflammatory mediators from mast cells and basophils and blocking the inflammatory effects of leukocytes in the nose. Local administration decreases the number of surface basophils and eosinophils, reduces vasodilatation and edema in the inflamed mucosa, stabilizes epithelial and endothelial membranes, reduces receptor sensitivity to irritants, and decreases the effect of cholinergic stimulation of intranasal glands. If the pretreatment period is sufficient, topical corticosteroids inhibit both immediate and delayed reactions to allergen challenge (Clissold and Heel, 1984). The mechanisms responsible for most of these actions are being elucidated.

Intranasal corticosteroids are safe and are the most effective agents available for prophylaxis and treatment of seasonal and chronic allergic rhinitis or for weaning patients with rhinitis medicamentosa from topical decongestants (Brogden et al, 1984; Clissold and Heel, 1984). Nonallergic nasal disorders, including nonallergic rhinitis with eosinophilia and vasomotor rhinitis also may respond to corticosteroids, although their effectiveness for the latter condition is usually limited. Because of their anti-inflammatory action, steroids are beneficial as adjuncts to nasal decongestants or alone when the latter drugs are ineffective. The efficacy of nasal spray preparations of dexamethasone [Decadron, Turbinaire], beclomethasone dipropionate [Beconase, Vancenase], flunisolide [Nasalide], and the investigational drugs, budesonide and fluocortin butyl, is similar.

Rhinorrhea, nasal pruritus, erythema, nasal congestion, postnasal drainage, and sneezing are relieved. Ocular symptoms usually are not improved. Patients with seasonal allergic rhinitis should be informed that, although significant relief of symptoms may be observed in one to three days, full effects may not occur for a week or longer. In chronic rhinitis, significant relief of symptoms may require at least one week and maximal improvement may not be observed for two to three weeks. Daily administration is required. These drugs should not be used in allergic rhinitis for more than three weeks if no response is attained.

Topical steroids often shrink nasal polyps and reduce nasal obstruction significantly; polyps may even disappear. However, when the corticosteroid is discontinued, the polyps can grow again. Even in patients requiring polypectomy, the reduction in size of the polyps facilitates surgery. After polypectomy, continued use of an intranasal steroid may prevent recurrence or slow regrowth.

Patients with severe rhinosinusitis and polyps or persistent middle ear effusion may not respond to these drugs. In some patients with nasal polyps, rhinitis medicamentosa, or other nasal diseases, severe nasal obstruction or congestion inhibits the access of intranasal steroid sprays and thus renders them ineffective. A few days of treatment with a topical nasal decongestant or a short course of oral corticosteroids (prednisone 10 mg two or three times a day for five to seven days) can reduce the obstruction and permit treatment with intranasal steroids (Busse, 1983).

In patients with severe turbinate dysfunction, intraturbinate injection of triamcinolone acetonide within each nostril may relieve severe nasal congestion within one to two hours and the effect lasts four to six weeks (Mabry, 1983; Ward and Berry, 1984). Adverse effects with this route include transient nasal bleeding, flushing of the cheeks, and a vasovagal reaction. Many authorities do not recommend intraturbinate injection of corticosteroids because intra-arterial embolization of drug particles occurs rarely and may cause unilateral transient or permanent blindness.

Depot injections or prolonged oral therapy may be effective in nonresponsive patients but can cause significant adrenocortical suppression (Phelan, 1984; Busse, 1983).

The need for an antihistamine or nasal decongestant is reduced in patients treated with a corticosteroid nasal spray. The combined use of an inhalant and intranasal corticosteroid in patients with a nasal disorder and asthma appears to be safe when recommended doses are employed (Norman, 1983). Intranasal beclomethasone or flunisolide are safer than other drugs in pregnant women and do not appear to affect the fetus.

Adverse Reactions and Precautions: Adverse reactions occur fairly frequently, are usually minor, and are probably due to the vehicle, since the incidence is the same as with a placebo. After initial application of an intranasal steroid, transient stinging and burning may occur but usually dissipates with continued use. Sneezing, headache, dry nose, and nasal bleeding have been reported. Beclomethasone or budesonide delivered from a Freon-propelled cannister has a drying, irritant effect on nasal mucous membranes. This can be avoided by using a nonFreon-containing preparation (eg, flunisolide), which is delivered by a mechanical pump. However, stinging and burning occur more frequently with flunisolide (probably due to the vehicle, propylene glycol). Nasal wetting agents may relieve minor bleeding and dryness of the nose.

Long-term adverse effects appear to be rare. Nasal candidiasis has not been reported. Mucosal atrophy has not been observed in patients using intranasal beclomethasone or flunisolide for up to five years and, in some studies with beclomethasone, for up to 12 years. Adrenocortical function is not affected when usual doses are employed. Dexamethasone nasal spray, the first intranasal corticosteroid available in this country, can suppress adrenocortical function with usual doses and is being used less frequently now that safer drugs are available.

The topical steroids should be used with caution or avoided in patients with active or quiescent tuberculosis, untreated bacterial infections, and systemic fungal or viral infections. They should be used with caution, if at all, in patients with a local nasal infection or ocular herpes simplex. See also Chapter 61, Adrenal Corticosteroids in Nonendocrine Diseases.

COUGH

Cough is a protective respiratory reflex by which foreign matter can be expelled from the tracheobronchial tree. As such, the cough is usually helpful and occurs occasionally in healthy people. However, in many conditions, coughing increases in frequency and severity and becomes troublesome rather than helpful, particularly when it prevents sleep.

The cough reflex is initiated by stimulation of mechanical receptors or chemoreceptors and is mediated by afferent pathways along the vagus, glossopharyngeal, and superior laryngeal nerves to a cough center located near the respiratory and vomiting centers in the hindbrain. An effective cough reflex requires an intact peripheral nerve pathway to the abdomen, thoracic muscles, diaphragm, and glottis and the muscles of these organs must be functional. Cough is severely impaired if any component in the reflex arc is inhibited, depressed, or malfunctioning.

Cough can be caused by conditions within the lower respiratory tract, as well as elsewhere in the body. Irritation of the trigeminal and glossopharyngeal nerves in the nose, sinuses, or pharynx; the vagal nerve in the ears, pleura, or stomach; or the phrenic nerve in the pericardium or diaphragm can produce coughing. Thus, cough can result from diseases in the head and abdomen as well as in the chest. Accordingly, an accurate diagnosis is required to select the most appropriate agents for cough therapy.

The self-limited character of most coughs associated with acute respiratory infection accounts for the popular conception that many cough preparations are effective and this explains their corresponding widespread use. Accordingly, patients who seek treatment for a cough expect some form of medication.

When evaluating the need for a cough suppressant, it is necessary to distinguish between acute and chronic cough. Symptomatic treatment is employed primarily for the self-limited acute nonproductive cough that accompanies mild upper respiratory infection or a common cold.

Chronic cough can be defined as that persisting for at least three weeks. Postnasal drip, bronchial asthma, or both accounts for over 70% of chronic coughs (Irwin, 1984). Significant causative factors in adults are chronic bronchitis and smoking. Bronchiectasis, tracheitis, gastrointestinal reflux with or without aspiration, sarcoidosis, congestive heart failure, chronic pulmonary infections, and pulmonary tumors cause cough rarely. Cough suppressants should be considered when their action will not interfere significantly with resolution of the underlying disease or when complications (eg, rib fracture, cough syncope) pose a danger to the patient (Irwin, 1984). Patients with productive cough generally should not be given cough suppressants.

Drug Selection

There are numerous prescription products and proprietary medicines available for the treatment of cough. These may contain a single ingredient or a combination of agents designed to suppress cough (antitussives), increase mucus excretion (expectorants), or liquefy secretions (hydrating or mucolytic agents) plus antihistamines, vasoconstrictors, analgesics, local antitussives or anesthetics, flavoring agents, and placebos.

Nonmedicated remedies, such as cough drops, lozenges, troches, rock candy, and horehound drops, are generally considered to be ineffective but are usually harmless. These may suffice as a placebo for brief episodes of self-limited cough or cough induced reflexly by pharyngeal irritation.

ANTITUSSIVES. Antitussives are usually classified as centrally or peripherally acting, depending upon whether they act on the medullary cough center or at the site of irritation. The centrally acting group includes the opium derivatives (eg, codeine, hydrocodone, hydromorphone [Dilaudid]) and the nonopioid, non-narcotic agent, dextromethorphan [Benylin DM, Cremacoat 1, Delsym]. The peripherally acting group includes agents with local anesthetic or analgesic activity, as well as expectorants and demulcents.

Reports on the effectiveness of various antitussive agents frequently conflict because of the difficulties in assessing their effects. Most currently available evaluations of single-entity antitussive drugs are based on subjective rather than objective methods, and the placebo effect is an important factor, particularly in self-limited conditions. Results of studies on patients with chronic cough are not necessarily applicable to those with acute cough, which often improves spontaneously and rapidly.

Centrally Acting Agents: Opioids. Narcotics decrease the sensitivity of the cough center to incoming stimuli. Results of experimental and clinical studies and many years of experience have shown that codeine is the most efficacious antitussive for acute cough caused by a variety of disease states or irritants. The related agent, hydrocodone, is also effective and is slightly more potent than codeine on a milligram basis, but it has greater dependence liability. Codeine and hydrocodone have been used widely to suppress cough and to allay anxiety in patients with congestive heart failure or with irritative nonproductive cough. However, the opioids can cause drying of the mucosa and release of histamine that may result in bronchospasm. In addition, because of the danger of depression of the respiratory center, the narcotic drugs must be used with great care in patients with pulmonary insufficiency. Their dependence potential also must be considered.

Other opioid analgesics (eg, morphine, ethylmorphine, hydromorphone, oxycodone, methadone, meperidine) probably have antitussive activity, but they may produce more adverse reactions and have a greater dependence liability with continued use than codeine. Thus, they are seldom used as general antitussives but are reserved for conditions in which cough is associated with pain, anxiety, and restlessness and for severe, nonproductive cough associated with tracheal irritation.

Nonopioids. A synthetic agent structurally related to codeine, dextromethorphan, is present in many over-the-counter cough preparations. It is as effective as codeine except for severe acute cough, and usual doses have no analgesic, sedative, or respiratory depressant effects. This drug has had more extensive clinical study than other nonopioid antitussives and is the safest antitussive available. Adverse effects are usually mild and may be similar to those produced by opioids (eg, nausea, drowsiness, dizziness).

Caramiphen has local anesthetic and anticholinergic effects, but its antitussive effect is erratic. This agent is available only as an ingredient of combination products. Such mixtures must be prescribed with caution in patients sensitive to atropine-like complications, such as glaucoma and prostatic hypertrophy.

The antitussive efficacy of carbetapentane is unproven. Sufficient evidence supports the efficacy of noscapine. Each of these two agents is available only in combination products. Some antihistamines, particularly diphenhydramine [Benadryl], also have antitussive activity; the mechanism of this action is unclear. Promethazine, a phenothiazine antihistamine, is an ingredient of some combination products for cough, but whether the drug has a specific antitussive effect is not known.

Some antihistamines have anticholinergic activity that has a drying effect on mucosal secretions. The long-held concept that anticholinergics should be avoided in asthmatics and other patients in whom thickening of secretions is undesirable is probably not valid.

Peripherally Acting Agents: Many types of cough can be alleviated by agents that act peripherally at the level of the cough receptors in the airway. These include expectorants, hydrating agents, local antitussives, local anesthetics, and bronchodilators.

Expectorants. In experimental studies, large doses of expectorants stimulate the flow of respiratory tract fluid and facilitate the movement of loosened material toward the pharynx by ciliary motion and coughing. These agents should be most useful in irritative, nonproductive cough associated with a small amount of secretion; increasing the quantity of secretion would facilitate removal of irritants and have a demulcent effect on the irritated mucosa, thus diminishing the tendency to cough.

The use of expectorants is based primarily on tradition and the widespread subjective impression among both patients and physicians that they are effective. Satisfactory techniques for proving that these drugs increase the secretion of respiratory tract fluid when administered in recommended doses must be developed.

Commonly used expectorants probably produce some of their effects through a local or reflex irritant action or an emetic effect that stimulates secretions by the respiratory tract secretory glands. Of the many agents promoted for their expectorant action, guaifenesin [Breonesin, Glycotuss, Robitussin, 2/G] is currently the most widely used. This agent, as well as ammonium salts, electrolytes, and iodide salts, are common ingredients of many cough mixtures. The efficacy of guaifenesin in recommended doses is questionable. Experimental and clinical studies have not clearly established its value.

Of the other commonly used expectorants, the iodides have produced the most positive results, but there is no evidence that they are effective in acute upper respiratory infection. The iodide salts have come into disfavor in recent years since their potential for thyroid suppression with prolonged administration became apparent; however, they are still useful in adults when prescribed judiciously and should not be used for more than a few weeks at a time. The American Academy of Pediatrics recommends that iodides not be used as expectorants in children (Committee on Drugs, American Academy of Pediatrics, 1976).

Ipecac syrup, ammonium chloride, and guaiacolsulfonate potassium may stimulate the secretion of respiratory tract fluid when subemetic doses are given. The available evidence on the effectiveness of these agents is equivocal. Terpin hydrate must be regarded as a placebo on the basis of evidence that it has no effect.

Hydrating Agents. The demulcent action of hydrating agents diminishes the frequency, severity, and duration of cough and also alleviates the symptoms of laryngotracheobronchitis. Hydrating agents are thought to thin bronchial secretions and may be more beneficial than expectorants. Some clinicians suggest that the most effective mucokinetic is the glass of water taken with the spoonful of cough mixture. Water given by inhalation, orally, or parenterally, appears to be very useful, particularly when secretions are thickened by dehydration.

The use of vaporizers is soothing for patients with upper airway, nasal, or sinus congestion and inflammation and may reduce the viscosity of secretions. However, they may be hazardous due to mold growth. Since little of the mist reaches the lower airways, this treatment has limited value in bronchial disorders but can be helpful in laryngotracheitis.

Water inhaled as a hot or cold steam mist appears to hydrate and soothe mucous membranes but may aggravate bronchospasm in patients with asthma or chronic bronchitis. Particles should be 1 to 5 microns to have a significant effect. Patients often report benefit from inhalation of water-saturated air, although the lack of particles may reduce its effectiveness. Although distilled or tap water can be used for inhalation to relieve disorders of the upper respiratory tract, normal and hypotonic saline solutions are often preferred for cold steam mist when the bronchial tree is affected.

Local Antitussives. Menthol is believed to have a local soothing or counterirritant effect when used in lozenge or ointment form for topical application. Camphor is also used in ointment form; its usefulness in solution is limited by the great danger of poisoning, especially in children.

Local Anesthetics. Local anesthetics may relieve irritation of pharyngeal receptors, particularly in cough accompanying sore throat or postnasal drip. These agents also may enhance cough by blocking pain that discourages coughing, as in postoperative patients. Local anesthesia of respiratory tract mucous membranes can be achieved with nebulization of lidocaine [Xylocaine]. The local anesthetic activity of benzonatate [Tessalon] and some other antitussive agents is claimed to be the basis for their effect, but their role in cough suppression has not been fully elucidated. In a limited number of studies, benzonatate appeared to be effective for some coughs; in addition to a local anesthetic action, it acts on pulmonary stretch receptors to inhibit transmission of afferent vagal impulses to the cough center. There is also evidence that benzonatate has a central antitussive effect.

Bronchodilators. Since cough may be caused or aggravated by bronchospasm, use of bronchodilators often diminishes cough, particularly in asthmatics whose earliest symptom is cough alone. In small children, bronchodilators often relieve the cough associated with asthma or with bronchospasm caused by viral respiratory infections.

Mucolytics. The solubilizing action of a mucolytic agent may make tenacious or inspissated secretions easier to eliminate but also may impair ciliary clearance. Acetylcysteine [Mucomyst] or hypertonic saline aerosol are reported to be effective for loosening secretions, thus leading to a productive cough. However, these agents are irritating and frequently trigger reflex bronchospasm. A major disadvantage of acetylcysteine is its sulfurous odor; a European product lacks this disadvantage and is also given orally.

Adverse Reactions and Precautions

Untoward effects produced by antitussives or expectorants occur infrequently, are generally mild, and usually subside promptly when the drugs are withdrawn. However, caution is indicated when opioid antitussives are used in sedated, debilitated, or hypoxic patients or those receiving other central nervous system depressants.

A productive cough is expected in patients with obstructive lung diseases, such as asthma, emphysema, or chronic bronchitis, and expulsion of respiratory tract secretions is desirable. Therefore, those with obstructive lung diseases and infants with pertussis should not, in general, receive cough suppressants since the correct treatment for cough in these patients is the appropriate management of the underlying conditions. Sedation associated with use of some cough suppressants also may cause retention of carbon dioxide in patients with severe asthma.

It should be borne in mind that the drugs administered postoperatively to relieve pain have cough suppressant properties and may cause retention of secretions, bronchial obstruction, atelectasis, and pneumonia.

Serious reactions, such as respiratory depression and excessive drowsiness, occur only rarely when usual doses of opioid preparations are given to children under 5 years, but poisoning and some deaths have followed ingestion of larger doses. Therefore, cough preparations containing opioids should rarely be prescribed for infants and should be used with great care in children. Tolerance to the antitussive effects of opioids may occur with chronic use.

The safety of most of these agents in pregnant or nursing women has not been established.

COLD REMEDIES

The common cold is an acute infection of the upper respiratory tract mucosa caused by many different types of viruses, particularly rhinoviruses and coronaviruses. Bacterial diseases that cause primarily nasal symptoms are nasal diphtheria, which is extremely rare, and infection by *Haemophilus* species or meningococci, in which nasal discharge is often purulent from the onset. In infants under 18 months, nasopharyngitis often is caused by group A streptococci and presents as a purulent nasal discharge.

Colds are transmitted chiefly by direct contact and rarely through exposure to aerosols generated by sneezing or coughing. Individuals with colds shed viruses in their respiratory secretions (especially nasal mucus); these contaminate hands or household objects, which may pass the viruses onto the hands of susceptible individuals who then inoculate their nasal mucosa. Handwashing (even without soap) removes cold viruses from hands and may limit transmission. A variety of factors affect an individual's susceptibility to cold viruses (Mills, 1983).

A viral upper respiratory infection can be diagnosed relatively easily. The major complaints are usually rhinorrhea, sneezing, and dry cough with or without mild sore throat. The chest is usually clear. Systemic symptoms include malaise, headache, and myalgia. Fever is unusual in adults, although mild to moderate fever is common in children and temperatures of 103 F or higher are not unusual in infants under 15 months. The nasal discharge is clear initially but may become purulent. Tenderness over frontal and maxillary sinuses is common but not pronounced. Ear discomfort may be present, particularly in children, because of blockage of the eustachian tubes, but eardrums usually are not inflamed.

The common cold is usually benign and self-limiting. Failure of symptoms to abate within one or two weeks or worsening symptoms suggests secondary bacterial infection of the paranasal sinuses, ears, tracheobronchial tree, or lungs. In such cases, administration of anti-infective agents may be warranted after appropriate diagnostic studies. Routine administration of antimicrobial agents to patients with colds has been shown to be completely useless.

Identification of the virus is unnecessary since specific therapy does not exist. Only symptoms can be relieved. That such relief is sought very frequently is attested to by the large number of patient visits for treatment of the common cold and the widespread use of prescription and nonprescription cold remedies.

No methods of prevention or cure are presently available. Vitamin C, the subject of many clinical studies, is ineffective. A single report showing a therapeutic effect of zinc gluconate lozenges (Eby et al, 1984) has not been confirmed. Topical interferon is effective prophylactically and therapeutically, but is potentially toxic and is not available yet.

Facial tissues impregnated with virucides are being investigated as a means of preventing transmission of colds. Studies have established their value in interrupting transmission for short periods in small groups, but their long-term value in large populations is not established.

SYMPTOMATIC TREATMENT. Cold remedies are designed to relieve nasal congestion, to dry the nasal mucous membranes, and, less often, to relieve fever and pain. Since no one drug serves all of these functions, various mixtures are employed but they are subject to the disadvantages of all mixtures: When a therapeutic amount of one agent is given, other drugs in the mixture may be administered at higher or lower than optimal therapeutic levels. In addition, some mixtures contain more than one ingredient from a pharmacologic group, often in subtherapeutic quantities of each. It appears doubtful that a combination of two fractional doses is more effective or even as effective as a full dose of a single ingredient from a given pharmacologic group. On the other hand, if the patient suffers from multiple symptoms, particularly during the early stages of a cold, use of a mixture provides a more convenient and sometimes less expensive means of providing relief than use of several single-entity products. In practice, both doctors and patients find them convenient and without serious disadvantages (see the section on Mixtures).

Nasal decongestants relieve nasal stuffiness in the common cold and also may help to maintain patency of the eustachian tubes and sinus ostia, thereby inhibiting the development of secondary infection. Topical sprays provide the greatest symptomatic relief and have a lower incidence of side effects than systemic preparations but have the disadvantage of producing rebound congestion. Therefore, topical decongestants should be used for no more than three to five days. Adverse effects with systemic administration of decongestants are due to the alpha-adrenergic properties of these drugs. (See Drug Selection in the section on Rhinitis.)

Antihistamines are frequently used in cold preparations. The traditional antihistamines are used for their atropine-like properties, which dry nasal secretions, and their sedating effect, which may be desirable at bedtime. Although their efficacy for symptomatic relief of colds has been documented statistically in double-blind, randomized trials, the degree of relief was minimal and drowsiness occurred in 20% of patients (Howard et al, 1979). See Chapter 58, Histamine and Antihistamines.

It has been claimed that the anticholinergic properties of some antihistamines dry and thicken lower respiratory tract secretions, thus leading to cough, particularly in infants and small children, but this is probably not true. Nevertheless, it is sometimes desirable to discontinue the use of drying medications.

Caffeine is present in some cold preparations, although it may not sufficiently counteract antihistamine-induced drowsiness. If a decongestant is present in the formulation, the additional cardiac stimulation provided by caffeine may be undesirable.

See the Table for a listing of commonly used cold remedy products.

Drug Evaluations

DRUGS USED FOR RHINITIS

Adrenergic Drugs

EPHEDRINE HYDROCHLORIDE
[Vatronol]

EPHEDRINE SULFATE
[Efedron]

This nasal decongestant is effective topically and orally but is now seldom used. Adverse effects include central nervous system stimulation with tremor, nervousness, and insomnia; transient hypertension; palpitations; and, with chronic use of large doses, cardiomyopathy.

Hypersensitivity to ephedrine occurs rarely and is a specific contraindication. This drug should be given with caution to patients with heart disease, diabetes, hypertension, or hyperthyroidism. Aqueous solutions are preferred; oily solutions are obsolete and hazardous, especially in children, because of the danger of lipid pneumonia.

For a more detailed discussion, see the section on Drug Selection in the Introduction.

DOSAGE AND PREPARATIONS.
Oral: Adults, 25 to 50 mg every three to four hours; *children,* 3 mg/kg/24 hours in four to six divided doses.

EPHEDRINE SULFATE:
Generic. Capsules 25 and 50 mg; syrup 10 and 20 mg/5 ml (nonprescription).

Topical: A 0.5% to 3% solution, generally as drops, is applied as needed; drops should be instilled with the head in the lateral, head-low position. The drug also may be applied as a pack or tampon for diagnostic or surgical procedures.

EPHEDRINE HYDROCHLORIDE:
Vatronol (Vicks). Solution 0.5% in 15 and 30 ml containers (nonprescription).

EPHEDRINE SULFATE:
Generic. Solution 3% in 30 ml containers (nonprescription).
Efedron (Hyrex). Jelly (menthol) 0.6% in 20 g containers (nonprescription).

EPINEPHRINE HYDROCHLORIDE
[Adrenalin Chloride]

Epinephrine stimulates both alpha and beta receptors. It is useful topically to control epistaxis or to facilitate nasal surgery but is only rarely used today as a nasal decongestant. This drug should be applied by a physician.

Like other topical nasal decongestants, epinephrine frequently causes rebound nasal congestion. Systemic adverse reactions include anxiety, tremor, vomiting, pallor, restlessness, weakness, dizziness, throbbing headache, and palpitations. Central nervous system stimulation occurs less frequently than with ephedrine. Adverse effects disappear quickly when the drug is discontinued. Epinephrine should be used only with extreme caution with cocaine hydrochloride.

For a more detailed discussion, see the section on Drug Selection in the Introduction.

DOSAGE AND PREPARATIONS.
Topical: A 0.1% aqueous solution, instilled as drops or spray, is applied as needed (maximum in healthy adults, 1 ml/15 minutes). Drops should be instilled with the head in the lateral, head-low position. Some solutions may sting slightly due to the presence of sodium bisulfite added as an antioxidant.

Generic. Solution (aqueous) 0.1% in 1 and 30 ml containers.
Adrenalin Chloride (Parke-Davis). Solution (aqueous) 0.1% in 30 ml containers (nonprescription).

NAPHAZOLINE HYDROCHLORIDE
[Privine]

Naphazoline is an imidazoline derivative used topically to relieve local swelling and congestion of nasal mucous membranes. This direct-acting alpha-adrenergic agonist constricts dilated nasal arterioles and has little or no effect on beta-adrenergic receptors. The onset of action occurs in less than ten minutes and the duration is two to six hours.

ADVERSE REACTIONS AND PRECAUTIONS. Adverse reactions include severe rebound congestion with irritation and swelling of the nasal mucosa from continued use. Swelling is generally alleviated a few days after the medication is discontinued. Naphazoline also may cause paralysis of the nasal cilia and, occasionally, anosmia, smarting, and sneezing.

Systemic adverse reactions include cardiac arrhythmias and transient hypertension, bradycardia, sweating, and drowsiness; rebound hypotension may follow hypertension and bradycardia. Systemic absorption after overdosage has caused deep sleep and, in children, coma. Because of these effects, naphazoline is not recommended for use in children younger than 6 years and should be used with particular caution in older children and patients with cardiovascular disease. Safer drugs are preferred in these patients.

The solution should not be used in atomizers containing any aluminum parts. For a more detailed discussion of nasal decongestants, see the section on Drug Selection in the Introduction.

DOSAGE AND PREPARATIONS.
Topical: Two drops or two spray inhalations in each nostril no more often than every three hours (drops) or four to six hours (spray). The drops should be instilled with the head in the lateral, head-low position.
Generic. Solution 0.05% in 473 ml containers (nonprescription).
Privine (CIBA). Solution 0.05% in 20 and 473 ml containers; spray 0.05% in 15 ml containers (nonprescription).

OXYMETAZOLINE HYDROCHLORIDE
[Afrin, Dristan, Neo-Synephrine 12-Hour]

USES. Oxymetazoline relieves nasal congestion associated with nonseasonal allergic rhinitis, hay fever, and other forms of acute and chronic rhinitis or sinusitis. It is somewhat longer acting than the other topical imidazoline derivatives. The onset of action occurs in less than ten minutes and effects may persist for five hours or longer.

ADVERSE REACTIONS AND PRECAUTIONS. Untoward effects are milder than with shorter acting nasal decongestants and include stinging, burning, and dryness of the nasal mucosa; sneezing; headache; lightheadedness; insomnia; and palpitations. Effects on the central nervous system or blood pressure have not been reported, but overdosage is presumed to produce side effects similar to those of other imidazolines. Rebound congestion may result from prolonged or excessive use.

For a more detailed discussion of nasal decongestants, see the section on Drug Selection in the Introduction.

DOSAGE AND PREPARATIONS.
Topical: Adults and children over 6 years, two to four drops or two or three squeezes of spray (0.05% concentration) in each nostril in the morning and at bedtime; *children 2 to 5 years,* two or three drops (0.025% concentration) in each nostril. Some patients may require more frequent administration.
Generic. Spray 0.05% in 15 ml containers (nonprescription).
Afrin (Schering). Solution (drops) 0.025% (pediatric) and 0.05% in 20 ml containers; spray 0.05% in 15 and 30 ml (regular) and 15 ml (menthol) containers (nonprescription).
Dristan Long Lasting Nasal Spray (Whitehall). Spray 0.05% in 15 and 30 ml (regular and menthol) containers (nonprescription).
Neo-Synephrine 12-Hour (Winthrop-Breon). Spray 0.05% in 15 and 30 ml (regular) and 15 ml (menthol) containers; solution (drops) 0.025% (pediatric) and 0.05% in 30 ml containers (all forms nonprescription).

PHENYLEPHRINE HYDROCHLORIDE
[Alconefrin, Coricidin Nasal Mist, Neo-Synephrine Hydrochloride]

ACTIONS AND USES. Phenylephrine is one of the most widely used topical nasal decongestants. It has purely alpha-adrenergic effects in contrast to epinephrine, which stimulates both alpha and beta receptors. Onset of action is rapid and the duration ranges from 30 minutes to four hours. Oral dosage forms available in combination with antihistamines in cold remedy preparations (see Table) are not as effective for nasal congestion as the topical drug when the suggested dose is used.

ADVERSE REACTIONS AND PRECAUTIONS. Adverse reactions include all of the untoward effects associated with ephedrine or epinephrine, except that phenylephrine causes little or no central nervous system stimulation. A concentration of 0.25% is usually effective; stronger concentrations cause chronic swelling of the nasal mucosa within a few days and probably should not be instilled except under the direct supervision of a physician.

For a more detailed discussion of nasal decongestants, see the section on Drug Selection in the Introduction.

DOSAGE AND PREPARATIONS.

Topical: Adults and older children, several drops of a 0.25% to 1% solution instilled in each nostril with the head in the lateral, head-low position. Administration may be repeated in three or four hours if needed. Alternatively, the nasal spray may be used or a small amount of the jelly may be placed in each nostril and inhaled. *Infants,* the 0.125% solution is used.

    Generic. Solution 0.25% and 1% in 500 ml containers (nonprescription).

    Alconefrin (Webcon). Solution (drops) 0.16% (pediatric), 0.25%, and 0.5% in 30 ml containers; spray 0.25% in 30 ml containers (both forms nonprescription).

    Coricidin Nasal Mist (Schering). Spray 0.5% in 20 ml containers (nonprescription).

    Neo-Synephrine Hydrochloride (Winthrop-Breon). Solution (drops) 0.125% (pediatric) in 30 ml containers, 0.25% and 0.5% in 30 ml containers, and 1% in 30 and 474 ml containers; spray 0.25% in 15 ml containers and 0.5% in 30 ml (regular) and 15 ml (menthol) containers; jelly (water-soluble) 0.5% in 18.75 g containers (all forms nonprescription).

PHENYLPROPANOLAMINE HYDROCHLORIDE
[Propagest, Sucrets Cold Decongestant Formula]

Phenylpropanolamine is one of the most frequently used oral nasal decongestants. Its pharmacologic properties are similar to those of ephedrine. Phenylpropanolamine is approximately equal in potency to ephedrine but usually causes less central nervous system stimulation. This agent can cause transient elevations in blood pressure.

For a more detailed discussion of nasal decongestants, see the section on Drug Selection in the Introduction.

This drug is a common ingredient of weight reduction preparations (see Chapter 51, Agents Used in Obesity).

DOSAGE AND PREPARATIONS.

Oral: Adults, 25 mg every four hours (maximum, 150 mg/day). *Children 6 to 12 years,* 12.5 mg every four hours (maximum, 75 mg/day). Not recommended for *children under 6 years* except under the direct supervision of a physician.

    Generic. Capsules (timed-release) 75 mg; tablets 25 and 50 mg (both forms nonprescription).

    Propagest (Carnrick). Tablets 25 mg (nonprescription).

    Sucrets Cold Decongestant Formula (Beecham). Lozenges 25 mg (nonprescription).

PROPYLHEXEDRINE
[Benzedrex]

ACTIONS AND USES. Propylhexedrine is used as a vapor for its nasal decongestant effect. It produces considerably less central nervous system stimulation than ephedrine. This drug is believed to act similarly to amphetamine; it stimulates alpha-adrenergic receptors indirectly and has some minor beta-adrenergic agonist activity. The onset of its vasoconstrictor activity is rapid (one to five minutes) and effects persist for 30 minutes to two hours. Because of its wider margin of safety and relative freedom from toxic effects, propylhexedrine may be used when an ephedrine-like pressor or stimulant action is undesirable. This nasal decongestant is considered safe for self-medication by adults, but children should not have unsupervised access to an inhaler. The vapor may dry the nasal mucosa and interfere with ciliary action.

For a more detailed discussion of nasal decongestants, see the section on Drug Selection in the Introduction.

DOSAGE AND PREPARATIONS.

Topical (inhalation): Two inhalations (0.6 to 0.8 mg) in each nostril as needed. The inhaler usually retains its effectiveness for two to three months after opening. If the inhaler is cold, it should be warmed in the hand before use.

    Benzedrex (Menley & James). Inhaler 250 mg (nonprescription).

PSEUDOEPHEDRINE HYDROCHLORIDE
[Novafed, Sudafed]

PSEUDOEPHEDRINE SULFATE
[Afrinol]

This drug is a stereoisomer of ephedrine with similar properties and uses, although pseudoephedrine is not effective in asthma. Pseudoephedrine is used orally, usually in combination with an antihistamine, in patients with vasomotor rhinitis or serous otitis media with eustachian tube congestion, but the value of this or any decongestant is questionable for the latter condition.

ADVERSE REACTIONS. Adverse reactions are similar to those of ephedrine and other nasal decongestants, but central nervous system stimulation and transient elevations in blood pressure occur less frequently and are less severe. There have been reports that antihistamine/pseudoephedrine combinations produced hallucinations in children, but dosages exceeding those usually recommended were administered or patients had predisposing factors, such as febrile conditions.

For a more detailed discussion of nasal decongestants, see the section on Drug Selection in the Introduction.

DOSAGE AND PREPARATIONS.

Oral: Adults, 60 mg three or four times daily; *children,* 4 mg/kg daily in four divided doses.

    PSEUDOEPHEDRINE HYDROCHLORIDE:

    Generic. Capsules (timed-release) 120 mg; liquid 30 mg/5 ml; tablets 30 and 60 mg (all forms nonprescription).

    Novafed (Merrell Dow). Capsules (timed-release) 120 mg; liquid 30 mg/5 ml (alcohol 7.5%) (nonprescription).

    Sudafed (Burroughs Wellcome). Capsules (timed-release) 120 mg; liquid 30 mg/5 ml; tablets 30 and 60 mg (all forms nonprescription).

PSEUDOEPHEDRINE SULFATE:
Afrinol (Schering). Tablets (timed-release) 120 mg (nonprescription).

TETRAHYDROZOLINE HYDROCHLORIDE
[Tyzine]

This imidazoline derivative is effective topically for temporary relief of nasal congestion. It acts within a few minutes and the duration of effect is four to eight hours.

ADVERSE REACTIONS. The most frequent adverse reactions are burning, stinging, and dryness of the mucosa; sneezing; headache; drowsiness; weakness; tremors; lightheadedness; insomnia; and palpitations. Prolonged or excessive use may cause rebound congestion. Adverse effects observed especially with overdosage include hypertension, bradycardia, severe drowsiness with sweating, rebound hypotension, and cardiac arrhythmias. Overdosage may produce severe drowsiness in young children. Because of these effects, tetrahydrozoline should be avoided in infants under 2 years and in patients with cardiovascular disease.

For a more detailed discussion of nasal decongestants, see the section on Drug Selection in the Introduction.

DOSAGE AND PREPARATIONS.
Topical: *Adults and children 6 years or older,* two to four drops of the 0.1% solution instilled in each nostril no more often than every three hours. Tetrahydrozoline should be used cautiously, if at all, in *children under 6 years* and should not be used in *infants under 2 years.* The manufacturer's suggested dosage is: *Children 2 to 6 years,* two to three drops of the 0.05% solution instilled in each nostril, with the head in the lateral, head-low position, at intervals of four to six hours.

Generic. Solution.
Tyzine (Key). Solution 0.05% (pediatric) in 15 ml containers and 0.1% in 15 and 474 ml containers.

XYLOMETAZOLINE HYDROCHLORIDE
[Neo-Synephrine II, Otrivin]

This imidazoline derivative is effective topically for temporary relief of nasal congestion. The onset of action is five to ten minutes and the duration of effect is five to six hours.

Untoward reactions are generally mild and infrequent and include local stinging or burning, sneezing, dryness of the nose, headache, insomnia, drowsiness, and palpitations.

Chronic swelling of the nasal mucosa has been reported with prolonged or excessive administration.

The solution should not be used in atomizers containing any aluminum parts. For a more detailed discussion of nasal decongestants, see the section on Drug Selection in the Introduction.

DOSAGE AND PREPARATIONS.
Topical: *Adults,* two or three drops of the 0.1% solution or one or two inhalations of the 0.1% nasal spray in each nostril every eight to ten hours. *Children 2 to 12 years,* two or three drops of the 0.05% solution in each nostril every four to six hours. *Children under 2 years,* not recommended.

Generic. Spray 0.1% (nonprescription).
Neo-Synephrine II (Winthrop-Breon). Solution (drops) 0.05% (pediatric) and 0.1% in 30 ml containers; spray (regular and menthol) 0.1% in 15 ml containers (all forms nonprescription).
Otrivin (Geigy). Solution (drops) 0.05% (pediatric) and 0.1% in 20 ml containers; spray 0.1% in 15 ml containers (both forms nonprescription).

Prophylactic Agent

CROMOLYN SODIUM
[Nasalcrom]

ACTIONS AND USES. The proposed mechanism of action of cromolyn is inhibition of the release of histamine and other allergic mediators from mast cells by blocking calcium transport across the mast cell membrane. Use of the nasal spray prevents symptoms of seasonal allergic rhinitis (runny nose and postnasal drip) but up to one week may be required before relief is obtained. Alleviation of sneezing, nasal congestion, and eye irritation is variable; throat irritation does not respond significantly. Cromolyn is usually less beneficial after symptoms have developed but, in some patients with mild symptoms, it may prevent severe nasal congestion. The presence of high preseasonal concentrations of IgE ragweed antibody correlates with significant reduction in symptoms and may predict the drug's effectiveness (Welsh et al, 1977).

Cromolyn's effectiveness in seasonal allergic rhinitis is similar to that of the antihistamines and is less than that of the topical corticosteroids. Patients with chronic allergic rhinitis are less likely to respond. The drug is ineffective in nonallergic rhinitis and conditions such as nasal polyps in which obstruction of nasal passages prevents access of the drug to its site of action (*Med Lett Drugs Ther*, 1983). The lack of serious adverse reactions is an advantage of cromolyn over other agents.

See also the section on Drug Selection in the Introduction.

ADVERSE REACTIONS AND PRECAUTIONS. Side effects

generally are mild and rarely require discontinuation of treatment. Local effects (nasal stinging, burning, irritation, or sneezing) occur in 2% to 10% of patients. Headache and an unpleasant taste have been reported in about 2% of patients. Postnasal drip and epistaxis are observed in less than 1% of patients. Rash and anaphylaxis are very rare.

Cromolyn should be used cautiously in pregnant and lactating women, for its safety in these patients has not been established unequivocally (FDA Pregnancy Category B).

Because cromolyn must be administered four to six times a day for maximal effectiveness, compliance is a problem. Patients should be informed that significant effects may not be observed for one week in patients with seasonal allergic rhinitis or for two to four weeks (if at all) in patients with chronic allergic rhinitis. Therefore, antihistamines and/or nasal decongestants may be required until the effects of cromolyn are noted, particularly in the latter condition. The dose of these drugs then may be reduced or their use discontinued.

PHARMACOKINETICS. Following application of the nasal spray, about 7% of the dose is absorbed into the blood stream, mainly through the gastrointestinal tract. About 80% of the unabsorbed portion is recovered from the feces. The plasma half-life is 1 to 1.5 hours.

Cromolyn is not metabolized. Approximately 50% of the amount absorbed is recovered in the urine and the remaining one-half in the bile.

DOSAGE AND PREPARATIONS.
Topical: Adults and children over 6 years, one spray (5.2 mg) in each nostril four to six times a day. The patient should inhale through the nose during administration of the spray. Nasal passages should be cleared (using a nasal decongestant if needed) prior to the use of cromolyn.

For seasonal allergic rhinitis, prophylactic therapy should be initiated at least one week before exposure to antigen or the expected occurrence of symptoms, and use should be continued throughout the period of exposure.

Nasalcrom (Fisons). Solution 40 mg/ml (5.2 mg/actuation) with a metered spray device.

Topical Corticosteroids

DEXAMETHASONE SODIUM PHOSPHATE
[Decadron Turbinaire]

Dexamethasone was the first intranasal corticosteroid available in this country and is as effective as the newer agents, beclomethasone and flunisolide, for the treatment of rhinitis and certain other nasal disorders. However, intranasal dexamethasone is absorbed and can cause systemic adverse effects, including mild adrenocortical suppression, if used for more than 30 days. Therefore, topical use of this drug is limited to a maximum of 30 days. Adrenocortical function usually returns to normal a few days after the nasal spray is discontinued but can be considerably delayed. Excessive intranasal application rarely causes nasal mucosal atrophy or ulceration.

The need for dexamethasone nasal spray has been greatly diminished by the availability of beclomethasone and flunisolide, which do not suppress adrenocortical function in recommended doses (Busse, 1983). See also the section on Drug Selection in the Introduction.

Dexamethasone is classified in FDA Pregnancy Category C.

DOSAGE AND PREPARATIONS.
Topical: Adults, two sprays in each nostril two or three times daily (maximum, 12 sprays). *Children 6 to 12 years,* one or two sprays in each nostril twice daily (maximum, eight sprays). When the maximal response is obtained (usually in one to two weeks), the dose is reduced to the lowest level that maintains symptomatic control.

Decadron Turbinaire (Merck Sharp & Dohme). Aerosol providing 84 mcg/actuation (equivalent to base).

BECLOMETHASONE DIPROPIONATE
[Beconase, Vancenase]

This halogenated corticosteroid has a marked anti-inflammatory effect when applied topically to the nasal mucosa. The nasal spray is effective and safe for seasonal and nonseasonal allergic rhinitis; for nonallergic disorders, such as nasal polyps and rhinitis medicamentosa; as well as for the rhinitis of pregnancy (Brogden et al, 1984). Nonallergic rhinitis with eosinophilia also may respond. This drug may be less useful for vasomotor rhinitis. Beclomethasone is more effective than antihistamines, decongestants, or cromolyn for prophylaxis and treatment of these disorders. Rhinorrhea, nasal pruritus, postnasal drainage, nasal congestion, and sneezing respond to therapy. Effectiveness is reduced when nasal congestion is severe, and a short course of topical nasal decongestants or an oral corticosteroid may be required prior to use of beclomethasone. Ocular symptoms are not relieved.

Significant relief of symptoms occurs in one to three days in patients with seasonal allergic rhinitis; full effects are not attained for a week or longer. In patients with nonseasonal rhinitis, relief may require one week and full effects are not observed for two to three weeks. Regular daily administration is required for maximal effectiveness.

An aqueous suspension of beclomethasone that contains no

Freon is being investigated. This nonpressurized aqueous form offers no advantages over the pressurized spray and transient nasal stinging occurs more often. However, some patients may tolerate the wet suspension better than the dry aerosol spray.

ADVERSE REACTIONS AND PRECAUTIONS. The incidence of minor adverse reactions is high; these effects probably are due to the vehicle, since the incidence is the same as with a placebo. Initial application produces nasal stinging, irritation, and burning that usually subside with continued use. Other adverse effects include sneezing, headache, dry nose, and nasal bleeding. Nasal candidiasis has not been reported.

Adrenocortical suppression does not occur with usual doses but is possible with large doses. Mucosal atrophy does not appear to occur after prolonged use.

Topical steroids should be used with caution or avoided in patients with active or quiescent tuberculosis, untreated bacterial infections, and systemic fungal or viral infections. Topical steroids should be used with caution, if at all, in patients with local nasal infections or ocular herpes simplex. It may inhibit wound healing and should be used with caution in patients with recent nasal trauma or surgery. Nasal polyps decrease in size during continuous use of this drug but may enlarge after cessation of therapy or in the presence of a respiratory infection.

If no significant response occurs, corticosteroid nasal sprays should be discontinued after three weeks when used for allergic rhinitis or after four or more weeks when used for nasal polyps.

This drug is classified in FDA Pregnancy Category C.

See also the section on Drug Selection in the Introduction.

PHARMACOKINETICS. Although some of the drug is absorbed from the nasal mucosa, beclomethasone is rapidly metabolized after absorption, primarily to inactive metabolites, which explains in part the low incidence of systemic side effects. Little unchanged drug is recovered in the urine or feces.

DOSAGE AND PREPARATIONS.

Topical: Adults and children 12 years and older, one inhalation (42 mcg) in each nostril two to four times daily (total dose, 168 to 336 mcg/day). When the maximal response is obtained (usually in one to two weeks), the dose is reduced to the lowest level that maintains symptomatic control. The intranasal spray must be placed properly to avoid localized deposition of drug on walls of the mucosa.

Beconase (Glaxo), **Vancenase** (Schering). Aerosol providing 42 mcg/actuation.

FLUNISOLIDE
[Nasalide]

The efficacy, indications, actions, adverse reactions, and precautions of flunisolide are similar to those of beclomethasone. Unlike beclomethasone, this preparation does not contain Freon and is delivered in a propylene glycol vehicle, which moistens the nasal mucosa and does not cause dryness.

ADVERSE REACTIONS. The most common adverse reactions of flunisolide nasal spray are stinging and burning (incidence, more than 40%) that last only a few seconds after application.

This drug is classified in FDA Pregnancy Category C.

See also the section on Drug Selection in the Introduction and the evaluation on Beclomethasone Dipropionate.

PHARMACOKINETICS. Flunisolide is well absorbed. Only 50% of a dose reaches the systemic circulation because of first-pass metabolism in the liver; the drug is converted rapidly to less active metabolites and conjugates. This explains in part the low incidence of systemic side effects. The plasma half-life is one to two hours. About one-half of the absorbed drug is recovered in the urine and one-half in the feces. The onset of action is usually two to five days.

DOSAGE AND PREPARATIONS.

Topical: Adults, initially, two sprays (50 mcg) in each nostril two times daily. If needed, this dose may be increased to two sprays in each nostril three times daily (maximum dose, 400 mcg/day). *Children 6 to 14 years,* initially, one spray (25 mcg) in each nostril three times daily or two sprays in each nostril two times daily (maximum dose, 200 mcg/day). This drug is not recommended in *children less than 6 years.* When the maximal response is obtained (usually in one to two weeks), the dose is then reduced to the lowest level that maintains symptomatic control.

Nasalide (Syntex). Spray providing 25 mcg/actuation.

BUDESONIDE

This investigational agent is similar to beclomethasone in efficacy, indications, actions, adverse reactions, and precautions (Clissold and Heel, 1984).

PHARMACOKINETICS. Budesonide is well absorbed. It undergoes significant first-pass metabolism in the liver and is converted rapidly to compounds with little systemic activity, which explains in part the low incidence of systemic side effects. The plasma half-life is approximately two hours. Little unchanged drug is recovered in the urine.

DOSAGE AND PREPARATIONS.

Topical: Adults, the usual dose for rhinitis is 100 mcg (two actuations) in each nostril twice daily (Clissold and Heel, 1984).

Budesonide (Merck Sharp & Dohme). (Investigational drug)

FLUOCORTIN BUTYL

This investigational agent is similar to beclomethasone in efficacy, indications, actions, adverse reactions, and precautions (Hartley et al, 1985). Following systemic absorption, it is metabolized rapidly by nonspecific tissue esterases to an inactive C-21 corticosteroid. Therefore, fluocortin butyl is highly active topically and almost inactive systemically.

The potential advantage of fluocortin butyl is that larger doses can be administered safely than is possible with beclomethasone, flunisolide, or budesonide (investigational agent) (all of which may suppress the HPA axis in large doses). (Investigational drug)

DRUGS USED FOR COUGH

Opioids

CODEINE PHOSPHATE

CODEINE SULFATE

Codeine, the reference compound with which other antitussives are compared, acts centrally to depress cough. This opioid is effective orally for acute cough associated with a variety of diseases and irritants. Codeine is more effective than dextromethorphan for severe acute cough.

This drug is metabolized more slowly than morphine. The plasma half-life is 2.5 to 3 hours.

ADVERSE REACTIONS AND PRECAUTIONS. Antitussive doses are generally well tolerated, but nausea, vomiting, constipation, dizziness, palpitations, drowsiness, pruritus, and, rarely, sweating and agitation have been reported.

Dependence is uncommon after antitussive use because of the short duration of therapy and the small doses required. However, codeine is sometimes abused since it is readily available in many cough mixtures. It is classified as a Schedule II drug under the Controlled Substances Act; mixtures containing codeine are classified as Schedule V substances.

Patients with productive cough generally should not be given cough suppressants. As with other narcotic analgesics, respiratory depression occurs with overdosage. This is a particular problem in children, especially those under 5 years, since the dosage schedule for the opioid antitussives has been established empirically. Infants may be especially sensitive to the respiratory depressant effects of narcotics. Respiratory depression can be reversed by the opioid antagonist, naloxone (see Chapter 80, Drugs Used in the Treatment of Poisoning).

This drug is classified in FDA Pregnancy Category C.

DOSAGE AND PREPARATIONS.

Oral: Adults, 10 to 20 mg every four to six hours (maximum, 120 mg/day) as necessary. *Children,* 1 to 1.5 mg/kg daily divided into four to six doses (maximum, 60 mg/day). For *children 6 to 12 years,* 5 to 10 mg every four to six hours (maximum, 60 mg/day); *2 to 6 years,* 2.5 to 5 mg every four to

six hours (maximum, 30 mg/day). Codeine is rarely indicated as a cough suppressant in children.

Generic. Tablets 15, 30, and 60 mg. The phosphate salt is much more soluble in water than the sulfate salt.

See the section on Mixtures for a listing of combination products containing codeine.

HYDROCODONE BITARTRATE

The usefulness of hydrocodone as an antitussive is similar to that of codeine; it is about three times more potent on a milligram basis. Accordingly, the dependence liability of hydrocodone is also greater than that of codeine. This antitussive is classified as a Schedule II drug under the Controlled Substances Act.

The most common adverse reactions are nausea, dizziness, and constipation. Dryness of the pharynx and occasional tightness of the chest have been reported. Other adverse reactions and precautions are the same as those reported for codeine. This drug is classified in FDA Pregnancy Category C.

DOSAGE AND PREPARATIONS.

Oral: Adults, 5 to 10 mg three or four times daily. *Children,* 0.6 mg/kg daily in three or four divided doses. Hydrocodone is rarely indicated as a cough suppressant in children.

Generic. Tablets 5 mg.

See the section on Mixtures for a listing of combination products containing hydrocodone.

Nonopiates

BENZONATATE
[Tessalon]

ACTIONS AND USES. Benzonatate is related structurally to tetracaine and has local anesthetic activity when applied topically to the mucosa. It is believed to exert its antitussive action by anesthetizing stretch or cough receptors in the respiratory tract, as well as by a central mechanism.

Benzonatate is safe and effective in relieving acute cough associated with a variety of diseases and irritants. Onset of action is 15 to 30 minutes after oral administration and the duration of effect is three to eight hours.

ADVERSE REACTIONS. Adverse reactions are mild and include rash, constipation, nasal congestion, slight vertigo, headache, nausea, drowsiness, and hypersensitivity reactions. The local anesthetic effect of benzonatate produces numbness of the mouth, tongue, and pharynx if the capsules are chewed. This drug should not be used in infants; because of the numbness produced, infants may have difficulty swallowing, and aspiration may result. Benzonatate has a very unpleasant taste.

DOSAGE AND PREPARATIONS.
Oral: Adults and children over 10 years, 100 to 200 mg three to six times daily; *under 10 years*, not recommended.
  Tessalon (DuPont). Capsules (liquid-filled) 100 mg.

DEXTROMETHORPHAN HYDROBROMIDE
[Benylin DM, Cremacoat I, Delsym]

This synthetic non-narcotic cough suppressant, the dextro-isomer of the codeine analogue of levorphanol, appears to be as effective as codeine except for severe acute cough and, like codeine, acts centrally to elevate the cough threshold. It does not have addictive, analgesic, or sedative actions and does not produce respiratory depression with usual doses. Dextromethorphan is the safest antitussive available and is present in most over-the-counter cough preparations. Timed-release preparations deliver the drug from liquid ion-exchange complexes over 9 to 12 hours.

ADVERSE REACTIONS. Adverse reactions are mild and occur infrequently. Slight drowsiness, nausea, and dizziness are most common. Central nervous system and respiratory depression may occur with very large doses, but no fatalities have been reported. Presumably, respiratory depression could be reversed by naloxone, but clinical data to substantiate this are not available.

DOSAGE AND PREPARATIONS.
Oral: (Regular preparation) *Adults,* 10 to 20 mg every four hours or 30 mg every six to eight hours (maximum, 120 mg/day). *Children,* 1 mg/kg daily in three or four divided doses. Alternatively, *children 6 to 12 years*, 5 to 10 mg every four hours or 15 mg every six to eight hours (maximum, 60 mg/24 hours); *2 to 6 years*, 2.5 to 5 mg every four hours or 7.5 mg every six to eight hours (maximum, 30 mg/day).
  (Timed-release preparation) *Adults,* 60 mg twice daily. *Children 6 to 12 years*, 30 mg twice daily; *2 to 6 years*, 15 mg twice daily.
  Generic. Powder; syrup 10 mg/5 ml (nonprescription).
  Benylin DM (Parke-Davis). Syrup 10 mg/5 ml (alcohol 5%) (nonprescription).
  Cremacoat 1 (Vicks). Syrup 10 mg/5 ml (alcohol 10%) (nonprescription).
  Delsym (McNeil). Suspension (timed-release) dextromethorphan polistirex equivalent to 30 mg/5 ml of hydrobromide (alcohol free) in 90 ml containers (nonprescription).
  See the section on Mixtures for a listing of combination products containing dextromethorphan.

DIPHENHYDRAMINE HYDROCHLORIDE
[Benylin]

Diphenhydramine is an amino alkyl ether antihistamine with limited central antitussive action. Like most antihistamines, it has a moderate sedative effect and some anticholinergic activity. Diphenhydramine is an effective antitussive only in doses that produce significant sedation. (See Chapter 58, Histamine and Antihistamines.)

DOSAGE AND PREPARATIONS.
Oral: Adults, 25 mg every four hours (maximum, 150 mg/24 hours). *Children 6 to 11 years,* 12.5 mg every four hours or 5 mg/kg/day in four divided doses (maximum, 75 mg/day). *Children 2 to 6 years,* dose must be individualized. This drug is not recommended for *children under 2 years* except under the direct supervision of a physician.
  Benylin (Parke-Davis), **Generic.** Syrup 12.5 mg/5 ml (alcohol 5% **[Benylin]**) (nonprescription).

Expectorant

GUAIFENESIN (Glyceryl Guaiacolate)
[Breonesin, Glycotuss, Robitussin, 2/G]

Guaifenesin is the most widely used expectorant. Doses up to ten times the usual amount probably act as an emetic, increase the volume of respiratory tract fluids, and may facilitate the transport of mucus. At lower doses, few beneficial effects have been demonstrated in patients with asthma, bronchitis, or other respiratory disorders (Medon and Holshouser, 1985). Also see the discussion of expectorants in the section on Cough in the Introduction.

Nausea and drowsiness occur rarely. Guaifenesin may produce a false-positive response for urinary 5-hydroxyindoleacetic acid (5-HIAA) and vanillylmandelic acid (VMA).

DOSAGE AND PREPARATIONS.
Oral: The dosage suggested by the manufacturers is: *Adults,* 200 to 400 mg every four hours (maximum, 2.4 g/day). *Children 6 to 12 years,* 50 to 100 mg every four to six hours (maximum, 600 mg/day). This drug should be given to *children under 2 years* only under the direct supervision of a physician.
  Generic. Syrup 100 mg/5 ml (nonprescription).
  Breonesin (Winthrop-Breon). Capsules 200 mg (nonprescription).
  Glycotuss (Vale). Tablets 100 mg; syrup 100 mg/5 ml (both forms nonprescription).

Robitussin (Robins), *2/G* (Merrell Dow). Syrup 100 mg/5 ml (alcohol 3.5%) (nonprescription).

See the section on Mixtures for a listing of combination products containing Guaifenesin.

MIXTURES

Single-entity products are preferred to mixtures for most patients with rhinitis or cough. Certain combination products are useful and convenient in patients with multiple symptoms who do not respond adequately to a single drug. If a mixture is to be used, it should meet the following criteria: (1) It contains no more than three active ingredients from different pharmacologic groups and no more than one active ingredient from each pharmacologic group. (2) Each active ingredient is present in an effective and safe concentration and contributes to the treatment for which the product is used. (3) The product is used only when multiple symptoms are present concurrently. (4) The product is therapeutically appropriate for the type and severity of symptoms being treated. (5) The possible adverse reactions of the components are taken into consideration.

Many mixtures popular with the lay public and physicians for treatment of upper respiratory tract disorders do not meet these criteria. Moreover, physicians should be aware that a product may be reformulated without a change in the brand name.

The mixtures listed in the following sections and in the Table are representative; no attempt has been made to include all available mixtures used for rhinitis or the common cold.

Mixtures Containing Nasal Decongestants

Mixtures combining a nasal decongestant with one or more other drugs are available for topical or oral use. Frequently, the added drug is an antihistamine, analgesic, or a second nasal decongestant. Other compounds occasionally present include atropine or other anticholinergic agents, various wetting compounds, and quaternary ammonium salts.

If relief of several respiratory symptoms is sought (eg, in hay fever), the combination of an antihistamine and adrenergic agent may be beneficial. When headache accompanies the nasal congestion, products containing an analgesic and a decongestant may be useful.

If nasal decongestion is the only desired effect, there is no good evidence that any of the available mixtures is more effective than a single-entity drug. Moreover, there is evidence that the other agents in the mixture either are detrimental or do not assist in relieving nasal decongestion and often increase the cost. For example, topical antihistamines provide limited added relief of nasal congestion when combined with decongestants and, even when administered orally, they produce little or no shrinkage of the engorged nasal mucosa. Topical mixtures are used and abused widely by both the medical profession and the lay public. Careful comparative evaluation of these mixtures with single-entity decongestants has not been made. However, because a mixture containing a nasal

decongestant cannot be expected to be more effective than the same quantity of the decongestant drug alone, the use of a mixture for relief of nasal congestion instead of a single-entity drug should be discouraged.

The preparation chosen and the total duration of use must be determined by the physician on the basis of experience and the response of the patient. Since individual tolerance and the tendency to develop chronic mucosal congestion with prolonged use vary among patients, administration of these agents should be regulated on an individual basis.

The following topical mixtures are listed for information only.

4-Way Nasal (Bristol-Myers). Spray containing phenylephrine hydrochloride 0.5%, naphazoline hydrochloride 0.05%, and pyrilamine maleate 0.2% in 15 and 30 ml containers (regular and menthol) (nonprescription).

Dristan Nasal Mist (Whitehall). Spray containing phenylephrine hydrochloride 0.5% and pheniramine maleate 0.2% in 15 and 30 ml containers (nonprescription).

For oral mixtures, see the Table.

Mixtures Containing Antitussives

Many of the preparations listed in this section appear to have been formulated for the symptomatic treatment of minor respiratory disorders rather than for specific relief of cough. Thus, in addition to an antitussive, these mixtures usually contain one or more ingredients classified as expectorants, one or more sympathomimetic agents as bronchodilators or nasal decongestants, and antihistamines. The effectiveness of such mixtures compared to single-entity preparations is not known. The physician should be aware of the ingredients in the formulation; for example, the brand name often does not indicate that the mixture contains codeine or other narcotic antitussives.

The following commonly used preparations are listed for information only; inclusion in the list does not indicate approval or recommendation for use.

Antitussive Mixtures Containing Codeine (All Schedule V Preparations)

Actifed W/Codeine (Burroughs Wellcome). Each 5 ml of syrup contains codeine phosphate 10 mg, pseudoephedrine hydrochloride 30 mg, and triprolidine hydrochloride 1.25 mg (alcohol 4.3%).

Ambenyl (Marion). Each 5 ml of syrup contains codeine phosphate 10 mg and bromodiphenhydramine hydrochloride 12.5 mg (alcohol 5%).

Calcidrine (Abbott). Each 5 ml of syrup contains codeine 8.4 mg and calcium iodide anhydrous 152 mg (alcohol 6%).

Cheracol (Upjohn). Each 5 ml of syrup contains codeine phosphate 10 mg and guaifenesin 100 mg (alcohol 4.75%).

Dimetane DC (Robins). Each 5 ml of syrup contains codeine phosphate 10 mg, brompheniramine maleate 2 mg, and phenylpropanolamine hydrochloride 12.5 mg (alcohol 0.95%).

Isoclor Expectorant (Fisons). Each 5 ml of syrup contains codeine phosphate 10 mg, guaifenesin 100 mg, and pseudoephedrine hydrochloride 30 mg (alcohol 5%).

Naldecon-CX (Bristol). Each 5 ml of suspension contains codeine phosphate 10 mg, phenylpropanolamine hydrochloride 18 mg, and guaifenesin 200 mg.

Novahistine Expectorant (Lakeside). Each 5 ml of liquid contains codeine phosphate 10 mg, guaifenesin 100 mg, and pseudoephedrine hydrochloride 30 mg (alcohol 7.5%).

Novahistine-DH (Lakeside). Each 5 ml of liquid contains codeine phosphate 10 mg, chlorpheniramine maleate 2 mg, and pseudoephedrine hydrochloride 30 mg (alcohol 5%).

Nucofed (Beecham). Each capsule or 5 ml of syrup contains codeine phosphate 20 mg and pseudoephedrine hydrochloride 60 mg.

Nucofed Expectorant (Beecham). Each 5 ml of syrup contains codeine phosphate 20 mg or 10 mg (pediatric), guaifenesin 200 mg or 100 mg (pediatric), and pseudoephedrine hydrochloride 60 mg or 30 mg (pediatric) (alcohol 12.5% or 7.5% [pediatric]).

Pediacof (Winthrop-Breon). Each 5 ml of syrup contains codeine phosphate 5 mg, chlorpheniramine maleate 0.75 mg, phenylephrine hydrochloride 2.5 mg, and potassium iodide 75 mg (alcohol 5%).

Penntuss (Pennwalt). Each 5 ml of liquid (timed-release) contains codeine polistirex equivalent to 10 mg of base and chlorpheniramine polistirex equivalent to 4 mg of maleate.

Phenergan Expectorant W/Codeine (Wyeth). Each 5 ml of syrup contains codeine phosphate 10 mg and promethazine hydrochloride 6.25 mg (alcohol 7%).

Phenergan-VC W/Codeine (Wyeth). Each 5 ml of expectorant contains same formulation as *Phenergan Expectorant W/Codeine* plus phenylephrine hydrochloride 5 mg.

Robitussin A-C (Robins). Each 5 ml of syrup contains codeine phosphate 10 mg and guaifenesin 100 mg (alcohol 3.5%).

Robitussin-DAC (Robins). Each 5 ml of syrup contains codeine phosphate 10 mg, guaifenesin 100 mg, and pseudoephedrine hydrochloride 30 mg (alcohol 1.4%).

SK-Terpin Hydrate and Codeine Elixir (Smith Kline & French). Each 5 ml of elixir contains codeine 10 mg and terpin hydrate 85 mg (alcohol 40%).

Triaminic Expectorant with Codeine (Dorsey). Each 5 ml of syrup contains codeine phosphate 10 mg, guaifenesin 100 mg, and phenylpropanolamine hydrochloride 12.5 mg (alcohol 5%).

Tussar-2, *Tussar SF* (USV). Each 5 ml of syrup contains codeine phosphate 10 mg, carbetapentane citrate 7.5 mg, chlorpheniramine maleate 2 mg, guaifenesin 50 mg, sodium citrate 130 mg, and citric acid 20 mg (alcohol 5%) (*Tussar-2*) or 12% (*Tussar-SF* [sugar-free]).

Tussi-Organidin (Wallace). Each 5 ml of liquid contains codeine phosphate 10 mg and iodinated glycerol 30 mg.

Antitussive Mixtures Containing Hydrocodone (All Schedule III Preparations)

Hycodan (DuPont). Each tablet or 5 ml of syrup contains hydrocodone bitartrate 5 mg and homatropine methylbromide 1.5 mg.

Hycomine (DuPont). Each 5 ml of syrup or 10 ml of pediatric syrup contains hydrocodone bitartrate 5 mg and phenylpropanolamine hydrochloride 25 mg.

Hycomine Compound (DuPont). Each tablet contains hydrocodone bitartrate 5 mg, phenylephrine hydrochloride 10 mg, chlorpheniramine maleate 2 mg, acetaminophen 250 mg, and caffeine 30 mg.

Hycotuss Expectorant (DuPont). Each 5 ml of syrup contains hydrocodone bitartrate 5 mg and guaifenesin 100 mg (alcohol 10%).

Ru-Tuss w/Hydrocodone (Boots). Each 5 ml of liquid contains hydrocodone bitartrate 1.67 mg, phenylpropanolamine hydrochloride 3.3 mg, phenylephrine hydrochloride 5 mg, pyrilamine maleate 3.3 mg, and pheniramine maleate 3.3 mg (alcohol 5%).

Tussend (Merrell Dow). Each tablet or 5 ml of liquid contains hydrocodone bitartrate 5 mg and pseudoephedrine hydrochloride 60 mg (alcohol 5%, liquid).

Tussend Expectorant (Merrell Dow). Each 5 ml of liquid contains same formulation as *Tussend* plus guaifenesin 200 mg (alcohol 12.5%).

Tussionex (Pennwalt). Each capsule, tablet, or 5 ml of suspension contains hydrocodone 5 mg and phenyltoloxamine 10 mg (as cationic exchange resin complexes).

Antitussive Mixtures Containing Dextromethorphan

Anatuss (Mayrand). Each 5 ml of syrup contains dextromethorphan hydrobromide 5 mg, phenylpropanolamine hydrochloride 12.5 mg, phenylephrine hydrochloride 5 mg, chlorpheniramine maleate 2 mg, guaifenesin 25 mg, and acetaminophen 130 mg (alcohol 12%); each tablet contains dextromethorphan hydrobromide 10 mg, phenylpropanolamine hydrochloride 25 mg, phenylephrine hydrochloride 5 mg, chlorpheniramine maleate 2 mg, guaifenesin 50 mg, and acetaminophen 300 mg.

Benylin DME (Parke-Davis). Each 5 ml of liquid contains dextromethorphan hydrobromide 5 mg and guaifenesin 100 mg (alcohol 5%) (nonprescription).

Cerose-DM Expectorant (Wyeth). Each 5 ml of syrup contains dextromethorphan hydrobromide 10 mg, phenylephrine hydrochloride 5 mg, phenindamine tartrate 5 mg, guaiacolsulfonate potassium 86 mg, sodium citrate 195 mg, citric acid 65 mg, and ipecac (alcohol 2.5%) (nonprescription).

Cheracol D (Upjohn). Each 5 ml of liquid contains dextromethorphan hydrobromide 10 mg and guaifenesin 100 mg (alcohol 4.75%) (nonprescription).

Dimacol (Robins). Each capsule or 5 ml of liquid contains dextromethorphan hydrobromide 15 mg, pseudoephedrine hydrochloride 30 mg, and guaifenesin 100 mg (alcohol 4.75% liquid) (nonprescription).

Dorcol Pediatric Cough Syrup (Dorsey). Each 5 ml of syrup contains dextromethorphan hydrobromide 5 mg, guaifenesin 50 mg, and pseudoephedrine hydrochloride 15 mg (alcohol 5%) (nonprescription).

Novahistine DMX (Lakeside). Each 5 ml of liquid contains dextromethorphan hydrobromide 10 mg, pseudoephedrine hydrochloride 30 mg, and guaifenesin 100 mg (alcohol 10%) (nonprescription).

Phenergan w/Dextromethorphan (Wyeth). Each 5 ml of syrup contains dextromethorphan hydrobromide 15 mg and promethazine hydrochloride 6.25 mg (alcohol 7%).

Robitussin-CF (Robins). Each 5 ml of syrup contains dextromethorphan hydrobromide 10 mg, guaifenesin 100 mg, and phenylpropanolamine hydrochloride 12.5 mg (alcohol 4.75%) (nonprescription).

Robitussin-DM (Robins). Each 5 ml of syrup contains dextromethorphan hydrobromide 15 mg and guaifenesin 100 mg (alcohol 1.4%) (nonprescription).

Rondec-DM (Ross). Each 5 ml of syrup contains dextromethorphan hydrobromide 15 mg, carbinoxamine maleate 4 mg and pseudoephedrine hydrochloride 60 mg (alcohol <0.6%); each milliliter of drops contains dextromethorphan hydrobromide 4 mg, carbinoxamine maleate 2 mg, and pseudoephedrine hydrochloride 25 mg (alcohol <0.6%).

Ry-Tuss Expectorant (Boots). Each 5 ml of liquid contains dextromethorphan hydrobromide 10 mg, guaifenesin 100 mg, and pseudoephedrine hydrochloride 30 mg (alcohol 10%).

Triaminic DM (Dorsey). Each 5 ml of liquid contains dextromethorphan hydrobromide 10 mg and phenylpropanolamine hydrochloride 12.5 mg.

Triaminicol Multisymptom (Dorsey). Each tablet or 5 ml of syrup contains dextromethorphan hydrobromide 10 mg, chlorpheniramine maleate 2 mg, and phenylpropanolamine hydrochloride 12.5 mg (nonprescription).

Tussagesic (Dorsey). Each tablet (timed-release) contains dextromethorphan hydrobromide 30 mg, acetaminophen 325 mg, pheniramine maleate 12.5 mg, phenylpropanolamine hydrochloride 25 mg, pyrilamine maleate 12.5 mg, and terpin hydrate 180 mg (nonprescription).

Tussar DM (USV). Each 5 ml of syrup contains dextromethorphan hydrobromide 15 mg, chlorpheniramine maleate 2 mg, and phenylephrine hydrochloride 5 mg (nonprescription).

Tussi-Organidin DM (Wallace). Each 5 ml of liquid contains dextromethorphan hydrobromide 10 mg and iodinated glycerol 30 mg.

Additional Antitussive Mixtures

Conar (Beecham). Each 5 ml of suspension contains noscapine 15 mg and phenylephrine hydrochloride 10 mg (nonprescription).

Conar A (Beecham). Each 5 ml of suspension contains noscapine 7.5 mg, acetaminophen 150 mg, guaifenesin 50 mg, and phenylephrine hydrochloride 5 mg; each tablet contains noscapine 15 mg, acetaminophen 300 mg, guaifenesin 100 mg, and phenylephrine hydrochloride 10 mg (both forms nonprescription).

Conar Expectorant (Beecham). Each 5 ml of syrup contains noscapine 15 mg, guaifenesin 100 mg, and phenylephrine hydrochloride 10 mg (nonprescription).

Rynatuss (Wallace). Each tablet contains carbetapentane tannate 60 mg, chlorpheniramine tannate 5 mg, ephedrine tannate 10 mg, and phenylephrine tannate 10 mg; each 5 ml of pediatric suspension contains carbetapentane tannate 30 mg, chlorpheniramine tannate 4 mg, ephedrine tannate 5 mg, and phenylephrine tannate 5 mg.

Tuss-Ornade (Smith Kline & French). Each capsule (timed-release) contains caramiphen edisylate 40 mg and phenylpropanolamine hydrochloride 75 mg; each 5 ml of liquid contains caramiphen edisylate 6.7 mg and phenylpropanolamine hydrochloride 12.5 mg (alcohol 5%).

Mixtures Containing Guaifenesin or Other Expectorants

(See previous lists for other combination products containing guaifenesin.)

Brexin (Savage). Each capsule or 5 ml of liquid contains guaifenesin 100 mg, carbinoxamine maleate 4 mg or 2 mg (liquid) and pseudoephedrine hydrochloride 60 mg or 30 mg (liquid).

Congess Sr, Congess Jr (Fleming). Each capsule contains guaifenesin 250 mg or 125 mg (Congess Jr) and pseudoephedrine hydrochloride 120 mg or 60 mg (***Congess Jr***).

Entex (Norwich Eaton). Each capsule contains guaifenesin 200 mg, phenylpropanolamine hydrochloride 45 mg, and phenylephrine hydrochloride 5 mg; each 5 ml of liquid contains guaifenesin 100 mg, phenylpropanolamine hydrochloride 20 mg, and phenylephrine hydrochloride 5 mg (alcohol 5%).

Entex LA (Norwich Eaton). Each tablet (timed-release) contains guaifenesin 40 mg and phenylpropanolamine hydrochloride 75 mg.

Phenergan VC (Wyeth). Each 5 ml of syrup contains promethazine hydrochloride 6.25 mg and phenylephrine hydrochloride 5 mg (alcohol 7%).

Robitussin-PE (Robins). Each 5 ml of syrup contains guaifenesin 100 mg and pseudoephedrine hydrochloride 30 mg (alcohol 1.4%) (nonprescription).

Triaminic Expectorant (Dorsey). Each 5 ml of liquid contains guaifenesin 100 mg and phenylpropanolamine hydrochloride 12.5 mg (alcohol 5%) (nonprescription).

COMPOSITION OF MIXTURES COMMONLY USED FOR RHINITIS OR THE COMMON COLD

Preparation	Decongestant†	Antihistamine†	Analgesic†
*Actifed (Burroughs Wellcome): capsules, tablets, syrup	pseudoephedrine HCl 60 mg (capsules, tablets), 30 mg (syrup)	triprolidine HCl 2.5 mg (capsules, tablets) 1.25 mg (syrup)	
*Actifed 12-Hour (Burroughs Wellcome): capsules (timed-release)	pseudoephedrine HCl 120 mg	triprolidine HCl 5 mg	
*Benadryl Decongestant (Parke-Davis): capsules	pseudoephedrine HCl 60 mg	diphenhydramine HCl 25 mg	
Comhist (Norwich Eaton): tablets	phenylephrine HCl 10 mg	phenyltoloxamine citrate 25 mg; chlorpheniramine maleate 2 mg	
Comhist LA (Norwich Eaton): capsules (timed-release)	phenylephrine HCl 20 mg	phenyltoloxamine citrate 50 mg; chlorpheniramine maleate 4 mg	
*Comtrex (Bristol-Myers): capsules, tablets, liquid	phenylpropanolamine HCl 12.5 mg (capsules, tablets), 4.2 mg (liquid)	chlorpheniramine maleate 1 mg (capsules, tablets), 0.33 mg (liquid)	acetaminophen 325 mg (capsules, tablets), 108.3 mg (liquid)

(continued on next page)

COMPOSITION OF MIXTURES COMMONLY USED FOR RHINITIS OR THE COMMON COLD *(continued)*

Preparation	Decongestant†	Antihistamine†	Analgesic†
*Contac (Menley & James): capsules (timed-release)	phenylpropanolamine HCl 75 mg	chlorpheniramine maleate 8 mg	
*Coricidin (Schering): tablets		chlorpheniramine maleate 2 mg	aspirin 325 mg
*Coricidin D (Schering): tablets	phenylpropanolamine HCl 12.5 mg	chlorpheniramine maleate 2 mg	aspirin 325 mg
*Coricidin Demilet (Schering): tablets	phenylpropanolamine HCl 6.25 mg	chlorpheniramine maleate 1 mg	acetaminophen 80 mg
*Coricidin Extra Strength Sinus Headache (Schering): tablets	phenylpropanolamine HCl 12.5 mg	chlorpheniramine maleate 2 mg	acetaminophen 500 mg
*CoTylenol (McNeil): tablets, liquid, pediatric liquid	pseudoephedrine HCl 30 mg (tablets), 10 mg (liquid), 6.25 mg (pediatric liquid)	chlorpheniramine maleate 2 mg (tablets), 0.67 mg (liquid), 1 mg (pediatric liquid)	acetaminophen 325 mg (tablets), 108.3 mg (liquid), 160 mg (pediatric liquid)
Deconamine (Berlex): tablets, elixir, syrup, capsules (timed-release)	pseudoephedrine HCl 60 mg (tablets), 30 mg (elixir, syrup), 120 mg (capsules)	chlorpheniramine maleate 4 mg (tablets), 2 mg (elixir, syrup), 8 mg (capsules)	
Dehist (Forest): capsules (timed-release)	phenylpropanolamine HCl 75 mg	chlorpheniramine maleate 12 mg	
*Demazin (Schering): tablets (timed-release), syrup	phenylephrine HCl 25 mg (tablets): phenylpropanolamine HCl 125 mg (syrup)	chlorpheniramine maleate 4 mg (tablets) 2 mg (syrup)	
*Dimetane (Robins): tablets, elixir	phenylephrine HCl 10 mg (tablets), 5 mg (elixir)	brompheniramine maleate 4 mg (tablets), 2 mg (elixir)	
Dimetane-DX (Robins): elixir	pseudoephedrine HCl 30 mg	brompheniramine maleate 2 mg	
*Dimetapp (Robins): elixir, tablets, tablets (timed-release)	phenylpropanolamine HCl 12.5 mg (elixir), 25 mg (tablets), 75 mg (timed-release tablets)	brompheniramine maleate 2 mg (elixir), 4 mg (tablets), 12 mg (timed-release tablets)	
*Disophrol (Schering): tablets, tablets (timed- release)	pseudoephedrine sulfate 60 mg (tablets), 120 mg (timed-release tablets)	dexbrompheniramine maleate 2 mg (tablets), 6 mg (timed-release tablets)	

(continued on next page)

COMPOSITION OF MIXTURES COMMONLY USED FOR RHINITIS OR THE COMMON COLD *(continued)*

Preparation	Decongestant†	Antihistamine†	Analgesic†
*Dristan-AF (Whitehall): tablets	phenylephrine HCl 5 mg	chlorpheniramine maleate 2 mg	acetaminophen 325 mg
*Drixoral (Schering) tablets (timed-release), syrup	pseudoephedrine sulfate 30 mg (syrup), 120 mg (tablets)	dexbrompheniramine maleate 6 mg (tablets); brompheniramine maleate 2 mg (syrup)	
*Entex (Norwich Eaton): capsules, liquid, tablets (timed-release)	phenylephrine HCl 5 mg; phenylpropanolamine HCl 45 mg (capsules), 20 mg (liquid), 75 mg (timed-release tablets)		
*Fiogesic (Sandoz): tablets	phenylpropanolamine HCl 25 mg	pheniramine maleate 12.5 mg; pyrilamine maleate 12.5 mg	calcium carbaspirin 382 mg (equivalent to 300 mg aspirin)
Histalet DM (Reid-Provident): syrup	pseudoephedrine HCl 45 mg	chlorpheniramine maleate 3 mg	
Histalet Forte (Reid-Provident): tablets (timed-release)	phenylpropanolamine HCl 50 mg; phenylephrine HCl 10 mg	chlorpheniramine maleate 4 mg; pyrilamine maleate 25 mg	
Isoclor (Fisons): tablets, liquid, capsules (timed-release)	pseudoephedrine HCl 60 mg (tablets), 30 mg (liquid), 120 mg (capsules)	chlorpheniramine maleate 4 mg (tablets), 2 mg (liquid), 8 mg (capsules)	
Naldecon (Bristol): syrup, tablets (timed-release)	phenylpropanolamine HCl 40 mg (tablets), 20 mg (syrup); phenylephrine HCl 10 mg (tablets), 5 mg (syrup)	phenyltoloxamine citrate 15 mg (tablets), 7.5 mg (syrup); chlorpheniramine maleate 5 mg (tablets), 2.5 mg (syrup)	
Nolamine (Carnrick): tablets (timed-release)	phenylpropanolamine HCl 50 mg	chlorpheniramine maleate 4 mg; phenindamine tartrate 24 mg	
Novafed A (Merrell Dow): capsules (timed-release), liquid	pseudoephedrine HCl 120 mg (capsules), 30 mg (liquid)	chlorpheniramine maleate 8 mg (capsules), 2 mg (liquid)	
Ornade (Smith Kline & French): capsules (timed-release)	phenylpropanolamine HCl 75 mg	chlorpheniramine maleate 12 mg	
Rondec (Ross): drops, syrup, tablets, tablets (timed-release) [Rondec-TR]	pseudoephedrine HCl 25 mg/ml (drops), 60 mg (syrup, tablets), 120 mg (timed-release tablets)	carbinoxamine maleate 2 mg/ml (drops), 4 mg (syrup, tablets), 8 mg (timed-release tablets)	

(continued on next page)

COMPOSITION OF MIXTURES COMMONLY USED FOR RHINITIS OR THE COMMON COLD *(continued)*

Preparation	Decongestant†	Antihistamine†	Analgesic†
Rynatan (Wallace): tablets, pediatric suspension	phenylephrine tannate 25 mg (tablets), 5 mg (suspension)	chlorpheniramine tannate 8 mg (tablets), 2 mg (suspension); pyrilamine tannate 25 mg (tablets), 12.5 mg (suspension)	
Singlet (Lakeside): tablets (timed-release)	phenylephrine HCl 40 mg	chlorpheniramine maleate 8 mg	acetaminophen 500 mg
Sinubid (Parke-Davis): tablets	phenylpropanolamine HCl 100 mg	phenyltoloxamine citrate 66 mg	acetaminophen 600 mg
*Sinulin (Carnrick): tablets	phenylpropanolamine HCl 37.5 mg	chlorpheniramine maleate 2 mg	acetaminophen 325 mg; salicylamide 250 mg
*Sinutab (Warner-Lambert): tablets	pseudoephedrine HCl 30 mg	chlorpheniramine maleate 2 mg	acetaminophen 325 mg
*Sinutab Maximum Strength (Warner-Lambert): capsules, tablets	pseudoephedrine HCl 30 mg	chlorpheniramine maleate 2 mg	acetaminophen 500 mg
*Sudafed Plus (Burroughs, Wellcome): tablets, liquid	pseudoephedrine HCl 60 mg (tablets), 30 mg (liquid)	chlorpheniramine maleate 4 mg (tablets), 2 mg (liquid)	
Tavist-D (Sandoz): tablets (timed-release)	phenylpropanolamine HCl 75 mg	clemastine fumarate 1.34 mg	
*Triaminic (Dorsey): tablets, tablets (chewable), syrup	phenylpropanolamine HCl 12.5 mg (syrup, tablets), 6.25 mg (chewable tablets)	chlorpheniramine maleate 2 mg (syrup, tablets), 0.5 mg (chewable tablets)	
*Triaminic Tablets (Dorsey): tablets, tablets (timed-release)	phenylpropanolamine HCl 25 mg (tablets), 75 mg (timed-release tablets)	chlorpheniramine maleate 4 mg (tablets) 12 mg (timed-release tablets)	
Trinalin (Schering): tablets (timed-release)	pseudoephedrine HCl 120 mg	azatadine maleate 1 mg	

*Nonprescription
†Per 5 ml of liquid (except drops)

Cited References

Cromolyn sodium nasal spray for hay fever. *Med Lett Drugs Ther* 25:89-90, 1983.

Decongestant-antihistamine judged ineffective in secretory otitis. *Pediatr Alert* 8:13-14, (Feb 17) 1983.

Ballow M: Allergic rhinitis and conjunctivitis. *Postgrad Med* 76:197-206, (July) 1984.

Bhambhani K, et al: Acute otitis media in children: Are decongestants or antihistamines necessary? *Ann Emerg Med* 12:13-16, 1983.

Brogden RN, et al: Beclomethasone dipropionate: Reappraisal of its pharmacodynamic properties and therapeutic efficacy after decade of use in asthma and rhinitis. *Drugs* 28:99-126, 1984.

Busse WW: Chronic rhinitis: Systematic approach to diagnosis and management. *Postgrad Med* 73:325-335, (Feb) 1983.

Cantekin EI, et al: Lack of efficacy of decongestant-antihistamine combination for otitis media with effusion ("secretory" otitis media) in children. *N Engl J Med* 308:297-301, 1983.

Clissold SP, Heel RC: Budesonide: Preliminary review of its pharmacodynamic properties and therapeutic efficacy in asthma and rhinitis. *Drugs* 28:485-518, 1984.

Committee on Drugs, American Academy of Pediatrics: Adverse reactions to iodide therapy of asthma and other pulmonary diseases. *Pediatrics* 57:272-274, 1976.

Crawford LV, Cohen RM: Therapy for allergic rhinitis: *Compr Ther* 11:60-69, (June) 1985.

Eby GA, et al: Reduction in duration of common colds by zinc gluconate lozenges in double-blind study. *Antimicrob Agents Chemother* 25:20-24, 1984.

Hardy JG, et al: Intranasal drug delivery by spray and drops. *J Pharm Pharmacol* 37:294-297, 1985.

Hartley TF, et al: Efficacy and tolerance of fluocortin butyl administered twice daily in adult patients with perennial rhinitis. *J Allergy Clin Immunol* 75:501-507, 1985.

Howard JC, et al: Effectiveness of antihistamines in symptomatic management of common cold. *JAMA* 242:2414-2417, 1979.

Irwin RS: That chronic cough: How to find the cause and treat it. *Mod Med* 111-123, (Dec) 1984.

Mabry RL: Corticosteroids in management of allergic rhinitis. *South Med J* 76:487-489, 1983.

Medon PJ, Holshouser MH: Self-medication: Antitussives. *Pharmacy Times* 80-90, (Jan) 1985.

Meltzer EO, et al: Chronic rhinitis in infants and children: Etiologic, diagnostic, and therapeutic considerations. *Pediatr Clin North Am* 30:847-871, 1983.

Mills J: Viral URIs: How to fight back. *Mod Med* 88-97, (Nov) 1983.

Norman PS: Review of nasal therapy: Update. *Allergy Clin Immunol* 72:421-432, 1983.

Phelan MJ: Prevention and treatment of hay fever. *Pharmaceut J* 232:711-712, (June) 1984.

Phillpotts R: Interferon prophylaxis of common cold. *TIPS* 5:466-468, 1984.

Proctor DF, Anderson I (eds): *The Nose, Upper Airway Physiology and the Atmospheric Environment.* Amsterdam, Elsevier Biomedical Press, 1982.

Simons FER: Chronic rhinitis. *Pediatr Clin North Am* 31:801-819, 1984.

Ward NO, Berry DW: Intranasal steroid treatment. *Ariz Med* 41:88-90, 1984.

Welsh PW, et al: Preseasonal IgE ragweed antibody level as predictor of response to therapy of ragweed hayfever with intranasal cromolyn sodium solution. *J Allergy Clin Immunol* 60:104-109, 1977.

Wood RP: Allergic rhinitis, in Cherniack RM (ed): *Current Therapy of Respiratory Disease, 1984-1985.* Philadelphia/St Louis, Decker/Mosby, 1984, 1-2.

Other Selected References

Establishment of monograph for OTC cold, cough, allergy, bronchodilator, and antiasthmatic products. *Federal Register* 41:38312-38424, (Sept 9) 1976.

Shatz M, et al: Allergic diseases during pregnancy: Management of mother and prevention in child, in Middleton E Jr, et al (eds): *Allergy Principles and Practice,* ed 2. St Louis, CV Mosby, 1983.

Drugs Used in Bronchial Disorders

22

Asthma is characterized by hyper-reactivity and narrowing of the bronchi in response to stimuli that do not produce narrowing to the same degree in the nonasthmatic. Mucosal edema and mucus plugging frequently are present. When asthma and bronchitis coexist, hypersecretion also may be present. Pulmonary parenchyma is normal. Airway narrowing may reverse spontaneously or with therapy. Type I (immediate) immune responses may play an important role in the development of asthma in children and many adults. When disease onset occurs in adulthood, allergic factors may be difficult to identify. Exposure to cold dry air, exercise, and other aggravating factors also may trigger asthma.

Emphysema and chronic obstructive bronchitis frequently coexist in what is commonly termed chronic obstructive pulmonary or lung disease (COPD or COLD). In emphysema, the primary pathology is parenchymal; airway collapse results from loss of elasticity. Clinically, it is difficult to assess the relative contributions of emphysema and chronic bronchitis to airway constriction. Environmental irritants, especially smoking, are closely linked etiologically. Response to therapy is partial at best.

In some individuals, asthma, emphysema, and chronic bronchitis may coexist.

ASTHMA

The most common symptoms of asthma are breathlessness and chest tightness. Wheezing (particularly with involvement of large airways), dyspnea, and cough also are prominent.

Reduced pulmonary function typical of obstructive rather than restrictive airway disease is usually observed. Asymptomatic periods often alternate with paroxysms. When maintenance drug therapy is essential to maintain an asymptomatic state and satisfactory pulmonary function between episodic exacerbations, most physicians arbitrarily classify the disease as chronic asthma.

Medical management is directed toward reversing or preventing bronchospasm, inflammation, and edema; eliminating mucus plugs; and correcting hypoxemia. Counseling to obtain patient understanding, cooperation, and compliance; early intervention at the first sign of an impending exacerbation; and avoiding pulmonary irritants, certain drugs, and allergens are critical to attain optimum results in treating asthma. In an acute exacerbation, the severity of symptoms, as well as response to drug therapy, vary considerably among patients and even in the same patient. The duration of therapy is guided as much by the patient's response to drug therapy as by the severity of symptoms. During a period of partial remission, the duration of treatment is determined by the signs and symptoms that interfere with daily functions and the results of appropriate pulmonary function tests if available.

PATHOPHYSIOLOGY. The bronchial muscles are controlled by the autonomic nervous system and parasympathetic fibers predominate in number and effect. Stimulation of parasympathetic nerves causes calcium-dependent constriction of the bronchi. Chemical mediators of bronchospasm, which include acetylcholine, histamine, serotonin, leukotrienes C and D, and prostaglandin $PGF_{2\alpha}$, are also thought to contribute to bronchoconstriction. The muscarinic receptors are closely related to cyclic guanosine monophosphate (cGMP). Sympathetic nerves are absent or sparse; animal experiments have shown that if present, they might cause local release of norepinephrine with subsequent relaxation. Beta-adrenergic receptors are closely related to adenylate cyclase, an enzyme in the plasma membranes of many cells, that indirectly controls the active secretion, transport, and storage of carbohydrates. This process involves cyclic adenosine monophosphate (cAMP), an intracellular mediator of adrenergic action that modifies enzyme activity and permeability barriers.

Nondrug Management

Patients with asthma must understand the nature of the illness and the role of each medication and treatment modality. Personal instructions by the physician and simple written directions are helpful. Psychological support, biofeedback, and breathing exercises may be beneficial adjuncts to specific therapy. Hydration is considered an important part of management, since adequate intake of fluids may minimize inspissation of bronchial secretions.

Portable peak flow meters may be provided for certain patients with severe disease for home use so that early signs of deterioration can be detected. The physician should be notified if there is a persistent reduction in peak expiratory flow rate (PEFR) that exceeds 20% to 25% or a sudden worsening of PEFR. Another early indication of impending trouble is the need for more frequent administration of bronchodilators with decreased therapeutic effect.

In moderately severe, recurrent asthmatic attacks, it is important that infectious and psychological elements be identified in order to develop a complete program of management. Management of any underlying allergic disorder also can be beneficial.

Nonsteroidal anti-inflammatory drugs, such as aspirin or indomethacin are contraindicated in some asthmatic patients. An aspirin-sensitive patient should avoid medications and in some cases foods containing tartrazine dye. Metabisulfites also may trigger asthma in some patients.

Acetylcysteine [Mucomyst] may aggravate bronchospasm and should not be used. Beta blockers administered systemically or even topically also may aggravate bronchospasm and should be given cautiously if deemed essential. Respiratory depressants should be avoided during an acute asthmatic attack.

Drug Therapy

GLOBAL TREATMENT. The goal of drug therapy for asthma is prevention of bronchospasm. Because it is usually not possible for either patient or physician to predict when bronchospasm may occur, patients with all but the most episodic and/or entirely seasonal attacks must realize that continuous therapy may be required. Observation over several months is required before it can be determined that intermittent or seasonal therapy may be sufficient.

Beta agonists stimulate beta$_2$-adrenergic receptors, increase intracellular cAMP, or inhibit the release of inflammatory mediators. Other useful drugs include theophylline and other xanthine drugs, which cause bronchodilation through unknown mechanisms; the biscromone, cromolyn [Intal], which prevents the release of mediator substances and blocks respiratory neuronal reflexes; and corticosteroids, which primarily decrease inflammation and edema. Anticholinergic drugs may relieve bronchospasm by blocking parasympathetic cholinergic impulses at the receptor level. Antihistamines occasionally prevent or abort allergic episodes, particularly in children.

Mild Asthma: In mild asthma, brief episodes of wheezing with or without dyspnea or cough occur. Episodes may be sporadic or occur daily and are easily controlled by inhalant beta-adrenergic drugs, which should be taken daily to prevent symptoms. Xanthine drugs are not effective when inhaled and have a slower onset of action after oral use; thus, they are less helpful for initial management of acute attacks.

If some signs and symptoms persist after treatment of the acute exacerbation, the combined use of an inhaled beta$_2$-adrenergic agonist and short-acting oral theophylline may be indicated.

Two or more inhalations of a longer acting beta$_2$ agonist (albuterol [Ventolin, Proventil]; terbutaline [Brethaire, Brethine, Bricanyl]; bitolterol [Tornalate]; the investigational agents, fenoterol [Berotec] and procaterol [Beta-Air]) at bedtime may be particularly useful for nocturnal asthma (Jenne, 1984). Nocturnal symptoms are often reduced when asthma is controlled during the day.

Moderate Asthma: Patients with moderate asthma experience wheezing and dyspnea, with or without cough and expectoration, that interfere with daily activities and/or sleep. When this pattern is apparent, daily therapy should include an inhalant beta$_2$ agonist and, if needed, oral theophylline. Inhalations of a beta$_2$ agonist up to a total of 12 to 16/day may be prescribed when control is not achieved with the usual dosage.

When drug delivery by metered-dose inhaler is inadequate for severe acute attacks, nebulized medications may be tried. If this approach is not feasible or is ineffective, two doses of terbutaline or epinephrine may be injected subcutaneously 15 or 30 minutes apart; a third dose of epinephrine is sometimes used. Patients may respond even when these beta agonists were ineffective prior to the acute episode (Rossing et al, 1983).

Intravenous aminophylline or theophylline is given when a severe exacerbation fails to respond adequately to a beta agonist. Even after initial improvement has occurred, intravenous therapy is usually continued. If the response is sustained, oral theophylline, possibly combined with inhalant or oral beta agonist therapy, can be given.

In the United States, timed-release theophylline is the most widely used drug for maintenance therapy in patients with moderate asthma. Long-acting inhaled beta$_2$-adrenergic agonists may be equally effective, especially in compliant patients. In some children and adults with asthma, cromolyn also may be equally effective and safer for prophylaxis. A five- to seven-day course of corticosteroid therapy may be required for severe exacerbations and to prevent status asthmaticus.

Repeated exacerbations suggest that corticosteroids are necessary for maintenance therapy.

Severe Asthma: Patients with severe asthma are incapacitated by dyspnea, unable to eat normally or sleep, very anxious, and exhausted. Signs of a potential life-threatening attack include a PaO_2 of less than 60 (at sea level); a $PaCO_2$ of more than 45 (at sea level) with increasing respiratory acidosis; poor air exchange and breath sounds; marked retraction of the accessory muscles of respiration; cyanosis; confusion and mental obtundation; pulsus paradoxus greater than 18 mm Hg; and signs of exhaustion.

A severe acute exacerbation of asthma is usually accompanied by hypoxia, and oxygen should be administered routinely. A flow rate of 2 to 4 L/minute by nasal cannula usually increases the arterial saturation of oxygen to 90% or greater. To reduce the thick mucous plugs in the airways and sputum viscosity, fluids should be administered intravenously. Oral intake may be limited by nausea and vomiting.

Drug therapy for a severe acute exacerbation should include an inhalant or subcutaneous beta agonist and intravenous aminophylline. If bronchodilators are not effective, intravenous steroids should be administered. A fatal outcome is much more likely from inadequate or inappropriate drug treatment than from the adverse effects of the drugs themselves. Fatalities have resulted from delay in instituting parenteral corticosteroid treatment or failure to employ adequate doses (Hetzel, 1984; Clarke and Newman, 1984; Paterson et al, 1983). Because of their slow onset of action (two to six hours) and time to maximal effects (24 to 96 hours), steroids must be administered early when physiologic improvement does not occur with bronchodilator therapy. Mechanical respiratory support is indicated when consecutive arterial blood gas determinations reveal progressive hypercapnia. Clinical signs of improvement (decreased dyspnea or wheezing) are notoriously unreliable. Intravenous isoproterenol occasionally is used in children with impending respiratory failure.

Once a severe acute exacerbation has been controlled, an inhalant beta$_2$ agonist and, if needed, an oral xanthine bronchodilator may be given.

When significant inflammation, mucous plugging, and hypersecretion have developed (particularly when an attack has developed over several days), bronchodilators are less effective alone. In such cases, once the acute exacerbation has resolved, the lowest effective dose of a short-acting corticosteroid, such as prednisone, may be taken daily for five to seven days or a single morning dose may be taken on alternate days for longer periods. In stable, well-controlled, compliant patients, an inhaled steroid is preferred.

Status Asthmaticus: Status asthmaticus is a medical emergency and requires intensive hospital care. A beta-adrenergic drug administered subcutaneously or by a nebulizer is an integral part of therapy. (Isoproterenol should be avoided in older patients because of its greater cardiovascular effects.) A loading dose of aminophylline is also administered by intravenous infusion over a 20-minute period while monitoring cardiovascular status and serum theophylline levels; adjustment in dose is necessary for patients with heart or liver disease and for those ingesting drugs or substances that affect theophylline

clearance (see the evaluation on Theophylline). Intravenous steroids must be given as soon as possible. All patients should receive oxygen for hypoxemia and intravenous fluids for dehydration. Antibiotics may also be required following appropriate cultures. Once the attack is controlled, parenteral drugs are withdrawn gradually and replaced by oral medication.

Exercise-induced Asthma: Some patients develop asthma five minutes or more after starting exercise. Rapid loss of heat and/or water from the respiratory passages may trigger bronchoconstriction. An inhalant beta$_2$-adrenergic agent is usually effective if used 15 minutes before exercise and offers protection for up to four hours (Sly, 1984). Cromolyn is effective for two hours after administration and may afford significant protection for up to four hours in some patients. Those whose wheezing prevents continuation of exercise should take medications regularly to improve their overall respiratory function.

Pregnancy: During pregnancy, severe bronchoconstriction is a greater danger to the fetus than the drugs used to combat it. Theophylline, corticosteroids, cromolyn, and beta-adrenergic agonists are probably safe in pregnant women, although many practitioners are reluctant to use selective beta$_2$ agonists during pregnancy because data demonstrating their safety in these patients are limited (Greenberger and Patterson, 1985). Systemic beta$_2$ agonists may inhibit labor and are contraindicated at term. For a review of precautions required in asthmatic patients during pregnancy and anesthesia, see Kingston and Hirshman, 1984.

Complications: Cough, nasal discharge, and other signs of *sinusitis* or *rhinitis* are often present in asthmatic patients, and appropriate symptomatic treatment may prevent acute exacerbations (see Chapter 21, Decongestant, Cough, and Cold Preparations). Acute or chronic *bacterial infection* may require the use of antibiotics; some patients who do not respond to conventional bronchodilator therapy may have unrecognized infection. *Gastroesophageal reflux* may accompany asthma and should be treated because it can precipitate or aggravate bronchospasm in some patients.

In patients with *heart disease,* the cardiovascular danger of any bronchodilator must be weighed against the greater risk of bronchoconstriction and hypoxemia.

Potassium depletion is the most common electrolyte disturbance in acute asthma. A potassium supplement (40 to 60 mEq/day or more) may be required, particularly in patients with vomiting or those taking steroids. The delay in instituting intravenous steroid and/or beta agonist therapy because of infusion of potassium is more likely to be hazardous for most patients than hypokalemia.

DRUG SELECTION. Primary factors in drug selection in asthmatic patients are the severity and status of the disease (ie, acute exacerbation, persistence of signs and symptoms between exacerbations, frequency and severity of previous exacerbations, prior response to therapy, cardiovascular-renal status, patient's age, current medications, drug allergies, associated disease). The availability of drugs with differing mechanisms of action and adverse drug reactions, as well as the availability of metered-dose inhalers, nebulizers, and timed-release preparations, are also important in drug selection.

Beta-Adrenergic Agonists: Actions and Uses. Beta agonists quickly reverse bronchoconstriction. These drugs also increase the rate of mucociliary clearance, which may be decreased in patients with obstructive lung disease (Clarke and Newman, 1984). Expectoration is often improved as a result of enhanced bronchodilation. In addition, these drugs prevent the release of inflammatory mediators and decrease the fatigability of diaphragmatic muscle (Galant, 1984).

Endogenous catecholamines, such as epinephrine, are readily metabolized by enzymes that are widely distributed throughout the body. Newer beta$_2$ agonists have been designed to better withstand enzyme degradation and, thus, are longer acting and useful orally. Adrenergic drugs can stimulate both beta$_1$ and beta$_2$ receptors to varying degrees; activation of beta$_2$ receptors relaxes bronchial smooth muscle, and activation of beta$_1$ receptors stimulates the heart. Newer compounds have been modified to emphasize beta$_2$ activity and minimize beta$_1$ activity.

The prototype of the adrenergic bronchodilators, epinephrine, stimulates beta$_2$ receptors but also has significant beta$_1$ and alpha-adrenergic activity. Since epinephrine acts within minutes after subcutaneous injection and side effects are short-lived, it is useful for the immediate management of acute bronchospasm. Often, tachycardia and hypertension associated with acute asthma resolve after respiratory status improves.

Ephedrine is less effective than epinephrine but can be given orally and has a longer duration of action. It appears to act indirectly by causing release of norepinephrine; however, its effect diminishes as intrinsic norepinephrine stores are depleted. This drug can cause central nervous system stimulation and cardiovascular side effects. Ephedrine is considered obsolete by some authorities and probably should not be used since selective beta$_2$ agonists are more potent and longer acting. Isoproterenol [Isuprel, Medihaler-Iso, Vapo-Iso] is a potent bronchodilator but has significant beta$_1$ receptor activity and can be dangerous in patients with cardiovascular disorders. Epinephrine or isoproterenol should not be used routinely by inhalation, particularly in patients with cardiac disease.

The adrenergic agents with greater specificity for beta$_2$ receptors include isoetharine [Bronkometer, Bronkosol], metaproterenol [Alupent, Metaprel], terbutaline [Brethaire, Brethine, Bricanyl], albuterol [Proventil, Ventolin], and bitolterol [Tornalate]. Metaproterenol, terbutaline, albuterol, and bitolterol are the most selective and are preferred to isoproterenol and isoetharine because they produce less direct cardiac stimulation and are longer acting. These drugs are effective when administered by metered-dose inhaler. Terbutaline and albuterol usually act for about four hours, bitolterol for about five hours, and metaproterenol for three to four hours (see Table).

A number of drugs are being studied, but thus far no clear advantage over presently available beta$_2$ agonists has been demonstrated. The investigational drugs, procaterol and fenoterol, are selective beta$_2$ agonists with efficacy comparable to that of albuterol; their duration of action is claimed to be slightly longer.

In acute airway obstruction, rapid relief of bronchospasm may be obtained by the subcutaneous injection of epinephrine or terbutaline. However, inhalant beta-adrenergic drugs may be as effective as subcutaneous epinephrine or terbutaline in many patients (Dwyer, 1984; Newman and Clarke, 1983). Each inhalation may improve the effectiveness of subsequent inhalations (Summers and Smith, 1984; Sly, 1984). For many patients, a metered-dose inhalant preparation of a beta$_2$ agonist may be the initial therapy; however, nebulization, which delivers larger doses and does not require the patient's cooperation for administration, is usually preferred for moderate to severe exacerbations. Failure to respond to therapy by metered-dose inhalation usually results from increasingly severe asthma or the development of tachyphylaxis.

Inhaled beta$_2$-adrenergic agonists may be inadequate alone in patients with severe asthma, steroid dependence, severe coughing, mucus hypersecretion, and/or inflammation.

ADRENERGIC AGONISTS FOR INHALATION

Drug	Potency	Beta$_2$ Selectivity	Peak Effect (min)	Duration of Effect* (hrs)	Dosage Forms†
Epinephrine	++++	0	>2	1-1.5	MDI, Solution
Isoproterenol	++++	0	5-15	1-2	MDI, Solution
Isoetharine	+++	++	15-60	2-3	MDI, solution
Metaproterenol	++++	+++	30-60	3-4	MDI, Solution
Terbutaline	++++	++++	60	4	MDI, Solution
Albuterol	++++	++++	30-60	4	MDI
Bitolterol	++++	++++	30-60	5	MDI

*May have longer duration of action in certain patients
†MDI = Metered dose inhaler
Solution = Solution for nebulization

Albuterol, metaproterenol, and terbutaline are often administered orally as maintenance therapy. Oral administration requires the use of much larger doses, produces more adverse reactions, and has a slower onset of action than inhalation. When given systemically, selective beta$_2$ agonists appear to lose some beta$_2$ specificity and produce significant tachycardia and other adverse effects as a result of stimulation of beta$_2$ receptors in cardiovascular as well as nonvascular tissues. Oral administration probably should be reserved for patients who cannot use the inhalant form correctly. A long-acting oral preparation may control nocturnal asthma.

Metered-Dose Inhalers. Many beta-adrenergic drugs are available in pressurized metered-dose inhalers (MDI), which deliver medication directly to the lung and allow use of much smaller doses, thus reducing the incidence and severity of adverse reactions. Patients must receive instructions on the correct use of this device. For very young children and some elderly patients, tube and reservoir spacers may be helpful (Newman and Clarke, 1983; Clarke and Newman, 1984).

For best results with any metered-dose inhaler, actuation should begin early in inspiration. Inspiration should be slow and complete and the breath should be held for ten seconds before exhalation. Administration is repeated once or twice at one- to five-minute intervals. This regimen may be repeated at three- to six-hour intervals. Children should be allowed to use handheld MDIs only under the supervision of a knowledgeable adult.

Overuse can occur during exacerbations of asthma, and patients should be instructed to seek immediate medical attention when symptoms worsen or when more frequent use of the inhaler is needed.

Nebulizer Devices. Nebulizers have no inherent advantages over metered-dose inhalers in maintenance therapy. Many practitioners prefer to deliver a beta-adrenergic agonist through a nebulizer in patients with an acute exacerbation of moderate to severe asthma because the delivered dose is more consistent and the patient's coordination and cooperation are not as critical. The chief disadvantages of a nebulizer are its expense, lack of portability (Newman, 1984), and the possibility of greater toxicity related to higher dosage.

A nebulizer can deliver almost any drug solution, including combinations of a beta-adrenergic drug, cromolyn, and/or other agents. More drug is available for absorption by the lungs with nebulizers than with metered-dose inhalers. The amount deposited in the lungs is about 10% to 15% of the delivered dose. The remainder of a nebulized dose is deposited within the nebulizer walls and apparatus.

Correct use of a nebulizer depends more on the set-up and operation of the unit than on the patient's technique (Newman and Clarke, 1983). A nebulizer solution should be administered slowly and intermittently over 15 to 30 minutes. Compressed air may be used to drive the unit. A final volume of 2 to 4 ml and a flow rate of 6 L/minute ensure a high aerosol outflow, small particle size, and short treatment period. Handheld bulbs can be used instead of gas-driven units but the amount of drug delivered to the lungs is variable.

To avoid bacterial contamination, the nebulizer unit should be cleaned frequently. Because beta-adrenergic drug solutions break down to inert reddish brown adrenochromes, only a freshly prepared solution should be used for nebulization. Ultrasonic nebulizer devices can cause bronchoconstriction and generally should be avoided.

Intermittent positive pressure breathing (IPPB) has no apparent benefit over other delivery systems and introduces the potential for pneumothorax.

Adverse Reactions and Precautions. All adrenergic drugs may cause anxiety, tremor, and restlessness. Older patients and those with long-standing chronic lung disease can be given epinephrine, but considerable caution is necessary to avoid tachycardia and other disturbances of cardiac rhythm and rate. These effects also may occur after parenteral administration or inhalation of epinephrine or isoproterenol. They occur less often after use of isoetharine, metaproterenol, terbutaline, albuterol, and bitolterol.

Tolerance, refractoriness, and even paradoxical bronchospastic reactions may develop with too frequent administration of epinephrine or isoproterenol, particularly when given by inhalation.

Central nervous system stimulation manifested by nervousness, irritability, and insomnia is common after oral administration of ephedrine, especially in adults. Less frequently, similar reactions follow the subcutaneous injection of epinephrine and the inhalation of isoproterenol.

Adrenergic drugs, particularly ephedrine, may cause urinary retention severe enough to necessitate catheterization in patients with bladder neck obstruction.

Skeletal muscle tremor resulting from beta$_2$ receptor stimulation is more common with oral agents. A reduction in the dosage usually eliminates this reaction and tolerance develops with continued use.

Beta agonist inhalers cannot control increasingly severe asthma. Excessive inhalation causes toxicity without additional benefit. A short course of oral corticosteroids frequently improves respiratory status and may enhance responsiveness to the beta agonist.

Tachyphylaxis or subsensitivity may develop after the regular use of beta$_2$-adrenergic bronchodilators but is often incomplete and usually does not necessitate a change in therapy. Responsiveness can be restored by parenteral administration of a corticosteroid (Jenne, 1984; Sly, 1984).

Inhalation of a selective beta$_2$ agonist usually has only slight effects on heart rate in normal patients. When palpitations do occur, they are generally observed within five minutes after an inhalant dose. Large doses delivered through a nebulizer not uncommonly produce tachycardia and tremor; rarely, hypokalemia, hypoxemia, and arrhythmias develop. Administration of oxygen during nebulization of a beta adrenergic agonist protects against the possibility of hypoxemia (Ziment, 1984; Williams, 1984).

Several fixed-dose combinations (eg, Bronkolixir, Marax, Tedral) contain sedating agent(s), as well as adrenergic drugs and other components. Since effective individual drugs are currently available, combinations are generally not advised (see the section on Mixtures).

Hyperthyroidism tends to accentuate all adrenergic side effects, particularly those of epinephrine, and may cause an exaggerated pressor effect.

Beta agonist preparations for use in metered-dose inhalers

do not contain sulfites, which can precipitate bronchospasm, but some solutions for nebulization or injection may.

It is not clear if inhalant beta-adrenergic drugs contributed to an increase in asthma deaths reported in England in the 1960s. The principal causes of these deaths were probably erroneous assessment of the severity of asthma, undertreatment (especially with corticosteroids), and delay in seeking additional therapy (Hetzel, 1984; Clarke and Newman, 1984; Paterson et al, 1983).

Interactions. Severe hypertension and, rarely, death may occur if epinephrine, ephedrine, or isoproterenol is administered with a monoamine oxidase (MAO) inhibitor (ie, isocarboxazid [Marplan], phenelzine [Nardil], tranylcypromine [Parnate]), because these agents block the metabolism of catecholamines. Ephedrine may antagonize the antihypertensive effect of guanethidine [Ismelin].

Adrenergic bronchodilators appear to be less effective in patients receiving beta blockers, such as propranolol [Inderal], or they may antagonize the action of these drugs. It may be necessary to increase the dose of the beta$_2$ agonist or substitute theophylline. The newer selective beta$_2$ agonists are less antagonistic.

Xanthine Drugs: *Actions.* Theophylline's mechanism of action is not precisely defined but may involve increased levels of cAMP, modulation of intracellular calcium transport, inhibition of adenosine receptors, and prostaglandin antagonism (Weinberger, 1984). Theophylline increases the contractility of diaphragmatic muscle and enhances its resistance to fatigue (Aubier et al, 1981). In patients with obstructive lung diseases associated with cor pulmonale, theophylline increases cardiac output and enhances right ventricular ejection fraction through its positive inotropic effects and reduction in pulmonary vascular resistance. Theophylline also may inhibit the release of inflammatory mediators. The respiratory center is stimulated primarily because the hypoxic drive is increased.

Uses. Theophylline is used to treat acute asthmatic episodes, to prevent attacks, or to minimize signs and symptoms during periods of remission. Extensive clinical experience has demonstrated that theophylline is effective and safe when care is taken to ensure that the optimum dose, formulation, and route of administration are employed.

In the United States, oral theophylline is the most widely used medication for maintenance therapy. The development of timed-release (sustained-release, SR) preparations and the availability of improved techniques to determine serum concentrations contribute to its current popularity. Some investigators believe that theophylline is more effective than a beta$_2$ agonist or cromolyn for maintenance therapy (Weinberger, 1984), but others stress that theophylline may not be as safe as inhalant beta$_2$ agonists and that it should be a secondary drug (Bukowskyj et al, 1984). Patients maintained on theophylline may experience breakthrough episodes of acute asthma. If this occurs, a beta$_2$ agonist or a short course of corticosteroid therapy usually is effective.

Intravenous aminophylline (theophylline) is utilized for the treatment of acute exacerbations of moderate to severe asthma. Since a number of studies have shown that little additional bronchodilation is produced beyond that obtained with maximum inhalant beta$_2$-agonist therapy, some practitioners recommend that intravenous aminophylline be given only when beta agonist drugs and steroids are inadequate (Rees, 1984 A). However, theophylline probably should be given to most patients with severe or prolonged airway obstruction to enhance the contractility of the diaphragm and increase its resistance to fatigue. Moreover, it provides sustained bronchodilation and protects patients who are subsensitive to the beta$_2$ agonists (Jenne, 1984).

The ethylenediamine component of aminophylline occasionally may be associated with allergic reactions. A parenteral theophylline preparation diluted in 5% dextrose that contains no ethylenediamine is now available for intravenous administration.

Another xanthine, dyphylline, is much less potent than theophylline. There is no xanthine preparation for inhalation.

Rectal suppositories of aminophylline are marketed but they are absorbed erratically and produce local irritation with prolonged use. A rectal solution is absorbed rapidly and reliably, although it too may cause local irritation. Although rectal preparations occasionally are useful, their misuse results in serious toxicity, especially when vomiting or dehydration develops.

Timed-Release Preparations. The serum concentration of theophylline varies considerably in those who metabolize the drug rapidly (especially smokers and children) when standard (rapidly absorbed) tablets are administered every four to six hours. To correct this problem and increase compliance, timed-release 8-hour, 12-hour, and 24-hour formulations were developed. These preparations are particularly useful in patients with nocturnal symptoms.

Preparations with at least a 12-hour dosing interval are preferred (Weinberger, 1984; Jenne, 1984). The 24-hour preparation is not recommended in patients who require more than 900 mg of theophylline per day. It is generally necessary to administer timed-release preparations more frequently in smokers and children.

Unfortunately, the absorption curves of timed-release forms still vary in the same individual (Jenne, 1984). Also, some 24-hour preparations administered within one hour of food or other ingested substances may be released prematurely (dumped) or, conversely, absorption may be delayed (Hendeles et al, 1985; Spector, 1985 A).

Before use, the package insert for any theophylline preparation should be consulted for more detailed information. See also the evaluation on Theophylline.

Standard (Rapidly Absorbed) Preparations. The availability of timed-release preparations has diminished the need for short-acting oral preparations (Weinberger, 1984). However, some nonsmoking adults and slow metabolizers can be maintained on standard oral forms (Weinstein and Brokaw, 1984).

Adverse Reactions and Precautions. Although serum concentrations of 8 to 20 mcg/ml are efficacious and safe for most patients, levels ranging from 10 to 15 mcg/ml may not be tolerated by an occasional patient. At serum concentrations above 20 mcg/ml, the risk of adverse effects sharply increases with little added benefit. Minor adverse reactions include nausea, vomiting and epigastric pain; these generally are preceded by headache and signs of central nervous system stimulation (dizziness, nervousness, and insomnia). Some minor reactions can be avoided if low doses are used initially and the amount increased gradually (Hendeles and Weinberger, 1983).

Serum concentrations above 20 mcg/ml increase the frequency and severity of the above symptoms and also produce tachycardia, fever, and hematemesis. At serum concentrations above 25 mcg/ml, life-threatening clonic and tonic convulsions or arrhythmias may develop. The seizures are often refractory to anticonvulsant therapy and may prove fatal.

Since the therapeutic blood level is close to the toxic one, careful evaluation of the patient is indicated and factors that alter the rate of elimination of this drug must be considered when adjusting dosage.

For a more detailed discussion of adverse reactions, precautions, factors affecting clearance, and interactions, see the evaluation on Theophylline.

Anti-inflammatory Corticosteroids: *Actions and Uses.* Systemic corticosteroids are the most effective antiasthmatic drugs available and should be considered in all patients with severe acute exacerbations of asthma. Because of adverse reactions, however, their long-term use should be restricted to patients who do not respond adequately to beta-adrenergic drugs, theophylline, cromolyn, or combinations of these drugs.

Steroids decrease the inflammatory component of asthma. Proposed mechanisms of antiasthmatic action include inhibition of the response to inflammation and prevention of the synthesis or action of inflammatory mediators. Steroids inhibit primarily intermediate (type III) hypersensitivity reactions and have little if any effect on immediate (type I) hypersensitivity. They do not stabilize mast cells. Corticosteroids stabilize lysosomal membranes, reduce cellular histamine stores, and restore the responsiveness of leukocytes and bronchial smooth muscle to beta-adrenergic drugs (Daniele, 1984; Spector, 1985 B).

A brief course of an oral corticosteroid (eg, prednisone given as a single morning dose or in divided doses for five to seven days or until symptoms are controlled) during an acute exacerbation of asthma may prevent status asthmaticus and avoid hospitalization. The total daily dose usually employed for adults is 20 to 40 mg; for children, 1 to 2 mg/kg/day is used. Some patients can be taught to recognize their need for additional medication and should be instructed to contact their physicians at the onset of increased dyspnea.

The short-term intravenous administration of a corticosteroid may be necessary in acute severe asthma. It is generally recommended that about 200 to 300 mg of hydrocortisone sodium succinate or the equivalent should be administered intravenously over 20 to 30 minutes every six hours until improvement has occurred as determined by FEV_1 and other pulmonary function tests. Higher doses have not been shown to be more effective in most patients. Some patients may require an intravenous corticosteroid for several days (Hiller and Wilson, 1983). When the patient has improved (often after 24 to 72 hours of intravenous steroid therapy), an oral steroid (eg, prednisone 40 to 60 mg daily in divided doses) is substituted. When symptoms are completely controlled, oral prednisone should be given if possible as a single daily dose at 8 AM.

Large oral or parenteral doses of short-acting corticosteroids can be used for up to two weeks with little risk of significant adrenal suppression or toxicity. Continuous, long-term therapy with a daily dose of prednisone at or above 10 mg/day (or the equivalent) may produce adrenal insufficiency. Hypothalamic-pituitary-adrenal (HPA) axis suppression and serious adverse reactions are unlikely during long-term therapy with lower daily doses, but few patients are helped by less than 10 mg/day.

Significant effects on the the HPA axis and most adverse reactions can be avoided if steroid-dependent patients are converted from daily therapy with a single morning dose of a short-acting corticosteroid (prednisone, methylprednisolone) to alternate-day therapy after symptoms have been controlled (Spector, 1985 B). Patients receiving more than 20 mg of prednisone or the equivalent per day are not easily converted to alternate-day therapy. In alternate-day therapy, three to four times the total daily dose is administered as a single dose every other morning at 8 AM. It may take considerable time to wean patients from daily to alternate-day therapy. Since the changeover is more difficult when divided daily doses have been used, patients must first be converted to a single morning dose.

Many steroid-dependent patients can be maintained on inhaled steroids without a serious risk of HPA axis suppression or other adverse reactions (Tse and Bernstein, 1984; Spector, 1985 B and following discussion).

A temporary period of stress (eg, surgery, infection) necessitates administration of larger oral or parenteral doses to patients already receiving oral steroids daily or on alternate days or to some patients taking inhalant steroids (Spector, 1985 B).

Asthma not controlled by large doses of oral prednisone and bronchodilators may respond to the combination of oral methylprednisolone and the macrolide antibiotic, troleandomycin. Combined use of these agents decreases steroid metabolism and may allow considerable reduction of the dose of steroid in children or adults (Weinstein and Brokaw, 1984; Eitches et al, 1985). This combination should be given only as a last resort, however, to avoid serious adverse reactions (eg, cholestatic jaundice, other severe hepatotoxicity, intensification of cushingoid side effects).

Long-acting steroids (eg, dexamethasone) should not be chosen to treat asthma, because severe withdrawal symptoms (eg, fever, myalgia, joint pain) are likely to follow their administration. Moreover, they can suppress the HPA axis even when given on alternate days. Corticotropin (ACTH) does not aid in HPA axis recovery.

Metered-dose Inhalers. A major advance in the therapy of asthma has been the development of inhalant corticosteroid preparations. Because a metered-dose inhaler (MDI) delivers the drug directly to the lung, small doses can be employed, thus reducing the incidence and severity of adverse reactions.

Inhalant corticosteroids are inactivated rapidly when absorbed systemically from the oropharynx and gut. The efficacy of currently available corticosteroid aerosol preparations (beclomethasone dipropionate [Beclovent, Vanceril], flunisolide [AeroBid], and triamcinolone acetonide [Azmacort]) appears to be similar. All are well absorbed, rapidly metabolized to inactive compounds, and highly active topically with low systemic activity. Recommended doses are safe in both adults and children. For severe childhood asthma, inhalant corticosteroids are much safer than systemic steroids and are preferable in those who are steroid-dependent. In England, inhaled steroids have been used safely in asthmatic children as young as 2 1/2 years.

In general, asthma should be controlled completely before a steroid inhaler is employed, and bronchodilators or other antiasthmatic agents should not be discontinued. The combination of an inhaled corticosteroid with oral prednisone or prednisolone permits a marked reduction of the oral dose in some patients (Tse and Bernstein, 1984). Most patients who require less than 10 mg of prednisone or its equivalent daily can be converted to inhalant corticosteroids alone. Those who require 20 mg or more of oral prednisone a day are not easily converted to inhalant steroids.

The use of an aerosol beta agonist five minutes prior to inhalation of a steroid may enhance the latter's distribution and effectiveness, as well as decrease the cough or wheezing produced by an inhalant steroid.

An inhalant corticosteroid also can be used as an alternative (or in addition) to cromolyn or an oral corticosteroid preparation in patients not adequately controlled by beta$_2$ agonists and/or theophylline (Clark, 1985).

For the patient with severe asthma who requires larger doses of inhaled steroids, a concentrated preparation would be advantageous. High-dose inhalant preparations of beclomethasone dipropionate (250 mcg/inhalation) and the investigational agent, budesonide (200 mcg/inhalation), may soon be available (Williams, 1984). These inhalers would allow reduction or discontinuation of oral doses in some patients and may reduce the frequency of administration to twice daily. The less frequent administration may increase patient compliance and reduce the incidence of oropharyngeal candidiasis (thrush).

Adverse Reactions and Precautions. The adverse reactions of systemic corticosteroids are discussed in detail in Chapter 61, Adrenal Corticosteroids in Nonendocrine Diseases.

The only significant adverse effects of inhaled corticosteroids are oropharyngeal candidiasis, dysphonia, and coughing or wheezing. The mouth should be rinsed with water immediately after inhalation. Slow inspiration for ten seconds and holding the breath for another ten seconds may improve delivery of the drug to the lungs and decrease adverse reactions. The use of a spacer (tube or reservoir chamber) increases the efficiency of drug delivery in patients using the MDI improperly and may allow doses to be increased severalfold without producing oral candidiasis.

Daily doses of up to 1.6 mg of beclomethasone dipropionate or the equivalent have been used without producing systemic adverse effects or effects on HPA axis function; doses between 1.6 and 2 mg/day may be safe but some systemic absorption is likely (Clark, 1985).

Patients who take inhalant steroids must be instructed to take oral steroids when acute attacks occur. The cough or wheezing produced by inhaled steroids can be minimized if a spacer is used or a beta agonist is inhaled prior to the steroid. Some patients may benefit from a few days of concomitant oral steroid therapy to improve the delivery of the inhaled drug into the bronchi.

Rhinitis and atopic dermatitis may be exacerbated after withdrawal of oral steroids.

Drug Interactions. Careful dosage adjustment is advised when barbiturates are administered to asthmatic patients receiving systemic corticosteroids, since the enzyme-inducing properties of the barbiturates may increase the metabolism of the steroids. Numerous other drug interactions have been noted. (See also Chapter 61, Adrenal Corticosteroids in Nonendocrine Diseases.)

The macrolide antibiotics, troleandomycin and erythromycin estolate, have a steroid-sparing action and also prolong the half-life of theophylline. When a macrolide antibiotic is used in patients receiving theophylline and a steroid, particularly for chronic illness, the doses of the latter two drugs must be reduced to prevent overdosage.

Biscromones: Unlike other drugs discussed in this chapter, cromolyn [Intal] is used only to prevent asthma. It has no adrenergic, antihistamine, or corticosteroid-like actions and little bronchodilator activity. This drug may inhibit the degranulation of mast cells and prevent release of the mediators of asthma that cause bronchospasm. It may also block respiratory neuronal reflexes. These actions may be due in part to inhibition of cellular calcium flux. The onset of action of cromolyn is delayed (generally two to six weeks) and other agents must be used in the interim. Daily administration is required for efficacy.

In several controlled clinical trials, cromolyn was as effective as theophylline for maintenance in children with chronic asthma (Bernstein, 1985; Shapiro and König, 1985). In England, it is the drug of choice for prophylaxis in children with mild to moderate chronic asthma, and an expanded role has been proposed in this country (Bernstein, 1985). Cromolyn prevents allergic asthma and some cases of nonallergic asthma and should be considered for patients with frequent wheezing, seasonal or occupational asthma, animal- or exercise-induced asthma, and asthma not controlled by beta-adrenergic drugs or theophylline or in those who cannot tolerate the latter drugs (Summers and Smith, 1984). In some patients who respond to cromolyn, it may be possible to reduce the dose of corticosteroids or eliminate their use (Daniele, 1984).

Cromolyn is currently available as an encapsulated powder that must be administered through a special device supplied by the manufacturer, in a 1% solution for nebulization, and in metered-dose inhalers.

Cromolyn causes minimal adverse reactions. Rapid inhalation is efficient for delivery of the dry powder, but there is considerable deposition of drug on the walls of the oropharynx, and only about 5% of the dose may reach the lungs (Newman and Clarke, 1983). Although hand-lung coordination is not required with a dry powder inhaler, some patients find it inconvenient to load a capsule into the device before use and improper technique can affect compliance.

Several oral biscromones with similar properties are being investigated. One of these, ketotifen, a tricyclic compound of the benzocycloheptathiopene class, is available in many countries. In addition to its cromolyn-like actions, it has antihistaminic activity and has been investigated as a long-acting (12 to 24 hours) oral alternative to cromolyn for maintenance in chronic asthma. The results of clinical studies have been variable and conflicting, and the ultimate efficacy of ketotifen for the prophylaxis of asthma remains to be established (Shapiro and König, 1985). Sedation and weight gain may occur after prolonged administration. Other common adverse effects include dizziness, nausea, headache, dry mouth, bronchospasm, and aggravation of asthma (Maclay et al, 1984).

Anticholinergic Drugs: Some elements of asthma may be due to vagal-mediated stimulation of bronchial muscle, which increases cholinergic tone in the airways and causes bronchospasm and mucus hypersecretion. Atropine and its congeners reduce bronchospasm associated with chronic bronchitis and their use in asthma has received renewed attention recently with the availability of atropine in inhalant form [Dey-Dose]. Some of the side effects (central nervous system stimulation, mydriasis, cycloplegia, dry mouth) that occur with subcutaneous administration of atropine are less severe after inhalation (Hemstreet, 1980). Nevertheless, adverse reactions may occur after inhalation even at the lowest effective dose.

An anticholinergic agent may be used when inhaled beta-adrenergic agonists or theophylline are ineffective or when cough is prominent; additive effects with beta$_2$ agonists have been observed. Anticholinergic drugs given by inhalation also may be useful when asthma is produced by beta-adrenergic blockade or specific stimuli (eg, cold air, excercise). These drugs may be beneficial in chronic bronchitis, particularly in patients not well controlled by beta-adrenergic drugs (Gross and Skorodin, 1984).

A congener of atropine, ipratropium bromide [Atrovent] (investigational), has been widely used overseas and in Canada. When inhaled, it is as effective as atropine but produces fewer adverse effects because it is a quaternary ammonium compound. Other quaternary ammonium drugs, such as atropine methonitrate, glycopyrrolate, and oxyphenonium, are being investigated for use in a nebulized solution for inhalation.

Calcium Channel Blocking Drugs: Calcium antagonists, such as verapamil [Calan, Isoptin] and nifedipine [Adalat, Procardia], selectively inhibit calcium ion influx across the cell membrane, thus suppressing calcium-dependent smooth muscle excitation. The secretion of histamine and other mediators may be initiated by movement of calcium into mast cells. Investigationally, calcium antagonists have been shown to prevent exercise-induced asthma. However, presently available calcium antagonists show little bronchodilating activity and do not appear likely to replace theophylline or beta-adrenergic agonists.

Mucokinetic Agents: Mucokinetic drugs, such as acetylcysteine [Mucomyst], guaifenesin, or potassium iodide, have limited value in patients with asthma (Ziment, 1984). Acetylcysteine induces expectoration through an irritant effect on bronchial mucosa, which causes bronchorrhea and stimulates coughing. However, pretreatment with a beta-adrenergic inhalant is necessary to protect against bronchospasm. Acetylcysteine has an unpleasant sulfurous odor and taste upon nebulization that can produce gagging, nausea, and vomiting. The efficacy of acetylcysteine in asthma is questionable and it should not be used.

Guaifenesin in recommended doses is of doubtful benefit for asthma. A saturated solution of potassium iodide may be a useful expectorant, but iodides can cause hypothyroidism and skin lesions (usually acneiform) and are not recommended for children or pregnant women. Isotonic saline is an effective expectorant. Inhalation of hypertonic saline also is effective but its use may be undesirable in patients who must restrict their intake of sodium and it may cause acute bronchospasm.

Patients who produce sputum chronically should be well hydrated. The value of water in inhalant therapy is considered to be due to its demulcent properties rather than its mucokinetic effects. Water can cause bronchospasm when inhaled. Some physicians do not believe that mucus becomes less viscid even with aggressive hydration.

CHRONIC BRONCHITIS

Two distinct forms of chronic bronchitis are recognizable clinically. The first is defined as the presence of cough and sputum for three or more months per year for at least two consecutive years. This form of the disease is characterized by mucus hypersecretion with an increase in bronchial mucus glands, but the air flow is not necessarily limited. Some investigators have coined the term, chronic simple bronchitis, to distinguish this benign entity from chronic obstructive bronchitis. It is unclear at the present time whether chronic simple bronchitis progresses to obstructive disease or is a separate entity.

In the second form, chronic obstructive bronchitis, there is a significant fixed obstruction in the small airways. Major ventilation/perfusion inequalities characterize the disease, and ultimately dyspnea, cyanosis, and cor pulmonale result.

Management of Chronic Obstructive Bronchitis: Hypersecretion is reduced by humidifying inspired air. Since removal of secretions markedly reduces the risk of upper respiratory infection, improved hydration to promote expectoration and postural drainage are thought to be beneficial. Because viral and bacterial infections increase airway hyperreactivity, antibiotics should be prescribed when appropriate to treat bacterial infections. Stress and bronchial irritants, particularly cigarette smoke, must be avoided; even passive smoking can aggravate or precipitate bronchospasm in these patients. Management of right heart failure may require oxygen, salt restriction, and diuretics.

Continuous oxygen therapy is the only treatment that prolongs survival in severely ill patients.

Chronic bronchitis responds to drug therapy, but the response is not as great as in patients with asthma. Nevertheless, therapy with a beta$_2$ agonist, theophylline, and/or an anticholinergic agent, such as atropine, should be tried even if results of pulmonary function tests indicate that airway obstruction is only partially reversible.

Some physicians recommend steroid therapy for two to four weeks in patients with chronic obstructive bronchitis to identify those patients with a significant asthmatic component. A history of wheezing, allergy, or increased eosinophils may predict the usefulness of steroids. Blood and sputum eosinophilia and responsiveness to adrenergic agents also may be predictive (Estepan and Libby, 1982).

A severe acute exacerbation of chronic obstructive bronchitis requires intravenous hydration, intravenous aminophylline, an inhalant or oral beta₂-adrenergic drug, controlled oxygen therapy, chest physical therapy with postural drainage, and usually antibiotics. Mechanical ventilatory support also may be necessary (Burton, 1984). Short-term steroid therapy is helpful to reduce bronchial edema and inflammation.

EMPHYSEMA

Emphysema is characterized by irreversible destruction and coalescence of alveolar septa with enlargement of the distal air spaces and loss of lung elasticity. The terminal airways tend to collapse during expiration increasing the work of breathing. Cor pulmonale and respiratory failure are observed less frequently in emphysema than in chronic obstructive bronchitis.

A small percentage of emphysema patients have a genetic deficiency of alpha-1-antitrypsin, the major component of plasma alpha-1-globulin in adults. In the absence of this factor, lung and blood proteases destroy lung parenchyma. Approximately 1% to 2% of patients with emphysema have a homozygous deficiency of alpha-1-antitrypsin and develop severe disease. Cigarette smoking and airborne irritants and pollutants increase the predisposition to emphysema in these patients. Mild emphysema may occur in patients with a heterozygous deficiency of this protein (Burton, 1984).

Management: Therapy for emphysema is aimed at relieving bronchospasm, reducing secretions, and managing infection, hypoxia, and heart failure if these occur.

Oxygen may be required for acute episodes and/or persistent hypoxia (see the evaluation). Continuous oxygen therapy is the only treatment that prolongs survival in patients with severe emphysema. In patients with cor pulmonale and pulmonary hypertension, continuous low-flow oxygen relieves hypoxemia, reduces pulmonary vascular resistance, and improves mental status and exercise tolerance. Home oxygen therapy should be considered for patients with a resting PaO₂ of less than 55 mm Hg with room air. Continuous oxygen is advisable if the PaO₂ is less than 50 mm Hg.

Theophylline enhances the contractility and decreases the fatigability of diaphragmatic muscle, provides chronotropic and inotropic stimulation of cardiac muscle, and lowers pulmonary and peripheral vascular resistance. In theory, these actions should be beneficial, especially in patients with cor pulmonale; however, theophylline may not relieve symptoms subjectively even when pulmonary function improves. A plasma concentration of 10 to 15 mcg/ml is adequate and safe in most patients (Jenne, 1984).

Exercise reconditioning improves exercise tolerance and permits performance of work with less oxygen consumption. Pursed lip breathing (inhaling through the nose with slow expiration through pursed lips) improves gas exchange and may relieve dyspnea, particularly during exercise.

Drug Evaluations

ADRENERGIC DRUGS

ALBUTEROL
[Proventil, Ventolin]

ALBUTEROL SULFATE
[Proventil, Ventolin]

$$HO-C_6H_3(CH_2OH)-CHCH_2NHC(CH_3)_3$$
(OH)

This potent, selective, beta₂-adrenergic agonist is closely related to terbutaline and is becoming the standard of this class of drugs for use in asthma. The catecholamine nucleus of albuterol has been modified to make it resistant to degradation by sulfatase and catechol-O-methyltransferase. This drug appears to stimulate the respiratory center.

The improvement in asthmatic patients is dose dependent (Spector and Gomez, 1977). Equieffective doses of albuterol cause fewer cardiovascular side effects than with most other adrenergic bronchodilators. Thus, it is safer in patients with myocardial ischemia. With intravenous use (investigational), albuterol produces minimal arrhythmia and is less likely to cause hypoxemia than isoproterenol and other nonselective beta agonists.

In recommended doses, the duration of action of the inhalant and oral forms is usually similar, about four hours, but significant relief of symptoms may persist for up to eight hours after an oral dose. In metered-dose inhaler form, albuterol is a drug of choice to prevent exercise-induced asthma (Sly, 1984). A solution for nebulization is expected to be available soon. A parenteral formulation for intravenous, intramuscular, and subcutaneous administration is available in Europe.

ADVERSE REACTIONS AND PRECAUTIONS. The most common side effect of oral or inhaled albuterol is fine finger tremor, which may interfere with precise hand work. Large doses of oral or intravenous albuterol can cause mild tachycardia and a slight fall in diastolic blood pressure. Serum potassium is reduced when albuterol is given intravenously and occasionally by other routes. Albuterol inhibits premature labor when given intravenously or orally. This drug is classified in FDA Pregnancy Category C.

For more information on indications, adverse reactions, and precautions, see the section on Drug Selection in the Introduction.

PHARMACOKINETICS. Most of an oral dose is conjugated in the intestinal mucosa and liver and excreted in the urine as unchanged drug and sulfate conjugates.

DOSAGE AND PREPARATIONS.
ALBUTEROL:
Inhalation: Adults and children over 12 years, two or three deep inhalations one to five minutes apart. This may be

repeated every four to six hours. The total daily dosage should not exceed 16 to 20 inhalations.

> *Proventil* (Schering), *Ventolin* (Glaxo). Metered aerosol 90 mcg/ actuation.

ALBUTEROL SULFATE:

Oral: (Tablets) *Adults and children over 12 years,* 2 to 4 mg three or four times daily. (Syrup) *Adults and adolescents over 14 years,* 2 to 4 mg three or four times daily; *children 6 to 14 years,* 2 mg three or four times daily; *2 to 6 years,* 0.1 mg/kg (maximum, 2 mg) three times daily.

> *Proventil* (Schering), *Ventolin* (Glaxo). Syrup 2 mg/5 ml; tablets 2 and 4 mg.

BITOLTEROL MESYLATE
[Tornalate]

The efficacy of this inhalant beta$_2$-adrenergic agonist in asthmatic patients is similar to that of albuterol but bitolterol is more potent (Walker et al, 1985; Orgel et al, 1985). It may be as effective as albuterol in preventing exercise-induced asthma.

When inhaled, this prodrug is activated primarily by lung esterases to the active catecholamine, colterol. Its relatively long duration of action (about five hours compared to four hours for albuterol) may be due to its greater potency and/or to the relatively slow activation process. In about 25% of patients, the duration of action of bitolterol is eight hours, which may make this drug useful in nocturnal asthma. It has been suggested that the duration of action may decrease with prolonged use, but this has not been shown in clinical studies.

In usual doses, bitolterol appears to produce few cardiovascular side effects. Tolerance is rare.

For indications, adverse reactions, and precautions, see the section on Drug Selection in the Introduction.

DOSAGE AND PREPARATIONS.

Inhalation: *Adults and children over 12 years,* two or three deep inhalations one to five minutes apart. This may be repeated every four to six hours. The total daily dosage should not exceed 16 to 20 inhalations.

> *Tornalate* (Winthrop-Breon). Metered aerosol 370 mcg/actuation.

EPINEPHRINE
[Primatene Mist, Sus-Phrine]

EPINEPHRINE BITARTRATE
[AsthmaHaler, Bronkaid Mist, Medihaler-Epi, Primatene Mist]

EPINEPHRINE HYDROCHLORIDE
[Adrenalin Chloride]

EPINEPHRINE HYDROCHLORIDE RACEMIC
[AsthmaNefrin, microNefrin, Vaponefrin]

ACTIONS AND USES. The principal therapeutic effect of epinephrine in asthma is bronchodilation; vasoconstriction and relief of bronchial edema also contribute to the improvement in vital capacity.

Epinephrine is widely used by subcutaneous injection to relieve acute asthma, but its continued use as a primary medication is questionable. This drug should not be given routinely to prevent exacerbations during periods of remission. It has a short duration of action by any route and its nonspecific adrenergic actions may cause a wide variety of adverse reactions, particularly in patients with cardiac decompensation or severe respiratory difficulties.

Effects occur immediately after subcutaneous injection, but administration may have to be repeated within 20 minutes. The duration may be extended to six to eight hours by using a suspension of crystalline epinephrine in glycerin [Sus-Phrine]. Since only about 80% of the epinephrine in this preparation is actually in suspension, the remaining 20% acts immediately. Sus-Phrine is useful after an initial dose of epinephrine hydrochloride has been administered subcutaneously and found to be effective.

A metered-dose inhaler and solution for nebulization can be employed for prophylaxis and treatment of bronchospasm, but selective beta$_2$ agonists are effective for a much longer period and are safer.

Rapid absorption in the respiratory tract may cause adverse effects. The short duration of action of epinephrine requires repeated use, which can lead to overdosage.

ADVERSE REACTIONS AND PRECAUTIONS. Adverse reactions due to systemic absorption of epinephrine include symptoms of excessive stimulation of alpha- and beta-adrenergic receptors (anxiety, tremors, palpitation, tachycardia, and headache). Such reactions are most common after parenteral administration. Rebound bronchospasm may occur, particularly after inhalation. Large doses or rapid intravenous injection may increase blood pressure with sequelae that include cerebral hemorrhage. Ventricular arrhythmias also may occur. Epinephrine generally is contraindicated in patients with hypertension, hyperthyroidism, ischemic heart disease, or cerebrovascular insufficiency. Geriatric patients and those with long-standing chronic lung disease may be given epinephrine only with considerable caution; however, despite the risk, this drug may have to be given since hypoxemia from uncontrolled bronchospasm can be life-threatening.

Refractoriness and tolerance may occur after too frequent

administration. Too frequent inhalation also irritates the pharyngeal and bronchial mucosa. Epinephrine should not be given with monoamine oxidase inhibitors.

This drug is considered to be safe in pregnant women (FDA Pregnancy Category C).

See also the section on Drug Selection in the Introduction.

DOSAGE AND PREPARATIONS.

Subcutaneous: *Adults,* 0.2 to 0.5 mg (0.2 to 0.5 ml of 1:1,000 solution) every 20 minutes as necessary up to three times; *children,* 0.01 mg/kg. In severe acute attacks of asthma, doses may be repeated for adults and children every 20 minutes for a maximum of three doses. Alternatively, 0.1 to 0.3 ml of an aqueous suspension of free base 1:200 [Sus-Phrine] for adults (maximum initial dose, 0.1 ml) or 0.005 ml/kg for children (maximum dose for children less than 30 kg, 0.15 ml) may be used when prolonged action is desired. Caution must be exercised, for this preparation is more concentrated than the standard preparation; administration generally should not be repeated within four hours.

EPINEPHRINE:
Generic. Suspension 1:1,000 (1 mg/ml) in 1, 2, and 30 ml containers.
Sus-Phrine (Forest). Suspension 1:200 (5 mg/ml) in 0.3 and 5 ml containers.
EPINEPHRINE HYDROCHLORIDE:
Adrenalin Chloride (Parke-Davis), **Generic.** Solution (sterile) 1:1,000 (1 mg/ml) in 1 and 30 ml containers.

Inhalation: 0.1% to 1% solution from a nebulizer or two inhalations from a metered-dose inhaler. However, epinephrine is not a preferred drug for this route of administration.

EPINEPHRINE:
Primatene Mist (Whitehall). Aerosol providing 0.2 mg/inhalation (alcohol 34%, nonprescription).
EPINEPHRINE BITARTRATE:
AsthmaHaler (Norcliff Thayer), **Bronkaid Mist** (Winthrop-Breon), **Medihaler-Epi** (Riker), **Primatene Mist** (Whitehall). Aerosol providing 0.3 mg (equivalent to 0.16 mg base)/inhalation (nonprescription).
EPINEPHRINE HYDROCHLORIDE:
Adrenalin Chloride (Parke-Davis). Solution (for nebulization) 1:100 (10 mg/ml) (nonprescription).
EPINEPHRINE HYDROCHLORIDE RACEMIC:
AsthmaNefrin (Norcliff Thayer), **microNefrin** (Bird), **Vaponefrin** (Fisons). Solution (for nebulization) 2.25% (nonprescription).

EPHEDRINE SULFATE

Ephedrine rarely should be used for the treatment of asthma. The actions of this nonselective adrenergic agonist are similar to those of epinephrine. However, ephedrine is given orally and is not as useful for severe attacks of asthma because of its weaker bronchodilator action. This drug is less effective and its duration of action is shorter than that of the selective beta$_2$ agonists in patients who require continuous medication. Tachyphylaxis develops quickly.

ADVERSE REACTIONS AND INTERACTIONS. Adverse reactions are similar to those caused by epinephrine (see also the section on Drug Selection in the Introduction and the evaluation on Epinephrine). Central nervous system stimulation, manifested by nervousness, excitability, and insomnia, is common. A sedative is not recommended to reduce these effects. An increase in peripheral vascular resistance may result in hypertension. Rarely, a patient may be allergic to ephedrine. Urinary retention may occur in men with prostatic hypertrophy. Ephedrine should not be given with monoamine oxidase inhibitors or guanethidine. This drug is classified in FDA Pregnancy Category C.

DOSAGE AND PREPARATIONS.

Oral: *Adults,* 25 to 50 mg every six hours; *children,* 3 mg/kg every 24 hours in four divided doses.
Generic. Capsules 25 and 50 mg; syrup 11 and 20 mg/5 ml (both forms nonprescription).

FENOTEROL HYDROBROMIDE
[Berotec]

This investigational agent is structurally related to metaproterenol and is a very specific beta$_2$ adrenergic agonist with a relatively long duration of action (Svedmyr, 1985). Fenoterol appears to have the same efficacy as albuterol and a similar duration of action (about four hours). It is the beta$_2$ agonist of choice in some European countries.

For indications, adverse reactions, and precautions, see the section on Drug Selection in the Introduction.
Berotec (Boehringer Ingelheim).
(Investigational drug)

ISOETHARINE HYDROCHLORIDE
[Bronkosol]

ISOETHARINE MESYLATE
[Bronkometer]

Isoetharine resembles isoproterenol structurally but has less beta$_1$-adrenergic activity and produces fewer adverse effects. It is widely used in metered-dose inhaler form but is less effective than the newer selective beta$_2$-adrenergic drugs. The onset of action is rapid and the duration of action is relatively short (two to three hours). Isoetharine is available only in aerosol form in the United States.

For indications, adverse reactions, and precautions, see the section on Drug Selection in the Introduction.

DOSAGE AND PREPARATIONS.

Inhalation: By hand nebulizer, isoetharine mesylate 0.61%, one or two inhalations. If the therapeutic response is inadequate after one minute, this dose may be repeated once and every two to four hours thereafter as needed.

When the isoetharine hydrochloride 1% solution is used with a hand nebulizer, two to four inhalations. When oxygen is used for nebulization, the usual dose is 5 mg inhaled over a period of 15 to 30 minutes.

ISOETHARINE HYDROCHLORIDE:
Generic. Solution (for nebulization) 0.08%, 0.1%, 0.125%, 0.14%, 0.167%, 0.2%, 0.25%, and 1%.
Bronkosol (Winthrop-Breon). Solution (for nebulization) 0.25% and 1%.

ISOETHARINE MESYLATE:
Bronkometer (Winthrop-Breon). Aerosol 0.61% providing 340 mcg/measured dose.

ISOPROTERENOL HYDROCHLORIDE
[Isuprel, Isuprel Mistometer, Vapo-Iso]

ISOPROTERENOL SULFATE
[Medihaler-Iso]

ACTIONS AND USES. Isoproterenol prevents and relieves bronchoconstriction. Because it has significant beta$_1$ activity, it also relaxes vascular smooth muscle and increases the rate and force of heart contractions.

The duration of action (one to two hours) is similar to that of epinephrine. For acute asthma, isoproterenol must be administered every one to two hours by inhalation. Absorption is erratic when isoproterenol is given sublingually.

Intravenous isoproterenol has been used in children in an attempt to avoid mechanical ventilation during status asthmaticus. It generally should be avoided in the elderly or patients with cardiovascular disorders.

ADVERSE REACTIONS AND PRECAUTIONS. Palpitation, tachycardia and other arrhythmias, hypotension, tremor, headache, and nervousness are especially frequent with excessive use. Angina has been reported. Excessive inhalation also can cause refractory bronchial obstruction that rarely is followed by sudden death, presumably from arrhythmia associated with hypoxemia. In sensitive patients, inhalation may cause a severe, prolonged attack of asthma.

The beta$_1$ effects are unopposed by alpha effects and vasodilation of the pulmonary blood vessels occurs; this increases blood flow and enhances systemic absorption, decreases the duration of action, and increases adverse reactions. Moreover, pulmonary vasodilation in poorly ventilated lung areas can increase ventilation perfusion abnormalities and cause a dangerous fall in PaO_2. This can also be seen with other beta agonists and with intravenous aminophylline.

Tolerance and refractoriness may develop with too frequent administration.

Isoproterenol should not be given with monoamine oxidase inhibitors or guanethidine.

See also the section on Drug Selection in the Introduction.

DOSAGE AND PREPARATIONS.

Inhalation: *Adults,* one or two deep inhalations every one to two hours from a handheld bulb, pressure-driven nebulizer, or metered-dose inhaler.

Children, for acute asthma, 5 to 15 deep inhalations from a hand nebulizer containing the 1:200 solution, repeated in 10 to 30 minutes if necessary, or three to seven deep inhalations of the 1:100 dilution. Some physicians prefer to limit the dose to five inhalations of the 1:200 solution and to avoid use of the 1:100 solution. Children should be allowed to use a metered-dose inhaler only if they are instructed in proper use and are aware of its limitations.

When a pressure-driven nebulizer is used, *adults,* up to 0.5 ml of the 1:200 solution or 0.3 ml of the 1:100 solution is delivered over 30 minutes with a flow of 5 to 10 L/min; however, a dilution of 1:2,000 may be preferable. Lower doses are recommended for children.

ISOPROTERENOL HYDROCHLORIDE:
Generic. Aerosol 1:400 (2.5 mg/ml).
Isuprel (Winthrop-Breon). Solution (for nebulization) 1:100 (10 mg/ml) and 1:200 (5 mg/ml).
Isuprel Mistometer (Winthrop-Breon). Aerosol providing 131 mcg/dose.
Vapo-Iso (Fisons). Solution (for nebulization) 1:200 (5 mg/ml).
ISOPROTERENOL SULFATE:
Medihaler-Iso (Riker). Aerosol 0.2% providing 80 mcg/measured dose.

Intravenous: This route is used only in intensive care units by experienced personnel and only with great caution. *Children* with respiratory failure caused by asthma, the initial infusion rate is 0.1 mcg/kg/min, increased by 0.1 mcg/kg/min at 15-minute intervals until a clinical response, a heart rate greater than 180, or an infusion rate of 0.8 mcg/kg/min is achieved.

ISOPROTERENOL HYDROCHLORIDE:
Generic. Solution 1:5,000 (0.2 mg/ml) in 5 and 10 ml containers.
Isuprel Hydrochloride (Winthrop-Breon). Solution (sterile) 1:5,000 (0.2 mg/ml) in 1 and 5 ml containers.

Sublingual: This route is not recommended because absorption is unpredictable. The manufacturer's suggested dosage is: *Adults,* 10 to 15 mg three or four times daily (maximum, 60 mg daily); *children,* 5 to 10 mg three or four times daily (maximum, 30 mg daily).

ISOPROTERENOL HYDROCHLORIDE:
Isuprel Hydrochloride (Winthrop-Breon). Tablets 10 and 15 mg.

METAPROTERENOL SULFATE
[Alupent, Metaprel]

ACTIONS AND USES. This selective beta$_2$ agonist is widely used in a nebulizer to treat acute asthma. Metaproterenol is also available in oral preparations and in a metered-dose inhaler.

When inhaled, metaproterenol often is as effective as albuterol or isoproterenol; onset of action is five minutes and duration is up to four hours.

Metaproterenol is often used orally; therapy should be

ly. This route is generally safe and the duration of action is three to four hours.

ADVERSE REACTIONS. Like other beta$_2$ agonists, the most common adverse reactions are tremor, nervousness and palpitations. This drug is classified in FDA Pregnancy Category C.

For further information on indications, adverse reactions, and precautions, see the section on Drug Selection in the Introduction.

DOSAGE AND PREPARATIONS.

Inhalation: Adults and children over 12 years, two or three deep inhalations every one to five minutes. This may be repeated at four-hour intervals, but the total daily dose should not exceed 16 inhalations.

　　Alupent (Boehringer Ingelheim), *Metaprel* (Dorsey). Powder (micronized) 225 mg (0.65 mg/measured dose) in metered-dose inhaler; solution (for nebulization) 0.6% premixed unit dose (*Alupent*) and 5%.

Oral: (Tablets and syrup) *Adults,* initially, 10 mg three or four times a day, increased gradually over two to four weeks to 20 mg three or four times daily, if needed. Limited data are available on use of the tablet form in *children.* (Syrup) *Children 6 to 9 years (under 27 kg),* 10 mg three or four times daily; *over 9 years (over 27 kg),* adult dose.

　　Alupent (Boehringer Ingelheim), *Metaprel* (Dorsey). Syrup 10 mg/5 ml; tablets 10 and 20 mg.

PROCATEROL

[Beta-Air]

This investigational beta$_2$-adrenergic agonist has a car-bostyril nucleus instead of the usual benzene ring. Procaterol was synthesized in Japan and is widely used in that country. It is used orally or by inhalation and appears to be more potent than albuterol. The duration of action also appears to be longer. Asthma may be controlled in some individuals with twice-daily dosing (Kemp et al, 1985).

The indications, adverse reactions, and precautions are the same as those of albuterol. The incidence of severe tremor is high initially, but, in general, procaterol is well tolerated.

　　Beta-Air (Parke-Davis).
　　(Investigational drug)

TERBUTALINE SULFATE

[Brethaire, Brethine, Bricanyl]

ACTIONS AND USES. The efficacy of this selective beta$_2$ agonist in asthma is similar to that of albuterol. It may be administered by metered-dose inhaler, subcutaneously, or orally. When inhaled in usual doses, terbutaline appears to have little or no effect on beta$_1$ receptors.

Inhaled terbutaline has a duration of action similar to that of albuterol (about four hours). In some studies, the oral form has had a slightly longer duration of action than oral albuterol. This preparation is as effective as oral metaproterenol, but both drugs cause more side effects than the inhaled form.

In general, the subcutaneous preparation resembles epinephrine in onset and effect, but the duration of action may be longer. The incidence and severity of adverse reactions also resemble those with subcutaneous epinephrine.

ADVERSE REACTIONS AND PRECAUTIONS. Oral terbutaline is generally safe and well tolerated, but tremor occurs frequently, especially in the elderly. Dizziness, nervousness, fatigue, tinnitus, and palpitations are rare. When inhaled, the incidence of these adverse reactions is low. This drug is classified in FDA Pregnancy Category B.

For more information on indications, adverse reactions, and precautions, see the section on Drug Selection in the Introduction.

DOSAGE AND PREPARATIONS.

Inhalation: Adults and children over 12 years, two or three deep inhalations one to five minutes apart. This may be repeated at four- to six-hour intervals. The total daily dosage should not exceed 16 to 20 inhalations.

　　Brethaire (Geigy). Aerosol 200 mcg/measured dose.

Oral: Adults, initially, 2.5 mg three times daily at approximately six-hour intervals, increased gradually over two to four weeks to 5 mg three times daily, if needed. *Children 12 years and over,* 1.25 to 2.5 mg three times daily at six- to eight-hour intervals; the dose may be increased, if needed and tolerated, to a maximum of 7.5 mg daily.

　　Brethine (Geigy), *Bricanyl* (Lakeside). Tablets 2.5 and 5 mg (equivalent to 2.05 and 4.1 mg of free base, respectively).

Subcutaneous: Adults, for acute exacerbations, 0.25 mg, repeated in 15 to 30 minutes if necessary; no more than 0.5 mg should be administered in any four-hour period. *Children,* 0.01 mg/kg (maximum total dose, 0.25 mg). The dose may be repeated once in 30 minutes if necessary but usually is effective for four hours.

　　Brethine (Geigy), *Bricanyl* (Lakeside). Solution (sterile) 1 mg (equivalent to 0.82 mg of free base)/ml in 2 ml containers.

XANTHINE DRUGS

THEOPHYLLINE

ACTIONS AND USES. Theophylline is the most widely prescribed bronchodilator in the United States for maintenance therapy in patients with moderate or severe asthma (Jenne, 1984; Weinberger, 1984; Bukowskyj et al, 1984). In addition to its bronchodilator effect, theophylline has positive cardiac inotropic, vasodilating, and diuretic actions. It also stimulates diaphragmatic contraction and increases its resistance to fatigue.

Indications for its use include treatment of moderate to severe exacerbations of asthma, prevention of attacks, or alleviation of signs and symptoms during periods of remission. Theophylline is especially useful in children and in those with acute asthma. It may be beneficial in patients with chronic bronchitis who have bronchospasm and, because of its stimulatory effects on the heart and diaphragmatic muscle, in some patients with emphysema. Theophylline stimulates the central nervous system at the medullary level and is given to treat apnea of prematurity (see Chapter 17, Adjuncts to Anesthesia).

The utilization of theophylline has increased with the availability of timed-release (sustained-release, SR) preparations and improved techniques for determining serum concentrations. Timed-release preparations may increase compliance and reduce fluctuations in serum concentrations. Satisfactory serum levels usually can be maintained for 12 to 24 hours. These forms can be especially helpful for nighttime use, a consideration in view of the predilection of asthma to increase in severity in late night and early morning hours. The use of standard (rapidly absorbed) oral preparations has decreased significantly with the availability of these timed-release forms.

Since the effective plasma level is close to the toxic concentration, periodic determinations of drug concentration are recommended if maximal doses are used. For most patients, adverse effects are rare if the serum concentration remains below 15 mcg/ml. The incidence of toxic effects increases greatly at concentrations higher than 20 mcg/ml.

The wide individual variation in theophylline plasma half-life (2 to 12 hours in adults) and the variety of factors that alter clearance (eg, drugs, diseases, diet) necessitate careful adjustment of dosage (Dwyer, 1984).

Because absorption kinetics of preparations vary, it is advisable for the physician to become familiar with only a few theophylline preparations.

ADVERSE REACTIONS AND PRECAUTIONS. Compliance may be a problem with use of theophylline and patients should be warned that doubling a dose after missing a dose can lead to serious toxicity. Side effects are primarily dose related and usually develop at serum levels exceeding 20 mcg/ml but occasionally occur at lower levels. Minor adverse effects include headache, dizziness, nervousness, insomnia, nausea, vomiting, and epigastric pain. Patients with pre-existing multifocal atrial tachycardia have been reported to experience an increase in the frequency of arrhythmias with serum levels in the normal range (Marchlinski and Miller, 1985). When adverse reactions occur, the drug should be withdrawn temporarily. During initial therapy, some authorities recommend gradual increases in dose every one to three weeks to reduce minor adverse effects and improve patient compliance (Hendeles and Weinberger, 1983).

The above adverse reactions intensify and increase in number with high serum concentrations. At a serum concentration above 35 mcg/ml, severe toxic reactions manifested by severe headache, hypokalemia, arrhythmias, persistent vomiting, agitation, hyperreflexia, fasciculations, and sometimes convulsions can occur regardless of the route of administration. Seizures, the first sign of toxicity in some patients, have been reported with serum concentrations as low as 25 mcg/ml and are often refractory to therapy; death or severe residual effects occur in a high percentage of these patients. Arrhythmias usually respond to lidocaine. In children, hematemesis, central nervous system stimulation, diaphoresis, and fever may be observed.

Aminophylline or theophylline must be injected or infused very slowly; rapid intravenous infusion has caused fatal cardiovascular reactions (Jenne, 1984). Because of occasional hypersensitivity to aminophylline, timed-release theophylline preparations are preferred for oral use.

Theophylline may relax the gastroesophageal sphincter, leading to reflux into the esophagus which may aggravate asthma. Theophylline compounds increase gastric acidity and should be used cautiously, if at all, in patients with gastrointestinal ulcers or significant reflux. Bladder relaxation may cause urinary retention when outflow from the urinary tract is already compromised.

The doses should be reduced in patients with overt liver disease or congestive heart failure.

Some reports have suggested that prolonged administration of theophylline in children occasionally produces behavioral and intellectual changes that interfere with learning and adversely affect personality (Furukawa et al, 1984; Selcow et al, 1983). In contrast, one study reported that theophylline enhanced fine motor coordination and did not produce significant detrimental effects on behavior or intellectual function (Joad et al, 1985).

There is no evidence that theophylline is unsafe for mothers, the fetus, or neonates. At usual blood levels, theophylline crosses the placenta and most infants tolerate theophylline levels that correspond to therapeutic levels in the mother. This drug is classified in FDA Pregnancy Category C. Theophylline is found in breast milk; a nursing infant could receive as much as 10% of the maternal dose of theophylline.

TREATMENT OF ACUTE OVERDOSE. Aggressive treatment is necessary to prevent seizures. Initial treatment with ipecac removes theophylline from the stomach, and further absorption is prevented by administering activated charcoal. Repeated use of activated charcoal enhances elimination of the drug. Concomitant administration of a cathartic, such as sodium sulfate, increases the elimination of charcoal and unabsorbed theophylline.

These procedures should be instituted when the serum concentration exceeds 40 mcg/ml (Weinberger, 1984) or at lower levels when symptoms occur. When theophylline serum concentrations exceed 50 mcg/ml, much of the administered dose of charcoal may be lost by vomiting (Sessler et al, 1985). In acute situations, extracorporeal hemoperfusion with charcoal clears theophylline more rapidly but requires special equipment and services, is costly, takes time to set up, and may be hazardous to the patient.

An acute single overdose of theophylline is better tolerated than sustained high levels occurring in chronic overdosage. Hemoperfusion may be used for an acute single overdose if the serum concentration of theophylline exceeds 100 mcg/ml. For chronic overdosage, hemoperfusion is recommended when serum levels exceed 60 mcg/ml and should be considered when serum levels exceed 40 mcg/ml (Olson et al, 1985). Since intravenous phenobarbital may raise the seizure threshold in patients with dangerously high serum theophylline concentrations prophylactic use of this drug is advisable, particularly in the agitated patient (Hendeles and Weinberger, 1983; Jenne, 1984).

PHARMACOKINETICS AND DRUG INTERACTIONS. Theophylline is metabolized by the liver and excreted by the kidneys. A small alteration in the percentage of theophylline metabolized can produce large differences in clearance. Since the volume of distribution is usually constant in adults and children, changes in elimination half-life are generally inversely parallel to changes in clearance.

The mean half-life of theophylline is about 8.7 hours in nonsmoking adults, 5.5 hours in smoking adults, and 3.7 hours in children. However, the half-life varies widely among individuals and is prolonged in premature infants, elderly patients, and patients with congestive heart failure, pulmonary edema, alcoholism, liver dysfunction, obesity, viral upper respiratory infections, pneumonia, and fever (Jenne, 1984).

Large doses of allopurinol and usual doses of cimetidine, oral contraceptives, and some macrolide antibiotics (eg, erythromycin, troleandomycin) may reduce the clearance and prolong the plasma half-life of theophylline, possibly leading to toxicity. For concurrent use with theophylline, ranitidine is preferable to cimetidine. A 50% reduction in dose of theophylline is indicated for patients receiving troleandomycin or cimetidine and for those with persistent high fever. Influenza virus vaccine, viral infections, furosemide, and beta-blocking agents also may prolong the half-life of theophylline. The dose of theophylline may need to be decreased when one or more of these factors is present.

The maintenance dose of theophylline should be decreased by 33% in patients also receiving erythromycin for over three days. Smoking may counteract the decreased rate of theophylline clearance induced by erythromycin or other agents.

Antibiotics that do not affect theophylline clearance include penicillin, ampicillin, tetracycline, rifampin, and cephalexin [Keflex]. Concomitant use of phenytoin, tobacco or marijuana smoking, or four weeks of phenobarbital therapy induce hepatic drug metabolizing enzymes and shorten the half-life of theophylline by increasing its clearance; the dose of theophylline may need to be increased in these patients.

Other methylxanthines consumed in the diet, such as caffeine and theobromine, compete with theophylline at sites of metabolism. These substances appear to decrease theophylline clearance but also may provide additional bronchodilator effects. It has been estimated that two to three cups of coffee are equivalent to 200 mg of theophylline. Patients who reduce their dietary intake of methylxanthines may need increased doses of theophylline.

Most preparations of theophylline are almost completely absorbed after oral administration. Once-a-day preparations are less completely absorbed. Some timed-release preparations may approach zero-order absorption kinetics. Aminophylline suppositories are erratically and unreliably absorbed; rectal solutions are well absorbed but may be irritating.

A fatty meal may cause the premature release (dumping) of theophylline from some timed-release preparations (primarily Theo-24) taken within one hour of eating (Hendeles et al, 1985). Dumping apparently does not occur with Theo-Dur, a 12-hour preparation. When Uniphyl, a 24-hour preparation, is administered with a meal, absorption may be enhanced significantly (Karim et al, 1985); when it is taken on an empty stomach, absorption may not be complete. Food has been shown to decrease the bioavailability of Theo-Dur Sprinkle. Serum concentrations may fluctuate in a single individual after prolonged treatment with any timed-release preparation.

Administration every 12 hours is preferable to once-daily dosing for maintenance therapy in children and adult smokers. In rapid metabolizers, 12-hour preparations may have to be given every 8 hours and 24-hour preparations every 12 hours. Nonsmoking adults generally can be managed with either a standard (rapidly absorbed) or timed-release form.

MONITORING OF SERUM CONCENTRATIONS. Monitoring the serum concentrations of theophylline is important for the following reasons: (1) The safe range of serum concentrations is narrow and individual requirements vary widely. (2) It is unclear to what extent drug interactions alter theophylline's rate of clearance. (3) The dosage can be adjusted to avoid toxicity if a serum concentration has been determined for at least the initial dose adjustment period.

Significant changes in serum concentration can result from small changes in dosage: An increment of 1 mg/kg raises the serum concentration by about 2 mcg/ml.

Steady-state levels are reached in five half-lives, and almost 90% of steady state is reached in three half-lives. In patients receiving long-term therapy, adjustment of serum concentration should be based on response to therapy and the disease's status.

The serum theophylline concentration should be measured when the patient's clinical condition changes. When tea, coffee, chocolate, acetaminophen, or cola drinks are ingested, serum concentrations of theophylline measured spectrophotometrically may be elevated unless these substances are separated out chromatographically.

In order to provide an adequate margin of safety and prevent toxic serum levels in both children and adults, it is generally recommended that a serum concentration of 10 to 15 mcg/ml be maintained (Jenne, 1984). Some individuals benefit from lower serum levels (5 to 10 mcg/ml). If carefully monitored, a serum concentration greater than 15 mcg/ml may be maintained if no toxicity develops.

DOSAGE AND PREPARATIONS. Theophylline may be administered orally (as theophylline, oxtriphylline, or aminophylline), rectally (as aminophylline), or intravenously (as theophylline or aminophylline). Oral preparations containing salts of theophylline, such as aminophylline and oxtriphylline, have no advantage over oral theophylline.

A number of dosing schedules are employed. Some of the most widely quoted schedules are discussed in this section.

The standard rapidly absorbed oral preparations must be given every four to six hours to sustain effective blood levels in patients in whom the theophylline half-life is short (children and adult smokers). *Timed-release preparations* provide adequate blood levels when given every 8, 12, or 24 hours. However, since the rates of absorption and metabolism vary widely among patients and in the same patient at different times (Dederich et al, 1981), use of timed-release preparations does not obviate the need for clinical and laboratory monitoring.

Many physicians do not routinely measure serum levels. If they are measured, the following guideline is suggested: The first serum determination can be made at least 72 hours after the initial dose. Ideally, the peak serum concentration should be determined 8 to 12 hours after the morning dose of a 24-hour preparation, four to six hours after the morning dose of a 12-hour preparation, or two hours after a standard rapidly absorbed preparation has been given. Some authorities measure only the trough concentration just before the next dose although, with a 12-hour preparation, the true trough may occur one to two hours later. Before serum concentrations are determined during long-term therapy, the patient should have taken the drug as prescribed with no missed or added doses for at least 48 hours. Determining the concentration 30 minutes after a loading dose of an intravenous xanthine is appropriate.

Rapid methods now available for determination of serum theophylline levels can help determine whether a loading dose is required for immediate induction of optimal theophylline therapy.

THEOPHYLLINE:

Dosages are expressed as milligrams of *anhydrous theophylline equivalents* per kilogram of ideal body weight for the elixir, syrup, liquid, oral suspension, tablet, chewable tablet, capsule, timed-release capsule, and tablet preparations (see below). The loading dose should be reduced or eliminated if the patient has received theophylline within 24 hours.

Oral: *(Standard Rapidly Absorbed Oral Formulations: Capsules, Tablets, and Liquids)* For an acute attack not requiring parenteral therapy, *adults,* initially, 5 mg/kg followed by a maintenance dose of 3 to 4 mg/kg every six hours to control symptoms. Single doses in excess of 4 mg/kg every six hours should not be given until the theophylline serum concentration is determined. However, in nonsmoking adults (in whom theophylline half-lives are longer), the total daily dose should be limited to 10 to 12 mg/kg/day initially, and a dose can be given every eight hours. The amount is even further reduced and closely monitored in patients with cardiac decompensation or liver disease. This initial dosage in the adult should usually result in mean theophylline serum concentrations of 10 to 15 mcg/ml. Further adjustments are made on the basis of measured serum concentrations. The same dosages and limitations are applicable for *children* except that the initial maintenance dose is 4 to 5 mg/kg every six hours.

(Oral Formulations Including Timed-Release Forms) For long-term prophylaxis, if there is no urgency and laboratory facilities for measurement of serum theophylline concentration are available, the following schedule for multistep titration of dosage has been recommended (Weinberger and Hendeles,

1983) to minimize the incidence and severity of side effects and toxic reactions.

Multistep Titration of Dosage: For *adults and children over 1 year,* the initial dose with either a standard or timed-release form (12- or 24-hour preparation) is 400 mg or 16 mg/kg daily *(whichever is less),* given in two or three divided doses at 8- or 12-hour intervals. This is inadequate for most patients but is unlikely to produce serious adverse effects. The dose should be increased *if tolerated* in increments of approximately 25% at three-day intervals, and the following limits should not be exceeded: *children less than 9 years,* 24 mg/kg/day; *9 to 12 years,* 20 mg/kg/day; *12 to 16 years,* 18 mg/kg/day; *over 16 years,* 13 mg/kg/day or 900 mg/day, whichever is less. (These limits represent the average therapeutic doses determined for these age groups.)

The final dosage adjustment (expressed as percentage change in total daily dose) is dependent upon the peak theophylline serum concentration (in mcg/ml) and assessment of clinical improvement. The dosing interval is more dependent on the trough serum level.

5 to 7.5: If the patient is asymptomatic, a drug-free period should be considered. Otherwise, the dose should be increased by 25% and the serum concentration measured again.

7.5 to 10: If the patient is asymptomatic, no increase is necessary; if symptoms occur during URI or exercise, the dose should be increased cautiously by 25%. If symptoms recur at the end of a dosing interval and the serum level is less than 10 mcg/ml, the drug should be given more frequently and a higher maintenance theophylline serum level may be necessary.

10 to 13: If the patient is asymptomatic, no increase is necessary; if symptoms occur during URI or exercise, the dose should be increased cautiously by 10%.

13 to 20: If "breakthrough" in asthmatic symptoms occurs at the end of a dosing interval with the standard short-acting form, a timed-release product is substituted and the serum level measurement is repeated. If side effects occur, the total daily dose is decreased by 10%.

20 to 25: Even if side effects are absent, the dose is decreased by 10%.

25 to 30: Even if side effects are absent, the next dose is omitted and the total daily dose is decreased by 25%; measurement of the serum concentration is repeated.

30 or above: The next two doses are omitted; the subsequent dose is decreased by at least 50% and the serum concentration is measured again.

After each dose adjustment, serum concentrations must be measured. When patients experience adverse effects, they should be advised to omit the next dose and, when the adverse effects disappear, to decrease the total daily dose upon resuming therapy. Once a satisfactory serum concentration has been established for long-term therapy, serum concentrations should be measured at least yearly or whenever it is suspected that theophylline's rate of elimination may be altered by factors that affect clearance.

Alternative to Multistep Titration of Dosage: Although the multistep titration of dosage described above is often quoted in the medical literature, some authorities believe that this approach is difficult to use chiefly because of intraindividual variables in theophylline absorption kinetics. An alternative simpler approach for adults is to begin therapy with 300 to 400 mg/24 hours (adaptation phase) for several days and then to increase to conservative full doses of 500 to 600 mg/day (depending on stature) in nonsmokers, patients with cor pulmonale, and the elderly, and to 800 to 900 mg/day in smokers. Following institution of a conservative full-dose schedule, the serum concentration is measured at least 48 hours after no missed doses and a final dose adjustment is made to achieve serum levels between 10 to 15 mcg/ml (Jenne, 1984). Thus, a distinction is made between smokers and nonsmokers in the initial dosing schedule. For some nonsmokers, doses above 10 to 12 mg/kg/day (ideal body weight) may occasionally produce high serum concentrations and toxicity (Jenne, 1984).

STANDARD PREPARATIONS:

Generic. Capsules 250 and 260 mg; elixir and solution 26.7 mg/5 ml; tablets 100, 200, and 300 mg.

Accubron (Merrell Dow). Elixir 50 mg/5 ml (alcohol 7.5%).

Aerolate (Fleming). Liquid 53.3 mg/5 ml.

Elixicon (Berlex). Suspension 100 mg/5 ml.

Elixophyllin (Forest). Capsules 100 and 200 mg; elixir 26.7 mg/5 ml (alcohol 20%).

Quibron-T (Mead Johnson). Tablets 300 mg.

Slo-Phyllin (Rorer). Syrup 26.7 mg/5 ml; tablets 100 and 200 mg.

Somophyllin-T (Fisons). Capsules 100, 200, and 250 mg.

Synophylate (Central). Elixir (theophylline sodium glycinate) 110 mg (equivalent to 50 mg of base)/5 ml (alcohol 20%).

Theolair (Riker). Liquid 26.7 mg/5 ml; tablets 125 and 250 mg.

TIMED-RELEASE PREPARATIONS:

Generic. Capsules 125, 200, 250, 260, and 300 mg (12 hours); tablets 100, 200, and 300 mg (12 hours).

Aerolate (Fleming). Capsules 65, 130, and 260 mg (8 to 12 hours).

Bronkodyl S-R (Winthrop-Breon). Capsules 300 mg (12 hours).

Constant-T (Geigy). Tablets 200 and 300 mg (8 to 12 hours).

Elixophyllin SR (Forest). Capsules 125 and 250 mg (12 hours).

Duraphyl (Forest). Tablets 100, 200 and 300 mg (12 hours).

LāBID (Norwich Eaton). Tablets 250 mg (12 hours).

Quibron-T/SR (Mead Johnson). Tablets 300 mg (12 hours).

Respid (Boehringer Ingelheim). Tablets 250 and 500 mg (8 to 12 hours).

Slo-bid (Rorer). Capsules 50, 100, 200, and 300 mg (12 hours).

Slo-Phyllin (Rorer). Capsules 60, 125, and 250 mg (8 to 12 hours).

Somophyllin-CRT (Fisons). Capsules 100, 200, 250, and 300 mg (12 hours).

Sustaire (Pfipharmecs). Tablets 100 and 300 mg (12 hours).

Theo-24 (Searle). Capsules 100, 200, and 300 mg (24 hours).

Theobid (Glaxo). Capsules 130 and 260 mg (12 hours).

Theo-Dur (Key). Tablets 100, 200, and 300 mg (12 to 24 hours).

Theo-Dur Sprinkle (Key). Capsules 50, 75, 125, and 200 mg (12 hours).

Theolair-SR (Riker). Tablets 200, 250, 300, and 500 mg (8 to 12 hours).

Theophyl-SR (McNeil). Capsules 125 and 250 mg (8 hours).

Theovent (Schering). Capsules 125 and 250 mg (12 hours).

Uniphyl (Purdue Frederick). Tablets 200 and 400 mg (12 to 24 hours).

NOTE FOR ONCE-A-DAY FORMS: Uniphyl should be taken with meals and at the same time each day. If doses of Theo-24 exceed 900 mg/day or 13 mg/kg/day (whichever is less), this product should be administered at least one hour before or after a meal. Fasting patients may not absorb the total daily dose of either Uniphyl or Theo-24 completely. Uniphyl and Theo-24 are usually administered at 8 AM. Some investigators suggest Uniphyl be given at bedtime to provide higher early morning serum levels for patients with nocturnal bronchospasm (Rivington et al, 1985).

Intravenous: See Aminophylline.

Theophylline and 5% Dextrose (Abbott, Travenol). 0.4 mg/ml in 1,000 ml containers, 0.8 mg/ml in 500 and 1,000 ml containers, 1.6 mg/ml in 250 and 500 ml containers, 2 mg/ml in 100 ml containers, and 4 mg/ml in 50 and 100 ml containers.

AMINOPHYLLINE:

Aminophylline formulations vary in their equivalence to anhydrous theophylline from 79% to 86%. Therefore, it is necessary to follow the manufacturers' recommended dose for the individual product or to calculate the appropriate dose on the basis of anhydrous theophylline equivalents: 100 mg of the 86% formulation = 86 mg anhydrous theophylline; 100 mg of the 79% formulation = 79 mg anhydrous theophylline. The following doses are given for milligrams of anhydrous theophylline per kilogram of body weight.

Intravenous: *Adults and children,* for an acute attack, a loading dose of 6 mg/kg aminophylline (5 mg/kg theophylline) is administered using a slow intravenous drip (rate no more than 25 mg/min). The loading dose should be reduced by 50% if the patient has received theophylline within the previous 24 hours.

After the loading dose, the following amounts of aminophylline (mg/kg/hr) are infused for maintenance: *children less than 9 years,* 1.0; *children 9 to 16 years and healthy adults who smoke,* 0.80; *healthy adults who do not smoke,* 0.5; *patients with cardiac decompensation or liver dysfunction,* 0.2. The maintenance dose should be reduced if nausea, vomiting, headache, tachycardia, or other toxic effects appear or the serum theophylline concentration exceeds 20 mcg/ml. Following the loading dose, measurement of serum concentrations will indicate the need for any adjustment in dose. Levels measured at 18 to 24 hours may warn of impending toxic levels before they occur (Jenne, 1984).

Generic. Solution (intravenous) 25 mg/ml in 10 and 20 ml containers; solution (intramuscular) 250 mg/ml in 2 ml containers.

Rectal: The rectal solution is absorbed reliably and rapidly and is safe for occasional use but routine administration cannot be recommended. Suppositories are not recommended because of their erratic absorption.

(Retention Unit) Adults, 5 ml (equivalent to 255 mg theophylline) one to three times daily. The total daily dose should not exceed the average therapeutic dose limits (see oral dosage for theophylline) or a serum theophylline concentration of 20 mcg/ml. *Children,* 5 mg/kg (as theophylline) administered no more often than every six hours. The total daily dose should be based on age and determined as for adults.

Generic. Suppositories 250 and 500 mg.

Somophyllin (Fisons). Solution 300 mg/5 ml in 90 and 150 ml containers.

Oral: Dosage is based on theophylline equivalents.

Generic. Liquid 105 mg/5 ml; tablets (plain, enteric-coated) 100 and 200 mg.

Phyllocontin (Purdue-Frederick). Tablets (timed-release) 225 mg (12 hours).

Somophyllin, Somophyllin-DF (Fisons). Liquid 105 mg/5 ml.

OXTRIPHYLLINE (Theophylline 64% with Choline 36%):

Oral: Dosage is based on theophylline equivalents.

Generic. Elixir 100 mg/5 ml; syrup (pediatric) 50 mg/5 ml; tablets 100 and 200 mg.

Choledyl (Parke-Davis). Elixir 100 mg/5 ml (alcohol 20%); syrup (pediatric) 50 mg/5 ml; tablets 100 and 200 mg; tablets (timed-release) 400 and 600 mg (**Choledyl SA**).

DYPHYLLINE
[Dilor, Lufyllin]

Dyphylline is much less potent than theophylline. Doses about five times those of theophylline are required to produce equivalent plasma drug concentrations (Lawyer et al, 1980), but theophylline serum assays cannot be used to monitor dyphylline levels (Bussey, 1981). Since the range of therapeutic plasma concentrations for dyphylline is not yet as clearly defined as that for theophylline, the latter is preferred for acute and chronic asthma, particularly when intravenous administration is required.

This drug may be administered orally, intramuscularly, or intravenously (investigational). It is rapidly eliminated unchanged in the urine; the half-life is about two hours (one-half that of theophylline). This may be extended by administering oral probenecid 1 g one-half hour before dyphylline is used (May and Jarboe, 1981).

Adverse reactions are similar to those produced by theophylline, although nervousness, dizziness, and palpitations may be less prominent.

DOSAGE AND PREPARATIONS. The following doses are recommended by the manufacturers.
Intramuscular: Adults, 250 to 500 mg every six hours; the dosage should be individualized on the basis of the condition and response of the patient. *Children,* dosage has not been established.

> **Dilor** (Savage), **Lufyllin** (Wallace), **Generic.** Solution (for intramuscular use only) 250 mg/ml in 2 (**Dilor** only) and 10 ml containers.

Intravenous (Investigational): 200 mg infused over 20 minutes, followed by 100 mg/hr. (This dose may require upward titration for relief of symptoms.)
Oral: Adults, 15 mg/kg every six hours; the dosage should be individualized on the basis of the condition and response of the patient. *Children,* dosage has not been established.

> **Dilor** (Savage). Elixir 53.3 mg/5 ml (alcohol 18%); tablets 200 and 400 mg.
> **Lufyllin** (Wallace). Elixir 33.3 mg/5 ml (alcohol 20%); tablets 200 and 400 mg.

ANTI-INFLAMMATORY CORTICOSTEROIDS

BECLOMETHASONE DIPROPIONATE
[Beclovent, Vanceril]

ACTIONS AND USES. Beclomethasone dipropionate is an esterified chlorinated analogue of betamethasone. This potent, lipid-soluble corticosteroid acts locally on the respiratory mucosa. Very low doses are delivered by a metered-dose inhaler (42 mcg/inhalation) and the absorbed drug is inactivated rapidly, which markedly reduces the incidence of hypothalamic-pituitary-adrenal (HPA) axis suppression or serious adverse reactions.

This potent inhalant corticosteroid is the standard to which other drugs of this class are compared (Brogden et al, 1984). Its use allows the elimination of oral steroids or a reduction in their dosage in some patients with severe steroid-dependent asthma. Symptoms of severe exercise-induced asthma are prevented in some patients.

Asthma should be brought under optimum control with an oral corticosteroid before an inhalant corticosteroid preparation is utilized. Patients who require less than 10 mg of oral prednisone or the equivalent often can be converted to an inhalant corticosteroid; conversion is usually much more difficult in patients who require 20 mg/day or more of the oral preparation.

Caution must be exercised in the transfer from an oral corticosteroid to an inhaled corticosteroid. Several asthmatic patients have died from adrenal crises during the transfer from oral to inhalation therapy, probably because the degree of adrenal suppression was not appreciated. Early morning cortisol levels may be monitored after slow withdrawal of the systemic steroid, but a normal level does not always indicate adequate adrenal responsiveness.

If patients undergo stressful situations (surgery, trauma, respiratory infection, or an exacerbation of severe asthma), a short course of an oral steroid in full therapeutic doses is indicated.

Inhalant corticosteroids are generally safe. Two inhalations three or four times a day are usually satisfactory in mild asthma. For severe asthma, more frequent administration of much larger doses (1 g/day or higher) may be tried but systemic effects may occur.

Beclomethasone inhalers are being developed that are inspiration- or actuator-activated. A high-dose beclomethasone inhaler that provides five times more drug (250 mcg/inhalation) is now available in Europe. Its introduction in this country may increase the percentage of patients who can be weaned from oral steroids.

ADVERSE REACTIONS AND PRECAUTIONS. Patients using beclomethasone aerosol occasionally complain of throat irritation. Dysphonia, sore throat, or dryness of the mouth may limit patient compliance. Use of an adrenergic aerosol about five minutes before inhalation of the steroid may enhance bronchial distribution and prevent cough and throat irritation. The reported incidence of candidal infection of the oropharynx or larynx varies considerably but may be as high as 15%. Patients should be instructed to gargle with water after inhalation to prevent candidiasis. Antifungal therapy and reduction of the dose may be required; discontinuation of beclomethasone therapy is rarely necessary. Adrenal suppression occurs frequently with daily doses above 2 mg and has been observed in adults receiving more than 1.6 mg.

The substitution of inhaled drug for oral corticosteroids can cause withdrawal symptoms, such as muscle and joint pain, lassitude, tiredness, headache, mental depression, nausea, vomiting, and anorexia (Brogden et al, 1984). Exacerbation of conditions previously controlled by systemic steroid therapy (eg, allergic rhinitis, eczema, nasal polyposis) has been observed. Most of these disorders respond to appropriate topical therapy.

For further discussion of indications, adverse reactions, and precautions, see the section on Drug Selection in the Introduction.

DOSAGE AND PREPARATIONS.

Oral Inhalation: Adults, two to four inhalations three or four times daily. The usual maximum recommended dose is 840 mcg/day, but doses up to 1.6 mg/day have been used without systemic reactions or effects on HPA axis function; higher doses (up to 2 mg/day) may be safe but some systemic absorption is more likely (Clark, 1985). *Children 6 to 12 years,* the usual dosage is one or two inhalations three or four times daily; the maximum recommended dose is 420 mcg/day. There are insufficient data to recommend a dosage for *children under 6 years.*

Effective relief of symptoms also can be obtained with twice-daily administration (Meltzer et al, 1985).

The use of a spacer attachment between the mouth and the metered-dose inhaler usually increases the efficiency of drug delivery in patients with improper technique and may decrease the occurrence or severity of oral candidiasis and throat irritation.

Beclovent (Glaxo), **Vanceril** (Schering). Aerosol providing 42 mcg/actuation.

BUDESONIDE

This investigational nonhalogenated corticosteroid has a higher ratio of topical to systemic activity and greater potency than beclomethasone dipropionate, triamcinolone acetonide, or flunisolide (Clissold and Heel, 1984). Doses of 200 to 800 mcg/day of inhaled budesonide are approximately as effective as 400 to 800 mcg/day of inhaled beclomethasone in adults and children with moderate to severe chronic asthma. Its only advantage over inhaled beclomethasone appears to be its effectiveness with twice-daily administration in a greater number of patients than with the latter drug. Otherwise, indications, adverse reactions, and precautions resemble those of beclomethasone dipropionate.

Budesonide (Merck Sharp & Dohme). (Investigational drug)

FLUNISOLIDE
[AeroBid]

The indications for this inhalant halogenated corticosteroid are similar to those for inhaled beclomethasone. Twice-daily administration appears to be effective in more patients and the incidence of oral candidiasis and dysphonia may be less than with inhaled beclomethasone (Orgel et al, 1983).

This drug is classified in FDA Pregnancy Category C.

For additional information on indications, adverse reactions, and precautions, see the evaluation on Beclomethasone Dipropionate and the section on Drug Selection in the Introduction.

DOSAGE AND PREPARATIONS.

Inhalation: Adults and children 6 years and older, two to four inhalations two or three times daily. The maximum daily dose should not exceed 2 mg. There are insufficient data to recommend a dosage for *children under 6 years.*

AeroBid (Key). Aerosol providing approximately 250 mcg/actuation.

TRIAMCINOLONE ACETONIDE
[Azmacort]

The indications for this inhalant halogenated corticosteroid are similar to those for inhaled beclomethasone. The spacer attachment provided with the unit may deliver a greater percentage of drug to the lungs and less to the oropharyngeal cavity, which may enhance the response in poorly coordinated patients who fail to show benefit when using a corticosteroid MDI without a spacer device.

This drug is classified in FDA Pregnancy Category D.

For additional information on indications, adverse reactions, and precautions, see the evaluation on Beclomethasone Dipropionate and the section on Drug Selection in the Introduction.

DOSAGE AND PREPARATIONS.

Oral Inhalation: Adults, two to four inhalations three or four times daily. The maximum daily dose should not exceed 1.6 mg. *Children 6 to 12 years,* one or two inhalations three or four times daily. The maximum daily dose should not exceed 1.2 mg. There are insufficient data to recommend a dosage for *children under 6 years.*

Azmacort (Rorer). Aerosol providing approximately 100 mcg/actuation.

BISCROMONE

CROMOLYN SODIUM
[Intal]

ACTIONS. Cromolyn inhibits both immediate and late asthmatic responses after exposure to a variety of allergens and appears to affect both large and small airways by a mechanism that is not clearly understood. Cromolyn has weak mast cell stabilizing properties. Major mechanisms may involve inhibition of mediator release from mast cells and attentuation or blockade of respiratory neuronal reflexes. These actions may in part be due to inhibition of calcium transport. Cromolyn may also inhibit neutrophil chemotaxis and thus may have anti-inflammatory effects.

USES. Cromolyn is safe and is as effective as theophylline for prophylaxis of mild to moderate asthma in children. Numerous well-controlled clinical trials, including large multicenter studies, have demonstrated that a large proportion of children with chronic asthma experience either partial or complete protection after oral inhalation of cromolyn (Bernstein, 1985; Shapiro and König, 1985). A smaller number of adults benefit from prophylactic use of this drug, but it may be effective in those with allergic asthma. Symptoms not controlled by bronchodilators may respond to cromolyn.

This drug may diminish the effects of reflex mediated asthma and diurnal swings of bronchial lability. It prevents allergic asthma, some cases of nonallergic asthma, and asthma induced by exercise, cold air, or sulfur dioxide. Prophylaxis for exercise- or irritant-induced bronchospasm may be enhanced by continuous therapy. Optimal effects are achieved by giving cromolyn 30 minutes before exposure to a known allergen, 15 minutes before exercise, and about one week before high allergen exposure.

In patients with severe asthma, who respond poorly to individual drugs, benefits may be enhanced by combining cromolyn with a bronchodilator (theophylline or a beta$_2$ agonist) and/or corticosteroid. If combined therapy is prescribed, the physician must individualize the dose of each drug to obtain maximal benefit with minimal adverse reactions. Patients who are able to receive lower doses of systemic steroid while taking cromolyn must be observed carefully when the latter drug is discontinued. If asthma worsens in these patients, the dose of systemic steroid may be increased temporarily and cromolyn therapy reinstituted for maintenance.

Cromolyn has limited value when asthma is associated with emphysema and/or chronic bronchitis. It is ineffective in acute asthma. If an acute attack occurs, conventional therapy should be instituted immediately and cromolyn discontinued.

Many therapeutic failures are due to incorrect inhalation technique utilizing the Spinhaler. With improved drug delivery, cromolyn's role in adults and possibly in the treatment of acute asthma may be re-examined. Wheezing and bronchospasm associated with use of the Spinhaler do not occur with the metered-dose inhaler or nebulizer. The latter devices are particularly useful in young children and patients who cannot tolerate the powder because of cough. Use of cromolyn and a beta-adrenergic drug in the same nebulizing solution is being investigated.

The three forms of cromolyn available for inhalant administration have similar efficacy. The metered-dose inhaler delivers 1 mg of cromolyn/inhalation, which is much less than the amount delivered with the Spinhaler. See also the section on Drug Selection in the Introduction.

ADVERSE REACTIONS AND PRECAUTIONS. Based on the extensive clinical experience that has accumulated in many countries, cromolyn appears to have achieved an unusual record of safety. Serious adverse effects are rare. Urticaria, maculopapular rashes, myositis, and gastroenteritis are rare and disappear when the drug is withdrawn. Reversible eosino-

philic pneumonia has been associated with administration of cromolyn in a few patients.

Occasionally, transient coughing, bronchospasm, throat irritation, dizziness, nausea, vomiting, hoarseness, and wheezing occur after oral inhalation. However, some of these symptoms also developed in patients inhaling a placebo and may be caused by the powder rather than by cromolyn. An inhaled beta agonist used five minutes prior to inhalation of cromolyn may be helpful for patients who develop coughing or wheezing following use of this drug. Throat irritation and hoarseness can be minimized by rinsing the mouth with water after inhalation.

No alterations in the results of hematologic, urinary, hepatic and renal function tests, chest roentgenograms, or electrocardiograms have been reported in patients receiving the drug continuously for as long as five years.

The safety of cromolyn during pregnancy has not been established unequivocally, but no damaging effects on the fetus have been reported. No teratogenic effects have been observed in animals, even after daily intravenous administration of enormous doses of cromolyn throughout pregnancy. However, increased fetal resorption and decreased fetal weight were observed with doses that produced toxic effects in the mother (FDA Pregnancy Category B).

Tolerance usually does not develop with long-term use.

PHARMACOKINETICS. Oral absorption of cromolyn sodium is minimal and the drug is not active by this route. After inhalation, 8% to 10% is absorbed into the blood stream (primarily by the lung but also by the gastrointestinal tract). The fraction of cromolyn absorbed following inhalation of 20 mg does not appear to exert any generalized systemic effects. Most of the absorbed portion is excreted unchanged in the bile and urine within a few days; none appears to undergo metabolic degradation. The unabsorbed portion (approximately 80%) is recoverable from the feces.

Following inhalation, the maximal plasma level is attained within several minutes, and the plasma half-life is 1 to 1.5 hours. The duration of action is four to six hours. Because of its slow onset of action, cromolyn may not be effective for two to six weeks after initiation of therapy and other drugs may be needed in the interim. In some patients, the total trial period can be extended from 8 to 12 weeks, and the dose can be doubled during the last six weeks (Bernstein, 1985).

DOSAGE AND PREPARATIONS. For prophylactic therapy of chronic asthma, regular administration of cromolyn is necessary. The physician must ensure that the patient is able to use the Spinhaler or metered dose inhaler effectively, for inefficient use will reduce the amount of drug reaching the site of action.

Inhalation: Adults and children over 5 years, initially, 20 mg (one Spinhaler capsule or nebulizer dose) or 1.6 mg (two inhalations from a metered-dose inhaler) should be inhaled four times per day at regular intervals. The number of doses should then be reduced to the minimum that will control symptoms. Any inhaled particulate matter may produce acute obstruction of pulmonary airflow in patients with hyperirritable airway; use of an inhaled adrenergic agonist five to ten minutes prior to cromolyn may lessen this problem.

One capsule is punctured in the special inhaler (Spinhaler).

The patient then inhales through the mouthpiece of the inhaler, thereby spinning and vibrating the capsule and introducing its contents into the stream of inspired air. The patient should remove the Spinhaler from his mouth and exhale into the air. This step is repeated until all of the powder is inhaled.

Only power-driven nebulizer devices with a suitable face mask or mouthpiece should be used; hand-operated units are not an acceptable alternative because they deliver too small a volume. The nebulizer solution is compatible with metaproterenol sulfate, 0.25% isoetharine hydrochloride, terbutaline sulfate, or 20% acetylcysteine solution for at least one hour after their admixture.

Intal (Fisons). Capsules 20 mg (**Spinhaler** supplied separately); solution (for nebulizer) 10 mg/ml in 2 ml containers; metered-dose inhaler 0.8 mg per actuation.

ANTICHOLINERGIC DRUGS

ATROPINE SULFATE

ACTIONS AND USES. This parasympathetic antagonist has particularly potent antimuscarinic effects. Inhaled atropine and other anticholinergic drugs inhibit the increase in cholinergic tone that occurs during reflex bronchoconstriction. These agents are more effective and may produce fewer adverse reactions when administered by inhalation.

Following inhalation, the peak effect occurs in 30 to 60 minutes; the duration of action is about three hours in young adults and may be considerably longer in children and the elderly.

Nebulized atropine may be useful in patients with acute asthma or status asthmaticus who do not respond satisfactorily to or cannot tolerate theophylline and/or inhaled beta-agonist drugs (Gross and Skorodin, 1984). It enhances the bronchodilation produced by beta-agonist drugs and may be a useful adjunct in some patients. The response to inhaled atropine is highly individualized.

At present, the primary use of inhaled atropine appears to be in patients with chronic bronchitis or asthma with a bronchitic component in which irritant-induced elevations in cholinergic tone contribute to reflex bronchoconstriction. It is more likely to be effective when cough is associated with the asthma or chronic bronchitis.

Atropine sulfate 1 to 2 mg by inhalation may be as effective as 100 to 200 mcg of albuterol.

ADVERSE REACTIONS. This tertiary amine crosses the blood-brain barrier; it enters the systemic circulation more readily and produces more adverse effects than ipratropium (investigational) and other quaternary ammonium agents. Dry mouth is common. Difficulty in urination and skin flushing have been reported occasionally. Other anticholinergic effects (eg, tachycardia, gastrointestinal complaints, blurred vision) are rare. Although it is often claimed that atropine increases the viscosity of bronchial secretions and impairs ciliary clearance, there is little evidence that such effects occur.

With massive overdoses, acute glaucoma, psychosis, hyperthermia, and fatalities may occur after inhalation of atropine.

For additional information, see the section on Drug Selection in the Introduction.

DOSAGE AND PREPARATIONS.
Oral Inhalation: Adults, 0.025 mg/kg diluted with 3 to 5 ml of saline and given by nebulizer three or four times daily.

A dose of 0.025 mg/kg is provided by diluting 0.1 to 0.2 ml of the 1% solution with isotonic saline to 3 to 5 ml. A dose of 0.05 mg/kg results in a maximal effect but causes more adverse effects. A total of 2.5 mg is the maximum single dose for most adults. For *children*, 0.05 mg/kg diluted in saline and given by nebulizer three or four times daily.

A 1% solution of atropine provides 10 mg/ml. Atropine can be prepared from a stock solution. It is also available commercially as a solution for nebulization.

Dey-Dose Atropine Sulfate (Dey). Solution (for nebulization) 0.2% (1 mg) and 0.5% (2.5 mg) in 0.5 ml containers.

IPRATROPIUM BROMIDE
[Atrovent]

This investigational quaternary ammonium drug is more effective and safer than atropine. It has been used as a bronchodilator in Europe for a number of years. Like inhaled atropine, ipratropium may be useful when theophylline and/or an inhaled beta₂ agonist is not adequate or not tolerated and in asthmatic patients with coexisting chronic bronchitis or cough as the predominant symptom. In England, nebulized ipratropium has been used in acute asthma and status asthmaticus when the response to inhaled beta-adrenergic drugs was inadequate (Rees, 1984 B). This drug is most effective in very young children and in older patients, especially for the treatment of chronic bronchitis; it is least useful in asthmatic patients in their teens or young adults.

Ipratropium 40 mcg delivered by metered-dose inhaler is reported to be as effective as albuterol 100 mcg or inhaled atropine 1 mg.

Ipratropium is absorbed poorly and blood levels are very low; thus, inhalation is safe and generally free of adverse effects (Gross and Skorodin, 1984). Peak onset of action occurs about one to two hours after inhalation and the duration of action is approximately three to five hours. Ipratropium does not cross the blood-brain barrier.

Inhaled ipratropium has no significant effects on mucus

viscosity, production, or clearance. It is probably safe for use in patients with glaucoma or bladder neck obstruction. Paradoxical bronchoconstriction occurs occasionally due to the hypotonicity of the inhalant solution but has not been observed with use of metered-dose inhalers. Tolerance has not developed in patients treated for up to five years.

Isotonic saline should be used to dilute the solution for nebulization because bronchospasm has occurred when water was used as the diluent.

For additional information, see the section on Drug Selection in the Introduction.

Atrovent (Boehringer Ingelheim).
(Investigational drug)

OXYGEN THERAPY

OXYGEN

Oxygen is transported in the blood primarily bound to hemoglobin. Available tissue stores are small and quickly exhausted when an increased demand for oxygen cannot be met by respiration. Tissue oxygen requirements increase during exercise and hypermetabolic states. The primary indication for oxygen therapy is to treat hypoxemia and to prevent hypoxia. As such, it should be regarded as a "drug" used to treat oxygen deficiency.

In emergencies, oxygen should be given without awaiting results of laboratory tests (arterial oxygen determination) when hypoxemia is apparent (eg, in shock, severe asthma, myocardial infarction). However, the use of oxygen is only supportive, and the cause of the hypoxemia must be determined and treated when possible.

USES. **Chronic Obstructive Pulmonary Disease (COPD):** Long-term home oxygen therapy is the only treatment that consistently improves survival in patients with severe emphysema and/or chronic obstructive bronchitis. Exercise tolerance improves, pulmonary hypertension and erythrocytosis decrease, and neuropsychologic function improves (Petty et al, 1979). Oxygen given for 15 hours/day was shown to prolong survival (Medical Research Council Working Party, 1981); continuous administration for 19 hours/day prolongs survival more than treatment for 12 hours (Nocturnal Oxygen Therapy Trial Group, 1980).

The primary aim of oxygen therapy in patients with COPD is to correct hypoxemia and thereby improve the quality of life, allow the patient to be ambulatory, and prolong survival. In COPD patients with pulmonary hypertension and cor pulmonale, continuous oxygen is particularly useful at night to prevent hypoxemia and increased pulmonary hypertension. The value of oxygen in preventing cor pulmonale has not been established.

Long-term oxygen therapy is indicated when the PaO_2 is below 55 mm Hg with the patient in the resting nonrecumbent position, and oxygen given for more than 12 hours/day may be useful when the PaO_2 falls below 55 mm Hg during exercise or sleep. Long-term oxygen therapy also should be considered when the PaO_2 exceeds 55 mm Hg and there is evidence of hypoxic organ dysfunction, such as cor pulmonale, pulmonary hypertension, secondary polycythemia, or impaired psychiatric function. The need for continued oxygen should be assessed every six months for the first year and at yearly intervals thereafter.

Hypoxemic patients with COPD should receive concentrations of oxygen sufficient to raise the arterial oxygen tension to 60 mm Hg or more than 90% oxygen saturation. A PaO_2 above this range may cause excessive carbon dioxide retention and respiratory acidosis and result in ventilatory depression or failure in patients with hypercarbia. The presence of hypercarbia and respiratory acidosis in patients with COPD are not contraindications to the initiation of prolonged oxygen therapy but patients should be monitored carefully. The gradual increase in carbon dioxide retention that occurs with chronic, controlled, low-flow oxygen is generally well tolerated. Patients with COPD should discontinue cigarette smoking prior to the initiation of oxygen therapy.

Oxygen is generally safe for use in nebulizers except when hypercarbia is present (Gunawardena et al, 1984). An oxygen concentrator delivering 95% oxygen at a flow rate of 0.5 to 3 L/minute is adequate for most patients with COPD.

Hypoxemia: Large doses of beta$_2$-adrenergic agonists administered by an air-driven nebulizer have the theoretical risk of increasing hypoxemia. The utilization of oxygen-driven nebulizers removes this hazard.

In most hypoxemic and normoxemic patients whose PaO_2 values worsen during exercise, exercise endurance and capacity improve following oxygen therapy.

Many patients with hypoxemic lung diseases develop disordered breathing during sleep, which is characterized by apnea or hypopnea and oxygen desaturation. Nocturnal oxygen therapy prevents desaturation and relieves the elevated pulmonary arterial pressure; however, the disordered breathing is not improved. In COPD patients who develop nocturnal desaturation without severe daytime hypoxemia, nighttime administration decreases morning headache, daytime sleepiness, and nocturnal arrhythmias. Patients with severe asthma should have oxygen available at home for use during an acute episode.

A maldistribution of ventilation and perfusion in the immediate postoperative period may produce a mild hypoxemia that requires inhaled oxygen. If the PaO_2 is not improved by oxygen, lung expansion techniques are usually necessary.

Acute Myocardial Infarction: Oxygen should be given to patients with uncomplicated myocardial infarction to reverse the mild hypoxemia often present. Measurement of arterial blood gases is necessary to determine the appropriate concentration.

Acute Anemia: In contrast to chronic anemia in which adaptive mechanisms occur, acute anemia is usually poorly tolerated. The administration of oxygen using a high FIO_2 (fraction of oxygen in inspired air) is useful temporarily until adequate blood replacement is available.

Dyspnea: Dyspnea is often present in patients without hypoxemia and is related to increased work of breathing. Any relief obtained by oxygen is associated with a decrease in ventilatory work rather than an increase in PO_2.

Miscellaneous Uses: Because arterial oxygen tension is often reduced in patients with hypotension and congestive heart failure, oxygen therapy is often recommended. The hypoxemia associated with adult respiratory distress syndrome is due to intrapulmonary shunting and responds poorly to oxygen.

Unestablished Uses: The usefulness of oxygen therapy for angina pectoris has not been determined in controlled studies. In patients with sickle cell disease, administration of 100% oxygen has been reported to decrease the number of sickle cells. However, in controlled studies, attempts to treat sickle-cell crises with oxygen have not been successful.

ADVERSE REACTIONS AND PRECAUTIONS. In an acute setting, use of the lowest concentration of oxygen for the shortest time minimizes serious lung damage (ACCP-NHLBI National Conference on Oxygen Therapy, 1984). The dose and duration of therapy that produce toxicity vary. Breathing 100% oxygen for less than 24 hours at atmospheric pressure has little adverse effect on the lungs, and exposure to 50% oxygen for two to seven days has no clinically significant effects. No specific index to allow early detection of oxygen toxicity exists, and no therapeutically useful way to use antioxidant substances to protect against lung damage produced by oxygen radicals is currently available. The benefits of therapy must be weighed against the serious and sometimes lethal effects of excessive oxygen.

Oxygen drawn from cylinders and piping systems is anhydrous and tends to dry the mucous membranes, which thickens secretions, reduces ciliary function, and causes discomfort. Dehydrating effects are accentuated when the gas is used by tube or catheter, which bypasses the humidifying functions of the mucosal surfaces. Careful use of a heated nebulizing apparatus reduces dryness, but the heated devices may produce condensation in the delivery tubing, particularly in infants. Ultrasonic nebulizers should not be used in COPD patients either with or without oxygen because bronchospasm frequently occurs.

Chronically high FIO_2 may decrease minute ventilation, produce absorption atelectasis, increase retention of carbon dioxide, or reverse compensatory hypoxic pulmonary vasoconstriction. Atelectasis may develop when the "nitrogen scaffold" is reduced by washout. The administration of high oxygen concentrations without mechanical support of respiration may induce apnea in patients with chronic hypercapnia, traumatic injury of the respiratory center, or barbiturate intoxication. Thus, high concentrations of supplemental oxygen may worsen hypoventilation in hypoxic patients with hypercarbia and may increase intrapulmonary shunting.

The intensity of fire in oxygen-enriched atmospheres is directly proportional to the concentration of oxygen supplied and is particularly great with oxygen tents. Smoking should be forbidden in areas in which oxygen is being used.

Cytotoxicity: Exposure to high concentrations of oxygen by lung cells can produce severe and fatal cytotoxic effects. It is generally believed that oxygen generates intracellular radicals as normal byproducts of metabolism, including the superoxide anion (O_2^-), activated hydroxyl radical ($OH-$), hydrogen peroxide (H_2O_2), and singlet oxygen (O_2). The most toxic is probably the hydroxyl radical not superoxide. These radicals apparently interact with DNA, proteins, carbohydrates, and lipids and disrupt transcription, cellular membrane integrity, enzyme activity, and other cell functions that alter structure and metabolism and cause cell death.

Within 24 hours after exposure to excessive oxygen, patients experience substernal discomfort, cough, and decreased vital capacity, which predict the development of pulmonary cytotoxicity. After one to four days of 100% oxygen, progressive dyspnea and hypoxemia occur in association with productive cough and a widened alveolar-arterial oxygen tension gradient (Ryerson and Block, 1984).

With continued exposure to excessive oxygen concentrations, extensive irreversible pathologic changes in lung structure occur. The early exudative phase is characterized by edema, hemorrhage, influx of inflammatory cells, destruction of type I alveolar pneumocytes, and necrosis of the capillary endothelium. If the patient survives this early exudative phase and more than 72 hours of exposure to hyperoxia, the proliferative phase begins. In this phase, early exudates are resorbed, the alveolar septa thicken, and type II alveolar pneumocytes hypertrophy and proliferate; lung scarring is sometimes permanent but may also regress; progressive loss of lung function occurs. The clinical pattern resembles pulmonary fibrosis and emphysema. It is often difficult to differentiate the effects of oxygen from those of the underlying disease. In the newborn exposed to excessive oxygen, manifestation of these pathologic changes is termed bronchopulmonary dysplasia.

Retrolental fibroplasia occurs in premature infants treated with oxygen concentrations above ambient air levels. The exact level or duration of elevated arterial oxygen that results in injury is unknown, but arterial oxygen partial pressure should be kept below 50 to 70 mm Hg. In this disorder, the immature retinal blood vessels are damaged. Scarring, retinal detachment, and permanent blindness can result. Hyperbaric oxygen causes similar effects in adults. The risk of hypoxia must be balanced against the risk of retrolental fibroplasia.

MIXTURES

The following mixtures contain an expectorant or decongestant and one or two bronchodilators. There is no evidence that expectorants or mucolytics are effective in acute asthma. Iodides are not recommended as expectorants for children or women of childbearing age by the Committee on Drugs of the American Academy of Pediatrics. A nasal decongestant is useful only temporarily when asthma is complicated by an acute upper respiratory infection. For these reasons, the use of the following combination products is not advised.

Asbron G (Sandoz). Each tablet or 15 ml of elixir contains theophylline sodium glycinate 300 mg (equivalent to 137 mg theophylline) and guaifenesin 100 mg (alcohol 15%, elixir).
Brondecon (Parke-Davis). Each tablet or 10 ml of elixir contains oxtriphylline 200 mg and guaifenesin 100 mg (alcohol 20%, elixir).
Dilor-G (Savage). Each tablet or 10 ml of liquid contains dyphyl-

line 200 mg and guaifenesin 200 mg.

Duo-Medihaler (Riker). Each measured dose of aerosol contains isoproterenol hydrochloride 0.16 mg and phenylephrine bitartrate 0.24 mg.

Elixophyllin-GG (Forest). Each 15 ml of liquid contains anhydrous theophylline 100 mg and guaifenesin 100 mg.

Elixophyllin-KI (Forest), **Generic**. Each 15 ml of elixir contains theophylline (anhydrous) 80 mg and potassium iodide 130 mg (alcohol 10%).

Lufyllin-GG (Wallace). Each tablet or 30 ml of elixir contains dyphylline 200 mg and guaifenesin 200 mg (alcohol 17%, elixir).

Mucomyst with Isoproterenol (Mead Johnson). Solution (for inhalation; sterile, aqueous) containing isoproterenol hydrochloride 0.05% and acetylcysteine 10%.

Quibron (Mead Johnson). Each capsule contains theophylline (anhydrous) 150 or 300 mg and guaifenesin 90 or 180 mg; each 15 ml of liquid contains theophylline (anhydrous) 150 mg and guaifenesin 90 mg.

Slo-Phyllin GG (Rorer). Each capsule or 15 ml of syrup contains theophylline (anhydrous) 150 mg and guaifenesin 90 mg.

Theo-Organidin (Wallace). Each 15 ml of elixir contains theophylline (anhydrous) 120 mg and iodinated glycerol 30 mg (alcohol 15%).

Theolair-Plus (Riker). Each 15 ml of liquid contains theophylline (anhydrous) 125 mg and guaifenesin 100 mg; each tablet contains theophylline (anhydrous) 125 or 250 mg and guaifenesin 100 or 180 mg.

Other types of mixtures used in asthma and bronchitis contain a barbiturate or antianxiety agent, one or more bronchodilators, and, in some preparations, an expectorant. Use of such fixed-dose combinations is inadvisable because the efficacy of barbiturates and antianxiety agents in bronchial disorders is not documented, and barbiturates may increase the metabolism of corticosteroids if the latter are given concomitantly.

Adrenergic drugs available in mixtures are those with the least beta$_2$ specificity. The undesirable central nervous system stimulant action of ephedrine may be synergistic with that of theophylline. Adjustment of the dose of theophylline is especially difficult or impossible with fixed-dose combination products.

Some physicians elect not to substitute single-entity products in chronic asthmatics who have responded satisfactorily for an extended period to one of the following combination products; however, the overall disadvantages of these types of mixtures should be considered before initiating therapy in newly diagnosed asthmatics.

Bronkolixir (Winthrop-Breon). Each 5 ml of elixir contains theophylline 15 mg, ephedrine sulfate 12 mg, phenobarbital 4 mg, and guaifenesin 50 mg (alcohol 19%) (nonprescription).

Bronkotabs (Winthrop-Breon). Each tablet contains theophylline 100 mg, ephedrine sulfate 24 mg, phenobarbital 8 mg, and guaifenesin 100 mg (nonprescription).

Marax (Roerig). Each tablet contains theophylline 130 mg, ephedrine sulfate 25 mg, and hydroxyzine hydrochloride 10 mg.

Mudrane GG (Poythress). Each 5 ml of elixir contains theophylline 20 mg, ephedrine hydrochloride 4 mg, phenobarbital 2.5 mg, and guaifenesin 26 mg (alcohol 20%); each tablet contains aminophylline 130 mg, ephedrine hydrochloride 16 mg, phenobarbital 8 mg, and guaifenesin 100 mg.

Quadrinal (Knoll). Each tablet contains theophylline calcium salicylate 130 mg (equivalent to 65 mg of theophylline anhydrous), ephedrine hydrochloride 24 mg, phenobarbital 24 mg, and potassium iodide 320 mg.

Quibron Plus (Mead Johnson). Each capsule or 15 ml of elixir contains theophylline 150 mg, ephedrine hydrochloride 25 mg, butabarbital 20 mg, and guaifenesin 100 mg (alcohol 15%, elixir).

Tedral (Parke-Davis). Each tablet contains theophylline 118 mg, ephedrine hydrochloride 24 mg, and phenobarbital 8 mg; each 5 ml of suspension and 10 ml of elixir contain theophylline 65 mg, ephedrine hydrochloride 12 mg, and phenobarbital 4 mg (alcohol 15%, elixir) (all forms nonprescription).

Tedral SA (Parke-Davis). Each tablet (timed-release) contains theophylline 180 mg, ephedrine hydrochloride 48 mg, and phenobarbital 25 mg.

Cited References

ACCP-NHLBI National Conference on Oxygen Therapy. *Chest* 86:234-247, 1984.

Aubier M, et al: Aminophylline improves diaphragmatic contractility. *N Engl J Med* 305:249-252, 1981.

Bernstein IL: Cromolyn sodium. *Chest* 87(suppl):68S-73S, 1985.

Brogden RN, et al: Beclomethasone dipropionate: Reappraisal of its pharmacodynamic properties and therapeutic efficacy after decade of use in asthma and rhinitis. *Drugs* 28:99-126, 1984.

Bukowskyj M, et al: Theophylline reassessed. *Ann Intern Med* 101:63-73, 1984.

Burton GG: Differential diagnosis of various obstructive pulmonary diseases and implications for therapy, in Burton GG, Hodgkin JE: *Respiratory Care: A Guide to Clinical Practice*. Chicago, Year Book Medical Publishers, 1984, 787-805.

Bussey HI: Theophylline toxicity after dyphylline therapy. *Am Rev Respir Dis* 124:504, 1981.

Clark TJH: Inhaled corticosteroid therapy: Substitute for theophylline as well as prednisolone? *J Allergy Clin Immunol* 76:330-334, 1985.

Clarke SW, Newman SP: Therapeutic aerosols 2: Drugs available by inhaled route, (editorial). *Thorax* 39:1-7, 1984.

Clissold SP, Heel RC: Budesonide: Preliminary review of its pharmacodynamic properties and therapeutic efficacy in asthma and rhinitis. *Drugs* 28:485-518, 1984.

Daniele RP: Chronic asthma, in Cherniack RM (ed): *Current Therapy of Respiratory Disease, 1984-1985*. Philadelphia/St Louis, Decker/Mosby, 1984, 107-111.

Dederich RA, et al: Intrasubject variation in sustained-release theophylline absorption. *J Allergy Clin Immunol* 67:465-471, 1981.

Dwyer JM: Pharmacological approach to management of asthma. *Ration Drug Ther* 18:1-8, 1984.

Eitches RW, et al: Methylprednisolone and troleandomycin in treatment of steroid-dependent asthmatic children. *Am J Dis Child* 139:264-268, 1985.

Estepan H, Libby DM: Glucocorticoid therapy of pulmonary disease. *Drug Ther* 12:109-118, (Oct) 1982.

Furukawa CT, et al: Learning and behaviour problems associated with theophylline therapy. *Lancet* 1:621, 1984.

Galant SP: β-adrenergic agonists. *West J Med* 141:513-514, 1984.

Greenberger PA, Patterson R: Management of asthma during pregnancy. *N Engl J Med* 312:897-902, 1985.

Gross NJ, Skorodin MS: Anticholinergic, antimuscarinic bronchodilators. *Am Rev Respir Dis* 129:856-870, 1984.

Gunawardena K, et al: Oxygen as driving gas for nebulizers: Safe or dangerous? *Br Med J* 288:272-274, 1984.

Hendeles L, Weinberger M: Theophylline: "State of the art" review. *Pharmacotherapy* 3:2-44, 1983.

Hendeles L, et al: Food-induced "dose-dumping" from once-a-day theophylline product as cause of theophylline toxicity. *Chest* 87:758-765, 1985.

Hemstreet MPB: Atropine nebulization: Simple and safe. *Ann Allergy* 44:138-141, 1980.

Hetzel M: More logical approach to asthma. *Postgrad Med J* 60:201-207, 1984.

Hiller FC, Wilson FJ Jr: Evaluation and management of acute asthma. *Med Clin North Am* 67:669-683, 1983.

Jenne JW: Theophylline use in asthma: Some current issues. *Clin Chest Med* 5:645-658, 1984.

Joad J, et al: Physiological and psychological variables during maintenance therapy with inhaled albuterol and theophylline used separately and in combination, (abstract). *J Allergy Clin Immunol* 75:113, 1985.

Karim A, et al: Food-induced changes in theophylline absorption from controlled-release formulations: Part I. Substantial increased and decreased absorption with Uniphyl tablets and Theo-Dur Sprinkle. *Clin Pharmacol Ther* 38:77-83, 1985.

Kemp J, et al: Therapeutic efficacy and equivalence of tablet and syrup formulations of procaterol hydrochloride in childhood asthma. *Ann Allergy* 55:588-592, 1985.

Kingston HGG, Hirshman CA: Perioperative management of patient with asthma. *Anesth Analg* 63:844-855, 1984.

Lawyer CH, et al: Utilization of intravenous dihydroxypropyl theophylline (dyphylline) in aminophylline-sensitive patient, and pharmacokinetic comparison with theophylline. *J Allergy Clin Immunol* 65:353-357, 1980.

Maclay WP, et al: Postmarketing surveillance: Practical experience with ketotifen. *Br Med J* 288:911-914, 1984.

Marchlinski FE, Miller JM: Atrial arrhythmias exacerbated by theophylline: Response to verapamil and evidence for triggered activity in man. *Chest* 88:931-934, 1985.

May DC, Jarboe CH: Inhibition of clearance of dyphylline by probenecid, (letter). *N Engl J Med* 304:791, 1981.

Medical Research Council Working Party: Long-term domiciliary oxygen therapy in chronic hypoxic cor pulmonale complicating chronic bronchitis and emphysema. *Lancet* 1:681-686, 1981.

Meltzer EO, et al: Effect of dosing schedule on efficacy of beclomethasone diproprionate aerosol in chronic asthma. *Am Rev Respir Dis* 131:732-736, 1985.

Newman SP: Therapeutic inhalation agents and devices: Effectiveness in asthma and bronchitis. *Postgrad Med* 76:194-207, (Oct) 1984.

Newman SP, Clarke SW: Therapeutic aerosols 1: Physical and practical considerations, (editorial). *Thorax* 38:881-886, 1983.

Nocturnal Oxygen Therapy Trial Group: Continuous or nocturnal oxygen therapy in hypoxemic chronic obstructive lung disease: Clinical trial. *Ann Intern Med* 93:391-398, 1980.

Olson KR, et al: Theophylline overdose: Acute single ingestion versus chronic repeated overmedication. *Am J Emerg Med* 3:386-394, 1985.

Orgel HA, et al: Flunisolide aerosol in treatment of steroid-dependent asthma in children. *Ann Allergy* 51:21-25, 1983.

Orgel HA, et al: Bitolterol and albuterol metered-dose aerosols: Comparison of two long-acting beta$_2$-adrenergic bronchodilators for treatment of asthma. *J Allergy Clin Immunol* 75:55-62, 1985.

Paterson JW, et al: Comment on β$_2$-agonists and their use in asthma. *TIPS* 67-69, (Feb) 1983.

Petty TL, et al: Outpatient oxygen therapy in chronic obstructive pulmonary disease: Review of 13 years experience and evaluation of modes of therapy. *Arch Intern Med* 139:28-32, 1979.

Rees J: Drug treatment in acute asthma. *Br Med J* 288:1747-1750, 1984 A.

Rees J: Treatment of chronic asthma. *Br Med J* 288:1819-1821, 1984 B.

Rivington RN, et al: Comparison of morning versus evening dosing with new once-daily oral theophylline formulation. *Am J Med* 79(suppl 6A):67-71, 1985.

Rossing TH, et al: Effect of outpatient treatment of asthma with beta agonists on response to sympathomimetics in emergency room. *Am J Med* 75:781-784, 1983.

Ryerson GG, Block AJ: Oxygen as drug: Chemical properties, benefits, and hazards of administration, in Burton GG, Hodgkin JE (eds): *Respiratory Care: A Guide to Clinical Practice.* Philadelphia, JB Lippincott, 1984, 395-415.

Selcow J, et al: Comparison of cromolyn and bronchodilators in patients with mild to moderately severe asthma in office practice. *Ann Allergy* 50:13-18, 1983.

Sessler CN, et al: Treatment of theophylline toxicity with oral activated charcoal. *Chest* 87:325-329, 1985.

Shapiro GG, König P: Cromolyn sodium: Review. *Pharmacotherapy* 5:156-170, 1985.

Sly RM: Beta-adrenergic drugs in management of asthma in athletes. *J Allergy Clin Immunol* 73:680-685, 1984.

Spector SL: Advantages and disadvantages of 24-hour theophylline. *J Allergy Clin Immunol* 76:302-311, 1985 A.

Spector SL: Use of corticosteroids in treatment of asthma. *Chest* 87(suppl):73S-79S, 1985 B.

Spector SL, Gomez MG: Dose-response effects of albuterol aerosol compared with isoproterenol and placebo aerosols. *J Allergy Clin Immunol* 59:280-286, 1977.

Summers R, Smith L: Asthma management: New perspectives, improved options. *Postgrad Med* 76:209-221, (July) 1984.

Svedmyr N: Fenoterol: Beta$_2$-adrenergic agonist for use in asthma; pharmacology, pharmacokinetics, clinical efficacy and adverse effects. *Pharmacotherapy* 5:109-126, 1985.

Tse CST, Bernstein IL: Corticosteroid aerosols in treatment of asthma. *Pharmacotherapy* 4:334-342, 1984.

Walker SB, et al: Bitolterol mesylate: Beta-adrenergic agent. *Pharmacotherapy* 5:127-137, 1985.

Weinberger M: Pharmacology and therapeutic use of theophylline. *J Allergy Clin Immunol* 73:525-540, 1984.

Weinberger M, Hendeles L: Slow release theophylline: Rationale and basis for production selection. *N Engl J Med* 308:760-764, 1983.

Weinstein AM, Brokaw A: Pharmacotherapy of asthma. *Ear Nose Throat J* 63:112-120, 1984.

Williams HO: Drug treatment of asthma. *Practitioner* 228:503-508, 1984.

Ziment I: Drugs used in respiratory therapy, in Burton GG, Hodgkin JE (eds): *Respiratory Care: A Guide to Clinical Practice.* Philadelphia, JB Lippincott, 1984, 456-492.

Agents Used To Treat Heart Failure

Heart failure has a poor prognosis regardless of etiology, and most cardiovascular deaths today are associated with left ventricular dysfunction. Two components of cardiac failure have been recognized: depressed myocardial contractility and circulatory congestion. The goals of treatment are to relieve congestive symptoms, improve functional capacity and the quality of life, and increase life expectancy.

The initial approach should be to correct treatable pressure or volume overloads, such as hypertension or aortic stenosis. Current drug therapy is directed toward ameliorating congestive symptoms by increasing myocardial contractility, reducing left ventricular filling pressure (preload) and systemic vascular resistance (aortic impedance), and normalizing heart rate and rhythm. The principal drugs used are the digitalis glycosides and other inotropic drugs, which increase myocardial contractility; diuretics, which reduce preload; vasodilators, which reduce aortic impedance and/or increase venous capacitance; and antiarrhythmic agents, which normalize cardiac rate and rhythm (see Chapter 24).

While drugs may relieve symptoms, they do not appear to reverse the underlying disease process or prolong life, although the effect of vasodilators on survival is currently being evaluated. Whether early intervention would improve prognosis is an important area for future research.

DIURETICS

Traditionally, chronic heart failure has been managed by restriction of activities, a low-sodium diet, digitalis, and diuretics. In recent years, the concept that digitalis should be given to all patients with heart failure has been questioned. Diuretics reduce preload and often relieve symptoms as effectively as digitalis, particularly when edema is the major manifestation. They also decrease left ventricular volume and wall tension and may thereby reduce myocardial oxygen demand. Diuretics are often used today as sole initial therapy in patients with mild congestive heart failure and normal sinus rhythm. When resting symptoms are controlled by the diuretic alone, the addition of digitalis does not appear to improve exercise capacity (McHaffie et al, 1978). Diuretics also are useful for treating acute pulmonary edema. Particular care should be taken to avoid excessive diuresis, which may cause a marked reduction in cardiac filling pressure and cardiac output, hypoperfusion of vital organs, and renal insufficiency. The long-term daily use of diuretics may be inadvisable in some patients; therefore, after the patient's weight has decreased to a stable baseline, the diuretic may be given intermittently to maintain stable weight or to sustain an edema-free state in selected patients.

For a more detailed discussion of diuretics, see Chapter 29.

DIGITALIS GLYCOSIDES

Actions

Digitalis has complex direct and indirect cardiovascular actions that are of value in the treatment of heart failure and most supraventricular tachyarrhythmias. In cardiac failure, its direct positive inotropic action may increase cardiac output and thereby decrease venous pressure, reduce heart size, and slow compensatory *reflex* tachycardia. Because digitalis decreases ventricular volume, it does not increase myocardial oxygen consumption in the failing heart. Improved renal hemodynamics promotes diuresis, thus reducing blood volume and relieving edema. The digitalis glycosides also have a mild direct diuretic action that is independent of changes in the glomerular filtration rate and renal blood flow. During long-term therapy, the effect of digitalis on resting hemodynamics is variable, whereas hemodynamic improvement during exercise is sustained (Arnold et al, 1980; Firth et al, 1980; Griffiths et al, 1982; Murray et al, 1983; Vogel et al, 1977). An increase in exercise *performance* has not been demonstrated, however.

The actions of digitalis that are of particular importance in antiarrhythmic therapy are the lengthening of A-V nodal conduction time and refractory period due to an increase in vagal tone, an antiadrenergic action, and, to a lesser extent, a direct effect. In addition, the direct positive inotropic effect of digitalis improves ventricular function and may thereby slow the sinus rate in patients with cardiac failure.

The direct actions of digitalis are believed to result from inhibition of (Na$^+$ + K$^+$)-ATPase, an enzyme system that provides the energy for active transport of sodium and potassium ions across the myocardial cell membrane (the "sodium pump"). Digitalis combines reversibly with (Na$^+$ + K$^+$)-ATPase on the cell membrane and thereby prevents the binding of ATP. Inactivation of the sodium pump increases intracellular sodium ions and decreases intracellular potassium ions; these effects are believed to underlie the *direct* electrophysiologic and toxic effects of the glycosides. Inhibition of the sodium-potassium transport system is accompanied by increased cellular uptake of calcium ions. Since calcium plays a central role in excitation-contraction coupling, the influx of calcium ions may explain the inotropic action.

Uses

Chronic Heart Failure: The positive inotropic effect of digitalis may be useful in patients with chronic heart failure, but the response to therapy depends upon the underlying etiology and the extent of myocardial damage. Digitalis is most effective when cardiac failure is caused by ischemic, hypertensive, valvular, or congenital heart disease or dilated cardiomyopathy. By slowing the ventricular response to atrial fibrillation, glycoside therapy reduces symptoms of heart failure by permitting adequate time for ventricular filling and emptying. To the degree that it decreases heart rate in conditions such as mitral stenosis, digitalis can relieve pulmonary congestion, but it is rarely useful in patients with mitral stenosis and normal sinus rhythm.

Approximately 90% of pediatric patients with cardiac failure are infants up to 3 months of age who have severe congenital anomalies that either obstruct ventricular outflow or reroute blood flow. These infants usually respond to digitalis and/or diuretics.

Glycoside therapy is of limited value in patients with heart failure associated with thyrotoxicosis, chronic anemia, beriberi, or A-V fistulas. Effective treatment of these disorders requires correction of the underlying cause.

Digitalis is usually ineffective in pulmonary heart disease unless left ventricular function is also impaired (Mathur et al, 1981); patients with pulmonary heart disease are also particularly susceptible to digitalis toxicity. Glycoside therapy often fails to restore compensation when congestive heart failure develops in conjunction with chronic constrictive pericarditis or myocarditis. Digitalis should be used cautiously in patients with hypertrophic cardiomyopathy, because it may increase the outflow obstruction.

Acute Myocardial Infarction: Cardiac glycosides are not generally used in the first 48 hours following acute myocardial infarction because they may precipitate ventricular arrhythmias. Supraventricular tachyarrhythmias that occur during the course of acute myocardial infarction may cause a marked deterioration in left ventricular function. DC cardioversion is the treatment of choice for terminating these arrhythmias; digitalis may be used later to prevent recurrences.

Mild congestive heart failure is common during the course of acute myocardial infarction. If pulmonary congestion develops, a diuretic is often used for initial treatment. A vasodilator, such as intravenous nitroglycerin or nitroprusside [Nipride, Nitropress], may be as useful or more useful than a diuretic in this setting, especially when heart failure is severe. Digitalis has been reported to improve hemodynamics in patients with moderate left ventricular dysfunction after myocardial infarction (Marchionni et al, 1985), but its use remains controversial.

Acute left ventricular failure with pulmonary edema represents an immediate threat to life that requires rapidly effective modes of treatment (ie, placing the patient in an upright position; administering morphine, furosemide [Lasix], vasodilators, and oxygen; applying tourniquets). If an inotropic agent is indicated to maintain cardiac output and sustain arterial pressure, a drug such as dobutamine [Dobutrex] may be safer and more effective than digitalis. Vasodilators probably represent the treatment of choice.

The treatment of cardiogenic shock is controversial and mortality is high. Digitalis does not appear to be useful for acute management of this syndrome, but other inotropic agents may be of value (see Chapter 27, Agents Used to Treat Shock).

Treatment with digitalis after discharge from the hospital was reported to increase mortality of myocardial infarct patients (Moss et al, 1981; Bigger et al, 1985), but a study in high-risk patients with severe coronary artery disease showed no deleterious effects attributable to glycoside therapy (Ryan et al, 1983).

Prophylactic Use: Patients with heart disease who do not have signs of overt failure sometimes are given digitalis prophylactically before cardiac surgery and in other stressful situations (eg, severe illness, pregnancy). There is considerable debate about the merits of prophylactic digitalization, because (1) it is difficult to determine an effective dose in patients who have no signs of congestive heart failure or a supraventricular tachyarrhythmia; (2) if postoperative arrhythmias occur, they may be treated more easily in nondigitalized patients; and (3) if the patient is not receiving digitalis, the drug cannot be implicated as a possible cause of postoperative arrhythmias.

Supraventricular Tachyarrhythmias: See Chapter 24.

Drug Selection

All digitalis glycosides possess the same pharmacologic actions, but they vary in potency, onset of action, rate of absorption, and rate and route of excretion. The physician should become thoroughly familiar with one or two preparations (usually digoxin and/or digitoxin) and use these agents exclusively.

The choice of preparation, dosage, and route of administration depends upon the clinical situation. A glycoside with a rapid onset of action (digoxin [Lanoxin], deslanoside [Cedilanid-D], or ouabain) may be given intravenously when prompt action is required, as in patients with acute congestive heart failure or a supraventricular arrhythmia with a rapid ventricular response. (Some cardiologists prefer verapamil [Calan, Isoptin] or a beta blocker alone or with digitalis to control the ventricular response in supraventricular arrhythmias.) Of the three glycosides, ouabain acts most rapidly, but its dosage is the most difficult to regulate for continued digitalization. Digoxin and deslanoside have a comparable onset (10 to 30 minutes) and time to peak action (one to four hours); digoxin is usually preferred because the oral maintenance dose is easily established after intravenous therapy and because its concentration in the serum can be measured, if necessary.

Digoxin and digitoxin are used orally for initial therapy in less critical situations and for maintenance. Rapid oral digitalization may be suitable for some patients with supraventricular tachyarrhythmias or acute heart failure, although the intravenous route is often preferred. Slower digitalization is indicated in chronic heart failure without acute symptoms and may be accomplished in two ways: by administering a loading dose followed by maintenance therapy or by giving the maintenance dose each day and allowing the patient to become fully digitalized over a longer period. The latter method is usually preferred.

Digoxin has the advantage of a relatively short half-life (36 to 40 hours), which makes toxic reactions easier to manage. In the past, digoxin tablets from different manufacturers varied greatly in bioavailability, and a change from one brand to another could result in intoxication or underdigitalization. Such differences among digoxin products appear to be less of a problem today because of new bioavailability standards (Greenblatt et al, 1976).

Some physicians prefer digitoxin for prolonged therapy because its longer half-life (five to nine days) provides a more sustained therapeutic effect. However, toxic effects are also more prolonged. If digitoxin is substituted for digoxin for maintenance therapy, slow redigitalization may be required because of the difference in duration of action of the two glycosides.

Factors Modifying Response to Therapy

The response to digitalis is influenced by many factors, including the nature and severity of the underlying heart disease; the patient's age; the status of renal function and electrolyte balance; the presence of noncardiac disorders; and the concomitant use of other drugs. Dosage must be individualized, and conditions that predispose to toxicity (eg, hypokalemia, hypercalcemia, hypothyroidism, hypomagnesemia) should be corrected. Impaired renal function (frequently seen in the elderly) necessitates a reduction in digoxin dosage because this glycoside is excreted largely unchanged in the urine. Digitoxin, on the other hand, is extensively metabolized before excretion and hepatic dysfunction may alter its pharmacokinetics.

In patients with atrial fibrillation or flutter, the optimal dose of digitalis is the smallest amount that controls the ventricular rate at rest and during mild exercise. An adequate therapeutic response depends in large measure upon the ability of digitalis to produce a relative degree of A-V block, and larger doses generally are required than for cardiac failure. It is more difficult to determine proper dosage for patients with heart failure and sinus rhythm. A satisfactory response is manifested by diuresis, weight loss, reduced pulmonary and systemic venous congestion, decreased heart size and/or rate, and relief of peripheral edema, fatigue, shortness of breath, and orthopnea. If digitalis is the initial and only therapeutic agent employed, these endpoints are useful in titrating dosage. However, rest, sodium restriction, and diuretic therapy also are prescribed for most patients with moderately severe heart failure. Since these measures reduce the load on the heart and relieve edema, the relative contribution of digitalis to the therapeutic response often cannot be assessed. If clinical improvement is not satisfactory, the dose of digitalis may be increased cautiously or the diuretic regimen altered.

Maintenance Therapy

Patients receiving maintenance therapy should be re-evaluated periodically to determine whether dosage should be adjusted or the drug discontinued. This precaution is particularly important in geriatric patients because of the high incidence and severity of toxic reactions in this age group.

Chronic atrial fibrillation with a rapid ventricular response is the most established indication for long-term therapy. Infants and children with heart failure associated with congenital anomalies also may require long-term digitalis treatment unless the underlying cause has been corrected.

Digitalis may not be required in patients with heart failure and/or arrhythmias associated with hypertension, anemia, beriberi, thyrotoxicosis, or valvular heart disease after treatment or correction of the underlying cause. Transient heart failure and arrhythmias that occur during the course of acute myocardial infarction also do not require long-term glycoside therapy.

In addition to individuals with correctable or transient disorders, many patients with a diagnosis of chronic heart failure may derive no lasting benefit from digitalis. Results of a number of studies have shown that digitalis can be withdrawn safely from many patients who have been taking it for long periods if they are compensated, in sinus rhythm, and have no history of chronic atrial tachyarrhythmias. (For review see Fleg and Lakatta, 1984, and Mulrow et al, 1984.) Those with mild episodic heart failure (Lee et al, 1982) and low serum levels (digoxin concentration less than 0.8 ng/ml) (Johnston and McDevitt, 1979) are least likely to deteriorate when digitalis is withdrawn.

These observations suggest that patients who tolerate withdrawal may have less cardiac impairment; may be controlled adequately by diuretics, vasodilators, or both; had questionable indications for digitalis in the first place; and may not be taking it regularly. Long-term digitalis therapy appears to benefit patients with more chronic and more severe heart failure that persists despite diuretic and/or vasodilator therapy, greater left ventricular dilation and ejection fraction depression, and an S_3 gallop (Lee et al, 1982).

Measurement of Serum Levels

Radioimmunoassay techniques for measuring serum levels of digoxin and digitoxin can be performed in most hospitals. A less commonly used method, the erythrocyte assay, is nonspecific for the various cardiac glycosides. The serum digitalis concentration may be useful to assess compliance, to detect underdigitalization, to determine whether digitalis has been ingested when this is in doubt, to monitor patients who may be predisposed to toxicity, and to detect problems in bioavailability caused by gastrointestinal disorders, concomitant use of other drugs, or poor tablet dissolution (Weintraub, 1977).

The experienced physician can usually evaluate the therapeutic effect of digitalis without measuring blood levels. The value of serum levels in diagnosing toxicity is also not established (Ingelfinger and Goldman, 1976). Serum levels do not correlate closely with clinical events and must be evaluated in conjunction with symptomatology, electrocardiographic changes, and results of laboratory tests. In the absence of other signs of toxicity, digitalis should not be discontinued solely on the basis of an elevated serum level. A serum concentration that is safe and effective for one patient may be excessive or inadequate for another. Infants and children may tolerate higher serum levels than adults.

Factors that may alter serum levels and/or the response to digitalis include electrolyte imbalance (particularly hypokalemia), renal impairment, age, thyroid disease, and drug interactions (Aronson, 1983). The time that the blood sample is obtained also must be taken into consideration, because levels are high during the absorptive and distributive phases (Weintraub, 1977). A delay of three to four hours after an intravenous dose of digoxin and six to eight hours after an oral dose is recommended (Doherty et al, 1978).

An endogenous substance that gives false-positive values on digoxin radioimmunoassay tests has been detected in the serum of nondigitalized patients with renal impairment, neo-

nates, pregnant women during the last trimester, and salt-loaded hypertensive patients. (See Pharmacokinetics in the evaluation on Digoxin.)

Interactions

Hypokalemia predisposes to digitalis toxicity; even a moderate reduction of the serum potassium concentration can precipitate serious arrhythmias. Hypokalemia is encountered most frequently in patients receiving long-term therapy with thiazide or loop diuretics and can usually be prevented by prescribing a potassium-sparing diuretic or potassium chloride supplement along with the potassium-wasting agent. In children, foods that are high in potassium and low in sodium may be preferable. Supplements and dietary sources are not as reliable as the potassium-sparing diuretics.

Quinidine increases serum digoxin levels by reducing renal and nonrenal clearance and altering volume of distribution. Gastrointestinal disturbances and ventricular arrhythmias have been attributed to this interaction (Leahey et al, 1978). It has been recommended that patients receiving both drugs should be monitored carefully for signs of digitalis toxicity, particularly during the first five days of combined therapy; that the dose of digoxin should be reduced by one-half before starting quinidine (Bigger, 1981); and that patients stabilized on both drugs should be evaluated for underdigitalization if quinidine is discontinued. Others doubt the clinical importance of this interaction because of controversial reports on the effect of quinidine on the inotropic action of digoxin.

Several other cardiovascular drugs may alter serum digoxin levels. Verapamil [Calan, Isoptin], amiloride [Midamor], amiodarone [Cordarone], and the investigational antiarrhythmic drug, propafenone, increase the serum digoxin concentration. Nifedipine [Procardia] and diltiazem [Cardizem] probably do not cause a clinically important increase in the serum concentration of digoxin. Symptomatic sinus bradycardia has been reported in patients receiving both digoxin and methyldopa [Aldomet]; however, methyldopa does not alter the disposition of digoxin. Spironolactone [Aldactone] has been reported to increase serum digoxin levels, but this apparent interaction now appears to be due to interference with digoxin radioimmunoassay by the spironolactone metabolite, canrenone. The acute administration of certain vasodilator drugs (nitroprusside [Nipride, Nitropress], hydralazine [Apresoline]) reduces serum digoxin levels by increasing renal clearance of the glycoside, and it may be necessary to adjust digoxin dosage during long-term vasodilator therapy.

Serum digoxin levels may be increased by quinine and hydroxychloroquine [Plaquenil] and reduced by rifampin [Rifadin, Rimactane]. In preterm infants, intravenous indomethacin [Indocin IV] decreases the renal excretion of digoxin.

Approximately 10% of patients convert substantial amounts of digoxin to inactive metabolites in the gut, and concurrent antibiotic therapy markedly increases serum digoxin levels in these individuals. The bioavailability of digoxin is reduced by antacid gels, kaolin-pectin preparations, cholestyramine resin [Questran], sulfasalazine [Azulfidine], neomycin, and cytotoxic drugs. Anticholinergic drugs may reduce the gastrointestinal absorption of slowly dissolving brands of digoxin tablets.

Studies on the effect of quinidine on serum digitoxin levels have yielded conflicting results. Serum concentrations of digitoxin may be reduced by drugs that increase hepatic microsomal enzyme activity (eg, barbiturates, phenytoin [Dilantin], rifampin). Cholestyramine resin and colestipol [Colestid] reduce the bioavailability of digitoxin.

Adverse Reactions and Precautions

The ratio between the full therapeutic and toxic dose of digitalis is narrow, and 5% to 20% of patients develop signs and symptoms of intoxication. Many of the manifestations of digitalis toxicity are difficult to distinguish from symptoms of the underlying disease. Digitalis intoxication usually results from too rapid loading, from accumulation of larger than necessary maintenance doses, from prescribing digitalis in doses beyond reasonable limits when it is not likely to be effective, from the presence of conditions that predispose to toxicity, or from intentional or accidental overdose.

Intoxication can usually be prevented by evaluating therapy frequently, by decreasing dosage in the presence of factors that tend to cause excessive accumulation (eg, impaired renal function), by correcting conditions that increase toxicity (eg, hypokalemia, alkalosis, hypercalcemia, hypoxia, hypomagnesemia), or by treating underlying diseases (eg, hypothyroidism, anemia, valvular heart disease). When the risk of intoxication is great, a short-acting glycoside should be used. Although intoxication cannot always be avoided by selecting one glycoside over another, digitoxin may be preferred in patients with elevated serum creatinine levels. In homes where young children reside with adults taking digitalis, the medication should be kept safely out of reach.

Newborn infants with heart disease, especially premature infants, are particularly susceptible to digitalis intoxication, and frequent electrocardiographic monitoring is essential in these patients. Similarly, special care must be exercised in elderly patients receiving digitalis because their body mass tends to be small and renal function is likely to be reduced. In addition, digitalis must be used with great caution in the presence of active heart disease, such as acute myocardial infarction or acute myocarditis. In patients with acute or unstable chronic atrial fibrillation, digitalis may not normalize the ventricular rate even when the serum concentration exceeds the usual "therapeutic" level. Although these patients may be less sensitive to the toxic effects of digitalis than those with sinus rhythm, it may be preferable to add propranolol [Inderal] to the regimen rather than to increase the dose of digitalis to potentially toxic levels.

All digitalis glycosides are classified in FDA Pregnancy Category C.

Extracardiac Reactions: Gastrointestinal and neurologic disturbances may be early signs of digitalis intoxication and serve as a warning that severe cardiotoxicity can result if the drug is not temporarily discontinued or the dosage reduced.

Anorexia, nausea, vomiting, and abdominal pain are the most common gastrointestinal symptoms; diarrhea is rare. The emetic effect of digitalis is probably of central origin and occurs after either oral or parenteral use. Gastrointestinal symptoms with digitalis leaf also may be due to direct gastric irritation.

Fatigue is the most frequent neurologic manifestation of toxicity. Other symptoms are depression, headache, drowsiness, weakness, lethargy, neuralgia, restlessness, nightmares, personality changes, vertigo, confusion, disorientation, and, rarely, hallucinations and other psychotic reactions. Ocular disturbances include mydriasis, photophobia, modified color perception (particularly yellow vision), visions of flashing or flickering lights, appearance of halos around lights, reduced visual acuity, and, rarely, temporary blindness. The reduction in visual acuity occurs in the form of bilateral central scotomata and appears to be caused by an effect of digitalis on the retinal receptor cells.

Gynecomastia, sexual dysfunction, sweating, and hypersensitivity reactions (urticaria, eosinophilia, thrombocytopenia, vasculitis) occur rarely and generally are not considered to be manifestations of overdosage.

Cardiac Reactions: A disturbance of cardiac rhythm may be the first evidence of digitalis intoxication. Almost any type of arrhythmia may occur; the most common are ventricular bigeminy or trigeminy, multiform premature ventricular complexes, atrial tachycardia with A-V block, and nonparoxysmal A-V junctional (nodal) tachycardia. The latter dysrhythmia is particularly likely to occur in the presence of pre-existing atrial fibrillation. Other digitalis-induced arrhythmias include sinus irregularities (sinus bradycardia, S-A block, sinus arrest), unifocal ventricular premature complexes, accelerated ventricular rhythm, and paroxysmal ventricular tachycardia. A-V dissociation may be induced by a combination of some degree of A-V block plus junctional (or ventricular) tachycardia. A bidirectional tachycardia, recently shown to be ventricular in origin, indicates an advanced stage of digitalis intoxication. Digitalis rarely causes atrial fibrillation or flutter.

Treatment of Toxicity: The management of digitalis intoxication consists of discontinuing glycoside therapy, determining serum potassium levels, and, if indicated, administering potassium chloride and/or antiarrhythmic drugs (see Chapter 24, Antiarrhythmic Agents). Potassium therapy is most effective in patients who have atrial tachycardia with A-V block, ventricular premature complexes, or ventricular tachycardia as a manifestation of digitalis intoxication. Potassium should be avoided in patients with hyperkalemia, severe renal impairment, or marked A-V conduction disturbances, because hyperkalemia may further impair A-V conduction.

Purified digoxin-specific antibody fragments (Fab fragments) recently became available for treatment of life-threatening, refractory digitalis intoxication. These Fab fragments bind with digoxin and digitoxin, and the resulting complexes are excreted rapidly by the kidney. This immunologic approach to treating advanced digitalis toxicity appears to be highly effective, and hypersensitivity reactions have not been reported. (Smith et al, 1982; Wenger et al, 1985).

Cholestyramine resin binds digitoxin in the gut and may be effective in treating intoxication caused by this glycoside. Alternatively, repeated doses of activated charcoal may be employed to interrupt the enterohepatic circulation of digitoxin.

Activated charcoal has also been used to treat digoxin intoxication. Hemoperfusion reduces serum digoxin levels but has little effect on tissue stores and is of no established value in treating toxicity.

Drug Evaluations

The dosage for all digitalis glycosides should be individualized and titrated in terms of the therapeutic response. The dose needed to increase myocardial contractility is generally smaller than that required to decrease the ventricular response in atrial fibrillation. The dose required to control the ventricular rate during various supraventricular tachyarrhythmias may differ. Generally, a larger amount is required to slow the ventricular rate during atrial flutter than during atrial fibrillation, and the ventricular response to atrial flutter is not easily controllable for prolonged periods.

DIGOXIN
[Lanoxin]

$(C_6H_{10}O_3)_3H$
(tridigitoxose)

Digoxin is a purified digitalis preparation derived from the leaves of *Digitalis lanata*. It is the most widely used digitalis glycoside. Onset of action is within 5 to 30 minutes after an intravenous dose and within one to two hours after oral administration. The maximal effect occurs within one to four hours after intravenous administration and two to six hours after oral administration. Many cardiologists prefer digoxin to other digitalis glycosides because its rapid onset of action makes it useful in emergency situations; its relatively short duration of action makes toxic reactions easier to manage; it can be administered both orally and parenterally, making the maintenance dosage easy to establish after emergency intravenous use; and a liquid preparation is available for oral therapy in infants and children.

See the Introduction for a discussion of indications, interactions, and toxicity.

PHARMACOKINETICS. Digoxin is absorbed from the upper small intestine. The bioavailability of Lanoxin tablets is 60% to 80% and that of Lanoxin elixir is 70% to 85%. Food reduces the rate, but not the total amount, absorbed. The absorption of tablets may be normal in many patients with limited absorptive surface due to mucosal disease or surgical resection but may be impaired in those with an extremely short length of functioning small intestine.

Digoxin has a high apparent volume of distribution (6 L/kg), which is decreased in elderly patients and in those with impaired renal function. It is widely distributed throughout body tissues, with high concentrations in skeletal muscle, liver, heart, brain, and kidneys. It does not accumulate in adipose tissue. For a given serum level, myocardial accumulation is greater in infants than in adults. Insignificant amounts of digoxin are removed by dialysis. Digoxin is 20% to 25% protein bound.

Digoxin crosses the placenta and, at delivery, the serum concentration in the newborn is similar to that in the mother. Approximately 50% to 75% of a dose is excreted unchanged in the urine of most patients but is more extensively metabolized to both active and inactive metabolites in a few. The half-life of digoxin is 1.5 to 2 days in patients with normal renal function. The half-life is prolonged in patients with impaired renal function, and dosage should be reduced on the basis of creatinine clearance (Aronson, 1980). The renal clearance of digoxin is lower in patients with congestive heart failure than in those with atrial fibrillation.

Therapeutic serum levels of digoxin generally range from 0.5 to 2.5 ng/ml. Sex hormones, bile salts, other digitalis glycosides, and, possibly, spironolactone and its metabolites may interfere with results of digoxin radioimmunoassay (Weintraub, 1977). In uremic patients, 6% to 42% of apparent digoxin in the serum may represent metabolites (Gibson and Nelson, 1980).

In addition, substantial variation has been noted in digoxin measurements obtained with different commercially available radioimmunoassay kits. Some of this variability may be caused by an endogenous substance that gives false-positive results on many digoxin radioimmunoassay tests. This substance, which has been termed digoxin-like factor (DLF), was detected in the serum of patients with renal impairment or liver disease, salt-loaded normal and hypertensive individuals, normal individuals during cardiovascular stress, neonates, and women during the last trimester of pregnancy (Graves et al, 1983, 1984; Valdes et al, 1983). Measured concentrations of DLF are higher in the blood of premature than in full-term newborns (Koren et al, 1984). DLF also has been found in amniotic fluid, where levels are higher in hypertensive than in normal pregnancies (Graves and Williams, 1984). These findings cast doubt on the accuracy of serum digoxin measurements in these patients unless baseline DLF levels are obtained and also may have implications regarding pharmacokinetics and dosage recommendations, particularly in neonates (Koren et al, 1984).

Results of recent investigations indicate that DLF is also present in the serum of normal controls but is highly protein-bound and does not interfere with immunoassays. The elevated values in certain clinical groups may be caused by a higher concentration of unbound or loosely bound DLF rather than an increase in total DLF (Valdes, 1985).

The physiologic activity of DLF is not known. Like digitalis, DLF appears to act by inhibiting the sodium pump, but whether it has the inotropic and electrophysiologic properties of digitalis has not been determined. It has been postulated that this substance plays a role in sodium and water homeostasis, may be a "natriuretic hormone," and may be involved in the pathogenesis of some forms of hypertension. (DLF should not be confused with "atrial natriuretic factor," a natriuretic and vasodilator substance produced by the atria. (See Chapter 29, Diuretics.)

BIOAVAILABILITY OF TABLET PREPARATIONS. Although digoxin is almost completely absorbed when administered in oral solution, tablets from different manufacturers have, in the past, varied in bioavailability. Peak serum levels as well as area under the serum time curve and urinary excretion varied widely with different tablet formulations, and this was reflected in the steady-state value. New regulations require all digoxin tablets to conform to an in vitro dissolution standard, and differences among preparations appear to be less of a problem today (Greenblatt et al, 1976).

DOSAGE AND PREPARATIONS. The following dosages are given to patients who have not received digitalis for at least two weeks. Smaller loading and maintenance doses should be used in small or elderly patients and in those with impaired renal function, electrolyte disturbances (particularly hypokalemia), or metabolic abnormalities (particularly hypothyroidism). *Oral: Adults,* the average digitalizing dose is 0.75 to 1.5 mg. For rapid digitalization, initially, 0.5 to 0.75 mg, followed by 0.25 to 0.5 mg every six to eight hours until full digitalization is achieved. For slow digitalization and maintenance, 0.125 to 0.5 mg daily (0.125 to 0.25 mg in the elderly), depending upon lean body weight and renal function as determined by creatinine clearance. The dose should be reduced as renal function decreases. *Institution of maintenance therapy without a loading dose is suitable for many patients with congestive heart failure.* Therapeutic serum levels are achieved after six to seven days of maintenance therapy in patients with normal renal function. Single daily doses are usually satisfactory for maintenance; however, it may be necessary to give two divided doses to some patients with recurrent supraventricular tachyarrhythmias.

For *children,* the following digitalizing doses are given in divided amounts at six-hour intervals. (To ensure adequate absorption, it may be desirable to initiate therapy by the intravenous route and then change to oral therapy, with the lower dose tested first.) *Premature infants,* 0.02 to 0.03 mg/kg; *full-term newborn infants,* 0.025 to 0.035 mg/kg; *1 month to 2 years,* 0.035 to 0.06 mg/kg; *2 to 5 years,* 0.03 to 0.04 mg/kg; *5 to 10 years,* 0.02 to 0.035 mg/kg; *over 10 years,* 0.01 to 0.015 mg/kg. The daily oral maintenance dose is 20% to 30% of the oral loading dose in premature infants and 25% to 35% of the oral loading dose in full-term infants and children. More gradual digitalization can be accomplished by initiating therapy with the appropriate maintenance dose.

  Generic. Tablets 0.25 mg.
  Lanoxin (Burroughs Wellcome). Elixir (pediatric) 0.05 mg/ml; tablets 0.125, 0.25, and 0.5 mg.

Intravenous: Adults, the average digitalizing dose is 0.5 to 1 mg. Initially, 0.25 to 0.5 mg, followed by 0.25 mg at four- to six-hour intervals if needed to a total dose of 1 mg. For maintenance, 0.125 to 0.5 mg daily.

For *children,* the following digitalizing doses of the pediatric solution are given in divided amounts at six-hour intervals: *Premature infants,* 0.015 to 0.025 mg/kg; *full-term newborn infants,* 0.02 to 0.03 mg/kg; *1 month to 2 years,* 0.03 to 0.05 mg/kg; *2 to 5 years,* 0.025 to 0.035 mg/kg; *5 to 10 years,* 0.015 to 0.03 mg/kg. The daily intravenous maintenance dose is 20% to 30% of the *oral* loading dose in premature infants and 25% to 30% of the *oral* loading dose in full-term infants and children.

  Generic. Solution 0.25 mg/ml in 1 and 2 ml containers.
  Lanoxin (Burroughs Wellcome). Solution (pediatric) 0.1 mg/ml in 1 ml containers and 0.25 mg/ml in 2 ml containers (alcohol 10%).

DIGOXIN SOLUTION IN CAPSULES
[Lanoxicaps]

The variable absorption of digoxin is caused primarily by the slow dissolution of various tablet formulations in the gut lumen. For this reason, a stable solution of digoxin within a soft gelatin capsule was developed for oral use. This new formulation is 90% to 100% bioavailable. The enhanced absorption is associated with reduced between-patient and within-patient variability in steady-state serum concentrations (Johnson et al, 1977). Because of this increased bioavailability, the dose of digoxin solution in capsules is smaller than the tablet dose.

For adverse reactions and precautions, see the Introduction.

DOSAGE AND PREPARATIONS. Dosage recommendations for digoxin solution in capsules are the same as those for intravenous digoxin.

  Lanoxicaps (Burroughs Wellcome). Capsules 0.05, 0.1, and 0.2 mg.

DIGITOXIN
[Crystodigin, Purodigin]

(C₆H₁₀O₃)₃H
(tridigitoxose)

Digitoxin is the chief active glycoside in digitalis leaf; 1 mg of digitoxin is therapeutically equivalent to approximately 1 g of digitalis leaf. Although digitoxin is administered less commonly today than formerly, it is very useful for maintenance therapy because of its long half-life (five to nine days), which provides a sustained therapeutic effect even if a dose is missed. This is a particular advantage in patients with recurrent supraventricular tachyarrhythmias and in those with compliance problems.

See the Introduction for a discussion of indications, interactions, and toxicity.

PHARMACOKINETICS. Digitoxin is almost completely absorbed from the gastrointestinal tract. Equivalent oral and intravenous doses produce essentially the same therapeutic effect, and intravenous administration is generally unnecessary unless the patient is unable to take medication orally. When given orally, the onset of action is one to four hours and the maximal effect is attained in 8 to 12 hours. Therapeutic serum levels range from 15 to 25 ng/ml and no variation in bioavailability has been encountered among different preparations. Some methods of measuring serum digitoxin do not differentiate cardioactive glycosides from inactive metabolites.

Digitoxin is 97% bound to plasma protein. Its tissue distribution is similar to that of digoxin. Digitoxin is extensively metabolized in the liver, excreted in the bile, recycled, and eventually excreted in the urine, 80% as inactive metabolites. Since little of the parent compound is eliminated by renal clearance, the half-life of digitoxin is not increased in patients with impaired renal function, and it may be the glycoside of choice in these patients. Insignificant amounts of digitoxin are removed by dialysis. Since the effects of impaired hepatic function on the pharmacokinetics of digitoxin are not clearly understood, the drug should be given with caution and, possibly, in reduced dosage to patients with hepatic dysfunction.

DOSAGE AND PREPARATIONS. The following dosages are given to patients who have not received digitalis for at least two weeks. Smaller loading and maintenance doses should be used in small or elderly patients or in those with electrolyte disturbances (particularly hypokalemia) or metabolic abnormalities (particularly hypothyroidism).

Oral: Adults, for rapid digitalization, initially 0.8 mg, then 0.2 mg every six to eight hours for two or three doses. For slower digitalization, 0.1 to 0.2 mg one to three times daily to a total of 1.2 to 1.8 mg. For maintenance, 0.1 mg daily (range, 0.05 to 0.2 mg). These doses may be given intravenously if the patient cannot take oral medication.

> **Generic.** Tablets 0.1 and 0.2 mg.
> **Crystodigin** (Lilly). Tablets 0.05, 0.1, 0.15, and 0.2 mg.
> **Purodigin** (Wyeth). Tablets 0.1 and 0.2 mg.

Oral, Intramuscular, Intravenous: For *children,* the following digitalizing doses are given in three or more divided doses at intervals of six hours or more: *Newborn infants,* 0.025 mg/kg; *2 weeks to 1 year,* 0.035 to 0.045 mg/kg; *1 to 2 years,* 0.04 mg/kg; *over 2 years,* 0.02 to 0.03 mg/kg. The maintenance dose is approximately 10% of the digitalizing dose.

> For oral preparations, see above.
> **Crystodigin** (Lilly). Solution 0.2 mg/ml in 1 ml containers (alcohol 49%).

> OTHER DIGITALIS GLYCOSIDES:
> **Digitalis Leaf:**
> **Generic.** Capsules and tablets 100 mg.
> **Ouabain:**
> **Generic.** Solution

DESLANOSIDE
[Cedilanid-D]

Deslanoside is derived from lanatoside C and has essentially the same pharmacologic properties but is available for parenteral use only. Deslanoside is used intravenously in emergencies, and oral glycosides are then substituted for maintenance therapy. The onset of action is 10 to 30 minutes and maximal effects are obtained in two to three hours. Because it may be difficult to transfer a patient from deslanoside to an oral agent, intravenous digoxin is usually preferred.

For a discussion of indications, interactions, and toxicity of digitalis glycosides, see the Introduction.

PHARMACOKINETICS. The half-life of deslanoside is approximately 33 hours. It is eliminated largely by renal excretion.

DOSAGE AND PREPARATIONS. The following dosages are given to patients who have not received digitalis for at least two weeks. Smaller doses should be used in small or elderly patients and in those with impaired renal function, electrolyte disturbances (particularly hypokalemia), or metabolic abnormalities (particularly hypothyroidism).

Intravenous: Adults, initially 0.8 mg, then 0.4 mg every two to four hours to a maximum of 2 mg. (The drug also may be given intramuscularly but the intravenous route is preferred for more immediate action.)

Intravenous, Intramuscular: For *children,* the following doses are given in two or three divided portions at three- or four-hour intervals: *Newborn infants,* 0.025 mg/kg; *2 weeks to 3 years,* 0.025 mg/kg; *over 3 years,* 0.02 mg/kg.

> **Cedilanid-D** (Sandoz). Solution 0.2 mg/ml in 2 ml containers (alcohol 9.8%).

Antidote

DIGOXIN IMMUNE FAB (OVINE)
[Digibind]

ACTIONS. Digoxin immune Fab consists of antigen-binding fragments derived from specific antidigoxin antibodies obtained from immunized sheep. These antibody fragments bind molecules of digoxin or digitoxin and the resulting Fab fragment-digitalis complex is excreted in the urine. Each 40 mg of Fab fragments (one vial) binds approximately 0.6 mg of digoxin or digitoxin.

USES. Digoxin immune Fab fragments are used to treat life-threatening digoxin intoxication. This product also has been used successfully to treat life-threatening digitoxin overdose.

ADVERSE REACTIONS AND PRECAUTIONS. Although allergic reactions have not been reported, the possibility of anaphylactic, hypersensitivity, or febrile reactions should be kept in mind, and facilities should be available for treating anaphylaxis. Skin testing may be appropriate for patients previously treated with these antibody fragments or in those allergic to sheep proteins.

The serum potassium level should be monitored closely during treatment because hypokalemia may develop rapidly and require correction. If possible, the serum glycoside concentration should be determined before treatment with digoxin immune Fab. An increase in the serum concentration may be observed during treatment, but the digitalis will be bound to the Fab fragments and thus will be unavailable to react with receptors.

Because withdrawal of the inotropic or antiarrhythmic action of digitalis may cause the patient's clinical condition to deteriorate, other modalities should be available to treat resulting heart failure or arrhythmias.

Excretion of the Fab fragment-digoxin complex is probably delayed when renal function is impaired.

DOSAGE AND PREPARATIONS.

Intravenous: Adults and children, see manufacturer's directions.

> **Digibind.** (Burroughs Wellcome). Powder (injection) 40 mg.

OTHER INOTROPIC DRUGS

The limited therapeutic efficacy of digitalis in severe heart failure led to a search for alternative inotropic drugs. Certain sympathomimetic agents and the phosphodiesterase inhibitor, amrinone [Inocor], and related investigational drugs have been tried. These drugs are usually reserved for patients with intractable heart failure refractory to digitalis, diuretics, and vasodilators.

The catecholamine, *dopamine* [Intropin], acts directly on beta₁ receptors and, to a lesser extent, releases norepinephrine from tissue stores. It also acts on dopamine receptors in the renal and mesenteric vascular beds and on alpha receptors. Small doses increase renal and mesenteric blood flow; larger doses increase myocardial contractility, heart rate, and cardiac output. With large doses, the alpha-adrenergic vasoconstrictor effect predominates. Dopamine has been used primarily to treat acute circulatory failure in patients with marked hypotension (see Chapter 27, Agents Used to Treat Shock), but it also may be useful in severe refractory chronic heart failure, particularly when combined with sodium nitroprusside [Nipride, Nitropress] (Miller et al, 1977) or nitroglycerin (Loeb et al, 1983).

The synthetic catecholamine, *dobutamine* [Dobutrex], increases myocardial contractility by stimulating beta₁ receptors, has a less pronounced effect on beta₂ and alpha receptors, and does not activate dopamine receptors. Dobutamine is usually preferred to dopamine in the presence of heart failure, especially when chronic. Dopamine tends to increase peripheral resistance and thus limit cardiac output while dobutamine tends to lower peripheral resistance and thus augment cardiac output. Dopamine is of greatest benefit when severe hypotension accompanies heart failure. In the absence of hypotension, dobutamine is preferable.

The sympathomimetic drug, *ephedrine,* is effective orally, has positive inotropic and chronotropic effects, and increases peripheral vascular resistance. Ephedrine has occasionally been used to treat severe refractory heart failure, usually in conjunction with a vasodilator. Its long-term efficacy has not been established and side effects may limit its usefulness.

Relatively selective beta₁ receptor agonists, such as *prenalterol,* may be useful for short-term treatment, but tolerance often develops to beta-adrenergic agonists during prolonged use, presumably due to a decrease in the density of beta-adrenergic receptors (Bristow et al, 1982; Colucci et al, 1981 A). Dopamine derivatives, such as ibopamine, and the dopamine precursor, levodopa, are also under investigation.

Amrinone [Inocor] is useful for short-term intravenous therapy, but absence of clear evidence of efficacy and a high incidence of adverse effects led to discontinuation of clinical studies on the oral form. A related agent, *milrinone*, appears to be better tolerated for long-term oral therapy. Several similar drugs in the early stages of investigation include piroximone, fenoximone, enoximone, and sulmazole.

Some authorities have expressed concern that long-term therapy with inotropic drugs may accelerate clinical deterioration in patients with severe heart failure, while others feel that apparent deterioration in such patients after drug withdrawal merely reflects progression of the underlying disease. This subject is currently highly controversial. It has been shown experimentally that prolonged inotropic stimulation damages the myocardium, and results of some clinical studies suggest that prolonged oral amrinone therapy may worsen the course of severe heart failure and increase mortality (Packer et al, 1984 A). Pooled results from a multicenter study showed no increase in morbidity and mortality attributable to the drug but also found no evidence that long-term therapy was beneficial (Massie et al, 1985).

Drug Evaluations

DOBUTAMINE HYDROCHLORIDE
[Dobutrex]

ACTIONS. This synthetic catecholamine was developed in a search for new inotropic agents with minimal chronotropic or vascular activity. Dobutamine acts primarily on myocardial beta₁ receptors, has less pronounced actions on beta₂ and alpha receptors, and does not activate dopamine receptors in the renal and mesenteric vascular beds. Moderate doses increase myocardial contractility without greatly increasing heart rate; large doses may increase the heart rate and blood pressure. In animal studies, equivalent inotropic doses of dobutamine had less than one-fourth the chronotropic effect of isoproterenol. This difference appeared to be independent of reflex hemodynamic effects and may reflect a relatively selective action on ventricular contractile tissue with a lesser effect on the S-A node.

USES. Dobutamine is used for short-term therapy to increase cardiac output in patients with severe chronic cardiac failure. In comparative studies, both dobutamine and dopamine increased cardiac output, but dobutamine was more effective in reducing left ventricular filling pressure (Loeb et al, 1977; Stoner et al, 1977). When infused in doses producing comparable increases in cardiac output, nitroprusside reduced systemic arterial and wedge pressures more than dobutamine and did not increase heart rate. Combined therapy with the two drugs produced a greater increase in cardiac output, a lower wedge pressure, and a greater reduction in systemic and pulmonary vascular resistance than either drug alone (Mikulic et al, 1977). Cardiac performance also improves when dobutamine is given with intravenous nitroglycerin (Awan et al, 1983). Preliminary data suggest that weekly or twice weekly dobutamine infusions may improve the clinical status of outpatients with advanced heart failure.

Dobutamine also has been used for inotropic support during emergence from cardiac surgery, and it appears to be as effective as isoproterenol in increasing cardiac output. It may cause less tachycardia and fewer arrhythmias than isoproterenol [Isuprel] in these patients, although some investigators have found no significant difference between the two drugs.

ADVERSE REACTIONS AND PRECAUTIONS. Tachycardia and hypertension are the most common adverse effects of dobutamine and usually can be controlled by reducing the dose. Nausea, headache, palpitations, anginal pain, dyspnea, and ventricular arrhythmias occur occasionally. Low doses may cause myocardial ischemia in patients with coronary artery disease who do not have heart failure. Since dobutamine facilitates A-V conduction, it may increase the ventricular response to atrial fibrillation. Dobutamine may increase insulin requirements in diabetics.

DOSAGE AND PREPARATIONS. Dobutamine is incompatible with alkaline solutions and should not be mixed with sodium bicarbonate injection. It may be reconstituted with sterile water or 5% dextrose injection by adding 10 to 20 ml of diluent to the vial containing 250 mg of dobutamine. This solution can be refrigerated for 48 hours or stored at room temperature for six hours. It must be diluted to at least 50 ml before infusion and should be used within 24 hours.

Intravenous: Adults, the rate of infusion required to increase cardiac output usually ranges from 2.5 to 10 mcg/kg/min. Rarely, infusion rates up to 40 mcg/kg/min may be required.

   Dobutrex (Lilly). Powder (sterile, lyophilized) 250 mg.

AMRINONE LACTATE
   [Inocor]

ACTIONS. This inotropic-vasodilator agent is a derivative of the anticholinergic drug, biperiden. Amrinone may act by inhibiting phosphodiesterase, thereby increasing intracellular concentrations of cyclic AMP, which increases calcium uptake in myocardial cells. It reduces left ventricular filling pressure and peripheral vascular resistance, increases myocardial contractility (although this has not been a consistent finding), and enhances cardiac output. Amrinone may cause a modest increase in heart rate, particularly when given in large doses.

The hemodynamic effects of amrinone are similar to those of dobutamine (Klein et al, 1981; Benotti et al, 1985). It is most effective in increasing cardiac output in patients with a marked elevation in left ventricular filling pressure, and its positive inotropic effect is less than that of isoproterenol (Firth et al, 1984). The inotropic effect of amrinone depends upon adequate stores of cyclic AMP, which may be depleted in patients with severe heart failure (Mancini et al, 1985).

USES. When given intravenously, amrinone improves cardiac performance in many patients with severe chronic heart failure refractory to digitalis, diuretics, and vasodilators (Ward et al, 1983). Its effects are additive to those of digitalis and diuretics. An acute beneficial effect of amrinone on exercise capacity was noted by some investigators (Siskind et al, 1981), but others reported that maximal exercise capacity did not im-

prove within 24 hours after drug administration (Weber et al, 1981).

Clinical studies on the oral form were discontinued because long-term therapy was ineffective and poorly tolerated (Massie et al, 1985).

ADVERSE REACTIONS, PRECAUTIONS, AND INTERACTIONS. Hypotension is a major and common dose-related side effect of intravenous amrinone. Fever and gastrointestinal disturbances (nausea, vomiting, anorexia, abdominal discomfort) have occurred occasionally. Dose-dependent thrombocytopenia has been reported in a few patients and appears to be due to decreased platelet survival time. Hepatotoxicity has occurred rarely. Arrhythmias have been reported but may be disease-related rather than drug-related. There is one report of excessive hypotension in a patient treated with amrinone and disopyramide.

Amrinone may cause discomfort at the infusion site.

PHARMACOKINETICS. Amrinone has a volume of distribution of 1.2 L/kg. Estimates of protein binding range from 10% to 49%. It is eliminated by urinary excretion of unchanged drug and by hepatic metabolism. The terminal elimination half-life is 5.8 hours in patients with congestive heart failure.

DOSAGE AND PREPARATIONS. The solution may be administered as supplied or diluted in 0.9 or 0.45 sodium chloride injection to a concentration of 1 to 3 mg/ml. It should not be diluted with dextrose-containing solutions or mixed with other drugs.

Intravenous: Adults, initially, a 0.75-mg/kg bolus is given over two to three minutes. For maintenance, the drug is infused at a rate of 5 to 10 mcg/kg/min. If needed, an additional bolus injection of 0.75 mg/kg may be given 30 minutes after initiation of therapy. The total daily dose should not exceed 10 mg/kg. Hemodynamic parameters should be monitored during therapy with amrinone.

   Inocor (Winthrop-Breon). Solution (lactate) 5 mg/ml in 20 ml containers.

MILRINONE

ACTIONS. Milrinone is a bipyridine derivative related to amrinone. Like amrinone, it appears to act by inhibiting phosphodiesterase. Milrinone is a more potent inotropic drug than amrinone and also has vasodilator action.

USES. Milrinone has been used for both acute intravenous and long-term oral therapy in patients with severe refractory heart failure. It produces acute hemodynamic improvement in most patients (Baim et al, 1983; Simonton et al, 1985) and symptomatic improvement in about 50% of patients during short-term maintenance therapy. Some patients who showed early hemodynamic and clinical improvement deteriorated during long-term milrinone therapy (Simonton et al, 1985). A favorable effect on mortality has not been demonstrated and, as with oral amrinone, worsening of mortality has been suggested (Timmis et al, 1985).

ADVERSE REACTIONS AND PRECAUTIONS. Headache,

ventricular ectopy and tachycardia, and worsening of myocardial ischemia have been reported. Fluid retention occurs frequently during long-term therapy, necessitating increased doses of diuretics.

DOSAGE AND PREPARATIONS.

Intravenous, Oral: Both an intravenous and an oral preparation are under study. Information is not sufficient to include dosage information.

    Milrinone (Winthrop-Breon).
    (Investigational drug)

VASODILATORS

Vasodilator drugs have assumed an important role as adjunctive agents in the management of severe refractory heart failure. They are particularly useful when heart failure is associated with hypertension, ischemic heart disease, congestive cardiomyopathy, or mitral or aortic insufficiency. When pump function fails, neurohumoral mechanisms are activated to maintain perfusion pressure, intravascular volume, and cardiac filling. The major compensatory response is an increase in sympathetic tone during the resting state, although the sympathetic response to exercise may be blunted (Francis et al, 1985). Other feedback mechanisms that may be activated in chronic heart failure are the renin-angiotensin-aldosterone system and the antidiuretic hormone system (Cohn et al, 1981).

These compensatory mechanisms may maintain circulatory homeostasis initially, but prolonged and excessive vasoconstriction may have deleterious effects on cardiac performance. Persistent arteriolar constriction increases aortic impedance (ventricular outflow resistance), thereby increasing cardiac work and reducing cardiac output, while excessive venoconstriction contributes to congestive symptoms. Plasma norepinephrine levels are directly related to subsequent mortality (Cohn et al, 1984).

Vasodilators reduce this excessive vasoconstriction. They differ in their relative effects on arterial (resistance) and venous (capacitance) vessels. Those that act primarily on resistance vessels reduce aortic impedance and thus increase stroke volume and cardiac output. Venodilators reduce left ventricular filling pressure, improve left ventricular diastolic compliance, and thereby relieve symptoms of pulmonary congestion. Vasodilators also differ in their effects on the regional distribution of blood flow. (See the Table for a summary of the actions, major adverse effects, and dosage of selected vasodilators.)

Agents Used For Short-term Therapy

Parenteral vasodilators are used to treat severe, acutely decompensated, chronic congestive heart failure refractory to digitalis and diuretics. They are also useful in patients with acute left ventricular failure and pulmonary edema. *Sodium nitroprusside* [Nipride, Nitropress] usually is preferred for short-term intravenous therapy in patients with marked pump dysfunction, elevated left ventricular filling pressure, and increased peripheral vascular resistance. Because it has a balanced vasodilator action on both the arterial and venous beds, nitroprusside reduces left ventricular filling pressure and increases cardiac output in these patients. It is more effective and more rapid-acting than furosemide [Lasix] in acutely decompensated chronic left ventricular failure (Franciosa and Silverstein, 1982). The increase in stroke volume induced by nitroprusside usually counterbalances the fall in peripheral vascular resistance so that arterial blood pressure is not greatly reduced. Heart rate usually is not increased and may decrease because of the improved hemodynamics.

Adrenergic inotropic agents, such as dopamine [Intropin] or dobutamine [Dobutrex], may enhance the effectiveness of nitroprusside. Combined inotropic-vasodilator therapy may be particularly useful when congestive heart failure is complicated by mild or moderate hypotension (Miller et al, 1977) (see also Chapter 27).

Intravenous nitroglycerin [Nitrobid IV, Nitrostat IV, Tridil] reduces preload as effectively as nitroprusside but has less effect on peripheral vascular resistance. It generally does not increase and may reduce cardiac output. Nitroglycerin has been used more often after acute myocardial infarction than in chronic heart failure. It is particularly useful for lowering elevated left ventricular filling pressure and relieving acute pulmonary edema. It also dilates epicardial coronary arteries, thereby improving the regional distribution of myocardial blood flow. (See also Chapters 25 and 27.)

Agents Used For Long-term Therapy

Nonparenteral vasodilators are used for long-term treatment of patients with severe, refractory chronic congestive heart failure. Direct-acting venous or arterial vasodilators, angiotensin antagonists, alpha blockers, and beta agonists have been employed.

Direct-acting Vasodilators: *Nitrates* act predominantly to increase venous capacitance and thus reduce preload and relieve pulmonary congestion. They do not increase cardiac output as effectively as arterial vasodilators. Partial tolerance to the circulatory and antianginal effects of oral nitrates has been reported but does not appear to be a significant clinical problem in patients with heart failure (Franciosa and Cohn, 1980; Leier et al, 1983). Oral isosorbide dinitrate [Isordil, Sorbitrate] improves hemodynamics, relieves symptoms, and improves exercise capacity in patients with severe refractory congestive heart failure (Franciosa and Cohn, 1980; Franciosa et al, 1980). It is well tolerated and has a relatively long duration of action (four to six hours). Beneficial hemodynamic effects have also been observed after administration of oral pentaerythritol tetranitrate [Duotrate, Pentritol, Peritrate], nitroglycerin ointment [Nitro-Bid, Nitrol, Nitrong], and chewable nitrate preparations. Sublingual nitrates are less useful because of their short duration of action, and oral nitroglycerin appears to be relatively ineffective. Although transdermal nitroglycerin patches [Nitrodisc, Nitrodur, Transderm-Nitro] produce beneficial hemodynamic effects for six hours, their

MAJOR VASODILATOR DRUGS USED TO TREAT REFRACTORY HEART FAILURE

Drug	Actions	Adverse Reactions*	Route, Usual Dosage, and Preparations
AGENTS USED FOR SHORT-TERM THERAPY			
Nitroprusside	Direct-acting vasodilator with balanced effect on arterial and venous beds and little effect on heart rate. Most commonly used agent for short-term therapy of chronic refractory heart failure.	Hypotension, increased blood levels of thiocyanate and cyanide	*Intravenous: Adults,* 15 to 200 mcg/min; *children,* 0.1 to 8 mcg/kg/min. *Nipride* (Roche), *Nitropress* (Abbott). Powder (for solution) 50 mg.
Nitroglycerin	Direct-acting vasodilator with predominant action on venous bed. Also improves regional distribution of myocardial blood flow in patients with coronary artery disease. Not as effective as nitroprusside in increasing cardiac output.	Hypotension, tachycardia, headache, and, rarely, bradycardia	See Chapter 27.
AGENTS USED FOR LONG-TERM THERAPY			
Captopril	Angiotensin-converting enzyme inhibitor that reduces peripheral vascular resistance and venous tone.	Hypotension, loss of taste, proteinuria, dermatologic reactions, neutropenia	*Oral: Adults,* initially, 25 mg three times daily. In volume-depleted or hyponatremic patients, initial dose should be 6.25 to 12.5 mg three times daily. Dosage may be titrated upward to 50 mg three times daily. Further increases should be delayed for at least two weeks (Maximal daily dose, 450 mg). *Children,* 5 to 10 mg/kg daily in four divided doses. *Capoten* (Squibb). Tablets 12.5, 25, 50, and 100 mg.
Enalapril	Angiotensin-converting enzyme inhibitor that reduces peripheral vascular resistance and venous tone.	Hirsutism, pruritus, rash, hypotension	*Oral: Adults,* 5 mg twice daily. *Vasotec* (Merck Sharp & Dohme). Tablets 5, 10, and 20 mg.
Isosorbide Dinitrate	Direct-acting vasodilator with predominant action on venous bed. Also improves regional distribution of myocardial blood flow in patients with coronary artery disease.	Orthostatic hypotension, headache, flushing, tachycardia	*Oral: Adults,* 10 to 80 mg three or four times daily. See Chapter 26 for preparations.
Hydralazine	Direct-acting vasodilator that reduces peripheral vascular resistance but has little or no effect on capacitance vessels. May be most useful when given with a nitrate for long-term therapy.	Tachycardia, hypotension, flushing, headache, myocardial ischemia, fluid retention, SLE syndrome	*Oral: Adults,* 200 to 400 mg daily in two to four doses. Dosage is variable and larger doses may be required in some patients. *Children,* 1 mg/kg every four to six hours. *Generic.* Tablets, 10, 25, and 50 mg. *Apresoline* (CIBA). Tablets 10, 25, 50, and 100 mg.

(continued on next page)

Drug	Actions	Adverse Reactions*	Route, Usual Dosage, and Preparations
AGENTS USED FOR LONG-TERM THERAPY (continued)			
Prazosin	Selective alpha-adrenergic blocking drug with arterial and venous dilator effects. Tolerance to effects on resting hemodynamics may develop during long-term therapy.	Orthostatic hypotension, syncope, fluid retention	*Oral: Adults,* 2 to 7 mg four times daily. Initial dose should not exceed 1 mg. *Children,* 0.1 mg/kg daily in divided doses. *Minipress* (Pfizer). Capsules 1, 2, and 5 mg
Trimazosin†	Similar to prazosin but also has direct vasodilator action.	Headache, dizziness, drowsiness, gastrointestinal disturbances, chest pain, fluid retention	*Oral: Adults,* 25 to 300 mg three times daily. *Cardovar* (Pfizer). Capsules 25, 50, 100 and 150 mg.

*See Chapter 25, Antianginal Agents, and Chapter 28, Antihypertensive Agents, for other adverse reactions.
†Investigational drug.

effects wane over the next 18 hours and hemodynamic rebound occurs after the patch is removed (Olivari et al, 1983). As currently constituted, these patches are unlikely to play a role in treating chronic heart failure.

Hydralazine [Apresoline] acts directly on resistance vessels. It improves hemodynamics (Chatterjee et al, 1980) and increases renal and limb blood flow but may not increase exercise capacity. Drug-specific tolerance develops in some patients (Packer et al, 1982), and long-term treatment with hydralazine alone may be ineffective (Franciosa et al, 1982). Reflex tachycardia occurs frequently when hydralazine is used to treat hypertension but is less common when the drug is used in congestive heart failure.

Combined *hydralazine-nitrate* therapy reduces left ventricular filling pressure and aortic impedance as effectively as nitroprusside and increases heart rate only slightly. The beneficial hemodynamic effect of this combination usually is accompanied by increased exercise capacity, and tolerance appears to be less common than with hydralazine alone (Massie et al, 1981).

The potent direct-acting arteriolar vasodilator, *minoxidil* [Loniten], improves hemodynamics and left ventricular function during long-term therapy. Minoxidil does not increase exercise capacity or improve symptomatology, however, and it may actually worsen prognosis (Franciosa et al, 1984).

Angiotensin-converting Enzyme Inhibitors: *Captopril* [Capoten] decreases venous tone and peripheral vascular resistance. It reduces angiotensin II and aldosterone levels by inhibiting the enzyme that converts the inactive angiotensin I to angiotensin II. When used to treat refractory heart failure, captopril acts predominantly to reduce left ventricular volume and filling pressure, but it also increases cardiac output. Heart rate may be reduced initially and blood pressure may be reduced markedly after the first few doses. During long-term therapy, renal plasma flow may increase.

Captopril has sustained therapeutic efficacy in many patients as determined by effects on hemodynamics, exercise

tolerance, ejection fraction, functional class, and symptomatology (Ader et al, 1980; Levine et al, 1980; Romankiewicz et al, 1983; Captopril Multicenter Research Group I, 1985). Although the initial hemodynamic effect is often sustained, other patterns of response are sometimes observed. These include a delayed response, an attenuated response, and a triphasic response consisting of initial responsiveness, a subsequent fall-off in response, followed by restoration of the initial hemodynamic effect (Packer et al, 1983). Although captopril is particularly effective in patients with initially high plasma renin levels, approximately 50% of those with low pretreatment plasma renin activity show long-term improvement; the development of reactive hyperreninemia during prolonged therapy may distinguish responders from nonresponders (Packer et al, 1984 B). Refractory edema often disappears when captopril is added to the regimen, and hypokalemia may be normalized (Captopril Multicenter Research Group I, 1985). Hyponatremia also is frequently corrected by captopril, particularly if furosemide is given concomitantly (Dzau and Hollenberg, 1984). The frequency of side effects can be reduced if the total daily dose does not exceed 150 mg, if the initial dose is small in volume-depleted or hyponatremic patients, and if the drug is not given to patients with a creatinine level exceeding 2.5 mg/100 ml.

Enalapril, a long-acting converting enzyme inhibitor, also appears to be effective for long-term therapy and may be better tolerated than captopril (Levine et al, 1984; Creager et al, 1985; Franciosa et al, 1985).

Alpha-adrenergic Blocking Agents: *Prazosin* [Minipress] has a balanced effect on the arteriolar and venous beds. Its hemodynamic effects are more prominent during exercise than at rest. Prazosin does not increase, and may decrease, the heart rate of patients with congestive heart failure. Symptomatic orthostatic hypotension may occur during initial therapy of hypertension but is rare in patients with congestive heart failure, presumably because these patients have higher filling pressures and are less susceptible to the venodilator actions of the drug.

With prolonged use, both hemodynamic and clinical tolerance to prazosin are relatively common (Awan et al, 1981; Markham et al, 1983). Measures that have been suggested to minimize tolerance include (1) instituting more intensive diuretic therapy; (2) increasing the dose of prazosin; or (3) substituting a different vasodilator.

Trimazosin (investigational) is related chemically to prazosin and has similar hemodynamic and therapeutic effects. Oral *phentolamine* [Regitine] has not been consistently effective.

Beta-adrenergic Agonists: These agents are of limited value for long-term therapy because of attenuation of their hemodynamic and clinical effects and their arrhythmogenicity. The loss of responsiveness is associated with a decreased density of beta-adrenergic receptors (Colucci et al, 1981 A and B; Bristow et al, 1982).

Calcium Antagonists: Although the calcium channel blocking agents have vasodilator properties, their direct negative inotropic effect limits their usefulness for treating cardiac failure. Nifedipine [Procardia] is a more potent vasodilator than verapamil or diltiazem and reflex sympathetic activity usually counteracts its negative inotropic effect. Nifedipine has improved hemodynamics in some patients with refractory heart failure, but severe myocardial depression has occurred in others.

Drug Selection

Short-term infusion of vasodilators often improves hemodynamics and relieves symptoms in patients with severe refractory cardiac failure. The efficacy of prolonged therapy with nonparenteral vasodilators is not as well established, and it is not known whether vasodilators increase life expectancy. It is also uncertain what measurements are most reliable for predicting the long-term clinical response (Franciosa, 1984). The only drugs that improve symptoms and exercise capacity during long-term therapy are those that possess venodilating ability (captopril and nitrates). Arteriolar dilators, such as hydralazine and minoxidil, have been ineffective when used alone. A large multicenter study is currently attempting to determine whether digitalis or captopril should be the next step when diuretics alone do not control congestive symptoms. Long-term studies are also in progress with other vasodilator drugs, including a nitrate-hydralazine combination and prazosin.

Adverse Reactions and Precautions

Patients with severe congestive heart failure may be more resistant to the hypotensive effect of vasodilators than patients without heart failure, but the dose should be titrated carefully to avoid a marked fall in blood pressure. Both supine and upright hemodynamic measurements should be used to guide drug selection and dosage but may not predict long-term therapeutic effects.

Although the fall in blood pressure induced by captopril usually is well tolerated, it occasionally is excessive, particularly in patients with volume depletion from excessive diuresis. Such patients should be monitored closely, usually in a hospital, and the initial dose should be small (12.5 mg or less). The patient should be followed closely during the first two weeks of treatment and whenever the dose of captopril and/or diuretic is increased. Persistent symptomatic hypotension occasionally prevents the long-term use of captopril in patients with heart failure. Since this drug may reduce renal function, continued close monitoring is advisable.

Symptomatic orthostatic hypotension may be a problem during treatment of ambulatory patients with prazosin, particularly during initial therapy. Nitrates also may cause orthostatic hypotension. Severe hypotension and vagally mediated sinus bradycardia have occurred rarely in patients treated with intravenous nitroglycerin.

Since the enhanced cardiac output induced by vasodilators leads to withdrawal of excessive sympathetic stimulation, reflex tachycardia usually is not a significant complication but may occur occasionally. Hydralazine may provoke myocardial ischemia in patients with congestive heart failure secondary to coronary artery disease. This complication may occur in the absence of reflex tachycardia and appears to be due to hydralazine's negligible effect on left ventricular preload (Packer et al, 1981).

Vasodilators with prominent pulmonary vascular effects (nitroprusside, phentolamine, and the combination of a nitrate and hydralazine) may cause mild hypoxemia. This is of little or no clinical importance because cardiac output is usually increased and the total oxygen-carrying capacity of the blood is enhanced despite the slight fall in PO_2; hypoxemia may be a problem rarely when the initial PO_2 is very low.

Long-term treatment with vasodilators may cause fluid retention and necessitate more intensive diuretic therapy.

Vasodilator therapy should be discontinued gradually because abrupt withdrawal of vasodilators, including nitroprusside, nitrates, prazosin, and hydralazine, occasionally has caused acute left ventricular failure.

Various mechanisms may contribute to the development of tolerance during long-term vasodilator therapy (Colucci et al, 1981 B). These include (1) activation of endogenous vasoconstrictor forces; (2) increased vascular stiffness due to sodium and water retention; (3) reduced affinity of the drug for a receptor; and (4) decreased number of drug receptors. When tolerance occurs, it is often drug-specific and responsiveness can be restored by substituting a different vasodilator.

Some types of heart failure do not respond favorably to vasodilator therapy. Patients with minimal left ventricular dysfunction occasionally experience hemodynamic deterioration. By reducing left ventricular filling pressure, vasodilators also may have detrimental effects in patients with stenotic valvular lesions or nondilated hypertrophic cardiomyopathy. Vasodilators are of no established value in patients with tricuspid regurgitation or infiltrative myocardial disorders (Packer and Meller, 1978).

For other adverse reactions and precautions, see Chapter 25 and Chapter 28.

Cited References

Ader R, et al: Immediate and sustained hemodynamic and clinical improvement in chronic heart failure by oral angiotensin-converting enzyme inhibitor. *Circulation* 61:931-937, 1980.

Arnold SB, et al: Long-term digitalis therapy improves left ventricular function in heart failure. *N Engl J Med* 303:1443-1448, 1980.

Aronson JK: Clinical pharmacokinetics of digoxin 1980. *Clin Pharmacokinet* 5:137-149, 1980.

Aronson JK: Indications for measurement of plasma digoxin concentrations. *Drugs* 26:230-242, 1983.

Awan NA, et al: Ambulatory prazosin treatment of chronic congestive heart failure: Development of late tolerance reversible by higher dosage and interrupted substitution therapy. *Am Heart J* 104:541-547, 1981.

Awan NA, et al: Effect of combined nitroglycerin and dobutamine in left ventricular dysfunction. *Am Heart J* 106:35-40, 1983.

Baim DS, et al: Evaluation of new bipyridine inotropic agent—milrinone—in patients with severe congestive heart failure. *N Engl J Med* 309:748-756, 1983.

Benotti JR, et al: Comparative vasoactive therapy for heart failure. *Am J Cardiol* 56:19B-24B, 1985.

Bigger JT Jr: Quinidine-digoxin interaction. *Int J Cardiol* 1:109-116, 1981.

Bigger JT Jr, et al: Effect of digitalis treatment on survival after acute myocardial infarction. *Am J Cardiol* 55:623-630, 1985.

Bristow MR, et al: Decreased catecholamine sensitivity and beta-adrenergic-receptor density in failing human hearts. *N Engl J Med* 307:205-211, 1982.

Captopril Multicenter Research Group I: Cooperative multicenter study of captopril in congestive heart failure: Hemodynamic effects and long-term response. *Am Heart J* 110:439-447, 1985.

Chatterjee K, et al: Oral hydralazine in chronic heart failure: Sustained beneficial hemodynamic effects. *Ann Intern Med* 92:600-604, 1980.

Cohn JN, et al: Neurohumoral control mechanisms in congestive heart failure. *Am Heart J* 102:509-514, 1981.

Cohn JN, et al: Plasma norepinephrine as guide to prognosis in patients with chronic congestive heart failure. *N Engl J Med* 311:819-823, 1984.

Colucci WS, et al: Decreased lymphocyte beta-adrenergic-receptor density in patients with heart failure and tolerance to beta-adrenergic agonist pirbuterol. *N Engl J Med* 305:185-190, 1981 A.

Colucci WS, et al: Mechanisms and implications of vasodilator tolerance in treatment of congestive heart failure. *Am J Med* 71:89-99, 1981 B.

Creager MA, et al: Acute and long-term effects of enalapril on cardiovascular response to exercise and exercise tolerance in patients with congestive heart failure. *J Am Coll Cardiol* 6:163-170, 1985.

Doherty JE, et al: Clinical pharmacokinetics of digitalis glycosides. *Prog Cardiovasc Dis* 21:141-158, 1978.

Dzau VJ, Hollenberg NK: Renal response to captopril in severe heart failure: Role of furosemide in natriuresis and reversal of hyponatremia. *Ann Intern Med* 100:777-782, 1984.

Firth BG, et al: Effect of chronic oral digoxin therapy on ventricular function at rest and peak exercise in patients with ischemic heart disease: Assessment with equilibrium gated blood pool imaging. *Am J Cardiol* 46:481-490, 1980.

Firth BG, et al: Assessment of inotropic and vasodilator effects of amrinone versus isoproterenol. *Am J Cardiol* 54:1331-1336, 1984.

Fleg JL, Lakatta EG: How useful is digitalis in patients with congestive heart failure and sinus rhythm? *Int J Cardiol* 6:295-305, 1984.

Franciosa JA: Long-term vasodilator therapy of chronic left ventricular failure: Does it work? *Int J Cardiol* 5:433-439, 1984.

Franciosa JA, Cohn JN: Sustained hemodynamic effects without tolerance during long-term isosorbide dinitrate treatment of chronic left ventricular failure. *Am J Cardiol* 45:648-654, 1980.

Franciosa JA, Silverstein SR: Hemodynamic effects of nitroprusside and furosemide in left ventricular failure. *Clin Pharmacol Ther* 32:62-69, 1982.

Franciosa JA, et al: Contrasting immediate and long-term effects of isosorbide dinitrate on exercise capacity in congestive heart failure. *Am J Med* 69:559-566, 1980.

Franciosa JA, et al: Hydralazine in long-term treatment of chronic heart failure: Lack of difference from placebo. *Am Heart J* 104:587-594, 1982.

Franciosa JA, et al: Minoxidil in patients with chronic left heart failure: Contrasting hemodynamic and clinical effects in controlled trial. *Circulation* 70:63-68, 1984.

Franciosa JA, et al: Effects of enalapril, new angiotensin-converting enzyme inhibitor, in controlled trial in heart failure. *J Am Coll Cardiol* 5:101-107, 1985.

Francis GS, et al: Relative attenuation of sympathetic drive during exercise in patients with congestive heart failure. *J Am Coll Cardiol* 5:832-839, 1985.

Gibson TP, Nelson HA: Question of cumulation of digoxin metabolites in renal failure. *Clin Pharmacol Ther* 27:219-223, 1980.

Graves SW, Williams GH: Endogenous ouabain-like factor associated with hypertensive pregnant women. *J Clin Endocrinol Metab* 59:1070-1074, 1984.

Graves SW, et al: Endogenous digoxin-like substance in patients with renal impairment. *Ann Intern Med* 99:604-608, 1983.

Graves SW, et al: Endogenous digoxin-immunoreactive substance in human pregnancies. *J Clin Endocrinol Metab* 58:748-751, 1984.

Greenblatt DJ, et al: Bioavailability of drugs: Digoxin dilemma. *Clin Pharmacokinet* 1:36-51, 1976.

Griffiths BE, et al: Maintenance of inotropic effect of digoxin on long-term treatment. *Br Med J* 284:1819-1822, 1982.

Ingelfinger JA, Goldman P: Serum digitalis concentration: Does it diagnose digitalis toxicity? *N Engl J Med* 294:867-870, 1976.

Johnson BF, et al: Comparability of dosage regimens of Lanoxin tablets and Lanoxicaps. *Br J Clin Pharmacol* 4:209-211, 1977.

Johnston GD, McDevitt DG: Is maintenance digoxin necessary in patients with sinus rhythm? *Lancet* 1:567-570, 1979.

Klein NA, et al: Hemodynamic comparison of intravenous amrinone and dobutamine in patients with chronic congestive heart failure. *Am J Cardiol* 48:170-176, 1981.

Koren G, et al: Significance of endogenous digoxin-like substance in infants and mothers. *Clin Pharmacol Ther* 36:759-764, 1984.

Leahey EB Jr, et al: Interaction between quinidine and digoxin. *JAMA* 240:533-534, 1978.

Lee DC-S, et al: Heart failure in outpatients: Randomized trial of digoxin versus placebo. *N Engl J Med* 306:699-705, 1982.

Leier CV, et al: Improved exercise capacity and differing arterial and venous tolerance during chronic isosorbide dinitrate therapy for congestive heart failure. *Circulation* 67:817-822, 1983.

Levine TB, et al: Acute and long-term response to oral converting enzyme inhibitor, captopril, in congestive heart failure. *Circulation* 62:35-41, 1980.

Levine TB, et al: Hemodynamic and clinical response to enalapril, long-acting converting-enzyme inhibitor, in patients with congestive heart failure. *Circulation* 69:548-553, 1984.

Loeb HS, et al: Superiority of dobutamine over dopamine for augmentation of cardiac output in patients with chronic low output cardiac failure. *Circulation* 55:375-381, 1977.

Loeb HS, et al: Beneficial effects of dopamine combined with intravenous nitroglycerin on hemodynamics in patients with severe left ventricular failure. *Circulation* 68:813-820, 1983.

Mancini D, et al: Intravenous use of amrinone for treatment of failing heart. *Am J Cardiol* 56:8B-15B, 1985.

Marchionni N, et al: Hemodynamic effects of digoxin in acute myocardial infarction in man: Randomized controlled trial. *Am Heart J* 109:63-68, 1985.

Markham RV Jr, et al: Efficacy of prazosin in management of chronic congestive heart failure: 6-month randomized, double-blind, placebo-controlled study. *Am J Cardiol* 51:1346-1352, 1983.

Massie BM, et al: Acute and long-term effects of vasodilator therapy on resting and exercise hemodynamics and exercise tolerance. *Circulation* 64:1218-1226, 1981.

Massie B, et al: Long-term oral administration of amrinone for congestive heart failure: Lack of efficacy in multicenter controlled trial. *Circulation* 71:963-971, 1985.

Mathur PN, et al: Effect of digoxin on right ventricular function in severe chronic airflow obstruction: Controlled clinical trial. *Ann Intern Med* 95:283-288, 1981.

McHaffie D, et al: Clinical value of digoxin in patients with heart failure and sinus rhythm. *Q J Med* 47:401-419, 1978.

Mikulic E, et al: Comparative hemodynamic effects of inotropic and vasodilator drugs in severe heart failure. *Circulation* 56:528-533, 1977.

Miller RR, et al: Combined dopamine and nitroprusside therapy in congestive heart failure: Greater augmentation of cardiac performance by addition of inotropic stimulation to afterload reduction. *Circulation* 55:881-884, 1977.

Moss AJ, et al: Digitalis-associated cardiac mortality after myocardial infarction. *Circulation* 64:1150-1155, 1981.

Mulrow CD, et al: Reevaluation of digitalis efficacy: New light on old leaf. *Ann Intern Med* 101:113-117, 1984.

Murray RG, et al: Evaluation of digitalis in cardiac failure. *Br Med J* 284:1526-1528, 1983.

Olivari MT, et al: Hemodynamic and hormonal response to transdermal nitroglycerin in normal subjects and in patients with congestive heart failure. *J Am Coll Cardiol* 2:872-878, 1983.

Packer M, Meller J: Oral vasodilator therapy for chronic heart failure: Plea for caution. *Am J Cardiol* 42:686-689, 1978.

Packer M, et al: Provocation of myocardial ischemic events during initiation of vasodilator therapy for severe chronic heart failure: Clinical and hemodynamic evaluation of 52 consecutive patients with ischemic cardiomyopathy. *Am J Cardiol* 48:939-946, 1981.

Packer M, et al: Hemodynamic characterization of tolerance to long-term hydralazine therapy in severe chronic heart failure. *N Engl J Med* 306:57-62, 1982.

Packer M, et al: Hemodynamic patterns of response during long-term captopril therapy for severe chronic heart failure. *Circulation* 68:803-812, 1983.

Packer M, et al: Hemodynamic and clinical limitations of long-term inotropic therapy with amrinone in patients with severe chronic heart failure. *Circulation* 70:1038-1047, 1984 A.

Packer M, et al: Efficacy of captopril in low-renin congestive heart failure: Importance of sustained reactive hyperreninemia in distinguishing responders from nonresponders. *Am J Cardiol* 54:771-777, 1984 B.

Romankiewicz JA, et al: Captopril: Update review of its pharmacological properties and therapeutic efficacy in congestive heart failure. *Drugs* 25:6-40, 1983.

Ryan TJ, et al: Effects of digitalis on survival in high-risk patients with coronary artery disease: Coronary Artery Surgery Study (CASS). *Circulation* 67:735-742, 1983.

Simonton CA, et al: Milrinone in congestive heart failure: Acute and chronic hemodynamic and clinical evaluation. *J Am Coll Cardiol* 6:453-459, 1985.

Siskind SJ, et al: Acute substantial benefit of inotropic therapy with amrinone on exercise hemodynamics and metabolism in severe congestive heart failure. *Circulation* 64:966-972, 1981.

Smith TW, et al: Treatment of life-threatening digitalis intoxication with digoxin-specific Fab antibody fragments: Experience in 26 cases. *N Engl J Med* 307:1357-1362, 1982.

Stoner JD III, et al: Comparison of dobutamine and dopamine in treatment of severe heart failure. *Br Heart J* 39:536-539, 1977.

Timmis AD, et al: Milrinone in heart failure: Effects of exercise haemodynamics during short term treatment. *Br Heart J* 54:42-47, 1985.

Valdes R Jr: Endogenous digoxin-like immunoreactive factors: Impact on digoxin measurements and potential physiological implications. *Clin Chem* 31:1525-1532, 1985.

Valdes R Jr, et al: Endogenous substance in newborn infants causing false positive digoxin measurements. *J Pediatr* 102:947-950, 1983.

Vogel R, et al: Short- and long-term effects of digitalis on resting and posthandgrip hemodynamics in patients with coronary artery disease. *Am J Cardiol* 40:171-176, 1977.

Ward A, et al: Amrinone: Preliminary review of its pharmacological properties and therapeutic use. *Drugs* 26:468-502, 1983.

Weber KT, et al: Amrinone and exercise performance in patients with chronic heart failure. *Am J Cardiol* 48:164-169, 1981.

Weintraub M: Interpretation of serum digoxin concentration. *Clin Pharmacokinet* 2:205-219, 1977.

Wenger TL, et al: Treatment of 63 severely digitalis-toxic patients with digoxin-specific antibody fragments. *J Am Coll Cardiol* 5:118A-123A, 1985.

Other Selected References

Braunwald E: Pathophysiology of heart failure, in Braunwald E (ed): *Heart Disease: A Textbook of Cardiovascular Medicine*, ed 2. Philadelphia, WB Saunders, 1984, 447-466.

Cohn JN (ed): *Drug Treatment of Heart Failure*. New York, Yorke Medical Books, 1983.

Cohn JN, Franciosa JA: Vasodilator therapy of cardiac failure. *N Engl J Med* 297:27-31, 254-258, 1977.

Firth BG: Southwestern Internal Medicine Conference: Chronic congestive heart failure; nature of problem and its management in 1984. *Am J Med Sci* 288:178-192, 1984.

Maskin CS, et al: Inotropic drugs for treatment of failing heart, in Conti CR (ed): *Cardiac Drug Therapy*. Philadelphia, FA Davis, 1984, 1-17.

Mason DT: Afterload reduction and cardiac performance: Physiologic basis of systemic vasodilators as new approach in treatment of congestive heart failure. *Am J Med* 65:106-125, 1978.

Schwartz AB, Chatterjee K: Vasodilator therapy in chronic congestive heart failure. *Drugs* 26:148-173, 1983.

Smith TW, et al: Digitalis glycosides: Mechanisms and manifestations of toxicity, parts I-III. *Prog Cardiovasc Dis* 26:413-458, 495-540; 27:21-56, 1984.

Smith TW, Braunwald E: Management of heart failure, in Braunwald E (ed): *Heart Disease: A Textbook of Cardiovascular Medicine*, ed 2. Philadelphia, WB Saunders, 1984, 503-559.

Sonnenblick EH, LeJemtel TH: Newer inotropic agents, in Braunwald E, et al (eds): *Congestive Heart Failure: Current Research and Clinical Applications*. New York, Grune & Stratton, 1982, 291-302.

Sonnenblick EH, et al: Rationale for inotropic therapy in heart failure. *Cardiovasc Rev Rep* 4:910-925, 1983.

Antiarrhythmic Agents *24*

MECHANISMS OF ARRHYTHMIAS

Cardiac arrhythmias are caused by disorders of electrical impulse formation, by disturbances in impulse conduction, or by a combination of these processes.

Disorders of Impulse Formation: Abnormal impulse generation may result from altered automaticity or from triggered activity. Abnormal automaticity is observed when the dominant pacemaker function of the sinus node is taken over by automatic cells in the atria, atrioventricular (A-V) junction, His-Purkinje system, or ventricles. Pacemaker discharge from these ectopic sites is initiated because the normal automaticity of the sinus node is depressed, as in some bradyarrhythmias, or because automaticity in other cells is enhanced, as in various types of premature ectopy and some tachyarrhythmias. Abnormal rhythms caused by altered automaticity also may occur when the sinus node is the dominant pacemaker but its rate of discharge is inappropriate.

Triggered activity, another cause of abnormal impulse formation, is initiated by delayed afterdepolarizations that reach threshold. Triggered activity has been demonstrated experimentally and has been proposed to be the mechanism of some digitalis-induced arrhythmias, although this has not been conclusively demonstrated in man.

Disorders of Impulse Conduction: When conduction is impaired, a normal cardiac impulse may be slowed or blocked at various points in the conduction system. Impaired conduction may lead to bradyarrhythmias such as sinus exit block, A-V nodal block, bundle branch block, intra- or infra-His bundle block. In special situations, unidirectional block may occur in one pathway, and the cardiac impulse may be conducted slowly through another pathway and re-enter the first in a retrograde direction. This establishes a single reentrant loop or a self-sustaining circus movement that is believed to be the mechanism underlying many tachycardias. A reentry loop may be fixed (anatomically determined) or variable (functionally determined). Both conduction velocity and the duration of the refractory period of cardiac cells are important in determining whether or not a reentrant arrhythmia will be perpetuated.

TABLE 1.
AGENTS USED TO TREAT TACHYARRHYTHMIAS

Drug/Class	Actions	Major Uses
Beta-adrenergic blocking agents (eg, propranolol)	Block cardiac beta receptors, thereby reducing sinus rate and myocardial contractility, lengthening A-V nodal conduction time and refractoriness, and depressing sinus node automaticity.	Atrial fibrillation and flutter; A-V nodal reentrant tachycardia; arrhythmias associated with the preexcitation syndrome; supraventricular and ventricular arrhythmias caused by increased sympathetic tone or circulating catecholamines and those associated with mitral valve prolapse syndrome; supraventricular arrhythmias in hypertrophic cardiomyopathy. Used for both acute control and maintenance therapy.
Calcium channel blocking agents (verapamil and diltiazem)	Prolong A-V nodal conduction time and refractoriness and decrease sinus node automaticity by interfering with calcium transport.	Supraventricular arrhythmias, particularly acute episodes of A-V nodal reentrant tachycardia; atrial fibrillation and flutter (to slow ventricular response); reciprocating tachycardia in the preexcitation syndrome.
Digitalis	Prolongs A-V nodal conduction time and functional refractory period, mainly by indirect (cholinergic and antiadrenergic) actions. Slows sinus rate, when ventricular function is impaired, by virtue of its direct positive inotropic effect, which leads to a reduction in sympathetic stimulation.	Atrial fibrillation and flutter (to slow ventricular response); A-V nodal reentrant tachycardia; arrhythmias associated with congestive heart failure. Used for both acute control and maintenance therapy.
Cholinesterase inhibitors (eg, edrophonium, neostigmine)	Increase vagal tone by preventing inactivation of acetylcholine.	Acute termination of A-V nodal reentrant tachycardia.
Vasoconstrictors (eg, phenylephrine, methoxamine)	Acutely increase blood pressure, thereby increasing vagal tone by reflex mechanisms.	Acute termination of A-V nodal reentrant tachycardia.
Adenosine*	Depresses sinus node automaticity and A-V nodal conduction.	Acute termination of A-V nodal reentrant tachycardia.
Quinidine	Has local anesthetic activity. Depresses automaticity, particularly at ectopic sites; slows conduction and increases refractoriness of atria, His-Purkinje system, accessory pathways, and ventricles. Has both direct and indirect (anticholinergic) actions.	Maintenance of sinus rhythm after conversion of atrial fibrillation and flutter; maintenance therapy in patients with A-V nodal reentrant tachycardia, automatic atrial tachycardia, and arrhythmias associated with the preexcitation syndrome; prevention of frequent ventricular premature complexes and ventricular tachycardia.
Disopyramide	Similar to quinidine	Similar to quinidine
Procainamide	Similar to quinidine	Acute termination of supraventricular and ventricular arrhythmias, particularly those associated with the preexcitation syndrome.
Amiodarone	Increases refractoriness of atria, A-V node, ventricles, His-Purkinje system, and accessory pathways; depresses sinus node automaticity; slows conduction in atria, A-V node, His-Purkinje system, and ventricles.	Prevention of ventricular and supraventricular arrhythmias, particularly ventricular tachycardia and fibrillation, atrial flutter and fibrillation in preexcitation syndrome, bradycardia-tachycardia syndrome (controls only tachycardia).
Lidocaine	Has local anesthetic properties. Depresses automaticity and reduces duration of refractory period in the His-Purkinje system and ventricles. In therapeutic doses, does not slow A-V nodal or intraventricular conduction, except in diseased myocardium.	Acute control of ventricular arrhythmias and prevention of these arrhythmias after acute myocardial infarction.

(Continued on next page)

Drug/Class	Actions	Major Uses
Phenytoin	Similar to lidocaine	Digitalis-induced arrhythmias
Mexiletine	Similar to lidocaine	Ventricular ectopy and tachycardia
Tocainide	Similar to lidocaine	Ventricular ectopy and tachycardia
Bretylium	After initial increase in automaticity (due to release of norepinephrine), increases refractory period of His-Purkinje system and ventricles without slowing conduction or depressing automaticity.	Prevention or acute control of ventricular tachycardia and fibrillation
Flecainide	Has local anesthetic properties. Slows conduction in atria, A-V node, ventricles, accessory pathways, and particularly in His-Purkinje system; to a lesser extent, increases atrial and ventricular refractoriness; suppresses sinus node automaticity.	Ventricular ectopy and tachycardia; arrhythmias associated with preexcitation syndrome; A-V nodal reentrant tachycardia
Encainide*	Similar to flecainide	Ventricular ectopy and tachycardia; arrhythmias associated with preexcitation syndrome; A-V nodal reentrant tachycardia
Lorcainide*	Similar to flecainide	Ventricular ectopy and tachycardia; arrhythmias associated with preexcitation syndrome
Propafenone*	Quinidine-like, with weak beta-blocking and calcium-blocking properties.	Ventricular arrhythmias, particularly ventricular tachycardia, and arrhythmias associated with the preexcitation syndrome
Acecainide*	Prolongs atrial and ventricular refractoriness.	Prevention of frequent premature ventricular complexes
Moricizine* (ethmozin)	Not fully characterized	Prevention of frequent premature ventricular complexes and ventricular tachycardia
Pirmenol*	Similar to quinidine	Prevention of frequent premature ventricular complexes

Investigational drug

GENERAL GUIDELINES FOR TREATMENT

The drugs used to treat tachyarrhythmias and premature complexes reduce automaticity in ectopic foci and/or affect reentrant conduction by altering conduction velocity and the duration of the refractory period. Agents that increase sinus rate and enhance A-V conduction are used occasionally in bradyarrhythmias. The actions and uses of these drugs are summarized in Tables 1 and 2. Antiarrhythmic agents also may be grouped into four categories on the basis of microelectrode studies in isolated cardiac cells (Table 3).

Electrophysiologic studies have facilitated drug selection for some supraventricular arrhythmias by revealing the pathways involved and the effect of different drugs on these pathways. The mechanisms of ventricular arrhythmias are not so well understood and the response to antiarrhythmic drugs is less predictable; therefore, it is often necessary to try various drugs and combinations (Zipes, 1985).

A therapeutic range has been described for many antiarrhythmic drugs. Measurement of the plasma drug concentration may be helpful to evaluate therapeutic failure; to assess compliance; and to facilitate dosage adjustment when age, disease states, or drug interactions alter drug absorption or disposition (Brown and Shand, 1982). It should be emphasized, however, that many patients will not respond to a particular drug even if its dosage is in the therapeutic range.

TABLE 2.
AGENTS USED TO TREAT BRADYARRHYTHMIAS

Drug/Class	Actions	Major Uses
Atropine	Increases sinus rate and A-V nodal conduction velocity and decreases effective refractory period of the A-V node by decreasing vagal tone.	Sinus bradycardia, sinoatrial arrest, sinoatrial block, type 1 second-degree A-V block
Isoproterenol	Increases sinus rate and myocardial contractility, enhances automaticity, and increases A-V nodal conduction velocity by stimulating cardiac beta receptors.	Second- or third-degree A-V block, prior to pacing

SUPRAVENTRICULAR TACHYARRHYTHMIAS

Sinus Tachycardia: Sinus tachycardia is common and usually benign. Generally, the underlying cause (eg, increased sympathetic tone, thyrotoxicosis, fever, congestive heart failure) should be determined and corrected rather than treating the sinus tachycardia as a primary disturbance. When therapy is indicated to control symptoms, a beta-adrenergic blocking agent (eg, propranolol [Inderal]) may be useful if heart failure is not present. Beta blockers slow a rapid sinus rate resulting from enhanced sympathetic tone or increased levels of circulating catecholamines. Digitalis may control sinus tachycardia associated with congestive heart failure but is not useful when the increased sinus rate is due to other causes.

Sinus Nodal and Atrial Reentrant Tachycardias: Paroxysmal supraventricular tachycardia is usually caused by A-V nodal reentry, but occasionally the reentrant circuit is confined to the sinus node, atria, or a bypass tract. Sinus nodal reentrant tachycardia, which may be difficult to distinguish from sinus tachycardia, is probably initiated by a premature atrial complex. If symptomatic, the measures used to terminate A-V nodal reentrant tachycardia (see below) may be tried.

Intra-atrial reentrant tachycardia also has been described but appears to be rare.

Automatic Atrial Tachycardia: This arrhythmia may be associated with acute myocardial infarction, cardiomyopathy, chronic lung disease, or metabolic derangements. Digitalis toxicity is also a frequent cause, particularly if A-V block is present. Automatic atrial tachycardia is believed to be caused

TABLE 3.
CLASSIFICATION OF ANTIARRHYTHMIC AGENTS*

Class	Actions†	Drugs
I	Have local anesthetic properties. Interfere with fast inward depolarizing current carried by sodium ions. These drugs subclassified into three categories:	
IA	Prolong refractoriness and slow conduction	Quinidine, procainamide, disopyramide
IB	Shorten duration of refractory period and have little effect on conduction in normal tissue	Lidocaine, phenytoin, tocainide, mexiletine
IC	Markedly slow conduction but have minimal effects on refractoriness	Encainide, flecainide, lorcainide, propafenone
II	Have antiadrenergic properties	Beta blockers, bretylium
III	Prolong refractoriness	Amiodarone, sotalol
IV	Block slow inward (calcium) current	Verapamil, diltiazem

*Adapted from Vaughan Williams, 1984; Harrison, 1985

†Based on drug's predominant electrophysiologic properties in normal tissue, usually Purkinje fibers. It should be emphasized that some drugs exhibit characteristics of more than one class, have important indirect actions, show different effects in abnormal tissue, or have active metabolites with electrophysiologic properties different from those of the parent drug.

by enhanced automaticity. In the absence of correctable precipitating factors (eg, digitalis toxicity), symptomatic patients may be treated with antiarrhythmic drugs that depress automaticity, such as quinidine, procainamide [Pronestyl, Pronestyl SR, Procan SR], or disopyramide [Norpace]. Vagal maneuvers or drugs that produce A-V nodal block usually are not effective.

Multifocal Atrial Tachycardia: This rhythm disturbance is most frequently encountered in patients with chronic pulmonary disease and is difficult to treat. Therapy is directed primarily toward the underlying disorder. Although multifocal atrial tachycardia is usually attributed to enhanced automaticity, it does not respond to antiarrhythmic drugs such as quinidine. In contrast, verapamil [Calan, Isoptin] reduces the atrial and ventricular rates and occasionally converts this arrhythmia to sinus rhythm.

Atrial Fibrillation and Flutter: These arrhythmias are most often observed in patients who have rheumatic heart disease with mitral valve involvement, cardiomyopathy, hypertensive heart disease, or coronary artery disease. Atrial fibrillation and flutter also may be encountered in patients with toxic or metabolic disturbances, such as alcoholism or thyrotoxicosis. Chronic atrial fibrillation is a common dysrhythmia; chronic atrial flutter is less common.

The goals in treatment are to reduce the ventricular rate by slowing A-V conduction and, if possible, to restore normal sinus rhythm. As with all arrhythmias, the choice of therapy depends upon the clinical situation, the condition of the patient, and the ventricular rate. DC cardioversion may be indicated for patients with hypotension, marked heart failure and/or angina, and a very rapid ventricular response. Drug therapy may be useful in less urgent situations. (For treatment of atrial fibrillation and flutter in patients with the Wolff-Parkinson-White syndrome, see the section on Preexcitation Syndrome.)

Digitalis prolongs A-V nodal conduction time and the functional refractory period. It is considered by many cardiologists to be the drug of choice for controlling the ventricular response to atrial fibrillation in adults and children. When therapeutic doses of digitalis are not effective, especially during stress or exertion when sympathetic tone is increased and parasympathetic tone is reduced, a beta blocker may added if significant heart failure is not present or is rate-related. Such combined therapy may provide better control of the arrhythmia and/or permit a reduction in glycoside dosage, particularly if the severity of the arrhythmia is out of proportion to the degree of cardiac decompensation. Intravenous verapamil also slows the ventricular response in most patients with atrial fibrillation. It has been used with digitalis (with careful monitoring for glycoside toxicity) and may be preferred to a beta blocker in some patients (eg, those with asthma or chronic bronchitis).

Atrial fibrillation may convert spontaneously to sinus rhythm during digitalis or verapamil therapy, particularly when the arrhythmia is of recent onset. If fibrillation persists and conversion to sinus rhythm is indicated, DC cardioversion is the method of choice and is effective in 80% to 90% of patients.

It is more difficult to decrease the ventricular rate during atrial flutter than during fibrillation. Digitalis, a beta blocker, or

verapamil may slow the ventricular response and may convert flutter to sinus rhythm or fibrillation, but the ventricular response may not be controlled for prolonged periods. Cardioversion is commonly required and is usually considered to be the treatment of first choice. Termination by rapid atrial pacing may be preferable if the patient has been receiving large doses of digitalis because of the possibility that cardioversion may induce ventricular fibrillation.

Quinidine, procainamide, or disopyramide may be used for long-term therapy to prevent recurrence of atrial fibrillation or flutter. Digitalis, propranolol, or verapamil should be given concomitantly to slow A-V conduction, because quinidine-like drugs may increase the ventricular response to rapid atrial rates when used alone. (However, concomitant use of disopyramide with propranolol or verapamil generally should be avoided because of potential adverse electrophysiologic and hemodynamic effects.)

Premature Supraventricular Complexes: Premature atrial or junctional complexes (extrasystoles) are usually innocuous and may only require reassurance and correction of precipitating causes, such as excess caffeine, nicotine, or alcohol. Propranolol, quinidine, procainamide, or disopyramide may be useful if the premature complexes cause intractable symptoms or presage sustained arrhythmias. Premature atrial complexes associated with heart failure may respond to digitalization.

A-V Nodal Reentrant Tachycardia (Paroxysmal Supraventricular Tachycardia): A-V nodal reentry is the most common cause of paroxysmal supraventricular tachycardia. The reentrant loop is believed to consist of dual pathways located within the A-V node; antegrade conduction usually occurs over the so-called slow pathway (the pathway with slow conduction but a short refractory period) and retrograde conduction occurs over the fast pathway (the pathway with fast conduction but a longer refractory period). The arrhythmia may be triggered by a premature atrial complex. A-V nodal reentrant tachycardia is usually not associated with underlying heart disease, but it frequently causes symptoms and hemodynamic changes.

Carotid sinus massage or other measures that increase vagal tone will often terminate an acute episode. If not effective as the initial approach, vagal maneuvers may be repeated after each pharmacologic intervention. Carotid sinus massage should be employed cautiously in elderly patients because it occasionally causes hypotension, syncope, asystole, ventricular arrhythmias, and stroke. It should be avoided in patients with cerebrovascular disease or a carotid bruit and is hazardous in those with sinus node dysfunction or digitalis intoxication.

When vagal maneuvers alone are ineffective, intravenous verapamil is usually preferred for acute termination of A-V nodal reentrant tachycardia provided that the patient does not have sinus node disease. Verapamil delays impulse conduction through the A-V node. If verapamil and vagal maneuvers are unsuccessful, a cholinesterase inhibitor, usually the short-acting edrophonium [Tensilon], is sometimes used in an attempt to terminate the arrhythmia by increasing parasympathetic activity. Edrophonium may not be successful if verapamil has failed. Intravenous digitalis or intravenous propranolol also may be tried. Both drugs slow conduction and prolong refractoriness in the A-V node. Propranolol generally should not be given intravenously in close temporal proximity to intravenous verapamil, however.

A vasoconstrictor (eg, phenylephrine [Neo-Synephrine], methoxamine [Vasoxyl]) is occasionally used to elevate blood pressure rapidly, thereby producing a reflex vagal discharge. Vasoconstrictors are most useful if the patient is hypotensive; they are hazardous in elderly patients and in those with hypertension, organic heart disease, hyperthyroidism, or acute myocardial infarction.

When the arrhythmia is established, DC cardioversion or atrial pacing maneuvers may be required. Attention should then be directed toward preventing recurrences by instituting long-term oral therapy with digitalis, adding or substituting propranolol or verapamil if necessary. In some patients, a drug that depresses conduction in the retrograde fast pathway (quinidine, procainamide, or disopyramide) may be required. Amiodarone is very effective in refractory cases.

In infants and young children, digitalis is often the preferred drug for terminating A-V nodal reentrant tachycardia; DC cardioversion is employed in emergencies. Since recurrence is most common during the first year of life, digitalis is usually given prophylactically until age 6 to 12 months. Propranolol may be added if additional control is needed.

Tachycardia Involving Reentry Over Concealed Pathway: Some cases of paroxysmal supraventricular tachycardia are caused by reentry over a concealed (not apparent on electrocardiogram) accessory pathway that conducts only in a retrograde direction. Vagal maneuvers and/or drugs that block A-V conduction may terminate an acute episode. Such drugs also may be given orally for long-term treatment. In some patients, an agent that depresses conduction and prolongs refractoriness in the accessory pathway (quinidine, procainamide, disopyramide) may be required. The bypass tract can be interrupted surgically when symptoms are not controlled by drugs.

PREEXCITATION SYNDROME (WOLFF-PARKINSON-WHITE SYNDROME)

Preexcitation is present when the atrial impulse bypasses the A-V node and His-Purkinje system to activate the ventricle. When it produces symptoms, the preexcitation syndrome is called the Wolff-Parkinson-White syndrome. The recurrent tachycardias associated with this disorder are caused by a reentrant circuit involving the normal A-V conduction system, an accessory pathway (Kent bundle) with a faster conduction velocity but a longer refractory period than the A-V node, the atria, and the ventricles. In most cases, antegrade conduction occurs over the normal pathway and retrograde over the bypass tract. The arrhythmia may be initiated by a premature atrial complex that blocks in the accessory pathway and is conducted to the ventricle over the A-V conducting system. The impulse then travels up the bypass tract in a retrograde direction to the atrium and re-enters the A-V node. Less

commonly, the accessory pathway serves as the antegrade limb and the A-V conduction system as the retrograde limb; rarely, multiple pathways are involved.

A reciprocating tachycardia is the most common arrhythmia in patients with the Wolff-Parkinson-White syndrome. Atrial fibrillation or flutter occurs less frequently and may be associated with a very rapid ventricular response because of rapid conduction over the accessory pathway. Ventricular fibrillation develops occasionally.

Vagal maneuvers may be tried as the initial approach to terminating an acute attack of reciprocating tachycardia. When vagal maneuvers alone are ineffective, intravenous verapamil is often the preferred drug for acute termination of the arrhythmia. If verapamil is not effective, propranolol or procainamide may be tried.

In treating atrial fibrillation or flutter complicating the Wolff-Parkinson-White syndrome, acute therapy with drugs that affect ventricular (bypass) conduction (usually intravenous procainamide) should be considered. A drug that prolongs A-V nodal refractoriness, such as intravenous propranolol, may be given concomitantly but generally should not be used alone because it has no significant effect on the accessory pathway. Digitalis should not be used as a single drug because it may enhance conduction in the accessory pathway and increase the ventricular rate. Verapamil also should be avoided because it may increase the ventricular response and induce hypotension. Amiodarone (intravenous form investigational), which slows conduction and increases refractoriness in both the A-V node and the accessory pathway, is useful in refractory cases. Cardioversion should be used initially if the ventricular rate is very rapid.

For maintenance, quinidine, disopyramide, or procainamide may be employed and, if not effective alone, propranolol or verapamil may be added to quinidine or procainamide. Amiodarone is particularly useful in patients who do not respond to standard therapy. Patients with frequent severe attacks should be referred for electrophysiologic testing to determine optimal drug therapy. Some may require surgical ablation of the accessory pathway or permanent pacing.

VENTRICULAR TACHYARRHYTHMIAS

Premature Ventricular Complexes: In individuals who have normal hearts, premature ventricular complexes are usually benign. Frequent or complex ventricular ectopy in patients with ischemic heart disease or cardiomyopathy may increase the risk of sudden death. After acute myocardial infarction, antiarrhythmic therapy is indicated when ventricular extrasystoles cause disturbing symptoms or predispose to ventricular tachycardia and fibrillation.

Ventricular Tachycardia: This arrhythmia usually occurs in the presence of organic heart disease and may progress to ventricular fibrillation, especially in patients with severe cardiac disease. Episodes may be paroxysmal or nonparoxysmal and may or may not result in syncope. Patients with underlying heart disease, sustained tachycardia, hemodynamic changes, or symptoms should be treated. DC cardioversion should be employed if the tachycardia causes hemodynamic deterioration. Intravenous antiarrhythmic therapy may be tried if the patient is hemodynamically stable.

Ventricular Flutter and Fibrillation: Immediate DC cardioversion is the treatment of choice for ventricular flutter and fibrillation. Antiarrhythmic drugs are used to treat persistent arrhythmias and to prevent recurrences.

Antiarrhythmic Therapy in Ventricular Arrhythmias: Because it acts rapidly and usually does not depress A-V conduction or myocardial contractility, lidocaine [Xylocaine] is the drug of choice for prevention or immediate control of serious ventricular arrhythmias, especially when these occur in association with acute myocardial infarction. If lidocaine is ineffective, intravenous procainamide or bretylium [Bretylol] may be tried. Intravenous preparations of amiodarone, disopyramide, encainide, flecainide, lorcainide, and mexiletine are under investigation for immediate control of refractory ventricular arrhythmias. The ability of an antiarrhythmic drug to prevent premature ventricular complexes is not necessarily correlated with its antifibrillatory activity. Bretylium appears to be more effective in preventing ventricular fibrillation than in suppressing ventricular ectopy.

Frequent premature ventricular complexes following acute myocardial infarction may occur in the presence of sinus bradycardia. Atropine 0.5 to 1 mg intravenously may abolish these ectopic beats by increasing the sinus rate, and no other antiarrhythmic agent may be needed.

Quinidine, procainamide, disopyramide, propranolol, tocainide [Tonocard], flecainide [Tambocor], mexiletine [Mexitil], or amiodarone [Cordarone] may be given orally for long-term suppression of symptomatic ventricular arrhythmias. Encainide, lorcainide, propafenone, moricizine (ethmozin), pirmenol, or cibenzoline (all investigational) may be useful if the standard drugs are ineffective.

Combination therapy (eg, propranolol or tocainide plus quinidine or procainamide) may reduce side effects by permitting a reduction in the dose of each drug (Zipes, 1985). Combination therapy may not prevent ventricular tachycardia induced by programmed electrical stimulation if the individual drugs have failed to control the arrhythmia (Ross et al, 1982; Duffy et al, 1983).

Long-term therapy with beta-blocking drugs decreases mortality in patients who have survived an acute myocardial infarction (see Chapter 25, Antianginal Agents). There is no conclusive evidence that empiric, long-term therapy with other antiarrhythmic drugs reduces mortality in high-risk patients.

BRADYARRHYTHMIAS

Sinus Bradycardia: Sinus bradycardia may not require treatment if cardiac output is adequate. A rate of 50 to 60 beats/minute is usually well tolerated. Marked bradycardia (less than 50 beats/minute) associated with acute myocardial infarction may have serious arrhythmogenic or hemodynamic consequences. If the slow sinus rate is accompanied by

hypotension or increased ventricular ectopy, atropine is usually indicated to increase the sinus rate; temporary pacing may be required in unresponsive patients. Because atropine occasionally causes myocardial ischemia and may precipitate severe ventricular arrhythmias, it should not be used routinely in asymptomatic patients.

Sinus Node Disorders: Drugs are of limited value for increasing the sinus rate in patients with sinus node disorders, such as sinoatrial block and bradycardia-tachycardia syndrome. Atropine or isoproterenol [Isuprel] may improve sinoatrial conduction for brief periods, and theophylline derivatives have occasionally been effective in mild cases. Long-term results generally have been disappointing. No drug is available that reliably increases heart rate on a long-term basis without producing side effects. Permanent demand pacing is usually preferred if severe symptoms are associated with the bradycardia. Digitalis and other antiarrhythmic drugs can then be used to control any associated tachyarrhythmias.

A-V Block and Intraventricular Block: First-degree A-V block rarely produces symptoms and does not require therapy. In more advanced conduction disturbances, treatment is necessary if the heart rate is not sufficient to maintain an adequate cardiac output during rest and exercise or if other arrhythmias are present.

Type I (Wenckebach) second-degree A-V block accompanying acute myocardial infarction is usually transient and does not require pacing. Atropine may improve conduction in symptomatic patients. Rarely, atropine worsens block by increasing the sinus rate without improving A-V conduction. It also may precipitate anginal attacks by increasing heart rate. *Chronic Type I second-degree A-V block* in older patients may have a similar prognosis to that of Type II second-degree A-V block, and patients with this disorder should be considered for pacing (Campbell, 1985).

Type II second-degree A-V block usually signifies a serious conduction disturbance in the His-Purkinje system and often requires temporary or permanent pacing. This conduction abnormality can progress rapidly to *third-degree (complete) A-V block*, and the resulting sudden reduction in cardiac output may cause syncope and seizures (Stokes-Adams syndrome). Atropine or isoproterenol may improve cardiac output initially in symptomatic patients, but beneficial effects are usually transient. Isoproterenol is most commonly used to maintain heart rate and cardiac output prior to insertion of a pacemaker. Some individuals with complete A-V block, particularly the congenital form, maintain an adequate lower escape rhythm without long-term drug or pacemaker therapy.

Patients who have acute anterior myocardial infarction and *bundle branch* or *fascicular block* may require temporary pacing if the block is acute or is associated with more severe conduction disturbances. Chronic intraventricular block does not require permanent pacing unless there is evidence of A-V block. Drugs are not useful for treatment.

In patients with acute myocardial infarction and a normal PR interval, commonly used antiarrhythmic drugs (lidocaine and/or procainamide, quinidine, digoxin, propranolol, or disopyramide) do not adversely affect A-V conduction. These drugs should be used cautiously, however, in patients with acute myocardial infarction accompanied by acute bundle branch block. Such patients have an increased risk of developing complete A-V block (Scheinman et al, 1980), and a temporary transvenous pacemaker should be inserted prior to drug administration.

DIGITALIS-INDUCED ARRHYTHMIAS

The most common arrhythmias produced by digitalis toxicity are ventricular bigeminy or trigeminy, multiform premature ventricular complexes, nonparoxysmal A-V junctional (nodal) tachycardia, and atrial tachycardia with block. However, almost any disorder of cardiac rhythm may occur (see Chapter 23, Agents Used to Treat Heart Failure). Temporarily discontinuing digitalis may be sufficient in patients with mild symptoms. Potassium replacement is indicated if hypokalemia is present, but routine replacement in normokalemic patients is not always advisable because hyperkalemia can intensify A-V block. Potassium therapy is most effective in patients who have atrial tachycardia with A-V block, ventricular premature complexes, or ventricular tachycardia as a manifestation of digitalis toxicity. It should be avoided in patients with hyperkalemia, severe renal impairment, or marked A-V conduction disturbances. Electrocardiographic monitoring and frequent determinations of serum potassium levels are essential during replacement therapy.

The drugs most commonly used to treat severe digitalis-induced tachyarrhythmias are lidocaine and phenytoin [Dilantin]. Lidocaine is usually preferred as the initial agent. Second- or third-degree A-V block is managed with atropine or temporary pacing. Antibody fragments against digitalis (investigational) have been effective in severe, life-threatening digitalis intoxication. (See Chapter 23.) Edetate disodium (EDTA) is rarely employed today to treat digitalis-induced arrhythmias because more effective drugs are available.

Since digitalis toxicity may predispose to postcountershock ventricular arrhythmias, DC cardioversion should be avoided unless other measures fail.

ANTIARRHYTHMIC DRUG THERAPY DURING AND AFTER DC CARDIOVERSION

Lidocaine should be available during DC cardioversion to prevent postconversion ventricular arrhythmias. Patients with atrial flutter or fibrillation may require maintenance therapy with quinidine, disopyramide, or procainamide prior to elective cardioversion to prevent immediate postcountershock arrhythmias and to prevent early relapse to atrial flutter and fibrillation. These drugs are then continued for at least three to six months to maintain normal sinus rhythm after conversion. However, many patients revert to the abnormal rhythm despite adequate blood levels of the drug, and some patients cannot tolerate prolonged antiarrhythmic therapy.

In the absence of overt glycoside toxicity, maintenance doses of digitalis are often continued to reduce the risk of heart failure or recurrence of a rapid ventricular rate after cardioversion. Digitalis does not appear to increase the risk of ventricular arrhythmias during cardioversion when serum concentrations do not exceed the therapeutic range (Mann et al, 1985). A low energy level should be employed initially and carefully titrated upward thereafter. If quinidine therapy is instituted prior to cardioversion, digitalis probably should be discontinued or the dosage reduced 24 to 48 hours prior to the procedure.

Drug Evaluations

AGENTS USED TO TREAT TACHYARRHYTHMIAS

ACECAINIDE HYDROCHLORIDE (N-acetylprocainamide) [NAPA]

ACTIONS. The electrophysiologic effects of this major metabolite of procainamide differ somewhat from those of procainamide and it may be less potent. Acecainide prolongs atrial and ventricular refractoriness but does not alter His-Purkinje conduction time. It does not appear to have a negative inotropic effect.

USES. Acecainide initially suppresses premature ventricular complexes in one-third to two-thirds of patients (Kluger et al, 1981 A; Winkle et al, 1981). Responsiveness to procainamide does not predict the therapeutic response to the metabolite (Roden et al, 1980). Unlike procainamide, acecainide does not readily induce ANA formation and it has been used in patients with previous procainamide-induced lupus whose symptoms then subsided or did not recur (Kluger et al, 1981 B). During long-term therapy, tolerance develops in many patients who initially responded favorably (Kluger et al, 1981 A), but others continue to respond to the drug (Atkinson et al, 1983).

ADVERSE REACTIONS, PRECAUTIONS, AND INTERACTIONS. Gastrointestinal disturbances (nausea, abdominal pain, vomiting, anorexia, diarrhea) are common and are most likely to occur in patients who reacted similarly to procainamide or quinidine. Blurred vision, lightheadedness, vivid dreams, and insomnia also may develop. Pruritic urticarial and maculopapular rashes have been reported. Rarely, lupus erythematosus-like reactions occur due to deacetylation of acecainide to procainamide (Kluger et al, 1981 B). Patients receiving large doses and those with severely impaired renal function may be particularly at risk, and symptoms may disappear if the dose is reduced. Torsades de pointes has also been reported.

Cimetidine may reduce the renal clearance of acecainide.

PHARMACOKINETICS. The bioavailability of acecainide is greater than 80%. Protein binding is 15%. Its elimination half-life is longer than that of procainamide and ranges from 6 hours in patients with normal renal function to 42 hours in functionally anephric patients (Stec et al, 1979). Therapeutic plasma levels have been reported to range from 9 to 32 mcg/ml. Low concentrations of procainamide (less than 1 mcg/ml) have been detected in the plasma of patients receiving acecainide, reflecting deacetylation of the metabolite.

DOSAGE AND PREPARATIONS.

Oral: Adults, initially 1 g every eight hours. After two to three days, if the arrhythmia is not controlled and if adverse effects are not severe, the dosage may be increased to 1.5 g every eight hours. Some patients may require further increments, but efficacy does not appear to be enhanced by raising trough plasma concentrations above 40 mcg/ml.

NAPA (Medco Research). Tablets 500 mg. (Investigational drug)

AMIODARONE HYDROCHLORIDE
[Cordarone]

ACTIONS. Amiodarone, an iodine-containing benzofuran derivative, is related structurally to thyroxine. It possesses antiadrenergic properties and exerts both antiarrhythmic and antianginal effects. After prolonged administration, the major electrophysiologic effect of amiodarone is an increase in refractoriness of the atria, A-V node, ventricles, His-Purkinje system, and bypass tracts. Amiodarone also depresses sinus node automaticity and slows conduction in the atria, A-V node, His-Purkinje system, and ventricles. After acute intravenous administration, the most prominent electrophysiologic effects of amiodarone are to slow conduction and prolong refractoriness of the A-V node. In contrast to many other antiarrhythmic agents, electrophysiologic testing does not always predict the response to this drug.

During prolonged therapy, amiodarone has mild negative inotropic and chronotropic effects and reduces peripheral and coronary vascular resistance. The negative inotropic effect may be marked following acute administration of intravenous amiodarone.

USES. Amiodarone is used to treat life-threatening ventricular and supraventricular arrhythmias that are refractory to other antiarrhythmic drugs. Given orally, it is often effective in suppressing recurrences of ventricular tachycardia or fibrillation (Podrid and Lown, 1981; Heger et al, 1983; Zipes et al, 1984), although severe side effects or recurrence of the arrhythmia may limit its long-term usefulness in some patients (Fogoros et al, 1983).

Amiodarone is also effective for preventing recurrences of atrial flutter and fibrillation and A-V nodal reentrant tachycardia. Because it prolongs refractoriness in both the A-V node and accessory pathways in addition to slowing A-V nodal conduction, it is particularly useful in patients with reciprocating tachycardia or atrial flutter and fibrillation associated with the Wolff-Parkinson-White syndrome (Zipes et al, 1984).

Amiodarone is being employed with increasing frequency to prevent both supraventricular and ventricular arrhythmias in patients with hypertrophic cardiomyopathy. It also may control episodes of tachycardia in patients with the bradycardia-tachycardia syndrome; because it may worsen bradycardia, a permanent pacemaker should be in place.

Intravenous amiodarone (investigational preparation) is often effective for acute termination of reentrant tachycardias (Holt et al, 1985) or for slowing the ventricular rate in patients with atrial fibrillation or flutter. It may convert atrial fibrillation to sinus rhythm (Strasberg et al, 1985). Amiodarone also has been used intravenously for acute suppression of severe refractory ventricular arrhythmias.

ADVERSE REACTIONS AND PRECAUTIONS. Amiodarone may cause anorexia, nausea, vomiting, abdominal pain, and constipation. Headache, weakness, myalgia, tremor, ataxia, paresthesias, depression, insomnia, nightmares, and hallucinations also have been reported. Amiodarone-induced peripheral neuropathy is associated with histologic changes in nerve fibers.

Lipofuscin deposits accumulate in the cornea of most patients during long-term therapy. These deposits, which are reported to be reversible, may cause photophobia, the appearance of colored halos around light, and, occasionally, reduced visual acuity. Anterior subcapsular lens opacities and isolated changes in the iris, ciliary body, choroid, and retina have also been reported but are not definitely linked to amiodarone therapy.

The drug often causes photosensitivity reactions, such as erythema and swelling of areas exposed to sunlight. It also may produce a persistent bluish discoloration of the skin and melanodermatitis due to deposition of crystals in the skin; petechiae, erythema nodosum, and other rashes also have been reported.

Amiodarone frequently alters thyroid hormone metabolism and occasionally induces clinical hypothyroidism or, less commonly, hyperthyroidism. The hypothyroidism may necessitate replacement therapy. Patients over the age of 60, those with high titers of antithyroid antibodies, or individuals with a family history of thyroid dysfunction may be at increased risk of hypothyroidism. Hyperthyroidism may lead to a worsening of arrhythmias and also may require treatment. Thyroid function should be monitored frequently during long-term amiodarone therapy.

Bradycardia, myocardial depression, hypotension, sinoatrial block, atropine-resistant A-V block, ventricular arrhythmias (including torsades de pointes) that may be refractory to cardioversion, fatal congestive heart failure, cardiogenic shock, and cardiac arrest have been reported. The drug should not be used in patients with severe sinus bradycardia or advanced A-V block. Transient ischemic attacks and stroke have been reported, but a cause-and-effect relationship has not been established.

Hypersensitivity pneumonitis and pulmonary fibrosis have developed in some patients taking amiodarone. These complications, which appear to be most common in those with pre-existing abnormalities of pulmonary function, may resolve if the drug is discontinued, but some patients have died from respiratory failure. In addition to drug withdrawal, a short course of corticosteroid therapy may be tried, although there is no clear evidence that this adverse effect is a steroid-responsive immunologic reaction. One case of severe alveolitis and polyarthropathy required additional therapy with an immunosuppressant drug and plasma exchange. Exacerbation of bronchial asthma has been reported rarely.

Serum aminotransferase levels are frequently elevated during amiodarone therapy and may remain so for many months after the drug is discontinued. Hepatic toxicity resembling alcoholic liver disease has been reported occasionally.

Elevated serum creatinine levels have been noted in some patients. Hyperglycemia and hypertriglyceridemia are uncommon side effects. Bone marrow depression has occurred in patients treated with amiodarone, but a cause-and-effect relationship has not been established. Epididymitis, vasculitis, polyserositis, and alopecia have been reported rarely.

Amiodarone crosses the placenta and has caused bradycardia in newborn infants of treated mothers. It is secreted in breast milk in concentrations estimated to be equivalent to a low maintenance dose.

DRUG INTERACTIONS. Amiodarone enhances the effect of warfarin, and the dose of the anticoagulant should be reduced by approximately 50% during concurrent therapy. This interaction may persist for several months after amiodarone is discontinued.

Amiodarone increases serum levels of digoxin, quinidine, procainamide, and phenytoin and the interaction may cause symptoms of toxicity. Ventricular arrhythmias (torsades de pointes) have been attributed to an interaction between amiodarone and quinidine, disopyramide, propafenone, or mexiletine. Hypokalemia also may increase the risk of ventricular arrhythmias. Symptomatic bradycardia or sinus arrest may occur if a beta blocker, digitalis, or verapamil is given to patients treated with amiodarone.

PHARMACOKINETICS.

Absorption: The absorption of amiodarone is variable. Bioavailability ranges from 20% to 80%.

Distribution: Amiodarone is widely distributed throughout the body with the highest concentrations in adipose tissue, liver, and lungs. It is 96% protein bound and the apparent volume of distribution ranges from 0.9 to 148 L/kg.

Metabolism: Amiodarone is extensively metabolized. The pharmacologic activity of its major metabolite, desethyl amiodarone, has not been determined. Amiodarone may be metabolized more rapidly in children than in adults. The terminal half-life of amiodarone is 13 to 107 days (after long-term treatment).

Elimination: Less than 1% of a dose is excreted unchanged in the urine. Total body clearance ranges from 0.10 to 0.77 L/min.

Monitoring: During long-term oral therapy, therapeutic serum concentrations for suppression of ventricular arrhythmias have been reported to range between 1.5 and 2 mcg/ml.

DOSAGE AND PREPARATIONS. Amiodarone has a slow onset of action. The full therapeutic response may not be evident for one week to three months, and effects may persist for one week to 50 days or more after the drug is discontinued.

Oral: Adults, for refractory ventricular arrhythmias, 800 mg to 1.6 g daily initially, followed by 600 to 800 mg daily after one or two weeks and then 400 to 600 mg daily. Thereafter the lowest effective dose should be given. For supraventricular arrhythmias, 600 mg daily in three divided doses for one week, followed by 200 to 400 mg daily. Thereafter, the lowest effective dose should be given to minimize side effects. A maintenance dose of 200 mg on alternate days may be effective in some patients. For the bradycardia-tachycardia syndrome (with a pacemaker in place), initially, 200 mg twice daily, followed by 200 to 600 mg daily. *Children,* 3 to 20 mg/kg daily.

Cordarone (Wyeth). Tablets 200 mg.

Intravenous: Adults, initially, up to 5 mg/kg given over a 5- to 15-minute period; this dose should *not* be repeated within 15 minutes. The drug may then be infused at a dosage of 600 mg to 1.2 g every 12 to 24 hours for several days.

Cordarone (Wyeth).
(Investigational preparation)

Beta-adrenergic Blocking Agents

Propranolol [Inderal] has been used more extensively than other beta blocking drugs in antiarrhythmic therapy, although other members of this group appear to have similar antiarrhythmic effects and potential uses (see Table 4).

PROPRANOLOL HYDROCHLORIDE
[Inderal]

ACTIONS. The antiarrhythmic effects of propranolol have been attributed to two actions: blockade of cardiac beta-adrenergic receptors and membrane-stabilizing activity. The former action is the most important, because the direct membrane effect occurs only at concentrations in excess of those usually employed clinically. The cardiac effects of beta blockade include a reduction in heart rate and myocardial contractility, lengthening of A-V conduction time and refractoriness, and suppression of automaticity.

USES. The major indications for propranolol as an antiarrhythmic agent are catecholamine-induced arrhythmias, atrial flutter and fibrillation, A-V nodal reentrant tachycardia, arrhythmias associated with the Wolff-Parkinson-White syndrome or

TABLE 4.
BETA-ADRENERGIC BLOCKING AGENTS

Drug	Characteristics	Oral Antiarrhythmic Dosage	Preparations
Propranolol	Prototype, nonselective	Effective dose varies widely. *Adults,* 10 to 80 mg 3 or 4 times daily. Larger doses (up to 640 mg daily) may be required to suppress chronic ventricular arrhythmias.* *Children,* 0.5 to 4 mg/kg daily in 4 divided doses. As much as 16 mg/kg daily has been used.	*Generic.* Tablets 10, 20, 40, and 80 mg. *Inderal* (Ayerst). Tablets 10, 20, 40, 60, 80, and 90 mg.
Acebutolol	Cardioselective with partial agonist activity	Initially, *adults,* 200 mg twice daily, increased gradually as needed. The usual maintenance dose ranges from 600 mg to 1.2 g daily. Doses larger than 800 mg daily should be avoided in elderly patients.	*Sectral* (Wyeth). Capsules 200 and 400 mg.
Atenolol	Long-acting, cardioselective	Initially, *adults,* 50 mg once daily. The dose may be increased to 100 to 200 mg daily. The dosage interval should be increased in patients with impaired renal function.	*Tenormin* (Stuart). Tablets 50 and 100 mg.
Metoprolol	Cardioselective	*Adults,* 100 mg twice daily.	*Lopressor* (Geigy). Tablets 50 and 100 mg.
Nadolol	Long-acting, nonselective	Initially, *adults,* 40 mg once daily. The dose may be increased gradually at weekly intervals as needed. The usual maintenance dose is 160 mg daily or less. The dosage interval should be increased in patients with impaired renal function.	*Corgard* (Squibb). Tablets 40, 80, 120, and 160 mg.
Pindolol	Nonselective with partial agonist activity	Insufficient information	*Visken* (Sandoz). Tablets 5 and 10 mg.
Timolol	Nonselective	Insufficient information	*Blocadren* (Merck Sharp & Dohme). Tablets 5, 10, and 20 mg.

For intravenous dose, see evaluation on Propranolol.

the mitral valve prolapse syndrome, and selected ventricular arrhythmias.

Propranolol prevents or terminates tachyarrhythmias caused by increased sympathetic tone or an excess of circulating catecholamines, including exercise-induced arrhythmias and those associated with pheochromocytoma. In the latter case, a beta blocker is used only after adequate alpha blockade has been established.

Because it increases the refractory period of the A-V node and prolongs A-V nodal conduction time, propranolol often slows the ventricular rate in patients with chronic atrial fibrillation or flutter who are not adequately controlled at rest and during exercise by therapeutic doses of digitalis. This combined therapy represents one of the most important uses of propranolol in the management of arrhythmias.

Propranolol also may be useful for short-term control and long-term treatment of A-V nodal reentrant tachycardia and for acute control of reciprocating tachycardia in patients with the Wolff-Parkinson-White syndrome. When atrial flutter or fibrilla-tion complicates the Wolff-Parkinson-White syndrome, propranolol should be given with a drug that affects bypass conduction (eg, procainamide).

Propranolol is usually less effective (but better tolerated) than quinidine or procainamide in suppressing chronic ventricular ectopic activity, although it may be useful in recurrent exercise-induced ventricular tachycardia. Plasma concentrations greater than those that produce beta blockade may be required to suppress chronic ventricular arrhythmias.

Propranolol is often used as initial therapy for both atrial and ventricular arrhythmias in patients with the mitral valve prolapse syndrome. It is useful for treating ventricular arrhythmias associated with a prolonged QT interval; when used for long-term therapy in patients with idiopathic long QT syndrome, propranolol appears to reduce the risk of syncope and sudden death (Moss et al, 1985). Supraventricular arrhythmias associated with hypertrophic cardiomyopathy may respond to beta blockers, but other antiarrhythmic drugs are often needed to control life-threatening ventricular arrhythmias. Propranolol also has been used to treat digitalis-induced arrhythmias, but lidocaine or phenytoin is preferred, especially if A-V block is present.

Long-term therapy with beta-blocking drugs may reduce the risk of reinfarction and sudden death and thus increase life expectancy of patients who survive the acute phase of myocardial infarction. It is not known whether this protective effect is due to antifibrillatory, anti-ischemic, or other actions of this class of drugs (see Chapter 25, Antianginal Agents).

ADVERSE REACTIONS AND PRECAUTIONS. Significant adverse effects include congestive heart failure, worsening of A-V conduction disturbances, and bronchospasm. Severe bradycardia and hypotension may occur, particularly when the drug is given intravenously. Adverse hemodynamic effects may develop when a beta blocker and verapamil are given intravenously in close temporal proximity. Propranolol should be discontinued if marked symptomatic bradycardia develops and should be used cautiously in patients with low sinus rates. Asymptomatic bradycardia (45 to 55 beats/minute) is common and should not be the sole cause for stopping the drug. In patients with coronary artery disease, sudden withdrawal of beta blockers has been implicated in the recurrence of unstable angina, ventricular tachycardia, myocardial infarction, and sudden death.

For a discussion of the pharmacology, pharmacokinetics, and additional adverse effects and interactions of propranolol and other beta-blocking drugs, see Chapter 25, Antianginal Agents.

TREATMENT OF TOXICITY. Atropine 0.5 to 1 mg intravenously controls excessive bradycardia when pronounced vagal tone is a major contributing factor. When myocardial depression is severe, isoproterenol should be given by slow intravenous infusion; the dose required may be large. A vasopressor, such as epinephrine or levarterenol, is used to treat severe hypotension. Heart failure is treated with digitalis and diuretics, and bronchospasm with a beta$_2$ agonist (eg, terbutaline) and/or theophylline.

DOSAGE AND PREPARATIONS.
Oral: See Table 4.
Intravenous: Adults, 0.1 to 0.15 mg/kg administered in increments of 0.5 to 0.75 mg every one to two minutes. *Children,* 0.01 to 0.15 mg/kg over three to five minutes. The electrocardiogram and blood pressure should be monitored continuously. Smaller doses should be used or the drug avoided if there is a risk of myocardial depression.
Inderal (Ayerst). Solution 1 mg/ml in 1 ml containers.

BRETYLIUM TOSYLATE
[Bretylol]

This quaternary ammonium compound was originally available as an oral preparation to treat hypertension, but it proved unsuitable for long-term therapy because of unpredictable gastrointestinal absorption, troublesome side effects (orthostatic hypotension and parotid pain), and frequent development of tolerance. The parenteral preparation was subsequently found to be useful in antiarrhythmic therapy.

ACTIONS. The major direct effect of bretylium is to prolong action potential duration and refractory period of the His-Purkinje system and ventricles without affecting conduction or automaticity. Bretylium also interacts with the sympathetic nervous system. It accumulates in sympathetic ganglia and postganglionic adrenergic neurons where it blocks adrenergic transmission by preventing the release of norepinephrine, thereby inducing a state resembling surgical sympathectomy. It does not antagonize (and may *increase*) sensitivity to circulating catecholamines. A transient increase in automaticity, heart rate, myocardial contractility, and blood pressure occurs prior to the onset of adrenergic neuron blockade; this effect is caused by the initial release of norepinephrine from sympathetic nerve terminals and can be prevented by propranolol. A temporal dissociation between the antiarrhythmic and antiadrenergic effects of bretylium has been noted.

USES. Bretylium is used for prophylaxis and treatment of ventricular fibrillation. It is also administered to treat ventricular tachycardia that has failed to respond to a first-line agent, such as lidocaine. The antifibrillatory effects of bretylium are usually noted within minutes, and it may terminate the arrhythmia, facilitate successful cardioversion, and prevent recurrences. Its effects appear to be comparable to those of lidocaine (Haynes et al, 1981).

Bretylium has a more delayed onset of action in suppressing ventricular ectopy and tachycardia; the maximal antiarrhythmic action may not be apparent for 20 minutes to 12 hours after injection. (See also Heissenbuttel and Bigger, 1979; Koch-Weser, 1979.)

ADVERSE REACTIONS AND PRECAUTIONS. The initial release of norepinephrine by bretylium may temporarily increase ventricular ectopic activity and elevate blood pressure. These effects may be enhanced if the patient is receiving vasopressor therapy or if the arrhythmia being treated is caused by digitalis toxicity. Bretylium generally should not be administered for digitalis-induced arrhythmias.

The initial pressor effect is followed (usually within one hour) by a fall in supine blood pressure, which is the most common (incidence, up to 66%) and most troublesome adverse reaction. Bretylium is particularly difficult to use in patients who are hypotensive. If the supine systolic pressure falls below 75 mm Hg, dopamine or norepinephrine may be infused, but the blood pressure should be monitored closely because bretylium enhances the pressor effect of catecholamines. Patients with severe aortic stenosis or pulmonary hypertension may be unable to compensate for a fall in peripheral resistance by increasing their cardiac output and, if possible, bretylium should be avoided in these patients. It may be given if the patient's survival is threatened by the arrhythmia, but the patient should be watched closely and vasoconstrictor amines given promptly if hypotension occurs.

Nausea and vomiting may occur, particularly when the drug is given rapidly; therefore, intravenous infusions in conscious patients should be administered slowly over a period of at least eight minutes. Less common adverse effects include bradycardia, anginal attacks, diarrhea, abdominal pain, hiccups, erythematous macular rash, flushing, fever, sweating, nasal congestion, and mild conjunctivitis.

PHARMACOKINETICS.

Distribution: Bretylium accumulates in sympathetic ganglia and postganglionic adrenergic neurons. Protein binding is negligible.

Elimination: Bretylium is eliminated entirely by renal excretion of unchanged drug; 70% to 80% of a dose is eliminated within 24 hours and an additional 10% during the next three days. No metabolites have been identified.

The half-life is 8 to 12 hours in normal volunteers and longer in patients with impaired renal function.

Monitoring: Plasma levels are not useful as a guide to therapy.

DOSAGE AND PREPARATIONS. The blood pressure and electrocardiogram should be monitored continuously during therapy. Bretylium is eliminated by the kidneys as unchanged drug, and the dosage should be reduced in patients with impaired renal function.

Intravenous: For immediate control of life-threatening ventricular arrhythmias (particularly ventricular fibrillation), *adults,* 5 mg/kg of undiluted drug is given rapidly. If fibrillation persists, dosage may be increased to 10 mg/kg and repeated as necessary. For immediate control of other ventricular arrhythmias, *adults,* the contents of one ampul should be diluted with at least 50 ml of dextrose injection or sodium chloride injection and 5 to 10 mg/kg infused slowly over eight minutes or more to avoid nausea; the dose may be repeated in one to two hours. For maintenance, *adults,* a dilute solution may be infused continuously at a rate of 1 to 2 mg/min, or 5 to 10 mg/kg may be given by slow intermittent infusion every six hours.

Bretylol (American Critical Care). Solution (sterile) 50 mg/ml in 10 ml containers.

Calcium Channel Blocking Agents (Calcium Antagonists)

These drugs selectively inhibit slow channel calcium ion transport in cardiac tissue. This slow inward current, which contributes to the plateau phase of the cardiac action potential, links myocardial excitation to contraction and controls energy storage and utilization. Action potentials from most specialized cardiac cells depend upon both fast (sodium) and slow (calcium) channels, but the pacemaker cells of the S-A node and cells in the proximal region of the A-V node are depolarized primarily by the calcium current. Some calcium channel blocking agents are useful in treating reentrant tachycardias that incorporate the sinus or A-V node. Verapamil is the most potent antiarrhythmic agent among the available calcium channel blockers. Diltiazem [Cardizem] has similar electrophysiologic properties, but it has not been widely used in antiarrhythmic therapy.

VERAPAMIL HYDROCHLORIDE
[Calan, Isoptin]

ACTIONS. This synthetic derivative of papaverine blocks the slow (calcium) channel and also has a slight nonspecific sympathetic depressant effect. The antiarrhythmic properties of verapamil derive from its ability to delay impulse transmission through the A-V node by a direct action. By prolonging A-V conduction time and increasing the refractory period of the A-V node, verapamil interrupts reentrant supraventricular tachycardias and slows the ventricular response to rapid atrial rates. It blocks A-V nodal conduction without significantly affecting conduction in accessory pathways. Verapamil also has a direct depressant effect on the sinus node. The negative inotropic effect of verapamil is not prominent with therapeutic doses, except in patients with significant congestive heart failure or those receiving other myocardial depressant drugs.

USES. Verapamil is highly effective when given intravenously to terminate an acute attack of A-V nodal reentrant tachycardia. It has a rapid onset of action (two to three minutes) and restores sinus rhythm in approximately 80% of patients. Intravenous verapamil also slows the ventricular response to atrial fibrillation or flutter; reversion to sinus rhythm is uncommon, except in patients whose arrhythmia is of recent origin and who have minimal left atrial enlargement (Singh et al, 1983). In multifocal atrial tachycardia, intravenous verapamil reduces both the atrial and ventricular rates and occasionally converts the arrhythmia to sinus rhythm (Levine et al, 1985).

Large oral doses of verapamil may prevent recurrences of A-V nodal reentrant tachycardia. The drug has not been consistently effective when used alone to prevent recurrence of atrial flutter or fibrillation, and it may be most useful when given with other agents, such as digitalis or quinidine.

Verapamil may or may not be indicated for arrhythmias associated with the Wolff-Parkinson-White syndrome. Through its action on the A-V node, verapamil terminates acute episodes of reciprocating tachycardia but it may be less effective in preventing recurrences (Harper et al, 1982). This drug should be avoided when atrial fibrillation or flutter complicates this syndrome because it may increase the ventricular response (Rinkenberger et al, 1980; Harper et al, 1982).

Verapamil is usually not effective in ventricular arrhythmias. See also Singh et al, 1980, 1983.

ADVERSE REACTIONS, PRECAUTIONS, AND INTERACTIONS. A transient, usually asymptomatic fall in blood pressure is the most common side effect of intravenous verapamil. The drug may cause severe hypotension, bradycardia, and asystole in patients with sick sinus syndrome or in those receiving an intravenous beta blocker. Intravenous verapamil generally should be avoided in these patients and in those with A-V conduction disturbances, cardiogenic shock, or advanced congestive heart failure (unless heart failure is secondary to a supraventricular tachyarrhythmia). A short run of ventricular ectopy may occur during conversion of A-V nodal reentrant tachycardia to sinus rhythm. Verapamil may increase the ventricular response to atrial fibrillation or flutter in patients with the Wolff-Parkinson-White syndrome.

Oral verapamil often causes constipation. Nausea, vomiting, lightheadedness, headache, flushing, nervousness, rashes, and pruritus also may occur. Orthostatic hypotension, pedal edema, A-V block (which may lead to A-V dissociation and accelerated junctional rhythms), pulmonary edema, and congestive heart failure have developed occasionally. Hepatitis has been reported occasionally.

Adverse hemodynamic effects have occurred occasionally during combined oral therapy with verapamil and a beta blocker; these drugs generally should not be used together if left ventricular function is compromised. Verapamil increases serum digoxin levels. Its concomitant administration with quinidine may cause hypotension. Calcium supplements may antagonize the effect of verapamil.

TREATMENT OF TOXICITY. Bradycardia, hypotension, A-V block, or asystole may respond to treatment with intravenous calcium salts (usually gluconate or chloride), atropine, or isoproterenol. Temporary ventricular pacing may be required in some cases. Persistent hypotension may require infusion of levarterenol. In patients with hypertrophic cardiomyopathy, an alpha-adrenergic agonist, such as phenylephrine, should be used to maintain blood pressure, and norepinephrine and isoproterenol should be avoided. If verapamil causes a marked increase in the ventricular rate (eg, in patients with the Wolff-Parkinson-White syndrome), DC cardioversion or procainamide may slow the ventricular response.

PHARMACOKINETICS.

Absorption: Oral verapamil is almost completely absorbed, but bioavailability ranges from 20% to 35% because of extensive first-pass metabolism. Bioavailability is reduced in elderly patients with atrial fibrillation and may be increased in those with cirrhosis.

Distribution: The steady-state volume of distribution is 6 L/kg; it is reduced in elderly patients with atrial fibrillation and increased in patients with cirrhosis. Verapamil is 90% protein bound.

Metabolism: Verapamil is extensively metabolized. Twelve metabolites have been identified; the major ones are N- and O-dealkylated products, including norverapamil, which has some vasodilator activity but does not affect A-V conduction. The elimination half-life of oral verapamil after repeated doses ranges from 4.5 to 12 hours; norverapamil has a longer half-life (10.3 to 16.5 hours). The half-life of verapamil is prolonged in patients with cirrhosis. Following intravenous infusion, the drug is eliminated biexponentially with a rapid early distribution phase (half-life, about four minutes) and a slower terminal elimination phase (half-life, two to five hours).

Elimination: Values for plasma clearance vary widely. Clearance is reduced in patients with cirrhosis and in elderly patients with atrial fibrillation. Approximately 3% to 4% of a dose is excreted unchanged.

Monitoring: The negative dromotropic effect of verapamil has been reported to correlate with the plasma concentration of the parent drug (therapeutic concentration, 100 ng/ml). Plasma verapamil levels are highest after bolus injection. Therapeutic concentrations can be sustained by maintenance infusion.

DOSAGE AND PREPARATIONS. The electrocardiogram and blood pressure should be monitored continuously.

Intravenous: Adults, 5 to 10 mg given over two minutes (or three minutes in elderly patients). An additional 10 mg may be given if necessary in 30 minutes. For maintenance, infusions of 0.005 mg/kg/min have been employed. *Infants up to 1 year,* 0.1 to 0.2 mg/kg over two minutes, repeated if necessary in 30 minutes. *Children 1 to 15 years,* 0.1 to 0.3 mg/kg, repeated if necessary in 30 minutes. No more than 10 mg should be given as a single dose.

Calan (Searle), *Isoptin* (Knoll). Solution 2.5 mg/ml in 2 and 4 ml containers.

Oral: Adults, 240 to 480 mg daily in three or four divided doses.

Calan (Searle), *Isoptin* (Knoll). Tablets 80 and 120 mg.

DIGITALIS GLYCOSIDES

ACTIONS. The digitalis glycosides have complex direct and indirect effects on the heart. The actions that are of particular importance in antiarrhythmic therapy are lengthening of A-V nodal conduction time and functional refractory period, which result from increased vagal tone, an antiadrenergic action, and, to a lesser extent, a direct effect. In addition, the direct positive inotropic effect of digitalis improves ventricular function, and may thereby slow the sinus rate in patients with cardiac failure.

USES. In atrial fibrillation or flutter, many cardiologists consider digitalis to be the agent of choice to slow the ventricular response. Generally, a larger dose is required to slow the ventricular rate during atrial flutter than during atrial fibrillation, and the ventricular response to atrial flutter is often not easily controllable for prolonged periods. Digitalis is more effective in patients with stable, chronic atrial fibrillation than in clinically unstable patients with acute atrial fibrillation (Goldman et al, 1975). Digitalis alone may not control the ventricular response to rapid atrial rates during exercise or stress; if additional control is needed, propranolol or verapamil may be given concurrently.

Digitalis may terminate A-V nodal reentrant tachycardia after vagal maneuvers and other antiarrhythmic drugs have failed; vagal maneuvers may be more effective after digitalization. Digitalis also may prevent recurrence of the arrhythmia. Sinus tachycardia associated with congestive heart failure also may respond to digitalis therapy.

The glycosides generally are contraindicated or must be used very cautiously in the presence of type I A-V block. Digitalis also should not be used as a single drug in patients with the Wolff-Parkinson-White syndrome because it may increase the ventricular response to atrial fibrillation or flutter.

For the treatment of digitalis-induced arrhythmias, see the Introduction.

The pharmacokinetics, adverse effects, and interactions of the digitalis glycosides are discussed in Chapter 23, Agents Used to Treat Heart Failure.

DOSAGE AND PREPARATIONS. See Chapter 23.

DISOPYRAMIDE PHOSPHATE
[Norpace, Norpace CR]

ACTIONS. The electrophysiologic effects of disopyramide are similar to those of quinidine. It also has both direct and anticholinergic actions and local anesthetic properties. Disopyramide has a significant negative inotropic effect, and in contrast to quinidine and procainamide, it causes peripheral vasoconstriction.

USES. Disopyramide is used orally for the same indications as quinidine. It prevents ventricular extrasystoles and ventricular tachycardia but may be less effective in supraventricular tachyarrhythmias (Heel et al, 1978). An intravenous preparation is currently under investigation.

ADVERSE REACTIONS, PRECAUTIONS, AND INTERACTIONS. The most common side effects are related to disopyramide's anticholinergic activity and include dryness of the mouth, blurred vision, constipation, and urinary retention. Efficacy is seldom achieved without mild anticholinergic side effects. Rarely, an attack of acute angle-closure glaucoma has been precipitated.

Nausea, vomiting, gastric pain, and diarrhea may occur, but these reactions are less common with disopyramide than with quinidine.

Disopyramide has both a negative inotropic action and a vasoconstrictor effect, and this combination may precipitate heart failure in poorly compensated patients, even those receiving digitalis and diuretics. Heart failure may be more common with disopyramide than with other antiarrhythmic agents (Podrid et al, 1980). Severe myocardial depression may lead to profound hypotension, sometimes associated with increased venous pressure and unexplained abdominal pain. Vasopressor amines should be available to treat this complication. Disopyramide should be used with extreme caution if at all in patients with cardiomegaly, uncompensated or marginally compensated congestive heart failure, and in those receiving beta blockers or other drugs with a negative inotropic effect.

Disopyramide may precipitate or worsen heart block. It probably should not be used in patients with second- or third-degree A-V block unless a ventricular pacemaker is in place. It also should be avoided in those with sinus node disorders because it may adversely affect sinus node function.

Like quinidine, disopyramide may increase the ventricular rate in nondigitalized patients with atrial flutter or fibrillation.

Prolongation of the QT interval, widening of the QRS complex, and a prominent U wave may be present on the electrocardiogram. Occasionally, these abnormalities may presage ventricular arrhythmias, including torsades de pointes; syncope may be the presenting symptom.

Adverse reactions reported rarely include nervousness, dizziness, fatigue, depression, headache, muscle weakness, acute psychosis, severe hypoglycemia, intrahepatic cholestasis, rash, and anaphylactoid reactions.

The safety of disopyramide in pregnant women and nursing mothers has not been definitely established. It was given to one pregnant woman from the twenty-sixth week without adverse effects on the fetus. The drug was reported to initiate uterine contractions in one patient. The drug and a metabolite are excreted in breast milk.

Disopyramide does not increase serum digoxin levels.

PHARMACOKINETICS.

Absorption: The bioavailability of disopyramide is 83%.

Distribution: The volume of distribution is 0.78 L/kg. Protein binding is 68% at 0.38 mcg/ml and 28% at 3.8 mcg/ml. Because of the drug's concentration-dependent protein-binding characteristics, an increase in dose results in a less than proportionate increase in *total* drug concentration, and it is difficult to estimate the free drug concentration when total drug is measured.

Metabolism: Approximately 20% of a dose is excreted as the mono-N-dealkylated metabolite and 10% as other metabolites. These metabolites do not appear to have significant antiarrhythmic activity. The half-life of disopyramide is 8 hours (regular preparation) or 12 hours (timed-release preparation) in patients with normal renal function. The half-life is increased in patients with impaired renal function.

Elimination: Clearance is 1.3 ml/min/kg (regular preparation). Approximately 50% of a dose is excreted unchanged. Renal and nonrenal elimination is variable in patients with impaired renal function.

Monitoring: Therapeutic plasma levels are reported to range from 2 to 4 mcg/ml or higher (up to 8 mcg/ml) for ventricular arrhythmias.

DOSAGE AND PREPARATIONS.

Oral: Adults, (Regular Preparation) initially, 100 to 150 mg every six hours (range, 400 to 800 mg daily). For patients with renal or hepatic insufficiency, the manufacturer recommends a maintenance dose of 100 mg with or without a loading dose of 150 mg at the following intervals: every 8 hours (creatinine clearance 30 to 40 ml/min); every 12 hours (creatinine clearance 15 to 30 ml/min); or every 24 hours (creatinine clearance less than 15 ml/min). Patients of small stature or those with hepatic insufficiency, cardiomyopathy, or cardiac decompensation also may require a smaller dose.

(Timed-release Preparation) 300 mg every 12 hours. Dosage should be reduced to 200 mg every 12 hours in patients with small stature or moderate renal insufficiency. The timed-release preparation should not be used in patients with severe renal insufficiency, cardiomyopathy, or cardiac decompensation.

For *children,* (Regular Preparation) a 1 to 10 mg/ml suspension can be prepared by adding the entire contents of disopyramide capsules to an appropriate volume of cherry syrup in an amber glass bottle. The suspension is stable for one month when refrigerated and should be thoroughly shaken before use. The suggested daily dosage for *children under 1 year* is 10 to 30 mg/kg; for *children 1 to 4 years,* 10 to 20 mg/kg; for *children 4 to 12 years,* 10 to 15 mg/kg; and for those *12 to 18 years,* 6 to 15 mg/kg.

    Norpace (Searle). Capsules 100 and 150 mg (equivalent to base); capsules (timed-release) 100 mg and 150 mg (equivalent to base) (*Norpace CR*).

EDROPHONIUM CHLORIDE
[Tensilon]

Edrophonium is a cholinesterase inhibitor that may be used to terminate A-V nodal reentrant tachycardia when vagal maneuvers fail. Because of its rapid onset and brief duration of action, edrophonium is usually preferred to neostigmine for this purpose. Edrophonium also has been given by intravenous infusion for up to 30 hours to maintain a slow ventricular response during atrial fibrillation or flutter (Frieden et al, 1971).

Cholinergic side effects (eg, miosis, sweating, increased bronchial and salivary secretion, gastrointestinal disturbances) are less common with edrophonium than with longer acting cholinesterase inhibitors. Edrophonium should be avoided in asthmatics and should be given cautiously to elderly patients, those receiving digitalis, and those with a history of cardiac disease, for it has caused sinus bradycardia, A-V block, and, rarely, cardiac arrest. Atropine is used to treat toxicity.

DOSAGE AND PREPARATIONS.
Intravenous: For A-V nodal reentrant tachycardia, administration of edrophonium should be followed by vagal maneuvers. *Adults,* 5 mg. If this dose is ineffective, an additional 5 to 10 mg may be given. An initial test dose of 1 to 2 mg may be advisable in elderly patients, in those receiving digitalis, and in those with a history of cardiac disease. *Children,* 2 mg administered slowly.

For atrial flutter or fibrillation, *adults,* if an initial bolus of 5 to 10 mg slows the ventricular response, a dilute solution may be infused at a rate of 0.25 to 2 mg/min to maintain the slow ventricular rate.

    Tensilon (Roche). Solution (sterile) 10 mg/ml in 1 and 10 ml containers.

ENCAINIDE
[Enkaid]

ACTIONS. Encainide is a benzanilide derivative with local anesthetic properties. When given intravenously, it slows conduction in the His-Purkinje system without greatly affecting conduction or refractoriness in other parts of the conduction system. After oral administration, encainide slows conduction in the A-V node, His-Purkinje system, and accessory pathways and increases refractoriness of the atria, ventricles, and accessory pathways (Jackman et al, 1982). These differences indicate the presence of active metabolites with electrophysiologic properties different from those of the parent drug. Encainide has a mild negative inotropic effect. It may suppress sinus node automaticity in patients with sinus node dysfunction.

USES. Encainide has been used most commonly to treat ventricular arrhythmias. Refractory ventricular tachycardia was controlled in about 54% of patients during six months of oral therapy and in approximately 29% of patients treated for longer periods (Mason and Peters, 1981). This drug may be more effective than quinidine in suppressing premature ventricular complexes (Harrison et al, 1980; Sami et al, 1981). Encainide also appears to be useful in preventing recurrences of reciprocating tachycardia in some patients with the Wolff-Parkinson-White syndrome (Prystowsky et al, 1984).

ADVERSE REACTIONS AND PRECAUTIONS. Encainide may cause lightheadedness, dizziness, headache, blurred vision, paresthesias, and, less commonly, gastrointestinal disturbances (nausea, vomiting, constipation). Worsening of ventricular arrhythmias (including torsades de pointes) is a relatively frequent dose-related adverse effect in patients receiving encainide for recurrent sustained ventricular tachycardia and/or fibrillation but occurs less commonly in those treated for ventricular ectopy. A-V block has developed rarely. Encainide may aggravate sinus node disorders.

PHARMACOKINETICS.
Absorption: There are wide individual differences in bioavailability (range, 7% to 82%).
Metabolism: Encainide is extensively metabolized and two active metabolites have been identified. The half-life of the parent drug is 1.9 to 3.8 hours; the active metabolites have much longer half-lives (up to 12 hours) and may be more important than the parent drug during prolonged therapy. Two pathways of metabolism are found that appear to be phenotypically determined. About 90% of patients metabolize the drug rapidly and form two active metabolites; in these patients, the half-life of encainide is one to three hours. The remaining 10% of patients metabolize the drug slowly (half-life, 8 to 12 hours).
Distribution: Encainide is 71% protein bound in rapid metabolizers and 78% in slow metabolizers. It has a small apparent volume of distribution.
Elimination: The total body clearance of encainide is 13.2 ml/min/kg.
Monitoring: Plasma concentrations of unchanged drug do not correlate closely with efficacy because of the contribution of active metabolites (Winkle et al, 1983).

DOSAGE AND PREPARATIONS.
Oral: Adults, 75 to 300 mg daily in three divided doses.
    Enkaid (Bristol-Myers). Capsules 10, 25, and 50 mg. (Investigational drug)

Intravenous: *Adults*, up to 1 mg/kg administered over 15 to 20 minutes.

> **Enkaid** (Bristol-Myers). Solution 10 mg/ml in 5 ml containers.
> (Investigational drug)

FLECAINIDE ACETATE
[Tambocor]

ACTIONS. Flecainide has local anesthetic properties. It depresses sinus node automaticity and prolongs conduction in the atria, A-V node, ventricles, accessory pathways, and particularly in the His-Purkinje system. To a lesser extent, it increases refractoriness of atrial and ventricular tissues (Estes et al, 1984). Flecainide exhibits a moderate negative inotropic effect.

USES. Flecainide is given orally to suppress chronic ventricular ectopy and runs of ventricular tachycardia (Anderson et al, 1984 A; Holmes and Heel, 1985; Vanhaleweyk et al, 1984). In short-term studies, flecainide was more effective than quinidine or disopyramide in preventing ventricular ectopy and complex arrhythmic events (Hodges et al, 1984; Kjekshus et al, 1984). The oral preparation also may be useful for long-term prophylaxis of reentrant tachycardias involving the A-V node or accessory pathways (Neuss, 1985).

Intravenous flecainide (investigational preparation) has been used to terminate A-V nodal reentrant tachycardia and reciprocating tachycardia associated with the Wolff-Parkinson-White syndrome (Camm et al, 1985; Hellestrand et al, 1983). It also may terminate atrial fibrillation but is less effective in atrial flutter (Camm et al, 1985). There is limited information on the use of the intravenous preparation in ventricular arrhythmias.

Divergent findings have been reported on the value of programmed electrical stimulation in predicting the long-term response to flecainide.

ADVERSE REACTIONS AND PRECAUTIONS. Blurred vision and dizziness are the most common side effects of flecainide. It also may cause headache, nausea, constipation, fatigue, nervousness, tremor, chest pain, dyspnea, paresthesias, and rash.

Flecainide increases sinus node recovery time and should be used cautiously in patients with sinus node dysfunction. Its negative inotropic effect may occasionally cause significant deterioration of cardiac function in patients with congestive heart failure. Worsening of congestive heart failure usually can be managed by adjusting the dose of digitalis and diuretic. Flecainide has occasionally precipitated bundle branch block or A-V block. It should be avoided in patients with advanced conduction disturbances unless a pacemaker is in place.

QT prolongation due to QRS complex widening, increased ventricular ectopy, and ventricular tachycardia or fibrillation have occurred in patients receiving flecainide. The drug has occasionally increased the ventricular response to atrial flutter. Proarrhythmic effects have been noted in 5% to 12% of patients and are most common in those with pre-existing left ventricular dysfunction or life-threatening ventricular arrhythmias.

Flecainide is classified in FDA Pregnancy Category C.

DRUG INTERACTIONS. Flecainide may slightly increase serum digoxin levels. During concomitant administration of flecainide and propranolol, plasma levels of both drugs may increase slightly.

PHARMACOKINETICS.

Absorption: The bioavailability of flecainide is greater than 90%.

Distribution: Flecainide has a large volume of distribution (10 L/kg) and is 40% protein bound.

Metabolism: Flecainide is extensively metabolized, but active metabolites have not been identified. The plasma half-life is 20 hours following multiple doses in patients with ventricular ectopy. The rate of elimination from the plasma is reduced in patients with congestive heart failure or renal failure.

Twenty-seven percent of a dose is excreted as unchanged drug in the urine and the balance as metabolites.

Monitoring: Therapeutic plasma levels appear to range from 0.2 to 1 mcg/ml. Plasma concentrations exceeding 1 to 1.5 mcg/ml have been associated with signs of toxicity.

DOSAGE AND PREPARATIONS.

Oral: *Adults,* initially, 100 mg every 12 hours. The dose may be increased by 50 mg twice daily every four days until efficacy is achieved or to a maximum dose of 200 mg every 12 hours (for patients with sustained ventricular tachycardia) or 300 mg every 12 hours (for those with ventricular ectopy or nonsustained ventricular tachycardia). (Because of flecainide's long half-life, four days may be required to reach steady state.) A maintenance dose of 100 mg twice daily may be effective in some patients (Flowers et al, 1985). The maximum dose for patients with congestive heart failure is 200 mg twice daily. Plasma level monitoring should guide dosage adjustments in patients with renal failure.

> **Tambocor** (Riker). Tablets 100 mg.

Intravenous: 1 to 2 mg/kg given as a slow injection or diluted with 5% dextrose and given as a slow infusion.

> **Tambocor** (Riker). Solution.
> (Investigational preparation)

LIDOCAINE HYDROCHLORIDE
[Xylocaine]

ACTIONS. Lidocaine is a local anesthetic that depresses automaticity and reduces refractory period duration in the His-Purkinje system and ventricles but has little effect on atrial tissue. Therapeutic doses do not slow A-V nodal or intraventricular conduction velocity except in the ischemic myocardium.

USES. Because it acts rapidly and moderate doses usually do not depress myocardial contractility or A-V conduction, intravenous lidocaine is the drug of choice for immediate suppression of ventricular ectopy and hemodynamically stable ventricular tachycardia occurring during acute myocardial infarction. It also is administered during cardioversion of ventricular fibrillation or symptomatic sustained ventricular tachycardia to prevent postconversion arrhythmias.

Since warning arrhythmias may be absent or undetected in up to 50% of patients who develop primary ventricular fibrillation after acute myocardial infarction, lidocaine is often administered prophylactically to patients hospitalized with acute chest pain (Harrison, 1978). This program was effective in some coronary care units (Lie et al, 1974; DeSilva et al, 1981), but other cardiologists have expressed doubts about the efficacy and safety of routine lidocaine prophylaxis (Kertes and Hunt, 1984). In a recent controlled study, lidocaine did not prevent serious ventricular arrhythmias or reduce mortality and caused significant side effects in some patients (Dunn et al, 1985).

The immediate prognosis of acute myocardial infarction was reported to be improved by intramuscular injection of lidocaine prior to hospitalization. This report was not confirmed in some subsequent studies.

In addition to its use in acute myocardial infarction, lidocaine may control ventricular arrhythmias caused by digitalis toxicity and those that develop during cardiac surgery or cardiac catheterization. It usually does not correct supraventricular arrhythmias and may increase the ventricular rate.

ADVERSE REACTIONS AND PRECAUTIONS. The major adverse effects of lidocaine are attributable to its action on the central nervous system and include drowsiness, slurred speech, paresthesias, muscle twitching, convulsions, coma, and respiratory depression. Large doses may depress myocardial contractility, automaticity, and A-V conduction, especially in the presence of conduction system disease. Untoward effects are most common in elderly patients and those with congestive heart failure. The high incidence of side effects in elderly patients can usually be avoided if a lower dose is employed. Lidocaine is in FDA Pregnancy Category B.

DRUG INTERACTIONS. Lidocaine clearance is reduced by concomitant administration of either cardioselective or nonselective beta blockers due to decreased cardiac output and hepatic blood flow. Cimetidine also reduces lidocaine clearance and increases its half-life. These interactions may be associated with symptoms of toxicity.

TREATMENT OF TOXICITY. Small increments of diazepam or an ultrashort-acting barbiturate are used to control severe convulsions. Vasopressors may be used to treat circulatory depression.

PHARMACOKINETICS.

Distribution: The volume of distribution is 1.1 ± .04 L/kg (increased in patients with hepatic dysfunction, decreased in those with congestive heart failure).

Although lidocaine has concentration-dependent protein-binding characteristics, it is not highly protein bound; therefore, changes in binding may not be an important problem during dose titration.

Metabolism: Ninety percent of a dose of lidocaine is metabolized. Two active metabolites have been identified. The half-life

of lidocaine is 80 to 108 minutes (after repeated doses or sustained infusion). The half-life is prolonged and plasma levels are increased in patients with hepatic dysfunction, reduced cardiac output, or after prolonged (more than 24 hours) infusion.

Elimination: Clearance is 9.2 ± 2.4 ml/min/kg and is reduced in patients with congestive heart failure or hepatic dysfunction. Urinary excretion is 10%.

Monitoring: Therapeutic plasma levels range from 1.2 to 5 mcg/ml.

DOSAGE AND PREPARATIONS.

Intravenous: *Adults,* for ventricular arrhythmias, a loading dose of 50 to 100 mg given over two to three minutes. This dose may be repeated in five minutes, or one or two supplemental doses of 25 to 50 mg may be given at five- or ten-minute intervals (up to 300 mg in a one-hour period). Following the loading dose, a solution is infused at a rate of 1 to 4 mg/min.

The following regimen has been recommended for prophylaxis after acute myocardial infarction: A loading dose of 200 mg is given as four 50-mg injections five minutes apart, or 20 mg/min is infused for ten minutes. Each bolus should be given slowly (over one to two minutes). Simultaneously with the loading dose, an infusion is started at a rate of 3 mg/min. The infusion should be continued for 24 to 36 hours or until a diagnosis of acute myocardial infarction is excluded.

Lidocaine and its metabolites accumulate in some patients during a constant maintenance infusion over 24 to 36 hours. Monitoring for early evidence of toxicity should be carried out and the dose reduced if toxic effects appear. If symptomatic ventricular arrhythmias occur during the first six hours of infusion, an additional smaller bolus may be given and the infusion rate increased.

In patients 70 years and older and those with congestive heart failure, cardiogenic shock, or hepatic disease, the loading dose should be decreased by about one-half and the infusion rate should be reduced to 1 to 2 mg/min. *Children,* 0.5 to 1 mg/kg every five minutes for a maximum of three doses, or a solution containing 5 mg/ml infused at a rate of 0.03 mg/kg/min.

Generic. Solution 10 mg/ml in 5 and 10 ml containers, 20 mg/ml in 5 ml containers, 40 mg/ml in 25 and 50 ml containers, 100 mg/ml in 10 ml containers, and 200 mg/ml in 5 and 10 ml containers.

Xylocaine Intravenous Injection for Cardiac Arrhythmias (Astra). Solution 20 mg/ml in 5 ml containers, 40 mg/ml in 25 and 50 ml containers, and 200 mg/ml in 5 and 10 ml containers.

Intramuscular: *Adults,* 300 mg (3 ml of a 10% solution) injected into the deltoid muscle.

Xylocaine Intramuscular Injection for Cardiac Arrhythmias (Astra). Solution 100 mg/ml in 5 ml containers.

LORCAINIDE

ACTIONS. Lorcainide is a local anesthetic-type antiarrhythmic drug. It slows atrial, His-Purkinje, and intraventricular conduction and slows conduction and increases refractoriness in the accessory pathways. It also may slow A-V nodal conduction and increase atrial and ventricular refractoriness. The effect on conduction is more pronounced in the His-Purkinje system and ventricles than in the atria or A-V node. This drug has a mild negative inotropic effect. It may prolong sinus node recovery in patients with sinus node dysfunction.

USES. Lorcainide is used to suppress chronic ventricular ectopy. When given intravenously, it may be superior to lidocaine in suppressing premature ventricular complexes (Anderson et al, 1985). With oral administration, it is comparable to quinidine in efficacy, but may cause more frequent side effects (Falk and O'Brien, 1984). Lorcainide may be useful in selected patients with ventricular tachycardia, but does not appear to be particularly effective in those with sustained ventricular tachycardia and fibrillation (Echt et al, 1985). It also may be of value in slowing conduction over the accessory pathway in patients with the Wolff-Parkinson-White syndrome (Eiriksson and Brogden, 1984).

ADVERSE REACTIONS AND PRECAUTIONS. Sleep disturbance is the most common and most troublesome adverse effect of oral lorcainide and may be accompanied by vivid dreams, sweating, chills, hot flashes, or anxiety. Oral lorcainide also may cause headache, tremor, slurred speech, ataxia, fatigue, nausea, vomiting, transient hyponatremia, and a metallic taste. Dizziness, headache, paresthesias, memory loss, and hallucinations have been associated with intravenous administration.

Lorcainide may worsen ventricular arrhythmias. It also may exacerbate congestive heart failure, aggravate sinus node dysfunction in patients with sinus node disorders, and cause bundle branch block or A-V block in those with pre-existing conduction disturbances. It should be used cautiously in patients with these disorders.

PHARMACOKINETICS.

Absorption: The bioavailability of a single dose is low due to extensive first-pass metabolism but increases after multiple doses.

Distribution: The volume of distribution of lorcainide is between 5 and 10 L/kg. It is 83% protein bound in normal subjects and 75% in those with congestive heart failure.

Metabolism: Lorcainide is extensively metabolized, and its major metabolite, norlorcainide, has antiarrhythmic activity. The half-lives are 8 hours (lorcainide) and 27 hours (norlorcainide).

Elimination: The clearance of lorcainide is 15 ml/min/kg. Less than 3% is excreted unchanged.

DOSAGE AND PREPARATIONS.

Oral: Adults, 100 mg twice daily. Because of the slow accumulation of its active metabolite, dosage should be increased no more frequently than at weekly intervals. The usual maintenance dose is 100 to 400 mg daily.

    Lorcainide (Janssen). Tablets 100 mg.
    (Investigational drug)

Intravenous: Adults, initially, 2 mg/kg administered over 10 to 20 minutes at a rate of 10 mg/min. For maintenance, 0.18 to 0.27 mg/kg/hr.

Lorcainide (Janssen). Solution 10 mg/ml in 10 ml containers. (Investigational drug)

MEXILETINE HYDROCHLORIDE
[Mexitil]

ACTIONS. Mexiletine is related structurally to lidocaine and has similar electrophysiologic properties, but, unlike lidocaine, is effective when given both intravenously and orally. It depresses automaticity in the ventricles but has little effect on atrial tissue and does not depress sinus node function except in patients with the sick sinus syndrome. In patients with normal A-V conduction, mexiletine does not appear to depress A-V nodal function, but A-V conduction time may be increased in those with pre-existing conduction disturbances. Mexiletine does not have a clinically important negative inotropic effect.

USES. Mexiletine is given orally to prevent or treat ventricular ectopy and tachycardia. It has been used frequently to suppress ventricular arrhythmias in survivors of acute myocardial infarction (Chew et al, 1979) and it appears to be as effective as procainamide for this purpose (Campbell et al, 1975). Mexiletine is less effective in patients with recurrent refractory ventricular arrhythmias, and side effects may limit its long-term usefulness (Heger et al, 1980). Concurrent administration of propranolol or quinidine may permit a reduction in the dose of mexiletine, provide better control of the arrhythmia, and reduce the incidence and severity of side effects (Leahey et al, 1980; Duff et al, 1983).

Mexiletine also has been given by the intravenous route (investigational preparation) to suppress early ventricular arrhythmias after acute myocardial infarction. It causes more adverse effects than lidocaine but may be useful in patients who are resistant to lidocaine. Mexiletine does not control supraventricular arrhythmias.

ADVERSE REACTIONS AND PRECAUTIONS. Extracardiac adverse reactions include nausea, vomiting, malaise, dizziness, tremor, diplopia, dysarthria, paresthesias, confusion, and ataxia.

Manifestations of cardiovascular toxicity include sinus bradycardia or tachycardia, atrial fibrillation, hypotension, dyspnea, and ventricular tachyarrhythmias, including torsades de pointes. Severe bradycardia and prolongation of the sinus node recovery time may occur if mexiletine is given to patients with the sick sinus syndrome. Mexiletine should be avoided in patients with severe bradyarrhythmias. Atropine controlled mexiletine-induced bradycardia in some patients. In one case of suicidal overdosage, ventricular asystole occurred and the myocardium was refractory to electrical pacing.

Mexiletine is excreted in breast milk. It is classified in FDA Pregnancy Category C.

DRUG INTERACTIONS. Phenytoin, rifampin, and probably other enzyme-inducing drugs decrease the half-life of mexiletine. Opiate analgesics may slow its absorption, while metoclopramide has been reported to accelerate absorption.

PHARMACOKINETICS.

Absorption: The bioavailability of mexiletine is 88%. Absorption is delayed and incomplete in patients with acute myocardial infarction, particularly in those who have received narcotic analgesics.

Distribution: Mexiletine is 70% protein bound. Its total volume of distribution is 5.5 L/kg.

Metabolism: Mexiletine is extensively metabolized. Several metabolites have been identified but do not appear to have antiarrhythmic activity. Plasma levels are increased in patients with chronic liver disease. The half-life of mexiletine is 8 to 12 hours in normal individuals and 18 hours in those with acute myocardial infarction. Since only 10% to 15% of the drug is excreted unchanged in the urine, renal insufficiency has little effect on drug clearance until creatinine clearance is 10 ml/min or less.

Elimination: The renal clearance of mexiletine is 6.5 ml/min/kg; 8% of the drug is excreted unchanged. Peak plasma levels are usually seen two to four hours after oral administration.

Monitoring: Therapeutic plasma levels appear to range between 0.5 and 2 mcg/ml.

DOSAGE AND PREPARATIONS. Mexiletine should be given with food or antacids.

Oral: Adults, initially, 200 mg every eight hours. If rapid control is essential, an initial loading dose of 400 mg may be administered, followed by a 200-mg dose in eight hours. Dosage may then be increased or decreased by 50 or 100 mg. A minimum of two to three days between dose adjustments is recommended. The usual maintenance dose is 200 to 300 mg every eight hours. If a satisfactory response is not achieved and the drug is well tolerated, 400 mg may be given every eight hours. Since the severity of central nervous system side effects increases with total daily dose, the dose should not exceed 1.2 g/day. If an adequate response is achieved with a dose of 300 mg or less every eight hours, the same total daily dose may be tried in divided doses every 12 hours while carefully monitoring the patient's response. This dose may be increased to a maximum of 450 mg every 12 hours if necessary.

　　Mexitil (Boehringer Ingelheim). Capsules 150, 200, and 250 mg.

Intravenous: Adults, initially, 200 to 300 mg infused over 30 minutes at a rate of 10 to 15 mg/min. For maintenance, the drug may be infused at a rate of 1 mg/min. The electrocardiogram and blood pressure should be monitored continuously. For maintenance, 500 mg to 1 g infused over 24 hours.

　　Mexitil (Boehringer Ingelheim). Solution 25 mg/ml in 10 ml containers.
　　(Investigational preparation)

MORICIZINE (Ethmozin)
　[Ethmozine]

ACTIONS. This phenothiazine derivative was developed in the Soviet Union and is currently under investigation in the United States. Its electrophysiologic properties have not been fully characterized, but it is usually classified as Type 1B (resembling lidocaine).

USES. The major use of oral moricizine is to suppress frequent premature ventricular complexes and ventricular tachycardia (Pratt et al, 1984). An intravenous preparation has been used abroad to terminate A-V nodal reentrant tachycardia and reciprocating tachycardia in patients with the Wolff-Parkinson-White syndrome.

ADVERSE REACTIONS AND PRECAUTIONS. The most common adverse effects of oral moricizine are dizziness, fatigue, nervousness, euphoria, perioral numbness, sleep disturbances, headache, nausea, palpitations, and chest pain. Tinnitus, dry mouth, and pruritus also have been reported.

DOSAGE AND PREPARATIONS.

Oral: Adults, 10 mg/kg daily in three divided doses.
　　Ethmozine (DuPont). Tablets 50, 100, 200, and 250 mg.
　　(Investigational drug)

PHENYTOIN
　[Dilantin]

PHENYTOIN SODIUM
　[Dilantin]

ACTIONS. Phenytoin depresses spontaneous depolarization in ventricular tissue. It usually does not alter intraventricular conduction and generally does not slow (and may improve) A-V conduction. Phenytoin has a mild negative inotropic effect and a peripheral vasodilator action.

USES. Phenytoin is not a first-line antiarrhythmic drug. Its major indication is to reverse some digitalis-induced arrhythmias (particularly ventricular arrhythmias) but, even for this purpose, lidocaine may be the drug of choice. Phenytoin may be useful to control postoperative ventricular arrhythmias in children and young adults after surgery for congenital heart disease and to treat ventricular arrhythmias associated with a prolonged QT interval.

ADVERSE REACTIONS, PRECAUTIONS, AND INTERACTIONS. Fatigue, dizziness, ataxia, nausea, vomiting, pruritus, and rash are common. Neurologic side effects progress in severity as the plasma concentration increases. Hepatitis, blood dyscrasias, and pseudolymphoma have occurred rarely. Rapid intravenous administration may cause myocardial depression, bradycardia, hypotension, paradoxical A-V block, and, rarely, cardiac arrest. During chronic therapy, phenytoin may cause a clinically important decrease in serum quinidine levels. This effect may persist for several weeks after phenytoin is discontinued.

Treatment of toxicity is nonspecific and may include assisted ventilation, oxygen, vasopressors, and possibly hemodialysis.

For other adverse reactions, drug interactions, and precautions, see Chapter 9, Antiepileptic Drugs.

PHARMACOKINETICS.
Absorption: Absorption from the gastrointestinal tract is slow and variable.
Distribution: The volume of distribution is 0.64 L/kg. Phenytoin is 93% bound to plasma protein. Patients with impaired hepatic function or uremia may respond to lower total plasma levels because the free drug concentration is increased.
Metabolism: Phenytoin is extensively metabolized before excretion. Plasma levels vary widely because of individual differences in the rate of metabolism resulting from genetic factors or concurrent administration of drugs that affect microsomal enzyme activity. No active metabolites have been identified. The half-life (8 to 60 hours) increases with increasing plasma concentration. Increases in the dose result in greater than proportionate changes in plasma concentration because of increasing saturation of metabolizing enzymes.
Elimination: Less than 5% of a dose is excreted unchanged. Plasma clearance is 0.3 ml/min/kg.
Monitoring: Antiarrhythmic blood levels usually range between 10 and 18 mcg/ml. Therapeutic plasma levels may be difficult to maintain because small increases in the maintenance dose may cause large increases in plasma levels.

DOSAGE AND PREPARATIONS.
Oral: Large initial doses may be required to achieve an effective plasma level rapidly. *Adults,* 1 g on the first day and 300 to 600 mg on the second and third days. For maintenance, 300 to 400 mg daily in one to four divided doses. *Children,* initially, 10 to 15 mg/kg in two or three doses over a 24-hour period. For maintenance, 5 to 10 mg/kg daily in two or three divided doses.

> PHENYTOIN:
> *Dilantin* (Parke-Davis). Suspension 30 (pediatric) and 125 mg/5 ml (alcohol >0.6%); tablets (pediatric, chewable) 50 mg.
> PHENYTOIN SODIUM:
> *Generic.* Capsules (plain, timed-release) 100 mg.
> *Dilantin* (Parke-Davis). Capsules (timed-release) 30 and 100 mg.
> **Additional Trademark.**
> *Diphenylan* (Lannett).

Intravenous: This route should be reserved for severe acute arrhythmias and should be used very cautiously with continuous monitoring of the electrocardiogram and blood pressure. The infusion rate should not exceed 25 to 50 mg/min. *Adults,* 100 mg every five minutes until the arrhythmia is reversed or toxicity is observed (maximum, 1 g).

> PHENYTOIN SODIUM:
> *Dilantin* (Parke-Davis), *Generic.* Solution 50 mg/ml in 2 and 5 ml containers.

PIRMENOL

ACTIONS. The electrophysiologic properties of pirmenol appear to be similar to those of quinidine. In laboratory studies, its antiarrhythmic effects were independent of the serum potassium concentrations. Pirmenol has a modest negative inotropic effect.

USES. Pirmenol has been used both orally and intravenously to prevent frequent premature ventricular complexes. It appeared to be effective and well tolerated in a short-term study (Anderson et al, 1984 B).

ADVERSE REACTIONS AND PRECAUTIONS. Information on adverse effects is limited. Dry mouth, bitter taste, nausea, and atrial flutter have been reported. Pirmenol may have myocardial depressant effects in patients with impaired left ventricular function.

PHARMACOKINETICS. The bioavailability of pirmenol is 83%. It is 87% protein bound and the half-life is approximately nine hours. Pirmenol is eliminated by both renal and nonrenal routes. Renal clearance is 100 ml/min.

DOSAGE AND PREPARATIONS.
Oral: Adults, 200 to 450 mg daily in two or three divided doses.

> *Pirmenol* (Warner-Lambert/Parke-Davis).
> (Investigational drug)

PROCAINAMIDE HYDROCHLORIDE
[Pronestyl, Pronestyl-SR, Procan SR]

ACTIONS AND USES. The electrophysiologic properties, hemodynamic effects, and antiarrhythmic actions of procainamide are similar to those of quinidine. Although the indications for the two drugs are the same, they do not always have the same effect in an individual patient. Quinidine is frequently preferred for prolonged oral therapy because of the high incidence of drug-induced lupus associated with long-term administration of procainamide.

For intravenous use, procainamide is often preferred to quinidine for terminating supraventricular or ventricular arrhythmias. It is particularly useful in patients with severe ventricular arrhythmias who do not respond to lidocaine. Atrial fibrillation of recent onset may convert to normal sinus rhythm during procainamide infusion; however, electrical cardioversion is usually required to convert chronic atrial fibrillation and is preferred in hemodynamically unstable patients. Because it slows conduction in accessory pathways, procainamide is useful for acute termination of arrhythmias associated with the Wolff-Parkinson-White syndrome.

ADVERSE REACTIONS AND PRECAUTIONS. Although procainamide may cause anorexia, nausea, and vomiting, gastrointestinal side effects occur less often than with quinidine. Its adverse cardiovascular effects are similar to those of quinidine (ie, hypotension, myocardial depression, A-V block, ventricular arrhythmias [including torsades de pointes], increased ventricular response to atrial flutter or fibrillation). QT prolongation and widening of the QRS complex may be early signs of toxicity.

The clinical usefulness of prolonged procainamide therapy is limited because of a reversible lupus erythematosus-like syndrome that develops in approximately 25% to 30% of patients. Manifestations may include polyarthralgia, arthritis, pleuritic pain, and, less commonly, fever, myalgia, rash, restrictive pericarditis, myocarditis, pleural effusion, thrombocytopenia, and hemolytic anemia. The titer of antinuclear antibodies (ANA) increases in 50% to 80% of patients after one year of therapy. Patients who develop elevated ANA titers should be watched closely because such an increase frequently precedes clinical symptoms. Acetylator status influences the rate, but not the frequency, of antibody development.

Manifestations of hypersensitivity unrelated to the lupus syndrome (fever, rash, urticaria, neutropenia, agranulocytosis, pancytopenia, and nephrotic syndrome) occur occasionally. A report that severe neutropenia and agranulocytosis may be more common in patients taking the timed-release preparation, Procan SR, than in those taking regular procainamide (Ellrodt et al, 1984) appears to reflect the current widespread use of this preparation. When the number of prescriptions for the two preparations is taken into consideration, there is no significant difference in the frequency of this adverse reaction (Meyers et al, 1985).

Rarely, mental disturbances (eg, depression, hallucinations, psychosis, cerebellar ataxia) have occurred in patients taking procainamide.

Cimetidine reduces the renal clearance of both procainamide and its active metabolite.

PHARMACOKINETICS.

Absorption: The bioavailability of procainamide is 75% to 95%.

Distribution: The volume of distribution is 2 L/kg. Protein binding is 15%.

Metabolism: The major metabolic pathway for biotransformation of procainamide is N-acetylation. The rate of acetylation is determined genetically and shows a bimodal distribution into slow and fast acetylators. The major active metabolite, N-acetylprocainamide, is currently under investigation as an antiarrhythmic drug (acecainide [NAPA]).

The elimination half-life of procainamide is approximately three hours in patients with normal renal function. The half-life is reduced in children and is prolonged in patients with renal insufficiency. Acecainide has a longer half-life than procainamide.

Elimination: Plasma clearance is 11.8 ml/min/kg. Urinary excretion is 50%.

Monitoring: Therapeutic blood levels range between 4 and 10 mcg/ml, but control of severe arrhythmias may require higher levels. Plasma levels of the active metabolite may rise disproportionately in patients with renal impairment, because acecainide is more dependent than procainamide on renal excretion for elimination.

DOSAGE AND PREPARATIONS. Dosage should be reduced in patients with impaired renal function.

Oral: (Regular Preparation) *Adults,* initially, 250 to 500 mg every three to six hours around the clock. A loading dose of 1 g produces an effective serum concentration quickly. *Children,* 50 mg/kg daily in four to six divided doses.

> **Pronestyl** (Squibb), **Generic**. Capsules and tablets 250, 375, and 500 mg.

Oral: (Timed-release Preparation) *Adults,* for maintenance

after initial treatment with the regular preparation, 1 g every six hours or 50 mg/kg daily in divided doses at six-hour intervals.

> **Pronestyl-SR** (Squibb). Tablets (timed-release) 500 mg.
> **Procan SR** (Parke-Davis). Tablets (timed-release) 250, 500, 750, and 1,000 mg.

Intravenous (slow): *Adults,* 25 to 50 mg/min until the arrhythmia is suppressed (maximum, 1 g). For maintenance, 2 to 4 mg/min. *Children,* 5 to 15 mg/kg given over 30 minutes.

> **Pronestyl** (Squibb), **Generic**. Solution (sterile, aqueous) 100 mg/ml in 10 ml containers and 500 mg/ml in 2 ml containers.

PROPAFENONE
[Rytmonorm]

ACTIONS. Propafenone is a local anesthetic-type antiarrhythmic drug that also possesses weak beta-blocking and calcium-blocking properties. It slows conduction in the atria, ventricles, A-V node, His-Purkinje system, and accessory pathways and increases atrial and ventricular refractoriness. It has a mild negative inotropic effect.

USES. Propafenone has been used intravenously and orally for acute termination or long-term suppression of ventricular arrhythmias, particularly recurrent ventricular tachycardia (Connolly et al, 1983; Shen et al, 1984; Chilson et al, 1985). It appears to be as effective as quinidine in suppressing frequent premature ventricular complexes, and the frequency of side effects is similar with the two drugs (Dinh et al, 1985). Because it depresses both A-V nodal and bypass tract conduction, propafenone also may prevent recurrences of arrhythmias associated with the Wolff-Parkinson-White syndrome.

ADVERSE REACTIONS AND PRECAUTIONS. Propafenone may cause nausea, constipation, dizziness, paresthesias, and taste disturbances. It may worsen congestive heart failure, cause A-V or intraventricular conduction disturbances, and aggravate ventricular arrhythmias. Rash, bronchospasm, acute pleuritis, and mania have also been reported.

DRUG INTERACTIONS. Propafenone increases serum digoxin levels.

PHARMACOKINETICS.

Absorption: Propafenone is 100% absorbed but its bioavailability is usually less than 20% because of extensive first-pass metabolism.

Distribution: The steady-state volume of distribution is 3.6 L/kg. Propafenone is more than 95% protein bound.

Metabolism: During chronic therapy, the elimination half-life of propafenone is approximately five to eight hours. The contribution of metabolites to its antiarrhythmic action is not known.

Elimination: Clearance is 11 ml/min/kg. Less than 1% is excreted unchanged.

DOSAGE AND PREPARATIONS.

Oral: *Adults,* initially 150 mg three times daily. If the arrhythmia is not controlled, dosage may be increased at weekly intervals to 300 mg twice daily, and then 300 mg three times daily.

> **Rytmonorm** (Knoll).
> (Investigational drug)

QUINIDINE SULFATE
[Cin-Quin, Quinidex]

QUINIDINE GLUCONATE
[Duraquin, Quinaglute]

QUINIDINE POLYGALACTURONATE
[Cardioquin]

ACTIONS. Quinidine has a direct action on the cell membrane and indirect (anticholinergic) effects. It possesses local anesthetic properties. Quinidine depresses automaticity, particularly in ectopic sites, and slows conduction and increases refractoriness of the atria, His-Purkinje system, accessory pathways, and ventricles. Because of its anticholinergic effect combined with the reduction in atrial impulses, quinidine may facilitate A-V conduction in patients with atrial fibrillation or flutter. It usually does not depress sinus node function except in patients with sick sinus syndrome. Quinidine dilates resistance and capacitance vessels and has a mild negative inotropic effect.

USES. Quinidine is useful in supraventricular and ventricular ectopy and tachyarrhythmias. Its major uses are to maintain sinus rhythm after conversion of atrial flutter or fibrillation and to prevent frequent premature ventricular complexes or ventricular tachycardia. It also is used for long-term prophylaxis in patients with A-V nodal reentrant tachycardia, automatic atrial tachycardia, and symptomatic premature supraventricular complexes.

Because it prolongs the refractory period of the accessory pathway and suppresses automaticity of ectopic pacemakers, quinidine may prevent recurrences of paroxysmal supraventricular tachycardia caused by reentry over a concealed pathway or reciprocating tachycardia associated with the Wolff-Parkinson-White syndrome. It also may slow the ventricular response over the accessory pathway to atrial flutter or fibrillation in the preexcitation syndrome.

Quinidine is often preferred to procainamide for long-term therapy because elevated ANA titers and drug-induced lupus are common during prolonged therapy with procainamide.

In the past, quinidine was often employed to convert atrial arrhythmias to normal sinus rhythm, but this use has declined in recent years because of the ready availability of cardioversion and the danger of using increasing doses of quinidine for this purpose.

ADVERSE REACTIONS AND PRECAUTIONS. The toxic effects of quinidine are generally dose related, but severe reactions may occur after small doses are given to patients hypersensitive to the drug. The oral route is preferred because serious cardiovascular reactions are more likely to occur after parenteral administration. Intramuscular injections are painful, increase serum creatine phosphokinase levels, and are erratically and incompletely absorbed.

Diarrhea, nausea, and vomiting (which may be due to a direct irritant effect) are the most common adverse effects of quinidine. Largely uncontrolled reports suggest that the gluconate and polygalacturonate salts are better tolerated by some patients. If gastrointestinal reactions become severe, procainamide or disopyramide may be substituted.

Fever, hepatitis, manifestations of cinchonism (eg, headache, vertigo, palpitations, tinnitus, visual disturbances, confusion, disorientation, memory loss, delirium, psychosis), and thrombocytopenic purpura may occur. Other blood dyscrasias (hemolytic anemia, nonthrombocytopenic purpura, Henoch-Schonlein syndrome, agranulocytosis) develop occasionally. (See also Cohen et al, 1977.) Dermatologic reactions to quinidine include urticaria, photosensitivity, eczematous dermatitis, morbilliform rashes, and lichen planus-like eruptions. Keratopathy, sicca syndrome, and anterior uveitis are uncommon ocular adverse effects. Rarely, quinidine has induced a lupus erythematosus-like syndrome. Quinidine may unmask or exacerbate myasthenia gravis. Quinidine is in FDA Pregnancy Category C.

In patients with atrial flutter or fibrillation, quinidine may increase the ventricular rate, but this complication generally can be avoided by prior and concomitant treatment with digitalis (with careful monitoring for glycoside toxicity), propranolol, or verapamil. Severe hypotension due to peripheral vasodilation may occur after rapid parenteral administration and should be treated with volume replacement and vasopressor amines. Large doses of quinidine may depress myocardial contractility and aggravate or induce heart failure in nondigitalized patients. However, the vasodilator effect usually compensates for the negative inotropic effect, and quinidine may not worsen (and may even improve) the condition of some patients with heart failure.

Quinidine may produce A-V block and should be used cautiously in patients with partial A-V block. It probably should not be used in the presence of high-grade second- or third-degree heart block unless a ventricular pacemaker is in place. Quinidine also may adversely affect sinus node function in patients with sinus node disorders.

Other manifestations of cardiac toxicity are prolongation of the QT interval, widening of the QRS complex, and ventricular arrhythmias, including torsades de pointes, a frequently self-terminating polymorphic ventricular tachycardia. These arrhythmias may occur at therapeutic or subtherapeutic plasma drug levels and are perhaps the most disconcerting of quinidine's adverse effects. Syncopal episodes and sudden death during quinidine therapy may be due to ventricular fibrillation. Other possible causes of syncope are hypotension and, rarely, an idiosyncratic reaction.

DRUG INTERACTIONS. Elevated serum digoxin levels have been noted in patients receiving both quinidine and digoxin. (See Chapter 23, Agents Used to Treat Heart Failure.) Procainamide and disopyramide are alternative antiarrhythmic drugs that do not increase serum digoxin levels. The concomitant administration of quinidine and verapamil may cause hypotension.

Occasionally nifedipine may alter the disposition of quinidine, and the serum quinidine concentration may increase when nifedipine is withdrawn.

Enzyme-inducing drugs, such as phenobarbital, phenytoin, and rifampin, may cause a clinically important reduction in the half-life of quinidine. Its half-life is increased by cimetidine and by drugs that alkalize the urine. The action of coumarin anticoagulants may be enhanced by quinidine. The cardiotoxic effect of quinidine is increased by hyperkalemia and decreased by hypokalemia. This agent should be used cautiously in patients receiving neuromuscular blocking drugs because the effects may be additive.

TREATMENT OF TOXICITY. There is no specific antidote and treatment is largely supportive. Rapid volume replacement and administration of sympathomimetic amines may control hypotension and correct some arrhythmias. Charcoal hemoperfusion may enhance quinidine clearance. Cardiovascular assistance with an intra-aortic balloon pump may improve hemodynamics and reverse oliguria. Phenytoin, lidocaine, propranolol, and bretylium have been used to treat quinidine-induced ventricular arrhythmias associated with a prolonged QT interval, but temporary overdrive pacing is often required. Molar sodium lactate has been suggested for treating cardiac toxicity but has not been consistently effective.

PHARMACOKINETICS.

Absorption: Bioavailability of the sulfate is 80% and of the gluconate is 70%. Food decreases the rate but not the extent of absorption and may reduce side effects. Differences in bioavailability have been reported between quinidine preparations from different manufacturers.

Distribution: The volume of distribution is 2 to 3.5 L/kg and is increased in patients with cirrhosis and reduced in those with congestive heart failure. Protein binding is 80% to 90% and is reduced in patients with cirrhosis or acute myocardial infarction.

Metabolism: Quinidine is 60% to 85% metabolized; some metabolites may have antiarrhythmic activity. The half-life of quinidine is 5 to 12 hours and is prolonged in elderly patients and those with cirrhosis.

Elimination: Clearance is 2.5 to 5 ml/min/kg and is reduced in the elderly and in patients with congestive heart failure. Quinidine is eliminated more rapidly in children than in adults. Urinary excretion is 20%.

Monitoring: Plasma concentrations vary according to the assay employed. With the method of Cramer and Isaakson, therapeutic plasma levels range from 2.3 to 5 mcg/ml.

DOSAGE AND PREPARATIONS. Elderly patients and those with congestive heart failure or impaired hepatic or renal function may require a reduction in dosage.

QUINIDINE SULFATE:

Oral: Adults, 200 to 400 mg every four to six hours. A loading dose of 400 to 1,000 mg produces an effective serum concentration quickly. Children, 6 mg/kg every four to six hours.

Generic. Capsules 200 mg; tablets 100, 200, and 300 mg.
Cin-Quin (Rowell). Capsules 200 and 300 mg; tablets 100, 200, and 300 mg.

Quinidex (Robins). Tablets (timed-release) 300 mg.

QUINIDINE GLUCONATE:

Oral: Adults, 324 to 972 mg every 8 to 12 hours. As with quinidine sulfate, a loading dose should be given if a rapid antiarrhythmic response is required.

Duraquin (Parke-Davis). Tablets (timed-release) 330 mg.
Quinaglute (Berlex), Generic. Tablets (timed-release) 324 mg.

Intramuscular: Intramuscular injections are erratically and incompletely absorbed. Adults, 400 mg is given initially and may be repeated every four to six hours. In emergencies, administration every two hours (for four or five doses) may be necessary.

Intravenous: This route is rarely used and should be employed only in hospitalized patients. Adults, 200 to 400 mg in dilute solution may be given very slowly (approximately 10 mg/min). Normal saline may be administered rapidly simultaneously to counteract the marked reduction in preload produced by quinidine. The electrocardiogram and blood pressure should be monitored continuously.

Generic. Solution 80 mg/ml in 10 ml containers.

QUINIDINE POLYGALACTURONATE:

Oral: The manufacturer's recommended dose for maintenance is: Adults, 275 mg two or three times daily.

Cardioquin (Purdue Frederick). Tablets 275 mg (equivalent to 200 mg of quinidine sulfate).

TOCAINIDE HYDROCHLORIDE
[Tonocard]

ACTIONS. Tocainide is active orally and has electrophysiologic properties similar to those of lidocaine (Anderson et al, 1978). It has a mild myocardial depressant effect and may increase peripheral and pulmonary vascular resistance slightly when given intravenously.

USES. Tocainide is given orally to prevent or treat ventricular ectopy and tachycardia (Engler et al, 1979; Winkle et al, 1980). Responsiveness to lidocaine is a fairly accurate method of selecting patients for therapy. Tocainide was reported to be effective in some patients with ventricular arrhythmias refractory to quinidine, disopyramide, procainamide, and propranolol, but, in a controlled study, quinidine was slightly more effective than tocainide in reducing the frequency of ventricular premature complexes. The long-term usefulness of tocainide may be limited by adverse reactions or late treatment failures. In this event, ventricular arrhythmias can sometimes be controlled by combined therapy with quinidine, propranolol, or disopyramide. Tocainide is not useful in supraventricular tachyarrhythmias.

Intravenous tocainide (not available commercially) has been used to prevent ventricular tachyarrhythmias after acute myocardial infarction. It reduces the incidence of premature ventricular complexes and ventricular tachycardia but has not been particularly effective in preventing primary ventricular fibrillation or improving survival. (See also Holmes et al, 1983.)

ADVERSE REACTIONS AND PRECAUTIONS. Tocainide has been discontinued in up to 20% of patients because of adverse reactions. The most common side effects are nausea, dizziness, tremor, paresthesias, and rash. Other gastrointestinal disturbances (anorexia, vomiting, abdominal pain, diarrhea), psychiatric or neurologic reactions (confusion, ataxia, anxiety, hallucinations), sweating, and blurred vision also may occur. These reactions are dose related and may respond to a reduction in dosage.

Adverse cardiovascular effects observed occasionally include aggravation of congestive heart failure, conduction disturbances, and ventricular arrhythmias.

Drug fever, pulmonary fibrosis, interstitial pneumonitis, alveolitis, hepatitis, elevated ANA titers, and blood dyscrasias (leukopenia, agranulocytosis, hypoplastic anemia, and thrombocytopenia) have been reported rarely. Tocainide is classified in FDA Pregnancy Category C.

PHARMACOKINETICS.

Absorption: The bioavailability of tocainide is approximately 100%.

Distribution: Tocainide is 10% to 20% protein bound. Its volume of distribution is 1.5 to 4 L/kg.

Metabolism: Tocainide is eliminated by both hepatic and renal mechanisms. No active metabolites have been identified. Its half-life is approximately 15 hours in patients with normal renal function and 17 to 43 hours in those with severe renal failure.

Elimination: The total body clearance of tocainide is 2.6 ml/min/kg. Approximately 30% to 50% of a dose is excreted as unchanged drug.

Monitoring: Therapeutic plasma levels usually range between 4 and 10 mcg/ml.

DOSAGE AND PREPARATIONS.

Oral: Adults, initially, 400 mg every eight hours. The usual maintenance dose is 1.2 to 1.8 g daily in three divided doses. Daily doses exceeding 2.4 g have been given infrequently. Patients who tolerate the drug when given three times daily may be tried on a twice-daily regimen with careful monitoring.

Smaller doses (less than 1.2 g daily) may be required in patients with renal or hepatic insufficiency.

Tonocard (Merck Sharp & Dohme). Tablets 400 and 600 mg.

AGENTS USED TO TREAT BRADYARRHYTHMIAS

ATROPINE SULFATE

ACTIONS. Atropine increases sinus rate and sinoatrial and A-V nodal conduction velocity and decreases the effective refractory period of the A-V node by blocking the effects of the parasympathetic neurotransmitter, acetylcholine. Small intra-venous doses (less than 0.4 mg) may cause a paradoxical decrease in the sinus rate, which may be followed by an increase. A biphasic response also may be seen immediately after administration of larger doses. The effects of atropine on conduction through the His-Purkinje system are variable and unpredictable (Schweitzer and Mark, 1980), but it usually has no effect.

USES. Atropine is used to treat certain reversible bradyarrhythmias that may accompany acute myocardial infarction, particularly marked symptomatic sinus bradycardia. Since a decrease in vagal tone may unmask sympathetic hyperactivity, atropine may precipitate severe ventricular arrhythmias. It is current practice, therefore, not to treat asymptomatic sinus bradycardia with atropine.

Atropine is also used to enhance A-V conduction in Wenckebach Type I second-degree A-V block. Rarely, a paradoxical worsening of A-V block may occur.

Atropine is the treatment of choice for bradycardia and hypotension associated with vasovagal episodes.

ADVERSE REACTIONS AND PRECAUTIONS. Therapeutic doses of atropine cause dryness of the mouth, cycloplegia, and mydriasis. Rarely, systemically administered anticholinergic drugs have induced acute angle-closure glaucoma in predisposed eyes. Large doses may cause hyperpyrexia, urinary retention, and central nervous system effects (eg, confusion, hallucinations).

Arrhythmias induced by atropine include atrial fibrillation and ventricular tachycardia and fibrillation. Rarely, A-V block may be worsened by atropine because doses that have little direct effect on the A-V node may increase the sinus rate, causing more sinus impulses to block. See also Chapter 17, Adjuncts to Anesthesia, and Chapter 53, Agents Used in Disorders of the Lower Intestinal Tract.

DOSAGE AND PREPARATIONS.

Intravenous: Adults, initially, 0.4 to 1 mg every one to two hours as needed; larger doses occasionally are required (maximum, 2 mg). *Children,* 0.01 to 0.03 mg/kg.

Generic. Solution 0.3 mg/ml in 1 ml containers; 0.4 mg/ml in 0.5, 1, 20, and 30 ml containers; 0.5 mg/ml in 1, 5, and 30 ml containers; 1 mg/ml in 1 and 10 ml containers; tablets (hypodermic) 0.3, 0.4, and 0.6 mg.

ISOPROTERENOL HYDROCHLORIDE

[Isuprel]

This adrenergic drug stimulates beta receptors in the heart, blood vessels, and bronchioles, thereby increasing heart rate and myocardial contractility, enhancing automaticity and conduction velocity, dilating resistance vessels (primarily in skeletal muscle), and causing bronchodilation. It has no significant effect on alpha receptors and therefore lacks the marked pressor effect of norepinephrine or epinephrine.

In patients with second- or third-degree A-V block, isoproterenol is used to maintain adequate heart rate and cardiac output prior to insertion of a pacemaker. It is particularly useful for the emergency treatment of Stokes-Adams attacks and also is indicated for severe myocardial depression induced by beta blockers.

Isoproterenol may cause tachycardia, extrasystoles, headache, dizziness, flushing, sweating, and tremors. Because it increases myocardial oxygen demand, it may precipitate anginal attacks in susceptible individuals. Severe tachyarrhythmias occur occasionally.

DOSAGE AND PREPARATIONS.

Intravenous: Adults, 1 to 2 mg (5 to 10 ml of a 1:5,000 solution) diluted in 500 ml of 5% dextrose injection in water is infused slowly at a rate of 0.5 to 2 ml/min with continuous monitoring of the electrocardiogram. The rate of infusion is determined by the chronotropic response. *Children,* 0.1 to 0.25 mcg/kg/min.

Generic. Solution 1:5,000 in 5 and 10 ml containers.

Isuprel (Winthrop-Breon). Solution (sterile) 1:5,000 (0.2 mg/ml) in 1 and 5 ml containers.

Cited References

Anderson JL, et al: Clinical electrophysiologic effects of tocainide. *Circulation* 57:685-691, 1978.

Anderson JL, et al: Proposal for clinical use of flecainide. *Am J Cardiol* 53:112B-119B, 1984 A.

Anderson JL, et al: Pirmenol for control of ventricular arrhythmias: Oral dose-ranging and short-term maintenance study. *Am J Cardiol* 53:522-527, 1984 B.

Anderson JL, et al: Comparison of intravenous lorcainide with lidocaine for acute therapy of complex ventricular arrhythmias: Results of randomized study with crossover option. *J Am Coll Cardiol* 5:333-341, 1985.

Atkinson AJ Jr, et al: Efficacy and safety of *N*-acetylprocainamide in long-term treatment of ventricular arrhythmias. *Clin Pharmacol Ther* 33:565-576, 1983.

Brown JE, Shand DG: Therapeutic drug monitoring of antiarrhythmic agents. *Clin Pharmacokinet* 7:125-148, 1982.

Camm AJ, et al: Clinical usefulness of flecainide acetate in treatment of paroxysmal supraventricular arrhythmias. *Drugs* 29(suppl 4):7-13, 1985.

Campbell RWF: Chronic Mobitz type I second degree atrioventricular block: Has its importance been underestimated? (editorial). *Br Heart J* 53:585-586, 1985.

Campbell RWF, et al: Comparison of procainamide and mexiletine in prevention of ventricular arrhythmias after acute myocardial infarction. *Lancet* 2:1257-1260, 1975.

Chew CYC, et al: Mexiletine: Review of pharmacological properties and therapeutic efficacy in arrhythmias. *Drugs* 17:161-181, 1979.

Chilson DA, et al: Electrophysiologic effects and clinical efficacy of oral propafenone therapy in patients with ventricular tachycardia. *J Am Coll Cardiol* 5:1407-1413, 1985.

Cohen IS, et al: Adverse reactions to quinidine in hospitalized patients: Findings based on data from Boston Collaborative Drug Surveillance Program. *Prog Cardiovasc Dis* 20:151-163, 1977.

Connolly SJ, et al: Clinical efficacy and electrophysiology of oral propafenone for ventricular tachycardia. *Am J Cardiol* 52:1208-1213, 1983.

DeSilva RA, et al: Lignocaine prophylaxis in acute myocardial infarction: Evaluation of randomized trials. *Lancet* 2:855-857, 1981.

Dinh H, et al: Efficacy of propafenone compared with quinidine in chronic ventricular arrhythmias. *Am J Cardiol* 55:1520-1524, 1985.

Duff HJ, et al: Mexiletine in treatment of resistant ventricular arrhythmias: Enhancement of efficacy and reduction of dose-related side effects by combination with quinidine. *Circulation* 67:1124-1128, 1983.

Duffy CE, et al: Inducible sustained ventricular tachycardia refractory to individual class I drugs: Effect of adding second class I drug. *Am Heart J* 106:450-458, 1983.

Dunn HM, et al: Prophylactic lidocaine in early phase of suspected myocardial infarction. *Am Heart J* 110:353-362, 1985.

Echt DS, et al: Treatment with oral lorcainide in patients with sustained ventricular tachycardia and fibrillation. *Am Heart J* 109:28-32, 1985.

Eiriksson CE, Brogden RN: Lorcainide: Preliminary review of its pharmacodynamic properties and therapeutic efficacy. *Drugs* 27:279-300, 1984.

Ellrodt AG, et al: Severe neutropenia associated with sustained-release procainamide. *Ann Intern Med* 100:197-201, 1984.

Engler R, et al: Assessment of long-term antiarrhythmic therapy: Studies on long-term efficacy and toxicity of tocainide. *Am J Cardiol* 43:612-618, 1979.

Estes NAM III, et al: Electrophysiologic properties of flecainide acetate. *Am J Cardiol* 53:26B-29B, 1984.

Falk RH, O'Brien JL: Lorcainide: Comparative trial with quinidine gluconate in patients with previously untreated ventricular arrhythmias. *Chest* 86:537-540, 1984.

Flowers D, et al: Flecainide: Long-term treatment using reduced dosing schedule. *Am J Cardiol* 55:79-83, 1985.

Fogoros RN, et al: Amiodarone: Clinical efficacy and toxicity in 96 patients with recurrent, drug-refractory arrhythmias. *Circulation* 68:88-94, 1983.

Frieden J, et al: Continuous infusion of edrophonium (Tensilon) in treating supraventricular arrhythmias. *Am J Cardiol* 47:294-297, 1971.

Goldman S, et al: Inefficacy of "therapeutic" serum levels of digoxin in controlling ventricular rate in atrial fibrillation. *Am J Cardiol* 35:651-655, 1975.

Harper RW, et al: Effects of verapamil on electrophysiologic properties of accessory pathway in patients with the Wolff-Parkinson-White syndrome. *Am J Cardiol* 50:1323-1330, 1982.

Harrison DC: Should lidocaine be administered routinely to all patients after acute myocardial infarction? *Circulation* 58:581-584, 1978.

Harrison DC: Antiarrhythmic drug classification: New science and practical applications. *Am J Cardiol* 56:185-187, 1985.

Harrison DC, et al: Encainide: New and potent antiarrhythmic agent. *Am Heart J* 100:1046-1054, 1980.

Haynes RE, et al: Comparison of bretylium tosylate and lidocaine in management of out of hospital ventricular fibrillation: Randomized clinical trial. *Am J Cardiol* 48:353-356, 1981.

Heel RC, et al: Disopyramide: Review of pharmacological properties and therapeutic use in treating cardiac arrhythmias. *Drugs* 15:331-368, 1978.

Heger JJ, et al: Mexiletine therapy in 15 patients with drug-resistant ventricular tachycardia. *Am J Cardiol* 45:627-632, 1980.

Heger JJ, et al: Clinical efficacy of amiodarone in treatment of recurrent ventricular tachycardia and ventricular fibrillation. *Am Heart J* 106:887-894, 1983.

Heissenbuttel RH, Bigger JT Jr: Bretylium tosylate: Newly available antiarrhythmic drug for ventricular arrhythmias. *Ann Intern Med* 91:229-238, 1979.

Hellestrand KJ, et al: Cardiac electrophysiologic effects of flecainide acetate for paroxysmal reentrant junctional tachycardias. *Am J Cardiol* 51:770-776, 1983.

Hodges M, et al: Flecainide versus quinidine: Results of multicenter trial. *Am J Cardiol* 53:66B-71B, 1984.

Holmes B, Heel RC: Flecainide: Preliminary review of its pharmacodynamic properties and therapeutic efficacy. *Drugs* 29:1-33, 1985.

Holmes B, et al: Tocainide: Review of its pharmacological properties and therapeutic efficacy. *Drugs* 26:93-123, 1983.

Holt P, et al: Intravenous amiodarone in acute termination of supraventricular arrhythmias. *Int J Cardiol* 8:67-76, 1985.

Jackman WM, et al: Electrophysiology of oral encainide. *Am J Cardiol* 49:1270-1278, 1982.

Kertes P, Hunt D: Prophylaxis of primary ventricular fibrillation in acute myocardial infarction: Case against lignocaine. *Br Heart J* 52:241-247, 1984.

Kjekshus J, et al: Double-blind, crossover comparison of flecainide acetate and disopyramide phosphate in treatment of ventricular premature complexes. *Am J Cardiol* 53:72B-78B, 1984.

Kluger J, et al: Long-term antiarrhythmic therapy with acetylprocainamide. *Am J Cardiol* 48:1124-1132, 1981 A.

Kluger J, et al: Acetylprocainamide therapy in patients with previous procainamide-induced lupus syndrome. *Ann Intern Med* 95:18-23, 1981 B.

Koch-Weser J: Bretylium. *N Engl J Med* 300:473-477, 1979.

Leahey EB Jr, et al: Combined mexiletine and propranolol treatment of refractory ventricular tachycardia. *Br Med J* 280:357-358, 1980.

Levine JH, et al: Treatment of multifocal atrial tachycardia with verapamil. *N Engl J Med* 312:21-25, 1985.

Lie KI, et al: Lidocaine in prevention of primary ventricular fibrillation: Double-blind randomized study of 212 consecutive patients. *N Engl J Med* 291:1324-1326, 1974.

Mann DL, et al: Absence of cardioversion-induced ventricular arrhythmias in patients with therapeutic digoxin levels. *J Am Coll Cardiol* 5:882-888, 1985.

Mason JW, Peters FA: Antiarrhythmic efficacy of encainide in patients with refractory recurrent ventricular tachycardia. *Circulation* 63:670-675, 1981.

Meyers DG, et al: Severe neutropenia associated with procainamide: Comparison of sustained release and conventional preparations. *Am Heart J* 109:1393-1395, 1985.

Moss AJ, et al: Long QT syndrome: Prospective international study. *Circulation* 71:17-21, 1985.

Neuss H: Long term use of flecainide in patients with supraventricular tachycardia. *Drugs* 29(suppl 4):21-25, 1985.

Podrid PJ, Lown B: Amiodarone therapy in symptomatic, sustained refractory atrial and ventricular tachyarrhythmias. *Am Heart J* 101:374-379, 1981.

Podrid PJ, et al: Congestive heart failure caused by oral disopyramide. *N Engl J Med* 302:614-617, 1980.

Pratt CM, et al: Comparative effect of disopyramide and ethmozine in suppressing complex ventricular arrhythmias by use of double-blind, placebo-controlled, longitudinal crossover design. *Circulation* 69:288-297, 1984.

Prystowsky EN, et al: Clinical efficacy and electrophysiological effects of encainide in patients with Wolff-Parkinson-White syndrome *Circulation* 69:278-287, 1984.

Rinkenberger RL, et al: Effects of intravenous and chronic oral verapamil administration in patients with supraventricular tachyarrhythmias. *Circulation* 62:996-1010, 1980.

Roden DM, et al: Antiarrhythmic efficacy, pharmacokinetics and safety of N-acetylprocainamide in human subjects: Comparison with procainamide. *Am J Cardiol* 46:463-468, 1980.

Ross DL, et al: Antiarrhythmic drug combinations in treatment of ventricular tachycardia: Efficacy and electrophysiologic effects. *Circulation* 66:1205-1210, 1982.

Sami M, et al: Antiarrhythmic efficacy of encainide and quinidine: Validation of model for drug assessment. *Am J Cardiol* 48:147-156, 1981.

Scheinman MM, et al: Effects of antiarrhythmic drugs on atrioventricular conduction in patients with acute myocardial infarction. *Circulation* 62:20-27, 1980.

Schweitzer P, Mark H: Effect of atropine on cardiac arrhythmias and conduction, parts I and II. *Am Heart J* 100:119-127, 255-261, 1980.

Shen EN, et al: Electrophysiologic and hemodynamic effects of intravenous propafenone in patients with recurrent ventricular tachycardia. *J Am Coll Cardiol* 3:1291-1297, 1984.

Singh BN, et al: New prospectives in pharmacologic therapy of cardiac arrhythmias. *Prog Cardiovasc Drugs* 22:243-301, 1980.

Singh BN, et al: Calcium antagonists: Clinical use in treatment of arrhythmias. *Drugs* 25:125-153, 1983.

Stec GP, et al: N-acetylprocainamide pharmacokinetics in functionally anephric patients before and after perturbation by hemodialysis. *Clin Pharmacol Ther* 26:618-628, 1979.

Strasberg B, et al: Efficacy of intravenous amiodarone in management of paroxysmal or new atrial fibrillation with fast ventricular response. *Int J Cardiol* 7:47-55, 1985.

Vanhaleweyk G, et al: Flecainide: One-year efficacy in patients with chronic ventricular arrhythmias. *Eur Heart J* 5:814-823, 1984.

Vaughan Williams EM: Classification of antiarrhythmic actions reassessed after decade of new drugs. *J Clin Pharmacol* 24:129-147, 1984.

Winkle RA, et al: Tocainide for drug-resistant ventricular arrhythmias: Efficacy, side effects, and lidocaine responsiveness for predicting tocainide success. *Am Heart J* 100:1031-1036, 1980.

Winkle RA, et al: Clinical pharmacology and antiarrhythmic efficacy of N-acetylprocainamide. *Am J Cardiol* 47:123-130, 1981.

Winkle RA, et al: Possible contribution of encainide metabolites to long-term antiarrhythmic efficacy of encainide. *Am J Cardiol* 51:1182-1183, 1983.

Zipes DP: Consideration of antiarrhythmic therapy, (editorial). *Circulation* 72:949-956, 1985.

Zipes DP, et al: Amiodarone: Electrophysiologic actions, pharmacokinetics and clinical effects. *J Am Coll Cardiol* 3:1059-1071, 1984.

Other Selected References

Akhtar M: Atrioventricular nodal reentrant tachycardia. *Med Clin North Am* 68:819-830, 1984.

Anderson JL: Rationale of combination antiarrhythmic drug therapy, in Dreifus LS (ed): *Cardiac Arrhythmias: Electrophysiologic Techniques and Management.* Philadelphia, FA Davis, 1985, 307-327.

Anderson JL, et al: Antiarrhythmic drugs: Clinical pharmacology and therapeutic uses. *Drugs* 15:271-309, 1978.

Bigger JT: Mechanisms and diagnosis of arrhythmias, in Braunwald E (ed): *Heart Disease: Textbook of Cardiovascular Medicine.* Philadelphia, WB Saunders, 1980, 630-690.

Bigger JT: Management of arrhythmias, in Braunwald E (ed): *Heart Disease: Textbook of Cardiovascular Medicine.* Philadelphia, WB Saunders, 1980, 691-743.

Bigger JT Jr: Perspectives on current treatment of cardiac arrhythmias. *Am J Cardiol* 54:2B-7B, 1984.

Block PJ, Winkle RA: Hemodynamic effects of antiarrhythmic drugs. *Am J Cardiol* 52:14C-23C, 1983.

Dreifus LS, Likoff W (eds): *Cardiac Arrhythmias.* New York, Grune & Stratton, 1973.

Harrison DC (ed): *Cardiac Arrhythmias: A Decade of Progress.* Boston, GK Hall, 1981.

Helfant RH: *Bellet's Essentials of Cardiac Arrhythmias,* ed 2. Philadelphia, WB Saunders, 1979.

Keefe DLD, et al: New antiarrhythmic drugs: Place in therapy. *Drugs* 22:363-400, 1981.

Morady F, et al: Mechanisms and management of paroxysmal supraventricular tachycardia. *Cardiovasc Rev Rep* 2:1014-1038, 1981.

Prystowsky EN, et al: Preexcitation syndromes: Mechanisms and management. *Med Clin North Am* 68:831-893, 1984.

Vetter VL: Management of arrhythmias in children: Unusual features, in Dreifus LS (ed): *Cardiac Arrhythmias: Electrophysiologic Techniques and Management.* Philadelphia, FA Davis, 1985, 329-358.

Zipes DP: Management of cardiac arrhythmias, in Braunwald E (ed): *Heart Disease: Textbook of Cardiovascular Medicine,* ed 2. Philadelphia, WB Saunders, 1984, 648-682.

Zipes DP: Specific arrhythmias: Diagnosis and treatment, in Braunwald E (ed): *Heart Disease: Textbook of Cardiovascular Medicine,* ed 2. Philadelphia, WB Saunders, 1984, 683-743.

Antianginal Agents

INTRODUCTION

NITRATES

BETA-ADRENERGIC BLOCKING AGENTS

CALCIUM CHANNEL BLOCKING AGENTS (CALCIUM ANTAGONISTS)

PROSTAGLANDINS AND RELATED AGENTS

The discomfort of angina pectoris is believed to reflect an imbalance between myocardial oxygen demand and supply. In classic, effort-induced angina, transient myocardial ischemia develops because the diseased coronary arteries cannot deliver sufficient oxygen to meet an increased demand. In contrast, Prinzmetal's variant (vasospastic) angina occurs at rest, may be accompanied by transient S-T segment elevation and arrhythmias, and appears to be caused by episodic reductions in myocardial oxygen supply due to coronary artery spasm. Vasospasm may be superimposed on fixed stenotic lesions or may occur in angiographically normal coronary arteries. Vascular spasm also may contribute to exertional angina in some patients and may play a role in the pathogenesis of unstable angina, myocardial infarction, and sudden death. Patients with mixed angina have underlying exercise-induced angina with episodes of myocardial ischemia occurring at rest.

Treatment with antianginal drugs should be part of a general program designed to alleviate symptoms and reduce risk factors that predispose to coronary artery disease. Cessation of smoking is particularly important, both to avoid the adverse effects of nicotine and carbon monoxide on anginal symptoms and to eliminate one factor that may accelerate atherosclerosis. In obese patients, improvement may follow weight reduction. Activities or events that precipitate anginal attacks should be recognized and avoided when possible; these factors include the consumption of heavy meals, undue emotional stress, strenuous unaccustomed exercise (particularly after meals), and exposure to cold air.

Many patients benefit both physically and psychologically from an individualized graduated exercise program. The improvement in physical fitness may enable the patient to exercise without increasing symptoms.

Conditions that aggravate angina (eg, hypertension, arrhythmias, congestive heart failure, anemia, hyperthyroidism) should be corrected. Control of hypertension reduces myocardial oxygen demand and alone may relieve angina.

The drugs used to treat angina alleviate symptoms by increasing blood flow to the ischemic myocardium and/or by reducing myocardial oxygen requirements. In classic angina of effort, sublingual nitrates are given intermittently to prevent or relieve acute attacks; beta-adrenergic blocking agents, oral and topical nitrates, and calcium channel blocking agents (calcium antagonists) are administered for long-term prophylaxis. Nitrates and calcium antagonists also are useful in variant and mixed angina; beta-blocking agents may improve symptoms but occasionally are detrimental when used alone. Intravenous nitroglycerin may alleviate symptoms in patients with unstable angina unresponsive to standard therapy, particularly in those with refractory variant angina. Digitalis and diuretics are useful occasionally in nocturnal angina, and digitalis also counters the tendency of beta blockers to exacerbate left ventricular dysfunction.

NITRATES

ACTIONS. Nitrates are direct-acting vasodilators. They reduce myocardial oxygen requirements through their effects on the systemic circulation. Their major systemic action is a reduction in venous tone, which leads to pooling of blood in peripheral veins, decreased venous return, and reduced ventricular volume and myocardial tension (preload). At higher doses, nitrates also cause a moderate decrease in peripheral vascular resistance, which reduces arterial blood pressure and ventricular outflow resistance (afterload).

Nitrates increase myocardial oxygen supply by improving regional myocardial blood flow to ischemic areas. They dilate the large epicardial (conductance) arteries but have little effect on intramyocardial (resistance) vessels. In the normal nonischemic myocardium, coronary blood flow may increase temporarily and then decrease because of the fall in central aortic pressure. In patients with coronary artery disease, nitrates dilate both normal and diseased coronary arteries and collateral vessels (Brown et al, 1981) and thus improve the *regional* distribution of myocardial blood flow even though overall coronary blood flow may decrease because of the fall in central aortic pressure (Abrams, 1980). Nitrates also relieve spasm of angiographically normal and diseased arteries.

Nitrates are believed to improve angina of effort through

their effects on the peripheral circulation; however, their hemodynamic actions are not always closely correlated with antianginal activity, and an increase in regional myocardial blood flow may contribute to the therapeutic response. Nitrates relieve variant angina primarily through their effect on the coronary circulation.

USES. Sublingual, oral, topical, and intravenous nitrates and a lingual aerosol spray are currently used in antianginal therapy. Amyl nitrite is rarely used today to treat angina and has become a drug of abuse.

Sublingual nitrates (nitroglycerin, isosorbide dinitrate, and erythrityl tetranitrate) are the mainstay of therapy in both classic and variant angina. They are given intermittently to prevent or relieve acute attacks (Goldstein et al, 1971; Klaus et al, 1973; Willis et al, 1976). Because of its more rapid action, long-established efficacy, and low cost, nitroglycerin is the drug of choice among these agents. When taken at the onset of ischemic pain in patients with classic or variant angina, it usually provides relief within one to three minutes. Since angina of effort frequently subsides spontaneously with cessation of activity, nitroglycerin is most useful when taken shortly before beginning activities that are likely to precipitate an attack. When exercise is not too strenuous, prophylaxis is effective for 20 to 30 minutes and occasionally for up to one hour. Sublingual isosorbide dinitrate may have a longer action (up to two hours).

Nitroglycerin lingual aerosol [Nitrolingual] appears to be as effective as sublingual nitroglycerin. It may be particularly useful in patients with dry mucous membranes who have problems with dissolution of sublingual preparations (Parker et al, 1986).

The *oral nitrates*, isosorbide dinitrate and nitroglycerin, and *nitroglycerin ointment* have a longer duration of action than sublingual preparations. When used for long-term prophylaxis of classic angina, they may improve exercise tolerance and reduce the requirements for sublingual nitrates. They are also used in variant angina and severe, intractable, chronic congestive heart failure (see Chapter 23). Because oral nitrates are metabolized rapidly by the liver, large doses may be required to achieve therapeutic effects (Abrams, 1978; Danahy et al, 1977; Elkayam and Aronow, 1982; Glancy et al, 1977; Lee et al, 1978 A; Winsor and Berger, 1975).

The efficacy of oral erythrityl tetranitrate and pentaerythritol tetranitrate in antianginal therapy has not been well established, although beneficial effects have been reported by a few investigators.

Antianxiety or sedative drugs may reduce the reaction to emotional stress in some patients, but they should be prescribed separately if needed. Combination products containing a nitrate and meprobamate [Miltrate] or a barbiturate are obsolete and are not recommended.

Transdermal nitroglycerin patches appear to be less effective than other long-acting nitrates. Absorption from the skin is variable, adequate plasma levels may not be achieved with low to moderate doses, and use of normally tolerated doses may lead to the rapid development of tolerance (Leier, 1985; Crean et al, 1984; Parker and Fung, 1984).

Intravenous nitroglycerin relieves refractory chest pain caused by myocardial ischemia (Mikolich et al, 1980). It is useful in hospitalized patients with severe unstable angina, particularly in those with refractory variant angina. Although ischemic episodes can be controlled in some of these patients by increasing doses of oral and topical nitrates, intravenous therapy provides more consistent control during the first 24 hours of treatment (Curfman et al, 1983). In some centers, intravenous nitroglycerin is given early in the course of acute myocardial infarction when tolerated; it reduces discomfort but studies to date have not provided conclusive evidence for improved mortality or myocardial preservation (see also Chapter 27, Agents Used to Treat Shock).

Intravenous nitroglycerin is also widely used to control perioperative hypertension during coronary revascularization surgery. Severe coronary artery spasm occurring immediately after bypass surgery may be refractory to intravenous therapy; intracoronary injection may relieve spasm in these patients.

ADVERSE REACTIONS. *Hypotension and Tachycardia:* Headache, flushing, and dizziness often are noted early during treatment but can be minimized by using small initial doses. Because of the pronounced action of nitrates on capacitance vessels, their therapeutic effect is enhanced but adverse effects are also increased when the patient is in the upright position. Marked orthostatic hypotension and rarely syncope may occur, particularly if doses are repeated at short intervals, but frequently can be diminished by reducing the dosage. The patient should be instructed to sit down after taking the tablet. Occasionally, generalized vasodilation may cause profound hypotension and reflex tachycardia, and the fall in perfusion pressure may worsen angina. Syncope and sweating may simulate acute myocardial infarction. Symptoms can be relieved by immediate assumption of the supine position with elevation of the legs. Excessive hypotension during intravenous infusion usually can be prevented by avoiding hypovolemia and titrating the dose carefully.

Bradycardia: Severe bradycardia is occasionally associated with hypotension. The bradycardia is, at least in part, vagally mediated, because it generally responds to atropine.

Cerebral Ischemia: Rarely, nitrates cause transient cerebral ischemia.

Alcohol Intoxication: The alcohol diluent in intravenous preparations has occasionally caused intoxication in patients receiving large doses. The alcohol also may have a depressant effect on the heart.

Miscellaneous: Allergic contact dermatitis has occasionally been associated with topical nitroglycerin (ointment or patches) therapy, and anaphylactoid reactions have occurred rarely. Precipitation or aggravation of peripheral edema occasionally has been reported with both oral and topical therapy.

PRECAUTIONS. *Tolerance:* There is a long-standing controversy concerning the use of short-acting versus long-acting nitrates (Abrams, 1983). A steady high level of nitrates leads to a readjustment of vascular tone that may be accompanied by loss of the therapeutic response. Because sublingual nitrates have a short duration of action, vascular tone is constantly changing and clinical tolerance does not develop. Some investigators have reported that the antianginal response to oral nitrates is sustained (Danahy et al, 1977; Lee et al, 1978 A and B). Others have found that, although plasma levels are higher during prolonged therapy, partial tolerance develops rapidly to circulatory effects and to effects on treadmill performance (Thadani et al, 1982). A clinically important reduction in the therapeutic response to oral nitrates does not appear to be common, however (Abrams, 1983).

When applied in doses that improve angina initially, transdermal nitroglycerin patches may be particularly likely to produce tolerance. Loss of responsiveness may occur because sustained drug delivery saturates receptors, depletes reduced sulfhydryl groups that convert the nitrate molecule into an active vasodilating molecule, or activates compensatory vasoconstrictor mechanisms (Abrams, 1984; Reichek et al, 1984; Leier, 1985). It has been reported that nitroglycerin ointment is less likely to induce tolerance than the patches (Reichek et al, 1974).

Dependence: Munitions workers exposed to high levels of nitroglycerin over prolonged periods have developed nitrate dependence. Anginal attacks and, rarely, myocardial infarction and sudden death occurred in some of these workers during withdrawal; these reactions appear to be caused by coronary artery spasm. Nitrate dependence is not common clinically, but rebound vasoconstriction has been documented, and a few fatalities have been reported after the drugs were discontinued abruptly. If nitrates are to be discontinued in patients who have been receiving large doses for prolonged periods, the dosage should be reduced gradually.

Cardioversion: Nitroglycerin patches should be removed before cardioversion to avoid formation of electrical arcs. Nitroglycerin ointment alters electrical resistance of the skin and should not be spread on areas where defibrillation paddles or ECG electrodes are placed.

Hypertrophic Cardiomyopathy: Nitrates should be avoided in patients with hypertrophic cardiomyopathy because they may increase outflow gradients (see the section on Hypertrophic Cardiomyopathy in Chapter 26, Agents Used in Miscellaneous Cardiovascular Disorders).

Methemoglobinemia: Patients with NADH-methemoglobin reductase deficiency may develop methemoglobinemia when exposed to oxidant drugs such as nitrates. Asymptomatic methemoglobinemia also has occurred in patients without this enzyme deficiency who received very large doses of intravenous nitroglycerin. Abuse of amyl nitrate has been associated with methemoglobinemia, hemolytic anemia, and immunologic abnormalities.

Glaucoma: There is no basis for warnings concerning the use of nitrates in patients with glaucoma. There is evidence that oral isosorbide dinitrate may actually *reduce* intraocular pressure.

Miscellaneous: The patient should be cautioned that nitroglycerin ointment or patches can be transferred to the skin of other individuals by direct contact.

DRUG INTERACTIONS. The hypotensive effect of nitrates may be enhanced by alcohol, beta blockers, calcium channel blocking agents, and tricyclic antidepressants.

Delayed dissolution of sublingual nitrates due to dry mouth may occur in patients taking drugs with anticholinergic properties. This is a common problem in the emergency room.

PHARMACOKINETICS. Organic nitrates are absorbed from the gut, and some also are absorbed from the buccal mucosa and skin. The hepatic enzyme, glutathione-organic nitrate reductase, rapidly converts nitroglycerin to inorganic nitrite and denitrated metabolites. These metabolites have little or no vasodilator activity. Nitroglycerin also undergoes significant vascular clearance.

After sublingual administration, peak plasma levels of nitroglycerin are attained in one to two minutes and the half-life is seven minutes. Plasma levels of 0.1 ng/ml may be detected 20 minutes after application of one inch of nitroglycerin ointment. Plasma concentrations increase with a larger area of application. Plasma concentrations achieved with nitroglycerin patches are considerably lower than those attained after use of the ointment, which covers a larger surface area (Curry et al, 1984).

Isosorbide dinitrate is metabolized by glutathione-organic nitrate reductase into 2-isosorbide mononitrate, which is inactive, and 5-isosorbide mononitrate, which has vasodilator activity. The latter compound is marketed in Europe and is under investigation in the U.S. for treatment of angina. The bioavailability of oral isosorbide dinitrate is approximately 30% and its half-life is brief; the active metabolite is 90% bioavailable and has a half-life of four hours. Chronic administration of isosorbide dinitrate results in prolonged high plasma levels of both parent drug and metabolites.

DOSAGE AND PREPARATIONS.

SUBLINGUAL NITRATES
NITROGLYCERIN:
Sublingual: Individual sensitivity varies and the dose must be individualized to relieve symptoms with minimal adverse effects. It is usually preferable to initiate therapy with the lowest dose. *Adults,* 0.15 to 0.6 mg. If symptoms are not relieved by a single dose, additional or larger doses may be taken at five-minute intervals, but no more than three tablets should be used within a 15-minute period.

Conventional nitroglycerin tablets gradually lose potency through volatilization; therefore, the drug must be packaged in glass containers with tightly fitting metal screw caps and with no more than 100 dose units in each container. It should be dispensed in the original unopened container, which should be closed tightly after each use. The tablets should not be exposed to heat. Stabilized tablets retain potency for a longer period than conventional tablets.

  Nitrostat (stabilized) (Parke-Davis), **Generic.** Tablets 0.15, 0.3, 0.4, and 0.6 mg.
ISOSORBIDE DINITRATE:
Sublingual: *Adults,* 2.5 to 5 mg.
  Isordil (Ives), **Sorbitrate** (Stuart), **Generic.** Tablets 2.5, 5, and 10 mg.
ERYTHRITYL TETRANITRATE:
Sublingual: *Adults,* 5 mg.
  Cardilate (Burroughs Wellcome). Tablets 5 and 10 mg.
NITROGLYCERIN LINGUAL AEROSOL:
Lingual: *Adults,* one or two doses are sprayed into the mouth, preferably onto or under the tongue. Administration may be repeated every three to five minutes, but no more than three doses should be given in a 15-minute period.
  Nitrolingual (Rorer). 0.4 mg/metered dose.

Tradename	Release Rate (mg/24 hr)	Surface Area (cm²)	Nitroglycerin Content (mg/unit)
Nitrodisc	5	8	16
(Searle)	10	16	32
Nitro-Dur	2.5	5	26
(Key)	5	10	51
	7.5	15	77
	10	20	104
Nitro-Dur II	2.5	5	20
(Key)	5	10	40
	7.5	15	60
	10	20	80
	15	30	120
Transderm-Nitro	2.5	5	12.5
(CIBA)	5	10	25
	10	20	50
	15	30	75

TOPICAL NITRATES

NITROGLYCERIN OINTMENT 2%:

Topical: The 2% ointment contains 15 mg/inch. Initially, 1/2 inch is spread in a thin uniform layer over a 6 X 6 inch area on the chest, back, abdomen, or anterior thighs. (It should not be spread on areas of the chest where defibrillation paddles or ECG electrodes are normally placed.) Plasma levels increase with a larger surface area of application. Dosage may be increased, if necessary, by 1/2 inch increments to the largest amount that does not cause headache. Rarely, 4 or 5 inches of ointment may be required. The ointment may be applied every four to eight hours. Dosage should be reduced gradually if the drug must be withdrawn.

  Generic. Ointment 2% in 20, 30, and 60 g containers.
  Nitro-Bid (Marion). Ointment 2% in 1, 20, and 60 g containers.
  Nitrol (Rorer). Ointment 2% in 3, 30 and 60 g containers.
  Nitrong (Wharton), *Nitrostat* (Parke-Davis). Ointment 2% in 30 and 60 g containers.

TRANSDERMAL NITROGLYCERIN PREPARATIONS:

Topical: These products consist of a nitroglycerin-impregnated polymer bonded to an adhesive bandage. The unit is applied to the skin where it provides controlled drug delivery over 24 hours. It should be applied to a site free of hair and should not be placed on the distal parts of the extremities. A new unit should be applied once daily and replaced after bathing or if the product loosens. The application site should be changed each time a new unit is applied to avoid irritation.

ORAL NITRATES

Dosage should be individualized and many patients need larger amounts than were used in the past. Patients whose pain is not relieved by a large dose of sublingual nitroglycerin are unlikely to benefit from oral nitrates. The dose should be reduced gradually if the drug must be withdrawn.

ISOSORBIDE DINITRATE:

Oral: Adults, 10 to 40 mg four times daily (or three times daily when timed-release preparations are used). Larger doses (up to 480 mg daily) have been effective in some patients who did not respond to lower doses.

  Generic. Capsules (plain, timed-release) 40 mg; tablets 5, 10, 20, 30, and 40 mg; tablets (timed-release) 40 mg.
  Dilatrate-SR (Reed & Carnrick). Capsules (timed-release) 40 mg.

Isordil (Ives). Tablets 5, 10, 20, 30, and 40 mg; capsules and tablets (timed-release) 40 mg; tablets (chewable) 10 mg.
Onset (Bock). Tablets (chewable) 5 and 10 mg.
Sorbitrate (Stuart). Tablets 5, 10, 20, 30, and 40 mg; tablets (timed-release) 40 mg; tablets (chewable) 5 and 10 mg.

NITROGLYCERIN:

Oral: Adults, 2.5 to 13 mg four times daily.
  Generic. Capsules (plain, timed-release) 2.5, 6.5, and 9 mg.
  Nitro-Bid (Marion), *Nitroglyn* (Key), *Nitro-Stat SR* (Parke-Davis). Capsules (timed-release) 2.5, 6.5, and 9 mg.
  Nitrong (Wharton). Tablets (timed-release) 2.6, 6.5, and 9 mg.
  Nitrospan (USV). Capsules (timed-release) 2.5 and 6.5 mg.

Information is insufficient to recommend a dosage for the following agents for prophylaxis in angina pectoris:

ERYTHRITYL TETRANITRATE:

Cardilate (Burroughs Wellcome). Tablets (oral) 5 and 10 mg; tablets (chewable) 10 mg.

PENTAERYTHRITOL TETRANITRATE:

  Generic. Capsules (timed-release) 30 and 80 mg; tablets 10, 20, 40, and 80 mg; tablets (timed-release) 80 mg.
  Pentritol (USV). Capsules (timed-release) 30 and 60 mg.
  Peritrate (Parke-Davis). Tablets 10, 20, and 40 mg; tablets (timed-release) 80 mg (*Peritrate SA*).

INTRAVENOUS NITROGLYCERIN:

Caution: Intravenous products of different manufacturers may differ in concentration and/or volume per vial. The manufacturers' literature should be consulted for dilution instructions, and care should be taken when substituting one preparation for another. Nitroglycerin should be diluted with dextrose 5% injection or sodium chloride injection 0.9% and should not be mixed with other drugs. *Glass* containers should be employed for dilution and storage. A solution containing 100 mcg/ml may be used for initial dosage titration; a more concentrated solution may be substituted if it is necessary to limit fluids.

Intravenous: Adults, initially 5 mcg/min of dilute solution is infused. Dosage may be increased gradually by 5 mcg/min every three to five minutes until a response is noted. If no response is observed with a dose of 20 mcg/min, increments of 10 and later 20 mcg/min may be employed. On occasion, it may be necessary to increase the infusion rate to 200 mcg/min or more to relieve chest pain, reduce pulmonary artery wedge pressure, and maintain near normal arterial perfusion pressure. Blood pressure and heart rate should be monitored continuously.

> **Nitroglycerin Injection** (Abbott). Solution (sterile) 5 mg/ml in 5 ml containers (alcohol 50%).
>
> **Nitro-Bid IV** (Marion). Solution (sterile) 5 mg/ml in 1, 5, and 10 ml containers (alcohol 70%).
>
> **Nitrostat IV** (Parke-Davis). Solution (sterile) 0.8 mg/ml in 10 ml containers (alcohol 5%) and 5 mg/ml in 10 ml containers (alcohol 30%) with or without delivery set.
>
> **Tridil** (American Critical Care). Solution (sterile) 5 mg/ml in 5 and 10 ml containers (alcohol 30%) with or without delivery set (**Tridilset**).

BETA-ADRENERGIC BLOCKING AGENTS

Effects of Beta Blockade: Beta-adrenergic receptors are located predominantly in the heart, in the arteries and arterioles of skeletal muscle, and in the bronchi, where they subserve cardiac excitation, peripheral vasodilation, and bronchial relaxation. Beta receptors are also present in the kidney, liver, and many other tissues. Beta-blocking drugs combine reversibly with these receptors to block the response to sympathetic nerve impulses or circulating catecholamines. Blockade of cardiac (beta$_1$) receptors reduces heart rate, myocardial contractility, and cardiac output. The atrioventricular (A-V) conduction time is slowed and, at the cellular level, automaticity is suppressed. Blood pressure also is reduced.

Blockade of noncardiac (beta$_2$) receptors increases airway resistance, inhibits catecholamine-induced glycogenolysis and lipolysis, and blocks the vasodilating effect of catecholamines on peripheral blood vessels. These noncardiac actions underlie some of the adverse effects of beta-blocking drugs (ie, bronchospasm, hypoglycemia, interaction with sympathomimetic amines, possibly aggravation of peripheral vascular insufficiency).

Beta-blocking agents differ in their relative affinity for beta$_1$ and beta$_2$ receptors. Propranolol [Inderal], nadolol [Corgard], timolol [Blocadren], pindolol [Visken], oxprenolol [Trasicor], and the investigational drugs, alprenolol, carteolol, penbutolol, and sotalol, block beta receptors at all sites and are classified as "nonselective." Metoprolol [Lopressor], atenolol [Tenormin], acebutolol [Sectral], and the investigational agents, betaxolol, bevantolol, and esmolol, are more cardioselective and may be safer in asthmatics, in patients prone to hypoglycemia, and possibly in those with peripheral vascular disease. However, all beta-blocking drugs should be used cautiously in these patients because cardioselectivity is not absolute and may not be apparent at higher dosages.

Ancillary Properties: Beta-blocking drugs also differ in partial agonist activity (PAA, intrinsic sympathomimetic activity, ISA) and membrane-stabilizing (local anesthetic) activity.

Beta blockers with PAA (pindolol, acebutolol, oxprenolol, alprenolol, carteolol, penbutolol) cause less resting bradycardia than those lacking this property; however, resting heart rate is largely under parasympathetic control (McDevitt, 1983). All beta blockers reduce heart rate during exercise, but agents with PAA may have a flatter exercise dose-response curve than those lacking this property. PAA may be undesirable in patients with angina occurring at rest and in those with severe exertional angina (Quyyumi et al, 1984). There is no convincing evidence that PAA protects against heart failure, bronchospasm, or peripheral vascular insufficiency.

Membrane-stabilizing activity is apparent only with large doses and probably does not contribute to the antiarrhythmic effect of beta blockers that possess this characteristic (propranolol, acebutolol, alprenolol, oxprenolol, pindolol).

Propranolol may inhibit platelet aggregation and cause a shift to the right of the oxyhemoglobin dissociation curve, but the clinical importance of these actions is unclear. There is limited information on the effects of other beta blockers.

Labetalol [Normodyne, Trandate] has both beta-blocking (nonselective) and alpha-blocking properties. It is used primarily to treat hypertension (see Chapter 28) but is occasionally used in angina, particularly in hypertensive patients.

Sotalol is unique among the beta blockers in its electrophysiologic effects. In addition to its beta-blocking properties, sotalol prolongs the effective refractory period of Purkinje fibers and atrial and ventricular muscle and is classified as a Type 3 (amiodarone-like) antiarrhythmic drug.

Pharmacokinetics: Plasma levels of beta blockers are not closely correlated with therapeutic response and are not useful as a guide to therapy. Hydrophilic beta blockers (eg, atenolol, nadolol, sotalol) are not as readily absorbed from the gastrointestinal tract as lipophilic agents (eg, propranolol, metoprolol, oxprenolol), are not extensively metabolized, and have relatively long plasma half-lives (Cruickshank, 1980). In patients with renal or hepatic impairment, these pharmacokinetic differences may be important for drug selection (Frishman, 1981). Hydrophilic beta blockers do not cross the blood-brain barrier as readily as lipophilic agents and are thought to be less likely to cause central nervous system side effects; however, there have been reports of central nervous system disturbances with these drugs. (See Table 1.)

Use in Angina Pectoris: The beneficial effect of beta-blocking drugs in angina of effort derives from their ability to decrease heart rate, myocardial contractility, and blood pressure, particularly during exercise. By attenuating the cardiac response to sympathetic stimulation, beta blockade reduces myocardial oxygen demand and thereby delays the onset of ischemic pain. The reduction in heart rate also may increase coronary blood flow and oxygen supply by prolonging the diastolic interval during which coronary flow occurs. The oxygen-sparing action of beta blockers usually overrides other effects that tend to increase myocardial oxygen consumption (ie, prolonged systolic ejection period, increased ventricular volume) and to decrease myocardial oxygen supply (ie, increased coronary vascular resistance).

Cardioselectivity, membrane-stabilizing properties, and hydrophilicity have no effect on the antianginal efficacy of beta blockers (Thadani et al, 1980). In patients with stable exertional angina, agents with PAA are as effective as those lacking this property (Thadani et al, 1980), but PAA may be associated with reduced efficacy in patients who have angina at rest or severe angina of effort (Quyyumi et al, 1984).

In the absence of specific contraindications, a beta blocker should be considered for trial in all patients with frequent attacks of classic angina, particularly those who have had a myocardial infarction. Sublingual nitrates should be continued,

TABLE 1.
PHARMACOKINETICS OF BETA-ADRENERGIC BLOCKING AGENTS

Drug	Bioavailability (%)	Half-life (Hours)	Lipid Solubility (Log Partition Coefficient Octanol/Water)	Protein Binding (%)	Urinary Excretion of Unchanged Drug (%)	Active Metabolites
Propranolol	30	2-3 (Increased in cirrhosis)	3.65	93	0.5	Yes
Acebutolol	40	3-4 (Active metabolite: 8-13)	1.87	26	30-40	Yes
Atenolol	40	6-7 (Increased in uremia)	0.23	5	85*	No
Metoprolol	50	3-4 (Increased in poor hydroxylators)	2.15	10	10	No
Nadolol	30	20-24 (Increased in uremia)	0.71	30	76*	No
Oxprenolol	30	2	2.18	80	5	No
Pindolol	75	3-4	1.75	57	30-40	No
Timolol	50	4	2.10	<10	15	No

*Dosage adjustment required in patients with renal failure.

as needed, to prevent or relieve symptoms, because nitrates and beta blockers reduce cardiac work by different mechanisms and may have an additive effect in reducing myocardial oxygen demand. Beta blockers attenuate the reflex tachycardia induced by nitrates, while nitrates counteract the increase in heart size, prolongation of ventricular systole, and increase in coronary vascular resistance that follow beta blockade. This combined regimen is often effective, even in patients with severe angina, and may avoid the need for bypass surgery in many patients.

The effect of beta-blocking drugs in variant angina is not always predictable. Both beneficial and detrimental effects have been reported. In general, beta-blocking drugs should be avoided as sole therapy in patients with documented vasospasm.

Beta blockade attenuates the cardiovascular response to exercise and may diminish exercise performance in normal volunteers, particularly during strenuous exercise. Beta blockers do not reduce the beneficial effects of exercise training in patients with coronary artery disease (Pratt et al, 1981; Vanhees et al, 1984; Fletcher, 1985; Froelicher et al, 1985). An increase in parasympathetic tone occurs during cardiovascular conditioning that contributes to training-induced bradycardia (Vanhees et al, 1984), and heart rate remains a useful guide for evaluating the effects of physical training in patients receiving beta blockers.

Use After Acute Myocardial Infarction: Several well-controlled clinical trials have shown that long-term therapy with a beta-blocking drug can reduce mortality after acute myocar-

dial infarction, particularly the incidence of sudden death, and decrease the reinfarction rate (Frishman et al, 1984; Yusuf et al, 1985). These trials utilized propranolol (β-Blocker Heart Attack Trial [BHAT] Research Group, 1982), timolol (Norwegian Multicenter Study Group, 1981), and metoprolol (Hjalmarson et al, 1981), and they confirmed results with practolol (no longer in clinical trials), sotalol, and alprenolol. The time when long-term therapy was begun and the follow-up periods were variable. A total of 18% to 28% of patients were excluded from these trials because of contraindications, and 9% to 21% were excluded because they needed or were already receiving a beta blocker for other indications. An overview of the results of these and other randomized trials demonstrated that long-term beta-blocker therapy reduces the risk of death from approximately 10% to 8% and of nonfatal reinfarction from 7.5% to 5.7% (Yusuf et al, 1985).

The cardioprotective effect of beta blockers is observed with both cardioselective and nonselective agents and is not affected by the presence or absence of membrane-stabilizing properties. Agents with partial agonist activity appear to be less effective (Frishman et al, 1984; Yusuf et al, 1985). The mechanism of the cardioprotective effect of beta blockers is uncertain, but antiarrhythmic, anti-ischemic, antihypertensive, and antiplatelet actions have been considered. An analysis of the BHAT data suggests that the antiarrhythmic action may play an important role (Lichstein et al, 1983). In particular, beta blockers may reduce the incidence of ventricular tachycardia and fibrillation.

It is currently recommended that all postinfarct patients in whom these drugs are not contraindicated should be *considered* for treatment with a beta blocker, although which subsets will benefit, when to institute treatment, and how long the protective effect lasts are still unresolved questions. In the absence of other clinical indications for a beta blocker, such as angina or arrhythmias, some cardiologists confine use of these drugs for secondary prevention to high-risk patients. Until further information becomes available, therapy probably should be instituted five days to four weeks after infarction and be continued for at least one to three years. Asymptomatic patients can then be re-evaluated to determine whether the drug should be continued or withdrawn.

Studies documenting the beneficial effect of beta blockers on cardiac mortality were conducted in patients with recent myocardial infarctions. Whether beta blockers can reduce mortality in patients with remote infarctions or in those with symptomatic coronary artery disease who have not yet had a myocardial infarction remains to be determined.

Use in the Early Stages of Acute Myocardial Infarction: Beta blockers also have been given during the evolution of acute myocardial infarction in an attempt to limit infarct size, relieve pain, reduce the frequency of arrhythmias, and improve mortality. In most trials utilizing an oral regimen, acute intervention did not improve prognosis (Frishman et al, 1984; Yusuf et al, 1985), and the currently preferred procedure is to begin treatment with an intravenous beta blocker.

Intravenous therapy followed by oral treatment with metoprolol, atenolol, or timolol reduced estimated infarct size (Herlitz et al, 1984; Yusuf et al, 1983; International Collaborative Study Group, 1984), but propranolol did not (Roberts et al, 1984). It is not certain whether these results reflect procedural variations or true differences among the drugs. A subsequent examination of all available data suggested that intravenous beta blockers may reduce infarct size and the frequency of ventricular arrhythmias if administered early, but not when given more than 12 hours after the onset of pain (Yusuf et al, 1985). There is no conclusive evidence that mortality is reduced.

Because beta$_2$ blockade may enhance the pressor effect of epinephrine (Houben et al, 1982), it has been argued that a selective beta blocker may be preferred in situations, such as acute myocardial infarction, in which plasma epinephrine levels are elevated. On the other hand, epinephrine may reduce the serum potassium level, an action that can be prevented by beta$_2$ blockade (Brown et al, 1983). Since hypokalemia increases the risk of ventricular arrhythmias in acute myocardial infarction, a nonselective beta blocker may have advantages (Johansson and Dziamski, 1984; Nordrehaug et al, 1985).

Adverse Reactions, Precautions, and Interactions

Cardiovascular Effects: Beta-blocking drugs may cause pronounced bradycardia and hypotension, most commonly with the intravenous route. These drugs should be discontinued if bradycardia is marked and symptomatic. Asymptomatic bradycardia (45 to 55 beats/minute) is common and should not be cause for stopping drug administration. Beta blockers with

PAA (eg, pindolol) may cause less resting bradycardia than those lacking this characteristic, but all beta blockers should be used cautiously in patients with slow sinus rates and they should be avoided in those with sick sinus syndrome.

Intravenous or intramuscular atropine controls the excessive bradycardia produced by beta blockers if pronounced vagal tone is a major contributory factor. If severe myocardial depression occurs, isoproterenol should be infused intravenously; because of the competitive nature of beta blockade, large doses may be needed.

Beta blockers may precipitate heart failure in patients with inadequate cardiac reserve and should be given with extreme caution to those with frank or incipient heart failure who depend upon sympathetic stimulation to remain compensated. If a beta-blocking drug must be used in such patients, therapy should be initiated with small doses and digitalis and/or a diuretic should be given concomitantly.

Beta-blocking agents may cause fatal cardiac slowing in patients with A-V block and are contraindicated in the presence of significant A-V conduction disturbances (ie, greater than first-degree A-V block). There is no convincing evidence that PAA reduces the risk of heart failure or conduction disturbances. Beta blockers potentiate the effects of other drugs with negative inotropic, chronotropic, and dromotropic actions.

Sudden withdrawal of large doses of a beta blocker has occasionally been followed within several days to two weeks by recurrence of unstable angina, ventricular tachycardia, fatal myocardial infarction, and sudden death (Harrison and Alderman, 1976). These complications are most common in patients with severe angina who are well stabilized on the drug. Milder withdrawal reactions include a rebound increase in heart rate, palpitations, tremor, and sweating. The beta blocker withdrawal syndrome has been attributed to an increase in the density and sensitivity of beta receptors.

If it becomes necessary to discontinue treatment, dosage should be reduced gradually over a one- to two-week period and physical activity should be restricted during this time. It is neither necessary nor desirable to discontinue beta blockers before surgery. Continued intraoperative and postoperative drug administration may reduce the risk of supraventricular arrhythmias after bypass surgery.

Beta blockers may cause cold extremities, precipitate or aggravate Raynaud's phenomenon, and worsen intermittent claudication. These reactions may be due to beta$_2$ blockade, reduced cardiac output, and/or a compensatory vasoconstrictor response to the reduced cardiac output. The effects of beta blockers and ergot alkaloids on the peripheral circulation may be additive. Beta blockers generally should be avoided in patients with chronic occlusive peripheral vascular disease.

Large doses of agents with PAA may paradoxically increase the blood pressure. Paradoxical hypertensive reactions also have occurred occasionally because of an interaction between propranolol and intravenous epinephrine or when propranolol was administered without prior alpha blockade to patients with pheochromocytoma. Hypertensive reactions also were reported when clonidine [Catapres] was withdrawn rapidly from patients receiving propranolol concurrently or when atenolol was abruptly substituted for clonidine. A hypertensive episode in one patient was attributed to an interaction between the methyldopa metabolite, alpha-methyl-norepinephrine, and intravenous propranolol. All of these interactions are caused by beta$_2$ blockade, which prevents beta-adrenergic vasodilation and thus permits unopposed alpha stimulation. An enhanced pressor response would therefore occur only with agents, such as epinephrine, that have mixed alpha and beta agonist actions. Although there have been reports that beta blockade also potentiates the pressor effect of the alpha agonist, phenylephrine, such an interaction would not be expected on a pharmacologic basis and was not supported by results of a controlled study (Myers, 1984).

Respiratory Effects: Blockade of beta$_2$ receptors increases airway resistance and may provoke asthmatic attacks in patients with a history of asthma or chronic bronchitis. Although a cardioselective beta blocker may be safer than a nonselective one in these patients, all beta blockers should be used cautiously because cardioselectivity may be lost at therapeutically effective dosage. A beta$_2$ agonist (eg, terbutaline [Brethine, Bricanyl]) given concomitantly reduces the risk of bronchospasm. If bronchospasm develops, a beta$_2$ agonist and aminophylline should be administered. Beta blockers also may worsen respiratory function in patients with nonasthmatic chronic obstructive lung disease.

Allergic Reactions: Severe, epinephrine-resistant anaphylactic reactions to drugs or allergy injections have occurred in patients receiving propranolol.

Metabolic Effects: Beta$_2$ blockade impairs the sympathetically mediated rebound response to hypoglycemia and may mask some hypoglycemic symptoms (primarily tachycardia). Although beta blockers are probably safe for use in most diabetics, they may potentiate and prolong insulin-induced hypoglycemia and may produce hypoglycemia in patients recovering from anesthesia, in those on dialysis, and in children during periods of restricted food intake. Beta blockers also occasionally induce hypoglycemia during prolonged exercise. In hypertensive patients, blood pressure may increase during hypoglycemic episodes.

Beta blockers may reduce HDL cholesterol and increase serum triglyceride and uric acid levels. The effect on serum lipids may be secondary to a reduction in lipoprotein lipase activity. The effects of thiazide diuretics on blood glucose, lipid, and urate levels may be enhanced by beta blockers.

Neurologic, Psychiatric, and Neuromuscular Effects: Fatigue and lethargy are the most common central side effects of beta blockers. Vivid dreams or nightmares (with or without insomnia), depression, and memory loss also occur frequently. Visual hallucinations, delirium, and psychotic reactions develop rarely. Paresthesias, arthropathy, and proximal myopathy also have been reported.

Central nervous system side effects are believed to be more common with lipophilic drugs, such as propranolol, but they also have occurred with hydrophilic agents, such as atenolol.

Sexual Dysfunction: Beta-blocking drugs may cause impotence and loss of libido.

Dermatologic Reactions: Various dermatologic reactions have been reported with beta blockers, including erythematous rashes, psoriasis, and pruritus. The severe oculomuco-

cutaneous syndrome caused by practolol has not been clearly associated with other beta-blocking drugs.

Sclerosing and Fibrosing Syndromes: Sclerosing peritonitis was one of the severe adverse effects of practolol that led to its eventual withdrawal. Despite occasional reports, there is no convincing evidence that other beta blockers cause this disorder.

Retroperitoneal fibrosis has been reported in patients receiving various beta blockers, but the available evidence suggests that these drugs may have been used to treat hypertension associated with the retroperitoneal fibrosis and were not causative. An association has also been reported between therapy with beta blockers and Peyronie's disease, a less severe fibrosing syndrome. It is now believed that this disorder is associated with chronic occlusive peripheral vascular disease and is not caused by beta-blocker therapy.

Pregnancy and Lactation: Beta blockers cross the placenta and have rarely caused bradycardia, hypotension, and hypoglycemia in the newborn. They are also excreted in breast milk. Atenolol, nadolol, propranolol, and timolol are classified in FDA Pregnancy Category C and metoprolol and pindolol in FDA Pregnancy Category B.

Miscellaneous Reactions: Beta blockers may cause gastrointestinal disturbances, blood dyscrasias, fever, cheilostomatitis, and alopecia. Very rarely, a reversible loss of hearing has been reported in patients receiving various beta blockers.

Beta blockade masks the signs and symptoms of hyperthyroidism, and latent thyrotoxicosis may become apparent when the drug is withdrawn.

Drug Evaluations

PROPRANOLOL HYDROCHLORIDE
[Inderal, Inderal LA]

ACTIONS. See Effects of Beta Blockade in the Introduction to this section.

USES. The prototype beta blocker, propranolol, has provided a significant advance in the long-term management of classic angina pectoris. During exercise tolerance tests, it usually delays the onset of anginal symptoms and the appearance of ischemic electrocardiographic changes. Long-term administration reduces the frequency of anginal attacks and decreases nitroglycerin requirements in many patients. Propranolol also reduces mortality and the risk of reinfarction when given for long-term therapy after acute myocardial infarction (β-Blocker Heart Attack Trial Research Group, 1982).

ADVERSE REACTIONS, PRECAUTIONS, AND INTERACTIONS. The adverse effects and interactions of propranolol that are secondary to blockade of beta$_1$ and beta$_2$ receptors are discussed in the Introduction.

Propranolol also may cause sexual dysfunction and gastrointestinal disturbances (nausea, vomiting, diarrhea, flatulence). Fever, rash, proximal myopathy, arthropathy, cheilostomatitis, alopecia, ocular inflammatory pseudotumor, and blood dyscrasias (thrombocytopenia, agranulocytosis) have occurred rarely.

Cimetidine may reduce the clearance of propranolol and inhibit its metabolism (for other interactions, see Chapter 28, Antihypertensive Agents).

PHARMACOKINETICS. See Table 1.

DOSAGE AND PREPARATIONS.

Oral: Adults, for angina, *regular preparation,* initially, 10 to 20 mg three or four times daily. The dosage may be increased gradually, as needed, to control symptoms. For maintenance, most patients require at least 160 to 240 mg daily, usually given in four divided doses. Some patients require up to 400 mg daily. Twice-daily administration may be effective in some patients with stable angina.

Long-acting preparation, initially, 80 mg once daily. The dosage should be increased gradually at three- to seven-day intervals until the optimal response is obtained. The average maintenance dose is 160 mg once daily.

Sublingual and long-acting nitrates should be continued as needed during therapy with propranolol.

For long-term prophylaxis after acute myocardial infarction, *regular preparation,* 180 to 240 mg daily in three divided doses.

> **Inderal** (Ayerst). Tablets 10, 20, 40, 60, 80, and 90 mg.
> **Inderal LA** (Ayerst). Capsules (timed-release) 80, 120, and 160 mg.

ACEBUTOLOL HYDROCHLORIDE
[Sectral]

ACTIONS. See Effects of Beta Blockade in the Introduction to this section.

USES. This relatively cardioselective beta-blocking drug appears to be useful in patients with stable angina of effort and it may be preferred to a nonselective agent in those with asthma or diabetes. Because acebutolol possesses partial agonist activity, it may be less useful in patients who have angina at rest or severe angina of effort.

ADVERSE REACTIONS, PRECAUTIONS, AND INTERACTIONS. The adverse effects of acebutolol that are secondary to beta blockade resemble those of other cardioselective beta blockers and the same precautions apply (see the Introduction). Acebutolol also may cause fatigue and other central nervous system disturbances, sexual dysfunction, gastrointestinal disturbances, and an increased incidence of antinuclear

antibody formation. Hypersensitivity pneumonitis, pleurisy, and pulmonary granulomas have been reported rarely.

PHARMACOKINETICS. See Table 1.

DOSAGE AND PREPARATIONS.

Oral: Adults, for angina, initially, 400 mg daily in two divided doses. Dosage may be increased gradually as needed to control symptoms. Sublingual and long-acting nitrates should be continued as needed.

> **Sectral** (Wyeth). Capsules 200 and 400 mg.

ATENOLOL
[Tenormin]

ACTIONS. See Effects of Beta Blockade in the Introduction to this section.

USES. The antianginal effect of this long-acting beta-blocking drug appears to be comparable to that of propranolol and other beta blockers and the same precautions apply (see the Introduction). Because of its relative cardioselectivity, atenolol may be preferred to a nonselective agent in asthmatics and diabetics.

ADVERSE REACTIONS, PRECAUTIONS, AND INTERACTIONS. The adverse effects and interactions of atenolol that are secondary to beta blockade are similar to those of other cardioselective beta-blocking drugs (see the Introduction) and the same precautions apply (including the importance of avoiding abrupt discontinuation of therapy, since withdrawal reactions have occurred with atenolol). Although atenolol does not readily cross the blood-brain barrier, central nervous system effects have been reported. It also may aggravate peripheral vascular insufficiency and cause gastrointestinal disturbances.

PHARMACOKINETICS. See Table 1.

DOSAGE AND PREPARATIONS.

Oral: For angina, *adults,* 50, 100, or 200 mg once daily. The dosage interval should be increased in patients with impaired renal function. Sublingual and long-acting nitrates should be continued as needed during therapy with atenolol.

> **Tenormin** (Stuart). Tablets 50 and 100 mg.

METOPROLOL TARTRATE
[Lopressor]

ACTIONS. See Effects of Beta Blockade in the Introduction to this section.

USES. The antianginal effect of metoprolol appears to be comparable to that of propranolol and other beta blockers (see the Introduction). Because of its relative cardioselectivity, metoprolol may be preferred to a nonselective agent in asthmatics and diabetics.

Metoprolol may reduce estimated infarct size when given intravenously in the early stages of acute myocardial infarction (Herlitz et al, 1984) and may decrease mortality when used for long-term therapy (Hjalmarson et al, 1981).

ADVERSE REACTIONS, PRECAUTIONS, AND INTERACTIONS. The adverse effects of metoprolol that are secondary to cardiac beta blockade, are comparable to those of other beta blockers (see the Introduction) and the same precautions apply (including the importance of avoiding abrupt discontinuation of therapy, since withdrawal reactions have occurred with metoprolol).

Despite metoprolol's relative cardioselectivity, clinically effective doses may increase airway resistance in asthmatics, although to a lesser extent than propranolol, and the increase may be more readily reversed by a beta$_2$ agonist, such as terbutaline. Cardioselective beta blockers may be preferred to nonselective agents in insulin-dependent diabetics; however, metoprolol occasionally potentiates the hypoglycemic effect of insulin and, in hypertensive patients, the blood pressure may increase during the hypoglycemic episode.

Aggravation of peripheral vascular insufficiency, rash, gastrointestinal disturbances, and central nervous system effects (fatigue, dizziness, headaches, nightmares, insomnia, and depression) may occur. Arthropathy and alopecia also have been reported. Cimetidine [Tagamet] may increase the bioavailability of metoprolol.

PHARMACOKINETICS. See Table 1.

DOSAGE AND PREPARATIONS.
Oral: Adults, for angina, 50 mg three or four times daily. Twice-daily administration may be effective in some patients with stable angina. Sublingual and long-acting nitrates should be continued as needed during therapy with metoprolol.

For long-term prophylaxis after acute myocardial infarction, 100 mg twice daily. For patients who received intravenous metoprolol therapy during the acute phase of myocardial infarction, oral therapy should be started 15 minutes after the last intravenous dose; initially, 25 or 50 mg is given orally every six hours for 48 hours, followed by maintenance therapy with 100 mg twice daily.
Lopressor (Geigy). Tablets 50 and 100 mg.
Intravenous: Adults, for early treatment of acute myocardial infarction, initially, three bolus injections of 5 mg are given at two-minute intervals. Blood pressure, heart rate, and the ECG should be monitored. Oral therapy may then be instituted 15 minutes after the last intravenous dose, provided that intravenous therapy was tolerated.
Lopressor (Geigy). Solution 1 mg/ml in 5 ml containers.

NADOLOL
[Corgard]

ACTIONS. See Effects of Beta Blockade in the Introduction to this section.

USES. The antianginal effect of this long-acting, nonselective, beta-blocking drug appears to be comparable to that of propranolol and other beta blockers (see the Introduction).

ADVERSE REACTIONS AND PRECAUTIONS. The adverse effects of nadolol that result from blockade of beta$_1$ and beta$_2$ receptors are similar to those of propranolol and other nonselective beta blockers and the same precautions apply. (See the Introduction.) Nadolol also may cause gastrointestinal disturbances, rash, central nervous system effects, and alopecia.

PHARMACOKINETICS. See Table 1.

DOSAGE AND PREPARATIONS.
Oral: Adults, for angina, initially, 40 mg once daily; the amount may be increased gradually by 40- to 80-mg increments at three- to seven-day intervals until the desired response is obtained. The usual maintenance dose is 40 or 80 mg once daily. Doses up to 240 mg once daily may sometimes be required. Sublingual and long-acting nitrates should be continued as needed during therapy with nadolol.

The dosage interval should be increased in patients with renal impairment. The following intervals are suggested:

Creatinine Clearance (ml/min/1.73 M^2)	Dosage Interval (hours)
>50	24
31-50	24-36
10-30	24-48
<10	40-60

Corgard (Squibb). Tablets 40, 80, 120, and 160 mg.

OXPRENOLOL

This beta blocker has been approved by the FDA but has not been marketed by the manufacturer, CIBA-Geigy Corporation.

PINDOLOL
[Visken]

ACTIONS. See Effects of Beta Blockade in the Introduction to this section.

USES. The therapeutic effect of pindolol in stable angina of effort appears to be comparable to that of propranolol and other beta-adrenergic blocking drugs (see the Introduction). Because pindolol has partial agonist activity, it may be less effective in patients with angina at rest or severe angina of effort.

ADVERSE REACTIONS AND PRECAUTIONS. Pindolol causes less resting bradycardia than beta blockers that lack PAA. Large doses may increase blood pressure. In other respects, its adverse effects are similar to those of other nonselective beta blockers and the same precautions apply. (See the Introduction.) Pindolol also may cause nausea, diarrhea, and abdominal discomfort. It is classified in FDA Pregnancy Category B.

PHARMACOKINETICS. See Table 1.

DOSAGE AND PREPARATIONS.

Oral: Adults, for angina, 10 mg four times daily (Kostis et al, 1982). Sublingual and long-acting nitrates should be continued as needed.

    Visken (Sandoz). Tablets 5 and 10 mg.

TIMOLOL MALEATE
[Blocadren]

ACTIONS. See Effects of Beta Blockade in the Introduction to this section.

USES. The antianginal effect of this nonselective beta-blocking drug appears to be comparable to that of propranolol and other beta blockers (see the Introduction). Timolol also may reduce mortality and the reinfarction rate when given for long-term therapy after acute myocardial infarction (Norwegian Multicenter Study Group, 1981).

ADVERSE REACTIONS AND PRECAUTIONS. The adverse effects of timolol that result from blockade of beta$_1$ and beta$_2$ receptors are similar to those of propranolol and other nonselective beta blockers and the same precautions apply (see the Introduction). Timolol also may cause gastrointestinal and central nervous system disturbances, rash, sexual dysfunction, and alopecia. It is classified in FDA Pregnancy Category C.

PHARMACOKINETICS. See Table 1.

DOSAGE AND PREPARATIONS.

Oral: Adults, for angina, 10 to 30 mg twice daily. Sublingual and long-acting nitrates should be continued as needed.

    For long-term prophylaxis after acute myocardial infarction, 10 mg twice daily.

    Blocadren (Merck Sharp & Dohme). Tablets 5, 10, and 20 mg.

CALCIUM CHANNEL BLOCKING AGENTS (CALCIUM ANTAGONISTS)

Electrophysiologic and Hemodynamic Effects: Calcium ions play a major role in the function of many tissues, including cardiac tissue and vascular smooth muscle. After the myocardial contractile cell has been depolarized by the rapid influx of sodium ions, a slow inward current develops that is largely calcium-dependent. This slow current, which contributes to the plateau phase of the cardiac action potential, links myocardial excitation to contraction and controls energy storage and utilization. Action potentials from most specialized cardiac cells depend upon both fast (sodium) and slow (calcium) channels, but the pacemaker cells of the S-A node and cells in the proximal region of the A-V node are depolarized primarily by the calcium current. Activation of the contractile process in vascular smooth muscle also depends upon calcium influx through two major systems, one of which resembles the slow calcium channel in myocardial cells (Robinson, 1985).

Calcium channel blockers inhibit calcium entry into cardiac cells and smooth muscle cells of the coronary and systemic arterial beds. By this action, they dilate peripheral arteries and arterioles and may reduce heart rate, decrease myocardial contractility, and slow A-V conduction. They are less active in veins than in arteries and thus do not increase venous capacitance. Calcium antagonists prevent increases in coronary artery tone but they have considerably less effect than nitroglycerin on basal tone (Chew et al, 1983; Hossack et al, 1984 A; Feldman et al, 1983).

The electrophysiologic and hemodynamic effects of the individual calcium antagonists vary according to their selectivity of action at different sites (particularly at the sinus and A-V nodes), their ancillary properties, and the degree to which afterload reduction and reflex increases in beta-adrenergic tone counteract their direct negative inotropic, chronotropic, and dromotropic effects (Braunwald, 1982; Lewis, 1983; Low et al, 1982; Singh et al, 1982; Stone et al, 1980; Zsoter and Church, 1983).

Nifedipine [Adalat, Procardia], verapamil [Calan, Isoptin], and diltiazem [Cardizem] are the only calcium channel blockers currently marketed in the United States. Lidoflazine, gallopamil, nicardipine, nitrendipine, tiapamil, felodipine, and others are under investigation. Long-acting formulations of the available calcium antagonists are also undergoing study.

Pharmacokinetics: See Table 2.

Use in Variant and Classic Angina: Calcium channel blockers alleviate symptoms of resting angina by relieving coronary artery spasm, thus increasing myocardial oxygen supply. In angina of effort, their beneficial effect appears to be due to both reduced myocardial oxygen demand and improved myocardial perfusion. The precise role of these agents in antianginal therapy has not yet been fully defined.

Nitrates and beta blockers remain the standard therapy for classic angina of effort. The cardioprotective effect of beta blockers is a particularly important consideration in patients who have had a myocardial infarction. A calcium antagonist may be useful if nitrates are ineffective or poorly tolerated or when beta blockers are contraindicated or produce intolerable side effects. Since calcium channel blockers do not adversely affect respiratory function, they are preferred to beta blockers in patients with bronchospastic disorders and also may be better tolerated in patients with peripheral vascular disease and possibly in diabetics. A calcium antagonist also may be added cautiously to the regimen of selected patients with

TABLE 2.
PHARMACOKINETICS OF CALCIUM CHANNEL BLOCKING AGENTS

Drug	Bioavailability (%)	Half-life (hours)	Protein Binding (%)	Urinary Excretion of Unchanged Drug (%)	Active Metabolites
Diltiazem	40	3-5	70-80	2-4	Yes
Nifedipine	65-70	2-5	90	Minimal	No
Verapamil	10-20	6-12 (increased in cirrhosis)	90	3-4	Yes

classic angina when maximal doses of a nitrate and beta-blocking drug are inadequate.

In angina occurring at rest (variant or unstable), calcium channel blockers are probably as effective as nitrates and may be preferred to beta blockers. Although resting angina may respond to a calcium antagonist alone, many patients will eventually require additional therapy with other antianginal drugs. Calcium channel blockers do not appear to reduce morbidity and mortality in these high-risk patients (Pepine et al, 1983).

Diltiazem, nifedipine, and verapamil control symptoms of both variant and classic angina. Nifedipine and verapamil appear to be equally effective in variant angina (Johnson et al, 1981; Winniford et al, 1982). In angina of effort, the two drugs may have comparable efficacy (Dawson et al, 1981) or verapamil may be more effective (Subramanian et al, 1982 A; Winniford et al, 1985). Data comparing all three calcium blockers are limited. In patients with classic angina, there appears to be no difference in frequency of attacks among patients treated with diltiazem, nifedipine, or verapamil, each given with propranolol (Johnston et al, 1985). The three drugs also may be of comparable efficacy when used alone in patients with resting angina (Pepine et al, 1983).

Clinically important differences among the calcium channel blockers in their effects on myocardial contractility, cardiac conduction, and the peripheral circulation may influence drug selection. Nifedipine is the most potent peripheral vasodilator of the three drugs and, unlike verapamil or diltiazem, has little or no depressant effect on S-A or A-V nodal function. It may, therefore, be preferred in patients with angina and coexisting sinus bradycardia or A-V conduction disturbances. Because its direct negative inotropic effect usually is masked by reflex sympathetic activity, nifedipine is safer than verapamil or diltiazem in patients with left ventricular dysfunction (and its afterload-reducing properties may be beneficial). It is also preferred to verapamil or diltiazem in patients receiving beta blockers. However, congestive heart failure and adverse interactions with beta blockers have occurred occasionally with all three calcium antagonists.

Reflex tachycardia occasionally leads to exacerbation of anginal symptoms in patients taking nifedipine. Verapamil and diltiazem usually cause mild bradycardia, which is beneficial in patients with angina. Verapamil has the most pronounced effect on A-V nodal conduction and is the calcium antagonist of choice in patients with a coexisting supraventricular tachyarrhythmia.

Drug Evaluations

DILTIAZEM
[Cardizem]

ACTIONS. Diltiazem is a benzothiazepine derivative with cardiovascular effects similar to those of verapamil. It dilates peripheral arteries and arterioles, depresses S-A and A-V nodal function, and prevents sympathetically mediated spasm of normal and diseased coronary arteries (Hossack et al, 1984 A). Diltiazem reduces heart rate to a lesser extent than verapamil, and it also decreases blood pressure. Diltiazem increases myocardial oxygen supply by relieving coronary artery spasm and reduces myocardial oxygen demand by decreasing heart rate and reducing afterload. Like other calcium antagonists, diltiazem has a direct negative inotropic effect, which could become prominent in patients with compromised left ventricular function or in those receiving other myocardial depressant drugs.

USES. In patients with variant angina, diltiazem reduces the frequency of anginal attacks and decreases nitroglycerin requirements (Rosenthal et al, 1980; Schroeder et al, 1982). It improves exercise performance and reduces the frequency of anginal attacks in those with angina of effort (Hossack et al, 1984 B; O'Hara et al, 1984). The efficacy of diltiazem is comparable to that of propranolol in stable angina of effort (O'Hara et al, 1984) and in unstable angina (Théroux et al, 1985). Diltiazem may have an additive beneficial effect with propranolol in reducing the frequency of attacks of exertional angina (Boden et al, 1985 A; Kenny et al, 1985; Strauss and Parisi, 1985), although the combination may be no more effective than diltiazem alone in some patients with stable effort-induced angina (Hung et al, 1983). For a guide to drug selection, see the Introduction.

ADVERSE REACTIONS, PRECAUTIONS, AND INTERAC-

TIONS. The incidence of side effects with diltiazem appears to be low. It occasionally may cause bradycardia, dizziness, weakness, headache, flushing, pedal edema, and gastrointestinal disturbances (pyrosis, anorexia, nausea, diarrhea, abdominal discomfort, constipation). Hypersensitivity reactions (rash, pruritus), shoulder and elbow pain, and akathisia have been reported.

Congestive heart failure, A-V conduction disturbances, and sinus arrest have occurred rarely. Severe sinus bradycardia, hypotension, and congestive heart failure may occur during combined treatment with a beta blocker. Excessive hypotension has also occurred in patients receiving diltiazem and timed-release nitroglycerin. Sinus arrest, hypotension, and oliguria occurred in one patient receiving diltiazem and amiodarone for an arrhythmia. Diltiazem should be avoided in patients with sick sinus syndrome and A-V conduction disturbances and should be given cautiously with other drugs (eg, beta blockers) that depress the myocardium or the S-A or A-V node. Diltiazem probably does not cause a clinically important increase in serum digoxin levels. Cimetidine may reduce the clearance of diltiazem. There is one report of acute renal failure attributed to diltiazem, but a cause-and-effect relationship was not clearly established. Worsening of myocardial ischemia has been reported rarely following sudden withdrawal of diltiazem but no evidence of a withdrawal reaction was found in a retrospective analysis of a crossover study.

Diltiazem is classified in FDA Pregnancy Category C. It is excreted in breast milk.

PHARMACOKINETICS. See Table 2.

DOSAGE AND PREPARATIONS.
Oral: Adults, initially, 30 mg four times daily before meals; the dose may be increased gradually to a maximum of 360 mg daily. Sublingual and long-acting nitrates should be continued as needed.

Cardizem (Marion). Tablets 30 and 60 mg.

NIFEDIPINE
[Adalat, Procardia]

ACTIONS. Nifedipine, a dihydropyridine derivative, has potent peripheral arterial vasodilator properties and little or no direct depressant effect on S-A or A-V nodal function. It may prevent increases in coronary artery tone but does not produce significant dilation of epicardial coronary arteries in patients without coronary artery spasm (Feldman et al, 1983). Although nifedipine usually relieves myocardial ischemia in patients with coronary stenosis, it occasionally promotes coronary steal and may fail to relieve or worsen angina in those with collateral vessels (Schulz et al, 1985).

Because nifedipine has a relatively selective action on

vascular smooth muscle, reflex sympathetic activity tends to counteract its direct negative inotropic effect. Its afterload-reducing properties may be useful in patients with mild left ventricular dysfunction, but negative inotropic effects may be evident in those with severe heart failure or aortic stenosis and in those who are receiving other myocardial depressant drugs. Nifedipine reduces blood pressure and may cause a reflex increase in heart rate. It increases myocardial oxygen supply by relieving coronary artery spasm and decreases myocardial oxygen demand by reducing afterload. The beneficial effect of nifedipine in classic angina appears to be due primarily to the latter action (Mueller et al, 1981).

USES. Nifedipine is more effective in patients whose anginal episodes are due to coronary vasospasm (including those with mixed angina) than in those with classic exertional angina (Stone et al, 1983). In refractory variant angina, it reduces the frequency of attacks, decreases nitroglycerin requirements, and blocks cold pressor- and ergonovine-induced coronary spasm (Antman et al, 1980; Ginsburg et al, 1982; Goldberg et al, 1979; Hill et al, 1982; Pepine et al, 1983). Nifedipine is as effective as oral isosorbide dinitrate (Ginsburg et al, 1982; Hill et al, 1982) or verapamil (Johnson et al, 1981) in variant angina and it enhances the effect of oral nitrates (Conti et al, 1985).

In angina of effort, nifedipine reduces the number of anginal episodes, decreases nitroglycerin requirements, and improves exercise tolerance (Moskowitz et al, 1979; Mueller and Chahine, 1981). Its efficacy in exertional angina is comparable to that of isosorbide dinitrate (Liang et al, 1985) and possibly verapamil (Dawson et al, 1981), although the latter drug was reported to be more effective in two studies (Subramanian et al, 1982 A; Winniford et al, 1985). Propranolol may be more effective than nifedipine in effort-induced angina (Lynch et al, 1980) but comparative data are very limited.

Nifedipine may provide additional benefit when added to the regimen of patients with stable or unstable angina who do not respond to maximum doses of nitrates and/or beta blockers (Dargie et al, 1981; Gerstenblith et al, 1982). Some patients with stable effort-induced angina may show greater improvement with the combination of nifedipine and a beta blocker than with all three drugs (Tolins et al, 1984). Close monitoring is advisable during initial dosage titration in patients receiving combination therapy because of the risk of heart failure, severe hypotension, and aggravation of myocardial ischemia.

For a guide to drug selection, see the Introduction to this section.

ADVERSE REACTIONS, PRECAUTIONS, AND INTERACTIONS. Nifedipine may cause headache, tachycardia, dizziness, weakness, nausea, flushing, transient hypotension, severe muscle cramps, and dermatologic reactions. Leg edema is relatively common; it usually is not caused by heart failure and may not respond to diuretics. Local vasodilation has been suggested as a possible cause of the edema. Periorbital edema has been reported rarely. Nifedipine shunts blood away from exercising muscle, which may exacerbate leg fatigue during exercise.

Nifedipine may worsen myocardial ischemia in some patients. This complication is more common in patients with angina of effort than in those with coronary artery spasm (Stone et al, 1983). Nifedipine-induced myocardial ischemia is associated with hypotension and appears to be caused by coronary steal. Some investigators have reported that the risk is increased by concomitant treatment with nitrates and beta blockers (Boden et al, 1985 B), but others feel that beta blockers reduce the incidence of this complication. If myocardial ischemia is worsened by nifedipine, the dose should be reduced or other antianginal drugs should be substituted.

Rarely, nifedipine has precipitated congestive heart failure or cerebral or retinal ischemia. Patients with aortic stenosis or those receiving beta blockers or other myocardial depressant drugs appear to be particularly at risk for development of heart failure. Coronary artery spasm has been reported rarely following rapid withdrawal of nifedipine.

Reversible renal dysfunction occasionally is associated with nifedipine therapy. This adverse reaction has been attributed to altered intrarenal hemodynamics. Immune complex glomerulonephritis has occurred rarely.

Glucose intolerance has been reported but has not been a consistent finding. Hepatitis, menorrhagia, erythromelalgia, and gingival hyperplasia have occurred rarely.

Nifedipine may increase serum digoxin levels, but to a lesser extent than verapamil. Several studies have shown no interaction between nifedipine and digoxin. Occasionally, nifedipine may alter the disposition of quinidine, possibly by its hemodynamic effects, and the serum quinidine concentration may increase when nifedipine is withdrawn. Cimetidine may reduce the clearance of nifedipine.

Nifedipine is classified in FDA Pregnancy Category C.

PHARMACOKINETICS. See Table 2.

DOSAGE AND PREPARATIONS.

Oral: Adults, initially, 10 mg three times daily. The usual effective dose range is 10 to 20 mg three times daily. Some patients, particularly those with variant angina, may require larger doses and/or more frequent administration, eg, 20 to 30 mg three or four times daily. Doses exceeding 180 mg daily are not recommended by the manufacturer. Titration should usually proceed over a 7- to 14-day period but the dosage may be adjusted more rapidly (eg, over a three-day period) if clinically indicated. In hospitalized patients under close observation, the dose may be increased in 10-mg increments over four- to six-hour periods, but a single dose should rarely exceed 30 mg. Sublingual and long-acting nitrates should be continued as needed.

Adalat (Miles), *Procardia* (Pfizer). Capsules 10 mg.

VERAPAMIL HYDROCHLORIDE
[Calan, Isoptin]

ACTIONS. Verapamil blocks calcium influx and also produces mild nonspecific sympathetic antagonism. It has antiarrhythmic, antianginal, and antihypertensive properties. Verapamil depresses S-A and A-V nodal functions and reduces peripheral vascular resistance. Both sympathetically mediated and ergonovine-induced coronary vasoconstriction are inhibited. Although it prevents coronary artery spasm, verapamil has only a minimal dilator action on normal or stenosed epicardial vessels in the basal state (Chew et al, 1983). This drug's direct negative inotropic effect is not prominent with therapeutic doses except in patients with compromised left ventricular function or in those who are receiving other myocardial depressant drugs. The major electrophysiologic action of verapamil is to slow A-V conduction and, for this reason, it is also useful as an antiarrhythmic agent (see Chapter 24).

Verapamil is not as active as nifedipine in its effects on vascular smooth muscle and, therefore, causes a less pronounced decrease in blood pressure and less reflex sympathetic activity. Mild bradycardia is common. Verapamil increases myocardial oxygen supply by relieving coronary artery spasm and reduces myocardial oxygen demand by decreasing heart rate and reducing afterload.

USES. In classic angina of effort, verapamil reduces the frequency of anginal attacks, decreases sublingual nitrate requirements, and improves exercise tolerance during long-term therapy. Its efficacy is comparable to or greater than that of nifedipine (Dawson et al, 1981; Subramanian et al, 1982 A; Winniford et al, 1985) and it is as effective as a beta-blocking drug (Livesley et al, 1973; Leon et al, 1981; Frishman et al, 1982; Sadick et al, 1982).

Combined therapy with verapamil and a beta blocker may relieve symptoms and improve exercise tolerance in carefully selected, closely monitored patients with refractory, effort-induced angina (Subramanian et al, 1982 B). However, verapamil may produce significant negative inotropic and chronotropic effects in patients receiving beta blockers (particularly large doses); an additive depressant effect on the A-V junction is another potential complication of combined therapy. Therefore, this combination should be used very cautiously and should be avoided in patients with compromised left ventricular function or A-V conduction disorders and in those receiving other myocardial depressant drugs (Packer et al, 1982; Subramanian et al, 1982 B).

In variant angina, verapamil reduces the frequency of attacks, the need for nitroglycerin, and the number of episodes of ST-segment elevation as effectively as nifedipine (Johnson et al, 1981; Winniford et al, 1982). The antianginal effect is sustained in many patients with variant or unstable angina (Scheidt et al, 1982). Verapamil appears to be more effective in treating angina before myocardial infarction than in the immediate postinfarction period, and it does not improve prognosis after acute myocardial infarction (Crea et al, 1985).

For a guide to drug selection, see the Introduction to this section.

ADVERSE REACTIONS, PRECAUTIONS, AND INTERACTIONS. Constipation is the most common side effect of verapamil. Headache, vertigo, weakness, nervousness, pruritus, flushing, rash, and gastric disturbances also may occur.

Orthostatic hypotension, A-V block, A-V dissociation, pedal edema, pulmonary edema, and congestive heart failure have occurred occasionally. Rebound angina has been reported rarely following sudden withdrawal of verapamil. Perceptual disorders (feelings of coldness and numbness), hyperprolactinemia, and galactorrhea also have been observed.

When given intravenously, verapamil may cause severe hypotension, bradycardia, and asystole in patients with sick sinus syndrome or in those who are also receiving a beta blocker. Severe hypotension, bradycardia, cardiac failure, and heart block also have developed during combined therapy with oral verapamil and a beta blocker (including timolol eyedrops); these drugs should not be used together if left ventricular function is compromised.

Verapamil generally should be avoided in patients with sick sinus syndrome, second- or third-degree A-V block, cardiogenic shock, or advanced congestive heart failure (except when cardiac failure is secondary to supraventricular tachyarrhythmia). Although verapamil is very effective in selected patients with hypertrophic cardiomyopathy, severe adverse reactions have occurred in others (see Chapter 26).

Verapamil increases serum digoxin levels. Hypotension has been reported to result from interaction between oral quinidine and intravenous verapamil. Rifampin, and probably other enzyme-inducing drugs, reduces the bioavailability of verapamil. Cimetidine may reduce its clearance. Calcium preparations have been effective in treating verapamil toxicity, and it is possible that the therapeutic response to verapamil (and perhaps to other calcium channel blockers) could be reduced in patients taking calcium supplements. Since calcium supplements are widely prescribed today to prevent postmenopausal osteoporosis, this is an important area for future research.

Elevated transaminase and alkaline phosphatase levels have been reported occasionally, and hepatitis has developed rarely.

Species-specific cataracts developed when large doses were given for prolonged periods to beagle dogs. Lens opacities did not occur in other species, and the drug does not appear to be cataractogenic in man.

Verapamil is classified in FDA Pregnancy Category C. It is excreted in breast milk.

For treatment of toxicity, see Chapter 24, Antiarrhythmic Agents.

PHARMACOKINETICS. See Table 2.

DOSAGE AND PREPARATIONS.
Oral: Adults, for angina, 240 to 480 mg daily in three or four divided doses. Patients with severely impaired hepatic function should receive approximately 30% of this dose. Sublingual and long-acting nitrates should be continued as needed.
    Calan (Searle), *Isoptin* (Knoll). Tablets 80 and 120 mg.

LIDOFLAZINE
[Angex]

ACTIONS. Lidoflazine is a piperazine derivative that interferes with both calcium and sodium transport and may potentiate the vasodilator effect of endogenous adenosine. Lidoflazine slows heart rate and A-V conduction velocity, dilates coronary and peripheral arteries and arterioles, and reduces venous tone.

USES. In patients with angina of effort, lidoflazine improves exercise performance and may reduce the frequency of anginal attacks and nitroglycerin requirements (Towse, 1980). When given for long-term therapy after acute myocardial infarction, the drug may reduce the reinfarction rate but does not improve mortality.

ADVERSE REACTIONS, PRECAUTIONS, AND INTERACTIONS. Headache, dizziness, and tinnitus may occur during initial therapy or when dosage is increased. Gastrointestinal disturbances (nausea, vomiting) also have been reported. Dermatologic reactions and central nervous system disturbances (depression, disturbing dreams, hallucinations) have been noted rarely.

Lidoflazine prolongs the QT interval and may induce ventricular tachycardia with syncopal episodes in patients with severe ischemic heart disease, conduction abnormalities, or preexisting arrhythmias. Digitalis, antiarrhythmic drugs, beta blockers, and potassium-wasting diuretics may increase this risk. Several deaths have been reported that may have been caused by drug-induced ventricular arrhythmias (Kennelly, 1977).

PHARMACOKINETICS. Lidoflazine is extensively metabolized. Its half-life is 16 to 24 hours.

DOSAGE AND PREPARATIONS. Lidoflazine has a slow onset of action and maximal therapeutic effects may not be achieved for several months. This drug should be taken after meals or with an antacid to reduce gastrointestinal side effects.
Oral: Adults, initially, 60 mg daily for one week. Dosage may be increased to 120 mg daily the second week, followed by 180 mg daily the third week and thereafter. If there is no significant improvement after two months, dosage may be increased gradually to a maximum of 360 mg daily. Sublingual and long-acting nitrates should be continued as needed.
    Angex (Janssen). Tablets 60 mg.
    (Investigational drug)

PROSTAGLANDINS AND RELATED AGENTS

The prostaglandin system is an important modulator of vascular tone and platelet aggregation, and its role in myocardial ischemia and infarction is currently being explored. The biosynthesis of prostaglandins is initiated by release of the polyunsaturated fatty acid, arachidonic acid, from membrane phospholipids. The enzyme, fatty acid cyclooxygenase, transforms arachidonic acid to the cyclic endoperoxides, PGG_2 and PGH_2, which then are converted to PGI_2 (prostacyclin, epoprostenol) and TXA_2 (thromboxane A_2) by the enzymes, prostacyclin synthase and thromboxane synthase.

PGI_2 and TXA_2 have opposing pharmacologic actions on vascular smooth muscle and platelet function. PGI_2, which is produced by blood vessels, dilates coronary, systemic, and pulmonary vascular beds and inhibits platelet aggregation. TXA_2, which is released by platelets, causes vasoconstriction and platelet aggregation (Pitt et al, 1983).

Recent studies have attempted to determine whether an imbalance in these modulators plays a role in coronary artery spasm, unstable angina, and myocardial infarction and whether interventions that increase PGI_2 or decrease TXA_2 are of therapeutic value. PGI_2 and TXA_2 have very short half-lives, but radioimmunoassay techniques have been developed to measure plasma levels of their longer-acting metabolites.

Although TXA_2 is released locally during coronary artery spasm, this phenomenon occurs late in ischemia and appears to be an effect rather than a cause. Suppression of TXA_2 synthesis by aspirin or indomethacin [Indocin] does not reduce the frequency or severity of variant anginal attacks (Robertson et al, 1981; Chierchia et al, 1982). Since these anti-inflammatory drugs act by inhibiting cyclooxygenase, they also suppress formation of PGI_2. Blood vessels are able to synthesize new cyclooxygenase, whereas platelets cannot, but whether PGI_2 levels are actually maintained may depend upon dosage.

Some traditional antianginal drugs, such as beta blockers and dipyridamole, may affect PGI_2-TXA_2 balance but it is not certain that this effect has clinical relevance. Selective inhibitors of thromboxane synthase, such as dazoxiben, are currently under investigation. Studies on the effect of dazoxiben in patients with angina have yielded variable results.

An intravenous formulation of PGI_2 (epoprostenol sodium) is under investigation for a number of indications, including variant angina and acute myocardial infarction, and orally active analogues are being developed (Lewis and Dollery, 1983). PGE_1 (alprostadil [Prostin VR Pediatric]), is used to maintain ductus arteriosus patency in certain congenital heart disorders (see Chapter 26, Agents Used in Miscellaneous Cardiovascular Disorders). Alprostadil has relieved symptoms in some patients with unstable angina.

Drug Evaluations

DIPYRIDAMOLE
[Persantine]

Dipyridamole is a coronary vasodilator and platelet inhibitor promoted for long-term prophylaxis of angina pectoris. It interferes with uptake of the vasodilator, adenosine, by erythrocytes and potentiates the effect of PGI_2. In contrast to nitrates (which dilate conductance vessels), dipyridamole di-

lates coronary resistance vessels, a phenomenon that may be associated with coronary steal. In double-blind studies, dipyridamole did not significantly decrease the incidence or severity of anginal attacks, and conclusive evidence of its efficacy in angina is lacking.

Because dipyridamole dilates coronary resistance vessels, it may worsen anginal symptoms if it causes coronary steal. Other adverse effects include dizziness, headache, syncope, gastrointestinal disturbances, and rash.

Efficacy has not been established; therefore, no dosage is suggested.

Persantine (Boehringer Ingelheim), **Generic**. Tablets 25, 50, and 75 mg.

EPOPROSTENOL SODIUM (Prostacyclin, PGI_2)
[Cyclo-Prostin]

ACTIONS AND USES. Prostacyclin is an arachidonic acid metabolite produced in the vascular endothelium. It is a potent coronary, systemic, and pulmonary vasodilator and inhibitor of platelet aggregation. Because of its very short half-life, continuous infusion is necessary to maintain the pharmacologic effect.

Prostacyclin has been tried for various indications in which its antithrombotic and/or vasodilator properties might prove useful, including variant angina, acute myocardial infarction, peripheral vascular disease, pulmonary hypertension, platelet consumption syndromes, and reduction of platelet loss in extracorporeal circuits (Lewis and Dollery, 1983). Experience with the drug is still limited for most of these uses. It has not been consistently effective in variant angina but may benefit selected patients (Pitt et al, 1983). It does not appear to reduce myocardial infarct size.

ADVERSE REACTIONS AND PRECAUTIONS. Prostacyclin may cause flushing, headache, restlessness, anxiety, nausea, vomiting, hypotension, and reflex tachycardia.

DOSAGE AND PREPARATIONS.

Intravenous: *Adults*, information is not sufficient to include a dosage.

Cyclo-Prostin (Upjohn) Powder (injection).
(Investigational drug)

Cited References

Abrams J: Usefulness of long-acting nitrates in cardiovascular disease. *Am J Med* 64:183-186, 1978.

Abrams J: Nitroglycerin and long-acting nitrates. *N Engl J Med* 302:1234-1237, 1980.

Abrams J: Does tolerance develop during long-acting nitrate therapy? Critical review, in Kaltenbach M, Kober G (eds): *Nitrates and Nitrate Tolerance in Angina Pectoris*. Frankfurt, Steinkopff Verlag Darmstadt, 1983, 13-23.

Abrams J: Brief saga of transdermal nitroglycerin discs: Paradise lost? (editorial). *Am J Cardiol* 54:220-224, 1984.

Antman E, et al: Nifedipine therapy for coronary-artery spasm: Experience in 127 patients. *N Engl J Med* 302:1269-1273, 1980.

β-Blocker Heart Attack Trial Research Group: Randomized trial of propranolol in patients with acute myocardial infarction. I. Mortality results. *JAMA* 247:1707-1714, 1982.

Boden WE, et al: Beneficial effects of high-dose diltiazem in patients with persistent effort angina on beta-blockers and nitrates: Randomized, double-blind, placebo-controlled cross-over study. *Circulation* 71:1197-1205, 1985 A.

Boden WE, et al: Nifedipine-induced hypotension and myocardial ischemia in refractory angina pectoris. *JAMA* 253:1131-1135, 1985 B.

Braunwald E: Mechanism of action of calcium-channel-blocking agents. *N Engl J Med* 307:1618-1627, 1982.

Brown BG, et al: Mechanisms of nitroglycerin action: Stenosis vasodilatation as major component of drug response. *Circulation* 64:1089-1097, 1981.

Brown MJ, et al: Hypokalemia from beta₂-receptor stimulation by circulating epinephrine. *N Engl J Med* 309:1414-1419, 1983.

Chew CYC, et al: Effects of verapamil on coronary hemodynamic function and vasomobility relative to its mechanism of antianginal action. *Am J Cardiol* 51:699-705, 1983.

Chierchia S, et al: Failure of thromboxane A₂ blockade to prevent attacks of vasospastic angina. *Circulation* 66:702-705, 1982.

Conti CR, et al: Isosorbide dinitrate and nifedipine in variant angina pectoris. *Am Heart J* 110:251-256, 1985.

Crea F, et al: Effects of verapamil in preventing early postinfarction angina and reinfarction. *Am J Cardiol* 55:900-904, 1985.

Crean PA, et al: Failure of transdermal nitroglycerin to improve chronic stable angina: Randomized, placebo-controlled, double-blind, double-crossover trial. *Am Heart J* 108:1494-1500, 1984.

Cruickshank JM: Clinical importance of cardioselectivity and lipophilicity in beta blockers. *Am Heart J* 100:160-178, 1980.

Curfman GD, et al: Intravenous nitroglycerin in treatment of spontaneous angina pectoris: Prospective, randomized trial. *Circulation* 67:276-282, 1983.

Curry SH, et al: Plasma nitroglycerin concentrations and hemodynamic effects of sublingual, ointment, and controlled-release forms of nitroglycerin. *Clin Pharmacol Ther* 36:765-772, 1984.

Danahy DT, et al: Sustained hemodynamic and anti-anginal effect of high dose oral isosorbide dinitrate. *Circulation* 55:381-387, 1977.

Dargie HJ: Nifedipine and propranolol: Beneficial drug interaction. *Am J Med* 71:676-682, 1981.

Dawson JR, et al: Calcium antagonist drugs in chronic stable angina: Comparison of verapamil and nifedipine. *Br Heart J* 46:508-512, 1981.

Elkayam U, Aronow WS: Glyceryl trinitrate (nitroglycerin) ointment and isosorbide dinitrate: Review of pharmacological properties and therapeutic use. *Drugs* 23:165-194, 1982.

Feldman RL, et al: Analysis of coronary responses to nifedipine alone and in combination with intracoronary nitroglycerin in patients with coronary artery disease. *Am Heart J* 105:651-658, 1983.

Fletcher GF: Exercise training during chronic beta blockade in cardiovascular disease. *Am J Cardiol* 55:110D-113D, 1985.

Frishman WH: β-adrenoceptor antagonists: New drugs and new indications. *N Engl J Med* 305:500-506, 1981.

Frishman WH, et al: Comparison of oral propranolol and verapamil for combined systemic hypertension and angina pectoris: Placebo-controlled double-blind randomized crossover trial. *Am J Cardiol* 50:1164-1172, 1982.

Frishman WH, et al: β-adrenergic blockade for survivors of acute myocardial infarction. *N Engl J Med* 310:830-837, 1984.

Froelicher V, et al: Can patients with coronary artery disease receiving beta blockers obtain training effect? *Am J Cardiol* 55:155D-161D, 1985.

Gerstenblith G, et al: Nifedipine in unstable angina: Double-blind, randomized trial. *N Engl J Med* 306:885-889, 1982.

Ginsburg R, et al: Randomized double-blind comparison of nifedipine and isosorbide dinitrate therapy in variant angina pectoris due to coronary artery spasm. *Am Heart J* 103:44-48, 1982.

Glancy DL, et al: Effect of swallowed isosorbide dinitrate on blood pressure, heart rate and exercise capacity in patients with coronary artery disease. *Am J Med* 62:39-46, 1977.

Goldberg S, et al: Nifedipine in treatment of Prinzmetal's (variant) angina. *Am J Cardiol* 44:804-810, 1979.

Goldstein RE, et al: Clinical and circulatory effects of isosorbide dinitrate: Comparison with nitroglycerin. *Circulation* 43:629-640, 1971.

Harrison DC, Alderman EL: Discontinuation of propranolol therapy: Cause of rebound angina pectoris and acute coronary events. *Chest* 69:1-2, 1976.

Herlitz J, et al: Göteborg metoprolol trial: Enzyme-estimated infarct size. *Am J Cardiol* 53:15D-21D, 1984.

Hill JA, et al: Randomized double-blind comparison of nifedipine and isosorbide dinitrate in patients with coronary arterial spasm. *Am J Cardiol* 49:431-438, 1982.

Hjalmarson A, et al: Effect on mortality of metoprolol in acute myocardial infarction. *Lancet* 2:823-827, 1981.

Hossack KF, et al: Diltiazem-induced blockade of sympathetically mediated constriction of normal and diseased coronary arteries: Lack of epicardial coronary dilatory effect in humans. *Circulation* 70:465-471, 1984 A.

Hossack KF, et al: Long-term study of high-dose diltiazem in chronic stable exertional angina. *Am Heart J* 107:1215-1220, 1984 B.

Houben H, et al: Effect of low-dose epinephrine infusion on hemodynamics after selective and nonselective β-blockade in hypertension. *Clin Pharmacol Ther* 31:685-690, 1982.

Hung J, et al: Effect of diltiazem and propranolol, alone and in combination, on exercise performance and left ventricular function in patients with stable effort angina: Double-blind, randomized, and placebo-controlled study. *Circulation* 68:560-567, 1983.

International Collaborative Study Group: Reduction of infarct size with early use of timolol in acute myocardial infarction. *N Engl J Med* 310:9-15, 1984.

Johnson SM, et al: Comparison of verapamil and nifedipine in treatment of variant angina pectoris: Preliminary observations in 10 patients. *Am J Cardiol* 47:1295-1300, 1981.

Johansson BW, Dziamski R: Malignant arrhythmias in acute myocardial infarction: Relationship to serum potassium and effect of selective and non-selective β-blockade. *Drugs* 28(suppl 1):77-85, 1984.

Johnston DL, et al: Clinical and hemodynamic evaluation of propranolol in combination with verapamil, nifedipine, and diltiazem in exertional angina pectoris: Placebo-controlled double-blind, randomized, crossover study. *Am J Cardiol* 55:680-687, 1985.

Kennelly BM: Comparison of lidoflazine and quinidine in prophylactic treatment of arrhythmias. *Br Heart J* 39:540-546, 1977.

Kenny J, et al: Beneficial effects of diltiazem and propranolol alone and in combination in patients with stable angina pectoris. *Br Heart J* 53:43-46, 1985.

Klaus AP, et al: Comparative evaluation of sublingual long-acting nitrates. *Circulation* 48:519-525, 1973.

Kostis JB, et al: Treatment of angina pectoris with pindolol: Significance of intrinsic sympathomimetic activity of beta blockers. *Am Heart J* 104:496-503, 1982.

Lee G, et al: Antianginal efficacy of oral therapy with isosorbide dinitrate capsules: Prolonged benefit shown by exercise testing in patients with ischemic heart disease. *Chest* 73:327-332, 1978 A.

Lee G, et al: Effects of long-term oral administration of isosorbide dinitrate on antianginal response to nitroglycerin: Absence of nitrate cross-tolerance and self-tolerance shown by exercise testing. *Am J Cardiol* 41:82-87, 1978 B.

Leier CV: Nitrate tolerance. *Am Heart J* 110:224-232, 1985.

Leon MB, et al: Clinical efficacy of verapamil alone and combined with propranolol in treating patients with chronic stable angina pectoris. *Am J Cardiol* 48:131-139, 1981.

Lewis JG: Adverse reactions to calcium antagonists. *Drugs* 25:196-222, 1983.

Lewis JP, Dollery CT: Clinical pharmacology and potential of prostacyclin. *Br Med Bull* 39:281-284, 1983.

Liang C-S, et al: Comparison of antianginal efficacy of nifedipine and isosorbide dinitrate in chronic stable angina: Long-term, randomized, double-blind, crossover study. *Am J Cardiol* 55:9E-14E, 1985.

Lichstein E, et al: Effect of propranolol on ventricular arrhythmia: Beta-Blocker Heart Attack Trial experience. *Circulation* 67(suppl I):5-10, 1983.

Livesley B, et al: Double-blind evaluation of verapamil, propranolol, and isosorbide dinitrate against placebo in treatment of angina pectoris. *Br Med J* 1:375-378, 1973.

Low RI, et al: Effects of calcium channel blocking agents on cardiovascular function. *Am J Cardiol* 49:547-553, 1982.

Lynch P, et al: Objective assessment of antianginal treatment: Double-blind comparison of propranolol, nifedipine, and their combination. *Br Med J* 281:184-187, 1980.

McDevitt DG: Beta-adrenoceptor blocking drugs and partial agonist activity: Is it clinically relevant? *Drugs* 25:331-338, 1983.

Mikolich JR, et al: Relief of refractory angina with continuous intravenous infusion of nitroglycerin. *Chest* 77:375-379, 1980.

Moskowitz RM, et al: Nifedipine therapy for stable angina pectoris: Preliminary results of effects on angina frequency and treadmill exercise response. *Am J Cardiol* 44:811-816, 1979.

Mueller HS, Chahine RA: Interim report of multicenter double-blind, placebo-controlled studies of nifedipine in chronic stable angina. *Am J Med* 71:645-657, 1981.

Mueller HS, et al: Nifedipine in treatment of cardiovascular disease. *Pharmacotherapy* 1:78-94, (Sept-Oct) 1981.

Myers MG: Beta adrenoceptor antagonism and pressor response to phenylephrine. *Clin Pharmacol Ther* 36:57-63, 1984.

Nordrehaug JE, et al: Effect of timolol on changes in serum potassium concentration during acute myocardial infarction. *Br Heart J* 53:388-393, 1985.

Norwegian Multicenter Study Group: Timolol-induced reduction in mortality and reinfarction in patients surviving acute myocardial infarction. *N Engl J Med* 304:801-807, 1981.

O'Hara MJ, et al: Comparison of diltiazem at two dose levels with propranolol for treatment of stable angina pectoris. *Am J Cardiol* 54:477-481, 1984.

Packer M, et al: Hemodynamic and clinical effects of combined verapamil and propranolol therapy in angina pectoris. *Am J Cardiol* 50:903-912, 1982.

Parker JO, Fung H-L: Transdermal nitroglycerin in angina pectoris. *Am J Cardiol* 54:471-476, 1984.

Parker JO, et al: Nitroglycerin lingual spray: Clinical efficacy and dose-response relation. *Am J Cardiol* 57:1-5, 1986.

Pepine CJ, et al: Clinical outcome after treatment of rest angina with calcium blockers: Comparative experience during initial year of therapy with diltiazem, nifedipine, and verapamil. *Am Heart J* 106:1341-1347, 1983.

Pitt B, et al: Prostaglandins and prostaglandin inhibitors in ischemic heart disease. *Ann Intern Med* 99:83-92, 1983.

Pratt CM, et al: Demonstration of training effect during chronic β-adrenergic blockade in patients with coronary artery disease. *Circulation* 64:1125-1129, 1981.

Quyyumi AA, et al: Effect of partial agonist activity in β blockers in severe angina pectoris: Double blind comparison of pindolol and atenolol. *Br Med J* 289:951-953, 1984.

Reichek N, et al: Sustained effects of nitroglycerin ointment in patients with angina pectoris. *Circulation* 50:348-352, 1974.

Reichek N, et al: Antianginal effects of nitroglycerin patches. *Am J Cardiol* 54:1-7, 1984.

Roberts R, et al: Effect of propranolol on myocardial-infarct size in randomized blinded multicenter trial. *N Engl J Med* 311:218-225, 1984.

Robertson RM, et al: Thromboxane A$_2$ in vasotonic angina pectoris: Evidence from direct measurement and inhibitor trials. *N Engl J Med* 304:998-1003, 1981.

Robinson BF: Functional differences in blood vessels determined from studies with calcium-channel blockers: Functional changes in forearm resistance vessels in men with primary hypertension. *Am J Cardiol* 55:24B-29B, 1985.

Rosenthal SJ, et al: Efficacy of diltiazem for control of symptoms of coronary artery spasm. *Am J Cardiol* 46:1027-1032, 1980.

Sadick NN, et al: Double-blind randomized trial of propranolol and verapamil in treatment of effort angina. *Circulation* 66:574-579, 1982.

Scheidt S, et al: Long-term effectiveness of verapamil in stable and unstable angina pectoris: One-year follow-up of patients treated in placebo-controlled double-blind randomized clinical trials. *Am J Cardiol* 50:1185-1190, 1982.

Schroeder JS, et al: Multiclinic controlled trial of diltiazem for Prinzmetal's angina. *Am J Med* 72:227-232, 1982.

Schulz W, et al: Relation of antianginal efficacy of nifedipine to degree of coronary arterial narrowing and to presence of coronary collateral vessels. *Am J Cardiol* 55:26-32, 1985.

Singh BN, et al: Electrophysiologic and hemodynamic effects of slow-channel blocking drugs. *Prog Cardiovasc Dis* 25:103-132, 1982.

Stone PH, et al: Calcium channel blocking agents in treatment of cardiovascular disorders. Part II: Hemodynamic effects and clinical applications. *Ann Intern Med* 93:886-904, 1980.

Stone PH, et al: Efficacy of nifedipine therapy in patients with refractory angina pectoris: Significance of presence of coronary vasospasm. *Am Heart J* 106:644-651, 1983.

Strauss WE, Parisi AF: Superiority of combined diltiazem and propranolol therapy for angina pectoris. *Circulation* 71:951-957, 1985.

Subramanian VB, et al: Randomized double-blind comparison of verapamil and nifedipine in chronic stable angina. *Am J Cardiol* 50:696-703, 1982 A.

Subramanian B, et al: Combined therapy with verapamil and propranolol in chronic stable angina. *Am J Cardiol* 49:125-132, 1982 B.

Thadani U, et al: Comparison of five beta-adrenoreceptor antagonists with different ancillary properties during sustained twice daily therapy in angina pectoris. *Am J Med* 68:243-250, 1980.

Thadani U, et al: Oral isosorbide dinitrate in angina pectoris: Comparison of duration of action and dose-response relation during acute and sustained therapy. *Am J Cardiol* 49:411-419, 1982.

Théroux P, et al: Randomized study comparing propranolol and diltiazem in treatment of unstable angina. *J Am Coll Cardiol* 5:717-722, 1985.

Tolins M, et al: "Maximal" drug therapy is not necessarily optimal in chronic angina pectoris. *J Am Coll Cardiol* 3:1051-1057, 1984.

Towse G (ed): *Myocardial Protection and Exercise Tolerance: The Role of Lidoflazine, A New Anti-anginal Agent.* London, Royal Society of Medicine, International Congress and Symposium Series, Number 29, 1980.

Vanhees L, et al: Influence of beta-adrenergic blockade on hemodynamic effects of physical training in patients with ischemic heart disease. *Am Heart J* 108:270-275, 1984.

Willis WH Jr, et al: Hemodynamic effects of isosorbide dinitrate versus nitroglycerin in patients with unstable angina. *Chest* 69:15-22, 1976.

Winniford MD, et al: Verapamil therapy for Prinzmetal's variant angina: Comparison with placebo and nifedipine. *Am J Cardiol* 50:913-918, 1982.

Winniford MD, et al: Propranolol-verapamil versus propranolol-nifedipine in severe angina pectoris of effort: Randomized double-blind, crossover study. *Am J Coll Cardiol* 55:281-285, 1985.

Winsor T, Berger HJ: Oral nitroglycerin as prophylactic antianginal drug: Clinical, physiologic, and statistical evidence of efficacy based on three-phase experimental design. *Am Heart J* 90:611-626, 1975.

Yusuf S, et al: Reduction in infarct size, arrhythmias, chest pain and morbidity by early intravenous β-blockade in suspected acute myocardial infarction. *Drugs* 25(suppl 2):303-307, 1983.

Yusuf S, et al: Beta blockade during and after myocardial infarction: Overview of randomized trials. *Prog Cardiovasc Dis* 27:335-371, 1985.

Zsoter TT, Church JG: Calcium antagonists: Pharmacodynamic effects and mechanism of action. *Drugs* 25:93-112, 1983.

Other Selected References

Hillis LD, Braunwald E: Coronary-artery spasm. *N Engl J Med* 299:695-702, 1978.

McDevitt DG, Harron DWG: Antianginal and beta-adrenoceptor blocking drugs, in Dukes MNG (ed): *Meyler's Side Effects of Drugs*, ed 10. Elsevier, 1984.

Paul O: Medical management of angina pectoris. *JAMA* 238:1847-1848, 1977.

Sostman HD, Langou RA: Contemporary medical management of stable angina pectoris. *Am Heart J* 95:775-788, 1978.

DUCTAL-DEPENDENT CONGENITAL HEART DISEASE

PATENT DUCTUS ARTERIOSUS

PULMONARY HYPERTENSIVE DISORDERS

Primary Pulmonary Hypertension

Secondary Pulmonary Hypertension

Persistent Pulmonary Hypertension of the Newborn

HYPERTROPHIC CARDIOMYOPATHY

PERIPHERAL VASCULAR DISEASE

Vasospastic Disorders

Chronic Occlusive Peripheral Vascular Disease

DUCTAL-DEPENDENT CONGENITAL HEART DISEASE

The ductus arteriosus, a fetal blood vessel connecting the pulmonary artery to the descending aorta, diverts blood away from the lungs to the placenta during fetal life. The ductus begins to constrict within one to two hours after birth and usually closes anatomically within one to several weeks in full-term neonates. Closure of an anatomically normal ductus may be delayed up to several months in premature newborns. Prostaglandins of the E series have been shown to dilate isolated rings of the ductus arteriosus and probably play a major role in maintaining ductal patency in the fetus. Persistently elevated serum concentrations of these substances may prevent normal constriction of the ductus in the neonate (Heymann, 1981; Heymann and Rudolph, 1981; Olley and Coceani, 1981).

Certain congenital heart disorders depend upon a patent ductus to provide adequate pulmonary blood flow, prevent systemic hypoperfusion, or, in selected cases, improve pulmonary-systemic arterial mixing. These anomalies include (1) cyanotic congenital heart disease with decreased pulmo-nary blood flow due to severe obstruction to right ventricular inflow or outflow (pulmonary atresia or stenosis, tetralogy of Fallot, tricuspid atresia); (2) cyanotic congenital heart disease with normal or increased pulmonary blood flow (d-transposition of the great arteries); and (3) congenital heart disease with decreased systemic blood flow due to aortic valve or aortic arch defects (interruption of the aortic arch, coarctation of the aorta, aortic atresia). Research into the pharmacology of the ductus arteriosus led to the clinical use of alprostadil (prostaglandin E_1) [Prostin VR Pediatric] in these disorders.

ALPROSTADIL (Prostaglandin E_1)
[Prostin VR Pediatric]

ACTIONS. Alprostadil is one of a family of naturally occurring compounds derived from fatty acids. It has a variety of pharmacologic actions; the most important are vasodilation, inhibition of platelet aggregation, and stimulation of intestinal and uterine smooth muscle. Alprostadil is a potent relaxant of the smooth muscle of the ductus arteriosus and preserves ductal patency in neonates when it is infused before anatomical closure has occurred. It also may dilate the pulmonary vascular bed.

USES. Alprostadil is used in neonates with ductal-dependent congenital heart disease to maintain patency of the ductus arteriosus until surgery can be performed. It has been employed most frequently and is most effective in cyanotic neonates with pulmonary atresia or stenosis, tetralogy of Fallot, or tricuspid atresia. The efficacy of alprostadil in these disorders is demonstrated by an increase in systemic arterial oxygen tension (PaO_2). In a large-scale collaborative study, the mean PaO_2 of infants in this group increased from 27.5 to 38.9 mm Hg during infusion. Beneficial effects usually were observed within 30 minutes. The greatest clinical improvement occurred in infants less than 4 days old and in those with an initial PaO_2 of less than 20 mm Hg (Freed et al, 1981).

Infants with d-transposition of the great arteries are managed initially by emergency cardiac catheterization and balloon septostomy to improve mixing of the pulmonary and systemic circulations. Alprostadil may be useful in two circumstances: prior to catheterization and septostomy in critically hypoxemic infants, and on a temporary basis when hypoxemia and acidosis persist despite adequate septostomy. The improvement in systemic oxygen saturation in these infants may be due to both ductal enlargement and decreased pulmonary vascular resistance (Benson et al, 1979). In the collaborative study, infants with transposition of the great arteries had a lower PaO_2 before and during infusion than those with other cyanotic congenital heart defects (mean, 22.9 mm Hg before and 31.8 mm Hg during infusion), but the overall increase in oxygenation was similar (Freed et al, 1981). Although PaO_2 returns toward the preinfusion level when alprostadil is discontinued, acidosis may not recur (Henry et al, 1981). If the infant does not improve or continues to require alprostadil, current practice is to perform early elective surgery (Mahony et al, 1982).

Alprostadil may improve systemic perfusion in infants with aortic arch abnormalities who depend upon a patent ductus to supply blood to the descending aorta. Cyanosis usually is not a prominent feature in these disorders; therefore, measurement of PaO_2 is not useful to determine whether alprostadil has dilated the ductus. Improvement is reflected by the return of palpable femoral pulses, amelioration of metabolic acidosis, increase in urinary output, and decrease in the pressure difference between the main pulmonary artery and the descending aorta (in those with aortic interruption) or between the ascending and descending aorta (in those with coarctation). Clinical improvement was reported in approximately 80% of infants with aortic arch abnormalities during infusion of alprostadil. The maximal response occurred later than in cyanotic infants (up to 4 hours in those with aortic interruption and up to 11 hours in those with coarctation). The ductus appeared to be closed irreversibly in some unresponsive patients (Freed et al, 1981). The temporary use of alprostadil has also been advocated for the infant with critical aortic stenosis.

ADVERSE REACTIONS AND PRECAUTIONS. **Respiratory:** Apnea has occurred in 10% to 12% of patients. It usually appears during the first hour of infusion and is most common in infants weighing less than 2 kg at birth (Lewis et al, 1981). Bradypnea, wheezing, hypercapnia, respiratory depression, respiratory distress, and tachypnea also have been reported. Respiratory status should be monitored throughout treatment and ventilatory assistance should be available. Alprostadil should not be used in infants with respiratory distress syndrome.

Cardiovascular: Flushing has been reported in about 10% of patients, bradycardia in 7%, hypotension in 4%, and tachycardia in 3%. Congestive heart failure, edema, conduction disturbances, and arrhythmias have occurred rarely. Prolonged infusion increases the fragility of the ductal and juxtaductal structures and may increase the risk of spontaneous or surgically induced rupture of the ductus (Cole et al, 1981). Among infants with transposition of the great arteries, prolonged ductal patency may be associated with congestive heart failure.

Central Nervous System: Seizures have occurred in approximately 4% of patients; hyperpyrexia in 14%; and cerebral bleeding, hyperextension of the neck, hyperirritability, hypothermia, jitteriness, lethargy, or stiffness in less than 1%.

Gastrointestinal: Diarrhea has occurred in 2% of patients and gastric regurgitation and hyperbilirubinemia in less than 1%.

Hematologic: Infusion of alprostadil rarely is associated with disseminated intravascular coagulation, anemia, thrombocytopenia, and bleeding. This agent should be used cautiously in infants with bleeding tendencies.

Renal: Anuria and hematuria have been reported rarely.

Skeletal: Cortical proliferation of the long bones was observed during prolonged infusion but regressed after drug withdrawal.

Metabolic: Hypokalemia, hyperkalemia, and hypoglycemia have been reported rarely.

PHARMACOKINETICS. Alprostadil is metabolized rapidly and must be infused continuously. Approximately 68% of circulating alprostadil is metabolized in one pass through the lungs, and the metabolites are excreted by the kidney. Excretion is complete within 24 hours. No unchanged alprostadil has been found in the urine.

DOSAGE AND PREPARATIONS. To prepare the infusion solution, 1 ml (500 mcg) should be diluted with sodium chloride or dextrose injection to a volume appropriate for the pump delivery system available. A fresh solution should be prepared every 24 hours.

Intravenous, Intra-arterial: *Infants,* continuous intravenous infusion is preferred, but the intra-arterial route may be employed. The lowest dose should be infused for the shortest time that will produce the desired effects. Prolonged infusion should be avoided. The initial infusion rate is 0.05 to 0.1 mcg/kg/min. If the initial dose is inadequate, the amount may be increased gradually to 0.2 mcg/kg/min. After a therapeutic response is obtained, the rate should be reduced to the lowest amount that maintains the response. The arterial blood pressure should be monitored continuously during infusion.

The intravenous preparation has been used orally with success in some patients who require prolonged (one to two months) treatment.

Prostin VR Pediatric (Upjohn). Solution (sterile) 500 mcg/ml in 1 ml containers. The ampuls should be stored in the refrigerator at 2 to 8 C.

PATENT DUCTUS ARTERIOSUS

In small preterm infants, a large left-to-right shunt through a persistently patent ductus arteriosus can cause severe congestive heart failure and deterioration of pulmonary function. Infants with respiratory distress syndrome or other pulmonary disorders are particularly susceptible to these complications, and administration of excessive fluid may aggravate symptoms. The presence of a large patent ductus may not become apparent until respiratory therapy is discontinued. If symptoms are not controlled with conventional medical measures, clinical improvement can often be obtained by closing the ductus. Active intervention is usually not indicated in asymptomatic preterm infants with small left-to-right shunts because spontaneous closure occurs eventually in most.

Surgical ligation is the usual method of closing a large patent ductus in symptomatic infants who are refractory to standard medical therapy. Since ductal patency appears to be mediated through prostaglandins of the E type, drugs that inhibit prostaglandin synthesis have been employed as an alternative to surgery. Most experience has been obtained with intravenous sodium indomethacin.

INDOMETHACIN SODIUM TRIHYDRATE
[Indocin IV]

ACTIONS. This nonsteroidal anti-inflammatory agent is a potent nonselective inhibitor of prostaglandin synthesis. It acts by interfering with formation of endoperoxides, the precursors of all prostaglandins. Its ability to constrict the patent ductus arteriosus in premature infants is believed to be due to this action. Indomethacin may affect the tone of the ductus arteriosus more than that of other blood vessels (Friedman et al, 1978).

USES. Indomethacin is used as a pharmacologic alternative to surgery in preterm infants with symptomatic patent ductus arteriosus and respiratory distress syndrome who are refractory to conventional medical therapy. It reduces clinical, radiographic, and echocardiographic signs of shunting in some infants after a single dose (Friedman et al, 1976; Heymann et al, 1976), but many require additional doses and some fail to respond (Freidman et al, 1976; Gersony et al, 1983; Heymann et al, 1976; Yanagi et al, 1981; Yeh et al, 1981).

Indomethacin appears to be equally effective whether given initially as an adjunct to conventional medical treatment or as backup therapy when conventional treatment alone is ineffec-

tive. The latter approach is associated with a lower incidence of bleeding and is therefore preferred. Surgery can then be reserved for infants who do not respond to drug therapy (Gersony et al, 1983). Indomethacin appears to be effective when given at any time up to 2 weeks of age and at all birth weights and gestational ages within the premature range (less than 1,500 g).

ADVERSE REACTIONS, PRECAUTIONS, AND INTERACTIONS. Indomethacin may cause a transient, dose-related decrease in renal function. Although sodium excretion is reduced, dilutional hyponatremia has been reported. Indomethacin should not be used in infants with renal impairment. If digoxin is given concomitantly, its dose should be reduced and serum glycoside levels should be monitored because indomethacin reduces digoxin clearance. A similar interaction with aminoglycoside antibiotics suggests that dosage of these drugs should be reduced as well (Zarfin et al, 1985).

Indomethacin may increase serum concentrations of unconjugated bilirubin by displacing bilirubin from albumin. It interferes with platelet function and has caused gastrointestinal bleeding. Indomethacin may impair the mesenteric circulation and may contribute to the development of necrotizing enterocolitis, although this complication also occurs in premature infants who have not received the drug. Indomethacin does not appear to increase the incidence of retinopathy of prematurity.

PHARMACOKINETICS. When indomethacin was given intravenously to premature infants with symptomatic patent ductus arteriosus, a twentyfold variation in plasma concentrations was observed. The median half-life was 32 hours and the clearance was 7 ml/kg/hr. Unsuccessful treatment was associated with lower plasma concentration (less than 250 ng/ml at 24 hours), shorter half-life, and more rapid clearance (Brash et al, 1981). However, other studies did not find a relationship between serum levels and therapeutic effects (Gersony et al, 1983).

DOSAGE AND PREPARATIONS. Indomethacin should be administered in a neonatal intensive care unit. The intravenous route is preferred, although the drug has also been given orally and rectally.

Intravenous: The drug is administered at 12-to-24 hour intervals for three doses unless closure occurs after the first or second dose or adverse effects appear. The following doses have been recommended:

Age	Dose 1	Doses 2 and 3
<48 hours	0.2 mg/kg	0.1 mg/kg
2 to 7 days	0.2 mg/kg	0.2 mg/kg
>7 days	0.2 mg/kg	0.25 mg/kg

This regimen may be repeated if the ductus reopens 48 hours or more after initial closure. Surgical ligation should be considered if the ductus does not close after the first course of treatment or if the second course fails and the infant still has cardiorespiratory embarrassment.

Indocin IV (Merck Sharp & Dohme). Each vial contains powder (sterile, lyophilized) equivalent to 1 mg of indomethacin.

PULMONARY HYPERTENSIVE DISORDERS

Primary Pulmonary Hypertension

Primary pulmonary hypertension is a rare disorder of unknown etiology that is seen in young people, particularly women. It is characterized by increased pulmonary artery pressure and pulmonary vascular resistance and eventually a reduced cardiac output. Primary pulmonary hypertension is probably minimally symptomatic until late in the course of the disease when right ventricular failure, exertional dyspnea, chest pain, and syncope develop. Death often occurs within three years after the onset of symptoms. There is marked variability in the course of the disease; therefore, interpretation of drug effects on survival is difficult.

The initial event in the development of primary pulmonary hypertension is believed to be an increase in pulmonary vasomotor tone that leads to fixed lesions as the disease progresses (Grossman et al, 1984; Weir, 1984). Although small vessel thromboemboli are commonly found at autopsy, their significance remains uncertain.

The goals of therapy are to improve functional status by reversing active vasoconstriction and to prevent progression of the disease. Ideally, treatment should improve oxygenation and increase cardiac output, but reduction of pulmonary artery pressure is the most important aim.

VASODILATOR THERAPY. Acute administration of various vasodilator drugs has decreased pulmonary vascular resistance, lowered pulmonary artery pressure, and increased cardiac output in selected patients with primary pulmonary hypertension. Salutary effects have been reported during infusion of direct-acting vasodilators, alpha-adrenergic blocking agents, beta agonists, and prostaglandins. Hemodynamic and symptomatic improvement were reported in a smaller number of patients during short-term therapy.

The beta-adrenergic agonist, isoproterenol [Isuprel], produced initial improvement when given sublingually to several patients with primary pulmonary hypertension (Daoud et al, 1978; Lupi-Herrera et al, 1981; Shettigar et al, 1976), but some showed reduced responsiveness during long-term therapy. Because it markedly increases cardiac output, isoproterenol often *increases* pulmonary artery pressure despite a fall in calculated pulmonary vascular resistance (Hermiller et al, 1982; Rich et al, 1983). Oral administration of the alpha-adrenergic blocking drug, phentolamine, reduced pulmonary artery pressure and relieved symptoms during exercise in one patient with primary pulmonary hypertension, but severe adverse effects occurred in others. There is limited experience with other alpha-blocking agents, such as phenoxybenzamine [Dibenzyline] and prazosin [Minipress]. The angiotensin antagonist, captopril [Capoten], appears to be ineffective in most patients.

Increased exercise tolerance and improved hemodynamics, both during exercise and at rest, have been reported in some patients during long-term oral therapy with the direct-acting vasodilators, hydralazine [Apresoline] (Lupi-Herrera et al, 1982; Rubin and Peter, 1980) and diazoxide [Proglycem] (Klinke and Gilbert, 1980; Wang et al, 1978). In a short-term study on patients with right ventricular failure and pulmonary hypertension, hydralazine reduced right ventricular end-diastolic pressure, increased cardiac output, and relieved symptoms without reducing pulmonary artery pressure (Rubin et al, 1982). Both hydralazine and diazoxide have sometimes caused severe adverse effects (Hermiller et al, 1982; Kronzon et al, 1982; Packer et al, 1982).

When given orally or sublingually, the calcium channel blocking agent, nifedipine [Adalat, Procardia], induced hemodynamic and clinical improvement in some patients during rest and exercise (El Allaf et al, 1984; Olivari et al, 1984; Rubin et al, 1983), but occasionally caused untoward effects. (A sublingual preparation of nifedipine is not available commercially. The drug can be administered by this route by puncturing the capsule with a pin and squeezing the contents under the tongue.) Verapamil [Calan, Isoptin] is usually not useful because of its negative inotropic effect and there has been limited experience with the other available calcium antagonist, diltiazem [Cardizem].

Some investigators feel that long-acting nitrates, such as nitroglycerin ointment, may be useful because they can reduce both pulmonary artery pressure and resistance without affecting systemic vascular resistance and blood pressure (Pearl et al, 1983).

One recent study evaluated the *long-term* effects of vasodilators in patients with primary pulmonary hypertension who responded acutely to nifedipine or hydralazine with a fall in pulmonary vascular resistance of greater than 20% (Rich et al, 1985). One-half of the patients with acute favorable drug responses were treated, while a similar group was not treated. No beneficial effect of vasodilator therapy, either on clinical course or survival, could be documented.

Drug Selection: Vasodilator therapy is probably useful only when pulmonary hypertension is detected before significant fixed obstruction has developed. There are no data showing that treatment prevents progression of the disorder or reduces mortality. There is also no evidence that one drug is consistently superior to others or that any (except oxygen) has a selective action on the pulmonary vessels.

Individual response to different vasodilators varies widely, and an agent that lowers pulmonary artery pressure in one patient may raise it in another (Rich et al, 1983). For this reason, the patient's response to different vasodilators should be determined by acute drug testing with hemodynamic monitoring before long-term therapy is instituted (Rich and Brundage, 1984; Weir, 1984). Most vasodilators lower pulmonary vascular resistance and increase cardiac output, but these effects may be accompanied by a decrease, an increase, or no change in pulmonary artery pressure. Spontaneous variability in pulmonary artery pressure from hour to hour and in systemic blood pressure and cardiac output should be taken into account when assessing the effects of therapy in individual patients (Rich et al, 1982). The ideal response is a dose-related reduction in pulmonary artery pressure and increase in cardiac output (Weir, 1984); however, a reduction in right ventricular afterload may lead to symptomatic improvement even in patients who show no change in pulmonary artery pressure (Rubin et al, 1982).

Adverse Reactions and Precautions: Vasodilators may cause adverse hemodynamic effects in patients who have pulmonary hypertension, particularly in those with advanced disease whose pulmonary vascular bed is unresponsive to the vasodilator. In these patients, the drug may cause a greater decrease in systemic vascular resistance than in pulmonary resistance. Since cardiac output is relatively fixed by the high pulmonary vascular resistance, the fall in systemic resistance results in hypotension. Tachycardia, arrhythmias, anginal pain, heart failure, and cardiac arrest are potential complications. Several fatalities have been reported.

For other adverse effects, see Chapters 28, Antihypertensive Agents; 27, Agents Used to Treat Shock; and 43, Agents Used to Regulate Blood Glucose.

ANTICOAGULANT THERAPY. The question of whether anticoagulation benefits patients with primary pulmonary hypertension has been debated for years. Obviously the theoretical benefits of anticoagulation, namely, reducing the incidence of fatal pulmonary emboli or "small vessel thromboemboli," must be weighed against the hazards of bleeding in these patients, particularly in light of their tendency to develop passive congestion of the liver and hepatic dysfunction. One recent retrospective study on the influence of long-term anticoagulation in a large series of patients with unexplained pulmonary hypertension identified a probable improvement in survival, particularly in patients who manifest small vessel thromboemboli at autopsy (Fuster et al, 1984).

Secondary Pulmonary Hypertension

Most forms of pulmonary hypertension are secondary to cardiac or lung disorders that increase pulmonary blood flow, pulmonary venous pressure, or pulmonary vascular resistance. Some congenital heart disorders, such as patent ductus arteriosus or ventricular septal defects, increase pulmonary blood flow and pulmonary artery pressure by shunting blood from the left side of the heart to the pulmonary circuit. When pulmonary hypertension is associated with an increase in pulmonary venous pressure, the most common causes are left ventricular failure or elevated left atrial pressure in conditions such as mitral stenosis. Increased pulmonary vascular resistance may result from obstruction (eg, emboli), obliteration of pulmonary vessels, or metabolic factors (particularly hypoxemia and acidosis, which are the major causes of pulmonary hypertension in patients with chronic obstructive lung disease).

Treatment of secondary pulmonary hypertension is directed toward correction of the underlying cause. Vasodilators have been used adjunctively in some forms, particularly in patients with chronic obstructive pulmonary disease and cor pulmonale unresponsive to conventional measures. The goal of vasodilator therapy in these patients is also to reduce right ventricular afterload by reducing pulmonary artery pressure (Rubin, 1984). Salutary effects have been reported after short-term administration of several vasodilators, including hydralazine (Rubin and Peter, 1981), nifedipine (Simonneau et al, 1981), nitrates, epoprostenol (prostacyclin, PGI₂), phentolamine, and isoproterenol. The beneficial effect of the latter drug may be due to its bronchodilator action (Rubin, 1984). Long-term efficacy has not been established.

Vasodilators have the potential for worsening hypoxemia, which can be particularly important in patients with chronic obstructive pulmonary disease (Brent et al, 1984). This adverse effect is probably caused by intrapulmonary shunting of blood to poorly ventilated areas. For this reason, systemic arterial oxygenation should be monitored closely when evaluating the clinical response.

Persistent Pulmonary Hypertension of the Newborn (PPHN, Persistent Fetal Circulation)

This syndrome occurs most commonly in full-term or postmature neonates without demonstrable cardiac or pulmonary parenchymal disease. It is characterized by elevated pulmonary vascular resistance and right-to-left shunting of unoxygenated blood through persisting fetal channels (ductus arteriosus and foramen ovale). Affected infants show marked cyanosis, tachypnea, and acidosis. Primary PPHN is believed to be caused by perinatal hypoxemia. Secondary PPHN has been associated with a variety of disorders that predispose to pulmonary vasoconstriction, including sepsis, primary pulmonary hypoplasia, and diaphragmatic hernia (Fox and Duara, 1983; Gersony, 1984; Heymann and Hoffman, 1984).

The goal in the treatment of PPHN is to reduce shunting by decreasing the ratio of pulmonary artery to systemic pressure. To this end, oxygen, mechanical hyperventilation, and, in some cases, a vasodilator (usually tolazoline [Priscoline]) are employed to reduce pulmonary vascular resistance. Systemic blood pressure is maintained by use of volume expanders and, if necessary, a pressor drug. Dopamine, which also improves cardiac function, is usually the preferred pressor drug. Metabolic abnormalities also should be corrected.

TOLAZOLINE HYDROCHLORIDE
[Priscoline]

ACTIONS. Tolazoline has a direct vasodilator action, produces transient alpha blockade, and also possesses histamine-like, sympathomimetic, and cholinergic properties. The effect of tolazoline on the pulmonary vasculature has been attributed to its action on histamine receptors, but there is no conclusive evidence that it selectively dilates pulmonary, as opposed to systemic, vessels. Tolazoline also increases cardiac output.

USES. Tolazoline is used to treat persistent pulmonary hypertension of the newborn when oxygen and mechanical hyperventilation do not relieve hypoxemia or when excessive ventilator settings are required. It initially increases arterial oxygen tension in some infants but does not appear to affect survival

(Drummond and Lock, 1984). Published studies have included both term and premature infants with PPHN of various etiologies, which may explain the variable responsiveness to tolazoline (Fox and Duara, 1983).

ADVERSE REACTIONS AND PRECAUTIONS. Adverse effects are common in neonates treated with tolazoline. Hypotension is the most frequent untoward effect, and high concentrations of dopamine may be required to counteract this effect. Oliguria develops in some infants. Thrombocytopenia is relatively common. Other adverse effects include hypochloremic alkalosis, gastrointestinal distension and hemorrhage, and pulmonary hemorrhage. Fatalities have been associated with gastrointestinal, pulmonary, and/or intracranial hemorrhage (Stevenson et al, 1979).

PHARMACOKINETICS. The half-life of tolazoline in neonates ranges from 3 to 10 hours, and is longest in infants with poor hemodynamic status.

DOSAGE AND PREPARATIONS.
Intravenous: Neonates, initially 1 to 2 mg/kg via scalp vein, followed by infusion of 1 to 2 mg/kg/hr. If the drug is effective, a response will usually occur within 30 minutes after the initial dose. There is little experience with infusions lasting longer than 36 to 48 hours.

Priscoline (CIBA). Solution 25 mg/ml in 10 ml containers.

HYPERTROPHIC CARDIOMYOPATHY

Hypertrophic cardiomyopathy (idiopathic hypertrophic subaortic stenosis) is a form of primary myocardial disease characterized by myocardial fiber hypertrophy and extensive fiber disarray. It is often familial but also may occur sporadically. The increase in myocardial mass is commonly associated with disproportionate involvement of the interventricular septum. Ventricular systolic volume is reduced, contraction is powerful, and ventricular diastolic compliance is markedly impaired. Hemodynamic abnormalities and symptoms have been attributed to dynamic obstruction to left ventricular outflow, impaired diastolic filling, or both. Dyspnea, angina, palpitations, and syncope are the most common symptoms. Arrhythmias occur frequently, are often asymptomatic, and are believed to be the most common cause of sudden death in these patients (Canedo and Frank, 1981; Canedo et al, 1980; Epstein et al, 1974; Goodwin, 1980; Goodwin and Oakley, 1983; McKenna et al, 1980; Maron et al, 1981; Savage et al, 1979).

Propranolol [Inderal] usually relieves symptoms and improves exercise tolerance. There has been less experience with other beta-blocking drugs, but all appear to be equally effective. The calcium channel blocking agent, verapamil [Calan, Isoptin], is frequently useful in patients refractory to beta blockers and is now being used by some investigators as primary therapy. However, it occasionally causes severe adverse effects. There has been limited experience with other calcium antagonists; nifedipine may benefit some patients but its vasodilating effect may cause severe adverse reactions in others and it should be used with care.

Antiarrhythmic drugs (and/or pacemaker insertion) are often required to control life-threatening arrhythmias (Canedo et al, 1980; McKenna et al, 1980). Amiodarone [Cordarone] is particularly effective (Goodwin, 1982; McKenna et al, 1984), but it should not be given with verapamil (Goodwin and Oakley, 1983). The place of implantable defibrillators is still under investigation. Digitalis may be used to control the ventricular rate if atrial fibrillation develops, but, by increasing myocardial contractility, it may increase gradients. The use of a beta blocker or verapamil usually obviates the need for digitalis.

Diuretics may be required to diminish congestive symptoms. Nitrates generally should be avoided because they may increase outflow gradients.

Surgery (myotomy-myectomy) reduces left ventricular outflow obstruction and relieves symptoms, but it is usually reserved for symptomatic patients who do not respond to aggressive medical therapy. Mitral valve replacement is indicated for severe mitral stenosis.

PROPRANOLOL HYDROCHLORIDE
[Inderal, Inderal LA]

ACTIONS. By blocking cardiac beta receptors, propranolol reduces heart rate and myocardial contractility. Its beneficial effect in hypertrophic cardiomyopathy has been attributed to reduced myocardial oxygen demand, longer diastolic filling periods, and a decrease in gradients during exercise.

USES. Propranolol relieves angina, dyspnea, palpitations, and syncope in patients with hypertrophic cardiomyopathy. It is more effective in improving symptoms during exercise than at rest. Propranolol may reduce the incidence of atrial tachyarrhythmias (McKenna et al, 1980) but may not prevent life-threatening ventricular arrhythmias, which should be managed with additional antiarrhythmic drugs (Canedo et al, 1980; Frank et al, 1978; McKenna et al, 1980).

PHARMACOKINETICS, ADVERSE REACTIONS, AND PRECAUTIONS. See Chapter 25, Antianginal Agents.

DOSAGE AND PREPARATIONS.
Oral: Adults, initially, 20 mg three or four times daily, increased by 20 mg at 24- to 48-hour intervals until symptoms improve, a resting heart rate of 50 to 60 beats/min is achieved, or side effects become evident. The effective dose usually ranges between 120 and 320 mg daily. If the timed-release preparation is used, the dose is 80 to 160 mg once daily.

Inderal (Ayerst), *Generic.* Tablets 10, 20, 40, 60, 80, and 90 *(Inderal* only) mg.

Inderal LA (Ayerst). Capsules (timed-release) 80, 120, and 160 mg.

VERAPAMIL HYDROCHLORIDE
[Calan, Isoptin]

ACTIONS. Verapamil interferes with the slow channel transport of calcium ions into myocardial cells and smooth muscle cells of the coronary and peripheral vasculature. Its beneficial effect in hypertrophic cardiomyopathy may be due to improved diastolic filling, decrease in gradients, and reduced myocardial oxygen demand.

USES. Verapamil relieves symptoms and improves exercise capacity in many patients with hypertrophic cardiomyopathy (Anderson et al, 1984; Bonow et al, 1983; Chatterjee et al, 1982; Kaltenbach et al, 1979; Rosing et al, 1985). It offers an important alternative to beta blockers in selected patients (Rosing et al, 1985).

ADVERSE REACTIONS AND PRECAUTIONS. The electrophysiologic and hemodynamic actions of verapamil may cause particularly severe adverse effects in patients with the obstructive form of hypertrophic cardiomyopathy. These include bradycardia, sinus arrest, A-V block, myocardial depression, orthostatic hypotension, and pulmonary edema. Fatalities have been reported, usually in patients with symptoms of pulmonary congestion or in those with pulmonary capillary wedge pressures exceeding 22 mm Hg. The concurrent administration of quinidine appeared to contribute to some hypotensive episodes (Epstein and Rosing, 1981; Rosing et al, 1985). See also Chapter 25, Antianginal Agents.

PHARMACOKINETICS. See Chapter 25.

DOSAGE AND PREPARATIONS.
Oral: Adults, initially, 20 to 40 mg three times daily, which may be increased gradually (if no adverse effects occur) to 80 mg three times daily for one week, then 120 mg three or four times daily. Some patients may require as much as 720 mg daily.
 Calan (Searle), *Isoptin* (Knoll). Tablets 80 and 120 mg.

PERIPHERAL VASCULAR DISEASE

Peripheral vascular diseases are usually classified as vasospastic or occlusive. In vasospastic disorders, such as Raynaud's disease, blood flow to the skin is reduced by reversible vasoconstriction and there is little or no organic involvement. Drugs that dilate blood vessels of the skin may be helpful in these patients. In chronic occlusive peripheral vascular disorders, blood flow is reduced by organic obstruction, and vasodilators do not improve blood flow to either skeletal muscle or skin.

Vasospastic Disorders

The attacks of digital pallor, cyanosis, and rubor that occur in patients with Raynaud's disease (primary Raynaud's phenomenon) are precipitated by exposure to cold or by emotional stress. Patients with this disorder have an abnormally small digital capillary blood flow. When sympathetic tone is increased, activation of alpha receptors in the blood vessels of the skin further decreases the blood flow (Coffman and Cohen, 1971). Attacks often can be prevented by avoiding precipitating factors. If such measures are ineffective, a vasodilator may improve digital capillary blood flow (Coffman and Cohen, 1971; Coffman and Davies, 1975; Coffman, 1979; Gifford, 1971; Halperin and Coffman, 1979).

In secondary Raynaud's phenomenon, episodic vasospasm involving the skin of the extremities occurs as a manifestation of collagen disease (especially scleroderma) or occlusive arterial disease (particularly thromboangiitis obliterans) or may be induced by trauma, certain drugs, and a number of other conditions (McGrath and Penny, 1974; Schatz et al, 1966). Raynaud's phenomenon may be the presenting symptom. Successful management depends upon identification and treatment of the underlying cause. Vasodilators improve cutaneous blood flow in some patients but are of marginal value in advanced cases with an obstructive component (Coffman and Davies, 1975; Halperin and Coffman, 1979).

In recent years, beta-adrenergic blocking drugs have become a relatively frequent cause of secondary Raynaud's phenomenon in patients with hypertension. This complication has occurred with both nonselective and cardioselective agents. A beta-adrenergic vasodilator mechanism has been identified in the cutaneous vascular bed. In the presence of increased levels of circulating catecholamines, beta blockers potentiate alpha-adrenergic mediated vasoconstriction by blocking this beta-adrenergic vasodilator mechanism (Cohen and Coffman, 1981). Other drugs that may precipitate Raynaud's phenomenon are ergot alkaloids, methysergide [Sansert], imipramine [Janimine, SK-Pramine, Tofranil, Tofranil-PM], bromocriptine [Parlodel], and the combination of vinblastine and bleomycin.

Other vasospastic peripheral vascular disorders include acrocyanosis and primary (idiopathic) livedo reticularis. These conditions are benign, do not progress significantly, and do not require vasodilator therapy.

Chronic Occlusive Peripheral Vascular Disease

Patients with arteriosclerosis obliterans often are asymptomatic at rest but experience pain during exercise (intermittent claudication), which indicates that skeletal muscle blood flow is not sufficient to meet an increase in metabolic requirements. Because skeletal muscle circulation is largely under autoregulatory control, vasodilators rarely increase blood flow beyond the level produced by maximal tolerated exercise, and they do not relieve intermittent claudication (Coffman and Mannick, 1972). A number of studies have demonstrated the benefits of exercise regimens for improving walking distance (eg, Clifford et al, 1980 A). The patient also must be encouraged to abstain from smoking and lose excessive weight (Verstraete, 1982).

Patients with advanced arteriosclerosis obliterans who have pain at rest or ischemic lesions need an increased blood supply to the skin. No vasodilator consistently increases cutaneous blood flow in the presence of significant organic obstruction. By dilating vessels in noninvolved areas, these drugs may actually divert blood from diseased to nondiseased areas and do more harm than good.

Cessation of smoking (which is a major risk factor), losing excess weight, avoiding exposure to cold and trauma, meticulous foot care, rest, and treatment of other risk factors (diabetes mellitus and hyperlipidemia) are more helpful than vasodilator therapy in these patients (Schatz, 1971). Drugs that adversely affect peripheral blood flow should be avoided (eg, beta blockers). Arterial surgery or angioplasty should be considered for patients with severe local ischemia.

Vasodilators are also of no benefit in thromboangiitis obliterans, except possibly in mild cases with considerable peripheral arterial spasm and minimal organic occlusion.

DRUG THERAPY. Several classes of drugs with vasodilator action have been used to treat peripheral vascular disorders. These include antiadrenergic drugs, direct-acting vasodilators, calcium channel blockers, angiotensin antagonists, beta agonists, and prostaglandins. Some of these drugs are potent hypotensive agents, and care should be taken to avoid a marked fall in blood pressure that may counterbalance the increase in blood flow, particularly in areas supplied by atherosclerotic vessels.

Reserpine [Sandril, Serpasil] dilates blood vessels in the skin by depleting catecholamine stores in sympathetic nerve terminals. It diminishes neurogenic vasoconstriction in Raynaud's disease and other peripheral arterial disorders in which episodes of peripheral ischemia are associated with increased sympathetic activity. Other antiadrenergic drugs, such as guanethidine [Ismelin] and methyldopa [Aldomet], also may be useful in vasospastic disorders.

The alpha-adrenergic blocking agent, phenoxybenzamine [Dibenzyline], acts selectively at alpha receptor sites to block the response to sympathetic nerve impulses or circulating catecholamines. Since alpha receptors are abundant in the resistance vessels of the skin, while skeletal muscle blood flow is largely controlled by local mechanisms, alpha blockade increases blood flow to skin but not to skeletal muscle. Phenoxybenzamine diminishes neurogenic vasoconstriction in primary and secondary Raynaud's phenomenon, although its usefulness is limited by pronounced side effects. Most of these side effects are evidence of alpha-blockade and may decrease as therapy is continued. The postsynaptic alpha-blocking drug, prazosin [Minipress], is better tolerated than phenoxybenzamine and has been helpful in some patients with primary or secondary Raynaud's phenomenon, but tolerance may develop.

The calcium channel blocking drug, nifedipine [Adalat, Procardia], has potent peripheral vasodilator properties. Nifedipine decreases the frequency and severity of attacks in many patients with primary Raynaud's phenomenon and in some

with the secondary form. Diltiazem [Cardizem] also may be effective but verapamil [Calan, Isoptin] is not.

Although nitrates have a more pronounced effect on veins than on arterioles, nitroglycerin ointment may be useful as an adjunct to oral antiadrenergic drugs in patients with Raynaud's phenomenon (Franks, 1982). Transdermal nitroglycerin does not appear to be of benefit (Sovijärvi et al, 1984).

Severe peripheral ischemia caused by ergot poisoning has been treated effectively by continuous infusion of sodium nitroprusside [Nipride, Nitropress] (Carliner et al, 1974) or nitroglycerin or by oral administration of captopril [Capoten] or prazosin. Captopril also has reversed peripheral vasospastic phenomena when used to control the severe hypertension associated with scleroderma (Lopez-Ovejero et al, 1979).

Pentoxifylline [Trental], a trisubstituted xanthine derivative that is classified as a hemorheologic agent, recently became available in the United States for the treatment of intermittent claudication. This drug has improved treadmill walking distance in some patients, but clinical results have been more variable.

Papaverine, isoxsuprine [Vasodilan], cyclandelate [Cyclospasmol], niacin [Nicobid], nicotinyl alcohol, and ethaverine [Ethatab, Ethaquin] have a nonspecific relaxant effect on vascular smooth muscle. They are not potent vasodilators when given orally, and their efficacy in peripheral vascular disorders has not been established.

Nylidrin [Arlidin] is usually classified as a beta-receptor stimulant, although animal studies have demonstrated that beta blockade only partially inhibits its vasodilator action. Nylidrin increases muscle blood flow under some circumstances, but it rarely increases calf muscle flow beyond the level produced by exercise to tolerance and is of no established value in relieving intermittent claudication. Its efficacy in treating Raynaud's phenomenon is also not established.

Other procedures are being tried abroad or are under investigation in the United States for treating peripheral vascular disorders. In Raynaud's phenomenon, prolonged symptomatic improvement has been reported after plasma exchange (O'Reilly et al, 1979) or intravenous infusion of alprostadil (prostaglandin E_1) (Clifford et al, 1980 B) or epoprostenol (prostacyclin, prostaglandin I_2) (Belch et al, 1983). Both of these prostaglandins induce vasodilation and inhibit platelet aggregation. Thromboxane synthetase inhibitors are not effective (Ettinger et al, 1984; Malamet et al, 1985).

Alprostadil does not appear to be useful in chronic occlusive vascular disease because it improves proximal, but not distal, blood flow in the legs (Nielsen et al, 1976). Epoprostenol was reported to improve rest pain and ischemic lesions in some patients with obstructive vascular disease, but negative results have been reported by others. Ketanserin, a serotonin (5-HT) antagonist that also possesses alpha-blocking properties, was reported to promote healing of digital ulcers in patients with Raynaud's phenomenon (Roald and Seem, 1984) and to improve treadmill walking distance in those with intermittent claudication (DeCree et al, 1984). Nafronyl oxalate, an investigational drug that is claimed to facilitate oxygen exchange and to enhance metabolism in ischemic tissues, does not appear to be effective in intermittent claudication (Ruckley et al, 1978).

Drug Evaluations

ANTIADRENERGIC DRUGS

RESERPINE
[Sandril, Serpasil]

ACTIONS AND USES. Reserpine depletes catecholamine stores in sympathetic nerve terminals, thereby reducing adrenergic vasoconstriction in the blood vessels of the skin. When given orally, it may be useful for long-term therapy in primary and secondary Raynaud's phenomenon (Coffman and Cohen, 1971; Kontos and Wasserman, 1969). Reserpine is inexpensive and convenient to use because it requires administration only once daily. Intra-arterial injection above the site of involvement has been reported to relieve symptoms for variable periods, but controlled studies have shown no clear-cut benefit over placebo injections (McFadyen et al, 1973; Surwit et al, 1983). Hematemesis, bradycardia, and orthostatic hypotension may occur with this route of administration.

Reserpine is not useful in chronic occlusive peripheral vascular disorders.

ADVERSE REACTIONS. Nasal congestion and bradycardia occur commonly with clinically effective doses of reserpine. More significant adverse effects include lethargy, nightmares, and mental depression, which may be insidious and occasionally is severe enough to require hospitalization or result in suicide. (See also Chapter 28, Antihypertensive Agents.)

DOSAGE AND PREPARATIONS.
Oral: Adults, initially, 0.25 mg daily, decreased or increased (maximum, 1 mg daily), depending upon symptomatic relief and side effects.

 Generic. Tablets 0.1, 0.25, and 1 mg.
 Sandril (Lilly), *SK-Reserpine* (Smith Kline & French). Tablets 0.25 mg.
 Serpasil (CIBA). Tablets 0.1 and 0.25 mg.

GUANETHIDINE MONOSULFATE
[Ismelin]

Guanethidine, which interferes with the release of norepinephrine from sympathetic nerve terminals, increases finger capillary blood flow in patients with Raynaud's phenomenon (LeRoy et al, 1971). Since guanethidine does not readily cross the blood-brain barrier, mental depression has not been a problem with its use, and it may be a suitable alternative to reserpine for patients with a history of depression. It is not useful in chronic occlusive peripheral vascular disorders.

Orthostatic hypotension and hypotension during exercise are the most common side effects. Other frequent adverse effects are fluid retention, bradycardia, diarrhea, and retrograde ejaculation. See also Chapter 28, Antihypertensive Agents.

DOSAGE AND PREPARATIONS.
Oral: Adults, 10 to 50 mg daily. The side effects of guanethidine are dose related and often limit its clinical usefulness. Some investigators have found that severe reactions can usually be avoided if the dose is limited to 10 mg daily and another agent, such as nitroglycerin or prazosin, is given concomitantly (Franks, 1982; Porter et al, 1981).
 Ismelin (CIBA), *Generic.* Tablets 10 and 25 mg.

METHYLDOPA
[Aldomet]

Methyldopa is an aromatic amino acid decarboxylase inhibitor that depresses sympathetic nervous system activity by an effect on the central nervous system. It reduces neurogenic vasoconstriction in some patients with Raynaud's phenomenon (Varadi and Lawrence, 1969). Methyldopa is not useful in chronic occlusive peripheral vascular disorders.

Drowsiness, dryness of the mouth, and fluid retention are common during methyldopa therapy. Severe reactions (eg, hemolytic anemia, hepatitis) are rare. (See also Chapter 28, Antihypertensive Agents.)

DOSAGE AND PREPARATIONS.
Oral: Adults, 1 to 2 g daily.
 Aldomet (Merck Sharp & Dohme). Suspension 250 mg/5 ml (alcohol 1%); tablets 125, 250, and 500 mg.

PHENOXYBENZAMINE HYDROCHLORIDE
[Dibenzyline]

Phenoxybenzamine dilates cutaneous blood vessels by blocking alpha-adrenergic receptors. It acts on both postsynaptic (alpha$_1$) and presynaptic (alpha$_2$) receptors. Phenoxybenzamine may be used to reduce neurogenic vasoconstriction in primary or secondary Raynaud's phenomenon. It does not increase skeletal muscle blood flow and is of no value in chronic occlusive peripheral vascular disease.

Side effects may limit the usefulness of phenoxybenzamine. Clinically effective doses produce orthostatic hypotension, reflex tachycardia, nasal congestion, inhibition of ejaculation, and miosis. These side effects are evidence of alpha blockade and vary according to the degree of blockade. They tend to decrease as therapy is continued. Gastrointestinal disturbances (nausea, vomiting, diarrhea) also may occur.

DOSAGE AND PREPARATIONS.
Oral: Adults, initially, 10 mg daily, increased by 10 mg at four-day intervals until the desired effect is achieved or adverse effects become intolerable. The usual maintenance dose is 20 to 60 mg daily. Only 20% to 30% of an oral dose is absorbed in active form.
   Dibenzyline (Smith Kline & French). Capsules 10 mg.

PRAZOSIN HYDROCHLORIDE
[Minipress]

Prazosin blocks postsynaptic (alpha$_1$) adrenergic receptors. It has been used to relieve neurogenic vasoconstriction in patients with Raynaud's disease (Nielsen et al, 1983) and Raynaud's phenomenon associated with systemic sclerosis (Surwit et al, 1984) or ergotamine-induced peripheral ischemia (Cobaugh, 1980). The response to prazosin may decrease after two months of therapy (Nielsen et al, 1983).

Prazosin is better tolerated than phenoxybenzamine but may cause symptomatic orthostatic hypotension during initial therapy ("first dose phenomenon"). It usually does not cause significant tachycardia. Dryness of the mouth, nasal congestion, and fluid retention have been reported. Urinary frequency, sexual dysfunction, febrile polyarthritis, hypothermia, and dermatologic reactions have occurred rarely (see also Chapter 28, Antihypertensive Agents).

DOSAGE AND PREPARATIONS.
Oral: Adults, 1 mg two or three times daily.
   Minipress (Pfizer). Capsules 1, 2, and 5 mg.

DIRECT-ACTING VASODILATORS

PAPAVERINE HYDROCHLORIDE

Papaverine is the prototype of the vasodilators that have a nonspecific relaxant effect on vascular smooth muscle. This drug is promoted for oral therapy in various obstructive and vasospastic peripheral vascular diseases, but no objective study has shown it to be effective despite many years of use. It is rarely used today for treatment of peripheral vascular disease.

Adverse reactions include nausea, abdominal discomfort, anorexia, constipation or diarrhea, malaise, drowsiness, vertigo, hyperhidrosis, headache, rash, facial flushing, and hepatic reactions due to hypersensitivity (jaundice, eosinophilia, abnormal results of liver function tests).

Because the role of this agent in the treatment of peripheral vascular disease has not been established, no dosage is suggested.
   PREPARATIONS.
   Generic. Capsules (timed-release) 150 mg; tablets 30, 60, 100, 150, 200, and 300 mg.
   Available Trademarks.
   Cerespan (USV), *P-200* (Boots) *Pavabid* (Marion) [all timed-release oral forms].

CYCLANDELATE
[Cyclospasmol]

Cyclandelate produces vasodilation by acting directly on vascular smooth muscle. It is promoted for the treatment of various vasospastic and obstructive peripheral vascular disorders, but its efficacy in these conditions has not been confirmed.

Cyclandelate may cause gastrointestinal disturbances (pyrosis, pain, eructation), flushing, tingling, headache, weakness, and tachycardia.

Because the role of this agent in the treatment of peripheral vascular disease has not been established, no dosage is suggested.
   PREPARATIONS.
   Generic. Capsules 200 and 400 mg.
   Cyclospasmol (Ives). Capsules 200 and 400 mg; tablets 100 mg.

ISOXSUPRINE HYDROCHLORIDE
[Vasodilan]

Isoxsuprine is often classified as a beta-receptor stimulant, although animal studies have shown that its vascular effect is not blocked by propranolol (Manley and Lawson, 1968). Isoxsuprine may increase muscle blood flow in normal individuals but does not significantly affect blood flow to the skin (Coffman, 1968). It does not improve calf muscle blood flow in patients with occlusive vascular disorders and does not relieve intermittent claudication (Coffman and Mannick, 1972; Zsoter and Baird, 1974). There is no convincing evidence that isoxsuprine is useful in vasospastic disorders.

Adverse effects include dizziness, hypotension, tachycardia, and, occasionally, severe rash.

Because the role of this agent in the treatment of peripheral vascular disease has not been established, no dosage is suggested.

> PREPARATIONS.
> *Generic.* Tablets 10 and 20 mg.
> *Vasodilan* (Mead Johnson). Solution (injection) 5 mg/ml in 2 ml containers; tablets 10 and 20 mg.

NIACIN (Nicotinic Acid)
[Nicobid]

NICOTINYL ALCOHOL TARTRATE

The pharmacologic actions of these weak vasodilators are similar; niacin is a metabolic product of nicotinyl alcohol. In clinical doses, these agents act primarily on dermal vessels in the blush area. They have little effect on the vessels of the lower extremities, and there is no convincing evidence that they are of any use in vasospastic disorders or other peripheral vascular diseases.

Adverse effects include transient flushing of the face and neck, pruritus, tingling, gastrointestinal disturbances, rash, and urticaria.

Because the role of these agents in the treatment of peripheral vascular disease has not been established, no dosage is suggested.

> PREPARATIONS.
> NIACIN:
> *Generic, Nicotinic Acid.* Capsules (timed-release) 125, 250, and 400 mg; tablets 25, 50, 100 (nonprescription), and 500 mg.
> *Nicobid* (USV). Capsules (timed-release) 125, 250, and 500 mg.
> NICOTINYL ALCOHOL TARTRATE:
> *Generic.* Tablets 50 mg; tablets (timed-release) 150 mg.

CALCIUM CHANNEL BLOCKING AGENT

NIFEDIPINE
[Adalat, Procardia]

Nifedipine inhibits calcium entry into cardiac cells and smooth muscle cells of the coronary and systemic arterial beds. It has a greater effect on blood vessels than on the heart. Recent evidence suggests that nifedipine also may inhibit platelet activation (Malamet et al, 1985).

Nifedipine reduces the frequency and severity of digital vasospasm in many patients with Raynaud's disease and may be effective in some with secondary Raynaud's phenomenon (Creager et al, 1984; Kahan et al, 1983; Rodeheffer et al, 1983; Smith and McKendry, 1982). Fingertip vascular resistance decreased 40% after nifedipine was given to patients with Raynaud's phenomenon who were in a cold environment. Healing of fingertip ulcerations also was observed (Creager et al, 1984). Nifedipine is not indicated for treatment of chronic occlusive peripheral vascular disorders and, by producing generalized vasodilation, it could worsen intermittent claudication by shunting blood away from leg muscles during exercise (Choong et al, 1985).

Nifedipine may cause headache, reflex tachycardia, dizziness, fatigue, nausea, flushing, hypotension, and edema. For other adverse effects, see Chapter 25, Antianginal Agents.

DOSAGE AND PREPARATIONS.
Oral: Adults, dosage should be individualized and adjusted over a 7- to 14-day period; initially, 10 mg three times daily for three days may be given. If no severe adverse effects occur at this dosage level, the amount may be increased to 20 mg three times daily. The maximal recommended dose is 180 mg.

> *Adalat* (Miles), *Procardia* (Pfizer). Capsules 10 mg.

BETA-ADRENERGIC STIMULANT

NYLIDRIN HYDROCHLORIDE
[Arlidin]

Nylidrin allegedly improves skeletal muscle blood flow by stimulating beta-adrenergic receptors; however, animal studies suggest that the vasodilator effect may be due in part to a direct action (Manley and Lawson, 1968). When measurements are taken at rest, nylidrin increases calf muscle blood flow in normal individuals (Coffman, 1963) and in some patients with arteriosclerosis obliterans (Coffman and Mannick, 1972). It rarely increases calf flow during exercise, however, and does not relieve intermittent claudication (Coffman and Mannick, 1972). Although nylidrin may increase blood flow to the skin (Coffman, 1963), there is no convincing evidence that it is useful in Raynaud's phenomenon.

Adverse effects include dizziness, tachycardia, hypotension, nausea, and vomiting.

Because the role of this agent in the treatment of peripheral vascular disease has not been established, no dosage is suggested.

> PREPARATIONS.
> *Arlidin* (USV), *Generic.* Tablets 6 and 12 mg.

HEMORHEOLOGIC AGENT

PENTOXIFYLLINE
[Trental]

ACTIONS. Pentoxifylline is a trisubstituted xanthine derivative that is classified as a hemorheologic agent. It is claimed to improve oxygenation of ischemic tissues by decreasing blood viscosity. Postulated mechanisms include an increase in erythrocyte flexibility, inhibition of platelet aggregation, and a reduction in plasma fibrinogen levels. At the cellular level, pentoxifylline increases the concentration of cyclic adenosine triphosphate (ATP) in erythrocytes. This agent also has mild vasodilator properties when given intravenously. In microelectrode studies, pentoxifylline increased oxygen tension in calf muscle of patients with chronic occlusive peripheral vascular disease.

USES. Pentoxifylline recently became available in the United States for the treatment of intermittent claudication associated with chronic occlusive peripheral arterial disease. Its effects on initial and absolute claudication distances (distance walked on a treadmill at which symptoms appear and maximal distance walked) were evaluated in a double-blind, placebo-controlled, multicenter study in which 82 patients were treated for 24 weeks (Porter et al, 1982). Pooled results showed a significant improvement in initial and, to a lesser extent, absolute claudication distances during the treatment period; however, marked variations in results were reported from the seven participating centers. There was a reduction in the incidence of paresthesias in the treated patients and a transient reduction in subjective reports of cold feet. In this study, the drug had no significant effect on other subjective variables or on the patients' evaluations of their condition. An improvement in treadmill walking distance was also reported in another controlled study (Accetto, 1982).

Pentoxifylline is not recommended for treatment of severe arterial obstructive disease manifested by rest pain, ischemic skin ulcers, and/or gangrene.

See also Aviado and Porter, 1984, and Dettelbach and Aviado, 1985.

ADVERSE REACTIONS. The adverse effects of pentoxifylline are dose related and usually involve the gastrointestinal tract. Nausea and dyspepsia are the most common side effects, and their incidence can be reduced by giving the drug with food. Flatulence, anorexia, and vomiting are less common.

Adverse effects involving the central nervous system or the cardiovascular system have been observed less frequently. Dizziness, headache, and flushing were noted most often. Nervousness, insomnia, drowsiness, anxiety, and confusion occurred occasionally, and palpitations, angina, arrhythmias, hypotension, dyspnea, and edema were reported rarely. Loss of consciousness, fever, agitation, and convulsions may occur with overdosage.

Blurred vision, rash, pruritus, urticaria, dry mouth, and nasal congestion have occurred occasionally in patients receiving pentoxifylline. Cholecystitis, hepatitis, jaundice, pancytopenia, thrombocytopenia, and purpura have been reported rarely but a cause-and-effect relationship has not been established.

PRECAUTIONS. Patients who are allergic to xanthines should not be treated with pentoxifylline.

Blood pressure should be monitored periodically in patients receiving concurrent antihypertensive therapy.

Pentoxifylline may reduce plasma fibrinogen levels. This drug is classified in FDA Pregnancy Category C.

PHARMACOKINETICS. Pentoxifylline is almost completely absorbed after oral administration but undergoes extensive first-pass metabolism. Food delays absorption from an immediate-release capsule (not marketed) but not the total amount absorbed. Plasma levels of metabolites exceed those of the parent drug. The plasma half-life of pentoxifylline is 0.4 to 0.8 hours; the half-lives of its metabolites range from 1 to 1.6 hours. Essentially no parent drug is excreted unchanged.

DOSAGE AND PREPARATIONS.
Oral: Adults, 400 mg three times daily with meals. The manufacturer recommends that treatment be continued for at least eight weeks if a beneficial effect is not apparent during the first few weeks of treatment. If gastrointestinal or central nervous system side effects develop, dosage should be reduced to 400 mg twice daily. If adverse effects persist, the drug should be discontinued.

Trental (Hoechst-Roussel). Tablets (timed-release) 400 mg. (NOTE: Clinical studies on this preparation were conducted abroad. A capsule formulation (not marketed) was employed in the U.S. multicenter study mentioned above.)

Cited References

Ductal-dependent Congenital Heart Disease

Benson LN, et al: Role of prostaglandin E₁ infusion in management of transposition of great arteries. *Am J Cardiol* 44:691-696, 1979.

Cole RB, et al: Prolonged prostaglandin E₁ infusion: Histologic effects on patent ductus arteriosus. *Pediatrics* 67:816-819, 1981.

Freed MD, et al: Prostaglandin E₁ in infants with ductus arteriosus-dependent congenital heart disease. *Circulation* 64:899-905, 1981.

Henry CG, et al: Treatment of d-transposition of great arteries: Management of hypoxemia after balloon atrial septostomy. *Am J Cardiol* 47:299-306, 1981.

Heymann MA: Pharmacologic use of prostaglandin E₁ in infants with congenital heart disease. *Am Heart J* 101:837-843, 1981.

Heymann MA, Rudolph AM: Neonatal manipulation: Patent ductus arteriosus, in Engle MA (ed): *Pediatric Cardiovascular Disease.* Philadelphia, FA Davis, 1981, 301-310.

Lewis AB, et al: Side effects of therapy with prostaglandin E₁ in infants with critical congenital heart disease. *Circulation* 64:893-898, 1981.

Mahony L, et al: Long-term results after atrial repair of transposition of great arteries in early infancy. *Circulation* 66:253-258, 1982.

Olley PM, Coceani F: Prostaglandins and ductus arteriosus. *Annu Rev Med* 32:375-385, 1981.

Patent Ductus Arteriosus

Brash AR, et al: Pharmacokinetics of indomethacin in neonate: Relation of plasma indomethacin levels to response of ductus arteriosus. *N Engl J Med* 305:67-72, 1981.

Friedman WF, et al: Pharmacologic closure of patent ductus arteriosus in premature infant. *N Engl J Med* 295:526-529, 1976.

Friedman WF, et al: Prostaglandins: Physiologic and clinical correlations. *Adv Pediatr* 25:151-204, 1978.

Gersony WM, et al: Effects of indomethacin in premature infants with patent ductus arteriosus: Results of national collaborative study. *J Pediatr* 102:895-906, 1983.

Heymann MA, et al: Closure of ductus arteriosus in premature infants by inhibition of prostaglandin synthesis. *N Engl J Med* 295:530-533, 1976.

Yanagi RM, et al: Indomethacin treatment for symptomatic patent ductus arteriosus: Double-blind control study. *Pediatrics* 67:647-652, 1981.

Yeh TF, et al: Intravenous indomethacin therapy in premature infants with persistent ductus arteriosus: Double-blind controlled study. *J Pediatr* 98:137-145, 1981.

Zarfin Y, et al: Possible indomethacin-aminoglycoside interaction in preterm infants. *J Pediatr* 106:511-513, 1985.

Pulmonary Hypertensive Disorders

Brent BN, et al: Relationship between oxygen uptake and oxygen transport in stable patients with chronic obstructive pulmonary disease: Physiologic effects of nitroprusside and hydralazine. *Am Rev Respir Dis* 129:682-686, 1984.

Daoud FS, et al: Isoproterenol as potential pulmonary vasodilator in primary pulmonary hypertension. *Am J Cardiol* 42:817-822, 1978.

Drummond WH, Lock JE: Neonatal 'pulmonary vasodilator' drugs. *Dev Pharmacol Ther* 7:1-20, 1984.

El Allaf D, et al: Nifedipine: Update of its therapeutic efficacy in pulmonary hypertension. *Cardiovasc Rev Rep* 5:1123-1128, 1984.

Fox WW, Duara S: Persistent pulmonary hypertension in neonates: Diagnosis and treatment. *Pediatrics* 103:505-514, 1983.

Fuster V, et al: Primary pulmonary hypertension: Natural history and importance of thrombosis. *Circulation* 70:580-587, 1984.

Gersony WM: Neonatal pulmonary hypertension: Pathophysiology, classification, and etiology. *Clin Perinatol* 11:517-524, 1984.

Grossman W, et al: Pulmonary hypertension, in Braunwald E (ed): *Heart Disease: Textbook of Cardiovascular Medicine*, ed 2. Philadelphia, WB Saunders, 1984, 823-848.

Hermiller JB, et al: Vasodilators and prostaglandin inhibitors in primary pulmonary hypertension. *Ann Intern Med* 97:480-489, 1982.

Heymann MA, Hoffman JIE: Persistent pulmonary hypertension syndromes in the newborn, in Weir EK, Reeves JT (eds): *Pulmonary Hypertension*. Mt Kisco, NY, Futura, 1984, 45-71.

Klinke WP, Gilbert JAL: Diazoxide in primary pulmonary hypertension. *N Engl J Med* 302:91-92, 1980.

Kronzon I, et al: Adverse effect of hydralazine in patients with primary pulmonary hypertension. *JAMA* 247:3112-3114, 1982.

Lupi-Herrera E, et al: Role of isoproterenol in pulmonary artery hypertension of unknown etiology (primary): Short- and long-term evaluation. *Chest* 79:292-296, 1981.

Lupi-Herrera E, et al: Role of hydralazine therapy for pulmonary arterial hypertension of unknown cause. *Circulation* 65:645-650, 1982.

Olivari MT, et al: Hemodynamic effects of nifedipine at rest and during exercise in primary pulmonary hypertension. *Chest* 86:14-19, 1984.

Packer M, et al: Deleterious effects of hydralazine in patients with pulmonary hypertension. *N Engl J Med* 306:1326-1331, 1982.

Pearl RG, et al: Acute hemodynamic effects of nitroglycerin in pulmonary hypertension. *Ann Intern Med* 99:9-13, 1983.

Rich S, Brundage BH: Primary pulmonary hypertension: Current update. *JAMA* 251:2252-2254, 1984.

Rich S, et al: Captopril as treatment for patients with pulmonary hypertension: Problem of variability in assessing chronic drug treatment. *Br Heart J* 48:272-277, 1982.

Rich S, et al: Reassessment of effects of vasodilator drugs in primary pulmonary hypertension: Guidelines for determining pulmonary vasodilator response. *Am Heart J* 105:119-127, 1983.

Rich S, et al: Effect of vasodilator therapy on clinical outcome of patients with primary pulmonary hypertension. *Circulation* 71:1191-1196, 1985.

Rubin LJ: Pulmonary hypertension secondary to lung disease, in Weir EK, Reeves JT (eds): *Pulmonary Hypertension*. Mt Kisco, NY, Futura, 1984, 291-320.

Rubin LJ, Peter RH: Oral hydralazine therapy for primary pulmonary hypertension. *N Engl J Med* 302:69-73, 1980.

Rubin LJ, Peter RH: Hemodynamics at rest and during exercise after oral hydralazine in patients with cor pulmonale. *Am J Cardiol* 47:116-122, 1981.

Rubin LJ, et al: Effects of oral hydralazine on right ventricular end-diastolic pressure in patients with right ventricular failure. *Circulation* 65:1369-1373, 1982.

Rubin LJ, et al: Treatment of primary pulmonary hypertension with nifedipine: Hemodynamic and scintigraphic evaluation. *Ann Intern Med* 99:433-438, 1983.

Shettigar UR, et al: Primary pulmonary hypertension: Favorable effect of isoproterenol. *N Engl J Med* 295:1414-1415, 1976.

Simonneau G, et al: Inhibition of hypoxic pulmonary vasoconstriction by nifedipine. *N Engl J Med* 304:1582-1585, 1981.

Stevenson DK, et al: Refractory hypoxemia associated with neonatal pulmonary disease. Use and limitations of tolazoline. *J Pediatr* 95:595-599, 1979.

Wang SWS, et al: Diazoxide in treatment of primary pulmonary hypertension. *Br Heart J* 40:572-574, 1978.

Weir EK: Diagnosis and management of primary pulmonary hypertension, in Weir EK, Reeves JT (eds): *Pulmonary Hypertension*. Mt Kisco, NY, Futura, 1984, 115-168.

Hypertrophic Cardiomyopathy

Anderson DM, et al: Hypertrophic obstructive cardiomyopathy: Effects of acute and chronic verapamil treatment on left ventricular systolic and diastolic function. *Br Heart J* 51:523-529, 1984.

Bonow RO, et al: Acute and chronic effects of verapamil on left ventricular function in patients with hypertrophic cardiomyopathy. *Eur Heart J* 4(suppl F):57-65, 1983.

Canedo MI, Frank MJ: Therapy of hypertrophic cardiomyopathy: Medical or surgical? Clinical and pathophysiologic considerations. *Am J Cardiol* 48:383-388, 1981.

Canedo MI, et al: Rhythm disturbances in hypertrophic cardiomyopathy: Prevalence, relation to symptoms and management. *Am J Cardiol* 45:848-855, 1980.

Chatterjee K, et al: Hypertrophic cardiomyopathy: Therapy with slow channel inhibiting agents. *Prog Cardiovasc Dis* 25:193-210, 1982.

Epstein SE, Rosing DR: Verapamil: Potential for causing serious complications in patients with hypertrophic cardiomyopathy. *Circulation* 64:437-441, 1981.

Epstein SE, et al: Asymmetric septal hypertrophy. *Ann Intern Med* 81:650-680, 1974.

Frank MJ, et al: Long-term medical management of hypertrophic obstructive cardiomyopathy. *Am J Cardiol* 42:993-1001, 1978.

Goodwin JF: Hypertrophic cardiomyopathy: Disease in search of its own identity. *Am J Cardiol* 45:177-180, 1980.

Goodwin JF: Frontiers of cardiomyopathy. *Br Heart J* 48:1-18, 1982.

Goodwin JF, Oakley CM: Medical and surgical treatment of hypertrophic cardiomyopathy. *Eur Heart J* 4(suppl F):209-214, 1983.

Kaltenbach M, et al: Treatment of hypertrophic obstructive cardiomyopathy with verapamil. *Br Heart J* 42:35-42, 1979.

Maron BJ, et al: Prognostic significance of 24 hour ambulatory electrocardiographic monitoring in patients with hypertrophic cardiomyopathy: Prospective study. *Am J Cardiol* 48:252-257, 1981.

McKenna WJ, et al: Arrhythmia in hypertrophic cardiomyopathy:

Exercise and 48 hour ambulatory electrocardiographic assessment with and without beta adrenergic blocking therapy. *Am J Cardiol* 45:1-5, 1980.

McKenna WJ, et al: Amiodarone for long-term management of patients with hypertrophic cardiomyopathy. *Am J Cardiol* 54:802-810, 1984.

Rosing DR, et al: Use of calcium-channel blocking drugs in hypertrophic cardiomyopathy. *Am J Cardiol* 55:185B-195B, 1985.

Savage DD, et al: Prevalence of arrhythmias during 24-hour electrocardiographic monitoring and exercise testing in patients with obstructive and nonobstructive hypertrophic cardiomyopathy. *Circulation* 59:866-875, 1979.

Peripheral Vascular Disease

Accetto B: Beneficial hemorheologic therapy of chronic peripheral arterial disorders with pentoxifylline: Results of double-blind study versus vasodilator-nylidrin. *Am Heart J* 103:864-869, 1982.

Aviado DM, Porter JM: Pentoxifylline: New drug for treatment of intermittent claudication: Mechanism of action, pharmacokinetics, clinical efficacy, and adverse effects. *Pharmacotherapy* 4:297-307, 1984.

Belch JJF, et al: Intermittent epoprostenol (prostacyclin) infusion in patients with Raynaud's syndrome: Double-blind controlled trial. *Lancet* 1:313-315, 1983.

Carliner NH, et al: Sodium nitroprusside treatment of ergotamine induced peripheral ischemia. *JAMA* 227:308-309, 1974.

Choong CYP, et al: Effects of nifedipine on systemic and regional oxygen transport and metabolism at rest and during exercise. *Circulation* 71:787-796, 1985.

Clifford PC, et al: Intermittent claudication: Is supervised exercise class worthwhile? *Br Med J* 280:1503-1505, 1980 A.

Clifford PC, et al: Treatment of vasospastic disease with prostaglandin E₁. *Br Med J* 281:1031-1034, 1980 B.

Cobaugh DS: Prazosin treatment of ergotamine-induced peripheral ischemia. *JAMA* 244:1360, 1980.

Coffman JD: Effects of dichlorisoproterenol, nylidrin, and placebo on peripheral blood flow. *J New Drugs* 3:356-361, 1963.

Coffman JD: Effect of vasodilator drugs in vasoconstricted normal subjects. *J Clin Pharmacol* 8:302-308, 1968.

Coffman JD: Vasodilator drugs in peripheral vascular disease. *N Engl J Med* 300:713-717, 1979.

Coffman JD, Cohen AS: Total and capillary fingertip blood flow in Raynaud's phenomenon. *N Engl J Med* 285:259-263, 1971.

Coffman JD, Davies WT: Vasospastic diseases: Review. *Prog Cardiovasc Dis* 18:123-146, 1975.

Coffman JD, Mannick JA: Failure of vasodilator drugs in arteriosclerosis obliterans. *Ann Intern Med* 76:35-39, 1972.

Cohen RA, Coffman JD: Beta-adrenergic vasodilator mechanism in the finger. *Circ Res* 49:1196-1201, 1981.

Creager MA, et al: Nifedipine-induced fingertip vasodilation in patients with Raynaud's phenomenon. *Am Heart J* 108:370-373, 1984.

DeCree J, et al: Placebo-controlled double-blind trial of ketanserin in treatment of intermittent claudication. *Lancet* 2:775-778, 1984.

Dettelbach HR, Aviado DM: Clinical pharmacology of pentoxifylline with special reference to hemorheologic effect for treatment of intermittent claudication. *J Clin Pharmacol* 25:8-26, 1985.

Ettinger WH, et al: Controlled double-blind trial of dazoxiben and nifedipine in treatment of Raynaud's phenomenon. *Am J Med* 77:451-456, 1984.

Franks AG Jr: Topical glyceryl trinitrate as adjunctive treatment in Raynaud's disease. *Lancet* 1:76-77, 1982.

Gifford RW Jr: Arteriospastic diseases: Clinical significance and management. *Cardiovasc Clin* 3:127-139, 1971.

Halperin JL, Coffman JD: Pathophysiology of Raynaud's disease. *Arch Intern Med* 139:89-92, 1979.

Kahan A, et al: Calcium entry blocking agents in digital vasospasm (Raynaud's phenomenon). *Eur Heart J* 4(suppl C):123-129, 1983.

Kontos HA, Wasserman AJ: Effect of reserpine in Raynaud's phenomenon. *Circulation* 39:259-266, 1969.

LeRoy EC, et al: Skin capillary blood flow in scleroderma. *J Clin Invest* 50:930-939, 1971.

Lopez-Ovejero JA, et al: Reversal of vascular and renal crises of scleroderma by oral angiotensin-converting-enzyme blockade. *N Engl J Med* 300:1417-1419, 1979.

Malamet R, et al: Nifedipine in treatment of Raynaud's phenomenon: Evidence for inhibition of platelet activation. *Am J Med* 78:602-608, 1985.

Manley ES, Lawson JW: Effect of beta adrenergic receptor blockade on skeletal muscle vasodilatation produced by isoxsuprine and nylidrin. *Arch Int Pharmacodyn Ther* 175:239-250, 1968.

McFadyen IJ, et al: Intraarterial reserpine administration in Raynaud syndrome. *Arch Intern Med* 132:526-528, 1973.

McGrath MA, Penny R: Mechanisms of Raynaud's phenomenon. *Med J Aust* 2:328-333, 367-375, 1974.

Nielsen PE, et al: Intra-arterial infusion of prostaglandin E₁ in normal subjects and patients with peripheral arterial disease. *Scand J Clin Lab Invest* 36:633-640, 1976.

Nielsen SL: Prazosin treatment of primary Raynaud's phenomenon. *Eur J Clin Pharmacol* 24:421-423, 1983.

O'Reilly MJG, et al: Controlled trial of plasma exchange in treatment of Raynaud's syndrome. *Br Med J* 2:1113-1115, 1979.

Porter JM, et al: Evaluation and management of patients with Raynaud's syndrome. *Am J Surg* 142:183-189, 1981.

Porter JM, et al: Pentoxifylline efficacy in treatment of intermittent claudication: Multicenter controlled double-blind trial with objective assessment of chronic occlusive arterial disease patients. *Am Heart J* 104:66-72, 1982.

Roald OK, Seem E: Treatment of Raynaud's phenomenon with ketanserin in patients with connective tissue disorders. *Br Med J* 289:577-579, 1984.

Rodeheffer RJ, et al: Controlled double-blind trial of nifedipine in treatment of Raynaud's phenomenon. *N Engl J Med* 308:880-883, 1983.

Ruckley CV, et al: Naftidrofuryl for intermittent claudication: Double-blind controlled trial. *Br Med J* 1:622-623, 1978.

Schatz IJ: Medical management of chronic occlusive arterial disease of extremities. *Cardiovasc Clin* 3:94-102, 1971.

Schatz IJ, et al: Thromboangiitis obliterans. *Br Heart J* 28:84-91, 1966.

Smith CD, McKendry RJR: Controlled trial of nifedipine in treatment of Raynaud's phenomenon. *Lancet* 2:1299-1301, 1982.

Sovijärvi ARA, et al: Transdermal nitroglycerin in treatment of Raynaud's phenomenon: Analysis of digital blood pressure changes after cold provocation. *Curr Ther Res* 35:832-839, 1984.

Surwit RS, et al: Intra-arterial reserpine for Raynaud's syndrome: Systemic reactions without therapeutic benefit. *Arch Dermatol* 119:733-735, 1983.

Surwit RS, et al: Double-blind study of prazosin in treatment of Raynaud's phenomenon in scleroderma. *Arch Dermatol* 120:329-331, 1984.

Varadi DP, Lawrence AM: Suppression of Raynaud's phenomenon by methyldopa. *Arch Intern Med* 124:13-18, 1969.

Verstraete M: Current therapy for intermittent claudication. *Drugs* 24:240-247, 1982.

Zsoter TT, Baird RJ: Isoxsuprine as oral vasodilator. *Can Med Assoc J* 110:1260-1261, 1974.

Agents Used to Treat Shock

27

PATIENT MONITORING

DRUG THERAPY

   Sympathomimetic Amines

   Vasodilators

   Other Agents

      Alkalizing Agents

      Digitalis Glycosides

      Adrenal Corticosteroids

      Opioid Antagonists

CLINICAL APPLICATIONS

   Hypovolemic Shock

   Cardiogenic Shock

   Septic Shock

DRUG EVALUATIONS

   Sympathomimetic Amines

   Vasodilators

Shock is caused by inadequate tissue perfusion and often is accompanied by increased sympathetic activity. Several of the following signs and symptoms usually are observed: mental obtundation, tachypnea, tachycardia, pallor, cold and clammy skin, oliguria, and metabolic acidosis. Most patients in shock are hypotensive, but the arterial pressure occasionally is normal, especially in those who were previously hypertensive. The goal of therapy is to ensure a sufficient blood flow for adequate perfusion of vital organs.

Hypotension usually does not require treatment unless there are signs or symptoms of tissue hypoperfusion. However, marked hypotension in the presence of coronary artery disease may lead to significant myocardial ischemia and arrhythmias. In such instances, arterial pressure should be raised to or toward normal levels.

The overriding concern of the clinician during management of shock states should be *maintenance of adequate intravascular volume.* Drug therapy is not the mainstay of treatment. Drugs should be used only when volume replacement and treatment of etiologic factors fail to maintain the circulation.

PATIENT MONITORING

Hemodynamic, metabolic, and respiratory variables should be monitored to detect potentially reversible disturbances and to assess the effectiveness of therapy. Hemodynamic measurements should include continuous electrocardiographic monitoring of cardiac rate and rhythm, intra-arterial pressure (preferably measured directly by an indwelling catheter), and pulmonary artery end-diastolic or pulmonary capillary wedge pressure using a Swan-Ganz flow-directed catheter. The pulmonary artery end-diastolic or wedge pressure usually provides a reliable estimate of left ventricular filling pressure and is particularly useful to evaluate the response to fluid challenge. Cardiac output can be increased in some patients by raising the wedge pressure to 18 to 20 mm Hg. Routine measurement of cardiac output is no longer considered mandatory (Weil and Shubin, 1974) but may be useful as wedge pressure is increased by plasma volume expansion.

Arterial blood gases, serum electrolytes and osmolality, skin and core temperature, fluid intake and output, urine osmolality, and plasma colloid osmotic pressure also should be monitored in some instances (Weil and Shubin, 1974; Weil et al, 1978). The arterial blood lactate level quantifies the extent of anaerobic metabolism and is useful as an indicator of perfusion failure. Patients who ultimately survive have been found to have normal or only slightly elevated blood lactate levels before therapy (Ruiz et al, 1979).

DRUG THERAPY

When shock is caused by inadequate circulating blood volume, blood or plasma volume expanders should be administered (see Chapter 35, Blood, Blood Components, and Blood Substitutes). In normovolemic patients and those who do not respond to adequate plasma volume expansion, sympathomimetic amines and other drugs may be indicated as a temporary expedient until definitive therapy becomes effective or the underlying pathologic state is corrected.

Sympathomimetic Amines

Except in patients with anaphylactic shock or life-threatening hypotension, sympathomimetic amines should not be the initial therapy. The purpose of employing these drugs is to improve tissue perfusion and not to keep the blood pressure at an arbitrary level. The need for and response to a sympathomimetic amine should be assessed on the basis of cerebral and myocardial function, urinary output, peripheral skin (toe) temperature, and the arterial blood lactate level. The rate of infusion must be regulated carefully so that the desired level of blood pressure is not exceeded. Generally, the systolic blood pressure should be maintained between 90 and 100 mm Hg or somewhat higher in previously hypertensive patients.

Actions and Uses: To be effective, sympathomimetic amines should maintain perfusion of the heart, brain, kidney, and other visceral organs by one or more of the following mechanisms: (1) enhancement of myocardial contractility, which increases cardiac output as long as venous return is adequate (however, in patients with coronary artery disease, myocardial oxygen demand may exceed supply if there is a marked increase in contractility); (2) constriction of capacitance vessels, which shifts venous blood centrally; and (3) dilation of resistance vessels, which increases blood flow to vital organs preferentially without affecting resistance vessels in nonvital organs.

Sympathomimetic amines mimic the effects of sympathetic nerve stimulation, and their effects vary according to their interaction with several types of cardiovascular adrenergic receptors. Three distinct receptors have been described: alpha-adrenergic, beta-adrenergic, and dopaminergic. These receptors differ in the actions they subserve and in their distribution in the cardiovascular system. Alpha-adrenergic receptors are present in most blood vessels but are most abundant in the resistance vessels of the skin, mucosa, intestine, and kidney. Drugs that activate peripheral alpha receptors produce greater vasoconstriction in these vascular beds. Two classes of peripheral alpha receptors have been identified pharmacologically: alpha$_1$ and alpha$_2$. Both types are found at postsynaptic sites where they mediate smooth muscle contraction. Alpha$_2$ receptors are also located on the presynaptic membrane where they regulate the release of norepinephrine from sympathetic nerve terminals. Stimulation of these receptors by high concentrations of norepinephrine in the synaptic cleft inhibits the subsequent release of norepinephrine by a negative feedback mechanism.

There are also two types of beta-adrenergic receptors: Beta$_1$ receptors subserve cardiac stimulation and beta$_2$ receptors subserve bronchial relaxation and vasodilation in peripheral arterioles. Drugs acting on beta$_1$ receptors increase myocardial contractility and heart rate, accelerate A-V conduction, and increase automaticity. Those acting on beta$_2$ receptors cause vasodilation, primarily in arterioles of skeletal muscles and mesenteric vascular beds, and bronchial relaxation. Dopaminergic receptors subserve vasodilation in the renal and mesenteric vascular beds and also are found in the coronary and cerebral circulations (Goldberg, 1972).

Sympathomimetic drugs act directly on adrenergic receptors or indirectly by liberating norepinephrine from tissue stores. Theoretically, indirect-acting agents (eg, metaraminol [Aramine]) may become ineffective after prolonged administration or during concomitant use of a catecholamine-depleting agent, such as reserpine or guanethidine [Ismelin].

Sympathomimetic amines used to treat shock include the endogenous catecholamines, norepinephrine (levarterenol) [Levophed], epinephrine [Adrenalin], and dopamine [Dopastat, Intropin], and the synthetic compounds, dobutamine [Dobutrex], isoproterenol [Isuprel], and metaraminol. Other sympathomimetic amines (ephedrine, mephentermine [Wyamine], methoxamine [Vasoxyl], and phenylephrine [Neo-Synephrine]) are used as pressor agents during anesthesia and cardiopulmonary resuscitation and are not generally employed in the treatment of most forms of shock.

Dopamine is the amine most commonly used as a temporary adjunct in the treatment of shock. It stimulates the heart primarily by a direct action on beta$_1$ receptors in the myocardium and, to a lesser extent, by releasing norepinephrine from tissue stores. Small doses may increase cardiac output by producing vasodilation in the renal and mesenteric vascular beds (action on dopaminergic receptors). Moderate doses activate beta receptors, which increases myocardial contractility, heart rate, and cardiac output. With large doses, the effect on alpha receptors is predominant, and arterial vasoconstriction increases arterial resistance and elevates blood pressure.

Norepinephrine stimulates the myocardium and increases cardiac output by acting on beta$_1$ receptors; it constricts the peripheral vessels by activating alpha receptors. With small doses, the inotropic action is predominant; with larger doses, the vasoconstrictor effect becomes more prominent. Cardiac work and myocardial oxygen consumption are increased, and blood flow may be reduced to all areas except the heart and brain. Norepinephrine is a more potent vasoconstrictor than dopamine.

Dobutamine acts primarily on beta$_1$ receptors and has less pronounced actions on beta$_2$ and alpha receptors. Moderate doses increase myocardial contractility and cardiac output without greatly increasing heart rate or altering blood pressure. This agent is used for inotropic support when cardiac decompensation is secondary to reduced myocardial contractility.

Metaraminol stimulates the myocardium and causes vasoconstriction, mainly by releasing norepinephrine from adrenergic nerve terminals. The hemodynamic actions and uses of metaraminol are similar to those of norepinephrine, but its duration of action is longer and it may be administered by either the intravenous or intramuscular route.

Isoproterenol acts on beta$_1$ receptors in the heart and beta$_2$ receptors in blood vessels, thereby elevating cardiac output and increasing blood flow, mainly in skeletal muscle. It usually produces pronounced tachycardia through a direct action on the heart and activation of baroreceptor reflexes. Small to moderate doses of isoproterenol increase systolic pressure and decrease diastolic pressure; the mean arterial pressure remains relatively unchanged. The increase in systolic pressure is caused by the drug's effect on myocardial contractility and cardiac output; the decrease in diastolic pressure is related to arteriolar dilation and reduction of peripheral vascular resistance. With large doses, systolic pressure also may decrease, despite the intense cardiac stimulation, because of the marked reduction in peripheral vascular resistance.

Isoproterenol is used primarily to treat bradyarrhythmias

prior to pacemaker insertion. It is no longer regarded as an appropriate agent for the management of low output states. The major disadvantages of isoproterenol are that it directs blood away from vital organs by its vasodilator action, it produces a disproportionate increase in myocardial oxygen requirements, and it may cause significant arrhythmias, particularly in the ischemic myocardium (Gunnar et al, 1967). Isoproterenol has been replaced by dobutamine and low-dose dopamine.

Epinephrine acts on beta$_1$ receptors in the heart and on both alpha and beta$_2$ receptors in peripheral blood vessels. Small doses dilate skeletal muscle and mesenteric arterial blood vessels and may decrease blood pressure, but even small amounts constrict cutaneous and renal blood vessels. When administered in large doses, the vasoconstrictor action predominates and blood pressure is increased. Epinephrine is used to enhance defibrillation during cardiopulmonary resuscitation and is a most useful inotropic drug after bypass surgery in which cold cardioplegia is used. Because it dilates constricted bronchioles (by acting on beta$_2$ receptors) and also raises blood pressure, epinephrine is the drug of choice for anaphylactic shock. (See Chapter 62, Agents for Active and Passive Immunity.)

The role of the nonadrenergic inotropic agent, amrinone, in shock is as yet unsettled.

Adverse Reactions and Precautions: It should be re-emphasized that vasopressor drugs are not a mainstay in the management of shock and conservative use of these agents is urged. Vasopressors are not clearly life-saving except when hypotension is associated with (1) life-threatening conduction defects or ventricular arrhythmias that respond to an increase in aortic, and thus coronary perfusion, pressure; (2) life-threatening pulmonary edema when an increase in aortic pressure is necessary to maintain renal perfusion pressure and diuresis; and (3) cerebral edema due to trauma, infection, or metabolic disease when brain viability must be secured by maintaining an arterial pressure/intracranial pressure perfusion gradient of at least 50 mm Hg.

Therapeutic doses of sympathomimetic amines may cause headache, restlessness, anxiety, weakness, pallor, dizziness, tremor, precordial pain, palpitations, and respiratory distress. Overdosage can induce convulsions, cerebral hemorrhage, and tachyarrhythmias. Excessive cardiac acceleration may reduce cardiac filling time, myocardial efficiency, coronary blood flow, and cardiac output. Fatal ventricular arrhythmias may be precipitated by sympathomimetic amines that have cardiac excitatory actions; therefore, the electrocardiogram should be monitored closely and the drug discontinued or the dosage reduced if an arrhythmia develops. Arrhythmias occur most frequently after administration of large doses, during the initial stage of infusion, and in patients with organic heart disease and/or severe shock complicated by extreme hypoxia and electrolyte imbalance. Digitalis therapy also may increase the risk of arrhythmias.

Prolonged administration of vasoconstrictor sympathomimetic amines may reduce plasma volume because constriction of the postcapillary vessels increases capillary pressure and facilitates transcapillary fluid loss. Renal blood flow and the glomerular filtration rate, already decreased by hypotension and compensatory vasoconstriction, may be reduced further by amines that constrict the renal vasculature. Severe metabolic acidosis and acute tubular necrosis may ensue.

Various pathologic changes have been attributed to the prolonged administration of large doses of sympathomimetic amines, particularly norepinephrine. These include edema, hemorrhage, and necrosis of the intestine, liver, and kidneys, as well as focal myocarditis, subpericardial hemorrhage, intravascular platelet aggregation, and local slough and gangrene of fingers or toes, especially in patients with pre-existing vascular disease. These changes are most common in patients in severe shock, and it is often difficult to determine whether they are caused by drug therapy or by the shock process alone. Prolonged administration of large doses of norepinephrine produces diffuse necrotic myocardial lesions in experimental animals, and similar lesions have been observed in patients who died after prolonged infusion (Haft, 1974).

Extravasation of norepinephrine or dopamine may produce local skin necrosis and slough involving subcutaneous and even muscle tissues. These effects can be minimized by prompt infiltration of phentolamine [Regitine] at the site of infusion (Zucker et al, 1960).

Recurrent hypotension may follow sudden withdrawal of sympathomimetic amines after several days or weeks of therapy, or sensitivity may be lost gradually during the infusion. The fall in arterial blood pressure may be due to generalized loss of vascular tone or, more probably, to hypovolemia that develops during the infusion. To avoid this complication, an attempt should be made to discontinue therapy as soon as possible. It may be necessary to accept a short period of hypotension if there is no evidence of tissue hypoperfusion. If there is difficulty in withdrawing the drug, appropriate fluids should be infused and the blood pressure and pulmonary artery wedge pressure should be monitored. Use of sympathomimetic amines should not be resumed until the systolic blood pressure falls close to the previous shock level and signs and symptoms of inadequate tissue perfusion are observed. If fluid replacement is unsuccessful, another attempt should be made to discontinue the drug five or ten minutes later. It may be necessary to repeat this procedure several times. A more gradual weaning process is recommended by some clinicians.

Vasodilators

Actions and Uses: Vasodilators are employed in selected patients with severe pump failure following acute myocardial infarction and in refractory chronic congestive heart failure (see Chapter 23). The objectives are to increase cardiac output by reducing peripheral vascular resistance (afterload reduction), to relieve pulmonary congestion by increasing venous capacitance (preload reduction), and to limit the extent of ischemic damage by reducing myocardial oxygen demand and increasing myocardial oxygen supply. Agents that produce both venodilation and arterial dilation are more useful than those with minimal action on veins. Vasodilators are generally not used alone in shock states but are sometimes given in conjunction with sympathomimetic amines.

The intravenously administered direct-acting vasodilators, nitroglycerin [Nitro-Bid IV, Nitrostat IV, Tridil] and sodium nitroprusside [Nipride, Nitropress], have been used most commonly. Both drugs may be given with dopamine or dobutamine to further enhance cardiac output. Nitroglycerin acts mainly on venous capacitance vessels and has less effect on resistance vessels. It also dilates the large epicardial (conductance) arteries in the coronary circulation.

Nitroprusside has a more pronounced effect on resistance vessels and is more effective in increasing cardiac output. In contrast to nitroglycerin, the primary action of nitroprusside in the coronary circulation is on resistance rather than conductance vessels. It may increase coronary arteriovenous shunting and theoretically may reduce myocardial perfusion by this action (coronary "steal"). Nitroprusside also may increase pulmonary arteriovenous shunting and consequently reduce arterial oxygen tension.

The alpha-adrenergic blocking drug, phentolamine, blocks both alpha$_1$ and alpha$_2$ receptors. It reduces peripheral resistance and venous tone, but tachycardia limits its usefulness and the drug is expensive.

Nonparenteral vasodilators are used mainly for long-term therapy in patients with severe, refractory, chronic congestive heart failure (see Chapter 23); sublingual, topical, and, occasionally, oral nitrates also have been administered after acute myocardial infarction. Angiotensin-converting enzyme inhibitors and calcium channel blocking agents may have beneficial hemodynamic effects in some patients with acute myocardial infarction, but their use is still experimental.

Adverse Reactions and Precautions: Hypotension is the major risk associated with use of vasodilator drugs, and constant hemodynamic monitoring is essential when these drugs are used in patients with signs of shock. When heart failure is not severe, vasodilators may diminish rather than increase cardiac output and thereby reduce coronary perfusion pressure and coronary blood flow and thus worsen myocardial ischemia. The use of vasodilators in acute myocardial infarction with shock may further reduce an already low coronary perfusion pressure to hazardous levels.

Reflex tachycardia is not usually a significant complication of therapy with nitroglycerin or nitroprusside, but it may occur occasionally with phentolamine. Severe hypotension with sinus bradycardia has been reported in patients receiving nitroglycerin. In patients with chronic congestive heart failure, rapid withdrawal of vasodilator drugs occasionally has precipitated acute left ventricular failure (see also Chapter 23).

Other Agents

Alkalizing Agents: Metabolic acidosis that occurs during shock is usually caused by perfusion failure and accumulation of acid metabolites. Measures that improve tissue perfusion generally correct the acidosis, and the use of sodium bicarbonate is falling into disfavor. The heart performs quite well during acidosis but does not respond well to alkalosis, and overcor-

rection with alkalizing agents can be more hazardous than undercorrection. Sodium bicarbonate may produce a paradoxical respiratory acidosis that affects both the brain and myocardial tissue; in the case of the myocardium, myocardial contractility may be reduced significantly and arrhythmias may develop. Even under the most extreme conditions of cardiac arrest, sodium bicarbonate is of unproven value. The possibility that organic buffers, such as tromethamine [THAM], may be more useful is under investigation.

Digitalis Glycosides: In cardiogenic shock, digitalis may improve left ventricular function if congestive heart failure continues after arterial pressure is established. The addition of digoxin to nitroprusside therapy may further increase cardiac output but does not further reduce the pulmonary capillary wedge pressure (Raabe, 1979). The rationale for using digitalis in other forms of shock is based on the observation that myocardial function is usually depressed during prolonged shock; its effectiveness in improving myocardial function in this setting is *not* established.

Adrenal Corticosteroids: Steroids are advocated by some investigators for treating septic shock because of experiments demonstrating that these agents stabilize lysosomal membranes and antagonize endotoxin. Steroids produce short-term improvement when very large doses are given for brief periods early in the course of septic shock, but they do not improve overall survival (Sprung et al, 1984). Steroids are specific treatment for patients in shock associated with adrenal insufficiency (addisonian crisis) and may have a supplemental role in anaphylactic shock (see Chapter 62, Agents for Active and Passive Immunity). There is no convincing evidence that they are useful in other forms of shock.

Opioid Antagonists: In laboratory animals, endogenous opioids are released in response to stress and may contribute to the pathogenesis of shock (Faden, 1984). The opioid antagonist, naloxone [Narcan], improves cardiovascular function and survival in experimental shock models, and several reports have described beneficial effects of naloxone infusion in patients with septic shock. Controlled studies are necessary to determine the safety and efficacy of this form of treatment.

CLINICAL APPLICATIONS

Hypovolemic Shock: Hypovolemic shock may result from external or internal loss of blood, plasma, or water following hemorrhage, trauma, burns, or protracted vomiting or diarrhea. Venous return and cardiac output are reduced and peripheral resistance is usually increased by compensatory mechanisms. Volume replacement is the only effective treatment, and fluid challenge should be guided by measurement of the pulmonary capillary wedge or pulmonary artery end-diastolic pressure in order to produce an optimal increase in cardiac output without causing pulmonary edema.

Vasodilators are occasionally used to estimate the adequacy of volume replacement and to permit administration of a larger volume of fluid without overloading the heart. Volume replacement should always precede administration of the vasodilator, and fluid should be available in case the drug causes an acute fall in arterial pressure. Vasoconstrictors may be necessary in patients with profound hypotension, especially if ventricular arrhythmias supervene, but they should not be used for prolonged periods because they may increase ischemic injury by further reducing blood flow through vital organs.

Cardiogenic Shock: The most common cause of cardiogenic shock is acute myocardial infarction, although myocardial depression also occurs in other forms of shock. The hemodynamic pattern is not always predictable but, in most patients, cardiac output is reduced, pulmonary wedge pressure is elevated, and peripheral vascular resistance is increased. Even under the best circumstances, cardiogenic shock is difficult to treat because of extensive myocardial necrosis, and mechanical cardiac assist systems and/or cardiac surgery are often required.

By increasing peripheral vascular resistance and arterial blood pressure, sympathomimetic amines may improve coronary perfusion. Some agents also improve blood flow to the renal and mesenteric vascular beds. Those that stimulate the myocardium may increase cardiac output, but sympathomimetic amines should be used with caution because they increase myocardial oxygen consumption by a direct effect on myocardial metabolism and by imposing extra pressure work on the heart. Whether the increased oxygen requirements are met by an adequate increase in coronary blood flow will ultimately depend upon the effect of the amine on the blood pressure, especially the diastolic pressure, which is the main determinant of perfusion through the coronary vessels.

Dopamine [Dopastat, Intropin] is often the preferred sympathomimetic drug for initial therapy provided that adequate perfusion pressure is maintained and heart rate does not increase too greatly. Dopamine produces less vasoconstriction than norepinephrine and is less likely to cause skin necrosis if extravasation occurs. It causes less vasodilation and tachycardia than isoproterenol and, in appropriate doses, it may increase blood flow to the kidneys and mesentery (Goldberg, 1972).

Because it acts rapidly and is the most potent pressor agent available, norepinephrine [Levophed] may be required in patients with severe hypotension. This drug should not be used for prolonged periods because it may cause ischemia of vital organs and may deplete the plasma volume.

Dobutamine [Dobutrex] is being employed with increasing frequency. Its hemodynamic effects in acute myocardial infarction are comparable to those attained with combined dopamine-nitroprusside therapy (Keung et al, 1981). Dobutamine may be useful in patients with acute circulatory collapse who have severely impaired pump function, low cardiac output, and elevated left ventricular filling pressure, provided that marked hypotension is not present (Francis et al, 1982). A combination of dopamine and dobutamine may be of value in selected patients (Leier and Unverferth, 1983).

In a minority of patients, hypotension accompanying acute myocardial infarction is associated with hypovolemia and a normal or low wedge pressure. The most common cause may be excessive vasoconstriction due to endogenous or exogenous adrenergic amines. Such patients may benefit from plasma volume expansion, but wedge pressure should be monitored closely (Figueras and Weil, 1979). A subset of patients who present with electrocardiographic signs of inferior infarction have infarction of the right ventricle. These patients are often hypotensive with normal or low wedge pressure and elevated central venous and right atrial pressures. Fluid administration usually improves their hemodynamic status.

Vasodilator drugs may be useful in selected patients with severe pump failure following acute myocardial infarction (Cohn and Burke, 1979). They appear to be most appropriate for patients with recurrent ischemic pain, increased vascular resistance, or a marked elevation of left ventricular filling pressure. Vasodilators generally are not used alone in shock states; they are most often added to a sympathomimetic amine, such as dopamine or dobutamine.

Therapy is initiated with an intravenous vasodilator; nitroglycerin [Nitro-Bid IV, Nitrostat IV, Tridil] and sodium nitroprusside [Nipride, Nitropress] have been used most frequently. In patients with ongoing ischemia, nitroglycerin is the drug of choice because it improves the regional distribution of myocardial flow and, in contrast to nitroprusside, does not produce coronary steal. In low output states, nitroprusside is preferred for initial use. When continued treatment is indicated, a nonparenteral nitrate may be substituted after about 72 hours. Sublingual or topical nitrates have been used occasionally for initial therapy.

If the systolic pressure falls below 90 mm Hg during vasodilator therapy, the drug should be discontinued or the dosage reduced. The fall in pressure may be abrupt; therefore, the arterial pressure should be monitored carefully.

Vasodilator therapy has improved short-term prognosis, but long-term prognosis remains unfavorable despite continued therapy with oral nitrates. Although the hemodynamic effects of combining a vasodilator with a sympathomimetic amine appear to be beneficial, there is no evidence that short-term prognosis is improved more with combined therapy than with a single agent.

Septic Shock: Shock may occur during the course of gram-negative or, less commonly, gram-positive bacterial infections. The most susceptible groups are patients receiving immunosuppressive therapy, elderly patients with chronic diseases, trauma or burn patients, and those who have undergone gastrointestinal or genitourinary surgery. The severity, hemodynamic changes, and response to therapy vary widely, depending upon the age of the patient, virulence of the bacteria, presence of concurrent disease or other factors (eg, diabetes mellitus, ischemic heart disease, surgery, trauma), and stage of the syndrome. Septic shock is associated with a defect in the distribution of blood flow and is classified as a distributive form of shock. In gram-negative bacteremia, the effective blood volume is reduced because of pooling in the venous capacitance bed; peripheral vascular resistance is usually low or normal. In gram-positive bacteremia, the perfusion deficit may be caused by fluid loss due to increased vascular permeability. Because arteriovenous shunting is increased, peripheral resistance is usually reduced.

Septic shock requires immediate drainage of pus, excision of necrotic tissue, and intensive antibiotic therapy. An adequate circulating volume should be maintained and blood gases monitored closely. Oxygen should be administered if there is evidence of hypoxemia. Whether sympathomimetic amines should be used adjunctively remains controversial. If a pressor or inotropic agent is employed, dopamine or dobutamine is usually preferred. If adequate perfusion pressure is not maintained with one of these agents, small doses of norepinephrine may be required for brief periods. Sympathomimetic amines should not be used routinely, because they may deplete intravascular volume, increase the workload of the heart, and increase myocardial oxygen demand.

Anaphylactic Shock: See Chapter 62, Agents for Active and Passive Immunity.

Drug Evaluations

SYMPATHOMIMETIC AMINES

DOPAMINE HYDROCHLORIDE
[Dopastat, Intropin]

ACTIONS. Dopamine exerts a positive inotropic effect through a direct action on beta-adrenergic receptors and release of norepinephrine from tissue storage sites. Hemodynamic effects vary with dosage. Small doses (less than 5 mcg/kg/min) activate dopaminergic receptors in the renal and mesenteric vascular beds to produce vasodilation. Slightly larger doses (5 to 10 mcg/kg/min) maintain the effect on dopaminergic receptors and also activate beta receptors; as a result, myocardial contractility, heart rate, and cardiac output are increased. With larger doses (more than 10 mcg/kg/min), vasoconstriction (alpha-adrenergic effect) predominates and renal blood flow may be reduced; when this occurs, urine output may decrease.

USES. Dopamine is usually the preferred sympathomimetic amine for treating shock when the marked vasoconstrictor activity of norepinephrine is unnecessary. It is a more potent pressor agent than dobutamine and is preferred to the latter drug in patients with marked hypotension and shock. Because of its unique hemodynamic effects, dopamine often is more beneficial than other sympathomimetic amines in patients with impaired renal function. Small doses (1 mcg/kg/minute) may promote diuresis in the early stages of acute oliguric renal failure.

In selected patients, a combination of dopamine with nitroprusside, nitroglycerin, or dobutamine may produce more beneficial hemodynamic effects than any of these drugs used alone. (See also Goldberg, 1972.)

ADVERSE REACTIONS AND PRECAUTIONS. Dopamine may cause nausea, vomiting, headache, central nervous system stimulation, tachyarrhythmias, and anginal pain. In cardiogenic shock, the improvement in hemodynamic status induced by dopamine may be accompanied by an increase in myocardial oxygen consumption (Mueller et al, 1978). Small doses occasionally precipitate a fall in blood pressure, which can be corrected by intravenous fluid challenge.

Dopamine is less likely than norepinephrine to cause tissue necrosis following extravasation but, if extravasation occurs, the site should be infiltrated with 10 ml of a solution containing 5 to 10 mg of phentolamine; a fine hypodermic needle should be used. Infusion of dopamine for long periods or in large doses has caused peripheral ischemia and gangrene, necessitating skin grafts and occasionally amputation of an extremity. Bilateral retinal infarction, attributed to dopamine-induced constriction of retinal vessels, has been reported. For further information on the adverse effects of sympathomimetic drugs, see the Introduction.

DRUG INTERACTIONS. Since dopamine is metabolized by monoamine oxidase, the dose should be reduced to one-tenth the usual amount in patients receiving monoamine oxidase inhibitors.

Cardiac arrest occurred in one patient who was treated with dopamine after receiving a small dose of tolazoline.

DOSAGE AND PREPARATIONS.
Intravenous: *Adults,* a solution, preferably containing 400 mcg/ml, is prepared by diluting the contents of an ampul, vial, or additive syringe with sterile sodium chloride injection or 5% dextrose injection. (This is a more dilute solution than that recommended by the manufacturer.) Initially, the dilute solution is infused at a rate of 2 to 5 mcg/kg/min. In more seriously ill patients, an initial infusion rate of 5 mcg/kg/min may be increased gradually by 5 to 10 mcg/kg/min to 20 to 30 mcg/kg/min. If larger doses are required, the urine output and electrocardiogram should be monitored closely. When dopamine is to be discontinued, protracted treatment with gradual reduction of the dose over hours or days should be avoided because a decrease in blood pressure may occur when the dose falls below the inotropic level. It is frequently necessary to add fluid as the drug is discontinued.

Generic. Solution 40 mg/ml in 5 and 10 ml containers and 80 mg/ml in 5 ml containers.
Dopastat (Parke-Davis). Solution 40 mg/ml in 5 ml containers.
Intropin (American Critical Care). Solution (aqueous) 40, 80, and 160 mg/ml in 5 ml containers.

DOBUTAMINE HYDROCHLORIDE
[Dobutrex]

ACTIONS AND USES. Dobutamine acts primarily on myocardial beta$_1$ receptors; it has balanced or less pronounced effects on beta$_2$ and alpha receptors and does not activate dopaminergic receptors. Moderate doses increase myocardial contractility and cardiac output and may reduce peripheral vascular resistance and ventricular filling pressure; large doses may increase heart rate and blood pressure. In animal studies, equivalent inotropic doses of dobutamine had less than one-fourth the chronotropic effect of isoproterenol.

Dobutamine is used primarily to treat severe, refractory, chronic congestive heart failure and for inotropic support after cardiac surgery (see Chapter 23, Agents Used to Treat Heart Failure). It may be useful in acute circulatory failure secondary to depressed myocardial contractility (Francis et al, 1982), but dopamine or norepinephrine is preferred when marked hypotension is present (Leier and Unverferth, 1983). In patients with acute myocardial infarction complicated by hypotension and severe left ventricular dysfunction, the hemodynamic effects of dobutamine are comparable to those obtained with combined dopamine and nitroprusside therapy (Keung et al, 1981).

ADVERSE REACTIONS AND PRECAUTIONS. Dobutamine occasionally causes nausea, headache, palpitations, anginal pain, and shortness of breath. Tachycardia and systolic hypertension, the most common adverse effects, usually can be controlled by reducing the dose. Ventricular arrhythmias occur occasionally. Since dobutamine facilitates A-V conduction, it may increase the ventricular rate in patients with atrial fibrillation.

DOSAGE AND PREPARATIONS. Dobutamine is incompatible with alkaline solutions and should not be mixed with sodium bicarbonate injection. It may be reconstituted with sterile water or 5% dextrose injection by adding 10 to 20 ml of diluent to the vial containing 250 mg of dobutamine. This solution can be stored for 48 hours when refrigerated or six hours at room temperature. It must be diluted to at least 50 ml before infusion and should be used within 24 hours.

Intravenous: Adults, potentially beneficial hemodynamic effects in patients with acute myocardial infarction have been reported with doses ranging from 8 to 24 mcg/kg/min.

Dobutrex (Lilly). Powder (sterile, lyophilized) 250 mg.

METARAMINOL BITARTRATE
[Aramine]

ACTIONS AND USES. The effects of metaraminol depend largely upon the release of norepinephrine from sympathetic nerve endings. Its hemodynamic effects and uses are similar to those of norepinephrine, except that metaraminol is less potent and has a more gradual onset and longer duration of action. In contrast to norepinephrine, it may be given intramuscularly as well as intravenously, for it does not cause tissue necrosis. In addition to its use in shock, metaraminol is used to treat paroxysmal atrial tachycardia, as are other pressor agents (see Chapter 24, Antiarrhythmic Agents).

ADVERSE REACTIONS AND PRECAUTIONS. Theoretically, the effect of metaraminol may lessen after prolonged adminis-

tration or with concomitant use of a catecholamine-depleting agent (eg, reserpine, guanethidine). If this complication occurs, norepinephrine should be substituted.

For a general discussion of adverse effects of sympathomimetic amines, see the Introduction.

DOSAGE AND PREPARATIONS.
Intravenous: Adults, 1.5 to 10 mcg/kg/min.
Intramuscular: Adults, 5 to 10 mg; *children,* 0.1 mg/kg.
Generic. Solution 1% (10 mg/ml) in 10 ml containers.
Aramine (Merck Sharp & Dohme). Solution (sterile) 1% (equivalent to 10 mg of base/ml) in 10 ml containers.

NOREPINEPHRINE BITARTRATE
[Levophed]

ACTIONS AND USES. This catecholamine has positive inotropic and chronotropic effects and a potent constrictor action on resistance and capacitance vessels. Its marked pressor effect is primarily due to increased peripheral resistance. Despite its direct positive chronotropic effects, norepinephrine may indirectly reduce the heart rate by reflex mechanisms. Norepinephrine has a prompt and reversible action and is used to treat shock when a potent vasoconstrictor is needed to maintain adequate tissue perfusion.

ADVERSE REACTIONS AND PRECAUTIONS. Norepinephrine can cause tissue necrosis at the site of injection. The risk of ischemic injury is reduced if the drug is infused via a catheter in a deeply seated vein and if a small amount of phentolamine is added to the solution. The infusion site should be changed when prolonged administration is necessary. If extravasation occurs, the site should be infiltrated with 10 ml of a solution containing 5 to 10 mg of phentolamine; a fine hypodermic needle should be used. To reduce the incidence of venous thrombosis, heparin may be added to the infusion solution in amounts supplying 100 to 200 units/hour.

For a general discussion of adverse effects of sympathomimetic amines, see the Introduction.

DOSAGE AND PREPARATIONS.
Intravenous: Adults, 0.03 to 0.15 mcg/kg/min.
Levophed (Winthrop-Breon). Solution (sterile, aqueous) equivalent to 1 mg of base/ml in 4 ml containers.

VASODILATORS

NITROGLYCERIN (for intravenous use)
[Nitro-Bid IV, Nitrostat IV, Tridil]

ACTIONS. Nitroglycerin is a direct-acting vasodilator with a greater effect on the venous than the arterial circulation. Its effect on coronary blood flow depends in part on the status of the coronary circulation. Nitroglycerin dilates the large epicardial (conductance) arteries but has little effect on intramyocardial (resistance) vessels. In the normal nonischemic myocardium, total coronary blood flow may increase temporarily and then may decrease if the central aortic pressure falls substantially. In patients with coronary artery disease, however, nitroglycerin improves the regional distribution of myocardial blood flow and oxygen supply by dilating large atherosclerotic coronary arteries and collateral vessels. Spasm of normal and diseased arteries may be decreased both in angina and in prolonged episodes of ischemia or infarction.

USES. Nitroglycerin is given intravenously to reduce myocardial ischemia and improve hemodynamics in patients with severe left ventricular dysfunction complicating acute myocardial infarction (Sorkin et al, 1984). It is indicated primarily in those who have recurrent ischemic pain or marked elevation of left ventricular filling pressure and pulmonary edema. Intravenous nitroglycerin relieves pulmonary congestion, decreases myocardial oxygen consumption, and reduces ST segment elevation. A decrease in infarct size or mortality is not established, but preliminary results suggest that these endpoints may be favorably affected if treatment is begun less than 10 hours after the onset of symptoms (Flaherty et al, 1983).

ADVERSE REACTIONS AND PRECAUTIONS. Nitroglycerin may cause headache, flushing, dizziness, hypotension, and tachycardia. Severe hypotension associated with sinus bradycardia has occurred in some patients. The bradycardia appears to be, at least in part, vagally mediated because it responds to atropine (Come and Pitt, 1976). Intravenous nitroglycerin preparations contain alcohol, and a considerable amount may be administered during prolonged infusion. See also the Introduction.

DOSAGE AND PREPARATIONS.
Caution: Several intravenous products are available that differ in concentration and/or volume per vial. The manufacturers' literature should be consulted for dilution instructions, and care should be taken when substituting one preparation for another. Nitroglycerin should be diluted with dextrose 5% injection or sodium chloride 0.9% injection and should not be mixed with other drugs. Dilution and storage should be made only in *glass* containers. (Plastic tubing will absorb considerable amounts of nitroglycerin until it becomes saturated.) A solution containing 100 mcg/ml may be used for initial dosage titration; a more concentrated solution may be substituted if it is necessary to limit fluids.

Intravenous: Adults, initially 5 mcg/min of dilute solution is infused. Dosage may be increased by 5 mcg/min every three to five minutes until a response is noted. If no response is observed with a dose of 20 mcg/min, increments of 10 and later 20 mcg/min may be used. On occasion, it may be necessary to increase the infusion rate to 200 mcg/min or more to relieve chest pain, reduce pulmonary artery wedge pressure, and maintain near normal arterial perfusion pressure. Blood pressure and heart rate should be monitored continuously.

Generic. Solution (sterile) 5 mg/ml in 5 ml containers (alcohol 50%).
Nitro-Bid IV (Marion). Solution (sterile) 5 mg/ml in 1, 5, and 10 ml containers (alcohol 70%).
Nitrostat IV (Parke-Davis). Solution (sterile) 0.8 mg/ml in 10 ml containers (alcohol 5%) and 5 mg/ml in 10 ml containers (alcohol 30%) with or without delivery set.
Tridil (American Critical Care). Solution (sterile) 5 mg/ml in 5 and 10 ml containers (alcohol 30%) with or without delivery set (*Tridilset*).

SODIUM NITROPRUSSIDE
[Nipride, Nitropress]

$$Na_2\left[Fe(CN)_5NO\right] \cdot 2H_2O$$

ACTIONS. This direct-acting vasodilator affects both the venous and arterial beds. It has a more pronounced effect on afterload than does nitroglycerin and therefore is more likely to increase cardiac output. Since the primary action of nitroprusside in the coronary circulation is on resistance rather than conductance vessels, it could precipitate coronary steal. Nitroprusside may increase both myocardial and pulmonary arterial venous shunts; therefore, increases in total blood flow, including coronary blood flow, may not be representative of the portion of the flow that contributes to improved perfusion.

USES. Nitroprusside is used to treat severe persistent pump failure in patients with markedly reduced cardiac output and increased peripheral vascular resistance (Cohn and Burke, 1979). It is particularly useful in treating severe, acutely decompensated, chronic congestive heart failure refractory to digitalis and diuretics (see Chapter 23). The role of nitroprusside in the management of acute myocardial infarction is controversial. It may have beneficial effects in patients with a persistent, moderately severe elevation in pulmonary wedge pressure but may have detrimental effects in those with only a slight or moderate elevation in wedge pressure (Cohn et al, 1982). Nitroprusside is not useful for treating the ischemia of acute myocardial infarction.

ADVERSE REACTIONS AND PRECAUTIONS. As with all vasodilators, hypotension is the major adverse effect of nitroprusside. Tachycardia occurs occasionally. Thiocyanate may accumulate during prolonged infusion. If the drug is infused for more than 72 hours, blood thiocyanate levels should be determined daily. High levels of blood cyanide also may develop during infusion of large amounts. Nitroprusside may precipitate coronary steal. (See also the Introduction and Chapter 28, Antihypertensive Agents, for a more detailed discussion of adverse reactions.)

DOSAGE AND PREPARATIONS.
Intravenous: Adults, initially, a dilute solution is infused at a rate of 16 mcg/min. The subsequent infusion rate should be determined by hemodynamic monitoring.
Nipride (Roche), *Nitropress* (Abbott), *Generic.* Powder equivalent to sodium nitroprusside dihydrate 50 mg.

PHENTOLAMINE MESYLATE
[Regitine]

Phentolamine is an alpha-adrenergic blocking drug that acts on both pre- and postsynaptic alpha receptors. It also has a direct relaxant effect on vascular smooth muscle. Both peripheral resistance and venous tone are reduced. Phentolamine has been used to improve left ventricular function in patients with acute myocardial infarction and to increase venous capacitance as an adjunct to volume replacement in hypovolemic shock.

Marked hypotension and tachycardia are the major side effects of phentolamine. The tachycardia, which has been attributed to enhanced release of norepinephrine resulting from presynaptic alpha blockade, limits this drug's usefulness in patients with acute myocardial infarction (see also Chapter 28, Antihypertensive Agents).

DOSAGE AND PREPARATIONS.

Intravenous: *Adults,* initially, a dilute solution is infused at a rate of 10 mcg/kg/min. The subsequent infusion rate should be determined by hemodynamic monitoring.

Regitine (CIBA). Powder (lyophilized, for solution) 5 mg.

Cited References

Cohn JN, Burke LP: Nitroprusside. *Ann Intern Med* 91:752-757, 1979.

Cohn JN, et al: Effect of short-term infusion of sodium nitroprusside on mortality rate in acute myocardial infarction complicated by left ventricular failure: Results of Veterans Administration cooperative study. *N Engl J Med* 306:1129-1135, 1982.

Come PC, Pitt B: Nitroglycerin-induced severe hypotension and bradycardia in patients with acute myocardial infarction. *Circulation* 54:624-628, 1976.

Faden AI: Opiate antagonists and thyrotropin-releasing hormone: I. Potential role in treatment of shock. *JAMA* 252:1177-1180, 1984.

Figueras J, Weil MH: Hypovolemia and hypotension complicating management of acute cardiogenic pulmonary edema. *Am J Cardiol* 44:1349-1411, 1979.

Flaherty JT, et al: Randomized prospective trial of intravenous nitroglycerin in patients with acute myocardial infarction. *Circulation* 68:576-588, 1983.

Francis GS, et al: Comparative hemodynamic effects of dopamine and dobutamine in patients with acute cardiogenic circulatory collapse. *Am Heart J* 103:995-1000, 1982.

Goldberg LI: Cardiovascular and renal action of dopamine: Potential clinical applications. *Pharmacol Rev* 24:1-29, 1972.

Gunnar RM, et al: Ineffectiveness of isoproterenol in shock due to acute myocardial infarction. *JAMA* 202:1124-1128, 1967.

Haft JI: Cardiovascular injury induced by sympathetic catecholamines. *Prog Cardiovasc Dis* 17:73-86, 1974.

Keung ECH, et al: Dobutamine therapy in acute myocardial infarction. *JAMA* 245:144-146, 1981.

Leier CV, Unverferth DV: Drugs five years later: Dobutamine. *Ann Intern Med* 99:490-496, 1983.

Mueller HS, et al: Effect of dopamine on hemodynamics and myocardial metabolism in shock following acute myocardial infarction in man. *Circulation* 57:361-365, 1978.

Raabe DS Jr: Combined therapy with digoxin and nitroprusside in heart failure complicating acute myocardial infarction. *Am J Cardiol* 43:990-994, 1979.

Ruiz CE, et al: Treatment of circulatory shock with dopamine: Studies on survival. *JAMA* 242:165-168, 1979.

Sorkin EM, et al: Intravenous glyceryl trinitrate (nitroglycerin): Review of its pharmacological properties and therapeutic efficacy. *Drugs* 27:45-80, 1984.

Sprung CL, et al: Effects of high-dose corticosteroids in patients with septic shock: Prospective, controlled study. *N Engl J Med* 311:1137-1143, 1984.

Weil MH, Shubin H: Monitoring and measurements during shock, in Schumer W, Nyhus LM: *Treatment of Shock: Principles and Practice.* Philadelphia, Lea & Febiger, 1974, 3-22.

Weil MH, et al: Relationship between colloid osmotic pressure and pulmonary artery wedge pressure in patients with acute cardiorespiratory failure. *Am J Med* 64:643-650, 1978.

Zucker G, et al: Treatment of shock and prevention of ischemic necrosis with levarterenol-phentolamine mixtures. *Circulation* 22:935-937, 1960.

Other Selected References

Amsterdam EA, et al: Vasodilators in myocardial infarction: Rationale and current status. *Drugs* 16:506-521, 1978.

Chatterjee K, Parmley WW: Vasodilator treatment for acute and chronic heart failure. *Br Heart J* 39:706-720, 1977.

Chatterjee K, et al: Effects of vasodilator therapy for severe pump failure in acute myocardial infarction on short-term and late prognosis. *Circulation* 53:797-802, 1976.

Cohn JN, Franciosa JA: Vasodilator therapy of cardiac failure. *N Engl J Med* 297:27-31, 254-258, 1977.

da Luz PL, et al: Current concepts on mechanisms and treatment of cardiogenic shock. *Am Heart J* 92:103-113, 1976.

Gunnar RM, et al: Cardiovascular assist devices in cardiogenic shock. *JAMA* 236:1619-1621, 1976.

Johnson SA, Gunnar RM: Treatment of shock in myocardial infarction. *JAMA* 237:2106-2108, 1977.

Kuhn LA: Management of shock following acute myocardial infarction. I. Drug therapy. II. Mechanical circulatory assistance. *Am Heart J* 95:529-534, 789-795, 1978.

Makabali C, et al: Update on therapy for shock: Current concepts on mechanisms and management of circulatory shock. *Cardiovasc Rev Rep* 3:899-922, 1982.

Moran NC: Evaluation of pharmacologic basis for therapy of circulatory shock. *Am J Cardiol* 26:570-577, 1970.

Smith TE, Forgacs P: Haemodynamic interventions and therapy in septic shock. *Drugs* 24:75-82, 1982.

Tarazi RC: Sympathomimetic agents in treatment of shock. *Ann Intern Med* 81:364-371, 1974.

Weil MH: Current understanding of mechanisms and treatment of circulatory shock caused by bacterial infections. *Ann Clin Res* 9:181-191, 1977.

Weil MH, et al: Treatment of circulatory shock: Use of sympathomimetic and related vasoactive agents. *JAMA* 231:1280-1286, 1975.

Antihypertensive Agents

Hypertension is a significant risk factor for the development of major cardiovascular complications, including congestive heart failure, stroke, coronary artery disease, and progressive renal failure. Many authorities believe that a high sodium intake and obesity play important roles in the pathogenesis of this disorder and that its prevalence would be reduced if genetically susceptible individuals severely restricted their sodium intake and attained ideal body weight (Freis, 1976).

28

EFFECT OF ANTIHYPERTENSIVE THERAPY ON MORBIDITY AND MORTALITY

Moderate to Severe Hypertension: The benefits of treating moderate to severe hypertension were well established by the Veterans Administration (VA) Cooperative Study Group on Antihypertensive Agents (1967, 1970). In men with pretreatment diastolic pressures averaging 105 mm Hg or higher, drug therapy reduced the prevalence of congestive heart failure, stroke, dissecting aneurysm, and renal failure but did not significantly lessen the risk of myocardial infarction.

Mild Hypertension: The effect of antihypertensive therapy on mild hypertension is less clear-cut. In the VA studies, treatment did not significantly affect morbidity and mortality in men with pretreatment diastolic pressures of 90 to 104 mm Hg

unless they had pre-existing cardiovascular or renal abnormalities or were over the age of 50. Results of a U.S. Public Health Service Study on men and women with pretreatment diastolic pressures of 90 to 115 mm Hg showed that antihypertensive therapy reduced the incidence of left ventricular hypertrophy, cardiomegaly, and retinopathy and prevented further increases in blood pressure, but had no significant effect on the major endpoints of death, myocardial infarction, and stroke (Smith, 1977).

The Hypertension Detection and Follow-up Program (HDFP) Cooperative Group (1979, 1982, 1984) found that patients given free, systematic, stepped-care drug therapy in special centers achieved better control of blood pressure and lower five-year mortality from all causes than patients referred to their usual source of medical care. It is not certain what aspect of the intensive care program was responsible for the reduction in mortality. The differences were most marked in patients over age 50, men, black women, and patients with initial diastolic blood pressures of 90 to 104 mm Hg. These results were confirmed for patients with diastolic blood pressures of 95 mm Hg or higher by an Australian study. In a study conducted by the Medical Research Council Working Party (1985) on patients with initial diastolic pressures of 90 to 109 mm Hg, active treatment reduced the incidence of strokes, but not of coronary events. Mortality (all causes) was reduced in men but increased in women. The Multiple Risk Factor Intervention Trial (MRFIT) (1982) showed no benefit on mortality from multifactor risk intervention and also introduced the possibility that diuretic therapy may have increased mortality in men with pre-existing electrocardiographic abnormalities.

Systolic Hypertension: Isolated systolic hypertension in the elderly (systolic pressure exceeding 160 mm Hg, diastolic pressure less than 90) also is associated with increased morbidity and mortality. This disorder is caused by reduced aortic distensibility due to atherosclerosis, but it is not known whether complications are caused by elevated systolic pressure or atherosclerosis (Gifford, 1982). A large multicenter study is currently in progress in the United States to determine if antihypertensive therapy improves prognosis.

GUIDELINES FOR TREATMENT

Prior to beginning life-long treatment, the patient with mildly or moderately elevated blood pressure should be seen on at least three separate visits to determine whether the elevation persists, but treatment should not be delayed in those with severe hypertension. The extent of organic changes, particularly those affecting the optic fundi, brain, heart, and kidneys, should be assessed. Baseline measurements of blood chemistry (serum potassium, creatinine, glucose, and cholesterol), a complete blood count, urinalysis (protein, blood, and glucose), and an electrocardiogram should be obtained. Measurements of plasma renin activity (PRA) and urinary aldosterone, intravenous urography or digital subtraction angiography, renal angiography, tests for pheochromocytoma, or other special tests should be performed only when specific indications are present. Although PRA values vary and antihypertensive drugs differ in their effects on PRA (diuretics and vasodilators increase and antiadrenergic drugs decrease PRA), "renin profiling" generally is not considered practical for routine use (Gifford, 1980; Kaplan, 1977).

The Joint National Committee (JNC) on Detection, Evaluation, and Treatment of High Blood Pressure (1984) currently recommends drug therapy for patients whose diastolic pressures consistently exceed 95 mm Hg and for those with lesser elevations who have target organ damage, a family history of major cardiovascular complications, or other important risk factors (eg, hypercholesterolemia, diabetes mellitus, male sex, black race, cigarette smoking, age over 50 years). The JNC suggests that nonpharmacologic methods be employed initially in patients with diastolic pressures of 90 to 94 mm Hg who are otherwise at low risk. Other authorities recommend nonpharmacologic measures initially when there are few risk factors and diastolic pressure is below 100 mm Hg (Freis, 1982; Kaplan, 1983). Nonpharmacologic management includes weight reduction in the obese, decreased sodium intake, regular exercise, and moderation of alcohol consumption (Kaplan, 1985). If the blood pressure is not decreased in three to six months by nonpharmacologic methods, drug therapy may be instituted.

The major drugs used to treat hypertension are (1) diuretics, (2) antiadrenergic agents, (3) direct-acting vasodilators, (4) angiotensin-converting enzyme inhibitors, and (5) calcium channel blocking drugs. (See Table 1 for listing of available and investigational agents.) The selection of an appropriate drug or combination depends upon the severity of the disease and the patient's response to a therapeutic trial. It is not yet known which drugs or combinations are most effective in reducing the cardiovascular complications of hypertension, and studies are currently in progress to determine whether true differences exist.

The goal of antihypertensive therapy is to reduce the diastolic blood pressure to the lowest level tolerated. The JNC suggests that the initial goal should be a diastolic pressure of less than 90 mm Hg. Because of differences in responsiveness, the regimen should be individualized, and it may be necessary to try various drugs or combinations until the optimal regimen is determined. Effective doses vary considerably from patient to patient. A slow, gradual reduction in blood pressure by step-wise increases in drug dosage is better tolerated than an abrupt reduction. Therapy usually should be initiated with a single drug and, if additional agents are needed, they should be added to the regimen one at a time using a stepped-care approach (see Table 2).

Approximately 80% of patients respond to a diuretic given alone or with an antiadrenergic drug. If more than one drug is required, use of a combination product may improve compliance and reduce costs, but a mixture should be substituted only if it contains nearly the same proportions of drugs found to be optimal by individual dose titration. Combination products may be unsuitable if the components have markedly different durations of action or if one component is potent, produces significant side effects, and/or has a wide range of effective dosage. Combinations should not be used if hypertension is difficult to control or if the dosage of one of the drugs requires frequent adjustment (Gifford, 1974).

After blood pressure has been maintained at normal levels for at least one year, it may be possible to "step down" therapy in some patients by first reducing the dose and then discontinuing one or more drugs (Finnerty, 1984; Levinson et al, 1982). These patients should be followed carefully because some may later require a stepping up of therapy to remain normotensive. Weight reduction and sodium restriction may increase the likelihood that the patient will remain normotensive after drug withdrawal (Langford et al, 1985).

Chronic Essential Hypertension

Step 1: For patients with mild to moderate hypertension (diastolic pressure 90 to 114 mm Hg), treatment is usually initiated with a diuretic or a beta blocker (or, less commonly, another antiadrenergic drug). If one of these drugs is ineffective or poorly tolerated, the other may be substituted before proceeding to Step 2 (Weber and Drayer, 1984).

If a diuretic is selected as initial therapy, a thiazide is usually preferred; loop diuretics are generally reserved for patients with impaired renal function. The lowest effective dose should be employed to reduce the risk of metabolic disturbances. Current practice is to add a Step 2 drug if the patient does not respond to the equivalent of 50 mg hydrochlorothiazide. Concurrent treatment with a potassium-sparing agent usually

TABLE 1.
ANTIHYPERTENSIVE AGENTS

Diuretics	Antiadrenergic Drugs		Direct-Acting Vasodilators	Angiotensin-Converting Enzyme Inhibitors	Calcium Channel Blocking Agents

Thiazide-type
  See Table 3
 	
Loop
  Furosemide
  Ethacrynic Acid
  Bumetanide
 	
Potassium-sparing
  Spironolactone
  Triamterene
  Amiloride
	Centrally Acting Agents
	  Clonidine
	  Methyldopa
	  Guanabenz
	  Guanfacine*
	  Lofexidine*
	
	Rauwolfia Alkaloids
	  Reserpine
	  (See text for
	  other alkaloids)
	
	Ganglionic Blockers
	  Trimethaphan
	  Mecamylamine
	
	Adrenergic Neuron Blockers
	  Guanethidine
	  Guanadrel
	  Debrisoquin*
		Beta Blockers
		  See Table 4
		
		Alpha-Blockers
		  Prazosin
		  Indoramin*
		  Terazosin*
		  Trimazosin*
		  Phenoxybenzamine
		  Phentolamine
		
		Alpha and Beta Blocker
		  Labetalol
		
		Agent that Blocks Catecholamine Synthesis
		  Metyrosine
		
		MAO Inhibitor
		  Pargyline
			Arterial Vasodilators
			  Hydralazine
			  Minoxidil
			  Diazoxide
			  Endralazine*
			
			Arterial and Venous Vasodilators
			  Sodium Nitro-
			  prusside
			  Nitroglycerin (IV)
				Captopril
				Enalapril
				Lisinopril*
					Diltiazem
					Nifedipine
					Verapamil
					Felodipine*
					Nicardipine*
					Nitrendipine*
					
					Dopamine Receptor Agonists
					
					Bromocriptine
					Fenoldopam*
					
					Serotonin Receptor Blocking Agent
					
					Ketanserin*

*Investigational

---

prevents hypokalemia, but these agents should not be used when renal function is impaired.

Diuretics generally are well tolerated. They control both supine and standing blood pressure in up to 50% of patients without additional therapy, and, if ineffective alone, are useful to counteract sodium retention and enhance the response to other antihypertensive drugs. Diuretics are more effective than beta-blocking drugs in blacks and elderly patients and are also preferred to beta blockers in patients with congestive heart failure, asthma, chronic bronchitis, or peripheral vascular disorders. A thiazide was usually part of the regimen in studies showing that drug treatment reduces morbidity and mortality in hypertensive patients. Although diuretics are still widely used for Step 1 therapy, concern about the hazards of hypokalemia and hypercholesterolemia has increased the use of alternative drugs.

A beta blocker is a suitable alternative for initial therapy, particularly in whites, patients with symptomatic coronary artery disease (especially after acute myocardial infarction) or arrhythmias, and young patients with hyperkinetic circulation. Beta blockers reduce the risk of reinfarction and improve mortality of patients who have survived an acute myocardial infarction. However, they may precipitate heart failure in patients with borderline cardiac reserve and bronchospasm in asthmatics and may mask the symptoms of hypoglycemia in insulin-dependent diabetics.

Step 2: The response to the Step 1 drug should be observed for four to eight weeks or up to six months in patients with mild hypertension. If a further reduction in blood pressure is indicated, an antiadrenergic agent is added as Step 2 in those initially receiving a diuretic and vice versa.

As with Step 1 therapy, a beta blocker is often the antiadrenergic drug selected. In addition to the advantages mentioned above, beta blockers may be preferred to other antiadrenergic

TABLE 2.
MODIFIED STEPPED-CARE APPROACH TO TREATMENT OF CHRONIC HYPERTENSION

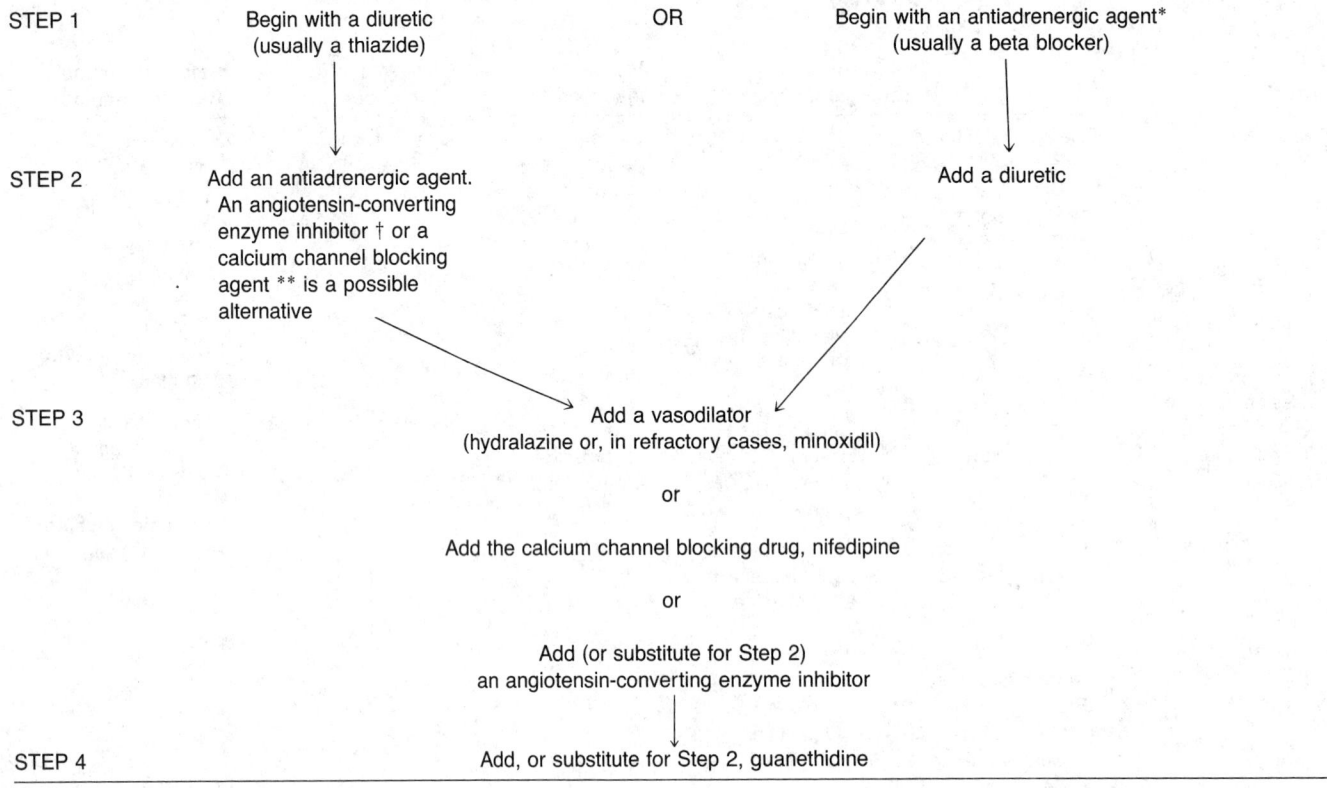

STEP 1   Begin with a diuretic   OR   Begin with an antiadrenergic agent*
                (usually a thiazide)   (usually a beta blocker)

STEP 2   Add an antiadrenergic agent.   Add a diuretic
                An angiotensin-converting
                enzyme inhibitor † or a
                calcium channel blocking
                agent ** is a possible
                alternative

STEP 3   Add a vasodilator
                (hydralazine or, in refractory cases, minoxidil)

                or

                Add the calcium channel blocking drug, nifedipine

                or

                Add (or substitute for Step 2)
                an angiotensin-converting enzyme inhibitor

STEP 4   Add, or substitute for Step 2, guanethidine

* *Beta blocker, reserpine, clonidine, methyldopa, guanabenz, prazosin, labetalol, or guanadrel*
† Captopril, enalapril
** Verapamil, diltiazem, nifedipine

agents because they do not cause orthostatic hypotension. Alternatively, reserpine; a centrally acting antiadrenergic (clonidine [Catapres], methyldopa [Aldomet], guanabenz [Wytensin]); the alpha-beta blocker, labetalol [Trandate, Normodyne]; the alpha$_1$ blocker, prazosin [Minipress]; or the adrenergic neuron blocker, guanadrel [Hylorel], may be used as Step 2.

A thiazide-reserpine regimen provides a simple, inexpensive, and reliable means for long-term control of hypertension. Because it depresses the central nervous system, reserpine may be poorly tolerated by some elderly patients and those whose work requires mental alertness and judgment. Individuals receiving reserpine should be observed for subtle or obvious symptoms of mental depression, and the drug should be discontinued if such symptoms appear.

Centrally acting antiadrenergic drugs are also useful for Step 2. Although they initially may cause drowsiness and dryness of the mouth, these side effects often subside with long-term use. Methyldopa may cause mental depression and rarely hepatitis or hemolytic anemia. The most severe adverse effect of clonidine is a withdrawal syndrome with rebound

hypertension that may occur if the drug is discontinued abruptly.

The alpha-beta blocker, labetalol, has the dual actions of a beta blocker and vasodilator. When used as the second drug in the regimen, it may eliminate the need for a third drug. The major adverse effects of labetalol are due to alpha blockade (orthostatic hypotension) or beta blockade (eg, bronchospasm). Labetalol should not be used when a beta blocker is contraindicated.

Prazosin may be used as the second or third drug in the regimen. It may be preferred to other Step 2 drugs when hypertension is complicated by congestive heart failure. Prazosin is less likely to cause central nervous system side effects than beta blockers, reserpine, or centrally acting antiadrenergics, but it may cause symptomatic orthostatic hypotension, particularly during initial therapy.

Although adrenergic neuron blocking drugs are usually reserved for Step 4, guanadrel has been used as the second or third drug in the regimen. It is not likely to cause central nervous system side effects but may produce orthostatic hypotension.

Alternative Step 2 drugs are the calcium channel blocking agents, nifedipine [Adalat, Procardia], diltiazem [Cardizem], and verapamil [Calan, Isoptin], and the angiotensin-converting enzyme inhibitors, captopril [Capoten] and enalapril [Vasotec]. The vasodilator, hydralazine [Apresoline], is also suitable as a Step 2 drug for elderly patients with blunted baroreceptor reflexes.

Step 3: Hydralazine is used most commonly as the third agent. It is better tolerated and more effective when given with other antihypertensive drugs than when used alone. The sodium retention that occurs with use of all vasodilator drugs generally can be counteracted by a diuretic, and reflex tachycardia can be minimized by a beta blocker. This three-drug regimen is usually well tolerated and is often effective in controlling severe hypertension (diastolic blood pressure 115 mm Hg or greater). Hydralazine does not cause CNS side effects or orthostatic hypotension. A drug-induced lupus syndrome may develop during long-term therapy, particularly when doses exceed 200 mg daily.

Minoxidil [Loniten] may be substituted for hydralazine if a more potent vasodilator is needed. Marked fluid retention and hypertrichosis are the most common adverse effects noted with minoxidil.

Captopril is often effective in patients refractory to other antihypertensive drugs. Like prazosin, captopril is useful in hypertensive patients with congestive heart failure. Rash and dysgeusia are common adverse effects, and a marked fall in blood pressure may occur with the initial dose, especially in volume depleted patients. Captopril should be used cautiously in patients with impaired renal function, particularly in those with severe bilateral renal artery stenosis or severe stenosis in an artery supplying a solitary kidney. Enalapril is also effective in severe hypertension. Rash and taste disturbances are less common with enalapril than with captopril.

The calcium channel blocker, nifedipine, is also often effective in resistant hypertension when given with a diuretic and antiadrenergic drug. Headache and ankle edema are common side effects.

Step 4: For patients who do not respond to these multiple-drug regimens or to large doses of captopril, the potent sympathetic depressant, guanethidine [Ismelin], may be given with a diuretic or added to a two- or three-drug regimen. The orthostatic hypotension produced by guanethidine may be troublesome, particularly when first arising in the morning, during hot weather, and after exertion. Because of the availability of other effective drugs, guanethidine is not commonly used today.

Hypertensive Urgencies and Emergencies

A severe or sudden elevation in blood pressure without impending complications requires prompt, but not immediate, treatment and is defined as a *hypertensive urgency*. Blood pressure usually can be reduced safely in less than 24 hours by oral antihypertensive drugs, such as clonidine, captopril, nifedipine, or a three-drug regimen consisting of a loop diuretic, beta blocker, and hydralazine or minoxidil. For a more rapid response, nifedipine may be given sublingually; the blood pressure begins to fall in about 15 minutes and the hypotensive effect is maximal in about 30 minutes.

A *hypertensive emergency* presents an immediate risk of cardiovascular complications or death and requires hospitalization and rapid reduction of blood pressure with parenteral antihypertensive drugs. An excessively rapid or severe reduction in pressure should be avoided because of the risk of cerebral and myocardial ischemia, particularly in elderly patients and those with long-standing, severe hypertension.

Among the causes of hypertensive emergencies are hypertensive encephalopathy; malignant hypertension; eclampsia; pheochromocytoma; hypertension complicated by congestive heart failure, dissecting aortic aneurysm, acute myocardial infarction, unstable angina, or intracranial hemorrhage; and hypertension caused by withdrawal of some antihypertensive drugs or by food or drug interactions with monoamine oxidase inhibitors. The drugs used to treat hypertensive emergencies may cause marked sodium and water retention; therefore, a loop diuretic (usually furosemide [Lasix] or bumetanide [Bumex]) should be given concomitantly by the intravenous route, and serum electrolyte levels should be monitored.

The vasodilator drug, sodium nitroprusside [Nipride, Nitropress], reduces both peripheral vascular resistance and venous tone. It is the most potent and consistently effective drug available to treat hypertensive emergencies and is the agent of choice for most patients. Because of its favorable hemodynamic effect on left ventricular function, nitroprusside is useful in hypertensive or normotensive patients with acutely decompensated chronic cardiac failure (see also Chapter 23, Agents Used to Treat Heart Failure). It also is used in selected patients with marked pump dysfunction, elevated left ventricular filling pressure, increased peripheral vascular resistance, and decreased cardiac output after acute myocardial infarction.

Intravenous nitroglycerin [Nitrostat IV, Nitro-Bid IV, Tridil] acts predominantly to reduce venous tone. At high infusion rates it also reduces peripheral vascular resistance. Nitroglycerin dilates epicardial coronary arteries and collaterals and improves the regional distribution of myocardial blood flow in patients with coronary artery disease. It is useful in hypertensive emergencies during and after cardiac surgery. Nitroglycerin also relieves refractory chest pain in patients with unstable angina (see Chapter 25, Antianginal Agents) and reduces myocardial ischemia and relieves pulmonary edema in those with severe left ventricular dysfunction following acute myocardial infarction (see Chapter 23, Agents Used to Treat Heart Failure, and Chapter 27, Agents Used to Treat Shock).

The alpha-beta blocker, labetalol, given intravenously, is now regarded as a first-line drug for managing many hypertensive emergencies including malignant hypertension, hypertensive encephalopathy, postoperative hypertension, hypertension associated with extensive burns, and hypertension in patients with coronary artery disease and acute myocardial infarction (Cressman et al, 1984; Wilson et al, 1983). Labetalol usually reduces blood pressure in 5 to 10 minutes without producing reflex tachycardia. During use of intravenous labetalol, the contribution of the postural component should be considered when positioning the patient and the patient should not be permitted to stand unaided until the ability to do so has been established.

The direct-acting vasodilator, diazoxide [Hyperstat I.V.], reduces blood pressure rapidly but is not as safe or consistently effective as nitroprusside. It should be administered by either repeated minibolus injections or continuous infusion rather than as a single large dose. Diazoxide has been used most commonly in patients with hypertensive encephalopathy, malignant hypertension, or hypertension associated with renal disease. Because marked reflex tachycardia may occur, this drug should not be used in patients with coronary artery disease, cardiac failure, or dissecting aortic aneurysm. It also should be avoided in those with cerebrovascular insufficiency because of the rapid reduction in blood pressure that it induces. Transient hyperglycemia is a relatively common side effect, and diazoxide should be given cautiously with constant monitoring of blood glucose levels to patients with known or suspected diabetes mellitus.

The blood pressure also can be reduced within minutes by intravenous administration of the ganglionic blocking drug, trimethaphan [Arfonad], but this agent is not commonly used today. Because trimethaphan may decrease myocardial contractility and cardiac output, it is sometimes employed for initial control of blood pressure in patients with acute dissecting aortic aneurysm. It also may be useful in hypertensive patients with cerebral or subarachnoid hemorrhage. Dosage must be adjusted carefully and the blood pressure monitored frequently to avoid excessive hypotension. Bladder and bowel atony and pseudotolerance (due to volume expansion) may occur with prolonged administration.

Hydralazine, given intramuscularly or intravenously, reduces blood pressure rapidly but is not as consistently effective as sodium nitroprusside or diazoxide. It is mainly used for eclampsia and hypertensive emergencies associated with acute or chronic glomerulonephritis. Methyldopa is available in parenteral form (as methyldopate hydrochloride) but is of limited value in most hypertensive emergencies because of its relatively slow onset of action and pronounced sedative effect. It is used primarily for postoperative hypertension.

The alpha-adrenergic blocking agents, phentolamine [Regitine] and phenoxybenzamine [Dibenzyline], and the tyrosine hydroxylase inhibitor, metyrosine [Demser], are used in hypertensive crises caused by pheochromocytoma. Phentolamine is used for intravenous therapy; phenoxybenzamine and metyrosine are given orally. The two alpha blocking drugs are also useful in hypertensive emergencies caused by the interaction between monoamine oxidase inhibitors and sympathomimetic amines and in the clonidine withdrawal syndrome. When given prophylactically, propranolol prevents severe paradoxical hypertension that often develops after repair of coarctation of the aorta.

Hypertension During Pregnancy

Chronic Hypertension: Most obstetricians consider methyldopa to be the drug of choice for treating chronic hypertension during pregnancy. There has been considerable long-term experience with its use in pregnant women, and controlled trials have shown it to be safe and effective. Controlled studies also have documented the efficacy and apparent fetal safety of beta blockers and labetalol. Hydralazine is also safe and effective during pregnancy and may be added when additional control is needed.

The use of diuretics remains controversial (see Chapter 29, Diuretics). Although many clinicians are reluctant to *initiate* diuretic therapy during pregnancy, thiazides often are continued when the patient was being treated prior to conception, and overall results have been favorable. Consideration should be given to the risk of adverse effects on the newborn (electrolyte disturbances, thrombocytopenia).

Pre-eclampsia, Eclampsia: Intravenous hydralazine is most commonly used to reduce blood pressure rapidly in patients with pre-eclampsia and is usually regarded as the agent of choice. Diazoxide may be given to patients who do not respond to hydralazine. Most obstetricians feel that diuretics should be avoided because an acute reduction in intravascular volume may impair uteroplacental perfusion. Magnesium sulfate is used to prevent or control eclamptic convulsions (see Chapter 17, Adjuncts to Anesthesia).

Drug Evaluations

DIURETICS

Thiazides and Related Compounds

ACTIONS. The thiazides and related compounds (see Table 3) inhibit sodium chloride reabsorption in the cortical thick ascending limb of Henle's loop and the early distal tubules. Their antihypertensive effect is associated with a reduction in plasma and extracellular fluid (ECF) volume (Bennett et al, 1977; Freis, 1983). Cardiac output is reduced and peripheral resistance is unchanged during initial therapy. During long-term therapy, cardiac output returns to control levels and total peripheral vascular resistance is reduced.

USES. A thiazide often serves as the basis of the antihypertensive regimen: as sole therapy in patients with mild or moderate hypertension or in combination with other antihypertensive drugs in patients not controlled by the diuretic alone. Thiazides are well tolerated and most are relatively inexpensive. They reduce both supine and standing blood pressure, and their antihypertensive effect is maintained during long-term administration. When used with other antihypertensive drugs, thiazides prevent secondary volume expansion and thus encourage continued responsiveness (Gifford, 1984). Such combined therapy also may permit a decrease in the dosage of other drugs, which reduces the number and severity of adverse reactions.

The various thiazides and related drugs differ primarily in their duration of action. When given in equipotent doses, no clear-cut differences in antihypertensive efficacy or toxicity have been demonstrated; however, metolazone and indapamide may be somewhat more effective than the other thiazides in patients with impaired renal function.

ADVERSE REACTIONS AND PRECAUTIONS. The thiazides may cause hypokalemia, hyperuricemia, hyperglycemia, hyponatremia, azotemia, and hypercholesterolemia. Dermatologic reactions, blood dyscrasias, and sexual dysfunction (decreased libido or impotence) also have been reported.

Mild hypokalemia seems to be well tolerated by most ambulatory patients with hypertension. Increased ventricular ectopic activity has been noted in some, but the role of hypokalemia in these disturbances has not been established conclusively. Restoration of normokalemia may not abolish these ectopic beats (see Chapter 29). Corrective measures (potassium-sparing diuretics or potassium supplements) are indicated if symptoms occur, if the serum potassium level falls below 3.5 mEq/L, if the electrocardiogram is abnormal, or if the patient is receiving digitalis. Potassium loss can be minimized by moderate sodium restriction.

The incidence of most biochemical disturbances increases with increasing dosage, whereas the antihypertensive effect is not clearly dose related. For this reason, therapy should be initiated with small daily doses (eg, 25 mg of hydrochlorothiazide or chlorthalidone or the equivalent of other thiazides). Elderly patients with reduced plasma volume may be particularly likely to develop orthostatic hypotension with diuretics, and initiation of therapy with smaller doses (eg, 12.5 mg hydrochlorothiazide) is especially important in this age group. Mild or moderate hypertension often can be controlled with doses that induce minimal biochemical changes (Materson et al, 1978; Tweeddale et al, 1977); however, the desire to avoid side effects should not lead to prescription of ineffective doses (Freis, 1984 A).

For further information on adverse reactions, see Chapter 29.

DOSAGE AND PREPARATIONS. See Table 3.

Loop Diuretics

FUROSEMIDE
[Lasix]

ETHACRYNATE SODIUM
[Sodium Edecrin]

ETHACRYNIC ACID
[Edecrin]

BUMETANIDE
[Bumex]

ACTIONS AND USES. The loop diuretics are chemically distinct but have similar pharmacologic actions. These drugs block active salt transport in the medullary and cortical thick ascending limb of Henle's loop. The loop diuretics have a more rapid onset of action and a greater diuretic effect than the thiazides. When given intravenously, they cause a rapid diuresis and are useful adjunctively in the treatment of hypertensive crises. Their use orally in chronic hypertension is usually reserved for patients with impaired renal function (creatinine clearance less than 30 ml/minute) because they are short acting and must be given at least twice and sometimes three times daily to control blood pressure. In addition, the acute diuresis that occurs in the first few hours after administration can be troublesome.

Furosemide has been used more commonly in antihypertensive therapy than the other loop diuretics. It is usually preferred to ethacrynic acid because it has a broader dose-response curve, is less ototoxic, produces fewer gastrointestinal disturbances, and is more convenient for intravenous use. Ethacrynic acid may be useful in patients sensitive to sulfonamides. There has been limited experience with bumetanide in antihypertensive therapy but it is frequently used in edematous states.

ADVERSE REACTIONS AND PRECAUTIONS. Proper use of the loop diuretics requires an understanding of the electrolyte and fluid derangements that they may induce. Overzealous therapy can cause dehydration, hypotension, and marked hypokalemia and hypochloremic alkalosis. Like the thiazides, the loop diuretics can cause prerenal azotemia, hyperuricemia, and hyperglycemia. Transient deafness has been reported following rapid administration of loop diuretics to azotemic or uremic patients. Permanent deafness has occurred rarely. Ethacrynic acid appears to be more ototoxic than furosemide or bumetanide. For other adverse effects, see Chapter 29, Diuretics.

DOSAGE AND PREPARATIONS.
FUROSEMIDE:
Intravenous: For hypertensive crises (in conjunction with other antihypertensive drugs), *adults* with normal renal function, 40 to 80 mg administered over one to two minutes. When the glomerular filtration rate is markedly reduced, larger doses may be required. The manufacturer suggests that large doses be given at a rate not exceeding 4 mg/min. An oral diuretic should be substituted for intravenous furosemide as soon as practical.
> *Lasix* (Hoechst-Roussel), **Generic.** Solution (sterile) 10 mg/ml in 2, 4, and 10 ml containers.

Oral: See Table 3.
ETHACRYNATE SODIUM:
Intravenous: For hypertensive crises (in conjunction with other antihypertensive drugs), *adults,* 50 mg or 0.5 to 1 mg/kg as a single dose; if a second dose is required, it should be injected at another site to avoid thrombophlebitis. An oral diuretic should be substituted for ethacrynate sodium as soon as practical.
> *Sodium Edecrin* (Merck Sharp & Dohme). Powder equivalent to 50 mg ethacrynic acid.

ETHACRYNIC ACID:
Oral: See Table 3.
BUMETANIDE:
Intravenous: For hypertensive crises (in conjunction with other antihypertensive drugs), *adults*, initially, 0.5 to 1 mg (maximum, 10 mg/day).
> *Bumex* (Roche). Solution 0.25 mg/ml in 2 ml containers.

TABLE 3.
ORAL DIURETICS

Drug	Usual Oral Dosage for Hypertension	Preparations
THIAZIDES		
Chlorothiazide	*Adults,* initially, 250 mg daily. May be increased to 500 mg daily. *Children,* 10 to 20 mg/kg daily in 2 divided doses.	*Diuril* (Merck Sharp & Dohme). Tablets 250 and 500 mg; suspension 250 mg/5 ml (alcohol 0.5%). *SK-Chlorothiazide* (Smith Kline & French), *Generic.* Tablets 250 and 500 mg
Hydrochlorothiazide	*Adults,* initially, 25 mg daily. May be increased to 50 mg daily. *Children,* 1 to 2 mg/kg daily in 2 divided doses.	*Esidrix* (CIBA), *HydroDIURIL* (Merck Sharp & Dohme), *Generic.* Tablets 25, 50, and 100 mg. *Oretic* (Abbott). Tablets 25 and 50 mg.
Bendroflumethiazide	*Adults,* initially, 2.5 mg daily. May be increased up to 5 mg daily. *Children,* initially, 0.1 mg/kg daily in 1 or 2 doses; for maintenance, 0.05 to 0.3 mg/kg daily in 1 or 2 doses.	*Naturetin* (Squibb). Tablets 2.5, 5, and 10 mg.
Benzthiazide	*Adults,* initially, 25 mg daily. May be increased to 50 mg daily. *Children,* 1 to 4 mg/kg daily in 3 doses.	*Aquatag* (Reid-Provident). Tablets 25 and 50 mg. *Exna* (Robins), *Proaqua* (Reid-Provident), *Generic.* Tablets 50 mg.
Cyclothiazide	*Adults,* initially, 1 mg daily. May be increased to 2 mg daily. *Children,* 0.02 to 0.04 mg/kg once daily.	*Anhydron* (Lilly). Tablets 2 mg.
Hydroflumethiazide	*Adults,* initially, 25 mg daily. May be increased to 50 mg daily. *Children,* 1 mg/kg daily.	*Diucardin* (Ayerst), *Saluron* (Bristol), *Generic.* Tablets 50 mg.
Methyclothiazide	*Adults,* initially, 2.5 mg daily. May be increased to 5 mg daily. *Children,* 0.05 to 0.2 mg/kg daily.	*Aquatensen* (Wallace). Tablets 5 mg. *Enduron* (Abbott), *Generic.* Tablets 2.5 and 5 mg.
Polythiazide	*Adults,* initially, 2 mg daily. May be increased to 4 mg daily. *Children,* 0.02 to 0.08 mg/kg daily.	*Renese* (Pfipharmecs). Tablets 1, 2, and 4 mg.
Trichlormethiazide	*Adults,* initially, 2 mg daily. May be increased to 4 mg once daily. *Children,* 0.07 mg/kg once daily or in divided doses.	*Metahydrin* (Merrell Dow), *Naqua* (Schering), *Generic.* Tablets 2 and 4 mg.
AGENTS RELATED TO THIAZIDES		
Chlorthalidone	*Adults,* initially, 25 mg daily. May be increased to 50 mg daily. *Children,* 1 mg/kg daily.	*Hygroton* (USV), *Generic.* Tablets 25, 50, and 100 mg. *Thalitone* (Boehringer Ingelheim). Tablets 25 mg.
Indapamide	*Adults,* initially, 2.5 mg daily. May be increased to 5 mg daily.	*Lozol* (USV). Tablets 2.5 mg.

(continued on next page)

Drug	Usual Oral Dosage for Hypertension	Preparations
Metolazone	*Adults,* initially, 2.5 mg daily. May be increased to 5 mg daily.	*Diulo* (Searle), *Zaroxolyn* (Pennwalt). Tablets 2.5, 5, and 10 mg.
Quinethazone	*Adults,* initially, 50 mg daily. May be increased to 100 mg daily.	*Hydromox* (Lederle). Tablets 50 mg.

LOOP DIURETICS

Drug	Usual Oral Dosage for Hypertension	Preparations
Bumetanide	*Adults,* initially, 0.5 mg daily. May be increased to 10 mg daily in 2 divided doses.	*Bumex* (Roche). Tablets 0.5 and 1 mg.
Furosemide	*Adults,* initially, 40 mg twice daily. If an adequate response is not obtained, dosage may be increased gradually up to 480 mg daily in 2 doses. *Children,* 1 to 2 mg/kg.	*Lasix* (Hoechst-Roussel). Solution (oral) 10 mg/ml; tablets 20, 40, and 80 mg. *SK-Furosemide* (Smith Kline & French). Tablets 20 and 40 mg. NOTE: Some generic products have been shown to have questionable bioavailability.
Ethacrynic Acid	*Adults,* initially, 25 mg twice daily. May be increased to 200 mg daily in 2 divided doses.	*Edecrin* (Merck Sharp & Dohme). Tablets 25 and 50 mg.

POTASSIUM-SPARING DIURETICS

Drug	Usual Oral Dosage for Hypertension	Preparations
Amiloride	*Adults,* initially, 5 mg daily. Dosage should be adjusted in accordance with the blood pressure and serum potassium level. Dosage should usually not exceed 10 mg daily.	*Midamor* (Merck Sharp & Dohme). Tablets 5 mg.
Amiloride and Hydrochlorothiazide	*Adults,* initially, 1 tablet daily. Dosage should be adjusted in accordance with the blood pressure and serum potassium level.	*Moduretic* (Merck Sharp & Dohme). Each tablet contains amiloride hydrochloride 5 mg and hydrochlorothiazide 50 mg.
Spironolactone	*Adults,* initially, 50 mg daily. May be increased to 100 mg daily in a single dose or 2 divided doses. The dosage should be adjusted in accordance with the blood pressure and serum potassium level. *Children,* 1 to 2 mg/kg daily in 2 doses.	*Aldactone* (Searle). Tablets 25, 50, and 100 mg. *Generic.* Tablets 25 mg.
Spironolactone and Hydrochlorothiazide	Initially, 1 tablet containing 25 mg of each component daily. May be increased to 50 mg of each component daily in a single dose or in divided doses. The dosage should be adjusted in accordance with the blood pressure and serum potassium level.	*Aldactazide* (Searle), *Generic.* Each tablet contains spironolactone 25 mg and hydrochlorothiazide 25 mg or spironolactone 50 mg and hydrochlorothiazide 50 mg (*Aldactazide* only).
Triamterene	*Adults,* initially, 50 mg daily. May be increased to 100 mg daily in a single dose or 2 divided doses should be given after meals. The dosage should be adjusted in accordance with the blood pressure and serum potassium level.	*Dyrenium* (Smith Kline & French). Capsules 50 and 100 mg.
Triamterene and Hydrochlorothiazide*	*Adults,* initially, 1 capsule of Dyazide daily. May be increased to 2 capsules Dyazide daily in single or divided doses or 1 capsule of Maxzide daily. The dosage should be adjusted in accordance with the blood pressure and serum potassium level.	*Dyazide* (Smith Kline & French), *Generic.* Each capsule contains triamterene 50 mg and hydrochlorothiazide 25 mg. *Maxzide* (Lederle). Each capsule contains triamterene 75 mg and hydrochlorothiazide 50 mg.

*Combination products containing triamterene and hydrochlorothiazide may vary in bioavailability. Both the triamterene and hydrochlorothiazide components of Maxzide are more bioavailable than those contained in Dyazide. In addition, Maxzide contains a larger dose of each component than Dyazide.

Potassium-Sparing Diuretics

SPIRONOLACTONE
[Aldactone]

TRIAMTERENE
[Dyrenium]

AMILORIDE HYDROCHLORIDE
[Midamor]

ACTIONS AND USES. Spironolactone, triamterene, and amiloride interfere with sodium reabsorption at the distal sites in the renal tubule where sodium reabsorption is related to the secretion of potassium and hydrogen ions. Spironolactone is an aldosterone antagonist; triamterene and amiloride act directly at the distal exchange sites in the renal tubules to reduce potassium excretion.

The potassium-sparing diuretics are not potent antihypertensive agents when used as sole therapy. They are usually employed as adjuncts to a thiazide or loop diuretic to prevent hypokalemia.

ADVERSE REACTIONS AND PRECAUTIONS. Careful monitoring of the serum potassium level is necessary during therapy with potassium-sparing diuretics because hyperkalemia may occur despite concomitant thiazide therapy. Precipitating factors are impaired renal function and/or a high potassium intake (dietary, supplements, salt substitutes). These drugs may increase blood urea nitrogen and possibly serum uric acid levels. For a more detailed discussion of actions, uses, interactions, and other adverse effects, see Chapter 29, Diuretics.

DOSAGE AND PREPARATIONS. See Table 3.
AVAILABLE MIXTURES.
Potassium-Sparing Diuretic and a Thiazide Diuretic: Since a potassium-sparing diuretic is most useful when given with a thiazide, these combination products are convenient, but occasionally it may be necessary to give the drugs separately for optimal potassium conservation (see Chapter 29).

For dosage and preparations, see Table 3.

ANTIADRENERGIC AGENTS

Centrally Acting Agents

CLONIDINE HYDROCHLORIDE
[Catapres]

ACTIONS. Clonidine inhibits sympathetic outflow from the brain by stimulating alpha$_2$ receptors in the vasomotor center of the medulla. Its hypotensive effect is associated with a fall in total peripheral resistance. Cardiac output is reduced initially but tends to return to baseline levels during prolonged therapy. Clonidine also slightly reduces heart rate, due in part to an increase in vagal tone. Activation of peripheral alpha$_1$ receptors (manifested by vasoconstriction and increased blood pressure) is not evident with therapeutic oral doses.

USES. Oral clonidine is useful in treating all degrees of chronic hypertension. It is most commonly added to the regimen as Step 2 when blood pressure is not controlled by a diuretic alone. Clonidine also may be useful in some hypertensive urgencies when an immediate reduction in blood pressure with parenteral drugs is not required. The "clonidine suppression test" utilizes oral clonidine to confirm a diagnosis of pheochromocytoma (Bravo and Gifford, 1984).

The transdermal preparation delivers clonidine through a rate-controlling membrane. The preparation is changed weekly by the patient and appears to have a sustained antihypertensive effect (Weber et al, 1984).

ADVERSE REACTIONS, PRECAUTIONS, AND INTERACTIONS. The most common side effects of clonidine are drowsiness, dryness of the mouth, and constipation. Orthostatic symptoms occur occasionally. These reactions may decrease in severity during long-term therapy. The transdermal preparation also may cause erythematous rashes at the site of application.

A pronounced withdrawal reaction with symptoms suggesting sympathetic overactivity may develop in 12 to 48 hours if clonidine is discontinued abruptly. Symptoms may be accompanied by a rapid rebound increase in blood pressure (to pretreatment levels or above) and, rarely, ventricular arrhythmias. Withdrawal reactions are associated with increased plasma and urinary catecholamine levels and are most likely to occur in patients who have been receiving large doses (over 1.2 mg daily). Clonidine should not be prescribed for patients who are unreliable about taking medication.

For a planned withdrawal, clonidine dosage should be decreased gradually over one week or more. If it is necessary to discontinue the drug prior to emergency surgery, blood pressure usually can be controlled intraoperatively and during the immediate postoperative period by sodium nitroprusside alone or with phentolamine. Intravenous methyldopa may be useful in selected patients.

Clonidine may increase bradycardia in patients with sinus node dysfunction. It also has been reported to potentiate the effect of digitalis on A-V conduction.

Overdosage usually leads to hypotension and bradycardia but occasionally the blood pressure may increase because of activation of alpha₁ receptors in the peripheral circulation. Other manifestations of toxicity are apnea, drowsiness, miosis, hypothermia, coma, and seizures. Atropine has been effective in treating the bradycardia, and volume replacement and vasopressors have been used to manage hypotensive reactions. Tolazoline, which has both central and peripheral alpha-adrenergic blocking properties, has been used to treat overdosage, but it has not been consistently effective.

Rarely, a paradoxical hypertensive response has developed during combined therapy with clonidine and a beta-blocking drug. Beta blockers also may exaggerate the rebound hypertension accompanying abrupt withdrawal of clonidine. Imipramine, desipramine, and probably other tricyclic antidepressants antagonize the antihypertensive effect of clonidine. Naloxone also may reverse the antihypertensive response.

Rashes, central nervous system disturbances (depression, hallucinations), sexual dysfunction, and gynecomastia have been reported. Psychosis has occurred rarely after withdrawal of clonidine in patients with pre-existing schizophrenia or manic-depressive illness. Clonidine may impair glucose tolerance after an acute glucose load but does not appear to adversely affect control of diabetes during long-term therapy. Clonidine accumulates in the choroid, but no adverse effects on the eye have been reported.

PHARMACOKINETICS. Clonidine is readily absorbed after oral administration and its bioavailability is 75%. The volume of distribution is 2.1 L/kg and the half-life is approximately 8.5 hours. Clonidine is eliminated largely as unchanged drug (62%); clearance is 3.1 ± 1.2 ml/min/kg.

DOSAGE AND PREPARATIONS. Dosage must be titrated carefully to provide an optimal therapeutic response with minimal side effects. Concomitant diuretic therapy enhances the antihypertensive effect.

Oral: Adults, initially, 0.1 mg once daily at bedtime for several weeks, followed by 0.1 mg twice daily. Dosage may be increased gradually by 0.1 or 0.2 mg. For maintenance, the usual daily dose ranges from 0.2 to 0.8 mg in divided amounts. Doses exceeding 1.2 mg daily are rarely required. If the patient complains of drowsiness, two-thirds of the total dose may be given at bedtime.

Catapres (Boehringer Ingelheim). Tablets 0.1, 0.2, and 0.3 mg.

Transdermal: Adults, initially, Catapres-TTS-1 is applied once weekly.

Catapres-TTS-1, -2, -3 (Boehringer Ingelheim). These devices are designed to deliver clonidine 0.1, 0.2, and 0.3 mg/day, respectively.

AVAILABLE MIXTURE.

Clonidine and Chlorthalidone: Successful regulation of blood pressure with clonidine requires careful titration of dosage, and an adjustment in dose may be required during continuous therapy. For these reasons, this fixed-dose combination of clonidine and a thiazide may be unsuitable for some patients.

Combipres (Boehringer Ingelheim). Each tablet contains clonidine hydrochloride 0.1, 0.2, or 0.3 mg and chlorthalidone 15 mg.

METHYLDOPA
[Aldomet]

METHYLDOPATE HYDROCHLORIDE
[Aldomet]

ACTIONS. Methyldopa is an aromatic amino acid decarboxylase inhibitor that depresses sympathetic nervous system activity through an effect on the central nervous system. The action of methyldopa is believed to be associated with its metabolism to alpha-methylnorepinephrine. This metabolite presumably lowers blood pressure by activating inhibitory alpha-adrenergic receptors in the central nervous system, thereby reducing sympathetic outflow (Frohlich, 1980). Methyldopa decreases total peripheral resistance with minimal reduction of heart rate and cardiac output. Renal, cerebral, and myocardial blood flow are maintained. Both supine and standing blood pressures are reduced.

USES. Methyldopa is useful in the treatment of all degrees of hypertension. It is most commonly added to the regimen as Step 2 when blood pressure is not controlled by a diuretic alone. Although methyldopa crosses the placenta and may slightly reduce blood pressure in newborn infants of treated mothers, it has been used in many pregnant women without serious adverse effects on the fetus and is often considered to be the drug of choice for treating chronic hypertension during pregnancy.

The intravenous preparation, methyldopate hydrochloride, is administered only rarely to treat hypertensive emergencies because of its delayed onset of action. In addition, the sedative effect may interfere with evaluation of mental status. It is used mainly to treat postoperative hypertension.

ADVERSE REACTIONS, PRECAUTIONS, AND INTERACTIONS. Drowsiness, a common side effect of methyldopa, often subsides with continued therapy. A reversible reduction in mental acuity has been observed in some patients. Mental depression is less common than with reserpine. Dryness of the mouth, nasal congestion, nausea, vomiting, diarrhea, and sexual dysfunction (decreased libido, impotence, and impaired ejaculation) also may occur. Excessive hypotension was the most common side effect reported in a study on hospitalized patients. Sodium and water retention may occur if methyldopa is administered without a diuretic. A reversible malabsorption syndrome associated with histologic abnormality of the small bowel has been reported rarely.

A positive Coombs' test has been noted in 10% to 20% of patients who received prolonged treatment. Hemolytic anemia occurs only rarely and is generally reversible when the drug is discontinued, but the Coombs' test may remain positive for several months. Since most patients having a positive Coombs' test do not develop hemolytic anemia, a positive test is not a contraindication to continued use of the drug.

Significant alterations in results of liver function tests (increased SGOT and alkaline phosphatase levels), indicative of drug-induced hepatitis, have been noted during the first 6 to 12 weeks of treatment. The hepatitis, which may or may not be accompanied by fever and malaise, is usually reversible. However, in a few instances, re-exposure to methyldopa caused fatal hepatic necrosis. Liver function tests probably should be performed at monthly intervals during the first four months of treatment or whenever an unexplained fever develops. Drug fever occurs in some patients without hepatic involvement.

Methyldopa may decrease HDL cholesterol levels. Uncommon effects that may or may not be drug-related include gynecomastia, reversible leukopenia, thrombocytopenia, lichenoid reactions, hypersensitivity myocarditis, acute colitis, pancreatitis, and extrapyramidal symptoms. Methyldopa may adversely affect sinus node function in patients with sinus node disorders.

Hypertensive reactions have been reported rarely after withdrawal of methyldopa or due to interaction with intravenous propranolol or with phenylpropanolamine and a beta blocker. Methyldopa may interfere with determination of urinary catecholamines by the fluorescent technique and thus may interfere with the diagnosis of pheochromocytoma. It also may interfere with measurement of serum creatinine (alkaline picrate method), uric acid (phosphotungstate method), and SGOT (colorimetric methods).

Methyldopa crosses the placenta and appears in breast milk but no significant adverse effects have been reported in the fetus or nursing infant.

PHARMACOKINETICS. The bioavailability of methyldopa is 50% and its volume of distribution is 0.37 ± 0.1 L/kg. Methyldopa is eliminated by renal excretion of active drug (63%) or conjugates, and its clearance is 3.1 ± 0.9 ml/min/kg. In the presence of renal insufficiency, delayed excretion may result in accumulation of drug and metabolites. The half-life of methyldopa is 1.8 hours and is increased in patients with uremia.

DOSAGE AND PREPARATIONS. Dosage must be titrated carefully to provide an optimal therapeutic response with minimal side effects. Concomitant diuretic therapy enhances the antihypertensive effect.

METHYLDOPA:

Oral: For chronic hypertension, *adults,* initially, 250 mg at bedtime; this dose may be increased to 250 mg twice daily after one week. Dosage then may be increased gradually until the blood pressure is controlled or a total daily dose of 2 g is reached. In most patients, the maximal antihypertensive effect is attained at a dose of 1 or 1.5 g/day. If the patient complains of drowsiness, a larger dose may be given at bedtime than in the morning. *Children,* initially, 10 mg/kg daily divided into two to four doses. The dose is then increased or decreased at two-day or longer intervals according to response (maximum, 65 mg/kg daily).

    Generic. Tablets 250 and 500 mg.
    Note: Some generic products may contain sulfites.
    Aldomet (Merck Sharp & Dohme). Suspension 250 mg/5 ml (alcohol 1%; contains sodium bisulfite); tablets 125, 250, and 500 mg.

METHYLDOPATE HYDROCHLORIDE:

Intravenous: For postoperative hypertension, *adults,* 250 to 500 mg every six to eight hours as required. *Children,* 20 to 40 mg/kg daily divided into four doses. After the blood pressure has been controlled, oral medication should be substituted.

    Aldomet (Merck Sharp & Dohme). Solution 50 mg/ml in 5 ml containers (contains sodium bisulfite).

AVAILABLE MIXTURES.

Methyldopa and a Thiazide: Successful regulation of blood pressure with methyldopa requires careful adjustment of dosage, and the effective dose may vary between 500 mg and 2 g daily. For this reason, fixed-dose combinations containing methyldopa and a thiazide may be unsuitable for some patients.

    Aldoclor-150, -250 (Merck Sharp & Dohme). Each tablet contains methyldopa 250 mg and chlorothiazide 150 or 250 mg.
    Aldoril-15, -25 (Merck Sharp & Dohme). Each tablet contains methyldopa 250 mg and hydrochlorothiazide 15 or 25 mg.
    Aldoril D30, D50 (Merck Sharp & Dohme). Each tablet contains methyldopa 500 mg and hydrochlorothiazide 30 or 50 mg.

GUANABENZ ACETATE
[Wytensin]

ACTIONS. This guanidine derivative reduces blood pressure by inhibiting sympathetic outflow from the brain through activation of central alpha-adrenergic receptors. It reduces both supine and standing blood pressure and heart rate. The hypotensive effect is more pronounced when the patient is in the erect position.

USES. Guanabenz has been studied in patients with mild to moderate hypertension. Although it may be effective as sole therapy in some patients, it is most useful and better tolerated when reduced doses are given with a diuretic. The antihypertensive effect of guanabenz appears to be comparable to that of other Step 2 drugs.

ADVERSE REACTIONS AND PRECAUTIONS. Sedation and dryness of the mouth are the most common and troublesome side effects of guanabenz. Weakness and orthostatic hypotension also may occur. Headache, palpitations, bradycardia, nasal congestion, blurred vision, urinary frequency, and gastrointestinal disturbances (nausea, vomiting, epigastric pain, diarrhea, constipation) have been reported occasionally. Anxiety, depression, insomnia, arrhythmias, sexual dysfunction, gynecomastia, and rashes have developed rarely. Withdrawal reactions have followed discontinuation of the drug in patients receiving large doses. (See evaluation on Clonidine Hydrochloride for description, precautions, and treatment of withdrawal reactions.)

This drug is classified in FDA Pregnancy Category C.

PHARMACOKINETICS. The bioavailability of guanabenz is 75%. The drug is 90% protein bound and is extensively metabolized. Less than 1% of unchanged drug is recovered in the urine. The half-life is 7 to 10 hours.

DOSAGE AND PREPARATIONS. Dosage should be titrated gradually to provide the optimal therapeutic response with minimal side effects. Concomitant administration of a diuretic enhances the antihypertensive effect.

Oral: Adults, initially, 4 mg twice daily. The dose may be increased gradually up to 32 mg twice daily.

Wytensin (Wyeth). Tablets 4 and 8 mg.

GUANFACINE

ACTIONS. This investigational guanidine derivative reduces blood pressure by stimulating central alpha-adrenergic receptors. It enters and leaves the brain more slowly than clonidine. The hypotensive effect is associated primarily with a fall in total peripheral resistance; heart rate and cardiac output also may be reduced.

USES. Guanfacine has been given alone and with oral diuretics, beta blockers, and vasodilators to patients with mild to severe hypertension. Like other centrally acting antiadrenergic agents, it is most useful as a Step 2 drug. When given in daily doses of 3 to 4 mg, the antihypertensive effect of guanfacine is comparable to that of clonidine 0.3 to 0.45 mg or small doses of guanethidine (20 mg), and it may be more effective than methyldopa 1.2 g.

ADVERSE REACTIONS, PRECAUTIONS, AND INTERACTIONS. The adverse effects of guanfacine resemble those of clonidine. Dryness of the mouth and sedation are most common. Constipation, orthostatic symptoms, sexual dysfunction, insomnia, and sweating also have been reported. Tolerance develops frequently if a diuretic is not given concomitantly.

A withdrawal syndrome with rebound hypertension has occurred when guanfacine was discontinued abruptly, most commonly in patients with severe hypertension receiving doses exceeding 4 mg daily. The withdrawal syndrome developed two to seven days after treatment was discontinued. (See the evaluation on Clonidine Hydrochloride for description, precautions, and treatment of withdrawal reactions.)

PHARMACOKINETICS. Guanfacine is rapidly and almost completely absorbed (90%) from the gastrointestinal tract. It has a large volume of distribution and a half-life of 16 to 20 hours in patients with normal renal function. Phenobarbital shortens its half-life. Guanfacine is eliminated both by renal excretion of unchanged drug and by hepatic metabolism. Plasma concentrations and the hypotensive effect are not increased in uremic patients.

DOSAGE AND PREPARATIONS. Dosage must be titrated carefully to provide an optimal therapeutic response with minimal side effects. Concomitant diuretic therapy enhances the antihypertensive effect.

Oral: Adults, initially, 0.5 mg twice daily, increased gradually as needed. A daily maintenance dose of 1 to 3 mg may be adequate in many patients and may be given as a single dose or in two divided doses.

Guanfacine (Robins). Capsules 0.5, 1, 2, and 3 mg. (Investigational drug)

Rauwolfia Alkaloids

RESERPINE

ACTIONS. Reserpine is regarded as the prototype of the rauwolfia alkaloids and is the most commonly used drug in this group. Its antihypertensive effect has been attributed to depletion of catecholamine stores in peripheral sympathetic nerve terminals and the central nervous system. Reserpine decreases total peripheral resistance, heart rate, and cardiac output; orthostatic hypotension occurs only rarely with currently recommended doses.

USES. Reserpine is used orally with a diuretic to treat mild or moderate hypertension, and it compares favorably to other Step 2 drugs (VA Cooperative Study Group on Antihypertensive Agents, 1977; Finnerty et al, 1979; Channick et al, 1981). It has a delayed onset of action and the patient should be observed for three to four weeks before other drugs are added to the regimen.

ADVERSE REACTIONS AND PRECAUTIONS. Lethargy, dryness of the mouth, nasal congestion, and bradycardia may occur with therapeutic doses; fluid retention may develop if a diuretic is not given concomitantly. Other adverse effects include diarrhea, nausea, vomiting, anorexia, sexual dysfunction (decreased libido, impotence, and impaired ejaculation), stress incontinence, and nightmares. Mental depression may be severe enough to require hospitalization or, rarely, may result in attempted suicide; this can occur with any amount but is most common with high-dose regimens (0.5 to 1 mg or more daily). Small doses of reserpine (less than 0.125 mg daily), combined with a diuretic, often control blood pressure and may produce fewer side effects than larger doses (Participating VA Medical Centers, 1982). The rauwolfia alkaloids should not be given to patients with a history of depression; if depressive symptoms appear, the drug should be discontinued. Barbiturates enhance the central nervous system depressant effects of rauwolfia alkaloids.

Gynecomastia has occurred rarely in patients receiving rauwolfia alkaloids. An association between long-term therapy and breast cancer was reported in three retrospective studies, but many subsequent investigations have shown no relationship, and the weight of evidence is now against any such association.

Rauwolfia alkaloids may adversely affect sinus node function in patients with sinus node disorders.

Reserpine may increase gastric acid secretion and should be used cautiously in patients with a history of peptic ulcer. If symptoms suggest recurrence of the ulcer, the drug should be discontinued. Because rauwolfia alkaloids increase gastrointestinal tone and motility, they should not be given to patients with a history of ulcerative colitis.

Reserpine passes through the placental circulation. When given parenterally (parenteral preparation no longer available) to treat eclampsia, it caused drowsiness, nasal congestion, cyanosis, and anorexia in the newborn infant.

Because rauwolfia alkaloids lower the convulsive threshold, they should be used cautiously in patients with epilepsy. Large doses may cause extrapyramidal reactions.

DOSAGE AND PREPARATIONS. The rauwolfia alkaloids have a slow onset and prolonged duration of action. Adjustments in dosage should not be made more frequently than every five to seven days. A diuretic should be given concomitantly to enhance the therapeutic response.

RESERPINE:

Oral: For chronic hypertension, *adults and children,* initially and for maintenance, 0.05 to 0.1 mg once daily. Dosage should be increased only if necessary and the daily dose should not exceed 0.25 mg.

    Generic. Tablets 0.1, 0.25, and 1 mg.
    Sandril (Lilly). Tablets 0.25 mg.
    Serpasil (CIBA). Tablets 0.1 and 0.25 mg.
    Additional Trademarks.
    Serpate (Vale), **SK-Reserpine** (Smith Kline & French).

OTHER RAUWOLFIA ALKALOIDS.

    RAUWOLFIA SERPENTINA:
    Raudixin (Squibb), **Generic.** Tablets 50 and 100 mg.
    ALSEROXYLON:
    Rauwiloid (Riker). Tablets 2 mg.
    DESERPIDINE:
    Harmonyl (Abbott). Tablets 0.1 and 0.25 mg.
    RESCINNAMINE:
    Moderil (Pfizer). Tablets 0.25 and 0.5 mg.

AVAILABLE MIXTURES.

Rauwolfia Alkaloid and an Oral Diuretic: The following oral combination products are convenient for patients who require both a thiazide and a rauwolfia alkaloid. Dosage requirements should be determined with the single-entity preparations before substituting the combination product.

    Diupres-250, -500 (Merck Sharp & Dohme). Each tablet contains chlorothiazide 250 or 500 mg and reserpine 0.125 mg.
    Diutensen-R (Wallace). Each tablet contains methylclothiazide 2.5 mg and reserpine 0.1 mg.
    Enduronyl (Abbott). Each tablet contains methyclothiazide 5 mg and deserpidine 0.25 or 0.5 (**Forte**) mg.
    Hydromox R (Lederle). Each tablet contains quinethazone 50 mg and reserpine 0.125 mg.
    Hydropres-25, -50 (Merck Sharp & Dohme). Each tablet contains hydrochlorothiazide 25 or 50 mg and reserpine 0.125 mg.
    Metatensin (Merrell Dow). Each tablet contains trichlormethiazide 2 or 4 mg and reserpine 0.1 mg.
    Naquival (Schering). Each tablet contains trichlormethiazide 4 mg and reserpine 0.1 mg.
    Rauzide (Squibb). Each tablet contains bendroflumethiazide 4 mg and rauwolfia serpentina 50 mg.
    Regroton (USV). Each tablet contains chlorthalidone 25 mg and reserpine 0.125 mg (**Demi-Regroton**) or chlorthalidone 50 mg and reserpine 0.25 mg.
    Renese-R (Pfipharmecs). Each tablet contains polythiazide 2 mg and reserpine 0.25 mg.
    Salutensin (Bristol). Each tablet contains hydroflumethiazide 25 mg and reserpine 0.125 mg (**Salutensin-Demi**) or hydroflumethiazide 50 mg and reserpine 0.125 mg.
    Serpasil-Esidrix No. 1, No. 2 (CIBA). Each tablet contains hydrochlorothiazide 25 mg (No. 1) or 50 mg (No. 2) and reserpine 0.1 mg.

Ganglionic Blocking Agents

Ganglionic blocking agents act on autonomic ganglia to inhibit both sympathetic and parasympathetic function. Oral preparations (mecamylamine [Inversine]) are rarely used today because of their untoward effects: severe orthostatic hypotension (due to blockade of sympathetic ganglia) and adynamic ileus and urinary retention (due to blockade of parasympathetic ganglia). The intravenous ganglionic blocking agent, trimethaphan, is still used occasionally to treat hypertensive emergencies, particularly acute dissecting aortic aneurysm.

TRIMETHAPHAN CAMSYLATE
[Arfonad]

USES. This short-acting ganglionic blocking drug is administered intravenously in hypertensive crises. It is particularly useful for the initial control of blood pressure in patients with acute dissecting aortic aneurysm. Trimethaphan also is used to produce controlled hypotension for short periods during some neurosurgical and cardiovascular operations in order to avoid excessive blood loss.

Continuous infusion is necessary to maintain the antihypertensive effect. The blood pressure should be monitored frequently while the rate of administration is established initially and every five minutes thereafter. The hypotensive effect is largely orthostatic, and if the blood pressure fails to decrease sufficiently with the patient in the supine position, the head of the bed should be elevated. If severe hypotension occurs, the blood pressure may be stabilized by use of the Trendelenburg position.

ADVERSE REACTIONS AND PRECAUTIONS. Trimethaphan may cause urinary retention and orthostatic hypotension. Adynamic ileus is usually not a problem unless the period of infusion exceeds 48 hours. Because prolonged treatment may be associated with sodium and water retention, pseudotolerance can be expected if a diuretic is not given concomitantly. Other adverse effects include anorexia, nausea, vomiting, dryness of the mouth, mydriasis, and cycloplegia. There is a risk of respiratory paralysis when the rate of administration exceeds 6 mg/minute.

DOSAGE AND PREPARATIONS.
Intravenous: Adults, a 0.1% solution (1 mg/ml) in 5% dextrose injection is infused continuously at a rate determined by the patient's response. Use of a variable rate infusion pump is recommended. The infusion may be started at a rate of 0.5 to 1 mg/min and increased gradually until the blood pressure falls 20 mm Hg or more. After several minutes, the rate can be increased again until the desired level is achieved. While stabilizing the blood pressure with trimethaphan, oral therapy with other antihypertensive drugs should be instituted.
Arfonad (Roche). Solution 50 mg/ml in 10 ml containers.

Agents That Block Neuroeffector Transmission

GUANADREL SULFATE
[Hylorel]

ACTIONS. This adrenergic neuron blocking drug has a mechanism of action and hemodynamic effects similar to those of guanethidine, but it has a more rapid onset and a shorter duration of action after withdrawal. Like guanethidine, guanadrel does not readily cross the blood-brain barrier.

USES. Although adrenergic neuron blocking drugs are usually reserved for patients with severe refractory hypertension, guanadrel has been used for Step 2 and Step 3 therapy. It has been compared with both methyldopa and guanethidine in patients who were receiving concurrent diuretic therapy. Guanadrel appears to be more effective than methyldopa and causes fewer central nervous system side effects but is more likely to cause orthostatic and postexercise hypotension and

diarrhea. It is as effective as guanethidine and may cause less diarrhea and less orthostatic hypotension on arising in the morning. Orthostatic symptoms during the rest of the day occur with equal frequency with the two drugs. Guanadrel may impair ejaculation to a lesser extent than guanethidine.

ADVERSE REACTIONS, PRECAUTIONS, AND INTERACTIONS. The adverse effects of guanadrel resemble those of guanethidine, with the exceptions noted above, and the same precautions apply. Drugs interacting with guanethidine also can be expected to interact with guanadrel.

PHARMACOKINETICS. Guanadrel is rapidly absorbed and peak plasma levels are attained 1.5 to 2 hours after ingestion. The maximal hypotensive effect occurs in four to six hours. Guanadrel is 20% protein bound. Forty percent of a dose is excreted in the urine as unchanged drug. Plasma drug levels indicate a two-compartment model. The half-life of the alpha phase is one to four hours and the half-life of the beta phase ranges from 5 to 45 hours.

DOSAGE AND PREPARATIONS. Guanadrel has a broad dose-response curve, and dosage should be titrated carefully to provide the desired therapeutic response with minimal untoward effects. A diuretic should be given concomitantly.
Oral: Adults, initially, 10 mg daily, increased daily or less frequently until the desired response is obtained. The usual maintenance dose is 25 to 75 mg daily. The total daily dose may be divided and taken in the morning and afternoon. Patients taking small doses may require only a morning dose.
Hylorel (Pennwalt). Tablets 10 and 25 mg.

GUANETHIDINE MONOSULFATE
[Ismelin]

ACTIONS. This adrenergic neuron blocking drug interferes with the release of norepinephrine from peripheral sympathetic nerve terminals. Its hypotensive effect is due to both a reduction in cardiac output (resulting from reduced venous return and negative chronotropic and inotropic effects) and a fall in total peripheral vascular resistance. Guanethidine has a marked effect on venous tone, and pronounced orthostatic effects occur frequently.

USES. Guanethidine is reserved for patients with severe hypertension who do not respond to other drug regimens. It is not commonly used today because the dosage is difficult to regulate without causing orthostatic hypotension or diarrhea, and other effective drugs, such as captopril and minoxidil, are now available for treating resistant hypertension.

ADVERSE REACTIONS, PRECAUTIONS, AND INTERACTIONS. Orthostatic hypotension (most prominent in the morning) and postexercise hypotension can be anticipated with use of guanethidine, and the patient should be warned of their possible occurrence. During initial therapy and whenever dosage is increased, blood pressure should be measured with the patient in the supine and standing positions and after mild exercise. Orthostatic hypotension may be minimized by cautioning the patient to arise slowly from the recumbent or seated position. Additional measures, such as elevating the head of the bed and using elastic support stockings, also may be helpful. Other common adverse effects are sodium retention (if a diuretic is not given concomitantly), bradycardia, diarrhea, and retrograde ejaculation.

Guanethidine should not be used in patients with pheochromocytoma, since severe hypertension may occur, possibly because of increased sensitivity of the adrenergic receptors to endogenous catecholamines. The response to exogenous catecholamines also may be enhanced. Sympathomimetic agents, such as amphetamines and ephedrine, as well as tricyclic antidepressants, methylphenidate, cocaine, and, to a lesser extent, chlorpromazine, may antagonize the antihypertensive effect of guanethidine.

PHARMACOKINETICS. Guanethidine is incompletely absorbed and less than 30% of an oral dose enters the systemic circulation. It is eliminated by renal excretion of unchanged drug (50%) and metabolites. Because of its long half-life, the maximal hypotensive effect may not be observed for 7 to 14 days. Effects may persist for seven to ten days or more after the drug is discontinued.

DOSAGE AND PREPARATIONS. Guanethidine has a very broad dose-response curve and dosage should be titrated carefully to provide the desired therapeutic effect with minimal untoward effects. A diuretic should be given concomitantly.
Oral: Adults, for ambulatory patients, initially, 10 to 12.5 mg once daily. The dose may be increased by 10 to 12.5 mg every seven days to 100 mg daily. If necessary, dosage can be increased further by 25-mg increments to a maximum of 300

mg daily; however, daily doses above 100 mg are rarely required because of the availability of newer drugs with fewer side effects. In hospitalized patients, treatment may be initiated with higher doses, eg, 25 to 50 mg daily. *Children,* initially, 0.2 mg/kg daily, increased by the same amount every seven to ten days if required.
   Ismelin (CIBA). Tablets 10 and 25 mg.
AVAILABLE MIXTURE.
Guanethidine and a Thiazide: Guanethidine is particularly unsuitable for incorporation in a fixed-dose product because it is potent, produces marked side effects, and has a wide range of effective dosage and long duration of action. Successful regulation of blood pressure with guanethidine requires careful titration of dosage, and adjustment is often required during continuous therapy. These considerations make use of a fixed-dose combination impractical and undesirable.
   Esimil (CIBA). Each tablet contains guanethidine monosulfate 10 mg (equivalent to 8.4 mg guanethidine sulfate) and hydrochlorothiazide 25 mg.

Beta-Adrenergic Blocking Drugs

Propranolol [Inderal], acebutolol [Sectral], atenolol [Tenormin], metoprolol [Lopressor], nadolol [Corgard], pindolol [Visken], and timolol [Blocadren] are the only beta-adrenergic blocking drugs that are marketed in the United States, but a number of others are currently under investigation. The pharmacology of these drugs is discussed in detail in Chapter 25, Antianginal Agents, and their properties are summarized in Table 4.

ACTIONS. Beta-adrenergic receptors are located primarily in the heart, arteries and arterioles of skeletal muscle, bronchi,

TABLE 4.
BETA-ADRENERGIC BLOCKING DRUGS

Drug	Tradename and Manufacturer	Cardio-selectivity	Partial Agonist Activity	Membrane Stabilizinig Properties
Acebutolol	Sectral (Wyeth)	+	+	+
Alprenolol*	Aptine (Astra)	−	+	+
Atenolol	Tenormin (Stuart)	+	−	−
Betaxolol	Betoptic** (Alcon)	+	−	−
Bevantolol*	—(Parke-Davis)	+	−	?
Carteolol*	Cartrol (Abbott)	−	+	−
Esmolol*	Brevibloc (American Critical Care)	+	−	−
Levobunolol	Betagan** (Allergan)	−	−	−
Metoprolol	Lopressor (Geigy)	+	−	−
Nadolol	Corgard (Squibb)	−	−	−
Oxprenolol+	Trasicor (CIBA)	−	+	+
Penbutolol*	—(Lilly)	−	+	−
Pindolol	Visken (Sandoz)	−	+	+
Propranolol	Inderal (Ayerst)	−	−	+
Sotalol*	Sotalex (Mead Johnson)	−	−	−
Timolol	Blocadren, Timoptic ** (Merck Sharp & Dohme)	−	−	−

   * *Investigational*
   + *Approved but not marketed*
   ** *Ophthalmic preparation*

pancreas, liver, kidney, and adipose tissue, where they subserve cardiac excitation, vasodilatation, and bronchial relaxation and mediate certain metabolic effects, such as lipolysis and glycogenolysis. Beta blocking agents combine reversibly with these receptors to block the response to sympathetic nerve impulses or circulating catecholamines. Blockade of cardiac (beta$_1$) receptors reduces heart rate and myocardial contractility, thus decreasing cardiac output. The atrioventricular (A-V) conduction time is slowed and automaticity is suppressed.

Blockade of noncardiac (beta$_2$) receptors increases airway resistance, inhibits catecholamine-induced glycogenolysis, and blocks the vasodilating effect of catecholamines on peripheral blood vessels. These noncardiac actions underlie some of the adverse effects of beta-blocking drugs (bronchospasm, hypoglycemia, interaction with sympathomimetic amines, and, possibly, aggravation of peripheral vascular insufficiency). Propranolol, nadolol, pindolol, and timolol are "nonselective" because they block beta receptors equally at all sites, whereas acebutolol, atenolol, and metoprolol are classified as "relatively cardioselective." Cardioselectivity is not absolute and may be apparent only at subtherapeutic doses.

Beta blockers also differ in partial agonist activity (PAA) and membrane stabilizing (local anesthetic) effect. These characteristics do not appear to influence safety or antihypertensive efficacy (Davidson et al, 1976), but agents with significant PAA (pindolol, acebutolol) cause less resting bradycardia than those lacking this property. Other potential benefits of PAA (eg, less depression of myocardial contractility, A-V conduction, and respiratory function) have not been clearly established (Frishman and Kostis, 1982).

Beta-blocking drugs reduce both supine and standing blood pressure during long-term therapy without causing orthostatic hypotension. Their antihypertensive effect has been attributed to various mechanisms: (1) Reduced cardiac output. Beta blockers may lower blood pressure by reducing cardiac output or through circulatory adjustments to a chronic reduction in cardiac output. More recently, it has been suggested that the antihypertensive mechanism of beta blockers (in patients who are also receiving diuretics) may be a reduction in cardiac output in the supine position and a reduction in total peripheral resistance in the upright position (Mulvihill-Wilson et al, 1985). (2) Effect on the central nervous system. Other investigators have suggested that beta blockers lower blood pressure by an effect on adrenergic receptors in the central nervous system, but this mechanism is unlikely because agents that readily enter the central nervous system are no more effective than those that do not. (3) Inhibition of renin release. This action is probably not involved because there is little or no relationship between the antihypertensive effect of beta-blocking drugs and changes in plasma renin activity, particularly in patients receiving diuretics and/or vasodilators. (4) Inhibition of norepinephrine release. In addition to blocking beta receptors postsynaptically, beta blockers may inhibit the release of norepinephrine from sympathetic nerve endings by presynaptic beta blockade.

Beta blockers may increase the serum potassium level slightly by decreasing the intracellular uptake of potassium or by suppressing plasma renin and serum aldosterone concentrations. This action is believed to be mediated by beta$_2$ receptors. Despite this effect, hypokalemia may still occur when a potassium-wasting diuretic is given concomitantly.

USES. A beta blocker is often given as the second drug in the antihypertensive regimen, but it may be a useful Step 1 drug in patients with symptomatic coronary artery disease (particularly after acute myocardial infarction) or arrhythmias and in young patients with hyperkinetic circulation. These drugs reduce the reinfarction rate and improve mortality of patients who have survived an acute myocardial infarction (see Chapter 25, Antianginal Agents).

Beta blockers are more effective in whites than in blacks (VA Cooperative Study Group on Antihypertensive Agents, 1982, part 1). Elderly patients may be less responsive to their antihypertensive effect than younger patients (Greenberg et al, 1984).

Plasma levels of the beta-blocking drugs do not correlate with the antihypertensive response and are not useful as a guide to therapy.

ADVERSE REACTIONS, PRECAUTIONS, AND INTERACTIONS. Beta blockers should be given with great caution to patients with borderline cardiac reserve because they may precipitate congestive heart failure. Concomitant diuretic therapy may reduce this risk, but it is usually advisable to prescribe digitalis also.

Beta blockers may cause A-V dissociation and even cardiac arrest in patients with A-V block and are contraindicated in the presence of severe A-V conduction disturbances (ie, greater than first-degree A-V block).

Beta blockers also may cause cold extremities, precipitate or aggravate Raynaud's phenomenon, and exacerbate intermittent claudication. The peripheral vascular effects have been attributed to beta$_2$ blockade, to the reduction in cardiac output, and/or to a compensatory vasoconstrictor response to the reduced cardiac output. Chronic occlusive peripheral vascular disease is a relative contraindication to use of these agents.

In patients with coronary artery disease, the sudden withdrawal of a beta blocker may be followed by recurrence of unstable angina, ventricular tachycardia, myocardial infarction, and, rarely, sudden death (see Chapter 25, Antianginal Agents). Symptoms suggesting sympathetic overactivity have been reported very rarely in patients with severe hypertension after withdrawal of large doses.

Large doses of agents with PAA may paradoxically increase the blood pressure. Hypertensive reactions have occurred occasionally because of an interaction between propranolol and intravenous epinephrine or when propranolol was administered without prior alpha blockade to patients with pheochromocytoma. Hypertensive reactions also were reported when clonidine was withdrawn rapidly from patients receiving propranolol concurrently. A hypertensive episode in one patient was attributed to an interaction between the methyldopa metabolite, alpha-methylnorepinephrine, and intravenous propranolol. All of these interactions are caused by beta$_2$ blockade, which prevents beta-adrenergic vasodilation and thus permits unopposed alpha stimulation.

Beta$_2$ blockade increases airway resistance and may provoke asthmatic attacks in patients with a history of asthma or chronic bronchitis. Although a cardioselective beta blocker may be safer than a nonselective one, all should be used cautiously. Beta blockers also may worsen respiratory function in patients with nonasthmatic chronic obstructive lung disease. Severe, epinephrine-resistant anaphylactic reactions also have been reported.

Beta$_2$ blockade may mask some of the warning symptoms of hypoglycemia and prolong the duration of hypoglycemia in those receiving insulin. Although beta blockers are probably safe for most diabetics, they may potentiate and prolong insulin-induced hypoglycemia and may produce hypoglycemia in patients recovering from anesthesia, in those on dialysis, and in children during periods of restricted food intake. Beta blockers also occasionally induce hypoglycemia during prolonged exercise. In hypertensive patients, blood pressure may increase during hypoglycemic episodes.

Beta-blocking drugs reduce serum HDL cholesterol, increase serum triglyceride and uric acid levels, and may enhance the effect of thiazide diuretics on blood glucose, urate, and lipid levels.

Neurologic and psychiatric adverse effects of beta blockers include fatigue, lethargy, vivid dreams, depression, memory loss, hallucinations, delirium, psychotic reactions, and paresthesias. Hydrophilic beta blockers (eg, atenolol, nadolol) do not cross the blood-brain barrier as readily as the more lipophilic agents (eg, propranolol, metoprolol, pindolol, timolol). Atenolol or nadolol may be worth a trial in patients who experience central nervous system disturbances from the lipophilic drugs, although the same effects have been reported occasionally with these agents.

Beta blockers also may cause sexual dysfunction (decreased libido and impotence), gastrointestinal disturbances, and, rarely, fever, rash, myopathy, arthropathy, cheilostomatitis, alopecia, and blood dyscrasias.

Beta blockers cross the placenta and have rarely caused bradycardia, hypotension, and hypoglycemia in the newborn. They are excreted in breast milk. Atenolol, metoprolol, nadolol, propranolol, and timolol are classified in FDA Pregnancy Category C and acebutolol and pindolol in FDA Pregnancy Category B.

The adverse effects and interactions of beta blockers are discussed in more detail in Chapter 25, Antianginal Agents.

PROPRANOLOL HYDROCHLORIDE
[Inderal]

USES. Propranolol is used as a Step 1 or Step 2 drug in the antihypertensive regimen. Its hypotensive effect is equivalent to that of a thiazide diuretic (Berglund and Andersson, 1981) or slightly less (VA Cooperative Study Group on Antihypertensive Agents, 1982, part 2). Combined thiazide/propranolol treat-

ment provides an enhanced therapeutic response (VA Cooperative Study Group on Antihypertensive Agents, 1977). Hydralazine may be added if a further reduction in blood pressure is required; this regimen is particularly useful in moderate to severe hypertension and is usually well tolerated by patients who have experienced disabling side effects with other regimens. Propranolol is more effective in preventing cardiovascular complications in nonsmokers than in smokers (Medical Research Council Working Party, 1985).

Propranolol may be added to an alpha-adrenergic blocking agent to prevent tachycardia and ventricular arrhythmias during the preoperative management of patients with pheochromocytoma and for prolonged treatment of patients who are not suitable candidates for surgery. A beta blocker should not be used in these patients without first administering adequate doses of the alpha-blocking drug, because it may increase blood pressure if used alone.

Propranolol also prevents the severe hypertension that often occurs after repair of coarctation of the aorta (Gidding et al, 1985). It is given orally for two weeks before surgery, intravenously during the immediate postoperative period, and orally for the first postoperative week.

ADVERSE REACTIONS AND PRECAUTIONS. See the Introduction and Chapter 25, Antianginal Agents.

PHARMACOKINETICS. See Chapter 25.

DOSAGE AND PREPARATIONS. Dosage must be titrated on the basis of the therapeutic response because the effective dose varies widely. Maximal effects may not be evident for several weeks.

Oral: For chronic hypertension (*regular preparation*), *adults,* initially, 40 mg twice daily. If the desired response is not obtained, the dosage should be increased to 80 mg twice daily. Further 80-mg increments may be added, if needed, to a maximum of 480 mg daily, usually in one or two divided doses. If control is not adequate, the drug should be given three times daily. The daily dose usually need not exceed 320 mg when propranolol is given with a diuretic and hydralazine.

Children, 1 mg/kg four times daily.

(*Long-acting preparation*), *adults,* initially, 80 mg once daily. For maintenance, 120 to 160 mg once daily. Occasionally, a daily dose of 480 mg may be required.

For pheochromocytoma, the dosage varies widely and must be individualized.

Generic. Tablets 10, 20, 40, and 80 mg.
Inderal (Ayerst). Tablets 10, 20, 40, 60, and 80 mg.
Inderal LA (Ayerst). Capsules (timed-release) 80, 120 and 160 mg.

AVAILABLE MIXTURES.

Propranolol and a Thiazide: Since the effective dose of propranolol varies widely, these combinations may not be suitable for all patients. A combination should not be used when large daily doses of propranolol are required because such use would lead to an excessive dose of the thiazide.

Inderide (Ayerst). Each tablet contains propranolol hydrochloride 40 or 80 mg and hydrochlorothiazide 25 mg.
Inderide LA (Ayerst). Each capsule (timed-release) contains propranolol hydrochloride 80, 120, or 160 mg and hydrochlorothiazide 50 mg.

ACEBUTOLOL HYDROCHLORIDE
[Sectral]

$$CH_3CH_2CH_2CNH$$
(structure: aromatic ring with acetyl group CCH_3, side chain OCH_2CHCH_2NHCH, OH, $(CH_3)_2$)

USES. Acebutolol has a relatively selective action on beta$_1$ receptors and mild partial agonist activity (PAA). Like other beta blockers, it is used as Step 1 or Step 2 in the antihypertensive regimen.

ADVERSE REACTIONS AND PRECAUTIONS. The adverse effects of acebutolol resemble those of other cardioselective beta blockers and the same precautions apply (see the Introduction and Chapter 25, Antianginal Agents). Because it possesses mild ISA, acebutolol may cause less resting bradycardia than beta blockers lacking this characteristic.

PHARMACOKINETICS. See Chapter 25, Antianginal Agents.

DOSAGE AND PREPARATIONS.
Oral: Initially, 400 mg as a single dose or in two divided doses. For maintenance, 200 to 800 mg daily. Some patients may require up to 1.2 g daily in two divided doses. Doses exceeding 800 mg daily should be avoided in elderly patients.
    Sectral (Wyeth). Capsules 200 and 400 mg.

ATENOLOL
[Tenormin]

(structure: H_2NCCH_2 attached to aromatic ring, side chain OCH_2CHCH_2NHCH, OH, $(CH_3)_2$)

USES. Atenolol is a long-acting beta blocker that acts primarily on beta$_1$ receptors. Like other beta blockers, atenolol is used as Step 1 or Step 2 in the antihypertensive regimen. Atenolol has been used to treat essential hypertension in pregnant women and early pre-eclampsia.

ADVERSE REACTIONS AND PRECAUTIONS. The adverse effects of atenolol resemble those of other cardioselective beta-blocking drugs and the same precautions apply (see the Introduction and Chapter 25, Antianginal Agents). Although atenolol does not readily cross the blood-brain barrier, central nervous system side effects have been reported with its use.

PHARMACOKINETICS. See Chapter 25, Antianginal Agents.

DOSAGE AND PREPARATIONS. Atenolol may be used as initial therapy or may be given with a diuretic as Step 2.
Oral: Adults, initially, 25 mg once daily. If the desired response is not obtained, dosage may be increased to 50 mg daily and then to 100 mg daily. A further increase is unlikely to produce further benefit. The following maximal doses are recommended for patients with renal impairment: 50 mg daily for patients with creatinine clearance of 15 to 35 mg/min/1.73 M^2; 50 mg on alternate days for patients with creatinine clearance of less than 15 ml/min/1.73 M^2.
    Tenormin (Stuart). Tablets 50 and 100 mg.
AVAILABLE MIXTURE.

Atenolol and a Thiazide: The following mixture may be useful if the dosage ratio meets the needs of the patient.
    Tenoretic 50, 100 (Stuart). Each tablet contains atenolol 50 or 100 mg and chlorthalidone 25 mg.

METOPROLOL TARTRATE
[Lopressor]

(structure: $CH_3OCH_2CH_2$ attached to aromatic ring, side chain $OCH_2CHCH_2\overset{+}{N}H_2CH$, OH, $(CH_3)_2$; with tartrate anion CO^-, $HCOH$, $HOCH$, COH, O)

USES. Metoprolol acts primarily on beta$_1$ receptors. Like other beta blockers, metoprolol is used as Step 1 or Step 2 in the antihypertensive regimen.

ADVERSE REACTIONS AND PRECAUTIONS. The adverse effects of metoprolol that are secondary to cardiac beta blockade are identical to those produced by propranolol and other beta blockers and the same precautions apply (see the Introduction and Chapter 25, Antianginal Agents).

Despite its relative cardioselectivity, effective doses may increase airway resistance in asthmatic patients (although to a lesser extent than propranolol) and may mask the warning symptoms of hypoglycemia in diabetics and delay the return to normoglycemia; blood pressure may increase during the hypoglycemic episode. Metoprolol also may aggravate peripheral vascular insufficiency.

See also Chapter 25.

PHARMACOKINETICS. See Chapter 25.

DOSAGE AND PREPARATIONS. The effective dose varies widely and must be titrated on the basis of the therapeutic response. Metoprolol may be used as initial therapy or may be given with a diuretic as Step 2.
Oral: Adults, initially, 50 mg daily. If the desired response is not obtained, the dosage may be increased gradually. The maintenance dose ranges from 100 to 300 mg daily, usually given in one or two doses. If control is not adequate, the drug should be given three times daily.
    Lopressor (Geigy). Tablets 50 and 100 mg.
AVAILABLE MIXTURE.

Metoprolol and a Thiazide: The following mixture may be useful if the dosage ratio meets the optimal needs of the patient.
    Lopressor HCT (Geigy). Each tablet contains metoprolol tartrate 50 or 100 mg and hydrochlorothiazide 25 mg or metoprolol tartrate 100 mg and hydrochlorothiazide 50 mg.

NADOLOL
[Corgard]

USES. Nadolol is a long-acting beta blocker that acts on both beta$_1$ and beta$_2$ receptors. Like other beta blockers, nadolol is used as Step 1 or Step 2 in the antihypertensive regimen (Freis, 1984 B).

ADVERSE REACTIONS AND PRECAUTIONS. See the Introduction and Chapter 25, Antianginal Agents.

PHARMACOKINETICS. See Chapter 25.

DOSAGE AND PREPARATIONS. The effective dose varies widely and dosage must be titrated according to the therapeutic response. Nadolol may be used as initial therapy or may be given with a diuretic as Step 2.

Oral: Adults, initially, 20 mg once daily. Dosage may be increased gradually to a usual maintenance dose of 40 to 80 mg. Up to 120 mg daily may be required rarely. The dosage interval should be increased as follows in patients with renal impairment:

Creatinine Clearance (ml/min/1.73 M²)	Dosage Interval (hrs)
>50	24
31-50	24-36
10-30	24-48
<10	40-60

Corgard (Squibb). Tablets 40, 80, 120, and 160 mg.
AVAILABLE MIXTURE.

Nadolol and a Thiazide: The following mixture may be useful if the dosage ratio meets the optimal needs of the patient.

Corzide (Squibb). Each tablet contains nadolol 40 or 80 mg and bendroflumethiazide 5 mg.

PINDOLOL
[Visken]

Pindolol acts on both beta$_1$ and beta$_2$ receptors and has partial agonist activity (PAA). Like other beta blockers, pindolol is used as Step 1 or Step 2 in the antihypertensive regimen.

ADVERSE REACTIONS. For adverse effects of nonselective beta blockers and precautions, see the Introduction and Chapter 25, Antianginal Agents. Because it possesses ISA, pindolol may cause less resting bradycardia than beta block-

ers lacking this characteristic. Also because of this feature, large doses may cause a paradoxical increase in blood pressure.

PHARMACOKINETICS. See Chapter 25.

DOSAGE AND PREPARATIONS. Pindolol may be used as initial therapy or may be given with a diuretic as Step 2.

Oral: Adults, initially, 10 mg twice daily or 5 mg three times daily. If a satisfactory response is not obtained in two to three weeks, the dosage may be increased by 10 mg/day at two- to three-week intervals up to 60 mg daily.

Visken (Sandoz). Tablets 5 and 10 mg.

TIMOLOL MALEATE
[Blocadren]

Timolol acts on both beta$_1$ and beta$_2$ receptors. Like other beta blockers, timolol is used as Step 1 or Step 2 in the antihypertensive regimen.

ADVERSE REACTIONS. For adverse effects of nonselective beta blockers and precautions, see the Introduction and Chapter 25, Antianginal Agents.

PHARMACOKINETICS. See Chapter 25.

DOSAGE AND PREPARATIONS. Timolol may be used as initial therapy or may be given with a diuretic as Step 2.

Oral: Initially, 10 mg twice daily. For maintenance, 20 to 40 mg daily. Some patients may require 60 mg daily in two divided doses.

Blocadren (Merck Sharp & Dohme). Tablets 5, 10, and 20 mg.
AVAILABLE MIXTURE.

Timolol Maleate and a Thiazide: The following mixture may be useful if the dosage ratio meets the optimal needs of the patient.

Timolide 10/25 (Merck Sharp & Dohme). Each tablet contains timolol maleate 10 mg and hydrochlorothiazide 25 mg.

Alpha- and Beta-Adrenergic Blocking Drug

LABETALOL HYDROCHLORIDE
[Normodyne, Trandate]

ACTIONS. Labetalol is a competitive antagonist at both alpha- and beta-adrenergic receptor sites and thus it reduces heart rate and myocardial contractility, slows A-V conduction, decreases total peripheral resistance, and lowers blood pressure. Labetalol selectively blocks alpha$_1$ receptors and is nonselective in its action on beta receptors. Following short-term administration, the antihypertensive effect of labetalol is largely due to vasodilation; during prolonged oral therapy, both peripheral resistance and heart rate are reduced.

USES. Oral labetalol is useful in patients with mild to severe hypertension. It is a preferred drug for the patient with coexisting angina and hypertension, although it has less antianginal activity than the beta blockers. The hypotensive effect of labetalol is enhanced by concomitant diuretic therapy, and it appears to be most suitable as a Step 2 drug. Its antihypertensive effect may be equivalent to that of a beta blocker and vasodilator combined and thus may obviate the need for a third drug.

The availability of both an oral and an intravenous preparation is convenient for converting a patient with a hypertensive crisis to oral therapy after initial control with the intravenous drug. Intravenous labetalol is used to treat various hypertensive emergencies, including malignant hypertension, hypertensive encephalopathy, postoperative hypertension, hypertension associated with extensive burns, and hypertension in patients with coronary artery disease or acute myocardial infarction. It has also been used in states of catecholamine excess such as severe tetanus, monoamine oxidase inhibitor-tyramine interaction, pheochromocytoma, and clonidine withdrawal syndrome but has occasionally caused a paradoxical hypertensive response in the two latter conditions. Some investigators have reported that intravenous labetalol is not consistently effective in patients concurrently receiving other antihypertensive drugs.

See also Wallin and O'Neill, 1983, and Prichard, 1984.

ADVERSE REACTIONS, PRECAUTIONS, AND INTERACTIONS. Labetalol may cause gastrointestinal disturbances (nausea, dyspepsia, abdominal pain, diarrhea), dryness of the mouth, tingling of the scalp, and fluid retention. Symptomatic orthostatic hypotension, occasionally with syncope, may occur, particularly during initial therapy or when larger than recommended doses are used. Excessive bradycardia has developed following overdosage. Bronchospasm, congestive heart failure, A-V conduction disturbances, and peripheral vascular reactions are less likely to occur with labetalol than with a beta-blocking drug but have been reported occasionally. All of the precautions and contraindications relating to use of beta blockers also pertain to labetalol, including the importance of avoiding rapid withdrawal in patients with angina.

Other reactions include lethargy, nervousness, urinary retention, nasal congestion, facial flushing, palpitations, sexual dysfunction (impotence, failure of ejaculation, decreased libido), paresthesias, muscle cramps or weakness, depression, nightmares, and reversible alopecia. Labetalol has occasionally produced a paradoxical increase in blood pressure in patients with pheochromocytoma or the clonidine withdrawal syndrome.

An increased titer of antinuclear antibodies has developed in some patients during long-term therapy, but a systemic lupus syndrome has been reported only rarely. Some patients also developed antimitochondrial antibodies. Elevated hepatic transaminase levels and, rarely, jaundice (usually cholestatic) have developed. Various types of rashes have occurred occasionally, including lichenoid skin eruptions, sometimes associated with increased antinuclear antibodies. Labetalol does not adversely affect blood lipid levels.

In animal studies, labetalol accumulated in tissue with high melanin content, such as the choroid; although the binding to eye pigment was reversible and no adverse ocular effects have been reported in humans, periodic eye examinations may be advisable during long-term therapy.

Labetalol crosses the placenta (FDA Pregnancy Category C) and is excreted in breast milk.

EFFECT ON LABORATORY TESTS. Labetalol has been reported to increase the excretion of catecholamines and their metabolites. This effect may be due to interference by labetalol or one of its metabolites with fluorometric and spectrophotometric methods of measuring catecholamine concentrations. A specific catecholamine radioenzymatic or high performance liquid chromatographic technique should be used to determine levels of catecholamines or their metabolites.

PHARMACOKINETICS. The bioavailability of labetalol is approximately 25% due to extensive first-pass metabolism. Food increases its bioavailability. Bioavailability also is increased in the elderly, in patients with liver disease, or in those taking cimetidine. Labetalol is widely distributed; during prolonged therapy, the volume of distribution is 9.4 L/kg and protein binding is 50%. This drug is moderately lipophilic. Labetalol is metabolized mainly by conjugation with glucuronic acid.

Less than 5% of a dose is excreted unchanged. The total body clearance is 33 ml/kg/min. The elimination half-life of oral labetalol is six to eight hours and is not affected by impaired renal function.

DOSAGE AND PREPARATIONS.
Oral: Adults, initially, 100 mg twice daily. For mild to moderate hypertension, the usual daily maintenance dose is 400 to 800 mg. Patients with severe hypertension may require up to 1.2 g daily in two or three divided doses. Concomitant diuretic therapy enhances the therapeutic response.

> ***Normodyne*** (Schering), ***Trandate*** (Glaxo). Tablets 100, 200, and 300 mg.

Intravenous: The patient should be kept in a supine position and blood pressure should be monitored during and after infusion or injection. Rapid or excessive reduction of either systolic or diastolic pressure should be avoided. *Adults,* initially, 20 mg may be given by slow intravenous injection over a two-minute period. Additional injections of 40 or 80 mg can be given at ten-minute intervals until the desired supine blood pressure is achieved or to a total dose of 300 mg. Alternatively, the drug may be given by slow continuous infusion; 200 mg (40 ml) is added to 160 or 250 ml of intravenous fluid and the solution is administered at a rate of 2 mg/min. The rate of infusion may be adjusted according to the blood pressure response.

Normodyne (Schering), *Trandate* (Glaxo). Solution 5 mg/ml in 20 ml containers.

Alpha-Adrenergic Blocking Drugs

Alpha-adrenergic receptors are found in most blood vessels but are most abundant in the resistance vessels of the skin, mucosa, intestine, and kidney. Stimulation of alpha receptors causes more vasoconstriction in these vascular beds. Alpha-adrenergic blocking agents block alpha receptors and thereby lower total peripheral resistance and decrease blood pressure.

Two alpha receptor subtypes have been identified pharmacologically: $alpha_1$ and $alpha_2$. Both types are found at postsynaptic sites where they mediate smooth muscle contraction. $Alpha_2$ receptors are also located on the presynaptic membrane where they regulate the release of norepinephrine from sympathetic nerve terminals. Stimulation of these receptors by high concentrations of norepinephrine in the synaptic cleft inhibits the subsequent release of norepinephrine by a negative feedback mechanism. $Alpha_2$ receptors also are found in the central nervous system, where they are involved in the central regulation of blood pressure (Frohlich, 1980; Hoffman and Lefkowitz, 1980; Van Zwieten et al, 1984).

Phentolamine [Regitine] blocks both $alpha_1$ and $alpha_2$ receptors, whereas prazosin [Minipress] selectively blocks $alpha_1$ receptors. Phenoxybenzamine [Dibenzyline] is a potent blocker of $alpha_1$ receptors and has a less pronounced but definite action on $alpha_2$ receptors. These differences, which were established in animal studies, are of questionable clinical importance during chronic therapy (Mulvihill-Wilson et al, 1983).

PRAZOSIN HYDROCHLORIDE
[Minipress]

ACTIONS. Prazosin is a quinazoline derivative that reduces total peripheral resistance by blocking $alpha_1$-adrenergic receptors. It dilates both arterioles and veins. Although prazosin decreases both supine and standing blood pressures, the hypotensive effect is most pronounced when the patient is standing. This drug has little effect on resting heart rate when the patient is supine or sitting; the heart rate increases when the patient is upright and during exercise. Prazosin has been reported to have no effect on plasma renin activity or to cause a slight increase.

USES. Since prazosin usually does not cause significant tachycardia, it may be used as a Step 2 or Step 3 drug. It is a preferred drug for treating patients with coexisting hypertension and congestive heart failure. When used in a three-drug regimen, prazosin and hydralazine were equally effective but side effects (dizziness, nightmares, sexual dysfunction) were more common with prazosin (VA Cooperative Study Group on Antihypertensive Agents, 1981). During long-term therapy, tolerance may develop to the antihypertensive effect of prazosin (Khatri et al, 1985).

ADVERSE REACTIONS AND PRECAUTIONS. Marked orthostatic hypotension and syncope, occasionally leading to collapse or loss of consciousness, may occur at the onset of treatment ("first dose phenomenon") or when dosage is increased. An associated tachycardia has been noted in some patients and chest pain has occurred rarely. Symptomatic orthostatic hypotension appears to be most common when the initial dose exceeds 2 mg and when the dose is increased rapidly. Patients receiving diuretics, beta blockers, and/or a low-sodium diet may be particularly susceptible. Although orthostatic hypotension may diminish during long-term therapy, rarely symptoms persist for at least six months (VA Cooperative Study Group on Antihypertensive Agents, 1981).

Prazosin may cause fluid retention and edema if a diuretic is not given concomitantly. Dryness of the mouth, nasal congestion, headache, nightmares, sexual dysfunction, and lethargy also may occur. Adverse effects rarely associated with prazosin therapy include urinary frequency, urinary incontinence, priapism, febrile polyarthritis, hypothermia, and dermatologic reactions (including urticaria and angioedema). Prazosin does not adversely affect blood lipid or blood glucose levels. In one study, antinuclear antibodies (ANA) were noted in one-third of patients taking prazosin; however, other investigators have found no relationship between prazosin therapy and ANA formation.

PHARMACOKINETICS. The bioavailability of prazosin ranges from 44% to 69%. Its absorption is not influenced by the presence of food in the gastrointestinal tract. The drug is 92% to 97% protein bound and its volume of distribution is 0.5 L/kg in hypertensive patients. Prazosin is extensively metabolized and less than 10% is excreted in the urine as unchanged drug. Clearance is 3 ± 0.3 ml/min/kg. The half-life of prazosin is approximately 2.5 hours and is prolonged in elderly patients and those with congestive heart failure.

DOSAGE AND PREPARATIONS. Rapid increases in dosage should be avoided. Prazosin should be added cautiously to the regimen of patients receiving a beta-blocking drug or other sympathetic depressants. When other antihypertensive drugs are added to the regimen, the dose of prazosin should be reduced to 1 or 2 mg and the optimal amount determined again on the basis of patient response.

Oral: Adults, to minimize the danger of a syncopal reaction, the first dose should not exceed 1 mg and should be given at bedtime. The patient should be instructed to remain in bed for several hours. Thereafter, 1 mg may be given two times daily, increased to three times daily later if required.

For maintenance, the dose may be increased gradually to 20 mg daily. Concomitant diuretic therapy enhances the therapeutic response. When administered with a diuretic and a beta blocker, relatively small doses may be sufficient for maintenance. *Children,* 0.1 mg/kg daily.

Minipress (Pfizer). Capsules 1, 2, and 5 mg.

AVAILABLE MIXTURE.

Prazosin and a Thiazide: The following combination is indicated only if the dosage ratio meets the optimal requirements of the patient.

Minizide 1, 2, 5 (Pfizer). Each capsule contains prazosin 1, 2, or 5 mg and polythiazide 0.5 mg.

INDORAMIN HYDROCHLORIDE
[Baratol]

ACTIONS. Indoramin is a selective alpha$_1$ blocker. In animal studies, it also exhibited membrane stabilizing, antihistamine, and slight antiserotonin properties. Like prazosin, indoramin reduces total peripheral resistance and venous tone but has little effect on heart rate and cardiac output.

USES. Indoramin has been used alone or with other drugs to treat mild to moderate hypertension. Its antihypertensive effect appears comparable to that of prazosin or methyldopa and is enhanced when a diuretic is given concomitantly.

ADVERSE REACTIONS AND PRECAUTIONS. Sedation is the most common adverse effect of indoramin. It also may cause dry mouth, nasal congestion, failure of ejaculation, depression, headache, and fluid retention. Dizziness may occur but syncopal reactions are rare. Overdosage has caused marked sedation, respiratory depression, hypotension, convulsions, and death.

PHARMACOKINETICS. Indoramin is well absorbed and undergoes extensive first-pass metabolism. It is 90% protein bound. The half-life is 5.5 hours and is increased in the elderly.

DOSAGE AND PREPARATIONS.
Oral: Adults, initially, 25 mg twice daily, increased gradually if necessary up to 200 mg daily in two or three doses. Diuretics enhance the therapeutic response.

Baratol (Wyeth). Tablets 25 and 50 mg.
(Investigational drug)

TERAZOSIN HYDROCHLORIDE
[Vasocard]

ACTIONS AND USES. Terazosin is a long-acting selective alpha$_1$-blocking agent that lowers blood pressure by reducing total peripheral resistance. Its antihypertensive efficacy has been demonstrated in patients with mild to moderate hypertension.

ADVERSE REACTIONS AND PRECAUTIONS. Adverse effects reported to date include lightheadedness, fatigue, headache, gastrointestinal disturbances, nasal congestion, tachycardia, and edema. Terazosin does not adversely affect blood lipids.

DOSAGE AND PREPARATIONS.

Oral: Adults, information is not sufficient to include dosage.
Vasocard (Abbott).
(Investigational drug)

TRIMAZOSIN HYDROCHLORIDE
[Cardovar]

ACTIONS. Trimazosin, a quinazoline derivative chemically related to prazosin, dilates both arterioles and veins. The effect of trimazosin on alpha$_1$ receptors is less pronounced than that of prazosin. It also has a direct action on vascular smooth muscle. The effects of trimazosin on heart rate are variable; heart rate usually is not affected during prolonged therapy. Trimazosin does not increase plasma renin activity.

USES. Trimazosin has been used alone and with a diuretic to treat mild to severe hypertension. Its efficacy appears to be comparable to that of other antiadrenergic drugs.

ADVERSE REACTIONS AND PRECAUTIONS. The adverse effects reported thus far are headache, orthostatic hypotension, drowsiness, weakness, fatigue, indigestion, nausea, edema, palpitations, chest pain, rash, flushing, and tinnitus. Trimazosin does not affect blood lipids.

PHARMACOKINETICS. The bioavailability of trimazosin is approximately 61%. It is 99% protein bound and is metabolized in the liver. The terminal elimination half-life of trimazosin is 2.7 hours; its major metabolite has a similar half-life.

DOSAGE AND PREPARATIONS.
Oral: Adults, 50 to 300 mg two or three times daily. In long-term studies, most patients responded to a total daily dose of 300 mg or less. Diuretics enhance the therapeutic response.

Cardovar (Pfizer). Capsules 25, 50, 100, and 150 mg.
(Investigational drug)

PHENOXYBENZAMINE HYDROCHLORIDE
[Dibenzyline]

PHENTOLAMINE MESYLATE
[Regitine]

ACTIONS. These alpha-adrenergic blocking agents reduce total peripheral resistance, venous tone, and blood pressure and may increase heart rate.

USES. Phenoxybenzamine and phentolamine are used to treat hypertensive states caused by an excess of circulating catecholamines. They are generally not useful in patients with uncomplicated essential hypertension, although phenoxybenzamine has occasionally been given to patients with severe, resistant hypertension who responded inadequately to various combination regimens.

Phenoxybenzamine is administered orally for the long-term treatment of patients with pheochromocytoma who are not suitable candidates for surgery; it also may be given preoperatively. A beta-adrenergic blocking agent may be used concomitantly to prevent excessive tachycardia.

Phentolamine mesylate is given intravenously to control blood pressure of patients with pheochromocytoma in the pre- and intraoperative periods, particularly when marked increases in blood pressure occur during surgical manipulation of the tumor. In the past, phentolamine was administered intravenously for diagnosis of pheochromocytoma, but measurement of plasma catecholamines and/or urinary catecholamine metabolites is now preferred (Bravo and Gifford, 1984). Phentolamine also is used to treat hypertensive crises caused by interaction between monoamine oxidase inhibitors and sympathomimetic amines and in the clonidine withdrawal syndrome.

ADVERSE REACTIONS AND PRECAUTIONS. On acute administration, reflex tachycardia and orthostatic hypotension are the most common untoward effects. Anginal pain and arrhythmias may occur, particularly with intravenous phentolamine. The tendency of these alpha blockers to cause reflex tachycardia has been attributed to their effect on alpha$_2$ receptors. However, during prolonged therapy in hypertensive patients, the effect of phenoxybenzamine on heart rate does not differ significantly from that of prazosin (Mulvihill-Wilson et al, 1983).

When phenoxybenzamine is used for long-term therapy, nasal congestion, sexual dysfunction (impaired ejaculation), gastrointestinal disturbances (nausea, vomiting, diarrhea), and stress incontinence may occur.

DOSAGE AND PREPARATIONS.
PHENOXYBENZAMINE HYDROCHLORIDE:
Oral: For pheochromocytoma, dosage varies widely and must be individualized.
   Dibenzyline (Smith Kline & French). Capsules 10 mg.
PHENTOLAMINE MESYLATE:
Intravenous: When used to control blood pressure immediately before or during surgery for pheochromocytoma, dosage varies widely and must be individualized.

For diagnosis of pheochromocytoma, *adults,* 5 mg dissolved in 1 ml of sterile water; *children,* 1 mg. A fall in blood pressure of more than 35 mm Hg systolic and 25 mm Hg diastolic suggests pheochromocytoma.

For hypertensive crises due to interaction of a monoamine oxidase inhibitor with sympathomimetic amines, *adults,* 5 to 20 mg.

For clonidine withdrawal syndrome, *adults,* 5 to 10 mg at five-minute intervals to a total dose of 20 to 30 mg.
   Regitine (CIBA). Powder (lyophilized) 5 mg with diluent.

Agent That Blocks Catecholamine Synthesis

METYROSINE
[Demser]

ACTIONS AND USES. Metyrosine blocks the first (and rate-limiting) step of catecholamine synthesis by inhibiting tyrosine hydroxylase, which catalyzes the conversion of tyrosine to DOPA. When administered to patients with pheochromocytoma, metyrosine reduces catecholamine production (as measured by excretion of catecholamines and metabolites) and usually decreases the frequency and severity of hypertensive attacks and associated symptoms (Engelman et al, 1968). It is useful for preoperative treatment and for long-term therapy when surgery is not feasible. Metyrosine has not been compared to the traditional treatment regimen for pheochromocytoma (combined therapy with alpha- and beta-blocking drugs). Phenoxybenzamine or prazosin should be added or substituted if the patient's condition is not adequately controlled by metyrosine. This drug is not indicated in essential hypertension.

ADVERSE REACTIONS, PRECAUTIONS, AND INTERACTIONS. Sedation is the most common adverse effect of metyrosine but usually lessens after the first week of therapy unless the dosage is increased. Anxiety and other central nervous system disturbances (depression, confusion, disorientation, hallucinations) also have been reported. Insomnia and psychic stimulation may occur when the drug is withdrawn. Extrapyramidal reactions have been reported in about 10% of patients, and the extrapyramidal effects of phenothiazines and butyrophenones may be potentiated.

Diarrhea has occurred in approximately 10% of patients and may be severe. Other gastrointestinal disturbances include nausea, vomiting, and abdominal pain.

Crystalluria and transient dysuria and hematuria have developed in some patients. To reduce the risk of nephrolithiasis, the patient should maintain a water intake sufficient to achieve a daily urine output of 2 L or more. The drug should be discontinued if crystalluria persists despite an increase in water intake.

Other adverse effects include breast swelling and galactorrhea, nasal congestion, dryness of the mouth, headache, sexual dysfunction (impotence, failure of ejaculation), eosinophilia, increased SGOT levels, peripheral edema, and hypersensitivity reactions (urticaria, pharyngeal edema).

PHARMACOKINETICS. Metyrosine is well absorbed from the gastrointestinal tract. Maximal biochemical effects occur one to three days after initiation of therapy, and the urinary concentration of catecholamines and metabolites usually returns to pretreatment levels three to four days after the drug is discontinued. Metyrosine is excreted in the urine largely as unchanged drug.

DOSAGE AND PREPARATIONS.

Oral: Adults and children over 12 years, initially, 250 mg four times daily, which may be increased by increments of 250 to 500 mg daily. The effective daily dose usually ranges between 2 and 3 g (maximum, 4 g). The optimal effective amount should be given for at least five to seven days before surgery. Dosage should be titrated by monitoring clinical symptoms, blood pressure, and catecholamine excretion. Phentolamine should be available during surgery, because metyrosine does not eliminate the danger of a hypertensive crisis caused by manipulation of the tumor.

Demser (Merck Sharp & Dohme). Capsules 250 mg.

Monoamine Oxidase Inhibitor

The monoamine oxidase inhibitor, pargyline [Eutonyl], and the combination of pargyline and a thiazide [Eutron] are seldom used because of the potential for serious adverse reactions following ingestion of foods containing high levels of tyramine or preparations containing sympathomimetic amines.

DIRECT-ACTING VASODILATORS

Arterial Vasodilators

HYDRALAZINE HYDROCHLORIDE
[Apresoline]

ACTIONS. Hydralazine reduces blood pressure by directly relaxing arteriolar smooth muscle; it has little effect on veins. Heart rate and cardiac output are increased. The tachycardia induced by hydralazine is greater than would be expected solely on a reflex basis and is poorly correlated with changes in blood pressure. Results of animal studies suggest that the cardiac effects may result from a combination of three actions: (1) a reflex response to the fall in blood pressure; (2) a direct effect on the myocardium; and (3) an effect on the central nervous system.

USES. Hydralazine is given orally for the management of chronic hypertension, usually as a Step 3 drug. Since it does not cause sedation or orthostatic hypotension, small doses may be useful as Step 2 therapy for elderly patients who experience unacceptable side effects with antiadrenergic drugs. These patients often have blunted baroreceptor reflexes and do not usually experience tachycardia with hydralazine.

Hydralazine, administered parenterally, is sometimes used to treat hypertensive emergencies and may be particularly useful in patients with acute glomerulonephritis or eclampsia. The antihypertensive effect begins within 15 minutes after intravenous administration and lasts three or four hours. However, sodium nitroprusside and diazoxide are generally preferred because of their more rapid onset of action, greater hypotensive potency, and more consistent effectiveness.

ADVERSE REACTIONS AND PRECAUTIONS. Like other vasodilators, hydralazine causes sodium and water retention if a diuretic is not given concomitantly. Headache and tachycardia are common when hydralazine is given alone and can be minimized by increasing the dose gradually. Tachycardia also can be reduced or controlled by prior and concomitant administration of an antiadrenergic drug, particularly a beta blocker. Although hydralazine may precipitate myocardial ischemia in patients with coronary artery disease, such patients can often be managed satisfactorily by the coadministration of a beta-blocking drug and a diuretic. Because it increases the velocity of left ventricular ejection, hydralazine is contraindicated in patients with dissecting aortic aneurysm. Gastrointestinal disturbances, flushing, and rash also may occur.

Hydralazine may produce an acute rheumatoid syndrome simulating systemic lupus erythematosus (SLE) with a positive antinuclear antibody test, fever, myalgia, arthralgia, splenomegaly, edema, and LE cells in the peripheral blood. This syndrome is most common in slow acetylators receiving 200 mg daily or more, occurs more frequently in women than in men, and is less prevalent in black patients (who tend to be rapid acetylators) than in whites. The effects are generally reversible when the drug is withdrawn. In contrast to spontaneously occurring SLE, renal disease is only rarely a feature of hydralazine-induced SLE. Hydralazine need not be withdrawn solely on the basis of a positive antinuclear antibody test, because test results frequently become positive during prolonged therapy in asymptomatic patients (Mansilla-Tinoco et al, 1982).

Rarely, hydralazine has caused peripheral neuropathy, blood dyscrasias (including neonatal thrombocytopenia), hepatotoxicity, and acute cholangitis. The neuropathy appears to result from pyridoxine deficiency and can be corrected by administration of pyridoxine. The tartrazine in some brands of hydralazine tablets may cause allergic reactions.

Hydralazine crosses the placenta. Negligible amounts are excreted in breast milk.

PHARMACOKINETICS. The bioavailability of hydralazine is 30% to 50%. It is 87% protein bound and the volume of distribution is 1.6 L/kg. The drug has a relatively short half-life (2.2 to 2.6 hours) and is eliminated by the kidney as active drug (12% to 14%) and metabolites. Its clearance rate is 8 to 10 ml/min/kg. Acetylation is one of the metabolic pathways for inactivation of the drug. Fast acetylators have lower plasma levels than slow acetylators; however, the rate of elimination from plasma does not differ greatly between the two groups, and other metabolic pathways also may be important.

DOSAGE AND PREPARATIONS.

Oral: For chronic hypertension (usually as the third agent in the regimen), *adults,* initially, 10 to 25 mg two or three times daily. Dosage then may be increased by 10 to 25 mg until the blood pressure is reduced to the desired level. Since the risk of drug-induced lupus increases with doses exceeding 200 mg, the maximal daily dose should generally not exceed this amount. *Children,* initially, 0.75 mg/kg daily in four divided doses. The dosage may be increased gradually over the next three to four weeks to a maximum of 7.5 mg/kg daily.

    Generic. Tablets 10, 25, and 50 mg.

    Apresoline (CIBA). Tablets 10, 25, 50, and 100 mg.

Intravenous: *Adults,* for pre-eclampsia or eclampsia, initially, 5 mg followed by boluses of 5 to 10 mg every 20 minutes as needed.

Intravenous (slow), Intramuscular: For hypertensive crises, *adults,* 10 to 20 mg, increased to 40 mg if necessary. The dose should be repeated as required. *Children,* 1.7 to 3.5 mg/kg daily divided into four to six doses. Oral antihypertensive therapy should be instituted while the blood pressure is being stabilized.

    Apresoline (CIBA). Solution 20 mg/ml in 1 ml containers.

AVAILABLE MIXTURES.

Hydralazine and Other Antihypertensive Agents: The products listed below are indicated only if the dosage ratio meets the optimal requirements of the patient. Because the central nervous system side effects of reserpine are dose related and increase if the total dose exceeds 0.25 mg daily, mixtures containing this drug may not be suitable for patients requiring large doses of hydralazine. If a hydralazine-reserpine mixture is used, a diuretic should be prescribed separately.

    Apresazide 25/25, 50/50, 100/50 (CIBA). Each capsule contains hydralazine hydrochloride 25 mg and hydrochlorothiazide 25 mg; or hydralazine hydrochloride 50 mg and hydrochlorothiazide 50 mg; or hydralazine hydrochloride 100 mg and hydrochlorothiazide 50 mg.

    Apresoline-Esidrix (CIBA). Each tablet contains hydralazine hydrochloride 25 mg and hydrochlorothiazide 15 mg.

    Hyserp (Reid-Provident), *Ser-Ap-Es* (CIBA), *Tri-Hydroserpine* (Rugby), *Unipres* (Reid-Provident), *Generic.* Each tablet contains hydralazine hydrochloride 25 mg, hydrochlorothiazide 15 mg, and reserpine 0.1 mg.

    Serpasil-Apresoline No. 1, No. 2 (CIBA). Each No. 1 tablet contains hydralazine hydrochloride 25 mg and reserpine 0.1 mg; each No. 2 tablet contains hydralazine hydrochloride 50 mg and reserpine 0.2 mg.

MINOXIDIL

[Loniten]

ACTIONS. Minoxidil acts directly on arterioles to reduce total peripheral resistance. It has little or no effect on the venous system. When given alone, the hypotensive effect of minoxidil is accompanied by a marked increase in heart rate and cardiac output.

USES. Minoxidil is more potent and longer acting than hydralazine and is useful for long-term therapy in patients with hypertension refractory to maximum tolerated doses of stan-

dard antihypertensive drugs given in combination. It is effective in patients with malignant or accelerated hypertension and advanced renal disease and thus provides an alternative to bilateral nephrectomy. Both a diuretic and a beta blocker or other sympathetic depressant drug should be given concomitantly to control fluid retention, prevent tachycardia, and enhance the therapeutic response. Other antihypertensive drugs also may be continued or added as necessary (see also Campese, 1981).

ADVERSE REACTIONS, PRECAUTIONS, AND INTERACTIONS. Fluid retention, manifested by weight gain and edema, is common, may be difficult to control, and does not always result in loss of blood pressure control. Although congestive heart failure may improve when minoxidil therapy is instituted, substantial volume overload can precipitate or worsen heart failure in some patients. If fluid retention occurs, patients who are receiving a thiazide should be given furosemide instead, and those already receiving furosemide should receive a larger dose. Combined therapy with a thiazide (especially metolazone) and furosemide may be effective in refractory cases. This combination should be administered under close supervision because it can cause marked diuresis, severe hypokalemia, and an increase in the serum creatinine level. Dialysis should be instituted or minoxidil discontinued if excessive fluid retention cannot be managed by these measures.

Approximately 3% of patients not receiving dialysis have developed pericardial effusion while taking minoxidil. This complication is most common in patients with severely impaired renal function and may be related to fluid retention; however, it often persists despite vigorous diuretic therapy. Echocardiography should be performed if pericardial effusion is suspected. The effusion usually abates when minoxidil is withdrawn. Cardiac tamponade has developed rarely and should be treated by pericardiocentesis or surgical drainage.

Reflex cardiac stimulation combined with reduced coronary perfusion occasionally may precipitate anginal attacks in patients receiving minoxidil, particularly if beta blockade is inadequate. Myocardial infarction has occurred rarely. Rebound hypertension has developed rarely when minoxidil was withdrawn abruptly and may be due in part to the high levels of angiotensin II that are frequently associated with minoxidil therapy.

Electrocardiographic abnormalities (flattening or inversion of T waves, sometimes accompanied by increased QRS voltage) are frequently observed. These changes are usually asymptomatic and reversible following discontinuation of minoxidil. During long-term therapy, T-wave abnormalities generally disappear and the increased QRS voltage is reduced.

Pulmonary hypertension has been reported as a complication of minoxidil therapy and may be secondary to increased cardiac output (hyperkinetic type) or marked fluid retention (congestive type) (Tarazi et al, 1976). Other investigators have found no relationship between minoxidil therapy and pulmonary hypertension (Klotman et al, 1977).

Minoxidil is usually not associated with orthostatic hypotension, but severe orthostatic effects have developed occasionally when minoxidil was administered with guanethidine. Whenever possible, guanethidine should be discontinued before instituting therapy with minoxidil. If the patient's condition does not permit withdrawal of guanethidine, it may be advisable to institute minoxidil therapy in the hospital.

Hypertrichosis develops in about 80% of patients after one or two months of therapy. This side effect can be particularly distressing to women and children but is easily controlled by shaving or use of a depilatory. The abnormal hair growth usually appears first on the face and later extends to other areas; it may be accompanied by darkening of the skin and coarsening of the facial features. The increased hair growth has not been associated with any definite endocrine abnormalities and disappears gradually when the drug is withdrawn.

Other side effects occasionally reported are nausea, headache, fatigue, dermatologic reactions (including Stevens-Johnson syndrome), and breast tenderness. Hemorrhagic cardiac lesions have developed in laboratory animals treated with minoxidil. Necrotic areas in the papillary muscles have been reported in patients who died from various causes after receiving minoxidil, but similar lesions also have been observed in patients with ischemic heart disease who never received the drug.

This drug is classified in FDA Pregnancy Category C.

PHARMACOKINETICS. The bioavailability of minoxidil is approximately 90%. The plasma half-life is about 4.2 hours, but therapeutic activity lasts considerably longer (about 24 hours). The drug is extensively metabolized, mainly to the inactive metabolite, minoxidil glucuronide. Parent drug (12%) and metabolites (88%) are eliminated primarily in the urine. Plasma levels do not correlate with the therapeutic response.

DOSAGE AND PREPARATIONS. A diuretic (usually furosemide) and a beta-blocking agent or other sympathetic depressant drug should be given concomitantly in adequate therapeutic doses.

Oral: Adults and children over 12 years, initially, 5 mg once daily. The dosage may be increased gradually to 10, 20, and then 40 mg daily in single or divided doses if necessary. Most patients require 10 to 40 mg daily (maximum, 100 mg). Dosage adjustments are usually made at intervals of three days or longer. When more rapid control of hypertension is required, dose adjustments can be made every six hours if the patient is monitored carefully. *Children under 12 years,* initially, 0.2 mg/kg daily as a single dose. Dosage may be increased if necessary in increments of 0.1 to 0.2 mg/kg until control is achieved or a maximum dose of 50 mg/day is given. The effective dose usually ranges between 0.25 and 1 mg/kg daily.

Loniten (Upjohn). Tablets 2.5 and 10 mg.

DIAZOXIDE
[Hyperstat I.V.]

ACTIONS. Diazoxide is a nondiuretic thiazide derivative that reduces blood pressure rapidly when given intravenously. The hypotensive effect is caused by a direct action on the arterioles; capacitance vessels are not affected. Heart rate and cardiac output are increased.

USES. Diazoxide is effective in many hypertensive emergencies but its action is not as predictable as that of nitroprusside. It may be useful in patients with hypertensive encephalopathy, malignant hypertension, and severe hypertension associated with acute or chronic glomerulonephritis. Diazoxide is also used for rapid control of blood pressure in patients with pre-eclampsia who are refractory to hydralazine; however, it usually abolishes spontaneous uterine contractions, necessitating use of oxytocin, and may cause neonatal hyperglycemia.

Diazoxide should be avoided in patients with coronary or cerebral vascular insufficiency in whom a rapid reduction in blood pressure could precipitate coronary or cerebral ischemia. Because it increases cardiac output and left ventricular ejection velocity, this agent is unsuitable for treating hypertension associated with dissecting aortic aneurysm.

ADVERSE REACTIONS AND PRECAUTIONS. Sodium and water retention, hyperglycemia, and hyperuricemia are the major side effects of diazoxide. Administration of adequate doses of furosemide will prevent fluid overload and may enhance the antihypertensive effect. This regimen is particularly important during repeated injections of diazoxide to avoid volume expansion and prevent drug resistance.

The hyperglycemic and hyperuricemic effects of diazoxide (which are more pronounced when a diuretic is given concomitantly) are usually mild and transitory; however, blood glucose levels should be monitored daily. Diabetic patients may require an adjustment of insulin dosage if repeated injections are necessary. Hyperglycemic, hyperosmolar, nonketoacidotic coma has been reported rarely following repeated administration of diazoxide; in one patient, hyperosmolar coma was associated with transient lens opacities. Neonatal hyperglycemia has occurred when diazoxide was given to the mother before delivery.

Diazoxide should be given by pulse administration of small doses or continuous infusion over 20 to 30 minutes because severe hypotension, anginal symptoms, cerebral ischemia, hemiplegia, and myocardial infarction have occurred after rapid injection of large (300 mg) doses. The risk of hypotension is enhanced in patients receiving other hypotensive agents concomitantly, particularly vasodilators.

Diazoxide also may cause gastrointestinal disturbances (nausea, vomiting, anorexia), headache, flushing, and temporary interruption of labor. Hypersensitivity reactions (rash, leukopenia, fever) are uncommon. Hemolytic episodes have occurred rarely. Extravasation causes severe local pain but tissue sloughing has not been reported.

Adverse effects reported after long-term oral therapy (eg, extrapyramidal symptoms, hypertrichosis) have not been noted after short-term intravenous use.

This drug is classified in FDA Pregnancy Category C.

PHARMACOKINETICS. Diazoxide is 90% bound to plasma protein, and it was formerly thought that the drug must be given as a bolus to exceed the binding capacity of serum albumin. Subsequent studies have shown that an adequate therapeutic response can be obtained with slow infusion (Garrett and Kaplan, 1982).

Diazoxide is eliminated by renal excretion, largely as unchanged drug. Its half-life is 28 ± 8 hours, but the duration of the therapeutic effect is variable. Clearance is 7 ml/min.

DOSAGE AND PREPARATIONS. Intravenous administration of furosemide will prevent fluid overload and ensure a continuing hypotensive response. Antihypertensive agents other than furosemide usually should not be given with diazoxide because of the risk of additive hypotensive effects, but oral therapy with other drugs may be instituted after the blood pressure has stabilized.

Intravenous: Adults, 1 to 3 mg/kg administered undiluted and rapidly up to a maximum of 150 mg in a single injection. This dose may then be repeated at intervals of 5 to 15 minutes until a satisfactory reduction in blood pressure has been achieved. This "minibolus" method of injection is as effective as the 300-mg dose formerly recommended and is safer. In pre-eclampsia and eclampsia, 30-mg miniboluses have been employed. Diazoxide also may be given by slow infusion over 20 to 30 minutes at a rate of 15 to 30 mg/min (Garrett and Kaplan, 1982). *Children,* 1 to 3 mg/kg.

Hyperstat I.V. (Schering). Solution 15 mg/ml in 20 ml containers.

Arterial and Venous Vasodilator

SODIUM NITROPRUSSIDE
[Nipride, Nitropress]

$$Na_2 \left[Fe(CN)_5 NO \right] \cdot 2H_2O$$

ACTIONS. This potent vasodilator acts directly to relax both resistance and capacitance vessels. Heart rate is usually increased by reflex mechanisms. Cardiac output generally is not increased because of the venodilation and reduction in venous return.

USES. Nitroprusside is the most rapid acting and consistently effective agent for treating hypertensive emergencies regardless of the cause. It reduces blood pressure immediately, but continuous infusion is necessary to maintain the hypotensive response. Because of its beneficial hemodynamic effects, nitroprusside is the drug of choice in the management of most hypertensive crises requiring parenteral therapy, including those associated with acute myocardial infarction and left ventricular failure. In hypertensive patients with cerebral or subarachnoid hemorrhage, nitroprusside infusion permits titration of the blood pressure to any desired level and restoration of a higher level in the event of neurologic deterioration.

ADVERSE REACTIONS AND PRECAUTIONS. Sodium nitroprusside may produce nausea, vomiting, headache, palpitations, restlessness, and sweating. These symptoms may be caused by the rapid fall in blood pressure and often are relieved by slowing the infusion rate or temporarily discontinuing the infusion.

Nitroprusside may cause muscle twitching, disorientation, delirium, and psychotic behavior. Hypothyroidism was ob-

served in one patient after infusion of 3.9 g over a period of 21 days. These adverse effects are usually attributed to the accumulation of thiocyanate during prolonged infusion, particularly in patients with renal insufficiency. If nitroprusside is infused for more than 72 hours (or less if renal failure is present), blood thiocyanate levels should be determined daily; if levels do not exceed 10 mg/dl, it is probably safe to continue administration.

High levels of blood cyanide may develop during infusion of large amounts, particularly in patients with inadequate endogenous thiosulfate or hepatic disease. Prolonged infusion should be avoided in patients with hepatic or renal disorders. Increased blood thiocyanate levels induce metabolic acidosis and also may occasionally cause tachyphylaxis. The blood thiocyanate level can be reduced by infusing sodium thiosulfate or hydroxocobalamin. Several deaths associated with use of nitroprusside during surgery have been attributed to cyanide poisoning. One case of methemoglobinemia has been reported.

Drug resistance has also been associated with an increase in cardiac output; if there is evidence of volume overload, responsiveness can be restored by administration of furosemide. A beta blocker may be useful if volume overload is not present (Rouby et al, 1982).

A rebound increase in blood pressure has occurred when nitroprusside was discontinued following its use to induce hypotension during anesthesia. Pretreatment with propranolol prevents this response. Nitroprusside may increase intracranial pressure in patients with brain tumors or metabolic encephalopathy. It decreases the platelet count and should be given cautiously to patients with bleeding tendencies or thrombocytopenia. Acute phlebitis has occurred rarely.

This drug is classified in FDA Pregnancy Category C.

PHARMACOKINETICS. Nitroprusside has a very brief half-life. It is converted by erythrocytes to cyanide, which is then transformed to the final metabolite, thiocyanate, by the hepatic enzyme, rhodanese. This reaction requires thiosulfate (which is derived endogenously from the amino acid, cysteine). Thiocyanate is eliminated by renal excretion. Its half-life is four to seven days in patients with normal renal function.

DOSAGE AND PREPARATIONS. Before using sodium nitroprusside, the manufacturer's prescribing information should be reviewed. Intravenous administration of furosemide will usually prevent fluid overload and ensure a continuing hypotensive response.

Intravenous: Sodium nitroprusside should be used only in an intensive care unit and the blood pressure should be monitored frequently during infusion. Administration with a variable rate infusion pump is preferred. The solution should be protected from light and, if used continuously, a fresh solution should be prepared every 24 hours.

Adults, 50 mg, dissolved in 250 to 1,000 ml of 5% dextrose injection in water, is infused at a rate of 0.5 to 10 mcg/kg/min. Oral therapy with other antihypertensive drugs should be instituted while the blood pressure is being stabilized with sodium nitroprusside. *Children,* 0.1 to 8 mcg/kg/min.

Nipride (Roche), *Nitropress* (Abbott), *Generic.* Powder (sterile) 50 mg.

ANGIOTENSIN-CONVERTING ENZYME INHIBITORS

Renin, a proteolytic enzyme produced and stored mainly in the kidney, is released in response to various stimuli, the most important being a reduction in renal perfusion pressure associated with hemorrhage, dehydration, chronic sodium depletion, or renal artery stenosis. The secretion of renin is also regulated by sympathetic nervous system activity and certain humoral factors.

In the circulatory system, renin reacts with a substrate formed in the liver to produce angiotensin I. This prohormone is then hydrolyzed to angiotensin II by a converting enzyme that is present in the lungs and to a lesser degree in other tissues. Angiotensin II acts on receptor sites in vascular smooth muscle, the central nervous system, and the adrenal cortex to constrict arterioles, increase sympathetic outflow from the central nervous system, reduce vagal tone, and induce secretion of aldosterone. These actions lead to an increase in total peripheral resistance, heart rate, and cardiac output, and to enhanced reabsorption of sodium and water. The resultant rise in blood pressure activates a feedback loop that reduces the secretion of renin. The renin-angiotensin-aldosterone system does not play an active role in maintaining circulatory homeostasis in the normovolemic, sodium-replete individual but is of major importance in maintaining blood pressure and intravascular volume during sodium deprivation or volume depletion.

Captopril and enalapril block the conversion of angiotensin I to angiotensin II by inhibiting the converting enzyme. These angiotensin-converting enzyme (ACE) inhibitors reduce blood pressure in both essential and renovascular hypertension. A correlation between initial plasma renin activity and the hypotensive response to ACE inhibitors is observed after short-term but not after long-term therapy; therefore, these agents do not appear to act solely through inhibition of the renin-angiotensin-aldosterone system. The ACE inhibitors may reduce sympathetic tone by inhibiting the action of angiotensin II on neurogenic vasoconstriction. They also prevent degradation of the vasodilator, bradykinin, and may increase production of vasodilator prostaglandins. However, these actions have not been shown to contribute to their therapeutic efficacy.

The competitive angiotensin antagonist, saralasin, is no longer marketed. Renin inhibitors (renin inhibitory peptides and renin-specific antibodies) are in the early stages of investigation (Cody, 1984).

CAPTOPRIL
[Capoten]

ACTIONS. Captopril is an orally active competitive inhibitor of angiotensin I-converting enzyme (ACE), which converts the inactive angiotensin I to angiotensin II. Inhibition of ACE by captopril leads to a decrease in circulating angiotensin II and aldosterone levels, which is accompanied by a compensatory increase in angiotensin I and renin concentrations. Because of the reduction in aldosterone secretion, less sodium-potassium exchange occurs in the distal renal tubules and the serum potassium concentration may increase slightly (Gavras et al, 1978; Johnston et al, 1979). Aldosterone secretion, which is influenced by other factors in addition to the renin-angiotensin system, may return to the pretreatment level during prolonged therapy.

The antihypertensive effect of captopril is associated with a decrease in total peripheral resistance. Blood pressure falls within two hours after therapy is instituted, but several weeks of treatment may be required before the optimal therapeutic response is attained. Captopril also reduces venous tone. It usually has little effect on heart rate.

Diuretics enhance the antihypertensive effect of captopril. During combined therapy, captopril reduces diuretic-induced hyperaldosteronism and hypokalemia, but the two drugs have additive effects on plasma renin levels.

USES. In small doses, captopril may be useful for treating mild to moderate hypertension, particularly when it is given with a thiazide diuretic (VA Cooperative Study Group on Antihypertensive Agents, 1984; Frohlich et al, 1984; Materson, 1984). Severe refractory hypertension often can be controlled by large doses of captopril given with a diuretic; other agents, such as a beta blocker, may be required in some patients. Captopril is more effective in whites than in blacks when used as sole therapy. It is a preferred drug for patients with coexisting hypertension and congestive heart failure.

Captopril also may be used for hypertensive urgencies when immediate reduction of blood pressure with parenteral drugs is not required.

ADVERSE REACTIONS, PRECAUTIONS, AND INTERACTIONS. Some adverse effects of captopril (rash, taste disturbances) resemble those of penicillamine and have been attributed to the sulfhydryl group in its molecule. Approximately 10% of patients have developed maculopapular or morbilliform rashes, sometimes accompanied by fever and/or pruritus. Pruritus also has occurred without rash. Urticaria, angioedema, lichenoid eruptions, pemphigus-like reactions, onycholysis, unexplained cough, erythroderma, exfoliative dermatitis, and alopecia have been reported rarely. Dermatologic reactions disappear when the drug is withdrawn and some erythematous rashes clear despite continued administration.

Loss or disturbance of taste occurs in approximately 7% of patients and is reversible, but it may be necessary to discontinue therapy if anorexia and weight loss develop. Rash and dysgeusia occur less frequently when low doses (150 mg daily or less) are used. Other gastrointestinal reactions include nausea, vomiting, gastric irritation, abdominal pain, flatulence, diarrhea, burning sensation of oral mucosa, and oral ulcerations. Reactivation of peptic ulcer also has been reported.

The initial dose of captopril may cause a precipitous symptomatic fall in blood pressure, particularly in patients who are volume depleted due to diuretic therapy (especially when recently instituted), in those on sodium-restricted diets or on dialysis, or in hyponatremic individuals. Such patients should be observed closely for several hours after the initial dose. Captopril should be used cautiously in those with coronary artery disease, particularly if beta blockers have been discontinued, because an acute fall in blood pressure may precipitate electrocardiographic changes and retrosternal chest pain.

A reversible elevation of BUN and serum creatinine levels may occur in volume-depleted patients or in those with renal disease; if this complication occurs, the dose of captopril should be reduced or the drug should be discontinued. Acute renal failure may develop if captopril is given to patients who have renal artery stenosis in both kidneys, in a solitary functioning kidney, or in a transplanted kidney, presumably because their renal blood flow depends upon high levels of endogenous angiotensin II.

Proteinuria has been reported in less than 2% of patients treated with captopril for three months or more; most of these patients had evidence of pre-existing renal disease. The proteinuria appears to be dose related and occasionally has regressed despite continued treatment, but a few patients developed nephrotic syndrome with biopsy evidence of membranous glomerulopathy. Glomerular changes also have been reported in patients without proteinuria.

Captopril may cause hyperkalemia (particularly in patients with impaired renal function) even when a potassium-wasting diuretic is given concomitantly. The risk of hyperkalemia is increased if potassium supplements or a potassium-sparing agent is given with captopril (Vidt et al, 1982).

Neutropenia has occurred in about 0.3% of patients receiving captopril. It tends to develop slowly during the first three months of therapy and has been observed most often in patients with renal failure or autoimmune disorders or in those receiving immunosuppressive therapy. Fatal agranulocytosis has occurred occasionally. If detected early, the neutropenia is reversible; therefore, white blood cell counts should be performed frequently during the first three months of captopril administration (at two-week intervals in high-risk patients) and periodically thereafter. Reversible lymphadenopathy has occurred rarely. Anemia has been reported in children. Headache and insomnia have developed occasionally.

Cholestatic jaundice has occurred rarely and appears to be an idiosyncratic reaction. There are a few reports of hypoglycemia when captopril was given to diabetics receiving insulin or oral hypoglycemic drugs.

Neurologic disturbances have been observed in patients receiving captopril and cimetidine concurrently. Indomethacin and aspirin antagonize the antihypertensive effect of captopril. Captopril may produce a false-positive urine test for acetone.

Captopril should not be given during pregnancy, for it may cause fetal growth retardation, fetal distress, and neonatal hypotension. There is one report of patent ductus arteriosus in an infant whose mother received the drug during pregnancy (FDA Pregnancy Category C).

PHARMACOKINETICS. Approximately 60% to 75% of an oral dose of captopril is absorbed. Bioavailability increases with prolonged administration. Captopril is 25% to 30% protein bound and its volume of distribution is 0.7 ± .04 L/kg. About 40% to 50% of a dose is excreted in the urine as unchanged drug, and renal impairment leads to drug retention. The elimination half-life of captopril is 1.7 hours.

DOSAGE AND PREPARATIONS. Captopril should be taken one hour before meals.

Oral: Adults, for mild to moderate hypertension, initially, 12.5 mg two or three times daily. For severe hypertension, initially, 25 mg two or three times daily, which may be increased to 50 mg two or three times daily after one or two weeks. If required, the dosage may be increased further at one- to two-week intervals to a maximum of 150 mg two or three times daily. Volume depleted patients and those with severe hypertension should be observed carefully for several hours after the initial dose. Dosage should be reduced in patients with impaired renal function. Diuretics enhance the therapeutic response.

Capoten (Squibb). Tablets 12.5, 25, 50, and 100 mg.
AVAILABLE MIXTURE.
The following combination is indicated only if the dosage ratio meets the optimal requirements of the patient.

Capozide 25/15, 25/25, 50/15, 50/25 (Squibb). Each tablet contains captopril 25 or 50 mg and hydrochlorothiazide 15 or 25 mg.

ENALAPRIL MALEATE
[Vasotec]

ACTIONS. This long-acting ACE inhibitor has pharmacologic actions similar to those of captopril. Enalapril is a prodrug that is de-esterified in the liver to the active diacid form, enalaprilat. It lacks the sulfhydryl group thought to be responsible for some of the adverse effects of captopril.

USES. Orally administered enalapril is effective in mild to severe essential hypertension and renovascular hypertension (Franklin and Smith, 1985; Herrera-Acosta et al, 1985). It may be particularly useful in hypertensive patients with coexisting congestive heart failure. Like captopril, enalapril is more effective in whites than in blacks when used alone; when combined with a diuretic, its antihypertensive effect is enhanced (Freier et al, 1984). Younger patients are more responsive to enalapril than older patients. An intravenous preparation, enalaprilat (not marketed in the United States), has been used in hypertensive emergencies.

ADVERSE REACTIONS AND PRECAUTIONS. Enalapril may cause headache, dizziness, nausea, diarrhea, hyperkalemia, and hyperesthesia of the oral mucosa. Severe, symptomatic hypotension may occur after the first dose, and acute renal failure has been reported. Angioedema has occurred rarely. Rash and taste disturbances are less common with enalapril than with captopril.

This drug is classified in FDA Pregnancy Category C.

PHARMACOKINETICS. The bioavailability of enalapril is 40%. The drug is extensively metabolized in the liver to its active form, enalaprilat. The accumulation half-life of enalaprilat following multiple doses is 11 hours and is increased in the presence of renal impairment.

DOSAGE AND PREPARATIONS.

Oral: Adults, initially, 2.5 mg for patients who are receiving a diuretic and those whose renal function is moderately to severely impaired (creatinine clearance ≤30 ml/min). An initial dose of 5 mg daily may be given to those who are not taking a diuretic and those with normal or mildly impaired renal function. For maintenance, 10 to 40 mg daily.

   Vasotec (Merck Sharp & Dohme). Tablets 5, 10, and 20 mg.

CALCIUM CHANNEL BLOCKING AGENTS

Calcium channel blocking drugs inhibit the entry of calcium into cardiac cells and smooth muscle cells of the coronary and systemic vasculature. These agents are useful in a number of cardiovascular disorders, including hypertension (Spivack et al, 1983). They are discussed in more detail in Chapter 25, Antianginal Agents.

NIFEDIPINE
[Adalat, Procardia]

ACTIONS. Nifedipine has potent peripheral arteriolar dilating properties. It reduces blood pressure and may reflexly increase heart rate. Although this drug exerts a negative inotropic effect on isolated myocardial tissue, myocardial depression is rarely seen in vivo because of the reflex response to the drug's vasodilating effect. Myocardial depression may be evident, however, in patients with severe heart failure or those receiving other myocardial depressant drugs.

USES. Nifedipine has been used more frequently to treat hypertension than the other calcium channel blocking drugs. It is effective for long-term therapy and appears to be particularly useful in patients with severe refractory hypertension when given with a diuretic and antiadrenergic drug, such as a beta blocker or methyldopa (Husted et al, 1982; Guazzi et al, 1980).

In hypertensive urgencies when parenteral drugs are not required, oral nifedipine may be useful; for more rapid action, the drug may be given sublingually (Frishman et al, 1984).

ADVERSE REACTIONS AND PRECAUTIONS. Nifedipine may cause headache, dizziness, fatigue, nausea, pedal edema, flushing, orthostatic hypotension, tinnitus, leg cramps, and dermatologic reactions. Tachycardia can be troublesome but is counteracted by concurrent administration of an antiad-

renergic drug. Rarely, nifedipine has worsened anginal symptoms or precipitated congestive heart failure or cerebral ischemia. Patients with aortic stenosis appear to be particularly at risk of heart failure with use of this drug.

Severe hypotension, heart failure, and myocardial infarction have occurred rarely in patients receiving nifedipine and a beta blocker for angina, but most authorities feel that this combination is well tolerated in the absence of heart failure. Excessive hypotension also has occurred when nifedipine was added to prazosin therapy.

Glucose intolerance has been reported occasionally and hepatitis has occurred rarely.

This drug is classified in FDA Pregnancy Category C.

See also Chapter 25, Antianginal Agents.

PHARMACOKINETICS. See Chapter 25.

DOSAGE AND PREPARATIONS.

Oral: Adults, for chronic hypertension, initially, 10 mg three times daily; this may be followed by doses of 20 mg three times daily. For hypertensive urgencies, 10 to 20 mg.

Sublingual: Adults, for hypertensive urgencies, initially, 10 or 20 mg is given by puncturing one or two capsules with a pin and squeezing the contents under the tongue. If necessary, a 10-mg dose (one capsule) can be repeated 30 to 60 minutes later.

   Adalat (Miles), *Procardia* (Pfizer). Capsules 10 mg.

VERAPAMIL HYDROCHLORIDE
[Calan, Isoptin]

ACTIONS. Verapamil blocks calcium influx and also produces mild nonspecific sympathetic antagonism. It depresses S-A and A-V nodal functions and reduces peripheral vascular resistance. Verapamil lowers blood pressure and reduces heart rate. It is not as active as nifedipine in its effects on vascular smooth muscle; therefore, its negative inotropic effect is less effectively counteracted by a reflex increase in sympathetic tone. Negative inotropic effects are not prominent with therapeutic doses, however, except in patients with compromised left ventricular function or in those receiving other myocardial depressant drugs.

USES. Verapamil has been studied primarily in patients with mild to moderate hypertension. The antihypertensive effect of oral verapamil appears to be comparable to that of a beta blocker, and it may be a useful alternative to the latter (Hornung et al, 1984).

ADVERSE REACTIONS, PRECAUTIONS, AND INTERACTIONS. Constipation is the most common side effect of verapamil. Headache, vertigo, weakness, nervousness, pruritus, flushing, rash, and gastric disturbances also may occur. Orthostatic hypotension, bradycardia, A-V block, A-V dissociation, pedal edema, pulmonary edema, and congestive heart failure have occurred occasionally. Perceptual disorders (feelings of coldness and numbness), hyperprolactinemia, and galactorrhea also have been observed.

When given intravenously, verapamil may cause severe hypotension, bradycardia, and asystole in patients with sick sinus syndrome or in those receiving a beta blocker concomitantly. Severe hypotension, bradycardia, cardiac failure, and arrhythmias also have developed during combined oral therapy with verapamil and a beta blocker; these drugs should not be used together, particularly the intravenous forms, if left ventricular function is compromised.

Verapamil generally should be avoided in patients with sick sinus syndrome, second- or third-degree A-V block, cardiogenic shock, or advanced congestive heart failure (unless heart failure is secondary to supraventricular tachyarrhythmia). Verapamil may increase serum digoxin levels.

Elevated transaminase and alkaline phosphatase levels have been reported occasionally, and hepatitis has developed rarely.

This drug is classified in FDA Pregnancy Category C.

See also Chapter 25, Antianginal Agents.

PHARMACOKINETICS. See Chapter 25.

DOSAGE AND PREPARATIONS.

Oral: *Adults*, for chronic hypertension, 80 to 120 mg three times daily.

Calan (Searle), *Isoptin* (Knoll). Tablets 80 and 120 mg.

DILTIAZEM HYDROCHLORIDE
[Cardizem]

ACTIONS. The cardiovascular effects of diltiazem are similar to those of verapamil. It dilates peripheral arteries and arterioles and depresses S-A and A-V nodal function. Diltiazem reduces heart rate, but to a lesser extent than verapamil, and also decreases blood pressure. Like other calcium antagonists, diltiazem has a direct negative inotropic effect, which could become prominent in patients with compromised left ventricular function or in those receiving other myocardial depressant drugs.

USES. In patients with mild to moderate hypertension, the effect of diltiazem is comparable to that of a thiazide diuretic (Inouye et al, 1984) or a beta blocker (Trimarco et al, 1984). Diuretic therapy enhances its therapeutic effect.

ADVERSE REACTIONS AND PRECAUTIONS. Diltiazem may cause bradycardia, dizziness, weakness, headache, flushing, dryness of the mouth, pedal edema, gastrointestinal disturbances, and dermatologic reactions.

Congestive heart failure, A-V conduction disturbances, and sinus arrest have occurred rarely. Diltiazem probably should be avoided in patients with sick sinus syndrome and A-V conduction disturbances and should be given cautiously with other drugs (eg, beta blockers) that depress the myocardium or the S-A or A-V node.

This drug is classified in FDA Pregnancy Category C.

See also Chapter 25, Antianginal Agents.

PHARMACOKINETICS. See Chapter 25.

DOSAGE AND PREPARATIONS.

Oral: *Adults*, 60 to 120 mg three times daily.

Cardizem (Marion). Tablets 30 and 60 mg.

SEROTONIN RECEPTOR BLOCKING AGENT

Serotonin (5HT) is synthesized in the gut from dietary tryptophan and is largely metabolized by the liver or deaminated by monoamine oxidase. The portion that escapes inactivation passes into the circulation where it is stored in platelets and released during platelet aggregation. Serotonin also has been demonstrated in the brain and in cardiac and vascular tissue.

Serotonin causes vasoconstriction in some vascular beds, bronchoconstriction, and further platelet aggregation; these effects are believed to be mediated by S_2 receptors. It also has vasodilator properties that may involve other types of receptors. Serotonin receptors and alpha-adrenergic receptors have many overlapping functions and may share a common binding site. Large doses of alpha-adrenergic blocking drugs also block serotonin receptors, and high concentrations of serotonin antagonists block alpha receptors (Marwood and Stokes, 1984).

KETANSERIN

ACTIONS. Ketanserin is a quinazoline derivative that blocks the effects of serotonin at peripheral S_2 receptor sites and thus prevents serotonin-induced vasoconstriction, bronchoconstriction, and platelet aggregation. It also has alpha-blocking properties, antihistamine activity, and is a weak dopamine antagonist (Marwood and Stokes, 1984). Blockade of $alpha_1$ receptors plays an important role in the antihypertensive action of ketanserin in laboratory animals (Marwood and Stokes, 1984). The relative role of alpha blockade and serotonin blockade in its hypotensive effect in man is still controversial (Fagard et al, 1984; Reimann and Frölich, 1983; Wenting et al, 1984).

Ketanserin lowers blood pressure by reducing total peripheral resistance. The acute hypotensive effect is accompanied by a transient reflex increase in heart rate and cardiac output. During long-term therapy, heart rate is unchanged or slightly reduced.

USES. Oral ketanserin has been used alone and with a diuretic or beta blocker to treat chronic hypertension. It appears to be effective and well tolerated. The parenteral preparation may be useful for treating hypertensive emergencies and hypertension during surgery.

ADVERSE REACTIONS AND PRECAUTIONS. Ketanserin may cause sedation, dizziness, headache, dryness of the mouth, and nausea.

DOSAGE AND PREPARATIONS.
Oral: Adults, initially, 20 mg two or three times daily. For maintenance, 40 mg twice daily.
   Ketanserin (Janssen). Tablets 20 and 40 mg.
Intravenous: Adults, 5 to 30 mg infused at a rate of 3 mg/min or given by repeated injection of 5 mg every few minutes.
   Ketanserin (Janssen). Solution 5 mg/ml in 2 and 10 ml containers.
   (Investigational drug)

Cited References

Bennett WM, et al: Do diuretics have antihypertensive properties independent of natriuresis? *Clin Pharmacol Ther* 22:499-504, 1977.

Berglund G, Andersson O: Beta-blockers or diuretics in hypertension? Six year follow-up of blood pressure and metabolic side effects. *Lancet* 1:744-747, 1981.

Bravo EL, Gifford RW Jr: Pheochromocytoma: Diagnosis, localization and management. *N Engl J Med* 311:1298-1303, 1984.

Campese VM: Minoxidil: Review of pharmacological properties and therapeutic use. *Drugs* 22:257-278, 1981.

Channick BJ, et al: Comparison of chlorthalidone-reserpine and hydrochlorothiazide-methyldopa as step 2 therapy for hypertension. *Clin Ther* 4:175-183, 1981.

Cody RJ: Haemodynamic responses to specific renin-angiotensin inhibitors in hypertension and congestive heart failure: Review. *Drugs* 28:144-169, 1984.

Cressman MD, et al: Intravenous labetalol in management of severe hypertension and hypertensive emergencies. *Am Heart J* 107:980-985, 1984.

Davidson C, et al: Comparison of antihypertensive activity of beta-blocking drugs during chronic treatment. *Br Med J* 2:7-9, 1976.

Engelman K, et al: Biochemical and pharmacologic effects of alpha methyltyrosine in man. *J Clin Invest* 47:577-594, 1968.

Fagard R, et al: Haemodynamic and humoral responses to chronic ketanserin treatment in essential hypertension. *Br Heart J* 51:149-156, 1984.

Finnerty FA Jr: Step-down treatment of mild systemic hypertension. *Am J Cardiol* 53:1304-1307, 1984.

Finnerty FA Jr, et al: Step 2 regimens in hypertension: Assessment. *JAMA* 241:579-581, 1979.

Franklin SS, Smith RD: Comparison of effects of enalapril plus hydrochlorothiazide versus standard triple therapy on renal function in renovascular hypertension. *Am J Med* 79(suppl 3C):14-23, 1985.

Freier PA, et al: Blood pressure, plasma volume, and catecholamine levels during enalapril therapy in blacks with hypertension. *Clin Pharmacol Ther* 36:731-737, 1984.

Freis ED: Salt, volume and prevention of hypertension. *Circulation* 53:589-595, 1976.

Freis E: Should mild hypertension be treated? (editorial). *N Engl J Med* 307:306-309, 1982.

Freis ED: How diuretics lower blood pressure. *Am Heart J* 106:185-187, 1983.

Freis ED: Advantages of diuretics. *Am J Med* 77:107-109, 1984 A.

Freis ED: Veterans Administration cooperative study on nadolol as monotherapy and in combination with diuretic. *Am Heart J* 108:1087-1091, 1984 B.

Frishman WH, Kostis J: Significance of intrinsic sympathomimetic activity in beta-adrenoceptor blocking drugs. *Cardiovasc Rev Rep* 3:503-512, 1982.

Frishman WH, et al: Calcium entry blockers for treatment of severe hypertension and hypertensive crisis. *Am J Med* 77(suppl 2B):35-45, 1984.

Frohlich ED: Methyldopa: Mechanisms and treatment 25 years later. *Arch Intern Med* 140:954-959, 1980.

Frohlich ED, et al: Review of overall experience of captopril in hypertension. *Arch Intern Med* 144:1441-1444, 1984.

Garrett BN, Kaplan NM: Efficacy of slow infusion of diazoxide in treatment of severe hypertension without organ hypoperfusion. *Am Heart J* 103:390-394, 1982.

Gavras H, et al: Antihypertensive effect of oral angiotensin-converting-enzyme inhibitor SQ 14225 in man. *N Engl J Med* 298:991-995, 1978.

Gidding SS, et al: Therapeutic effect of propranolol on paradoxical hypertension after repair of coarctation of aorta. *N Engl J Med* 312:1224-1228, 1985.

Gifford RW Jr: Drug combinations as rational antihypertensive therapy. *Arch Intern Med* 133:1053-1057, 1974.

Gifford RW Jr: Is renin-sodium profile helpful in evaluating hypertension? *JAMA* 244:35-37, 1980.

Gifford RW Jr: Isolated systolic hypertension in the elderly: Some controversial issues. *JAMA* 247:781-785, 1982.

Gifford RW Jr: Role of diuretics in treatment of hypertension. *Am J Med* 77:102-106, 1984.

Greenberg G, et al: Effects of diuretic and beta-blocker therapy in Medical Research Council trial. *Am J Med* 76:45-51, 1984.

Guazzi MD, et al: Short- and long-term efficacy of calcium-antagonist agent (nifedipine) combined with methyldopa in treatment of severe hypertension. *Circulation* 61:913-919, 1980.

Herrera-Acosta J, et al: Enalapril in essential hypertension. *Drugs* 30(suppl 1):35-46, 1985.

Hoffman BB, Lefkowitz RJ: Alpha-adrenergic receptor subtypes. *N Engl J Med* 302:1390-1396, 1980.

Hornung RS, et al: Propranolol versus verapamil for treatment of essential hypertension. *Am Heart J* 108:554-560, 1984.

Husted SE, et al: Long-term therapy of arterial hypertension with nifedipine given alone or in combination with beta-adrenoceptor blocking agent. *Eur J Clin Pharmacol* 22:101-103, 1982.

Hypertension Detection and Follow-up Program Cooperative Group: Five-year findings of hypertension detection and follow-up program: I. Reduction in mortality of persons with high blood pressure, including mild hypertension. II. Mortality by race, sex and age. III. Reduction in stroke incidence among persons with high blood pressure. *JAMA* 242:2562-2571, 2572-2577, 1979; 247:633-638, 1982.

Hypertension Detection and Follow-up Program Cooperative Research Group: Effect of antihypertensive drug treatment on mortality in presence of resting electrocardiographic abnormalities on baseline: HDFP experience. *Circulation* 70:996-1003, 1984.

Inouye IS, et al: Antihypertensive therapy with diltiazem and comparison with hydrochlorothiazide. *Am J Cardiol* 53:1588-1592, 1984.

Joint National Committee on Detection, Evaluation, and Treatment of High Blood Pressure: 1984 report. *Arch Intern Med* 144:1045-1057, 1984.

Johnston CI, et al: Long-term effects of captopril (SQ 14 225) on blood-pressure and hormone levels in essential hypertension. *Lancet* 2:493-496, 1979.

Kaplan NM: Renin profiles: Unfulfilled promises. *JAMA* 238:611-613, 1977.

Kaplan NM: Mild hypertension: When and how to treat. *Arch Intern Med* 143:255-259, 1983.

Kaplan NM: Non-drug treatment of hypertension. *Ann Intern Med*

102:359-373, 1985.

Khatri IM, et al: Initial and long-term effects of prazosin on sympathetic vasopressor responses in essential hypertension. *Am J Cardiol* 55:1015-1018, 1985.

Klotman PE, et al: Effects of minoxidil on pulmonary and systemic hemodynamics in hypertensive man. *Circulation* 55:394-400, 1977.

Langford HG, et al: Dietary therapy slows return of hypertension after stopping prolonged medication. *JAMA* 253:657-664, 1985.

Levinson PD, et al: Persistence of normal BP after withdrawal of drug treatment in mild hypertension. *Arch Intern Med* 142:2265-2268, 1982.

Mansilla-Tinoco R, et al: Hydralazine, antinuclear antibodies, and lupus syndrome. *Br Med J* 284:936-939, 1982.

Marwood JF, Stokes GS: Serotonin (5HT) and its antagonists: Involvement in cardiovascular system. *Clin Exp Pharmacol Physiol* 11:439-456, 1984.

Materson BJ: Monotherapy of hypertension with angiotensin-converting enzyme inhibitors. *Am J Med* 77:128-134, 1984.

Materson BJ, et al: Dose response to chlorthalidone in patients with mild hypertension: Efficacy of lower dose. *Clin Pharmacol Ther* 24:192-198, 1978.

Medical Research Council Working Party: MRC trial of treatment of mild hypertension: Principal results. *Br Med J* 291:97-104, 1985.

Multiple Risk Factor Intervention Trial Research Group: Multiple risk factor intervention trial: Risk factor changes and mortality results. *JAMA* 248:1465-1477, 1982.

Mulvihill-Wilson J, et al: Hemodynamic and neuroendocrine responses to acute and chronic alpha-adrenergic blockade with prazosin and phenoxybenzamine. *Circulation* 67:383-392, 1983.

Mulvihill-Wilson J, et al: Single and combined therapy for systemic hypertension with propranolol, hydralazine and hydrochlorothiazide: Hemodynamic and neuroendocrine mechanisms of action. *Am J Cardiol* 56:315-320, 1985.

Participating Veterans Administration Medical Centers: Low doses v standard dose of reserpine: Randomized, double-blind, multiclinic trial in patients taking chlorthalidone. *JAMA* 248:2471-2477, 1982.

Prichard BNC: Combined α- and β-receptor inhibition in treatment of hypertension. *Drugs* 28(suppl 2):51-68, 1984.

Reimann IW, Frölich JC: Mechanism of antihypertensive action of ketanserin in man. *Br Med J* 287:381-383, 1983.

Rouby J-J, et al: Resistance to sodium nitroprusside in hypertensive patients. *Crit Care Med* 10:301-304, 1982.

Smith WM: Treatment of mild hypertension: Results of ten-year intervention trial (U.S. Public Health Service Hospitals Cooperative Study Group). *Circ Res* 40(suppl 1):98-105, (May) 1977.

Spivack C, et al: Calcium antagonists: Clinical use in treatment of systemic hypertension. *Drugs* 25:154-177, 1983.

Tarazi RC, et al: Vasodilating drugs: Contrasting hemodynamic effects. *Clin Sci Molecul Med* 51(suppl 3):575-578, 1976.

Trimarco B, et al: Diltiazem in treatment of mild or moderate essential hypertension: Comparison with metoprolol in crossover double-blind trial. *J Clin Pharmacol* 24:218-227, 1984.

Tweeddale MG, et al: Antihypertensive and biochemical effects of chlorthalidone. *Clin Pharmacol Ther* 22:519-527, 1977.

Van Zwieten PA, et al: Role of alpha adrenoceptors in hypertension and in antihypertensive drug treatment. *Am J Med* 77:17-25, 1984.

Veterans Administration Cooperative Study Group on Antihypertensive Agents: Effects of treatment on morbidity in hypertension: Results in patients with diastolic blood pressures averaging 115 through 129 mm Hg. *JAMA* 202:1028-1034, 1967.

Veterans Administration Cooperative Study Group on Antihypertensive Agents: Effects of treatment on morbidity in hypertension: Results in patients with diastolic blood pressures averaging 90 through 114 mm Hg. *JAMA* 213:1143-1152, 1970.

Veterans Administration Cooperative Study Group on Antihypertensive Agents: Propranolol in treatment of hypertension. *JAMA* 237:2303-2310, 1977.

Veterans Administration Cooperative Study Group on Antihypertensive Agents: Comparison of prazosin with hydralazine in patients receiving hydrochlorothiazide: Randomized, double-blind clinical trial. *Circulation* 64:772-779, 1981.

Veterans Administration Cooperative Study Group on Antihypertensive Agents: Comparison of propranolol and hydrochlorothiazide for initial treatment of hypertension. I. Results of short-term titration with emphasis on racial differences in response. II. Results of long-term therapy. *JAMA* 248:1996-2003, 2004-2011, 1982.

Veterans Administration Cooperative Study Group on Antihypertensive Agents: Low-dose captopril for treatment of mild to moderate hypertension. I. Results of 14-week trial. *Arch Intern Med* 144:1947-1953, 1984.

Vidt DG, et al: Captopril. *N Engl J Med* 306:214-238, 1982.

Wallin JD, O'Neill WM Jr: Labetalol: Current research and therapeutic status. *Arch Intern Med* 143:485-490, 1983.

Weber MA, Drayer JIM: Single-agent and combination therapy of essential hypertension. *Am Heart J* 108:311-316, 1984.

Weber MA, et al: Transdermal administration of clonidine for treatment of high BP. *Arch Intern Med* 144:1211-1213, 1984.

Wenting GJ, et al: 5-HT, alpha-adrenoreceptors, and blood pressure: Effects of ketanserin in essential hypertension and autonomic insufficiency. *Hypertension* 6:100-109, 1984.

Wilson DJ, et al: Intravenous labetalol in treatment of severe hypertension and hypertensive emergencies. *Am J Med* 75(suppl 4A):95-102, 1983.

Other Selected References

Chervenak FA, Berkowitz RL: Hypertension in pregnancy. *Mt Sinai J Med* 52:46-58, 1985.

Frohlich ED: Newer concepts in antihypertensive drugs. *Prog Cardiovasc Dis* 20:385-402, 1978.

Kaplan NM: *Clinical Hypertension*, ed 4. Baltimore, Williams & Wilkins, 1986.

Lindheimer MD, Katz AI: Hypertension in pregnancy. *N Engl J Med* 313:675-680, 1985.

Stevenson JC, Umstead GS: Sexual dysfunction due to antihypertensive agents. *Drug Intell Clin Pharm* 18:113-121, 1984.

Vidt DG: Antihypertensive agents, in Wang IH: *Practical Drug Therapy*. Philadelphia, JB Lippincott, 1979.

Vidt DG, Gifford RW Jr: Compendium for treatment of hypertensive emergencies. *Cleve Clin Q* 51:421-430, (Summer) 1984.

Wollam GL, et al: Antihypertensive drugs: Clinical pharmacology and therapeutic use, in Avery GS (ed): *Cardiovascular Drugs*. New York, ADIS Press, vol 4, 1979, 1-67.

Wollam GL, et al: Clinical pharmacology of antihypertensive drugs, in Wollam GL, Hall WD (eds): *Hypertension Management*. Baltimore, Williams & Wilkins, in press.

Zuspan FP: Chronic hypertension in pregnancy. *Clin Obstet Gynecol* 27:854-873, 1984.

Diuretics

29

RENAL REGULATION OF SODIUM AND WATER
BALANCE

SITE AND MECHANISM OF ACTION OF DIURETICS

MAJOR USES OF DIURETICS

DRUG EVALUATIONS

Thiazides and Related Compounds

Loop Diuretics

Potassium-sparing Diuretics

Osmotic Diuretics

Carbonic Anhydrase Inhibitors

Diuretics reduce the volume of extracellular fluid and thereby prevent or alleviate edema. They enhance the urinary excretion of salt and secondarily of water by directly or indirectly impairing sodium chloride reabsorption in the renal tubules. The resulting diuresis is influenced by the drug's site of action in the nephron and, to a lesser extent, by hemodynamic and hormonal regulatory mechanisms that promote the reabsorption of sodium, other ions, and water. The selection and proper use of a diuretic require familiarity with the renal regulation of salt and water balance and with the site and mechanism of action of the different classes of diuretics.

RENAL REGULATION OF SODIUM AND WATER BALANCE

Glomerulus and Proximal Tubule: Approximately 180 liters of plasma are filtered through the glomeruli daily. Under normal conditions, over 99% of this protein-free filtrate is reabsorbed. The largest portion of filtered sodium (50% to 60%) is reabsorbed isosmotically in the proximal convoluted tubule. In the early proximal convoluted tubule, sodium reabsorption occurs by active transport and is coupled electrogenically to reabsorption of glucose and amino acids and nonelectrogenically to reabsorption of bicarbonate. Glucose, amino acids, and phosphate compete for the available sodium electrochemical gradient (Jacobson, 1982). The transport of sodium bicarbonate, which is a major determinant of acid-base balance, is linked to hydrogen ion secretion and is mediated largely by the enzyme, carbonic anhydrase. Since bicarbonate is the principal anion accompanying the reabsorbed sodium, fluid leaving the early proximal convoluted tubule contains a high concentration of chloride, which diffuses passively out of

the lumen with additional sodium in the late proximal convoluted tubule.

The straight proximal tubule (pars recta) also reabsorbs tubular fluid isosmotically, but is less involved in the transport of bicarbonate, glucose, and amino acids than the convoluted segment. The pars recta is the site at which most diuretics are secreted into the renal tubule.

Sodium reabsorption in the proximal tubule is related directly to the glomerular filtration rate and inversely to extracellular fluid volume; it also may be altered by humoral agents, including parathyroid hormone and catecholamines. Although these and other factors may markedly alter proximal sodium reabsorption, the more distal segments of the nephron can reabsorb sodium that has been rejected by the proximal tubule. For this reason, diuretics that inhibit sodium reabsorption only in the proximal tubules are relatively ineffective.

Loop of Henle and Early Distal Tubule: The portion of glomerular filtrate that is not reabsorbed in the proximal tubule passes into the loop of Henle. Sodium chloride reabsorption in the loop provides the driving force for concentration or dilution of the urine. The descending limb is highly permeable to water and impermeable to solutes. Its primary function is to equilibrate the tubular fluid osmotically (Kokko, 1982). Since the medullary interstitium contains high concentrations of salt and urea, the tubular fluid becomes hypertonic as it approaches the tip of the loop due to outflow of water down its concentration gradient.

The thin ascending limb is highly permeable to sodium chloride and impermeable to water; consequently, sodium chloride diffuses into the interstitium. Transport processes in this segment are principally passive (Kokko, 1982).

Approximately 15% to 20% of the filtered load of sodium and chloride is reabsorbed in the water-impermeable thick ascend-

541

ing limb of Henle's loop. This segment absorbs salt by a cotransport mechanism whereby secondary active chloride transport depends upon the presence of sodium and potassium ([1 Na$^+$, 1 K$^+$, 2 Cl$^-$] cotransport process). The energy for this process is provided by the sodium gradient across the luminal membrane. In the medullary portion of the thick ascending limb, sodium chloride is deposited in the medullary interstitium, creating an increasing concentration of solute from cortex to medulla, which provides the osmotic driving force for urinary concentration.

Further reabsorption of sodium chloride without water occurs in the cortical thick ascending limb and early distal tubule (cortical diluting segment). Salt reabsorption at this site does not contribute to medullary hypertonicity and thus permits urinary dilution when ADH is not present (Burg, 1982; DuBose and Kokko, 1977; Hebert and Andreoli, 1984).

Specialized epithelial cells in the ascending limb of the loop of Henle and the juxtaglomerular apparatus are in close proximity to the glomerular arterioles (macula densa). The transport of sodium chloride into or across these cells appears to activate a feedback mechanism that adjusts the glomerular filtration rate (GFR) to the reabsorptive capacity of the nephron. This system is believed to be one of the mechanisms that regulates salt and water excretion in accordance with body requirements and protects against volume depletion when the tubular reabsorptive mechanisms fail (Blantz and Pelazo, 1984; Kahn et al, 1974; Thurau and Boylan, 1976; Wright and Briggs, 1979). The reduction in GFR that occurs in response to renal hypoperfusion also may prevent regional renal hypoxia. The medullary thick ascending limb is particularly sensitive to oxygen deprivation. By reducing the need for solute reabsorption at this site, the fall in GFR decreases oxygen requirements and may thereby prevent anoxic injury (Brezis et al, 1984).

Late Distal Tubule and Collecting Tubule: In the late distal convoluted and the cortical collecting tubules, sodium reabsorption is related to the secretion of potassium and hydrogen ions, a process that is under the permissive influence of the adrenal mineralocorticoid, aldosterone. The cortical collecting tubule is the main site of action of this hormone. The final regulation of sodium excretion probably occurs in the papillary collecting tubule (Stokes, 1982).

Several interrelated factors influence sodium reabsorption in the distal and collecting tubules. These include the rate of delivery of tubular fluid and electrolytes, the level of circulating aldosterone, the acid-base balance of the body, the serum potassium level, the relative concentrations of potassium and hydrogen ions in the tubular cell, the concentrations of reabsorbable and nonreabsorbable anions in the glomerular filtrate, and the extracellular fluid volume.

Humoral Factors: *Renin-Angiotensin-Aldosterone System.* Renin, a proteolytic enzyme produced and stored in the kidney, is released in response to various stimuli, the most important being a reduction in renal perfusion pressure. Renin secretion is also regulated by sympathetic nervous system activity and certain humoral factors.

In the circulatory system, renin reacts with a substrate formed in the liver to produce angiotensin I. This prohormone is then hydrolyzed to angiotensin II by a converting enzyme that is present in highest concentrations in the lungs. Angiotensin II acts on receptor sites in vascular smooth muscle, the central nervous system, and the adrenal cortex to constrict arterioles, increase sympathetic outflow from the central nervous system, reduce vagal tone, and induce secretion of aldosterone. These actions result in increased peripheral vascular resistance, elevated heart rate and cardiac output, and increased reabsorption of sodium and water. The resultant rise in blood pressure activates a feedback loop that reduces the secretion of renin. The renin-angiotensin-aldosterone system does not play an active role in maintaining circulatory homeostasis in the normovolemic, sodium-replete individual but is of major importance in maintaining blood pressure and intravascular volume during sodium deprivation or volume depletion.

Antidiuretic Hormone (ADH). The cortical collecting tubule is the site of action of ADH, which is released from the posterior pituitary when there is a need to conserve body water. Under the influence of ADH, the collecting tubules become more permeable to water, which diffuses into the hypertonic medulla, enters the capillaries, and is returned to the general circulation. This process results in formation of a concentrated urine. ADH also facilitates the diffusion of urea out of the medullary collecting tubule into the medullary interstitium, which contributes to the hypertonicity of the medulla. In the absence of ADH, the hypotonic tubular fluid delivered out of the cortical diluting segment is excreted as dilute urine.

Natriuretic Hormone. A circulatory substance, termed "natriuretic hormone" or "third factor," has been postulated to explain the natriuresis that follows "escape" from aldosterone action and other sodium-retaining states. Among the substances that have been considered is a peptide(s) identified in mammalian atria, atrial natriuretic factor (ANF). Infusion of atrial extracts or purified atrial peptides into laboratory animals induces rapid diuresis and natriuresis and a fall in arterial blood pressure (Beasley and Malvin, 1985; Palluk et al, 1985; Maack et al, 1985). Similar effects followed injection of a synthetic human atrial natriuretic peptide in man (Richards et al, 1985). The major renal effect of ANF is to markedly increase the glomerular filtration rate and possibly to increase inner medullary blood flow and "wash out" the medullary gradient. Whether it has an additional direct tubular action or affects the renin-angiotensin-aldosterone system is controversial.

ANF is released during episodes of A-V nodal reentrant (paroxysmal supraventricular) tachycardia and probably causes the polyuria observed during these attacks (Schiffrin et al, 1985). Plasma concentrations of ANF are also elevated in volume-expanded states such as severe congestive heart failure (Tikkanen et al, 1985) and chronic renal failure (Rascher et al, 1985). Clinical studies are beginning (under sponsorship of Merck) to determine ANF's role in the normal regulation of volume and blood pressure and its possible therapeutic value in disorders such as heart failure and hypertension.

ANF should not be confused with digoxin-like factor (DLF), which is discussed in Chapter 23, Agents Used to Treat Heart Failure.

SITE AND MECHANISM OF ACTION OF DIURETICS

All diuretics interfere with sodium chloride reabsorption in the renal tubules but, because they act at different sites, each class has distinctive effects on the pattern of electrolyte excretion, acid-base balance, and the concentrating and diluting capacities of the kidney (see Table 1). Most clinically useful diuretics act from within the renal tubule to inhibit sodium transport mechanisms in the luminal membrane.

Carbonic Anhydrase Inhibitors: Carbonic anhydrase inhibitors (eg, acetazolamide [Diamox]) enhance sodium excretion by reducing sodium bicarbonate reabsorption in the early proximal convoluted tubule. Passive sodium chloride reabsorption in the late proximal convoluted tubule is consequently decreased, but excess chloride (with accompanying sodium) is subsequently reabsorbed in the loop of Henle. Thus, sodium bicarbonate is excreted predominantly and the total diuretic effect is minimal. Potassium excretion is increased during initial therapy with carbonic anhydrase inhibitors due to the increased distal tubular flow rate and sodium concentration, the elevated pH of the tubular fluid, and possibly the presence of a nonreabsorbable anion in the distal tubular fluid (which increases electronegativity of the tubular lumen). Clinically significant hypokalemia is seldom a problem, because excess hydrogen ions in the extracellular fluid tend to diffuse into the cells and displace potassium ions, which move into the extracellular compartment. After several days of continuous administration, a mild hyperchloremic acidosis develops, which decreases the diuretic effect.

Osmotic Diuretics: These agents are believed to produce diuresis by more than one mechanism, and species differences have been noted (Buerkert et al, 1981; Gennari and Kassirer, 1974). Mannitol [Osmitrol], the most widely used osmotic diuretic, is freely filtered at the glomerulus and is not reabsorbed or secreted by the renal tubules. Because of its osmotic action in the proximal tubule, mannitol prevents the reabsorption of water and secondarily of sodium. In the loop of Henle, mannitol reduces medullary hypertonicity by increasing medullary blood flow. Sodium and water reabsorption in the collecting tubule is subsequently reduced because of papillary washout (and loss of concentration gradient), high flow rate, or other factors.

Loop Diuretics and Thiazides: The *loop diuretics*, furosemide [Lasix], ethacrynic acid [Edecrin], and bumetanide [Bumex], block sodium chloride reabsorption in both the medullary and cortical portions of the thick ascending limb of Henle's loop by inhibiting the luminal cotransport system. Their primary effect appears to be inhibition of the secondary active chloride transport mechanism. This action reduces the osmotic gradient in the renal medulla and impairs both the concentrating and diluting capacities of the kidney.

Thiazide-type diuretics block the reabsorption of sodium chloride in the cortical thick ascending limb of Henle's loop and the early distal tubule. These diuretics thus interfere with urinary dilution but do not affect the concentrating mechanism. (In large doses, the thiazides, furosemide, and possibly bumetanide also have slight, clinically unimportant, carbonic anhydrase inhibitory activity in the proximal tubules.)

Thiazides and loop diuretics increase the rate of delivery of tubular fluid and electrolytes to the distal sites of hydrogen and potassium ion secretion, and plasma volume contraction increases the production of aldosterone via the renin-angiotensin-aldosterone system (secondary hyperaldosteronism). The combination of increased delivery and high aldosterone levels promotes sodium reabsorption at the distal sites and thus increases the loss of potassium and hydrogen ions. These changes may be associated with hypokalemia and mild hypochloremic alkalosis with or without an effective

TABLE 1.
SITE AND MECHANISM OF ACTION OF DIURETICS

Drug	Major Site of Action	Mechanism of Action
Thiazides	Cortical thick ascending limb of loop of Henle and early distal tubule	Inhibition of sodium chloride reabsorption
Loop	Medullary and cortical thick ascending limb of loop of Henle	Inhibition of luminal cotransport system (1 Na^+, 1 K^+, 2 Cl^-), major action being to inhibit the secondary active chloride transport mechanism
Potassium-sparing	Cortical collecting tubule	Inhibition of sodium reabsorption and potassium secretion by competitive antagonism of aldosterone (spironolactone) or by direct action (triamterene and amiloride)
Osmotic	(1) Proximal tubule	Inhibition of sodium and water reabsorption by osmotic action
	(2) Loop of Henle	Inhibition of sodium and water reabsorption because of reduction in medullary hypertonicity
	(3) Collecting tubule	Inhibition of sodium and water reabsorption because of papillary washout, high flow rate, or other factors
Carbonic Anhydrase Inhibitors	Early proximal convoluted tubule	Inhibition of sodium bicarbonate reabsorption

diuresis. The reduction in extracellular fluid volume also activates compensatory mechanisms that increase sodium reabsorption in the proximal tubules, thereby limiting the amount of sodium reaching the distal sites. A high sodium intake may increase potassium loss by counteracting this sodium-conserving mechanism (Tucker et al, 1980).

Potassium-sparing Diuretics: Spironolactone [Aldactone] and related steroids, triamterene [Dyrenium], and amiloride [Midamor] interfere with sodium reabsorption in the cortical collecting tubule, thereby promoting sodium excretion while conserving potassium. Spironolactone is a competitive antagonist of aldosterone; triamterene and amiloride interfere directly with electrolyte transport. Amiloride (which also acts in the late distal convoluted tubule) prevents sodium from gaining access to the sodium pump by blocking the sodium channel at the apical membrane. These agents are not potent diuretics when used alone because of the small volume of tubular fluid reaching their sites of action. When given with a more proximally acting diuretic, they reduce potassium loss, enhance sodium excretion, and minimize alkalosis.

MAJOR USES OF DIURETICS

Chronic Congestive Heart Failure: The kidney plays an important role in the pathogenesis of congestive heart failure. By reducing the extracellular fluid volume, diuretics decrease preload and relieve pulmonary congestion and peripheral edema. The traditional approach is to initiate therapy with digitalis, a low-sodium diet, and restriction of activities; a diuretic is given concomitantly or added later if symptoms are not adequately controlled. Today, diuretics often are used for initial therapy in patients who have mild congestive failure and normal sinus rhythm.

A thiazide is often the preferred diuretic if renal function is well preserved. When the glomerular filtration rate is less than 30 ml/minute, thiazides (with the exception of metolazone and indapamide) are usually ineffective, but a loop diuretic will frequently produce a diuresis. Potassium-sparing agents are particularly appropriate when given with a thiazide or loop diuretic to digitalized patients, because hypokalemia may predispose to or accentuate digitalis intoxication.

If cardiac failure is difficult to control with a diuretic and moderate doses of digitalis, the possibility of sodium abuse should be considered. Refractory cardiac edema often can be controlled by digitalis and a thiazide if sodium intake is restricted to 50 to 70 mEq daily. Excessive diuretic therapy is another possible cause of "refractory" edema. Intermittent (eg, three days/week) or alternate-day administration of the diuretic may be more effective than continuous daily treatment. (See also Chapter 23, Agents Used to Treat Heart Failure.)

Acute Pulmonary Edema: The loop diuretics have replaced the mercurials in treating acute cardiogenic pulmonary edema. Furosemide [Lasix] is usually preferred for the initial management of patients with pulmonary congestion following acute myocardial infarction. In addition to its diuretic effect, furosemide reduces venous tone, which relieves symptoms before the onset of diuresis. During reversal of acute pulmo-nary edema with a single dose of furosemide, intravascular volume is replenished at a rate that equals or exceeds the volume removed by diuresis (Schuster et al, 1984).

Hypertension: Diuretics initially lower blood pressure by reducing the plasma volume; during long-term therapy, peripheral resistance also is decreased. Thiazides are used as sole therapy in patients with mild or moderate hypertension or in combination with other antihypertensive drugs in patients who are not controlled by the diuretic alone. The loop diuretics are usually reserved for patients with markedly impaired renal function unless an immediate action is required (ie, in hypertensive crisis). A potassium-sparing diuretic may be given concurrently to minimize potassium wasting when hypokalemia is a problem. (See Chapter 28, Antihypertensive Agents.)

Nephrotic Syndrome: In treating the nephrotic syndrome, major emphasis should be placed on diagnosis so that the underlying disease process may be treated, if possible. Restriction of dietary sodium is important in managing edema associated with this disorder, and diuretics should be considered ancillary agents. Vigorous diuresis should be avoided because the effective arterial blood volume is already reduced in these patients. Some clinicians initiate diuretic therapy with a thiazide alone or in combination with spironolactone or amiloride. Nephrotic edema may be more difficult to control than cardiac edema, and a satisfactory diuresis often can be obtained only with a loop diuretic, usually given with spironolactone. The potassium-sparing diuretic should be discontinued if renal function deteriorates; otherwise, serious hyperkalemia may occur.

Chronic Renal Failure: Patients with stable chronic renal failure may remain in sodium balance on a normal salt intake but may not readily adapt to a marked deficiency or excess of dietary sodium. Management of these patients requires careful attention to salt and water balance. If a diuretic is needed to control edema or hypertension, a loop diuretic (usually furosemide or bumetamide) is preferred because thiazides (with the exception of metolazone and indapamide) are usually ineffective in patients with a GFR less than 30 ml/minute. To avoid excessive sodium depletion, careful dosage adjustment is necessary, and daily diuretic therapy may not be advisable.

Potassium-sparing diuretics should not be used in patients with chronic renal failure because they may cause severe hyperkalemia. Aldosterone may play a major role in maintaining potassium homeostasis in these patients (Berl et al, 1978).

Acute Oliguric Renal Failure: In oliguric patients, mannitol and/or furosemide have been used diagnostically, prophylactically, and therapeutically. These diuretics are sometimes used adjunctively to differentiate prerenal azotemia from acute tubular necrosis, but some nephrologists feel that urinalysis and clinical evaluation are safer and more accurate (Levinsky et al, 1981). A careful assessment of the extracellular volume status is always necessary. Many clinicians feel that all patients who have oliguria should receive isotonic sodium chloride (0.9%) prior to initiation of diuretic therapy, as long as there is no evidence of volume overexpansion.

The value of diuretics in preventing or reversing acute renal failure is also not clearly established. The rationale for use of a diuretic in patients at risk for developing acute tubular necrosis is to increase renal blood flow and prevent tubular obstruction. Mannitol may reduce the risk of acute tubular necrosis when administered prior to or immediately after some types of renal insult (eg, during aortic aneurysm surgery). Furosemide also has been used for prophylaxis but, if administered to volume-depleted patients, it may further reduce the effective blood volume and precipitate rather than prevent acute renal failure. If a satisfactory diuresis is achieved (in the absence of cardiopulmonary overload), fluid losses must be replaced carefully to avoid dehydration.

Furosemide may convert established acute oliguric renal failure to the nonoliguric form and, unlike mannitol, it does not cause volume expansion if it fails to produce a diuresis. Although furosemide may reduce the need for dialysis, there is no convincing evidence that the underlying pathologic picture is changed. The value of increasing urine volume in these patients has been questioned (Tiller and Mudge, 1980).

Renal Tubular Acidosis (RTA): In proximal RTA, impaired bicarbonate reabsorption in the proximal tubule leads to a hyperchloremic hypokalemic acidosis. Thiazides are given in conjunction with bicarbonate supplementation to reduce extracellular fluid volume and thus enhance proximal bicarbonate reabsorption. A potassium-sparing diuretic may be given concomitantly to prevent further potassium wasting.

Diuretics also are used in Type 4 RTA, which is characterized by hyperkalemia and hyperchloremic acidosis. Patients with hyporeninemic hypoaldosteronism, hypertension, and extracellular fluid volume expansion may be treated with furosemide in conjunction with a mineralocorticoid to lower the serum potassium level and enhance distal hydrogen ion secretion. Mineralocorticoid-resistant hyperkalemia with salt retention and hypertension may be caused by enhanced reabsorption of chloride in the distal tubule. This disorder has been successfully treated with salt restriction and/or prolonged thiazide therapy (Cogan, 1982; Sebastian et al, 1982).

Disorders Characterized by Hypokalemic Alkalosis: Spironolactone normalizes blood pressure and corrects hypokalemia in patients with primary hyperaldosteronism. It is used preoperatively or for long-term therapy (Ganguly and Donohue, 1983).

Hypertension and hypokalemic alkalosis in Liddle's syndrome are corrected by potassium-sparing diuretics that act directly on the renal tubules (triamterene and amiloride). Spironolactone is ineffective in this rare familial disorder, which may be caused by an unidentified mineralocorticoid (Sebastian et al, 1982). Neither spironolactone nor other treatment modalities have been consistently effective in reversing hypokalemia and metabolic alkalosis in Bartter's syndrome.

Cirrhosis with Ascites: Peripheral edema is easily and safely mobilized in patients with chronic liver disease. Reabsorption of ascitic fluid is strictly rate limited (probably 1 to 1.5 L/day). If sodium restriction and bedrest are ineffective, diuretic therapy may be initiated very cautiously. The goal should be a weight loss of 1 to 2 pounds daily in patients with both ascites and edema or 0.3 pounds daily in those with ascites only (Linas et al, 1983). Vigorous treatment of ascites should be avoided because it may lead to intravascular volume depletion with resultant azotemia and electrolyte disturbances (particularly hypokalemia and metabolic alkalosis), which may precipitate hepatic coma.

Secondary hyperaldosteronism is common and usually severe in cirrhotics, but hormonal mediators other than aldosterone may play an important role in the sodium retention observed in this disorder (Epstein, 1983). Spironolactone [Aldactone] often is given for initial therapy and is effective alone in 40% to 75% of patients (Frakes, 1980). If the therapeutic response is inadequate, a thiazide may be given concurrently. In very resistant cases, a loop diuretic may be substituted for the thiazide, but extreme care must be taken to avoid electrolyte imbalance and volume depletion.

Edema of Pregnancy: In the past, thiazide diuretics were often prescribed routinely, along with dietary salt restriction, to prevent or relieve edema of pregnancy and pre-eclampsia. Enthusiasm for diuretic therapy and/or sodium restriction in pregnant women has lessened in recent years. Dependent or generalized edema develops in up to 80% of normotensive women during uncomplicated pregnancy. The phenomenon is thus physiologic and well tolerated, and attempts to mobilize mild edema with diuretics may compromise uteroplacental perfusion. Consideration also should be given to the risk of adverse effects on the newborn, such as electrolyte disturbances and neonatal thrombocytopenia (Lindheimer and Katz, 1973).

The role of diuretics in the prevention and treatment of pre-eclampsia is controversial. Some clinicians believe that, by decreasing the sensitivity of vascular receptors to endogenous pressor substances, diuretics may be beneficial. Others feel that diuretic therapy does not influence the course of the disease and, since intravascular volume is decreased in pre-eclampsia, may further impair uteroplacental perfusion. Even when diuretics relieve edema and lower elevated blood pressure, there is no conclusive evidence that they have either a beneficial or an adverse effect on perinatal mortality (Collins et al, 1985).

Idiopathic Edema: This poorly understood condition occurs primarily in women. Treatment has included avoidance of precipitating causes (eg, prolonged standing), mild salt restriction, periods of recumbency in the afternoon, use of elastic stockings, diuretic therapy (including potassium-sparing agents), and administration of sympathomimetic amines. It must be emphasized that many cases of idiopathic edema appear to be caused or aggravated by diuretic abuse (MacGregor et al, 1979). Women with this disorder are often overly concerned about weight and appearance and become habitual users of diuretics, which may be taken surreptitiously. Hypokalemia induced by thiazides or loop diuretics tends to aggravate the edema. These patients often resist efforts to discontinue the drug because excessive sodium retention, weight gain, and edema develop for a number of days after withdrawal of diuretics. Successful long-term treatment involves complete abstinence from diuretics with eventual reestablishment of normal sodium and water homeostasis (MacGregor et al, 1979). Other causes that have been considered are fluctuations in sodium and carbohydrate intake, laxative abuse, self-induced vomiting, capillary leak of albumin, and hormonal disturbances.

Brain Edema: Osmotic agents are given intravenously (mannitol or urea) or orally (glycerin) to reduce intracranial pressure temporarily in neurosurgical patients. Mannitol is usually preferred to urea for short-term intravenous therapy because it does not diffuse into cells and, therefore, has less tendency to produce a rebound effect. The efficacy of prolonged maintenance therapy with glycerin has not been established. Glucocorticoids are the most effective agents for long-term treatment (see Chapter 61, Adrenal Corticosteroids in Nonendocrine Diseases).

Acute Hypercalcemia: Loop diuretics increase the urinary excretion of calcium and are useful (in conjunction with saline infusion) for the emergency treatment of acute hypercalcemia. Furosemide has been used most commonly for this purpose. Thiazides should not be used because they may increase the serum calcium concentration. (See Chapter 49, Agents Affecting Calcium Metabolism.)

Idiopathic Calcium Urolithiasis: Since thiazides decrease urinary calcium excretion, they may prevent recurrence of calcium-containing renal calculi in patients with idiopathic calcium urolithiasis whether hypercalciuria is present or not. Loop diuretics should not be used for this purpose because they increase calcium excretion. (See Chapter 31, Agents Used to Treat Urologic Disorders.)

Diabetes Insipidus: The thiazides have a paradoxical antidiuretic action in patients with diabetes insipidus and are useful in both the nephrogenic and central forms. The mechanism whereby these agents reduce urine volume appears to involve mild sodium and extracellular volume depletion, which increases sodium and water reabsorption in the proximal tubules and thus reduces delivery of glomerular filtrate to the diluting segment. (See Chapter 30, Agents Affecting Water Homeostasis.)

Acute Mountain Sickness: Acute exposure to high altitude induces respiratory alkalosis, which may be accompanied by symptoms of acute mountain sickness (headache, irritability, lassitude, malaise, anorexia, nausea, vomiting, and insomnia). During acclimatization, an increase in the renal excretion of bicarbonate returns the blood pH to normal and symptoms usually subside. Acute mountain sickness and its severe complications (pulmonary and cerebral edema) usually can be prevented or diminished by gradual ascent.

Acetazolamide [Diamox], taken before and during initial exposure to high altitude, ameliorates symptoms (Greene et al, 1981; Hackett and Rennie, 1976) but does not reduce the risk of pulmonary or cerebral edema (which mandate rapid descent and administration of oxygen) or the incidence of retinal hemorrhages (Meehan and Zavala, 1982). Acetazolamide appears to act by inducing metabolic acidosis, which increases tissue oxygenation by increasing respiratory drive.

Glaucoma Therapy and Intraocular Surgery: Carbonic anhydrase inhibitors reduce intraocular pressure by decreasing the production of aqueous humor. They are used for the long-term treatment of patients with primary open-angle glaucoma and other chronic glaucomas that cannot be controlled by topical therapy alone. They also are administered for preoperative treatment of acute angle-closure and congenital glaucoma. The osmotic agents are used to reduce intraocular pressure and vitreous volume rapidly prior to iridectomy and other ocular surgical procedures. They also are of temporary benefit in some secondary glaucomas. (See Chapter 18, Agents Used to Treat Glaucoma.)

Acne and Hirsutism: Spironolactone has antiandrogen effects and is under investigation for the treatment of acne and hirsutism (see Chapters 39 and 56).

Drug Evaluations

Individual and class evaluations are presented in the following order: Thiazides and Related Compounds, Loop Diuretics, Potassium-sparing Diuretics, Osmotic Diuretics, and Carbonic Anhydrase Inhibitors. The clinical uses, biochemical side effects, and adverse interactions of diuretics are summarized in Tables 2, 3, and 4.

THIAZIDES AND RELATED COMPOUNDS

The prototype thiazide, chlorothiazide, was introduced in 1958 and was the first reliable, well tolerated, orally effective diuretic. A number of derivatives and four similarly acting nonthiazide agents (chlorthalidone, quinethazone, metolazone, and indapamide) were developed subsequently. The major differences among the various agents involve dosage and duration of action (see Table 5). Indapamide may have vasodilator properties in addition to its diuretic effect, but there is no conclusive evidence that vasodilation contributes to its antihypertensive effect (Chaffman et al, 1984).

ACTIONS AND USES. Thiazide-type diuretics increase the urinary excretion of sodium chloride and water by inhibiting sodium reabsorption in the cortical thick ascending limb of Henle's loop and the early distal tubules (cortical diluting segment). They also increase the urinary excretion of potassium, magnesium, and, to a small extent, bicarbonate ions (the latter effect is due to their slight carbonic anhydrase inhibitory action). During long-term therapy, urinary calcium excretion is reduced.

When renal function is normal, the thiazides are often preferred for maintenance therapy in ambulatory patients with cardiac edema or benign essential hypertension. They may be given with a potassium-sparing diuretic to reduce potassium loss and enhance the therapeutic response. Such combined therapy also may be effective in patients with nephrotic edema or cirrhotic edema and ascites. In addition, thiazides are used to control edema associated with corticosteroid or estrogen therapy.

Thiazide-type diuretics are usually ineffective in patients with impaired renal function (GFR less than 30 ml/min) and may cause further deterioration of renal function. Metolazone is effective in these patients when given in large doses, which suggests that its site and mechanism of action may differ in some respects from those of the other thiazide-type diuretics. Nevertheless, a loop diuretic is usually preferred to very large doses of metolazone. Indapamide has also been reported to be effective in patients with impaired renal function.

ADVERSE REACTIONS AND PRECAUTIONS. Thiazides

TABLE 2.
CLINICAL USES OF DIURETICS

Disorder	Drug	Comments
Hypertension	Thiazide-type	Preferred diuretic in patients with normal renal function
	Loop	Used when renal function is impaired or when immediate action is required
	Potassium-sparing	Used in conjunction with thiazide or loop diuretic when hypokalemia is a problem and renal function is normal
Chronic Congestive Heart Failure	Thiazide-type	Used in patients with normal renal function
	Loop	Particularly useful in patients with impaired renal function
	Potassium-sparing	Used in conjunction with thiazide or loop diuretic when hypokalemia is a problem and renal function is normal
Acute Pulmonary Edema	Loop	Reduces venous tone in addition to diuretic effect
Nephrotic Syndrome	Thiazide-type or loop, often with spironolactone	
Chronic Renal Failure	Loop; metolazone or indapamide may be effective in some patients	The combination of a loop diuretic and metolazone may produce a diuresis when the loop diuretic alone is ineffective. Serum electrolytes should be closely monitored.
Acute Renal Failure	Mannitol and/or furosemide	If diuresis is successful, fluid volume must be replaced carefully.
Cirrhosis with Ascites	Spironolactone	Used if renal function is normal
	Spironolactone and thiazide	Used if renal function is normal
	Spironolactone and loop	All diuretics, particularly loop diuretics, should be used cautiously.
Brain Edema	Osmotic	
Hypercalcemia	Furosemide	
Renal Calculi	Thiazide-type	
Diabetes Insipidus	Thiazide-type	
Open-angle Glaucoma	Carbonic anhydrase inhibitor	Used for long-term therapy
Acute Angle-closure Glaucoma	Osmotic and carbonic anhydrase inhibitor	Used preoperatively

may cause dizziness, weakness, fatigue, orthostatic hypotension, and leg cramps, which may reflect electrolyte imbalance. Serum sodium, potassium, chloride, bicarbonate, and magnesium levels should be determined periodically, and the lowest effective dose should be employed to avoid electrolyte disturbances. Some authorities believe that the short-acting thiazides cause less severe electrolyte disturbances than the long-acting agents.

The serum potassium frequently falls to a level of 3 to 3.5 mEq/L during long-term therapy; mild hypochloremic alkalosis also may develop. Since a further decrease in the serum potassium concentration may occur during episodes of diarrhea, vomiting, or anorexia, patients should be instructed to report any such occurrence promptly. In addition, careful

consideration should be given to the effect of sodium abuse on the potassium-wasting action of diuretics. Diuretic-induced potassium loss often can be reduced by moderate sodium restriction (Ram et al, 1981).

Corrective measures should be instituted if symptoms develop, if the serum potassium level falls below 3.5 mEq/L, or if the patient has an irritable myocardium, is receiving digitalis, or has cirrhosis. Thiazide-induced hypokalemia can be prevented or corrected by concurrent administration of a potassium-sparing diuretic or large doses of potassium chloride. Potassium loss can also be reduced by acute parenteral administration of magnesium, but prolonged use of oral magnesium supplements does not affect potassium balance.

The need for routine potassium replacement in healthy,

TABLE 3.
BIOCHEMICAL SIDE EFFECTS OF DIURETICS

Side Effect							
Hypokalemia and Hypochloremic alkalosis	+	+	+	+	0	0	0
Hyperkalemia	0	0	0	0	+	+	+
Hyperglycemia	+	+	Rare	Rare?	0	Rare	Rare
Azotemia	+	+	+	+	+	+	+
Hyperuricemia	+	+	+	+	+	+	+
Hyponatremia	+	+	+	+	+	?	+
Hypercalcemia	+	0	0	0	0	0	0

ambulatory patients with hypertension has been questioned. Mild hypokalemia is generally well tolerated and is not associated with a clinically important deficiency of total body potassium. An increase in ventricular ectopic activity has been noted in some patients receiving thiazides (Holland et al, 1981), particularly during long-term therapy (Whelton, 1984) and subgroup analysis of the results of a multifactor intervention trial revealed a trend toward increased coronary events in diuretic-treated hypertensive patients with resting electrocardiographic abnormalities (Multiple Risk Factor Intervention Trial Research Group, 1985). Restoration of normokalemia was reported to abolish diuretic-induced ectopic activity by one group of investigators (Holland et al, 1981), but others failed to confirm these observations (Papademetriou et al, 1983). Because of the danger of hyperkalemia in patients with renal insufficiency or insulin-dependent diabetes, routine potassium replacement in these groups should be strictly avoided.

Thiazides increase fasting blood glucose levels and decrease glucose tolerance during long-term therapy. Thiazide-induced glucose intolerance is sometimes attributed to potassium loss; however, concomitant therapy with triamterene does not prevent it (Amery et al, 1978). The effect on glucose tolerance is readily reversed when the drug is discontinued (Murphy et al, 1982) and is not clinically important except in patients with pre-existing or subclinical diabetes who may require an adjustment in dosage of hypoglycemic drugs. In the rare instances in which hyperglycemia is difficult to control, it may be advisable to substitute a diuretic less likely to cause carbohydrate intolerance. Ethacrynic acid appears to be the best choice. Although the potassium-sparing diuretics may be less likely to decrease glucose tolerance than the thiazides, these agents may cause severe hyperkalemia in patients with moderate to severe diabetes and should be avoided, particularly when there is associated renal insufficiency.

A reversible elevation of the blood urea nitrogen level may occur during thiazide therapy. This prerenal azotemia is caused by a decrease in renal blood flow and glomerular filtration rate secondary to the reduction of blood volume induced by the diuretic. The thiazides also may directly depress renal blood flow.

Thiazides produce an asymptomatic hyperuricemia, which may be caused by decreased secretion of uric acid by the tubular cells into the lumen of the tubule or increased renal tubular reabsorption of uric acid. Asymptomatic hyperuricemia does not appear to produce any long-term deleterious effects and need not be treated. The development of acute gouty arthritis is rare, except in patients with chronic renal failure or a hereditary predisposition to gout. Patients with a history of gout may continue to take the thiazide if colchicine is administered with a uricosuric agent (probenecid, sulfinpyrazone).

Since thiazides block sodium reabsorption in the diluting segment of the nephron, hyponatremia may occur if water intake is excessive. The hyponatremia is caused by the combined effects of a disorder of water excretion and excessive intake of sodium-free solutions. This complication is usually encountered in markedly edematous patients with severe congestive heart failure, cirrhosis, or the nephrotic syndrome who are refractory to diuretics and it may be more common in women than in men. Hyponatremia can sometimes be prevented by restricting fluids during periods of active diuresis in markedly edematous patients. Correction depends upon discontinuing the diuretic, improving circulatory status, restricting fluid intake, and temporarily liberalizing salt intake or, if hyponatremia is severe and symptomatic, by infusing 3% sodium chloride solution. Occasionally, severe symptomatic hyponatremia has developed in nonedematous, normally hydrated patients treated with thiazide diuretics (Fichman et al, 1971; Ashraf et al, 1981).

Thiazides frequently increase the serum calcium level by increasing the protein-bound fraction (hemoconcentration effect). True hypercalcemia (increased ionized calcium) caused by a decrease in calcium excretion is a rare complication usually associated with latent primary hyperparathyroidism; in these patients, the serum calcium level may decrease when the thiazide is discontinued. If not, further evaluation is necessary to rule out the presence of a parathyroid adenoma. Thiazides also may induce a transient hypercalcemia in patients who are taking calcium-containing medications (eg, antacids) concurrently and in hypoparathyroid patients taking vitamin D, particularly if renal function is impaired.

Studies on the effects of thiazide-type diuretics on serum lipid levels have yielded highly divergent results, which were analyzed in a recent review (Ballantyne and Ballantyne, 1983). The authors concluded that short-term therapy may increase

TABLE 4.
CLINICALLY IMPORTANT ADVERSE INTERACTIONS OF DIURETICS

Agent	Diuretic	Effect
Adrenal Corticosteroids	Thiazides Loop	Enhanced hypokalemia
Amantadine	Triamterene with Thiazide	Neurotoxicity
Aminoglycosides	Loop	Increased ototoxicity
Aminoglycosides	Loop	Increased nephrotoxicity?
Anticoagulants (oral)	Thiazides Possibly others	Decreased anticoagulant effect due to concentration of clotting factors
Anticonvulsants	Furosemide	Possible decrease in natriuretic response
Beta blockers	Thiazides	Enhanced effect on blood lipid, urate, and glucose levels
Chlorpropamide	Thiazides Amiloride with Thiazide	Hyponatremia
Diazoxide	Thiazides Furosemide	Hyperglycemia
Digitalis	Thiazides Loop	Increased digitalis toxicity (if hypokalemia occurs)
Indomethacin	Potassium-sparing	Hyperkalemia Nephrotoxicity
Indomethacin and probably other inhibitors of renal prostaglandin synthesis	Thiazides Loop	Attenuation of natriuretic, antihypertensive, and potassium-wasting effect of the diuretic
Lithium	Thiazides Loop Possibly others	Increase in serum lithium levels
Potassium supplements	Potassium-sparing	Life-threatening hyperkalemia
Succinylcholine	Loop	Increased neuromuscular blocking effect
Tetracyclines	Probably all	Increased azotemia in patients with pre-existing renal disease
Trimethoprim	Amiloride with Thiazide	Hyponatremia
Tubocurarine	Thiazides Loop	Increased neuromuscular blocking effect
Vitamin D, Calcium products	Thiazides	Hypercalcemia

total cholesterol, triglyceride, and LDL-cholesterol concentrations but probably does not affect HDL levels. No firm conclusions were drawn on the effects of long-term therapy, but two of three studies showed no significant elevation after a year or more of treatment. Triglyceride levels were consistently elevated when a thiazide was given with a beta blocker for 4 to 16 weeks, but conflicting results were obtained in two long-term studies.

Factors that may be associated with thiazide-induced changes in serum lipid levels have not been clearly defined, but obesity, glucose intolerance, and hyperuricemia have been mentioned. A lipid-lowering diet may prevent the increase in serum lipid concentrations.

Thiazides may cause nausea, constipation, and sexual dysfunction. Blood dyscrasias (leukopenia, aplastic anemia, thrombocytopenic purpura, immune hemolysis, and agranulocytosis) and hypersensitivity reactions (eg, pneumonitis, rash, photosensitivity) occur occasionally. Rarely, photosensitivity has persisted after drug withdrawal. Acute pancreatitis has been reported infrequently. An association between thiazide use and acute cholecystitis has been noted by some investigators but denied by others. Necrotizing vasculitis of the skin and kidney has occurred in elderly patients, but its relationship to thiazide therapy is still unproved.

Electrolyte disturbances and thrombocytopenia have been reported in neonates whose mothers were treated with thiazides. Negligible amounts of hydrochlorothiazide and chlorothiazide are excreted in breast milk. These diuretics probably can be given safely to nursing mothers without adverse effects on the infant.

Reactions that have occurred rarely with specific thiazides are idiosyncratic pulmonary edema (allergic pneumonitis?) and anaphylactoid reactions (hydrochlorothiazide) and episodes of acute muscle cramps followed by syncope and epileptiform movements (metolazone).

Thiazides displace bilirubin from albumin and should be used cautiously in jaundiced infants.

Since small bowel lesions (stenosis with or without ulceration) have occurred in patients who received enteric-coated preparations of potassium chloride, these products (which are sometimes available in combination with a thiazide) should not be used.

DRUG INTERACTIONS. See Table 4.

PHARMACOKINETICS. Pharmacokinetic data are not available for all thiazide diuretics. Hydrochlorothiazide, metolazone, bendroflumethiazide, and indapamide are absorbed rapidly from the gastrointestinal tract, and their bioavailability ranges from approximately 65% (hydrochlorothiazide and metolazone) to 93% (indapamide) and 100% (bendroflumethiazide). The bioavailability of hydrochlorothiazide is increased to 75% when it is taken with food. Chlorothiazide tablets are absorbed erratically and poorly and bioavailability is not proportional to dose.

The onset of diuretic action occurs within one hour after administration of most thiazides. All are actively secreted in the proximal tubules, and their duration of action appears to be determined by the degree of protein binding and tubular reabsorption (Beermann and Groschinsky-Grind, 1980). Hy-

drochlorothiazide, hydroflumethiazide, and chlorothiazide are eliminated largely by renal excretion of unchanged drug, whereas bendroflumethiazide and indapamide undergo extensive metabolism. Only 7% of a dose of indapamide is excreted as unchanged drug.

DOSAGE AND PREPARATIONS. See Table 5.

LOOP DIURETICS

The loop diuretics, furosemide [Lasix], ethacrynic acid [Edecrin], and bumetanide [Bumex], block active sodium chloride transport in the thick ascending limb of Henle's loop. The loop diuretics have a much greater diuretic effect than the thiazides. Unlike the mercurials, they remain effective even in the presence of electrolyte and acid-base disturbances. Their proper use requires an understanding of the electrolyte and fluid derangements that they may induce. These potent agents are generally reserved for patients with impaired renal function, acute pulmonary edema, or hypertensive crises.

FUROSEMIDE
[Lasix]

ACTIONS AND USES. Furosemide is a potent, short-acting, sulfonamide diuretic that is chemically similar to the thiazides. When administered orally, the onset of action occurs within 30 to 60 minutes and the diuretic effect lasts six to eight hours; with parenteral administration, the diuretic effect is immediate and persists for about two hours. Furosemide has a very wide dose-response curve, and dosage can be adjusted to produce a graded response. In addition to sodium and chloride, furosemide increases the renal excretion of potassium, magnesium, calcium, and, to a lesser extent, bicarbonate ions.

Furosemide is usually preferred to ethacrynic acid because it (1) has a broader dose-response curve; (2) is less ototoxic; (3) causes fewer gastrointestinal side effects; (4) is more convenient for intravenous use; (5) may be less likely to cause alkalosis; and (6) is available as an oral solution.

Oral furosemide is usually effective in patients with cardiac edema who do not respond to thiazides. It is of particular value in treating edema associated with impaired renal function because it is effective even when the glomerular filtration rate is greatly reduced. Although some patients with the nephrotic syndrome may respond to less potent diuretics, edema and hypertension in patients with chronic renal failure often can be controlled only with the loop diuretics; large doses may be required but care should be taken to avoid further depletion of the blood volume. Furosemide should be administered very cautiously to patients with resistant cirrhotic edema and ascites; intensive diuretic therapy may not be desirable in these patients, especially if plasma volume is borderline.

When fluid retention is refractory to furosemide, the addition

TABLE 5.
THIAZIDES AND RELATED DIURETICS

Drug and Chemical Structure	Usual Diuretic Dosage*	Duration of Action (hours)	Preparations

THIAZIDES
Chlorothiazide
	Oral:
	Adults, 500 mg to 1 g once or twice daily; *children,* 22 mg/kg daily in 2 divided doses; *infants under 6 months,* up to 33 mg/kg daily in 2 divided doses.
		6 to 12	*SK--Chlorothiazide* (Smith Kline & French), *Generic.*
			  Tablets 250 and 500 mg.
			Diuril (Merck Sharp & Dohme).
			  Tablets 250 and 500 mg; suspension 250 mg/5 ml.

Chlorothiazide Sodium	*Intravenous:* *Adults,* 500 mg twice daily.	6 to 12	*Diuril [Sodium]* (Merck Sharp & Dohme). Powder (injection) equivalent to 500 mg chlorothiazide.

Hydrochlorothiazide	*Oral:*
	Adults, initially, 25 to 200 mg once or twice daily for several days; for maintenance, 25 to 100 mg daily or intermittently.
	Children, 2 mg/kg daily in 2 doses; *infants under 6 months,* up to 3 mg/kg daily in 2 doses.
		6 to 12	*Esidrix* (CIBA), *HydroDIURIL* (Merck Sharp & Dohme), *Generic.*
			  Tablets 25, 50 and 100 mg.
			Oretic (Abbott), *SK-Hydrochlorothiazide* (Smith Kline & French).
			  Tablets 25 and 50 mg.
			Zide (Reid-Provident).
			  Tablets 50 mg.

Bendroflumethiazide	*Oral:* *Adults,* initially, 5 mg daily, preferably in the morning; dose may be increased to 20 mg as a single dose or in 2 divided doses. For maintenance, 2.5 to 15 mg once daily or intermittently. *Children,* initially, up to 0.4 mg/kg daily in 2 divided doses. For maintenance, 0.05 to 0.1 mg/kg daily in a single dose.	More than 18	*Naturetin* (Squibb). Tablets 2.5, 5 and 10 mg.

Benzthiazide	*Oral:*
	Adults, initially, 50 to 200 mg daily for several days, depending upon patient's response. For maintenance, dosage is reduced gradually to minimum effective amount.
	Children, initially, 1 to 4 mg/kg daily in 3 divided doses. For maintenance, dose is reduced as needed.
		12 to 18	*Aquatag* (Reid-Provident).
			  Tablets 25 and 50 mg.
			Exna (Robins), *Generic.*
			  Tablets 50 mg.

*See Chapter 28 for antihypertensive doses.

(continued on next page)

TABLE 5.
THIAZIDES AND RELATED DIURETICS (continued)

Drug and Chemical Structure	Usual Diuretic Dosage*	Duration of Action (hours)	Preparations
Cyclothiazide	*Oral:* *Adults,* initially, 1 to 2 mg daily, preferably in the morning; for maintenance, 1 mg on alternate days or 2 or 3 times weekly. *Children,* initially, 0.02 to 0.04 mg/kg daily; for maintenance, dose is reduced as needed.	18 to 24	*Anhydron* (Lilly). Tablets 2 mg.
Hydroflumethiazide	*Oral:* *Adults,* initially, 50 to 100 mg daily; for maintenance, 25 to 200 mg in divided amounts, depending upon response. *Children,* initially, 1 mg/kg daily; for maintenance, dose is adjusted as needed.	18 to 24	*Diucardin* (Ayerst). *Saluron* Bristol), *Generic.* Tablets 50 mg.
Methyclothiazide	*Oral:* *Adults,* initially, 2.5 to 10 mg once daily; same dose range is used for maintenance. *Children,* 0.05 to 0.2 mg/kg daily.	More than 24	*Aquatensen* (Wallace). Tablets 5 mg. *Enduron* (Abbott), *Generic.* Tablets 2.5 and 5 mg.
Polythiazide	*Oral:* *Adults,* initially, 1 to 4 mg daily, depending upon response and severity of the condition; for maintenance, 0.5 to 8 mg daily adjusted for optimal response. *Children,* initially, 0.02 to 0.08 mg/kg daily; for maintenance, dose is adjusted according to response.	24 to 48	*Renese* (Pfizer) Tablets 1, 2 and 4 mg.
Trichlormethiazide	*Oral:* *Adults,* initially, 2 to 4 mg after breakfast daily or twice daily if needed; for maintenance, 1 to 2 mg once daily. *Children,* 0.07 mg/kg daily in single or divided doses.	Up to 24	*Metahydrin* (Merrell Dow), *Naqua* (Schering), *Generic.* Tablets 2 and 4 mg.
RELATED COMPOUNDS Chlorthalidone	*Oral:* *Adults,* initially, 50 to 100 mg after breakfast daily or 100 mg on alternate days or 3 times weekly; some patients may require 200 mg. Maintenance doses should be adjusted individually. *Children,* 2 mg/kg 3 times weekly; maintenance dose should be adjusted individually.	24 to 72	*Hygroton* (USV), *Generic.* Tablets 25, 50 and 100 mg.
Indapamide	*Oral:* *Adults,* initially, 2.5 mg daily. The dose may be increased to 5 mg daily.	24	*Lozol* (USV). Tablets 2.5 mg.

*See Chapter 28 for antihypertensive doses

(continued on next page)

Drug and Chemical Structure	Usual Diuretic Dosage*	Duration of Action (hours)	Preparations
Quinethazone	*Oral:* *Adults,* 50 to 100 mg daily, depending upon response and severity of the condition. Some patients may require as much as 150 or 200 mg daily, on alternate days, or 3 times weekly.	18 to 24	*Hydromox* (Lederle). Tablets 50 mg.
Metolazone	*Oral:* *Adults,* 5 to 20 mg daily, depending upon response and severity of the condition. Doses as large as 150 mg daily may be required in patients with chronic renal failure.	12 to 24	*Diulo* (Searle), *Zaroxolyn* (Pennwalt). Tablets 2.5, 5 and 10 mg.

*See Chapter 28 for antihypertensive doses

of metolazone or another thiazide-type diuretic may promote diuresis. Serum electrolytes, blood pressure, and renal function should be monitored frequently during such combined therapy because massive fluid and electrolyte losses and fatal circulatory collapse may occur.

Patients with cardiogenic pulmonary edema respond rapidly to intravenous furosemide, and it is often preferred for the initial management of pulmonary congestion following acute myocardial infarction. Since relief of symptoms may precede the diuretic action, a vascular effect (ie, reduced venous tone) has been postulated. Excessive diuresis should be avoided because of the danger of precipitating shock. Moderate doses reverse acute pulmonary edema without depleting plasma volume (Schuster et al, 1984).

The use of furosemide in premature infants with respiratory distress syndrome is controversial. It may improve pulmonary function and decrease ventilator requirements (Green et al, 1983 A; Yeh et al, 1984), but does not prevent bronchopulmonary dysplasia or affect mortality (Yeh et al, 1984) and has caused adverse effects (see Adverse Reactions and Precautions).

In oliguric patients, furosemide is used by some nephrologists for diagnosis and prophylaxis of acute renal failure. In patients with established acute tubular necrosis, furosemide may reduce the need for dialysis, but a favorable effect on the mortality rate has not been reported. The value of increasing urine flow in these patients has been questioned. If diuresis is

successful, careful fluid replacement is necessary to prevent dehydration and further renal insult.

ADVERSE REACTIONS AND PRECAUTIONS. Because of its potency, therapy with furosemide must be instituted cautiously and dosage should be individualized to avoid excessive diuresis. Overzealous therapy can cause volume depletion, hypotension, and marked hypokalemia and hypochloremic alkalosis; therefore, it is advisable to begin therapy with small doses and increase the amount gradually if necessary. During rapid mobilization of edema, serum electrolytes should be monitored carefully and prophylactic measures may be indicated to prevent severe hypokalemia; fluids should be restricted to prevent dilutional hyponatremia.

Serum electrolyte levels also should be determined periodically in patients receiving long-term therapy. A potassium-sparing diuretic or potassium supplements may be indicated in digitalized or cirrhotic patients. In addition, all patients receiving furosemide should be instructed to report promptly any events that might further reduce the serum potassium level (eg, diarrhea, vomiting, anorexia). Like the thiazides, furosemide may cause azotemia, hyperuricemia, and hyperglycemia. Hyponatremia occurs less frequently than with the thiazides.

Furosemide stimulates the renal synthesis of prostaglandin E_2 and may increase the incidence of patent ductus arteriosus in preterm infants with respiratory distress syndrome (Green et al, 1983 B). The increased urinary loss of calcium induced by furosemide may lead to secondary hyperparathyroidism, osteopenia, and renal calcification in these infants (Hufnagle et al, 1982; Venkataraman et al, 1983). The concurrent use of chlorothiazide was reported to prevent the renal calcifications. An association has been reported between furosemide therapy and the development of gallstones in premature infants.

Dermatologic reactions (urticaria, erythema multiforme, photosensitivity), hematologic disturbances (agranulocytosis, anemia, thrombocytopenia), allergic interstitial nephritis, nonspecific chronic aortitis, and acute pancreatitis have been reported rarely.

Transient deafness has occurred following rapid intravenous administration of large doses and occasionally after administration of small doses and/or during oral therapy. Permanent deafness is rare. Most affected patients had concomitant renal disease or were receiving other ototoxic drugs (aminoglycoside antibiotics or ethacrynic acid).

When furosemide is used for long-term therapy of edematous conditions, rapid withdrawal may be followed by rebound edema, a complication that may result from diuretic-induced secondary hyperaldosteronism. Spironolactone may aid in weaning these patients from furosemide (Chan et al, 1979).

DRUG INTERACTIONS. See Table 4.

PHARMACOKINETICS. The bioavailability of oral furosemide (Lasix tablets) is 60% to 69% in normal subjects but is reduced to 43% to 46% in patients with end-stage renal disease. Some generic products may show lower bioavailability. Food slows the rate of absorption but does not alter the total amount of furosemide absorbed. Absorption is also slowed in patients with decompensated congestive heart failure. Furosemide is 91% to 99% bound to serum albumin, but protein binding is reduced in those with uremia and nephrosis. This drug is eliminated largely by renal excretion of unchanged drug. The half-life is prolonged in newborn infants, elderly patients, and those with renal or hepatic impairment (Cutler and Blair, 1979).

DOSAGE AND PREPARATIONS.

Oral: For edema, *adults,* initially, 20 to 80 mg as a single dose, preferably in the morning. If an adequate diuretic response is not achieved, the dose may be increased gradually at intervals of six to eight hours. The effective maintenance dose varies widely and no definite upper limit has been established; however, 600 mg daily is the maximum amount recommended by the manufacturer. The frequency of administration also must be determined individually. Furosemide reaches the site of action within the tubular lumen by glomerular filtration and tubular secretion, and one or two large doses appear to be more effective than small doses administered frequently, especially in patients with renal insufficiency. Furosemide may be administered daily, on alternate days, or for two to four consecutive days per week. In some patients, intermittent therapy may be the most efficient method of mobilizing refractory edema. *Infants and children,* initially, 2 mg/kg given as a single dose. If an adequate response is not obtained, the dose may be increased gradually in increments of 1 or 2 mg/kg/dose no sooner than six to eight hours after the previous dose (maximum, 6 mg/kg).

Lasix (Hoechst-Roussel). Solution (oral) 10 mg/ml; tablets 20, 40, and 80 mg.

SK-Furosemide (Smith Kline & French). Tablets 20 and 40 mg.

Intravenous: *Adults,* for acute pulmonary edema, the usual initial dose is 40 mg, which may be repeated in 60 to 90 minutes. *Infants and children,* initially, 1 mg/kg given slowly. If an adequate response is not obtained, the amount may be increased in increments of 1 mg/kg no sooner than two hours after the previous dose (maximum, 6 mg/kg). *Premature and full-term newborn infants,* 1 mg/kg given no more frequently than twice daily. (Furosemide also may be administered intramuscularly, but the intravenous route is usually preferred.)

For acute renal failure, *adults,* initially, 40 to 80 mg. The amount may then be increased until a diuretic response is obtained, but the total dose should rarely exceed 500 mg in a 24-hour period. *Large intravenous doses should be given at a rate not exceeding 4 mg/min.* If diuresis fails to ensue, the drug should be discontinued. It is important to ascertain that the plasma volume is adequate before furosemide is administered to the oliguric patient. In prerenal azotemia, even large doses may not produce a diuresis without volume replacement. In the event of successful diuresis and in the absence of edema or cardiopulmonary overload, total fluid losses should be replaced every two to four hours to maintain adequate plasma volume and renal perfusion.

Lasix (Hoechst-Roussel), *Generic*. Solution (sterile) 10 mg/ml in 2, 4, and 10 ml containers.

ETHACRYNIC ACID
[Edecrin]

ETHACRYNATE SODIUM
[Sodium Edecrin]

ACTIONS AND USES. Ethacrynic acid, a derivative of aryloxyacetic acid, is a potent, short-acting diuretic with an onset and duration of action similar to furosemide. The two drugs have the same therapeutic applications, but furosemide is usually preferred.

ADVERSE REACTIONS AND PRECAUTIONS. The electrolyte and fluid derangements induced by ethacrynic acid are identical to those caused by furosemide, and the same precautions should be observed. Ethacrynic acid also may cause azotemia and hyperuricemia. Since hyperglycemia occurs only rarely, this drug may be preferred for use in diabetics.

Transient deafness (occasionally accompanied by nystagmus) has been reported, most commonly following rapid intravenous administration of large doses to azotemic or uremic patients or in those receiving other ototoxic drugs (eg, aminoglycoside antibiotics). Permanent deafness has occurred rarely but is much more common than with furosemide.

When given orally, ethacrynic acid may cause watery diarrhea and other gastrointestinal disturbances. If these develop, the drug should be discontinued. Gastrointestinal bleeding occurred in some patients during intravenous therapy. Dermatologic reactions, jaundice, abnormal results of liver function tests, agranulocytosis, thrombocytopenia, neutropenia, Henoch-Schönlein purpura, and acute pancreatitis have been reported rarely.

DRUG INTERACTIONS. See Table 4.

DOSAGE AND PREPARATIONS.

Oral: For edema, *adults,* initially, 50 to 100 mg daily. If an adequate response is not obtained, the daily dosage may be increased, usually in increments of 25 or 50 mg. For maintenance, the dose and frequency of administration must be determined individually. Patients with refractory edema may require 400 mg daily (usually in two divided doses); in such patients, intermittent therapy may be the most efficient method of mobilizing edema. *Children,* initially, 25 mg daily. Dosage may be increased gradually by increments of 25 mg.

ETHACRYNIC ACID:
Edecrin (Merck Sharp & Dohme). Tablets 25 and 50 mg.

Intravenous: For acute pulmonary edema, *adults,* initially, 50 mg or 0.5 to 1 mg/kg *injected slowly; children,* initially, 1 mg/kg. These doses may be increased if necessary.

ETHACRYNATE SODIUM:
Sodium Edecrin (Merck Sharp & Dohme). Powder equivalent to 50 mg ethacrynic acid.

BUMETANIDE
[Bumex]

ACTIONS AND USES. Bumetanide is a metanilamide derivative. Its onset and duration of action, diuretic efficacy, and biochemical effects are comparable to those of furosemide, but bumetanide is more active on a weight basis. Given orally, 1 mg of bumetanide is equivalent to approximately 40 mg of furosemide.

Oral bumetanide is effective in patients with chronic congestive heart failure, chronic renal failure, cirrhosis with ascites, and the nephrotic syndrome. In most comparative studies, it was as effective as furosemide during both short-term and long-term therapy. Bumetanide also is useful when given intravenously to treat acute pulmonary edema (Brogden et al, 1975).

ADVERSE REACTIONS AND PRECAUTIONS. The fluid and electrolyte changes induced by bumetanide are similar to those of furosemide and the same precautions apply (see the evaluation on Furosemide). Bumetanide also may cause azo-

temia, hyperuricemia, and, rarely, impaired glucose tolerance. In patients with renal failure, large doses may cause myalgia, which may be severe. Nausea, vomiting, abdominal pain, and rashes, including one case of Stevens-Johnson syndrome, have been reported. Blood dyscrasias (granulocytopenia, thrombocytopenia) have occurred rarely.

Bumetanide is ototoxic in laboratory animals. Although deafness has not been reported clinically, the potential danger should be kept in mind.

DRUG INTERACTIONS. See Table 4.

PHARMACOKINETICS. The bioavailability of bumetanide is 95%. It is 95% protein bound and the volume of distribution is 12 to 35 L. Approximately 45% of an oral dose is excreted as unchanged drug. The half-life is 1 to 1.5 hours and is prolonged in patients with renal failure.

DOSAGE AND PREPARATIONS.

Oral: Adults, for edema, initially, 1 mg daily in the morning. A second dose may be given if required six to eight hours later. Dosage may be increased in refractory cases but usually need not exceed 4 mg except in patients with severe renal failure who may require up to 15 mg daily.
Bumex (Roche). Tablets 0.5 and 1 mg.

Intravenous: Adults, for pulmonary edema, initially, 0.5 to 1 mg. The dose may be repeated if necessary after 20 minutes.
Bumex (Roche). Solution 0.25 mg/ml in 2 ml containers.

POTASSIUM-SPARING DIURETICS

The potassium-sparing diuretics interfere with sodium reabsorption at the distal sites in the renal tubules where sodium reabsorption is related to the secretion of potassium and hydrogen ions. These agents thereby promote sodium excretion while conserving potassium. They also appear to be magnesium-sparing. Agents in this group include the aldosterone antagonists, spironolactone [Aldactone] and related investigational steroids (canrenone, canrenoate potassium, and mexrenoate potassium), and the direct-acting agents, triamterene [Dyrenium] and amiloride [Midamor].

Since only a small fraction of filtered sodium normally is reabsorbed at the distal sites, the potassium-sparing agents are not potent diuretics when used alone. Their major use is in conjunction with the thiazides or loop diuretics. Such combined therapy reduces potassium excretion, minimizes alkalosis, and may have an additive diuretic effect. Because hypokalemia predisposes to digitalis toxicity, combined therapy is particularly useful in digitalized patients.

The potassium-sparing diuretics are far better tolerated than potassium supplements and are much more reliable in raising and maintaining the serum potassium level during diuretic therapy. Because they block the renal regulatory mechanisms that control potassium excretion, these agents are often effective in patients who do not respond to potassium supplements. Also for this reason, their dosage may be more difficult to manipulate in accordance with changes in the serum potassium level, and they are more prone to cause hyperkalemia, particularly when renal function is impaired or potassium intake is excessive. Because renal function decreases with age, these drugs should be used extremely cautiously in elderly patients.

Potassium-sparing diuretics generally should be avoided in diabetics. Many patients with moderate to severe diabetes and mild to moderate renal insufficiency have a defect in the renin-angiotensin-aldosterone axis. This defect, in addition to insulin deficiency, makes them particularly prone to life-threatening hyperkalemia. Those with mild diabetes, normal renal function, and a normally responsive renin-angiotensin-aldosterone system do not appear to be at risk.

SPIRONOLACTONE
[Aldactone]

SPIRONOLACTONE AND HYDROCHLOROTHIAZIDE
[Aldactazide]

ACTIONS AND USES. Spironolactone is a steroid that acts as a competitive antagonist of the potent endogenous mineralo-corticoid, aldosterone. Although aldosterone must be present for spironolactone to act, it need not be present in large amounts. Spironolactone has a slower onset of action than triamterene or amiloride but its natriuretic effect is slightly greater during long-term therapy. During combined treatment with a thiazide, the potassium-sparing effect of spironolactone is comparable to that of triamterene and may be greater than that of amiloride.

Spironolactone is used to treat edema associated with chronic congestive heart failure, cirrhosis, and the nephrotic syndrome. It is sometimes administered as the sole diuretic agent, particularly in cirrhosis with ascites, but is most effective when given with a thiazide or loop diuretic.

ADVERSE REACTIONS AND PRECAUTIONS. Careful monitoring of the serum potassium level is necessary during therapy with spironolactone because hyperkalemia may occur even when a potassium-wasting diuretic is given concomitantly. Precipitating factors are a high intake of potassium (supplements, salt substitutes, or dietary) and/or impaired renal function. Spironolactone should be used very cautiously, if at all, in patients with a reduced glomerular filtration rate and only if the serum potassium level is monitored closely. It generally should be avoided in diabetics. The concurrent use of potassium-sparing diuretics and potassium supplements and/or salt substitutes can be hazardous.

Spironolactone may increase blood urea nitrogen and serum uric acid levels. Its effects on serum lipid levels are not clearly defined. Hyponatremia may occur following excessive

ingestion of water. Serum bicarbonate levels should be measured periodically in patients with chronic liver disease because hypochloremic acidosis may develop during treatment.

Daily doses of 100 mg or more often cause gynecomastia in men, which may be related to binding of the active metabolite, canrenone, to tissue androgen receptors. Decreased libido and impotence also have been reported. Menstrual disturbances and breast tenderness may occur in women. Breast cancer has developed in some patients during or after spironolactone therapy, but a cause-and-effect relationship has not been established.

Gastrointestinal disturbances occur occasionally and gastric ulceration rarely. Rashes and neurologic disturbances also have been reported. Agranulocytosis has rarely been associated with spironolactone therapy. There is one report of a possible association between spironolactone therapy and elevated liver enzyme levels in a patient with primary hyperaldosteronism.

DRUG INTERACTIONS. See Table 4.

EFFECT ON LABORATORY TESTS. Spironolactone interferes with plasma cortisol determinations by the fluorometric method. Spironolactone and its metabolites may interfere with some radioimmunoassay tests for digoxin.

PHARMACOKINETICS. Spironolactone is rapidly and extensively metabolized in the liver, and approximately 79% of its activity is due to the metabolite, canrenone. Food increases the bioavailability of this active metabolite. Canrenone is 98% bound to plasma proteins and has a half-life of 10 to 35 hours. Canrenone and other metabolites are excreted in the urine and feces. Steady-state plasma levels of spironolactone and its metabolites are not increased in patients with renal or hepatic impairment (Karim, 1978).

DOSAGE AND PREPARATIONS.

SPIRONOLACTONE:
The onset of action of spironolactone is relatively slow and maximal effects usually do not occur until the third day of therapy. When discontinued, effects diminish gradually over two or three days. Spironolactone is usually given with a thiazide or loop diuretic. Serum potassium and creatinine levels should be monitored.
Oral: Adults, for edema, 50 to 100 mg daily in single or divided doses. Larger doses cause little additional elevation of serum potassium levels and frequently produce side effects. *Children,* 1 mg/kg three times daily.

For primary hyperaldosteronism, see Chapter 37, Agents Used to Treat Adrenal Dysfunction.
Generic. Tablets 25 mg.
Aldactone (Searle). Tablets 25, 50, and 100 mg.

SPIRONOLACTONE AND HYDROCHLOROTHIAZIDE:

The serum potassium response to spironolactone varies sevenfold in patients receiving a thiazide; therefore, this combination may not be suitable for some patients. The serum potassium level should be monitored.
Oral: Adults, for edema, one tablet one to four times daily.
Aldactazide (Searle), *Generic.* Each tablet contains spironolactone 25 mg and hydrochlorothiazide 25 mg or spironolactone 50 mg and hydrochlorothiazide 50 mg (*Aldactazide* only).

TRIAMTERENE
[Dyrenium]

TRIAMTERENE AND HYDROCHLOROTHIAZIDE
[Dyazide, Maxzide]

ACTIONS AND USES. Triamterene is a pteridine derivative that is chemically related to folic acid. It interferes with sodium reabsorption and potassium and hydrogen ion secretion in the cortical collecting tubule by a direct action. Triamterene is used primarily for its potassium-sparing effect. It is given with a thiazide or loop diuretic to treat edema associated with congestive heart failure, cirrhosis, or the nephrotic syndrome. Triamterene has a more rapid onset of action than spironolactone but is less effective when used alone. When given with a thiazide, the potassium-sparing effect of 200 mg triamterene is equivalent to that of 50 mg spironolactone (Jackson et al, 1982).

ADVERSE REACTIONS AND PRECAUTIONS. Like spironolactone, triamterene can cause hyperkalemia and the same precautions should be observed (see the evaluation on Spironolactone). Glucose intolerance and hyperkalemia may occur in patients with moderate to severe diabetes mellitus. Triamterene may increase blood urea nitrogen and serum uric acid levels. Gastrointestinal disturbances, rashes, and photosensitivity occur occasionally.

Patients receiving triamterene (usually as Dyazide) have passed urinary stones composed of triamterene and a metabolite, sometimes with other constituents, such as calcium oxalate or uric acid. It is not definitely known whether triamterene initiates stone formation or becomes incorporated in a pre-existing stone, but patients that form these stones appear to absorb, metabolize, and excrete triamterene normally (Carey et al, 1984). Although a prior episode of renal lithiasis has not been shown to increase the risk of triamterene calculi, the drug should probably be avoided in patients with such a history. Acute interstitial nephritis has rarely been associated with triamterene or Dyazide therapy. One patient developed nephrogenic diabetes insipidus while taking Dyazide.

Megaloblastic anemia has been reported in cirrhotic patients, but a cause-and-effect relationship has not been definitely established. Anaphylactic reactions have occurred rarely.

DRUG INTERACTIONS. See Table 4.

EFFECT ON LABORATORY TESTS. Triamterene interferes with the fluorescent measurement of quinidine.

PHARMACOKINETICS. Triamterene is rapidly absorbed and excreted. Its bioavailability is 52%. The onset of action of a single dose occurs within one hour and reaches a peak in two to three hours. Diuresis usually declines gradually in seven to nine hours. The urinary recovery of triamterene varies among individuals and in the same individual tested on different days.

Approximately 20% is excreted unchanged and 80% is recovered as various metabolites. The major metabolite, hydroxytriamterene sulfate, is pharmacologically active. The half-life of triamterene is 100 to 120 minutes. The excretion of triamterene and its active metabolite is reduced in patients with impaired renal function or cirrhosis.

DOSAGE AND PREPARATIONS.
TRIAMTERENE:
Triamterene is usually given with a thiazide or loop diuretic. Serum potassium and creatinine levels should be monitored.
Oral: Adults, for edema, 100 mg twice daily after meals; the maximal dose is 300 mg daily. *Children,* 2 to 4 mg/kg daily in divided doses.
   Dyrenium (Smith Kline & French). Capsules 50 and 100 mg.
TRIAMTERENE AND HYDROCHLOROTHIAZIDE:
Combination products containing triamterene and hydrochlorothiazide may vary in bioavailability. Both the triamterene and the hydrochlorothiazide components of Maxzide are more bioavailable than those contained in Dyazide. In addition, it should be noted that Maxzide contains a larger dose of each component than Dyazide.
Oral: Adults, for edema, one tablet of Maxzide daily or one or two capsules of Dyazide twice daily after meals. Serum potassium levels should be monitored.
   Dyazide (Smith Kline & French). Each capsule contains triamterene 50 mg and hydrochlorothiazide 25 mg.
   Maxzide (Lederle). Each tablet contains triamterene 75 mg and hydrochlorothiazide 50 mg.

AMILORIDE HYDROCHLORIDE
[Midamor]

AMILORIDE HYDROCHLORIDE AND HYDROCHLOROTHIAZIDE
[Moduretic]

ACTIONS AND USES. This pteridine compound inhibits sodium reabsorption and potassium and hydrogen ion secretion in the distal convoluted tubule and cortical collecting tubule by a direct action. Amiloride is used primarily for its potassium-sparing effect. It is given with a thiazide or loop diuretic to treat edema associated with chronic congestive heart failure or cirrhosis. Amiloride has a more rapid onset of action than spironolactone. During long-term therapy, its natriuretic and potassium-sparing effects are less, but amiloride may be more effective in correcting metabolic alkalosis. Amiloride has a longer duration of action than triamterene.

ADVERSE REACTIONS AND PRECAUTIONS. Like the other potassium-sparing diuretics, amiloride may cause hyperkalemia and the same precautions apply (see the evaluation on Spironolactone). Patients with moderate to severe diabetes mellitus may develop glucose intolerance and hyperkalemia during therapy. Amiloride also may cause azotemia, hyponatremia, and hyperuricemia. Gastrointestinal disturbances (nausea, vomiting, anorexia, diarrhea) and dizziness also have been reported.

DRUG INTERACTIONS. See Table 4.

PHARMACOKINETICS. In fasting subjects, 61% of a 10- to 20-mg dose was recovered in the urine after 48 hours. Bioavailability is decreased when the drug is given with food. Unlike spironolactone and triamterene, amiloride is excreted unchanged by the kidneys. Its half-life is six hours, but is prolonged in patients with impaired renal function.

DOSAGE AND PREPARATIONS.

AMILORIDE HYDROCHLORIDE:

Amiloride is usually given with a thiazide or loop diuretic. Serum potassium and creatinine levels should be monitored.

Oral: Adults, 5 to 10 mg daily.

> *Midamor* (Merck Sharp & Dohme). Tablets 5 mg.

AMILORIDE HYDROCHLORIDE AND HYDROCHLOROTHIAZIDE: Some investigators found amiloride to be less effective in preventing hypokalemia when given in a fixed-dose combination with hydrochlorothiazide than when the drugs were given separately in the same dosage ratio (5:50). When both products are given once daily in fixed-dose combination, the antihypertensive effect of amiloride and hydrochlorothiazide (5:50) is comparable to that of triamterene and hydrochlorothiazide (50:25) but the former causes greater potassium loss due to the larger dose of thiazide.

Oral: Adults, for edema, one or two tablets daily. Serum potassium levels should be monitored.

> *Moduretic* (Merck Sharp & Dohme). Each tablet contains amiloride hydrochloride 5 mg and hydrochlorothiazide 50 mg.

OSMOTIC DIURETICS

Osmotic diuretics inhibit sodium and water reabsorption in the proximal tubule, loop of Henle, and collecting duct. With the exception of mannitol, which is used for diagnosis and prophylaxis of acute renal failure, osmotic agents are not used as diuretics. Their main clinical applications are to reduce intraocular pressure and vitreous volume prior to ocular surgery and to reduce intracranial pressure pre- and postoperatively in neurosurgical patients.

Mannitol is preferred to urea because it is more convenient to use, less irritating, less likely to cause thrombophlebitis, does not cause tissue necrosis following extravasation, is longer acting, and is safer in patients with renal failure. It is also less likely than urea to cause a rebound increase in intracranial pressure in patients with brain edema.

MANNITOL
[Osmitrol]

$$\begin{array}{c} CH_2OH \\ | \\ HOCH \\ | \\ HOCH \\ | \\ HCOH \\ | \\ HCOH \\ | \\ CH_2OH \end{array}$$

USES. This osmotic diuretic is used by some nephrologists for diagnosis and prophylaxis of acute renal failure. It also is used to reduce intraocular pressure and vitreous volume prior to ocular surgery, to reduce intracranial pressure temporarily in patients with brain edema, and to promote urinary excretion of toxic substances.

ADVERSE REACTIONS AND PRECAUTIONS. Headache, nausea, vomiting, chills, dizziness, polydipsia, lethargy, confusion, and sensations of constriction or pain in the chest have been observed following infusion of mannitol. Hyponatremia is a common problem. Fatalities have occurred after large doses. Too rapid administration of large amounts draws intracellular water into the extracellular space, causing cellular dehydration and overexpansion of the intravascular space and resulting in congestive heart failure and pulmonary edema. Hyperkalemia may result from movement of potassium from the intracellular to the extracellular space. Rarely, massive infusion of mannitol has caused reversible acute oliguric renal failure.

Mannitol may increase cerebral blood flow and thus the risk of postoperative bleeding in neurosurgical patients. Although mannitol crosses the blood-brain barrier less readily than urea, a rebound increase in intracranial pressure has occurred occasionally in patients with Reye's syndrome.

Anaphylactoid reactions have occurred rarely with use of this drug. Hemodialysis is the most effective treatment for mannitol intoxication.

DOSAGE AND PREPARATIONS. Hypertonic solutions of mannitol should not be added to whole blood for transfusion because increased osmotic pressure will cause crenation and agglutination of red blood cells.

Intravenous: To promote diuresis in oliguric patients, after restoration of plasma volume, *adults,* 300 to 400 mg/kg of a 20% or 25% solution may be given as a single dose (sometimes in conjunction with furosemide). *Children,* 750 mg/kg. If diuresis ensues, fluid losses should be replaced at two- to four-hour intervals to maintain intravascular fluid volume. Doses should not be repeated in patients with persistent oliguria, since this can cause a hyperosmolar state and precipitate congestive heart failure and pulmonary edema due to volume overload.

To reduce intracranial pressure, *adults and children,* 1.5 to 2 g/kg of a 15%, 20%, or 25% solution infused over a period of 30 to 60 minutes.

To promote urinary excretion of toxic substances, *adults,* a 5% to 25% solution may be infused as long as indicated if the urinary output remains high. The concentration will depend upon the fluid requirement and urinary output. Water and electrolytes should be given intravenously to replace the loss of these substances in urine, sweat, and expired air. If benefits are not observed after 200 g has been infused, the drug should be discontinued. *Children,* 2 g/kg of a 5% to 10% solution.

> *Mannitol should not be confused with mannitol hexanitrate, an antianginal drug.*
> *Generic.* Solution 5%, 10%, 15%, 20%, and 25%.
> *Osmitrol* (Travenol). Solution (aqueous) 5% in 1,000 ml containers, 10% in 500 and 1,000 ml containers, 15% in 150 and 500 ml containers, and 20% in 250 and 500 ml containers.

CARBONIC ANHYDRASE INHIBITORS

Following the observation in 1949 that large doses of sulfanilamide produced diuresis in edematous patients with congestive heart failure and the recognition that the diuresis resulted from inhibition of carbonic anhydrase in the renal tubules, acetazolamide, the first orally administered sulfonamide diuretic, was introduced. Because tolerance develops rapidly, this drug and its analogues proved to be of limited value in diuretic therapy and were soon supplanted by the thiazides. Their major use today is as an adjunct in glaucoma therapy (see Chapter 18).

ACETAZOLAMIDE
[Diamox]

ACTIONS AND USES. Acetazolamide inhibits sodium bicarbonate reabsorption in the proximal tubule. There is no significant increase in chloride excretion and, after several days of continuous administration, a mild hyperchloremic acidosis occurs. Tolerance develops to the diuretic action in the presence of this acid-base disturbance.

Given before and for a short time after acute exposure to high altitude, acetazolamide may reduce the incidence and severity of acute mountain sickness (Greene et al, 1981; Hackett and Rennie, 1976). It is indicated in individuals who are susceptible to acute mountain sickness and in those who must ascend rapidly. Since acetazolamide does not prevent the life-threatening complications of pulmonary and cerebral edema, it should not be used routinely as a substitute for gradual ascent (Meehan and Zavala, 1982).

For use in glaucoma therapy, see Chapter 18. For use in the periodic paralyses, see Chapter 12, Drugs Used in Disorders Affecting Skeletal Muscle.

ADVERSE REACTIONS AND PRECAUTIONS. Acetazolamide may cause paresthesias, gastrointestinal disturbances, anorexia, drowsiness, fatigue, and transient myopia. The serum potassium level may fall during the first few weeks of therapy but this decrease is not sustained. No serious problems (eg, enhanced digitalis toxicity) have been associated with the initial hypokalemia.

Carbonic anhydrase inhibitors reduce the excretion of uric acid, and there is one report of an exacerbation of gout associated with acetazolamide therapy. Acetazolamide may promote formation of renal calculi by reducing the urinary excretion of citrate. A few patients have died in acute renal failure during acetazolamide therapy; a sulfonamide-like nephropathy may be involved in these cases. Urticaria, drug fever, and blood dyscrasias have occurred rarely.

DOSAGE AND PREPARATIONS.
Oral: Adults, for acute mountain sickness, 250 mg twice daily (or 500 mg of timed-release preparation once daily) beginning three to four days before arrival at high altitude and continuing for a short time thereafter.
Generic. Tablets 250 mg.
Diamox (Lederle). Capsules (timed-release) 500 mg; tablets 125 and 250 mg.

Cited References

Amery A, et al: Glucose intolerance during diuretic therapy. *Lancet* 1:681-683, 1978.

Ashraf N, et al: Thiazide-induced hyponatremia associated with death or neurologic damage in outpatients. *Am J Med* 70:1141-1163, 1981.

Ballantyne D, Ballantyne FC: Thiazides, beta blockers and lipoproteins. *Postgrad Med J* 59:483-488, 1983.

Beasley D, Malvin RL: Atrial extracts increase glomerular filtration rate in vivo. *Am J Physiol* 248:F24-F30, 1985.

Beermann B, Groschinsky-Grind M: Clinical pharmacokinetics of diuretics. *Clin Pharmacokinet* 5:221-245, 1980.

Berl T, et al: Role of aldosterone in control of sodium excretion in patients with advanced chronic renal failure. *Kidney Int* 14:228-235, 1978.

Blantz RC, Pelazo JC: Functional role for tubuloglomerular feedback mechanism. *Kidney Int* 25:739-746, 1984.

Brezis M, et al: Renal ischemia: New perspective. *Kidney Int* 26:375-383, 1984.

Brogden RN, et al: Bumetanide: Preliminary report of its pharmacological properties and therapeutic efficacy in oedema. *Drugs* 9:4-18, 1975.

Buerkert J, et al: Role of deep nephrons and the terminal collecting duct in mannitol-induced diuresis. *Am J Physiol* 240:411-422, 1981.

Burg MB: Thick ascending limb of Henle's loop. *Kidney Int* 22:454-464, 1982.

Carey RA, et al: Triamterene and renal lithiasis: Review. *Clin Therapeut* 6:302-309, 1984.

Chaffman M, et al: Indapamide: Review of its pharmacodynamic properties and therapeutic efficacy in hypertension. *Drugs* 28:189-235, 1984.

Chan MK, et al: Diuretic escape and rebound oedema in renal allograft recipients. *Br Med J* 2:1604-1605, 1979.

Cogan MG: Disorders of proximal nephron function. *Am J Med* 72:275-288, 1982.

Collins R, et al: Overview of randomised trials of diuretics in pregnancy. *Br Med J* 290:17-23, 1985.

Cutler RE, Blair AD: Clinical pharmacokinetics of frusemide. *Clin Pharmacokinet* 4:279-296, 1979.

DuBose TD, Kokko JP: Renal chloride transport and control of extracellular fluid volume. *Cardiovasc Med* 2:967-981, 1977.

Epstein M: Renal sodium hardening in cirrhosis in Epstein M (ed): *The Kidney in Liver Disease*, ed 2. New York, Elsevier, 1983, 25-53.

Fichman MP, et al: Diuretic-induced hyponatremia. *Ann Intern Med* 75:853-863, 1971.

Frakes JT: Physiologic considerations in medical management of ascites. *Arch Intern Med* 140:620-623, 1980.

Ganguly A, Donohue JP: Primary aldosteronism: Pathophysiology, diagnosis and treatment. *J Urol* 129:241-242, 1983.

Gennari FJ, Kassirer JP: Osmotic diuresis. *N Engl J Med* 291:714-720, 1974.

Green TP, et al: Furosemide promotes patent ductus arteriosus in premature infants with respiratory-distress syndrome. *N Engl J Med* 308:743-748, 1983 A.

Green TP, et al: Diuresis and pulmonary function in premature infants with respiratory distress syndrome. *J Pediatr* 103:618-623, 1983 B.

Greene MK, et al: Acetazolamide in prevention of acute mountain sickness: Double-blind controlled cross-over study. *Br Med J* 283:811-813, 1981.

Hackett PH, Rennie D: Incidence, importance, and prophylaxis of acute mountain sickness. *Lancet* 2:1149-1154, 1976.

Hebert SC, Andreoli TE: Control of NaCl transport in thick ascending limb. *Am J Physiol* 246:F745-F756, 1984.

Holland OB, et al: Diuretic-induced ventricular ectopic activity. *Am J Med* 70:762-768, 1981.

Hufnagle KG, et al: Renal calcifications: Complication of long-term furosemide therapy in preterm infants. *Pediatrics* 70:360-363, 1982.

Jackson PR, et al: Relative potency of spironolactone, triamterene, and potassium chloride in thiazide-induced hypokalaemia. *Br J Clin Pharmacol* 14:257-263, 1982.

Jacobson HR: Transport characteristics of in vitro perfused proximal convoluted tubules. *Kidney Int* 22:425-433, 1982.

Kahn T, et al: Factors influencing sodium reabsorption in distal nephron. *Proc Soc Exp Biol Med* 145:737-742, 1974.

Karim A: Spironolactone: Disposition, metabolism, pharmacodynamics, and bioavailability. *Drug Metab Rev* 8:151-188, 1978.

Kokko JP: Transport characteristics of thin limbs of Henle. *Kidney Int* 22:449-453, 1982.

Levinsky NG, et al: Acute renal failure, in Brenner BM, Rector FC Jr: *The Kidney,* ed 2. Philadelphia, WB Saunders, 1981, vol 1, 1181-1236.

Linas SL, et al: Rational use of diuretics in cirrhosis, in Epstein M (ed): *The Kidney in Liver Disease,* ed 2. New York, Elsevier, 1983, 555-567.

Lindheimer MD, Katz AI: Sodium and diuretics in pregnancy. *N Engl J Med* 288:891-894, 1973.

Maack T, et al: Atrial natriuretic factor: Structure and functional properties. *Kidney Int* 27:607-615, 1985.

MacGregor GA, et al: Is "idiopathic" edema idiopathic? *Lancet* 1:397-400, 1979.

Meehan RT, Zavala DC: Pathophysiology of acute high-altitude illness. *Am J Med* 73:395-403, 1982.

Multiple Risk Factor Intervention Trial Research Group: Baseline rest electrocardiographic abnormalities, antihypertensive treatment, and mortality in Multiple Risk Factor Intervention Trial. *Am J Cardiol* 55:1-15, 1985.

Murphy MB, et al: Glucose intolerance in hypertensive patients treated with diuretics; fourteen-year follow-up. *Lancet* 2:1293-1295, 1982.

Palluk R, et al: Atrial natriuretic factor. *Life Sci* 36:1415-1425, 1985.

Papademetriou V, et al: Diuretic-induced hypokalemia in uncomplicated systemic hypertension: Effect of plasma potassium correction on cardiac arrhythmias. *Am J Cardiol* 52:1017-1022, 1983.

Ram CVS, et al: Moderate sodium restriction and various diuretics in treatment of hypertension: Effects of potassium wastage and blood pressure control. *Arch Intern Med* 141:1015-1019, 1981.

Rascher W, et al: Atrial natriuretic peptide in plasma of volume-overloaded children with chronic renal failure. *Lancet* 2:303-305, 1985.

Richards AM, et al: Renal, haemodynamic, and hormonal effects of human alpha atrial natriuretic peptide in healthy volunteers. *Lancet* 1:545-547, 1985.

Schiffrin EL, et al: Plasma concentration of atrial natriuretic factor in patient with paroxysmal atrial tachycardia, (letter). *N Engl J Med* 312:1196-1197, 1985.

Schuster C-J, et al: Blood volume following diuresis induced by furosemide. *Am J Med* 76:585-592, 1984.

Sebastian A, et al: Disorders of distal nephron function. *Am J Med* 72:289-307, 1982.

Stokes JB: Ion transport by the cortical and outer medullary collecting tubule. *Kidney Int* 22:473-484, 1982.

Tikkanen I, et al: Plasma atrial natriuretic peptide in cardiac disease and during infusion in healthy volunteers. *Lancet* 2:66-69, 1985.

Thurau K, Boylan JW: Acute renal success: Unexpected logic of oliguria in acute renal failure. *Am J Med* 61:308-315, 1976.

Tiller DJ, Mudge GH: Pharmacologic agents used in management of acute renal failure. *Kidney Int* 18:700-711, 1980.

Tucker RM, et al: 7. Diuretics: Role of sodium balance. *Mayo Clin Proc* 55:261-266, 1980.

Venkataraman PS, et al: Secondary hyperparathyroidism and bone disease in infants receiving long-term furosemide therapy. *Am J Dis Child* 137:1157-1161, 1983.

Whelton PK: Diuretics and arrhythmias in medical research council trial. *Drugs* 28(suppl 1):54-65, 1984.

Wright FS, Briggs JP: Feedback control of glomerular blood flow, pressure, and filtration rate. *Physiol Rev* 59:958-1006, 1979.

Yeh TF, et al: Early furosemide therapy in premature infants (<2000 gm) with respiratory distress syndrome: Randomized controlled trial. *J Pediatr* 105:603-609, 1984.

Other Selected References

Burg MB: Renal handling of sodium chloride, water, amino acids, and glucose, in Brenner BM, Rector FC Jr (eds): *The Kidney,* ed 2. Philadelphia, WB Saunders, 1981, vol 1, 328-370.

Cannon PJ: The kidney in heart failure. *N Engl J Med* 296:26-32, 1977.

Cannon PJ: Diuretics: Their mechanism of action and use in hypertension. *Cardiovasc Rev Rep* 4:649-666, 1983.

Cannon PJ: Pharmacology of diuretics, in Rosen MR, Hoffman BF (eds): *Cardiac Therapy.* Boston, Martinus Nijhoff, 1983, 413-434.

Cannon PJ, Martinez-Maldonado M: Pathogenesis of cardiac edema. *Semin Nephrol* 3:211-224, 1983.

Cogan MG, et al: Acid-base disorders, in Brenner BM, Rector FC Jr (eds): *The Kidney,* ed 2. Philadelphia, WB Saunders, 1981, 841-907.

De Wardener HE, Clarkson EM: Concept of natriuretic hormone. *Physiol Rev* 65:658-759, 1985.

Francisco LL, Ferris TF: Use and abuse of diuretics. *Arch Intern Med* 142:28-32, 1982.

Gifford RW Jr: Guide to practical use of diuretics. *JAMA* 235:1890-1893, 1976.

Jacobson HR, Kokko JP: Diuretics: Sites and mechanisms of action. *Annu Rev Pharmacol Toxicol* 16:201-214, 1976.

Kleit SA, et al: Diuretic therapy: Current status. *Am Heart J* 79:700-712, 1970.

Kokko JP: Site and mechanism of action of diuretics. *Am J Med* 77:11-17, 1984.

Lant A: Diuretics: Clinical pharmacology and therapeutic use, parts I and II. *Drugs* 29:57-87, 162-188, 1985.

Reineck HJ, Stein JH: Mechanisms of action and clinical uses of diuretic drugs, in Brenner BM, Rector FC Jr (eds): *The Kidney,* ed 2. Philadelphia, WB Saunders, 1981, vol 1, 1097-1131.

Stein JH, Reineck HJ: Effect of alterations in extracellular fluid volume on segmental sodium transport. *Physiol Rev* 55:127-141, 1975.

Suki WN, Ng RCK: Renal actions and uses of diuretics, in Massry SG, Glassock RJ (eds): *Textbook of Nephrology.* Baltimore, Williams & Wilkins, 1983, vol 1, 3.158-3.173.

Agents Affecting Water Homeostasis

Body fluid osmolality is maintained within a narrow range by hypothalamic osmoreceptors that regulate water intake and excretion by controlling thirst and secretion of antidiuretic hormone (ADH). ADH is synthesized in supraoptic and paraventricular nuclei of the hypothalamus and incorporated into granules that also contain its carrier protein, neurophysin. The granules are transported along axons that terminate in the median eminence and posterior pituitary where they are stored in the terminal bulbs. ADH and other granular contents are secreted in response to physiologic stimuli processed by the osmoreceptors. An increase in plasma osmolality is the most important stimulus for ADH secretion. Nonosmotic stimuli for release of ADH include hypotension and decreased plasma volume.

ADH has osmotic and, in higher concentrations, vasoactive properties. It interacts with specific receptors on the collecting tubules of the nephron to increase their permeability to water and urea, thus permitting an increase in water reabsorption. ADH also increases the contractility of smooth muscle but the amount released by the usual osmotic stimuli is probably not sufficient to cause vasoconstriction. Sodium excretion is increased during continuous infusion or inappropriate secretion of ADH, because the filtered load of sodium is increased and fractional sodium reabsorption is reduced in response to the expanded plasma volume.

DIABETES INSIPIDUS

Diabetes insipidus is a disorder of water metabolism characterized by polyuria, nocturia, polydipsia, low urine osmolality, and hypernatremia. It is caused by partial or complete deficiency of ADH (central diabetes insipidus) or by inability of the kidney to respond to the hormone (nephrogenic diabetes insipidus). Clinically, diabetes insipidus may resemble primary polydipsia, a disorder in which abnormal regulation or perception of thirst leads to excessive water intake. In contrast, increased water intake in patients with diabetes insipidus reflects an appropriate response to osmotic or volume stimuli.

Etiology: Central diabetes insipidus may be idiopathic, familial, or acquired as the result of head trauma, neurosurgery, neoplasms, infection, granulomatous disease, or other conditions that damage the hypothalamus or posterior pituitary. In some patients with idiopathic diabetes insipidus, autoantibodies to ADH-secreting cells have been identified in hypothalamic tissue. Depending on the location and extent of the lesion, ADH deficiency may be partial or complete and, under certain circumstances (eg, postoperatively), it may be transient. In some cases of central diabetes insipidus, particularly post-traumatic, the thirst center also may be damaged.

Primary nephrogenic (vasopressin-resistant) diabetes insipidus is a rare hereditary disorder that most frequently affects males. In this disease, the renal response to ADH is absent, although the hormone is secreted in adequate amounts. Recently, a form of nephrogenic diabetes insipidus with partial sensitivity to ADH has been described in women (Moses et al, 1984). Resistance to ADH may accompany thyrotoxicosis, the nephropathies of hypercalcemia and severe potassium depletion, obstructive uropathy, sickle cell anemia, methoxyflurane toxicity, and the distal tubular form of renal tubular acidosis, or it may develop during late pregnancy or in response to certain drugs, particularly lithium and demeclocycline [Declomycin].

Diagnosis: A dehydration test should be employed to establish the etiology of polydipsia/polyuria, especially when ADH or one of its analogues is being considered for prolonged therapy. The procedure both stimulates endogenous ADH and evaluates renal responsiveness to exogenous hormone. This test should be conducted under close medical supervision in the hospital because unsupervised patients may develop life-threatening complications.

The first step, water deprivation, establishes an osmotic stimulus for release of endogenous ADH. Since polyuria of any cause tends to "wash out" the renal medullary concentration gradient, the reliability of this test can be increased by infusing sodium chloride prior to dehydration. If urinary osmolality rises after water deprivation, endogenous ADH is present and renal responsiveness is established. If urinary osmolality fails to increase, ADH is either absent (complete central diabetes insipidus) or ineffective (nephrogenic diabetes insipidus). Variable increases in urinary osmolality occur in patients with partial ADH deficiency.

The second step is administration of exogenous ADH. When ADH is given to patients who failed to concentrate their urine in Step 1, an increase in urine osmolality suggests central diabetes insipidus, whereas no change suggests the nephrogenic variant. When ADH is given to patients who concentrated their urine in Step 1, a further increase in urine osmolality suggests partial central diabetes insipidus. If urinary osmolality rises no further, primary polydipsia is the presumptive diagnosis.

Occasionally, measurement of blood or urinary ADH by radioimmunoassay may be necessary to distinguish central diabetes insipidus with severe long-standing polyuria from nephrogenic diabetes insipidus or to distinguish partial central diabetes insipidus from primary polydipsia (Miller and Moses, 1977; Zerbe and Robertson, 1981).

Therapy: The central form of diabetes insipidus is treated by hormone replacement with preparations containing natural or synthetic ADH (desmopressin, vasopressin, lypressin). When central diabetes insipidus is partial, nonhormonal drugs that promote release of endogenous ADH or enhance its peripheral action (eg, chlorpropamide, clofibrate) may be used.

Aqueous vasopressin [Pitressin Synthetic] is a short-acting preparation that is given intramuscularly or subcutaneously. It is useful when brief antidiuresis is desirable, as in initiation of therapy following hypophysectomy, neurosurgery, or head injuries, or to assess the renal response to ADH in Step 2 of the dehydration test (see Diagnosis). The injectable form of desmopressin acetate [DDAVP Injection, Stimate] has a longer duration of action than aqueous vasopressin. This preparation also may be used for short-term replacement therapy after head trauma or surgery or when conditions such as nasal congestion preclude use of the intranasal preparation.

Vasopressin tannate in oil [Pitressin Tannate] is effective for the long-term treatment of moderate to severe central diabetes insipidus, but the intramuscular injections are inconvenient and may be painful, and large doses may cause cardiovascular and gastrointestinal reactions and water intoxication. Lypressin nasal spray [Diapid] is used in mild to moderate disease. It is better tolerated than the obsolete posterior pituitary powder; however, its brief duration of action may result in episodes of abrupt, severe polyuria.

Intranasal desmopressin [DDAVP] is long-acting, effective, and has no significant pressor activity. It is generally regarded as the agent of choice for long-term therapy of most patients with central diabetes insipidus.

The orally administered nonhormonal agents, chlorpropamide [Diabinese] and clofibrate [Atromid-S], are useful in mild to moderate partial central diabetes insipidus but may not provide adequate control in patients with severe disease. They may be given singly or in combination with each other or with a thiazide. The tricyclic compound, carbamazepine [Tegretol], also has antidiuretic activity but toxicity limits its usefulness.

By impairing the renal excretion of free water, thiazide diuretics have a paradoxical antidiuretic action in patients with diabetes insipidus. They are rarely effective alone in the central form of the disease but are sometimes useful as sole therapy in nephrogenic diabetes insipidus when given in conjunction with sodium restriction. Indomethacin [Indocin] and other nonsteroidal anti-inflammatory agents also may reduce free water clearance in the nephrogenic form of the disease (Blachar et al, 1980; Chevalier and Rogol, 1982).

Precautions: Patients with diabetes insipidus who have developed a pattern of excessive water drinking must limit their fluid intake when therapy is initiated, because water retention with resultant hyponatremia has been observed with all forms of antidiuretic therapy. In patients with marked polyuria and polydipsia, fluid intake and output should be monitored during the first few days of therapy. When the renal excretion of water is impaired and water intake continues, the body fluid volume expands. An increase in sodium excretion also may contribute to the hyponatremia.

Signs and symptoms of water intoxication (ie, headache, nausea and vomiting, confusion, lethargy, ataxia, coma, convulsions) occur with movement of fluid from the extracellular into the intracellular space. Water intoxication is most likely to be observed in patients with hypothalamic dysfunction and disordered regulation of thirst, in those receiving hypotonic fluids intravenously, or in infants who cannot voluntarily adjust their water intake. It is uncommon when thirst regulation is normal and water is available. Water intoxication is managed by water restriction, temporary withdrawal of the antidiuretic agent, and sometimes by administration of hypertonic sodium chloride with or without furosemide [Lasix].

For adverse drug reactions, see the evaluations.

SYNDROME OF INAPPROPRIATE SECRETION OF ANTIDIURETIC HORMONE (SIADH)

Etiology: Under certain abnormal conditions, ectopic production or sustained pituitary secretion of ADH or ADH-like substances may lead to hyponatremia and water intoxication (syndrome of inappropriate secretion of ADH, SIADH). Ectopic production is observed most commonly in patients with neoplasms (particularly oat cell carcinoma of the lung) in which the tumor itself synthesizes ADH. SIADH due to sustained pituitary secretion may be associated with central nervous system lesions, nonmalignant pulmonary disease, pain, trauma, emotional stress, surgery, and psychiatric disorders (Bartter, 1973). ADH secretion that occurs in response to alterations in effective plasma volume or stimulation of the renin-angiotensin system may play a role in the hyponatremia observed in patients with advanced congestive heart failure or cirrhosis. "Idiopathic" SIADH is usually caused by an age-related decline in osmoreceptor function that leads to failure to inhibit ADH secretion in response to hypotonicity and volume expansion. Hyponatremia also may occur in response to drugs, including many that stimulate ADH secretion or enhance its peripheral action (see Table).

The diagnosis of SIADH is made by exclusion. All conditions promoting the *appropriate* secretion of ADH must be ruled out. The presence of cardiac, renal, or central nervous system disease may make it difficult to establish the presence of SIADH.

Therapy: The management of hyponatremia depends on

DRUGS CAUSING HYPONATREMIA

HYPOGLYCEMIC AGENTS
  Chlorpropamide [Diabinese]
  Tolbutamide [Orinase]

PSYCHOPHARMACOLOGIC AND NEUROLOGIC DRUGS
  Amitriptyline [Elavil, Endep, SK-Amitriptyline]
  Barbiturates
  Carbamazepine [Tegretol]
  Fluphenazine [Permitil, Prolixin]
  Haloperidol [Haldol]
  Narcotics
  Thioridazine [Mellaril]
  Thiothixene [Navane]
  Tranylcypromine [Parnate]

DIURETICS
  Thiazide-type
  Spironolactone [Aldactone]

ANTINEOPLASTIC AGENTS
  Cyclophosphamide [Cytoxan]
  Vinblastine [Velban]
  Vincristine [Oncovin]

MISCELLANEOUS AGENTS
  Clofibrate [Atromid-S]
  Lorcainide [investigational]
  Nicotine

whether it is acute or chronic and on its severity. When hyponatremia is acute and severe (serum sodium 115 mEq/L or less), the mortality from neurologic complications is high, especially among malnourished or alcoholic patients. Rapid correction of hyponatremia to between 120 to 130 mEq/L at a rate of 1 to 2 mEq/L/hour seems to offer the best chance for survival (Arieff, 1984). This usually requires infusion of hypertonic sodium chloride (3% solution) at a rate that does not cause volume overload yet achieves the desired rate of increase in the serum sodium concentration. Furosemide (initially 1 mg/kg intravenously with intravenous replacement of excreted electrolytes) may be a useful adjunct to hypertonic sodium chloride when a more rapid diuresis or a less concentrated urine is desired (Adlard and George, 1978).

Acute mild to moderate hyponatremia (serum sodium greater than 115 mEq/L) usually responds to water restriction and to discontinuation of all medications that cause hyponatremia. Hypertonic sodium chloride and/or furosemide may be used to increase the serum sodium to between 120 and 130 mEq/L in patients who are slow to respond to conservative measures.

Chronic hyponatremia is better tolerated and usually can be managed by restricting fluids to 500 to 1,500 ml daily. Several drugs have been used for the long-term treatment of patients who cannot tolerate prolonged fluid restriction or are unable to maintain their serum sodium above 125 to 130 mEq/L. When this approach is employed, the drug should be discontinued periodically to determine whether the syndrome is still present, particularly when the underlying disorder is treatable. Lithium and demeclocycline interfere with the action of ADH on the renal tubules and may be useful in patients who require

prolonged therapy (Bartter, 1973; Moses and Miller, 1974). Demeclocycline 600 mg to 1.2 g daily is usually preferred because it is more effective and less toxic than lithium (Forrest et al, 1978); however, it should not be used in young children, because of adverse effects on bones and teeth, or in patients with congestive heart failure or cirrhosis, because it may cause renal damage.

Several narcotics with kappa agonist activity inhibit the release of ADH from the neurohypophysis and may be of value in patients with SIADH of central nervous system origin (Miller, 1980; Miller and Moses, 1977). It has been reported that urea rapidly corrects hyponatremia in patients with SIADH by decreasing urinary sodium loss while producing an osmotic water diuresis. Oral administration of urea 30 g daily may be useful for long-term therapy (Decaux et al, 1980). Oral furosemide 40 to 80 mg daily also has been used in refractory cases (Decaux et al, 1982). Vasopressin analogues with anti-ADH activity are in the early stage of investigation.

Drug Evaluations

ANTIDIURETIC HORMONE AND ANALOGUES

VASOPRESSIN INJECTION
[Pitressin Synthetic]

VASOPRESSIN TANNATE INJECTION
[Pitressin Tannate]

ACTIONS AND USES. These preparations are used in central diabetes insipidus; they are usually not effective in the nephrogenic form. The units used to describe antidiuretic activity are defined by a pressor assay in anesthetized animals; vasopressin contains 20 pressor units and not more than 1 oxytocic unit per milliliter.

The rapid onset of action and brief (two to eight hours) antidiuretic effect produced by intramuscular or subcutaneous administration of vasopressin injection (aqueous vasopressin) make this agent useful for diagnosis of diabetes insipidus and for initiating therapy following hypophysectomy, brain surgery, or trauma and in acutely ill or unconscious patients with the central form of disease. It also has been applied topically to the nasal mucous membranes by cotton pledgets, spray, or dropper, but this route is rarely used today because of the availability of desmopressin and lypressin.

Vasopressin tannate in peanut oil suspension has a long duration of action and is useful for long-term therapy in patients with moderate to severe central diabetes insipidus. The antidiuretic effect of a single intramuscular dose may last one to three days or longer. Vasopressin tannate is therefore not a desirable agent to use in patients who are undergoing surgery and/or receiving intravenous fluids. If intravenous fluids are required in a patient who has been treated with this preparation, the patient should be closely monitored to minimize the risk of water intoxication.

The duration of antidiuretic action of vasopressin tannate

occasionally is decreased after prolonged therapy, which may be caused by antibody formation. However, a high titer of antibodies without a decrease in response to the hormone also has been observed.

ADVERSE REACTIONS AND PRECAUTIONS. Because of its long duration of action, excessive water retention is more likely to occur with use of vasopressin tannate than with other preparations. Patients receiving this preparation should be made aware of the early clinical symptoms of hyponatremia and water intoxication such as fatigue, nausea, and confusion (see the Introduction).

Although the official name for ADH, vasopressin, implies primarily vasoconstrictor activity, only doses much larger than those usually given to treat diabetes insipidus increase blood pressure in conscious patients. Even large doses elevate the blood pressure only slightly (10 to 20 mm Hg) in conscious patients and this is of brief duration.

Vasopressin may cause significant constriction of the coronary arteries. Angina, electrocardiographic evidence of myocardial ischemia, and myocardial infarction have been reported after injection of 20 units; a latent period of several hours may precede chest pain. Ventricular arrhythmias have occurred when vasopressin was given by the intravenous or intra-arterial route, and cutaneous gangrene has developed after peripheral infusion. Patients with ischemic heart disease should receive the minimal dose needed to control polyuria. If cardiac symptoms occur, desmopressin or an oral antidiuretic agent should be substituted.

Large doses of vasopressin (5 to 20 units) stimulate gastrointestinal smooth muscle and may produce nausea, abdominal cramps, diarrhea, and the urge to defecate. These reactions are more common in women than in men. Uterine cramps also may occur after large doses. Allergic reactions to vasopressin tannate (urticaria, bronchial constriction, anaphylaxis) are encountered infrequently, and alternative therapy should be selected for patients who have experienced these effects.

Repeated injections of vasopressin tannate at the same site may cause a severe local inflammatory reaction requiring surgical drainage or excision. For this reason, it is particularly important to vary the site of injection.

DOSAGE AND PREPARATIONS.

VASOPRESSIN INJECTION:

Intramuscular, Subcutaneous: Adults, for treatment of central diabetes insipidus, 5 to 10 units (0.25 to 0.5 ml) three or four times daily; for diagnosis of polyuria, 5 units. *Children,* for treatment, 2.5 to 10 units (0.125 to 0.5 ml) three or four times daily.

    Pitressin Synthetic (Parke-Davis). Solution (sterile) 20 pressor units/ml in 0.5 and 1 ml containers.

VASOPRESSIN TANNATE INJECTION:

Errors in dosage are common unless separation of the active principle from the oil vehicle is avoided by warming the vial in the hand or under hot water and shaking the warmed vial vigorously until the brown powder is evenly dispersed. An absolutely dry syringe should be used for injection.

Intramuscular: Adults, 1.25 to 5 units (0.25 to 1 ml) and *children,* 1.25 to 2.5 units (0.25 to 0.5 ml), as required. These amounts usually are administered every one to three days but not until the effect of the previous dose has worn off.

Pitressin Tannate (Parke-Davis). Suspension (in peanut oil) 5 pressor units/ml in 1 ml containers.

DESMOPRESSIN ACETATE
[DDAVP, DDAVP Injection, Stimate]

ACTIONS AND USES. Desmopressin was developed in a search for vasopressin analogues with more specific and prolonged antidiuretic effects. In comparison with the naturally occurring human hormone, arginine vasopressin, the structural alterations of the desmopressin molecule have increased the antidiuretic/pressor ratio from 0.9 to 2,000 and prolonged the duration of action from a maximum of 6 to 20 hours.

Intranasal desmopressin is effective for long-term treatment of adults and children with central diabetes insipidus. It is preferred to vasopressin tannate in oil for long-term management of severe disease. Since desmopressin is expensive, it may not completely replace other treatment modalities for mild to moderate disease, although it does offer advantages over both the short-acting lypressin and the less effective (and sometimes more toxic) oral agents. Desmopressin is considerably longer acting and more effective than lypressin. After a single dose, the antidiuretic effect persists for 8 to 20 hours; in comparison, the duration of action of lypressin is only three to four hours (Cobb et al, 1978; Robinson, 1976).

Desmopressin is usually not effective in nephrogenic diabetes insipidus but large doses (20 to 40 mcg) of the nasal spray every four hours may be useful in treating women with a variant of the disorder who exhibit partial responsiveness to ADH.

A transient (one to two day) reduction in the duration of response to intranasal desmopressin has been noted occasionally and may be associated with periods of increased physical activity. Rarely, resistance has developed after prolonged therapy (Cobb et al, 1978). When resistance develops, the addition of an oral antidiuretic agent to the regimen may be beneficial.

The injectable form of desmopressin is a suitable alternative to aqueous vasopressin for use after head trauma or surgery. It also may be substituted for the intranasal preparation when upper respiratory infection, allergy, or changes in the nasal mucosa impair absorption of the latter.

Desmopressin has been used occasionally instead of aqueous vasopressin to evaluate renal concentrating capacity.

ADVERSE REACTIONS AND PRECAUTIONS. Desmopressin is well tolerated. Large doses may cause headache, nausea, and a slight increase in blood pressure, which disappear upon reduction of the dose. Nasal congestion, mild abdominal cramps, and vulval pain have occurred rarely. Fluid intake should be adjusted during therapy to avoid hyponatremia and water intoxication, particularly in infants, elderly patients, and during initiation of therapy. Undertreatment, which may permit occasional polyuria, is preferable to overtreatment, which could cause water intoxication. Although the safety of desmopressin during pregnancy has not been definitely established, no adverse effects occurred in several pregnant women given the drug (FDA Pregnancy Category B).

DOSAGE AND PREPARATIONS.

Topical (intranasal): Desmopressin is administered through a flexible calibrated nasal tube. Therapy should be initiated with a small dose, and the amount is then adjusted on the basis of changes in urine volume and osmolality and control of nocturia. For central diabetes insipidus, the usual dose for *adults* is 0.1 ml twice daily (range, 0.1 to 0.4 ml daily as a single dose or divided into two or three doses). For *children 3 months to 12 years,* the usual dosage range is 0.05 to 0.3 ml daily as a single dose or in two divided doses.

   DDAVP (USV). Solution (for intranasal administration) 0.1 mg/ml in 2.5 ml containers.

Intravenous, Subcutaneous: For central diabetes insipidus, *adults,* 0.5 to 1 ml daily, usually in two divided doses. Morning and evening doses should be adjusted separately on the basis of changes in urine volume and osmolality and control of nocturia. For patients who are switched from intranasal to injectable desmopressin, the dose of the injectable form is approximately one-tenth that of the intranasal dose.

   DDAVP Injection (USV). Solution (for injection) 4 mcg/ml in 1 ml containers.

   Stimate (Armour). Solution (for injection) 4 mcg/ml in 10 ml containers.

LYPRESSIN
[Diapid]

Cys—Tyr—Phe—Gln—Asn—Cys—Pro—Lys—Gly—NH$_2$

ACTIONS AND USES. Lypressin solution contains synthetic lysine-8-vasopressin, a polypeptide that occurs in swine and is similar to arginine-8-vasopressin, the antidiuretic hormone found in the posterior pituitary of man. It has an activity of 50 posterior pituitary (pressor) units per milliliter.

Lypressin is rapidly absorbed from the nasal mucosa. It is effective as sole therapy in mild to moderate central diabetes insipidus if administered frequently. In more severe disease, treatment may be complicated by episodes of abrupt, severe polyuria that result from the short duration of action of lypressin. Desmopressin or vasopressin tannate is more satisfactory in these patients. Lypressin is not effective in the nephrogenic form of diabetes insipidus.

ADVERSE REACTIONS AND PRECAUTIONS. No significant local or systemic reactions have been reported, although hypersensitivity, manifested by a positive skin test, occurs rarely. In the presence of edema of the nasal mucosa, which may occur during an upper respiratory tract infection or as a result of allergy, there may be impaired absorption of lypressin with loss of antidiuretic effect.

DOSAGE AND PREPARATIONS.

Topical (intranasal): One or more sprays in one or both nostrils. The dose and interval between applications must be determined individually. Each spray delivers approximately 2 pressor units, but the exact amount depends upon how vigorously the bottle is squeezed. Four sprays in each nostril provide the maximal amount that can be absorbed at one time without waste. Administration three or four times daily usually is necessary. A bottle commonly lasts five to seven days; if it lasts a shorter or longer period, the patient may not be receiving the proper dosage.

   Diapid (Sandoz). Solution (spray) 50 pressor units/ml (0.185 mg/ml) in 8 ml containers. [This product has an expiration date of 36 months.]

ORALLY ADMINISTERED AGENTS WITH ANTIDIURETIC ACTIVITY

CLOFIBRATE
[Atromid-S]

ACTIONS AND USES. The hypolipidemic agent, clofibrate, has antidiuretic action in patients with mild to moderate central diabetes insipidus (Moses et al, 1973). Daily doses of 2 g reduce urine volume by approximately 50% (Thompson et al, 1977). Clofibrate appears to act by increasing the release of ADH from the neurohypophysis; there is no evidence that the peripheral action of ADH is enhanced. Clofibrate is a less effective antidiuretic agent than chlorpropamide. If clofibrate alone does not provide an adequate response, some patients may benefit from the addition of small doses of chlorpropamide to the regimen. Like chlorpropamide, clofibrate is less effective in patients with severe central diabetes insipidus and is ineffective in those with complete central diabetes insipidus or the nephrogenic form of the disease.

ADVERSE REACTIONS AND PRECAUTIONS. Gastrointestinal disturbances (nausea, vomiting, diarrhea, dyspepsia, and flatulence) are the most common side effects of clofibrate. Clofibrate increases the risk of cholelithiasis. For other adverse reactions, see Chapter 50, Agents Used to Treat Hyperlipidemia.

DOSAGE AND PREPARATIONS.

Oral: Adults, 1.5 to 2 g daily in divided doses.

   Atromid-S (Ayerst). Capsules 500 mg.

CHLORPROPAMIDE
[Diabinese]

ACTIONS AND USES. The hypoglycemic agent, chlorpropamide, has an antidiuretic action in many patients with central diabetes insipidus. It is most effective in those with less severe disease in whom, presumably, there are small amounts of ADH present in the hypothalamus (Miller and Moses, 1970). Chlorpropamide and some of its degradation products reduce free-water clearance by increasing the sensitivity of the renal tubular epithelium to ADH or by increasing the renal osmotic gradient for water reabsorption. It also may increase ADH release. Urine volume is decreased by approximately 60% with a daily dose of 250 mg. If an adequate therapeutic response is not obtained with chlorpropamide alone, better control often can be achieved when clofibrate or a thiazide is given concomitantly. Chlorpropamide is not effective in patients with nephrogenic diabetes insipidus.

ADVERSE REACTIONS AND PRECAUTIONS. Chlorpropamide reduces fasting blood glucose in patients with diabetes insipidus, and significant, symptomatic hypoglycemia is not uncommon (Thompson et al, 1977). This effect can be minimized by reducing the dose and adding another oral antidiuretic agent to the regimen. Hypoglycemic reactions are most common in children, in patients with associated anterior pituitary deficiency, and in those with reduced food intake. Patients should be informed of the importance of not missing meals and warned to avoid alcoholic beverages since disulfiram-like effects may occur. The effects of long-term therapy on the beta cells of the normal pancreas have not been studied (see also Chapter 43, Agents Used to Regulate Blood Glucose).

DOSAGE AND PREPARATIONS.
Oral: Adults, 250 to 500 mg daily; 125 mg daily may be sufficient when another oral antidiuretic agent is given concomitantly.
    Diabinese (Pfizer), *Generic.* Tablets 100 and 250 mg.

THIAZIDE DIURETICS

ACTIONS AND USES. The thiazide diuretics have a paradoxical antidiuretic action in patients with diabetes insipidus (Earley and Orloff, 1962; Lant and Wilson, 1971). By producing mild volume depletion, thiazides enhance proximal tubular reabsorption of glomerular filtrate. This action reduces delivery of water to the ADH-dependent sites of water reabsorption in the distal nephron. Thiazides are used primarily for nephrogenic diabetes insipidus and are usually the only effective agents available for treating this disorder. In central diabetes insipidus, thiazides are rarely useful as sole therapy but may be given with other oral agents, such as chlorpropamide. *Thiazides are not effective unless dietary sodium is restricted.*

ADVERSE REACTIONS AND PRECAUTIONS. Thiazide diuretics are generally well tolerated. Mild symptomatic hypokalemia is common during long-term therapy and can be controlled by addition of a potassium-sparing diuretic to the regimen. Thiazides increase serum uric acid and may enhance the hyperuricemia observed in some adults with primary nephrogenic diabetes insipidus. For other adverse effects, see Chapter 29, Diuretics.

DOSAGE AND PREPARATIONS.
Oral: The same dosage as that used to control edema is given (see Chapter 29).

Cited References

Adlard JM, George JM: Hyponatremia. *Heart Lung* 7:587-593, 1978.
Arieff AI: Central nervous system manifestations of disordered sodium metabolism. *Clin Endocrinol Metab* 132:269-294, 1984.
Bartter FC: Syndrome of inappropriate secretion of antidiuretic hormone (SIADH). *DM* 1-47, Nov 1973.
Blachar Y, et al: Effect of inhibition of prostaglandin synthesis on free water and osmolar clearances in patients with hereditary nephrogenic diabetes insipidus. *Int J Pediatr Nephrol* 1:48-52, 1980.
Chevalier RL, Rogol AD: Tolmetin sodium in management of nephrogenic diabetes insipidus. *J Pediatr* 101:787-789, 1982.
Cobb WE, et al: Neurogenic diabetes insipidus: Management with dDAVP (1-desamino-8-D arginine vasopressin). *Ann Intern Med* 88:183-188, 1978.
Decaux G, et al: Treatment of syndrome of inappropriate secretion of antidiuretic hormone by urea. *Am J Med* 69:99-106, 1980.
Decaux G, et al: Inappropriate secretion of antidiuretic hormone treated with frusemide. *Br Med J* 285:89-90, 1982.
Earley LE, Orloff J: Mechanism of antidiuresis associated with administration of hydrochlorothiazide to patients with vasopressin-resistant diabetes insipidus. *J Clin Invest* 41:1988-1997, 1962.
Forrest JN, et al: Superiority of demeclocycline over lithium in treatment of chronic syndrome of inappropriate secretion of antidiuretic hormone. *N Engl J Med* 298:173-177, 1978.
Lant AF, Wilson GM: Long-term therapy of diabetes insipidus with oral benzothiadiazine and phthalimidine diuretics. *Clin Sci* 40:497-511, 1971.
Miller M: Role of endogenous opioids in neurohypophyseal function of man. *J Clin Endocrinol Metab* 50:1018-1020, 1980.
Miller M, Moses AM: Mechanism of chlorpropamide action in diabetes insipidus. *J Clin Endocrinol Metab* 30:488-496, 1970.
Miller M, Moses AM: Clinical states due to alteration of ADH release and action, in Moses AM, Share L (eds): *Neurohypophysis,* Proceedings of the International Conference on the Neurohypophysis. Basel, S Karger, 1977, 153-166.
Moses AM, Miller M: Drug-induced dilutional hyponatremia. *N Engl J Med* 291:1234-1239, 1974.
Moses AM, et al: Clofibrate-induced antidiuresis. *J Clin Invest* 52:535-542, 1973.
Moses AM, et al: Marked hypotonic polyuria resulting from nephrogenic diabetes insipidus with partial sensitivity to vasopressin. *J Clin Endocrinol Metab* 59:1044-1049, 1984.
Robinson AG: DDAVP in treatment of central diabetes insipidus. *N Engl J Med* 294:507-511, 1976.
Thompson P, et al: Comparison of clofibrate and chlorpropamide in vasopressin-responsive diabetes insipidus. *Metabolism* 26:749-762, 1977.
Zerbe RL, Robertson GL: Comparison of plasma vasopressin measurements with standard indirect test in differential diagnosis of polyuria. *N Engl J Med* 305:1539-1546, 1981.

Other Selected References

Bartter FC: Antidiuretic hormone: Its role in urinary concentration, in Schwartz AB, Lyons H (eds): *Acid Base Balance and Electrolyte Disorders.* New York, Grune & Stratton, 1977, 135-148.
Cobb WE: Management of neurogenic diabetes insipidus with dDAVP and other agents, in Reichlin S (ed): *The Neurohypophysis.* New York, Plenum Publishing, 1984, 139-163.
Fitzsimons JT: Physiological basis of thirst. *Kidney Int* 10:3-11, 1976.
Jamison RL, Oliver RE: Disorders of urinary concentration and dilution. *Am J Med* 72:308-322, 1982.
Moses AM: Long-standing posttraumatic diabetes insipidus. *Med Grand Rounds* 2:117-128, 1983.
Moses AM: Clinical and laboratory features of central and nephrogenic diabetes insipidus and primary polydipsia, in Reichlin S (ed): *The Neurohypophysis.* New York, Plenum Publishing, 1984, 115-138.
Moses AM, et al: Pathophysiologic and pharmacologic alterations in release and action of ADH. *Metabolism* 25:697-721, 1976.
Schrier RW, Berl T: Nonosmolar factors affecting renal water excretion. *N Engl J Med* 292:81-88, 141-145, 1975.
Share L: Blood pressure, blood volume, and release of vasopressin, in Knobil E, Sawyer WH (eds): *Handbook of Physiology. IV. The Pituitary Gland and Its Neuroendocrine Control,* part 1. Washington, DC, American Physiological Society, 1974, 243-255.

Agents Used to Treat Urologic Disorders

Drugs that stimulate or inhibit smooth muscle activity are useful in some disorders of the lower urinary tract. The goals of therapy are to improve the storage and emptying functions of the urinary bladder and to prevent renal complications.

Urinary bladder dysfunction may be manifested as recurrent urinary tract infection, recurrent or persistent retention of urine, urinary frequency, or incontinence. It is of paramount importance to examine the patient thoroughly and, if indicated, to perform appropriate urodynamic tests before instituting therapy (Mundy et al, 1984). Urodynamic tests also are useful to document drug efficacy prior to instituting long-term therapy.

PHYSIOLOGY

Storage and elimination of urine are accomplished by coordinated activity of the smooth muscle of the bladder wall (detrusor muscle), the smooth muscle of the bladder neck and the proximal urethra (the "internal sphincter"), the striated muscle of the urethra (the intrinsic rhabdosphincter), and the periurethral striated muscle of the urogenital diaphragm and levator ani, which constitute the "external sphincter." The bladder stores urine by virtue of its property of accommodation, and continence is maintained by the tonicity of the internal sphincter. Voluntary contraction of the external sphincter can be used to terminate micturition abruptly. In males, the preprostatic urethra is surrounded by sympathetically innervated smooth muscle that is continuous with the capsule of the prostate. Contraction of this muscle in the bladder neck prevents the retrograde propulsion of seminal fluid into the bladder during ejaculation.

The afferent nerve impulses generated in stretch receptors of the bladder wall are activated by bladder distention. These nerve impulses are relayed to the central nervous system and through the efferent arm of the reflex arc, the pelvic parasympathetic nerves, which activate the detrusor muscle. At the same time, motor activity in the pudendal motor nerves is inhibited, relaxing the periurethral striated muscles of the external sphincter. This "micturition reflex" is integrated in the rostral pons. Volitional control of the reflex is maintained by excitatory and inhibitory pathways originating in the cerebral cortex (Fletcher and Bradley, 1978). Bladder neck resistance is decreased by suppression of alpha receptors in the internal sphincter during voiding. Although sympathetic tone is presumed to be of minor importance in normal urinary function, it may be a major element of outlet resistance in pathologic conditions. In normal micturition, the first urodynamic event is cessation of sphincter EMG activity accompanied by a decrease in outlet resistance. This is followed by contraction of the detrusor. When the detrusor contracts, the bladder neck opens concurrently.

UROLOGIC DISORDERS

Incontinence in Adults

Incontinence represents a failure in the storage phase of bladder function. Various factors may be responsible for incontinence and the specific cause must be determined in order to select the appropriate therapy.

Urge Incontinence: The terms motor urge incontinence, uninhibited neurogenic bladder, unstable bladder, and detrusor instability refer to the presence of involuntary detrusor contractions. When these contractions are caused by neurologic lesions, the condition is termed detrusor hyperreflexia. Detrusor hyperreflexia is encountered commonly in patients with lesions superior to the micturition reflex center in the basal ganglia (Parkinson's disease), brainstem (atherosclerosis or cerebrovascular insult), or spinal cord (tumor, multiple sclerosis, or congenital anomalies). In these disorders, the bladder undergoes involuntary contractions during filling; the contractions may be demonstrated by cystometric examination. Depending upon the location of the lesion, there also may be dysfunction of the sphincters (Blaivas et al, 1981). Urgency usually is present in those patients with a normal sensorium. Frequency and nocturia also may be present. Dysuria usually does *not* occur unless there is concurrent infection.

Irritation of the bladder mucosa caused by infection, stones, irradiation, interstitial cystitis, or carcinoma, as well as unstable bladder secondary to prostatic hypertrophy or obstruction of the bladder neck, should be ruled out. Acute vaginitis, estrogen-responsive mucosal atrophy of the urethra and vagina in postmenopausal women, and chronic constipation should be corrected, since these conditions may be associated with urge incontinence. Iatrogenic causes should be corrected if possible by (1) including more appropriate toilet facilities for patients with reduced mobility or physical handicaps and (2) modifying drug regimens, particularly those employing neuroleptic agents such as phenothiazines or haloperidol [Haldol] (Ambrosini, 1984).

Excessive detrusor activity can be suppressed in some patients by anticholinergic agents (eg, propantheline [Pro-Banthīne]) or antispasmodics (eg, oxybutynin [Ditropan]) (Finkbeiner and Bissada, 1980; Lloyd, 1979; Wein, 1979). Dry mouth and constipation are the side effects most commonly cited by patients for lack of acceptance. One-half of the usual dose may control urge incontinence in the elderly and markedly reduces the severity of side effects (Diokno, 1983). Urinary retention may occur in some patients, particularly in those with coexistent asymptomatic prostatism or other forms of outlet obstruction. These patients may be managed with intermittent self-catheterization.

Detrusor control may improve significantly by instituting a regular voiding schedule (bladder retraining drill) and this may be the initial treatment of choice (Jarvis, 1981; Weiss, 1983); however, a good initial response may not be sustained (Ferrie et al, 1984). Although anticholinergic drugs are usually employed simultaneously, there is some evidence that they do not enhance the benefits of reflex training (Fantl et al, 1981). Therefore, the role of these drugs may be limited to patients who are unable or unwilling to participate in retraining or in whom it is ineffective.

Results have been promising in elderly patients with urge incontinence given imipramine [Janimine, SK-Pramine, Tofranil] orally as a single dose at bedtime.

Because bladder wall activity may be increased by the prostaglandins, inhibitors of prostaglandin synthesis (eg, indomethacin [Indocin]) are being evaluated for use in urge incontinence (Cardozo and Stanton, 1980). Baclofen [Lioresal] (Tay-lor and Bates, 1979) and the calcium channel blocking agents (eg, verapamil [Calan, Isoptin], nifedipine [Procardia]) also are undergoing clinical investigation for this use.

Stress Incontinence: Stress incontinence is manifested by the involuntary loss of urine following a sudden increase in intra-abdominal pressure, as may occur during coughing, sneezing, laughing, change to a standing position, or physical exercise (walking, running), usually *without* other urinary symptoms. It is caused by sphincter incompetence rather than detrusor dysfunction and may be of neurogenic or non-neurogenic origin. *Neurogenic stress incontinence* results from a lesion in the sympathetic nerves supplying the vesical neck. It is seen commonly in myelodysplasia (McGuire et al, 1981; Barbalias and Blaivas, 1983) and after radical pelvic surgery (eg, hysterectomy, abdominoperineal resection of the rectum) (Blaivas and Barbalias, 1983). *Non-neurogenic stress incontinence* is a common disorder of older, particularly multiparous, women. The mechanism of urine loss is still controversial and includes shortening of the functional urethral length, loss of the urethrovesical angle, or descent of the proximal urethra below the pelvic diaphragm. Elevations in intra-abdominal pressure are transmitted inadequately to the upper urethra where it descends below the pelvic diaphragm (Cantor, 1979). Another form of non-neurogenic stress incontinence may result from increased urethral rigidity caused by aging, injury, inflammation, or scarring from instrumentation and surgery, particularly multiple surgical procedures for stress incontinence.

The striated muscle tone of the external sphincter cannot be enhanced by drugs, but proximal urethral resistance can be increased by agents that activate alpha-adrenergic receptors in the smooth muscle of the internal sphincter. For this reason, alpha-adrenergic drugs, such as ephedrine (usually the drug of choice), phenylpropanolamine, and pseudoephedrine, sometimes may be used to treat stress incontinence if surgical correction, which is the usual treatment (particularly in women), is not appropriate or must be deferred. In hypertensive patients who must avoid alpha-adrenergic drugs, propranolol [Inderal] 10 mg four times daily has been used (Awad and Downie, 1981), but it does not appear to be very effective. Propranolol also has been tried in stress incontinence associated with partial detrusor denervation. Very mild (grade I) stress incontinence in women may be improved by the conscientious performance of modified Kegel exercises (Mohr et al, 1983).

Stress incontinence associated with urgency, particularly in women, may be encountered in patients with a history of frequently postponed voiding. Other than an increased bladder capacity and an irregular voiding pattern, urodynamic findings are normal and neurologic disease is absent. These patients may respond to a timed voiding pattern at frequent intervals (eg, every two hours), even in the absence of a voiding urge (Godec, 1984). If no benefit is produced within two weeks, drugs or surgery may be instituted.

Overflow Incontinence: Overflow (paradoxical) incontinence is caused by inadequate emptying of the bladder. This condition may result from outflow obstruction (eg, due to prostatic enlargement), hypotonicity of the detrusor muscle (particularly in women), or loss of bladder sensation to filling (sensory neurogenic [paralytic] bladder) that may occur in diabetic visceral neuropathy or tabes dorsalis. Surgical relief of obstruction or periodic self-catheterization is required. In the absence of obstruction, drug therapy similar to that for urinary retention (eg, bethanechol [Duvoid, Myotonachol, Urecholine], phenoxybenzamine [Dibenzyline]) may be instituted but often is unsuccessful. The infusion of dinoprostone (prostaglandin E_2) (Desmond et al, 1980) or the 15(S)-15 methyl derivative of prostaglandin $F_{2\alpha}$ (Vaidyanathan et al, 1981) into the bladder was reported to provide prolonged relief in selected patients, but the beneficial effects could not be duplicated by another group of investigators (Delaere et al, 1981).

Postprostatectomy Incontinence: Mild to moderate incontinence due to injury of smooth and skeletal muscle during prostatectomy is sometimes improved by drug therapy. Adrenergic drugs (phenylpropanolamine) or mixed function drugs (imipramine) are used if sphincter incompetence is the primary dysfunction, and anticholinergic drugs (oxybutynin, propantheline) are used if detrusor instability is present. Ancillary measures, particularly sphincter exercises, can be instituted. Incontinence due to edema or loss of elasticity of the bladder neck usually improves with time. If drug therapy does not control incontinence after one year, insertion of an inflatable sphincter should be considered.

Shy-Drager Syndrome: This disorder is characterized by progressively severe orthostatic hypotension, anhidrosis, parkinsonian signs, impotence, and bladder and anorectal dysfunction. The urologic symptoms occur early and begin with nocturia, followed by incontinence and urinary retention. There are large, uninhibited contractions during bladder filling, but the patient is unable to maintain a sustained reflex bladder contraction during attempts at voiding. An anticholinergic agent (eg, propantheline) is given to suppress the uninhibited filling contractions and thus improve urine storage. Intermittent self-catheterization or use of an indwelling catheter also may be necessary (Lockhart et al, 1981; Wulfsohn and Rubenstein, 1981).

Urinary Retention

Neurogenic disorders of the lower urinary tract may result from trauma, congenital defects, ischemia, tumors, infection, neurologic disease, or a defect in corticoregulatory control without a detectable organic lesion. There may be an associated malfunction of the detrusor muscle, the internal sphincter, or the external sphincter; the disorders may exist alone or with coordinated or uncoordinated bladder-sphincter function (dyssynergia).

The agents used to treat neurogenic bladder disorders may enhance detrusor contractions (cholinergic agents, dinoprostone) or decrease internal sphincter tonus (alpha-adrenergic blocking drugs). In addition, a regimen of frequent, periodic voiding by clean, intermittent self-catheterization often is the treatment of choice. High pressure voiding techniques, such as external compression (Credé maneuver), are generally ineffective.

The cholinergic drug, bethanechol, has been used to enhance intravesical pressure and thus facilitate bladder emptying in patients with spinal cord lesions above S_2-S_4 (*reflex neurogenic bladder*) during the recovery phase after spinal shock. However, its use remains controversial (Downie, 1984; Finkbeiner, 1985). This drug is not effective during spinal shock. It also may reduce residual urine volume in patients with lesions involving the afferent limb of the micturition reflex arc (*sensory paralytic bladder*) and in those with incomplete lower motor neuron impairment (*motor paralytic bladder*). Bethanechol should not be used unless bladder and external sphincter function are coordinated, ie, involuntary detrusor contractions occur concomitantly with relaxation of the external sphincter (Diokno and Koppenhoefer, 1976; Sonda et al, 1979).

Regardless of the etiology of urine retention, efforts to facilitate bladder emptying with bethanechol have been disappointing (Barrett, 1981; Wein, 1983; Blaivas, 1985). *It is recommended that the drug's effectiveness be documented during a short trial before committing a patient to long-term therapy* (Wein, 1979; Wein et al, 1980).

Results of studies to determine the usefulness of instilling dinoprostone into the bladder of patients with inactive or hypotonic detrusor function have been promising. The patient must be free of organic or functional outlet obstruction and must have an intact sacral reflex arc (absence of complete lower neuron lesion). Approximately one-half of patients showed sustained (months) improvement in mean urine flow rate and decreased residual volume (Desmond et al, 1980). Bethanechol may be continued during therapy with dinoprostone or added to the regimen later. A prostaglandin analogue, 15(S)-15 methyl prostaglandin $F_{2\alpha}$, produces urinary bladder contractions of greater amplitude than dinoprostone and has a longer half-life than prostaglandin $F_{2\alpha}$. In a study to define which patients would benefit from the intravesical instillation of this drug (Vaidyanathan et al, 1981), it was shown that reflex voiding could be achieved in patients with incomplete suprasacral lesions. It was not possible to induce reflex voiding in patients with complete denervation, in those with spinal cord injuries during the spinal shock phase, or in patients with detrusor-striated sphincter dyssynergia. Not all investigators have reported success with use of dinoprostone (Delaere et al, 1981).

The alpha-adrenergic blocking agent, phenoxybenzamine, relaxes the internal sphincter and has been used to treat various neurogenic bladder disorders in which residual urine volume is increased because of functional outlet obstruction or internal sphincter dyssynergia (Smey et al, 1980). It may be given with bethanechol (Mobley, 1976; Raz and Smith, 1976). In spinal cord injury, phenoxybenzamine is effective only for patients with incomplete lesions (Graham, 1981).

In an effort to reduce the incidence of side effects encountered with phenoxybenzamine, particularly reflex tachycardia and orthostatic hypotension, agents with selective receptor blocking activity have been tested (Wein, 1983). Of these, prazosin [Minipress] showed some promise during early clinical evaluation in adults with lower motor neuron lesions and autonomous bladder. A dose of 0.5 mg was given twice daily and increased gradually over one week (to avoid first dose phenomenon hypotension) to 2 mg twice daily. The only side effect reported was nasal congestion in one patient

(Andersson et al, 1981). Suppression of ejaculation by prazosin appears to be far less of a problem than with phenoxybenzamine. The clinical experience to date indicates that prazosin is as effective as phenoxybenzamine.

Detrusor-striated sphincter dyssynergia is a functional obstruction involving the external urethral sphincter. It develops most often in patients with neurologic damage above the level of the sacral spinal cord (Blaivas et al, 1981). It also has been reported in patients with no apparent structural or neurologic abnormality, particularly young children. This may represent a learned behavior for inappropriate sphincter contractions and not true dyssynergia. When no neurologic basis is apparent, diazepam [Valium] may be effective because of its antianxiety action (Wein, 1983); the dose should not exceed that used for anxiety (for use in adults, see Gleason, 1978, and Kaplan et al, 1980; for use in children, see Firlit and Cook, 1977, and Smey et al, 1978).

Diazepam is not effective in detrusor-striated sphincter dyssynergia due to suprasacral lesions. This condition may be secondary to mass reflex activity following acute spinal cord injury and may persist for two years or more after the initial trauma. A substantial number of patients with multiple sclerosis, transverse myelitis, and other upper motor lesions also exhibit external sphincter dyssynergia.

No drug acts selectively on the external sphincter to relieve spasticity, but dantrolene [Dantrium] and baclofen [Lioresal] are being investigated for this purpose (Wein, 1979; Wein, 1983; Leyson et al, 1980). Dantrolene is presumed to act by promoting the inactivation of excitation-contraction coupling in muscle. Urination patterns have improved, but the drug's use is limited by its potential hepatotoxicity. Baclofen acts by enhancing polysynaptic inhibition in the spinal cord. It appears to be more effective than dantrolene in external sphincter spasm and dyssynergias, but its safety and efficacy have not been evaluated fully. Treatment with either drug may result in satisfactory reflex voiding in males, but incontinence will continue to be a major problem in women (McGuire, 1980).

Patients with chronic aseptic prostatitis (Siroky et al, 1981) or prostatodynia (Osborn et al, 1981) who experience hesitancy, weak stream, infrequent voiding, and terminal dribbling but who have no demonstrable neurologic abnormality may benefit from diazepam, baclofen, or phenoxybenzamine. Despite extensive urodynamic investigations, the criteria for drug selection have not been established.

Chronic *psychogenic urinary retention* is a relatively uncommon condition occurring almost exclusively in women. Management of the urologic component is by intermittent self-catheterization and bladder training. Drugs are employed only as required for management of the psychiatric component.

Female Urethral Syndrome

The symptoms of female urethral syndrome are urinary frequency, urgency, dysuria, pressure sensations, and low back pain. These symptoms may be present regardless of the etiology of the disorder (infectious cystitis, urethritis, or vaginitis; carcinoma in situ; early interstitial cystitis; postmenopausal atrophy; external sphincter dysfunction; and neuropathic blad-

der) (Gleason, 1978; Graham, 1980; Komaroff and Friedland, 1980; Schmidt, 1985). In most instances, the symptoms are produced by treatable infections (Stamm et al, 1981); see Chapter 65, Antimicrobial Therapy and Chemoprophylaxis of Infectious Diseases, for treatment.

Urethral syndrome without bacteriuria or pyuria sometimes requires cystoscopy to rule out carcinoma in situ or interstitial cystitis and/or urodynamic testing to determine the appropriate pharmacologic or surgical intervention. Patients with dysuria not associated with frequency should be evaluated for vaginitis or genital herpes simplex infection.

Interstitial Cystitis

Interstitial cystitis is a bladder disorder of unknown etiology; it is more common in women than in men (Walsh, 1978) and is characterized by urgency, frequency, nocturia, dysuria, and suprapubic or perineal pain, which is diminished by voiding. Submucosal edema and vasodilation are characteristic histologic findings, and cystoscopic examination may reveal glomerulations, reduced bladder capacity, and ulceration (Messing and Stamey, 1978). Before therapy is initiated, care should be taken to rule out diffuse carcinoma of the bladder.

Interstitial cystitis has been treated by hydrodilation, surgery, and various drugs, including corticosteroids and anticholinergic agents. Irrigation with oxychlorosene [Clorpactin WCS-90] (Messing and Stamey, 1978) or dimethyl sulfoxide (DMSO) [Rimso-50] (Shirley et al, 1978; Fowler, 1981) has been useful in some patients. An experimental protocol using oral sodium pentosanpolysulfate, a sulfated polysaccharide, appears promising (Parsons, 1985).

Enuresis and Unstable Bladder of Childhood

Enuresis is repeated involuntary urination in children over 6 years old; the condition is classified as primary if it has persisted since birth. Nocturnal enuresis is the most common form, although some children also suffer from urgency, frequency, and urge incontinence during the day. Numerous causative factors have been proposed (Kass et al, 1979). Regardless of therapy, if any, this condition usually resolves with maturation. If treatment is indicated, motivational conditioning or conditioning with a waking device is usually tried initially. However, for short-term management or for those who do not respond to conditioning, oxybutynin (Redman, 1982) or imipramine may be effective (Kass et al, 1979; Mikkelsen and Rapoport, 1980).

Children who have no daytime urinary symptomatology, neurologic or anatomic abnormalities, or infection usually have normal bladders and do not require urodynamic tests, intravenous pyelography (IVP), or endoscopy. Those with persistent day- and nighttime wetting (with or without recurrent urinary infection) may benefit from more extensive diagnostic evaluation. This "unstable bladder of childhood" has been categorized further into four distinct syndromes (Bauer et al, 1980): small capacity hypertonic bladder, hyperreflexic bladder (uninhibited neurogenic bladder), large capacity hypotonic bladder (lazy bladder), and external sphincter dyssynergia (non-neurogenic neurogenic bladder, pseudoneurogenic bladder, occult neuropathic bladder).

Children with daytime incontinence who have anatomically small bladders and normal sphincter function may respond to alpha-adrenergic blocking agents (eg, phenoxybenzamine). Anticholinergic agents (propantheline, belladonna tincture, and flavoxate [Urispas]) are somewhat less effective.

Children with hyperreflexic bladder have premature detrusor contractions during filling with frequency, urgency, urge incontinence, and posturing to avoid enuresis. With maturation, the uncontrolled contractions characteristic of infant voiding disappear and adult patterns of urinary control develop. Until this occurs, the goal is elimination of unstable contractions without interfering with normal voiding (Koff, 1984). Anticholinergic agents significantly improve this condition in most children. Hyperreflexic (uninhibited) bladder appears to be a common cause of recurrent urinary infection in girls 3 to 8 years, and anticholinergic agents, eg, oxybutynin 5 mg three times daily (Koff et al, 1978), are often useful as adjuncts to antibacterial therapy, a regular voiding schedule, and moderate fluid restriction.

Patients with the lazy bladder syndrome, usually girls, void infrequently and experience stress or overflow incontinence secondary to an overdistended bladder. This secondary enuresis (occurring after toilet training) requires alteration of voiding habits (frequent, every two to three hours, timed voiding). If detrusor activity is inadequate, intermittent catheterization may be required.

Dysfunctional voiding in children secondary to external sphincter dyssynergia may be primary or secondary to day- and nighttime enuresis. It is characterized by infrequent voiding associated with urgency and stress incontinence. Recurrent urinary infection and constipation are common. Radiographs show a trabeculated, large-capacity bladder; large residual volumes of urine; and, frequently, hydronephrosis and reflux. Voiding retraining, intermittent catheterization, or biofeedback techniques are instituted to reduce the external sphincter dyssynergia (Hanna et al, 1981). This may be supplemented with diazepam to relax the external sphincter (Smey et al, 1978). Phenoxybenzamine (to reduce outflow resistance) and bethanechol (in an attempt to enhance detrusor contractility) may be added as needed.

In many children over age 3 years with neurogenic bladder (caused by spina bifida, meningocele, or traumatic paraplegia), continence may be maintained with intermittent catheterization by either the parent or the patient. This can be supplemented with an alpha-adrenergic stimulant (eg, ephedrine) and/or a bladder relaxant (eg, propantheline, oxybutynin), particularly if urodynamic assessment indicates uninhibited detrusor contractions (Mulcahy and James, 1979).

Giggle incontinence is abrupt, involuntary, uncontrollable, complete emptying of the bladder associated with giggling or laughter. It is distinct from the slight wetting that may occur during laughter in stress incontinence. Giggle incontinence is probably familial, usually begins about age 5 to 7 years, and is more common in girls. Urodynamic and neurologic evaluations generally show no abnormalities. The condition usually resolves gradually, rarely persisting into adulthood. Symptomat-

ic relief was reported in two preadolescent boys following a short course of propantheline (Brocklebank and Meadow, 1981). Giggle incontinence also may be associated with focal seizures; incontinence in these patients responds to anticonvulsant therapy (Rogers et al, 1982). Rarely, giggle incontinence may be a variant of stress incontinence (Sawczuk and Blaivas, 1984).

Retrograde Ejaculation

Reduction of sympathetic tone in the bladder neck may prevent adequate closure of the internal sphincter during ejaculation, which allows retrograde ejection of semen into the urinary bladder. This interruption of normal sympathetic activity may occur after instrumentation or surgery (transurethral resection of the prostate, bilateral lumbar sympathectomy, retroperitoneal lymph node dissection, and abdominoperineal resection of the rectum), administration of certain drugs (eg, guanethidine [Ismelin]), or in those with diabetic visceral neuropathy. Aspermia usually is caused by absence of ejaculation, but if retrograde ejaculation can be demonstrated, alpha-adrenergic agents (ephedrine, phenylpropanolamine) or tricyclic drugs (imipramine) may be beneficial.

Autonomic Hyperreflexia

The syndrome of hyperreflexia is a medical emergency occurring in quadriplegic or paraplegic patients with complete or incomplete spinal lesions above T-6. It is characterized by symptoms of reflex sympathetic discharge: hypertension, headache, bradycardia, diaphoresis, flushing, cutis anserina, and nausea. The hypertensive episode may result in retinal or cerebrovascular hemorrhage, seizures, heart failure, and death. In approximately 90% of patients, the symptoms are induced by manipulation or irrigation of the bladder. In most of the remaining 10%, symptoms occurred after distention of the bowel or rectal examination.

When this syndrome is caused by bladder distention, it is treated by immediate drainage of the bladder. If the response is inadequate, alpha-adrenergic blocking agents or direct-acting vasodilators (eg, sodium nitroprusside [Nipride, Nitropress]) should be administered. The oral administration of guanethidine 10 mg three times a day has protected patients against subsequent episodes (Brown et al, 1979). Phenoxybenzamine 30 mg/day is an alternative drug but may be slightly less effective (Scott and Morrow, 1978).

Malacoplakia

Malacoplakia is an uncommon, acquired, inflammatory granuloma that can affect any part of the urinary tract in men or women of any age. It is encountered most commonly in the bladder of middle-aged women, frequently in association with diabetes or other systemic disease. This lesion often is associated with chronic infection, commonly *Escherichia coli*. The lesions may ulcerate, causing hematuria.

Routine antibiotic therapy may be ineffective because of intracellular infection. Surgical reduction, excision of massive lesions, or vesical fulguration may be necessary. Malacoplakia in renal transplant patients may respond to reduction or discontinuation of immunosuppressive agents and initiation of long-term antibiotic therapy (Streem, 1984).

Drug Evaluations

AGENTS USED TO TREAT URINARY INCONTINENCE

Anticholinergic Drugs

Anticholinergic drugs block the action of acetylcholine at postganglionic cholinergic sites, thereby increasing bladder capacity by reducing the number of motor impulses reaching the detrusor muscle. The response of the detrusor muscle to parasympathetic stimulation is relatively resistant to cholinergic blockade; therefore, doses that inhibit the urinary bladder produce the usual anticholinergic side effects (eg, constipation, dryness of the mouth).

A large number of anticholinergic agents are available commercially (see Chapter 53, Agents Used in Disorders of the Lower Intestinal Tract), but there is no evidence that any one is more effective or better tolerated than propantheline bromide. Both the natural belladonna alkaloids (atropine, belladonna tincture, and hyoscyamine [Anaspaz, Cystospaz, Levsin]) and various synthetic substitutes (eg, propantheline [Pro-Banthīne]) have been used in urologic disorders. Because quaternary ammonium compounds are not as well absorbed orally as the natural belladonna alkaloids, they may have a slightly longer duration of action.

Other urinary antispasmodics (dicyclomine [Bentyl], flavoxate [Urispas], and oxybutynin [Ditropan]) relax the detrusor and other smooth muscle by cholinergic blockade, as well as by a direct relaxant effect on muscle fibers, but they do not offer any clinical advantage over the anticholinergic agents.

BELLADONNA TINCTURE

Because this preparation is administered as a liquid, it is used primarily in children with nocturnal enuresis who also experience urgency, frequency, and urge incontinence during the day.

Belladonna produces antimuscarinic effects on the salivary glands, heart, eye, and gastrointestinal tract; large doses may cause flushing, fever, and marked central nervous system effects (eg, excitement, hallucinations, delirium). See also Chapter 53, Agents Used in Disorders of the Lower Intestinal Tract.

DOSAGE AND PREPARATIONS.

Oral: Children over 5 years, initially, 0.25 to 0.5 ml (10 to 20 drops) three times daily. Dosage may be increased gradually, if necessary, to 1 ml/dose. The dose should be reduced if flushing or other signs of toxicity occur. *Adults* (usually reserved for those who cannot take solid preparations), 0.4 to 1 ml (15 to 40 drops) four times daily.

    Generic. Tincture 0.3 mg/ml in 120 and 474 ml containers (alcohol 67%). Available with graduated droppers 40 drops/ml.

DICYCLOMINE HYDROCHLORIDE
[Bentyl]

This drug has anticholinergic and antispasmodic properties. It has been reported to increase bladder capacity in adults with detrusor hyperreflexia.

Dicyclomine can produce anticholinergic side effects and is contraindicated in the presence of urinary outflow obstruction (eg, prostatic hypertrophy) or intestinal atony and in patients who cannot tolerate tachycardia. For more detailed discussion, see Chapter 53, Agents Used in Disorders of the Lower Intestinal Tract.

DOSAGE AND PREPARATIONS.

Oral: Adults, 20 to 30 mg three times daily (Wein, 1984 B).

    Generic. Capsules 10 and 20 mg; syrup 10 mg/5 ml; tablets 20 mg.

    Bentyl (Merrell Dow). Capsules 10 mg; tablets 20 mg; syrup 10 mg/5 ml.

FLAVOXATE HYDROCHLORIDE
[Urispas]

ACTIONS AND USES. Flavoxate has local anesthetic, analgesic, and slight anticholinergic properties. It also may have a direct relaxant effect on smooth muscle. Urinary excretion of the drug with resultant local action may play an additional role. The relative contribution of each of these characteristics to the antispasmodic effect is difficult to appraise.

Flavoxate has been used to reduce dysuria, nocturia, suprapubic pain, and urinary frequency, urgency, and incontinence associated with cystitis, prostatitis, urethritis, and trigonitis. Despite its various actions, flavoxate has not proved to be more effective in these disorders than an anticholinergic drug (Benson et al, 1977; Finkbeiner and Bissada, 1980) and is considered to be no better than a placebo by some authorities. It should not be considered a drug of first choice for incontinence.

ADVERSE REACTIONS AND PRECAUTIONS. Adverse reactions are relatively uncommon; nausea, vomiting, dryness of the mouth, nervousness, vertigo, headache, drowsiness, blurred vision, disturbed visual accommodation, increased intraocular pressure, urticaria and other dermatoses, confusion (especially in the elderly), dysuria, tachycardia, fever, eosinophilia, and reversible leukopenia (one case) have been reported. Some of these reactions resemble anticholinergic effects; therefore, the same precautions and contraindications should apply (see Chapter 53, Agents Used in Disorders of the Lower Intestinal Tract).

DOSAGE AND PREPARATIONS.

Oral: Adults, 100 or 200 mg three or four times daily; the dose may be reduced when symptoms improve. Dosage has not been established for *children under 12 years.*

    Urispas (Smith Kline & French). Tablets 100 mg.

HYOSCYAMINE
[Cystospaz]

HYOSCYAMINE SULFATE
[Anaspaz, Cystospaz-M, Levsin]

Hyoscyamine has the same actions and side effects as the other belladonna alkaloids. Its most common use in urology has been to treat bladder spasm associated with infection, inflammation, or use of a retention catheter, although these conditions are less responsive to anticholinergic medication than neurogenic bladder disorders.

Adverse effects are similar to those observed with other anticholinergic agents (see Chapter 53, Agents Used in Disorders of the Lower Intestinal Tract). Hyoscyamine is classified in FDA Pregnancy Category C.

DOSAGE AND PREPARATIONS.

Oral: Adults, 0.15 to 0.3 mg of the base three or four times daily or 0.375 mg of the sulfate twice daily.

    HYOSCYAMINE:
    Cystospaz (Webcon). Tablets 0.15 mg.
    HYOSCYAMINE SULFATE:
    Anaspaz (Ascher). Tablets 0.125 mg.
    Cystospaz-M (Webcon). Capsules (timed-release) 0.375 mg.
    Levsin (Kremers-Urban). Capsules (timed-release) 0.375 mg (**Levsinex**); drops 0.125 mg/ml (alcohol 5%); elixir 0.125 mg/5 ml (alcohol 20%); tablets 0.125 mg.

OXYBUTYNIN CHLORIDE
[Ditropan]

ACTIONS AND USES. Oxybutynin has both anticholinergic and direct antispasmodic actions and also may possess mild analgesic properties. In a limited number of clinical trials, oxybutynin increased bladder capacity and improved urinary frequency, urgency, and urge incontinence in adults and children (Koff et al, 1978) with uninhibited bladder contractions; it also increased bladder capacity and reduced incontinence in those with reflex neurogenic bladder. It has not consistently relieved bladder spasm following transurethral surgical procedures.

Ditropan syrup is an acceptable alternative to tincture of belladonna in young children for whom a liquid preparation improves compliance.

ADVERSE REACTIONS AND PRECAUTIONS. Adverse reactions reflect this agent's anticholinergic activity. Severe dryness of the mouth is most common; nausea, blurred vision, flushing, and tachycardia also have been observed. Hallucinations have been reported in young children. The contraindications to oxybutynin are the same as for other drugs with anticholinergic properties (see Chapter 53, Agents Used in Disorders of the Lower Intestinal Tract).

DOSAGE AND PREPARATIONS.

Oral: Adults, 5 mg two or three times daily (maximum, 20 mg daily); up to 10 mg four times a day (maximum, 40 mg/day) has been recommended by some urologists. *Children over 5 years,* 5 mg two times daily (maximum, 15 mg daily).

    Ditropan (Marion). Syrup 5 mg/5 ml; tablets 5 mg.

PROPANTHELINE BROMIDE
[Pro-Banthīne]

ACTIONS AND USES. This quaternary ammonium compound is a synthetic anticholinergic agent with both antimuscarinic and ganglionic blocking properties. Its therapeutic effects are usually attributed to the antimuscarinic component.

Propantheline is given orally to increase bladder capacity and to reduce urinary frequency, urgency, and urge incontinence associated with uninhibited neurogenic bladder. It has been used more commonly for this purpose than other anticholinergic drugs. It may be given in combination with imipramine. In paraplegic patients with lesions above the sacral spinal cord (reflex neurogenic bladder), propantheline also may control reflex detrusor activity and thus preserve continence in the interval between catheterizations.

ADVERSE REACTIONS AND PRECAUTIONS. The adverse reactions produced by propantheline are common to all anticholinergic drugs. Doses that inhibit detrusor contractions also suppress salivation, interfere with ocular accommodation, dilate pupils, increase heart rate, and reduce gastrointestinal motility to cause constipation. Quaternary ammonium compounds do not readily cross the blood-brain barrier; therefore, central nervous system effects are rare. Because of their ganglionic blocking properties, large doses can cause orthostatic hypotension and impotence. See also Chapter 53, Agents Used in Disorders of the Lower Intestinal Tract.

DOSAGE AND PREPARATIONS. To improve bioavailability, propantheline should be administered one hour prior to meals.

Oral: To improve bladder capacity in patients with uninhibited neurogenic bladder, *adults,* initially, 15 mg every four to six hours; the amount may be increased by 15 mg/dose at weekly intervals until side effects become intolerable (particularly visual) to a maximum of 90 mg four times daily (Mundy et al, 1984). *Children,* 7.5 mg every four to six hours.

To maintain continence between catheterizations in patients with reflex neurogenic bladder, *adults,* 15 to 30 mg every four to six hours; *children,* 7.5 to 15 mg every four to six hours.

Pro-Banthine (Searle). Tablets 7.5 and 15 mg.

SK-Propantheline Bromide (Smith Kline & French), *Generic.* Tablets 15 mg.

Tricyclic Drug

IMIPRAMINE HYDROCHLORIDE
[Janimine, SK-Pramine, Tofranil]

USES. Imipramine is used routinely to treat nocturnal enuresis in children; however, some children are refractory to its effects and some develop a tolerance to its action. Improvement may not be sustained when the drug is discontinued. Reported rates of cure range from 10% to over 50% (Stewart, 1975; McKendry et al, 1975) and appear to be related to the patient's response to drug therapy (Mikkelsen and Rapoport, 1980; Mikkelsen et al, 1980). Imipramine's mechanism of action in enuresis is unclear, but may be related to direct inhibition of bladder muscle and increased outlet resistance.

Imipramine is useful in urge incontinence, particularly in elderly patients, and may be combined with an anticholinergic agent, such as propantheline. It can be tried in the postprostatectomy patient with mild incontinence in whom sphincter weakness appears to be the primary deficit and can be utilized prior to intercourse in patients with demonstrable retrograde ejaculation.

ADVERSE REACTIONS AND PRECAUTIONS. A transient "dull feeling" may be noted for the first one to two weeks of therapy. Drowsiness, dryness of the mouth, nausea, vomiting, constipation, blurred vision, restlessness, sleep disturbances, and mood changes are common adverse effects. Overdosage can cause convulsions, coma, and severe cardiovascular reactions, including A-V block and marked hypotension. The most common source of imipramine poisoning in children is nonsecured medication belonging to an older, enuretic sibling.

Parents should be given adequate warning of this potential danger. Withdrawal reactions (nausea, headache, and malaise) have been reported following abrupt discontinuation of long-term therapy.

See also Chapter 7, Drugs Used in Affective Disorders. To avoid misunderstandings, it is recommended that the patient be informed that the drug is *not* being given for its antidepressant action, which requires a much larger dose.

PHARMACOKINETICS. About 30% to 70% of the drug is absorbed from the gastrointestinal tract into the systemic circulation. The amount may vary because of the wide range of first-pass metabolism. Peak plasma levels occur approximately three hours after a single oral dose. The volume of distribution is 15 L/kg, and the drug is 89% to 94% protein bound. Imipramine (half-life, 13 to 28 hours) is biotransformed to the active metabolite, desipramine (half-life, 18 hours). No dosage adjustment is required in the presence of renal disease.

DOSAGE AND PREPARATIONS.

Oral: For nocturnal enuresis, *children 6 to 12 years,* 25 mg daily; if a satisfactory response is not apparent in one week, the dose should be increased to 50 mg daily; *children over 12 years,* up to 75 mg daily. The drug may be administered after dinner or up to one hour before bedtime. Some early nighttime bedwetters may benefit from administration in divided doses given at midafternoon and bedtime. When optimal effects are obtained, administration is continued for two to three months; the dose is then reduced gradually over three to four months.

For urge incontinence in *adults,* the following dosage has been proposed: Initially, 25 mg is given at bedtime and increased by 25 mg every third day until the patient is continent or experiences side effects (eg, orthostatic hypotension) to a maximum of 150 mg (Castleden et al, 1981). About 5 to 10 days are required to obtain a maximum effect. This dosage should be reduced by one-half in the elderly (Wein, 1985). In *children,* smaller doses given every eight hours seem to be more effective in urge incontinence than a single bedtime dose.

For postprostatectomy incontinence, up to 75 mg three times daily. For retrograde ejaculation, 25 mg three to four times daily.

Janimine (Abbott), **SK-Pramine** (Smith Kline & French), **Tofranil** (Geigy), **Generic.** Tablets 10, 25, and 50 mg.

Alpha-Adrenergic Drugs

EPHEDRINE SULFATE

This adrenergic drug has both alpha- and beta-stimulating properties and is often preferred to other sympathomimetic agents because it is effective orally, is generally well tolerated, and has a relatively long duration of action. By increasing urethral resistance, ephedrine improves urine storage in patients with mild to moderate stress incontinence of neurogenic or non-neurogenic origin, but it is of little value if the periurethral striated muscle is completely denervated or severely damaged or if there is severe damage to the posterior urethra (Diokno and Taub, 1975).

Since ephedrine increases blood pressure and stimulates the heart, it should be used cautiously in patients with hypertension and other cardiovascular disorders and in those with hyperthyroidism. It also stimulates the central nervous system and may cause insomnia and anxiety.

DOSAGE AND PREPARATIONS.
Oral: For stress incontinence, *adults,* 25 to 50 mg four times daily; *children,* 11 to 20 mg four times daily. For retrograde ejaculation, 50 mg one to two hours before intercourse.

> **Generic.** Capsules 25 and 50 mg (nonprescription); syrup 11 (alcohol 12%) and 20 mg/5 ml (nonprescription).

PHENYLPROPANOLAMINE HYDROCHLORIDE AND CHLORPHENIRAMINE MALEATE

> [Ornade, Triaminic-12]

USES. Women with mild to moderate stress incontinence may respond to this mixture, which contains an alpha-adrenergic stimulant (phenylpropanolamine) and an antihistamine (chlorpheniramine). It is less satisfactory in men with postprostatectomy incontinence, although a few patients with mild symptoms may improve (Stewart et al, 1976). This preparation had the advantage of being in a timed-release form that permitted twice-a-day use, but can be replaced by the single-entity phenylpropanolamine timed-release preparations available now.

ADVERSE REACTIONS AND PRECAUTIONS. Any combination of sympathomimetic, antihistaminic, and anticholinergic side effects may occur. Drowsiness, dryness of the mouth and nasal passages, and tachycardia are most common. If these effects are troublesome, the dose should be reduced or a single-entity preparation of phenylpropanolamine should be substituted. This mixture should be used cautiously in patients with hypertension and other cardiovascular disorders and in those with hyperthyroidism. It is classified as an FDA Pregnancy Category C substance. See also the evaluation on Phenylpropanolamine Hydrochloride.

DOSAGE AND PREPARATIONS.
Oral: For incontinence, *adults,* one capsule twice daily. For retrograde ejaculation, one capsule twice daily.

> **Ornade** (Smith Kline & French). Capsules (timed-release) containing phenylpropanolamine hydrochloride 75 mg and chlorpheniramine maleate 12 mg.
> **Triaminic-12** (Dorsey). Tablets (timed-release) containing phenylpropanolamine hydrochloride 75 mg and chlorpheniramine maleate 12 mg (nonprescription).

PHENYLPROPANOLAMINE HYDROCHLORIDE

USES. Phenylpropanolamine, marketed for use as an appetite suppressant and nasal decongestant, is effective in stress incontinence (Awad et al, 1978). Use of the single-entity agent is preferable to combination agents containing the substance.

Any beneficial response that occurs is apparent immediately or within a few days. An excellent response can be expected in mild stress incontinence; good response, but rarely total dryness, is observed in moderate to severe incontinence. Incontinence usually recurs if several doses are omitted or if therapy is discontinued.

ADVERSE REACTIONS AND PRECAUTIONS. The incidence of side effects is low and generally related to the size of the dose. Reactions include dizziness and headache; central nervous system stimulation is much less marked than with ephedrine, and nervousness and insomnia are rarely a problem. Hypertensive episodes are uncommon.

The drug should be used with caution in patients with hypertension, other cardiovascular disease, hyperthyroidism, and diabetes mellitus. Elderly patients may be more sensitive to large doses.

Phenylpropanolamine is contraindicated in patients receiving monoamine oxidase inhibitors. The antihypertensive effectiveness of guanethidine may be reduced.

PHARMACOKINETICS. About 80% to 90% of the dose is eliminated unchanged in the urine within 24 hours. Approximately 10% is metabolized to an active metabolite.

DOSAGE AND PREPARATIONS.
Oral: Adults, for incontinence, 50 mg three times a day. The dosage may be increased if required to 75 mg three times a day. Some patients may be able to omit the evening dose without a notable decrease in effectiveness. A single 75-mg timed-release preparation each morning may be adequate.

> **Generic.** Capsules (timed-release) 75 mg; tablets 25 and 50 mg (both forms nonprescription).

PSEUDOEPHEDRINE HYDROCHLORIDE

Pseudoephedrine hydrochloride, marketed for use as a nasal decongestant, is effective for stress incontinence. It acts similarly to ephedrine but causes less central nervous system stimulation and hypertension. For additional details, see Chapter 21, Decongestant, Cough, and Cold Preparations.

DOSAGE AND PREPARATIONS.
Oral: Adults, 30 to 60 mg four times daily (Wein, 1984 A).
> **Generic.** Capsules (timed-release) 120 mg; tablets 30 and 60 mg; syrup 30 mg/5 ml (nonprescription).

AGENTS USED TO TREAT URINARY RETENTION

The drugs used to treat urinary retention facilitate bladder emptying by increasing detrusor muscle contractility (cholinergic agents) or by reducing outlet resistance (alpha-adrenergic blocking drugs). Bethanechol [Duvoid, Myotonachol, Urecholine] is the cholinergic agent most commonly recommended for management of chronic hypotonic bladder and for short-term treatment of postoperative urinary retention in selected patients. The cholinesterase inhibitor, neostigmine methylsulfate [Prostigmin], also can be used for the latter purpose. The alpha-adrenergic blocking drug, phenoxybenzamine [Dibenzyline], facilitates voiding by relaxing the internal sphincter and is used in certain neurogenic bladder disorders. It may be given with bethanechol. Relaxants used primarily to combat spasticity, dantrolene [Dantrium] and baclofen [Lioresal], reduce urinary retention secondary to spasm of the external sphincter.

Cholinergic Drugs

BETHANECHOL CHLORIDE
[Duvoid, Myotonachol, Urecholine]

$$H_2NCOCHCH_2\overset{+}{N}(CH_3)_3 \quad Cl^-$$
$$\underset{CH_3}{|}$$

ACTIONS AND USES. Bethanechol is a choline ester that acts directly on effector cells. Its effects are similar to those of acetylcholine but are more prolonged because bethanechol is relatively resistant to hydrolysis by cholinesterase. Effects on autonomic ganglia are minimal. The action on the urinary bladder and gastrointestinal tract is more pronounced than that on the cardiovascular system. However, most investigators have shown that bethanechol has little or no beneficial effect in any voiding dysfunction.

Bethanechol is used in conjunction with clean intermittent self-catheterization to facilitate emptying of the hypotonic neurogenic bladder. It is sometimes employed during the recovery phase after spinal shock to enhance weak detrusor contractions in patients with spinal cord lesions above the vesical reflex arc (S_2-S_4) and coordinated bladder-external sphincter function (Diokno and Koppenhoefer, 1976). If tolerated, it also may be used for long-term therapy in patients with sensory paralytic bladder or in those with incomplete motor lesions and coordinated sphincter function (Sonda et al, 1979). Its effectiveness should be documented during a short trial before committing a patient to long-term therapy (Wein, 1979; Wein et al, 1980; Wein, 1983).

Bethanechol also is used to restore normal micturition in selected patients with acute urinary retention associated with surgery or parturition.

ADVERSE REACTIONS AND PRECAUTIONS. Bethanechol may cause flushing, headache, salivation, sweating, nausea, abdominal cramps, diarrhea, asthmatic attacks, and a fall in blood pressure. Some patients cannot tolerate prolonged therapy because of these reactions. Side effects may be counteracted immediately by atropine (children to age 12, 0.01 mg/kg; adults, 0.6 mg); the subcutaneous route is used except in emergencies and administration may be repeated every two hours if needed. Atropine should be available during the subcutaneous administration of bethanechol.

Bethanechol must not be given intravenously or intramuscularly because acute severe muscarinic effects, including acute circulatory failure and cardiac arrest, may result.

CONTRAINDICATIONS. Bethanechol is contraindicated in the presence of anatomic or functional urinary tract obstruction. This drug also should be avoided in patients with detrusor-external sphincter dyssynergia (involuntary detrusor contractions accompanied by contraction of the external sphincter) unless an effective external sphincter relaxant is given concomitantly, because prolonged therapy has caused bladder trabeculation, diverticula, and vesicoureteral reflux. Although dyssynergia resulting from internal sphincter overactivity may be less common, the possibility of adverse effects in such cases should be considered.

Bethanechol also is contraindicated in patients with bronchial asthma because it may cause bronchospasm. It may reduce blood pressure and generally should be avoided in patients with hypotension, bradycardia, or coronary artery disease and during therapy with ganglionic blocking agents (eg, mecamylamine, trimethaphan). Additional contraindications include hyperthyroidism, hypertension, and atrioventricular conduction defects.

Because it increases gastrointestinal motility, bethanechol should not be given to patients with peptic ulcer and other gastrointestinal lesions or to those with intestinal obstruction. It should not be employed following recent gastrointestinal resection and anastomosis.

EFFECTS ON LABORATORY TESTS. Serum amylase, lipase, and transaminase (SGOT) levels may be increased secondary to pancreatic stimulation and contraction of the sphincter of Oddi.

DOSAGE AND PREPARATIONS. The dosage and route of administration must be individualized. The drug should be given before meals to avoid nausea and vomiting. A subcutaneous dose of 5 mg is considered equivalent to an oral dose of 200 mg.

In neurogenic bladder disorders, bethanechol may be used in conjunction with surgery or other drugs (phenoxybenzamine) to reduce anatomic or functional outlet obstruction.

Subcutaneous: For acute postoperative and postpartum urinary retention in selected adults, 5 mg (1 ml). If this dose is ineffective, the patient should be catheterized. Bethanechol should not be used unless the patient is alert and there is no outlet obstruction.

Subcutaneous, Oral: For patients with incomplete spinal cord lesions above the reflex arc and voluntary control of the external sphincter, initially, 2.5 to 5 mg subcutaneously every four to six hours. The patient should be catheterized once or twice daily; when residual urine is less than 50 ml, oral therapy may be substituted (50 mg every six hours) or subcutaneous therapy may be continued (2.5 mg every six hours). This regimen should be continued for at least one week and, if the amount of residual urine remains low, the drug may be discontinued following a gradual reduction in dosage. Some patients may require several weeks or months of therapy.

In sensory paralytic bladder and partial motor paralytic bladder with coordinated sphincter function, initially, 5 to 10 mg subcutaneously every four hours around the clock. (An initial dose of 5 mg may be advisable in very frail patients.) The patient should be asked to try to urinate 20 to 30 minutes after the drug is administered. This voiding program may be initiated with an indwelling catheter, which is removed after the first few doses. When the amount of residual urine is less than 50 ml for three days, each dose may be reduced by 2.5 mg. If the response remains satisfactory, dosage may be reduced to a minimum of 5 mg every four hours. Oral therapy (50 mg four times daily) may be substituted when complete bladder emptying is achieved over a three-day period. The drug may be discontinued when the sensory paralytic bladder is rehabilitated, but patients with incomplete motor lesions generally require life-long treatment.

For *children* with lazy bladder syndrome and inadequate detrusor activity, 0.2 mg/kg or 6.7 mg/M² orally three times a day or 0.15 to 0.2 mg/kg or 5 to 6.7 mg/M² subcutaneously three times a day. The drug should be discontinued when voiding retraining is accomplished.

Oral: For patients with lesions above the sacral reflex arc and coordinated bladder and sphincter function, initially, 25 mg every six hours. Dosage may be increased or decreased depending upon the response (the usual adult dose is 50 to 100 mg four times a day), and the drug should be discontinued if reflex voiding is established.

> **Generic.** Tablets 5, 10, 25, and 50 mg.
> **Duvoid** (Norwich Eaton). Tablets 10, 25, and 50 mg.
> **Myotonachol** (Glenwood). Tablets 10 and 25 mg.
> **Urecholine** (Merck Sharp & Dohme). Solution (for injection) 5 mg/ml; tablets 5, 10, 25, and 50 mg.

Alpha-adrenergic Blocking Agent

PHENOXYBENZAMINE HYDROCHLORIDE
[Dibenzyline]

ACTIONS AND USES. By blocking alpha receptors in the smooth muscle of the bladder neck and proximal urethra, phenoxybenzamine relaxes the internal sphincter. It may improve voiding efficiency in patients with functional outlet obstruction and obviate or delay the need for transurethral surgery. Phenoxybenzamine has been effective in patients with reflex, autonomous, and motor paralytic bladders when urinary retention could not be prevented by other methods, such as reflex voiding, Credé maneuver, or bethanechol (Kleeman, 1977; Mobley, 1976; Scott and Morrow, 1978). It is particularly useful in rehabilitating decompensated or atonic bladders when administered with bethanechol (Finkbeiner and Bissada, 1980). Phenoxybenzamine has no effect on striated muscle and therefore is ineffective in urinary retention caused by excessive or inappropriate activity of the external sphincter. Phentolamine has been employed to identify patients who are likely to benefit from long-term phenoxybenzamine therapy (Olsson et al, 1977).

In addition to its use in neurogenic bladder dysfunction, phenoxybenzamine has been employed to treat voiding disturbances in patients with prostatic obstruction who are not suitable candidates for surgery or those who have only occasional, transient, acute episodes of retention (Caine et al, 1981; Waterfall and Williams, 1980). As an alternative to catheterization of the bladder, phenoxybenzamine can be employed to relieve postoperative retention of urine. A dose of 10 mg orally may be given prophylactically 6 and 18 hours after surgery or if signs of obstruction become evident (Leventhal and Pfau, 1978).

ADVERSE REACTIONS AND PRECAUTIONS. The major side effects of phenoxybenzamine, orthostatic hypotension and reflex tachycardia, result from blockade of alpha receptors in the peripheral circulation. Elastic stockings may counteract hypotension. Other adverse reactions include nasal congestion, transient lassitude, nausea, diarrhea, miosis, and inhibition of ejaculation.

A two-year study in rats showed a high dose-related proliferation of basal cells in the nonglandular portion of the stomach. For this reason, the manufacturer currently recommends that this drug be reserved for emergency, short-term use, such as the preoperative management of pheochromocytoma.

PHARMACOKINETICS. The gastrointestinal absorption of phenoxybenzamine is erratic; about 20% to 30% of orally administered drug appears in the systemic circulation. The volume of distribution has not been reported. Phenoxybenzamine has high lipid solubility and accumulates in body fat. About 50% of an intravenous dose is excreted in 12 hours and over 80% in 24 hours.

DOSAGE AND PREPARATIONS.
Oral: Adults, initially, 10 mg once daily. If larger amounts are needed, the dosage may be increased by 10-mg increments every four to five days to a maximum of 60 mg daily. Daily doses larger than 10 mg should be divided evenly and given every 8 to 12 hours. The maximum effect usually becomes apparent only after one week following initiation or change in dosage (Wein, 1984 A). During long-term therapy, some patients may require as little as 10 mg two or three times a week. *Children,* similar to the adult protocol, to a maximum of 10 mg three times daily (Diokno and Sonda, 1984).

> **Dibenzyline** (Smith Kline & French). Capsules 10 mg.

PRAZOSIN HYDROCHLORIDE
[Minipress]

This antihypertensive agent has relatively specific adrenergic blocking activity for alpha₁ receptor sites. In contrast to phenoxybenzamine, it has not demonstrated mutagenic or carcinogenic action, and its use as a subsitute for that drug is under investigation.

Marked orthostatic hypotension and syncope that occasionally leads to collapse and unconsciousness may occur at the onset of treatment (first-dose phenomenon). An associated tachycardia has been noted occasionally and chest pain has occurred rarely. Symptomatic orthostatic hypotension appears to be most common when the initial dose exceeds 2 mg and when dosage is increased rapidly. Patients receiving diuretics, a beta blocker, and/or a low-sodium diet may be particularly susceptible. Prazosin may cause edema if a diuretic is not given concomitantly.

For additional information on side effects, precautions, and pharmacokinetics, see Chapter 28, Antihypertensive Agents.

DOSAGE AND PREPARATIONS.
Oral: Adults, initially, 1 mg at bedtime, then 1 mg three times daily. This may be increased at weekly intervals by 1 mg/dose until an adequate effect is produced, the side effects become unacceptable, or a maximum of 20 mg daily is given. The dose equivalency to phenoxybenzamine has not been established (Wein, 1984 B).

Minipress (Pfizer). Capsules 1, 2, and 5 mg.

External Sphincter Relaxants

BACLOFEN
[Lioresal]

ACTIONS AND USES. Baclofen reduces polysynaptic reflex activity in the spinal cord. Its primary indication is spasticity resulting from upper motor neuron lesions (see Chapter 12, Drugs Used in Disorders Affecting Skeletal Muscle). It may be useful in the management of external sphincter hypertonicity or detrusor-external sphincter dyssynergia. Patients with concurrent bladder hypotonicity who demonstrate weak or poorly sustained detrusor contraction on voiding also may require a cholinergic agent, such as bethanechol, to attain the optimal effect. Baclofen apparently is a more potent relaxant of the external sphincter than diazepam or dantrolene.

ADVERSE REACTIONS AND PRECAUTIONS. Baclofen usually is well tolerated. Drowsiness (incidence 10% to 63%), dizziness (incidence 5% to 15%), and muscle weakness may occur but often disappear with continued administration and may be minimized by avoiding abrupt increases in dosage. Occasional reactions include nausea, constipation, insomnia, and headache. Baclofen may increase the frequency of seizures in epileptic patients. Abrupt discontinuation of long-term, high-dose therapy may be associated with visual and auditory hallucinations and agitated behavior. The safety of baclofen during pregnancy or in children has not been established. Alcohol and other central nervous system depressants should be avoided.

Baclofen may increase blood glucose, serum alkaline phosphatase, and serum transaminase (SGOT) values.

PHARMACOKINETICS. Absorption from the gastrointestinal tract is rapid and complete; peak plasma levels are obtained one to two hours after oral administration. The volume of distribution is not known. About 85% of orally administered drug is excreted unchanged by the kidney. The major metabolite has a hydroxy group substituted for the amino group. The half-life is two to four hours. Dosage should be adjusted if renal impairment is present.

DOSAGE AND PREPARATIONS. The dosage should be titrated, and therapy should be discontinued slowly over a one- to two-week period to avoid precipitating hallucinations and/or agitated behavior.
Oral: In *adults,* initially, 5 mg three times a day, increased by 15 mg/day every fourth day until the desired effect is achieved. The manufacturer's literature specifies that most patients respond to a total daily dose of 40 to 80 mg and that doses in excess of 80 mg daily should not be used. In one study, however, most patients required an average daily dose of 120 mg to reduce external urethral sphincter spasticity significantly (Leyson et al, 1980). Usually a minimum of five weeks is required to assess the effectiveness of therapy.

Lioresal (Geigy). Tablets 10 and 20 mg.

DANTROLENE SODIUM
[Dantrium]

ACTIONS AND USES. Dantrolene acts directly on skeletal muscle to produce relaxation by interfering with the release of calcium ions from the sarcoplasmic reticulum. This action is helpful in relieving spasticity secondary to upper motor neuron lesions (see Chapter 12, Drugs Used in Disorders Affecting Skeletal Muscle) and for the pre- and intraoperative management of malignant hyperthermia (see Chapter 17, Adjuncts to Anesthesia). Dantrolene is of some benefit in patients with external sphincter hypertonicity who have excessive residual urine volume and high urethral pressure. Its action may be enhanced by the concomitant administration of diazepam, but the combination may produce significant sedation. In patients with concurrent bladder hypotonicity who demonstrate weak or poorly sustained detrusor contraction on voiding, a cholinergic agent, such as bethanechol, also may be required for an optimal effect.

ADVERSE REACTIONS AND PRECAUTIONS. Minor side effects, which usually disappear with continued treatment, are drowsiness and dizziness, nausea, vomiting, and diarrhea. The only adverse reaction that occurs commonly during long-term therapy is an acne-like skin eruption. The incidence of these and less common untoward effects has been reviewed (Pinder et al, 1977).

The limiting reaction at the dosage levels required to manage external sphincter spasm is generalized muscle weakness. Patients with brain stem or high cervical lesions, amyotrophic lateral sclerosis, or multiple sclerosis may not tolerate large doses of dantrolene because of severe muscle weakness. The drug should be used with caution in patients with impaired pulmonary function, particularly obstructive lung disease or respiratory weakness caused by motor neuron disease. Alcohol should be avoided.

Dantrolene is contraindicated in patients with active liver disease, for it may produce dose-related, fatal, hepatocellular injury in susceptible patients. This has been observed most frequently in patients over 30 years of age, usually women (particularly those receiving estrogens), when total daily doses greater than 300 mg were used for 60 days or longer. Most cases occur between the second and sixth month of therapy. Baseline and monthly measurements of SGOT and SGPT levels are usually recommended; however, these values may increase temporarily in about 10% of patients exposed to the drug regardless of dosage.

PHARMACOKINETICS. About 70% of an oral dose is absorbed, but there may be a threefold difference among patients. Peak plasma levels occur in four to six hours. The volume of distribution is not known. Dantrolene is metabolized in the liver, principally by hydroxylation but also by reduction of the nitro group, followed by acetylation. The metabolites are excreted by the kidney. There is no evidence that metabolism is affected significantly by hepatic impairment or by enzyme-inducing drugs. The hydroxylated derivative exhibits a weak dantrolene-like action. A total of 40% to 45% of the oral dose is excreted unchanged in the bile. The half-life is 8.7 hours in normal adults and 7.3 hours in spastic children.

DOSAGE AND PREPARATIONS. The dosage should be titrated. On a theoretical basis, the urethral pressure can be decreased only by 50%. The risks of dantrolene therapy must be weighed against the potential benefit in patients with incomplete neurologic lesions. The drug is not a substitute for external sphincterotomy in male patients with complete spinal cord lesions. Usually five to seven weeks are required to assess the value of therapy.

Oral: Adults, initially, 25 mg once daily; 25 mg is added every fourth day until the desired effect is attained or until a maximum dose of 400 mg/day is reached. The manufacturer's literature specifies that most patients respond to a total daily dose of 400 mg or less and that only rarely should doses larger than this be given. However, in one study, most patients required 600 mg daily (Hackler et al, 1980). *Children,* a similar schedule should be used, beginning with 0.5 mg/kg twice daily, increased to a maximum of 3 mg/kg four times daily. Doses larger than 400 mg/day should not be given.

Dantrium (Norwich Eaton). Capsules 25, 50, and 100 mg.

DIAZEPAM
[Valium]

ACTIONS AND USES. Diazepam has an antispastic action in addition to its sedative and antianxiety properties. This effect is believed to be the result of combined presynaptic inhibition in the spinal cord and suppression of the lateral reticular system that is facilitative to the gamma motor neurons. Its beneficial action in voiding, however, is ascribed by many solely to its antianxiety action.

Diazepam is useful as a supplement to voiding retraining or intermittent catheterization in children with external sphincter dyssynergia (non-neurogenic neurogenic bladder of childhood) and as a supplement to anticholinergic agents in women with urethral syndrome due to spasm of the external sphincter. The drug is less effective in spastic external sphincter secondary to upper motor neuron lesions.

For a discussion of adverse reactions, precautions, and pharmacokinetic data, see Chapter 5, Drugs Used for Anxiety and Sleep Disorders.

DOSAGE AND PREPARATIONS. The half-life is prolonged in premature infants, elderly patients, and in those with hepatic disease; the latter require a reduction in dosage. Dosage adjustment is not required in those with renal disease.

Oral: The dosage for urologic disorders should not exceed the usual amount given for anxiety. *Children,* 0.2 to 0.4 mg/kg three or four times a day; *adults,* 2 to 5 mg/day. This amount is continued for two to six months and then is reduced slowly.

Valium (Roche), **Generic**. Tablets 2, 5, and 10 mg.

AGENTS USED TO TREAT INTERSTITIAL CYSTITIS

DIMETHYL SULFOXIDE (DMSO)
[Rimso-50]

USES. DMSO is available as a 50% solution for direct instillation into the bladder to treat interstitial cystitis. It relieves symptoms in many patients and may improve the endoscopic appearance of the bladder. However, some patients do not respond and others may relapse after initial improvement (Shirley et al, 1978).

ADVERSE REACTIONS AND PRECAUTIONS. No serious adverse effects have occurred after intravesical instillation of the 50% solution. The most common side effect of DMSO, which results from systemic absorption, is a garlic-like taste and odor on the breath and skin for as long as 72 hours; this is without clinical significance. Other side effects are self-limiting and include suprapubic discomfort, headache, lethargy, and nausea. A stronger concentration (100%) has caused severe, transient, chemical cystitis.

When applied to the skin, dimethyl sulfoxide has caused urticaria, severe allergic reactions (including shortness of breath and anaphylactoid facial swelling), gastrointestinal disturbances, headache, nausea, diarrhea, photophobia, and transient disturbances in color vision. Lens opacities have occurred following prolonged administration to animals, but this is species specific and has not occurred in man. Dimethyl sulfoxide is classified as an FDA Pregnancy Category C substance.

PHARMACOKINETICS. The portion of dimethyl sulfoxide that is absorbed into the systemic circulation after intravesical instillation is tightly protein bound and can be detected for 36 to 48 hours. A portion is reduced to dimethyl sulfide, which is responsible for the garlic-like taste and odor on the breath. The principal metabolite is an oxidation product, dimethyl sulfone, which may be detected in the serum for longer than two weeks after a single intravesical instillation.

DOSAGE AND PREPARATIONS.

Intravesical Instillation: Following local anesthesia of the urethra, 50 ml of a 50% solution is instilled slowly by catheter directly into the bladder. An anticholinergic drug may be given to prevent bladder spasm. DMSO is retained in the bladder for 20 minutes and then eliminated by spontaneous voiding. Instillation may be repeated at two-week intervals in patients with severe symptoms or at three- to six-month intervals in those with milder symptoms.

Rimso-50 (Research Industries). Solution (sterile) 50% in 50 ml containers.

WARNING: The preparation, *Cryoserv* (formerly *Rimso-100*), which is used for cryogenic preparations, is not intended for human use. The instillation of *Cryoserv* into the bladder would cause a tissue-damaging exothermic reaction.

OXYCHLOROSENE SODIUM
[Clorpactin WCS-90]

This topical antiseptic is a mixture of the sodium salt of hypochlorous acid and alkylbenzene sulfonates (see Chapter 56, Dermatologic Preparations). It is employed to relieve the symptoms of interstitial cystitis. General or spinal anesthesia is required for instillation.

Neither side effects attributable to this agent nor injury to the bladder has been reported. Oxychlorosene may, however, produce ureteral fibrosis in patients with vesicoureteral reflux (Messing and Freiha, 1979). In these patients, the ureteral orifice should be occluded before instillation. An intensification of symptoms (lasting up to 72 hours) may occur immediately following each treatment. Concentrations greater than 0.4% should not be exceeded.

DOSAGE AND PREPARATIONS.

Intravesical Instillation: A 0.4% solution of oxychlorosene sodium is prepared immediately prior to use. After the patient is anesthetized, the solution is instilled through a large urethral catheter under low pressure (10 cm water) until the bladder is full. The bladder then is emptied and instillations are repeated until 1,000 ml has been utilized. The patient is observed for four weeks after both the first and second instillation. If symptoms do not subside, four additional consecutive weekly instillations are performed. If improvement is attained during a treatment course, no more is given until symptoms recur. A six-month interval is allowed to elapse prior to a second course of therapy if this is required (Messing and Stamey, 1978).

Clorpactin WCS-90 (Guardian). Powder (water-soluble) in 2 g containers.

UROLITHIASIS

The factors that influence the formation of most renal stones are unknown (Drach, 1978; Coe and Favus, 1979). Urolithiasis occurs more often in men than women and in white than nonwhite (particularly black) individuals. The incidence increases with age, becoming maximal in the 40- to 60-year-old group in whites and somewhat later in blacks. After age 60, the prevalence declines and is almost zero in those over age 80. About 0.5% to 1% of the population is affected. In general, the earlier the age of onset, the greater the likelihood of recurrence. The recurrence rate in untreated patients probably is 50% to 80%. The incidence also varies with geographic location, water intake, diet, occupation, and season (Drach, 1978).

In North America, the principal kidney stones are calcium 70% to 80% (as calcium oxalate, calcium phosphate [apatite or brushite], or mixtures of these salts), uric acid 10%, cystine 1%, and "struvite" 10% (magnesium ammonium phosphate or a mixture of struvite and carbonate apatite, calcium phosphate carbonate).

Following the onset of renal or ureteral colic, the diagnosis of urolithiasis usually can be confirmed by urinalysis (which generally shows gross or microscopic hematuria and, sometimes, crystals of the same type as those comprising the stone) and radiographic examination of the kidneys, ureter, and bladder (KUB, computed tomography, ultrasonography, intravenous urogram). The intravenous urogram may be needed to determine the degree of obstruction in the acute episode.

The acute condition is managed with narcotic analgesics (meperidine [Demerol] 50 to 100 mg or morphine 10 to 15 mg, depending on body size, age, coexisting disease, and severity of pain). Most stones smaller than 0.5 cm pass; stones 0.5 to 0.7 cm may pass, and stones larger than 0.7 cm probably will not pass (Drach, 1978). Most patients do not require immediate surgery or percutaneous ultrasonic lithotripsy unless there is an obstruction of the kidney or an active infection that does not respond quickly to antibiotics. Extracorporeal shock wave lithotripsy (ESWL) is being used increasingly in the management of patients with stones located in the kidney or upper ureter.

To improve the specificity of therapy, an attempt should be made to determine the underlying metabolic abnormality (Pak, 1982; Smith, 1983). An effort also should be made to recover the calculus for analysis. If indicated by the urinalysis, the urine should be cultured. Most clinicians believe a serum biochemical profile (calcium, phosphorus, uric acid, and blood urea nitrogen) and complete blood count should be obtained on all patients. Opinions vary regarding the need for serum immunoreactive parathyroid hormone studies, creatinine clearance determinations, and measurements of a variety of urinary products in 24-hour specimens. These decisions often are based on the frequency and severity of disease in the individual patient (Kosko and Resnick, 1985).

Urolithiasis may be categorized as metabolically active or inactive (Smith, 1979). Patients with inactive disease require a large fluid intake and follow-up examinations. Those who experience metabolically active disease over the course of a year (as indicated by radiologic evidence of new stone formation, stone growth, or documented passage of gravel) are candidates for long-term therapy. Any anatomic or systemic disease predisposing to stone formation should be diagnosed and corrected, and urinary tract infections should be treated with appropriate antimicrobial agents. Drug selection for the management of urolithiasis is shown in the Table. It is emphasized that many patients with urolithiasis will have more than one of the abnormalities shown in the Table. If necessary, several agents or therapeutic approaches may be used simultaneously to manage a patient's particular problem.

The fundamental principle of management, regardless of the type of calculus, is fluid intake sufficient to maintain a urine volume above 2.5 L/24 hours (Smith et al, 1978; Pak et al, 1980).

Calcium Oxalate and Calcium Phosphate Urolithiasis:
Therapy for calcium urolithiasis is aimed at identification and management of the underlying metabolic defect (see the Table and Chapter 49, Agents Affecting Calcium Metabolism). These include hyperparathyroidism, sarcoidosis, multiple myeloma, hypervitaminosis D, hyperoxaluria of any etiology, pyridoxine deficiency, hyperthyroidism, and metastatic malignant neoplasms (Drach, 1978). Hypercalciuria also may result from abrupt immobilization (casts, traction, or quadriplegia) and distal renal tubular acidosis.

Most patients have hypercalciuria (absorptive or renal) and another abnormality related to oxalate or uric acid metabolism. A large fluid intake to maintain a urine output above 2.5 L/day is initiated in all patients. If this does not prevent active stone formation or growth, dietary restrictions are added if indicated: (1) low oxalate intake (eg, limited ingestion of tea, nuts, spinach) and, if high calcium absorption is present, (2) low calcium intake (limited ingestion of milk, milk products, and calcium-enriched cereals and breads). If this is inadequate, patients with hyperabsorption of calcium (absorptive hypercalciuria Type I) may be treated with sodium cellulose phosphate or a thiazide diuretic. The former decreases the intestinal absorption of calcium and enhances the inhibitory property of the urine by increasing the excretion of pyrophosphate. Patients with gastrointestinal malabsorption syndromes (eg, chronic diarrhea) and calcium urolithiasis may not excrete enough magnesium and citrate (both inhibitors of stone formation) and may benefit from supplemental amounts of these substances (Rudman et al, 1980; Johansson et al, 1980).

The incidence of frequently recurring calcium stones, which appear to develop whether hypercalciuria is present or not, can be reduced by daily administration of a thiazide diuretic (Coe, 1981; Graziani et al, 1981); chlorothiazide [Diuril] 500 mg twice daily or the equivalent of other thiazides is employed (Yendt and Cohanim, 1978). Supplementation with potassium citrate 10 to 20 mEq three times a day is recommended to prevent hypocitraturia, which may result from thiazide treatment. Usually, the hypocalciuric effect begins within two days, is maximal within six days, and is sustained. The effectiveness of the thiazide is abolished by a high sodium or potassium intake. Furosemide [Lasix] and diazoxide [Hyperstat I.V.] do not have a hypocalciuric effect.

When the 24-hour calcium excretion exceeds 4 mg/kg (or 300 mg in men and 250 mg in women) but uric acid excretion is less than 800 mg in men or 750 mg in women (renal leak hypercalciuria), a thiazide alone may be used. If hyperuricosuria also is present, dietary restriction of purine intake and/or allopurinol [Lopurin, Zyloprim] 150 to 300 mg daily is added. If the excretion of calcium and/or uric acid is excessive, a follow-up 24-hour urine collection should be performed in about eight weeks to assess the effectiveness of the dosage.

Patients with hyperoxaluria associated with loss of function of the small intestine (eg, surgery for Crohn's disease) may benefit from a low-fat diet (maximum, 50 g daily) and limited intake of oxalate. If the urinary excretion of calcium is low (less than 100 mg/24 hours), supplementing the diet with up to 1 g of calcium may be helpful. However, recent evidence has shown that the empiric use of calcium may be hazardous and it is preferable to monitor calcium excretion. For patients with hyperoxaluria due to intestinal bypass, corrective surgery is indicated, although a combination of calcium (1.1 g as lactate or phosphate daily), a low-oxalate diet, and magnesium has reduced the rate of new stone formation in some patients (Holm and Hessov, 1981). In Crohn's disease and after intestinal bypass, urinary citrate and the pH are lower; supplementation with potassium citrate may be helpful.

Primary hyperoxaluria is a rare genetic disease. If untreated, urolithiasis progresses to renal failure. Large doses of pyridoxine (200 mg/day) decrease oxalate excretion in some patients. Oral orthophosphate (2 g elemental phosphorus) or magnesium (as magnesium oxide or magnesium hydroxide) can be used concomitantly. Orthophosphate supplementation plus pyridoxine is currently preferred (Smith, 1980).

Struvite (Magnesium Ammonium Phosphate) Lithiasis:
Struvite stones are formed in association with infection by urea-splitting bacteria (usually *Proteus*), often but not necessarily in conjunction with anatomic abnormalities or foreign bodies in the urinary tract. Stones that produce obstruction, pain, bleeding, and infections must be removed surgically. Multiple approaches can be used; these include traditional open surgery, percutaneous lithotripsy, or extracorporeal shock wave lithotripsy. Appropriate bactericidal antibiotic therapy is instituted 48 hours prior to surgery and is continued for 10 to 14 days thereafter. This may be followed by long-term suppressive treatment with trimethoprim/sulfamethoxazole [Bactrim, Septra] (Coe and Favus, 1979). Alternatively, methenamine mandelate [Mandelamine] 1 g and ammonium chloride 500 mg are given four times a day (Smith, 1979). Care must be taken to avoid calcium loss from bone that can result from long-term ammonium chloride administration.

Restriction of dietary phosphate and administration of aluminum hydroxide gel to decrease the intestinal absorption of phosphate may reduce the growth and recurrence of stones, but may result in a syndrome of hypercalciuria and phosphorus depletion. A more modest restriction of dietary phosphate without the antacid may be necessary. Bacterial urease inhibitors, such as acetohydroxamic acid [Lithostat], also prevent new stone formation. The use of acetohydroxamic acid should be restricted to patients (1) with chronic disease due to urease-producing organisms not responsive to antimicrobial agents, and (2) with adequate renal function (serum creatinine

DRUG SELECTION FOR UROLITHIASIS

Type of Stone and Metabolic Abnormality	Therapy
CALCIUM OXALATE/PHOSPHATE	
Calcium urolithiasis with no demonstrable metabolic abnormality	Dietary oxalate restriction and high fluid intake
Renal hypercalciuria	Thiazide diuretics
Absorptive hypercalciuria Type I	Sodium cellulose phosphate with magnesium supplement and moderate oxalate restriction, thiazide diuretic
Hyperuricosuric calcium oxalate	Allopurinol, purine-restricted diet
Absorptive hypercalciuria Type II	Dietary calcium restriction and high fluid intake, thiazide diuretic
Absorptive hypercalciuria Type III (Hypophosphatemic absorptive hypercalciuria)	Orthophosphate
Hypocitraturic calcium urolithiasis	Potassium citrate*
Resorptive hypercalciuria (Primary hyperparathyroidism)	Surgery
Hyperoxaluria, enteric	Dietary restriction of fats and oxalate; management of underlying GI disorder; calcium salts; cholestyramine*; potassium citrate*
Hyperoxaluria, primary Type I or II	Pyridoxine, orthophosphate; magnesium oxide
Distal renal tubular acidosis	Sodium or potassium citrate or bicarbonate
CYSTINE	
Cystinuria	Alkalization with citrate or bicarbonate; penicillamine; tiopronin**; acetylcysteine; tromethamine
STRUVITE (Magnesium ammonium phosphate)	
Infection with urea-splitting organisms	Antibacterial agents; acetohydroxamic acid; moderate restriction of dietary phosphate; surgical removal of stone
URIC ACID	
Hyperuricosuria	Alkalization with citrate or bicarbonate; allopurinol; fluid
XANTHINE	
Xanthinuria	Alkalization with citrate or bicarbonate and high fluid intake

*Investigational use
**Investigational drug

concentration below 3 mg/dl) (Williams et al, 1984). As with other forms of urolithiasis, a large fluid intake should be maintained.

Various irrigation solutions and procedures are available to dissolve struvite stones in patients who are not candidates for surgery (Drach, 1978) or to remove stone fragments post-surgically. Failure to remove even minute fragments during surgery may result in recurrent infection and new stone formation. Irrigation of the renal pelvis with a 10% solution of Renacidin dissolves all traces of struvite stones (Nemoy, 1980). *Sterile urine and normal kidney function are prerequisites* to the use of Renacidin. Once these are assured, the renal pelvis is irrigated with saline on the fourth or fifth postoperative day at a rate of 120 ml/hour for 24 to 48 hours. If no leakage, fever, or flank pain occurs, 10% Renacidin is instilled at the same rate. In the absence of visible fragments in plain film tomograms of the kidney, irrigation is continued for 24 to 48 hours. If visible fragments are present, irrigation is continued until stones are dissolved. During irrigation, serum magnesium and creatinine levels should be monitored. Because hypermagnesemia is potentially fatal, infusion should be discontinued if the serum magnesium level exceeds 5 to 6 mEq/L. Hyperphosphatemia occasionally is produced. Urine cultures should be obtained daily and, if positive, the irrigation must be discontinued until the infection is eradicated.

Uric Acid Lithiasis: Treatment of hyperuricosuria is aimed at increasing the solubility of uric acid by maintaining an adequate urine output and by increasing urinary pH. Patients should test their urine at each voiding to adjust alkali intake. If there are no restrictions for sodium, this is accomplished most easily by taking sodium bicarbonate 2 to 4 g/day or more in divided doses two hours after each meal and at bedtime. Sodium citrate is an alternative alkalizing agent that is available in palatable liquid form (eg, Bicitra, Polycitra). Potassium citrate is also an excellent alkalizing agent.

Urinary alkalization may be enhanced by direct irrigation with a sodium bicarbonate solution 167 mEq/L in normal saline utilizing a percutaneous or urethral catheter (Rodman et al, 1984) or by the intravenous administration of 1/6 M sodium lactate (Kursh and Resnick, 1984). Alkalization may decrease uric acid stones, but may induce calcium stones. Although its value is controversial, a low-purine diet may be considered. Weak uricosuric drugs (salicylates, thiazides) should be avoided. Allopurinol is often prescribed for patients at high risk for developing uric acid calculi, but there is no significant relationship between the serum level of uric acid and subsequent stone formation (Fessel, 1979).

Cystine Lithiasis: Cystinuria is inherited as an autosomal recessive trait and causes excessive urinary excretion of the dibasic amino acids, cystine, ornithine, lysine, and arginine; only cystine forms stones, for the other amino acids are readily soluble. Patients who excrete less than 800 mg cystine/day usually are managed by measures to achieve a urinary output of 3 to 4 L/day and by alkalization of the urine, which must be above pH 7.5 and is best accomplished with potassium citrate. Excessive methionine in the diet should be avoided, but low-methionine diets rarely are acceptable to patients.

If these measures are inadequate or if therapy is directed toward increasing the rate of dissolution of cystine calculi, penicillamine [Cuprimine, Depen] or the investigational drug, tiopronin (alpha-mercaptopropionylglycine), can be employed.

Penicillamine, tiopronin, tromethamine, and acetylcysteine have been employed to dissolve cystine calculi by pelvicaliceal irrigation. Of these, the most effective is acetylcysteine in an alkaline solution or tromethamine-E infusion (Dretler et al, 1984). Irrigation may be combined with shock wave lithotripsy (Schmeller et al, 1984).

Drug Evaluations

ACETOHYDROXAMIC ACID
[Lithostat]

$$CH_3-\overset{\overset{\displaystyle O}{\|}}{C}-\underset{\underset{\displaystyle H}{|}}{N}-OH$$

ACTIONS AND USES. This urease inhibitor is employed to prevent the formation of struvite stones that develop in the presence of urea-splitting bacteria (usually *Proteus*). The drug is ineffective for nonurease-producing organisms. Its use should be restricted to chronic infections not responsive to antibacterial therapy or surgery.

ADVERSE REACTIONS AND PRECAUTIONS. Acetohydroxamic acid should be used only in patients with adequate renal function (serum creatinine concentration below 3 mg/dl). It is contraindicated in women who are pregnant or who may become pregnant (FDA Pregnancy Category X). Pregnant patients exposed to this drug should be advised of its potential teratogenic effects.

In approximately 15% of patients, laboratory findings are characteristic of a Coombs'-negative hemolytic anemia. Some patients experience associated nausea, vomiting, anorexia, and malaise. A greater number exhibit mild reticulocytosis. These responses are reversible with discontinuation of therapy. Since acetohydroxamic acid chelates iron, hypochromic anemia should be managed by iron administration timed not to coincide with acetohydroxamic acid administration. Large doses of acetohydroxamic acid produce bone marrow depression in animals (leukopenia, thrombocytopenia), but this has not been encountered with clinical doses in man.

Mild, usually transient, headache responsive to salicylates is common during the first 48 hours of treatment. The drug has been associated with depression, anxiety, and tremulousness severe enough to warrant interrupting or discontinuing therapy in about 6% of patients.

Nausea, anorexia, and vomiting are common during initial therapy and usually do not persist. A nonpruritic, maculopapular rash of the upper extremities and face occurred, particularly with long-term therapy and in patients using alcoholic beverages. Avoidance of alcoholic beverages is recommended.

Superficial phlebitis of the lower extremities, sometimes with secondary pulmonary embolus, has been observed, particularly in patients with poor renal function. A history of thrombophlebitis should be considered a relative contraindication to the use of this agent.

DOSAGE AND PREPARATIONS.
Oral: *This drug should be taken on an empty stomach. Adults,* initially, 12 mg/kg/day administered in divided doses at six- to eight- hour intervals. The maximum daily dose should not exceed 1.5 g. *Children,* 10 mg/kg/day administered in divided doses two to three times a day.

Lithostat (Mission). Tablets 250 mg.

ALLOPURINOL
[Lopurin, Zyloprim]

Allopurinol is employed in urolithiasis associated with hyperuricemia and hyperuricosuria and in idiopathic calcium urolithiasis associated with hyperuricosuria (Tiselius, 1980). This latter condition may be benefited further if a thiazide is added to the regimen (Coe, 1978).

ADVERSE REACTIONS. The most common adverse reaction with allopurinol is maculopapular rash, frequently preceded by pruritus. Side effects that appear occasionally include nausea, vomiting, diarrhea, abdominal discomfort, drowsiness, headache, and a metallic taste.

For a more complete discussion of side effects and toxic reactions, see Chapter 60, Agents Used in Gout and Hyperuricemia. Large quantities of alcohol or vitamin C (ascorbic acid) may interfere with the action of allopurinol.

PHARMACOKINETICS. Oral bioavailability is about 80%. The volume of distribution is unknown. Allopurinol is not bound to protein. About 70% to 90% is metabolized rapidly (half-life, less than one hour) to the active metabolite, oxypurinol (alloxanthine), which has a half-life of 18 to 30 hours. Oxypurinol is excreted entirely by the kidney. When renal disease is present, the dose or dosing interval should be modified.

DOSAGE AND PREPARATIONS. Dosage should be individualized to obtain the desired urate level in hyperuricemic patients; the daily uric acid excretion should be less than 800 mg in men and 750 mg in women.

Oral: The usual *adult* dosage for urolithiasis is 300 mg once daily, and this dose should not be exceeded; 150 to 200 mg daily may be adequate. Allopurinol is better tolerated if taken after a meal. A high urine output (>2.5 L/day) must be maintained and urine should be kept alkaline.

> *Lopurin* (Boots), *Zyloprim* (Burroughs Wellcome), *Generic*. Tablets 100 and 300 mg.

ORTHOPHOSPHATES
[K-Phos Neutral, Neutra-Phos]

Orthophosphates used in urolithiasis consist of monobasic potassium phosphate with or without dibasic potassium phosphate, monobasic sodium phosphate, and dibasic sodium phosphate. The monobasic salts are known also as potassium acid phosphate and sodium acid phosphate, respectively. The combination salts are used to decrease the tendency for calcium to crystallize in the urine (see the Table and Chapter 49, Agents Affecting Calcium Metabolism). Acid phosphate salts should not be administered alone, since this may increase stone formation.

The most common adverse effect of phosphate salts is diarrhea. Patients with kidney stones may pass old stones when phosphate therapy is started and should be warned of this possibility. Phosphates are contraindicated in patients with infected stones and in those with renal function less than 30% of normal.

DOSAGE AND PREPARATIONS.

Oral: The average dosage for *adults* is 500 mg three or four times a day. An exact dosage does not appear to be critical, as long as the patient receives 1.5 to 2 g of elemental phosphorus in divided doses per 24 hours.

> *K-Phos Neutral* (Beach). Tablets containing dibasic sodium phosphate anhydrous 852 mg, monobasic potassium acid phosphate 155 mg, and monobasic sodium phosphate 130 mg (13 mEq sodium, 1.1 mEq potassium). This supplies 250 mg phosphorus per tablet.

> *Neutra-Phos* (Willen). Capsules containing monobasic and dibasic sodium phosphate 164 mg and monobasic and dibasic potassium phosphate 278 mg (7.125 mEq sodium, 7.125 mEq potassium). This supplies 765 mg phosphorus per capsule.

PENICILLAMINE
[Cuprimine, Depen]

$$CH_3 - \underset{\underset{CH_3}{|}}{\overset{\overset{SH}{|}}{C}} - \underset{\underset{H}{|}}{\overset{\overset{NH_2}{|}}{C}} - \overset{O}{\overset{||}{C}}OH$$

ACTIONS AND USES. This chelating agent forms a water-soluble mixed disulfide with cystine, which may prevent the formation of cystine stones and permit the dissolution of stones already formed. Because of its inherent toxicity, penicillamine should be used only if hydration with a urine output greater than 2 L/day and alkalization have been unsuccessful. A dilute, alkaline urine should be maintained during penicillamine therapy.

ADVERSE REACTIONS AND PRECAUTIONS. The incidence of side effects is high with penicillamine, and some reactions are potentially fatal. Therefore, long-term use demands adequate medical supervision. Most reactions occur shortly after therapy is begun.

Various types of rashes with different characteristics may develop. Erythematous maculopapular or morbilliform rashes with pruritus are common (incidence, 5%) and are considered to be hypersensitivity reactions; they often can be alleviated by concomitant administration of cyproheptadine or hydroxyzine. This rash usually disappears shortly after discontinuing medication and seldom recurs when therapy is resumed at a lower dosage. Less frequently, rash may occur after six or more months of treatment. This type usually appears on the trunk and is accompanied by intense pruritus. Following discontinuation of penicillamine, the rash may persist for many weeks and usually recurs if therapy is reinstituted.

Some patients may exhibit drug fever, usually two or three weeks after initiation of therapy, which may be accompanied by a macular eruption. Therapy should be discontinued temporarily until this reaction subsides and reinstituted at a lower dosage with the amount increased gradually. Systemic steroid therapy is usually helpful if the reaction recurs. Purpuric or vesicular ecchymoses or rashes accompanied by fever, leukopenia, thrombocytopenia, eosinophilia, arthralgia, and lymphadenopathy may indicate the onset of a penicillamine-induced autoimmune syndrome or bone marrow suppression. Therapy must be discontinued and adrenal corticosteroids administered if necessary.

If oral mucosal ulcers resembling aphthae and gastrointestinal upset occur, they usually respond to a reduction in dosage. Oral mucosal ulcers characterized by bullous lesions require discontinuation of penicillamine and treatment with corticosteroids.

Impairment of taste (hypogeusia) develops in some patients (incidence, 12%) and may progress to a total loss of taste. The effect is transient and normal sensitivity usually returns after two or three months of therapy. The administration of copper salts to overcome this effect is without benefit.

Anorexia, nausea, vomiting, and epigastric pain may occur (incidence, 17%). Isolated cases of cholestatic jaundice and pancreatitis, which presumably were induced by penicillamine, have been reported.

The two most common symptoms of serious toxicity are bone marrow suppression and immune disorders. Thrombocytopenia (incidence, 4%) and leukopenia (incidence, 2%) are early signs of impending bone marrow aplasia, which may be manifested by agranulocytosis, selective red cell aplasia, or erythromyeloid aplasia. Leukopenia is of the granulocytic type and sometimes is associated with an increase in the number of eosinophils. Thrombocytopenia, with decreased megakaryocytes in the marrow, is part of the aplastic anemia syndrome. If the marrow content of megakaryocytes is normal or increased, it is presumed that the thrombocytopenia is an immune reaction.

Autoimmune or immune complex disorders that are presumed to be caused by penicillamine include dermatomyositis, polymyositis, lupus erythematosus, diffuse alveolitis, obliterative bronchiolitis, and myasthenia gravis.

Nephrotic syndrome may occur after several months of treatment. When reversible proteinuria develops during therapy (incidence, 6%), the dosage should not be increased further and quantitative urinary protein determinations should be performed periodically. Therapy should be terminated if proteinuria exceeds 2 g/24 hours or if hematuria occurs. The development of abnormal urinary findings suggestive of glomerulonephritis, hemoptysis, and pulmonary infiltrates (Goodpasture's syndrome) occurs rarely and requires immediate discontinuation of penicillamine therapy.

Optic neuropathy has been observed in patients given racemic penicillamine but has not been reported with use of the D isomer; the neuropathy disappeared after administration of pyridoxine.

Careful examination of the skin, as well as urinalysis, differential and white blood cell counts, direct platelet counts, and hemoglobin determinations should be performed every three days during the first two weeks of therapy, at least every ten days for three or four months, and monthly thereafter for the duration of treatment. If the white blood count falls below 3,500/microliter or the platelet count below 100,000/microliter, penicillamine should be discontinued until these values return to normal. When therapy is resumed, the initial dose should be small and the amount increased cautiously.

It is recommended that the drug be withheld from pregnant patients with cystinuria. If continued therapy with penicillamine is considered necessary, the dosage should be limited to 1 g/day if possible. If cesarean section is planned, the dose should be reduced to 250 mg/day during the last six weeks of pregnancy and during the immediate postoperative period until healing has occurred.

Cross sensitivity between penicillin and penicillamine does not always occur; therefore, penicillamine can be given cautiously to patients who are hypersensitive to penicillin.

DOSAGE AND PREPARATIONS. Penicillamine should be given on an *empty stomach* at least one hour before meals, and other medication should not be taken concurrently.

The interruption of therapy for even a few days may cause sensitivity reactions when treatment is reinstituted. *This must be stressed to the patient.* If therapy is interrupted, it should be reinstituted at a lower dosage, which is increased gradually to the full amount.

Oral: For cystinuria, *adults,* initially 1 g (increasing gradually to 2.5 g, if necessary) daily in four divided doses; *young children and infants,* 30 mg/kg/day in four divided doses. If the patient cannot tolerate the full calculated dosage of penicillamine, a daily dose of 250 mg may be given initially and increments added gradually. If equal doses are not possible or if adverse reactions necessitate a reduction in dosage, the largest amount should be given at bedtime. High fluid intake also is required (about 500 ml of water at bedtime and another 500 ml during the night when the urine is more concentrated and more acidic than during the day). Effective therapy is indicated by the urinary excretion of less than 100 to 200 mg of cystine/L.

Because of the drug's effects on collagen and elastin, the dosage is reduced to 250 mg/day prior to elective oral or general surgery.

Patients should be given supplemental pyridoxine 25 mg/day during long-term penicillamine therapy because of increased requirements for this vitamin. Iron deficiency may develop, particularly in children or menstruating women. Since preparations containing iron may interfere with the action of penicillamine, at least two hours should elapse between the administration of the drug and iron salts.

Cuprimine (Merck Sharp & Dohme). Capsules 125 and 250 mg.
Depen (Wallace). Tablets 250 mg.

POTASSIUM CITRATE
[Polycitra-K, Urocit-K]

ACTIONS AND USES. Potassium citrate is metabolized to potassium bicarbonate; the induced alkali load increases renal clearance of citrate. This preparation decreases the saturation and spontaneous nucleation of calcium oxalate. It is useful in patients with hypocitraturic calcium urolithiasis with hypocitraturia as the sole abnormality and to correct hypocitraturia occurring with other metabolic abnormalities, such as absorptive hypercalciuria, renal tubular acidosis, and enteric hyperoxaluria (Pak et al, 1983). It may be combined with a thiazide and/or allopurinol to treat hypercitraturic or hyperuricosuric calcium oxalate urolithiasis. Potassium citrate also may be used to alkalize the urine in patients with stones composed of cystine, uric acid, or xanthine.

ADVERSE REACTIONS AND PRECAUTIONS. Some patients complain of gastroenteric discomfort, bad taste, and a laxative effect when taking the liquid preparation, which may be minimized by diluting the preparation in water and taking it after meals. These side effects are less common with the tablet form. Potassium citrate should not be used in the presence of active urinary tract infection or severe renal impairment. The concurrent administration of other potassium-containing medications or potassium-sparing diuretics, especially in the presence of renal disease, may lead to serious hyperkalemia and systemic alkalosis. The tablet preparation should not be used in patients with active peptic ulcer. In patients who require a potassium-restricted diet, sodium citrate and citric acid solution [Bicitra] should be substituted.

DOSAGE AND PREPARATIONS.

Oral: (Syrup) *Adults,* 15 to 30 ml; *children,* 5 to 15 ml. This amount is diluted in water and taken four times a day after meals and at bedtime.

(Tablets) *Adults*, two to four tablets three times daily within one-half hour of meals.

Polycitra-K (Willen). Each 5 ml of syrup contains potassium citrate monohydrate 1.1 g and citric acid monohydrate 334 mg. Each 5 ml contains 10 mEq potassium (approximately equivalent to 10 mEq bicarbonate).

Urocit-K (Mission). Each tablet contains 5 mEq potassium citrate.

SODIUM CELLULOSE PHOSPHATE
[Calcibind]

ACTIONS AND USES. This agent is taken with meals to reduce the absorption of dietary and secreted calcium from the intestinal tract. It is indicated *only* for absorptive hypercalciuria Type I associated with recurrent calcium oxalate or calcium phosphate urolithiasis. Sodium cellulose phosphate 5 g reduces urinary calcium by approximately 50 mg.

ADVERSE REACTIONS AND PRECAUTIONS. This drug is contraindicated in patients with primary or secondary hyperparathyroidism, including renal hypercalciuria; hypocalcemic states (hypoparathyroidism, intestinal malabsorption); bone disease (osteoporosis, osteomalacia, osteitis); hypomagnesemia (serum magnesium less than 1.5 mg/dl); or enteric hyperoxaluria and in patients with seriously impaired renal function (glomerular filtration rate less than 40 ml/minute).

Sodium cellulose phosphate also reduces the intestinal absorption of dietary magnesium. The resulting hypomagnesemia responds to supplementation with magnesium. Since less calcium is available to bind oxalate, urinary oxalate increases, but the level is reduced by a moderate restriction of dietary oxalate and the use of sodium cellulose phosphate 10 to 15 g/day.

Because of the increased need for dietary calcium, sodium cellulose phosphate should not be used in children less than 16 years or during pregnancy (FDA Pregnancy Category C).

As the result of the decreased intestinal absorption of calcium, parathyroid function may increase and lead to bone disease. Therefore, parathyroid function, serum calcium, and serum magnesium should be assessed at three- to six- month intervals. If there is an increase in serum parathyroid hormone, the drug should be stopped or the dosage adjusted. If there is an inadequate hypocalciuric response to the drug (a reduction in urinary calcium of less than 30 mg/5 mg sodium cellulose phosphate while patients are on a moderate calcium-restricted diet), therapy should be considered ineffective and the agent discontinued. Urinary excretion of oxalate in excess of 55 mg/day also is reason to reassess therapy. Although the continued use of sodium cellulose phosphate does not seem to affect trace elements, copper, zinc, and iron, these elements should be measured periodically until more experience with this drug has accumulated.

A dose of 15 g contains 23 to 48 mEq of exchangeable sodium, which should be considered before sodium cellulose phosphate is used in patients with congestive heart failure or ascites. Some patients complain of loose bowel movements or diarrhea.

DOSAGE AND PREPARATIONS.

Oral: The drug is suspended in water, a soft drink, or fruit juice for ingestion during or within 30 minutes of each meal. The initial dose in patients on a moderate calcium-restricted diet with a 24-hour urinary excretion of calcium greater than 300 mg is 15 g/day. In patients with a lower initial calcium excretion but greater than 200 mg/day, the dose is 10 g/day.

Patients receiving 15 g/day should receive 1.5 g magnesium gluconate before breakfast and at bedtime at least one hour before or after ingestion of sodium cellulose phosphate. The dose of supplemental magnesium gluconate for patients receiving 10 g/day of sodium cellulose phosphate is 1 g twice daily.

Calcibind (Mission). Powder 2.5 g (sodium content 11%).

THIAZIDES

The thiazide diuretics are used to reduce the urinary calcium level in patients with hypercalciuria. These drugs may be combined with allopurinol to treat calcium urolithiasis associated with hyperuricemia.

For precautions and adverse effects, see Chapter 29, Diuretics. Hypokalemia should be avoided by potassium supplementation as needed to prevent hypocitraturia.

DOSAGE AND PREPARATIONS.

Oral: Hydrochlorothiazide 50 mg twice daily or the equivalent of other thiazides. It is important to avoid a high dietary intake of sodium or potassium, since this can negate the hypocalciuric response to the thiazides.

For preparations, see Chapter 29.

TIOPRONIN (Alpha-Mercaptopropionylglycine)
[Thiola]

$$CH_3CHCNHCH_2COH$$

This investigational drug forms a water-soluble mixed disulfide with cystine and is used to dissolve cystine calculi. The toxicity of tiopronin has been reported to be lower than that of penicillamine, although both drugs produce a dose-related nephrotic syndrome. For this reason, routine monitoring of urinary protein excretion is recommended. Other adverse effects include urticaria, fever, lymphadenopathy, and essentially all of the side effects of penicillamine, although to a lesser degree.

DOSAGE AND PREPARATIONS. Tiopronin should be given on an *empty stomach* at least one hour before meals, and other medication should not be taken concurrently.

Oral: The dosage should be less than 50 mg/kg/day; hydration to maintain a urine output above 2 L/day and alkalization to a urinary pH of 6.8 to 7.0 are essential during therapy.

Thiola (Santen Pharmaceutical Company, Japan).
(Investigational drug)

Cited References

Ambrosini PJ: Pharmacological paradigm for urinary incontinence and enuresis. *J Clin Psychopharmacol* 4:247-253, 1984.

Andersson K-E, et al: Effects of prazosin on isolated human urethra and in patients with lower motor neuron lesions. *Invest Urol* 19:39-42, 1981.

Awad SA, Downie JW: Pharmacologic therapy, in McGuire EJ (ed): *Urinary Incontinence.* New York, Grune & Stratton, 1981, 87-111.

Awad SA, et al: Alpha-adrenergic agents in urinary disorders of proximal urethra: Part 1. Sphincteric incontinence. *Br J Urol* 50:332-335, 1978.

Barbalias GA, Blaivas JG: Neurologic implications of pathologically open bladder neck. *J Urol* 129:780-782, 1983.

Barrett DM: Effect of oral bethanechol chloride on voiding in female patients with excessive residual urine: Randomized double-blind study. *J Urol* 126:640-642, 1981.

Bauer SB, et al: Unstable bladder of childhood. *Urol Clin North Am* 7:321-336, 1980.

Benson GS, et al: Bladder muscle contractility: Comparative effects and mechanisms of action of atropine, propantheline, flavoxate, and imipramine. *Urology* 9:31-35, 1977.

Blaivas JG: Pathophysiology of lower urinary tract dysfunction. *Clin Obstet Gynecol* 12:11-25, 1985.

Blaivas JG, Barbalias GA: Characteristics of neural injury after abdomino-perineal resection. *J Urol* 129:84-87, 1983.

Blaivas JG, et al: Detrusor-external sphincter dyssynergia: Detailed electromyographic study. *J Urol* 125:545-548, 1981.

Brocklebank JT, Meadow SR: Cure of giggle micturition. *Arch Dis Child* 56:232-234, 1981.

Brown BT, et al: Guanethidine sulfate in prevention of autonomic hyperreflexia. *J Urol* 122:55-57, 1979.

Caine M, et al: Phenoxybenzamine for benign prostatic obstruction: Review of 200 cases. *Urology* 27:542-546, 1981.

Cantor EB (ed): *Female Urinary Stress Incontinence.* Springfield, IL, Charles C Thomas, 1979.

Cardozo LD, Stanton SL: Comparison between bromocriptine and indomethacin in treatment of detrusor instability. *J Urol* 123:399-401, 1980.

Castleden CM, et al: Imipramine: Possible alternative to current therapy for urinary incontinence in the elderly. *J Urol* 125:318-320, 1981.

Coe FL: Hyperuricosuric calcium oxalate nephrolithiasis. *Kidney Int* 13:418-426, 1978.

Coe FL: Prevention of kidney stones. *Am J Med* 71:514-516, 1981.

Coe FL, Favus MJ: Renal calculi, in Conn HF (ed): *Current Therapy.* Philadelphia, WB Saunders, 1979, 530-535.

Delaere KPJ, et al: Value of intravesical prostaglandin E$_2$ and F$_{2\alpha}$ in women with abnormalities of bladder emptying. *Br J Urol* 53:306-309, 1981.

Desmond AD, et al: Clinical experience with intravesical prostaglandin E$_2$: Prospective study of 36 patients. *Br J Urol* 52:357-366, 1980.

Diokno AC: Practical approach to management of urinary incontinence in the elderly. *Compr Ther* 9:67-75, (July) 1983.

Diokno AC, Koppenhoefer R: Bethanechol chloride in neurogenic bladder dysfunction. *Urology* 8:455-458, 1976.

Diokno AC, Sonda LP: Pharmacological management of neuropathic bladder and urethra, in Caine M (ed): *The Pharmacology of the Urinary Tract.* New York, Springer-Verlag, 1984, 77-99.

Diokno AC, Taub M: Ephedrine in treatment of urinary incontinence. *Urology* 5:624-625, 1975.

Downie JW: Bethanechol chloride in urology: Discussion of issues. *Neurourol Urodynam* 3:211-222, 1984.

Drach GW: Urinary lithiasis, in Harrison JH, et al (eds): *Campbell's Urology,* ed 4. Philadelphia, WB Saunders, 1978, 779-878.

Dretler SP, et al: Percutaneous catheter dissolution of cystine calculi. *J Urol* 131:216-219, 1984.

Fantl JA, et al: Detrusor instability syndrome: Use of bladder retraining drills with and without anticholinergics. *Am J Obstet Gynecol* 140:885-890, 1981.

Ferrie BG, et al: Experience with bladder training in 65 patients. *Br J Urol* 56:482-484, 1984.

Fessel WJ: Renal outcomes of gout and hyperuricemia. *Am J Med* 67:74-82, 1979.

Finkbeiner AE: Is bethanechol chloride clinically effective in promoting bladder emptying? Literature review. *J Urol* 134:443-449, 1985.

Finkbeiner AE, Bissada NK: Drug therapy for lower urinary tract dysfunction. *Urol Clin North Am* 7:3-16, 1980.

Firlit CF, Cook WA: Voiding pattern abnormalities in children. *Urology* 10:25-29, 1977.

Fletcher TF, Bradley WE: Neuroanatomy of bladder-urethra. *J Urol* 119:153-160, 1978.

Fowler JE Jr: Prospective study of intravesical dimethyl sulfoxide in treatment of suspected early interstitial cystitis. *Urology* 18:21-26, 1981.

Gleason DM: Female urologic disorders, in Devine CJ Jr, Stecker JF Jr (eds): *Urology in Practice.* Boston, Little, Brown and Company, 1978, 201-230.

Godec CJ: "Timed voiding": Useful tool in treatment of urinary incontinence. *Urology* 23:97-100, 1984.

Graham JB: Female urethral syndrome? *Urol Clin North Am* 7:59-62, 1980.

Graham SD: Present urological treatment of spinal cord injury patients. *J Urol* 126:1-4, 1981.

Graziani G, et al: Do thiazides prevent recurrent idiopathic renal calcium stones, (letter). *Lancet* 2:578-579, 1981.

Hackler RH, et al: Clinical experience with dantrolene sodium for external urinary sphincter hypertonicity in spinal cord injured patients. *J Urol* 124:78-81, 1980.

Hanna MK, et al: Urodynamics in children: Part II. Pseudoneurogenic bladder. *J Urol* 125:534-537, 1981.

Holm CN, Hessov I: Effect of calcium treatment on urinary stone index after intestinal bypass for obesity. *Digestion* 22:255-258, 1981.

Jarvis GJ: Controlled trial of bladder drill and drug therapy in management of detrusor instability. *Br J Urol* 53:565-566, 1981.

Johansson G, et al: Biochemical and clinical effects of prophylactic treatment of renal calcium stones with magnesium hydroxide. *J Urol* 124:770-774, 1980.

Kaplan WE, et al: Female urethral syndrome: External sphincter spasm as etiology. *J Urol* 124:48-49, 1980.

Kass EJ, et al: Enuresis: Principles of management and result of treatment. *J Urol* 121:794-796, 1979.

Kleeman FJ: Use of phenoxybenzamine poorly defined. *Urology* 9:708, 1977.

Koff SA: Non-neuropathic vesico-urethral dysfunction in children, in Mundy AR, et al (eds): *Urodynamics: Principles, Practice and Application.* New York, Churchill Livingstone, 1984, 311-325.

Koff SA, et al: Uninhibited bladder in children: Cause for urinary obstruction, infection, and reflux, in Hodson J, Kinkaid-Smith P (eds): *Reflux Nephropathy.* New York, Masson, 1978, 161-170.

Komaroff AL, Friedland G: Dysuria-pyuria syndrome. *N Engl J Med* 303:452-454, 1980.

Kosko J, Resnick MI: Urinary calculi: Evaluation and medical management, in Resnick MI (ed): *Current Trends in Urology.* Baltimore, Williams & Wilkins, 1985, vol 3, 59-68.

Kursh ED, Resnick MI: Dissolution of uric acid calculi with systemic alkalization. *J Urol* 132:286-287, 1984.

Leventhal A, Pfau A: Pharmacologic management of postoperative overdistention of bladder. *Surg Gynecol Obstet* 146:347-348, 1978.

Leyson JFJ, et al: Baclofen in treatment of detrusor-sphincter dyssynergia in spinal cord injury patients. *J Urol* 124:82-84, 1980.

Lloyd LK: Neurogenic bladder dysfunction. *Cont Educat* 11:21-42, 1979.

Lockhart JL, et al: Neurogenic bladder dysfunction in Shy-Drager syndrome. *J Urol* 126:119-121, 1981.

McGuire EJ: Upper motor neuron lesions; lower motor neuron lesions, in Kaufman JJ (ed): *Current Urologic Therapy.* Philadelphia, WB Saunders, 1980, 236-243.

McGuire EJ, et al: Prognostic value of urodynamic testing in myelodysplastic patients. *J Urol* 126:205-209, 1981.

McKendry JBJ, et al: Primary enuresis: Relative success of three methods of treatment. *Can Med Assoc J* 113:953-955, 1975.

588

Messing EM, Freiha FS: Complication of Clorpactin WCS90 therapy for interstitial cystitis. *Urology* 13:389-392, 1979.

Messing EM, Stamey TA: Interstitial cystitis. *Urology* 12:381-392, 1978.

Mikkelsen EJ, Rapoport JL: Enuresis: Psychopathology, sleep stage, and drug response. *Urol Clin North Am* 7:361-377, 1980.

Mikkelsen EJ, et al: Childhood enuresis: I. Sleep patterns and psychopathology. II. Psychopathology, tricyclic concentration in plasma, and antienuretic effect. *Arch Gen Psychiatry* 37:1139-1145, 1146-1152, 1980.

Mobley DF: Phenoxybenzamine in management of neurogenic vesical dysfunction. *J Urol* 116:737-738, 1976.

Mohr JA, et al: Stress urinary incontinence: Simple and practical approach to diagnosis and treatment. *J Am Geriatr Soc* 31:476-478, 1983.

Mulcahy JJ, James HE: Management of neurogenic bladder in infancy and childhood. *Urology* 13:235- 240, 1979.

Mundy AR, et al (eds): *Urodynamics: Principles, Practice and Application*. New York, Churchill Livingston, 1984.

Nemoy NJ: Renacidin in treatment of infection stones, in Kaufman JJ (ed): *Current Urologic Therapy*. Philadelphia, WB Saunders, 1980, 145-146.

Olsson CA, et al: Phentolamine test in neurogenic bladder dysfunction. *J Urol* 117:481-485, 1977.

Osborn DE, et al: Prostatodynia: Physiological characteristics and rational management with muscle relaxants. *Br J Urol* 53:621-623, 1981.

Pak CYC: Medical management of nephrolithiasis. *J Urol* 128:1157-1164, 1982.

Pak CYC, et al: Evidence justifying high fluid intake in treatment of nephrolithiasis. *Ann Intern Med* 93:36-39, 1980.

Pak CYC, et al: Physiological and physicochemical correction and prevention of calcium stone formation by potassium citrate therapy. *Trans Assoc Am Phys* 96:294-305, 1983.

Parsons CL: Urinary tract infections in female patient. *Urol Clin North Am* 12:355-360, 1985.

Pinder RM, et al: Dantrolene sodium: Review of its pharmacologic properties and therapeutic efficacy in spasticity. *Drugs* 13:3-23, 1977.

Raz S, Smith RB: External sphincter spasticity syndrome in female patients. *J Urol* 115:443-446, 1976.

Redman JF: Pharmacologic management of nocturnal enuresis, in Finkbeiner AE, et al (eds): *Pharmacology of the Urinary Tract and Male Reproductive System*. New York, Appleton-Century-Crofts, 1982, 273-284.

Rodman JS, et al: Dissolution of uric acid calculi. *J Urol* 131:1039-1044, 1984.

Rogers MP, et al: Giggle incontinence. *JAMA* 247:1446-1448, 1982.

Rudman D, et al: Hypocitraturia in patients with gastrointestinal malabsorption. *N Engl J Med* 303:657-661, 1980.

Sawczuk I, Blaivas JG: Successful surgical treatment of giggle incontinence: Case report. *Neurourol Urodynam* 3:63-66, 1984.

Schmeller NT, et al: Combination of chemolysis and shock wave lithotripsy in treatment of cystine renal calculi. *J Urol* 131:434-438, 1984.

Schmidt RA: Urethral syndrome. *Urol Clin North Am* 12:349-354, 1985.

Scott MB, Morrow JW: Phenoxybenzamine in neurogenic bladder dysfunction after spinal cord injury. II. Autonomic dysreflexia. *J Urol* 119:483-484, 1978.

Shirley SW, et al: Dimethyl sulfoxide in treatment of inflammatory genitourinary disorders. *Urology* 11:215-220, 1978.

Siroky MB, et al: Functional voiding disorders in men. *J Urol* 126:200-204, 1981.

Smey P, et al: Voiding pattern abnormalities in normal children: Results of pharmacologic manipulation. *J Urol* 120:574-577, 1978.

Smey P, et al: Dysfunctional voiding in children secondary to internal sphincter dyssynergia: Treatment with phenoxybenzamine. *Urol Clin North Am* 7:337-347, 1980.

Smith LH: Urolithiasis, in Earley LE, Gottschalk CW (eds): *Strauss and Welt's Diseases of the Kidney*, ed 3. Boston, Little, Brown and Company, 1979, 893-931.

Smith LH: Enteric hyperoxaluria and other hyperoxaluric states, in Coe FL, et al (eds): *Contemporary Issues in Nephrology*. New York, Churchill Livingston, 1980, vol 5, 136-164.

Smith LH: Medical treatment of idiopathic calcium urolithiasis. *Kidney* 16:9-15, (March) 1983.

Smith LH, et al: Nutrition and urolithiasis. *N Engl J Med* 298:87-89, 1978.

Sonda LP, et al: Further observations on cystometric and uroflowmetric effects of bethanechol chloride on the human bladder. *J Urol* 122:775-777, 1979.

Stamm WE, et al: Treatment of acute urethral syndrome. *N Engl J Med* 304:956-958, 1981.

Stewart MA: Treatment of bedwetting. *JAMA* 232:281-283, 1975.

Stewart BH, et al: Stress incontinence: Conservative therapy with sympathomimetic drugs. *J Urol* 115:558-559, 1976.

Streem SB: Genitourinary malacoplakia in renal transplant recipients: Pathogenic, prognostic and therapeutic considerations. *J Urol* 132:10-12, 1984.

Taylor MC, Bates CP: Double-blind crossover trial of baclofen: New treatment for unstable bladder syndrome. *Br J Urol* 51:504-505, 1979.

Tiselius H-G: Inhibition of calcium oxalate crystal growth in urine during treatment with allopurinol. *Br J Urol* 52:189-192, 1980.

Vaidyanathan S, et al: Study of intravesical instillation of 15(S)-15 methyl prostaglandin F_2-alpha in patients with neurogenic bladder dysfunction. *J Urol* 126:81-85, 1981.

Walsh A: Interstitial cystitis, in Harrison JH, et al (eds): *Campbell's Urology*, ed 4. Philadelphia, WB Saunders, 1978, 693-707.

Waterfall NB, Williams G: Effects of phenoxybenzamine on bladder neck opening. *J R Soc Med* 73:345-347, 1980.

Wein AJ: Pharmacologic approaches to management of neurogenic bladder dysfunction. *J Contin Educat Urol* 18:17-34, 1979.

Wein AJ: Non-surgical treatment of lower urinary tract dysfunction in the female, in Raz S (ed): *Female Urology*. New York, WB Saunders, 1983, 161-168.

Wein AJ: Pharmacology of bladder and urethra, in Mundy AR, et al (eds): *Urodynamics: Principles, Practice and Application*. New York, Churchill Livingstone, 1984 A, 26-41.

Wein AJ: Pharmacological treatment of non-neurogenic voiding dysfunction, in Caine M (ed): *The Pharmacology of the Urinary Tract*. New York, Springer-Verlag, 1984 B, 100-134.

Wein AJ: Pharmacologic treatment of lower urinary tract dysfunction in the female patient. *Urol Clin North Am* 12:259-269, 1985.

Wein AJ, et al: Effects of bethanechol chloride on urodynamic parameters in normal women and in women with significant residual urine volumes. *J Urol* 124:397-399, 1980.

Weiss BD: Unstable bladder in elderly patients. *Am Fam Physician* 28:243-247, (Oct) 1983.

Williams JJ, et al: Randomized double-blind study of acetohydroxamic acid in struvite nephrolithiasis. *N Engl J Med* 311:760-764, 1984.

Wulfsohn MA, Rubenstein A: Management of Shy-Drager syndrome with propantheline and intermittent self-catheterization: Case report. *J Urol* 126:122-123, 1981.

Yendt ER, Cohanim M: Prevention of calcium stones with thiazides. *Kidney Int* 13:397-409, 1978.

Agents Used to Treat Deficiency Anemias

IRON DEFICIENCY ANEMIAS

   Iron Compounds

MEGALOBLASTIC ANEMIAS

   Vitamin B$_{12}$ Compounds

   Folates

SIDEROBLASTIC ANEMIAS

REFRACTORY ANEMIAS

MIXTURES

Anemia, defined as a hemoglobin concentration below that considered normal for the individual, is indicative of underlying disease and should be investigated. It often is secondary to chronic blood loss, increased hemolysis, replacement or incompetence of marrow, nutritional deficiency, infection, inflammation, chronic diseases, endocrine deficiencies, or malignancy.

A definitive diagnosis is essential for the treatment of anemia and, if possible, its underlying cause. History, physical examination, and laboratory studies should be done. The initial laboratory screening tests include red cell indices, particularly mean corpuscular volume (MCV); blood smear; leukocyte count and differential; reticulocyte count; and platelet count. If the underlying cause of anemia is not apparent after these tests have been performed, further investigation of the pathophysiologic states associated with decreased red cell production and life span is indicated. The discussion in this chapter is limited to anemias caused by deficiency in which replacement of the specific nutrient elicits normal production and lifespan of erythrocytes.

In nutritional anemias, the production of red cells is impaired by dietary deficiency of substances essential for erythropoiesis: iron, folate, and cobalamin. In the United States, iron deficiency is the most common dietary cause of anemia in children and young women (Dallman et al, 1984); in men and postmenopausal women, the cause usually is abnormal bleeding. Folic acid deficiency is less common and anemias caused by deficiencies of vitamin B$_{12}$ or other hematopoietic nutrients are rare.

IRON DEFICIENCY ANEMIAS

Iron Distribution: Iron is present in every cell. It is a constituent of hemoglobin, myoglobin, and a number of enzymes necessary for oxygen transfer. Iron is stored as ferritin or hemosiderin, primarily in hepatic cells and reticuloendothelial cells of the spleen and marrow.

Iron is absorbed through the intestinal mucosa into the blood where, bound to transferrin, it is transported to the marrow and all other tissues. Absorption is most efficient in the duodenum and decreases progressively throughout the intestinal tract. Many factors influence utilization but, for the most part, hemoglobin synthesis controls the rate of plasma iron turnover. Reticuloendothelial reserves are derived from both dietary sources and red blood cell destruction. Stored iron can be mobilized for hemoglobin synthesis.

Iron is rigidly conserved. Only small amounts are lost through sloughing of epithelial cells from the skin or gastrointestinal, genitourinary, and respiratory systems. Homeostasis is maintained by control of iron absorption in response to body iron needs. Absorption is increased in iron deficiency and during periods of increased erythropoiesis (Savin and Cook, 1980).

Iron Depletion: Deficiency results from acute or chronic blood loss and inadequate intake during periods of accelerated growth in infants and children or increased demands in pregnant women. Menstruation is the most common cause of bleeding in women and they require more iron than men. When rapid growth or pregnancy does not appear to underlie iron deficiency, it is prudent to conclude that blood loss is the cause (almost no diet is so poor in iron that it cannot offset the obligatory metabolic loss of 1 mg daily). Therefore, the treatment of iron deficiency anemia requires that the source of blood loss be identified and that hemoglobin be replenished. The first requirement is often most important, particularly in men and postmenopausal women. Blood loss and iron deficiency in men result only from disease. Cancer is the cause in at least 2% of adults with iron deficiency anemia. In tropical and subtropical areas, the most common cause of chronic bleeding is hookworm infestation.

When bleeding is slow and chronic, the hemoglobin concentration is maintained by mobilization of tissue iron stores, and anemia develops only after reserves are depleted. Thus, anemia is not a sensitive indicator of iron depletion. Although hypochromic microcytic red blood cells usually signify iron deficiency, they may result from abnormal hemoglobin synthesis.

Early iron depletion produces few recognizable changes in red cell morphology but can be confirmed by decreased or absent marrow hemosiderin. Reliable estimates also can be determined without marrow aspiration. When the saturation of serum transferrin is 15% or less (less than 10% in young children) and the total iron binding capacity (TIBC) is increased (more than 400 mcg/dl), iron deficiency is present. However, a serum ferritin level of less than 12 mcg/L is diagnostic of iron deficiency and the other tests help to determine the severity of depletion (Cook, 1982). Because liver disease, infection, or other chronic diseases may be associated with elevated serum ferritin levels, a value in the normal range does not exclude iron deficiency anemia.

Iron Compounds

Prophylactic use of iron preparations should be reserved for individuals at high risk of developing iron deficiency, pregnant and lactating women, low-birth-weight infants, and infants maintained on unsupplemented milk formulas. Iron supplements also may be indicated in rapidly growing children whose diets contain little meat and in adults with chronic blood loss (eg, heavy menses, hereditary hemorrhagic telangiectasia). The inappropriate prophylactic use of iron should be avoided in adults because excessive accumulation may damage tissues (Olsson et al, 1978). Prophylactic use of iron also may mask iron loss associated with occult malignancy and delay diagnosis.

Therapeutic doses of iron are used only to treat iron deficiency anemia. Oral administration is preferred. Because they are absorbed more easily, ferrous salts (sulfate, fumarate, gluconate) are preferred to ferric salts, including chelated compounds.

Formulations and Dosage: Ferrous sulfate is the standard for other oral iron preparations. Most patients respond to this form and those who do not are unlikely to benefit from any iron salt. Therefore, when ferrous sulfate is well tolerated, there is seldom justification for use of more complex and expensive preparations. Timed-release and enteric-coated preparations are designed to prevent the release of iron in the stomach, where it is irritating, and to maximize iron release in the duodenum. However, some of these products transport iron past the sites of maximal absorption and actually reduce the amount available.

Gastrointestinal tolerance of any iron preparation depends on the amount of ionized elemental iron present. Despite claims to the contrary, substitution of one form for another may not relieve untoward effects if equivalent amounts of elemental iron are given.

Because the iron content varies greatly among preparations, the dosage should be calculated in terms of elemental iron. For iron-deficient adults, manufacturers recommend 50 to 100 mg of elemental iron (one 300-mg ferrous sulfate tablet contains 60 mg of elemental iron) three times daily to replenish body iron stores within six months. However, 30 mg of elemental iron daily appears to correct most uncomplicated anemias rapidly, although iron stores are replenished more slowly. Iron is absorbed best when taken between meals, but the usual dosage provides an excess and the preparation can be taken with meals to reduce intolerance. However, iron should not be taken with carbonate antacids or tetracyclines. Traditionally, one tablet daily is given initially with a meal to minimize side effects and increase compliance.

In most adults with severe iron deficiency anemia (hemoglobin less than 6 g/dl), 100 mg of elemental iron daily corrects uncomplicated deficiency rapidly and produces maximum repletion of iron stores with minimum adverse effects; larger doses are unnecessary and undesirable. The therapeutic response is limited by the amount of erythropoietic marrow, which does not enlarge very rapidly after therapy begins. Thus, additional iron cannot hasten repletion (Crosby, 1984). Larger doses do not increase hemoglobin regeneration appreciably but do increase side effects (Savin, 1982).

The hematologic response to oral iron becomes evident after two weeks. In iron-deficient patients, adequate oral treatment increases hemoglobin production by 0.1 to 0.2 g/dl of blood daily or 2 g/dl in the first three weeks of treatment; values usually become normal after two months in uncomplicated cases. To replenish depleted iron stores when blood loss has stopped, oral therapy should continue for four to six months after the hemoglobin level has returned to normal. When bleeding cannot be controlled (eg, heavy menses), iron should be given indefinitely or until bleeding stops (eg, at menopause).

If the response is not satisfactory after three weeks of therapy, it is probable that (1) the diagnosis of iron deficiency anemia is incorrect, (2) the dosage regimen is not being followed, (3) blood loss is occurring simultaneously, or (4) complicating factors (eg, defective iron absorption or utilization, infection, chronic disease) are present. If the patient is assimilating iron while blood loss continues, the reticulocyte count may be elevated. When relapse occurs after therapy is withdrawn, abnormal blood loss is continuing. Iron deficiency need not be corrected rapidly if bleeding has stopped or is known not to be harmful (eg, menorrhagia) and iron metabolism is in positive balance.

Parenteral iron (iron dextran injection [Imferon]) acts similarly to oral iron but is rarely indicated for the treatment of iron deficiency. Because serious reactions may develop, parenteral iron should be reserved for patients with a confirmed diagnosis of iron deficiency who do not respond to oral therapy (eg, continuing loss greater than can be replaced because of limitations to intestinal absorption), when immediate replacement is necessary, or when patients refuse to take iron orally.

Malabsorption syndromes (eg, tropical sprue, celiac disease, partial gastrectomy) and apparent intolerance to iron usually do not constitute valid indications for parenteral iron therapy. Marked malabsorption of iron is rare. Following gastric resection, rapid transit past the duodenum may reduce absorption. However, even in these patients, absorption usually is adequate to produce a therapeutic response, particularly if a liquid preparation is used. Intolerance probably is dose related and may be corrected by decreasing the size of each dose.

For a discussion on combination products containing iron, see the section on Mixtures.

Adverse Reactions and Precautions: Iron compounds are contraindicated in patients with primary or secondary hemochromatosis, including thalassemia major and transfusion siderosis. Iron overload and siderosis may occur if iron is given to patients with chronic inflammation or chronic renal disease. These preparations should not be used to treat hemolytic anemias unless iron deficiency also exists, since storage of excess iron may cause secondary hemochromatosis. Iron overload is particularly likely in patients given excessive amounts of parenteral iron, in those taking both oral and parenteral preparations, and in patients with refractory anemias erroneously diagnosed as iron deficiency anemia. Iron should not be given to patients receiving repeated blood transfusions, since transfused red blood cells contain approximately 0.5 mg of iron/ml of blood. Prolonged administration of therapeutic doses should be avoided, except in patients with continued bleeding, copious menstrual periods, or repeated pregnancies.

Patients with paroxysmal nocturnal hemoglobinuria may become deficient from urinary losses of iron. Treatment with large doses of iron may result in dangerous hemolytic crises. To avoid this complication, erythropoiesis may be limited by using very small oral doses. Many hematologists recommend blood transfusion prior to administration of iron to further reduce erythropoiesis, thus suppressing production of complement-sensitive red cells.

Oral iron therapy is preferred because toxic reactions, including hemosiderosis with tissue damage, are more likely with parenteral administration that bypasses intestinal regulatory mechanisms. Fever, lymphadenopathy, nausea and vomiting, arthralgias, urticaria, and fatal anaphylactic reactions also have occurred after parenteral therapy.

Parenteral iron should not be administered concomitantly with oral iron preparations, particularly since the primary indication for parenteral iron therapy is a pre-existing condition that precludes the use of oral iron.

Excessive iron storage rarely results from oral administration except in patients with increased iron absorption (eg, those with Laennec's cirrhosis, hemochromatosis, or sideroblastic anemia). In any case, iron should be given only to treat demonstrated iron deficiency. Gastrointestinal disturbances, particularly nausea, epigastric pain, diarrhea, or constipation, may occur with oral administration, and pre-existing gastrointestinal diseases (eg, chronic ulcerative colitis, regional enteritis) may be aggravated by the standard large doses of iron.

Timed-release preparations may incorporate the iron into matrices that are eliminated intact. These preparations should not be used in patients with Crohn's disease or other disorders in which intestinal strictures may entrap the insoluble matrix.

Infants and children appear to tolerate therapeutic doses better than adults. Although pregnant women are particularly susceptible to gastrointestinal disturbances, there is no absolute intolerance for oral iron. These untoward effects tend to subside with continuation of therapy, ingestion of iron with meals, and, if necessary, reduction of the individual dose.

Brightly coated tablets and flavored syrups are particularly hazardous because they are attractive to children. Parents should be warned that iron is toxic and can be fatal if excessive amounts are ingested by children. All iron-containing products should be labeled as potentially hazardous and kept away from children.

For a discussion of iron poisoning, see the evaluation on Deferoxamine Mesylate in Chapter 80, Drugs Used in the Treatment of Poisoning.

Drug Evaluations

ORAL IRON PREPARATIONS

The usual therapeutic doses cited in the evaluations follow the traditional regimens; however, smaller doses are preferred, particularly if gastrointestinal upset is a problem. Some clinicians recommend one tablet daily initially with a meal to minimize side effects and increase compliance. If this is tolerated, two and then three or four tablets can be given daily but such massive doses are indicated rarely if ever (Crosby, in press). About 30 mg of elemental iron daily replenishes iron stores in most adults. Larger doses do not increase hemoglobin regeneration appreciably but do increase side effects and may result in storage of excess iron (Crosby, 1984).

FERROUS SULFATE
[Feosol, Fer-In-Sol, Fero-Gradumet, Mol-Iron, Slow Fe]

Ferrous sulfate is the agent of choice to treat uncomplicated iron deficiency anemia. Since conditions for iron absorption are favorable only in the duodenum and upper jejunum, timed-release or enteric-coated preparations should be used only if objective bioavailability data have shown that the particular preparation is absorbed adequately and the supposed benefits outweigh the disadvantage of added cost. Any iron preparation that is likely to pass intact beyond the upper gastrointestinal tract is less effective.

ADVERSE REACTIONS AND PRECAUTIONS. Adverse effects are generally dose dependent; in 10% of patients, they are severe enough to be intolerable. Gastrointestinal disturbances (usually nausea, bloating, constipation or diarrhea, anorexia, pyrosis) are most common. Ferrous sulfate is absorbed best when taken between meals, but gastrointestinal symptoms may be minimized by reducing the dose and/or giving it in divided amounts with meals or shortly thereafter. Iron should not be given with carbonate antacids or tetracyclines, and its absorption may be markedly inhibited when given with meals containing predominantly grain products. In some patients, administration of one-half the total daily dose at bedtime improves tolerance. As with other oral iron salts, large doses of ferrous sulfate may aggravate existing gastrointestinal disease (eg, peptic ulcer, regional enteritis, ulcerative colitis).

Acute severe iron poisoning is uncommon in adults but does occur in children who ingest formulations intended for adults. In young children, as little as 400 mg of elemental iron is potentially fatal. Initial toxic effects include nausea, vomiting, and shock. Death has resulted from acute circulatory failure, gastric necrosis, and acute hepatic necrosis.

DOSAGE AND PREPARATIONS.

Therapeutic:

The manufacturers' recommended doses are given (see also the discussion on Formulations and Dosage in the Introduction).

Oral: Adults, initially, 30 to 60 mg of elemental iron, increased if necessary by 30-mg increments to a maximum of 180 mg daily in three or four divided doses; *children 6 to 12 years,* 24 to 120 mg (3 mg/kg) of elemental iron daily in three or four divided doses (elixir or syrup); *children 2 to 5 years,* 15 to 45 mg (3 mg/kg) of elemental iron daily in three or four divided doses (elixir or syrup); *children 6 months to two years,* up to 6 mg/kg of elemental iron daily in three or four divided doses (elixir or syrup); *infants,* a quantity of a pediatric preparation sufficient to provide 10 to 25 mg of elemental iron daily given in three or four divided doses. See also the Introduction to this section.

Prophylactic (supplementation):

Oral: Women of childbearing age, adolescents, and children, approximately 20 mg of elemental iron daily; *pregnant and lactating women,* 25 mg of elemental iron daily. *Men and postmenopausal women* should not receive iron supplements routinely, because iron loss may be masked and diagnosis of occult gastrointestinal malignancy may be delayed. Prophylactic iron should be given only if well documented risk factors for iron deficiency are present (eg, frequent blood donation, heavy menses). *Low-birth-weight infants and infants with low iron stores,* initially, 2 mg/kg of elemental iron daily, decreased gradually to approximately 1 mg/kg daily; *normal infants,* 10 to 15 mg of elemental iron daily during the first year. Many infant formulas contain iron, and this should be considered when determining whether supplementation is necessary. Mixtures containing iron usually are given for prophylaxis. (See the section on Mixtures and Chapter 47, Vitamins and Minerals.)

Generic. Capsules (timed-release) 150, 225, and 250 mg (30, 45, and 50 mg elemental iron, respectively); elixir 220 mg (44 mg elemental iron)/5 ml; tablets 195 and 300 mg (39 and 60 mg elemental iron, respectively); tablets (plain, enteric-coated) 325 mg (65 mg elemental iron) (all forms nonprescription).

Feosol (Menley & James). Capsules (exsiccated, timed-release) 167 mg (50 mg elemental iron); elixir 220 mg (44 mg elemental iron)/5 ml (alcohol 5%); tablets (exsiccated) 200 mg (65 mg elemental iron) (all forms nonprescription).

Fer-In-Sol (Mead Johnson). Capsules (exsiccated) 190 mg (60 mg elemental iron); drops 75 mg (15 mg elemental iron)/0.6 ml (alcohol 0.2%); syrup 90 mg (18 mg elemental iron)/5 ml (alcohol 5%) (all forms nonprescription).

Fero-Gradumet (Abbott). Tablets (timed-release) 525 mg (105 mg elemental iron) (nonprescription).

Mol-Iron (Schering). Tablets 195 mg (39 mg elemental iron) (nonprescription).

Slow Fe (CIBA). Tablets (exsiccated, timed-release) 160 mg (50 mg elemental iron) (nonprescription).

FERROUS FUMARATE
[Feostat, Ircon]

FERROUS GLUCONATE
[Fergon]

These compounds are as effective as ferrous sulfate in iron deficiency anemia and are claimed to be less irritating when equal amounts are administered because they dissolve slowly. Because of poor solubility, these salts may be ineffective in patients with achlorhydria; ferrous sulfate should be used in these patients.

Gastrointestinal disturbances are usually mild and can be minimized by reducing the dose and taking the drug with meals. Like ferrous sulfate, ferrous fumarate or gluconate may aggravate existing gastrointestinal disease (eg, regional enteritis, ulcerative colitis). Overdosage has caused acute severe iron poisoning, especially in children.

DOSAGE AND PREPARATIONS.

FERROUS FUMARATE:

Therapeutic:

The manufacturers' recommended doses are given (see also the discussion on Formulations and Dosage in the Introduction).

Oral: Adults, 100 to 400 mg (approximately 33 to 133 mg of elemental iron) daily in one to four doses; *children 6 to 12 years,* 100 to 300 mg (33 to 100 mg of elemental iron) daily in one to four doses (suspension); *children 1 to 5 years,* initially, a quantity of a pediatric preparation sufficient to provide 15 mg of elemental iron (12 drops or 1/2 teaspoon of the suspension), increased gradually to a maximum of 45 mg of elemental iron daily, if necessary, in three or four divided doses; *infants,* 10 to 20 mg of elemental iron daily (5 to 16 drops) divided into two to four doses. See also the Introduction to this section.

Prophylactic:

Same as for Ferrous Sulfate.

Generic. Tablets 300 and 325 mg (99 and 108 mg elemental iron, respectively) (nonprescription).

Feostat (Forest). Drops 45 mg (15 mg elemental iron)/0.6 ml; suspension 100 mg (33 mg elemental iron)/5 ml; tablets (chewable) 100 mg (33 mg elemental iron) (all forms nonprescription).

Ircon (Key). Tablets 200 mg (66 mg elemental iron) (nonprescription).

FERROUS GLUCONATE:

Therapeutic:

The manufacturers' recommended doses are given (see also the discussion on Formulations and Dosage in the Introduction).

Oral: Adults, 320 to 640 mg (38 to 77 mg of elemental iron) three times daily. *Children,* 100 to 300 mg (12 to 36 mg of elemental iron) three times daily. *Infants,* initially, 120 mg (30 drops of elixir equivalent to 15 mg of elemental iron); this amount may be increased gradually to 300 mg (36 mg of elemental iron) daily. See also the Introduction to this section.

Prophylactic:

Same as for Ferrous Sulfate.

> **Generic.** Capsules 325 mg (38 mg elemental iron); tablets 300 and 325 mg (35 and 38 mg elemental iron, respectively) (both forms nonprescription).
>
> **Fergon** (Winthrop-Breon). Capsules 435 mg (50 mg elemental iron); elixir 300 mg (35 mg elemental iron)/5 ml; tablets 320 mg (37 mg elemental iron) (all forms nonprescription).

IRON-POLYSACCHARIDE COMPLEX
[Niferex-150]

This ferric iron preparation is not absorbed as well as the soluble ferrous salts, which are preferred for the treatment of iron deficiency anemia.

Mild gastrointestinal disturbances are the most common adverse effects. Although this complex appears to be less toxic on a weight basis than the ferrous salts, this reflects the smaller quantity of ionic iron reaching the gastric and intestinal mucosa. Equal amounts of ionic iron from iron-polysaccharide complex and the ferrous salts are probably equally toxic. The danger of severe iron poisoning still exists, particularly in children. Like other iron preparations, iron-polysaccharide complex may aggravate gastrointestinal disease.

DOSAGE AND PREPARATIONS.

Oral: Adults, to correct iron deficiency anemia, 330 to 660 mg (40 to 80 mg of elemental iron) three times daily; *children,* 1.5 to 2 mg of elemental iron/kg daily. *Infants,* for prophylaxis, 1 to 1.5 mg of elemental iron/kg daily. See also the Introduction to this section.

> Strengths are expressed in terms of elemental iron.
>
> **Niferex-150** (Central). Capsules 150 mg; elixir 100 mg/5 ml (alcohol 10%); tablets 50 mg (all forms nonprescription).

PARENTERAL IRON PREPARATION

IRON DEXTRAN INJECTION
[Imferon]

ACTIONS AND USES. Iron dextran injection should be used only after iron deficiency anemia has been confirmed. This drug is indicated only when oral therapy has failed or may further irritate gastrointestinal disease (eg, regional enteritis, ulcerative colitis), when iron loss exceeds the amount absorbable from oral ferrous sulfate (more than 500 to 1,000 ml of blood per week [McCurdy, 1977]), when immediate replace-

ment is necessary (eg, severe anemia in late pregnancy), when a patient is not capable of compliance, or when an infant will not receive iron at home.

Iron dextran complex is dissociated by the reticuloendothelial cells to make the iron biologically available; a small proportion may remain complexed for three or four months, particularly after intramuscular injection. Complexed iron may persist in bone marrow reticuloendothelial cells and mask relapse of iron deficiency in previously treated patients, since stainable iron (complexed) may be found in the marrow despite total depletion of available iron stores.

ADVERSE REACTIONS AND PRECAUTIONS. Serious toxic effects (eg, anaphylactic shock, acute circulatory failure, cardiac arrest) have occurred. Iron dextran injection also may cause urticaria, arthralgia, headache, fever, nausea, vomiting, and regional lymphadenopathy.

Because the rate of intravenous administration and thus the rate of absorption can be controlled, the risk of anaphylaxis is decreased compared to intramuscular injection. It is recommended that a small test dose (one to two drops of solution) be given initially to detect sensitivity. Epinephrine and emergency resuscitative equipment should be readily available, since severe anaphylactic reactions have occurred with doses as small as 0.01 ml. (See Chapter 62, Agents for Active and Passive Immunity, for treatment of anaphylaxis.)

Intramuscular injection can cause painful persistent irritation and skin discoloration that may last for months; divided doses given by deep intramuscular injection (Z-track technique) minimize this possibility. Although the animal data are not conclusive, sarcomas have been reported at the site of intramuscular injection. For these reasons and because absorption is unpredictable, the intramuscular route should not be used.

Fetal abnormalities have occurred in animals following use of iron dextran injection during early pregnancy. Therefore, this parenteral form of iron should not be used during early pregnancy or in patients who may become pregnant unless the benefits outweigh the possible risk. *Parenteral and oral iron preparations should not be used concomitantly.*

DOSAGE AND PREPARATIONS. Dosages are expressed in terms of elemental iron. The patient's response should be monitored closely to determine the effectiveness of therapy. The total dose required to reconstitute the hemoglobin mass may be calculated by a number of formulas, one of which follows:

$$0.66 \times \text{body weight (kg)} \times \left(100 - \left[\frac{\text{patient's Hg(g/dl)} \times 100}{14.8}\right]\right) = \text{total grams of iron}$$

The value computed by this formula represents the amount of elemental iron needed to restore blood hemoglobin levels to normal and to replenish iron stores. An adult who is not bleeding should receive no more than 2 g as a total dose for one course of therapy. Once determined, the total estimated dose should not be exceeded. If the hemoglobin response is insufficient, other causes of anemia must be sought. See also the manufacturer's literature.

Intravenous: *Adults and children, (undiluted)* one or two drops followed in about 15 minutes by an additional test dose of 0.5 ml (25 mg). If no allergic reactions are evident, a total of 100 mg (2 ml) of undiluted drug may be given daily at a rate not exceeding 50 mg (1 ml)/min. If larger doses are indicated, most authorities believe that infusion of the total calculated amount as a single dose is the safest method of administering iron dextran injection to the adult (Savin, 1982). *Adults and children, (diluted)* after dilution with 500 to 1,000 ml of physiologic saline or 5% dextrose in water, a test dose of a few milliliters should be infused slowly. After 10 to 15 minutes, the diluted solution may be administered at a rate of 1 L/four to six hours. In elderly or severely anemic patients, the large volume may result in pulmonary edema unless a diuretic (eg, furosemide [Lasix]) is given concomitantly.

Because of the risk of fatal anaphylactic reactions, patients should be observed constantly during the first 30 to 60 minutes of the infusion and at frequent intervals thereafter. As noted earlier, emergency drugs and resuscitative equipment should be readily available during infusion.

Intramuscular (deep): This route of administration is not advocated. See the manufacturer's literature for dosage information. Experiments using iron dextran injection radioisotope indicate that approximately 30% of an intramuscular dose remains at the site of injection for more than 30 days.

> **Generic.** Powder; solution 50 mg/ml of elemental iron in 10 ml containers.
>
> **Imferon** (Merrell Dow). Solution equivalent to 50 mg of elemental iron/ml in 2 ml (intramuscular, intravenous) and 10 ml (intramuscular) containers with phenol 0.5%.

MEGALOBLASTIC ANEMIAS

Folic Acid and Vitamin B₁₂ Deficiency: Since both folic acid and vitamin B_{12} are essential cofactors for DNA synthesis, a deficiency of either nutrient causes defective nuclear maturation, which inhibits normal hematopoiesis. The erythroblast nucleus cannot accumulate sufficient DNA to permit normal cell division, resulting in large cells in both marrow and blood (Wyngaarden et al, 1985). Leukopenia and thrombocytopenia also are commonly present. The rate of erythrocyte destruction in bone marrow and, to a lesser degree, in blood is increased in megaloblastic anemia. In other proliferating cells, particularly in the alimentary tract, defective DNA synthesis results in secondary diminution and abnormality of epithelial cells of the tongue, stomach, and small intestine. This may result in malabsorption that contributes to the deficiency.

In pernicious anemia, which is rare in patients younger than 30 years, the cause of vitamin B_{12} deficiency is lack of gastric intrinsic factor, which chelates the vitamin to form a complex necessary for absorption. The primary defect is gastric atrophy due to autoimmune gastritis in which parietal cells no longer secrete intrinsic factor.

Folate deficiency is more common because folate stores are depleted rapidly in the presence of dietary deficiency, whereas

vitamin B_{12} reserves may last for several years. Maximal absorption of vitamin B_{12} occurs primarily in the lower one-half of the ileum and of folic acid in the upper one-third of the small intestine. Therefore, an intact small intestine is essential for normal absorption of these vitamins.

Megaloblastic anemias may be caused by nutritional deficiency of folic acid, vitamin B_{12}, or both. Also, conditions such as malabsorption (eg, in tropical sprue, celiac disease, blind loop syndrome); impaired utilization; competition for the vitamins by intestinal parasites (eg, fish tapeworm); or increased losses in association with other diseases, chronic infection, or drugs may either produce anemia or exacerbate it. The increased incidence of congestive heart failure may be secondary to severe anemia. Existing anemias also may be aggravated by conditions that increase the requirements for vitamin B_{12}, folate, or both (eg, hemolytic anemias, hyperthyroidism, pregnancy). Primary abnormalities of DNA synthesis also occur in some refractory anemias and preleukemic disorders, causing megaloblastic anemia that does not respond to vitamin B_{12} or folic acid.

Diagnosis: Although hematologic findings produced by folic acid or vitamin B_{12} deficiency may be identical and large doses of one may overcome, at least temporarily, the metabolic blockade in hematopoiesis produced by a deficiency of the other, vitamin B_{12} and folic acid are not interchangeable therapeutic agents. Large doses of folic acid may correct the anemia of vitamin B_{12} deficiency, but neurologic damage progresses and becomes irreversible unless specific replacement therapy is initiated promptly.

For diagnosis of folic acid and vitamin B_{12} deficiencies, initial tests should include complete blood count, reticulocyte count, blood smear, and mean corpuscular volume (MCV). The combination of macro-ovalocytosis and increased hypersegmented polymorphonuclear leukocytes on the blood smear is strong evidence of megaloblastosis. A Schilling's test performed after oral administration of intrinsic factor can help delineate the mechanism of the absorption abnormality (Gilman et al, 1985). Assay of serum vitamin B_{12}, serum folic acid, and red cell folic acid are diagnostic of the deficiency. A therapeutic trial is confirmatory. However, vitamin B_{12} and folic acid deficiency may coexist.

Therapy: Only rarely is therapy required before the diagnosis is established. However, when severe thrombocytopenia associated with bleeding, severe leukopenia associated with infection, severe anemia, marked neurologic damage, or other serious complications make immediate therapy necessary, both vitamin B_{12} 1,000 mcg and folic acid 15 mg are given intramuscularly or intravenously, followed by daily oral administration of folic acid 5 mg and vitamin B_{12} 1,000 mcg for one week. Folate deficiency may occur in poorly nourished, critically ill patients even when the serum folate concentration is normal. This is common in patients with severe infections, and life-threatening granulocytopenia or thrombocytopenia may develop unless these patients receive folic acid therapy.

The vitamin B_{12} or folate deficiency anemia usually responds so rapidly to specific therapy that transfusion of red cell concentrate is indicated only when severe anemia is associated with impending or actual cardiac failure. In these patients, plasmapheresis to reduce the plasma volume with the cautious administration of red blood cell concentrate may produce rapid and dramatic relief. Since the risk of hepatitis increases with the number of units administered, the dose should be kept as low as practical.

In addition to hematologic abnormalities, patients with pernicious anemia commonly have associated disorders that may require medical attention. These include thyroiditis resulting in hypothyroidism, late-onset immunoglobulin deficiency, and gastric carcinoma. The latter may develop in as many as 20% of patients despite replacement therapy with vitamin B_{12}. Because of the high risk of carcinoma of the stomach, patients with pernicious anemia should be evaluated at regular intervals throughout their lives by appropriate studies to detect early gastric carcinoma.

Vitamin B_{12} Compounds

Vitamin B_{12} Metabolism: Vitamin B_{12} is the common name for several cobalt-containing compounds (cobalamins). These are synthesized by microorganisms ingested from soil and water by animals, absorbed by them, and made available to humans through consumption of meat, fish, and dairy products. Because plants do not provide vitamin B_{12}, strict lactovegetarians (vegans) may develop a deficiency. However, the deficiency may not appear for many years, since most vitamin B_{12} is reabsorbed in the enterohepatic circulation and depletion of body stores is gradual. Vitamin B_{12}, in contrast to other B-complex vitamins, is stored mainly in the liver.

The average diet supplies 5 to 15 mcg/day of vitamin B_{12} in a protein-bound form that is available for absorption after normal digestion. Vitamin B_{12} is bound to intrinsic factor during transit through the alimentary tract; absorption occurs on the surface of the terminal ileum in the presence of calcium. Vitamin B_{12} enters the mucosal cell for absorption and is then transported by specific binding proteins, transcobalamins. These delivery proteins for vitamin B_{12} function like transferrin does for iron. In addition, a small amount of vitamin B_{12} (approximately 1% to 3% of the total amount ingested) is absorbed by simple diffusion, but this mechanism is significant only with large doses.

In pernicious anemia, the lack of intrinsic factor reduces the absorption of vitamin B_{12}, and deficiency occurs two to five years after onset of intrinsic factor deficiency. The total cobalamin deficit has been estimated to be 4,000 to 5,000 mcg.

Rarely, congenital transcobalamin deficiency has been reported and causes vitamin B_{12} deficiency in infants. Unless vitamin B_{12} (1,000 mcg injected twice weekly) is administered promptly, mental development may be impaired (Chanarin, 1983).

Subnormal intestinal absorption of vitamin B_{12} is often present in tropical sprue, celiac disease, regional enteritis, and other malabsorption syndromes or following total gastric resection. Patients undergoing peritoneal or hemodialysis and those with renal transplants appear to maintain normal serum vitamin B_{12} levels (Milman, 1980).

Formulations and Uses: Hydroxocobalamin has hematopoietic activity identical to that of the antianemia factor in purified liver extract. Cyanocobalamin, the stable pharmaceutical form, is equally active after it loses its cyanide adduct. It is effective in vitamin B_{12} deficiency states but has no proven therapeutic value (except as a placebo) in any of the nonhematologic conditions for which it has been used (eg, acute viral hepatitis, trigeminal neuralgia and other neuropathies, multiple sclerosis, delayed growth, poor appetite, certain dermatologic and psychiatric disorders, allergies, amblyopia, aging, sterility, thyrotoxicosis, malnutrition).

Hydroxocobalamin [alphaRedisol] is closely related chemically to cyanocobalamin. This agent is more highly bound to blood proteins than cyanocobalamin and thus is retained in the body a little longer. However, this is not usually an important clinical consideration and hydroxocobalamin has no advantage over cyanocobalamin. Furthermore, some patients develop antibodies to the complex of hydroxocobalamin and transcobalamin II. Thus, cyanocobalamin is preferred.

Massive doses of hydroxocobalamin have been used experimentally as an antidote in cyanide poisoning (see Chapter 80, Drugs Used in the Treatment of Poisoning) and are alleged to be of value in tobacco amblyopia. Cyanocobalamin cannot be used for these purposes.

Because absorption is unreliable, refractoriness often develops, and allergic sensitization may occur, preparations containing vitamin B_{12} and intrinsic factor concentrate are not recommended for treatment of megaloblastic anemia. Also, these preparations are ineffective in patients with structural or functional disorders of the small intestine.

Preparations of liver for injection provide a source of vitamin B_{12} activity but are outmoded and should not be used. Also, they may cause allergic reactions.

Administration: The intramuscular or subcutaneous injection of crystalline cyanocobalamin or hydroxocobalamin solutions may be preferred for pernicious anemia or other forms of defective absorption (eg, tropical sprue, celiac disease, regional enteritis, gastric resection). Oral administration usually is reserved for *nutritional* deficiency when gastrointestinal absorption is normal. (See also Chapter 47, Vitamins and Minerals.) However, large oral doses (1,000 mcg once or twice weekly) induce and maintain remission in patients with pernicious anemia (Crosby, 1980; Lacroce, 1981).

Vitamin B_{12}-deficient patients respond dramatically to therapy with cyanocobalamin or hydroxocobalamin. Normoblastic hematopoiesis is evident 48 to 72 hours following intramuscular injection. Depression and other affective disorders caused by vitamin B_{12} deficiency usually improve in 24 hours. *However, the patient with pernicious anemia or other permanent defects in absorption must understand that lifelong vitamin B_{12} therapy is required to prevent irreversible neurologic damage.* If treatment is discontinued, vitamin B_{12} deficiency recurs in six months to two years. Demonstrable neurologic damage from pernicious anemia that is not reversed after 12 to 18 months of adequate therapy must be considered irreversible.

Drug Evaluations

CYANOCOBALAMIN

HYDROXOCOBALAMIN
[alphaRedisol]

The primary clinical uses of these drugs are to treat confirmed deficiency of vitamin B_{12} and to perform Schilling's test for pernicious anemia or other malabsorption disorders. A third occasional use is in suspected cases of severe pernicious anemia when the patient refuses bone marrow examination, Schilling's test is not available, and analysis of serum vitamin B_{12} is not completed before therapy is begun. Oral vitamin B_{12} supplements should be given to vegetarians (see Chapter 47).

Hydroxocobalamin has a somewhat longer duration of action than cyanocobalamin. However, antibodies may develop to the complex of hydroxocobalamin and transcobalamin II and thus cyanocobalamin is preferred for treatment of megaloblastic anemia. Doses of either cyanocobalamin or hydroxocobalamin exceeding 30 mcg daily have no therapeutic advantage, but do increase vitamin stores to a degree, although the amount excreted in the urine increases proportionately.

No toxicity has been reported following use of either preparation. Allergic reactions to impurities in the preparation occur rarely. Injection causes little or no pain, and no adverse local effects have been reported.

DRUG INTERACTIONS. Absorption from the intestine may be decreased by aminoglycoside antibiotics, chloramphenicol, colchicine, anticonvulsants, timed-release potassium preparations, aminosalicylic acid, and long-term excessive alcohol intake.

DOSAGE AND PREPARATIONS.
Intramuscular, Subcutaneous (deep): The following regimen is usually recommended: For treatment of uncomplicated pernicious anemia or defective absorption of vitamin B_{12}, *adults,* 100 mcg daily for five to ten days, followed by 100 to 200 mcg monthly until remission is complete; thereafter, 100 mcg monthly will maintain remission. For serious complications requiring immediate therapy, both vitamin B_{12} 1,000 mcg and folic acid 15 mg are given intramuscularly or intravenously, followed by daily oral administration of folic acid 5 mg and vitamin B_{12} 1,000 mcg for one week. *Children,* a total of 1,000 to 5,000 mcg given in divided doses of 30 to 50 mcg/day for two or more weeks. Thereafter, 100 mcg every four weeks will maintain remission. *Infants,* for congenital transcobalamin deficiency, 1,000 mcg twice weekly. *Therapy must be lifelong in order to maintain remissions.*

Intramuscular: For a therapeutic trial to establish diagnosis of vitamin B_{12} deficiency, 1 mcg/day for ten days plus low dietary folic acid and vitamin B_{12}. The flushing dose for Schilling's test is 1,000 mcg.

CYANOCOBALAMIN:
Generic. Solution 30 mcg/ml in 30 ml containers, 100 mcg/ml in 10 and 30 ml containers, 120 mcg/ml in 30 ml containers, and 1,000 mcg/ml in 10 and 30 ml containers.
Available Trademarks.
Berubigen (Upjohn), *Betalin 12* (Lilly), *Redisol* (Merck Sharp & Dohme), *Rubramin PC* (Squibb).
HYDROXOCOBALAMIN:
Generic. Solution 1,000 mcg/ml in 10 and 30 ml containers (intramuscular only).
alphaRedisol (Merck Sharp & Dohme). Solution 1,000 mcg/ml in 10 ml containers (intramuscular only).

Oral: (therapeutic) For maintenance of remission in pernicious anemia, *adults and children,* 1,000 mcg twice weekly (Crosby, 1980; Lacroce, 1981).
CYANOCOBALAMIN:
Generic. Tablets 500 and 1,000 mcg (nonprescription).

Oral: (dietary supplements) For dietary vitamin B_{12} deficiency, *adults and children,* 6 mcg daily (in vegans); *infants up to 1 year,* 2 to 3 mcg daily.
For oral dietary supplements, see the section on Mixtures in Chapter 47, Vitamins and Minerals. Single-entity preparations are available in 50-mcg concentrations only.

VITAMIN B_{12} WITH INTRINSIC FACTOR CONCENTRATE
[Biopar Forte]

This oral preparation is a mixture of vitamin B_{12} and dried stomach or duodenum from hogs or other food animals. Hematopoietic activity is measured in oral units of activity, 1 oral unit being equivalent to not more than 15 mcg of cyanocobalamin. Since no more than approximately 1% of the administered dose is absorbed, this is a costly method of treatment. Furthermore, this preparation is useless in patients with functional or structural intestinal disease. Refractoriness often develops. Allergic sensitization from hog or other animal protein also may occur. Therefore, this preparation is not recommended for treatment of megaloblastic anemia.

Biopar Forte (USV). Tablets 0.5 N.F. units with intrinsic factor concentrate and cobalamin 25 mcg.

LIVER INJECTION

The crude, soluble vitamin B_{12} activity of liver is available generically as a single-entity preparation and in vitamin mixtures for injection. Because crystalline cyanocobalamin for injection is superior to all liver preparations, the latter should not be used.

Adverse reactions include local hypersensitivity, allergy, anaphylactic reactions, and brownish discoloration of the skin at the injection site.

No dosage regimen is given since use of liver injection is now obsolete.

Folates

Folic acid is widely distributed in nature as a conjugate (usually, heptaglutamate) with one or more molecules of glutamic acid. These forms of folates are present in nearly all foodstuffs. They are destroyed by prolonged cooking and other types of processing.

Naturally occurring folates must be reduced to mono- and diglutamates by conjugases in the gut before they can be efficiently absorbed from the proximal small intestine. Folates are transported to the liver where they are stored and transformed into 5-methyltetrahydrofolate, the principal form circulating in the blood. Enterohepatic recirculation of folate is significant.

The circulating 5-methyltetrahydrofolate enters tissue cells where a vitamin B_{12}-dependent conversion to the metabolically active form, tetrahydrofolate, occurs. Tetrahydrofolate is the substrate for intracellular polyglutamate forms, which function as coenzymes in DNA synthesis. 5-methyltetrahydrofolate is the only folate entering the central nervous system; folate concentrations three to four times those in serum are found in cerebrospinal fluid. In the fetus, folates play a role in blood formation and early development of the central nervous system, but their function in the central nervous system in adults has not been clarified. Exogenous folic acid bypasses the metabolic step requiring vitamin B_{12} for conversion to tetrahydrofolate; thus DNA synthesis and cell growth proceed normally and mask vitamin B_{12} deficiency.

The minimal adult requirement for folic acid is estimated to be 50 mcg daily. The average store of folate in adults is approximately 7.5 mg. Since the free folate content of the average daily diet in the United States is 200 to 300 mcg, dietary sources are generally adequate. Folate deficiency is common in intestinal diseases that interfere with absorption of folic acid, in chronic diseases (eg, renal, inflammatory, neoplastic), and in alcoholics who have reduced food intake and increased folate requirement. In alcoholics, impaired release of folate from hepatic stores may cause deficiency despite adequate dietary intake. Withdrawal from alcohol without exogenous folate supplementation may be all that is needed to treat such patients.

When folate deficiency anemia is of dietary origin, correction of the diet is preferred to supplemental medication. The addition of one fresh uncooked fruit or vegetable or glass of fruit juice to the diet each day often constitutes adequate correction. Folate requirements are particularly high during pregnancy and lactation and pregnant women receiving no prenatal folate supplements are especially vulnerable to folate deficiency anemia.

The sodium salt of folic acid (folate sodium) may be given by intramuscular, intravenous, or deep subcutaneous injection. Parenteral administration has no advantage over the oral route, but it may be preferred when this drug is a constituent of hyperalimentation infusion.

Indications: Folate-deficient patients with megaloblastic anemia generally respond rapidly to folic acid; reticulocytosis usually begins in two to five days.

Folic acid alleviates the megaloblastic anemias that occur during pregnancy and infancy and those associated with most cases of tropical sprue or celiac disease. Folates also are used to treat hematologic diseases in which deficiency is associated with a fast turnover of red cells (hemolytic disease), especially in children with thalassemia major, in patients with sickle cell disease, and in older patients with myelofibrosis and myeloid metaplasia. In these patients, weekly prophylactic doses may reduce the need for transfusions.

Severely ill hospitalized patients may develop subclinical folate deficiency when maintained on unsupplemented intravenous fluids. Even in the absence of overt megaloblastic anemia, these individuals have reduced bone marrow reserves that may limit production of granulocytes, platelets, and red cells. Inclusion of folic acid in the hyperalimentation fluid is essential.

Folate deficiency is thought by some investigators to have a causative role in neurologic and psychiatric disorders, especially in the elderly. Complaints such as fatigue, irritability, forgetfulness, depression, insomnia, and chronic constipation have been ascribed to folate deficiency and are reported to be alleviated by folic acid therapy. Peripheral neuropathy has been reported but in only a few cases has the response to folic acid therapy been documented with electrophysiologic testing (Rivey et al, 1984).

Folic acid and folates may correct the anemia of pernicious anemia and other types of vitamin B_{12} deficiency but should not be used in these disorders unless adequate doses of vitamin B_{12} are given concomitantly, because they neither arrest nor prevent the neurologic damage. Their indiscriminate prophylactic use may mask symptoms of pernicious anemia and make diagnosis difficult. Before folic acid is given, serum and red cell concentrations of folic acid should be measured to confirm deficiency. The sample must be handled carefully to prevent consumption of folate during transit.

A daily prophylactic dose of folic acid should be given routinely during pregnancy and lactation, since dietary intake cannot meet the increased demands. In pregnant women with epilepsy taking anticonvulsants, daily doses up to 1 mg apparently do not affect seizure control (Hiilesmaa et al, 1983). In one study, folate treatment before conception may have prevented neural tube defects in infants of women who had previously delivered one child with neural tube defect (Laurence et al, 1981). Larger doses may be indicated in women with marked absorption defects or chronic hemolytic anemia (eg, hereditary spherocytosis), but the dose should not interfere with the absorption of dietary zinc. Fetal storage of folate occurs primarily during the latter part of pregnancy; consequently, premature infants have smaller stores and are more likely to develop deficiency.

Individuals taking certain anticonvulsant, antimalarial, or contraceptive drugs may develop folic acid deficiency. Long-term use of analgesics, steroids, or large doses of sulfasalazine (more than 2 g/day) also may increase folate requirements. The mechanisms of the deficiency are not understood completely but include reduction of folic acid absorption by some anticonvulsants and inhibition of dihydrofolate reductase by some antimalarial agents that block the reduction of folic acid to its metabolically active form. Folic acid deficiency can be corrected by withdrawing the offending drug. Supplementing the diet with folic acid may overcome the deficiency when the mechanism is not enzyme inhibition.

If supplementation fails to correct the deficiency or when dihydrofolate reductase deficiency is present (eg, in patients with severe hepatic damage; after administration of the folate antagonists, pyrimethamine, trimethoprim, or triamterene), leucovorin calcium (folinate calcium) should be tried. This agent is already in the reduced state beyond the metabolic step that requires dihydrofolate reductase.

In pilot studies, therapeutic doses (10 mg/day) of folic acid reduced the progression of cervical dysplasia in women taking combination oral contraceptives (Check, 1980).

Drug Evaluations

FOLIC ACID
[Folvite]

FOLATE SODIUM
[Folvite Solution]

These synthetic agents are specific for the correction of folic acid deficiency. They should never be used as the sole agent in pernicious anemia or other vitamin B_{12} deficiency states. Such use may complicate diagnosis by correcting the anemia, and irreversible neurologic damage may occur if vitamin B_{12} is not given promptly. The efficacy of folic acid therapy in various psychiatric disorders has not been proven and its use is advocated only when folic acid deficiency exists.

Although most patients with malabsorption cannot adequately absorb food folates, they are able to absorb oral synthetic folic acid. Thus, oral administration is preferred. Parenteral administration is reserved for those with unresponsive malabsorption syndromes and those receiving parenteral or enteral alimentation.

When severe thrombocytopenia and other serious complications of deficiency anemia occur and immediate therapy is indicated, both folic acid and vitamin B_{12} are given intramuscularly or intravenously, followed by daily oral administration for one week.

Oral doses exceeding 0.1 mg should not be used unless vitamin B_{12} deficiency anemia has been ruled out or is being treated with a cobalamin or unless folate deficiency is accompanied by infection, uremia, arthritis, ulcerative colitis, hepatitis, or other conditions that may suppress hematopoiesis. Daily doses exceeding 1 mg do not enhance the hematologic effect, and most of the excess is excreted unchanged in the urine.

Except for one questionable report of an allergic reaction, folic acid is essentially nontoxic in man. There is evidence that the anticonvulsant action of phenytoin is antagonized by folic acid and increased doses may be required to prevent convulsions if folic acid is given concurrently.

DOSAGE AND PREPARATIONS.
Therapeutic:
Intramuscular, Intravenous, Subcutaneous: Adults and children, 0.5 to 1 mg daily for most deficiencies. When symptoms subside and blood tests become normal, a maintenance dose of 0.1 to 0.25 mg daily should be given orally if possible. For severe anemia requiring immediate therapy, folic acid 15 mg with vitamin B_{12} 1,000 mcg, followed by oral administration of folic acid 5 mg and vitamin B_{12} 1,000 mcg daily for one week.
Oral: The manufacturers' recommended oral replacement dose for *adults and children* is 0.25 to 1 mg daily. In most patients with uncomplicated folate deficiency, doses as small as 0.1 mg produce an adequate hematologic response and avoid masking concomitant vitamin B_{12} deficiency.
Prophylactic:
Oral: Adults and children, during periods of increased demand (eg, hemolytic disease, alcoholism, infection), 0.5 to 1 mg daily. *During pregnancy,* 0.8 mg daily; *during lactation,* 0.6 mg daily. These are RDA recommendations, but 1 mg daily may be given for all indications. *Low-birth-weight infants and those fed goat milk formulas,* 0.05 mg daily.

FOLIC ACID:
Generic. Tablets 0.1, 0.4, 0.8, and 1 mg.
Folvite (Lederle). Tablets 1 mg.
FOLATE SODIUM:
Generic. Solution (injection) equivalent to folic acid 10 mg/ml in 10 ml containers.
Folvite Solution (Lederle). Solution (injection) equivalent to folic acid 5 mg/ml in 10 ml containers.
For additional preparations, see the section on Mixtures in Chapter 47, Vitamins and Minerals, and the section on Infant Formulas in Chapter 48, Parenteral and Enteral Nutrition.

LEUCOVORIN CALCIUM (Folinate Calcium)
[Wellcovorin]

ACTIONS. Leucovorin calcium (citrovorum factor, 5-formyl tetrahydrofolic acid) is a metabolically active, reduced form of folic acid and has the same actions and interactions. It is absorbed rapidly and metabolized to 5-methyltetrahydrofolate in the liver without requiring reduction by dihydrofolate reductase. Onset of action is 20 to 30 minutes following oral administration and 10 to 20 minutes following intramuscular injection. The peak plasma concentration is attained after 1.5 to 2 hours. The duration of action is three to six hours, and 80% to 90% is eliminated by renal excretion.

USES. Although leucovorin calcium may be administered parenterally to treat megaloblastic anemias when oral therapy is not feasible, folic acid is much less expensive and is preferred.

This drug is useful to treat overdosage of folate antagonists (antifols) (see the discussion on methanol and ethylene glycol poisoning in Chapter 80, Drugs Used in the Treatment of Poisoning). It also is used adjunctively in patients with disseminated cancer receiving large doses of methotrexate or vincristine (Frei et al, 1980; Grush and Morgan, 1979). (See Chapter 64, Drugs Used in Cancer Chemotherapy.)

Leucovorin is classified in FDA Pregnancy Category C. It rarely produces hypersensitivity reactions (eg, urticaria, rash, pruritus, wheezing).

DOSAGE AND PREPARATIONS.

Oral, Intramuscular*: Adults and children*, for megaloblastic anemia, no more than 1 mg daily.
> ***Generic****.* Powder for injection (cryodesiccated, preservative-free) 50 mg; solution (injection) 3 mg/ml in 1 ml containers.
> ***Wellcovorin*** (Burroughs Wellcome). Solution (injection) 5 mg/ml in 1 and 5 ml containers; tablets 5 and 25 mg.

SIDEROBLASTIC ANEMIAS

Sideroblastic anemias are characterized by normoblasts containing a perinuclear ring of stainable iron granules (ring sideroblasts), which represent an accumulation of nonheme iron in and around the mitochondria. This excess iron has been transported into the cell but cannot be incorporated into porphyrin to form heme. When erythroblasts show megaloblastic features indicative of folic acid deficiency, this should be corrected. Sideroblastic anemia is uncommon and may be hereditary (primary) or acquired (secondary). Alcoholism is the most common cause; abstinence from alcohol and administration of folic acid usually are curative. Alcoholic patients in whom formation of pyridoxal phosphate is impaired also should be given pyridoxine 50 mg daily for two to four weeks.

If hereditary or neoplastic sideroblastic anemia responds to pyridoxine, treatment should be continued indefinitely to prevent relapse, because retreatment is less effective.

Since pyridoxal phosphate functions as a coenzyme in porphyrin synthesis, deficiency of pyridoxine or administration of drugs that antagonize its action (eg, isoniazid, chloramphenicol, cycloserine, immunosuppressive agents, lead) also may cause sideroblastic anemias. Some rare, genetic disorders (eg, hyperirritability and convulsions in infants, homocystinuria) may be accompanied by anemia that responds to pyridoxine or pyridoxal phosphate. Although there is no dietary deficiency of pyridoxine in these and other familial sideroblastic anemias, hemoglobin concentrations improve in some patients given 100 to 300 mg daily. Therefore, pyridoxine may be tried in patients with familial refractory anemias. However, even when the anemia improves, hemoglobin levels remain subnormal and morphologic abnormalities of red blood cells persist.

The sideroblastic anemia associated with preleukemic states and many idiopathic acquired sideroblastic anemias rarely respond to the therapies discussed above. This type of anemia usually occurs in elderly men, accompanies many diseases (eg, neoplasm, infection, inflammatory diseases), and is associated with ingestion of various drugs and toxins. All of these agents and conditions appear to interfere with the heme synthetic pathway. Clinically, the condition may resemble iron deficiency, but serum iron and ferritin are elevated. Blood transfusions may be necessary if the anemia seriously impairs the patient's functional ability. Administration of iron is contraindicated in any patient with sideroblastic anemia. Young patients requiring maintenance blood transfusions probably should be considered for chelation therapy to treat iron overload (see Chapter 80, Drugs Used in the Treatment of Poisoning).

REFRACTORY ANEMIAS

Androgens have been used to treat some types of anemia refractory to other therapy. Testosterone sometimes stimulates erythropoiesis, and large doses of androgens have been used to treat refractory anemias caused by inadequate production of erythrocytes. Although not all patients benefit from such therapy and results usually are not dramatic, those with aplastic and refractory myelophthisic anemias (anemias associated with space-occupying lesions of the bone marrow, such as myelofibrosis) may require fewer transfusions. In some instances, remission has been sustained (see also Chapter 38, Androgens and Anabolic Steroids). Cobaltous chloride 60 to 150 mg daily also has been given to treat refractory anemias. However, cobalt is potentially toxic and may cause adverse effects.

Discussion of other procedures (eg, transfusion, splenectomy) used to treat anemia is beyond the scope of this book.

MIXTURES

Deficiency anemias must be diagnosed accurately before therapy is initiated. Once a diagnosis has been established, the condition generally responds rapidly to a specific single-entity drug unless there are multiple deficiencies.

Except in nutritional anemias resulting from very poor diets for which a multiple vitamin supplement may be considered rational therapy, use of mixtures to treat anemias is strongly discouraged. Combination therapy is indicated only when it can be clearly demonstrated that one type of deficiency anemia is superimposed upon another. Even under these circumstances, however, use of the specific agents required is preferred. Avoidance of mixtures not only is better therapy, but may be an absolute necessity when the preferred routes of administration for two therapeutic agents are different. For example, in anemia caused by deficiencies of iron and vitamin B_{12}, the oral route is preferred for iron and the parenteral route for vitamin B_{12}.

Mixtures are an added expense when an adequate, less expensive regimen is available. For example, although a tablet containing an iron salt and a large dose of ascorbic acid may constitute acceptable therapy in the patient having difficulty absorbing iron (ascorbic acid enhances iron absorption), ingestion of one 300-mg ferrous sulfate tablet represents a more than sufficient dose of iron despite poor absorption.

The supplemental vitamins or minerals present in many iron preparations in no way improve the therapeutic effect of the iron and are not necessary unless other deficiencies also are present. The response to iron alone will confirm the diagnosis; addition of other agents may complicate determination of the degree of iron deficiency. Mixtures of iron with folic acid, cyanocobalamin, and pyridoxine generally should not be used to treat anemia, although a combination of folic acid and iron is a reasonable prophylactic supplement during pregnancy. There is no scientific basis for the inclusion of trace metals (eg, copper, molybdenum, cobalt) in any preparation used to treat anemia.

Available mixtures contain almost every imaginable combination of two or more of the following compounds or groups of compounds: iron salts, all vitamins including folic acid and cyanocobalamin, all trace minerals, liver extract, and intrinsic factor. The bioavailability of some components in the mixtures is questionable.

A partial listing of some widely used preparations is provided below. For a discussion of the multiple vitamin and vitamin with mineral preparations used to treat deficiency states not related to anemia, see Chapter 47, Vitamins and Minerals.

Cevi-Fer (Geriatric). Each capsule contains ferrous fumarate 60 mg (equivalent to elemental iron 20 mg), ascorbic acid 300 mg, and folic acid 1 mg.

Chromagen Capsules (Savage). Each capsule contains ferrous fumarate 200 mg (equivalent to elemental iron 66 mg), cyanocobalamin 10 mcg, ascorbic acid 250 mg, and desiccated stomach substance 100 mg.

Feosol Plus (Menley & James). Each capsule contains ferrous sulfate dried 200 mg (equivalent to ferrous sulfate 325 mg, elemental iron 65 mg), vitamin B_{12} activity equivalent 5 mcg, folic acid 0.2 mg, thiamine hydrochloride 2 mg, riboflavin 2 mg, pyridoxine hydrochloride 2 mg, ascorbic acid 50 mg, and niacin 20 mg (nonprescription).

Ferancee (Stuart). Each tablet (chewable) contains ferrous fumarate 200 mg (equivalent to elemental iron 67 mg), ascorbic acid 49 mg, and sodium ascorbate 114 mg (nonprescription).

Fergon Plus (Winthrop-Breon). Each capsule contains ferrous gluconate 500 mg (equivalent to elemental iron 58 mg), vitamin B_{12} with intrinsic factor concentrate NF 1/2 unit, and ascorbic acid 75 mg.

Fermalox (Rorer). Each tablet contains ferrous sulfate 200 mg and magnesium-aluminum hydroxide 200 mg (nonprescription).

Fero-Folic-500 (Abbott). Each tablet (timed-release) contains ferrous sulfate 525 mg (equivalent to elemental iron 105 mg), folic acid 0.8 mg, and sodium ascorbate 500 mg.

Fero-Grad-500 (Abbott). Each tablet (timed-release iron) contains ferrous sulfate 525 mg (equivalent to elemental iron 105 mg) and sodium ascorbate 500 mg (nonprescription).

Ferro-Sequels (Lederle). Each capsule (timed-release) contains ferrous fumarate 150 mg (equivalent to elemental iron 50 mg) and docusate sodium 100 mg (nonprescription).

Heptuna Plus (Roerig). Each capsule contains ferrous sulfate dried 311 mg (equivalent to elemental iron 100 mg), undefatted desiccated liver 50 mg, vitamin B_{12} cobalamin concentrate 5 mcg, intrinsic factor concentrate 25 mg, sodium ascorbate 150 mg, thiamine mononitrate 3.1 mg, riboflavin 2 mg, pyridoxine hydrochloride 1.6 mg, niacinamide 15 mg, calcium pantothenate 0.9 mg, copper 1 mg, molybdenum 0.2 mg, calcium 37.4 mg, iodine 0.05 mg, manganese 0.033 mg, magnesium 2 mg, phosphorus 29 mg, and potassium 1.7 mg.

Iberet (Abbott). Each tablet (timed-release iron) or 20 ml of liquid contains ferrous sulfate 525 mg (equivalent to elemental iron 105 mg), cyanocobalamin 25 mcg, ascorbic acid 150 mg, thiamine mononitrate 6 mg, riboflavin 6 mg, niacinamide 30 mg, pyridoxine hydrochloride 5 mg, and calcium pantothenate 10 mg (tablet) or dexpanthenol 10 mg (liquid) (both forms nonprescription).

Iberet-500 (Abbott). Each tablet (timed-release) or 20 ml of liquid contains same formulation as **Iberet** except sodium ascorbate 500 mg (both forms nonprescription).

Iberet-Folic-500 (Abbott). Each tablet (timed-release) contains same formulation as **Iberet-500** plus folic acid 0.8 mg.

Iberol (Abbott). Each tablet contains ferrous sulfate 525 mg (equivalent to elemental iron 105 mg), cyanocobalamin 12.5 mcg, sodium ascorbate 75 mg, thiamine mononitrate 3 mg, riboflavin 3 mg, niacinamide 15 mg, pyridoxine hydrochloride 1.5 mg, and calcium pantothenate 3 mg (nonprescription).

Ircon-FA (Key). Each tablet contains ferrous fumarate 250 mg (equivalent to elemental iron 82 mg) and folic acid 1 mg.

Iromin-G (Mission). Each tablet contains ferrous gluconate 333.3 mg (equivalent to 38.6 mg elemental iron), vitamin B_{12} (crystalline or resin) 2 mcg, ascorbic acid 100 mg, thiamine mononitrate 5 mg, riboflavin 2 mg, pyridoxine hydrochloride 25 mg, niacinamide 10 mg, folic acid 0.8 mg, calcium pantothenate 1 mg, vitamin A acetate 4,000 IU, vitamin D_2 400 IU, calcium carbonate 70 mg, calcium gluconate 100 mg, calcium lactate 100 mg, and calcium 50 mg (nonprescription).

Niferex Forte (Central). Each capsule contains iron-polysaccharide complex 150 mg, vitamin B_{12} 25 mcg, and folic acid 1 mg; each 5 ml of elixir contains iron-polysaccharide complex 100 mg, vitamin B_{12} 25 mcg, and folic acid 1 mg.

Nu-Iron Plus (Mayrand). Each 5 ml of elixir contains iron-polysaccharide complex 100 mg, vitamin B_{12} 25 mcg, and folic acid 1 mg (alcohol 10%).

Perihemin (Lederle). Each capsule contains ferrous fumarate 168 mg (equivalent to elemental iron 55 mg), vitamin B_{12} 5 mcg, intrinsic factor concentrate 25 mg, folic acid 0.3 mg, and ascorbic acid 50 mg.

Peritinic (Lederle). Each tablet contains ferrous fumarate (equivalent to elemental iron 100 mg), cyanocobalamin 50 mcg, thiamine monohydrate 7.5 mg, riboflavin 7.5 mg, pyridoxine hydrochloride 7.5 mg, ascorbic acid 200 mg, niacinamide 30 mg, folic acid 0.05 mg, pantothenic acid 15 mg, and docusate sodium 100 mg (nonprescription).

Pronemia (Lederle). Each capsule contains ferrous fumarate 350 mg (equivalent to elemental iron 115 mg), vitamin B_{12} (as cobalamin concentrate) 15 mcg, intrinsic factor concentrate 75 mg, ascorbic acid 150 mg, and folic acid 1 mg.

Reticulogen (Lilly). Each milliliter of solution (for injection) contains cyanocobalamin 20 or 40 mcg (**Forte**) and thiamine 5 mg in 5 ml containers.

Simron (Merrell Dow). Each capsule contains ferrous gluconate 86 mg (equivalent to elemental iron 10 mg) and polysorbate 20 400 mg (nonprescription).

Simron Plus (Merrell Dow). Each capsule contains ferrous gluconate 86 mg (equivalent to elemental iron 10 mg), cyanocobalamin 3.3 mcg, polysorbate 20 400 mg, sodium ascorbate 50 mg, pyridoxine hydrochloride 1 mg, and folic acid 0.1 mg (nonprescription).

Stuartinic (Stuart). Each tablet contains ferrous fumarate 300 mg (equivalent to elemental iron 100 mg), ascorbic acid 300 mg, sodium ascorbate 225 mg, cyanocobalamin 25 mcg, thiamine mononitrate 6 mg, riboflavin 6 mg, pyridoxine hydrochloride 1 mg, niacinamide 20 mg, and calcium pantothenate 10 mg (nonprescription).

Tabron (Parke-Davis). Each tablet contains ferrous fumarate 304.2 mg (equivalent to 100 mg elemental iron), ascorbic acid 500 mg, cyanocobalamin 25 mcg, folic acid 1 mg, thiamine mononitrate 6 mg, riboflavin 6 mg, pyridoxine hydrochloride 5 mg, niacinamide 30 mg, calcium pantothenate 10 mg, vitamin E 30 IU, and docusate sodium 50 mg.

Theragran Hematinic (Squibb). Each tablet contains ferrous fumarate equivalent to elemental iron 66.7 mg, cyanocobalamin 50 mcg, folic acid 0.33 mg, sodium ascorbate 100 mg, thiamine mononitrate 3.3 mg, riboflavin 3.3 mg, niacinamide 33.3 mg, pyridoxine hydrochloride 3.3 mg, vitamin A acetate 2.5 mg (8,333 IU), ergocalciferol 3.3 mg (133 IU), vitamin E 5 mg (5 IU), calcium pantothenate 11.7 mg, copper sulfate 0.67 mg, and magnesium carbonate 41.7 mg.

TriHemic 600 (Lederle). Each tablet contains ferrous fumarate 350 mg (equivalent to elemental iron 115 mg), cyanocobalamin 25 mcg, intrinsic factor concentrate 75 mg, folic acid 1 mg, ascorbic acid 600 mg, vitamin E 30 IU, and docusate sodium 50 mg.

Trinsicon (Glaxo). Each capsule contains ferrous fumarate equivalent to elemental iron 110 mg, vitamin B$_{12}$ activity (from liver-stomach concentrate or cobalamin concentrate) 15 mcg, intrinsic factor concentrate 240 mg, folic acid 0.5 mg, and ascorbic acid 75 mg.

Vitron-C (Fisons). Each tablet (chewable) contains ferrous fumarate 200 mg (equivalent to elemental iron 66 mg) and ascorbic acid 125 mg (nonprescription).

Cited References

Chanarin I: Management of megaloblastic anemia in the very young. *Br J Haematol* 53:1-3, 1983.

Check WA: Folate for oral contraceptive users may reduce cervical cancer risk. *JAMA* 244:633-634, 1980.

Cook JD: Clinical evaluation of iron deficiency. *Semin Hematol* 19:6-18, 1982.

Crosby WH: Improvisation revisited: Oral cyanocobalamin without intrinsic factor for pernicious anemia. *Arch Intern Med* 140:1582, 1980.

Crosby WH: Rationale for treating iron deficiency anemia, (editorial). *Arch Intern Med* 144:471-472, 1984.

Crosby WH: Overtreatment of deficiency anemias. *Arch Intern Med* (in press).

Dallman PR, et al: Prevalence of anemia. *Am J Clin Nutr* 39:437-445, 1984.

Frei E III, et al: High dose methotrexate with leucovorin rescue: Rationale and spectrum of antitumor activity. *Am J Med* 68:370-376, 1980.

Gilman AG, et al (eds): *The Pharmacological Basis of Therapeutics*, ed 7. New York, Macmillan, 1985.

Grush OC, Morgan SK: Folinic acid rescue for vincristine toxicity. *Clin Toxicol* 14:71-78, 1979.

Hiilesmaa V, et al: Serum folate concentrations during pregnancy in women with epilepsy: Relation to antiepileptic drug concentrations, numbers of seizures, and fetal outcome. *Br Med J* 287:577-579, 1983.

Lacroce V: Oral crystalline cyanocobalamin available, (letter). *Arch Intern Med* 141:1558, 1981.

Laurence KM, et al: Double-blind randomised controlled trial of folate treatment before conception to prevent recurrence of neural-tube defects. *Br Med J* 282:1509-1511, 1981.

McCurdy PR: Microcytic hypochromic anemias. *Postgrad Med* 61:147-151, (June) 1977.

Milman N: Serum vitamin B$_{12}$ and erythrocyte folate in chronic uraemia and after renal transplantation. *Scand J Haematol* 25:151-157, 1980.

Olsson KS, et al: Preclinical hemochromatosis in a population on high-iron-fortified diet. *JAMA* 239:1999-2000, 1978.

Rivey MP, et al: Phenytoin-folic acid: Review. *Drug Intell Clin Pharm* 18:292-301, 1984.

Savin MA: Anemia due to iron deficiency, in Conn HF (ed): *Current Therapy, 1982*. Philadelphia, WB Saunders, 1982, 249-252.

Savin MA, Cook JD: Mucosal iron transport by rat intestine. *Blood* 56:1029-1035, 1980.

Wyngaarden JB, et al (eds): Hematologic diseases, in: *Cecil Textbook of Medicine*, ed 17. Philadelphia, WB Saunders, 1985, 866-900.

Other Selected References

Baker SJ, DeMaeyer EM: Nutritional anemia: Its understanding and control with special reference to work of World Health Organization. *Am J Clin Nutr* 32:368-417, 1979.

Bothwell TH, et al: *Iron Metabolism in Man*. Oxford, Blackwell Scientific, 1980.

Chanarin I: *The Megaloblastic Anaemias*, ed 2. Oxford, Blackwell Scientific, 1979.

Cook JD (ed): *Methods in Hematology: Iron*. New York, Churchill Livingstone, vol 1, 1980.

Das KC, et al: Unmasking covert folate deficiency in iron-deficient subjects with neutrophil hypersegmentation: dU suppression tests on lymphocytes and bone marrow. *Br J Haematol* 39:357-375, 1978.

Erbe RW: Inborn errors of folate metabolism. *N Engl J Med* 293:753-757, 807-812, 1975.

Herbert V: Nutritional anemias. *Hosp Pract* 15:65-89, (March) 1980.

Herbert V, et al: Nutritional anemias overview; megaloblastic anemia, in Gordon AS, et al (eds): *The Year in Hematology, 1977*. New York, Plenum Press, 1977.

Kellermeyer RW: General principles of evaluation and therapy of anemias. *Med Clin North Am* 68:533-543, 1984.

Provisor AJ: Childhood anemia. *Am Fam Physician* 14:124-134, (Oct) 1976.

Shojania AM: Problems in diagnosis and investigation of megaloblastic anemia. *Can Med Assoc J* 122:999-1004, 1980.

Williams WJ, et al: *Hematology*, ed 3. New York, McGraw-Hill, 1982.

Wintrobe MM: *Clinical Hematology*, ed 8. Philadelphia, Lea & Febiger, 1981.

Agents Used for Anticoagulant Therapy

Thromboembolic disorders are a significant cause of morbidity and mortality. Venous thromboembolism occurs as a complication of other diseases, including cancer, diabetes, heart failure, previous episodes of thromboembolism, varicose veins, and obesity. Smoking, pregnancy, trauma, surgery, and immobilization following stroke, paraplegia, or myocardial infarction also are established risk factors. Estrogen-containing oral contraceptives are associated with a small but definite risk of venous thrombosis. Arterial thromboembolism often accompanies rheumatic heart disease or disorders affecting the coronary, cerebral (intra- and extracranial), or peripheral arteries.

Appropriate drug therapy for thromboembolism depends upon an understanding of the major factors of thrombogenesis, the mechanisms of coagulation, and the pharmacology of drugs used for prophylaxis or therapy. Some knowledge of the complexities of blood coagulation is particularly useful in evaluating the therapeutic effects of anticoagulants and interpreting the laboratory tests required to control therapy.

Blood Coagulation

MECHANISMS. A system of integrated actions and reactions maintains the normal fluidity of blood and promotes the prompt, appropriate response to imbalances to protect the body from traumatic blood loss (see the figure). In response to injury, local blood vessels constrict and platelets form a hemostatic plug. The end point of the coagulation pathway is the fibrin clot, which reinforces an initial platelet plug. The fibrinolytic system may be activated simultaneously with coagulation. Its purpose is to restore normal hemostasis by digesting the fibrin clot. (See Chapter 34, Thrombolytics.)

Prothrombin (factor II) is converted to thrombin (factor II$_a$) in two separate pathways. In the extrinsic system, tissue factor (tissue thromboplastin), a large lipoprotein complex not normally found in the blood, reacts with factor VII and directly activates factor X to factor X$_a$ in the presence of calcium. This complex also activates factor IX in the intrinsic system (see below). Thrombin then is formed by the prothrombin-

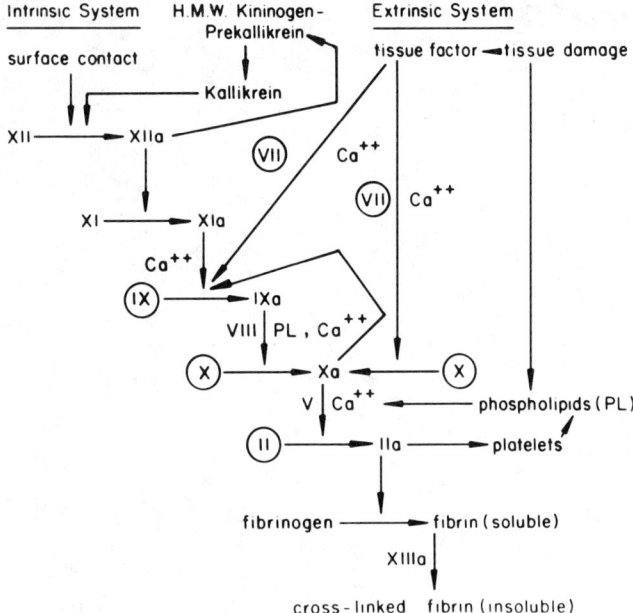

Factors circled are coumarin-sensitive and vitamin K-dependent.

converting activity developed by a complex of factor X_a, factor V, and calcium ions adsorbed onto phospholipid micelles of platelets. Factor X_a is responsible for the proteolytic cleavage of thrombin, but the other factors accelerate the conversion.

Thrombin initiates actual coagulation through its action on fibrinogen (factor I). Two peptides are removed from each of the alpha (fibrinopeptides A) and beta (fibrinopeptides B) chains; a specific arginyl-glycine bond is cleaved in each. The removal of these peptides from fibrinogen leads to spontaneous gelation of fibrin monomers (factor I_a), which are then stabilized only by noncovalent forces and may still be dispersed. The gel is stabilized further by cross linkage when covalent bonds are formed by a transglutaminase (factor XIII_a); this confers relative resistance to the action of proteolytic enzymes (eg, plasmin).

In the intrinsic system, despite the fact that all the factors necessary for coagulation are present in circulating blood, it takes several minutes for whole blood to clot. This is in contrast to the extrinsic system in which the time-consuming early reactions are bypassed and clotting occurs in seconds. (An example of extrinsic system coagulation in the test tube is the Quick one-stage prothrombin time test.)

Coagulation is initiated in the intrinsic system when Hageman factor (factor XII) binds to a negatively charged surface (eg, glass tube, silica, subendothelial collagen of a disrupted blood vessel). This contact induces a conformational change, which makes Hageman factor more susceptible to activation by small concentrations of kallikrein or factor XII_a (activated Hageman factor). In addition to Hageman factor, HMW-kininogen-prekallikrein and HMW-kininogen-factor XI complexes also bind to negatively charged surfaces through the HMW-kininogen moiety. Factor XII_a activates both prekallikrein and factor XI. The kallikrein generated then activates additional factor XII. In the presence of calcium ions, the resulting factor XI_a transforms factor IX to an active serine

protease, factor IX_a. Factor X is then activated by a complex of factor IX_a, factor VIII (antihemophilic globulin), and calcium ions adsorbed onto platelet phospholipid surfaces. The rest of the coagulation sequence is identical to that of the extrinsic system.

Tissue factor-factor VII reaction product, with calcium ions, directly activates both factor IX in the intrinsic pathway and factor X in the extrinsic pathway. This activation is of the same order of magnitude as that induced by factor XI_a and may explain why hereditary factor XI deficiency produces only mild bleeding while hereditary factor IX deficiency causes severe bleeding (Østerud and Rapaport, 1980).

This complicated and repetitive pattern serves as a biologic amplifier to enhance activity severalfold at each stage. The chain reaction sequence is mandatory, since a gradual generation of thrombin with slow conversion of fibrinogen to fibrin is hemostatically ineffective as isolated platelet aggregates and fibrin threads are washed away by the blood stream. The extent of coagulation also is limited by the rapid hepatic clearance of many of the activated products.

Inactive zymogens are converted to activated forms by limited proteolysis. They participate at various stages of coagulation as serine proteases, for each has a serine residue in the enzymatically active site. Only factors V and VIII do not appear to exert a proteolytic effect in blood coagulation but, in the presence of calcium ions, they form complexes with other activated coagulation factors as described above.

Antithrombin III (AT-III), formerly known as heparin cofactor, is the principal physiologic inhibitor of thrombin and other activated clotting factors (serine proteases). Normal levels of AT-III and its binding to activated coagulation factors appear to be necessary to maintain blood fluidity and prevent thrombosis. A few families have been reported to have hereditary AT-III deficiency resulting in recurrent venous thromboembolism. In normal individuals, levels may be decreased following surgery or in the presence of disseminated intravascular coagulation (DIC), hepatic cirrhosis, nephrotic syndrome, and, infrequently, acute thrombosis. Although AT-III levels are unaffected by estrogen therapy, the reaction of AT-III and factor X_a is retarded. Usually only focal activation of the coagulation mechanism occurs and hemostasis is normal outside the affected area.

Other coagulation inhibitors, protein C and protein S, depend on vitamin K for synthesis, and they regulate the induction of thrombosis. Protein C is present in blood and bound to endothelial cell surfaces by thrombomodulin; it is activated from zymogen to enzyme by thrombin, which is bound to the receptor thrombomodulin on endothelial cells. This generation of thrombin leads not only to coagulation but, by binding to thrombomodulin present on the endothelial surfaces, activates zymogens that then inhibit coagulation. Protein C cleaves activated factors V:C and VIII:C to eliminate their procoagulant activity and prevent coagulation away from the site of vessel injury. The net action of the protein C system is to limit the size and growth of a thrombus by inhibiting formation and enhancing dissolution of fibrin (Marlar, 1985). Hereditary deficiency of protein C is associated with an increased risk of thrombosis (Broekmans et al, 1983). Homozygous protein C deficiency is fatal; infants develop catastrophic thrombosis and do not survive the neonatal period without protein C replacement (Marlar, 1985). Acquired deficiency may occur in patients with vitamin K deficiency, liver disease, or disseminated intravascular coagulation and in those taking oral anticoagulants.

Protein S acts as a cofactor to accelerate the anticoagulant activity of activated protein C. Persons with normal protein C levels but reduced levels of protein S may be prone to thrombosis.

DISSEMINATED INTRAVASCULAR COAGULATION (DIC). This condition results from excessive activation of both the blood coagulation process and the fibrinolytic factors that normally counteract coagulation. Thus, clinical signs of bleeding and clotting may be observed concurrently. Continuous coagulation may coat the vascular system with fibrin, which often occludes small vessels and imperils adequate perfusion of vital organs. As long as acute DIC persists (unless initial levels of coagulation factors are abnormally high or losses are rapidly compensated by synthesis that may occur in subacute or chronic DIC), the normal concentrations of prothrombin, fibrinogen, and factors II, V, VII, and X decrease in the circulation, as do platelets that aggregate on the fibrin masses. Antithrombin III levels frequently are reduced. Also, fibrinogen/fibrin degradation products are increased and further interfere with hemostasis by inhibiting fibrin polymerization to produce unclottable complexes.

Because clotting factors and platelets are being "consumed," this condition occasionally is termed "consumptive coagulopathy." Hemorrhage can occur spontaneously or after needle puncture, surgery, or other trauma and usually is widespread, but a tendency to bleed may be the only sign. Excessive oozing of blood should be investigated in any patient who has been severely ill for several weeks.

Conditions that precipitate DIC include (1) excessive activation of the intrinsic system (massive endothelial damage, deposition and depletion of platelets) caused by sepsis, endotoxin shock, and antigen-antibody complexes; (2) excessive activation of the extrinsic system (introduction of tissue factor into the system) produced by transplant rejection, neoplasms, obstetrical accidents (eg, amniotic fluid embolism, abruptio placentae, retention of dead fetus), massive tissue injury (especially brain), snakebite, and hemolytic transfusion reaction; and (3) decreased hepatic clearance of activated clotting factors (acute circulatory failure) caused by hepatic failure, pulmonary embolism, congestive heart failure, and giant hemangiomas.

Clinical symptoms are those of the primary disorder and coagulation abnormalities are most frequently observed in patients with acute onset DIC. No single test is specific but the combination of bleeding in the presence of a small friable clot; schistocytes on a red cell smear; low and steadily decreasing platelet count; prolonged prothrombin, partial thromboplastin, and thrombin times; and serum fibrinogen/fibrin degradation product (FDP) levels exceeding 80 mcg/ml is strongly diagnostic of DIC. Abnormalities in three or more of these parameters are suggestive.

Extreme caution is required when treating DIC; continuous laboratory monitoring and the assistance of an experienced hematologist are essential. Thrombin time, fibrinogen assay,

and serum FDP levels should be determined frequently to ascertain if further replacement therapy is required. The primary aims are to reverse the underlying disorder and maintain supportive therapy. Associated conditions (eg, acidosis, anemia, hypotension) also should be treated. If these aims cannot be accomplished, success in elimination of DIC is limited.

Treatment: Suggested therapy (Wyngaarden and Smith, 1982) includes administration of fresh frozen plasma 2 to 10 units/day to replace depleted clotting factors and various plasma serine protease inhibitors. Platelet concentrates (6 to 10 platelet packs given once or twice) should be administered if the platelet count is less than 50,000/ml. Cryoprecipitated antihemophilic factor (factor VIII) may be given to increase the fibrinogen level, particularly if it is less than 100 mg/dl. One container of cryoprecipitate raises the fibrinogen level by 2 to 5 mg/dl. However, replacement of clotting factors may accelerate DIC and administration of an excessive amount of platelets or fibrinogen may lead to their rapid consumption and exacerbate microvascular thrombosis.

Heparin therapy is controversial and is seldom used to treat DIC except in patients with leukemia. Because the risk of hemorrhage, thrombocytopenia, and paradoxical thrombosis is substantial, heparin should not be administered unless a platelet count of 30,000/mm^3 can be maintained (Corash, 1980). Heparin also should not be used when hemorrhage occurs within the central nervous system or in patients with uncontrolled hypertension or severe liver disease.

Prophylaxis with heparin is indicated in acute promyelocytic leukemia before beginning chemotherapy. The incidence of DIC is very high and pretreatment with heparin has prevented DIC in most patients.

Aminocaproic acid [Amicar] has been given with heparin to prevent thrombus formation when the fibrinolytic system is active. If bleeding becomes more severe, antifibrinolytic drugs are not useful and may even increase the risk of thrombosis. Protamine should not be given even when hemorrhage persists, since complete coagulation of the circulating blood may result.

Thrombus Formation

MECHANISMS. Damage to blood vessels initiates coagulation when formed elements of blood and clotting factors are exposed to extravascular tissues. The extrinsic pathway is activated by tissue thromboplastin (from fibroblasts and damaged endothelial cells), which accelerates platelet aggregation at the injured surface and results in the immediate formation of an unstable plug. The intrinsic pathway is activated simultaneously by contact between the collagen of the damaged area and factor XII, and coagulation is accelerated by phospholipid from platelet surfaces. Thrombin is generated, which then converts fibrinogen to fibrin (see the figure); fibrin stabilizes platelet aggregates at the site of injury. The hemostatic plug is largely extravascular and is digested slowly by leukocytes and plasma fibrinolysis. Meanwhile, its surface becomes covered with endothelium.

Thrombus formation resembles the process of hemostasis but occurs intravascularly. The thrombus consists of cellular material and a fibrin network; the precise composition depends upon its age and the conditions of formation. Venous thrombi frequently occur in the absence of detectable intimal damage and usually develop in regions of slow or disturbed blood flow (eg, valve pockets of deep leg veins). Increased turnover of both platelets and fibrinogen reflects activation of the coagulation mechanism. Small deposits of platelets become interspersed with fibrin and extend in the direction of blood flow. As the thrombus grows, a red tail (mainly fibrin interspersed with red cells) forms; this often occludes the vein or may separate and migrate as an embolus.

In contrast, arterial thrombi have a greater platelet component and are called white thrombi. They develop at sites of vascular narrowing or irregularity in areas of rapid blood flow, and symptoms are determined by the location rather than by the size of the thrombus. Platelets aggregate on the surface of damaged vessels or prostheses and become interspersed with fibrin and blood cells; thrombus formation reflects reactions between platelets and the blood vessel wall. However, arterial thrombi do not cause occlusion as readily as venous thrombi. Instead, they tend to remain fixed, acting as a focus for further accumulation. The resulting mass can interfere with blood flow and cause infarctions or it may become an embolus.

Platelets are directly involved in the coagulation process and play a major role in thrombus formation and embolization, especially in the arterial system. Platelets adhere to damaged endothelium, undergo marked alterations in shape and membrane kinetics, and secrete chemicals (eg, adenosine diphosphate, serotonin, fibrinogen) that cause the platelets to aggregate. Adenosine diphosphate (ADP) has a positive feedback effect that promotes further aggregation. Serotonin may cause smooth muscle contraction, which facilitates vascular constriction.

The initial change in the platelet membrane also activates phospholipases, which causes release of arachidonic acid from platelet membrane phospholipid. Arachidonic acid is converted by cyclo-oxygenase to cyclic endoperoxides (PGG_2 and PGH_2), which are then converted by thromboxane synthetase to thromboxane A_2 (TXA_2) in the platelets. Thromboxane A_2 is a vasoconstrictor that induces platelets to undergo a release reaction that discharges the contents of intracellular storage granules and results in their aggregation. In vessel walls, PGG_2 and PGH_2 are converted by prostacyclin synthetase to prostacyclin (PGI_2), a vasodilator and potentiator of adenyl cyclase. When platelets are exposed to PGI_2, platelet cyclic AMP (cAMP) levels rise and platelet aggregation is impaired. Therefore, the balance between the generation of TXA_2 and PGI_2 is important in regulating platelet function.

ANTIPLATELET THERAPY. Many drugs interfere with platelet function, including clofibrate [Atromid-S], tricyclic antidepressants, penicillin and related antibiotics, chloroquine [Aralen], nitroprusside [Nipride, Nitropress], and alcohol. Drugs used for their antiplatelet effect are aspirin, dipyridamole [Persantine], and sulfinpyrazone [Anturane].

Aspirin 325 mg decreases the synthesis of TXA_2 and PGI_2 by irreversibly inhibiting cyclo-oxygenase for the life of the platelet, but this enzyme can be regenerated by endothelial cells. The net effect is to reduce the release reaction and subsequent aggregation and thus inhibit platelet function.

Indomethacin [Indocin] and the investigational agent, flurbiprofen, have effects similar to aspirin. Very low doses of aspirin (20 to 40 mg) markedly reduce the production of platelet TXA_2 for up to 96 hours; there is less effect on PGI_2, but results appear to be similar to those with aspirin 325 mg (Eichner, 1984).

Dipyridamole inhibits phosphodiesterase, the enzyme that degrades cAMP; this increases cAMP levels, stimulates PGI_2 biosynthesis, and inhibits platelet function. Because the doses required for this effect also cause flushing and headache in about 10% of patients, smaller amounts of dipyridamole often are given with aspirin. The action of sulfinpyrazone is not known, but, like aspirin, it is thought to competitively inhibit prostaglandin synthesis, although to a lesser degree.

In patients with venous thrombosis, drugs that impair platelet function cannot restore platelet and fibrinogen turnover to normal. However, in some patients with arterial disease, dipyridamole restores platelet turnover to normal (Deykin, 1982).

Multicenter trials have been conducted to evaluate the effects of these drugs in patients with arterial thrombosis and embolism, transient ischemic attacks (TIA), unstable angina, or recurrent myocardial infarction (MI) and after insertion of prosthetic heart valves. One analysis of data pooled from six trials indicated that aspirin significantly reduced total deaths (p <0.05) and cardiovascular mortality (p <0.01) during the first year of administration in postmyocardial infarction patients (Canner, 1983). Although most studies have not yielded definitive information, some general statements may be made.

Among survivors of myocardial infarction, there is some evidence that aspirin protects against acute recurrence and reduces mortality somewhat. However, the evidence is not conclusive with regard to benefits from dipyridamole or sulfinpyrazone. The Aspirin Myocardial Infarction Study Research Group (1980) concluded that aspirin increased the incidence of hemorrhage. The Persantine-Aspirin Reinfarction Study Research Group reported that aspirin reduced recurrence in patients who experienced an attack within six months before entry into the trial (Krol, 1980). However, defects in the design of this study may invalidate the conclusion. The Anturane Reinfarction Trial Research Group/Policy Committee reports (1980, 1982) suggested that the incidence of sudden death was reduced during the first six months after acute myocardial infarction in patients receiving sulfinpyrazone. However, the results of this study remain controversial, and the efficacy of sulfinpyrazone is not established (Temple and Pledger, 1980; Eichner, 1984). The Canadian Cooperative Study Group (1978) studied the effects of aspirin and sulfinpyrazone in patients with threatened stroke and concluded that aspirin reduced the incidence of TIAs, associated strokes, and death in men, but that sulfinpyrazone had no prophylactic value. Also, concurrent use of aspirin and sulfinpyrazone may reduce the uricosuric action of sulfinpyrazone and result in formation of uric acid stones in the kidney.

Further studies may provide more definitive information. Meanwhile, low doses of aspirin (325 mg or less/day) may be indicated for prophylaxis after testing to eliminate patients who cannot tolerate this drug (Elwood, 1984). Patients most likely to benefit from this therapy are those who have survived a myocardial infarct and those at high risk of thrombosis. Therapy with aspirin 25 to 75 mg/day should be initiated early after myocardial infarction. In patients with prosthetic heart valves, a combination of warfarin and dipyridamole 25 to 75 mg three times daily has been found to reduce the incidence of thromboembolism. The combination of warfarin and aspirin probably should not be used under these circumstances because of the increased risk of bleeding; increased intracranial bleeding was reported in one study (Chesebro et al, 1983).

In patients undergoing coronary artery bypass surgery, dipyridamole 25 to 75 mg three times daily administered several hours prior to surgery and postoperatively in combination with aspirin has been found to reduce the incidence of graft closure. Additional benefits may be obtained if dipyridamole 400 mg/day is begun two days before bypass surgery. Individuals with valvular disease and atrial fibrillation may benefit from prophylaxis with sulfinpyrazone 200 to 400 mg/day (Mehta and Roy, 1984).

Several drugs that actively inhibit platelet aggregation are being investigated. Anagrelide decreases platelet count and shortens platelet survival. It is probably not useful for long-term prophylaxis, but may be of value to reduce the platelet count in disorders such as polycythemia vera and thrombocythemia. Dazoxiben is a selective inhibitor of thromboxane synthetase and thus TXA_2, but it has no effect on cyclooxygenase. However, pharmacologic blockade of TXA_2 in platelets may not be a critical functional pathway and its therapeutic value does not appear to be promising. Epoprostenol (prostacyclin, PGI_2), which inhibits platelet aggregation, is being used to increase the circulating levels of prostacyclin in an attempt to reduce the incidence of thrombus formation. However, it has a short half-life, must be given by continuous intravenous infusion, and causes side effects (eg, headache, nausea, vomiting, anxiety, gastrointestinal complications) (see the evaluation in Chapter 25, Antianginal Agents). Ticlopidine is a platelet inhibitor that prolongs the bleeding time, but its therapeutic efficacy has not been determined.

Beta-blocking agents (eg, propranolol [Inderal]) are claimed to prevent the recurrence of myocardial infarction; a proposed mechanism for this cardioprotective effect is an antiplatelet action. For discussion of these agents, see Chapter 25, Antianginal Agents.

Other agents that interfere with the ability of platelets to initiate or perpetuate thrombus formation are being studied. Dextrans inhibit platelet adhesiveness and decrease vascular stasis by affecting blood flow. A low-molecular-weight dextran [Gentran 40, 10% LMD, Rheomacrodex] has been used prophylactically in patients undergoing surgery who are at high risk of developing thromboembolic complications. Dextrans have not been shown to be more useful than oral anticoagulants or heparin in patients undergoing general surgery but appear to be beneficial in those having hip surgery. (For adverse reactions and precautions, see Chapter 35, Blood, Blood Components, and Blood Substitutes.)

ANTICOAGULANT THERAPY. Oral anticoagulants and heparin inhibit fibrin formation and are used prophylactically to reduce the incidence of venous thromboembolism. Because they do not alter platelet adhesion or aggregation, these agents are less likely to affect arterial thrombi. Once a thrombus has occurred, anticoagulants are given to prevent further growth and diminish the likelihood of embolization, but these agents do not alter the size of the original thrombus or limit subsequent vascular damage. (See also the following section on Anticoagulants.) Streptokinase [Kabikinase, Streptase] and urokinase [Abbokinase] dissolve existing fresh thrombi and emboli by diffusing into clots to activate trapped plasminogen (see Chapter 34, Thrombolytics). Anticoagulants are then given to prevent recurrence.

SURGERY. Surgical interruption of veins may prevent pulmonary embolization, but benefits may last for only a few weeks because of the rapid enlargement of collateral veins. Surgery is considered when anticoagulants cannot be used or when adequate anticoagulant therapy does not prevent embolus formation.

ANTICOAGULANTS

The anticoagulants used therapeutically are heparin, the coumarin derivatives (dicumarol, phenprocoumon [Liquamar], warfarin sodium [Coumadin, Panwarfin], and warfarin potassium [Athrombin-K]), and the indandione derivative, anisindione [Miradon].

Mechanism of Action: Heparin accelerates the formation of complexes involving antithrombin III (AT-III), a normal plasma alpha-2-globulin, and several coagulation proteases, primarily thrombin and factor X_a. The onset of action of heparin is immediate. Biochemical data suggest that the primary prophylactic effect may be mediated by the anti-X_a mechanism rather than by inactivation of thrombin. Commercial preparations contain both low- and high-molecular-weight fractions. The low-molecular-weight fraction (less than 6,000) has potent anti-X_a activity and moderate antithrombin properties; the reverse is true for the high-molecular-weight fraction (more than 25,000). Heparin is administered intravenously or subcutaneously.

Heparin calcium [Calciparine] was formulated as an alternative to the sodium salt for subcutaneous administration in low doses to prevent postoperative thromboembolism. The calcium salt has been claimed to produce lower blood levels of heparin and thus reduce the incidence of hemorrhagic disturbances. No substantial difference between the calcium and sodium preparations has been documented with regard to incidence of bleeding, hematoma formation, or discomfort at the site of injection.

The mechanism of action of all coumarin and indandione anticoagulants is identical. These compounds block the post-translational modification of factors II, VII, IX, and X by impairing the vitamin K-dependent reactions. A vitamin K-dependent mechanism converts several glutamate residues in these factors to gamma carboxyglutamic acid residue. Vitamin K undergoes a cycle of oxidation and reduction in the liver to produce the active form. The coumarins prevent the reduction of vitamin K once it is oxidized. Since the oxidized form of vitamin K is ineffective, the coumarins indirectly impair gamma carboxylation. Normally, resulting carboxylated residues bind calcium and facilitate orientation of clotting factors on a phospholipid surface, thus accelerating their interaction and promoting generation of thrombin. With prolonged administration of warfarin, carboxylation of vitamin K-dependent factors is impeded, binding of calcium is depressed, coagulation is retarded, and thrombin formation is reduced.

The coumarin derivatives and the indandione, anisindione, are administered orally. Warfarin sodium also can be given intravenously, but parenteral administration usually has no advantage except in patients who should not or cannot take drugs orally. The full anticoagulant effect is achieved in about three days. Although the development of individual peak effects is variable, any of these drugs can maintain the therapeutic response established by another. Both abnormal resistance and increased sensitivity to anticoagulant action have been reported.

Dosage Requirements: The former custom of giving a large loading dose, which then is decreased immediately or gradually to the maintenance dose is no longer recommended. The initial effect of a loading dose primarily reflects depression of factor VII, which has a rapid half-life of four to six hours. Factors IX and X decrease more slowly but at the same rate whether a single large loading dose or smaller doses of 10 to 15 mg/day are administered.

Evidence suggests that the benefits of warfarin in preventing formation or extension of thrombi are related largely to depression of factors IX and X. Therefore, initiation of therapy with 15 mg, 10 mg, and 10 mg on the first three days is preferred (Deykin, 1982). Prothrombin time should be determined daily and the dosage adjusted according to the rate of degradation of warfarin. This supervised regimen has the advantage of avoiding hyperresponse and a precipitous decrease in factor VII, which minimize the risks of major bleeding and skin necrosis that is probably due to warfarin-induced depression of protein C (McGehee et al, 1984). Protein C is a vitamin K-dependent inhibitor of factors V and VIII. Depletion of protein C before depletion of factors IX, X, and II actually renders the patient hypercoagulable. Avoiding a loading dose also minimizes the danger of hemorrhage in patients with diminished tolerance or unusual sensitivity to the anticoagulant (eg, those who have recently undergone major surgery; elderly, malnourished, or debilitated patients; those with infections, liver disease, or congestive heart failure).

Indications: *Heparin* reduces fibrin formation by inhibiting several early steps in the intrinsic coagulation cascade. One major clinical use is to help maintain extracorporeal circulation during open heart surgery and renal hemodialysis. It also is given when immediate hypocoagulability is required, as in massive deep venous thrombosis or pulmonary infarction. For these purposes, standard full doses generally are administered intravenously. Heparin also is administered to treat DIC but should be given only if the diagnosis is unequivocal, there is evidence of ongoing thrombosis, or there is evidence that treatment will be clinically useful and the patient can be monitored carefully. (See the section on Disseminated Intravascular Coagulation.) Routine use of heparin for DIC is not indicated since it can cause serious bleeding.

The efficacy of small subcutaneous doses for prophylaxis of venous thromboembolism is well documented. The incidence of pulmonary embolism is reduced in patients over 40 years who have undergone abdominal-thoracic surgery under general anesthesia lasting longer than 30 minutes. A few reports suggest that this procedure does not increase intracranial or intraspinal bleeding when spinal or epidural anesthesia is employed. This regimen has not proved to be uniformly efficacious in patients who have undergone prostatic surgery, and its use in orthopedic surgery is controversial. Minidose therapy should not be used in patients undergoing ocular surgery and is inadequate for those experiencing an active thrombotic process. Low-dose heparin prophylaxis also should be considered for patients who are immobilized for long periods.

Although data are inconclusive, it has been suggested that small doses of heparin may reduce the incidence of postoperative acute myocardial infarction. The effect of heparin on the incidence of mural thrombi or systemic embolism has not yet been determined.

The usefulness of inhalation of aerosol preparations of heparin has not been established. Prolonged subcutaneous self-administration by pregnant patients with prosthetic heart valves or a history of major thromboembolism is feasible but may cause spinal collapse. Therefore, this method of administration should be used cautiously. However, heparin, unlike warfarin, does not cross the placenta and is less likely to cause embryopathy.

Oral anticoagulants are generally used for long-term prophylaxis. The use of anticoagulants in deep venous thrombosis (DVT) and pulmonary embolism (PE) is established. Since clinical signs are not sufficient to establish a diagnosis of DVT, objective documentation (eg, venography, impedance plethysmography, Doppler ultrasonography) is necessary before treatment is begun. For confirmed deep venous thrombosis of the proximal veins, initial heparin therapy to establish rapid hypocoagulability should be followed by oral anticoagulant treatment for a minimum of six weeks to three months (Lagerstedt et al, 1985). Treatment may be continued (usually for a total of six months) in patients with extensive disease or pulmonary embolism. Recurrent thromboses after six months of oral anticoagulant therapy indicate the need for lifelong use of these drugs, particularly if the underlying cause is deficiency of antithrombin III, protein C, or protein S. For treatment of massive pulmonary embolism, see Chapter 34, Thrombolytics.

Despite the lack of stringently controlled trials, most clinicians prescribe oral anticoagulants when mitral valve disease is associated with atrial fibrillation, even if surgical correction has been attempted or no embolism is present in the cerebral or limb arteries.

Anticoagulants often are given to reduce the incidence of systemic embolism after cardioversion in patients with chronic atrial fibrillation. Controlled clinical trials have shown that these drugs decrease the incidence of thromboembolism in patients with prosthetic heart valves; this effect is enhanced significantly in some patients with concomitant use of dipyridamole [Persantine] 400 mg daily. However, combined use of an oral anticoagulant and aspirin increases the risk of bleeding. No definitive clinical study has been published demonstrating that oral anticoagulants can prevent the occlusion of an aortocoronary bypass.

Studies on the use of oral anticoagulants in patients with

peripheral artery disease or after bypass surgery of a limb artery have been uncontrolled or limited to small numbers of patients, but the results suggest that the preventive role of anticoagulants in peripheral vascular disease is minimal.

The indications for use of anticoagulants in patients with cerebrovascular insufficiency are restricted to those with transient ischemic attacks (TIAs). These agents are beneficial during the first few months of treatment but do not alter mortality. Their use for more than one year during a trial at the Mayo Clinic was associated with a substantial risk of intracranial hemorrhage. Morbidity and mortality are reduced in patients with recurrent cerebral embolization if anticoagulants are given after the diagnosis is established unequivocally.

Contraindications: Anticoagulants are absolutely contraindicated after cerebral hemorrhage and have no place in the treatment of thrombotic cerebral infarction. Therapy to prevent recurrences should not be started for several days after a cerebral embolism; however, if CAT scanning techniques have been used, anticoagulants may be started within 24 to 48 hours.

Other contraindications include initiation of oral anticoagulant therapy during pregnancy; use in patients with aortic aneurysm, infective endocarditis, acute pericarditis, or other potential bleeding sites; and use in patients with moderate to severe hypertension.

Anticoagulants also should not be used in patients with active ulcerative disease of the gastrointestinal tract, hemorrhagic blood dyscrasias, severe liver or kidney disease, open ulcerative wounds, or recent surgery of the eye or spinal cord. Other factors that may constitute contraindications are unwillingness or inability of the patient to understand therapy, absence of a reliable laboratory to perform monitoring tests, or serious risk of drug interactions.

Prolonged therapy in outpatients should never be prescribed unless the patient or someone in the household can assume responsibility for competent care.

Drug Selection: Anticoagulants are potentially toxic and their use should be carefully considered in conditions in which efficacy has not been confirmed. The choice between heparin and an oral drug depends on the purpose of therapy.

Heparin is the drug of choice for initial therapy when the risk of thrombosis is high. However, it must be administered parenterally. The coumarins may be preferred after the effects of heparin have been established and when long-term oral anticoagulant therapy is indicated; anisindione may be given if the coumarins are not tolerated. Initially, heparin often is given to assure rapid depression of clotting factor activity and to maintain anticoagulation while stepwise replacement with the oral drugs is accomplished, since patients may not be well regulated with these agents for six or seven days.

The selection of the most appropriate oral anticoagulant in a given situation is influenced both by individual and class characteristics. Dicumarol, phenprocoumon, and anisindione are so long acting that they may be hazardous if hemorrhage occurs, although maintenance therapy can be better controlled and alternate-day therapy may be feasible. The dosage of dicumarol is somewhat difficult to control because it is incompletely absorbed and has a dose-dependent half-life of one to four days. Phenprocoumon has a long half-life (approximately

six and one-half days), which may be dangerous in the presence of hemorrhage. Therefore, warfarin is usually the oral anticoagulant of choice. It is rapidly and completely absorbed and has a half-life between 1 and 1.5 days.

Because the rate of degradation varies among patients, the dose of all anticoagulants must be individualized to provide effective therapeutic levels with minimal complications. Although most patients require 5 to 7 mg of warfarin daily, the range may be between 2 and 12 mg daily.

Monitoring Therapy: Anticoagulation induced by heparin or oral agents must be sufficient to maintain the equilibrium between the desired antithrombotic protection and actual bleeding. This requires not only careful calculation of the dose but also multiple control sampling and reliable laboratory testing.

Present evidence indicates that small doses of heparin given subcutaneously to prevent venous embolism do not require repeated blood sampling, even in most high-risk patients. However, the response to heparin varies and one or two tests for heparin activity probably should be performed at the start of therapy. Laboratory monitoring may be required when standard doses of heparin are administered by intermittent intravenous injection (usually at four-hour intervals) or by continuous intravenous infusion.

The various tests recommended to monitor heparin therapy are whole blood clotting time (Lee-White clotting time test), partial thromboplastin time (PTT), or activated partial thromboplastin time (APTT). The APTT test is most widely accepted. Experimental thrombosis is prevented in laboratory animals at values one and one-half to two times normal (60 to 80 seconds if the control value is 40 seconds).

The Quick one-stage prothrombin time test or a modification is used to regulate the dose of oral anticoagulants. Results of this test may be regarded as estimates of the combined activities of the complex of prothrombin, factor V, factor VII, factor X, and, to a minor extent, fibrinogen. Prothrombin, factor VII, and factor X are functionally depressed when anticoagulants are given orally. (Factor IX is vitamin K-dependent and coumarin-sensitive but is not measured by any one-stage prothrombin test.) Since the depression of each of these factors is not additive and each has a markedly different half-life, the factor depressed most quickly and profoundly (usually factor VII) acts as the determinant of a routine prothrombin time during the first few days of therapy. During prolonged therapy, factor X ultimately shows the lowest activity in the steady state. With usual oral anticoagulant doses, the Quick one-stage prothrombin time test has a value one and one-half to two times greater than the control when expressed in seconds.

To adjust the dose of oral anticoagulants, prothrombin time should be determined three times during the first week, twice the second week, and weekly thereafter until the maintenance dose is established. The maintenance dose should be reevaluated monthly and more often in patients with impaired liver function, congestive heart failure, or frequent diarrhea; when the vitamin K content of the diet is drastically changed; or when new drugs are added to or withdrawn from the regimen. (See also Chapter 3, Drug Interactions and Adverse Drug Reactions.)

Caution must be exercised when interpreting the results of the one-stage prothrombin time test in a patient receiving both full-dose heparin therapy and an oral anticoagulant. Heparin may prolong the one-stage prothrombin time, and the estimated doses of the oral anticoagulant may be insufficient to maintain the clinical effect when heparin is discontinued.

Treatment of Overdosage: The action of heparin can be antagonized by the intravenous administration of protamine sulfate, but there are hazards associated with use of this compound (see the evaluation). The anticoagulant effect of coumarin derivatives and anisindione can be overcome by administration of phytonadione (vitamin K_1), but effects are not apparent for four to eight hours. When anticoagulant therapy is then resumed, larger than usual doses may be required initially. If the effects of the oral anticoagulants must be counteracted quickly, fresh or frozen single-donor human plasma may be used; three units of plasma usually is adequate to correct prothrombin time. In patients who metabolize warfarin at a slow rate, secondary prolongation of the prothrombin time may occur (in 10 to 12 hours) after the effects of plasma have worn off. Caution is required because plasma products may produce hepatitis and hypervolemia.

Adverse Reactions: Hemorrhage is a hazard of treatment with any anticoagulant and is the main complication of therapy, but the frequency and severity can be minimized by careful management. The incidence of bleeding depends on the intensity of anticoagulation, the duration of administration, the compliance of the patient, the reliability of laboratory tests, and the occurrence of drug interactions. Hemorrhage also is more likely to occur in patients who have an underlying medical or surgical problem that prevents the use of anticoagulants. If gastrointestinal or urinary tract bleeding occurs in patients receiving an anticoagulant and the cause cannot be determined, an occult lesion may be present. Cerebral or adrenal hemorrhage, corpus luteum hemorrhage and rupture, subdural hematoma, intestinal submucosal hemorrhage with adynamic ileus or colitis, acute hemorrhagic pancreatitis, and cutaneous hemorrhagic necrosis are possible serious complications. When the prothrombin time is greatly prolonged, the incidence of hemopericardium after myocardial infarction is greater in patients receiving anticoagulants.

Intravenous or subcutaneous injection of heparin seldom produces serious adverse reactions (see the evaluation), but intramuscular administration may cause local capillary rupture and should not be employed.

Heparin-associated thrombocytopenia has been reported in as many as 5% of patients (King and Kelton, 1984). It usually occurs 6 to 12 days after initiation of treatment. If the thrombocytopenia is associated with arterial thrombosis, stroke, myocardial infarction, and death may ensue. Diagnosis is difficult because most patients receiving anticoagulants have other conditions that cause thrombocytopenia. However, in patients with thrombocytopenia plus an acute thrombotic event, a platelet count less than 50,000/microliter, or bleeding, immediate discontinuation of heparin is indicated. Depending on the location of the thrombus, antithrombotic therapy may be necessary (eg, vena caval interruption, defibrinating agent). Since heparin-associated thrombocytopenia is a delayed phenomenon, the incidence may be reduced by treating patients with acute venous thrombosis or pulmonary embolism with both heparin and oral anticoagulants initially, discontinuing heparin as soon as the oral anticoagulant becomes effective (5 to 7 days). For patients with acute arterial thrombus, other specific treatment may include surgical removal of the thrombus and treatment with antiplatelet agents (eg, aspirin).

Severe, sometimes fatal, hepatic, renal, hematologic, and cutaneous reactions developed in some patients who received phenindione, which is no longer marketed. Although these effects have not been reported with the other indandione derivative, anisindione, this drug must be considered potentially toxic because of its chemical similarity to phenindione.

The coumarin compounds have been given for prolonged periods without producing signs of toxicity. Occasional adverse reactions include gastrointestinal disturbances (especially diarrhea with dicumarol), elevated transaminase levels, urticaria, dermatitis, leukopenia, and alopecia. These reactions have not been observed with all coumarin drugs (eg, leukopenia has not been reported with warfarin). Necrotic lesions that are not the result of hemorrhage but are probably due to depression of protein C also have developed; the lesions are most commonly observed in overweight women given a large loading dose, usually at sites rich in fat tissue, such as the breasts, abdomen buttocks, thighs, and calves.

Precautions: If major hemorrhagic complications occur, all anticoagulants should be discontinued immediately. Bleeding episodes of any kind indicate the need for immediate reappraisal of the patient's condition.

Anticoagulants should be used with caution in the presence of mild liver or kidney disease, mild hypertension, alcoholism, infective endocarditis, drainage tubes in any orifice, or a history of gastrointestinal ulcers and in those with occupations that may be hazardous.

If treatment of ulcers is indicated during warfarin therapy, ranitidine [Zantac] or antacids alone should be given rather than cimetidine [Tagamet], which enhances the anticoagulant actions of warfarin.

Anisindione should be discontinued promptly if fever or rash develops. Because severe adverse effects may occur, this drug should be reserved for patients who cannot tolerate the coumarins.

The maintenance dose of oral anticoagulants may require adjustment in the presence of conditions that interfere with their actions. Patients receiving anticoagulant therapy have experienced increased prothrombin times when they adhere to certain fad diets low in vitamin K_1 (eg, when grapefruit are consumed as essentially the only nutritional item). Also, excessive intake of vitamin E may prolong warfarin-induced changes in prothrombin time. Careful supervision and use of the one-stage prothrombin time test are mandatory in the presence of such conditions.

Pregnancy and Lactation: If anticoagulants must be used during pregnancy (eg, in those with severe thrombophlebitis, pulmonary emboli, prosthetic valves), heparin, given subcutaneously, is the agent of choice. Although the incidence of maternal hemorrhage is increased, as are stillbirths and prematurity (Hall et al, 1980 A), when heparin is given to a hemostatically competent pregnant patient in doses limited to

10,000 units twice daily, the risk of intrauterine hemorrhage appears to be very low.

Because oral anticoagulants cross the placenta and have been associated with birth defects, particularly those involving the central nervous system, any woman of childbearing age who is taking oral anticoagulants should be advised to postpone pregnancy. If pregnancy occurs, the patient should be informed of the risks and termination of pregnancy should be considered. About one-third of infants are stillborn or abnormal if born alive. (See also the evaluation on Warfarin.)

Warfarin may appear in the milk of lactating women but does not appear to be hazardous to the nursing infants.

Interactions: Although many drugs affect the action of oral anticoagulants in laboratory animals, a much smaller number have been *clearly* demonstrated to produce such effects in man. Drugs shown to significantly *prolong* or *intensify* the action of oral anticoagulants clinically include sulfinpyrazone [Anturane], phenylbutazone [Azolid, Butazolidin], oxyphenbutazone [Oxalid], disulfiram [Antabuse], clofibrate [Atromid-S], thyroid drugs, anabolic steroids, large daily doses of aspirin (more than 3 g), metronidazole [Flagyl, Protostat], trimethoprim/sulfamethoxazole [Bactrim, Septra], and cimetidine [Tagamet] (O'Reilly, 1980).

The barbiturates, glutethimide [Doriden], and rifampin [Rifadin, Rimactane] are the primary drugs that *diminish* the response, although carbamazepine [Tegretol], oral contraceptives, diuretics, allopurinol [Lopurin, Zyloprim], antacids, laxatives, narcotic analgesics, cholestyramine resin [Questran] and other bile acid sequestrants, griseofulvin [Fulvicin, Grifulvin V, Grisactin, Gris-PEG], and anticholinergic drugs also have been implicated.

Dicumarol may cause tolbutamide [Orinase, SK-Tolbutamide] and phenytoin [Dilantin] to accumulate in the body. Therefore, doses of these drugs should be reduced when they are given with coumarins, or anisindione can be substituted. See also Chapter 3, Drug Interactions and Adverse Drug Reactions.

Drug Evaluations

HEPARIN CALCIUM
[Calciparine]

HEPARIN SODIUM

ACTIONS. Endogenous heparin, a sulfated mucopolysaccharide, is chemically heterogeneous. It is synthesized in mast cells and is particularly abundant in the lungs. The physiologic function of heparin is not fully understood, but its sudden release into the blood following anaphylactic shock indicates that it may play a role in immunologic reactions. Since the distribution of heparin in tissues was shown to correspond to the distribution of mast cells within the same tissues, it has been assumed that an injection has the same effect as release of heparin from mast cells. However, evidence now indicates that endogenous and exogenous heparin are handled differently within the body.

Commercial preparations consist of straight chain anionic polysaccharides of variable molecular weight (usually 7,000 to 40,000). Heparin prepared from different tissues also appears to vary: More protamine is required to neutralize a unit of beef lung heparin than porcine mucosal heparin, and plasma lipolytic activity, antifactor X_a activity, and activated partial thromboplastin time ratio are significantly different.

Heparin binds to the lysine residue of antithrombin III (AT-III), which produces a complex with greater affinity for serine proteases than AT-III alone. Thus, heparin functions as an anticoagulant by accelerating AT-III neutralization of activated clotting factors. Small amounts of heparin with AT-III inactivate factor X_a and prevent development of a hypercoagulable state by preventing conversion of prothrombin to thrombin. Larger amounts of heparin with AT-III inhibit coagulation by inactivating thrombin and earlier clotting factors, thus preventing conversion of fibrinogen to fibrin.

USES. Heparin is the only anticoagulant commonly used parenterally (warfarin also may be given intramuscularly or intravenously) and is the drug of choice when a rapid effect is desired. A major clinical application of heparin is to help maintain extracorporeal circulation during open heart surgery and renal hemodialysis. It also is given when immediate anticoagulation is required, such as in the treatment of massive deep venous thrombosis or pulmonary embolism with or without infarction. It can be used in place of sodium citrate as an anticoagulant for donor blood during cardiovascular surgery or hemodialysis. Heparin may be beneficial in the treatment of unequivocal DIC in patients who have acute leukemia (usually of the promyelocytic type). There are no data that support its use in other patients with DIC. (See the discussion on Disseminated Intravascular Coagulation in the Introduction.)

There is evidence that the subcutaneous administration of low doses of heparin greatly diminishes massive postoperative pulmonary embolism in patients at risk who are over age 40 (see the Introduction). Subcutaneous doses of 20,000 units/24 hours were as effective as warfarin in preventing recurrent thigh vein thromboses (Hull et al, 1982), but prolonged administration of this dose may cause osteoporosis. The routine use of low-dose heparin in general surgical patients at risk who are younger than 40 years is not advocated, for the possibility of hemorrhage and wound complications may exceed the risk of embolism. However, low-dose heparin may be indicated in women under forty years who are taking oral contraceptives.

When full-dose heparin is indicated in patients at high risk of bleeding, low-dose subcutaneous administration is not a satisfactory alternative to intravenous administration. Low-dose heparin does not prevent pulmonary embolism when thrombophlebitis is established, and it does not halt propagation of a thrombus distal to an arterial embolus (Deykin, 1982).

Small amounts of heparin calcium have been given subcutaneously to prevent postoperative thromboembolism. Claims that this salt produces lower blood levels, thereby reducing the incidence of bleeding, hematoma formation, or discomfort at the site of injection, have not been substantiated.

Heparin reduces postprandial lipemia by activating lipoprotein lipase and has a slight antihistaminic effect. Because of these actions, it has been claimed that heparin also may be useful as a hypolipidemic or anti-inflammatory agent, but there is no evidence of its efficacy for such purposes.

ADVERSE REACTIONS AND PRECAUTIONS. Subcutaneous injection seldom produces serious adverse reactions, although absorption may be irregular and unpredictable and hematoma or cumulative effects may occur after multiple doses. Skin necrosis, which may be severe enough to require grafting, can occur at sites of subcutaneous injection (Hall et al, 1980 B).

Clinically significant bleeding is related to numbers of units given/24 hours and occurs more frequently with larger than usual doses. Bleeding seldom is a problem if dosage is regulated on the basis of the results of clotting tests and continuous infusion is utilized. Major bleeding may be more common in elderly patients, severely ill patients, alcoholics, or those given antiplatelet drugs concomitantly. Bleeding also is increased when aspirin and small bolus doses of heparin are given concurrently or to patients with a predisposing condition (eg, recent surgery). The risk of hemorrhage is greater in those with thrombocytopenia or in those receiving intramuscular injections. The effects of therapy should be monitored by the activated partial thromboplastin time (APTT) test and the value maintained at one and one-half times normal.

Thrombocytopenia also may be induced by heparin, even with low-dose regimens. Early appearance of this complication (within two or three days after therapy is initiated) is usually not serious. However, delayed thrombocytopenia, which develops after 9 to 12 days of therapy, may be severe. In this form, the risk of hemorrhage and paradoxical thromboembolism is substantially increased. Therefore, a platelet count should be obtained before heparin therapy is initiated and at frequent intervals during treatment. If severe thrombocytopenia develops (platelet count less than 50,000/microliter), heparin should be discontinued and other measures instituted to manage the thrombosis. (See also the discussion in the Introduction.)

Fever, urticaria, and anaphylaxis occur occasionally after administration of heparin, and myalgia, bone pain, and osteoporosis may be noted with prolonged use. The latter has developed with doses larger than 20,000 units/day given for four months or possibly for shorter periods. Alopecia or a burning sensation in the feet occurs rarely.

Local capillary rupture with subsequent ecchymoses in the area of injection must be anticipated. This has occurred after both subcutaneous and intramuscular injection but is most likely after the latter. Therefore, intramuscular administration should never be used.

Heparin given subcutaneously is used to treat women who have experienced significant thromboembolism during pregnancy. However, the benefits must be weighed against potential risk to the fetus (FDA Pregnancy Category C). The use of heparin during pregnancy is associated with an increased incidence of maternal hemorrhage, stillbirth, and prematurity (Hall et al, 1980 A).

PHARMACOKINETICS. Heparin is metabolized mainly in the liver and is excreted by the kidneys. Up to 50% may be eliminated unchanged, particularly when large doses are injected. The duration of action is dose dependent: Intravenous doses of 100, 200, and 400 units/kg have half-lives of 56, 96, and 152 minutes, respectively. Subcutaneous administration produces a more prolonged but unpredictable effect.

ADMINISTRATION. Because of its immediate onset of action, heparin often is given for seven to ten days and an oral anticoagulant is added during the last three or four days using stepwise doses until the desired depression of clotting factor activity is achieved. Administration of heparin probably should be continued for six or seven days after satisfactory depression of prothrombin complex activity is obtained. Since significant quantities of circulating heparin prolong the prothrombin time, prothrombin time determinations should be made just before administering the next dose of heparin or with concomitant administration of an oral anticoagulant.

Full-dose heparin may be administered by intermittent subcutaneous or intravenous injection, by continuous intravenous drip, or by use of a constant infusion pump. This agent is inactive orally. The intravenous route is preferred; continuous infusion and intermittent injection appear to be equally effective in preventing thromboembolism, but continuous infusion prolongs clotting time more consistently.

The onset of anticoagulant effect is immediate following an intravenous bolus injection of full therapeutic doses and occurs approximately 20 to 30 minutes after subcutaneous injection. When the continuous infusion method is used, the two- to three-hour delay in anticoagulant effect may be avoided by injecting 5,000 units of heparin directly into the tubing after the infusion has been started.

DOSAGE AND PREPARATIONS. The dosage of heparin should be prescribed in units rather than milligrams. The U.S.P. standard for minimal potency is 120 units/mg of dry material derived from lung tissue and 140 units/mg of dry material derived from other sources. The potency of commercial preparations ranges from 140 to 190 units/mg. Thus, doses expressed in milligrams have no practical therapeutic meaning, since 100 mg of heparin may represent between 12,000 and 19,000 units of effect. Also, the U.S.P. unit is approximately 10% greater than the international unit (IU) and the difference should be taken into account.

Small doses usually are given to prevent thromboembolism. Larger doses are required to prevent propagation of an established thrombus. Still larger doses are necessary to block the thrombin-platelet interaction in acute pulmonary embolism. *Intravenous Infusion: Adults,* initially 5,000 units into the tubing after infusion is started, then 20,000 to 30,000 units daily at an initial rate of 0.5 unit/kg/min in 5% dextrose injection or isotonic sodium chloride injection. The rate is subsequently adjusted according to the results of clotting time tests. *Children,* 50 units/kg initially, followed by 100 units/kg every four hours.

An intravenous drip system or an infusion pump can be used to control the dosage. Although the infusion pump is the most accurate of the two methods, the pump must be monitored carefully since it will continue to force fluid extravascularly if the needle is dislodged, whereas an extravasating intravenous drip will usually stop within a reasonable period.

Intravenous (Intermittent): Adults, 5,000 units initially, followed by 5,000 to 10,000 units every four to six hours. Suitable laboratory testing is necessary to regulate the dose. For disseminated intravascular coagulation, one suggested regimen is, *adults,* 50 units/kg initially, and *children,* 25 units/kg every six hours or by continuous infusion. (See also the Introduction.)

Subcutaneous: For low-dose prophylaxis, *adults,* 5,000 units two hours before surgery and every 12 hours thereafter until the patient is discharged or is fully ambulatory. For usual full-dose effects, *adults,* 10,000 to 12,000 units every eight hours or 14,000 to 20,000 units every 12 hours. Different sites around the iliac crest or over the lower abdomen, a small needle (–27), and the smallest volume possible should be used to prevent massive hematoma.

Intramuscular: This route should not be used because of the likelihood of tissue irritation, local bleeding, or hematoma. Hematoma may not be clinically apparent until 1,000 ml or more has accumulated. In addition, absorption is unpredictable after intramuscular administration.

> HEPARIN CALCIUM:
> *Calciparine* (American Critical Care). Solution (sterile) 5,000, 12,500, and 20,000 units (from porcine intestinal mucosa).
> HEPARIN SODIUM:
> *Generic.* Solution 1,000, 2,500, 5,000, 7,500, 10,000, 15,000, 20,000, and 40,000 units/ml.
> **Available Trademark.**
> *Liquaemin Sodium* (Organon).

PROTAMINE SULFATE

ACTIONS AND USES. Protamine sulfate binds and inactivates heparin because of its strong electropositive charge. It combines ionically with heparin to form a stable complex. Paradoxically, it has anticoagulant action of its own and prolongs clotting time in the absence of heparin.

Protamine is indicated for treatment of heparin overdose that causes hemorrhage or increases the risk of hemorrhage. If hemorrhage is severe, transfusion of blood or plasma also may be required. Each milligram of protamine neutralizes 80 to 100 U.S.P. units of heparin activity, depending on the source of heparin. The reaction is almost instantaneous and effects persist for approximately two hours. However, since the effect of heparin may last longer than that of protamine, bleeding may recur, particularly in postoperative patients, and another injection of protamine may be needed.

ADVERSE REACTIONS AND PRECAUTIONS. Protamine is usually well tolerated. Large intravenous doses (up to 200 mg in two hours) have been administered without untoward effects, but no more than 50 mg should be administered as a single bolus. This drug must be used cautiously to prevent thrombotic complications.

Diabetic patients receiving protamine zinc insulin may be sensitized to protamine and experience a severe reaction when this agent is administered intravenously. Rarely, protamine hypersensitivity has occurred and repeated doses may result in anaphylactic reactions. Hypersensitivity also may occur in patients allergic to fish since protamine is obtained from fish of the salmon family. When protamine is used, facilities to treat shock and anaphylaxis should be available. Toxic manifestations include acute hypotension, dyspnea, and bradycardia. Occasionally, a feeling of warmth and flushing of the face may be observed.

Prolonged monitoring of patients is necessary following administration of large doses of heparin (eg, during cardiopulmonary bypass operations, dialysis) to determine requirements for additional doses of protamine. Suggested tests are the activated clotting time (ACT), activated partial thromboplastin time (APTT), or thrombin time (TT).

DOSAGE AND PREPARATIONS.
Intravenous: Total dosage is determined by the amount of heparin given over the previous three to four hours (each milligram of protamine sulfate, calculated as dry material, neutralizes not less than 80 U.S.P. units of heparin activity derived from lung tissue and not less than 100 U.S.P. units of heparin activity derived from intestinal mucosa). A solution containing 10 mg/ml is injected slowly over one to three minutes, not to exceed 50 mg in any ten-minute period.
> *Generic.* Powder; solution 10 mg/ml in 5 and 25 ml containers.

COUMARIN DERIVATIVES

DICUMAROL

Dicumarol has the same actions and uses as other oral anticoagulants and can usually maintain the effect established by other anticoagulants. It is long acting and, in the usual dosage range, three to five days are required for peak action. Once hypoprothrombinemia is established, the anticoagulant effect persists for two to ten days following discontinuation of therapy. Dicumarol is incompletely absorbed from the gastrointestinal tract and has a dose-dependent plasma half-life; therapy is therefore somewhat difficult to control; frequent monitoring is usually indicated. If overdosage occurs, it can be counteracted by phytonadione (vitamin K_1).

Dicumarol frequently causes flatulence and diarrhea. For other adverse reactions, precautions, interactions, and general class characteristics of the coumarin compounds, see the Introduction and the evaluation on Warfarin.

DOSAGE AND PREPARATIONS.
Oral: Adults, 200 to 300 mg on the first day, followed by 25 to 200 mg daily using prothrombin time determinations as a guide. Frequent dosage adjustments may be necessary during the first 7 to 14 days of therapy. Prothrombin time should be determined daily during this period and dosage adjusted to maintain prothrombin activity at approximately one and one-half times normal. The maintenance dose varies between 25 and 150 mg daily, depending on the results of these determinations.
> *Generic.* Tablets 25 and 50 mg.

PHENPROCOUMON
[Liquamar]

The actions and uses of this long-acting agent are qualitatively similar to those of other coumarin derivatives. The onset of a full anticoagulant effect is 48 to 72 hours after administration of the initial dose. Recovery may take up to seven days after the last dose is given. Phenprocoumon usually will maintain the anticoagulant effect established by other anticoagulants. Phytonadione (vitamin K_1) counteracts overdosage.

For adverse reactions, interactions, precautions, and general class characteristics of coumarin compounds, see the Introduction and the evaluation on Warfarin.

DOSAGE AND PREPARATIONS.
Oral: Adults, 24 mg on the first day. Maintenance dosage is individualized on the basis of prothrombin time determinations and varies between 0.75 and 6 mg; the exact amount may have to be adjusted to within 0.5 mg.
  Liquamar (Organon). Tablets 3 mg.

WARFARIN POTASSIUM
[Athrombin-K]

WARFARIN SODIUM
[Coumadin, Panwarfin]

ACTIONS. Like other coumarin compounds, warfarin depresses prothrombin activity. The results of the one-stage prothrombin time test and the activated partial thromboplastin time test are prolonged. The oral, intramuscular, and intravenous routes may be employed but parenteral administration offers no advantage over oral use except in patients who cannot tolerate oral therapy.

USES. Warfarin is the drug of choice when an oral anticoagulant is indicated.
  Deep Venous Thrombosis (DVT): After unequivocal diagnosis, a single episode should be treated with warfarin for three to six months. Patients with recurrent DVT require lifelong treatment. If these patients, particularly younger individuals, also have decreased platelet survival times, dipyridamole should be given concomitantly.
  Ischemic Heart Disease: Although the risk of hemorrhage is high and routine anticoagulant therapy is not advocated, warfarin has been given for three to six months following acute myocardial infarction to reduce the incidence of recurrent thromboembolism in selected patients. However, patients with unstable angina do not appear to benefit from long-term use of anticoagulants.

  Atrial Fibrillation (AF): Although data are from uncontrolled trials, long-term use of warfarin appears to reduce the risk of embolism in patients with AF due to mitral stenosis, chronic sinoatrial disease, congestive cardiomyopathy, or thyrotoxicosis. However, in patients with mitral valve prolapse, routine anticoagulation is not indicated.
  Cardiac Surgery: Lifelong use of warfarin is necessary for patients with artificial (metal, plastic) aortic or mitral valve prostheses. Routine anticoagulation probably is not needed in patients with tissue aortic valves but may be indicated in those with tissue mitral valves, especially if AF persists. Evidence that oral anticoagulants are beneficial after coronary artery bypass surgery is unconvincing.
  Transient Ischemic Attacks: Although oral anticoagulants are widely used, data have not shown that their prophylactic use reduces the incidence of subsequent cerebral infarction and antiplatelet agents are preferred.
  Peripheral Vascular Disease: There is no evidence that oral anticoagulants are of benefit in peripheral vascular disease.

ADVERSE REACTIONS AND PRECAUTIONS. As with all anticoagulants, hemorrhagic complications may occur during therapy. If bleeding develops, the decision to use vitamin K should be based on a balance between antithrombotic protection and the severity of bleeding. If use of vitamin K is considered necessary, warfarin should be discontinued immediately and phytonadione (vitamin K_1) administered to counteract the anticoagulant effect: For mild bleeding, a single dose of 1 to 5 mg intravenously or 10 to 20 mg orally; for severe bleeding, 20 to 40 mg intravenously with additional doses at four-hour intervals, as necessary. The peak effect of phytonadione usually occurs within four to eight hours after oral administration (see also Chapter 36, Hemostatics). Administration of phytonadione, particularly in doses greater than 2.5 mg, results in rebound hypercoagulability and resistance to oral anticoagulants may develop. If hemorrhage is severe, concomitant administration of whole blood or single-donor plasma may be necessary.

Untoward reactions occur infrequently with coumarin derivatives and include dermatitis; necrosis of the breast, buttocks, thighs, abdomen, calves, and skin; purple toes syndrome; alopecia; gastrointestinal irritation; urticaria; and elevated transaminase levels. Unlike other coumarin derivatives, leukopenia has not been noted with warfarin.

The recurrent skin necrosis occurring during warfarin therapy has been associated with protein C deficiency. When necrosis occurs during initial oral anticoagulant therapy, the possibility of protein C deficiency should be considered and tests to verify its presence should be performed (Griffin, 1984).

TERATOGENICITY. When given during the first trimester (especially the sixth to ninth week) of pregnancy, warfarin is associated with embryopathy characterized most commonly by nasal hypoplasia and stippled epiphyses. Other abnormalities, including central nervous system and eye defects (eg, blindness), are thought to result from longer exposure, probably during the second and third trimesters. Review of case histories reveals that about one-third of infants exposed to coumarin derivatives are stillborn or abnormal if born alive.

INTERACTIONS. See the Introduction and Chapter 3, Drug Interactions and Adverse Drug Reactions.

PHARMACOKINETICS. Warfarin is intermediate acting; a peak effect is achieved in 36 to 72 hours and the action lasts two to five days. The drug is readily absorbed from the gastrointestinal tract, is highly fat soluble, and is transported in blood loosely bound to albumin. Some tissue binding occurs, particularly in the liver. However, only the unbound drug is active and available for hydroxylation in the liver. Metabolites probably are inactive in man and, together with a small amount of unchanged drug, are excreted by the kidneys. The rate of degradation is independent of the dose and, although constant for an individual, varies widely among patients.

DOSAGE AND PREPARATIONS.
Oral, Intravenous: The preferred dosage is 15 mg, 10 mg, and 10 mg on the first three days. Usually, there is little change in prothrombin time during the first 24 hours, followed by a slow rise to 16 to 20 seconds (assuming control values of between 12 and 15 seconds) by the third day. The usual maintenance dose is 5 to 7.5 mg daily thereafter. However, variations in induction response may require doses (after the first 24 hours) of approximately 5 to 20 mg, with maintenance doses of less than 5 to at least 10 mg, respectively. (See the Introduction.)

Prothrombin time should be determined before the initial dose is given and every day thereafter until the response is stabilized. After a steady state is achieved, prothrombin time should be determined at regular intervals.

WARFARIN POTASSIUM:
Athrombin-K (Purdue Frederick). Tablets 5 mg.
WARFARIN SODIUM:
Coumadin (DuPont). Tablets 2, 2.5, 5, 7.5, and 10 mg; powder (lyophilized, for injection) 50 mg with 2 ml of diluent.
Panwarfin (Abbott), ***Generic.*** Tablets 2, 2.5, 5, 7.5, and 10 mg.

INDANDIONE DERIVATIVE

ANISINDIONE
[Miradon]

ACTIONS AND USES. This long-acting agent has actions and uses similar to those of the coumarins; however, since anisindione is potentially dangerous, it should be reserved for patients who cannot tolerate the coumarins. See the Introduction.

After the initial dose, the peak effect is reached in 48 to 72 hours, and coagulation factors gradually return to normal 24 to 72 hours after the drug is discontinued. As with other oral anticoagulants, both resistance and sensitivity have been reported. Phytonadione (vitamin K_1), fresh whole blood, or single-donor plasma counteracts the effect of anisindione, but blood or plasma should be administered only if hemorrhagic complications are severe.

ADVERSE REACTIONS AND PRECAUTIONS. Dermatitis is the only untoward reaction consistently associated with anisindione therapy. However, since the related indandione, phenindione (no longer marketed), produced serious and sometimes fatal adverse effects (eg, agranulocytosis, jaundice, nephropathy), anisindione must be assumed to have the potential to cause serious complications. The drug should be discontinued promptly if fever, sore throat, or rash appears, for these symptoms may signal the onset of severe toxicity.

Anisindione occasionally discolors alkaline urine orange; this can be differentiated from hematuria by its disappearance on acidification of the urine. The patient should be advised of this possibility.

DOSAGE AND PREPARATIONS.
Oral: *Adults,* 300 mg on the first day, 200 mg on the second day, and 100 mg on the third day. For maintenance, the amount that maintains prothrombin time values at 2 to 2.5 times normal should be given; the usual dose ranges from 25 to 250 mg daily.
Miradon (Schering). Tablets 50 mg.

Cited References

Anturane Reinfarction Trial Research Group: Sulfinpyrazone in prevention of sudden death after myocardial infarction. *N Engl J Med* 302:250-256, 1980.

Anturane Reinfarction Trial Policy Committee: Anturane reinfarction trial: Reevaluation of outcome. *N Engl J Med* 306:1005-1008, 1982.

Aspirin Myocardial Infarction Study Research Group: Randomized, controlled trial of aspirin in persons recovered from myocardial infarction. *JAMA* 243:661-669, 1980.

Broekmans AW, et al: Congenital protein C deficiency and venous thromboembolism: Study of three Dutch families. *N Engl J Med* 309:340-344, 1983.

Canadian Cooperative Study Group: Randomized trial of aspirin and sulfinpyrazone in threatened stroke. *N Engl J Med* 299:53-59, 1978.

Canner PL: Aspirin in coronary heart disease: Comparison of six clinical trials. *Isr J Med Sci* 19:413-423, 1983.

Chesebro JH, et al: Trial of combined warfarin plus dipyridamole or aspirin therapy in prosthetic heart valve replacement: Danger of aspirin compared with dipyridamole. *Am J Cardiol* 51:1537-1541, 1983.

Corash L: Disseminated intravascular coagulation. *Primary Care* 7:423-438, 1980.

Deykin D: Thrombosis and anticoagulant therapy, in Isselbacher KJ, et al (eds): *Update II. Principles of Internal Medicine,* ed 9. New York, McGraw-Hill, 1982, 51-73.

Eichner ER: Platelets, carotids, and coronaries: Critique on antithrombotic role of antiplatelet agents, exercise, and certain diets. *Am J Med* 77:513-523, 1984.

Elwood PC: Aspirin in prevention of myocardial infarction: Current status. *Drugs* 28:1-5, 1984.

Griffin JH: Clinical studies of protein C. *Semin Thromb Hemostas* 10:162-166, 1984.

Hall JG, et al: Maternal and fetal sequelae of anticoagulation during pregnancy. *Am J Med* 68:122-140, 1980 A.

Hall JC, et al: Heparin necrosis: Anticoagulation syndrome. *JAMA* 244:1831-1832, 1980 B.

Hull R, et al: Adjusted subcutaneous heparin versus warfarin sodium in long-term treatment of venous thrombosis. *N Engl J Med* 306:189-194, 1982.

King DJ, Kelton JG: Heparin-associated thrombocytopenia. *Ann Intern Med* 100:535-540, 1984.

Krol WF: Persantine and aspirin in coronary heart disease. *Circulation* 62:449-461, 1980.

Lagerstedt CI, et al: Need for long-term anticoagulant treatment in symptomatic calf-vein thrombosis. *Lancet* 2:515-518, 1985.

Marlar RA: Protein C in thromboembolic disease. *Semin Thromb Hemostas* 11:387-393, 1985.

McGehee WG, et al: Coumarin necrosis associated with hereditary protein C deficiency. *Ann Intern Med* 100:59-60, 1984.

Mehta J, Roy L: Platelet-suppressive therapy in cardiovascular disease. *Cardiovasc Clin* 14:211-234, 1984.

O'Reilly RA: Anticoagulant, antithrombolytic, and thrombolytic drugs, in Gilman AG, et al (eds): *The Pharmacological Basis of Therapeutics,* ed 6. New York, Macmillan, 1980, 1347-1366.

Østerud B, Rapaport S: Activation of ^{125}I-factor IX and ^{125}I-factor X: Effect of tissue factor and factor VII, factor X_a and thrombin. *Scand J Haematol* 24:213-226, 1980.

Temple R, Pledger GW: FDA's critique of Anturane reinfarction trial. *N Engl J Med* 303:1488-1492, 1980.

Wyngaarden JB, Smith LH Jr (eds): *Cecil Textbook of Medicine,* ed 16. Philadelphia, WB Saunders, 1982.

Other Selected References

Breckenridge A: Oral anticoagulant drugs: Pharmacokinetic aspects. *Semin Hematol* 15:19-26, 1978.

Brozovic M: Oral anticoagulants in clinical practice. *Semin Hematol* 15:27-34, 1978.

Deykin D: Heparin therapy: Regimens and management. *Drugs* 13:46-51, 1977.

Deykin D: Current status of anticoagulant therapy. *Am J Med* 72:659-664, 1982.

Didisheim P, Fuster V: Actions and clinical status of platelet-suppressive agents. *Semin Hematol* 15:55-72, 1978.

Fuster V, Chesebro JH: Antithrombotic therapy: Role of platelet-inhibitor drugs. I. Current concepts of thrombogenesis: Role of platelets. II. Pharmacologic effects of platelet-inhibitor drugs. III. Management of arterial thromboembolic and atherosclerotic disease. *Mayo Clin Proc* 56:102-112, 185-195, 265-273, 1981.

Hirsch J: Role of aspirin and antithrombotic agents in cardiovascular disease. *Cardiovasc Rev Rep* 5:1003-1013, 1984.

Salem HH: Current status of anticoagulants. *Drug Ther* 13:57-66, (Oct) 1983.

Thomas DP: Heparin in prophylaxis and treatment of venous thromboembolism. *Semin Hematol* 15:1-17, 1978.

Verstraete M, Verwilghen R: Haematological disorders, in Avery GS (ed): *Drug Treatment: Principles and Practice of Clinical Pharmacology,* ed 2. New York, ADIS Press, 1980, 889-952.

Weiss HJ: Platelet physiology and abnormalities of platelet function. *N Engl J Med* 293:531-541, 1975.

Weiss HJ: Antiplatelet therapy. *N Engl J Med* 298:1403-1406, 1978.

Wessler S: Anticoagulant dilemma: Prescription for its resolution. *Am J Med Sci* 274:106-117, 1977.

Thrombolytics

The coagulation system is activated to maintain the integrity of vascular function following injury to the blood vessels. The consequent formation of fibrin clots proceeds through an interdependent series of coagulation reactions (see Chapter 33, Agents Used for Anticoagulant Therapy). The fibrinolytic system provides the physiologic mechanism for repair by digesting the fibrin clot, and it may be activated simultaneously with the coagulation system to prevent inappropriate or excessive thrombosis. However, when a thrombus obstructs an artery or vein, permanent damage in the ischemic area may occur before physiologic fibrinolysis can take place.

Anticoagulants prevent the extension and propagation of existing thrombi, and thrombolytic agents dissolve existing thrombi through a proteolytic action on the supporting fibrin network. Rapid lysis of the clot promptly decreases pulmonary hypertension and restores hemodynamic disturbances to normal in patients with pulmonary emboli. Thrombolytics are used when rapid dissolution of the clot is required to preserve organ and limb function (arterial occlusion) or valve function of the veins (venous occlusion). Anticoagulants should then be given to prevent recurrence. The thrombolytic agents used for dissolution of thrombi are streptokinase [Kabikinase, Streptase] and urokinase [Abbokinase]. They are agents of choice for treating pulmonary embolism and deep vein thrombosis in selected patients (*Ann Intern Med*, 1980).

Thrombolysis also is being employed frequently to treat acute myocardial infarction (AMI). This use has been studied extensively since coronary artery thrombi were reported to occur in 70% to 90% of patients with AMI, and coronary occlusion usually does not resolve spontaneously during the initial 24 hours of transmural infarction (De Wood et al, 1980, 1983). Reports (eg, Rentrop et al, 1979) that rapid reperfusion

of the infarcted artery could be accomplished by intracoronary infusion of streptokinase have stimulated continuing research. The focus has been on limiting the extent of myocardial damage during the acute occlusion. Clinical strategy is based on the concept that early restoration of adequate myocardial perfusion will limit damage at the site of occlusion and protect the tissue at risk of necrosis distal to the occluded area. Although many cardiologists believe thrombolysis to be beneficial in acute myocardial infarction, effects on long-term morbidity and mortality have not been determined.

Before discussing the pharmacologic activities of thrombolytic agents, the function of the fibrinolytic system should be considered.

Mechanisms of Thrombolysis: The fibrinolytic system consists of three main components: (1) the circulating proenzyme, plasminogen; (2) plasminogen activators, which are enzymes present in blood, vascular endothelium, and numerous tissues (the most important is tissue-type plasminogen activator [tPA] that originates in the endothelial wall); and (3) natural inhibitors, which rapidly neutralize plasmin or inhibit the action of tPA.

Plasminogen, a single-chain protein with multiple isoelectric forms, is normally present in human plasma and is activated primarily by plasminogen activators originating in the vascular wall or tissues.

The activators of plasminogen, particularly tPA, are released from tissues in response to local trauma, thrombi, or certain other stimuli (eg, neurohumoral factors). Inhibitors limit tPA's activity in circulating blood.

Plasmin, the active serine protease converted from plasminogen, digests fibrin and fibrinogen to produce degradation products (FDP). FDP inhibit thrombin's conversion of fibrinogen to fibrin and thereby become circulating anticoagulants themselves. Plasmin also hydrolyzes a number of other proteins, including prothrombin; factors V, VIII, and XII; the first component of complement; and prekallikrein. However, natural inhibitors in the blood, particularly α_2-antiplasmin, rapidly limit plasmin's action and prevent the massive systemic proteolysis and fibrinolysis that would occur if it were allowed to circulate freely. Free plasmin is not normally detectable in blood, probably because the inhibitor capacity exceeds the activation potential.

Both tPA and plasminogen bind to fibrin at lysine binding sites. In the presence of fibrin, tPA has a greatly enhanced ratio of activation for plasminogen. The plasmin that is formed is inhibited relatively slowly by α_2-antiplasmin because the lysine binding sites of plasmin are occupied by fibrin. This allows time for plasmin to exert its thrombolytic effect on the clot before inhibition can occur. As fibrin is lysed, activator and plasmin are released into blood where they are bound by their inhibitors to prevent fibrinolysis in circulating blood. Therefore, the selective fibrinolysis of thrombi without proteolysis of circulating proteins is regulated by localization of plasminogen activator-plasminogen complex on the surface of forming fibrin.

Diagnosis of Thrombotic Disorders: Angiographic demonstration is necessary for diagnosis of occlusion in acute AMI. The decision to use thrombolytics should be based on definitive evidence of thrombotic disease and determination of its severity. Demonstration of deep vein thrombosis by venography and pulmonary embolism by pulmonary angiography is necessary. Although radioisotope perfusion or lung scans are widely used and a normal scan eliminates the diagnosis of pulmonary embolism, lung scans and some noninvasive tests also may be abnormal in various nonthrombotic disorders. Arterial blood gas measurements are inadequate for diagnosis.

For thrombophlebitis, combined impedance plethysmography and ^{125}I-fibrinogen leg scanning are safe and detect deep venous thrombosis in approximately 90% of patients (Hull et al, 1981).

Monitoring Therapy: When treating conditions other than evolving myocardial infarction, the activity of the fibrinolytic system should be confirmed by performing the thrombin time (TT) test three or four hours after infusion of the thrombolytic agent is begun. The test does not, however, reliably predict fibrinolytic efficacy or risk of bleeding. A hematocrit value also should be determined at this time. If essential, venipuncture with a 22- or 23-gauge needle may be performed for arterial blood gas studies but only in patients confined to strict bedrest. The arm should be used and digital compression of the puncture site for at least 30 minutes is mandatory. Vital signs should be assessed every four hours during infusions. To avoid dislodging deep vein thrombi, blood pressure measurements should not be taken in the legs.

Therapy: Although several techniques for initiating thrombolysis have been investigated, the only currently practical means is by activation of the fibrinolytic system with streptokinase or urokinase. Both are proteins that convert plasminogen to plasmin, resulting in digestion of fibrin and lysis of blood clots.

Because these agents cause systemic lysis (depletion of plasminogen and fibrinogen, consumption of circulating α_2-antiplasmin, increase in circulating fibrinogen degradation products) that may result in bleeding, a second generation of substances with some clot selectivity is being developed. The most promising compound under clinical investigation is tissue-type plasminogen activator (tPA), a natural enzyme that is being produced by recombinant DNA technology (rtPA). Since this agent has a high affinity for fibrin and fibrin-bound plasminogen, clot-selective fibrinolysis occurs. However, because clot selectivity is not absolute, modest fibrinogenolysis may occur. Further studies are needed to determine whether such recanalization produces long-term benefits.

Pro-UK, a kidney plasminogen activator, also has been produced by recombinant DNA techniques and is claimed to be fibrin-specific in that fibrinogen is not degraded by fibrinolytic concentrations of pro-UK. It is being tested clinically.

Another investigational approach to thrombolytic therapy involves the use of modified enzyme precursors (eg, acylated derivatives of plasmin, streptokinase-plasmin complex) to provide controlled clot breakdown (Smith et al, 1981). The acylated enzymes are able to bind to fibrin clots but are protected while in the circulation from interaction with the inhibitor α_2-antiplasmin. As the acyl group dissociates from the plasmin, the enzyme becomes proteolytically active and degrades the fibrin clot. In the presence of a fibrin clot, the acyl-streptokinase group dissociates, leaving the plasmin close to the fibrin clot. These chemically modified enzyme precursors theoretically can be given in doses calculated to provide the steady-state fibrin-bound concentrations necessary to achieve the required rate of thrombolysis. However, according to some investigators, patients given acylated streptokinase plasminogen complex experienced significant dose-related fibrinolysis that was modified by streptokinase antibodies (Walker et al, 1984).

Currently, it appears that all available fibrinolytic agents should be used only in patients who can be treated promptly and should not be used indiscriminately in patients with evolving infarction.

Myocardial Infarction

Pathophysiology of Myocardial Infarction and Coronary Reperfusion: When occlusion of a coronary artery occurs, the affected muscle is paralyzed immediately and recovery depends on the duration, magnitude, and severity of ischemia. The size of the infarct depends on the duration of the ischemia, presence or absence of collaterals, and myocardial oxygen requirements.

Initially, myocardial ischemia causes reversible cellular injury that becomes irreversible if myocardial blood flow is not restored. Myocyte injury progresses rapidly in the subendocardial region and continuing ischemia affects more cells in a wavefront effect spreading toward the subepicardial region to become a transmural infarct (Jennings and Reimer, 1983). Vascular injury also occurs but at a slower rate.

In most patients, acute damage progresses to necrosis during the first three to six hours following total occlusion. To prevent myocyte death, reperfusion must occur before irreversible necrosis. Reperfusion accelerates disintegration of irreversibly damaged cells; if vascular integrity is compromised, a no-flow phenomenon results and hemorrhage into irreversibly damaged tissue may occur.

Following experimental coronary occlusion in dogs, ischemia in the subendocardial region was found to be reversible during the first 20 minutes; after that time, only cells in the subepicardial region could be reperfused successfully. In these animal studies, subepicardial cells were salvageable for up to three hours; after five to six hours, limitation of infarct size could not be demonstrated. Results of these studies probably cannot be extrapolated directly to humans, although progression of necrosis is similar. In man, a thrombotic coronary occlusion often is superimposed on severe atherosclerotic plaque that has narrowed the artery. In patients with long-standing atherosclerosis, collateral vessels may have developed in this area and occlusion may be more gradual. Therefore, reperfusion may salvage jeopardized myocardium in the subepicardial region for periods longer than six hours. Nevertheless, the sooner that reperfusion can be achieved, the more likely that the effects will be beneficial.

The ultimate goal of reperfusion is to restore left ventricular function. The rate of recovery of contractile function after reperfusion is inversely related to the duration of ischemia (Kloner et al, 1983 A). In multicenter studies (Rentrop et al, 1981 A and B; Rentrop et al, 1983), left ventricular ejection fraction improved in patients permanently reperfused within six hours after onset of AMI symptoms. However, the ischemic myocardium requires several days before function, biochemical characteristics, and ultrastructure return to normal and measurement of left ventricular function should be postponed for 10 to 14 days after AMI. This transient postischemic dysfunction is called the stunned myocardium phenomenon. The hemorrhagic condition of the necrotic area does not appear to affect the recovery rate, because the bleeding is confined within tissue that was already necrotic at the time of reperfusion (Kloner, 1983 B).

Thrombolytics in Acute Myocardial Infarction: Following acute myocardial infarction, therapy to restore patency of occluded coronary arteries in ischemic but not yet necrotic myocardial tissue appears promising. The only intervention that reduces damage is one that includes reperfusion of the ischemic area. None of the drugs that reduce oxygen demand have routinely reduced infarct size, although selected beta blockers (eg, timolol [Blocadren], metoprolol [Lopressor], atenolol [Tenormin]) may slow the rate of myocardial necrosis when given intravenously within two to four hours after onset of symptoms of AMI (see Chapter 25, Antianginal Agents). Such agents may be beneficial in patients with residual flow to the infarct zone (Gersh, 1985). Hyaluronidase [Wydase], which has no negative inotropic activity, had no significant effect on the incidence of infarction, infarct size, or survival following AMI (Jaffe, 1985).

Both streptokinase and urokinase can reperfuse occluded coronary arteries in patients with AMI. Because of its lower cost, streptokinase has been used most commonly. However, urokinase is equally effective. Results of a randomized study comparing the two drugs indicated that patients receiving

urokinase had less systemic fibrinolysis (Tennant et al, 1984). Also, urokinase is nonantigenic and may be preferred in patients with high antibody titers to streptokinase.

Thrombolytics have been given by the intracoronary route in an attempt to provide high local concentrations while minimizing systemic fibrinolysis. However, whether given intravenously or by intracoronary infusion, both streptokinase and urokinase activate the fibrinolytic system in the general circulation at the doses required for successful thrombolysis of coronary arteries. Data from numerous studies indicate that intracoronary infusion of streptokinase recanalizes infarct-related occlusion of coronary arteries in approximately 75% of patients. Although immediate thrombolytic therapy appears to be a rational means of achieving reperfusion, reperfusion per se is not the ultimate goal. Rescue of at least a portion of the jeopardized myocardium is necessary to limit infarct size, achieve recovery of left ventricular function (LVF), and improve survival. There is some indication that early reperfusion limits infarct size. Electrocardiographic changes and elevation of CK-MB were reported in some successfully reperfused patients. Improved LVF has been reported, but results are inconsistent. In one study, improvement occurred only in patients with subtotal stenosis and/or extensive collateral circulation in the ischemic area (Rodgers et al, 1984), but the mean time to initiation of thrombolytic therapy was seven hours after onset of symptoms, and the effects of early reperfusion could not be assessed. In another study on factors relating to recovery of LVF (Sheehan et al, 1985), it was suggested that reperfusion must provide adequate flow (minimum stenosis diameter greater than 0.4 mm) and therapy must be instituted within 2.5 hours after onset of symptoms if LVF is to be improved in patients with total occlusion of the left anterior descending coronary artery without collaterals.

Data on long-term survival after successful reperfusion also are meager and equivocal. Results of the Western Washington thrombolytic trial showed significantly improved survival during the first 30 days in patients successfully reperfused with intracoronary streptokinase (Kennedy et al, 1983). After one year, the reduced mortality in this group was still significantly different from those who had either unsuccessful or partial reperfusion (Kennedy et al, 1985). When mortality was calculated on the basis of data from eight prospective randomized trials using intracoronary streptokinase (Furberg, 1984), the difference between treated groups and controls was not significant. However, the trials varied considerably in design and the pooled data should be interpreted cautiously.

There may be important differences in risks and benefits of thrombolytic therapy for various subgroups of patients. Those with transmural infarction are more likely to benefit from early reperfusion than patients with nontransmural infarctions in whom total coronary occlusion is less common. In patients with collateral circulation, reperfusion more than six hours after onset of symptoms may salvage some myocardium. However, when the occlusion is of longer duration, myocardial blood flow is not restored to normal by reperfusion and the no-flow phenomenon may occur. Although late application of thrombolytic agents may reperfuse arteries, reperfusion in a necrotic area may produce a hemorrhagic infarct even though it does not increase infarct size (Laffel and Braunwald, 1984).

Reperfusion of the artery can only re-establish blood flow; it cannot reverse the underlying disease. Blood flow may remain suboptimal after lysis due to residual stenosis, which is correlated with risk of reocclusion. Because the effects of streptokinase or urokinase dissipate within a few hours, subsequent adequate anticoagulation is necessary.

To decrease the risk of recurrence, thrombolytic therapy usually is continued for 30 to 60 minutes after reperfusion, anticoagulation is maintained with heparin for 2 to 12 days, and warfarin or antiplatelet agents are given for three months thereafter. Despite effective anticoagulation, some patients develop reocclusion and more definitive procedures, such as percutaneous transluminal coronary angioplasty (PTCA) or coronary artery bypass grafting (CABG), may be necessary.

Complications, such as hemorrhage, are usually localized and arrhythmias that occur upon reperfusion in a substantial number of patients (and may be considered a marker for successful reperfusion) usually can be controlled by standard therapy.

Successful thrombolysis provides the time needed to implement definitive procedures (PTCA or CABG) in patients with severe residual stenosis and provides immediate benefits, such as reduction in severity of angina, resolution of ST-segment abnormalities, and possibly improvement in ventricular function. However, there are several limitations and disadvantages to use of intracoronary streptokinase or urokinase. Thrombolysis must be started early (within two to four hours) following onset of symptoms of AMI if it is to be effective. Thus, emergency cardiac catheterization facilities must be available and staffed by skilled personnel 24 hours a day. At present in the United States, the technical expertise and specialized equipment required are available to only approximately 10% of the patients with evolving myocardial infarction.

Treatment with intravenous streptokinase or urokinase is available to most patients with evolving myocardial infarction and has been considered an alternative. Use of this method avoids the complications associated with catheterization and can be started more promptly. This could theoretically salvage more ischemic myocardium and is less hazardous than intracoronary thrombolysis because coronary arteriography is not involved. Successful recanalization has been reported in 30% to 70% of patients receiving intravenous streptokinase. The wide variability in results may be due to inclusion of patients with incomplete obstruction, since there was no documentation of degree of occlusion in some studies. The large doses necessary (usually 1,500,000 units within a one-hour period) increase the risk of hemorrhage. However, this form of therapy has been considered promising and is being used with increasing frequency.

Preliminary results of Phase I of the Thrombolysis in Myocardial Infarction (TIMI) Trial indicate that intravenous streptokinase is effective in approximately 35% of patients. All patients had angiographic confirmation of at least 50% reduction in the diameter of the infarct-related artery after administration of 200 mcg of intracoronary nitroglycerin before being given thrombolytic therapy (TIMI Study Group, 1985). Data from previous trials have indicated a recanalization rate of approximately 75% in patients receiving intracoronary streptokinase. Therefore, it appears that intravenous streptokinase is approximately one-half as effective as intracoronary streptokinase for reperfusion of infarct-related occluded arteries following AMI. Because studies have not shown that this therapy influences mortality, use of the intravenous route for coronary artery reperfusion should be considered investigational.

Other Indications

Pulmonary Embolism: A panel of experts convened by the National Institutes of Health has determined that streptokinase and urokinase are the agents of choice for treating pulmonary embolism and deep vein thrombosis in selected patients (*Ann Intern Med*, 1980). These agents are safe, more effective than conventional anticoagulants in carefully selected patients, and provide greater long-term benefit than heparin. Bleeding is a serious complication, but advantages may outweigh the risk when patients are properly selected and treatment is carefully monitored. (See section on Selection of Patients below.)

A major indication includes patients with acute, massive, and severe life-threatening pulmonary emboli (ie, emboli large enough to occlude two-thirds or more of the main branches of the pulmonary artery or the equivalent in other pulmonary blood supply that cause acute right side heart failure with or without shock, dyspnea, and progressive deterioration). Patients with pre-existing lung or heart disease with severe pulmonary hypertension due to less extensive emboli also may be considered for thrombolytic therapy. Those with an unstable hemodynamic condition caused by major residual circulatory obstruction may be suitable candidates if the thrombosis has occurred no more than 48 hours previously.

Although immediate mortality is high and thrombolytic treatment is urgent, these drugs should be used only after pulmonary embolism is confirmed by pulmonary angiography. While the diagnosis is being confirmed, heparin may be given but should be discontinued prior to infusion of the thrombolytic agent.

Urokinase or streptokinase dissolve a major portion of the acute embolus and decrease pulmonary hypertension, improve perfusion of the pulmonary capillary bed, and correct other hemodynamic disturbances. Although disputed by many investigators, prompt thrombolytic therapy has been reported to have long-term beneficial effects on pulmonary microcirculation (Sharma et al, 1980). Acute morbidity may be decreased because right heart strain and breathlessness are relieved, but mortality is not reduced and surgical embolectomy (usual mortality of 50%) followed by caval interruption may be necessary. Furthermore, thrombolytics are useful only within five to seven days after embolism has occurred. For subacute, chronic, or small emboli or during pregnancy, heparin is preferred.

In a limited number of patients, angiographically localized infusion utilizing lower doses was effective and did not cause bleeding.

Deep Venous Thrombosis: Streptokinase and urokinase are useful in patients with an established diagnosis of deep venous thrombosis that has developed within 72 hours (Goldhaber et al, 1984). Approximately two-thirds of such thrombi can be dissolved. Older thrombi become increasingly resistant to lysis. Potential beneficial effects include reduction of edema, induration, and pain and preservation of valvular function. Thrombolytic treatment may be indicated in patients with recent occlusive iliofemoral thrombosis. However, those with thrombosis distal to the popliteal vein may be managed adequately by anticoagulants.

Patients with thrombi in deep veins of the upper extremity also may be candidates for thrombolytic therapy. Anticoagulant treatment alone has caused a high incidence of chronic symptoms of venous hypertension in these patients (Rubin, 1983).

Low doses of thrombolytic agents have been infused intra-arterially in a small number of patients for localized treatment of deep venous thrombosis (Taylor et al, 1984). However, complications are the same as with larger doses and more investigation is necessary before this therapy can be recommended.

Occluded Arteriovenous Cannulae: Instillation of streptokinase into occluded arteriovenous cannulae in patients on chronic renal dialysis has salvaged most occluded cannulae and avoided surgery. This technique should be reserved for use after conventional mechanical measures have failed.

Peripheral Artery Thrombosis: In acute thromboembolism of peripheral arteries, embolectomy using a Fogarty balloon catheter is preferred if the artery is normal. In arteries with major atheromatous changes, thrombolytic therapy may be effective if the occlusion is less than 72 hours old. However, restoration of circulation also depends on the location of the occlusion, the amount of collateral circulation, and the extent of irreversible tissue damage. Initial surgical treatment precludes subsequent use of thrombolytics for at least ten days. Thrombolytic agents are not indicated for superficial thrombophlebitis; thrombolysis is considered only if the thrombus extends into the femoral vein.

Miscellaneous Uses: Other uses of thrombolytic agents have included severe unstable angina pectoris, renal artery thrombosis, prosthetic heart valve thrombosis, vein graft thrombosis, retinal artery or vein occlusion, and impending renal cortical necrosis. However, more data are needed before thrombolytics can be recommended for these disorders.

Selection of Patients

Patients with evolving myocardial infarction who experience chest pain for at least one-half hour but less than four hours and who exhibit ST-segment elevation of a least 0.1 mV in two electrocardiographic leads that is unresponsive to nitroglycerin may be considered candidates for thrombolytic therapy. They should be excluded from thrombolytic therapy according to the guidelines outlined below, which were developed by the NIH panel of experts for all patients receiving such therapy:

1. Since thrombolytics lyse fibrin at any source, whether pathologic thrombi or hemostatic plugs, invasive procedures (eg, puncture of noncompressible vessels) should not be performed ten days before or during treatment to minimize the possibility of bleeding. For exceptions, see the discussion on Monitoring Therapy.

2. Because cerebral hemorrhage has been associated with thrombolytic therapy, absolute contraindications are active internal bleeding, stroke or other cerebrovascular accident within the past two months, and intracranial neoplasm.

3. Relative contraindications are severe hypertension, major surgery, delivery of a child, organ biopsy, serious gastrointestinal bleeding, and serious trauma within the previous ten days.

4. Precautions include recent cardiopulmonary resuscitation, subacute bacterial endocarditis, mitral disease with atrial fibrillation, hemostatic defects associated with hepatic or renal disease, diabetic retinopathy, pregnancy, septic thrombophlebitis, occluded A-V cannula at a seriously infected site, prior severe allergic reaction to the thrombolytic agent, or advanced age (over 75).

5. Since thrombi become increasingly resistant to lysis with time, those present for more than seven days should be treated with heparin; thrombolytic agents should not be administered.

6. If pulmonary angiography must be performed, the arm should be used. Otherwise, diagnostic procedures were not discussed by the NIH panel. However, after initial diagnosis and before therapy is begun, the following laboratory tests are recommended to provide baseline data and determine whether a bleeding diathesis exists: thrombin time (TT), activated partial thromboplastin time (APTT), prothrombin time (PT), hematocrit, fibrinogen concentration, and platelet count. The TT and APTT values should be less than twice the normal control times before therapy is started. Heparin should be discontinued.

Generally, the potential benefits should be weighed against the risk of bleeding. Intramuscular injections or unnecessary handling of the patient should be avoided during therapy. Relative contraindications not mentioned by the NIH group are dissecting aneurysm, visceral carcinoma, active tuberculosis with cavitation of recent onset, or systemic infections.

Thrombolytic agents should not be used during the first 18 weeks of pregnancy because the fetus and its membranes are attached to the uterus mainly by fibrin, and there is a theoretical risk of premature separation of the placenta. (Streptokinase is classified in FDA Pregnancy Category A and urokinase in FDA Pregnancy Category B.)

Spontaneous bleeding from internal sites not accessible to control by pressure may occur in patients with abnormalities in platelet count, prothrombin time, partial thromboplastin time, or bleeding time. Therefore, the condition of these patients should be assessed carefully before initiating treatment.

Adverse Reactions and Precautions

Bleeding is the most common and serious complication of thrombolytic therapy. The incidence of major bleeding is no higher than that following full-dose heparin therapy, but bruising and oozing of blood at sites of needle puncture, invasive procedures, trauma, or recent wounds are more likely. Streptokinase and urokinase impair hemostasis by increasing fibrinolytic activity. Also, fibrinogen/fibrin degradation products may interfere with platelet function and impede fibrin polymerization. Proteolysis of plasma proteins other than fibrin is induced, including splitting of the C-terminal end of the A chains of fibrinogen, which then are more sensitive to digestion by plasmin.

If bleeding from an invasive site is not serious, local pressure is usually sufficient and thrombolytic therapy may be continued under close supervision. If serious spontaneous bleeding occurs, treatment should be discontinued and plasma volume expanders administered to replace the deficit. If blood loss has been extensive, administration of red blood cells or whole blood may be necessary. For rapid reversal of the fibrinolytic state, fibrinolysis inhibitors, such as aminocaproic acid 100 mg/kg, can be given by slow intravenous injection. (See the evaluation on Aminocaproic Acid in Chapter 36, Hemostatics.) However, fresh frozen plasma is preferred because it replaces clotting factors.

A moderate reduction in the hematocrit level not related to clinical bleeding occurs in 20% to 30% of patients receiving thrombolytic drugs.

Streptokinase is a foreign protein but rarely produces antigenic (eg, chills, bronchospasm, rash, malaise) or anaphylactoid reactions. Minor allergic reactions can be avoided if the initial dose is given over a period of about 30 minutes. If allergic reactions are severe, streptokinase should be discontinued and hydrocortisone 40 to 80 mg may be given intravenously. In hypersensitive individuals, premedication with corticosteroids (eg, prednisolone 25 mg or equivalent) or chlorpheniramine [Chlor-Trimeton] given intravenously may prevent reactions such as fever. Urokinase occurs naturally in urine and is derived from embryonic human kidney cells; thus, it is not antigenic. However, minor allergic reactions have been reported.

After infusion of streptokinase or urokinase, anticoagulants should be withheld until prothrombin time is less than twice normal, usually three or four hours. Heparin is then given in conventional doses to reduce the risk of reocclusion.

Drug Evaluations

STREPTOKINASE
[Kabikinase, Streptase]

Streptokinase, a nonenzymatic protein (molecular weight 47,000 daltons), is a catabolic product secreted by Group C beta-hemolytic streptococci. Although it is antigenic, commercial products are so highly purified that pyrogenic or allergic reactions are rarely serious. Most individuals have some sensitivity as a result of previous streptococcal infections; a delayed reaction manifested by fever occurs in about one-third of patients. Because immune antibodies inactivate streptokinase, a loading dose is given initially. When the resistance level to streptokinase exceeds 1,000,000 IU, this agent is probably inactive and should not be used. Similarly, high antibody titers during or immediately following streptococcal infections or in patients recently treated with streptokinase rule out further use of this agent for three to six months.

Streptokinase activates plasminogen in a complex manner: It combines with plasminogen in a 1:1 stoichiometric complex to produce a conformational alteration in plasminogen. The plasminogen thus activated then converts the complex to plasmin-streptokinase from which the streptokinase is fragmented into lower molecular weight products.

See the Introduction for information on mechanism of action, indications, adverse reactions, and precautions.

PHARMACOKINETICS. The half-life of streptokinase is biphasic: a "fast" half-life of approximately 11 to 13 minutes (due to the action of antibodies) and a "slow" half-life of 83 minutes in the absence of antibodies. Activity ceases shortly after therapy is discontinued.

DOSAGE AND PREPARATIONS. The powder should be reconstituted with isotonic sodium chloride injection or 5% dextrose for injection, usually to a total volume of approximately 45 ml, and should be used within 24 hours after preparation. Shaking should be avoided to minimize foaming and/or flocculation. The reconstituted solution should be stored at 2 to 4 C.

Intravenous: Adults, in acute myocardial infarction, the total dose is 1 to 1.5 million IU; 750,000 IU is given during the first 10 to 15 minutes and the remainder is given over 60 minutes. For other indications, initially, a loading dose of 250,000 IU of reconstituted solution is infused over 30 minutes, followed by 100,000 IU/hr (usually for 24 hours in patients with pulmonary embolism, 24 to 72 hours in patients with arterial thrombosis or embolism, and 72 hours in patients with deep vein thrombosis). After treatment is discontinued and the thrombin time has decreased to less than twice the normal control value (usually after two to four hours), heparin is given by continuous infusion in a dose that prolongs the APTT by 20 to 30 seconds. An oral anticoagulant may be substituted later, if warranted.

Intra-arterial: This route of administration is not recommended for local perfusion of an occluded vessel.

For local instillation into occluded arteriovenous cannulae after pulling and flushing have been ineffective, 250,000 IU diluted to 2 ml into each occluded limb of the cannula over 30 minutes, followed by clamping of the cannula for two hours. Cannula contents then are aspirated and the cannula is flushed with normal saline and reconnected.

Intracoronary: Prior to angiography, 5,000 to 10,000 units of heparin is administered intra-arterially. After the obstructed vessel is identified by angiography, streptokinase is started, usually by ostial infusion through the initial angiographic catheter. Some systems allow a catheter to be passed down the coronary artery to the site of the clot, and infusion at this site is possible; 20,000 IU is administered initially, then 2,000 units/min are infused with interruption of infusion every 15 minutes to monitor the progress of clot lysis (by administration of dye). Infusion is continued until reperfusion occurs (usually to a total dose of 150,000 to 250,000 units) and for 30 to 60 minutes thereafter; total infusion time is generally 60 to 90 minutes. Following this treatment, heparin is administered intravenously and the dosage is adjusted to maintain a clotting time two to three times normal. Warfarin and dipyridamole or aspirin or dipyridamole can be substituted when anticoagulation can be maintained orally, and therapy is continued for three months. Warfarin should not be used with aspirin because bleeding is increased.

Kabikinase (Pharmacia). Powder (lyophilized) 250,000, 600,000, and 750,000 IU.
Streptase (Hoechst-Roussel). Powder (lyophilized) 250,000 and 750,000 IU.

UROKINASE
[Abbokinase]

Urokinase is an enzyme isolated from human urine or tissue cultures of human kidneys. Two molecular forms exist: S_1, the most active form, has a molecular weight of 34,500 ± 2,000 daltons. The S_2 form has a molecular weight of 54,000 daltons. The S_1 form probably represents a breakdown product of urokinase formed during purification procedures; its amino acid sequence is very similar to the B-chain of thrombin and plasmin. Unlike streptokinase, urokinase is a direct activator of plasminogen. It can be purified to a high degree but rarely may cause variable transient hypercoagulation; low doses may induce platelet aggregation. However, urokinase is nonantigenic and does not cause the allergic reactions encountered with streptokinase. It may be used if streptokinase resistance is high or when a second course of treatment is required.

See the Introduction for information on mechanism of action, indications, adverse reactions, and precautions.

DOSAGE AND PREPARATIONS. The powder should be reconstituted only with sterile water for injection and used immediately. Any unused portion of the reconstituted material should be discarded. The unreconstituted powder should be stored at 2 to 8 C.

Intravenous: Adults, 4,400 IU/kg infused over a period of ten minutes, followed by continuous infusion of 4,400 IU/kg/hr for 12 to 24 hours. As with streptokinase, its use should be followed by administration of heparin and later by use of oral anticoagulants.

Intracoronary: The contents of three reconstituted vials are added to 500 ml of 5% dextrose in water (1,500 IU/ml). After a bolus dose of 2,500 to 10,000 units of heparin and angiography, urokinase 6,000 IU/min (4 ml/min of solution) is given for up to two hours. The average dose required to achieve lysis of thrombi is 500,000 IU. Progress should be monitored by angiography at 15-minute intervals.

For occluded intravenous catheters, 5,000 IU/ml is *gently* instilled by tuberculin syringe in amounts equal to the internal volume of the catheter. Aspiration of the clot and urokinase solution is attempted after five to ten minutes. The procedure may be repeated until catheter patency is restored.

Abbokinase (Abbott). Powder (lyophilized) 250,000 IU with mannitol 25 mg and sodium chloride 45 mg.

Abbokinase Open-Cath (Abbott). Powder (lyophilized) 5,000 IU with mannitol 15 mg and sodium chloride 1.7 mg.

Investigational Drug

RECOMBINANT HUMAN TISSUE-TYPE PLASMINOGEN ACTIVATOR (tPA)
[TPA]

Tissue-type plasminogen activator (tPA) is a naturally occurring serine protease that is now produced by recombinant DNA technology. Recombinant human tissue-type plasminogen activator has the same characteristics as tissue plasminogen activator generated locally by endothelial cells of the vessel wall as part of the normal physiologic mechanism for digesting fibrin clots.

ACTIONS. tPA has a high affinity for fibrin and activates fibrin-bound plasminogen to plasmin to a much greater extent than it activates circulating plasminogen. Thus, when tPA is given in doses that are capable of dissolving clots, plasmin does not accumulate in plasma in amounts sufficient to deplete α_2-antiplasmin and cause systemic fibrinolysis. However, this clot-selective fibrinolysis is not absolute. When large doses are given for prolonged periods, tPA can overwhelm the inhibitory mechanisms in the circulation and induce systemic fibrinolysis.

tPA has a short half-life of approximately eight minutes in circulating plasma. It is taken up and degraded by the liver and then excreted.

USES. Studies in animals showed that tPA can reperfuse occluded coronary arteries. In one placebo-controlled trial, intravenous doses of 0.5 mg/kg given in 30 minutes plus 0.25 mg/kg given over the next 90 minutes (total dose of 0.75 mg/kg) achieved recanalization in 75% (33 of 45) of patients with angiographically confirmed complete coronary occlusion following acute myocardial infarction (Collen et al, 1984). In other patients, similar results were obtained after intracoronary infusion of tPA 0.375 mg/kg in 15 to 30 minutes. In this study, fibrinogen levels decreased less than 10% (in no case below 100 mg/dl) and fibrinogen degradation products (FDP) increased moderately. No hemorrhagic complications requiring transfusion were encountered. However, reocclusion occurred soon after termination of infusion in approximately 20% of patients who were successfully recanalized. Results of other studies (Van de Werf et al, 1984; Williams, 1985) on a small number of patients suggest that both intravenous and intracoronary tPA induce thrombolysis without systemic lysis.

tPA is undergoing investigation in a multicenter trial (Thrombolysis in Myocardial Infarction [TIMI] Study Group, 1985) under the auspices of the National Heart, Blood, and Lung Institute. In Phase I, intravenous TPA 80 mg has been compared to intravenous streptokinase 1.5 million units. TPA was given over three hours (40 mg, 20 mg, 20 mg during the first, second, and third hours, respectively) and streptokinase over a one-hour period, since it appears to be most effective when infused rapidly in large doses. Since tPA has a short half-life, it was given for a longer period to reduce the risk of reocclusion. Lysis was measured 90 minutes after initiation of infusion in both groups. Preliminary reports of this trial indicate that the thrombolytic effect of intravenous tPA is twice that of intravenous streptokinase. Results of the European Cooperative Study are similar (Verstraete et al, 1985). Data from numerous trials employing intracoronary streptokinase (Rentrop et al, 1981 A; Anderson et al, 1983; Khaja et al, 1983; Kennedy et al, 1983; Rentrop et al, 1984) show that intravenous streptokinase is slightly more than half as effective as intracoronary streptokinase. Although intravenous tPA and intracoronary streptokinase have not been compared directly, some investigators suggest that, when given by these routes, these agents are of approximately equal efficacy for reperfusion of occluded coronary arteries.

ADVERSE REACTIONS AND PRECAUTIONS. Although no hemorrhage requiring transfusion was encountered, hematoma at the catheterization site was common and gastrointestinal tract bleeding was noted in 6% of the TPA group and 10% of the streptokinase group. Thus, hemorrhagic complications were similar in both groups.

Because the protocol for Phase I of the TIMI trial required coronary catheterization and angiographic documentation of total occlusion, TPA and streptokinase were not administered until approximately five hours following onset of symptoms of AMI, and all patients had evidence of myocardial necrosis.

Phase II of the TIMI trial will compare the effects of intravenous TPA with conventional therapy on morbidity and mortality. Because catheterization will not be required, TPA can be administered earlier and may be more effective in limiting the size of the infarct. However, the relatively high rate of reocclusion that followed thrombolysis despite adequate anticoagulation during the Phase I period is likely to be observed in Phase II studies also.

TPA (Genentech).
(Investigational drug)

Cited References

Thrombolytic therapy in thrombosis: National Institutes of Health consensus development conference. *Ann Intern Med* 93:141-144, 1980.

Anderson JL, et al: Randomized trial of intracoronary streptokinase in treatment of acute myocardial infarction. *N Engl J Med* 308:1312-1318, 1983.

Collen D, et al: Coronary thrombolysis with recombinant human tissue-type plasminogen activator: Prospective, randomized, placebo-controlled trial. *Circulation* 70:1012-1017, 1984.

DeWood MA, et al: Prevalence of total coronary occlusion during early hours of transmural myocardial infarction. *N Engl J Med* 303:897-902, 1980.

DeWood MA, et al: Coronary arteriographic findings in acute transmural myocardial infarction. *Circulation* 68(suppl I):I39-I49, 1983.

Furberg CD: Clinical value of intracoronary streptokinase, (editorial). *Am J Cardiol* 53:626-627, 1984.

Gersh BJ: Role of thrombolytic therapy in evolving myocardial infarction. *Mod Concepts Cardiovasc Dis* 54:13-17, (March) 1985.

Goldhaber SZ, et al: Pooled analyses of randomized trials of streptokinase and heparin in phlebographically documented acute deep venous thrombosis. *Am J Med* 76:393-397, 1984.

Hull R, et al: Replacement of venography in suspected venous thrombosis by impedance plethysmography and ^{125}I-fibrinogen leg scanning. *Ann Intern Med* 94:12-15, 1981.

Jaffe AS: Administration of hyaluronidase to patients with acute myocardial infarction: Results of MILIS study, (abstract). *J Am Coll Cardiol* 5:447, 1985.

Jennings RB, Reimer KA: Factors involved in salvaging ischemic myocardium: Effect of reperfusion of arterial blood. *Circulation* 68(suppl I):I25-I36, 1983.

Kennedy JW, et al: Western Washington randomized trial of intracoronary streptokinase in acute myocardial infarction. *N Engl J Med* 309:1477-1482, 1983.

Kennedy JW, et al: Western Washington randomized trial of intracoronary streptokinase in acute myocardial infarction: 12-month follow-up report. *N Engl J Med* 312:1073-1078, 1985.

Khaja F, et al: Intracoronary fibrinolytic therapy in acute myocardial infarction: Report of prospective randomized trial. *N Engl J Med* 308:1305-1311, 1983.

Kloner RA, et al: Studies of experimental coronary artery reperfusion: Effects on infarct size, myocardial function, biochemistry, ultrastructure and microvascular damage. *Circulation* 68(suppl I):I8-I15, 1983 A.

Kloner RA, et al: Coronary reperfusion for treatment of acute myocardial infarction: Postischemic ventricular dysfunction. *Cardiology* 70:233-246, 1983 B.

Laffel GL, Braunwald E: Thrombolytic therapy: New strategy for treatment of acute myocardial infarction, parts 1 and 2. *N Engl J Med* 311:710-717, 770-776, 1984.

Rentrop KP, et al: Acute myocardial infarction: Intracoronary application of nitroglycerin and streptokinase. *Clin Cardiol* 2:354-363, 1979.

Rentrop P, et al: Selective intracoronary thrombolysis in acute myocardial infarction and unstable angina pectoris. *Circulation* 63:307-317, 1981 A.

Rentrop P, et al: Changes in left ventricular function after intracoronary streptokinase infusion in clinically evolving myocardial infarction. *Am Heart J* 102:1188-1193, 1981 B.

Rentrop P, et al: Changes in left ventricular ejection fraction after intracoronary thrombolytic therapy: Results of Registry of European Society of Cardiology. *Circulation* 68(suppl I):I55-I60, 1983.

Rentrop KP, et al: Effects of intracoronary streptokinase and intracoronary nitroglycerin infusion on coronary angiography patterns and mortality in patients with acute myocardial infarction. *N Engl J Med* 311:1457-1463, 1984.

Rodgers WJ, et al: Return of left ventricular function after reperfusion in patients with myocardial infarction: Importance of subtotal stenoses or intact collaterals. *Circulation* 69:338-349, 1984.

Rubin RN: Fibrinolysis and its current usage. *Clin Therapeut* 5:211-222, 1983.

Sharma GC, et al: Effect of thrombolytic therapy on pulmonary capillary blood volume in patients with pulmonary embolism. *N Engl J Med* 303:842-845, 1980.

Sheehan FH, et al: Factors that determine recovery of left ventricular function after thrombolysis in patients with acute myocardial infarction. *Circulation* 71:1121-1128, 1985.

Smith RAG, et al: Fibrinolysis with acyl-enzymes: New approach to thrombolytic therapy. *Nature* 290:505-508, 1981.

Taylor LM Jr, et al: Intraarterial streptokinase infusion for acute popliteal and tibial artery occlusion. *Am J Surg* 147:583-588, 1984.

Tennant SN, et al: Intracoronary thrombolysis in patients with acute myocardial infarction: Comparison of efficacy of urokinase with streptokinase. *Circulation* 69:756-760, 1984.

Thrombolysis in Myocardial Infarction Study Group: Thrombolysis in myocardial infarction (TIMI) trial. *N Engl J Med* 312:932-936, 1985.

Van de Werf F, et al: Coronary thrombolysis with tissue-type plasminogen activator in patients with evolving myocardial infarction. *N Engl J Med* 310:609-613, 1984.

Verstraete M, et al: Randomised trial of intravenous recombinant tissue-type plasminogen activator versus intravenous streptokinase in acute myocardial infarction. *Lancet* 1:842-847, 1985.

Walker ID, et al: Acylated streptokinase: Plasminogen complex in patients with acute myocardial infarction. *Thromb Haemostas* 51:204-206, 1984.

Williams DO: Intravenous recombinant tissue type plasminogen activator (r-tPA) in acute myocardial infarction. *J Am Coll Cardiol* 5:495, 1985.

Other Selected References

Greater use of fibrinolytic agents urged. *JAMA* 243:2275-2276, 1980.

Fenster PE, Kern KB: Streptokinase in acute myocardial infarction. *Drug Ther (Hosp)* 7:41-48, (May) 1982.

Harrington JT: Thrombolytic therapy in renal vein thrombosis, (editorial). *Arch Intern Med* 144:33-34, 1984.

Sherry S: Setting thrombolysis in action. *Drug Ther* 7:23-26, (Aug) 1977.

Sherry S: Streptokinase: Use it to lyse clots. *Mod Med* 46:93-98, (May 30-June 15) 1978.

Sullivan JM: Streptokinase and myocardial infarction. *N Engl J Med* 301:836-837, 1979.

Verstraete M: Biochemical and clinical aspects of thrombolysis. *Semin Hematol* 15:35-54, 1978.

Blood, Blood Components, and Blood Substitutes

35

Transfusion of blood provides temporary support during treatment of an underlying condition. However, a blood transfusion is potentially hazardous and should not be given unless the risk/benefit ratio is favorable. Viral infections, particularly hepatitis and, rarely, acquired immunodeficiency syndrome (AIDS) may be transmitted.

Whole blood is obtained from a donor and collected into a bag containing an acidified anticoagulant preservative solution (usually CPDA-1). Blood components are produced from single units of blood by centrifugation or freezing. Utilization of a closed system of presterilized, interconnected bags prevents bacterial contamination but does not affect parasites or viruses present in the donor's blood. Blood derivatives (eg, albumin, plasma protein fraction) are prepared from large pools of plasma and are sterilized and filtered; some are heat-treated to minimize the potential for transmission of infectious agents. Blood derivatives, unlike blood components, can be assayed and standardized.

The availability and proper use of component preparations have minimized risks and markedly reduced the need for whole blood transfusions. The required component (eg, red cells, platelets) usually can be administered without burdening the circulation; exposure to donor alloantibodies, potentially harmful cations, and metabolites is reduced; and utilization of each unit of blood is maximized, since components not needed by one patient are available for other recipients.

For a detailed discussion of donor selection, transfusion procedures, and current accepted standards, see publications on blood banking, such as *Standards for Blood Banks and Transfusion Services* (Schmidt, 1984), *Clinical Practice of Blood Transfusion* (Petz and Swisher, 1981) and *The Technical Manual* (Huestis et al, 1985).

When acute bleeding occurs, attempts should be made to maintain (1) blood volume at 100% of normal, (2) hemoglobin level of at least 8 g/dl and hematocrit at 24% to allow adequate oxygen transport to tissues, (3) total serum protein level of at least 60% of normal, (4) plasma coagulation factors above 35% of normal, except factor VIII at 50% of normal, and (5) platelets above 25% (50,000/mm^3) of normal. To achieve these levels, the following is suggested: When blood loss is 20% or less of total volume, a crystalloid solution (eg, balanced electrolyte solution) usually is adequate. With further blood loss, nonprotein plasma volume expanders may be preferred and red cell concentrates should be added. When blood loss exceeds 50%, whole blood is given if available; albumin or plasma protein fraction may be necessary if whole blood is unavailable. When the total blood volume is replaced in less than 24 hours, hemodilution may result in thrombocytopenia and reduction of plasma coagulation factors. Platelet concentrates and fresh frozen plasma then may be necessary, but, to avoid the risk of hepatitis, they usually are administered only when platelets and coagulation factors must be replaced.

Autologous Transfusion: This type of transfusion is particularly valuable in patients with rare blood types who have antibodies to common blood group antigens, those who experience severe reactions to homologous blood products, or those in whom transmission of disease (eg, hepatitis) would be especially hazardous.

Techniques utilized for transfusion of autologous blood include prior collection and storage, preoperative phlebotomy with artificial hemodilution during surgery and postoperative retransfusion, intraoperative blood salvage and retransfusion, and postoperative collection of shed blood or salvage and reinfusion of blood from the pleural cavity following trauma. In nonemergencies, prior collection of blood is preferred.

The advantages of autologous transfusion are avoidance of immunologic mismatch and disease transmission and conservation of available blood stores. Anticoagulants must be added and the blood can be reinfused after filtration or saline washing. A major disadvantage of autologous transfusion is the risk of reinfusing contaminants.

Apheresis: Because each blood component has a different specific gravity, apheresis techniques employing centrifugation may be used to separate the various elements. The desired fraction is retained and the remaining fractions are recombined and returned to the donor.

Two types of apheresis are used: (1) With *cytapheresis*, one or more cellular elements are withdrawn and the plasma and remaining cellular elements are returned to the donor. Leukapheresis and thrombocytapheresis (plateletpheresis) represent types of cytapheresis. Thrombocytapheresis separates platelets from donor blood, and plasma and red cells are returned to the donor. With continuous or intermittent flow centrifugation, the equivalent of up to ten platelet concentrates can be obtained from one donor in a single session. Platelets obtained by thrombocytapheresis must be administered within 24 hours if an open system procedure is used because of the risk of bacterial contamination. In a closed system procedure, the platelets may be stored for five days.

(2) With *plasmapheresis*, plasma is removed from the cellular constituents, which are then suspended in an equivalent volume of another fluid (eg, electrolytes, fresh frozen plasma, albumin) and retransfused. It is performed on healthy donors whose plasma contains a commercially desirable substance for manufacture of immune globulins or other products (eg, blood bank reagents). When large volumes of abnormal plasma are replaced by normal plasma or other proteins and an equal volume of fluid, the process is known as plasma exchange. Plasma exchange separates plasma from the cellular elements, which are then suspended in another fluid.

Newer plasma perfusion techniques remove undesirable components (eg, cholesterol, toxic materials, immune complexes). Many of these approaches are experimental, but new and increasingly specific technology is being developed.

Because it is relatively safe compared to other therapeutic modalities, apheresis has been considered in diseases for which no specific therapy exists, such as those associated with high levels of circulating antibody or antigen-antibody complexes. However, therapy is very expensive, must be repeated frequently, and results are often disappointing.

Plasmapheresis or a variant may be used as standard therapy in hyperviscosity syndrome, myasthenia gravis, rapidly progressive glomerulonephritis, Goodpasture's syndrome without anuria, Refsum's disease, thrombotic thrombocytopenic purpura, acute severe polyradiculoneuropathy, thyrotoxic crisis, symptomatic or presurgical thrombocytosis (by thrombocytapheresis), and sickle-cell syndromes (by erythrocytapheresis) (Council on Scientific Activities, 1985).

Leukapheresis has been used in patients with malignant myelo- or lymphoproliferative diseases to reduce the circulating tumor cell burden and provide time for chemotherapeutic drugs to exert an effect. Benefits are temporary and serial cytapheresis is required to maintain lowered cell counts (Sandler, 1980). Leukapheresis is used to collect granulocytes (leukocytes) from normal donors for management of infection in granulocytopenic patients.

In the following diseases, apheresis should be withheld until more conventional therapy has failed: systemic lupus erythematosus, vasculitis without renal disease, cryoglobulinemia, hemophilia with inhibitor, maternal-fetal incompatibility, renal transplant rejection, renal failure with myeloma, posttransfusion purpura, cholestasis with severe pruritus, and severe familial hypercholesterolemia (type IIa). Rheumatoid arthritis and multiple sclerosis have responded to lymphocytapheresis (sometimes combined with plasmapheresis).

For other diseases (eg, progressive systemic sclerosis, Raynaud's disease, polymyositis and dermatomyositis, amyotrophic lateral sclerosis, multiple sclerosis, autoimmune hemolytic anemia, aplastic anemia, acquired immunodeficiency syndrome (AIDS), burn shock, psoriasis, juvenile rheumatoid arthritis, psoriatic arthritis, chronic polyradiculoneuropathies, Goodpasture's syndrome with anuria, idiopathic thrombocytopenic purpura, pemphigus, liver diseases, angiokeratoma corporis diffusum), apheresis has not shown reasonable evidence of efficacy and is not currently recommended.

Side effects occur in about 15% of patients and are usually mild, but deaths have been reported in patients with impaired cardiovascular function. Contamination, mechanical problems, coagulation disorders, thrombophlebitis, electrolyte imbalance, pulmonary or cerebral embolism, paresthesias, hematoma or nerve damage at the access site, and hypersensitivity reactions to components of the replacement fluid may occur.

Leukocyte donors may be given steroids before collection to increase the harvest of white cells. Because granulocytes do not separate readily from red blood cells, a sedimenting agent (hydroxyethyl starch) may be added and can be retransfused in the donor. Thus, side effects attributable to these substances may occur in the donor.

Exchange Transfusions: Exchange transfusions of whole blood are widely used to treat hemolytic disease of the newborn and other neonatal disorders, some red cell disorders, and various other diseases. Plasma exchanges remove some poisons when dialysis is not applicable. Automated red cell exchanges have replaced manual exchange transfusion in many nonpediatric patients.

Red cell exchanges using a cell separator have been effective in sickle cell anemia during crises or prior to surgery. Operative mortality is reduced greatly when sickle cells are replaced with normal red cells, but red cell transfusion alone is not as effective as exchange transfusions. Cell separators have been used to separate young red cells (neocytes) from older ones in donor blood. Neocytes survive longer after transfusion, and have been used in the treatment of thalassemias to reduce the frequency of transfusion and thereby diminish the iron load, but the procedure is still considered experimental.

Some autoimmune diseases can be treated by plasma exchange (see above). Since it is difficult to remove only immune globulins, the entire plasma portion of blood is replaced. If only 1 or 2 L is exchanged, the substitute fluid may be crystalloid (eg, saline, electrolyte solutions). However, using crystalloids to replace large volumes may cause severe hypotension because of changes in osmotic pressure. For exchanges of approximately 4 L (equivalent to one volume exchange in a 70-kg adult), a protein such as 5% albumin is satisfactory. If large volumes (eg, 10 L) are required, fresh frozen plasma should be used to replace coagulation factors. The disease also may help to determine which replacement solution is most suitable.

Therapeutic plasma exchange has been effective in hemophilia with inhibitors to factor VIII, and may be considered during a severe bleeding episode or when surgery is planned if more conventional therapy (large doses of factor VIII and/or activated prothrombin complex) has failed. Each procedure should consist of at least one plasma volume exchange (2 to 3 L), if possible. Preliminary data in patients with malignant tumors, aplastic anemia, pure red cell aplasia, and similar diseases have been encouraging, but further study is necessary before recommendations can be made.

Whole Blood or Red Blood Cell Transfusion: During storage of blood, changes in red cell metabolism and hemoglobin structure and function occur. The pH, glucose, adenosine triphosphate (ATP), and 2,3-diphosphoglycerate (DPG) decrease and lactic acid accumulates. These changes reduce the survival time of transfused red cells and decrease hemoglobin function. Current standards require that a mean of 75% of erythrocytes be viable 24 hours after transfusion.

Whole blood may be preferred when there is acute loss of a substantial portion of blood volume, as in surgical or medical catastrophes, but appropriate components can be used instead.

When the sole aim of transfusion is to increase oxygen-carrying capacity, red cell concentrate should be used. Transfusion of red cell concentrate with a hematocrit of 70% to 80% reduces the danger of hypervolemia and associated congestive heart failure and is preferred in patients with cardiac disease and chronic anemia. (Red blood cells, adenine-saline added, have a hematocrit of 55% to 65%, and may need to be concentrated by centrifugation or sedimentation before use in patients at risk for circulatory overload [*Circular of Information for the Use of Human Blood and Blood Components*, 1984].) Separation of plasma immediately prior to transfusion reduces the amount of sodium, potassium, and ammonium ions administered. (The routinely stocked red cell concentrates prepared shortly after collection and stored will not have reduced amounts of these ions.) During dire emergencies, red cell concentrate should be used if out-of-group transfusion is necessary because of the reduced amounts of anti-A and

anti-B alloantibodies in the volume of red cell concentrate required. However, the risk of transmitting hepatitis is not reduced.

Most blood banks now routinely stock red cell concentrates, which may contain additives or lack various cellular components. When packed in a closed sterile system, their shelf-life is the same as that of whole blood. After the hermetic seal is broken, the shelf-life is 24 hours. Requirements for crossmatching and method of administration are the same as for whole blood.

Frozen red blood cells are now prepared in a number of blood centers. The high cost of preparation and storage, the time required to thaw and wash the cells (to remove cryoprotective agent) before they can be transfused, and the limited post-thaw shelf-life (24 hours) preclude their routine use. The risk of bacterial contamination during preparation, thawing, and washing also is somewhat greater than for red blood cells or whole blood, because a closed system cannot be used. Furthermore, the risk of post-transfusion hepatitis is not eliminated (Alter et al, 1978; Haugen, 1979).

After thawing and transmembrane washing (deglycerolizing), frozen red cells contain very little cellular debris from leukocytes or platelets, thus minimizing febrile nonhemolytic transfusion reactions. Saline-washed or recentrifuged and suitably filtered red cells may be satisfactory for this purpose. Thawed, deglycerolized red cells should be reserved for patients who continue to experience reactions to saline-washed or leukocyte-poor red cells, for individuals with paroxysmal nocturnal hemoglobinuria (PNH), or for those who have had anaphylactoid transfusion reactions.

Frozen red blood cells of rare types can be prepared for either autologous or homologous transfusion. Hemolytic disease in newborn infants caused by maternal antibodies against high-incidence antigens can be treated with frozen red blood cells obtained from the mother during early pregnancy. If necessary, the blood can be collected after delivery and washed prior to transfusion. Autologous frozen red blood cells may be accumulated to meet anticipated needs in selected persons. However, logistics preclude their use for routine autologous blood transfusion.

Frozen red blood cells were once preferred for patients scheduled to undergo organ transplantation, but most data now suggest that survival of renal transplants is decreased when only frozen red blood cells are employed. Prior transfusion of whole blood enhances renal homograft survival but appears to have a deleterious effect in patients who undergo bone marrow transplantation.

Platelet Transfusion: Platelet transfusions are indicated when severe acute thrombocytopenia is associated with active or imminent bleeding, especially that resulting from decreased platelet production. Thrombocytopenia may be caused by decreased production or increased destruction of platelets, and dilutional thrombocytopenia can develop following massive transfusion of stored blood. Spontaneous bleeding usually does not occur unless the platelet count is less than 20,000/microliter. Patients with leukemia and other malignancies who are receiving intensive chemotherapy may require platelet transfusions to maintain counts greater than 20,000/

microliter. During major surgery and the postoperative period, the platelet count should be maintained at greater than 50,000/microliter.

Patients with aplastic anemia and some other conditions characterized by prolonged suppression of bone marrow function who have low (less than 20,000/microliter) but stable platelet counts do not require maintenance platelet transfusions unless hemorrhage occurs. Prophylactic platelet transfusions should be avoided because these patients usually develop alloantibodies that decrease the effectiveness of the transfusions.

Platelet transfusions are less likely to be effective in conditions associated with increased platelet destruction (eg, sepsis, fever, active bleeding). They are not recommended when platelet destruction is caused by systemic consumption (disseminated intravascular coagulation [DIC]) or an antibody (idiopathic thrombocytopenic purpura [ITP]). Patients with splenomegaly may require large doses of platelets because of splenic sequestration.

Platelet concentrate is defined as the platelets collected from a single donor by differential centrifugation of never refrigerated, fresh, whole blood and suspended in 50 to 70 ml of the original plasma. Platelets from one unit of blood (one random-donor platelet concentrate) should increase the platelet count of a 70-kg adult by at least 5,000/microliter. The usual adult dose necessary to achieve hemostasis is six to eight such concentrates (Snyder, 1983).

Viable platelets form hemostatic plugs that seal small openings in blood vessels. This capacity is lost during storage if the pH is permitted to drop below 6.0 due to the glycolytic production of lactic acid. Platelets stored at room temperature (20 to 24 C) must be buffered with 50 to 70 ml of suspending plasma. Gentle agitation during storage is essential to supply oxygen and facilitate gas exchange, which prevent the deleterious changes associated with reduced pH. Under these conditions, platelets can be kept for up to seven days (in plastic containers designed to permit gas exchange) after collection and have adequate survival in vivo. Bacterial contamination has not been a problem, and most blood banks now store platelets at 20 to 24 C. Platelets preserved at 4 C appear to be effective only if transfused within 24 hours. Storage at 4 C for longer than 48 hours causes irreversible disc-to-sphere transformation. At either temperature, the sooner that platelets are administered after donation, the better in vivo recovery will be.

Prolonged preservation by freezing with a cryoprotective agent has been accomplished but currently is not practical as a routine measure. Cryopreserved platelets obtained during remissions from patients with hematologic malignancies have been used to combat hemorrhage during subsequent relapse (Schiffer, 1977). Cryopreservation may be particularly important if the patient does not respond to HLA-matched single-donor platelets obtained by plateletpheresis.

Refractoriness to repeated administration of random-donor platelets is not uncommon. This usually is caused by antibodies directed against histocompatibility antigens (HLA) or, less frequently, against specific platelet antigens. For this reason, some workers have advocated that prophylactic platelet transfusion not be given to nonbleeding patients.

HLA-matched platelets may increase the platelet increment and survival time after immunization has developed. Transfusion of platelets from the "preferred" donor, an HLA-matched sibling, can provide long-term support but is contraindicated when marrow transplantation from that sibling or another family member is contemplated. Larger centers have developed lists of HLA-typed donors for rapid matching to thrombocytopenic patients who are refractory to random-donor platelets.

Although platelet concentrates contain a few erythrocytes, they also contain large amounts of plasma, and administration on the basis of ABO plasma compatibility is desirable. Although platelets do not contain the $Rh_o(D)$ antigen, the small quantity of red cells present can cause primary immunization. Infusion of platelets from an Rh-positive donor into an Rh-negative woman could result in Rh immunization. Therefore, Rh-negative female children and women of childbearing age should be given $Rh_o(D)$ immune globulin immediately after receiving platelets from an Rh-positive donor.

Granulocyte Transfusion: Severe thrombocytopenia and leukopenia caused by marrow hypoplasia frequently result from aggressive cancer chemotherapy, but platelet transfusion has decreased mortality from thrombocytopenic hemorrhage in these patients. As a result, infections, particularly those caused by gram-negative organisms, rather than hemorrhage, are now the leading case of death in patients with bone marrow failure.

The incidence of infection increases as the granulocyte count falls below 500/microliter. Although antibiotics have been helpful, the patient remains at serious risk until marrow function returns. In some patients who remain febrile despite adequate antibiotic therapy for at least 48 hours, granulocyte transfusion has improved survival. Granulocytes can be given only to a level approximately 10% of the normal daily production, but this appears to provide enough white cells to overcome infection in responsive patients. However, this therapy is controversial and should not be used when recovery of marrow function is unlikely.

Although some data support therapeutic granulocyte transfusion, its prophylactic use is not recommended. In one study, the rate of infection was not reduced in leukemia patients, but serious pulmonary toxicity occurred in those receiving granulocyte transfusions (Strauss et al, 1981). Another large controlled trial in patients with documented infections failed to show substantial benefit from granulocyte transfusion over optimal use of antibiotics alone (Winston et al, 1982). However, this study has been criticized for using doses lower than those currently recommended (Winton et al, 1983).

Since granulocyte preparations also contain red cells, ABO compatibility should be assured. Compatible granulocytes may be required in alloimmunized patients.

Plasma Transfusion: Plasma, the cell-free portion of anticoagulated blood, constitutes approximately 60% of blood volume and contains most of the blood proteins, electrolytes, coagulation factors, and other elements, including immunoregulatory factors. When a unit of whole blood is converted to red blood cells, plasma is removed. Plasma also can be obtained by plasmapheresis. The plasma can be fractionated into blood derivatives (eg, albumin, plasma protein fraction) or used as a source of procoagulants. Fresh plasma and thawed fresh frozen plasma may be used as a source of all the coagulation factors. Supernatant plasma remaining after removal of cryoprecipitate, platelets, or both is useful to replace the stable clotting factors (II, VII, IX, X, XI, XII).

Plasma is employed primarily in the management of bleeding associated with liver disease and massive blood transfusion or dilutional coagulopathies caused by administration of more than 15 units of stored blood. Because the activity of labile clotting factors (V and VIII) stored in plasma decreases during storage, fresh frozen single-donor plasma generally is preferred to correct deficiencies of factor V; factor VIII deficiency preferably is treated by replacement of the specific factor (see Chapter 36, Hemostatics). Although plasma is useful in factor IX deficiency, as well as in multiple coagulation factor deficiencies, large volumes usually are required to achieve hemostatic levels of these factors.

Plasma is indicated in conjunction with therapeutic plasma exchange for thrombotic thrombocytopenic purpura, for infants with protein-losing enteropathy, and for selected patients with other immune deficiencies (National Institutes of Health Consensus Conference, 1985). It may be useful adjunctively to control bleeding associated with oral anticoagulant or antiplatelet therapy, particularly prior to emergency surgery. Plasma also has been used to maintain circulating blood volume but is not currently recommended for this use (except in burn patients with infection) or for parenteral nutrition because of the risk of hepatitis.

Single-donor or fresh frozen plasma carries the same risk of transmitting hepatitis as a single unit of whole blood and contains anti-A (found in type O and type B donor) and/or anti-B alloagglutinins (found in type O and type A donor) if not obtained from an AB donor. Because of the great risk of viral hepatitis, pooled plasma is no longer licensed by the Food and Drug Administration.

Plasma Volume Expanders: If temporary maintenance of blood volume is the sole therapeutic objective, plasma volume expanders should be used instead of whole blood, and crystalloid solutions can be used if the estimated volume deficit is small. Plasma should not be used for this purpose. Albumin (human) [Albuminar, Albutein, Buminate, Plasbumin] and plasma protein fraction (PPF) [Plasmanate, Plasma-Plex, Plasmatein, Protenate] are processed from liquid plasma (normal human plasma) and may be indicated in the emergency treatment of shock or to correct hypoproteinemia. However, severe hypotension developed in some patients undergoing cardiopulmonary bypass who were treated with this product before prekallikrein activator (PKA) levels of the product were controlled. These preparations are sterile-filtered and heated for ten hours at 60 C, which eliminates the risk of hepatitis.

Plasma substitutes (eg, dextran 70 [Macrodex], dextran 75 [Gentran 75], hetastarch [Hespan]) support the circulation in hypovolemic states (eg, cardiogenic shock, respiratory distress syndrome). They can be given to restore blood volume after hemorrhage while typing and crossmatching of blood is being done, to correct the oligemia of burn shock, or to maintain colloidal osmotic pressure temporarily in emergen-

cies or during certain types of cardiovascular surgery. They are not substitutes for blood components in the treatment of anemia or hypoproteinemia. Dextran 40 [Gentran-40, Rheomacrodex, 10% LMD] solutions may be used as adjuncts in the treatment of shock, but the effects are of shorter duration than those of higher molecular weight dextran.

Dextrans and hetastarch have been associated with histamine release and major anaphylactoid reactions. Dextrans also have been associated with increased bleeding tendencies and renal failure. Because of these hazards, the use of dextran solutions has declined.

Most physicians now believe that moderate hypovolemia and hemoconcentration can be treated by temporary replacement with a balanced electrolyte solution (in amounts three or four times the estimated blood loss). Sodium chloride and 5% dextrose in water solutions also can be used, but the effects of all crystalloid solutions last two hours or less. (See Chapter 46, Replenishers and Regulators of Water and Electrolytes.)

$Rh_o(D)$ Immune Globulin: This sterile gamma globulin preparation is obtained by fractionating the plasma of donors who are nonreactive for hepatitis B surface antigen and who have high titers of antibodies to $Rh_o(D)$. It is used to prevent active immunization against $Rh_o(D)$ in the $Rh_o(D)$-negative, D^u-negative mother who has delivered an $Rh_o(D)$-positive infant or abortus. It also should be given when the Rh status of the abortus is unknown, in tubal pregnancy, following amniocentesis, and to prevent alloimmunization when $Rh_o(D)$-positive blood, platelet concentrate, or granulocyte concentrate is given to an $Rh_o(D)$-negative female before or during the childbearing period, especially during pregnancy. (See the evaluation in Chapter 63, Immunomodulators.)

Immune Globulins: These specially prepared concentrates of globulins do not transmit hepatitis. They protect against hepatitis A when administered before or within two weeks after exposure and against non-A, non-B hepatitis and hepatitis B when administered before exposure. Treated patients experience a reduced incidence of chronic active hepatitis. Immune globulins should not be used in patients known to have anti-IgA antibodies, for they contain small amounts of IgA. Because of low antibody titers (1:100), immune globulin, when given after exposure, is unlikely to reduce the incidence of transfusion-associated hepatitis.

Some preparations with high specific antibody titers provide postexposure prophylaxis against hepatitis B, pertussis, rabies, and tetanus (see the evaluations in Chapter 62, Agents for Active and Passive Immunity).

Hemin for Injection: Hemin is an enzyme inhibitor derived from processed red blood cells. It is used to ameliorate attacks of acute intermittent porphyria associated with the menstrual cycle. Similar results are obtained following acute attacks of any of the inducible hepatic porphyrias (acute intermittent porphyria, variegate porphyria, hereditary coproporphyria). Hemin blocks the induction of delta-aminolevulinic acid synthetase in the liver (elevated levels of this enzyme are associated with acute attacks of hepatic porphyrias). However, the exact mechanism of action has not been determined and hemin therapy is contraindicated in other porphyrias (porphyria cutanea tarda, congenital erythropoietic porphyria, erythropoietic protoporphyria).

Perfluorochemicals: Studies in animals have demonstrated that perfluorochemicals transport oxygen and remove carbon dioxide, thus enabling these compounds to act as hemoglobin substitutes. They are effective only when high concentrations of oxygen are inhaled by patients with severely depleted hemoglobin and do not provide platelets or coagulation factors. Although perfluorochemicals dissolve approximately three times as much oxygen as an equivalent amount of plasma, this gas is in solution and released only when oxygen tensions are higher than oxygen bound to hemoglobin. Also, some of the material accumulates in the reticuloendothelial system, liver, spleen, and other organs and is retained for long periods.

Fluosol-DA, a mixture of perfluorodecalin and perfluorotripropylamine, has been used in Japan as a blood substitute. It is useful for perfusion of organs to prolong viability before transplantation and is promising for the management of carbon monoxide intoxication. It also has been administered in the emergency treatment of patients with rare blood types when replacement blood was not immediately available and has been used experimentally in a few patients who refused blood for religious reasons.

Fluosol-DA is relatively unstable and must be stored at -10 to -30 C to prevent enlargement of the average particle size. The chemical material has a half-life of approximately 65 days or less in the body; the half-life of its oxygen-carrying capacity is several hours.

Perfluorochemicals are being investigated in animals in the United States and development of preparations with greater emulsion stability and more rapid clearance is being attempted. Fluosol-DA is supplied by Alpha Therapeutic, Inc, in the United States and is available only for research.

Blood Substitute: Chemically altered hemoglobin solutions are prepared by hemolyzing outdated red blood cells and removing all the contaminating stroma, which is nephrotoxic. This material is stable, may be stored for up to 18 months, has no incompatibilities, and produces no adverse reactions following repeated doses in laboratory animals. However, these solutions have an intravascular half-life of less than 100 minutes and are eliminated rapidly in the urine; thus, they have not yet proved clinically acceptable as red blood cell substitutes.

Coagulation Factor Concentrates: These blood components are discussed in Chapter 36, Hemostatics.

Adverse Reactions and Precautions

Viral Hepatitis: This is the most common serious adverse reaction associated with transfusion therapy and may occur after the use of all blood and blood component preparations, whole blood, red cell concentrates, and plasma (eg, platelets, granulocytes, cryoprecipitated antihemophilic factor, antihemophilic and prothrombin complex concentrates). Since hepatitis virus cannot be eliminated totally from these preparations, components prepared from the blood of volunteer donors should be used whenever possible and all blood *must* be screened by sensitive tests for hepatitis B antigens.

Hepatitis B surface antigen (HBsAg) is specific for hepatitis B virus. Testing of donor blood for this antigen is required by the Office of Biologic Research and Review of the Food and Drug Administration, the American Red Cross, and the American Association of Blood Banks. A positive test or a history of hepatitis precludes donation. A complete list of products licensed for use in testing is available from the Office of Biologic Research and Review, Division of Blood and Blood Products, Bethesda, MD, 20205.

The exclusion of HBsAg-positive donors has markedly reduced this cause of post-transfusion hepatitis. However, hepatitis B virus causes only 10% or less of post-transfusion hepatitis. The remaining 90% is caused primarily by agent(s) designated non-A, non-B for which no tests are available. Type A (infectious) hepatitis is rarely transmitted by blood transfusion because it has a short lifespan in blood. Other viruses (eg, cytomegalovirus, Epstein-Barr virus) can be transmitted by transfusion and may also cause a type of hepatitis.

The precise incidence of post-transfusion hepatitis appears to be grossly underestimated; the incidence can be determined only if blood recipients are followed prospectively and serum aminotransferases are measured periodically. Two large-scale prospective studies indicate that 5% of patients receiving multiple transfusions of volunteer donor blood develop hepatitis (estimated risk is 2%/unit transfused). Most cases are subclinical and anicteric, but even icteric cases may not be reported to the institution that provided the blood. Despite the benign course of the acute phase of anicteric hepatitis, it predisposes to chronic liver disease and a carrier state.

In general, although type B hepatitis tends to be more severe acutely, non-A, non-B hepatitis more frequently progresses to chronic liver disease. Liver biopsy specimens frequently show histologic findings consistent with chronic active hepatitis. The development of a serologic test to detect the agent(s) responsible for non-A, non-B hepatitis prior to transfusion remains a major goal, which would further reduce the incidence of post-transfusion hepatitis.

Other Infectious Diseases: Many infections can be transmitted by blood transfusion, including cytomegalovirus, Epstein-Barr virus, infectious mononucleosis, syphilis, herpes simplex, malaria, Chagas' disease, and brucellosis. Cytomegalovirus and Epstein-Barr infection are usually asymptomatic and self-limited, but associated fever and hepatosplenomegaly may be hazardous in pregnant women, immunosuppressed patients, and premature infants. Blood products processed to reduce the risk of cytomegalovirus transmission are recommended for these patients.

Acquired immunodeficiency syndrome (AIDS) is caused by human T-lymphotropic virus type III (HTLV-III), although infection with HTLV-III does not always cause AIDS. However, infected persons may be capable of transmitting infection for many years, although they remain asymptomatic. This persistence of the HTLV-III infection results in a population of persons at risk for development of AIDS for several years. Currently, the incubation period between infection and onset of symptoms in adults is thought to be from months to six years or more and in infants from six weeks to five years or more.

HTLV-III infection is transmitted by infected sexual partners through exchange of body fluids, by shared equipment used to administer intravenous drugs of abuse, and from infected mothers to infants. Although uncommon, AIDS also can be transmitted by transfusion of contaminated blood and blood products. Hemophilics receiving heat-treated antihemophilic concentrates have a 0.001% chance of contracting AIDS (Curran, 1984), although a large number have positive tests for HTLV-III antibody. The probability of contracting AIDS has been as high as 0.27% from use of either antihemophilic concentrate or cryoprecipitate that had been administered prior to development of donor screening tests (*Morbid Mortal Week Rep*, 1985). Blood banks have initiated programs to restrict donation of blood from persons in high-risk groups (eg, homosexual men, bisexual men and their female partners, recent immigrants from Haiti). Detection and exclusion of any donors with HTLV-III antibodies should markedly reduce the transmission of AIDS. Increased use of autologous transfusion also may be valuable in patients not requiring repeated blood replacement.

Hypersensitivity Reactions: Donor blood causes allergic responses in 1% to 3% of recipients. Most of these reactions (eg, urticarial rashes, generalized pruritus) are mild and transitory, but severe effects (eg, bronchospasm, angioedema) occur occasionally and cause death rarely. Antihistamines may control mild reactions, but epinephrine or corticosteroids may be necessary for serious ones. (For treatment, see Chapter 62, Agents for Active and Passive Immunity.) Patients who lack IgA may become sensitized and experience anaphylactic reactions with subsequent transfusions. These patients require blood products from IgA-deficient donors or thoroughly saline-washed or thawed, deglycerolized red cells.

Febrile Reactions: Fever may exceed 39.4 to 40 C (103 to 104 F) and usually occurs within 15 minutes after transfusion is begun, although fever may develop two hours or more after completion of transfusion. It frequently is accompanied by chills, headache, and malaise. When fever develops, the transfusion should be stopped and the cause investigated, since increased temperature may be an early manifestation of a more serious problem, especially hemolytic transfusion reaction or bacterial contamination. However, most febrile reactions are of unknown cause or are attributable to antibodies directed against HLA or other antigens located on granulocytes and platelets. After at least two consecutive febrile, nonhemolytic reactions, administration of leukocyte-poor preparations (saline-washed red cells; red cells filtered to remove leukocytes; thawed, deglycerolized red cells) is indicated.

Hemolysis: This potentially fatal complication results from the administration of incompatible blood and usually is caused by clerical error (eg, mislabeling of specimens, misidentification of recipients). Only rarely does it result from technical errors in blood typing and crossmatching. The transfusion of as little as 10 to 50 ml of ABO- and other antigen-incompatible blood may cause flushing, nausea, hypotension, tachycardia, restlessness, dyspnea, chills, fever, headache, substernal

and/or flank pain, and vomiting. Hemoglobinemia and hemoglobinuria occur and often are followed by oliguria and acute renal failure. Hemorrhagic diathesis with thrombocytopenia and spontaneous bleeding may be observed and is caused by disseminated intravascular coagulation (DIC). Hypotension and unexpected bleeding from a surgical wound may be the only findings in an anesthetized patient. Extreme caution is required in treating DIC. (See Chapter 33, Agents Used for Anticoagulant Therapy.) Rarely, shock and death occur shortly after initiating the transfusion.

If a hemolytic reaction is suspected, the transfusion must be stopped immediately and the container and tubing saved for study. Prompt intravenous administration of fluids and furosemide [Lasix] or a suitable osmotic diuretic (eg, mannitol) may prevent acute renal failure. The transfusion service should be consulted immediately and supplied with both clotted and anticoagulated samples of the patient's blood together with all containers and attachments used.

Delayed hemolytic transfusion reactions sometimes are observed in patients who do not have serologically detectable antibodies at the time of transfusion but who later develop an increased antibody titer anamnestically. Since the hallmark of the delayed transfusion reaction is a transiently positive direct antiglobulin test, this type of reaction may mimic autoimmune hemolytic anemia.

Reactions from Contaminated Products: Administration of whole blood, blood components, or plasma contaminated by bacteria or bacterial endotoxins is a rare cause of catastrophic transfusion reactions. A severe reaction, manifested by nausea and vomiting, chills, fever, profound shock with marked cutaneous erythema (red shock), coma, convulsions, and, frequently, death, may occur after the injection of the first 50 to 100 ml of a product contaminated by gram-negative bacilli. Management must be prompt and aggressive. Treatment should include management of shock and administration of a broad spectrum antibiotic, followed by use of the most specific antibiotic for the organism once it has been identified and sensitivity tests performed. Administration of systemic corticosteroids lessens the severity of the reactions. Proper preparation and storage should prevent contamination, which is extremely rare in the United States.

Hypervolemia: Hypervolemia can be a serious consequence of transfusions with whole blood, plasma, or plasma substitutes, particularly in the elderly, the very young, and patients with pulmonary or cardiac disease. The use of red blood cells greatly reduces but does not eliminate this hazard. Hematocrit determinations are commonly used as guides for transfusion therapy but do not detect hypervolemia. The monitoring of central venous or pulmonary wedge pressure is useful to detect volume overexpansion. When serious hypervolemia occurs, prompt intravenous administration of a suitable diuretic (eg, furosemide) and/or phlebotomy may be indicated.

Immunization: The recipient of transfusions may become immunized to one or a combination of red blood cell, white blood cell, platelet, and protein antigens. Although symptoms do not develop, red cell compatibility testing is more difficult and provision of blood products is more hazardous when subsequent transfusions are necessary.

Miscellaneous Adverse Effects: When more than 80% of a patient's original blood volume is replaced within a short time, dilution of hemostatic factors may occur and result in a bleeding tendency. Since banked blood is deficient in platelets and coagulation factors V and VIII, the hemorrhagic diathesis in these patients may be treated with factor VIII concentrate or cryoprecipitate and platelet concentrate. Rapid administration of citrate during massive transfusions may produce muscle tremors, circulatory depression, and electrocardiographic changes consistent with hypocalcemia. To neutralize the citrate load, a source of ionized calcium (10 ml of a 10% calcium gluconate solution/two units of blood) may be administered in special circumstances (eg, in patients with impaired liver function or hypothermia). This is not advocated routinely in massive transfusion because administration of excessive calcium may occur.

Hemosiderosis develops after repeated transfusions in patients with some chronic anemias (eg, sickle cell anemia, thalassemia major, aplastic anemia). Hemosiderosis appears to be less common in other patients receiving chronic transfusion therapy. In patients with thalassemia or sideroblastic anemias, iron overload may be life-threatening as a result of organ damage associated with secondary hemochromatosis (eg, arrhythmias, congestive heart failure, cirrhosis, diabetes). Iron chelating agents have been employed to forestall this process. Iron excretion may be increased if deferoxamine [Desferal] 1 g is given by slow intravenous infusion before each transfusion or 120 mg daily is given by continuous infusion over a 12-hour period several times each week (Weatherall et al, 1977). Automated delivery systems for continuous subcutaneous administration of deferoxamine also have been used.

Drug Evaluations

BLOOD AND BLOOD COMPONENTS

CPD WHOLE BLOOD

CP2D WHOLE BLOOD

CPDA-1 WHOLE BLOOD

HEPARINIZED WHOLE BLOOD

Whole blood is drawn from a selected donor under aseptic conditions and ABO and Rh types are identified. The content (eg, hemoglobin levels, number of viable erythrocytes) of a unit of blood varies according to the donor. Except for heparinized blood, citrate ion (usually as a citrate-phosphate-dextrose-adenine mixture [CPDA-1] or citrate-phosphate-dextrose mixture [CPD or CP2D]) is used as the anticoagulant.

Following crossmatching, blood is administered through a recipient set with a 170 to 180 mesh filter.

Whole blood is stored between 1 and 6 C, except during shipment when the temperature may vary from 1 to 10 C. The expiration date is not later than 21 days after collection if a CPD or CP2D formulation is used and 42 days if CPDA-1 is used. Units on which the hermetic seal is broken are outdated within 24 hours.

Heparinized whole blood contains all of the normal constituents of whole blood, but heparin solution is employed as the anticoagulant instead of CPD, CP2D, or CPDA-1. Heparinized whole blood is contraindicated for routine transfusions. This product has been used to prime pump oxygenators during cardiac surgery but is no longer advocated. Red blood cells in additive solutions (eg, adenine-saline) or CPD whole blood less than five days old, modified by the addition of heparin and calcium chloride immediately prior to use, are preferred.

The routine use of whole blood is wasteful, may produce hypervolemia, and provides excessive ions or metabolites that could be deleterious in some patients. Whole blood transfusion should be reserved for patients with massive bleeding (greater than 20% of the blood volume) or when the need for oxygen-carrying capacity is combined with a need for volume expansion. Conventional cell-free resuscitation fluids cannot restore circulating red cell volume and do not provide sufficient oxygen following severe hemorrhage. In all other instances, red cell concentrates alone, with electrolyte solutions, or with a specific component should be utilized. (See also the Introduction.)

After 24 hours of storage, blood contains few functioning platelets. Coagulation factors V and VIII decrease to about 50% of normal after five to seven days, but factor IX is more stable. Massive blood transfusions utilizing old bank blood may produce significant dilutional thrombocytopenia. Rarely, factor V and VIII deficiencies also may occur, usually in patients with congenital deficiency of these factors or DIC. Infusion of platelet concentrates and fresh frozen plasma may be needed to correct these deficits, but they are indicated only when definite evidence of dilutional coagulopathy is present.

DOSAGE AND PREPARATIONS.

Intravenous: One unit (450 ± 45 ml with 63 ml of CPD, CP2D, or CPDA-1), repeated as needed. Units must be administered through a standard 170-micron filter. Other medications should not be added.

Available through hospital blood banks.

MODIFIED WHOLE BLOOD

Modified whole human blood is prepared in a closed system of containers. Plasma is removed from a fresh unit of whole blood, platelets are separated by differential centrifugation, and/or antihemophilic factor is removed by cryoprecipitation. The remaining platelet- and/or factor VIII-poor plasma then is reintroduced into the original container. Units from which cryoprecipitate has been removed should not be used to promote or maintain coagulation. Otherwise, side effects, hazards, dosage, storage, and dating period are the same as for whole blood. This product is given infrequently and its use is not encouraged.

RED BLOOD CELLS CPD OR CP2D

RED BLOOD CELLS CPDA-1

Human red blood cell concentrates are prepared by removing most of the plasma from whole blood at any time during the dating period; the ABO and Rh types are identified, and the hematocrit of the final product usually ranges from 70% to 80%.

Characteristics of this product may vary with the donor, the process used, and the duration of storage of the whole blood before red cell extraction. The characteristics of red cells contained in a unit may not be apparent from the label, but the product may contain platelet or leukocyte debris and products of red cell metabolism and hematocrit levels may vary.

Unfrozen red cell concentrate should be stored at 1 to 6 C. The expiration date for unfrozen cells is not later than that of the whole blood from which it was derived or 24 hours after the hermetic seal is broken.

Red blood cell concentrate provides the same hemoglobin content and oxygen-carrying capacity as the whole blood from which it was derived in approximately 50% of the volume. It is the product of choice when an increased red cell mass is required (except in patients with massive hemorrhage who also require volume replacement and who may require coagulation factor replacement). Red cell concentrates less than seven days old are preferable to whole blood to prevent hypervolemia in seriously ill neonates.

Red blood cell concentrate may be mixed with 50 to 100 ml of 0.9% sodium chloride injection to increase the flow rate, but it should not be mixed with other solutions (eg, dextrose causes hemolysis unless sufficient sodium chloride is added to prevent osmotic lysis; lactated Ringer's injection may cause clotting in the unit of blood or tubing by providing a source of ionized calcium, although lactated Ringer's solution without calcium is available).

For adverse reactions and precautions, see the Introduction.

DOSAGE AND PREPARATIONS.
Intravenous: One unit usually elevates the venous hematocrit level by approximately 3% in a 70-kg recipient; 50 to 100 ml of 0.9% sodium chloride injection may be added to a unit of packed red blood cells through a standard Y-administration set.

Available through hospital blood banks.

RED BLOOD CELLS, ADENINE-SALINE

Most of the plasma and possibly platelet and/or leukocyte fractions from whole blood, collected in CPD or CP2D anticoagulant, are removed, and an additive solution is mixed with the red blood cells to provide a product with a hematocrit of 55% to 65%. Typical additive solutions are dextrose and adenine in physiologic saline solution with mannitol (AS-1) or without mannitol but with additional citrate and phosphate (AS-2) plus additional dextrose and adenine (AS-3). These products are labeled to identify the anticoagulant and additive solution. They have approximately the same flow rate as whole blood and no further dilution is required.

The actions, indications, and contraindications are the same as for CPD or CPDA-1 Red Blood Cells. However, use of more than 40 units of AS-1 could produce the side effects of mannitol. Furthermore, because of the dilution with saline, large amounts of these solutions should not be used in patients at risk of circulatory overload.

DOSAGE AND PREPARATIONS. The dosage is the same as for Red Blood Cells CPD or CPDA-1.
AS-1.
Adsol (Pennwalt).
AS-2, AS-3.
Neutracil (Cutter).

RED BLOOD CELLS LEUKOCYTES REMOVED

Many patients experience nonhemolytic febrile reactions following transfusion of red blood cells or whole blood. These reactions may result from alloimmunization to antigens associated with white blood cells, platelets, plasma proteins, and other nonerythrocyte elements; most often there is no clear explanation. More than 80% of patients who develop febrile reactions to a single transfusion do not react to subsequent transfusions. Therefore, most patients do not require leukocyte-poor preparations unless at least two successive transfusions have caused febrile reactions. However, febrile reactions are common in patients who received multiple transfusions (particularly those with diseases such as leukemia or aplastic anemia) and immunosuppressed or immunodeficient individuals. These patients should receive preparations from which leukocytes have been removed.

Leukocyte-poor or buffy coat-poor concentrates can be prepared simply by removing the sedimented buffy coat after centrifugation of whole blood. Removal of leukocytes is more efficient from blood stored for more than 10 days. Preparations from which at least 70% of the original white cells are removed are usually adequate for uncomplicated situations. However, in persons with high titers of leukoagglutinins or HLA antibodies, further removal of white blood cell and platelet debris may be necessary. Several techniques involving filtration, inverted centrifugation, or sedimentation are utilized. Newer bedside spin-filter techniques are commonly used.

DOSAGE AND PREPARATIONS. Same as for Red Blood Cells CPD or CPDA-1.

RED BLOOD CELLS SALINE-WASHED

Significant amounts of leukocytes, platelets, plasma, and other debris are removed by washing, especially when automated blood cell processors are used. The red blood cells are washed with normal saline within 24 hours before transfusion, but products vary according to the shelf-age before washing. The more efficient batch washing process removes approximately 90% of leukocytes, almost all plasma, and about 20% of erythrocytes. Although contamination is reduced slightly less than with frozen, deglycerolized red blood cells, these preparations can be used in most alloimmunized patients with recurrent nonhemolytic febrile transfusion reactions.

DOSAGE AND PREPARATIONS. Same as for Red Blood Cells CPD or CPDA-1.

RED BLOOD CELLS FROZEN

A unit of red cells less than six days old is frozen rapidly after addition of a cryoprotective agent, usually glycerol, and stored at -65 C or colder. The expiration date is three years, but units have demonstrated adequate in vivo recovery after storage for more than ten years. Transfusion must be preceded by thawing and deglycerolizing to replace the cryoprotectant with saline. Thawed red cells are outdated in 24 hours. These preparations contain about 2% of the original leukocytes and almost no measurable plasma protein, platelets, or plasma. The method used to deglycerolize cells must be compatible with the procedure used for freezing. If glycerol has not been removed sufficiently, intravascular hemolysis may result.

Although processing is expensive and time consuming, frozen erythrocytes can be kept for long periods. This type of preparation is particularly useful for storing erythrocytes of rare phenotypes and predeposits for autotransfusion in special circumstances (eg, anticipated needs during pregnancy, elective surgery, or neonatal exchange transfusions). (See also the Introduction.)

Thawed, deglycerolized red blood cells are reserved for patients with confirmed severe febrile or allergic transfusion reactions who continue to experience reactions to saline-washed or unfrozen leukocyte-poor red cells or individuals with paroxysmal nocturnal hemoglobinuria.

DOSAGE AND PREPARATIONS. Same as for Red Blood Cells CPD or CPDA-1.

PLASMA FRESH FROZEN

This preparation is the liquid portion of a single unit of citrated (CPD, CPDA-1) whole blood that has been separated from the cells within four hours and frozen within six hours of donation. It may be stored at -18 C or lower for up to one year after the date of collection. The unit is thawed in a water bath at 37 C (with gentle agitation to facilitate thawing), and it must be used shortly afterward. The product usually contains 70% or more of the coagulation factors present in fresh plasma.

USES. Fresh frozen plasma may be used to replace coagulation factor II, VII, IX (mild), X, or XI deficiencies and is the agent of choice to replace coagulation factor V deficiency. Although fresh frozen plasma also contains factor VIII, antihemophilic factor preparations (cryoprecipitate and concentrates) are preferred for deficiency of this factor. Plasma should not be used routinely to treat hemophilia but is reserved for patients with acute blood loss. Cryoprecipitated factor VIII preparations also are preferred to treat hypofibrinogenemia or, experimentally, for fibronectin deficiency. Plasma may be used prior to surgery in patients with severe liver disease and multiple clotting factor deficiencies.

Fresh frozen plasma or plasma from donors known to be deficient in IgA is indicated for the treatment and prophylaxis of immunoglobulin deficiencies when class-specific anti-IgA antibodies are present and may provide the only source of IgG and IgM currently available. These patients may have anaphylactic reactions to transfusion of IgA-containing materials, including albumin and immune globulin. Fresh frozen plasma is indicated for the treatment of infants with secondary immunodeficiency associated with severe protein-losing enteropathy.

When plasmapheresis is used to treat thrombotic thrombocytopenic purpura, the replacement fluid of choice is fresh frozen plasma. Its usefulness in congenital thrombocytopenia is controversial, but plasma transfusions may be beneficial in selected patients with documented deficiencies of immunoglobulins or complement (Sandler, 1980). When bleeding is caused by anticoagulants, fresh frozen plasma is indicated for rapid hemostasis (eg, prior to emergency surgery). Plasma can be used in antithrombin III deficiency, particularly before surgery or in patients who require heparin for the treatment of thrombosis. Also, the use of plasma for its oncotic properties in burn patients with infection appears to be promising.

ADVERSE REACTIONS AND PRECAUTIONS. Plasma may cause circulatory overload and carries a risk of hepatitis. It should not be used when blood volume can be adequately replaced by crystalloids or colloids (eg, albumin, plasma protein fraction).

DOSAGE AND PREPARATIONS.
Intravenous: Dosage is determined by clinical response and, when possible, by laboratory assays of appropriate coagulation factors. ABO compatibility is desirable, but crossmatching is not necessary.

PLASMA

Plasma is the liquid portion of a single unit of citrated (CPD, CPDA-1) whole blood separated during the dating period (21 days [CPD] or 35 days [CPDA-1]). It is the liquid remaining after removal of cryoprecipitate and/or platelets when separation is carried out within four to six hours after blood is collected. Plasma also may be obtained by plasmapheresis. It may be stored at 1 to 6 C for no more than 26 days (CPD) or 40 days (CPDA-1) after collection of the whole blood. This product contains variable amounts of stable coagulation factors depending on the duration of storage before separation, but labile clotting factors and platelets decrease during the first few days of blood storage and are not present in the plasma prepared from stored blood. It also contains significant quantities of cellular debris, adenine, citrate, sodium, potassium, and other ions, which increase the metabolic burden in a bleeding patient. It has all the disadvantages of fresh frozen plasma and no compensating advantages.

Plasma may be used to treat mild deficiencies of stable clotting factors (eg, II, VII, IX, X, XI, XIII). It may be of value to counteract anticoagulant overdose in patients who are bleeding or require emergency surgery. This product should not be used as a plasma volume expander because of the risk of hepatitis.

DOSAGE AND PREPARATIONS.

Intravenous: Dosage is determined by clinical response and, when possible, by laboratory assays of appropriate coagulation factors. ABO compatibility is desirable, but crossmatching is not required.

PLATELETS

Platelet concentrate (one of the primary products obtained from routine conversion of whole blood into red cell concentrate) is prepared by centrifugation of citrated (CPD or CPDA-1) whole blood at 20 to 24 C within four hours after collection. An average unit of random-donor platelets obtained from whole blood contains more than 5.5×10^{10} platelets suspended in 20 to 70 ml of the original plasma. Single-donor platelets may be obtained by automated apheresis techniques and multiple units may be obtained from one donor by manual thrombocytapheresis. The dating period of random-donor platelets is up to seven days depending on the plastic container used after collection when stored at 20 to 24 C and no longer than 48 hours when stored at 1 to 6 C (see the Introduction). Those preserved at room temperature must be agitated gently and continuously.

Ordinarily, ABO-identical platelets are used but, when unavailable, platelets from non-ABO-identical donors may be administered if not grossly contaminated with red cells. However, large volumes of the suspending incompatible plasma should not be given to children. If necessary, some of the incompatible plasma may be removed just prior to administration. Rh-negative platelets should be used in Rh-negative females before and during the childbearing period to prevent Rh alloimmunization by contaminating red blood cells.

For indications, see the Introduction.

DOSAGE AND PREPARATIONS.

Intravenous: Units must be administered through a 170-micron filter *(microaggregate filters must not be used)*. Adults, initially, 1 unit/10 kg; the appropriate number (usually 8 to 10) of units is pooled immediately prior to infusion. In patients without platelet antibodies, splenomegaly, sepsis, or disseminated intravascular coagulation, this dose should increase the platelet count by approximately 35,000/microliter in a 70-kg person. See also the section on Platelet Transfusion in the Introduction.

GRANULOCYTES

It was only after technology for obtaining granulocytes by continuous or intermittent flow centrifugation or by filtration (leukapheresis) was developed that granulocyte transfusion became practical. Steroids may be given to the donor and a sedimenting agent (eg, hydroxyethyl starch) may be used to increase the harvest of granulocytes. With mechanical leukapheresis, a single donor can provide at least 1×10^{10} granulocytes in two to three hours. Although this quantity is only about 10% of the normal daily granulocyte production, it may be sufficient to combat infection in the recipient. However, some authorities believe the minimum effective adult dose may be 1.5×10^{10} granulocytes.

Unless the patient is in critical condition, a one- to two-day trial with broad spectrum antibiotics may control the infection and obviate the need for granulocyte transfusion.

USES. Granulocytes may be transfused to treat sepsis if (1) the patient's granulocyte count is less than 500/microliter, and (2) fever persists for 48 hours despite appropriate antibiotic therapy. Granulocytes should be administered for at least three or more consecutive days in conjunction with appropriate antibiotics (Schiffer, 1977). Additionally, there should be a reasonable likelihood for recovery and significant improvement after recovery from the infection. Granulocytes should not be given to patients with widespread malignant disease that is unresponsive to chemotherapy. If recovery of bone marrow function is unlikely, granulocyte transfusion will not alter the course of the disease and may cause additional problems (eg, pulmonary toxicity) because of sensitization to the infused cellular infiltrates.

The prophylactic use of granulocyte transfusions is not recommended. However, HLA-matched granulocytes have been beneficial in patients recovering from bone marrow transplants. (It is advisable to irradiate all blood products given to bone marrow recipients to suppress graft-versus-host disease.)

Results of in vitro tests suggest that granulocytes from normal donors may retain some phagocytic and microbicidal functions for as long as 48 hours. However, they should be used within six hours after collection to assure maximum benefit.

ADVERSE REACTIONS AND PRECAUTIONS. Fever often follows granulocyte transfusion and can be ameliorated by an antipyretic.

Pulmonary reactions (eg, respiratory insufficiency) may result from sequestration of granulocytes in the pulmonary capillaries. The reaction may be particularly severe in those with pulmonary infections or congestive heart failure.

Serious pulmonary reactions also have been reported in patients given amphotericin B concomitantly with granulocyte transfusions. Respiratory deterioration characterized by acute dyspnea, hypoxemia, and interstitial infiltrates were reported to contribute to death in a few patients (Wright et al, 1981), but these observations have not been confirmed by other investigators (Forman et al, 1981; DeGregorio et al, 1981). Combined therapy is not precluded but should be administered cautiously in patients with gram-negative bacteremia. If signs of pulmonary distress are noted, the transfusion should be discontinued, hydrocortisone 100 to 500 mg given intravenously, and symptomatic treatment initiated (Higby and Burnett, 1980).

Cytomegalovirus infection and toxoplasmosis occasionally are observed following granulocyte transfusions because these organisms are concentrated in granulocytes.

DOSAGE AND PREPARATIONS.

Intravenous: A minimum of 1.5×10^{10} granulocytes is administered slowly once daily on at least three or more consecutive days (Conrad, 1981). The optimum dose and frequency of administration have not been determined, but one suggested regimen is administration over a two-hour period via standard blood administration sets. Micropore filters should *not* be used (Ritchey, 1983).

ALBUMIN HUMAN (Normal Human Serum Albumin)
[Albuminar, Albutein, Buminate, Plasbumin]

This sterile plasma protein preparation is obtained by fractionating plasma nonreactive for hepatitis B surface antigen (HBsAg) and anti-HTLV III in a series of controlled precipitations with cold ethanol. Human albumin contains no coagulation factors or blood group antibodies. Sterile filtration and heating for ten hours at 60 C appear to remove the hazard of viral hepatitis. Albumin preparations contain sodium caprylate and/or acetyltryptophanate as stabilizers. Unopened preparations can be stored for approximately three years at temperatures not exceeding 37 C. All albumin preparations should be used within four hours after the container has been opened. Unused portions should be discarded.

USES. Albumin 25 g is equivalent osmotically to about 500 ml of fresh frozen plasma (*Med Lett Drugs Ther*, 1979). This preparation is used to restore the colloidal osmotic pressure of plasma in hypovolemic states (eg, burns, hemorrhage, surgical procedures, during plasmapheresis).

Albumin binds bilirubin and has been used adjunctively during exchange transfusion to treat hyperbilirubinemia, most frequently that associated with hemolytic disease in the newborn. It has been given to patients with nephrosis and hepatic cirrhosis, but most authorities consider these uses to be questionable and of temporary benefit at best.

The 5% solution is preferred for most indications. The 25% preparation is hypertonic and may cause hypervolemia.

ADVERSE REACTIONS AND PRECAUTIONS. Since albumin is a constituent of human blood, it usually can be given with relative safety, although chills, fever, urticaria, and variable effects on blood pressure, pulse, and respiration have been noted. This preparation does not interfere with normal coagulation mechanisms or promote clotting. Albumin preparations contain 100 to 160 mEq/L of sodium, and this should be considered when salt intake must be restricted. Patients with heart failure should not be given albumin. Because patients with low cardiac reserve or severe anemia and those not deficient in albumin are more likely to develop hypervolemia and congestive heart failure, they should not receive large amounts of albumin.

Albumin should not be administered if the solution is turbid or contains sediment.

DOSAGE AND PREPARATIONS.

Intravenous: Dosage should be determined by monitoring the pulmonary artery, wedge, or central venous pressure during administration to avoid hypervolemia. No more than 250 g/48

hours should be given. When more than this is necessary, whole blood or plasma should be given.

The 5% solution is given undiluted, usually at a rate of 2 to 4 ml/min. The 25% solution can be administered undiluted or it can be diluted with sterile, nonpyrogenic sodium chloride injection or 5% dextrose injection. (In the presence of edema, the undiluted 25% concentrate should be used, but 5% dextrose injection may be employed if dilution is necessary.)

Albumin must be administered slowly (1 ml/min) to patients with low cardiac reserve to prevent rapid expansion of plasma volume and possible pulmonary edema. For shock caused by diminished plasma volume, it may be given as rapidly as desired, preferably diluted (an approximately isotonic solution can be prepared by diluting each 20 ml of 25% solution to a volume of 100 ml).

For shock, *adults and older children,* 25 g initially, repeated in 15 to 30 minutes if necessary. Whole blood may be required if the patient is hemorrhaging.

For burns, the extent of burn determines the amount and duration of administration. The dose should be sufficient to restore plasma volume and to decrease hemoconcentration. Initially, 500 ml of 5% solution or 100 ml of 25% solution has been used in addition to electrolyte solutions. For nonemergency treatment of *children,* 6.25 to 12.5 g.

> *Generic.* Solution 5% in 50 ml containers and in 250 and 500 ml containers with intravenous administration set; 25% in 20 ml containers and in 50 and 100 ml containers with intravenous administration set.
>
> *Albuminar-5, Albuminar-25* (Armour), *Albutein 5% and 25%* (Alpha Therapeutic), *Buminate 5%, 25%* (Hyland), *Plasbumin-5, Plasbumin-25* (Cutter). Solution (aqueous) 5% in 50 ml containers (*Albuminar-5, Plasbumin-5*), 250 and 500 ml containers with intravenous administration sets (*Albuminar-5, Albutein 5%, Buminate 5%*), and 1,000 ml containers (*Albuminar-5*); solution (aqueous) 25% in 20, 50, and 100 ml containers (*Albuminar-25, Albutein 25%, Buminate 25%, Plasbumin-25*). The 50 and 100 ml containers are supplied with intravenous administration sets. Use of 4% and 20% solutions is permitted by the Code of Federal Regulations. These concentrations are produced by some manufacturers in the United States for export; they are not generally available in this country.

PLASMA PROTEIN FRACTION (Human Plasma Protein Fraction)
[Plasmanate, Plasma Plex, Plasmatein, Protenate]

Plasma protein fraction (PPF) is a 5% solution of stabilized human plasma proteins (at least 83% albumin, no more than 17% globulin, and no more than 1% of total protein as gamma globulin) in sodium chloride injection. The material is prepared from large pools of normal human plasma nonreactive for hepatitis B surface antigen (HBsAg) and anti-HTLV III by fractionation involving a series of controlled precipitations with cold ethanol (Cohn process). Products are heated at 60 C for 10 hours to minimize the risk of transmitting viral disease.

Plasma protein fraction is used to treat hypovolemic shock and to provide protein in patients with hypoproteinemia. It also is effective for the initial treatment of shock in infants and small children with dehydration, hemoconcentration, and electrolyte deficiency caused by diarrhea. PPF does not provide labile clotting factors and should not be given to correct coagulation defects.

ADVERSE REACTIONS AND PRECAUTIONS. Chills, fever, urticaria, nausea, and vomiting have occurred. Serious hypotension was reported in surgical patients undergoing extracorporeal circulation following transfusion of earlier preparations of PPF. Contamination of some of these lots with prekallikrein activator (PKA) was implicated as the cause of bradykinin-induced peripheral vasodilation. This usually could have been avoided by slowing the rate of infusion to less than 10 ml/minute. PKA levels have been reduced in all preparations and hypotension has been rare since this change was made. Nevertheless, PPF probably should not be given when rapid intravenous infusion is necessary.

All patients should be observed carefully for signs of hypervolemia (eg, pulmonary edema) or cardiac failure. Administration of large quantities to patients with impaired renal function has caused electrolyte imbalances resulting in metabolic alkalosis (Rahilly and Berl, 1979).

Solutions should not be mixed with or administered through the same sets as other intravenous fluids. Administration is contraindicated if the preparation is turbid or a precipitate forms.

DOSAGE AND PREPARATIONS.
Intravenous: The following amounts serve as guides; the total amount administered must be adjusted to meet the needs of each patient. *Adults,* for hypoproteinemia, 1 to 1.5 L of solution containing 50 to 75 g of protein infused at a rate of 5 to 8 ml/min, repeated as necessary. *Infants and young children,* for dehydration, 33 ml/kg infused at a rate of 5 to 10 ml/min.

> **Plasmanate** (Cutter), **Generic.** Solution 5% in 50 ml containers and in 250 and 500 ml containers with intravenous administration set.
> **Plasma Plex** (Armour), **Plasmatein** (Alpha Therapeutic), **Protenate** (Hyland). Solution 5% in 250 and 500 ml containers with intravenous administration set.

BLOOD SUBSTITUTES

DEXTRAN 40
[Gentran-40, Rheomacrodex, 10% LMD]

DEXTRAN 70
[Macrodex]

DEXTRAN 70 WITH 10% DEXTROSE
[Hyskon]

DEXTRAN 75
[Gentran-75]

Dextran 70 or 75 is a water-soluble glucose polymer biosynthesized by *Leuconostoc mesenteroides* from sucrose. The mean molecular weight is 70,000 and 75,000, respectively. When these high-molecular-weight products are treated further by partial acid hydrolysis and differential fractionation, a finished product of lower and more uniform molecular weight (dextran 40) is obtained. This has a mean molecular weight of approximately 40,000 and effects last two to four hours.

USES. Because they remain in the intravascular space for about 12 hours, the high-molecular-weight preparations may be used as plasma volume expanders to increase filling pressure in shock. They also may be used to correct the oligemia of burn shock or to maintain colloidal osmotic pressure temporarily during certain types of cardiovascular surgery.

Dextran 40 is used as a priming fluid (alone or as an additive) for pump-oxygenators during extracorporeal circulation and as an adjunct in the treatment of shock or impending shock. More recently, dextran 40 has been administered to prevent venous thrombosis and thromboembolism (see Chapter 33, Agents Used for Anticoagulant Therapy).

Another dextran product, 32% dextran 70 in 10% dextrose, is used in hysteroscopy to help distend and irrigate the uterine cavity. Since it may be absorbed, adverse reactions are the same as those encountered after intravenous administration.

ADVERSE REACTIONS. Hypersensitivity reactions (rash, pruritus, nasal congestion, dyspnea, chest tightness, and mild hypotension) are the most common untoward effects. The incidence is very low and reactions generally are mild when adequately hydrolyzed and refined preparations are used. Dextran 40 has considerably less antigenic potential than the higher molecular weight products. Nevertheless, both forms of dextran have produced urticaria, angioedema, bronchospasm, and anaphylactic reactions. Patients also may develop nausea, vomiting, and, occasionally, acute hypotension.

Discontinuation of therapy usually relieves the milder reactions. More serious adverse effects may require the immediate subcutaneous administration of 1:1,000 epinephrine 0.5 ml, followed if necessary by intravenous injection of 0.25 to 0.5 ml of a 1:10,000 solution. Antihistamines, steroids, and other supportive measures also may be required to counteract shock and hypotension. (See also Chapter 62, Agents for Active and Passive Immunity, for treatment of anaphylaxis.) Equipment for emergency resuscitation should be readily available. Because death from anaphylactic reactions has occurred after intravenous administration of as little as 10 ml of dextran 75 solution, blood pressure should be monitored and the patient observed closely during at least the first 30 minutes of infusion of any dextran preparation.

Increased bleeding time caused by interference with platelet function occurs in many patients receiving dextran, especially when the higher molecular weight products are used and the dose exceeds 1 to 1.5 L. This reaction may not appear for six to nine hours following infusion, and bleeding may occur, especially if there is a pre-existing coagulation defect.

Since the renal threshold for dextran is at a molecular weight of about 55,000, more dextran 40 than dextran 70 or 75 is filtered by the glomerulus (approximately 75% of dextran molecules below 50,000 appear in the urine within 24 hours). Dextran 70 or 75 is degraded enzymatically to glucose; the average rate of metabolism is 70 to 90 mg/kg daily. In patients with adequate urine flow, dextran has little effect on urine viscosity. However, when urine flow is diminished, dextran markedly increases urine viscosity and specific gravity, and possibly causes subsequent acute tubular failure.

EFFECTS ON LABORATORY TESTS, PRECAUTIONS, AND CONTRAINDICATIONS. Any dextran preparation may induce rouleaux formation, thus interfering with crossmatching techniques; therefore, if blood is to be administered subsequently, the crossmatch specimen should be drawn prior to dextran infusion. Dextran also may interfere with certain tests of renal and hepatic function.

Because of adverse reactions and the availability of alternative treatments, clinical use of dextran has declined. The potential hazards must be considered before dextran is selected in lieu of safer (although more expensive) products, such as albumin.

Dextran is contraindicated in patients with known hypersensitivity, severe congestive heart failure, renal failure, hypervolemic conditions, or severe bleeding disorders. It should be used with caution in patients with chronic liver disease or impaired renal function or in those likely to develop pulmonary edema or congestive heart failure.

DOSAGE AND PREPARATIONS. Dextran may precipitate from solution on storage. It can be redissolved by heating in a water bath for a short time at the minimal temperature required to effect solution.

DEXTRAN 40:

Intravenous: Adults and children, for shock, the first 10 ml/kg of 10% solution may be infused as rapidly as necessary to effect improvement; the remainder of the dose is given more slowly. Monitoring of the central venous pressure is strongly recommended as a guide to dosage. The total dosage during the first 24 hours should not exceed 20 ml/kg. If therapy is continued for more than 24 hours, the total daily dose should not exceed 10 ml/kg. Therapy should not be continued for more than five days.

> *Dextran 40* (American McGaw), *Gentran-40* (Travenol), *Rheo-macrodex* (Pharmacia), *10% LMD* (Abbott). Solution 10% in 0.9% sodium chloride solution or 5% dextrose in 500 ml containers.

DEXTRAN 70, DEXTRAN 75:

Intravenous: Adults, in an emergency, 500 ml of 6% solution may be infused at a rate of 20 to 40 ml/min. *Children,* the best guide to dosage is the body weight or surface area of the patient. The total dosage should not exceed 20 ml/kg during the first 24 hours.

> DEXTRAN 70:
> *Dextran 70* (American McGaw). Solution 6% in 0.9% sodium chloride solution in 250 and 500 ml containers.
> *Macrodex* (Pharmacia). Solution 6% in 0.9% sodium chloride solution or 5% dextrose in water in 500 ml containers.
> DEXTRAN 75:
> *Dextran 75* (Abbott). Solution 6% in 0.9% sodium chloride solution or 5% dextrose solution in 500 ml containers.
> *Gentran-75* (Travenol). Solution 6% in 0.9% sodium chloride solution in 500 ml containers.

DEXTRAN 70 WITH 10% DEXTROSE:

Intrauterine Instillation: Hyskon Hysteroscopy Fluid should be introduced into the uterine cavity through the cannula of a hysteroscope at approximately 100 mm Hg pressure until the uterus is distended enough to permit adequate visualization. Instillation is continued throughout the examination. The infusion should be maintained at a rate that does not produce pressure in excess of 150 mm Hg.

> *Hyskon Hysteroscopy Fluid* (Pharmacia). Solution 32% in 10% dextrose in 100 and 250 ml containers.

HETASTARCH
[Hespan]

Hetastarch (hydroxyethyl starch, HES) is an artificial colloid. The molecular weight of at least 80% of the polymer units ranges from 10,000 to 2,000,000.

A 6% solution of hetastarch has approximately the same osmotic properties as 5% albumin at physiologic concentration. The pH is approximately 5.5 (range, 4.5 to 7.0) and the osmolality is approximately 310 mOsm/L. Following intravenous infusion of hetastarch, the plasma volume is expanded slightly in excess of the actual volume given. This effect is observed for 24 to 36 hours after infusion; 40% of a dose is eliminated within 24 hours (*Med Lett Drugs Ther*, 1981). The larger molecules (over 50,000) are removed from the circulation and stored temporarily in various body tissues, principally the liver and spleen. These larger molecules are degraded by amylase. About 64% of the dose is eliminated within eight days, and approximately 90% in 42 days; the average half-life is 17 days. The remaining 10% is eliminated in 48 days. Additional doses have additive effects.

USES. Hetastarch is used to expand plasma volume in the treatment of hypovolemia, shock, or impending shock caused by hemorrhage, burns, surgery, sepsis, or other trauma.

Studies comparing hetastarch and other plasma volume expanders (eg, albumin) indicate that the hemodynamic effects of this agent are similar to those of albumin (Lazrove et al, 1980; Diehl et al, 1981). One study in England indicated that hetastarch and dextran 70 had similar hemodynamic effects, but hetastarch had less potential to induce anaphylaxis or coagulation abnormalities. However, other studies indicate that hetastarch may have approximately the same potential as dextran for producing anaphylactoid reactions (Ring and Messmer, 1977).

Hetastarch also is useful as a sedimenting agent in the preparation of granulocytes by leukapheresis (continuous and intermittent flow cytapheresis). In these healthy donors, the main concern is the delayed excretion of hetastarch.

ADVERSE REACTIONS AND PRECAUTIONS. Nausea, vomiting, mild febrile reactions, chills, pruritus, and urticaria have occurred. Rarely, anaphylactoid reactions have been reported (incidence, less than 0.1% according to the manufacturer's literature). Excessive doses decrease the hematocrit, dilute plasma proteins, and interfere with platelet function. Thus, hetastarch is contraindicated in patients with severe bleeding disorders.

Because hetastarch is excreted relatively slowly, primarily by the kidneys, hypervolemia is a potential danger, particularly in patients with impaired renal function. Accordingly, this agent is contraindicated in patients with severe congestive heart failure and renal failure with oliguria or anuria.

No teratogenic effects were demonstrated during studies in mice, but extrapolation of animal data to humans may not be applicable and the risk/benefit potential must be considered carefully before this drug is used in pregnant women. Similarly, no data are available on the use of hetastarch in children.

DOSAGE AND PREPARATIONS.

Intravenous Infusion: Adults, for plasma volume expansion, total dosage and rate of infusion depend upon the amount of blood lost and the resultant hemoconcentration. The usual amount administered is 500 to 1,000 ml. The total dosage does not usually exceed 1,500 ml per day or approximately 20 ml/kg for the typical 70-kg patient, but doses of 3 to 4 L are not uncommon in severe hypovolemia (eg, trauma).

In acute hemorrhagic shock, a rate approaching 20 ml/kg/hr may be used; in burn or septic shock, the rate is usually slower. For leukapheresis in continuous flow centrifugation (CFC) procedures, 250 to 700 ml is typically infused at a constant fixed ratio to venous whole blood, usually 1:8.

Multiple CFC procedures of up to two per week to a total of seven to ten have been reported to be safe and effective. Adequate data are not available to establish the safety of more frequent or a greater number of procedures.

> **Hespan** (American Critical Care). Solution 6% in 0.9% sodium chloride solution in 500 ml containers.

PORPHYRIAS

Porphyrias are a relatively rare, heterogeneous group of metabolic diseases characterized by derangements in heme biosynthesis; the forms are differentiated by the specific enzyme defects. Enzyme activity is reduced to 50% or less of normal in affected individuals and at least one parent. Except for porphyria cutanea tarda, in which the genetic determination is obscure, the porphyrias are inborn errors of metabolism manifested by neurologic (hepatic porphyrias) and/or cutaneous (erythroid porphyrias) dysfunction resulting from increased production and excretion of porphyrins or their precursors. The types of porphyria may be identified by characteristic enzyme deficiencies and the pattern of porphyrin excretion in urine and feces.

In most susceptible individuals, the disease is latent until clinical expression is precipitated by environmental, metabolic, or chemical factors.

Congenital erythropoietic porphyria (CEP) is very rare. Photosensitivity results in severe cutaneous lesions with scarring and hypertrichosis. The disease also is characterized by hemolytic anemia and erythrodontia. The skin must be protected from sunlight (sunscreens are ineffective) and skin trauma must be avoided. Splenectomy or oral beta carotene may be helpful.

Erythropoietic protoporphyria (EPP) is more common than CEP (4 or possibly more/100,000 population). Most patients have mild to moderate photosensitivity but little or no hemolysis. However, a few patients develop progressive liver damage due to hepatic deposition of protoporphyrin; also, the inci-

dence of cholelithiasis is increased. The skin must be protected from sunlight and beta carotene 15 to 180 mg/day is given orally to increase tolerance to sunlight. Other therapeutic regimens (high carbohydrate intake, administration of cholestyramine or hematin) are being studied.

Acute intermittent porphyria (AIP) occurs in 3 or 4/100,000 population. Precipitating factors (drugs, starvation, sex hormones, infection) induce delta-aminolevulinic acid synthetase, the rate-limiting enzyme necessary for hepatic heme biosynthesis. Photosensitivity does not occur. Symptoms of the acute attack result from neurologic damage caused by porphyrin precursors and may involve any part of the nervous system. Abdominal pain, labile hypertension, painful extremities, depression and organic brain syndrome, tachycardia, and paresthesia often occur. Neuropathy may progress to hypothalamic dysfunction, respiratory paralysis, and death. Although patients may recover completely from an acute attack, neurologic deficits may persist. AIP is more prevalent in women and often recurs prior to the onset of menstruation.

Hereditary coproporphyria (HCP) is much less common than AIP and similar but milder neurovisceral symptoms occur during an acute attack. Photosensitivity can develop but usually does not persist after the acute attack.

During an acute attack, *variegate porphyria* (VP) produces symptoms common to those of the hepatic porphyrias (AIP, VP, HCP) in which there is increased hepatic production and increased fecal or urinary excretion of the porphyrin precursors, delta-aminolevulinic acid (ALA) and porphobilinogen (PBG). However, cutaneous disease resembling porphyria cutanea tarda can occur either simultaneously or separately. Variegate porphyria is less prevalent than AIP in the United States but is much more common in South African whites.

The same treatment is required as for hepatic porphyrias. Of primary importance is avoidance of precipitating factors. This may be difficult in females whose exacerbations are associated with their menstrual cycles. When an attack occurs, large amounts of carbohydrate (450 to 500 g daily) are given to decrease the excretion of porphyrin precursors by blocking the hepatic induction of delta-aminolevulinic acid synthetase. Hemin (hematin) apparently acts in the same fashion. Also important is supportive care of neurologic dysfunction, which may include phenothiazines and/or propranolol for autonomic symptoms, strong analgesics for pain, and antiemetics or anticonvulsants. Assisted ventilation may be indicated for impaired pulmonary function. Long-term occupational and physical therapy may be needed for established neuropathy.

Porphyria cutanea tarda (PCT) is the most common form of porphyria, and usually appears sporadically in middle life or later, more frequently in males than in females. Cutaneous manifestations are prominent with scarring, hirsutism, and pigmented or depigmented areas; disfiguring changes occur in severe untreated disease. Liver disease often is present and common predisposing factors are excessive alcohol or iron intake and use of estrogens or oral contraceptives. PCT is differentiated from the hepatic porphyrias (AIP, HCP, and VP) by the absence of acute neurovisceral symptoms and by normal PBG excretion. In PCT, there is increased excretion of urinary uroporphyrin with a lesser increase in coproporphyrin excretion. The opposite is true in VP and this distinguishes the two diseases, which are treated differently. When iron is elevated, PCT is treated by phlebotomy to decrease iron levels and induce remissions. Patients should avoid precipitating factors.

HEMIN FOR INJECTION
[Panhematin]

ACTIONS. This iron-containing metalloporphyrin is an enzyme inhibitor derived from processed red blood cells (approximately 1.8 g of hemin is obtained from 250 ml of packed red cells). It limits the hepatic and/or bone marrow synthesis of porphyrin, probably by inhibiting delta-aminolevulinic acid synthetase. The exact mechanism by which hematin improves symptoms in patients with acute attacks of the hepatic porphyrias is not known.

Following intravenous injection in nonicteric patients, fecal urobilinogen increases in amounts roughly proportional to the dose of hemin. This suggests an enterohepatic pathway as one route of elimination. Bilirubin metabolites also are excreted in the urine following hemin administration.

USES. Hemin is indicated for the amelioration of recurrent attacks of acute intermittent porphyria temporally related to the menstrual cycle in susceptible women. Pain, hypertension, tachycardia, abnormal mental status, and neurologic signs may be controlled in selected patients with this disorder. Similar response has been reported in patients with other hepatic porphyrias (variegate porphyria and hereditary coproporphyria).

During an acute attack, prompt administration is essential to prevent progression of porphyria and avoid irreversible neuronal damage (pre-existing neuronal damage is not affected). However, therapy should not be started until alternative therapy (ie, 400 g of dextrose/day) given for one to two days has failed.

Hemin therapy is not curative. After discontinuation of treatment, symptoms generally return, although remission may be prolonged. Some neurologic symptoms improved weeks to months after therapy was terminated, although little or no response was noted at the time of treatment.

ADVERSE REACTIONS. One case of reversible renal shutdown occurred when an excessive amount (12.2 mg/kg) was administered as a single dose. Phlebitis with or without leukocytosis and pyrexia occurred when hemin was administered through small veins. There has been one report of coagulopathy with prolonged prothrombin and partial thromboplastin times, thrombocytopenia, mild hypofibrinogenemia, mild elevation of fibrin split products, and a 10% reduction in hematocrit.

Teratogenicity has not been studied (FDA Pregnancy Category C). Effects on nursing mothers and children are not known.

PRECAUTIONS. Diagnosis of acute porphyria should be made by evaluating symptoms and performing a Watson-Schwartz or Hoesch test before hemin therapy is started.

Hemin for injection should be used only by physicians experienced in the management of porphyrias and in hospitals where the recommended clinical and laboratory diagnostic and monitoring techniques are available. It is contraindicated in patients with known hypersensitivity to the drug and in those with porphyria cutanea tarda.

Since hemin is thought to act by inhibiting delta-aminolevulinic acid synthetase, drugs that increase the activity of this enzyme should be avoided. These include estrogens, barbiturates, and steroids.

Mild, transient anticoagulant effects have been noted during clinical studies. Therefore, concomitant anticoagulant therapy should be avoided.

Reversible renal shutdown may result if recommended dosage levels are exceeded.

MONITORING THERAPY. The efficacy of treatment is demonstrated by decreased urinary concentrations of one or more of the following compounds: aminolevulinic acid (ALA), uroporphyrinogen (UPG), and porphobilinogen (PBG).

DOSAGE AND PREPARATIONS.

Intravenous: A large arm vein or central venous catheter must be used to avoid phlebitis. No drug or chemical agent should be added unless its effect on the chemical and physical stability of hemin has been determined.

For acute attacks of porphyria that do not respond to dextrose, infusion of 1 to 4 mg/kg/day over 10 to 15 minutes for 3 to 14 days may be given. Based on the clinical signs in more severe cases, this dose may be repeated no more often than every 12 hours. No more than 6 mg/kg should be infused in any 24-hour period.

Reconstituted material is not transparent and should be administered through a sterile 0.45-micron or smaller filter to prevent administration of particulate material. For information regarding preparation of solution, stability, and storage, see the manufacturer's literature.

>**Panhematin** (Abbott). Powder (313 mg/container after reconstitution with 43 ml sterile water for injection).
>
>Because Panhematin is unstable and is suitable for only a limited number of patients, it is available only from Abbott Laboratories, Chicago distribution center. Abbott ships the drug on the next available commercial airline flight. To order, call collect: 312-937-5558, Monday through Friday, from 7:00 AM to 4:00 PM. In emergencies after business hours, call collect: 312-937-7970.

Cited References

Blood products. *Med Lett Drugs Ther* 21:93-96, 1979.

Changing patterns of acquired immunodeficiency syndrome in hemophilia patients: United States. *Morbid Mortal Week Rep* 34:214-243, (May 3) 1985.

Circular of Information for the Use of Human Blood and Blood Components, (pamphlet). AABB, CCBC, American Red Cross, 1984.

Hetastarch (Hespan): New plasma expander. *Med Lett Drugs Ther* 23:16, 1981.

Alter HJ, et al: Transmission of hepatitis B virus infection by transfusion of frozen-deglycerolized red blood cells. *N Engl J Med* 298:637-642, 1978.

Conrad ME: Blood transfusions: Uses, abuses, and practices. *Semin Hematol* 18:81-83, 1981.

Council on Scientific Activities: Current status of therapeutic plasmapheresis and related techniques: Report of AMA Panel on Therapeutic Plasmapheresis. *JAMA* 253:819-825, 1985.

Curran JW: Acquired immunodeficiency syndrome associated with transfusions: Evolving perspective. *Ann Intern Med* 100:298-300, 1984.

DeGregorio MW, et al: Pulmonary reactions associated with amphotericin B and leukocyte transfusions, (letter). *N Engl J Med* 305:585, 1981.

Diehl JT, et al: Clinical comparison of hetastarch and albumin in postoperative cardiac patients. *Surg Forum* 32:260-262, 1981.

Forman SJ, et al: Pulmonary reactions associated with amphotericin B and leukocyte transfusions, (letter). *N Engl J Med* 305:585, 1981.

Haugen RK: Hepatitis after transfusion of frozen red cells and washed red cells. *N Engl J Med* 301:393-395, 1979.

Higby DJ, Burnett D: Granulocyte transfusions: Current status. *Blood* 55:2-8, 1980.

Huestis DW, et al: *The Technical Manual.* Washington, DC, AABB, 1985.

Lazrove S, et al: Hemodynamic, blood volume, and oxygen transport responses to albumin and hydroxyethyl starch infusions in critically ill postoperative patients. *Crit Care Med* 8:302-306, 1980.

National Institutes of Health Consensus Conference: Fresh-frozen plasma: Indications and risks. *JAMA* 253:551-553, 1985.

Petz LD, Swisher SN (eds): *Clinical Practice of Blood Transfusion.* New York, Churchill Livingstone, 1981.

Rahilly GT, Berl T: Severe metabolic alkalosis caused by administration of plasma protein fraction in end-stage renal failure. *N Engl J Med* 301:824-826, 1979.

Ring J, Messmer K: Incidence and severity of anaphylactoid reactions to colloid volume substitutes. *Lancet* 1:466-469, 1977.

Ritchey BE: Apheresis, in Pittiglio DH, et al (eds): *Modern Blood Banking and Transfusion Practices.* Philadelphia, FA Davis, 1983, 349-359.

Sandler SG: Recent advances in practice and technology of blood transfusion. *Primary Care* 7:347-367, 1980.

Schiffer CA: Principles of granulocyte transfusion therapy. *Med Clin North Am* 61:1119-1131, 1977.

Schmidt PJ (ed): *Standards for Blood Banks and Transfusion Services,* ed 11. Arlington, VA, AABB, 1984.

Snyder EL (ed): *Blood Transfusion Therapy: A Physician's Handbook.* Washington, DC, AABB, 1983.

Strauss RG, et al: Controlled trial of prophylactic granulocyte transfusions during initial induction chemotherapy for acute myelogenous leukemia. *N Engl J Med* 305:587-603, 1981.

Weatherall DJ, et al: Iron loading and thalassemia: Experimental successes and practical realities. *N Engl J Med* 297:445-446, 1977.

Winston DJ, et al: Therapeutic granulocyte transfusions for documented infections: Controlled trial in ninety-five infectious granulocytopenic episodes. *Ann Intern Med* 97:509-515, 1982.

Winton EF, et al: Dose in granulocyte transfusion, (letter). *Ann Intern Med* 98:257, 1983.

Wright DG, et al: Lethal pulmonary reactions associated with combined use of amphotericin B and leukocyte transfusion. *N Engl J Med* 304:1185-1189, 1981.

Other Selected References

Code of Federal Regulations, section 21, parts 600-1299. Supt of Documents, US Government Printing Office, Washington, DC, 20402.

Granulocyte transfusions: Established or still experimental therapeutic procedure? *Vox Sang* 38:40-58, 1980.

Transfusion problems in hematology. *Semin Hematol* 18:81-176, 1981.

Alving BM, et al: Hypotension associated with prekallikrein activator (Hageman-factor fragments) in plasma protein fraction. *N Engl J Med* 299:66-70, 1978.

Barton JC: Nonhemolytic, noninfectious transfusion reactions. *Semin Hematol* 18:95-121, 1981.

Blajchman MA, et al: Clinical use of blood, blood components and blood products. *Can Med Assoc J* 121:33-42, 1979.

Conrad ME: Diseases transmissible by blood transfusion: Viral hepatitis and other infectious disorders. *Semin Hematol* 18:122-146, 1981.

Gould SA, et al: Red cell substitutes: Update. *Ann Emerg Med* 14:798-803, 1985.

Greenwalt TJ: Pathogenesis and management of hemolytic transfusion reactions. *Semin Hematol* 18:84-94, 1981.

Guttman RD: Renal transplantation. *N Engl J Med* 301:1038-1048, 1979.

Leitman SF, Holland PV: Irradiation of blood products: Indications and guidelines. *Transfusion* 25:293-303, 1985.

Oberman HA (ed): *General Principles of Blood Transfusion.* Chicago, American Medical Association, 1985.

Ring J, Messmer K: Incidence and severity of anaphylactoid reactions to colloid volume substitutes. *Lancet* 1:466-469, 1977.

Storb R, Weiden PL: Transfusion problems associated with transplantation. *Semin Hematol* 18:163-176, 1981.

Stump DC, et al: Effects of hydroxyethyl starch on blood coagulation, particularly factor VIII. *Transfusion* 25:349-354, 1985.

Tullis JL: Albumin. 1. Background and use. 2. Guidelines for clinical use. *JAMA* 237:355-363, 460-463, 1977.

Wenz B, Barland P: Therapeutic intensive plasmapheresis. *Semin Hematol* 18:147-161, 1981.

Hemostatics

Defects in the interaction of blood vessels with platelets and circulating clotting factors or abnormal synthesis or activation of clotting factors may cause excessive bleeding. Bleeding disorders may be hereditary or acquired and may be caused by a single or by multiple defects. An understanding of the mechanisms of blood clotting and fibrinolysis is essential to determine the etiology of bleeding and to select an appropriate hemostatic agent.

If bleeding results from a specific hereditary deficiency (eg, factor VIII), diagnosis may be relatively simple and only replacement treatment may be required. Conversely, acquired deficiencies of multiple coagulation factors can be difficult to diagnose and may respond poorly to treatment. Such disorders may result from deficient factor formation, disseminated intravascular coagulation (DIC), or fibrinolysis.

Initially, a detailed clinical history must be obtained to identify significant mucocutaneous or deep bleeding, particularly following surgery or trauma. A drug history also should be taken, since thrombocytopenia or platelet dysfunction often follows the use of certain drugs. Screening tests that usually are adequate for presumptive diagnosis of a coagulopathy are platelet count, bleeding time, one-stage prothrombin time, activated partial thromboplastin time, and plasma fibrinogen concentration. Any abnormality in these tests indicates the need for referral to a specialist for more detailed diagnostic procedures. A clinical history of significant bleeding also may be sufficient for referral to a coagulation disorder center, even if screening tests are normal (the results of all these laboratory tests are normal in patients with factor XIII deficiency or mild von Willebrand's disease).

A specialized center for hemophilia is preferred when surgery, dental extractions, and treatment of major bleeding episodes are required in patients with hemophilia or other severe bleeding disorders. For routine maintenance in hemophilics, factor replacement therapy may be administered at the center, by the patient's primary care physician, or by the patient or a trained family member. Hemophilic patients should exercise regularly to maintain joint flexibility and muscle strength, perform frequent routine dental hygiene measures to minimize the need for extensive restorations and extractions, and avoid taking aspirin or other drugs that inhibit platelet function.

Frequent, severe, and spontaneous hemorrhages occur in patients with factor VIII or factor IX activities less than 1% of normal. A factor activity of 2% to 5% usually is associated with hemarthroses only after trauma, and a concentration above 5% usually precludes bleeding except after trauma or surgery. In general, therapy to raise the factor activity to 25% to 30% is adequate for normal hemostasis; a higher percentage is necessary during special circumstances (eg, surgery, trauma, prolonged external bleeding). Also, the presence of an inhibitor should be excluded before any intervention is undertaken even if no inhibitor has been demonstrated previously. The amount of factor needed is determined by the severity and location of bleeding and the baseline activity of the deficient factor.

Most hemostatics are administered systemically to overcome specific coagulation defects. Concentrates prepared from human blood include lyophilized antihemophilic factor concentrate (factor VIII, AHF) [Factorate, Hemofil, Koāte-HT, Profilate], cryoprecipitated antihemophilic factor (human), and factor IX complex (plasma thromboplastin component) [Konȳne-HT, Profilnine, Proplex, Prothar]. Fibrinogen is no longer prepared from pooled plasma because of the high risk of hepatitis. Cryoprecipitate or single donor plasma is now used as a source of fibrinogen when necessary.

Intravenous desmopressin [DDAVP, Stimate] is given to increase the concentration of factor VIII complex temporarily. Rarely, aminocaproic acid [Amicar] is administered to inhibit fibrinolysis.

Systemic hemostatics used to augment synthesis of normal coagulation factors in patients with vitamin K deficiency or those receiving warfarin are vitamin K preparations (phytonadione [AquaMEPHYTON, Konakion, Mephyton], menadione, menadione sodium bisulfite, and menadiol sodium diphosphate [Synkayvite]).

Hemostatics also are applied locally to control surface bleeding and capillary oozing. These absorbable agents, which assist in fibrin stabilization, include absorbable gelatin film [Gelfilm], absorbable gelatin sponge [Gelfoam], oxidized cellulose [Oxycel], oxidized regenerated cellulose [Surgicel], microfibrillar collagen hemostat [Avitene], and thrombin (bovine source) [Thrombinar, Thrombostat]. Absorbable gelatin film also is implanted as a substitute membrane following thoracic, ocular, or neurosurgery.

Estrogens are claimed to control postoperative bleeding when given intravenously, but current evidence does not substantiate this effect and they may cause thrombosis.

The synthetic androgen, danazol [Danocrine], has been given to some patients with factor VIII or factor IX deficiency. In preliminary clinical trials, the drug increased the activity of these factors and allowed use of reduced amounts of factor VIII or IX concentrates. However, subsequent data have indicated that factor activities were not affected and that bleeding episodes increased (Garewal and Corrigan, 1985). The long-term effects of danazol therapy have included liver dysfunction and use for factor VIII or IX deficiency is not warranted.

HEMOPHILIC DISORDERS

Hemorrhage requiring specific factor replacement therapy occurs most frequently in inherited factor VIII or IX deficiency.

Factor VIII is a complex molecule consisting of the procoagulant protein (VIII:C, antihemophilic factor) and the related protein multimers, VIIIR (VIII:vWF, von Willebrand factor). VIII:C is the procoagulant property of normal plasma and is measured in standard coagulation assays or by its antigenic determinants (VIII:CAg) in immunoassays utilizing human antibodies. VIIIR is necessary for normal platelet adhesion to subendothelial collagen (smaller multimers are less able to support platelet adhesion) and normal bleeding time. It is measured by its antigenic determinants (VIIIR:Ag) detected by heterologous antibodies and by the ability of normal VIIIR to support ristocetin-induced agglutination of washed normal platelets (VIIIR:RC, VIIIR:Cof). Evidence suggests that, in addition to plasma von Willebrand factor, subendothelial von Willebrand factor is an essential component for primary hemostasis (Stel et al, 1985; Turitto et al, 1985). Furthermore, plasma von Willebrand multimers serve as transport proteins for factor VIII (Deykin, 1983). VIII:C accelerates coagulation through its role as a cofactor in the enzymatic activation of factor X by factor IXa.

Characteristics: Patients with hemophilia have VIII:C deficiency that, in the inherited form, is transmitted by X chromosomes; these individuals have normal VIIIR. The severity of bleeding that results from congenital deficiency of factor VIII:C (classical hemophilia) varies markedly; it may even be minor or absent, and there may be no family history of this sex-linked disorder. Definitive diagnosis must be established by a specific plasma assay for factor VIII activity.

In von Willebrand's disease, an autosomally inherited disorder that usually is characterized by mild to moderate bleeding and a prolonged bleeding time, factor VIII procoagulant activity and factor VIII-von Willebrand protein complex are reduced. In the most common form of the disease (type I), bleeding from mucous membranes is the principal manifestation. In the homozygous form of von Willebrand's disease (rare), hemorrhagic diathesis is pronounced and bleeding time is markedly prolonged because factor VIII is not released from its site of synthesis in the absence of plasma VIIIR. In variant forms of von Willebrand's disease, VIII:C, VIIIR:Ag, and VIIIR:RC may be reduced to varying degrees; some, but not all, may even be normal.

Type I is characterized by a reduced amount of normal VIIIR; in type II, the components in the complex also are abnormal. In type IIA, the ability to form large multimers of VIIIR is reduced; larger multimers are absent from plasma and platelets and the response to ristocetin is reduced. In type IIB, the sensitivity of platelets to ristocetin is increased despite low activity of VIIIR:RC.

Factor IX deficiency (plasma thromboplastin component deficiency, Christmas disease) is a sex-linked disorder that is clinically similar to hemophilia.

Hereditary deficiency of factor XI (plasma thromboplastin antecedent [PTA]) is a rare, usually mild, autosomally inherited disorder that may require transfusion therapy during hemorrhagic episodes and surgery. Since factor XI is stable in stored plasma, infusion of small amounts of plasma may be effective.

Other hereditary hemorrhagic disorders associated with clotting factor deficiencies are exceedingly rare, and a specialized text should be consulted for details of treatment.

Therapy: Replacement therapy is required in hemophilics with active bleeding, whether spontaneous or traumatic, and just prior to surgery. The factor activity in plasma should be monitored carefully after infusion.

Before lyophilized or cryoprecipitated plasma concentrates became available, bleeding in hemophilics required frequent infusion of large volumes of plasma or, rarely, whole blood. However, hypervolemia resulted and plasma activities of factor VIII were inadequate during severe hemorrhage. The development of cryoprecipitated or heat treated, concentrated antihemophilic factor (AHF) preparations has virtually eliminated the need for other products to treat factor VIII deficiency. However, patients with an undefined bleeding disorder can be treated with blood group-specific fresh frozen plasma 15 ml/kg while diagnostic studies are being performed (Gill, 1984). This also is useful to treat bleeding episodes in patients with multiple factor deficiencies (eg, in liver disease).

Lyophilized AHF concentrates are most frequently used to treat severe hemophilia and are preferred for life-threatening hemorrhage, as well as for therapy at home and during travel. Cryoprecipitated antihemophilic factor (human) obtained from plasma is recommended for young patients and those with mild to moderate hemophilia. Cryoprecipitated AHF also is useful in von Willebrand's disease, because it contains VIIIR, which is usually degraded during processing of commercial factor VIII preparations (Blatt et al, 1976). Smaller amounts of cryoprecipitate are needed in patients with von Willebrand's disease than in those with hemophilia, for infusion increases endogenous factor VIII activity. Fresh frozen plasma also may be used.

Selected patients with hemophilia who are under close medical supervision may use AHF at home to reduce cost, allow a more normal life, and provide prompt therapy to prevent serious complications when bleeding occurs. Commercial factor VIII concentrates sometimes are preferred for home use because they are stable, easier to handle and store, and contain a standardized amount of AHF. However, such concentrates may be more expensive than cryoprecipitated AHF and are theoretically more likely to cause hepatitis, since they are prepared from pooled plasma derived from a large number of donors. The heat treated concentrates of factor VIII or factor IX are less likely to transmit retrovirus infections. Despite current programs of home use of these preparations, however, new arthropathy occurs or progresses, particularly in children 3 to 8 years. These patients often do not report hemorrhagic episodes promptly, and bone damage may progress rapidly.

Each of the many schedules for administration of AHF concentrates is based upon the severity of the bleeding diathesis. The major portion of transfused factor VIII remains in the intravascular space, and its biological half-life is approximately 12 hours. Hemophilic patients with factor VIII activities 2% to 5% of normal usually do not experience spontaneous bleeding. Bleeding in a confined area (eg, joint) may be controlled with an activity as low as 15% to 20% of normal, but the specific concentration needed to stop bleeding in a given joint has not been determined. Hemostasis during and after major surgery requires maintenance of a plasma AHF concentration at least 40% to 50% of normal for seven to ten days. See the Table for general guidelines for treatment of bleeding related to factor VIII deficiency. One unit/kg of factor VIII increases the plasma activity of factor VIII by 2% (50 units/kg increase it to 100% of normal activity).

Intravenous desmopressin [DDAVP, Stimate] markedly increases factor VIII activity in patients with moderate or mild hemophilia, uremic bleeding, and type I von Willebrand's disease. Desmopressin causes few adverse effects and does not transmit hepatitis. Thus, it may be a promising adjunct to cryoprecipitated AHF concentrates in selected patients with mild hemophilia or type I von Willebrand's disease. However, this drug may cause platelets to agglutinate in type IIB and platelet type variants of von Willebrand's disease and should not be used in patients with these subtypes of von Willebrand's disease.

Plasma is preferred in young patients with factor IX deficiency or in those with mild deficiency to avoid thrombotic episodes and hepatitis. Because plasma cannot provide levels exceeding 20%, heat treated, stable, dried, purified preparations of factor IX complex [Konȳne-HT, Profilnine, Proplex, Prothar] are necessary for patients with severe bleeding or those undergoing major surgery. *AHF preparations are not effective in factor IX deficiency.* Fresh frozen plasma also is the agent of choice in acquired coagulation disorders and in most patients with deficiency of factors II, V, VII, X, XI, or XIII. For these single-factor deficiencies, the dose of plasma is calculated on the basis of 1 unit of factor IX activity/1 ml of plasma; 10 to 20 ml/kg usually is given in one to two hours, with administration repeated every 12 hours until bleeding stops. Factors II, VII, and X (the other vitamin K-dependent factors) also are present in factor IX complex preparations. These preparations have been used to treat deficiency of any of the factors in the complex (eg, congenital deficiency, anticoagulant-induced vitamin K deficiency), but the risk of hepatitis and thrombosis is high. Factor IX complex preparations should not be administered to treat the multifactor deficiencies of acquired coagulation disorders, for these conditions usually are associated with increased fibrinolysis and/or circulating endogenous anticoagulants.

Resistance: Circulating antibodies called anticoagulants or inhibitors directed against factor IX occur in 2% to 3% of patients with hereditary factor IX deficiency, and a few patients with lupus erythematosus appear to have an acquired factor IX inhibitor. Thus, when bleeding occurs in patients with lupus erythematosus, the presence and identification of an inhibitor must be established prior to treatment.

About 15% of patients with factor VIII deficiency develop an immunoglobulin inhibitor that inactivates infused factor VIII and its anamnestic response to factor VIII makes treatment of subsequent bleeding episodes more difficult. When inhibitor concentrations remain below 5 Bethesda units, larger amounts of factor VIII usually are effective; higher concentrations of

GENERAL GUIDELINES FOR TREATMENT
OF BLEEDING EPISODES IN FACTOR VIII DEFICIENCY*

Condition	Prophylaxis Replacement Activity	Treatment Replacement Activity	Comments
MINOR HEMORRHAGE			
Joint hemorrhage			
Single acute		30% (single infusion)	Use cold compresses and immobilize the joint.
Chronic		30% (two or more infusions)	Use cold compresses and immobilize the joint.
Skin or subcutaneous bleeding		30% (if suturing is required and when they are removed)	
Muscle hemorrhage without nerve compression		30%–50% until bleeding stops	Use cold compresses and immobilize the affected part. Exercises and physical therapy may be necessary. Do *not* administer aminocaproic acid.
Hematuria			
Nontraumatic		30% (if bleeding persists after several days of bedrest)	
Traumatic		50% until bleeding stops and injury heals (infusion repeated at 12-hour intervals)	
Epistaxis		30%–50% (single infusion)	Blood transfusions may be necessary.
Mouth bleeding		30%–50% (usually single infusion)	Aminocaproic acid 6 g every six hours should be administered orally. Topical thrombin powder also may be applied to the site of hemorrhage. Aminocaproic acid should *not* be given in the presence of hematuria or within eight hours after administering factor IX concentrate or anti-inhibitor coagulant complex.
Tonsil inflammation		50% until tonsils heal	
MAJOR HEMORRHAGE			
Intracranial trauma			
Without neurologic symptoms		100% (single infusion)	
With symptoms	100%	50% for at least five days (infusion repeated at 12-hour intervals)	Perform CT scan.
With persistent neurologic symptoms	100%	>30% for two weeks after bleeding stops	Perform CT scan, brain scan, and EEG.
Epidural bleeding		100% (prior to lumbar puncture)	

(Continued on next page)

Condition	Prophylaxis Replacement Activity	Treatment Replacement Activity	Comments
MAJOR HEMORRHAGE (continued)			
Retroperitoneal bleeding		100% initially, then >50% for five to eight days	Perform ultrasound and CT scan. Administer red cell transfusions as necessary.
Muscle bleeding with nerve compression		70% initially, >30% until tissue is healed, and 50% on the first ambulatory day	Fasciotomy should be performed if necessary. Physical therapy is required after tissues have healed.
Retropharyngeal hemorrhage, airway threatened		100% initially, >30% until bleeding stops (infusion repeated at 12-hour intervals)	Rarely, endotracheal intubation or tracheostomy is required.
Gastrointestinal hemorrhage		70%–100% initially, >30% for several days after bleeding has stopped	
Surgery in patients without inhibitor	70%–100%	30%–50% at completion and in eight hours, then every 12 hours for at least two weeks (up to three weeks for major surgery and during physical therapy following joint surgery)	Antifibrinolytic agents are *contraindicated* during abdominal surgery.
Dental restorations with local anesthesia	30%		
Dental extractions	50%–100%	50% if oozing persists	Topical thrombin should be applied to the socket. Aminocaproic acid should be given on the day prior to extraction and for ten days afterward. Antibiotics may be required. Aminocaproic acid should *not* be administered in the presence of hematuria or within eight hours after administering factor IX concentrate or anti-inhibitor coagulant complex.

*The presence of an inhibitor should be excluded before treatment of a bleeding episode is started. Factor VIII preparations may contain anti-A and anti-B agglutinins. Therefore, ABO-compatible units are preferred. If hemolysis occurs, administration of ABO-compatible red cell concentrate may be necessary.

inhibitor require a massive volume of factor VIII preparations to correct the deficiency. When an acquired inhibitor, usually monoclonal IgG, has been demonstrated, therapy with factor VIII should be withheld unless life-threatening hemorrhage occurs. Assay for this inhibitor should be performed periodically in all hemophilics, especially before surgery. These inhibitors also develop rarely in healthy individuals, elderly patients, postpartum women, and patients with systemic lupus erythematosus, autoimmune disorders, drug hypersensitivity, or paraproteinemia.

Factor IX concentrates may be useful in patients with acquired factor VIII inhibitor (see the evaluation on Factor IX Complex). Also, an activated factor IX complex (anti-inhibitor coagulant complex) [Autoplex, Feiba Immuno] with factor VIII inhibitor bypassing activity has been developed. Various mechanisms for such activity have been proposed, but they are ill-defined and complex. Patients with high titers of antibody against antihemophilic factor (some patients receiving aggressive therapy have high titers) have been treated with these activated concentrates. Beneficial effects have been observed, but the antibody titer increased in some patients and a few cases of mild disseminated intravascular coagulation (DIC) were observed. At present, these products should be reserved for patients refractory to nonactivated factor IX concentrates.

Purified porcine factor VIII concentrate, which has less cross reactivity with factor VIII antibodies than the human product, has been used in Europe but may be immunogenic. It may, however, have some efficacy in treating hemophilia in patients with low-titer antibodies who cannot be managed effectively with human factor VIII preparations.

Plasma exchange is only temporarily effective but may be

helpful in life-threatening circumstances. Immunosuppressive therapy is of limited benefit.

Adverse Reactions and Precautions: Hepatitis is the most common adverse effect of concentrated preparations of plasma products. Screening of donors for hepatitis B surface antigen (HBsAg) has markedly decreased the risk of transmitting type B hepatitis. Also, manufacturers of these highly purified, dried products made from pooled plasma screen each plasma unit for HBsAg and eliminate those that are positive. Unfortunately, however, this does not guarantee freedom from type B or non-A non-B hepatitis, and all factor VIII or IX preparations can transmit these viruses. The hazard with use of cryoprecipitated AHF is the same as with single units of whole blood. Nevertheless, cryoprecipitate prepared from single-donor plasma is recommended for patients who do not require frequent treatment. Factor IX complex is also derived from human plasma and may transmit viral hepatitis. Immune globulin (gamma globulin) does not attenuate hepatitis virus and intramuscular injections are dangerous in any patient with a bleeding disorder. Hepatitis B vaccine should be given to all hemophilics who do not already have antihepatitis B surface antibody (see Chapter 62, Agents for Active and Passive Immunity).

Opportunistic infections and acquired immunodeficiency syndrome (AIDS) are more likely to occur in older patients who have received frequent factor replacement therapy. By 1984, AIDS was the second most frequent cause of death in hemophilics. In 1985, approximately 1% of all AIDS victims were those with hemophilia or other coagulation disorders, and at least 85% of the hemophilic population was seropositive for HTLV-III. Testing donated blood for HTLV-III and heat treatment of clotting factor concentrates should markedly reduce the danger of transmitting AIDS to the hemophilic community.

All preparations of factor IX complex have a significant potential to produce thrombotic complications, including disseminated intravascular coagulation. To reduce this risk, the smallest effective dose should be given slowly and plasma should be utilized for mild bleeding. Intravascular thrombosis has occurred most frequently in surgical patients who received large doses of factor IX complex. It is thought that the high levels of prothrombin and factor X produced may contribute to the development of thrombosis. These complications have been particularly severe in patients with underlying liver disease; therefore, factor IX complex or activated prothrombin complex concentrates should be used with great caution in patients with significant liver function abnormalities. Concomitant use of aminocaproic acid [Amicar] is not advocated, as this may increase the risk of thrombosis.

Hemolytic anemia may occur when AHF fractions are given to individuals with group A, B, or AB red blood cell antigens, because anti-A or anti-B antibodies may be present in the precipitated fraction. The anemia is usually mild and abates after discontinuation of AHF therapy. Spherocytosis of peripheral red blood cells may be the initial sign of hemolysis. Patients who develop hemolysis should be treated with cryoprecipitate from type-matched or type O donors who have low anti-A and anti-B titers. Type-specific blood is preferred if hemolysis is severe and immediate transfusion is required, but type O blood with low anti-A and anti-B titers can be used.

AHF preparations may cause severe hyperfibrinogenemia that interferes with the results of several laboratory tests. Although the increase may not be clinically significant, it has been implicated as a cause of an increased bleeding tendency due to platelet malfunction. Transient proteinuria with deposits of fibrin and fibrinogen in the kidneys also has been noted rarely.

Aspirin should not be used in patients with hemophilia. Analgesics that do not interfere with platelet aggregation (eg, acetaminophen) should be substituted.

Intramuscular injections should be avoided, and firm pressure should be applied directly to the site of intravenous injection for two or three minutes after venipuncture.

Drug Evaluations

ANTIHEMOPHILIC FACTOR
[Factorate, Hemofil, Koāte-HT, Profilate]

CRYOPRECIPITATED ANTIHEMOPHILIC FACTOR

COMPOSITION AND STORAGE. Commercially prepared antihemophilic factor concentrates (factor VIII:C, AHF) are lyophilized from the pooled plasma of as many as 2,000 to 5,000 donors by a variety of techniques. Each lot is standardized and contains a known amount of factor VIII:C. Depending on the batch, a unit of concentrate contains 250 to 1,500 IU of factor VIII:C, but little fibrinogen or factor VIIIR. These preparations may be stored up to four weeks (Koāte-HT, Factorate, and Hemofil may be kept for six months) at room temperature and for longer periods at 2 to 8 C.

A single unit of cryoprecipitated antihemophilic factor is made from the plasma of one unit of whole blood centrifuged and frozen within six hours after donation or from one or more units of single-donor fresh frozen plasma, which is thawed slowly to yield a solution rich in factor VIII and fibrinogen. Each shelf unit contains 80 to 125 IU of VIII:C, depending on the donor and the efficiency of processing. The cryoprecipitate contains a higher percentage of non-AHF plasma factors, including fibronectin 4 mg/ml, VIIIR, and fibrinogen 250 to 300 mg, than the dried material. The cryoprecipitated product must be kept frozen; storage usually should not exceed 12 months at temperatures of -18 C.

Cryoprecipitated preparations represent the most efficient use of community blood resources, since they are inexpensive to prepare in the blood bank laboratory of most hospitals, can be stored in the freezer until needed, and the material remaining in the plasma can be used to process other components.

USES. All AHF preparations can be used in patients with hemophilia (factor VIII deficiency) or acquired factor VIII inhibitors. Commercial lyophilized concentrates are most frequently used to treat severe hemophilia and are preferred for life-threatening hemorrhage, since high activities can be achieved and maintained for long periods. They are preferred for home therapy and during travel because of ease of storage and reconstitution. Since commercial preparations contain little factor VIII:vWF or fibrinogen, they should not be used to treat hypofibrinogenemia or von Willebrand's disease.

Cryoprecipitate is preferred in factor VIII- deficient patients who are young or have mild to moderate disease in whom maintenance of high titers of AHF is not required. Cryoprecipitate also may be used to treat hypofibrinogenemia, von Willebrand's disease, or fibronectin deficiency.

Plasma fibronectin (cold-insoluble globulin) is a circulating opsonic glycoprotein that selectively filters antigenic and toxic particulate matter to protect the reticuloendothelial system. Fibronectin concentrations often are severely deficient in critically ill patients, particularly following trauma or surgery, and in those with clinical syndromes resulting in disseminated intravascular coagulation (DIC). Fibronectin is stable in whole blood, plasma, platelet concentrate, and cryoprecipitate and is present in concentrated form in cryoprecipitated antihemophilic factor preparations. Some investigators have reported beneficial results following infusion of cryoprecipitate to provide fibronectin to severely ill patients (eg, Rodgers and Heymach, 1984).

Although dialysis is the principal therapy to treat uremia in patients with prolonged bleeding times, cryoprecipitate may be used to reverse bleeding temporarily in patients who require invasive procedures. Although the specific defect is not known, abnormalities of factor VIII complex are thought to be major determinants in the altered primary hemostasis that accompanies uremic bleeding (Deykin, 1983).

ADVERSE REACTIONS AND PRECAUTIONS. Headache may occur if the dried preparations are employed, and hyperfibrinogenemia may result when cryoprecipitated preparations are administered rapidly. Neither the dried nor cryoprecipitated preparations cause hypervolemic reactions.

Since the dried forms are prepared from large pools of fresh human plasma, they frequently cause hepatitis B even when screened for HBsAg. In addition, non-A non-B hepatitis can be transmitted. Although there is less danger with the cryoprecipitated material, results of some studies suggest that the cumulative risk over long periods of frequent use is probably the same as with the commercial lyophilized products. Nevertheless, hemophilics who require infrequent treatment should receive the cryoprecipitated product to reduce the risk of exposure to hepatitis virus.

Transaminase levels are elevated in the majority of treated hemophilics. Chronic liver disease, possibly caused by non-A non-B hepatitis, occurs in approximately 20% to 25% of hemophilics (Hay et al, 1985).

Heat treatment to reduce the risk of transmitting retroviruses has been applied to some products, but its efficacy has not yet been determined by extensive use. Eighteen patients who received heat-treated factor VIII [Hemofil-T] exclusively were followed for one year or more; none developed antibodies against the AIDS virus (Rouzioux et al, 1985). However, non-A non-B hepatitis developed in 11 of 13 previously untreated patients with hemophilia A given heat-treated factor VIII lyophilized concentrates (Colombo et al, 1985).

Over 85% of hemophilics have seropositive tests for HTLV-III. Symptoms of AIDS have been documented in hemophilics with no other known risk factors, and immune deficiencies have been demonstrated in many asymptomatic hemophilics

(eg, increased number of suppressor T-cells, decreased number of helper T-cells), particularly in patients receiving the lyophilized products.

AHF preparations also contain small amounts of groups A and B isohemagglutinins and are usually labeled with the ABO group of the donor. Administration of compatible units is preferred, because large amounts given to patients with blood groups A, B, or AB may cause hemolysis.

Chills or mild fever may occur shortly after administration of AHF.

PHARMACOKINETICS. The normal half-life of AHF is biphasic. There is a short phase (four to eight hours) consistent with equilibrium within the extravascular space and a longer, second phase (12 to 15 hours) consistent with biodegradation.

DOSAGE AND PREPARATIONS. Cryoprecipitated AHF should be thawed in a water bath at 37 C (higher temperatures result in loss of factor VIII activity), kept at room temperature after thawing, and used within three hours. The bag should be gently agitated to assure dissolution and the material then administered through a filter.

Lyophilized concentrates should be reconstituted with the sterile diluent supplied.

Intravenous: Various formulas are available to estimate dosage, and details appear in the manufacturers' literature. Based on experimental evidence, approximately 1 unit/kg increases activity about 2%; to maintain the desired level, doses should be repeated every 12 hours. Regardless of the therapeutic guide, factor VIII assays should be performed frequently, if proper techniques are available, to ensure achievement and maintenance of adequate factor VIII activities. These determinations may be imperative when using cryoprecipitated AHF, because there is no uniformity in the concentration of AHF from one plasma donor to the next. If several single-donor units are infused, cryoprecipitate from different donors should be used. A test for factor VIII inhibitors also should be performed prior to infusion.

A circulating AHF activity 20% to 30% of normal usually controls hemarthrosis in hemophilics. Usually, a single dose of 15 to 20 units/kg given at a rate of 10 to 15 ml/min achieves hemostasis and maintains activities sufficient for clotting. For mild bleeding into muscles or soft tissues in noncritical areas, a single dose of 10 units/kg is usually sufficient to achieve the necessary circulating AHF activity of 15% to 20% of normal. For surgery, an activity at least 60% of normal is necessary preoperatively for effective hemostasis; postoperatively, it is desirable to maintain a circulating activity 40% to 50% of normal for up to 14 days.

For patients with retroperitoneal, retropharyngeal, or central nervous system bleeding, severe trauma, or spontaneous bleeding into a body cavity, hospitalization is necessary and hemostasis is achieved with initial doses of 40 to 50 units/kg and subsequent doses of 20 to 25 units/kg repeated at 12-hour intervals until hemorrhage is controlled or the wound is healed. Bleeding recurs if treatment is discontinued prematurely.

For hypofibrinogenemia, usually four containers of cryoprecipitate/10 kg will raise the fibrinogen concentration by 150 mg/dl.

Generic. 250, 500, 1,000, and 1,500 units.

Factorate, Factorate Generation II, HT-Factorate, HT-

Factorate Generation II (Armour), *Hemofil, Hemofil T* (Hyland), *Koāte-HT* (Cutter), *Profilate, Profilate Heat-Treated* (Alpha Therapeutic). Each container is labeled with the number of units it contains (200 to 1,700 units/container). One unit is the antihemophilic factor activity present in 1 ml of average, normal, human plasma pooled from at least ten donors and tested within three hours after collection. These materials must be reconstituted with the diluent supplied to a volume dependent upon final container assay of potency and dosage/ml desired.

Cryoprecipitated Antihemophilic Factor (Human) can be prepared by the hospital blood bank as a byproduct of blood banking. This product cannot be standardized, but each bag usually contains between 80 and 125 units of factor VIII in a volume of 15 ml.

DESMOPRESSIN ACETATE
[DDAVP, Stimate]

ACTIONS. Desmopressin, a synthetic analogue of arginine vasopressin, is used to treat diabetes insipidus (see the evaluation in Chapter 30, Agents Affecting Water Homeostasis). Intravenous desmopressin temporarily increases the concentrations of factor VIII:C, VIIIR (von Willebrand factor), and, to a lesser extent, the other components of factor VIII complex. The effect is evident within 30 minutes. The maximum increase is three- to fivefold above initial concentrations, occurs in 90 to 120 minutes, and persists for up to six hours. Administration of desmopressin more often than every two or three days frequently diminishes the response. The drug also causes release of tissue-type plasminogen activator, but bleeding problems have not been reported.

USES. Desmopressin may be used in patients with mild or moderate factor VIII deficiency who have baseline concentrations of at least 5% factor VIII and in those with type I von Willebrand's disease. The drug controls minor bleeding in these patients but may not maintain normal coagulation after major surgery. Therefore, it should be given only when a short-term increase in factor VIII is required (eg, hemarthroses, mucosal bleeding, dental extractions). Because desmopressin causes release of von Willebrand factor multimers from storage sites (endothelial cells) into plasma and shortens bleeding time in uremic patients, it may be used to reverse uremic bleeding temporarily in patients who require urgent invasive procedures (Deykin, 1983). Use of desmopressin avoids the risk of hepatitis and AIDS associated with blood products.

CONTRAINDICATIONS. Desmopressin should not be given to patients with factor VIII:C activities less than 5% or to those with factor IX deficiency. In patients with type IIB von Willebrand's disease, desmopressin may cause release of an abnormal factor VIII complex that has platelet-aggregating properties and can induce thrombocytopenia. Therefore, it should not be used to treat type IIB von Willebrand's disease.

ADVERSE REACTIONS AND PRECAUTIONS. Rarely, headache, nausea, facial flushing, mild abdominal cramps, and pain and swelling at the site of injection occur. Slight elevations in blood pressure have been reported, and the drug should be used with caution in patients with coronary artery insufficiency or hypertension. Because of the antidiuretic effects of the drug, water intake should be limited, particularly in very young and elderly patients, to prevent water intoxication and hyponatremia.

DOSAGE AND PREPARATIONS. The dose should be diluted in physiologic sodium chloride solution. In adults and children weighing more than 10 kg, 50 ml of diluent is used; for children under 10 kg, 10 ml of diluent is used. Blood pressure and pulse should be monitored during infusion.

Intravenous: 0.3 mcg/kg infused slowly over a period of 15 to 30 minutes. Dosage should not be repeated within 24 hours.

DDAVP (USV). Solution 4 mcg/ml in 1 ml containers.
Stimate (Armour). Solution 4 mcg/ml in 10 ml containers.

FACTOR IX COMPLEX (HUMAN)
[Konȳne-HT, Profilnine Heat-Treated, Proplex, Prothar]

COMPOSITION AND STORAGE. Factor IX complex (prothrombin complex, plasma thromboplastin component) concentrates are prepared from pooled plasma. These stable, dried, purified plasma fractions contain the vitamin K-dependent coagulation factors (II, VII, IX, and X), as well as small amounts of other plasma proteins. Products are alleged to be free of thrombin, thromboplastin-like activity, anticomplement activity, and depressor activity. Konȳne and Profilnine contain no heparin; heparin is added to Proplex and Prothar to help prevent the formation of thrombin after the manufacturing process (eg, with increased temperature during storage). Because amounts of anti-A and anti-B agglutinins are clinically insignificant, factor IX complex (human) may be used without typing or crossmatching. Hypervolemic reactions do not occur because of the concentrated nature of these products and the small amount of fluid needed for administration.

Most dried preparations must be refrigerated at 2 to 8 C (Konȳne, Profilnine, Proplex, and Prothar may be stored for up to one month at temperatures below 37 C). Freezing should be avoided to prevent breakage of the diluent bottle. Although factor IX complex (human) is stable after reconstitution for at least 12 hours at room temperature, it should be administered promptly. It is diluted with sterile water for injection and the concentration must not exceed 50 units/ml.

USES. Factor IX complex (human) may be used to treat bleeding associated with factor IX deficiency (Christmas disease) or deficiency of one or more of the other factors contained in this preparation. However, plasma is preferred when bleeding is not severe. When large amounts of factor IX are required, the addition of heparin (5 units/ml) is recommended by some clinicians to reduce the likelihood of disseminated intravascular coagulation (DIC) (Eyster, 1978).

Factor IX complex also is useful in about 50% of patients with factor VIII deficiency who develop an inhibitor, presumably because it supplies activated factors that participate in the coagulation process beyond the steps where factor VIII is needed. These preparations should be used in newborn infants only when life-threatening hemorrhagic disease is caused by proven deficiency of factor II, VII, IX, or X. They should almost never be given to nonhemophilic patients (ie, those with anticoagulant-induced deficiency of vitamin K-dependent coagulation factors). Such patients should receive plasma if administration of vitamin K alone is not sufficient.

Rarely, factor IX complex may be useful in patients with compromised cardiovascular function who are unresponsive to plasma. Also, when rapid reversal of factor IX deficiency is critical in patients with severe hemorrhage, these concentrates may be used despite the risk of hepatitis to avoid the large volumes of plasma required. In these cases, the risk of hepatitis and/or thrombosis must be weighed against the benefits.

ADVERSE REACTIONS AND PRECAUTIONS. Because they are prepared from pooled plasma, there is substantial risk of inducing viral hepatitis or other retrovirus infection (eg, AIDS) when factor IX complex concentrates are given. Heat treatment of factor IX products may help reduce transmission of retroviruses.

Thromboembolic disease has been reported frequently, possibly as a result of decreased antithrombin III (AT III) activity and AT III complex formation. Factor IX complex concentrates are contraindicated in patients with severe liver disease or with milder liver disease when there is any suspicion of DIC or fibrinolysis, for both these patients and neonates have low circulating concentrations of antithrombin III and do not efficiently remove the activated clotting factors.

Transient fever, chills, urticaria, nausea and vomiting, headache, flushing, or tingling can occur shortly after administration of factor IX complex, particularly if the injection is given rapidly. Myocardial infarction has been reported in three young patients with factor VIII inhibitors who received large doses of Konȳne repeatedly (Lusher et al, 1980; Fuerth and Mahrer, 1981; Gruppo et al, 1983). Rarely, severe hypersensitivity reactions (eg, anaphylactic shock) have been observed.

If no response is evident after three to four doses of factor IX complex, other therapy should be tried. Concomitant use of aminocaproic acid or other antifibrinolytic agents is contraindicated.

PHARMACOKINETICS. The immediate recovery of factor IX is between 20% and 60% of the infused dose. The biological half-life is biphasic, with a short first phase (four to six hours) consistent with equilibration within the extravascular space and a longer second phase (22.5 hours) consistent with biodegradation.

DOSAGE AND PREPARATIONS. Factor IX complex should be given within three hours after reconstitution and the rate of administration should not exceed 10 ml/min to avoid vasomotor reactions.

Intravenous: The amount of factor IX complex (human) required depends upon the patient and the nature of the deficiency. Each unit contains the factor IX activity of 1 ml of normal fresh plasma; 1 unit/kg increases factor IX activity 1% and, for maintenance of a desired activity, doses should be repeated every 24 hours. Overdosage should be avoided because the long postinfusion half-life of factors II and X can produce unnecessarily high levels. Specific dosage is similar to the lowest dose employed in factor VIII deficiency (see the evaluation on Antihemophilic Factor). Following surgery, a factor IX level 40% to 50% of normal should be maintained for four days, with a level 30% to 40% of normal maintained on days five to eight.

For nonlife-threatening bleeding in patients with hemophilia who have factor VIII inhibitors, initially, 75 units/kg, repeated once after 8 to 12 hours if necessary. If bleeding persists, alternative therapy, eg, anti-inhibitor coagulant complex (AICC, activated prothrombin complex), may be used. In life-threatening hemorrhage, these patients should receive AICC as the initial therapy.

> ***Generic.*** 500 and 1,000 units.
>
> ***Konȳne-HT*** (Cutter). Contains 500 units of factors IX and amounts of factors II, VII, and X approximately proportionate to their respective levels in average fresh plasma (heparin-free).
>
> ***Profilnine Heat-Treated*** (Alpha Therapeutic). Contains factors II, VII, IX, and X; amount of factor IX stated on container (heparin-free).
>
> ***Proplex, Proplex SX, Proplex SX-T*** (Hyland). Contains factors II, VII, IX, and X; amounts of factor IX stated on container. ***Proplex SX*** contains up to 1.5 units of heparin/ml of reconstituted material. The amount of factor VII in ***Proplex SX*** is significantly lower than that in ***Proplex***.
>
> ***Prothar*** (Armour). Contains factors II, VII, IX, and X; amounts of factor IX stated on container. Prothar contains up to 3 units of heparin/ml of reconstituted material.

ANTI-INHIBITOR COAGULANT COMPLEX
[Autoplex, Feiba Immuno]

Anti-inhibitor coagulant complex is prepared from pooled human plasma by a process of controlled activation. It contains variable amounts of activated and precursor clotting factors associated with the prothrombin complex plus factors of the kinin generating system. The active ingredients are unknown except for activated coagulation factors VIIa and IXa, and the duration of effectiveness has not been determined.

Although the mechanism of action is not clear, it is postulated that these activated factors exert their effect at a level beyond factor VIII in the coagulation cascade to achieve fibrin formation and hemostasis.

USES. This preparation is indicated as an alternative treatment for active bleeding in patients with high titers of factor VIII inhibitors.

Elective surgery for hemophilic patients with inhibitor has been contraindicated, but a report (Hutchinson et al, 1983) on two patients in whom hemostasis was achieved with use of Autoplex following synovectomy for hemophilic arthropathy and the experience of many hemophilia centers have shown that this preparation can achieve hemostasis when surgery is essential.

CONTRAINDICATIONS, ADVERSE REACTIONS, AND PRECAUTIONS. Anti-inhibitor coagulant complex should be used only in patients who have or who had inhibitor levels exceeding 5 Bethesda units (Abildgaard et al, 1980). It should not be given when signs of fibrinolysis or DIC are present. Thrombotic complications and DIC have not been reported but these possibilities should be kept in mind, particularly following repeated administration. Repeated administration also appears to predispose patients to an anamnestic response (Laurian et al, 1984).

Transient hypofibrinogenemia has been observed in two children; therefore, fibrinogen levels should be monitored in young patients receiving repeated doses (Abildgaard et al, 1980).

The rate of infusion should not exceed 10 ml/min and may have to be decreased if headache, flushing, or changes in pulse rate or blood pressure are noted. If these reactions are severe, the infusion should be stopped until symptoms disappear and then resumed at a rate of approximately 2 ml/min.

DOSAGE AND PREPARATIONS. This complex is standardized by its ability to correct the clotting time of factor VIII-deficient plasma, and each vial is labeled with factor VIII correctional units. (Each unit is that quantity of activated prothrombin complex which, when added to an equal volume of factor VIII-deficient plasma, will correct the clotting time to 35 seconds by the ellagic acid-APTT test.) The reconstituted product contains a maximum of 2 units/ml of heparin and 0.02 M sodium citrate. The material should be reconstituted with sterile water for injection immediately before injection and the solution should be given at a rate of no more than 10 ml/min.
Intravenous: 50 to 100 units/kg, depending on the severity of hemorrhage. Early treatment of minor bleeding problems may respond to lower doses (25 units/kg). Dosage should be adjusted according to the APTT determined 30 minutes after infusion. If hemostasis is not observed after six hours, the dose should be repeated. Subsequent treatment should be adjusted according to the patient's response.

There are no reliable laboratory tests to measure the effect of anti-inhibitor coagulant complex. Some investigators limit dosage to the amount capable of reducing the prothrombin time below eight seconds (Abildgaard et al, 1980).

   Autoplex (Hyland). Powder in 30 ml containers (each container labeled with factor VIII correctional activity) with sterile diluent (contains up to 2 units heparin/ml).

   Feiba Immuno (Immuno U.S.). Freeze-dried powder (each container labeled with factor VIII inhibitor bypassing activity) with sterile diluent (heparin-free).

HYPOFIBRINOGENEMIA

Fibrinolysis is regulated by activator(s) of plasminogen and inhibitors of plasmin (predominantly α_2-antiplasmin) in the nonpathologic state. Hypofibrinogenemia usually is associated with acquired hemorrhagic disorders and is most commonly caused by liver disease, in which increased destruction and decreased synthesis occur, and by intravascular coagulation. Excessive fibrinolytic activity once was thought to be the primary cause of acquired hemorrhagic disorders, but it is now known to be a defense mechanism against intravascular fibrin deposition and should not be inhibited (Hoyer, 1981). Hypofibrinogenemia also occurs rarely as an autosomal disorder that is manifested clinically in homozygotes. Bleeding is similar to that produced by factor XIII deficiency; umbilical hemorrhage

is noted early and cerebral hemorrhage is the major cause of death.

In acute conditions, fibrinogen may not only have no effect on hemostasis but, by increasing the available substrate, may increase the level of degradation products and aggravate intravascular clotting. Fibrinogen preparations also carried a great risk for transmitting hepatitis. Thus, their manufacture has been discontinued in the United States.

If fibrinogen is required, ABO-compatible cryoprecipitated antihemophilic factor (human) is the agent of choice. A dose sufficient to raise the fibrinogen concentration to 100 to 200 mg/dl is recommended (see the evaluation in previous section). However, initial therapy should be directed toward control of the underlying disease. Aminocaproic acid is an alternative but should not be used in patients with DIC or in those who are thrombosis-prone.

Although aminocaproic acid has been used in subarachnoid hemorrhage, no long-term benefit has been noted. The investigational antifibrinolytic agent, tranexamic acid, was tested in 479 patients with subarachnoid hemorrhage in a multicenter, double-blind, controlled trial. Adequate fibrinolytic action (rebleeding was significantly reduced) was counterbalanced by increases in ischemic complications (eg, cerebral infarction); therefore, it was concluded that tranexamic acid was of no benefit in patients with subarachnoid hemorrhage (Vermeulen et al, 1984).

Drug Evaluation

AMINOCAPROIC ACID
   [Amicar]

$$H_2NCH_2(CH_2)_3CH_2\overset{\overset{\textstyle O}{\|}}{C}OH$$

ACTIONS. Aminocaproic acid may help to control serious hemorrhage associated with excessive fibrinolysis caused by increased plasminogen (profibrinolysin) activation. This mono-amino carboxylic acid is a potent competitive inhibitor of plasminogen activators and inhibits plasmin (fibrinolysin) to a lesser degree. Therefore, aminocaproic acid prevents formation of the excessive plasmin responsible for the destruction of fibrinogen, fibrin, and other important clotting components. Its use as a specific antidote for overdoses of streptokinase or urokinase has been suggested. However, administration of aminocaproic acid has produced endocardial hemorrhage and myocardial fat degeneration in animals. Therefore, caution is advocated if this use is considered, because many patients receiving thrombolytic agents have pre-existing cardiac disease.

Since this drug inhibits the dissolution of clots, it may interfere with normal mechanisms for maintaining the patency of blood vessels, particularly in thrombosis-prone patients. Before this hemostatic is used, it is important to understand the role of the fibrinolytic system in maintaining the patency and integrity of the vascular system, the laboratory procedures used to determine coagulation defects, and the mechanism of action of aminocaproic acid.

QUALIFICATIONS FOR USE. A pathologic fibrinolytic state may be suspected in patients with a predisposing clinical condition when results of laboratory tests suggest increased fibrinolytic activity, prolonged thrombin and prothrombin times, hypofibrinogenemia, or decreased plasminogen levels. However, these conditions and some of the laboratory findings usually are associated with diffuse intravascular coagulation (DIC). If aminocaproic acid is given to patients with DIC, it may cause serious or even fatal thrombus formation. For this reason, *most experts do not use aminocaproic acid to treat "fibrinolytic" hemorrhage unless there is definitive proof that DIC is not the underlying cause.* If such proof is lacking, the following criteria may assist in distinguishing between DIC and primary fibrinolysis but are not diagnostic. In DIC, the platelet count is reduced, the protamine paracoagulation test may be positive, and euglobulin clot lysis (a measure of the fibrinolytic potential of plasma) may be normal or reduced. In primary fibrinolysis, the platelet count is normal, the protamine paracoagulation test is negative, and euglobulin clot lysis is reduced. However, isolated fibrinolysis is rare and almost always secondary to DIC.

USES. Although cryoprecipitated AHF is preferred for treatment of hypofibrinogenemia, aminocaproic acid may be useful in surgical and nonsurgical hematuria arising from the bladder, prostate, or urethra. In patients undergoing transurethral and suprapubic prostatectomy, postoperative hematuria has been reduced significantly. However, use of aminocaproic acid should be restricted to patients who are seriously threatened by hemorrhage for whom a correctable cause of bleeding from the prostatic bed has been excluded.

Because aminocaproic acid inhibits C'_1 esterase, it has been used to prevent or control attacks of hereditary angioedema. It has been given following subarachnoid hemorrhage and also before and during surgery for ruptured intracranial aneurysms, but is of questionable value in these conditions.

Results of isolated case reports suggest that hemorrhagic cystitis may be controlled within 24 hours when aminocaproic acid is given both systemically and intravesically.

Aminocaproic acid does not control hemorrhage caused by thrombocytopenia or most other coagulation defects, although it has been very useful in hemophilics prior to and following tooth extraction and for other traumatic bleeding in the mouth and nasopharynx. When multiple hemostatic defects exist, other therapeutic measures (eg, fresh frozen plasma, cryoprecipitated antihemophilic factor, vitamin K) may be required. Since the drug does not control bleeding caused by loss of vascular integrity, valuable time may be wasted if it is used in patients with post-tonsillectomy bleeding, gastrointestinal hemorrhage from ulcers or ruptured esophageal varices, hemoptysis due to bronchiectasis, open surgical wounds, or functional uterine bleeding.

ADVERSE REACTIONS AND PRECAUTIONS. The most common untoward effects of aminocaproic acid are nausea, diarrhea, and vomiting. Less common are dizziness, pruritus, erythema, rash, hypotension, headache, dyspepsia, inhibition of ejaculation, conjunctival erythema, arrhythmias, fatigue, and nasal congestion. Inflammatory myopathy with myoglobinuria has been reported in a few patients who received doses of 24 to 38 g/day for more than a month (Brodkin, 1980) and in another patient with underlying skeletal muscle disease who received a single dose of 3 g (Morris et al, 1983). Painful urination or urinary frequency has occurred, and one patient developed acute renal failure that required hemodialysis (Biswas et al, 1980). The most serious adverse effect is generalized thrombosis; therefore, hemostatic mechanisms should be monitored. Liver failure has been reported in patients with cirrhosis.

Cardiac and hepatic necroses were found at postmortem examination in one patient who received therapeutic doses of aminocaproic acid. Since subendocardial hemorrhages and myocardial depression have occurred in several animal species, the drug should be used with caution in patients with cardiac disease. It may transiently alter protein metabolism by inhibiting the utilization of lysine.

Use of aminocaproic acid in women taking oral contraceptives or estrogens may increase the potential for thromboses.

Teratogenic studies in animals have produced variable results, but no significant abnormalities have been noted clinically. Nevertheless, the drug should not be used during the first and second trimester unless absolutely essential. It may be given during the last trimester if specifically indicated and if the potential benefit outweighs the possible hazards to the mother and fetus.

When aminocaproic acid is given during surgery, care must be taken to free the bladder of blood clots, since the drug accumulates in these clots and inhibits their dissolution. Also, aminocaproic acid should not be used when renal or ureteral bleeding is suspected, for ureteral clot formation and, possibly, obstruction may result.

PHARMACOKINETICS. Aminocaproic acid is well absorbed orally and also can be given intravenously. It is widely distributed throughout the body. This drug is concentrated in the urine and is excreted rapidly (most within 12 hours), largely unchanged. Peak plasma levels are obtained about two hours after a single oral dose.

DOSAGE AND PREPARATIONS. Further evidence is needed to determine the safety of prolonged use of aminocaproic acid in the following doses. This drug should not be used undiluted or injected rapidly.

Intravenous, Oral: *Adults,* initially, 4 to 5 g orally or by *slow* intravenous infusion (in 250 ml of physiologic sodium chloride, sterile water, 5% dextrose, or Ringer's solutions), then 1 g (in 50 ml of diluent if given intravenously) at hourly intervals or 4 to 5 g every four hours if renal function is normal (maximum, 30 g/24 hours). This dosage produces effective plasma concentrations of approximately 13 mg/dl. The manufacturer recommends that the dose be reduced to 25% in patients with renal disease or oliguria. After prostatic surgery, a dose of 6 g/24 hr is effective because the drug is concentrated in the urine. *Children,* initially, 100 mg/kg followed by 33 mg/kg/hr (maximum total dose, 18 g/M² /24 hours). The patient's condition should be re-evaluated after 8 hours of continuous therapy.

Generic. Solution (injection) 250 mg/ml in 20 ml containers.
Amicar (Lederle). Solution (injection) 250 mg/ml in 20 ml containers; syrup 1.25 g/5 ml; tablets 500 mg.

VITAMIN K DEFICIENCY

Vitamin K is an essential cofactor for the hepatic microsomal enzyme system that converts multiple glutamic acid residues to gamma-carboxyglutamic acid residues in factors II, VII, IX, X, and protein C. Through the gamma-carboxyglutamic acid residues, these proteins bind calcium, which allows them to bind to phospholipid surfaces and thus function in the clotting cascade. If vitamin K deficiency occurs, the blood concentration of these procoagulant factors decreases and a hemorrhagic disorder develops.

The vitamin K compounds are fat-soluble naphthoquinones. Phytonadione (vitamin K_1) occurs in a variety of foods and also is prepared synthetically. Vitamin K_2 is produced by bacteria in the gastrointestinal tract. Like phytonadione, menadione (vitamin K_3) can be prepared synthetically.

Vitamin K_2 accumulates in the liver, spleen, and lungs, but significant amounts are not stored in the body for long periods. The daily requirement for vitamin K is estimated to be 1 to 5 mcg/kg for infants and 0.03 mcg/kg for adults. Dietary sources usually satisfy these requirements and adults, even those with inadequate diets, are unlikely to develop a deficiency on the basis of an unbalanced diet alone. However, uptake of vitamin K is diminished during prolonged oral antibiotic therapy, cleansing of the bowel prior to colonic surgery, or when a malabsorption syndrome exists (eg, pancreatic insufficiency, dysentery, celiac disease, intestinal fistula, blind loop syndrome). In young infants, deficiency may result from acute diarrhea, even of short duration. An existing deficiency of vitamin K may be accentuated by alteration of intestinal flora during treatment of infectious diarrhea with antibiotics. Deficiency also can develop rapidly following surgery, particularly if renal failure develops.

The K vitamins, except for the water-soluble salts of menadione (menadione sodium bisulfite, menadiol sodium diphosphate), are absorbed from the gastrointestinal tract only in the presence of adequate quantities of bile salts and pancreatic lipase. Thus, steatorrhea may cause deficiency of vitamin K and consequently of factors II, VII, IX, and X. Also, oral anticoagulants that inhibit vitamin K-dependent factor formation induce deficiency of these factors.

Phytonadione and the water-soluble sodium diphosphate salt of menadione can be given orally and by all parenteral routes; menadione is given orally and menadione sodium bisulfite is given parenterally. Intravenous administration should be used only in emergencies, because serious and occasionally fatal anaphylactoid reactions have occurred following use of this route.

Appropriate therapy in cases of apparent vitamin K deficiency requires that true deficiency be differentiated from defective synthesis of vitamin K-dependent clotting factors. For example, in liver disease with severe cellular damage (eg, cirrhosis, hepatitis, hemochromatosis, porphyria cutanea tarda, Wilson's disease), the vitamin K-dependent clotting factors may be reduced significantly despite the presence of adequate vitamin K, and replacement therapy is ineffective. Although treatment may be unsatisfactory, these patients should receive whole blood or fresh frozen plasma if bleeding occurs. The one-stage prothrombin time test is used routinely to monitor the efficacy of vitamin K therapy.

Therapy: Phytonadione, the natural fat-soluble vitamin K_1, is preferred in hypoprothrombinemia (particularly to control oral anticoagulant-induced bleeding), during the last weeks of pregnancy, or in hemorrhagic disease of the newborn. The water-soluble salts of menadione (vitamin K_3) are useful in hypoprothrombinemias caused by conditions that limit the absorption or synthesis of vitamin K (eg, celiac disease, ulcerative colitis). Because menadione can combine with tissue sulfhydryl groups to produce hemolytic anemia and liver damage, phytonadione is generally preferred when large doses or prolonged therapy is indicated. None of the vitamin K preparations counteract the anticoagulant effects of heparin, and they are generally ineffective when hypoprothrombinemia is secondary to liver disease.

Coumarin derivatives inhibit vitamin K activity in the liver and are among the most common causes of iatrogenic hypocoagulability in man. Coagulation factor activities often are markedly decreased in patients treated with these drugs. A single oral dose of phytonadione often corrects the defect. Alternatively, stored plasma can be used for mild or moderate bleeding, since the vitamin K-dependent clotting factors are relatively stable. However, if severe bleeding occurs, the anticoagulant may have to be discontinued and intravenous phytonadione therapy initiated. Because the response to vitamin K does not develop for 4 to 24 hours, concomitant transfusion of fresh frozen plasma is essential in life-threatening hemorrhage. The prothrombin time should be measured frequently to monitor the effects of the oral anticoagulant and natural decay of the clotting factors in the transfused plasma. Adults usually require two to three units of plasma. When time is critical (eg, central nervous system hemorrhage), use of factor IX complex may be necessary despite the risk of hepatitis and/or thrombosis.

In vitamin K deficiency caused by poor nutrition or malabsorption, a single loading dose of phytonadione frequently stops bleeding within a few hours, and additional doses replenish vitamin K stores in the body. If an absorptive defect cannot be localized, small parenteral doses should be given at regular intervals until the defect is corrected. When malabsorption of vitamin K is caused by biliary disease (obstructive jaundice, atresia, fistulas), the prothrombin time increases gradually. If hepatic cell damage also is present, hypoprothrombinemia and the associated deficiency of other vitamin K-dependent factors may become even more severe.

Patients with hereditary hypoprothrombinemia or hereditary deficiency of factors VII, IX, or X do not respond to vitamin K therapy.

Vitamin K supplementation should be routine in patients receiving long-term intravenous feeding and in debilitated patients who may have experienced long periods of inadequate diet; deficiency develops rapidly during parenteral feeding, especially if broad spectrum antibiotics are given concomitantly.

The prothrombin activity in newborn infants is substantially lower than that in adults, but this may not be reflected in prothrombin time determinations. Prothrombin time often is prolonged in infants at birth and may increase during the next two to four days if vitamin K is not available. Spontaneous hemorrhage caused by deficiency of vitamin K-dependent clotting factors is unlikely after the sixth day, particularly if cow's milk (maternal milk contains virtually no vitamin K) is used for feeding. The enzyme systems that synthesize these factors may not be fully developed at birth, and administration of vitamin K usually does not increase levels in infants to the same extent as in adults.

Other conditions that may contribute to defective hepatic synthesis of vitamin K-dependent clotting factors in neonates are a lack of vitamin K-producing bacteria in the gastrointestinal tract (which decreases the amount of vitamin K absorbed), reduced stores of vitamin K, and maternal drug ingestion (eg, oral anticoagulants). If anticonvulsants (phenobarbital, phenytoin) are taken during the third trimester, severe hemorrhagic disease may occur in the neonate. Bleeding often can be prevented by administration of phytonadione to the mother before delivery and to the infant immediately after birth.

In pregnant women with vitamin K deficiency or in those who undergo prolonged labor, the administration of phytonadione 12 to 24 hours before delivery may prevent hemorrhagic disease in the neonate. More commonly, a single intramuscular dose of 0.5 to 1 mg is administered to the infant within 24 hours after birth. Because large doses of menadione or its salts may cause kernicterus due to hemolysis, phytonadione is the only acceptable preparation for this purpose. Kernicterus has not been reported with use of this agent, and small doses do not hemolyze red cells deficient in glucose-6-phosphate dehydrogenase.

In small premature infants with immature liver function or infants with hepatocellular disease, phytonadione may not prevent bleeding and plasma may be required. Doses exceeding 1 mg may cause hemolytic anemia due to glycolytic enzyme deficiencies in these infants (Machin, 1980).

Adverse Reactions and Precautions: Adverse reactions are observed only rarely in adults after oral administration of vitamin K. However, serious reactions, including fatalities, have occurred during and immediately following intravenous injection, even when dilute solutions are infused slowly. These reactions resemble hypersensitivity or anaphylaxis and may be associated with shock, respiratory arrest, or both. They may occur in some patients receiving vitamin K for the first time. Therefore, the intravenous route should be used only when other routes are not feasible or the potential risk is justified. Other parenteral routes also may be hazardous. One patient developed indurated erythematous plaques with persistent intermittent pruritus at the injection site following intramuscular administration of phytonadione (Robison and Odom, 1978).

When vitamin K is used to treat hemorrhagic diseases in infants, it can increase hemolysis and the plasma levels of unbound bilirubin, resulting in kernicterus, hemolytic anemia, and hemoglobinuria. However, hyperbilirubinemia has been observed only rarely after use of phytonadione, and this drug has not yet been implicated in causing kernicterus. The hemolytic potential of vitamin K is greatest in infants with

relatively low activity of glucose-6-phosphate dehydrogenase (G6PD) but also is observed in adults with this deficiency. Plasma concentrations of free bilirubin may increase in premature infants if the mother has received large (more than recommended) doses of menadione sodium bisulfite, although moderate doses are relatively safe and often necessary.

Patients with liver disease should not be given large doses of vitamin K repeatedly if the response to initial administration is unsatisfactory. Patients receiving large doses of vitamin K (25 to 50 mg) may be resistant to coumarin drugs given later, making effective anticoagulant therapy difficult until the vitamin is metabolized and excreted. It may be necessary to reinstitute anticoagulant therapy with larger doses to overcome resistance, or to use heparin.

Drug Evaluations

PHYTONADIONE (Vitamin K₁)
[AquaMEPHYTON, Konakion, Mephyton]

USES. Phytonadione is used either prophylactically or during bleeding episodes and is the only preparation that reverses the hypoprothrombinemia produced by oral anticoagulants. It does not combat hemorrhage caused by overdosage of heparin.

This preparation also is used to prevent or treat hemorrhagic disease in neonates and hypoprothrombinemia caused by poor nutrition, inadequate absorption of vitamin K, inadequate synthesis of vitamin K in the gastrointestinal tract, or the toxic action of certain drugs (eg, salicylates) given with anticoagulants.

Phytonadione has a more prompt, potent, and prolonged effect than the vitamin K analogues and is generally preferred when large doses or long-term therapy is indicated. In contrast to menadione-type drugs, it does not hemolyze red cells in patients who are deficient in glucose-6-phosphate dehydrogenase (G6PD) and is generally safe for use in newborn infants if recommended doses are not exceeded.

Phytonadione reverses moderately excessive anticoagulation caused by warfarin overdose. Doses ranging from 0.5 to 10 mg partially correct the prothrombin time in approximately four to six hours and full correction usually occurs within 24 hours. When further warfarin therapy is not required, up to 10 mg of phytonadione may be used (large doses make the patient resistant to warfarin for several days thereafter); in patients requiring subsequent warfarin maintenance therapy, doses should be limited to 0.5 to 1 mg. The oral and subcutaneous routes are less likely to cause adverse reactions and are preferred for nonemergency situations. Since control of hypoprothrombinemia re-exposes the patient to the same hazards of intravascular clotting that existed prior to anticoagulant therapy, the dose of phytonadione should be as low as possible and prothrombin times should be determined frequently. Heparin's anticoagulant effect is not impaired by large amounts of phytonadione, and it should be readily available if needed to counteract incipient hypercoagulability.

When immediate correction of hypoprothrombinemia is necessary (eg, overdose of oral anticoagulants), transfusion of plasma or plasma concentrates rich in stable vitamin K-dependent clotting factors is indicated. Fresh frozen plasma or blood component therapy may be needed if bleeding is severe and factors V and VIII are depleted. The slow (not to exceed 1 mg/min) intravenous injection of phytonadione also may be indicated (AquaMEPHYTON only; Konakion is given intramuscularly only). Concomitant use of phytonadione and plasma three units (15 ml/kg) is recommended initially. However, hypervolemia may result and precipitate pulmonary edema in patients with limited cardiac reserve. If rapid reversal of hypoprothrombinemia is necessary in these patients, factor IX complex concentrates may be administered to avoid transfusing large volumes of plasma despite the risk of hepatitis and/or thrombosis.

ADVERSE REACTIONS AND PRECAUTIONS. Intravenous injection of phytonadione can cause flushing of the face, hyperhidrosis, a feeling of chest constriction, cyanosis, acute peripheral vascular failure, shock, and hypersensitivity or anaphylactic-type reactions. Fatalities have occurred (see the Introduction to this section). Following subcutaneous and intramuscular administration, the action is more prolonged than with the intravenous route; delayed nodule formation and pain may occur at the site of injection. Intramuscular injection may produce hemorrhage in hypoprothrombinemic patients.

Parenteral administration in neonates can increase unbound plasma bilirubin significantly and cause hemolytic anemia and hemoglobinuria. These reactions are less likely with phytonadione than with the water-soluble analogues (menadiol sodium diphosphate, menadione sodium bisulfite) and occur rarely if recommended doses are not exceeded. Kernicterus has not yet been reported.

DOSAGE AND PREPARATIONS.

Oral, Subcutaneous, Intramuscular: For hypoprothrombinemic states, *adults and children,* 2.5 to 25 mg; rarely, doses as large as 50 mg may be needed.

    Mephyton (Merck Sharp & Dohme). Tablets 5 mg.
    For parenteral preparations, see below.

Intravenous, Intramuscular, Subcutaneous: The preparation may be diluted with 5% dextrose, 0.9% sodium chloride, or 5% dextrose and sodium chloride injection. Other diluents should not be used. When intravenous administration is necessary, the rate of injection should not exceed 1 mg/min. For prophylaxis of hemorrhagic disease in the newborn, 0.5 to 1 mg immediately after birth; although less desirable, 1 to 5 mg may be given to the mother 12 to 24 hours before delivery. For treatment of hemorrhagic disease in the newborn, 1 mg intramuscularly or subcutaneously. If no improvement occurs within six hours, the condition of the infant should be re-evaluated.

Whenever possible, the subcutaneous or intramuscular route is preferred to intravenous administration.

Intravenous (slow): The intravenous route should be used only when other routes are not feasible and the risk is justified. Initially, for mild overdose of oral anticoagulants, 0.5 to 5 mg; for moderate overdose, up to 10 mg; for severe hemorrhage, 25 mg (rarely up to 50 mg). The frequency of administration and amount of additional doses should be determined by the prothrombin time or the patient's condition. If prothrombin time is not satisfactory after six to eight hours, the dose should be repeated. The smallest effective dose should be used to prevent temporary refractoriness to further anticoagulant therapy. If shock occurs or blood loss is excessive, fresh frozen plasma or component therapy is essential.

    AquaMEPHYTON (Merck Sharp & Dohme). Solution 2 mg/ml in 0.5 ml (1 mg/0.5 ml) containers and 10 mg/ml in 1, 2.5, and 5 ml containers.
    Konakion (Roche). Solution (intramuscular only) 2 mg/ml in 0.5 ml containers and 10 mg/ml in 1 ml containers.

MENADIONE (Vitamin K$_3$)

Menadione has the same actions and uses as phytonadione, although it is not as active on a weight basis (see the Introduction and the evaluation on Phytonadione). Because it may produce hemolytic anemia and liver damage, menadione should not be given in large doses or for long-term therapy. This preparation is almost insoluble in water and is used orally; the presence of bile salts is required for intestinal absorption.

The incidence of adverse reactions is low when usual therapeutic doses are used, and reactions are similar to those produced by phytonadione. In addition, menadione hemolyzes red blood cells in patients with G6PD deficiency, as well as in newborn (especially premature) infants. Therefore, it probably should not be given to newborn infants or to women during the last few weeks of pregnancy.

DOSAGE AND PREPARATIONS.
Oral: 2 to 10 mg daily.
    Generic. Tablets 5 mg.

MENADIOL SODIUM DIPHOSPHATE
    [Synkayvite]

MENADIONE SODIUM BISULFITE

These water-soluble salts of menadione have actions and uses similar to those of phytonadione (see the evaluation); however, they should not be given to prevent or treat hemorrhagic disease in the newborn or to treat hypoprothrombinemia caused by overdosage of oral anticoagulants. These salts and esters are converted to menadione in the liver. Concomitant administration of bile salts is not necessary for intestinal absorption. Because menadione can produce hemolytic anemia and liver damage, these menadione salts should not be given when large doses or prolonged therapy is necessary. Their use is not recommended in patients with obstructive jaundice or biliary fistula.

Adverse reactions are similar to those produced by phytonadione, but the incidence is low when usual therapeutic doses are used. Nevertheless, parenteral forms of vitamin K-related compounds should be used only when there is a definite indication for them, since these routes (particularly intramuscular injection) may cause serious toxicity. Like menadione, these salts hemolyze red blood cells in patients with G6PD deficiency, as well as in newborn (especially premature) infants. Therefore, they probably should not be given to newborn infants or to women during the last few weeks of pregnancy.

DOSAGE AND PREPARATIONS.
MENADIOL SODIUM DIPHOSPHATE:
Oral, Subcutaneous, Intramuscular, Intravenous: *Adults,* for secondary hypoprothrombinemia, 5 to 15 mg once or twice daily; *children,* 5 to 10 mg once or twice daily. Doses may be repeated if prothrombin levels do not return to normal.
  Synkayvite (Roche). Solution (injection) 5 and 10 mg/ml in 1 ml containers and 37.5 mg/ml in 2 ml containers; tablets 5 mg.
MENADIONE SODIUM BISULFITE:
Subcutaneous, Intramuscular, Intravenous: 2.5 to 10 mg daily, depending upon the route and indications for use. Larger doses may be needed in patients with severe vitamin K deficiency. Intravenous administration produces the most rapid response, but effects may last longer when the other routes are used.
  Generic. Bulk.

LOCAL BLEEDING

The absorbable hemostatics for local use are absorbable gelatin sponge [Gelfoam], oxidized cellulose [Oxycel], oxidized regenerated cellulose [Surgicel], microfibrillar collagen hemostat [Avitene], and thrombin [Thrombinar, Thrombostat]. Absorbable gelatin film [Gelfilm] is not a hemostatic but is used surgically as an absorbable implant. These agents may help to control surface bleeding and capillary oozing and tend to be fairly innocuous. However, if significant contamination is present at the site of application, these substances may exacerbate infections.

In dermatologic procedures, caustic agents, such as ferric subsulfate (Monsel's solution) and aluminum chloride solution, produce hemostasis during limited superficial surgery by coagulating skin proteins. Excessive use of ferric subsulfate may result in tattoo marks, especially if electrocautery is used after it is applied.

Drug Evaluations

ABSORBABLE GELATIN FILM
[Gelfilm]

This sterile, thin film is used in neurologic and thoracic surgery for nonhemostatic purposes to repair defects in the dura and pleural membranes. It is also used in ocular surgery. Depending upon the site and size of implant, eight days to six months are required for absorption.

DOSAGE AND PREPARATIONS.
Topical (in operative site): The film is soaked in sterile saline solution until pliable and cut to desired size and shape. The minimal amount required to cover the area should be applied.
  Gelfilm (Upjohn). Film 25 x 50 mm (ophthalmic) and 100 x 125 mm.

ABSORBABLE GELATIN SPONGE
[Gelfoam]

This sterile, gelatin-base surgical sponge is applied locally to help control both capillary oozing and mild to moderate hemorrhage. Highly vascular areas that are difficult to suture are primary sites of application. Absorbable gelatin sponge is insoluble in water and is usually moistened with sterile sodium chloride or thrombin solution before application (a compressed form is available specifically for dry application).

This preparation may be left in place following closure of a surgical wound. When it is packed into cavities or closed tissue spaces, care should be exercised to avoid overpacking, because the material expands on absorbing fluid and may press on neighboring structures. This caution is particularly important when nerve tissue is involved. Absorption is complete in four to six weeks and there is no excessive scar tissue formation or cellular reaction.

Information is insufficient to determine its teratogenic potential, but absorbable gelatin sponge should be used with caution in pregnant women. It should not be used to control postpartum bleeding or menorrhagia.

This material should not be applied in closure of skin incisions (since it may interfere with healing of skin) or when infection is present.

ADVERSE REACTIONS. Absorbable gelatin sponge may form a nidus for infection or abscess. Giant-cell granuloma has been reported at the site of absorbable gelatin products implanted in the brain. Accumulation of sterile fluid has caused compression of brain and spinal cord.

DOSAGE AND PREPARATIONS.

Topical (in wound or at operative site): The minimal amount required to cover the area and control hemorrhage should be applied.

Gelfoam (Upjohn). Blocks 20 x 60 x 3 mm and 20 x 60 x 7 mm (general and neurologic surgery), 80 x 62.5 x 10 mm and 80 x 125 x 10 mm (general surgery), 80 x 250 x 10 mm (packing for cavities or dead spaces); pleated surgical packs 40 x 2 cm (general packing and filling), 40 x 6 cm (gynecologic and rectal surgery), 10 x 20 x 7 mm and 20 x 20 x 7 mm (dental packing blocks); compressed blocks 125 x 80 mm (dry applications); powder 1 g (sterile); prostatectomy cones 13 and 18 cm in diameter.

OXIDIZED CELLULOSE
[Oxycel]

OXIDIZED REGENERATED CELLULOSE
[Surgicel]

ACTIONS. These celluloses are absorbable fabrics prepared by the controlled oxidation of cellulose or regenerated cellulose. The gauze does not enter into the normal physiologic clotting mechanism but, when exposed to blood, expands and is converted to a reddish brown or black gelatinous mass that forms an artificial clot. Oxidized cellulose products have a very low pH and possess some cauterizing action. The hemostatic action of these celluloses is not enhanced by other hemostatic agents (thrombin is destroyed by the low pH of this material).

The rate of absorption depends upon the size of the implant, the adequacy of blood supply to the area, and the degree of chemical degradation of the material. Two to seven days are usually required, but complete absorption of large amounts of blood-soaked material may take six weeks or longer. Under optimal conditions, absorption from a body cavity occurs without cellular reaction or fibrosis. However, some stenosis of arterial anastomoses may occur, apparently from cicatricial contraction.

USES. Oxidized cellulose or oxidized regenerated cellulose is useful in surgical procedures to control moderate bleeding when suturing or ligation is technically impractical or ineffective. Such situations include control of capillary, venous, or small arterial hemorrhage encountered in biliary tract surgery; partial hepatectomy; resections or injuries of the pancreas, spleen, or kidneys; amputations; resection of the bowel, breast, thyroid, or prostate; oral surgery and exodontia; certain types of neurologic and otolaryngologic surgery; and as a wrap to control the anastomotic bleeding that occurs in vascular surgery.

PRECAUTIONS. These products should not be used for permanent packing or implantation in fractures because they may interfere with bone regeneration and cause cyst formation. They are less effective on surfaces treated by chemical cautery. The Oxycel brand should not be used as a surface dressing except for immediate control of hemorrhage, since it inhibits epithelialization; silver nitrate or other corrosive chemicals should not be applied prior to its use.

Information is insufficient to determine the teratogenic po-

tential of these celluloses, and they should be used with caution in pregnant women.

DOSAGE AND PREPARATIONS.

Topical (in wound or at operative site): The minimal amount required to control hemorrhage should be used to facilitate absorption. This material should be placed on the bleeding site and held firmly until hemostasis is obtained.

OXIDIZED CELLULOSE:
Oxycel (Parke-Davis). Pads (gauze type) 7.6 x 7.6 cm 8 ply; pledgets (cotton type) 5.1 x 2.5 x 2.5 cm; strips (gauze type) 12.7 x 1.3 cm 4 ply, 45.7 x 5.1 cm 4 ply, 91.4 x 1.3 cm 4 ply.

OXIDIZED REGENERATED CELLULOSE:
Surgicel (Johnson & Johnson). Knitted fabric strips 1.3 x 5.1, 5.1 x 7.6, 10.2 x 20.3, and 5.1 x 35.6 cm.

MICROFIBRILLAR COLLAGEN HEMOSTAT
[Avitene]

ACTIONS AND USES. This water-insoluble fibrous material is prepared from purified bovine corium collagen. When applied directly on the bleeding surface, it attracts and entraps platelets to initiate formation of the platelet plug; a natural clot results. Microfibrillar collagen hemostat is assimilated within seven weeks, leaving very little residue.

This material is indicated as an adjunct during surgical procedures when ligature and/or cautery are ineffective or impractical. However, it should not be used instead of ligation or resection to control large vessel bleeding during surgery or for routine surgical bleeding.

Microfibrillar collagen hemostat is beneficial in diffuse capillary bleeding (eg, from friable tissues or highly vascular organs). It controls hepatic bleeding, such as that following cholecystectomy, lacerations, biopsy, or resections of hepatic tumors and capillary bleeding from splenic tears or superficial splenic injuries. This material also is used around vascular anastomoses where only minimal suturing is possible and to control oozing from cancellous bone. However, it should not be used on bone surfaces to which prosthetic materials are to be attached with methylmethacrylate adhesives. This hemostatic appears to retain its effectiveness in heparinized patients and also may be useful in patients with moderate thrombocytopenia but not in those with clinical thrombasthenia. Microfibrillar collagen hemostat is a useful adjunct for bleeding in the oral cavity of patients with hemophilia, in those receiving coumarin derivatives, and in patients with inhibitors to coagulation factors.

APPLICATION. Microfibrillar collagen hemostat adheres to tissue surfaces to form a firm flexible film; since it also will adhere to any moist surface (eg, gloves, instruments), dry, smooth, sterile forceps should be used for handling. Surfaces to be treated should first be compressed with dry sponges and then covered with microfibrillar collagen hemostat; moderate pressure with a dry sterile sponge should then be exerted. Pressure for one minute may control superficial capillary bleeding, but five minutes or more may be needed when high-pressure leaks from artery suture holes or other pronounced bleeding is encountered. If oozing is not controlled, additional microfibrillar collagen hemostat may be used. However, only the amount needed to produce hemostasis should be used and excess material should be removed by teasing or irrigating. This usually can be done without a recurrence of bleeding.

ADVERSE REACTIONS AND PRECAUTIONS. Since it is a foreign protein, microfibrillar collagen hemostat may exacerbate infection; abscess formation; dehiscence of cutaneous incisions, where collagen may form a mechanical barrier between opposed skin edges; mediastinitis; and adhesion formation. By sealing the surface, it may conceal deep hemorrhage or hematoma in penetrating wounds. Use of this hemostatic is contraindicated for skin closure, because healing of the wound edges is deterred. However, it does not interfere with epidermal or bone healing.

No systemic allergic reactions or beef antibody responses have been reported. Although weak positive reactions to bovine serum albumin have occurred occasionally, significant IgE antibodies have not developed following use of this product.

Microfibrillar collagen hemostat must be kept dry, since moisture impairs its hemostatic capacity. It is inactivated by autoclaving and should not be resterilized. Sterility is not guaranteed once the container is opened; therefore, the unused portion should be discarded. Care should be taken to avoid spillage on nonbleeding surfaces, particularly in abdominal or thoracic viscera.

Information is insufficient to determine its teratogenic potential, and this preparation should be used with caution in pregnant women.

DOSAGE AND PREPARATIONS.
Topical: For capillary bleeding, 1 g is usually sufficient for a 50-cm^2 area. Thicker coverage is required for more pronounced bleeding. To control oozing from cancellous bone, the preparation should be firmly packed into the spongy bone surface and compressed for 5 to 10 minutes.

> ***Avitene*** (Avicon). Fibrous form (sterile) in 1 and 5 g jars contained in a sealed can; nonwoven web (sterile) 70 x 35 x 1 and 70 x 70 x 1 mm.

THROMBIN
[Thrombinar, Thrombostat]

ACTIONS AND USES. This sterile plasma protein substance is prepared from bovine prothrombin. It is applied topically to control capillary oozing in operative procedures and also has shortened the duration of bleeding from puncture sites in heparinized patients (eg, after hemodialysis). Thrombin may clot whole blood, plasma, or a solution of fibrinogen without the addition of other substances; it also may be combined with gelatin sponge but should not be used to moisten microfibrillar collagen hemostat. Thrombin alone does not control arterial bleeding.

When applied to denuded tissue, thrombin is neutralized rapidly by antithrombins, and its activity is reduced as a result of absorption on fibrin. There is little danger of thrombin being absorbed into the vascular system. It has been used successfully as an adjunct for oral bleeding following dental extractions in patients with hemophilia.

Thrombin has been instilled into the stomach in an effort to hasten hemostasis in ulcerative disease, but activity is limited because of its rapid transit. In addition, thrombin becomes inactive below pH 5.0.

This compound is stable as a dry powder if stored between 2 and 8 C. In solution, it begins to lose activity within eight hours at room temperature or within 48 hours if refrigerated.

PRECAUTIONS. Thrombin should never be injected, particularly intravenously, for there is danger of thrombosis and death within a few minutes. Antigenic reactions have occurred in animals, and allergic reactions may develop in persons sensitive to bovine material.

DOSAGE AND PREPARATIONS.
Topical (in wound or at operative site): Thrombin is dusted on as a powder, applied as a solution by flooding or spraying the site, or combined with a suitable sponge matrix (eg, absorbable gelatin sponge). The usual amount applied is 5,000 units.

> ***Thrombinar*** (Armour). Powder (bovine origin) in 1,000, 5,000, 10,000, 20,000, and 50,000 unit containers. The 5,000-unit container is supplied with 10 ml of diluent. The 10,000- and 20,000-unit containers are supplied with 20 ml of diluent.
> ***Thrombostat*** (Parke-Davis). Powder (bovine origin) 1,000, 5,000, and 10,000 unit containers. The 5,000-unit container is supplied with 5 ml of sterile isotonic sodium chloride as diluent with phemerol 0.02 mg/ml as preservative.

Cited References

Abildgaard CF, et al: Anti-inhibitor coagulant complex (Autoplex) for treatment of factor VIII inhibitors in hemophilia. *Blood* 56:978-984, 1980.

Biswas CK, et al: Acute renal failure and myopathy after treatment with aminocaproic acid. *Br Med J* 281:115-116, 1980.

Blatt PM, et al: Antihemophilic factor concentrate therapy in von Willebrand disease. *JAMA* 236:2770-2772, 1976.

Brodkin HM: Myoglobinuria following epsilon-aminocaproic acid (EACA) therapy: Case report. *J Neurosurg* 53:690-692, 1980.

Colombo M, et al: Transmission of non-A, non-B hepatitis by heat-treated factor VIII concentrate. *Lancet* 2:1-4, 1985.

Deykin D: Uremic bleeding. *Kidney Int* 24:698-705, 1983.

Eyster ME: Hemophilia: Guide for primary care physician. *Postgrad Med* 64:75-81, (Nov) 1978.

Fuerth JH, Mahrer P: Myocardial infarction after factor IX therapy. *JAMA* 245:1455-1456, 1981.

Garewal HS, Corrigan JJ Jr: Danazol in hemophilia, (letter). *JAMA* 254:754-755, 1985.

Gill FM: Congenital bleeding disorders: Hemophilia and von Willebrand's disease. *Med Clin North Am* 68:601-615, 1984.

Gruppo RA, et al: Fatal myocardial necrosis associated with prothrombin-complex-concentrate therapy in hemophilia A. *N Engl J Med* 309:242-243, 1983.

Hay CRM, et al: Progressive liver disease in haemophilia: Understated problem? *Lancet* 1:1495-1498, 1985.

Hoyer LW: Factor VIII complex: Structure and function. *Blood* 58:1-13, 1981.

Hutchinson RJ, et al: Anti-inhibitor coagulant complex (Autoplex) in hemophilia inhibitor patients undergoing synovectomy. *Pediatrics* 71:631-633, 1983.

Laurian Y, et al: Incidence of immune responses following 102 infusions of Autoplex in 18 hemophilic patients with antibody to factor VIII. *Blood* 63:457-462, 1984.

Lusher JM, et al: Prothrombin complex concentrates in hemophilia with inhibitors: Multicenter therapeutic trial. *N Engl J Med* 303:421-425, 1980.

Machin SJ: The bleeding patient. *Br J Hosp Med* 24:152-158, 1980.

Morris CDW, et al: Epsilon-aminocaproic acid-induced myopathy: Case report. *South Afr Med J* 64:363-366, 1983.

Robison JW, Odom RB: Delayed cutaneous reaction to phytonadione. *Arch Derm* 114:1790-1792, 1978.

Rodgers GP, Heymach GJ III: Cryoprecipitate therapy in amniotic fluid embolization. *Am J Med* 76:916-920, 1984.

Rouzioux C, et al: Absence of antibodies to AIDS virus in haemophiliacs treated with heat-treated factor VIII concentrate, (letter). *Lancet* 1:271-272, 1985.

Stel HV, et al: von Willebrand factor in vessel wall mediates platelet adherence. *Blood* 65:85-90, 1985.

Turitto VT, et al: Factor VIII/von Willebrand factor in subendothelium mediates platelet adhesion. *Blood* 65:823-831, 1985.

Vermeulen M, et al: Antifibrinolytic treatment in subarachnoid hemorrhage. *N Engl J Med* 311:432-437, 1984.

Other Selected References

Vitamin-K-type coagulants: Proposed bioequivalence requirements. *Federal Register* 45:14063-14067, (March 4) 1980.

Aledort LM: *The Management of Hemophilia.* Manual available without charge from the National Hemophilia Foundation, 25 W 39th St, New York, NY, 10018.

Aledort LM: Methods of care, products available, complications of therapy. *Mt Sinai J Med* 44:332-338, 1977.

Aledort LM: Factor IX and thrombosis. *Scand J Haematol* 30(suppl):40-42, 1977.

Ambritz R, et al: Danazol in hemophilia, (letter). *JAMA* 254:754, 1985.

Hilgartner MW: Management of hemophilia: Routine and crises. *Drug Ther* 8:141-154, (Feb) 1978.

Hilgartner MW, Sergis E: Current therapy for hemophilics: Home care and therapeutic complications. *Mt Sinai J Med* 44:316-331, 1977.

Hruby MA: Bleeding disorders in children. *Compr Ther* 3:26-34, (Sept) 1977.

Jason J, et al: Immune status of blood product recipients. *JAMA* 253:1140-1145, 1985.

Jones P, et al: AIDS and haemophilia: Morbidity and mortality in well defined population. *Br Med J* 291:695-699, 1985.

Mannuci PM, et al: 1-Deamino-8-D-arginine vasopressin: New pharmacological approach to management of hemophilia and von Willebrand's disease. *Lancet* 1:869-872, 1977.

Ratnoff OD: Antihemophilic factor (factor VIII). *Ann Intern Med* 88:403-409, 1978.

Telfer MC, Chediak J: Factor VIII-related disorders and their relationship to pregnancy. *J Reprod Med* 19:211-222, 1977.

Verstraete M: Clinical application of inhibitors of fibrinolysis. *Drugs* 29:236-261, 1985.

Agents Used to Treat Adrenal Dysfunction

PHYSIOLOGY AND PHARMACOLOGY

Secretion: The adrenal cortex secretes glucocorticoids and mineralocorticoids, which have 21 carbon atoms, and androgens, which have 19 carbon atoms. It also secretes small amounts of progesterone, 17-α hydroxyprogesterone (21 carbon atoms), and estrogens (18 carbon atoms). Under basal conditions, 15 to 25 mg (12 $\pm$ 3 mg/M^2) of cortisol and 1.5 to 4 mg of corticosterone, the major natural glucocorticoids, are secreted daily. The amount of aldosterone, the most important mineralocorticoid, secreted is 30 to 150 mcg daily; its rate of secretion is related inversely to the dietary intake of sodium and is constant at all ages. (In contrast, the rate of cortisol secretion is related to body size.) Although a similar quantity of the mineralocorticoid, desoxycorticosterone, is secreted daily, it has only 3% to 5% of the sodium-retaining activity of aldosterone on an equimolar basis.

The principal androgens secreted by the adrenal cortex are dehydroepiandrosterone (DHEA), DHEA sulfate, and androstenedione. Adrenal androgens usually do not have a potent masculinizing effect: In men, testosterone secreted by the testes has the greatest androgenic effect. However, in women, a portion of adrenal androstenedione is converted in peripheral tissues to testosterone, which is responsible for sexual hair development, support of normal libido, and possibly the slight masculinization that sometimes occurs after menopause. Adrenal androgen production increases during the early stages of puberty (adrenarche) in both sexes and is an integral part of normal maturation.

In hypersecretory states or with certain adrenal tumors, overproduction of adrenal androgens, estrogens, or their metabolites can produce typical effects on responsive tissues (see also Chapter 38, Androgens and Anabolic Steroids).

The adrenal cortex does not store appreciable amounts of glucocorticoids; glucocorticoid steroidogenesis and secretion are rapidly stimulated by adrenocorticotropin (ACTH). The steroidogenic and trophic actions of ACTH on the adrenal cortex are mediated by activation of adenylate cyclase and increased production of cyclic adenosine monophosphate (cAMP). The response to stimulation by ACTH occurs within two minutes and is complete in less than one hour.

ACTH is produced in the basophilic cells of the anterior pituitary gland; its secretion is stimulated by corticotropin-releasing hormone (CRH), which has been identified as a polypeptide (Vale et al, 1981). CRH is synthesized in the hypothalamus and transported to the anterior pituitary gland by the hypophyseal portal blood vessels. Secretion of ACTH is inhibited by a negative feedback effect of glucocorticoids, probably at both the hypothalamus (decreasing CRH secretion) and directly at the anterior pituitary gland.

Stimulation of CRH and, therefore, of ACTH secretion occurs in response to two types of extrahypothalamic central nervous system signals: The first neural signal comes from the anterior areas of the brain, including the amygdala, and results in basal secretion with circadian rhythmicity. In individuals maintaining a normal sleep-activity cycle, peak blood levels occur between 4 AM and 8 AM and periodic bursts of secretion are superimposed upon the basic pattern. The nadir occurs in the late evening or early sleep period. This circadian rhythm is absent or blunted in patients with Cushing's disease and is accentuated in those with partial adrenal insufficiency. The inhibitory effect of glucocorticoids (endogenous or exogenous) on ACTH secretion also has circadian periodicity; suppression is least when the steroid is given about the time of peak cortisol secretion, early in the morning. The time of maximal ACTH secretion in response to stress is in the evening coincident with the nadir of cortisol secretion.

The second type of neural input occurs in response to stressful stimuli (eg, trauma, anxiety, severe infections, hypoglycemia, surgery). The signals enter the hypothalamus from both anterior and posterior brain areas, the latter probably arising from the reticular formation.

The amount of ACTH secreted at any time is influenced by the integration of negative feedback from circulating glucocorticoids and the neural signals associated with circadian secretion and the response to stress. Severe stress is the most potent stimulus for ACTH secretion and can increase cortisol secretion tenfold.

Glucocorticoids exert two types of negative feedback control on ACTH secretion, which differ in the time required for inhibitory effect. The fast feedback system acts almost immediately and is responsible for normal minute-to-minute physiologic control. The delayed feedback system suppresses ACTH secretion when pharmacologic doses of glucocorticoids are administered.

As with glucocorticoids, appreciable amounts of aldosterone are not stored in the adrenal cortex, and the rates of synthesis and secretion are essentially equal. Secretion has a slight circadian rhythmicity and levels are maximal after arising in the morning. Aldosterone secretion is controlled primarily by the renin-angiotensin system and partially by ACTH. It also is stimulated directly by elevated serum potassium levels. When the effective circulating plasma volume and plasma sodium levels are decreased, renin production and, ultimately, aldosterone secretion are stimulated. The central nervous system also may stimulate renin production directly via sympathetic fibers to afferent arterioles and the juxtaglomerular apparatus. When large doses of ACTH are administered, aldosterone secretion increases initially but returns to baseline or lower levels even when ACTH stimulation is maintained. Aldosterone does not exert a significant negative feedback effect on ACTH production.

ACTH stimulates adrenal androgen as well as cortisol secretion. Another, as yet unidentified, substance secreted by the pituitary may stimulate secretion of adrenal androgens but not other adrenocortical hormones. Pituitary gonadotropins probably stimulate only the secretion of gonadal sex steroids.

Adrenal sex steroids do not exert feedback control on ACTH secretion.

Mechanism of Action: Like other steroid hormones, corticosteroids exert their cellular effects through interaction with steroid receptors and the eventual production of proteins that carry out the steroid-specific function for cells of that particular tissue. Cortisol forms a complex with a specific receptor protein in the cytoplasm of responsive cells, which eventually binds to nuclear chromatin. This is followed by transcription of specific genes of the DNA into corresponding messenger RNA and RNA translation into proteins, usually enzymes. In tissues in which corticosteroids have a catabolic effect, it is not known whether enzyme production is inhibited by a similar process or whether synthesized cellular proteins are responsible for catabolism. Corticosteroids accomplish their biological functions within hours.

Transport and Metabolism: The major portion of cortisol is transported in the blood, reversibly bound to corticosteroid-binding globulin (CBG) and albumin. It is generally accepted that the unbound portion is the active form. Some synthetic corticosteroids, such as prednisone, compete for binding to CBG; others, like dexamethasone, do not bind to CBG. Aldosterone has low affinity for CBG. More than 90% of plasma cortisol is protein bound, mainly to CBG, while only 50% of circulating aldosterone is protein bound, principally to albumin. The synthetic corticosteroids vary in their affinity and capacity for protein binding. These factors, as well as differences in clearance rates, affect the proportion of steroid available to exert a therapeutic effect and may explain why relatively small doses of some synthetic preparations cause cushingoid effects.

In certain conditions associated with high concentrations of total blood corticosteroids, the negative feedback mechanism maintains normal functional levels of the free fraction. For example, during pregnancy or in patients taking estrogens, the concentration of CBG and thus total plasma levels of corticosteroid are elevated, but the physiologically active, unbound portion remains at functionally normal levels. The effect that a disease or drug has on protein binding must be taken into account when interpreting the results of certain adrenal function tests.

Natural corticosteroids have relatively short plasma half-lives, ranging from 30 minutes for aldosterone to 90 minutes for cortisol. The tissue half-life of cortisol, which determines the duration of biological effectiveness, is approximately 8 to 12 hours.

Most endogenous cortisol is metabolized in the liver, where physiologically inactive, water-soluble conjugates are formed. These are excreted in the bile and most are reabsorbed so that 90% of cortisol metabolites are excreted in the urine and the remaining 10% in the feces.

EFFECTS OF PHYSIOLOGIC CONCENTRATIONS

Intermediary Metabolism: Glucocorticoids affect carbohydrate, protein, and fat metabolism; in contrast, mineralocorticoids have no effect on intermediary metabolism. In general, the glucocorticoids enhance glucose availability and stimulate protein catabolism and lipolysis. They increase glucose availability by (1) stimulating hepatic gluconeogenesis and inducing transaminases involved in gluconeogenesis and amino acid metabolism; as a result of protein catabolic processes, urinary excretion of nitrogen is increased; (2) decreasing glucose utilization (anti-insulin effect); and (3) stimulating glycogen storage, particularly by the liver. Glucocorticoid insufficiency results in glucose being less readily available and may result in hypoglycemia (eg, during stress or prolonged fasting).

The mobilization of fatty acids from adipose tissue is enhanced by glucocorticoids, probably through facilitation of the lipolytic response to cAMP. However, there is no consistent change in blood lipid levels.

Water and Electrolyte Balance: The effects of adrenal corticosteroids on water and electrolyte balance are exerted mainly by aldosterone through control of the renal excretion of cations. Although 98% of filtered sodium is absorbed by active and passive mechanisms before reaching the distal tubules, mineralocorticoids promote reabsorption of small but significant portions of filtered sodium here. The renal excretion of potassium and hydrogen ions is enhanced by mineralocorticoids. Therefore, severe mineralocorticoid deficiency produces excessive sodium loss resulting in a hypo-osmotic intracellular compartment, decreased extracellular fluid volume, hyperkalemia, mild acidosis, and, eventually, circulatory and renal failure and death. Mineralocorticoids also stimulate sodium reabsorption across other epithelial tissues (eg, colonic mucosa, exocrine pancreatic ducts, sweat and salivary glands).

Cortisol also is involved in the regulation of water balance. In glucocorticoid deficiency, the glomerular filtration rate decreases and the concentration of antidiuretic hormone (ADH) increases; inability to excrete a water load results. Administration of a glucocorticoid restores normal function.

The glucocorticoids also affect calcium balance by decreasing intestinal uptake and increasing renal excretion.

Cardiovascular System and Blood: Both glucocorticoids and mineralocorticoids are important in supporting normal cardiovascular function. Although the mechanism is poorly understood, glucocorticoids appear to be necessary for the vasoconstrictor action of adrenergic stimuli on small vessels. In the absence of glucocorticoids, the vasomotor response is inadequate, blood pressure is decreased, and capillary permeability is increased. Mineralocorticoids help to maintain normal blood volume by stimulating sodium retention. In deficiency states, hypotension and circulatory failure may result from decreased volume.

Glucocorticoids increase hemoglobin, erythrocytes, and polymorphonuclear leukocytes in the blood and elevate the total white blood cell count. In contrast, they decrease eosinophils, basophils, monocytes, and lymphocytes. The observation that daily fluctuations in blood eosinophil levels occur is of historical interest because it led to the discovery of the circadian rhythm of glucocorticoid secretion.

Central Nervous System: In general, the role of the corticosteroids in central nervous system function is poorly defined but, in part, it is secondary to their effects on carbohydrate metabolism, electrolyte balance, and cerebral blood flow. Corticosteroids also influence mood, sleep patterns, and EEG activity. Adrenal insufficiency is associated with changes in mood (irritability and depression) and with greater than usual EEG slow wave activity. Both conditions are relieved by hydrocortisone. Seizure thresholds are lowered by glucocorticoids and elevated by mineralocorticoids. The net effect in adrenalectomized animals is to lower the threshold (increase excitability) to various seizure-inducing stimuli.

Skeletal Muscle: Corticosteroids are required to maintain normal skeletal muscular strength. The muscular weakness associated with adrenal insufficiency probably is caused primarily by circulatory incompetence and, to a lesser extent, by disorders of carbohydrate metabolism and electrolyte balance.

Stress: Although the mechanisms involved have never been determined definitively, two observations support the probable protective nature of increased glucocorticoid secretion in response to stressful stimuli: (1) Cortisol secretion is immediately and greatly enhanced at the initiation of stress. (2) Patients experiencing severe stress (eg, surgery) who are incapable of secreting additional glucocorticoids require exogenous hormones to prevent circulatory failure.

Two characteristics of severe stress in patients with adrenal insufficiency are hypoglycemia and hypotension. During most stress situations, both adrenal medullary and glucocorticoid secretion are increased, and these hormones act synergistically to increase blood glucose levels and blood pressure.

EXCESSIVE SECRETION OF ADRENOCORTICAL HORMONES

Cushing's Syndrome

Cushing's syndrome results from excessive glucocorticoids and is usually iatrogenic. Cushing's syndrome is also caused by adrenal hypersecretion. This hypersecretion of glucocorticoids is due to either a primary adrenal source (ie, benign adenoma, carcinoma) or to excessive ACTH. In Cushing's disease (as distinguished from syndrome), increased secretion of ACTH results from pituitary and/or hypothalamic dysfunction, which is often associated with basophilic hyperplasia or pituitary adenomas. Cushing's syndrome also may result from ectopic ACTH-producing tumors (eg, carcinoma of lung, thyroid, esophagus, islet cell, ovary, breast, or prostate; bronchial adenoma; carcinoid).

The manifestations of Cushing's syndrome (osteoporosis, myopathy, skin atrophy and striae, bleeding tendency, abnormal fat distribution, abnormal glucose tolerance, euphoria and other behavioral abnormalities, and growth suppression in children) are qualitatively similar to some side effects of pharmacologic doses of glucocorticoids administered for nonendocrine disorders (see Chapter 61, Adrenal Corticosteroids in Nonendocrine Diseases).

DIAGNOSIS. Cortisol suppression tests (eg, dexamethasone) and measurement of urinary free cortisol are used to diagnose Cushing's syndrome. Measurement of plasma ACTH and radiography or computed tomography of the pituitary, adrenal glands, or chest (to detect the source of ectopic ACTH) also may be required for differential diagnosis. (See also Chapter 42, Agents Related to Anterior Pituitary and Hypothalamic Function.)

TREATMENT. Treatment of Cushing's syndrome is directed toward the cause. Transsphenoidal adenectomy or hypophysectomy or pituitary irradiation are used to treat pituitary-hypothalamic dysfunction. Adrenal sources and certain other conditions are treated surgically. Drugs are most useful as adjuncts to pituitary surgery or irradiation or as palliative treatment for adrenal carcinoma or ectopic ACTH-producing tumors.

Surgery: Transsphenoidal microsurgery is used frequently when pituitary or hypothalamic disorders cause Cushing's syndrome. Microadenectomy is the treatment of choice for most adults even in the absence of tomographic evidence of microadenoma, because tumors are often found on exploration. Complications of surgery include transient diabetes insipidus, hemorrhage, or, more rarely, rhinorrhea, optic nerve damage, and meningitis.

Surgery is successful in 50% to 90% of patients; hypercortisolism is corrected rapidly and other pituitary function is preserved. Return of normal pituitary-adrenal function may require months; the situation is analogous to removal of a glucocorticoid-producing tumor or abrupt cessation of prolonged pharmacologic treatment with glucocorticoids. During this period, the patient is treated for secondary adrenal insufficiency and appropriate precautions should be observed: increased doses of glucocorticoid should be given during stress (eg, febrile illness, surgical or other trauma), and the patient should wear medical identification and carry an emergency supply of injectable glucocorticoid (see also Chapter 61, Adrenal Corticosteroids in Nonendocrine Diseases).

If partial removal of the pituitary is followed by recurrence of symptoms, a second operation may be performed to remove the remaining pituitary tissue partially or completely, or pituitary irradiation may be undertaken.

Hypophysectomy also may be employed for Nelson's syndrome, which develops in some patients following bilateral adrenalectomy for Cushing's syndrome; removal of the adrenal glands is followed by the appearance of a pituitary adenoma, which secretes ACTH and is accompanied by severe hyperpigmentation.

Hypophysectomized patients require replacement therapy with thyroid hormone, sex steroids, and (assuming a pituitary disorder caused Cushing's syndrome) glucocorticoids.

Adrenalectomy for Cushing's disease has been superseded by pituitary surgery but may be preferred in patients requiring an immediate cure because of progressive conditions, such as hypertension or severe osteoporosis. Bilateral adrenalectomy is also appropriate in the presence of inoperable, ectopic, ACTH-producing tumors. One or both adrenal glands may be removed for benign adenoma or adrenal carcinoma. Patients undergoing bilateral adrenalectomy require replacement of both glucocorticoids and mineralocorticoid.

Pituitary Irradiation: Irradiation of the pituitary as the primary treatment of Cushing's disease improves or cures 50% to 85% of patients. However, 12 to 18 months may be required before therapeutic results are complete. Patients under age 18 respond more rapidly than adults. Normal pituitary function is restored (after transient hypoadrenalism), growth resumes, and sexual development is normal. However, there is concern that complications may develop years after irradiation in childhood. Pituitary irradiation also is indicated in young adults with mild disease and no radiographic evidence of tumor, in patients at high risk for surgery, following unsuccessful or successful pituitary surgery (the latter to prevent recurrence of disease), and following bilateral adrenalectomy to prevent Nelson's syndrome.

Drug Therapy: Use of drugs as the primary treatment for Cushing's syndrome has been only partially successful. Mitotane [Lysodren] (an adrenolytic agent), enzyme inhibitors (metyrapone [Metopirone], aminoglutethimide [Cytadren], trilostane [Modrastane]), and centrally acting agents (cyproheptadine [Periactin], bromocriptine [Parlodel]) are generally used as adjuncts to prepare patients for adrenal surgery, in conjunction with pituitary irradiation, to control ectopic ACTH-producing tumors, for medical adrenalectomy, or rarely as primary treatment of Cushing's disease.

Mitotane destroys adrenocortical cells and thus has the potential to control hypercortisolism permanently. Enzyme inhibitors and centrally acting agents control cortisol secretion only temporarily, and relapse occurs after discontinuation of treatment. All drugs used to treat Cushing's syndrome have unpleasant and serious side effects that limit their usefulness.

The enzyme inhibitors block the biosynthetic pathway for cortisol production. In pituitary-dependent disease, however, removal of the negative feedback control of cortisol on the pituitary causes even greater secretion of ACTH, which overcomes the metabolic blockade and renders the drug less effective after several days. Cyproheptadine, a serotonin antagonist, may act directly on the microadenoma cells to inhibit ACTH secretion, but adequate sustained suppression has been reported in only 10% to 40% of patients (Orth, 1983). Bromocriptine, a dopaminergic agent, decreases ACTH secretion in some patients, but normal cortisol levels are not obtained.

Enzyme inhibitors are most useful for ectopic ACTH-producing tumors or other autonomous tumors when the neoplasm is inoperable or metastatic. Unlike pituitary-dependent ACTH secretion in which the synthetic blockade is not overcome, enzyme inhibitors effectively block cortisol synthesis from ectopic sites where negative feedback control is absent.

Enzyme inhibitors also are used to reduce cortisol secretion temporarily in patients being prepared for adrenal surgery who are at high risk due to hypercortisolism. These agents may be used separately or together as palliative treatment of metastatic adrenal carcinoma. Aminoglutethimide, which blocks sex steroid synthesis in the gonads and adrenal glands, may be particularly useful when virilization results from excessive androgen production by the adrenal tumor. The enzyme inhibitors are generally less toxic and therefore preferable to mitotane, which achieves palliative control of cortisol secretion in adrenal carcinoma by destroying adrenal cortical cells. Trilostane also has general steroid-inhibiting potential and appears to be less toxic than aminoglutethimide, but experience is inadequate to determine its relative effectiveness.

Enzyme inhibitors or cyproheptadine are used to control hypercortisolism until the effects of pituitary irradiation are realized months later and when irradiation is only partially effective. Mitotane may be considered if other drugs are ineffective.

All patients receiving drugs to control Cushing's syndrome should be monitored to detect adrenal insufficiency that may develop as therapy becomes effective.

Primary Hyperaldosteronism

Conn's syndrome, as described in 1955, is caused by an aldosterone-producing adrenal adenoma that increases plasma aldosterone and decreases plasma renin values and is associated with hypokalemia, metabolic alkalosis, and hypertension. Hypokalemia causes electrocardiographic changes and neuromuscular symptoms (eg, muscle weakness and fatigue, particularly of the lower extremities). There also are other forms of primary hyperaldosteronism. Increased production of aldosterone due to bilateral adrenal hyperplasia may account for 10% to 15% of cases. Rarely, primary hyperaldosteronism is associated with adrenal carcinoma. Reviews of the subject are available (Horton and Hsueh, 1983; Tuck, 1983; Adler and Williams, 1985).

DIAGNOSIS. Primary hyperaldosteronism is diagnosed by the demonstration of hypokalemia with excessive urinary excretion of potassium, decreased plasma renin, and increased plasma aldosterone not suppressed by volume expansion (eg, infusion of saline, administration of fludrocortisone). When the diagnosis of hyperaldosteronism has been established, the cause must be differentiated before appropriate treatment can be given, for the management of disease due to adrenal adenoma differs from that due to bilateral adrenal hyperplasia. The latter tends to produce milder disease with less severe electrolyte aberrations. Diagnostic techniques to differentiate the two conditions include adrenal radioiodocholesterol scan, CAT scan of the adrenal glands, and simultaneous catheterization of the adrenal veins.

TREATMENT. When disease is caused by an adrenal adenoma, simple resection of the adenoma or removal of the entire adrenal is curative. Potassium levels should be normal before surgery. This can be accomplished with large doses of spironolactone [Aldactone], a potassium-sparing diuretic and aldosterone antagonist, given for several weeks before surgery in conjunction with a low-sodium diet. Some physicians add oral potassium chloride to this regimen for one week prior to surgery.

Hyperaldosteronism caused by bilateral adrenal hyperplasia is usually not cured by partial resection of the glands, and persistent hypertension in the presence of corrected electrolyte balance is common. This form of disease is controlled medically. Despite several drawbacks, spironolactone is the agent of choice. The serum potassium level may become normal within two weeks, although renin levels continue to increase for several months. Normalization of blood pressure may require the addition of another diuretic. In addition to antagonizing the effect of aldosterone, spironolactone also

may inhibit its synthesis directly; an eventual reduction in dose may be possible. Spironolactone has antiandrogenic side effects that may limit its long-term use in some individuals, particularly males.

Other potassium-sparing diuretics also can be used to treat this condition. Triamterene [Dyrenium] 100 to 300 mg daily or amiloride [Midamor] 40 mg/day inhibits potassium excretion by a direct effect on the renal tubules (see Chapter 29, Diuretics). Trilostane also has been used to treat primary hyperaldosteronism.

In one form of primary hyperaldosteronism, aldosterone secretion depends on secretion of ACTH or possibly another pituitary factor. Treatment with a glucocorticoid suppresses aldosterone and corrects hypertension and other aberrations caused by hyperaldosteronism (Ganguly and Donohue, 1983).

Drug Evaluations

AMINOGLUTETHIMIDE
[Cytadren]

ACTIONS. Aminoglutethimide reversibly inhibits adrenal steroid secretion by blocking enzymatic conversion of cholesterol to Δ^5-pregnenolone. The blockade is at an earlier point on the synthetic pathway than that produced by metyrapone. Aminoglutethimide blocks the first step in the biosynthesis of steroids and decreases the secretion of glucocorticoids, mineralocorticoids, and sex steroids. Other steroid-producing tissues also may be affected. In addition, aminoglutethimide inhibits aromatase activity in other tissues, which decreases conversion of androstenedione to estrogens.

USES. Aminoglutethimide is used alone or with other agents to control cortisol secretion in Cushing's syndrome: as an adjunct to pituitary irradiation; to prepare high-risk patients for adrenalectomy; as palliative treatment for metastatic adrenal carcinoma; and for ectopic ACTH-producing tumors. In pituitary-dependent Cushing's syndrome, drug efficacy may decrease as negative feedback of cortisol is reduced and ACTH secretion is thus increased enough to overcome the enzyme blockade. Aminoglutethimide is not curative; relapse occurs upon cessation of therapy.

For the use of aminoglutethimide to treat breast carcinoma, see Chapter 64, Drugs Used in Cancer Chemotherapy.

ADVERSE REACTIONS. Frequent and reversible effects include drowsiness, morbilliform skin rash, nausea, and anorexia. Less common reactions include headache and dizziness, fever and bone marrow depression, hypothyroidism, masculinization and hirsutism in females, and precocious sexual development in males.

666

As the drug becomes effective, adrenal insufficiency with deficiency of both glucocorticoids and mineralocorticoid may result. Hypotension may develop. The incidence of side effects appears to be higher with aminoglutethimide than with metyrapone.

PRECAUTIONS. Adrenal and thyroid function should be monitored, and replacement therapy should be provided if necessary. Aminoglutethimide should not be used in patients hypersensitive to it or to glutethimide.

TERATOGENICITY. Aminoglutethimide is a teratogen in rats. When this drug was administered with anticonvulsants to pregnant women, pseudohermaphroditism was reported in female infants, but normal pregnancies also occurred (FDA Pregnancy Category D).

DRUG INTERACTIONS. If adrenocortical hormone replacement therapy is required, dexamethasone should not be used because its metabolism is accelerated by aminoglutethimide. Hydrocortisone should be used instead.

DOSAGE AND PREPARATIONS.
Oral: Adults, for Cushing's syndrome, 250 mg every six hours initially, increased by 250 mg daily every one to two weeks if necessary to 2 g daily. Plasma cortisol levels are monitored until the desired level of suppression is achieved. Dosage reduction or discontinuation of therapy may be necessary if adverse effects develop.
    Cytadren (CIBA). Tablets 250 mg.

CYPROHEPTADINE HYDROCHLORIDE
[Periactin]

ACTIONS. Cyproheptadine is a serotonin antagonist and antihistamine with anticholinergic and sedative effects. The drug may act directly on pituitary microadenoma cells to decrease ACTH secretion and induce remission in Cushing's disease or Nelson's syndrome.

USES. Cyproheptadine has been used investigationally to control excessive ACTH secretion in Cushing's disease and Nelson's syndrome either as primary treatment or as an adjunct to pituitary irradiation. The drug induces remission in 10% to 50% of patients, and effectiveness may last several years. Discontinuation of therapy usually results in relapse. Cyproheptadine is more effective in adults than in children.

ADVERSE REACTIONS AND PRECAUTIONS. Cyproheptadine causes the adverse effects typical of antihistamines (see Chapter 58, Histamine and Antihistamines). In addition, this drug stimulates the appetite and the potential weight gain would be superimposed on the obesity associated with Cushing's syndrome.

Because of its atropine-like effects, cyproheptadine should be used with caution in patients with bronchial asthma, increased intraocular pressure, hyperthyroidism, cardiovascular disease, or hypertension.

DRUG INTERACTIONS. The anticholinergic effects of cyproheptadine may be increased and prolonged by monoamine oxidase inhibitors. The drug may have additive effects with central nervous system depressants.

PREGNANCY AND LACTATION. Animal studies have revealed no teratogenic effects or evidence of impaired fertility. There are inadequate data to determine the safety of this drug in pregnant women (FDA Pregnancy Category B). It is not known whether cyproheptadine is excreted in human milk.

DOSAGE AND PREPARATIONS.
Oral: Adults, for selected cases of Cushing's disease and Nelson's syndrome, initially 4 mg three times daily increased over a two-week period to 4 mg every four hours. Effectiveness is not increased by larger doses.
    Periactin (Merck Sharp & Dohme), **Generic.** Syrup 2 mg/5 ml; tablets 4 mg.
    (Investigational indication)

METYRAPONE
[Metopirone]

ACTIONS. Metyrapone blocks cortisol production by reversibly blocking 11β-hydroxylase activity in the adrenal cortex. Although the drug also inhibits aldosterone secretion, the production of desoxycorticosterone, a mineralocorticoid, is increased and mineralocorticoid deficiency usually does not occur.

USES. Metyrapone is used investigationally alone or with other agents to control cortisol secretion in Cushing's syndrome. Its use in this disorder is similar to that of aminoglutethimide (see evaluation). The effectiveness of this drug also is overcome by the increased secretion of ACTH in pituitary-dependent disease.

For the use of metyrapone to test anterior pituitary function, see Chapter 42, Agents Related to Anterior Pituitary and Hypothalamic Function.

ADVERSE REACTIONS AND PRECAUTIONS. Side effects of metyrapone include nausea, abdominal distress, drowsiness, headache, dizziness, and skin rash.

Since adrenal insufficiency may occur, especially when metyrapone is given with another adrenal suppressant, such as aminoglutethimide, adrenal function should be monitored. Replacement therapy may be instituted if necessary, or the dose of the drug(s) may be reduced.

PREGNANCY AND LACTATION. When metyrapone is administered to pregnant women during the second and third trimesters, the drug may cause enzymatic blockade in the fetus (FDA Pregnancy Category C). It is not known whether this drug is excreted in human milk.

PHARMACOKINETICS. Metyrapone is well absorbed after oral administration. The drug is excreted in the urine, mostly as glucuronides, and has an elimination half-life of 1 to 2.5 hours.

DOSAGE AND PREPARATIONS.

Oral: For selected patients with Cushing's syndrome, 250 to 500 mg three times daily. Up to 2 g/day has been suggested.
  Metopirone (CIBA). Tablets 250 mg.
  (Investigational indication)

MITOTANE
[Lysodren]

ACTIONS. Mitotane is a relatively specific adrenolytic agent; it rapidly destroys adrenal cortical cells, which decreases the synthesis of adrenal steroid. Peripheral metabolism of steroids also is altered; 17-hydroxysteroid is decreased and 6-β-hydroxycortisol is increased.

USES. Mitotane is used as palliative treatment for metastatic adrenal carcinoma (see Chapter 64, Drugs Used in Cancer Chemotherapy). It has been used investigationally as an adjunct to pituitary irradiation to temporarily inhibit or permanently destroy (depending on dose) adrenal tissue in selected patients with Cushing's syndrome.

ADVERSE REACTIONS AND PRECAUTIONS. Mitotane is relatively toxic and most patients experience adverse effects. Gastrointestinal disturbances (eg, nausea, vomiting, diarrhea) are most common and occur in 80% of patients; central nervous system effects (eg, lethargy, somnolence, dizziness, vertigo) are observed in 40% of patients and dermatitis in 15% of patients. Infrequent effects include visual problems, genito-urinary disturbances (eg, hematuria, cystitis, albuminuria), and cardiovascular effects (eg, flushing, hypertension, orthostatic hypotension).

The effects of mitotane may occur rapidly, and patients should be monitored and treated for adrenal insufficiency (both glucocorticoid and mineralocorticoid replacement) when appropriate. All possible tumor tissue should be removed before administration of the drug to prevent infarction and hemorrhage in the tumor following the rapid adrenolytic action of the drug.

Prolonged administration of mitotane may cause brain damage and behavioral and neurologic impairment.

The safety of mitotane in pregnant and lactating women has not been established.

DOSAGE AND PREPARATIONS.

Oral: Adults, for palliative treatment of metastatic adrenal carcinoma, the total daily dose is divided into three or four amounts. Initially, 3 to 4 g is given daily; the amount is increased after three to six days to 6 to 8 g daily and after another week to 10 g daily. The drug can be continued as long as clinical benefit is evident and adverse effects are tolerable. See also Chapter 64, Drugs Used in Cancer Chemotherapy.

For adjunctive therapy with pituitary irradiation in selected patients with Cushing's syndrome (investigational indication), initially, 4 g daily in divided doses; for maintenance, 1.5 to 2 g daily.
  Lysodren (Bristol). Tablets 500 mg.

SPIRONOLACTONE
[Aldactone]

ACTIONS. This steroidal aldosterone antagonist promotes natriuresis and inhibits potassium excretion by acting directly on the distal renal tubule. Doses exceeding 100 mg/day may inhibit biosynthesis and block the peripheral action of testosterone by competing for androgen receptor sites.

USES. Spironolactone is used to treat primary hyperaldosteronism and to correct potassium depletion prior to surgery in patients with an aldosterone-producing adrenal adenoma. The drug also is used for the long-term treatment of hyperaldosteronism due to bilateral adrenal hyperplasia.

For other uses of spironolactone, see Chapter 28, Antihypertensive Agents, and Chapter 29, Diuretics.

ADVERSE REACTIONS. Spironolactone may cause decreased libido, impotence, tenderness of the breast, and gynecomastia in males. Breast tenderness and menstrual irregularity may occur in females. These side effects may limit the long-term usefulness of the drug, particularly in males. Other effects of spironolactone include diarrhea, rash, urologic disturbances, and increased blood urea nitrogen and serum uric acid levels. Patients with chronic renal failure or those taking potassium supplements concurrently may develop hyperkalemia.

DOSAGE AND PREPARATIONS.

Oral: To prepare patients with aldosterone-producing adrenal adenoma for surgery, *adults,* 300 to 600 mg/day in four divided doses for three to four weeks before surgery. For prolonged treatment of hyperaldosteronism due to bilateral adrenal hyperplasia, initially, 200 to 400 mg daily. The dosage may subsequently be reduced to 75 to 100 mg daily.
  Generic. Tablets 25 mg.
  Aldactone (Searle). Tablets 25, 50, and 100 mg.

TRILOSTANE
[Modrastane]

ACTIONS. This synthetic steroid has no inherent hormonal activity. Trilostane inhibits adrenal 3-β-hydroxysteroid dehydrogenase activity and decreases the secretion of cortisol and aldosterone. When given alone in therapeutic doses, the drug does not suppress adrenal secretion below normal levels, depress testicular testosterone production significantly, or cure the underlying disease process.

Studies in monkeys demonstrated that the peak plasma concentration occurs four hours after oral administration. The metabolites are excreted mainly as glucuronides in the urine.

USES. Trilostane is used in selected patients with Cushing's syndrome to control hypersecretion of glucocorticoids. It has been used investigationally to treat hyperaldosteronism.

ADVERSE REACTIONS AND PRECAUTIONS. Adverse reactions are reported in about one-fourth of patients; they are seldom severe and generally do not necessitate discontinuation of therapy. They can be minimized by using small doses initially and increasing the amount gradually. Gastrointestinal reactions (eg, diarrhea, abdominal discomfort, nausea) occur in about 20% of patients. Effects observed in less than 10% of patients include oral or nasal burning sensation, flushing, and headache.

Although trilostane alone does not produce adrenal insufficiency, the adrenal response to severe stress may be impaired. The therapeutic response to the drug should be monitored. Trilostane should not be given to patients with severe renal or liver disease.

DRUG INTERACTIONS. Because trilostane inhibits aldosterone secretion, the potassium-wasting effect of thiazides or loop diuretics is reduced.

PREGNANCY AND LACTATION. Trilostane should not be given to pregnant patients (FDA Pregnancy Category X), because it inhibits fetal steroidogenesis. It has terminated pregnancy in rats, monkeys, and women through an interceptive mechanism. Concurrent administration of progesterone overcame this effect in monkeys. Skeletal teratogenesis was observed in rats.

It is not known whether trilostane is excreted in human milk but, because of the potential for adrenal suppression in the infant, lactating mothers should not take this drug.

DOSAGE AND PREPARATIONS.
Oral: For selected *adults* with Cushing's syndrome, 30 mg four times a day for at least three days. Thereafter, the dosage may be adjusted at three- to four-day intervals according to the patient's response. The usual range is 120 to 360 mg daily. Doses above 480 mg/day are not recommended.
Modrastane (Winthrop-Breon). Capsules 30 and 60 mg.

REPLACEMENT OF ADRENOCORTICAL HORMONES

Corticosteroid replacement is required when there is a defect at any level of the hypothalamic-pituitary-adrenal axis. Conditions requiring therapy include those associated with destruction of the adrenal glands, inadequate secretion of ACTH or CRF, or congenital defects in steroidogenesis. The goal of therapy is to provide enough exogenous hormone to maintain normal function in dependent body systems. The doses used are small compared to those employed in nonendocrine diseases; thus, many adverse reactions encountered with use of pharmacologic amounts do not occur.

Replacement therapy for primary, secondary, or tertiary adrenal insufficiency should simulate normal glucocorticoid secretory patterns. Administration of two-thirds of the daily dose in the morning and one-third in the afternoon approximates this pattern satisfactorily. When a mineralocorticoid is needed, it is customarily given once daily. Children with congenital adrenal hyperplasia require not only replacement of

cortisol but also suppression of ACTH secretion; for the optimum schedule, see the discussion on Congenital Adrenal Hyperplasia Syndromes.

PRIMARY ADRENOCORTICAL INSUFFICIENCY. Addison's disease is associated with adrenal atrophy, which may be idiopathic or caused by autoimmune disease or destruction of the cortex by tuberculosis, histoplasmosis, metastatic carcinoma, or hemorrhage. It also may be induced by etomidate [Amidate], an anesthetic, which has been reported to inhibit adrenal steroidogenesis and may produce hypoadrenalism by blocking steroid biosynthetic enzyme activities (Fry and Griffiths, 1984; Wagner et al, 1984).

Signs and symptoms include weakness, weight loss, hyperpigmentation, anorexia, nausea, vomiting, hypoglycemia, hypotension, hyponatremia, and hyperkalemia. Since production of both cortisol and aldosterone is deficient, mineralocorticoid and glucocorticoid replacement is necessary. The goals of therapy are to re-establish strength, weight, normal mental processes, normal blood pressure, and electrolyte balance.

Hydrocortisone and cortisone (which is converted to cortisol, the active steroid) are preferred because they possess both glucocorticoid and weak mineralocorticoid activity. A more potent mineralocorticoid often is added to the regimen; if orthostatic hypotension persists despite cortisol replacement therapy and liberal salt intake, the dose of the mineralocorticoid is increased. The mineralocorticoid most commonly used for this purpose is fludrocortisone [Florinef], which is the only oral preparation available; desoxycorticosterone acetate [Doca Acetate, Percorten] also can be used but must be administered intramuscularly. Neither compound has significant glucocorticoid activity in the doses employed to achieve sodium balance.

SECONDARY AND TERTIARY ADRENOCORTICAL INSUFFICIENCY. *Secondary adrenocortical insufficiency* is caused by inadequate secretion of ACTH resulting from surgical ablation of the pituitary, pituitary disease, or prolonged administration of pharmacologic doses of glucocorticoids (see Chapter 61). *Tertiary adrenocortical insufficiency* is caused by inadequate secretion of CRH (see Chapter 42, Agents Related to Anterior Pituitary and Hypothalamic Function). The secondary and tertiary forms have similar symptoms and cannot easily be distinguished. Mineralocorticoid secretion is generally not impaired, but dilutional hyponatremia may result from glucocorticoid insufficiency. Symptoms are characteristic of glucocorticoid insufficiency and include fasting hypoglycemia, malaise, anorexia, vomiting, and inability to handle stress. Hyperpigmentation does not occur.

Replacement therapy is the same for secondary and tertiary adrenal insufficiency. The dose of glucocorticoid (usually hydrocortisone, cortisone, or prednisone) must be individualized. Mineralocorticoid replacement usually is not required.

Panhypopituitarism requires replacement of thyroid as well as adrenal hormones. The glucocorticoid should be administered alone until normal adrenal function is re-established. If thyroid hormone is administered first, acute adrenal insufficiency may be precipitated. Children also require replacement of growth hormone and gonadotropins (or androgens or estrogens).

Isolated *hypoaldosteronism* has been described in patients

with moderate renal impairment. Renin levels are reduced, possibly due to expanded extracellular fluid volume or damage to the juxtaglomerular apparatus, and decreased aldosterone secretion and hyperkalemia result. Fludrocortisone [Florinef] corrects the hyperkalemia.

ACUTE ADRENAL INSUFFICIENCY (CRISIS). Adrenal (addisonian) crisis can be caused by acute adrenal or pituitary failure (following neurosurgery, head trauma, or hemorrhagic shock), failure to maintain adrenal replacement therapy, rapid withdrawal of large doses of corticosteroids, or failure to provide additional corticosteroids to dependent patients subjected to stress. Occasionally, patients with borderline adrenal insufficiency are diagnosed after an unusual stress (eg, severe infection, surgery) induces adrenal crisis. Symptoms include fever, hypotension, dehydration, weakness, vomiting, and diarrhea. If untreated, this condition proceeds to shock and death. Crisis of the classic addisonian type results from deficiencies of both cortisol and aldosterone leading to sodium loss and marked dehydration.

Rapid replacement of salt, fluids, and glucocorticoids is required; a mineralocorticoid also may be administered. Initially, hydrocortisone is given intravenously as a bolus, followed by normal (0.9%) saline with dextrose in amounts sufficient to correct the blood pressure, and then by slow intravenous infusion of hydrocortisone. Intramuscular injection of cortisone acetate generally should not be given because absorption may be erratic and insufficient. The amount of saline administered in the first 24 hours depends upon the degree of dehydration and is generally less than 5% of ideal body weight but may exceed 10%, particularly in children. The total dose of hydrocortisone in adults during the first 24 hours is about 200 mg/M^2. The amount is reduced gradually to replacement levels during the next several days. The underlying condition (eg, infection, hemorrhage) is treated concurrently.

CONGENITAL ADRENAL HYPERPLASIA SYNDROMES (CAH). In these syndromes, the synthesis of cortisol and sometimes aldosterone is partially or completely deficient due to an inherited enzyme deficiency. Clinical manifestations depend upon the specific enzyme(s) involved but, in all patients, the initial low plasma cortisol levels increase the secretion of ACTH by the pituitary because of lack of negative feedback control; adrenal hyperplasia results. If the enzyme deficiency is partial, the increased ACTH secretion may raise cortisol levels to normal. In all patients, hypersecretion of the steroids occurs prior to the enzyme block or overproduction of steroids occurs from an alternate pathway. Therefore, symptoms may be related to either a hormone deficiency or an excess of a related steroid.

In 21-hydroxylase deficiency, which accounts for up to 95% of cases, hypersecretion of ACTH (in response to low cortisol levels) results in excessive secretion of adrenal androgen, particularly androstenedione, which is partially metabolized peripherally to testosterone, causing virilization. The pathways to cortisol and, in severe cases, to aldosterone, are partially or completely blocked. The 21-hydroxylase deficiency can occur as the simple virilizing form or as the salt-losing form. The two conditions may represent extremes of a continuum of severity of enzyme deficiency.

The salt-losing form develops in about two-thirds of patients

with 21-hydroxylase deficiency (Fife and Rappaport, 1983). The enzyme deficiency is most severe in this form and affects both cortisol and aldosterone synthesis. It has been suggested that the deficiency is limited to the zona fasciculata in the simple virilizing form, but also involves the zona glomerulosa in the salt-losing form (Kuhnle et al, 1981). Salt loss is exacerbated by the natriuretic effect of progesterone and 17-hydroxyprogesterone, which accumulate in large quantities as a result of the enzyme block. All patients with 21-hydroxylase CAH probably develop some degree of mineralocorticoid deficiency and progesterone natriuresis with a resultant decrease in total body sodium, and, possibly, increased plasma renin activity. However, the defect may not be severe enough to warrant treatment or classification as the salt-losing form.

In 21-hydroxylase CAH, impairment of cortisol secretion is partially compensated by increased ACTH secretion; plasma cortisol may be low in the salt-losing form or normal in the simple virilizing form. Therefore, initial cortisol deficiency may not be of major clinical significance if compensation is adequate. However, the cortisol response to stress may be diminished, and these patients may require supplementary doses of corticosteroids to avoid addisonian crisis during stress.

The ultimate result of 21-hydroxylase deficiency is lack of inhibitory feedback control of cortisol, which increases the secretion of ACTH and leads to hyperplasia of the adrenal cortex. Excessive secretion of adrenal androgens by the fetus ensues, causing masculinization of the external genitalia in female neonates; in affected infants, sexual ambiguity may result and necessitate surgical correction. The excessive androgens do not, however, affect either the gonads or the internal ducts. Therefore, female infants have normal ovaries, fallopian tubes, and uterus despite ambiguous external genitalia. Excessive androgen production is not always apparent in male infants, but may be manifested by phallic enlargement and scrotal pigmentation. Virilization in females is more severe in the salt-losing form. In untreated cases, signs of progressive masculinization occur in both sexes.

Rarer forms of CAH are associated with deficiencies of other enzymes. Deficiency of 11-β-hydroxylase results in hypersecretion of androgen, which causes masculinizing effects, and of desoxycorticosterone, which causes salt retention and hypertension. Administration of sufficient hydrocortisone to control the secretion of ACTH suppresses the secretion of androgen and desoxycorticosterone and normalizes blood pressure.

In 3-β-hydroxysteroid dehydrogenase deficiency, the synthesis of cortisol and aldosterone is impaired (leading to salt loss), but masculinizing effects on female fetuses are minimal because the androgen that is secreted in excess, dehydroepiandrosterone, has weak biological activity. A similar enzyme defect in the testes prevents formation of testosterone, and the genitalia of male infants are incompletely masculinized. This condition has a high mortality rate during infancy.

In 17-hydroxylase deficiency, androgen and estrogen synthesis are impaired in the adrenal glands and gonads. This may affect the development of the male external genitalia and result in male pseudohermaphroditism. The adrenals secrete excessive amounts of desoxycorticosterone, which causes hypertension. Secretion of corticosterone also is increased to compensate for decreased cortisol output.

Complete block of steroid synthesis by the adrenal glands and gonads occurs in cholesterol 20-, 22-desmolase deficiency. If the enzymatic deficiency is marked, early death often results. In less severe cases, there is salt loss as well as cortisol deficiency. The effect on the development of genitalia is similar to that in 17-hydroxylase and 3-β-hydroxysteroid dehydrogenase deficiencies. In these three deficiencies, pubertal development must be induced in both sexes.

Late onset or attenuated (previously designated "acquired") CAH has been diagnosed in late childhood to adulthood (Bongiovanni, 1981; Migeon, 1981; Bartter, 1983). Deficiency of 21-hydroxylase may be detected around the time of puberty in females who present with hirsutism, acne, and possibly clitoral enlargement. In addition to these characteristics, patients with 11-hydroxylase deficiency may develop hypertension and hypokalemia. Both attenuated deficiencies may be associated with polycystic ovarian disease and/or infertility in females. Fertility can be restored when adrenal activity is suppressed by glucocorticoid therapy or, in some cases, glucocorticoid plus clomiphene [Clomid] (Birnbaum and Rose, 1984).

The excess androgen secretion associated with these disorders may not be noticed in puberal males. However, early hypertension with hypokalemia in males suggests 11-hydroxylase deficiency. Late onset of an incomplete form of 3-β-hydroxysteroid dehydrogenase deficiency is characterized by hirsutism and oligomenorrhea in adult women. Reports of serum androgen levels are somewhat inconsistent, but Δ^5-steroids (eg, dehydroepiandrosterone sulfate) appear to be increased more than Δ^4-steroids (eg, androstenedione, testosterone) (Lobo and Goebelsmann, 1981; Pang et al, 1985).

Treatment: The goals of treatment are to correct the hormonal imbalance and allow growth to normal height, prevent virilism in girls or prepubertal sexual development in boys, and allow normal puberty and fertility. As in other types of adrenocortical insufficiency, cortisol is replaced (as hydrocortisone or cortisone). In patients with salt-losing CAH, a mineralocorticoid is prescribed. Mineralocorticoids also are sometimes used in patients not losing salt who are difficult to control and have high plasma renin levels. In patients with hypertensive forms of CAH, hormone replacement is provided by a glucocorticoid with minimal mineralocorticoid activity (eg, prednisone), and salt restriction is required rarely. Potent preparations (eg, dexamethasone) may be used if the dose is monitored carefully to avoid overdosage, which can cause growth retardation and iatrogenic Cushing's syndrome.

Dosage must be individualized on the basis of clinical and laboratory assessments of the patient's condition. Enough corticosteroid is given to suppress ACTH secretion (and thus excess androgen production), but not enough to cause cushingoid changes or inhibit growth. Usually, the dose is equivalent to about twice the amount of cortisol secreted daily. One-third may be given in the morning and two-thirds in the evening. Thus, the larger portion of hormone is taken late in the day, which theoretically provides maximum suppression of peak ACTH secretion early in the morning. Alternatively, the steroid is administered in three equal doses evenly spaced throughout the day.

The necessity for glucocorticoid replacement is life-long. If therapy is withdrawn before growth is complete, height may be compromised due to premature epiphyseal closure. Later in life, lack of adrenal suppression causes virilization and menstrual disorders in females. In adult males, however, excessive adrenal androgen secretion does not interfere significantly with the normal feedback control of gonadotropins. Hence, untreated adult males have normal plasma testosterone levels despite slightly, but not abnormally, low serum LH levels and normal fertility. CAH patients who discontinue glucocorticoid therapy later in life are at risk of inadequate adrenal response to stress (infections, surgery, or trauma).

In patients with the salt-losing forms of CAH, desoxycorticosterone or fludrocortisone is administered for mineralocorticoid replacement. Desoxycorticosterone is given parenterally as pellets or by intramuscular injection and fludrocortisone is given orally. Although the salt-losing tendency is most severe early in life, most physicians continue mineralocorticoid and glucocorticoid therapy throughout life. If the mineralocorticoid is discontinued, there is a greater risk of adrenal insufficiency, especially in the presence of salt deprivation. Furthermore, it has been suggested that prolonged replacement of mineralocorticoid may allow use of smaller doses of glucocorticoids.

Careful, frequent (every three months) monitoring of young patients is required to adjust the dose of glucocorticoid to the size and individual requirements of the growing child. Both overtreatment and undertreatment can compromise adult height, the former by directly inhibiting growth and the latter by allowing excessive androgen secretion and premature epiphyseal closure. Follow-up examination should include assessment of growth rate (most important single parameter) including bone age, monitoring for signs of virilization, and testing for hypertension, which indicates mineralocorticoid overdosage in salt-losing CAH. Laboratory analyses of electrolytes and appropriate steroids also are performed at regular intervals, although some practitioners believe plasma steroid values to be of limited value in monitoring the effectiveness of treatment.

In 21-hydroxylase deficiency, elevated urinary 17-ketosteroids and pregnanetriol levels indicate undertreatment. Although the assay of plasma 17-hydroxyprogesterone has largely replaced measurement of urinary steroids and obviates the inconvenience of 24-hour urine collection, levels of this steroid fluctuate with a circadian rhythmicity. Therefore, serial samples should be taken or measurements should be standardized for time of day. It has been suggested that plasma androstenedione levels correlate best with urinary steroid excretion. Newer assays for salivary 17-hydroxyprogesterone and androstenedione also are used to monitor patients with CAH. However, it has been suggested that biochemical measurements appear to be more effective in detecting undertreatment than in distinguishing between optimal and overtreatment. This is because overtreated patients may not exhibit a corresponding decrease in serum levels of diagnostic steroid (Hendricks et al, 1982).

Measurements of appropriate steroids to monitor other CAH syndromes depend on the associated enzyme deficiency.

Salt-Losing Crisis: Infants with diagnosed CAH or those with ambiguous genitalia should be observed closely for signs of salt-losing crisis. This generally occurs between the first and third weeks of life, but may be seen earlier or later. Affected infants eat poorly, vomit, and are dehydrated; death occurs rapidly without adequate treatment. Fluids containing normal saline and hydrocortisone are administered intravenously, and intramuscular desoxycorticosterone is given initially. Potassium is avoided because hyperkalemia may be present, but it may be needed later in the course of treatment. Serum electrolytes and hematocrit values should be monitored until the condition of the infant stabilizes. Following the crisis, maintenance therapy is initiated.

Precautions: All patients receiving glucocorticoid replacement therapy require supplemental doses (two to three times replacement amounts) during physical stress. The dose must be increased in proportion to the severity of the stress. Temporary, excessive doses are preferred to inadequate replacement. During mild illness, such as upper respiratory infections, doubling the maintenance dose usually is sufficient. When the oral intake of steroids is not possible for any reason, including vomiting, a parenteral preparation (hydrocortisone, cortisone acetate, prednisolone phosphate or succinate, or dexamethasone sodium phosphate) should be given intramuscularly. When mineralocorticoids are required, the dose also must be increased and adequate salt replacement assured or hyponatremia may result; desoxycorticosterone should be given intramuscularly if the child is vomiting, has diarrhea, or experiences severe dehydration.

Patients receiving replacement therapy who are undergoing major surgery require about five times the replacement dose during, immediately before, and, after the procedure. Replacement of salt, fluid, and mineralocorticoid is prescribed as necessary. If adequate amounts of steroids are administered, salt and fluid replacement is similar to that for any patient undergoing similar surgery. If the postoperative course is uncomplicated, the dose can be reduced gradually over two to five days to the usual replacement amount. The physician and patient should be aware that prolonged overtreatment will result in the gradual development of cushingoid symptoms.

The steroid dependence and increased dosage requirement under widely variable conditions of stress are of utmost importance and should be understood by the patient or parents. All such patients should carry an identification card and bracelet indicating their dependence on steroid medication. In addition, care should be taken to assure that an adequate supply of steroids is available at all times for emergencies. This should include oral medication and a glucocorticoid suitable for intramuscular injection. An injectable mineralocorticoid also should be available for patients who require it. Older patients should be taught to self-administer injections and parents should be trained to administer these injections to their children.

Drug Evaluations

Except when noted, the choice of preparation depends largely on the relative mineralocorticoid/glucocorticoid poten-

cy desired, the route of administration preferred, and the appropriate duration of action. Drugs with similar relative potencies and durations of action generally are considered to be equivalent therapeutically (see the table in Chapter 61, Adrenal Corticosteroids in Nonendocrine Diseases). Factors such as cost, preference for older drugs for which cumulative experience is greater, and commercial availability often dictate the selection.

Oral preparations are used most commonly. Parenteral preparations are employed when oral medication cannot be used, during emergencies, and for critically ill patients.

See also Chapter 61, Adrenal Corticosteroids in Nonendocrine Diseases.

HYDROCORTISONE
[Cortef, Hydrocortone]

HYDROCORTISONE CYPIONATE
[Cortef]

HYDROCORTISONE SODIUM PHOSPHATE
[Hydrocortone Phosphate]

HYDROCORTISONE SODIUM SUCCINATE
[A-hydroCort, Solu-Cortef]

USES. Hydrocortisone is a preferred drug for replacement therapy in acute or chronic adrenocortical insufficiency and salt-losing forms of congenital adrenal hyperplasia because it has both glucocorticoid and weak mineralocorticoid activities and is chemically identical to cortisol, the endogenous glucocorticoid.

The oral preparations (base and cypionate salt) are often used for replacement therapy. The water-soluble forms (sodium phosphate, sodium succinate) are given intravenously or intramuscularly in emergencies, such as acute adrenocortical insufficiency (addisonian crisis); for salt-losing crisis in congenital adrenal hyperplasia; or to prepare patients who require replacement therapy for major surgery.

DOSAGE AND PREPARATIONS.

Oral: For chronic adrenocortical insufficiency, 12 to 15 mg/M^2 daily. The daily dosage may be divided, with two-thirds given in the morning upon arising and one-third in the afternoon, to simulate normal adrenocortical secretion.

For congenital adrenal hyperplasia, the dosage must be carefully individualized according to the requirement of each patient. The following dosages are suggested: 25 mg/M^2/24 hours (one-third given every eight hours) or one-third given in the morning and two-thirds in the evening for maximum suppression of the early morning surge of corticotropic secretion.

HYDROCORTISONE:
Cortef (Upjohn). Tablets 5, 10, and 20 mg.
Hydrocortone (Merck Sharp & Dohme), *Generic*. Tablets 10 and 20 mg.
HYDROCORTISONE CYPIONATE:
Cortef (Upjohn). Oral suspension equivalent to hydrocortisone 10 mg/5 ml.

Intravenous: The dosage depends on the size of the patient; smaller doses are appropriate for infants. In emergencies, initially, 100 mg, repeated if necessary. Larger doses have been suggested for shock (50 mg/kg). For salt-losing crisis in congenital adrenal hyperplasia, 50 to 100 mg with intravenous fluids for one to two days until the crisis is controlled.

Intramuscular: The dosage depends on the size of the patient; smaller doses are appropriate for infants. For emergencies when the intravenous route is not feasible, initially, 100 to 250 mg, repeated if necessary.

HYDROCORTISONE SODIUM PHOSPHATE:
Hydrocortone Phosphate (Merck Sharp & Dohme). Solution 50 mg/ml in 2 and 10 ml containers.
HYDROCORTISONE SODIUM SUCCINATE:
A-hydroCort (Abbott), *Solu-Cortef* (Upjohn), *Generic*. Powder 100, 250, and 500 mg and 1 g.

CORTISONE ACETATE
[Cortone Acetate]

USES. Cortisone acetate is readily converted in the body to cortisol, the naturally occurring active form. Like hydrocortisone, it is a preferred drug for replacement therapy in chronic adrenocortical insufficiency and for most patients with salt-losing forms of congenital adrenal hyperplasia because it has both glucocorticoid and mild mineralocorticoid effects. In anti-inflammatory effect, 25 mg of cortisone acetate is equivalent to 20 mg of hydrocortisone; the mineralocorticoid activity of the two drugs is approximately equal.

See the Introduction for specific indications and precautions.

DOSAGE AND PREPARATIONS.

Oral: For chronic adrenocortical insufficiency, 12 to 15 mg/M^2 daily. The daily dosage may be divided, with two-thirds given in the morning upon arising and one-third in the afternoon, to simulate normal adrenocortical secretion.

For congenital adrenal hyperplasia, 20 to 30 mg/M^2 daily. The dosage is divided as for hydrocortisone (see the evaluation). The dosage must be carefully individualized according to the requirements of each patient.

Generic. Tablets 5, 10, and 25 mg.
Cortone Acetate (Merck Sharp & Dohme). Tablets 25 mg.

Intramuscular: Initially, 20 to 300 mg daily, depending upon the disorder being treated, with the highest doses used for severe shock or cardiovascular collapse. The dose is adjusted

until the patient's response is satisfactory within a reasonable period of time. Maintenance dosage is determined by gradually decreasing the initial dose to the lowest dose that maintains adequate clinical response. Cortisone generally should not be given intramuscularly for acute adrenal insufficiency because absorption may be erratic and insufficient.

Cortone Acetate (Merck Sharp & Dohme), *Generic*. Suspension 25 mg/ml in 10 and 20 ml containers (*Cortone Acetate* 20 ml only) and 50 mg/ml in 10 ml containers.

DESOXYCORTICOSTERONE ACETATE
[Doca Acetate, Percorten Acetate]

DESOXYCORTICOSTERONE PIVALATE
[Percorten Pivalate]

ACTIONS AND USES. Desoxycorticosterone, a mineralocorticoid, primarily affects the metabolism of sodium, potassium, and water. When given to treat adrenal insufficiency, it decreases the hematocrit and the excretion of sodium and increases blood volume, extracellular fluid, and excretion of potassium.

Desoxycorticosterone is of historic interest because it was the first corticosteroid synthesized and available for clinical use. This mineralocorticoid has almost no glucocorticoid activity and is available for parenteral administration as replacement therapy in chronic primary adrenocortical insufficiency and salt-losing forms of congenital adrenal hyperplasia when the patient is unable to take oral medication. It is administered with appropriate doses of a glucocorticoid, such as hydrocortisone. Desoxycorticosterone is available in oil solution, aqueous suspension, or pellets for subcutaneous implantation. These preparations are usually not given for maintenance therapy if oral medication can be taken.

ADVERSE REACTIONS. If the dose, treatment period, or intake of dietary sodium is excessive, adverse reactions result from sodium and water retention and potassium loss (eg, hypertension, edema, hypokalemia, cardiac enlargement, congestive heart failure).

DOSAGE AND PREPARATIONS.

Intramuscular: For chronic primary adrenocortical insufficiency, initially, 1 to 2 mg desoxycorticosterone acetate (solution in oil) daily. For salt-losing congenital adrenal hyperplasia, 1 to 2 mg daily for the first three or four days; thereafter, dosage is adjusted on the basis of clinical response and the serum electrolyte level. In contrast to the dosage of glucocorticoid, which must be adjusted to body size, the dosage of mineralocorticoid is similar at all ages. After the maintenance dose is determined (usually 1 mg), the long-acting, microcrystalline aqueous suspension of desoxycorticosterone pivalate should be given at a rate of 1 ml (25 mg) for each milligram of desoxycorticosterone acetate solution in oil; the pivalate suspension is injected intramuscularly through a 20-gauge needle into the upper outer quadrant of one or both buttocks. The average dose is 25 mg every four weeks.

DESOXYCORTICOSTERONE ACETATE:
Doca Acetate (Organon). Solution (in sesame oil) 5 mg/ml in 10 ml containers.
DESOXYCORTICOSTERONE PIVALATE:
Percorten Pivalate (CIBA). Suspension (repository) 15 mg/ml in 4 ml containers.

Subcutaneous Implantation: After the patient has been maintained on desoxycorticosterone acetate for at least two to three months, pellet implantation may be substituted. Once every 8 to 12 months, one pellet is implanted for each 0.5 mg of solution required daily for maintenance.
DESOXYCORTICOSTERONE ACETATE:
Percorten Acetate (CIBA). Pellets containing approximately 125 mg.

FLUDROCORTISONE ACETATE
[Florinef Acetate]

USES. Fludrocortisone is a halogenated derivative of cortisol. It has very potent mineralocorticoid and moderate glucocorticoid effects and is, therefore, useful for mineralocorticoid replacement therapy in primary chronic adrenocortical insufficiency, salt-losing forms of congenital adrenal hyperplasia, and hyperkalemia associated with isolated hypoaldosteronism. This is the only oral mineralocorticoid available. It is not suitable for use as an anti-inflammatory agent.

ADVERSE REACTIONS. Adverse reactions include hypertension, edema, hypokalemia, and cardiac hypertrophy. Salt intake must be adjusted to meet individual requirements.

DOSAGE AND PREPARATIONS.
Oral: For chronic primary adrenocortical insufficiency, 0.05 to 0.1 mg (50 to 100 mcg) daily (range, 0.05 to 0.2 mg daily). For salt-losing forms of congenital adrenal hyperplasia, initially, up to 0.2 mg (200 mcg) daily; this can be reduced gradually to 0.05 to 0.1 mg (50 to 100 mcg) daily over several months.
Florinef Acetate (Squibb). Tablets 0.1 mg.

PREDNISOLONE
[Delta-Cortef, Sterane]

PREDNISONE
[Deltasone, Meticorten, Orasone, SK-Prednisone]

USES. Prednisolone and prednisone are Δ-1 analogues of hydrocortisone and cortisone, respectively. They are available as oral and parenteral preparations (see Chapter 61). Prednisone is converted in the body to the active compound, prednisolone.

Because they have little mineralocorticoid activity, neither drug is suitable as the sole agent in primary adrenocortical insufficiency. However, they can be used for replacement therapy in secondary adrenocortical insufficiency or hypertensive (salt-retaining) forms of congenital adrenal hyperplasia. When given with a mineralocorticoid, prednisolone or prednisone also can be used in primary adrenocortical insufficiency or salt-losing forms of congenital adrenal hyperplasia. These agents are sometimes preferred for congenital adrenal hyperplasia because they are longer acting than hydrocortisone or cortisone and more readily induce adrenocortical suppression throughout the day.

DOSAGE AND PREPARATIONS.
Oral: For replacement therapy, 4 mg/M² daily. The daily dosage may be divided, with two-thirds given in the morning upon arising and one-third in the afternoon, to simulate normal glucocorticoid secretion. For congenital adrenal hyperplasia, 5 mg/M² daily given in two or three divided doses.

PREDNISOLONE:
Delta-Cortef (Upjohn), *Sterane* (Pfipharmecs), *Generic.* Tablets 5 mg.
PREDNISONE:
Generic. Tablets 1, 2.5, 5, 10, 20, 25, and 50 mg.
Deltasone (Upjohn). Tablets 2.5, 5, 10, 20, and 50 mg.
Meticorten (Schering). Tablets 1 mg.
Orasone (Rowell). Tablets 1, 5, 10, 20, and 50 mg.
SK-Prednisone (Smith Kline & French). Tablets 5 mg.

Cited References

Adler GK, Williams GH: Primary aldosteronism, in Krieger DT, Bardin CW (eds): *Current Therapy in Endocrinology and Metabolism 1985-1986.* St Louis, CV Mosby, 1985, 116-121.

Bartter FC: Late-onset virilizing congenital adrenal hyperplasia, in Krieger DT, Bardin CW (eds): *Current Therapy in Endocrinology, 1983-1984.* St Louis, CV Mosby, 1983.

Birnbaum MD, Rose LI: Late onset adrenocortical hydroxylase deficiencies associated with menstrual dysfunction. *Obstet Gynecol* 63:445-451, 1984.

Bongiovanni AM: Acquired adrenal hyperplasia: With special reference to 3β-hydroxysteroid dehydrogenase. *Fertil Steril* 35:599-608, 1981.

Fife D, Rappaport EB: Prevalence of salt-losing among congenital adrenal hyperplasia patients. *Clin Endocrinol* 19:259-264, 1983.

Fry DE, Griffiths H: Inhibition by etomidate of the 11β-hydroxylation of cortisol. *Clin Endocrinol* 20:625-629, 1984.

Ganguly A, Donohue JP: Primary aldosteronism: Pathophysiology, diagnosis and treatment. *J Urol* 129:241-247, 1983.

Hendricks SA, et al: Urinary and serum steroid concentrations in management of congenital adrenal hyperplasia: Lack of physiologic correlations. *Am J Dis Child* 136:229-232, 1982.

Horton R, Hsueh WA: Primary aldosteronism, in Krieger DT, Bardin CW (eds): *Current Therapy in Endocrinology 1983-1984*. St Louis, CV Mosby, 1983, 127-130.

Kuhnle U, et al: 21-hydroxylase activity in glomerulosa and fasciculata of adrenal cortex in congenital adrenal hyperplasia. *J Clin Endocrinol Metab* 52:534-544, 1981.

Lobo RA, Goebelsmann U: Evidence for reduced 3β-ol-hydroxysteroid dehydrogenase activity in some hirsute women thought to have polycystic ovary syndrome. *J Clin Endocrinol Metab* 53:394-400, 1981.

Migeon CJ: Physiology and pathology of adrenocortical function in infancy and childhood, in Collu R, et al (eds): *Pediatric Endocrinology*. New York, Raven Press, 1981.

Orth DN: Cushing's syndrome, in Krieger DT, Bardin CW (eds): *Current Therapy in Endocrinology 1983-1984*. St Louis, CV Mosby, 1983.

Pang S, et al: Late-onset adrenal steroid 3β-hydroxysteroid dehydrogenase deficiency. I. Cause of hirsutism in pubertal and postpubertal women. *J Clin Endocrinol Metab* 60:428-439, 1985.

Tuck ML: Disorders of aldosterone secretion, in Carlson HE (ed): *Endocrinology*. New York, John Wiley & Sons, 1983, 143-155.

Vale W, et al: Characteristics of 41-residue ovine hypothalamic peptide that stimulates secretion of corticotropin and β-endorphin. *Science* 213:1394-1397, 1981.

Wagner RL, et al: Inhibition of adrenal steroidogenesis by anesthetic etomidate. *N Engl J Med* 310:1415-1421, 1984.

Other Selected References

Batlle DC, Kurtzman NA: Syndromes of aldosterone deficiency and excess. *Med Clin North Am* 67:879-902, 1983.

Hughes IA: Congenital and acquired disorders of adrenal cortex. *Clin Endocrinol Metab* 11:89-125, 1982.

Krieger DT: Physiopathology of Cushing's disease. *Endocrinol Rev* 4:22-43, 1983.

Androgens and Anabolic Steroids

Physiology

Androgens and proandrogens are secreted by the testes in males, the ovaries in females, and the adrenal cortex in both sexes. In males, androgens are responsible for the development and maintenance of secondary sexual characteristics, normal reproductive function, and sexual performance ability, as well as for stimulating the growth and development of the skeleton and skeletal muscle during puberty. In women, androgens are responsible for growth of pubic hair and possibly for stimulation of libido. They also act as estrogen precursors, particularly after menopause. Excessive production of androgens from the ovary or adrenal cortex causes masculinizing effects ranging from acne, hirsutism, hoarseness, and menstrual irregularities to baldness, permanent deepening of the voice, and clitoral enlargement.

Men: Testosterone is the principal androgen secreted by the steroidogenic Leydig cells, which are located in the interstitial spaces of the testis. Men produce 2.5 to 10 mg of testosterone daily and plasma concentrations are 350 to 1,000 ng/dl. Plasma levels fluctuate in a circadian pattern in young men and are maximal in the early morning. Superimposed on this rhythm are shorter, smaller, secretory peaks that follow elevated luteinizing hormone secretion within hours. These variations in plasma hormone levels demonstrate the importance of multiple blood sampling in some experimental and diagnostic situations.

In males, about half of the 17-ketosteroids (testosterone precursors or proandrogens) are secreted by the adrenal cortex. However, since the rate of conversion to testosterone is low, adrenal androgens are not as important functionally as the smaller amount of testosterone produced by the testis. If Leydig cell function is lost or markedly impaired, the amount of testosterone produced by conversion of the adrenocortical proandrogens, androstenedione and dehydroepiandrosterone, is inadequate to maintain normal male function.

The anterior pituitary hormone, luteinizing hormone (LH), originally called interstitial cell-stimulating hormone (ICSH), stimulates steroidogenesis in the Leydig cells. Follicle-stimulating hormone (FSH) is necessary to initiate spermatogenesis. A negative feedback system involving the hypothalamus, the anterior pituitary, and the testis controls hormone secretion. Testosterone suppresses secretion of LH and, to a lesser extent, FSH. Inhibin, a peptide probably elaborated by the Sertoli cells of the seminiferous tubules, also inhibits release of FSH. Estradiol, which is secreted by the testis and produced by the peripheral conversion of testosterone and other androgens, also participates in the negative feedback control of LH and FSH. Synthetic androgens that cannot be aromatized to estrogen (eg, oxandrolone, mesterolone) are less effective in suppressing gonadotropins than testosterone, which can be aromatized.

In men, approximately 98% of circulating testosterone is bound to protein, primarily to sex hormone-binding globulin (SHBG, testosterone-estradiol-binding globulin) and albumin. As with other steroid hormones, the biologically active portion is the free (dialyzable, unbound) fraction. The hepatic synthesis of SHBG is decreased by androgens and elevated by estrogens. Consequently, men have higher levels of free circulating testosterone than women, both proportionately and in total amount. In contrast, because of their high total estradiol secretion, women have higher free estradiol concentrations even though a smaller fraction of plasma estradiol is unbound.

The half-life of endogenous free testosterone in the blood is 10 to 20 minutes. Testosterone is metabolized primarily in the liver and is excreted mainly in the urine as the metabolites, androsterone and etiocholanolone. Small amounts of testosterone glucuronide and sulfate also are excreted. About 6% of the hormone is excreted unaltered in the feces. Synthetic androgens are also metabolized by reduction of the Δ4-3 keto function and oxidation elsewhere on the molecule, but their plasma half-lives are longer because they are metabolized more slowly. Synthetic androgens may be excreted as unaltered hormone or as metabolites.

The steroidogenic activity of LH is mediated through stimulation of cyclic adenosine monophosphate (cAMP) and calmodulin synthesis. The androgenic action of testosterone in some tissues (eg, prostate, seminal vesicle, external genitalia) normally depends upon the intracellular reduction of testosterone to 5α-dihydrotestosterone (DHT), which binds to the specific androgen receptor in the cytoplasm of these tissues. In other tissues (eg, skeletal muscle, bone marrow, Sertoli cells), testosterone itself is probably the active intracellular hormone. In the central nervous system, the hormonal effects of testosterone may result in part from its aromatization to estradiol. The ultimate effect of the steroid-receptor complex is to influence production of messenger RNA to direct protein synthesis in the cell.

Women: Under normal conditions, the ovaries and adrenal cortex secrete relatively little testosterone in women. Instead, they secrete primarily preandrogens, such as 4-androstenedione and dehydroepiandrosterone, which are metabolized to testosterone in most peripheral tissues. The overall production of testosterone in women averages 0.23 mg daily and normal plasma concentrations are 15 to 65 ng/dl. About one-half of plasma testosterone is produced by peripheral conversion of androstenedione, and the other one-half is derived equally from other ovarian and adrenal secretory products. Adrenal dehydroepiandrosterone sulfate is the androgen secreted in greatest quantity after adrenarche, but it is less important functionally because of its low rate of conversion to testosterone.

Secretion of androgen by the adrenal cortex is stimulated principally by corticotropin (ACTH), while ovarian androgens are secreted in response to LH. Probably because 50% of androstenedione is of adrenal origin, the small amplitude circadian periodicity found in its secretion coincides with that of cortisol. Also, plasma concentrations of ovarian androgens, including androstenedione and testosterone, increase slightly around midcycle.

Certain pathologic conditions of the adrenal cortex or ovaries (eg, hyperplasia, adenoma, carcinoma) markedly increase the production of testosterone and its precursors. Precocious puberal development, virilism, or amenorrhea may result if the overproduction is great and sustained. In hirsutism, the total plasma testosterone level may be slightly high or normal but the amount of unbound hormone is usually elevated.

The mechanism of action of androgens in women is the same as that in men. Testosterone or dihydrotestosterone is the active intracellular androgen, depending upon the target tissue. Androgen-sensitive hair follicles in women require DHT for stimulation.

Aging: Increasing age in men has been correlated with decreased Leydig cells, reduced sperm production, and elevated serum concentrations of LH and FSH. Elevation of FSH is greater and correlates with lowest sperm production (Neaves et al, 1984). In addition, free plasma testosterone declines with advancing age and correlates with reduction of various aspects of sexuality (eg, frequency of activity, erectile and orgasmic function, level of enjoyment). Hormonal changes are thought to be responsible for only a small part of declining sexual activity with age (Davidson et al, 1983).

There is no male hormonal climacteric analogous to that in women. However, when serum testosterone levels decrease abruptly at any age (eg, following surgical trauma or orchiectomy), vasomotor flushing can occur. This may be alleviated by testosterone replacement therapy.

Behavior: Because of complex and interacting variables involved in the determination of human behavior, it is not surprising that clinical studies have failed to describe consistent hormonal profiles for certain behavioral patterns in men (ie, homosexuality, aggressive behavior). Data from different studies are difficult to compare because procedures have not been standardized (eg, measurement of total versus free testosterone, sampling at different amplitudes of the circadian cycle, lack of information on ratio of free estrogen:testosterone). Furthermore, reported differences in hormone level may be a cause, an effect, or unrelated to behavior.

Based on results obtained in animals, behavior may be influenced by hormonal imprinting at a critical stage in development rather than by hormones present later. In some animals, for example, androgens program the brain in fetal or neonatal life and set patterns of gonadotropic hormone secretion and sexual behavior. It has been suggested that similar influences are operative in humans (Magee, 1983). Psychosexual orientation that may have been influenced by prenatal hormone exposure has been described (eg, some females with virilizing congenital adrenal hyperplasia, genetic males with 5-α-reductase deficiency) but not proved (Pardridge et al, 1982).

In one study, men with lifelong homosexual orientation demonstrated a serum LH response to LHRH administration that was intermediate between that of women and heterosexual men; the group observation could not be extrapolated to individuals, however (Gladue et al, 1984).

Antiandrogens (eg, cyproterone acetate) have been used in other countries to treat individuals who demonstrate paraphilic behavior. Although pharmacologic treatment of such behavior is controversial, medroxyprogesterone acetate (a progestin with antiandrogenic activity) is sometimes used for this purpose in the United States. These agents depress LH secretion and antagonize peripheral androgen action.

Indications

Androgens are used for replacement therapy in hormone deficiency states in males and for certain gynecologic conditions and metastatic breast cancer in women (see also Chapter 39, Estrogen, Progestins, and Other Agents Used to Treat Gynecologic Conditions, and Chapter 64, Drugs Used in Cancer Chemotherapy). Androgens or anabolic steroids are used in certain circumstances to increase growth and to stimulate hematopoiesis in some refractory anemias.

Constitutional Delay of Growth: This condition occurs in approximately 2.5% of normal children and more frequently causes concern in boys than in girls. Family history may reveal similar growth retardation in parents, siblings, or other relatives. The diagnosis is made by exclusion and is conclusive after normal but late and prolonged adolescent development. Medical attention is frequently sought because of short stature rather than lack of sexual development, in contrast to patients with primary or hypogonadotropic hypogonadism whose height is often normal. Characteristics of constitutional delayed growth include normal birth weight, growth curve parallel to normal, low bone age for chronological age but normal for the stage of development (bone age is normal in genetic short stature), and low levels of plasma gonadotropins and adrenal androgens for age but normal for size and stage of sexual development (Rosenfeld et al, 1982; Kelley and Ruvalcaba, 1982; Kulin, 1983).

Bone age is determined at the initial evaluation. Family history of growth development is obtained and nonendocrine causes of growth retardation are considered. In girls, a karyotype to detect Turner's syndrome should be performed. Further testing may be postponed during a six-month observation period unless the child is three or more standard deviations below average height or there is no sexual maturation by bone

age of 12 to 13 or chronological age of 13 in girls and 14 in boys. Extreme anxiety of the patient and parents also may stimulate earlier evaluation. Serum thyroxine and gonadotropins are measured and, if normal, the adequacy of growth hormone secretion may be determined.

Drug therapy is not required to achieve normal growth in constitutional delay of growth and puberty; normal development occurs by 18 years and full adult height is usually within the normal range, although linear growth may not be complete until after age 20. However, when delayed growth and puberty cause significant emotional stress despite reassurance, treatment with androgenic agents may be considered in boys.

The goal of therapy is to accelerate initiation of a growth spurt that would otherwise occur later. Patients should be 12 to 14 years or older with a bone age at least two years behind the chronological age before treatment is attempted. However, consideration may be given to using lower dosages in younger children experiencing severe constitutional delay of growth. Care must be taken to avoid doses that produce premature epiphyseal closure, which would compromise adult height. Usually, hormone treatment is employed for three to six months, followed by a drug-free observation period of six months. Bone age should be determined roentgenographically before initiation of therapy and at intervals during and after treatment. The increase in bone age should not exceed the increase in height age. Since stimulation of bone maturation may persist for six months after therapy is discontinued, steroids should be withdrawn well before the skeletal age reaches the norm for the chronological age. Often the puberal changes initiated by treatment proceed spontaneously after one course of therapy, but a second course may be employed if necessary.

Any anabolic steroid or androgen may be prescribed for constitutional delay of growth. The choice of preparation depends upon the balance of growth stimulation and sexual maturation desired. The route of administration preferred also may influence drug selection. Usually an oral anabolic steroid, such as oxandrolone [Anavar], is selected. The activity of this preparation has a favorable anabolic to androgenic ratio. However, a preparation with greater androgenic activity, usually an intramuscular testosterone ester (eg, testosterone enanthate [Andryl, Delatestryl]), may be chosen if stimulation of sexual development is desired and growth potential is achieved or nearly so.

Although small doses of anabolic steroids may stimulate growth in girls with constitutional delay of growth, these preparations are rarely used for this purpose. They must be used cautiously because of their potential to cause virilization and to accelerate epiphyseal closure.

Growth Hormone Deficiency: Prepuberal children with growth hormone deficiency have been treated experimentally with androgen or an anabolic steroid (usually oxandrolone) in combination with growth hormone. The rationale for utilizing the combination is that the linear growth-promoting effects of these agents are synergistic and use of the combination allows conservation of growth hormone. Some success in achieving both goals has been reported, but the most advantageous regimens with respect to prior growth hormone therapy, dosage, preparation, and schedule of treatment have not been determined. There is disagreement on whether combined use is most beneficial as initial therapy or after the first or second year of growth hormone therapy when response to this hormone alone decreases (see also Chapter 42, Agents Related to Anterior Pituitary and Hypothalamic Function). However, the use of growth hormone and an anabolic steroid is not favored by some clinicians. Recently, human growth hormone made from recombinant DNA technology (somatrem [Protropin]) became available commercially, and this eventually may obviate the need for regimens designed to conserve growth hormone.

Hypogonadism: Decreased Leydig cell function can result from abnormality of the testis (primary hypogonadism) or from lack of gonadotropic stimulation (hypogonadotropism) caused by hypothalamic or pituitary failure (secondary hypogonadism). Disorders associated with primary Leydig cell failure include chromosomal defect (eg, Klinefelter's syndrome), trauma, irradiation, or testicular failure associated with disease (eg, myotonic dystrophy, mumps orchitis). Serum gonadotropin levels are high in primary failure (due to lack of negative feedback by androgen) and low in secondary hypogonadism. Patients with primary or secondary hypogonadism may seek help because of failure of normal puberal development or because impotence, lack of libido, infertility, or decreased beard growth developed after puberal development was complete.

The time to initiate replacement therapy depends on the time that clinical manifestations appear and not on whether hypogonadism is primary or secondary. For example, patients with primary testicular failure may not seek medical attention until adulthood. A patient with Klinefelter's syndrome may have normal height, incomplete virilization, and eunuchoid body proportions but may not consult a physician until infertility becomes apparent in adulthood.

Regardless of the cause of hypogonadism, the dose and schedule for replacement therapy depend upon age and developmental stage at presentation and the severity of the deficit. Therapy may be directed toward induction of puberty, maintenance of secondary sexual characteristics and sexual behavior, or treatment of infertility. When *induction of puberty* is undertaken, a parenteral preparation (eg, testosterone enanthate, testosterone cypionate [Andro-Cyp, Depo-Testosterone, T-Ionate-P.A.]) achieves best results. Replacement dosages are generally increased to induce progressive changes of puberty, and full sexual development is usually attained in three to four years. Priapism can be alleviated by adjusting the dose. Although oral therapy with fluoxymesterone [Halotestin] or methyltestosterone [Metandren, Oreton Methyl, Testred] may be more convenient for maintenance therapy in patients with hypogonadism, the parenteral testosterone esters are preferred for long-term use because of their greater potency and the hepatotoxicity associated with 17α-alkylated compounds.

Human chorionic gonadotropin (HCG) may be used diagnostically to test the testicular response to gonadotropin. If HCG stimulates testosterone secretion markedly, primary gonadal failure or insensitivity to gonadotropin is ruled out. HCG also can be used to stimulate testicular function, but treatment is inconvenient and expensive and generally is not used except for infertility (see Chapter 41).

When *infertility* is a manifestation of secondary hypogonadism, replacement therapy with gonadotropins is required to stimulate and maintain normal spermatogenesis. A combination of menotropins (HMG) plus HCG may be successful (see Chapter 41).

Testosterone has been used to treat infertility caused by idiopathic oligospermia, but such therapy is not effective (see Chapter 41).

Micropenis can occur in association with hypospadias, hypogonadotropic or primary hypogonadism, androgen insensitivity, or as an idiopathic condition. Penile growth may occur after intramuscular administration of testosterone. Alternatively, topical application of testosterone to the penis may be employed, although some authorities feel that the response is better after parenteral administration. It is generally agreed that the action of topical androgen is mediated, at least partly, through systemic absorption of the hormone. It has been suggested that topical application may simplify management and reduce expense. Side effects (eg, pubic hair development) can be minimized by using low concentrations (ie, 1.25% and 2.5% testosterone) (Sokol and Swerdloff, 1983). This type of preparation is not available commercially and must be compounded. Treatment of micropenis is usually limited to three to six months to avoid epiphyseal maturation.

Oxandrolone, fluoxymesterone, or oxandrolone combined with growth hormone has been used in some centers to treat patients with *Turner's syndrome*. Acceleration of linear growth and greater ultimate height have been reported, but androgenic side effects, such as acne, may occur. Dosage must be controlled carefully to avoid clitoral enlargement. Treatment precedes administration of estrogens to induce puberal development. This type of treatment is not endorsed by some practitioners.

Gynecologic Conditions: The most common indication for large-dose, long-term androgen therapy in women is advanced or metastatic *breast carcinoma*. The dosage required to induce remissions is larger than that used for replacement therapy in males, and patients should be advised that virilizing side effects will occur. The short-acting preparations (eg, testosterone propionate, methyltestosterone, fluoxymesterone) are preferred initially, since prompt withdrawal is necessary if symptomatic hypercalcemia develops. Various derivatives of testosterone have been reported to induce remissions with fewer virilizing effects, and testolactone [Teslac] is free of androgenic activity (see Chapter 64, Drugs Used in Cancer Chemotherapy). Androgens are contraindicated in male breast cancer.

Breast pain, tenderness, and nodularity are relieved partially or completely in most women with *fibrocystic breast disease* (FBD) after administration of danazol [Danocrine], an impeded androgen. Several months of daily treatment may be required. Symptoms may recur within one year after cessation of therapy, and another course may then be initiated (see the evaluation in this chapter and Chapter 39, Estrogens, Progestins, and Other Agents Used to Treat Gynecologic Conditions).

Women with *lichen sclerosus* may have deficient 5α-reductase activity in the perineal skin, thus limiting tissue conversion of testosterone to dihydrotestosterone (DHT). Topical application of testosterone may induce further enzyme activity, normalizing DHT formation and producing clinical improvement (Friedrich and Kalra, 1984). Treatment with testosterone ointment alleviates pruritus and normalizes the gross and histologic appearance of the skin. (A 2% ointment may be compounded by mixing 30 ml of testosterone propionate [100 mg/ml] with 120 g of petrolatum.) The condition eventually reappears after cessation of treatment. Corticosteroid cream may be used concurrently for prompt relief of pruritus but should not be employed for long periods (Friedrich, 1976).

Small doses of androgens, alone or with estrogen, have been used to *restore libido*, especially in menopausal women. However, results are equivocal. Administration of even small amounts of androgen for prolonged periods may produce masculinization in sensitive women; such use must be monitored closely.

Androgen in combination with estrogen [Deladumone] has been given intramuscularly at delivery to *suppress lactation* postpartum; however, use of hormonal preparations often is followed by rebound lactation, and administration of estrogen is discouraged because of the risk of thromboembolism (see Chapter 39). If drug therapy is desired to suppress lactation, bromocriptine [Parlodel] is preferred (see Chapter 42).

For use of the impeded androgen, danazol, in the treatment of *endometriosis*, see Chapter 41, Agents Used to Treat Infertility.

Osteoporosis: Androgens and anabolic steroids have been used to treat postmenopausal women with osteoporosis. It has been suggested that these agents not only inhibit loss of calcium (like estrogens) but also promote reformation of bone tissue (Chestnut, 1981; Chestnut et al, 1983). However, because there is no objective evidence that they are superior to estrogens and because of their masculinizing effects, these agents have not been used commonly for this indication (see also Chapter 39).

Hereditary Angioedema: In this autosomal dominant disorder, a deficiency of Cl esterase inhibitor leads to uncontrolled activation of the complement system, production of vasoactive substances, and angioedema. Androgens are useful for prophylaxis in this potentially fatal condition. Danazol or anabolic steroids, such as stanozolol [Winstrol], are preferred, especially in women, because of their effectiveness and low androgenic activity. Remission of symptoms and increased hepatic production of the deficient serum α-globin, Cl inhibitor (Gelfand et al, 1976), are noted after treatment (see also Chapter 63, Immunomodulators). (For the dose of danazol, see the evaluation.) The dose of stanozolol is 2 mg three times a day; after a favorable response, the amount is reduced gradually to 2 mg/day or on alternate days.

Anemias: Experimental evidence suggests that androgens and anabolic steroids support erythropoiesis by stimulation of renal production of erythropoietin, as well as by direct, dose-related stimulation of the erythropoietin-sensitive elements in bone marrow. Androgens also increase erythrocytic 2-3 diphosphoglycerate levels, which decreases hemoglobin-oxygen affinity and makes oxygen more readily available to the tissues. Accordingly, large doses of these agents are used to treat some *refractory anemias* caused by defective production of erythrocytes (eg, aplastic anemia, sideroblastic anemia), hereditary conditions (eg, Fanconi's anemia), or associated with disorders such as myelofibrosis and systemic lupus erythematosus. Androgenic-anabolic agents also may alleviate leukopenia and thrombocytopenia, but longer treatment is required and results are inconsistent.

Only 25% of patients with severe aplastic anemia improve with androgen therapy, and the remissions may be spontaneous. Histocompatible bone marrow transplantation or antilymphocyte globulin therapy is more effective than androgen therapy in these patients. Androgens may be more effective when there is some residual erythropoietic and myelopoietic activity, as in mild aplastic anemia or myeloproliferative disease, although this is not proven. If there are no signs of improvement after three months of therapy or if the drug is no longer effective, it should be discontinued. Relapses occur in 20% to 50% of responsive patients after the androgen is discontinued, but a second course of therapy is often effective. Some patients become dependent on androgen therapy to support adequate hematopoiesis (Najean, 1981).

Seventy percent of children with Fanconi's syndrome initially respond to androgen therapy. Continued use of smaller doses is required for maintenance. Eventually, androgen therapy fails to sustain adequate hematopoiesis.

There is little convincing evidence that one androgen is more effective than another for stimulating hematopoiesis. Oral preparations may be preferable in patients with severe thrombocytopenia because intramuscular injection can cause deep hematoma. Androgenic preparations that lack a 17α-alkyl group (eg, testosterone and derivatives, nandrolone phenpropionate [Androlone, Durabolin, Nandrolin], nandrolone decanoate [Androlone-D, Deca-Durabolin]) may be preferred for high-dose, long-term therapy, since liver dysfunction may occur less frequently with their use (see the section on Adverse Reactions and Precautions).

Androgens are useful in anemia secondary to acute or chronic *renal failure* and are particularly effective in acute renal failure of pregnancy. These agents stimulate production of erythropoietin even in anephric patients, but the response is better if some functional renal tissue remains. Treatment is most successful when patients are adequately nourished and dialyzed concomitantly. Drug therapy increases erythrocyte mass and reduces the transfusion requirement. The latter effect is a less compelling basis for androgen therapy than formerly thought, since it has been shown that prior transfusion improves renal transplant survival.

Anabolic steroids combat myelosuppression induced by cytostatic agents (Huys and Van Vaerenbergh, 1976; Spiers et al, 1981). Danazol may be effective for idiopathic or autoimmune hemolytic anemia associated with nonmalignant diseases and has been used with glucocorticoids for severe conditions or as the sole agent when hemolysis lessens (Ahn et al, 1985). Danazol also was reported to induce remissions in patients with idiopathic thrombocytopenic purpura and appeared to reduce the need for glucocorticoids (Ahn et al, 1983).

Protein Anabolism: Anabolic steroids reverse the negative nitrogen and calcium balance associated with high-dose glucocorticoid therapy. Although this use of anabolic steroids is a rational approach to prevent some side effects of corticosteroids (eg, muscle wasting and weakness, demineralization of bone), their long-term efficacy has not been established.

Defective protein metabolism with loss of tissue protein may occur in patients with chronic debilitating illnesses and in those convalescing from severe infections, surgery, burns, trauma, irradiation, or cytotoxic drug therapy. Testosterone or related anabolic steroids decrease or reverse negative nitrogen balance, seem to provide a feeling of well-being, and sometimes stimulate appetite; however, there is no evidence that they shorten the period of recovery. Their effectiveness depends upon adequate protein and caloric intake. Although there are no adequate clinical trials proving efficacy, use of anabolic agents as adjunctive or supportive therapy in such conditions, particularly in terminal patients, may be helpful.

Anabolic steroids do not alleviate the symptoms or alter the progress of *muscular dystrophy*. Masculinizing effects occurred when these agents were used in children with this disorder.

Athletic Performance: The use of anabolic steroids to improve athletic performance is "contrary to the ethical principles of athletic competition and is deplored" (American College of Sports Medicine, 1984). It was thought that steroids do not significantly increase muscle mass in healthy young men beyond that due to physical conditioning. However, some studies suggest that steroid increases lean muscle mass, although the tissue may be phosphate-poor and have ultrastructural abnormalities (Mellion, 1984). Body weight increases with steroid treatment, but much of the gain is due to fluid retention. Studies designed to identify changes in strength in athletes who took steroids have yielded equivocal results (Ryan, 1981; American College of Sports Medicine, 1984; Haupt and Rovere, 1984).

Regardless of objective evidence supporting or refuting the claim that anabolic steroids enhance athletic performance, many athletes feel that they benefit from ingesting large quantities of these agents. Perceived effects include increased muscular strength, heightened aggressive tendencies, more energy, and the ability to train more intensively. The use of anabolic steroids by athletes is apparently widespread, particularly among weight lifters, shot-putters, discus throwers, and football players. Such drug use is increasing among younger athletes, even junior high school students (Dyment, 1984). Some female athletes also use anabolic steroids, virilizing effects notwithstanding.

Not only is the use of anabolic steroids for improving athletic strength a medically trivial indication, but adverse effects, some serious, are associated with steroid use. The potential for adverse effects is presumably highest in athletes who consume quantities far in excess of therapeutic doses or in those who "stack" drugs (ie, ingest large doses of several steroids simultaneously).

The 17α-alkylated compounds are commonly used and may alter liver function tests and cause other abnormalities (see the section on Adverse Reactions and Precautions). Death from liver cancer has been reported recently in an athlete taking steroids (Overly et al, 1984). Other adverse effects include reduced serum gonadotropin and endogenous testosterone

levels, decreased testicular size, and depressed spermatogenesis. Gynecomastia may occur with some steroid preparations. Retention of salt and fluid may cause hypertension. Blood lipid patterns show potentially atherogenic changes: HDL cholesterol is decreased while LDL cholesterol concentrations rise (Webb et al, 1984). Irritability may occur.

Anabolic steroids may stimulate skeletal muscle in female athletes more than in males. In a study of women competitors in strength sports, subjects reported lowering of voice pitch, facial hair, clitoral enlargement, increased aggressiveness, and menstrual irregularities (Strauss et al, 1985). The development of such effects emphasizes the undesirability of these steroids in women athletes.

Use of anabolic steroids in juvenile athletes is of particular concern. Puberty may be induced in sexually immature boys, and final adult height may be compromised by premature epiphyseal closure. The possibility of other effects on the maturing hypothalamic-pituitary-gonadal axis also must be considered.

Alcohol-induced Hepatitis: In a cooperative placebo-controlled study of alcohol-induced hepatitis, oxandrolone given for 30 days enhanced survival from the end of the treatment period up to 1.5 years in patients with moderate disease. When prednisolone was used instead of oxandrolone, no consistent effect on survival was observed (Mendenhall et al, 1984).

Hyperlipidemia: See Chapter 50.

Adverse Reactions and Precautions

When androgens and anabolic steroids are used for indications other than androgen deficiency, their most common undesirable effect is virilism. Although some agents are less likely to produce these reactions, all steroidal anabolic agents cause masculinizing effects when taken in sufficient quantities. Because such effects are of greater concern in women and children, the less androgenic preparations are preferred in these patients.

Signs of virilism in prepubertal children are pubic hair development, phallic enlargement and increased frequency of erections in boys, and clitoral enlargement in girls. In boys, there is a risk of priapism; any increase in erectile frequency is an indication for reducing the dose. In aging men, androgens may stimulate prostatic hyperplasia, causing urinary obstruction. In women, hirsutism, deepening of the voice, oily skin, alopecia, acne, clitoral enlargement, stimulation of libido, and menstrual irregularities may occur; voice change and clitoral enlargement are often irreversible, but hirsutism may be reversible. Acne and facial hair may be among the earliest manifestations in women and may warrant re-evaluation of therapy. Combined estrogen and androgen therapy does not significantly delay or prevent signs of virilism. Paradoxically, androgens may cause gynecomastia, particularly in children (eg, when used for constitutional delay of growth), or in men after administration of large doses or in the presence of liver disease. This is probably due to the aromatization of testosterone to estrogen and does not occur with use of steroids that are reduced in the 5α position.

Anabolic steroids should not be used to stimulate growth in children who are small but otherwise normal and healthy, except in selected cases of constitutional delayed growth. When they are used, the rate of skeletal maturation may exceed the rate of linear growth, thereby inducing premature closure of the epiphyses and reducing the attainable adult height. The extent to which this complication occurs depends upon the child's bone age, the drug used, dosage, and duration of therapy. The decision to administer anabolic steroids to children for a specific growth problem should be made only after careful evaluation by an experienced pediatric endocrinologist.

Androgenic and anabolic steroids with an alkyl group substituted in the alpha position on carbon 17 (ie, methyltestosterone [Metandren, Oreton Methyl, Testred], fluoxymesterone [Halotestin], ethylestrenol [Maxibolin], methandrostenolone (no longer marketed in the United States), oxandrolone [Anavar], oxymetholone [Anadrol-50], stanozolol [Winstrol]), as well as the impeded androgen, danazol [Danocrine], have produced signs of liver dysfunction. Increased sulfobromophthalein (BSP) retention and SGOT levels appear to be dose related and are relatively unimportant. Increased serum bilirubin and alkaline phosphatase values indicating excretory dysfunction are rare but important idiosyncratic reactions. Clinical jaundice is unusual and reversible when the drug is discontinued. The histologic findings consist of intrahepatic cholestasis with little or no cellular damage. Therefore, these drugs should be used with caution in all patients and particularly those with pre-existing liver disease. Long-term administration of 17α-alkylated androgens and anabolic steroids should be avoided.

Rarely, hepatocellular and endothelial malignancies, as well as intrahepatic hemorrhage associated with peliosis hepatis, have developed, particularly in anemic patients treated for long periods with large doses of 17α-alkylated steroids. Hepatocellular adenomas or carcinomas may regress when androgens are discontinued. Patients with Fanconi's syndrome experience more severe liver toxicity from androgen therapy than other patients with anemia; it is not known whether this is due to prolonged androgen therapy or increased susceptibility to liver dysfunction in these patients (Camitta et al, 1982). Patients receiving prolonged androgen therapy should be monitored for functional and structural liver abnormalities.

Abnormal liver function tests are thought to occur less frequently with the intramuscular preparations of testosterone and its derivatives, nandrolone phenpropionate and nandrolone decanoate, which lack the 17α-alkylated group.

Women receiving androgen therapy for disseminated breast carcinoma may develop hypercalcemia. If symptoms occur, the patient should be hydrated, appropriate drugs administered (see Chapter 49, Agents Affecting Calcium Metabolism), and the androgen discontinued.

Large doses of androgens and anabolic steroids cause potentially deleterious changes in blood lipids. Athletes taking these drugs showed a 50% reduction in HDL cholesterol and increased LDL cholesterol concentrations compared to levels measured during a steroid-free period. Patterns associated with large doses (ie, 50 to 100 mg methandrostenolone daily plus testosterone 100 to 200 mg and nandrolone decanoate 100 to 200 mg weekly) are potentially atherogenic (Webb et al, 1984).

Salt and fluid retention are usually not serious but can be undesirable in elderly patients, patients with congestive heart failure, or those with a tendency to develop edema from other causes (eg, cirrhosis, hypoproteinemia).

Care should be taken when 17α-alkylated preparations are used in patients on hemodialysis because these drugs may increase blood fibrinolytic activity.

Androgens and anabolic steroids are contraindicated in pregnant women (except in acute renal failure of pregnancy) because of possible masculinization of the female fetus (FDA Pregnancy Category X). Their use in premature and newborn infants is not recommended, since evidence of beneficial effect is lacking. They also are contraindicated in men with carcinoma of the prostate or breast.

Drug Interactions

Caution is required when 17α-alkylated androgens are administered to patients receiving anticoagulants. Methandrostenolone and ethylestrenol increase the potency of coumarin and indandione anticoagulants, and thus increase the risk of hemorrhage (see Chapter 3, Drug Interactions and Adverse Drug Reactions). Therefore, when any androgenic steroid is added to or withdrawn from a regimen that also includes an anticoagulant, more frequent prothrombin determinations and adjustments in dose of the anticoagulant should be made.

Methandrostenolone may decrease the metabolism of oxyphenbutazone [Oxalid] resulting in a longer, more intense, and unpredictable response to the latter. Therefore, it is advisable to avoid the concomitant use of these drugs. Methandrostenolone also has been reported to increase both the therapeutic and toxic effects of corticosteroids.

The requirement for antidiabetic agents may be decreased when anabolic steroids are added to the regimen, because the steroids may reduce blood sugar levels directly in diabetics.

Effects on Laboratory Tests

Androgens reduce the level of circulating thyroxine-binding globulin, thereby decreasing thyroid hormone levels and increasing triiodothyronine resin uptake. However, the free T_3 and T_4 are unaffected and there is no evidence of thyroid dysfunction. Androgens enhance blood fibrinolytic activity, increase hematocrit and serum haptoglobin levels, and have variable effects on serum lipids. Administration of testosterone, but not the 17α-alkylated derivatives, elevates urinary 17-ketosteroids.

Preparations

Testosterone and its derivatives have anabolic and somatic growth effects. Attempts to separate the anabolic from the androgenic effects by modifying the testosterone molecule have been only partially successful and have resulted in the development of a number of synthetic analogues, termed anabolic steroids. These include the oral preparations, ethylestrenol [Maxibolin], oxandrolone [Anavar], oxymetholone [Anadrol-50], and stanozolol [Winstrol]. All are 17α-alkylated compounds. Parenteral preparations for intramuscular administration include nandrolone phenpropionate [Androlone, Durabolin, Nandrolin] and nandrolone decanoate [Androlone-D, Deca-Durabolin], which are not alkylated in the 17α position.

All anabolic steroids have androgenic activity, and masculinizing side effects occur if sufficient doses are given for a prolonged period. Information is insufficient to compare the anabolic potencies of the various compounds in man. Results of animal bioassays do not necessarily predict the results when these preparations are used clinically.

Unaltered testosterone is not suitable for therapeutic use except, perhaps, topically because its half-life in the blood is short and absorption and hepatic degradation are rapid after oral or parenteral administration. Esterification of testosterone has produced less polar molecules that are soluble in oil vehicles and in fatty tissue. Generally, the longer the carbon chain of the ester substituent, the more slowly the hormone is released into the circulation. The esters are hydrolyzed to testosterone, which can be assayed in the blood when monitoring therapy. Testosterone esters are administered as the propionate, cypionate [Andro-Cyp, Depo-Testosterone, T-Ionate-P.A.], and enanthate [Andryl, Delatestryl]. Testosterone propionate is injected two to four times weekly, while the longer-acting cypionate and enanthate are administered every two to four weeks. The latter two preparations are drugs of choice for hypogonadism, which requires long-term therapy.

Methyltestosterone [Metandren, Oreton Methyl, Testred] and fluoxymesterone [Halotestin] are alkylated in the 17α position, which retards hepatic degradation and renders these preparations effective after oral administration. They must be given daily and their androgenic potency, milligram-for-milligram, is less than that of the parenteral forms of testosterone. Also, 17α-alkylated androgens may be more hepatotoxic (see the section on Adverse Reactions and Precautions).

Newer preparations that provide greater ease of administration and effectiveness are being developed. Siloxane capsules containing testosterone are implanted subcutaneously and provide relatively constant blood levels over a long period. The undecanoate ester (marketed in other countries) and a preparation of microparticulate testosterone that are effective orally also are being investigated.

Drug Evaluations

FLUOXYMESTERONE
[Halotestin]

This short-acting preparation (half-life about ten hours) is used orally. It is less effective for replacement therapy than the long-acting esters of testosterone. Full sexual maturation in patients with prepuberal hypogonadism cannot be achieved easily with fluoxymesterone, but it is sometimes used for replacement therapy when hypogonadism begins in adult life or after secondary sexual characteristics have developed

following therapy with a parenteral preparation. However, because of its potential hepatotoxicity, this androgen should not be used for long periods.

Fluoxymesterone also can be given for its anabolic properties (see the Table) and for the palliative treatment of certain cases of metastatic breast carcinoma in women. See the introduction for other indications and adverse reactions.

DOSAGE AND PREPARATIONS.
Oral: For androgen deficiency, 10 to 20 mg daily. For metastatic breast carcinoma in *women,* 10 to 30 mg daily in divided doses. For anabolic therapy, see the Table.
    Halotestin (Upjohn), *Generic.* Tablets 2, 5, and 10 mg.

METHYLTESTOSTERONE
[Metandren, Oreton Methyl, Testred]

This short-acting preparation (half-life about 2.5 hours) is used orally and buccally. Although absorption is more variable, the bioavailability is greater with buccal administration, probably because the hepatic circulation is bypassed. However, the oral route is used more commonly for convenience.

Methyltestosterone is much less effective for replacement therapy than the long-acting esters of testosterone. Although methyltestosterone does not produce full sexual maturation in patients with prepuberal hypogonadism, it is sometimes used for replacement therapy when hypogonadism begins in adult life or after secondary sexual characteristics have developed following therapy with testosterone. However, because of its potential hepatotoxicity, this androgen should not be used for long periods.

Methyltestosterone also can be given for its anabolic properties (see the Table) and for the palliative treatment of certain cases of metastatic breast carcinoma in women. See the introduction for other indications and adverse reactions.

DOSAGE AND PREPARATIONS.
Oral: For androgen deficiency, 10 to 50 mg daily. For metastatic breast carcinoma in *women,* the average daily dose is 50 to 200 mg. Because of marked variation in sensitivity, signs of virilism may occur in women even when small doses are given. The dosage must be individualized and the daily amount should be given in divided doses. For anabolic therapy, see the Table.
    Metandren (CIBA), *Oreton Methyl* (Schering), *Generic.* Tablets 10 and 25 mg.
    Testred (ICN). Capsules 10 mg.
Buccal: *Adults,* one-half of oral dosage (rate of absorption is variable).
    Metandren (CIBA). Tablets (buccal) 5 and 10 mg.
    Oreton Methyl (Schering), *Generic.* Tablets (buccal) 10 mg.

TESTOSTERONE CYPIONATE
[Andro-Cyp, Depo-Testosterone, T-Ionate-P.A.]

TESTOSTERONE ENANTHATE
[Andryl, Delatestryl]

These long-acting, potent esters of testosterone are given intramuscularly to develop or maintain secondary sexual char-

STEROIDS USED FOR ANABOLIC THERAPY

Drug and Chemical Structure	Usual Dosage	Preparations

TESTOSTERONE ESTERS
Testosterone Cypionate
 	
Testosterone
	Intramuscular: Adults, 200 mg every 2 weeks or 400 mg every 4 weeks.	*Generic.*
		    Solution (in oil) 100 and 200 mg/ml in 10 ml containers.
		Andro-Cyp (Keene).
		    Solution (in oil) 100 and 200 mg/ml in 10 ml containers.
		Depo-Testosterone (Upjohn).
		    Solution (in cottonseed oil) 50 mg/ml in 10 ml containers and 100 and 200 mg/ml in 1 and 10 ml containers.
		T-Ionate-P.A. (Reid-Provident).
		    Solution (in cottonseed oil) 200 mg/ml in 10 ml containers.

Testosterone Enanthate	*Intramuscular: Adults,* 200 mg every 2 weeks or 400 mg every 4 weeks.	*Generic.*
		    Solution (in oil) 100 and 200 mg/ml in 10 ml containers.
		Andryl (Keene).
		    Solution (in sesame oil) 200 mg/ml in 10 ml containers.
		Delatestryl (Squibb).
		    Solution (in sesame oil) 200 mg/ml in 1 and 5 ml containers.

Testosterone Propionate	*Intramuscular: Adults,* 10 to 25 mg daily.	*Generic.* Solution (in cottonseed oil) 25 mg/ml in 10 ml containers and 50 and 100 mg/ml in 10 and 30 ml containers.
17α-ALKYLATED COMPOUNDS Ethylestrenol 	*Oral: Adults,* 8 to 16 mg daily; for growth stimulation in *children,* 0.1 to 0.2 mg/kg daily.	*Maxibolin* (Organon). Elixir 2 mg/5 ml (alcohol 10%); tablets 2 mg.
Fluoxymesterone 	*Oral: Adults,* 4 to 10 mg daily; for growth stimulation in boys, 2.5 to 10 mg daily; to stimulate erythropoiesis, 0.4 to 1 mg/kg daily.	*Halotestin* (Upjohn), *Generic.* Tablets 2, 5, and 10 mg.

Methyltestosterone
 	
	Oral: Adults, 10 to 20 mg daily; for growth stimulation in boys, 10 to 20 mg daily.
	
	Buccal: Adults, one-half oral dosage; absorption variable.
		Metandren (CIBA), *Oreton Methyl* (Schering), *Generic.*
		    Tablets 10 and 25 mg.
		Testred (ICN).
		    Capsules 10 mg.
		Metandren (CIBA).
		    Tablets (buccal) 5 and 10 mg.
		Oreton Methyl (Schering), *Generic.*
		    Tablets (buccal) 10 mg.

(Continued on next page)

STEROIDS USED FOR ANABOLIC THERAPY (Continued)

Drug and Chemical Structure	Usual Dosage	Preparations
17α-ALKYLATED COMPOUNDS (Continued) Oxandrolone	*Oral: Adults,* 5 to 10 mg daily; for growth stimulation in *children,* 0.1 to 0.25 mg/kg daily.	*Anavar* (Searle). Tablets 2.5 mg.
Oxymetholone	*Oral:* For erythropoiesis, *adults and children,* 1 to 5 mg/kg daily. (maximum, 100 mg daily).	*Anadrol-50* (Syntex). Tablets 50 mg.
Stanozolol	*Oral: Adults,* 6 mg daily. *Children 6 to 12 years,* 2 to 6 mg daily; *under 6 years,* 2 mg daily.	*Winstrol* (Winthrop-Breon). Tablets 2 mg.
OTHER COMPOUNDS *Nandrolone Decanoate*	*Intramuscular* (deep): *Adults,* 50 to 100 mg every 3 to 4 weeks. *Children 2 to 13 years,* 25 to 50 mg every 3 to 4 weeks. For anemia of renal disease, *women,* 50 to 100 mg/week; *men,* 100 to 200 mg/week; *children 2 to 13 years,* 25 to 50 mg every 3 to 4 weeks.	*Generic.* Solution (in oil) 50 and 100 mg/ml in 2 ml containers and 20 mg/ml in 1 ml containers. *Androlone-D* (Keene). Solution (in sesame oil) 50 and 100 mg/ml in 2 ml containers. *Deca-Durabolin* (Organon). Solution (in sesame oil) 50 and 100 mg/ml in 1 and 2 ml containers and 200 mg/ml in 2 ml containers.
Nandrolone Phenpropionate	*Intramuscular* (deep): *Adults,* 25 to 50 mg weekly. *Children 2 to 13 years,* 12.5 to 25 mg every 2 to 4 weeks. For erythropoiesis, up to 100 mg weekly.	*Generic.* Solution (in oil) 25 mg/ml in 5 ml containers and 50 mg/ml in 2 ml containers *Androlone* (Keene). Solution (in sesame oil) 25 mg/ml in 5 ml containers and 50 mg/ml in 2 ml containers. *Durabolin* (Organn). Solution (in sesame oil) 25 mg/ml in 1 and 5 ml containers and 50 mg/ml in 2 ml containers. *Nandrolin* (Reid-Provident). Solution (in sesame oil) 25 mg/ml in 5 ml containers.

acteristics and other physiologic functions in androgen-deficient males. These agents are preferred to induce full sexual development in eunuchoidal males when testicular disease has interfered with normal puberal development and to treat postpuberal Leydig cell failure. Peak blood levels are achieved within one day after administration and decline to baseline levels after seven to nine days depending on the dose. Intramuscular administration of these preparations thus results in uneven serum levels of testosterone, and it is recommended that the dosing interval not exceed two to three weeks to avoid long periods without androgen support (Sokol and Swerdloff, 1983).

Either ester may be used for the palliative treatment of breast carcinoma in women who have responded favorably to initial treatment with a short-acting preparation. Some clinicians prefer to use short-acting preparations for the entire treatment period because it is possible to discontinue therapy quickly if adverse effects occur.

These preparations also may be given for three to six months as anabolic agents (see the Table) and to initiate puberty in selected boys with constitutional delay of growth.

See the Introduction for information on other indications and adverse reactions.

DOSAGE AND PREPARATIONS.
Intramuscular: For induction of puberty in *boys,* 25 to 50 mg/M^2/month closely simulates the first year of puberty; 100 mg/M^2/month simulates normal midpuberty sexual development and growth spurt. Alternatively, 50 to 100 mg is given every three weeks to accommodate growth, followed in the second or third year by 100 to 150 mg every four weeks. Dosage is increased gradually thereafter to the following maintenance schedule for adults. For maintenance therapy in androgen deficiency, *adults,* 100 mg/M^2 or 150 to 200 mg every two weeks or 300 mg every three weeks.

For metastatic breast carcinoma in *women,* 200 to 400 mg every two to four weeks. Because of marked variation in sensitivity, signs of virilism may occur in some females even with lower doses.

For anabolic therapy, see the Table.
> TESTOSTERONE CYPIONATE:
> *Generic.* Solution (in oil) 100 and 200 mg/ml in 10 ml containers.
> *Andro-Cyp* (Keene). Solution (in cottonseed oil) 100 and 200 mg/ml in 10 ml containers.
> *Depo-Testosterone* (Upjohn). Solution (in cottonseed oil) 50 mg/ml in 10 ml containers and 100 and 200 mg/ml in 1 and 10 ml containers.
> *T-Ionate-P.A.* (Reid-Provident). Solution (in cottonseed oil) 200 mg/ml in 10 ml containers.
> TESTOSTERONE ENANTHATE:
> *Generic.* Solution (in oil) 100 and 200 mg/ml in 10 ml containers.
> *Andryl* (Keene). Solution (in sesame oil) 200 mg/ml in 10 ml containers.
> *Delatestryl* (Squibb). Solution (in sesame oil) 200 mg/ml in 1 and 5 ml containers.

TESTOSTERONE PROPIONATE

Testosterone propionate can be used to induce or maintain secondary sexual characteristics and other physiologic func-

tions in androgen-deficient males. This relatively short-acting preparation produces a steady response when used parenterally, but this route is not practical for long-term therapy. However, in older patients, the prostate gland may be sensitive to androgen and bladder neck obstruction may develop; this complication is more easily corrected if a short-acting preparation is used initially.

The short duration of action also makes testosterone propionate useful initially for the palliative treatment of breast carcinoma in women, because prompt withdrawal of the androgen is necessary if hypercalcemia develops. The propionate ester also may be used parenterally for anabolic purposes.

See the Introduction for other indications and adverse reactions.

DOSAGE AND PREPARATIONS.
Intramuscular: For androgen deficiency, 50 mg three times weekly.

For metastatic breast carcinoma in *women,* 50 to 100 mg three times weekly. Because of marked variation in sensitivity, signs of virilism may occur in women when less than the virilizing dose cited by the manufacturers (300 mg per month) is given.

For anabolic therapy, see the Table.
> *Generic.* Solution (in oil) 25 mg/ml in 10 ml containers and 50 and 100 mg/ml in 10 and 30 ml containers.

IMPEDED ANDROGEN

DANAZOL
[Danocrine]

ACTIONS. This impeded androgen, a synthetic derivative of 17α-ethinyl testosterone (ethisterone), has mild androgenic activity. Danazol does not exhibit estrogenic or progestational properties and suppresses the midcycle surge of LH and FSH. In animals, danazol was shown to bind to androgen receptor and was translocated to the nucleus. Clinical studies have demonstrated that it probably directly inhibits gonadal and adrenal enzymes involved in steroidogenesis, although adrenal function is unaffected except after acute stimulation by exogenous ACTH (Stillman et al, 1980).

Decreased levels of plasma HDL cholesterol and increased levels of other lipoproteins were reported to be associated with danazol, although total cholesterol was unaffected. Effects were reversible after treatment was discontinued (Allen and Fraser, 1981).

USES. Danazol is useful when suppression of gonadal function is desirable.
Fibrocystic Breast Disease: Breast pain and tenderness may be relieved during the first month of danazol therapy, and

nodularity may disappear after four to six months of daily administration (Greenblatt et al, 1980) in up to 80% of patients. Irregular menses or amenorrhea is common, especially with larger doses. Symptoms recur in more than one-half of patients within one to two years after cessation of medication, and another course of therapy may then be initiated. Although dosages employed for this indication are probably associated with nonovulatory cycles and an atrophic endometrium, nonhormonal contraception is recommended during danazol therapy.

Hereditary Angioedema: Danazol is a drug of choice in the long-term prophylaxis of hereditary angioedema but is not effective for acute attacks.

Miscellaneous Uses: Danazol has been used investigationally for other indications. The drug may be effective in precocious puberty in both sexes, although LH-releasing hormone analogues may prove to be preferable for this indication. Regression of secondary sexual characteristics occurs and girls become amenorrheic. However, the accelerated bone maturation is unaffected.

Danazol also has been used investigationally to treat hemophilia A and B. However, there is conflicting evidence as to whether this agent is beneficial or is associated with greater risks than benefits (Hathaway, 1985).

Danazol was reported to relieve symptoms of systemic lupus erythematosus in some women. It also has been used in males to treat gynecomastia and as a component of an experimental oral contraceptive.

ADVERSE REACTIONS AND PRECAUTIONS. Most adverse reactions caused by danazol are related to its weak androgenic and anabolic activity. They include weight gain, edema, acne, oily skin, decreased breast size, and hirsutism. Other hypoestrogenic symptoms (flushing, sweating, vaginitis) also occur in women.

Therapy should begin during menstruation, or a pregnancy test should be performed to rule out that possibility. Pseudohermaphroditism may occur in female infants whose mothers received danazol during early pregnancy.

As with other 17α-alkylated steroids, danazol has been associated with abnormal liver function tests and jaundice. This drug should not be used in patients with markedly impaired hepatic, renal, or cardiac function or in women with abnormal genital bleeding.

PHARMACOKINETICS. After administration of danazol 400 mg, peak plasma levels of 80 to 100 ng/ml are attained in one to two hours. The half-life in plasma is about 4.5 hours (Dmowski, 1979). Unaltered steroid appears to be biologically active. Danazol is metabolized to conjugates, sulfates, and glucuronides and is excreted predominantly in the urine but also in feces.

DOSAGE AND PREPARATIONS.
Oral: For fibrocystic breast disease, 100 to 400 mg daily in two divided doses, depending upon the severity of symptoms and the patient's response.

For angioedema, the initial dose is 400 to 600 mg daily given in divided amounts, with step-down titration to determine the lowest effective amount. Treatment can be reinstituted if symptoms recur upon cessation of therapy.

Danocrine (Winthrop-Breon). Capsules 50, 100, and 200 mg.

MIXTURES

Androgen-Estrogen Preparations

Short-term administration of androgen-estrogen mixtures has been used for postpartum suppression of lactation, but bromocriptine [Parlodel] is preferred for this indication when a pharmacologic agent is appropriate (see also Chapter 39). Combined therapy also has been employed empirically to restore libido in postmenopausal women and to relieve a variety of symptoms that accompany aging, but there is no evidence that the addition of small amounts of androgen to estrogen retards such symptoms. The use of fixed-dose combinations for any of these indications is not encouraged. Masculinizing effects may occur.

FOR POSTPARTUM SUPPRESSION OF LACTATION:
Deladumone OB (Squibb). Each milliliter contains estradiol valerate 8 mg and testosterone enanthate 180 mg in sesame oil.
FOR MENOPAUSAL AND POSTMENOPAUSAL WOMEN:
Deladumone (Squibb), *Teev* (Keene). Each milliliter contains estradiol valerate 4 mg and testosterone enanthate 90 mg in sesame oil.
Depo-Testadiol (Upjohn), *Duo-Cyp* (Keene). Each milliliter contains estradiol cypionate 2 mg and testosterone cypionate 50 mg in cottonseed oil.
Halodrin (Upjohn). Each tablet contains fluoxymesterone 1 mg and ethinyl estradiol 0.02 mg.
Premarin with Methyltestosterone (Ayerst). Each tablet contains conjugated estrogens 0.625 or 1.25 mg and methyltestosterone 5 or 10 mg.

Preparations Containing Androgens, Estrogens, and Other Ingredients

Mixtures containing androgens and estrogens combined with vitamins, minerals, progesterone, sedatives, stimulants, and other drugs are available. Many are advocated for use in geriatric patients, but none of these preparations can be considered desirable therapy.

Mediatric (Ayerst). Each tablet or capsule contains conjugated estrogens 0.25 mg, methyltestosterone 2.5 mg, methamphetamine hydrochloride 1 mg, ascorbic acid (capsules) or sodium ascorbate (tablets) 100 mg, cyanocobalamin 2.5 mcg, thiamine mononitrate 10 mg, riboflavin 5 mg, niacinamide 50 mg, pyridoxine hydrochloride 3 mg, pantothenate calcium 20 mg, and ferrous sulfate dried 36 mg.
Mediatric Liquid (Ayerst). Each 15 ml contains conjugated estrogens 0.25 mg, methyltestosterone 2.5 mg, thiamine hydrochloride 5 mg, cyanocobalamin 1.5 mcg, and methamphetamine hydrochloride 1 mg (alcohol 15%).

Cited References

Ahn YS, et al: Danazol for treatment of idiopathic thrombocytopenic purpura. *N Engl J Med* 308:1396-1399, 1983.
Ahn YS, et al: Danazol therapy for autoimmune hemolytic anemia. *Ann Intern Med* 102:298-301, 1985.
Allen JK, Fraser IS: Cholesterol, high density lipoprotein and danazol. *J Clin Endocrinol Metab* 53:149-152, 1981.

American College of Sports Medicine: Position stand on use of anabolic-androgenic steroids in sports. *Am J Sports Med* 12:13-18, 1984.

Camitta BM, et al: Aplastic anemia: Pathogenesis, diagnosis, treatment, and prognosis. *N Engl J Med* 306:712-718, 1982.

Chestnut CH III: Treatment of postmenopausal osteoporosis: Some current concepts. *Scott Med J* 26:72-80, 1981.

Chestnut CH III, et al: Stanozolol in postmenopausal osteoporosis: Therapeutic efficacy and possible mechanisms of action. *Metabolism* 32:571-580, 1983.

Davidson JM, et al: Hormonal changes and sexual function in aging men. *J Clin Endocrinol Metab* 57:71-77, 1983.

Dmowski WP: Endocrine properties and clinical application of danazol. *Fertil Steril* 31:237-251, 1979.

Dyment PG: Drugs and adolescent athlete. *Pediatr Ann* 13:602-604, 1984.

Friedrich EG Jr: Lichen sclerosus. *J Reprod Med* 17:147-154, 1976.

Friedrich EG Jr, Kalra PS: Serum levels of sex hormones in vulvar lichen sclerosus, and effect of topical testosterone. *N Engl J Med* 310:488-491, 1984.

Gelfand JA, et al: Treatment of hereditary angioedema with danazol: Reversal of clinical and biochemical abnormalities. *N Engl J Med* 295:1444-1448, 1976.

Gladue BA, et al: Neuroendocrine response to estrogen and sexual orientation. *Science* 225:1496-1499, 1984.

Greenblatt RB, et al: Treatment of benign breast disease with danazol. *Fertil Steril* 34:242-245, 1980.

Hathaway WE: Danazol and hemophilia, (editorial). *JAMA* 253:1167, 1985.

Haupt HA, Rovere GD: Anabolic steroids: Review of literature. *Am J Sports Med* 12:469-484, 1984.

Huys J, Van Vaerenbergh PM: Effect of nandrolone decanoate on bone marrow suppression induced by cytostatic agents. *Clin Oncol* 2:207-214, 1976.

Kelley VC, Ruvalcaba RHA: Use of anabolic agents in treatment of short children. *Clin Endocrinol Metab* 11:25-39, 1982.

Kulin HE: Delayed puberty in male, in Krieger DT, Bardin CW (eds): *Current Therapy in Endocrinology 1983-1984.* St Louis, CV Mosby, 1983.

Magee MC: Physiology of sexual behavior: Embryologic organization and adult activation. *Urology* 22:467-478, 1983.

Mellion MB: Anabolic steroids in athletics. *Am Fam Physician* 30:113-119, (July) 1984.

Mendenhall CL, et al: Short-term and long-term survival in patients with alcoholic hepatitis treated with oxandrolone and prednisolone. *N Engl J Med* 311:1464-1470, 1984.

Najean Y: Long-term follow-up in patients with aplastic anemia: Study of 137 androgen-treated patients surviving more than two years. *Am J Med* 71:543-551, 1981.

Neaves WB, et al: Leydig cell numbers, daily sperm production, and serum gonadotropin levels in aging men. *J Clin Endocrinol Metab* 55:756-763, 1984.

Nieschlag E: Endocrine function of human testis in regard to sexuality, in: *Sex Hormones and Behavior.* Ciba Foundation Symposium 62, Excerpta Medica, 1979.

Overly WL, et al: Androgens and hepatocellular carcinoma in athlete, (letter). *Ann Intern Med* 100:158-159, 1984.

Pardridge WM, et al: Androgens and sexual behavior. *Ann Intern Med* 96:488-501, 1982.

Rosenfeld RG, et al: Prospective, randomized study of testosterone treatment of constitutional delay of growth and development in male adolescents. *Pediatrics* 69:681-687, 1982.

Ryan AJ: Anabolic steroids are fool's gold. *Fed Proc* 40:2682-2688, 1981.

Sokol RZ, Swerdloff RS: Hypogonadism: Androgen therapy, in: Krieger DT, Bardin CW (eds): *Current Therapy in Endocrinology 1983-1984.* St Louis, CV Mosby, 1983.

Spiers ASD, et al: Beneficial effects of anabolic steroid during cytotoxic chemotherapy for metastatic cancer. *Am J Med* 12:433-445, 1981.

Stillman RJ, et al: Inhibition of adrenal steroidogenesis by danazol in vivo. *Fertil Steril* 33:401-406, 1980.

Strauss RH, et al: Anabolic steroid use and perceived effects in ten weight-trained women athletes. *JAMA* 253:2871-2874, 1985.

Webb OL, et al: Severe depression of high-density lipoprotein cholesterol levels in weight lifters and body builders by self-administered exogenous testosterone and anabolic-androgenic steroids. *Metabolism* 33:971-975, 1984.

Estrogens, Progestins, and Other Agents Used to Treat Gynecologic Conditions

PHYSIOLOGY. Estradiol 17-β (hereafter referred to as estradiol) is the major estrogen in premenopausal women. A total of 100 to 600 mcg is secreted daily by the ovary. Androstenedione, an androgen precursor, also is secreted by the ovary, where it is converted to testosterone, which then is demethylated and aromatized to estrogen. Androstenedione also may be converted to estrone and then to estradiol. Estradiol and estrone (which is about one-half as potent as estradiol) thus are secreted by the ovary, while estriol (a much weaker estrogen) is formed by the peripheral metabolism of ovarian estrogens. Estradiol and estrone are extensively interconverted in the body.

Estrone also is produced by peripheral conversion of androstenedione in a variety of tissues. In premenopausal women, this conversion accounts for about 25% of the estrone produced; the balance is secreted directly by the ovary. In postmenopausal women, peripheral conversion of androstenedione to estrone is the principal source of this estrogen. Although circulating levels of total estrogens decrease and androstenedione levels are about one-half or less of those in premenopausal women, the daily production of estrone remains similar (about 45 mcg), because of a compensatory increase in the conversion rate of androstenedione. Before menopause, androstenedione is derived almost equally from ovarian and adrenal secretion; after menopause, the principal source of androstenedione is the adrenal cortex.

Progesterone is produced primarily by direct secretion from the ovary (from the corpus luteum after ovulation); a very small amount is secreted by the adrenal cortex. Preovulatory progesterone production is about 1 to 3 mg daily; during the luteal phase, 20 to 30 mg is secreted daily. A small quantity of testosterone is produced by the ovary in normal women. About one-half of the testosterone present is derived from peripheral conversion of androstenedione, and the balance is secreted directly by the ovary and adrenal cortex.

Ovarian estrogen (estradiol) in the premenopausal years is secreted during the follicular and luteal phase of the cycle, while progesterone is secreted almost entirely during the luteal phase. In the follicular phase, FSH interacts with receptors on the granulosa cells and LH with receptors on the thecal cells. The latter results in production of androstenedione and testosterone by the thecal cells. These androgens diffuse into the granulosa cells where aromatizing enzymes (stimulated by FSH) convert them to estrone and estradiol. The combination of FSH and estradiol stimulates growth of new granulosa cells and LH receptors on these cells. During the luteal phase, LH stimulates production of progesterone as well as estrogen in the granulosa cells. Overstimulation of LH receptors is avoided by down-regulation, that is, the number of receptors decreases as LH levels increase.

The increasing levels of estrogen before ovulation act as a positive feedback, modulating the effect of luteinizing hormone releasing hormone (LH-RH), also called gonadotropin releasing hormone (GnRH), and enhancing the pituitary response to LH-RH. This results in a midcycle surge of gonadotropin secretion from the anterior pituitary gland. The high level of luteinizing hormone (LH) is responsible for ovulation of the mature follicle(s). Estrogen and progesterone produced during the luteal phase exert a negative feedback effect on the hypothalamus and anterior pituitary, and gonadotropin secretion during this time is low.

In the perimenopausal years, ovulatory cycles decrease in frequency and the production of ovarian steroids by the follicle and corpora lutea becomes less efficient; this may be due partly to the relative insensitivity of the remaining follicles to the effects of gonadotropin. After menopause, ovarian secretion of estrogen and progesterone essentially ceases, and circulating estrogen (estrone) is produced primarily by peripheral conversion of androstenedione.

The placenta produces enormous quantities of estrogens and progesterone during pregnancy resulting in high levels of steroids in the maternal circulation. These values rise steadily as pregnancy progresses. Since the placenta does not possess the enzyme systems to accomplish this alone, precursors for progesterone must be supplied from the maternal circulation and precursors for estrogen from the fetal adrenal cortex (the fetoplacental unit for steroid production). The latter relationship is the basis for measuring the maternal urinary excretion of estriol daily as one test for fetal well-being in late pregnancy. The functions of the high levels of estrogen and progesterone during pregnancy are not completely understood, but several are probable: Progesterone may suppress the maternal immune response to allow implantation of the blastocyst; it may maintain myometrial quiescence and lack of irritability; and it may serve as a precursor for fetal adrenal corticosteroids. Estrogen stimulates uterine growth and uteroplacental blood flow.

In nonpregnant women, estrogen and progesterone support physiologic processes that ultimately result in release of an ovum and preparation of the uterine endometrium to support a conceptus. The interaction of steroid hormones and gonadotropins, the influence of steroids on ovum and sperm transport, and the stimulation by steroids of endometrial growth and glycogen secretion are all directed toward this end.

Estrogen and progesterone stimulate puberal changes (eg, growth and maturation of uterus, breasts, and other hormone-responsive tissues; stimulation and eventual limitation of linear skeletal growth) and later maintain the integrity of responsive tissues (eg, breast, uterus, vaginal and urethral mucosa). These hormones also have widespread effects on metabolism (eg, transport protein, electrolyte balance). The reduction of circulating estrogen levels following menopause often is associated with symptoms referable to these target tissues (eg, atrophic vagina, urethral irritation, osteoporosis).

The cellular mechanism of action of all steroid hormones is similar. Most evidence has been obtained with estrogen. Steroid hormones cross cell membranes by simple diffusion and bind to intracellular receptors. The hormone-receptor complex penetrates the nuclear membrane, binds to chromatin, and activates selective messenger RNA synthesis. The message undergoes maturation in the nucleus and is transferred to the ribosomes, where enzymes and other proteins are manufactured and carry out the specific cellular function of the hormone.

Estradiol circulates in the blood bound to protein transport carriers. Part is bound to sex-hormone-binding globulin (SHBG), a beta globulin that is also the carrier protein for testosterone; part is loosely bound to albumin, and a small amount is unbound. Progesterone is bound largely to corticosteroid-binding globulin (CBG), which also binds cortisol. For all steroid hormones, including estrogen and progesterone, only the relatively small portion that is unbound or not tightly bound is biologically active.

The steroids are metabolized to inactive forms in the liver and then excreted in the urine and bile. Estrogens are converted to sulfates and glucuronides, and progesterone is metabolized to a number of products, including pregnanediol, and then conjugated. A urine assay for pregnanediol was once widely used to measure progesterone production, but more sensitive, accurate radioimmunoassays and competitive protein binding assays now are widely utilized to measure many of the circulating steroids.

THERAPEUTIC PREPARATIONS. Most of the agents used therapeutically are synthetic or naturally occurring analogues of endogenous hormones. Therapy may provide hormones in unphysiologic patterns to the tissues, and certain tissues may have relatively greater exposure to exogenous hormone compared to normal secretory patterns. For example, with the commonly used oral preparations, the hepatic-portal circulation carries a greater concentration of the hormone than under conditions of normal physiologic secretion.

Estrogens, progesterone, and progestins (synthetic compounds possessing progestational activity) are available in a variety of preparations for oral, parenteral, or topical administration. Natural estrogen and progesterone generally are not useful orally because of rapid deactivation by the liver. An exception is the micronized preparation of estradiol [Estrace] in which particle size is greatly reduced, total surface area is increased, and satisfactory absorption is obtained. Natural estradiol and progesterone are effective when given parenterally. Progesterone also is used as vaginal or rectal suppositories to treat selected patients with infertility (see Chapter 41, Agents Used to Treat Infertility).

All natural estrogen products are steroidal. These include estradiol (see above), estrone compounds, and preparations of conjugated estrogens that are usually prepared from the urine of pregnant mares. Synthetic estrogens may be steroidal or nonsteroidal. The addition of a 17α-ethinyl group to estradiol increases potency and enhances oral activity by impeding hepatic degradation. Quinestrol [Estrovis], which is closely related to ethinyl estradiol [Estinyl, Feminone], is stored in adipose tissue, thus prolonging its action. Esters of estradiol (benzoate, cypionate, valerate) in oily solutions or aqueous suspensions for intramuscular injection have more prolonged activity than oral preparations (see the evaluation).

Most nonsteroidal estrogens are related to stilbene in chemical structure. Diethylstilbestrol (DES), a stilbene, was the first to be synthesized and has potent estrogenic activity. Further modifications in structure yielded other nonsteroidal compounds (eg, dienestrol [DV], methallenestril, chlorotrianisene [TACE]) with varying potency. Clomiphene [Clomid, Serophene], which is related structurally to chlorotrianisene, possesses both estrogenic and antiestrogenic activity and is used to treat infertility (see Chapter 41).

Synthetic progestins are derived from two sources: (1) from modification of the testosterone molecule (norethindrone [Norlutin], norethindrone acetate [Aygestin, Norlutate], and other progestins used only in oral contraceptives), and (2) from 17α-hydroxy-progesterone (hydroxyprogesterone caproate [Delalutin], medroxyprogesterone acetate (MPA) [Amen, Curretab, Depo-Provera, Provera], megestrol acetate [Megace]). Depending upon the parent compound and the chemical alterations employed, these agents have varying degrees of progestational, estrogenic, or androgenic potency.

The biological activities of the synthetic estrogens and progestins are similar, but not identical, to those of the natural compounds. Potency and side effects vary according to the chemical structure or route of administration employed.

Indications

Hormones are administered therapeutically to mimic or accentuate the biological effects of endogenous hormones: to supplement inadequate endogenous production (eg, Turner's syndrome, menopause), to correct hormonal imbalance (eg, dysfunctional bleeding), to reverse an abnormal process (eg, hirsutism, endometriosis), and for contraception (see Chapter 40, Contraceptive Agents).

AMENORRHEA. Estrogen and progestins are used both to determine the etiology of amenorrhea and to treat it, if appropriate. Amenorrhea may be primary or secondary, but generally the same diagnostic approach is employed in either case. A complete medical history and physical examination are necessary to exclude causes outside the reproductive system.

Amenorrhea secondary to hyper- or hypofunction of the adrenal cortex or thyroid or to diabetes mellitus may be corrected by treating the primary disorder. Functional aberrations of neurotransmitters (ie, dopamine, norepinephrine) and/or the endorphin system probably interfere with normal LH-RH secretion, causing amenorrhea (Kase, 1983). Other possible etiologies may be referable to dysfunction at any level of the hypothalamic-pituitary-gonadal axis: hypothalamic/pituitary disorders (eg, prolactin-secreting tumors; hypogonadotropism, including craniopharyngioma and Kallmann's syndrome; functional causes); ovarian defects (eg, premature ovarian failure, Turner's syndrome); or uterine/vaginal defects (eg, congenital absence, Asherman's syndrome, imperforate hymen). Amenorrhea also can result from hyperandrogenic disorders (eg, polycystic ovarian disease, ovarian tumor, adrenal hyperfunction or tumor). Hormones and hormone assays are useful to establish the source of the defect (ie, ovary, endometrium, anterior pituitary, hypothalamus, thyroid, adrenal).

Secondary amenorrhea, particularly in adolescents, may result from inadequate nutrition, excessive exercise, or psychological stress. Amenorrhea also occurs in thin women who engage in regular endurance athletic training (eg, running, dancing, swimming). The cause is unknown but may be related to low body fat or the repeated stress of exercise (Bullen et al, 1985). Another hypothesis suggests that chronic endurance training causes a series of events progressing from increased cardiac output and increased metabolic clearance of gonadal hormones that interferes with normal hypothalamic/pituitary feedback mechanisms to menstrual dysfunction (Casper et al, 1984). This condition is of concern because of the long-term potential for osteoporosis associated with hypoestrogenism. Vertebral bone was reduced in women with amenorrhea from various causes, including that associated with exercise; estrogen levels were in the low normal range (Cann et al, 1984). Cortical bone loss may be less prevalent when amenorrhea is caused by exercise than by other factors (Drinkwater et al, 1984; Jones et al, 1985). It appears that, although exercise enhances bone development, the effect may be inadequate to compensate for low estrogen levels. Amenorrheic athletes should be evaluated for hormonal status after four to six months of missed menses. Patients with evidence of anovulation and unopposed estrogen secretion are given a progestin only, while hypoestrogenic patients are given estrogen plus progestin (Shangold, 1982). Usual replacement doses of an estrogen and progestin or a low-dose oral contraceptive may be given. Some authorities suggest calcium alone for therapy.

Diagnostic Tests: To test for the presence of estrogenic stimulation and ability of the endometrium to respond, intramuscular progesterone in oil (75 to 100 mg) or oral medroxyprogesterone acetate (MPA) (10 mg daily for five days) is administered. *Pregnancy must always be ruled out before exogenous hormones are used for diagnosis.* An oral preparation is often preferred for convenience and to avoid the discomfort associated with injection of progesterone. Withdrawal bleeding three to five days after treatment indicates adequate estrogenic stimulation of the endometrium and probable anovulation; it suggests inadequate production or abnormal temporal pattern of secretion of gonadotropin (hypothalamic-pituitary-ovarian axis dysfunction). Absence of withdrawal bleeding suggests lack of endogenous estrogen stimulation, ovarian failure (high levels of serum gonadotropins support this diagnosis), obstruction of outflow from the uterus, or ovulation within the last two weeks. If bleeding does not occur, a course of estrogen therapy is given with a progestin added at the end of the cycle (withdrawal bleeding demonstrates uterine competence).

If the estrogen-progestin challenge fails to produce withdrawal bleeding, a defect in the outflow tract or endometrium is suggested. The latter may be a result of Asherman's syndrome (uterine synechiae); surgical correction by hysteroscopy and lysis of adhesions is followed by insertion of an IUD (left in place for approximately one month). Alternatively, following surgery, a pediatric Foley catheter filled with 3 ml of fluid is placed in the uterus and allowed to remain for seven days. An antibiotic is given concurrently. Estrogen-progestin therapy designed to rebuild a normal endometrium follows either of these procedures. Suggested postoperative regimens include (1) conjugated estrogens 2.5 mg daily for three weeks plus MPA 10 mg daily during the last ten days of estrogen therapy, repeated monthly for three months, or (2) conjugated estrogens 5 mg daily for three weeks plus MPA 10 mg daily for the last ten days of estrogen therapy, repeated monthly for three cycles.

Drug Therapy: Ovarian failure may be congenital (eg, Turner's syndrome, presence of Y chromosome, mosaicism) or caused by premature menopausal changes. Estrogen replacement therapy should be considered to stimulate or maintain secondary sex characteristics and to prevent osteoporosis. A progestin is given concurrently when the uterus is in situ to prevent unopposed endometrial stimulation. Suggested regimens include conjugated estrogens 0.625 to 1.25 mg daily for 25 days per month with oral MPA 10 mg daily during the last ten days of estrogen therapy. (Atypical adenomatous hyperplasia has developed in women taking conjugated estrogens with seven days or less of MPA therapy.) Each cycle can begin on the first of each month for convenience. The adequacy of such therapy is indicated by the relief of symptoms. Oral contraceptives are generally not used for replacement therapy because they contain pharmacologic, not physiologic, quantities of hormones.

Preliminary results of a study utilizing various estrogen regimens to treat Turner's syndrome suggested that standard treatment may not be ideal. Estrogen therapy has a biphasic effect, and linear growth is stimulated by small doses (about 4 mcg daily) and inhibited by standard dosages (20 to 50 mcg daily) (Ross et al, 1983).

The treatment of amenorrhea caused by dysfunction of the hypothalamic-pituitary-ovarian (HPO) axis depends upon the goals of the patient. After excluding the presence of a pituitary adenoma, other life-threatening disease, and ovarian failure and if the patient desires pregnancy, induction of ovulation may be attempted (see Chapter 41). If pregnancy is not desired and the patient has sufficient endogenous estrogen to promote endometrial stimulation, intermittent progestin therapy should be administered (after pregnancy has been excluded) to interrupt this steady-state estrogen effect and prevent endometrial hyperplasia. MPA 10 mg daily for ten days monthly will serve this purpose and produce withdrawal bleeding.

Patients with HPO axis dysfunction may unknowingly experience return of spontaneous cyclicity and therefore may be at risk of pregnancy if they are sexually active. Nonhormonal contraceptives are generally preferred in these patients, but low-dose OCs are sometimes administered. It has been suggested, but not proven, that OCs further suppress or alter already abnormal HPO axis function. A discussion of the management of amenorrhea and other dysfunction related to anovulation is available (Olive and Hammond, 1985).

DYSFUNCTIONAL UTERINE BLEEDING. Abnormal uterine bleeding may be of organic origin (eg, endometrial cancer, coagulation defects, chronic endometritis, polyps, myomas, complications of pregnancy) or may be dysfunctional, that is, caused by estrogen and progesterone imbalance unassociated with organic pathology. Dysfunctional bleeding is often associated with anovulatory cycles, which are most common during adolescence and the perimenopausal years. This type of cycle produces an estrogen-dominated, fragile, hyperplastic endometrium characterized by periodic profuse bleeding or irregular, possibly chronic, spotting. These abnormalities result from relatively constant, low-level estrogen stimulation uninterrupted by the action of progesterone. Dysfunctional bleeding also may be caused by an atrophic endometrium secondary to progestin dominance. A history of combined OC use with a progressively decreasing volume of withdrawal bleeding or progestin-only (minipill or depot preparation) contraception helps in diagnosing the latter type of bleeding. Endometrial biopsy and medical history assist in determining the rationale of drug therapy. Before hormonal therapy or surgical intervention is initiated, pregnancy should be excluded.

Drug Therapy: If the endometrium is proliferative or hyperplastic, progesterone (50 to 100 mg in oil intramuscularly) or an oral progestin (MPA 10 mg daily for 10 to 20 days) is useful. Alternatively, norethindrone acetate (5 mg daily) or norethindrone (10 mg daily) may be given.

The patient with a denuded endometrium benefits from administration of a high-potency estrogen-progestin combination or estrogen alone to build up a structurally stable endometrium (see Chapter 40 for a listing of oral contraceptive preparations). Conjugated estrogens rarely is used intravenously initially to control acute bleeding. Suggested oral regimens for initial control or following intravenous estrogen include (1) three oral contraceptive pills daily (taken after meals) for seven to ten days; (2) ethinyl estradiol 50 to 100 mcg plus MPA 10 mg daily for seven to ten days; (3) conjugated estrogens 2.5 to 3.75 mg plus MPA 10 mg daily for seven to ten days or conjugated estrogens 5 mg daily for one week with a progestin added the last five days (MPA 10 mg or norethindrone acetate 5 mg daily).

The patient should be prepared for heavy withdrawal bleeding with dysmenorrhea following treatment. The bleeding is usually self-limited and ceases within one to three days; if it continues, curettage may be necessary. Subsequent cycles are regulated by administering OCs for one year or, if contraception is not required, a progestin alone (MPA 10 mg or norethindrone acetate 5 mg daily for ten days preceding expected withdrawal bleeding) can be used during the second six months. Some physicians prefer long-term nonhormonal contraception for young anovulatory patients based on the theoretical possibility (not supported by experimental evidence) of suppressing the already compromised HPO feedback control axis (see also the discussion on Amenorrhea). Clomiphene [Clomid] may be used to induce ovulation in patients who desire pregnancy. If pregnancy fails to ensue, the ovulatory cycle produced will likely produce normal menses.

Uterine prostaglandin levels normally increase during the luteal phase of the cycle, and dysfunctional bleeding is associated with high levels of uterine prostaglandins, particularly prostacyclin. This substance inhibits platelet aggregation and is a vasodilator, actions that are consistent with causing menorrhagia in ovulatory cycles (Strickler, 1985). Nonsteroidal anti-inflammatory agents that are prostaglandin synthetase inhibitors, such as mefenamic acid [Ponstel] or ibuprofen [Advil, Motrin, Nuprin, Rufen], given in the usual therapeutic doses may reduce excessive menstrual fluid loss and dysmenorrhea (Mishell et al, 1984).

DYSMENORRHEA. Dysmenorrhea may be primary or secondary to other conditions (eg, endometriosis), in which case the specific cause is treated. Primary dysmenorrhea probably results from the increased production of prostaglandin (PG) by the secretory endometrium during the luteal phase. Therefore, agents that inhibit ovulation, steroidogenesis, or PG production are often effective. Patients who require contraception as well as relief from primary dysmenorrhea often benefit from treatment with OCs. See Chapter 40 for list of preparations. If dysmenorrhea is not relieved by OCs, endometriosis or another organic cause should be considered. Several types of PG inhibitors that combine effectiveness with safety include fenamates (eg, mefenamic acid, flufenamic acid) and phenylpropionic acid derivatives (eg, ibuprofen [Advil, Medipren, Motrin, Nuprin, Rufen], naproxen [Naprosyn], naproxen sodium [Anaprox], suprofen [Suprol]). These agents are taken at the onset of menstrual discomfort and are particularly useful when concurrent contraception is unnecessary. Treatment is continued only as long as needed to relieve symptoms, usually two to five days. If a patient fails to respond to one agent, another preparation may be successful. Indomethacin [Indocin] also is effective, but adverse effects are reported more commonly (Budoff, 1982; Roy, 1983; Wenzloff and Shimp, 1984; Dawood, 1985). See Chapter 4, General Analgesics, for preparations.

PREMENSTRUAL SYNDROME (PMS). This syndrome is characterized by complaints such as irritability, depression, anxiety, abdominal bloating and fluid retention, headache, and enlargement and tenderness of breasts; these symptoms occur premenstrually and not at other times in the menstrual cycle. PMS may occur in any menstruating woman, but the incidence increases in those over 30 years. Interpretation of studies is difficult because of lack of standard criteria and different measures used to determine efficacy. Patterns of symptoms are variable, and the probability of several distinct types of premenstrual syndrome with separate etiologies seems likely. It is, therefore, not surprising that none of the wide variety of pharmacologic treatments suggested for PMS has been universally effective. Most have not been proved effective by controlled studies and there are conflicting reports of efficacy among those most widely recommended (Havens, 1985).

Drug Therapy: Progesterone has been used in severe PMS for many years (Dalton, 1984). The drug may be administered parenterally but vaginal or rectal suppositories are more convenient; an intranasal cream is being investigated. Its trial is based on the theoretical premise that a relative progesterone deficiency or an increased estrogen:progesterone ratio causes PMS. However, the validity of this etiology has not been demonstrated universally, and controlled studies have yielded conflicting results. Nevertheless, this drug is widely used and is claimed to be effective for selected patients. In one study, PMS patients who responded to progesterone had different cyclic characteristics than nonresponders and the possibility of selecting responders based on cyclic patterns was suggested (Richter et al, 1984).

An agonist of LH-RH suppressed cyclic function, including menses and symptoms of PMS, in some patients. However, it is unlikely that this agent would be appropriate for chronic therapy because of the long-term effects of low estrogen levels (eg, osteoporosis) (Muse et al, 1984).

Pyridoxine (vitamin B_6) has alleviated depression associated with oral contraceptive use. In such instances, contraceptive hormones are believed to cause a relative vitamin B deficiency, alter tryptophan metabolism, and decrease serotonin production, which causes depression. The suggestion that a similar hormone-related etiology is responsible for depression in PMS has led to the use of pyridoxine for this indication. One study demonstrated that doses of 100 mg daily given from the tenth day of the cycle to the third day of the following cycle were more effective than placebo (Barr, 1984). Other uncontrolled studies have produced variable results.

Because prolactin is involved in osmoregulation in lower animals and some symptoms of PMS appear to be related to fluid retention, it has been suggested that this hormone may be a causative factor in PMS. However, no consistent differences in serum prolactin have been observed in symptomatic and normal women. Bromocriptine [Parlodel], a dopaminergic agent that inhibits prolactin secretion, has been used to treat PMS. Although relief of breast tenderness, abdominal bloating, and depression has been reported, favorable responses are not universal.

Diuretics also are used to treat PMS and may relieve symptoms related to fluid retention. It was hypothesized that aldosterone levels, which are elevated during the luteal phase of the cycle, may be responsible for fluid retention premenstrually. Spironolactone [Aldactone], an aldosterone inhibitor, relieved premenstrual symptoms in a double-blind study. However, because serum levels of aldosterone were no higher in symptomatic women, it was suggested that the effect of spironolactone was related to its nonspecific diuretic action (O'Brien et al, 1979).

Oral contraceptives, which are effective in dysmenorrhea, have been reported to relieve PMS in some patients but generally are not considered useful for this indication.

Definitive studies are necessary to define all etiologic factors more clearly and assist in the development of rational treatment for PMS.

HIRSUTISM. Plasma androgen levels are elevated in most hirsute women. Although the total testosterone concentration may be in the normal range, the combination of decreased protein binding of testosterone and elevation of free (biologically active) testosterone may be sufficient to cause hirsutism. In one study on 138 hirsute women, the free plasma testosterone level was elevated in 82% and dehydroepiandrosterone sulfate (DHEA-S) was increased in 59% of patients (Wild et al, 1983). Conditions such as Cushing's syndrome, congenital adrenal hyperplasia, and ovarian or adrenal neoplasms must be considered in the differential diagnosis and treated appropriately if present. It should also be recognized that greater than average hair growth may be a normal characteristic of certain ethnic groups (eg, those of Mediterranean descent).

Diagnostic Tests: Diagnostic tests include measurements of serum total testosterone (unbound or free testosterone determination is more expensive and probably not necessary) and DHEA-S. The latter yields the same information as the less convenient measurement of 24-hour 17-ketosteroids. Determination of serum prolactin is also useful because hyperprolactinemia is sometimes associated with hyperandrogenism (Glickman et al, 1982). Androstanediol glucuronide also is elevated in hirsutism (Greep et al, 1986). Thyroid function is tested and treated if abnormal. Endometrial biopsy is useful to evaluate anovulation, which is frequently present. Rapidly progressing signs of masculinization and very high serum androgen concentrations (ie, greater than 200 ng/dl testosterone, greater than 700 mcg/dl DHEA-S) suggest tumor of the ovary or adrenal gland, respectively. Lower levels usually represent ovarian and/or adrenal dysfunction.

It was once thought that hypersecretion of ovarian androgen due to elevated LH was the most common cause of hirsutism, but the frequent findings of slightly elevated serum DHEA-S and decreased androgen levels in response to glucocorticoid therapy suggest that the adrenal gland also is affected. Some hirsute women show hyperresponsiveness to corticotropin similar to that in patients with Cushing's disease (Meikle et al, 1984). Whether the primary defect is ovarian or adrenal, or whether this can be readily determined or is critical in the choice of therapy, is not understood completely.

Drug Therapy: Various pharmacologic agents have been used to treat hirsutism (Braithwaite and Jabamoni, 1983). A combination oral contraceptive preparation is selected most often. The progestin suppresses ovarian steroidogenesis secondary to LH while the estrogen component increases sex hormone-binding globulin, which binds to testosterone and decreases the quantity of free hormone. If estrogen is contraindicated, a progestin may be used instead (eg, medroxyprogesterone acetate: oral 30 mg/day, intramuscular depot 150 mg every three months).

In patients who do not respond after several months, particularly those with persistently elevated DHEA-S levels, a trial of glucocorticoid (eg, dexamethasone 0.5 mg daily before bedtime) may be used. Adrenal androgen production is stimulated by ACTH, and low doses of glucocorticoid may suppress excessive androgen secretion. The selection of patients who would benefit from this therapy has been largely on an empiric basis. One study suggested a dichotomy of response in hirsute patients. Patients who responded to a glucocorticoid with a decrease in serum testosterone greater than 50% also demonstrated lower LH levels with long-term glucocorticoid therapy. In patients whose serum testosterone was decreased less than 50% after glucocorticoid administration, prolonged therapy failed to reduce circulating LH (Karpas et al, 1984). Until it is possible to predict whether a patient is most likely to respond to sex steroids or glucocorticoid therapy, the latter probably should be used as an alternative to sex steroid therapy, and the usual precautions associated with glucocorticoid administration should be taken (see Chapter 61, Adrenal Corticosteroids in Nonendocrine Diseases).

With either type of therapy, up to one year of treatment may be required before effects are apparent. Although hormones suppress new hair growth, normal androgen levels maintain hair that is already present. Electrolysis is useful to hasten the cosmetic results.

Other agents are also administered to treat hirsutism. Bromocriptine may be used when hirsutism is secondary to hyperprolactinemia. Cyproterone acetate, an agent with antiandrogen and progestin activity, is not marketed in the United States but is available in some European countries and Canada. This agent inhibits binding of androgen to intracellular binding protein and also has antigonadotropic activity. Successful treatment of hirsutism with a "reverse sequential" regimen (cyclic administration of cyproterone and estrogen followed by estrogen alone) has been reported (Garner and Poznanski, 1984). Side effects may include loss of libido and depression.

Spironolactone [Aldactone], an antihypertensive agent, also appears to be useful for treating hirsutism. It inhibits ovarian androgen synthesis and competes for androgen receptors in susceptible hair follicles (Cumming et al, 1982). Diuresis may occur for several days after initiating therapy, and there is the potential for hyperkalemia. Cimetidine [Tagamet] also has been administered to treat hirsutism, and probably acts by a peripheral mechanism because serum androgen levels are not reduced (Vigersky et al, 1980).

See also Speroff et al, 1983, for a discussion of diagnosis and treatment of hirsutism.

ENDOMETRIOSIS. Treatment of endometriosis depends partly on whether the patient desires immediate or future pregnancy (see Chapter 41, Agents Used to Treat Infertility). Endometriosis may be treated surgically, ranging from a conservative procedure, in which the reproductive organs are preserved for future pregnancy, to total hysterectomy with removal of both ovaries. In general, the latter approach is used if other methods have failed.

Various pharmacologic regimens offer some degree of effectiveness. Danazol inhibits ovarian steroidogenesis by inhibiting gonadotropin secretion and, probably, by a direct action on the ovary. Without hormonal support, growth of endometrial implants is prevented. The drug does not possess significant estrogenic or progestational activity. The mild androgenic effect of this agent is responsible for its side effects (eg, weight gain, oily skin and acne, hypoestrogenic symptoms). Although danazol is expensive compared to other drug regimens, it is probably the agent most frequently used when hormonal therapy is indicated.

Since endometrial implants undergo decidualization, necrosis, and reabsorption during pregnancy, induction of a pseudopregnant state by the continuous (noncyclic) administration of combination OCs (low-dose OCs are effective; see Chapter 40 for preparations) for six to nine months also may be of benefit. If estrogens are contraindicated, oral or depot MPA may be employed. The depot form has a variable duration of action and may cause amenorrhea that lasts for months or occasionally years. Other progestins also may be used to treat endometriosis. Because a progestin alone produces an atrophic endometrium rather than decidual progression, irregular bleeding may occur.

Methyltestosterone 10 mg daily also may relieve symptoms but has little histologic effect on implants and is not commonly used.

LH-RH analogues are being used investigationally to treat endometriosis. These agents induce a hypoestrogenic state, but do not have androgenic side effects.

See Chapter 41 for a more detailed discussion of endometriosis.

ABERRANT GROWTH PATTERNS. Puberty may be delayed by associated disorders or may represent constitutional delay of puberty (CDP), a variant of normal. Short stature is a feature in abnormal states, such as growth hormone deficiency and gonadal dysgenesis. Girls with CDP may be short but have a height appropriate for the bone age. Differentiation between CDP and hypogonadotropic hypogonadism may be difficult and remain unresolved for years. If there is severe psychological stress due to lack of development in the interim, brief treatment designed to stimulate development without advancing bone age is sometimes instituted. Ethinyl estradiol 5 to 10 mcg daily or conjugated estrogens 0.6 to 1.25 mg daily can be given for three months. The course may be repeated in six months if lack of development persists. If there is no spontaneous activity by 17 years of age, a gonadotropin deficiency probably exists, and replacement therapy can be undertaken after this has been documented.

Puberty can be induced in girls with sexual infantilism from any cause that requires treatment with the above regimen. Therapy can be initiated at age 12 or, when concomitant growth hormone deficiency exists, may be delayed until several years after treatment with growth hormone is undertaken. When secondary sexual characteristics appear (the dosage may be doubled if development does not progress), estrogen is given for 21 to 25 days per month. When breakthrough bleeding occurs, MPA 5 or 10 mg daily is administered concurrently during the last ten days of the cycle. This regimen is repeated monthly.

The diagnosis of *constitutional precocious puberty* is likely in girls who experience puberal changes before age 8 after ovarian, adrenal, hypothalamic, pineal, or HCG-producing tumors have been ruled out. Large doses of depot MPA suppress gonadotropin secretion. Breast size decreases (but may subsequently increase during treatment) and menses cease. However, epiphyseal closure is not prevented, and adult height may be limited. Suggested regimens include 400 mg intramuscularly once every three months, 100 to 200 mg/M² intramuscularly weekly, or 20 to 40 mg orally daily. Danazol [Danocrine], cyproterone acetate, and a long-acting analogue of LH-RH have been used investigationally to treat precocious puberty.

When otherwise normal girls have a predicted adult height (from tables based on present stature and bone age) of greater than six feet and when realization of this growth potential is severely threatening to the child, estrogen therapy is sometimes employed to *suppress the growth rate* and the eventual height attained. Estrogens inhibit production of somatomedin and are effective even though growth hormone levels increase during treatment. Therapy is more effective when begun early, but this principle has limitations. Treatment at age 8 or 9 may be undesirable because of the psychological impact of the long-term regimen (usually one to two years) and the puberal changes, including induced menses, that result. On the other hand, if therapy is not begun until after the adolescent growth spurt (usually premenarcheal), suppression of growth is often minimal. There is usually an initial acceleration of growth before suppression occurs. If therapy is discontinued before epiphyseal closure, further growth will occur.

When estrogen treatment is initiated by bone age of 11 or 12 years (or early to midpuberty), adult height averages 2 to 3 inches less than the predicted height. Dosages are approximately ten times those used for replacement therapy. Suggested regimens include conjugated estrogens 5 to 10 mg (or the equivalent) daily and continuously, with a progestin (eg, MPA 10 mg, norethindrone 10 mg daily) added for ten days each month to induce withdrawal bleeding and thus avoid overstimulation of the endometrium. Bromocriptine [Parlodel] has been suggested as a safe and effective alternative treatment for this indication. The drug reduces the growth hormone response to protirelin and, after 6 to 12 months of therapy, the predicted adult height was reduced in most patients (Evain-Brion et al, 1984).

The potential hazards of estrogen therapy must be considered, and the long-term effects of therapy are unknown. The HPO axis apparently is not suppressed, however, since almost all patients experience spontaneous regular menses two to six months after cessation of treatment. Decreased antithrombin levels (but not clinical signs of thrombosis) have been observed, and it was suggested that serum antithrombin levels should be monitored during treatment (Blombäck et al, 1983). Some clinicians feel that the risks of therapy outweigh the benefits of attempting to restrict linear growth.

CANCER. Hormonal therapy is employed commonly in *metastatic breast cancer*. Demonstration of estrogen receptors in the neoplasm is necessary when selecting patients who will benefit from hormonal treatment. Their absence is an excellent predictor of failure, but their presence is not an entirely reliable predictor of success (about 60% of estrogen receptor-positive patients respond to therapy). Patients with both progesterone and estrogen receptors in the neoplasm may have higher response rates (McGuire, 1982). Patients with estrogen-negative receptors or those who fail to respond to hormonal management may receive chemotherapy.

Large doses of estrogen may be used in selected patients with metastatic breast cancer ten or more years after menopause. Progestins or androgens also are sometimes employed. The latter appear to be more effective in peri- than in postmenopausal women and when bone metastases occur. This type of hormonal therapy may be employed when relapse occurs after initial response to hormonal manipulation (eg, tamoxifen).

Progestin therapy may benefit up to 40% of patients with metastatic *endometrial carcinoma*. Best results usually are observed in younger patients, those with well-differentiated tumors, and patients with progesterone and/or estrogen receptors in the neoplastic tissue (Kauppila, 1984). Large doses produce endometrial atrophy; in addition, tumor nodules may decrease in size and pulmonary metastases may disappear. Regression or arrest may be only temporary, although some patients have experienced long-term remissions. One to two months of treatment may be necessary before an objective response becomes evident. Although response to therapy is not related to site of metastases, undifferentiated tumors or those displaying a papillary growth pattern are less responsive than tumors demonstrating squamous metaplasia.

Megestrol acetate has induced remission of advanced recurrent *ovarian carcinoma* in almost one-half of patients treated (Geisler, 1983).

Hormone-sensitive disseminated *prostatic carcinoma* is

treated with estrogens, bilateral orchiectomy, or, more recently, leuprolide [Lupron]. Hormonal manipulation induces histologic remission of the tumor and regression of bone metastases. The effectiveness of estrogen therapy is partly due to suppression of LH secretion with resultant suppression of testosterone production, and that of castration is due to removal of the primary source of this androgen. Estrogen also may act by directly suppressing the growth of tumor cells and by nonspecific stimulation of the immune response.

Signs of improvement occur in 80% of patients and include decreased gland size with subsequent relief of urinary obstruction, rapid relief of ostealgia, and increased feeling of well-being. The effect is palliative but may last several years, although survival may not be prolonged. Undesirable side effects include loss of libido, impotence, gynecomastia, thromboembolic phenomena, and congestive heart failure due to fluid retention.

Other hormonal agents to treat metastatic prostatic cancer are being investigated (Geller and Albert, 1983). The combination of a large dose of megestrol acetate with a small amount of DES may provide greater therapeutic benefit than either agent alone (Canetta et al, 1983).

See also Chapter 64, Drugs Used in Cancer Chemotherapy.

MENOPAUSE. The menopause is often accompanied by vasomotor symptoms (ie, hot flushes, sweating) that respond best to estrogen replacement. Subjective complaints are associated with decreased skin resistance and core temperature, increased skin temperature, perspiration on the upper part of the body, and increased pulse rate. Although the onset of flushing occurs just prior to pulsatile secretion of ACTH, LH, and growth hormone from the pituitary, these secretions are not causative (Meldrum et al, 1984); flushes also occur in women who have undergone hypophysectomy. Both flushes and pulsatile pituitary secretion are probably due to hypothalamic neurotransmitter release.

Evidence suggests that decreased endogenous opioids in the hypothalamus and brain stem may trigger increased noradrenergic activity that in turn stimulates neurons involved in thermoregulation and releasing hormone production (Casper and Yen, 1985). The hypothalamic thermoregulatory set point is lowered, resulting in increased peripheral blood flow and sweating, which facilitate heat loss. Transient changes in plasma catecholamines (increased epinephrine, decreased norepinephrine) have been observed within minutes of a flush and are consistent with increased heart rate and finger blood flow (Kronenberg et al, 1984). Objectively measured hot flushes correlate with waking episodes during sleep, which suggests that menopausal flushes are associated with chronic sleep disturbances. Both the number of flushes and nocturnal waking episodes decrease with estrogen therapy (Erlik et al, 1981).

Manifestations of vaginal and urethral atrophy (eg, vaginitis, dyspareunia, urinary frequency) may occur after menopause and usually respond to estrogen therapy. The presence of estrogen receptors in the lower urinary tract support the use of estrogens to treat urinary stress incontinence in postmenopausal women (Iosif et al, 1981). Changes in vaginal physiology at menopause (ie, increased pH; decreased blood flow, fluid, transvaginal potential difference) also are reversed by estrogen therapy (Semmens and Wagner, 1982).

Emotional complaints (eg, irritability, anxiety, depression), fatigability, and headache sometimes occur and may be secondary to other, particularly vasomotor, disturbances. However, significant improvement in memory and reduction of anxiety have been observed after estrogen therapy in women who did not report vasomotor flushing (Campbell, 1976).

Aging is accompanied by loss of elasticity and wrinkling of the skin. Although a cosmetic benefit from estrogen replacement therapy has not been demonstrated clearly, some observations are of interest. Estrogen receptors in skin increase in number when oophorectomized women are given estrogen. Estrogen reportedly helped to maintain epidermal thickness (Nichols et al, 1984), and postmenopausal women with implants of estrogen and testosterone had higher skin collagen content than untreated women (Brincat et al, 1985).

In general, other agents are less effective in relieving estrogen-responsive menopausal symptoms. However, when estrogen is contraindicated, alternative agents, which are less effective or have unpleasant side effects at effective doses, may relieve some symptoms. Progestins, clonidine [Catapres], or methyldopa [Aldomet] may be tried for vasomotor symptoms. In a placebo-controlled, double-blind, crossover study, MPA relieved hot flushes and reduced the amplitude and frequency of LH pulses (Albrecht et al, 1981). In addition to relieving vasomotor symptoms, MPA may retard bone resorption (Lobo et al, 1984). Although effectiveness in clinical trials has not been universal, the preponderance of studies have shown that clonidine reduces the number of flushes by at least 50% (Hammar and Berg, 1985). In another double-blind, placebo-controlled study, propranolol [Inderal] reduced the frequency and severity of vasomotor symptoms (Alcoff et al, 1981). Lubricants may be tried for relief of dyspareunia but are generally not effective.

Preparations and Regimens for Menopausal Therapy: Oral estrogen preparations are most often recommended to treat menopausal symptoms and conjugated estrogens are most commonly used. Other natural and synthetic oral preparations are also effective, and the superiority of a particular type has not been demonstrated conclusively.

Effectiveness and side effects are influenced by the route of administration, pattern of delivery (cyclic or continuous), and dosage, as well as by the specific compound or preparation. For example, the hepatic circulation has greater exposure to hormone absorbed orally; thus, the metabolic effects with this route may differ from those exerted with parenteral administration. Natural estrogens (ie, conjugated estrogens, micronized estradiol, piperazine estrone sulfate) cause less hepatic response relative to their ability to suppress FSH than the synthetic estrogens, ethinyl estradiol and diethylstilbestrol (Mashchak et al, 1982). Relatively more estradiol is converted to estrone when estradiol is given by the oral compared to parenteral route (Nichols et al, 1984). However, equivalent amounts of ethinyl estradiol given orally or vaginally produced similar hepatic effects, suggesting that the 17α-ethinyl group in this compound produces adverse hepatic effects regardless of the route of administration (Goebelsmann et al, 1985).

Vaginal estrogen preparations are readily absorbed and produce higher blood levels than the same quantity given orally. They are effective for systemic as well as local symptoms but should not be prescribed when estrogen is contraindicated. If symptoms of atrophic urogenital changes are the only indication for postmenopausal estrogen therapy, intermittent courses of estrogen in low doses administered intravaginally may be appropriate.

With injection of long-acting preparations, exposure to the hormone is uninterrupted; injections are also inconvenient and usually expensive. If these preparations are used when the uterus is in place, a progestin also should be prescribed. Complete protection of the endometrium under conditions of steady estrogen levels may require progestin therapy for one-half of each month (Thom et al, 1979).

Sublingual, intranasal, and transdermal methods of estrogen delivery are being investigated (Nichols et al, 1984; Place et al, 1985; Powers et al, 1985). A transdermal estradiol preparation [Estraderm] may be marketed soon. Subcutaneous implants provide relatively steady plasma estrogen levels and may be particularly useful for surgical menopause. However, they are difficult to remove in case of overdosage. Easily removable vaginal rings avoid this problem.

In general, the goal of menopausal estrogen therapy is to relieve specific symptoms with the lowest effective dosage. Not all target organs are restored to the normal premenopausal condition, but most symptoms can be controlled by conjugated estrogens 0.625 mg or the equivalent given daily and cyclically. Bone loss and fractures are also prevented by this amount of conjugated estrogens or by 20 mcg of ethinyl estradiol (Hammond, 1984; Lindsay et al, 1984). Initial control of symptoms may require larger doses than those used for maintenance. Eventually, withdrawal of medication is recommended in the absence of continuing symptoms or other indications (ie, prophylaxis or treatment of osteoporosis). Vasomotor symptoms usually diminish, and the dose can be reduced gradually or discontinued eventually.

Certain risks, including endometrial cancer (see the section on Metabolic Effects, Adverse Reactions, and Precautions), must be considered in patients receiving estrogen therapy. These women should be re-evaluated at 6- to 12-month intervals to confirm the continuing need for medication, as well as to monitor status. Blood pressure, breast, and pelvic examinations should be included. Endometrial biopsy or another method of endometrial sampling should be performed annually if an estrogen alone is administered cyclically or there are other risk factors for endometrial cancer. Papanicolaou smears should include material from the endocervical canal. Any episode of abnormal bleeding should be investigated promptly and thoroughly.

Current recommendations are for cyclic administration of estrogen when the uterus is in situ to avoid uninterrupted stimulation of the endometrium. The addition of a progestin reduces the incidence of endometrial hyperplasia and carcinoma (see below). With the combined regimen, estrogen is administered daily for three weeks and a progestin (usually MPA 10 mg) is administered daily for the last 10 to 13 days of each estrogen cycle. This regimen is followed by one week with no hormonal therapy during which withdrawal bleeding occurs. The hormonal regimen then is resumed whether or not bleeding has ceased. Whether the same level of endometrial protection can be afforded by a dose of progestin that does not cause bleeding has not been determined. For convenience, each cycle of therapy can be initiated on the first of the month. Other estrogen-progestin regimens also are being investigated. In one study, continuous administration of various oral estrogen/progestin combinations resulted in endometrial atrophy without withdrawal bleeding (Magos et al, 1985).

A similar schedule is followed if estrogen is given without a progestin (three weeks on therapy, one week off). Some physicians recommend endometrial sampling if any bleeding occurs with estrogen-only therapy. Cyclic therapy is advised even in women who have undergone hysterectomy, since this pattern more closely simulates premenstrual secretion of estrogen and avoids continuous stimulation of other target tissues. Opinion is divided on the advisability of adding progestin to the estrogen regimen in hysterectomized women. Those in favor cite possible protection from breast cancer as a benefit of combined therapy.

The rationale for use of the combination regimen is based on the effects of a progestin on estrogen-primed tissue: Progestin decreases estrogen receptors and enhances conversion of estradiol to estrone, thus inhibiting the ultimate growth-stimulating effect of the hormone. Secretory changes are induced and the endometrial lining regresses, making endometrial conditions unfavorable for the development of hyperplasia. One study showed that after one year of replacement therapy with estrogen only, there was a high incidence of endometrial hyperplasia after both continuous and cyclic therapy. The addition of a progestin was recommended (Schiff et al, 1982). Other studies have shown that fewer endometrial carcinomas occurred in women who used a combined regimen (Hammond et al, 1979, part II); fewer endometrial carcinomas also occurred in menopausal women given estrogen and progestin than in women who did not receive any hormonal replacement (Gambrell et al, 1983 A).

A progestin challenge test has been suggested to reduce the risk of endometrial carcinoma in estrogen-treated women and postmenopausal women with high endogenous estrogen production. The test consists of administering a progestin (eg, MPA 10 mg, norethindrone acetate 5 mg) for 10 to 13 days each month as long as withdrawal bleeding occurs. The procedure may be repeated annually after negative results are obtained (Gambrell et al, 1980). Careful monitoring is always required, and abnormal bleeding requires investigation of endometrial status.

If long-term estrogen therapy is considered in postmenopausal women, the expected benefits must outweigh the risks and the patient should understand the factors involved and participate in the decision. For a discussion of the cardiovascular effects of estrogen replacement therapy, see the section on Metabolic Effects, Adverse Reactions, and Precautions below. More accurate assessment of the risk/benefit ratio will become possible with use of diagnostic improvements, such as single photon absorptiometry (Wasnich et al, 1985), that permit early identification of women likely to become osteoporotic, and as cost-effective methods for endometrial sampling become available to ensure early detection of endometrial pathology.

For further discussion of the menopause and the management of related problems, see Judd et al, 1983; Hammond and Maxson, 1982; Upton, 1982, 1984; Council on Scientific Affairs, American Medical Association, 1983; and Gambrell, 1982.

OSTEOPOROSIS. This disorder occurs frequently after menopause and is a more serious problem in women who have earlier loss of ovarian function (eg, surgical menopause, gonadal dysgenesis). It is uncommon in men and black women. Thin, small-framed, Caucasian women and women who smoke are more susceptible. Immobilization, high alcohol ingestion, low calcium intake, and malabsorption of calcium also enhance the risk. Thirty-five to forty percent of postmenopausal women develop osteoporosis, and about 25% of white women over 60 years of age have vertebral compression fractures. Fractures of the radius and neck of the femur also are common in osteoporotic women. Hip fractures have high associated morbidity and mortality (one-sixth of elderly patients with hip fractures die within three months of injury). Only 25% to 30% of elderly white women do not experience appreciable bone loss.

The development of osteoporosis is more closely related to estrogen deficiency than to advancing age per se; estrogens are believed to inhibit bone resorption. Onset of osteoporosis is more rapid after bilateral oophorectomy than after natural menopause, possibly because the decline of estrogen levels in the former situation is rapid, whereas the decline is more gradual in natural menopause. Because there are no estrogen receptors in bone tissue, the hormone's effect on bone is believed to be secondary and may involve inhibition of bone sensitivity to PTH and stimulation of calcitonin secretion. Although differences in plasma calcitonin are not observed, less calcitonin is secreted in response to calcium infusion in osteoporotic women than in normal women (Judd et al, 1983). Studies on the use of calcitonin [Calcimar] to treat osteoporosis are in progress but results thus far have been disappointing (see also Chapter 49, Agents Affecting Calcium Metabolism).

Unfortunately, routine radiographic procedures detect osteoporosis only after considerable bone loss has occurred. Diagnostic techniques, such as quantitative computed tomography, dual photon absorptiometry, and neutron activation analysis, are being developed; these may be sensitive enough to detect asymptomatic early bone loss and to monitor the effectiveness of therapy. Single photon absorptiometry is becoming increasingly available at an affordable cost (about $50) and is useful for screening purposes. The other procedures are relatively expensive and/or availability is limited.

Drug Therapy: Estrogen replacement therapy is particularly effective in preventing osteoporosis in women who have undergone oophorectomy before natural menopause. However, estrogen also retards bone loss after natural menopause. Several studies have demonstrated that the risk of fractures is reduced in menopausal women given estrogen replacement therapy (Hammond et al, 1979, part I; Hutchinson et al, 1979; Weiss et al, 1980; Paganini-Hill et al, 1981; Jensen et al, 1982). Withdrawal of estrogen therapy after four years was

followed by rapid bone loss and the end result was similar to that in women who did not receive estrogen (Lindsay et al, 1978). However, another study showed that after two years with an estrogen-progestin regimen followed by one year of placebo, the bone mineral content was still higher than among women treated for the entire period with placebo (Christiansen et al, 1981). In another study, at the end of an average of 14 years of estrogen replacement therapy followed by 3.6 years of additional observation, postmenopausal women treated with estrogen experienced only one-half the fractures and had greater bone mineral content by several measures than untreated controls (Ettinger et al, 1985).

Estrogen alone prevents bone loss and may result in slight net gain of bone tissue if given in adequate doses (Horsman et al, 1983). The addition of a progestin to the regimen appears to afford even more protection (Upton, 1982). In clinical studies utilizing combined estrogen-progestin regimens, bone resorption decreased and bone mass increased (Nachtigall et al, 1979; Christiansen et al, 1981, 1982). In one study, a progestin alone prevented bone mineral loss in postmenopausal women treated continuously for one year. The mechanism appeared to be different from that of estrogen (Abdalla et al, 1985). However, no agent available reverses bone changes of the magnitude of those observed in osteoporosis.

The most effective use of estrogen is in prophylaxis of osteoporosis when treatment is begun before significant bone loss has occurred; administration must be continued to maintain the effect. In one study, bone loss was retarded for an average of nine years (Lindsay et al, 1980).

Because of the serious consequences of osteoporosis, long-term estrogen therapy should be considered for high-risk or symptomatic women, for those who have undergone early hysterectomy (in whom the possibility of endometrial cancer is obviated), and for patients in whom bone loss has been confirmed by single and/or dual photon absorptiometry. It has been suggested that prophylactic therapy also be administered to postmenopausal women who have high urinary excretion of hydroxyproline, which is correlated with bone loss (Nordin, 1979). The possibility of a predictive test for osteoporosis was suggested by a study in which perimenopausal women with increased bone alkaline phosphatase were shown to experience more fractures during an eight-year follow-up (Collins et al, 1984).

Weight-bearing exercise should be encouraged, and adequate intake of calcium should be assured through diet and dietary supplements if necessary. Postmenopausal women treated with estrogen require a total of 1 g of calcium daily, and those not receiving replacement therapy require 1.5 g daily. Premenopausal women in their mid-thirties or early forties may begin to supplement calcium in their diet to assure 1 g of calcium intake daily. (See also Chapter 49, Agents Affecting Calcium Metabolism.)

Calcium alone does not prevent loss of bone mineral content (Nilas et al, 1984), although it probably reduces the amount lost (National Institutes of Health Consensus Conference, 1984). A regimen of estrogen, calcium, and fluoride prevented vertebral fractures in postmenopausal osteoporotic patients better than other combinations of these agents or estrogen or calcium alone. The addition of vitamin D to any of these regimens did not increase effectiveness. Some patients discontinued the fluoride regimens because of side effects (Riggs et al, 1982).

Androgens and anabolic steroids are sometimes used, and preliminary evidence suggests that bone loss is slowed and bone mass is increased (Chestnut, 1984). However, masculinizing side effects may occur in postmenopausal women, and this treatment is not generally favored. There are no studies comparing the effectiveness of anabolic steroids to that of estrogen plus progestin.

For preparations and regimens used for osteoporosis, see the discussion on Menopause and Chapter 49, Agents Affecting Calcium Metabolism.

PREVENTION OF POSTPARTUM LACTATION. Lactation eventually ceases without drug intervention in the absence of suckling, but breast engorgement and pain (which can be relieved at least partially by analgesics) are common. Estrogens, alone or with an androgen, often have been used to prevent lactation and the discomforts associated with its suppression. However, there is an increased risk of thromboembolic phenomena, and rebound lactation often occurs after withdrawal of medication. Androgens are often only partially effective and masculinizing side effects are possible even with brief use. Following parturition, prolactin levels usually remain elevated for only two to three weeks.

When bromocriptine [Parlodel] is used for 14 days postpartum to prevent lactation, discontinuation of medication does not usually increase prolactin secretion or cause lactation to persist. Once secretion is inhibited and the suckling stimulus is absent, the hormonal conditions necessary to reinitiate lactation are no longer present. Therefore, bromocriptine is the drug of choice when pharmacologic intervention is deemed desirable to suppress postpartum lactation.

In controlled studies, bromocriptine was more effective and safer than estrogens or androgens in preventing breast engorgement, discomfort, and lactation. Normal prolactin levels are achieved within one day after initiating therapy. This drug also is more effective in suppressing established lactation; rebound lactation occurs only infrequently in this subgroup of patients (Rolland, 1979; Duchesne and Leke, 1981).

HYPOVENTILATION. Endogenous progesterone stimulates respiration during the luteal phase and pregnancy. MPA administered to normal men has the same effect. This property has proved useful in the treatment of selected patients with the obesity-hypoventilation (pickwickian) syndrome. Patients are predominantly male and demonstrate extreme obesity, hypoventilation (with resultant hypoxemia and hypercapnia), polycythemia, and cor pulmonale. A prominent feature is hypersomnolence caused by multiple episodes of nighttime apnea (possibly caused by prolapse of the tongue against the posterior pharynx) that cause sleep deprivation. Life-threatening arrhythmias may occur during apneic episodes. Diagnosis is aided by demonstration of normalization of blood gases after voluntary hyperventilation.

Surgery (uvulopalatopharyngoplasty or, in severe cases, tracheostomy) or treatment with digitalis and diuretics may be necessary. Those with milder symptoms respond to weight reduction, but this is generally difficult to achieve in these patients. MPA stimulates respiration and improves blood gases in awake patients, but does not benefit patients with mechanical airway obstruction during sleep (Block, 1985). The hematocrit also is reduced.

MPA also has been used to stimulate respiration in patients with chronic obstructive pulmonary disease. Treatment improves oxygenation and stimulates CO_2 expiration more in awake patients than during sleep (Dolly and Block, 1983). MPA is usually administered sublingually (20 mg three times daily); oral administration has not been tested. Some male patients become impotent as a result of therapy.

THREATENED ABORTIONS. Although estrogens have been used to treat *habitual* and *threatened abortions* in the past, such treatment has not been effective. Estrogens now are contraindicated during pregnancy, largely because of the teratogenic effects produced by diethylstilbestrol (DES) and other estrogens in both female and male offspring (see the section on Metabolic Effects, Adverse Reactions, and Precautions).

Progestins also have been used to prevent abortion of established pregnancies but are no longer administered for this indication because proof of efficacy is lacking and there is concern about teratogenicity. However, progesterone and hydroxyprogesterone [Delalutin] are used for certain indications during pregnancy: Progesterone is used to treat luteal phase dysfunction from ovulation through early pregnancy (see also Chapter 41, Agents Used to Treat Infertility), and hydroxyprogesterone has prevented premature births in some high-risk women when given from the sixteenth week of pregnancy (after organogenesis has been completed); thus far, no adverse effects have been reported in the offspring (Johnson et al, 1975, 1979 A). Another study in which patients were treated from the twelfth gestational week yielded similar results (Yemini et al, 1985) (see Chapter 41).

SEX OFFENDERS. Intramuscular injection of MPA in large doses (average, 300 mg weekly) has been used as an adjunct to psychiatric or psychological counseling in men with a variety of paraphilias. Treatment decreased serum testosterone and LH and helped some men to control deviant behavior. Sperm count was not appreciably depressed. Adverse effects observed in some patients included weight gain, decreased glucose tolerance, elevated blood pressure, and gallbladder disease (Meyer et al, 1985).

Metabolic Effects, Adverse Reactions, and Precautions

In general, some side effects of estrogen and progestin resemble those of hormonal contraceptives (see Chapter 40, Contraceptive Agents). The dosages prescribed for replacement therapy, the most common noncontraceptive indication for estrogen and progestin, generally are smaller than those prescribed for contraception and hence the incidence and intensity of effects are lower.

Nausea occurs relatively often initially when estrogen is administered but can be minimized by taking medication with food. This reaction usually disappears with continued administration, even when large doses are used to treat cancer.

Fullness or tenderness of breasts and edema caused by sodium and water retention may occur with estrogen treatment (less likely with cyclic administration); if they occur during replacement therapy, these effects may indicate excessive dosage.

METABOLISM. Estrogen replacement therapy usually does not adversely affect glucose tolerance. Effects on serum lipids are variable and may be related to the route of administration as well as the preparation (Fahraeus and Wallentin, 1983).

The preponderance of evidence shows that the total cholesterol level is reduced slightly but the triglyceride level is increased. Administration of oral estrogens is associated with decreased levels of low density lipoproteins (LDL) and increased levels of high density lipoproteins (HDL), which are inversely related to the incidence of coronary heart disease (Wahl et al, 1983; Nichols et al, 1984). Progestins that are derivatives of 19-nortestosterone appear to decrease HDL levels in a dose-dependent relationship (larger doses are associated with lower HDL levels), thus possibly reversing the beneficial effect of estrogen. MPA (a derivative of hydroxyprogesterone) does not appear to have this effect (Hirvonen et al, 1981).

Usual replacement doses of conjugated estrogens exert minimal effects on protein synthesis and elevate CBG levels only slightly. In postmenopausal women treated with replacement doses of estrogen, changes in hepatic excretory function result in greater cholesterol saturation in the bile, thus predisposing to gallstone formation. The risk of gallbladder surgery is increased 2.5 times in these women. Estrogens should not be given to patients with severe acute (active) liver disease.

If hypercalcemia occurs when estrogens are administered as chemotherapy to patients with breast cancer and bone metastases, the estrogen should be discontinued and the serum calcium level reduced by appropriate means (see Chapter 49, Agents Affecting Calcium Metabolism).

CARDIOVASCULAR EFFECTS. Although there are conflicting reports on whether replacement dosages of estrogen increase some clotting factors, the risk of thromboembolism is not increased. The risk also is not affected by a combined estrogen-progestin regimen (Notelovitz et al, 1983). Nevertheless, estrogens usually are not administered to menopausal patients with thromboembolic disease or a past history of such disease because they are presumably at higher risk. The likelihood of thromboembolic phenomena has been reported to be increased when pharmacologic doses of estrogen are used to treat breast or prostatic cancer. Administration of estrogen to suppress postpartum lactation is associated with a higher incidence of thromboembolism, and this use of estrogen is no longer preferred (see the section on Indications).

Premenopausal women have a lower incidence of coronary heart disease than men of comparable age, but this advantage is lost after natural menopause or after oophorectomy. The possibility that this difference is ascribable to the higher levels of estrogen in premenopausal women and that coronary heart disease may be prevented in men and older women by administration of estrogen is being considered. On the other hand, mortality from myocardial infarction (MI) was increased in men with a history of MI who were treated with conjugated estrogens 5 mg daily. Cardiovascular deaths also increased in men receiving DES 5 mg daily for prostatic carcinoma but not at lower dosages. It should be noted that these doses are much higher than those currently used for replacement therapy, treatment was studied in men, and these men had previously documented arteriosclerotic disease. Therefore, these data do not provide an appropriate standard for determination of possible beneficial effects in postmenopausal women.

There are reports suggesting that premenopausal hysterectomy, particularly bilateral oophorectomy, increases the risk of coronary artery disease (Centerwall, 1981; Rosenberg et al, 1981). Hypoestrogenic women treated for at least five years with estrogen had fewer new diagnoses of cardiovascular disease and hypertension than untreated younger women (less than 40 years) (Hammond et al, 1979, part I). The risk of death from any cause was lower in women aged 40 to 69 years who received estrogen replacement therapy than in nonusers; the reduction in risk was thought to be partly due to increased HDL levels in estrogen users (Bush et al, 1983). On the other hand, it has been reported that the associated risk of developing angina pectoris almost doubled in women given postmenopausal estrogen therapy, although mortality was not increased (Ryan, 1976; Gordon et al, 1978).

The risk of myocardial infarction is not increased and may be decreased (Ross et al, 1981) with estrogen treatment for menopause. Although the incidence of hypertension generally is not increased, this may occur in sensitive individuals. If hypertension develops or worsens with estrogen therapy, medication should be discontinued. The risk of stroke was not elevated in postmenopausal women given estrogen replacement therapy in one study (Judd et al, 1983).

Two reports published simultaneously presented different conclusions regarding the cardiovascular effects of postmenopausal estrogen therapy. One study found an increased risk of cardiovascular morbidity and cerebrovascular disease from estrogen use with no increase in mortality (Wilson et al, 1985). The second study found a decreased risk of coronary artery disease among subjects taking postmenopausal estrogen therapy (Stampfer et al, 1985). Although the populations and experimental designs of the studies were different, the opposing conclusions and other conflicts suggest that the cardiovascular benefits or risks of estrogen replacement therapy have not been determined conclusively. The subject of cardiovascular effects of postmenopausal replacement therapy has been reviewed (Mishell, 1985).

Estrogens should be administered with caution to patients with migraine and discontinued if attacks increase in number or become more severe.

TERATOGENICITY. Synthetic progestins should not be administered during pregnancy because of their teratogenic potential (see also Chapter 40, Contraceptive Agents). Hormonal pregnancy tests are outmoded for this reason and because accurate immunologic assays of serum or urine HCG concentration are available.

Most teratogenic effects of progestins have been observed with agents with high androgenic potency, some of which are no longer marketed. A study of progestin (mostly medroxyprogesterone) use during the first trimester of pregnancy showed no increased risk of teratogenicity (Katz et al, 1985). Although congenital malformations have occurred rarely with use of

21-carbon compounds (ie, hydroxyprogesterone caproate [D-elalutin], progesterone), the incidence is no greater than from chance (Resseguie et al, 1985). It is believed that these agents are safe for specific appropriate indications during pregnancy, including prevention of premature birth (hydroxyprogesterone caproate) and treatment of luteal phase dysfunction (progesterone). See the section on Indications and Chapter 41, Agents Used to Treat Infertility.

DES Daughters: The administration of any estrogen is contraindicated during pregnancy. The use of synthetic hormones to treat threatened abortion is ineffective and carries the risk of teratogenicity. Administration of DES (or other chemically related, nonsteroidal, synthetic estrogens, such as dienestrol) for this indication is associated with reproductive tract anomalies, including vaginal adenosis in more than one-third and cervical ectropion in two-thirds of affected patients; rarely, vaginal clear cell carcinoma (adenocarcinoma) in female offspring; and reproductive tract abnormalities and oligospermia in male offspring.

Postpuberal girls whose mothers received DES during pregnancy should be examined yearly for early detection of abnormalities. Management of adenosis is conservative; no treatment is generally given but regular examinations are continued. Recommendations for the identification and management of exposed individuals (male and female) are available (National Cancer Institute, 1983).

During normal female development, vaginal columnar epithelium of müllerian origin is replaced by squamous epithelium and the squamocolumnar junction is located in the cervix. In females exposed to DES in utero, columnar epithelium persists (adenosis) and the junction is located in the vagina. The incidence of cervical dysplasia and vaginal and cervical carcinoma in situ is increased in DES-exposed daughters compared to unexposed cohorts (1.6% versus 0.8%); the highest rates are in women with the greatest areas of squamous metaplasia. As in earlier studies, a venereal relationship was observed with cervical dysplasia, but this did not account for the difference between women exposed and not exposed to DES (Robboy et al, 1984).

Vaginal adenosis and other structural abnormalities may decline or disappear with time (Robboy et al, 1979; Antonioli et al, 1980; Jeffries et al, 1984). This may be due to continuing metaplasia at the junction. The extent of the teratogenic effect is related to the time at which DES was given to the mother: Effects are most severe when the drug was given during embryonal development of müllerian structures. Structural abnormalities (eg, cockscomb, collar, pseudopolyp, hypoplastic cervix) occurred most often when exposure was between weeks 13 to 22 (Jeffries et al, 1984). Steroidal estrogens apparently do not have this effect (Johnson et al, 1979 B). The incidence of urinary tract anomalies is not increased in DES-exposed daughters.

Vaginal adenocarcinoma occurs in less than 0.1% of exposed female offspring, peaks in incidence at age 19, and declines to a very low level by age 30. This pattern of incidence is temporally related to the declining incidence of abnormally located vaginal tissue with age. Although malignant transformation of vaginal adenosis is thought to be rare, two cases have been reported in DES-exposed patients.

These patients had been under observation for two and four years for adenosis and had been found free of malignancy in previous examinations (Veridiano et al, 1981). It is not known whether DES-exposed females will be at higher risk for adenocarcinoma later in life when this form of cancer appeared most commonly before DES was employed in pregnancy.

Structural and functional abnormalities of the female reproductive tract also result from in utero exposure to DES. In one study, two-thirds of exposed patients had reproductive tract anomalies demonstrable by hysterosalpingogram (Kaufman et al, 1980). Functional abnormalities include an increased incidence of infertility and early and late complications of pregnancy. There is an increased incidence of ectopic pregnancy, spontaneous abortion (first and second trimester), incompetent cervix, prematurity, and perinatal deaths. However, approximately 80% of DES-exposed daughters who desire children eventually have a live birth (Barnes et al, 1980; Berger and Goldstein, 1980; Herbst et al, 1980).

DES Sons: The reproductive tracts of male offspring exposed to DES were reported to be affected in some studies (Gill et al, 1979; Whitehead and Leiter, 1981). In the latter study, only one-third of DES-exposed patients had normal semen. In general, there was a higher than normal incidence of testicular hypoplasia (often including a history of cryptorchidism), varicocele, and epididymal cyst. DES exposure in males may explain reproductive abnormalities, including infertility. There appears to be no associated risk of cancer (except, possibly, that secondary to cryptorchidism), although testicular cancer has been reported. In contrast to the above reports, one cohort study found no increased risk of urogenital abnormalities in DES-exposed males (Leary et al, 1984).

DES Mothers: The possibility that women who took DES during pregnancy (ie, DES mothers) may have suffered adverse effects has been considered. The risk of developing breast cancer 20 years or more after exposure was increased slightly (relative risk 1.5) (Greenberg et al, 1984). The results of this study of over 3,000 exposed women with more than 85,000 woman-years of follow-up in both exposed and unexposed groups differ from the negative or equivocal results of earlier, smaller studies (Bibbo et al, 1978; Brian et al, 1980). A British study reported no increased risk of breast cancer in 650 DES mothers (Vessey et al, 1983).

CARCINOGENICITY. Women should be examined for breast and genital carcinoma before estrogen therapy is instituted and periodically during administration. Therapy should be withdrawn if estrogen-dependent carcinoma is found or suspected. Most available evidence indicates that menopausal estrogen therapy does not increase the risk of breast cancer (Kaufman et al, 1984). In a seven-year study of over 5,000 women, postmenopausal estrogen replacement therapy was associated with no increased risk of breast cancer, and the addition of a progestin to the regimen appeared to decrease the risk (Gambrell et al, 1983 B). Greater caution is advised in women with a strong family history or in those who are otherwise at increased risk of the disease (Ross et al, 1980).

In several studies, an increase in the risk of endometrial carcinoma has been associated with estrogen therapy in postmenopausal women. Generally the risk increases with increasing dosage and duration of use and is higher in women who did *not* have conditions previously identified with a higher risk of endometrial cancer (eg, obesity, diabetes, hypertension). The relative risk varied from 4 to 15 times (Stavraky et al, 1981; see references in Hulka, 1980). Endometrial cancer associated with estrogen therapy is usually an early stage malignancy. The latent period between estrogen administration and development of cancer is relatively short (three to six years) and the risk of cancer is reduced after an estrogen-free interval of two years (Hulka et al, 1980). These observations are consistent with the hypothesis that estrogen acts as a tumor promoter rather than as a carcinogen in endometrial carcinoma. However, resolution of this point would not necessarily assist in making therapeutic decisions about estrogen usage.

Addition of a progestin to a cyclic estrogen treatment program reduces the risk of hyperplasia and endometrial carcinoma (see the discussion under Menopause).

DRUG INTERACTIONS. Estrogens and progestins presumably have drug interactions that are qualitatively similar to those observed with oral contraceptives (see Chapter 40, Contraceptive Agents). However, at the low dosages used for replacement therapy, therapeutic effectiveness might be compromised more easily by drugs that increase metabolism (eg, anticonvulsants, barbiturates, rifampin [Rifadin, Rimactane]) or decrease enterohepatic circulation of hormones (eg, certain antibiotics).

Drug Evaluations

ESTROGENS

Steroidal Estrogens

ESTRADIOL
  [Estrace]

ESTRADIOL BENZOATE

ESTRADIOL CYPIONATE
  [Depo-Estradiol, E-Ionate P.A.]

ESTRADIOL VALERATE
  [Delestrogen]

Estradiol is the principal and most biologically potent ovarian estrogen. It is usually injected intramuscularly as esters in oil or aqueous suspension. The onset of action is gradual and uncertain and the duration is variable (three or four days to three or four weeks).

Oral therapy is generally ineffective because of rapid inactivation. However, the oral micronized form [Estrace] is effective because the reduced particle size increases surface area, dissolution, and rate of absorption; estradiol is quickly converted to estrone after absorption of this product. The recommended daily oral dose for menopausal symptoms (1 to 2 mg) is five to ten times the amount of estradiol produced daily by the normal premenopausal ovary. It is not yet known whether long-term therapy with this relatively large quantity of estradiol will have undesirable physiologic effects.

A sublingual dose of only 0.5 mg produced serum levels of estrogen similar to those achieved with a 2-mg oral dose. Conversion to estrone also occurs with the sublingual route. Vaginal administration of 0.5 mg every other day has produced acceptable results, although conversion to estrone does not occur with this route (Burnier et al, 1981).

See the Introduction for specific indications and adverse reactions. Estrogens used for replacement therapy are frequently given with a progestin.

DOSAGE AND PREPARATIONS.
Intramuscular: For replacement therapy, (estradiol benzoate) 0.5 to 1.5 mg two or three times weekly; (estradiol cypionate) 1 to 5 mg weekly for two or three weeks; (estradiol valerate) 10 to 20 mg every four to six weeks.

  ESTRADIOL BENZOATE:
  Generic. Powder 1 and 5 g.
  ESTRADIOL CYPIONATE:
  Generic. Solution 5 mg/ml (in oil) in 10 ml containers.
  Depo-Estradiol (Upjohn). Solution (sterile, in cottonseed oil) 1 mg/ml in 10 ml containers and 5 mg/ml in 5 ml containers.
  E-Ionate P.A. (Reid-Provident). Solution (in cottonseed oil) 5 mg/ml in 10 ml containers.
  ESTRADIOL VALERATE:
  Generic. Solution (in oil) 10, 20, and 40 mg/ml in 10 ml containers.
  Delestrogen (Squibb). Solution (in sesame oil) 10 mg/ml in 5 ml containers; solution (in castor oil) 20 and 40 mg/ml in 5 ml containers.
  Additional Trademarks.
  Estraval (Reid-Provident), **Gynogen LA** (Forest).

Oral: For menopausal symptoms, 1 to 2 mg daily for three weeks, then one week without medication; a progestin may be added the last ten days (see also the section on Indications).
  ESTRADIOL:
  Estrace (Mead Johnson). Tablets (micronized) 1 and 2 mg.
Topical (vaginal): For atrophic vaginitis or kraurosis vulvae, 2 to 4 g daily and cyclically, depending on the severity of the condition.
  Estrace (Mead Johnson). Cream 0.1 mg/g in 42.5 containers.

ESTRONE

ESTROPIPATE (Estrone Piperazine Sulfate)
  [Ogen]

ESTRONE AND ESTRONE POTASSIUM SULFATE

Estrone is an ovarian estrogenic hormone available in aqueous suspension. The mixture contains water-insoluble estrone and water-soluble estrone potassium sulfate and is claimed to have a more prompt effect than insoluble estrone suspensions. The potency of most oral mixtures of estrogenic substances is expressed in terms of the estrone sodium sulfate content.

See the Introduction for specific indications and adverse reactions. Estrogens used for replacement therapy are frequently given with a progestin.

DOSAGE AND PREPARATIONS.
ESTRONE:
Intramuscular: For menopausal symptoms, 0.1 to 2 mg weekly in single or divided doses. For prostatic carcinoma, 2 to 4 mg two or three times weekly.
> ***Generic.*** Suspension (aqueous) 2 and 5 mg/ml in 10 and 30 ml containers.

ESTROPIPATE:
Oral: For replacement therapy, 0.35 to 1.5 mg daily, cyclically; a progestin may be added the last ten days (see also the section on Indications).
> ***Ogen*** (Abbott). Tablets 0.75, 1.5, 3, and 6 mg (equivalent to estrone sodium sulfate activity 0.625, 1.25, 2.5, and 5 mg, respectively).

Topical (vaginal): For atrophic vaginitis or kraurosis vulvae, 2 to 4 g daily and cyclically, depending on the severity of the condition.
> ***Ogen*** (Abbott). Cream 1.5 mg/g in 45 g containers.

ESTRONE AND ESTRONE POTASSIUM SULFATE:
Intramuscular: For replacement therapy, 0.25 to 1 ml one or two times weekly.
> ***Generic.*** Each milliliter of suspension (aqueous) contains estrone 2 mg and estrone potassium sulfate 1 mg in 10 ml containers.

CONJUGATED ESTROGENS, U.S.P.
[Premarin]

This is a combination of the sodium salts of the sulfate esters of estrogenic substances, principally estrone and equilin; the esters are similar to the type excreted by pregnant mares. The various preparations contain 50% to 65% estrone sodium sulfate and 20% to 35% equilin sodium sulfate. They are effective orally, parenterally, and vaginally. There is disagreement on whether the parenteral preparation controls spontaneous capillary bleeding rapidly and reduces capillary bleeding during surgery.

See the Introduction for specific indications and adverse reactions. Estrogens used for replacement therapy are frequently given with a progestin.

DOSAGE AND PREPARATIONS.
Oral: For menopausal symptoms, 0.3 to 1.25 mg daily, cyclically; a progestin may be added the last ten days. (See also the section on Indications.)

For replacement therapy in hypogonadism, 0.625 to 1.25 mg daily, cyclically (25 days each month with a progestin added during the last ten days) (see the section on Indications).

For dysfunctional uterine bleeding due to atrophic endometrium, 2.5 to 5 mg daily in divided doses for one week with a progestin added to the regimen. See also the section on Indications.

For breast carcinoma in women more than five years after menopause, 10 mg three times daily for at least three months.

For prostatic carcinoma, 1.25 to 2.5 mg three times daily.
> ***Premarin*** (Ayerst), **Generic**. Tablets 0.3, 0.625, 0.9 (***Premarin*** only), 1.25, and 2.5 mg.

Intravenous: For emergency treatment of dysfunctional uterine bleeding when there is a denuded endometrium, 25 mg initially every four hours for three doses; oral treatment with an estrogen progestin combination is then initiated. See also the section on Indications.
> ***Premarin*** (Ayerst). Powder (sterile, lyophilized) 25 mg with 5 ml of diluent.

Vaginal: For atrophic vaginitis or kraurosis vulvae, 2 to 4 g daily intravaginally or topically cyclically, depending on the severity of the condition.
> ***Premarin*** (Ayerst). Cream 0.625 mg/g in 42.5 g containers.

ESTERIFIED ESTROGENS, U.S.P.
[Estratab, Menest]

This is a combination of the sodium salts of the sulfate esters of estrogenic substances, principally estrone; the esters are similar to the type excreted by pregnant mares. Preparations of esterified estrogens contain 75% to 85% estrone sodium sulfate and 6% to 15% equilin sodium sulfate, in such proportion that the total of these two components is not less than 90%.

See the Introduction for indications and adverse reactions.

DOSAGE AND PREPARATIONS. For dosage, see the evaluation on Conjugated Estrogens.
> ***Estratab*** (Reid-Provident), **Menest** (Beecham). Tablets 0.3, 0.625, 1.25, and 2.5 mg.

ETHINYL ESTRADIOL
[Estinyl, Feminone]

This potent, orally effective steroid is related to estradiol, the principal ovarian estrogen. It is used alone and as a component of some estrogen/progestin oral contraceptives (see

Chapter 40). Recent evidence suggests that ethinyl estradiol 5 mcg may be equivalent to conjugated estrogens 0.625 mg for menopausal replacement therapy, particularly with respect to effects on bone and vaginal epithelium (Mandel et al, 1982). However, this amount is less than that supplied by available preparations.

See the Introduction for specific indications and adverse reactions.

DOSAGE AND PREPARATIONS.

Oral: For menopausal symptoms, 0.02 to 0.05 mg daily, cyclically; a progestin may be added the last ten days (see also the section on Indications).

For dysfunctional uterine bleeding, 0.05 to 0.1 mg given with a progestin for ten days (see the section on Indications).

For progressive breast carcinoma in selected postmenopausal women, 1 mg three times daily.

For prostatic carcinoma, 0.15 to 2 mg daily.

Estinyl (Schering). Tablets 0.02, 0.05, and 0.5 mg.
Feminone (Upjohn). Tablets 0.05 mg.

SIMILAR PREPARATION:
Estraderm (Ciba-Geigy). Transdermal preparation (investigational).

Nonsteroidal Estrogens

CHLOROTRIANISENE
[TACE]

Chlorotrianisene is a proestrogen with a long-acting effect; estrogenic activity has been found in adipose tissue up to one month after cessation of therapy. The drug is used most frequently for the palliative treatment of prostatic carcinoma. Its long duration of action makes chlorotrianisene unsuitable for the treatment of menstrual disorders and for replacement when cyclic therapy is desired.

See the Introduction for indications and adverse reactions.

DOSAGE AND PREPARATIONS.

Oral: For prostatic carcinoma, 12 to 25 mg daily.
TACE (Merrell Dow). Capsules 12, 25, and 72 mg.

DIENESTROL
[DV]

This nonsteroidal estrogen is related chemically to diethylstilbestrol. It is applied topically to relieve symptoms of hypoestrogenic vaginal atrophy. Dienestrol is contraindicated during pregnancy.

See the Introduction and the evaluation on Diethylstilbestrol for indications and adverse reactions.

DOSAGE AND PREPARATIONS.

Topical (vaginal): For atrophic and senile vaginitis, the preparation is applied one or two times daily for one to two weeks; the application is then reduced gradually to a maintenance level of one to three times a week.

DV (Merrell Dow). Cream 0.01% in 90 g containers.

DIETHYLSTILBESTROL

DIETHYLSTILBESTROL DIPHOSPHATE
[Stilphostrol]

Diethylstilbestrol (DES) is the most potent nonsteroidal estrogen and has been used extensively. It is given orally, topically, and intravenously. Since the drug is inactivated slowly, it can be given in single daily doses even when large amounts are required.

DES is generally believed to cause a greater incidence of nausea than some other estrogen preparations and occasionally causes pigmentation (facies, nipples).

This estrogen is contraindicated in pregnant women, especially during the first 16 weeks, for vaginal adenosis has occurred in 30% to 90% of postpuberal females whose mothers received DES or a closely related congener during pregnancy. Vaginal adenocarcinoma also has been reported rarely. Yearly examination of patients with this history is recommended. Epididymal cysts and impaired fertility have been reported in some postpuberal males whose mothers received DES during pregnancy.

See the Introduction for specific indications and adverse reactions. For contraceptive use of DES, see Chapter 40.

DOSAGE AND PREPARATIONS.

DIETHYLSTILBESTROL:

Oral: For hypogonadism or replacement therapy, 0.2 to 0.5 mg daily and cyclically. A progestin may be added the last ten days.

For breast carcinoma in selected postmenopausal women, initially, 15 mg daily, increased according to the tolerance of the patient.

For prostatic carcinoma, initially, 1 to 3 mg daily; dosage is increased in advanced cases.

Generic. Tablets (plain, enteric-coated) 0.1, 0.25, 0.5, 1, and 5 mg.

Topical (vaginal): For replacement therapy, a maximum of 7 mg weekly.

Generic. Suppositories 0.1 and 0.5 mg.

DIETHYLSTILBESTROL DIPHOSPHATE:

Intravenous: For prostatic carcinoma, 250 to 500 mg one or two times weekly.

Stilphostrol (Miles). Solution 250 mg/ml in 5 ml containers.

Oral: For prostatic carcinoma, 50 mg three times daily; the dose may be increased to 200 mg or more three times daily.
  Stilphostrol (Miles). Tablets 50 mg.

QUINESTROL
[Estrovis]

Quinestrol is the 3-cyclopentyl ether of ethinyl estradiol. After gastrointestinal absorption, it is stored in adipose tissue, slowly released, and metabolized principally to the parent compound. Because of this property, an effective drug level is maintained with once weekly administration after an initial priming regimen.

In one multicenter, double-blind, controlled study, quinestrol was superior to placebo and equivalent to conjugated estrogens in relieving vasomotor flushes in menopausal women (Baumgardner et al, 1978). There is concern because of the depot nature of the drug; the patient is potentially exposed to constant estrogenic stimulation, although hormonal levels are variable. Therefore, the risk of endometrial hyperstimulation may be increased. There are no data on the effect of concurrent progestin therapy with this agent.

ADVERSE REACTIONS. In general, side effects occur infrequently and are similar to those observed with other estrogens. Nausea, breast tenderness, headache, dizziness, blurred vision, vaginal discharge, and spotting have been reported.

Endometrial hyperplasia has occurred in patients taking doses in the upper range or higher (Greenblatt and Zarate, 1967; Ober and Bronstein, 1967). A thorough study of the endometrial (particularly long-term) effects of quinestrol at the recommended dosage has not been published.

DOSAGE AND PREPARATIONS.
Oral: For replacement therapy, 100 mcg once daily for seven days, followed by 100 mcg weekly beginning two weeks after initiating treatment.
  Estrovis (Parke-Davis). Tablets 100 mcg.

Estrogens Combined with Other Drugs

ESTROGENS AND ANDROGENS

This type of mixture generally should not be used in women, since prolonged administration of androgens may cause masculinization. However, small doses of androgen given with estrogens may decrease stimulation of the breasts and endometrium and may enhance libido during the menopause.

See Chapter 38, Androgens and Anabolic Steroids, for preparations.

ESTROGENS WITH ANTIANXIETY AGENTS

This type of mixture is used to treat menopausal symptoms. Vasomotor flushes and atrophic vaginitis usually respond readily to estrogen alone. Anxiety may occur secondary to discomfort from these estrogen-responsive complaints. Under these circumstances, when anxiety is not relieved by estrogen therapy, antianxiety agents may be helpful. Therefore, if one of the available combinations contains ingredients appropriate both quantitatively and qualitatively for an individual patient, the use of these mixtures may be acceptable for a *limited* period. Administration of the separate components is preferred, however.

  AVAILABLE MIXTURES.
  Menrium (Roche). Each tablet contains esterified estrogens 0.2 or 0.4 mg and chlordiazepoxide 5 mg or esterified estrogens 0.4 mg and chlordiazepoxide 10 mg.
  Milprem (Wallace). Each tablet contains conjugated estrogens 0.45 mg and meprobamate 200 or 400 mg.

HORMONE COSMETIC PREPARATIONS

Hormones used topically on the skin are marketed principally as quasi-cosmetic rejuvenating creams. Topical preparations containing physiologic amounts of estrogens or natural progesterone have no effect on human sebaceous glands and oil secretion. There is no evidence that hormone creams are any more effective than simple emollients in relieving dryness of the skin, increase the amount of water that the skin can hold, or restore fat to the subcutaneous layer. However, there is some evidence that certain topically applied steroid hormones (both active and inactive biologically) may cause slight histologic thickening in some areas of the epidermis of aged skin. Estrogen can increase dermal thickness slightly, but it is unlikely that this alters facial appearance.

Because of the current FDA restrictions on the concentrations of ovarian hormones permitted in such products, there is little likelihood that the amount is sufficient to produce any systemic effects with ordinary use. However, systemic effects have followed *excessive* use of hormone creams.

An FDA Advisory Review Panel concluded that concentrations higher than 1 mg estrone or the equivalent produce systemic effects and should not be available without prescription. Progesterone in concentrations up to 5 mg/30 g is probably safe for daily use when the total amount does not exceed 60 g per month. Higher concentrations of progesterone were not tested (*Federal Register*, 1982).

PROGESTERONE AND PROGESTINS

PROGESTERONE

This natural progestational substance acts on target genital tissues and endocrine glands and also has general systemic effects. Parenteral preparations in oil are used primarily to diagnose and treat menstrual disorders; responsiveness of the target organ depends upon the priming action of estrogen. The drug is ineffective when given orally.

Progesterone is also available in an IUD [Progestasert] (see Chapter 40).

See the Introduction for indications and adverse reactions.

DOSAGE AND PREPARATIONS.

Intramuscular: For diagnostic use in amenorrhea, 100 or 200 mg in oil; for dysfunctional uterine bleeding, 50 to 100 mg in oil.

Generic. Powder 5 g; suspension (in oil) 25 and 50 mg/ml in 10 and 30 ml containers and 100 mg/ml in 10 ml containers.

HYDROXYPROGESTERONE CAPROATE
[Delalutin]

This derivative of progesterone is administered parenterally. Its duration of action is about 9 to 17 days. Since hydroxyprogesterone has no estrogenic activity, priming with estrogen is necessary before a response is noted.

See the Introduction for indications and adverse reactions.

DOSAGE AND PREPARATIONS.

Intramuscular: For menstrual disorders, 125 to 250 mg per cycle.

Generic. Solution 125 mg/ml in 10 ml containers and 250 mg/ml in 5 ml containers.

Delalutin (Squibb). Solution (in sesame oil) 125 mg/ml in 10 ml containers and 250 mg/ml (in castor oil) in 5 ml containers.

MEDROXYPROGESTERONE ACETATE (MPA)
[Amen, Curretab, Depo-Provera, Provera]

Medroxyprogesterone is effective both orally and parenterally. The duration of action of the depot preparation is variable and occasionally prolonged; therefore, this preparation may be inappropriate in women desiring pregnancy in the imminent future. Since the drug has no inherent estrogenic activity, priming with estrogen is necessary before a response is noted.

See the Introduction for indications and adverse reactions. For use of the parenteral preparation as a contraceptive, see Chapter 40.

DOSAGE AND PREPARATIONS.

Oral: For amenorrhea and dysfunctional uterine bleeding, 5 to 10 mg daily for ten days, depending upon the indication.

For endometriosis, 30 mg daily.

For menopausal replacement therapy, 10 mg for the last ten days of estrogen administration (see the section on Indications).

Amen (Carnrick), **Curretab** (Reid-Provident), **Generic.** Tablets 10 mg.

Provera (Upjohn). Tablets 2.5 and 10 mg.

Intramuscular: For endometriosis, 150 mg every three months. For endometrial carcinoma, 400 mg to 1 g weekly initially.

Depo-Provera (Upjohn). Suspension (sterile, aqueous) 100 mg/ml in 5 ml containers and 400 mg/ml in 1, 2.5, and 10 ml containers.

MEGESTROL ACETATE
[Megace]

This progestin is used in the palliative treatment of advanced carcinoma of the breast or endometrium. See Chapter 64, Drugs Used in Cancer Chemotherapy.

DOSAGE AND PREPARATIONS.

Oral: For breast carcinoma, 160 mg daily in four divided doses; for endometrial carcinoma, 40 to 320 mg daily in divided doses. At least two months of continuous therapy is considered adequate to determine the efficacy of this agent. In women with recently diagnosed breast carcinoma (in whom estrogen is contraindicated), 40 to 80 mg daily may relieve menopausal symptoms. Higher dosages are used investigationally for several types of malignancies.

Megace (Bristol-Myers). Tablets 20 and 40 mg.

NORETHINDRONE
[Norlutin]

NORETHINDRONE ACETATE
[Aygestin, Norlutate]

This derivative of nortestosterone is a potent oral progestational agent. Its androgenic effects are minor and variable. For therapeutic purposes, the acetate salt is considered to be approximately twice as potent as the base. Norethindrone is given alone or with estrogens for many indications, including contraception (see Chapter 40). See the Introduction for indications and adverse reactions.

DOSAGE AND PREPARATIONS.

NORETHINDRONE:

Oral: For amenorrhea and dysfunctional uterine bleeding, 5 to 20 mg daily, starting on the fifth day of the cycle and ending on the twenty-fifth day.

For endometriosis, initially, 10 mg daily for two weeks, increased by 5 mg daily every two weeks until a dose of 30 mg daily is reached, then 30 mg daily for maintenance. Maintenance therapy may be continued for six to nine months or until breakthrough bleeding necessitates temporary discontinuation.

For menopausal replacement therapy, 5 mg for the last ten days of estrogen administration.

See also the section on Indications in the Introduction.

Norlutin (Parke-Davis). Tablets 5 mg.

NORETHINDRONE ACETATE:

Oral: For amenorrhea and dysfunctional uterine bleeding, 2.5 to 10 mg, starting on the fifth day of the cycle and ending on the twenty-fifth day.

For endometriosis, initially, 5 mg daily for two weeks, increased by 2.5 mg daily every two weeks until a dose of 15 mg daily is reached, then 15 mg daily for maintenance. Maintenance therapy may be continued for six to nine months or until breakthrough bleeding necessitates temporary discontinuation of therapy.

For menopausal replacement therapy, 2.5 mg for the last ten days of estrogen administration.

See also the section on Indications in the Introduction.

Aygestin (Ayerst), ***Norlutate*** (Parke-Davis). Tablets 5 mg.

Cited References

Topically applied hormone-containing drug products for over-the-counter human use. *Federal Register* 47:429-434, (Jan 5) 1982.

Abdalla HI, et al: Prevention of bone mineral loss in postmenopausal women by norethisterone. *Obstet Gynecol* 66:789-792, 1985.

Albrecht BH, et al: Objective evidence that placebo and oral medroxyprogesterone acetate therapy diminish menopausal vasomotor flushes. *Am J Obstet Gynecol* 139:631-635, 1981.

Alcoff JM, et al: Double-blind, placebo-controlled, crossover trial of propranolol as treatment for menopausal vasomotor symptoms. *Clin Ther* 3:356-364, 1981.

Antonioli DA, et al: Natural history of diethylstilbestrol-associated genital tract lesions: Cervical ectopy and cervicovaginal hood. *Am J Obstet Gynecol* 137:847-853, 1980.

Barnes AB, et al: Fertility and outcome of pregnancy in women exposed in utero to diethylstilbestrol. *N Engl J Med* 302:609-613, 1980.

Barr W: Pyridoxine supplements in premenstrual syndrome. *Practitioner* 228:425-427, 1984.

Baumgardner SB, et al: Replacement estrogen therapy for menopausal vasomotor flushes: Comparison of quinestrol and conjugated estrogens. *Obstet Gynecol* 51:445-452, 1978.

Berger MJ, Goldstein DP: Impaired reproductive performance in DES-exposed women. *Obstet Gynecol* 55:25-27, 1980.

Bibbo M, et al: Twenty-five year follow-up study of women exposed to diethylstilbestrol during pregnancy. *N Engl J Med* 298:763-767, 1978.

Block J: Sleep apnea and related disorders. *DM* 3:6-53, 1985.

Blombäck M, et al: Estrogen treatment of tall girls: Risk of thrombosis? *Pediatrics* 72:416-419, 1983.

Braithwaite SS, Jabamoni R: Hirsutism, (editorial). *Arch Dermatol* 119:279-284, 1983.

Brian DD, et al: Breast cancer in DES-exposed mothers: Absence of association. *Mayo Clin Proc* 55:89-93, 1980.

Brincat M, et al: Long-term effects of menopause and sex hormones on skin thickness. *Br J Obstet Gynaecol* 92:256-259, 1985.

Budoff PW: Zomepirac sodium in treatment of primary dysmenorrhea syndrome. *N Engl J Med* 307:714-719, 1982.

Bullen BA, et al: Induction of menstrual disorders by strenuous exercise in untrained women. *N Engl J Med* 312:1349-1353, 1985.

Burnier AM, et al: Sublingual absorption of micronized 17β-estradiol. *Am J Obstet Gynecol* 140:146-150, 1981.

Bush TL, et al: Estrogen use and all-cause mortality: Preliminary results from Lipid Research Clinics Program follow-up study. *JAMA* 249:903-906, 1983.

Campbell S: Double blind psychometric studies on effects of natural estrogens on post-menopausal women, in Campbell S (ed): *The Management of the Menopause and Post-Menopausal Years.* Baltimore, University Park Press, 1976, 149-172.

Cann CE, et al: Decreased spinal mineral content in amenorrheic women. *JAMA* 251:626-629, 1984.

Canetta R, et al: Megestrol acetate. *Cancer Treat Rev* 10:141-157, 1983.

Casper RF, Yen SSC: Neuroendocrinology of menopausal flushes: Hypothesis of flush mechanism. *Clin Endocrinol* 22:293-312, 1985.

Casper RF, et al: Effect of increased cardiac output on luteal phase gonadal steroids: Hypothesis for runners' amenorrhea. *Fertil Steril* 41:364-368, 1984.

Centerwall BS: Premenopausal hysterectomy and cardiovascular disease. *Am J Obstet Gynecol* 139:58-61, 1981.

Chestnut CH III: Treatment of postmenopausal osteoporosis. *Compr Ther* 10:41-47, (July) 1984.

Christiansen C, et al: Bone mass in postmenopausal women after withdrawal of oestrogen/gestagen replacement therapy. *Lancet* 1:459-461, 1981.

Christiansen C, et al: Pathophysiological mechanisms of estrogen effect on bone metabolism: Dose-response relationships in early postmenopausal women. *J Clin Endocrinol Metab* 55:1124-1130, 1982.

Collins DP, et al: Possible prediction of accelerated osteoporosis by alkaline phosphatase isoenzymes. *Am J Obstet Gynecol* 149:304-310, 1984.

Council on Scientific Affairs, American Medical Association: Estrogen replacement in menopause. *JAMA* 249:359-361, 1983.

Cumming DC, et al: Treatment of hirsutism with spironolactone. *JAMA* 247:1295-1298, 1982.

Dalton K: *The Premenstrual Syndrome and Progesterone Therapy,* ed 2. Chicago, Year Book Medical Publishers, 1984.

Dawood MY: Dysmenorrhea. *J Reprod Med* 30:154-167, 1985.

Dolly FR, Block AJ: Medroxyprogesterone acetate and COPD: Effect on breathing and oxygenation in sleeping and awake patients. *Chest* 84:394-398, 1983.

Drinkwater BL, et al: Bone mineral content of amenorrheic and eumenorrheic athletes. *N Engl J Med* 311:277-281, 1984.

Duchesne C, Leke R: Bromocriptine mesylate for prevention of postpartum lactation. *Obstet Gynecol* 57:464-467, 1981.

Erlik Y, et al: Association of waking episodes with menopausal hot flushes. *JAMA* 245:1741-1744, 1981.

Ettinger B, et al: Long-term estrogen replacement therapy prevents bone loss and fractures. *Ann Intern Med* 102:319-324, 1985.

Evain-Brion D, et al: Studies in constitutionally tall adolescents: II. Effects of bromocriptine on growth hormone secretion and adult height prediction. *J Clin Endocrinol Metab* 58:1022-1026, 1984.

Fahraeus L, Wallentin L: High density lipoprotein subfractions during oral and cutaneous administration of 17α-estradiol to menopausal women. *J Clin Endocrinol Metab* 56:797-801, 1983.

Gambrell RD Jr: Menopause: Benefits and risks of estrogen-progestogen replacement therapy. *Fertil Steril* 37:457-474, 1982.

Gambrell RD Jr, et al: Use of progestogen challenge test to reduce risk of endometrial cancer. *Obstet Gynecol* 55:732-738, 1980.

Gambrell RD Jr, et al: Role of estrogens and progesterone in etiology and prevention of endometrial cancer: Review. *Am J Obstet Gynecol* 146:696-707, 1983 A.

Gambrell RD Jr, et al: Decreased incidence of breast cancer in postmenopausal estrogen-progestin users. *Obstet Gynecol* 62:435-443, 1983 B.

Garner PR, Poznanski N: Treatment of severe hirsutism resulting from hyperandrogenism with reverse sequential cyproterone acetate regimen. *J Reprod Med* 29:232-236, 1984.

Geisler HE: Megestrol acetate for palliation of advanced ovarian carcinoma. *Obstet Gynecol* 61:95-98, 1983.

Geller J, Albert JD: Comparison of various hormonal therapies for prostatic carcinoma. *Semin Oncol* 10(suppl 4):34-41, 1983.

Gill WB, et al: Association of diethylstilbestrol exposure in utero with cryptorchidism, testicular hypoplasia, and semen abnormalities. *J Urol* 122:36-39, 1979.

Glickman SP, et al: Multiple androgenic abnormalities, including elevated free testosterone, in hyperprolactinemic women. *J Clin Endocrinol Metab* 55:251-257, 1982.

Goebelsmann U, et al: Comparison of hepatic impact of oral and vaginal administration of ethinyl estradiol. *Am J Obstet Gynecol* 151:868-877, 1985.

Gordon T, et al: Menopause and coronary heart disease: Framingham study. *Ann Intern Med* 89:157-161, 1978.

Greenberg ER, et al: Breast cancer in mothers given diethylstilbestrol in pregnancy. *N Engl J Med* 311:1393-1398, 1984.

Greenblatt RB, Zarate A: Endometrial studies following quinestrol administration. *Int J Fertil* 12:187-202, 1967.

Greep N, et al: Androstanediol glucuronide plasma clearance and production rates in normal and hirsute women. *J Clin Endocrinol Metab* 62:22-27, 1986.

Hammar M, Berg G: Clonidine in treatment of menopausal flushing. *Acta Obstet Gynecol Scand* Suppl 132:29-31, 1985.

Hammond MG: Managing menopausal signs and symptoms. *Drug Ther* 14:38-45, (Dec) 1984.

Hammond CB, Maxson WS: Current status of estrogen therapy for menopause. *Fertil Steril* 37:5-25, 1982.

Hammond CB, et al: Effects of long-term estrogen replacement therapy. I. Metabolic effects. II. Neoplasia. *Am J Obstet Gynecol* 133:525-536, 537-547, 1979.

Havens C: Premenstrual syndrome: Tactics for intervention. *Postgrad Med* 77:32-37, (May) 1985.

Herbst AL, et al: Comparison of pregnancy experience in DES-exposed and DES-unexposed daughters. *J Reprod Med* 24:62-69, 1980.

Hirvonen E, et al: Effects of different progestogens on lipoproteins during postmenopausal replacement therapy. *N Engl J Med* 304:560-563, 1981.

Horsman A, et al: Effect of estrogen dose on postmenopausal bone loss. *N Engl J Med* 309:1405-1407, 1983.

Hulka BS: Effect of exogenous estrogen on postmenopausal women: Epidemiologic evidence. *Obstet Gynecol* 35:389-399, 1980.

Hulka BS, et al: Predominance of early endometrial cancers after long-term estrogen use. *JAMA* 244:2419-2422, 1980.

Hutchinson TA, et al: Postmenopausal oestrogens protect against fractures of hip and distal radius: Case-control study. *Lancet* 2:705-709, 1979.

Iosif CS, et al: Estrogen receptors in human female lower urinary tract. *Am J Obstet Gynecol* 141:817-820, 1981.

Jefferies JA, et al: Structural anomalies of cervix and vagina in women enrolled in the Diethylstilbestrol Adenosis (DESAD) Project. *Am J Obstet Gynecol* 148:59-66, 1984.

Jensen GF, et al: Fracture frequency and bone preservation in postmenopausal women treated with estrogen. *Obstet Gynecol* 60:493-496, 1982.

Johnson JWC, et al: Efficacy of 17 alpha-hydroxyprogesterone caproate in prevention of premature labor. *N Engl J Med* 293:675-680, 1975.

Johnson JWC, et al: High risk prematurity: Progestin treatment and steroid studies. *Obstet Gynecol* 54:412-418, 1979 A.

Johnson LD, et al: Vaginal adenosis in stillborns and neonates exposed to diethylstilbestrol and steroidal estrogens and progestins. *Obstet Gynecol* 53:671-679, 1979 B.

Jones KP, et al: Comparison of bone density in amenorrheic women due to athletics, weight loss, and premature menopause. *Obstet Gynecol* 66:5-8, 1985.

Judd HL, et al: Estrogen replacement therapy: Indications and complications. *Ann Intern Med* 98:195-205, 1983.

Karpas AE, et al: Effect of acute and chronic androgen suppression by glucocorticoids on gonadotropin levels in hirsute women. *J Clin Endocrinol Metab* 59:780-784, 1984.

Kase NG: Neuroendocrinology of amenorrhea. *J Reprod Med* 28:251-255, 1983.

Katz Z, et al: Teratogenicity of progestogens given during first trimester of pregnancy. *Obstet Gynecol* 65:775-780, 1985.

Kaufman RH, et al: Upper genital tract changes and pregnancy outcome in offspring exposed in utero to diethylstilbestrol. *Am J Obstet Gynecol* 137:299-308, 1980.

Kaufman DW, et al: Noncontraceptive estrogen use and risk of breast cancer. *JAMA* 252:63-67, 1984.

Kauppila A: Progestin therapy of endometrial, breast and ovarian cancer. *Acta Obstet Gynecol Scand* 63:441-450, 1984.

Kronenberg F, et al: Menopausal hot flashes: Thermoregulatory, cardiovascular, and circulating catecholamine and LH changes. *Maturitas* 6:31-43, 1984.

Leary FJ, et al: Males exposed in utero to diethylstilbestrol. *JAMA* 252:2984-2989, 1984.

Lindsay R, et al: Bone response to termination of oestrogen treatment. *Lancet* 1:1325-1327, 1978.

Lindsay R, et al: Prevention of spinal osteoporosis in oophorectomised women. *Lancet* 2:1151-1153, 1980.

Lindsay R, et al: Minimum effective dose of estrogen for prevention of postmenopausal bone loss. *Obstet Gynecol* 63:759-763, 1984.

Lobo RA, et al: Depo-medroxyprogesterone acetate compared with conjugated estrogens for treatment of postmenopausal women. *Obstet Gynecol* 63:1-5, 1984.

Magos AL, et al: Amenorrhea and endometrial atrophy with continuous oral estrogen and progestin therapy in postmenopausal women. *Obstet Gynecol* 65:496-499, 1985.

Mandel FP, et al: Biologic effects of various doses of ethinyl estradiol in postmenopausal women. *Obstet Gynecol* 59:673-679, 1982.

Mashchak CA, et al: Comparison of pharmacodynamic properties of various estrogen formulations. *Am J Obstet Gynecol* 144:511-518, 1982.

McGuire WL: Hormone receptors and hormonal treatment of breast cancer, in Carter SK, et al (eds): *Principles of Cancer Treatment.* New York, McGraw-Hill, 1982, 352-357.

Meikle AW, et al: Adrenal corticoid hyperresponsiveness in hirsute women. *Fertil Steril* 41:575-579, 1984.

Meldrum DR, et al: Pituitary hormones during menopausal hot flush. *Obstet Gynecol* 64:752-756, 1984.

Meyer WJ III, et al: Physical, metabolic, and hormonal effects on men of long-term therapy with medroxyprogesterone acetate. *Fertil Steril* 43:102-109, 1985.

Mishell DR Jr (ed): Estrogen replacement therapy: Measuring benefit v cardiovascular risk. *J Reprod Med* 30:795-826, 1985.

Mishell DR Jr, et al: Menorrhagia: Symposium. *J Reprod Med* 29:763-782, 1984.

Muse KN, et al: Premenstrual syndrome: Effects of "medical ovariectomy." *N Engl J Med* 311:1345-1349, 1984.

Nachtigall LE, et al: Estrogen replacement therapy: I. 10-year prospective study in the relationship to osteoporosis. *Obstet Gynecol* 53:277-281, 1979.

National Cancer Institute: Prenatal diethylstilbestrol (DES) exposure: Recommendations of Diethylstilbestrol-Adenosis (DESAD) Project for identification and management of exposed individuals. *Clin Pediatr* 22:139-143, 1983.

National Institutes of Health Consensus Conference: Osteoporosis. *JAMA* 252:799-802, 1984.

Nichols KC, et al: 17β-estradiol for postmenopausal estrogen replacement therapy. *Obstet Gynecol Surv* 39(suppl):230-245, 1984.

Nilas N, et al: Calcium supplementation and postmenopausal bone loss. *Br Med J* 289:1103-1106, 1984.

Nordin BEC: Treatment of postmenopausal osteoporosis. *Drugs* 18:484-492, 1979.

Notelovitz M, et al: Combination estrogen and progestogen replacement therapy does not adversely affect coagulation. *Obstet Gynecol* 62:596-600, 1983.

Ober WB, Bronstein SB: Endometrial morphology following oral administration of quinestrol. *Int J Fertil* 12:210-228, 1967.

O'Brien PMS, et al: Treatment of premenstrual syndrome by spironolactone. *Br J Obstet Gynecol* 86:142-147, 1979.

Olive DL, Hammond CB: Evaluation of anovulatory patient: When to proceed, when to refer. *Postgrad Med* 77:205-216, (April) 1985.

Paganini-Hill A, et al: Menopausal estrogen therapy and hip fractures. *Ann Intern Med* 95:28-31, 1981.

Place VA, et al: Double-blind comparative study of Estraderm and Premarin in amelioration of postmenopausal symptoms. *Am J Obstet Gynecol* 152:1092-1099, 1985.

Powers MS, et al: Pharmacokinetics and pharmacodynamics of transdermal dosage forms of 17β-estradiol: Comparison with conventional oral estrogens used for hormone replacement. *Am J Obstet Gynecol* 152:1099-1106, 1985.

Ressegiue LJ, et al: Congenital malformations among offspring exposed in utero to progestins, Olmsted County, Minnesota, 1936-1974. *Fertil Steril* 43:514-519, 1985.

Richter MA, et al: Progesterone treatment of premenstrual syndrome. *Curr Ther Res* 36:840-850, 1984.

Riggs BL, et al: Effect of fluoride/calcium regimen on vertebral fracture occurrence in postmenopausal osteoporosis: Comparison with conventional therapy. *N Engl J Med* 306:446-450, 1982.

Robboy SJ, et al: Pathologic findings in young women enrolled in National Cooperative Diethylstilbestrol Adenosis (DESAD) Project. *Obstet Gynecol* 53:309-317, 1979.

Robboy SJ, et al: Increased incidence of cervical and vaginal dysplasia in 3,980 diethylstilbestrol-exposed young women: Experience of National Collaborative Diethylstilbestrol Adenosis Project. *JAMA* 252:2979-2983, 1984.

Rolland R: Use of bromocriptine in inhibition of puerperal lactation. *Drugs* 17:326-336, 1979.

Rosenberg L, et al: Early menopause and risk of myocardial infarction. *Am J Obstet Gynecol* 139:47-51, 1981.

Ross RK, et al: Case-control study of menopausal estrogen therapy and breast cancer. *JAMA* 243:1635-1639, 1980.

Ross RK, et al: Menopausal oestrogen therapy and protection from death from ischaemic heart disease. *Lancet* 1:858-860, 1981.

Ross JL, et al: Preliminary study of effect of estrogen dose on growth in Turner's syndrome. *N Engl J Med* 309:1104-1106, 1983.

Roy S: Double-blind comparison of propionic acid derivative (ibuprofen) and fenamate (mefenamic acid) in treatment of dysmenorrhea. *Obstet Gynecol* 61:628-632, 1983.

Ryan KJ: Estrogens and atherosclerosis. *Clin Obstet Gynecol* 19:805-815, 1976.

Schiff I, et al: Endometrial hyperplasia in women on cyclic or continuous estrogen regimens. *Fertil Steril* 37:79-82, 1982.

Semmens JP, Wagner G: Estrogen deprivation and vaginal function in postmenopausal women. *JAMA* 248:445-448, 1982.

Shangold MM: Update: Advising patients about exercise. *Fertil News* 16:3-5, (Summer) 1982.

Speroff L, et al: Hirsutism, in: *Clinical Gynecologic Endocrinology and Infertility*, ed 3. Baltimore, Williams & Wilkins, 1983.

Stampfer MJ, et al: Prospective study of postmenopausal estrogen therapy and coronary heart disease. *N Engl J Med* 313:1044-1049, 1985.

Stavraky KM, et al: Comparison of estrogen use by women with endometrial cancer, gynecologic disorders, and other illnesses. *Am J Obstet Gynecol* 141:547-555, 1981.

Strickler RC: Dysfunctional uterine bleeding in ovulatory women. *Postgrad Med* 77:235-246, (Jan) 1985.

Thom MH, et al: Prevention and treatment of endometrial disease in climacteric women receiving oestrogen therapy. *Lancet* 2:455-457, 1979.

Upton GV: Perimenopause: Physiologic correlates and clinical management. *J Reprod Med* 27:1-28, 1982.

Upton GV: Therapeutic considerations in management of climacteric: Critical analysis of prevalent treatments. *J Reprod Med* 29:71-79, 1984.

Veridiano NP, et al: Delayed onset of clear cell adenocarcinoma of vagina in DES-exposed progeny. *Obstet Gynecol* 57:395-398, 1981.

Vessey MP, et al: Randomized double-blind clinical controlled trial of value of stilbestrol therapy in pregnancy: Long-term follow-up of mothers and their offspring. *Br J Obstet Gynaecol* 90:1007-1017, 1983.

Vigersky RA, et al: Treatment of hirsute women with cimetidine: Preliminary report. *N Engl J Med* 303:1042, 1980.

Wahl P, et al: Effect of estrogen/progestin potency on lipid/lipoprotein cholesterol. *N Engl J Med* 308:862-867, 1983.

Wasnich RD, et al: Prediction of postmenopausal fracture risk with use of bone mineral measurements. *Am J Obstet Gynecol* 153:745-751, 1985.

Weiss NS, et al: Decreased risk of fractures of hip and lower forearm with postmenopausal use of estrogen. *N Engl J Med* 303:1195-1198, 1980.

Wenzloff NJ, Shimp L: Therapeutic management of primary dysmenorrhea. *Drug Intell Clin Pharm* 18:22-26, 1984.

Whitehead ED, Leiter E: Genital abnormalities and abnormal semen analyses in male patients exposed to diethylstilbestrol in utero. *J Urol* 125:47-50, 1981.

Wild RA, et al: Androgen parameters and their correlation with body weight in one hundred thirty-eight women thought to have hyperandrogenism. *Am J Obstet Gynecol* 146:602-606, 1983.

Wilson PWF, et al: Postmenopausal estrogen use, cigarette smoking, and cardiovascular morbidity in women over 50: Framingham study. *N Engl J Med* 313:1038-1043, 1985.

Yemini M et al: Prevention of premature labor by 17α-hydroxyprogesterone caproate. *Am J Obstet Gynecol* 151:574-577, 1985.

Contraceptive Agents

Throughout history, since the relationship between coitus and pregnancy became known, efforts have been made to limit the number of children conceived and to abort unwanted pregnancies. Early attempts centered on various vaginal treatments and abortion methods; they were sometimes crude and dangerous and often were ineffective. Some of the earliest ideas have survived, however, and appear in our culture in the form of condoms, vaginal spermicides, and intravaginal abortifacients.

Contraception can be accomplished at any point from gametogenesis in both sexes to endometrial implantation. Combination oral contraceptives (OCs) and intramuscular depot progestins prevent ovulation and render cervical mucus incompatible to passage of sperm. Oral agents that suppress spermatogenesis (eg, gossypol) are being investigated. Sperm are destroyed by vaginal spermicides, but there is no agent available to destroy released ova. Methods to prevent the union of sperm and ovum utilize timing (eg, natural family planning, periodic abstinence using calendar methods), surgery (eg, tubal ligation, hysterectomy, vasectomy), mechanical devices (eg, condom, diaphragm, cervical cap, sponge), or chemical agents (eg, spermicidal foams, gels, creams). Even after fertilization has occurred, pregnancy may be prevented with interceptive ("morning after") methods that alter the uterine environment to prevent nidation (eg, high-dose estrogens, some OCs, intrauterine devices [IUDs]).

Agents that interfere with the function of the corpus luteum and placenta are being sought, but a clinically effective luteolytic agent is not yet available. Immunologic approaches are directed toward development of a vaccine to neutralize human chorionic gonadotropin or progesterone. Analogues of luteinizing hormone-releasing hormone, given intranasally, may have contraceptive activity by inhibiting ovulation in women and by interfering with normal gonadotropic stimulation in men. New delivery systems for hormonal contraceptives, such as vaginal rings containing an estrogen and progestin and subcutaneous capsules containing a progestin, are in use in other countries or are being tested clinically.

CHOICE OF CONTRACEPTIVE

The best contraceptive for an individual depends upon its use-effectiveness for that individual, its relative safety, and the patient's age, parity, and medical history. For example, patients with menorrhagia or dysmenorrhea may benefit from the endometrial suppression or inhibition of ovulation produced by combination OCs.

Effectiveness: The effectiveness of contraceptive techniques usually is measured by life table methods, which determine the probability of pregnancy with use of a specific contraceptive method within a given time interval. Failure rates also have been expressed by the Pearl index, which is defined as the number of pregnancies/100 woman-years of use. It is important to distinguish between theoretical effectiveness and use-effectiveness: The former measures efficacy after consistent correct usage and the latter after actual conditions of use. The higher failure rates shown by the use-effectiveness index may be due to improper technique (barrier methods), forgetting to take pills (OCs), and failure to limit coitus to nonfertile times of the cycle (periodic abstinence). Generally, the theoretical and use-effectiveness rates for IUDs are similar because, once inserted, little is required of the patient. However, the use-effectiveness rate may be decreased if the device is inserted improperly, is too small for the uterus, has been expelled spontaneously without the patient's knowledge, or is not replaced (medicated device) at the recommended interval.

Estimates of effectiveness for the various contraceptive methods as reported in several sources of the literature appear in Table 1. For barrier methods (ie, diaphragm, condom), simultaneous use of a vaginal spermicide may enhance efficacy. Failure rates for IUDs and diaphragms decline after the first year of use and with increasing age of the user.

Safety: In general, OCs probably are associated with the widest variety of adverse effects, but complications caused by IUDs more often result in hospitalization and may be more likely to decrease future fertility. The mortality rates are lower with use of OCs, IUDs, traditional barrier forms, or first trimester abortion than with pregnancy that results from failure to use contraception. An exception is use of OCs in women over 35 years who smoke; mortality is higher in these patients than with other methods or when no contraception is employed. When comparison is limited to women using a contraceptive method, mortality (including that associated with pregnancies resulting from contraceptive failures) is comparable with all methods until age 30, when the risk for smokers who take OCs increases. After age 35, the risk of death even among nonsmokers taking OCs may be greater than for patients relying on abortion or using IUDs. Women who used barrier contraceptive methods and had an abortion when contraception was unsuccessful have the lowest mortality at all ages (Tietze and Lewit, 1979). These data were based on use of OC formulations that contained greater amounts of estrogen than is usually prescribed today. Therefore, risk

assessments may not apply to women taking low-dose OCs, particularly in the absence of known risk factors.

The risk of pelvic inflammatory disease (PID) is increased in the three following groups: (1) IUD users, especially those having multiple sexual partners; (2) those with a history of gonorrhea; and (3) possibly younger women. Contraceptives other than IUDs are preferred in these patients. In contrast, the risk of PID is decreased in women who use OCs compared to those using other or no contraception. Because PID may cause infertility, some physicians prefer not to use IUDs in young nulliparous women who eventually wish to bear children. Older patients are good candidates for IUDs or barrier methods because of the relatively greater risk of mortality associated with OCs in this age group. Also, OCs mask menopausal symptoms and contraception may be continued needlessly. Patients who have completed their families may prefer sterilization (for either the male or female partner) to continuing use of a contraceptive.

Because of the recent withdrawal of the Lippes Loop and the copper-containing IUDs from the market, Progestasert is the only IUD available in the United States. Women who do not wish to undergo the yearly replacement necessary with the Progestasert will be forced to choose another contraceptive method. Current users of other IUDs may follow the usual medical guidelines for eventual removal of the device.

Patient Variables: Other conditions affecting the choice of contraceptive include the patient's age, attitude toward various methods, frequency of coitus, extent of male participation in contraception, level of protection desired (ie, absolute versus spacing children), possibility of benefits in addition to contraception (eg, menstrual regularity, decreased dysmenorrhea with OCs), attitude toward contraceptive failure (ie, would response to failure be abortion or unwanted pregnancy), and compliance (eg, unreliability in taking OCs or in utilizing coitus-related methods favors use of an IUD). Low-dose OCs are often used by teenage patients who have a continuing need for contraception.

In women who engage in sporadic sexual activity, a condom, diaphragm, or spermicide might be more appropriate than OCs; furthermore, compliance with an OC regimen may

TABLE 1.
ESTIMATES OF CONTRACEPTIVE EFFICACY

Method	Pregnancy Rate per Year	
	Theoretical Effectiveness	Use-Effectiveness
Oral Contraceptives (combined regimen)	0.1%	2–3%
"Minipill" (progestin only)	1%	2.5–4%
Intrauterine Devices	1–3%	4–9%
Vaginal Spermicides	3%	2–30%
Condoms, Diaphragms	3%	3–20%
Rhythm	5%	25–30%
Contraceptive Sponge	–	9–27%
No Contraception	Pregnancy would occur in 80% to 85% of women	

be lax during periods of abstinence and contraceptive protection would be unreliable. Such patients might be encouraged to plan ahead, to carry contraceptive foam and/or a condom, or to insert a diaphragm or contraceptive sponge prior to a possible sexual encounter. Barrier contraceptive methods with spermicides offer some protection against sexually transmitted diseases and are particularly useful in individuals who have multiple sexual partners.

Proper instruction in contraceptive use is of utmost importance; methods with a potentially high failure rate (eg, diaphragm) may be very effective (failure rate, 3%) in highly motivated, properly instructed patients.

Patient preference is paramount when selecting a contraceptive method. A difference in effectiveness of 1% between two methods may be significant on a population basis, but unimportant to a given patient. OCs, IUDs, and barrier methods are all effective, and the best choice among them may be the one that the patient feels most comfortable with and which she will use consistently, even though its theoretical effectiveness is not the highest.

VAGINAL SPERMICIDES

Formulations: Spermicidal agents for topical vaginal application are available as creams, gels, foams, suppositories, effervescent suppositories, and sponges (see Table 2). All can be obtained without prescription, are easily applied, and, when used correctly (particularly in combination with a diaphragm or condom), offer good protection. Some creams, gels, and foams are designed for use only with a diaphragm. Higher concentrations and total amount of active ingredients are necessary for greatest effectiveness when a vaginal spermicide is used alone.

Formulations differ in speed of distribution and degree of surface coverage, and some require special applicators. Suppositories are inserted high into the vagina and require a melting and/or effervescence time of 10 to 15 minutes for maximum coverage. In general, aerosol foams are easy to apply, cover the cervix almost immediately, and are distributed over a larger surface area. Effervescent vaginal suppositories are designed to provide similar coverage without the need for a special applicator.

Most vaginal spermicides marketed in the United States contain nonoxynol-9 or octoxynol-9 as the active ingredient. These nonionic surfactants are effective and generally safe, but local irritation (which may be due to the inactive ingredients, such as perfume) may affect either partner. Selection of another product with different components may alleviate irritation.

Proper usage of these agents enhances their effectiveness. They should be applied before coitus (from minutes to one hour, as directed) and must be reapplied before each ejaculation. Douching should be avoided for six to eight hours following coitus, since this may dilute the spermicide. Douching is not effective for contraception.

Several new vaginal spermicides are being investigated clinically. In one type, the spermicide is incorporated into squares of water-soluble film resembling plastic wrap. The product can be applied to the erect penis or inserted into the vagina, where it dissolves. Spermicide-releasing vaginal rings are also being developed.

Another novel investigational approach to contraception is the use of propranolol oral tablets inserted vaginally. The drug immobilizes sperm through its membrane-stabilizing property. A higher serum concentration is achieved after vaginal compared to oral administration. Therefore, to avoid systemic effects, the D isomer, which has low beta-blocker activity, will probably be utilized for further investigation (Patel et al, 1983).

Contraceptive Sponge: The newest type of vaginal contraceptive available is a disposable polyurethane sponge containing a spermicide [Today]. The sponge has a concave surface designed to be placed over the cervix. It acts as a mechanical barrier to sperm, absorbs seminal fluid, and releases the spermicide that is incorporated into the sponge. A wide range of effectiveness has been reported. In one study, the pregnancy rate among parous women who used the sponge was higher than in those who used a diaphragm (Edelman et al, 1984). The sponge offers potential advantages: It requires no fitting, it is not messy, the spermicide is immediately available, and it may be left in place and is effective for multiple coital encounters over a 24-hour period.

Adverse effects include vaginal irritation and dryness. Insertion and/or removal may be difficult. Nonmenstrual and menstrual toxic shock syndrome (TSS) has been reported, but it is not known if the risk of TSS is increased with sponge use (Faich et al, 1985). Although the sponge was left in place for up to 48 hours in early studies, current instructions recommend that use not exceed 24 hours.

Safety: The results of several studies have suggested that vaginal spermicides may increase the risk of congenital abnormalities. These can be divided into chromosomal effects and other types of abnormalities. A study of aborted zygotes showed an excess of postfertilization chromosomal errors in women who had used spermicidal agents around the time of conception (Strobino et al, 1980). An excess of Down's syndrome was associated with vaginal spermicide use in a study of infants with heart defects (Rothman, 1982). The risk of chromosomal and other abnormalities (eg, limb reduction deformities, neoplasms, hypospadias) doubled and the incidence of spontaneous abortions may have increased among presumed users of vaginal spermicides (Jick et al, 1981). Presumed use was ascertained on the basis of prescriptions filled for vaginal spermicides, but actual use was not determined. None of these studies differentiated time of exposure to spermicide (before, at the time of, or after conception). An increased risk of hypospadias and limb reduction defects with spermicide use after the last menstrual period was suggested, but not statistically significant in another study (Polednak et al, 1982).

One study reported 25% more female births in women who used spermicides around the time of conception and double the number of fetal losses in women who used these agents after the month of conception (Scholl et al, 1983). The cause of fetal loss could not be determined, and it seems unlikely that spermicidal exposure the month after conception could be related to chromosomal effects.

A report of the Oxford/Family Planning Association also

TABLE 2.
VAGINAL SPERMICIDES (NONPRESCRIPTION)

Product and Manufacturer	Active Ingredient	Other Ingredients[1]
Creams		
Conceptrol (Ortho)	nonoxynol 9, 5%	oil-in-water emulsion[3]
Koromex Cream[2] (Youngs)	octoxynol, 3%	propylene glycol, stearic acid, sorbitan stearate, polysorbate 60, boric acid, fragrance
Ortho Creme[2] (Ortho)	nonoxynol 9, 2%	oil-in-water emulsion[3]
GELS		
Conceptrol Disposable Gel (Ortho)	nonoxynol 9, 4%	[3]
Gynol II[2] (Ortho)	nonoxynol 9, 2%	[3]
Koromex Gel[2] (Youngs)	nonoxynol 9, 2%	propylene glycol, cellulose gum, boric acid, sorbitol, simethicone, fragrance
Koromex II A Jelly[2] (Youngs)	nonoxynol 9, 3%	same as Koromex Gel
Ortho-Gynol[2] (Ortho)	p-diisobutylphenoxypoly-ethoxyethanol, 1%	aqueous gel[3]
Ramses Vaginal Jelly (Schmid)	nonoxynol 9, 5%	boric acid 1%, ethyl alcohol 5%, jelly base
FOAMS		
Delfen Foam (Ortho)	nonoxynol 9, 12.5%	oil-in-water foam[3]
Emko[1] (Schering)	nonoxynol 9, 8%	same as Emko Because
Emko Because[2] (Schering)	nonoxynol 9, 8%	benzethonium chloride 0.2%, stearic acid, triethanolamine, glyceryl monostearate, poloxamer 188, polyethylene glycol 600, substituted adamantane, dichlorodifluoromethane, dichlorotetrafluoroethane
Koromex (Youngs)	nonoxynol 9, 12.5%	propylene glycol, isopropyl alcohol, laureth 4, cetyl alcohol, polyethylene glycol stearate, fragrance, dichlorodifluoromethane, dichlorotetrafluoroethane
SPONGE		
Today (VLI)	nonoxynol 9, 1 g	none
SUPPOSITORIES		
Encare (Thompson)	nonoxynol 9, 2.27%	effervescent, water-soluble base[3]
Intercept Inserts (Ortho)	nonoxynol 9, 10%	[3]
Semicid (Whitehall)	nonoxynol 9, 10%	polyethylene glycol[3]

[1] *It is anticipated that inactive ingredients will be listed on the package early in 1986.*
[2] *Used with diaphragm*
[3] *No further information available from manufacturer*

suggested that the risk of congenital malformations may increase slightly with vaginal spermicide use, especially when conception resulted from contraceptive failure; the rate of spontaneous abortion was not affected (Huggins et al, 1982). However, the preponderance of evidence does not support an association between congenital abnormalities and vaginal spermicides (Shapiro et al, 1982; Bracken and Vita, 1983; Cordero and Layde, 1983; Bracken, 1985). In one study, exposure to various spermicides with different active ingredi-

ents before or after the last menstrual period was unrelated to malformations in general or specific defects or organ systems (Mills et al, 1982).

In another study, there was no increased risk of malformations related to contraceptive methods in women who reported contraceptive failures. Furthermore, malformations cited by Jick were found less often in spermicide users than in those who used other forms of contraception or no contraception (Linn et al, 1983). In a large prospective study, there was no increase in congenital malformations, spontaneous abortion, or low birth weight or premature delivery in women who used vaginal spermicides before or after the last menstrual period prior to pregnancy (Mills et al, 1985). Studies on nonoxynol-9 and octoxynol-9 in rats have shown no teratogenic effects (*Popul Rep [H]*, 1984).

The absence of a single teratogenic syndrome makes the relationship of spermicide use with other types of malformations even less tenable. The marginal and conflicting data suggest that any possible risk of congenital malformations associated with vaginal spermicide use would be very slight. Nevertheless, continuing investigation and concern are warranted concerning these agents that were previously judged to be without significant adverse effects. As with other medications, suspected pregnancy should be verified and spermicide use discontinued if pregnancy is confirmed.

Noncontraceptive Benefits of Spermicides/Barrier Methods: Vaginal contraception may reduce the risk of sexually transmitted diseases (STDs). In vitro and in vivo studies suggest that spermicides kill the causative microorganisms and offer some protection from gonorrhea, genital herpes, trichomoniasis, and other STDs. Pelvic inflammatory disease resulting from such infections also was reduced after use of barrier contraceptives (Kelaghan et al, 1982). The mechanical barrier provided by diaphragms, cervical caps, sponges, and condoms may contribute to this anti-infective effect and also may protect against organisms that may initiate or promote cervical cancer (*Popul Rep [H]*, 1984). Vaginal contraception thus may be particularly useful for women with multiple sexual partners or those who are otherwise at increased risk of contracting an STD. On the other hand, these findings should *not* be interpreted to mean that spermicides and/or barrier methods provide reliable protection from STDs, although regular use appears to reduce the risk somewhat.

INTRAUTERINE DEVICES

In 1985 and 1986, the Lippes Loop and copper-containing devices [Cu-7, Tatum-T] were withdrawn from the United States market by their manufacturers. These actions were taken voluntarily by the manufacturers based on economic considerations and were not the result of defects in the products. Many of these products remain in use, and their eventual removal from wearers presumably will be governed by the same medical criteria that were applicable before product withdrawal. At the time of publication, only one IUD, Progestasert, is marketed in the United States. The Progestasert system containing progesterone requires replacement yearly.

An IUD is most easily inserted during menses when the cervical os is dilated and the absence of pregnancy can be presumed, but it may be inserted at any time during the cycle if a nonpregnant state is assured. The chance of involuntary expulsion appears to be lowest when insertion takes place after day 11 of the cycle (White et al, 1980). After a term pregnancy, insertion generally is delayed until involution is complete to decrease the risk of uterine perforation or spontaneous expulsion; a barrier method of contraception may be used in the interim. The risk of perforation is increased for at least eight weeks postpartum, probably because of variations in the time required to complete involution. Women who breast feed are reported to be at substantially greater risk of perforation (Heartwell and Schlesselman, 1983). In one study, immediate postpartum insertion of IUDs modified for such use did not increase infection or uterine perforation, but expulsion rates were higher than after insertion at other times (Cole et al, 1984). The uterus is smaller when abortion is induced during the first trimester, perforation is less likely, involution occurs sooner than after full-term delivery, and insertion usually can take place immediately afterward.

IUDs have been used as an interceptive measure within three days after unprotected midcycle intercourse. (See also the section on Postcoital Contraceptives.)

Mechanism of Action

IUDs prevent implantation of the blastocyst by altering the biochemical milieu of the endometrium. Leukocytic infiltration occurs soon after insertion, and a sterile inflammatory reaction in the endometrial cavity releases substances toxic to the sperm. The serum immunoglobulin level is elevated and may interfere with the normal immunologic tolerance that allows successful nidation. Sperm transport to the oviducts also is inhibited.

Medicated IUDs have the additional effects of the active agent. Inert models of these devices are ineffective. The addition of copper increases leukocytic infiltration, which enhances efficacy. Prostaglandin production is greater with copper than with an inert device, and this probably stimulates the inflammatory reaction. Copper also may decrease sperm motility directly. In addition to enhancing contraceptive efficacy, copper inhibits the growth of gonococci in vitro, but the clinical usefulness of this effect has not been demonstrated. Blood copper levels are not altered.

The Progestasert device continuously releases small quantities (65 mcg daily) of progesterone into the endometrial cavity; glandular atrophy and a chronic decidual reaction that is unfavorable for implantation result. Progesterone also may directly inhibit metabolism, capacitation, and swimming speed of sperm. The volume of menstrual blood loss (compared to preinsertion cycles or cycles in which a copper device was used) is decreased, and dysmenorrhea may be reduced compared to non-IUD cycles. Results of research suggest that the risk of PID was decreased with progesterone-containing IUDS (see section on Adverse Reactions and Contraindications). The progesterone device requires yearly replacement, and spotting may occur throughout the cycle. Normal cyclic function, including ovulation, continues as it does with other IUDs. The amount of progesterone absorbed systemically does not affect carbohydrate or lipid metabolism.

Precautions

Although leukocytic infiltration begins shortly after insertion of an IUD, it is not known exactly when contraceptive protection is assured. Therefore, a barrier method may be used around the time of expected ovulation for the first month for the greatest possible protection. High fundal placement maximizes efficacy; low placement may be followed by partial expulsion and is associated with decreased effectiveness and increased risk of infection. Spontaneous expulsion may be undetected and usually occurs within six months (highest incidence is in the first month). Insertion of another device is usually successful.

The uterus should be sounded carefully before insertion and a device of appropriate size should be used. Insertion into a uterus of less than 6.5 cm may cause discomfort, bleeding, and expulsion. The presence of the IUD string should be confirmed after each menses. Missing strings usually are not associated with serious causes, but require prompt investigation: The possibility of pregnancy should first be ruled out (the string can be drawn into the enlarging uterine cavity) and then the presence and location of the device should be confirmed by a uterine sound (the string may be coiled in the endocervical canal); ultrasound also may be used.

Perforation of the uterine wall and translocation of the device may occur at insertion. IUDs also may become embedded in the endometrium without perforation. Surgical removal, usually by laparoscopy, is required if the IUD is in the peritoneal cavity, particularly when the device contains copper, because tenacious adhesions to the omentum may develop.

If pregnancy occurs with an IUD in situ and the patient elects to complete the pregnancy, the risk of spontaneous first trimester abortion is increased (up to 50%). If the device can be removed without undue resistance, this should be done whether the pregnancy is to be continued or not. Congenital abnormalities probably are not increased when an IUD (medicated or inert) remains in place.

Fatal septic abortions in patients wearing Dalkon Shields resulted in the withdrawal of this device from the U.S. market. Evidence suggests that the multifilament tail acted as a wick to carry pathogens into the uterine cavity, which usually is separated from the vaginal flora by the cervical mucus. Other devices also have been associated with sepsis during pregnancy and it is possible that any IUD with a string appendage (this includes all IUDs in use in the United States) may present some degree of risk. Patients wearing IUDs who become pregnant should be informed of the risk and instructed to report symptoms of infection promptly (Mishell, 1984). Because the Dalkon Shield especially has been associated with this serious complication and with an increased risk of pelvic inflammatory disease, these devices should be removed even in asymptomatic women who are still wearing them (see the discussion of pelvic inflammatory disease under Adverse Reactions and Contraindications).

Adverse Reactions and Contraindications

Insertion of an IUD usually causes discomfort. A transient vasovagal response (ie, syncope, bradycardia) may occur. Cramps and bleeding are common for up to 24 hours following insertion. Dysmenorrhea may be more severe with other devices, but with the Progestasert device, dysmenorrhea and average blood loss actually decrease; however, spotting may be more of a problem.

IUDs should not be used during pregnancy, in the presence of genital bleeding of unknown etiology, or in patients with suspected or diagnosed uterine carcinoma. Their use generally is not recommended when the uterine cavity is distorted from any cause, when the uterus is less than 6.5 cm, or when the cervical canal is severely stenotic. See the manufacturer's guidelines for a complete list of contraindications.

Pelvic Inflammatory Disease: The incidence of pelvic inflammatory disease (PID) is increased two to ten times when IUDs are employed (Ory, 1978; Kaufman et al, 1980 A, 1983; Vessey et al, 1981; Burkman, 1981; Lee et al, 1983). In contrast, the risk is decreased with use of other contraceptives, including oral contraceptives (Burkman, 1981). The Dalkon Shield is associated with a higher risk of PID than other IUDs (Kaufman et al, 1983; Lee et al, 1983), and patients still wearing these devices should have them removed.

In one study on fallopian tube specimens obtained at elective sterilization, one-half of specimens from users of nonhormonal IUDs demonstrated sterile salpingitis, while specimens from women using the Progestasert device did not show histologically detectable salpingitis. It was suggested that inflammation may predispose to bacterial invasion and that users of progesterone-releasing IUDs may have less risk of PID than those using other types of IUDs (Soderstrom, 1983). Results of a multicenter study showed that the relative risk of PID was similar in users of various nonmedicated devices and slightly higher in those employing medicated devices (Cu7 or Progestasert) (Lee et al, 1983). Another study showed that copper-containing devices were associated with the lowest relative risk of PID of any type of IUD (Kaufman et al, 1983). Two other studies demonstrated increased risk of primary tubal infertility with IUD use; copper-containing IUDs showed the lowest risk, followed by inert devices, and the Dalkon Shield had the highest risk (Cramer et al, 1985; Daling et al, 1985). The former study found no increased risk in women who reported only one sexual partner. In summary, IUDs in general have a higher relative risk of PID, and the Dalkon Shield repeatedly has been shown to have the highest associated risk of PID. However, study results are inconsistent regarding comparative risk of other types of devices.

Age appears to be inversely related to risk of PID, but there is no consensus on the influence of parity. Although the risk appears to be greater for short-term IUD users, long-term users (five years or longer) are more likely to develop PID requiring hysterectomy or bilateral adnexal surgery. This observation remained statistically significant when Dalkon Shields were excluded from the analysis (Stadel and Schlesselman, 1984).

If abdominal pain or tenderness, abnormal vaginal discharge, and fever occur, PID should be considered. If the infection is mild and responds to antibiotic therapy within one or two days, some practitioners leave the IUD in place. Severe infection requires removal of the device, possibly hospitalization, and prompt, vigorous antibiotic therapy. An IUD should not be inserted in the presence of acute pelvic infection from any cause. Furthermore, women at high risk for PID (eg, history of PID, multiple sexual partners) are not good candidates for initial or continuing IUD use. Since IUDs increase the risk of primary tubal infertility, other contraceptive methods should be considered first for nulliparous women. However, the IUD may be appropriate for some nulliparous women, such as those with one sexual partner for whom OCs are contraindicated and who do not wish to use barrier methods.

Bacterial Infection: *Actinomyces* organisms may be a normal part of the flora in the genital tract of healthy women (Persson and Holmberg, 1984). Colonization of these organisms in the upper genital tract appears to be related to long-term IUD use and may cause problems ranging from mild symptoms of infection to endometritis, tubo-ovarian abscess, and, rarely, death. One study found that the incidence of this infection was much higher in patients using inert plastic IUDs than in those using copper IUDs (Duguid et al, 1980). Calcium encrustations form on plastic IUDs and may serve as a site for *Actinomyces* culture. Copper IUDs have a smaller surface area and are replaced more frequently; fewer positive cultures of *Actinomyces* would thus be expected.

In asymptomatic patients, routine Pap smears should be tested for *Actinomyces*; if positive, the IUD probably should be removed until the organisms disappear from the smear (Mishell, 1984). A Progestasert device may be inserted if replacement is elected.

Ectopic Pregnancy: Ectopic pregnancy is less likely to occur in women using any contraceptive method, including IUDs, than in women not using a contraceptive. More ectopic pregnancies result from failure of barrier methods and IUDs than from OC failures (Ory, 1981). IUDs act primarily by preventing intrauterine rather than extrauterine (tubal and ovarian) pregnancy. If a patient conceives while using an IUD, the possibility of an ectopic pregnancy (3% to 9%) should be considered (Mishell, 1984). The incidence of ectopic pregnancy is the same for copper-containing and inert devices but may be higher with the Progestasert system.

Although the incidence of ectopic pregnancy in IUD users remains constant (about 1/1,000 women-years of use), the likelihood of ectopic pregnancy increases with duration of use, probably because of a parallel decline in intrauterine pregnancy (Vessey et al, 1979). Since the greatest risk may be immediately after removal of the device, it may be preferable to defer pregnancy for three months after removal. Women with a history of ectopic pregnancy should not use IUDs thereafter.

Diabetes: A high failure rate with copper or inert IUDs was reported in insulin-dependent diabetic women (Gosden et al, 1982), although this has not been confirmed by others. No difference in the pattern of copper corrosion or contraceptive efficacy was observed in insulin-dependent diabetic women compared to nondiabetic controls (Skouby et al, 1984).

PREPARATION.

> ***Progestasert*** (Alza). 36 mm tubular vertical stem containing progesterone 38 mg initially (32 mm horizontal crossarms). Replacement required yearly.

ORAL CONTRACEPTIVES

Oral contraceptives (OCs) are highly effective in preventing pregnancy. The most common are mixtures of a synthetic estrogen (ethinyl estradiol or mestranol) and a progestin (norethindrone, norethindrone acetate, ethynodiol diacetate, norethynodrel, norgestrel, or levonorgestrel). Other preparations contain a progestin alone. For the chemical structure of the steroids and the composition of OCs, see the Figure (page 722) and Table 3. Ethinyl estradiol, norethindrone, and norethindrone acetate also are available as single-entity drugs for noncontraceptive indications (see Chapter 39, Estrogens, Progestins, and Other Agents Used to Treat Gynecologic Conditions). Natural steroids are not used because very large oral doses are required to achieve the desired pharmacologic effect. The addition of a 17 α-ethinyl group enhances the oral activity of the steroids used in OCs by inhibiting hepatic degradation.

Combination products are available in "low dose" (less than 50 mcg estrogen), "regular" (50 mcg estrogen or more), or "phasic" (variable dose depending on the day of the cycle) preparations. Variable dose products are "biphasic" or "triphasic" depending on the number of dosage regimens in a cycle. "Minipills" contain a progestin only (norethindrone or norgestrel).

Combination OCs are taken for 21 days of the cycle (usually days 5 through 24), followed by one week without medication during which withdrawal bleeding occurs. Most preparations are available in "memory packets" containing 21 active pills and 7 inert pills. Some preparations contain iron in the nonhormonal pills. Minipills are taken daily and continuously.

Administration of combination OCs may be started two to four weeks after full-term pregnancy. Ovulation does not occur before this time and the theoretic danger of associated thromboembolism following delivery probably is reduced by waiting at least two weeks. If bromocriptine is taken to suppress postpartum lactation, ovulation may occur early and OCs can be resumed two weeks after delivery. The risk of thromboembolic phenomena following abortion is not great, but the chance of early ovulation is high; therefore, OCs may be initiated within 48 hours after a first trimester abortion and within one week after a second trimester abortion. Minipills may be started immediately after full-term pregnancy or abortion.

In general, combination OCs are effective within the first cycle of use if started by the fifth day of the cycle. However, some practitioners suggest use of additional contraceptive protection initially or throughout the first cycle with low-dose or phasic preparations. The manufacturer's recommendations should be consulted. Some physicians recommend concomitant utilization of a barrier method during the first month of OC use or until compliance is established. Substituting one combination formulation for another may be accomplished easily at the initiation of a new cycle or immediately after the last pill of the previous regimen. Contraceptive effectiveness is not interrupted.

Noncontraceptive Benefits: Oral contraceptives provide the most effective nonsurgical contraception. Although numer-

TABLE 3.
ORAL CONTRACEPTIVES AVAILABLE IN THE UNITED STATES:
CONTENT AND RELATIVE POTENCIES[1]
(Listed within classes according to decreasing estrogenic potency)

Progestin	Mg	Estrogen	Mcg	Trademarks and Manufacturers
PRODUCTS CONTAINING LESS THAN 50 MCG ESTROGEN				
Norethindrone	0.5	Ethinyl estradiol	35	Brevicon (Syntex)
Norethindrone	0.5	Ethinyl estradiol	35	Modicon (Ortho)
Norethindrone	0.4	Ethinyl estradiol	35	Ovcon-35 (Mead Johnson)
Norethindrone	1.0	Ethinyl estradiol	35	Ortho Novum 1/35 (Ortho)
Norethindrone	1.0	Ethinyl estradiol	35	Norinyl 1 + 35 (Syntex)
Levonorgestrel	0.15	Ethinyl estradiol	30	Nordette (Wyeth)
Norgestrel	0.3	Ethinyl estradiol	30	Lo/Ovral (Wyeth)
Norethindrone Acetate	1.5	Ethinyl estradiol	30	Loestrin 1.5/30 (Parke-Davis)
Norethindrone Acetate	1.0	Ethinyl estradiol	20	Loestrin 1/20 (Parke-Davis)
Ethynodiol Diacetate	1.0	Ethinyl estradiol	35	Demulen 1/35 (Searle)
BIPHASIC				
Norethindrone	0.5; 1	Ethinyl estradiol	35	Ortho Novum 10/11 (Ortho)
TRIPHASIC				
Norethindrone	0.5; 0.75; 1	Ethinyl estradiol	35	Ortho Novum 7/7/7 (Ortho)
Norethindrone	0.5; 1; 0.5	Ethinyl estradiol	35	Tri-Norinyl (Syntex)
Levonorgestrel	0.5; 0.075; 0.125	Ethinyl estradiol	30; 40; 30	Tri-Levlen (Berlex)
Levonorgestrel	0.5; 0.075; 0.125	Ethinyl estradiol	30; 40; 30	Triphasil (Wyeth)
PRODUCTS CONTAINING 50 MCG ESTROGEN				
Norethindrone	1.0	Ethinyl estradiol	50	Ovcon-50 (Mead Johnson)
Norgestrel	0.5	Ethinyl estradiol	50	Ovral (Wyeth)
Norethindrone Acetate	1.0	Ethinyl estradiol	50	Norlestrin 1/50 (Parke-Davis)
Norethindrone	1.0	Mestranol	50	Norinyl 1 + 50 (Syntex)
Norethindrone	1.0	Mestranol	50	Ortho Novum 1/50 (Ortho)
Ethynodiol Diacetate	1.0	Ethinyl estradiol	50	Demulen (Searle)
Norethindrone Acetate	2.5	Ethinyl estradiol	50	Norlestrin 2.5/50 (Parke, Davis)
PRODUCTS CONTAINING MORE THAN 50 MCG ESTROGEN				
Norethynodrel	2.5	Mestranol	100	Enovid E (Searle)
Ethynodiol Diacetate	1.0	Mestranol	100	Ovulen (Searle)
Norethindrone	2.0	Mestranol	100	Norinyl 2 (Syntex)
Norethindrone	2.0	Mestranol	100	Ortho Novum 2 (Ortho)
Norethindrone	1.0	Mestranol	80	Norinyl 1 + 80 (Syntex)
Norethindrone	1.0	Mestranol	80	Ortho Novum 1/80 (Ortho)

Number of Tablets (Active and Inert)[2]	Potency Estimates (0 to +4)			Endometrial Activity [1,3]
	Estrogenic	Progestational	Androgenic	
21, 28	+2	+1	+1	14.6*
21, 28	+2	+1	+1	14.6*
21, 28	+2	+1	+1	11.0
21, 28	+2	+2	+2	14.7*
21, 28	+2	+2	+2	14.7*
21, 28	+1	+1	+2	14.0
21, 28	+1	+1	+2	9.6
21, 28 Fe	+1	+3	+3	25.6
21, 28 Fe	+1	+2	+2	30.9
21, 28	+1	+2	+1	37.4
21, 28	+2	+2	+2	19.6*
21, 28	+2	+1	+1	12.2
21, 28	+2	+1	+1	14.7
21, 28	+1	+1	+2	5.7
21, 28	+1	+1	+2	15.1
21, 28	+2	+2	+2	11.9
21, 28	+2	+2	+3	4.5
21, 28, 28, Fe	+2	+2	+2	13.6
21, 28	+2	+2	+2	10.6*
21, 28	+2	+2	+2	10.6*
21, 28	+1	+2	+1	13.9
21, 28 Fe	+1	+3	+4	5.1
21	+3	+1	0	10.9
21, 28	+3	+2	+1	7.7
20	+2	+3	+3	6.1
21	+2	+3	+3	6.1
21, 28	+2	+2	+2	4.8
21, 28	+2	+2	+2	4.8

(Continued on next page)

TABLE 3 (Continued)

Progestin	Mg	Estrogen	Mcg	Trademarks and Manufacturers
PRODUCTS FOR THERAPEUTIC USE ONLY				
Norethynodrel	9.85	Mestranol	150	Enovid 10 (Searle)
Norethynodrel	5.0	Mestranol	75	Enovid 5 (Searle)
PRODUCTS CONTAINING PROGESTIN ONLY (for continuous administration; all tablets active)				
Norethindrone	0.35			Micronor (Ortho)
Norethindrone	0.35			Nor Q.D. (Syntex)
Norgestrel	0.075			Ovrette (Wyeth)

[1]Adapted from Dickey, 1984
[2]20, 21, 42, 50 and 100, all active; 28 (21 active, 7 inert); 28 Fe (21 active, 7 ferrous fumarate 75 mg)
[3]Percentage spotting and bleeding in third cycle of use; information submitted to Food and Drug Administration by manufacturers, adapted from Dickey, 1984. These rates are derived from separate studies conducted by different investigators in several population groups; therefore, a precise comparison cannot be made.

ous adverse effects have been described, the risks of benign fibrocystic breast disease, ovarian cyst, menorrhagia, endometrial or ovarian cancer, endometriosis, and iron deficiency anemia appear to be reduced (Mishell, 1982). The incidence and severity of dysmenorrhea may be reduced by certain formulations (Milsom and Andersch, 1984). The severity of the first episode of salpingitis was reduced in women using OCs compared to those using IUDs or neither contraceptive (Svensson et al, 1984). The risk of severe pelvic inflammatory disease associated with gonococcal infections is evidently reduced with OC use. However, it was hypothesized that OCs may afford no protection and may even increase the risk of *Chlamydia trachomatis* cervical infections, which have a milder course but are associated with subsequent infertility in many patients (Washington et al, 1985). Recent data refute the suggestion that OCs protect against rheumatoid arthritis (del Junco et al, 1985).

Mechanism of Action

Combination OCs inhibit ovulation through a negative feedback effect on the hypothalamus. This alters the normal pattern of gonadotropin secretion by the anterior pituitary; both follicular phase FSH and the midcycle surge of gonadotropins are inhibited. The cervical mucus thickens (except with the most estrogenic preparations), which renders it unfavorable to penetration by sperm even if ovulation occurs. In addition, the quality of the endometrium may be unfavorable for nidation and tubal transport may be affected.

Inhibition of ovulation is not a prominent feature of contraception with progestin-only minipills. These agents cause formation of a thick cervical mucus that is relatively impenetrable to sperm; they may increase tubal transport time and also cause endometrial involution.

Choice of Oral Contraceptive

The numerous combination OC preparations on the market (see Table 3) differ in the type and quantity of estrogen and progestin present in the formulation. Their effectiveness is equivalent with certain exceptions. For example, preparations containing the smallest amount of estrogen (35 mcg or less) may be less effective in women taking drugs that enhance the metabolism, and thus decrease blood levels, of the estrogen (see the discussion on Drug Interactions). Theoretically, low-dose estrogen preparations may not provide effective drug concentrations in large women, and the risk of failure may be greater when pills are missed.

As a general rule, preparations containing the smallest quantity of steroid consistent with efficacy and tolerable side effects are preferred. This means selection of a product containing less than 50 mcg of estrogen for a first-time user. Changing to lower dose preparations is recommended even for patients successfully maintained on older, higher dose estrogen products. The phasic preparations are designed to reduce the total progestin content in the menstrual cycle and to provide contraceptive effectiveness comparable to higher dose regimens. Although this makes these preparations theoretically attractive, it is too early to determine if they offer significant benefits over other low-dose OCs. Discussions on selection and management of patients receiving OCs are available (Block and Rulin, 1985; Mishell, 1985).

The progestin-only minipill frequently causes menstrual irregularities and is not as widely used (see the section on Metabolic Effects, Adverse Reactions, and Contraindications). Although minipills are slightly less effective than combination OCs, they may be suitable for patients who accept the inconvenience of menstrual irregularities, do not require the most effective protection, and should avoid estrogen-containing medications (eg, older women, those with a history of migraine headaches or hypertension, patients who experienced estrogen-related side effects from combination OCs). The following discussion on selection of OC is devoted to combination products.

Relative Potency: There is disagreement about whether the various formulations available provide real therapeutic alternatives (Edgren and Sturtevant, 1976). Attempts have been made to assess the biological activities of the ingredients in order to tailor the OC to the patient's unique hormonal balance.

Number of Tablets (Active and Inert)[2]	Potency Estimates (0 to +4)			Endometrial Activity [1,3]
	Estrogenic	Progestational	Androgenic	
50	+4	+3	0	4.0
20	+4	+2	0	7.4
28	+1	+3	+1	42.3
42	+1	+3	+1	42.3
28	0	+1	+1	34.9

In comparative studies within the same population group, the endometrial activity of norethindrone 1 mg plus ethinyl estradiol 35 mcg was equal to norethindrone 1 mg plus mestranol 50 mcg and greater than norethindrone 0.5 mg plus ethinyl estradiol 35 mcg or norethindrone 0.5/1 mg plus ethinyl estradiol 35 mcg, a biphasic preparation.

However, numerous considerations complicate interpretation of available data. These include interaction between the estrogen and progestin components and the complex activities of some synthetic progestins, which possess varying degrees of progestational, estrogenic, and androgenic activities. Furthermore, results of the variety of assays available to measure each activity differ, and animal models are not completely analogous to man. Although different assay systems may show significant differences in potency, they may be unimportant at the dosage ranges employed clinically.

The estrogen component of combination OCs marketed in the United States is either ethinyl estradiol or mestranol (3-methylether ethinyl estradiol). Ethinyl estradiol is 50% more potent than mestranol in animal assays, but clear-cut differences have not been demonstrated clinically. Comparison of the two steroids in doses of 50 mcg or more reveals little difference in their effects on the reproductive system, including endometrial histology, inhibition of ovulation, and gonadotropin secretion (Goldzieher et al, 1975). Similar data comparing effects of doses lower than 50 mcg on the reproductive system are not available.

The progestin component of an OC may be one of four derivatives of 19-nortestosterone (norethynodrel, norethindrone, norethindrone acetate, ethynodiol diacetate) or of gonane (norgestrel and levonorgestrel). The latter two have the most potent progestational activity (Dorflinger, 1985). All the progestins except norgestrel and levonorgestrel possess slight estrogenic activity. Norgestrel is a racemic mixture of levonorgestrel and an inactive isomer, with one-half the potency of levonorgestrel. Levonorgestrel and norgestrel have the strongest androgenic, antiestrogenic, and progestational effects. All the progestins except norethynodrel have androgenic activity. Norethynodrel has only progestational and estrogenic activity. Because of these differences, comparison of OC formulations on the basis of weight of components alone is meaningless.

A plan for initial selection of an oral contraceptive and management of side effects has been suggested. The relative potencies of OC formulations (based on animal and clinical data) can be considered in conjunction with the patient's menstrual history or known sensitivities to hormones (eg, response to exogenous administration or pregnancy) (Dickey, 1984) (see Table 3). Ideally, the preparation chosen would closely mimic the balance of the patient's endogenous hormones or minimize problems with her specific hormone sensitivities. For example, a patient with symptoms of estrogen sensitivity (eg, nausea, fluid retention, increased menstrual flow) should be given a preparation with low estrogen content and potency (see also the section on Metabolic Effects, Adverse Reactions, and Contraindications). Patients with androgen sensitivity (eg, oily skin and scalp, acne) or progestin sensitivity (eg, depression, noncyclic weight gain) should receive a combination low in androgenic and progestational activities, respectively. Symptoms of estrogen deficiency (eg, vasomotor flushes, atrophic vagina, spotting in the first week of the cycle, no withdrawal bleeding) or progestin deficiency (eg, delayed withdrawal bleeding, heavy flow with clots, spotting in latter part of cycle) might benefit from a preparation with an appropriate combination of potencies. Comparison of commercial products on the basis of their estimated relative hormonal activities provides a rational but theoretical approach for selection of an OC preparation. This method probably has less application with low-dose preparations than with the higher dose preparations used formerly.

Precautions

Patients should be warned that the risk of pregnancy is increased if pills are missed during the cycle. Pills missed early in the cycle probably place the patient at higher risk than pills missed later in the cycle. If only one or two is omitted, an extra pill should be taken for one or two days, respectively, following the lapse. If two pills are missed, a barrier method of contraception should be used in addition to OCs for the rest of the cycle. A pregnancy test should be performed if menstruation does not occur on time. If three or more pills are omitted, another cycle should be initiated. A barrier contraceptive should be used for the first two weeks of the new cycle (Hatcher et al, 1984).

The risk of pregnancy from missed medication may be

ESTROGENS AND PROGESTINS IN ORAL CONTRACEPTIVES

ESTROGENS

Ethinyl Estradiol

Mestranol

PROGESTINS

Norethindrone

Norgestrel

Norethindrone Acetate

Ethynodiol Diacetate

Norethynodrel

greater when low-dose estrogen or phasic preparations are used, although clinical evidence to support this assumption is unavailable. Manufacturers' recommendations for missed pills are similar with the exception that back-up contraception is sometimes recommended when even one pill is missed. The progestin-only minipill is less effective than combination OCs, and pregnancies are more likely to occur during the first six months of use. Therefore, a barrier method should be used around the time of expected ovulation, particularly during the first month of minipill use. Patients taking combination or minipill contraceptives should be encouraged to take the pills at the same time every day to enhance compliance and to avoid wide fluctuations in levels of circulating steroids.

Patients taking OCs should be monitored regularly. Biannual blood pressure measurement and annual physical examination, including urinalysis, liver palpation, and breast and pelvic examinations with Papanicolaou smear should be performed. Other laboratory tests, such as measurement of serum glucose and lipid levels, also should be performed when appropriate (OC users over 35 years, younger women at risk of diabetes or cardiovascular disease on the basis of personal or family history). Patients should be encouraged to examine their breasts monthly.

A periodic pill-free interval is not recommended, since it appears to provide no therapeutic advantage and does not enhance the resumption of ovulatory cycles after cessation of OC therapy. Such intervals may, on the other hand, result in noncompliance with the substituted contraceptive and unwanted pregnancies.

Metabolic Effects, Adverse Reactions, and Contraindications

The pharmacologic quantities of synthetic hormones present in OC preparations have numerous metabolic effects, some of which resemble those experienced during pregnancy. Effects may be minor, tolerable, or temporary but can be serious and even life-threatening. The patient's medical history must be examined carefully to identify contraindications. This is even more compelling with use of OCs than with other drugs, because most patients are healthy before therapy is initiated and alternative contraceptive methods are available.

Most adverse effects associated with OCs are believed to be due to the estrogen component, but cardiovascular changes may be due to either component. Although it appears that the progestin-only minipill is devoid of the most deleterious effects of the combination preparations, more experience is necessary for confirmation. Low-dose estrogen and progestin preparations probably produce fewer cardiovascular complications than products containing more steroid, and it is reasonable to expect that other adverse effects attributable to steroid might be influenced similarly.

The use of progestin-only products has been limited by lack of patient acceptance. The endometrium lacks the structural stability imparted by estrogen, and menstrual irregularities, ranging from intermenstrual spotting to amenorrhea, result. Anxiety about possible pregnancy also is common. When pregnancy occurs during minipill use, the ectopic/intrauterine ratio is higher than when other agents are employed.

Common complaints associated with use of combination OCs include nausea sometimes accompanied by vomiting, breast tenderness, and water retention. The nausea is similar to that experienced by some women during early pregnancy and is more common if medication is taken in the early morning or without food. These effects usually develop during the first two or three months of therapy and diminish after that time.

Effects on Reproductive System: Ovarian size is reduced because large follicles and corpora lutea are absent. Gonadotropic stimulation is diminished and resembles that occurring in the early follicular phase of a normal cycle. Likewise, endogenous steroid production is low. Some growth of follicles occurs, but is followed by early atresia. Storage of ova and reproductive life span are not increased. The endometrium rapidly progresses from a proliferative to a secretory phase, and glandular atrophy and possibly stromal decidualization then occur, which accounts for decreased or even absent withdrawal bleeding. Regression of the endometrium after a few cycles may be a factor in short-term amenorrhea. Breakthrough bleeding and spotting are common during the first few cycles of use (particularly with low-dose preparations). Therapeutic intervention with estrogen and/or progestin may be necessary if bleeding is heavy or prolonged (see Chapter 39, Estrogens, Progestins, and Other Agents Used to Treat Gynecologic Conditions, for a discussion of dysfunctional bleeding).

Cyclic menses usually resume one to three months after cessation of OC therapy, although the interval from contraception to conception was reported to be longer in OC users than in women who used other contraceptive methods (Linn et al, 1982). Occasionally, failure of cyclicity persists for 6 to 12 months. If pregnancy is desired, the condition should be treated in the same manner as other cases of secondary amenorrhea; usually clomiphene [Clomid] or bromocriptine [Parlodel] (if hyperprolactinemia is present) is utilized (see Chapter 41, Agents Used to Treat Infertility). Results of ovulation induction are similar regardless of contraceptive background (Hull et al, 1981).

Although some controversy exists, it is generally felt that there is no causal relationship between use of OCs and subsequent amenorrhea (postpill amenorrhea). In most studies, this effect is reported in less than 1% of patients who take OCs. The incidence of spontaneous secondary amenorrhea in women who do not take OCs is similar. It does not appear to be related to dosage of either component or to duration of use. Amenorrhea occurring after cessation of OC therapy may represent progression of an unidentified prior disease with manifestations masked by the regular cycle imposed by OCs. The cause also may be unrelated to contraception (eg, stringent dieting, excessive exercise, underweight or overweight).

On the other hand, abnormally increased serum prolactin (defined in this study as more than 20 ng/ml serum) was observed in 30% of patients taking OCs (Reyniak et al, 1980). The risk of hyperprolactinemia was increased in OC users, especially women who began use before age 25 (Badawy et al, 1981). The risk of galactorrhea, usually associated with elevated prolactin levels, was increased in women after discontinuation of OCs, particularly for the first year after cessation (Taler et al, 1985). Amenorrhea and menstrual irregularities are common in the presence of hyperprolactinemia and galactorrhea.

The incidence of prolactinomas appears to be increasing in the population, but is not influenced by OC use per se (Maheux et al, 1982; Pituitary Adenoma Study Group, 1983). The increase may be accounted for, at least partially, by advances in diagnostic technology. In one study, the risk of prolactinoma was higher in women who had used OCs for menstrual regulation compared to nonusers or those who had used OCs for birth control only (Shy et al, 1983). This evidence supports the possibility that OCs may exacerbate underlying pathology. Because of these observations, some physicians may prefer to use another form of contraception in patients with a history of irregular menstrual cycles.

The quality and quantity of milk produced during lactation may be adversely affected by some OC preparations, especially the older, high-dose formulations. The steroids are found in the milk with even low-dose preparations, and, although no adverse effects have been described with use of current formulations, their long-range effects on the nursing infant are not known. The amount of estrogen ingested by the suckling infant is similar whether the source is endogenous production by the lactating mother or estrogen from a combination OC. The progestin component is also found in milk, whereas natural progesterone is not (Committee on Drugs, American Academy of Pediatrics, 1981). Nonhormonal contraception is preferable for nursing mothers but, when steroid contraception is elected, a progestin-only minipill (which contains less progestin than combination pills) or a low-dose combination formulation is preferred.

Hepatic Effects: The incidence of *gallbladder disease* and gallstones is increased when OCs are used; this is probably related to increased cholesterol concentrations in bile. Women who developed jaundice during pregnancy or nulliparous women with a genetic predisposition are at risk of developing *cholestatic jaundice* during therapy. The observation that gallbladder disease tends to occur more frequently in younger women and less frequently with increasing duration of OC use suggests that there is a subpopulation of women who are metabolically susceptible to gallstone formation. These women are more likely to be affected shortly after hormone exposure (eg, OCs, pregnancy) (Wingrave and Kay, 1982; Scragg et al, 1984). Results of laboratory tests are similar to those in patients with recurrent jaundice of pregnancy (eg, increased bilirubin, alkaline phosphatase, 5-nucleotidase activity; reduced BSP clearance). Biopsies reveal cholestasis and, sometimes, minimal hepatocellular degeneration and necrosis. Upon cessation of OC use, jaundice and pruritus disappear and liver function tests return to normal without residual effects. Patients with this history and those with active liver disease should not take OCs; those who have recovered from liver disease (eg, hepatitis, mononucleosis) may receive this medication after hepatic function studies are normal for one full year. In a clinical study using an OC containing 35 mcg ethinyl estradiol, the incidence of abnormal liver function tests was lower than previously reported for products containing 50 to 100 mcg estrogen (Dickerson et al, 1980).

Benign *hepatic adenomas* and focal nodular hyperplasia are rare adverse effects of OC use. Peliosis may accompany the adenoma or may be present independently. The relative risk of adenomas increases greatly after three years of OC use (Rooks et al, 1979), although the absolute (attributable) risk remains low. The tumors are potentially serious because of the danger of rupture. About one-half of patients present with abdominal pain (sometimes associated with a liver mass) but almost one-third are asymptomatic at the time of diagnosis. One-quarter remain asymptomatic until a sudden life-threatening hemorrhage occurs. Palpation of the liver should be performed during every periodic examination of patients taking OCs. If a mass is present, appropriate diagnostic procedures (eg, scintiscanning, ultrasonography, computer assisted tomography, hepatic angiography) should be undertaken. Needle biopsy is not used because of the vascularity of the tumors. Cessation of OC use is mandatory and spontaneous regression usually occurs. Budd-Chiari syndrome also has been associated with oral contraceptive use (Lockhat et al, 1981).

Carbohydrate, Lipid, and Protein Metabolism: The effect of combination OCs on *carbohydrate metabolism* is complex. Utilization of glucose may be retarded with a compensatory increase in insulin secretion. A peripheral anti-insulin effect of growth hormone may be involved during the first year of use, since OCs increase the pituitary secretion of growth hormone in some patients. After one year, growth hormone secretion appears to return to normal in some individuals. If alterations in glucose tolerance continue, other diabetogenic factors may be responsible.

Both the estrogen and progestin components probably affect carbohydrate metabolism, the latter apparently having the greater influence. Studies of selected combination OC preparations containing different progestins and progestins alone have shown that all of these agents may elevate blood glucose and insulin levels. Norethindrone and ethynodiol diacetate appear to be the weakest and norgestrel the strongest in this respect. The decreased numbers and affinity of insulin receptors observed in women using a low-dose OC containing norgestrel are consistent with these effects on carbohydrate metabolism (Spellacy, 1982). More data are necessary to define the optimal selection of progestin and dosage of progestin that will best combine desirable progestational effects (eg, suppression of gonadotropin secretion, effect on endometrium) with least disturbance of carbohydrate and lipid metabolism.

Patients who have had gestational diabetes are particularly likely to develop abnormal glucose tolerance with OCs. Also, patients who eventually develop diabetes mellitus (eg, those with a strong family history) may become clinically diabetic earlier than without the diabetogenic influence of OCs. Other forms of contraception should be encouraged in these women.

Although increased blood glucose levels can be controlled by adjusting the dose of hypoglycemic agent, some physicians do not use OCs in diabetics who require hypoglycemic medication. However, the decision must be made on an individual basis. Consideration should be given to the possible increased risk of atherosclerosis in young diabetic patients taking OCs, the risks associated with pregnancy, and the acceptability of other contraceptive methods. Many physicians prescribe low-dose or triphasic OCs for their diabetic patients. These preparations also may be considered for diabetic patients currently using copper-containing IUDs if use of a Progestasert is not desired at the time of usual replacement.

Serum lipids also are affected by OCs. Triglyceride levels increase by an average of 50%; the increase in low density lipoproteins (LDL) is smaller and the effect on high density lipoproteins (HDL) varies depending on the preparation. The estrogen component of combination OCs elevates HDL levels, while the progestin component may reduce them (Wynn and Niththyananthan, 1982; Briggs and Briggs, 1981). The effect of progestin on HDL appears to be dose and potency dependent (higher dose associated with lower HDL levels). There appears to be no progression of changes in lipid metabolism with continued OC use (Fotherby, 1984).

Increased levels of HDL are associated with a lower risk of coronary artery disease; increased levels of LDL are associated with a higher risk. It has been suggested that progestin-dominant OC preparations should be avoided in women at risk for cardiovascular disease (Brooks, 1984). Periodic measurements of serum triglyceride and cholesterol should be performed in women with a strong family history of coronary disease who are taking OCs. If abnormal levels are found, a complete lipid profile should be obtained and another form of contraception should be used. The patient's lipid levels should be monitored subsequently.

Changes in *serum protein* levels during OC use are qualitatively similar to those that occur during pregnancy, but they are generally of less magnitude. Alterations in clotting factors occur (see the discussion on Cardiovascular and Hematologic Effects); alpha-2 globulins (including angiotensinogen) and beta globulins are increased and serum albumin levels are decreased.

OCs also increase circulating corticosteroid-binding globulin (CBG, transcortin), which elevates the amount of protein-bound cortisol in peripheral blood. The slight rise in the free (biologically active) cortisol level is probably partly due to the reduced rate of cortisol metabolism. The effect of prolonged elevation of cortisol concentrations is unknown. Pituitary-adrenal response to stress remains normal. The level of thyroxine-binding globulin (TBG) is also greater but, since the concentration of free thyroxine is unchanged, thyroid function is not altered. Sex hormone-binding globulin increases with the estrogen level of OCs. Other binding proteins, such as transferrin and ceruloplasmin, also are increased.

Cardiovascular and Hematologic Effects: The preponderance of data from both prospective and retrospective studies reveals that the relative risk of developing idiopathic *thrombo-embolic phenomena* (including deep vein thrombosis and pulmonary embolism) is approximately 4 to 11 times greater and the relative risk of superficial thrombosis is two to three times greater among women who use OCs. It appears that OC use is associated with about 80 new cases of deep vein thrombosis or pulmonary embolism per 100,000 previously healthy current OC users per year. Presumably, the risk is greater in women with conditions that predispose to thromboembolic disease. The risk of postoperative venous thrombosis is doubled in OC users. Although the magnitude of this relative

risk is small, the absolute risk attributable to OCs, which is more meaningful clinically, is high (61/10,000 surgical procedures) because of the high incidence of this postoperative complication even without the influence of OCs (Stadel, 1981, part 1).

The risk of thromboembolic phenomena in OC users increases rapidly during the first month of use and declines at the same rate after discontinuation of treatment. The major risk factor is a history of thromboembolic disease.

Intravascular clot formation may be enhanced by increased numbers of platelets or platelet adhesiveness, higher levels of blood clotting factors, decreased fibrinolysis, or inflammatory changes in the blood vessel wall. OCs may alter the concentration of various clotting factors (increased prothrombin and factors VII, VIII, IX, and X; decreased antithrombin III). Larger numbers of platelets and increased adhesiveness are sometimes observed, although decreases or no change in adhesiveness also have been reported. The hematocrit and plasma fibrinogen levels are elevated, which increases blood viscosity (Lowe et al, 1980). These changes may be related to the greater risk of thromboembolic phenomena in patients taking OCs.

The increased risk of deep vein thrombosis is believed to be related to the estrogen content of OCs, although progestin may be related to occlusion of superficial veins (Dalen and Hickler, 1981). The incidence of thromboembolic disease was reported to be less among users of preparations containing smaller amounts of estrogen (Royal College of General Practitioners, 1974; Böttiger et al, 1980).

Preparations containing the least amount of estrogen (usually 35 mcg or less) that will provide reliable contraception with a minimum of untoward effects (eg, breakthrough bleeding, spotting) should be utilized. Women with a history of or those with active thromboembolic disease, thrombophlebitis, or hypercoagulable state should not take OCs. In addition, OCs should not be employed within one month before or after elective surgery or immediately postpartum because of the greater risk of thromboembolism at these times. When OCs cannot be discontinued prior to surgery, as in acute trauma, prophylactic low-dose heparin therapy should be considered.

The risk of cardiovascular disease is increased with OC usage, particularly in smokers and women over 35 years (Stadel, 1981, parts 1 and 2; Dalen and Hickler, 1981). The risk of death due to circulatory diseases (primarily ischemic heart disease and subarachnoid hemorrhage) is increased about fourfold in OC users (Royal College of General Practitioners, 1981).

Although other studies have not found that past use of OCs affects the incidence of *myocardial infarction,* one large case-control study determined that past OC users between 40 and 49 years may be at continued risk of myocardial infarction (up to ten years after discontinuation) and that the risk increased with duration of use (Slone et al, 1981). In another study, the risk of death (mostly cardiovascular) was reported to be higher among former OC users, but there was no relationship between duration of OC use and cardiovascular deaths (Royal College of General Practitioners, 1981). Later data demonstrated continued risk of only cerebrovascular disease in former OC users (Layde et al, 1983).

OC use appears to be an independent risk factor. However, the greatest influence of OCs is in their ability to multiply the effect of other risk factors (ie, age, smoking, hypertension, diabetes, obesity, hyperlipidemia). Because of its prevalence, cigarette smoking has the greatest impact. Most myocardial infarctions associated with OC use could probably be prevented by not prescribing these agents for women with known risk factors or a family history of premature coronary artery disease.

The incidence of fatal and nonfatal *stroke* may be increased in OC users. In current users, the risk of thrombotic stroke is increased about tenfold and that of hemorrhagic stroke is increased almost twofold. An increased risk of subarachnoid hemorrhage also has been found in past OC users. In one study, nonhemorrhagic stroke was related to OC dosage; no strokes were reported in women using low-dose (less than 50 mcg estrogen) pills (Vessey et al, 1984). Of the small percentage of fatal strokes among OC users, most are caused by subarachnoid hemorrhages. In addition to oral contraceptive use, other risk factors include hypertension, cigarette smoking, and age over 35 years (Longstreth and Swanson, 1984). The combination of OC use and hypertension increases the risk of both thrombotic and hemorrhagic stroke synergistically. Smoking has been suggested to synergize with OCs to increase the risk of subarachnoid hemorrhage.

The pathogenesis of both myocardial infarction (Engel et al, 1983) and stroke associated with current OC use usually is not atheromatous in nature. Myocardial infarctions in young women, whether or not associated with OCs, are usually caused by obstructive coronary artery disease (the left anterior descending coronary artery is a frequent site of the lesion). OCs may contribute to the progression of subclinical thrombosis and to coronary occlusion by their effects on clotting mechanisms. Autopsies on women who died from stroke associated with OC use reveal a common pattern: Thrombi are found at sites of endothelial proliferation and subendothelial fibrosis. These structural characteristics and the increased tendency for clotting may account for occlusion of cerebral arteries (with or without hemorrhage) in affected women. If cardiovascular risk persists in past OC users, it may be related to the effects of prolonged elevation of serum lipids and blood pressure and decreased glucose tolerance, which accelerate atherogenesis (Dalen and Hickler, 1981; Stadel, 1981, part 2).

Both the estrogen and progestin components of OCs may contribute to the increased risk of cardiovascular disease. Increases in clotting factors are usually attributed to estrogens, and decreasing the estrogen content may reduce the incidence of ischemic heart disease. However, in one study, increasing the dose of progestins elevated the incidence of ischemic heart disease (norethindrone acetate) and strokes (norethindrone acetate and levonorgestrel) (Meade et al, 1980). If this observation is confirmed, it might be expected that other closely related progestins have similar effects.

Because of the epidemiologic evidence that OCs increase the occurrence of cardiovascular disease, women with other risk factors (eg, smoking, diabetes, hyperlipidemia, hypertension, family history of premature coronary artery disease) should use another form of contraception or be given OCs with caution and close monitoring. Age is an independent risk factor; therefore, women over 35 years preferably should use other contraceptive measures, but flexibility can be exercised before age 45 if no additional risk factors exist.

Cigarette smoking is a serious risk factor and the risk associated with cigarette smoking and OC use increases synergistically with age. Women over 35 years who smoke should not take OCs, and it is preferable that smoking and OC use not be combined at any age.

Increases in both systolic (about 5 mm Hg) and diastolic (1 to 2 mm Hg) *blood pressure* have been reported, but are usually within the normal range. However, women who use OCs are about three to six times more likely to develop hypertension than nonusers (see references in Dalen and Hickler, 1981). In one study, small increases in systolic and diastolic blood pressure were similar to the above, and the diastolic pressure continued to increase 0.5 mm Hg for each year of OC use. Blood pressure returned to approximately pretreatment levels when OCs were discontinued (Cook et al, 1985). Other evidence suggests that the probability of hypertension increases with duration of OC use and age and is most prominent in women over 35 years. The increase in blood pressure that normally occurs after age 40 apparently is accelerated in current OC users, and women who are already hypertensive may experience a further rise. In women using a low-dose OC preparation, 8.2% of high-risk patients (past history of hypertension) discontinued therapy because of recurrent hypertension. However, although the mean baseline blood pressure was higher in the high-risk group than in controls with no hypertensive history, there was no increase in mean blood pressure compared to baseline in either group (Tsai et al, 1985).

Estrogen alone alters blood pressure and progestins also probably increase blood pressure. In one study employing ethinyl estradiol 50 mcg and norethindrone acetate 1, 3, and 4 mg, the incidence of hypertension increased with the progestin content (Royal College of General Practitioners, 1977).

Changes in blood pressure are usually reversible within one to six months after cessation of therapy. The mechanism of this effect probably involves the renin-angiotensin system. Angiotensinogen (renin substrate) levels increase and the negative feedback control of renin production is impaired; elevated levels of angiotensin, a potent vasoconstrictor, and aldosterone result. Since these changes occur in OC users whether or not they become hypertensive, it appears that individual sensitivity or predisposition is important in the blood pressure response to OCs.

The blood pressure should be monitored after three months of OC therapy and every 6 to 12 months thereafter. If hypertension develops, another form of contraception should be utilized. Other contraceptives are preferred in women who are already hypertensive; if OCs are employed, careful monitoring of blood pressure is necessary. Several cases of pulmonary hypertension have been reported in women using OCs, although most of these individuals had predisposing conditions.

OCs have been associated with changes in the pattern of *migraine headache*. Attacks that occur frequently during the interval when steroids are not taken may be due to fluid retention and are not dangerous. However, if migraine is first experienced after beginning OC medication or the frequency or intensity increases during treatment, therapy should be discontinued since they may be prodromal symptoms of stroke.

Teratogenicity: Sex steroids and related compounds may produce teratogenic effects on genital tissues. Large doses of diethylstilbestrol (and possibly other estrogens) produce defects in the reproductive tracts of both female and male offspring (see Chapter 39, Estrogens, Progestins, and Other Agents Used to Treat Gynecologic Conditions). Masculinization of female fetuses has occurred when some progestins were taken during early pregnancy (eg, therapy for threatened abortion).

Among women who discontinue use of OCs, the risk of spontaneous abortion; congenital abnormalities, including any of the VACTERL anomalies (vertebral, anal, cardiac, tracheal, esophageal, renal, or limb); or Down's syndrome in liveborn infants is not increased. Some studies have found a higher risk of nongenital malformations among infants exposed to sex steroids, including inadvertent continuation of OCs, during susceptible periods in embryogenesis. Cardiovascular and other defects in the VACTERL group have been described (Nora et al, 1978; Heinonen et al, 1977; Janerich et al, 1980), mostly in male infants. In general, the increased risk of nongenital congenital malformations associated with OC use is small, and the likelihood of a causal association has been questioned (Wilson and Brent, 1981) and refuted (Nora et al, 1982). It has been suggested that the nonrandom association of VACTERL anomalies (regardless of cause) may be explained on the basis of defective mesodermal development during embryogenesis (Khoury et al, 1983). Because OCs rarely may cause such abnormalities, therapy should be discontinued as soon as pregnancy is confirmed.

Fibrocystic Breast Disease: Women with fibrocystic breast disease showing proliferative lesions on biopsy (especially those with atypia) have an increased risk of breast cancer (Dupont and Page, 1985). Several studies have shown that there is no increased (Franceschi et al, 1984) or decreased risk of *benign breast disease* in women who use combination OCs (Hislop and Threlfall, 1984). The fact that OCs often are not prescribed for women with a history of benign breast disease may account for the higher incidence among control subjects.

Breast Cancer: Most studies agree that there is no general increase in the incidence of *breast cancer* with OC use. However, some have suggested higher risk for certain groups of users. Until recently, there was particular concern that women who use OCs for several years before their mid-twenties or prior to first-term pregnancy may be at increased risk of breast cancer by their late thirties to mid-forties (Pike et al, 1983; McPherson et al, 1983; Olsson et al, 1985). In one study (Pike et al, 1983), an increase in breast cancer by the late thirties was associated with long-term use of OCs with high progestin activity before age 25; the methods used to rank OCs by progestin activity have since been widely criticized. Recently, data from a large case-control study showed no alteration in the incidence of breast cancer up to age 45 for any group of OC users. The risk was not increased with long-term use (greater than four years), even when initial

administration began before age 20 or prior to first-term pregnancy. The risk of breast cancer by the mid-thirties was unrelated to use of OCs with high progestin activity before age 25, even when the duration exceeded six years (Stadel et al, 1985). In an early report (Paffenbarger et al, 1977), OC use for more than six years was associated with increased breast cancer among women with a prior history of benign breast disease; however, when more data were collected, the association largely disappeared (Paffenbarger et al, 1980). Other studies show no increased risk for OC users with prior benign breast disease (Centers for Disease Control Cancer and Steroid Hormone Study, 1983 A; Rosenberg et al, 1985). One small study (Jick et al, 1980) suggested a possible increase in breast cancer for premenopausal women who continue using OCs after age 45; this has not been confirmed. Use of OCs is not recommended for women in this age group (see section on Adverse Reactions) and is currently uncommon.

In general, overall conclusions of large studies do not support a causal relationship between OCs and breast cancer. Data suggesting increased risk in certain subgroups are often based on small numbers and are not always consistent among studies. Epidemiologic studies continue to monitor this issue. Since estrogen can stimulate growth of pre-existing cancerous breast lesions, OCs are contraindicated in women with known or suspected breast carcinoma, and caution must be exercised if they are prescribed for patients at high risk of breast cancer.

Other Carcinogenicity: An increased incidence of *endometrial cancer* was observed in women who took the sequential type of OC, which had a relatively high estrogen content unopposed by progestin. Sequential OCs have been removed from the market in the United States.

The risk of endometrial carcinoma among women who have used combined OCs appears to be about one-half that of nonusers overall; the protective effect increases with duration of use and persists for at least ten years after discontinuation of OCs (Weiss and Sayvetz, 1980; Kaufman et al, 1980 B; Hulka et al, 1982; Centers for Disease Control Cancer and Steroid Hormone Study, 1983 B). However, since estrogen may stimulate the growth of existing endometrial cancer, OCs should not be prescribed for women with undiagnosed abnormal genital bleeding.

The incidence of cervical dysplasia, carcinoma in situ, and invasive *cervical cancer* has been reported to increase with OC use. However, differences between OC users and nonusers with respect to age at commencement of regular intercourse and total number of sexual partners appear to explain at least some of this increase. In one study, the incidence of cervical dysplasia and neoplasia increased in OC compared to IUD users, and there was a trend toward increased risk with increasing duration of OC use. However, the lack of data on venereal factors precluded consideration of this confounding variable (Vessey et al, 1983). It is widely believed that cervical cancer may be caused by a sexually transmitted virus.

Women taking OCs appear to have a reduced risk of ovarian cancer, which further decreases with duration of use (Casagrande et al, 1979; Rosenberg et al, 1982). It has been estimated that 1,700 cases of ovarian cancer are avoided each year because of past or current OC use in the United States

(Centers for Disease Control Cancer and Steroid Hormone Study, 1983 C).

Firm conclusions about the carcinogenicity of OCs are not yet possible because of the long latent period (up to 15 years) between the administration of a carcinogen and the development of cancer.

Miscellaneous Reactions: *Melasma* similar to that observed during pregnancy sometimes develops in women who use OCs. Those with dark complexions or a history of melasma of pregnancy or those exposed to excessive amounts of sunlight are most susceptible. Decreasing the quantity of estrogen may reduce pigmentation. However, even after cessation of medication, a long time may be required before pigmentation disappears.

Hair loss and changes in hair growth and texture may be related to either the androgenic potency of the progestin component or a decrease in estrogen activity relative to previous endogenous levels. Rarely, a male pattern of hair growth may appear on the face and body or recession of temporal hair may occur. Other manifestations of androgenicity include oily skin and scalp and acne. A preparation containing a progestin with lower androgenicity or a higher estrogen/progestin potency ratio may be considered. Androgen-producing ovarian or adrenal pathology should be ruled out. The effects of changes in drug regimen on hair growth may not be apparent for several months.

Rarely, *chorea* is associated with oral contraceptives, particularly in women with disorders of the basal ganglia. One-half of affected patients have a history of chorea, often associated with rheumatic fever. Symptoms generally resolve upon discontinuation of OCs (Nausieda et al, 1979).

Some women (most commonly those with a history of a psychological disorder) may experience mood changes or develop *depression* while taking OCs; this may be related to changes in tryptophan metabolism that decrease brain serotonin production. Administration of pyridoxine (vitamin B_6) is sometimes effective in women with a deficiency of this vitamin.

Alterations in *libido* sometimes occur with OCs. These changes may be in either direction and may be unrelated to steroidal effects (eg, libido may increase because of lack of fear of pregnancy). If decreased libido is a problem, a preparation containing a small amount of estrogen and an androgenic progestin may be helpful.

Changes in blood levels of vitamins and minerals have been observed. Plasma folate, pyridoxine, vitamin B_{12}, carotene, calcium, magnesium, manganese, zinc, and phosphorus levels may decrease while ascorbic acid, vitamin A, iron, and copper levels increase. The clinical significance of these changes is not apparent and decreased levels do not result in deficiency. Vitamin supplementation is unnecessary in women with adequate diets.

Ocular abnormalities (eg, retinal vascular occlusion, retinal edema, optic neuropathy, retinal vasculitis) have been associated rarely with use of OCs. Symptoms may appear during therapy, disappear on withdrawal, and reappear upon resumption of the drugs. OCs should be discontinued if there is an unexplained decrease in vision or color vision or other serious symptoms, and appropriate diagnostic and therapeutic measures should be taken. Some ophthalmologists recommend discontinuing OCs in women with retinitis pigmentosa because of the impression that pregnancy accelerates peripheral field loss and the similarity between the hormonal milieu of pregnancy and OC therapy (Petursson et al, 1981). Results of controlled studies indicate that OCs probably do not affect *contact lens* tolerance as was thought earlier.

Drug Interactions: OCs may decrease the hypoprothrombinemic response to coumarin anticoagulants, and larger doses of the latter may be required. The metabolic clearance of acetaminophen may be accelerated in women taking OCs, and larger doses of acetaminophen may be required to achieve the desired response (Baciewicz, 1985). There have been reports of pregnancies and breakthrough bleeding when OCs were taken with barbiturates, anticonvulsants, griseofulvin, and particularly rifampin [Rifadin, Rimactane]. This is probably due to the increased metabolism of estrogen by mixed-function oxidases when these drugs are taken with OCs. An increased absolute bioavailability of imipramine, consistent with inhibition of hepatic imipramine oxidation, was observed in regular OC users. It was suggested that the dose of imipramine be reduced to achieve desired steady-state plasma concentrations in OC users (Abernethy et al, 1984). OCs may reduce the metabolism of theophylline and patients taking this combination should be monitored for theophylline toxicity (Baciewicz, 1985).

A few isolated interactions with antibiotics, including ampicillin and tetracycline, decreased contraceptive effectiveness (eg, breakthrough bleeding, pregnancy). The probable mechanism is decreased enterohepatic circulation of hormones due to destruction of bacterial flora in the gut (Hansten and Horn, 1985). Normally, bacterial enzymes hydrolyze hormone conjugates, freeing the steroid for reabsorption by the gut (Back et al, 1981). A study of the effect of gut flora on digoxin metabolism suggested that antibiotic suppression of these organisms may continue for weeks (Lindenbaum et al, 1981).

The wide range of steady-state plasma concentrations of OC steroids observed may partly explain why few individuals (those with low plasma concentrations) experience decreased contraceptive efficacy with fairly common drug combinations (Back and L'E Orme, 1984). Because of the limited number of reports, an accurate assessment of the frequency of clinically significant interactions is not possible. However, some physicians advise patients taking antibiotics to watch for signs of decreased OC efficacy (eg, breakthrough bleeding), to use an additional form of contraception during antibiotic therapy, or to use another contraceptive method during long-term antibiotic treatment.

When OCs and pharmacologic amounts of corticosteroids are administered concurrently, the metabolism of the latter is reduced and may allow reduction of the corticosteroid dosage. In one study, women taking OCs or postmenopausal estrogen therapy were given prednisolone concurrently. Alterations in metabolism of prednisolone, including increased half-life, were consistent with a potential for enhanced pharmacologic effect or toxicity when prednisolone was added to an estrogen regimen (Gustavson et al, 1986). Because estrogen increases the synthesis of thyroxine-binding globulin (TBG), an increase in the dosage of exogenous thyroid hormone may be required when OCs are taken concurrently.

The blood levels of unbound chlordiazepoxide [Librium] may be increased in OC users, but differences in clinical effect have not been observed. Low-dose OCs may have a differential effect on benzodiazepine metabolism: metabolism of some agents metabolized by conjugation may be accelerated and that of some agents metabolized by oxidation may be inhibited (Stoehr et al, 1984).

The combination of aminocaproic acid and oral contraceptives may produce a hypercoagulable state.

Ingestion of ascorbic acid 1 g daily elevates plasma levels of ethinyl estradiol. This implies that the patient who initiates OC therapy while taking regular megadoses of vitamin C could experience reduction of estrogen levels in the blood upon withdrawal of the vitamin. Conversely, initiating vitamin C intake while taking OCs may elevate the effective estrogen levels. Clinical manifestations are theoretically possible (ie, reduced contraceptive efficacy, estrogen excess) in either case. Further verification of this effect and its clinical significance is required.

Effects on Laboratory Tests: Reversible sulfobromophthalein (BSP) retention may occur during administration of OCs. The defect is in the transfer of BSP from liver cells to bile; storage is not affected.

Estrogens raise the level of thyroxine-binding globulin (TBG), which increases values for total thyroxine (T_4) and decreases values for the T_3 resin uptake test. The free thyroxine index (FTI) and direct measurements of T_3 or T_4 by radioimmunoassay remain unchanged. Thyroid function test results return to pretreatment levels within two months after discontinuing therapy.

OCs may elevate plasma triglycerides and otherwise alter lipid levels. Glucose tolerance may be decreased. Serum iron and copper levels may increase because of higher concentrations of their respective transport proteins, transferrin and ceruloplasmin. OCs may cause a false-positive test for LE cells and/or antinuclear antibodies. Urinary 17-hydroxycorticosteroids may be decreased. See also the section on Metabolic Effects, Adverse Reactions, and Contraindications.

POSTCOITAL CONTRACEPTION

When coitus has occurred without contraceptive protection and pregnancy is not desired, interceptive (ie, postfertilization) measures may eliminate unwanted pregnancy and avoid abortion. Postcoital techniques are often referred to as "morning after" contraception. Various estrogen regimens (see Table 4) or IUDs may be used for this purpose.

Extensive clinical experience and documentation of effectiveness have been obtained with diethylstilbestrol (DES). Large doses are administered within 72 hours after unprotected midcycle sexual exposure. The estrogen may change the sequence of hormonal influences on the fallopian tubes, thereby disturbing the passage of the ovum. Estrogen also may alter the endometrial milieu and interfere with nidation.

Ethinyl estradiol and conjugated estrogens were used as postcoital contraceptives (see Table 4 for doses) in a multicenter study. Ethinyl estradiol appeared to be more effective. Both drugs substantially reduced the pregnancy rates, which were lower when treatment was instituted within 24 hours rather than 24 to 72 hours after coitus (Dixon et al, 1980).

The patient who seeks postcoital contraception should understand that high-dose estrogen regimens should be used infrequently or in emergencies (eg, rape, incest), for the presumed risk of serious side effects after frequently repeated large doses is unacceptable. Breast tenderness is noted frequently. Nausea and vomiting occur routinely. Five days of therapy are commonly employed, and the severe nausea that results may require discontinuation of treatment or concurrent use of an antiemetic. If vomiting is severe, the interceptive regimen may be ineffective.

Excellent results (0.6% to 1.9% failures per cycle) were reported with a regimen of 100 mcg ethinyl estradiol and 1 mg norgestrel (two Ovral tablets) taken 12 hours apart within 72 hours of a single midcycle coital exposure (Yuzpe, 1984). This regimen compared favorably with the standard ethinyl estradiol regimen in a comparative study (Van Santen and Haspels, 1985). The total amount of estrogen used with the combination estrogen-progestin method is much lower than when estrogen alone is administered and treatment is completed in one day. The frequency and severity of adverse effects are reduced. Thus, the combination method is preferable to other high-dose hormonal regimens.

Because of the teratogenic potential of estrogens, a preexisting pregnancy must be ruled out before treatment is begun. Administration of DES during the first trimester of pregnancy is associated with a high incidence of vaginal adenosis and, rarely, adenocarcinoma in female offspring, as well as effects on the male urogenital tract (see Chapter 39, Estrogens, Progestins, and Other Agents Used to Treat Gynecologic Conditions). Adenosis also has been reported following the use of estrogens other than DES. However, there is no information on the effects of any estrogen given as an interceptive contraceptive on a pregnancy that may ensue in the event of contraceptive failure. If interceptive therapy fails and pregnancy results, some women will elect abortion simply because the pregnancy is unwanted. However, abortion need not be recommended solely on the basis of the teratogenic effects of the estrogen. The patient should be given a realistic assessment of the potential, but uncertain, risks involved before determining the fate of the pregnancy.

IUDs also have been employed for interceptive contraception. The IUD is inserted within one day but may be inserted within five days after unprotected intercourse and left in place, if appropriate, for continuing contraception. Most experience has been achieved with the copper-containing devices, which are no longer marketed in the United States.

DEPOT PREPARATIONS

Several long-lasting depot preparations are under clinical investigation for use as contraceptives. These products may contain both an estrogen and a progestin but a progestin is usually used alone. Norethisterone enanthate is being investigated in several countries. Medroxyprogesterone acetate (DMPA) [Depo-Provera] has received most attention and is widely utilized throughout the world. A dose of 150 mg is

TABLE 4.
POSTCOITAL CONTRACEPTIVE REGIMENS

Estrogen	Dosage
Ethinyl Estradiol and Norgestrel (combination available as Ovral)	100 mcg ethinyl estradiol and 1 mg norgestrel (two Ovral tablets) taken twice 12 hours apart
Ethinyl Estradiol	2.5 mg twice daily for five days
Conjugated Estrogens	10 mg three times daily for five days
Estrone	5 mg three times daily for five days
Diethylstilbestrol	25 mg twice daily for five days

injected intramuscularly every three months, although the effect usually extends beyond this period. Usually, the drug is measurable in plasma for six to eight months after the last injection. The contraceptive protection provided is as effective as combination OCs. Intramuscular injection of 400 mg every six months also has been used with only a slight decrease in efficacy.

DMPA inhibits ovulation by suppressing the midcycle surge of LH secretion and also causes thickening of cervical mucus and development of an atrophic endometrium that may not be conducive to nidation. Gonadotropin suppression is not complete, and there is some follicular development; estrogen production is slightly less than in a normal follicular phase.

Fertility is delayed following contraceptive use of DMPA. For this reason, the drug is not recommended for young women whose contraceptive needs are to space children. Average time to conception after the last injection is about one year but may be as long as two and one-half years. This may be related to persistent plasma levels of the drug, continuing pituitary suppression after clearance of the progestin, or coincidental pathologic changes. There is considerable variation in rate of absorption and metabolism, which could account for the prolonged effect.

Adverse Reactions: Side effects include weight gain, depression, headache, and abdominal bloating. The most common problems are irregular menstrual cycles and spotting or amenorrhea, and most patients who discontinue therapy do so because of these complaints. In glucose tolerance tests, an exaggerated insulin response to glucose has been observed but is milder than that observed with OCs. If bleeding persists and requires correction, steroidal therapy may be attempted (see Chapter 39, Estrogens, Progestins, and Other Agents Used to Treat Gynecologic Conditions, for a discussion on dysfunctional bleeding). However, the routine use of estrogens to "normalize" the menstrual cycle is not advocated. An atrophic endometrium develops progressively, and total amenorrhea is common 6 to 12 months after therapy is begun. Studies of DMPA's effect on blood pressure have yielded equivocal results but most often no effect or a decrease in blood pressure has been reported.

DMPA has glucocorticoid properties, particularly when given in large doses (eg, to treat endometrial carcinoma). In contraceptive doses, plasma cortisol levels are sometimes decreased and the response to metyrapone may be diminished, but there is no clinical evidence of adrenal insufficiency.

Large doses of DMPA are teratogenic in rabbits; this effect is probably related to the glucocorticoid properties of DMPA. DMPA does not appear to have a teratogenic effect in man. However, administration of progestins during pregnancy is generally not recommended, and fetal exposure may be prolonged if a depot preparation is administered during an existing pregnancy or if contraceptive failure occurs.

Large doses of DMPA have caused malignant mammary tumors in beagle dogs, but there is no evidence of a similar effect in other test animals (including monkeys) or in women. This effect appears to be peculiar to the beagle and the appropriateness of this animal model has been questioned. An increased risk of cervical carcinoma in situ also has been investigated, but firm evidence to either support or reject this relationship does not exist. Endometrial carcinoma was reported in long-term studies on monkeys given 50 times the clinical contraceptive dosage.

In a study of 5,000 women followed for 4 to 13 years after initial DMPA injection, there was no increased risk of breast, uterine, or ovarian cancer (Liang et al, 1983).

The DMPA Controversy: The contraceptive use of DMPA has been scientifically and politically controversial for over a decade. DMPA is used as a contraceptive in more than 70 countries. In 1984, Great Britain approved labeling of the drug as a second-line contraceptive. Scientific panels of the World Health Organization (WHO), International Planned Parenthood Federation (IPPF), and the U.S. Agency for International Development (USAID) have endorsed its use in developing countries (Gold and Willson, 1981). The U.S. Food and Drug Administration (FDA) has refused to label the drug for contraception (it is commonly used in the United States to treat breast and endometrial cancer). The FDA concluded that the benefit/risk assessment differs among areas of the world and, with the advanced health care system in the United States, that the concerns of potential adverse effects (see above) outweigh the need for this contraceptive. A Public Board of Inquiry in 1983 recommended that further epidemiologic evidence of safety be obtained before the labeling change is approved. The issues involved in this long-standing debate with the FDA have been discussed extensively (Rosenfield et al, 1983).

Conclusions: In spite of the foregoing problems, DMPA may be an appropriate contraceptive in special situations. Its main values lie in its great effectiveness and the need for infrequent administration. The latter property is a drawback in the event of side effects, however. Although the contraceptive use of DMPA remains controversial in this country, it is an option for consideration. It is particularly justified in patients who are unable to use other forms of contraception, in those who are noncompliant in methods requiring cooperation, when estrogens are contraindicated (eg, previous thromboembolic disease), and in intellectually or psychologically impaired patients.

Cited References

New developments in vaginal contraception. *Popul Rep [H]* 12:H159-190, (Jan-Feb) 1984.

Abernethy DR, et al: Imipramine disposition in users of oral contraceptive steroids. *Clin Pharmacol Ther* 35:792-797, 1984.

Baciewicz AM: Oral contraceptive drug interactions. *Therapeut Drug Monitor* 7:26-35, 1985.

Back DJ, L'E Orme M: Interindividual variability in oral contraceptive disposition. *TIPS* 480-483, (Nov) 1984.

Back DJ, et al: Interindividual variation and drug interactions with hormonal steroid contraceptives. *Drugs* 21:46-61, 1981.

Badawy SZA, et al: Relation between oral contraceptive use and subsequent development of hyperprolactinemia. *Fertil Steril* 36:464-467, 1981.

Block M, Rulin MC: Managing patients on oral contraceptives. *Am Fam Physician* 32:154-168, (Aug) 1985.

Böttiger LE, et al: Oral contraceptives and thromboembolic disease: Effects of lowering oestrogen content. *Lancet* 1:1097-1101, 1980.

Bracken MB: Spermicidal contraceptives and poor reproductive outcomes: Epidemiologic evidence against association. *Am J Obstet Gynecol* 157:552-556, 1985.

Bracken MB, Vita K: Frequency of nonhormonal contraception around conception and association with congenital malformations in offspring. *Am J Epidemiol* 117:281-291, 1983.

Briggs M, Briggs M: Randomized study of metabolic effects of four low-estrogen oral contraceptives. I. Results after 6 cycles. *Contraception* 23:463-471, 1981.

Brooks PG: Relationship of estrogen and progesterone to breast disease. *J Reprod Med* 29(suppl):530-538, (July) 1984.

Burkman RT: Association between intrauterine device and pelvic inflammatory disease. *Obstet Gynecol* 57:269-276, 1981.

Casagrande JT, et al: "Incessant ovulation" and ovarian cancer. *Lancet* 2:170-173, 1979.

Centers for Disease Control Cancer and Steroid Hormone Study: Long-term oral contraceptive use and risk of breast cancer. *JAMA* 249:1591-1595, 1983 A.

Centers for Disease Control Cancer and Steroid Hormone Study: Oral contraceptive use and risk of endometrial cancer. *JAMA* 249:1600-1604, 1983 B.

Centers for Disease Control Cancer and Steroid Hormone Study: Oral contraceptive use and risk of ovarian cancer. *JAMA* 249:1596-1599, 1983 C.

Cole LP, et al: Postpartum insertion of modified intrauterine devices. *J Reprod Med* 29:677-682, 1984.

Committee on Drugs, American Academy of Pediatrics: Breast feeding and contraception. *Pediatrics* 68:138-140, 1981.

Cook NR, et al: Regression analysis of changes in blood pressure with oral contraceptive use. *Am J Epidemiol* 121:530-540, 1985.

Cordero JF, Layde PM: Vaginal spermicides, chromosomal abnormalities and limb reduction defects. *Fam Plann Perspect* 15:16-18, 1983.

Cramer DW, et al: Tubal infertility and intrauterine device. *N Engl J Med* 312:941-947, 1985.

Dalen JE, Hickler RB: Oral contraceptives and cardiovascular disease. *Am Heart J* 101:626-639, 1981.

Daling JR, et al: Primary tubal infertility in relation to use of intrauterine device. *N Engl J Med* 312:937-941, 1985.

del Junco DJ, et al: Do oral contraceptives prevent rheumatoid arthritis? *JAMA* 254:1938-1941, 1985.

Dickerson J, et al: Liver function tests and low-dose estrogen oral contraceptives. *Contraception* 22:597-603, 1980.

Dickey RP: *Managing Contraceptive Pill Patients*, ed 4. Minneapolis, Creative Infomatics, 1984.

Dixon GW, et al: Ethinyl estradiol and conjugated estrogens as postcoital contraceptives. *JAMA* 244:1336-1339, 1980.

Dorflinger LJ: Relative potency of progestins used in oral contraceptives. *Contraception* 31:557-570, 1985.

Duguid HLD, et al: *Actinomyces*-like organisms in cervical smears from women using intrauterine contraceptive devices. *Br Med J* 281:534-537, 1980.

Dupont WD, Page DL: Risk factors for breast cancer in women with proliferative breast disease. *N Engl J Med* 312:146-151, 1985.

Edelman DA, et al: Comparative trial of Today contraceptive sponge and diaphragm. *Am J Obstet Gynecol* 150:869-876, 1984.

Edgren RA, Sturtevant FM: Potencies of oral contraceptives. *Am J Obstet Gynecol* 125:1029-1038, 1976.

Engel H-J, et al: Coronary atherosclerosis and myocardial infarction in young women: Role of oral contraceptives. *Eur Heart J* 4:1-8, 1983.

Faich G, et al: Toxic shock syndrome and vaginal contraceptive sponge. *JAMA* 255:216-218, 1985.

Fotherby K: New look at progestogens. *Clin Obstet Gynaecol* 11:701-722, 1984.

Franceschi S, et al: Oral contraceptives and benign breast disease: Case-control study. *Am J Obstet Gynecol* 149:602-606, 1984.

Gold RB, Willson PD: Depo-Provera: New development in decade-old controversy. *Fam Plann Perspect* 13:35-39, 1981.

Goldzieher JW, et al: Comparative studies of ethynyl estrogens used in oral contraceptives. I. Endometrial response. II. Antiovulatory potency. III. Effect on plasma gonadotropins. *Am J Obstet Gynecol* 122:615-636, 1975.

Gosden C, et al: Intrauterine contraceptive devices in diabetic women. *Lancet* 1:530-534, 1982.

Gustavson LE, et al: Impairment of prednisolone disposition in women taking oral contraceptives or conjugated estrogens. *J Clin Endocrinol Metab* 62:234-237, 1986.

Hansten PD, Horn JR: Inhibition of oral contraceptive efficacy. *Drug Interact Newslett* 5:7-10, 1985.

Hatcher RA, et al: *Contraceptive Technology 1980-1983*, ed 12. New York, Irvington Publishers, 1984.

Heartwell SF, Schlesselman S: Risk of uterine perforation among users of intrauterine devices. *Obstet Gynecol* 61:31-36, 1983.

Heinonen OP, et al: Cardiovascular birth defects and antenatal exposure to female sex hormones. *N Engl J Med* 296:67-70, 1977.

Hislop TG, Threlfall WJ: Oral contraceptives and benign breast disease. *Am J Epidemiol* 120:273-280, 1984.

Huggins G, et al: Vaginal spermicides and outcome of pregnancy: Findings in large cohort study. *Contraception* 25:219-230, 1982.

Hulka BS, et al: Protection against endometrial carcinoma by combination-product oral contraceptives. *JAMA* 247:475-477, 1982.

Hull MGR, et al: Normal fertility in women with post-pill amenorrhoea. *Lancet* 1:1329-1332, 1981.

Janerich DT, et al: Oral contraceptives and birth defects. *Am J Epidemiol* 112:73-79, 1980.

Jick H, et al: Oral contraceptives and breast cancer. *Am J Epidemiol* 112:577-585, 1980.

Jick H, et al: Vaginal spermicides and congenital disorders. *JAMA* 245:1329-1332, 1981.

Kaufman DW, et al: Intrauterine contraceptive device use and pelvic inflammatory disease. *Am J Obstet Gynecol* 136:159-162, 1980 A.

Kaufman DW, et al: Decreased risk of endometrial cancer among oral-contraceptive users. *N Engl J Med* 303:1045-1047, 1980 B.

Kaufman DW, et al: Effect of different types of intrauterine devices on risk of pelvic inflammatory disease. *JAMA* 250:759-762, 1983.

Kelaghan J, et al: Barrier-method contraceptives and pelvic inflammatory disease. *JAMA* 248:184-187, 1982.

Khoury MJ, et al: Population study of VACTERL association: Evidence for etiologic heterogeneity. *Pediatrics* 71:815-820, 1983.

Layde PM, et al: Incidence of arterial disease among oral contraceptive users: Royal College of General Practitioners' Oral Contraception Study. *J R Coll Gen Pract* 33:75-82, 1983.

Lee NC, et al: Type of intrauterine device and risk of pelvic inflammatory disease. *Obstet Gynecol* 62:1-6, 1983.

Liang AP, et al: Risk of breast, uterine corpus, and ovarian cancer in women receiving medroxyprogesterone injections. *JAMA* 249:2909-2912, 1983.

Lindenbaum J, et al: Inactivation of digoxin by gut flora: Reversal by antibiotic therapy. *N Engl J Med* 305:789-794, 1981.

Linn S, et al: Delay in conception for former "pill" users. *JAMA* 247:629-632, 1982.

Linn S, et al: Lack of association between contraceptive usage and congenital malformations in offspring. *Am J Obstet Gynecol* 147:923-928, 1983.

Lockhat D, et al: Oral contraceptives and liver disease. *Can Med Assoc J* 124:993-999, 1981.

Longstreth WT Jr, Swanson PD: Oral contraceptives and stroke. *Stroke* 15:747-750, 1984.

Lowe GDO, et al: Increased blood viscosity in young women using oral contraceptives. *Am J Obstet Gynecol* 137:840-842, 1980.

Maheux R, et al: Oral contraceptives and prolactinomas: Case-control study. *Am J Obstet Gynecol* 142:134-138, 1982.

McPherson K, et al: Oral contraceptives and breast cancer, (letter). *Lancet* 2:1414-1415, 1983.

Meade TW, et al: Progestogens and cardiovascular reactions associated with oral contraceptives and comparison of safety of 50- and 30-mcg oestrogen preparations. *Br Med J* 280:1157-1161, 1980.

Mills JL, et al: Are spermicides teratogenic? *JAMA* 248:2148-2151, 1982.

Mills JL, et al: Are there adverse effects of periconceptional spermicide use? *Fertil Steril* 43:442-446, 1985.

Milsom I, Andersch B: Effect of various oral contraceptive combinations on dysmenorrhea. *Gynecol Obstet Invest* 17:284-292, 1984.

Mishell DR Jr: Noncontraceptive health benefits of oral steroid contraceptives. *Am J Obstet Gynecol* 142:809-816, 1982.

Mishell DR Jr: Intrauterine devices. *Clin Obstet Gynaecol* 11:679-699, 1984.

Mishell DR Jr (ed): Update on oral contraceptives. *J Reprod Med* 30(suppl):689-713, (Sept) 1985.

Nausieda PA, et al: Chorea induced by oral contraceptives. *Neurology* 29:1605-1609, 1979.

Nora JJ, et al: Exogenous progestogen and estrogen implicated in birth defects. *JAMA* 240:837-843, 1978.

Nora JJ, et al: Exogenous sex hormones and birth defects: Continuing the dialogue, (letter). *Am J Obstet Gynecol* 144:860-862, 1982.

Olsson H, et al: Oral contraceptive use and breast cancer in young women in Sweden. *Lancet* 1:748-749, 1985.

Ory HW: Review of association between intrauterine devices and acute pelvic inflammatory disease. *J Reprod Med* 20:200-204, 1978.

Ory HW: Ectopic pregnancy and intrauterine contraceptive devices: New perspectives. *Obstet Gynecol* 57:137-144, 1981.

Paffenbarger RS Jr, et al: Cancer risk as related to use of oral contraceptives during fertile years. *Cancer* 39(suppl):1887-1891, (April) 1977.

Paffenbarger RS Jr, et al: Characteristics that predict risk of breast cancer before and after menopause. *Am J Epidemiol* 112:258-268, 1980.

Patel LG, et al: Propranolol concentrations in plasma after insertion into vagina. *Br Med J* 287:1247-1248, 1983.

Persson E, Holmberg K: Longitudinal study of *Actinomyces israelii* in female genital tract. *Acta Obstet Gynecol Scand* 63:207, 1984.

Petursson GJ, et al: Pharmacology of ocular drugs: 6. Oral contraceptives. *Ophthalmology* 88:368-371, 1981.

Pike MC, et al: Breast cancer in young women and use of oral contraceptives: Possible modifying effect of formulation and age at use. *Lancet* 2:926-929, 1983.

Pituitary Adenoma Study Group: Pituitary adenomas and oral contraceptives: Multicenter case-control study. *Fertil Steril* 39:753-760, 1983.

Polednak AP, et al: Birth weight and birth defects in relation to maternal spermicide use. *Teratology* 26:27-38, 1982.

Reyniak JV, et al: Incidence of hyperprolactinemia during oral contraceptive therapy. *Obstet Gynecol* 55:8-11, 1980.

Rooks JB, et al: Epidemiology of hepatocellular adenoma: Role of oral contraceptive use. *JAMA* 242:644-648, 1979.

Rosenberg L, et al: Epithelial ovarian cancer and combination oral contraceptives. *JAMA* 247:3210-3212, 1982.

Rosenberg L, et al: Breast cancer and oral contraceptive use. *Am J Epidemiol* 119:167-176, 1985.

Rosenfield A, et al: Food and Drug Administration and medroxyprogesterone acetate: What are the issues? *JAMA* 249:2922-2928, 1983.

Rothman KJ: Spermicide use and Down's syndrome. *Am J Public Health* 72:399-401, 1982.

Royal College of General Practitioners: *Oral Contraceptives and Health: Interim Report.* New York, Pitman, 1974.

Royal College of General Practitioners: Effect on hypertension and benign breast disease of progestagen component in combined oral contraceptives. *Lancet* 1:624, 1977.

Royal College of General Practitioners: Further analyses of mortality in oral contraceptive users. *Lancet* 1:541-546, 1981.

Scholl TO, et al: Effects of vaginal spermicides on pregnancy outcome. *Fam Plann Perspect* 15:244-250, 1983.

Scragg RKR, et al: Oral contraceptives, pregnancy, and endogenous oestrogen in gall stone disease: Case control study. *Br Med J* 288:1795-1799, 1984.

Shapiro S, et al: Birth defects and vaginal spermicides. *JAMA* 247:2381-2384, 1982.

Shy KK, et al: Oral contraceptive use and occurrence of pituitary prolactinoma. *JAMA* 249:2204-2207, 1983.

Skouby SO, et al: Consequences of intrauterine contraception in diabetic women. *Fertil Steril* 42:568-572, 1984.

Slone D, et al: Risk of myocardial infarction in relation to current and discontinued use of oral contraceptives. *N Engl J Med* 305:420-424, 1981.

Soderstrom RM: Will progesterone save the IUD? *J Reprod Med* 28:305-309, 1983.

Spellacy WN: Carbohydrate metabolism during treatment with estrogen, progestogen, and low-dose oral contraceptives. *Am J Obstet Gynecol* 142:732-734, 1982.

Stadel BV: Oral contraceptives and cardiovascular disease, parts 1 and 2. *N Engl J Med* 305:612-618, 672-677, 1981.

Stadel BV, Schlesselman S: Extent of surgery for pelvic inflammatory disease in relation to duration of intrauterine device use. *Obstet Gynecol* 63:171-178, 1984.

Stadel BV, et al: Oral contraceptives and breast cancer in young women. *Lancet* 2:970-973, 1985.

Stoehr GP, et al: Effect of oral contraceptives on triazolam, temazepam, alprazolam, and lorazepam kinetics. *Clin Pharmacol Ther* 36:683-690, 1984.

Strobino B, et al: Exposure to contraceptive creams, jellies, and douches and their effect on zygote, (abstract). *Am J Epidemiol* 112:434, (Sept) 1980.

Svensson L, et al: Contraceptives and acute salpingitis. *JAMA* 251:2553-2555, 1984.

Taler SJ, et al: Case-control study of galactorrhea and its relationship to use of oral contraceptives. *Obstet Gynecol* 65:665-668, 1985.

Tietze C, Lewit S: Life risks associated with reversible methods of fertility regulation. *Int J Gynaecol Obstet* 16:456-459, 1979.

Tsai CC, et al: Low-dose oral contraception and blood pressure in women with past history of elevated blood pressure. *Am J Obstet Gynecol* 151:28-32, 1985.

Van Santen MR, Haspels AA: Comparison of high-dose estrogens versus low-dose ethinylestradiol and norgestrel combination in postcoital interception: Study in 493 women. *Fertil Steril* 43:206-213, 1985.

Vessey MP, et al: Risk of ectopic pregnancy and duration of use of intrauterine device. *Lancet* 2:501-502, 1979.

Vessey MP, et al: Pelvic inflammatory disease and intrauterine device: Findings in large cohort study. *Br Med J* 282:855-857, 1981.

Vessey MP, et al: Neoplasia of cervix uteri and contraception: Possible adverse effect of the pill. *Lancet* 2:930-934, 1983.

Vessey MP, et al: Oral contraceptives and stroke: Findings in large prospective study. *Br Med J* 289:530-531, 1984.

Washington AE, et al: Oral contraceptives, *Chlamydia trachomatis* infection, and pelvic inflammatory disease: Word of caution about protection. *JAMA* 253:2246-2250, 1985.

Weiss NS, Sayvetz TA: Incidence of endometrial cancer in relation to use of oral contraceptives. *N Engl J Med* 302:551-554, 1980.

White MK, et al: Intrauterine device termination rates and menstrual cycle day of insertion. *Obstet Gynecol* 55:220-224, 1980.

Wilson JG, Brent RL: Are female sex hormones teratogenic? *Am J Obstet Gynecol* 141:567-580, 1981.

Wingrave SJ, Kay CR: Oral contraceptives and gallbladder disease: Royal College of General Practitioners' Oral Contraception Study. *Lancet* 2:957-959, 1982.

Wynn V, Niththyananthan R: Effect of progestins in combined oral contraceptives on serum lipids with special reference to high-density lipoproteins. *Am J Obstet Gynecol* 142:766-772, 1982.

Yuzpe AA: Postcoital contraception. *Clin Obstet Gynaecol* 11:787-797, 1984.

Agents Used to Treat Infertility

Approximately 15% of couples who wish to have children experience some type of infertility that precludes pregnancy unless treatment is instituted; another 10% have less than the desired number of children. Successful pregnancy is achieved in about one-half of the couples who seek medical attention.

Couples who embark on a program of treatment for infertility should be selected carefully. They should be fully aware of the potential side effects of drug therapy and the extended treatment period that may be required. They also should be prepared for the anxiety, frustration, and disappointment that may accompany unsuccessful cycles of treatment and realize that these problems are common to many couples in this circumstance.

Requirements for Fertility: Fertility depends upon a complex and integrated hormonal milieu and the anatomic integrity of the reproductive organs. The responsibility and contribution of the male reproductive system are, in general, the production and delivery of mature, motile sperm in sufficient number and quality to effect fertilization. The role of the female extends beyond gamete production to encompass the elegant life support system that nurtures the developing fetus until viability in the external environment is assured.

In both sexes, the physiologic stimulus for gametogenesis emanates from gonadotropins produced and secreted by the anterior pituitary gland. The anterior pituitary releases both follicle-stimulating hormone (FSH) and luteinizing hormone (LH) in response to pulsatile production of luteinizing hormone-releasing hormone (LH-RH, gonadotropin-releasing hormone, GnRH) by the hypothalamus. FSH and LH are named for their actions in the female, although they are also necessary for normal reproductive function in the male. In females, LH stimulates the production of testosterone and its derivatives by the thecal cells of the follicle before ovulation; these hormones are then transported to the granulosa cells where aromatization to estradiol takes place. LH also stimulates estrogen and progesterone production by the converted granulosa cells of the corpus luteum (CL) after ovulation. FSH stimulates the growth of graafian follicles in the ovary and induces the aromatase enzyme in the granulosa cells.

A slight surge in FSH coupled with a marked surge of LH secretion occurs at midcycle. LH stimulates ovulation of the prepared follicle, and FSH induces formation of LH receptors on the granulosa cells, thus assuring luteal response to LH. Estrogen and progesterone produced by the CL prepare the endometrium for nidation. Progesterone is necessary to support the uterine lining during the early weeks of pregnancy before the placenta assumes its steroidogenic function.

Although fluctuations in gonadotropin secretion occur in males, there is apparently nothing analogous to the midcycle surge of LH and FSH secretion that occurs in females. LH (originally called ICSH or interstitial cell-stimulating hormone and found to be identical to LH) stimulates production of androgen, principally testosterone, by the Leydig cells. The initiation of spermatogenesis is stimulated by the sequential action of testosterone and FSH. The high local concentration of testosterone in the seminiferous tubules facilitates maturation of primary to secondary spermatocytes, while FSH appears to induce maturation of late spermatids to mature spermatozoa. Testosterone and FSH also stimulate the Sertoli cells to produce the putative transport molecule, androgen-binding protein (ABP), which is probably responsible for maintaining a greater concentration of testosterone in the seminiferous tubules than in the serum. Further maturational events occur in the epididymis; at ejaculation, the mature, motile sperm are mixed with secretions from the prostate and seminal vesicles and released. Even when the germinal epithelium is able to produce sperm at the constant enormous rate required for normal function, a compatible epididymal environment (temperature and chemical composition) and a patent ductal system are necessary to ensure fertility. Testosterone also is important for maintenance of libido and potency.

Even in the presence of two perfectly functioning reproductive systems, coitus must occur during the time when the fertile lives of the sperm (36 to 72 hours) and the ovum (12 to 24 hours) overlap. If coitus is spaced evenly every 48 hours, sperm capable of fertilization are almost always present in the woman's reproductive tract.

Diagnosis of Infertility: Evaluation of infertility should involve both partners. A detailed description of diagnostic procedures is beyond the scope of this book. The appropriate selection and sequence of tests can maximize the amount of information gained and eventually may spare the couple the time and expense of further testing, the possibility of inappropriate drug therapy, and unwarranted hopefulness. An accurate medical history, including determination of frequency and timing of coitus, may suggest the need for education rather than infertility tests. A likely cause of infertility deserving early evaluation (eg, mumps orchitis in the male, pelvic inflammatory disease in the female) also may be revealed. There is some evidence that habitual abortion is sometimes associated with a high degree of HLA antigen sharing between the partners (Thomas et al, 1985).

In addition, it should be recognized that a variety of agents affect fertility in both females and males (see the Table). The effects may be reversible in some cases upon discontinuation of the drug. For more detailed discussion, see reviews by Beeley, 1984, and Buchanan and Davis, 1984.

Because the male is the sole partner affected in about 30% of infertile couples, or because both partners may have impaired reproductive capacity, the simple semen analysis is reasonably the initial diagnostic procedure employed. A postcoital test immediately preceding or at ovulation measures the quality of cervical mucus and evaluates the interaction between sperm and cervical secretions. Basal body temperature patterns, measurement of serum progesterone levels, and/or endometrial biopsy provide presumptive evidence of ovulatory function. Patency of the fallopian tubes can be demonstrated by hysterosalpingography. Optimal timing of tests allows almost complete evaluation in the first cycle (ie, postcoital tests and hysterosalpingogram just before ovulation, endometrial biopsy just before menses, temperature chart throughout cycle). Measurement of serum prolactin and thyroid stimulating hormone (TSH) are useful to rule out hyperprolactinemia and hypothyroidism, respectively.

When these measures fail to determine the source of infertility, laparoscopy may reveal an initially unsuspected

EFFECTS OF DRUGS ON FERTILITY

Drug	Reported Effect	
	Females	**Males**
Busulfan [Myleran]	Amenorrhea	Possible sterility, azoospermia, and testicular atrophy
Chlorambucil [Leukeran]	---	Oligospermia; azoospermia
Cimetidine [Tagamet]	---	Decreased sperm count
Colchicine	---	Azoospermia
Cyclophosphamide [Cytoxan, Neosar]	Amenorrhea	Azoospermia
Diethylstilbestrol (use in pregnancy)	*Daughters:* Reduced fertility; increased spontaneous abortions	*Sons:* Epididymal cysts; questionable increase in cryptorchidism and infertility
Ethyl Alcohol	---	Decreased serum testosterone; impaired sperm motility
Heroin	Oligomenorrhea; amenorrhea	---
Levothyroxine [Levothroid, Synthroid]	Anovulation	---
Marijuana	Abnormal menstruation; anovulation	Decreased serum testosterone; decreased sperm count; impaired sperm motility; abnormal morphology
Methadone [Dolophine]	---	Decreased serum testosterone
Methotrexate [Folex, Mexate]	---	Oligospermia
Prednisolone	---	Oligospermia
Spironolactone [Aldactone]	Irregular menses or amenorrhea	---
Sulfasalazine [Azulfidine, S.A.S.-500]	---	Decreased sperm count
Thioridazine [Mellaril]	Amenorrhea	Slightly decreased serum testosterone

Adapted from Lipman, 1984

cause (eg, endometriosis, peritubal abnormalities) in up to 40% of women. Usually this procedure is delayed for two to three months after hysterosalpingography because of the increased incidence of pregnancy during this interval.

Drug Therapy: Drug therapy is directed primarily toward stimulating or enhancing ovulation and facilitating sperm transport in women and stimulating spermatogenesis in men. Pharmacotherapy currently is more advanced and successful in women than in men, but regimens are being refined continually to treat specific causes of infertility in both sexes.

Since FSH and LH are necessary to support gametogenesis in both females and males, clomiphene [Clomid, Serophene], menotropins (HMG) [Pergonal], and human chorionic gonadotropin (HCG) [A.P.L., Follutein, Pregnyl, Profasi HP] can be used to treat both anovulation and male infertility secondary to inadequate secretion or abnormal patterns of secretion of these gonadotropic hormones. Clomiphene stimulates secretion, while HMG and HCG provide replacement therapy.

Clomiphene requires an intact anterior pituitary gland and hypothalamus to be effective, because endogenous secretion of gonadotropin is stimulated by this agent. Clomiphene induces ovulation in most women and stimulates spermatogenesis in some men. Menotropins, a preparation of human menopausal gonadotropins (HMG), contains both FSH and LH activity. It is indicated when the pituitary gland cannot secrete these hormones in response to stimulation. HCG has the biological activity of LH and stimulates ovulation of prepared follicles (assuming prior stimulation by endogenous or exogenous FSH). In women, it is used primarily with HMG and sometimes after administration of clomiphene. In men, HCG may be used to treat hypogonadotropic hypogonadism. In addition to its use as a diagnostic agent in males and females, gonadorelin (LH-RH) [Factrel] has been used investigationally to induce ovulation.

Agents prescribed to treat other types of infertility include estrogens, oral contraceptives, danazol [Danocrine], progestins, and bromocriptine [Parlodel]. In women, estrogen is used to improve the quality of poor cervical mucus that occurs spontaneously or after treatment with clomiphene. Danazol or oral contraceptives may be used to treat infertility due to endometriosis. Bromocriptine reduces the secretion of abnormally high levels of prolactin and often normalizes cyclic function and ovulation.

FEMALE INFERTILITY

Female infertility can result from any interference with the necessary delicate hormonal integration that results in failure of ovulation, impairment of the life and function of the CL, or impediment in the access of the sperm to the ovum. Female infertility also may result from anatomical or physiologic conditions that prevent normal transport of the fertilized ovum through the fallopian tubes or interfere with the ability of the uterus to provide adequate nutrition and support of the fetus.

The primary causes of female infertility are organic (eg, adrenal, thyroid, pituitary/hypothalamic disorders) or anatomic (eg, obstruction of the fallopian tubes). Disorders that are at least partly amenable to drug therapy include unfavorable cervical mucus, anovulation, luteal phase defect, hyperprolactinemia, and endometriosis.

Unfavorable Cervical Mucus

Copious quantities of thin, watery cervical mucus are characteristic of normal estrogenic stimulation around the time of ovulation. If instead the mucus is scant and/or thick, transport of sperm through the cervix is inhibited. Favorable cervical mucus can be demonstrated by the spinnbarkeit test of viscosity, which is performed by drawing out a strand of cervical mucus between two slides. A strand of 10 to 15 cm indicates that conditions are favorable for sperm penetration. Test results are valid only during the periovulatory period when the effect of the estrogen peak on the cervical mucus can be seen. However, sperm survival, as demonstrated by a periovulatory postcoital test, is more important and may occur even when the quality of the cervical mucus does not appear to be ideal.

Unfavorable cervical mucus develops spontaneously or is sometimes caused by the antiestrogenic effect of clomiphene, especially when large doses are given. If poor cervical mucus is associated with failure to ovulate in a clomiphene-treated cycle, a change in drug regimen may be indicated (see the discussion on Clomiphene). If the quantity of cervical mucus is inadequate in an ovulatory cycle during clomiphene treatment, estrogen supplementation may be indicated.

Drug Therapy: Treatment of spontaneous or clomiphene-associated poor cervical mucus is similar: For spontaneous unfavorable cervical mucus, ethinyl estradiol 0.02 to 0.08 mg is given daily in divided doses starting on day 6 to 8 of the cycle and continuing to day 12 or 13. An alternative regimen is conjugated estrogens 2.5 to 5 mg given from day 5 to 15 of the cycle. Some practitioners achieve successful results with lower doses (conjugated estrogens 0.625 or 1.25 mg) given on a similar schedule. When used with clomiphene, estrogen is begun the day following the last dose of clomiphene and continued for a total of 10 days. Clomiphene and estrogen should not be given concurrently because they compete for binding sites and the therapeutic action of clomiphene is blocked. Estrogen should not be given during the luteal phase when it may be luteolytic, and it should not be added to a clomiphene regimen unless the condition of the cervical mucus warrants it.

A recent approach to improving cervical mucus is the use of guaifenesin, which may have a mucolytic action in the endocervix as well as the respiratory system. Usual therapeutic doses given from day 3 of the cycle through ovulation sometimes improves the liquidity and volume of cervical mucus.

Appropriate antibiotic or other local therapy can be prescribed if the thickened mucus is due to chronic cervicitis. Cervicitis due to chlamydia infection should be ruled out if mucopurulent cervical discharge is present. Cervical cryosurgery may be indicated for severe chronic cervical infections.

The management of sperm antibodies in cervical mucus is discussed in the section on Immunologic Infertility.

Anovulation and Oligo-ovulation

Clomiphene (alone or with other agents), HMG, and HCG are used to treat ovulatory failure; the latter agents are used in combination. Gonadorelin (LH-RH or GnRH) has been used investigationally to induce ovulation. Clomiphene stimulates the endogenous secretion of gonadotropins or corrects abnormal patterns of secretion by an antiestrogenic mechanism, while HMG and HCG replace inadequate quantities of gonadotropins. Gonadorelin, the synthetic form of LH-RH, directly stimulates gonadotropin secretion just as the endogenous hormone does. Dosage regimens must be based on the expected and actual response to treatment. There may be considerable discrepancy between the apparent ovulatory rates and the number of pregnancies achieved. There is no evidence that these drugs improve fertility in normally ovulating women.

Tamoxifen [Nolvadex] has been used investigationally as an alternative to clomiphene. More clinical experience is necessary to determine if the two agents are equivalent or have clinically relevant differences.

Clomiphene: The ideal patients for clomiphene therapy secrete gonadotropins and estrogen but fail to ovulate because of an abnormality in the cycling mechanism that controls gonadotropin secretion. Menstruation is a demonstration of gonadotropin production, ovarian responsiveness to gonadotropin (ie, secretion of estrogen), and endometrial responsiveness to ovarian steroids. In women with amenorrhea, a normal endometrium and estrogenic stimulation can be demonstrated by a positive (ie, bleeding within one or two weeks) response to a progesterone withdrawal test (preferably one intramuscular injection of progesterone 100 to 200 mg or oral medroxyprogesterone acetate [Provera] 10 mg daily for ten days). A negative progesterone withdrawal test and high concentrations of serum gonadotropins indicate ovarian failure, which is not responsive to clomiphene. Abnormally low levels of gonadotropins suggest pituitary failure that is unlikely to be affected by clomiphene, although this agent should be tried.

Women who respond to clomiphene usually have low to normal FSH levels, normal estrogen concentrations, and normal to high LH levels. Pregnancy should be ruled out with an immunologic assay for HCG before a synthetic progestin is administered for the progesterone withdrawal test because of the alleged teratogenic potential of these preparations (see Chapter 39, Estrogens, Progestins, and Other Agents Used to Treat Gynecologic Conditions).

Small doses of clomiphene usually induce ovulation in women with polycystic ovaries who often have high LH and estrogen levels. These women may have associated endometrial hyperplasia and, in obese women with abnormal bleeding patterns, endometrial hyperplasia and carcinoma should be ruled out by biopsy and/or dilatation and curettage (D and C) before ovulation is induced.

Before beginning clomiphene therapy, pregnancy should be ruled out, a semen analysis completed, and an endometrial biopsy and/or D and C performed in patients with long-term anovulation to identify possible endometrial hyperplasia or carcinoma. Serum prolactin measurement can identify hyper-prolactinemic patients who are unlikely to respond to clomiphene therapy. Any remaining tests can be performed as needed during the early treatment cycles.

Although the ovulation rate in properly selected patients approaches 90% with use of clomiphene, the pregnancy rate may be only 25% to 65%. Several possibilities may explain this apparent discrepancy: (1) About one-third of clomiphene-treated ovulatory cycles result in either inadequate progesterone production by the corpus luteum or an inadequately stimulated endometrium that does not support implantation (luteal phase dysfunction). (2) The antiestrogenic effect of large doses of clomiphene occasionally thickens cervical mucus, making it unfavorable to sperm penetration. (3) Luteinization of an unruptured follicle may produce presumptive signs of ovulation secondary to progesterone secretion, but the ovum is not available for fertilization. (4) Using life-table analysis, the pregnancy rate is close to that expected in normal cycles.

Menotropins (HMG): Therapy with HMG is complex and should be undertaken only by a physician experienced in its use and with the patient's full understanding and cooperation. Furthermore, monitoring of the patient during treatment requires laboratory facilities capable of completing estrogen assays (urinary or serum) within 24 hours (preferably less) after collection. The utilization of ultrasonography is desirable.

Induction of ovulation with HMG is reserved for patients who require exogenous supplementation of gonadotropins to achieve pregnancy. It is the only therapy that can stimulate ovulation in hypophysectomized patients or in those with primary hypopituitarism. Anovulatory patients with deficient production of gonadotropins and estrogen also are likely to respond to therapy. Some patients who are able to produce estrogen but fail to ovulate with clomiphene may respond to HMG.

Patients with ovarian failure, as demonstrated by high levels of serum gonadotropins, are generally not suitable candidates for HMG. However, apparent ovarian failure has been overcome in some women; estrogen plus progestin was used for one or more cycles to suppress FSH. Menotropins given thereafter may stimulate ovulation with subsequent pregnancy (Check and Chase, 1984).

Patients with polycystic ovary (PCO) may be hypersensitive to this agent. Those who do not respond to clomiphene and HCG may be given HMG with caution, and estrogen levels should be monitored daily on initiation of treatment. Ovulation may occur before administration of HCG (Wang and Gemzell, 1980). Patients with PCO and associated hyperprolactinemia may respond to bromocriptine.

Because of the expense and the potential for complications (eg, multiple births, hyperstimulation syndrome), complete infertility testing should be performed prior to initiating HMG treatment to rule out and treat other causes of infertility. The cost of the drug may be $250 to $750 per cycle excluding laboratory and physician's fees. A course of clomiphene is usually given before HMG therapy is begun, because some hypogonadotropic patients will respond to the former agent.

As with clomiphene, there is a discrepancy between the ovulatory and pregnancy rates with HMG. In properly selected patients, ovulatory rates approach 100%, but only 40% to 70% of treated women become pregnant. Multiple gestations due to ovulation of multiple ova occur in 15% to 30% of pregnancies, and twins are delivered in up to 75% of these pregnancies. Spontaneous abortion is observed in about 25% of pregnancies and is more likely with multiple gestations. Miscarriages occur less frequently in second gonadotropin-induced pregnancies (Ben-Rafael et al, 1983). The incidence of congenital abnormalities is not increased with HMG.

Combination Therapy: Selected patients who fail to respond to standard ovulation-inducing regimens may benefit from combinations of the above agents. Women who appear to ovulate in response to clomiphene but who fail to develop favorable cervical mucus may become pregnant when estrogen is added to the regimen. HCG may be added to a clomiphene regimen when patients fail to ovulate with clomiphene alone but show evidence of follicular development. These patients may be lacking only the LH surge, which HCG replaces. Other failures with clomiphene may be due to a short luteal phase after ovulation, and this also may respond to HCG. (See the evaluation on Clomiphene Citrate for dosages.)

Some candidates for HMG therapy who exhibit some degree of hypothalamic-pituitary-ovarian function (withdrawal bleeding after administration of progesterone indicating estrogen effect) may benefit from the combined actions of clomiphene, HMG, and HCG. Partial follicular maturation is induced by clomiphene so that smaller doses of HMG may be used. HCG is employed as usual to stimulate ovulation. Monitoring is the same as with HMG-HCG therapy, and the possibility of ovarian hyperstimulation and multiple gestations also is similar. The rationale for this regimen is based on economic, not physiologic, considerations. Preliminary results suggest that the dose of HMG may be reduced by one-half, thus providing financial relief for this costly therapy (see the evaluation on Menotropins for dosage).

Gonadorelin (LH-RH): This peptide hormone may be used to induce ovulation in patients with hypothalamic amenorrhea. Such use is considered investigational in the United States. Usually the patients selected do not have polycystic ovaries and have not responded to clomiphene and HMG. Gonadorelin must be administered parenterally and, because of its short half-life, requires frequent administration. Ovulation has been induced and pregnancies have been achieved using portable infusion pumps delivering 1 to 10 mcg every 90 to 120 minutes (Miller et al, 1983; Corenblum et al, 1985). Subcutaneous infusion also has been utilized because it is potentially less hazardous than the intravenous route. Although some investigators have reported inconsistency and lack of success with subcutaneous infusion, others have reported excellent results. All 28 patients in one study conceived within six treatment cycles using 10- to 25-mcg pulses (the majority received 15 mcg) delivered at 90-minute intervals (Mason et al, 1984). Successful pregnancies were achieved in 11 of 14 patients receiving subcutaneous pulses of 5 to 15 mcg gonadorelin every 90 minutes (Hurley et al, 1984). Gonadorelin infusion is usually discontinued when ovulation is verified, and HCG is administered to provide luteal support.

Although hyperstimulation (Schweditsch et al, 1984) and

multiple births may occur (Heineman et al, 1984), their frequencies appear to be lower than with HMG therapy. The frequency of spontaneous abortions is not increased. Gonadorelin infusion appears to be an effective option for ovulation induction when conventional methods fail and may have advantages over HMG therapy. The intranasal route is also being investigated. See the evaluation in Chapter 42, Agents Related to Anterior Pituitary and Hypothalamic Function.

The subject of ovulation induction with gonadorelin has been reviewed (Zacur, 1985).

Androgen Excess

Disorders involving abnormal androgen production are associated with female infertility. The most common hyperandrogenic condition is polycystic ovary (PCO), which is characterized by anovulation and, frequently, by amenorrhea, obesity, and hirsutism. The ovaries may be enlarged with multiple cystic follicles in a thickened capsule. Although the etiology varies, pathophysiologic events probably include lack of sufficient follicular stimulation by FSH leading to increased androgen secretion by the follicle; peripheral conversion of the excess androgen (particularly in adipose tissue of obese patients) to estrone; increased intraovarian androgens contributing to accelerated follicular atresia; and increased tonic LH secretion, due to slightly elevated estrogen (increased LH:FSH ratio), causing stimulation of ovarian stroma and further androgen secretion. Peripherally, the elevated levels of serum androgens decrease sex hormone-binding globulin, which may increase the amount of biologically active free serum testosterone in the presence of normal total serum testosterone.

The patient's history often suggests onset of PCO at puberty, perhaps due to excess adrenal androgen production in a disordered adrenarche. Late-onset congenital adrenal hyperplasia also has been suggested to elevate adrenal androgen secretion. The presence of hyperprolactinemia in some patients with PCO is consistent with estrogen-induced decrease in hypothalamic dopamine and increased LH secretion. Prolactin may stimulate adrenal androgen secretion and inhibit ovarian steroidogenesis directly.

The diagnosis of PCO may be apparent from the history and physical findings. Although the serum testosterone may be normal, elevated testosterone or androstenedione suggests an ovarian source, while increased dehydroepiandrosterone sulfate (DHEAS) is of adrenal origin. If testosterone or DHEAS is grossly elevated, ovarian or adrenal tumors, respectively, must be ruled out.

Drug Therapy: Clomiphene is the usual choice to induce ovulation in PCO patients (see the section on Anovulation and Oligo-ovulation). If clomiphene alone is unsuccessful, HCG or rarely menotropins (HMG) plus HCG is added to the regimen. However, PCO patients may be sensitive to these agents and the risks of multiple births and hyperstimulation may be higher, although these side effects tend to be idiosyncratic.

PCO patients with marginal or slightly elevated DHEAS may benefit from treatment with clomiphene plus dexamethasone

(Lobo et al, 1982 A). The glucocorticoid suppresses pituitary ACTH and adrenal androgen secretion. This regimen may be successful when clomiphene or clomiphene plus HCG is ineffective, thus obviating the need to use HMG. It has been suggested that dexamethasone be used empirically even without evidence of excess adrenal androgen. The rationale is that normalization of the total androgen pool (regardless of the source of excess) may be conducive to induction of ovulation. This approach is indirect and nonspecific, however, and generally not favored.

Because the LH:FSH ratio is elevated in PCO patients, treatment with a purified FSH preparation (instead of HMG, which contains approximately equal amounts of FSH and LH) seems a reasonable approach to normalize gonadotropic balance. Overall results of studies on a preparation of urinary FSH, Metrodin (not yet marketed in the United States), were as good as those obtained with HMG. However, spontaneous LH surges were unpredictable and may have caused luteinization of immature follicles or ovarian hyperstimulation (Flamigni et al, 1985; García et al, 1985). Reducing the amount of FSH and increasing the duration of administration were suggested to increase spontaneous LH surges and ovulation and reduce multiple births and ovarian hyperstimulation (Seibel et al, 1985). Demonstration of a clear advantage of FSH treatment over HMG awaits development of modified regimens that yield superior clinical results and decrease adverse effects.

PCO patients who do not respond to pharmacologic intervention may ovulate after ovarian wedge resection. By reducing the volume of ovarian tissue, ovarian androgen production is decreased. However, ovulation does not always result and postoperative adhesions may preclude conception even in the presence of ovulation.

Luteal Phase Defect

Luteal phase defect is a general term describing compromise of corpus luteum function, either in the amount of progesterone produced or in the progesterone:estradiol ratio in the luteal phase. Infertility or repeated fetal wastage may result. About 4% of infertile women, 25% to 35% of patients with recurrent spontaneous abortion, and about 35% of clomiphene-treated cycles may be affected. The defect is probably caused by a deficiency or an abnormal pattern of secretion of FSH and/or LH, causing inadequate follicular stimulation. The abnormal secretion of gonadotropin may be spontaneous or secondary to hyperprolactinemia or clomiphene administration.

A short luteal phase can be suspected if the duration of luteal function is subnormal (basal temperature elevated for less than 10 days). Inadequate secretion of progesterone as determined by single or serial measurements of serum progesterone during the luteal phase, or evidence of an abnormal endometrium, as determined by endometrial biopsy taken within two days of the next expected menses, is diagnostic. Endometrial biopsy is more accurate. The results of the biopsy must be more than two days out of phase with the normal histologic appearance for the appropriate stage of the cycle (with reference to the onset of the next menses) (Noyes et al, 1950). Serum progesterone levels are also used to detect inadequate luteal function, but interpretation of results (especially of a single sample) is complicated by the pulsatile nature of progesterone secretion, which causes wide excursions in serum concentration. Since episodes of luteal dysfunction sometimes occur in women with normal function, drug therapy should be reserved for abnormalities documented in more than one cycle.

Drug Therapy: Pharmacotherapy is directed either toward treating the cause of the abnormality or replacing progesterone. Therapy should be initiated in the intended cycle of conception rather than after the first missed menses, and efficacy should be verified by endometrial biopsy during the first treatment cycle.

Luteal defect associated with hyperprolactinemia may be treated with bromocriptine [Parlodel] (see the section on Prolactin-related Reproductive Dysfunction). Clomiphene, which causes luteal phase deficiency in certain patients, may be effective in spontaneous luteal dysfunction resulting from inadequate FSH secretion (eg, short luteal phase, long follicular phase). Clomiphene is most effective in patients whose defects are most severe as judged by endometrial histology (Downs and Gibson, 1983).

HCG appears to be luteotropic and may be effective when supplementary support of the corpus luteum is needed. The initial dose may serve as the trigger if ovulation is being induced and also supports the corpus luteum. Less desirable aspects of treatment with HCG include the necessity for parenteral administration, the delay of menses for up to one week if pregnancy does not ensue, and interference with the interpretation of a pregnancy test. Rarely, the corpus luteum may resist stimulation by HCG and fails to produce adequate progesterone.

Progesterone replacement therapy has generally been the treatment of choice because it is effective regardless of the etiology of luteal dysfunction. Unlike HCG or clomiphene, efficacy does not depend upon a secondary response. Natural progesterone must be used because a synthetic progestin may be luteolytic and/or teratogenic (see also Chapter 39, Estrogens, Progestins, and Other Agents Used to Treat Gynecologic Conditions).

Progesterone 12.5 mg daily may be administered intramuscularly, but this is inconvenient and painful. Progesterone vaginal or, less commonly, rectal suppositories (25 mg twice daily) are preferred. Suppositories are not available commercially but may be compounded by a pharmacist (see the evaluation). Suppositories are more convenient and the small doses (physiologic) do not delay menses for more than two days if the patient is not pregnant. Intranasal and oral progesterone preparations are being tested clinically.

Administration of progesterone is begun after ovulation has occurred (as judged by basal body temperature) in the intended cycle of conception and is continued until placental steroidogenesis is fully functional at about eight to ten weeks of gestation. A shorter course of therapy may be adequate, but data are insufficient to support a more restricted regimen (Soules et al, 1981).

Endometriosis

Endometriosis occurs when endometrial tissue exists in ectopic sites (possibly initiated by retrograde menstruation). It is found most frequently around the ovaries, the peritoneum of the cul-de-sac, the uterosacral and/or round ligaments, the oviducts, and the serosal surface of the uterus. Rarely, cells may travel via blood vessels and lymphatics and form implants at distant sites. Endometriosis is characterized by pelvic or lower back pain that increases during menstruation; dysmenorrhea, particularly if it first appears in the late twenties or thirties and becomes progressively worse; dyspareunia and/or pain on defecation, particularly during menses; and infertility. The disease occurs predominantly during the childbearing years, for the stimulation of endometrial implants and the associated discomfort depend upon cyclic hormonal stimulation. It also may develop in adolescents as well as in fertile, asymptomatic older women. The ectopic implants respond to normal cyclic hormonal stimulation similarly to normally located endometrium.

The pathogenesis and treatment of endometriosis have been reviewed (Schmidt, 1985).

The pain of endometriosis is probably related to peritoneal irritation or involvement of other structures that results from scarring, bleeding from the implants during menstruation, or increased production of prostaglandins. The severity of pain is not necessarily related to the extent of the disease. Use of standardized staging criteria for endometriosis helps to determine appropriate therapy and provides a basis for comparing various therapeutic modalities. A revised classification is available (American Fertility Society, 1985).

Endometriosis may be the single cause of infertility in 10% of infertile women and is a major factor in 25% to 40%. It is a frequent finding upon laparoscopy in those with previously unexplained infertility. When pregnancy is achieved in women with untreated endometriosis, spontaneous abortion may occur in up to one-half of cases (Groll, 1984). Mild endometriosis was associated with a higher incidence of spontaneous abortion than moderate or severe disease in one study (Wheeler et al, 1983), but other investigators have not observed this correlation.

Infertility associated with endometriosis may result from ovarian or tubal adhesions that interfere with ovum transport. In many cases of mild endometriosis, however, there is no visible cause. The prostaglandin concentration and total volume of peritoneal fluid may be increased, but the mechanism by which these conditions influence fertility is unknown. In patients with endometriosis, a decreased number of ovulatory stigmata was observed at laparoscopy compared to controls. Therefore, unruptured but luteinized follicles may cause infertility in some women (Brosens et al, 1978).

Endometriosis responds to surgery or drug therapy but lesions tend to recur after cessation of the drug. Surgery is most often curative, but both modes of treatment can relieve symptoms and enhance fertility.

Surgery: Surgery is usually indicated if the ovaries are greatly enlarged or disease is extensive. Older patients with severe disease who do not wish to become pregnant frequent-

ly undergo more radical surgery (removal of the uterus and ovaries). In patients desiring pregnancy, conservative surgery preserves and enhances reproductive function; pregnancy rates of 40% to 80% have been reported and probably reflect the severity of the disease. The greatest chance of pregnancy is in the first 16 to 18 months after surgery. Surgery may be postponed if pregnancy is desired at a later time.

The role of surgery is questionable in mild disease. In a study of 90 patients, those treated with conservative surgery at the time of diagnostic endoscopy had virtually the same pregnancy rate (about 75%) at the end of one year as patients who received endoscopy with no additional treatment (Schenken and Malinak, 1982).

Drug Therapy: Drugs are utilized as the sole treatment for endometriosis or as an adjunct to surgery in more severe cases. The agent most frequently used is danazol [Danocrine], an androgen derivative. This drug has antigonadotropic (inhibits midcycle surge) and mild anabolic and androgenic activity. Other effects probably include alteration of ovarian steroidogenesis and, perhaps, a direct effect upon the implants. Symptoms are suppressed, endometrial implants regress promptly, and pregnancy occurs in some previously infertile patients after cessation of medication. Results of many uncontrolled studies indicate that danazol is effective, and one controlled study demonstrated its superiority to an oral contraceptive regimen: The cure or improvement rate, as well as the pregnancy rate, was higher; fewer patients discontinued therapy because of adverse effects; and fewer patients required surgery (Noble and Letchworth, 1979).

Neither surgery nor danazol may be beneficial in patients with mild disease. In a study of 65 patients, danazol did not improve and may have impaired the pregnancy rate compared to patients who received no treatment after diagnostic laparoscopy (Seibel et al, 1982). Other investigators also reported low pregnancy rates when danazol was used to treat mild endometriosis (Butler et al, 1984).

Danazol often is given after radical surgery in women not desiring pregnancy. This drug also may be administered to older women until menopause occurs to avoid the necessity for more radical surgery. A disadvantage of this drug is its expense (up to $240 monthly).

Oral contraceptives were preferred for endometriosis until danazol became available, and many practitioners continue to prescribe them for this indication, particularly when cost is a limiting factor. Oral contraceptives are given continuously (not cyclically) for six to nine months and produce a pseudopregnant state in which the uterine endometrium and ectopic implants undergo a decidual reaction, necrosis, and eventual atrophy. Although oral contraceptives with a high estrogen content have been used in the past, experience has shown that preparations with less estrogen (eg, less than 50 mcg ethinyl estradiol) are equally effective. If breakthrough bleeding occurs, the frequency of administration may be increased temporarily. Symptoms may increase before improvement is noted, and the usual adverse effects of oral contraceptives or estrogens may occur (see Chapters 40, Contraceptive Agents, and 39, Estrogens, Progestins, and Other Agents Used to Treat Gynecologic Conditions). Oral contraceptives should be employed with caution in the presence of myomas, since these agents may stimulate growth.

Progestins alone have often been used for endometriosis, particularly when estrogens should be avoided. Medroxyprogesterone acetate (MPA) 30 mg daily for three months has been beneficial (Moghissi and Boyce, 1976). A depot preparation of MPA acetate is sometimes administered unless pregnancy is desired; its extended duration of action causes infertility (see Chapter 39 for preparation information). Progestins induce endometrial atrophy and breakthrough bleeding may be a problem.

Androgens have been used to treat endometriosis, but such use is uncommon and generally not preferred. These hormones may provide temporary relief, but no microscopic changes are observed in ectopic implants. Androgens may be useful when dyspareunia is a problem and stimulation of libido is desirable. However, ovulation is not inhibited and pregnancy may occur during treatment. Caution must be exercised and the drug discontinued as soon as pregnancy is documented to avoid masculinization of a female fetus.

LH-RH analogues are being investigated for the treatment of endometriosis. The agents inhibit pituitary gonadotropin secretion and suppress normal cyclic ovarian steroid production. They cause a hypoestrogenic state but do not have the androgenic side effects of danazol. One LH-RH antagonist marketed in the United States for the treatment of prostatic carcinoma is leuprolide [Lupron]; the preparation must be injected subcutaneously. Another LH-RH analogue, nafarelin (investigational drug), has been administered intranasally and was reported to be effective for endometriosis (Shriock et al, 1985).

Combination Treatment: Danazol therapy before conservative surgery initiates regression and softens implants, thus potentially limiting the extent of surgery. Some practitioners recommend that conservative surgery be followed by three to six months of danazol therapy before pregnancy is attempted. The rationale is that small, unresected endometriomas will regress postoperatively, producing a relatively disease-free state in which to attempt pregnancy. In one study on patients with severe endometriosis, danazol was administered for three to six months after surgery; 79% of patients became pregnant compared to 30% who had surgery alone (Wheeler and Malinak, 1981). In other studies, results have been less favorable and the investigators believe that drug therapy during the immediate postoperative period is not beneficial and may actually waste the time in which pregnancy is most likely to succeed.

Hyperprolactinemia in Females

Amenorrhea or oligomenorrhea with or without galactorrhea is often associated with elevated levels of plasma prolactin. Hyperprolactinemic states are often associated with impaired fertility, whether it is a normal physiologic condition (postpartum lactation) or is caused by a pathologic disorder (eg, pituitary tumor). Luteal dysfunction may be secondary to elevated prolactin secretion.

The mechanisms underlying the effects of hyperprolactinemia are not completely understood but probably involve central derangement of normal gonadotropin secretion, as well as peripheral actions of secondary importance that block the gonadotropic effect on target tissue (gonad). Both males and females may be affected, but interference with reproductive function is more definitely established in the female.

Drug Therapy: Bromocriptine [Parlodel], a dopaminergic agent, has a direct action on the dopamine receptors of prolactin-secreting cells in the anterior pituitary to decrease the secretion of prolactin. When used in women with hyperprolactinemic disorders, the reduction in serum prolactin level is usually followed by normalization of menstrual cycles and return of fertility. Up to 80% of hyperprolactinemic women with no pituitary pathology or microadenomas and more than one-third with macroadenomas achieve ovulation induction with bromocriptine (Reyniak, 1983). Bromocriptine generally does not restore ovulatory function in amenorrheic women with normal prolactin levels (Coelingh Bennink and van der Steeg, 1983), although treatment has been successful in some patients.

During normal pregnancy, rising estrogen levels are associated with anterior pituitary hyperplasia and elevated prolactin secretion. The potential for prolactinoma expansion in the hormonal milieu of pregnancy is therefore of concern. However, clinical evidence is reassuring and the presence of a prolactin-secreting tumor is not a contraindication to pregnancy (Ruiz-Velasco and Tolis, 1984). Although 35% to 40% of untreated patients with macroadenomas may experience complications due to tumor expansion, only 5% of patients treated before pregnancy with bromocriptine experience such difficulties.

When ovulation has been induced and pregnancy occurs, bromocriptine is withdrawn for the duration of pregnancy. Although teratogenicity or other adverse effects on mother or fetus are not apparent (Turkalj et al, 1982), bromocriptine should not be taken routinely during pregnancy because safety cannot be assured. When bromocriptine is withdrawn at the beginning of pregnancy, serum prolactin increases to a similar level in normal patients and those with prolactinomas.

If visual field impairment or other neurologic symptoms appear during pregnancy, bromocriptine therapy may be reinstated. Bromocriptine reduces prolactin secretion and tumor size and reverses the neurologic effects of suprasellar tumor expansion (see also Chapter 42, Agents Related to Anterior Pituitary and Hypothalamic Function). If bromocriptine is continued or resumed during pregnancy to control symptoms, prolactin secretion is decreased to an amount lower than during normal pregnancy (Ruiz-Velasco and Tolis, 1984). Surgical removal of the adenoma is usually not necessary, but remains an option if bromocriptine therapy fails to control tumor growth.

Following delivery, the patient may nurse if desired. Otherwise bromocriptine is used to suppress lactation. If future pregnancy is desired, bromocriptine therapy may be continued. Successful long-term (five to nine years) bromocriptine therapy without tumor progression has been reported (Corenblum and Taylor, 1983).

In a study comparing bromocriptine and pergolide (investigational drug), a long-acting dopaminergic agent, the drugs appeared to be equally effective, had similar adverse effects, and produced similar outcomes after cessation of therapy. It is not known whether patients who are refractory or who develop tolerance to one drug may respond to the other. The once-daily pergolide regimen may be preferable for convenience (Blackwell et al, 1983).

In Vitro Fertilization (IVF) and Embryo Transfer (ET)

The first human birth resulting from IVF occurred in 1978; since then, more than 2,000 births have been achieved utilizing variations of that initial process. Ethical issues continue to arise as technical advances offer new treatment options and the ramifications are realized. Guidelines have been offered for some of these concerns (American Fertility Society, 1984). A discussion of relevant legal issues is also available (Quigley and Andrews, 1984).

The majority of candidates for IVF have irreparable tubal damage, but some patients have severe endometriosis or other causes of infertility. Male infertility (eg, decreased sperm count or motility) unresponsive to conventional treatment also may be an indication. The procedure is expensive, costing several thousand dollars per transfer attempt, and usually is not covered by medical insurance.

Earliest IVF methods utilized a single oocyte retrieved from the patient during a normal ovulatory cycle. Most centers today use regimens that induce superovulation to obtain a larger number of oocytes in a single treatment cycle. In general, ovulation is induced by clomiphene alone; clomiphene and HCG; clomiphene, menotropins (HMG), and HCG; FSH [Metrodin] and HCG; or FSH, HMG, and HCG. Although the agents used are the same as for conventional induction of ovulation, the treatment schedule, details of monitoring follicular development, and timing of HCG administration may differ. Details of regimens currently in use and considerations in their selection can be found elsewhere (Lopata, 1983; Jones, 1984). The goal is to develop multiple follicles for IVF; in contrast, only a single mature follicle is desired in ovulation induction. Monitoring for increased serum estradiol, measuring follicular size via ultrasound, and other patterns of response to HMG guide the critical timing of HCG injection. Timing also is critical for oocyte aspiration, in vitro fertilization, and embryo transfer.

Although 80% to 90% of recovered oocytes are fertilized, only 75% of these continue to grow to an appropriate stage for transfer (usually a four- to eight-cell conceptus). The greatest inefficiency in IVF-ET occurs after transfer. Only 15% to 25% of transferred embryos implant, and the spontaneous abortion rate may be as high as 50%. Transfer of several embryos increases the chance of successful implantation but also the risk of multiple births. Transfer of three or four embryos per attempt is considered an acceptable compromise. Pooled data from 58 IVF programs showed that transfer of one, two, or three embryos resulted in successful pregnancies in 10%, 15%, and 19%, respectively, of attempted transfers (Soules, 1985). There appears to be no increased risk of congenital abnormalities in successful pregnancies.

Several variations of the IVF-ET procedure with respect to source of oocyte, sperm, and embryo, have been utilized: (1) Wife's oocyte and husband's sperm fertilized in vitro with embryo transfer to the wife; (2) same as above except that donor sperm is used; (3) "embryo adoption" in which an unused embryo is implanted into another recipient; (4) donor oocyte is fertilized in vivo using artificial insemination with the husband's sperm. The embryo is flushed from the donor before implantation and transferred to the wife (Bustillo et al, 1984). This procedure allows a woman to be a "gestational mother" of her husband's child if she is the carrier of a genetic disease or is unable to produce retrievable oocytes. (5) Embryo freezing for future use is the newest technique and may be valuable when extra viable embryos are available after an embryo transfer. If the implantation is unsuccessful, an embryo may be thawed and transferred later. The expense and risks of subsequent laparoscopy could thus be avoided. It has been suggested that ET in a later, normal cycle might have a greater chance of success because of the more natural hormonal milieu at the time of implantation. Frozen embryos also may be donated to an unrelated recipient in an "embryo adoption" procedure.

MALE INFERTILITY

Almost one-half of cases of infertility are at least partially due to reproductive dysfunction in the male partner. Whatever the etiology, male infertility may be manifested by an alteration in sperm density, motility, or morphology or abnormalities of seminal fluid viscosity or volume. The cause may be an anatomic abnormality (eg, varicocele, cryptorchidism); obstruction of the ductal system due to inflammatory disease (eg, tuberculosis, gonorrhea); genetic (eg, Klinefelter's syndrome); destruction of the germinal epithelium (eg, mumps orchitis, irradiation, drugs); environmental factors (eg, increased scrotal temperature from hot baths, certain pesticides); immunologic (eg, sperm antibodies); ejaculatory dysfunction (eg, retrograde ejaculation); marijuana, which may decrease testosterone levels and cause abnormal spermatogenesis (eg, motility, morphology, sperm count); or acute infection as suggested by leukocytes in the semen. Only a small proportion of male infertility is caused by a recognized endocrinologic disorder.

Varicocele

About 20% to 40% of infertile males are found to have varicocele. Left varicoceles are most common; bilateral involvement occurs less often and a right varicocele is rare. Surgical or venographic correction of venous reflux may be appropriate in patients with oligospermia, which is usually associated with altered motility or morphology. Semen quality may improve in the majority, and pregnancies may be achieved in 30% to 55% of previously childless couples (Saypol, 1984). In one study, men in whom sperm density improved postoperatively also showed normalization of hormonal parameters. An exaggerated response to LH-RH and decreased seminal dihydrotestosterone also were altered toward normal after surgery in some patients (Hudson et al, 1985).

Adjunctive drug therapy with HCG (Dubin and Amelar, 1977; Mehan and Chehval, 1982) or clomiphene (Check, 1980; Cockett et al, 1984) has been suggested for patients with preoperative sperm counts of less than 10,000,000/ml.

Hypogonadotropic Hypogonadism

Hypogonadotropic infertility is uncommon in males. However, spermatogenesis can be initiated and pregnancies achieved in one-half of properly selected patients. Definitive diagnostic tests include those that exclude other causes of infertility in both partners; measurement of serum gonadotropins, prolactin, and testosterone; and testicular biopsy.

Hormonal therapy for male infertility caused by hypogonadotropic hypogonadism depends on the severity of the defect. When there is only partial gonadotropin deficiency, HCG alone often increases sperm counts and produces normal ejaculates. In patients with severe deficiency, androgen therapy stimulates virilization during adolescence (see Chapter 38, Androgens and Anabolic Steroids). Maximum stimulation of spermatogenesis requires three to four years of gonadotropin replacement; therefore, androgen therapy may be discontinued and gonadotropin therapy begun when the patient reaches his early twenties. Alternatively, gonadotropin therapy may be postponed until the patient desires fertility.

In complete hypogonadotropic hypogonadism, HCG stimulates testicular development only partially despite complete virilization. After 18 to 24 months of treatment with no further testicular growth and persistent azoospermia, menotropins (HMG) is added to the regimen (see the evaluations on HCG and Menotropins). After successful treatment, most patients with complete hypogonadotropic hypogonadism achieve adequate, testicular size and produce ejaculates containing 2,000,000 to 5,000,000 sperm. Pregnancies have been achieved at this low sperm level when the female partner has normal fertility. When maximal stimulation of germinal tissue and sperm output have been achieved, menotropins is withdrawn but HCG is continued to maintain sperm production (Sherins, 1984).

In the future, treatment of hypogonadotropic hypogonadism may include use of luteinizing hormone-releasing hormone (LH-RH), since the pituitary is usually responsive to this stimulus. However, long-acting analogues must become commercially available before this therapy is feasible.

Hyperprolactinemia in Males

Since both men and women require gonadotropic support for gametogenesis, it seems reasonable to expect that the male reproductive system also may be subject to various inhibitions associated with elevated prolactin levels. Galactorrhea sometimes occurs in males with prolactin-secreting tumors, and impotence is often, but not invariably, present. In some men, LH concentration and pulse frequency, sperm counts, and testosterone levels are increased following bromocriptine-induced normalization of serum prolactin levels (Winters and Troen, 1984). Hyperprolactinemia may account for refractoriness in some men whose hormonal profile indicates that they are candidates for clomiphene or HCG therapy. Identification and treatment of selected patients with bromocriptine may improve pregnancy rates in patients who would otherwise be treatment "failures."

Idiopathic Male Infertility

Probably 25% to 40% of all infertile males have no identifiable anatomic or endocrine defect. Therapy in these cases is empiric and nonspecific. Clomiphene is commonly employed to treat subfertile males (see the evaluation). However, the lack of controlled studies, standardized patient selection, and treatment regimens makes interpretation of clinical results difficult; consequently, this therapy is not enthusiastically endorsed by all experts.

As in women, clomiphene stimulates endogenous gonadotropin secretion. Criteria for patient selection include serum gonadotropin and testosterone levels usually within the normal range. If a testicular biopsy is performed, it may indicate presence of all germinal elements, although decreased in number (hypospermatogenesis). Clomiphene usually increases serum testosterone levels and may increase the number and motility of sperm. Successful treatment of some men with idiopathic infertility was reported in an uncontrolled study utilizing tamoxifen [Nolvadex], another antiestrogenic agent (Buvat et al, 1983). However, the initial increase in sperm count may be followed by a decline. Patients with primary testicular failure (increased serum FSH, hyalinization, or other evidence of permanent epithelial damage) or ductal obstruction are not suitable candidates for gonadotropin or gonadotropin-stimulating therapy (Paulson, 1977).

Gonadotropins (HCG or a combination of HCG and HMG) also have been used investigationally to treat idiopathic male infertility, particularly that unresponsive to clomiphene. Although success has been reported in some men (Mehan and Chehval, 1982), results generally have been disappointing. The necessity for repeated intramuscular injections is inconvenient, and treatment, particularly when HMG is employed, is expensive. The effectiveness of gonadotropin therapy in males with a normal sperm count is doubtful. Unless such regimens eventually produce results superior to those achieved with clomiphene, they probably will be reserved, as in women, for patients refractory to clomiphene.

Testosterone rebound has been employed sporadically since its introduction 30 years ago. A depot preparation (testosterone enanthate or cypionate 200 mg) is injected intramuscularly once weekly for 12 to 20 weeks. The negative feedback effect of testosterone suppresses pituitary gonadotropin output and azoospermia ensues. Following cessation of therapy, there have been some reports of a rebound phenomenon in which the germinal epithelium recovers function and sperm production is increased to a level compatible with fertility. The action has been ascribed to the release of gonadotropin that was stored in the pituitary during the period of testosterone suppression. Success rates are variable but do not exceed 40%, and there are several disadvantages: (1) The treatment period is long and rebound sperm production is delayed for three to four months after cessation of therapy. (2) In most men, the improvement in sperm production lasts only two to three months. (3) Treatment may be followed by permanent depression of the sperm count (Charny and Gordon, 1978). Because of these problems and the uncertainty of success, the testosterone suppression method is best reserved for patients with severe idiopathic oligospermia who do not respond to other therapy and who understand the consequences of treatment.

Few causes of male infertility are amenable to drug therapy alone. In the past, thyroid and adrenal supplements were used empirically; however, more sensitive diagnostic endocrine tests are available today, and such treatment cannot be recommended unless thyroid or adrenal hormone deficiency has been documented.

In uncontrolled studies, improved sperm motility with an increase in the number of pregnancies has been reported following administration of low doses of androgen to infertile males with a defect of sperm motility but normal sperm counts, morphology, and serum testosterone levels (Brown, 1975). These results have not been confirmed and such use of testosterone is now not generally recommended.

Infertile men with poor sperm motility and low seminal zinc concentration responded more favorably to administration of zinc and fluoxymesterone [Halotestin] than to either agent alone. However, pregnancy rates were not reported (Takihara et al, 1983).

Prostaglandin inhibitors have improved sperm count, motility, and fertilizing capacity in oligospermic infertile men (Barkay et al, 1984). In the presence of infection, appropriate antibiotic therapy may be effective.

Immunologic Infertility

Agglutinating or immobilizing sperm antibodies may cause infertility in 5% of males and up to 13% of females who are infertile. Antibodies are present in the serum and seminal plasma of males and in the serum and cervical mucus of females. There is much debate about the significance of immunologic problems as an etiologic factor in infertility, and enthusiasm for methods of treatment is variable.

When the female partner is affected, use of a condom reduces exposure to sperm antigens and often decreases antibody levels. Unprotected coitus at the time of ovulation may then be successful. When the male partner develops autoimmunity to sperm, the semen can be washed to remove antibodies and then used for insemination. However, this technique has not proved particularly helpful. Alternatively, artificial insemination of donor semen may be attempted.

Immunosuppressive therapy with large doses of corticosteroids (prednisolone 60 mg/day for 7 or 14 days) also has been

suggested (Alexander et al, 1983). Pregnancies were achieved within four months in 45% of treated couples compared to 12% of untreated couples. Regimens using larger amounts of corticosteroids have been reported (Shulman and Shulman, 1982). The couple must weigh the possibility of adverse effects from this experimental treatment against the importance of a possible pregnancy (see also Bronson et al, 1984).

Drug Evaluations

BROMOCRIPTINE MESYLATE
[Parlodel]

ACTIONS AND USES. The clinical usefulness of this semisynthetic ergot alkaloid depends primarily upon its dopaminergic activity. Bromocriptine inhibits the secretion of prolactin at the anterior pituitary gland and may be used to correct female infertility secondary to hyperprolactinemic states (eg, menstrual irregularities with or without galactorrhea, hyperprolactinemic form of luteal phase defect).

Impotence, hypogonadism, or infertility in males associated with elevated prolactin levels sometimes responds to bromocriptine. The drug is not effective in psychogenic impotence or that caused by conditions other than hyperprolactinemia. Symptoms frequently recur upon cessation of therapy.

Bromocriptine suppresses hypersecretion of prolactin caused by a pituitary adenoma and may inhibit tumor growth and reduce tumor size. In selected cases, the drug may be used during pregnancy to stop growth of an enlarging prolactinoma. However, bromocriptine is not a substitute for surgery or radiation if either measure is appropriate because of pressure from or growth of the tumor. Otherwise, bromocriptine may be used to induce ovulation in infertile women with hyperprolactinemia.

The natural course of prolactin-secreting microadenomas (less than 1 cm diameter) is not clearly understood, but these neoplasms may prove to be relatively common (asymptomatic microadenomas have been found during routine autopsies) and without threat of morbidity other than that associated with their endocrine function. Resumption of hyperprolactinemia after cessation of bromocriptine may be expected in virtually all cases within a year. See also the section on Prolactin-Related Reproductive Dysfunction.

ADVERSE REACTIONS AND PRECAUTIONS. The doses employed for reproductive dysfunction generally do not cause severe side effects. Nausea is most common, but vomiting, constipation, dizziness, and orthostatic hypotension also occur. These untoward effects can be minimized by taking the medication with food and at bedtime and by initiating therapy with small doses and gradually increasing the amount to effective levels.

Although there appears to be no increased risk of teratogenic effects in humans, cleft lip has occurred in the offspring of rabbits treated with bromocriptine. Until more evidence of safety in human pregnancy is obtained, the drug ordinarily should be discontinued as soon as pregnancy is documented.

Following pregnancy, if contraception is desired, oral contraceptives should not be used because the estrogen component may further stimulate growth of the prolactinoma.

DOSAGE AND PREPARATIONS. Bromocriptine should be taken with food.

Oral: For amenorrhea-galactorrhea and related conditions, initially, 1.25 to 2.5 mg once daily at bedtime, increased after two or three days to 2.5 mg twice daily. If necessary, dosage may be increased by 2.5 mg every two or three days. Other doses and treatment schedules also have been employed.

In appropriately selected males with elevated plasma prolactin, 2.5 mg twice daily.

   Parlodel (Sandoz). Capsules 5 mg; tablets 2.5 mg.

CLOMIPHENE CITRATE
[Clomid, Serophene]

ACTIONS AND USES. This nonsteroidal agent is a mixture of two isomers in approximately a 1:1 ratio and is related chemically to chlorotrianisene. It is antiestrogenic in man and mildly estrogenic in animals. Clomiphene competes with endogenous estrogen for hypothalamic estrogen receptors; this produces a low estrogen signal, which, in turn, increases the secretion of LH-RH and the levels of LH and FSH. Ovarian stimulation results. Clomiphene also may affect the anterior pituitary and ovary directly (Adashi, 1984).

Clomiphene may stimulate ovulation in anovulatory and oligo-ovulatory women with potentially functional hypothalamic-pituitary-ovarian axes and adequate endogenous estrogens. Incremental doses are given until an ovulatory dose is reached. If ovulation is achieved but pregnancy does not occur, the ovulatory dose can be repeated cyclically; it should not be exceeded (this may actually decrease the probability of pregnancy). Because the patient may not respond identically in different cycles, a dose that has not produced ovulation may be repeated before advancing to the next level. This conservative approach (repetition of a nonovulatory dosage) is not advocated by many physicians, however, especially with lower amounts (50 to 100 mg). Although 75% of clomiphene-induced pregnancies occur in the first three cycles of treatment (ie, with low doses), a significant number (15%) occur after 150 to 200 mg has been given. The use of 25-mg increments may be necessary to achieve an ovulatory dose.

Body weight and obesity were positively correlated with the ovulatory dose in one study. Although 85% of women under 110 pounds ovulated with 50 mg of clomiphene, only 20% of women over 200 pounds did. However, the variability in response related to body weight precluded precise prediction of ovulatory dosage (Lobo et al, 1982 B).

The patient who fails to ovulate at a given dose and has poor cervical mucus may benefit from a longer duration of therapy rather than an increase in dose. The appearance of adequate cervical mucus in the absence of ovulation suggests that follicular maturation has occurred but the LH surge has not (ultrasonography may be used to demonstrate the presence of a mature follicle). In this case, HCG can be administered to replace the LH surge and stimulate ovulation. Other patients refractory to the effects of clomiphene alone may respond to a regimen of clomiphene-HMG-HCG. With this combination, less HMG may be required than when it is used alone to stimulate follicular development. (See the section on Unfavorable Cervical Mucus and the discussion on Combination Therapy in the Introduction and the evaluation on Menotropins.)

Monitoring is necessary during each treatment cycle to evaluate the dosage in terms of ovulatory response and side effects. Ovulation is assumed to occur if the basal body temperature is at least 0.5 F higher than during the follicular phase, if an endometrial biopsy during the luteal phase shows a secretory effect, and/or if serum progesterone levels achieved during the midluteal phase are consistent with a functioning corpus luteum. When therapy is successful, ovulation usually occurs five to ten days after the last dose. Therefore, patients should have intercourse approximately every other day during this period. Before a subsequent cycle of therapy is begun, the patient should be examined to determine if ovarian enlargement (hyperstimulation) or pregnancy has occurred.

Clomiphene also is used to stimulate sperm production in selected male patients (see the section on Male Infertility for patient selection).

ADVERSE REACTIONS AND PRECAUTIONS. Ovarian cysts form in 5% to 15% of patients. The most serious, although rare, adverse reaction of clomiphene is massive cystic enlargement of the ovaries (hyperstimulation syndrome). Maximal enlargement occurs about one week after ovulation and regression is usually spontaneous after several days or weeks. Additional therapy should not be given until the ovaries return to pretreatment size (usually within one month). The patient then may be given a lower dose of clomiphene plus HCG when the cervical mucus appears favorable.

When clomiphene induces ovulation, luteal phase defect may occur in up to one-half of the cycles in some patients. This can be treated by adding progesterone or HCG to the regimen. (See the section on Luteal Phase Defect.)

The incidence of multiple gestations is about 8% or six times normal but is lower than with HMG. Multiple births are almost always twins; larger multiple gestations have been reported rarely. Spontaneous abortions (mostly early miscarriages) occur in approximately 20% of clomiphene-induced pregnancies, which may be slightly higher than normal but the incidence is not higher than in a previously infertile population.

Blurred vision and scintillating scotomata are dose related and reversible when the drug is discontinued. Objective signs are rarely found, although measurable loss of visual acuity, definable scotomata, and changes in retinal cell function have been reported. Some physicians consider visual abnormalities to be a contraindication to further use, while others continue therapy with lower doses.

Other adverse reactions include hot flushes resembling menopausal vasomotor symptoms (10% to 40%) and, less commonly, nausea, headache, breast engorgement, and abdominal bloating. Symptoms disappear when therapy is stopped. Untoward effects may occur at the lowest dosages in sensitive individuals (see also the Introduction).

TERATOGENICITY. Although there is no evidence that the incidence of fetal anomalies is increased clinically, aberrations have been observed in the offspring of some subprimate animals given clomiphene *during* pregnancy. Since clomiphene is excreted slowly, there is at least theoretical reason for concern about teratogenicity in man. Clomiphene should not be administered to pregnant women; there is no indication for clomiphene therapy once conception has been achieved.

PHARMACOKINETICS. About one-half of the ingested dose is excreted in five days; traces appear in the feces up to six weeks after administration. Clomiphene is excreted mainly in the feces; small amounts appear in the urine.

DOSAGE AND PREPARATIONS.

Oral: To induce ovulation, initially, 50 mg daily for five days starting on the fifth day of the cycle (spontaneous or induced bleeding) or at any time in patients who have not menstruated recently provided that pregnancy has been ruled out. Lower doses or a shorter duration of treatment is recommended if unusual sensitivity to pituitary gonadotropin is suspected. If ovulation (monitored by basal body temperature and possibly serum progesterone or endometrial biopsy) without conception occurs, the same dosage is given cyclically (and should not be exceeded) until conception or for six to eight cycles. If conception fails to occur after three ovulatory cycles in which cervical mucus is unfavorable prior to ovulation, estrogen may be added to the regimen (see the section on Unfavorable Cervical Mucus).

If ovulation does not occur, the dosage is increased by 50 mg in each cycle until 200 mg/day for five days is given. Alternatively, lower doses can be given for 7 to 10 days (see the section on Female Infertility in the Introduction).

If doses of 150 to 200 mg daily for five days fail to stimulate ovulation, if there is evidence of ovulatory failure due to lack of an LH surge, or if there is evidence of a short luteal phase, HCG may be added to the regimen. A dose of 10,000 IU is given intramuscularly 12 to 14 days after starting clomiphene if a mature follicle is present or 5,000 IU is given initially, followed by 5,000 IU five days later. Various protocols for clomiphene regimens appear in the literature (Gysler et al, 1982; García-Flores and Vazquez-Méndez, 1984; Hammond, 1984).

For oligospermia in selected male patients, 25 mg daily is frequently used. Medication is continued for 6 to 12 months or until pregnancy is achieved. If serum hormone levels are in the normal range and the quality of semen does not improve after at least three months of therapy, the dosage may be increased to 50 mg daily. Other regimens have also been suggested (Ross et al, 1980).

Clomid (Merrell Dow), **Serophene** (Serono). Tablets 50 mg.

DANAZOL
[Danocrine]

ACTIONS. This synthetic derivative of 17α-ethinyl testosterone (ethisterone) is used to treat pelvic endometriosis. This agent does not exhibit significant estrogenic or progestational properties but acts at several levels of the hypothalamic-pituitary-ovarian axis. It binds to androgen, progesterone, and glucocorticoid (but not estrogen) receptors and to sex hormone-binding and corticosteroid-binding globulins. Danazol inhibits the midcycle gonadotropin surge and multiple enzymes of ovarian steroidogenesis (Barbieri and Ryan, 1981). It causes atrophy of endometrial tissue in the uterus as well as in ectopic sites and amenorrhea often results. Ovulation and menstruation are re-established promptly on cessation of therapy, and pregnancy may be achieved in the first cycle before menstruation occurs (see Adverse Reactions and Precautions).

USES. Danazol is indicated for endometriosis amenable to hormonal management; it is generally thought to be more effective than estrogen-progestin regimens and is generally preferable to these preparations, especially when estrogens are contraindicated. A definitive diagnosis of endometriosis should be established before danazol therapy is begun. The drug may be used as sole therapy or preoperatively and/or postoperatively in severe disease. Most patients experience relief of symptoms and show objective improvement upon laparoscopy. Pregnancy rates generally are improved. However, patients with mild disease may not benefit from danazol therapy (see section on Endometriosis). Endometriosis may recur after discontinuing treatment.

Danazol is not indicated when surgery alone is the treatment of choice and should not be given to women with underlying abnormal genital bleeding or markedly impaired hepatic, renal, or cardiac function. This agent is considerably more expensive than therapeutically equivalent courses of other medication.

ADVERSE REACTIONS AND PRECAUTIONS. Adverse reactions include weight gain, edema, and androgenic and anabolic effects (acne, mild hirsutism, oily skin or hair, decreased breast size). Danazol treatment is associated with a decrease in high-density lipoprotein cholesterol level but no change in triglyceride concentration in the serum. Sequelae of a hypoestrogenic state (vasomotor flushing, sweating, atrophic vaginitis) may occur with lower dosage, but androgenic effects usually are not a problem when less than 600 mg is administered daily.

Danazol should not be administered to pregnant or lactating women. Masculinization of the external genitalia of female neonates has been reported when danazol was taken during the first trimester of pregnancy (Duck and Katayama, 1981; Peress et al, 1982). Lower doses of danazol may not inhibit ovulation. The possibility of inadvertent administration during pregnancy may be reduced by initiating therapy after several days of a normal menstrual period.

In one study, the incidence of second and third trimester intrauterine fetal deaths was high (4 of 39 pregnancies) among pregnancies begun within three menstrual cycles after cessation of treatment with danazol. It was postulated that the atrophic effects of the drug may have caused inadequate placentation (Dmowski and Cohen, 1978). A cautious approach would be to postpone pregnancy following use of danazol until the endometrium has recovered normal function as evidenced by a normal menstrual period.

Abnormal liver function tests and jaundice have been reported. Danazol should not be taken in the presence of acute liver disease, congestive heart failure, severe hypertension, or renal disease. Danazol may potentiate the action of anticoagulants. Lowering of voice pitch, which may return only partially to the pretreatment level, has been reported (Mercaitis et al, 1985).

DOSAGE AND PREPARATIONS.
Oral: Dosage is determined on the basis of severity of disease and is adjusted according to response and the occurrence of adverse reactions. Some cases of endometriosis are treated adequately with 200 mg daily. The majority of patients are given 400 to 600 mg daily, and those with more severe disease may require 800 mg daily. The appropriate amount is given daily in two to four divided doses for three to nine months. Serum estradiol is depressed more effectively with the more frequent administration of the same total dose (Dickey et al, 1984). Treatment can be reinstituted if symptoms recur upon cessation of therapy.

> *Danocrine* (Winthrop-Breon). Capsules 50, 100, and 200 mg.

HUMAN CHORIONIC GONADOTROPIN (HCG)
[A.P.L., Follutein, Pregnyl, Profasi HP]

Human chorionic gonadotropin (HCG) is a placental hormone extracted from the urine of pregnant women. It is a glycoprotein with a molecular weight of 30,000. In most radioimmunoassay systems, there is a cross reaction between HCG and LH; however, substantial differences in the sequence of protein and carbohydrate exist. Biologically, HCG mimics the actions of LH. HCG has two half-lives for disappearance from plasma, 11 hours and approximately 24 hours.

USES. HCG is used to treat infertility in women and men. It serves as a substitute for the LH surge to stimulate ovulation of a prepared follicle when used with clomiphene and/or menotropins (HMG). HCG also may be utilized to supplement deficient amounts of endogenous LH in women with luteal

phase defect. The effectiveness of treatment depends upon the ability of the corpus luteum to respond to HCG stimulation.

HCG, alone or with menotropins, is used to restore or stimulate full spermatogenesis in men with hypogonadotropic infertility. Similar regimens have been used investigationally with limited success in men with idiopathic infertility.

DOSAGE AND PREPARATIONS.
Intramuscular: To stimulate ovulation, see the evaluations on Clomiphene Citrate and Menotropins.

For luteal phase defect, treatment must begin in the intended cycle of conception; 5,000 IU is injected three days after the elevation in basal body temperature and again three days later, or 2,500 to 5,000 IU is given initially and every two to three days for four injections.

For hypogonadotropic infertility in men, 2,000 IU two or three times per week. If after 18 to 24 months, there is no further testicular growth and azoospermia persists, menotropins may be added to the regimen. When maximal spermatogenesis is established, sperm production usually continues as long as HCG (2,000 IU three times/week) is given.

> *A.P.L.* (Ayerst), *Generic*. Powder 5,000, 10,000, and 20,000 U.S.P. units with 10 ml of diluent.
> *Follutein* (Squibb), *Pregnyl* (Organon). Powder (lyophilized) 10,000 U.S.P. units with 10 ml of diluent.
> *Profasi HP* (Serono). Powder (sterile, lyophilized) 5,000 and 10,000 U.S.P. units with 10 ml of diluent.

MENOTROPINS (HMG)
[Pergonal]

ACTIONS AND USES. Menotropins is a preparation of human menopausal gonadotropin (HMG) extracted from the urine of postmenopausal women. FSH and LH activity are present in a 1:1 ratio. The goal of therapy is to replace gonadotropins and stimulate follicular development. Therapeutic effects are achieved by combination with HCG or clomiphene and HCG.

In anovulatory women judged suitable for gonadotropin therapy (see the Introduction), menotropins is given initially in doses sufficient to induce follicular growth and maturation as determined by serial measurements of serum or urinary estrogens or by ultrasonography of the developing follicle. Following follicular maturation, HCG is given to induce ovulation. Since ovulation of properly prepared follicles usually occurs within two days after HCG administration, the couple is instructed to have coitus on the evening of the injection and for the next two or three days. Three to five cycles of treatment usually constitute an adequate trial. Therapy beyond five cycles is not likely to increase the success rate.

Induction of ovulation with gonadotropins is difficult and expensive and should be carried out only by physicians with specialized training and experience. Proper administration of menotropins requires individualization of dosage based on the patient's response.

Menotropins is sometimes used with HCG to treat hypogonadotropic male infertility, and it has been used investigationally in idiopathic male infertility. Such treatment is prolonged and very expensive (see the section on Male Infertility).

ADVERSE REACTIONS AND PRECAUTIONS. Symptoms of

ovarian hyperstimulation occur in 10% to 20% of patients and may be observed after any dose but are most common after use of large doses. Mild hyperstimulation is manifested by ovarian enlargement and abdominal discomfort, lasts seven to ten days, and requires no treatment. Severe hyperstimulation is life-threatening and necessitates hospitalization. Ovarian enlargement is accompanied by weight gain, ascites, pleural effusion, oliguria, hypotension, and hypercoagulability. Treatment is largely supportive, although rarely ovarian rupture with intraperitoneal hemorrhage may require surgical intervention.

Multiple gestations occur frequently (incidence, 15% to 20%) in gonadotropin-induced pregnancies and are not predictable on the basis of the estrogen levels produced alone, but may be predicted on the basis of ultrasound.

Menotropins is contraindicated in patients with ovarian failure, which can be diagnosed by elevated FSH and LH levels.

MONITORING THERAPY. Monitoring patient response is crucial to determine that adequate stimulation is not accompanied by ovarian hyperstimulation and to reduce the likelihood of multiple gestations. Monitoring is required in each cycle of therapy because the patient's response may vary from cycle to cycle. The basal body temperature should be recorded daily.

Ideally, the patient should be examined daily to monitor changes in ovarian size, cervical mucus, and estrogen production, although this may not be necessary during the first several days except in patients with polycystic ovarian disease. Daily examinations and estrogen determinations are required when there is clinical evidence of improvement (ie, the spinnbarkeit test demonstrates follicular maturation and estrogen production).

Because the appearance of cervical mucus and vaginal cytology are not sensitive enough to determine the timing of HCG injection, measurement of 24-hour urinary estrogens or serum estrogen assays are used. When estrogen levels are approximately double the normal value for the preovulatory peak (absolute values may vary among laboratories), HCG should be given within 24 hours or up to 36 hours after the last dose of menotropins. When follicular maturation has reached this stage of active estrogen secretion, the rate of estrogen production can be expected to double daily. Acceptable estrogen levels for HCG-induced ovulation vary slightly, depending upon the time elapsed between the collection of the sample and administration of HCG. If estrogen production is lower than optimum, administration of menotropins should be continued. If estrogen production is three to four times greater than the preovulatory level, HCG should not be administered because of the risk of ovarian hyperstimulation.

Follicular maturation occasionally proceeds without the usual signs of estrogen production and, for this reason, estrogen secretion should be measured one week after beginning administration of menotropins even if the quality of cervical mucus does not improve. HCG should never be given to induce ovulation unless estrogen production has been measured for the previous 24 hours.

Ultrasonography is being used with increasing frequency to determine follicle size and to identify multiple follicles. Follicles between 19 and 23 mm generally are ready for ovulation induction.

DOSAGE AND PREPARATIONS.
MENOTROPINS AND HCG:
Intramuscular: For induction of ovulation, the dosage requirement may vary in the same individual and therefore is determined according to the patient's response in each cycle of treatment. Usually patients are initially given one to two ampuls (each containing 75 IU FSH and 75 IU LH) daily. Dosage may be continued at this level if there is evidence of estrogen production; if such evidence is lacking, the amount may be increased after the first seven days. Up to six ampuls per day may be required to stimulate follicular development.

When the patient has reached the appropriate level of follicular development as judged by serum estrogen measurement and ultrasonography (see the discussion on Monitoring Therapy), a single injection of 10,000 IU of HCG is administered about 24 hours after the last injection of menotropins; alternatively, 5,000 IU of HCG is administered, followed by 5,000 IU three to five days later. Other variations in the amount and timing of HCG have been employed and are designed not only to provide ovulatory stimulus but also to support corpus luteum function at a critical stage (particularly if there is evidence of luteal phase defect).

For hypogonadotropic infertility in males or idiopathic male infertility unresponsive to clomiphene (to be given with HCG; see the evaluation on HCG), 75 IU is given three times a week. (One-half of patients respond to 25 IU three times per week. Therefore, lower dosages may be attempted if desired.) Effectiveness of therapy is determined after six to nine months at a specific dosage level. When maximal stimulation of the germinal tissue and sperm output has been achieved, menotropins can be discontinued; sperm production continues as long as HCG (2,000 IU three times/week) is given.
MENOTROPINS, CLOMIPHENE, AND HCG:
Oral, Intramuscular: For induction of ovulation, this regimen may be tried in properly selected patients (see the Introduction) to reduce the cost of therapy. Clomiphene is given orally on the fifth day of the cycle (spontaneous or induced); 100 mg is given for five to seven days or 200 mg is given for five days. Two ampuls of menotropins then are given intramuscularly each day for four days, followed by one ampul daily for two days. HCG 10,000 IU is given intramuscularly 24 hours after the last dose of menotropins. As with menotropins-HCG therapy, estrogen levels are monitored and, along with ultrasonography, serve as a guide for modification of dosage and duration of drug administration.

Pergonal (Serono). Each 2-ml ampul contains 75 IU each of follicle-stimulating hormone (FSH) activity and luteinizing hormone (LH) activity (with 10 mg lyophilized lactose).

PROGESTERONE

USES. Progesterone is the drug of choice to treat luteal phase dysfunction that results in infertility or repeated early spontaneous abortion. This disorder should be documented before progesterone therapy is undertaken. Treatment is begun in the intended cycle of conception and generally is continued until placental production of steroids is established (eight to ten weeks). A synthetic progestin should not be administered for this indication.

Progesterone may be given intramuscularly, which is painful and inconvenient, or in suppository form. Suppositories are not available commercially but may be compounded by a pharmacist using the following formulation: 44 g progesterone powder, 2,096 g polyethylene glycol 400, 1,392 g polyethylene glycol 6,000 (makes 1,760 suppositories containing 25 mg progesterone each). See also the Introduction.

DOSAGE AND PREPARATIONS.

Intramuscular: For support of pregnancy in luteal phase dysfunction, 12.5 mg daily beginning as soon as ovulation can be diagnosed and continuing, if needed, to the eleventh week of gestation.

    Generic. Solution (in oil) 25 and 50 mg/ml in 10 and 30 ml containers and 100 mg/ml in 10 ml containers.

Vaginal, Rectal: For support of pregnancy in luteal phase dysfunction, one 25-mg suppository inserted twice daily beginning as soon as ovulation can be diagnosed and continuing, if needed, up to the eleventh week of gestation.

    Not available commercially; see above for preparation of suppositories.

Cited References

Adashi EY: Clomiphene citrate: Mechanism(s) and site(s) of action: Hypothesis revisited. *Fertil Steril* 42:331-344, 1984.

Alexander NJ, et al: Pregnancy rates in patients treated for antisperm antibodies with prednisone. *Int J Fertil* 28:63-67, 1983.

American Fertility Society: Ethical statement on in vitro fertilization. *Fertil Steril* 41:12-13, 1984.

American Fertility Society: Revised classification of endometriosis. *Fertil Steril* 43:351-352, 1985.[Copies may be ordered from The American Fertility Society, 2131 Magnolia Avenue, Suite 201, Birmingham, AL 35256.]

Barbieri RL, Ryan KJ: Danazol: Endocrine pharmacology and therapeutic applications. *Am J Obstet Gynecol* 141:453-463, 1981.

Barkay J, et al: Prostaglandin inhibitor effect of antiinflammatory drugs in therapy of male infertility. *Fertil Steril* 42:406-411, 1984.

Beeley L: Drug-induced sexual dysfunction and infertility. *Adv Drug React Acc Pois Rev* 3:23-42, 1984.

Ben-Rafael Z, et al: Abortion rate in pregnancies following ovulation induced by human menopausal gonadotropin/human chorionic gonadotropin. *Fertil Steril* 39:157-161, 1983.

Blackwell RE, et al: Comparison of dopamine agonists in treatment of hyperprolactinemic syndromes: Multicenter study. *Fertil Steril* 39:744-748, 1983.

Bronson R, et al: Sperm antibodies: Their role in infertility. *Fertil Steril* 42:171-183, 1984.

Brosens IA, et al: Study of plasma progesterone, oestradiol-17β, prolactin and LH levels, and of luteal phase appearance of ovaries in patients with endometriosis and infertility. *Br J Obstet Gynaecol* 85:246-250, 1978.

Brown JS: Effect of orally administered androgens on sperm motility. *Fertil Steril* 26:305-308, 1975.

Buchanan JF, Davis LJ: Drug-induced infertility. *Drug Intell Clin Pharm* 18:122-132, 1984.

Bustillo M, et al: Nonsurgical ovum transfer as treatment in infertile women. *JAMA* 251:1171-1181, 1984.

Butler L, et al: Collaborative study of pregnancy rates following danazol therapy of stage I endometriosis. *Fertil Steril* 41:373-376, 1984.

Buvat J, et al: Increased sperm count in 25 cases of idiopathic normogonadotropic oligospermia following treatment with tamoxifen. *Fertil Steril* 39:700-703, 1983.

Charny CW, Gordon JA: Testosterone rebound therapy: Neglected modality. *Fertil Steril* 29:64-68, 1978.

Check JH: Improved semen quality in subfertile males with varicocele-associated oligospermia following treatment with clomiphene citrate. *Fertil Steril* 33:423-426, 1980.

Check JH, Chase JS: Ovulation induction in hypergonadotropic amenorrhea with estrogen and human menopausal gonadotropin therapy. *Fertil Steril* 42:919-922, 1984.

Cockett ATK, et al: Varicocele. *Fertil Steril* 41:5-11, 1984.

Coelingh Bennink HJT, van der Steeg HJ: Failure of bromocriptine to restore menstrual cycle in normoprolactinemic post-pill amenorrhea. *Fertil Steril* 39:238-240, 1983.

Corenblum B, Taylor PJ: Long-term follow-up of hyperprolactinemic women treated with bromocriptine. *Fertil Steril* 40:596-599, 1983.

Corenblum B, et al: Ovulation induction and pregnancy in women with hypothalamic amenorrhea treated with intermittent gonadotropin-releasing hormone. *J Reprod Med* 30:736-740, 1985.

Dickey RP, et al: Serum estradiol and danazol: I. Endometriosis response, side effects, administration interval, concurrent spironolactone and dexamethasone. *Fertil Steril* 42:709-716, 1984.

Dmowski WP, Cohen MR: Antigonadotropin (danazol) in treatment of endometriosis. *Am J Obstet Gynecol* 130:41-48, 1978.

Downs KA, Gibson M: Clomiphene citrate therapy for luteal phase defect. *Fertil Steril* 39:34-38, 1983.

Dubin L, Amelar RD: Varicocelectomy: 986 cases in twelve year study. *Urology* 10:446-449, 1977.

Duck SC, Katayama KP: Danazol may cause female pseudohermaphroditism. *Fertil Steril* 35:230-231, 1981.

Flamigni C, et al: Use of human urinary follicle-stimulating hormone in infertile women with polycystic ovaries. *J Reprod Med* 30:184-188, 1985.

García N, et al: Induction of ovulation with purified urinary follicle-stimulating hormone in patients with polycystic ovarian syndrome. *Am J Obstet Gynecol* 151:635-640, 1985.

García-Flores RF, Vazquez-Méndez J: Progressive dosages of clomiphene in hypothalamic anovulation. *Fertil Steril* 42:543-547, 1984.

Groll M: Endometriosis and spontaneous abortion. *Fertil Steril* 41:933-935, 1984.

Gysler M, et al: Decade's experience with individualized clomiphene treatment regimen including effect on postcoital test. *Fertil Steril* 37:161-167, 1982.

Hammond MG: Monitoring techniques for improved pregnancy rates during clomiphene ovulation induction. *Fertil Steril* 42:499-509, 1984.

Heineman MJ, et al: Quadruplet pregnancy following ovulation induction with pulsatile luteinizing hormone-releasing hormone. *Fertil Steril* 42:300-302, 1984.

Hudson RW, et al: Hormonal parameters of men with varicoceles before and after varicocelectomy. *Fertil Steril* 43:905-910, 1985.

Hurley DM, et al: Induction of ovulation and fertility in amenorrheic women by pulsatile low-dose gonadotropin-releasing hormone. *N Engl J Med* 310:1069-1074, 1984.

Jones GS: Update on in vitro fertilization. *Endocr Rev* 5:62-75, (Winter) 1984.

Lipman AG: Be aware of drugs that may cause infertility. *Mod Med* 231-232, (Sept) 1984.

Lobo RA, et al: Clomiphene and dexamethasone in women unresponsive to clomiphene alone. *Obstet Gynecol* 60:497-501, 1982 A.

Lobo RA, et al: Clinical and laboratory predictors of clomiphene response. *Fertil Steril* 37:168-174, 1982 B.

Lopata A: Concepts in human in vitro fertilization and embryo transfer. *Fertil Steril* 40:289-301, 1983.

Mason P, et al: Induction of ovulation with pulsatile luteinising hormone releasing hormone. *Br Med J* 288:181-185, 1984.

Mehan DJ, Chehval MJ: Human chorionic gonadotropin in treatment of infertile man. *J Urol* 128:60-63, 1982.

Mercaitis PA, et al: Effect of danazol on vocal pitch: Case study. *Obstet Gynecol* 65:131-135, 1985.

Miller DS, et al: Pulsatile administration of low-dose gonadotropin releasing hormone: Ovulation and pregnancy in women with hypothalamic amenorrhea. *JAMA* 250:2937, 1983.

Moghissi KS, Boyce CR: Management of endometriosis with oral medroxyprogesterone acetate. *Obstet Gynecol* 47:265-267, 1976.

Noble AD, Letchworth AT: Medical treatment of endometriosis: Comparative trial. *Postgrad Med J* 55(suppl 5):37-39, 1979.

Noyes RW, et al: Dating the endometrial biopsy. *Fertil Steril* 1:3-25, 1950.

Paulson DF: Clomiphene citrate in management of male hypofertility: Predictors for treatment selection. *Fertil Steril* 28:1226-1229, 1977.

Peress MR, et al: Female pseudohermaphroditism with somatic chromosomal anomaly in association with in utero exposure to danazol. *Am J Obstet Gynecol* 142:708-709, 1982.

Quigley MM, Andrews LB: Human in vitro fertilization and the law. *Fertil Steril* 42:348-355, 1984.

Reyniak JV: Modern management of prolactinoma. *J Reprod Med* 28:257-263, 1983.

Ross LS, et al: Clomiphene treatment of idiopathic hypofertile male: High-dose, alternate-day therapy. *Fertil Steril* 33:618-623, 1980.

Ruiz-Velasco V, Tolis G: Pregnancy in hyperprolactinemic women. *Fertil Steril* 41:793-805, 1984.

Saypol DC: Varicocele, in Garcia C-R, et al (eds): *Current Therapy of Infertility 1984-1985*. Toronto, Decker/Mosby, 1984.

Schenken RS, Malinak LR: Conservative surgery versus expectant management for infertile patient with mild endometriosis. *Fertil Steril* 37:183-186, 1982.

Schmidt CL: Endometriosis: Reappraisal of pathogenesis and treatment. *Fertil Steril* 44:157-173, 1985.

Schriock E, et al: Treatment of endometriosis with potent agonist of gonadotropin-releasing hormone (nafarelin). *Fertil Steril* 44:563-588, 1985.

Schweditsch MO, et al: Ovarian hyperstimulation during chronic pulsatile GnRH therapy. *Gynecol Obstet Invest* 17:276-277, 1984.

Seibel MM, et al: Effectiveness of danazol on subsequent fertility in minimal endometriosis. *Fertil Steril* 38:534-537, 1982.

Seibel MM, et al: Ovulation induction in polycystic ovary syndrome with urinary follicle-stimulating hormone or human menopausal gonadotropin. *Fertil Steril* 43:703-708, 1985.

Sherins RJ: Evaluation and management of men with hypogonadotropic hypogonadism, in Garcia C-R, et al (eds): *Current Therapy of Infertility 1984-1985*. Toronto, Decker/Mosby, 1984.

Shulman JF, Shulman S: Methylprednisolone treatment of immunologic infertility in male. *Fertil Steril* 38:591-599, 1982.

Soules MR: In vitro fertilization pregnancy rate: Let's be honest with one another, (editorial). *Fertil Steril* 43:511-512, 1985.

Soules MR, et al: Function of corpus luteum of pregnancy in ovulatory dysfunction and luteal phase deficiency. *Fertil Steril* 36:31-36, 1981.

Takihara H, et al: Effect of low-dose androgen and zinc sulfate on sperm motility and seminal zinc levels in infertile men. *Urology* 22:160-164, 1983.

Thomas ML, et al: HLA sharing and spontaneous abortion in humans. *Am J Obstet Gynecol* 151:1053-1058, 1985.

Turkalj I, et al: Surveillance of bromocriptine in pregnancy. *JAMA* 247:1589-1591, 1982.

Wang CF, Gemzell C: Use of human gonadotropins for induction of ovulation in women with polycystic ovarian disease. *Fertil Steril* 33:479-486, 1980.

Wheeler JM, Malinak LR: Postoperative danazol therapy in infertility patients with severe endometriosis. *Fertil Steril* 36:460-463, 1981.

Wheeler JM, et al: Relationship of endometriosis to spontaneous abortion. *Fertil Steril* 39:656-660, 1983.

Winters SJ, Troen P: Altered pulsatile secretion of luteinizing hormone in hypogonadal men with hyperprolactinaemia. *Clin Endocrinol* 21:257-263, 1984.

Zacur HA: Ovulation induction with gonadotropin-releasing hormone. *Fertil Steril* 44:435-448, 1985.

Other Selected References

AMA Council on Scientific Affairs Report: Marijuana. *JAMA* 246:1823-1827, 1981.

Amelar RD, Dubin L: Infertility in the male, in Kendall AR, Kerafin L (eds): *Practice of Surgery: Urology*. Philadelphia, Harper & Row, vol 2, 1985.

Archer DF (ed): Ovulation induction. *Clin Obstet Gynecol* 27:917-1016, 1984.

Lee RD, Lipshultz LI: Male infertility, in Resnick MI (ed): *Current Trends in Urology*. Baltimore, Williams & Wilkins, 1985, vol 3, 30-58.

Lipshultz LI, Howards SS (eds): *Infertility in the Male*. New York, Churchill Livingstone, 1983.

Moghissi KS, Wallach EE: Unexplained infertility. *Fertil Steril* 39:5-21, 1983.

Moltich ME: Pregnancy and hyperprolactinemic woman. *N Engl J Med* 312:1364-1370, 1985.

Ross LS: Diagnosis and treatment of infertile men: Clinical perspective. *J Urol* 130:847-854, 1983.

Speroff L, et al: *Clinical Gynecologic Endocrinology and Infertility*, ed 3. Baltimore, Williams & Wilkins, 1983.

Agents Related to Anterior Pituitary and Hypothalamic Function

42

INTRODUCTION

GROWTH HORMONE

THYROTROPIN

CORTICOTROPIN

BETA-LIPOTROPIN

GONADOTROPINS

PROLACTIN

Anterior Pituitary Hormones: The anterior pituitary gland synthesizes and secretes polypeptide and glycoprotein hormones. The polypeptides include (1) growth hormone (GH, somatotropin), which has growth-promoting and anabolic properties; (2) prolactin (PRL), which plays a primary role in stimulating lactation, is involved in regulating gonadal function, and may have additional, as yet unidentified, metabolic actions; (3) corticotropin (ACTH), which stimulates glucocorticoid secretion by the adrenal cortex; and (4) β-lipotropin (β-LPH, lipotropin, lipotropic hormone), which contains within its structure several biologically active hormones whose functions are being investigated. GH and PRL are similar in size, and ACTH and LPH have a common precursor molecule.

The glycoprotein hormones are (1) thyrotropin (TSH, thyroid-stimulating hormone), which regulates thyroid function and the synthesis and release of thyroid hormones; (2) luteinizing hormone (LH), which stimulates ovulation, promotes formation of the corpus luteum, and, in men, is the primary regulator of Leydig cell function; and (3) follicle-stimulating hormone (FSH), which stimulates follicular growth and maturation in the ovary and is essential for spermatogenesis. The glycoprotein hormones contain alpha (α) and beta (β) subunits that have carbohydrate and sialic acid moieties. The specificities of these hormones result from the unique structure of the β subunits and carbohydrate groups; their α subunits are identical.

Because only a portion of these complex molecules exhibit biological activity, the synthesis of active compounds that are smaller than those produced by the anterior pituitary gland is being explored. The amino acid sequence of all anterior pituitary hormones is known, and several have been synthesized either partly or completely.

Pituitary hormones can be divided into three groups according to similarities in chemical structure and biologic function.

ACTH, LPH, and the derivatives of LPH form one group; the larger polypeptides, GH and PRL, form the second, and the glycoprotein hormones, LH, FSH, and TSH, form the third.

Electron microscopy and immunocytochemical staining show that morphologically distinct cells produce the various anterior pituitary hormones. In some tumors, GH and PRL may be synthesized by the same cell.

Releasing Hormones: The synthesis and release of anterior pituitary hormones are regulated largely by factors or hormones that are synthesized in the hypothalamus and transported to the anterior pituitary via the hypothalamic-hypophyseal portal system.

Several hypothalamic hormones affect the release and/or synthesis of individual hormones by the anterior pituitary. Each hormone is named for what was initially postulated to be its biological function, although other actions may be significant. For example, the tripeptide, thyrotropin-releasing hormone (TRH, protirelin), was named for its role in inducing release of TSH, but it is now also known to be a potent stimulator of PRL secretion. Abnormal secretion of growth hormone and ACTH occurs in some patients with acromegaly and Cushing's disease, respectively. Similarly, the decapeptide, luteinizing hormone-releasing hormone (LH-RH, gonadotropin-releasing hormone, GnRH, gonadorelin), stimulates the release of LH and FSH. PRL secretion is controlled primarily by a prolactin-inhibiting factor (PIF, which is probably dopamine), but a stimulating factor probably also plays a role. Corticotropin-releasing factor (CRH), a 41-amino acid peptide, stimulates ACTH secretion (Vale et al, 1981). Growth hormone secretion is regulated by a releasing factor (GH-RH) and an inhibiting factor (GH-RIH, somatostatin).

Pituitary releasing hormones are not limited to the hypothalamus, however. TRH is also present in the gastrointestinal tract, islets of Langerhans, male reproductive system, placenta, and retina, but most of the total content is found in other areas of the central nervous system (eg, spinal cord, pineal gland) (Jackson, 1982).

TRH, LH-RH, somatostatin, CRH, and GH-RH have been purified, isolated, sequenced, and characterized as polypeptides. TRH and LH-RH are available commercially as protirelin [Relefact TRH, Thypinone] and gonadorelin [Factrel], respectively; analogues with longer half-lives that act as agonists or antagonists have been synthesized and are under investigation. Leuprolide [Lupron], an LH-RH agonist, became available in 1985 for the treatment of prostatic carcinoma.

Feedback Control: Regulation of hypothalamic releasing factors and pituitary secretion is complex. In most instances, there is a negative feedback control mechanism. For instance, autonomous hypersecretion or exogenous administration of cortisol decreases CRH release, which reduces ACTH secretion, and inhibits release of ACTH by the pituitary in response to CRH. Administration of GH stimulates release of somatostatin, which in turn decreases release of endogenous growth hormone. In other segments of the hypothalamic-hypophyseal system, a positive feedback mechanism is involved, that is, tropic hormone levels increase with elevations of the target organ hormone. An example of positive feedback is the elevation of plasma LH levels (midcycle "surge") induced by increasing amounts of plasma estrogen during the late follicular phase of the ovarian cycle. Also, the pituitary's response to releasing hormones is modulated by hormones produced by the target organ (eg, thyroid, adrenal, ovary, testis).

The concepts of negative and positive feedback have limited applicability in some hypothalamic-hypophyseal phenomena. The importance of the central nervous system for the integration of environmental influences on anterior pituitary hormone levels (eg, the diurnal variation in corticotropin levels) has been well documented. Pituitary function may be altered by stimuli originating within the central nervous system (eg, the nocturnal elevation of LH secretion during puberty).

Regulatory Peptides: In addition to the pituitary hormones, their derivatives, and the hypothalamic-releasing hormones discussed above, other peptides (eg, vasoactive intestinal peptide [VIP], cholecystokinin [CCK], substance P) have been identified that are synthesized in the central nervous system and other tissues (eg, gastrointestinal tract, pancreas). These peptides probably act as neurotransmitters or neuromodulators and have regulatory functions in the peripheral tissues where they are found.

Immunochemical studies have shown that neuropeptides and conventional neurotransmitters can coexist in the same neuron (eg, serotonin, substance P, and TRH in medullary neurons). Peptides are synthesized by similar mechanisms in different tissues. For example, there is evidence that somatostatin, a tetradecapeptide (containing 14 amino acids), is synthesized from a larger precursor molecule in the brain, gut, and pancreas; its function differs in each tissue. Peptides mediate different functions at different sites. For example, TRH ultimately stimulates thyroid function and metabolic rate, is involved in stimulation of motor activity via the central nervous system, and modifies autonomic effects consistent with increased metabolic rate (eg, increased blood pressure, heart rate, and catecholamine level). In diseases involving functional imbalance of these peptides, peptide analogues may be useful as diagnostic or therapeutic agents (Krieger, 1983; Brown and Fisher, 1984).

GROWTH HORMONE

PHYSIOLOGY. The hormones that are particularly important for normal growth and development are growth hormone (GH, somatotropin), thyroid hormones, insulin, androgen in boys, and estrogen in girls. GH circulates in three identifiable forms of different molecular weights (Stolar et al, 1984), although the monomer is believed to be the biologically important form. The 24-hour integrated GH secretion is higher in children than in adults, and GH is secreted in a pulsatile pattern with the highest peaks observed in children during early nocturnal sleep.

Growth hormone has widespread metabolic effects. It stimulates amino acid uptake by muscle cells and protein synthesis, which increase nitrogen balance and decrease urea production. Growth hormone also stimulates lipolysis and fatty acid oxidation and decreases utilization of glucose in tissue (eg, muscle, adipocytes), which tends to increase blood glucose levels.

Some effects of GH on growth are mediated by somatomedins, a group of intermediate growth factors elaborated by the liver and, probably, by the kidney, muscle, and other tissues. Normal somatomedin levels increase with age up to the second decade of life; no diurnal variation has been observed. Low somatomedin production is associated with GH deficiency and other conditions (eg, malnutrition, malabsorption, anorexia nervosa, liver disease, Laron-type dwarfism) (Clemmons and Van Wyck, 1984; Hall and Sara, 1984). However, a low serum somatomedin C concentration is not a reliable diagnostic index by itself. Serum somatomedin levels are usually high in acromegaly.

Somatostatin: Somatostatin (Growth-Hormone-Inhibiting Hormone; GH-IH), a tetradecapeptide, is the first neuropeptide hormone synthesized by recombinant DNA techniques. It is found in the hypothalamus, other areas of the central and peripheral nervous system, the gastrointestinal tract (stomach antrum, small intestine, D cells of pancreatic islets), the adrenal medulla, and thyroid C cells. Somatostatin inhibits the secretion of GH, TSH, gastrin, glucagon, insulin, and other hormones and exocrine pancreatic secretion. It does not inhibit secretion of gonadotropins, prolactin, or ACTH. Somatostatin is involved in the regulation of GH secretion and possibly that of TSH and may have a role as a neurotransmitter in the central nervous system. Its presence in pancreatic tissue suggests participation in paracrine control of insulin and glucagon secretion (Wass, 1983). Research is being directed toward the development of long-acting analogues with separate activities to treat diabetes, acromegaly, and peptic ulcer (to control gastrointestinal bleeding). (See reviews by Gomez-Pan and Rodriguez-Arnao, 1983; Reichlin, 1983; Wass, 1983.)

Growth Hormone-Releasing Hormone (GH-RH): A peptide isolated from a pancreatic tumor in an acromegalic patient has been found to have the properties of, and is identical to, hypothalamic GH-RH (Guillemin et al, 1982; Spiess et al, 1982; Rivier et al, 1982). Synthetic GH-RH derivatives contain

40 or 44 amino acids, have similar biological potency, and stimulate the secretion of growth hormone but not other pituitary hormones (Gelato et al, 1983; Rosenthal et al, 1983; Thorner et al, 1983; Vance et al, 1984 A). GH-RH has half-lives of 7.6 and 52 minutes for the fast and slow distribution components in human plasma (Frohman et al, 1984). On the basis of GH-RH stimulation tests, it has been suggested that a deficiency of hypothalamic GH-RH may cause growth hormone deficiency (Borges et al, 1984; Rogol et al, 1984; Schriock et al, 1984). GH-RH shows promise as a diagnostic (Rogol et al, 1984; Takano et al, 1984) and therapeutic (Thorner et al, 1985) agent for GH deficiency. It does not appear to be useful for the diagnosis of acromegaly, however (Gelato et al, 1985). Long-acting analogues may be useful in some forms of GH deficiency.

GROWTH HORMONE DEFICIENCY. **Complete Growth Hormone Deficiency:** Deficient secretion of GH during childhood may be idiopathic or secondary to a central nervous system lesion (eg, tumor) or physical or emotional trauma, and may involve other tropic hormones as well. If untreated, hypopituitary dwarfism may result. True GH deficiency as a cause of growth failure can be treated only with human GH; animal GH is ineffective.

Rarely, patients with growth retardation (eg, Laron-type dwarfism) cannot produce adequate amounts of somatomedin, have high endogenous blood levels of GH, and do not respond to exogenous GH.

The diagnosis of GH should be demonstrated by results of at least two GH stimulation tests (insulin hypoglycemia, oral levodopa, intravenous arginine, clonidine). Growth hormone treatment is not effective in patients with closed or closing epiphyses, individuals with bone age of 15 years or more, or those who cannot produce somatomedin after stimulation with GH. It also should not be given to patients with an enlarging intracranial lesion until 12 months after treatment of the lesion. Treatment of growth hormone deficiency has been reviewed (Preece, 1982; Frasier, 1983; Rosenfeld and Hintz, 1983).

Growth hormone is sometimes administered with an anabolic steroid (eg, oxandrolone) to conserve the supply of GH. Theoretically, the steroid accelerates linear growth. Steroids should be withheld if the bone age is greater than height age before or during therapy, because the final adult height may be limited by early closure of the epiphyses. Some practitioners do not favor use of an anabolic steroid with GH. If somatrem becomes plentiful and expense is reduced, the problem of GH conservation, and thus the underlying rationale for adding an anabolic steroid to a GH regimen, may be obviated. See also Chapter 38, Androgens and Anabolic Steroids.

Partial Growth Hormone Deficiency: Several studies have described short children who appeared to have a mild form of GH deficiency (Rudman et al, 1981; Frazer et al, 1982; Van Vliet et al, 1983; Gertner et al, 1984; Spiliotis et al, 1984). Some may previously have been designated as having constitutional delay of growth. These children produced normal quantities of GH after standard pharmacologic stimuli, but responded to GH administration with accelerated growth rates. One explanation of these observations is that the GH produced by these patients may be biologically defective, as demonstrated by the lower GH concentrations measured by a discriminating radioreceptor compared to those measured by radioimmunoassay (Rudman et al, 1981; Frazer et al, 1982). Another explanation is that these patients represent a point on the continuum between normal and classical GH deficiency. In blood samples collected every 20 minutes for 24 hours, total GH secretion, number of secretory pulses, and peak amplitude of GH pulses were lower in the short children subsequently diagnosed with "neurosecretory dysfunction" than in children of normal height (Spiliotis et al, 1984). These explanations have different mechanisms but are not mutually exclusive.

Unfortunately, practical diagnostic criteria for partial GH deficiency responsive to GH treatment have not been determined. Several tests have been claimed to predict successful GH treatment in short children (eg, basal serum somatomedin concentration, size of somatomedin increase in response to short-term GH administration, estimations of nocturnal GH peaks), but none is supported by a consensus by experts.

More research is needed to define the diagnostic criteria for partial GH deficiency and other conditions that may respond to GH (eg, Turner's syndrome, intrauterine growth retardation). Optimal dosage regimens also must be determined. It is not known whether GH treatment in these children will increase height or simply achieve predicted height earlier.

At present, GH should be given only to children who do not respond to standard GH provocative stimuli (American Academy of Pediatrics, 1983; *Med Lett Drugs Ther*, 1984) or to patients in controlled research studies that offer psychological as well as medical evaluation and support (Underwood, 1984). The use of GH in fractures, serious burns, osteoporosis, aging, and other conditions requires investigation.

Preparations: Somatrem (methionyl-human growth hormone) is human growth hormone produced in bacteria by recombinant DNA technology. One preparation [Protropin] is now available commercially.

Somatropin [Asellacrin, Crescormin] is human GH purified from pituitaries obtained at necropsy. One year of therapy requires approximately 25 to 40 pituitaries. Somatropin preparations have been withdrawn from distribution because of the possibility that contaminated preparations caused Creutzfeldt-Jakob disease in several patients (see the evaluation). The hormone previously could be obtained free of charge under special circumstances from the National Hormone and Pituitary Program and also from commercial sources (see the evaluation on Somatropin).

Ethical Considerations: The imminent likelihood of unlimited availability of GH underlines the need for guidelines for GH use. Already there have been reports of GH abuse by athletes, and numerous ethical questions have arisen. GH therapy currently is uncomfortable and prolonged (injections three times weekly for six months or more until puberty or epiphyseal closure). Is such treatment justified for what may be trivial medical or psychological indications? Should GH therapy be available for children with genetic short stature in the normal range; for children of those parents who foresee an athletic or business advantage for a taller child; for any patients who consider short stature a functional handicap? Would the eventual result be an increase in average height or less variability in the height of the population? Since there is no guarantee that GH treatment will be effective, what psychological effect would GH treatment failure have in a child who has undergone prolonged therapy to correct a perceived defect that otherwise might have been accepted as normal (Benjamin et al, 1984; Underwood, 1984)? Answers to these and other questions should be provided by thoughtful and responsible clinical investigations.

GROWTH HORMONE EXCESS. Hypersecretion of GH produces gigantism in children and acromegaly in adults. Acromegaly is most commonly caused by a GH-producing adenoma but may result from pituitary hyperplasia or from GH-RH- or GH-secreting neoplasms (eg, pancreatic tumor). Serum somatomedin C also is elevated in acromegaly.

Acromegaly may be treated surgically, by irradiation, or medically. Transsphenoidal adenomectomy is often the initial treatment for small tumors. Surgical removal of large tumors may be followed by irradiation and/or drug therapy. Surgery alone is curative in 25% to 50% of patients and is most effective when tumors are small without extrasellar extension and the plasma GH level is less than 40 ng/ml (Baskin et al, 1982). Irradiation is not used as widely as formerly, primarily because the full effects take several years to develop. After ten years, the GH level is controlled adequately in about 75% of patients. Radiation therapy is still useful after excision of large tumors or following surgical failure.

Acromegaly also is treated with the dopaminergic agent, bromocriptine [Parlodel]. The investigational agents, lisuride and pergolide, also have been used. A long-acting analogue of somatostatin is being investigated for this indication in Europe. Drugs may be employed as primary treatment of microadenomas but are more often adjuncts to surgery or irradiation (Nelson, 1984). (See the evaluation on Bromocriptine Mesylate in the section on Prolactin.)

Drug Evaluations

SOMATREM
[Protropin]

Somatrem is a preparation of human growth hormone made using recombinant DNA technology. The product contains 192 amino acid residues, has a molecular weight of approximately 22,000, and is identical to natural GH except for the addition of methionine on the N-terminus of the molecule. The biological effects appear to be identical to those of GH from pituitary glands (somatropin).

Potency of growth hormone preparations is determined by bioassay in hypophysectomized rats. Although the serum half-life of growth hormone is only 20 minutes, the effects on target tissues are long-lasting.

USES. Somatrem is indicated for the treatment of proven GH deficiency in children. It is the only GH available for this purpose since somatropin was withdrawn from distribution (see the evaluation). Growth hormone deficiency must be documented before somatrem is administered. It is not known whether this preparation induces growth in children with short stature not attributable to GH deficiency; therefore, such use is not recommended except under investigational circumstances.

Growth hormone usually has been administered intramuscularly. However, the subcutaneous route appears to be safe, effective, and produces less pain (Russo and Moore, 1982), and it is currently thought to be interchangeable with or preferable to (Wilson et al, 1985) the intramuscular route.

When growth hormone (somatropin) was administered daily in the evening by the subcutaneous route, better growth response was obtained than when the same amount was given in two or three intramuscular injections weekly (Kastrup et al, 1983).

If growth does not exceed 2.5 cm in a six-month period, dosage may be doubled for six months. Therapy is usually continued until epiphyseal closure occurs or there is no further response to treatment. If therapy is unsuccessful after six months, treatment should be discontinued and the patient re-evaluated.

ADVERSE REACTIONS AND PRECAUTIONS. Antibodies to somatrem are found in approximately 30% of patients, ranging from 5% in patients previously treated with pituitary GH to 40% in those who received no prior GH. With one exception, the antibodies did not interfere with growth stimulation. It is not known whether antibody formation neutralizes endogenous GH activity in nondeficient short children.

Growth hormone preparations are diabetogenic and may cause hyperglycemia and ketosis. Particular caution should be exercised when they are administered to diabetic patients or those with a family history of diabetes. Tests for glycosuria should be performed in all patients.

Growth retardation is a side effect of glucocorticoid therapy and these agents may inhibit the response to somatropin. Daily doses exceeding 10 to 15 mg/M^2 of hydrocortisone or the equivalent should not be given with a growth hormone preparation.

Patients should be evaluated periodically for hypothyroidism, which should be treated with full replacement dosage (Frasier, 1983).

DOSAGE AND PREPARATIONS.
Intramuscular: Dosage must be individualized. The maximum dosage is 0.1 mg/kg (0.2 I.U./kg) three times per week.

Treatment with somatrem is expensive. The cost of somatrem will vary depending on the child's requirement, but it can be expected to be in the range of $10,000 to $20,000 per year. For further information, contact Genentech, Inc, 460 Point San Bruno Blvd, South San Francisco, CA 94080. Telephone (415) 266-1015

Protropin (Genentech). Powder (sterile, lyophilized) 5 mg (approximately 10 I.U.)/container.

SOMATROPIN
[Asellacrin, Crescormon]

(NOTE: This preparation of GH has been withdrawn from distribution for an undetermined period of time. See Adverse Reactions.)

Somatropin, a single-chain polypeptide consisting of 191

amino acid residues, has a molecular weight of 22,000. This preparation of growth hormone is extracted from human pituitary glands obtained from cadavers, sterilized, and lyophilized.

USES. Somatropin is indicated for the treatment of GH deficiency in children. Growth hormone deficiency must be documented before somatropin is administered.

ADVERSE REACTIONS AND PRECAUTIONS. Several cases of Creutzfeldt-Jakob disease (a fatal neurodegenerative disorder) have been identified that were probably due to contaminated pituitary extract (Brown et al, 1985; Committee on Growth Hormone Use, 1985; Gibbs et al, 1985; Koch et al, 1985). The affected patients were treated with hormone supplied by the National Hormone and Pituitary Program (NHPP) that was probably prepared prior to 1978. Distribution from NHPP and from commercial sources of GH, which are prepared from human pituitaries, was halted in 1985 for an indefinite period.

Purification methods employed since 1978 probably destroy the Creutzfeldt-Jakob pathogen, but this is not known with certainty. It is estimated that a year will be required to determine if current purification procedures are adequate and three years to determine if GH supplies on hand are safe for use.

Antibodies develop in less than 5% of patients and are not a problem with current preparations. High-titer growth-inhibiting antibody is now rarely seen.

DOSAGE AND PREPARATIONS.
Intramuscular, Subcutaneous: Initially, 2 I.U. or 0.06 to 0.1 I.U./kg three times weekly with a minimum of 48 hours between injections. The site of injection should be rotated.

Prior to the discontinuation of the product, the cost of somatropin obtained commercially for one year of treatment ranged from $5,000 to $10,000, depending upon the regimen. For further information, contact Serono Laboratories, Inc, 11 Brooks Drive, Braintree, MA 02184, (617) 848-8404 or Pharmacia Laboratories, 800 Centennial Avenue, Piscataway, NJ 08854, (201) 457-8000.

For research projects conducted by qualified investigators, a similar preparation of human GH was supplied without cost from the National Hormone and Pituitary Program (NHPP), 210 W. Fayette St, Suite 503-7, Baltimore, MD 21201. Similar criteria were employed for patient selection.

> **Asellacrin** (Serono). Powder (sterile, lyophilized) 2 I.U. with mannitol 20 mg and 10 I.U. with mannitol 40 mg with diluent.
> **Crescormon** (Pharmacia). Powder (sterile, lyophilized) 4 I.U. with 2 ml of diluent.

THYROTROPIN

Normal thyroid function requires an intact hypothalamic-hypophyseal axis and adequate iodine intake. Sensitive, precise methods for measuring circulating thyroid hormone levels (free and bound T_4 and T_3) are available to assess biological effect.

The anterior pituitary gland secretes thyrotropin (TSH), a double-chain glycoprotein hormone with about 96 amino acid residues in the α chain, 113 amino acid residues in the β chain, and a molecular weight of 28,000. Radioimmunoassay of TSH is used to distinguish among primary (thyroid failure), secondary (pituitary failure), and tertiary (hypothalamic) hypothyroidism.

Serum TSH levels increase after thyroid ablation (surgical or radioiodide), destruction of the thyroid by autoimmune thyroiditis, or other causes of primary hypothyroidism and precede the clinical manifestations of hypothyroidism. However, serum TSH may also be elevated in the presence of high thyroxine levels in patients with TSH-producing pituitary adenomas or pituitary resistance to thyroid hormone. In contrast, serum TSH levels are low when sufficient thyroid hormone is administered to correct hypothyroidism or when high levels of endogenous thyroid hormone are present in autoimmune or autonomous thyrotoxic states. (See also Chapter 44, Agents Used to Treat Thyroid Disease.)

Some hypothyroid patients with low serum T_4 and normal TSH levels may not have pituitary dysfunction. These patients may secrete TSH in response to stimulation by thyrotropin-releasing hormone (TRH). This disorder has been referred to as tertiary hypothyroidism, and the defect is thought to be in the hypothalamus, in contrast to secondary hypothyroidism (defect in the pituitary).

Drug Evaluations

PROTIRELIN (TRH)
[Relefact TRH, Thypinone]

Synthetic thyrotropin-releasing hormone (TRH) (pyroglutamyl-histidyl-proline amide) was the first hypothalamic-releasing hormone to become commercially available in the United States. After intravenous injection, protirelin has a plasma half-life of about five minutes.

ACTIONS AND USES. Protirelin stimulates the release of TSH from the pituitary and can be administered to test pituitary, and, indirectly, hypothalamic and thyroid function. Patients taking thyroid preparations should discontinue taking those containing liothyronine (T_3) at least three weeks before and those containing thyroxine (T_4) at least six weeks before undergoing diagnostic testing with protirelin.

Thyrotropin (TSH) levels are measured before intravenous protirelin is given and 30, 60, 90, and 120 minutes later. In suspected thyrotoxicosis with borderline elevation of serum thyroid hormone levels, a normal TSH response to protirelin stimulation excludes thyrotoxicosis; a suppressed response indicates thyrotoxicosis. However, some patients with multinodular goiters or other conditions (eg, renal failure, liver failure, severe illness, starvation, alcoholism, Cushing's syndrome) or those taking corticosteroids, dopamine, or levodopa may have a suppressed response to protirelin but are clinically euthyroid. Suppressed response also occurs in some patients with major depression, and this effect is used as an adjunct to clinical observation in the diagnosis of depression (Gold et al, 1981).

Protirelin may be used adjunctively to distinguish between secondary (pituitary) and tertiary (hypothalamic) hypothyroidism, although this test is not as definitive as initially hoped. If deficiency is due to pituitary failure, TSH secretion is not stimulated in approximately 60% of patients; if the deficiency is caused by hypothalamic dysfunction, a delayed but quantitatively normal or increased elevation of TSH commonly occurs.

Protirelin is given to test the adequacy of thyroid suppressive or replacement therapy. In these cases, administration of thyroid hormone is *not* discontinued prior to testing. In patients receiving thyroxine to suppress thyroid activity in nodular thyroid diseases or thyroid carcinoma, the absence of a TSH response to protirelin indicates adequate suppression.

Protirelin can be utilized as part of a general evaluation of pituitary function when hypothalamic or pituitary lesions are suspected. The TSH response distinguishes primary (high TSH) from secondary (low TSH) hypothyroidism, but this also may be accomplished by measuring the basal serum TSH level. The normal response to protirelin may be slightly lower in older men and higher in women.

Protirelin is useful in distinguishing thyrotoxicosis due to TSH-producing tumors (no TSH response) from pituitary resistance to thyroid hormone (normal or exaggerated response). Protirelin also may be used to diagnose generalized resistance to thyroid hormone, in which serum levels of T_4 and T_3 are elevated but there are no clinical features of hyperthyroidism. Serum TSH and response to protirelin are normal or elevated in those with this condition.

Because protirelin is a potent stimulator of prolactin secretion by the anterior pituitary gland, it is sometimes administered to evaluate hyperprolactinemic disorders. However, its usefulness is minimal because of overlapping values among normal and abnormal subjects. In hyperprolactinemic conditions, including idiopathic hyperprolactinemia and prolactin-secreting pituitary tumors, serum prolactin concentrations are high but there is little or no further increase after protirelin stimulation. A normal response is a two- to eightfold increase in the baseline plasma prolactin level. However, a few patients with prolactin-producing pituitary adenoma with elevated prolactin levels also exhibit a normal response. A prolactin (but not TSH) response to protirelin suggests isolated TSH deficiency. The prolactin response to protirelin is inhibited by high levels of thyroid hormone or glucocorticoids.

The growth hormone level does not increase after injection of protirelin in normal individuals, but an increase occurs in approximately one-third of patients with acromegaly. This finding is of diagnostic value. ACTH also responds to protirelin injection in some patients with Cushing's disease.

Because of the wide distribution of TRH in the central nervous system and peripheral tissues, protirelin is being investigated for a variety of uses. Protirelin was reported to reverse hypotension in endotoxic, hemorrhagic, and anaphylactic shock and to aid in neurologic recovery after spinal trauma in animals (Holaday and Bernton, 1984). In one study,

protirelin briefly (about one hour) improved motor function of patients with amyotrophic lateral sclerosis (Engel et al, 1983).

ADVERSE REACTIONS. The intravenous injection of protirelin is usually followed by a metallic taste in the mouth, nausea, and flushing. An urge to urinate has been reported in both sexes and, in some women, a vaginal sensation similar to mild sexual arousal may occur. These effects develop almost immediately after injection and last up to several minutes.

Alterations in blood pressure (usually increased) may occur immediately after protirelin administration, and elderly patients or those with hypertension or other cardiovascular disorders should be monitored carefully. Severe hypotensive episodes may be avoided by placing the patient in a supine position during testing.

The TSH response to protirelin may be inhibited by aspirin, thyroid hormone, glucocorticoids, levodopa, or other dopaminergic drugs.

The safety of protirelin in pregnant women is unknown and use of this agent during pregnancy should be avoided. In lactating women, breast enlargement and leakage may occur for several days.

DOSAGE AND PREPARATIONS.

Intravenous: TSH levels are measured in serum samples taken immediately before and 30, 60, 90, and 120 minutes after a bolus injection of 200 to 500 mcg administered over 10 to 15 seconds. For *children 6 years and older*, 7 mcg/kg (maximum, 500 mcg) is given. (Since thyroid hormones suppress the response to TSH, thyroid replacement therapy must be discontinued three to six weeks before administration unless the purpose of the test is assessment of replacement or suppressive therapy.) The same procedure is followed for measurement of serum prolactin levels. Serum samples are obtained at the time of the expected prolactin peak (15 to 20 minutes after injection). Prolactin response also is suppressed (but to a lesser extent) in the presence of high levels of thyroid hormone.

Relefact TRH (Hoechst-Roussel), **Thypinone** (Abbott). Solution (sterile) 500 mcg/ml in 1 ml containers.

THYROTROPIN (TSH)
[Thytropar]

ACTIONS AND USES. Thyrotropin is isolated from bovine anterior pituitary glands. It stimulates thyroidal iodine uptake and the formation and secretion of thyroid hormones.

TSH is used to increase the uptake of radioactive iodine in patients with toxic adenomatous goiters, to demonstrate differentiated thyroid carcinoma or metastases in thyroid carcinoma, and to show the presence of normal thyroid tissue (using a scan) in patients with toxic nodule.

This hormone once was used to differentiate primary from secondary hypothyroidism but, because of adverse reactions and the greater reliability and wide availability of radioimmunoassay of serum TSH, it is *not* used for this purpose today. Thyrotropin also is inappropriate in the treatment of either secondary or tertiary hypothyroidism.

ADVERSE REACTIONS AND PRECAUTIONS. Thyrotropin can induce hyperthyroidism, especially after repeated injections; thus, it should be used with extreme caution in patients with cardiovascular disease who might not tolerate even mild thyrotoxicosis (eg, those with congestive heart failure or coronary artery disease with or without angina). Thyrotropin also must be administered cautiously to patients with primary (adrenal) or secondary (pituitary) adrenocortical insufficiency because of the danger of precipitating acute adrenocortical crisis. These patients should receive replacement corticosteroid therapy before and during administration of TSH.

Minor untoward effects include nausea, vomiting, headache, and urticaria. Hypotension, arrhythmias, thyroid swelling, and a few anaphylactic reactions have been reported. Repeated injection can elicit antibody formation with allergic reactions, false elevation of TSH, or resistance to subsequent administration of thyrotropin.

To avoid repeated administration, thyroid hormone replacement may be withdrawn to allow endogenous TSH secretion to rise and stimulate radioiodine uptake by thyroid tissue or metastases.

DOSAGE AND PREPARATIONS.

Intramuscular, Subcutaneous: To increase the uptake of radioactive iodine, 10 I.U. is given daily for three to five days prior to a tracer or therapeutic dose of iodine.

> Thytropar (Armour). Powder (sterile, lyophilized) 10 I.U. of thyrotropic activity with diluent.

CORTICOTROPIN

Physiology: Secretion of adrenal corticosteroids, particularly glucocorticoids, depends upon stimulation by corticotropin (adrenocorticotropin, ACTH). Secretion of ACTH, in turn, is modulated by hypothalamic corticotropin-releasing hormone (CRH) and glucocorticoid negative feedback.

ACTH is secreted in a circadian pattern: In normal individuals maintaining a normal day-night schedule, ACTH and cortisol concentrations are maximal before and upon awakening and are lowest in the late evening. This periodicity appears to be controlled by the central nervous system. Since the periodicity of plasma corticosteroid concentrations is secondary to that of plasma corticotropin levels, knowledge of the time of day when the blood sample was obtained is important in interpreting measurements of plasma corticotropin or cortisol. Pronounced episodic fluctuations of ACTH and cortisol also occur.

Hypothalamic corticotropin-releasing hormone (CRH), a 41-amino acid polypeptide, has been isolated from ovine hypothalami and synthesized (Vale et al, 1981). Ovine CRH stimulates ACTH in a variety of animals and stimulates ACTH, β-endorphin, and lipotropin in man (Jackson et al, 1984). CRH and vasopressin may act synergistically to stimulate ACTH secretion in man (Lamberts et al, 1984). Ovine CRH displays a biexponential decay curve in human plasma; half-lives range from 6.1 to 11.6 minutes for the fast distribution component and from 55 to 73 minutes for the slow component (Nicholson et al, 1983; Schulte et al, 1984). The half-life of human CRH has been reported to be considerably more rapid (Chrousos et al, 1985).

CRH has been used investigationally to test the pituitary response to ACTH in the differential diagnosis of adrenal insufficiency and Cushing's syndrome. The variability in ACTH and cortisol responses has thus far hampered definitive interpretations. CRH testing may supplant other dynamic tests of pituitary function (eg, dexamethasone suppression) if it can better discriminate etiologies of adrenal malfunction.

Corticotropin-releasing factor activity has also been identified in the brain outside of the hypothalamus and in tissues outside of the central nervous system. Experiments in rats suggest that this "tissue CRF" may be released from traumatized tissue and may stimulate prolonged release of ACTH.

Pathology: Excessive pituitary secretion of ACTH in the presence of intact adrenal cortices causes Cushing's disease. The negative feedback mechanisms that control pituitary secretion of ACTH are set at a higher level in such instances. Hypersecretion of ACTH also can occur when the negative feedback mechanism is normal, as in patients with uncontrolled Addison's disease. This is due to lack of inhibition of ACTH by glucocorticoid feedback. The skin pigmentation characteristic of Addison's disease or Nelson's syndrome may be caused by ACTH and related peptides, such as β- and γ-LPH, which have intrinsic skin-darkening properties.

In hypopituitarism, deficient ACTH secretion markedly reduces the production of glucocorticoids and adrenal androgens, but mineralocorticoid synthesis is not affected significantly because of continuing stimulation by the renin-angiotensin system. Patients may be asymptomatic under normal circumstances, but may develop acute adrenocortical insufficiency during severe stress. A hypothalamic defect also may be present. See also Chapter 37, Agents Used to Treat Adrenal Dysfunction.

Chemistry: Corticotropin is a straight-chain polypeptide consisting of 39 amino acids. The sequence of the first 24 amino acids is common to man, cattle, pigs, and sheep, and this segment contains the biological activity of the molecule. The arrangement of the remaining amino acids varies among species. These heterologous segments may stimulate production of antibodies and cause allergic reactions when corticotropin of animal origin is used in man. More importantly, animal preparations contain other antigenic proteins or peptides. Corticotropin is used diagnostically and therapeutically (see the evaluation).

Synthetic corticotropin analogues containing subunits of the 39-amino acid polypeptide have been prepared. Cosyntropin [Cortrosyn], which contains the first 24 amino acids and possesses the biological activity of the hormone, is used as a diagnostic agent (see the evaluation).

Diagnosis of Adrenal Insufficiency: Tests designed to stimulate secretion of adrenal steroids are used to diagnose adrenal insufficiency. In primary adrenocortical insufficiency, the plasma level of ACTH is elevated and that of cortisol is depressed, whereas both are decreased in hypopituitarism. Corticotropin preparations are used for diagnosis (ACTH stimulation test).

In primary adrenocortical insufficiency, steroid secretion is not stimulated by exogenous ACTH. In hypopituitarism, the adrenal response to ACTH is retained, although repeated administration may be necessary to initiate steroidogenesis. Plasma ACTH may be measured directly by radioimmunoassay. When cortisol levels are low, high plasma levels of ACTH indicate primary adrenal insufficiency and low levels indicate that the deficiency is secondary to pituitary or hypothalamic failure.

Diagnosis of Adrenocortical Hyperfunction: The tests most frequently used to diagnose adrenocortical hyperfunction are designed to suppress ACTH secretion. The overnight dexamethasone test is used to screen patients for unsuppressed adrenal activity. Most false-positive responses can be eliminated by measuring urinary free cortisol (UFC). A low-dose followed by a high-dose dexamethasone suppression test is then given to patients with elevated UFC levels (see the evaluation). Excessive secretion of ACTH by the pituitary is suggested if adrenal secretion is suppressed by a high-dose but not by a low-dose dexamethasone test. Unsuppressed adrenal activity in the presence of elevated plasma ACTH indicates an ectopic source of ACTH (eg, lung tumor). Unsuppressed adrenal activity in the presence of low plasma ACTH suggests a benign adrenal adenoma or adrenal carcinoma.

Adrenal stimulation tests also have been used to identify the cause of adrenal hypersecretion. In Cushing's syndrome secondary to adrenocortical hyperplasia, the corticosteroid response is exaggerated following administration of corticotropin. The response is usually decreased or absent (but may be increased) when the disease is secondary to a hypersecreting adrenal adenoma and usually is absent when adrenal carcinoma is the underlying disorder. However, this test is not discriminating because of the variability and overlap of response.

Metyrapone [Metopirone] has been used in the differential diagnosis of both adrenocortical insufficiency and Cushing's syndrome. This agent blocks cortisol synthesis and indirectly stimulates ACTH secretion. Adrenal metabolites before the enzymatic block are measured in the urine or plasma. The drug determines pituitary ACTH reserve and assists in distinguishing pituitary from nonpituitary causes of adrenal insufficiency or Cushing's syndrome. However, metyrapone is now used less frequently because of nonspecific results and the ability to measure plasma ACTH directly.

Drug Evaluations

CORTICOTROPIN (ACTH)
[Acthar, Cortrophin Gel, Cortrophin-Zinc]

ACTIONS AND USES. Corticotropin is prepared from animal pituitaries and is bioassayed against a standard preparation. It stimulates the adrenal cortex to secrete cortisol, desoxycorticosterone, androgens, and other steroids. Corticotropin can be used to determine the competence of the hypophyseal-adrenal axis, although the synthetic analogue cosyntropin is preferred because of the lower risk of allergic reactions.

Corticotropin also may be used to treat glucocorticoid-responsive diseases in patients with functional adrenal glands; however, treatment with this agent is less predictable, less convenient, more expensive, and usually possesses no advantages over use of a glucocorticoid. Some investigators prefer corticotropin to glucocorticoids in patients with ulcerative colitis, but objective evidence of superiority is lacking. It has been reported that corticotropin does not inhibit growth to the same extent as glucocorticoids when given to children with chronic diseases responsive to long-term glucocorticoid therapy, but these results have not been confirmed.

In one study, patients with progressive multiple sclerosis treated with intravenous cyclophosphamide and corticotropin were stabilized more effectively than those treated with (1) a combination of low-dose oral cyclophosphamide, intravenous corticotropin, and plasma exchange or (2) intravenous corticotropin alone (Hauser et al, 1983).

Although corticotropin causes adrenal hyperplasia rather than atrophy, prolonged therapy impairs the ability of the hypophyseal-adrenal axis to respond to stress. Its use during glucocorticoid withdrawal does not hasten, and may even impair, the establishment of hypothalamic-hypophyseal-adrenal responsiveness.

The activity of corticotropin is destroyed by proteolytic enzymes in the gastrointestinal tract; therefore, the drug is administered intramuscularly and, occasionally, subcutaneously or intravenously.

ADVERSE REACTIONS. In addition to the adverse effects caused by increased secretion of glucocorticoids, corticotropin also can produce electrolyte disturbances and acne, hirsutism, and amenorrhea in women. Acute allergic reactions have occurred in sensitized patients. Corticotropin is classified in FDA Pregnancy Category C.

DOSAGE AND PREPARATIONS. Since adrenal glands vary in their response to corticotropin, the dosage must be individualized to obtain a satisfactory therapeutic effect with minimal dosage and alteration in metabolism. The gel form delays uptake from tissues, thereby prolonging the hormone's action.
Intramuscular: For therapeutic use, 40 units of aqueous solution daily in four divided doses (10 units every six hours) or 40 units of gel (repository) or aqueous suspension with zinc hydroxide (repository) every 12 to 24 hours.

For diagnostic use, 40 to 80 units of gel daily for one to three successive days.

Available generically and as ACTH: Gel (repository) 40 and 80 units/ml in 5 ml containers; powder 40 units.
Acthar (Armour). Powder (sterile, lyophilized) 25 and 40 units; gel (repository) 40 and 80 units/ml in 1 and 5 ml containers (**H.P. Acthar Gel**).
Cortrophin Gel (Organon). (intramuscular, subcutaneous) Gel (repository) 40 and 80 units/ml in 5 ml containers.
Cortrophin-Zinc (Organon). Suspension (repository for intramuscular use only) 40 units with 2 mg of zinc/ml in 5 ml containers.
Additional Trademarks.
Cortigel-40, -80 (Savage), **Cotropic Gel 40, 80** (Reid-Provident).

COSYNTROPIN
[Cortrosyn]

Cosyntropin is a synthetic corticotropin analogue. It contains the first 24 amino acids of the corticotropin molecule and possesses the biological activity of the hormone. Cosyntropin is used diagnostically when adrenocortical insufficiency is suspected and is preferred to corticotropin for this purpose. This preparation is not used therapeutically.

Hypersensitivity reactions are uncommon and the previous occurrence of one is the only contraindication to use of cosyntropin. Caution should be exercised when giving cosyntropin to patients who are hypersensitive to natural corticotropin.

DOSAGE AND PREPARATIONS.

Intramuscular, Intravenous: For diagnostic use, *adults and children older than 5 years*, 0.25 mg (equivalent to 25 units of corticotropin); *children 1 to 5 years*, 0.15 mg; *1 year or less*, 0.1 mg. Plasma cortisol levels are determined before and 30 or 60 minutes after intramuscular injection; in most patients, a normal response is a doubling of the basal cortisol level. A cortisol level that exceeds 18 mcg/dl 30 minutes after injection and that is at least 10 mcg/dl above the basal level is considered normal. Lack of a normal response indicates adrenal insufficiency of adrenal, pituitary, or hypothalamic origin. In patients with long-standing and severe pituitary or hypothalamic hypoadrenalism, cosyntropin may be given for several days to ensure the maximum chance of adrenal stimulation.

To distinguish between adrenal and pituitary adrenal insufficiency when assay of plasma ACTH is unavailable, cosyntropin 0.25 mg to 0.75 mg is infused intravenously over a period of four to eight hours. This dosage may elicit a response in patients with functional adrenal cortical tissue. The response can be determined by measuring plasma cortisol levels. The diagnosis of hypopituitarism in responsive patients can be confirmed by other tests of pituitary function. Little or no response is obtained in patients with Addison's disease.

> **Cortrosyn** (Organon). Powder (lyophilized) 0.25 mg with mannitol 10 mg in 1 ml containers with diluent.

DEXAMETHASONE
[Decadron, Dexone, Hexadrol]

Dexamethasone, a fluorinated derivative of prednisolone, is a high-potency glucocorticoid used primarily to treat inflammatory or allergic conditions. It also is used to diagnose endogenous hypercortisolism. In normal individuals, dexamethasone exerts a negative feedback effect on the anterior pituitary and suppresses ACTH and cortisol secretion. Failure to suppress cortisol secretion or suppression only after administration of a large dose of dexamethasone, in conjunction with other tests, suggests the cause of adrenal hypersecretion (see Diagnosis of Adrenocortical Hyperfunction in the Introduction to this section).

The overnight dexamethasone test is used initially to screen patients for Cushing's syndrome. The low- and high-dose dexamethasone tests identify patients with Cushing's disease or other causes of endogenous hypercortisolism.

DOSAGE AND PREPARATIONS.

Oral: *Overnight Dexamethasone Test:* To screen patients for Cushing's syndrome, 1 mg is administered at 11 PM, and the cortisol concentration is determined from a blood sample drawn at 8 AM the next morning before breakfast. Plasma cortisol concentrations less than 5 mcg/dl indicate normal cortisol suppression and exclude Cushing's syndrome. Plasma cortisol concentrations above 10 mcg/dl suggest Cushing's disease. Values between these concentrations are indeterminate. False-positive results may occur in the presence of alcoholism, depression, or obesity or if the patient is taking estrogen or phenytoin.

Low-dose Dexamethasone Test: This is a more accurate test to diagnose Cushing's syndrome. A dose of 0.5 mg is administered every six hours for eight doses. On the second day of administration, an 8 AM plasma cortisol and a 24-hour urine collection are obtained. The normal response is 19 to 25 mcg or less of urinary free cortisol/24 hours. Findings in these ranges excludes Cushing's syndrome. False-positive results (failure to suppress) may occur infrequently, particularly in depressed patients.

High-dose Dexamethasone Test: To identify the etiology of Cushing's syndrome, 24-hour urine collections are analyzed on two successive days prior to testing to determine control levels of urinary free cortisol, and 8 AM plasma is obtained for measurement of cortisol. Dexamethasone 2 mg is then given every six hours for two days. On the second day of administration, an 8 AM plasma cortisol and 24-hour urine collection are obtained. Suppression of urinary-free cortisol by at least 50% suggests adrenal hyperplasia as the cause of Cushing's syndrome. Suppression is less than 50% in those with Cushing's syndrome due to adrenal adenoma or carcinoma or to an ectopic ACTH source. False-positive results may occur infrequently in these latter conditions, however.

> **Generic.** Tablets 0.25, 0.5, 0.75, 1, 1.5, 2, and 4 mg; elixir 0.05 mg/5 ml; oral solution 0.5 mg/ml (alcohol free) and 0.5 mg/0.5 ml (alcohol 1%).
> **Decadron** (Merck Sharp & Dohme). Tablets 0.25, 0.5, 0.75, 1.5, 4, and 6 mg; elixir 0.5 mg/ml (alcohol 5%).
> **Dexone** (Rowell). Tablets 0.5, 0.75, 1.5, and 4 mg.
> **Hexadrol** (Organon). Tablets 0.5, 0.75, 1.5, and 4 mg; elixir 0.05 mg/5 ml (alcohol 5%).

BETA-LIPOTROPIN

Beta-lipotropin (β-LPH) is found in the pituitary gland in the intermediate lobe of animals (in humans, an intermediate lobe can be identified only during fetal life and pregnancy) and in the anterior lobe of man and animals. Unlike other pituitary hormones, chemical isolation and identification (91 amino acid residues) preceded description of its function. The hormone was named after discovery of its lipolytic activity, but this does not appear to be its primary function. In fact, although much has been learned about the biologically active peptides present within the molecule, β-LPH remains a "hormone in search of a function."

β-LPH contains within its structure the amino acid sequences for β-melanocyte stimulating hormone (β-MSH), β-endorphin, and met-enkephalin (methionine enkephalin). Although β-MSH is important in animals, it probably does not exist as a separate hormone in man. Rather, it is a byproduct of β-LPH during pituitary extraction procedures. Melanocyte-stimulating activity in man may be attributable to ACTH. β-endorphin, in turn, contains within its structure the pentapeptide, met-enkephalin. Both peptides exhibit opiate-like activities (analgesia, catatonia, hypothermia) and cross tolerance to morphine. Their effects are blocked by the narcotic antagonist, naloxone [Narcan]. The peptides are found within neurons in the central nervous system in areas involved with transmission of pain and expression of anxiety and emotion (limbic system).

The neurons that contain β-endorphin and their distribution are distinct from those containing met-enkephalin. β-endorphin neurons are generally concentrated in periventricular areas, whereas enkephalin neurons are in the basal ganglia and substantia nigra. Pituitary β-LPH is probably not the source of enkephalins found in the central nervous system; these are synthesized in situ and separate precursors have been identified. Although β-endorphin is generally not active when injected systemically, the blood-brain barrier is probably incomplete.

Endogenous opioids are distributed in tissues other than the pituitary and central nervous system. β-endorphin is found in the pancreas, placenta, male reproductive tract, and semen. Enkephalins are found in the gut, placenta, adrenal medulla, and in carcinoid tumors of the thymus and lung. Dymorphins, a third group of opioid peptides, are found in gut, posterior pituitary, hypothalamus, and brain stem (Akil et al, 1984).

The synthesis and release of pituitary β-LPH are closely linked to those of ACTH. Both hormones have a common precursor (pro-opiomelanocortin), both are secreted by the same cell, and the secretion of both is controlled in parallel by positive (eg, stress, CRF stimulation) and negative (eg, dexamethasone) feedback mechanism. The parallel between ACTH and β-LPH secretion suggests that they function in the generalized stress response. The adrenal medulla contains enkephalins, which may mediate endogenous opioid stress analgesia (Lewis et al, 1982).

β-endorphin also may affect the physiologic secretion of pituitary hormones: Prolactin secretion is stimulated, and gonadotropin secretion is inhibited. Hypothalamic opioid activity may be increased in women taking oral contraceptives (Casper et al, 1984) and in women with hypothalamic hypogonadotropic amenorrhea, including exercise-induced amenorrhea.

β-LPH may serve as a prohormone, releasing its biologically active fragments after cleavage by proteolytic enzymes in the pituitary. Additional functions may be unrelated to the opioid properties of the smaller molecules in β-LPH. However, the central nervous system endorphins probably modulate functions that respond to the administration of opiates.

Numerous studies are currently in progress to elucidate the role of β-endorphin and related peptides in normal physiology. In addition to hypothalamic regulation of pituitary function, endogenous opioid peptides may play a role in the hypothalamic control of body temperature, respiration, and cardiovascular activity. They are probably important for pain perception and tolerance. When administered by intrathecal or intraventricular injection, β-endorphin relieved intractable pain associated with disseminated carcinoma. β-endorphin has been administered intrathecally during labor and has produced analgesia without affecting uterine contractions. The placenta contains β-endorphin-like material, and plasma levels of β-endorphin increase during labor and delivery. Administration

of β-endorphin to animals induces analgesia and behavioral effects, such as catatonia, which are reversed by naloxone. It has been suggested that "runners' high" and the euphoria reported in near-death experiences may involve β-endorphin.

Endogenous opioid peptides also may be involved in the pathophysiology of certain diseases. β-endorphin has been identified immunochemically in normal human pancreatic islet cells but not in a similar preparation from a diabetic patient. Synovial fluid has greater concentrations of β-endorphin than serum and may be capable of synthesizing the peptide. Arthritic patients may have lower than normal levels of β-endorphin.

Synthetic β-endorphin is being investigated clinically. Many analogues of enkephalin have been synthesized. Some are active when administered intravenously, intramuscularly, and orally. It is anticipated that this hormone or its analogues or derivatives may be useful in a wide spectrum of disorders.

GONADOTROPINS

The ovaries and testes have dual functions: Each produces gametes as well as steroid hormones essential for the establishment and maintenance of secondary sexual characteristics. The glycoproteins, follicle-stimulating hormone (FSH) and luteinizing hormone (LH), were first named for their most prominent action upon the ovary. FSH is essential for follicular maturation and LH for the formation and maintenance of the corpus luteum. FSH enhances estrogen secretion and LH, estrogen and progesterone secretion. In addition, a surge of LH at midcycle triggers ovulation.

These glycoproteins also have effects on the testis. LH, once called interstitial cell stimulating hormone (ICSH) in the male, stimulates the production of testosterone by the Leydig cells and elevates serum estrogen levels in men. Both LH and FSH are essential for spermatogenesis, although FSH appears to be more critical for the final stages.

FSH and LH are secreted by anterior pituitary gonadotrophs and are double-chain glycoproteins. Their α chains contain about 96 amino acid residues, while their β chains contain 115; molecular weights are 29,000 (FSH) and 28,000 (LH). Preparations of human gonadotropins purified from pituitaries obtained at autopsy are available in limited amounts for investigational use.

Negative feedback is important in regulating gonadotropin production. The high serum levels of LH and FSH seen after castration and in gonadal dysgenesis result from lack of negative feedback from gonadal steroids. However, control of gonadotropin secretion is much more complex. In women, the manner in which estradiol affects serum gonadotropin levels depends upon the stage of the ovarian cycle during which it is given. In men, estradiol is probably a more potent suppressant of gonadotropin than testosterone, although it is not as important as testosterone physiologically because estradiol levels are low in males. Also, a protein substance, inhibin, is produced in the germinal epithelium of the testis and is distinct from androgen-binding protein. Inhibin selectively inhibits FSH secretion, as demonstrated by the elevation of FSH levels in men with azoospermia. A similar follicular inhibin is produced in the ovary.

Luteinizing Hormone-Releasing Hormone: Luteinizing hormone-releasing hormone (LH-RH, gonadotropin-releasing hormone, GnRH) stimulates release of LH and to a lesser extent FSH. LH-RH is synthesized mainly in the hypothalamus but has been found in other tissues, including the placenta, pancreatic islet cells, ovary, and adrenal gland; high concentrations also occur in breast milk. Its function in nonhypothalamic tissues is unknown. LH-RH has a short half-life in plasma (two to eight minutes).

Although a separate FSH-releasing hormone may exist, LH-RH is the only hypothalamic hormone known to be of importance in regulating pituitary LH and FSH secretion. The differential patterns of release of these hormones probably result from interactions at the anterior pituitary level, changing patterns of LH-RH secretion, and feedback from gonadal steroids and inhibin-like products.

Pulsatile release of LH-RH is necessary for normal cyclic gonadotropic activity in females (Knobil, 1980). Delivery of a steady supply of LH-RH or the chemically identical synthetic substance, gonadorelin, to the pituitary results in desensitization or down regulation after initial stimulation of gonadotropin receptors.

Gonadorelin is used as a diagnostic agent in patients with suspected gonadotropin deficiency and to assess pituitary gonadotropin function following pituitary ablative therapy (see the evaluation).

Leuprolide [Lupron], an LH-RH agonist, is used to treat prostatic carcinoma. After initial stimulation, serum testosterone decreases, symptoms are alleviated, and bone pain is relieved in metastatic disease. Treatment is as effective as orchiectomy in relieving pain and delaying disease progression. Thus, leuprolide may effect medical castration without increasing the cardiovascular risk associated with estrogens. LH-RH analogues may also be useful in hormone-dependent breast cancer. See the evaluation in Chapter 64, Drugs Used in Cancer Chemotherapy.

Investigational Uses and Agents: Gonadorelin [Factrel], a decapeptide, and numerous analogues are being tested for use as fertility or contraceptive agents, as well as to treat conditions such as delayed puberty, endometriosis, prostate cancer, precocious puberty, and cryptorchidism (see references in reviews by Fraser, 1984; Ory, 1983; Yen, 1983). The super agonists (usually nonapeptides) are more potent and have been more effective than the antagonists. However, when gonadotropin suppression is required, agonists, which induce down regulation of LH-RH receptors, are as effective as antagonists, which competitively bind to receptors.

Synthetic LH-RH preparations have been used when gonadotropin stimulation was desired. Ovulation has been induced in patients with hypothalamic amenorrhea, Kallmann's syndrome, hyperprolactinemia, and clomiphene-refractory polycystic ovarian disease after subcutaneous or intravenous pulse injection of LH-RH. Ovarian hyperstimulation and multiple ovulation occurred after use of large doses.

Male patients with *delayed puberty* or *hypogonadotropic hypogonadism* have been treated with LH-RH preparations.

Although isolated successes have been reported in experimental situations, the necessity for long-term pulsatile administration makes this treatment impractical. Stimulatory effects decline when the hormone is discontinued. Formation of antibodies to LH-RH with consequent lack of response has occurred when the hormone was given subcutaneously. In *cryptorchidism*, intranasal LH-RH produced partial or complete descent of testes in almost two-thirds of patients.

LH-RH agonists are being tested clinically to treat reproductive disorders requiring suppression of gonadotropin or gonadal steroid secretion. Preparations have been administered by injection or intranasally. *Female contraception* may be achieved with an LH-RH agonist that induces amenorrhea and blocks ovulation. However, a preparation and regimen must be developed to avoid potential problems, ranging from hypoestrogenism and irregular vaginal bleeding to unopposed estrogenic stimulation of the endometrium. Another approach to female contraception is to use an LH-RH analogue to inhibit postovulatory LH secretion and produce luteolysis. These effects have been achieved in normal cycles. However, if conception occurs, placental HCG provides the necessary support for continued luteal function, thus precluding contraceptive action. Attempts to utilize an LH-RH agonist as a *male contraceptive* have produced mixed results similar to those noted with danazol. Daily administration of an LH-RH agonist decreases serum testosterone and sperm density and motility. However, an androgen must be given to overcome the lack of libido and impotence that also occur.

Endometriosis may be controlled by LH-RH agonists and few side effects have occurred. Serum estrogens are reduced to menopausal levels, and endometrial atrophy and relief of pain are observed. Pregnancies have occurred in previously infertile patients. Although alleviation of symptoms may continue temporarily after discontinuing the drug, it is not curative and disease tends to recur when therapy is withdrawn (Lemay et al, 1984). The possible adverse effects on bone (eg, osteoporosis) of prolonged hypoestrogenism have yet to be evaluated. Comparative studies with danazol [Danocrine] and an LH-RH agonist to determine tolerance and effectiveness for implant suppression and enhancement of fertility would be useful.

Promising results have been obtained in the treatment of *precocious puberty* with LH-RH agonists. Nocturnal gonadotropin secretion is suppressed, serum estradiol is reduced, menstruation ceases, and breast size and pubic hair development regress in girls. Growth velocity is decreased in boys and girls, which may ultimately increase adult height. This is an apparent advantage over treatment with medroxyprogesterone and cyproterone, which are relatively ineffective in preventing premature epiphyseal closure. Discontinuation of therapy reverses the beneficial effects; therefore, treatment may be necessary until the desired results are obtained (Luder et al, 1984; Mansfield et al, 1983).

In summary, use of gonadorelin to achieve stimulatory effects is limited at this time by the impracticality of pulsatile dosing regimens. For LH-RH and its analogues, interpretation and comparison of results of investigational studies are difficult because of differences in experimental agents, regimens, and routes of administration. In general, the most beneficial and reproducible effects are achieved in decreasing order when LH-RH preparations are administered by the intravenous, subcutaneous, or intranasal route. The latter is obviously more convenient than parenteral forms. The difficulties of overcoming proteolytic degradation have not been surmounted and oral preparations are not available. For both stimulatory and inhibitory uses of LH-RH and its analogues, equivalence or superiority to current treatments remains to be demonstrated.

Other Agents: Other drugs available to treat dysfunction of the hypothalamic-pituitary-gonadal axis include human chorionic gonadotropin (HCG), human menopausal gonadotropin (menotropins, HMG [Pergonal]), and clomiphene [Clomid, Serophene]. These drugs are used almost exclusively to treat infertility in women and men (see Chapter 41, Agents Used to Treat Infertility, for further discussion and evaluations on Menotropins and Clomiphene). A drug that possesses anti-gonadotropic activity, danazol [Danocrine], is also available.

Drug Evaluations

HUMAN CHORIONIC GONADOTROPIN (HCG)
[A.P.L., Follutein, Pregnyl, Profasi HP]

ACTIONS AND USES. Human chorionic gonadotropin (HCG) is a placental hormone extracted from the urine of pregnant women. Its biological activity is the same as that of luteinizing hormone and it is used as a substitute for human LH, which is available only in small quantities for investigational studies. HCG has some intrinsic thyroid-stimulating properties, which accounts for the thyrotoxic state that occurs in patients with HCG-secreting neoplasms.

HCG is indicated for the medical treatment of cryptorchidism. If this condition is not treated, little spontaneous testicular descent occurs after 12 months of age and progressive and irreversible tubular damage may begin by age 5; therefore, treatment should begin early. Initiation of drug therapy is usually recommended by age 2. However, in one study of 153 cryptorchid boys, testicular descent failed to occur in 81% of patients treated before age 3 years. Among treated patients age 3 to 4 years, 55% failed to respond and 45% experienced complete or partial testicular descent (Garagorri et al, 1982). Some testicular function may be preserved even when treatment is started in prepuberal boys; delay until puberty results in inability to produce sperm. Even after testicular descent, normal spermatogenesis may not occur. Success rates are slightly higher in bilateral cryptorchidism than in unilateral cryptorchidism. Hormonal stimulation is less likely to be effective when the testes are located high in the inguinal canal. Even when complete descent is not accomplished, HCG stimulates scrotal development and facilitates surgical correction (orchiopexy).

If hormonal therapy is unsuccessful, surgical correction (or removal if this fails) should be performed. Cryptorchid testes have a high potential for malignancy that is reduced by hormonal or surgical correction. However, orchiopexy does not always avoid malignancy; in unilateral cryptorchidism, malignancy has occurred in the contralateral, normal testis. Correction of cryptorchidism facilitates detection if malignancy does occur.

Androgen production may be compromised due to testicular fibrosis. Deficient androgen production in uncorrected bilateral cryptorchidism may be apparent after 6 years of age (Anoussakis et al, 1983).

HCG is sometimes used diagnostically in males with delayed puberty or when there is doubt about the steroidogenic ability of the testes to respond to gonadotropin stimulation (see also Chapter 38, Androgens and Anabolic Steroids). It also has been used occasionally in hirsute females to locate the source of excess androgen (ie, ovary or adrenal). However, the test is unreliable because a lack of androgen secretion after administration of HCG does not exclude an ovarian source and adrenal androgen production may be stimulated by HCG.

Daily injections of HCG have been used in conjunction with a low-calorie diet in weight reduction programs. Results of a controlled double-blind study comparing subjects on such a regimen to those on the same diet but receiving saline instead of HCG demonstrated no difference in weight loss, body measurements, hunger appeasement, and various metabolic measurements (Shetty and Kalkhoff, 1977). There is no evidence that HCG causes weight reduction beyond that due to caloric restriction. Therefore, it is not indicated in the treatment of obesity.

For use of HCG in the treatment of infertility, see the evaluation in Chapter 41, Agents Used to Treat Infertility.

DOSAGE AND PREPARATIONS.

Intramuscular: In cryptorchidism, for rapid response and minimal sexual development, 5,000 units every other day for four injections; to achieve a greater degree of sexual development, the more prolonged regimen of 500 units three times weekly for three weeks, or, for *boys 10 years or older,* 1,000 units three times weekly for three weeks is used.

In males, for diagnosis of responsiveness to gonadotropin stimulation, 2,000 units daily for three days. Blood levels of testosterone are measured at baseline and on the fourth day (day following last injection). An approximate doubling of testosterone levels is normal. It may be possible to obtain the same amount of information using a single HCG injection (Saez and Forest, 1979) or a shorter postinjection interval (Glass and Vigersky, 1980), but standardized protocols have not been developed.

    A.P.L. (Ayerst), **Generic.** Powder 5,000, 10,000, and 20,000 U.S.P. units with 10 ml of diluent.
    Follutein (Squibb), **Pregnyl** (Organon). Powder (lyophilized) 10,000 U.S.P. units with 10 ml of diluent.
    Profasi HP (Serono). Powder (sterile, lyophilized) 5,000 and 10,000 U.S.P. units with 10 ml of diluent.

GONADORELIN
[Factrel]

USES. Gonadorelin is a synthetic preparation of LH-RH that is identical to the endogenous hormone. It is used to diagnose and monitor hypothalamic-pituitary gonadotropin function.

Gonadorelin is employed as an adjunct to clinical observation in the diagnosis of gonadotropin deficiency but it cannot reliably distinguish pituitary from hypothalamic dysfunction. Theoretically, gonadorelin should bypass hypothalamic dysfunction and stimulate LH release without affecting pituitary dysfunction; however, overlapping results may occur. Repeated administration may improve the specificity of this test.

Gonadorelin also may be used to monitor gonadotropic function in patients who have undergone partial or complete hypophysectomy or pituitary irradiation.

ADVERSE REACTIONS AND PRECAUTIONS. Adverse effects generally are infrequent and not serious. Headache, nausea, abdominal discomfort, lightheadedness, and flushing may occur. Hypersensitivity has not been reported. Repeated use of large doses may cause luteolysis and inhibit spermatogenesis.

Drugs that may affect serum levels or pituitary control of gonadotropins (eg, androgens, progestins, estrogens, spironolactone, levodopa, digoxin, phenothiazines) should not be used while performing gonadorelin tests. There are no indications for use of gonadorelin during pregnancy and its safety during pregnancy is unknown (FDA Pregnancy Category B).

DOSAGE AND PREPARATIONS.

Intravenous, Subcutaneous: *Adults*, 100 mcg. In females, the test should be administered between the first and seventh day of the menstrual cycle if that can be established. Venous blood samples are drawn 15 minutes before, immediately before (these two samples are averaged to obtain a baseline value), and 15, 30, 45, 60, and 120 minutes after administration. For interpretation of results, see the manufacturer's literature.

Factrel (Ayerst). Powder (lyophilized) 100 and 500 mcg.

PROLACTIN

Prolactin (PRL) was known to exist in animals but was not identified as a separate hormone in humans until 1970. Before then, it was thought that lactogenic activity in humans was produced solely by growth hormone (GH). Human PRL is a linear polypeptide with 198 amino acid residues and a molecular weight of 23,000. Human GH also has lactogenic activity, and 16% of its amino acid sequence is identical to that of human prolactin.

As with other anterior pituitary hormones, the secretion of prolactin is controlled by hypothalamic substances. However, unlike these other hormones, the predominant hypothalamic influence is inhibitory (prolactin-inhibiting factor, PIF). Dopamine inhibits prolactin secretion and is probably the major PIF. A still unidentified prolactin-releasing factor (PRF) is involved in regulating the production and secretion of this hormone. Indirect evidence suggests that serotonin stimulates the release of prolactin. Thyrotropin-releasing hormone (TRH), which is used to stimulate thyrotropin (TSH) and prolactin secretion diagnostically, may not be important in the normal regulation of prolactin production. In the absence of normal hypothalamic control (eg, stalk section), hypersecretion of prolactin occurs but secretion of other anterior pituitary hormones is decreased.

The only well-defined function of prolactin in humans is stimulation of milk production after parturition. The function of prolactin in males is not understood but it may have some role in normal reproduction. In certain lower animals, prolactin affects metamorphosis and salt balance and, particularly in birds, prolactin stimulates parental behavior in both sexes.

Although the function of prolactin appears to be quite restricted in humans, increased amounts are secreted in a wide variety of physiologic circumstances: Secretion is increased in both sexes during sleep, exercise, and in response to stress and in women throughout pregnancy, in the early postpartum period (even in the absence of suckling), and in association with orgasm in some women. The most effective and specific stimulus for prolactin secretion is suckling. Prolactin is also increased in the fetus and is responsible for milk secretion (witch's milk) in some neonates.

In nonphysiologic states, prolactin levels may be increased by a prolactin-secreting pituitary adenoma, hypothalamic damage, and drugs (eg, neuroleptics, estrogens, antihistamines, antihypertensive agents); levels also may be elevated without identifiable hypothalamic-pituitary disease (idiopathic hyperprolactinemia) and occasionally in those with hypothyroidism, renal or hepatic failure, chest wall disease, and spinal cord injury.

Other than rare cases of isolated prolactin deficiency that prevent normal postpartum lactation, no symptoms result from prolactin deficiency. However, hypersecretion is associated with a variety of symptoms that affect reproductive function in men and women.

Hyperprolactinemia: Hyperprolactinemic reproductive dysfunction may be manifested in women by amenorrhea, galactorrhea, and/or infertility. Any or all of these symptoms may occur concomitantly. Even during the physiologic hyperprolactinemia associated with lactation, reproductive capacity is partially or wholly compromised. Bone loss has been observed in amenorrheic women with hyperprolactinemia. Lack of estrogen may be contributory, but prolactin may directly stimulate bone resorption under certain circumstances (Schlechte et al, 1983; Cann et al, 1984). Delayed puberty has been associated with hyperprolactinemia in both sexes (Patton and Woolf, 1983). Elevated prolactin levels in men can decrease libido and potency and rarely cause galactorrhea.

Functional hyperprolactinemia of unknown cause may be an early manifestation of a pathologic continuum that eventually results in a pituitary adenoma.

Prolactinomas: Radiologic evidence of prolactin-secreting micro- or macroadenomas is present in 30% or more of patients with hyperprolactinemia. These adenomas are often associated with amenorrhea or oligomenorrhea in women, impotence in men, and galactorrhea and infertility in both sexes. Neurologic symptoms (eg, visual field defects, bitemporal headaches) may be present. Tumors tend to be smaller and are discovered about ten years earlier in women than in men and probably reflect the appearance of clinical effects at an earlier stage of tumor development in women (Franks and

Jacobs, 1983). It is estimated that asymptomatic prolactinomas occur in 10% to 25% of adults based on autopsy evidence from patients who died of unrelated causes.

Diagnosis of prolactinomas is based on endocrine function studies, neurologic assessment (eg, visual field testing), and radiologic evidence. Computerized tomography provides more accurate diagnosis than polytomography. Management of an adenoma depends on its size, the level of discomfort, and considerations of future fertility. Intervention may be unnecessary when a microadenoma causes tolerable symptoms and fertility is not desired. Such patients may be monitored for further increase in serum prolactin levels and worsening of symptoms.

Pituitary tumors are often removed surgically. Bromocriptine [Parlodel], a dopaminergic agent that inhibits prolactin secretion, is used with or instead of ablative therapy and usually reduces prolactin secretion of any etiology. There is increasing evidence that tumor growth is retarded or reversed in many patients. However, the effect depends on continuous use of the drug; discontinuation has been associated with tumor regrowth (see the evaluation).

The investigational agent, pergolide, has actions similar to those of bromocriptine but it is more potent by weight and has a longer duration of action. In clinical studies, pergolide inhibited prolactin secretion in patients with hyperprolactinemia and growth hormone secretion in some patients with acromegaly (Franks et al, 1983; L'Hermite et al, 1983; Kleinberg et al, 1983).

Drug Evaluation

BROMOCRIPTINE MESYLATE
[Parlodel]

ACTIONS. Bromocriptine is a synthetic ergot alkaloid that acts directly on dopaminergic receptors of pituitary cells. It also may exert a central effect on prolactin secretion, but this has not yet been fully established.

USES. Bromocriptine is employed in a variety of conditions in which dopaminergic activity is useful (eg, hyperprolactinemic reproductive dysfunction, prolactin-secreting adenomas, suppression of postpartum lactation, acromegaly, Parkinson's disease) (see Chapters 11, Drugs Used in Extrapyramidal Movement Disorders; 39, Estrogens, Progestins, and Other Agents Used to Treat Gynecologic Conditions; and 41, Agents Used to Treat Infertility).

Bromocriptine reduces elevated prolactin levels caused by physiologic, pathologic, or iatrogenic (eg, drug ingestion)

conditions, but the levels usually increase on cessation of therapy unless the underlying disorder is corrected. Bromocriptine also inhibits prolactin secretion in normal individuals, but the reduction is less pronounced than when the secretory rate is abnormally high.

Prolactinomas: Bromocriptine is the preferred initial therapy for microadenomas. For macroadenomas, the drug may be used to control symptoms and avoid surgery or to reduce tumor size to facilitate surgery. Management with bromocriptine compared to surgery allows maximum preservation of other anterior pituitary secretion.

Transsphenoidal removal of the adenoma may be employed if bromocriptine therapy fails or chronic drug therapy is not desired. Surgical removal reduces prolactin secretion to normal in 60% to 90% of patients with microadenomas but in less than 50% of patients with macroadenomas. Bromocriptine may be used when surgery fails to normalize prolactin secretion.

Irradiation of prolactinomas has been abandoned in some centers because several years may be required to achieve the desired control of tumor size and activity (Reyniak, 1983; Vance et al, 1984 B).

Bromocriptine rapidly reduces prolactin secretion. The greatest decrease is observed within four weeks, although more time may be required to reduce secretion to normal in patients with a macroadenoma.

Bromocriptine shrinks prolactin-producing adenomas in 40% to 80% of patients (Barbieri and Ryan, 1983). The suppression often continues for the duration of drug therapy. Decrease in tumor size is due to reduction in cytoplasmic volume and not the number of cells (Tindall et al, 1982; Bassetti et al, 1984). Although suppression of adenoma activity occasionally continues after cessation of therapy, effects are usually reversed: prolactin secretion increases (although not always to the previous level) and regrowth of the adenoma eventually may occur (Johnston et al, 1983). The pattern of prolactin secretion following bromocriptine withdrawal is variable, but plateau occurs after about six weeks (Maxson et al, 1984).

Hyperprolactinemia in Males: Four to eight percent of men who complain of impotence have hyperprolactinemia (Braunstein, 1983; Slag et al, 1983). Decreased libido is common, and testosterone deficiency may occur. Several reports suggest that bromocriptine may alleviate these problems by decreasing prolactin secretion; however, therapy has not been uniformly effective. For best results, both reduction of serum prolactin and treatment of testosterone deficiency (if this is not corrected by bromocriptine) are required. Bromocriptine is ineffective when impotence is not due to hyperprolactinemia (see also Chapter 41).

Acromegaly: Bromocriptine provides a medical alternative for the treatment of acromegaly, which once was treatable only by surgery or irradiation. The drug is usually employed as an adjunct to an ablative procedure, particularly irradiation. Bromocriptine is sometimes used alone in mild cases or when the patient is unable or unwilling to undergo surgery or irradiation, but it should not be used as the sole treatment when there is suprasellar extension of the tumor.

In most studies, about 25% of patients experienced a major

decrease in growth hormone levels and even more patients reported amelioration of symptoms. However, the drug's effects on glucose tolerance and plasma insulin levels usually persist for the duration of treatment. GH levels generally are not reduced to normal, and abnormal patterns of secretion may persist. Some patients show clinical improvement (eg, remission of soft tissue swelling) in the presence of decreased somatomedin C, but other patients improve in the absence of changes in either serum GH or somatomedin C (Nortier et al, 1985). It has been suggested that the monomeric, most biologically active form of GH is decreased more than less active oligomeric forms, which are nevertheless measured by immunoassay (Wass and Besser, 1983).

The response to bromocriptine is rapid; blood levels of GH are decreased within hours and the drug's effectiveness may be assessed within weeks. Some investigators believe that the response to a single dose may correlate with long-term effectiveness and can predict the ultimate usefulness of bromocriptine therapy (Oppizzi et al, 1984).

Indicators of a favorable response include improved glucose tolerance; reduced insulin requirements in diabetics; decreased sweating, urinary hydroxyproline levels, and incidence of headaches; and improved libido in men. The latter may be due to concomitant inhibition of prolactin secretion (hyperprolactinemia is associated with acromegaly in one-third of patients). Improvements in morphologic features include softening of facial features, decreased skin and tongue thickness, and decreased hand and foot size. Regression of early visual defects and radiologic improvement suggest that bromocriptine may reduce the growth and mass of some GH-producing tumors. However, tumor regression is not as common with GH-secreting tumors as with prolactinoma or mixed prolactin- and GH-producing tumors (Odell, 1984).

In spite of the good results reported, bromocriptine is not curative. If the cause of acromegaly (ie, pituitary tumor) is not eliminated, increased secretion of growth hormone resumes after cessation of treatment.

In summary, the advantage of bromocriptine in acromegaly is that it affects only the secretion of growth hormone and prolactin. It appears to be useful as an adjunct to surgery or irradiation, in the treatment of persistent endocrinopathy after surgery, or to hasten relief of clinical symptoms in the interim between irradiation and realization of its effects. Although most patients appear to benefit, bromocriptine usually suppresses GH only partially and is a temporary noncurative measure.

Cushing's Disease: Bromocriptine has been used investigationally to treat Cushing's disease. Although plasma ACTH may decrease in some patients, plasma ACTH and cortisol concentrations do not return to normal.

ADVERSE REACTIONS. Adverse reactions are common when bromocriptine therapy is initiated. Thereafter, their incidence and severity depend upon the dosage and its rate of increase. Common untoward effects include nausea, vomiting, dizziness, and orthostatic hypotension. Nausea usually disappears after three to four days and may be minimized by taking the medication with food and at bedtime. Rarely, orthostatic hypotension appeared to be associated with fainting or collapse in sensitive individuals, even after ingestion of a single dose.

Postpartum hypertension, seizures, and stroke have been associated with use of bromocriptine to suppress lactation. Other drugs that may have contributed to the hypertensive effects were taken concomitantly in some cases and causation remains unproven. However, postpartum hypertension or eclampsia has been reported with use of other ergot alkaloids.

Rhinorrhea developed during treatment of a pituitary tumor with bromocriptine and may have been due to exposure of a defective sella floor as the tumor tissue retracted (Wilson et al, 1983).

Patients taking larger doses (eg, acromegalic patients) may experience decreased alcohol tolerance, constipation, dyspepsia, dryness of the mouth, nasal congestion, nocturnal leg cramps, and peripheral digital vasospasm on exposure to cold.

The risk of spontaneous abortions or neonatal malformations did not appear to increase when bromocriptine was taken during the first eight weeks of pregnancy (Turkalj et al, 1982).

PHARMACOKINETICS. Bromocriptine is absorbed rapidly after oral administration; peak plasma levels are attained in about one hour. First-pass metabolism occurs with over 90% of the absorbed dose. The plasma half-life is three hours. About 98% is excreted in the feces, and the remaining 2% is eliminated in the urine.

DOSAGE AND PREPARATIONS.
Oral: For all indications, initially, 1.25 to 2.5 mg is given in the evening for two or three days. This dose may be increased by 2.5 mg on alternate days until tolerance and the maintenance level are reached.

For hyperprolactinemic reproductive functional disorders, 2.5 mg two or three times daily is usually sufficient. If pregnancy occurs, the medication should be discontinued.

For prevention of postpartum lactation, 2.5 mg one to three times daily is the usual dosage. Therapy is started at least four hours after delivery when vital signs have stabilized and is continued for 14 days. If rebound lactation occurs, 2.5 mg daily may be taken for an additional week.

For acromegaly, the most commonly used dosages are 15 to 20 mg daily in three or four divided doses. Depending upon clinical response, the amount may be increased to 60 mg daily in four divided doses.

Parlodel (Sandoz). Capsules 5 mg; tablets 2.5 mg.

Cited References

Growth hormone. *Med Lett Drugs Ther* 26:80-81, 1984.

Akil H, et al: Endogenous opioids: Biology and function. *Ann Rev Neurosci* 7:223-255, 1984.

American Academy of Pediatrics: Growth hormone in treatment of children with short stature. *Pediatrics* 72:891-894, 1983.

Anoussakis C, et al: Effect of surgical repair of cryptorchidism on endocrine testicular function. *J Pediatr* 103:919-921, 1983.

Barbieri RL, Ryan KJ: Bromocriptine: Endocrine pharmacology and therapeutic applications. *Fertil Steril* 39:727-741, 1983.

Baskin DS, et al: Transsphenoidal microsurgical removal of growth hormone-secreting pituitary adenomas. Review of 137 cases. *J Neurosurg* 56:634, 1982.

Bassetti M, et al: Bromocriptine treatment reduces cell size in human macroprolactinomas: Morphometric study. *J Clin Endocrinol Metab* 58:268-273, 1984.

768

Benjamin M, et al: Short children, anxious parents: Is growth hormone the answer? *Hastings Center Rep* 14:5-9, (April) 1984.

Borges JLC, et al: Stimulation of growth hormone (GH) and somatomedin C in idiopathic GH-deficient subjects by intermittent pulsatile administration of synthetic human pancreatic tumor GH-releasing factor. *J Clin Endocrinol Metab* 59:1-6, 1984.

Braunstein GD: Endocrine causes of impotence. *Postgrad Med* 74:207-217, (Oct) 1983.

Brown P, et al: Potential epidemic of Creutzfeldt-Jakob disease from human growth hormone therapy. *N Engl J Med* 313:728-731, 1985.

Brown MR, Fisher LA: Brain peptides as intercellular messengers: Implications for medicine. *JAMA* 251:1310-1315, 1984.

Cann CE, et al: Decreased spinal mineral content in amenorrheic women. *JAMA* 251: 626-629, 1984.

Casper RF, et al: Prolonged elevation of hypothalamic opioid peptide activity in women taking oral contraceptives. *J Clin Endocrinol Metab* 58:582-584, 1984.

Chrousos GP, et al: Clinical applications of corticotropin-releasing factor. *Ann Intern Med* 102:344-358, 1985.

Clemmons DR, Van Wyk JJ: Factors controlling blood concentration of somatomedin C. *Clin Endocrinol Metab* 13:113-143, 1984.

Committee on Growth Hormone Use: Degenerative neurologic disease in patients formerly treated with growth hormone. *J Pediatr* 107:10-12, 1985.

Engel WK, et al: Effect on weakness and spasticity in amyotrophic lateral sclerosis of thymotropic-releasing hormone. *Lancet* 2:73-75, 1983.

Franks S, Jacobs HS: Hyperprolactinaemia. *Clin Endocrinol Metab* 12:641-668, 1983.

Franks S, et al: Effectiveness of pergolide mesylate in long term treatment of hyperprolactinaemia. *Br Med J* 286:1177-1179, 1983.

Fraser HM: GnRH and its analogues: Current therapeutic applications and new prospects. *Drugs* 27:187-193, 1984.

Frasier SD: Human pituitary growth hormone (hGH) therapy in growth hormone deficiency. *Endocrin Rev* 4:155-170, 1983.

Frazer T, et al: Growth hormone-dependent growth failure. *J Pediatr* 101:12-15, 1982.

Frohman LA, et al: Metabolic clearance and plasma disappearance rates of human pancreatic growth hormone-releasing factor in man. *J Clin Invest* 73:1304-1311, 1984.

Garagorri J-M, et al: Results of early treatment of cryptorchidism with human chorionic gonadotropin. *J Pediatr* 101:923-927, 1982.

Gelato MC, et al: Effects of growth hormone-releasing factor in man. *J Clin Endocrinol Metab* 57:674-676, 1983.

Gelato MC, et al: Effects of growth hormone-releasing factor on growth hormone secretion in acromegaly. *J Clin Endocrinol Metab* 60:251-257, 1985.

Gertner JM, et al: Prospective clinical trial of human growth hormone in short children without growth hormone deficiency. *J Pediatr* 104:172-176, 1984.

Gibbs CJ Jr, et al: Clinical and pathological features and laboratory confirmation of Creutzfeldt-Jakob disease in recipient of pituitary-derived human growth hormone. *N Engl J Med* 313:734-738, 1985.

Glass AR, Vigersky RA: Correlation of acute and chronic increases in serum gonadal steroid levels after administration of human chorionic gonadotropin. *Fertil Steril* 34:41-45, 1980.

Gold MS, et al: Diagnosis of depression in 1980's. *JAMA* 245:1562-1564, 1981.

Gomez-Pan A, Rodriguez-Arnao: Somatostatin and growth hormone releasing factor: Synthesis, location, metabolism and function. *Clin Endocrinol Metab* 12:469-507, 1983.

Guillemin R, et al: Growth hormone-releasing factor from human pancreatic tumor that caused acromegaly. *Science* 218:585-587, 1982.

Hall K, Sara VR: Somatomedin levels in childhood, adolescence and adult life. *Clin Endocrinol Metab* 13:91-111, 1984.

Hauser SL, et al: Intensive immunosuppression in progressive multiple sclerosis: Randomized, three-arm study of high dose intravenous cyclophosphamide, plasma exchange, and ACTH. *N Engl J Med* 308:173-180, 1983.

Holaday JW, Bernton EW: Protirelin (TRH): Potential neuromodulator with therapeutic potential. *Arch Intern Med* 144:1138-1139, 1984.

Jackson IMD: Thyrotropin-releasing hormone. *N Engl J Med* 306:145-155, 1982.

Jackson RV, et al: Synthetic ovine corticotropin-releasing hormone: Simultaneous release of proopiolipomelanocortin peptides in man. *J Clin Endocrinol Metab* 58:740-743, 1984.

Johnston DG, et al: Hyperprolactinemia: Long-term effects of bromocriptine. *Am J Med* 75:868-874, 1983.

Kastrup KW, et al: Increased growth rate following transfer to daily sc administration from three weekly im injections of hGH in growth hormone deficient children. *Acta Endocrinol* 104:148-152, 1983.

Kleinberg DL, et al: Pergolide for treatment of pituitary tumors secreting prolactin or growth hormone. *N Engl J Med* 309:704-709, 1983.

Knobil E: Neuroendocrine control of menstrual cycle. *Rec Prog Horm Res* 36:53-88, 1980.

Koch K, et al: Creutzfeldt-Jakob disease in young adult with idiopathic hypopituitarism: Possible relation to administration of cadaveric human growth hormone. *N Engl J Med* 313:731-733, 1985.

Krieger DT: Brain peptides: What, where, and why? *Science* 222:975-985, 1983.

Lamberts SWJ, et al: Corticotropin-releasing factor (ovine) and vasopressin exert synergistic effect on adrenocorticotropin release in man. *J Clin Endocrinol Metab* 58:298-303, 1984.

Lemay A, et al: Reversible hypogonadism induced by luteinizing hormone-releasing hormone (LH-RH) agonist (Buserelin) as new therapeutic approach for endometriosis. *Fertil Steril* 41:863-871, 1984.

Lewis JW, et al: Adrenal medullary enkephalin-like peptides may mediate opioid stress analgesia. *Science* 217:557-559, 1982.

L'Hermite M, et al: Treatment of hyperprolactinemia with pergolide. *Acta Endocrinol* 103:441-445, 1983.

Luder AS, et al: Intranasal and subcutaneous treatment of central precocious puberty in both sexes with long-acting analog of luteinizing hormone-releasing hormone. *J Clin Endocrinol Metab* 58:966-972, 1984.

Mansfield MJ, et al: Long-term treatment of central precocious puberty with long-acting analogue of luteinizing hormone-releasing hormone: Effects on somatic growth and skeletal maturation. *N Engl J Med* 309:1286-1290, 1983.

Maxson WS, et al: Hyperprolactinemic response after bromocriptine withdrawal in women with prolactin-secreting pituitary tumors. *Fertil Steril* 41:218-223, 1984.

Nelson DH: Growth hormone secreting tumors, in Odell WD, Nelson DH (eds): *Pituitary Tumors*. New York, Futura, 1984.

Nicholson WE, et al: Plasma distribution, disappearance half-time, metabolic clearance rate, and degradation of synthetic ovine corticotropin-releasing factor in man. *J Clin Endocrinol Metab* 57:1263-1269, 1983.

Nortier JWR, et al: Bromocriptine therapy in acromegaly: Effects on plasma GH levels, somatomedin-C levels and clinical activity. *Clin Endocrinol* 22:209-217, 1985.

Odell WD: Further considerations of therapy of pituitary tumors, in Odell WD, Nelson DH (eds): *Pituitary Tumors*. New York, Futura, 1984.

Oppizzi G, et al: Dopaminergic treatment of acromegaly: Different effects on hormone secretion and tumor size. *J Clin Endocrinol Metab* 58:988-992, 1984.

Ory SJ: Clinical uses of luteinizing hormone-releasing hormone. *Fertil Steril* 39:577-591, 1983.

Patton ML, Woolf PD: Hyperprolactinemia and delayed puberty: Report of three cases and their response to therapy. *Pediatrics* 71:572-575, 1983.

Preece MA: Diagnosis and treatment of children with growth hormone deficiency. *Clin Endocrinol Metab* 11:1-24, 1982.

Reichlin S: Somatostatin, Parts I and II. *N Engl J Med* 309:1495-1501, 1556-1563, 1983.

Reyniak JV: Modern management of prolactinoma. *J Reprod Med*

28:257-263, 1983.

Rivier J, et al: Characterization of growth hormone-releasing factor from human pancreatic islet tumor. *Nature* 300:276-278, 1982.

Rogol AD, et al: Growth hormone release in response to human pancreatic tumor growth hormone-releasing hormone-40 in children with short stature. *J Clin Endocrinol Metab* 59:580-586, 1984.

Rosenfeld RG, Hintz RL: Diagnosis and management of growth disorders. *Drug Ther* 13:61-76, (May) 1983.

Rosenthal SM, et al: Synthetic human pancreas growth hormone-releasing factor (hpGRF, $_{1-44}$NH2) stimulates growth hormone secretion in normal men. *J Clin Endocrinol Metab* 57:677-679, 1983.

Rudman D, et al: Children with normal-variant short stature: Treatment with human growth hormone for six months. *N Engl J Med* 305:123-131, 1981.

Russo L, Moore WV: Comparison of subcutaneous and intramuscular administration of human growth hormone in therapy of growth hormone deficiency. *J Clin Endocrinol Metab* 55:1003-1006, 1982.

Saez JM, Forest MG: Kinetics of human chorionic gonadotropin-induced steroidogenic response of human fetus. I. Plasma testosterone: Implication for human chorionic gonadotropin stimulation test. *J Clin Endocrinol Metab* 49:278-283, 1979.

Schlechte JA, et al: Bone density in amenorrheic women with and without hyperprolactinemia. *Obstet Gynecol Surv* 39:35-36, 1983.

Schriock EA, et al: Effect of growth hormone (GH)-releasing hormone (GRH) on plasma GH in relation to magnitude and duration of GH deficiency in 26 children and adults with isolated GH deficiency or multiple pituitary hormone deficiencies: Evidence for hypothalamic GRH deficiency. *J Clin Endocrinol Metab* 58:1043-1049, 1984.

Schulte HM, et al: Corticotropin-releasing factor: Pharmacokinetics in man. *J Clin Endocrinol Metab* 58:192-196, 1984.

Shetty KR, Kalkhoff RK: Human chorionic gonadotropin (HCG): Treatment of obesity. *Arch Intern Med* 137:151-155, 1977.

Slag MF, et al: Impotence in medical clinic outpatients. *JAMA* 249:1736-1740, 1983.

Spiess J, et al: Sequence analysis of growth hormone releasing factor from human pancreatic islet tumor. *Biochemistry* 21:6037-6040, 1982.

Spiliotis BE, et al: Growth hormone neurosecretory dysfunction: Treatable cause of short stature. *JAMA* 251:2223-2230, 1984.

Stolar MW, et al: Plasma "big" and "big-big" growth hormone (GH) in man: Oligomeric series composed of structurally diverse GH monomers. *J Clin Endocrinol Metab* 59:212-218, 1984.

Takano K, et al: Plasma growth hormone (GH) response to GH-releasing factor in normal children with short stature and patients with pituitary dwarfism. *J Clin Endocrinol Metab* 58:236-241, 1984.

Thorner MO, et al: Human-pancreatic growth-hormone-releasing factor selectively stimulates growth hormone secretion in man. *Lancet* 1:24-28, 1983.

Thorner MO, et al: Acceleration of growth in two children treated with human growth hormone-releasing factor. *N Engl J Med* 312:4-9, 1985.

Tindall GT, et al: Human prolactin-producing adenomas and bromocriptine: Histological, immunocytochemical, ultrastructural, and morphometric study. *J Clin Endocrinol Metab* 55:1178-1183, 1982.

Turkalj I, et al: Surveillance of bromocriptine in pregnancy. *JAMA* 247:1589-1591, 1982.

Underwood LE: Report of Conference on Uses and Possible Abuses of Biosynthetic Human Growth Hormone. *N Engl J Med* 311:606-608, 1984.

Vale W, et al: Characterization of 41-residue ovine hypothalamic peptide that stimulates secretion of corticotropin and β-endorphin. *Science* 213:1394-1397, 1981.

Vance ML, et al: Human pancreatic tumor growth hormone-releasing factor: Dose-response relationships in normal man. *J Clin Endocrinol Metab* 58:838-844, 1984 A.

Vance ML, et al: Bromocriptine. *Ann Intern Med* 100:78-91, 1984 B.

Van Vliet G, et al: Growth hormone treatment for short stature. *N Engl J Med* 309:1016-1022, 1983.

Wass JAH: Growth hormone neuroregulation and clinical relevance of somatostatin. *Clin Endocrinol Metab* 12:695-724, 1983.

Wass JAH, Besser GM: Medical management of hormone-secreting tumors of pituitary. *Ann Rev Med* 34:283-294, 1983.

Wilson JD, et al: Cerebrospinal fluid rhinorrhea during treatment of pituitary tumors with bromocriptine. *Acta Endocrinol* 103:457-460, 1983.

Wilson DM, et al: Subcutaneous versus intramuscular growth hormone therapy: Growth and acute somatomedin response. *Pediatrics* 76:361-364, 1985.

Yen SSC: Clinical applications of gonadotropin-releasing hormone and gonadotropin-releasing hormone analogues. *Fertil Steril* 39:257-266, 1983.

Agents Used To Regulate Blood Glucose

43

DIABETES MELLITUS

Diabetes mellitus is a disorder with metabolic and vascular components that are interrelated. A relative or absolute deficiency of insulin activity is associated with hyperglycemia and altered lipid and protein metabolism. Vascular components consist of accelerated atherosclerosis and microangiopathy that primarily affects the renal and retinal microcirculation. Associated peripheral and autonomic neuropathies are probably secondary to metabolic abnormalities, especially hyperglycemia. Subgroups of patients with diabetes have different clinical and genetic characteristics.

Classification

The current classifications and nomenclature for diabetes and other types of glucose intolerance were established by an international workgroup sponsored by the National Diabetes Data Group of the National Institutes of Health (National Diabetes Data Group, 1979). Diabetes mellitus is classified as insulin-dependent diabetes mellitus (IDDM, Type I), noninsulin-dependent diabetes mellitus (NIDDM, Type II), or diabetes mellitus associated with other conditions (eg, pancreatic disease, hormonal, drugs), formerly known as secondary diabetes.

IDDM was once termed juvenile onset diabetes, because the age of onset is predominantly before adulthood, or ketosis-prone diabetes. Patients with IDDM require insulin to prevent ketosis and to sustain life. Islet cell antibodies are common early in the disease. The onset of diabetes sometimes follows viral infection. A strong positive correlation exists between IDDM and the presence of HLA antigens DR3 and/or DR4. Siblings who are HLA-identical to IDDM patients have a higher risk of developing the disease than siblings who are not HLA-identical (Gorsuch et al, 1982). Based on retrospective analysis, it appears that children of IDDM fathers are at greater risk of developing IDDM than children of IDDM mothers (Warram et al, 1984). There is some evidence that women with gestational diabetes are more likely to have diabetic mothers than diabetic fathers.

NIDDM was previously identified as maturity-onset (MOD), adult-onset (adulthood is the most common time of onset), or ketosis-resistant diabetes. NIDDM is further subdivided into nonobese and obese types; the latter is more common. Although insulin may be used to control hyperglycemia, patients with NIDDM are not prone to ketosis and have either relatively low insulin levels or normal to high insulin levels associated with peripheral tissue resistance to the hormone. Antagonism to insulin may occur at the receptor level due to down regulation of receptors secondary to hyperinsulinemia or at intracellular sites (Davidson, 1985). Diet therapy and exercise, alone or in conjunction with oral hypoglycemic agents or insulin, are appropriate to treat this form of diabetes.

The special classification of gestational diabetes mellitus (GDM) remains the same. It includes women who experience the *onset* or first recognition of glucose intolerance during pregnancy. GDM must be reclassified after pregnancy if glucose intolerance persists. Blood sugar must be controlled during pregnancy; insulin is used when dietary management is not successful. The role of exercise during pregnancy is being evaluated, and no firm recommendations are yet available.

Selected patients are characterized as nondiabetic with impaired glucose tolerance (IGT) and further subdivided into nonobese, obese, and IGT associated with certain conditions (eg, pancreatic disease, hormonal, drugs). An oral glucose tolerance test is necessary to establish a diagnosis of IGT. Only approximately 20% of patients with IGT develop diabetes and test results return to normal in approximately 30% of patients. Although atherosclerosis is accelerated in patients with IGT, other complications of diabetes (eg, retinopathy, nephropathy) do not develop.

Two additional statistical risk categories were established by the National Diabetes Data Group: previous abnormality of glucose tolerance (Prev AGT) and potential abnormality of glucose tolerance (Pot AGT). The former includes patients with normal glucose tolerance who have experienced diabetic hyperglycemia (eg, gestational diabetics whose glucose tolerance reverted to normal after parturition; formerly obese diabetics whose glucose tolerance became normal after weight loss; patients who were hyperglycemic under stress of infection, myocardial infarction, or surgery). The Pot AGT class includes individuals with no history of glucose intolerance who are at increased risk of developing IDDM (eg, those with islet cell antibodies; monozygotic twins; other siblings; first-degree relatives or offspring of IDDM diabetics) or NIDDM (eg, monozygotic twins, first-degree relatives, mothers of large neonates, members of certain American Indian tribes, individuals with cystic fibrosis, individuals with alpha-1 antitrypsin deficiency). Patients in these latter risk categories should be monitored for impaired glucose tolerance or frank diabetes mellitus, and the importance of avoiding obesity should be stressed.

The diagnostic criteria for diabetes mellitus and related disorders of glucose intolerance are summarized in Table 1. It is emphasized that a glucose tolerance test is not indicated to establish the diagnosis of diabetes mellitus if the fasting plasma glucose repeatedly exceeds 140 mg/dl. In addition, patients with the classic symptoms of uncontrolled diabetes (ie, polyuria, polydipsia) and random blood glucose concentrations greater than 200 mg/dl have diabetes and no formal testing is required.

Treatment

Dietary Therapy: Adherence to an appropriate diet is fundamental in the management of all types of diabetes. A caloric intake that attempts to achieve and maintain ideal body weight consonant with age, sex, height, and build, with reasonable adjustments to fit the individual's living habits, should be prescribed initially for both symptomatic and asymptomatic patients.

The goals, strategies, and priorities vary for the different types of diabetes. In IDDM, composition and timing of meals and snacks must be relatively constant because of the constraints of the insulin program. Adequate quantities of carbohydrate and protein are needed at each meal to accommodate growth and variable amounts of exercise, particularly in juveniles. Three meals a day plus midmorning, midafternoon, and bedtime snacks may facilitate treatment. Rarely, hypoglycemia occurs if meals are delayed even 15 to 30 minutes. In middle-aged, overweight patients with NIDDM not treated with insulin, precise timing of meals is relatively unimportant and secondary to caloric restriction to achieve ideal body weight.

The guidelines of the American Diabetes Association recommend 12% to 20% of total energy intake as protein, 50% to 60% as carbohydrates, and up to 30% as fats (no more than 10% as saturated fat). In the absence of definitive evidence, it is reasonable to restrict cholesterol and saturated fats and to substitute unsaturated fats when possible to impede the progression of atherosclerosis. These guidelines allow relatively more carbohydrate and less fat than previous diabetic diets (American Diabetes Association, 1979 A).

TABLE 1.
CRITERIA FOR THE DIAGNOSIS OF DIABETES MELLITUS

Condition	Plasma Glucose (mg per dl)			
	Fasting	One hour	Two hours	Three hours
Normal	<115	<200	<140	
Impaired glucose tolerance	115–140	>200	140–200	
Diabetes mellitus	>140	>200	>200	
Gestational diabetes mellitus	>105	>190	>165	>145

Standard oral glucose load is 75 g in adults, 100 g during pregnancy and 1.75 g per kg in children. At least two specimens must be elevated for diagnosis, if classic symptoms are not present. The ambulatory patient should receive a high-carbohydrate diet for three days before the test. The test is done in the morning, after a 10- to 16-hour fast. No exercise, smoking or medication is allowed during the test. The patient should not be experiencing physical or emotional stress and should not be recovering from recent illness, pregnancy, trauma or myocardial infarction.

Reprinted from Moss JM: New diagnostic classification of diabetes mellitus. Am Fam Physician 23:180, (Feb) 1981 (by permission of the American Academy of Family Physicians).

Previous dietary guidelines stressed avoidance of monosaccharides and disaccharides and preference for complex carbohydrates, such as starch. This was based on the belief that simple sugars were absorbed rapidly and caused postprandial hyperglycemia. Studies of specific carbohydrate-containing foods have documented numerous exceptions to these rules. Sugars vary in the rapidity with which they affect serum glucose levels: with maltose, the rise is rapid; with sucrose, intermediate; with lactose and fructose, slow. White potatoes, white or whole wheat bread, and corn increase glucose levels markedly, while pasta, legumes, rice, sweet potatoes, and ice cream elevate glucose moderately (Kolata, 1983; American Diabetes Association, 1984). Preference should be given to foods that cause the least increase in serum glucose. The identification of additional foods that cause small increases in blood glucose awaits further nutritional evaluation.

Dietary fiber decreases postprandial plasma glucose levels and may be beneficial. The ADA suggests that high-fiber, unrefined carbohydrates be substituted for highly refined carbohydrates with low fiber content. This may reduce insulin requirements. For special dietary considerations in controlled diabetics with hyperlipidemia, see Chapter 50, Agents Used to Treat Hyperlipidemia.

Control of Blood Glucose: The desirability of strict, rather than flexible, control of the blood glucose concentration primarily stems from the evidence in animals and humans that maintaining near normal levels of blood glucose prevents the progression of diabetic complications (Kilo, 1985). There is strong evidence to support this belief. Most experts agree that hyperglycemia is a major risk factor in the development of the nephropathy, neuropathy, and retinopathy of diabetes. A causal association between hyperglycemia and macrovascular complications has not yet been established (O'Sullivan, 1982; University Group Diabetes Program, 1982). However, poor control of blood glucose is associated with known or probable risk factors for atherosclerosis (ie, increased total cholesterol, total triglycerides, and LDL lipoproteins in plasma) (Sosenko et al, 1980).

Observations that support the causal association of hyperglycemia and microvascular and neuronal complications include development of glomerular abnormalities in normal kidneys transplanted into diabetic patients (Mauer et al, 1983); reversal of glomerular pathology in rats after beta cell transplants; and slowing of nerve conduction velocity associated with hyperglycemia, which improved after correction of hyperglycemia. The elevated sorbitol concentration in neurons caused by the conversion of glucose by aldose reductase may play a role in the pathogenesis of diabetic neuropathy (Brown and Asbury, 1984). Pain tolerance is decreased in the presence of hyperglycemia (Morley et al, 1984). Diabetic patients who developed retinopathy during a seven-year observation period were more poorly controlled than those who did not develop this complication (Howard-Williams et al, 1984). However, rapid improvement in glycemic control by multiple injections or continuous infusion of insulin was accompanied by worsening of retinopathy during the first year; this effect was transient in most patients and was not seen in the second year of observation (Dahl-Jørgensen et al, 1985).

There are well-recognized metabolic differences between IDDM and NIDDM, and the progression of complications also may be influenced differently. However, most observers believe that the reduction of blood glucose concentration is of primary importance. Attempts must be made to normalize glucose levels if this does not require unreasonable therapeutic measures. However, less stringent control may be acceptable in patients who are asymptomatic and uncooperative or unsuccessful with a weight reduction diet, have a tendency toward severe hypoglycemic episodes, are unresponsive to drug therapy, or are older than 65 years. Furthermore, severe hypoglycemia should be avoided in all patients, especially when mental alertness is compromised or the circulatory system is impaired.

HYPOGLYCEMIC AGENTS

Choice of Therapy

Patients with IDDM do not respond to oral hypoglycemic agents and require insulin. Insulin also should be used in NIDDM patients with severely impaired renal or hepatic function; during stress (eg, infection, surgery); when corticosteroid therapy is given concomitantly; and during pregnancy when blood glucose regulation is required. Patients taking oral agents or those controlled adequately by diet and exercise alone may require insulin if these complications arise.

Most patients with NIDDM are obese and have normal to elevated levels of endogenous insulin, but the target tissues are resistant to the hormone. There is a negative feedback between insulin levels and the concentration of insulin receptors in target tissues, and tissue responsiveness to insulin is correlated with the receptor concentration. The treatment of choice in these patients is caloric restriction, weight reduction, and exercise, which increases sensitivity to insulin by increasing the concentration of insulin receptors and reducing postreceptor insulin resistance. It has been suggested that the use of any hypoglycemic agent that increases insulin levels may worsen insulin insensitivity when a weight reducing diet and exercise program are not followed (ie, physiologic resistance, nonimmune type). This is because the lipogenic action of insulin theoretically could enhance further weight gain and thus increase insulin resistance. However, this explanation is not accepted by all practitioners.

Weight reduction and exercise are the foundation and most important aspects of therapy in obese diabetic patients. A team approach (physician, nurse, dietitian, patient, person responsible for food preparation) is recommended to achieve and maintain a successful weight control program.

An adequate and documented trial of diet therapy alone is essential before any hypoglycemic agent is prescribed in NIDDM (except in certain symptomatic patients or when the fasting blood sugar is more than 160 mg/dl). If a hypoglycemic agent is then deemed necessary, it should be considered *only a supplement* to continuing caloric restriction and exercise rather than a substitute for weight reduction. Opinions differ on when hypoglycemic therapy should be instituted in mildly symptomatic or asymptomatic NIDDM patients. Generally, if the fasting blood glucose remains above 160 to 200 mg/dl despite dietary compliance, drug therapy should be instituted. Some practitioners utilize drug therapy for patients whose fasting blood sugar is less than 150 mg/dl but whose postprandial levels exceed 200 mg/dl. Since the trend is toward closer control of hyperglycemia, drug therapy may be initiated when glucose levels are lower (eg, more than 140 mg/dl), particularly in younger, lean patients.

When a hypoglycemic agent is necessary to treat NIDDM, a choice between insulin and an oral sulfonylurea (acetohexamide [Dymelor], chlorpropamide [Diabinese], glipizide [Glucotrol], glyburide [DiaBeta, Micronase], tolazamide [Ronase, Tolinase], tolbutamide [Orinase, SK-Tolbutamide]) must be made. (The only biguanide available in the United States, phenformin, may be obtained only under special circumstances; see the evaluation.) The choice between an oral agent and insulin is complicated by the decade-old controversy about the findings of the University Group Diabetes Program (UGDP), and practice varies widely in the United States. In Europe, where the impact of the UGDP study was minimal, the clinical use of oral agents (sulfonylureas and biguanides) has always been more liberal. However, guidelines for the selection of a hypoglycemic agent can be suggested.

When properly used, insulin is probably more effective in controlling blood glucose on a long-term basis. Primary and secondary (after initial control) failures do occur with oral hypoglycemic agents, but these drugs are more convenient and easier to administer than insulin. This is particularly important in elderly patients who have poor vision and in whom injection of incorrectly measured doses may cause hypoglycemia. Ease of administration is also important for patients with a strong aversion to injecting insulin. Oral agents also are sometimes used in NIDDM patients who are allergic to insulin and unwilling or unable to undergo desensitization.

Any attempt to control hyperglycemia in asymptomatic NIDDM patients should be preceded by an adequate trial of diet therapy. If this fails, many physicians routinely prescribe oral hypoglycemic agents initially because of their convenience, reserving insulin for those in whom primary or secondary failure occurs. However, other physicians prescribe oral hypoglycemic agents rarely, if ever, preferring insulin if a hypoglycemic agent is needed. Still other physicians prefer insulin when dietary therapy fails for certain types of patients (eg, under 40 years, lean, cardiovascular risk factors). Insulin is preferred for initial control if blood glucose levels are very high. It has been suggested that low C-peptide levels identify NIDDM patients who are likely to require insulin therapy (Rendell, 1983). Patients stabilized on a low daily dose of insulin sometimes may be placed on oral therapy or diet alone for maintenance. In summary, although insulin has greater overall effectiveness, the physician must assess other factors that may favor use of an oral agent (Advisory Panel on Oral Hypoglycemic Drugs, American Medical Association, 1980). Discussions of the pathophysiology and management of NIDDM are available (Bernstein, 1983; Beaser, 1984; Lipson and Lipson, 1984; Ward et al, 1984).

Combined regimens of oral hypoglycemic agents and insulin control blood glucose in some NIDDM patients. Studies suggest that such a combination may improve glycemic control at least temporarily in selected patients characterized by leanness, short duration of NIDDM, and residual endogenous insulin secretion. However, more research is necessary before this combination can be recommended (Burke et al, 1984; Osei et al, 1984; *Diabetes Care*, 1985).

UGDP Study

The UGDP study was initiated to determine whether the development and progression of vascular complications in asymptomatic patients with mild NIDDM could be avoided or mitigated by controlling the blood glucose level, but did not answer this question. The study was discontinued because of the emerging pattern of a higher incidence of cardiovascular deaths in certain groups treated with oral agents. The assumption was widely made that oral antidiabetic drugs were cardiotoxic and inappropriate for use in patients with NIDDM and cardiovascular risk factors. Subsequent to the publication of these results, various aspects of the UGDP (eg, study design and interpretation, inappropriate treatment of some groups by current standards) have been criticized. Compelling arguments have been offered on both sides by recognized authorities (Biometric Society, 1975; Boyden and Bressler, 1979; Feinstein, 1979; Kilo et al, 1980 A and B).

Further analysis of the UGDP data has revealed the following: (1) The cardiovascular death rate in the placebo group that was compared to the tolbutamide group may have been spuriously low. (2) Baseline cardiovascular risk factors were higher in the tolbutamide group. (3) Excess cardiovascular deaths in the tolbutamide group occurred primarily in patients whose fasting blood glucose exceeded 200 mg/dl. By current standards, the failure to control hyperglycemia constitutes inappropriate use of tolbutamide (Kilo et al, 1980 A and B).

Other studies that differed substantially in design from the UGDP do not confirm the increased mortality from cardiovascular disease with long-term use of tolbutamide and phenformin. Evidence of the cardiotoxicity of oral hypoglycemic drugs, therefore, appears to be less tenable than a decade ago. The American Diabetes Association reassessed its original support of the UGDP results and suggested that "any formal recommendations on the use of tolbutamide in maturity-onset diabetes that are based on the initial findings of the UGDP study should be held in abeyance" (American Diabetes Association, 1979 B).

On the other hand, the possibility that tolbutamide has detrimental cardiovascular effects is consistent with evidence demonstrating its inotropic effect on the myocardium. In addition, a pharmacogenetic study of tolbutamide metabolism demonstrated a ninefold variation in plasma half-life in almost one-fourth of the subjects studied, which appeared to be an inherited autosomal trait. If tolbutamide does have cardiotoxic properties, this pharmacogenetic finding may account for the manifestation of this complication in "slow inactivators" (Scott and Poffenbarger, 1978).

Unfortunately, the emphasis on the putative cardiotoxicity of the sulfonylureas has diverted attention from other considerations in the selection of hypoglycemic drugs (eg, relative efficacy, proper use of oral agents). See also the section on Oral Hypoglycemic Agents.

INSULINS

Preparations, Regimens, and Delivery Systems

Insulins available in the United States differ in concentration, time of onset and duration of action, purity, and species of origin, and clinically significant differences among them have been reviewed (Galloway, 1980; Deckert, 1980). Insulin U100 (100 units/ml) is the most commonly used concentration. (The production of U80 preparations was discontinued in 1980.)

Insulins may be divided into rapid-, intermediate-, and long-acting groups (see Table 2). Insulin injection (crystalline zinc insulin, regular insulin) has a rapid onset and short duration of action. Isophane (NPH) (intermediate-acting) and protamine zinc (long-acting) insulins are conjugated with large protein molecules, which delays absorption and prolongs their duration of action. (These preparations have an isoelectric point at physiologic pH, which reduces solubility and contributes to their long action.)

The large particle size and crystalline form of extended insulin zinc suspension (ultralente insulin) also delay absorption and prolong the duration of action. Because of its small particle size and amorphous structure, prompt insulin zinc suspension (semilente insulin) is more rapidly absorbed and shorter acting. The combination of 70% ultralente and 30% semilente insulin produces insulin zinc suspension (lente insulin), which has an intermediate duration of action and approximates the general characteristics of isophane insulin.

Advances in industrial chemistry continue to improve the stability and purity of insulin. Unbuffered regular insulin with neutral pH (7.4) has been termed Neutral Regular Insulin (NRI). Patients may keep the bottle currently in use (usually a two- to four-week supply) at room temperature but protected from excessive heat and sunlight. Additional bottles should be refrigerated until needed.

In 1980, the FDA ordered the purity of insulin products to be designated as "conventional" and "purified." Purified preparations contain less than 10 ppm proinsulin (the most antigenic protein contaminant); "single component" and "monocomponent" were terms formerly used to distinguish preparations of this purity. In general, since 1980, insulins of much higher purity have become available from several manufacturers.

Conventional insulins usually are mixtures of bovine-porcine origin, although conventional single species insulins are available. Purified preparations are usually of either bovine or porcine origin. Human insulin is also available. All human insulin preparations are purified.

Isophane and lente insulin have been considered comparable preparations, but experimental evidence has shown some differences in their course of action, compatibility with other insulins, and immunogenicity. Although both insulins are intermediate acting, the time of peak action is slightly earlier for NPH (see Table 2).

Lente insulin appears to be more immunogenic than isophane and may exacerbate zinc allergy in sensitive individuals. On the other hand, the protamine contained in isophane may augment insulin allergy or, rarely, may sensitize the patient to protamine and cause an allergic response at a later time (eg, when protamine is used to neutralize the anticoagulant action of heparin).

Mixing Insulins: Regular insulin may be mixed with other insulins subject to certain limitations. Regular insulin mixed with NPH should be used immediately or within five minutes; the regular insulin may be altered slightly, resulting in more prolonged action. With preparations containing greater amounts of protamine than NPH (ie, protamine zinc insulins), the degree to which regular insulin loses solubility (and becomes longer acting) depends on the amount of excess protamine. The action of regular insulin may be delayed when it is mixed with lente insulin (Heine et al, 1984). When regular insulin is mixed with ultralente insulin or in a ratio of 1:3 (regular to lente), the excess zinc may complex with regular insulin and decrease its solubility. This effect may increase with time (Nolte et al, 1983). Such mixtures should be injected immediately to minimize changes in the time course of action of the regular insulin. These observations suggest reexamination of the procedure when premixed syringes containing a short-acting and a longer acting preparation are prepared for later use.

Human Insulin: The goal of producing the purest insulins possible has led to methods of synthesizing insulin identical to that produced by the human pancreas. Two approaches have been utilized. The first technique uses recombinant DNA technology and resulted in the introduction of human insulin as the first marketed product of this technology. Synthetic genes for insulin A and B chains are spliced to *Escherichia coli* genes for beta-galactosidase. The insulin chains are cleaved from the beta-galactosidase and joined with sulfide bonds to form the insulin molecule. Alternatively, the proinsulin gene may be introduced into *E. coli* and the resulting proinsulin then converted to insulin.

The second method utilizes an enzymatic process that converts porcine to human insulin. In this process, threonine is substituted for the single amino acid that differs from human insulin, the terminal alanine on the B-chain.

In some patients, human insulin may have a more rapid onset and shorter duration of action compared to a comparable pork product. As with purified pork insulin, questions about clinical importance must be resolved (see the section on Choice of Insulin Preparation).

Purified Insulin Preparations: The clinical significance of pure versus conventional insulin preparations has not been determined. Although purified preparations produce lower antibody titers, the species of origin is more important to immunogenicity than the purity. Pork insulin differs from human insulin by only one amino acid and is less immunogenic than beef preparations. Purified pork insulin and human insulin are least immunogenic.

Insulin antibodies are minimal in patients treated solely with purified pork insulin or human insulin. Lipodystrophies are unusual in these patients, and lipoatrophy improves after treatment with purified pork insulin.

The relationship between insulin antibody formation and dosage requirements has been considered. Early experiments using relatively impure preparations suggested that the dose could be reduced by 10% to 20% by substituting a purified pork preparation (such dosage reductions are undertaken

TABLE 2.
INSULIN PREPARATIONS AVAILABLE IN THE UNITED STATES[1]

Preparation (Tradename)	Source	Purified[2]	Concentration[3] (units/ml)	Hours After Subcutaneous Administration[4]		
				Onset of Action[5]	Maximum Effect	Duration of Action[5]
RAPID ACTING						
Insulin Injection (Regular, Crystalline Zinc)						
Regular Iletin I (Lilly)	Bovine-porcine	No	40 & 100	½–1	2–4	6–8
Regular Insulin (Squibb-Novo)	Porcine	No	100	½	2½–5	8
Pork Regular Iletin II (Lilly)	Porcine	Yes	100	½–1	2–4	6–8
Beef Regular Iletin II (Lilly)	Bovine	Yes	100	½–1	2–4	6–8
Velosulin (Nordisk-USA)	Porcine	Yes	100	½	1–3	8
Purified Pork Insulin (Squibb-Novo)	Porcine	Yes	100	½	2½–5	8
Humulin R (Lilly)	Human[6]	NA	100	½–1	2–4	6–8
Novolin R (Squibb-Novo)	Human[7]	NA	100	½	2½–5	8
Regular (Concentrated) Iletin II,[1] U-500 (Lilly)	Pork	Yes	500	½	---	24
Prompt Insulin Zinc Suspension (Semilente)						
Semilente Iletin I (Lilly)	Bovine-porcine	No	40 & 100	1–3	3–8	10–16
Semilente Insulin (Squibb-Novo)	Bovine	No	100	1½	5–10	16
Semilente Purified Pork Prompt Insulin (Squibb-Novo)	Porcine	Yes	100	1½	5–10	16
INTERMEDIATE ACTING						
Isophane (NPH) 70% Regular Insulin 30%						
Mixtard (Nordisk-USA)	Porcine	Yes	100	½	4–8	24
Isophane (NPH) Insulin Suspension						
NPH Iletin I (Lilly)	Bovine-porcine	No	40 & 100	2	6–12	18–26
NPH Insulin (Squibb-Novo)	Bovine	No	100	1½	4–12	24
Beef NPH Iletin II (Lilly)	Bovine	Yes	100	2	6–12	18–26
Pork NPH Iletin II (Lilly)	Porcine	Yes	100	2	6–12	18–26
NPH Purified Pork Isophane Insulin (Squibb-Novo)	Porcine	Yes	100	1½	4–12	24
Insulatard NPH (Nordisk-USA)	Porcine	Yes	100	1½	4–12	24
Humulin N (Lilly)	Human[6]	NA	100	1–2	6–12	18–24
Novolin N (Squibb-Novo)	Human[7]	NA	100	1½	4–12	24
Insulin Zinc Suspension (Lente)						
Lente Iletin I (Lilly)	Bovine-porcine	No	40 & 100	2–4	6–12	18–26
Lente Insulin (Squibb-Novo)	Bovine	No	100	2½	7–15	24
Beef Lente Iletin II (Lilly)	Bovine	Yes	100	2–4	6–12	18–26
Pork Lente Iletin II (Lilly)	Porcine	Yes	100	2–4	6–12	18–26
Lente Purified Pork Insulin (Squibb-Novo)	Porcine	Yes	100	2½	7–15	22
Humulin L (Lilly)	Human[6]	NA	100	1–3	6–12	18–24
Novolin L (Squibb-Novo)	Human[7]	NA	100	2½	7–15	22

(Continued on next page)

Preparation (Tradename)	Source	Purified[2]	Concentration[3] (units/ml)	Hours After Subcutaneous Administration[4]		
				Onset of Action[5]	Maximum Effect	Duration of Action[5]
LONG ACTING						
Protamine Zinc Insulin Suspension						
Protamine Zinc & Iletin I (Lilly)	Bovine-porcine	No	40 & 100	4–8	14–24	28–36
Beef Protamine Zinc & Iletin II (Lilly)	Bovine	Yes	100	4–8	14–24	28–36
Pork Protamine Zinc & Iletin II (Lilly)	Porcine	Yes	100	4–8	14–24	28–36
Extended Insulin Zinc Suspension (Ultralente)						
Ultralente Iletin I (Lilly)	Bovine-porcine	No	40 & 100	4–8	14–24	28–36
Ultralente Insulin (Squibb-Novo)	Bovine	No	100	4	10–30	36
Ultralente Purified Beef Insulin (Squibb-Novo)	Bovine	Yes	100	4	10–30	36

[1]All preparations are nonprescription except Regular (Concentrated) Iletin II U-500, a concentrated (500 units/ml) purified pork preparation for use in severe insulin resistance. This preparation may show activity over a 24-hour period.

[2]Less than 10 ppm proinsulin contamination.

[3]In 10 ml containers

[4]The duration of action is for a single injection. With daily injections, the duration of the longer acting insulins is longer than indicated.

[5]Onset and duration of action vary among patients and are influenced by such factors as concentration and volume, site and depth of injection.

[6]Biosynthetic; recombinant DNA origin

[7]Semisynthetic; conversion from pork insulin

gradually due to the long half-life of IgG). However, although the insulin antibody titer usually decreases, the dosage requirement is reduced in only 12% to 43% of patients; some patients require no change or even an increase in dose of the purified preparation. Human insulin preparations are comparable in this respect to purified pork insulins.

The long-term importance of using purified preparations or human insulin to reduce antibody formation in patients who are controlled satisfactorily with conventional preparations is unknown.

Choice of Insulin Preparation: There appears to be no compelling reason to substitute a purified pork or human preparation for a conventional insulin if control of diabetes is satisfactory. However, theoretically, human insulin should be preferred to the closest animal-derived alternative. Human insulin is also slightly less antigenic than purified pork insulin; therefore, when a purified preparation is being considered, human insulin appears to be preferable if other factors are equal.

Clinical situations in which purified pork or human insulin may be used to advantage include: (1) Patients with local insulin allergy, immunologic insulin resistance, or injection site lipodystrophies. (2) When insulin treatment is temporary (eg, gestational diabetes, NIDDM patients treated intermittently with insulin during infection or surgery, insulin given as part of total parenteral nutrition). Patients with systemic insulin allergy or immunologic resistance frequently have a history of interrupted insulin therapy. (3) Newly diagnosed patients, especially if they are young, in whom any potential benefits of

long-term treatment with low immunogenic insulin might be realized (*Diabetes Care*, 1980; Sonnenberg and Berger 1983).

Because of the wide variability in purity, patients should use the same preparation continuously to avoid a change in dosage requirement: Patients *should not arbitrarily change* to insulin of a different *degree of purity* or of a *different species of origin* without careful supervision.

Insulin Pumps: The importance of strict regulation of serum glucose is becoming more widely accepted. Portable insulin infusion pumps that provide constant, smoother control of glucose levels have been developed, and several devices that deliver insulin subcutaneously, intramuscularly, intraperitoneally, or intravenously are being tested clinically. Subcutaneous infusion pumps are "open-loop" devices that permit regulation of the infusion rate manually or by preprogrammed control. The patient must be willing and able to monitor blood glucose at home. More sophisticated "closed-loop" devices contain a built-in glucose sensor that automatically regulates the dose of insulin; these pumps are currently available for bedside use in hospitals to manage ketoacidosis and to regulate glucose during surgery, labor, and delivery. These devices require constant sampling of blood and are currently used only for acute situations (up to two days). An implantable or portable "artificial endocrine pancreas" of this capability requires further technologic refinements, such as miniaturization of components. Numerous functional problems (eg, optimal route of administration, insulin precipitation, power supply, biocompatibility of components) also must be solved before production and general use become feasible.

Although not proven conclusively, it is generally believed that strict control of blood glucose levels will reduce the chronic micro- and possibly macrovascular complications of diabetes. More clinical experience is necessary before the comparative benefits and risks of using continuous subcutaneous insulin infusion (CSII) versus conventional intensive insulin therapy to achieve this end can be determined with assurance. However, CSII is probably at least as effective as conventional intensive insulin therapy in properly selected patients. Use of CSII requires the participation and backup of a skilled professional team, as well as a highly motivated patient (American Diabetes Association, 1985 A).

Patient characteristics and circumstances in which CSII might be utilized include: (1) Acute situations, such as surgery, treatment of ketoacidosis, and labor and delivery; (2) if the patient can be expected to derive long-term benefits from close control of blood glucose; (3) when the patient is planning to become pregnant or from the beginning of pregnancy; (4) in motivated adolescents, particularly those with growth retardation; (5) in patients who respond poorly to conventional intensive insulin therapy; and (6) in patients who may prefer or benefit from the increased flexibility in meal scheduling that may result from CSII. Patients who are not good candidates for CSII include those unable or unwilling to monitor their blood glucose levels; those not expected to derive long-term benefit due to age or life expectancy; those at risk of unrecognized hypoglycemia; those with renal insufficiency not corrected by a kidney transplant; and those with severe autonomic neuropathy (Bonner, 1985; Felig and Bergman, 1983; Tamborlane and Press, 1984).

Insulin pumps are associated with certain adverse effects. *Infection* at the site of needle insertion is the most common and the incidence may be increased in patients who are nasal carriers of *Staphylococcus aureus* (Mecklenburg et al, 1984). Proper preparation and care of the infusion site is important, and the infusion set should be changed every other day. *Ketoacidosis* may occur more frequently with CSII than conventional intensive insulin therapy. This may be caused by mechanical malfunction of the pump, battery, or tubing. Furthermore, ketoacidosis may occur within hours of pump failure; the lack of an insulin depot probably contributes to the rapidity of this effect. Unexplained increases in blood glucose should alert the patient to check the integrity of the infusion line. If blood glucose levels remain elevated, the infusion set should be changed (Bonner, 1985). Hypoglycemia also occurs with CSII, but rarely results from pump malfunction, and the frequency is no greater than with conventional intensive insulin therapy. There appears to be no increased risk of death due to CSII compared to conventional intensive insulin therapy (Teutsch et al, 1984).

Transplantation: Human transplantation of pancreatic islet tissue is being investigated. Numerous variations have been attempted from transplanting part or all of a pancreas (some attached to the duodenum) to transplanting islets via injection into various sites. Major obstacles include obtaining an adequate supply of transplantable tissues, graft rejection, and for pancreas grafts, the disposition of pancreatic exocrine secretions. The latter problem possibly can be managed by suppressing exocrine secretion with synthetic polymers injected into the duct or by allowing the secretions to drain into the gut through the attached duodenum (Sutherland et al, 1984). If these obstacles are resolved and techniques become generally available, the need for exogenous insulin and delivery systems eventually may be obviated. However, if there is a persistent autoimmune response, the transplanted islets or pancreas may fail.

Other Recent Developments: Routes of administration other than by injection would simplify insulin administration and be more convenient and comfortable for the patient. Intranasal application of aerosolized insulin was studied as a possible adjunct to subcutaneous administration. Nasal irritation occurred in most patients, and five to ten times the usual dose was required. The potential effect of inflamed nasal membranes due to viral infections on the amount of insulin absorbed is not known (Salzman et al, 1985). The possibility of enclosing insulin within a chemical complex that resists digestion, thus allowing oral administration, also is being investigated.

Management

An intermediate-acting preparation plus regular insulin is chosen for *initial treatment* of IDDM. In the absence of ketosis or other acute complications, the initial dose for adults may be 10 to 20 units given (in combination) before breakfast. Depending upon the response, postprandial blood glucose levels, and urine tests, this dose may be increased by 5 to 10 units weekly until control is satisfactory. Some practitioners recommend initiating insulin therapy with two injections per day to establish better control of blood glucose (see below). The initial insulin dosage range for young diabetic patients is 0.7 to 1.5 units/kg.

Blood glucose measurements before meals and at bedtime pinpoint the timing of hyperglycemia. Capillary glucose determinations performed by the patient at home using glucose reagent strips should be used to adjust the insulin dose. Self-monitoring of blood glucose is recommended for all diabetic patients who require insulin, but is most important for those using insulin pumps or receiving multiple injections daily, pregnant (or planning to be pregnant) patients, and those who become hypoglycemic without the usual warning symptoms (American Diabetes Association, 1985 B). However, urine testing (using second-voided specimens) is preferable to no testing and may be adequate for some patients (eg, an NIDDM patient whose renal threshold for glucose is normal); urine testing remains useful for detecting ketones.

Glycosylated hemoglobin assays provide information on the average blood glucose levels during the previous two months, but they are not helpful for adjusting day-to-day insulin requirements. These assays performed three to four times yearly are an adjunct to the primary method of monitoring blood glucose and validate the patient's home measurements. Because values vary among laboratories, a single laboratory should be used for a given patient (Baynes et al, 1984; Health and Public Policy Committee, American College of Physicians, 1984).

Although some NIDDM patients who take insulin can be managed with one daily injection, regulation of the dosage for most IDDM patients is usually achieved with (at least) two injections daily, one before breakfast and the other before the evening meal. Increasing the morning dose of intermediate-acting insulin generally corrects hyperglycemia occurring before the evening meal or at bedtime; prebreakfast hyperglycemia that is not a sequel of nocturnal hypoglycemia is often controlled by reducing the size of the bedtime snack and/or giving an additional dose of an intermediate-acting preparation before the evening meal; alternatively, the intermediate-acting preparation can be given at bedtime to avoid prebreakfast hyperglycemia due to the dawn phenomenon.

Regular insulin is often added to the intermediate-acting preparation to control blood glucose before the latter becomes effective. With twice daily injections (split-dose regimens), regular insulin added to the prebreakfast dose of the intermediate-acting preparation (given in the same injection) prevents hyperglycemia before lunch; also, regular insulin added to the intermediate-acting preparation before the evening meal prevents hyperglycemia before the bedtime snack. Most commonly, the total dose is divided to provide two-thirds to three-fourths in the morning; this injection should be given 15 to 30 minutes before breakfast. This interval allows the peak of carbohydrate absorption to coincide more closely with the peak activity of regular insulin.

Three or more daily injections of insulin or continuous subcutaneous insulin injection (CSII) are sometimes used to provide optimum control. These intensified insulin regimens require the patient to monitor blood glucose several times daily. In these cases, an intermediate- or long-acting insulin is used (before the evening meal or at bedtime) in combination with regular insulin, which is added before meals and in the evening as required to achieve optimum control (Skyler et al, 1981).

A growing number of physicians recommend divided doses as the standard regimen, and single-dose therapy only in certain situations (eg, patients over 65 years, patients adequately controlled on one injection/day). Divided doses are especially indicated (1) when diabetes is otherwise difficult to control; (2) when severe prebreakfast hyperglycemia cannot be corrected by one dose daily; and (3) when more than 100 units daily is required (ordinary insulin syringes do not hold more than 100 units). In these patients, dietary carbohydrate is often divided into six or seven feedings.

A between-meal snack containing 15 to 25 g of carbohydrate plus additional protein and fat may be necessary at the time of peak action of the insulin preparation being used, and a bedtime snack also is often needed. These snacks help to prevent hypoglycemic reactions that occur at night, between meals, or before exercise; along with regular exercise, this permits insulin dosage to be tailored to the patient's specific needs.

Vigorous exercise after appropriate training and conditioning is important in diabetic management because it increases utilization of glucose by muscle and decreases insulin requirements. It also provides a healthy sense of well-being. Exercise achieves this effect partially by increasing the binding of insulin to receptors. The patient may find it helpful to take a small snack before exercise to prevent hypoglycemia. Because exercise may increase the rate of absorption of insulin, it may be advisable to avoid exercise immediately after insulin is injected.

Newly diagnosed IDDM patients may experience a partial or, infrequently, a complete but temporary remission and may not require insulin during this period ("honeymoon phase"). Immunosuppressive therapy has been investigated to delay or prevent further islet cell destruction that may be due to immune mechanisms in early IDDM. In one study, over 50% of newly diagnosed diabetic patients treated with cyclosporine [Sandimmune] became insulin-independent during treatment, while only 3% of patients not given cyclosporine had a complete remission. Best results were obtained in patients with the shortest duration of disease (Stiller et al, 1984). In the future, early detection of IDDM coupled with some form of immunotherapy may prevent full expression of IDDM. However, the long-term dangers of immunosuppressants must be recognized, especially in patients with a life expectancy of 30 to 50 years.

Use in Special Situations

Prompt recognition and appropriate management of the complications of insulin therapy are essential for the safety of the patient and the effective control of diabetes mellitus. Patients who have intercurrent illness, emotional stress, or trauma or those hospitalized for major illness may require, at least temporarily, multiple injections of a rapid-acting human insulin. Almost invariably, a temporary increase in total requirements will have been created by the complication. The degree of glycosuria, ketonuria, and hyperglycemia occurring subsequently determines the timing, type, and amount of insulin needed.

Every diabetic patient taking insulin should carry some form of readily available carbohydrate, as well as an identification card containing pertinent information. The availability of glucagon and instruction in its proper use (family members and close friends) are mandatory for all patients who require insulin.

Pregnancy: The most common form of diabetes in pregnancy (90% of diabetic pregnancies) is gestational diabetes (GDM), in which diagnosis is made during pregnancy (often in the third trimester). It occurs in 1% to 2% of pregnancies. These patients commonly have a family history of diabetes and one-half may develop overt diabetes within 15 years of onset of GDM.

The diabetogenic effects of the hormones produced during pregnancy (eg, human placental lactogen, estrogen, progesterone) increase insulin requirements, while the placenta simultaneously promotes insulin catabolism. If symptoms do not respond to diet therapy alone, insulin is required. An oral agent should not be used because these agents cross the placenta and decrease fetal blood glucose levels late in pregnancy. Use of a purified insulin preparation or human insulin may preclude potential insulin sensitization and related problems if overt diabetes develops subsequently.

In diabetic pregnancies, the risk of many fetal and neonatal complications is increased and is generally related to the severity of the disease. The risk of prematurity, perinatal death, and congenital anomalies is three to four times greater in pregnant IDDM patients with vascular complications. The risk of spontaneous abortion also appears to be higher in those with IDDM (Miodovnik et al, 1984). Poorly controlled diabetes (as determined by hemoglobin A_{1c} levels) in early pregnancy is associated with an increased risk of major structural malformations in neonates (Miller et al, 1981). These observations lend support to the advice that diabetic women plan their pregnancies and that close control of blood glucose should be established *before* conception and maintained throughout the critical period of organogenesis, as well as later in pregnancy (Cousins, 1983; Simpson et al, 1983). The efficacy of such a program has not yet been proved, but investigations are in progress to evaluate the beneficial effects of such control.

Macrosomia occurs commonly in newborns of diabetic mothers. It has been assumed that macrosomia is related to maternal hyperglycemia and that stricter control of maternal blood glucose would reduce the incidence. However, clinical evidence of a cause-and-effect relationship has been conflicting.

More stringent control of blood glucose levels during pregnancy may require more frequent injections. The usual schedule includes two injections (before breakfast and the evening meal) of a combination of short- and intermediate-acting insulins. A third or even fourth daily injection may be required for ideal control. In the pregnant IDDM patient, insulin needs may be quite different than before pregnancy and may vary throughout the course of the pregnancy. It is particularly important to avoid ketoacidosis, coma, and hypoglycemia, which tend to occur in the second or third trimester, since these complications may cause fetal death. Self-monitoring of capillary blood glucose is preferred to facilitate accurate dosage adjustments. Urine testing is usually not sensitive enough to maintain close control; results are usually negative in reasonably well-controlled pregnant diabetics. However, the renal threshold in pregnancy may decrease so much that glycosuria is present (eg, after meals) even when the patient is satisfactorily controlled. Maternal blood sugar should be regulated as close to normal pregnancy levels as possible (60 to 120 mg/dl plasma). Insulin dosage should be adjusted if the fasting plasma glucose exceeds 120 mg/dl or the postprandial glucose exceeds 140 mg/dl. CSII is also used to achieve close blood glucose control during pregnancy. In one study of 22 pregnant diabetic women, both intensive conventional insulin therapy and CSII provided excellent metabolic control and there were no differences in outcome between the two methods (Coustan et al, 1986).

Insulin requirements generally are unchanged or even decreased slightly during the first trimester but increase during the second and third trimesters. One study showed a disparity between the increased need for insulin in pregnant IDDM and NIDDM patients. Pregnant IDDM patients required 38% more insulin from the second to third trimester (similar to normal pregnant women), while pregnant NIDDM patients required a 98% increase (Rigg et al, 1980). During the last month of pregnancy, insulin needs may decrease slightly, but a 50% decrease may indicate placental malfunction and fetal distress.

Close control of blood glucose and fluctuations in insulin requirement during labor can be managed by constant intravenous infusion of dextrose and insulin. The insulin requirement is reduced or even absent during labor, as in other forms of strenuous exertion. Neonatal hypoglycemia, believed to be caused by fetal insulinemia, was not avoided by maintaining euglycemia with an insulin infusion during labor (Golde et al, 1982). Oral feeding in the first few hours of life is important to avoid severe hypoglycemia.

Delivery of the infant and placenta abruptly ends diabetogenic stress; in the first day postpartum, the insulin requirement may decrease precipitously to one-half to two-thirds of the prepregnancy level. Thereafter, there is a gradual increase until about three to five days postpartum when the usual prepregnancy level of insulin is needed. In GDM patients, insulin may not be required postpartum. If premature labor ensues, corticosteroids (to enhance pulmonary maturity) and/or a uterine relaxant, such as ritodrine [Yutopar] to inhibit labor, may be used. Supplemental insulin may be necessary to offset the hyperglycemic effects of these agents.

See reviews by Freinkel, 1985, and Freinkel et al, 1985, for general management of diabetic pregnancy.

Surgery: Diabetic patients should be prepared for the stress of surgery and maintained intraoperatively with appropriate measures. Patients with long-standing diabetes should be evaluated for renal and cardiovascular function, neuropathy and retinopathy, infection, or other conditions that could adversely affect surgical outcome or recovery. Correction of serious problems may necessitate delay of surgery. For example, intraoperative changes in blood pressure or coagulation may cause retinal hemorrhage in a patient with severe retinopathy, which may be better treated before surgery (Gallina et al, 1983).

Insulin for the operative period may be given as an intermediate-acting preparation before and immediately after surgery in the recovery room. Glucose levels must be monitored during the procedure and additional regular insulin may be given intravenously if required. Alternatively, an infusion pump may be utilized to deliver regular insulin in saline.

In IDDM patients, inadequate intraoperative monitoring increases the risk of hyperglycemia, ketoacidosis, and electrolyte imbalance. Those with NIDDM may develop hyperglycemia and hyperosmolarity. If a diabetic patient requires emergency surgery, glycemic control must be established; blood glucose and electrolytes should be monitored. If the patient is hyperglycemic, insulin infusion may result in a rapid and dangerous decrease in serum potassium unless appropriate replacement is given.

Postoperatively, the usual insulin regimen and normal diet may be resumed at the same time. If food intake is restricted, the amount of insulin administered is reduced proportionately.

Diabetic Ketoacidosis: This potentially life-threatening emergency requires prompt diagnosis, accurate estimation of severity, and treatment of any precipitating factor, as well as skillful administration of insulin, fluids, and electrolytes (particularly potassium) and prompt treatment of any coexisting condition. Although there may be intracellular depletion of potassium, serum levels initially may be normal or high. Replacement of potassium should be started as soon as the serum potassium level begins to decline, even though it may still be above normal levels.

Ketoacidosis is now treated with much smaller doses of insulin than were formerly utilized. Older regimens utilized 200 to 800 units of insulin to control an episode, whereas less than 100 units may be needed using new, low-dose regimens (see the evaluation on Insulin Injection). When low-dose infusions are used, the insulin dose should be increased if the blood glucose level is not decreased by 5% to 10%/hour. A decrease in serum glucose of approximately 70 mg/dl/hour indicates adequate insulin therapy (Alberti, 1977; Heber et al, 1977; Kreisberg, 1978). Initially, 0.9% (normal) saline is administered for the first one to two hours; 0.45% (half-normal) saline then is given. This prevents too rapid reduction in osmolality, which may increase the risk of cerebral edema.

Potassium salts may be given as potassium chloride and potassium phosphate. The addition of phosphate has the theoretical advantage of enhancing tissue oxygenation. In ketoacidosis, erythrocyte 2, 3-diphosphoglycerate (2, 3-DPG) is reduced, which increases the affinity of hemoglobin for oxygen and less oxygen is released to tissues. Acidosis itself favors oxygen release, but with correction of the pH to normal, the reduced 2, 3-DPG may adversely affect oxygen supply to the tissues. Administration of phosphate salts speeds replacement of 2, 3-DPG, which otherwise may take several days. However, it has been suggested that this treatment, although theoretically advantageous, has little practical effect on tissue oxygenation (Fisher and Kitabchi, 1983). Phosphate must be given cautiously to avoid hypocalcemia.

Although bicarbonate rapidly corrects pH, its use in ketoacidosis is generally not recommended because the resulting shift of potassium to the intracellular compartment may cause hypokalemia. Bicarbonate may be used in severe acidosis to correct the pH to 7.1 but should not be used beyond that point. In one study, the use of bicarbonate, even for severe acidosis, was not advantageous when a low-dose insulin regimen was used (Lever and Jaspan, 1983). (See reviews by Felts, 1983, and Sperling, 1984.)

Hyperosmolar (Nonketotic) Coma: This condition may be confused initially with stroke or a severe hypoglycemic reaction. It is observed most often in individuals over 60 years and may complicate pre-existing diabetes or it may present as the initial manifestation of diabetes. It rarely occurs in younger diabetics. Hyperosmolar coma represents an incomplete manifestation of the metabolic derangement seen in diabetic ketoacidosis. Although hyperglycemia occurs, lipolysis is not increased and ketosis and acidosis do not result or are present to a slight degree.

Associated illness, physiologic stress, or a history of taking a drug(s) that inhibits insulin secretion or elevates blood glucose is common. The mortality rate is high (10% to 20%) and the cause of death is usually the complicating illness rather than the metabolic abnormality. Polydipsia and polyuria are present for several days to several weeks previously. Weight loss, stupor or coma, severe dehydration, and very high levels of glucose (800 to 1,500 mg/dl plasma or more) are observed. Azotemia and hyperosmolarity are present. The insulin requirement is usually less than for diabetic ketoacidosis and more fluid may be needed. There is some disagreement about

the most appropriate replacement fluid; 10 or more liters of hypotonic electrolyte solution (eg, 0.45% sodium chloride) may be given during the first 12 to 36 hours to correct hyperosmolarity (urine output is monitored). Alternatively, 0.9% saline may be preferred initially if there is severe intravascular volume depletion, and hypotonic solution is administered thereafter. Potassium replacement must be monitored carefully, particularly since cardiac complications may be present in older patients. Morbidity and central nervous system complications are common in survivors and are usually due to arterial or venous thrombotic occlusions from the severe dehydration in the early phase of the syndrome.

Insulin Resistance: Historically, the term, "insulin resistance," has been applied to patients who require more than 200 units daily for several days or more in the absence of ketoacidosis or intercurrent complications. It is sometimes caused by unusually high titers of IgG antibodies to insulin. Changing the species source from beef or mixed beef-pork to pork or human insulin may reduce hyperglycemia. If this is tried and the patient still requires more than 200 units daily, corticosteroids may be administered. Prednisone 40 to 80 mg daily is given until the insulin requirement decreases or for a maximum of one month. An increased duration of action is associated with IgG binding of regular insulin. The corticosteroid may decrease IgG production or reduce the binding of insulin to the antibody. The usual adverse effects of high-dose corticosteroid therapy may occur. Steroid therapy should be initiated in the hospital or with careful outpatient observation because insulin requirements may increase initially due to the hyperglycemic effect of the corticosteroid.

Since insulin resistance is self-limited, lasting from several months to years, many physicians avoid corticosteroid therapy by using highly concentrated insulin (U500) in large enough quantities to avoid ketoacidosis even though the level of control may be unsatisfactory. The patient must be monitored carefully when hypoglycemia signals the gradual (several weeks) return of sensitivity. Both reduction of IgG antibody titers and release of bound insulin contribute to the rapid decrease in insulin requirements (Davidson, 1981).

Other conditions also may cause insulin insensitivity by different mechanisms. Obese patients are insulin resistant because the number of insulin receptors in adipose tissue is reduced or there is a postreceptor defect; weight reduction improves insulin sensitivity. Antibodies to insulin receptors cause insulin resistance in patients with acanthosis nigricans, while insulin receptors are structurally abnormal in those with leprechaunism. NIDDM patients have reduced numbers of receptors, probably due to obesity when present, and down regulation of insulin receptors caused by hyperinsulinemia. These patients also have a postreceptor defect that may impair the cellular glucose transport system in target tissues. Insulin reportedly reverses the postreceptor defect in adipose and possibly other tissues (Scarlett et al, 1983; Garvey et al, 1985). A postreceptor defect may account for the insulin resistance observed during infection (Drobny et al, 1984).

In another form of insensitivity to insulin, patients respond to intravenous but are relatively insensitive to subcutaneous administration. Insulin antibody titers are not elevated, circulatory distribution of hormone appears to be normal, and there is no serious receptor defect. The probable cause is excessive protease activity in subcutaneous tissue, which degrades insulin at the injection site. Intramuscular injection may improve insulin absorption. Intraperitoneal injection through a subcutaneously implanted catheter or intravenous infusion with an insulin pump also may be tried. Insulin mixed with aprotinin, an investigational protease inhibitor, has been effective in some patients, but toxic reactions, including anaphylaxis, may occur (Schade et al, 1983).

Hypoglycemia: This may be observed in any patient receiving insulin and is commonly caused by altered food intake followed by unanticipated exercise. It often occurs near the time of maximal activity of the particular preparation used and at almost the same time of the day or night. It may occur with intensified insulin regimens (conventional or pump). Common manifestations are hunger, anxiety, warmth and sweating, tremulousness, weakness, confusion, emotional lability, palpitation, pallor, abnormal behavior, fatigue, paresthesias, and hyperesthesias of the lips, nose, or fingers. The specific cluster of symptoms varies with the individual patient and tends to recur with hypoglycemic episodes.

In severe hypoglycemia, profound cerebrocortical dysfunction may occur, manifested by convulsions, coma, and eventually death. Autonomic signs and symptoms may result from the *rate* of decrease in blood glucose, and central nervous system effects are related to the absolute blood glucose concentration. Therefore, if glucose levels decrease slowly, autonomic symptoms may not precede central nervous system depression.

The symptoms of hypoglycemia are quite variable in children: A child may have a voracious appetite, tremors, and pallor or simply be faint, easily fatigued, or have a headache. Appearance may be apathetic or sleepy and the parent may mistakenly assume the child wishes to sleep longer.

Causes of hypoglycemia are (1) reduction or change in diet (eg, omission or delay of a meal), especially decreased intake of carbohydrate; (2) alleviation of stress; (3) insulin or sulfonylurea overdosage; (4) weight reduction; (5) termination or completion of pregnancy; (6) exercise; (7) correction of disorders associated with hyperglycemia; or (8) onset of disorders associated with hypoglycemia, such as overindulgence in alcohol without food. Hypoglycemia also may be caused by errors in insulin administration (eg, failure to agitate the container before use, improper measurement, improper injection technique), remission of the diabetic state, or institution of medication (for an unrelated disorder) that may produce hypoglycemia. (See the section on Hyperglycemic Agents for treatment.) Patient education is an integral part of initiating insulin therapy. Patients and family members should be taught to recognize an insulin reaction and how to treat it.

Dawn Phenomenon, Somogyi Effect: The *dawn phenomenon* is an increase in fasting blood glucose levels and insulin requirements before breakfast. It has been observed in both IDDM and NIDDM patients (Bolli and Gerich, 1984). The principal cause appears to be an inability to respond to normal nocturnal surges of growth hormone secretion (Campbell et al, 1985). Nondiabetic individuals also exhibit the dawn phenomenon but are able to respond to the glucose challenge by increasing insulin secretion, which reduces the elevation of

blood glucose (Bolli et al, 1984 A; Schmidt et al, 1984). In diabetic patients, adjustment of the dosage regimen should control the fasting hyperglycemia.

For IDDM patients, the second dose of intermediate-acting insulin may be given at bedtime instead of before the evening meal so that peak activity occurs closer to the time of expected hyperglycemia. A programmable insulin pump also may be set to increase insulin delivery at the appropriate time. NIDDM patients may also benefit from administration of insulin in the evening as the sole or second dose of the day (Riddle, 1985).

The *Somogyi effect* consists of rebound hyperglycemia in response to secretion of glucogenic substances (ie, epinephrine, norepinephrine, growth hormone, cortisol) during unrecognized hypoglycemic episodes. Although the Somogyi effect has been demonstrated in diabetic patients (Bolli et al, 1984 B), it is probably not responsible for prebreakfast hyperglycemia (as formerly thought) but may be contributory if nocturnal hypoglycemia results from excessive doses of insulin. This can be confirmed by measuring nocturnal blood glucose; if nocturnal hypoglycemia occurs, a gradual reduction in the dose of insulin may correct the problem.

Adverse Reactions and Precautions

Allergic Reactions: Although patients treated with insulin have both IgE and IgG antibodies to insulin, serious allergic problems are rare. Allergic reactions to insulin can be either systemic or local; the latter occur about ten times more frequently than the former, and both forms may be observed in some patients.

Local allergy occurs more commonly with the older, less pure preparations. It is manifested by an erythematous, indurated area at the site of injection that develops within hours and may persist for several days. The reaction often begins a few weeks after starting insulin treatment. If it commences within the first few days after initiation of therapy, previous sensitization to beef or pork protein may be causative. Local reactions are thought to be produced by noninsulin or large-molecular-weight materials present in some preparations.

Local inflammatory responses (which some consider irritant and others allergic) or infection may result from improper cleansing of the skin, contamination of the injection site, use of a sensitizing antiseptic, or accidental intradermal rather than subcutaneous injection. These reactions usually subside spontaneously.

Generalized reactions begin immediately after injection and are characterized by urticarial skin eruptions with or without systemic manifestations that may include angioedema, respiratory symptoms (eg, asthma, dyspnea), and, very rarely, hypotension, shock, and death. These reactions have been ascribed to sensitivity to the insulin molecule itself. Patients with systemic allergy have high titers of IgE antibody to insulin and commonly have a history of (1) intermittent treatment with insulin, in which case allergy is manifested one or two weeks after resumption of therapy; (2) allergy to other materials (eg, penicillin); or (3) increased serum antibody titers to beef insulin. Pork and human insulins are less antigenic than the beef product and are used for desensitization and subsequent treatment. Human and purified pork insulin appear to be comparably low in antigenicity. However, even though antigenicity is low, cutaneous allergy to human recombinant DNA insulin has been reported.

Desensitization is indicated in patients with symptoms of systemic allergy who require insulin (a desensitization kit is available from Eli Lilly and Company). The patient may be desensitized to a mixed or single species preparation. In general, the process involves injection of small amounts of human or pork insulin initially, gradually increasing the dosage. These small amounts are bound to IgE antibody-mast cell combinations, and degranulation of the mast cells releases histamine and other inflammatory substances. However, the amounts released by small increments of insulin do not cause symptoms, and eventually all IgE antibodies are bound by insulin. The patient can then tolerate therapeutic doses (Davidson, 1981). Occasionally, treatment with an antihistamine also may be needed.

Lipodystrophies: Some patients may be susceptible to lipodystrophy (atrophy or hypertrophy). In lipoatrophy, a depression in the skin underlying the site of insulin injection is due to atrophy of fat tissue. This condition may be due to an immune phenomenon and tends to occur more frequently in young female patients and when less pure insulin preparations are used. The injection of a purified pork or human preparation directly into the atrophic area for two to four weeks will cause subcutaneous fat to accumulate. Unless insulin is injected into affected areas every two to four weeks, atrophy may recur. Return to the use of a less purified preparation also may cause recurrence.

Lipohypertrophy is an accumulation of subcutaneous fat that sometimes develops at sites of repeated insulin injection and is a lipogenic tissue response to insulin. Regression occurs gradually if the affected sites are not used for injections.

Vision Changes: In uncontrolled diabetes, a transient loss of accommodation has been attributed to changes in the physical properties of the lens secondary to hyperglycemia; this condition is reversed during the early phase of effective management. Since alterations in osmotic equilibrium between the lens and vitreous and aqueous fluids may not stabilize for a few weeks after initiating therapy, evaluation for new corrective lenses should be delayed for three to six weeks.

Interactions: Hormones that tend to counteract the hypoglycemic effect of insulin include growth hormone (somatotropin), glucocorticoids, thyroid hormone, estrogens, progestins, and glucagon. Epinephrine inhibits insulin secretion and stimulates glycogenolysis. Excessive levels of these hormones should be considered when assessing insulin therapy.

Guanethidine [Ismelin] decreases blood glucose levels, and the dose of insulin may require adjustment when this agent is added to or omitted from the regimen. Certain antibiotics (eg, chloramphenicol, tetracyclines), salicylates, and phenylbutazone [Azolid, Butazolidin] increase the duration of serum insulin levels and also may have a direct hypoglycemic effect. Hypoglycemia has occurred in diabetics also taking beta blockers, which may mask the tachycardia associated with hypoglycemia. The hypoglycemic effect of insulin also may be potentiated by monoamine oxidase inhibitors, anabolic steroids, captopril [Capoten], disopyramide [Norpace], and fenfluramine [Pondimin].

Drug Evaluations

INSULIN INJECTION (Crystalline Zinc Insulin, Regular Insulin)
[*Unpurified:* Regular Insulin, Regular Iletin I; *Purified:* Purified Pork Insulin, Regular Iletin II, Velosulin]

This rapid-acting agent has a relatively short duration of action and is the only insulin preparation that may be given intravenously and intramuscularly, as well as subcutaneously (see Table 2).

Insulin injection is widely used to supplement intermediate- and long-acting preparations, and it is the insulin used with infusion pumps. Insulin mixtures provide more flexibility in delivering appropriate amounts of insulin at the time of food intake (see the section on Mixing Insulins).

Insulin injection is the preparation of choice in unstable diabetes when complications, such as infection, shock, or surgical trauma, occur. It may be administered intravenously in the presence of ketoacidosis or during surgery. There may be substantial adherence of insulin to in-line intravenous filters. However, this is not a problem if the infusion tubing is initially flushed with 100 to 200 ml of the insulin solution.

See the introduction to this section for further information.

DOSAGE AND PREPARATIONS.
Subcutaneous: Dosage must be individualized. As an adjunct to intermediate-acting preparations, 5 to 10 units given in the same syringe (except with protamine zinc insulin) before breakfast or the evening meal; this dose must be adjusted according to blood or urine glucose measurements at the appropriate times (ie, after breakfast and before lunch for the morning dose of regular insulin; after supper and before the bedtime snack for the before supper dose of regular insulin).
Intravenous: For ketoacidosis, *adults,* 6 to 10 units/hr given by infusion. *Children,* 0.1 unit/kg/hr (limitation up to the adult dose above) given as a continuous infusion.
Intramuscular: For ketoacidosis when facilities for continuous intravenous infusion are limited, initially, 10 to 20 units as an intravenous bolus, followed by 5 to 10 units hourly intramuscularly.

Insulin injection is available from single or mixed species sources and in conventional or purified preparations (see Table 2). These should not be considered equivalent to, nor should they be substituted for, one another by the patient.

PROMPT INSULIN ZINC SUSPENSION
[*Unpurified:* Semilente Iletin I, Semilente Insulin; *Purified:* Semilente Purified Pork Prompt Insulin]

This rapid-acting preparation is used most commonly to supplement lente and ultralente forms when their duration of action is not quite appropriate for a specific patient. A mixture of prompt insulin zinc suspension 30% and long-acting extended insulin zinc suspension (ultralente insulin) 70% has an intermediate duration of action (lente) (see the evaluations on Insulin Zinc Suspension and Extended Insulin Zinc Suspension). Insulins of the lente series can be mixed in any proportion to obtain the desired dose without altering the activity of any component.

DOSAGE AND PREPARATIONS.
Subcutaneous (should never be given intravenously): No standard dose can be cited. For patients with newly diagnosed mild diabetes, initially, 10 to 20 units 30 minutes before breakfast. At least two doses daily may be necessary.

This preparation is most frequently used in combination with lente insulin to modify the time of peak insulin action.

> Prompt insulin zinc suspension is available from single or mixed species sources and in conventional or purified preparations (see Table 2).

ISOPHANE INSULIN SUSPENSION
[*Unpurified:* NPH Iletin I, NPH Insulin; *Purified:* Insulatard NPH, NPH Iletin II, NPH Purified Pork Isophane Insulin; *Mixture:* Mixtard (70% NPH isophane, 30% regular)]

Isophane insulin is an intermediate-acting preparation (see Table 2). Absorption is delayed because the insulin is conjugated with protamine in a complex of reduced isoelectric solubility. This preparation contains less protamine than protamine zinc insulin and is useful in all forms of diabetes except the initial treatment of diabetic ketoacidosis or in emergencies. Isophane insulin or insulin zinc suspension (usually in combination with regular insulin) is often used for previously untreated diabetic patients who require insulin. Isophane insulin may be mixed in the same syringe with other insulin preparations subject to certain limitations (see the section on Mixing Insulins).

Hypoglycemic reactions in mid to late afternoon may be less obvious in onset, more prolonged, and more common than with rapid-acting preparations because of the prolonged effect of the dose. See the introduction to this section for additional information.

DOSAGE AND PREPARATIONS.
Subcutaneous (should never be used intravenously): Dosage must be individualized. Initially, 10 to 20 units (often in combination with regular insulin) 30 to 60 minutes before breakfast. If needed, a combination of this preparation and regular insulin may be given in divided doses to provide approximately one-third of the daily amount 30 minutes before the evening meal or at bedtime.

> Isophane insulin suspension is available from single or mixed species sources and in conventional or purified preparations (see Table 2).

INSULIN ZINC SUSPENSION
[*Unpurified:* Lente Iletin I, Lente Insulin; *Purified:* Lente Iletin II, Lente Purified Pork Insulin]

This intermediate-acting preparation is a mixture of 30% prompt insulin zinc suspension (semilente insulin) and 70% extended insulin zinc suspension (ultralente insulin) (see Table 2). Insulin zinc suspension or isophane insulin (usually in combination with regular insulin) is often used for previously untreated diabetics who require insulin. Insulin zinc suspension is not a suitable substitute for insulin injection (regular insulin) in emergencies because of its delayed onset of action. Insulins of the lente series can be mixed in any proportion without changing the activity of the components.

Hypoglycemic reactions in mid or late afternoon may be less obvious in onset, more prolonged, and more common than with rapid-acting preparations because of the more prolonged effect of the dose. Insulins in the lente series do not contain a modifying protein and can be mixed in any ratio. See the introduction to this section for additional information on adverse reactions.

Pharmacologically, insulin zinc suspension is equivalent to isophane insulin on a unit-for-unit basis. However, responses vary and some patients may have a hypersensitivity reaction to one of these insulins but not the other. In patients who previously received only regular insulin, the total amount should be reduced by one-third for the first two or three days. Similarly, when protamine zinc insulin was the preparation used formerly, the dose may be decreased gradually to one-half the previous amount.

DOSAGE AND PREPARATIONS.
Subcutaneous (should never be given intravenously): See the dosage for Isophane Insulin Suspension.

> Insulin zinc suspension is available from single or mixed species sources and in conventional or purified preparations (see Table 2).

PROTAMINE ZINC INSULIN SUSPENSION
[*Unpurified:* Protamine, Zinc & Iletin I; *Purified:* Protamine, Zinc, & Iletin II]

This long-acting preparation contains more modifying protein (protamine) and zinc than isophane insulin (see Table 2). Combining regular insulin with protamine zinc insulin is complicated by the conversion of a portion of the unmodified insulin to an insoluble form. In the past, mixtures of the two in ratios of 2 or more to 1 were utilized; however, use of insulin in the lente series is much more flexible. Like extended insulin zinc suspension (ultralente insulin), protamine zinc insulin suspension has limited usefulness when given alone; it is usually administered with a shorter acting preparation. Long-acting preparations are less adaptable than intermediate-acting forms given in divided doses.

The long duration of action of protamine zinc insulin may result in recurrent hypoglycemic reactions if the dosage is not properly adjusted. A readily available carbohydrate (eg, sweetened orange juice) may be given to prevent such reactions, but the carbohydrate content of the meal following injection may have to be limited to avoid hyperglycemia. Between-meal snacks may be needed and bedtime snacks are essential. The long delay in onset of action makes this form unsuitable for emergencies. Protamine zinc insulin suspension is rarely used today.

See the introduction to this section for additional information on adverse reactions.

DOSAGE AND PREPARATIONS.

Subcutaneous (should never be given intravenously): See the dosage for Isophane Insulin Suspension.

Protamine zinc insulin is available from single or mixed species sources and in conventional and purified preparations (see Table 2).

EXTENDED INSULIN ZINC SUSPENSION

[*Unpurified:* Ultralente Iletin I, Ultralente Insulin; *Purified:* Ultralente Purified Beef Insulin]

The actions, indications, and potential for hypoglycemic reactions of this long-acting preparation resemble those of protamine zinc insulin. (See Table 2 and the previous evaluation.) Like prompt insulin zinc suspension (semilente insulin), this form contains no modifying protein to which patients may be sensitive. Like protamine zinc insulin, it has limited usefulness when given alone. This insulin preparation is usually administered in combination with a shorter acting form. In slightly reduced doses, it may be combined with insulin zinc suspension (lente insulin) when blood glucose levels are not adequately controlled during the daytime. Insulins of the lente series can be mixed in any proportion without changing the activity of the components. Extended zinc insulin suspension is not suitable for use in emergencies because of its delayed onset of action.

DOSAGE AND PREPARATIONS.

Subcutaneous (should never be given intravenously): See the dosage for Isophane Insulin Suspension.

Extended insulin zinc suspension is available from bovine or mixed species sources and in conventional or purified preparations (see Table 2).

REGULAR HUMAN INSULIN INJECTION (Biosynthetic and Semisynthetic)

[Humulin R, Novolin R]

This rapid-acting form of human insulin is produced by recombinant DNA techniques (biosynthetic) or enzymatic conversion (semisynthetic) of pork insulin. It may be administered subcutaneously, intravenously, intramuscularly, or through an infusion pump.

Therapeutically, this preparation is probably equivalent to purified pork insulin injection. Human regular insulins are absorbed faster than the corresponding purified pork product in some patients. Although the peak serum concentration of human insulin injection after subcutaneous administration is slightly higher than that of purified pork insulin injection, the time to peak concentration and overall bioavailability are similar and control of blood glucose appears to be equivalent. No differences are apparent in binding, actions, metabolism, or potency.

As with purified pork insulin, patients receiving only human insulin subcutaneously have been reported to produce insulin-specific IgG and IgE antibodies. When human insulin was substituted for mixed beef-pork insulin, antibody levels and insulin binding to antibodies decreased. Insulin binding to antibodies decreased slightly when human insulin was substi-

tuted for purified pork insulin. No antibodies to *Escherichia coli* peptides have been found in biosynthetic products. Systemic insulin allergy, lipoatrophy, and lipohypertrophy have occurred only rarely in patients receiving only human insulin.

It is not known whether the slight differences between purified pork and human insulin will prove to be clinically significant. Until more information is available, human insulin will probably be used in clinical situations where purified pork insulin would be appropriate.

These preparations may be mixed with other insulins subject to certain limitations (see the section on Mixing Insulins).

DOSAGE AND PREPARATIONS.

Subcutaneous, Intramuscular, Intravenous: Some patients require a different dose than with animal-source insulins. The adjustment may be needed with the first dose or over a period of several weeks.

For dosage guidelines, see the evaluation on Insulin Injection.

For preparations, see Table 2.

NPH ISOPHANE HUMAN INSULIN SUSPENSION (Biosynthetic and Semisynthetic)

[Humulin N, Novolin N]

This intermediate-acting form of human insulin is produced by recombinant DNA techniques (biosynthetic) or enzymatic conversion (semisynthetic) of pork insulin. It is administered subcutaneously and should not be given intravenously. Absorption is delayed because the insulin is conjugated with protamine in a complex of reduced isoelectric solubility.

Therapeutically, this preparation is probably comparable to purified pork insulin. However, human NPH insulin may have a slightly shorter duration of action than comparable purified pork products. In patients who receive only one injection of the human preparation daily, this may decrease glycemic control slightly and increase fasting serum glucose and ketonuria slightly.

It is not known whether the differences between purified pork and human insulin will prove to be clinically significant. Until more information is available, human insulin probably will be used in clinical situations where purified pork insulin would be appropriate (see section on Choice of Insulin Preparation). This insulin may be mixed with other insulins subject to certain limitations (see section on Mixing Insulins). Human insulin preparations are more expensive than other insulin preparations.

DOSAGE AND PREPARATIONS.

Subcutaneous: Some patients will require a different dosage than with animal-source insulins. The adjustment may be needed with the first dose or over a period of several weeks.

For dosage guidelines, see the evaluation on Isophane Insulin Suspension.

For preparations, see Table 2.

HUMAN INSULIN ZINC SUSPENSION (Biosynthetic and Semisynthetic)

[Humulin L, Novolin L]

This intermediate-acting form of human insulin is produced

by recombinant DNA techniques (biosynthetic) or enzymatic conversion of pork insulin (semisynthetic). It is administered subcutaneously and should not be given intravenously.

Therapeutically, this preparation is probably comparable to purified pork insulin. No difference in bioavailability has been observed.

It is not known whether the slight differences between purified pork and human insulin will prove to be clinically significant. Until more information is available, human insulin will probably be used in clinical situations where purified pork insulin would be appropriate.

DOSAGE AND PREPARATIONS.

Subcutaneous: Some patients require a different dosage than with animal-source insulins. The adjustment may be needed with the first dose or over a period of several weeks. Insulins of the lente series may be mixed without changing the activity of the components.

For dosage guidelines, see the evaluation on Insulin Zinc Suspension.

For preparations, See Table 2.

ORAL HYPOGLYCEMIC AGENTS

The first generation sulfonylurea compounds are acetohexamide [Dymelor], chlorpropamide [Diabinese, Glucamide], tolazamide [Ronase, Tolinase], and tolbutamide [Orinase, SK-Tolbutamide]. The second generation compounds (glyburide [DiaBeta, Micronase], glipizide [Glucotrol]) are now approved for use in the United States. Gliclazide is an investigational agent. These agents reduce the blood glucose level in selected patients with diabetes (see the section on Choice of Therapy). The second generation agents are more potent than other sulfonylureas (see Table 3). The biguanide compound, phenformin, is available in the United States only under special circumstances (see the evaluation).

Pharmacokinetics: The absorption of all sulfonylureas is fairly rapid and complete. These agents are weakly acidic and circulate bound to protein (70% to 99%), principally albumin. All are metabolized in the liver to inactive (tolbutamide, tolazamide, glipizide, glyburide) or active compounds that are excreted in the urine, mainly by tubular secretion. The primary therapeutic differences among the sulfonylureas are in duration of action, elimination half-life, and relative potencies (see Table 3). The maximal hypoglycemic effect is similar for all agents, however. Plasma levels vary widely and dose-response relationships generally are weak, although responsive patients usually have higher mean plasma levels of drug (Balant, 1981; Jackson and Bressler, part I, 1981).

Mechanism of Action: Although the sulfonylureas are sulfonamide derivatives, they have no antibacterial action. Functional pancreatic tissue must be present for activity. Sulfonylureas appear to act initially by stimulating the release of insulin from pancreatic islet tissue by increasing the sensitivity of the beta cells to glucose, which stimulates insulin secretion. These agents also may suppress the secretion of glucagon and the production of hepatic glucose. They potentiate insulin-stimulated glucose transport in adipose tissue and across skeletal muscle membrane. Sulfonylureas also act peripherally at postreceptor intracellular sites to increase insulin activity (Cader Asmal and Marble, 1984). In a comparison of second generation sulfonylureas, glipizide reduced

TABLE 3.
SULFONYLUREA ORAL HYPOGLYCEMIC AGENTS IN THE UNITED STATES

Drug and Tradename	Daily Dose Range (Average in Parentheses)	Elimination Half-life (Hours)	Duration of Action (Hours)
FIRST GENERATION			
Acetohexamide Dymelor (Lilly)	500 mg–1.5 g (1 g)	1.3–6 (including metabolite)	12–24
Chlorpropamide Diabinese (Pfizer)	50 mg–500 mg (250 mg)	30–36	1–3 days
Tolazamade Ronase (Rowell) Tolinase (Upjohn)	100 mg–1 g (250 mg)	4.7–8	12–24
Tolbutamide Orinase (Upjohn) SK-Tolbutamide (Smith Kline & French) Generic	500 mg–3 g (2 g)	4–8	6–12
SECOND GENERATION			
Glipizide Glucotrol (Roerig)	2.5 mg–40 mg (20–15 mg)	2–4	12–24
Glyburide DiaBeta (Hoechst-Roussel) Micronase (Upjohn)	1.25 mg–20 mg	4.6–12	12–24

postprandial blood glucose more effectively, while glyburide was more effective in decreasing fasting blood glucose levels (Frederiksen and Mogensen, 1982). However, there is no universal agreement with this assessment.

The sulfonylureas decrease blood glucose levels in nondiabetic as well as in diabetic individuals. Conversely, usual therapeutic doses of the biguanide, phenformin, have no hypoglycemic effect in individuals without diabetes, because increased peripheral glucose utilization is compensated by increased hepatic release of glucose.

A placebo-controlled study of patients with impaired glucose tolerance suggested that early treatment with glipizide may reverse diabetic microangiographic changes (Camerini-Davalos et al, 1983), but further investigation is necessary to substantiate this observation. Furthermore, similar studies with other oral agents are necessary to determine whether these drugs might have similar effects.

Management

Adequate time should be allowed for the patient to learn and practice the necessary dietary habits before other modes of therapy for NIDDM are introduced. Failure to emphasize the necessity and principles of continuous dietary management is perhaps the primary shortcoming in the present treatment of NIDDM. Mild elevation of blood glucose levels (up to 160 mg/dl) during this initial period is not life-threatening, and administering a hypoglycemic agent before the principles of dietary compliance are understood is not the wisest course for long-term management. If hyperglycemia continues after an appropriate trial with diet alone, an oral agent or insulin may be needed.

Oral hypoglycemic agents fail to control hyperglycemia in 15% to 30% of patients, depending on compliance with dietary restrictions. Even when initial control is established with an oral agent, secondary failure occurs in 5% of patients/year. After three years, the blood glucose remains controlled in up to 50% of patients; after six or seven years, only 6% to 12% of patients remain well controlled. If primary or secondary failure occurs, principles of dietary therapy should be re-emphasized. Another preparation may be administered, although the probability of success is reduced when there is a history of failure with a similar agent (unless therapeutic failure was due to bioinequivalence; see the evaluation on Tolbutamide). The circumstances concomitant with the change in drug (eg, renewed dietary compliance) may be more important to the success of therapy than the specific preparation substituted.

Asymptomatic patients in whom blood glucose levels remain elevated despite dietary compliance should be given an oral agent (or insulin). When an oral agent is given, blood glucose is monitored every one to two weeks until the dosage is established and monthly thereafter; therapy is continued if the response is satisfactory. If the response is unsatisfactory, the dose is increased gradually to the maximum effective amount; if this fails to control blood glucose, another oral agent may be substituted. Symptomatic patients or those with a fasting blood glucose exceeding 160 mg/dl may be given an oral agent simultaneously with dietary therapy (without prior dietary trial).

Dosage adjustments may be required (see the evaluations).

Patients who have had NIDDM for less than ten years usually respond most favorably to oral agents. When NIDDM patients do not respond to sulfonylurea agents, lack of dietary compliance should be considered. If weight reduction, dietary restriction, exercise, and an oral agent fail to control hyperglycemia, insulin must be substituted.

Once control of hyperglycemia is achieved with an oral agent and the dose is reduced to the lowest effective amount, a trial of diet only should be attempted. Control often can be maintained with diet and exercise alone.

If substitution of an oral agent for insulin is considered, an insulin-free interval should be established with careful monitoring to determine whether dietary regulation alone is effective. If moderate to severe ketonuria occurs within 12 to 24 hours after withdrawal of insulin, control cannot be maintained without this agent.

Choice of Oral Hypoglycemic Agent: Short-acting preparations facilitate initial control, and a long-acting agent can then be substituted for convenience and to improve compliance. However, many physicians initiate oral hypoglycemic therapy with the agent they intend to use for prolonged treatment. Long-acting agents should be used with caution in the elderly. Patients in cardiac failure should avoid chlorpropamide (and, to a lesser degree, tolbutamide) because of the possibility of water retention.

The second generation sulfonylureas, glipizide and glyburide, appear to be at least as effective as other oral hypoglycemic agents and resemble each other in their ability to control blood glucose. They do not cause water retention or flushing upon ingestion of alcohol or interact with acidic drugs that tend to displace protein-bound drugs. However, they probably offer no clear advantage in patients already controlled by a first generation oral hypoglycemic agent.

Relative potency alone does not determine drug selection because maximal effectiveness is similar for all agents. A single daily dose of any sulfonylurea (except tolbutamide) is often adequate to control blood glucose in NIDDM patients.

Adverse Reactions and Precautions

Acute toxic effects appear to be relatively rare, but the combined use of more than one oral hypoglycemic agent increases the risk of untoward reactions.

Hypoglycemic reactions have been reported after use of all sulfonylureas but are more common with the long-acting agent, chlorpropamide. Severe reactions are rare, but fatalities have occurred. Hypoglycemia also has developed in nondiabetic individuals who received sulfonylureas for other diseases on an investigational basis. Hypoglycemia may persist for several days and require repeated administration of intravenous dextrose; the severity of this reaction fluctuates during such episodes. Hospitalization should be considered for patients who develop severe hypoglycemia after taking their usual dose of an oral hypoglycemic agent because the precipitating condition (eg, inability to eat, decreased renal excretion of the drug) may continue after acute treatment and hypoglycemia may recur until the blood level of the drug is reduced.

Hypoglycemic reactions have occurred after one dose of a sulfonylurea, after two or three days of therapy, or after many months of previously uneventful treatment. Hypoglycemia may develop after treatment with a single sulfonylurea, after substitution of one oral drug for another, or after an oral drug is substituted for insulin. It may occur in patients who receive an inappropriately large dose, in those who do not eat properly, or in those who fail to metabolize or excrete the drug because of impaired hepatic or renal function. Thus, these agents generally should not be used in patients with renal (or possibly hepatic) disease, because they are more vulnerable to the hypoglycemic effects. These factors become even more significant in the elderly whose counterregulatory mechanisms may be diminished and who may be more likely to have insufficient food intake. Furthermore, hypoglycemia in the elderly may develop insidiously and may be manifested as brain dysfunction and, ultimately, coma. A decreased rate of excretion is likely to intensify the hypoglycemia.

Allergic skin reactions (pruritus, erythema, urticaria, morbilliform or maculopapular rash, lichenoid reactions) have been noted after use of sulfonylureas and phenformin. Most of these effects are transient; if they persist, the drug should be discontinued. Gastrointestinal disturbances (eg, nausea, vomiting, gastritis) are most common with phenformin and are unusual with sulfonylureas. They are alleviated by taking the drug with meals, adjusting the dosage, or dividing the medication into two or three smaller doses each day. If symptoms persist, the drug should be discontinued at least temporarily.

Water retention and dilutional hyponatremia (syndrome of inappropriate secretion of antidiuretic hormone, SIADH) have been reported with administration of chlorpropamide to patients with diabetes mellitus, particularly those with a tendency to retain water (eg, patients with congestive heart failure or hepatic cirrhosis, those receiving diuretics). Tolazamide, glipizide, and glyburide are mildly diuretic.

Signs of hyponatremia include serum hypo-osmolarity, continued sodium excretion despite hyponatremia, and impaired ability to dilute urine and to excrete a water load. Chlorpropamide may potentiate endogenous antidiuretic hormone activity at the renal tubular level and augments the hypothalamic-pituitary release of ADH. These abnormalities have been corrected by withdrawing the drugs but have recurred with readministration (see Chapter 30, Agents Affecting Water Homeostasis).

Leukopenia, thrombocytopenia, agranulocytosis, aplastic anemia, hemolytic anemia, acute intermittent porphyria, and jaundice caused by reversible intrahepatic cholestasis have been reported rarely after use of the sulfonylureas but not after use of phenformin.

The oral hypoglycemic agents have not yet been shown to cause teratogenic effects in man, but such effects have been observed after use of large doses in animals. These agents are not recommended for diabetic women who may become pregnant. Insulin is used during pregnancy, principally because the transplacental passage of oral agents may cause neonatal hypoglycemia.

The sulfonylureas are contraindicated in *nondiabetic* patients with renal glycosuria, since their hyperresponsiveness to these agents may result in prolonged or fatal hypoglycemia.

The possible cardiotoxicity of sulfonylureas is discussed in the section on the UGDP Study.

Interactions: Agents that aggravate the diabetic state by increasing blood glucose levels include glucocorticoids, estrogens, thiazides and other diuretics, and beta-adrenergic agonists. Phenobarbital and rifampin [Rifadin, Rimactane] induce hepatic enzymes that increase metabolism of oral hypoglycemic agents. Concomitant use may require adjustment of the dose of the hypoglycemic agent. The dosage requirements for oral hypoglycemic agents may be increased in those receiving chlorpromazine [Thorazine], thiazides, or phenytoin [Dilantin], since these drugs inhibit the release of endogenous insulin and may cause hyperglycemia.

Drugs that may increase the risk of hypoglycemia in patients taking the sulfonylureas include insulin, alcohol, phenformin, sulfonamides, large doses of salicylates, phenylbutazone [Azolid, Butazolidin], dicumarol, chloramphenicol [Chloromycetin], monoamine oxidase inhibitors, guanethidine [Ismelin], anabolic steroids, fenfluramine [Pondimin], and clofibrate [Atromid-S]. Glipizide and glyburide are less easily displaced from protein binding sites than other oral agents, and the risk of hypoglycemia when taken with drugs such as salicylates, which are highly protein bound, is probably lower.

Propranolol [Inderal] and other beta blockers inhibit tachycardia and tremors (but not sweating) induced by hypoglycemia from any cause, including oral hypoglycemic agents. Chlorpropamide may decrease tolerance to alcohol; this is manifested by unusual flushing of the skin, particularly of the face and neck, similar to that caused by disulfiram [Antabuse]. Patients taking chlorpropamide may be more likely to develop hyponatremia if thiazide diuretics are taken concomitantly (Kadowaki et al, 1983).

Other discussions of adverse effects and interactions with oral hypoglycemic agents are available (Jackson and Bressler, part II, 1981; Paice et al, 1985).

Drug Evaluations

SULFONYLUREA COMPOUNDS

ACETOHEXAMIDE
[Dymelor]

Acetohexamide is similar to other oral hypoglycemic agents in the sulfonylurea class. However, since it is the only one with uricosuric properties, some clinicians prefer this agent for diabetic patients with gout. Acetohexamide is hydroxylated in the liver to hydroxyhexamide, a metabolite having 2.5 times the hypoglycemic effect of the parent compound.

Differences in bioequivalence of certain generic products may be a problem. Some of these differences are due to variations in dissolution rates of tablets or effects of storage area and relative humidity on dissolution rate.

The incidence of untoward effects is low and reactions are reversible when acetohexamide is discontinued. Relatively severe hypoglycemic reactions have been observed occasionally in patients given large doses for prolonged periods without close observation. Rarely, hypoglycemic reactions due to hyperresponsiveness have occurred in patients given usual therapeutic doses. Since the active metabolite is excreted by the kidneys, this drug should be avoided in patients with renal dysfunction.

See also the introduction to the section on Oral Hypoglycemic Agents.

DOSAGE AND PREPARATIONS.
Oral: Dosage should be individualized. The usual range is 500 mg to 1.5 g daily. Doses in excess of this amount will not improve control. Most patients receiving 1 g or less per day can be given the full amount once daily; however, the drug should be given in divided doses before the morning and evening meals if more than 1 g is required. Those who have recently discontinued use of a long-acting insulin preparation should be given relatively small doses initially.
   Dymelor (Lilly). Tablets 250 and 500 mg.

CHLORPROPAMIDE
[Diabinese, Glucamide]

Chlorpropamide has essentially the same actions, uses, and limitations as the other sulfonylureas. It has the longest duration of action (one to three days). Primary and secondary failures have been reported less frequently than with tolbutamide. (See also the introduction to this section.)

Differences in bioequivalence of certain generic products may be a problem. Some of these differences are due to variations in dissolution rates of tablets or effects of storage area and relative humidity on dissolution rate.

ADVERSE REACTIONS AND PRECAUTIONS. Untoward reactions have been reported more frequently with chlorpropamide than with other sulfonylureas. In a few older patients, hypoglycemic reactions have been severe. Water retention with hyponatremia is rare but can be life-threatening in patients with a tendency to retain water (eg, those with congestive heart failure or hepatic cirrhosis). Elderly patients and those taking thiazide diuretics may be more likely to develop this complication. This drug should not be used in patients with renal insufficiency, because the duration of action is greatly prolonged.

Facial flushing after ingestion of alcohol occurs in up to one-third of patients taking chlorpropamide. The mechanism, like that of the disulfiram reaction, probably involves inhibition of the oxidation of acetaldehyde, a metabolite of ethanol. Chlorpropamide-alcohol flushing (CPAF) may be genetically determined. The plasma concentration of chlorpropamide may be correlated with CPAF (Jerntorp et al, 1983; Groop et al, 1984). CPAF may be associated with a lower risk of micro- and macrovascular complications, but better methods of measuring flush and distinguishing CPAF from alcohol flushing alone

are necessary to evaluate this possibility (Hillson and Hockaday, 1984; Johnston et al, 1984; Waldhäusl, 1984).

See also the introduction to this section.

PHARMACOKINETICS. Chlorpropamide is metabolized by the liver and unchanged drug and metabolites are excreted by the kidneys; 80% to 90% of a single oral dose is excreted within four days.

DOSAGE AND PREPARATIONS.
Oral: Dosage should be individualized; the total amount is usually given once daily with breakfast. For *middle-aged patients,* initially, up to 250 mg daily, depending on the severity of hyperglycemia; *older patients,* 100 mg daily. After five to seven days, the blood glucose level reaches a plateau and the dose may be increased or decreased by 50 to 125 mg at weekly intervals. The maintenance dose depends upon the response of the patient and the severity of the disease; the usual range is 100 to 500 mg daily. Patients who do not respond adequately to 500 mg daily usually will not respond to larger doses.
   Diabinese (Pfizer), *Glucamide* (Lemmon), **Generic.** Tablets 100 and 250 mg.

GLIPIZIDE
[Glucotrol]

Glipizide is similar to other oral hypoglycemic agents in the sulfonylurea class. This second generation sulfonylurea is at least 100 times as potent as tolbutamide, but the maximal hypoglycemic effect is similar to that produced by the other sulfonylureas.

ACTIONS. A single morning dose of glipizide stimulates insulin secretion after three meals over a 12-hour period. Fasting insulin levels are not elevated. Peripheral effects include increased glucose uptake and suppression of hepatic glucose output (Lebovitz, 1985). These effects on insulin secretion persist for more than three years. Long-term control (more than six years) has been reported in more than two-thirds of patients with NIDDM who responded initially. Glipizide has a mild diuretic effect.

ADVERSE REACTIONS. Glipizide is relatively free of serious adverse effects and only approximately 1.5% of patients discontinued this drug because of adverse reactions. Gastrointestinal disturbances are most common (incidence, 1.7% to 3.7%); skin rashes occur in up to 1.4% of patients. There are no reports of adverse effects on liver, kidney, or bone marrow. This drug is classified in FDA Pregnancy Category C.

See also the introduction to this section.

PHARMACOKINETICS. Glipizide is rapidly and completely absorbed after oral administration and peak serum concentrations are observed 1 to 3.5 hours after ingestion. Because the presence of food delays absorption, the drug should be taken approximately 30 minutes prior to a meal. Glipizide is 98.4% nonionically bound to plasma albumin. The drug is metabolized in the liver to inactive metabolites. These metabolites, as well as less than 10% of unchanged drug, are excreted in the urine. Peak blood levels occur two to six hours after a single dose.

DOSAGE AND PREPARATIONS.

Oral: Dosage should be individualized. The drug should be given 30 minutes before a meal for greatest efficacy. The usual initial dose is 5 mg given before breakfast. Elderly patients or those with liver disease may be given 2.5 mg initially. Several days should elapse before the dose is increased, and the amount should be based on the blood glucose level. Increments of 2.5 to 5 mg may be used. Daily doses exceeding 15 mg should be divided and given before meals. The maximum recommended daily dose is 40 mg.

    Glucotrol (Roerig). Tablets 5 and 10 mg.

GLYBURIDE
[DiaBeta, Micronase]

ACTIONS AND USES. Glyburide (often referred to in the European literature as glibenclamide) has actions and uses similar to those of the other sulfonylureas. The drug is 200 times more potent than tolbutamide on a weight basis, but the maximal hypoglycemic effect is similar to that of the other sulfonylureas. Glyburide stimulates secretion of insulin but also increases peripheral sensitivity to insulin by a post-receptor mechanism. Inhibition of hepatic glucose production is an important factor in glycemic control (Simonson et al, 1984). The drug has mild diuretic activity.

    Primary and secondary therapeutic failures occur, and the overall failure rate after 1.5 years is approximately 21%.

ADVERSE REACTIONS. The incidence of serious side effects with glyburide is low. Gastrointestinal disturbances develop in 1.8% of patients. Skin rashes occur in 1.5% of patients and may disappear with continued use. Glyburide does not appear to adversely affect the liver, kidney, or bone marrow. This drug is classified in FDA Pregnancy Category B.

PHARMACOKINETICS. Glyburide is absorbed rapidly and the peak serum concentration occurs 4 to 5.3 hours after ingestion. More than 97% of the drug is nonionically bound to serum proteins. Glyburide is metabolized by the liver; about 50% of the metabolites are excreted in the urine, and the rest are excreted in feces. Glyburide is generally effective when given once daily. When administration is discontinued, the drug is cleared from the serum in approximately 36 hours.

    See also the introduction to this section. Review articles on glyburide are available (Krall, 1984; Feldman, 1985).

DOSAGE AND PREPARATIONS.

Oral: Dosage should be individualized. The drug should be taken with breakfast. The usual initial dose is 2.5 mg to 5 mg daily, but 1.25 mg may be adequate in more responsive patients. The dose may be increased by maximal increments of 2.5 mg at weekly intervals and should be based on the blood glucose level. The usual maintenance dose is 1.25 to 20 mg daily. Amounts larger than 10 mg daily may be divided into two doses.

    DiaBeta (Hoechst-Roussel), *Micronase* (Upjohn). Tablets 1.25, 2.5, and 5 mg.

TOLAZAMIDE
[Ronase, Tolinase]

Tolazamide is similar to other oral hypoglycemic agents in the sulfonylurea class. However, since this potent agent lacks antidiuretic activity (and may have a mild diuretic action), it may be especially useful in patients with a tendency to retain water.

Tolazamide is metabolized in the liver to several substances, three of which have much weaker hypoglycemic activity. The metabolites are excreted by the kidney.

Differences in bioequivalence of certain generic products may be a problem. Some of these differences are due to variations in dissolution rates of tablets or effects of storage area and relative humidity on dissolution rates.

Generally, the untoward effects associated with tolazamide are the same as those noted with the other sulfonylureas; the incidence is low and reactions are reversible when tolazamide is discontinued. Hypoglycemia has been reported occasionally.

See also the introduction to this section.

DOSAGE AND PREPARATIONS.

Oral: Dosage should be individualized. Initially, 100 to 250 mg daily is given with breakfast; the amount then is adjusted every four to six days as needed. A single daily dose is effective in most patients; if 500 mg or more is required daily, the drug should be given in two doses. Amounts larger than 1 g daily probably will not improve control.

    Ronase (Rowell), *Tolinase* (Upjohn), *Generic.* Tablets 100, 250, and 500 mg.

TOLBUTAMIDE
[Orinase, SK-Tolbutamide]

Tolbutamide has the same actions, uses, and limitations as other sulfonylurea compounds. It is metabolized in the liver mainly to two inactive metabolites, which are excreted in the urine.

Differences in bioequivalence of certain generic products may be a problem. Some of these differences are due to variations in dissolution rates of tablets or effects of storage area and relative humidity on dissolution rates.

The toxicity of tolbutamide appears to be low, and reactions are similar to those observed with other sulfonylureas.

See also the introduction to this section.

DOSAGE AND PREPARATIONS.

Oral: Dosage should be individualized. Initially, 500 mg is given twice daily; the dose then is adjusted gradually until the minimal effective amount is established. The maintenance dose is 250 mg to 3 g daily. The total daily dose is given in divided amounts throughout the day. Doses exceeding 3 g daily are no more effective than smaller amounts; more than 2 g daily is seldom required.

Orinase (Upjohn). Tablets 250 and 500 mg.

SK-Tolbutamide (Smith Kline & French), **Generic.** Tablets 500 mg.

TOLBUTAMIDE SODIUM
[Orinase Diagnostic]

In patients with pancreatic islet cell tumor, the blood glucose level drops quickly after intravenous injection of tolbutamide sodium and remains low for three hours. Since other hypoglycemic states usually are not affected, tolbutamide sodium may be used in conjunction with estimates of plasma insulin to rule out this condition. The hypoglycemia produced can be severe and may be fatal if not treated. It is reversed with intravenous dextrose.

This agent also has been used during ulcer surgery to verify the completeness of vagus nerve section (by measurement of gastric acid secretion after tolbutamide-stimulated insulin release).

Thrombophlebitis has occurred in 0.8% to 2.4% of patients; no important sequelae have been reported.

DOSAGE AND PREPARATIONS.

Intravenous (diagnostic): 1 g.

Orinase Diagnostic (Upjohn). Powder (sterile, for diagnostic use only) 1 g (present as 1.081 g tolbutamide sodium) with diluent.

BIGUANIDE COMPOUND

PHENFORMIN HYDROCHLORIDE

STATUS. This drug was removed from the general United States market by the FDA in 1978 because of the lactic acidosis associated with its use. This complication usually occurs in diabetic patients who are seriously ill with conditions accompanied by hypoxia (eg, cardiac failure, hypotension, liver or kidney disease), in those who take the drug with alcohol, or following severe anorexia or vomiting and ketosis, although lactic acidosis may develop without predisposing conditions. The mortality rate is approximately 50%. Probably very few, if any, patients who cannot be managed by other therapeutic measures require phenformin. However, this agent may be obtained under special circumstances for use in selected patients.

Phenformin is now available only under an Investigational New Drug Application (IND) exemption under conditions set forth by the FDA. These conditions include documentation that the patient is nonketotic and has not responded to diet or diet plus sulfonylureas; sulfonylureas cannot be tolerated; the

patient has responded to phenformin treatment in the past; there is no contraindication to the use of phenformin; and insulin cannot be taken. Informed consent must be obtained from the patient or guardian. Physicians may request further information in writing from Ciba-Geigy Corporation or the Division of Metabolism and Endocrine Drug Products (HFD-130), Food and Drug Administration, 5600 Fishers Lane, Rockville, MD 20857.

ACTIONS. Phenformin is not related chemically to the insulins or the sulfonylureas. It does not stimulate insulin secretion from the islet cells. Possible mechanisms of action include inhibition of hepatic gluconeogenesis, decreased intestinal absorption of glucose, up regulation of insulin receptors, and increased anaerobic glycolysis, which increases glucose utilization. Large doses appear to inhibit the conversion of alanine to glucose (gluconeogenesis) and lactate to glucose, whereas small doses enhance glycolysis without inhibiting gluconeogenesis or the conversion of lactate to glucose in vitro. However, it is not known if these effects are responsible for the hypoglycemic action noted with usual doses.

Although some physicians believe that phenformin may cause weight loss in the obese, mildly diabetic patient, some double-blind studies have not confirmed this finding. In addition to inducing anorexia, phenformin may retard the absorption of food. This agent inhibits the uptake of glucose by isolated, full-thickness human ileum.

Occasionally, patients in whom normal blood glucose concentrations are maintained by phenformin may experience weight loss, asthenia, and "starvation" ketonuria unless insulin also is administered. Phenformin alone rarely causes hypoglycemia, but this has occurred when it was given with another oral hypoglycemic agent.

(Investigational drug)

HYPERGLYCEMIC AGENTS

Hypoglycemic reactions may follow the use of alcohol and many drugs (eg, large doses of salicylates or acetaminophen, dicumarol, phenylbutazone [Azolid, Butazolidin], propranolol [Inderal] and other beta-adrenergic blocking agents) but probably are most common after administration of insulin or the sulfonylureas. (See the sections on Hypoglycemia under Insulin Use in Special Situations, and Adverse Reactions and Precautions under Oral Hypoglycemic Agents.) The diabetic patient must be aware of the earliest manifestations of hypoglycemia so that a readily available carbohydrate (eg, fruit juice, sugar) can be taken immediately.

For severe hypoglycemia and in unconscious or stuporous patients, intravenous 50% dextrose is preferred, but glucagon may be given intramuscularly (for increased rate of absorption) or subcutaneously before the physician arrives. Upon rousing, carbohydrate is given orally. Subsequent management of severe hypoglycemia depends upon the patient's clinical status and the blood glucose levels.

Hyperglycemic agents counteract the effects of increased insulin secretion in pathologic states. Diazoxide [Proglycem] blocks insulin secretion and is sometimes given preoperatively for insulinomas. Therapy may be prolonged in mild cases of islet cell tumors or when tumors cannot be found at surgery. This agent is sometimes used with streptozocin [Zanosar]. The latter destroys the beta cells of the islet tissue and is used for malignant insulinomas (see also Chapter 64, Drugs Used in Cancer Chemotherapy).

Leucine-sensitive hypoglycemia, often a familial condition occurring in young children with islet cell pathology or hyperinsulinemia, usually improves by age 3 to 6 years. Excessive insulin secretion is avoided by restricting leucine intake, and hypoglycemic effects are counteracted by supplementing carbohydrate intake and administering diazoxide.

Treatment of idiopathic reactive (functional) hypoglycemia is primarily dietary. Hyperglycemic agents are not indicated in this condition.

Drug Evaluations

DIAZOXIDE
[Proglycem]

ACTIONS AND USES. This nondiuretic thiazide is used for its hyperglycemic actions when given orally [Proglycem] and antihypertensive effects when given intravenously [Hyperstat I.V.] (see Chapter 28, Antihypertensive Agents). It produces a prompt, dose-related increase in blood glucose by directly inhibiting insulin secretion and, possibly, by inhibiting peripheral glucose utilization and stimulating hepatic glucose production. Diazoxide is used to counteract hyperinsulinism in conditions such as insulinoma or leucine-sensitive hypoglycemia. It is not indicated in the treatment of functional hypoglycemia.

ADVERSE REACTIONS, PRECAUTIONS, AND INTERACTIONS. Although diazoxide is a thiazide, it causes sodium and water retention that may necessitate concurrent administration of a diuretic; however, thiazide diuretics may intensify the drug's hyperglycemic and hyperuricemic effects. Oral diazoxide may potentiate the effects of other antihypertensive drugs, although the effect on blood pressure is not marked when this agent is used alone orally. The hyperglycemic action of diazoxide is antagonized by alpha-adrenergic blocking agents.

Diazoxide also may cause gastrointestinal irritation, thrombocytopenia, eosinophilia, neutropenia, and tachycardia. Excessive hair growth of a lanugo type occurs most frequently in children.

Diazoxide is teratogenic in animals (cardiovascular and skeletal deformities) and causes degeneration of fetal beta islet cells. The safety of this drug in pregnant women has not been established (FDA Pregnancy Category C).

PHARMACOKINETICS. Over 90% of diazoxide is bound to plasma proteins in the blood. The half-life of the oral form is 24 to 36 hours but may be prolonged after overdosage or in those with impaired renal function. Because of its long half-life, prolonged observation of patients is necessary. Overdosage

can cause marked hyperglycemia sometimes associated with ketoacidosis or nonketotic hyperosmolar coma.

DOSAGE AND PREPARATIONS.
Oral: *Adults and children,* 3 to 8 mg/kg daily; *infants,* 8 to 15 mg/kg daily. The drug is given in two or three equally divided doses.

Proglycem (Medical Market Specialties). Capsules 50 mg; oral suspension 50 mg/ml (alcohol 7.25%).

GLUCAGON

ACTIONS AND USES. Glucagon is a polypeptide produced by the alpha cells of the pancreas. Like insulin, its normal function appears to be to control the homeostasis of glucose, amino acids, and possibly free fatty acids. However, in contrast to insulin, glucagon has potent glycogenolytic and gluconeogenic activity and these effects form the basis for its clinical usefulness. Glucagon also reduces gastric and pancreatic secretions. It increases myocardial contractility but relaxes smooth muscle.

Glucagon is given principally to treat severe hypoglycemia in diabetic patients. It is often administered by a member of the family at home when a severe hypoglycemic episode occurs and the patient is unable to ingest sugar or simple carbohydrates or is unconscious.

Glucagon also has been used to diagnose insulinoma and pheochromocytoma. It increases the blood glucose concentration by mobilizing hepatic glycogen and thus is effective only when hepatic glycogen is available. Patients with reduced glycogen stores (eg, starvation, adrenal insufficiency, alcoholic hypoglycemia) cannot respond to glucagon.

Other uses of glucagon (eg, cardiovascular emergencies, meat impaction in the esophagus, beta blocker overdose) have been reviewed (Hall-Boyer et al, 1984).

ADMINISTRATION. Glucagon is effective only when administered parenterally. Its hyperglycemic effect is more gradual than that of dextrose and is of relatively brief duration. However, the blood glucose level is elevated enough to rouse the unconscious patient to take oral carbohydrate (first simple sugars, then complex carbohydrates for sustained effect), which restores hepatic glycogen and prevents secondary hypoglycemia. If carbohydrate is not ingested, blood glucose levels usually fall to normal or hypoglycemic levels in 60 to 90 minutes. An additional sugar source is especially important in juveniles, since their response is less pronounced than that of adults with stable diabetes. If there is no response within 20 minutes, dextrose should be given intravenously to avoid the deleterious effects of cerebral hypoglycemia.

ADVERSE REACTIONS. Nausea and vomiting have occurred occasionally after injection of glucagon; these effects also develop, but less frequently, with hypoglycemia. Hypersensitivity reactions are possible. This drug is classified in FDA Pregnancy Category B.

DOSAGE AND PREPARATIONS.
Intramuscular, Intravenous, Subcutaneous: *Adults and children,* 0.5 to 1 mg (usually subcutaneously, but intramuscu-

larly or intravenously if desired) every 15 to 20 minutes for two or three doses. (See the manufacturer's literature for directions on preparing the solution.)

The manufacturer's literature also contains instructions for the administration of glucagon by a family member; however, the drug should be used only under the direction of the physician. If it is used in an emergency, the physician should be notified. Any patient receiving insulin therapy should have glucagon available. Adult family members or a responsible friend should be instructed on the proper administration of glucagon.

Glucagon (Lilly). Powder (lyophilized) 1 and 10 mg with diluent.

Cited References

Combined sulfonylurea and insulin therapy in insulin-dependent diabetes: Research or clinical practice? (editorial). *Diabetes Care* 8:511-514, 1985.

Plethora of insulins, (editorial). *Diabetes Care* 3:638-639, 1980.

Advisory Panel on Oral Hypoglycemic Drugs, American Medical Association. *JAMA* 243:2078-2079, 1980.

Alberti KGMM: Low-dose insulin in treatment of diabetic ketoacidosis. *Arch Intern Med* 137:1367-1376, 1977.

American Diabetes Association: Principles of nutrition and dietary recommendations for individuals with diabetes mellitus: 1979. *Diabetes* 28:1027-1030, 1979 A.

American Diabetes Association: Policy statement: UGDP controversy. *Diabetes* 28:168-170, 1979 B.

American Diabetes Association: Policy statement: Glycemic effects of carbohydrates. *Diabetes Care* 7:607-608, 1984.

American Diabetes Association: Policy statement: Continuous subcutaneous insulin infusion. *Diabetes* 34:946-947, 1985 A.

American Diabetes Association: Policy statement: Self-monitoring of blood glucose. *Diabetes* 34:945, 1985 B.

Balant L: Clinical pharmacokinetics of sulphonylurea hypoglycaemic drugs. *Clin Pharmacokinet* 6:215-241, 1981.

Baynes JW, et al: National diabetes data group: Report of expert committee on glucosylated hemoglobin. *Diabetes Care* 7:602-606, 1984.

Beaser RS: Oral hypoglycemics: Optimizing benefits of new drugs and old. *Consultant* 82-98, (Oct) 1984.

Bernstein RS: Obesity and diabetes mellitus. *Cardiovasc Rev Rep* 4:813-819, 1983.

Biometric Society: Report of Committee for Assessment of Biometric Aspects of Controlled Trials of Hypoglycemic Agents. *JAMA* 231:583-608, 1975.

Bolli GB, Gerich JE: "Dawn phenomenon": Common occurrence in both non-insulin-dependent and insulin-dependent diabetes mellitus. *N Engl J Med* 310:746-750, 1984.

Bolli GB, et al: Demonstration of dawn phenomenon in normal human volunteers. *Diabetes* 33:1150-1153, 1984 A.

Bolli GB, et al: Glucose counterregulation and waning of insulin in Somogyi phenomenon (posthypoglycemic hyperglycemia). *N Engl J Med* 311:1214-1219, 1984 B.

Bonner RA: Insulin infusion therapy: Potential benefits and risks. *Postgrad Med* 77:153-164, (June) 1985.

Boyden T, Bressler R: Oral hypoglycemic agents. *Adv Intern Med* 24:53-70, 1979.

Brown MJ, Asbury AK: Diabetic neuropathy. *Ann Neurol* 15:2-12, 1984.

Burke BJ, et al: Improved diabetic control in insulin-dependent diabetes treated with insulin and glibenclamide. *Acta Endocrinol* 107:70-77, 1984.

Cader Asmal A, Marble A: Oral hypoglycaemic agents: Update. *Drugs* 28:62-78, 1984.

Camerini-Davalos RA, et al: Drug-induced reversal of early diabetic microangiopathy. *N Engl J Med* 309:1551-1556, 1983.

Campbell PJ, et al: Pathogenesis of dawn phenomenon in patients with insulin-dependent diabetes mellitus: Accelerated glucose production and impaired glucose utilization due to nocturnal surges in growth hormone secretion. *N Engl J Med* 312:1473-1479, 1985.

Cousins L: Congenital anomalies among infants of diabetic mothers: Etiology, prevention, prenatal diagnosis. *Am J Obstet Gynecol* 147:333-338, 1983.

Coustan DR, et al: Randomized clinical trial of insulin pump vs intensive conventional therapy in diabetic pregnancies. *JAMA* 255:631-636, 1986.

Dahl-Jørgensen K, et al: Rapid tightening of blood glucose control leads to transient deterioration of retinopathy in insulin dependent diabetes mellitus: Oslo study. *Br Med J* 290:811-815, 1985.

Davidson MB: *Diabetes Mellitus: Diagnosis and Treatment.* New York, John Wiley & Sons, 1981.

Davidson MB: Pathogenesis of impaired glucose tolerance and type II diabetes mellitus: Current status. *West J Med* 142:219-229, 1985.

Deckert T: Intermediate-acting insulin preparations: NPH and lente. *Diabetes Care* 3:623-626, 1980.

Drobny EC, et al: Insulin receptors in acute infection: Study of factors conferring insulin resistance. *J Clin Endocrinol Metab* 58:710-716, 1984.

Feinstein AR: How good is statistical evidence against oral hypoglycemic agents? *Adv Intern Med* 24:71-95, 1979.

Feldman JM: Glyburide: Second-generation sulfonylurea hypoglycemic agent; history, chemistry, metabolism, pharmacokinetics, clinical use and adverse effects. *Pharmacotherapy* 5:43-62, 1985.

Felig P, Bergman M: Insulin pump treatment of diabetes: Decision-making without definitive data. *JAMA* 250:1045-1047, 1983.

Felts PW: Ketoacidosis. *Med Clin North Am* 67:831-843, 1983.

Fisher JN, Kitabchi AE: Randomized study of phosphate therapy in treatment of diabetic ketoacidosis. *J Clin Endocrinol Metab* 57:177-180, 1983.

Frederiksen PK, Mogensen EF: Clinical comparison between glipizide (Glibenese) and glibenclamide (Daonil) in treatment of maturity onset diabetes: Controlled double-blind cross-over study. *Curr Ther Res* 32:1-7, 1982.

Freinkel N (ed): Summary and recommendations of Second International Workshop-Conference on Gestational Diabetes Mellitus. *Diabetes* 34(suppl 2):123-126, 1985.

Freinkel N, et al: Care of pregnant woman with insulin-dependent diabetes mellitus. *N Engl J Med* 313:96-101, 1985.

Gallina DL, et al: Surgery in diabetic patient. *Compr Ther* 9:8-16, (Feb) 1983.

Galloway JA: Insulin treatment for the early 80s: Facts and questions about old and new insulins and their usage. *Diabetes Care* 3:615-622, 1980.

Garvey WT, et al: Effect of insulin treatment on insulin secretion and insulin action in type II diabetes mellitus. *Diabetes* 34:222-234, 1985.

Golde SH, et al: Insulin requirements during labor: Reappraisal. *Obstet Gynecol* 144:556-559, 1982.

Gorsuch AN, et al: Can future type I diabetes be predicted? Study in families of affected children. *Diabetes* 31:862-866, 1982.

Groop L, et al: Chlorpropamide-alcohol flush: Significance of body weight, sex and serum chlorpropamide level. *Eur J Clin Pharmacol* 26:723-725, 1984.

Hall-Boyer K, et al: Glucagon: Hormone or therapeutic agent? *Crit Care Med* 12:584-589, 1984.

Health and Public Policy Committee, American College of Physicians: Glycosylated hemoglobin assays in management and diagnosis of diabetes mellitus. *Ann Intern Med* 101:710-713, 1984.

Heber D, et al: Low-dose continuous insulin therapy for diabetic ketoacidosis. Prospective comparison with "conventional" insulin therapy. *Arch Intern Med* 137:1377-1380, 1977.

Heine RJ, et al: Absorption kinetics and action profiles of mixtures of short- and intermediate-acting insulins. *Diabetologia* 27:558-562, 1984.

Hillson RM, Hockaday TDR: Chlorpropamide-alcohol flush: Critical reappraisal. *Diabetologia* 26:6-11, 1984.

Howard-Williams J, et al: Retinopathy associated with higher glycaemia in maturity-onset type diabetes. *Diabetologia* 27:198-202, 1984.

Jackson JE, Bressler R: Clinical pharmacology of sulphonylurea hypoglycaemic agents, parts I and II. *Drugs* 22:211-245, 295-320, 1981.

Jerntorp P, et al: Plasma chlorpropamide: Critical factor in chlorpropamide-alcohol flush. *Eur J Clin Pharmacol* 24:237-242, 1983.

Johnston C, et al: Chlorpropamide-alcohol flush: Case in favour. *Diabetalogia* 26:1-5, 1984.

Kadowaki T, et al: Chlorpropamide-induced hyponatremia: Incidence and risk factors. *Diabetes Care* 6:468-471, 1983.

Kilo C: Value of glucose control in preventing complications of diabetes. *Am J Med* 79(suppl 2B):33-37, 1985.

Kilo C, et al: Achilles heel of University Group Diabetes Program. *JAMA* 243:450-457, 1980 A.

Kilo C, et al: Crux of UGDP: Spurious results and biologically inappropriate data analysis. *Diabetologia* 18:179-185, 1980 B.

Kolata G: Dietary dogma disproved. *Science* 220:487-488, 1983.

Krall LP: Glyburide (DiaBeta): New second-generation hypoglycemic agent. *Clin Therapeut* 6:747-762, 1984.

Kreisberg RA: Diabetic ketoacidosis: New concepts and trends in pathogenesis and treatment. *Ann Intern Med* 88:681-695, 1978.

Lebovitz HE: Glipizide: Second-generation sulfonylurea hypoglycemic agent: Pharmacology, pharmacokinetics and clinical use. *Pharmacotherapy* 5:63-77, 1985.

Lever E, Jaspan JB: Sodium bicarbonate therapy in severe diabetic ketoacidosis. *Am J Med* 75:263-268, 1983.

Lipson LG, Lipson M: Therapeutic approach to obese maturity-onset diabetic patient. *Arch Intern Med* 144:135-138, 1984.

Mauer SM, et al: Development of lesions in glomerular basement membrane and mesangium after transplantation of normal kidneys to diabetic patients. *Diabetes* 32:948-952, 1983.

Mecklenburg RS, et al: Acute complications associated with insulin infusion pump therapy: Report of experience with 161 patients. *JAMA* 252:3265-3269, 1984.

Miller E, et al: Elevated maternal hemoglobin A$_{1c}$ in early pregnancy and major congenital anomalies in infants of diabetic mothers. *N Engl J Med* 304:1331-1334, 1981.

Miodovnik M, et al: Spontaneous abortion among insulin-dependent diabetic women. *Am J Obstet Gynecol* 150:372-376, 1984.

Morley GK, et al: Mechanism of pain in diabetic peripheral neuropathy: Effect of glucose on pain perception in humans. *Am J Med* 77:79-82, 1984.

National Diabetes Data Group: Classification and diagnosis of diabetes mellitus and other categories of glucose intolerance. *Diabetes* 28:1039-1057, 1979.

Nolte MS, et al: Reduced solubility of short-acting soluble insulins when mixed with longer-acting insulins. *Diabetes* 32:1177-1181, 1983.

Osei K, et al: Concomitant insulin and sulfonylurea therapy in patients with type II diabetes: Effects on glucoregulation and lipid metabolism. *Am J Med* 77:1002-1009, 1984.

O'Sullivan JB: Epidemiology of cardiovascular disease and diabetes mellitus in perspective. *Mt Sinai J Med* 49:163-168, 1982.

Paice BJ, et al: Undesired effects of sulphonylurea drugs. *Adv Drug React Acc Pois Rev* 1:23-36, 1985.

Rendell M: C-peptide levels as criterion in treatment of maturity-onset diabetes. *J Clin Endocrinol Metab* 57:1198-1206, 1983.

Riddle MC: New tactics for type 2 diabetes: Regimens based on intermediate-acting insulin taken at bedtime. *Lancet* 1:192-195, 1985.

Rigg L, et al: Effects of exogenous insulin on excursions and diurnal rhythm of plasma glucose in pregnant diabetic patients with and without residual β-cell function. *Am J Obstet Gynecol* 136:537-544, 1980.

Salzman R, et al: Intranasal aerosolized insulin: Mixed-meal studies and long-term use in type I diabetes. *N Engl J Med* 312:1078-1084, 1985.

Scarlett JA, et al: Insulin treatment reverses postreceptor defect in adipocyte 3-0-methylglucose transport in type II diabetes mellitus. *J Clin Endocrinol Metab* 56:1195-1201, 1983.

Schade DS, et al: Unstable diabetes and insulin resistance, in: *Intensive Insulin Therapy*. Princeton, Medical Examination Publishing, 1983.

Schmidt MI, et al: Fasting early morning rise in peripheral insulin: Evidence of dawn phenomenon in nondiabetics. *Diabetes Care* 7:32-35, 1984.

Scott J, Poffenbarger PL: Pharmacogenetics of tolbutamide metabolism in humans. *Diabetes* 28:41-51, 1978.

Simonson DC, et al: Mechanism of improvement in glucose metabolism after chronic glyburide therapy. *Diabetes* 33:838-845, 1984.

Simpson JL, et al: Diabetes in pregnancy, Northwestern University series (1977-1981): I. Prospective study of anomalies in offspring of mothers with diabetes mellitus. *Am J Obstet Gynecol* 146:263-270, 1983.

Skyler JS, et al: Algorithms for adjustment of insulin dosage by patients who monitor blood glucose. *Diabetes Care* 4:311-318, 1981.

Sonnenberg GE, Berger M: Human insulin: Much ado about one amino acid? (editorial). *Diabetologia* 25:457-459, 1983.

Sosenko JM, et al: Hyperglycemia and plasma lipid levels: Prospective study of young insulin-dependent diabetic patients. *N Engl J Med* 302:650-669, 1980.

Sperling MA: Diabetic ketoacidosis. *Pediatr Clin North Am* 31:591-610, 1984.

Stiller CR, et al: Effects of cyclosporine immunosuppression in insulin-dependent diabetes mellitus of recent onset. *Science* 223:1362-1367, 1984.

Sutherland DER, et al: Pancreas transplantation. *Pediatr Clin North Am* 31:735-750, 1984.

Tamborlane WV, Press CM: Insulin infusion pump treatment of type I diabetes. *Pediatr Clin North Am* 31:721-733, 1984.

Teutsch SM, et al: Mortality among diabetic patients using continuous subcutaneous insulin-infusion pumps. *N Engl J Med* 310:361-368, 1984.

University Group Diabetes Program: Effects of hypoglycemic agents on vascular complications in patients with adult-onset diabetes. I. Design, methods, and baseline results. II. Mortality results. *Diabetes* 19(suppl):747-783, 785-830, 1970. III. Clinical implications of UGDP results. *JAMA* 218:1400-1410, 1971. IV. Preliminary report on phenformin results. *JAMA* 217:777-784, 1971. V. Evaluation of phenformin therapy. *Diabetes* 24(suppl 1):65-184, 1975. VI. Supplementary report on nonfatal events in patients treated with tolbutamide. *Diabetes* 25:1129-1153, 1976. VII. Mortality and selected nonfatal events with insulin treatment. *JAMA* 240:37-42, 1978. VIII. Evaluation of insulin therapy; final report. *Diabetes* 31(suppl 5):1-18, 1982.

Waldhäusl W: To flush or not to flush? Comments on chlorpropamide-alcohol flush. *Diabetologia* 26:12-14, 1984.

Ward WK, et al: Pathophysiology of insulin secretion in non-insulin-dependent diabetes mellitus. *Diabetes Care* 7:491-502, 1984.

Warram JH, et al: Differences in risk of insulin-dependent diabetes in offspring of diabetic mothers and diabetic fathers. *N Engl J Med* 311:149-152, 1984.

Agents Used to Treat Thyroid Disease

Physiology

Thyroid hormones principally affect metabolism, growth, and development. Their most fundamental metabolic actions are calorigenic and protein anabolic; thyroid hormones accelerate the rate of cellular oxidation to increase energy expenditure and heat production. This, in turn, affects the metabolism of vitamins, proteins, carbohydrates, lipids, electrolytes, and water and the activity of hormones and drugs. The protein anabolic effect of thyroid hormones is important in growth and development.

The two metabolically important thyroid hormones are triiodothyronine (T_3) and tetraiodothyronine (T_4, thyroxine). (The synthetic preparations used clinically are, respectively, liothyronine [Cytomel] and levothyroxine [Levothroid, Synthroid]. Occasionally, a mixture of the two, liotrix [Euthroid, Thyrolar], is employed.) All of the T_4 and 10% to 20% of the T_3 produced daily are secreted by the thyroid; the remainder of T_3 results from monodeiodination of T_4.

In the thyroid follicular cells, iodide (the rate-limiting substrate for hormone synthesis) from the blood is concentrated 20 to 50 times by an active membrane transport process.

Other tissues (eg, salivary glands, placenta, mammary glands, parts of the gastrointestinal tract) also actively transport iodide from the blood against a concentration gradient but cannot synthesize thyroid hormone. This "trapping" of iodide can be blocked by inhibitors of oxidative metabolism, by agents that uncouple oxidative phosphorylation (eg, 2-4-dinitrophenol), by inadequate oxygen, and by certain monovalent anions (eg, perchlorate, thiocyanate).

After trapping, the iodide is oxidized ("activated") and then incorporated into mono- and diiodotyrosines (MIT and DIT) within the thyroglobulin molecule. DIT then couples with MIT or another DIT molecule to form T_3 or T_4, respectively. Thyrotropin (thyroid stimulating hormone, TSH) stimulates iodide trapping and each step of hormone synthesis, as well as release of hormones from the gland.

T_3 and T_4 are stored within thyroglobulin in the follicular lumina of the gland. In the presence of adequate iodide substrate, as in North America, the thyroid stores 10 to 20 times more T_4 than T_3 and releases about 1% daily. Thyroglobulin is transported by endocytosis back into the epithelial follicular cell, where it is degraded by proteolytic lysosomal enzymes to release T_3, T_4, MIT, and DIT. The T_4 and T_3 thus freed are secreted into the blood stream. Most of the MIT and DIT is deiodinated within the follicular cells; the iodide released is reincorporated into protein and represents an important source of iodine. Approximately 70 to 90 mcg of T_4 and 25 to 35 mcg of T_3 are produced daily by the thyroid gland. The remaining circulating T_3 (about 100 mcg) is formed by mono-deiodination of T_4 in peripheral tissues.

T_3 and T_4 are transported bound to serum proteins. About 70% of T_4 is bound to thyroxine-binding globulin (TBG), about 15% to thyroxine-binding prealbumin (TBPA), and about 15% to albumin. T_3 also is bound to TBG, but less firmly than T_4, as well as to TBPA and albumin. It has a shorter half-life in the circulation. Only the minute proportions of free thyroid hormones are biologically active and determine true thyroid status. Although exact figures are disputed, the free T_4 level is probably several times larger than the free T_3 concentration. Both are probably metabolically active, although, on a molar basis, T_3 is three to five times more potent calorigenically than T_4, and tissue receptors within the cell nucleus have predominant affinity for T_3. The protein-bound hormone serves principally as a reservoir.

Circulating thyroid hormone levels are regulated through a feedback system involving the thyroid, anterior pituitary, and hypothalamus. As the blood levels and, secondarily, tissue levels of free thyroid hormones increase, the secretion of TSH from the pituitary is inhibited, thereby decreasing thyroid secretion. Conversely, in the presence of subnormal levels of thyroid hormones, release of TSH is increased, which stimulates the secretion of thyroid hormones. In primary hypothyroidism, secretion of TSH is increased and serum TSH levels are elevated; in hyperthyroidism (except in the rare secondary or TSH-induced form), serum TSH levels are decreased. The major negative feedback effect occurs within the anterior pituitary where conversion of T_4 to T_3 precedes the inhibitory effect. TSH secretion also is stimulated by hypothalamic thyrotropin-releasing hormone (TRH), and the tonic level of thyroid gland activity appears to be maintained by hypothalamic TRH. Hypothalamic somatostatin and dopamine appear to inhibit TSH secretion. An intrathyroidal autoregulatory system also exists in which increased concentrations of iodide transiently inhibit the iodination of tyrosine; iodide also directly inhibits release of hormones from the gland.

In certain conditions, TBG levels may be altered, thus changing the total extrathyroidal pool of thyroid hormones. For example, TBG levels are physiologically elevated during pregnancy in response to high estrogen levels; this increases the serum concentrations of both protein bound and total T_4 and T_3 but not the amount of free hormones. The biologically active moieties are kept within normal limits and thyroid function is not affected. The opposite situation occurs during androgen therapy, when TBG levels are reduced. Increased binding of thyroxine to a serum albumin-like protein may be a familial trait, and failure to recognize this may lead to misdiagnosis of hyperthyroidism.

The half-life of T_4 in blood is about six days and that of T_3 is one and one-half days in euthyroid individuals. The half-life of T_4 is shortened in hyperthyroid patients (to as little as three days) and may be prolonged in hypothyroid patients (up to ten days). Conditions associated with elevated amounts of binding protein (eg, pregnancy, treatment with estrogen) increase the half-life, while those associated with reduced amounts of binding protein (eg, kidney or liver disease) may decrease the half-life. A significant degradative pathway for thyroid hormones is through conjugation in the liver. About 10% of secreted hormone, both conjugated and free, is excreted in the feces via the hepatobiliary system.

Approximately 85% to 90% of thyroid hormones is deiodinated in tissues, and the iodine released is available for reincorporation into new thyroid hormone; the portion of the hormone that is not reutilized is excreted in the urine. Deiodination of the outer ring (relative to the alanine side chain) of T_4 occurs at the 5′ position to form the active metabolite, T_3. Deiodination at the 5 position forms the inert metabolite, reverse T_3 (rT_3); a small amount of rT_3 probably is secreted directly by the thyroid. The serum concentrations of T_3 and rT_3 often assume a reciprocal relationship. The latter is increased in certain pathologic conditions (eg, starvation, acute debilitating disease, cachexia, surgery, cirrhosis, renal failure). In such cases, reduced 5′-deiodination of T_4 reduces T_3 production and rT_3 degradation, thus decreasing serum T_3 and increasing serum rT_3. rT_3 is the major circulating metabolite in the fetus and neonate.

Thyroid hormones increase oxygen utilization by the tissues through mechanisms involving cell nuclei and mitochondria. They bind to the nuclear nonhistone protein receptor (about 85% of iodothyronine bound to nuclei is T_3; 15% is T_4), stimulate synthesis of messenger RNA, and increase production of enzymes and proteins that carry out the metabolic effects of the hormone. These enzymes increase adenosine triphosphate (ATP) production and mitochondrial oxygen consumption. Other enzymes and proteins mediate effects on metabolism, growth, and development. Thyroid dysfunction thus has profound effects on many body systems, but effective treatment is available for most dysfunctional states.

Thyroid Function Tests

Although some thyroid diseases are recognized easily after a careful history and physical examination, appropriate diagnosis and therapy usually require laboratory confirmation of the type and severity of the disorder. Thyroid function tests can define the pathophysiologic state but should be used selectively and results should be consistent with clinical judgment.

The *serum T_4* determination is used as the initial screening test; total serum T_4 (protein-bound and unbound) preferably is measured by radioimmunoassay (T_4RIA) and is closely correlated with overall thyroid activity. This test alone is not sufficient for diagnosis, however, and is subject to misinterpretation if TBG levels are abnormal. In addition, levels may be low in patients with chronic illness or as a result of drug effects and may be either high or low in patients with severe nonthyroidal illness. Total serum T_4 also may be temporarily elevated in euthyroid patients with acute psychiatric disorders.

Misinterpretation is sometimes avoided by performing a serum free thyroxine (FT$_4$) or *free thyroxine index (FTI)* to screen for abnormal TBG levels. The FTI is expressed as a unitless number, since it does not represent a specific quantity of hormone. It is obtained by multiplying the serum T_4 concentration by the results of a resin T_3 uptake test. The *resin T_3 uptake test* (RT$_3$U) does *not* measure serum T_3 levels but instead provides an indirect estimate of serum TBG levels by indicating the number of available binding sites for thyroid hormones in serum. It is useful only in conjunction with measurement of total circulating T_4 levels. Ideally, the RT$_3$U is performed with a standard control serum pool and the result is reported relative to the control serum (value = 1). The fractional RT$_3$U value x total T_4 performed by RIA = "corrected T_4" value.

When the T_4 is elevated and the RT$_3$U is low, excess TBG is suggested. A low T_4 and high RT$_3$U suggest TBG deficiency or drug effects, since some drugs (eg, aspirin, phenytoin, diazepam, heparin) occupy serum protein sites normally occupied by thyroid hormone. In either instance, the "corrected T_4" value is normal. When both values are high or low, there is a true disturbance in the thyroid status and the "corrected T_4" value is abnormal. A high T_4 value suggests hyperthyroidism (or thyrotoxicosis); a low T_4 value suggests hypothyroidism. TBG levels may be determined directly by radioimmunoassay, which may detect abnormalities in binding not diagnosed by the resin T_3 uptake test.

The *protein-bound iodine* (PBI) test is used only rarely now but may be of value to determine the amount of serum non-T_4 iodoprotein in certain pathologic states (eg, thyroiditis, inborn defects in thyroid hormone synthesis).

The *serum T_3* radioimmunoassay test measures the total serum T_3 concentration and is useful to detect hyperthyroidism, T_3-thyrotoxicosis, or autonomous hyperfunctioning thyroid nodules since, in these conditions, T_3 may become elevated earlier and more markedly than T_4. However, modestly increased levels of T_3 also are observed rarely in iodine deficiency hypothyroidism or following radioiodine therapy. Serum T_3 levels are decreased or normal in hypothyroidism and decreased in patients with acute or chronic disease. In the latter patients, conversion of T_4 to T_3 in peripheral tissues is reduced; this clinical condition is referred to as low T_3 syndrome or euthyroid sick syndrome.

The determination of *serum TSH* by radioimmunoassay may be used to distinguish between primary (thyroidal) and secondary (pituitary) hypothyroidism. In these conditions, the serum TSH levels are elevated or undetectable, respectively, in the presence of low T_4 concentrations. Measurement of serum TSH also is useful to assess thyroid hormone replacement in the hypothyroid patient (see the section on Monitoring Therapy).

Dynamic tests of thyroid function also are utilized. *TRH* (thyrotropin-releasing hormone) may be used adjunctively to differentiate hypothalamic hypothyroidism (TSH secretion increased) from pituitary hypothyroidism (TSH secretion not increased), although the test is not as definitive as originally hoped. TRH is useful in confirming the diagnosis of thyrotoxicosis when determinations of both FT$_4$ and serum T_3 yield conflicting results. In the absence of pituitary disease, TSH responsiveness to TRH is absent in thyrotoxic patients. The test is especially useful in the diagnosis of hyperthyroidism in patients with cardiovascular disease or serious illness in whom thyroid hormone suppression tests would be unsafe (Chopra, 1983). Alternatively, a suppressed TSH concentration may be detected by a sensitive TSH radioimmunoassay.

In a *thyroid scan*, a small amount of radioactive iodine or technetium is given and the morphology of the areas of radioactive uptake and hence active thyroid tissue is outlined. Scanning is used (1) to determine whether hyperthyroidism is caused by Graves' disease, thyroid adenoma, or multinodular goiter, and (2) to help distinguish between malignant and nonmalignant nodules. Ultrasonography is used in the evaluation of hypofunctioning nodules to differentiate cystic nodules from solid lesions. Magnetic resonance imaging provides a better means for differentiating tumors and lymph nodes than computerized tomography but is still considered experimental. The *radioactive iodine uptake test* assists in determining the dosage for radioactive iodide ablation therapy and in differentiating Graves' disease from hyperthyroidism caused by thyroiditis.

Tests also are available to detect abnormal thyroid-stimulating immunoglobulins present in Graves' disease (see the section on Hyperthyroidism), although they are employed primarily as research tools. Antibodies against thyroid cell components and thyroglobulin present in Graves' disease, Hashimoto's (autoimmune) thyroiditis, or primary myxedema also can be measured. Their presence indicates an active autoimmune process but does not identify the specific disease.

For detailed descriptions of these and other tests and their interpretation, see specialty texts.

HYPOTHYROIDISM

Symptoms: Clinical manifestations of hypothyroidism include the classical myxedema facies with its round, puffy, sleepy appearance; dry, rough skin and brittle hair; bradycardia; and slightly elevated diastolic blood pressure. Myalgias and arthralgias are common. Fatigue, somnolence, irritability or apathy, constipation, hyperlipidemia, nonpitting peripheral edema, or intolerance to cold also may be observed. However, the severity of symptoms may not correlate with the severity of the disease (Utiger, 1983). When hypothyroidism occurs congenitally or during early infancy (ie, cretinism), there may be inadequate development of the brain, bones, teeth, and muscles; mental retardation; and delayed skeletal maturation.

Since thyroid hormone affects most organ systems, clinically dominant symptoms may not necessarily indicate thyroid disease (Klein and Levey, 1984). Such symptoms include anemia, coagulopathy, myopathy, and cardiomegaly.

Etiology: Clinical hypothyroidism is usually of thyroidal origin (primary); it may be idiopathic or follow destruction of the thyroid gland by radioactive iodine therapy, surgical removal, or autoimmune disease (goitrous, chronic lymphocytic [Hashimoto's] thyroiditis, nongoitrous atrophic thyroiditis). Hypothyroidism also may result from hypopituitarism (secondary) or hypothalamic injury (tertiary) produced by conditions such as tumor or trauma. The manifestations of severe hypothyroidism in adults (myxedema) may develop gradually over many years. Another cause of hypothyroidism is tissue resistance to thyroid hormone.

Hypothyroidism also may be induced by drugs (eg, lithium, antithyroid compounds, preparations with high iodine content), and withdrawal of the causative agent usually cures the condition. If these agents must be continued, thyroid replacement therapy may be given concomitantly.

Cretinism results from thyroid hormone deficiency during infancy or early childhood. It usually is caused by failure of the thyroid to develop normally, but may result from TSH deficiency, genetic defects in thyroid hormonogenesis, or extreme deficiency of iodine. Maternal ingestion of antithyroid drugs may produce transient neonatal hypothyroidism, and respiratory difficulties due to thyroid enlargement can occur. Hypothyroid infants who are breast fed may receive enough thyroid hormone in the milk to alleviate the deficiency partially (Bode et al, 1978). Juvenile hypothyroidism develops after 3 years of age in children who apparently were normal previously; it usually is produced by autoimmune mechanisms, but errors in thyroid hormonogenesis with delayed decompensation also may be causative.

Indications for Treatment

Regardless of the etiology or severity of hypothyroidism, replacement therapy with thyroid hormone is necessary. The only exception is drug-induced hypothyroidism in which withdrawal of the offending agent is indicated.

Early diagnosis and adequate treatment are mandatory for the management of *cretinism*. Screening programs for congenital hypothyroidism in neonates are now in widespread use and ensure the earliest possible detection. Screening programs are important, since only 5% of hypothyroid neonates identified by screening programs exhibit clinical manifestations. Hypothyroid neonates tend to have longer gestations (two to three weeks beyond term) and thus greater birth weights than normal (La Franchi, 1979). The incidence in female infants is about twice that in males.

Most of the permanent sequelae of cretinism can be minimized or avoided when appropriate treatment is begun immediately after birth. When treatment is initiated in the first weeks of life and maintained thereafter, intellectual ability is almost always normal. Treatment initiated after about 3 months of age does not reverse all of the intellectual impairment that has already occurred but does reverse the physical effects. Hypothyroidism that develops after age 2 to 3 years is not associated with mental retardation but usually is characterized by growth retardation, delayed epiphyseal maturation, and delayed dentition.

Because of its severity, *myxedema coma* should be treated as soon as a definitive diagnosis is made. Treatment is threefold: (1) Levothyroxine [Levothroid, Synthroid], liothyronine [Cytomel], or a combination of the two drugs, liotrix [Euthroid, Thyrolar], may be used. The combination may be advantageous in myxedema coma because peripheral conversion of T$_4$ to T$_3$ may be attenuated. Relatively large initial doses are given orally or intravenously, followed by oral therapy after the first day. (2) Appropriate supportive measures should be provided (ventilatory assistance, regulation of fluids and electrolytes, and administration of dextrose if hypoglycemia is present). (3) Intravenous corticosteroids should be given because adrenal insufficiency is difficult to rule out immediately.

Thyroid hormones are indicated to treat *large multinodular goiter* and *chronic lymphocytic (Hashimoto's) thyroiditis,* since replacement therapy may reduce the size of the goiter by suppressing secretion of TSH and avoids the occurrence of hypothyroidism.

Thyroid hormones also are indicated to prevent the growth of adenomatous goiters and to ameliorate the goitrogenic effects of some drugs (eg, lithium, aminosalicylic acid, some sulfonamides).

Rarely, transient hypothyroidism occurs during the course of *subacute thyroiditis.* Symptomatic improvement can be achieved with thyroid replacement during prolonged hypothyroid phases.

Thyroid hormones are used in the management of *thyroid carcinoma* and may produce a demonstrable regression of metastatic papillary lesions. All patients with papillary or follicular carcinoma require thyroid replacement therapy to minimize TSH stimulation. Such patients also require appropriate surgery and/or ablative radioiodine therapy. Prophylactic use of thyroid hormones after neck irradiation may be indicated to inhibit development of thyroid gland carcinoma.

In patients with cardiovascular disease (particularly arrhythmias), propranolol [Inderal] given with thyroid replacement therapy has been reported to decrease the risk of arrhythmia and angina and to allow greater tolerance of levothyroxine.

Hypothyroidism may occur during pregnancy and may increase the incidence of stillbirth. Full replacement doses of levothyroxine are administered to achieve plasma hormone levels in the normal range for pregnancy. Since little thyroid hormone crosses the placenta, the thyroid status of the fetus is not affected.

Since *abnormalities of reproductive function* (amenorrhea, menorrhagia, dysmenorrhea, premenstrual tension, sterility, habitual abortion, and oligospermia) may be associated with hypothyroidism, thyroid preparations have been used empirically in these disorders. There is no evidence that such therapy is beneficial unless the patient is proven to be hypothyroid.

Thyroid hormones have been given to treat so-called *metabolic insufficiency* without adequate laboratory documentation that thyroid hormone deficiency exists. Vague symptoms suggesting hypometabolism (eg, dry skin, fatigue, slight anemia, constipation, apathy) should not be treated indiscriminately with thyroid hormone. Since specific and precise tests of thyroid function are available, administration of thyroid preparations without proper documentation cannot be justified.

Thyroid hormones also have been used inappropriately to effect *weight loss* in euthyroid obese individuals. Since it is necessary to induce a state of hyperthyroidism to produce weight loss, such treatment can be harmful. Thus, preparations containing thyroid hormones should not be used for this purpose (see Chapter 51, Agents Used in Obesity).

Drug Therapy

Although synthetic levothyroxine is the preferred drug and thyroid, U.S.P., is considered obsolete, the latter is the proto-type of substances used to treat hypothyroidism. It is derived from the desiccated thyroid gland of animals and contains the active hormonal substances (T_3 and T_4), iodotyrosines, and other organic materials. Other preparations include thyroglob-ulin [Proloid], a substance prepared from animal thyroid glands; synthetic salts of the pure thyroid hormones, T_4 (levothyroxine sodium [Levothroid, Synthroid]) and T_3 (liothy-ronine sodium [Cytomel]); and a mixture of levothyroxine and liothyronine (liotrix [Euthroid, Thyrolar]). All produce similar metabolic and clinical effects, but they differ in potency and duration of action.

Thyroid preparations usually are administered orally. Paren-teral preparations are used in emergencies and when oral administration is impossible.

Relative Potency: The clinical response to 60 mg of thyroid, U.S.P., or 60 mg of thyroglobulin is approximately equal. The relative potency of synthetic preparations compared to desic-cated thyroid has been re-evaluated. Once it was thought that desiccated thyroid 60 mg was equivalent to synthetic prepara-tions of T_4 100 mcg, but recent evidence indicates that synthetic preparations of T_4 are considerably more potent. It is suggested that synthetic preparations of T_4 60 mcg are ap-proximately equivalent to desiccated thyroid 60 mg (Sawin et al, 1978). Theoretically, assuming that T_3 is three times more potent biologically than T_4, 25 mcg of synthetic preparations of T_3 is equivalent to 75 mg of desiccated thyroid. Preparations of liotrix containing 50 or 60 mcg of T_4 and 12.5 or 15 mcg of T_3, respectively, would be approximately equivalent to 90 to 100 mg of desiccated thyroid, respectively.

All desiccated thyroid preparations are standardized using high pressure liquid chromatography to identify content of levothyroxine and liothyronine and to determine the ratio of T_4 to T_3. However, batch-to-batch variability may occur and potency may vary from 90% to 110% of labeled amounts of levothyroxine and liothyronine. (See also the evaluation on Thyroid.)

Drug Selection: The thyroid preparation preferred for re-placement therapy is synthetic T_4 (levothyroxine sodium). It also is the drug of choice for congenital hypothyroidism (Committee on Drugs, American Academy of Pediatrics, 1978) and allows more precise assessment of clinical progress (see the section on Monitoring Therapy). Levothyroxine produces normal blood levels of both T_3 and T_4, although there may be slight fluctuations partly due to bioavailability problems en-countered with tablet formulations. However, patients who have been maintained for years on desiccated animal thyroid may not require newer, purer products. Use of desiccated thyroid in all other patients is considered obsolete (Smith, 1984).

Synthetic T_3 (liothyronine sodium) generally is not preferred for maintenance therapy, since it is difficult to monitor plasma levels of the hormone. Wider oscillations in plasma concentra-tion occur because of its shorter half-life. Since there is a long latent period between the appearance of both thyroid hor-mones in blood and the occurrence of biologic effects in the tissues, it is not known if fluctuations in plasma T_3 levels affect the physiologic results when liothyronine is taken for prolonged periods. Some physicians prefer liothyronine for initial therapy in myxedema and myxedema coma because of its short half-life. Liothyronine also has better absorption characteris-tics (80% to 100% absorbed compared to approximately 70% for T_4) and may be preferred when the reliability of gastroin-testinal absorption is in doubt.

When preparations containing a physiologic ratio of both T_4 and T_3 (liotrix) were introduced, it was thought that they would produce a physiologic ratio of the two hormones in the blood. However, since most circulating T_3 is formed by peripheral monodeiodination of T_4, the T_3 component is not needed. Therefore, the combination products offer no therapeutic ad-vantage over levothyroxine alone for the routine treatment of hypothyroidism. The possibility that combination products may be useful when the peripheral conversion of T_4 to T_3 is reduced has not been evaluated, and the importance of this variation in T_3 availability in nonthyroid disorders is as yet unknown.

The slight difference in cost among the various thyroid replacement products makes this factor unimportant in drug selection.

Dosage: The dosage of thyroid preparations must be indi-vidualized and varies with the severity of hypothyroidism and the age of the patient; therapy usually must be life-long. In cretinism, treatment is begun with full replacement doses. In adults, the initial dose generally is small and the amount is increased gradually until an optimal response is produced. The dose required to maintain this response then is given once daily for an indefinite period. However, since thyroid require-ments decrease with age, thyroid status should be evaluated periodically to determine whether an adjustment in mainte-nance dosage is required. If liothyronine is used, it should be given in divided doses two or three times daily.

Hypothyroid patients have increased sensitivity to thyroid hormones, and determination of the optimum maintenance dose should be based on apparent clinical status, age, and the results of appropriate laboratory tests (see the following section on Monitoring Therapy). Maintenance doses for adults are lower (100 to 200 mcg of levothyroxine daily) than those formerly utilized. If a patient currently receives larger amounts, the dose may be reduced gradually to the minimum required to suppress serum TSH or to maintain normal serum levels of T_4.

Mild hypothyroidism can be treated initially with one-half the expected maintenance dosage, with full replacement amounts given after one to two months. In myxedema, the dose is increased more gradually because these patients are very sensitive to thyroid hormone; four to six months of therapy may be required to achieve euthyroidism. Factors that favor conser-vatism in treatment include coronary artery disease; severe, prolonged thyroid disease; and advanced age. The half-life of thyroid hormones is increased in the latter; therefore, elderly patients, particularly those with arterial disease, require a small initial dose, gradual dosage increments, and a lower maintenance dose than younger adults. In children, maintenance levels are relatively higher than in adults; adolescents usually require adult levels for replacement. In general, dose is related to lean body mass but has no relationship to total body mass in obese subjects.

Monitoring Therapy: Assessment of therapy requires monitoring of signs and symptoms as well as laboratory data. It is important that the physician understand the difficulties of interpreting thyroid function tests when patients are taking thyroid medication. Even when standard assay kits are employed, results from different laboratories may vary; thus, a single laboratory should be employed.

The optimal serum T_4 levels vary, depending upon the preparation used. In adequately treated euthyroid patients, plasma levels of T_4 are in the normal range when levothyroxine is used (this is about 20% higher than with liotrix). When liothyronine is employed, plasma T_4 levels remain low.

Measurement of serum TSH, a highly specific test, is useful for monitoring thyroid therapy in patients with primary hypothyroidism. TSH levels begin to decrease within hours after initiating therapy and correlate inversely with thyroid hormone levels. Elevated levels of TSH indicate inadequate replacement dosage. The TRH test also should be normal when replacement of thyroid hormone is adequate; inadequate replacement is associated with a normal to elevated TSH response to TRH.

Measurement of the serum TSH concentration is unreliable as the sole indicator of adequate thyroid therapy, however. This is particularly true in congenital hypothyroidism, because serum TSH levels may remain elevated for months or years when appropriate or even excessive doses are given. In these patients, the set point for T_3 feedback control of TSH appears to be abnormal as a result of the intrauterine hypothyroxinemia. In these cases, serum T_4 should be monitored by radioimmunoassay and maintained in the upper half of the normal range for the age of the infant or child (serum FTI also may be used). This ensures sufficient hormone for the growing child between changes in regimen.

Adverse Reactions: If the appropriate amount of thyroid hormone is provided for replacement, no adverse reactions occur. However, overdosage of any thyroid preparation causes thyrotoxicosis. Signs and symptoms include tachycardia, palpitations, wide variations in pulse pressure, angina pectoris, tremor, nervousness, insomnia, headache, change in appetite, diarrhea, weight loss, hyperhidrosis, heat intolerance, and fever. The dose of thyroid hormone that produces thyrotoxicosis varies widely from patient to patient.

The suggestion that the incidence of breast cancer was increased in women receiving thyroid replacement therapy has been evaluated and the evidence was found to be tenuous. There was no increased risk associated with long-term use of thyroid hormone, and it is recommended that patients with a documented need for thyroid medication continue their therapeutic program (Education Committee, American Thyroid Association, 1977; Shapiro et al, 1980).

Precautions: Since hypothyroid patients may discontinue medication when euthyroidism has been attained, it is important to stress (1) that their need for thyroid replacement therapy is life-long, and (2) that they must inform any new physician of their condition.

Hypothyroid patients respond rapidly to replacement doses of thyroid hormones. In adults, it is important that the dose not be increased too rapidly when there is underlying arteriosclerosis or myocardial disease. In such patients, the capacity of the heart to handle the increased metabolic demands of the body may be exceeded. If cardiovascular symptoms appear, the dose must be reduced. On the other hand, for patients with myxedema coma or severe myxedema with bowel obstruction, it may be lifesaving to accept the hazard associated with rapid replacement. In younger patients, the dose may be increased to the full replacement amount more rapidly without undue risk.

When hypothyroidism and adrenal insufficiency coexist, as in pituitary insufficiency (secondary hypothyroidism), adequate amounts of cortisone or hydrocortisone should be given before attempting thyroid replacement therapy, since thyroid hormones increase the metabolic turnover and degradation of adrenocortical hormones and may precipitate acute adrenocortical insufficiency.

Drug Interactions: Thyroid hormones enhance the effect of coumarin anticoagulants by increasing catabolism of vitamin K-dependent clotting factors. If levothyroxine and a coumarin anticoagulant are given concomitantly, the dose of the latter may have to be decreased.

Cholestyramine [Questran] binds orally administered thyroid hormone in the intestine, delaying or preventing absorption. To prevent this interaction, there should be a four- to five-hour interval between administration of cholestyramine and an oral thyroid drug.

Initiation of thyroid therapy in diabetic patients may increase the requirement for insulin or oral hypoglycemic agents. In digitalized patients, the requirement for digoxin [Lanoxin] may be increased.

Drug Evaluations

LEVOTHYROXINE SODIUM
[Levothroid, Synthroid]

ACTIONS AND USES. This synthetic sodium salt of the levorotatory isomer of T_4 (thyroxine) is used most commonly for replacement therapy in hypothyroidism. In myxedema coma, levothyroxine should be given intravenously with hydrocortisone to prevent adrenal crisis (Jordan, 1983). These patients should be treated in the intensive care unit and electrocardiographic monitoring is necessary since this therapy may cause ventricular arrhythmias.

Other uses of levothyroxine include the treatment of simple nonendemic goiter, chronic lymphocytic (Hashimoto's) thyroiditis, and thyrotropin-dependent carcinoma of the thyroid (see the Introduction). It also may prevent the goitrogenic effects of other therapeutic agents (eg, lithium, aminosalicylic acid, some sulfonamide compounds). *For most indications requiring thyroid replacement, levothyroxine is the drug of choice.*

PHARMACOKINETICS. Levothyroxine is less completely absorbed from the gastrointestinal tract than liothyronine and has a slower onset of action when given orally. The half-life of levothyroxine is approximately one week. Thus, the change in serum thyroxine levels is slow when the oral dosage is increased or decreased. A steady-state level is achieved in about one month.

See the Introduction for adverse reactions and precautions with use of levothyroxine.

DOSAGE AND PREPARATIONS. Levothyroxine usually is administered orally, but the intravenous route is used in myxedema coma or when oral administration is impractical. In general, the intravenous dosage for levothyroxine is one-half the oral dosage.

Oral: For mild hypothyroidism, *young and middle-aged adults,* initially, 50 to 100 mcg daily, increased by 50 mcg or less at three- to four-week intervals until the desired response is maintained. (The average maintenance dose is 125 to 150 mcg/day.) For severe hypothyroidism, initially, 25 mcg daily, increased by 25 mcg at two-week intervals to 100 mcg daily. Further increases by increments of 50 to 100 mcg may be made at two-week intervals until the desired response is maintained. Most patients can be maintained in a euthyroid state with 100 to 200 mcg daily. Patients receiving suppressive therapy for goiter or thyroid cancer may require larger doses. *Older adults,* initially, 12.5 to 50 mcg daily for three to six weeks, increased by 12.5 to 25 mcg every three to eight weeks until the desired response is maintained.

For otherwise normal *infants 0 to 6 months,* initially, 25 to 50 mcg or 8 to 10 mcg/kg daily in a single oral dose (usually, 37.5 mcg is appropriate). *Premature infants less than 2 kg and infants at risk of cardiac failure,* initially, 25 mcg daily. The dose usually can be increased to 50 mcg daily in four to six weeks. *Infants 6 to 12 months,* 50 to 75 mcg or 6 to 8 mcg/kg daily. *Children 1 to 5 years,* 75 to 100 mcg or 5 to 6 mcg/kg daily. *Children 6 to 12 years,* 100 to 150 mcg or 4 to 5 mcg/kg daily, which may be continued with adjustments until midadolescence when adult dosage (usually 2.3 mcg/kg/day) is sufficient. The maintenance dose should produce serum T_4 and T_3 concentrations in the upper half of the normal range for the child's age.

　　Generic. Tablets 100, 200, and 300 mcg.
　　Levothroid (USV), *Synthroid* (Flint). Tablets 25, 50, 75, 100, 125, 150, 175 (*Levothroid* only), 200, and 300 mcg.

Intravenous: For *newborn infants* unable to take oral medication, 50% of the oral dose (see above) is given daily. For myxedema coma, *adults,* 1.5 to 5 ml of a solution containing 100 mcg/ml (150 to 500 mcg but usually 400 mcg); 1 to 3 ml may be given on the second day if necessary. Hydrocortisone is given concomitantly; the dose is 300 mg/day in divided doses; decreased gradually over the next four to five days (Jordan, 1983). After the patient's condition has stabilized, levothyroxine is given orally for maintenance.

　　Levothroid (USV). Powder (lyophilized) 200 or 500 mcg with mannitol 15 mg.
　　Synthroid (Flint). Powder (lyophilized) 200 or 500 mcg with mannitol 10 mg.

LIOTHYRONINE SODIUM
[Cytomel]

ACTIONS AND USES. This drug is the synthetic sodium salt of the levorotatory isomer of T_3. On a weight basis, liothyronine is 2.5 to 3.3 times more potent than levothyroxine. Although less is bound to TBG than is thyroxine, about 99% is protein bound to both TBG and albumin. It is readily available to tissues and is rapidly metabolized and excreted. Therefore, the onset and duration of action are short. Monitoring is difficult because blood levels fluctuate after each dose. Thus, liothyronine is not as useful as levothyroxine for maintenance therapy. However, it may be preferred to levothyroxine if intestinal absorption of T_4 is impaired. Liothyronine also may be used for short-term suppression of a solitary thyroid nodule, prior to radioiodine scanning, or when thyroid therapy must be interrupted periodically, such as in patients with thyroid cancer who require ablative radioiodine therapy. However, liothyronine should not be used for long-term replacement in these patients because it is less effective than levothyroxine in suppressing TSH production.

Liothyronine may be given intravenously to treat myxedema coma, since its rapid action facilitates the adjustments in dosage often required. However, levothyroxine is the drug of choice for intravenous administration. (See the Introduction.) Although liothyronine is not available commercially in a form suitable for intravenous use, the manufacturer will supply a kit, upon request, for parenteral administration. Alternatively, crushed tablets are sometimes given through a nasogastric tube.

See the Introduction for adverse reactions and precautions.

DOSAGE AND PREPARATIONS.

Oral: Liothyronine should be given in divided doses two or three times daily. For mild hypothyroidism, *young and middle-aged adults,* initially, 25 mcg daily, increased by 12.5 to 25 mcg at intervals of one to two weeks until the desired response is maintained. For severe hypothyroidism, initially, 5 mcg daily, increased by 5 to 10 mcg at intervals of one to two weeks until a daily dose of 25 mcg is reached; thereafter, this amount is increased by 12.5 to 25 mcg at one- to two-week intervals until the desired response is maintained. The usual maintenance dose is up to 75 mcg/day. *Older adults,* initially, 2.5 to 5 mcg daily for three to six weeks; the amount is then doubled every six weeks until the desired response is maintained.

　　Cytomel (Smith Kline & French). Tablets 5, 25, and 50 mcg.

Intravenous: For myxedema coma, no specific dosage recommendations are made, since the initial dose should be determined by the patient's condition. Initial doses for *adults* have ranged from 10 to 100 mcg. Subsequent doses are regulated by response of the patient to the initial dose. Hydrocortisone is given concomitantly (see the evaluation on Levothyroxine Sodium for dosage). Liothyronine is given orally for maintenance.

Cytomel (Smith Kline & French). Powder (for solution). When reconstituted, 100 mcg/ml of liothyronine is present as the free acid. Parenteral preparation not available commercially; manufacturer will supply kit, upon request, for use in myxedema coma.

LIOTRIX
[Euthroid, Thyrolar]

Liotrix is a mixture of levothyroxine sodium and liothyronine sodium in a ratio of 4:1, respectively. The indications, adverse reactions, and precautions are the same as those for levothyroxine (see the Introduction and the evaluation on Levothyroxine Sodium). The mixture is equivalent to but offers no clinical advantage over levothyroxine, since conversion of T_4 to T_3 in peripheral tissue usually results in a normal physiologic ratio of the two hormones. Plasma levels of T_3 increase several hours after an oral dose. However, in myxedema coma, in which peripheral conversion of T_4 to T_3 may be reduced, use of the combination may be advantageous.

Liotrix tablets are designated in sizes 1/4, 1/2, 1, 2, and 3, indicating approximate biologic potency compared to that quantity of desiccated thyroid expressed in grains. It should be noted that the same potency designations used by the two manufacturers actually indicate different quantities of hormone. For example, Euthroid-1/2 contains 30 mcg levothyroxine and 7.5 mcg liothyronine, while Thyrolar-1/2 contains 25 mcg levothyroxine and 6.25 mcg liothyronine. These variations in hormone levels may cause clinically significant differences in response, and this should be considered before substituting one brand for the other.

Newer estimates of potency suggest that liotrix preparations are more potent than indicated by the size designation (eg, 1/2, 1, 2). See also the discussion on Relative Potency in the Introduction. Usual replacement dosages of this preparation produce serum FTI levels that are more typically normal.

DOSAGE AND PREPARATIONS.

Oral: For hypothyroidism, *young and middle-aged adults,* initially, one tablet daily containing either 30 mcg of levothyroxine sodium and 7.5 mcg of liothyronine sodium [Euthroid] or 25 mcg of levothyroxine sodium and 6.25 mcg of liothyronine sodium [Thyrolar]. Depending upon the response, the dose is increased by one tablet every two weeks. For maintenance, tablets that conveniently provide optimal therapy as determined by results of laboratory tests and clinical status are given. The final maintenance dose may be greater in children than in adults. *Older adults,* initially, one-fourth to one-half the amount prescribed for younger adults; the dose is doubled at six- to eight-week intervals until the desired response is achieved.

Euthroid (Parke-Davis). Tablets (**Euthroid-1/2, -1, -2,** and **-3)** containing, respectively, levothyroxine sodium and liothyronine sodium: 30/7.5, 60/15, 120/30, and 180/45 mcg.

Thyrolar (USV). Tablets (**Thyrolar-1/4, -1/2, -1, -2,** and **-3)** containing, respectively, levothyroxine sodium and liothyronine sodium: 12.5/3.1, 25/6.25, 50/12.5, 100/25, and 150/37.5 mcg.

THYROID, U.S.P.
[Armour Thyroid, S-P-T, Thyrar, Thyroid Strong]

This preparation is the cleaned, dried, powdered thyroid gland of domesticated animals. The U.S.P. standards for all thyroid products from animal sources require that the sum of the contents of levothyroxine and liothyronine is not less than 0.095% and not more than 0.125%, by weight, of thyroid and that the ratio of levothyroxine to liothyronine is not less than 5:1 (thyroid tablet). The content of inorganic iodide is limited to 0.004% or less (*U.S.P. XXI*, 1985). These standards reduce variability, but batch-to-batch differences may occur and the label should be consulted. (Thyroid tablets contain not less than 90% and not more than 110% of the labeled amounts of thyroid and levothyroxine.) The variable potency could be harmful, especially in infants and children or adults with angina pectoris and hypothyroidism. Some of the variations due to tablet texture can be obviated by chewing the tablet.

Thyroid has the same indications, adverse reactions, and precautions as levothyroxine (see the Introduction). However, desiccated thyroid is considered obsolete and is recommended only for those who have been maintained for years on this product. Desiccated thyroid often produces postabsorptive T_3 elevations above the normal range and could be hazardous in patients with cardiovascular disease or in the elderly. See the Introduction.

DOSAGE AND PREPARATIONS. Thyroid hormone should be taken on an empty stomach to enhance absorption. For replacement therapy, the dose must be individualized. The optimal amount is determined primarily by the clinical response and confirmed by results of laboratory tests. The initial dose is usually small and the amount is increased gradually until a euthyroid state is obtained; the patient is then maintained on this dose.

Oral: For *younger adults,* the common practice has been to give 15 to 30 mg daily initially, increased by increments of 15 to 30 mg at two-week intervals until the desired response is obtained; however, some authorities start younger patients on nearly full replacement doses. The usual maintenance dose is 60 to 120 mg daily in a single dose. *Older adults,* initially, 7.5 to 30 mg daily; the dose is doubled at two- to eight-week intervals until an optimal response is obtained.

For suppressive therapy, as for replacement therapy, the initial dose for *adults* should be lower than the maintenance dose (eg, 60 mg) and is increased as indicated by the response; for maintenance, 90 to 180 mg daily.

Generic. Tablets 16, 32, 65, 130, 195, 260, and 325 mg corresponding to 1/4, 1/2, 1, 2, 3, 4, and 5 grains, respectively; tablets (enteric-coated) 32, 65, and 130 mg, corresponding to 1/2, 1, and 2 grains, respectively.

Armour Thyroid Tablets (USV). Tablets (pork extract) 16, 32, 65, 98, 130, 195, 260, and 325 mg, corresponding to 1/4, 1/2, 1, 1 1/2, 2, 3, 4, and 5 grains, respectively.

S-P-T (Fleming). Capsules (liquid) 65, 130, 195, and 325 mg, corresponding to 1, 2, 3, and 5 grains, respectively.

Thyrar (USV). Tablets (beef extract) 32, 65, and 130 mg, corresponding to 1/2, 1, and 2 grains, respectively.

Thyroid Strong (Marion). Tablets 32, 65, 130, and 195 mg corresponding to 1/2, 1, 2, and 3 grains, respectively (50% stronger than Thyroid, U.S.P.).

THYROGLOBULIN

[Proloid]

Thyroglobulin is obtained from a purified extract of frozen hog thyroid. It is standardized according to U.S.P. requirements for thyroid and tablets contain not less than 90% or more than 110% of the labeled amounts of thyroglobulin and levothyroxine. Also, the ratio of levothyroxine to liothyronine is not less than 2.8:1. On a weight basis, the potency of this preparation is equal to that of thyroid, and the indications, adverse effects, precautions, and doses are the same (see the Introduction and the evaluation on Thyroid, U.S.P.).

Generic. Powder 100 mg.

Proloid (Parke-Davis). Tablets 32, 65, 100, 130, and 200 mg, corresponding to 1/2, 1, 1 1/2, 2, and 3 grains, respectively.

HYPERTHYROIDISM

Thyrotoxicosis results from the excessive secretion of thyroid hormones and may be caused by Graves' disease (toxic diffuse goiter), toxic multinodular goiter, thyroiditis, single hyperfunctioning thyroid nodules, or other less common causes. In each case, the ratio of T_4:T_3 secreted may vary from normal. If T_3 predominates, T_3 thyrotoxicosis may occur. In this condition, the serum level of T_3 is increased but the serum level of T_4 may be normal or only slightly increased. The deviation appears to be important only diagnostically, since the symptoms of T_3 thyrotoxicosis resemble those of other forms of hyperthyroidism and the treatment is similar.

Thyrotoxicosis is characterized by hypermetabolism manifested by effects on temperature regulation (eg, increased heat production with intolerance to heat; warm, moist, flushed skin); cardiovascular effects (eg, rapid, strong heartbeat; in older patients, angina, arrhythmias, heart failure); skeletal muscle weakness and wasting; tremor; emotional instability; general overactivity; hypercalcemia, hypercalciuria, and osteopathy; and increased appetite with weight loss if caloric requirements are not met by adequate food intake.

Evidence suggests that Graves' disease, the most common form of hyperthyroidism, is an autoimmune disorder in which circulating humoral stimulators act on the thyroid gland. These immunoglobulins are designated TSI (thyroid stimulating immunoglobulins) or TSAb (thyroid stimulating antibodies). They are distinct from TSH and occur in the serum of most patients with this disease. Other designations for these immunoglobulins based on the method of their assay include LATS (long-acting thyroid stimulator), HTSI (human thyroid-stimulating immunoglobulin, formerly LATS-protector), or HTACS (human thyroid adenylate cyclase stimulator).

It is believed that TSI bind to TSH receptors on thyroid follicular cell membranes, resulting in stimulation of the thyroid gland. TSI mimic the actions of TSH and stimulate production of T_4 and T_3. However, their precise role in the pathogenesis of Graves' disease is still uncertain. The presence of TSI in the blood indicates disease activity, and their persistence after a course of antithyroid therapy is predictive of relapse. The absence of TSI does not guarantee that relapse will not occur, however (Zakarija et al, 1980; Bech and Madsen, 1980).

Graves' disease is approximately six times more common in women than in men. The disease may develop at any age but most often appears during the third or fourth decade. Vitiligo, myasthenia gravis, and pernicious anemia are observed more frequently in patients with Graves' disease.

The ophthalmopathy associated with Graves' disease may improve with effective treatment or may worsen, especially if hypothyroidism develops. The unpredictability of the ophthalmopathy must be emphasized to the patient. Pretibial myxedema, which is uncommon, usually is observed simultaneously with exophthalmos; correction of the thyroid state does not control either disorder. Severe exophthalmos may be relieved by high-dose oral glucocorticoid therapy and pretibial myxedema may be ameliorated with topical steroids. Cyclosporine [Sandimmune] was reported to improve the ophthalmopathy in two patients (Weetman et al, 1983). However, until more experience has accumulated, its efficacy cannot be determined.

Potentially fatal thyrotoxic crisis (thyroid storm) may occur in hyperthyroid patients who experience trauma or infection or who are not adequately prepared for surgery. It is manifested by hyperthermia, extreme tachycardia, profound asthenia, high-output heart failure, and, finally, syncope and coma. Treatment should be started immediately without waiting for laboratory confirmation and includes antithyroid medication (initially), iodine, propranolol, hydrocortisone or dexamethasone, fluids and electrolytes, and digitalis glycosides if necessary. Other standard supportive measures (eg, sedation, oxygen, cooling of the patient) should be employed. This potentially dangerous state can be reversed rapidly by charcoal hemodialysis. Plasmapheresis has been used when conventional therapy fails.

Neonatal thyrotoxicosis may occur, particularly in infants of thyrotoxic mothers, and is presumed to be caused by placental transfer of maternal TSI. The mortality rate is high and this complication is treated with antithyroid drugs, propranolol, sedation, and digitalization, as well as with appropriate supportive measures. Neonatal thyrotoxicosis typically resolves within two months and medication can be withdrawn gradually.

Resistance to thyroid hormones may be confused with hyperthyroidism. Patients with global resistance to thyroid hormones (GRTH) may have elevated levels of free T_4 and T_3, normal or slightly elevated TSH levels, and preservation of the TSH response to TRH; the usual symptoms of hyperthyroidism may be absent and goiter may be present. Indiscriminate measures to reduce elevated thyroid hormone levels should be avoided, for the resulting damage may be irreversible in infants or children (Refetoff et al, 1983).

Heart disease often complicates hyperthyroidism. Arrhythmias are common and heart failure may occur, especially in the elderly. If congestive heart failure develops, it must be treated conventionally at the same time that control of thyro-toxicosis is initiated. However, digitalis preparations are less effective than usual in these patients unless hyperthyroidism is corrected. Also, in the aged, hyperthyroidism may exist without the classical signs and often appears as "apathetic" hyperthy-roidism in which cardiac abnormalities may be the predomi-nant manifestation.

The treatment of hyperthyroidism is directed toward reduc-ing the excessive production of thyroid hormones. This can be accomplished with antithyroid drugs (which render the patient euthyroid until a spontaneous remission occurs), radiation, or surgery; the latter two procedures are more definitive. Since many of the signs and symptoms of hyperthyroidism reflect increased cellular sensitivity to adrenergic stimulation, the beta-adrenergic blocking drug, propranolol [Inderal], may be used adjunctively. Accurate diagnosis is essential before treatment is started, and the choice of therapy depends upon careful evaluation of each patient.

Choice of Therapy

The choice of antithyroid drugs, radiation, or surgery (after antithyroid drugs) to treat hyperthyroidism is influenced by the patient's age and sex, cardiovascular status, degree of hyper-thyroidism, and history of previous management of the dis-ease. Opinions vary on which therapeutic modality is best.

Antithyroid drugs of the thioamide type (propylthiouracil and methimazole [Tapazole]) are frequently utilized for the initial treatment of Graves' disease since spontaneous and, possi-bly, permanent remission may occur during therapy. However, the rate of remission now appears to be lower than reported formerly (30% to 40% each two to three years rather than 50%), which may be due to the increased intake of dietary iodine in recent years. Because of this, many physicians and patients choose to employ radioactive iodine or subtotal thyroidectomy for initial and definitive treatment. Response times to antithyroid drugs and irradiation are similar. Thioam-ides remain the usual initial choice for management of hyper-thyroidism and are preferred for children and adolescents, pregnant women, patients being prepared for surgery, and those with cardiac disease being prepared for radiation thera-py.

If antithyroid drugs are ineffective in children after two to four years, surgery might be selected (the risk decreases with increasing age). Surgery also is appropriate for a large disfig-uring goiter. In these cases, antithyroid drugs are employed initially to induce euthyroidism preoperatively, since surgical complications are increased in hyperthyroid patients.

Irradiation is used in patients who are poor surgical risks or who have undergone previous thyroid surgery (the risk of complications is greater if thyroid surgery is repeated). Some physicians prefer irradiation (even in children) to antithyroid drugs for Graves' disease because the course and outcome are more predictable. Radioiodine or surgery also may be selected to treat toxic nodular goiter, because remission is uncommon.

Hyperthyroidism tends to improve during pregnancy. If treatment is appropriate, an antithyroid drug is used in early pregnancy. Surgery may be performed in the second trimester if drug therapy is ineffective.

Complications may occur after either surgery or radiation therapy. Although both carry a long-term potential for the development of hypothyroidism, this is more likely after radia-tion; recurrent hyperthyroidism is more likely after surgery. Patients receiving either form of ablative treatment should be monitored periodically for thyroid status.

Morbidity and mortality are greater after surgery, but they are greatly reduced when the surgeon is experienced in performing these operations. In general, radiation is relatively safe, although thyrotoxic manifestations occasionally increase for seven to ten days following high doses of sodium iodide I 131 [Iodotope]. This could compromise patients with limited cardiac reserve. Also of concern is the possibility that irradia-tion may be carcinogenic or injurious to gametes. Recent review of large numbers of treated patients after two to three decades of follow-up has shown no increase in the incidence of other malignancy and no evidence of gamete injury in offspring. Therefore, most physicians advocate modification of the age limits (ie, only for those over 40 years) formerly used to select patients for radiation therapy. However, radioiodine is contraindicated during pregnancy because of the risk of fetal thyroid ablation. Because data on long-term effects in children are limited, most physicians avoid irradiation in younger pa-tients.

Drug Therapy

THIOAMIDE DERIVATIVES. The principal agents used to suppress the production of thyroid hormone are thioamide derivatives. The drugs used in this country are propylthiouracil (PTU) and methimazole [Tapazole], which have replaced the more toxic parent compound, thiouracil. They inhibit the incor-poration of iodide into thyroglobulin, but do not inactivate or interfere with the release of thyroid hormone previously formed and stored in the gland. There is no permanent effect upon the thyroid gland. These drugs are used primarily to prepare patients for surgery (thyroid or other) or irradiation (if hyperthy-roidism is severe) or in the long-term suppression of hyperthy-roidism in children and selected adults.

Propylthiouracil is more widely used and appears to offer some therapeutic advantages. PTU, but not methimazole, decreases the peripheral conversion of T_4 to T_3; the serum level of the physiologically inactive rT_3 also increases. This drug crosses the placenta less readily during pregnancy than methimazole. Although methimazole is more potent than PTU and thus smaller doses are needed, this is not particularly advantageous because the incidence of adverse effects is similar with therapeutically equivalent doses of the two drugs. Methimazole has the advantage of a longer half-life, which makes once-daily administration possible in some patients.

The clinical effects of these drugs are not apparent until the thyroid hormone reserve has been utilized, and several weeks may elapse before signs of decreased thyroid activity are observed. Since patients with severe hyperthyroidism dissi-pate their stores rapidly, they may respond to therapy more quickly than those with mild hyperthyroidism. Moreover, as the abnormally high metabolic state is corrected, the half-life of

PTU and methimazole may increase, resulting in reduced dosage requirements.

An antithyroid agent sometimes is given with thyroid replacement therapy to minimize the possibility of hypothyroidism. However, the accurate determination of clinical status by frequent measurements of serum T_4 levels is complicated by administering thyroid hormone. The proponents of combined antithyroid-thyroid therapy feel that this regimen eliminates the possibility of hypothyroidism and obviates the need for precise regulation of antithyroid dosage. These advantages are more important in adolescents who tend to be labile. The implications of combined antithyroid-thyroid therapy during pregnancy are more complex (see below).

Thioamide derivatives have short half-lives (one to nine hours). However, their duration of action is longer than is suggested by the plasma half-lives and is correlated with the intrathyroidal concentration. The interval between doses should be no more than eight hours, particularly during initial therapy. Many so-called treatment failures probably result from inadequate frequency of administration. If the patient does not respond to a given dose, a shorter interval (eg, four hours) may be tried before increasing the total dose. This procedure also avoids dose-related side effects. For maintenance, the drug can be administered less frequently; once-daily administration sometimes is successful (eg, for maintenance after the patient is rendered euthyroid) but is generally not recommended.

In *Graves' disease*, the goal of long-term antithyroid drug therapy is to inhibit hormone synthesis and secretion until spontaneous remission occurs. This takes six months to one year in responsive patients, although there is considerable variability. Long-term antithyroid drug treatment is commonly employed in adolescents in whom the half-time of remission approximates three years. Thioamides also appear to have an immunosuppressive effect, since they reduce TSI and thyroid antibodies. Decrease in the size of the gland during therapy indicates the likelihood of remission. Early remission is less likely in patients with large goiters, in those who experienced relapse after previous remissions, or in patients with persistently high serum TSI levels. If there is doubt about whether a remission has occurred, serum TSI can be measured.

When hyperthyroidism occurs initially during *pregnancy* (incidence, about 0.2%), moderate doses of PTU may be relatively safe, but this drug crosses the placenta and may cause neonatal goiter and hypothyroidism (FDA Pregnancy Category D). Intellectual ability is not impaired in neonates thus affected (Burrow et al, 1978). When pregnant women were maintained on only 100 to 200 mg of PTU daily, neonatal thyroxine levels were reduced and TSH levels were elevated but the concentrations normalized within five days after birth (Cheron et al, 1981).

Some physicians have proposed administration of an antithyroid-thyroid combination during pregnancy, theorizing that exogenous thyroid hormone crosses the placenta and may retard the effect of PTU on the fetus. However, it is now known that thyroid hormones do not readily cross the placenta. Also, larger doses of antithyroid drug are required to maintain euthyroidism in pregnant women receiving combination therapy (Mestman et al, 1974). Therefore, it is prudent to use PTU alone in the lowest effective dosage, erring on the side of slight maternal hyperthyroidism if necessary. Treatment reduces the incidence of prematurity.

Antithyroid drugs have not been administered to lactating mothers because of possible detrimental effects on the suckling infant. However, one study demonstrated that the concentration of PTU in milk is only 10% of that in maternal serum. The amount ingested by an infant is minimal (ie, 150 mcg daily when PTU 600 mg/day is taken by the mother) and is thought to be clinically insignificant (Kampmann and Hansen, 1981). However, methimazole is more lipid soluble than PTU and levels in milk would be expected to be closer to maternal serum concentrations.

Adverse Reactions and Precautions of Thioamides: If the vascularity and size of the thyroid gland increase during thioamide treatment, the dose may need to be reduced.

In general, the adverse reactions produced by antithyroid drugs are similar (see the evaluation on Propylthiouracil) and cross sensitivity sometimes occurs. Since some mild reactions (eg, rash) disappear spontaneously with continued treatment, another drug often is not substituted unless the reaction fails to clear promptly. On the other hand, if a severe reaction necessitates withdrawal of one drug, the other may be tried cautiously, although there is an increased risk of recurrence with administration of the related agent. Agranulocytosis and granulocytopenia are the most serious toxic effects but are reversible if detected promptly. Since neutropenia also may be produced by Graves' disease, baseline determinations should be done before antithyroid drugs are administered.

ADRENERGIC BLOCKING AGENTS. These agents may be beneficial adjunctively in the initial treatment of hyperthyroidism and during exacerbations. The beta-blocking agent, propranolol [Inderal], is most widely prescribed for this purpose and is preferred to reserpine and guanethidine [Ismelin], which produce general sympathetic blockade. Propranolol rapidly controls tachycardia and is, therefore, useful as an adjunct to other appropriate therapy for thyrotoxic crisis and neonatal thyrotoxicosis. It is given with antithyroid drugs preoperatively (thyroid or other surgery) and in patients with limited tolerance to antithyroid drugs. Generally, propranolol is not used alone but is sometimes given to control signs and symptoms associated with painless subacute thyroiditis in which the hyperthyroid state is transient. Propranolol should not be discontinued abruptly, for exacerbations of the hyperthyroidism may occur.

Investigationally, propranolol also has been administered as the sole agent for the preoperative preparation of hyperthyroid patients and for the long-term control of thyrotoxic symptoms. However, this agent probably does not significantly affect total thyroid secretion (but does inhibit conversion of T_4 to T_3), does not alter goiter or exophthalmos, and does not correct metabolic effects (increased oxygen consumption). Continued high oxygen demand combined with the drug's negative inotropic effect may produce congestive heart failure. Propranolol may increase uterine irritability during pregnancy.

IODINE. Iodine, once the only substance available for the management of hyperthyroidism, inhibits the synthesis and release of thyroid hormones and may suppress iodide trapping by the thyroid follicular cell membrane. Iodine usually is only partially effective and control often is not sustained (iodine escape). Therefore, its use as an antithyroid drug is now limited to special circumstances: to treat potentially fatal thyrotoxic crisis (thyroid storm) or neonatal thyrotoxicosis and preoperatively to decrease the vascularity of the thyroid gland. Since the irradiated thyroid is more sensitive to the effects of iodine, this agent controls hyperthyroidism after radioiodine therapy. It should not be given alone. Its use is not recommended during pregnancy because it crosses the placenta and may block the synthesis of thyroid hormones by the fetal thyroid. High dietary intake and other sources of iodine (eg, iodine douches) also should be avoided in pregnant hyperthyroid patients.

LITHIUM. The observation that some patients receiving lithium for psychiatric disorders developed hypothyroidism led to the trial of this drug in the treatment of hyperthyroidism. In a limited number of patients, lithium ameliorated thyrotoxicosis and decreased circulating thyroid hormone levels. However, its effect is transient unless used with a thioamide. Also, lithium frequently causes adverse effects. It offers no advantage over iodine and its role in hyperthyroidism has not been defined.

ORAL CHOLECYSTOGRAPHIC AGENTS. Ipodate [Oragrafin] and iopanoic acid [Telepaque] suppress thyroid function in euthyroid and hyperthyroid individuals. Ipodate is more potent in this respect and has been used to treat hyperthyroidism; 1 g once daily causes a rapid decline in serum T_3 and T_4, increases rT_3, and appears to be more potent than PTU in inhibiting extrathyroidal conversion of T_4 to T_3. Another mechanism probably involves the slower inhibition of thyroid hormone secretion caused by release of iodine after metabolism of ipodate. The use of ipodate and similar agents is investigational but appears promising for short-term early treatment of hyperthyroidism or as an adjunct to thioamide drugs (Wu et al, 1982; Hartzband and Solomon, 1981).

Radiation Therapy

Administration of sodium iodide I 131 [Iodotope] is effective in the treatment of hyperthyroidism caused by Graves' disease, multinodular goiter, or a single toxic adenoma. Radioactive iodine accumulates in thyroid tissue and partially destroys the gland.

Since radioiodine also destroys the fetal thyroid, pregnancy should be ruled out before treatment is begun and women who elect to receive radiation therapy should be advised to avoid pregnancy during the next year, for retreatment may be required during that time.

A radioactive iodine uptake test should be performed prior to therapy to determine the dosage that will ensure adequate thyroidal accumulation of the radioisotope. A single dose is often sufficient but repeated administration may be required, especially in patients with large nodular goiters. In multinodular goiter, the initial dose may be considerably larger than that needed in Graves' disease.

The release of thyroid hormones occasionally may be increased several days after irradiation, which could aggravate the thyrotoxic state; thus, some physicians recommend that elderly patients or those with severe hyperthyroidism or cardiac disease be treated initially with propylthiouracil or methima-

zole. The antithyroid drug must be discontinued two to four days before irradiation to avoid interference with isotope uptake. Some physicians resume drug therapy after two to ten days to hasten the return to euthyroidism, although this approach is not accepted by all. If antithyroid medication is administered too soon, the rate of release of I 131 from the gland may be increased, diminishing the therapeutic effect. The onset of action of radioiodine is gradual; two to three months may be required before clinical effects are significant. Therefore, iodine therapy started 10 days after I 131 treatment has been recommended by some clinicians to control toxic symptoms until radiation becomes effective.

Radioactive iodine also is used to treat metastatic thyroid carcinoma. However, this treatment is beneficial only when the lesions have an affinity for iodine (papillary and follicular carcinoma).

Hypothyroidism often develops after thyroid irradiation. Reducing the dose of radioisotope decreases the incidence of early onset of hypothyroidism but does not avoid this complication completely. Thyroid insufficiency may become evident clinically years after therapy; 50% to 80% of patients develop hypothyroidism within 15 years. Replacement therapy may be given when the patient approaches euthyroidism to avoid hypothyroidism. This may be particularly useful if there is a problem in ready access to follow-up care. The possibility that thyroid failure is the natural progression of Graves' disease may account for some cases of hypothyroidism. Hypothyroidism is seen only occasionally after radiation for toxic nodular goiter. Long-term follow-up is necessary to identify these patients.

Surgery

When surgery is used to treat hyperthyroidism, propylthiouracil or methimazole should be administered initially to induce euthyroidism. Propranolol also may be given with the antithyroid agent to reduce symptoms. About ten days before surgery, Strong Iodine Solution, U.S.P. (Lugol's solution), potassium iodide, or sodium iodide usually is added to the regimen to promote involution and decrease vascularity of the thyroid gland, thus reducing the tendency toward excessive bleeding during surgery.

Subtotal thyroidectomy controls hyperthyroidism in a high percentage of patients. The principal drawbacks to surgery, in addition to cost and operative morbidity and mortality, are the complications that can occur (eg, permanent hypothyroidism, hypoparathyroidism, recurrent laryngeal nerve damage with vocal cord paralysis and altered voice quality) and the propensity for recurrence of hyperthyroidism (5% to 20%). If there is a recurrence, radiation or an antithyroid drug is employed because the incidence of complications is higher after subsequent operations.

Drug Evaluations

POTASSIUM IODIDE

POTASSIUM IODIDE SOLUTION

SODIUM IODIDE

STRONG IODINE SOLUTION (Lugol's Solution)

Iodine is commonly administered as Strong Iodine Solution, U.S.P. (Lugol's solution) or Potassium Iodide Solution, U.S.P.; solutions of sodium iodide also are used occasionally. Iodine is given orally with an antithyroid drug to prepare hyperthyroid patients for thyroidectomy or to control hyperthyroidism after radioiodine therapy, and intravenously to treat thyrotoxic crisis or neonatal thyrotoxicosis. It should not be administered alone.

If an accident were to occur at a nuclear power reactor, large quantities of radionuclides, including isotopes of radioiodine, could be released into the atmosphere. Administration of potassium iodide blocks the accumulation of radioiodine by the thyroid gland. The risk associated with short-term use of relatively low doses of potassium iodide in a radiation emergency (projected radiation dose, 25 rem or greater) is judged to be less than that of radioiodine-induced thyroid nodules or cancer (Food and Drug Administration, 1982).

ADVERSE REACTIONS AND PRECAUTIONS. The adverse effects of iodine (iodism) usually include the unpleasant (brassy) taste of iodine and burning in the mouth, sore mouth and throat, hypersalivation, painful sialadenitis, acne and other rashes, diarrhea, and productive cough. In patients with nontoxic nodular goiter, iodide administration may be followed by an increase in plasma thyroid hormones and thyrotoxic symptoms (Jodbasedow phenomenon). Conversely, iodide-induced hypothyroidism and goiter may occur. The use of iodine during pregnancy is not recommended, for fetal hypothyroidism may result (FDA Pregnancy Category C).

Acute poisoning is relatively rare but can occur in very sensitive individuals immediately or several hours after administration. Angioedema with swelling of the larynx may lead to dyspnea. Manifestations of serum sickness also may develop.

DOSAGE AND PREPARATIONS.
Oral: Adults and children, to prepare hyperthyroid patients for thyroidectomy, a common practice is to administer Strong Iodine Solution, U.S.P. (2 to 6 drops three times daily) or Potassium Iodide Solution, U.S.P. (5 drops three times daily) for ten days before surgery. For thyrotoxic crises, one hour after thiocarbamide and as part of the medical emergency treatment, two drops of strong iodide solution or 50 to 100 mg of Potassium Iodide Solution, U.S.P., every 12 hours (DeGroot et al, 1984). Other clinicians recommend dosage as high as 1 g/day.

Individuals likely to receive a projected radiation dose of 25 rem or greater from radioiodines released into the environment may be given the following amounts of potassium iodide: *adults and children over 1 year,* 130 mg/day; *children under 1 year,* 65 mg/day. This dose is administered for three to ten days.

POTASSIUM IODIDE:
Generic. Tablets 300 mg.
POTASSIUM IODIDE SOLUTION:
Generic. Solution 1 g/ml.

SODIUM IODIDE:
Generic. Bulk (crystals, granules, powder).
STRONG IODINE SOLUTION:
Generic. Solution containing iodine 5% and potassium iodide 10%. Also marketed under the name Lugol's Solution.
Intravenous: For thyrotoxic crisis, 250 to 500 mg of Sodium Iodide, U.S.P., daily, beginning one hour after an initial dose of PTU and propranolol, has been administered. Other appropriate agents and procedures are described in the Introduction to this section.
SODIUM IODIDE:
Generic. Bulk (crystals, granules); solution 10%.

PROPYLTHIOURACIL

ACTIONS AND USES. Propylthiouracil (PTU), the prototype of the antithyroid drugs, is used to manage hyperthyroidism, to prepare hyperthyroid patients for thyroidectomy, and to treat thyrotoxic crisis. It also may be given before or after radioactive iodine. (See also the section on Radiation Therapy.) The serum half-life of PTU is one to two hours, but the duration of action is more prolonged.

PTU inhibits the synthesis of thyroid hormones by preventing the iodination of tyrosine residues in thyroglobulin. Because it also inhibits the conversion of T_4 to T_3, PTU is preferred to methimazole in elderly patients, in those with cardiac disease, and in thyrotoxic crisis. PTU probably crosses the placenta less readily than methimazole and thus is also preferred for pregnant women. However, both drugs are classified in FDA Pregnancy Category D. The concentration of PTU in human milk is low and a lactating mother may breast feed with close supervision of the infant.

ADVERSE REACTIONS AND PRECAUTIONS. Granulocytopenia and agranulocytosis occur rarely and are the most serious adverse reactions of propylthiouracil. These effects require immediate cessation of therapy and institution of supportive measures. Most cases are observed during the first two months of treatment, and the incidence gradually declines thereafter. Since neutropenia also may be caused by Graves' disease, baseline determinations should be done before an antithyroid drug is administered. Periodic blood cell counts, although helpful to detect gradual reductions in the leukocyte count, should not be relied upon to detect agranulocytosis because of the rapidity with which this complication can develop. Patients should be instructed to report sore throat or fever immediately, for these symptoms may signal the development of agranulocytosis. Milder leukopenias develop when doses exceeding 400 mg/day are used, but discontinuing therapy or reducing the dose is not necessary if blood cell counts are performed periodically and the leukopenia does not become severe.

A lupus erythematosus-like polyserositis syndrome occurs rarely and requires discontinuation of antithyroid drug treatment.

Pruritus is common and may be caused by the drug or by the disease. Rash, usually urticarial or papular, is observed in approximately 3% of patients; it can be severe but usually is quite mild. Patients occasionally experience nausea, abdominal discomfort, arthralgia, headache, dizziness, paresthesia, and drowsiness. Temporary ageusia may occur with PTU, but has not been observed following use of methimazole.

DOSAGE AND PREPARATIONS. The plasma half-life of propylthiouracil is only about 1.5 hours; therefore, frequent administration is necessary, especially initially, to achieve maximal clinical effectiveness. When large doses are required, a dosing interval of four to six hours may provide more constant suppression of thyroid activity.

Oral: For hyperthyroidism, *adults,* initially, 300 to 600 mg daily in divided doses every six to eight hours; as much as 1.2 g daily may be required for initial control. These doses are given until the patient is euthyroid. For maintenance, 100 to 300 mg is given daily in three divided doses. *Children 10 years and over,* initially, 150 to 300 mg daily in divided doses every six to eight hours. The usual maintenance dose is 100 to 300 mg daily divided into two doses at 12-hour intervals. *Children 6 to 10 years,* initially, 50 to 150 mg daily in divided doses every six to eight hours. *Children under 6 years*, initially, 120 to 175 mg/M^2 daily in divided doses every eight hours. Monthly checkups are advised; dosage is gradually decreased and then withdrawn after one to two years.

For neonatal thyrotoxicosis, 10 mg/kg daily in divided doses.

For preoperative preparation of the thyroidectomy patient, the drug is given to *adults and children* in the same doses used for hyperthyroidism until the patient is euthyroid; iodine then is added to the regimen for ten days before surgery.

For thyrotoxic crisis, *adults,* 600 mg to 1.2 g daily in divided doses; the tablets can be taken orally or crushed and delivered by nasogastric tube. The initial dose is followed in one hour by administration of iodine. (See the evaluation on the iodine salts.)

Generic. Tablets 50 mg.

METHIMAZOLE
[Tapazole]

Methimazole has the same actions and indications as propylthiouracil (PTU) (see the Introduction to this section and the evaluation on Propylthiouracil) but is approximately ten times more potent. The onset of action, degree of response, and incidence of adverse reactions depend upon dosage. The plasma half-life of methimazole (three to nine hours) is longer than that of PTU. However, methimazole does not have any effect on peripheral thyroid hormone conversion, and PTU may be preferred for treatment of thyrotoxic crisis (Jordan, 1983). Effectiveness sometimes can be achieved with less frequent administration, and a single daily dose may be adequate for maintenance therapy in some patients.

In general, adverse reactions are similar to those caused by PTU. There is some indication that agranulocytosis occurs less frequently with methimazole but that the overall incidence of adverse reactions is higher; however, these differences have not been established conclusively. Cross sensitivity to PTU may occur in susceptible patients.

This drug is classified in FDA Pregnancy Category D.

DOSAGE AND PREPARATIONS.

Oral: Adults, initially, 15 to 60 mg in divided doses every six to eight hours until the patient is euthyroid. For maintenance, 10 to 30 mg daily in one to three doses. *Children 6 to 10 years,* initially, 0.4 mg/kg daily in divided doses every six to eight hours. *Children under 6 years*, 12 to 17.5 mg/M^2 daily in divided doses every eight hours. Monthly checkups are advised; dosage is decreased gradually and then withdrawn after one to two years.

For preoperative preparation of the thyroidectomy patient, the drug is given to *adults and children* in the same doses used for hyperthyroidism until the patient is euthyroid; iodine is then added to the regimen for ten days before surgery.

For thyrotoxic crisis, *adults,* 60 to 120 mg daily in divided doses; the tablets are taken orally or crushed and delivered by nasogastric tube. The initial dose is followed in one hour by the dose of iodine (see the evaluation on the iodine salts).

Tapazole (Lilly). Tablets 5 and 10 mg.

PROPRANOLOL HYDROCHLORIDE
[Inderal]

ACTIONS AND USES. Propranolol acts peripherally on effector organs to suppress the clinical symptoms of hyperthyroidism, particularly tachycardia, hyperhidrosis, tremors, nervousness, anxiety, weakness, spasticity, heat intolerance, and hyperreflexia. Although the drug usually does not significantly affect total thyroid secretion (occasionally, increases in T_4 have been observed), serum levels of T_3 are decreased and those of rT_3 are increased; this is probably due to inhibition of monodeiodination of T_4. This beta-adrenergic blocking agent is preferred to reserpine or guanethidine, which act as general adrenergic blocking agents.

The main advantage of propranolol is its rapid control of symptoms until more definitive therapy (antithyroid drugs or radioactive iodine) takes effect; this may be two or three weeks with antithyroid drugs or as long as three months with radiation therapy. Its adjunctive use prior to thyroidectomy and in neonatal thyrotoxicosis hastens the control of symptoms. Propranolol is sometimes given as the sole agent to control signs and symptoms of transient hyperthyroidism (eg, painless subacute thyroiditis). Investigationally, propranolol also has been given alone for preoperative preparation of hyperthyroid patients and for long-term control of thyrotoxic symptoms. However, this drug should be used cautiously in these patients, for it may produce congestive heart failure.

Unless contraindicated by the presence of congestive heart failure, propranolol should be administered immediately either orally or intravenously as an adjunct in the treatment of thyrotoxic crisis. Dosage depends on the patient's clinical status (DeGroot, 1984). If appropriate, the patient should be digitalized to counteract the decreased myocardial contractility produced by propranolol, for the combined effect of increased oxygen requirement and decreased heart rate may precipitate heart failure.

PRECAUTIONS. Propranolol should be avoided or used very cautiously in patients with asthma or chronic bronchitis. (See also the section on Drug Therapy.) This drug should not be administered during pregnancy because it may increase uterine irritability and impair adaptation of the fetus to extrauterine life. It also should be avoided in patients who experience episodes of spontaneous hypoglycemia.

Abrupt withdrawal of propranolol from hypertensive patients may be followed by symptoms of hyperthyroidism due to increased serum levels of T_3 (but not T_4 or total thyroid hormones), which occur simultaneously with decreased blood levels of propranolol (Kristensen et al, 1978).

Propranolol appears to be better tolerated by hyperthyroid than euthyroid patients. For further discussion of adverse reactions and precautions, see the evaluation in Chapter 25, Antianginal Agents.

DOSAGE AND PREPARATIONS.
Oral: 40 to 240 mg daily in divided doses. For thyrotoxic crisis, 20 to 200 mg every six hours.
    Generic. Tablets 10, 20, 40 and 80 mg.
    Inderal (Ayerst). Tablets 10, 20, 40, 60, 80, and 90 mg.
    Inderal LA (Ayerst). Capsules (timed-release) 80, 120, and 160 mg.
Intravenous: A maximum of 5 mg is administered cautiously at a rate not exceeding 1 mg/min. The dose may be repeated, if necessary, in four to six hours; the electrocardiogram should be used to monitor the patient. For thyrotoxic crisis, 1 to 3 mg every four to six hours.
    Inderal (Ayerst). Solution 1 mg/ml in 1 ml containers.

SODIUM IODIDE I 131
[Iodotope]

ACTIONS AND USES. This radioactive isotope of iodine accumulates in the thyroid gland where its ionizing beta radiation destroys the functional and regenerative capacities of thyroid cells within weeks. It also emits gamma radiation, which contributes relatively little to biological activity but provides an accurate dosage and uptake measurement.

Radioactive iodine is used to treat hyperthyroidism and carcinoma of the thyroid when uptake of the nuclide is sufficient (see also the discussion on Radiation Therapy in the Introduction). Tracer amounts also are used to evaluate thyroid pathology. These procedures are believed to be virtually without hazard if test doses are small (eg, infants and small children, 1 microcurie; adults, less than 10 microcuries).

For use of other radioactive isotopes in the diagnosis of thyroid disease (eg, I-123, mTc-99), see specialty texts.

ADVERSE REACTIONS AND PRECAUTIONS. Ablative treatment with radioactive iodine occasionally induces temporary but potentially serious thyrotoxic reactions during the first few days or weeks following therapy; these complications are of special significance in patients with severe thyrotoxic heart disease. The area over the thyroid gland may become tender and painful as a result of radiation thyroiditis, but this usually is alleviated by analgesics. Antithyroid drugs should be discontinued three days before administration of radioactive iodine.

Permanent hypothyroidism is a common complication of ablative therapy. The incidence is about 10% in the first year and is increased by approximately 2% to 3% each year following treatment. Since follow-up studies of ten years or longer do not reveal any evidence of a plateau, most patients treated with radioactive iodine eventually develop hypothyroidism and require replacement therapy. Long-term observation is needed to avoid the deleterious effects of unrecognized hypothyroidism. However, since many patients cannot be followed adequately after radioiodine therapy, some clinicians recommend the use of replacement doses of thyroid hormones prior to the advent of hypothyroidism in anticipation of this complication.

If greater than 30 millicuries are administered as a single dose, appropriate precautions for care of the patient and disposal of body wastes should be observed.

Before treating carcinoma of the thyroid with high doses of radioiodine (100 to 200 microcuries), the residual thyroid should be ablated either surgically or by pretreatment with low doses of the radioiodine. If thyroid tissue is present, large doses of radioiodine may cause severe laryngitis with necrosis.

Sodium iodide I 131 is contraindicated during pregnancy and nursing. Most physicians avoid irradiation in younger patients.

DOSAGE AND PREPARATIONS.
Oral: For selected patients with Graves' disease and other types of hyperthyroidism, the usual therapeutic dose is that which results in the retention of 75 to 120 microcuries/g of gland at 24 hours. This can be calculated using an estimate of the weight of the gland and the percentage of uptake in a radioactive iodine uptake test. Further refinements of dosage can be determined (DeGroot et al, 1984). However, the use of a standard dose of radioiodine (4 to 10 millicuries) is sometimes preferred. If initial treatment is not successful, retreatment after three to four months is usually recommended. Larger doses are required for patients with toxic nodular goiter.

For thyroid carcinoma, 50 millicuries (range, 30 to 100 millicuries) for ablation of normal thyroid tissue; 100 to 200 millicuries is the usual subsequent therapeutic dose for metastases.

For the use of radioactive iodine in diagnostic procedures, see specialty texts.
    Generic. Capsules ranging from 0.8 to 100 millicuries; oral solution ranging from 3.5 to 150 millicuries/ml.
    Iodotope (Squibb). Capsules ranging from 1 to 50 millicuries; oral solution 7.05 millicuries/ml.

Cited References

USP XXI: *The United States Pharmacopeia*, ed 21. Rockville, MD, United States Pharmacopeial Convention, 1985.

Bech K, Madsen SN: Influence of treatment with radioiodine and propylthiouracil on thyroid stimulating immunoglobulins in Graves' disease. *Clin Endocrinol* 13:417-424, 1980.

Bode HH, et al: Mitigation of cretinism by breast-feeding. *Pediatrics* 62:13-16, 1978.

Burrow GN, et al: Intellectual development in children whose mothers received propylthiouracil during pregnancy. *Yale J Biol Med* 51:295-296, 1978.

Cheron RG, et al: Neonatal thyroid function after propylthiouracil therapy for maternal Graves' disease. *N Engl J Med* 304:525-528, 1981.

Chopra IJ: Challenges in diagnosis of hyperthyroidism. *Drug Ther* 13:70-78, (Nov) 1983.

Committee on Drugs, American Academy of Pediatrics: Treatment of congenital hypothyroidism. *Pediatrics* 62:413-417, 1978.

DeGroot LJ, et al: *The Thyroid and Its Diseases,* ed 5. New York, John Wiley & Sons, 1984.

Education Committee, American Thyroid Association: ATA statement on breast cancer and thyroid hormone therapy. *J Pediatr* 90:683-684, 1977.

Food and Drug Administration: Final Recommendations. Potassium as thyroid-blocking agent in radiation emergency: Recommendations on use. April, 1982. [Complete text available from Food and Drug Administration, Bureau of Radiological Health, 5600 Fishers Lane, Rockville, MD 20857.]

Hartzband PI, Solomon DH: *The Treatment of Hyperthyroidism.* Chicago, Year Book Medical Publishers, 1981.

Jordan RM: Endocrine emergencies. *Med Clin North Am* 67:1193-1213, 1983.

Kampmann JP, Hansen JM: Clinical pharmacokinetics of antithyroid drugs. *Clin Pharmacokinet* 6:401-428, 1981.

Klein I, Levey GS: Unusual manifestations of hypothyroidism. *Arch Intern Med* 144:123-128, 1984.

Kristensen BO, et al: Propranolol withdrawal and thyroid hormones in patients with essential hypertension. *Clin Pharmacol Ther* 23:624-629, 1978.

La Franchi SH: Hypothyroidism. *Pediatr Clin North Am* 26:33-51, 1979.

Mestman JH, et al: Hyperthyroidism and pregnancy. *Arch Intern Med* 134:434-439, 1974.

Refetoff S, et al: Consequences of inappropriate treatment because of failure to recognize the syndrome of pituitary and peripheral tissue resistance to thyroid hormone. *Metabolism* 32:822-834, 1983.

Sawin CT, et al: Comparison of thyroxine and desiccated thyroid in patients with primary hypothyroidism. *Metabolism* 27:1518-1525, 1978.

Shapiro S, et al: Use of thyroid supplements in relation to risk of breast cancer. *JAMA* 244:1685-1687, 1980.

Smith SR: Desiccated thyroid preparations: Obsolete therapy, (editorial). *Arch Intern Med* 144:926-927, 1984.

Utiger RD: When and how to treat hypothyroidism. *Drug Ther* 13:55-69, (Nov) 1983.

Weetman AP, et al: Cyclosporin improves Graves' ophthalmopathy. *Lancet* 2:486-489, 1983.

Wu S-Y, et al: Comparison of sodium ipodate (Oragrafin) and propylthiouracil in early treatment of hyperthyroidism. *J Clin Endocrinol Metab* 54:630-634, 1982.

Zakarija M, et al: Clinical significance of assay of thyroid-stimulating antibody in Graves' disease. *Ann Intern Med* 93:28-32, 1980.

Other Selected References

Brennan MD: Thyroid hormone. *Mayo Clin Proc* 55:33-44, 1980.

DeVisscher M (ed): *The Thyroid Gland*. New York, Raven Press, 1980.

Haynes RC Jr, Murad F: Thyroid and antithyroid drugs, in Gilman AG, et al (eds): *The Pharmacological Basis of Therapeutics*, ed 6. New York, Macmillan, 1980, 1397-1419.

Hershman JM, Bray GA (eds): *The Thyroid: Physiology and Treatment of Disease*. New York, Pergamon Press, 1978.

Larsen PR: Thyroid-pituitary interaction: Feedback regulation of thyrotropin secretion by thyroid hormones. *N Engl J Med* 306:23-32, 1982.

Selenkow HA, et al: Autoimmune thyroid disease: Integrated concept of Graves' and Hashimoto's diseases. *Compr Ther* 10:48-56, (April) 1984.

Solomon DH: Pregnancy and PTU, (editorial). *N Engl J Med* 304:538-539, 1981.

Sperling MA: How to recognize and treat thyroid disorders in children. *Drug Ther* 12:179-204, (Nov) 1982.

Stoffer SS, Szpunar WE: Potency of brand name and generic levothyroxine products. *JAMA* 244:1704-1705, 1980.

Werner SC, Ingbar SH (eds): *The Thyroid*, ed 4. Hagerstown, MD, Harper & Row, 1978.

Uterine Stimulants and Relaxants

UTERINE STIMULANTS

Oxytocic agents stimulate contraction of the myometrium and are used to induce labor at term, to induce abortion, to prevent or control postpartum or postabortion hemorrhage, and to assess fetal status in high-risk pregnancies. Drugs used clinically include the neurohypophyseal hormone, oxytocin [Pitocin, Syntocinon]; the prostaglandins, carboprost tromethamine [Prostin/15M], dinoprost tromethamine [Prostin F$_2$ alpha], and dinoprostone [Prostin E2]; hypertonic saline or urea [Ureaphil]; and the ergot alkaloids, ergonovine [Ergotrate] and methylergonovine [Methergine]. The choice for a specific use is based upon the drug's oxytocic and other pharmacologic properties.

PHYSIOLOGY OF LABOR. The myometrium is capable of contraction at any time; however, the integrated effects of factors involved in the physiologic status of uterine smooth muscle result in a state of relative quiescence throughout most of pregnancy. As pregnancy advances, the myometrium becomes more sensitive to contractile stimulation by oxytocin. Like other smooth muscle, it exhibits spontaneous, repetitive action potentials but tension is generated only in the presence of synchronized electrical discharge. Contractions are noticeable weeks before labor begins and initially are weak, uncoordinated, and involve few muscle fibers. Eventually, the strong, synchronous, propagating contractions characteristic of full-term labor begin.

Physiologic and pharmacologic factors favoring contraction include estrogen, prostaglandins, and oxytocin, as well as stretching of muscle fibers. Factors favoring quiescence include progesterone and beta-adrenergic stimulation.

Progesterone production increases throughout most of pregnancy and generally maintains the uterus in a nonexcitable state. Mechanisms of action may include hyperpolarization of the muscle cell membrane, limitation of impulse conduction among cells, and increased binding of calcium to the sarcoplasmic reticulum, which reduces the cytoplasmic concentration of calcium available for contractile processes. The muscle fibers of the nonpregnant uterus have a resting membrane potential of -40 mv; during pregnancy, the cells are hyperpolarized (-60 mv). In rabbits and possibly in humans, myometrial cells underlying the placenta are hyperpolarized (resistant to stimulation) compared to those in other areas of the uterus; this may be due to relatively high local concentrations of progesterone produced by the placenta. As pregnancy progresses, the myometrial area under the placenta becomes proportionately smaller and factors enhancing excitability become dominant.

Estrogen production increases throughout pregnancy and may be partly responsible for this shift in dominance, but high estrogen levels are not obligatory for initiation of labor. Enlargement of the uterine content during pregnancy results in stretching of myometrial muscle fibers, which stimulates smooth muscle activity and results in the muscle fibers approaching resting length (the length at which maximum tension can be generated with contraction). The stretching of these fibers is also associated with the production of prostaglandins by the uterus.

Although there is a gradual increase in maternal plasma oxytocin during pregnancy, the concentration does not change markedly preceding labor. However, the concentration of oxytocin *receptors* in the myometrium increases, which allows greater responsiveness to the relatively low concentrations of oxytocin available. The concentration of oxytocin receptors is also elevated in the uterine decidua where high levels of prostaglandin synthetase are present. Since oxytocin stimulates uterine prostaglandin production in animals, a similar mechanism may be operable in humans. Prostaglandins may diffuse into the myometrium and enhance the effect of oxytocin on uterine contractions (Fuchs et al, 1982).

During the second trimester, uterine muscle is resistant to stimulation. Large doses of prostaglandins can overcome this resistance and are useful to induce labor at this time. Conversely, the myometrium is relatively resistant to the effects of oxytocin at this stage of pregnancy, and this agent is not effective in inducing labor. The changes in myometrial sensitivity to prostaglandins and oxytocin as pregnancy progresses result from the interaction of these agents with cell membrane receptors and their effects on transmembrane ionic fluxes, membrane potential, and intracellular calcium concentrations. The ability to inhibit binding of calcium to sarcoplasmic reticulum in the myometrial cell increases 10,000 times for oxytocin and only 100 times for prostaglandins during pregnancy. Also, the increasing production of estrogen may be partly responsible for increased uterine sensitivity to oxytocin with time, since estrogen increases both the number of binding sites and the affinity of uterine oxytocin receptors.

Although the autonomic nervous system probably is not involved in the initiation of labor, uterine contractions can be influenced by autonomic drugs. Beta-adrenergic drugs inhibit uterine contractions and have been used to delay premature labor (see the section on Uterine Relaxants). The effect is mediated by increased production of cyclic adenosine monophosphate (cAMP) but may also affect calcium channels. It is not known if changes in cAMP levels are required for changes in contractility, however.

Indications

INDUCTION OF TERM LABOR. Labor should be induced when the risks of continuing the pregnancy are greater than the risks of induction. Premature rupture of the membranes probably is the most common indication. Other indications include some instances of antepartum bleeding, intrauterine growth retardation, erythroblastosis fetalis, and placental insufficiency, which may result from diabetes mellitus, pre-eclampsia, or eclampsia. In these situations, induction of labor may reduce maternal and neonatal morbidity and mortality. See relevant texts for management of obstetrical emergencies.

Intravenous infusion of oxytocin is preferred to induce or augment labor. Small doses stimulate uterine contractility at term, and the pattern of contractions approximates that of natural labor. Oxytocin also is used to augment dysfunctional labor (eg, hypotonic myometrial contractions) except that caused by cephalopelvic disproportion.

Although only oxytocin is labeled for the induction of labor, several prostaglandins are being evaluated for this indication. These agents produce both uterine stimulation and cervical ripening and do not cause neonatal jaundice (Davey, 1980) or water retention, which may be dangerous in certain patients (eg, in those with pre-eclampsia, hypertension, or kidney disease). However, although clinical studies have demonstrated that their efficacy is equivalent to that of oxytocin, the prostaglandins can cause hyperstimulation of the uterus, which compromises uteroplacental blood flow, and they have a longer duration of action than oxytocin. These adverse reactions have reduced enthusiasm among many specialists for the use of prostaglandins in labor.

Intravenous dinoprost tromethamine (PGF$_{2\alpha}$THAM) [Prostin F$_2$ alpha] is effective, but a localized erythematous reaction may develop at the site of infusion and other side effects limit the useful dosage range. The dose of dinoprost required to achieve a given uterine response is ten times larger than that of dinoprostone (PGE$_2$) [Prostin E2]; for this reason, the latter is preferred by some obstetricians for this indication. Dinoprostone has received more extensive investigation as an inducing agent. Since the myometrium is extremely sensitive to prostaglandins at term, small doses should be used to avoid tetanic contractions. The use of lower doses greatly reduces the gastrointestinal side effects and hyperpyrexia, which often develop with the larger doses used for abortion.

Although the oral form is regarded as safe and effective in the low doses employed to induce term labor (Porreco and Watson, 1983), intravaginal forms (eg, gel, suppository) show the most promise of effectiveness with diminished side effects (effective dose at term less than or equal to 3 mg); however, the response may be unpredictable with this route (Jagani et al, 1984) and, in many patients, augmentation of labor with oxytocin is required. (Only a 20-mg suppository is commercially available in this country.)

When oxytocin is given after dinoprostone, the contractile response is enhanced. For this reason, prostaglandins and oxytocin should never be given simultaneously because of the increased risk of uterine hypercontractility and rupture (Claman et al, 1984). A period of "washout" (until regular contractions have dissipated) should elapse before oxytocin is administered and the lowest pump setting should be used initially.

In general, induction of labor with oxytocics should not be attempted in cases of cephalopelvic disproportion, malpresentation, complete placenta previa, or vertical uterine scar from previous cesarean section, hysterotomy, or myomectomy. In patients with previous low transverse section delivery, oxytocin has not been shown to increase the risk of uterine rupture. Extreme caution should be observed in patients with abruptio placentae, partial placenta previa, and uterine overdistension. In women of high parity (five or more), labor should be induced only with great caution because of the risk of uterine rupture.

During induced labor, the mother and fetus should be

monitored continuously to determine fetal and maternal heart rate, maternal blood pressure, and strength of uterine contractions. If uterine hyperstimulation occurs (hypertonus and abnormally frequent contractions), the uterine stimulant should be withdrawn immediately. Although oxytocin (intravenous) and the prostaglandins (dinoprost and dinoprostone) have very short plasma half-lives, the uterine contractions induced by prostaglandins may be prolonged. For tetanic contractions secondary to prostaglandins, an intravenous bolus of terbutaline [Brethine, Bricanyl] 250 mcg or magnesium sulfate 3 to 4 g may be used if there are no contraindications. Short-term administration of a tocolytic agent is not contraindicated in a diabetic patient.

Other oxytocic agents are not suitable for induction or augmentation of labor. Quinine and quinidine are unreliable in safe doses, and there is considerable danger of eighth nerve damage in the infant. The ergot alkaloids and sparteine, a plant alkaloid with oxytocic properties, are too long acting and produce excessive, unphysiologic uterine contractions with the potential to cause fetal bradycardia; sparteine is no longer available in the United States.

CERVICAL RIPENING. Failure of induction of labor can be attributed partly to an unfavorable cervical condition. The state of the cervix is a critical factor in successful induction (Lange et al, 1982 A). Various agents (eg, prostaglandins, relaxin, estrogen, oxytocin, laminaria) are being investigated to ripen the cervix before induction of term labor or dilation and evacuation (D and E) abortion.

Prostaglandins are currently the most widely used pharmacologic agents for softening and dilating unfavorable cervices before labor is induced. Small doses of dinoprostone in a viscous gel administered extra-amniotically, intracervically, or intravaginally (pessary) are effective (Jagani et al, 1984; Buchanan et al, 1984; Ulmsten et al, 1983; Sørensen et al, 1985; Gordon and Calder, 1983), and there is evidence that the incidence of cesarean deliveries is decreased (Porreco and Watson, 1983; Gordon and Calder, 1983). There currently is disagreement on the effect of dinoprostone on the duration of induced labor (see the evaluation). Local administration appears to be more effective than systemic use and causes fewer side effects. Ideally, local application of dinoprostone should produce only cervical ripening, but labor has been induced in a significant number of patients with the accompanying risk of fetal distress. Therefore, external fetal monitoring is recommended during the ripening process, particularly in high-risk pregnancies (Buchanan et al, 1984). This lack of site specificity has stimulated the search for more selective ripening agents.

The use of laminaria sticks (natural and synthetic) to ripen the cervix before induction of labor is controversial. They are effective (Cross and Pitkin, 1978) and do not stimulate uterine contractions (Johnson et al, 1985), but may increase the risk of maternal and neonatal infectious morbidity (Kazzi et al, 1982), although this has not been reported in some studies (Gower et al, 1982). Laminaria sticks are also employed to dilate the cervix in first trimester abortions.

One study employing intracervical instillation of relaxin showed significant improvement in the cervical state without uterine contractions and decreased induction-to-delivery time (Evans et al, 1983). Further studies are needed to confirm these findings.

ELECTIVE ABORTION. In general, abortions performed during the *first trimester* (up to 12 weeks after the last menstrual period [LMP]) utilize a suction procedure and, if done four to six weeks after the LMP (menstrual extraction or minisuction), require little or no cervical dilation. As pregnancy progresses in the first trimester, cervical dilation becomes necessary.

As an alternative to a suction procedure, prostaglandin analogues (vaginal or intramuscular) are being investigated for use during early pregnancy. Overall, suction appears to be superior to prostaglandins during the first trimester because it is relatively rapid and eliminates the necessity of undergoing labor. In addition, it can be performed earlier than instillation techniques that require amniocentesis, thereby reducing the complications associated with abortion as pregnancy progresses.

When *cervical dilation* (with or without concomitant administration of uterine stimulants) is required, laminaria tents may be useful. These sticks of seaweed are placed in the cervical canal 4 to 12 hours before the anticipated procedure. As the sticks absorb fluid and expand, the cervix is dilated gradually, usually with less damage than from other methods of mechanical dilation. The dose of oxytocic drugs required is often reduced and the drug-to-abortion time is sometimes decreased.

Prostaglandins and combinations of agents for intra-amniotic instillation are used in *second trimester* abortions. However, dilation and evacuation is the most common method of elective abortion to 16 weeks after the LMP and is sometimes used to 20 weeks. Evaluation of procedures is complicated by the wide variety utilized and the lack of standardization. If an instillation method is employed, a choice must be made between a hypertonic agent (ie, hypertonic saline, urea) and dinoprost.

Although there is considerable debate, D and E appears to be preferred for early second trimester abortions, while instillation methods are used more often as pregnancy progresses (Bhatt et al, 1978; Grimes and Cates, 1979; Robins and Surrago, 1980; Grimes et al, 1980).

Hypertonic Solutions: Hypertonic solutions (usually saline 20% or urea 40% to 50%), instilled intra-amniotically act as chemical poisons on the placenta and fetus. Instillation requires amniocentesis and is usually limited to pregnancies of 16 weeks from the LMP or longer when the amniotic cavity is adequate in size.

Hypertonic saline is effective in more than 90% of cases, and the mean abortion time is about 36 hours. However, major complications result from inadvertent myometrial or intravascular injection. The former causes uterine damage and the latter produces hypernatremia, which may cause disseminated intravascular coagulation (DIC) that can be fatal. Intravascular injection may be avoided by not injecting saline into bloody amniotic fluid. By withholding general anesthetics and analgesics, the patient can report symptoms of hypernatremia promptly. Hypertonic saline should not be used in patients whose ability to handle a sodium load is compromised (eg, those with impaired renal or cardiac function, hypertension).

Experience with hypertonic urea is not as extensive; it appears to be less effective but safer than hypertonic saline. Inadvertent intravascular injection does not cause serious complications. The mean abortion time is about 43 hours. Urea can produce dehydration and coagulation defects have been reported. It should not be used in patients with impaired renal or hepatic function.

Prostaglandins: These agents are preferred to oxytocin for second trimester induction of labor, since large doses of oxytocin (with the attendant risk of water intoxication) are necessary to induce labor prior to term and are often ineffective. Prostaglandins stimulate labor at any time during gestation, but elective abortion preferably should be performed before 20 weeks of pregnancy. Several prostaglandin preparations and routes of administration have been compared (Lauersen, 1979).

Dinoprost, administered by the intra-amniotic route, has been widely used and may be the preferred prostaglandin when the uterus is large enough to perform amniocentesis (later than 16 weeks). However, there is evidence that it is not superior to saline (Grimes and Cates, 1979). Disadvantages of dinoprost are a higher incidence of live births, incomplete abortions, and abortion failures. Although dinoprost does not produce hypernatremia or DIC, the overall incidence of serious complications (eg, hemorrhage, endometritis, fever, convulsions) is high (see evaluation). Abortion times are generally shorter than with saline.

Prostaglandins also may be administered by the extra-amniotic (extraovular) route (dinoprost) (more frequently in Europe), as a vaginal suppository (dinoprostone), or by intramuscular injection (15-methyl $PGF_{2\alpha}$, carboprost) to induce second trimester abortions. Extraovular administration is accomplished by placing a catheter through the cervix and instilling the medication between the fetal membranes and the uterine wall. The intra-amniotic route is preferred because systemic absorption is reduced, thus decreasing the incidence of adverse effects. If the uterus is too small for amniocentesis or if this procedure has failed, extraovular administration can be used, but there is a risk of intrauterine infection caused by insertion of the catheter. The incidence of incomplete abortions is generally higher after extraovular instillation of dinoprost.

Dinoprostone vaginal suppositories are useful over a wide range of gestational ages, are more convenient than intra-amniotic or extraovular methods, and have a high success rate. This prostaglandin was preferred for abortion of up to 20 weeks' gestation in one report (Robins and Surrago, 1980). It also can be used when other abortion methods fail. However, dinoprostone is not useful when there is vaginal hemorrhage and is not recommended in the presence of previous uterine scar. A major drawback is the occurrence of live births (3%) (Surrago and Robins, 1982).

The newest prostaglandin abortifacient, carboprost [Prostin/15M], is longer acting than other available prostaglandins, is easily administered by intramuscular injection, and also can be used over a wide range of gestational ages. It is particularly useful when other methods of abortion have failed and is preferred to dinoprostone when vaginal bleeding is present. The gastrointestinal side effects are more prominent with systemic administration, however.

All methods of abortion using prostaglandins cause a high incidence of adverse effects (nausea, vomiting, diarrhea) and there is the possibility of delivering a live fetus. Dinoprost and carboprost are more likely to cause bronchospasm in asthmatic patients than dinoprostone, but the incidence of febrile reactions is significant with the latter agent.

Combination Regimens: Oxytocin is sometimes used as an *adjunct* to other abortifacients to stimulate contractions and shorten the abortion time (Horowitz, 1978; Hachamovitch et al, 1979; Cates and Schulz, 1980). *Caution must be exercised when such combinations are used because effects are often additive and the incidence of adverse effects (DIC, cervical detachments, and uterine rupture) is increased* (Cederqvist and Birnbaum, 1980). Also, when larger doses of oxytocin are used, as in second trimester abortion, the risk of water intoxication is increased. Therefore, the addition of oxytocin to other abortifacient regimens is preferably limited to specific indications (eg, prolonged abortion time, prolonged rupture of membranes, incomplete abortion).

Other combination regimens employ a hypertonic agent and dinoprost administered intra-amniotically (Wellman and Jacobson, 1976; King et al, 1977). This combination has several advantages: The abortion time is shorter than with a hypertonic agent alone; lower doses of dinoprost (5 or 10 mg total) are effective, thus reducing the gastrointestinal reactions; and use of a hypertonic agent minimizes the likelihood of a live fetus. Combination methods have the potential to maximize effectiveness and minimize side effects. On the other hand, there is the risk of complications from untried regimens. Lack of standardization of treatments also complicates analysis of results.

OTHER INDICATIONS FOR INDUCTION OF LABOR. A *hydatidiform mole* increases the risk of pre-eclampsia, uterine hemorrhage, infection, and choriocarcinoma and should be removed promptly on diagnosis. Oxytocic agents have been used to stimulate expulsion, but evacuation of the uterine cavity by suction curettage is preferred. The large doses of oxytocin required for this indication increase the risk of water intoxication. Dinoprostone vaginal suppositories can be used to stimulate expulsion of the mole, but D and C also should be performed to assure complete evacuation. Intra-amniotic dinoprost is not suitable because of the lack of amniotic fluid; furthermore, the relatively large doses required may result in severe systemic reactions. It should be noted that there is an increased risk of trophoblastic embolization with any oxytocic agent.

Fetal death in utero often is followed by spontaneous labor within two to three weeks, but labor may be delayed. Prolonging such pregnancies increases the risk of DIC. All methods employed to induce delivery of the dead fetus, including surgical evacuation, may cause excessive bleeding.

A conservative approach is to wait for spontaneous delivery for one to two weeks after fetal death if this does not represent an extreme emotional burden on the patient. Dinoprostone vaginal suppositories are a good noninvasive choice to induce delivery (Lauersen et al, 1980) but there is the potential for uterine rupture, particularly in multigravid women, with advanced gestation, in the presence of previous uterine scar (nonlongitudinal), or with concomitant use of oxytocin, which is discouraged (Schulman et al, 1979). Extraovular or intra-amniotic dinoprost sometimes is effective, but the latter route is impractical if resorption of amniotic fluid has occurred. Carboprost can induce delivery of the dead fetus in a shorter time than delivery of a live fetus in elective terminations of pregnancy, but gastrointestinal side effects are more prominent (Wallenburg et al, 1980). Intra-amniotic instillation of saline further increases the risk of DIC, which can be fatal, and increases the possibility of intravascular injection. Large doses of oxytocin are necessary for this indication.

Preliminary reports of induction of preterm labor for *anencephalic fetus* have indicated that dinoprostone is effective but usually requires a long time to ripen the cervix due to lack of estrogen priming. For this reason, some clinicians recommend slow serial induction with dinoprostone suppositories. Previous procedures to encourage early delivery in such cases (ie, oxytocin, cesarean section) have not been entirely satisfactory. Induction of labor avoids the continuing emotional strain on the patient once the diagnosis has been made, particularly in view of the possibility of prolonged gestation in these cases, and reduces the possibility of delivery of a live infant.

OXYTOCIN CHALLENGE TEST. This test of fetal well-being is used in certain high-risk obstetrical patients (eg, those with diabetes mellitus, prolonged pregnancy, pre-eclampsia). It may be employed to clarify the clinical condition after a nonreactive nonstress test. This test is usually performed in a hospital at weekly intervals during late pregnancy, and the method is similar to that employed for induction of labor at term (see the evaluation on Oxytocin). A diagnosis of chronic fetal distress (fetal hypoxia, placental insufficiency) may be inferred if late decelerations of fetal heart rate (FHR) occur after each uterine contraction of equal amplitude. A positive test is an indication for interrupting pregnancy if the fetal lungs are mature (lecithin/sphingomyelin ratio more than 2). A negative finding is usually accurate, but one-third of positive test results may be false. Therefore, optimal management requires consideration of other factors (more detailed assessment of FHR patterns) before the decision to terminate pregnancy is made (Braly and Freeman, 1977). Theoretically, this test may increase the risk of premature labor but results of one prospective study that followed patients for up to five days indicated that the risk was not increased over that reported with a nonstress test or that expected in the general population (Braly et al, 1981).

POSTPARTUM USES. Oxytocin may be used to produce firm uterine contractions and decrease uterine bleeding after term delivery or following abortion. The need for oxytocic stimulation is increased if general anesthesia is employed, since this usually decreases spontaneous uterine contractility. It may be most convenient to administer oxytocin by slow intravenous infusion during the immediate postpartum period. Rapid intravenous infusion should be avoided because transient hypotension and increased heart rate may occur and could be life-threatening, particularly in patients with fixed cardiac output or hypotension resulting from hemorrhage.

Ergot alkaloids (ergonovine [Ergotrate], methylergonovine [Methergine]) also can be used postpartum and usually are administered intramuscularly. These drugs are preferred when sustained action is required, since they are effective for several hours. Oral tablets are sometimes given prophylactically for one or two days to patients who have undergone abortion. Ergot alkaloids generally should not be given intravenously because of the danger of increasing blood pressure, particularly in hypertensive patients. Methylergonovine has less hypertensive activity than ergonovine.

Prostaglandins also are used postpartum by intramyometrial or intramuscular injection to treat postpartum hemorrhage refractory to usual measures and to correct uterine atony (see the evaluation on Carboprost Tromethamine). Other uses for prostaglandins are delayed postpartum hemorrhage (Andrinopoulos and Mendenhall, 1983) and recurrent puerperal uterine inversion (Heyl et al, 1984).

STIMULATION OF MILK LET-DOWN REFLEX. The suckling infant stimulates sensory receptors around the nipple, which initiate separate neuroendocrine reflexes that release prolactin from the anterior pituitary and oxytocin from the posterior pituitary. Prolactin is important in initiating and maintaining milk production and oxytocin stimulates myoepithelial cells in the mammary gland, which causes milk ejection, commonly termed the milk let-down reflex. Oxytocin is not galactopoietic. Milk ejection also can be initiated by psychic stimuli (eg, seeing the infant, hearing the infant cry). When failure of the neuroendocrine reflex is responsible for insufficient breast milk, intranasal oxytocin may be useful.

Adverse Reactions

All oxytocic agents are potentially dangerous and patients receiving these drugs must be monitored closely. Their injudicious use may cause injury or death of the mother or infant. Hyperstimulation during labor may progress to uterine tetany with marked impairment of uteroplacental blood flow, uterine rupture, cervical laceration, amniotic fluid embolism, or trauma to the infant (eg, hypoxia, intracranial hemorrhage). See also the previous section and evaluations.

Drug Evaluations

OXYTOCIN
[Pitocin, Syntocinon]

Oxytocin is a cyclic octapeptide synthesized in the paraventricular nucleus of the hypothalamus. Weakly bound to neurophysin within granules, oxytocin is transported in this form down the axons of the hypothalamic neurons to the posterior pituitary gland where it is stored. Oxytocin circulates in the blood as the free peptide and has a plasma half-life of 12 to 17 minutes. Inactivation occurs principally in the liver and kidneys. All available commercial preparations are synthetic.

USES. Oxytocin is the drug of choice to induce labor at term and may be given to augment labor in selected patients with uterine dysfunction. This agent also may be used in inevitable or incomplete abortion after 20 weeks of gestation, although prostaglandins are preferred because they are more effective during the second trimester. Oxytocin may be given after term delivery or abortion to prevent or control hemorrhage and to correct uterine hypotonicity. It also is administered to test fetal-placental function in high-risk obstetric patients (oxytocin challenge test). For more information, see the section on Indications in the Introduction.

Depending upon the indication, oxytocin is administered intravenously, intramuscularly, or intranasally. For induction of labor, intravenous infusion with an electric pump is preferred because the dosage can be controlled precisely and increased gradually while the patient's response is observed. Intramuscular injections or intravenous infusions may be employed to control postpartum bleeding and uterine hypotonus. Nasal application has been used to stimulate the milk let-down reflex.

ADVERSE REACTIONS AND PRECAUTIONS. Hypofibrinogenemia and postpartum bleeding have been observed following use of oxytocin during labor, but these disorders are probably related to the underlying problem rather than to the drug. Water intoxication with convulsions caused by the inherent antidiuretic effect of oxytocin may occur if large doses (40 to 50 milliunits/min) are infused for long periods. However, this complication should not be a problem at the low concentrations employed to induce labor at term. The risk of water intoxication (even with the larger doses used when oxytocin is administered as an adjunct to another abortifacient for second trimester abortion) can be minimized by infusing the drug intravenously in an electrolyte solution (physiologic saline or Ringer's solution) or in a combination of dextrose 5% and a physiologic electrolyte solution instead of dextrose 5% alone. Increasing the concentration of oxytocin rather than the volume of solution infused also minimizes the risk of water intoxication.

Injudicious use of oxytocin may provoke uterine rupture, anaphylactoid and other allergic reactions, and maternal death. Induced uterine contractions of long duration may cause sinus bradycardia, premature ventricular contractions and other arrhythmias in the fetus, and fetal deaths. A higher incidence of jaundice has been reported in neonates whose mothers were given oxytocin infusions during labor, but one prospective study has shown that jaundice results from fetal immaturity and not oxytocin (Lange et al, 1982 B).

Oxytocin should not be used simultaneously by more than one route. *If it is given with another oxytocic agent, caution must be exercised to prevent additive myometrial hypertonia* (Claman et al, 1984; Cederqvist and Birnbaum, 1980). During induction of labor, uterine contractility, maternal pulse and

blood pressure, and fetal heart rate should be monitored, the latter by external or internal fetal monitor. Administration should be discontinued immediately if tetany occurs.

Contraindications for induction of labor are cephalopelvic disproportion, malpresentation, complete placenta previa, and hysterotomy. Except in unusual circumstances, labor should not be induced in the presence of a vertical uterine scar from previous cesarean section or myomectomy. With the increasing acceptance of a trial of labor in second pregnancies with previous cesarean deliveries, the benefits and risks of administering oxytocin to augment labor must be weighed. Results of one large study have shown that, in women with a previous low transverse section, oxytocin did not increase the incidence of dehiscence, hemorrhage, uterine atony, or hysterectomy when the patient was monitored carefully (Horenstein and Phelan, 1985).

DOSAGE AND PREPARATIONS.

Intravenous Infusion: For induction of labor, a dilute solution (10 milliunits/ml) is administered, preferably with a constant rate infusion pump (counting drops is less reliable). An initial infusion rate of 0.5 milliunits/min, increased by 1 to 2 milliunits/min every 20 to 30 minutes, has been recommended. However, recent studies indicate that approximately 40 minutes are required to reach a steady-state plasma concentration. Based on this information, it has been suggested that the dose be increased only every 40 minutes to reduce the possibility of overstimulation and fetal distress (Seitchik et al, 1984). The dosage is increased until an optimal uterine response is obtained (three or four contractions similar to normal labor in ten minutes) without evidence of fetal distress. Approximately 90% of patients respond to a final infusion rate of less than or equal to 5 milliunits/min (Seitchik et al, 1984). Physiologic saline, Ringer's solution, or a combination of dextrose 5% and a physiologic electrolyte solution should be used as the diluent, especially if a faster rate of infusion is used. As labor progresses, the dose required to maintain contractions often decreases or the drug may be withdrawn altogether.

For the oxytocin challenge test, a dilute solution is infused intravenously starting at the lowest pump setting (approximately 0.5 milliunits/min), and the dose is doubled every 20 to 30 minutes until three contractions are observed every ten minutes (maximum rate, 20 milliunits/min) unless repetitive late deceleration or fetal bradycardia occurs earlier. If either occurs, oxytocin should be discontinued immediately.

For prevention of postpartum uterine atony and hemorrhage, 20 to 40 milliunits/ml in an electrolyte solution is given at the rate of 40 milliunits/min or a rate sufficient to control uterine atony. The higher concentration assures adequate dosage without excessive fluid. Bolus injection should be avoided because untoward cardiovascular effects (eg, hypotension, tachycardia) may occur even in young healthy patients.

Intramuscular: To control postpartum bleeding, 3 to 10 units (0.3 to 1 ml).

Generic. Solution 10 units/ml in 1 and 10 ml containers.
Pitocin (Parke-Davis). Solution (sterile, aqueous) 5 units/ml in 0.5 ml containers and 10 units/ml in 0.5, 1, and 10 ml containers.
Syntocinon (Sandoz). Solution (sterile, aqueous) 10 units/ml in 1 ml containers.

Topical (nasal spray): To promote milk ejection, one spray into one or both nostrils two or three minutes before nursing.

    Syntocinon (Sandoz). Nasal spray 40 units/ml (40,000 milliunits/ml) in 2 and 5 ml containers.

ERGOT ALKALOIDS

ERGONOVINE MALEATE
[Ergotrate Maleate]

METHYLERGONOVINE MALEATE
[Methergine]

USES. These drugs are used after delivery of the placenta and following suction curettage or instillation abortion to produce firm uterine contractions and decrease uterine bleeding. Both drugs have a rapid onset of action, which varies according to the route of administration (intravenous, 40 seconds; intramuscular, 7 to 8 minutes; oral, 10 minutes). Their usefulness is further enhanced by their prolonged duration of action (several hours).

ADVERSE REACTIONS AND PRECAUTIONS. The adverse effects produced by ergonovine and methylergonovine are similar but are more severe after intravenous administration; for this reason, the intramuscular and oral routes are preferred. Intravenous injection often produces transient hypertension, which is more prominent in patients with chronic hypertension or pre-eclampsia. Hypertensive episodes may be asymptomatic or associated with nausea, vomiting, blurred vision, headaches, and possibly convulsions and death. The intravenous administration of methylergonovine has less tendency to cause hypertension than ergonovine, but neither agent should be given to patients with hypertension.

Ergot alkaloids should not be used in pregnant patients or to induce labor, because of their long duration of action and the unphysiologic uterine contractions that they induce. They also should not be given to those with a history of hypersensitivity

to ergot alkaloids. Both drugs should be administered cautiously to patients with cardiac, hepatic, renal, or obliterative vascular disease.

DOSAGE AND PREPARATIONS.

Intramuscular: To control uterine hemorrhage, 0.2 mg (1 ml); the dose may be repeated in two to four hours if bleeding is severe.

Intravenous: In emergencies to control excessive uterine bleeding, 0.2 mg (1 ml).

    ERGONOVINE MALEATE:
    Ergotrate Maleate (Lilly), **Generic.** Solution 0.2 mg/ml in 1 ml containers.
    METHYLERGONOVINE MALEATE:
    Methergine (Sandoz). Solution 0.2 mg/ml in 1 ml containers.

Oral: 0.2 or 0.4 mg two to four times daily, usually for two days.

    ERGONOVINE MALEATE:
    Ergotrate Maleate (Lilly), **Generic.** Tablets 0.2 mg.
    METHYLERGONOVINE MALEATE:
    Methergine (Sandoz). Tablets 0.2 mg.

PROSTAGLANDINS

CARBOPROST TROMETHAMINE
[Prostin/15M]

ACTIONS AND USES. Carboprost (15-methyl $PGF_{2\alpha}$) is a synthetic analogue of the naturally occurring $PGF_{2\alpha}$. Addition of a methyl group at C-15 produced a compound with a longer duration of action. This agent stimulates uterine contractions similar to those observed during term labor and is used to induce abortion between 13 and 20 weeks after the LMP.

The successful abortion rate is 96%, including 78% complete abortions (ie, complete passage of fetal products without surgical intervention). The mean time to abortion is about 16 hours, the mean total dose is 2.4 mg, and the mean total blood loss is 140 ml. Time to abortion and total dose increase with greater gestational age but decrease with greater gravidity or parity. Incomplete or failed abortions usually can be completed by D and C or suction curettage.

Although a suppository form is not commercially available, intravaginal carboprost has been used to induce cervical ripening prior to D and E in first trimester abortions (Kent et al, 1983; Arias, 1984).

Carboprost has several advantages over other prostaglandin abortifacients. Intramuscular injection is technically less difficult and avoids the potential problems inherent in the invasive intra-amniotic or extraovular techniques. Like dinoprostone, carboprost is easily utilized for abortion between 12 and 15 weeks after the LMP and can be used when the membranes have ruptured. An additional advantage of intramuscular carboprost over intravaginal dinoprostone is that the intramuscular route can be used in the presence of profuse vaginal bleeding that could lead to expulsion of a vaginal suppository.

Carboprost has been shown to control persistent postpartum hemorrhage secondary to uterine atony unresponsive to oxytocin and ergonovine or methylergonovine (Herbert and Cefalo, 1984; Nelson, 1980). In view of the life-threatening nature of this condition, the risk/benefit relationship favors use of carboprost, since the recommended dose (0.25 to 0.5 mg every 1.5 hours) is similar to that used for abortion and the need for surgery may be eliminated. In one study, most patients responded to one dose and the average time to increased uterine tone and decreased bleeding was 45 minutes (Hayashi et al, 1984). The intramuscular route is usually employed, but the intramyometrial route also can be utilized. See also the Introduction.

ADVERSE REACTIONS AND PRECAUTIONS. Adverse effects are common but usually not serious. Vomiting and diarrhea occur in over 60% of patients, and the concurrent administration of antiemetic and antidiarrheal agents is recommended. Fever (more than 2 F) occurs in over 10% of patients, and care must be taken to differentiate drug-induced pyrexia from that due to endometritis.

Carboprost should not be administered to patients who are hypersensitive to the drug or to those with acute pelvic inflammatory disease or active cardiac, pulmonary, renal, or hepatic disease. Patients with a history of asthma; hypertension; cardiovascular, renal, or hepatic disease; anemia; jaundice; diabetes; or epilepsy and those who have undergone uterine surgery, including previous cesarean section, should receive this drug only with caution. Measures should be taken to ensure complete abortion. Although cervical trauma is unusual, the cervix should be examined after abortion.

As with other prostaglandins, abortion induced by carboprost may result in delivery of a live fetus. Because of the teratogenic potential of certain prostaglandins in animals, pregnancy should be terminated by another method if abortion cannot be induced by carboprost.

Carboprost should be administered only by qualified medical personnel in hospitals with obstetric intensive care and surgical facilities.

DOSAGE AND PREPARATIONS.
Intramuscular: To induce abortion, initially, 250 mcg deep in the muscle, repeated at intervals of 1.5 to 3.5 hours, depending upon the response. Dosage may be increased to 500 mcg if contractility is inadequate after several 250-mcg doses. The total dose should not exceed 12 mg.

    Prostin/15M (Upjohn). Solution (sterile) 250 mcg carboprost and 83 mcg tromethamine/ml in 1 ml containers.

DINOPROST TROMETHAMINE
[Prostin F2 alpha]

ACTIONS AND USES. Dinoprost tromethamine ($PGF_{2\alpha}THAM$) stimulates uterine contractility and is usually given intra-amniotically to induce abortion when the size of the uterus and the amount of amniotic fluid are adequate, usually after 15 weeks of gestation. It is injected transabdominally into the amniotic sac, transferred slowly across the fetal membranes, and acts directly on the myometrium. Although systemic absorption is least with this route of administration, low levels of the drug are found in maternal plasma, which accounts for the adverse effects observed. From 60% to 100% of abortions are complete (ie, passage of all fetal products without surgical intervention), and the mean abortion time is approximately 20 hours.

The extra-amniotic (extraovular) method of administration is not widely used in the United States. This method requires placement of an indwelling catheter between the uterine wall and the fetal membranes. It probably should be reserved for termination of pregnancies between 12 and 14 weeks (when the intra-amniotic method is technically difficult to perform) or when amniocentesis has failed. The extraovular technique uses much smaller doses than the intra-amniotic method, but the potential for rapid systemic absorption of the drug is probably greater. Incomplete abortion (usually retention of placenta) is more common with the extraovular technique, and the risk of intrauterine infection is greater because of the indwelling transcervical catheter.

Oxytocin is sometimes employed adjunctively to shorten the abortion time. Since effects are additive, the danger of uterine hyperstimulation and rupture is greater (Cederqvist and Birnbaum, 1980). There is no universal agreement on the advisability of this practice; if employed, caution should be exercised.

Several other routes of administration and regimens have been used investigationally. Continuous intravenous infusion, intramuscular and subcutaneous administration, and oral or intravaginal tablets and solution-soaked tampons have had variable success. The incidence and severity of adverse effects, which are related directly to the circulating level of prostaglandin, are generally unacceptable with these routes.

Investigational uses of dinoprost include induction of labor and stimulation of contractions in early rupture of membranes, missed abortion, intrauterine fetal death, hydatidiform mole, and postpartum hemorrhage. Intramyometrial dinoprost has been effective in controlling severe postpartum hemorrhage (Tagaki et al, 1976).

ADVERSE REACTIONS AND PRECAUTIONS. Cervical or lower uterine laceration or rupture, retention of the placenta, and hemorrhage are the most dangerous effects of dinoprost in second trimester abortion. The drug should be used cautiously in women with a history of cesarean section, hysterotomy, uterine fibroids, or cervical stenosis. Intra-amniotic dinoprost should be used with caution in nulliparous women; laminaria should be used concomitantly to avoid abortion through the lower uterine segment.

Nausea or vomiting occurs in most patients but can be ameliorated or prevented by antiemetics. Breast engorgement and lactation are more frequent after use of dinoprost than after suction curettage, intra-amniotic saline or oxytocin, and other methods of abortion. Fever, hypotension and syncope, hypertension, headache, and pain and erythema at the site of injection are noted less frequently. Bronchospasm may be observed in asthmatic patients. Seizures probably occur only in patients with epilepsy. Vasomotor reactions, arrhythmias, atrioventricular conduction disturbances, hyperventilation, paresthesias and hyperesthesias, chest pain, hiccups, and dysuria have developed after intrauterine administration.

Inadvertent intravenous administration produces immediate bronchospasm, uterine tetanic contraction, and hypotension or hypertension that could proceed to shock, severe cramping, vomiting, and diarrhea. Because of this, the establishment of an intravenous line is recommended before intra-amniotic instillation of dinoprost. Since prostaglandins are metabolized rapidly, reactions seldom last longer than 15 to 30 minutes.

DOSAGE AND PREPARATIONS.

Intra-amniotic Instillation: Following the establishment of a peripheral intravenous line, a spinal needle (No. 18 to 22) is used for transabdominal intra-amniotic tap; 1 or more ml of fluid is removed to determine alkalinity and 40 mg (8 ml) of dinoprost tromethamine is injected slowly if the amniotic fluid is not bloody. The first milliliter should be injected over one to two minutes to determine sensitivity and to confirm correct needle placement. If there is minimal or no response, a second dose of 10 to 20 mg is given after six hours.

Extra-amniotic (Extraovular) Instillation: (Investigational route) A 14 or 16 Foley catheter with a 30-ml balloon is placed into the lower uterine segment posteriorly in the extraovular space. Suggested dosages include (1) 0.5 mg initially, followed by 0.75 mg every two hours until abortion; (2) 0.25 mg initially, followed by 0.75 mg in five minutes, 1 mg in 30 minutes, and 1 mg every six hours until abortion; (3) 0.1 mg/ml infused continuously at the rate of 1 mg/hr; or (4) 5-mg bolus injections every two or three hours to a total dose of 15 mg.

Intramyometrial: For severe postpartum hemorrhage, 1 mg transabdominally with a spinal needle.

> ***Prostin F2 alpha*** (Upjohn). Solution (as tromethamine) 5 mg/ml in 4 and 8 ml containers.

DINOPROSTONE
[Prostin E2]

ACTIONS AND USES. Dinoprostone (PGE_2) occurs naturally in mammalian tissues, human seminal plasma, and menstrual fluid.

Termination of Pregnancy: This prostaglandin is used in suppository form to induce labor in intrauterine fetal death (less than 28 weeks gestation), missed abortion, hydatidiform mole, anencephalic fetus, or elective abortion. It also is useful when uterine perforation has occurred before completion of suction curettage. Uterine contractions are qualitatively similar to those that occur during term labor.

Pregnancy can be interrupted with dinoprostone before 15 weeks of gestation. This is an advantage over intra-amniotic dinoprost because transabdominal amniocentesis is avoided, fewer complications occur with earlier abortion, and elective abortion or evacuation of the fetus in intrauterine death need not be delayed.

Vaginal administration concentrates drug action at the target tissue and is noninvasive. Vaginal application of dinoprostone induces myometrial contractions that usually empty the uterus. It also enhances cervical softening, which facilitates cervical dilatation. Generally, the total dose required to induce delivery declines with advancing gestation so that only a fraction of the 20-mg suppository is needed (Macer et al, 1984).

Like dinoprost, dinoprostone can induce uterine contractions when administered orally, intramuscularly, intravenously, or intra- and extra-amniotically, but use of these routes is still investigational in this country. The effective half-life of prostaglandin action on the uterus is approximately 30 to 60 minutes.

The success rate for elective abortion before 20 weeks of pregnancy is 92%, including 74% complete abortions. Mean time to abortion is about 17 hours, and the mean dose required is 90 mg. Blood loss averages 170 ml.

When dinoprostone is used to stimulate labor in intrauterine fetal death, the success rate is almost 100% (including 95% to 99% complete abortions). The time to abortion is 11 hours, and the total dose is about 60 mg. The average blood loss (200 ml) is slightly higher than in elective abortion and may be due to coagulation defects and hypofibrinogenemia, which are more likely to occur with retention of a dead fetus.

For expulsion of benign hydatidiform mole, the average dose is 70 mg and the time to evacuation varies widely (1 to 80 hours, mean 16 hours). Blood loss averages 645 ml and nearly one-half of patients require blood transfusion.

Uses in Term Labor: There are a number of favorable reports on the use of dinoprostone as a cervical ripening agent before induction of labor with oxytocin or as an alternative to oxytocin (Ulmsten et al, 1983; Porreco and Watson, 1983); the use of dinoprostone in cervical ripening is investigational, however. Dinoprostone-induced cervical ripening seems to be associated with increased collagenolysis (Ekman et al, 1983) similar to the normal ripening process (Uldbjerg et al, 1983) and ripening is not dependent upon uterine contractions (Goeschen et al, 1985).

Dinoprostone is preferred to carboprost and dinoprost when induction of labor is necessary but the cervix is unfavorable (eg, following spontaneous rupture of membranes). Intravaginal or intracervical administration of small doses of dinoprostone suppository or gel produces significant cervical softening (increased Bishop scores) (Graves et al, 1985; Buchanan et al, 1984; MacKenzie and Embrey, 1977; Jagani et al, 1984) and reduces the number of failed inductions (Buchanan et al, 1984; Lange et al, 1984). Although the optimal dose has not been determined, dinoprostone gel 0.4 to 0.5 mg extra-amniotically or intracervically (Gordon and Calder, 1983; Ulmsten et al, 1983) and intravaginal suppositories 1 mg were effective (Jagani et al, 1984). The incidence of gastrointestinal adverse reactions is greatly reduced with these doses.

Whether the cervical ripening produced by dinoprostone

significantly decreases the induction-to-delivery time has been the subject of a number of studies. In some studies, no significant difference in duration of oxytocin-induced labor with dinoprostone or placebo was reported (Buchanan et al, 1984; Jagani et al, 1984) despite significant dinoprostone-induced cervical ripening (as measured by increased Bishop score) and uniform timing of amniotomy with subsequent oxytocin initiation. No differences in fetal distress or maternal complications were observed. In contrast to these results, pretreatment with dinoprostone gel was reported to reduce the duration of oxytocin-induced labor and the incidence of cesarean delivery in primigravidae with low Bishop scores (unfavorable cervices) (Fenton et al, 1985; Gordon and Calder, 1983; Porreco and Watson, 1983; MacKenzie and Embrey, 1977). These conflicting results complicate determination of the benefit of cervical ripening on the duration of induced labor. More clinical trials are needed to resolve this question.

Cervical ripening with even low doses of dinoprostone is not without risk of fetal distress, since uterine contractions are stimulated in many patients. The fetus should be monitored during the ripening process; if hyperstimulation occurs, intravenous terbutaline 250 mcg can be employed or magnesium sulfate 3 to 4 g given by slow intravenous push.

As an alternative to oxytocin for induction of labor, dinoprostone has the advantage of inducing both cervical ripening and uterine contractions. Dinoprostone suppositories or pessaries are used routinely in some countries to induce labor and have been reported to be most useful when the cervix is unfavorable, especially in primigravidae (Hunter et al, 1984). Successful induction was reported in 73% of patients with average Bishop scores of 5. A 3-mg suppository is commonly administered intravaginally (Hunter et al, 1984; Macer et al, 1984; Lange et al, 1984; Magos et al, 1983). The incidence of hypertonicity is dose related (Graves et al, 1985) and patients receiving 3 mg or more should be monitored closely. Oral dinoprostone 0.5 to 1.5 mg every hour also has been demonstrated to induce regular uterine contractions two to three hours after administration with rapid cervical softening and dilation (3 cm/hour) (Ueland and Conrad, 1983). In multiparous patients, induction-to-delivery time was about seven hours. Subsequent augmentation with oxytocin is required in most patients to maintain the established pattern of contractions, but the two oxytocics should not be given simultaneously.

In one study comparing oxytocin- and dinoprostone-initiated labor, successful vaginal deliveries occurred in 95% of 85 patients with favorable cervical states after use of either drug (Bishop score greater than or equal to 5) (Macer et al, 1984). The same study showed that dinoprostone significantly decreased the amount of oxytocin required; side effects (gastrointestinal reactions, fever, uterine hypertonus, and postpartum hemorrhage) were not significantly different with either agent.

ADVERSE REACTIONS AND PRECAUTIONS. Adverse reactions are common with abortive doses of dinoprostone but generally are not serious. Gastrointestinal disturbances are reported most frequently and are related to contractile effects on smooth muscle. Vomiting occurs in approximately two-thirds and diarrhea in one-half of patients treated. These symptoms can be alleviated by antiemetics and antidiarrheal agents and by increasing the interval between doses.

Fever (more than 2 F), frequently with chills, occurs in up to one-half of patients. Drug-induced fever must be differentiated from pyrexia due to endometritis, particularly in intrauterine fetal death when there is a greater risk of sepsis. Also, when the combination of fever and hypotension suggests sepsis, the possibility of drug-induced fever and hypotension due to blood loss associated with uterine rupture should be considered.

Headache and decreased diastolic blood pressure (mean, 29 mm Hg in elective abortion patients) occur in 10% of patients. Blood loss resulting from the procedure may contribute to reduced blood pressure. Unlike abortion induced by hypertonic saline, there is no risk of hypernatremia and the incidence of DIC is not increased; however, there is a higher risk of hemorrhage from retained placentas.

Uterine hypertonicity and rupture have been reported (Claman et al, 1984). Rupture of the amniotic and chorionic membranes is not a contraindication to continued use of dinoprostone as it is for intra- or extra-amniotic administration of prostaglandins, but wash-out of the suppository can occur. Profuse vaginal bleeding also may cause expulsion of the suppository.

Unlike abortion induced by hypertonic saline or urea, that induced by prostaglandins may result in delivery of a live fetus, particularly with increasing gestational age. This agent is not labeled for use beyond 28 weeks and should be employed cautiously in fetal death in utero during the third trimester because of the increased risk of uterine rupture.

In animal studies, certain prostaglandins have been shown to have teratogenic potential. Therefore, if treatment with dinoprostone fails to abort the fetus, the pregnancy should be terminated by appropriate measures (eg, suction, curettage).

Dinoprostone should be used cautiously in patients with cervicitis, infected endocervical lesions, or acute vaginitis and in those with a history of asthma; hypertension or hypotension; cardiovascular, renal, or hepatic disease; anemia; jaundice; diabetes; or epilepsy. It should not be given to patients with acute pelvic inflammatory disease, uterine scars, or hypersensitivity to the drug. The concomitant use of oxytocin in abortion is generally not advised because of the increased risk of uterine rupture.

Dinoprostone should be administered only by qualified medical personnel in hospitals with obstetric intensive care and surgical facilities.

DOSAGE AND PREPARATIONS. Suppositories must be stored at or below -20 C (-4 F) and brought to room temperature just before use.

Vaginal: To induce abortion, one 20-mg suppository is inserted high in the vagina, and the patient should remain supine for ten minutes following insertion. Subsequently, suppositories are inserted at intervals of three to five hours until abortion occurs. Within this interval, administration time is determined by uterine contractility and patient tolerance. If abortion is incomplete, administration may be continued to completion if blood loss is not excessive and adverse reactions are not severe.

For doses used for cervical ripening and to induce labor (investigational indications), see Actions and Uses.

Prostin E2 (Upjohn). Vaginal suppositories 20 mg.

HYPERTONIC SOLUTIONS

SALINE

USES. Hypertonic saline is used to induce second trimester abortion. It was once the most commonly used agent for this indication but has been replaced to some extent by prostaglandins and urea. Some practitioners prefer saline, and the choice among agents depends on several factors (see the discussion on Elective Abortion in the Introduction).

Hypertonic saline is usually administered by transabdominal amniocentesis. It is effective in about 90% of patients; the mean abortion time is approximately 36 hours. Sometimes saline is administered with another agent, such as oxytocin or dinoprost, to reduce abortion time. However, care must be taken when more than one uterine stimulant is used because the effects are additive.

PRECAUTIONS. Saline abortion should not be attempted in patients whose ability to handle a sodium load is compromised (eg, those with renal or cardiac failure, hypertension). Inadvertent intravascular injection causes hypernatremia and possibly disseminated intravascular coagulation. Accidental instillation into the uterine wall destroys uterine tissue.

DOSAGE AND PREPARATIONS.
Intra-amniotic Instillation: Following the establishment of an intravenous line and amniocentesis with a properly placed needle for aspiration of amniotic fluid, 200 ml of a 20% salt solution (40 g sodium chloride) is instilled via a catheter threaded through the needle into the amniotic cavity. No more than 40 g of salt should be left in the uterus. It may be possible to produce fetal death and expulsion in early gestations (ie, 14 weeks) with only 100 ml of a 20% solution if some exchange infusion is done beforehand. However, inadequate salt concentration could result in failure to produce fetal death or delayed or failed expulsion. The patient should feel nothing or only a sensation of fullness when the salt solution is injected. Subcutaneous, intraperitoneal, or intramyometrial injection produces severe pain and burning (Neubardt and Schulman, 1977).

   Sodium Chloride 20% (Abbott). Solution 20% in 250 ml containers.

UREA
[Ureaphil]

USES. A hypertonic solution of urea is used as an alternative to hypertonic saline, dinoprost, dinoprostone, or carboprost to induce second trimester abortions. Like dinoprost and saline, urea is administered by transabdominal amniocentesis. The abortion time is longer (43 versus 36 hours) than with saline but urea is theoretically safer.

Oxytocin is sometimes administered after instillation of urea to shorten the abortion time. A solution of urea and dinoprost has been administered intra-amniotically, and the combination appears to reduce abortion time (16 to 17 hours) and the likelihood of live births compared to dinoprost alone. The combination decreases the adverse effects of both drugs because of the smaller doses employed. However, a combination of urea and oxytocin is preferred in patients with a history of asthma or epilepsy. Care must be taken when more than one uterine stimulant is used because the effects are additive. See also the section on Indications in the Introduction.

ADVERSE REACTIONS AND PRECAUTIONS. Urea may cause hyponatremia, hypokalemia, or hyperkalemia. It should not be used in patients with severely impaired renal or hepatic function, intracranial bleeding, or dehydration. Patients should be encouraged to drink fluids and should receive intravenous fluid during the procedure to enhance excretion of urea. Nausea, vomiting, and headaches also may occur. Inadvertent intravascular spill can cause headache, nausea, uterine cramps, and a feeling of warmth.

DOSAGE AND PREPARATIONS.
Intra-amniotic Instillation: 80 g is reconstituted to a volume of 135 to 200 ml with 5% dextrose solution to make a 40% to 50% solution. It is recommended that a peripheral intravenous line be established initially and then, following amniocentesis with a properly placed needle for aspiration of amniotic fluid, the solution is instilled by gravity via a suitably attached administration set connected to the needle.

   Ureaphil (Abbott). Powder (nonpyrogenic) 40 g in 150 ml single-dose containers. The desired diluent can be added directly to the contents.

UTERINE RELAXANTS

Uterine relaxants are used to treat premature labor until the fetus has matured sufficiently for survival. They also may be employed briefly to delay delivery while treatment with corticosteroids is instituted. Use of selective beta$_2$ adrenergic agents (to relax uterine smooth muscle) is replacing older, less specific approaches, such as infusion of alcohol. The use of combination tocolysis, which consists of adjuvant therapy with magnesium sulfate or prostaglandin inhibitors, is increasing but controlled studies are needed to determine efficacy, maternal tolerance, and neonatal outcome compared to use of beta-adrenergic therapy alone. Corticosteroids may be given concurrently to stimulate production of fetal lung surfactant (see also Chapter 61, Adrenal Corticosteroids in Nonendocrine Diseases).

Choice of Therapy: Uterine contractions may cease spontaneously after conservative treatment with hydration, bed rest, or sedation or may progress to premature labor. Uterine relaxants are more likely to inhibit labor earlier in pregnancy and before labor is far advanced.

When the diagnosis of premature labor is established, the benefits of therapy may outweigh the risks if gestation is less than 34 weeks, if the cervix is dilated less than 4 cm, and if there are no contraindications to the drugs. The incidence of fetal respiratory distress syndrome was reduced significantly when beta-adrenergic therapy was given to women with intact membranes (Curet et al, 1984). Contraindications include any condition in which treatment and continuation of the pregnancy represent the greater hazard (eg, eclampsia, severe preeclampsia, hemorrhage, intrauterine fetal death, chorioamnionitis, maternal cardiovascular disease).

Beta-adrenergic agents are most commonly used to prevent premature delivery. They are usually administered intravenously until contractions are inhibited. After discharge from the hospital, the patient may be maintained on oral medication until delivery of a mature infant is assured. However, tachyphylaxis occurs with long-term therapy and some authorities believe a shorter course of treatment (eg, five days) is equally effective and avoids prolonged exposure of mother and fetus to the drug. If premature labor recurs, intravenous therapy may be repeated.

Ritodrine [Yutopar] is the only agent currently labeled for tocolysis and has been used extensively throughout the world. Terbutaline [Brethine, Bricanyl], commonly used as a bronchodilator, has not been employed as extensively, but data indicate that it is therapeutically equivalent to ritodrine (Caritis et al, 1984). Protocols for the use of terbutaline to interrupt premature labor are available (for intravenous administration, Haller, 1980; for subcutaneous administration, Stubblefield and Heyl, 1982). Because isoxsuprine [Vasodilan], which is used to treat peripheral vascular disorders, has relatively less specific beta$_2$-adrenergic effects, the incidence and severity of undesirable cardiovascular effects (ie, tachycardia, hypotension) are greater (Caritis, 1983). Other beta$_2$-adrenergic drugs used investigationally to arrest premature labor are albuterol (salbutamol) [Proventil, Ventolin] (available in the United States for treatment of asthma as oral and nasal spray preparations only); fenoterol and hexoprenaline (not available in the United States); and nylidrin [Arlidin].

Hyperglycemia, hypokalemia, angina, and other cardiovascular complications have occurred after use of beta-adrenergic agents. Adult respiratory distress syndrome and pulmonary edema also have developed with and without concurrent corticosteroid therapy (for fetal lung maturation). Although it has been recommended that potent general anesthetics that depress the myocardium be avoided when beta-adrenergic agents are used, there is little clinical data to support this view.

Intravenous alcohol, once widely used to inhibit premature labor, has been replaced by beta-adrenergic therapy. The proposed mechanism of alcohol-induced uterine relaxation involves the indirect inhibition of the myometrium by preventing oxytocin's release from the posterior pituitary gland (Lauersen et al, 1981). Intravenous alcohol causes inebriation and, if general anesthesia is required for delivery, care must be taken to prevent aspiration of gastric contents, since alcohol is a gastric secretagogue. Alcohol postpones labor for only a few hours or days, thus limiting its usefulness.

Magnesium sulfate prevents convulsions in pre-eclampsia and inhibits uterine contractions by a direct effect on the myometrial cells. Excitation and contraction are uncoupled, which decreases the frequency and force of contractions. This drug is administered intravenously and appears to be more effective than alcohol. Repeated administration may inhibit premature labor for one week or longer. The drug is generally safe but can cause temporary loss of deep tendon reflexes in the mother and may depress skeletal muscle activity in the neonate (Caritis, 1983). It should not be used in patients with heart disease or severely impaired renal function but may be preferred to beta-adrenergic agonists for diabetic, hyperthyroid, or hypertensive patients. The uterine inhibitory action and

relative safety of magnesium sulfate have been appreciated for many years, and a number of protocols are available (Caritis, 1983; Carpenter, 1982).

Diazoxide [Hyperstat IV], a potent antihypertensive agent, is used to control blood pressure in hypertensive patients in labor. This agent also inhibits uterine contractions and has been employed investigationally to arrest premature labor. Because it is not more effective than beta agonists and may cause severe hypotension, marked maternal hyperglycemia, and neonatal hypoglycemia, its use for this indication is generally not favored (Huddleston, 1982).

Prostaglandins probably play a role in stimulating uterine contractions during normal labor, and their concentrations increase in amniotic fluid and serum during active labor. Prostaglandin inhibitors, particularly indomethacin [Indocin], have been used investigationally to delay preterm labor. However, prostaglandins are necessary to maintain a patent ductus arteriosus in the fetus, and prostaglandin inhibitors may cause premature closure. In a large retrospective study utilizing combined suppository and oral indomethacin for 24 to 48 hours to delay premature labor, premature closure of the ductus arteriosus did not occur (Dudley and Hardie, 1985). The incidence of imminent premature labor was decreased from 59% in controls to 29% in treated patients, but the incidence of spontaneous abortion was not decreased. Further clinical trials are necessary before the use of prostaglandin inhibitors can be recommended.

In women at high risk of premature delivery (ie, history of premature deliveries or spontaneous abortions), hydroxyprogesterone caproate [Delalutin] was reported to be more effective than placebo in maintaining pregnancy (Yemini et al, 1985). The drug was given prophylactically from the twelfth to thirty-seventh weeks of pregnancy or until delivery. The possibility of late teratogenic effects must be determined and more experience is necessary before hydroxyprogesterone can be recommended routinely (see also the discussion on alternative therapies for premature labor in Caritis et al, 1979, and Huddleston, 1982).

Drug Evaluations

RITODRINE HYDROCHLORIDE
[Yutopar]

ACTIONS. Ritodrine decreases the frequency, intensity, and duration of uterine contractions by direct stimulation of beta$_2$ receptors through activation of adenyl cyclase. Its effect is antagonized by beta blockers, such as propranolol. Although ritodrine selectively stimulates beta$_2$ receptors, it also has some beta$_1$ activity, which is responsible for cardiovascular side effects.

USES. This beta$_2$-adrenergic agonist is used to prevent the progress of premature labor in selected patients (eg, gestation of 20 weeks or more, labor that is not far advanced, intact or ruptured membranes, absence of contraindications). Therapy may be initiated as soon as the diagnosis is established and contraindications are ruled out. Delivery has been delayed for several days to enhance fetal lung maturity with corticosteroid therapy or for weeks to achieve a near normal gestation period. Intravenous administration stops contractions, and oral therapy is given for maintenance. Intravenous therapy may be repeated if further episodes of premature labor occur.

Although results of studies have been variable, ritodrine is superior to control therapies when premature labor begins before 33 weeks: Neonatal mortality decreased (13% to 5%), the incidence of respiratory distress syndrome was reduced (20% to 11%), the mean gestational age at birth increased (35.5 versus 34.5 weeks), the number of days to delivery increased (32.6 versus 21.3 days), and the number of infants with birth weights exceeding 2,500 g increased (58% versus 43%). However, if gestation exceeds 33 weeks when premature labor begins, overall advantages cannot be demonstrated statistically due to small numbers. Since morbidity is rarer after 33 weeks, many more cases are needed to prove the benefit of any treatment (Finkelstein, 1981). Ritodrine is less likely to be effective in advanced labor when the cervix is effaced more than 80% and dilated more than 4 cm.

ADVERSE REACTIONS. Cardiovascular and metabolic effects are observed in both mother and fetus. Adverse effects are most severe after intravenous administration and usually are controlled by reducing the dose, although discontinuation of therapy may be required. Theoretically, overdosage can be managed with a beta blocker (Feely et al, 1983), but there is little clinical evidence that this is necessary.

Intravenous infusion has caused tachycardia in almost all patients (mean maximum increase, 40 beats/min); increased systolic blood pressure (mean, 12 mm Hg); and decreased diastolic blood pressure (mean, 23 mm Hg). Hemoglobin concentrations decline in some patients. Blood glucose and insulin levels increase temporarily and return toward normal within 48 to 72 hours, even with continued infusion. Ketoacidosis has been reported. Serum potassium levels decrease and free fatty acid levels may increase. About one-third of patients experience palpitations, and up to 15% have chest pains, shortness of breath, tremor, nausea and vomiting, headache, or erythema. Less common reactions include nervousness, anxiety, malaise, and cardiovascular effects. Rarely, pulmonary edema occurs even after the drug is withdrawn. Attributing pulmonary edema to the combination of ritodrine and a corticosteroid with low mineralocorticoid activity has been questioned (Benedetti, 1983). Ritodrine unmasked latent myotonic muscular dystrophy in one patient (Sholl et al, 1985).

Intravenous administration also may cause tachycardia in the fetus. The concentration of insulin in cord blood may be elevated, resulting in neonatal hypoglycemia. Neonatal hypocalcemia has been reported. Before delivery, the fetus may be affected by maternal ketoacidosis. Infusion should be discontinued as soon as labor appears to be irreversible to allow metabolic recovery before delivery.

Fewer and less severe side effects have been reported after *oral* administration. The maternal heart rate may increase, but the blood pressure is not affected significantly. Carbohydrate and electrolyte balance do not appear to be affected. Tremors,

palpitations, nausea, nightmares, arrhythmias, or nervousness occur infrequently and are dose related.

Animal studies have shown no teratogenic effects and no impairment of reproductive function. Follow-up studies for two years revealed no deleterious effects on growth, development, or maturation in 7- to 9-year-old children exposed to ritodrine prenatally (Polowczyk et al, 1984). However, there are no well-controlled studies on the use of ritodrine prior to 20 weeks' gestation.

DRUG INTERACTIONS. Ritodrine and corticosteroids have additive diabetogenic effects. Insulin requirements may increase greatly during intravenous administration of ritodrine. Pulmonary edema also occurs rarely when ritodrine and corticosteroids are given concurrently, but the contribution of the corticosteroid has not been determined (Benedetti, 1983). The combination of ritodrine and magnesium sulfate has been reported to cause cardiac disturbances that necessitated withdrawal of tocolytic therapy (Ferguson et al, 1984).

Ritodrine may potentiate the effects of other sympathomimetic amines and may have an additive hypotensive effect with drugs such as anesthetics. The possibility of an additive effect with potassium-depleting diuretics also should be considered.

PRECAUTIONS AND CONTRAINDICATIONS. Fluid balance and serum glucose and potassium levels should be monitored during infusion, particularly in diabetic patients or those taking potassium-wasting diuretics. Because cardiovascular effects are most pronounced during intravenous infusion, maternal blood pressure and maternal and fetal heart rate should be monitored. Cerebral ischemia has been reported during beta-adrenergic therapy in two women with a history of migraine, and caution probably should be observed when ritodrine is used in these patients (Benedetti, 1983). If pulmonary edema develops, infusion should be discontinued and appropriate therapy instituted.

Ritodrine should not be used in pregnancies of less than 17 weeks' gestation because of lack of experience. It also should not be used when continuation of the pregnancy is hazardous to the mother or fetus, as in eclampsia, severe pre-eclampsia, antepartum hemorrhage, chorioamnionitis, and maternal cardiovascular disease. Caution should be observed in patients with hyperthyroidism or diabetes. This drug is classified in FDA Pregnancy Category B.

PHARMACOKINETICS. After intravenous infusion in normal nonpregnant women, ritodrine exhibited three half-lives: (1) six to nine minutes in the distribution phase, (2) 1.7 to 2.6 hours in the elimination phase, and (3) greater than 10 hours in the third phase (Gandar et al, 1980). Oral administration to male subjects produced peak serum concentrations in 20 to 40 minutes. Two phases of distribution (half-lives, 1.3 and 12 hours) occurred.

About 30% of an oral dose of ritodrine is bioavailable. Approximately 32% circulates bound to albumin. Up to 90% is excreted in the urine within 24 hours. Ritodrine crosses the placenta, and the cord blood concentration may equal that in the maternal circulation (Finkelstein, 1981).

DOSAGE AND PREPARATIONS. Treatment is individualized and the optimal dosage is determined by the balance between desired uterine response and undesirable effects. The patient should remain in the left lateral recumbent position to minimize hypotension. Three ampuls or one vial (150 mg) in 500 ml of diluent (eg, 5% dextrose) yield a final concentration of 300 mcg/ml (0.3 mg/ml). Because of the increased risk of pulmonary edema, saline diluents should not be used unless dextrose solution is less desirable (eg, diabetes mellitus) (Philipsen et al, 1981). The solution should be used promptly and discarded after 48 hours or if discoloration or particulate matter is observed.

Intravenous: Initially, 100 mcg/min (0.1 mg/min), increased by 50 mcg/min (0.05 mg/min) every ten minutes until contractions stop or a rate of 350 mcg/min (0.35 mg/min) is reached. The lowest dose that maintains uterine quiescence is continued for 12 hours after contractions are controlled. At the recommended rate of infusion, a maximum of approximately 840 ml of fluid would be administered in 12 hours. Repeated intravenous administration may be employed if there are subsequent episodes of premature labor.

   Yutopar (Astra). Solution (sterile, aqueous) 10 mg/ml in 5 ml containers and 15 mg/ml in 10 ml containers.

Oral: After premature labor is controlled by intravenous administration, oral therapy is initiated and continued as long as it is desirable to prolong pregnancy or until intravenous therapy is required again. One tablet (10 mg) is given 30 minutes before intravenous administration is terminated and repeated every two hours for the first 24 hours; subsequently, one to two tablets (10 to 20 mg) are taken every four to six hours to a maximum total daily dose of 120 mg. Treatment may be continued as long as it is desirable to prolong pregnancy.

   Yutopar (Astra). Tablets 10 mg.

TERBUTALINE SULFATE
[Brethine, Bricanyl]

ACTIONS AND USES. Like ritodrine, this drug is predominantly a beta$_2$-receptor agonist with some beta$_1$ activity, which causes cardiovascular side effects. Although terbutaline is not marketed for prevention of premature labor, it was employed by a number of physicians before ritodrine was introduced and is still preferred by some. Terbutaline and ritodrine have equivalent effectiveness and similar side effects with intravenous administration. However, in patients with intact membranes, the incidence of tachycardia (more than 130 beats/min) was reported to be greater with ritodrine and the incidence of hyperglycemia was greater with terbutaline (Caritis et al, 1984). Oral maintenance therapy with terbutaline 30 mg/day prolonged pregnancy by 40 ± 25 days compared to 22 ± 24 days for oral ritodrine 120 mg/day (Caritis et al, 1984). Labor recurred in fewer women given oral terbutaline for maintenance than with ritodrine.

See the evaluation on Ritodrine Hydrochloride for uses, adverse reactions, interactions, precautions, and contraindications of beta-adrenergic therapy.

DOSAGE AND PREPARATIONS.

Intravenous: Initially, 2.5 mcg/min (0.125 ml/min), increased by 2.5 mcg/min every 20 minutes until contractions stop or a rate of 17.5 mcg/min is reached. After contractions are controlled, the rate is reduced by 2.5 mcg/min every 20 minutes until the minimum effective infusion rate is established. This rate is then maintained for 12 hours. If labor recurs during this time, the rate can again be increased by 2.5 mcg/min every 20 minutes to re-establish control.

   Brethine (Geigy). Solution 1 mg/ml in 1 and 2 ml containers.

Oral: For maintenance therapy, 5 mg is given 30 minutes before discontinuing intravenous infusion; subsequent doses are given every four hours (maximum, 30 mg daily).

   Brethine (Geigy), *Bricanyl* (Lakeside). Tablets 2.5 and 5 mg.

Cited References

Uterine Stimulants

Andrinopoulos GC, Mendenhall HW: Prostaglandin F$_{2\alpha}$ in management of delayed postpartum hemorrhage. *Am J Obstet Gynecol* 146:217-218, 1983.

Arias F: Efficacy and safety of low-dose 15-methyl prostaglandin F$_{2\alpha}$ for cervical ripening in first trimester of pregnancy. *Am J Obstet Gynecol* 149:100-101, 1984.

Bhatt RV, et al: Midtrimester abortion with prostaglandin and hypertonic saline: Comparative study. *Int J Gynaecol Obstet* 16:254-258, 1978.

Braly P, Freeman RK: Significance of fetal heart rate reactivity with positive oxytocin challenge test. *Obstet Gynecol* 50:689-693, 1977.

Braly P, et al: Incidence of premature delivery following oxytocin challenge test. *Am J Obstet Gynecol* 141:5-8, 1981.

Buchanan D, et al: Cervical ripening with prostaglandin E$_2$ vaginal suppositories. *Obstet Gynecol* 63:659-663, 1984.

Cates W Jr, Schulz KF: Oxytocin augmentation of second trimester abortion: Safe or hazardous? *Contraception* 22:513-525, 1980.

Cederqvist LL, Birnbaum SJ: Rupture of uterus after midtrimester prostaglandin abortion. *J Reprod Med* 25:136-138, 1980.

Claman P, et al: Uterine rupture with use of vaginal prostaglandin E$_2$ for induction of labor. *Am J Obstet Gynecol* 150:889-890, 1984.

Cross WC, Pitkin RM: Laminaria as adjunct in induction of labor. *Obstet Gynecol* 51:606-608, 1978.

Davey DA: Induction of labor. *Clin Obstet Gynecol* 7:481-509, 1980.

Ekman G, et al: Increased postpartum collagenolytic activity in cervical connective tissue from women treated with prostaglandin E$_2$. *Gynecol Obstet Invest* 16:292-298, 1983.

Evans MI, et al: Ripening of human cervix with porcine ovarian relaxin. *Am J Obstet Gynecol* 147:410-414, 1983.

Fenton DW, et al: Does cervical ripening with PGE$_2$ affect subsequent uterine activity in labour? *Acta Obstet Gynecol Scand* 64:27-30, 1985.

Fuchs A-R, et al: Oxytocin receptors and human parturition: Dual role for oxytocin in initiation of labor. *Science* 215:1396-1398, 1982.

Goeschen K, et al: Effect of β-mimetic tocolysis on cervical ripening and plasma prostaglandin F$_{2\alpha}$ metabolite after endocervical application of prostaglandin E$_2$. *Obstet Gynecol* 65:166-171, 1985.

Gordon AJ, Calder AA: Cervical ripening. *Br J Hosp Med* 30:52-58, 1983.

Gower RH, et al: Laminaria for preinduction cervical ripening. *Obstet Gynecol* 60:617-619, 1982.

Graves GR, et al: Effect of vaginal administration of various doses of prostaglandin E$_2$ gel on cervical ripening and induction of labor. *Am J Obstet Gynecol* 151:178-181, 1985.

Grimes DA, Cates W Jr: Comparative efficacy and safety of intra-amniotic prostaglandin F$_{2\alpha}$ and hypertonic saline for second-trimester abortion: Review and critique. *J Reprod Med* 22:248-254, 1979.

Grimes DA, et al: Midtrimester abortion by dilatation and evacuation versus intra-amniotic instillation of prostaglandin F$_{2\alpha}$: Randomized clinical trial. *Am J Obstet Gynecol* 137:785-790, 1980.

Hachamovitch M, et al: Saline-instillation abortion with laminaria and megadose oxytocin. *Am J Obstet Gynecol* 135:327-330, 1979.

Hayashi RH, et al: Management of severe postpartum hemorrhage with prostaglandin F$_{2\alpha}$ analogue. *Obstet Gynecol* 63:806-808, 1984.

Herbert WNP, Cefalo RC: Management of postpartum hemorrhage. *Clin Obstet Gynecol* 27:139-147, 1984.

Heyl PS, et al: Recurrent inversion of puerperal uterus managed with 15 (S)-15-methyl prostaglandin F$_{2\alpha}$ and uterine packing. *Obstet Gynecol* 63:263-264, 1984.

Horenstein JM, Phelan JP: Previous cesarean section: Risks and benefits of oxytocin usage in trial of labor. *Am J Obstet Gynecol* 151:564-569, 1985.

Horowitz AJ: Midtrimester abortion utilizing intra-amniotic prostaglandin F$_{2\alpha}$, laminaria, and oxytocin. *J Reprod Med* 21:236-240, 1978.

Hunter IWE, et al: Induction of labor using high-dose or low-dose prostaglandin vaginal pessaries. *Obstet Gynecol* 63:418-420, 1984.

Jagani N, et al: Role of prostaglandin-induced cervical changes in labor induction. *Obstet Gynecol* 63:225-229, 1984.

Johnson IR, et al: Comparison of Lamicel and prostaglandin E$_2$ vaginal gel for cervical ripening before induction of labor. *Am J Obstet Gynecol* 151:604-607, 1985.

Kazzi GM, et al: Efficacy and safety of laminaria digitata for preinduction ripening of cervix. *Obstet Gynecol* 60:440-443, 1982.

Kent DR, et al: Preoperative cervical dilation with single long-acting prostaglandin analog suppository: Alternative to traumatic mechanical dilatation before surgical evacuation. *J Reprod Med* 28:778-780, 1983.

King TM, et al: Intra-amniotic urea and prostaglandin F$_{2\alpha}$ for midtrimester abortion: Clinical and laboratory evaluation. *Am J Obstet Gynecol* 129:817-824, 1977.

Lange AP, et al: Prelabor evaluation of inducibility. *Obstet Gynecol* 60:137-147, 1982 A.

Lange AP, et al: Neonatal jaundice after labour induced or stimulated by prostaglandin E$_2$ or oxytocin. *Lancet* 1:991-994, 1982 B.

Lange IR, et al: Effect of vaginal prostaglandin E$_2$ pessaries on induction of labor. *Am J Obstet Gynecol* 148:621-625, 1984.

Lauersen NH: Investigation of prostaglandins for abortion. *Acta Obstet Gynaecol Scand* Suppl 81:1-36, 1979.

Lauersen NH, et al: Management of intrauterine fetal death with prostaglandin E$_2$ vaginal suppositories. *Am J Obstet Gynecol* 137:753-772, 1980.

Macer J, et al: Induction of labor with prostaglandin E$_2$ vaginal suppositories. *Obstet Gynecol* 63:664-668, 1984.

MacKenzie IZ, Embrey MP: Cervical ripening with intravaginal prostaglandin E$_2$ gel. *Br Med J* 2:1381-1384, 1977.

Magos AL, et al: Controlled study comparing vaginal prostaglandin E$_2$ pessaries with intravenous oxytocin for stimulation of labour after spontaneous rupture of membranes. *Br J Obstet Gynaecol* 90:726-731, 1983.

Nelson GH: Prostaglandins and reproduction, in Goldstein DP, et al (eds): *Current Problems in Obstetrics and Gynecology*. Chicago, Year Book Medical Publishers, 1980.

Neubardt S, Schulman H: *Techniques of Abortion*, ed 2. Boston, Little, Brown and Company, 1977.

Porreco RP, Watson JD: Induction of labor: 1983. *Hosp Drug Ther* 8:45-65, (April) 1983.

Robins J, Surrago EJ: Alternatives in midtrimester abortion induction. *Obstet Gynecol* 56:716-722, 1980.

Schulman H, et al: Mechanism of failed labor after fetal death and treatment with prostaglandin E$_2$. *Am J Obstet Gynecol* 133:742-752, 1979.

Seitchik J, et al: Oxytocin augmentation of dysfunctional labor: IV. Oxytocin pharmacokinetics. *Am J Obstet Gynecol* 150:225-228, 1984.

Sørensen SS, et al: Induction of labor and cervical ripening by intracervical prostaglandin E$_2$. *Obstet Gynecol* 65:110-114, 1985.

Surrago EJ, Robins J: Midtrimester pregnancy termination by intravaginal administration of prostaglandin E$_2$. *Contraception* 26:285-294, 1982.

Takagi et al: Effects of intramyometrial injection of prostaglandin F$_{2\alpha}$ on severe postpartum hemorrhage. *Prostaglandins* 12:565, 1976.

Ueland K, Conrad JT: Characteristics of oral prostaglandin E$_2$-induced labor. *Clin Obstet Gynecol* 26:87-94, 1983.

Uldbjerg N, et al: Ripening of human uterine cervix related to changes in collagen, glycosaminoglycans, and collagenolytic activity. *Am J Obstet Gynecol* 147:662-666, 1983.

Ulmsten U, et al: Local application of prostaglandin E$_2$ for cervical ripening or induction of term labor. *Clin Obstet Gynecol* 26:95-105, 1983.

Wallenburg HCS, et al: Intramuscular administration of 15(S)-15-methyl prostaglandin F$_{2\alpha}$ for induction of labour in patients with fetal death. *Br J Obstet Gynaecol* 87:203-209, 1980.

Wellman L, Jacobson A: Intra-amniotic prostaglandin F$_{2\alpha}$ and urea for midtrimester abortion. *Fertil Steril* 27:1374-1379, 1976.

Uterine Relaxants

Benedetti TJ: Maternal complications of parenteral β-sympathomimetic therapy for premature labor. *Am J Obstet Gynecol* 145:1-6, 1983.

Caritis SN: Treatment of preterm labor: Review of therapeutic options. *Drugs* 26:243-261, 1983.

Caritis SN, et al: Pharmacologic inhibition of preterm labor. *Am J Obstet Gynecol* 133:557-578, 1979.

Caritis SN, et al: Double-blind study comparing ritodrine and terbutaline in treatment of preterm labor. *Am J Obstet Gynecol* 150:7-14, 1984.

Carpenter RJ Jr: Preterm labor: Cause and management. *Compr Ther* 8:37-46, (June) 1982.

Curet LB, et al: Association between ruptured membranes, tocolytic therapy, and respiratory distress syndrome. *Am J Obstet Gynecol* 148:263-268, 1984.

Dudley DKL, Hardie MJ: Fetal and neonatal effects of indomethacin used as tocolytic agent. *Am J Obstet Gynecol* 151:181-184, 1985.

Feely J, et al: Beta-blockers and sympathomimetics. *Br Med J* 286:1043-1047, 1983.

Ferguson JE II, et al: Adjunctive use of magnesium sulfate with ritodrine for preterm labor tocolysis. *Am J Obstet Gynecol* 148:166-171, 1984.

Finkelstein BW: Ritodrine. *Drug Intell Clin Pharm* 15:425-433, 1981.

Gandar R, et al: Serum level of ritodrine in man. *Eur J Clin Pharmacol* 17:117-122, 1980.

Haller DL: Use of terbutaline for premature labor. *Drug Intell Clin Pharm* 14:757-764, 1980.

Huddleston JF: Preterm labor. *Clin Obstet Gynecol* 25:123-136, 1982.

Lauersen NH, et al: Inhibitory effect of ethanol on oxytocin-induced labor at term. *J Reprod Med* 26:547-550, 1981.

Philipsen T, et al: Pulmonary edema following ritodrine-saline infusion in premature labor. *Obstet Gynecol* 58:304-308, 1981.

Polowczyk D, et al: Evaluation of seven- to nine-year-old children exposed to ritodrine in utero. *Obstet Gynecol* 64:485-488, 1984.

Sholl JS, et al: Myotonic muscular dystrophy associated with ritodrine tocolysis. *Am J Obstet Gynecol* 151:83-86, 1985.

Stubblefield PG, Heyl PS: Treatment of premature labor with subcutaneous terbutaline. *Obstet Gynecol* 59:457-462, 1982.

Yemini M, et al: Prevention of premature labor by 17 α-hydroxyprogesterone caproate. *Am J Obstet Gynecol* 151:574-577, 1985.

Other Selected References

Petrie RH: Pharmacology and use of oxytocin. *Clin Perinatol* 8:35-47, 1981.

Population Information Program: Use of prostaglandins in human reproduction. *Popul Rep [G]* 8:77-118, (March) 1980.

Tepperman HM, et al: Drugs affecting myometrial contractility in pregnancy. *Clin Obstet Gynecol* 20:423-445, 1977.

Replenishers and Regulators of Water and Electrolytes

MAINTAINING HYDRATION

ABNORMAL STATES OF HYDRATION

ACID-BASE DISTURBANCES

POTASSIUM IMBALANCES

MAGNESIUM IMBALANCES

DRUG EVALUATIONS

Agents Used in Abnormal States of Hydration

Agents Used in Acid-Base Disturbances

Agents Used in Potassium Imbalances

Agents Used in Hypomagnesemia

The rational prescription of fluids and electrolytes requires understanding of the physiology and pathophysiology of fluid and electrolyte balance and the requirements of the patient. In this chapter, the preparations used in fluid and electrolyte therapy are discussed in broad groups according to major indications, and the discussion is limited to general information on therapy for larger children and adults. For more detailed information, the following references are suggested: Maxwell and Kleeman, 1980; Levinsky, 1980; Mudge, 1980; Schrier, 1980; and Andreoli, 1985. More specialized references (eg, Finberg et al, 1982) should be consulted for information on therapy in infants and smaller children, who are much more vulnerable than adults to fluid and electrolyte imbalances.

When drugs are added to parenteral solutions, the possibility of physical, chemical, and pharmacologic incompatibilities should be considered (Trissel, 1983). Some are well known, but subtle incompatibilities also may occur, for example, the inactivation of buffered penicillin G by parenteral solutions containing vitamin B complex with ascorbic acid. No more than one drug should be added to a single intravenous solution unless it is known that each additional drug is compatible.

Because of fluid restrictions or lack of additional intravenous sites, occasionally it is necessary to admix drugs for which no compatibility data are available. Decisions should then be based on the drugs' physiochemical properties. Close monitoring of the intravenous solutions and tubings for evidence of gross incompatibilities (eg, visible crystallization, color change) is recommended.

Maintaining Hydration

Patients (especially those requiring hospitalization) often have conditions that preclude the oral intake of food or fluids. To maintain homeostasis, they must receive sufficient parenteral fluids and electrolytes to match their daily output from urine, feces, and insensible losses. An unstressed adult in a comfortable climate requires approximately 25 to 40 ml/kg/day of fluid to maintain a urine output within the physiologic range. Electrolyte needs generally can be met for short periods by giving sodium 70 to 140 mEq/day and potassium 40 to 80 mEq/day slowly over 24 hours.

Various regimens have been recommended to maintain fluid and electrolyte balance in unstressed patients. These include (1) 1,000 ml of dextrose 10% with potassium chloride 20 mEq over 12 hours, followed by 1,000 ml of dextrose 5% and sodium chloride 0.45% with potassium chloride 20 mEq over the next 12 hours (Freitag and Miller, 1980); (2) 1,000 ml of dextrose 5% in Ringer's lactate or sodium chloride 0.9% with potassium chloride or potassium acetate 20 to 40 mEq, followed by 1,500 to 2,000 ml of dextrose 5% with potassium chloride or potassium acetate 30 to 60 mEq over 24 hours (Kopple and Blumenkrantz, 1980); and (3) 1,000 ml of dextrose 5% with potassium chloride 40 mEq over 12 hours, followed by 1,000 ml of sodium chloride 0.9% with potassium chloride 40 mEq over the next 12 hours (Lawson and Henry, 1977). These regimens probably are equally effective to maintain fluid and electrolyte balance for most unstressed patients, because normally functioning kidneys are able to modify the internal milieu within the desired limits.

Abnormal States of Hydration

Because of the dynamic interrelationship between solute and fluid volume control, sodium and water depletion must be considered together. Abnormal states of hydration may be characterized by (1) loss of sodium and water in isotonic proportions, (2) loss of water in excess of sodium, (3) loss of sodium in excess of water, and (4) volume excess.

Isotonic loss of sodium and water (extracellular volume depletion) may be caused by gastroenteric losses (vomiting, diarrhea, nasogastric suctioning) or renal losses (diuretics, kidney disease, adrenal disorders). Sodium chloride injection 0.9% may be used to restore the extracellular fluid volume. Actual fluid losses and changes in weight should be measured. The volume should be replaced gradually to avoid pulmonary edema and volume overload. Serum electrolytes should be monitored and the exact composition of the infusion modified as indicated.

Although "balanced" isotonic electrolyte solutions are available, usually it is preferable to tailor the composition of the infusion to the needs of the patient. Dextrose 5% injection should not be used alone, because it is metabolized rapidly to carbon dioxide and water and its infusion is physiologically equivalent to that of free water. Whole blood is the only complete replacement therapy when intravascular volume depletion is caused by hemorrhage (see Chapter 35, Blood, Blood Components, and Blood Substitutes). For the treatment of hypovolemic shock, see Chapter 27, Agents Used to Treat Shock.

Loss of water in excess of sodium, which causes hypernatremia, may result primarily from inadequate water intake (seen in patients with central nervous system disease who cannot report thirst sensations or in infants given excessively concentrated foods) and also from hyperhidrosis, extensive skin damage caused by burns, and osmotic diuresis (hyperglycemia, high protein tube feeding) with concomitant deficiency of water intake.

Initially, it may be important to correct hypertonicity by providing fluid without electrolytes or with reduced levels of electrolytes; water should be given orally or dextrose 5% intravenously for this purpose. Fluid should be administered over several hours until about one-half of the calculated deficit is replaced; the remaining one-half should be given over the next 24 to 48 hours (Feig, 1981). Frequently, a substantial salt deficit is present as well and requires early treatment with sodium chloride injection 0.9% or 0.45%. Electrolyte levels should be monitored closely.

Hypertonic dehydration pulls water from within the cells to the extracellular fluid compartment, resulting in intracellular dehydration. However, the brain produces new intracellular solutes (idiogenic osmoles) that prevent it from seriously dehydrating, which is potentially fatal. The rate at which idiogenic osmoles can be removed or inactivated after hypertonicity has been corrected is unknown. Therefore, when administering fluids to treat loss of water in excess of sodium, it is important to monitor the patient for evidence of deteriorating sensorium or appearance of neurologic signs, for such signs may result from brain cell overhydration and cerebral edema when fluids are infused too rapidly.

For the treatment of diabetes insipidus, see Chapter 30, Agents Affecting Water Homeostasis.

Loss of sodium in excess of water, which causes hyponatremia, may occur when the kidneys are unable to conserve sodium appropriately (diuretic therapy, salt-wasting nephropathies, adrenocortical insufficiency), when there is excessive water retention (syndrome of inappropriate secretion of antidiuretic hormone [SIADH]), or when isotonic or hypotonic losses (eg, gastrointestinal losses, excessive sweating) are replaced by water without sufficient salt.

When the serum sodium concentration is moderately reduced and there is clinical evidence of reduced extracellular fluid volume, administration of sodium chloride 0.9% is the treatment of choice and often is all that is required to expand the extracellular fluid volume and normalize the serum concentration of sodium. In severe hypo-osmolal hyponatremia (ie, symptoms of central nervous system dysfunction, such as confusion, stupor, or convulsions, are present and appear to be due to hyponatremia), sodium chloride injection 3% may be administered cautiously for as long as 24 hours until a serum sodium concentration of 125 to 130 mEq/L is achieved (Ayus et al, 1982). Full correction should not be attempted rapidly (Schwartz, 1979; Goldberg, 1981). One liter of sodium chloride injection 3% contains 513 mEq of sodium; thus, the number of liters to be infused over 24 hours can be approximated by dividing the total amount of sodium needed by 500. A formula to calculate the amount of sodium required is:

$$\text{Sodium (mEq)} = [130 \text{ mEq/L} - \text{the observed serum sodium concentration (mEq/L)}] \times 0.5 \text{ body weight (kg)}$$

The fluid status should be monitored by checking for the appearance of peripheral edema, pulmonary congestion, and distended neck veins and the degree of skin turgor. Patients susceptible to volume overload should be given a bolus of furosemide [Lasix] to initiate diuresis prior to administration of sodium chloride. Each milliliter of urine should be replaced by 1 ml of hypertonic sodium chloride.

Hyponatremia caused by adrenocortical insufficiency also should be treated with hormone replacement therapy and sodium chloride 0.9% to support the extracellular and intracellular compartments (see Chapter 37, Agents Used to Treat Adrenal Dysfunction). Hyponatremia associated with inappropriate secretion of antidiuretic hormone (SIADH) is caused primarily by water retention, and restriction of water intake usually corrects the imbalance. Drugs used to treat SIADH are discussed in Chapter 30, Agents Affecting Water Homeostasis.

Volume excess (edema) is observed in patients with congestive heart failure, nephrotic syndrome, or cirrhosis with ascites. Drugs used to treat edema are discussed in Chapter 23, Agents Used to Treat Heart Failure, and Chapter 29, Diuretics. Restriction of dietary sodium is important in the management of this imbalance. Water restriction is necessary only when hyponatremia occurs.

Acid-Base Disturbances

Acute Metabolic Acidosis: Metabolic acidosis may be caused by excessive production of lactic acid (lactic acidosis) or ketoacids (ketoacidosis), chronic renal failure, a defect in the ability of the kidney to acidify the urine (renal tubular acidosis), diarrhea, or ingestion of certain drugs or toxins (eg, salicylates, ethylene glycol, methanol, paraldehyde). Treatment of the underlying disease usually corrects the acid-base and fluid derangements. If the plasma bicarbonate level falls below 10 to 12 mEq/L or the blood pH below 7.15, an alkalizing agent, preferably intravenous sodium bicarbonate, usually may be given, but therapy must be individualized. The amount of bicarbonate required may be calculated as follows:

Bicarbonate (mEq) = (15 mEq - observed plasma bicarbonate [mEq/L]) x 0.5 x body weight (kg)

If the arterial pH is less than 7.1, 0.8 rather than 0.5 should be used in this equation (Kaehny and Gabow, 1980). This formula does not take into account ongoing acid production.

Potassium concentrations should be monitored during short-term alkali administration. Elevating the plasma pH drives extracellular potassium into the cells and can result in severe symptomatic hypokalemia.

Chronic Metabolic Acidosis: Patients with chronic renal failure or renal tubular acidosis usually have chronic metabolic acidosis. Mild to moderate acidosis does not require treatment. When the plasma bicarbonate concentration drops below 15 to 20 mEq/L, oral alkali therapy with sodium bicarbonate or sodium citrate should be initiated. The goal is to maintain the plasma bicarbonate concentration at about 20 mEq/L (Quintanilla and Qureshi, 1981). Most patients tolerate oral bicarbonate well but they must be monitored for evidence of sodium overload, hypertension, and tetany. Those with symptoms of gastric irritation often can be treated with Shohl's solution.

Metabolic Alkalosis: Metabolic alkalosis is associated with numerous diseases and is characterized by primary elevations of the plasma pH and bicarbonate concentration. This condition can be separated into sodium chloride-responsive and sodium chloride-resistant types. Sodium chloride-responsive metabolic alkalosis is caused by excessive loss of hydrogen ion (eg, in patients with intractable vomiting or gastric suctioning), overaggressive treatment with certain diuretics (eg, ethacrynic acid [Edecrin], furosemide [Lasix]), abrupt relief of chronic hypercapnia, or excessive fecal loss of chloride ion (eg, congenital chloridorrhea, villous adenoma of the colon). Treatment of sodium chloride-responsive metabolic alkalosis should be aimed at reversing the underlying condition.

Infusing sodium chloride injection 0.9% and potassium chloride allows the kidneys to excrete bicarbonate and retain sodium, potassium, and chloride, thus normalizing the systemic pH. Patients who cannot tolerate volume expansion (eg, those with congestive heart failure) may benefit from a trial of a carbonic anhydrase inhibitor, such as acetazolamide [Diamox]. Cimetidine [Tagamet] or ranitidine [Zantac] may be useful in patients with Zollinger-Ellison syndrome or in those undergoing nasogastric suction (Kaehny and Gabow, 1980). Rarely, acid may be administered as dilute hydrochloric acid, ammonium chloride, or arginine or lysine (currently preferred) hydrochloride. The latter forms of therapy should be used cautiously and only when alkalosis is severe (serum bicarbonate over 40 mEq/L, pH 7.6 or greater) and the patient is refractory to more conventional therapy. A large volume of hydrochloric acid must be infused into a large bore vein, and dextrose or sodium chloride should be administered concomitantly. Ammonium chloride is absolutely contraindicated in patients with severe parenchymal liver disease because it can precipitate hepatic encephalopathy. L-arginine hydrochloride can cause life-threatening hyperkalemia.

Potassium Imbalances

Hypokalemia: Hypokalemia is defined as a serum potassium concentration less than or equal to 3.5 mEq/L. It can be caused by a shift of potassium from the extracellular to the intracellular fluid (eg, in metabolic alkalosis, as a result of insulin therapy or beta-adrenergic stimulation), decreased intake (eg, anorexia nervosa), increased gastrointestinal losses (eg, diarrhea, vomiting, laxative abuse, villous adenoma), and increased renal losses (eg, increased mineralocorticoid activity; renal tubular acidosis; delivery of large nonabsorbable anions, such as carbenicillin, and sodium to the distal nephron; hypomagnesemia). Thiazide and loop diuretics are the most common causes of hypokalemia. They act by increasing delivery of sodium to the distal nephron where sodium is actively exchanged for potassium, thereby increasing the amount of potassium excreted in the urine.

The form of therapy used to treat hypokalemia depends on the severity of the condition and its underlying cause. Pharmacologic therapy may not be needed when the decrease in serum potassium is due to a shift from extracellular to intracellular fluid or when the deficiency is mild. See Table 1 for guidelines on prescribing potassium supplements. Most patients receiving diuretics maintain a serum potassium concentration above 3.5 mEq/L. Unless they are receiving digitalis glycosides, have an abnormal electrocardiogram, or are otherwise at risk from hypokalemia and therefore require pharmacologic potassium therapy, these patients generally require only an increase in dietary potassium intake (Bear and Neil, 1983).

When the potassium concentration drops below 3.5 mEq/L, potassium supplements or potassium-sparing diuretics may be prescribed. However, potassium supplements should not be taken in conjunction with potassium-sparing diuretics, except in rare circumstances, because of the risk of hyperkalemia. Potassium-sparing diuretics are more effective and may be preferred in high-risk patients (see Chapter 29, Diuretics).

Oral replacement therapy is indicated whenever feasible to avoid sudden large increases in serum potassium. Potassium chloride solution is preferred to other salts because, if there is an associated metabolic alkalosis, this salt may correct both the hypokalemia and the metabolic alkalosis. There is little evidence that other salts are tolerated better than potassium chloride. Other salts are used in rare instances in which hypokalemia is associated with acidosis (eg, renal tubular acidosis). Since potassium supplements are not retained well in patients receiving diuretics (Down et al, 1972), large doses may be required (Schwartz and Swartz, 1974). Patients with hypomagnesemia and hypokalemia may require magnesium therapy in conjunction with potassium supplementation to correct the potassium imbalance.

If correction is indicated in patients unable to take potassium orally, potassium chloride is given intravenously. The electrocardiogram should be monitored frequently, because the dangerous effects of hyperkalemia can be detected more rapidly by changes in the electrocardiogram than by measuring serum potassium levels; however, the electrocardiogram is *not* a substitute for the determination of serum potassium. An adequate urinary output also must be assured.

Hyperkalemia: Hyperkalemia is usually the result of impaired potassium excretion in patients with decreased renal function or impaired secretion of mineralocorticoids (Addison's disease, hypoaldosteronism) and is particularly prevalent in those taking large amounts of potassium with potassium-sparing diuretics. It also may be caused by the rapid intravenous administration of potassium-containing solutions or by shift of potassium out of the cells (eg, acidosis, tissue breakdown, familial periodic paralysis). (See Whang, 1976, or Alvo and Warnock, 1984, for other causes.)

The measures used for treatment depend upon the degree of hyperkalemia and the severity of its manifestations. In all cases, potassium intake should be discontinued. When the electrocardiogram is distinctly abnormal (eg, absence of P-wave, widening of QRS complex, S-T segment changes with high peaked T waves) or the serum potassium rises rapidly to more than 6.5 mEq/L, the intravenous infusion of dextrose injection 5% or 10% to which one to three ampuls (44 mEq/ampul) of sodium bicarbonate have been added is indicated. Ten to fifteen units of regular insulin also may be added to each liter of dextrose injection 5%. Sodium bicarbonate and insulin reduce the serum potassium level by causing potassium to shift into cells. In patients with hyponatremia and volume contraction, 5% dextrose in 0.9% sodium chloride may be preferred for replacement therapy because it also counteracts the cardiotoxic effect of potassium. A hypertonic sodium chloride solution may be indicated in patients with severe hyponatremia.

If cardiotoxicity is extreme and the patient is not receiving digitalis, 10 to 30 ml of calcium gluconate 10% may be injected intravenously over a three- to five-minute period; this dose may be repeated once. The electrocardiogram should be monitored constantly.

An exchange resin (eg, sodium polystyrene sulfonate [Kayexalate]) may be given orally or rectally to promote the gastrointestinal elimination of potassium. Oral therapy is effective only after many hours, but an enema containing 30 to 50 g of the resin suspended in 150 ml of 20% to 70% sorbitol will reduce serum potassium in about one hour. In oliguric patients, hemodialysis or peritoneal dialysis may be indicated to remove large amounts of potassium from the blood, but this treatment is too slow for emergency management.

Magnesium Imbalances

Hypomagnesemia: Hypomagnesemia may accompany malabsorption, prolonged diarrhea, prolonged intravenous feeding without magnesium, chronic alcoholism, diuretic therapy, renal tubular damage, and other disorders often associated with hypocalcemia or hypokalemia. It occurs in approximately 20% of patients receiving digitalis therapy (Whang et al, 1985). Oral administration of magnesium gluconate, magnesium hydroxide, or milk of magnesia may be used for supplementation. Magnesium sulfate may be given intramuscularly for treatment of hypomagnesemia. Alternatively, it may be given intravenously in low concentrations alone or as a constituent of multiple electrolyte solutions to prevent iatrogenic deficiency during routine fluid and electrolyte therapy. Magnesium sulfate should be administered cautiously if renal function is impaired.

Hypermagnesemia: Most patients can tolerate moderately elevated plasma levels of magnesium, but toxicity may occur with prolonged administration of magnesium (eg, in antacid preparations or cathartics) in patients with severe renal impairment. In such patients, hypermagnesemia may result in nausea, vomiting, refractory hypotension, and muscle weakness. Occasionally, third-degree atrioventricular block and respiratory arrest occur. The intravenous administration of 5 to 10 mEq of calcium salts counteracts the depression of the respiratory muscles. As in the treatment of hyperkalemia, dextrose and insulin also may be infused to cause an influx of magnesium into the cells (Parfitt and Kleerekoper, 1980). Dialysis is indicated in severe hypermagnesemia with coexistent renal insufficiency and/or refractory hypotension.

Drug Evaluations

AGENTS USED IN ABNORMAL STATES OF HYDRATION

Sodium chloride injection or dextrose injection may be used to treat most abnormal states of hydration. Other solutions have been developed for balanced maintenance or replacement of fluid and electrolytes. In addition to sodium and chloride, these solutions provide potassium, magnesium, and bicarbonate precursors, such as acetate. In general, it is preferable to individualize therapy. A partial list of the available formulations appears in Tables 2, 3, and 4.

SODIUM CHLORIDE

SODIUM CHLORIDE INJECTION

USES. Sodium chloride is used to correct extracellular volume depletion. It should be administered orally as table salt for replacement therapy whenever possible. A solution containing 3 to 4 g of sodium chloride (1 g of sodium chloride contains

TABLE 1.
SUGGESTED GUIDELINES FOR POTASSIUM SUPPLEMENTATION IN SOME COMMON CLINICAL SITUATIONS THAT MAY PRODUCE IMBALANCE

Prophylactic Potassium Therapy Indicated	Potassium Therapy Indicated Only When Serum Level <3.5 mEq/L
Patient receiving the following drugs	Patient receiving the following drugs
—Intravenous alkali —Thiazide or loop diuretic in addition to digitalis glycosides —Thiazide or loop diuretic in patient with hepatic cirrhosis —Insulin during rehydration for diabetic ketoacidosis —Prolonged high-dose carbenicillin, ticarcillin, or penicillin G sodium	—Thiazide or loop diuretic for essential hypertension —Thiazide or loop diuretic for cardiac failure NOT treated with digitalis glycosides
	Chronic Laxative Abuser
Acute Myeloid Leukemia	Acute or Chronic Vomiting or Diarrhea
	Elderly Patient
Severe Pseudomembranous Colitis	Patient with Poor Nutrition

Regular monitoring of serum/plasma potassium concentration is necessary for all patients in both groups.
Adapted from Lawson, 1981.

17.1 mEq of sodium) and 1.5 to 3 g of sodium bicarbonate/L (1 g of sodium bicarbonate contains 11.9 mEq of sodium) also is satisfactory for oral use if solid foods cannot be ingested.

Isotonic sodium chloride injection is a 0.9% solution containing 154 mEq of sodium and chloride/L. (In comparison, plasma contains 137 to 147 mEq of sodium and 98 to 106 mEq of chloride/L.) Concentrations of 0.11% to 0.45% are hypotonic and concentrations of 3% and 5% are hypertonic. The concentration and tonicity of sodium chloride solutions determine their usefulness in different disorders.

Sodium chloride injection 0.9% is infused when sodium and water have been depleted in isotonic proportions. It may be used to maintain effective extracellular fluid volume and a stable circulation during and after surgery in patients with normal cardiovascular and renal function and to maintain plasma volume, thus temporarily postponing the need for blood transfusions in emergencies. Hypertonic sodium chloride injection should be reserved for the treatment of severe symptomatic hyponatremia (serum sodium less than 120 mEq/ml) and should be used only during the critical phase. Hypotonic solutions (usually 0.45% containing 77 mEq sodium and chloride/L) generally are given with dextrose for maintenance therapy in patients who are unable to take fluid and nutrients orally for one to three days and are administered without dextrose in the management of hyperosmolar diabetes mellitus.

PRECAUTIONS. Sodium chloride must be infused with great caution, particularly in patients with congestive heart failure, renal failure, or hypoproteinemia. Signs and symptoms of excessive therapy are peripheral edema and pulmonary congestion (rales, edema). Hypertonic solutions should be given slowly and cautiously in small volumes (200 to 400 ml) because of the danger of volume excess, pulmonary edema,

and hyperosmolarity. Hyperosmolarity may cause confusion, stupor, or coma.

PREPARATIONS.
Generic. Solution 0.45%, 0.9%, 3%, and 5%.

BALANCED ELECTROLYTE INJECTION

RINGER'S LACTATE

USES. The indications for these hypotonic and isotonic electrolyte formulations are similar to those for sodium chloride injection 0.45% and 0.9%. Although these solutions more closely approximate normal extracellular electrolyte concentrations, additional electrolytes may be necessary to meet the specific needs of the patient (eg, to correct acidosis, alkalosis, or deficits of individual electrolytes). In general, specific formulations of intravenous fluids are preferred to these premixed formulations. These solutions are not indicated to replace blood or plasma volume expanders when the latter are indicated, except for the temporary maintenance of plasma volume in emergencies.

PREPARATIONS. See Tables 2, 3, and 4.

DEXTROSE INJECTION

DEXTROSE AND SODIUM CHLORIDE INJECTION

USES. Dextrose is administered intravenously to provide nutrient and water when oral feeding is not feasible. It usually

TABLE 2.
MULTIPLE ELECTROLYTE INTRAVENOUS SOLUTIONS

Tradename (Manufacturer)	mOsm/L	Na$^+$	K$^+$	Ca^{++}	Mg^{++}	Cl$^-$	HCO$_3^-$ Precursor	Volume Available (ml)
Plasma-Lyte 56 (Travenol)	110	40	13	—	3	40	Acet 16	1,000
Ringer's Injection (Various)	309	147	4	4	—	155	—	250, 500, & 1,000
Normosol-R, Normosol-R pH 7.4 (Abbott)	295	140	5	—	3	98	Acet 27 Glu 23	500 & 1,000
Isolyte S, Isolyte S pH 7.4 (American McGaw)	295	140	5	—	3	98	Acet 28 Glu 23	500 & 1,000
Isolyte E (American McGaw)	315	140	10	5	3	103	Acet 49 Cit 8	1,000
Plasma-Lyte 148, Plasma-Lyte A pH 7.4 (Travenol)	294	140	5	—	3	98	Acet 27 Glu 23	500 & 1,000
Plasma-Lyte R (Travenol)	312	140	10	5	3	103	Acet 47 Lac 8	1,000
Ringer's Lactate (Various)	273	130	4	3	—	109	Lac 28	250, 500, & 1,000
Ringer's Acetate (Various)	275	131	4	3	—	109	Acet 28	1,000

is administered as a 5% aqueous infusion, which is approximately isotonic compared to blood (277 mOsm/L) and provides about 170 calories/L. Dextrose injection 5% or sodium chloride injection 0.11% to 0.45% with dextrose 5% in water may be used intravenously when there is loss of water in excess of sodium. Solutions containing 10% dextrose provide more nutrient in less volume, but this concentration may be irritating to the veins and, in newborns, may cause hyperglycemia. The immediate intravenous administration of 50 ml (25 g) of 50% dextrose solution is recommended for comatose patients when the cause of depression is unknown *without waiting for the blood glucose determination* in order to prevent brain damage from hypoglycemia. A solution containing 20% to 50% dextrose (often with insulin added) is used to promote the shift of potassium into cells. Hypertonic dextrose is infused in a high-flow vein to provide calories in total parenteral nutrition (TPN). (See Chapter 48, Parenteral and Enteral Nutrition.)

The rate of utilization of dextrose varies considerably. As an approximate guide, however, the average maximal rate is 500 mg/kg/hr (10 ml/kg/hr of dextrose injection 5%) over periods of less than 24 hours. If the patient's capacity to utilize dextrose is exceeded, hyperglycemia, glycosuria, and excessive diuresis will occur.

ADVERSE REACTIONS AND PRECAUTIONS. Dextrose solutions are acidic (pH 3.5 to 5.0) and may produce thrombophlebitis. Subcutaneous administration is very irritating, may distend tissue, and may lead to necrosis. Therefore, this route is never employed. Dextrose injection should not be used as a diluent for blood because it causes clumping of red blood cells and, possibly, hemolysis.

PREPARATIONS.

DEXTROSE INJECTION:
Generic. Solution 2.5%, 5%, 10%, 20%, 25%, 30%, 38%, 40%, 50%, 60%, and 70%; 5% with alcohol 5% or 10%.

DEXTROSE AND SODIUM CHLORIDE INJECTION:
Generic. Solution containing dextrose 2.5% with sodium chloride 0.45%; dextrose 5% with sodium chloride 0.11%, 0.2%, 0.225%, 0.3%, 0.33%, 0.45%, 0.9%; dextrose 10% with sodium chloride 0.45%, 0.9%.

FRUCTOSE INJECTION

FRUCTOSE AND SODIUM CHLORIDE INJECTION

INVERT SUGAR INJECTION (containing equal parts of dextrose and fructose)

Fructose offers no advantages over dextrose injection and possesses some disadvantages. It may increase serum levels of lactate and urate if given rapidly, and it is considerably more expensive than dextrose. Infusion of fructose has been associated with increased production of uric acid and hyperuricemia. In patients with hereditary fructose intolerance (aldolase deficiency), fructose can cause severe reactions (hypoglycemia, nausea, vomiting, tremors, coma, convulsions) and is contraindicated.

TABLE 3.
CONCENTRATED MULTIPLE ELECTROLYTE INTRAVENOUS SOLUTIONS*

Tradename (Manufacturer)	mOsm/L†	mEq/Single Vial							Volume Available (ml)
		Na+	K+	Ca++	Mg++	Cl−	HPO₃⁻ Precursor	HPO₄⁼	
Hyperlyte (American McGaw)	6050	25	40.5	5	8	33.5	Glu 5 Acet 40.6	10	25 ml in 50 ml vial
Hyperlyte CR (American McGaw)	5500	25	20	5	5	30	Acet 30	—	150 & 250 ml vial
Hyperlyte R (American McGaw)	4200	25	20	5	5	30	Acet 25	—	25 ml in 50 ml vial
Lypholyte (LyphoMed)	7562	25	40.5	5	8	33.5	Glu 5 Acet 40.6	—	20 ml vial

*Must be diluted before administration. NOT for direct intravenous administration.
†Osmolality of concentrated solution

AGENTS USED IN ACID-BASE DISTURBANCES

SODIUM BICARBONATE

USES. Sodium bicarbonate is the drug of choice in the treatment of metabolic acidosis secondary to actual loss of bicarbonate from the body. However, its efficacy in hypoxic lactic acidosis secondary to increased generation of organic acids is unsettled and further laboratory and clinical study is necessary (Graf et al, 1985; Hale et al, 1984; Lever and Jaspan, 1983).

In acute mild to moderate acidosis, oral treatment is preferable to intravenous therapy; tablets (325 mg, 650 mg, and 1 g), oral solutions (2% to 5%), or a solution containing sodium bicarbonate 0.15% to 0.3% and sodium chloride 0.3% to 0.4% may be used. In severe acute acidosis, sodium bicarbonate may be given intravenously. Commercial solutions are generally hypertonic (4.2%, 7.5%, and 8.4%) and require dilution. The 7.5% solution, commonly employed in cardiac resuscitation, contains 44.6 mEq/50 ml (892 mEq/L).

ADVERSE REACTIONS AND PRECAUTIONS. Excessive amounts of sodium bicarbonate may cause metabolic alkalosis and hypernatremia. Rapid alkalization may precipitate tetany in hypocalcemic patients and cause cardiotoxicity and paralysis in hypokalemic patients. In addition, too rapid administration produces a transient elevation of PCO_2, and CO_2 diffuses into the cells and cerebrospinal fluid more rapidly than bicarbonate, resulting in intracellular and central nervous system acidosis. Sodium bicarbonate should be given cautiously to patients with congestive heart failure or other edematous or sodium-retaining conditions, oliguria, or anuria.

PREPARATIONS.
ORAL:
Generic. Tablets 325 and 650 mg (11.9 mEq/g).

INTRAVENOUS:
Generic. Solution 4%, 4.2%, 5%, 7.5%, and 8.4%.

SODIUM CITRATE AND CITRIC ACID SOLUTION (Shohl's Solution)
[Bicitra]

Shohl's solution contains sodium citrate and citric acid equivalent to 1 mEq sodium and bicarbonate/ml. After absorption, the citrate is metabolized to bicarbonate. This systemic alkalizer is used most frequently in renal tubular acidosis, but it may be employed in chronic metabolic acidosis of other etiologies. It must be used with care in the presence of renal insufficiency or conditions requiring sodium restriction.

This preparation may be preferred by patients because it does not cause belching. It may, however, cause diarrhea and large doses may produce nausea and vomiting.

DOSAGE AND PREPARATIONS.
Oral: Adults, for renal tubular acidosis, 0.5 to 2 mEq/kg in four or five divided doses daily. The total dose should be increased until acidosis and hypercalciuria are eliminated. Serum chloride and carbon dioxide content and urinary calcium excretion should be determined approximately twice yearly. The dosage requirement may be increased during intercurrent illness.
Bicitra (Willen). Solution containing sodium citrate dihydrate 500 mg and citric acid monohydrate 334 mg/5 ml in 120, 473, and 3,792 ml containers.

SODIUM LACTATE

Sodium lactate is metabolized to sodium bicarbonate in the liver and has been used to treat metabolic acidosis. Sodium bicarbonate is preferred for this purpose, however, because

TABLE 4.
DEXTROSE AND MULTIPLE ELECTROLYTE INTRAVENOUS SOLUTIONS

Tradename (Manufacturer)	Calories/L	mOsm/L	Na$^+$	K$^+$	Ca^{++}	Mg^{++}	Cl$^-$	HPO$_4$$^=$	HCO$_3^-$ Precursor	NH$_4^+$	Volume Supplied
Ringer's Acetate Dextrose 5% (American McGaw)	170	535	131	4	3	—	122	—	Acet 28	—	1,000 ml
Ringer's Lactate ½ Str. Dextrose 2.5% (Various)	85	265	65	2	1	—	55	—	Lact 14	—	250, 500, & 1,000 ml
Ringer's Lactate Dextrose 5% (Various)	170	525	130	4	3	—	111	—	Lact 28	—	250, 500, & 1,000 ml
Ringer's Lactate Dextrose 10% (American McGaw)	340	775	130	4	3	—	111	—	Lact 28	—	1,000 ml
Ringer's ½ Str. Dextrose 2.5% (Various)	85	280	74	2	2	—	78	—	—	—	500 ml
Ringer's Dextrose 5% (Various)	170	560	147	4	4	—	155	—	—	—	500 & 1,000 ml
Electrolyte No. 48 Dextrose 5% (Travenol)	170	347	25	20	—	3	24	3	Lact 23	—	250, 500, & 1,000 ml
Ionosol MB Dextrose 5% (Abbott)	170	350	25	20	—	3	22	3	Lact 23	—	250, 500, & 1,000 ml
Electrolyte No. 75 Dextrose 5% (Travenol)	170	402	40	35	—	—	48	15	Lact 20	—	250, 500, & 1,000 ml
Ionosol T Dextrose 5% (Abbott)	170	406	40	35	—	—	40	15	Lact 20	—	250, 500, & 1,000 ml
Ionosol B Dextrose 5% (Abbott)	170	423	57	25	—	5	49	13	Lact 25	—	500 & 1,000 ml
Ionosol G Dextrose 10% (Abbott)	340	812	63	17	—	—	151	—	—	71	1,000 ml
Ionosol D-CM Dextrose 5% (Abbott)	170	573	138	12	5	3	108	—	Lact 50	—	
Isolyte E Dextrose 5% (American McGaw)	180	565	140	10	5	3	103	Cit 8	Acet 47	—	1,000 ml
Isolyte G Dextrose 5% (American McGaw)	170	555	65	17	—	—	150	—	—	70	1,000 ml
Isolyte G Dextrose 10% (American McGaw)	340	805	65	17	—	—	150	—	—	70	1,000 ml
Isolyte H Dextrose 5% (American McGaw)	170	370	40	13	—	3	40	—	Acet 16	—	1,000 ml
Normosol M Dextrose 5% (Abbott)	170	368	40	13	—	3	40	—	Acet 16	—	500 & 1,000 ml
Plasma-Lyte 56 Dextrose 5% (Travenol)	170	362	40	13	—	3	40	—	Acet 16	—	500 & 1,000 ml

(Continued on next page)

TABLE 4.
DEXTROSE AND MULTIPLE ELECTROLYTE INTRAVENOUS SOLUTIONS (continued)

Tradename (Manufacturer)	Calories/L	mOsm/L	Na^+	K^+	Ca^{++}	Mg^{++}	Cl^-	$HPO_4^=$	HCO_3^- Precursor	NH_4^+	Volume Supplied
Isolyte M Dextrose 5% (American McGaw)	175	405	38	35	—	—	40	15	Acet 20	—	250, 500, & 1,000 ml
Isolyte P Dextrose 5% (American McGaw)	175	350	25	19	—	3	23	3	Acet 23	—	250, 500, & 1,000 ml
Isolyte R Dextrose 5% (American McGaw)	170	380	40	16	5	3	40	—	Acet 24	—	1,000 ml
Isolyte S Dextrose 5% (American McGaw)	185	550	140	5	—	3	98	—	Glu 23 Acet 27	—	1,000 ml
Normosol-R Dextrose 5% (Abbott)	185	552	140	5	—	3	98	—	Glu 23 Acet 27	—	500 & 1,000 ml
Plasma-Lyte 148 Dextrose 5% (Travenol)	185	547	140	5	—	3	98	—	Glu 23 Acet 27	—	500 & 1,000 ml
Plasma-Lyte R Dextrose 5% (Travenol)	170	564	140	10	5	3	103	—	Lact 8 Acet 47	—	1,000 ml
Plasma-Lyte M Dextrose 5% (Travenol)	170	376	40	16	5	3	40	—	Lact 12 Acet 12	—	500 & 1,000 ml

the conversion of lactate to bicarbonate may be impaired in severely ill patients and those with hepatic disease.
PREPARATIONS.
Generic. Solution 167 mEq/L (M/6).

SODIUM ACETATE

Sodium acetate is often used in total parenteral nutrition as a bicarbonate precursor. Acetate is converted to bicarbonate on almost an equimolar basis. It is readily metabolized outside the liver and its conversion is not impaired in severely ill patients or in those with hepatic disease.

AGENTS USED IN POTASSIUM IMBALANCES

POTASSIUM CHLORIDE

USES. Since hypokalemia is usually accompanied by metabolic alkalosis, potassium chloride is the agent of choice for treatment. It is used to counteract the potassium-wasting effect of thiazide and loop diuretics in those at risk from hypokalemia, such as digitalized or cirrhotic patients (see Chapter 29, Diuretics). In addition, it may be indicated in those with inadequate dietary intake of potassium, excessive gastrointestinal losses, renal tubular disorder with potassium-wasting primary adrenal disease, or in those receiving corticosteroids. Potassium chloride also is used to treat digitalis intoxication and hypokalemic periodic paralysis. See also Table 1.

FORMULATIONS. The liquid form of potassium chloride is the preparation of choice for oral therapy. Most commercial preparations contain 10 to 40 mEq of potassium chloride/15 ml and are flavored to mask the disagreeable taste. Such preparations *must be diluted* before ingestion to minimize gastric irritation, and administration after meals is advisable.

For patients who find the liquid solutions unpalatable or intolerable, a timed-release preparation may be prescribed. The two primary forms of timed-release preparations are a tablet containing potassium chloride in a wax matrix and a capsule containing small microencapsulated particles of potassium chloride. Both forms are designed to release potassium slowly in the gastrointestinal tract; this prevents local exposure to high concentrations of potassium and chloride ions, thus reducing the risk of gastric irritation. Although timed-release preparations are safer than uncoated products, they occasionally cause small bowel lesions, esophageal ulceration and stricture, and perforation of gastric ulcer. There is no conclusive evidence that the microencapsulated capsule is safer or causes fewer side effects than the wax matrix form (Skoutakis et al, 1984).

The intravenous route is indicated in emergencies or when patients cannot take drugs orally. The electrocardiogram and serum potassium concentration should be monitored frequently, and adequate urinary output must be assured. Concentrated potassium chloride solutions may cause pain on injection into a small vein.
PRECAUTIONS. Potassium preparations should be given very cautiously to patients with impaired renal function, for severe hyperkalemia may occur. Potassium supplements are particularly dangerous in patients who are also receiving potassium-sparing diuretics.

DOSAGE AND PREPARATIONS.

Oral: Adults, 10 to 15 mEq three or four times daily. Patients receiving thiazide or loop diuretics may require 80 to 100 mEq daily.

For trademark preparations, see Table 5, Oral Potassium Preparations.

Intravenous: Potassium chloride injection must be diluted before infusion. *Adults,* if serum potassium is greater than 2.5 mEq/L, neuromuscular and cardiac abnormalities are minimal, and renal function is not impaired, potassium is given in concentrations usually no greater than 40 mEq/L at a rate not exceeding 10 to 15 mEq/hr. The total dosage usually should not exceed 100 to 300 mEq/day. If the serum potassium level is less than 2 mEq/L in the presence of cardiovascular abnormalities or muscle paralysis, potassium may be given very cautiously in concentrations as high as 60 mEq/L at a rate of up to 40 mEq/hr. Total dosage usually should not exceed 400 mEq/day. Infusions must be regulated carefully on the basis of results of continuous electrocardiographic monitoring and repeated serum and urinary potassium determinations.

Generic. Solutions 1.5 mEq/ml in 20 ml, 2.4 mEq/ml in 12.5 ml, and 3.2 mEq/ml in 12.5 ml containers (Abbott); 2.0 mEq/ml in 5, 10, 15, and 20 ml containers (Abbott, Cutter, Travenol). These preparations are extremely concentrated and *must* be diluted prior to use.

AVAILABLE MIXTURES OF DILUTE SOLUTIONS:

Generic. Potassium chloride 10, 20, 30, and 40 mEq/L with dextrose 5% in 500 and 1,000 ml containers.

Potassium chloride 10, 20, 30, and 40 mEq/L with sodium chloride 0.9%.

Potassium chloride 10, 20, 30, and 40 mEq/L with sodium chloride 0.2%, 0.225%, and 0.45% with dextrose 5% in 250, 500, and 1,000 ml containers.

Potassium chloride 20 mEq/L with sodium chloride 0.33% in dextrose 5% in 1,000 ml containers.

POTASSIUM BICARBONATE AND CITRATE
[K-Lyte]

POTASSIUM GLUCONATE
[Kaon]

POTASSIUM TRIPLEX (Potassium acetate, bicarbonate, and citrate)
[Trikates]

These preparations are used to treat hypokalemia associated with hyperchloremia (eg, renal tubular acidosis). If they are

TABLE 5.
ORAL POTASSIUM PREPARATIONS

Tradename (Manufacturer)	Potassium (mEq)[1]	Anion (mEq)[1]	Formulation
LIQUID POTASSIUM CHLORIDE PRODUCTS			
Generic	20	Cl-20	Liquid
	40	Cl-40	Liquid
Kaochlor 10% Liquid[2,3] (Adria)	20	Cl-20	Liquid
Kaochlor S-F 10% Liquid[2] (Adria)	20	Cl-20	Liquid (sugar-free)
Kaon-Cl 20%[2] (Adria)	40	Cl-40	Liquid (sugar-free)
Kay Ciel[2] (Berlex)	20	Cl-20	Liquid (sugar-free)
Klorvess 10%[2] (Sandoz)	20	Cl-20	Liquid
Rum-K (Fleming)	30	Cl-30	Liquid (sugar-free)
SK-Potassium Chloride[2] (Smith Kline & French)	20	Cl-20	Liquid (sugar-free)
	40	Cl-40	Liquid (sugar-free)
POTASSIUM CHLORIDE PRODUCTS FOR RECONSTITUTION			
Generic	20	Cl-20	Powder
Kato (ICN)	20	Cl-20	Powder
Kay Ciel Powder (Berlex)	20	Cl-20	Powder (sugar-free)
K-Lor (Abbott)	20	Cl-20	Powder
Klor-Con (Upsher-Smith)	20	Cl-20	Powder
Klor-Con/25 (Upsher-Smith)	25	Cl-25	Powder
Klorvess Effervescent Granules (Sandoz)	20	Cl-20	Effervescent powder (sugar-free)

(Continued on next page)

TABLE 5.
ORAL POTASSIUM PREPARATIONS (continued)

Tradename (Manufacturer)	Potassium (mEq)[1]	Anion (mEq)[1]	Formulation
Klorvess (Sandoz)	20	Cl-20	Effervescent tablet (sugar-free)
K-Lyte/Cl (Mead Johnson)	25	Cl-25	Effervescent tablet
K-Lyte/Cl 50 (Mead Johnson)	50	Cl-50	Effervescent tablet
K-Lyte/Cl (Mead Johnson)	25	Cl-25	Powder
Potage (Lemmon)	20	Cl-20	Powder
TIMED-RELEASE POTASSIUM CHLORIDE PRODUCTS			
Generic	4	Cl-4	Enteric-coated tablet
Kaon Cl[3] (Adria)	6.7	Cl-6.7	Wax-matrix tablet
Kaon Cl-10 (Adria)	10	Cl-10	Wax-matrix tablet
Klotrix (Mead Johnson)	10	Cl-10	Wax-matrix tablet
K-Tab (Abbott)	10	Cl-10	Wax-matrix tablet
Micro-K (Robins)	8	Cl-8	Microencapsulated capsule
Micro-K 10 (Robins)	10	Cl-10	Microencapsulated capsule
Slow-K (CIBA)	8	Cl-8	Wax-matrix tablet
OTHER POTASSIUM PRODUCTS			
Generic	20	Gluc-20	Liquid
Bi-K (USV)	20	Gluc-14.8 Citrate-5.2	Liquid
Kaon[2] (Adria)	20	Gluc-20	Liquid (sugar-free)
Kaon Tablets (Adria)	5	Gluc-5	Tablet
K-Lyte (Mead Johnson)	25	Bicarbonate & Citrate	Efferverscent tablet
K-Lyte DS (Mead Johnson)	50	Bicarbonate & Citrate	Effervescent tablet
Kolyum (Pennwalt)	20	Cl-3.4 Gluc-16.6	Liquid (sugar-free)
Kolyum (Pennwalt)	20	Cl-3.4 Gluc-16.6	Powder (sugar-free)
Twin-K (Boots)	20	Gluconate & Citrate	Liquid
Twin-K-Cl (Boots)	15	Cl-4 Gluconate & Citrate	Liquid

[1]*Per 15 ml, packet, or tablet*   [2]*Contains alcohol*   [3]*Contains tartrazine*

used in patients with hypokalemic hypochloremic alkalosis, chloride ion also must be provided. There is no convincing evidence that any of these products is better tolerated than potassium chloride.

DOSAGE AND PREPARATIONS. See Table 5, Oral Potassium Preparations, and evaluation on Potassium Chloride.

SODIUM POLYSTYRENE SULFONATE
[Kayexalate]

ACTIONS AND USES. This exchange resin is used occasionally to treat hyperkalemia. It acts by exchanging sodium ion for potassium in the intestine; the potassium-containing resin is then excreted in the feces. In clinical use, much of the exchange capacity is utilized for other cations and, possibly, lipids and proteins; therefore, in vivo exchange of potassium is estimated to be about 0.5 to 1 mEq of potassium/g of resin. Because its action is not evident for 2 to 24 hours, sodium polystyrene sulfonate is most useful when serum potassium levels are not life-threatening or when other measures have reduced the immediate danger.

ADVERSE REACTIONS AND PRECAUTIONS. Adverse reactions usually involve the gastrointestinal tract. The most common are constipation, anorexia, nausea, and vomiting. Fecal impaction may occur in elderly patients when large oral doses are given without concomitant administration of a laxative (eg, sorbitol). Intestinal obstruction due to concretions of aluminum hydroxide coadministered with sodium polystyrene sulfonate have been reported.

Hypokalemia may occur as a result of therapy with sodium polystyrene sulfonate. The risk can be minimized if the serum potassium concentration is monitored at least daily during therapy and the dose is decreased or therapy discontinued when the level falls to 4 or 5 mEq/L. Sodium polystyrene sulfonate should be used with caution in patients receiving digitalis, since hypokalemia enhances digitalis toxicity. Hypocalcemia also may occur.

Sodium polystyrene sulfonate exchanges sodium for potassium and, therefore, should be used cautiously in patients who require salt restriction, since volume overload may occur. Because of this problem, calcium and hydrogen ion exchange resins have been used experimentally, but the former may cause hypercalcemia and the latter acidosis.

DRUG INTERACTIONS. Concomitant use of sodium polystyrene sulfonate with antacids containing magnesium or calcium should be undertaken with caution, especially in patients with renal failure (Mangini, 1983). Sodium polystyrene sulfonate is thought to bind to magnesium and calcium, thus preventing these cations from combining with bicarbonate in the small intestine and resulting in systemic alkalosis (Hansten, 1979).

DOSAGE AND PREPARATIONS. Oral administration is generally preferred to rectal use because enemas are not as reliable and often are difficult to recover unless the resin is placed in a dialysis bag. However, patients with impaired coordination during swallowing or with nausea and vomiting because of uremia have been reported to aspirate the suspension when

administered orally. Rectal administration may be preferable for these patients (Haupt and Hutchins, 1982).

Oral: Adults, 15 g suspended in 45 to 60 ml of water, syrup, fruit juice, or a soft drink one to four times daily. The preparation may be administered by stomach tube. To prevent constipation, 10 to 20 ml of 70% sorbitol or 30 ml of 50% sorbitol is given every two to three hours until a loose stool is passed, then once or twice daily as needed to avoid constipation.

Rectal: Adults, 30 to 50 g suspended in 100 ml of aqueous vehicle, such as sorbitol, is given every six hours initially (enemas may be given every one to two hours if the circumstances dictate); the frequency of administration may be decreased on succeeding days. The preparation should be retained as long as possible and should be followed by a cleansing enema. Some authorities believe that the preferred method of rectal administration is to place the drug in a sealed dialysis bag which is inserted into the rectum.

Kayexalate (Winthrop-Breon). Powder in 454 g containers [sodium content: approximately 100 mg (4.1 mEq)/g].

AGENTS USED IN HYPOMAGNESEMIA

MAGNESIUM GLUCONATE

MAGNESIUM HYDROXIDE (Milk of Magnesia)

MAGNESIUM SULFATE

USES. Magnesium sulfate is used to treat severe hypomagnesemia, to prevent hypomagnesemia during total parenteral nutrition (TPN), and in convulsive states, especially eclampsia. When the gluconate and hydroxide salts are administered orally, they act as cathartics. The duration of action of an intramuscular dose of magnesium sulfate is several hours; intravenous doses last only 30 minutes.

PRECAUTIONS AND INTERACTIONS. Magnesium sulfate interacts with succinylcholine and the nondepolarizing neuromuscular blocking agents. It should be given cautiously to patients with impaired renal function and to those receiving digitalis and is contraindicated in patients with heart block. A calcium salt (eg, calcium gluconate) should be available for intravenous injection to counteract the potential hazard of respiratory muscle depression.

DOSAGE AND PREPARATIONS.
Oral: Adults and older children, for magnesium supplementation, 5 mg of magnesium/kg/day. Magnesium gluconate or magnesium hydroxide tablets are generally used. If an oral liquid is preferred, magnesium hydroxide (milk of magnesia) four times/day is recommended (Flink, 1985).
MAGNESIUM GLUCONATE:
Generic. Tablets 500 mg.
MAGNESIUM HYDROXIDE (MILK OF MAGNESIA):
Generic. Tablets 325 mg; liquid 7.75%.
Intramuscular, Intravenous: Adults and older children, for severe hypomagnesemia, 2 to 4 g (4 to 8 ml of 50% solution or 16 to 32 mEq) daily intramuscularly in divided doses; adminis-

tration is repeated daily until serum levels have returned to normal. If the deficiency is not severe, 1 g (2 ml of 50% solution) can be given once or twice daily. Serum magnesium levels should serve as a guide to continued treatment. Magnesium sulfate 10% may be infused intravenously at a rate not exceeding 1.5 ml/min. It also may be added to TPN solution (see Chapter 48, Parenteral and Enteral Nutrition).

For pre-eclampsia and eclampsia, see Chapter 17, Adjuncts to Anesthesia.

MAGNESIUM SULFATE:
Generic. Solution 10% in 10 and 20 ml containers, 12.5% in 8 and 20 ml containers, 25% in 150 ml containers, 50% in 2, 5, and 10 ml containers.

Cited References

Alvo M, Warnock DG: Hyperkalemia. *West J Med* 141:666-671, 1984.

Andreoli TE: Disorders of fluid volume, electrolyte, and acid-base balance, in Wyngaarden JB, Smith LH (eds): *Cecil Textbook of Medicine*, ed 17. Philadelphia, WB Saunders, 1985, 515-544.

Ayus JC, et al: Rapid correction of severe hyponatremia with intravenous hypertonic saline solution. *Am J Med* 72:43-48, 1982.

Bear RA, Neil GA: Clinical approach to common electrolyte problems: 2. Potassium imbalances. *Can Med Assoc J* 129:28-31, 1983.

Down PF, et al: Fate of potassium supplements in six outpatients receiving long-term diuretics for oedematous disease. *Lancet* 2:721-724, 1972.

Feig PU: Hypernatremia and hypertonic syndromes. *Med Clin North Am* 65:271-290, 1981.

Finberg L, et al: *Water and Electrolytes in Pediatrics: Physiology, Pathophysiology and Treatment.* Philadelphia, WB Saunders, 1982.

Flink EB: Hypomagnesemia in patient receiving digitalis. *Arch Intern Med* 145:625-626, 1985.

Freitag JJ, Miller LW: *Manual of Medical Therapeutics*, ed 23. Boston, Little, Brown and Company, 1980.

Goldberg M: Hyponatremia. *Med Clin North Am* 65:251-269, 1981.

Graf H, et al: Evidence for detrimental effect of bicarbonate therapy in hypoxic lactic acidosis. *Science* 227:754-756, 1985.

Hale PJ, et al: Metabolic effects of bicarbonate in treatment of diabetic ketoacidosis. *Br Med J* 289:1035-1038, 1984.

Hansten PD: *Drug Interactions*, ed 4. Philadelphia, Lea & Febiger, 1979.

Haupt HM, Hutchins GM: Sodium polystyrene sulfonate pneumonitis. *Arch Intern Med* 142:379-381, 1982.

Kaehny WD, Gabow PA: Pathogenesis and management of metabolic acidosis and alkalosis in, Schrier RW (ed): *Renal and Electrolyte Disorders*, ed 2. Boston, Little, Brown and Company, 1980, 115-157.

Kopple JD, Blumenkrantz MJ: Total parenteral nutrition and parenteral fluid therapy, in Maxwell MH, Kleeman CR (eds): *Clinical Disorders of Fluid and Electrolyte Metabolism*, ed 3. New York, McGraw-Hill, 1980, 413-498.

Lawson AAH: Potassium replacement: When is it necessary? *Drugs* 21:354-361, 1981.

Lawson DH, Henry DA: Drug therapy reviews: Intravenous fluid therapy. *Am J Hosp Pharm* 34:1332-1338, 1977.

Lever E, Jaspan JB: Sodium bicarbonate therapy in severe diabetic ketoacidosis. *Am J Med* 75:263-268, 1983.

Levinsky NG: Fluids and electrolytes, in Isselbacher KJ, et al (eds): *Harrison's Principles of Internal Medicine*, ed 9. New York, McGraw-Hill, 1980, 435-443.

Mangini RJ (ed): *Drug Interaction Facts.* St Louis, MO, Facts and Comparisons Division, JB Lippincott, 1983, 430a.

Maxwell MH, Kleeman CR (eds): *Clinical Disorders of Fluid and Electrolyte Metabolism*, ed 3. New York, McGraw-Hill, 1980.

Mudge GH: Agents affecting volume and composition of body fluids, in Gilman AG, et al (eds): *The Pharmacological Basis of Therapeutics*, ed 6. New York, Macmillan, 1980, 848-884.

Quintanilli AP, Qureshi N: Renal acidoses. *Comp Ther* 7:51-55, (March) 1981.

Parfitt AM, Kleerekoper M: Clinical disorders of calcium, phosphorus, and magnesium metabolism, in Maxwell MH, Kleeman CR (eds): *Clinical Disorders of Fluid and Electrolyte Metabolism*, ed 3. New York, McGraw-Hill, 1980, 947-1151.

Schrier RW (ed): *Renal and Electrolyte Disorders*, ed 2. Boston, Little, Brown and Company, 1980.

Schwartz WB: Disorders of fluid, electrolyte, and acid-base balance, in Beeson PB, et al (eds): *Textbook of Medicine*, ed 15. Philadelphia, WB Saunders, 1979, 1950-1969.

Schwartz AB, Swartz CD: Dosage of potassium chloride elixir to correct thiazide-induced hypokalemia. *JAMA* 230:702-704, 1974.

Skoutakis VA, et al: Liquid and solid potassium chloride: Bioavailability and safety. *Pharmacotherapy* 4:392-397, 1984.

Trissel LA: *Handbook on Injectable Drugs*, ed 3. Washington, DC, American Society of Hospital Pharmacists, 1983.

Whang R: Hyperkalemia: Diagnosis and treatment. *Am J Med Sci* 272:19-29, 1976.

Whang R, et al: Frequency of hypomagnesemia in hospitalized patients receiving digitalis. *Arch Intern Med* 145:655-656, 1985.

Vitamins and Minerals

Vitamins and some minerals are essential for normal metabolism and maintenance of health. Food is the best source of vitamins and minerals, and healthy persons consuming an adequate balanced diet will not benefit from additional vitamins. However, individuals on low-calorie diets (less than 1,200 calories/day) often do not ingest adequate vitamins and may require a supplement. Purified or synthetic products are available individually or in various combinations. Products intended for prophylactic use should be distinguished from those preparations suitable only for therapeutic purposes.

Uses: Although there are few valid indications for vitamin or mineral supplements, almost 40% of adults in the United States are thought to take such preparations. Approximately 4% of those taking vitamin A ingest more than five times the RDA; 25% of vitamin E users and 21% of vitamin C users ingest more than ten times the RDA. The danger of toxic effects from excessive amounts of vitamin A or D and all minerals, particularly in infants and children, should be considered (Reuter and Hellriegel, 1983; Lewis, 1980; Marshall, 1983). Massive-dose therapy usually is justified only in patients who cannot utilize nutrients properly, in those with certain diseases, or in those with inborn errors of metabolism that respond to pharmacologic doses of vitamins (see the evaluations).

Vegetarian diets utilizing multiple food sources can provide essential nutrients if milk products or eggs are added to supply vitamin B_{12}. As these diets become more restrictive, the risk of nutritional inadequacies increases greatly, especially deficiencies of protein, vitamin B_{12}, calcium, vitamin D, and riboflavin. Because some restricted diets consist of high-bulk foods, they provide few calories. The higher levels of Zen macrobiotic diets can endanger health. For example, infants fed Kokoh (a Zen macrobiotic food mixture for infant feeding) grow poorly, and children consuming this type of diet have experienced protein-calorie undernutrition, which may progress to death from extreme malnutrition.

The toxic substances known as vitamin B_{15} (pangamic acid) and vitamin B_{17} (laetrile) are neither nutrients nor vitamins. Laetrile contains 6% cyanide by weight and has caused chronic cyanide poisoning and death (Herbert, 1980; Moertel et al, 1982). Pangamic acid or pangamate may be mutagenic (Herbert, 1979). Neither substance has any established nutritional or other usefulness.

Allowances: The Recommended Dietary Allowances (RDA) for vitamins and minerals established by the Food and Nutrition Board of the National Academy of Sciences-National Research Council provide authoritative information to assist the physician in evaluating the formulas of multivitamin preparations (see also the section on Multivitamin Preparations With or Without Minerals). These allowances (see Table 1) exceed the minimum requirements necessary to prevent deficiency and are not absolute nutritional standards or recommendations for an ideal diet. They are formulated to encompass individual variability and represent amounts that will maintain good nutrition in practically all healthy persons. (The allowances for calories and protein also are shown in Table 1.) RDA should not be confused with the United States Recommended Daily Allowances (U.S. RDA), which is the largest amount of each nutrient recommended for any age group as determined by the National Academy of Sciences/National Research Council in 1968 (see Table 2). The U.S. RDA is used by the Food and Drug Administration for labeling purposes. The RDA is used throughout this chapter for comparison, except in the section on Multivitamin Preparations With or Without Minerals, in which the U.S. RDA is used. The FDA has authority to regulate the vitamin and mineral content of supplements only for use in children under 12 years and in pregnant or lactating women. However, the labels provide information on the proportion of established allowances that are supplied by a product and permit the consumer to judge the appropriateness of the product (see the section on Multivitamin Preparations With or Without Minerals for discussion of recommended composition).

Requirements of Infants: Full-term infants breast fed by well-nourished mothers generally receive adequate amounts of vitamins and minerals, except vitamin K and vitamin D. Vitamin K deficiency has been reported during the first week of life before the intestinal flora become established. Therefore, newborns should be given 0.5 to 1 mg of vitamin K_1 (phytonadione) intramuscularly immediately after birth to prevent hemorrhage and loss of vitamin K-dependent coagulation factors.

The quantity of vitamin D in breast milk may be insufficient for some infants, especially those protected from sunlight or nursed by malnourished mothers, to maintain adequate 25(OH)-D concentrations and reduced bone mineralization may result (Tsang, 1983). A daily supplement of 400 IU is safe and effective for breast-fed infants.

Supplemental administration of vitamin A or E is rarely indicated. The rationale for adding vitamin A to most supplements containing vitamin D is historical; both vitamins are contained in cod liver oil. Supplemental doses of water-soluble vitamins also are rarely indicated. Infants fed a strict vegan diet

TABLE 1.
RECOMMENDED DAILY DIETARY ALLOWANCES

	Age (years)	Weight (kg)	Weight (lb)	Height (cm)	Height (in)	Protein (g)	A (mcg RE)[2]	D (mcg)[3]	E (mg α-TE)[4]
Infants	0.0-0.5	6	13	60	24	kg×2.2	420	10	3
	0.5-1.0	9	20	71	28	kg×2.0	400	10	4
Children	1-3	13	29	90	35	23	400	10	5
	4-6	20	44	112	44	30	500	10	6
	7-10	28	62	132	52	34	700	10	7
Males	11-14	45	99	157	62	45	1000	10	8
	15-18	66	145	176	69	56	1000	10	10
	19-22	70	154	177	70	56	1000	7.5	10
	23-50	70	154	178	70	56	1000	5	10
	51+	70	154	178	70	56	1000	5	10
Females	11-14	46	101	157	62	46	800	10	8
	15-18	55	120	163	64	46	800	10	8
	19-22	55	120	163	64	44	800	7.5	8
	23-50	55	120	163	64	44	800	5	8
	51+	55	120	163	64	44	800	5	8
Pregnant						+30	+200	+5	+2
Lactating						+20	+400	+5	+3

[1]The allowances take into account individual variations among most normal persons living in the United States under usual environmental stresses. Diets should be based on a variety of common foods to provide other nutrients for which human requirements have been less well defined.

[2]Retinol Equivalents (1 RE = 1 mcg retinol or 6 mcg beta carotene)

[3]As cholecalciferol (10 mcg cholecalciferol = 400 IU vitamin D)

[4]alpha-Tocopherol Equivalents (1 mg d-alpha tocopherol = 1 alpha-TE)

[5]1 NE (Niacin Equivalent) = 1 mg niacin or 60 mg dietary tryptophan

[6]Folacin allowances refer to dietary sources as determined by Lactobacillus casei assay after treatment with enzymes (conjugases) to make polyglutamyl forms of the vitamin available to the test organism.

may require vitamin B_{12} supplementation. Formula-fed infants should receive supplemental amounts of ascorbic acid if less than 30 mg of this vitamin is ingested daily.

Iron deficiency seldom occurs before age 4 to 6 months and usually can be managed by adding iron-fortified cereal to the diet. Iron supplements may be necessary if the infant receives an inadequate quantity from iron-fortified foods.

Fluoride supplementation for infants should take the infant's age and nutritional source into account. Breast-fed infants should receive fluoride supplements (0.25 mg/day) shortly after birth. For formula-fed infants, the dose depends upon the type of formula used. Powdered and concentrated formulas are mixed with water from the local water supply; therefore, dosage recommendations are based on the concentration of fluoride in the local water (see Table 3). Ready-to-use formulas are required by federal law to be manufactured using water with low fluoride levels; therefore, infants receiving these products should receive the same dose of fluoride as breast-fed infants (ie, 0.25 mg/day).

Commercial infant formulas sold in the United States must contain vitamins and minerals in quantities established by the FDA. Healthy infants fed proprietary formulas usually do not require supplementation during the first six months. Supplementation may be required during the second six months of life if the amount of formula ingested is inadequate.

Preterm infants should receive vitamin and mineral supplementation during the first weeks of life. The dosage should supply the equivalent of the RDA for term infants and also should contain vitamin E and folic acid. The prescription of iron should be delayed until after the first weeks.

When parenteral preparations of vitamin E are necessary, only those licensed by the FDA should be utilized.

Requirements of Children: Normal children usually receive adequate amounts of vitamins and minerals from their diet and do not require supplementation. An important exception is fluoride, which should be supplemented when there are insufficient quantities in the local water supply. Children and adolescents from deprived families, those who are neglected or abused, or those with poor eating habits are considered to be at high risk for vitamin and mineral deficiency and should receive supplementation as shown in Table 4.

Requirements of Pregnant and Lactating Women: The

Water-Soluble Vitamins							Minerals					
C (mg)	Thiamin (mg)	Riboflavin (mg)	Niacin (mg NE)[5]	B_6 (mg)	Folacin[6] (mg)	B_{12} (mcg)	Calcium (mg)	Phosphorus (mg)	Magnesium (mg)	Iron (mg)	Zinc (mg)	Iodine (mcg)
35	0.3	0.4	6	0.3	30	0.5[7]	360	240	50	10	3	40
35	0.5	0.6	8	0.6	45	1.5	540	360	70	15	5	50
45	0.7	0.8	9	0.9	100	2.0	800	800	150	15	10	70
45	0.9	1.0	11	1.3	200	2.5	800	800	200	10	10	90
45	1.2	1.4	16	1.6	300	3.0	800	800	250	10	10	120
50	1.4	1.6	18	1.8	400	3.0	1200	1200	350	18	15	150
60	1.4	1.7	18	2.0	400	3.0	1200	1200	400	18	15	150
60	1.5	1.7	19	2.2	400	3.0	800	800	350	10	15	150
60	1.4	1.6	18	2.2	400	3.0	800	800	350	10	15	150
60	1.2	1.4	16	2.2	400	3.0	800	800	350	10	15	150
50	1.1	1.3	15	1.8	400	3.0	1200	1200	300	18	15	150
60	1.1	1.3	14	2.0	400	3.0	1200	1200	300	18	15	150
60	1.1	1.3	14	2.0	400	3.0	800	800	300	18	15	150
60	1.0	1.2	13	2.0	400	3.0	800	800	300	18	15	150
60	1.0	1.2	13	2.0	400	3.0	800	800	300	10	15	150
+20	+0.4	+0.3	+2	+0.6	+400	+1.0	+400	+400	+150	[8]	+5	+25
+40	+0.5	+0.5	+5	+0.5	+100	+1.0	+400	+400	+150	[8]	+10	+50

[7]The recommended dietary allowance for vitamin B_{12} in infants is based on the average concentration of the vitamin in human milk. The allowances after weaning are based on energy intake (as recommended by the American Academy of Pediatrics) and consideration of other factors, such as intestinal absorption.

[8]The increased requirement during pregnancy cannot be met by the iron content of usual American diets or by the existing iron stores in many women; therefore, 30 to 60 mg of supplemental iron is recommended. Iron needs during lactation are not substantially different from those of nonpregnant women, but continued supplementation for the mother for two to three months after parturition is advisable to replenish stores depleted by pregnancy.

Adapted from Recommended Dietary Allowances, *1980.*

TABLE 2.
U.S. RDA FOR DIETARY SUPPLEMENTS[1]

	Units of Measurement	Infants (birth–1 yr)	Children (1–4 yrs)	Adults and Children Over 4 yrs	Pregnant and Lactating Women
VITAMINS					
A	RE[2] (IU)	450 (1,500)	750 (2,500)	1,500 (5,000)	2,400 (8,000)
D	mcg[3] (IU)	10 (400)	10 (400)	10 (400)	10 (400)
E	mg[4] (IU)	3.3 (5)	6.7 (10)	20 (30)	20 (30)
C	mg	35	40	60	60
Thiamin	mg	0.5	0.7	1.5	1.7
Riboflavin	mg	0.6	0.8	1.7	2.0
Niacin	mg	8.0	9.0	20	20
B_6	mg	0.4	0.7	2.0	2.5
B_{12}	mcg	2.0	3.0	6.0	8.0
Folic Acid	mg	0.1	0.2	0.4	0.8
Biotin	mg	0.5	0.15	0.3	0.3
Pantothenic Acid	mg	3.0	5.0	10	10
MINERALS					
Calcium	mg	600	800	1,000	1,300
Iron	mg	15	10	18	18
Phosphorus	mg	500	800	1,000	1,300
Iodine	mcg	45	70	150	150
Magnesium	mg	70	200	400	450
Zinc	mg	5	8	15	15
Copper	mg	0.6	1	2	2

[1]These values usually represent the highest allowance for any age group within the broad category and are the amounts judged necessary to maintain health.
[2]RE = Retinol Equivalents (1 RE = 3.3 IU vitamin A)
[3]As cholecalciferol (10 mcg cholecalciferol = 400 IU vitamin D)
[4]As d-alpha tocopherol (1 mg d-alpha tocopherol = 1.5 IU vitamin E)

routine prescription of multivitamin and mineral supplements for pregnant and lactating women is common but generally unnecessary. A well-balanced diet designed to meet the needs of pregnant and lactating women minimizes the need for supplementation. However, there are some exceptions (see Table 4).

During pregnancy and for two to three months postpartum, the requirements for iron exceed the level normally available from dietary intake; 30 to 60 mg of elemental iron daily is recommended. Therapeutic doses of iron should be considered for women at risk of developing iron deficiency anemia (ie, packed cell volume less than 30%, hemoglobin less than

TABLE 3.
SUPPLEMENTAL FLUORIDE DOSE (MG FLUORIDE ION/DAY)
BASED ON FLUORIDE CONCENTRATION IN DRINKING WATER*

Age (years)	Concentration of Fluoride in Water (ppm)		
	<0.3	0.3–0.7	>0.7
Birth to 2	0.25	0	0
2 to 3	0.50	0.25	0
3 to 13	1.00	0.50	0

Adapted from Accepted Dental Therapeutics, 1984

TABLE 4.
GUIDELINES FOR VITAMIN AND MINERAL SUPPLEMENTATION IN
HEALTHY INFANTS AND CHILDREN AND PREGNANT OR LACTATING WOMEN*

	Multivitamins/Minerals	Vitamins			Minerals	
		D	E	Folate	Iron	Fluoride[1]
PRETERM INFANT[2]						
Breast-fed	+	+	0[3]	0	+	0
Formula-fed	+	+	0[3]	0	+[4]	0
TERM INFANT						
Breast-fed	−	0	−	−	0[4]	+
Formula-fed	−	−	−	−	−	+
OLDER INFANT (6 mos)						
Normal	−	−	−	−	0[4]	+
High-risk[5]	+	−	−	−	0	+
CHILD						
Normal	−	−	−	−	−	+
High-risk	+	−	−	−	−	+
PREGNANT AND LACTATING WOMEN	+	−	−	+	+	+/−

+: Supplement usually indicated
0: Supplement sometimes indicated
−: Supplement not usually indicated

[1]Fluoride supplements should be started shortly after birth in term infants and continued throughout life. The dose depends upon the concentration in the water supply. Ready-to-use formulas are manufactured with water low in fluoride.
[2]Multivitamin supplement (plus added folate) is usually needed primarily when the calorie intake is <300 kcal/day or when the infant weighs <2.5 kg. Vitamin D should be supplemented in breast-fed infants until at least age 6 months. Iron should be started at age 2 months.
[3]Vitamin E should be in a preparation that is well absorbed by preterm infants. Breast-fed preterm infants are less susceptible to vitamin E deficiency.
[4]Iron supplements are usually unwarranted before age 4 to 6 months. After age 6 months, iron should be supplemented either by adding iron-fortified cereal to the diet (preferred) or by prescribing an iron supplement.
[5]Multivitamin and mineral preparations (with iron) are preferred to the use of iron alone.
*Adapted from Committee on Nutrition, American Academy of Pediatrics, 1980.

11 mg/dl). Iron should be administered orally whenever feasible; if the patient is unable to ingest sufficient iron due to side effects or is likely to be noncompliant, parenteral administration may be necessary.

Prophylactic folic acid supplementation is recommended in pregnant women with (1) a history of megaloblastic anemia not attributable to other causes during a previous pregnancy; (2) multiple pregnancies; (3) conditions associated with a high turnover of erythrocytes; (4) inadequate dietary intake; and (5) inpatients receiving phenytoin (Dwyer, 1982). Some experts also recommend that all pregnant women receive supplemental folic acid 300 to 800 mcg during the second half of pregnancy.

Women who cannot tolerate milk may require calcium supplementation. There are a few special conditions in which other vitamins and minerals should be prescribed to supplement the diet of pregnant and lactating women.

Requirements of Vegetarians: Patients who consume a vegan-vegetarian diet may require both vitamin B_{12} and vitamin D. Lacto-ovo vegetarians, who consume some animal foods, need only iron supplements to maintain a normal dietary intake of the essential vitamins and minerals.

Requirements of Elderly Individuals: It has not been substantiated that elderly persons consuming an adequate diet have higher requirements for vitamins or minerals than other healthy adults. However, since many elderly individuals do not eat an adequate diet, especially those living alone, many physicians recommend a multiple vitamin and mineral supplement.

Requirements of Patients on Hemodialysis: Hemodialysis removes circulating coenzymatic compounds derived from folacin, pyridoxine, and ascorbic acid; therefore, compensatory amounts (100% to 300% of the RDA) of these vitamins should be prescribed. The requirement for other vitamins, with the possible exception of vitamin E, apparently is not increased.

Parenteral Administration: Vitamins and minerals should be administered parenterally only in certain special circumstances (see the discussion on Therapeutic Multivitamin Preparations and Table 5). They should not be combined with other intravenous medications unless admixture is specified in the labeling. Compatibility data are available in most hospital pharmacies and should be consulted.

FAT-SOLUBLE VITAMINS

The fat-soluble vitamins (A, D, E, and K) are absorbed by complex processes that parallel the absorption of fat. Thus, any condition that causes malabsorption of fat (eg, bile acid deficiency, obstructive jaundice, celiac disease, tropical sprue, regional enteritis) may result in deficiency of one or all of these vitamins. Fat-soluble vitamins affect permeability or transport in various cell membranes and act as oxidation-reduction agents, coenzymes, or enzyme inhibitors. Vitamin A has some, and vitamin D has extensive, hormonal activity. Fat-soluble vitamins are stored principally in the liver and are excreted in the feces. Since these vitamins are metabolized very slowly, overdosage may produce toxic effects.

Drug Evaluations

VITAMIN A (Retinol)

Vitamin A is essential for growth and bone development in children, for vision (particularly in dim light), for integrity of mucosal and epithelial surfaces, and for reproduction.

SOURCES. Vitamin A includes several active compounds, of which retinol is the major naturally occurring form. Precursor carotenoid pigments, especially beta-carotene, may be obtained from green and yellow vegetables, but only about one-sixth is absorbed and converted to vitamin A in man. Preformed vitamin A (retinols) is acquired primarily from animal sources (eggs, dairy products, and liver). Dietary fat is necessary for effective absorption of carotene, and protein is required for absorption of retinols. Sufficient vitamin A to satisfy requirements for several months is stored in the liver of well-nourished people. Protein and possibly zinc may be required to mobilize hepatic reserves.

Human milk supplies sufficient vitamin A for infants unless the maternal diet is grossly inadequate, in which case enough vitamin A should be given during the first six months after birth to provide a daily total of 420 retinol equivalents (1,400 IU). Healthy children and adults consuming a well-balanced diet do not require supplementation.

VITAMIN A DERIVATIVES. Several vitamin A derivatives have been developed in an attempt to reduce toxicity and increase biological activity. Retinoic acid (eg, tretinoin, isotretinoin), in which the alcohol group of retinol has been oxidized, promotes growth, differentiation, and maintenance of epithelial tissue in vitamin-A deficient animals. However, it does not restore visual, auditory, or reproductive function in the latter. Retinoic acid is absorbed from the gut via the portal vein and transported in plasma complexed with albumin. Unlike the retinols, it is not stored in the liver, but is rapidly excreted.

Tretinoin has been applied topically in the treatment of skin diseases, such as acne, Darier's disease, and ichthyosis. This route is safe and effective but oral administration may cause hypervitaminosis A. Various newer retinoids, such as isotretinoin [Accutane], are equally efficacious in skin disorders and do not appear to be toxic to the vitamin A target organs. (See also Chapter 56, Dermatologic Preparations.)

Vitamin A also has been prescribed to treat or prevent hyperkeratotic dermatoses, including severe acne, psoriasis, lichen planus, ichthyosis, and pityriasis rubra pilaris. The response in severe acne has been mixed and appears to be dose dependent. In a recent study, the intake of massive doses (90,000 to 150,000 retinol equivalents daily for three to four months) was very effective against cystic acne (Kligman et al, 1981). However, the risk of toxicity associated with the required doses makes this an unacceptable form of therapy.

Deficiency of vitamin A reportedly enhances the susceptibility of epithelial tissues to carcinogenesis, and large doses of retinoids have been shown to prevent certain forms of experimental cancer in animals. Studies are being conducted employing synthetic retinoids to prevent cancer in certain high-risk human populations, but results are not yet available. The evidence at this time does not support the use of supplemental vitamin A for the prevention of cancer.

HYPOVITAMINOSIS A. Vitamin A deficiency occurs when the dietary intake is inadequate, when intestinal absorption is impaired (eg, cystic fibrosis, steatorrhea, biliary obstruction), when the ability to store or transport vitamin A is impaired (eg, hepatic cirrhosis, abetalipoproteinemia), when metabolic requirements are increased (eg, in growing infants, pregnant and lactating women), or when hyperthyroidism is present.

The initial manifestation of hypovitaminosis A is night blindness (nyctalopia), which may progress to xerophthalmia and keratomalacia with corneal perforation and, eventually, blindness, particularly in young children. Hyperkeratosis of the skin and metaplasia of mucous membranes, which impair local defenses against infection, also may occur.

HYPERVITAMINOSIS A. Toxicity of vitamin A usually results from ingestion of more than 210 to 900 retinol equivalents/kg/day for several months to years. However, liver damage has resulted from ingestion of as little as the adult RDA for years by a child and as little as five times the RDA for seven to ten years by an adult (Herbert, 1982). Acute intoxication has followed the ingestion of a single dose of 450,000 retinol equivalents (1,500,000 IU) in adults and 90,000 retinol equivalents (300,000 IU) in infants. In adults, the symptoms of acute intoxication include dizziness, nausea, vomiting, and erythema with eventual desquamation that persists for several weeks; in infants, the symptoms include transient hydrocephalus and vomiting.

Chronic hypervitaminosis A in infants and children produces pseudotumor cerebri, tinnitus, bulging fontanelles, increased cerebrospinal fluid pressure, bone pain, lethargy, pruritus, exfoliative dermatitis, angular stomatitis, hyperostosis, metaphyseal cupping, and paronychia. Diplopia and papilledema occur; in long-standing cases, optic atrophy and blindness may result. Common symptoms in adults are vomiting, skin changes, irritability, headache, hypomenorrhea, and weakness. Psychiatric symptoms also may be observed, and such patients rarely have been placed in psychiatric hospitals with a diagnosis of severe depression or schizophrenia. Hepatic dysfunction, often associated with hepatosplenomegaly, may occur and marked hypercalcemia and ascites have been reported. In children and adults, chronic hypervitaminosis A may cause dryness of the skin and mucous membranes, alopecia, anorexia, brittle nails, myalgia, ostealgia, arthralgia, abdominal pain, splenomegaly, and hypoplastic anemia with leukopenia. Most symptoms disappear when the vitamin is discontinued, but growth retardation caused by premature epiphyseal closure may occur in children.

TERATOGENICITY. Overdosage of vitamin A in animals has produced malformations of the central nervous system, eye, palate, and urogenital tract. The maximal nonteratogenic dose is somewhat species dependent, ranging from 40,000 retinol equivalents/kg in rats to 750 retinol equivalents/kg in mice. The relative sensitivity of humans is unknown (*Federal Register*, 1983). Because of possible teratogenic effects on the human fetus, doses exceeding the RDA should not be administered during pregnancy.

DOSAGE AND PREPARATIONS.
THERAPEUTIC:
Doses exceeding 7,500 retinol equivalents (25,000 IU) daily should not be prescribed unless the deficiency is severe. The safety of doses exceeding 1,800 retinol equivalents (6,000 IU) daily during pregnancy and lactation has not been established. Oral administration is preferred; the intramuscular route may be used for short-term therapy when absorption is grossly impaired, ocular symptoms are prominent, or oral administration is not feasible.

Intramuscular: In severe deficiency, *adults and children over 8 years,* 15,000 to 30,000 retinol equivalents (50,000 to 100,000 IU) daily for three days, followed by 15,000 retinol equivalents (50,000 IU) daily for two weeks; *1 to 8 years,* 1,500 to 4,500 retinol equivalents (5,000 to 15,000 IU) daily for ten days; *infants,* 1,500 to 3,000 retinol equivalents (5,000 to 10,000 IU) daily for ten days.

   Aquasol A (Armour). Solution 50,000 IU/ml in 2 ml containers.

Oral: In deficiency, *adults and children over 8 years,* 1,500 to 3,000 retinol equivalents (5,000 to 10,000 IU) daily for one to two weeks. In severe deficiency, 30,000 retinol equivalents (100,000 IU) daily for three days, followed by 15,000 retinol equivalents (50,000 IU) daily for two weeks, then 3,000 to 6,000 retinol equivalents (10,000 to 20,000 IU) daily for another two months.

   Generic. Capsules (nonprescription) 10,000, 25,000, and 50,000 IU; tablets (chewable, nonprescription) 25,000 IU.

   Available Trademarks.
   Alphalin (Lilly) (fat-soluble), *Aquasol A* (Armour) (water-dispersible).

DIETARY SUPPLEMENTATION OR PROPHYLAXIS:
The dosage should not exceed the RDA after evaluation of the patient's diet. The diet should be corrected or the dose adjusted on the basis of the RDA. No single-entity preparations are available; see the section on Multivitamin Preparations With or Without Minerals.

VITAMIN D

Vitamin D is the generic designation for several sterols and their metabolites that have antirachitic properties. Ergocalciferol (vitamin D_2), derived from yeast and fungal ergosterol, is the usual active ingredient supplied commercially. Irradiation of the provitamin, 7-dehydrocholesterol, in the skin or irradiation of food produces cholecalciferol (vitamin D_3).

METABOLISM AND FUNCTIONS. Vitamin D is stored mainly in the liver but also in adipose tissue and muscle and is excreted slowly. The vitamin is stable and is well absorbed from the gastrointestinal tract. Following absorption, it is hydroxylated in the liver to form 25-hydroxy-vitamin D (25-(OH)-D_3 or calcifediol). Further hydroxylation occurs in the kidney in response to the need for calcium and phosphorus, and 1,25-dihydroxy-vitamin D (1,25-$(OH)_2D_3$ or calcitriol) is produced. In conjunction with calcitonin and parathyroid hormone, calcitriol regulates calcium and phosphorus metabolism in the intestine, bone, and possibly kidney; it facilitates the intestinal absorption of calcium and may initiate phosphorus transport, thus increasing serum calcium and phosphorus levels to allow normal mineralization of the skeleton. Paradoxically, vitamin D also mobilizes calcium from bone to maintain proper plasma levels of calcium. It may act in the kidney to suppress parathyroid hormone secretion, thus preventing phosphaturia, and may have a direct action on the proximal tubules to promote phosphorus retention.

REQUIREMENTS. Although vitamin D is essential, the daily requirement in adults is very small and may be obtained by adequate exposure to sunlight or in the diet. Products containing more than 10 mcg (400 IU) should be used only when deficiency is documented.

Premature infants and those fed unfortified formulas should receive enough supplemental vitamin D to provide a daily intake of 10 mcg. Infants and children receiving adequate amounts of vitamin D-fortified food require no supplementation; in fact, use of a supplement can result in overdosage. Members of dark-skinned races inhabiting northern climates have a slightly higher requirement for vitamin D because melanin interferes with irradiation. Because of increased calcium requirements, pregnant and lactating women may need supplementation if their diet does not supply 10 to 12.5 mcg (400 to 500 IU) daily. However, use of excessive amounts during pregnancy may produce hypercalcemia, which is potentially teratogenic; supravalvular aortic stenosis, vascular injury, and suppression of parathyroid function may occur in the neonate.

HYPOVITAMINOSIS D. Primary nutritional deficiency of vitamin D is rare in the United States. An absolute or relative deficiency may occur secondary to malabsorption syndromes, in individuals not exposed to the sun, or in patients with metabolic disorders. Deficiency causes hypocalcemia and hypophosphatemia, which stimulates parathyroid hormone secretion to restore plasma calcium levels at the expense of bone. This causes rickets in infants and children and osteomalacia in adults. When produced by dietary deficiency, these conditions respond rapidly to adequate doses of vitamin D, but treatment of other disorders may depend upon blood levels of calcium, phosphate, and parathyroid hormone, as well as the degree of derangement of vitamin D metabolism. See Chapter 49, Agents Affecting Calcium Metabolism, for discussion of the therapeutic uses of vitamin D.

In all deficiency states, the dose of vitamin D should be reduced to the RDA after symptoms are relieved and before normal biochemical levels are achieved or bone healing is complete. When bone healing has occurred, the requirement may decrease suddenly and, since the action of vitamin D may persist long after administration is discontinued, hypercalcemia and renal damage may result.

Administration of vitamin D to treat lupus vulgaris is obsolete, and its topical use for other dermatoses is not justified.

HYPERVITAMINOSIS D. Vitamin D is very toxic in large doses. In infants and children, the margin of safety between prophylactic or therapeutic and toxic doses is narrow. Hyper-

calcemia may develop in hypersensitive infants at doses very close to 10 mcg. In addition, large amounts may be ingested inadvertently by children who consume a great variety of foods fortified with vitamin D.

Prolonged hypervitaminosis D in infants causes mental and physical retardation, elfin facies, renal failure, and death. Symptoms of toxicity may occur with doses greater than 25 mcg (1,000 IU) daily, and retardation of linear growth has been reported after daily doses of 45 mcg (1,800 IU) (Beeson et al, 1979). Amounts exceeding 1.25 mg (50,000 IU) daily produce hypercalcemia in normal adults and children. Initial manifestations of toxicity are associated with symptoms of hypercalcemia (eg, weakness, anorexia, vomiting, diarrhea, polydipsia, polyuria, mental changes). Proteinuria may indicate renal impairment, and prolonged hypercalcemia may result in soft tissue calcifications (calcinosis universalis). Prolonged use of massive doses ultimately results in irreversible renal failure and death.

Vitamin D intoxication usually is reversible after administration is discontinued unless renal impairment is severe. Some patients also require a low-calcium diet, glucocorticoids, and other measures to reduce plasma calcium levels to normal.

DOSAGE AND PREPARATIONS. Dosage for vitamin D is preferably expressed in terms of cholecalciferol (10 mcg of cholecalciferol equals 400 IU).

PROPHYLACTIC:

Oral: Premature or breast-fed infants when maternal milk is inadequate or infants given unfortified formulas, 10 mcg (400 IU) daily. *Infants abnormally susceptible to rickets* (eg, malabsorption syndrome, born to mothers with vitamin D deficiency), up to 750 mcg (30,000 IU) daily for a short period. In *adults,* based on dietary intake and exposure to sunlight, supplementation may be needed during pregnancy and lactation and in the elderly to assure a daily intake of 10 mcg. If larger doses are used for prolonged periods, blood calcium levels and 24-hour urine specimens should be monitored frequently. Blood calcium levels should be maintained at 9 to 10 mg/dl.

Generic. Capsules, 25,000 and 50,000 IU; tablets 50,000 IU.

THERAPEUTIC:

See Chapter 49, Agents Affecting Calcium Metabolism.

VITAMIN E (Tocopherol)

Vitamin E refers to a group of fat-soluble substances occurring in plants. Alpha-tocopherol is the most active and abundant form; soybean products contain gamma-tocopherol, which is less potent but contributes somewhat to vitamin E intake. When only the amount of alpha-tocopherol is reported on the labeling, total milligrams of alpha-tocopherol equivalents may be calculated by increasing the value in milligrams by 20% to account for other tocopherols present in a mixed diet.

FUNCTIONS. Vitamin E is considered to be an essential nutrient, but its biochemical functions are not completely understood; 50% to 80% is absorbed and transported by lipoprotein in essentially the same manner as fats. It is stored in adipose tissue and is thought to stabilize the lipid portions of cell membranes. Vitamin E protects polyunsaturated fatty acids (PUFA) from oxidation and appears to influence the synthesis of heme, porphyrin, and heme proteins. Other functions attributed to vitamin E are enhancement of vitamin A utilization, inhibition of prostaglandin production, and stimulation of an essential cofactor in steroid metabolism. A number of other substances that occur naturally in foods (eg, selenium, sulfur amino acids, coenzyme Q) can function as partial substitutes for vitamin E in certain metabolic reactions.

REQUIREMENTS. Surveys indicate that adequate amounts of vitamin E are supplied by the usual diet, that human requirements are small, and that the RDA exceeds the actual needs of normal persons. The requirement for vitamin E increases as the intake of PUFA increases. However, foods that supply PUFA (vegetable oils, shortenings, and margarine) also are good sources of vitamin E. Nevertheless, consumption of excessive amounts of PUFA (more than 20 g/day over normal dietary intake) may warrant supplementation with vitamin E, particularly if the PUFA intake is discontinued abruptly, thus producing a relative deficiency of the vitamin.

Vitamin E requirements may be increased in people exposed to high-oxygen environments or in those taking therapeutic doses of iron or large doses of thyroid hormone. Skin lesions, hematologic changes, and edema have developed in premature infants receiving formulas high in PUFA and low in vitamin E; the deficiency of vitamin E may be aggravated by the large iron supplements given these infants. Recovery followed administration of 25 to 50 mg of alpha-tocopherol equivalent (37.5 to 75 IU) daily.

USES. **Deficiency States:** Vitamin E therapy should be restricted to deficiency states demonstrable by low serum vitamin E levels and/or increased fragility of red cells to hydrogen peroxide. These may occur in patients who have malabsorption syndromes with steatorrhea (eg, celiac disease, tropical sprue, gastrointestinal resections) and other conditions characterized by prolonged malabsorption of fats (eg, cystic fibrosis, hepatic cirrhosis, biliary obstruction, excessive ingestion of mineral oil).

Retinopathy of Prematurity: Because of advances in neonatal intensive care, more premature infants of extremely low birth weight are surviving. In infants weighing less than 1,500 g and of less than 31 weeks' gestational age at birth, the risk of retinopathy of prematurity remains high. In an effort to reduce the incidence and severity of retinopathy of prematurity, large oral doses of vitamin E (100 mg/kg/day) have been given to premature infants beginning within hours of birth until the eyes mature or for as long as active neovascularization continues. One double-blind study indicated that vitamin E does not prevent retinopathy of prematurity but does reduce its severity. Thus, the incidence of blindness is decreased when vitamin E is given from the first day of life (Hittner et al, 1981). However, infants with plasma vitamin E concentrations greater than 3.5 mg/dl may be at increased risk of necrotizing enterocolitis and

sepsis; therefore plasma concentrations should be maintained between 1.2 and 3.5 mg/dl (Hittner et al, 1984).

Intermittent Claudication: When combined with active muscular training, vitamin E may be a useful adjunct for treatment of intermittent claudication. A study reported that 73% of patients given both muscular training and vitamin E 100 mg three times daily had improved arterial bloodflow in the affected limb compared to 19% of control patients undergoing muscular training only (Haeger, 1982); however, the response may not be noticeable for several months. Previous studies that found no significant improvement probably used inadequate doses or measured response for too short a time (Bieri et al, 1983).

Unsubstantiated Uses: There is no evidence to support the efficacy of vitamin E in the numerous conditions for which it is popularly used. Large doses do not protect against arteriosclerosis, cancer, pulmonary damage from air pollution, or deterioration from aging, and vitamin E is ineffective in inflammatory skin disorders, habitual abortion, heart disease, menopausal syndrome, infertility, peptic ulcer, burns, and porphyria.

ADVERSE REACTIONS AND PRECAUTIONS. Because excessive amounts of other fat-soluble vitamins (A and D) are known to be toxic, large doses of vitamin E should be used cautiously. In anemic children, the hematologic response to parenteral iron is suppressed by large doses of alpha-tocopherol. Excessive use of vitamin E may deplete vitamin A stores and inhibit the absorption or action of vitamin K, although adverse effects (eg, increased hypoprothrombinemic response to oral anticoagulants) occur only rarely when 200 to 270 mg daily is taken for prolonged periods. However, the long-term use of doses as low as 270 to 540 mg daily has been reported to produce nausea, muscular weakness, fatigue, headache, and blurred vision in a few patients, and very large doses (1.3 to 8 g daily) have been reported to cause gastrointestinal upset, decreased gonadal function, and creatinuria (Hayes and Hegsted, 1973). Symptoms disappeared within a few weeks when excessive doses were discontinued.

DOSAGE AND PREPARATIONS.

Oral, Intramuscular: For deficiency in *adults and children,* four to five times the RDA. Commercial formulas for infant feeding that are high in polyunsaturated fats should contain at least 3.3 mg/L (5 IU/L). For low-birth-weight or premature infants, the formula should contain 4.7 mg/L (7 IU/L); the Committee on Nutrition of the American Academy of Pediatrics (1980) has recommended an additional oral supplement of 3.3 mg (5 IU) of water-soluble alpha-tocopherol.

Oral: For prophylaxis for retinopathy of prematurity, 100 mg/kg/day from birth until eyes mature or for as long as active neovascularization continues.

> Available generically under the name Vitamin E. Capsules 50, 100, 200, 400, 600, and 1,000 IU (nonprescription); solution (injection) 200 IU/ml in 10 and 30 ml containers; tablets 100, 200, 400, 600, and 1,000 IU (nonprescription); chewable tablets 100, 200, and 400 IU (nonprescription).
> *Aquasol E* (Armour). Capsules (tocopheryl acetate) 100 and 400 IU; drops 50 IU/ml (both forms nonprescription).
> *E-ferol* (Forest). Capsules (tocopheryl succinate) 200 to 400 IU (nonprescription).
> *Eprolin* (Lilly). Capsules (tocopheryl acetate) 50 and 100 IU (nonprescription).

VITAMIN K

In normal individuals, synthesis of vitamin K provides about one-half the estimated daily requirement; the remainder is supplied by the average diet.

Hypoprothrombinemia due to vitamin K deficiency may be secondary to malabsorption of fats, prolonged hyperalimentation, or inhibition of intestinal bacterial biosynthesis (eg, long-term administration of antibiotics). Relative deficiency also may result from an imbalance of fat-soluble vitamins following excessive doses of one or all of the other fat-soluble vitamins (A, D, E). Newborn infants, especially those who are premature, have low concentrations of vitamin K-dependent clotting factors that decrease for a few days after birth. Small doses (0.5 to 1 mg) of phytonadione (vitamin K_1) administered either intramuscularly or intravenously immediately after birth are advocated for all newborn infants. This dose may be repeated if required.

Oral liquid nutritional products that contain vitamin K can be purchased at health food stores, and patients who require oral anticoagulants should be warned that these products may interfere with the hypoprothrombinemic response.

For a detailed discussion on the therapeutic and prophylactic uses of vitamin K, see Chapter 36, Hemostatics.

WATER-SOLUBLE VITAMINS

The water-soluble vitamins include ascorbic acid and the B-complex vitamins, biotin, folic acid (folacin), niacin (nicotinic acid), pantothenic acid, pyridoxine (B_6), riboflavin (B_2), thiamine (B_1), and cyanocobalamin (B_{12}). Since cyanocobalamin and folic acid are used principally to treat deficiency anemias (see Chapter 32), they are discussed only briefly in this chapter.

Water-soluble vitamins are structurally diverse and act as coenzymes or as oxidation inhibitors. Metabolism is rapid, any excess is excreted in the urine, and, except for niacin and pyridoxine, overdosage seldom causes toxic effects in individuals with normal renal function.

Drug Evaluations

ASCORBIC ACID

ASCORBATE CALCIUM

ASCORBATE SODIUM

Ascorbic acid (vitamin C) acts as a coenzyme and, under certain conditions, as a reducing agent and antioxidant. It is indicated to prevent and treat scurvy.

REQUIREMENTS. Like other primates, man lacks the microsomal enzyme necessary to convert L-gulonolactone to ascorbic acid; therefore, vitamin C must be supplied exogenously. Intake of 60 to 75 mg of vitamin C daily produces a serum ascorbate concentration of approximately 0.75 mg/dl (7.5 mg/L) and a total body pool of approximately 1.5 g in the average healthy adult male. Requirements are increased during pregnancy and lactation, as reflected in the RDA (see Table 1). Environmental stresses (eg, extremes in temperature, surgery, thermal burns, trauma) also increase the daily requirement by 300% to 500%. Cigarette smokers are estimated to require as much as 50% more ascorbic acid to maintain serum concentrations within the normal range (Sauberlich, 1984). Women taking oral contraceptives also have decreased serum ascorbate concentrations, but the clinical relevance of this is unknown.

SOURCES. Vitamin C is present in relatively high concentrations in citrus fruits, tomatoes, potatoes, and leafy vegetables.

HYPOVITAMINOSIS C. Clinical scurvy occurs after three to five months on an ascorbic acid-free diet and is relatively rare in the United States. In adults, scurvy usually occurs in elderly or chronically ill individuals, alcoholics, and dietary cultists. Infants fed diets deficient in ascorbic acid are also susceptible.

Pathology is manifest in most body tissues, especially those of mesodermal origin (ie, collagen, growing bones, teeth, blood vessels). Defective ground substance is formed and formation of scar tissue is delayed. Capillary fragility combined with defective calcification of cartilage causes subperiosteal hemorrhages and, eventually, bone resorption, abnormal bone development, and defective development of teeth in growing children. Ecchymoses appear and hemorrhages into muscles and joints may occur. A normocytic or macrocytic anemia, which is multifactorial in origin, is common. Rarely, megaloblastic anemia is observed (most often associated with deficiency of both ascorbic and folic acids). If untreated, convulsions, coma, hypotension, and death occur.

OTHER USES. Vitamin C is used to treat a number of syndromes not associated with deficiency. However, efficacy in most of the purported uses is unfounded, unproven, or unsubstantiated. Vitamin C does not affect the incidence of colds, although it may attenuate the severity and duration of the symptoms slightly. There is good evidence that pharmacologic doses of ascorbic acid have no beneficial effect in patients with advanced cancer (Moertel et al, 1985).

Other conditions treated with megadoses of vitamin C that have been studied and found to be unaffected include atherosclerosis, healing of wounds, and schizophrenia.

There are a variety of diseases for which vitamin C may be indicated, but further research is required. Among these are asthma, pressure sores, male infertility due to nonspecific spermagglutination, osteogenesis imperfecta, and adjunctive therapy in narcotic withdrawal (Ovesen, 1984).

ADVERSE REACTIONS. The incidence of adverse reactions from even megadoses of vitamin C is low. Doses exceeding 1 g/day may cause diarrhea due to direct irritation of the intestinal mucosa that results in increased peristalsis. The irritant action also may cause nonspecific urethritis with dysuria and clear watery discharge that is primarily limited to the distal urethra (Fong, 1981).

Ascorbic acid increases iron absorption and, thus, large doses may be dangerous in patients with hemochromatosis, thalassemia, or sideroblastic anemia. Mild hemolysis has been reported in patients with G6PD deficiency receiving large doses of vitamin C; in one patient, acute hemolysis resulted in disseminated intravascular coagulation, acute renal failure, and death (Campbell et al, 1975). Megadoses of ascorbic acid also may produce sickle cell crisis by converting oxidized SS hemoglobin to reduced SS hemoglobin. In megadoses, parenteral ascorbic acid has caused severe renal damage (Balcke et al, 1984; Schwartz et al, 1984).

INTERACTIONS. In doses of 1 g/day, ascorbic acid has been reported to increase ethinyl estradiol plasma levels. This interaction may cause breakthrough bleeding and contraceptive failure when women taking oral contraceptives containing ethinyl estradiol abruptly discontinue ascorbic acid (Morris et al, 1981).

INTERFERENCE WITH LABORATORY TEST RESULTS. Large doses of ascorbic acid can affect results of the enzyme dip test for glycosuria used by many diabetics to regulate the dosage of hypoglycemic drugs. The Testape test is falsely negative, and the Clinitest is falsely positive. Megadoses also can cause false-positive results when Benedict's solution is used as a test for glycosuria. Tests for occult blood in the stool may be falsely negative in patients with carcinoma of the colon.

DOSAGE AND PREPARATIONS. For prophylaxis or correction of deficiency, vitamin C may be given as fresh or frozen orange juice (contains approximately 0.5 mg of ascorbic acid/ml). Crystalline ascorbic acid is a suitable alternative; oral administration is preferred, but the vitamin also may be injected intramuscularly or intravenously.

PROPHYLACTIC:

Oral, Intramuscular: For the first few weeks of life, *infants on formula feedings,* 35 mg daily or, if the formula contains two or three times the amount of protein in human milk, 50 mg daily. *Older infants, children, and adults,* at least 60 to 120 ml of orange juice or other source of vitamin C or 50 to 100 mg of crystalline ascorbic acid daily. During pregnancy and lactation, an additional 20 to 40 mg of ascorbic acid is recommended. During periods of increased requirement (eg, infections, trauma), 150 mg daily.

THERAPEUTIC:

Oral, Intramuscular, Intravenous: Adults and children, the diet should be corrected by ingesting at least 60 to 120 ml of orange juice or other source of vitamin C daily. For treatment of scurvy, 100 mg three times daily for one week, followed by 100 mg daily for several weeks until tissue saturation is normal. For severe burns, 200 to 500 mg daily until healing has occurred or grafting operations are completed.

ASCORBIC ACID:

Generic. Capsules (timed-release) 500 mg and 1 g; solution (injection) 50 mg/ml in 2 ml containers, 100 mg/ml in 10 ml containers, 200 mg/ml in 5 and 10 ml containers, 250 mg/ml in 2, 10, 30, and 50 ml containers, and 500 mg/ml in 30 and 50 ml containers; syrup 20 and 100 mg/ml; tablets 25, 50, 100, 250, and 500 mg and 1 and 1.5 g; tablets (chewable) 100, 250, and 500 mg and 1 g; tablets (timed-release) 500 mg and 1 and 1.5 g (all oral forms and sizes nonprescription).

Cecon (Abbott). Drops 100 mg/ml (nonprescription).

Cevalin (Lilly). Solution (intramuscular) 100 mg/ml in 10 ml containers and 500 mg/ml in 1 ml containers; tablets 250 and 500 mg (nonprescription).

Cevi Bid (Geriatric). Capsules (timed-release) 500 mg (nonprescription).

Ce-Vi-Sol (Mead Johnson). Drops (pediatric) 35 mg/0.6 ml (alcohol 5%, nonprescription).

ASCORBATE CALCIUM:

Oral form available only in multivitamin preparations.

ASCORBATE SODIUM:

Cenolate (Abbott). Solution (injection) equivalent to ascorbic acid 500 mg/ml in 1 and 2 ml containers.

BIOTIN

This member of the B-complex group of vitamins is a coenzyme essential for fatty acid and carbohydrate metabolism and other carboxylation reactions and is synthesized by intestinal bacteria. Persons with multiple carboxylase deficiency, an inborn error of biotin-dependent enzyme systems, respond to 10 mg of biotin given once or twice daily (Nyhan, 1980). Deficiency can be produced by prolonged ingestion of large amounts of raw egg white, which contains the inactivating protein, avidin. Biotin deficiency also may occur during long-term parenteral nutrition.

In adults, symptoms of deficiency include alopecia, anorexia, mental depression, partial memory loss, and dermatitis. In young infants, deficiency causes seborrheic dermatitis, and the Committee on Nutrition of the American Academy of Pediatrics (1980) recommends that formulas contain 15 mcg/1,000 kcal. Because the amounts produced by intestinal microorganisms are not well defined, no firm RDA has been determined.

FOLIC ACID (Folacin)

Folacin is the generic term for several compounds having folic acid activity. Adequate varied diets provide sufficient amounts for normal individuals. Chronic alcoholics are susceptible to folacin deficiency; 40% to 87% of alcoholics admitted to municipal hospitals have low serum folate concentrations (Wagner, 1984).

Amounts present in human or cow's milk are adequate to fulfill infant requirements. Supplementation may be needed in low-birth-weight infants, those who are breast-fed by mothers with folic acid deficiency (50 mcg daily), infants who do not receive solid foods until quite late, or those with infections or prolonged diarrhea. During pregnancy and lactation, folic acid requirements are markedly increased and deficiency will result in fetal damage.

In patients with megaloblastic anemia, the diagnosis of vitamin B_{12} deficiency should be excluded before therapeutic doses of folic acid are prescribed. Patients with pernicious anemia who receive more than 400 mcg of folic acid daily and who are inadequately treated with vitamin B_{12} may show reversion of hematologic parameters to normal, while neurologic damage due to vitamin B_{12} deficiency progresses.

Doses of folic acid exceeding the RDA should not be included in multivitamin preparations; if therapeutic amounts are necessary, folic acid should be given separately.

For a more detailed discussion of folic acid, see Chapter 32, Agents Used to Treat Deficiency Anemias.

NIACIN (Nicotinic Acid)

NIACINAMIDE (Nicotinamide)

FUNCTIONS. Niacin, including niacinamide and tryptophan, is converted to physiologically active diphosphopyridine nucleotide (DPN or NAD) and triphosphopyridine nucleotide (TPN or NADP). As coenzymes of numerous dehydrogenases, these nucleotides are functional groups of electron transfer agents active in cellular respiration, glycolysis, and lipid synthesis.

SOURCES AND METABOLISM. Chief dietary sources of niacin are proteins of animal origin, yeast, and green vegetables. Bound forms, which are unavailable for conversion to nucleotides, are present in many foods, especially cereals. The conversion of dietary tryptophan to NAD and NADP requires thiamine, riboflavin, and pyridoxine; approximately 60 mg of precursor tryptophan is equivalent to 1 mg of niacin. Thus, the dietary requirement for niacin is influenced by the protein content of the diet. Larger amounts are needed during periods of increased metabolism (eg, pregnancy, lactation, prolonged infection, hyperthyroidism, burns).

DEFICIENCY. Primary dietary deficiency is rare in the United States except in areas where corn (which is low in tryptophan) is the main constituent of the diet. Secondary deficiency may occur in those with malabsorption syndromes, in alcoholics, or in dietary cultists.

Deficiency causes pellagra, which is characterized by erythematous lesions on areas of the skin exposed to sun, friction, or pressure. As lesions become chronic, pigmentation and hyperkeratinization occur. Diarrhea and abdominal pain are prominent. Other symptoms include mental depression or apathy, headache, insomnia, atrophy of sebaceous glands and hair follicles, inflammation and atrophy of mucous membranes, angular stomatitis, sialorrhea, and glossitis. As pellagra progresses, psychoses (eg, hallucinations, disorientation) often occur. The condition may be complicated by thiamine deficiency with associated peripheral neuritis. The macrocytic anemia that sometimes accompanies pellagra probably is related to concomitant folic acid deficiency. Therefore, patients treated for pellagra also should receive small doses of all B-complex vitamins and consume a well-balanced diet with adequate protein to provide tryptophan.

Pellagra may be associated with isoniazid therapy (competitive inhibition of niacin incorporation into NAD), carcinoid syndrome (deviation of precursor tryptophan for conversion by tumor to serotonin), Hartnup disease (a genetic disorder characterized by impaired absorption of tryptophan), or hepatic cirrhosis (decreased hepatic dehydrogenases leading to decreased niacin activity).

OTHER USES. The vasodilating effect of niacin is of doubtful therapeutic value (see Chapter 26, Agents Used in Miscellaneous Cardiovascular Disorders). The large doses used in psychiatric disorders lack any beneficial effect (Petrie and Ban, 1985). Niacin (but not niacinamide) reduces blood lipid levels, although adverse effects may limit its usefulness (see Chapter 50, Agents Used to Treat Hyperlipidemia).

ADVERSE REACTIONS. Therapeutic doses of niacin may cause pruritus, flushing, headache, paresthesias, nausea, and other symptoms of gastrointestinal irritation. Large doses may activate peptic ulcer, impair glucose tolerance, or produce liver damage and hyperuricemia. These reactions are usually reversible when therapy is discontinued. Rarely, anaphylaxis has been reported following intravenous administration.

DOSAGE AND PREPARATIONS.

Oral (preferred): For pellagra, *adults,* initially, 300 to 500 mg niacinamide daily in divided doses; *children,* initially, 100 to 300 mg daily in divided doses. For maintenance, a preparation containing RDA amounts of niacinamide, thiamine, riboflavin, and pyridoxine should be given daily. Associated anemia may require the use of iron, folic acid, or vitamin B_{12}. For less severe deficiency, 50 to 100 mg daily.

As dietary supplement, 10 to 20 mg daily.

Intravenous (preferred parenteral route): For pellagra, initially, 25 to 100 mg niacinamide every two or three hours to a maximum of 1 g/day. The vitamin must be given very slowly at a concentration of no more than 10 mg/ml or it may be diluted in 500 ml of 0.9% sodium chloride injection and given at a rate of 2 mg/min. The oral route and a well-balanced diet should be initiated as soon as possible.

Intramuscular: For pellagra, *adults and children,* 50 to 100 mg niacinamide daily in five or more divided doses.

NIACIN:
Generic, Nicotinic Acid. Capsules (timed-release) 125, 250, and 400 mg; tablets 50, 100 (nonprescription), and 500 mg; solution

(injection, sodium salt) 50 mg/ml in 2 ml containers and 100 mg/ml in 30 ml containers.
Nicobid (Armour). Capsules (timed-release) 125, 250, and 500 mg (nonprescription).
Nico-400 (Marion). Capsules (timed-release) 400 mg (nonprescription).
Nicotinex (Fleming). Elixir 50 mg/5 ml (alcohol 14%) (nonprescription).
NIACINAMIDE (Nicotinamide):
Generic. Tablets 50, 100, and 500 mg (nonprescription); solution (injection) 100 mg/ml in 30 ml containers.

PANTOTHENIC ACID

As a precursor of coenzyme A, pantothenic acid is essential in the intermediary metabolism of fats, carbohydrates, and proteins and in the synthesis of steroids, porphyrins, acetylcholine, and other substances. The RDA has not been established, but a daily intake of 4 to 7 mg is recommended for adults. A balanced diet containing 2,500 calories supplies about 10 mg.

Spontaneous clinical deficiency has not been observed, presumably because pantothenic acid is present in almost all plant and animal tissues and also is produced by intestinal bacteria. Deficiency is unlikely except in association with other B-vitamin deficiencies (eg, pellagra, beriberi, alcoholism), and there is no indication for use of this vitamin alone.

Large doses are ineffective in the prevention or treatment of graying hair, adynamic ileus, diabetic neuropathy, or psychiatric states.

Pantothenic acid is largely nontoxic, although large doses reportedly cause liver disease in rats.

DOSAGE AND PREPARATIONS.
Oral: Pantothenic acid is considered suitable for inclusion in multivitamin preparations in amounts of 5 to 20 mg.

PYRIDOXINE HYDROCHLORIDE (Vitamin B₆)

The vitamin B₆ group is composed of three compounds (pyridoxine, pyridoxal, pyridoxamine) that are metabolically and functionally interrelated. These compounds are converted to pyridoxal phosphate and, to a lesser extent, pyridoxamine phosphate, which function principally in protein and amino acid metabolism (eg, as coenzymes for decarboxylations or transaminations).

REQUIREMENTS. The requirement for pyridoxine appears to parallel protein intake (approximately 0.02 mg/g of protein compound). Most balanced diets provide adequate amounts, but home-prepared artificial formulas for infants should be fortified with pyridoxine. Intake must be increased during pregnancy and lactation and in some women taking oral contraceptives.

DEFICIENCY. Dietary deficiency is rare except in combination with other vitamin B-complex deficiencies (eg, in alcoholism, malabsorption syndromes). However, inadequate utilization of pyridoxine due to inborn errors of metabolism has been implicated in pyridoxine-dependent seizures, pyridoxine-responsive anemia, homocystinuria, xanthinuric aciduria, and cystathioninuria. Pyridoxine-dependent seizures should be considered in all infants with intractable convulsions. The proposed biochemical pathology is decreased affinity of the enzyme, glutamic acid decarboxylase, which converts glutamic acid to GABA, for pyridoxal phosphate. Thus, larger than usual amounts of pyridoxine are required to overcome the depressed enzyme binding and maintain normal GABA, an inhibitory neurotransmitter, in the central nervous system.

USES. Pyridoxine-responsive anemia (usually sideroblastic) is uncommon and may occur in patients without deficiency. It cannot be induced in normal persons either by deficiency in the diet or administration of pyridoxine antagonists. Therefore, a genetic defect is presumed to be the cause (see also Chapter 32, Agents Used to Treat Deficiency Anemias).

Pyridoxine is indicated to prevent or treat peripheral neuritis caused by certain drugs (eg, isoniazid, cycloserine, hydralazine, penicillamine) that act as pyridoxine antagonists and/or increase its excretion in the urine. Pyridoxine may be given prophylactically in doses 300% to 500% higher than the RDA during therapy with pyridoxine antagonists.

Patients with homocystinuria, xanthinuric aciduria, and cystathioninuria require large doses of pyridoxine to overcome inborn errors of metabolism.

This agent has been reported to improve symptoms, such as cheilosis, seborrheic dermatitis, glossitis, and stomatitis, that do not respond to thiamine, riboflavin, and niacin and to relieve the symptoms associated with premenstrual tension.

ADVERSE REACTIONS. Pyridoxine can cause sensory neuropathy or neuropathic syndromes when given in doses exceeding 500 mg to 2 g daily over prolonged periods (Schaumburg et al, 1983; Berger and Schaumberg, 1984). The initial findings are unstable gait and numb feet, followed by numbness and awkwardness of the hands and perioral numbness. Pinprick and temperature sensations are less affected. Symptoms gradually resolve over a period of months once the intake of pyridoxine is stopped.

DRUG INTERACTIONS. Pyridoxine supplements should not be given to patients receiving levodopa, because the action of the latter is antagonized. However, this vitamin may be used concurrently with a preparation containing both carbidopa and levodopa.

Pyridoxine 80 to 400 mg daily has been reported to enhance the hepatic metabolism of phenobarbital or phenytoin by 40% to 50% in some patients, which reduces serum drug concentrations. These findings have not been substantiated.

DOSAGE AND PREPARATIONS.
Oral (preferred), Intramuscular, Intravenous: In pyridoxine dependency syndromes, *infants,* 2 to 15 mg daily; *adults and children,* 10 to 250 mg daily. For drug-induced peripheral

neuritis, *adults and children,* 50 to 200 mg daily. For prophylaxis in patients taking drugs that affect pyridoxine disposition, 25 to 50 mg daily. For deficiency, *adults and children,* 5 to 25 mg daily for three weeks, followed by 1.5 to 2.5 mg daily in a multivitamin preparation for maintenance. During pregnancy and lactation, same dose as for deficiency.

Generic. Solution (injection) 100 mg/ml in 10 and 30 ml containers; tablets 5, 10, 25, 50, 100, 200, 250, and 500 mg (nonprescription).

Hexa-Betalin (Lilly). Solution (injection) 100 mg/ml in 10 ml containers.

RIBOFLAVIN (Vitamin B₂)

FUNCTIONS AND REQUIREMENTS. Riboflavin functions as the coenzyme for flavin adenine dinucleotide (FAD) and flavin mononucleotide (FMN), which primarily influence hydrogen transport in oxidative enzyme systems (eg, cytochrome C reductase, succinic dehydrogenase, xanthine oxidase).

This vitamin is readily absorbed from the intestine and is distributed to all tissues, but little is stored. A well-balanced diet provides adequate amounts for normal individuals. A minimum of 1.2 mg/day is recommended for persons with low caloric intake. Requirements parallel carbohydrate intake and are increased during pregnancy, lactation, and possibly in women taking oral contraceptives. The requirement also is reported to be increased by prolonged administration of phenothiazines and derivatives or tricyclic antidepressants.

DEFICIENCY. Ariboflavinosis is characterized by cheilosis, angular stomatitis, glossitis, seborrheic dermatitis of the nose and scrotum, and corneal vascularization (injection and proliferation of capillaries in the limbic plexus). Ocular symptoms include pruritus, burning, blepharospasm, photophobia, and visual impairment. The lesions of the skin and mucous membranes also are noted in other B-complex deficiencies.

Riboflavin deficiency seldom occurs alone; it often is associated with pellagra and other vitamin B-complex deficiency states (eg, alcoholism, malabsorption syndromes). Therefore, ariboflavinosis should be treated with multivitamin B preparations.

There is no acceptable evidence that riboflavin has any effect other than in the treatment or prevention of its deficiency state. No toxic effects have been reported clinically.

DOSAGE AND PREPARATIONS.

Oral: For deficiency, 5 to 25 mg daily, preferably in a preparation containing the other B-complex vitamins.

Generic. Tablets 5, 10, and 25 mg (nonprescription).

THIAMINE HYDROCHLORIDE (Vitamin B₁)

Thiamine is an essential coenzyme for carbohydrate metabolism. Requirements parallel caloric intake, particularly of carbohydrate, and are increased during pregnancy and lactation.

DEFICIENCY. Thiamine deficiency occurs in the United States, although severe deficiency (beriberi) is relatively rare. Mild deficiency may occur even with apparently adequate diets, especially when energy needs are increased (eg, in hyperthyroidism, during heavy manual labor). Elderly persons should maintain an intake of 1 mg/day, for impaired utilization of thiamine has been reported in this age group.

Beriberi is most common in alcoholics, in pregnant women receiving inadequate diets, or in patients with malabsorption syndromes, prolonged diarrhea, or hepatic diseases causing defective utilization of thiamine. Beriberi has two principal forms: (1) chronic dry beriberi characterized mainly by polyneuropathy, and (2) acute wet beriberi, in which edema and serous effusions predominate.

Chronic dry beriberi occurs most often in adults and usually is associated with malabsorption or multiple vitamin deficiencies. It also may occur during long-term dialysis or parenteral feeding. In chronic alcoholism with associated malnutrition, Wernicke's encephalopathy may develop. The characteristic symptoms (ophthalmoplegia, ataxia, polyneuropathy, mental deterioration) often are accompanied by Korsakoff syndrome (amnestic confabulatory psychosis). This condition is considered a medical emergency and immediate parenteral administration of thiamine is necessary to limit permanent damage of the central nervous system.

Wet beriberi is endemic in areas where polished, unenriched rice forms a large part of the diet. In adults, it may progress from anorexia, muscle weakness, and personality changes to severe circulatory disturbances with edema and high-output heart failure. Severe deficiency in infants may cause death within 24 hours after the onset of symptoms (anorexia, vomiting, convulsions, cyanosis) unless intensive treatment is begun immediately.

There is no evidence that thiamine is of value for anything other than deficiency. Oral administration corrects most uncomplicated deficiencies, but the parenteral route may be utilized in severe, acute situations. In all individuals, the absorptive capacity is limited; the maximum individual oral dose absorbed probably is 5 mg.

ADVERSE REACTIONS. Thiamine produces no toxic effects when given orally and the excess is excreted rapidly in the urine. Anaphylactoid reactions, a few of which were fatal, have occurred rarely after intravenous administration of large amounts in sensitive patients.

DOSAGE AND PREPARATIONS.

Oral, Intramuscular, Intravenous: For deficiency, 5 to 10 mg three times daily. Larger parenteral doses have been recommended in severe cases, but no satisfactory evidence exists to show that an increased response occurs with doses larger than 30 mg daily. After signs of deficiency have been corrected, the dose should be no greater than the RDA as supplied by correction of the diet, if possible, or by a daily supplement. Unless evidence indicates that the deficiency is clearly one of thiamine alone or a therapeutic test is being employed, administration of a vitamin B-complex preparation is preferred until a well-balanced diet is restored.

> *Generic.* Tablets 5, 10, 25, 50, 100, 250, and 500 mg (nonprescription); elixir 1 mg/5 ml (nonprescription); solution (injection) 100 mg/ml in 1, 2, 10, and 30 ml containers.
>
> **Available Trademark.**
> *Betalin S* (Lilly).
>
> **Similar Preparation.**
> *Thiamine Mononitrate, U.S.P.* Used in some multivitamin preparations.

VITAMIN B₁₂ (Cyanocobalamin)

Vitamin B₁₂ is a generic term for several cobalt-containing compounds. As a component of various coenzymes, it is important in the synthesis of nucleic acid, thereby influencing cell maturation and maintenance of the integrity of neuronal tissue. Animal products are the primary food sources, and dietary deficiencies are rare except in strict vegetarians. Since milk is a relatively good source of vitamin B₁₂, supplementation is unnecessary in infants unless artificial formulas lacking this vitamin are used.

The absorption of vitamin B₁₂ depends upon the presence of sufficient intrinsic factor and calcium ions. Intrinsic factor deficiency causes pernicious anemia, which may be associated with demyelination of the spinal cord, as may occur with any form of vitamin B₁₂ deficiency. Prompt parenteral administration of vitamin B₁₂ prevents progression of neurologic damage. Oral dietary supplements are inadequate to treat this disorder, except in very large doses, and should be reserved for patients in whom pernicious anemia has been ruled out.

Supplemental amounts of vitamin B₁₂ may be necessary during pregnancy and lactation or in vegetarians. A daily intake of 0.15 mcg/100 kcal for all infants receiving commercial formulas is now required. Vitamin B₁₂ should be included in B-complex preparations that also contain folic acid.

See Chapter 32, Agents Used to Treat Deficiency Anemias, for a more detailed discussion of vitamin B₁₂.

MINERALS

Many mineral elements function as essential constituents of enzymes, regulate a variety of physiologic functions (eg, maintenance of osmotic pressure, oxygen transport, muscle contraction, central nervous system integrity), and are required for growth and maintenance of tissues and bones. Some elements (calcium, phosphorus, sodium, potassium, magnesium, sulfur, and chloride) are present in relatively large amounts, while others appear only in trace quantities. Trace elements recognized as essential in man are cobalt (as vitamin B₁₂), copper, fluorine, iodine, iron, zinc, chromium, selenium, manganese, and molybdenum. Because of their effects in experimental animal species, nickel, tin, silicon, and arsenic also are considered essential.

Unless absorption is impaired, severe mineral deficiency is uncommon in the United States, since most minerals (except zinc) are widely distributed in foods. However, iron deficiency is relatively common in infants, children, and women. Marginal zinc and copper deficiencies also occur frequently. A balanced, varied diet supplies adequate amounts of most trace elements, and dietary supplements containing minerals should be used only when there is evidence of deficiency or when demands are known to be increased (eg, during pregnancy and lactation).

Trace element deficiencies may develop during prolonged total parenteral nutrition (TPN). The suggested daily intravenous dose of trace minerals for maintenance of adults in stable condition is zinc 2.5 to 4 mg, copper 0.5 to 1.5 mg, chromium 10 to 15 mcg, manganese 0.15 to 0.8 mg, iron 1 mg, and iodine 75 mcg. For administration of potassium, magnesium, calcium, and phosphorus, see Chapter 48, Parenteral and Enteral Nutrition. Minerals should be given routinely when the need for supplementation is anticipated (eg, patients with Crohn's disease, ileal bypass surgery or other resections, malabsorption syndromes). In patients with renal disease or biliary tract obstruction, caution is necessary to avoid excessive dosage.

Minerals Present in Relatively Large Amounts

Calcium: This element is present in the body in greater amounts than any other mineral. Its metabolism, functions, and uses are discussed in Chapter 49, Agents Affecting Calcium Metabolism.

Vitamin D is required for efficient absorption of calcium. Quantities of calcium greater than those required to maintain equilibrium have no beneficial effects. Dietary requirements are increased in growing children, during pregnancy and lactation, and in postmenopausal women. Infants fed artificial formulas require supplementation. Intake of calcium also should be increased when high-protein and/or high-phosphorus diets are consumed. Various investigators have suggested intake of approximately 1.2 g/day of calcium for alcoholics, patients with malabsorption syndromes, and those receiving corticosteroids, isoniazid, tetracycline, or aluminum-containing antacids.

Magnesium: Magnesium activates many enzyme systems (alkaline phosphatase, enolases, leucine aminopeptidase) and is an essential cofactor in oxidative phosphorylation, thermoregulation, muscular contractility, and nerve excitability. Deficiency is uncommon in normal individuals eating a varied diet, but the requirement for magnesium parallels the amount of protein, calcium, and phosphorus ingested.

Hypomagnesemia increases neuronal excitability and neuromuscular transmission; severe deficiency may result in tetany and convulsions. Hypomagnesemia has been observed in alcoholics; in patients with kwashiorkor, infantile tetany, diabetes, malabsorption syndromes, hyper- or hypoparathyroidism, and renal diseases; during diuretic therapy; in burn patients treated with daily saline baths; in patients receiving total parenteral nutrition without adequate magnesium supplements; in patients receiving cisplatin [Platinol]; and postoperatively.

Hypermagnesemia produces peripheral vasodilation and loss of tendon reflexes; it has a curare-like effect at the myoneural junction and blocks release of catecholamine from the adrenal glands. Respiratory failure and cardiac arrest occur after very large doses.

For a more detailed discussion of magnesium imbalances, see Chapter 46, Replenishers and Regulators of Water and Electrolytes.

Phosphorus: This mineral is necessary for utilization of many B-complex vitamins. It is present in bones and teeth in amounts nearly equal to those of calcium, is a prominent component of all body tissues, and is very important as a buffer in body fluids. Lipids, proteins, carbohydrates, and various enzymes involved in energy transfer contain phosphorus.

A varied diet supplies sufficient phosphorus. The calcium:phosphorus ratio also is important. If an appropriate amount of vitamin D is ingested, diets supplying excess phosphorus in relation to calcium are tolerated. Deficiency does not occur in adults unless there is prolonged excessive use of alcohol or nonabsorbable antacids, prolonged vomiting, liver disease, or, less commonly, hyperparathyroidism.

For further discussion of the therapeutic use of phosphorus, see Chapter 49, Agents Affecting Calcium Metabolism.

Potassium: The differential concentration of potassium (the principal cation of intracellular fluid) and sodium (the principal cation of extracellular fluid) across the cell wall regulates the excitability of the cell, nerve impulse conduction, and body fluid balance and volume.

Although dietary deficiency is rare in individuals consuming an adequate diet, hypokalemia may occur in children whose diet lacks protein. The most common cause of hypokalemia is diuretic therapy, especially when thiazides or furosemide are given. Other causes of hypokalemia include prolonged diarrhea, particularly in infants; hyperaldosteronism; inappropriate

or inadequate parenteral fluid therapy; and long-term use of adrenal corticosteroids or laxatives. The most serious consequences of hypokalemia are neuromuscular disorders that may progress to areflexic paralysis of the skeleton, gut, and heart.

Hyperkalemia most commonly is caused by impaired renal excretion of potassium, which may occur in patients with adrenocortical insufficiency, acute renal failure, or terminal chronic renal failure; inappropriate vitamin K supplementation; or use of aldosterone antagonists. Severe arrhythmias and conduction defects are the most serious sequelae. Other manifestations include weakness and paresthesias.

For the therapeutic uses of potassium, see Chapter 29, Diuretics, and Chapter 46, Replenishers and Regulators of Water and Electrolytes.

Sodium: Sodium helps to maintain fluid balance and volume. Its concentration in body fluids is under homeostatic control. Imbalances occur only when these mechanisms fail or losses are greater than the compensatory abilities of adaptive mechanisms. Sodium often is added during the processing of food. Most individuals consume more sodium than necessary. Dietary restriction often is recommended in patients with congestive heart failure, hepatic cirrhosis, and hypertension. Intake of less than usual amounts of sodium starting in childhood and continuing throughout adult life may aid in preventing hypertension in susceptible individuals. However, dietary restriction of sodium in healthy women during pregnancy is not recommended.

Hyponatremia is encountered rarely in normal individuals but may occur after prolonged diarrhea or vomiting, particularly in infants; in renal disorders, cystic fibrosis, or adrenocortical insufficiency; or with use of diuretics. Excessive sweating may cause pronounced sodium loss, and replacement therapy should include both water and sodium chloride.

Chloride: Chloride is the most important anion in the maintenance of electrolyte balance. Hypochloremic metabolic alkalosis may develop following prolonged vomiting or excessive use of diuretics. Excessive loss may accompany excessive loss of sodium and, when sodium intake is curtailed, substitution of another source of chloride may be necessary. If potassium chloride is used, the possibility of hyperkalemia and its associated dangers should be considered.

Sulfur: Several essential amino acids, thiamine, and biotin contain sulfur. Although this mineral is known to be essential for man, its precise function other than as an atom in the above essential molecules is not known and no daily requirements have been established.

Trace Elements

Chromium: Trivalent chromium plays a role in a cofactor complex for insulin and thus is involved in normal glucose utilization. The organic form of chromium exists in a dinicotino-glutathionine complex in natural foods and appears to be absorbed better than the inorganic form.

Deficiency has been reported in a few patients receiving total parenteral nutrition for five months to three years. These patients had peripheral neuropathy and/or encephalopathy that was alleviated by administration of chromium 150 mcg daily. Symptoms included a diabetes-like condition with impaired utilization of glucose. Other patients with similar symptoms of glucose intolerance also had protein-calorie malnutrition.

Marginal levels of chromium have been associated with decreased glucose utilization during pregnancy and in the elderly. In these patients, administration of the metal improved glucose tolerance. However, the clinical significance of these findings requires further clarification. Supplemental amounts of chromium do not have a hypoglycemic effect in normal individuals. Excessive chromium is toxic.

Cobalt: Cobalt is a component of vitamin B_{12}; it has no other known function in human nutrition. The daily requirement is easily obtained from a balanced, varied diet.

Cobalt salts have been used with dubious success to treat certain types of anemias refractory to other therapy; they appear to act via selective toxicity. In massive doses (ie, 20 mg to 30 mg daily), cobalt can produce polycythemia, thyroid hyperplasia, and cardiomyopathy.

Copper: Copper is absorbed in the proximal portion of the small intestine and then transported to the liver bound loosely to albumin and other proteins. In the liver, copper is incorporated into ceruloplasmin, its major blood carrier protein. Copper is an essential component of a number of proteins (eg, erythrocuprein, hepatocuprein) and enzymes (eg, lysyl, hydroxylase, dopamine beta-hydroxylase). This mineral is thought to act as a catalyst in the storage and release of iron to form hemoglobin. It is believed to be essential for connective tissue formation, hematopoiesis, and central nervous system function.

Most unprocessed foods are excellent sources of copper and deficiency was thought to be rare. However, a typical American diet may supply only one-half the RDA for copper (Patterson et al, 1984). Copper deficiency has also been reported in malnourished children with anemia and neutropenia. Hypocupremia has been observed in adults with sickle cell anemia who received large doses of zinc for several months. In addition, the administration of zinc in doses slightly in excess of the RDA reduces the absorption of copper and increases its fecal excretion (Festa et al, 1985). Competitive inhibition of copper by iron and certain sugars has been demonstrated in experimental animals and possibly in a premature infant receiving an iron-fortified formula.

Copper supplements should be given during prolonged parenteral or enteral alimentation: The intravenous dose for adults is 0.3 mg, and that for children is 0.2 mg daily.

Hypocupremia unrelated to nutritional factors may result from reduced or defective formation of ceruloplasmin; this occurs in newborn infants (especially premature infants) and in the rare genetic disorder, Wilson's disease (hepatolenticular degeneration). In Menkes' syndrome (kinky hair disease), an inherited disease, there is abnormal copper transport by intestinal cells. Although hypocupremia has been observed in patients with protein-calorie malnutrition, tropical sprue, celiac disease, and nephrotic syndrome, it is thought to be secondary to disturbances of protein metabolism with loss of copper-protein complexes.

Elevated serum levels of copper occur in various diseases and are produced by some drugs (eg, estrogens, thyroid, corticotropin), but associated abnormalities are rare. Acute toxicity has occurred following the oral ingestion of as little as 10 to 15 mg of inorganic copper and may be manifested by nausea and vomiting, epigastric pain, diarrhea, malaise, and, in more severe poisoning, acute hemolysis and renal tubular disorders. For the treatment of hypercupremia, see the evaluation on Penicillamine in Chapter 80, Drugs Used in the Treatment of Poisoning.

Fluoride: Fluoride is incorporated into teeth and decreases the incidence of dental caries, especially in children. There is evidence that it also aids in retention of calcium in bones. However, evidence regarding fluoride supplementation as a means of preventing or alleviating bone diseases, such as osteoporosis, especially in the elderly, remains controversial. (See Chapter 49, Agents Affecting Calcium Metabolism.) The need for fluoride persists throughout life.

Fluoridation of the water supply (optimum concentration, 0.7 to 1.2 ppm) is the most efficient and economical method of assuring adequate intake. For maximal anticariogenic effects, fluoride should be ingested daily from birth throughout life. Dietary supplements should be used only when water supplies contain less than 0.7 ppm, and the dose should be adjusted according to the amount of fluoride in the water (see Table 3). Approximately one-half the daily dose is recommended when drinking water contains between 0.3 and 0.7 ppm fluoride. Use of fluoride should be reviewed if the family moves or when the fluoride content of the water changes. In trace quantities, fluoride is a nutrient; in large quantities, it is a poison.

Chronic toxicity (fluorosis) usually results from prolonged exposure to insecticides or industrial dusts or from prolonged daily ingestion of water containing more than 4 ppm. Mottled enamel (dental fluorosis) may occur if teeth are developing, and osteomalacia and osteosclerosis may be induced in older people. Considerable mottling of teeth and bone disorders occur when more than 8 ppm are present in the water supply or with combined intake from water and fluoride supplements. Except for orthopedic and supportive measures, there is no treatment for fluorosis; therefore, all efforts should be directed at prevention.

Claims that persons residing in areas where water supplies are fluoridated have experienced a higher incidence of cancer have been refuted by the National Cancer Institute (*J Am Diet Assoc*, 1977) and in a more recent review (Clemmesen 1983).

Iodine: Iodine is an integral part of the thyroid hormones, tetraiodothyronine (thyroxine) and triiodothyronine. Deficiency results in compensatory hyperplasia and hypertrophy of the thyroid gland (endemic goiter). Endemic goiter occurs in areas where the soil is deficient in iodine and was common before the iodization of table salt. It no longer appears to be a problem in the United States, where recent nutrition surveys suggest that iodine intake exceeds requirements. Iodate in bread and use of iodophores as antiseptics by the dairy industry are the main source of iodide in most diets. Iodized table salt is another economical and efficient source of iodine. Seafoods are a reliable food source.

Amounts of 100 to 300 mcg daily are desirable and up to 1 mg daily may be consumed safely. Requirements for iodine are increased in growing children and in pregnant or lactating women. However, the prolonged ingestion of large amounts of iodides during pregnancy may result in neonatal thyroid enlargement, hypothyroidism, or cretinism.

Manifestations of acute iodine intoxication are related to the organ systems that incorporate iodine (eg, thyroid gland, salivary apparatus, eye) and include edema, fever, and conjunctivitis. Laryngeal edema resulting in airway obstruction is potentially fatal. Local reactions in the gastrointestinal tract include abdominal pain, vomiting, and diarrhea (sometimes bloody), which may lead to dehydration and shock.

Chronic iodine poisoning (iodism) is more common. There is considerable individual variation in sensitivity to iodine, and 6 mg or more daily may inhibit thyroid activity and lead to development of hypothyroidism. Hypersensitivity reactions include rash and dermatoses (which appear to be dose related), nausea, edema of the face and eyes, headache, cough, and gastric irritation.

For therapeutic use of iodine, see Chapter 44, Agents Used to Treat Thyroid Disease, and Chapter 56, Dermatologic Preparations.

Iron: Ionic iron is an essential component of a number of enzymes necessary for energy transfer and also is present in compounds required for oxygen transport and utilization. On the average, 10% of inorganic and food iron is absorbed when given orally; increased absorption (up to 20%) occurs in iron-deficient individuals. Absorption of nonheme iron also is increased by concomitant use of ascorbic acid. Iron from meat (heme iron) is absorbed an average of five times better than that from vegetables (primarily nonheme iron).

Requirements are increased in infants and young children, adolescents, and menstruating, pregnant, and lactating women. They are greatest during infancy and, because of the low iron content of milk, formulas should supply 10 to 15 mg of iron daily during the first year of life. Pregnant women cannot obtain sufficient iron from a normal diet unless large amounts of meat are consumed or iron pots are used for cooking. This deficit can be corrected only by supplementation (usually 30 mg of elemental iron daily). Supplements should be continued for two to three months after parturition to increase iron stores depleted during pregnancy.

Tannins, phosphates, and antacids bind iron in relatively insoluble complexes and thus decrease its absorption, inorganic iron in food also is often bound in these poorly absorbed insoluble complexes.

Bleeding associated with gastrointestinal disease (eg, hemorrhoids, peptic ulcer, ulcerative colitis, neoplasms) frequently produces iron deficiency, and malabsorption of iron may occur in those with tropical sprue or celiac disease, gastrectomy, prolonged diarrhea, or achlorhydria. Deficiency may increase the absorption of other elements, which may lead to chronic lead, cobalt, and manganese poisoning. Copper deficiency decreases iron mobilization and, if uncorrected, causes anemia even in the presence of abundant iron stores, which cannot be adequately utilized. After iron stores in ferritin and hemosiderin are depleted, hemoglobin production is reduced and anemia results. See Chapter 32, Agents Used to Treat Deficiency Anemias.

Excess iron is stored in the liver, kidneys, heart, and other organs, and iron overload can be hazardous, particularly in patients with certain diseases (eg, primary and secondary hemochromatosis, porphyria cutanea tarda). Acute iron poisoning is most common in children under 5 years. Iron-containing medications should be labeled as hazardous, kept out of the reach of children, and packaged in childproof containers. For treatment of iron poisoning, see Chapter 80, Drugs Used in the Treatment of Poisoning.

Manganese: This element is concentrated in cell mitochondria, mostly in the pituitary gland, liver, pancreas, kidney, and bone. It influences the synthesis of mucopolysaccharides, stimulates hepatic synthesis of cholesterol and fatty acids, and is a cofactor in many enzymes, including arginase and alkaline phosphatase in the liver. Manganese is abundant in many foods. Deficiency is unknown clinically, but a daily intake of 2.5 to 5 mg is thought to be safe and adequate for adults. Manganese should be supplemented during long-term total parenteral nutrition.

Chronic manganese intoxication by inhalation is an occupational hazard in mining and industrial areas, although manganese released into the atmosphere from its many industrial uses has not been a general hazard. In cases of exposure, the onset of parkinsonian symptoms is subtle and may progress unless the exposure ends quickly. Levodopa may relieve rigidity or dystonia.

Molybdenum: This element is an essential constituent of many enzymes. It is well absorbed and is present in the bones, liver, and kidneys. Deficiency is rare. Ingestion of 0.15 to 0.5 mg/day for adults has been estimated to be safe and adequate, and this apparently is provided by the usual diet.

Intake of 10 to 15 mg of molybdenum daily has been associated with a gout-like syndrome, and a moderate excess of 0.54 mg/daily may be associated with significant urinary loss of copper. Therefore, ingestion of amounts in excess of normal dietary intake is not recommended.

Selenium: Deficiency of selenium decreases the fertility and survival rates of the offspring of pigs and cattle and causes muscular dystrophy in sheep and cattle, pancreatic degeneration in poultry, and liver necrosis in rats. Glutathione peroxidase, a selenium-dependent enzyme present in most tissues, has peroxidase-destroying capabilities, which explains much of the biological activity of selenium. There appears to be a close relationship between vitamin E and selenium.

Evidence that selenium is an essential trace element in man is provided by a study of Keshan disease (a fatal cardiomyopathy of children and young women) in China. The incidence of this disease is high in children living in areas where selenium levels in the staple food are low. Large-scale selenium supplementation in children has practically abolished Keshan disease. A similar cardiomyopathy has been found in a few patients after long-term parenteral feeding and may be due, at least partially, to selenium deficiency. However, more information is needed before definite requirements are known.

It is assumed that the dietary intake of selenium is adequate, since dietary deficiency has not been encountered in this country. Tolerance in humans has not been determined, but 0.05 to 0.2 mg/day appears to be safe for adults. Its use for either life extension or the prevention of cancer is not supported by currently available data. Selenium is toxic in massive quantities and may cause alopecia, loss of nails, fatigue, nausea, vomiting, and sour-milk breath (Jensen et al, 1984).

Zinc: Zinc is a cofactor for over 100 enzymes and is important in nucleic acid metabolism and protein synthesis. It is necessary for growth, sexual maturation and function (primarily in males), appetite and taste acuity, and wound healing.

The absorption of zinc is a saturable process involving an active transport mechanism facilitated by low-molecular-weight ligands of pancreatic origin. About 20% to 30% of orally administered zinc is absorbed, primarily in the duodenum and proximal small intestine. The percentage absorbed depends upon a number of factors, including the source of the element. Zinc from animals generally is better absorbed than that from plant sources, probably due to the presence of phytates and fiber in plants that bind to zinc in the intestine, thus rendering it unavailable. Phosphates, iron, copper, lead, cadmium, and calcium also inhibit zinc absorption. Absorption is enhanced by pregnancy, corticosteroids, endotoxin, and leukocyte endogenous mediator (Jeejeebhoy, 1984).

Zinc is distributed throughout the body. The highest concentrations appear in the choroid of the eye, spermatozoa, hair, nails, prostate, and bone. In the plasma, most zinc is protein bound, predominately to albumin, alpha 2-macroglobulin, and transferrin. Human breast milk contains about 3 mg/L immediately after delivery, but the concentration tends to decrease over time.

The major route of excretion is intestinal, with fecal loss accounting for approximately two-thirds of the normal dietary intake. Only about 2% of the daily intake is excreted in the urine. Patients with diarrhea or drainage from a stoma or fistula can lose a large amount of zinc that must be replaced.

Zinc deficiency may be due to inadequate dietary intake (eg, debilitated or elderly patients, alcoholics with cirrhosis and poor diets), decreased absorption (eg, malabsorption syndrome, cystic fibrosis), increased excretion (eg, sickle cell disease, major burns, draining fistulas), or an inherited defect in metabolism (ie, acrodermatitis enteropathica). Evidence of marginal to mild deficiency has been found among some groups of children, but severe deficiency in this country probably occurs only secondary to malabsorption syndromes. It has been suggested that maternal zinc deficiency during pregnancy may have teratogenic effects, since malformation and behavioral disturbances have been reported in animal offspring.

Cutaneous manifestations of deficiency resembling acrodermatitis enteropathica have been reported following long-term parenteral nutrition. Patients on total parenteral nutrition should receive zinc supplements (2.5 to 4 mg of elemental zinc as the sulfate added to the solution daily) after about one month of therapy. When enterally administered defined formula diets are the sole source of nutrients, 100% of the RDA for zinc should be given.

Symptoms of deficiency include disturbances in taste and smell, anorexia, and suboptimal growth in children. More severe deficiency results in delayed bone maturation, hepatosplenomegaly, hypogonadism, testicular hypofunction, and decreased growth or dwarfism. Other manifestations are alopecia, rashes, multiple cutaneous lesions, glossitis, stomatitis, blepharitis, and paronychia.

Gonadal dysfunction and impotence in patients with renal disease can sometimes be corrected partially by administering zinc.

During dialysis, zinc chloride may be added to the dialysate in sufficient quantities (400 mcg/L) to maintain the plasma concentrations between 100 and 150 mg/dl.

Evidence suggesting that zinc may promote healing of wounds or chronic ulcers is controversial; accelerated healing following zinc administration probably occurs only in those with deficiency.

Plasma concentrations of zinc may be decreased in patients with acute or chronic infection, myocardial infarction, neoplastic disease, alcoholism with liver disease, and pernicious or sickle cell anemia.

Increased concentrations of zinc may occur in those with hypertension, hyperthyroidism, or polycythemia and following irradiation.

Zinc is notable for its large margin of safety. In one case, oral ingestion of 12 g of elemental zinc (800 times the RDA) resulted only in pronounced lethargy. Doses required to treat zinc deficiency (ie, elemental zinc 1 mg/kg/day) cause essentially no adverse reactions. However, ingestion of excessive doses for prolonged periods is not recommended. High concentrations alter the immune response by inhibiting neutrophil migration and accumulation. Excessive intake also may induce copper and iron deficiency by interfering with their absorption and utilization and may cause nausea, vomiting, headache, chills, fever, malaise, and abdominal pain (*Med Lett Drugs Ther*, 1978).

Miscellaneous Elements: Deficiencies of elements such as nickel, tin, silicon, and vanadium have been produced in animals under rigid experimental conditions, but their importance in human nutrition is unknown.

MULTIVITAMIN PREPARATIONS WITH OR WITHOUT MINERALS

Clinically apparent vitamin deficiencies are rare in the United States, and subclinical deficiencies are difficult to detect. Excessive use of one or more vitamins may cause relative deficiencies of other essential micronutrients, and large doses of all minerals, fat-soluble vitamins, and some water-soluble vitamins are toxic. Also, multivitamin preparations used by adequately nourished individuals may grossly exceed nutrient needs and represent unnecessary expense.

When needed, properly formulated multivitamin preparations are useful, since clinical vitamin deficiencies are frequently multiple. Such preparations should contain only those ingredients essential for human nutrition in amounts proportional to the U.S. RDA. Additional components, such as liver, yeast, and wheat germ, do not confer any special advantage over the pure chemical ingredients, and inclusion of agents that have no proved value (eg, choline, methionine, lecithin, bioflavonoids, inositol) is unwarranted. The amount of vitamin D in the preparation should not exceed the U.S. RDA (10 mcg, 400 IU) because of the dangers of hypervitaminosis D. Quantities of folic acid should not exceed the U.S. RDA. Although excessive amounts produce a satisfactory hematologic response in pernicious anemia, they do not prevent progression

TABLE 5.
SUGGESTED COMPOSITION FOR INTRAVENOUS MULTIVITAMIN FORMULATIONS

Vitamin[1]	Units of Measurement	Infants/Children (<11 years)	Adults
A	RE[2] (IU)	690 (2,300)	990 (3,300)
D	mcg[3] (IU)	10 (400)	5 (200)
E	mg[4] (IU)	4.7 (7)	6.7 (10)
K₁ (Phylloquinone)	mg	0.2	—
Ascorbic Acid	mg	80	100
Folacin	mg	0.14	0.4
Niacin	mg	17	40
Riboflavin	mg	1.4	3.6
Thiamin	mg	1.2	3.0
B₆ (Pyridoxine)	mg	1.0	4.0
B₁₂ (Cyanocobalamin)	mcg	1.0	5.0
Pantothenic Acid	mg	5.0	15.0
Biotin	mcg	20.0	60.0

[1] *May be provided in appropriate salt or ester form in equivalent potency*
[2] *RE: = Retinol Equivalents (1 RE = 3.33 IU vitamin A)*
[3] *As cholecalciferol (10 mcg cholecalciferol = 400 IU vitamin D)*
[4] *As d-alpha tocopherol (1 mg d-alpha tocopherol = 1.5 IU vitamin E)*

of the neurologic symptoms of this disorder and, in fact, may mask these symptoms, rendering diagnosis difficult.

Caution is necessary when selecting multivitamin preparations because many manufacturers use the same general trademark for several preparations having very different formulas. Additionally, some manufacturers make drastic changes in product formulation while maintaining the same trademark. Until multivitamin preparations are brought into greater conformity with current nutritional knowledge, the physician should make an effort to prescribe only those having a rational quantitative basis. There seems to be little logic in a formulation containing less than 50% of the U.S. RDA for some vitamins and more than 500% of the U.S. RDA for others (particularly the interrelated B vitamins). Dosage should take into account the contribution of the patient's diet, especially vitamins A and D and all minerals.

Supplemental Multivitamin Preparations (With or Without Minerals)

Prophylactic multivitamin preparations may reasonably contain 50% to 150% of the U.S. RDA (except that vitamin D should not exceed the U.S. RDA) and should be chosen to fit the needs of the individual. These preparations may be useful during periods of increased requirements (eg, pregnancy, lactation), during relatively brief illnesses that impair absorption of nutrients, and in patients who are not eating properly. They should be discontinued after recovery or when correction of the diet has been assured. Preparations containing 150% of the U.S. RDA may be useful to supplement therapeutic, but nutritionally inadequate, diets (eg, in allergy) or when food intake is reduced drastically (eg, in rapid weight reduction programs, during prolonged illness). During pregnancy and lactation, supplemental preparations should contain folic acid, cyanocobalamin, and iron, for these nutrients probably cannot be supplied adequately by the diet.

Supplemental amounts of a particular vitamin are sometimes contraindicated. For example, vitamin D supplements should be avoided in individuals, especially infants and children, who have adequate exposure to sunlight or a normal diet. Pyridoxine may interfere with the effectiveness of levodopa in the treatment of parkinsonism and, therefore, amounts exceeding the U.S. RDA should be avoided in these patients.

The individual preparations are not listed because the formulations are often changed by the manufacturers, frequently without notice, while the tradenames are unaltered.

Therapeutic Multivitamin Preparations (With or Without Minerals)

Therapeutic multivitamin preparations should be labeled as such and prescribed only to treat deficiency states and for supportive therapy in pathologic conditions that markedly increase nutritional requirements (eg, alcoholism, postoperative cachexia). *They should not be used as dietary supplements,* and medical supervision is important when such amounts are administered.

Multivitamin preparations for therapeutic use may contain as much as five times the U.S. RDA. If the required dose for a vitamin exceeds 500% of the U.S. RDA, that vitamin should be given separately. Therapeutic multivitamin preparations should not contain more than the U.S. RDA of vitamin D. In addition, the intake of vitamin A must be limited in order to avoid hypervitaminosis A.

Multivitamin preparations for parenteral administration are essential during long-term total parenteral nutrition (TPN) or to treat conditions in which oral intake or absorption of vitamins is inadequate. Guidelines for formulations of intravenously administered vitamins were established by an Expert Panel of the Nutrition Advisory Group, AMA Department of Foods and Nutrition in December, 1975 (see Table 5). It was recommended that a pediatric formulation be prepared for infants and children to age 10 and an adult formulation be prepared for those age 11 and older.

The preparations used during TPN should be incorporated into daily intravenous feedings and include the fat-soluble vitamins. When parenteral administration is necessary in other conditions, intramuscular injection is usually preferred. For intramuscular use, the same formulation shown in Table 5 for water-soluble vitamins only is recommended; when the fat-soluble vitamins are also needed, they should be given separately as single entities in an appropriate form for intramuscular administration. The fat-soluble vitamins are not indicated for routine use except in patients with specific deficiencies.

Ideally, all essential minerals should be included during long-term TPN. The following should be added to intravenous alimentation fluids or given as separate intravenous injections at appropriate intervals: iron, iodine, cobalt (as vitamin B_{12}), zinc, copper, chromium, selenium, and manganese. The dose should be based on the patient's age and clinical and metabolic status.

Daily doses suggested for stable adults by the Expert Panel are zinc 2.5 to 4 mg, copper 0.5 to 1.5 mg, chromium 10 to 15 mcg, selenium 50 to 200 mcg, and manganese 0.15 to 0.8 mg. Frequent monitoring of blood levels and adjustment of dose are essential. (See also Chapter 48, Parenteral and Enteral Nutrition.) Other clinicians suggest that iron 1 to 5 mg and iodine 70 to 150 mcg be given daily or that appropriate doses be given once weekly if desired.

Cited References

Fluoride compounds, in: *Accepted Dental Therapeutics,* ed 40. Chicago, American Dental Association, 1984, 395-420.

National nutrition consortium endorses fluoridation. *J Am Diet Assoc* 10:354, 1977.

Recommended Dietary Allowances, ed 9. Washington, DC, National Academy of Sciences, 1980.

Vitamin A; proposed affirmation of Gras status as direct human food ingredient. *Federal Register* 48:1745-1758, (Jan 14) 1983.

Zinc. *Med Lett Drugs Ther* 20:57-59, 1978.

Balcke P, et al: Ascorbic acid aggravates secondary hyperoxalemia in patients on chronic hemodialysis. *Ann Intern Med* 101:344-345, 1984.

Beeson PB, et al (eds): Diseases of nutrition. *Textbook of Medicine,* ed 15. Philadelphia, WB Saunders, 1979, 1670-1691.

Berger A, Schaumburg HH: More on neuropathy from pyridoxine abuse, (letter). *N Engl J Med* 311:986-987, 1984.

Bieri JG, et al: Medical uses of vitamin E. *N Engl J Med* 308:1063-1071, 1983.

Campbell GD Jr, et al: Ascorbic acid-induced hemolysis in G-6-PD deficiency. *Ann Intern Med* 82:810, 1975.

Clemmesen J: Alleged association between artificial fluoridation of water supplies and cancer: Review. *Bull WHO* 61:871-883, 1983.

Committee on Nutrition, American Academy of Pediatrics: Vitamin and mineral supplementation in normal children in the United States. *Pediatrics* 66:1015-1021, 1980.

Dwyer J: Nutritional support during pregnancy and lactation. *Primary Care* 9:475-496, 1982.

Festa MD, et al: Effect of zinc intake on copper excretion and retention in man. *Am J Clin Nutr* 41:285-292, 1985.

Fong T: Problems associated with megadose vitamin C therapy, (letter). *West J Med* 134:264, 1981.

Haeger K: Long-term study of alpha-tocopherol in intermittent claudication. *Ann NY Acad Sci* 82:369-375, 1982.

Hayes KC, Hegsted DM: Toxicity of vitamins, in *Toxicants Occurring Naturally in Foods,* ed 2. Washington, DC, National Academy of Sciences, 1973, 235-253.

Herbert V: Pangamic acid ("vitamin B_{15}"). *Am J Clin Nutr* 32:1534-1540, 1979.

Herbert V: The vitamin craze. *Arch Intern Med* 140:173-176, 1980.

Herbert V: Toxicity of 25,000 IU vitamin A supplements in "health" food users. *Am J Clin Nutr* 36:185-186, 1982.

Hittner HM, et al: Retrolental fibroplasia: Efficacy of vitamin E in double-blind clinical study of preterm infants. *N Engl J Med* 305:1365-1371, 1981.

Hittner HM, et al: Retrolental fibroplasia and vitamin E in preterm infant: Comparison of oral versus intramuscular:oral administration. *Pediatrics* 73:238-249, 1984.

Jeejeebhoy KN: Zinc and chromium in parenteral nutrition. *Bull NY Acad Med* 60:118-124, 1984.

Jensen R, et al: Selenium intoxication: New York. *Morbid Mortal Week Rep* 33:157-158, 1984.

Kligman AM, et al: Oral vitamin A in acne vulgaris: Preliminary report. *Int J Dermatol* 20:278-285, 1981.

Lewis JG: Adverse reactions to vitamins. *Adverse Drug React Bull* 82:296-299, (June) 1980.

Marshall CW: *Vitamins and Minerals: Help or Harm?* Philadelphia, Stickley, 1983.

Moertel CG, et al: Clinical trial of amygdalin (Laetrile) in treatment of human cancer. *N Engl J Med* 306:201-206, 1982.

Moertel CG, et al: High-dose vitamin C versus placebo in treatment of patients with advanced cancer who have had no prior chemotherapy. *N Engl J Med* 312:137-141, 1985.

Morris JC, et al: Interaction of ethinyloestradiol with ascorbic acid in man, (letter). *Br Med J* 283:503, 1981.

Nyhan WL: Understanding inherited metabolic disease: Treatment. *Clin Symp* 32:30-31, 1980.

Ovesen L: Vitamin therapy in absence of obvious deficiency: What is the evidence? *Drugs* 27:148-170, 1984.

Patterson KY, et al: Zinc, copper, and manganese intake and balance for adults consuming self-selected diets. *Am J Clin Nutr* 40:1397-1403, 1984.

Petrie WM, Ban TA: Vitamins in psychiatry: Do they have a role? *Drugs* 30:58-65, 1985.

Reuter H, Hellriegel KP: Vitamins, in Dukes MNG (eds): *Side Effects of Drugs Annual 7*. Amsterdam, Excerpta Medica, 1983, 370-373.

Sauberlich HE: Ascorbic acid, in *Nutrition Reviews' Present Knowledge in Nutrition*, ed 5. Washington, DC, The Nutrition Foundation, 1984, 260-272.

Schaumberg H, et al: Sensory neuropathy from pyridoxine abuse: New megavitamin syndrome. *N Engl N Med* 309:445-448, 1983.

Schwartz RD, et al: Hyperoxaluria and renal insufficiency due to ascorbic acid administration during total parenteral nutrition. *Ann Intern Med* 100:530-531, 1984.

Tsang RC: Quandary of vitamin D in newborn infant. *Lancet* 1:1370-1372, 1983.

Wagner C: Folic acid, in *Nutrition Reviews' Present Knowledge in Nutrition*, ed 5. Washington, DC, The Nutrition Foundation, 1984, 332-346.

Other Selected References

Committee on Nutrition, American Academy of Pediatrics: *Pediatric Nutrition Handbook*, ed 2. American Academy of Pediatrics, Elk Grove Village, IL, 1985.

DeLuca HF: Vitamin D endocrinology. *Ann Intern Med* 85:367-377, 1976.

Goodhart RS, Shils ME (eds): *Modern Nutrition in Health and Disease*, ed 6. Philadelphia, Lea & Febiger, 1980.

Herbert V: *Nutrition Cultism: Facts and Fictions*. Philadelphia, Stickley, 1981.

Herbert V, Barrett S: *Vitamins and "Health" Foods: The Great American Hustle*. Philadelphia, Stickley, 1981.

James MB, et al: Hypervitaminosis A: Case report. *Pediatrics* 69:112-115,1982.

Memon AS: Role of vitamin C in causation and outcome of cancer. *Res Staff Physician* 30:63-71, 1984.

Schneider HA, et al (eds): *Nutritional Support of Medical Practice*. Philadelphia, Harper & Row, 1977.

Ulmer DD: Trace elements. *N Engl J Med* 297:318-321, 1977.

Parenteral and Enteral Nutrition

The products discussed in this chapter are used to supply nutrients to patients unable to ingest and absorb amounts adequate to meet their fluid, mineral, caloric, and protein requirements. In addition, information on formulas for healthy infants is given.

Nutritional support is indicated (1) to correct existing malnutrition; (2) to prevent malnutrition that will occur unless there is intervention (eg, in comatose patients; in those with serious intestinal obstruction, major burns, trauma, severe prolonged infection, or other persistent hypermetabolic states); (3) when bowel rest is required (eg, in those with acute symptomatic inflammatory bowel disease, acute pancreatitis, intestinal fistulae); (4) during the perioperative period; (5) when serious gastrointestinal disturbances occur during cancer chemotherapy or radiotherapy; (6) after massive bowel resection or other disorders resulting in serious malabsorption; and (7) when mechanical problems exist (dysphagia, surgery of the head or neck).

Protein-calorie malnutrition (PCM) occurs in 10% to 50% of patients in city-run hospitals. In the United States, malnutrition generally results from anorexia, increased metabolic rate, and malabsorption rather than from lack of adequate food supplies as in developing countries.

The patient's nutritional status must be evaluated to determine the prognosis and to develop a rational nutritional regimen. A thorough history and physical examination are necessary initially. Measuring nitrogen balance directly or by urinary urea and determining nitrogen excretion initially and at weekly intervals are useful in selected patients. In addition, the following determinations have been recommended: (1) plasma protein concentrations (eg, albumin, transferrin, thyroxine-binding prealbumin), which reflect visceral protein status; (2) creatinine/height index and upper arm muscle circumference, which reflect the status of muscle protein; (3) lymphocyte count and cell-mediated immunity, which indicate immune competence; and (4) triceps skin fold, which is used to estimate fat stores. However, these data are complex and expensive to gather and, although epidemiologically useful, have not been shown necessary to detect the presence of malnutrition (Baker et al, 1982). Standard laboratory tests are indicated serially to ensure the adequacy of parenteral or enteral nutritional support.

PARENTERAL NUTRITION

Parenteral nutrition is indicated in patients who are unable to ingest, digest, and absorb sufficient nutrients in the alimentary tract to maintain normal nutritional status or replace lost nutrients.

Peripheral Parenteral Nutrition

Peripheral parenteral nutrition is recommended to supply nutrients for a limited period to patients without severe deficits when oral or enteral intake is insufficient. Since intravenous sites must be changed every 24 to 48 hours and large volumes must be infused (ie, 3 to 4 L/day), administration is not appropriate for long-term total parenteral nutrition in most patients.

A solution containing 3.5% to 4.25% amino acids, 5% to 10% dextrose, and maintenance doses of electrolytes, vitamins, and trace elements is commonly used. Most of the calories are supplied by concomitantly administered fat emulsions (10% to 20%).

Intravenous fat decreases the final osmolality of the mixture entering the vein and prevents phlebitis. In addition, the amount of potassium chloride and calcium salts added to the mixture should be kept to a minimum to reduce venous irritation. The infusion line employed to administer peripheral parenteral nutrition should not be used for other drugs.

Central Parenteral Nutrition

Central venous infusion is indicated when serious protein and calorie deficits exist or are anticipated, as in patients with serious gastrointestinal disease or hypermetabolic states; when enteral feeding is contraindicated or inadequate in those with severe nausea, vomiting, diarrhea, or mucositis secondary to cancer chemotherapy; or pre- and postoperatively in debilitated patients when repletion is desirable to improve surgical risk. By providing essential and nonessential amino acids with adequate calories, lean body mass is preserved and repletion of lean body mass and wound healing may be enhanced. Some investigators also have noted improvement of an impaired immune response and a decrease in postoperative morbidity and mortality.

Total parenteral nutrition (TPN) is administered to hospitalized patients and also may be given at home by trained patients or family members. A home TPN program may be indicated for persistent gastrointestinal hypomotility or obstruction, massive bowel resection, severe radiation enteritis and other malabsorption states, or high-output fistulas or stromas located in the upper intestine. Home TPN also may be employed for short-term therapy when use of the gastrointestinal tract must be stopped temporarily. It is much less expensive than similar therapy in a hospital and is safe provided the patient is in a reasonably stable condition and the home situation is conducive to this technique. Most importantly, home TPN often permits patients to maintain normal activities.

PREPARATION AND ADMINISTRATION OF SOLUTIONS. TPN solutions are prepared from commercially available parenteral solutions by mixing hypertonic dextrose, most commonly a 50% or 70% concentration, with an amino acid solution [Aminosyn, FreAmine III, Novamine, Travasol] and appropriate amounts of electrolytes, trace elements, and vitamins. By using different base solutions, almost any concentration of dextrose and amino acids and volume of fluid can be obtained. In the United States, fat emulsions are not routinely mixed with the TPN solution but are given through a separate peripheral vein or a Y-connector via the same vein.

To reduce the possibility of bacterial contamination, TPN solutions are prepared aseptically under a laminar air flow hood, refrigerated, and administered within 24 to 48 hours. Home TPN solutions not containing perishable vitamins can be premixed under aseptic conditions and stored in a refrigerator for up to a month. Darkened or cloudy solutions should be discarded. Drugs should not be added to TPN solutions unless compatibility and stability have been established.

TPN solutions containing more than 10% to 15% dextrose must be infused into a central vein with a high blood flow for rapid dilution. The percutaneous approach to the superior vena cava via the subclavian vein is preferred, although tunneled catheters are being used more often in hospitalized

and home TPN patients. The solution is generally administered continuously with an infusion pump at a constant rate. Alternatively, it may be infused intermittently over a 9- to 16-hour period (depending on a patient's needs) with the patient on a "heparin lock" or heparin-flushed Hickeman or Broviac catheter during the remainder of the day. With the cycling technique, it is generally advisable to decrease the rate of infusion by one-half for 60 to 90 minutes before discontinuing administration to avoid hypoglycemia induced by the insulin response to dextrose infusion. Bolus TPN administration is dangerous because it causes hyperglycemia, glycosuria, and osmotic diuresis with eventual dehydration.

COMPONENTS OF TPN. The following components may be added to the amino acid solutions and hypertonic dextrose to supply specific needs in adults.

Electrolytes and Minerals: The nutrients in TPN may produce hyperglycemia or elevate the blood urea nitrogen level if the dose exceeds the patient's ability to metabolize the components. Hyperglycemia increases the osmotic load and may cause osmotic diuresis. Repletion of body mass results in increased demand for intracellular minerals such as phosphate and magnesium. Potassium enters cell with glucose, thus increasing potassium requirements.

Adults with no abnormal electrolyte loss or retention and with normal renal function require approximately 80 to 120 mEq of sodium and 60 to 100 mEq of potassium daily. Sodium and potassium are generally added to TPN solutions as mixtures of chloride or acetate salts to achieve a proper anion/cation ratio and to provide an acidifying or alkalizing effect as necessary. Potassium or sodium phosphate is essential; requirements for phosphate are increased when glycolytic activity is increased or urinary losses are high (eg, persistent acidosis, proximal renal tubular defect). Approximately 200 to 400 mg (6.5 to 13 mM) of phosphorus is required daily for maintenance, but larger amounts are often needed when initiating TPN to maintain the serum phosphate level above 2.5 mg/dl. For each 500 ml of 50% dextrose in water infused, 12 mM of phosphorus has been recommended.

Hypomagnesemia develops after eight to ten days unless the TPN solution contains magnesium sulfate. The recommended amount is 8 to 12 mEq of magnesium/L of TPN solution; some commercial solutions provide 5 mEq/L, which is probably suboptimal. Usually 10 to 24 mEq daily is adequate, but more may be needed in the presence of extensive gastrointestinal fluid loss or increased urinary loss, which accompanies continued use of diuretics, alcoholism, or renal tubular damage. Magnesium and potassium should be administered cautiously (with monitoring of serum levels) to patients with impaired renal function.

The average adult requires 200 to 400 mg (10 to 20 mEq) of elemental calcium daily, usually supplied as calcium gluconate. (Calcium and phosphate requirements are increased in children for bone growth.) Calcium losses in urine are related to the amount of amino acids administered. Currently, there is no evidence that calcium is related to metabolic bone disease. The need for calcium during prolonged TPN varies. Many adult patients experience problems with bone metabolism for reasons that are not well understood (Klein et al, 1981; Shike et al, 1980; Seligman et al, 1984).

Trace Elements: These should be included in parenteral feeding from the beginning, especially in malnourished patients or in those with extensive gastrointestinal fluid losses (see Table 1).

Zinc and copper deficiencies may develop within six to seven weeks unless adequate amounts are included in TPN solutions. The zinc and copper requirements are correlated with fecal loss and small bowel fluid loss (Wolman et al, 1979; Shike, 1984). If less than 300 ml is lost, the daily requirement is approximately 1.5 to 6 mg for zinc and 0.3 mg for copper; if the loss is great, as much as 12 mg/day zinc and 0.5 mg/day copper are necessary. Manganese, chromium, selenium, and iron also are essential during long-term therapy. Administration of chromium corrects or prevents deficiency and related glucose intolerance. Molybdenum and iodine also may be needed, but exact amounts have not been determined (see Table 1).

Copper and manganese may accumulate in patients with significant biliary obstruction and should be given cautiously and serum levels should be monitored. Iron stores should be monitored by measuring serum iron/total iron binding capacity or ferritin levels. Patients requiring TPN often have received blood transfusions and thus have very high total iron stores. Iron should be withheld from these patients until iron stores become normal. When iron is indicated, it can be infused intravenously in the TPN solution after testing for sensitivity.

Crystalline amino acid preparations contain variable amounts of zinc and, like other large volume parenteral solutions, contain very low levels of other trace elements. Salts of zinc, copper, manganese, selenium, molybdenum, and chromium or a single element are available commercially.

Vitamins: All vitamins may be depleted in malnourished patients, especially those with prolonged malabsorption. Requirements may be increased during stress, such as severe trauma, major surgery, or serious illness, but quantitative data are lacking. A parenteral multivitamin preparation that includes appropriate fat-soluble vitamins should be added to the intravenous solution on a regular schedule (see Table 5 in Chapter 47, Vitamins and Minerals). Because water-soluble vitamins are excreted quickly when given too rapidly, bolus administration should be avoided.

Care should be taken to avoid overdosage of vitamin A and D because they are toxic, and vitamin A overdose may impair the utilization of vitamin E. Vitamin A is adsorbed rapidly onto both plastic and glass and may be destroyed on exposure to light. The claim that administration of vitamin D is associated with metabolic bone disease in some patients on long-term TPN remains unproven.

Folic acid and vitamin B_{12} may be given as components of multiple vitamin preparations or separately. Vitamin K should be administered separately in adults (5 to 10 mg intramuscularly once weekly). In children, vitamin K should be incorporated into daily feedings to provide approximately 0.2 mg/day. Alternatively, weekly administration of 0.2 to 1.5 mg, depending on age, may be used if there are no contraindications. See also Chapter 47, Vitamins and Minerals.

Biotin deficiency has been demonstrated.

Fat: Essential fatty acid deficiency may develop during prolonged TPN. Intravenous fat emulsions [Intralipid, Liposyn II, McGaw I.V. Fat Emulsion, Soyacal, Travamulsion] prevent or correct essential fatty acid deficiencies when infused in amounts that provide 3% to 5% of the total caloric input as linoleic acid. The 10% preparations provide 1.1 calories/ml and the 20% preparations provide 2 calories/ml. Thus, 500 ml of a 10% fat emulsion two or three times weekly usually prevents deficiency. Since they are isotonic, these preparations can be administered through a peripheral vein.

Intravenous fat emulsions also have been infused peripherally as a major source (30% to 50%) of non-nitrogen calories during TPN in patients whose daily requirement does not exceed 1,800 calories and who are not under metabolic stress. However, since a fat emulsion should provide no more than 60% of the total daily caloric input, a central vein catheter usually is also needed for infusion of hypertonic dextrose to supply the remainder of calories needed.

Hypermetabolic patients receiving balanced TPN regimens

TABLE 1.
TRACE ELEMENTS: RECOMMENDED DAILY INTAKES DURING NUTRITIONAL SUPPORT[1]

Trace Minerals	Adults	Pediatric
Chromium	10–20 mcg	0.14–0.2 mcg/kg
Copper[2]	0.5–1.5 mg	15–20 mcg/kg
Iodine[3]	60 mcg	2–3 mcg/kg
Manganese[2]	0.15–0.5 mg	—
Molybdenum	300 mcg	—
Selenium	25–50 mcg	3.15 mcg/kg
Zinc[4]	1.5–2.5 mg	100–300 mcg/kg (below age 6)

[1]Patients should be monitored for signs and symptoms of deficiency or excess of each component, and appropriate changes made to assure optimum level of intake.
[2]Not routinely administered to those with significant liver impairment.
[3]Iodine may not be necessary in patients taking some food orally or in patients treated with dermal preparations of povidone-iodine.
[4]Additional zinc may be required in patients losing bowel fluids.

(ie, regimens in which intravenous fats provide a significant proportion of nonprotein calories) can achieve positive nitrogen balance. When fat is administered as a source of calories, it must replace glucose calories; otherwise hypertriglyceridemia occurs.

Fat emulsions may cause hyperlipidemia in patients with impaired fat metabolism; hyperlipidemia may be treated with small doses of heparin (1,000 units), which stimulates lipoprotein lipase and clears triglycerides from blood. Another disadvantage of these emulsions is their high cost compared to 50% dextrose.

Carbohydrate: Hyperglycemia and glycosuria can be prevented by limiting the amount of dextrose given initially (1,000 to 1,200 kcal/day or 300 to 350 g/day), usually as a 12.5% solution, and gradually increasing the dose by 500 to 1,000 kcal every one to two days as tolerance is demonstrated. As amounts are increased, a more concentrated solution (eg, 25%) may be used. This precaution is essential in known or suspected diabetics and elderly patients. No adaptation is required if one-half the calories are given as fat emulsion.

Fractional urine sugar and blood glucose levels should be determined every six hours for the first two or three days. If urine levels correlate poorly with blood levels, the amount in the blood should be used as a guide and should be determined frequently by the finger-stick method. The blood glucose level should be monitored until glucose tolerance is demonstrated (usually in two to three days as endogenous insulin production increases). If the blood glucose level remains greatly elevated, regular insulin may be given intravenously in the TPN solutions, starting with 5 to 10 units/liter of TPN solution. Some studies suggest that approximately 50% of insulin adheres to glass or plastic, but the remainder is stable for 24 to 48 hours.

Accurate charting of intake and output is essential, together with daily weights. In addition, fractional urine or blood glucose levels should be determined and supplemental amounts of regular insulin given subcutaneously if needed until the optimum level of insulin has been attained. When an adequate ratio of exogenous insulin to glucose has been determined, any increase in the amount of carbohydrate (glucose) administered should be accompanied by proportional increases in the dose of insulin and monitoring should continue. However, as the underlying illness resolves, the resistance to insulin may disappear and lower the insulin requirements.

The carbohydrate requirement is reduced in severely malnourished patients to avoid edema and cardiovascular overload. Weight gain of more than 0.5 kg/24 hours may signify fluid retention. If overhydration occurs, it may be treated with diuretics or by restricting sodium and/or fluid intake.

Excessive infusion of glucose calories increases carbon dioxide production and oxygen consumption, which can complicate weaning of hypermetabolic patients from respirators or precipitate respiratory distress in patients with pulmonary abnormalities (Askanazi et al, 1980).

Other Requirements: Acute or symptomatic anemia is treated by transfusion of packed red cells.

In most patients receiving TPN, the serum albumin level decreases initially due to dilution and then increases gradually (estimated half-life of albumin, 16 to 20 days) when adequate amino acids and calories are given and no underlying pathologic condition impairs synthesis or increases catabolism of albumin. The routine administration of albumin for the sole purpose of increasing albumin levels above 2.5 to 2.8 g/dl should be avoided. Patients with symptomatic, severe hypoalbuminemia accompanied by hypovolemia or peripheral edema that requires diuretics may receive albumin early in the course of TPN; 12.5 to 50 g of albumin daily (to maintain a serum level of approximately 2.8 g/dl) is given intravenously to increase the blood pressure and improve fluid status. Albumin also is administered to restore plasma oncotic pressure. No benefit will be obtained if capillary permeability is increased, as occurs during sepsis.

MONITORING OF TPN. Bedside examinations and determinations of serum and urine chemistries should be performed initially and at frequent intervals for several days after initiating TPN. Serum electrolytes and blood urea nitrogen or creatinine levels should be measured three times weekly or more often if the patient is metabolically unstable. If initial values are within a reasonable range, liver function studies and measurement of serum albumin, calcium, phosphorus, and magnesium levels may be performed once or twice weekly. Additions or deletions to the solutions should be made as necessary to correct any electrolyte or fluid imbalance.

The efficacy of nutritional support is determined most simply by weight measurements assessed in relation to possible edema formation.

ADVERSE REACTIONS AND PRECAUTIONS. The major complications of TPN are catheter-related sepsis and metabolic abnormalities; mechanical problems related to the catheter and infusion apparatus also may occur. The cause of an elevated temperature, particularly the spiking type, during TPN should be investigated immediately. Blood should be obtained by venipuncture and from the TPN line and cultured for bacterial growth, and a search for infectious foci distant from the catheter tip should be undertaken (Vanhuynegem et al, 1985). Rarely, the solution may be contaminated. If the temperature remains elevated for 24 hours, especially in association with rigor, and no other explanation can be found, the catheter may be incriminated empirically as a source of infection; it should be removed and replaced at a new site or aseptically exchanged over a sterile guide wire. The tip of the removed catheter should be cultured, and appropriate antibiotic therapy initiated if defervescence does not occur rapidly.

TPN administration should be discontinued gradually over 60 to 90 minutes because the pancreatic insulin response does not necessarily cease once the dextrose infusion is stopped and insulin levels are often elevated during infusion. If 50% of calories are supplied as fat, this is not necessary. If TPN must be stopped suddenly, 10% dextrose should be infused peripherally for one to two hours to prevent hypoglycemia.

Prior to major surgery with general anesthesia, consideration should be given to discontinuing TPN therapy. Accidental or emergency cessation of TPN during anesthesia may cause hypoglycemia, which may be unrecognized and result in irreversible brain damage or death.

Hyperglycemia, glycosuria, and osmotic diuresis may occur with excessive dextrose infusion. Hyperammonemia had been associated with infusion of protein hydrolysates and Nephramine, but occurs less frequently with crystalline amino acid solutions that contain arginine.

Liver disease in premature infants receiving long-term parenteral nutrition has been attributed to many factors, including essential fatty acid deficiency and protein hydrolysate toxicity; however, this complication also has occurred in infants receiving amino acids and Intralipid.

Drug Evaluations

AMINO ACID SOLUTIONS
[Aminosyn, FreAmine III, Novamine, ProcalAmine, Travasol]

COMPOSITION AND USES. These solutions contain a mixture of essential and nonessential crystalline amino acids with or without electrolytes. They are indicated for intravenous administration when there is interference with ingestion, digestion, or absorption of protein for long periods or when parenteral supplementation of oral protein intake is required. Parenterally administered free amino acids are utilized more efficiently than the peptides produced by enzymatic cleavage of protein hydrolysates. Consequently, crystalline amino acid solutions have replaced protein hydrolysates for TPN.

Low concentrations (3% or 3.5%) of these amino acid solutions also have been used instead of or with 5% to 10% dextrose for short-term peripheral intravenous therapy in surgical patients, but the high cost without accompanying advantages has prevented their widespread use for this purpose. These solutions are useful as substitutes for 5% dextrose in some marginally depleted patients with diabetes, but they are not safe for use in insulin-dependent diabetics.

ADVERSE REACTIONS AND PRECAUTIONS. Mild thrombophlebitis has occurred rarely during infusion of amino acid solutions. Flushing, fever, and nausea also have been reported. Because amino acids increase the blood urea nitrogen level, they should be given cautiously and in restricted amounts to patients with impaired renal function.

In patients with chronic or acute liver disease, hepatic coma may be precipitated because of accumulation of nitrogenous substances in the blood. For this reason, standard amino acid solutions should be used cautiously in patients with cirrhosis, severe viral hepatitis, and major involvement of the liver by cancer.

Amino acid solutions containing significant amounts of sodium should be used cautiously in patients who must restrict sodium intake, and those containing significant amounts of potassium and magnesium generally should be avoided in patients with renal failure not on dialysis. Monitoring of the latter patients is necessary to avoid potassium imbalances.

PREPARATIONS. See Tables 2 and 3.

AMINO ACID SOLUTIONS: RENAL FAILURE FORMULAS
[Aminess Aminosyn-RF, NephrAmine, RenAmin]

COMPOSITION AND USES. Renal failure formulas (RFF) predominantly contain eight essential amino acids plus histidine, which is considered essential in patients with chronic renal failure, in hypertonic dextrose solution. When mixed with appropriate vitamins, minerals, and electrolytes, these formulas provide about 1,200 calories in 750 to 800 ml.

Initially, these preparations were recommended to supply the needed amino acids and energy in all patients with renal failure who were unable to eat and could not tolerate enteral feeding. However, the indications for RFF have narrowed sharply because these formulas appear to have no significant advantage over standard amino acid solutions in most patients with renal failure. Currently, they are indicated in patients with acute renal failure in whom dialysis is dangerous or contraindicated and who have very low blood urea nitrogen levels. The use of RFF and hypertonic dextrose may reduce the frequency of dialysis in these patients. Additionally, some nephrologists recommend infusing essential amino acid solutions (without dextrose) near the end of dialysis therapy as a protein supplement. However, most dialysis patients have decreased total nitrogen and energy balance in addition to depressed essential amino acid balance; therefore, it may be preferable to administer a parenteral solution containing essential and nonessential amino acids in hypertonic dextrose.

ADVERSE REACTIONS AND PRECAUTIONS. Large amounts of Nephramine cause hyperammonemia leading to central nervous system disorders, and coma may result from lack of arginine. For further information on adverse reactions and precautions, see the evaluation on Amino Acid Solutions.

DOSAGE. Renal failure formulas that are prepared with 70% dextrose are infused into a central vein because of their high osmolality. The dosage must be individualized.

PREPARATIONS. See Table 4.

AMINO ACID SOLUTIONS: BRANCHED CHAIN AMINO ACID-ENRICHED FORMULAS
[BranchAmin, FreAmine HBC, HepatAmine]

COMPOSITION. HepatAmine is designed specifically to supply nutrients to patients who have hepatic disease with portacaval shunting and impending or actual encephalopathy. It contains reduced quantities of aromatic amino acids (phenylalanine, tyrosine, and tryptophan) and methionine and increased quantities of arginine. FreAmine HBC and BranchAmin are designed for use in patients with trauma and sepsis. These products contain high concentrations of branched chain amino acids (leucine, isoleucine, and valine). FreAmine HBC also contains standard quantities of phenylalanine, tryptophan, and methionine and relatively low quantities of glycine. BranchAmin contains only these amino acids and must be admixed with standard amino acid solutions.

USES. *Hepatic Formula:* The rationale for use of HepatAmine

TABLE 2.
AMINO ACID SOLUTIONS

	Aminosyn (Abbott)				
	3.5%	5%	7%	8.5%	10%
NORMALIZED AMINO ACID CONTENT (mg/1%)					
Essential (% Nitrogen)					
Isoleucine (10.7)	72	72	73	73	72
Leucine (10.7)	94	94	94	95	94
Lysine (19.2)	72	72	73	73	72
Methionine (9.4)	40	40	40	40	40
Phenylalanine (8.5)	44	44	44	45	44
Threonine (11.8)	52	52	53	54	52
Tryptophan (13.7)	16	16	17	18	16
Valine (12.0)	80	80	80	80	66
TOTAL EAA	470	470	474	478	470
Nonessential (% Nitrogen)					
Alanine (15.7)	128	128	129	129	128
Arginine (32.2)	98	98	99	100	98
Histidine (27.1)	30	30	30	31	30
Proline (12.2)	86	86	87	88	86
Serine (13.3)	42	42	43	44	42
Tyrosine (7.7)	9	9	6	5	4
Glycine (18.9)	128	128	129	129	128
Cysteine (11.6)	—	—	—	—	—
TOTAL NEAA	521	521	523	526	516
ELECTROLYTES (mEq/L)					
Sodium	7	—	—	—	—
Potassium	—	5.4	5.4	5.4	5.4
Magnesium	—	—	—	—	—
Chloride	—	—	—	35	—
Acetate	46	86	105	90	148
Phosphate (mM/L)	—	—	—	—	—
EAA/TAA%	47	47	48	48	48
BCAA/EAA%	52	52	52	52	52
BCAA/TAA%	25	25	25	25	25

to treat hepatic encephalopathy is based on the neurotransmitter amino acid hypothesis, which presumes that hepatic encephalopathy is caused, at least in part, by elevated concentrations of aromatic amino acids (AAA) that result in overproduction of the false neurotransmitters, octopamine, tyramine, and the putative neurotransmitter, serotonin, in the central nervous system. These false neurotransmitters then replace the true neurotransmitters, dopamine and norepinephrine, and hepatic encephalopathy ensues. The role of branched chain amino acids (BCAA) is to compete with AAA for entry into the central nervous system, reduce abnormal neurotransmitter production, and resolve the encephalopathy.

Although BCAA may be useful, the vast majority of patients with hepatic encephalopathy can be successfully treated with a more traditional approach. Furthermore, as additional experimental evidence has accrued, it is controversial whether this formula is superior to more conventional therapy (Wahren et al, 1983; Millikan et al, 1983; Cerra et al, 1985). HepatAmine should be reserved for patients with impending or actual portal systemic encephalopathy and altered plasma BCAA concentrations, those with gastrointestinal dysfunction when more traditional therapy is not feasible, or those with cirrhosis in whom standard amino acid solutions produce encephalopathy at doses that are insufficient to provide adequate nutritional support (McCullough et al, 1983).

Stress Formula: The other claimed role for branched chain amino acid-enriched solutions is as a nutritional supplement to prevent peripheral muscle catabolism following trauma or sepsis. The rationale for stress formula is based on the different response of metabolism during stress compared to that during starvation. Stress and trauma increase skeletal muscle catabolism and nitrogen loss. The ability of the liver and possibly the heart and skeletal muscle to oxidize fatty acids is impaired. Skeletal muscle protein catabolism gene-

	FreAmine III (American McGaw)		Travasol (Travenol)			Novamine (KabiVitrum)	
	8.5%	10%	5.5%	8.5%	10%	8.5%	11.4%
	69	69	48	48	60	49	50
	91	91	62	62	73	69	69
	73	73	58	58	58	79	79
	53	53	58	58	40	49	50
	56	56	62	62	56	69	69
	40	40	42	42	42	49	50
	15	15	18	18	18	16	17
	66	66	46	46	58	65	64
	463	463	394	394	405	445	448
	71	71	207	207	207	146	145
	95	95	103	104	115	99	98
	28	28	44	44	48	59	60
	112	112	42	42	68	59	60
	59	59	—	—	50	40	39
	—	—	4	4	4	2	3
	140	140	207	207	103	69	69
	<3	<3	—	—	—	—	—
	508	508	608	608	595	553[a]	553[b]
	10	10	—	—	—	—	—
	—	—	—	—	—	—	—
	—	—	—	—	—	—	—
	<3	<3	22	35	—	—	—
	72	89	48	73	87	88	114
	10	10	—	—	—	—	—
	48	48	39	39	41	45	45
	49	49	40	40	47	41	41
	23	23	16	16	19	18	18

[a]*Includes 29 mg aspartic acid and 49 mg glutamic acid*
[b]*Includes 29 mg aspartic acid and 50 mg glutamic acid*

rates both free aromatic and branched chain amino acids (BCAA); alanine and glutamine are utilized for glucose synthesis even though patients often are hyperglycemic.

FreAmine HBC contains standard amounts of essential and nonessential amino acids (with an increased quantity of BCAA) and is claimed to be beneficial for septic and traumatized patients. When combined with hypertonic fat, dextrose, and insulin, this formula may decrease nitrogen loss or even produce positive nitrogen balance and improve protein and energy metabolism during stress (Fischer and Freund, 1983). This is an area of active investigation, and the value of additional BCAA above that supplied in standard formulations remains unsettled. BranchAmin contains only BCAA and must be admixed with standard amino acid solutions in order to promote protein synthesis. For adverse reactions and precautions, see the evaluation on Amino Acid Solutions.

PREPARATIONS. See Table 4.

AMINO ACID SOLUTION: PEDIATRIC FORMULA
[TrophAmine]

COMPOSITION AND USES. This mixture of essential and nonessential amino acids, taurine, and N-acetyl-L-tyrosine is designed specifically for use in infants and young children. It produces plasma amino acid patterns similar to those found in breast-fed infants, and its use may result in increased weight

TABLE 3.
AMINO ACID SOLUTIONS WITH ELECTROLYTES

	Aminosyn (Abbott)			FreAmine III (American McGaw)	ProcalAmine[1] (American McGaw)	Travasol (Travenol)		
	3.5%	7%	8.5%	3%	3%	3.5%	5.5%	8.5%
NORMALIZED AMINO ACID CONTENT (mg/1%)								
Essential (% Nitrogen)								
Isoleucine (10.7)	72	73	73	70	70	48	48	48
Leucine (10.7)	94	94	95	90	90	62	62	62
Lysine (19.2)	72	73	73	73	73	58	58	58
Methionine (9.4)	40	40	40	53	53	58	58	58
Phenylalanine (8.5)	44	44	45	57	57	62	62	62
Threonine (11.8)	52	53	54	40	40	42	42	42
Tryptophan (13.7)	16	17	18	15	15	18	18	18
Valine (12.0)	80	80	80	67	67	46	46	46
TOTAL EAA	470	474	478	465	465	394	394	394
Nonessential (% Nitrogen)								
Alanine (15.7)	128	129	129	70	70	208	207	207
Arginine (32.2)	98	99	100	97	97	104	104	104
Histidine (27.1)	30	30	31	28	28	44	44	44
Proline (12.2)	86	87	88	113	113	42	42	42
Serine (13.3)	42	43	44	60	60	--	--	--
Tyrosine (7.7)	9	6	5	--	--	4	4	4
Glycine (18.9)	128	129	129	140	140	208	207	207
Cysteine (11.6)	--	--	--	<3	<7	--	--	--
TOTAL NEAA	521	523	526	575	575	610	608	608
ELECTROLYTES (mEq/L)								
Sodium	47	70	70	35	35	47	70	70
Potassium	13	66	66	24	24	13	60	60
Magnesium	3	10	10	5	5	3	10	10
Chloride	40	96	98	41	41	40	70	70
Acetate	58	124	142	47	47	58	102	141
Phosphate (mM/L)	3.5	30	30	3.5	3.5	3.5	30	30
EAA/TAA%	47	48	48	47	47	39	39	39
BCAA/EAA%	52	52	52	49	49	40	40	40
BCAA/TAA%	25	25	25	23	23	16	16	16

[1]*Also contains 3% glycerin equivalent to 130 nonprotein calories/1,000 ml*

gain and positive nitrogen balance with less protein than that supplied in standard formulas. However, further studies are needed to determine its role in the nutritional support of infants and children.

For adverse reactions and precautions, see the evaluation on Amino Acid Solutions.

PREPARATIONS. See Table 4.

FAT EMULSIONS
[Intralipid, Liposyn, McGaw I.V. Fat Emulsion, Soyacal, Travamulsion]

USES. Intravenous fat emulsions are used to prevent or correct essential fatty acid deficiency and to provide calories in high density form on a regular basis during prolonged TPN. They also are used to feed patients with chronic obstructive pulmonary disease. Substituting carbohydrate calories for fat calories lowers the respiratory quotient and may help to decrease the arterial CO_2 concentrations. Since they are isotonic with plasma, these preparations are suitable for peripheral infusion and, if sufficient calories can be provided by this method, the administration of hypertonic (greater than 10%) dextrose via a central vein catheter may sometimes be avoided. In peripheral TPN, fat emulsions are infused continuously through a Y-adapter to decrease the frequency of phlebitis. A total of 500 ml of 20% emulsions provides 1,000 calories; the same volume of 10% emulsions provides 550 calories.

Weight gain, healing of fistulas, and increased serum protein levels have been observed in some patients during long-term TPN utilizing fat emulsions as the main nonprotein calorie source.

When administered to prevent essential fatty acid deficiency, 3% to 5% of the total caloric intake should be provided by intravenous fat emulsions. When administered to correct fatty acid deficiency, 8% to 10% of the caloric intake should be supplied by intravenous fat emulsions to provide adequate linoleic acid. When used as a source of calories, they should comprise no more than 60% of the total caloric intake in adults and children and 40% in newborn infants; the remainder should be supplied by dextrose and a source of amino acids.

PHARMACOLOGY. In usual doses, intravenous fats are metabolized in the same manner as natural chylomicrons, and a transient increase in plasma triglycerides occurs after infusion. Some patients, however, experience more prolonged hypertriglyceridemia due to impaired metabolism of infused fat. The triglycerides are hydrolyzed to free fatty acids and glycerol by lipoprotein lipase. Free fatty acids then enter the tissues (where they may be oxidized or resynthesized into triglycerides and stored) or circulate in the plasma bound to albumin. In the liver, circulating free fatty acids are oxidized or converted to very low density lipoproteins that re-enter the blood stream.

ADVERSE REACTIONS AND PRECAUTIONS. In contrast to older products, currently available fat emulsions rarely cause severe adverse reactions.

Hyperlipidemia may occur if these preparations are infused too rapidly, given to patients with impaired fat metabolism, or administered with an excessive amount of dextrose. Excessive accumulation can be recognized by visual inspection of the plasma six to eight hours after infusion is completed, determination of triglyceride concentrations, or measurement of plasma light-scattering activity by nephelometry. These preparations are contraindicated in patients with pathologic hyperlipidemic states.

Newborn infants, particularly those who are premature, small, or acutely ill, may metabolize intravenous fat emulsions slowly; infusion at a constant slow rate over 20 to 24 hours may reduce the risk of hyperlipidemia in these patients. Since free fatty acids compete with bilirubin for albumin binding sites, intravenous fats may increase the risk of kernicterus in infants with hyperbilirubinemia and may interfere with estimation of serum bilirubin. Deaths have been reported following too rapid infusion in preterm infants; fat-engorged capillaries were found in the lungs of these infants (Levene et al, 1980). However, these were related to overinfusion without proper pumping controls.

The fat particles do not aggregate, and there appears to be no risk of fat embolism if the recommended infusion technique is followed. After prolonged therapy, there may be a proliferation of Kupfer cells in the liver and deposition of a brown pigment (intravenous fat pigment) throughout the reticuloendothelial system, but this is of no clinical significance.

Thrombophlebitis, vomiting, pain in the chest or back, and hypersensitivity reactions have occurred rarely. Hepatomegaly, thrombocytopenia, anemia, transient abnormalities in liver function tests, and decreased pulmonary diffusing capacity also have been reported rarely. The "overloading syndrome" (focal seizures, fever, leukocytosis, thrombocytopenia, splenomegaly, and shock) associated with use of earlier fat emulsions is also rare following infusion of currently available preparations. However, caution is advised when administering fat emulsion to patients with severe liver disease, anemia, or blood coagulation disorders.

Periodic liver function tests, plasma lipid profile, hemogram, and blood coagulation tests and frequent platelet counts should be performed during long-term therapy. The lipemia must clear between daily infusions. These preparations should be discontinued if a significant abnormality in these parameters is attributable to fat infusion.

DOSAGE AND PREPARATIONS. Intravenous fat emulsions may be infused via a peripheral or central vein. Compatibility should be verified before admixing with other solutions, drugs, or vitamins. Three-in-one systems, in which fats, amino acids, and dextrose are admixed in one container, are available. They should be infused over 24 hours. Intravenous fats may be infused into the same vein as the dextrose-amino acid solution by means of a Y-connector on the patient side of any in-line filter, because the emulsions contain particles that are too large to pass through any bacterial or particulate filter. The contents of any partly used bottle must be discarded. Bottles should be stored at less than 25 C prior to use; if accidentally frozen, the bottle must be discarded.

Intravenous: *Adults,* the initial infusion rate should not exceed 1 ml/min (10%) or 0.5 ml/min (20%) for 15 to 30 minutes. If no adverse effects occur, the rate may be increased to provide a maximum of 500 ml over a period of two to four hours (10%) or eight hours (20%). Only 500 ml of the 20% preparations should be given on the first day of therapy. On the following day, the dosage may be increased but should not provide more than 2.5 g of fat/kg of body weight daily.

In *children,* the initial infusion rate is 0.1 ml/min (10%) or 0.05 ml/min (20%) for 10 to 15 minutes; if tolerated, the rate then may be increased to provide 1 g of fat/kg in four hours. The amount of fat should not routinely exceed 3 g/kg/day. Even smaller doses should be used in patients with infection, compromised pulmonary function, and/or hyperbilirubinemia.

In *newborn infants,* intravenous fat emulsions should be infused at a constant rate over 20 hours with a maximal daily dose calculated to provide 2 to 4 g of fat/kg and no more than 1 g/kg in four hours. The lipemia should be monitored and must clear between daily infusions.

PREPARATIONS. See Table 5.

ENTERAL NUTRITION

Enteral nutrition is indicated for patients with a patent alimentary tract who cannot or will not ingest adequate amounts of food or who have a digestive or absorptive disorder not amenable to modification of a normal oral diet. Enteral feeding may comprise part of the total daily diet for those who can ingest and absorb some nutrients, or it may comprise the total intake for those unable to ingest or absorb anything. The contraindications for enteral feeding are (1) severe malabsorption in which tube feeding exacerbates diarrhea uncontrollably, (2) total bowel obstruction, (3) persistent and uncontrolled vomiting, and (4) tendency to aspirate (de-

TABLE 4.
AMINO ACID SOLUTIONS FOR SPECIFIC SITUATIONS

	Renal Failure Formulations			
	Aminess (KabiVitrum)	Aminosyn–RF (Abbott) 5.2%	NephrAmine (American McGaw) 5.4%	RenAmin (Travenol) 6.5%
NORMALIZED AMINO ACID CONTENT (mg/1%)				
Essential (% Nitrogen)				
Isoleucine (10.7)	101	89	104	77
Leucine (10.7)	159	140	163	92
Lysine (19.2)	115	103	119	69
Methionine (9.4)	159	140	163	77
Phenylalanine (8.5)	159	140	163	75
Threonine (11.8)	72	63	74	58
Tryptophan (13.7)	36	32	37	25
Vallne (12.0)	115	102	119	126
TOTAL EAA	995[2]	892[2]	988[2]	664[2]
Nonessential (% Nitrogen)				
Alanine (15.7)	–	–	–	86
Arginine (32.2)	–	115	–	97
Histidine (27.1)	79	83[2]	46[2]	65[2]
Proline (12.2)	–	–	–	54
Serine (13.3)	–	–	–	46
Tyrosine (7.7)	–	–	–	6
Glycine (18.9)	–	–	–	46
Cysteine (11.6)	–	–	–	–
TOTAL NEAA	0	115[2]	0[2]	335[2]
ELECTYROLYTES (mEq/L)				
Sodium	–	–	5	–
Potassium	–	5.4	–	–
Magnesium	–	–	–	–
Chloride	–	–	<3	–
Acetate	50	105	44	–
Phosphate (mM/L)	00	–	–	–
EAA/TAA%	100	89	100	66
BCAA/EAA%	38	37	39	44
BCAA/TAA%	38	33	39	30

[1]Must be admixed with a complete amino acid solution. BranchAmin does not contain all of the essential amino acids.
[2]Histidine is an essential amino acid for patients in renal failure. This is reflected in the total EAA, total NEAA, and ratios.

spite placement of the feeding tube tip in the small bowel), especially in the presence of serious pulmonary disease.

Enteral formulas differ in digestibility; caloric density; palatability; lactose, protein, and fat content; osmolality; viscosity; and expense. Some products contain minimally altered foods and others contain processed or chemically isolated food derivatives. Formulas containing meat or meat products have medium residue; most other formulations provide low residue. Preparations containing intact proteins are more palatable than those made from hydrolyzed protein or crystalline amino acids, and the former should be used for oral enteral feeding when tolerated. Formulations containing large amounts of milk provide high levels of lactose, calcium, and phosphorus when used in the volumes necessary to meet total nutritional and caloric requirements.

Components of Enteral Formulas

Carbohydrates: These constitute the main source of calories in most enteral formulations. Carbohydrates are available as dextrose, sucrose, lactose, dextrins, starch, and glucose oligosaccharides. Dextrose, sucrose, and lactose contribute to high osmolality and are more likely to produce diarrhea than the more complex forms. The absorptive and digestive capacity of the mucosa also should be considered when selecting a source of carbohydrates. Complex carbohydrates (ie, dextrins, starch) require a larger segment of functional gastrointestinal tract for absorption than simple sugars. Glucose oligosaccharides have low osmolality but are readily hydrolyzed to simple sugars and easily absorbed even in patients with moderate gastrointestinal dysfunction. On a per gram basis, they pro-

Stress Formulations		Hepatic Formulation	Pediatric Formulation
BranchAmin[1] (Travenol) 4%	FreAmine HBC (American McGaw) 6.9%	HepatAmine (American McGaw) 8%	TrophAmine (American McGaw) 6%
345	110	113	82
345	199	138	140
—	59	76	82
—	36	13	33
—	46	13	48
—	29	56	42
—	13	8	20
310	127	105	78
1,000	619	522	599[3]
—	58	96	53
—	84	75	122
—	23	30	48[3]
—	91	100	68
—	48	63	38
—	—	—	23[3]
—	48	113	—
—	<3	<3	<3[3]
0	355	480	403[3,4]
—	10	10	5
—	—	—	—
—	—	—	—
—	<3	<3	<3
—	57	62	56
—	—	10	—
100	64	52	60
100	70	68	50
100	45	36	30

[3]Histidine and cysteine are essential amino acids for infants. This is reflected in the total EAA, total NEAA, and ratios.
[4]Includes 37 mg aminoacetic acid, 32 mg L-aspartic acid, 50 mg L-glutamic acid, and 3 mg taurine

duce glucose and insulin responses indistinguishable in time and magnitude from those produced by simple glucose.

Lactose intolerance is common in many adolescents and adults, particularly blacks, Orientals, Mexicans, American Indians, and those of Jewish descent and often is associated with diseases of malabsorption (eg, celiac disease, tropical sprue, regional enteritis) or short bowel syndrome. In individuals with genetic lactase deficiency, formulations containing large amounts of milk or milk products should be given cautiously. Patients with severe malabsorption secondary to disease or resection also may have deficiency of other disaccharidases and large amounts of sucrose should be avoided. Although these products may be tolerated if given in small amounts (less than 8 g of lactose daily) or slowly, formulas containing maltodextrins or glucose oligosaccharides have lower osmolality and are preferred. These carbohydrates can be mixed with small amounts of sucrose or fructose to increase palatability.

The carbohydrate content of enteral formulations must be considered when treating diabetics. Adjustment of insulin or oral hypoglycemic dosage may be required.

Amino Acids: These are available as intact proteins (eg, eggs, milk, puréed meat), protein isolates (eg, casein from milk, egg whites, soy isolates), hydrolyzed proteins (eg, casein) fortified with tryptophan and methionine, protein dipeptides, and free amino acids.

Relatively few studies have been performed to determine the digestibility of these proteins in various diseases. Although

TABLE 5.
COMPOSITION OF INTRAVENOUS FAT EMULSIONS

Preparation	Oil Source	Fatty Acids				
		Linoleic	Oleic	Palmitic	Linolenic	Stearic
Intralipid (KabiVitrum)						
10%	Soybean	50%	26%	10%	9%	3.5%
20%	Soybean	50%	26%	10%	9%	3.5%
Liposyn II (Abbott)						
10%	Safflower 5% and soybean 5%	65.8%	17.7%	8.8%	4.2%	3.4%
20%	Safflower 10% and soybean 10%	65.5%	17.7%	8.8%	4.2%	3.4%
McGaw IV Fat Emulsion (McGaw)						
10%	Soybean	49–60%	21–26%	9–13%	6–9%	3–5%
20%	Soybean	49–60%	21–26%	9–13%	6–9%	3–5%
Soyacal (Alpha Therapeutic)						
10%	Soybean	49–60%	21–26%	9–13%	6–9%	3–5%
20%	Soybean	49–60%	21–26%	9–13%	6–9%	3–5%
Travamulsion (Travenol)						
10%	Soybean	56%	23%	11%	6%	—
20%	Soybean	56%	23%	11%	6%	—

protein absorption is relatively rapid in the upper jejunum, short-chain oligopeptides (as such or in the form of hydrolyzed protein) are somewhat less active osmotically than free amino acids, do not require pancreatic proteolytic enzymes for digestion, and some are absorbed more rapidly than free amino acids (Adibi, 1977; Silk et al, 1980).

Dipeptides or tripeptides may be especially useful in patients with a reduced absorptive surface, cystinuria, or Hartnup's disease; such patients are able to absorb dipeptides but not free amino acids. Some formulations supply the majority of nitrogen as dipeptides and tripeptides (eg, Criticare HN).

Selection of a formula that provides sufficient total nitrogen as protein or amino acids is essential for all patients. However, low-protein formulations are indicated for patients with severe renal failure. Mixtures of amino acids with altered ratios may be useful for patients with impending or actual encephalopathic symptoms secondary to portacaval shunting. Also, for those with chronic renal insufficiency, adequate protein intake is necessary to prevent malnutrition. Increased amounts of protein or amino acids (100 g or more daily) are indicated when the nitrogen requirement is increased, as in those with trauma, burns, or sepsis. The efficient utilization of amino acids for tissue synthesis depends upon adequate caloric intake.

The rationale for selecting specific enteral formulas for stressed patients or those with renal, hepatic, or pulmonary disease parallels the rationale for selecting similar TPN formulas, and is equally controversial. See the evaluations on Amino Acid Solutions: Renal Failure Formulas and Amino Acid Solutions: Branched Chain Amino Acid-Enriched Formulas for further discussion.

Fat: Fat has a higher caloric density than carbohydrate (9 versus 4 kcal/g), does not increase the osmolality of the formula as much as simple sugars, and improves palatability. The amount of fat in these preparations varies considerably. Most commercial formulas contain a high percentage of polyunsaturated fat, but some have a very low total fat content. Those included most commonly (corn oil, soy oil, safflower oil) are long-chain fats. The triglycerides of all long-chain fats (LCT) are absorbed efficiently by patients with normal digestive and absorptive capabilities and no one oil has any significant advantage over others.

A few formulas contain medium-chain triglycerides (MCT), with some of these preparations containing relatively small amounts of MCT compared to LCT. More data are needed to determine whether there is any advantage to the use of various combinations and proportions of MCT and LCT in individuals with normal bowel function. MCT has a lower caloric density (8.4 kcal/g) than LCT (9 kcal/g). There are ample data to indicate that MCT are absorbed better than LCT when (1) the endothelium of the intestinal mucosa is damaged, resulting in inhibition of fat synthesis; (2) transport of fat from epithelial cells into the lymphatic system is impaired or lymphatic flow is obstructed, causing impaired fat absorption; or (3) amounts of conjugated bile salts are decreased. Products containing only MCT do not provide essential fatty acids; when used as a principal source of fat, supplements high in linoleic acid must be given. Large amounts of MCT can lead to acidosis because of rapid metabolism. MCT should be used with caution in patients with advanced hepatic cirrhosis.

Unless the patient has maldigestion and/or malabsorption of fat or respiratory failure, formulas with a normal range of fat

Phospholipids	Glycerol	Calories/ml	mOsm/L
1.2%	2.25%	1.1	260
1.2%	2.25%	2	268
1.2%	2.5%	1.1	—
1.2%	2.5%	2	—
1.2%	2.21%	1.1	—
1.2%	2.21%	2	—
1.2%	2.21%	1.1	280
1.2%	2.21%	2	315
1.2%	2.25%	1.1	270
1.2%	2.25%	2	300

content are preferred. When a low-fat formulation is used and there is a need for increased calories or a decreased carbohydrate load, the appropriate type and amount of fat should be added if tolerated. To prevent fatty acid deficiency, especially during long-term use, the low-fat formulations should contain some source of linoleic acid; in *adults,* the amount of essential fatty acids should approximate 1% to 2% and, in *children,* 2% to 4% of total calories fed.

If malabsorption is severe, a low-fat formulation is recommended initially with LCT or MCT added gradually as tolerated. In patients with hepatic cirrhosis or portacaval shunts, excessive blood levels of fatty acids of any chain length may act synergistically with high levels of ammonia and other toxins to exacerbate or cause hepatic encephalopathy. Patients with pulmonary dysfunction may benefit from a high-fat preparation (eg, Pulmocare) because carbohydrates are metabolized with a respiratory quotient of 1, while LCT is metabolized with a respiratory quotient of 0.7.

Residue: The amount of residue provided largely determines fecal bulk. Some residue is produced from intestinal cell sloughing or bacteria even when no food or very low-residue food is ingested orally. Physicians' attitudes toward prescribing low-residue diets for patients with chronic intestinal disease vary, but it is generally felt that patients with chronic partial bowel obstruction should consume low-residue preparations. One enteral preparation (Enrich) contains additional residue and is designed for patients on long-term enteral nutrition who are prone to constipation and impaction.

Flavoring: Flavored oral preparations are preferred by most patients, and the medical staff should be aware of the taste characteristics of these formulations, since the flavor may be important to patient acceptance. Some oral formulations are best tolerated when kept in an ice bath at the patient's bedside where they may be consumed regularly in small amounts. Flavorings can be added to some enteral formulas; however, this may alter the pH and osmolality of the supplement. Initially, hyperosmolar diets should be given at half strength to determine tolerance, particularly in gastrectomized patients.

Diets given by tube should be unflavored, particularly when used in infants.

Fluid and Electrolytes: Water must be available to satisfy fluid requirements, especially for patients who are completely dependent on these formulations or those who have impaired renal concentrating ability. To prevent dehydration, sufficient water must be given to replace insensible water loss, sweat, a reasonable amount of urine, and gastrointestinal losses. Additional electrolytes may be required in patients with some salt-losing nephropathies, diarrhea, fistulas, burns, or other conditions in which there is excessive electrolyte loss.

Vitamins and Minerals: A minimum volume has to be ingested to provide 100% of all micronutrients (see Table 6). Some formulas provide inadequate amounts of minerals, particularly zinc, potassium, and magnesium, for patients with large gastrointestinal losses, and these must be added if enteral alimentation is the sole source of nutrition and is prolonged (see Table 1). Manufacturers now are adding a variety of trace elements to the formulations. The label should be checked to ensure adequacy for long-term use. To avoid hypoprothrombinemia, vitamin K also should be present if administration is prolonged. However, patients receiving oral anticoagulants should be monitored, for the vitamin K content of some preparations has been reported to interfere with anticoagulation.

Indications

Nutritional requirements vary with different diseases. Anorexia or mechanical obstruction of the gastrointestinal tract may result in inadequate intake. Frequent vomiting, draining fistulas, and malabsorption increase nutrient losses. Hypermetabolism, often associated with stress, severe injury, or burn, may increase the requirements for nutrients severalfold to prevent rapid decrease of lean body mass. Deficiency of any nutrient may occur, but protein and calorie deficiencies are most common.

Many enteral formulations are promoted for use in conditions associated with impaired digestion or absorption, but very little basic work has been done to determine the optimum requirements for many of these formulations in different disease states or to compare the efficacy of various preparations in a given disease. Formulations with special ingredients (ie, crystalline amino acids) are expensive and are indicated only for patients with digestive or absorptive problems and/or hepatic, renal, or pulmonary disease; even in such situations, they may be less effective than those containing hydrolyzed protein. For patients with normal digestion and absorption, placement of the feeding tube tip in the upper small bowel permits adequate digestion.

Oral Feeding: Nutritionally complete, liquified food and defined formulas supplemented with a complex carbohydrate source are indicated for patients with no special nutritional requirements and those with mild to moderate impairment of absorptive surface area or digestive enzyme activities who are capable of digesting intact protein, long-chain fats, or complex branched-chain polysaccharides. If oral ingestion is feasible, enteral formulas can be given to supplement increased nutrient intake in patients with trauma, malignancies, cachexia, or protein-calorie malnutrition when the gastrointestinal tract is intact.

Tube Feeding: Tube feedings using nasogastric, nasoduodenal, nasojejunal, esophagostomy, gastrostomy, or jejunostomy tubes may be necessary for infants, patients having mechanical problems chewing or swallowing, comatose patients, and those with impaired gastrointestinal function or anorexia.

Commercial formulations of natural foodstuffs are so finely suspended that they pass through small bore tubes. These preparations are indicated when tube feeding is necessary. Food blended in ordinary kitchen equipment is not suitable because the larger particles may clog small bore tubes.

Nasogastric tubes should be placed with care to ensure proper positioning of the tip and to prevent dislodgement with resulting aspiration. Enteral formulas are administered through a fine (5F to 8F) nasogastric catheter positioned into the stomach (if appropriate gastric motility is present) or duodenum and checked by air insufflation (or by lateral chest x-ray in neonates). Long, fine bore nasal tubes may be passed into the distal duodenum or upper jejunum with radiographic confirmation of tube position. The latter two positionings are necessary when aspiration may be a problem, gastric retention occurs, or intragastric administration is contraindicated. For long-term feeding, surgical placement of an esophagostomy, gastrostomy, or jejunostomy tube may be necessary.

Dosage should be individualized, based on the patient's condition, the specific formula administered, and the method of administration. Hyperosmolar formulations should be started at 0.33 to 0.5 kcal/ml and infused at 30 to 50 ml/hr. Jejunal feeding should be initiated at iso-osmolar concentrations (270 to 300 mOsm/L) and the osmolality gradually increased.

For slow-drip feeding, use of an automated infusion pump is recommended; absorption and tolerance are improved and the incidence of adverse reactions is reduced by slow constant feeding over many hours rather than repeated bolus feedings. This method of administration prevents the dumping syndrome, which occurs when hyperosmolar solutions are introduced rapidly into the small intestine. The rate should be increased gradually and, if gastric retention, diarrhea, or glycosuria is not encountered, the concentration is increased until the full strength is given, typically within 24 to 36 hours. The volume administered is then increased to provide the total caloric input desired. Patient tolerance generally is reached when 1,800 to 3,500 ml/24 hours is given. If a solution containing 1 kcal/ml is used, maximum volume in a 70-kg patient is 3,500 ml. These levels can be attained only if hyperglycemia or glycosuria does not occur. Free access to water should be permitted and additional water or electrolyte supplements may be administered if needed.

All patients receiving enteral tube feeding should be monitored frequently for difficulties associated with refeeding during malnutrition. Initially, serum glucose concentrations should be monitored and determination of serum glucose, electrolytes, pH, and osmolarity is recommended every two or three days. After the dose and measurements are stable, the monitoring interval can be extended gradually to once or twice weekly.

Adverse Reactions and Precautions

Overall, 10% of patients receiving enteral nutrition through a nasogastric tube experience some type of complication (Cataldi-Betcher et al, 1983). Gastrointestinal disturbances, including diarrhea, inadequate gastric emptying, vomiting, and gastrointestinal bleeding, account for over one-half of the complications. The frequency of these adverse effects can be minimized by using a slow initial infusion rate and diluting the formula to a maximum of one-half strength. The infusion rate is then increased gradually and, if gastric retention, diarrhea, or hyperglycemia is not encountered, the concentration is increased to full strength, commonly within 24 to 36 hours. Severely malnourished patients with hypoproteinemia may develop edema in the gut secondary to decreased colloid osmotic pressure, leading to malabsorption. About one-half of patients experiencing gastrointestinal complications will require TPN, at least temporarily. An overlooked cause of gastrointestinal disturbances is coadministration of oral electrolyte solutions and certain medications through the enteral feeding tube (Niemiec et al, 1983). This problem can be minimized by diluting oral medications tenfold with water.

The most serious mechanical complication of tube feeding is aspiration pneumonitis. Patients should be kept in a semisitting position (head of the bed elevated 30°) during feeding and for one hour thereafter. A 30° angle should be maintained for the elderly, infants, those with decreased gastric motility (eg, postoperative, septic, or trauma patients; patients with diabetes mellitus), or those who are comatose. The loss of gag reflex, hiccuping, a tendency to vomit, or significant pulmonary dysfunction is a contraindication to bolus feeding through a nasopharyngeal tube and even feeding by slow drip should be undertaken with great caution. The tube should be inserted into the duodenum or jejunum for slow-drip feeding; otherwise, intravenous feeding should be instituted. When tube feeding is used cautiously, aspiration occurs in less than 1% of patients.

Metabolic complications secondary to enteral feeding can be minimized by close monitoring of the serum electrolyte and glucose concentrations. Hyperglycemia progressing to non-ketotic coma can result from administration of excessive carbohydrate and protein. Caution is required in patients prone to hyperglycemia (eg, those with pancreatitis or diabetes mellitus; those taking glucocorticoids, adrenergic drugs, or potent diuretics). Large amounts of carbohydrates with inadequate phosphate also can cause significant hypophosphatemia in three to seven days. Phosphate supplements should be given intravenously because administration through the tube may cause diarrhea.

Preparations containing large amounts of electrolytes should be given cautiously to patients with cardiovascular, renal, or hepatic disease. Some commercial defined formula diet preparations contain excessive amounts of sodium and potassium (and magnesium for those with renal disease). The label should be examined prior to use. In patients with excessive intestinal fluid loss (eg, fistula, diarrhea), additional sodium and potassium administered orally or intravenously may be required.

The occurrence of rashes following more than a year of enteral feeding with diets low in fat is thought to be caused by fatty acid deficiency.

After dry preparations are mixed with water or concentrates are diluted, they must be refrigerated and used within 24 hours. Dry preparations may be kept for extended periods at temperatures less than 60 F (see the manufacturers' literature). Once water is added, they serve as excellent culture media and should be refrigerated promptly.

The enteral route should not be used in patients with intractable vomiting, severe gastrointestinal bleeding, or intestinal obstruction in which a feeding tube cannot be placed distal to the site of obstruction (eg, adynamic ileus, hernia, volvulus). The use of enteral feeding formulas in patients with chronic diarrhea will depend on the cause of the diarrhea.

Available Formulations

Nutritionally Complete Formulas: These preparations (see Table 6) contain high-molecular-weight protein, complex carbohydrates, and long-chain fats. The source of protein is generally casein, soy protein, or egg albumin. A few formulas contain lactose as a source of carbohydrate. Complex fats provide approximately 30% of the nonprotein calories and improve the palatability of nutritionally complete formulas compared to defined formula diets. They supply total nutritional requirements when given in the appropriate concentration and volume (at least 2 L/day in adults).

Nutritionally complete formulas are indicated for patients who have no special nutritional requirement, for patients with an obstruction above the small bowel, and for those with mild to moderate impairment of the absorptive surface area or digestive enzyme activities who are capable of digesting intact proteins, long-chain fats, and complex branched-chain polysaccharides. Patients with obstruction can be fed via tube if the tip of the tube is located past the obstruction. Most nutritionally complete formulas are flavored and are accepted by patients when administered orally. They are generally iso-osmolar and are less expensive than defined formula diets.

Defined Formula Diets: DFD are monomeric formulas with moderate to high osmolalities. They flow easily through a small-bore tube directly into the stomach, duodenum, or jejunum. Many are composed of chemically isolated food derivatives that may or may not require digestion and may be well absorbed in the jejunum and upper ileum. The degree of absorption depends upon the efficacy of the absorption processes and the amount of normal absorptive surface present. (For listing, see Table 6.)

DFD are indicated only when luminal hydrolysis or absorption is impaired (eg, in patients with inflammatory bowel disease, dysphagia secondary to radiation or surgery, severe exocrine pancreatic enzyme deficiency, or short bowel syndrome). They should be used as adjuncts to or instead of parenteral nutrition when enteral feeding can provide adequate calories.

DFD decrease gastric secretions and reduce stool bulk. They have some advantage over standard feeding with nutritionally complete formulas in patients with the following conditions: (1) Fistulas of the alimentary tract (particularly the lower portion); spontaneous closure of fistulas has occurred with the use of DFD. (2) Pancreatitis complicated by alcoholism or gallstones when oral feeding is not feasible. DFD should be administered through a tube with the tip in the small bowel. In chronic pancreatic insufficiency, steatorrhea has been reduced by feeding DFD with MCT and decreased LCT or supplemented with pancreatic enzyme preparations. However, patients with pancreatic disorders also may have diabetes mellitus, and the additional glucose load imposed by DFD may require adjustment of the dose of hypoglycemic drug. (3) Inflammatory bowel disease (eg, Crohn's disease, ulcerative colitis, radiation enteritis); in children with Crohn's disease, excessive diarrhea may be controlled and an anabolic response achieved both pre- and postoperatively by the use of DFD (Hartline, 1977). (4) Serious malabsorption and short bowel syndrome, especially when the DFD is administered as a slow drip over many hours following the initial period using TPN. This stimulates luminal absorption and encourages growth of intestinal mucosa. (5) After rectal surgery; the reduced residue and decreased fecal bulk may assist healing. (6) For individuals with galactosemia, lactase deficiency, allergy to milk protein, and glycogen storage disease and to assist in diagnosing food allergy.

TABLE 6.
NUTRITIONALLY COMPLETE ENTERAL FORMULATIONS

Preparations	Per 1,000 Kcal					
	Protein (g)	Fat (g)	Carbohydrate (g)	Phosphorus (mg)	Sodium (mg)	Potassium (mg)
LACTOSE-CONTAINING FORMULATIONS						
Compleat-B (Sandoz Nutrition)	40	40	120.4	1,250	1,187	1,314
Meritene Liquid (Sandoz Nutrition)	60	33.3	115	1,250	1,915	1,670
Sustacal & Milk (Mead Johnson)	60	27	128	1,330	920	2,815
Sustagen & Water (Mead Johnson)	60	9	172	920	920	2,111
LACTOSE-FREE FORMULATIONS						
(1 kcal/ml, standard protein content)						
Criticare HN (Mead Johnson)	36.0	3.2	210.0	500	598	1,251
Enrich (Ross)	36.1	33.8	147.3	654	770	1,423
Ensure (Ross)	35.1	35.1	136.7	519	798	1,474
Ensure HN (Ross)	31.4	33.5	133	718	879	1,474
High Nitrogen Vivonex (Norwich Eaton)	44.4	0.9	210	333	529	1,173
Osmolite (Ross)	35.1	36.3	136.7	519	517	954
Osmolite HN (Ross)	41.9	34.7	133	718	879	1,474
Precision High Nitrogen (Sandoz Nutrition)	41.7	1.2	205.7	333	934	864
Precision Isotonic (Sandoz Nutrition)	30	31.3	150	667	801	1,001
Precision LR (Sandoz Nutrition)	23.7	1.4	223.2	526	632	790
Standard Vivonex (Norwich Eaton)	21.8	1.5	230.7	556	469	1,173
Travasorb (Travenol)	33	35	136.4	500	699	1,204
Travasorb HN (Travenol)	45	13.3	175	500	920	1,173
Travasorb STD (Travenol)	30	13.4	190	500	920	1,173
Vital High Nitrogen (Ross)	41.7	10.8	185	667	467	1,333
Vivonex T.E.N. (Norwich Eaton)	38.2	2.8	206	500	460	782

mOsm/kg	Volume to Supply 1,000 Kcal (ml)	Kcal to Supply 100% of RDA for Vitamins	Comment
405	938	1,500	Tube feeding, moderate residue
505–570[a]	1,042	1,255	Oral and tube feeding, low residue
1,000[b]	769	1,090	Oral and tube feeding, moderate residue
625	990	1,725	Oral and tube feeding, low residue
650	943	2,000	Fat free, low residue
480[c]	910	1,538	Contains fiber, moderate residue
450[c]	943	2,000	Low residue
470[c]	943	1,389	Low residue
810[d]	1,000	3,000	Oligomeric, fat free, low residue
300	943	2,000	Isotonic, low residue
310	943	1,389	Isotonic, low residue
525	950	3,030	Oligomeric, fat free, low residue
300	1,040	1,500	Isotonic, low residue
480–510[e]	890	1,900	Oligomeric, fat free, low residue
550[d]	1,000	1,786	Oligomeric, fat free, low residue
486	1,000	2,000	Low residue
560	1,000	2,000	Oligomeric, low fat, low residue
560	1,000	2,000	Oligomeric, low fat, low residue
450	1,000	1,500[f]	Oligomeric, low fat, low residue
630	1,000	2,000	Oligomeric, fat free, protein content is high in branched chain amino acids (33% of total amino acids)

(Continued on next page)

TABLE 6.
NUTRITIONALLY COMPLETE ENTERAL FORMULATIONS (continued)

Preparations	Per 1,000 Kcal					
	Protein (g)	Fat (g)	Carbohydrate (g)	Phosphorus (mg)	Sodium (mg)	Potassium (mg)
LACTOSE-FREE FORMULATIONS (continued)						
(1.5 kcal/ml)						
Ensure Plus (Ross)	36.7	35.6	133.4	423	761	1,552
Ensure Plus (Ross)	41.7	33.3	133.3	705	789	1,212
Sustacal HC (Mead Johnson)	40	38	125	560	552	977
Traumacal (Mead Johnson)	55	46	95	500	782	938
Travasorb MCT (Travenol)	50	34	125	500	529	1,001
(2 kcal/ml)						
Isocal HCN (Mead Johnson)	38	45	113	330	414	704
Magnacal (Chesebrough-Pond's)	35	40	125	500	499	626
Two Cal (Ross)	41.7	45.3	108.2	526	529	1,165
SPECIALIZED FORMULAS						
Renal Failure Formulas						
Amin-Aid (American McGaw)	10	23.6	186.5	0	169	<3
Travasorb Renal (Travenol)	17.1	13.3	202.7	0	0	0
Hepatic Encephalopathy Formulas						
Hepatic-Aid II (American McGaw)	37.5	31	143	0	201	3
Travasorb Hepatic (Travenol)	26.4	13.2	193.2	435	405	1,036
Formulas for Trauma Patients						
BCAA Stresstein (Sandoz Nutrition)	58.4	23.4	141.7	417	543	919
Traum-Aid HBC (American McGaw)	56	12.4	166	400	530	1,170
MISCELLANEOUS FORMULAS						
Lonalac (Mead Johnson)	53	55	75	1,560	39	1,564
Lofenalac (Mead Johnson)	33	39	129	700	460	1,017

mOsm/kg	Volume to Supply 1,000 Kcal (ml)	Kcal to Supply 100% of RDA for Vitamins	Comment
600	666.7	2,857	Oral and tube feeding, low residue
650[c]	666.7	1,428	Oral and tube feeding, low residue
650	654	1,785	Oral and tube feeding, low residue
550	667	3,000	Oral and tube feeding, high protein, low residue
312	670	2,000	High protein, oral and tube feeding, isotonic, low residue
690	500	3,000	Tube feeding, low residue
590	500	2,000	Oral and tube feeding, low residue
750[c]	500	1,901	Oral and tube feeding, low residue
850	510	—	2 kcal/ml, oral and tube feeding, protein content is 100% essential amino acids
590	750	—	1.33 kcal/ml, oral and tube feeding, protein content is 100% essential amino acids
560	850	—	1.2 kcal/ml, oral and tube feeding, protein content is high in branched chain amino acids and low in aromatic amino acids and methionine
690	926	2,270	1.1 kcal/ml, oral and tube feeding. Protein content is high in branched chain amino acids and arginine, low in aromatic amino acids and methionine
910	833	2,400	1.2 kcal/ml, tube feeding, high protein content consisting of 44% branched chain amino acids
675	1,000	3,000	1 kcal/ml, oral and tube feeding, high protein content is 50% branched chain amino acids
—	1,480[g]	—	Contains lactose, 0.7 kcal/ml, oral and tube feeding, high protein. For sodium-restricted adults as a milk substitute
—	1,500[g]	641	0.7 kcal/ml, oral and tube feeding. For infants and children up to 2 years of age with phenylketonuria

(Continued on next page)

TABLE 6.
NUTRITIONALLY COMPLETE ENTERAL FORMULATIONS (continued)

Preparations	Per 1,000 Kcal					
	Protein (g)	Fat (g)	Carbohydrate (g)	Phosphorus (mg)	Sodium (mg)	Potassium (mg)
MISCELLANEOUS FORMULAS (continued)						
Pulmocare (Ross)	41.7	61.4	70.4	705	874	1,271
Ross SLD (Ross)	53.6	0.7	195	1,193	1,194	1,193
Special Formula S-14 (Wyeth)	16	54.5	105	469	373	704
Special Formula S-29 (Wyeth)	25	34	149.5	250	11	469
Special Formula S-44 (Wyeth)	25	34	149.5	250	11	469

[a]Depending on flavor
[b]Mixed with whole milk to a dilution of 40 kcal/30 ml
[c]Add 15 to 30 mOsm/kg per flavor packet
[d]Add 45 mOsm/kg per flavor packet

[e]30 kcal/30 ml
[f]3,448 kcal are required to supply 100% of vitamin E
[g]Standard dilution of 20 kcal/30 ml

Adapted from Heimburger and Weinsier, 1985.

Commercial defined formula diets are formulated for adults but can be used in infants and children if the concentration and rate of administration are reduced and the patient is observed closely and monitored carefully. Infants do not tolerate initial concentrations greater than 10%. However, if the concentration is increased gradually, strengths up to 18% may be used ultimately. Close monitoring of infants and children is necessary to prevent hyperosmolar dehydration. In one study (Hartline, 1977), a 3 1/2 French feeding tube inserted nasogastrically was used with an infusion pump in infants. Initially, 50 ml/kg/day was infused, with the amount increased gradually to 165 ml/kg/day over 40 to 96 hours. Supplemental fluid was provided by peripheral intravenous injection until an adequate enteral volume was tolerated. The concentration was increased from 0.5 cal/ml to 0.67 cal/ml and 1 to 2 ml of safflower oil (72% linoleic acid) was added daily to provide essential fatty acids. Vitamins A, C, and D; fluoride; and iron also were added daily. For infants and children on long-term feeding without oral supplements, a source of essential fatty acids with linolenic acid and linoleic acid is advisable.

Modular Formulas: Modular formulas are used as supplements or as base formulas to which specified components are added as needed. They are not intended to be the sole source of nutrients and must be combined with a nutritionally complete formula or ordinary foods to provide essential nutrition. Familiarity with the composition of these products before prescription is essential, since they may provide some nutrients in excess of requirements for certain patients.

Specialized Formulas for Specific Diseases: Special nutritional formulations are available for use in specific diseases

(see Table 6). Lofenalac is indicated only for patients with phenylketonuria. The manufacturer recommends its use in infants and children up to 2 years, with ingestion of a phenylalanine-free product [Phenylfree (Mead Johnson)] thereafter. With use of the latter, a wider choice of supplemental foods containing phenylalanine is possible; intake should be adjusted to the level necessary to support physical and mental development. Other low-protein foods should be added, as required, to provide calories. For children, sufficient Phenylfree and other foods to provide 15 to 30 mg/kg of phenylalanine daily appears to be most beneficial. Frequent monitoring of blood and urine levels of phenylalanine and tyrosine is essential during prolonged use, with subsequent adjustment of diet as necessary.

Isomil, MBF, Nursoy, Nutramigen, Pregestimil, ProSobee, Soyalac, and i-Soyalac are suitable substitutes for cow's milk in individuals with galactosemia, lactase deficiency, allergy to milk protein, milk-induced steatorrhea, or glycogen storage disease. They may be useful in newborn infants with a family history of allergy to cow's milk and to diagnose intolerance to milk. However, about one-third of the infants sensitive to cow's milk protein have cross-sensitivity to soy protein. i-Soyalac and Nursoy contain no corn products and may be useful if sensitivity to corn is suspected or to diagnose intolerance to corn.

These products are made hypoallergenic by substituting either hydrolyzed casein, soy flour, soy protein isolate, aqueous extracts of whole soybeans, or homogenized beef for the protein in cow's milk. Intolerance to galactose and lactose is avoided by substituting sucrose, maltose, dextrose, dextrins,

mOsm/kg	Volume to Supply 1,000 Kcal (ml)	Kcal to Supply 100% of RDA for Vitamins	Comment
490[c]	666.7	1,429	1.5 kcal/ml, oral and tube feeding, low carbohydrate, high fat. For patients with impaired pulmonary function
545	1,429	840	0.7 kcal/ml, oral and tube feeding, high protein, fat free. For patients requiring a clear liquid or fat-restricted diet
280	1,479	5,000	Contains lactose, high protein. For patients with leucine-sensitive hypoglycemia
359	1,479	5,000	Contains lactose. For sodium-restricted diet
359	1,479	—	Contains lactose. For idiopathic hypercalcemia

corn syrup solids, arrowroot starch, or tapioca dextrins. These products usually are diluted to provide 0.67 kcal/ml. They are used in infants, children, and adults in amounts that supply adequate fluid and nutrients.

Formulas for Normal Infants: These formulas may be used to provide nutrients for normal premature or full-term bottle-fed infants or as a supplement for breast-fed infants. They have been formulated to provide nutrients in proportions similar to those present in human breast milk and are available as ready-to-feed formulations or as concentrated liquid or powder for dilution with water. Most formulas are nutritionally complete, although some do not contain iron and others do not provide sufficient iron for older infants. If the formula contains insufficient iron, supplemental amounts should be given; the American Academy of Pediatrics recommends at least 1 mg iron/100 kcal of formula. Most formulas provide 0.67 kcal/ml.

In 1985, the FDA established guidelines for the composition of commercially available formulas for healthy infants sold through interstate commerce. The guidelines were originally developed by the Committee on Nutrition of the American Academy of Pediatrics (1976).

Cited References

Adibi SA: Oligopeptides as carriers of amino acids for chemically defined diets, in Shils ME (ed): *Defined Formula Diets for Medical Purposes.* Chicago, American Medical Association, 1977, 15-20.

Askanazi J, et al: Respiratory changes induced by large glucose loads of total parenteral nutrition. *JAMA* 243:1444-1447, 1980.

Baker JP, et al: Nutritional assessment: Comparison of clinical judg-ment and objective measurements. *N Engl J Med* 306:969-972, 1982.

Cataldi-Betcher EL, et al: Complications occurring during enteral nutrition support: Prospective study. *J Parent Ent Nutr* 7:546-552, 1983.

Cerra FB, et al: Disease-specific amino acid infusion (F080) in hepatic encephalopathy: Prospective, randomized, double-blind, con-trolled trial. *J Parent Ent Nutr* 9:288-295, 1985.

Committee on Nutrition, American Academy of Pediatrics: Commen-tary on breast-feeding and infant formulas, including proposed standards for formulas. *Pediatrics* 57:278-285, 1976.

Fischer JE, Freund HR: Central hyperalimentation, in Fischer JE (ed): *Surgical Nutrition.* Boston, Little, Brown and Company, 1983, 663-702.

Hartline JV: Continuous intragastric infusion of elemental diet: Experi-ences with ten infants having small intestine disease. *Clin Pediatr* 16:1105-1109, 1977.

Heimburger DC, Weinsier RL: Guidelines for evaluating and categoriz-ing enteral feeding formulas according to therapeutic equiva-lence. *J Parent Ent Nutr* 9:61-67, 1985.

Klein GL, et al: Reduced serum levels of 1α, 25-dihydroxyvitamin D during long-term parenteral nutrition. *Ann Intern Med* 94:638-643, 1981.

Levene MI, et al: Pulmonary fat accumulation after Intralipid infusion in preterm infant. *Lancet* 2:815-818, 1980.

McCullough AJ, et al: Branched-chain amino acids as nutritional therapy in liver disease: Dearth or surfeit? *Hepatology* 3:269-271, 1983.

Millikan WJ Jr, et al: Total parenteral nutrition with F080 in cirrhotics with subclinical encephalopathy. *Ann Surg* 197:294-304, 1983.

Niemiec PW Jr, et al: Gastrointestinal disorders caused by medication and electrolyte solution osmolality during enteral nutrition. *J Parent Ent Nutr* 7:387-389, 1983.

Seligman JV, et al: Metabolic bone disease in patient on long-term total parenteral nutrition: Case report with review of literature. *J Parent Ent Nutr* 8:723-727, 1984.

Shike M: Copper in parenteral nutrition. *Bull NY Acad Med* 60:132-143, 1984.

Shike M, et al: Metabolic bone disease in patients receiving long-term total parenteral nutrition. *Ann Intern Med* 92:343-350, 1980.

Silk DBA, et al: Use of peptide rather than free amino acid nitrogen source in chemically defined 'elemental' diets. *J Parent Ent Nutr* 4:548-553, 1980.

Vanhuynegem L, et al: Detection of central venous catheter-associated sepsis. *Eur J Clin Microbial* 4:46-48, 1985.

Wahren J, et al: Is intravenous administration of branched chain amino acids effective in treatment of hepatic encephalopathy? Multicenter study. *Hepatology* 3:475-480, 1983.

Wolman SL, et al: Zinc in total parenteral nutrition: Requirements and metabolic effects. *Gastroenterology* 76:458-467, 1979.

Other Selected References

Department of Foods and Nutrition, American Medical Association: Guidelines for essential trace elements for parenteral use: Statement by expert panel. *JAMA* 241:2051-2054, 1979.

Wan KK, Tsallas G: Dilute iron dextran formulation for addition to parenteral nutrient solutions. *Am J Hosp Pharm* 37:206-210, 1980.

Agents Affecting Calcium Metabolism

49

INTRODUCTION

DISORDERS OF CALCIUM METABOLISM

Hypercalcemia

Hypocalcemia

Osteomalacia and Rickets

Renal Osteodystrophy

Osteoporosis

Paget's Disease of Bone

DRUG EVALUATIONS

Calcium is essential to support neuromuscular transmission, muscle cell contraction, blood coagulation, cardiac function, and cell membrane permeability. Calcium homeostasis is maintained by the interaction of intrinsic factors that control the continuous remodeling of bone, and regulatory mechanisms that modify the absorption, excretion, and exchange of calcium. The metabolic role of calcium has priority over its structural function, and maintenance of calcium ion homeostasis will occur, if necessary, at the expense of bone. The concentration of total calcium in the serum is maintained within the narrow range of 8.6 to 10.5 mg/dl.

The amount of calcium absorbed is related to the quantity ingested; 50% of calcium may be absorbed during conditions of low calcium intake, while only 20% may be absorbed with intake of 1.5 g/day. More than 98% of endogenous calcium is present in skeletal tissue as part of the hydroxyapatite crystal; 1% is in soft tissue and only 0.1% is in extracellular fluid where it may be ionized, protein bound, or complexed with various ions (eg, phosphate, carbonate, citrate, sulfate). Ionized calcium in extracellular fluid and plasma is in constant equilibrium with the small fraction of skeletal calcium (4 to 6 g) available for rapid exchange. The protein bound fraction of serum calcium is mostly bound to albumin; on the average, 1 g of serum albumin binds approximately 0.8 mg of calcium. Only unbound, ionized serum calcium is physiologically active and its concentration is controlled by interactions with the homeostatic agents: parathyroid hormone (PTH, parathyrin, parathormone), vitamin D, and calcitonin.

The serum calcium concentration usually is controlled by a negative feedback mechanism involving ionized serum calcium, PTH, and calcitonin secretion. A *fall* in ionized serum calcium stimulates secretion of PTH, which, in turn, promotes the renal tubular reabsorption of calcium, decreases the renal reabsorption of phosphate, and if the decrement is large,

increases osteoclastic mobilization of calcium from bone. In addition, PTH stimulates the renal synthesis of 1,25-dihydroxy-vitamin D_3 (1,25-$(OH)_2D_3$), a biologically active metabolite of vitamin D. Synthesis of 1,25-$(OH)_2D_3$ also is stimulated by a decrease in the serum concentration of inorganic phosphate caused by PTH effects on renal phosphate excretion. This metabolite is the major hormonal regulator of calcium (and possibly phosphate) absorption in the intestine. It also has a permissive effect on PTH-induced stimulation of bone resorption.

The major actions of calcitonin are to inhibit bone resorption and renal tubular reabsorption of calcium, thus promoting hypocalcemia. Although the secretion of calcitonin from the parafollicular cells of the thyroid gland is inhibited by decreasing serum calcium levels, the relative significance of reduced calcitonin levels in normalizing hypocalcemia in man is unclear.

A *rise* in the level of ionized serum calcium inhibits the release of PTH and, secondarily, the renal production of 1,25-$(OH)_2D_3$; the effects are opposite those noted above. An increased concentration of calcium also stimulates the secretion of calcitonin, which inhibits the mobilization of calcium from bone and increases the renal excretion of not only calcium, but phosphate, sodium, chloride, magnesium, and potassium as well. In infants and children, enhanced calcitonin secretion after feeding may modulate postabsorptive hypercalcemia. Under normal conditions, calcitonin's long-term effect on the skeleton is to reduce bone remodeling.

Other hormones (eg, glucocorticoids, growth hormone, thyroid hormone, insulin, androgens, estrogens) also affect calcium balance and bone metabolism either directly or by influencing the secretion and/or action of the primary regulators. The subject of bone formation has been reviewed extensively (Canalis, 1983; Raisz and Kream, 1983).

885

Several adjustments in calcium metabolism occur during pregnancy. Increased secretion of PTH helps to balance the tendency toward lower maternal serum calcium concentration caused by expansion of extracellular fluid volume and the active transport of calcium from mother to fetus. The concentration in the fetus is high relative to that in the mother until parturition when the neonate's calcium source ends abruptly. Neonatal serum calcium drops before recovering to normal levels about two days after delivery (Pitkin, 1985).

Changes in biochemical variables associated with disorders of calcium metabolism are summarized in Table 1. The mechanism of action of certain drugs used in these disorders and the indications for their use appear in Table 2. Disorders of calcium homeostasis have been reviewed (Agus et al, 1982).

DISORDERS OF CALCIUM METABOLISM

Hypercalcemia

Most hypercalcemic patients are asymptomatic. When symptoms occur, they frequently include polyuria, nausea and vomiting, constipation, and neuropsychiatric disturbances. Hypercalcemia may affect the kidneys (eg, renal vasoconstriction, decreased concentrating ability, nephrocalcinosis), cen-

tral nervous system (eg, depression, lethargy, confusion), gastrointestinal tract (eg, anorexia, peptic ulcer, pancreatitis), and heart (eg, arrhythmias, ECG changes). Abnormal deposition of calcium also may occur (eg, cornea, conjunctiva, other soft tissues).

Life-threatening hypercalcemia is most commonly caused by neoplasms; breast and squamous cell lung carcinoma are the most frequent types but hypercalcemia also is associated with a variety of hematologic cancers or solid tumors with or without bone metastases. Certain tumors synthesize and release substances that stimulate bone resorption in areas of skeletal metastasis or generally in the absence of metastases. These substances may include osteoclast-activating factors (cytokines), prostaglandins, and transforming growth factors. A substance(s) with activity common to PTH but immunologically distinct from it also may be secreted by some tumors (Mundy et al, 1984).

Hyperparathyroidism also commonly causes hypercalcemia, which may be intermittent and is usually mild compared to that produced by neoplasms. Sarcoidosis and other granulomatous diseases (eg, tuberculosis, fungal infections, berylliosis, leprosy), hypervitaminosis D, hyperthyroidism, milk-alkali syndrome, and thiazide therapy also cause hypercalcemia. Less commonly, hypercalcemia may be associated with hypervitaminosis A, hypothyroidism in children, acute adrenocortical

TABLE 1.
CHEMICAL CHANGES IN DISORDERS OF CALCIUM HOMEOSTASIS

	Ca	Phos	Mg	Bone Alk Phos	PTH	25 (OH)D	Hb	BUN	Cl	Urine Ca	Tubular Reab Phos
Primary Hyperparathyroidism	↑	↓(N)	(↓)	N(↑)	↑	N	N	N(↑)	>102	↑(N)	↓(N)
Ectopic Parathyroid Hormone	↑	↓(N)	N↓	N	↑(N)	N	↓(N)	(N)↑	<102	↑(N)	↓(N)
Vitamin D Intoxication	↑	↑	↑	N	↓	↑	N	N(↑)	N	↑	↑
Sarcoidosis	↑	↑	↑	N	↓	N	N	N	N	↓(N)	↑
Milk-Alkali Syndrome	↑	↑	N	N	↓	N	N	↑	↓	↓(N)	↑
Multiple Myeloma	N(↑)	↑(N↓)	N	N(↑)	↓	N	↓	N(↑)	N	↑	↑(N↓)
Hyperthyroidism	N(↑)	↑	N	N(↑)	↓	N	N	N	N	↑	↑
Idiopathic Hypercalciuria	N	↓(N)	N	N	↓(N↑)	N	N	N	N	↑	N↓
Hypoparathyroidism	↓	↑	N	N	↓	N	N	N	N(↓)	↓	↑
Pseudohypoparathyroidism	↓	↑	N	N(↑)	↑	N	N	N	N(↓)	↓	↑
Magnesium Deficiency	↓	N(↓)	↓	N	N	N(↓)	N	N	N	↓	N
Osteomalacia (Vit. D deficiency)	↓	↓(N)	N(↓)	↑(N)	↑	↓	N	N	N(↑)	↓	↓(N)
Osteomalacia (Renal Phos Leak)	N	↓	N	↑	N	N	N	N	N	N(↑)	↓
Osteomalacia (Antacid Abuse)	N	↓	N	↑(N)	N(↓)	N	N	N	N	↑(N)	↑

From Hahn TJ: Parathyroid hormone, calcitonin, vitamin D, mineral and bone: Metabolism and disorders, in Mazzaferri EL (ed): Endocrinology: Review of Clinical Endocrinology, ed. 2. New Hyde Park, NY, Medical Examination Pub. Co., Inc, 1980, 461. Reprinted by permission.

TABLE 2.
ACTIONS AND INDICATIONS FOR DRUGS
USED TO TREAT DISORDERS OF CALCIUM METABOLISM

| Drug | Actions | | | | Indications for Use |
	Calcium Excretion	Calcium Intestinal Absorption	Bone Mineral-ization	Bone Resorption	
Adrenal Corticosteroids		−			Certain types of hypercalcemia
Calcitonin				−	Paget's disease, hypercalcemic states associated with high bone mineral loss
Calcium Preparations		+			Hypocalcemia
Edetate Disodium (rarely used)	+				Life-threatening hypercalcemia
Estrogens				−	Postmenopausal osteoporosis
Etidronate Disodium			−	−	Paget's disease, heterotopic ossification due to spinal cord injury or total hip replacement
Furosemide	+				Hypercalcemia
Plicamycin				−	Severe hypercalcemia associated with carcinoma, Paget's disease
Phosphates	−		+		Hypophosphatemic rickets or osteomalacia, hypercalciuria, hypercalcemia
Thiazides	−				Hypercalciuria with renal calculi
Vitamin D Preparations		+			Vitamin D deficiency, hypopara-thyroidism, osteomalacia, rickets

− *decreases* + *increases*

insufficiency, pheochromocytoma, and immobilization. A familial syndrome of idiopathic hypercalcemia also must be considered in the differential diagnosis.

Hypercalcemia and hypokalemia enhance digitalis toxicity and may necessitate a reduction in dose.

Therapy: The primary objective of treatment is to control the underlying disease. Definitive diagnosis and conservative therapy (including maintenance of hydration) may be adequate in asymptomatic patients with mild hypercalcemia, but intervention generally is indicated when total serum calcium exceeds 12 mg/dl. Levels above 15 mg/dl require immediate intensive treatment to avoid a hypercalcemic crisis. There is no consistent correlation between the total serum calcium concentration and symptoms. Some symptoms (eg, mental changes) may occur in older individuals even with mild hypercalcemia.

The drugs used to treat hypercalcemia reduce serum calcium levels (1) by increasing the renal excretion of calcium (saline and loop diuretics), (2) by promoting calcium uptake by bone and other tissues (phosphates), (3) by inhibiting bone resorption (plicamycin [Mithracin], calcitonin [Calcimar], phosphates, etidronate [Didronel] or other diphosphonates, and

corticosteroids), (4) by reducing gastrointestinal absorption of calcium (phosphates, corticosteroids, cellulose phosphate), or (5) by chelating calcium. Therapy depends upon the severity of hypercalcemia, the etiology, the status of renal function, and the response to prior therapy. Blood calcium levels should be measured frequently so that therapy can be modified as needed.

Symptomatic patients usually are dehydrated because of reduced fluid intake, vomiting, and polyuria; therefore, hydration is the first step in treatment. Calcium intake should be restricted, intravenous fluids (usually isotonic sodium chloride) infused, and other electrolyte deficits (eg, potassium, magnesium) corrected. Ambulation is encouraged to reduce bone resorption resulting from immobility. The saline infusion may be continued in patients with adequate renal and cardiovascular function to increase sodium excretion and maintain volume expansion, since both factors enhance a calcium diuresis. When overexpansion of plasma volume is accomplished, a loop diuretic (furosemide [Lasix] or ethacrynic acid [Edecrin]) may be given cautiously (with monitoring to prevent electrolyte imbalance and hypovolemia) in low doses at two- to four-hour intervals to promote calciuresis. (Thiazides should not be used for this purpose because, unlike the loop diuretics, they increase the tubular reabsorption of calcium.)

Patients with severe renal insufficiency may undergo hemodialysis and peritoneal dialysis (using calcium-free dialysis fluids) to remove large amounts of calcium. Other methods to promote calciuresis are largely obsolete. The chelating agent, edetate disodium (EDTA) [Chealamide, Endrate], should not be used except in the emergency treatment of refractory cases when the ionized calcium level must be reduced substantially within 30 minutes. Infusion of sodium sulfate or citrate increases calciuresis but has no significant advantage over sodium chloride.

Elevated serum calcium levels also can be reduced by phosphate, which promotes the deposition of calcium in bone and soft tissues. Phosphate may be used in the presence of hypophosphatemia but is contraindicated in the presence of hyperphosphatemia. The oral route is safest and is preferred. If renal function is normal, oral phosphate can be given daily for prolonged periods without loss of effectiveness. Phosphate may be administered intravenously in emergencies, but it is not as effective or rapid-acting as sodium chloride and furosemide. Furthermore, intravenous phosphate is potentially dangerous and may cause severe hypocalcemia and acute renal failure. Deposition of calcium in the kidney, lungs, and blood vessels may be fatal. Too rapid infusion can cause acute renal failure.

Phosphate should not be used until the serum phosphorus level and renal function have been determined. Serum calcium and phosphate levels should be monitored closely to avoid hypocalcemia and hyperphosphatemia; serum phosphate concentrations should not exceed 6 mg/dl (Elliott and McKenzie, 1983). Adequate hydration should be maintained during treatment.

Calcitonin [Calcimar] is useful in most forms of acute, severe hypercalcemia associated with increased bone resorption and is the only treatment devoid of serious side effects. Transient reductions (1 to 3 mg/dl) in the serum calcium concentration are usually achieved safely. Lack of effectiveness may reflect inadequate doses. The drug's main limitation is its transient efficacy. Loss of efficacy may be due to calcitonin-induced reductions of serum phosphate levels, but unidentified factors are also involved. Responsiveness may be restored or possibly enhanced in some patients by adding glucocorticoids or oral phosphate supplements.

Glucocorticoids may be effective in hypercalcemia associated with production of osteoclast-activating and other factors (eg, myeloma) and probably act directly on the tumor cells rather than through an antivitamin D effect. Patients with both hematologic and solid tumors vary in their response to steroids, but those with skeletal metastases usually experience some reduction in serum calcium levels. Since the prolonged use of moderate doses of glucocorticoids may produce serious adverse effects, these drugs should be administered only for short periods when other therapy is inadequate. Reviews of the characteristics, diagnosis, and management of hypercalcemia are available (Avioli, 1982; Elliott and McKenzie, 1983; Smith, 1984; Jamieson, 1985).

Plicamycin (mithramycin), a cytotoxic agent, reduces elevated serum calcium concentrations. This drug is usually not administered for initial therapy but is particularly useful in recurrent hypercalcemia associated with advanced neoplastic disease. Plicamycin may cause hemorrhagic complications due to platelet deficiency; the effect is dose related and occurs rarely with the small doses used for hypercalcemia. Transient or permanent renal impairment also is rare. In most responsive patients, serum calcium is significantly reduced the morning after a single plicamycin infusion. Additional courses may be required (see the evaluation). The serum calcium level must be measured daily during therapy, and the patient should be monitored for hematologic and renal complications before administering the next dose.

The diphosphonate, etidronate, has been used investigationally to treat persistent hypercalcemia due to malignancy. Moderate doses given by intravenous infusion (preparation not available commercially) over a two-hour period for one to four days has reduced calcium levels (Ryzen et al, 1985). Since the drug is known to reduce osteoclastic bone resorption in Paget's disease, the same mechanism is probably responsible for reducing hypercalcemia. Other investigational diphosphonates, such as disodium aminohydroxypropylidene diphosphonate (APD), have shown promise in the treatment of hypercalcemia associated with neoplasms, Paget's disease, or hyperparathyroidism. They also suppress the mobilization of skeletal calcium by inhibiting osteoclast activity.

Measures that reduce the gastrointestinal absorption of calcium are important in treating hypercalcemia associated with the milk-alkali syndrome, sarcoidosis, hypervitaminosis D, and idiopathic hypercalcemia. Reduction of calcium intake alone may be effective, especially in the milk-alkali syndrome. The next measure to be employed depends upon the disease state and its severity. Phosphate may be effective in the presence of hypophosphatemia (eg, hyperparathyroidism) by enhancing the deposition of calcium, primarily in bone. A third measure is use of large doses of corticosteroids, which appear to inhibit the intestinal absorption of calcium. They are particularly effective in hypervitaminosis D and hypercalcemia associated with sarcoidosis or certain malignant diseases, but are not useful in hyperparathyroidism.

Hypocalcemia

Hypocalcemia results primarily from a deficiency of PTH or vitamin D (or its active metabolites), although isolated cases may be due to other factors. The differential diagnosis of hypocalcemia is facilitated by distinguishing that associated with hyperphosphatemia from that associated with hypophosphatemia. In the former, hypocalcemia may be due to PTH deficiency, resistance to PTH (pseudohypoparathyroidism), or advanced renal insufficiency. Hypocalcemia with hyperphosphatemia also may occur when there is a large influx of phosphate into the circulation, as in leukemia or lymphoma after chemotherapy induces rapid tissue lysis, when large amounts of phosphate are administered, and when phosphate enemas are used in children.

Hypocalcemia with hypophosphatemia usually indicates deficiency or altered metabolism of vitamin D or an intestinal malabsorption syndrome. Prolonged administration of anticonvulsants (eg, primidone [Mysoline], phenytoin [Dilantin], barbiturates), rifampin [Rifadin, Rimactane], glutethimide [Doriden], and probably other drugs also may induce hypocalcemia and hypophosphatemia secondary to increased metabolism of vitamin D. Marked hypocalcemia with hypophosphatemia may occur during the acute phase of hemorrhagic pancreatitis and may be secondary to extraskeletal deposition of calcium. The low serum calcium level encountered occasionally in conditions associated with hypomagnesemia is believed to be secondary to decreased release of PTH with impaired tissue responsiveness to PTH. Replenishment of magnesium stores usually corrects this condition.

In severe alcoholism, hypocalcemia is frequently secondary to inadequate intake of calcium, magnesium, and vitamin D; transient malabsorption; and excessive urinary excretion of calcium and magnesium. Osteoblastic metastases rarely cause hypocalcemia.

In most chronic hypocalcemic disorders (except those associated with primary hypoparathyroidism and hypomagnesemia), there is a compensatory increase in the secretion of PTH (secondary hyperparathyroidism), which mobilizes mineral from bone. As a result, the serum calcium level may be raised toward normal at the expense of bone, and there may be evidence of excessive PTH.

A low total serum calcium level also may be secondary to decreased serum albumin (as in chronic liver disease) but, since the ionized calcium concentration is normal, this is not true hypocalcemia and does not require treatment. A frequently used guideline is to allow a decrease in serum calcium of 0.8 mg/dl for each 1 g/dl decrement in serum albumin from a baseline albumin level of 4 g/dl.

Therapy: Regardless of etiology, treatment is necessary to prevent complications (eg, convulsions, tetany, laryngospasm, respiratory and other muscle spasms). The initial treatment of severe symptomatic hypocalcemia is intravenous infusion of a source of rapidly available calcium ion, such as 10% calcium gluconate. (There is no evidence that parenteral proprietary mixtures of calcium salts have any advantages over single-entity agents.) For maintenance, an oral calcium salt is given orally. The calcium content of available oral calcium salts ranges from 9% (calcium gluconate) to 40% (calcium carbonate).

Calcitriol [Rocaltrol] is indicated for hypocalcemia and bone disease caused by defective conversion of vitamin D to 1,25-$(OH)_2D_3$, as in patients undergoing renal dialysis and those with postsurgical or idiopathic hypoparathyroidism or pseudohypoparathyroidism (Chan et al, 1985).

If functional or actual vitamin D deficiency exists, the vitamin or its active metabolites should be administered after acute hypocalcemic symptoms have been controlled. When the deficiency is severe, the increase in serum calcium concentration after treatment may be delayed, and additional oral and/or intravenous calcium may be required to ameliorate symptoms. Vitamin D itself also can be employed to increase the serum calcium level in hypoparathyroidism. This is often accompanied by a reciprocal decline in serum phosphate levels. The

effects of vitamin D on calcium and phosphate metabolism are similar to those of PTH except that renal phosphate excretion is stimulated markedly with PTH. Parathyroid injection is no longer used therapeutically, but is still employed to distinguish pseudohypoparathyroidism from idiopathic and postsurgical hypoparathyroidism.

Osteomalacia and Rickets

Osteomalacia and rickets (severe osteomalacia in children causing deformities) are characterized by impaired mineralization of bone and accumulation of uncalcified osteoid or cartilage. The osseous changes are associated with low or normal serum calcium and phosphorus levels, increased serum alkaline phosphatase, and sometimes secondarily elevated PTH. Backache, diffuse bone pain, muscle weakness, bowing of the legs, fractures of the long bones, kyphosis (particularly when associated with osteoporosis), and waddling gait are clinical features of osteomalacia. In children, epiphyseal changes are dominant; delayed bone development, skeletal deformity, growth retardation, and muscle weakness are the principal manifestations.

Vitamin D deficiency (actual or functional), renal and gastrointestinal disorders associated with fat malabsorption, and hypophosphatemia (including vitamin D-resistant or familial hypophosphatemic rickets) are the most common causes of osteomalacia and rickets. When hypophosphatemia is the primary abnormality, best results are achieved when phosphate is added to the vitamin D regimen. Calcitriol plus phosphate was more effective in improving phosphate homeostasis and bone mineralization than vitamin D_2 (ergocalciferol) plus phosphate in patients with X-linked hypophosphatemic rickets (Chesney et al, 1983). Selected patients with renal hypophosphatemic rickets (due to renal wastage of phosphate) may benefit from the addition of hydrochlorothiazide and amiloride [Moduretic] to the calcitriol/phosphate regimen. The renal threshold for phosphate is raised and the serum phosphate concentration is increased; therefore, smaller doses of supplemental phosphate are required, thus avoiding the diarrhea that often accompanies phosphate administration (Alon and Chan, 1985).

Osteomalacia also may result from increased metabolism of vitamin D caused by the prolonged administration of anticonvulsants (Hahn, 1980 A). Inadequate diet or limited exposure to sunlight contributes to the osteomalacia commonly seen in elderly, bedridden patients and institutionalized individuals of all ages. These deficiencies usually respond to physiologic (or slightly larger) doses of vitamin D; pharmacologic doses are required in patients with vitamin D-dependent rickets, malabsorption syndromes, and renal or hepatic disorders. See also the following section on Renal Osteodystrophy.

Renal Osteodystrophy

Osteodystrophy often accompanies end-stage renal disease and has been attributed to hormonal and metabolic responses to loss of functioning nephrons and to accumulation of uremic toxins. In many patients, the histologic and radiologic manifestations of renal osteodystrophy include some degree of osteomalacia, osteitis fibrosa, and osteosclerosis, while others may present with nearly "pure" osteitis fibrosa or osteomalacia. Renal osteodystrophy also is often accompanied by osteoporosis, which may progress despite treatment. Hyperphosphatemia and elevated serum alkaline phosphatase levels are common, but the serum calcium level may be low, normal, or high depending upon the stage of the disease. Phosphate retention, secondary hyperparathyroidism, impaired vitamin D metabolism, calcium malabsorption, and chronic acidosis are important in the pathogenesis of this disorder.

Osteitis fibrosa, a common lesion in renal osteodystrophy, is caused by severe secondary hyperparathyroidism. PTH secretion is increased because of the fall in the serum calcium level, which occurs in response to phosphate retention, impaired vitamin D metabolism, and decreased intestinal calcium absorption. Serum PTH levels (as measured by radioimmunoassay) also may be elevated because of impaired renal clearance or degradation of the hormone and the presence of inactive PTH fragments that are cleared slowly. The increase in parathyroid hormone activity helps to restore homeostasis by decreasing renal phosphate reabsorption and increasing renal calcium retention; however, prolonged parathyroid stimulation eventually may cause hyperparathyroid bone disease with or without hypercalcemia. Hypercalcemia may appear or persist after renal transplantation due to persistent hyperplasia of the parathyroid glands (sometimes requiring surgery) despite the removal of factors that cause resistance to PTH stimulation (Hahn, 1980 B).

Osteomalacia probably results largely from decreased renal conversion of vitamin D to its active metabolite, 1,25-$(OH)_2D_3$. Because circulating levels of this metabolite are reduced, the intestinal absorption of calcium is impaired and insufficient calcium is available for mineralization. However, this cannot be the only causative factor because anephric patients do not necessarily develop osteomalacia. Serum levels of the major circulating vitamin D metabolite, 25-OHD_3, are variable. This metabolite is produced in the liver and is important largely as the precursor of 1,25-$(OH)_2D_3$. Supraphysiologic amounts also probably affect bone metabolism directly.

Aluminum deposition in bone is a major cause of osteomalacia in long-term dialysis patients. Aluminum is deposited at the mineralization front and thus prevents normal calcium deposition (see below). Other factors that may contribute to osteomalacia in patients with chronic renal failure are metabolic acidosis and hypophosphatemia due to excessive use of phosphate-binding antacids.

Therapy: An understanding of the pathophysiology of renal osteodystrophy provides a rational approach to therapy. The goals are (1) to decrease serum phosphate levels with dietary measures and phosphate-binding agents, and (2) to improve calcium balance with calcium and vitamin D or its active metabolites, calcitriol [Rocaltrol] (1,25-$(OH)_2D_3$) and calcifediol [Calderol] (25-OHD_3). Although there are no controlled trials demonstrating clear superiority of any agent, both calcitriol and calcifediol have some advantages over other vitamin D preparations for this indication (see the evaluations) but are more expensive. An investigational vitamin D_3 analogue, alfacalcidol (1-α-hydroxycholecalciferol, 1-α-OHD_3), also is used to treat renal osteodystrophy. The serum calcium level should be monitored carefully during therapy with vitamin D preparations, because severe hypercalcemia may occur and is especially dangerous if there is associated hyperphosphatemia.

In early renal failure, secondary hyperparathyroidism may be avoided by progressively reducing phosphate absorption in proportion to the decrease in glomerular filtration rate. This is accomplished by restricting protein and (since dietary phosphate levels cannot be decreased below 400 mg daily without adhering to an intolerable diet) by giving antacids, such as aluminum hydroxide, that bind phosphate in the gut and prevent absorption. Aluminum hydroxide gel 30 ml may be given three times daily. The dose should be adjusted to maintain serum phosphate levels between 4 and 5 mg/dl; further depletion may induce or worsen osteomalacia. Mixed aluminum and magnesium gels are not used because of the potential for hypermagnesemia.

The high levels of aluminum found in the brain tissue of uremic patients who died are thought to be the cause of dialysis encephalopathy. Aluminum in the water supply and in phosphate binding gels is the likely source. Aluminum toxicity also is manifested by abnormal accumulation in bone. Osteomalacia is rare when aluminum-free dialysate is used and oral aluminum ingestion is minimized. The toxic effects of aluminum related to dialysis and other conditions have been reviewed (Wills and Savory, 1983).

Calcium carbonate may be used to bind phosphate, especially in patients taking more than 6 g/day of aluminum hydroxide gel or in those experiencing aluminum toxicity. Calcium carbonate given with meals forms insoluble complexes with dietary phosphates, and doses should be proportional to the amount of phosphate in the meal. Although the risk of hypercalcemia is small, patients should be monitored for this possibility (Norris and Coburn, 1985).

Calcium may be administered by high calcium dialysis or orally (1 to 2 g daily). Small doses of calcitriol, calcifediol, or alfacalcidol improve calcium absorption, increase serum calcium levels, decrease parathyroid hormone secretion, and improve radiologic and histologic signs of osteitis fibrosa with or without osteomalacia. Osteomalacia due to aluminum toxicity is frequently unresponsive to vitamin D preparations. The chelating agent, deferoxamine, has been effective in removing aluminum during hemodialysis (Coburn and Henry, 1984).

Osteoporosis

Osteoporosis is characterized by a reduction in the total amount of bone tissue with a normal ratio of unmineralized to mineralized matrix. The pathologic process may involve an increased rate of bone resorption without a compensating increase in bone formation or depressed bone formation with normal or depressed resorption. Progressive loss of bone mass is reflected by pain, especially of the spine; loss of height and kyphosis as vertebral compression and collapse develop; and susceptibility to peripheral fractures. Two patterns of fractures occur in postmenopausal women. The first type is vertebral crush fracture, which is associated with an early deficit of trabecular bone and occurs at a relatively early age (around 65 years). The second type is hip fracture in which there is a deficit of both trabecular and cortical bone but not necessarily a greater deficit than in patients of the same age who do not have fractures. These fractures tend to occur later (over age 70 or 80 years) (Johnston et al, 1985 A; Raisz and Smith, 1985). Patients with osteoporosis also may develop osteomalacia, which contributes to structural weakness and pain.

Involutional (postmenopausal or senile) osteoporosis is the most common metabolic bone disorder; 25% of women over age 60 experience vertebral compression fractures. This disorder also affects a smaller number of Caucasian males in the same age range. Involutional osteoporosis appears to be as common in orientals as in whites but is uncommon in blacks. Other types of osteoporosis include a rare, idiopathic disorder affecting younger individuals and secondary forms associated with immobilization, corticosteroid therapy, or hyperthyroidism and occasionally with malabsorption or chronic liver or kidney disease. Prolonged amenorrhea from any cause, including strenuous exercise, also may contribute to bone loss and theoretically increases the long-term risk of osteoporosis.

The etiology of involutional osteoporosis is not completely known, but estrogen deficiency accounts for the great majority of cases. Genetic factors, inactivity, inadequate dietary calcium and vitamin D, excessive alcohol consumption, smoking, and increased sensitivity of bone to PTH stimulation also may be causative. Calcium absorption is reported to be impaired in osteoporotic women, perhaps because of decreased synthesis of $1,25\text{-}(OH)_2D_3$ (Aloia et al, 1985 A). This possibility is supported by the results of one study, in which long-term administration of small doses of calcitriol (synthetic $1,25\text{-}(OH)_2D_3$) corrected the calcium absorption defect in osteoporotic women (Riggs and Nelson, 1985).

Therapy: Patients with inadequate dietary calcium should receive oral calcium supplements, and small doses of vitamin D (400 or 1,000 IU) also may be indicated if there is a deficiency or lack of exposure to sunlight. Postmenopausal women given estrogen replacement therapy should ingest 1 g of calcium daily, and those not taking estrogen should receive 1.5 g daily. Although there is some evidence that bone resorption is decreased by estrogen replacement, skeletal mass does not appear to increase, possibly because of a secondary decrease in bone formation.

The association between menopause, osteoporosis, and early bone loss in patients with premature surgical menopause suggests that estrogen deficiency plays a role in the pathogenesis of this disorder. Osteoporosis is more closely related to estrogen deficiency than to advancing age per se. Gradual decline of estrogen production prior to menopause may be associated with bone loss, particularly from the vertebrae (Johnston et al, 1985 B). Estrogens reduce the response of bone to PTH by an unknown mechanism, although calcitonin reserve may be increased. Estrogens have been used for many years to prevent or treat osteoporosis, but there is still uncertainty about patient selection, optimal dosage, and dura-

tion of treatment. Regular weight-bearing exercise should be encouraged whether or not replacement therapy is prescribed.

Women who have undergone oophorectomy and hysterectomy in the pre- or perimenopausal period are prime candidates for prophylactic therapy, because (1) there is a relationship between early loss of ovarian function and subsequent osteoporosis; (2) estrogen prevents bone loss in this group; (3) symptoms of estrogen deficiency (eg, senile vaginitis, vasomotor disturbances) are likely to develop; and (4) these patients are not at risk of endometrial carcinoma. Since bone loss is most rapid during the first few years after oophorectomy, therapy should be initiated promptly. Postmenopausal oophorectomy is not associated with rapid loss of bone.

In patients with natural menopause, the indications for replacement therapy are less clear-cut, particularly when there are no symptoms of estrogen deficiency. Until more definitive guidelines become available, the patient's age, race, bone mass, body build, and muscle mass should be considered in assessing the potential benefits of prophylactic estrogen therapy.

The risk of osteoporosis is greatest in small-framed, thin, Caucasian women. Other factors that increase risk include family history of osteoporotic fractures, previous wrist or Colles fracture, low bone mass, nulliparity, early menopause, history of gastrectomy or prolonged corticosteroid therapy, smoking, and ingestion of large amounts of alcohol. Newer methods of measuring bone mass in vivo (single and double photon beam absorptiometry, neutron activation, and quantitative computed tomography) may detect osteoporosis before severe symptoms result (Genant et al, 1983). Routine radiography has proved inadequate in this regard. Some centers screen women at menopause, particularly those at high risk, using tests such as single beam absorptiometry to select patients for estrogen replacement therapy.

The minimum effective dose for prevention of bone loss is 0.625 mg of conjugated estrogens or the equivalent daily (Lindsay et al, 1984; National Institutes of Health Consensus Conference, 1984). The estrogen is given cyclically with the addition of a progestin preferred during the last part of the cycle in women with an intact uterus; some practitioners recommend this schedule even after hysterectomy. Larger doses are used to treat established osteoporosis. See also Chapter 39, Estrogens, Progestins, and Other Agents Used to Treat Gynecologic Conditions, for preparations, dosage, adverse reactions, and contraindications.

Several studies have shown that the risk of fractures in postmenopausal women was decreased by estrogen replacement therapy (Hammond et al, 1979; Hutchinson et al, 1979; Paganini-Hill et al, 1981). When estrogen therapy was withdrawn, bone loss resumed (Lindsay et al, 1978). Estrogen is most effective when given before significant bone loss has occurred, and bone loss has been retarded for an average of nine years (Lindsay et al, 1980). Data beyond that length of time are not available. There is some evidence that a combination of estrogen and progestin provides additional protection from osteoporosis and increases bone mass (Nachtigall et al, 1979; Upton, 1982; Christiansen et al, 1981). Progestin probably minimizes the risk of endometrial carcinoma when given in a cyclic regimen with estrogen.

Estrogen reduces bone resorption in older women who have already experienced spinal compression fractures. However, this effect is partially offset by the secondary decrease in bone formation that occurs during long-term therapy. For this reason, estrogen therapy may slow the progression of osteoporosis, but it does not restore skeletal quality to normal (Heaney, 1976).

Results of some population surveys have suggested that the incidence of osteoporosis may be reduced in areas with a high fluoride content in the drinking water; no information is available to contradict this observation. Fluoride increases bone mass and skeletal density, but large doses cause skeletal fluorosis, osteomalacia, and may increase the incidence of fractures in elderly patients. In one study, the combination of estrogen, calcium, and fluoride was most effective in preventing fractures in postmenopausal women. Other regimens, in order of effectiveness, were estrogen and calcium, calcium and fluoride, and calcium alone. The addition of vitamin D to these regimens did not increase effectiveness (Riggs et al, 1982). Fluoride should never be used in patients with renal insufficiency because toxic levels may accumulate.

The role of calcitonin in the prevention or treatment of osteoporosis is receiving renewed attention. Patients of both sexes who had undergone total thyroidectomy had lower bone mineral content (BMC) than controls, which suggests that calcitonin deficiency plays a role (McDermott et al, 1983). Data on serum levels of calcitonin in osteoporotic patients are conflicting. In one study, serum calcitonin concentrations were lower in osteoporotic compared to normal subjects, and also were positively correlated with BMC (Jensen et al, 1984). However, in another study, basal serum levels of calcitonin were higher in osteoporotic patients than in controls (Tiegs et al, 1985). In a study that used a specific monomeric calcitonin assay, women had lower plasma levels of calcitonin than men of comparable age, and men had a greater calcitonin secretory response to calcium than women (Body and Heath, 1983). Serum calcitonin increases following estrogen replacement therapy in postmenopausal women, and this may partially explain the effectiveness of estrogen in retarding bone loss in these individuals (Avioli, 1982).

Calcitonin has been shown to increase BMC (Wallach et al, 1977; Gennari et al, 1985; Mazzuoli et al, 1986). However, there was only preliminary (Gennari et al, 1985) or no evidence (Gruber et al, 1984; Aloia et al, 1985 B) that the incidence of fractures decreased. The decision to use calcitonin, a relatively safe drug, to prevent or treat osteoporosis must be weighed against the uncertain benefits, the high cost of treatment, and the inconvenience of parenteral administration. However, calcitonin may be particularly useful for older osteoporotic patients, those in whom estrogen is contraindicated, or in osteoporotic patients with high bone turnover. Long-term investigations to study the potential benefit of calcitonin in the treatment of osteoporosis are in progress.

Preliminary evidence suggests that anabolic steroids may slow bone loss and increase bone mass (Chestnut, 1981), but side effects, including masculinization, may be a problem in postmenopausal women. No studies comparing the effectiveness of anabolic steroids to an estrogen/progestin regimen are available. These agents may be appropriate for osteoporotic men, but there are no controlled studies to support their efficacy in these patients.

Although inorganic phosphates directly decrease bone resorption and stimulate bone formation, phosphorus supplementation has the opposite effect upon osteoporotic bone, possibly because of secondary hyperparathyroidism induced during long-term therapy (Goldsmith et al, 1976). Patients given etidronate [Didronel] for osteoporosis have developed hyperphosphatemia and defective mineralization.

Bone loss was delayed for six months in postmenopausal women treated with thiazide diuretics (Transbøl et al, 1982). One study showed that hypertensive elderly men taking thiazide diuretics for an average of seven years had greater BMC than hypertensive or normotensive subjects who did not take thiazides (Wasnich et al, 1983). This slight, if temporary, benefit may favor selection of thiazides for postmenopausal women who also need a diuretic.

In summary, no currently available drug restores the 30% to 40% loss of bone mass that occurs in symptomatic osteoporosis. Most of the agents studied inhibit bone resorption and had less effect on bone formation. Thus, they are probably of greater use in prophylaxis and stabilization than in restoration of bone mass. Agents that enhance bone formation have not prevented (sodium fluoride) fractures or are of questionable benefit (calcitonin) in preventing fractures. Until a more potent stimulant of bone formation becomes available, efforts should be made to develop precise methods of identifying susceptible individuals and detecting osteoporosis in its early stages.

Paget's Disease of Bone

Paget's disease of bone (osteitis deformans) is a chronic disorder that occurs primarily in persons over age 40. Although the etiology is unknown, there is some evidence that a slow viral infection is causative (Hosking, 1981). Paget's disease is characterized by increased bone resorption, formation of structurally abnormal replacement bone, and increased vascularity in the affected regions. The rate of progression, degree of disability, and extent of involvement vary. Patients with mild disease are often asymptomatic, and pagetic lesions may be localized. In about 25% of patients, the disease is moderate to severe and bone pain and osteoarthritic changes in joints adjacent to affected areas are common; local or generalized skeletal deformity also may be present. Thickening of the skull can be extensive. Complications include fractures and neurologic defects resulting from compression of the spinal cord, spinal nerves, and cranial nerves (including deafness). Rarely, high-output congestive heart failure develops when extensive skeletal involvement is associated with greatly increased blood flow to bone. Osteogenic sarcoma also occurs rarely and usually is fatal within two years.

The serum calcium level is normal in ambulatory patients with Paget's disease but may be elevated if the patient is immobilized. When active disease involves a significant proportion of the skeleton, the increased bone turnover is reflected by elevated serum alkaline phosphatase and urinary hydroxyproline levels.

The diagnosis, pathophysiology, and treatment of Paget's

disease of bone have been reviewed (Ryan, 1983; Siris, 1983; Strewler, 1984).

Therapy: Asymptomatic patients with small areas of bone involvement are usually not treated, although those with early hearing loss are candidates for immediate therapy. Mild pain often can be managed with analgesics and anti-inflammatory agents. In symptomatic patients with more extensive skeletal involvement, agents that inhibit excessive bone turnover are employed to relieve symptoms and perhaps retard progression of the disease (Wallach, 1982). Salmon, porcine, and human calcitonin have been used for this purpose. The salmon preparation [Calcimar] has the longest duration of action and highest potency and is the only form that is currently available commercially in the United States. A synthetic preparation of human calcitonin may be available in the future. Because of the apparent safety of calcitonin, it has been suggested that administration to asymptomatic patients might delay complications, such as fractures, bone deformities, and premature deafness. However, because the effectiveness of calcitonin treatment may decrease with time, the usual practice is to reserve it for more severely affected patients.

Serum alkaline phosphatase and urinary hydroxyproline levels usually decrease and bone pain is relieved during calcitonin therapy. Neurologic symptoms may be alleviated and functional capacity may increase; improved bone histology and radiologic evidence of regression of abnormalities have been reported in a few patients. Calcitonin must be administered parenterally but is generally well tolerated. Although its effectiveness may decrease over time, it appears to be safe for long-term therapy.

Diphosphonates inhibit bone resorption and formation by interfering with calcium phosphate crystal formation and dissolution (Hosking, 1981). They decrease the rate of formation and activity of osteoclasts. Etidronate [Didronel], the only diphosphonate currently available in the United States, decreases bone pain, improves biochemical abnormalities, and, unlike calcitonin, is effective orally. A major disadvantage of etidronate is that large doses (10 to 20 mg/kg/day) inhibit mineralization of osteoid, but this effect is dose- and time-dependent; it rarely occurs with lower therapeutic doses (5 mg/kg/day) and is reversible upon discontinuation of therapy. The investigational agent, disodium aminohydroxypropylidene diphosphonate (APD), also appears to be effective in Paget's disease, and therapeutic doses do not produce defective mineralization. However, the effects of larger doses on mineralization of osteoid are unknown.

Plicamycin is sometimes used to treat symptomatic patients unresponsive to other agents. It is also useful when a rapid response is desired, as in spinal cord compression. However, toxicity and the need for intravenous administration limit this drug's usefulness.

Calcitonin and etidronate have not been compared in controlled clinical trials. Calcitonin is the drug of choice for rapid relief of pain. Because administration is more convenient, etidronate is often preferred for patients with less severe disease. A regimen of etidronate followed by calcitonin (each agent administered for six months) produced a larger decrement in alkaline phosphatase levels than when the two agents were given in reverse order (Perry et al, 1984).

Nephrolithiasis

For a discussion of the pathogenesis and management of nephrolithiasis, see Chapter 31, Agents Used to Treat Urologic Disorders.

Drug Evaluations

ADRENAL CORTICOSTEROIDS

Glucocorticoids reduce the intestinal absorption of calcium by antagonizing the action of vitamin D. They are effective in hypercalcemia due to hypervitaminosis D, sarcoidosis, and adrenocortical insufficiency. Because of additional direct or indirect effects on bone resorption, they are also useful in some patients with hypercalcemia due to myeloma, leukemia, and lymphoma and in some patients with solid tumors. Large doses may be necessary initially. The onset of action varies, but improvement may occur within 24 to 72 hours.

The adverse effects of prolonged glucocorticoid therapy are an important consideration (see Chapter 61, Adrenal Corticosteroids in Nonendocrine Diseases).

DOSAGE AND PREPARATIONS.
Intravenous, Intramuscular: Adults, for severe hypercalcemia, parenteral preparations are preferred (hydrocortisone sodium succinate 100 to 500 mg daily or prednisolone sodium phosphate 20 to 100 mg daily); these drugs may be given intramuscularly, intravenously, or, preferably, by intravenous infusion.
Oral: Adults, initially, 40 to 80 mg of prednisone or the equivalent daily until the serum calcium level is controlled. Dosage then is reduced gradually; final dosage is determined by the results of serum calcium determinations.

See Chapter 61 for preparations.

CALCITONIN (SALMON)
[Calcimar]

ACTIONS AND USES. This synthetic polypeptide derived from salmon reduces bone resorption and thereby controls symptoms, prevents complications, and possibly halts progression of Paget's disease of bone. It is indicated primarily in symptomatic patients with moderate to severe involvement and is the drug of choice for rapid relief of pain. In approximately two-thirds of patients, calcitonin reduces increased levels of serum alkaline phosphatase and urinary hydroxyproline and relieves bone pain. Neurologic defects caused by compression of the spinal cord, spinal nerves, or cranial nerves may be relieved and functional capacity increased. Calcitonin does not reverse deafness but may prevent further hearing loss. If cardiac output is elevated because of increased blood flow to bone, calcitonin may relieve the congestive symptoms. There is radiologic evidence that abnormalities in some affected bones regress in a few patients, but it is not yet known whether long-term calcitonin therapy will prevent bony overgrowth and deformities and improve skeletal structure.

After about one year of calcitonin therapy, a partial loss of effectiveness has been noted in approximately 20% of patients with Paget's disease who initially responded well. The biochemical parameters (serum alkaline phosphatase and urinary hydroxyproline) are affected more often than the symptomatology and the hypocalcemic effect is maintained. In some cases, loss of response is probably related to high titers of neutralizing antibodies to salmon calcitonin. However, low antibody titers occur in up to two-thirds of patients, most of whom do not become resistant to the drug. Some of these patients have been successfully treated with human calcitonin. However, it is not known if resistance not due to antibody formation will be overcome by the use of the human preparation.

Calcitonin also has been used to treat hypercalcemic states associated with high rates of bone mineral loss, such as hyperparathyroidism, immobilization (particularly in association with Paget's disease), and malignancies. Calcitonin is useful in emergencies because it usually produces a rapid but small anticalcemic effect. However, it should not be the sole agent used in hypercalcemic states. Effectiveness may decrease after several days of use; the addition of oral phosphate or corticosteroids may restore responsiveness.

Calcitonin has been used as an adjunct to chemotherapy and anabolic steroids in the treatment of multiple myeloma. Relief of pain was noted a few weeks after initiating therapy and before chemotherapy began; the analgesic effect occurred prior to reduction in tumor size and was therefore independent of the drug's antiresorptive effect. Calcitonin probably contributes to repair of bone lacunae, although new osteolytic lesions may continue to form (Fremiotti et al, 1984).

Calcitonin also may be used to treat osteoporosis, especially in elderly patients, those in whom estrogen is contraindicated, or in those with high bone turnover (see the section on Osteoporosis).

ADVERSE REACTIONS. Calcitonin is generally well tolerated, but rash, nausea, vomiting, diarrhea, facial flushing, and malaise may occur. The gastrointestinal and skin reactions usually diminish with continued therapy. A transient, marked increase in sodium and water excretion has been noted during initial therapy and is probably related to both a direct renal effect and to improved circulatory dynamics. Soreness and inflammation at the site of injection may occur. This drug is classified in FDA Pregnancy Category C.

DOSAGE AND PREPARATIONS.
Subcutaneous, Intramuscular (subcutaneous generally preferred): For Paget's disease, *adults,* 50 to 100 IU daily or three times a week until a satisfactory clinical or biochemical response is obtained. For maintenance, 50 IU three times a week. For relapse, larger doses should be tried but do not consistently improve the clinical response.

For hypercalcemia, 4 IU/kg every 12 hours. If response is unsatisfactory in one or two days, the dose may be increased to 8 IU/kg every 12 hours. If response is still unsatisfactory after two more days, a maximum of 8 IU/kg may be administered every six hours.

For postmenopausal osteoporosis, 100 IU daily.
   Calcimar (USV). Solution (sterile) 200 IU/ml in 2 ml containers.

CALCIUM CARBONATE
[Caltrate 600, Os-Cal 500, Titralac, Tums]

This oral calcium salt (40% elemental calcium) may be used for initial and maintenance therapy of mild hypocalcemia. It is also the preferred calcium salt for supplementation in patients with osteomalacia, rickets, osteoporosis, and renal osteodystrophy. Calcium carbonate is converted in the stomach to soluble calcium salts by interaction with hydrochloric acid. Although absorption is impaired in patients with achlorhydria when calcium carbonate is taken in the fasting state, absorption is similar to normal patients when the agent is taken with meals (Recker, 1985).

Hypercalcemia may occur during long-term therapy, particularly in patients who are also receiving vitamin D. Calcium carbonate may cause constipation.

DOSAGE AND PREPARATIONS.
Oral: *Adults,* 1 to 2 g (equivalent to 400 to 800 mg elemental calcium) three times daily with meals; the powder preparation may be mixed with water or sprinkled on food if this is preferable to tablets.
   Generic. Powder; tablets 650 mg (equivalent to 260 mg elemental calcium) (nonprescription).
   Caltrate 600 (Lederle). Tablets 1.5 g (equivalent to 600 mg elemental calcium) (nonprescription).
   Os-Cal 500 (Marion). Tablets 1.25 g (equivalent to 500 mg elemental calcium) (nonprescription).
   Titralac (3 M). Tablets 420 mg and 1 g (nonprescription).
   Tums (Norcliff Thayer). Tablets (chewable) 650 mg and 750 mg (*Tums E-X*) (nonprescription).

CALCIUM CHLORIDE

Calcium chloride (27.2% elemental calcium) is effective intravenously in severe hypocalcemia. However, other salts are usually preferred because calcium chloride is more irritating to the veins and subcutaneous tissue, and care must be taken to avoid extravasation. It should never be administered intramuscularly. Since this salt is irritating to the gastrointestinal tract, it is rarely given orally.

Hypercalcemia may occur during long-term therapy, particularly in patients who are also receiving vitamin D. Intravenous calcium should be administered cautiously to digitalized patients, because calcium enhances the effect of digitalis and may precipitate arrhythmias.

This drug is classified in FDA Pregnancy Category C.

DOSAGE AND PREPARATIONS.
Intravenous (slow): *Adults,* 5 to 10 ml of a 10% solution.
   Generic. Solution 10% in 10 ml containers (each ml contains 27.2 mg elemental calcium).

CALCIUM CITRATE
[Citracal]

This oral calcium salt (21% elemental calcium) may be used as a dietary supplement. It is more soluble and is absorbed more effectively than calcium carbonate in fasting normal

(Nicar and Pak, 1985) and achlorhydric subjects. However, in nonfasting patients with achlorhydria, absorption of calcium is similar with either calcium carbonate or calcium citrate (Recker, 1985). The incidence of achlorhydria increases with age and thus may affect postmenopausal women who are at risk for osteoporosis. A preliminary report suggested that urinary calcium oxalate crystal and kidney stone formation may be decreased when this preparation is used for calcium supplementation (Harvey et al, 1985).

Hypercalcemia may occur during long-term therapy, particularly in patients who are also receiving vitamin D.

DOSAGE AND PREPARATIONS.
Oral: 950 mg to 1.9 g (equivalent to 200 to 400 mg elemental calcium) three to four times daily.
>   *Citracal* (Mission). Tablets 950 mg (equivalent to 200 mg elemental calcium) (nonprescription).

CALCIUM GLUCEPTATE

Intravenous calcium gluceptate (8.2% elemental calcium) is effective in the treatment of severe hypocalcemia. A transient tingling sensation and metallic taste may be noted after use of this route. Calcium gluceptate also may be given intramuscularly to infants and other patients in whom intravenous administration is not feasible. This salt is well tolerated, although mild local reactions may occur.

Intravenous calcium usually should not be administered to digitalized patients, because it may cause severe bradycardia. These patients should receive oral calcium supplements and/or calcitriol depending on the etiology of the hypocalcemia. If intravenous administration of calcium is necessary in digitalized patients because of severe hypocalcemia (ie, tetany), the infusion should be given very slowly.

DOSAGE AND PREPARATIONS.
Intravenous: *Adults,* 5 to 20 ml. *Newborn infants,* to prevent hypocalcemia during exchange transfusions, 0.5 ml after every 100 ml of blood exchanged.
Intramuscular: 2 to 5 ml in gluteal region or, in *infants,* in the lateral thigh.
>   *Generic.* Solution 220 mg/ml (18 mg/ml elemental calcium) in 5 and 50 ml containers.

CALCIUM GLUCONATE
[Kalcinate]

CALCIUM GLUBIONATE
[Neo-Calglucon]

Calcium gluconate (9.3% elemental calcium) is a source of rapidly available calcium ions; it is administered intravenously and is the treatment of choice in severe hypocalcemia. The gluconate salt is not irritating to the veins but has been reported to cause skin necrosis and sloughing in infants. The intramuscular route should not be used because it is irritating, painful, and may cause abscess formation.

Intravenous calcium usually should not be administered to digitalized patients, because it may cause severe bradycardia. These patients should receive oral calcium supplements and/or calcitriol depending on the etiology of hypocalcemia. If intravenous administration of calcium is necessary because of severe hypocalcemia (ie, tetany), the infusion should be given very slowly.

Calcium gluconate tablets are also available but their use is impractical because of the large number of tablets needed to achieve a therapeutic effect.

The oral preparation, calcium glubionate (6.6% elemental calcium), provides 115 mg calcium in each 5 ml (teaspoon). Calcium glubionate 1.8 g (one teaspoon) provides the same amount of calcium as calcium gluconate 1.2 g. This agent may cause diarrhea.

Hypercalcemia may occur during long-term therapy with either agent, particularly in patients who are also receiving vitamin D.

DOSAGE AND PREPARATIONS.
CALCIUM GLUCONATE:
Intravenous: *Adults,* initially, 20 ml of a 10% solution injected slowly, followed by slow infusion of a 0.3% to 0.8% solution (30 to 40 ml of 10% solution in 500 ml to 1 L of isotonic sodium chloride or 5% dextrose injection) over 3 to 12 hours. *Infants,* 2 ml/kg of 10% solution.
>   *Generic.* Solution 10% in 10 and 20 ml containers (each ml contains 9.3 mg elemental calcium).
>   *Kalcinate* (Kay). Solution 10% in 10 ml containers (each ml contains 9 mg elemental calcium).
CALCIUM GLUBIONATE:
Oral: *Adults,* 15 g daily in divided doses; *children,* 500 mg/kg daily in divided doses.
>   *Neo-Calglucon* (Sandoz). Syrup 1.8 g/5 ml (each ml contains 23.8 mg elemental calcium) (nonprescription).

CALCIUM LACTATE

This oral calcium salt (anhydrous salt containing 13% elemental calcium) is readily absorbed and may be used to treat mild hypocalcemia and for maintenance therapy. However, use of the tablets is impractical because of the large number needed to achieve a therapeutic effect.

Hypercalcemia may occur during long-term administration, particularly in patients who are also receiving vitamin D.

DOSAGE AND PREPARATIONS. See manufacturers' literature for dosage recommendations.
>   *Generic.* Tablets 325 and 650 mg (containing 42 and 84 mg elemental calcium respectively) (nonprescription).

EDETATE DISODIUM (EDTA)
[Chealamide, Endrate]

This chelating agent forms soluble complexes with calcium in the blood that are filtered by the glomeruli and not reabsorbed by the renal tubules. Although edetate disodium is very effective in the treatment of acute hypercalcemia, its nephrotoxic potential limits its use to dire emergencies when death from hypercalcemic crisis is judged to be imminent. Renal tubular damage has occurred after prolonged use or administration of doses larger than 3 g. Other adverse reactions are pain at the site of infusion and hypotension. Marked hypocalcemia may occur if the drug is not diluted sufficiently or is administered too rapidly. Other therapeutic modalities should be instituted simultaneously so that treatment with this agent will not exceed 48 hours.

A preparation containing calcium (edetate calcium disodium [Calcium Disodium Versenate]) for use in lead poisoning is already chelated to calcium and therefore is useless in the treatment of hypercalcemia. See also Chapter 80, Drugs Used in the Treatment of Poisoning.

DOSAGE AND PREPARATIONS.
Intravenous: Adults, for emergency treatment of severe hypercalcemia, 40 mg/kg infused over four to six hours (maximum, 3 g in 24 hours).

Chealamide (Vortech), **Endrate** (Abbott), **Generic.** Solution 150 mg/ml in 20 ml containers.

ESTROGENS

Estrogens are used in postmenopausal women (natural or surgical menopause) for prophylaxis of osteoporosis or to prevent progression of established disease. Although any estrogen may be used, conjugated estrogens are most widely prescribed in the United States.

In women with intact uteri, estrogens are given cyclically, often with a progestin added during the third week of medication to prevent endometrial hyperplasia and carcinoma.

DOSAGE AND PREPARATIONS.
Oral: For prophylaxis of osteoporosis in menopausal women, 0.625 mg conjugated estrogens or the equivalent daily for 24 days each month. A progestin may be added during the last week of medication, especially in women with an intact uterus. (See also Chapter 39, Estrogens, Progestins, and Other Agents Used to Treat Gynecologic Conditions.)

CONJUGATED ESTROGENS:
Premarin (Ayerst), **Generic.** Tablets 0.3, 0.625, 0.9 (**Premarin** only), 1.25, and 2.5 mg.
See Chapter 39 for other estrogen preparations.

ETIDRONATE DISODIUM
[Didronel]

$$\overset{+\ -}{Na}\ O-\overset{\overset{OH}{|}}{\underset{\overset{||}{O}}{P}}-\overset{\overset{OH}{|}}{\underset{\overset{|}{CH_3}}{C}}-\overset{\overset{OH}{|}}{\underset{\overset{||}{O}}{P}}-O^-\overset{+}{Na}$$

ACTIONS AND USES. This diphosphonate compound slows osteoblastic and osteoclastic activity and is used to treat symptomatic patients with Paget's disease of bone. The oral route of administration for this drug is more convenient than the parenteral route required with calcitonin.

Like calcitonin, etidronate lowers serum alkaline phosphatase and urinary hydroxyproline levels, reduces cardiac output by decreasing bone vascularity, and may improve bone histology and reduce bone pain. One to three months of therapy may elapse before biochemical improvement occurs (60% of patients show symptomatic improvement). Maximal effects are achieved within six months, and bone turnover may be reduced to one-half the pretreatment rate. Elevated osteoclast counts decrease, and resorption surfaces are reduced (Johnston et al, 1980). Long-term intermittent treatment over a period of years may reduce the fracture rate.

The greatest effectiveness and longest remissions are achieved in patients with moderate disease. Although biochemical remission may persist for 18 months or more after a single course of therapy, the serum alkaline phosphatase and urinary hydroxyproline levels may increase when the drug is discontinued. When relapse occurs, subsequent courses should be given intermittently because the safety of long-term continuous therapy has not been established. The use of etidronate to treat Paget's disease has been reviewed (Krane, 1982; Altman, 1985).

Etidronate also is given to prevent and treat heterotopic ossification due to spinal cord injury and total hip replacement. It has been used investigationally in selected patients with hypercalcemia due to malignancy (see the section on Hypercalcemia).

ADVERSE REACTIONS AND PRECAUTIONS. Etidronate is usually well tolerated, but nausea and diarrhea have been reported, particularly in patients receiving doses of 10 to 20 mg/kg/day. These effects are often alleviated by dividing the total daily dose. The serum phosphate level may increase when 10 to 20 mg/kg/day is given, presumably because of increased renal reabsorption, but therapy should not be discontinued. This elevation usually does not occur when 5 mg/kg/day is employed. Elevated serum phosphate levels generally return to normal two to four weeks after therapy ceases. Patients with impaired renal function (reduced glomerular filtration rates) should receive smaller doses and should be monitored closely.

The most serious adverse effect of etidronate is inhibition of bone mineralization. Accumulation of unmineralized osteoid is common in patients receiving large doses (10 to 20 mg/kg daily) but also may occur when lower doses (5 mg/kg/day) are given for long periods. New episodes of incapacitating bone pain and fractures have occurred during a six-month period of treatment with 10 to 20 mg/kg daily, but not with 2.5 to 5 mg/kg daily (Canfield et al, 1977). Bone pain alone occurs in up to 20% of patients receiving 5 mg/kg daily.

Since effects on serum alkaline phosphatase and urinary hydroxyproline levels may be disease- or treatment-related and may not occur in all patients receiving etidronate, these biochemical indices cannot be used as the sole guide to therapy.

This drug is classified in FDA Pregnancy Category B.

PHARMACOKINETICS. Approximately 1% of an oral dose of 5 mg/kg/day is absorbed and the amount is increased to about 2.5% at 10 mg/kg/day and to 6% at 20 mg/kg/day. The rest is excreted unchanged in the feces. Approximately 50% of the absorbed dose is chemisorbed to bone; the rest is excreted unchanged in the urine.

DOSAGE AND PREPARATIONS.

Oral: Adults, for Paget's disease, etidronate should be given as a single daily dose with water. Eating should be avoided for two hours before and after taking the medication. Initially, 5 mg/kg is given daily for no longer than six months. Larger doses should be reserved for use when there is a need for rapid suppression of increased bone turnover or prompt reduction of elevated cardiac output. When more than 10 mg/kg daily is given (maximum, 20 mg/kg), the treatment period should not exceed three months. Increased or recurrent bone pain and/or pain at previously asymptomatic sites has been reported. If therapy is continued, pain may resolve in some patients but persist in others. If fractures occur, the drug should be withheld until signs of callus formation are evident. Serum alkaline phosphatase and/or urinary hydroxyproline levels should be monitored during and after therapy. Treatment may be initiated again after a drug-free period of at least three months if there is biochemical, symptomatic, or other evidence of active disease.

For heterotopic ossification due to spinal cord injury, initially, 20 mg/kg daily for two weeks, followed by 10 mg/kg daily for ten weeks (total treatment period, 12 weeks). For heterotopic ossification following total hip replacement, 20 mg/kg daily for one month before and three months after surgery (four months total).

Didronel (Norwich Eaton). Tablets 200 and 400 mg.

FUROSEMIDE
[Lasix]

ACTIONS AND USES. Furosemide reduces the serum calcium concentration by increasing calcium excretion. This diuretic blocks active chloride transport in the thick ascending limb of Henle's loop, thereby interfering with the passive reabsorption of sodium. Since the calcium ion is handled like the sodium ion in this segment of the nephron, a parallel increase in calcium excretion occurs due to blocked resorption of calcium.

Furosemide is given intravenously in conjunction with isotonic sodium chloride to reduce the serum calcium level rapidly in the emergency treatment of hypercalcemia. The saline solution should be administered before the diuretic to ensure adequate expansion of the extracellular fluid volume. During diuresis, urinary loss of water and electrolytes (including sodium, potassium, and magnesium) should be measured carefully and replaced. If these measures are not followed, severe fluid and electrolyte disturbances may occur. In addition, volume contraction may increase reabsorption of calcium in the proximal tubules and reduce the therapeutic response.

ADVERSE REACTIONS AND PRECAUTIONS. See Chapter 29, Diuretics.

DOSAGE AND PREPARATIONS.

Intravenous: Large doses should be given at a rate not exceeding 4 mg/min to avoid ototoxic reactions. Maintenance of extracellular fluid volume to avoid hypovolemia and exacerbation of hypercalcemia is essential. *Adults,* for severe hypercalcemia, 80 to 100 mg every one or two hours, after infusion of isotonic sodium chloride, until an adequate response is obtained and other therapeutic modalities can be instituted. Smaller doses may be given every two to four hours in those less severely affected. *Children,* 25 to 50 mg every four hours.

Lasix (Hoechst-Roussel), **Generic.** Solution 10 mg/ml in 2, 4, and 10 ml containers.

PHOSPHATE SALTS

Inorganic phosphates (monobasic or dibasic sodium or potassium phosphate) may be effective in hypercalcemia regardless of the etiology; the increase in serum phosphorus levels reduces the serum calcium level. They are most effective and safe when the serum phosphate concentration is reduced. The mechanism is not well understood but may involve all of the following: decreased bone resorption, increased bone formation, and reduced calcium absorption secondary to decreased renal synthesis of $1,25\text{-}(OH)_2D_3$.

Phosphates are used orally to treat mild to moderate hypercalcemia. They also are used for the long-term treatment of patients with hypophosphatemic rickets or osteomalacia.

Intravenous administration is effective but can be dangerous. Hypocalcemia, hypotension and shock, myocardial infarction, tetany, and acute renal failure have occurred, and several deaths have been reported. Ectopic calcification also may occur if phosphate is administered by the intravenous route without proper monitoring to detect an increase in the serum phosphate concentration. For these reasons, intravenous therapy is justified only rarely (eg, when rapid reduction of serum calcium would be lifesaving) and should never be the first treatment modality employed.

Oral administration is safer, but careful monitoring of serum electrolyte levels and renal function is necessary. Nausea, vomiting, and diarrhea may occur and may be dose dependent. Concomitant use of antacids containing aluminum and/or magnesium should be avoided, because they may bind phosphate and prevent its absorption (calcium antacids also may bind phosphate, and it is assumed that these agents are not given to hypercalcemic patients).

Phosphate should not be given to patients with impaired renal function or hyperphosphatemia. They should not be given to patients with alkaline urine due to urinary tract infections because increased calcium and phosphate concentrations in the alkaline urine increase the risk of calcium phosphate stones.

DOSAGE AND PREPARATIONS.

Oral: Adults, 1 to 2 g of phosphorus daily in divided doses. The sodium-free preparations (K-Phos Original, Neutra-Phos K) should be used in patients on a sodium-restricted diet. Following remission, the dose should be reduced to maintain a normal serum calcium concentration.

Preparations available generically; compounding necessary for prescription.

K-Phos Neutral (Beach). Each tablet contains phosphorus 250 mg, sodium 298 mg, and potassium 45 mg.

K-Phos Original (Sodium Free) (Beach). Each tablet contains potassium acid phosphate 500 mg.

K-Phos M.F. (Beach). Each tablet contains potassium acid phosphate 155 mg and sodium acid phosphate 350 mg.

K-Phos No. 2 (Beach). Each tablet contains potassium acid phosphate 305 mg and sodium acid phosphate 700 mg.

Neutra-Phos (Willen). Each 75 ml of solution (after reconstitution) or capsule contains phosphorus 250 mg, sodium 164 mg, and potassium 278 mg (both forms nonprescription).

Neutra-Phos K (Willen). Each 75 ml of solution (after reconstitution) or capsule contains phosphorus 250 mg and potassium 556 mg (sodium-free) (both forms nonprescription).

Intravenous: Adults, 1.5 g of phosphorus infused over six to eight hours. The dose may be repeated daily, but no more than two infusions are usually required.

Preparations available generically; compounding necessary for prescription.

PLICAMYCIN (Mithramycin)
[Mithracin]

ACTIONS AND USES. Plicamycin is a cytotoxic antibiotic used primarily to treat testicular neoplasms. It decreases serum calcium levels in both hypercalcemic and normocalcemic individuals, possibly by a direct toxic effect on osteoclasts in bone. Plicamycin also is used to treat severe hypercalcemia associated with carcinoma (with or without bony metastases) and is more effective than glucocorticoids for this purpose. In some patients, a single infusion reduces serum calcium levels within 24 hours without serious toxic effects; in others, a satisfactory response may require several consecutive daily infusions. The duration of action may be only a few days but occasionally persists for three weeks or longer, especially if three or four consecutive daily infusions are given.

Plicamycin has been used in Paget's disease of bone, but calcitonin and etidronate are less toxic. Occasionally, plicamycin is used in patients with severe disease who are unresponsive to other therapy.

ADVERSE REACTIONS AND PRECAUTIONS. In addition, to anorexia, nausea, and vomiting, plicamycin can produce se-

vere thrombocytopenia and abnormalities in multiple clotting factors that may progress to a hemorrhagic diathesis. Abnormal results of hepatic and renal function tests have also been reported. Although lower doses are used for hypercalcemia than for neoplasms, the same precautions and contraindications apply (see Chapter 64, Drugs Used in Cancer Chemotherapy). It is also important to monitor serum calcium levels closely. Plicamycin generally should not be used in patients with renal or hepatic disease, bone marrow depression, thrombocytopathy, thrombocytopenia, coagulation disorders, or increased susceptibility to bleeding from other causes.

DOSAGE AND PREPARATIONS.

Intravenous: 25 mcg/kg is added to 5% dextrose in water or isotonic saline and infused over four to six hours. If serum calcium levels are not reduced by the next morning, 25 mcg/kg may be given daily for two to four days. Additional courses may be administered if hypercalcemia is not controlled, but this increases potential toxicity. Alternatively, one to three doses may be given weekly, depending upon the patient's response. The drug should be discontinued after three infusions or sooner when a favorable effect has been achieved.

Mithracin (Miles). Powder (cryodesiccated) 2,500 mcg with mannitol 100 mg and sufficient disodium phosphate to adjust to pH 7.

THIAZIDES

Although most diuretics that promote renal sodium loss also increase renal calcium loss, the thiazide diuretics reduce urinary calcium excretion. The mechanism is not clearly understood but appears to involve a dissociation between sodium and calcium reabsorption in the distal tubules.

Thiazides (in conjunction with a low-sodium diet) have been recommended as adjuncts to calcium and vitamin D in hypoparathyroidism, but their efficacy in this condition must be confirmed. It is unlikely that the thiazides alone will be effective in patients with severe hypoparathyroidism (eg, serum calcium less than 7.5 mg/dl), because urinary calcium excretion is already minimal in such patients. However, thiazides may reduce the amount of vitamin D needed to maintain serum calcium in the desired range and may be particularly useful when control is difficult.

Because thiazides reduce urinary calcium excretion temporarily, it has been suggested that selection of a thiazide when a diuretic is needed may help prevent bone loss in older individuals. However, thiazides are not suggested as a treatment per se for osteoporosis (see the section on Osteoporosis).

The adverse effects of prolonged thiazide therapy are discussed in Chapter 29, Diuretics.

DOSAGE AND PREPARATIONS. See Chapter 29.

VITAMIN D PREPARATIONS

Vitamin D is obtained by ingestion of vitamin D_2 (ergocalciferol) or D_3 (cholecalciferol) or by ultraviolet irradiation of 7-dehydrocholesterol to vitamin D_3 in the skin. Vitamin D_3 (or D_2) is hydroxylated at C-25 in the liver to produce 25-hydroxy-vitamin D_3 (or D_2), which is the major metabolite circulating in the plasma. This compound is available commercially as calcifediol [Calderol]. The metabolite is further hydroxylated in the kidney to 1,25-dihydroxy-vitamin D_3 (or D_2), the most active metabolite in initiating intestinal transport of calcium and phosphate and mobilization of mineral from bone. $1,25(OH)_2D_3$ is available commercially as calcitriol [Rocaltrol]. An analogue of this metabolite, alfacalcidol (1-α-OHD_3), is used in Europe, Canada, and Japan to treat renal osteodystrophy and is under investigation in this country. Alfacalcidol is converted in the liver to calcitriol and is easier to produce and less expensive (although the relative cost when it becomes available in the United States cannot be predicted accurately). Another metabolite of vitamin D, $24,25$-$(OH)_2D_3$, is formed in the kidney and bone, but its metabolic actions are uncertain.

In general, the onset of action of vitamin D is slow and the duration of action is long. The newer metabolites act more rapidly (a calcemic response may be obtained with calcitriol in one or two days) and have shorter biological half-lives.

VITAMIN D_2 (Ergocalciferol)

ACTIONS AND USES. Vitamin D is used in hypoparathyroidism, vitamin D deficiency states (eg, simple and conditioned deficiencies, genetic vitamin D-dependent rickets, malabsorption, impaired renal or hepatic metabolism), and as an adjunct in osteomalacia associated with hypophosphatemia and renal tubular disorders. In parathyroid hormone deficiency, large doses of vitamin D increase serum calcium levels and there may be a moderate reciprocal decrease in serum phosphorus levels. Large doses may be associated with phosphaturia, increase mobilization of mineral from bone, and increase intestinal absorption of calcium, phosphate, and magnesium; these effects account for the elevation of serum calcium concentrations.

Rickets and osteomalacia caused by dietary deficiency of vitamin D and inadequate exposure to sunlight respond rapidly to physiologic doses of vitamin D, but larger doses are required to treat vitamin D-dependent and resistant rickets. In malabsorption disorders, effective treatment of the primary cause usually cures associated osteomalacia or rickets, but if the underlying condition does not respond to therapy, life-long administration of large doses of vitamin D and calcium may be necessary. In hypophosphatemic states (vitamin D-resistant or familial hypophosphatemic rickets) and renal tubular disorders, large doses of vitamin D may be needed, but correction of hypophosphatemia or acidosis is of primary importance.

The low serum levels of 25-OHD_3 observed in patients receiving long-term anticonvulsant, rifampin, or glutethimide therapy have been attributed to drug-induced stimulation of hepatic microsomal enzymes, which is presumed to accelerate the metabolism of vitamin D_3 to inactive metabolites. For this reason, prophylactic doses of vitamin D may be desirable during prolonged therapy with these drugs. Pharmacologic doses are indicated when overt bone disease is associated with impaired hepatic or renal metabolism of vitamin D.

The lag between initiation of vitamin D therapy and onset of effectiveness is 10 to 14 days or longer, depending upon the preparation used. The onset of action of ergocalciferol is somewhat slower than that of dihydrotachysterol and the duration of effect is more prolonged.

The dose of vitamin D should be based on measurement of the serum calcium concentration (in the early treatment period, weekly; with chronic treatment, about every three months). Urinary calcium (the amount excreted in 24 hours) should be used as a guide, since this parameter often increases before the serum calcium concentration.

ADVERSE REACTIONS AND PRECAUTIONS. Vitamin D is potent and potentially harmful. Overdosage can cause gastrointestinal and central nervous system disturbances and soft tissue calcification. Renal complications may be severe and death may result; the possibility of renal damage persists long after discontinuing the drug. Adverse effects occasionally result from increased sensitivity in patients not receiving excessive doses.

Vitamin D should be given cautiously to digitalized patients because hypercalcemia may precipitate arrhythmias.

This drug is classified in FDA Pregnancy Category C. (See also Chapter 47, Vitamins and Minerals.)

DOSAGE AND PREPARATIONS.

Oral: For hypoparathyroidism, *adults,* initially, 50,000 to 200,000 IU daily as soon as acute tetany is controlled with an intravenous calcium preparation. The maintenance dose is usually 25,000 to 100,000 IU daily. *Children,* 10,000 to 25,000 IU daily.

For osteomalacia and rickets caused by dietary deficiency of vitamin D, *adults,* initially, 1,000 to 2,000 IU daily; for maintenance, 400 IU daily. *Children,* initially, 1,000 to 4,000 IU daily; for maintenance, 400 IU daily.

For genetic vitamin D-dependent rickets, *children,* 5,000 to 50,000 IU daily.

For familial hypophosphatemia (vitamin D-resistant rickets), *children,* 25,000 to 100,000 IU daily in conjunction with a high phosphate intake and calcium supplements. For sporadic hypophosphatemia, *adults,* 40,000 to 100,000 IU daily in conjunction with a high phosphate intake.

For osteomalacia in malabsorption syndromes, *adults,* 10,000 to 50,000 IU daily. *Children,* 10,000 to 25,000 IU daily. For osteomalacia in hepatobiliary disease, *adults,* 10,000 to 40,000 IU daily. *Children,* 10,000 to 25,000 IU daily. For osteomalacia associated with anticonvulsant therapy, *adults and children,* 1,000 IU daily.

For renal osteodystrophy (rarely used now in chronic renal failure), *adults,* 20,000 to 50,000 IU daily.

For multiple renal tubular defects, *adults,* 40,000 to 100,000 IU daily; *children,* 25,000 to 50,000 IU daily.

VITAMIN D_2 (ERGOCALCIFEROL):

Available generically under names Vitamin D (capsules 25,000 and 50,000 IU) and Calciferol (tablets 50,000 IU).
Deltalin (Lilly). Capsules 50,000 IU.
Drisdol (Winthrop-Breon). Capsules 50,000 IU; liquid 8,000 IU/ml.

DIHYDROTACHYSTEROL (DHT)
[Hytakerol]

This form of vitamin D is hydroxylated in the liver but does not require renal activation. It acts somewhat more rapidly than the D_2 and D_3 forms. In comparison to ergocalciferol, the phosphate diuresis produced by dihydrotachysterol is almost as great, the intestinal absorption of calcium is less (on a molar basis), and the serum calcium concentration rises more rapidly. Because its duration of action is shorter, the hazards of hypercalcemia are less with dihydrotachysterol than with ergocalciferol. (See the evaluation on Vitamin D for adverse reactions and precautions.)

Dihydrotachysterol has only weak antirachitic activity (about 1/450 that of vitamin D).

DOSAGE AND PREPARATIONS.

Oral: For hypoparathyroidism, *adults,* initially, 0.75 to 2.5 mg daily; specific dosage is determined by frequent estimations of serum calcium levels. For maintenance, 0.25 to 1.75 mg weekly has been given, but larger doses may be required in some patients.

For prevention of renal osteodystrophy, *adults,* initially, 0.1 to 0.25 mg daily. *Children,* initially, 0.01 mg daily. For patients on long-term hemodialysis, *adults,* initially, 0.25 to 0.375 mg daily. Some patients may require doses as large as 1 mg daily.
Generic. Solution 0.2 mg/ml (alcohol 20%); tablets 0.125, 0.2, and 4 mg.
Hytakerol (Winthrop-Breon). Capsules 0.125 mg; solution (in oil) 0.25 mg/ml.

CALCITRIOL
[Rocaltrol]

ACTIONS. Calcitriol is the synthetic preparation of $1,25(OH)_2D_3$. The endogenous product is produced in the kidney and is sometimes classified as a renal hormone. It is the most active vitamin D metabolite in initiating the intestinal transport of calcium and phosphate and the mobilization of mineral from bone. Conversion to this active metabolite is enhanced by the presence of parathyroid hormone and/or a decrease in serum inorganic phosphate levels. The major advantages of calcitriol are its efficacy in patients with renal failure, its rapid onset of action, and its short half-life (less than one day contrasted to three to four weeks for vitamin D), which makes toxic reactions easier to manage. On the other hand, the extreme potency and rapid onset of action of calcitriol necessitate caution in dosage regulation, for toxicity can occur very rapidly. Moreover, calcitriol is much more expensive for equivalent therapeutic effects than ergocalciferol.

USES. Calcitriol has been used primarily in patients with chronic renal failure or renal tubular disease. It was more effective than vitamin D in elevating the serum calcium level and reducing parathyroid hormone secretion (Berl et al, 1978). The serum calcium level may not increase for several weeks, however, particularly if skeletal disease is severe. When renal osteodystrophy is present, calcitriol often relieves bone pain, permits increased physical activity, and may improve bone histology.

Calcitriol is effective in the treatment of hypoparathyroidism following thyroidectomy or parathyroid surgery. Idiopathic hypoparathyroidism also responds to calcitriol. Larger doses may be required during episodes of malabsorption and diarrhea. Pseudohypoparathyroidism is also treated with this agent.

Calcitriol is used in various forms of rickets and osteomalacia. Phosphate may be added to the regimen when hypophosphatemia is also present (see the section on Osteomalacia and Rickets).

ADVERSE REACTIONS. Calcitriol stimulates intestinal absorption of both calcium and phosphate, which are utilized in remineralization of the skeleton initially. A decrease in serum alkaline phosphatase serves as a warning of an impending increase in serum calcium. Metastatic calcification, decreased renal function, and increased serum phosphate concentrations are possible consequences. These complications may be avoided by decreasing the dose of calcitriol when the serum alkaline phosphatase concentration declines, by administering phosphate-binding agents to combat hyperphosphatemia, and by monitoring serum calcium and phosphate levels. (See the section on Renal Osteodystrophy.) For other adverse reactions and precautions, see the evaluation on Vitamin D.

DOSAGE AND PREPARATIONS.

Oral: Initially, 0.25 mcg/day. If the response is not adequate, the dosage may be increased by 0.25 mcg/day at two- to four-week intervals for hypoparathyroid patients and at four- to eight-week intervals for dialysis patients. Serum calcium concentrations should be measured at least twice weekly and the drug should be discontinued if hypercalcemia occurs. Treatment may be reinstituted when the serum calcium concentration is normal. Patients with normal or only slightly reduced serum calcium levels may respond to 0.25 mcg every other day. Most patients undergoing hemodialysis require 0.5 or 1 mcg/day.

Most adults and children 6 years and older with hypoparathyroidism have responded to 0.5 to 2 mcg daily. Hypoparathyroid children 1 to 5 years are usually given 0.25 to 0.75 mcg daily.

Rocaltrol (Roche). Capsules 0.25 and 0.5 mcg.

CALCIFEDIOL
[Calderol]

ACTIONS AND USES. Calcifediol is the synthetic preparation of 25-OHD$_3$. The endogenous product is formed in the liver from hydroxylation of vitamin D$_3$ and is the major form of vitamin D circulating in the blood. Levels of 25-OHD$_3$ can be monitored readily. Calcifediol is useful therapeutically because it is converted to the potent metabolite, 1,25(OH)$_2$D$_3$ (calcitriol) and has some intrinsic activity. It is used in metabolic bone diseases associated with chronic renal failure in patients undergoing dialysis. This agent increases serum calcium and may decrease alkaline phosphatase and parathyroid hormone levels. Bone resorption, signs of hyperparathyroid bone disease, and mineralization defects are reduced. Calcifediol also may be used to treat osteopenia caused by prolonged glucocorticoid therapy (Hahn, 1980 A). It is used investigationally in osteomalacia secondary to hepatic disease when endogenous production of 25-OHD$_3$ is impaired. Because vitamin D metabolites other than 1,25(OH)$_2$D$_3$ may have direct effects on bone, calcifediol, the common precursor, may prove to be more advantageous than calcitriol in patients with osteomalacia and in children with renal osteodystrophy or hypoparathyroidism who have not achieved full bone growth. In such cases, a mixture of calcifediol and calcitriol may be used.

ADVERSE REACTIONS AND PRECAUTIONS. As with all vitamin D metabolites, excessive doses of calcifediol may result in hypercalcemia and possibly hypercalciuria. Serum calcium should be monitored at least weekly during dosage adjustment, and the drug should be discontinued if hypercalcemia develops.

There are no well-controlled studies on use of calcifediol in pregnant women, but teratogenic effects were observed in experimental animals.

For other adverse reactions and precautions, see the evaluation on Vitamin D.

PHARMACOKINETICS. Calcifediol is rapidly absorbed and a peak serum concentration is attained in four to eight hours. It is transported bound to protein and has a half-life of about 16 days.

DOSAGE AND PREPARATIONS.

Oral: Dosage must be individualized and adequate intake of calcium assured. In patients with chronic renal failure on dialysis, initially, 50 mcg daily or 100 mcg on alternate days.

Dosage may be increased at four-week intervals if a satisfactory response is not obtained. Serum calcium should be measured at least weekly during dosage adjustment. Most patients respond to doses of 50 to 100 mcg daily or 100 to 200 mcg on alternate days.

Calderol (Organon). Capsules 20 and 50 mcg.

Cited References

Agus ZS, et al: Disorders of calcium and magnesium homeostasis. *Am J Med* 72:473-488, 1982.

Aloia JF, et al: Risk factors for postmenopausal osteoporosis. *Am J Med* 78:95-100, 1985 A.

Aloia JF, et al: Treatment of osteoporosis with calcitonin, with and without growth hormone. *Metabolism* 34:124-129, 1985 B.

Alon U, Chan JCM: Effects of hydrochlorothiazide and amiloride in renal hypophosphatemic rickets. *Pediatrics* 75:754-763, 1985.

Altman RD: Long-term follow-up therapy with intermittent etidronate disodium in Paget's disease of bone. *Am J Med* 79:583-590, 1985.

Avioli LV: Calcitonin therapy for bone disease and hypercalcemia, (editorial). *Arch Intern Med* 142:2076-2078, 1982.

Berl T, et al: 1,25 dihydroxycholecalciferol effects in chronic dialysis: Double-blind controlled study. *Ann Intern Med* 88:774-780, 1978.

Body J-J, Heath H III: Estimates of circulating monomeric calcitonin: Physiological studies in normal and thyroidectomized man. *J Clin Endocrinol Metab* 57:897-903, 1983.

Canalis E: Hormonal and local regulation of bone formation. *Endocr Rev* 4:62-77, 1983.

Canfield R, et al: Diphosphonate therapy of Paget's disease of bone. *J Clin Endocrinol Metab* 44:96-106, 1977.

Chan JCM, et al: Calcium and phosphate metabolism in children with idiopathic hypoparathyroidism or pseudohypoparathyroidism: Effects of 1,25-dihydroxyvitamin D$_3$. *J Pediatr* 106:421-426, 1985.

Chesney RW, et al: Long-term influence of calcitriol (1,25-dihydroxyvitamin D) and supplemental phosphate in X-linked hypophosphatemic rickets. *Pediatrics* 71:559-567, 1983.

Chestnut CH III: Treatment of postmenopausal osteoporosis: Some current concepts. *Scott Med J* 26:72-80, 1981.

Christiansen C, et al: Bone mass in postmenopausal women after withdrawal of oestrogen/gestagen replacement therapy. *Lancet* 1:459-461, 1981.

Coburn JW, Henry DA: Renal osteodystrophy. *Adv Intern Med* 387-424, 1984.

Elliott GT, McKenzie MW: Treatment of hypercalcemia. *Drug Intell Clin Pharm* 17:12-22, 1983.

Fremiotti A, et al: Effect of calcitonin on skeleton and bone pain in multiple myeloma. *Curr Ther Res* 36:627-640, 1984.

Genant HK, et al: Osteoporosis: Part I. Advanced radiologic assessment using quantitative computed tomography. *West J Med* 139:75-84, 1983.

Gennari C, et al: Comparative effects on bone mineral content of calcium and calcium plus salmon calcitonin given in two different regimens in postmenopausal osteoporosis. *Curr Ther Res* 38:455-464, 1985.

Goldsmith RS, et al: Effects of phosphorus supplementation on serum parathyroid hormone and bone morphology in osteoporosis. *J Clin Endocrinol Metab* 43:523-532, 1976.

Gruber HE, et al: Long-term calcitonin therapy in postmenopausal osteoporosis. *Metabolism* 33:295-303, 1984.

Hahn TJ: Drug-induced disorders of vitamin D and mineral metabolism. *Clin Endocrinol Metab* 9:107-129, 1980 A.

Hahn TJ: Parathyroid hormone, calcitonin, vitamin D, mineral and bone: Metabolism and disorders, in Mazzaferri EL (ed): *Endocrinology: A Review of Clinical Endocrinology,* ed 2. Excerpta Medica, 1980 B, 425-558.

Hammond CB, et al: Effects of long-term estrogen therapy. I. Metabolic effects. *Am J Obstet Gynecol* 133:525-536, 1979.

Harvey JA, et al: Calcium citrate: Reduced propensity for crystallization of calcium oxalate in urine resulting from induced hypercalciuria of calcium supplementation. *J Clin Endocrinol Metab* 61:1223-1225, 1985.

Heaney RP: Estrogens and postmenopausal osteoporosis. *Clin Obstet Gynecol* 19:791-803, 1976.

Hosking DJ: Paget's disease of bone. *Br Med J* 283:686-688, 1981.

Hutchinson TA, et al: Postmenopausal oestrogens protect against fractures of hip and distal radius: Case-control study. *Lancet* 2:705-709, 1979.

Jamieson MJ: Hypercalcaemia. *Br Med J* 290:378-382, 1985.

Jensen GF, et al: Calcitonin: Pathogenic factor in postmenopausal osteoporosis? in Cohn DV, et al (eds): *Endocrine Control of Bone and Calcium Metabolism.* Elsevier Science, 1984, 22-25.

Johnston CC Jr, et al: Use of etidronate (EHDP) in Paget's disease of bone. *Arthritis Rheum* 23:1172-1176, 1980.

Johnston CC, et al: Heterogeneity of fracture syndromes in postmenopausal women. *J Clin Endocrinol Metab* 61:551-556, 1985 A.

Johnston CC Jr, et al: Early menopausal changes in bone mass and sex steroids. *J Clin Endocrinol Metab* 61:905-911, 1985 B.

Krane SM: Etidronate disodium in treatment of Paget's disease of bone. *Ann Intern Med* 96:619-625, 1982.

Lindsay R, et al: Bone response to termination of oestrogen treatment. *Lancet* 1:1325-1327, 1978.

Lindsay R, et al: Prevention of spinal osteoporosis in oophorectomised women. *Lancet* 2:1151-1153, 1980.

Lindsay R, et al: Minimum effective dose of estrogen for prevention of postmenopausal bone loss. *Obstet Gynecol* 63:759-763, 1984.

Mazzuoli GE, et al: Effects of salmon calcitonin in postmenopausal osteoporosis: Controlled double-blind clinical study. *Calcif Tissue Int* 38:3-8, 1986.

McDermott MT, et al: Reduced bone mineral content in totally thyroidectomized patients: Possible effects of calcitonin deficiency. *J Clin Endocrinol Metab* 56:936-939, 1983.

Mundy GR, et al: Hypercalcemia of cancer: Clinical implications and pathogenic mechanisms. *N Engl J Med* 310:1718-1727, 1984.

Nachtigall LE, et al: Estrogen replacement therapy. I. 10-year prospective study in relationship to osteoporosis. *Obstet Gynecol* 53:277-281, 1979.

National Institutes of Health Consensus Conference: Osteoporosis. *JAMA* 252:799-802, 1984.

Nicar MJ, Pak CYC: Calcium bioavailability from calcium carbonate and calcium citrate. *J Clin Endocrinol Metab* 61:391-393, 1985.

Norris KC, Coburn JW: Rocaltrol (calcitriol): Guidelines for management. *Dialysis Transplant* Suppl 1-8, (July) 1985.

Paganini-Hill A, et al: Menopausal estrogen therapy and hip fractures. *Ann Intern Med* 95:28-31, 1981.

Perry HM III, et al: Alternate calcitonin and etidronate disodium therapy for Paget's bone disease. *Arch Intern Med* 144:929-933, 1984.

Pitkin RM: Calcium metabolism in pregnancy and perinatal period: Review. *Am J Obstet Gynecol* 151:99-109, 1985.

Raisz LG, Kream BE: Regulation of bone formation, parts 1 and 2. *N Engl J Med* 309:29-35, 83-89, 1983.

Raisz LG, Smith J: Prevention and therapy of osteoporosis. *Ration Drug Ther* 19:1-6, (Aug) 1985.

Recker RR: Calcium absorption and achlorhydria. *N Engl J Med* 313:70-73, 1985.

Riggs BL, Nelson KI: Effect of long term treatment with calcitriol on calcium absorption and mineral metabolism in postmenopausal osteoporosis. *J Clin Endocrinol Metab* 61:457-461, 1985.

Riggs BL, et al: Effect of fluoride/calcium regimen on vertebral fracture occurrence in postmenopausal osteoporosis: Comparison with conventional therapy. *N Engl J Med* 306:446-450, 1982.

Ryan WG: Pathophysiology and modern management of Paget's disease. *Compr Ther* 9:64-69, (Sept) 1983.

Ryzen E, et al: Intravenous etidronate in management of malignant hypercalcemia. *Arch Intern Med* 145:449-452, 1985.

Siris ES: Diagnosis and treatment of Paget's disease of bone. *Compr Ther* 9:47-53, (Sept) 1983.

Smith R: Hypercalcaemia. *Br J Hosp Med* 174-184, (March) 1984.

Strewler GJ: Paget's disease of bone. *West J Med* 140:763-768, 1984.

Tiegs RD, et al: Calcitonin secretion in postmenopausal osteoporosis. *N Engl J Med* 312:1097-1100, 1985.

Transbøl I, et al: Thiazide for postponement of postmenopausal bone loss. *Metabolism* 31:383-386, 1982.

Upton GV: Perimenopause: Physiologic correlates and clinical management. *J Reprod Med* 27:1-28, 1982.

Wallach S: Treatment of Paget's disease. *Adv Intern Med* 27:1-43, 1982.

Wallach S, et al: Effect of salmon calcitonin on skeletal mass in osteoporosis. *Curr Ther Res* 22:556-572, 1977.

Wasnich RD, et al: Thiazide effect on mineral content of bone. *N Engl J Med* 309:344-347, 1983.

Wills MR, Savory J: Aluminum poisoning: Dialysis encephalopathy, osteomalacia, and anaemia. *Lancet* 2:29-33, 1983.

Agents Used to Treat Hyperlipidemia

Atherosclerosis, the basic pathophysiology responsible for most ischemic heart disease, has many causes. Any factor(s) that contributes to endothelial injury, thickening of the arterial intima, accumulation of connective tissue within the intima, and deposition of lipids or blood constituents may narrow the lumen and decrease blood flow. Such factors increase the biochemical and pathophysiologic abnormalities that predispose to atherosclerosis.

The potential for developing atherosclerosis is increased by elevated levels of serum cholesterol or low density lipoprotein (LDL) cholesterol, low levels of high density lipoprotein (HDL) cholesterol, hypertension, cigarette smoking, sedentary habits, diabetes mellitus, marked overweight, advancing age, male sex, or a family history of premature coronary artery disease (before age 55 to 60). These factors are additive, have complex interactions, and have no categorical threshold of abnormality. HDL (inversely) and LDL (positively) are linearly related to coronary artery disease (Castelli et al, 1983). Also, all factors have significant familial aggregation either genetically or through shared environmental influences (Glueck et al, 1985).

Once heart disease has become clinically manifest, the status and function of the myocardium are highly predictive of short-term survival, and the presence of risk factors is predictive of coronary artery disease progression (Arntzenius et al,

1985; Campeau et al, 1984). Because prognosis for long-term survival of symptomatic patients is not encouraging, the ultimate goal should be primary prevention. The potential for secondary prevention is less promising, although results of some reports suggest that progression of disease can be decreased (Campeau et al, 1984; Nikkila et al, 1984; Levy et al, 1984). Reducing risk factors, especially reduction of cholesterol, cessation of smoking, and control of hypertension, is a rational long-term approach to retard progression of atherosclerosis, even in patients with established coronary disease and especially following coronary artery bypass surgery.

Elevated concentrations of LDL cholesterol and reduced levels of HDL cholesterol are independent risk factors that accelerate the progression of atherosclerosis and its complications (eg, coronary artery disease, angina, myocardial infarction, sudden death, stroke, peripheral or renal arterial disease). Furthermore, at any LDL cholesterol value, risk is influenced greatly by the LDL:HDL ratio.

Reduction of plasma lipids by diet delayed the development of atherosclerosis and its clinical manifestations in a Norwegian study on primary prevention (Hjermann et al, 1981). Data extrapolated from epidemiologic information and animal experiments support this observation. Furthermore, results of the Lipid Research Clinics Coronary Primary Prevention Trial (LRC-CPPT) using diet plus cholestyramine [Questran] therapy in high-risk hypercholesterolemic men demonstrated that for each 1% reduction in blood cholesterol, myocardial infarction and/or mortality from coronary artery disease can be reduced 2% (*JAMA*, 1984, parts I and II). The decrease in coronary artery disease progression seen in hypercholesterolemic patients is entirely due to the increased HDLC and decreased TC and LDLC concentrations induced by cholestyramine (Levy et al, 1984).

The presence of more than one risk factor, especially a family history of premature atherosclerotic complications, makes active intervention more urgent, particularly in younger patients. When a family member experiences a myocardial infarct or stroke before age 55 in males or age 60 in females, has essential hypertension, or has documented hypercholesterolemia, other family members should be tested for presence of risk factors. Since the efficacy of reducing cholesterol has been proved in primary and secondary CHD prevention trials (*JAMA*, 1984, parts I and II; Arntzenius et al, 1985; Levy et al, 1984) and since atherosclerosis begins in childhood (Glueck, 1984, 1986; Glueck and Lewis, 1984; Newman et al, 1986), many investigators believe that all children should routinely be screened for abnormal lipid levels, that primary prevention and modification of risk factors should begin early in life, and that treatment, at least by dietary alterations, may delay the development of atherosclerosis.

Lipid Components

The major plasma lipids (cholesterol, triglycerides, phospholipids, and free fatty acids) are insoluble in aqueous plasma. Except for free fatty acids, which are bound to albumin, they circulate as soluble protein complexes (lipoproteins).

Lipoproteins: Lipoproteins consist of an inner core of nonpolar lipids (cholesteryl ester and triglycerides) surrounded by a surface coat of hydrophilic water-soluble components, including protein and polar lipids (phospholipids and unesterified cholesterol). The lipoproteins involved in lipid transport are metabolically interrelated and alterations in plasma lipids usually result from abnormal lipoprotein metabolism. All lipoproteins contain cholesterol in differing proportions, but their atherogenicity varies considerably. Thus, a precise diagnosis of atherogenic hyperlipidemia requires determination of specific lipoprotein abnormalities, and therapy should be directed toward correcting the lipoprotein aberrations rather than simply reducing total plasma cholesterol and/or triglyceride levels.

Because the various lipoproteins differ in electric charge and density, they can be separated by ultracentrifugation, chemical precipitation, or electrophoresis into five major groups:

(1) Chylomicrons, the largest lipoproteins, contain over 90% triglycerides (dietary, exogenous) and less than 5% cholesterol by weight. They transport dietary triglyceride to adipose tissue and skeletal muscle and dietary cholesterol to the liver. Since chylomicrons are rapidly catabolized, their presence in plasma after a 12- to 14-hour fast is considered abnormal. Although chylomicrons are not atherogenic, severe hyperchylomicronemia and hypertriglyceridemia frequently cause pancreatitis.

(2) Very low density lipoproteins (VLDL, prebeta lipopro-

teins) contain about 60% triglycerides (endogenous) and 10% to 15% cholesterol. They transport triglyceride and cholesterol away from the liver. VLDL are synthesized primarily in the liver from precursors such as free fatty acids (FFA). Since FFA and glycerol can be synthesized from carbohydrates, ingestion of large amounts of carbohydrates may transiently increase the hepatic synthesis of VLDL. VLDL synthesis also may be altered by changes in caloric intake and body weight, ingestion of alcohol, stress, and exercise. Although not clearly independently atherogenic, hypertriglyceridemia may be a marker for low HDL cholesterol and often is associated with obesity, glucose intolerance, essential hypertension, and hyperuricemia. Occasionally, hypertriglyceridemia in those with familial type V hyperlipoproteinemia has been reported to cause peripheral sensory neuropathy, which improves when triglyceride levels are reduced.

(3) Intermediate density lipoproteins (IDL, broad-beta) contain successively less triglyceride, more cholesterol, and relatively more B and E apoproteins as the catabolic conversion of VLDL to LDL progresses. IDL are normal intermediates in the conversion of VLDL to LDL, but they are not present in large concentrations unless further catabolism is delayed.

(4) Low density lipoproteins (LDL, beta lipoproteins) contain almost 50% cholesterol and less than 10% triglyceride by weight. They are derived from the metabolic breakdown of VLDL. LDL deliver cholesterol to peripheral tissues or liver. The transfer from LDL via cell receptors is a major route by which cells obtain cholesterol. LDL carry 60% to 75% of plasma cholesterol and have the highest atherogenic potential. Their concentration in plasma depends upon many factors, including dietary intake of cholesterol and saturated fat and the rate of production and removal of LDL and VLDL.

(5) High density lipoproteins (HDL, alpha lipoproteins) contain about 20% cholesterol, less than 5% triglyceride, and 50% protein by weight. They appear to be important for clearance of triglyceride and cholesterol and for transport and metabolism of cholesteryl ester in plasma. HDL normally carry 20% to 25% of the cholesterol in blood. Males and females have approximately the same levels until puberty, when the HDL concentrations in males decrease and thereafter remain about 20% lower than in females. In individuals with normal lipid values, the HDL concentrations remain relatively constant throughout adult life (approximately 45 mg/dl in males and 54 mg/dl in females).

HDL may be subdivided into fractions, lipid-rich HDL_2 and protein-rich, lipid-poor HDL_3, which vary in size, density, and apoprotein composition. Transfer of surface components from chylomicrons or VLDL to HDL_3 during hydrolysis generates HDL_2, which transports cholesterol from the periphery to the liver for degradation. These activities may help explain why increased concentrations of total HDL are associated with a reduced incidence of atherosclerotic events, while low levels of total HDL are associated with increased prevalence, morbidity, and mortality from atherosclerosis.

Also, a subclass of HDL rich in apo E may compete with LDL for receptor-mediated uptake and thereby reduce the uptake of LDL cholesterol by peripheral cells.

Familial hypoalphalipoproteinemia is characterized by low concentrations of HDL cholesterol as the predominant lipoprotein defect, is inherited as a dominant trait, and is closely associated with premature ischemic heart disease and stroke (Third et al, 1984; Borecki et al, in press). Low levels of HDL often are seen in association with poorly controlled diabetes mellitus or use of steroids. Whether familial or acquired, persons with low HDL often have normal total cholesterol and LDL levels. It is premature to assume that elevating HDL levels would reduce the incidence of atherosclerosis. It may be speculated, however, that an ability to increase HDL concentrations may be the mechanism of action of drugs that are effective in reducing the risk of CHD (Saku et al, 1985).

Large amounts of total HDL may increase total plasma cholesterol, and HDL levels must be determined to assess the risk of atherosclerosis in patients with mild or moderate hypercholesterolemia. This is particularly important in childhood. An LDL:HDL ratio exceeding 5 suggests increased risk and the need for intervention.

HDL levels may be elevated in those with familial hyperalphalipoproteinemia, following exposure to hepatic toxins (eg, chlorinated hydrocarbon pesticides), after moderate ingestion of alcohol, and after exercise. They are decreased by obesity, smoking, poorly controlled diabetes, beta-adrenergic blocking agents, probucol [Lorelco], and some estrogen/progestin combinations. Decreased concentrations of plasma HDL also have been associated with sedentary life style and hypertriglyceridemia.

Apoproteins: Apoproteins are the protein moieties of the lipoproteins. These heterogeneous groups of proteins often combine with phospholipids to provide a stable complex for solubilizing and transporting plasma lipids and have at least three essential functions. (1) They play a role in maintaining the structure of lipoproteins (apo A-II in HDL, apo B-48 in chylomicrons, and apo B-100 in VLDL, IDL, and LDL). (2) They serve as binding ligands or recognition sites for receptors on the surface of cells to facilitate the removal of lipoproteins from circulation for catabolism. For instance, apo E serves as a recognition site for receptors in the liver; LDL receptors recognize both apo B-100 and apo E (B,E receptors); and a specific apo E receptor recognizes chylomicron remnants and apo E-HDL, does not recognize normal LDL, and is resistant to modulation or regulation under a variety of metabolic conditions (Mahley et al, 1981; Angelin et al, 1983). (3) Apoproteins act as cofactors to the enzymes involved in the metabolism of lipoprotein lipid in the circulation. During the conversion of chylomicrons or VLDL to HDL, the catabolic process is regulated by lipoprotein lipase (LPL) and lecithin:cholesterol acyltransferase (LCAT). Both enzymes require apoprotein cofactors to exert their effects. Apo A-I and apo C-I activate LCAT, the major enzyme responsible for esterification of plasma cholesterol. Apo C-II is the specific cofactor for activation of LPL, the enzyme responsible for hydrolysis of triglycerides. See also Table 1.

Lipid Transport

Lipid transport mechanisms shuttle cholesterol and triglyceride among the liver, intestine, and other tissues. In individuals with normal plasma lipids, lipoprotein cholesterol is contin-

uously and efficiently cycled into and out of plasma and does not accumulate extensively in artery walls. The ability to metabolize lipoproteins and lipoprotein cholesterol may be altered by hormonal and genetic factors that influence the concentration of enzymes involved in lipid transport, the apoprotein content, and the number and activity of lipoprotein receptors. Because the concentration of cholesterol in plasma is not a simple product of dietary intake and hepatic synthesis, understanding the lipoprotein transport system helps explain why individuals vary in their response to dietary cholesterol intake (Brown and Goldstein, 1980).

Lipids are transported by both exogenous and endogenous pathways. In the intestinal epithelium, ingested fats (often more than 100 g triglycerides and 400 to 600 mg cholesterol per day) are incorporated into chylomicrons along with apoproteins B-48 and A-I. These are secreted into lymph and then into plasma where they receive C and E apoproteins from HDL and bind to the surface of endothelial cells on capillary walls in adipose tissue or muscle.

The chylomicrons are composed of a triglyceride and cholesterol core with A, B-48, and C apoproteins on the surface. Apoprotein C-II activates lipoprotein lipase on the endothelial cell surface, which then hydrolyzes the triglyceride core of the chylomicron, releasing free fatty acids and monoglycerides. The fatty acids enter cells where they are oxidized for energy or re-esterified for storage. As the triglyceride core is depleted, the chylomicron shrinks and excess surface materials (mainly phospholipids and free cholesterol plus C and A apoproteins) are transferred to HDL, with esterification of cholesterol by LCAT; apoprotein E is received in exchange. The resulting E-containing chylomicron remnant with its intact cholesteryl esters dissociates from the epithelium, re-enters the circulation, and is cleared rapidly from plasma by the liver (plasma half-life of chylomicrons and remnants is four to five minutes). The remnants are bound to receptors on hepatic cells, which resemble receptors that take up LDL particles, except that these hepatic receptors appear to recognize only apo E and the apo E-containing particles are cleared more efficiently. By feedback inhibition of 3-hydroxy-3-methylglutaryl coenzyme A reductase (HMG-CoA reductase), a cholesterol-synthesizing enzyme, chylomicron remnant catabolism regulates the formation of cholesterol in the liver. The chylomicron remnants are transported into the liver much more rapidly than LDL or HDL, and cholesterol derived from chylomicrons effectively inhibits hepatic cholesterol synthesis. Some of the cholesterol in the hepatocyte is derived from receptor-mediated uptake of chylomicron remnants. When this source is insufficient, the liver synthesizes cholesterol by increasing the activity of a rate-controlling enzyme, HMG-CoA reductase.

Some hepatic cholesterol is converted to bile acids and excreted into the intestine. Another portion is secreted into the bile as unesterified cholesterol. Most of the cholesterol (and bile acids) is reabsorbed from the intestine and used to form endogenous lipoproteins, and a small portion is excreted in the feces.

Endogenous lipid transport originates in the liver where ingested carbohydrate is converted to fatty acids, which then are esterified into triglycerides. Together with apoprotein B-100 and apoprotein E, which are synthesized in the liver, the

TABLE 1.
APOPROTEIN COMPONENTS OF LIPOPROTEINS

| Apoprotein | Chylomicron | Lipoprotein in which present | | | | Function |
		VLDL	IDL	LDL	HDL	
A-I	major	minor	—	trace	major (more in HDL$_2$ than in HDL$_3$)	LCAT[1] activator Acceptor of peripheral cholesterol (?)
A-II	minor	minor	—	trace	major (more in HDL$_3$ than in HDL$_2$)	Structural role in HDL
A-III (see D)						
A-IV	major	trace	—	—	minor	Structural role and transport of chylomicrons
B-48	major	—	—	—	minor	Structural role and transport of chylomicrons
B-100	—	major	major	major	minor	Structural role for VLDL, IDL, LDL Binding protein for primary LDL (apo B, E) receptor (both hepatic and extrahepatic)
C-I	major	major	minor	trace	minor	LCAT[1] activator
C-II	major	major	minor	trace	minor	LPL[2] activator (for chylomicron and VLDL triglyceride hydrolysis)
C-III[3]	major	major	minor	trace	minor	LPL[2] weak inhibitor (for chylomicron and VLDL triglyceride hydrolysis)
D (also called A-III)	—	minor	—	trace	minor (in HDL$_3$)	Cholesterol ester transport
E[4] (also called arginine-rich)	minor	major	major	—	minor	Binding protein at apo B, E receptors and apo E receptors (involved in chylomicron remnant removal) Acceptor of peripheral cholesterol (?)

[1]*LCAT = lecithin:cholesterol acyltransferase*
[2]*LPL = lipoprotein lipase*
[3]*Further subdivision of apoprotein C-III according to the number of sialic acid residues present is C-III$_0$, C-III$_1$, C-III$_2$, and C-III$_3$.*
[4]*Several isoelectric forms exist. Major isoform in normal individuals is E-III.*

triglycerides are incorporated into VLDL and secreted into the plasma where they receive C apoproteins from HDL. Secretion of VLDL is stimulated whenever synthesis of triglycerides and free fatty acids is increased, as after high carbohydrate intake.

VLDL contain about five times more triglyceride than cholesteryl esters in their core and have approximately the same surface components as chylomicrons. VLDL enter the capillaries of adipose tissue or muscle where they interact with lipoprotein lipase (as do chylomicrons) and are cleared from the plasma in one to three hours. As triglyceride is removed, the size of the particle decreases, density increases, and an IDL particle is formed. As the excess surface material, including C apoproteins, is transferred to HDL, cholesteryl ester is exchanged from the HDL and new particles are formed with a core containing mostly cholesteryl esters. As a result of the almost continuous lipolysis and exchanges, most of the re-

maining triglycerides are removed and all apoproteins (except B) are lost, thus forming LDL. A portion of IDL is cleared rapidly by the liver. The process is mediated by hepatic LDL receptors that recognize either apo E or B-100. When the number of LDL receptors is decreased, more IDL remains in plasma and is converted to LDL. Thus, a decrease in hepatic LDL receptors not only impairs LDL catabolism but also causes an apparent slight overproduction of LDL by the shunt mechanism (Goldstein and Brown, 1983; Goldstein et al, 1983).

LDL delivers cholesterol to extrahepatic cells (eg, adrenals, gonads, muscle, lymphocytes) and to the liver. The LDL in plasma bind to high affinity receptors (apo B,E receptors) located in regions of the cell membrane called coated pits. The pits invaginate and internalize the LDL by endocytosis and lysosomal hydrolytic enzymes (eg, acid cholesterol esterase) degrade apoprotein B to amino acids and liberate free cholesterol for membrane synthesis or (as a precursor) for steroid hormone synthesis. The receptors are recycled to the surface of the cell. Some free cholesterol is esterified for storage by acyl CoA cholesterol acyl transferase (ACAT) in the cell. Intracellular free cholesterol regulates the number of high affinity receptors for LDL as well as the activity of HMG-CoA reductase, thus limiting both cholesterol entry from the blood and synthesis. In normal individuals, 33% to 66% of the LDL cholesterol is degraded in this way.

LDL also can be degraded by phagocytosis via macrophages of the reticuloendothelial system, but this mechanism is less efficient. As the plasma concentration of LDL rises, increasing amounts are degraded by these scavenger cells, which store the cholesteryl esters. When macrophages become overloaded with lipid, foam cells typical of the atherosclerotic plaque develop and cholesterol may be deposited in arterial walls, tendons, or skin (Brown and Goldstein, 1985).

HDL circulate for five to six days, function in reverse cholesterol transport, and may be considered the central storage site for lipoprotein apoproteins for exchange where needed to assure lipid catabolism. They bind the cholesterol released from cells and esterify it through interaction of their apoprotein A-I with LCAT. The C apoproteins are transferred from HDL to chylomicrons or VLDL to initiate catabolism of triglycerides and are transferred back to HDL during VLDL-IDL catabolism. Some HDL have apo E as their only protein component, contain 50% cholesterol, and are known as apo E-HDL (Mahley and Innerarity, 1983).

With continuing study of the apoproteins, more complete understanding of lipid transport will occur. It is already apparent that apoprotein content and metabolism help explain the interrelationships of the lipoprotein families in normal lipid transport and the altered mechanisms in most forms of hyperlipidemia. Disturbances of lipoprotein metabolism often can be explained by alterations of apoproteins.

Genetic defects in apoprotein structure have the following effects: (1) Severe HDL deficiency caused by defective apo A-I characterizes homozygous Tangier disease. (2) In apo A-I/C-III deficiency, HDL levels are markedly reduced and severe coronary artery disease develops (Krause and Newton, 1984). (3) In patients with no detectable normal apo C-II, hyperchylomicronemia (type I or V hyperlipoproteinemia) or severe hypertriglyceridemia occurs. The incidence of cardiovascular disease does not appear to be increased but pancreatitis is common. (4) In patients who lack apo B-100 but have normal amounts of apo B-48, dietary fats are absorbed normally but LDL and VLDL are not present in plasma (Krause and Newton, 1984). (5) Some patients with coronary artery disease have normal concentrations of LDL but the LDL contain elevated levels of apo B-100. (6) The major apo E isoform found in most patients with type III hyperlipoproteinemia may be apo E-II and the apo E-III found in normal individuals is absent. (7) Some patients with type V hyperlipoproteinemia have increased levels of apo E-IV. (8) Some patients with familial xanthelasma but no hypercholesterolemia are reported to have either elevated apo B or decreased apo E-III levels (Douste-Blazy et al, 1982). (9) Abnormal apo E components, apo E-V and apo E Suita, which may be mutations and are not present in normal individuals, have been identified in patients with ischemic heart disease, although a causal relationship has not been confirmed (Yamamura et al, 1984).

Types of Hyperlipoproteinemia

Five major types of hyperlipoproteinemia have been described, based on which lipoproteins are abnormally increased, and they may be either primary or secondary; occasionally both forms occur in the same individual. Lipoprotein levels normally vary with age and sex and can be altered markedly by changes in weight or diet and by concurrent illness.

Primary hyperlipoproteinemias are genetically determined or sporadic and vary in clinical manifestations, prognosis, and response to treatment. Secondary hyperlipoproteinemias may be associated with poorly controlled diabetes mellitus, alcoholism, hypothyroidism, obstructive liver disease, nephrotic syndrome, uremia, glycogen storage disease, or dysproteinemias (multiple myeloma, macroglobulinemia, lupus erythematosus). Successful treatment of the underlying disease, when feasible, usually corrects the hyperlipoproteinemia. The acquired hyperlipoproteinemias also may result from diet or administration of corticosteroids, estrogens, androgens, diuretics, or beta-blocking drugs.

In addition to atherosclerosis, hyperlipoproteinemia may produce lipid deposits (xanthomas) in the skin and tendons. Hypertriglyceridemia may induce abdominal pain, hepatosplenomegaly, eruptive xanthomas, and pancreatitis.

Lipoprotein patterns (types I to V, see Table 2 and below) do *not* define a specific disease mechanism but help to identify the site of the abnormality in the complex area of lipid transport. Hyperlipoproteinemia may result from malfunction in any of the numerous metabolic steps during synthesis, transport, interconversion, or catabolism. An etiologic diagnosis is not always possible but the lipoprotein and apoprotein patterns, which are purely descriptive, may aid in assessing prognosis and management. Furthermore, each type of hyperlipoproteinemia may represent several different disorders. Although the present classification is imperfect, differential diagnosis is important since treatment and response vary significantly.

Type I is characterized by massive fasting hyperchylomicronemia induced even by normal dietary fat intake. It usually is caused by deficiency of a lipoprotein lipase needed to metabolize chylomicrons. Also, a few families who lack normal apoprotein C-II have been reported to have an identical symptom complex. Serum triglycerides are markedly elevated, and the cholesterol:triglyceride ratio is usually less than 0.2:1.

Patients with type I usually are symptomatic before age 10 (often within the first year of life); colic, recurrent abdominal pain, eruptive xanthomas, and hepatosplenomegaly often develop in early childhood. Adults also may experience pain (pancreatitis) that mimics acute abdominal crises and is often accompanied by fever, leukocytosis, anorexia, and vomiting. Acute hemorrhagic pancreatitis is the most severe, and often fatal, complication of primary type I hyperlipoproteinemia.

TABLE 2.
CHARACTERISTICS OF TYPES OF HYPERLIPOPROTEINEMIA*

	Type I	Type II	
	Exogenous Hyperlipemia (Hyperchylomicronemia)	a. Hyperbetalipoproteinemia (Hypercholesterolemia)	b. Combined Hyperlipidemia (Mixed Hyperlipidemia)
Lipoprotein characteristics of plasma	Chylomicrons markedly increased LDL, VLDL, and HDL usually decreased	LDL increased VLDL normal Chylomicrons absent	LDL increased VLDL increased Chylomicrons absent
Metabolic defect	Clearance of chylomicrons decreased by lipoprotein lipase deficiency or apo C-II abnormality	Synthesis increased and clearance of LDL decreased by deficiency in primary LDL receptors or defective LDL receptors	Same as Type IIa plus elevated VLDL LDL may contain increased amounts of apo B
Appearance of plasma after standing overnight at 4 C (sample taken after 12-14 hr fast)†	Cream layer on top, clear infranate	Clear (no cream layer on top)	No cream layer on top, clear to turbid infranate (depending on VLDL level)
Cholesterol: triglyceride ratio	<0.2:1	>1.5:1	Variable
Other laboratory abnormalities	Fat tolerance markedly abnormal PHLA low		
Clinical manifestations	Eruptive xanthomas Hepatosplenomegaly Lipemia retinalis Abdominal pain Pancreatitis	Tendon xanthomas, occasionally associated with polyarthritis Xanthelasma Arcus corneae juvenilis Tuberous xanthomas	
Secondary causes (to be evaluated and, if possible, eliminated before treating for hyperlipoproteinemia)	Dysgammaglobulinemia Diabetic acidosis	Hypothyroidism Obstructive liver disease Macroglobulinemia Multiple myeloma Nephrotic syndrome Excess dietary cholesterol Excess saturated fat in diet	
Incidence	Rare	Common	
Usual age at detection	Early childhood	Infancy or early childhood	
Ischemic heart disease risk	No association	Greatly accelerated	

*VLDL—very low density lipoproteins (pre-β-lipoproteins) represent endogenous triglyceride concentration.
LDL—low density lipoproteins (β-lipoproteins) represent major portions of cholesterol concentration
IDL—intermediate density lipoproteins (floating β-lipoproteins) represent intermediates in VLDL metabolism or VLDL remnants.
Chylomicrons—represent exogenous triglyceride concentration
HDL—high density lipoproteins (α-lipoproteins) are not included in the chart.

Type III Broad Beta Pattern (Dysbetalipoproteinemia)	Type IV Endogenous Hyperlipidemia (Hypertriglyceridemia)	Type V Mixed Hyperlipidemia
IDL increased Chylomicrons may be present	VDL increased LDL normal (or decreased) Chylomicrons absent	VLDL increased Chylomicrons increased LDL normal (or decreased)
Either production of IDL increased or clearance of IDL decreased. Total plasma apo E (as apo E-II isoform) increased plus apo E-III deficiency. Possibly deficiency of hepatic lipase	Production of VLDL increased, clearance of VLDL decreased, or both. Possibly abnormal apo A-I/C-III complex	Either production of chylomicrons and VLDL increased or clearance of both is decreased. Possibly imbalance between apo C-II and C-III. Possibly abnormal apo E (apo E-IV isoform present in E-III deficiency)
Faint cream layer on top, turbid infranate	No cream layer on top, clear to turbid infranate (depending on VLDL level)	Cream layer on top, turbid infranate
Often 1:1, but may vary from 0.3 to 2.0:1	Variable	0.15 to 0.6:1
Carbohydrate sensitivity and glucose tolerance often abnormal Uric acid levels often elevated	Carbohydrate sensitivity and glucose tolerance often abnormal Uric acid levels often elevated	Carbohydrate sensitivity and glucose tolerance usually abnormal Uric acid levels usually elevated Fat tolerance abnormal PHLA sometimes low
Planar xanthomas Tuberoeruptive xanthomas Tendon xanthomas Occasionally, arcus corneae juvenilis Rarely, xanthelasma	Usually none	Eruptive xanthomas Abdominal pain Pancreatitis Hepatosplenomegaly Lipemia retinalis Occasionally, tuberoeruptive xanthomas, paresthesias
Hypothyroidism Dysgammaglobulinemia Diabetic acidosis Multiple myeloma	Nephrotic syndrome Juvenile diabetes Multiple myeloma Alcoholism Von Gierke disease Werner syndrome Use of OCs or estrogens Obesity Acute metabolic stress	Hypothyroidism Nephrotic syndrome Diabetic acidosis Multiple myeloma Alcoholism Von Gierke disease Use of OCs or estrogens
Relatively uncommon	Common	Relatively uncommon
Early adulthood	Adulthood (middle age)	Early adulthood
Peripheral and coronary vascular disease accelerated	Probably accelerated	Data inadequate to determine association

PHLA—postheparin lipolytic activity represents a group of enzymes necessary for metabolism of triglycerides.
Chylomicrons represent exogenous triglyceride concentration.
†Cream layer indicates elevated chylomicron concentration; turbid infranate indicates elevated triglycerides (VLDL).

However, premature atherosclerotic heart disease is not associated with this form of lipidemia.

Type II is characterized by elevated LDL and apoprotein B-100 concentrations with normal (IIa) or moderately elevated (IIb) VLDL. In individuals in whom increased cholesterol and saturated fat intake elevates plasma LDL concentrations, dietary restriction of cholesterol and saturated fats controls the hyperbetalipoproteinemia (LDL).

Familial type II hyperlipoproteinemia is manifested clinically in early childhood in homozygous individuals, but symptoms usually do not appear before age 20 in the heterozygote. Both homozygous and heterozygous disorders can be diagnosed in childhood by measuring LDL cholesterol. The most common form of familial type II is caused by decreased numbers of high affinity LDL receptors. In other primary abnormalities, receptors have reduced affinity for LDL or have aberrant locations, which permit binding but prevent internalization of LDL. Heterozygotes have approximately one-half the number of normal receptors and homozygotes have few, if any, functional primary receptors. This block in degradation causes LDL to accumulate in the plasma and increases their deposition in the artery wall.

Xanthomas of the tuberous or tendinous type occur in both homozygotes and heterozygotes; planar lesions often are evident in homozygotes. In homozygous patients, ischemic heart disease is almost inevitable before age 20; in male heterozygotes, the probability is at least 60% by age 50. Therefore, early detection is important. If genetically determined type II hyperbetalipoproteinemia is present, about one-half of first-degree family members will be affected; thus, blood relatives should be screened.

Type III is characterized by the accumulation of IDL, possibly because of a partial block in metabolism of VLDL to LDL, rapid production of apoprotein B, or abnormal apoprotein E levels. In some patients with familial type III disorder, one isoelectric form of apoprotein E, apo E-III for which the liver has a high affinity, is absent or deficient and isoform E-II is present. In these patients, the hepatic uptake of VLDL and chylomicron remnants is blocked because receptors do not recognize the apo E-II isoform and IDL accumulate in blood and tissues. Serum cholesterol and triglyceride concentrations are similarly elevated (350 to 800 mg/dl) in those with this disorder.

Symptoms may appear by early adulthood, especially in males. Palmar planar xanthomas and tuberoeruptive lesions on the elbows, knees, or buttocks are characteristic. Accelerated coronary and peripheral vascular disease frequently occur in the fourth and fifth decades, and glucose intolerance and hyperuricemia are observed in about 40% of patients.

Type IV is characterized by elevated VLDL levels with resulting hypertriglyceridemia and reciprocal depression of HDL. This genetically diverse disorder is a common form of hyperlipoproteinemia and signs usually appear in middle age. About one-half of those at genetic risk exhibit elevated triglyceride levels by age 25 (Glueck, 1982). The mechanisms of the familial disorder are uncertain, but acquired type IV often is secondary to other diseases or to excessive intake of alcohol or carbohydrates and patients are frequently obese. Ischemic heart disease may occur (although less frequently than in familial type II) during the fourth decade or later in patients with familial type IV hyperlipoproteinemia; there usually are no prior external signs. Many patients have carbohydrate intolerance with an excessive insulin response to a carbohydrate load and more than 40% have hyperuricemia.

Type V is characterized by accumulation of VLDL and chylomicrons, probably caused by defective catabolism of endogenous and exogenous triglycerides. Since all lipoproteins contain cholesterol, cholesterol concentrations may be elevated if triglyceride levels are very high. This disorder is relatively uncommon and may be genetically heterogeneous. Patients with the familial disorder usually do not become symptomatic until after age 20. Obesity greatly exacerbates this lipid transport disorder. These patients have fat and carbohydrate intolerance and usually have hyperuricemia. An association between type V disorder and premature ischemic heart disease has not been established unequivocally, but triglyceride levels should be reduced to decrease the likelihood of eruptive xanthomas, pancreatitis, and abdominal pain.

TREATMENT

Atherosclerosis is characterized by the accumulation and deposition of cholesteryl esters in the arterial wall; the rate of deposition depends in part on the presence and interaction of risk factors. Elevated LDL concentration in blood is an independent risk factor: The higher the level of LDL, the faster the rate of accumulation in arteries even in the absence of other risk factors. Although an elevated triglyceride concentration apparently is not an independent risk factor, it often indicates lipid derangements (particularly in HDL metabolism) and helps identify persons at increased risk for coronary artery disease (National Institutes of Health Consensus Conference, 1984).

Long-term controlled studies suggest that decreasing blood lipid levels may reduce morbidity and mortality in patients with established ischemic heart disease who have experienced at least one myocardial infarction. However, these studies have been criticized for various reasons. Furthermore, once atherosclerotic complications have occurred, it is probable that the coronary artery disease is sufficiently advanced and the myocardium already damaged so that reducing lipid levels may be less effective because of the presence of muscle damage and other factors. Nevertheless, secondary prevention has been shown to retard progression of coronary artery disease (Levy et al, 1984) and is particularly important following coronary bypass surgery.

The value of reducing lipid levels in the primary prevention of atherosclerosis has been proved. The National Institutes of Health Consensus Conference on reducing cholesterol (1985) concluded that decreasing elevated blood cholesterol levels, especially LDL cholesterol, reduces the risk of coronary artery disease. Although the data from the LRC-CPPT (*JAMA*, 1984, parts I and II) apply only to men with type IIa hyperlipoproteinemia given cholestyramine with a low-cholesterol, low-saturated-fat diet, the results establish that the risk of coronary artery disease can be reduced by appropriate diet and drug therapy. It is reasonable to assume that early therapy before sequelae have developed may be more beneficial than late intervention. A Norwegian study provides some evidence that diet and cessation of smoking reduce expected rates of morbidity and mortality in normotensive men who have no signs of ischemic heart disease but are at risk because of hypercholesterolemia and/or cigarette smoking (Hjermann et al, 1981).

Type I hyperlipoproteinemia is quite rare, types III and V are uncommon, and types II and IV are relatively common. Since hyperlipoproteinemia is often genetically determined and is associated with a high risk of ischemic heart disease (especially types II, III, and IV), family members (particularly younger siblings and children) should be screened for abnormal lipid levels so that treatment can be initiated before irreversible vascular damage has occurred. Because manifestations of type IV are uncommon in children, early detection may be difficult.

Therapeutic Guidelines

Differential Diagnosis: Rational treatment of lipid disorders depends upon definitive differential diagnosis. Definite diagnostic levels have been established for lipids.

The National Institutes of Health Consensus Conference on lowering cholesterol (1985) concluded that cholesterol levels of most Americans are higher than optimum and that levels exceeding 200 mg/dl indicate increased risk. Individuals at moderate risk were defined as those age 20 to 29 with cholesterol levels 200 mg/dl, 30 to 39 with cholesterol levels 220 mg/dl, and 40 or older with cholesterol levels 240 mg/dl. These individuals should be evaluated and receive diet therapy; adjunctive drug therapy should be prescribed if they are unresponsive to diet and have other risk factors. High-risk cholesterol levels (>90th percentile) for the same age groups were defined as 220, 240, and 260 mg/dl, respectively. Individuals at high risk often require both dietary modification and drug therapy, particularly those with hereditary hypercholesterolemia.

The National Institutes of Health Consensus Conference on hypertriglyceridemia (1984) stated that, in the absence of other risk factors, triglyceride levels below 250 mg/dl do not indicate increased risk for cardiovascular disease and do not require treatment. Triglyceride levels between 250 and 500 mg/dl increase the risk of cardiovascular disease when associated with other risk factors (eg, obesity, hypertension, hypercholesterolemia, low HDL, low apo A-I, high apo B, family history of premature coronary artery disease). Other diseases (eg, diabetes mellitus, hypothyroidism, chronic renal disease) and factors (eg, acute stress, alcoholism, certain drugs) causing secondary elevation of triglycerides also indicate increased risk. Dietary therapy to reduce triglyceride levels is of primary importance; treatment for any underlying cause, weight control, increased physical activity, and alcohol restriction also are necessary. Drugs may be given adjunctively only when these measures are ineffective. The danger of pancreati-

tis increases in proportion to the degree of hypertriglyceridemia and patients with triglyceride levels exceeding 600 mg/dl should be treated aggressively.

Proper evaluation for a lipid transport disorder includes complete personal, dietary, and family history; thorough physical examination; and laboratory evaluation, including tests of carbohydrate tolerance and thyroid, hepatic, and renal function. Total cholesterol and triglyceride determinations are adequate for initial screening, but elevated values do not identify the specific lipid transport disorder. Cholesterol is present in all lipoproteins, and hypercholesterolemia may result from an increased level of any lipoprotein. In nonfasting patients, cholesterol levels are relatively reliable and triglyceride values above 300 mg/dl indicate abnormality and the need for further testing. (Since they complicate interpretation of test results, intake of hypolipidemic drugs, estrogens, contraceptive agents, or steroids should be discontinued, if feasible, at least three weeks prior to diagnostic determinations.)

After at least one week on a conventional American diet, cholesterol and triglyceride analyses should be performed on blood samples acquired after a 12- to 14-hour fast. If cholesterol and/or triglyceride levels are elevated, at least two further measurements, including HDL (and LDL cholesterol), should be obtained at two-week intervals to confirm the diagnosis of hyperlipidemia and to establish a pretreatment baseline. Office kits are unsatisfactory for these purposes, and one should insist that the laboratory doing the lipid determinations is appropriately standardized and can provide precise and accurate lipid values. Many authorities recommend that HDL cholesterol also be measured during initial screening, since low HDL is a major risk factor for coronary artery disease and stroke (Glueck et al, 1982).

If hypercholesterolemia is present, examination of the fasting plasma after overnight refrigeration identifies the type of hyperlipoproteinemia in about two-thirds of cases. (VLDL and chylomicrons refract light and produce turbidity in hyperlipidemic plasma, but LDL and HDL do not; see Table 2.) However, type IIb, III, and mild type IV cannot be differentiated by this procedure. Direct determination of HDL by simple precipitation techniques distinguishes increased LDL from increased HDL and also may be used to calculate the level of LDL cholesterol (LDL_C) in fasting plasma according to the formula:

$$LDL_C = total\ cholesterol - \frac{triglycerides}{5} - HDL\ cholesterol$$

Except in type III, this formula is accurate when chylomicrons are not present and the triglyceride concentration is 400 mg/dl or less; at concentrations above 400 mg/dl, ultracentrifugation is necessary to determine LDL_C.

Serum triglyceride levels usually increase and serum cholesterol levels decrease immediately after acute myocardial infarction or stroke; therefore, determination of lipoprotein type should be postponed until serum lipids have stabilized (usually after two months), although some data indicate that levels may be measured during the first 24 hours following a myocardial infarction.

After the type of abnormality has been established, periodic measurements of cholesterol, triglyceride, HDL cholesterol, and a derived LDL cholesterol may be required to monitor the effects of diet and drug therapy.

Thiazide-type diuretics or beta-blocking drugs may elevate serum lipids, principally VLDL, particularly in patients with type IV or type V hyperlipoproteinemia. When this occurs, other medication can be substituted and dietary changes and/or withdrawal of these drugs may be advisable to prevent potential acceleration of atherogenesis. For patients who must continue diuretic or antihypertensive therapy, a weight reduction program and a diet low in saturated fat/cholesterol should be followed.

Dietary Management: Manipulation of diet is the initial treatment for primary hyperlipoproteinemias. The response to any corrective diet differs among patients and the variations in response are determined both by the environment (diet is a major factor) and by genetic variables. Therefore, diets should be individualized according to the type of hyperlipoproteinemia being treated (see Table 3). For outpatients, understanding of and adherence to a diet may require several months of adjustment with frequent follow-up and encouragement by the physician.

Strong patient motivation is a prerequisite if prolonged dietary modification is to succeed, and it is usually necessary to be specific about foods to be avoided. In general, consumption of meat and dairy fat should be decreased and egg yolks, butter, cooking oils rich in saturated fat, and baked goods, such as cakes and cookies, should be avoided. Consumption of fruits, vegetables, fiber, whole grains, seafood (except shrimp), and skim milk should be increased. Diets employing fish three to four times per week have been reported to reduce coronary artery disease. Use of fish oils containing high levels of eicosapentaenoic and decasapentaenoic acids as the source of unsaturated fats has been suggested. However, they often contain cholesterol and may increase bleeding time by inhibiting platelet aggregation. Also, excessive amounts of fish oils contain sufficient quantities of vitamins A and D to cause toxic effects.

For overweight patients with primary hypertriglyceridemia (lipoprotein phenotypes IIb, III, IV, and V), weight reduction to attain ideal body weight is the therapy of choice; this decreases triglycerides to normal levels in 60% to 75% of those with type IV disorder and aids in reducing triglycerides in those with

TABLE 3.
GENERAL DIETARY RESTRICTIONS IN TREATMENT OF HYPERLIPOPROTEINEMIAS

	Type I	Type II a	Type II b
General prescription	Low fat Supplement with medium-chain triglycerides High carbohydrate	Low cholesterol Low saturated fat supplemented with unsaturated fat	Low cholesterol Low saturated fat supplemented with unsaturated fat Weight reduction when necessary Moderate alcohol restriction
Weight reduction	Has little effect	Has little effect	To ideal body weight may be necessary
Calories	Not restricted Patients with high energy requirements may have difficulty maintaining weight	Not restricted	Restricted to maintain ideal body weight
Protein	Not restriced; 15%-20% (50-100 g daily)	Not restricted; 15%-20% (50-100 g daily)	
Fat	Adults, less than 25 g/day; children 6 to 12 years of age, less than 15 g/day. May be either saturated or unsaturated fats. Supplement with medium-chain triglycerides according to caloric requirement	Restricted to 30% or less daily. Low saturated fat (less than 5% of calories) supplemented with unsaturated fat to increase P/S ration to >1.1	
Cholestrol	Not restricted	Low. Adults, less than 300 mg daily; children, less than 200 mg daily	
Carbohydrate	Not restricted Substitute carbohydrate for fat	Not restricted	
Alcohol	None allowed	Not restricted	
Remarks	Diet should reduce chylomicrons to normal	Diet should lower LDL 15%-30%	

types IIb, III, and V. Reduction of triglycerides also may normalize decreased HDL concentrations typical of hypertriglyceridemia. When ideal body weight is attained or when maximal beneficial effects have been achieved, the diet appropriate for the type of hyperlipoproteinemia should then be started.

Some authorities believe that a single diet is appropriate in all hyperlipidemias (except for the very rare, genetically determined, lipoprotein lipase deficiency in type I). The National Institutes of Health Consensus Conference on reducing cholesterol advocates the American Heart Association fat-controlled diet for all Americans. In this diet, initially, 30% of calories is derived from fat, with less than 10% of total calories from saturated fats (polyunsaturated fats and carbohydrates are substituted for saturated fats). However, caloric intake from polyunsaturated fats should not exceed 10% until their relationship to HDL metabolism has been defined and the claims that increased deposition of polyunsaturates in tissues increases cellular damage have been clarified. Cholesterol intake also should be reduced to less than 300 mg daily.

Data from long-term studies on children with heterozygous hypercholesterolemia suggest that dietary intervention does not affect normal growth and weight gain (Glueck et al, in press). However, the Committee on Nutrition of the American Academy of Pediatrics does not advocate dietary changes for *all* children, since data on long-term effects are inadequate to justify widespread alterations.

Acquired elevation of LDL often can be normalized by strict adherence to the prescribed diet and weight control. Type II heterozygotes rarely attain the normal range of LDL on diet alone and homozygotes never do. Diet therapy with weight control may reduce lipids to normal concentrations in types III, IV, and sometimes V.

Drug Therapy: *Drugs are indicated only when dietary restrictions, including weight reduction when necessary, are unsuccessful and the risk of atherosclerotic (eg, transient ischemic attacks, intermittent claudication, myocardial infarction, stroke) or other complications (eg, pancreatitis, abdominal pain, xanthomas) justifies their use. Dietary regulation must continue during drug therapy, since effects are additive.*

Following initiation of drug treatment, plasma lipid levels should be measured monthly until they become stable and at

Type III	Type IV	Type V
Weight reduction to ideal body weight Low cholesterol Balanced, modified fat and carbohydrate Low alcohol intake	Weight reduction to ideal body weight Controlled carbohydrate Modified fat Low alcohol intake	Weight reduction to ideal body weight High protein Moderate fat and carbohydrate reduction No alcohol intake
To ideal body weight is necessary	To ideal body weight is necessary	To ideal body weight is necessary
Restricted to maintain ideal body weight	Restricted to maintain ideal body weight	Restricted to maintain ideal body weight
Moderate; 18%-21% (75-125 g daily)	Moderate; 18%-21% (75-125 g daily)	High; 21%-24% (90-145 g daily)
Restricted to 30% daily with unsaturated fat substituted for a portion of saturated fat	Restricted to control calories; substitution of unsaturated fat for a portion of saturated fat	Restricted to 20% or less daily, with unsaturated fat substituted for a portion of saturated fat
Low. Less than 300 mg daily	Moderate restriction. Less than 500 mg daily	Moderate restriction. Less than 500 mg daily
Controlled to 40% daily	Controlled to 40% daily	Controlled. Less than 50% daily
Restricted to 2 servings daily Substitute for carbohydrate	Restricted to 2 servings daily Substitute for carbohydrate	None allowed

TABLE 4.
CHANGES INDUCED BY ADMINISTRATION OF HYPOLIPIDEMIC DRUGS

	Cholestyramine	Clofibrate	Colestipol	Dextrothyroxine
Cholestrol	↓	↔ ↓	↓	↓
Triglycerides	↔ ↑	↓	↔ ↑	↔ ↓
Chylomicrons				
VLDL	↔ ↑	↓	↔ ↑	↔ ↓
IDL		↓		
LDL	↓	↔ ↓ or ↑	↓	↓
HDL	↑ (slight)	↔ ↑	↑ (slight)	
HDL cholesterol Total cholesterol	↑		↑	
HDL$_2$: HDL$_3$	↑ (slight)			
Apo A-I	↑	↑		
A-II				
A-III (see D)				
B	↓		↓	↓
C-I				
C-II				
C-III				
D				
E				

gradually longer intervals thereafter. In most instances, the dose should be modified or another drug substituted or added if lipoprotein levels are not reduced significantly after an adequate trial (usually two to three months). Drug therapy must be continuous and lifelong in the primary hyperlipoproteinemias, since plasma lipid levels usually return to pretreatment concentrations if treatment is discontinued. In addition, the patient must be monitored indefinitely at regular intervals since dosage adjustments are required if diet or body weight changes, if concomitant medications are used, or if adverse reactions occur.

Several drugs lower elevated plasma cholesterol and/or triglycerides (see Table 4), but no single drug is effective in all types of hyperlipoproteinemia and their long-term effects have not been established. At present, the agents advocated for treatment of hyperlipidemias are cholestyramine resin [Questran], clofibrate [Atromid-S], colestipol [Colestid], gemfibrozil [Lopid], niacin (nicotinic acid) [Nicobid, Nicolar], and probucol [Lorelco]. Dextrothyroxine [Choloxin], neomycin [Mycifradin], norethindrone [Aygestin, Norlutate], and oxandrolone [Anavar] are used occasionally. Estrogens are no longer advocated because they may increase the incidence of cardiovascular complications. See the discussion on Treatment of Hyperlipoproteinemia Types and the evaluations.

Several agents with hypolipidemic activity have been used investigationally but require further study. Aminosalicylic acid (PAS), a drug used to treat tuberculosis, decreases cholesterol and triglycerides by reducing LDL and VLDL. However, it is not well tolerated because of gastrointestinal disturbances. A highly purified preparation (PAS-C) with similar hypolipidemic activity produces fewer side effects but rarely may cause hypersensitivity reactions or goiter.

Halofenate, which is structurally similar to clofibrate, reduces VLDL but has caused severe gastrointestinal bleeding. In limited studies, bezafibrate, an analogue of clofibrate, has been shown to have actions resembling those of clofibrate but does not affect bile composition; it rarely causes a myositis-like syndrome and impotence. Bezafibrate and other analogues of clofibrate (fenofibrate, ciprofibrate) may elevate HDL and reduce triglycerides to a greater extent than clofibrate. Also, the toxicity seen following use of clofibrate has not yet been encountered with these other fibric acid derivatives.

An investigational condensation product of clofibrate and niacin, etofibrate, is reported to have the combined action of its two components but is less toxic than either drug.

The investigational agents, compactin (mevastatin) and mevinolin, are competitive inhibitors of HMG-CoA reductase. They stimulate the fractional catabolic rate of LDL by increas-

Gemfibrozil	Neomycin	Niacin	Probucol	Sitosterols
↔↓	↓	↓	↓	↓
↓	↔	↓	↔	
		↔↓		
↓	↔	↓	↔	
↓	↔	↓	↔	
↔↓ or ↑	↓	↓	↓	↓
↑	↔	↑	↓	
↑		↑	↓ (slight)	
↑		↑		
↑		↑	↓	
↑			↓	
	↓	↓		

ing the production of LDL receptors in the liver. (See the evaluation on Compactin and Mevinolin.)

Table 5 summarizes the drug therapy for the five major types of hyperlipoproteinemia, listed in order of preference (see also the evaluations). These drugs should be discontinued if acute myocardial infarction occurs, because they may interfere with other drugs used for treatment. Drug therapy may be reinstituted cautiously, if at all, during the first month after myocardial infarction.

Most therapeutic failures are due to inability of the patient to follow the diet and/or to take drugs regularly. However, even with ideal therapy, plasma lipid levels remain elevated in some patients. Many investigators are studying the concomitant use of two hypolipidemic drugs in such individuals. For example, corrective diet plus cholestyramine and niacin, which act by different mechanisms, have been useful in patients with severe heterozygous or homozygous type II hyperlipoproteinemia relatively refractory to diet and cholestyramine alone.

When severe hyperlipidemia causes abdominal pain (this occurs fairly often in types I and V), complete fasting for 24 to 48 hours and, when necessary, intravenous administration of electrolyte solutions without dextrose usually relieve pain and reduce triglyceride levels dramatically. This is the only therapy recommended for type I, since drugs are not effective. Repeat-

ed isovolumetric plasmapheresis may be useful for acute removal of chylomicrons to reduce the risk of pancreatitis. In type V, triglyceride concentrations may be decreased further when drugs are added to a dietary regimen designed to reduce or abolish attacks of abdominal pain and/or pancreatitis.

The serum cholesterol level increases by approximately 35% during the last trimester of pregnancy independent of diet. The use of hypolipidemic drugs during pregnancy is not advocated, because their effect on the fetus has not been established.

Other Lipid-Lowering Regimens: Partial bypass of the terminal ileum has been performed to reduce refractory hypercholesterolemia in patients with type II who are unable or unwilling to take drugs. This surgery may aggravate hyperlipidemia in patients with other types of hyperlipoproteinemia. It should be considered investigational and used with extreme caution. Intermittent plasmapheresis reduces plasma cholesterol levels (LDL) in patients with homozygous type IIa hyperlipidemia but also is considered investigational. Chelation therapy has been advocated by some physicians to treat atherosclerosis but has not been shown to be effective (*JAMA*, 1983). Data are anecdotal and there is no supporting clinical evidence; thus, chelating agents have no place in the treatment of atherosclerosis with or without hyperlipidemia.

TABLE 5.
DRUG THERAPY IN HYPERLIPOPROTEINEMIA*

	Type II	
	a	b

HETEROZYGOTES
  Cholestyramine resin (Questran)
    Initial dose: 4 g two times a day for the first week,
      8 g two times daily the second week.
    Maintenance dose: 12 g twice daily after the second week.
    LDL levels should decrease 20%-40% over diet alone.
      In IIb, there may be a variable increase in VLDL.
  Alternatively,
  Colestipol hydrochloride (Colestid)
    Adults: 15-30 g daily divided into 2-4 doses with meals.
- -

  Niacin (Nicobid, Nicolar), particularly in type IIb
    Initial dose: 100 mg three times a day.
    Maintenance dose: 1-3 g three times a day with meals.
    LDL levels should decrease 15%-35%. VLDL levels should
    decrease 40% over diet alone. HDL levels should increase.
  **Probucol (Lorelco)
    Adults: 500 mg twice daily with morning and evening meal.
    LDL should decrease 10%-20% over diet alone. HDL may decrease 10%-40%.

- -

  Neomycin sulfate (Mycifradin Sulfate)
    Initial dose: 0.5 g/day
    Maintenance dose: 1-2 g/day.
    LDL levels should decrease 20%-25% over diet alone.
      Ineffective for lowering VLDL levels. Potential adverse effects limit usefulness.

- -

Dextrothyroxine sodium (Choloxin)	Cholestyramine resin (Questran)
Initial dose: 1 mg/day.	12 g twice a day or Colestipol (Colestid) 15-30 g daily
Maintenance dose: 4-8 mg/day.	in 2 to 4 doses with meals and niacin 1-3 g twice a day.
LDL levels should decrease 15%-30% over diet alone.	The sequestrant component should decrease LDL
Should not be used in patients with coronary artery	25%-35%; niacin will have some effect on LDL
disease, organic heart disease, or arrhythmias.	(15%-30%) and should decrease VLDL 35%-50%.

HOMOZYGOTES
  Cholestyramine resin (Questran)
    4-8 g four times a day and niacin 1.2-3 g 3 times a day with meals.
    Should be started in childhood before vascular damage becomes too severe.

No drug therapy is effective for type I.
**Less effective than cholestyramine resin or colestipol in patients with familial type IIa disorder.*

Treatment of Hyperlipoproteinemia Types

In familial *type I* (rare) and in secondary hyperchylomicrone-mia not responsive to treatment of the underlying disease, restriction of dietary fat (25 g/day or less) markedly decreases triglyceride levels, resolves eruptive xanthomas, and relieves abdominal pain, although moderate lipemia may persist. A fat-free diet may be required initially when the disorder is very severe. At least 1% of total calories should consist of linoleic acid to meet essential fatty acid requirements, and fat-soluble vitamins should be prescribed if they are not provided in the diet. The addition of medium-chain triglycerides (MCT), which are transported directly to the liver without chylomicron formation, increases palatability and caloric intake. To supply adequate calories, carbohydrate should be substituted for fat. Alcohol consumption should be avoided to prevent abdominal pain. None of the currently available hypolipidemic drugs is effective in type I.

Type III	Type IV	Type V

Niacin (Nicobid, Nicolar)
  Initial dose: 100 mg three times a day.
  Maintenance dose: 1 g three times a day.
  Given with meals.
  VLDL levels should decrease 40%-80% over diet alone. HDL levels should increase
	Niacin (Nicobid, Nicolar)
	  Initial dose: 100 mg three times a day.
	  Maintenance dose: 1-3 g three times a day.
	  Both LDL and VLDL levels should decrease more than 30%. HDL levels should increase. Side effects may limit usefulness.
		Niacin (Nicobid, Nicolar)
		  Initial dose: 100 mg three times a day.
		  Maintenance dose: 1-3 g three times a day.
		  LDL levels should decrease 30%.
		    VLDL levels should decrease as much as 70% over diet alone. HDL levels should increase. More effective than clofibrate but side effects may limit usefulness.

Clofibrate (Atromid-S)
  Dose: 500 mg three or four times daily.
  VLDL levels should decrease 40%-80% over diet alone.
  Cholelithiasis is a major adverse effect.
	Gemfibrozil (Lopid)
	  Dose: 600 mg twice a day with meals.
	  Should decrease VLDL levels more than 30%. Should increase HDL levels.
		Gemfibrozil (Lopid)
		  Dose: 600 mg twice a day with meals.
		  VLDL levels should decrease more than 30%. HDL levels should increase.

		Clofibrate (Atromid-S)
		  Dose: 500 mg three or four times daily.
		  VLDL levels may decrease 10%-50%.
		  Cholelithiasis is a major adverse effect.
		  Use of clofibrate in type V usually is not indicated because of undesirable side effects.

Gemfibrozil (Lopid)
  Dose: 600 mg twice a day with meals.
  VLDL levels should decrease more than 30%. HDL levels should increase.
	Clofibrate (Atromid-S)
	  Dose: 500 mg three to four times daily.
	  VLDL levels may decrease 10%-50%, but LDL levels may increase more than 50%.
	  Use of clofibrate in type IV usually is not indicated because of undesirable side effects.
		Norethindrone acetate
		  (Aygestin, Norlutate)
		  For use only in women, initial and maintenance doses: 5 mg/day (premenopausal women should receive the drug 21 days/month to permit regular menses).
		  VLDL levels should decrease 10%-50%.

		Oxandrolone (Anavar)
		  For use only in men.
		  Dose: 2.5 mg three times a day (investigational use).
		  VLDL and triglyceride levels should decrease 60%. Chylomicron levels decrease.

In *type II* hyperlipoproteinemia, the cholesterol intake should be low (less than 300 mg/day) and saturated fat should be restricted, while polyunsaturated fat should be increased to provide a P:S ratio of approximately 2:1. Weight reduction often is important in type IIb. In most individuals, elevated LDL levels are caused by subtle aberrations of many genes whose detrimental effects are elicited by environmental cofactors (eg, high intake of cholesterol or dietary fat, excessive calories). Dietary modification, increased exercise, and treatment of other risk factors (eg, obesity, diabetes) usually reduce LDL concentrations.

In the familial type II disorder, elevated LDL levels are caused by defective clearance due to genetic deficiency of LDL receptors and patients often require both dietary and drug therapy. One-half of LDL receptors are normal in heterozygous type II disorders; these receptors can be stimulated to increased activity when hepatic levels of cholesterol are depleted. Since bile acid sequestrants (cholestyramine, colestipol) stimulate cholesterol degradation and excretion from the liver, they increase the activity of hepatic LDL receptors and are the agents of choice to treat heterozygous type II patients. If the response is inadequate, niacin may be added to the regimen. Although niacin also decreases VLDL production and thus is especially useful in type IIb, side effects may limit its usefulness. Probucol may be substituted for cholestyramine or colestipol but is less effective in patients with familial type II. Also, probucol decreases HDL cholesterol proportionately more than LDL cholesterol, which may increase the risk of atherosclerosis (Mellies et al, 1980). Dextrothyroxine may reduce LDL concentrations but should not be given to patients with arrhythmias or known or suspected atherosclerotic heart disease. These contraindications limit the use of dextrothyroxine, since many patients with type II have latent coronary artery disease. Neomycin has been effective in some patients with type IIa. Clofibrate reduces LDL only moderately and is usually inadequate in familial type IIa. It may be beneficial in type IIb and nonhereditary type IIa disorders. Gemfibrozil has LDL-lowering effects similar to those of clofibrate but reduces triglycerides and elevates HDL more effectively. Both drugs should be tried only when the response to more effective hypocholesterolemic drugs is inadequate.

Familial homozygous type II is the most malignant form of hyperlipoproteinemia; untreated patients seldom live beyond early adulthood. Homozygous type II patients have no functional LDL receptors; thus, no response can be expected from therapy designed to increase LDL receptor activity. This form is particularly resistant to treatment, although some success has been reported with a combination of diet, cholestyramine, and niacin. Repeated isovolumetric plasmapheresis decreases the blood lipid concentration in type II homozygotes (Stein et al, 1981).

In type III, dietary restriction to achieve ideal body weight, followed by adherence to a low-cholesterol, low-saturated fat diet, frequently is the only therapy needed. In some patients, restriction of carbohydrate and alcohol also may be required. If this does not normalize lipid concentrations, concomitant administration of clofibrate usually reduces serum lipids to the normal range and causes regression of xanthomas. Because of its similarity to clofibrate, gemfibrozil may be considered an alternative for the treatment of type III disorder. Niacin is very effective in type III and is considered a drug of choice because of the side effects (eg, cholelithiasis) encountered with clofibrate. Cholestyramine is not useful in this type of hyperlipoproteinemia and may even worsen it.

Weight reduction to achieve ideal body weight is of primary importance in the management of type IV, and patients should be maintained on a low-carbohydrate, low-alcohol diet. Excess carbohydrates should be replaced by unsaturated fats (especially omega-3 fatty acids) and cholesterol should be restricted (less than 500 mg/day). Adherence to this regimen produces normal triglyceride concentrations in many patients. The American Heart Association diet does not restrict carbohydrates, and advocates of this regimen suggest that liberal intake of carbohydrates is well tolerated if calories are restricted during weight loss and/or if an isocaloric diet is substituted during subsequent maintenance. Cautious use of adjunctive drugs may be considered only when the triglyceride concentration remains elevated. Clofibrate, gemfibrozil, and niacin reduce VLDL, but clofibrate and possibly gemfibrozil may cause a reciprocal rise in LDL cholesterol. Gemfibrozil is particularly effective in elevating depressed HDL cholesterol levels in those with hypertriglyceridemia, probably by increasing synthesis of apo A-I, A-II, HDL_2, and HDL_3.

Since most patients with type V are overweight, the first step in management is weight reduction. The maintenance diet should be as high in protein and low in fat as can be tolerated; carbohydrate content also should be controlled. Restriction of alcohol consumption often is necessary, especially to prevent abdominal pain. These measures frequently control symptoms and reduce lipid levels. If concomitant drug administration is needed to decrease these levels further, clofibrate or gemfibrozil may be prescribed but neither drug is uniformly effective. Niacin is more effective but may aggravate hyperglycemia and hyperuricemia. Norethindrone [Aygestin, Norlutate] may be used in women and oxandrolone [Anavar] in men; either may prevent attacks of abdominal pain even when plasma lipids remain relatively high. In fact, oxandrolone may reduce triglyceride and VLDL levels in men with type V disorder.

Drug Evaluations

CHOLESTYRAMINE RESIN
[Questran]

ACTIONS. Cholestyramine binds bile acids in the small intestine and prevents their reabsorption; the reduced level of bile acids increases the rate of conversion of cholesterol to bile acids in the liver, thereby increasing LDL receptor activity and apoprotein B catabolism.

USES. Cholestyramine is a drug of choice for type IIa (hyperbetalipoproteinemia) to reduce the risks of atherosclerotic coronary artery disease and myocardial infarction. When used as an adjunct to dietary control, it reduces LDL an additional 20% to 40%; 90% of the effect is noted in 7 to 14 days and the maximum effect is apparent within 28 days. In type IIb, usual doses decrease LDL but may elevate VLDL somewhat. For heterozygous type II disorder, the combination of cholestyramine and niacin has reduced cholesterol, triglycerides (in IIb), and LDL concentrations more than maximal doses of cholestyramine alone.

In the usual dosage range, cholestyramine is ineffective in hyperprebetalipoproteinemia and is of little benefit in types III, IV, or V; in fact, this drug may aggravate these conditions.

ADVERSE REACTIONS AND PRECAUTIONS. Cholestyramine probably is one of the safest drugs currently available to treat hyperlipoproteinemia. It is not absorbed from the gastrointestinal tract and has no significant systemic toxic effects. Nevertheless, because of the large doses required, the drug is unpleasant to take. The most frequent untoward effects are bloating, mild nausea, and constipation, which usually subside with continued therapy. One case of intestinal impaction has followed the use of cholestyramine, and most patients require treatment for constipation (eg, large fluid intake, regular use of a mild laxative). The drug should be used cautiously in patients with anorectal disease. Other adverse reactions include epigastric distress and diarrhea. Rarely, vomiting and irritation of the tongue and perianal region have been reported.

Cholestyramine occasionally interferes with the absorption of fat; deficiency of the fat-soluble vitamins (A, D, and E) may occur and supplementation may be required. Vitamin K deficiency also may develop and result in bleeding due to hypoprothrombinemia. Large doses may cause hyperchloremia in young children. Some investigators suggest that folate deficiency occurs during long-term treatment, and patients, especially children, should receive 5 mg of folic acid daily, if necessary.

Steatorrhea, weight loss, and malabsorption syndrome may be noted with excessive doses.

DRUG INTERACTIONS. Since cholestyramine may adsorb other drugs given concomitantly (particularly thiazides, thyroid, digitalis, iron compounds, phenylbutazone, antibiotics, barbiturates, and warfarin), these drugs should be given at least one hour before or four hours after cholestyramine. The prothrombin time may be slightly prolonged but bleeding has not been reported; nevertheless, the dose of concomitantly administered anticoagulants should be monitored closely.

DOSAGE AND PREPARATIONS.
Oral: Initially, *adults,* 4 g (one packet or one rounded teaspoonful) two times daily for the first week, increased to 8 g twice daily the second week and 12 g twice daily thereafter. Dosage should be reduced temporarily if symptoms such as bloating or constipation are troublesome. Although the dosage in *children over 6 years* has not been definitively established, the usual dose is 8 g twice daily with meals; often 8 to 12 g/day is adequate. *Children under 6 years,* dosage has not been established.

The drug should never be swallowed dry because of the hazard of esophageal irritation or blockage. It should be mixed with 120 to 180 ml of water, fruit juice, preferred liquids, soups, or pulpy fruit just before ingestion.

Questran (Mead Johnson). Powder in packets and cans (378 g) providing 4 g of anhydrous cholestyramine resin per packet or per 9 g scoopful.

CLOFIBRATE
[Atromid-S]

ACTIONS. The mechanism of action is unclear, but clofibrate may inhibit the hepatic release of lipoproteins (particularly VLDL), interferes with the binding of serum free fatty acids to albumin, increases the fecal excretion of neutral sterols, inhibits cholesterol biosynthesis, and affects the metabolism of some lipoprotein apoproteins. It reportedly potentiates lipoprotein lipase activity, increases apo A-I levels, and may increase HDL concentration (Nestel et al, 1980). A few studies indicate that clofibrate accelerates the catabolism of VLDL and IDL.

The major effect of clofibrate in hyperlipoproteinemia is to reduce VLDL; the hypocholesterolemic effect usually is moderate and variable. A rebound increase in cholesterol and triglyceride concentrations often is observed after clofibrate is discontinued.

USES. When used with appropriate dietary regulation, clofibrate decreases IDL levels and is useful in type III hyperlipoproteinemia; no untoward lipoprotein shift occurs in these patients. Xanthomas have regressed and patients with peripheral vascular disease associated with type III have improved. However, clofibrate has no effect on the apoprotein E-III deficiency associated with this disorder. The benefits of the drug outweigh its hazards in patients with type III.

The usefulness of clofibrate in other types of hyperlipoproteinemia is limited by the observation in the large European clofibrate trial of excess mortality from noncardiac causes (see Precautions). This drug may reduce VLDL levels in type IV and V abnormalities, but a reciprocal increase in LDL has been noted in some patients; this increase may be caused by increased lipoprotein lipase activity produced by clofibrate. Although patients with homozygous type II and heterozygous type IIa usually do not respond adequately to clofibrate, this drug appears to reduce VLDL levels in type IIb heterozygotes since the VLDL concentration also is increased. Clofibrate also has been reported to reduce serum fibrinogen levels and may diminish platelet adhesiveness.

ADVERSE REACTIONS. Gastrointestinal disturbances (nausea, vomiting, diarrhea, dyspepsia, and flatulence) occur in about 10% of patients but are usually transient and disappear with continued therapy. Less frequently, leukopenia, rash, drowsiness, and alopecia areata have been noted.

Potentially serious effects on skeletal and cardiac muscle are rare; creatine phosphokinase levels may increase and frank myositis with asthenia, myalgia, and malaise may develop. Elevated levels may persist when other serum enzymes return to normal and the patient is asymptomatic. In patients with chest pain, increased transaminase and creatine phosphokinase levels may be caused by clofibrate rather than by myocardial infarction.

Clofibrate causes hepatomegaly in animals, but similar changes have not been observed in man. However, reversible elevations in serum transaminase levels have been noted, and SGOT, SGPT, and creatine phosphokinase values should be determined periodically in all patients receiving clofibrate.

PRECAUTIONS. Patients receiving long-term therapy must be supervised closely. Clofibrate should be used with caution and in reduced doses in those with impaired renal or hepatic function, since delayed detoxification and excretion make the duration of action unpredictable.

Clofibrate is contraindicated during pregnancy and should not be given to nursing mothers, for it may be excreted in milk. This drug is not recommended for children, since data are insufficient to determine its safety in this age group.

The Coronary Drug Project utilized clofibrate for the long-term management of men with established ischemic heart disease. There was no definitive evidence that this agent reduced total mortality or cardiovascular morbidity and mortality. Furthermore, the incidence of peripheral vascular disease, pulmonary embolism, thrombophlebitis, angina pectoris, increased heart size, arrhythmias, and intermittent claudication were all significantly increased. The incidence of cholelithiasis also increased twofold or more, and feminizing effects (decreased libido, breast tenderness) were noted occasionally (Coronary Drug Project Research Group, 1975). Therefore, clofibrate should not be given indiscriminately to patients who have experienced a myocardial infarction but should be reserved for those with marked hypercholesterolemia and hypertriglyceridemia who are at high risk of ischemic heart disease.

The large primary prevention trial of clofibrate conducted in Europe further confirms the need for caution in the use of this drug (*Br Heart J*, 1978). A report on the approximately eight-year follow-up indicates that excessive mortality related to noncardiac causes was entirely related to clofibrate administration (Oliver et al, 1984). Because of the risks, most clinicians suggest restricting its use to patients with type III hyperlipoproteinemia.

DRUG INTERACTIONS. Clofibrate potentiates the action of coumarin anticoagulants, phenytoin, and tolbutamide. The dose of anticoagulants must be reduced (by at least one-half for most patients) and prothrombin times should be determined frequently, especially during initiation of therapy.

PHARMACOKINETICS. Clofibrate undergoes rapid hydrolysis to an active metabolite, chlorophenoxyisobutyric acid (CPIB). Peak concentrations of CPIB are usually attained in three to six hours; the mean half-life is 1.7 hours, but there are wide individual variations. At doses up to 2 g/day, absorption is complete. The mean plasma elimination half-life of CPIB is 15.1 hours. Plasma binding decreases as the dose increases and is associated with increased plasma clearance. Approximately 40% to 70% is recovered in the urine as a glucuronide ester of CPIB (Gugler, 1978).

DOSAGE AND PREPARATIONS.
Oral: Adults, 500 mg three or four times daily.
  Atromid-S (Ayerst). Capsules 500 mg.

COLESTIPOL HYDROCHLORIDE
[Colestid]

The action and indications for this odorless, tasteless, bile-sequestering agent are similar to those of cholestyramine. Although there is less experience with its use, colestipol is considered to be interchangeable with cholestyramine in type IIa patients. In patients with heterozygous type II disorder, the combination of colestipol and niacin reduces cholesterol, triglycerides (in IIb), and LDL levels more than maximal doses of colestipol alone.

Like cholestyramine, colestipol is probably one of the safest drugs currently available to treat hyperlipoproteinemia. For specific adverse reactions, precautions, and drug interactions, see the evaluation on Cholestyramine Resin.

DOSAGE AND PREPARATIONS.
Oral: Adults, 15 to 30 g daily (mixed with 120 to 180 ml of suitable liquid) in two to four divided doses with meals. This drug should be given at least one hour before or four hours after other drugs. Although the safety and effectiveness of colestipol in *children* has not been definitively established, it appears to be safe and effective and 10 to 15 g daily divided into two doses (mixed with fluids at the morning and evening meals) has been used in children with familial type II hyperlipidemia.

  Colestid (Upjohn). Granules in 5-g packets and in 500 g containers with scoop providing 5 g per level scoopful.

CONJUGATED ESTROGENS

ETHINYL ESTRADIOL

Estrogens were used to treat hyperlipidemia after it was found that, compared to men, women have lower serum beta lipoprotein (LDL), higher alpha lipoprotein (HDL, particularly HDL_2), and decreased susceptibility to atherosclerosis and ischemic heart disease until after the menopause. However, estrogens are unsuitable in men because they have feminizing effects, elevate VLDL and triglyceride concentrations, and increase the levels of several blood clotting factors.

In a long-term trial in men with established ischemic heart disease, estrogens increased the incidence of thromboembolism and cardiovascular complications. They also have been reported to increase mortality from cancer. In women, estrogens may elevate VLDL levels and decrease postheparin lipoprotein lipase activity (PHLA). They also are reported to cause abdominal pain and pancreatitis in women with type V hyperlipoproteinemia.

Although a study in Finland (Tikkanen et al, 1978) reported that estrogens reduced LDL in women with type II hyperlipoproteinemia, these observations require confirmation.

See Chapter 39, Estrogens, Progestins, and Other Agents Used to Treat Gynecologic Conditions, for preparations.

DEXTROTHYROXINE SODIUM
[Choloxin]

ACTIONS AND USES. Of the thyroid analogues, dextrothyroxine has the highest ratio of hypolipidemic:calorigenic activity. The drug reduces LDL by increasing LDL receptor activity in both euthyroid and hypothyroid patients. It also may increase the rate of conversion of cholesterol to bile acid by limiting bile acid synthesis through stimulation of the enzyme, 7α-hydroxylase. The decrease in serum cholesterol may range from 15% to 30% and is greatest in patients with the highest baseline concentrations. Maximal effects appear in one to two months.

Dextrothyroxine is indicated only in type IIa hyperlipoproteinemia. It has no consistent effect on VLDL in the usual dosage range and thus is seldom useful in patients with types III, IV, or V patterns. Because it increases mortality in patients with established ischemic heart disease, dextrothyroxine currently should be used only in patients with severe type II hyperlipidemia who are at high risk and cannot tolerate more conventional therapy.

ADVERSE REACTIONS AND PRECAUTIONS. Untoward effects occur frequently, are usually caused by metabolic stimulation, and generally mimic the symptoms of hyperthyroidism. Weight loss appears to be the first sign of hypermetabolism. Related effects include nervousness, insomnia, tremors, hyperhidrosis, and menstrual irregularity. Some patients report altered taste sensations, vertigo, and diarrhea during the first six weeks of therapy, but these reactions subside spontaneously. Rash and pruritus may develop in patients who are hypersensitive to iodine.

Dextrothyroxine should be used judiciously, if at all, in pregnant women and nursing mothers, because effects on the fetal and neonatal thyroid gland are unknown. The drug also must be given cautiously to patients with hypertension or hepatic or renal disease.

The use of dextrothyroxine in a long-term trial (Coronary Drug Project) in men with established ischemic heart disease was discontinued because of increased mortality in patients with arrhythmias, angina pectoris, or multiple infarctions. Therefore, dextrothyroxine should not be given to patients with pre-existing ischemic heart disease or arrhythmias, especially ventricular premature contractions.

DRUG INTERACTIONS. In some diabetic patients, prolonged use of dextrothyroxine decreases glucose tolerance, which may necessitate increasing the dose of hypoglycemic agents. Since this drug augments the effect of oral anticoagulants (probably by increasing receptor affinity), the dose of the latter may require reduction by approximately one-third and prothrombin times should be determined more frequently. Dextrothyroxine should be withdrawn two weeks before elective surgery if use of anticoagulants is contemplated.

PHARMACOKINETICS. The pharmacokinetics of dextrothyroxine are essentially the same as those of levothyroxine. (See Chapter 44, Agents Used to Treat Thyroid Disease.)

DOSAGE AND PREPARATIONS.

Oral: Euthyroid adults, initially, 1 mg daily for one month; the daily dose may be increased by increments of 1 to 2 mg at intervals of at least one month until a satisfactory reduction of serum cholesterol has been achieved or a maximal daily dose of 8 mg is reached. In patients receiving digitalis, the maximal dose is 4 mg daily. *Children,* initially, 0.05 mg/kg daily; this dose may be doubled after one month. The dose is increased by increments of 0.05 mg/kg at monthly intervals until satisfactory reduction of serum cholesterol has been observed or a maximal dose of 4 mg daily has been attained.

Choloxin (Flint). Tablets 1, 2, 4, and 6 mg.

GEMFIBROZIL
[Lopid]

ACTIONS. Gemfibrozil is a chemical homologue of clofibrate. This drug appears to reduce incorporation of long-chain fatty acids into newly formed triglycerides, thus reducing VLDL production in the liver. Also, it potentiates lipoprotein lipase (LPL) activity and increases the rate of synthesis of apo A-I and A-II (by about 30%).

The effects of gemfibrozil are similar to those of clofibrate on cholesterol, triglycerides, and LDL cholesterol. However, this drug is considerably more effective in elevating the HDL cholesterol (15% to 25%) and the HDL cholesterol:total cholesterol ratio. In one study on 300 patients, mostly men with type IIa or IIb hyperlipoproteinemia, six-year follow-up data showed that plasma lipids were significantly improved in 90% of patients. Also, apoproteins A-I and A-II were slightly increased and the HDL_2:HDL_3 ratio was increased (Manninen, 1981).

In animal studies, intermediates of cholesterol synthesis did not accumulate and fibrinogen levels were not affected. The drug inhibited platelet aggregation but had less effect on unbound warfarin levels than an equivalent dose of clofibrate. However, frequent determinations of prothrombin time are advised if gemfibrozil and warfarin are given concomitantly. Hepatocellular enlargement with no change in liver function was found in some species.

USES. Gemfibrozil may be used in selected high-risk patients with types III, IV, or V hyperlipoproteinemia (triglyceride concentrations exceeding 750 mg/dl) who do not respond to diet and drugs for which more data on long-term use is available. Gemfibrozil is given with niacin to increase HDLC concentrations in subjects with familial hypoalphalipoproteinemia. However, it is not indicated for the sole purpose of raising HDL cholesterol levels in those with hyperlipoproteinemia.

ADVERSE REACTIONS AND PRECAUTIONS. Although gemfibrozil is structurally similar to clofibrate, occult toxicity has not yet been demonstrated. Side effects are similar to those of clofibrate; gastrointestinal disturbances and rash occur most frequently. In type IV patients, LDL cholesterol commonly is increased.

Transient elevations in serum transaminase levels have been noted. Gemfibrozil is contraindicated in patients with severe renal dysfunction or hepatic disease, including primary biliary cirrhosis. Cholesterol saturation indices after administration of clofibrate and gemfibrozil were reported to be similar or less for gemfibrozil, which suggests that the risk of cholelithiasis is theoretically similar for both drugs (Hall et al, 1981). Gemfibrozil is contraindicated in patients with pre-existing gallbladder disease.

Although doses of 800 mg/day do not impair the control of diabetes when an oral hypoglycemic agent or insulin is administered, blood glucose levels may be elevated. Therefore, the drug should be used with caution in diabetics.

This drug is classified in FDA Pregnancy Category B.

PHARMACOKINETICS. Peak plasma levels are attained in one to two hours. Plasma levels are proportional to the dose and there is no evidence of accumulation. The half-life is estimated to be 1.5 hours; 70% of a dose is excreted unchanged, primarily in the urine.

DOSAGE AND PREPARATIONS.

Oral: *Adults,* 600 mg twice daily (one-half hour before breakfast and dinner).

Lopid (Parke-Davis). Capsules 300 mg.

NEOMYCIN SULFATE
[Mycifradin Sulfate]

ACTIONS AND USES. Neomycin is absorbed only minimally from the gastrointestinal tract. It reduces the absorption of cholesterol by precipitating it from micellar solution. Like cholestyramine, it is thought to act by forming insoluble complexes with bile acids, thereby increasing excretion of bile acids and cholesterol. Small doses given for several years reduce LDL levels an average of 22% without serious adverse effects. Neomycin has variable effects on VLDL.

Until additional information on safety and efficacy is available, use of this agent should be reserved for patients with type IIa hyperlipoproteinemia who have failed to respond to conventional therapy and who have a high risk of ischemic heart disease.

ADVERSE REACTIONS AND PRECAUTIONS. Malabsorption syndrome, acute suprainfection, nephropathy, and permanent damage to the eighth nerve have occurred after neomycin was given parenterally or in large oral doses. It is claimed that these reactions do not develop with the oral doses used to treat hyperlipidemia. Diarrhea and abdominal cramps, which usually subside spontaneously during continued treatment, have been reported with use of hypolipidemic doses. Anorexia and metallic taste may occur.

Neomycin is contraindicated in patients with renal insufficiency, for excessive levels may accumulate and cause nephrotoxicity and ototoxicity.

Because neomycin may potentiate coumarin anticoagulants, concomitant use requires frequent monitoring of the prothrombin time.

For other adverse reactions, see Chapter 70, Aminoglycosides.

DOSAGE AND PREPARATIONS.

Oral: *Adults,* 0.5 to a maximum of 2 g daily.

Generic. Tablets 500 mg.

Mycifradin Sulfate (Upjohn). Solution 125 mg/5 ml and tablets 500 mg equivalent to 85.7 mg and 350 mg of the base, respectively.

NIACIN (Nicotinic Acid)
[Nicobid, Nicolar]

ACTIONS AND USES. In contrast to other hypolipidemic agents, studies suggest that niacin reduces the rate of synthesis of LDL and apoprotein B by depressing the synthesis of VLDL. VLDL and LDL cholesterol decrease and HDL cholesterol increases as a result. Therefore, niacin may be effective in all types of hyperlipoproteinemia except type I. It often is more effective than other drugs in lowering the triglyceride concentration in patients with severe type V disorder. In type III hyperlipoproteinemia, lipids are reduced to normal but the apoprotein E-III defect is not affected. This drug may be useful in patients with primary familial type II who do not respond adequately to cholestyramine or colestipol alone. When given with other hypolipidemic drugs, smaller doses may be adequate and the drug may be better tolerated.

ADVERSE REACTIONS AND PRECAUTIONS. Niacin often produces potentially troublesome side effects but is usually well tolerated in patients who respond to 4 g/day or less. Flushing (mediated through prostaglandin release) occurs initially in almost all patients and persists in 10% to 15%. This effect often can be ameliorated by concomitant use of aspirin 300 mg daily. Other common untoward effects are pruritus, dry skin with scaling, acanthosis nigricans, and gastrointestinal irritation (eg, nausea, vomiting, flatulence, diarrhea). The latter symptoms may subside with continued therapy. Use of small initial doses that are increased gradually reduces the severity of these reactions in most patients.

More serious reactions are activation of peptic ulcer, impaired glucose tolerance, hyperuricemia, and liver dysfunction, including cholestatic jaundice. These effects are usually reversible when the drug is discontinued. However, irreversible chronic hepatitis has been reported in a few patients. Many patients with type III, IV, and V have pre-existing hyperglycemia and hyperuricemia that may be aggravated by niacin. Toxic amblyopia also has been reported.

Liver function tests should be performed periodically in all patients receiving niacin, and the drug should be discontinued if significant elevation of any liver enzyme occurs. Niacin should not be given to patients with hepatic disease, peptic ulcer, gouty arthritis, or diabetes mellitus. This drug is classified in FDA Pregnancy Category C.

Niacin was used in the Coronary Drug Project trial for the long-term management of men with established ischemic heart disease, but when the original results were reported there was no definitive evidence that this agent reduced total mortality. It appeared to decrease the incidence of recurrent nonfatal myocardial infarction significantly, but the incidence of atrial fibrillation and other arrhythmias was increased. However, follow-up after nine years has revealed a statistically significant reduction in mortality in the group treated with niacin, including an 11% decrease in the death rate from cardiac causes (Canner, 1985).

DRUG INTERACTIONS. Niacin potentiates the effects of ganglionic blocking agents and, when used with these drugs in hypertensive patients, it may cause orthostatic hypotension.

PHARMACOKINETICS. Niacin is absorbed rapidly; peak concentrations are achieved in about 45 minutes. It has been reported that 88% of a 3-g dose is recovered in the urine, which suggests that intestinal absorption is almost complete. Niacin disappears rapidly from blood and is concentrated mainly in the liver, but it also appears in adipose tissue and kidneys. It has a high hepatic extraction ratio and plasma clearance may be reduced in patients with hepatic impairment. Renal clearance depends on plasma concentration and may be decreased with high therapeutic concentration (Gugler, 1978).

DOSAGE AND PREPARATIONS.
Oral: Adults, initially, 100 mg three times daily, increased to 3 to 9 g given in three or four divided doses with or after meals. Although more than 7 g is seldom prescribed, doses as high as 12 g daily have been used.

> NIACIN:
> Available generically and under the name Nicotinic Acid: Capsules (timed-release) 125, 250, and 400 mg; tablets 25, 50, 100 (nonprescription), and 500 mg.
> **Nicobid** (USV). Capsules (timed-release) 125, 250, and 500 mg (nonprescription).
> **Nicolar** (USV). Tablets 500 mg.

NORETHINDRONE ACETATE
[Aygestin, Norlutate]

ACTIONS AND USES. Results of recent studies have shown that this progestational agent, when used in conjunction with appropriate diet, decreases VLDL and chylomicrons but decreases HDL and apoprotein A in some women with type V hyperlipoproteinemia. There is a concurrent increase in postheparin lipolytic activity (PHLA), and abdominal pain and pancreatitis are ameliorated. Norethindrone also has been tried in women with types III, IV, or V in whom estrogens or combination oral contraceptives caused undesirable effects (hypertriglyceridemia and decreased PHLA). However, recent studies have shown that progestins may elevate serum cholesterol levels. Therefore, until more experience has accumulated, norethindrone should be reserved for women with type V hyperlipoproteinemia who are refractory to established

therapy. Its use in men is not advocated because of its estrogenic activity.

For adverse reactions, see Chapter 39, Estrogens, Progestins, and Other Agents Used to Treat Gynecologic Conditions.

DOSAGE AND PREPARATIONS.
Oral: Women, 5 mg daily. Premenopausal women should receive the drug 21 days per month to permit regular menses.
> **Aygestin** (Ayerst), **Norlutate** (Parke-Davis). Tablets 5 mg.

OXANDROLONE
[Anavar]

ACTIONS AND USES. Oxandrolone, an anabolic steroid with weak androgenic properties, is a synthetic derivative of testosterone. It reduces triglyceride levels (affecting both VLDL and chylomicrons) by increasing postheparin lipoprotein lipase activity (PHLA) but has little effect on cholesterol and LDL, although LDL cholesterol increased slightly in a few patients. HDL cholesterol is decreased, apparently through stimulation of hepatic lipase and increased LDL catabolism.

The use of oxandrolone in hyperlipidemia is investigational and should be reserved for men with severe symptomatic hypertriglyceridemia who are refractory to more conventional agents.

ADVERSE REACTIONS AND PRECAUTIONS. Oxandrolone should not be used in women because of its virilizing effect or in children because it may cause premature epiphyseal closure and alter sexual development.

Since oxandrolone may induce edema, it should be used cautiously in men with cardiac, renal, or hepatic disease and should not be given with adrenal corticosteroids or corticotropin. The dosage of anticoagulants may have to be reduced in patients receiving oxandrolone.

For further information on adverse reactions and precautions, see Chapter 38, Androgens and Anabolic Steroids.

DOSAGE AND PREPARATIONS.
Oral: Men, 2.5 mg three times daily.
> **Anavar** (Searle). Tablets 2.5 mg.
> (Investigational indication)

PROBUCOL
[Lorelco]

ACTIONS. Probucol, a *bis*-phenol, is structurally unrelated to other hypolipidemic agents. It decreases elevated serum cholesterol levels by reducing LDL concentrations. It does not reduce serum triglyceride levels appreciably in most patients. HDL concentrations are reduced proportionately more than LDL, resulting in an unfavorable LDL:HDL ratio. Studies indicate that probucol increases the fractional rate of catabolism of LDL but the enhanced removal apparently does not involve the primary LDL receptors. This action may be responsible for the increased excretion of fecal bile acids that has been observed. Probucol also reduces the synthesis of apo A-I and apo A-II.

USES. Probucol appears to be effective primarily in type IIa hyperlipoproteinemia. Results of limited studies indicate that probucol is less effective than cholestyramine or colestipol in patients with familial type IIa, although it may increase the optimal effect of diet by 14%. When used with bile acid-binding resins, probucol may have an additive hypocholesterolemic effect and the constipation produced by the resins may be decreased when they are given in combination with probucol.

This drug also may be used with agents that decrease serum triglyceride levels in types IIb, III, and IV when hypercholesterolemia persists. Since a low HDL cholesterol level is at least as great a risk factor for atherogenesis as an increased LDL level, the decrease in HDL caused by probucol may reduce its usefulness. Until further data accumulate, probucol should be used only when more effective hypocholesterolemic drugs are inadequate or contraindicated.

ADVERSE REACTIONS AND PRECAUTIONS. The most common adverse reactions are mild gastrointestinal disturbances (diarrhea, flatulence, abdominal pain, and nausea), which are usually transient. Less common reactions include excessive or fetid perspiration, angioedema, headache, dizziness, paresthesias, and eosinophilia. Transient elevations of serum transaminases, alkaline phosphatase, creatine phosphokinase, bilirubin, uric acid, blood urea nitrogen, and blood glucose levels have occurred occasionally.

Administration of probucol to rhesus monkeys and dogs fed high-cholesterol, high-fat diets produced cardiotoxic effects, especially dysrhythmias, in some of these animals. Although similar cardiovascular effects have not yet been encountered in man, prolongation of the QT interval may occur, and probucol is not advocated for patients with arrhythmias.

Because probucol may decrease HDL levels, HDL determinations should be performed periodically and the drug discontinued if HDL levels decrease.

Clinical experience does not indicate that probucol has an adverse effect on the fetus. Nevertheless, it should not be used in pregnant women, and women of childbearing age should exercise strict birth control both during and for six months after therapy is discontinued, since the half-life of this drug is prolonged. It is not known whether probucol is excreted in human milk, but mothers receiving this drug should not breast-feed their infants.

No interactions have been reported to date between probucol and insulin, oral hypoglycemic agents, or anticoagulants.

PHARMACOKINETICS. Absorption is limited, but peak blood levels are higher when probucol is administered with meals.

Blood levels increase gradually for three or four months with continuous oral administration and remain relatively constant thereafter. There is no correlation between blood concentrations and hypocholesterolemic effect.

With prolonged treatment, this fat-soluble agent accumulates slowly in fatty tissues. The major pathway of excretion is through the biliary system into the feces; renal clearance is negligible.

DOSAGE AND PREPARATIONS.
Oral: Adults, 500 mg with the morning and evening meal. The safety and efficacy of probucol in *children* have not been established. Some investigators have given 250 mg twice daily with meals to children weighing less than 27 kg and 500 mg twice daily with meals to children weighing more than 27 kg.
Lorelco (Merrell Dow). Tablets 250 mg.

Investigational Drugs

COMPACTIN (Mevastatin)

MEVINOLIN

ACTIONS AND USES. Compactin and mevinolin are fungal derivatives that inhibit hepatic and extrahepatic cholesterol synthesis. The prototype, compactin, is a metabolite isolated from *Penicillium citrinum*. Mevinolin is a similar compound isolated from a strain of *Aspergillus*.

Both drugs are reversible competitive inhibitors of HMG-CoA reductase, the rate-limiting enzyme of cholesterol synthesis. They reduce LDL cholesterol by stimulating the production of LDL receptors in the liver, thereby increasing the uptake of LDL. As a consequence, the fractional catabolic rate for LDL is increased.

In one clinical trial on 13 patients with heterozygous familial hypercholesterolemia, mevinolin reduced serum LDL cholesterol by 20% to 40%. These patients were maintained on a low-cholesterol (less than 300 mg/day), low-saturated fat (less than 10%/day) diet; previous drug therapy failed to reduce serum cholesterol to below 300 mg/dl. The response was not significantly greater with doses of 80 mg/day than with doses of 10 to 40 mg/day (Illingworth and Sexton, 1984). Limited clinical trials using compactin have produced similar results. Mevinolin, but not compactin, also decreased plasma triglyceride levels when larger doses (40 to 80 mg/day) were used and some studies suggest that mevinolin causes modest increases in HDL concentrations. Serum uric acid levels were decreased following use of compactin, but the clinical significance of this action is unknown.

Mevinolin and compactin are promising investigational agents for the treatment of selected adults with or without a genetic defect. However, their long-term safety has not yet been evaluated.

Studies in animals have demonstrated that mevinolin and compactin act synergistically with bile acid sequestrants to lower LDL. This combination would be appropriate for patients with primary hypercholesterolemia, including those with familial heterozygous type IIa hyperlipoproteinemia, since these individuals have the genetic capacity to produce LDL receptors. Clinical trials in a limited number of patients using compactin and cholestyramine (Mabuchi et al, 1983; Yamamota et al, 1984) or mevinolin and colestipol (Illingworth, 1984) substantiated the usefulness of combined therapy.

ADVERSE REACTIONS. Compactin and mevinolin are well tolerated. Occasionally, insomnia, headache, and elevation (usually transient) of alkaline phosphatase levels have been reported. Results of other liver function tests were normal except for increased SGOT levels in two patients. No long-term studies employing these drugs have yet been conducted.

Cited References

Chelation therapy. *JAMA* 250:672, 1983.

Co-operative trial in primary prevention of ischaemic heart disease using clofibrate: Report from Committee of Principal Investigators. *Br Heart J* 40:1069-1118, 1978.

Lipid Research Clinics Coronary Primary Prevention Trial results: I. Reduction in incidence of coronary heart disease. II. Relationship of reduction in incidence of coronary heart disease to cholesterol lowering. *JAMA* 251:351-364, 365-374, 1984.

Angelin B, et al: Regulation of hepatic lipoprotein receptors in the dog: Rapid regulation of apolipoprotein B,E receptors but not of apolipoprotein E receptors, by intestinal lipoproteins and bile acids. *J Clin Invest* 71:816-831, 1983.

Arntzenius AC, et al: Diet, lipoproteins, and progression of coronary atherosclerosis. *N Engl J Med* 312:805-811, 1985.

Borecki IB, et al: Major gene for familial hypoalphalipoproteinemia. *Am J Hum Genet* (in press).

Brown MS, Goldstein JL: Hyperlipoproteinemias and other disorders of lipid metabolism, in Isselbacher K, et al (eds): *Principles of Internal Medicine*, ed 9. New York, McGraw-Hill, 1980, 507-530.

Brown MS, Goldstein JL: Drugs used in treatment of hyperlipoproteinemias, in Goodman AG, et al (eds): *The Pharmacological Basis of Therapeutics*, ed 7. New York, Macmillan, 1985, 827-845.

Campeau L, et al: Relation of risk factors to development of atherosclerosis in saphenous-vein bypass grafts and progression of disease in native circulation: Study 10 years after aortocoronary bypass surgery. *N Engl J Med* 311:1329-1332, 1984.

Canner PL: Mortality in coronary drug project patients during nine-year post-treatment period, (abstract). *J Am Coll Cardiol* 5:442, 1985.

Castelli WP, et al: Summary estimates of cholesterol used to predict coronary heart disease. *Circulation* 67:730-734, 1983.

Coronary Drug Project Research Group: Clofibrate and niacin in coronary heart disease. *JAMA* 231:360-381, 1975.

Douste-Blazy P, et al: Increased frequency of apo E-ND phenotype and hyperapobetalipoproteinemia in normolipidemic subjects with xanthelasmas of the eyelids. *Ann Intern Med* 96:164-169, 1982.

Glueck CJ: Colestipol and probucol: Treatment of primary and familial hypercholesterolemia and amelioration of atherosclerosis. *Ann Intern Med* 96:475-582, 1982.

Glueck CJ: Therapy of familial and acquired hyperlipoproteinemia in children and adolescents. *Prevent Med* 12:835-847, 1984.

Glueck CJ: Pediatric primary prevention of atherosclerosis, (editorial). *N Engl J Med* 314:175-177, 1986.

Glueck CJ, Lewis B: Summary and recommendations of conference on blood lipids in children: Optimal levels for early prevention of coronary-artery disease. *Prevent Med* 12:731-737, 1984.

Glueck CJ, et al: Pediatric victims of unexplained stroke and their families: Familial lipid and lipoprotein abnormalities. *Pediatrics* 69:308-316, 1982.

Glueck CJ, et al: Familial aggregations of coronary risk factors, in Connor W, et al (eds): *Coronary Heart Disease*. Philadelphia, JB Lippincott, 1985, 173-193.

Glueck CJ, et al: Efficacy and safety of long-term diet and intervention

in children heterozygous for familial hypercholesterolemia, in Hetzel BS, Berenson G (eds): *Reduction of Cardiovascular Risk Factors in Childhood*. Amsterdam, Elsevier, (in press).

Goldstein JL, Brown MS: Low-density lipoproteins and atherosclerosis. *Cardiovasc Rev Rep* 17-22, (Jan) 1983.

Goldstein JL, et al: Defective lipoprotein receptors and atherosclerosis: Lessons from animal counterpart of familial hypercholesterolemia. *N Engl J Med* 309:288-296, 1983.

Gugler R: Clinical pharmacokinetics of hypolipidaemic drugs. *Clin Pharmacokinet* 3:425-439, 1978.

Hall MJ, et al: Gemfibrozil: Effect on biliary cholesterol saturation of new lipid-lowering agent and comparison with clofibrate. *Atherosclerosis* 39:511-516, 1981.

Hjermann I, et al: Effect of diet and smoking intervention on incidence of coronary heart disease: Report from Oslo Study Group of randomised trial in healthy men. *Lancet* 2:1303-1310, 1981.

Illingworth DR: Mevinolin plus colestipol in therapy for severe heterozygous familial hypercholesterolemia. *Ann Intern Med* 101:598-604, 1984.

Illingworth DR, Sexton GJ: Hypocholesterolemic effects of mevinolin in patients with heterozygous familial hypercholesterolemia. *J Clin Invest* 74:1972-1978, 1984.

Krause BR, Newton RS: Plasma apolipoproteins and drug discovery. *TIPS* 384-387, (Sept) 1984.

Levy RI, et al: Influence of changes in lipid values induced by cholestyramine and diet on progression of coronary artery disease: Results of NHLBI Type II Coronary Intervention Study. *Circulation* 69:325-337, 1984.

Mabuchi H, et al: Reduction of serum cholesterol in heterozygous patients with familial hypercholesterolemia: Additive effects of compactin and cholestyramine. *N Engl J Med* 308:609-613, 1983.

Mahley RW, Innerarity TL: Lipoprotein receptors and cholesterol homeostasis. *Biochimica Biophysica Acta* 737:197-222, 1983.

Mahley RW, et al: Two independent lipoprotein receptors on hepatic membranes of dog, swine, and man: APO-B,E and APO-E receptors. *J Clin Invest* 68:1197-1206, 1981.

Manninen V: Treatment of dyslipidemia. Hyperlipoproteinemia and coronary artery disease: Atherogenic connection, (symposium). Dallas, 1981.

Mellies MJ, et al: Effects of probucol on plasma cholesterol, high and low density lipoprotein cholesterol, and apolipoproteins A1 and A2 in adults with primary familial hypercholesterolemia. *Metabolism* 29:956-964, 1980.

National Institutes of Health Consensus Conference: Treatment of hypertriglyceridemia. *JAMA* 251:1196-1200, 1984.

National Institutes of Health Consensus Conference: Lowering blood cholesterol to prevent heart disease. *JAMA* 253:2080-2086, 1985.

Nestel PJ, et al: Clofibrate raises plasma apoprotein A-I and HDL-cholesterol concentrations. *Atherosclerosis* 37:625-629, 1980.

Newman WP III, et al: Relation of serum lipoprotein levels and systolic blood pressure to early atherosclerosis: Bogalusa Heart Study. *N Engl J Med* 314:138-144, 1986.

Nikkila EA, et al: Prevention of progression of coronary atherosclerosis by treatment of hyperlipidemia: Seven year prospective angiographic study. *Br Med J* 289:220-223, 1984.

Oliver MF, et al: WHO cooperative trial of primary prevention of ischaemic heart disease with clofibrate to lower serum cholesterol: Final mortality follow-up: Report of committee of principal investigators. *Lancet* 2:600-604, 1984.

Saku K, et al: Mechanism of action of gemfibrozil on lipoprotein metabolism. *J Clin Invest* 75:1702-1712, 1985.

Stein EA, et al: Repetitive intermittent flow plasma exchange in patients with severe hypercholesterolemia. *Atherosclerosis* 38:149-164, 1981.

Third JHLC, et al: Primary and familial hypoalphalipoproteinemia. *Metabolism* 33:136-146, 1984.

Tikkanen MJ, et al: Natural oestrogen as effective treatment for type-II hyperlipoproteinaemia in postmenopausal women. *Lancet* 2:490-491, 1978.

Yamamura T, et al: New mutants of apolipoprotein E associated with atherosclerotic diseases but not to type III hyperlipoproteinemia. *J Clin Invest* 74:1229-1237, 1984.

Yamamota A, et al: Combined drug therapy—cholestyramine and compactin—for familial hypercholesterolemia. *Int J Clin Pharmacol Ther Toxicol* 22:493-497, 1984.

Other Selected References

Berman M, et al: Metabolism of apoB and apoC lipoproteins in man: Kinetic studies in normal and hyperlipoproteinemic subjects. *J Lipid Res* 19:38-56, 1978.

Brown WV, et al: Treatment of common lipoprotein disorders. *Prog Cardiovasc Dis* 27:1-20, 1984.

Davignon J: Lipid hypothesis: Pathophysiological basis. *Arch Surg* 113:28-34, 1978.

Day CE: Pharmacologic regulation of serum lipoproteins, in Clarke FH (ed): *Annual Reports in Medicinal Chemistry.* New York, Academic Press, 1978, vol 13, 184-195.

Eder HA, Roheim PS: Plasma lipoproteins and apolipoproteins. *Ann NY Acad Sci* 275:169-179, 1976.

Franklin FA Jr, Margolis S: Drug therapy for hyperlipidemia. *Cardiovasc Clin* 14:265-284, 1984.

Gotto AM Jr: Hyperlipidemia: Finding patient at risk. *Mod Med* 46:62-74, (March 30) 1978.

Gotto AM Jr: High-density lipoproteins: Biochemical and metabolic factors. *Am J Cardiol* 52:2B-4B, 1983.

Harlan WR, Stross JK: Educational view of national initiative to lower plasma lipid levels. *JAMA* 253:2087-2090, 1985.

Heiss G, et al: Lipoprotein-cholesterol distributions in selected North American populations: Lipid Research Clinics Program Prevalence Study. *Circulation* 61:302-315, 1980.

Lees RS, Lees AM: Therapy of hyperlipidemias. *Postgrad Med* 60:99-107, (Sept) 1976.

Levy RI: Effect of hypolipidemic drugs on plasma lipoproteins. *Annu Rev Pharmacol Toxicol* 17:499-510, 1977.

Levy RI: Cholesterol, lipoproteins, apoproteins, and heart disease: Present status and future prospects. *Clin Chem* 27:653-662, 1981.

Levy RI: Mechanisms of action of lipid-lowering drugs. *Cardiovasc Rev Rep* 8:1167-1170, 1982.

Lewis B: Relation of high-density lipoproteins to coronary artery disease. *Am J Cardiol* 52:5B-8B, 1983.

Lipid Research Clinics Program Epidemiology Committee: Plasma lipid distributions in selected North American populations: Lipid Research Clinics Program Prevalence Study. *Circulation* 60:427-439, 1979.

Morrison JA, et al: Parent-offspring and sibling lipid and lipoprotein associations during and after sharing of household environments: Princeton School District Family Study. *Metabolism* 31:158-167, 1982.

Schaefer EJ, Levy RI: Pathogenesis and management of lipoprotein disorders. *N Engl J Med* 312:1300-1310, 1985.

Agents Used in Obesity 51

Obesity is often defined as weight more than 20% in excess of "ideal" weight (based on actuarial data on height and body build/weight at various ages), but the excess may be as little as 10% in persons with small body build. However, the body mass index (W/H^2) is more closely related to the amount of body fat (Bray, 1984). Obesity may impair both cardiac and pulmonary function, modify endocrine function, and cause emotional problems. It is a major independent risk factor for atherosclerotic heart disease, and may contribute to morbidity and mortality in people with hypertension, stroke, diabetes mellitus type II (NIDDM), some types of cancer, and gallbladder disease. Metabolic abnormalities induced by weight gain and reversed after weight reduction include insulin resistance and hypertriglyceridemia. Obesity is a serious health problem in the United States; approximately 24% of male and 27% of female Americans age 18 to 74 are significantly overweight (National Institutes of Health Consensus Development Panel, 1985).

Patterns of eating and physical activity usually develop during childhood. Although controversy exists, many experts believe that fat children usually become fat adults. Since some proportion of fat children do become fat adults, intervention during childhood is an important preventive measure. Among family members, social factors, shared environment, and genetic influences produce similarities in excess weight. Of these, environment usually is most influential but genetic factors also are important because they determine the biochemical and physiologic mechanisms activated by environmental factors to lead to obesity (Bray, 1979). Thus, two persons of the same age, sex, and body characteristics with the same level of physical activity may gain weight at different rates while consuming the same amount and type of food.

Whether the cause of obesity is physiologic, psychological, metabolic, or any combination of these, body weight is often resistant to change. Obesity, particularly massive obesity (100% or greater than ideal weight), is a complex condition and treatment must be based upon the patient's personal habits, motivations, and life style. Most authorities agree that the safest way to lose weight is to consistently eat a balanced diet that supplies fewer calories than the body uses. Weight reduction is a prolonged procedure and instruction in sound nutrition is essential.

Proponents claim that techniques of behavior modification are more successful than other programs for many patients (Stuart and Davis, 1972). After one year, patients adhering to such a program had regained less weight than those receiving drugs or a combination of drugs and behavior modification techniques (Craighead et al, 1981).

A discussion of the radical treatment of obesity by starvation regimens in the hospital, plastic surgery, destruction of the lateral hypothalamus, gastric bypass, gastroplasty, and intestinal bypass surgery is beyond the scope of this presentation.

DIETARY TREATMENT

The fundamental treatment of obesity is caloric restriction. Calories ingested must be decreased to a level below the calories expended.

Research has shown that balanced diets composed of foods familiar to the patient are as conducive to weight loss as those that are high in fat and protein and these balanced diets can be maintained for extended periods. Balanced diets also are safer than fad diets, very low calorie diets, or total starvation. Diets rich in fat and protein provide a high proportion of saturated fat and cholesterol and may induce hyperlipidemia. Such diets are low in carbohydrate, are ketogenic, and are particularly dangerous for patients with diabetes or kidney disease. Other fad diets may cause deficiencies of calcium, trace elements, vitamins, and protein; amino acid imbalance; and hypokalemia or other electrolyte imbalance. Long-term compliance with fad diets is not only unlikely, but may produce serious hazards, such as cardiac arrhythmias.

In general, a daily intake of 1,500 calories for men and 1,000 calories for women over an extended period induces satisfactory weight loss. To provide a steady weight loss of approximately one to two pounds per week, the total calories ingested should be decreased to about 1,000/day less than caloric expenditure. To prevent imbalances, the diet should contain approximately 40% carbohydrate, 25% to 30% protein, and 30% to 35% fat. Exceptions should be made only under careful supervision by the physician. Diets predesigned for each week, with weekly or biweekly evaluation by trained personnel, are desirable. Diet planning should not be left to the patient until adequate training in caloric equivalence has been learned. Excellent nutrition management guides are available (American Diabetes Association, 1976; Pennington and Church, 1980; Neimark, 1980; Department of Dietetics, University of Alabama Hospitals, 1981; Committee on Dietetics, Mayo Clinic, 1981).

The nutritional management team also should provide emotional support. After one or two weeks on a diet program, there is a compensatory increase in metabolic efficiency reflected by decreased oxygen consumption, which slows the rate of weight loss. Many patients then require encouragement to continue a program of caloric restriction.

It is essential for an overweight person to make a permanent change in eating habits and behavior and to increase physical activity if long-term maintenance of weight loss is to succeed. The intake of foods containing natural fiber should be increased and the intake of foods containing refined carbohydrates (eg, sugar, white flour) should be reduced. Fresh fruits, vegetables, and whole grain products with a high proportion of fiber are absorbed more slowly and thus are postulated to satisfy hunger longer than the refined carbohydrate equivalent.

ANOREXIANT THERAPY

Usage

Use of drugs to promote weight loss should be discouraged. All anorexiants have side effects, encourage reliance on drugs, and produce only modest weight loss in most patients. These agents do not change the behavior that caused obesity.

Anorexiant therapy should be reserved for *adults* and used only as an adjunct to caloric restriction, exercise, and behavior modification. Anorexiants reduce hunger temporarily, which provides psychological support initially. If significant weight loss is not achieved after four to six weeks, drug therapy should be discontinued. If weight loss continues, these agents may be given for a longer period. Some clinicians prefer diet therapy initially, followed by short-term use of anorexiants only when weight loss has reached a plateau. Other clinicians believe that anorexiants can be employed for longer periods to prevent weight gain even when further loss does not occur (Bray, 1982; Stunkard, 1980, 1982). Although extensive studies on the long-term use of anorexiants have not been conducted, there have been several reports on such use. When diethylpropion was administered for 25 weeks, it did not appear to produce tolerance or dependence (Sullivan and Comai, 1978). Similar results were obtained when diethylpropion was used for more than 12 months in ten patients (Craddock, 1985). Fenfluramine [Pondimin], given for one year, induced weight loss of approximately 25 pounds during a five- to-seven month period that was maintained during the remaining time. However, prolonged mazindol [Mazanor, Sanorex] therapy may cause hyperinsulinemia that reduces its long-term effectiveness (Bray, 1984). Since the safety of long-term treatment has not been established conclusively, after 12 weeks of anorexiant therapy, it may be preferable to use some of these drugs intermittently (except fenfluramine, which should not be given in intermittent courses) to achieve additional weight loss when a plateau is reached despite good dietary habits, exercise, and other measures. However, weight loss may be no greater than that achieved by a good diet and exercise program alone. Even with short-term use, the average total amount of weight lost remains modest and may not be sustained after the medication is discontinued.

Prolonged use of some drugs, especially those listed in Schedule II, may cause dependence and reinforces a drug habit rather than proper eating habits. Abrupt discontinuation of treatment after the prolonged administration of therapeutic doses or the short-term use of large doses of anorexiants (especially fenfluramine) is sometimes followed by temporary fatigue, marked lethargy, paranoid psychosis, and mental depression that may be severe.

Some anorexiants increase blood pressure and produce central nervous system stimulation with insomnia (except fenfluramine), which limits their administration after 4 PM.

Drugs should not be prescribed for the treatment of obesity in *growing children*. Although data are conflicting, growth impairment has been reported with use of fenfluramine (Pinder et al, 1975), mazindol (Collipp et al, 1977), and possibly other anorexiants. In some *adolescents*, short-term therapy may be helpful temporarily if there is close supervision. Anorexiants should not be used in pregnant women.

Amphetamines: The amphetamines (amphetamine, dextroamphetamine [Dexedrine], and methamphetamine [Desoxyn]) were the first drugs prescribed widely for appetite suppression, and they are still the standard to which newer drugs are compared. However, they are no longer recommended for the treatment of obesity because the risk of dependence is great. The FDA Bureau of Drugs has concluded that the amphetamines have no advantage over other safer anorexiants (*Federal Register*, 1979), and a few states and Canada have prohibited their use for weight control.

Other Anorexiants: Benzphetamine [Didrex], diethylpropion [Tenuate, Tepanil], fenfluramine [Pondimin], mazindol [Mazanor, Sanorex], phendimetrazine [Bacarate, Plegine, Prelu-2, Statobex], phenmetrazine [Preludin], phentermine hydrochloride [Adipex-P, Fastin, Phentrol], and phentermine resin [Ionamin] have some actions similar to those of the amphetamines, although their potency and spectrum of action vary considerably. These drugs were developed in the hope that they would produce a similar anorexiant effect with fewer untoward reactions than the amphetamines. Despite differences in pharmacologic actions and untoward effects, none of these drugs is more effective than dextroamphetamine.

All anorexiants induce about the same degree of weight loss, but the increase in locomotor activity and stimulation of the central nervous system differ greatly. Unlike amphetamines, which have been used for their stimulant effect in other conditions (eg, narcolepsy, attention deficit disorder), the other anorexiant agents have been promoted only for suppression of appetite. See the evaluations for more specific information and the Table for a comparison of anorexiants.

Nonprescription Drugs: An FDA Advisory Panel considers two OTC drugs to be safe and effective as aids in weight reduction. The first, phenylpropanolamine, has almost no stimulant properties but may cause other adverse effects, particularly when the dose exceeds 75 mg/day, and should not be used indiscriminately. Benzocaine, the other drug used in proprietary preparations, has no particular merit as an anorexiant. (See the discussion on Nonprescription Drugs Used as Anorexiants in the Drug Evaluations section.)

Miscellaneous Drugs: Many drugs have been misused as anorexiants including digitalis, thyroid, diuretics, chorionic gonadotropin, antispasmodics, and laxatives. Use of any of these agents as an aid to weight reduction is unjustified.

Digitalis may induce arrhythmias, and the anorexia that it produces is a symptom of potentially fatal intoxication. Drugs with thyroid hormone activity are ineffective in overweight euthyroid patients when doses within the range of usual hormone requirements are given. Larger doses act as anorexiants but may suppress endogenous thyroid secretion and have potentially dangerous effects on cardiac function including cardiomegaly and tachyarrhythmias. Weight loss associated with use of thyroid hormone is attributed primarily to increased metabolism, which may increase protein catabolism and could lead to myopathy or osteomalacia if protein intake is inadequate. The Food and Drug Administration now requires that the labeling for thyroid, digitalis, or related drugs warn against use of these agents in the treatment of obesity.

Diuretics are of no use in decreasing adipose tissue in normally hydrated persons, although they may cause transient fluid loss. In numerous studies, human chorionic gonadotropin (HCG) was shown to have no greater effect on weight reduction than placebo injections. Starch blockers, promoted for weight loss by preventing digestion of starch, may produce diarrhea and have not been proved effective. Antispasmodics have no effect on body fat or caloric balance.

Laxatives used in doses large enough to produce diarrhea can result in loss of water, but potentially fatal hypokalemia and/or dehydration also may occur after prolonged administration. Also, malabsorption of vitamins and minerals may be induced by prolonged use or administration of large doses of laxatives. Bulk-producing agents, such as methylcellulose, cause gastric distention, inducing a transient sensation of satiety. Although these agents relieve hunger briefly when given with water, they may cause gastrointestinal disturbances (eg, flatulence, possible intestinal obstruction or fecal impaction), particularly if used for prolonged periods in excessive doses. Occasional use to provide short-term (one-half hour or so) support is not associated with adverse reactions.

Pharmacology

All anorexiant drugs except mazindol share the phenethylamine nucleus and thus are structurally similar to the amphetamines. They decrease appetite by stimulating the hypothalamus to release catecholamines in the central nervous system. With the exception of fenfluramine, which affects the central nervous system primarily through serotonin metabolism, anorexiant action is mediated by norepinephrine and dopamine metabolism. Anorexiant drugs (except fenfluramine) increase physical activity, and all of these agents have metabolic effects involving fat (inhibiting lipogenesis, enhancing lipolysis) and carbohydrate metabolism, but these probably are secondary to suppression of appetite.

Adverse Reactions

Most anorexiants are directly or indirectly related to amphetamine and produce central nervous system stimulation. Manifestations include nervousness, irritability, insomnia, decreased sense of fatigue, increased alertness and ability to concentrate, and euphoria. (With usual doses, mazindol does not appear to cause euphoria and fenfluramine has sedative effects; with overdosage or at conventional doses in sensitive patients, fenfluramine may have stimulant effects.) As the stimulant actions decline, fatigue and depression occur with most anorexiant agents. The central nervous system effects may be severe enough to require discontinuing the drug.

Sympathetic nervous system effects include dryness of the mouth, blurred vision and mydriasis, dizziness and lightheadedness, tachycardia and palpitations, hypertension, and sweating.

These agents have adrenergic effects on heart rate and may potentiate arrhythmias in patients with cardiovascular disease.

Nausea, vomiting, and, occasionally, diarrhea or constipation occur. Severe vomiting and/or diarrhea with abdominal pain has been reported with use of fenfluramine.

For additional adverse effects, see the evaluations.

Teratogenicity: Conclusive evidence of teratogenicity has not been observed when these agents were taken during pregnancy, although an infant born to a mother who abuses amphetamines may be agitated and hyperglycemic at birth. A few studies have suggested that the incidence of cleft palate or congenital heart defect was increased (Milkovich and Van Den Berg, 1978). Therefore, use of anorexiants during pregnancy is inappropriate. Furthermore, they are of little value for control of weight during pregnancy. (See also the discussion on use of drugs during pregnancy in Chapter 3.)

Tolerance: Some loss of anorexiant effect may occur within 6 to 12 weeks, and subsequent cross tolerance to other anorexiants usually occurs. The dose should not be increased to compensate for this loss of effect because larger amounts produce marked nervous system effects and increase the danger of psychological or physical dependence.

Intoxication and Abuse: Susceptible patients may develop dependence with use of anorexiant agents. Accordingly, amphetamine, dextroamphetamine, methamphetamine, phenmetrazine, and mixtures containing amphetamine compounds are classified as Schedule II drugs under the Controlled Substances Act. Because of the risk of dependence, Schedule II drugs have no place in the treatment of obesity. Benzphetamine and phendimetrazine are classified as Schedule III drugs, and diethylpropion, fenfluramine, mazindol, and phentermine as Schedule IV drugs. The risk of dependence is proportional to the stimulant effect in decreasing order: amphetamine, dextroamphetamine (or methamphetamine), phentermine, mazindol, diethylpropion, and fenfluramine (Craddock, 1976). See also the section on Prescribing Controlled Psychotropic Drugs in Chapter 1, Prescription Practices and Regulatory Agencies.

Individuals who abuse an amphetamine frequently inject as much as several grams daily; polyarteritis nodosa (necrotizing angiitis) has been associated with the intravenous administration of large doses of methamphetamine and amphetamine in these individuals. In general, chronic abuse of large intravenous doses produces a distinctive amphetamine psychosis characterized by paranoia, stereotyped behavior, picking at the skin, preoccupation with one's own thoughts, and auditory and visual hallucinations.

Withdrawal of amphetamines or other anorexiants from abusers may unmask symptoms of chronic fatigue (mental depression, asthenia, tremors, and gastrointestinal disturbances), which may be followed by drowsiness and prolonged sleep or lethargy and paranoid psychosis. Such reactions are now accepted as being a true withdrawal syndrome. Sudden withdrawal of fenfluramine may cause severe depression whether or not the patient has a history of depression.

Acute Overdosage (Poisoning): Rarely, acute poisoning occurs in those who use anorexiants irregularly, usually in conjunction with strenuous physical activity during hot weather. In general, acute overdosage accentuates the usual pharmacologic effects of excitement, agitation, hypertension, tachycardia, mydriasis, slurred speech, ataxia, tremor, chills, hyperreflexia, tachypnea, fever, headache, and toxic psychoses characterized by auditory and visual hallucinations and paranoid delusions. If these reactions appear, the drug should be discontinued permanently, sedatives prescribed, and custodial care and psychotherapy employed when needed. In severe cases, overdosage may cause hyperpyrexia, chest pain, acute circulatory failure, convulsions, and coma; fatalities have been reported. Fenfluramine poisoning appears to have some specific characteristics, including rotary nystagmus and continuous tremor of the lower jaw. Either pronounced drowsiness or agitation may occur.

Chlorpromazine [Thorazine] may be of value in blocking the central nervous system effects. If an anticholinergic drug has been taken recently, another antipsychotic drug that lacks prominent anticholinergic action (eg, haloperidol [Haldol]) may be substituted. Ammonium chloride facilitates excretion of amphetamine by acidifying the urine. If symptoms are severe and amphetamine ingestion is verified, gastric lavage or induced vomiting may be considered (Council on Scientific Affairs, 1978).

Precautions

Before prescribing any anorexiant, the patient's medical history must be ascertained to determine whether there is any tendency to abuse drugs, including alcohol, or evidence of pathologic depression. Anorexiants should not be given to such patients. Because of the dangers of drug abuse, use of amphetamine, dextroamphetamine, methamphetamine, or phenmetrazine is not advocated except in patients who previously found them to be effective and who did not experience side effects.

Anorexiant therapy should be supervised closely by a physician, and the amount of drug prescribed should be limited to that sufficient for a two-week period. It is advisable to schedule visits for these intervals, and anorexiants should be given at subsequent consultations only if the patient continues to comply with the program. The physician should see the patient personally at each visit to determine whether euphoria, irritability, or depression is present. If so, continuation of anorexiant therapy is inadvisable.

Because of their stimulant effects on the cardiovascular system, amphetamines and most other anorexiants should not

AVAILABLE ANOREXIANTS*

Generally Preferred Drugs	Alternative Drugs	Drugs Not Recommended for Weight Loss
Diethylpropion+ (IV) Mazindol+ (IV) Phentermine+ (IV)	Fenfluramine (IV) Benzphetamine (III) Phendimetrazine (III)	Amphetamine (II) Dextroamphetamine (II) Methamphetamine (II) Phenmetrazine (II)

See the evaluations for specific comments.
+Except in patients with severe hypertension or heart disease.*
Numbers within parentheses indicate Controlled Substances Act Schedule.

be used in persons with ischemic heart disease, hyperthyroidism, or advanced arteriosclerosis (see the evaluations).

Since amphetamines have the potential for increasing prolactin levels, they should be used with caution in patients with breast cancer (see also Chapter 42, Agents Related to Anterior Pituitary and Hypothalamic Function).

Interactions: Most anorexiants theoretically release norepinephrine and/or dopamine from adrenergic neurons and also impair re-entry of some hypotensive drugs into the adrenergic neuron. However, interference with the action of antihypertensive drugs probably is clinically unimportant with usual doses of anorexiants, because their action is offset by the fall in blood pressure that accompanies weight loss. Nevertheless, blood pressure should be monitored weekly for the first four to six weeks of therapy.

Since anorexiants can precipitate a hypertensive crisis when used with monoamine oxidase inhibitors, they should not be given within 14 days after administration of any monoamine oxidase inhibitor.

Blood levels of anorexiant drugs are increased by agents that alkalize the urine and are decreased by those that acidify the urine.

Drug Evaluations

Schedule IV Drugs

DIETHYLPROPION HYDROCHLORIDE
[Tenuate, Tepanil]

Diethylpropion is comparable to the amphetamines in suppressing the appetite. Although mild restlessness, dryness of the mouth, and constipation are common, the overall incidence of central nervous system side effects (nervousness, excitability, euphoria, and insomnia) is considerably lower. Psychic and physical dependence may occur, but the incidence is low despite common worldwide use. In one study, administration of diethylpropion for 25 weeks did not produce tolerance or dependence (Sullivan and Comai, 1978).

Diethylpropion is considered to be the safest of the anorexiant drugs for patients with mild to moderate hypertension even when myocardial ischemia is present. No adverse cardiovascular effects have been reported to date in patients with angina pectoris or hypertension, but use of this drug in patients with severe cardiovascular disease or marked hypertension generally is inadvisable. Diethylpropion should not be used in patients who are tense or nervous unless a mild antianxiety agent (preferably small doses of a benzodiazepine) is given concomitantly.

The safety and efficacy of diethylpropion during pregnancy and lactation have not been established; therefore, this anorexiant should not be given to women who are or are likely to become pregnant.

DOSAGE AND PREPARATIONS.
Oral: Adults, 25 mg three times daily one hour before meals. An additional 25 mg may be taken in the evening if needed. Alternatively, one timed-release preparation is taken once daily in midmorning.

Tenuate (Lakeside), **Tepanil** (Riker), **Generic.** Tablets 25 mg; tablets (timed-release) 75 mg.

FENFLURAMINE HYDROCHLORIDE
[Pondimin]

ACTIONS AND USES. This agent, a substituted phenethylamine, has some sympathomimetic properties but differs from other available anorexiants in that it usually depresses rather than stimulates the central nervous system.

Fenfluramine is comparable to dextroamphetamine in its ability to suppress the appetite, but drowsiness occurs frequently. Therefore, it is useful in nervous or tense patients or when central nervous system stimulant effects are undesirable. Fenfluramine should not be given to patients with depression or a history of it or to those receiving other central nervous system depressants. The effects in an individual patient are unpredictable. Fenfluramine, given for one year, induced loss of approximately 25 pounds during a five- to seven-month period that was maintained during the remaining time (Bray, 1984).

Fenfluramine may be beneficial when taken before the evening meal by patients who snack excessively in the evening. Also, when taken late in the day, its sedative effects would be less disruptive for patients who must remain alert during the day (Weintraub, 1981).

This drug improves glucose tolerance in some patients, probably by increasing glucose uptake in muscle or decreasing gastric emptying. However, fenfluramine should not be used to treat glucose intolerance. It is considered the anorexiant of choice for patients with diabetes mellitus type II (NIDDM) who do not have depression and/or have not responded to other types of therapy. Fenfluramine also has a slight hypotensive effect and can be used in patients with hypertension.

ADVERSE REACTIONS AND PRECAUTIONS. Occasionally, severe vomiting and/or diarrhea with abdominal pain has occurred during use of fenfluramine. One case of reversible pulmonary hypertension has been reported (Douglas et al, 1983).

Fenfluramine appears to be mildly hallucinogenic in some individuals and has become a drug of abuse in drug dependent persons in South Africa. Because the depth of sleep often is decreased, patients may be more aware of vivid dreaming. Fenfluramine may cause physical dependence with prolonged use and should not be discontinued abruptly in any patient. Sudden withdrawal can cause depression, which may be severe. Reinstitution of therapy followed by gradual reduction of the dose appears to be satisfactory for such patients. However, fenfluramine should not be used in intermittent courses for treatment of obesity. Fenfluramine is classified as a Schedule IV drug under the Controlled Substances Act.

Overdosage produces amphetamine-like symptoms and some specific characteristics (rotary nystagmus, continuous tremor of the lower jaw). Convulsions, coma, and a few deaths have been reported. Ventricular extrasystoles culminating in irreversible ventricular fibrillation have been fatal in several patients. Standard supportive measures are effective in most cases of overdosage; forced diuresis with acidification of the urine and/or large doses of diazepam may be helpful in severe cases.

An interaction between halothane and fenfluramine has been reported; it is suggested that fenfluramine be discontinued one week prior to elective surgery (Bennett and Eltringham, 1977).

The safety and efficacy of fenfluramine during pregnancy and lactation have not been established; therefore, this anorexiant should not be given to women who are or are likely to become pregnant (FDA Pregnancy Category D).

DOSAGE AND PREPARATIONS.
Oral: Adults, initially, 20 mg three times daily one hour before meals. Dosage may be increased to 40 mg three times daily one hour before meals. The drug should not be discontinued abruptly; dosage should be decreased gradually to prevent withdrawal reactions.
Pondimin (Robins). Tablets 20 mg.

MAZINDOL
[Mazanor, Sanorex]

ACTIONS AND USES. Mazindol is an imidazoisoindole and lacks the phenethylamine structure of the amphetamines and other anorexiant agents. It appears to act principally by blocking the neuronal reuptake of norepinephrine and synaptically released dopamine.

Mazindol is comparable to dextroamphetamine and diethylpropion in suppressing the appetite.

ADVERSE REACTIONS AND PRECAUTIONS. Mazindol does not appear to produce euphoria; therefore, its abuse potential is low. Otherwise, the stimulant effects are similar to those of the amphetamines, but the incidence is much lower and reactions are less severe. However, the incidence of central nervous system stimulation (eg, insomnia, dizziness, agitation) is greater with use of mazindol than diethylpropion, particularly during the first two weeks of treatment.

Psychological and physical dependence have not been reported, but the possibility of their occurrence remains.

Although the only cardiovascular action attributed to mazindol is an increase of 10 beats/minute in the orthostatic heart rate, use of this drug in patients with severe cardiovascular disease, including marked hypertension, is inadvisable. There is some evidence that mazindol may be safe for use in patients with stable atherosclerotic heart disease or mild to moderate hypertension. Control of diabetes mellitus or rheumatic diseases does not appear to be affected adversely by mazindol. Although both dextroamphetamine and mazindol cause hyperinsulinemia, this effect is probably counterbalanced by the increased lipogenesis that also may occur. However, hyperinsulinemia may reduce the effectiveness of mazindol during long-term therapy (Bray, 1984).

In one patient, the concomitant use of mazindol and lithium increased the toxicity of the latter drug (*Clin Alert*, 1980). Mazindol is a tricyclic compound and can potentiate the effects of catecholamines. Therefore, extreme care is needed during concomitant use of pressor amines.

The safety and efficacy of mazindol during pregnancy and lactation have not been established; therefore, this drug should not be given to women who are or are likely to become pregnant.

DOSAGE AND PREPARATIONS.
Oral: Adults, 1 to 2 mg daily with the first meal.
Mazanor (Wyeth). Tablets 1 mg.
Sanorex (Sandoz). Tablets 1 and 2 mg.

PHENTERMINE HYDROCHLORIDE
[Adipex-P, Fastin, Phentrol]

PHENTERMINE RESIN
[Ionamin]

Phentermine is available as the hydrochloride salt and as a complex of the base with an ion exchange resin. It is comparable to dextroamphetamine in suppressing the appetite.

Intermittent courses of treatment consisting of six weeks of phentermine followed by four weeks without drug administration are as effective as continuous drug use.

The incidence and severity of central nervous system stimulation are less than with dextroamphetamine, but the incidence of insomnia is higher than with diethylpropion and is unacceptable to some patients. Although insomnia is rare when phentermine resin is given, both forms may increase blood pressure, produce tachycardia, and commonly cause dryness of the mouth. Therefore, phentermine is not advocated for patients with hypertension and cardiovascular disease.

The safety and efficacy of phentermine during pregnancy and lactation have not been established; therefore, this drug should not be given to women who are or are likely to become pregnant. Because euphoria is rare, the abuse potential is low.

DOSAGE AND PREPARATIONS.

PHENTERMINE HYDROCHLORIDE:

Oral: *Adults,* 8 mg three times daily one-half hour before meals or 24 to 30 mg once daily two hours after breakfast. Since the half-life of phentermine is reported to be 20 hours, timed-release products have no advantage. Administration during the evening should be avoided to decrease insomnia.

    Generic. Capsules 8, 15, 18.75, 30, and 37.5 mg; tablets 8, 15, 30, and 37.5 mg.

    Adipex-P (Lemmon). Tablets 37.5 mg; capsules 37.5 mg (equivalent to 30 mg of base).

    Fastin (Beecham). Capsules 30 mg (equivalent to 24 mg of base).

    Phentrol (Vortech). Capsules 30 mg (equivalent to 24 mg of base); capsules (timed-release) 30 mg (equivalent to 24 mg of base); tablets 8 mg (equivalent to 6.4 mg of base).

PHENTERMINE RESIN:

Oral: *Adults,* 15 to 30 mg before breakfast or 10 to 14 hours before bedtime. Consistent bioavailability of the resin has been demonstrated.

    Ionamin (Pennwalt). Capsules 15 and 30 mg.

Schedule III Drugs

BENZPHETAMINE HYDROCHLORIDE
[Didrex]

Benzphetamine is comparable to dextroamphetamine in suppressing the appetite and causes similar, but fewer, untoward effects. Psychotic episodes are rare when recommended doses are used.

Benzphetamine is a secondary agent for use in obesity because it may produce euphoria and, thus, dependence in susceptible individuals. The safety and efficacy of benzphetamine during pregnancy and lactation have not been established; therefore, this drug should not be given to women who are or are likely to become pregnant.

DOSAGE AND PREPARATIONS.

Oral: *Adults,* 25 to 50 mg one to three times daily.

    Didrex (Upjohn). Tablets 25 and 50 mg.

PHENDIMETRAZINE TARTRATE
[Bacarate, Plegine, Prelu-2, Statobex]

Phendimetrazine is comparable to dextroamphetamine in its ability to suppress the appetite and stimulate the central nervous system. This drug is a secondary agent for use in obesity because it produces euphoria with the potential for abuse and because the degree of central nervous stimulation is unacceptable to some patients.

Cardiovascular effects occur infrequently. Phendimetrazine should be used with caution in patients with even mild hypertension and is contraindicated in those with moderate or severe hypertension. It also should not be given to patients with other cardiovascular disorders, hyperthyroidism, or glaucoma.

Glossitis, stomatitis, abdominal cramps, headache, and dysuria are noted occasionally. Phendimetrazine may decrease the hypotensive effect of guanethidine and may alter insulin requirements in diabetics.

The safety and efficacy of phendimetrazine during pregnancy and lactation have not been established; therefore, this anorexiant should not be given to women who are or are likely to become pregnant.

DOSAGE AND PREPARATIONS. The dosage cited by the manufacturers follows.

Oral: *Adults,* 35 mg (range, 17.5 to 70 mg) two or three times daily one hour before meals. Alternatively, one capsule (timed-release) in the morning.

    Generic. Capsules 35 mg; capsules (timed-release) 105 mg; tablets 35 mg.

    Bacarate (Reid-Provident), *Plegine* (Ayerst). Tablets 35 mg.

    Prelu-2 (Boehringer Ingelheim). Capsules (timed-release) 105 mg.

    Statobex (Lemmon). Capsules, tablets 35 mg.

    Additional Trademarks.

    Melfiat, SPRX-105 (Reid-Provident), *Wehless* (Hauck).

Schedule II Drugs (Not Recommended))

AMPHETAMINE SULFATE

This drug is the racemic form of amphetamine. It is less effective as an appetite suppressant and has more pronounced cardiovascular effects than the dextrorotatory isomer, but neither isomer is advocated for use in obesity. The danger of dependence is great in susceptible individuals.

PREPARATIONS.

Generic. Tablets 5 and 10 mg.

DEXTROAMPHETAMINE SULFATE
[Dexedrine]

USES. Dextroamphetamine is a more potent appetite suppressant than amphetamine, and its effect on the cardiovascular system is slightly less pronounced but may be severe. The drug should be discontinued immediately if chest pain or arrhythmias develop. Because dextroamphetamine may produce euphoria and the danger of dependence is great in susceptible individuals, it is not recommended as an appetite suppressant.

ADVERSE REACTIONS AND PRECAUTIONS. Dextroamphetamine causes marked central nervous system stimulation, which may be manifested by dystonic movements of the head, neck, and extremities. Severe depression or psychotic reactions may follow prolonged use, and toxic psychoses may occur after administration of large doses.

The safety and efficacy of dextroamphetamine during pregnancy and lactation have not been established; therefore, this anorexiant should not be given to women who are or are likely to become pregnant (FDA Pregnancy Category C).

DOSAGE AND PREPARATIONS. The dosage cited by the manufacturers follows.

Oral: Adults, 5 to 10 mg three times daily at least one hour before a meal. Alternatively, a timed-release preparation (10 to 15 mg) is taken once daily in the morning.

Generic. Capsules 10 mg; capsules (timed-release) 15 mg; tablets 5 and 10 mg.

Dexedrine (Smith Kline & French). Capsules (timed-release) 5, 10, and 15 mg; elixir 5 mg/5 ml (alcohol 10%); tablets 5 mg.

METHAMPHETAMINE HYDROCHLORIDE
[Desoxyn]

Methamphetamine is essentially equivalent to dextroamphetamine in its effect on the central nervous and cardiovascular systems, as well as in its ability to suppress the appetite. The danger of dependence is also equivalent and methamphetamine is not recommended for use in obesity.

The safety and efficacy of methamphetamine during pregnancy and lactation have not been established; therefore, this drug should not be given to women who are or are likely to become pregnant.

DOSAGE AND PREPARATIONS. The dosage cited by the manufacturer follows.

Oral: Adults, 2.5 to 5 mg three times daily 30 to 60 minutes before each meal. Alternatively, a timed-release tablet (10 or 15 mg) is taken once daily in the morning.

Desoxyn (Abbott). Tablets 5 mg; tablets (timed-release) 5, 10, and 15 mg.

PHENMETRAZINE HYDROCHLORIDE
[Preludin]

Phenmetrazine is comparable to dextroamphetamine in suppressing the appetite and produces similar untoward effects. The danger of dependence is also comparable to that observed with dextroamphetamine. Psychoses and changes in the electrocardiogram have been reported. This agent is not advocated for use in obesity; equally effective alternative drugs are available that are less likely to produce dependence. Also, phenmetrazine has become an agent of abuse as a replacement for less readily obtainable amphetamines (Mellar and Hollister, 1982).

The safety and efficacy of phenmetrazine during pregnancy and lactation have not been established; therefore, this drug should not be given to women who are or are likely to become pregnant.

DOSAGE AND PREPARATIONS. The dosage cited by the manufacturer follows.

Oral: Adults, one timed-release tablet once daily in midmorning or 25 mg two or three times daily one hour before meals.

Preludin (Boehringer Ingelheim). Tablets 25 mg; tablets (timed-release) 75 mg.

NONPRESCRIPTION DRUGS USED AS ANOREXIANTS

Benzocaine is available without prescription for use in weight control. Its appetite suppressant effect theoretically results from numbness of the oral cavity and gastrointestinal mucosa that modifies taste sensitivity and thus discourages "snacking." There are no conclusive data to support benzocaine's effectiveness as an anorexiant, but an FDA Advisory Panel considers this local anesthetic to be safe and effective as an aid in weight reduction. Cyanotic reactions have been reported rarely.

Phenylpropanolamine is an adrenergic agent related to ephedrine but has less pronounced stimulant properties. It is available without prescription in various proprietary products as an aid in weight reduction. An FDA Advisory Panel concluded that phenylpropanolamine is safe and effective as an aid in weight reduction. However, this drug is no more effective than any other anorexiant and it should not be used indiscriminately.

Side effects may occur with any dose, but particularly when the amount exceeds 75 mg/day. These include nervousness, restlessness, insomnia, dizziness, tinnitus, headache, nausea, and excessive elevation of blood pressure (Horowitz et al, 1980). Because of its adrenergic properties, phenylpropanolamine also may cause cardiac stimulation and elevate blood glucose levels. This drug should not be used in individuals with diabetes, heart disease, hypertension, or hyperthyroidism unless a physician supervises therapy. Dosage reduction may be necessary in patients with kidney disease.

There is evidence that phenylpropanolamine is being ingested in excessive doses, both as an appetite suppressant and as a substitute for the less readily available amphetamines. Reactions that result from cerebral stimulation and vasoconstriction have been reported, including hemiparesis, grand mal seizures, and psychotic reactions (eg, mania, hallucinations, paranoid reactions). Chest pain, myocardial damage, and arrhythmias also have been noted. These reactions also may occur with use of usual doses by individuals hypersensitive to phenylpropanolamine.

Formulations previously contained caffeine, which may have contributed to central nervous system stimulation.

One death caused by ventricular arrhythmia has been reported in a schizophrenic patient taking thioridazine who ingested a single capsule containing phenylpropanolamine 50 mg and chlorpheniramine 4 mg.

Two cases of acute renal failure and rhabdomyolysis have been reported following ingestion of diet pills containing phenylpropanolamine, but a cause-and-effect relationship has not been established.

Phenylpropanolamine may interact with monoamine oxidase inhibitors and indomethacin or other drugs that inhibit prostaglandin synthesis (eg, aspirin, other anti-inflammatory agents) to cause severe hypertensive episodes (Lee et al, 1979). Reserpine and guanethidine may interfere with the action of phenylpropanolamine.

Since serious adverse reactions occur and long-term effectiveness of the drug has not been demonstrated, the usefulness of phenylpropanolamine as an aid to weight reduction is limited *(Med Lett Drugs Ther,* 1984).

MIXTURES

The mixtures available for weight control combine more than one amphetamine (which may be considered essentially a single-entity drug). They are classified as Schedule II drugs under the Controlled Substances Act.

The following products are listed for information only.

Biphetamine (Pennwalt). Each capsule contains resin complexes equivalent to dextroamphetamine 6.25 or 10 mg and amphetamine 6.25 or 10 mg.

Obetrol (Obetrol). Tablets containing 2.5 or 5 mg each of dextroamphetamine sulfate, dextroamphetamine saccharate, amphetamine aspartate, and amphetamine sulfate.

Cited References

Amphetamines: Drugs for human use; drug efficacy study implementation. *Federal Register* 44:41552-41571, (July 17) 1979.

Mazindol: Precipitation of lithium toxicity. *Clin Alert* 104, (May 30) 1980.

Phenylpropanolamine for weight reduction. *Med Lett Drugs Ther* 26:55-56, 1984.

American Diabetes Association: *Exchange Lists for Meal Planning*, (booklet). New York, American Diabetes Association, 1976.

Bennett JA, Eltringham RJ: Possible dangers of anaesthesia in patients receiving fenfluramine: Results of animal studies following case of human cardiac arrest. *Anaesthesia* 32:8-13, 1977.

Bray GA: Obesity. *DM* 26:1-85, (Oct) 1979.

Bray GA: Obesity. *Current Concepts.* The Upjohn Company, 1982.

Bray GA: Treating obesity with drugs. *Drug Ther* 14:93-100, (July) 1984.

Collipp PJ, et al: Effects of mazindol on growth and growth hormone, (abstract). *Pediatr Res* 11:424, 1977.

Committee on Dietetics, Mayo Clinic: *Mayo Clinic Diet Manual: A Handbook of Dietary Practices.* Philadelphia, WB Saunders, 1981.

Council on Scientific Affairs: Clinical aspects of amphetamine abuse. *JAMA* 240:2317-2319, 1978.

Craddock D: Anorectic drugs: Use in general practice. *Drugs* 11:378-393, 1976.

Craddock D (personal communication), 1985.

Craighead LW, et al: Behavior therapy and pharmacotherapy for obesity. *Arch Gen Psychiatry* 38:763-768, 1981.

Department of Dietetics, University of Alabama Hospitals: *Manual for Nutritional Management.* Birmingham, University of Alabama, 1981.

Douglas JG, et al: Long-term efficacy of fenfluramine in treatment of obesity. *Lancet* 1:384-386, 1983.

Horowitz JD, et al: Hypertensive responses induced by phenylpropanolamine in anorectic and decongestant preparations. *Lancet* 1:60-61, 1980.

Lee KY, et al: Severe hypertension after ingestion of appetite suppressant (phenylpropanolamine) with indomethacin. *Lancet* 1:1110-1111, 1979.

Mellar J, Hollister LE: Phenmetrazine: Obsolete problem drug. *Clin Pharmacol Ther* 32:671-675, 1982.

Milkovich L, Van Den Berg BJ: Amphetamines in pregnancy: Excess of cleft palates found. *Mod Med* 46:145, (March 30) 1978.

National Institutes of Health Consensus Development Panel: Health implications of obesity. *Ann Intern Med* 103:147-151, 1985.

Neimark PG: *A Doctor's Approach to Sensible Dieting and Weight Control.* Chicago, Budlong Press, 1980.

Pennington JAT, Church HN: *Food Values of Portions Commonly Used*, ed 13. Philadelphia, JB Lippincott, 1980.

Pinder RM, et al: Fenfluramine: Review of its pharmacological properties and therapeutic efficacy in obesity. *Drugs* 10:241-323, 1975.

Stuart RB, Davis B: *Slim Chance in a Fat World.* Champaign, IL, Research Press, 1972.

Stunkard AJ (ed): *Obesity.* Philadelphia, WB Saunders, 1980.

Stunkard AJ: Anorectic agents lower body weight set point. *Life Sci* 30:2043-2055, 1982.

Sullivan AC, Comai K: Pharmacological treatment of obesity. *Int J Obes* 2:167, 1978.

Weintraub M: New look at obesity. *Drug Update* 15-17, (Oct) 1981.

Other Selected References

Bernstein E, Diskant BM: Phenylpropanolamine: Potentially hazardous drug. *Ann Emerg Med* 11:311-315, 1982.

Bierman EL: Obesity, in Beeson PB, et al (eds): *Textbook of Medicine,* ed 15. Philadelphia, WB Saunders, 1979, 1692-1698.

Bray GA: *The Obese Patient.* Philadelphia, WB Saunders, 1976, 353-410.

Connell PH: Central nervous system stimulants and anorectic agents, in Dukes MNG (ed): *Side Effects of Drugs. Annual 2.* Amsterdam, Excerpta Medica, 1978.

Craddock D: *Obesity and Its Management,* ed 3. Edinburgh, Churchill Livingstone, 1978, 92-109.

Friedman RB, et al: What to tell patients about weight-loss methods. *Postgrad Med* 72:85-88, (Oct) 1982.

Goldrick RB: Management of obesity. *Drugs* 12:301-304, 1976.

Guggenheim FG: Basic considerations in treatment of obesity. *Med Clin North Am* 61:781-796, 1977.

Hafen BQ (ed): *Overweight and Obesity: Causes, Fallacies, Treatment.* Provo, UT, Brigham Young University Press, 1975.

Morgan JP, Kagan DV (eds): Phenylpropanolamine: Risks, benefits, and controversies, in: *Clinical Pharmacology and Therapeutics.* New York, Praeger, 1985

Salans LB, Wise JK: Metabolic studies of human obesity. *Med Clin North Am* 54:1533-1542, 1970.

Samuel PD, Burland WL: Drug treatment of obesity, in *Obesity in Perspective,* part 2. Fogarty International Center Series on Preventive Medicine, Washington, DC, US Dept Health, Education and Welfare, 1975, vol 2, 419-428.

Scoville BA: Review of amphetamine-like drugs by Food and Drug Administration: Clinical data and value judgments, in *Obesity in Perspective,* part 2. Fogarty International Center Series on Preventive Medicine, Washington, DC, US Dept Health, Education and Welfare, 1975, vol 2, 441-443.

Tan T-L, et al: Current therapy of eating disorders: II. Obesity. *Ration Drug Ther* 18:1-7, (Feb) 1984.

Van Itallie TB, Yang M-U: Current concepts in nutrition: Diet and weight loss. *N Engl J Med* 297:1158-1161, 1977.

Weil WB Jr: Current controversies in childhood obesity. *J Pediatr* 91:175-187, 1977.

PEPTIC ULCER DISEASE

Peptic (esophageal, gastric, and duodenal) ulcers occur in areas of the gastrointestinal tract exposed to acid and pepsin and result from an imbalance between the erosive action of acid and pepsin on the one hand and the gastroduodenal mucosal defense system on the other. In patients with gastric ulcer, the acid output is normal or reduced, suggesting that mucosal resistance is a primary factor in development; in contrast, high acid output appears to be an important causative factor in duodenal ulcers (Shearman and Finlayson, 1982). The etiology of chronic peptic ulcers is unclear, but environmental and genetic factors contribute to their development; aspirin and other nonsteroidal anti-inflammatory drugs also may be causative.

The goals of peptic ulcer therapy are to decrease or abolish symptoms, to hasten healing, to prevent serious complications (hemorrhage, perforation, and obstruction), and to prevent recurrences. These goals usually can be achieved with drug therapy and avoidance of precipitating or aggravating substances.

Nondrug Management

Dietary Measures: There is little evidence that any single dietary factor influences the healing of peptic ulcers, and the so-called "ulcer diet" consisting of bland soft foods with milk or cream does not affect the rate of healing or recurrence. However, foods, spices, and liquids that provoke or worsen symptoms should be avoided, and patients should eat three meals a day that comprise a balanced diet of their choosing.

Eating small meals every two or three hours may minimize variations in intragastric pH, but may not be necessary in patients receiving antiulcer medications. Unless an H$_2$-receptor antagonist is taken concomitantly, a small snack at bedtime may be harmful, since it stimulates nocturnal acid secretion.

Although the ingestion of milk is advocated by some authorities (Lewis, 1983), its value is controversial. Consumption of alcohol on an empty stomach may delay healing and is not recommended, but moderate alcohol intake with meals does not aggravate symptoms or delay healing. It is sometimes recommended that coffee (both caffeinated and decaffeinated), tea, cola drinks, and acid juices be avoided, but there is no good evidence that they are harmful.

Avoidance of Irritating Drugs: There is evidence that nonsteroidal anti-inflammatory drugs (eg, ibuprofen, salicylates, indomethacin, phenylbutazone) aggravate mucosal damage, delay healing, and/or predispose to bleeding. Therefore, they should be avoided in patients with peptic ulcer. Low doses of corticosteroids may be used in patients with peptic ulcer, although it should be borne in mind that steroids may mask symptoms of perforation and other complications (Shearman and Finlayson, 1982).

Control of Emotional Factors: The high placebo response in patients with peptic ulcers suggests that emotional factors (anxiety, stress) contribute to the development of peptic ulcers in some patients (Peters and Richardson, 1983), but they are not a primary cause. However, anxiety and stress may hasten recurrence of active peptic ulcer disease. The resolution of problems that contribute to emotional distress may reduce the extent and frequency of pain. The physician's reassurance often relieves anxiety and promotes compliance.

Treatment of serious emotional disorders should be independent of peptic ulcer treatment. Adjunctive use of diazepam [Valium] or another antianxiety agent may be useful (Gillespie et al, 1983).

Avoidance of Smoking: Smoking should be avoided by patients with peptic ulcers. The incidence of peptic ulcer is higher in smokers than in nonsmokers. Moreover, cigarette smoking delays healing, may increase the rate of recurrence, and may decrease the effectiveness of cimetidine and other antiulcer medications (McCarthy, 1984).

Drug Therapy

Peptic ulcers usually have a benign prognosis and may be self-limiting. Almost all patients can be treated successfully with drugs and alteration of lifestyle; surgery may be required for those refractory to drug therapy. Most therapeutic failures are due to inadequate therapy, noncompliance, or incorrect diagnosis. Before drug therapy is initiated, the possibility that gastric carcinoma and other serious diseases are present must be considered.

Drugs known to promote healing in acid peptic disorders reduce gastric acidity or enhance mucosal defense systems (Grossman et al, 1981). Peptic ulcers usually can be controlled by single-drug therapy with antacids, H_2 blockers (eg, cimetidine [Tagamet], ranitidine [Zantac]), or sucralfate [Carafate]. Combination therapy using an H_2 antagonist with adjunctive medications (eg, antacids, anticholinergic agents, sucralfate) is being investigated for patients resistant to single-drug therapy and those with the Zollinger-Ellison syndrome (Grossman et al, 1981; Jadhav and Freston, 1983; Richardson and Peterson, 1982).

Peptic ulcers recur within one year in 40% to 80% of patients when drug therapy is discontinued or they may recur even during maintenance therapy. Cimetidine and ranitidine are drugs of choice to prevent recurrence of gastric or duodenal ulcer; ranitidine may be more effective. Sucralfate may prevent recurrence of a duodenal ulcer.

Guidelines for Therapeutic Management of Uncomplicated Peptic Ulcers: Assessment of the effectiveness of drug therapy is more difficult in gastric than duodenal ulcers. Evidence from many controlled studies suggests that the rate of healing of gastric ulcers equals that of duodenal ulcers when patients follow prescribed regimens (Isenberg et al, 1983; Jadhav and Freston, 1983). The chief differences in therapy involve frequency of administration, dosage, and the end point of treatment. The following guidelines are for patients with uncomplicated gastric and duodenal ulcers:

1. Discontinue all ulcerogenic drugs and cigarette smoking.
2. Prescribe cimetidine, ranitidine, sucralfate, or antacids (for four to six weeks in patients with duodenal ulcer, 8 to 12 weeks in those with gastric ulcer).
3. Patients are usually asymptomatic long before healing occurs. In duodenal ulcer, discontinue drug therapy after six weeks if all symptoms have disappeared, although healing may not be complete in some patients. However, for patients with gastric ulcers, confirm healing after eight weeks of therapy by x-ray or endoscopy. Unhealed gastric ulcers are presumed to be malignant until proved otherwise.

The results of radiologic examinations and the improvement of symptoms do not always reflect the extent of healing of peptic ulcer. Unhealed ulcers can be observed endoscopically in asymptomatic patients and healed peptic ulcers may be seen in patients still experiencing pain and other symptoms (Isenberg et al, 1983). Although relief of pain from peptic ulcer can occur rapidly after drug treatment, results of numerous well-controlled studies have demonstrated endoscopically confirmed healing of duodenal ulcer only after 4 to 6 weeks of daily treatment with the above agents in most patients; healing of gastric ulcer generally requires 8 to 12 weeks.

4. Further treatment depends on whether the ulcer does not produce symptoms, heals completely, or recurs. Patients with benign gastric ulcer can be evaluated annually but are more generally evaluated upon recurrence of symptoms. In the absence of recurrence, re-evaluation is not necessary for patients with duodenal ulcer. If the ulcer recurs during the first three or four months, prescribe a full course of drug therapy for four weeks. After healing, evaluate the patient at three-month intervals for one year. If the ulcer does not heal, recurs frequently, or enlarges, substitute another drug or combination of drugs. In therapeutic failures, evaluate compliance, adequacy of dosage, and the possibility of a wrong diagnosis (eg, gastric cancer, Zollinger-Ellison syndrome, use of nonsteroidal anti-inflammatory drugs).

5. Bleeding stops spontaneously in approximately 90% of patients with bleeding ulcers. Surgery may be required for intractable bleeding.

Maintenance Therapy to Prevent Recurrence: Whether maintenance therapy should be instituted or drugs withdrawn after peptic ulcer has healed is unclear. Maintenance therapy with cimetidine, ranitidine, or sucralfate usually prevents recurrence of a duodenal ulcer as long as treatment continues (success rate, 65% to 90%). Therapy beyond one year is recommended in elderly, debilitated, or other poor-risk patients. It is less clear if maintenance therapy with cimetidine or ranitidine for gastric ulcer has significant value beyond one year; in one study, cimetidine had significant prophylactic effect after one year, but there was little benefit beyond two years (Barr et al, 1983). The adverse effects of long-term use of cimetidine or ranitidine (more than three or four years) are unknown.

In uncomplicated duodenal or gastric ulcer, cimetidine 400 mg once at bedtime (duodenal ulcer) or in the morning and at bedtime (gastric or duodenal ulcer) prevented recurrences in more than 80% of patients for at least one year (Barr et al, 1983; Jadhav and Freston, 1983). A single bedtime dose of ranitidine 150 mg maintained remission for one year in 65% of patients with duodenal ulcer and 90% of patients with gastric ulcer (Alstead et al, 1983). For relapses of duodenal ulcer occurring after three to four months of therapy in patients experiencing fewer than two or three recurrences a year, some practitioners recommend intermittent, full-dose treatment with cimetidine or ranitidine; neither drug is given between relapses.

Combination Therapy: For most patients with uncomplicated gastric or duodenal ulcer, the use of cimetidine, ranitidine, sucralfate, or an anticholinergic in any combination is costly and yields no additional therapeutic advantage while subjecting the patient to possible additional adverse effects of combination regimens.

In about 20% of patients with intractable peptic ulcers, the Zollinger-Ellison syndrome, multiple endocrine adenomas, systemic mastocytosis, or other gastric acid hypersecretory states, the use of single drugs is unsatisfactory and various combinations have been tried. Studies have shown that the combined use of cimetidine or ranitidine in larger than usual doses with an anticholinergic agent (propantheline [Pro-Banthine], pirenzepine (investigational), or isopropamide [Darbid]) appears to produce additive acid antisecretory effects and enhance effectiveness in the above conditions (Richardson and Peterson, 1982; DiMario et al, 1984).

DRUG SELECTION. No single drug is most efficacious in the treatment of peptic ulcer disease. Similar rates of healing (75% to 85%) are reported for cimetidine, ranitidine, sucralfate, antacids, and a number of investigational agents (eg, carbenoxolone, tripotassium dicitrato bismuthate [colloidal bismuth compound]). The rate of healing has been reported to be 100% after four weeks of therapy with the investigational drug, omeprazole. Factors to consider when selecting a specific drug include ease of administration, incidence and severity of adverse effects, availability, and cost.

Antacids: In several controlled studies, an adequate antacid regimen was as effective as cimetidine in patients with gastric or duodenal ulcer. For uncomplicated duodenal ulcer, an intensive course of liquid antacid (144 mEq one and three hours after meals and at bedtime, total 1,008 mEq/day) may be required (Peterson et al, 1977), although considerably smaller amounts are often effective. Tablets appear to be as effective as liquid preparations. In one study, a low-dose regimen of antacid tablets (14 tablets, 280 mEq total daily dose) was as effective as ranitidine in healing duodenal ulcers (Berstad et al, 1982). When antacids are used for initial healing, however, the frequent administration required, lack of palatability, and side effects (diarrhea, constipation) reduce patient compliance significantly, particularly when ulcer symptoms are absent.

Because of the low gastric acidity usually associated with gastric ulcer, relatively low-dose regimens (275 to 375 mEq) of a liquid antacid containing aluminum and magnesium hydroxides heal a significant percentage of gastric ulcers (Romankiewicz and Reidenberg, 1981; Isenberg et al, 1983).

Antacids also are often prescribed intermittently with cimetidine, ranitidine, or sucralfate to alleviate pain rapidly in patients with uncomplicated peptic ulcer.

Poorly absorbed antacids are preferred in the treatment of peptic ulcer. Certain highly concentrated aluminum, magnesium, and calcium compounds appear to have a prolonged duration of action and beneficial effects on pH. Mixtures of aluminum oxide-hydroxide and magnesium oxide-hydroxide are used most frequently. Calcium carbonate has a greater neutralizing capacity, but its utilization has decreased because of absorption of calcium, concern regarding possible acid rebound, and the formation of kidney stones.

Sodium bicarbonate, which is an active ingredient of some proprietary preparations, is very soluble and has an immediate and pronounced neutralizing effect, but its duration of action is extremely brief. Because sodium bicarbonate produces meta-bolic alkalosis when used excessively or in patients with impaired renal function, it must not be taken for long periods. This antacid should not be used routinely in the management of peptic ulcer and is contraindicated in patients requiring a low-sodium diet.

For additional information on available antacid preparations, see the discussion on Antacids in the evaluation section.

Histamine$_2$ Receptor Antagonists: Cimetidine and ranitidine are currently among the drugs of choice for initial treatment and maintenance therapy in most patients with uncomplicated gastric or duodenal ulcer. They have little value in bleeding peptic ulcers. Cimetidine is currently the most widely used antiulcer medication, but approximately 20% of patients fail to respond and another drug or surgery may be needed (Richardson and Peterson, 1982; Shearman and Finlayson, 1982). Studies indicate that a single bedtime dose of cimetidine 800 mg or ranitidine 300 mg may be as efficacious as presently recommended regimens (Gledhill et al, 1983).

The overall incidence of adverse reactions to cimetidine is low. Elderly and debilitated individuals, patients with impaired renal function, and those who require prolonged therapy with large doses (eg, Zollinger-Ellison syndrome) are the most likely to experience side effects (see the evaluation). Ranitidine may be a preferred drug for these patients and those who do not respond or become refractory to cimetidine. Ranitidine is 4 to 13 times more potent than cimetidine, has little antiandrogenic activity (and thus produces gynecomastia only rarely), does not significantly inhibit hepatic drug metabolizing enzymes, and causes fewer drug interactions (Konturek, 1982; Brogden et al, 1982); larger doses can be used in refractory patients because of the lower incidence of adverse reactions. Although reactions to ranitidine are rare, more experience must be obtained before the effects of long-term use can be assessed.

Sucralfate: Sucralfate, a sulfated disaccharide, is as effective as cimetidine in healing a duodenal ulcer and may prevent recurrence. Preliminary studies indicate that sucralfate also is useful in healing gastric ulcer, but its prophylactic value in long-term maintenance therapy is unclear. Its chief advantage is lack of significant absorption and, hence, the absence of systemic adverse reactions; constipation and other minor gastrointestinal disturbances are noted infrequently. Sucralfate is being employed increasingly as an alternative to cimetidine, particularly in the elderly and debilitated.

Unlike H$_2$ receptor antagonists, sucralfate may not be useful for refractory peptic ulcers (Spiro, 1982; Brogden et al, 1984).

Anticholinergic Agents: Anticholinergic drugs should be used only adjunctively with H$_2$ receptor antagonists or other agents in peptic ulcer disease. The antisecretory action of the antimuscarinic anticholinergic drugs is less pronounced than that of the H$_2$ antagonists and they produce more side effects; thus, their use has declined.

The development of the selective anticholinergic drug, pirenzepine (investigational), which causes fewer significant side effects, may further limit the role of less selective antimuscarinic agents in peptic ulcer disease.

Investigational Agents: A number of drugs currently under clinical trial in this country show some promise. Included among these agents are the following.

The H$_2$ receptor antagonist, *famotidine,* is about 50 times more potent than cimetidine, has a longer duration of action, and dissociates more slowly from the H$_2$ receptor.

Pirenzepine, a tricyclic anticholinergic drug, selectively inhibits M$_1$ subtype muscarinic receptors in the gastric mucosa. Doses that inhibit gastric acid secretion do not cause significant ocular, bladder, or salivary (M$_2$ subtype muscarinic receptors) side effects. Although studies show that pirenzepine heals gastric and duodenal ulcers, it may be less effective than cimetidine. This drug may be useful in maintenance programs to prevent recurrence. Its chief indication will probably be in combination with other antiulcer drugs in the Zollinger-Ellison syndrome and refractory peptic ulcers (Farini et al, 1983; Collen et al, 1982; DiMario et al, 1984).

Tripotassium dicitrato bismuthate (colloidal bismuth compound) has no significant acid neutralizing activity. At acid pH, it binds protein at the ulcer site and has a demulcent effect that forms a barrier against acid and pepsin. This compound may be effective in gastric and duodenal ulcers (Wilson and Alp, 1982; Richardson and Peterson, 1982). Adverse reactions are minimal; the stool is darkened and liquid preparations smell of ammonia.

Prostaglandin derivatives (eg, *arbaprostil, misoprostol, enprostil, trimoprostil*) have an antisecretory action and a protective effect on gastric and duodenal mucosa. These agents have been effective in clinical trials for healing duodenal and gastric ulcers (Bond, 1984, 1985; Henahan, 1985). They also show promise for prevention of peptic ulcer and bleeding in patients receiving aspirin and other nonsteroidal anti-inflammatory drugs.

Omeprazole represents a new class of gastric acid inhibitors, the substituted benzimidazoles. It markedly inhibits gastric acid secretion by inhibiting the K$^+$/H$^+$ ATPase proton pump in parietal cells. A single daily dose inhibits the production of gastric acid. Oral omeprazole taken once daily has healed duodenal ulcers and controlled gastric acid secretion in patients with the Zollinger-Ellison syndrome. This drug may be particularly effective in reflux esophagitis. Data on its effectiveness in gastric ulcers are limited. A dose ten times greater than the largest amount used in clinical trials produced benign gastric carcinoid tumors in rats. Significant adverse effects have not been observed during short-term clinical studies, but long-term effects remain to be established.

The *tricyclic antidepressants* (eg, trimipramine [Surmontil]) were as effective as cimetidine in healing gastric and duodenal ulcers in a number of controlled studies (Richelson, 1983; Ries et al, 1984). Another tricyclic antidepressant, doxepin [Adapin, Sinequan], also may be useful in peptic ulcer disease. Doses one-third to one-sixth of those used to treat depression are effective. Because of their long half-lives and potency, a single daily dose appears to be adequate in peptic ulcer disease. Although the overall incidence of adverse effects produced by these agents is low, dry mouth and drowsiness may be troublesome in some patients. The mechanism of action is unclear; their anticholinergic activity may account for the antisecretory effect.

Carbenoxolone, a triterpenoid licorice derivative, accelerates the healing of gastric and duodenal ulcers (Nagy, 1978).

The precise mechanism of action is unknown, but it appears to enhance mucosal defense. Adverse reactions (eg, hypertension, fluid retention, hypokalemia) have delayed the marketing of this drug in the United States. Moreover, the availability of numerous other effective agents with fewer adverse reactions may limit the role of carbenoxolone in the treatment of peptic ulcer disease (Richardson and Peterson, 1982).

ESOPHAGEAL DISORDERS

The only esophageal disorder that responds significantly to drug treatment is reflux esophagitis (gastroesophageal reflux disease). Achalasia and diffuse esophageal spasm respond poorly to drugs, although several agents are being used investigationally.

REFLUX ESOPHAGITIS. The factors thought to be important in the pathogenesis of reflux esophagitis and heartburn include lower esophageal sphincter (LES) incompetence, repeated relaxation of the LES not associated with swallowing (Dent, 1981; Holloway et al, 1981), impaired ability of the esophagus to clear refluxed material, low intraesophageal pH, and impaired resistance of the esophageal mucosa to injury.

Initial management should include elevation of the head of the bed; weight reduction in obese patients; elimination of tight garments; avoidance of heavy lifting; avoidance of large meals and of lying down three to four hours after eating; and elimination of smoking and coffee, alcohol, chocolate, and other foods known to exacerbate symptoms.

Drug Therapy: Antacids or an antacid/alginic acid combination relieve symptoms in many patients. Systemic agents are used concomitantly when the response to the above measures is inadequate. Presently available drugs relieve symptoms but do not cure esophagitis. Results of controlled studies suggest that cimetidine [Tagamet], ranitidine [Zantac], bethanechol [Duvoid, Myotonachol, Urecholine], and metoclopramide [Reglan] are more effective than placebo (Holloway and McCallum, 1983; Wu and Castell, 1983; Wesdorp et al, 1983). Sucralfate [Carafate] also was more effective than placebo and as effective as alginate/antacid combination [Gaviscon] (Laitinen et al, 1985). Omeprazole, an investigational agent, may be particularly effective for reflux esophagitis.

The H$_2$ antagonists, cimetidine and ranitidine, are often drugs of first choice to relieve symptoms. They reduce gastric acid secretion but have no effect on LES pressure or esophageal motility; antacid consumption is reduced significantly more than with a placebo. The rate of healing, as determined by endoscopy and biopsy, is not increased as much as relief of symptoms.

Bethanechol increases LES pressure in some patients with chronic reflux, which is purported to explain its additive effect with antacids. The addition of bethanechol (10 to 25 mg) before meals and at bedtime was reported to accelerate healing (Thanik et al, 1982), although this finding has not been consistent (Saco et al, 1982).

Metoclopramide elevates LES pressure, improves esophageal acid clearance, and enhances gastric emptying. It may be particularly useful in patients with delayed gastric emptying.

However, usual doses cause drowsiness, lassitude, and extrapyramidal reactions in a significant number of patients.

Since anticholinergic and calcium channel blocking agents facilitate reflux, they have no value in reflux esophagitis and are contraindicated in patients with this disorder.

ACHALASIA AND DIFFUSE ESOPHAGEAL SPASM. Dysphagia is a primary symptom of these disorders of motility. Because chest pain is prominent in patients with diffuse esophageal spasm, stress, anxiety, and fear that the pain is cardiac in origin are common and patient reassurance is important. The dysphagia that accompanies motor disorders must be differentiated from that caused by mechanical obstruction of the esophagus due to rings, webs, strictures, and benign or malignant tumors (Meyer and Castell, 1981).

Achalasia is much easier to diagnose and treat than diffuse esophageal spasm. Heller myotomy or pneumatic dilation is successful in most patients with achalasia. Bougie dilation, which may be repeated at intervals, relieves symptoms in many patients with diffuse esophageal spasm, but myotomy should be avoided because it may predispose to severe reflux and esophagitis.

Drug Therapy: The calcium channel blocking agents have been investigated in patients with these disorders of esophageal motility. Results of open clinical studies (Blackwell et al, 1981; Berger and McCallum, 1982) demonstrate that nifedipine [Procardia] reduced LES pressure (mean decrease, 58% to 70%), the frequency of spontaneous esophageal contractions, and the amplitude of distal peristaltic esophageal contractions in some patients with achalasia; this drug decreased LES pressure and the amplitude and frequency of spasm in patients with diffuse esophageal spasm. Gastric emptying was not affected. Verapamil [Calan, Isoptin] and diltiazem [Cardizem] also are being evaluated for use in these disorders (Richter et al, 1984). Nifedipine 10 to 20 mg sublingually (investigational route) has aborted painful esophageal spasm; 20 mg orally 30 minutes before each meal has been useful for prophylaxis (Traube et al, 1984). For additional information on calcium channel blocking drugs, see Chapter 25, Antianginal Agents.

Isosorbide dinitrate [Isordil, Sorbitrate] has been evaluated in patients with achalasia or diffuse esophageal spasm. An open study (Gelfond et al, 1982) comparing isosorbide dinitrate 5 mg and nifedipine 20 mg in achalasia revealed that both drugs relieved dysphagia subjectively after sublingual administration. Isosorbide dinitrate reduced LES pressure more promptly and eliminated a radionuclide test meal from the esophagus more consistently, but side effects (dizziness, flushing, headache, fainting) were more troublesome.

Anticholinergic agents may be somewhat useful in achalasia, particularly in patients who exhibit sensitivity in the Mecholyl test, although these drugs are of limited benefit even in this group.

STRESS ULCERATION AND HEMORRHAGE

The incidence of stress ulcers is high in critically ill, high-risk patients with hepatic, respiratory, or renal failure; sepsis; burns over more than 35% of body surface; head injury; and multiple trauma. In addition, many patients develop stress ulcers postoperatively. In critically ill patients, hemorrhage from stress ulcers is a serious complication. The major factor underlying the development of stress ulceration appears to be decreased gastric mucosal blood flow that impairs mucosal defenses. Many affected patients have increased gastric acid output, which also favors the development of ulcers. Although the net gastric acid output may be normal or low in some patients with altered metabolic states, significant back diffusion of hydrogen ion can occur (Zinner et al, 1981).

Prophylaxis: The incidence of upper gastrointestinal tract bleeding in critically ill patients can be decreased by prevention of anemia, hypovolemia, sepsis, hypoalbuminemia, and malnutrition. Patients receiving enteral nutrition are less susceptible to gastrointestinal hemorrhage and may not require prophylactic drug therapy (Pingleton, 1983). The incidence of bleeding in intensive care units has decreased with good general management and it is now a minor problem.

Pharmacologic prophylaxis is aimed at maintaining the intragastric pH above 5.0. Antacid therapy is more effective than placebo in both low-risk and critically ill high-risk patients. However, large doses must be administered by nasogastric intubation every one to two hours, and a high percentage of patients at risk cannot tolerate antacids because of severe diarrhea, hypophosphatemia, and metabolic alkalosis (Pingleton, 1983).

Most well-controlled studies indicate that cimetidine is superior to placebo and equivalent to intensive antacid therapy for prophylaxis of stress ulcer in low-risk patients. Its value in high-risk patients is controversial (Myerson, 1984; Babb, 1984). In one major study, cimetidine was useful in low-risk patients but no more effective than placebo in high-risk critically ill patients, even when the dosage was increased (Priebe et al, 1980). In contrast, other reports indicate that cimetidine administered as an intravenous bolus dose every four to six hours (McElwee et al, 1979; Halloran et al, 1980; Peura and Johnson, 1985) or as a continuous intravenous infusion (Ostro et al, 1984; Siepler and Trudeau, 1984) may be effective in high-risk critically ill patients. Although this drug causes few adverse reactions, critically ill patients are particularly susceptible. Cimetidine and an antacid are often combined for prophylactic therapy, but any additional benefit over use of a single agent is unproved.

Sucralfate may be as effective as antacids in preventing stress ulceration and hemorrhage. Its ease of administration, low incidence of adverse effects, and low cost may make sucralfate a useful alternative to antacids (Borrero et al, 1985; Bresalier et al, 1985).

Treatment: It is difficult to assess the efficacy of drugs used to control hemorrhage since bleeding usually is self-limited. Antacids may be useful in some patients. Evidence suggests that the intermittent intravenous administration of cimetidine is ineffective in acute gastrointestinal bleeding due to stress ulcers, although continuous intravenous infusion may be helpful (Spiro and Peppercorn, 1982; *Intern Med Alert*, 1984). The role of ranitidine and sucralfate in stress ulceration and hemorrhage is under investigation.

DISORDERS OF GASTRIC EMPTYING

A variety of conditions are associated with disorders of gastric emptying, gastric atony, and/or gastric outlet obstruction; they include diabetic gastroparesis, vagotomy or partial gastric resection, reflux esophagitis, active duodenal or pyloric ulcer, bile reflux gastritis, collagen diseases, primary anorexia nervosa, and electrolyte imbalance. All produce nausea, vomiting, and abdominal distress (flatulence, bloating, epigastric fullness, or pain), which complicate management of the underlying diseases.

The pathophysiology of the deficit in gastric emptying is unclear. Various abnormalities in gastric muscle function at the cellular level, failure of neurohormonal feedback mechanisms (primarily vagal dysfunction), and psychogenic influences are involved in most disorders of gastric emptying (Malagelada, 1982; Heading, 1982; Domstad and Deland, 1982). Delayed emptying of solids due to absent or abnormal gastric antral contractions is characteristic of these disorders. Gastric emptying of liquids often is normal.

In diabetic gastroparesis, the most common disorder of gastric emptying, vomiting can result in insulin overdosage. Gastroparesis is probably due to neural regulatory dysfunction caused by enhanced sympathetic or decreased parasympathetic input to the gastric antrum. Most of these patients have long-standing insulin-dependent diabetes that has been poorly controlled for many years. In some patients, however, gastroparesis may be the only diabetic complication.

Therapy: Management of diabetic gastroparesis and other disorders of gastric emptying is similar. Hospitalization may be required if symptoms are frequent or severe. Nonpharmacologic measures include avoidance of anticholinergic drugs and ingestion of a liquid diet.

In most patients with mild symptoms, metoclopramide enhances gastric emptying and is the drug of choice. It is less useful for severe symptoms. This drug improves gastric motility, and acts centrally as an antiemetic (Harrington et al, 1983; Albibi and McCallum, 1983). (See the evaluation.)

Domperidone (investigational), an antidopaminergic drug with actions similar to those of metoclopramide, also has been used in disorders of delayed gastric emptying. It may be less effective than metoclopramide but causes fewer central nervous system effects and is less likely to cause extrapyramidal reactions (Malagelada, 1982). Bethanechol, a cholinergic drug, is being investigated as another alternative to metoclopramide.

ASPIRATION PNEUMONITIS

Aspiration pneumonitis may occur during regurgitation or vomiting when the glottal reflex is obtunded. Surgical patients especially at risk include those undergoing obstetrical procedures, those who are morbidly obese, or those who require emergency surgery. During delivery, the aspiration of gastric acid during general anesthesia is known as Mendelson's syndrome and is the chief cause of maternal death. Chronic aspiration occurs in children and adults with asthma, nocturnal cough or achalasia, and in other patients susceptible to reflux.

Treatment: Once aspiration has occurred, aggressive prompt measures are required because pulmonary damage occurs in seconds. Recommended measures include removal of particulate matter, oxygenation and positive pressure ventilation with or without positive end expiratory pressure, use of bronchodilators and other measures to maintain the airway, and replacement of intravascular volume (Cohen, 1982; Kallos et al, 1983; Wynne and Modell, 1977).

Prophylaxis: All of the following measures to decrease the risk of aspiration should be utilized when possible: Oral intake before surgery or during labor should be limited to small amounts of water. Proper anesthetic technique is essential, including adequate preoxygenation, rapid induction, and use of a muscle relaxant to facilitate endotracheal intubation. After anesthesia has been induced and a cuffed endotrachial tube is in place, a nasogastric tube can reduce the risk of aspiration during recovery (Scott, 1981; Cohen, 1982; Kallos et al, 1983; Wynne and Modell, 1977). Anesthesia itself delays gastric emptying and inhibits gastric acid secretion.

Prophylactic measures that increase the pH of the gastric contents above 2.5 have been useful in preventing aspiration pneumonitis. Reduction of gastric volume is employed much less frequently (Cohen, 1982; Kallos et al, 1983). Drugs used for prophylaxis include antacids, cimetidine, and ranitidine.

Recent studies indicate that antacids decrease morbidity but have little effect on mortality, which may reflect their inability to raise gastric pH sufficiently. Because an oral antacid is more rapid acting than cimetidine or ranitidine, it is more useful for emergency surgery. Antacids raise the gastric pH in 10 to 30 minutes. Many practitioners advocate use of a single oral dose prior to anesthesia (Cohen, 1982; Wheatley et al, 1979) or administration every two hours during labor (Wynne and Modell, 1977), but the value of frequent administration is unclear.

Magnesium trisilicate is as efficacious as aluminum-magnesium mixtures for prophylaxis of aspiration pneumonitis and is safer (Crawford and Potter, 1984), but large volumes must be used.

The clear nonparticulate antacid, sodium citrate, is preferred by many physicians for oral prophylaxis. Sodium citrate (0.3 M) has a more rapid effect than particulate antacids, mixes with gastric contents better, and there is no hazard of aspirating colloidal particles. A single dose administered 10 to 45 minutes prior to anesthesia significantly decreases the risk of aspiration (Cohen, 1982; Wrobel et al, 1982; Gibbs et al, 1982; Abboud et al, 1984).

Disadvantages of antacid administration have been demonstrated. Antacids increase gastric volume and thus increase the risk of aspiration. The presence of particulate antacids or an alkaline food mixture and uneven mixing of particulate antacids with the stomach contents increase the severity of aspiration pneumonitis.

Single-entity aluminum antacids delay gastric emptying and repeated doses may cause significant accumulation of gastric contents and subsequent aspiration (Cohen, 1982); they should not be used to prevent aspiration pneumonitis.

Disadvantages of sodium citrate include its lack of palatability and the need to prepare solutions because commercial single-entity products are not available. One commercial product, Bicitra, contains sodium citrate (0.34 M) with citric acid (0.32 M); although its buffering capacity is less than that of sodium citrate 0.3 M, preliminary results in the prophylaxis of aspiration pneumonitis are encouraging (Gibbs and Banner, 1984).

A number of controlled studies have shown that cimetidine (Cohen, 1982; Durrant and Strunin, 1982; Kallos et al, 1983; Manchikanti et al, 1982; Morison et al, 1982) or ranitidine (Durrant and Strunin, 1982; Manchikanti et al, 1984; McAuley et al, 1983; Morison et al, 1982) raises the pH of gastric contents significantly more than antacids, decreases morbidity significantly, and may decrease mortality. The use of these drugs in emergency surgery is limited because effects do not occur for 45 to 60 minutes. This lag apparently reflects the time required for pre-existing gastric acid to be emptied from the stomach.

Because existing stomach acid is unaffected by cimetidine or ranitidine, some practitioners recommend two doses: an oral dose at bedtime the night before elective surgery and another dose intramuscularly, intravenously, or orally 60 minutes before anesthesia is induced; in some studies, parenteral administration just prior to surgery produced a higher gastric pH than oral administration. To ensure continued protection during labor, cimetidine may be administered every two hours. Ranitidine's longer duration of action may obviate the need for additional doses (Durrant and Strunin, 1982; McAuley et al, 1983; Morison et al, 1982).

Combination therapy with an antacid and cimetidine or ranitidine shows promise of increasing the level of protection in both elective and emergency obstetric surgery (Gillett et al, 1984; Moir, 1983; Okasha et al, 1983).

The anticholinergic agents, atropine, glycopyrrolate [Robinul], and pirenzipine (investigational), may be useful adjuncts to antacids or H$_2$ blockers (Cohen, 1982; Dewan et al, 1982).

It is not clear if metoclopramide significantly decreases gastric volume when given with antacids (Schmidt and Jørgenson, 1984) or if it has additive actions with H$_2$ blockers or antacids (Cohen, 1982; Manchikanti et al, 1984). Nevertheless, some investigators believe that it is probably wise to administer this drug adjunctively to patients at high risk from aspiration (Cohen et al, 1984).

Drug Evaluations

H$_2$ RECEPTOR ANTAGONISTS

CIMETIDINE
[Tagamet]

CIMETIDINE HYDROCHLORIDE
[Tagamet]

ACTIONS. Cimetidine markedly reduces the volume and concentration of acid secreted both in the resting state and after stimulation by food, histamine, pentagastrin, insulin, and caffeine (Wastell and Lance, 1979). This agent protects the gastric mucosa from aspirin-induced damage as measured microscopically and by mucosal potential differences. Results of animal studies suggest that chemical erosive gastritis produced by bile salts, alcohol, antiarthritic drugs, aspirin, and urea may be diminished or prevented by cimetidine. The drug does not appear to exert a clinically significant effect on gastric motility or emptying, on lower esophageal sphincter pressure, or on secretion by the pancreas or gallbadder.

USES. Cimetidine heals gastric and duodenal ulcer. Small daily doses prevent the recurrence of duodenal ulcer in most patients as long as the drug is taken. The value of maintenance therapy in preventing recurrences of gastric ulcer for more than one year is unclear (Barr et al, 1983). The adverse effects of cimetidine when given for more than three or four years are not known.

Because the incidence of adverse effects is increased by the large doses necessary to treat Zollinger-Ellison syndrome and other gastric acid hypersecretory states (eg, systemic mastocytosis), cimetidine may be less useful than ranitidine in these disorders (Helman and Ou Tim, 1983). A few patients with Zollinger-Ellison syndrome required as much as 10.8 g daily to heal peptic ulcer and prevent recurrence (Jensen et al, 1983).

Cimetidine was as effective as an intensive course of antacids in numerous controlled comparative studies on patients with gastric ulcer and duodenal ulcer. Like antacids, it relieves symptoms but does not heal lesions in reflux esophagitis. Cimetidine is a preferred alternative for many patients who cannot or will not tolerate an intensive, prolonged antacid regimen.

Gradually decreasing responsiveness after prolonged use has been reported occasionally, but the clinical significance of this phenomenon awaits further study. Basal and postprandial serum gastrin levels increase slightly and progressively during six months of continuous therapy; however, this finding does not appear to have clinical significance, because "acid rebound" has not been reported in patients with duodenal ulcer after abrupt cessation of cimetidine.

Cimetidine has been used investigationally for stress ulcers and bleeding. It is more useful for prophylaxis than for treatment. Its value may be enhanced significantly by the use of continuous intravenous infusion (Ostro et al, 1984; Siepler and Trudeau, 1984).

Cimetidine is a useful alternative to antacids in preventing aspiration pneumonitis during childbirth and elective surgical procedures. It is less useful than antacids during emergency surgery because of its slow onset of action. This drug has been used to prevent alkalosis in patients subjected to prolonged nasogastric aspiration, especially those secreting large amounts of acid.

In patients with pancreatic insufficiency, claims have been made that the reduction in hydrochloric acid secretion induced by cimetidine enhances the efficacy of oral pancreatic enzymes. However, cimetidine is effective only in patients with low rates of gastric acid secretion, and such patients rarely require cimetidine or other adjuvants. Well-controlled studies have demonstrated that cimetidine is ineffective in acute pancreatitis and it may actually increase and prolong hyperamylasemia.

ADVERSE REACTIONS. The overall incidence of adverse reactions is low. Untoward effects during short-term trials include diarrhea, dizziness, myalgia, or rash (which is usually transient). Confusion and more severe central nervous system reactions have occurred, usually after ingestion of excessive doses, in elderly patients, or in those with renal impairment (Larsson et al, 1982); these symptoms were reversed when the drug was discontinued. Some dementia-like symptoms may reflect interaction between cimetidine and concomitantly administered psychotropic drugs or may be primary side effects.

Drug-related elevations of serum transaminase levels have been noted; no other signs of hepatic dysfunction were observed. Rarely, unexplained elevations in alkaline phosphatase levels have been reported. Slight elevations of creatinine concentrations without evidence of renal dysfunction occur during treatment; appreciable increases associated with interstitial nephritis that cleared upon discontinuation of the drug have been documented occasionally (Pitone et al, 1982; Rudnick et al, 1982).

Cimetidine is transformed to an N-nitroso compound in the stomach; in initial studies, the latter's carcinogenic potential appeared to be low but long-term studies are required.

No endocrine dysfunction was encountered, but prolactin levels may be elevated transiently after intravenous administration of cimetidine. Gynecomastia and impotence have developed in patients treated with standard doses for prolonged periods or with larger than usual doses for hypersecretory states or duodenal ulcer. Swelling and nipple tenderness were mild and did not progress after several months of therapy. In one study, a reversible reduction (but within the normal range) in sperm counts, complete impotence, and/or gynecomastia were noted in men taking cimetidine for more than two months. The effects were dose dependent in 7 of 19 patients with hypersecretion of gastric acid who received large doses of cimetidine (mean, 4.5 g/day; range, 1.2 to 10.8 g/day) for at least 12 months. They did not recur when equieffective doses of ranitidine were given (Allende et al, 1982). The proposed mechanism of these effects is antagonism of androgen receptors.

A few cases of neutropenia, leukopenia, and thrombocytopenia have been reported, and the incidence of delayed hypersensitivity reactions increased after six weeks of treatment. Fever, bradycardia, and other arrhythmias have occurred, but a direct causal relationship is difficult to verify.

In animals, cimetidine crosses the placenta and is excreted in maternal milk, but toxicity has not been found. Clinical experience is insufficient to assure the drug's safety during pregnancy.

DRUG INTERACTIONS. Antacids and metoclopramide reduce the oral bioavailability of cimetidine by 20% to 30% (Gugler et al, 1981; Sorkin and Darvey, 1983). These interactions may not be clinically significant (Hansten, 1985), but an interval of at least one hour should be maintained between the administration of either the antacid or metoclopramide and oral cimetidine.

The absorption of ketoconazole is reduced by approximately one-half when administered with cimetidine; ketoconazole should be given two hours before cimetidine (Sorkin and Darvey, 1983).

Cimetidine inhibits drug metabolizing microsomal enzymes in the liver (Hansten, 1983), which increases the plasma half-life of warfarin and similar anticoagulants, theophylline and caffeine (Broughton and Rogers, 1981), phenobarbital, phenytoin, carbamazepine, propranolol, diazepam, chlordiazepoxide, and probably prazepam and clorazepate. Benzodiazepines that are eliminated almost entirely by glucuronidation (eg, oxazepam, lorazepam) are not affected. Reduced hepatic blood flow has been reported, but the indirect methods used for measurement have been questioned and the significance of this effect is unproven. Cimetidine also impairs the disposition and elevates the serum concentrations of lidocaine and nifedipine (Hansten, 1983). Cimetidine is incompatible with aminophylline or barbiturates in intravenous solutions.

PHARMACOKINETICS. The oral bioavailability of cimetidine is approximately 70%; younger patients usually absorb the drug better than elderly individuals. Bioavailability is essentially the same after intravenous or intramuscular administration. Plasma binding is limited to about 20%.

Food delays the rate, but not the extent, of absorption; therefore, cimetidine should be administered with or just after meals to take advantage of the acid buffering effect of food and to prolong the drug's effect during the postprandial period. Peak absorption occurs in 60 to 90 minutes, and the volume of distribution is 1 L/kg. Blood levels correlate poorly with peptic ulcer healing.

Cimetidine distributes well into the central nervous system; the cerebrospinal fluid concentration is 10% to 20% of the serum concentration.

About 50% to 80% of an intravenous dose is excreted as unchanged drug; 40% of an oral dose is excreted unchanged in the urine in patients with peptic ulcer disease. Most of the remainder of the drug appears in the urine as 5-hydroxymethyl or sulfoxide metabolites. The plasma elimination half-life is about two hours; renal clearance is 400 to 600 ml/minute (Somogyi and Gugler, 1983).

DOSAGE AND PREPARATIONS.
Oral: For gastric or duodenal ulcer and reflux esophagitis, *adults*, 300 mg with or immediately after meals and at bedtime (total, 1.2 g daily) for four to six weeks. Duodenal ulcer usually heals in 4 to 6 weeks with daily treatment; gastric ulcer healing generally requires 8 to 12 weeks.

For duodenal ulcer, alternative schedules include 200 mg with meals and 400 mg at bedtime (Graham et al, 1981), 400 mg in the morning and 400 mg at bedtime (Delattre et al, 1982), or 800 mg at bedtime (Lacerte et al, 1984). Endoscopy or x-rays are used to verify healing of a gastric ulcer. Some authorities do not recommend repeated x-rays or endoscopy in patients with duodenal ulcer and consider relief of symptoms after four to six weeks the endpoint of initial therapy. For maintenance therapy, 400 mg once daily at bedtime prevents recurrence of gastric or duodenal ulcer in about 60% to 80% of patients.

Patients with the Zollinger-Ellison syndrome require indefinite treatment and the dosage must be individualized. Most responsive patients have been managed with less than 2.4 g/day (Jensen et al, 1983), but up to 10.8 g/day has been used in refractory patients. Efficacy is usually established by determining that acid output is less than 10 mEq/hr one hour before the next dose. The drug is usually administered every six to eight hours. When the total daily dose exceeds 5 or 6 g, substitution of ranitidine may be considered.

Antacids may be taken as needed to control pain with an interval of at least one hour between the administration of antacid and cimetidine.

For prevention of aspiration pneumonitis in surgical patients, see the discussion of this disorder in the Introduction.

Children, 20 to 40 mg/kg daily in divided doses has been given; however, clinical experience in children is limited, and the benefit/risk ratio should be considered carefully.

CIMETIDINE:
Tagamet (Smith Kline & French). Tablets 200, 300, and 400 mg.
CIMETIDINE HYDROCHLORIDE:
Tagamet (Smith Kline & French). Liquid 300 mg/5 ml (alcohol 2.8%).

Intravenous, Intramuscular: For short-term use in patients with severe gastric acid hypersecretory conditions (eg, Zollinger-Ellison syndrome) or peptic ulcer disease refractory to oral medication or in patients who refuse to take or cannot tolerate oral medication, the following dosages are suggested: *Adults* (intravenous), 1 to 4 mg/kg/hr is infused or 300 mg is diluted and injected over a two-minute period or infused over a 15- to 20-minute period; (intramuscular) 300 mg is given every six hours. When feasible, the dosage should be adjusted to maintain an intragastric pH greater than 5.0. Dosage should be reduced in patients with impaired renal function; if the impairment is severe, 300 mg twice daily is suggested. Oral administration should be substituted as soon as possible (eg, when signs of bleeding have been absent for 48 hours).

For prevention of aspiration pneumonitis in surgical patients, see the discussion of this disorder in the Introduction.

For prophylaxis and treatment of stress ulcers and bleeding (investigational indication), 300 to 400 mg is injected intravenously every six hours or up to 50 mg/hr (1.2 g/day) is infused (Ostro et al, 1984).

Children, see oral dosage.

CIMETIDINE HYDROCHLORIDE:
Tagamet (Smith Kline & French). Solution 150 mg/ml in 2 and 8 ml containers.

RANITIDINE HYDROCHLORIDE
[Zantac]

$$(CH_3)_2NCH_2 \underset{O}{\diagup\diagdown} CH_2SCH_2CH_2NHCNHCH_3 \quad (\overset{CHNO_2}{\underset{\|}{})}$$

ACTIONS. This H_2 blocking agent is a competitive antagonist of histamine-induced gastric acid secretion. It is 4 to 13 times more potent than cimetidine in antagonizing pentagastrin-stimulated gastric acid secretion (Helman and Ou Tim, 1983;

Hirschowitz et al, 1982). Like cimetidine, ranitidine inhibits both the volume and concentration of gastric acid induced nocturnally and by food but does not affect gastric mucus or its production and does not affect lower esophageal sphincter pressure.

USES. Ranitidine is effective for the treatment of duodenal or gastric ulcer. Investigationally, it has relieved symptoms of reflux esophagitis and prevented aspiration pneumonitis during surgery. Its value in the prophylaxis of stress ulcers and bleeding is also under investigation.

Many patients with peptic ulcers refractory to cimetidine have responded to ranitidine (Helman and Ou Tim, 1983; Danilewitz et al, 1982; Zeldis et al, 1983). Because of its greater potency and the lower incidence of adverse effects compared to cimetidine, ranitidine is the drug of choice for patients with the Zollinger-Ellison syndrome and other gastric acid hypersecretory states. The gynecomastia and impotence that occur during high-dose cimetidine therapy in patients with the Zollinger-Ellison syndrome may disappear promptly when ranitidine is substituted (Zeldis et al, 1983; Jensen et al, 1983) but may take 12 to 24 months to regress in some patients. Up to 6 g/day has been used in these patients without untoward effects.

Ranitidine is preferred to cimetidine in patients taking multiple drugs (particularly drugs whose metabolism is affected by cimetidine), patients who require very large doses of cimetidine, individuals refractory to cimetidine, those who cannot tolerate cimetidine's adverse effects, geriatric patients, and patients with severe liver or kidney dysfunction.

ADVERSE REACTIONS. Minor adverse effects occur infrequently (incidence less than 3%) and include headache and skin rashes that usually subside with continued therapy, malaise, nausea, constipation, dizziness, and abdominal pain (Zeldis et al, 1983; Helman and Ou Tim, 1983). Usual doses of ranitidine only rarely produce confusion, gynecomastia, hyperprolactinemia, sexual dysfunction, bradycardia, or hepatitis. All of these adverse effects are seen more frequently with cimetidine.

In contrast to cimetidine, ranitidine binds minimally to the hepatic mixed-function oxidase system, androgen receptors, or peripheral lymphocytes. Serum transaminase and plasma creatinine levels increase but return to normal with continued treatment. Ranitidine appears in breast milk and should be used with caution in nursing mothers.

Neither cimetidine nor ranitidine is carcinogenic in animals. The N-nitroso derivatives of ranitidine are not mutagenic, but long-term studies are required to rule out carcinogenic effects in man.

Hypersensitivity is uncommon, and no cross reaction occurred when ranitidine was given to a patient who experienced erythema annulare induced by cimetidine.

DRUG INTERACTIONS. Although ranitidine interacts with other medications much less frequently than does cimetidine, an increasing number of drug interactions is being reported (Kirch et al, 1984). Interactions with midazolam, fentanyl, nifedipine, warfarin, theophylline, and metoprolol have been observed. Mechanisms other than inhibition of P-450 hepatic drug metabolizing systems may be involved. Ranitidine may decrease the absorption of diazepam and reduce its plasma concentration by 25% (Hansten, 1983); these drugs should be administered at least one hour apart.

The concurrent administration of antacids with neutralizing capacity above 40 mEq may decrease the bioavailability of ranitidine; lower doses of antacid may not affect bioavailability. Propantheline and other anticholinergic drugs may delay the absorption and increase the peak serum concentration and bioavailability of ranitidine. Although these interactions may not be clinically significant, it is probably wise to allow at least one hour between administration of antacids or anticholinergic drugs and ranitidine.

PHARMACOKINETICS. The oral bioavailability of ranitidine is about 50% and is increased in patients with liver disease. The plasma half-life is approximately 1.7 to 3 hours in adults and is prolonged in geriatric patients and those with liver or kidney disease. Peak plasma concentrations occur within one to three hours after an oral dose of 150 mg. The apparent volume of distribution is 1.2 to 1.9 L/kg. Plasma protein binding is only 15%.

Ranitidine undergoes significant first-pass metabolism after oral administration. It is metabolized in the liver to the pharmacologically inactive desmethylranitidine, ranitidine-N-oxide, and ranitidine-S-oxide.

Less than 10% of an intravenous or oral dose is excreted as metabolites; 68% to 79% of an intravenous dose and 30% of an oral dose appear in the urine as unchanged drug. The drug and its metabolites are excreted principally in the urine; the remainder is recovered in the feces (Helman and Ou Tim, 1983; Zeldis et al, 1983). In healthy individuals, renal clearance is approximately 500 ml/minute. Ranitidine is removed by dialysis.

DOSAGE AND PREPARATIONS.
Oral: For gastric or duodenal ulcer and reflux esophagitis, *adults*, 150 mg twice daily. For duodenal ulcer, 300 mg once daily at bedtime is as effective as twice daily administration (Ireland et al, 1984). Duodenal ulcer usually heals in four to six weeks with daily treatment; gastric ulcer healing generally requires 8 to 12 weeks. Endoscopy or x-rays are used to verify healing of a gastric ulcer. Some authorities do not recommend repeated x-rays or endoscopy in patients with duodenal ulcer and consider relief of symptoms after four to six weeks the endpoint of initial therapy.

For maintenance, 150 mg at bedtime inhibits nocturnal acid secretion and prevents recurrence of gastric or duodenal ulcer (Alstead et al, 1983). Antacids may be taken as needed to control pain if an interval of at least one hour has elapsed between the administration of antacid and ranitidine.

For the Zollinger-Ellison syndrome and other gastric acid hypersecretory conditions, 150 mg twice daily or more frequently; up to 6 g/day has been given to patients with severe disease. Dosage should be individualized and continued indefinitely.

For prevention of aspiration pneumonitis in surgical patients, see the discussion of this disorder in the Introduction.

Because ranitidine is excreted primarily by the kidney, adults with impaired renal function should not receive more than 150 mg every 24 hours. Dosage may be increased with caution to 150 mg every 12 hours or more frequently if necessary. Hemodialysis reduces the level of circulating ranitidine; therefore, the timing of administration should coincide with the end of hemodialysis.

Zantac (Glaxo). Tablets 150 mg.
Intravenous: For temporary use in patients with the Zollinger-Ellison syndrome or other gastric acid hypersecretory conditions or peptic ulcer disease refractory to oral medication, or in patients who refuse to take or cannot tolerate oral medication, 50 mg every six to eight hours.

For prevention of aspiration pneumonitis in surgical patients, see the discussion of this disorder in the Introduction.

Zantac (Glaxo) Solution 25 mg/ml in 2 and 10 ml containers.

ANTACIDS

Actions: The clinically useful antacids are basic aluminum, calcium, and magnesium salts that react with hydrochloric acid to form neutral, less acidic, or poorly soluble salts. Adequate doses increase the pH of the gastric contents to 5.0 or more, thus decreasing pepsin activity and facilitating healing of peptic ulcer.

Liquid preparations are thought to be more effective than tablets. However, it has been demonstrated that some tablets have equal acid neutralizing capacity. The liquid formulation is preferred in patients with duodenal ulcer who would require a large number of tablets daily.

The acid neutralizing effect of different antacids varies widely. Antacids with high neutralizing potency in vitro are generally more efficacious in vivo. The appropriate antacid should be determined individually on the basis of patient response and acceptance. If a generic preparation is prescribed, its neutralizing capacity should be known. The dose should be determined by the mEq of hydrochloric acid neutralized rather than by the total amount of antacid ingested. See Tables 1 and 2 for the acid neutralizing capacities of antacid products.

A recent report (Hollander et al, 1984) suggests that antacids may have a cytoprotective action on gastric mucosa mediated by the release of endogenous prostaglandins. However, the precise mechanism by which antacids relieve pain has not been explained completely. They do not provide a beneficial coating on or around the ulcer crater.

Uses: For specific indications for antacids, see the discussion of the disorders in the Introduction.

Antacids also are commonly taken to treat functional symptoms, such as dyspepsia, heartburn, or so-called acid indigestion. However, hydrochloric acid is not always responsible for these symptoms, which may occur in patients with achlorhydria. There are no well-controlled studies demonstrating the effectiveness of antacids in the treatment of these functional disorders.

Aluminum hydroxide and basic aluminum carbonate are used to treat renal calculi and to control hyperphosphatemia encountered early in the course of chronic renal failure (see Chapter 49, Agents Affecting Calcium Metabolism).

Adverse Reactions and Precautions: The adverse reactions and drug interactions of antacids have been reviewed (Henry and Langman, 1981). The most common reactions associated with prolonged use are diarrhea and constipation. Magnesium salts cause diarrhea and large, frequently administered doses are not tolerated. Conversely, constipation may occur when large doses of calcium or aluminum preparations are given too often. Doses of 20 to 40 g of calcium carbonate daily are reported to cause fecal impaction; however, these amounts are well above the manufacturers' maximum recommended daily dose of 8 g. Disruption of normal bowel function can be minimized by teaching the patient how to determine the necessary balance of magnesium salts with calcium or aluminum preparations. Very few patients achieve perfect regulation of bowel function with high-dose regimens of available fixed-ratio mixtures, and further supplementation with laxative or constipating antacids is often required.

Adverse systemic effects of aluminum and magnesium occur in patients with renal insufficiency; nephrolithiasis has been encountered. Magnesium compounds can produce hypermagnesemia in patients with renal failure. Because aluminum-containing antacids delay gastric emptying, they should not be used to prevent aspiration pneumonitis (Cohen, 1982). Aluminum antacids may rarely produce intestinal obstruction in the elderly and in patients with decreased bowel motility, dehydration, or restricted fluid intake. Hemodialysis and renal transplant patients appear to be at high risk for fecal impaction when using aluminum hydroxide preparations (see the evaluations).

All antacids produce a temporary compensatory increase in the secretion of hydrochloric acid, probably because the increased gastric pH induced by antacids enhances the release of antral gastrin (Clayman, 1980; Schrumpf, 1980). Frequent administration during the early painful period maintains acid neutralization and mitigates the effect of acid rebound.

A number of aluminum or magnesium antacid preparations can be used cautiously in patients requiring a low-sodium diet; however, the exact amounts of sodium should be known when antacids are prescribed for these patients (see Tables 1 and 2).

Drug Interactions: Antacids reduce the oral bioavailability of concomitantly administered cimetidine or ranitidine (Hansten, 1985). Although this interaction may not be clinically significant, these drugs probably should be given one hour apart. Because the simultaneous administration of antacids may impair the binding of sucralfate to the ulcerated mucosa, at least 30 minutes should elapse between administration of the antacid and sucralfate.

By altering gastric and renal pH and thus the ionization of drugs, antacids may interfere with the dissolution, absorption, and excretion of concomitantly used medications. Antacids containing calcium, magnesium, or especially aluminum interfere with the absorption of the tetracyclines and possibly digoxin. Nonchelating antacids, such as sodium bicarbonate, may decrease tetracycline absorption by decreasing dissolution. If the urine is sufficiently alkalized by the aluminum-magnesium antacids, blood concentrations of quinidine may increase and concentration of aspirin may decrease because of variations in renal excretion.

Aluminum Compounds

ALUMINUM HYDROXIDE GEL

DRIED ALUMINUM HYDROXIDE GEL

ACTIONS AND USES. Aluminum hydroxide is the prototype and most commonly used aluminum compound for acid peptic disorders. The gel is a poorly soluble antacid-buffer that reacts slowly with hydrochloric acid and has low neutralizing capacity. This antacid adsorbs and temporarily inactivates pepsin, which may contribute to healing of peptic ulcer (Sepelyak et al, 1984). Aluminum ions relax gastric smooth muscle and delay gastric emptying, which prolong the duration of action. Rapid gastric emptying decreases the efficacy of more slowly reactive preparations. Preparations vary in neutralizing potency.

Aluminum hydroxide has demulcent properties that do not contribute to its effect in peptic ulcer. Its astringent action may cause release of prostaglandins. Aluminum hydroxide probably should be reserved for peptic ulcer patients who cannot tolerate magnesium-containing antacids.

ADVERSE REACTIONS AND PRECAUTIONS. The most common adverse reaction is dose-related constipation, and combined therapy with a magnesium compound is required almost invariably. The astringent action or taste of this agent may produce nausea and vomiting. If phosphate intake is low, patients receiving large doses for long periods may develop hypophosphatemia and osteomalacia.

Adverse central nervous system effects ("dialysis dementia") may occur when aluminum hydroxide is given for prolonged periods to dialysis patients. High levels of aluminum in the water of the dialysis bath have been implicated in some cases. Aluminum encephalopathy has not been described in patients taking aluminum antacids who are not being dialyzed, although patients with uremia who do not receive dialysis are at risk for aluminum intoxication if they are given aluminum-containing preparations. The concomitant use of calcium carbonate allows reduction of the dose of aluminum antacid in these patients (Alfrey, 1984).

Neutron activation analysis has demonstrated that the intestinal barrier is permeable to a heavy aluminum load and that aluminum may be deposited in the bones of patients with normal renal function.

Antacids containing aluminum should not be used to prevent aspiration pneumonitis.

DRUG INTERACTIONS. Aluminum hydroxide complexes with the tetracyclines and can interfere with the absorption or excretion of warfarin, digoxin, quinine, and quinidine. Therefore, the therapeutic effect of these drugs may be affected when antacids containing aluminum are used concomitantly.

DOSAGE AND PREPARATIONS.
Oral: The dose and frequency of administration depend upon

the disorder being treated, the frequency and severity of pain, and the degree of relief obtained.

For peptic ulcer, *adults*, 80 and 40 mEq of gel per dose for duodenal and gastric ulcer, respectively, one and three hours after meals and at bedtime. For severe symptoms, 120 mEq of gel every 30 minutes may be required; this may be given by continuous intragastric drip after dilution with two to three parts water. Similar doses should be employed for other acid peptic disorders.

Generic. Liquid and suspension (gel); tablets 500 mg (dried gel) (all forms nonprescription).
See Table 1 for trademark preparations.

BASIC ALUMINUM CARBONATE GEL

This gel reacts slowly with hydrochloric acid and is rarely used today as an antacid. It is prescribed primarily in conjunction with a low-phosphate diet to reduce elevated phosphate levels and demineralization of bones in patients with renal insufficiency and to prevent the formation of phosphatic urinary stones.

Patient compliance usually is poor, since the quantities required cause gastrointestinal discomfort, taste intolerance, and constipation. Serum levels of calcium and phosphorus should be monitored periodically in patients with impaired renal function. As with other amphoteric gels, absorption of the tetracyclines is prevented when these drugs are used concomitantly.

See also Chapter 49, Agents Affecting Calcium Metabolism.

DOSAGE AND PREPARATIONS.
Oral: For peptic ulcer, see the evaluation on Aluminum Hydroxide Gel.
See Table 1 for trademark preparations.

DIHYDROXYALUMINUM SODIUM CARBONATE

This aluminum compound is claimed to have properties of both sodium carbonate and aluminum hydroxide; sodium carbonate reacts rapidly while aluminum hydroxide has a more prolonged effect. Results of a limited number of studies have shown that this agent temporarily neutralizes gastric acid; however, there are no convincing comparative data to demonstrate its superiority to solid dosage forms of other aluminum compounds.

Constipation may occur with large doses.

DOSAGE AND PREPARATIONS.
Oral: The dose and frequency of administration depend upon the disorder being treated and the degree of relief obtained. A suggested dosage for duodenal and gastric ulcer is 80 and 40 mEq per dose, respectively. The traditional dose recommendation is *adults,* one or two tablets four or more times daily.
See Table 1 for trademark preparation.

Calcium Compounds

The calcium compound used most commonly as an antacid is calcium carbonate. Tribasic calcium phosphate has been used occasionally, but its neutralizing action is weak and of brief duration; its principal indication is as a source of calcium and phosphate in deficiency states (see Chapter 49, Agents Affecting Calcium Metabolism).

CALCIUM CARBONATE

ACTIONS AND USES. Calcium carbonate has a rapid onset of action, very high neutralizing capacity, and a relatively prolonged effect. Its use as an antacid has been abandoned, perhaps prematurely, by many gastroenterologists because of emphasis on the acid rebound and the elevation in serum gastrin level that occur after single doses. However, the calcium specificity of gastrin-stimulated acid rebound has not been proved (Clayman, 1980; Schrumpf, 1980). In the alkaline intestinal milieu, this compound may be reconstituted as insoluble calcium soaps or calcium phosphate resulting in minimal systemic absorption. Significant hypercalcemia occurs in some patients, but usually only when the recommended dosage is exceeded.

ADVERSE REACTIONS AND PRECAUTIONS. Lack of palatability is a frequent complaint of patients using the hourly regimen for active ulcer. Dose-related constipation is common when 20 to 40 g is taken daily, which is well above the manufacturers' maximum recommended daily dose of 8 g. Hemorrhoids, painful and bleeding anal fissures, or fecal impaction also may occur. Acute appendicitis has been produced by impacted calcium carbonate fecoliths. Liberation of carbon dioxide in the stomach may cause eructation and flatulence. Constipation can be minimized by substituting sufficient amounts of a magnesium preparation; a mixture of one part magnesium oxide to five parts calcium carbonate produces relatively normal stools in many patients.

The milk-alkali syndrome may occur after prolonged administration of calcium carbonate with sodium bicarbonate and/or homogenized milk containing vitamin D. This relatively rare syndrome is characterized by hypercalcemic alkalosis with normal or elevated phosphorus levels, azotemia, and normal alkaline phosphatase levels. Renal failure and metastatic calcinosis also occur; the urinary excretion of calcium is generally not increased but the calcium nephropathy that occurs suggests a relationship between hypercalciuria and calcium carbonate ingestion. Conjunctival and episcleral suffusion accompany the alkalosis, and calcium deposits (manifested by band keratopathy) are noted. Nausea is a common symptom, in part reflecting the hypercalcemia. Symptoms subside gradually following discontinuation of the antacid and/or the milk. Predisposing factors are hypertension, sarcoidosis, dehydration and electrolyte imbalance due to vomiting or aspiration of gastric contents with inadequate intravenous fluid replacement, and renal dysfunction caused by primary renal disease. Magnesium and aluminum salts have not been implicated in this syndrome.

DOSAGE AND PREPARATIONS.
Oral: The dose and frequency of administration depend upon whether an active ulcer or an interval phase is being treated. *Adults,* 1 to 4 g one and three hours after meals and at

TABLE 1.
COMPOSITION OF COMMONLY USED NONPRESCRIPTION SINGLE-ENTITY ANTACID PREPARATIONS
(per capsule, tablet, or 5 ml)

Product (Manufacturer)	Dosage Form	Acid Neutralizing Capacity OTC Method (mEq)	Active Ingredients			Sodium Content	
			Al(OH)$_3$ (mg)	Calcium Carbonate (mg)	Other (mg)	(mg)	(mEq)
ALternaGEL (Stuart)	Suspension	16	600	—		<2.5	0.109
Amphojel (Wyeth)	Suspension	40	320	—		2.3	0.1
	Tablets (0.6 g)	16	600	—		3.1	0.13
	(0.3 g)	8	300	—		1.9	0.08
Basaljel (Wyeth)	Suspension	11.5	400*	—		2.9	0.13
	Extra-Strength	11	1,000*	—		23.6	1.03
	Capsules	12	500*	—		2.7	0.12
	Tablets	12.5	500*	—		2.7	0.12
Dicarbosil (Norcliff Thayer)	Tablets	10	—	500		<2.3	<0.1
Milk of Magnesia (Glenbrook)	Suspension	13.9	—	—	Mg(OH)$_2$ 405	0.12	0.005
	Tablets	10.9	—	—	Mg(OH)$_2$ 311	0.26	0.011
Rolaids (Warner Lambert)	Tablets	7.5	—	—	Dihydroxy-aluminum Sodium Carbonate 334	53	2.30
Titralic (3M Personal Care)	Suspension	19	—	1,000	Glycine	11	0.416
	Tablets	7.5	—	420		0.3	0.013
Tums (Norcliff Thayer)	Tablets	10	—	500		<3.0	<0.130
	Extra Strength	15	—	750		<4.5	<0.19

Aluminum hydroxide equivalent, present as basic aluminum carbonate

bedtime; 2 to 4 g every hour may be required to relieve pain. The tablets should be chewed before swallowing.

> *Generic.* Powder; tablets 650 mg (both forms nonprescription). See Table 1 for trademark preparations.

Magnesium Compounds

The carbonate, hydroxide, oxide, phosphate, and trisilicate salts of magnesium are used as antacids, usually in combination with aluminum hydroxide. Magnesium trisilicate reacts slowly in gastric juice, and the stomach may empty before much of the acid is neutralized.

Magnesium salts have a laxative effect; therefore, their correct proportion in combination products will prevent or reduce the constipating effect of aluminum or calcium salts, which reciprocally control the diarrheal effect of magnesium salts. Because large doses must be given frequently to control ulcer pain, most available antacid combinations must be supplemented with aluminum or calcium salts to avoid diarrhea. Magnesium compounds are rarely tolerated as the sole antacid, because the laxative effect occurs at doses only slightly greater than those that produce the antacid effect.

Antacids containing magnesium seldom produce serious toxic effects; however, some compounds may cause hypermagnesemia in patients with severely impaired renal function.

MAGNESIUM HYDROXIDE

MAGNESIUM OXIDE

MILK OF MAGNESIA

These antacids have the same properties because magnesium oxide is hydrolyzed to the hydroxide in water. They have a high neutralizing capacity with a rapid onset of action.

For adverse reactions, see the preceding discussion on Magnesium Compounds.

DOSAGE AND PREPARATIONS.

Oral: Like all antacids with laxative properties, the dose and frequency of administration are determined by the number of substitutions for aluminum or calcium salts that result in normal stool consistency.

MAGNESIUM HYDROXIDE:
Generic. Powder (nonprescription).
MAGNESIUM OXIDE:
Generic. Capsules 140 mg; tablets 250 and 500 mg; powder in both heavy and light forms (light form suspends more readily in liquid) (all forms nonprescription).
MILK OF MAGNESIA:
Generic. Liquid, suspension, tablets (all forms nonprescription).

MAGNESIUM CARBONATE

The effect of magnesium carbonate is similar to that of the hydroxide and oxide salts, but this compound liberates carbon dioxide in the stomach during neutralization. It has a high neutralizing capacity but is rarely used alone for peptic ulcer. See Table 2 for antacid mixtures containing this agent.

For adverse reactions and precautions, see the preceding discussion on Magnesium Compounds.

Generic. Powder in both heavy and light forms (light form suspends more readily in liquid) (nonprescription).

MAGNESIUM PHOSPHATE

The action of this alkaline powder is similar to that of other magnesium preparations. Its neutralizing capacity is less than that of magnesium carbonate.

For adverse reactions and precautions, see the preceding discussion on Magnesium Compounds.

Generic. Powder (nonprescription).

Sodium Compound

SODIUM CITRATE

SODIUM CITRATE WITH CITRIC ACID

Sodium citrate is the antacid of choice for prophylaxis of aspiration pneumonitis during childbirth (Mendelson's syndrome) and other surgical procedures (Abboud et al, 1984; Gibbs et al, 1982); 30 ml of a 0.3 M solution of this clear nonparticulate antacid is rapid acting and safe in emergency surgery. Its chief drawback is lack of palatability. Commercial products containing sodium citrate alone are not available. However, a preparation of Shohl's solution containing sodium citrate with citric acid [Bicitra] has been adapted for this use (Gibbs and Banner, 1984).

Bicitra (Willen). Solution containing sodium citrate dihydrate 500 mg (0.34 M) and citric acid monohydrate 334 mg (0.32 M)/5 ml in 15, 120, 473, and 3,792 ml containers (sodium, 1 mEq/ml, equivalent to 1 mEq bicarbonate).

MIXTURES OF ANTACIDS

Products containing aluminum and/or calcium compounds with magnesium salts are more commonly used to treat peptic ulcer than single-entity antacids. The antacid effect of these combination products usually is the sum of effects of the individual components, but supplemental amounts of aluminum, calcium, or magnesium often are required to reduce constipation or diarrhea when large doses are employed. Newer formulations have been prepared in an attempt to provide a greater neutralizing action.

PREPARATIONS. See Table 2.

MIXTURES OF ANTACIDS WITH OTHER INGREDIENTS

Several products containing antacid and nonantacid ingredients are claimed to provide additional benefits. The alginic acid in *Gaviscon* forms a foam that acts as a carrier for antacids. The foam purportedly floats on top of the gastric contents and thus brings the antacids in contact with the mucosa, especially during reflux. The amount of antacid in these formulations is much less than the usual dose. The antacids do not neutralize the gastric contents but rely more on local action to produce their effect. There is no evidence that the effects of Gaviscon are more beneficial than those of conventional antacids, although some studies demonstrate that Gaviscon is at least as effective as other antacids in relieving heartburn. However, adverse effects may occur less frequently with Gaviscon than with more potent antacids. Alginic acid has no demonstrable effect on reflux esophagitis produced by acid peptic or bile reflux.

The *simethicone* present in some mixtures is claimed to alleviate symptoms of gas; however, its efficacy is doubtful and the rationale for its mechanism of action is dubious (see the evaluation on Simethicone). Simethicone has, however, been designated "safe and effective" by the FDA-OTC Antacid and Antiflatulent Review Panel (*Federal Register*, 1974). There is no convincing evidence that mixtures containing this apparently safe agent have beneficial effects other than those provided by the antacid.

PREPARATIONS. See Table 2.

MISCELLANEOUS AGENTS

METOCLOPRAMIDE
[Reglan]

ACTIONS. Metoclopramide is related structurally to procainamide but has a different spectrum of pharmacologic activity. This drug stimulates the motility of the upper gastrointestinal tract and increases the rate of gastric emptying. The exact

TABLE 2.
COMPOSITION OF COMMONLY USED NONPRESCRIPTION ANTACID MIXTURES
(per capsule, tablet, or 5 ml)

Product (Manufacturer)	Dosage Form	Acid Neutralizing Capacity OTC Method (mEq)	Active Ingredients Al(OH)$_3$ (mg)	Mg(OH)$_2$ (mg)	Mg Trisilicate (mg)	Other (mg)	Sodium Content (mg)	(mEq)
Aludrox (Wyeth)	Suspension	12	307	103	—	—	2.2	0.1
	Tablets	9.5	233	83	—	—	1.3	0.06
Calcitrel (Glenbrook)						Calcium Carbonate		
	Suspension	15.8	—	120	—	585	2.2	0.01
	Tablets	15.5	—	120	—	558	2.2	0.01
Camalox (Rorer)						Calcium Carbonate		
	Suspension	18	225	200	—	250	1.2	0.05
	Tablets	18	225	200	—	250	1.0	0.4
Delcid (Lakeside)	Suspension	42	600	665	—	—	<15	0.53
Di-Gel (Plough)	Tablets	9	282[1]	85	—	Simethicone 25	<5	0.22
	Suspension	10.5	282[2]	87	—	Simethicone 20	8.5	0.37
Gaviscon (Marion)	Suspension	3.8	31.7	—	—	Sodium Alginate 135.8 Magnesium Carbonate 137.3	39.1	1.7
	Tablets	0.5	80	—	20	Alginic Acid 200	19	0.8
Gaviscon-2 (Marion)	Tablets	—	160	—	40	Alginic Acid 400	38.3	1.6
Gelusil (Parke-Davis)	Suspension	12.0	200	200	—	Simethicone 25	0.7	0.030
	Tablets	11.0	200	200	—	Simethicone 25	0.8	0.035
Gelusil-M (Parke-Davis)	Suspension	15.0	300	200	—	Simethicone 25	1.2	0.052
	Tablets	12.5	300	200	—	Simethicone 25	1.3	0.057
Gelusil-II (Parke-Davis)	Suspension	24.0	400	400	—	Simethicone 30	1.3	0.057
	Tablets	21.0	400	400	—	Simethicone 30	2.1	0.09
Kolantyl (Lakeside)	Gel	10.5	150	150	—	—	2.2	0.095
	Wafers	10.8	180	170	—	—	2.0	0.086
Kudrox (Kremers-Urban)	Suspension	25	565	180	—	Sorbitol	<1.5	0.065
Maalox (Rorer)	Suspension	13.3	225	200	—	—	1.35	0.06
	Tablets							
	(No. 1)	9.7	200	200	—	—	0.7	0.03
	(No. 2)	11.7	400	400	—	—	1.4	0.06

(Continued on next page)

TABLE 2 (continued)

Product (Manufacturer)	Dosage Form	Acid Neutralizing Capacity OTC Method (mEq)	Active Ingredients				Sodium Content	
			Al(OH)₃ (mg)	Mg(OH)₂ (mg)	Mg Trisilicate (mg)	Other (mg)	(mg)	(mEq)
Maalox Plus (Rorer)	Suspension	13.3	225	200	—	Simethicone 25	1.2	0.05
	Tablets	11.4	200	200	—	Simethicone 25	0.8	0.03
Maalox Therapeutic Concentrate (Rorer)	Suspension	27.2	600	300	—	—	0.8	0.069
	Tablets	28.0	600	300	—	—	0.5	0.02
Mylanta (Stuart)	Suspension	12.7	200	200	—	Simethicone 20	0.68	0.03
	Tablets	11.5	200	200	—	Simethicone 20	0.77	0.03
Mylanta II (Stuart)	Suspension	25.4	400	400	—	Simethicone 40	1.14	0.06
	Tablets	23.0	400	400	—	Simethicone 40	1.3	0.06
Remegel (Warner Lambert)	Squares (chewable)	13.2	—	—	—	Aluminum Hydroxide-Magnesium Carbonate Codried Gel 476	25	1.1
Riopan (Ayerst)	Tablets	13.5	—	—	—	Magaldrate³ 480	<0.1	0.004
	Suspension	15	—	—	—	540	<0.1	0.004
Riopan Extra Strength (Ayerst)	Suspension	30	—	—	—	Magaldrate³ 1,080	0.3	0.01
Riopan Plus (Ayerst)	Tablets	13.5	—	—	—	Simethicone 20 Magaldrate³ 480	<0.1	0.004
	Suspension	15	—	—	—	Simethicone 20 Magaldrate³ 540	<0.1	0.004
Riopan Plus Extra Strength (Ayerst)	Suspension	30	—	—	—	Magaldrate³ 1,080 Simethicone 30	0.3	0.01
Silain Gel (Robins)	Suspension	15	282²	285	—	Simethicone 25	4.8	0.21
Simeco (Wyeth)	Suspension	22	365²	300	—	Simethicone 30	6.9-13.8 (usual value 9 mg)	0.3-0.6 (usual value 0.39 mEq)
WinGel (Winthrop)	Suspension	12.2	180	160	—	—	<2.5	
	Tablets	12.2	180	160	—	—	<2.5	

[1] As a coprecipitate with magnesium carbonate
[2] Equivalent to dried gel
[3] A complex of aluminum and magnesium hydroxides

mechanism of action of this dopamine antagonist has not been fully clarified. Upper gastrointestinal transit time is accelerated by increased contractions of the esophageal body, increased gastric (especially antral) contractions with coordination of antral and duodenal peristalsis, and enhanced pyloric activity and pressure. The antiemetic action may contribute to the effectiveness of metoclopramide in gastroparesis (Snape et al, 1982). Effects in the small intestine are similar to those in the esophagus and stomach. Gastric acid secretion is not affected. Gallbladder and bile duct pressure are increased, the sphincter of Oddi is relaxed, and pancreatic secretion is unaffected. No significant effect on colorectal function has been noted.

Therapeutic levels of some drugs that are absorbed primarily in the small intestine are achieved more rapidly, because metoclopramide increases the rate of gastric emptying (Harrington et al, 1983). The clinical significance of this effect has not been determined.

USES. Oral metoclopramide may relieve symptoms of mild diabetic gastroparesis; it may be less useful in patients with severe symptoms. Several studies indicate that this agent may be useful in the treatment of gastric atony occurring after vagotomy and gastric resection for peptic ulcer disease and for idiopathic gastric stasis. Investigationally, it has been used adjunctively to improve gastric emptying and prevent aspiration pneumonitis in surgical patients before and during anesthesia (Albibi and McCallum, 1983; Harrington et al, 1983; Cohen et al, 1984).

When long-term therapy is needed, intravenous administration of metoclopramide may be required initially for a few days because inadequate gastric emptying prevents passage of the drug from the stomach and inhibits absorption.

In one study, metoclopramide was effective in 60% of patients with gastroparesis. Only 25% of patients with prior gastric surgery responded to this drug; most of these patients had undergone antrectomy, which suggests that an intact antrum is important to metoclopramide's action (Pellegrini et al, 1983).

The dosage may be increased in unresponsive patients, but the incidence of adverse effects also increases. Lack of response may be due to other factors, such as concomitant treatment with narcotics or other analgesics or drugs that impair gastric motility. Mechanical obstruction contributes to delayed emptying (Pellegrini et al, 1983).

Very large doses of metoclopramide have an antiemetic effect but do not prevent motion sickness (see Chapter 14).

Intravenous metoclopramide facilitates intubation and biopsy of the small intestine and has also been used adjunctively in the radiologic examination of the stomach and small intestine in individuals with delayed gastric emptying. Its value for the latter indication is unproven in clinical trials.

Since metoclopramide increases lower esophageal sphincter pressure and enhances gastric emptying, it has been used orally to treat reflux esophagitis. It may be particularly valuable in patients with slow gastric emptying. However, data from long-term studies to establish its safety and role in the treatment of this condition are lacking.

ADVERSE REACTIONS. Usual doses cause adverse reactions in up to 20% of patients; however, the effects often are mild and are reversible after metoclopramide is withdrawn. Drowsiness and lassitude are common. Constipation, diarrhea, urticarial or maculopapular rash, brief episodes of agitation or anxiety, restlessness, dryness of the mouth, glossal or periorbital edema, hirsutism, and methemoglobinemia have been noted. A hypertensive crisis has been reported when this drug was given to a patient with pheochromocytoma.

Extrapyramidal reactions occur infrequently but are more common in the elderly and in children. They are identical to the reactions produced by phenothiazine and butyrophenone drugs. Parkinsonism, dystonic movements, and tardive dyskinesia may occur, especially after therapeutic doses are taken daily for many months (Grimes et al, 1982). Unlike parkinsonism, tardive dyskinesia is not always reversible when the drug is discontinued.

Markedly increased prolactin levels have stimulated lactation, and metoclopramide may be contraindicated in patients with breast cancer who have undergone radiation or chemotherapy.

Particular caution should be employed when metoclopramide is given to elderly or young patients. The safety of metoclopramide during pregnancy has not been established (FDA Pregnancy Category B), but its short-term use to prevent aspiration pneumonitis during childbirth (investigational indication) is apparently safe.

DRUG INTERACTIONS. The action of metoclopramide on gastrointestinal motility may be impaired by the concomitant administration of atropine or other anticholinergic agents. Metoclopramide should not be given with thioxanthene, phenothiazine, or butyrophenone compounds or to patients with extrapyramidal symptoms or epilepsy, although it has been used safely in patients with parkinsonism. Therapy should not be initiated in patients who have received tricyclic antidepressants, adrenergic agents, or monoamine oxidase inhibitors within the previous two weeks. Metoclopramide may impair the vascular effect of dopamine.

Metoclopramide reduces the oral bioavailability of cimetidine by 25% to 30% (Gugler et al, 1981); therefore, at least one hour should elapse between administration of the two drugs. The dose of cimetidine may be increased when the two drugs are administered concomitantly, but this is not preferred.

PHARMACOKINETICS. Metoclopramide is well absorbed orally; the time to peak effect is 30 to 60 minutes. The volume of distribution is 2 to 3 L/kg. The range of plasma half-life is 2.6 to 5 hours. About 85% of an oral dose appears in the urine, one-half as free drug and sulfate and glucuronide conjugates and the remainder as a major and a few minor metabolites.

DOSAGE AND PREPARATIONS.

Oral: To relieve symptoms of diabetic gastroparesis and other disorders of gastric emptying, *adults*, 10 mg given 30 minutes before meals and at bedtime. *Children and young adults*, a maximum of 0.5 mg/kg is given daily in three divided doses. *Children under 6 years* should not receive more than 0.1 mg/kg as a single dose.

   Reglan (Robins). Syrup 5 mg/5 ml (monohydrochloride); tablets 10 mg (monohydrochloride).

Intravenous, Intramuscular: The following dosages are used for severe symptoms of diabetic gastroparesis when oral administration is not practical. Intravenous injection should be carried out over one to two minutes. *Adults*, 10 mg is given 30 minutes before meals and at bedtime. *Children over 6 years and young adults*, a maximum of 0.5 mg/kg is given daily in three divided doses. *Children under 6 years* should not receive more than 0.1 mg/kg as a single dose.

Intravenous: To facilitate small bowel intubation or when delayed gastric emptying interferes with x-ray examination of the upper gastrointestinal tract or small bowel, the manufacturer's suggested dose for *adults* is 10 mg (2 ml) injected over a one- to two-minute period. For *children 6 to 14 years*, 2.5 to 5 mg; *under 6 years*, 0.1 mg/kg.

For the dosage of metoclopramide as an antiemetic, see Chapter 14, Drugs Used in Vertigo and Vomiting.

> *Reglan* (Robins). Solution 5 mg/ml (monohydrochloride) in 2, 10, and 30 ml containers.

MISOPROSTOL
[Cytotec]

ACTIONS AND USES. Misoprostol and other investigational prostaglandins are alternatives to H_2 receptor blocking drugs in refractory patients (Bond, 1984, 1985; Henahan, 1985). This PGE_1 methyl ester has both antisecretory and protective actions in the gastric mucosa. In clinical trials, misoprostol was as effective as cimetidine for short-term treatment of duodenal ulcer and appeared to be effective for healing gastric ulcer. In addition, the rate of duodenal ulcer recurrence was significantly lower in patients treated with this drug than in patients treated with cimetidine. Misoprostol has shown promise in preventing gastrointestinal irritation and peptic ulcer in patients receiving long-term therapy with aspirin or other nonsteroidal anti-inflammatory agents. Other studies are under way to determine its value in reflux esophagitis, gastritis, stress ulcers, upper gastrointestinal bleeding, and bile reflux.

ADVERSE REACTIONS AND PRECAUTIONS. This drug is generally well tolerated. Minor adverse effects include diarrhea, mild nausea, abdominal discomfort, dizziness, and headaches. Misoprostol should not be used in pregnant women or women of childbearing age. In one clinical trial, bleeding occurred in about 50% of pregnant women in the first trimester, and complete or incomplete abortion was induced in 7% of the women.

DOSAGE AND PREPARATIONS.

Oral: For duodenal ulcer, *adults*, 200 mcg four times a day or 400 mcg twice daily.

> *Cytotec* (Searle).
> (Investigational drug)

SUCRALFATE
[Carafate]

$$R = SO_3 \left[Al_2(OH)_2(H_2O)_y \right]$$

ACTIONS. Sucralfate is a complex of sulfated sucrose and aluminum hydroxide. Its healing effect for gastric and duodenal ulcers has been attributed to its ability to form a complex with proteins (primarily albumin and fibrinogen) that adheres to the ulcer to form a relatively persistent barrier against acid, pepsin, and bile acid penetration. Gastric mucosal protective actions mediated by prostaglandins (Hollander et al, 1985) and/or other endogenous compounds also may contribute to its healing effects. In addition, the sucralfate suspension adsorbs bile acids and pepsin; the enzyme activity of pepsin is reduced by about 30%.

The site of these actions is entirely local; only 2% to 5% of the sulfated disaccharide is absorbed (even in patients with mucosal lesions) and excreted in the urine. No gastric acid antisecretory action, acid-neutralizing effect, or direct stimulation of healing at ulcer sites has been demonstrated.

An earlier report (Hurwitz et al, 1982) that gastric emptying is prolonged significantly following administration of sucralfate with a liquid meal has not been corroborated (Marano et al, 1985).

USES. In controlled clinical trials, sucralfate was as effective as cimetidine or antacids in healing duodenal and gastric ulcers. When it was given prophylactically, the rate of recurrence of duodenal ulcers was decreased. Its effect in preventing recurrences of gastric ulcers is unclear (Brogden et al, 1984) but it may do so (Marks et al, 1985). This drug may be particularly valuable in uremic patients with peptic ulcers.

Sucralfate also may be useful in reflux esophagitis (Brogden et al, 1984) and in hyperphosphatemia in uremic patients (Leung et al, 1983).

In some studies (Borrero et al, 1985; Bresalier et al, 1985), administration of sucralfate by nasogastric tube was as effective as antacids in preventing stress ulcers and bleeding during the first 40 to 48 hours after hospital admission.

ADVERSE REACTIONS. The overall incidence of adverse reactions was 4.7% in studies involving 2,500 patients. The most common side effect was constipation (2.2%). Other untoward effects (no single reaction occurred in more than 0.3% of patients) were similar to those in placebo groups.

No toxicity was reported in animals after the short-term administration of maximum oral doses, and no tumorigenicity was observed after 12 times the human dose was given to animals for 24 months. Likewise, administration of 50 times the human dose to mice, rats, and rabbits revealed no teratogenic, fetotoxic, reproductive, or fertility effects. Sucralfate has not been studied in pregnant women and should be used during pregnancy only if the potential benefits outweigh the possible risks (FDA Pregnancy Category B).

DRUG INTERACTIONS. Various unconfirmed reports suggest that sucralfate may interfere with the absorption of tetracyclines, warfarin, phenytoin, cimetidine, or digoxin (*Med Lett Drugs Ther*, 1984). Sucralfate and these drugs should be given two hours apart to minimize this possibility.

DOSAGE AND PREPARATIONS.

Oral: Adults, for treatment of duodenal and peptic ulcer, 1 g four times a day (one hour before meals and at bedtime). The suggested dose for prophylaxis is 2 g daily. Antacids may be prescribed as needed for relief of pain, but they should not be taken within one-half hour before or after sucralfate. When used for reflux esophagitis, the tablets must be crushed and chewed.

> ***Carafate*** (Marion). Tablets 1 g.

SIMETHICONE

[Mylicon, Silain]

This combination of dimethylpolysiloxanes and silica gel is available as a single-entity product and in mixtures containing antacids, belladonna alkaloids, and/or digestive enzymes. Simethicone has an antifoaming action by virtue of its effect on the surface tension of gas bubbles. It is promoted to relieve the symptoms of gaseous distention occurring postoperatively or as a result of aerophagia; however, evidence from controlled studies to prove that symptoms of intestinal gas are relieved by use of this agent, alone or in combination products, is inconclusive. Simethicone eliminates mucus-embedded bubbles that interfere with visualization during gastroscopy. It does not reduce intestinal gas that may interfere with radiologic or ultrasound examination of the abdomen. No adverse reactions have been reported.

> ***Mylicon*** (Stuart). Drops 40 mg/0.6 ml; tablets (chewable) 40 and 80 mg (both forms nonprescription).
>
> ***Silain*** (Robins). Tablets 50 mg (nonprescription).

Cited References

Antacid and antiflatulent products, part II. *Federal Register* 39:19862-22140, 1974.

Medical therapy for active upper GI bleeding and prevention of rebleeding. *Intern Med Alert* 6:25-27, 1984.

Sucralfate for peptic ulcer: Reappraisal. *Med Lett Drugs Ther* 26:43-44, 1984.

Abboud TK, et al: Efficacy of clear antacid prophylaxis in obstetrics. *Acta Anaesthesiol Scand* 28:301-304, 1984.

Albibi R, McCallum RW: Metoclopramide: Pharmacology and clinical application. *Ann Intern Med* 98:86-95, 1983.

Alfrey AC: Aluminum intoxication. *N Engl J Med* 310:1113-1115, 1984.

Allende HD, et al: Cimetidine-induced impotence and gynecomastia: Reversal with ranitidine, (abstract). *Gastroenterology* 82:1007, 1982.

Alstead EM, et al: Ranitidine in prevention of gastric and duodenal ulcer relapse. *Gut* 24:418-420, 1983.

Babb RR: Cimetidine in preventing or treating acute upper gastrointestinal tract hemorrhage. *West J Med* 140:478-482, 1984.

Barr GD, et al: Two-year prospective controlled study of maintenance cimetidine and gastric ulcer. *Gastroenterology* 85:100-104, 1983.

Berger K, McCallum RW: Nifedipine in treatment of achalasia. *Ann Intern Med* 96:61-63, 1982.

Berstad A, et al: Controlled clinical trial of duodenal ulcer healing with antacid tablets. *Scand J Gastroenterol* 17:953-959, 1982.

Blackwell JN, et al: Effect of nifedipine on oesophageal motility and gastric emptying. *Digestion* 21:50-56, 1981.

Bond WS: Prostaglandins: Next generation of antiulcer agents, part I. *Facts Compar Drug Newslett* 3:89-91, 1984.

Bond WS: Prostaglandins: Next generation of antiulcer agents, part II. *Facts Compar Drug Newslett* 4:1-3, 1985.

Borrero E, et al: Comparison of antacid and sucralfate in prevention of gastrointestinal bleeding in patients who are critically ill. *Am J Med* 79(suppl 2C):62-64, 1985.

Bresalier RS, et al: Sucralfate suspension vs antacids for prophylaxis of stress-related bleeding in critically ill patients, (abstract). *Gastroenterology* 88:1334, 1985.

Brogden RN, et al: Ranitidine: Review of its pharmacology and therapeutic use in peptic ulcer disease and other allied diseases. *Drugs* 24:267-303, 1982.

Brogden RN, et al: Sucralfate: Review of its pharmacodynamic properties and therapeutic use in peptic ulcer disease. *Drugs* 27:194-209, 1984.

Broughton LJ, Rogers HJ: Decreased systemic clearance of caffeine due to cimetidine. *Br J Clin Pharmacol* 12:155-159, 1981.

Clayman CB: The carbonate affair: Chalk one up, (editorial). *JAMA* 244:2554, 1980.

Cohen SE: Aspiration syndrome. *Clin Obstet Gynecol* 9:235-254, 1982.

Cohen SE, et al: Does metoclopramide decrease volume of gastric contents in patients undergoing cesarean section? *Anesthesiology* 61:604-607, 1984.

Collen MJ, et al: Beneficial effects of pirenzepine, selective anticholinergic agent, in patients with Zollinger-Ellison syndrome, (abstract). *Gastroenterology* 82:1035, 1982.

Crawford JS, Potter SR: Magnesium trisilicate mixture BP: Its physical characteristics and effectiveness as prophylactic. *Anaesthesia* 39:535-539, 1984.

Danilewitz M, et al: Ranitidine suppression of gastric hypersecretion resistant to cimetidine. *N Engl J Med* 306:20-22, 1982.

Delattre M, et al: Treatment of duodenal ulceration: Comparative trial of cimetidine (Tagamet) at daily dosages of 800 mg (400 mg b.i.d.) and 1000 mg (250 mg q.i.d.). *Clin Trials J* 19:94-105, 1982.

Dent J: What's new in the esophagus. *Digest Dis Sci* 26:161-169, 1981.

Dewan DM, et al: Antacid anticholinergic regimens in patients undergoing elective caesarean section. *Can Anaesth Soc J* 29:27-30, 1982.

DiMario F, et al: Combined ranitidine and pirenzepine in treatment of highly recurrent duodenal ulcer. *Clin Trials J* 21:258-264, 1984.

Domstad PA, Deland FH: Management of gastric outlet obstruction. *Compr Ther* 8:17-20, (Aug) 1982.

Durrant JM, Strunin L: Comparative trial of effect of ranitidine and cimetidine on gastric secretion in fasting patients at induction of anaesthesia. *Can Anaesth Soc J* 29:446-451, 1982.

Farini R, et al: Pirenzepine and cimetidine in long-term treatment of duodenal ulcer. *Clin Trials J* 20:71-76, 1983.

Gelfond M, et al: Isosorbide dinitrate and nifedipine: Treatment of achalasia, clinical, manometric and radionuclide evaluation. *Gastroenterology* 83:963-969, 1982.

Gibbs CP, Banner TC: Effectiveness of Bicitra as preoperative antacid. *Anesthesiology* 61:97-99, 1984.

Gibbs C, et al: Effectiveness of sodium citrate as antacid. *Anesthesiology* 57:44-46, 1982.

Gillespie IE, et al: The stomach, in Gillespie IE, Thompson TJ (eds): *Gastroenterology, An Integrated Course.* New York, Churchill Livingstone, 1983, 46-91.

Gillett GB, et al: Prophylaxis against acid aspiration syndrome in obstetric practice. *Anesthesiology* 60:525, 1984.

Gledhill T, et al: Single nocturnal dose of H₂ receptor antagonist for treatment of duodenal ulcer. *Gut* 24:904-908, 1983.

Graham DY, et al: Double-blind multicenter comparison of 1,200 mg and 1,000 mg cimetidine in hospitalized and ambulatory duodenal ulcer patients. *Am J Gastroenterol* 76:500-505, 1981.

Grimes JD, et al: Adverse neurologic effects of metoclopramide. *Can Med Assoc J* 126:23-25, 1982.

Grossman MI, et al: Peptic ulcer: New therapies, new diseases. *Ann Intern Med* 95:609-627, 1981.

Gugler R, et al: Impaired cimetidine absorption due to antacids and metoclopramide. *Eur J Clin Pharmacol* 20:225-228, 1981.

Halloran LG, et al: Prevention of acute gastrointestinal complications after severe head injury: Controlled trial of cimetidine prophylaxis. *Am J Surg* 139:44-48, 1980.

Hansten PD: Drug interactions of ranitidine vs cimetidine. *Drug Interact Newslett* 3:31-34, 1983.

Hansten PD: Interactions between antiulcer medications. *Drug Interact Newslett* 5:11-14, 1985.

Harrington RA, et al: Metoclopramide: Updated review of its pharmacological properties and clinical use. *Drugs* 25:451-494, 1983.

Heading RC: Gastric emptying: Clinical perspective. *Clin Sci* 63:231-235, 1982.

Helman CA, Ou Tim L: Pharmacology and clinical efficacy of ranitidine, new H_2-receptor antagonist. *Pharmacotherapy* 3:185-192, 1983.

Henahan J: Laboratory devised prostaglandin derivatives offer antiulcer promise. *JAMA* 253:617-620, 1985.

Henry DA, Langman MJS: Adverse effects of anti-ulcer drugs. *Drugs* 21:444-459, 1981.

Hirschowitz BI, et al: Inhibition of basal acid, chloride, and pepsin secretion in duodenal ulcer by graded doses of ranitidine and atropine with studies of pharmacokinetics of ranitidine. *Gastroenterology* 82:1314-1326, 1982.

Hollander D, et al: Cytoprotective action of antacids against alcohol-induced gastric mucosal injury: Morphologic, ultrastructural and functional time sequence analysis. *Gastroenterology* 86:1114, 1984.

Hollander D, et al: Protective effect of sucralfate against alcohol-induced gastric mucosal injury in rat: Macroscopic, histologic, ultrastructural, and functional time sequence analysis. *Gastroenterology* 88:366-374, 1985.

Holloway RH, McCallum RW: Practical approach to gastroesophageal reflux. *Drug Ther* 13:151-160, 1983.

Holloway RH, et al: Upper gastrointestinal motility. I. Pathophysiologic approach to management of reflux esophagitis. *Am J Gastroenterol* 76:280-290, 1981.

Hurwitz A, et al: Prolongation of gastric emptying by sucralfate in man, (abstract). *Gastroenterology* 82:1088, 1982.

Ireland A, et al: Ranitidine 150 mg twice daily vs 300 mg nightly in treatment of duodenal ulcers. *Lancet* 2:274-276, 1984.

Isenberg JI, et al: Healing of benign gastric ulcer with low-dose antacid or cimetidine: Double-blind, randomized, placebo-controlled trial. *N Engl J Med* 308:1319-1324, 1983.

Jadhav GR, Freston JW: Peptic ulcers: Can maintenance therapy prevent relapse? *Drug Ther* 13:183-188, 1983.

Jensen RT, et al: Cimetidine-induced impotence and breast changes in patients with gastric hypersecreting states. *N Engl J Med* 308:883-887, 1983.

Jensen RT, et al: Zollinger-Ellison syndrome: NIH combined clinical staff conference. *Ann Intern Med* 98:59-75, 1983.

Kallos T, et al: Pulmonary aspiration of gastric contents, in Orkin FK, Cooperman LH (eds): *Complications in Anesthesiology*. Philadelphia, JB Lippincott, 1983, 152-164.

Kirch W, et al: Interactions and non-interactions with ranitidine. *Clin Pharmacokinet* 9:943-510, 1984.

Konturek SJ: Pharmacology and clinical use of ranitidine. *Mt Sinai J Med* 49:370-382, 1982.

Lacerte M, et al: Single daily dose of cimetidine for treatment of symptomatic duodenal ulcer. *Curr Ther Res* 35:777-782, 1984.

Laitinen S, et al: Sucralfate and alginate/antacid in reflux esophagitis. *Scand J Gastroenterol* 20:229-232, 1985.

Larsson R, et al: Pharmacokinetics of cimetidine and sulphoxide metabolite in patients with normal and impaired renal function. *Br J Clin Pharmacol* 13:163-170, 1982.

Leung ACT, et al: Aluminum hydroxide versus sucralfate as phosphate binder in uraemia. *Br Med J* 286:1379-1381, 1983.

Lewis JH: Treatment of gastric ulcer. *Arch Intern Med* 143:264-274, 1983.

Malagelada JR: Gastric emptying disorders: Clinical significance and treatment. *Drugs* 24:353-359, 1982.

Manchikanti L, et al: Cimetidine and related drugs in anesthesia. *Anesth Analg* 61:595-608, 1982.

Manchikanti L, et al: Ranitidine and metoclopramide for prophylaxis of aspiration pneumonitis in elective surgery. *Anesth Analg* 63:903-910, 1984.

Marano AR, et al: Effect of sucralfate and aluminum hydroxide gel on gastric emptying of solids and liquids. *Clin Pharmacol Ther* 37:629-632, 1985.

Marks IN, et al: Maintenance therapy with sucralfate reduces rate of gastric ulcer recurrence. *Am J Med* 79(suppl 2C):32-35, 1985.

McAuley DM, et al: Ranitidine as antacid before elective caesarean section. *Anaesthesia* 38:108-114, 1983.

McCarthy DM: Smoking and ulcers: Time to quit, (editorial). *N Engl J Med* 311:726-728, 1984.

McElwee HP, et al: Cimetidine affords protection equal to antacids in prevention of stress ulceration following thermal injury. *Surgery* 86:620-626, 1979.

Meyer GW, Castell DO: Evaluation and management of diseases of esophagus. *Am J Otolaryngol* 2:336-344, 1981.

Moir DD: Cimetidine, antacids, and pulmonary aspiration. *Anesthesiology* 59:81-83, 1983.

Morison DH, et al: Double-blind comparison of cimetidine and ranitidine as prophylaxis against gastric aspiration syndrome. *Anesth Analg* 61:988-992, 1982.

Myerson RM: Enhancing gastric mucosal defense: Possible new role for cimetidine. *Infect Surg* 3:901-907, 1984.

Nagy GS: Evaluation of carbenoxolone sodium in treatment of duodenal ulcer. *Gastroenterology* 74:7-10, 1978.

Okasha AS, et al: Cimetidine-antacid combination as premedication for elective caesarean section. *Can Anaesth Soc J* 30:593-597, 1983.

Ostro MJ, et al: Control of gastric pH with cimetidine: Boluses versus primed infusions, (abstract). *Gastroenterology* 86:1203, 1984.

Pellegrini CA, et al: Diagnosis and treatment of gastric emptying disorders: Clinical usefulness of radionuclide measurements of gastric emptying. *Am J Surg* 145:143-151, 1983.

Peters MN, Richardson CT: Stressful life events, acid hypersecretion, and ulcer disease. *Gastroenterology* 84:114-119, 1983.

Peterson WL, et al: Healing of duodenal ulcer with antacid regimen. *N Engl J Med* 297:341-345, 1977.

Peura DA, Johnson LF: Cimetidine for prevention and treatment of gastroduodenal mucosal lesions in patients in intensive care unit. *Ann Intern Med* 103:173-177, 1985.

Pingleton SK: Gastrointestinal hemorrhage. *Med Clin North Am* 67:1215-1231, 1983.

Pitone JM, et al: Cimetidine-induced acute interstitial nephritis. *Am J Gastroenterol* 77:169-171, 1982.

Priebe JH, et al: Antacid versus cimetidine in preventing acute gastrointestinal bleeding. *N Engl J Med* 302:426-430, 1980.

Richardson CT, Peterson WL: New agents for peptic ulcer. *Drug Ther* 12:145-151, 1982.

Richelson E: Tricyclic antidepressants: Therapy for ulcer and other novel uses. *Mod Med* 74-86, (Oct) 1983.

Richter JE, et al: Effects of oral calcium blocker, diltiazem, on esophageal contractions. *Digest Dis Sci* 29:649-656, 1984.

Ries RK, et al: Tricyclic antidepressant therapy for peptic ulcer disease. *Arch Intern Med* 144:566-569, 1984.

Romankiewicz JA, Reidenberg MM: Current status of cimetidine in acid-peptic disorders. *Ration Drug Ther* 15:1-5, (May) 1981.

Rudnick MR, et al: Cimetidine-induced acute renal failure. *Ann Intern Med* 96:180-182, 1982.

Saco LS, et al: Double-blind controlled trial of bethanechol and antacid versus placebo and antacid in treatment of erosive esophagitis. *Gastroenterology* 82:1369-1373, 1982.

Schmidt JF, Jørgenson BC: Effect of metoclopramide on gastric contents after preoperative ingestion of sodium citrate. *Anesth Analg* 63:841-843, 1984.

Schrumpf E: Effects of antacids on gastrin release. *Scand J Gastroenterol* 15:25-28, 1980.

Scott DB: Mendelson's syndrome, in Rugheimer E, Zindler M (eds): *Anaesthesiology. Proceedings of the 7th World Congress of Anaesthesiologists*. Princeton, Excerpta Medica, 1981, 799-801.

Sepelyak RJ, et al: Adsorption of pepsin by aluminum hydroxide. II: Pepsin inactivation. *J Pharmaceut Sci* 73:1517-1521, 1984.

Shearman DJC, Finlayson NDC: *Peptic Ulceration in Diseases of the Gastrointestinal Tract and Liver*. New York, Churchill Livingstone, 1982, 134-168.

Siepler J, Trudeau W: Treatment of UGIH by constant versus intermittent infusion of cimetidine in intensive care unit. *Gastroenterology* 86:1251, 1984.

Snape WJ Jr, et al: Metoclopramide to treat gastroparesis due to diabetes mellitus: Double-blind, controlled trial. *Ann Intern Med* 96:444-446, 1982.

Somogyi A, Gugler R: Clinical pharmacokinetics of cimetidine. *Clin Pharmacokinet* 8:463-495, 1983.

Sorkin EM, Darvey DL: Review of cimetidine drug interactions. *Drug Intell Clin Pharm* 17:110-120, 1983.

Spiro HM: Pharmacology, clinical efficacy, and adverse effects of sucralfate, nonsystemic agent for peptic ulcer. *Pharmacotherapy* 2:67-71, (March/April) 1982.

Spiro AH, Peppercorn MA: Evaluation and medical therapy of acute gastrointestinal bleeding. *Pharmacotherapy* 2:235-241, 1982.

Thanik K, et al: Bethanechol or cimetidine in treatment of symptomatic reflux esophagitis. *Arch Intern Med* 142:1479-1481, 1982.

Traube M, et al: Effects of nifedipine in achalasia and in patients with high-amplitude peristaltic esophageal contractions. *JAMA* 252:1733-1736, 1984.

Wastell C, Lance P: *Cimetidine: The Westminster Hospital Symposium 1978.* London, Churchill Livingstone, 1979.

Wesdorp ICE, et al: Reflux esophagitis: Another indication for ranitidine? *Gut* 24:921-924, 1983.

Wheatley RG, et al: Milk of magnesia is effective preinduction antacid in obstetric anesthesia. *Anesthesiology* 50:514-519, 1979.

Wilson P, Alp MH: Colloidal bismuth subcitrate tablets and placebo in chronic duodenal ulceration: Double-blind randomised trial. *Med J Aust* 1:222-223, 1982.

Wrobel J, et al: Sodium citrate: Alternative antacid for prophylaxis against aspiration pneumonitis. *Anaesth Intens Care* 10:116-119, 1982.

Wu WC, Castell DO: Gastroesophageal reflux. *Compr Ther* 9:57-63, (Nov) 1983.

Wynne JW, Modell JH: Respiratory aspiration of stomach contents. *Ann Intern Med* 87:466-474, 1977.

Zeldis JB, et al: Ranitidine: New H_2-receptor antagonist. *N Engl J Med* 309:1368-1373, 1983.

Zinner MJ, et al: Prevention of upper gastrointestinal tract bleeding in patients in intensive care unit. *Surg Gynecol Obstet* 153:214-220, 1981.

Agents Used in Disorders of the Lower Intestinal Tract

DIARRHEAL DISORDERS

Diarrhea is characterized by excessive fluidity, decreased consistency, and increased weight (more than 200 g/day) of the stool. It is almost always associated with more frequent defecation (more than three times/day) and may be acute or chronic. Causes include infection, intoxication, ischemia of the bowel, maldigestion, malabsorption, inflammation, functional disorders, tumors of the bowel, and, rarely, allergy or certain extraintestinal hormone-producing neoplasms. The readiness with which diarrhea subsides depends largely upon the underlying cause. Appropriate therapy, if indicated, depends upon proper diagnosis.

Acute severe diarrhea causes water and salt depletion that may lead to dehydration and/or electrolyte imbalance, especially hypokalemia. Even mild chronic diarrhea may produce hypokalemia with profound weakness and malaise. Cramping from intermittent spasm and gas produced by fermentation can occur. The frequency of defecation may cause unbearable discomfort when the number of bowel movements exceeds ten per day. Perianal irritation is common and hemorrhoids may be irritated.

Treatment with nonspecific antidiarrheal agents to alleviate acute, self-limited diarrhea is optional and may prolong the course of an enteric infection. Symptomatic treatment of severe acute or chronic diarrhea is justified to provide temporary relief until the cause is identified.

Dehydration can be prevented by the judicious use of fluids and electrolytes soon after symptoms appear. Patients with mild uncomplicated diarrhea should drink clear liquids to replace fluids lost in the stools and vomitus. Severely ill patients and infants require oral or intravenous rehydration with a balanced electrolyte solution containing sodium chloride and dextrose. Children should be given small amounts of oral fluids frequently. Depending on the level of dehydration, it may be necessary to administer parenteral fluids initially: 50 to 100 ml/kg over four hours, followed by 100 ml/kg every 24 hours for maintenance (Skirrow, 1984).

If commercial oral electrolyte solutions (eg, Infalyte, Lytren, Pedialyte) are not available, a mixture of 1 level teaspoon of table salt and 10 teaspoons of sugar in one quart of water is satisfactory. Potassium chloride (1/4 teaspoon) and sodium bicarbonate (1/2 teaspoon of baking soda) also may be included in this home remedy (Swedberg and Steiner, 1983; Gaginella, 1983).

Infectious Diarrhea: A variety of organisms cause acute diarrhea, and appropriate therapy depends on the diagnosis. For mild cases, antispasmodic anticholinergics, heat applied to the abdomen, and food restriction may relieve cramps and diarrhea. The intake of foods with a high fiber content (unrefined cereals, fruits, and vegetables) should be reduced and milk products and lactose-containing foods should be avoided. More vigorous efforts (eg, use of antibiotics) to treat or prevent diarrhea may lengthen the period of morbidity.

For self-limited infectious diarrhea, if antidiarrheal therapy is used, only nonspecific agents should be prescribed to prevent the development of asymptomatic carriers or antibiotic-resistant organisms. However, even nonspecific agents are seldom required except in the elderly and infants or when diarrhea is severe; dehydration may be life-threatening in these patients. The temporary avoidance of food and the use of oral or intravenous dextrose/electrolyte solutions usually maintains hydration. For severe diarrhea, hospitalization may be required to avoid or correct dehydration, electrolyte disturbances, and inadequate nutrition.

Infections with enterotoxigenic *Escherichia coli* are a common cause of brief (24 to 48 hours) self-limited diarrhea. Rotavirus and Norwalk virus also commonly cause infectious diarrhea, but antimicrobial drug therapy is *not* effective in viral infections.

Staphylococcal food poisoning produces diarrhea infrequently. Acute gastroenteritis produced by *Salmonella* infections other than typhoid is often self-limited but may be serious, especially in older patients. The use of antibiotics does not shorten the duration of illness and may even prolong the excretion of infectious organisms; however, appropriate antibiotic therapy is advisable in recurrent or severe *Salmonella* infections, particularly in patients with associated chronic illnesses, in infants, or in the elderly. Supportive therapy (replacement of fluids and electrolytes) and specific antimicrobial agents are recommended for infectious diarrhea caused by *Shigella*. *Campylobacter* causes diarrhea more often than *Salmonella* or *Shigella*; most infections resolve spontaneously, but specific drug therapy is recommended in severely ill patients who do not respond to symptomatic treatment. Isolated epidemics of diarrhea caused by *Yersinia*, salt-dependent *Vibrio parahaemolyticus*, or more common pathogens should be treated after identification of the causative organism.

There is evidence that the toxin(s) of *Clostridium difficile* cause pseudomembranous (antibiotic-associated) colitis, which is potentially fatal. Elderly patients, chronically ill debilitated individuals, or those who have undergone surgery are most vulnerable. Drug therapy is effective, but pseudomembranous colitis also has occurred during or after therapy with many antibacterial agents.

Most cases of travelers' diarrhea are due to enterotoxigenic *Escherichia coli*. Other important pathogens include *Shigella, Salmonella, Giardia*, and *Campylobacter*. Antimicrobial prophylaxis is not generally recommended because of the potential for drug resistance and adverse reactions. Prophylaxis with bismuth subsalicylate or other nonspecific antidiarrheal agents is useful only in selected individuals for whom infection poses a high risk. Most infectious disease experts prefer early treatment rather than prophylaxis. Although prompt antimicrobial therapy decreases the severity and duration of illness in most patients, many physicians question the need to treat mild infections with these drugs.

For a discussion of giardiasis and amebiasis, see Chapter 77, Antiprotozoal Agents. For a more detailed discussion on the treatment of infectious diarrhea, see Chapter 65, Antimicrobial Therapy and Chemoprophylaxis of Infectious Diseases.

Maldigestion and Malabsorption Syndromes: Patients with disaccharidase deficiencies and gluten-induced enteropathy require specific diet therapy. Individuals with symptomatic lactase deficiency often respond to lactase enzyme replacement [LactAid, Lactrase]; these products are taken in or with milk or milk products.

Dietary restriction of fat may ameliorate diarrhea associated with postsurgical vagotomy, hyperthyroidism, or lymphangiectasia and other steatorrheas. Medium-chain triglycerides are a more readily absorbable substitute for fat.

Most patients with maldigestive diarrhea caused by pancreatic insufficiency respond to replacement therapy with pancreatic enzymes (see Chapter 55, Agents Used in Disorders of the Liver, Biliary Tract, and Pancreas).

Patients who have undergone limited ileal resection (less than 100 cm) may experience diarrhea caused by bile salt malabsorption with increased colonic secretion and reduced colonic absorption of water and electrolytes. Such patients often benefit from therapy with cholestyramine resin [Questran], which binds bile acids. Patients with more extensive resection often develop short bowel syndrome with severe steatorrhea (greater than 20 g daily). These patients are not usually helped by cholestyramine but may respond to a low-fat diet with medium-chain triglycerides.

Hormonal Diarrheas: A number of hormonal or humoral substances produced in excess by certain tumors can cause moderate to severe secretory diarrhea (eg, serotonin in carcinoid syndrome; calcitonin and prostaglandins in medullary carcinoma of the thyroid; calcitonin, gastric inhibitory polypeptide, and/or vasoactive intestinal peptide in the watery diarrhea syndrome [pancreatic nonbeta cell tumors, often referred to as pancreatic cholera]; gastrin in Zollinger-Ellison syndrome; histamine in mastocytosis). Temporary intravenous parenteral nutrition may be required until surgery and/or cancer chemotherapy is initiated.

Concomitant use of indomethacin [Indocin] and prednisolone has helped control secretory diarrhea produced by pancreatic nonbeta cell tumors in a few patients (Jaffee et al, 1977). Trifluoperazine [Stelazine] (Donowitz et al, 1980) and lithium carbonate (Pandol et al, 1980) also have been utilized. Other agents that have been effective investigationally in pancreatic cholera include aspirin, clonidine [Catapres], lidamidine hydrochloride (investigational drug), and somatostatin. Indomethacin, somatostatin, or bromocriptine [Parlodel] may be useful for diarrhea associated with medullary carcinoma of the thyroid and cromolyn sodium has been given for diarrhea associated with systemic mastocytosis (Krejs and Fordtran, 1983).

INFLAMMATORY BOWEL DISEASE

Inflammatory bowel disease generally includes Crohn's disease (regional enteritis, granulomatous or Crohn's colitis) and ulcerative colitis. Focal transmural lesions in the small intestine and/or colon with extraintestinal manifestations are the principal features of Crohn's disease. Diffuse colonic mucosal lesions that extend proximally from the rectum are characteristic of ulcerative colitis. Although diarrhea is associated with both disorders, bloody diarrhea is more common in ulcerative colitis. Inflammatory bowel disease is characterized by unpredictable relapses. Intercurrent infections, possible nonessential antibiotic use, or excessive stress often increase the frequency and severity of attacks.

Individualized medical management that includes dietary control, nutritional and emotional support, and antidiarrheal and anti-inflammatory medication often controls ulcerative colitis and Crohn's disease despite the tendency to recurrence.

Surgery is indicated for ulcerative colitis when complications are severe, the response to maximal medical therapy is poor, or side effects of drugs (eg, steroids) are excessive. Colectomy and ileostomy or colectomy and ileal pouch-anal anastomosis cures ulcerative colitis. Physiologic adjustment of the bowel after ileoanal surgery may require many months and the ultimate status of this procedure is yet to be determined. Ileorectal anastomosis may be feasible when the rectum is unaffected or mildly affected.

Surgery is indicated for Crohn's disease when persistent intestinal obstruction, uncontrollable bleeding, or perforation occurs. Total colectomy and ileostomy may be required for severe colonic disease. However, surgery does not cure Crohn's disease; the recurrence rate is approximately 80% after intestinal resection and anastomosis and about 15% after colectomy and ileostomy.

Inflammatory bowel disease in children may be severe. Growth retardation is more frequent and pronounced in children with Crohn's disease than in ulcerative colitis and sometimes is permanent; many children require surgery. Nutritional intake must be increased 30% to 50% to achieve growth, but compliance may be a problem. Steroid therapy is required to allow growth in some children with active inflammation, but may retard growth if steroid-free intervals are not introduced. Alternate-day steroid therapy may control symptoms without aggravating growth retardation.

Nutritional Therapy: The usefulness of defined formula diets (DFD) and total parenteral nutrition (TPN) in patients with inflammatory bowel disease is controversial. Although it is widely used, there is little evidence that dietary therapy has any lasting benefits other than to ensure adequate nutrition (Spiro, 1983). However, the improved nutrition enhances healing capacity, immune function, and response to drugs.

Drug Therapy: Sulfasalazine [Azulfidine] is effective in acute attacks of mild to moderate ulcerative colitis, but is less effective in severe disease. Because sulfasalazine also prevents relapses of ulcerative colitis, it should not be discontinued prematurely in patients without signs of active disease.

In the National Cooperative Crohn's Disease study, the drug's usefulness for acute disease appeared to be limited to patients with colitis or ileocolitis; it did not prevent relapses in Crohn's disease. However, many physicians prescribe sulfasalazine for ileal disease and maintain therapy after remissions are achieved (Sack and Peppercorn, 1983).

Sulfasalazine is metabolized by colonic bacteria to sulfapyridine and 5-aminosalicylic acid (Azad Khan and Truelove, 1982). Current evidence suggests that 5-aminosalicylic acid is the active moiety and that most adverse reactions are due to sulfapyridine.

A variety of 5-aminosalicylic acid formulations are being investigated for use in ulcerative colitis; timed-release formulations may be more useful than standard preparations because they deliver more drug to the colon and are being investigated as alternatives to sulfasalazine in nonresponsive refractory patients or in those who cannot tolerate this drug (Dew et al, 1984). Both 5-aminosalicylic acid and 4-aminosalicylic acid (investigational agents) appear to be equally effective when administered as retention enemas in patients with distal ulcerative colitis (Selby et al, 1984).

Disodium azodisalicylic acid (investigational agent) contains two molecules of 5-aminosalicylic acid linked by an azo bond. It is cleaved by bacteria and high concentrations of 5-aminosalicylic acid are released in the distal colon. This agent appears to be effective in ulcerative colitis (Jewell and Truelove, 1981). Significant absorption of the intact diazo compound does not occur (Willoughby et al, 1982). Secretory diarrhea may be a limiting side effect.

Corticotropin (ACTH) or adrenal corticosteroids are combined with sulfasalazine to treat acute exacerbations of ulcerative colitis, and many physicians use these combinations in acute Crohn's disease despite lack of supportive evidence of their effectiveness from controlled clinical trials. Corticosteroids also are useful alone in these conditions and are usually required for moderate disease not responsive to sulfasalazine. Oral and parenteral hydrocortisone, prednisone, prednisolone, and methylprednisolone are employed. Triamcinolone and certain other fluorinated corticosteroids are not used because effective doses produce rapid, profound nitrogen loss. Most studies show that steroid maintenance therapy does not prevent relapses (Sack and Peppercorn, 1983). These agents should be withdrawn very gradually when remission has occurred. Patients with Crohn's disease may be more resistant to complete withdrawal than those with ulcerative colitis.

Severe ulcerative colitis in hospitalized patients usually requires the use of parenteral steroids, but oral forms can be effective. Large doses of prednisolone or methylprednisolone (40 to 60 mg/day) should be used initially. These drugs are less effective when courses are repeated after incomplete responses.

Some physicians utilize corticotropin (ACTH) intramuscularly in selected patients. However, corticosteroids are more effective than corticotropin in patients previously treated with these drugs. Corticotropin is more useful in patients without prior exposure to corticosteroids (Meyers, 1983), since adrenal cortical function has not been suppressed.

Judgment and experience are required to minimize the almost inevitable occurrence of adverse reactions, which are sometimes serious and increase with prolonged systemic use. Both sulfasalazine and steroids are safe for use in pregnant or nursing women.

Enema preparations containing hydrocortisone [Cortenema] or methylprednisolone [Medrol Enpak] are useful in patients with distal ulcerative colitis or proctitis, and occasionally they obviate the added need for oral steroids. Combined oral and enema steroid therapy often permits reduction of the oral dose. Moreover, the extent of adrenal suppression and other systemic adverse effects is much less with enema preparations (Sack and Peppercorn, 1983).

An open study utilizing an enema preparation of beclomethasone dipropionate showed this preparation to be as beneficial as betamethasone in patients with ulcerative colitis and hypothalamic-pituitary-adrenal suppression did not occur (Kumana et al, 1982).

An enema preparation of tixocortol pivalate (investigational agent) was as effective as glucocorticoid enemas and did not produce significant adverse effects. This steroidal agent has no glucocorticoid or mineralocorticoid actions (Friedman, 1985).

The role of immunosuppressive agents in the treatment of severe inflammatory bowel disease is controversial. Azathioprine [Imuran] and its congener, mercaptopurine [Purinethol], have been effective in the treatment and maintenance therapy of active and chronic Crohn's disease (Present et al, 1980; Sack and Peppercorn, 1983; Korelitz, 1983) and in chronic ulcerative colitis (Korelitz, 1983). Three to six months may elapse before these agents become effective when used initially. Subsequent courses of therapy produce effects more rapidly. These drugs are ineffective alone in acute active disease. Both drugs have a steroid-sparing effect and allow reduction of steroid dosage. Mercaptopurine may facilitate closure of perianal fistulas in patients with Crohn's disease.

Because the long-term safety of these drugs is unclear, it has been recommended that their use be restricted to patients with severe disease refractory to other drugs, steroid-dependent patients, patients in whom surgery is inappropriate, patients in whom surgery has been recommended, or as adjuncts to sulfasalazine, steroids, or both (Sack and Peppercorn, 1983). However, many physicians do not use immunosuppressive agents because of their potential adverse effects.

Metronidazole [Flagyl, Protostat] may be as effective as sulfasalazine in colonic Crohn's disease and is particularly useful for perianal complications (Frank et al, 1983). It should be limited to patients who do not respond to sulfasalazine or those who cannot tolerate it. The primary adverse effect is dose-related peripheral neuropathy; the possible occurrence of this disorder necessitates regular re-examination of the patient, even in the absence of symptoms. Change in taste sensation may be the earliest subjective indication of toxicity. Mutagenic, teratogenic, and carcinogenic effects have occurred in animals but not in man.

The nonspecific antidiarrheal agents (eg, codeine, loperamide [Imodium], diphenoxylate with atropine [Lomotil], bulk-forming agents) should be used only for mild disease. They are often ineffective in acute inflammatory bowel disease and may precipitate ileus or toxic megacolon if prescribed in large amounts for ill, undernourished patients.

IRRITABLE BOWEL SYNDROME

The irritable bowel syndrome is a common, recurrent, often self-limiting, physiologic or functional disorder characterized by diarrhea or constipation with abdominal pain. Gaseous distention of the bowel is not uncommon. Impaired neural coordination of colonic contractions may be responsible for this disorder (Snape, 1978). There are no objective pathologic signs and a complete history and examination should be performed, since the diagnosis often is made by exclusion.

Emotional stress aggravates this disorder and may precipitate acute episodes in many patients. The alterations in normal motility may be an exaggerated response to stress resulting from a generalized autonomic disturbance (Shearman and Finlayson, 1982). Many investigators consider the etiology to be psychological. The placebo response is high and symptoms often abate without treatment.

At least two forms of this disorder have been observed: Spastic colon (spastic colitis) is characterized by abdominal pain and constipation. In another form, painless diarrhea occurs (Shearman and Finlayson, 1982; Langman, 1982). Many patients experience alternating episodes of diarrhea and constipation and mixed forms are common.

Treatment: No diet or drug therapy is consistently more effective than placebo in the irritable bowel syndrome. The efficacy of drug therapy is difficult to demonstrate because the placebo response is high.

The value of dietary fiber is unclear. Many physicians believe that spastic colon associated with constipation or "pellet" stools may be improved by bulk-forming agents, such as psyllium, or bran. In contrast, reduction in unrefined fiber products is often helpful in patients with a tendency toward excess gas or diarrhea.

Anticholinergic drugs are widely used alone or with an antianxiety agent, but their effectiveness in irritable bowel syndrome is variable. Antianxiety drugs may block stress-induced increases in colonic motility (Narducci et al, 1982). Although anticholinergic drugs provide only short-term benefits and their adverse effects may outweigh their usefulness, small doses may be helpful. The milder anticholinergic drugs (eg, tincture of belladonna, dicyclomine) often are quite effective and produce few side effects. Potent anticholinergic drugs, such as propantheline, are undesirable. Patients most likely to respond to anticholinergic drugs have postprandial abdominal pain and constipation that are relieved when the medication is administered before meals, but these patients constitute only a relatively small portion of cases (Thompson, 1984).

Nonspecific antidiarrheal drugs, such as loperamide, may be effective in patients with loose stools, frequent bowel movements, and urgency. Loperamide also is useful in patients with alternating constipation and diarrhea (Cann et al, 1984).

NONSPECIFIC ANTIDIARRHEAL AGENTS

Opioids

Actions and Uses: The opioids are the most effective and prompt-acting nonspecific antidiarrheal agents. They probably act by slowing gastrointestinal motility and prolonging the transit time of the fecal mass to allow more time for absorption of water and electrolytes from the intestinal lumen. Codeine also interacts with central opiate receptors that regulate intestinal motility. Loperamide [Imodium] may decrease intestinal secretion by inactivating calmodulin, the calcium-dependent regulatory protein (Merritt et al, 1982). It is not known if opioids have an antisecretory action that enhances fluid and electrolyte absorption from the intestinal lumen (Gaginella, 1983; Schiller et al, 1984).

Opium tincture and paregoric (camphorated opium tincture) are much more widely used in this country than the purified alkaloids (eg, codeine), which are equally effective in equivalent doses. Paregoric may be preferable to opium tincture since the dose of the former is measured by teaspoon, while the dose of the latter is in drops. Because usual doses produce neither euphoria nor analgesia, these preparations may be prescribed for acute, self-limited diarrhea with little or no risk of dependence. However, dependence may develop if opioids are used indefinitely to treat chronic diarrhea or diarrhea associated with inflammatory bowel disease.

In a double-blind crossover study in patients with chronic diarrhea, codeine, loperamide, and diphenoxylate with atropine [Lomotil] were equally efficacious in reducing the frequency of bowel movements. However, loperamide and codeine were superior to diphenoxylate with atropine in producing a solid stool and reducing rectal urgency (Palmer et al, 1980).

Because loperamide or diphenoxylate with atropine have little abuse potential, they have become the most widely used nonspecific antidiarrheal preparations. Physical dependence has not been documented clinically for loperamide or diphenoxylate in therapeutic doses, and large doses given for long periods did not produce dependence in animals. Nevertheless, these drugs should not be prescribed for long-term, unsupervised use in dependence-prone patients.

Adverse Reactions and Precautions: The more serious untoward effects of these drugs (see Chapter 4, General Analgesics) are not encountered with usual antidiarrheal doses. The opioids, loperamide, and diphenoxylate may precipitate toxic megacolon in patients with active inflammatory bowel disease or acute colitis caused by bacteria, amebae, schistosomes, or ischemia. Although these agents may alleviate cramping and reduce the number of bowel movements in patients with acute infectious diarrhea, fluid may be sequestered in dilated loops of bowel, most often in children and adolescents. Hepatic coma has developed in patients with severe liver disease, presumably from prolonged exposure of colonic contents to urea-splitting bacteria with formation of ammonia and diminished hepatic detoxification.

It is often recommended that opioids be avoided in acute diarrheas caused by antibiotics, poisons, infectious organisms, or exotoxins until mural infection has subsided and/or it can be assumed that most of the toxic material has been eliminated. However, it is presently believed that these agents are safe when given for brief periods to patients with infectious diarrhea if significant fever and dysentery are absent (DuPont, 1983 A).

The safety of nonspecific antidiarrheal agents during pregnancy and in infants less than 1 month has not been determined. Respiratory depression has been reported after overdose of diphenoxylate with atropine in infants and young children.

Other Agents

Antisecretory Agents: Salicylates and other inhibitors of prostaglandin synthesis often have marked antisecretory effects in experimental animals. Bismuth subsalicylate stimulates absorption of fluid and electrolytes across the intestinal wall and is effective in secretory diarrhea produced by enterotoxigenic *Escherichia coli*, as well as for nonspecific diarrhea.

Lidamidine hydrochloride (investigational agent) may be the prototype for a new class of antidiarrheal agents with a unique mechanism of action. It is postulated that lidamidine, like clonidine, stimulates alpha$_2$-adrenergic receptors in the intestinal mucosa that mediate the absorption of electrolytes (Gaginella, 1983).

Hydrophilic Substances: Polycarbophil, methylcellulose, and various psyllium seed derivatives bind water and bile salts and may be effective in the symptomatic treatment of watery diarrhea. Fewer, bulkier stools may be passed more comfortably but the amount of stool is not decreased. (See also Chapter 54, Laxatives and Cathartics.)

Adsorbent Powders: The use of preparations containing bismuth subcarbonate, subgallate, subnitrate, or subsalicylate to treat diarrhea is empiric. It has been claimed that these salts adsorb intraluminal toxins, bacteria, and viruses or provide a protective coating for the mucosa, but proof of these actions has not been established.

Poorly absorbed powders, such as calcium carbonate, also retain fluid to produce a bulkier stool. However, if diarrhea subsides, impaction may follow quickly unless ample fluid intake is maintained.

Activated charcoal has been used empirically to treat diarrhea, but there are no controlled studies confirming its efficacy for this purpose. This preparation is used in poisoning caused by certain drugs (see Chapter 80, Drugs Used in the Treatment of Poisoning).

Kaolin and other hydrated aluminum silicate clays (eg, activated attapulgite) combined with pectin have been claimed to act as adsorbents and protectants. Only a few adequately controlled clinical studies demonstrate their efficacy. Results of animal studies suggest that the fluidity of the stool is decreased but total water loss appears to be unchanged and sodium and potassium loss may be exacerbated (McClung et al, 1980). Small amounts of other ingredients often are present in mixtures of kaolin and pectin, but they too are of unproved efficacy.

The adsorbents are generally quite safe, but they may interfere with the absorption of other therapeutic agents; a two- to three-hour interval is recommended between the oral administration of adsorbent powders and other drugs. Adsorbents are contraindicated in patients with suspected obstructive lesions of the bowel and in children less than 3 years of age.

The anion exchange resin, cholestyramine, binds bile acids and the toxin of *Clostridium difficile*. Cholestyramine relieves diarrhea due to excessive bile salts and may be effective for antibiotic-induced pseudomembranous colitis.

Lactobacillus: Viable *Lactobacillus* cultures [Bacid, Lactinex] are promoted for the treatment of diarrhea caused by antibiotics, and are reported to be useful in the prophylaxis of ampicillin-associated diarrhea (Gotz et al, 1979). Additional well-controlled studies to support their effectiveness are needed. It is anticipated that most of the organisms are killed by the normal gastric acidity.

Anticholinergic Antispasmodics: These drugs have been used as antidiarrheal agents, but their primary effect is to relieve cramps by reducing contractile activity. They are used most commonly as adjuncts in the treatment of the irritable bowel syndrome. Their effect on diarrhea is negligible. There is no conclusive evidence that any drug in this class exerts a selective effect on the gastrointestinal tract, although dicyclomine [Bentyl] has been promoted in such a manner.

Amebicides: Clioquinol (iodochlorhydroxyquin) and iodoquinol (diiodohydroxyquin) [Yodoxin] have been used in the prophylaxis of travelers' diarrhea but proof of their efficacy is lacking. Subacute myelo-optic neuropathy (SMON) has occurred. Since amebae cause only a small percentage of the diarrheas encountered while traveling, the indiscriminate use of such potentially toxic agents is unjustified. Clioquinol is no longer available for systemic use in the United States.

Drug Evaluations

NONSPECIFIC ANTIDIARRHEAL AGENTS

BISMUTH SUBSALICYLATE
[Pepto-Bismol]

ACTIONS AND USES. Bismuth subsalicylate binds toxins produced by *Vibrio cholerae* and *Escherichia coli*; an antimicrobial action has been demonstrated both in vitro and in vivo. It also has been suggested that the subsalicylate salt is hydrolyzed by coliforms to liberate salicylic acid, which inhibits synthesis of a prostaglandin responsible for intestinal inflammation and hypermotility. Salicylate also may have antisecretory actions and stimulate absorption of fluid and electrolytes across the intestinal wall.

This agent is useful for the symptomatic treatment of nonspecific diarrhea. Bismuth subsalicylate administered prophylactically as a suspension (DuPont et al, 1977, 1980) or as tablets (Graham et al, 1983) also reduces travelers' diarrhea. When this agent is taken shortly after the onset of diarrhea, the frequency of bowel movements is reduced and stomach cramps are relieved in diarrhea caused by enterotoxigenic *Escherichia coli* and viral infections. However, the large volume of suspension required (240 ml) and the amount of salicylate ingested (2.1 g) daily (Tolle and Elliot, 1984) may be hazardous. With a recommended daily dose of 240 ml, serum salicylate concentrations equivalent to eight aspirin tablets may result (DuPont, 1983 B). To avoid the large volume, tablets may be used (Graham et al, 1983); however, each tablet contains 350 mg of calcium carbonate, and up to 2 g of calcium is ingested daily, which occasionally causes hypercalcemia (Levine, 1983).

ADVERSE REACTIONS, PRECAUTIONS, AND INTERACTIONS. Bismuth may produce impaction in infants and elderly debilitated patients. Grayish black discoloration of the stool should not be confused with melena. Bismuth is radiopaque and may interfere with radiologic examination of the gastrointestinal tract.

Bismuth subsalicylate decreases the bioavailability of doxycycline and should be given at least two hours after this antibiotic (Ericsson et al, 1982).

DOSAGE AND PREPARATIONS.
Oral: Adults, 30 ml or two tablets; *children 3 to 6 years,* 5 ml or one-third tablet; *6 to 9 years,* 10 ml or two-thirds tablet; *9 to 12 years,* 15 ml or one tablet. This dose is repeated every 30 minutes if needed until eight doses are taken. The amount is doubled for severe diarrhea (DuPont et al, 1977). A dose of 60 ml four times daily has been administered prophylactically for three weeks to young adults.

    Generic. Powder.
    Pepto-Bismol (Procter & Gamble). Suspension 262 mg/15 ml in 120, 240, 360, and 474 ml containers; tablets (chewable) 262 mg (both forms nonprescription).

CODEINE PHOSPHATE

CODEINE SULFATE

Codeine is a purified opium alkaloid used for the short-term symptomatic treatment of mild diarrhea. Indications and contraindications are identical to those of diphenoxylate, loperamide, and the opium extracts. Drug dependence is a small but definite risk with prolonged use. Adverse reactions are similar to those produced by other opioids but are seldom encountered with usual antidiarrheal doses.

DOSAGE AND PREPARATIONS.
Oral: Adults, 15 to 60 mg every four to eight hours as needed. Codeine should not be used in *children under 12 years.*
Intramuscular: 15 to 30 mg every two to four hours as needed.
    CODEINE PHOSPHATE:
    Generic. Solution 30 mg/ml in 1, 2, and 20 ml containers and 60

mg/ml in 1 and 2 ml containers; tablets (soluble) 15, 30 and 60 mg; powder.
CODEINE SULFATE:
Generic. Powder; tablets (oral, soluble) 15, 30, and 60 mg.

DIPHENOXYLATE HYDROCHLORIDE WITH ATROPINE SULFATE
[Lomotil]

ACTIONS AND USES. This opioid is as effective as the other opium derivatives in relieving diarrhea. It limits peristalsis by inhibiting mucosal receptors, which abolishes the local mucosal peristaltic reflex, and by stimulating segmental contraction. In one controlled study, this preparation decreased frequency of bowel movements and stool volume without affecting sphincter tone or rectal continence in patients with chronic diarrhea and fecal incontinence (Harford et al, 1980).

ADVERSE REACTIONS AND PRECAUTIONS. Diphenoxylate with atropine has minimal dependence liability in recommended doses and is classified as a Schedule V substance under the Controlled Substances Act. The presence of atropine helps to prevent abuse but adds the potential for its own unpleasant side effects.

The incidence of adverse reactions is relatively low. Those reported include abdominal distention, intestinal obstruction, dilation of the colon, rash, drowsiness, dizziness, mental depression, restlessness, nausea, headache, and blurred vision.

Toxic megacolon or ileus may occur in patients with idiopathic, infectious, or ischemic colitis and may be precipitated by anticholinergic and narcotic medications; the complication is more likely in severely ill and undernourished patients. Investigationally, large doses (40 to 60 mg) of diphenoxylate have produced a morphine-like euphoria, and toxic doses may cause respiratory depression and coma. Narcotic antagonists are effective antidotes (see Chapter 80, Drugs Used in the Treatment of Poisoning). Side effects of atropine generally occur after overdosage. This preparation should be used cautiously in patients with liver disease, since delayed intestinal transport has precipitated hepatic coma in patients with cirrhosis.

DRUG INTERACTIONS. Diphenoxylate may potentiate the actions of barbiturates, opioids, and other central nervous system depressants.

DOSAGE AND PREPARATIONS.
Oral: Adults, 5 mg (two tablets) or 10 ml three or four times daily. The manufacturer recommends that Lomotil tablets not be used in *children 2 to 12 years*, and neither tablets nor liquid be used in those *under 2 years*. The dosage suggested for the liquid in *children 8 to 12 years* is 10 mg (20 ml) daily in five divided doses; *5 to 8 years*, 8 mg (16 ml) daily in four divided

doses; and *2 to 5 years*, 6 mg (12 ml) daily in three divided doses.
Lomotil (Searle), *Generic.* Each tablet or 5 ml of liquid contains diphenoxylate hydrochloride 2.5 mg and atropine sulfate 0.025 mg.

LOPERAMIDE HYDROCHLORIDE
[Imodium]

ACTIONS. This opioid is a derivative of haloperidol and resembles meperidine structurally. It has much less effect on the central nervous system than haloperidol and meperidine when effective antidiarrheal doses are used. The exact mechanism(s) and site of action have not been determined. In animal studies, loperamide's influence on gastrointestinal contractile activity resembles that of diphenoxylate and other opioids. In addition, loperamide may decrease intestinal secretion by inactivating the calcium-dependent regulatory protein, calmodulin (Merritt et al, 1982), or enhance the rate of absorption of water and electrolytes from the intestinal lumen (Sandhu et al, 1983). In man, transit time is prolonged, fecal volume is reduced, and loss of water and electrolytes is decreased; this results in decreased frequency of bowel movements and improved consistency of stools.

USES. In open clinical trials and double-blind crossover comparisons with placebo, diphenoxylate, and other opioids, loperamide was shown to be effective and had a prompt and prolonged action in both acute and chronic diarrhea. However, codeine and the opium extracts are less expensive.

Loperamide is often used for the prophylaxis and treatment of travelers' diarrhea. Large doses are often effective in acute and chronic infectious diarrhea; abdominal pain is relieved and diarrhea is reduced in patients with infection due to enterotoxigenic *Escherichia coli* and other bacteria. The usefulness of loperamide for acute infectious diarrhea in infants is unclear. One report suggests that loperamide can be life-saving in some infants with severe prolonged diarrhea unresponsive to other treatment (Sandhu et al, 1983). Opioids are not as safe or as effective as antibiotics in severe infectious diarrhea; their use should be limited to patients with mild to moderate illness who are not dehydrated (DuPont, 1983 A).

Loperamide may help to control chronic diarrhea in patients with the irritable bowel syndrome, colostomy, ileostomy, and malabsorption. This drug has been advocated to reduce the volume of ileostomy effluent, decrease the frequency of bowel movements, and improve the consistency of stools in patients with ulcerative colitis and Crohn's disease, but it should not be considered for routine use in these patients.

In patients who have undergone colectomy for ulcerative colitis (in whom no risk of recurrence exists, unlike patients with Crohn's disease), loperamide may be of value when dietary measures alone cannot control the liquidity of the effluent or when renal electrolyte loss is increased and added intestinal loss would be hazardous.

ADVERSE REACTIONS AND PRECAUTIONS. No significant adverse reactions or drug interactions have been reported. Loperamide does not potentiate the central nervous system depressant effects of barbiturates or alcohol. Toxic megacolon may be precipitated in patients with acute colitis. Opioids should not be used to treat bacterial or parasitic infection of the bowel wall when significant fever or dysentery is present because they may worsen symptoms, prolong the illness, or cause perforation. This agent should be used with caution in the presence of hepatic insufficiency or other conditions in which constipation should be avoided. No teratogenic effects have been reported.

Overdose should be treated with naloxone [Narcan] if morphine-like signs and symptoms occur.

PHARMACOKINETICS. About 40% of an oral dose of loperamide is absorbed. Experimentally, a considerable proportion of the remaining drug also is absorbed into the intestinal wall where it is desmethylated and secreted back into the lumen of the intestine (Miyazaki et al, 1982).

DOSAGE AND PREPARATIONS. The manufacturer's suggested dosages are:

Oral: For acute and chronic diarrhea, *adults,* 4 mg, followed by 2 mg after each diarrheal stool. Subsequent dosage is individualized but is usually 2 to 4 mg once or twice daily (maximum, 16 mg daily). Loperamide should be discontinued after 48 hours if no improvement is observed in patients with acute diarrhea. Chronic diarrhea is unlikely to be relieved if symptoms are not alleviated in ten days with doses of 16 mg daily.

Children 2 to 12 years, the recommended first-day dosage schedule for acute diarrhea is: (liquid only) *2 to 5 years* (13 to 20 kg), 1 mg three times; *5 to 8 years* (20 to 30 kg), 2 mg twice; *8 to 12 years* (more than 30 kg), 2 mg three times. Subsequently, 1 mg/10 kg should be administered only after a loose stool. The total daily dose should not exceed the recommended first-day dose. The pediatric dosage for chronic diarrhea has not been established. Use of loperamide in *children under 2 years* is not recommended.

Imodium (Janssen). Capsules 2 mg; liquid 1 mg/5 ml.

OPIUM TINCTURE

USES. Opium tincture is prompt-acting and useful for the symptomatic treatment of diarrhea. It is less widely used today than paregoric because the latter, despite an unpleasant taste, is more dilute and teaspoonful doses are more convenient to measure than the dropper quantities of opium tincture prescribed. However, the prescription of the tincture may be smaller in volume and the number of drops adjusted more precisely to the needs of the patient.

PRECAUTIONS. Opioids should not be used in patients with bacterial or parasitic infection of the bowel wall when significant fever or dysentery is present because they may worsen symptoms, prolong the illness, or cause perforation.

Effective antidiarrheal doses do not relieve pain or produce euphoria or dependence; however, larger doses or prolonged use may cause dependence (see Chapter 4, General Analgesics). Opium tincture is classified as a Schedule II drug under the Controlled Substances Act and is classified in FDA Pregnancy Category C.

DOSAGE AND PREPARATIONS.

Oral: 0.6 ml (range, 0.3 to 1 ml) four times daily. The maximal single dose is 1 ml every two to four hours, and no more than 6 ml should be taken in 24 hours.

Generic. Tincture 10% in 120 and 474 ml containers (alcohol 19%).

PAREGORIC

Paregoric (camphorated opium tincture) is as effective as opium tincture in equivalent doses and provides the convenience of teaspoonful dosage. It frequently is combined with other antidiarrheal agents of unproven effectiveness, thus exposing the patient to the adverse effects of the other constituents at greater expense and with no additional benefit (see the section on Mixtures).

ADVERSE REACTIONS AND PRECAUTIONS. Adverse effects are rare, but nausea and other gastrointestinal disturbances occur occasionally. Usual oral doses do not produce euphoria or analgesia, but prolonged use has produced physical dependence despite the drug's unappealing taste. Paregoric is classified as a Schedule III drug under the Controlled Substances Act.

Opioids should not be used to treat patients with bacterial or parasitic infection of the bowel wall when high fever or dysentery is present because they may worsen symptoms, prolong the illness, or cause perforation.

This drug is classified in FDA Pregnancy Category C.

DOSAGE AND PREPARATIONS.

Oral: Adults, 5 to 10 ml one to a maximum of four times daily until diarrhea is controlled. *Children,* 0.25 to 0.5 ml/kg one to a maximum of four times daily. The amount usually recommended per prescription is 30 or 60 ml.

Generic. Tincture (camphorated) containing morphine 0.4 mg/ml in 5, 60, 120, 474, and 3,792 ml containers (alcohol 45%).

SPECIFIC ANTIDIARRHEAL AGENTS

ANTI-INFECTIVE AGENTS

See the appropriate chapters of Section XI, Anti-Infective Agents. For dosages, see Chapter 65.

CHOLESTYRAMINE RESIN
[Questran]

USES. Cholestyramine may be useful when diarrhea is caused by increased concentrations of certain bile acids in the colon resulting from defective ileal reabsorption of bile acids or by deconjugation of bile acids by colonic flora in the upper small intestine. In patients with extensive ileal resections (short bowel syndrome) or those with postvagotomy diarrhea who are consuming a normal diet, cholestyramine may reduce the fluidity of diarrhea slightly but may increase steatorrhea due to excessive binding of bile salts (Duncombe et al, 1977). If steatorrhea is a problem, small amounts of cholestyramine given with a diet low in animal fats supplemented with medium-chain triglycerides and a hydrophilic colloid may control diarrhea while permitting caloric balance. Patients with severe steatorrhea (more than 20 g daily) are unlikely to respond.

Cholestyramine binds the toxin of *Clostridium difficile* and thus may be used to treat antibiotic-induced pseudomembranous colitis, although metronidazole or vancomycin is preferred in patients with moderate to severe involvement.

ADVERSE REACTIONS AND PRECAUTIONS. Cholestyramine resin may cause constipation or perianal irritation. Reduction of serum folate has been reported with long-term administration; folate, vitamin A, and vitamin D supplements may be required. For a more detailed discussion, see the evaluation on Cholestyramine Resin in Chapter 50, Agents Used to Treat Hyperlipidemia.

DOSAGE AND PREPARATIONS.
Oral: Adults, initially, 2 to 4 g three times daily; for maintenance, 4 g four times daily before meals and at bedtime. In many patients with ileal resection, the maintenance dose can be reduced to 4 g before breakfast or to 2 g before other meals. The preparation is suspended in 120 to 180 ml of water or, when necessary, in pulpy juices, mashed banana, applesauce, gelatin, or cooked cereal. The drug should never be swallowed dry because of the hazard of esophageal irritation or blockage.

Cholestyramine resin should be administered at least four hours before or one hour after other oral medications (eg, thyroid hormones, anticoagulants, digitalis glycosides) because the absorption of concurrently administered oral drugs may be decreased or delayed; moreover, when cholestyramine is withdrawn, sudden increased absorption of these drugs can produce toxicity.

> *Questran* (Mead Johnson). Powder 4 g/packet or scoopful in 9 g single-dose containers and 378 g containers.

ANTI-INFLAMMATORY DRUGS

ADRENAL CORTICOSTEROIDS (SYSTEMIC)

See the Introduction and Chapter 61, Adrenal Corticosteroids in Nonendocrine Diseases.

HYDROCORTISONE
[Cortenema]

METHYLPREDNISOLONE ACETATE
[Medrol Enpak]

USES. Retention enemas containing one of these adrenal corticosteroids are useful in the treatment of nonspecific ulcerative proctitis, proctosigmoiditis, ulcerative colitis, and Crohn's disease. They also may be of value in proctitis caused by radiation. Combined use of oral and enema preparations often permits reduction of the oral steroid dose.

Approximately 50% of the steroid is absorbed from noninflamed mucosa, but larger amounts may be absorbed if acute inflammation is present. Colonic absorption is approximately 16% of an oral dose. A beneficial effect is usually noted within 48 hours.

ADVERSE REACTIONS AND PRECAUTIONS. All of the serious toxic reactions produced by systemic adrenal corticosteroids may occur with use of these rectal preparations (see Chapter 61, Adrenal Corticosteroids in Nonendocrine Diseases). Accordingly, the same precautions should be observed. However, the extent of adrenal suppression and other systemic adverse effects is much less with enema preparations (Sack and Peppercorn, 1983).

DOSAGE AND PREPARATIONS.
Rectal: A retention enema containing hydrocortisone 100 mg or methylprednisolone acetate 40 mg is instilled once or twice daily. The enema is inserted with the patient in the left Sims's position. Since optimal absorption is achieved with prolonged retention, the patient should lie quietly for at least 30 minutes after instillation. Dosage usually is reduced over a period of weeks as improvement occurs.

> HYDROCORTISONE:
> *Cortenema* (Rowell). Retention enema 100 mg in 60 ml single-dose containers.
> METHYLPREDNISOLONE ACETATE:
> *Medrol Enpak* (Upjohn). Retention enema 40 mg.

SULFASALAZINE
[Azulfidine]

ACTIONS. The actions of sulfasalazine in inflammatory bowel disease are due to one of its constituents, 5-aminosalicylic acid. Less than 30% of an oral dose of sulfasalazine is absorbed, almost all of which re-enters the intestine with bile. Thus, the major proportion of a dose reaches the colon and is converted to sulfapyridine and 5-aminosalicylic acid by colonic bacteria (Azad Khan and Truelove, 1982). Sulfapyridine is inactive but completely absorbed and partially metabolized. The high blood levels of sulfapyridine account for almost all of the adverse reactions of sulfasalazine. Less than 50% of 5-aminosalicylic acid is absorbed; it is acetylated and eliminated rapidly in the urine. The mechanism of action of 5-aminosalicylic acid has been tentatively ascribed to inhibition of arachidonic acid cascade (prostaglandin and thromboxane metabolites). Sulfasalazine and 5-aminosalicylic acid block the lipoxygenase pathway in neutrophils, inhibit the production of prostaglandin-like agents, and may inhibit the migration of neutrophils and other inflammatory cells into the bowel wall (Sack and Peppercorn, 1983).

USES. Sulfasalazine is most effective in acute exacerbations of mild to moderate ulcerative colitis. It appears to be less effective in severe disease. Results of controlled clinical studies indicate that prophylactic use of sulfasalazine decreases the rate of recurrence in patients with chronic, idiopathic, ulcerative colitis. Because patients without overt symptoms may still have active disease, its use should not be discontinued prematurely.

This drug also may be useful as an adjunct in about 50% of patients with acute Crohn's disease; the colon appears to be more responsive than the small intestine (Sack and Peppercorn, 1983; Summers et al, 1979; Van Hees et al, 1981). A trial in recurrent Crohn's disease may be worthwhile, although most studies show that sulfasalazine does not prevent relapses.

ADVERSE REACTIONS, PRECAUTIONS, AND INTERACTIONS. Patients who acetylate sulfapyridine slowly may require smaller doses and are more likely to develop untoward effects. Generalized adverse reactions to sulfasalazine, such as nausea and vomiting, headache, abdominal discomfort, malaise, arthralgia, and anorexia, are common and often persistent, especially when daily doses exceed 2 g (Singleton et al, 1979; Azad Khan et al, 1980) or the drug is taken on an empty stomach. A reduction of dose or discontinuation of therapy may be necessary. Most patients with mild allergic reactions, such as fever or skin rash, can undergo desensitization by gradually increasing the dose (Korelitz et al, 1984; Taffett and Das, 1983).

Hypersensitivity pneumonitis, a lupus-like syndrome, and toxic hepatitis have been reported. Agranulocytosis and other blood dyscrasias occur rarely and are sometimes fatal. Both immune and nonimmune hemolytic anemia develop; the latter is more common in G6PD-deficient patients. Macrocytic anemias may be related to impaired absorption of folic acid. Desensitization should not be attempted in patients who experience serious adverse reactions. Complete blood counts should be performed periodically, particularly during the first few weeks of therapy.

A retrospective review of 531 pregnant patients suggests that prospects for normal pregnancies in women with inflammatory bowel disease who take sulfasalazine and/or steroids are better than those for patients with untreated disease and similar to those for the general population (Mogadam et al, 1981). Another study demonstrates that the prognosis for a successful pregnancy improves when the disease is controlled or in remission (Baiocco and Korelitz, 1984). Sulfasalazine is safe for use in nursing mothers.

Reversible oligospermia and infertility have been described in men treated with sulfasalazine (Rachmilewitz, 1982). These problems also have been observed in undernourished patients not receiving sulfasalazine.

Folate deficiency is common in patients treated with sulfasalazine. Therefore, adequate dietary intake of folate should be assured (Halsted et al, 1981). Sulfasalazine can impair the absorption of digoxin. An interval of two to three hours between the oral administration of these drugs is recommended.

DOSAGE AND PREPARATIONS.
Oral: Adults, initially, 0.5 g daily, increased by 0.5 g/day until a maximum of 4 g daily in divided doses is reached. For maintenance, 2 to 4 g daily is given in divided doses. *Children over 2 years,* initially, 40 to 60 mg/kg daily in four to six divided doses; for maintenance, 30 mg/kg daily in four divided doses.

The enteric-coated tablet may be used to reduce gastric irritation.

   Generic. Tablets (plain, enteric-coated) 500 mg.
   Azulfidine (Pharmacia). Suspension 250 mg/5 ml; tablets 500 mg; tablets (enteric-coated) 500 mg (*Azulfidine-EN*).

ANTICHOLINERGIC ANTISPASMODICS

ANTICHOLINERGIC COMPOUNDS

ACTIONS. Atropine, the prototype of the *naturally occurring anticholinergic agents,* competitively antagonizes the effect of acetylcholine at muscarinic sites. It does not block transmission either at the neuromuscular junction or at autonomic ganglia unless it is administered in toxic doses. This tertiary amine is readily absorbed from the gastrointestinal tract and crosses the blood-brain barrier.

Atropine reduces both the motility and secretory activity of the gastrointestinal tract. It has much less effect on the smooth muscle of the bile ducts, gallbladder, ureter, urinary bladder, and myometrium. Usual doses have only modest inhibitory action on gastric secretion. Salivary secretions are generally inhibited at doses lower than those required to affect gastrointestinal motility and gastric secretion.

The *quaternary ammonium compounds* are ionized and rarely affect the central nervous system, because they do not readily cross the blood-brain barrier. Their ionization is largely responsible for the wide individual variability in absorption noted after oral administration. Most of their actions are attributable to the antimuscarinic effect of usual therapeutic doses. Some antispasmodic actions of quaternary ammonium compounds may be due to their relatively specific ganglionic blocking effects in the gastrointestinal tract.

The *synthetic tertiary amine derivatives* have a more uniform oral bioavailability than the naturally occurring belladonna alkaloids, and central nervous system effects generally are less prominent. Although all of these derivatives have anticholinergic properties, some exhibit an additional or primary noncholinergic gastrointestinal antispasmodic effect experimentally; the mechanism of action is unknown.

Unfortunately, there are no clinically significant, clear-cut differences among the anticholinergic antispasmodics to aid in drug selection and, on a practical basis, no available anticholinergic drug has a particular advantage over others.

USES. Anticholinergic antispasmodics are occasionally useful as adjuncts in the treatment of irritable bowel syndrome, usually when postprandial abdominal pain and constipation are prominent (Ivey, 1975; Thompson, 1984). Because of a

ANTICHOLINERGIC ANTISPASMODICS

Drug	Usual Initial Dosage	Preparations
NATURALLY OCCURRING COMPOUNDS *Belladonna Alkaloids* Atropine Sulfate	*Oral, Subcutaneous: Adults*, 0.3 to 1.2 mg every 4 to 6 hours. *Subcutaneous: Children*, 0.01 mg/kg every 4 to 6 hours.	*Generic.* Solution (for injection) 0.05 mg/ml in 5 ml containers; 0.1 mg/ml in 5 and 10 ml containers; 0.3 mg/ml in 1 ml containers; 0.4 mg/ml in 0.5, 1, 20, and 30 ml containers; 0.5 mg/ml in 1, 5, and 30 ml containers; 1 mg/ml in 1 and 10 ml containers; 1.2 mg/ml in 1 ml containers; tablets (oral, soluble) 0.3, 0.4, and 0.6 mg.
l-Hyoscyamine Sulfate	*Oral: Adults*, 0.125 to 0.25 mg every 4 to 6 hours. *Children 2 to 10 years*, one-half above dosage range; *under 2 years*, one-fourth above dosage range. *Intramuscular, Subcutaneous, Intravenous: Adults*, 0.25 to 0.5 mg every 4 to 6 hours. When symptoms are controlled, oral medication is substituted. *Children*, dosage not established.	*Anaspaz* (Asher). Tablets 0.125 mg. *Levsin* (Kremers-Urban). Drops 0.125 mg/ml (alcohol 5%); elixir 0.125 mg/5 ml (alcohol 20%); tablets 0.125 mg; tablets (timed-release) [*Levsinex*] 0.375 mg; solution (for injection) 0.5 mg/ml in 1 and 10 ml containers.
Scopolamine Hydrobromide	*Oral: Adults*, 0.4 to 0.8 mg 3 or 4 times daily. *Intramuscular, Intravenous, Subcutaneous: Adults*, 0.3 to 0.6 mg as a single dose.	*Generic.* Solution (for injection) 0.3, 0.4, and 1 mg/ml in 1 ml containers.
Belladonna Extract	*Oral: Adults*, 15 mg 3 times daily.	*Generic.* Tablets 15 mg.
Belladonna Leaf	*Oral: Adults*, 30 to 200 mg.	No single-entity dosage form available; compounding necessary for prescription.
Belladonna Leaf Fluidextract	*Oral: Adults*, 0.06 ml 3 times daily.	*Generic.* Fluidextract in pint containers.
Belladonna Tincture	*Oral: Adults*, 0.6 to 1 ml 3 or 4 times daily. *Children*, 0.03 ml/kg in 3 or 4 divided doses.	*Generic.* Tincture in 120 ml and pint and gallon containers.
Bellafoline (total levorotatory alkaloids of belladonna as malates)	*Oral: Adults*, 1 or 2 tablets 3 times daily. *Children over 6 years*, ½ to 1 tablet 3 times daily. *Subcutaneous: Adults*, 0.5 to 1 ml once or twice daily.	*Bellafoline* (Sandoz). Tablets 0.25 mg; solution (for injection) 0.5 mg/ml in 1 ml containers.
QUATERNARY AMMONIUM DERIVATIVES OF NATURAL OR SEMISYNTHETIC BELLADONNA ALKALOIDS Homatropine Methylbromide	*Oral: Adults*, 2.5 to 10 mg 4 times daily. *Children*, 3 to 6 mg 4 times daily. *Infants*, 0.3 mg dissolved in water 5 or 6 times daily.	*Generic.* Powder.
Methscopolamine Bromide	*Oral: Adults*, 2.5 to 5 mg 4 times daily. Total daily dose may be increased to 30 mg, if necessary. *Children*, 0.2 mg/kg daily in 4 doses. *Intramuscular, Subcutaneous: Adults*, 0.25 to 1 mg every 6 to 8 hours until acute symptoms are controlled and patient can take oral medication. *Children*, dosage not established.	*Available generically under the name Scopolamine Methylbromide.* Solution; tablets. *Pamine* (Upjohn). Tablets 2.5 mg.

(Continued on next page)

ANTICHOLINERGIC ANTISPASMODICS (continued)

Drug	Usual Initial Dosage	Preparations
OTHER SYNTHETIC QUATERNARY AMMONIUM COMPOUNDS		
Anisotropine Methylbromide	*Oral: Adults,* 50 mg 3 times daily.	*Generic, Valpin 50* (DuPont). Tablets 50 mg.
Clidinium Bromide	*Oral: Adults,* 2.5 to 5 mg 3 or 4 times daily before meals and at bedtime. For the aged and debilitated, 2.5 mg 3 times daily before meals is recommended. *Children,* dosage not established.	*Quarzan* (Roche). Capsules 2.5 and 5 mg.
Glycopyrrolate	*Oral: Adults,* initially, 1 or 2 mg 3 times daily; for maintenance, 1 mg 2 times daily. *Children,* dosage not established. *Intramuscular, Intravenous, Subcutaneous: Adults,* 0.1 or 0.2 mg at 4-hour intervals 3 or 4 times daily. *Children,* dosage not established.	*Generic.* Tablets 1 and 2 mg. *Robinul* (Robins). Tablets 1 and 2 mg *(Forte)*; solution (for injection) 0.2 mg/ml in 1, 2, 5, and 20 ml containers.
Hexocyclium Methylsulfate	*Oral: Adults,* 25 mg 4 times daily before meals and at bedtime or timed-release preparation twice daily. Not recommended for *children.*	*Tral* (Abbott). Tablets 25 mg; tablets (timed-release) 50 mg.
Isopropamide Iodide	*Oral: Adults and children over 12 years,* initially, 5 mg every 12 hours; for patients with severe symptoms, 10 mg every 12 hours. Not recommended for *children under 12 years.*	*Darbid* (Smith Kline & French). Tablets 5 mg.
Mepenzolate Bromide	*Oral: Adults,* 1 or 2 tablets 3 times daily, preferably with meals, and 1 or 2 tablets at bedtime. Not recommended for *children.*	*Cantil* (Merrell Dow). Tablets 25 mg.
Methantheline Bromide	*Oral: Adults,* initially, 50 to 100 mg every 6 hours; dose reduced to 25 mg for patients who cannot tolerate larger doses. For maintenance, generally one-half initial dose. *Children,* 5 to 10 mg/kg daily in 4 divided doses.	*Banthine* (Searle). Tablets 50 mg.
Oxyphenonium Bromide	*Oral: Adults,* the average dose is 10 mg 4 times daily. Dosage is reduced, if indicated, depending on patient response. Initial dosage may need to be reduced in elderly and debilitated patients.	*Antrenyl* (CIBA). Tablets 5 mg.
Propantheline Bromide	*Oral: Adults,* 15 mg 3 times daily and 30 mg at bedtime. *Children,* 1.5 mg/kg daily in 4 divided doses.	*Generic.* Tablets 15 mg. *Pro-Banthine* (Searle). Tablets 7.5 and 15 mg.
SYNTHETIC TERTIARY AMINE COMPOUNDS		
Dicyclomine Hydrochloride	*Oral Intramuscular: Adults,* 10 to 20 mg 3 or 4 times daily. Solution should not be given intravenously. *Children,* 10 mg 3 or 4 times daily. *Infants,* 5 mg 3 or 4 times daily. For infants, dose diluted with equal volume of water.	*Generic.* Capsules 10 and 20 mg; syrup 10 mg/5 ml; tablets 20 mg; solution (for injection) 10 mg/ml in 2 and 10 ml containers. *Bentyl* (Merrell Dow). Capsules 10 mg; syrup 10 mg/5 ml; tablets 20 mg; solution (for injection) 10 mg/ml in 2 and 10 ml containers.
Oxyphencyclimine Hydrochloride	*Oral: Adults,* 10 mg twice daily; gradually increased to 50 mg if side effects are absent. *Children,* dosage not established.	*Daricon* (Beecham). Tablets 10 mg.

high placebo effect, it is difficult to assess their value in most patients. (See the section on Irritable Bowel Syndrome.)

Opinion is divided on the usefulness of anticholinergic antispasmodics in Crohn's disease and acute ulcerative colitis (see the section on Inflammatory Bowel Disease).

ADVERSE REACTIONS, PRECAUTIONS, AND INTERACTIONS. Untoward effects associated with therapeutic doses of anticholinergic agents include dryness of the mouth, anhidrosis, mydriasis, cycloplegia, tachycardia, constipation, dysuria, and acute urinary retention. Tolerance to some of these reactions develops with continued use and/or administration of smaller doses, but effectiveness also may be reduced. Hypersensitivity, usually manifested as rash, occurs infrequently.

Toxic doses may produce extreme dryness of the mouth accompanied by a burning sensation, dysphagia, thirst, marked photophobia, flushing in the blush area, fever, leukocytosis, rash, nausea, vomiting, tachycardia, and hypotension or hypertension. Ileus or toxic megacolon has been reported in some patients with severe inflammatory, ischemic, or amebic colitis. Physostigmine may counteract this complication (see Chapter 80, Drugs Used in the Treatment of Poisoning).

Large doses of the naturally occurring anticholinergic compounds may produce signs of central nervous system excitation (eg, restlessness, tremor, irritability, delirium, hallucinations), which may be followed by respiratory depression and death from medullary paralysis. Children are more susceptible to these toxic effects than adults.

Large doses of the quaternary ammonium compounds may cause ganglionic blockade, as evidenced by orthostatic hypotension and impotence, and toxic doses may cause respiratory arrest as a result of neuromuscular blockade. Since quaternary ammonium compounds do not readily cross the blood-brain barrier, central nervous system effects occur only rarely.

Anticholinergic drugs are contraindicated in patients with reflux esophagitis because they decrease both esophageal and gastric motility and relax the lower esophageal sphincter. They should be used with caution in patients with prostatic hypertrophy, pyloric obstruction, obstruction of the bladder neck, and congestive heart failure with tachycardia. The anticholinergic drugs may precipitate an attack of acute glaucoma in patients predisposed to angle closure because of their mydriatic effect. This has occurred occasionally after parenteral administration but only rarely after oral use. Anticholinergic drugs can be given safely to patients with open-angle glaucoma who are being treated with miotics.

Since antacids may interfere with the absorption of anticholinergic agents, these drugs should not be given concomitantly; an interval of at least one hour is suggested.

DOSAGE AND PREPARATIONS. Dosage requirements vary markedly among patients and may differ from those recommended by the manufacturers. The doses suggested in the Table are guidelines for initial therapy. The dose is usually determined by increasing the amount to just below that which causes mild adverse effects (eg, dryness of the mouth, blurred vision). It is not useful to give large doses to maximize the effect; lower doses also improve patient compliance.

Anticholinergic agents usually are administered orally before meals and at bedtime; timed-release preparations are given less frequently.

For suggested doses and preparations, see the Table.

MIXTURES

Antidiarrheal Preparations

The use of antidiarrheal mixtures containing opiates or poorly absorbed antibacterial agents (often in inadequate dosage) with adsorbents and protectants (most commonly, kaolin and pectin) and antispasmodic agents is unwarranted, since additional benefits beyond those afforded by the single effective agent are questionable and the patient is subjected to the added expense and the combined adverse effects of the individual ingredients.

The following mixtures are popular with some physicians and the laity and provide varying degrees of symptomatic relief. Preparations containing opium are classified as Schedule V substances under the Controlled Substances Act.

Corrective Mixture (Beecham). Each 5 ml of suspension contains zinc sulfocarbolate 10 mg, phenyl salicylate 22 mg, bismuth subsalicylate 85 mg, and pepsin 45 mg (alcohol 1.5%, sodium 0.13 mEq/5 ml) (nonprescription).

Corrective Mixture W/Paregoric (Beecham). Each 15 ml of suspension contains the same formulation as *Corrective Mixture* plus paregoric 1.8 ml (alcohol 2%, sodium 10.38 mEq/15 ml).

Donnagel (Robins). Each 30 ml of suspension contains kaolin 6 g, pectin 142.8 mg, hyoscyamine sulfate 0.1037 mg, atropine sulfate 0.0194 mg, and scopolamine hydrobromide 0.0065 mg (alcohol 3.8%) (nonprescription).

Donnagel PG (Robins). Each 30 ml of suspension contains the same formulation as *Donnagel* plus powdered opium 24 mg (alcohol 5%).

Kaolin with Pectin (various manufacturers). Suspension; liquid (both forms nonprescription).

Kaopectate (Upjohn). Each 30 ml of suspension contains kaolin 5.85 g and pectin 130 mg; tablets containing attapulgite 600 mg (both forms nonprescription).

Kaopectate Concentrate (Upjohn). Each 30 ml of concentrate contains kaolin 8.7 g and pectin 190 mg (nonprescription).

Parepectolin (Rorer). Each 30 ml of suspension contains opium 15 mg (paregoric equivalent 3.7 ml), pectin 162 mg, and kaolin 5.5 g (alcohol 0.69%).

Polymagma (Wyeth). Each tablet contains activated attapulgite 500 mg and pectin 45 mg (nonprescription).

Mixtures Containing Anticholinergic Antispasmodics

Many widely promoted mixtures contain anticholinergic antispasmodics and antianxiety agents (ie, benzodiazepines, hydroxyzine, meprobamate, barbiturates). Combinations containing antispasmodics and antianxiety agents may aid in the relief of the irritable bowel syndrome. If an antianxiety agent is needed, the benzodiazepines appear to be the most efficacious and safest (see Chapter 5, Drugs Used for Anxiety and Sleep Disorders). Some products also contain ergotamine, but controlled studies have not shown that this drug has any special value in gastrointestinal disorders.

Anticholinergic compounds require greater individualization of dosage than most drugs to be effective and to minimize side effects. Since the need for adjustments in the dose of the individual ingredients is seldom parallel, it often is impractical, especially during initial therapy, to utilize combination products.

The following list of commonly used preparations is for information only; inclusion in the list does not indicate approval or recommendation for use.

ANTICHOLINERGIC ANTISPASMODIC PLUS ANTIANXIETY AGENT

BENZODIAZEPINE (CHLORDIAZEPOXIDE):
Librax (Roche). Each capsule contains clidinium bromide 2.5 mg and chlordiazepoxide hydrochloride 5 mg.
HYDROXYZINE:
Enarax (Beecham). Each tablet contains oxyphencyclimine hydrochloride 5 or 10 mg and hydroxyzine hydrochloride 25 mg.
MEPROBAMATE:
Milpath (Wallace), *Pathibamate* (Lederle). Each tablet contains tridihexethyl chloride 25 mg and meprobamate 200 or 400 mg.
PHENOBARBITAL OR BUTABARBITAL:
Generic. Each tablet contains hyoscyamine hydrobromide or sulfate 0.1037 mg, atropine sulfate 0.0194 mg, scopolamine hydrobromide 0.0065 mg, and phenobarbital 16.2 mg.
Anaspaz PB (Ascher). Each tablet contains hyoscyamine sulfate 0.125 mg and phenobarbital 15 mg.
Belap (Lemmon). Each tablet contains belladonna extract 10.8 mg and phenobarbital 16.2 mg.
Belladenal (Sandoz). Each tablet or timed-release tablet (*Belladenal-S*) contains levorotatory alkaloids of belladonna as malates 0.25 mg and phenobarbital 50 mg.
Butibel (Wallace). Each tablet or 5 ml of elixir contains belladonna extract 15 mg, butabarbital sodium 15 mg, and alcohol 7% (elixir).
Chardonna-2 (Rorer). Each tablet contains belladonna extract 15 mg and phenobarbital 15 mg.
Daricon PB (Beecham). Each tablet contains oxyphencyclimine hydrochloride 5 mg and phenobarbital 15 mg.
Donnatal (Robins). Each capsule, tablet, or 5 ml of elixir contains hyoscyamine sulfate 0.1037 mg, atropine sulfate 0.0194 mg, scopolamine hydrobromide 0.0065 mg, phenobarbital 16.2 mg, and alcohol 23% (elixir); each No. 2 tablet contains same formulation as *Donnatal* except phenobarbital 32.4 mg; each tablet (timed-release) contains hyoscyamine sulfate 0.3111 mg, atropine sulfate 0.0582 mg, scopolamine hydrobromide 0.0195 mg, and phenobarbital 48.6 mg.
Kinesed (Stuart). Each tablet (chewable) contains hyoscyamine sulfate 0.12 mg, atropine sulfate 0.02 mg, scopolamine hydrobromide 0.007 mg, and phenobarbital 16 mg.
Levsin w/Phenobarbital (Kremers-Urban). Each tablet or 5 ml of elixir contains hyoscyamine sulfate 0.125 mg, phenobarbital 15 mg, and alcohol 20% (elixir); each 1 ml of drops (*Levsin-PB Drops*) contains the same formulation as elixir except alcohol 5%; each timed-release capsule (*Levsinex w/Phenobarbital*) contains hyoscyamine sulfate 0.375 mg and phenobarbital 45 mg.

ANTICHOLINERGIC ANTISPASMODIC PLUS PHENOBARBITAL PLUS ERGOTAMINE

Bellergal (Sandoz). Each tablet contains levorotatory alkaloids of belladonna as malates 0.1 mg, ergotamine tartrate 0.3 mg, and phenobarbital 20 mg; each tablet (timed-release) (*Bellergal-S*) contains levorotatory alkaloids of belladonna as malates 0.2 mg, ergotamine tartrate 0.6 mg, and phenobarbital 40 mg.

ANORECTAL PREPARATIONS

Hemorrhoids, anal fissures, and cryptitis are common and often associated with pruritus, bleeding, mucus seepage, and pain, which may become severe, especially during or just after defecation.

Composition: Some topical anorectal preparations afford symptomatic relief but none are curative (*Federal Register*, 1980). Most of these preparations contain protectants or emollients, often in combination with a local anesthetic and, sometimes, a corticosteroid, which is included for its anti-inflammatory effect. Some preparations also contain ingredients of questionable value, such as belladonna, opium, vitamins, vasoconstrictors, weak antiseptics, and astringents. Convincing data to prove that any one mixture is superior to another are lacking. The more bland, simple formulations probably are safest. None controls bleeding and none is a substitute for personal hygienic measures to keep the affected areas as clean as possible.

The local anesthetics commonly incorporated into these preparations include benzocaine, tetracaine, dibucaine, diperodon, dyclonine, lidocaine, and pramoxine. The base forms of local anesthetics can be absorbed through unbroken skin, but salt forms are absorbed only through mucosa or abraded surfaces. In some preparations, the concentration of the base is too low to be effective. Benzocaine, one of the most widely used topical anesthetics, is not absorbed through the mucosa in concentrations of less than 5% and is poorly soluble in many aqueous vehicles. (See also Chapter 15, Local Anesthetics.)

Dosage Forms: The suppository is the most common dosage form available. Some products may be applied by introduction of a multiple aperture tip into the anal canal. Thus, the medication is more likely to be applied at the site of the lesion. This overcomes the disadvantage produced when the suppository slips into the rectum to melt. However, the danger of self-inflicted trauma from misdirection of the applicator must be considered. The effectiveness of creams or ointments may be enhanced by intra-anal application up to the distal joint of the rubber-cotted finger.

Adverse Reactions: Untoward systemic effects may result from the absorption of local anesthetics, corticosteroids, or other ingredients from the anal or rectal mucosa or excoriated perianal skin. Hypersensitivity reactions with severe dermatitis may occur after topical application of local anesthetics, antiseptics, and some other drugs present in these preparations. Symptoms of overdosage are uncommon because of the small quantity of the drugs in the formulation. Fatalities have occurred when certain of these products have been ingested by infants.

Preparations: The preparations listed below are those most commonly prescribed or widely used. Those with multiple ingredients are not necessarily preferred to preparations containing topical local anesthetics with or without hydrocortisone.

Americaine (American Critical Care). Ointment containing benzocaine 20% and benzethonium chloride 0.1%; solution containing benzocaine 20% (both forms nonprescription).

Anusol (Parke-Davis). Each gram of ointment contains pramoxine hydrochloride 10 mg, benzyl benzoate 12 mg, Peruvian balsam 18 mg, and zinc oxide 110 mg; each suppository contains bismuth subgallate 2.25%, bismuth resorcin compound 1.75%, benzyl benzoate 1.2%, Peruvian balsam 1.8%, and zinc oxide 11% (both forms nonprescription).

Anusol-HC (Parke-Davis). Each gram of cream contains bismuth subgallate 22.5 mg, bismuth resorcin compound 17.5 mg, benzyl benzoate 12 mg, Peruvian balsam 18 mg, zinc oxide 110 mg, and hydrocortisone acetate 5 mg; each suppository contains same formulation as ***Anusol*** suppositories plus hydrocortisone acetate 10 mg.

Corticaine (Glaxo). Each gram of cream contains dibucaine 5 mg and hydrocortisone acetate 5 mg in a washable base.

Preparation H (Whitehall). Ointment or suppositories containing shark liver oil 3%, live yeast cell derivative (supplying 2,000 units of skin respiratory factor/30 g of ointment or suppository base), and phenylmercuric nitrate 0.01% (preservative); cleansing pads containing witch hazel 50% and glycerin 10% (all forms nonprescription).

Proctocort Cream (Reid-Rowell). Each gram of cream (buffered) contains hydrocortisone 10 mg.

Proctofoam HC (Reed & Carnrick). Aerosol foam containing pramoxine hydrochloride and hydrocortisone acetate 1% in a mucoadhesive base.

Rectal Medicone (Medicone). Each suppository contains benzocaine 130 mg, 8-hydroxyquinoline sulfate 16 mg, menthol 9 mg, zinc oxide 195 mg, and Peruvian balsam 65 mg in cocoa butter-vegetable and petroleum oil base (nonprescription).

Rectal Medicone-HC (Medicone). Each suppository contains the same formulation as ***Rectal Medicone*** plus hydrocortisone acetate 10 mg.

Tronolane (Abbott). Cream or suppositories containing pramoxine hydrochloride 1% (both forms nonprescription).

Tucks (Parke-Davis). Pads containing witch hazel 50% and glycerin 10% (nonprescription).

Wyanoids (Wyeth). Each suppository contains belladonna extract 15 mg, ephedrine sulfate 3 mg, zinc oxide, boric acid, bismuth oxyiodide, bismuth subcarbonate, and Peruvian balsam in cocoa butter and beeswax (nonprescription).

Cited References

Anorectal drug products for over-the-counter human use; establishment of monograph. *Federal Register* 45:35576-35677, 1980.

Azad Khan AK, Truelove SC: Disposition and metabolism of sulphasalazine (salicylazosulphapyridine) in man. *Br J Clin Pharmacol* 13:523-528, 1982.

Azad Khan AK, et al: Optimum dose of sulphasalazine for maintenance treatment in ulcerative colitis. *Gut* 21:232-240, 1980.

Baiocco PJ, Korelitz BI: Influence of inflammatory bowel disease and its treatment on pregnancy and fetal outcome. *J Clin Gastroenterol* 6:211-216, 1984.

Cann PA, et al: Role of loperamide and placebo in management of irritable bowel syndrome. *Digest Dis Sci* 29:239-247, 1984.

Dew MJ, et al: 5-aminosalicylic acid for treatment of inflammatory bowel disease. *Gastroenterology* 87:480-481, 1984.

Donowitz M, et al: Trifluoperazine reversal of secretory diarrhea in pancreatic cholera. *Ann Intern Med* 93:284-285, 1980.

Duncombe VM, et al: Double-blind trial of cholestyramine in postvagotomy diarrhoea. *Gut* 18:531-535, 1977.

DuPont HL: Using OTC drugs for acute diarrhea. *Drug Ther* 13:127-136, (Feb) 1983 A.

DuPont HL: Traveler's diarrhea, (letter response). *N Engl J Med* 308:464, 1983 B.

DuPont HL, et al: Symptomatic treatment of diarrhea with bismuth subsalicylate among students attending Mexican university. *Gastroenterology* 73:715-718, 1977.

DuPont HL, et al: Prevention of traveler's diarrhea (emporiatric enteritis): Prophylactic administration of subsalicylate bismuth. *JAMA* 243:237-241, 1980.

Ericsson C, et al: Influence of subsalicylate bismuth on absorption of doxycycline. *JAMA* 247:2266-2267, 1982.

Frank MS, et al: Pharmacotherapy of inflammatory bowel disease. Part 2: Metronidazole. *Postgrad Med* 74:155-160, (Dec) 1983.

Friedman G: New drugs in gastroenterology. *Mt Sinai J Med* 52:484-489, 1985.

Gaginella TS: Diarrhea: Some new aspects of pharmacotherapy. *Drug Intell Clin Pharm* 17:914-916, 1983.

Gotz V, et al: Prophylaxis against ampicillin-associated diarrhea with lactobacillus preparation. *Am J Hosp Pharm* 36:754-757, 1979.

Graham DY, et al: Double-blind comparison of bismuth subsalicylate and placebo in prevention and treatment of enterotoxigenic *Escherichia coli*-induced diarrhea in volunteers. *Gastroenterology* 85:1017-1022, 1983.

Halsted CH, et al: Sulfasalazine inhibits absorption of folates in ulcerative colitis. *N Engl J Med* 305:1513-1517, 1981.

Harford WV, et al: Acute effect of diphenoxylate with atropine (Lomotil) in patients with chronic diarrhea and fecal incontinence. *Gastroenterology* 78:440-443, 1980.

Ivey KJ: Are anticholinergics of use in irritable colon syndrome? *Gastroenterology* 68:1300-1307, 1975.

Jaffee BM, et al: Indomethacin-responsive pancreatic cholera. *N Engl J Med* 297:817-821, 1977.

Jewell DP, Truelove SC: Disodium azodisalicylate in ulcerative colitis. *Lancet* 2:1168-1169, 1981.

Korelitz BI: Role of immunosuppressives. *Mt Sinai J Med* 50:144-147, 1983.

Korelitz BI, et al: Desensitization to sulfasalazine after hypersensitivity reactions in patients with inflammatory bowel disease. *J Clin Gastroenterol* 6:27-31, 1984.

Krejs GJ, Fordtran JA: Diarrhea, in Sleisenger MH, Fordtran JS (eds): *Gastrointestinal Disease*. Philadelphia, WB Saunders, 1983, 257-280.

Kumana CR, et al: Beclomethasone dipropionate enemas for treating inflammatory bowel disease without producing Cushing's syndrome or hypothalamic pituitary adrenal suppression. *Lancet* 1:579-583, 1982.

Langman MJS: Large bowel disease, in: *A Concise Textbook of Gastroenterology*. New York, Churchill Livingstone, 1982, 84-98.

Levine RA: Risk of hypercalcemia from prophylaxis of traveler's diarrhea. *JAMA* 249:1151-1152, 1983.

McClung HJ, et al: Effect of kaolin-pectin adsorbent on stool losses of sodium, potassium and fat during lactose-intolerance diarrhea in rats. *J Pediatr* 96:769-771, 1980.

Merritt JE, et al: Loperamide and calmodulin, (letter). *Lancet* 1:283, 1982.

Meyers S: Role of corticosteroids. *Mt Sinai J Med* 50:141-143, 1983.

Miyazaki H: Loperamide in rat intestines: Unique disposition. *Life Sci* 30:2203-2206, 1982.

Mogadam M, et al: Pregnancy in inflammatory bowel disease: Effect of sulfasalazine and corticosteroids on fetal outcome. *Gastroenterology* 80:72-76, 1981.

Narducci F, et al: Stimulation of colonic myoelectric activity by emotional stress in healthy subjects and irritable bowel syndrome: Effect of pretreatment with librium. *Gastroenterology* 82:1137, 1982.

Palmer KR, et al: Double-blind cross-over study comparing loperamide, codeine and diphenoxylate in treatment of chronic diarrhea. *Gastroenterology* 79:1272-1275, 1980.

Pandol SJ, et al: Beneficial effect of oral lithium carbonate in treatment of pancreatic cholera syndrome. *N Engl J Med* 302:1403-1404, 1980.

Present DH, et al: Treatment of Crohn's disease with 6-mercaptopurine. *N Engl J Med* 302:981-987, 1980.

Rachmilewitz D: Sulphasalazine-induced infertility. *Gastroenterology* 82:996-997, 1982.

974

Sack DM, Peppercorn MA: Drug therapy of inflammatory bowel disease. *Pharmacotherapy* 3:158-176, 1983.

Sandhu BK, et al: Loperamide in severe protracted diarrhoea. *Arch Dis Child* 58:39-43, 1983.

Schiller LR, et al: Mechanism of antidiarrheal effect of loperamide. *Gastroenterology* 86:1475-1480, 1984.

Selby WS, et al: Topical treatment of distal ulcerative colitis with 4-amino-salicylic acid enemas. *Digestion* 29:231-234, 1984.

Shearman DJC, Finlayson NDC: Structure and function of the large intestine: Irritable bowel syndrome, in Shearman DJC, Finlayson NDC (eds): *Diseases of the Gastrointestinal Tract and Liver*. New York, Churchill Livingstone, 1982, 807-815.

Singleton JW, et al: National Cooperative Crohn's Disease Study: Adverse reactions to study drugs. *Gastroenterology* 77:870-882, 1979.

Skirrow MB: Three Rx steps to calming acute diarrhea. *Mod Med* 235-238, (March) 1984.

Snape WS Jr: Disorders of colonic motility, in Brooks FP (ed): *Gastrointestinal Pathophysiology,* ed 2. New York, Oxford University Press, 1978, 317-326.

Spiro HM: *Clinical Gastroenterology*, ed 3. New York, Macmillan, 1983, 789-828.

Summers RW, et al: National Cooperative Crohn's Disease Study: Results of drug treatment. *Gastroenterology* 77:847-869, 1979.

Swedberg J, Steiner FJ: Oral rehydration therapy in diarrhea. *Postgrad Med* 74:335-354, (Nov) 1983.

Taffet SL, Das KM: Sulfasalazine: Adverse effects and desensitization. *Digest Dis Sci* 28:833-842, 1983.

Thompson WG: Irritable bowel. *Gut* 25:305-320, 1984.

Tolle SW, Elliot DL: Evaluation and management of acute diarrhea. *West J Med* 140:293-297, 1984.

Van Hees PAM, et al: Effect of sulphasalazine in patients with active Crohn's disease: Controlled double-blind study. *Gut* 22:404-409, 1981.

Willoughby CP, et al: Distribution and metabolism in healthy volunteers of disodium azodisalicylate, potential therapeutic agent for ulcerative colitis. *Gut* 23:1081-1087, 1982.

Index

Primary headings appear in boldface type and may be drug names (generic and trademark), indications, or adverse reactions. Drug names followed by (M) are mixtures. Boldface page numbers denote individual evaluations.

As Antiemetic-Antivertigo Agent   254   **262**
As Antihistamine   **1046**
In Anxiety   **107**
Teratogenicity   260
HY-FLOW (polyvinyl alcohol)   365
HYGROTON (chlorthalidone)   514   552
HYLOREL (guanadrel)   521
HYMENOLEPIASIS   1604
HYPOSENSITIZATION   1158
HYOSCYAMINE
As Antispasmodic   **969**
In Urinary Incontinence   **573**
HYPERAB (rabies immune globulin)   1132
HYPERALDOSTERONISM   665
Laxative-induced   977
Spironolactone In   545
HYPERALIMENTATION (see NUTRITION)
HYPERAMMONEMIA
Drug-induced
total parenteral nutrition   867
HYPERBILIRUBINEMIA
Drug-induced
antipsychotics   119
phenol   1527
Treatment
albumin   636
barbiturates   94
HYPERCALCEMIA   886
Drug-induced
anabolic/androgenic steroids   681   1212
edetate calcium disodium   1638
estramustine   1212
estrogens   700   1211
progestins   1210
tamoxifen   1213
thiazides   548
vitamin A   847
vitamin D   847
Treatment
diuretics   546   547
HYPERCALCIURIA   581
HYPERCHOLESTEROLEMIA (see also HYPERLIPIDEMIA)
Apheresis In   626
HYPERFIBRINOGENEMIA
AHF-induced   648
HYPERGLYCEMIA (see also SOMOGYI EFFECT)
Drug-induced
amiodarone   444
asparaginase   1206
beta-adrenergic agents   822
captopril   536
diazoxide   533
enteral nutrition   877
furosemide   553
glycerin   339
somatrem   756
thiabendazole   1612
total parenteral nutrition   867
HYPERGLYCEMIC AGENTS   741
HYPERHEP (hepatitis B immune globulin)   1127
HYPERHIDROSIS   1025
HYPERKALEMIA   830

Drug-induced
alprostadil   484
analgesics   68
arginine   829
enalapril   536
laxatives   978
penicillin G potassium   1304
piroxicam   1068
potassium-sparing diuretics   516   556
urea   821
HYPERKINETIC SYNDROME (see ATTENTION DEFICIT DISORDER)
HYPERLIPIDEMIA   903
Diagnosis   911
Drug-induced
adrenal corticosteroids   1095
amiodarone   444
anabolic/androgenic steroids   681
fat emulsions   871
isotretinoin   1010
oral contraceptives   725
thiazides   548
Lipid Components
apoproteins   905   906
lipoproteins   904
Lipid Transport   905
Treatment   910
diet   912
drugs   913   914   918
other regimens   915
Types   907   908
HYPERLIPOPROTEINEMIA (see HYPERLIPIDEMIA)
HYPERLYTE PREPARATIONS   833
HYPERMAGNESEMIA   830
Antacid-induced   947
Laxative-induced   978
HYPERMETABOLIC STATES
Parenteral Nutrition In   864
HYPERNATREMIA   828
HYPEROSMOLARITY
Sodium Chloride-induced   831
HYPEROSTOSIS
Etretinate-induced   1014
Isotretinoin-induced   1010
HYPEROXALURIA   581
HYPERPARATHYROIDISM
Drug-induced
furosemide   553
sodium cellulose phosphate   586
HYPERPHOSPHATEMIA
Drug-induced
calcitriol   900
laxatives   978
HYPERPIGMENTATION   1017
Drug-induced
busulfan   1189
clofazimine   1550
dactinomycin   1200
estrogens   1215
fluorouracil   1195   1196
plicamycin   1203
procarbazine   1209
tetracyclines   1413
HYPERPROLACTINEMIA   742   744   765

As Laxative 979
SORBITRATE (isosorbide dinitrate) 465 466
SOTALEX (sotalol) 522
SOTALOL
In Hypertension 522
In Tremor 215
SOUTH AMERICAN BLASTOMYCOSIS (see PARACOCCIDIOIDOMYCOSIS)
SOYACAL 870 874
SPARINE (promazine hydrochloride) 268
SPARTEINE 813
SPASM
Biliary
opioid-induced 56
Coronary Artery
nifedipine-induced 476
Esophageal **941**
Urinary
opioid-induced 56
SPASM, ACCOMMODATION
Atropine In 346
SPASTICITY
Muscle **227**
SPECIAL FORMULA PREPARATIONS 882
SPECTAZOLE (econazole nitrate) 1515
SPECTINOMYCIN 1475
SPECTROBID (bacampicillin hydrochloride) 1319
SPECTROCIN (M) 1505
SPERMATOGENESIS DECREASED
Drug-induced 736
alkylating agents 1150
antineoplastic agents 1184
ketoconazole 1560
nitrofurantoin 1480
sulfasalazine 968
SPERMICIDES 713 714
Sponge 713
SPIDER BITE 1142
SPIRAMYCIN
In Cryptosporidiosis 1568
In Toxoplasmosis 1574
SPIRO 32 (spirogermanium) 1221
SPIROGERMANIUM
As Antineoplastic Agent **1221**
SPIRONOLACTONE
Adverse Reactions 548
hyponatremia 563
Drug Interactions
digoxin 422
Effects On Fertility 736
Uses
acne 1007
diuretic **556**
hirsutism 694
hyperaldosteronism **667**
hypertension **516**
premenstrual syndrome 693
SPIRONOLACTONE AND HYDROCHLOROTHIAZIDE 556
SPLENOMEGALY
Drug-induced
fat emulsions 871
vitamin A 847

SPONDYLITIS, ANKYLOSING 1053
SPORICIDIN (M) 1524
SPOROTRICHOSIS 1553 1554 1557
SPRX-105 (phendimetrazine tartrate) 933
S-P-T (thyroid USP) 802
STADOL (butorphanol tartrate) 65
STANOZOLOL 684
STAPHCILLIN (methicillin sodium) 1312
STARCH BLOCKERS
As Anorexiants 929
STATICIN (erythromycin) 1008
STATOBEX (phendimetrazine tartrate) 933
STATROL OPHTHALMIC OINTMENT, SOLUTION (M) 1501
STATUS ASTHMATICUS 395
Timolol-induced 336
STATUS EPILEPTICUS 174 175
STATUS MIGRAINOSUS 319
STEARIC ACID, STEARYL ALCOHOL 1027
STEATORRHEA
Nutritional Formulas In 882
STELAZINE (trifluoperazine hydrochloride) 124
STENOSIS, IDIOPATHIC HYPERTROPHIC SUBAORTIC (see CARDIOMYOPATHY Hypertrophic)
STERANE (prednisolone) 673 1102
STERCULIA GUM (see KARAYA GUM)
STEVENS-JOHNSON SYNDROME
Drug-induced
antiepileptic drugs 179
barbiturates 94
bumetanide 555
carbamazepine 198
diflunisal 1060
Fansidar 1587
minoxidil 533
penicillins 1303
pentamidine 1581
sulindac 1069
sulfonamides 1453
thiabendazole 1612
trimethoprim/sulfamethoxazole 1463
STIBOCAPTATE
As Anthelmintic 1599-1600
STIBOGLUCONATE
In Leishmaniasis **1585**
STILPHOSTROL (diethylstilbestrol diphosphate) 704
STIMAMIZOL (levamisole) 1599-1600
STIMATE (desmopressin) 564 650
STIMULANTS
Central Nervous System **141**
Respiratory **322**
in sleep apnea 86
Uterine **811**
STOXIL (idoxuridine) 1500
STREPTASE (streptokinase) 622
STREPTOBACILLUS INFECTION 1261
STREPTOKINASE
As Thrombolytic **622**
STREPTOMYCIN 1445
Teratogenicity 44 46
Uses 1431
mycobacterial infections **1544**

Laxatives and Cathartics

54

Most active, healthy people eating a balanced diet have no problem with bowel function and usually have at least three bowel movements per week. Normal consistency, frequency, and quantity of stool can be maintained by eating adequate amounts of high-residue, natural laxative foods (fruit, vegetables, high-fiber cereals) and drinking an ample amount of liquid. Proper toilet habits and regular exercise also contribute to normal bowel function.

The normal stool is neither hard nor loose and can be passed with minimal straining. The consistency of the stool rather than the frequency of elimination determines the extent of constipation. For instance, once daily elimination of a small, hard, "rabbit-like" stool is considered to be constipation.

The most common causes of constipation are poor dietary habits, inadequate dietary fiber, and ignoring the defecatory urge; the latter diminishes the rectal response to distention leading to reabsorption of water and electrolytes from the feces. Increasing the amount of dietary fiber and obedience to normal defecatory urges often relieve simple constipation. Bowel retraining procedures improve function in many patients in one to two weeks (Stratton and Mackeigan, 1982). Laxative or cathartic agents may be necessary in certain patients (see Indications).

Actions

Laxatives and cathartics promote and/or ease defecation by accelerating the passage of feces through the large intestine, by influencing the consistency and amount of stool, and by facilitating its elimination from the rectum. The terms, laxative and cathartic, reflect the intensity and latency of effect. A cathartic produces prompt fluid evacuation, while a laxative produces a soft formed stool over a protracted period. Enemas cause fragmentation, liquefaction, or lubrication of the feces and fluid distention of the bowel wall with resultant reflex elimination.

The traditional concept that the primary mechanism of action of the stimulant cathartics is to enhance intestinal motility is not accurate. Laxative-cathartics promote net fluid accumulation within the bowel lumen by a hydrophilic effect, an osmotic action, and/or a direct action on mucosal cells to decrease absorption and/or enhance secretion of water and electrolytes. These effects are mediated by alterations in the synthesis of sodium-potassium ATPase, adenylate cyclase, and prostaglandin. The complex effects of fluid accumulation and the influence of the laxative-cathartics on intestinal motility are not completely understood.

See also Drug Selection.

Indications

Laxative-cathartics are used (1) to ease the pain of elimination in patients with episiotomy wounds, painful thrombosed hemorrhoids, anal fissures, or perianal abscesses; (2) to ease elimination and thereby reduce excessive straining and intra-abdominal pressure in those with body wall and diaphragmatic hernias, anorectal stenosis, aneurysm, or other diseases of the cerebral or coronary arteries; (3) to relieve constipation during pregnancy or the puerperium; (4) in geriatric patients with poor eating habits whose abdominal and perineal muscles have lost their tone; (5) in children with congenital or acquired megacolon; (6) when bowel motility has been altered by drugs (eg, anticholinergic agents, narcotics); (7) to prevent or decrease colonic absorption of ammonia and other neurotoxins in patients with hepatic encephalopathy; (8) to prepare the bowel prior to surgery and radiologic, proctoscopic, or colonoscopic procedures; (9) to provide a fresh stool for parasitologic examination; (10) to accelerate excretion of various parasites, including nematodes, after anthelmintic therapy; (11) to hasten excretion of poisonous substances; and (12) to modify the effluent in patients with an ileostomy or colostomy.

Enemas may be indicated (1) to relieve impaction, (2) to empty the rectum and colon prior to radiographic or endoscopic procedures; (3) to cleanse the large bowel prior to surgery or delivery; (4) for patients with fecal incontinence or colostomies; and (5) occasionally, as substitutes for glycerin suppositories to re-establish the rectal reflex in constipated patients.

Most patients with colonic inertia or atony respond poorly to laxatives or enemas.

Laxative Habit: In most instances, laxatives should be used only temporarily, and the agent chosen should not empty the bowel completely. With few exceptions, there is no justification for prescribing or self-administering drugs that perpetuate and intensify the condition for which they are used initially.

Some laxatives may cause evacuation from the ascending colon in addition to the usual site, the distal descending or sigmoid colon. After such overemptying, two to five days usually elapse before the normal fecal mass can be re-established. Worry regarding the lack of bowel movement during this period provokes repeated use of the laxative, and a vicious cycle can be established: Spontaneous bowel function is reduced, laxatives are used in larger doses, and the laxative habit becomes fixed. Unfortunately, many people have misconceptions concerning the necessity for daily bowel movements. Because a variety of laxative preparations are available and are advertised aggressively, overuse of laxatives is a problem and often leads to dependence, especially with excessive use of agents that overempty the bowel.

In general, laxatives should be avoided in children. Some parents give laxatives to their children in the mistaken belief that a daily bowel movement is essential; laxative-dependent constipation is created in this manner.

Fecal Impaction: Impaction occurs when the fecal mass becomes too large to pass through the anal sphincter. It results from prolonged incomplete evacuation due to prolonged immobility, debility, and the use of constipating drugs. A variety of treatment regimens are employed. The softening and lubricating effects of mineral oil and minimal manual disimpaction often relieve impaction (see the evaluation on Mineral Oil).

Prevention: Constipation can be prevented or alleviated in most patients who are at risk and/or cannot tolerate constipation, including women during pregnancy or the puerperium, chronically bedridden or immobilized patients, individuals taking constipating drugs, and those with hemorrhoids, anal fissures, or cerebrovascular or cardiovascular disease. Psyllium or another bulk-forming agent, small doses of senna pod, and/or mineral oil taken daily are usually safe and effective (Godding, 1984 A; Klein, 1982).

Drug Selection

A single appropriate laxative produces the best results in most patients. Ideally, selection should be based on a laxative's mechanism and site of action. Although data on laxative-cathartics are insufficient for precise classification, these drugs can be divided into three groups on the basis of the intensity and latency of their effect (Fingl, 1980): agents that usually produce a soft formed stool within one to three days, a soft semifluid stool within 6 to 12 hours, or a watery stool within two to six hours (see Table 1). This descriptive classification is more useful than the traditional pharmacologic classification (ie, bulk-forming agents, stimulants, saline cathartics, wetting agents, lubricants), because the latter no longer adequately reflects current knowledge.

The choice of the most appropriate drug is based on the indication, the effect desired, the idiosyncrasies of the individual patient, and the differences among the types of laxative-cathartics. A laxative should never be given to patients with undiagnosed abdominal pain or intestinal obstruction. Laxatives other than mineral oil should be avoided in the initial management of fecal impaction. Constipation that reflects a change in bowel habits must be investigated thoroughly because it may be a symptom of colon cancer or other serious diseases.

Laxatives have been reviewed by an Advisory Panel of the FDA as part of the Drug Efficacy Study Implementation project and a monograph on these agents was published (*Federal Register*, 1985). The Committee on FDA-related Matters of the American College of Gastroenterology also has reviewed the use of laxatives (Tedesco et al, 1985).

Dietary Fiber: Dietary fiber is the portion of plant food that escapes digestion and is composed of lignin and polysaccharides (ie, cellulose, hemicelluloses, pectins, gums, alginates). Two distinct mechanisms are proposed for the laxative effect of dietary fiber (Stephen and Cummings, 1980): (1) Cereal fibers generally possess small cells with highly lignified cell walls that resist digestion and retain water within their cellular structure. (2) Other types of dietary fiber (eg, apple, carrot, guar, pectin) are digested extensively by and stimulate the growth of colonic flora, which increases fecal mass. Osmotically active metabolites also may contribute to the laxative effect.

Patients with poor dietary habits might consider adding raw bran (2 to 6 tablespoons with each meal) to soft or liquid foods and a glass of water or another beverage. Raw bran changes the texture but not the flavor of food, requires no refrigeration, and is unaffected by heat. A significant laxative effect is not observed for three to five days, and several weeks may be required to relieve chronic constipation. Raw vegetables and fruits have a low fiber content and are not adequate substitutes for raw bran. Many patients take too much bran with too little fluid, however. Large amounts of bran can cause nausea, abdominal bloating, or gas and can interfere with the absorption of magnesium, calcium, iron, zinc, and other minerals. These effects can be decreased by using a very small amount initially and slowly increasing the number of tablespoonsful ingested daily.

TABLE 1.
CLASSIFICATION AND COMPARISON OF REPRESENTATIVE LAXATIVES*

Type of Laxative-Cathartic Effect and Latency

Softening of Formed Stool (1 to 3 days)	Soft-Semifluid Stool (6 to 12 hours)	Watery Stool (2 to 6 hours)

Bulk-Forming Agents
  Dietary fiber
  Methylcellulose
  Psyllium Preparations
  Calcium Polycarbophil
	Saline Laxatives
	  (low dose)
	  Milk of Magnesia
	  Magnesium Sulfate
		Saline Laxatives
		  (high dose)
		  Milk of Magnesia
		  Magnesium Citrate
		  Magnesium Sulfate
		  Sodium Phosphates
		  Sodium Sulfate

Ducosate Salts
  Sodium, Potassium,
  or Calcium Salts of
  Dioctylsulfosuccinate
	Diphenylmethane
	Derivatives
	  Phenolphthalein
	  Bisacodyl
		Castor Oil

Lactulose	Anthraquinone Derivatives Senna	Polyethylene Glycol- Electrolyte Preparations
Sorbitol	Cascara Sagrada Danthron	

* Adapted from Fingl, 1980.

Bulk-Forming Drugs: Psyllium, methylcellulose, and other bulk-forming agents are more refined and concentrated than bran and generally are more effective, but they are also considerably more expensive. The bulk-forming drugs should be well diluted to ensure adequate mixing with the food bolus and should be ingested shortly after a meal. When taken with adequate amounts of liquid, these drugs increase the water content and bulk volume of the stool, which decreases intestinal transit time. The response usually begins in 12 to 24 hours but up to three days may be required for the fecal mass to reach the rectum in patients who use laxatives chronically.

Bulk-forming agents are generally not absorbed and are safe when adequate quantities of liquids are ingested concomitantly. They are used most commonly by patients with diverticulosis or the irritable bowel syndrome. Some bulk-forming agents have been used to improve fecal consistency in patients with disease of the terminal ileum or to modify the effluent in patients with ileostomy or colostomy in order to relieve maceration or discomfort and to reduce the number of evacuations.

Claims that the bulk-forming preparations are effective in the treatment of obesity have not been substantiated.

Impaction or obstruction may occur if the bulk-forming laxatives are arrested in their passage through the alimentary canal; water is absorbed and the bolus can become inspissated within the bowel lumen. Thus, abnormal narrowing of the lumen at any level represents a hazard. Inspissation does not occur in the normal bowel if one or more glasses of water are taken concurrently with the laxative.

Bloating and gas are observed less frequently with psyllium and other commercial bulk-forming agents than with bran. Allergic reactions (urticaria, nonseasonal rhinitis, dermatitis, and bronchial asthma) may be a serious consequence of the use of karaya and other plant gums, as well as other bulk-forming agents; this is less likely to occur with the synthetic agents, carboxymethylcellulose sodium and calcium polycarbophil. Digitalis, salicylates, and nitrofurantoin are bound by cellulose, but this interaction is not usually clinically significant. The sugar added to some psyllium preparations to improve their palatability can be hazardous in diabetics, but sugar-free preparations are available (see the evaluation).

Sodium intake is increased substantially with use of carboxymethylcellulose sodium, which contains 2.7 to 4 mEq/g. Marked fluid retention has been reported when carboxymethylcellulose sodium was used as an anorexiant.

Contact Laxatives: Many practitioners believe that contact laxatives should be used only when milder laxatives or tap water enemas are ineffective. Since contact laxatives are most often abused, some clinicians recommend that these drugs not be used regularly for longer than one week.

The precise mechanism(s) of action for each drug in this group has not been established, but, in general, they produce a net luminal accumulation of fluid and electrolytes. Direct stimulation of intramural nerve plexuses has not been proved. There is no conclusive evidence that contact laxatives have a direct mucosal stimulant or irritant effect, but morphologic changes of the surface epithelium occur and water and electrolyte transport is altered.

The continuous use of contact laxatives infrequently produces an irritable bowel-like diarrhea that is severe or prolonged enough to cause hyponatremia, hypokalemia, dehydration, hyperaldosteronism, protein-losing gastroenteropathy with hypoalbuminemia, steatorrhea, and osteomalacia. Changes in the radiologic appearance of the colon can simulate megacolon or ulcerative colitis.

Elderly patients who are being prepared for diagnostic

procedures must be monitored closely, because weakness, incoordination, and even orthostatic hypotension (often resulting in falls) can be exacerbated by electrolyte loss.

When contact laxatives are used in suppository form or as enemas, the same problems of dependence, habituation, and tolerance observed with oral use occur.

Castor oil is hydrolyzed in the upper small intestine to ricinoleic acid, a long-chain fatty acid that markedly affects the mucosal transport systems to cause a net luminal accumulation of water and electrolytes resulting in watery stools. Its use is principally limited to preparation of the bowel before radiologic procedures when prompt, complete evacuation is desired.

The stimulation of anion secretion probably is ricinoleic acid's most important action to alter fluid movement. However, some studies indicate that this agent may erode villous tips, disorganize the microvillous surface of the small intestine, and increase mucosal permeability to molecules with molecular weights as large as 16,000 (eg, dextran).

The anthraquinone-containing laxatives (eg, senna [Senokot], cascara sagrada, danthron [Dorbane, Modane]) are widely used and abused. These agents usually act within 6 to 12 hours. Cascara has the mildest action and produces a soft or formed stool with little or no colic. Standardized senna (senna pod) may be particularly helpful in patients with severe constipation and is apparently safe even in large doses. When combined with psyllium or other bulk-forming agents, smaller amounts of senna pod may be employed (Godding, 1984 B). Neither senna pod nor cascara is absorbed significantly or excreted in breast milk when recommended doses are administered. Crude senna also produces a soft or formed stool, but usually causes more muscle contraction with cramping. Danthron, a synthetic compound containing free anthraquinone, is only effective in large doses. Rhubarb and aloe are the most potent, but should not be used because they almost always produce colic.

It should be noted that although most anthraquinone-containing laxatives discolor the urine and colonic mucosa (melanosis coli), this effect is presumed to be innocuous and is reversible. Anthraquinones are excreted in the milk of lactating mothers but, at recommended doses, the concentration is rarely sufficient to exert a laxative effect in the infant. If there is concern, a laxative of a different class should be prescribed.

Reflex peristalsis following stimulation of sensory nerves only partly explains the effect of the diphenylmethane laxatives, bisacodyl [Dulcolax, Fleet Bisacodyl] and phenolphthalein. Both agents alter active electrolyte transport and thus affect fluid movement. Although bisacodyl produces a soft to formed stool usually with little or no colic, an enteric coating is required to minimize gastric irritation; the suppository preparation may cause stinging, tenesmus, and mild proctitis in a few patients. Phenolphthalein is more likely to produce a semifluid stool with little or no colic. Because of significant enterohepatic circulation, its action may be prolonged (three to four days) in sensitive patients.

Docusate sodium [Colace, Doss, Doxinate, Modane Soft], docusate potassium [Dialose, Kasof], and docusate calcium [Surfak] are presumed to soften the feces by an emollient action that reduces surface tension, thus permitting penetration of the fecal mass by intestinal fluids. There also is evidence that these agents increase mucosal permeability, inhibit water absorption in the jejunum and colon, and/or increase accumulation of intraluminal water and electrolytes (Gullikson et al, 1977; Moriarity et al, 1982). In these respects, the docusate drugs act like bile salts, which are anionic detergents, and also may be considered contact laxatives. Docusate salts usually produce a soft formed stool.

The calcium and sodium salts of docusate (and probably the potassium salt) are absorbed to some extent in the duodenum and proximal jejunum. Their metabolic fate, the bioavailability of drugs taken with them, and the significance of their absorption are unknown and require further study. Morphologic changes and increased mucosal permeability have been noted in vitro. These contact laxatives should be prescribed in the smallest effective amounts.

Dihydroxy bile acids induce colonic secretion of water and electrolytes, which results in a net accumulation of luminal fluid that produces a mild laxative action. Dehydrocholic acid [Decholin], a synthetic derivative of cholic acid, also has a hydrocholeretic action, but controlled studies to prove that this effect is beneficial are lacking.

Saline Laxatives: Each of these agents is a salt, one or both ions of which are poorly and slowly absorbed. Commonly used preparations are magnesium carbonate, oxide, citrate, hydroxide, or sulfate; sodium sulfate or phosphate; and mixed sodium and potassium tartrate. A hypertonic solution may draw a substantial volume of fluid into the intestinal lumen by osmosis and stimulate stretch receptors to increase propulsive movements. Release of cholecystokinin (CCK) from the intestinal wall, which enhances intestinal secretory and motor activity, has been proposed as an additional mechanism of action for the magnesium salts.

Large doses of saline laxatives are used as cathartics to hasten the evacuation of worms or toxic materials. They provide a liquid stool for examination of parasites without rupture of trophozoites. They also are given to empty the bowel before various diagnostic and surgical procedures are performed. In larger doses, saline laxatives usually act within two to six hours. Smaller doses usually produce a soft semifluid stool in 6 to 12 hours.

Congestive heart failure has been precipitated through indiscriminate use of saline laxatives, and coma or death from hyperkalemia and hypermagnesemia has been observed in patients with renal insufficiency who used these drugs. Oral sodium phosphate salts administered to normal volunteers significantly decreased serum calcium levels and increased serum phosphate levels. Therefore, phosphate salts should be used with caution in individuals with cardiac disease, convulsive disorders, or hypocalcemia. Tetany (resulting from hypocalcemia) and hyperphosphatemia may develop when phosphate salts are used by patients with impaired renal function. Sodium phosphate-biphosphate preparations may also cause sloughing of the surface epithelium of the rectum.

Lubricant: Mineral oil (liquid petrolatum), which is indigestible, is used orally to prevent injury to hemorrhoidal tissue or further irritation of anal fissures and to lessen the strain of evacuation (eg, in patients with hernia or cardiovascular disease) by virtue of its emollient action. It is particularly effective in relieving fecal impaction. Lipid pneumonia caused by aspiration and deposition of mineral oil in the liver have been reported. Anal seepage may occur.

Miscellaneous Agents: Electrolyte preparations containing polyethylene glycol [Colyte, GoLYTELY] produce a liquid stool within hours and are useful to cleanse the bowel prior to colonoscopy. However, when administered on the same day as a barium enema, polyethylene glycol preparations can interfere with barium coating of the bowel wall.

Net electrolyte excretion in the bowel is minimal, even when the large volumes (four liters) needed to cleanse the bowel are administered. This increases their safety in elderly patients, in those with cardiovascular or renal disorders, and in those who are poorly hydrated. These preparations are as or more effective and convenient than the usual regimen of diet combined with oral laxatives, suppositories, or enemas used for cleansing the bowel. Adverse effects are generally infrequent; nausea, abdominal bloating or fullness, cramps, or vomiting occur occasionally but usually subside rapidly.

Kits for cleansing the gastrointestinal tract prior to diagnostic examination also are available [Dulcolax Bowel Prep Kit, Evac-Q-Kit, Evac-Q-Kwik]. The solutions, tablets, and suppositories present in these kits are administered sequentially on the afternoon, evening, and/or morning prior to the examination.

Sorbitol and lactulose are poorly absorbed sugars that are not digested by intestinal enzymes. They are, however, hydrolyzed in part to lactic, acetic, and formic acids by coliforms. Accumulation of fluid in the colon is stimulated by the mild osmotic effect of these acid metabolites, and this usually produces soft formed stools. Large amounts of gas and an acid pH also result; the latter may have an additional effect on colonic transport of water and electrolytes. For the use of lactulose in portal systemic encephalopathy, see Chapter 55, Agents Used in Disorders of the Liver, Biliary Tract, and Pancreas.

Although belladonna tincture is used as an adjunct for constipation-induced cramping associated with irritable colon, it aggravates constipation in some patients.

Because of its hyperosmolarity, glycerin in suppository form promotes defecation by producing tissue dehydration and reflex rectal contraction; it also lubricates and softens inspissated fecal material. The suppository is safe for temporary use to re-establish proper bowel habits in patients who have lost the rectal reflex. Rectal instillation of hypertonic sorbitol also stimulates defecation but appears to have no advantage over glycerin.

Enemas: Most enemas act by increasing volume. Because enemas or suppositories act locally in the rectum and probably the sigmoid colon and have little effect on the more proximal colon and small bowel, they may be preferred to contact laxatives. Although they can contain saline, mineral oil, and hypertonic fluids, an enema containing only warm tap water relieves constipation in most individuals. Patients who fail to respond to oral laxatives and who have no spontaneous bowel movements can self-administer tap water enemas every three

to four days. The addition of laxatives or other substances to an enema solution may have little therapeutic value and is potentially harmful. However, the small-volume prepackaged lubricant (mineral oil), hypertonic (sorbitol, sodium phosphate-biphosphate), or detergent (docusate potassium, bisacodyl) enema kits are convenient and fairly safe for self-administration. Some elderly patients may require a commercial small-volume enema occasionally (Sparberg, 1984), particularly when the stool is not excessively hard.

Numerous complications are associated with either the solution employed or the mode of administration. Most enema solutions irritate the mucosa, sometimes producing excessive mucus in the stool. Early changes of ulcerative proctosigmoiditis are simulated. Peroxide, household detergents, and hypertonic solutions (sodium phosphate-biphosphate) are most irritating. If the rectum must be cleansed before proctoscopy, a saline enema is least likely to alter the appearance of the mucosa. If a question regarding the mucosa remains, the examination should be repeated without prior use of an enema.

Weakness, excessive perspiration, shock, convulsions, and/or coma may result with the use of enemas from water intoxication and dilutional hyponatremia. Children and the elderly are most vulnerable. This syndrome can also occur in patients with megacolon given a tap water enema even in the customary volume (500 ml). Tap water or soapsuds enemas have caused weakness and incoordination in elderly patients. Severe hypokalemia may follow the use of a tap water enema, especially in patients also receiving thiazides or more potent congeners as antihypertensive agents or diuretics. Convulsions with hypocalcemia have occurred after absorption of large amounts of phosphate by children given sodium phosphate-biphosphate enemas.

Isotonic sodium chloride solution (one level teaspoon/pint of water) is commonly employed in older individuals but should be used cautiously in patients with sodium and fluid retention (eg, in those with congestive heart failure, cirrhosis, or nephrosis). Significant absorption of sodium does not occur when sodium phosphate-biphosphate enemas are employed in patients who must restrict sodium intake (Zumoff and Hellman, 1978). In these patients, small-volume disposable kits containing sorbitol or a detergent (wetting agent) (eg, docusate potassium) may be used instead.

Methemoglobinemia, colitis with toxic megacolon, severe serosanguineous fluid loss, anaphylaxis, and rectal gangrene have followed the use of concentrated soap solutions. Alkaline soapsuds enemas should be avoided; they are particularly hazardous in the presence of portal systemic encephalopathy, since they increase diffusion of ammonia into the portal circulation. Therefore, only pure castile soap should be used (20 ml of soap solution to 1 or 1.5 liters of water).

Rectal abrasion and laceration have been produced by aggressive insertion of a hard enema tip, and bleeding or draining pus may result. Perforation may cause ischiorectal abscess. The rectal wall is insensitive above the pectinate line, and the patient may be unaware of the injury. Free perforation with fecal peritonitis occurs when the transmural tear is above the peritoneal reflection. Inflamed sigmoidal diverticula are vulnerable to rupture if water pressure is increased even slightly. Syringes should be avoided to prevent high intraluminal pressure. The enema fluid level should be no higher than 18 to 20 inches above the anus, and no more than 750 ml of fluid should be instilled over a ten-minute period. Only soft plastic or rubber tubes with side openings should be inserted and only gentle pressure should be applied. The anus should be well lubricated with petroleum jelly or similar preparations to avoid injury.

In view of the risks, enemas should be administered only when there is a clear indication for their use and when no adequate substitute can be provided.

Drug Evaluations

BULK-FORMING AGENTS

CARBOXYMETHYLCELLULOSE SODIUM

R=H or $CH_2CO^- Na^+$

METHYLCELLULOSE
[Cologel]

These cellulose derivatives are indigestible and nonabsorbable. When mixed with water, a bulky hydrophilic colloid is formed. Softening of the formed stool usually occurs within one to three days. These agents have been used to decrease the fluidity of stools in patients with chronic watery diarrhea.

For adverse reactions and precautions, see the Introduction. Fluid retention caused by the substantial amounts of sodium in carboxymethylcellulose has occurred after use of this preparation as an anorexiant.

DOSAGE AND PREPARATIONS.
CARBOXYMETHYLCELLULOSE SODIUM:
Oral: Adults, 4 to 6 g daily; *children over 6 years,* 1 to 1.5 g daily. The drug should be taken with one or two glasses of water and ingested rapidly.
    Generic. Bulk (nonprescription).
METHYLCELLULOSE:
Oral: Adults, initially, 5 to 20 ml (450 mg to 1.8 g) with one glass of water three times daily. For severe cases, 30 ml (2.25 g) with one glass of water twice daily. For maintenance, 5 to 15 ml (450 mg to 1.35 g) with one glass of water daily. *Children,* the dose is in proportion to size.
    Generic. Bulk (powder); capsules 500 mg; tablets 500 mg (all forms nonprescription).
    Cologel (Lilly). Oral liquid 450 mg/5 ml (alcohol 5%, nonprescription).

KARAYA GUM (Sterculia Gum)

This indigestible, nonabsorbable vegetable gum contains hydrophilic polysaccharides that act like other bulk-forming laxatives. Allergic reactions and urticaria have been reported rarely. For general adverse reactions and precautions, see the discussion on bulk-forming agents in the Introduction.

DOSAGE AND PREPARATIONS.
Oral: 5 to 10 g daily taken with an adequate amount of fluid.
    Generic. Bulk (powder, nonprescription).

PLANTAGO SEED (Psyllium Seed)

PSYLLIUM HYDROPHILIC COLLOID
[Effersyllium, Konsyl, Metamucil, Naturacil, Perdiem Plain]

The whole or powdered seeds of the three species of *Plantago* or the refined colloid obtained from psyllium seeds are rich in mucilage (a hemicellulose). These preparations increase bulk by imbibing water and are indigestible and nonabsorbable.

Psyllium preparations are commonly used in patients with diverticulosis or the irritable bowel syndrome and may be useful in patients with hemorrhoids to relieve painful defecation. Choleretic diarrhea caused by small bowel resection or disease of the terminal ileum may be alleviated by psyllium hydrophilic colloid, but cholestyramine resin is more effective. Psyllium also is useful when combined with senna pod, with or without mineral oil, to prevent constipation in patients at risk or in those who cannot tolerate constipation.

Plantago psyllium and *P. indica* but not *P. ovata* produce pigmentation of renal tubules in animals. No abnormalities in renal function have been noted in men receiving large doses of plantago seed for two to seven years. For general adverse reactions and precautions, see the discussion on bulk-forming agents in the Introduction.

DOSAGE AND PREPARATIONS.
PLANTAGO SEED:
Oral: Adults, 2.5 to 30 g daily; *children over 6 years,* 1.25 to 15 g daily. The preparation should be added to a glass of water and ingested rapidly.
    Available generically under the name Psyllium Seed. Powder (nonprescription).
PSYLLIUM HYDROPHILIC COLLOID:
Oral: Adults, 1 rounded teaspoonful (7 g) or one packet (instant mix) is mixed with a glass of water or other suitable fluid and ingested rapidly one to three times daily. A second glass of water enhances the effect. *Children over 6 years,* 1.25 to 15 g daily.
    Generic. Powder.
    Effersyllium (Stuart). Powder (effervescent) 3 g/dose (sodium <5 mg) (nonprescription).
    Konsyl (Lafayette). Powder (sugar-free) 6 g/dose (sodium, <4 mg) (nonprescription).
    Metamucil (Searle). Powder 3.4 g/dose (sodium 1 mg); powder (sugar-free) 3.5 g/dose (sodium <10 mg); powder (effervescent) 3.6 g/dose (sodium 7 mg) (all forms nonprescription).
    Naturacil (Mead Johnson). Chewable pieces 3.4 g/two-piece dose (sodium 14 mg) (nonprescription).
    Perdiem Plain (Rorer). Granules 4.03 g/dose (sodium 1.8 mg) (nonprescription).
    Additional Trademarks.
    Fiberall (Rydelle), *Hydrocil Instant* (Rowell), *Konsyl-D* (Lafayette), *Modane Bulk* (Adria), *Mucilose* (Winthrop), *Syllact* (Wallace).

CALCIUM POLYCARBOPHIL
[Mitrolan]

Polycarbophil, a hydrophilic polyacrylic resin, is indigestible, nonabsorbable, and metabolically inert. It has more water-binding activity than the other bulk-forming agents, absorbing 60 to 100 times its weight in water. Because of this property, polycarbophil is an effective laxative and may modify the effluent in chronic watery diarrhea. The preparation has a low sodium content (0.02 mEq/tablet) and thus may be useful in patients who must restrict the intake of sodium. No toxicity has been observed in animal studies.

Calcium polycarbophil releases free calcium after ingestion and should not be used with tetracyclines or in patients who must restrict the intake of calcium. For general adverse reactions and precautions, see the discussion on bulk-forming agents in the Introduction.

DOSAGE AND PREPARATIONS.
Oral: Adults, two tablets four or more times daily (maximum, 12 tablets); *children 6 to 12 years,* one tablet three or more times daily (maximum, six tablets); *children 3 to 6 years,* one tablet two or more times daily (maximum, three tablets). Each dose should be taken with one glass of liquid.
  Mitrolan (Robins). Tablets (chewable) equivalent to 500 mg of base (nonprescription).

CONTACT LAXATIVES

BISACODYL
[Dulcolax, Fleet Bisacodyl]

Bisacodyl may produce a soft to formed stool usually within six hours after oral ingestion and 15 to 60 minutes after rectal administration. However, its strong purgative action can be difficult to control. Emptying is sufficient to prepare patients for proctoscopic or colonoscopic procedures.

The tablets must be swallowed whole to avoid gastric irritation. They should not be taken within one hour after ingestion of milk or antacids to prevent premature dissolution of the enteric coating and resultant dyspepsia.

The suppository may produce mild smarting or tenesmus, and continued rectal administration may cause proctitis. Sloughing of the surface epithelium of the rectum also has been observed (Meisel et al, 1977). Inflammatory changes that occur after the short-term use of bisacodyl suppositories may resemble those seen in mild idiopathic ulcerative proctitis. Hence, prolonged use of this dosage form is undesirable.

DOSAGE AND PREPARATIONS.
Oral: Adults, 10 mg (range, 5 to 15 mg); up to 30 mg may be given to prepare the lower gastrointestinal tract for special procedures. *Children 6 years and older,* 5 mg.
  Generic. Tablets (plain, enteric-coated) 5 mg (nonprescription).
  Dulcolax (Boehringer Ingelheim), **Fleet Bisacodyl** (Fleet). Tablets (enteric-coated) 5 mg (nonprescription).

Rectal: Adults and children over 2 years, 10 mg (suppository) or 30 ml (enema); *under 2 years,* 5 mg (one-half suppository).
  Dulcolax (Boehringer Ingelheim), **Generic.** Suppositories and enema preparations 10 mg (nonprescription).
  Fleet Bisacodyl (Fleet). Suppositories 10 mg (nonprescription).

CASCARA SAGRADA

Cascara is one of the mildest anthraquinone-containing laxatives. Its effect on the small intestine is insignificant or slight, but it stimulates mass peristalsis in the large intestine. A soft or formed stool is produced, usually in six to eight hours, with little or no colic. Casanthranol, a derivative of cascara sagrada, is present in some proprietary mixtures.

Prolonged use of cascara may produce benign pigmentation of the colonic mucosa (melanosis coli) that may regress after therapy is discontinued. This agent imparts a yellowish brown color to acid urine and a reddish color to alkaline urine.

In recommended doses, cascara is safe for use in nursing mothers and poses little danger to the infant.

DOSAGE AND PREPARATIONS.
Oral: Adults, 200 to 400 mg of extract, 0.5 to 1.5 ml of fluid extract, or 5 ml of aromatic fluid extract. *Infants and children up to 2 years,* 1 to 2 ml of the aromatic fluid extract as one dose only. *Children 2 years and older,* 2.5 ml of the aromatic fluid extract as one dose only; the dose is adjusted for patient size and need.
  Generic. Tablets 325 mg; fluid extract (plain, aromatic) (all forms nonprescription).

CASTOR OIL

CASTOR OIL, EMULSIFIED
[Neoloid]

ACTIONS AND USES. Castor oil has been classified as a contact cathartic because lipolysis in the small intestine liberates ricinoleic acid. This long-chain fatty acid inhibits the absorption of water and electrolytes, resulting in fluid accumulation in vitro, and these changes are presumed to account for the marked net fluid accumulation in vivo.

Castor oil produces one or more copious, watery evacuations two to six hours after ingestion. The colon is emptied so completely that passage of normal stool may be delayed for two days or more. Since castor oil thoroughly empties gas and feces from the intestine, it is used to prepare patients for radiologic examination. This strong cathartic should not be used to treat common constipation.

Palatability is improved by administering chilled castor oil with fruit juice or by consuming a carbonated beverage immediately thereafter. A flavored emulsion of castor oil, such as Neoloid, also may be more palatable.

ADVERSE REACTIONS AND PRECAUTIONS. Castor oil causes morphologic changes in the small intestine and alters mucosal permeability. Colic, dehydration, and electrolyte imbalance may occur.

DOSAGE AND PREPARATIONS.
CASTOR OIL:
Oral: Adults, 15 to 60 ml; *children,* 5 to 15 ml; *infants under 2 years,* 1 to 5 ml.
 Generic. Capsules; liquid (both forms nonprescription).
CASTOR OIL, EMULSIFIED:
Oral: Adults, 30 to 60 ml; *infants,* 2.5 to 7.5 ml; *children,* dose is adjusted between that used for infants and adults.
 Neoloid (Lederle). Emulsion 36.4% (nonprescription).

DANTHRON
[Dorbane, Modane]

This synthetic anthraquinone has a mode of action similar to that of other contact laxatives (see the Introduction). It produces a soft to semifluid stool in six to eight hours.

Melanosis coli has been reported after prolonged use; this benign pigmentation gradually disappears after the drug is discontinued. Danthron also imparts a pink color to alkaline urine.

Danthron is excreted in breast milk and should not be given to lactating mothers.

A combination containing danthron with a stool softener, such as docusate sodium, should be avoided because their combined use may damage the intestinal mucosa or liver.

DOSAGE AND PREPARATIONS.
Oral: Adults and children over 12 years, 75 to 150 mg as a single dose. This contact laxative should be used sparingly if at all in *children under 12 years.*
 Dorbane (3M Personal Care), *Generic.* Tablets 75 mg (nonprescription).
 Modane (Adria). Liquid 37.5 mg/5 ml (alcohol 5%); tablets 37.5 (Mild) and 75 mg (all forms nonprescription).

DOCUSATE CALCIUM
[Surfak]

DOCUSATE POTASSIUM
[Dialose, Kasof]

DOCUSATE SODIUM
[Colace, Doss, Doxinate, Modane Soft]

ACTIONS AND USES. In vitro studies suggest that these salts of dioctylsulfosuccinic acid lower the surface tension of the stool to permit water and lipids to enter more readily and thus soften the feces. However, more recent evidence indicates that they may stimulate the secretion of water and electrolytes on contact with the mucosa. Water absorption may be inhibited in the small and large bowel. One to two days or more may be required for full effect, since it may be that long before the softened fecal bolus reaches the rectum.

In usual doses, the docusate salts are probably marginally effective (Kallman, 1983). These mild contact laxatives lessen the strain of defecation (eg, in persons with hernia or cardiovascular disease) and relieve constipation caused by delayed rectal emptying. The calcium or potassium salt may be preferred in patients who must restrict sodium intake.

ADVERSE REACTIONS AND PRECAUTIONS. Docusate salts can cause diarrhea. Morphologic damage to the intestine has been observed in rats. They also may be hepatotoxic (Kallman, 1983; Sparberg, 1984).

These agents are often combined with other laxatives with little justification. They enhance the absorption and, hence, the toxicity of several other laxatives (see the section on Mixtures).

DOSAGE AND PREPARATIONS.
DOCUSATE CALCIUM, DOCUSATE SODIUM:
Oral: Adults and children over 12 years, 50 to 360 mg daily; *2 to 12 years,* 50 to 150 mg daily of the sodium salt. It is suggested that 240 to 300 ml of water be taken with each dose.
DOCUSATE CALCIUM:
 Generic. Capsules 240 mg.
 Surfak (Hoechst-Roussel). Capsules 50 mg (alcohol 1.3%) and 240 mg (alcohol 3%) (nonprescription).
DOCUSATE SODIUM:
 Generic and under the name Dioctyl Sodium Sulfosuccinate: Capsules 50, 100, and 250 mg; liquid; syrup 16.67 and 20 mg/5 ml; tablets 100 mg (all forms nonprescription).
 Colace (Mead Johnson). Capsules 50 and 100 mg; solution for drops 10 mg/ml; syrup 20 mg/5 ml (all forms nonprescription).
 Doss (Ferndale). Capsules 300 mg (*Doss 300*); syrup 20 mg/5 ml (both forms nonprescription).
 Doxinate (Hoechst-Roussel). Capsules 240 mg; solution 50 mg/ml (alcohol 5%) (both forms nonprescription).
 Modane Soft (Adria). Capsules 100 mg (nonprescription).
DOCUSATE POTASSIUM:
Oral: The manufacturers' recommended dosage is, *adults,* 240 mg once daily. Some clinicians believe that administration twice daily is more effective.
 Dialose (Stuart). Capsules 100 mg (nonprescription).
 Kasof (Stuart). Capsules 240 mg (nonprescription).

PHENOLPHTHALEIN

ACTIONS. Phenolphthalein acts primarily on the large intestine to produce a semifluid stool in four to eight hours with little or no colic. The claim that yellow phenolphthalein is three times more potent than the white form has not been substantiated. The action of a single dose may persist for three to four days as a result of enterohepatic circulation. This drug is the active agent in many over-the-counter laxative preparations.

ADVERSE REACTIONS. Serious adverse effects are rare but can occur with excessive doses. Phenolphthalein should be avoided in the elderly because its prolonged action may deplete water and electrolytes severely.

Dermatitis (fixed drug eruptions, pruritus, burning, vesiculation, and residual pigmentation) may occur in hypersensitive patients. Fatal anaphylactic reactions have been reported, but an absolute causal relationship with phenolphthalein has not been established. Nonthrombocytopenic purpura has been reported occasionally, while dehydration from excessive laxative action or electrolyte imbalance after prolonged use occurs infrequently. Phenolphthalein imparts a pink color to alkaline urine or feces.

DOSAGE AND PREPARATIONS.
Oral: Adults, 30 to 270 mg daily; *children 6 years and older,* 30 to 60 mg daily; *2 to 5 years,* 15 to 20 mg daily.
  Generic. Bulk (powder) (nonprescription).
  Available Trademarks.
  Alophen (Parke-Davis), *Ex-Lax* (Ex-Lax), *Feen-a-Mint* (Plough), *Phenolax* (Upjohn) (all nonprescription).

SENNA WHOLE LEAF PREPARATIONS

SENNA POD PREPARATIONS
[Senokot]

CALCIUM SALTS OF SENNOSIDES A AND B
[Nytilax]

The actions and uses of this anthraquinone-type contact laxative are similar to those of cascara, but senna is more potent. Senna increases transit time and the frequency of defecation, softens the stool, and increases stool weight. A soft semifluid stool is produced 6 to 12 hours after ingestion.

Senna is available as the crude drug (Senna, Senna Fluidextract, Senna Syrup) and as a standardized, purified concentrate [Senokot]. The purified preparations are used most often and are claimed to produce colic and watery stools only rarely when administered in the recommended dosage.

Low doses of senna are usually effective and are not appreciably absorbed. Senna pod is believed to have the most physiologic action of all the contact laxatives. Colonic bacterial enzymes cleave senna and release the active anthrone metabolite gradually, which may explain the mild action of small doses (Godding, 1984 C). This laxative may inhibit the activity of cyclic sodium-potassium ATPase, and gastrointestinal regulatory peptides may be involved in its action. There is evidence that senna decreases colonic and jejunal water absorption independently of histologic alterations or effects on cyclic adenosine monophosphate; other effects on ion transport also occur (Donowitz et al, 1984).

Senna is particularly useful in patients with severe constipation (Godding, 1984 C). Minimal doses should be used and the drug should be discontinued as soon as normal bowel function is restored. Large doses of the purified preparations appears to be safe but should not be used chronically. Senna pod is also useful in combination with a psyllium preparation with or without mineral oil to prevent constipation in patients at risk or in those who cannot tolerate constipation because of debility or disease. Mixtures containing senna and a docusate salt are less useful because the latter agent may enhance the absorption of senna (see the section on Mixtures).

Senna is safe for use during pregnancy and the puerperium. In recommended doses, it is not excreted in breast milk and poses no danger to the infant.

Melanosis coli has not been reported with use of senna products despite the fact that senna is an anthracene derivative. Crude senna preparations may impart a yellowish brown color to acid urine and a reddish color to alkaline urine.

DOSAGE AND PREPARATIONS.
SENNA WHOLE LEAF PREPARATIONS:
Oral: Adults, 0.5 to 2 g (senna), 2 ml (senna fluidextract), or 8 ml (senna syrup). *Children 6 to 12 years,* one-half adult dose; *2 to 5 years,* one-quarter adult dose; *under 2 years,* one-eighth adult dose.
  Generic. Leaves; powder (both forms nonprescription).
SENNA POD PREPARATIONS:
Oral: (Granules) *Adults,* 1 level teaspoonful to a maximum of 2 level teaspoonsful two times daily; *geriatric, obstetric, or gynecologic patients and children over 27 kg,* dosage reduced by one-half. (Syrup) *Adults,* 2 to 3 teaspoonsful one or two times daily; *geriatric, obstetric, or gynecologic patients,* dosage reduced by one-half; *children 5 to 15 years,* 1 to a maximum of 2 teaspoonsful two times daily; *1 to 5 years,* one-half to a maximum of 1 teaspoonful two times daily; *1 month to 1 year,* one-quarter to a maximum of one-half teaspoonful twice daily. (Tablets) *Adults,* two to a maximum of four tablets two times daily; *geriatric, obstetric, or gynecologic patients and children over 27 kg,* dosage reduced by one-half.
  Senokot (Purdue Frederick). Granules, syrup, tablets (all forms nonprescription).
  Available Mixture.
  Perdiem (Rorer). Granules in 100 and 250 g containers (0.74 g senna and 3.25 g psyllium/6 g dose; sodium content, 1.8 mg/dose) (nonprescription).
Rectal: Adults, one suppository; if necessary, a second suppository may be administered two hours later. *Children over 27 kg,* one-half suppository.
  Senokot (Purdue Frederick). Suppositories (nonprescription).
CALCIUM SALTS OF SENNOSIDES A AND B:
Oral: Adults, one to three tablets (usually two) at bedtime.
  Nytilax (Mentholatum). Tablets (nonprescription).

SALINE LAXATIVES

MAGNESIUM, POTASSIUM, AND SODIUM SALTS

ACTIONS AND USES. Many salts having essentially the same actions are used as laxatives or cathartics. They usually produce a watery evacuation in two to six hours when doses at the upper range of effectiveness are used and are most effective if taken with substantial amounts (at least 240 ml) of fluid on an empty stomach. Magnesium-containing laxatives cause the release of cholecystokinin from duodenal mucosa, which may contribute to their osmotic action by stimulating colonic motility. Milk of magnesia or magnesium sulfate, in doses at the lower range of effectiveness, usually produces a soft semifluid stool in six to eight hours.

These preparations are given to empty the bowel prior to surgical, radiographic, proctoscopic, or colonoscopic procedures and to remove toxic material in some cases of poisoning. They also are useful to eliminate parasites and toxic vermifuge after anthelmintic therapy. The watery diarrhea produced does not destroy the osmotically sensitive trophozoites of *Entamoeba histolytica* or *Giardia lamblia*. Thus, these preparations are suitable for the collection of fresh stool specimens for parasite examination. The same laxative used as an enema destroys the trophozoites but not the cyst forms of *E. histolytica*.

ADVERSE REACTIONS AND PRECAUTIONS. Saline laxatives should be given with large amounts of liquids to prevent dehydration and maximize their effects. Magnesium salts should be avoided in patients with simple constipation. Up to 20% of magnesium may be absorbed and enter the systemic circulation. Magnesium and potassium salts are contraindicated in patients with impaired renal function. The bitter taste of magnesium sulfate may cause nausea. Sodium salts are contraindicated in patients with heart disease who have edema or congestive heart failure or in those on a low-sodium diet. The sodium phosphate-biphosphate preparations may cause sloughing of the surface epithelium of the rectum.

DOSAGE AND PREPARATIONS. See Table 2.

LUBRICANT

MINERAL OIL (Liquid Petrolatum)

ACTIONS AND USES. Mineral oil is an indigestible liquid hydrocarbon of limited absorbability. When used in recommended doses, mineral oil is safe and is particularly effective when used rectally in the management of fecal impaction. Mineral oil can be used in combination with a psyllium preparation and/or senna pod to prevent constipation in patients at risk or in those who cannot tolerate constipation because of debility or disease. It has been used orally to lessen the strain of evacuation of inspissated stool (eg, patients with hernia or cardiovascular disease).

The emulsified preparations are claimed to reduce seepage through the anal sphincter and to be more effective than nonemulsified preparations, but conclusive evidence from controlled studies is not available. Mineral oil is preferable to contact laxatives because it is safer and tolerance does not occur (Klein, 1982; Sparberg, 1984).

TABLE 2.
SALINE CATHARTICS

Preparations	Usual Dose (Adults) [1,2]
Fleet Enema (Fleet) (solution containing 19 g sodium biphosphate and 7 g sodium phosphate/delivered dose)	120 ml (rectal only)
Magnesium carbonate	8 g
Magnesium citrate solution (1.55 to 1.9 g/100 ml magnesium oxide with citric acid anhydrous and potassium bicarbonate for effervescence)	200 ml
Milk of Magnesia (7% to 8.5% magnesium hydroxide suspension)	15 to 30 ml (low) 30 to 60 ml (high)
Magnesium oxide	4 g
Magnesium sulfate	10 to 30 g
Phospho-Soda (Fleet) (aqueous solution containing 48 g sodium biphosphate and 18 g sodium phosphate/100 ml)	10 to 20 ml
Potassium bitartrate	2 g
Potassium phosphate	4 g
Potassium sodium tartrate	5 to 10 g
Sodium phosphate	3.6 to 7.2 g
Sodium phosphate, effervescent, dried	10 g
Sodium phosphate solution	7.5 g
Seidlitz powders (blue powder paper, sodium bicarbonate 2.5 g and potassium sodium tartrate 7.5 g; white powder paper, tartaric acid 2.2 g)	contents of one blue and one white powder paper, mixed in about 60 ml of water.

[1]Dosage is reduced for children (see Table in Chapter 2).
[2]Except where indicated, all doses are administered orally. Flavored preparations of various saline cathartics are marketed, but usually are more expensive than the generic preparations.

ADVERSE REACTIONS AND PRECAUTIONS. In recent years, the oral use of mineral oil has not been advocated because of the possibility of interference with the absorption of fat-soluble vitamins and the danger of pulmonary aspiration. The dose required for the former effect exceeds that normally used in clinical practice. Advising the patient to remain upright for at least two hours after administration reduces the danger of lipid pneumonia. Seepage of oil from the rectum can be avoided by reducing the dose.

Hepatic infiltration can result from absorption of mineral oil. Because concurrent use of the docusate salts may further increase the absorption of mineral oil, their concomitant administration is not recommended.

Mineral oil is still prescribed by some surgeons after anorectal surgery despite the fact that it sometimes causes pruritus ani. Laceration of the area from scratching or rubbing can interfere with healing because droplets of the inert material act in the wound as a foreign body.

DOSAGE AND PREPARATIONS.
Oral: Adults, 15 to 45 ml two times daily; *children over 6 years*, 10 to 15 ml of plain mineral oil at bedtime or 10 to 15 ml of emulsion two times daily.

For fecal impaction, 30 ml is administered hourly while the patient is awake until oil seeps from the rectum (usually within 24 to 48 hours) or the obstruction is relieved. At this point, after most of the softened feces has been removed manually, several tap water enemas are administered followed by an oral cathartic dose of a saline laxative to flush out the rectum (Klein, 1982; Sparberg, 1984).

Patients should not lie down for at least two hours after taking mineral oil to avoid pulmonary aspiration of oil droplets. Large amounts of fluid should be administered to prevent dehydration.
Rectal: Adults, 120 ml; *children over 6 years*, 60 ml.
  Generic. Liquid (nonprescription).
  Available Trademarks.
  Agoral Plain (Parke-Davis), *Fleet Mineral Oil Enema* (Fleet), *Kondremul Plain* (Fisons), *Milkinol* (Kremers-Urban), *Petrogalar Plain* (Wyeth) (all nonprescription).

MISCELLANEOUS AGENTS

GLYCERIN SUPPOSITORIES

Glycerin suppositories promote fecal evacuation in 15 to 30 minutes by stimulating rectal contraction through hyperosmotic and irritant actions. This preparation also may be used to soften and lubricate inspissated fecal material. It is often used temporarily to re-establish normal bowel function in laxative-dependent patients. Glycerin suppositories are often useful in bowel retraining regimens and in individuals with intermittent constipation.

DOSAGE AND PREPARATIONS.
Rectal: Adults, 3 g; *children under 6 years*, 1 to 1.5 g.
  Generic. Suppositories (nonprescription).

LACTULOSE
[Chronulac]

ACTIONS AND USES. Lactulose, a synthetic disaccharide, is not hydrolyzed by gastrointestinal enzymes and is not absorbed significantly in the small intestine. As a result, lactulose reaches the colon unchanged where it is metabolized by colonic bacteria to short-chain organic acids (eg, lactic, acetic, and formic acids). The increased osmotic activity of these nonabsorbable acid metabolites results in a modest net fluid accumulation in the colon. A soft formed stool usually is produced in one to three days but, in some patients, a semifluid stool is produced in 6 to 24 hours. Lactulose [Cephulac] also is used to treat portal systemic encephalopathy (see Chapter 55).

In several double-blind controlled studies, lactulose was effective in patients with chronic constipation and markedly reduced the incidence of fecal impaction in the elderly. Large doses (30 to 60 ml/day) are usually required, and 24 to 48 hours may elapse before normal bowel function is reestablished. Because of its nonsystemic, colon-specific action, lactulose avoids the potentially harmful effects that result from the absorption of many laxatives. However, many patients receiving lactulose experience cramping and flatulence that may persist with continued therapy. Because of its adverse effects, relatively high cost and lack of proof that it is more efficacious than conventional laxatives, lactulose probably should be reserved for patients who do not respond to other medications (Sparberg, 1984).

ADVERSE REACTIONS AND PRECAUTIONS. Initial administration frequently produces flatulence and intestinal cramps, which are usually transient. Excessive doses can produce watery stools.

Patients may not tolerate the extremely sweet taste. Because lactulose contains galactose (less than 2.2 g/15 ml) and lactose (less than 1.2 g/15 ml), it should be used with caution in diabetics. Lactulose can produce nausea, and elderly patients may have difficulty swallowing large volumes of the diluted drug (Kallman, 1983).

Serum electrolytes should be measured periodically in elderly debilitated patients who receive lactulose for more than six months.

DOSAGE AND PREPARATIONS.
Oral: Adults, 15 to 30 ml (10 to 20 g of lactulose) daily, increased to 60 ml daily if necessary. There is insufficient experience to recommend a dose in *children.*
  Chronulac (Merrell Dow). Each 15 ml of syrup contains lactulose 10 g, galactose less than 2.2 g, lactose less than 1.2 g, and other sugars 1.2 g or less.

POLYETHYLENE GLYCOL ELECTROLYTE PREPARATIONS
[Colyte, GoLYTELY]

ACTIONS AND USES. Each liter of these isosmotically balanced solutions contains about 60 g of polyethylene glycol (PEG-3350), a nonabsorbable osmotic agent, plus smaller amounts of sodium sulfate, potassium chloride, sodium chloride, and sodium bicarbonate. Absorption of sodium is inhibited by sulfate, and the other electrolytes prevent net absorption or secretion of other ions. The solutions cleanse the bowel rapidly by producing a voluminous liquid stool without significant changes in water and electrolyte balance or mucosal histology (Michael et al, 1985).

When administered four to five hours before a diagnostic procedure, these preparations are as or more effective than the usual regimen of diet and oral laxatives, suppositories, or enemas for cleansing the bowel. In addition, they act more rapidly and cause less discomfort (*Med Lett Drugs Ther*, 1985). Up to one liter of the fluid may be retained in the colon but can be removed by suctioning during colonoscopy. However, some physicians consider these solutions unsatisfactory for barium enema examination because they may interfere with barium coating of the bowel wall using the double-contrast technique. Addition of bisacodyl to the regimen evacuates residual fluid and may significantly improve coating with barium (Girard, 1984).

These solutions are generally safe for elderly patients; those with cardiovascular, hepatic, or renal disorders; or those who are poorly hydrated.

ADVERSE REACTIONS AND PRECAUTIONS. Nausea, vomiting, abdominal bloating or fullness, and cramps occur occasionally but are transient and usually well tolerated. Metoclopramide does not prevent any of these effects. Chilling the solution improves the unpleasant salty taste but may cause hypothermia. Sugar, other sweetening agents, or any additive should not be included in the solution.

Potential problems include gastrointestinal bleeding and aspiration due to obstruction. The same precautions observed with other laxatives apply to use of polyethylene glycol electrolyte preparations. The solutions should not be used in patients with intestinal obstruction or perforation, toxic colitis, or megacolon. If given through a nasogastric tube, the patient should be observed closely to prevent regurgitation and aspiration. These agents are not recommended for children, and their safety for pregnant women and the fetus has not been established (FDA Pregnancy Category C).

DOSAGE AND PREPARATIONS.

Oral: Adults, 200 to 300 ml (7 to 10 oz) orally every 10 minutes or through a nasogastric tube at a rate of 20 to 30 ml/min. Administration should begin four to five hours before the examination and continue until the rectal discharge is clear. This generally requires 4 L. The first bowel movement usually commences about one hour after administration of the initial dose. In patients who are to receive a barium enema, the solution can be given the evening before the examination. Patients should ingest only clear liquids for two to four hours before the examination and until it is complete.

Colyte (Reed & Carnrick). Powder containing polyethylene glycol 3350 with sodium sulfate, sodium bicarbonate, sodium chloride, and potassium chloride in 120 g (2 L), 227.1 g (4 L), and 360 g (6 L) containers.
GoLYTELY (Braintree). Powder containing polyethylene glycol 3350 with sodium sulfate, sodium bicarbonate, sodium chloride, and potassium chloride in 236 g (4.8 L) containers.

MIXTURES

There is no satisfactory evidence that laxative-cathartic mixtures are advantageous. The concomitant use of two or more laxatives does not enhance efficacy sufficiently to justify the additional hazards. With a knowledge of the mechanism of action of the various laxatives and an understanding of the patient's problem, the need for mixtures should be minimized. Too often, constipation caused by delay in passage of fecal material through the colon, delay in evacuating the rectum, or simply insufficient quantity of stool may be converted to a more serious condition by injudicious use of a combination of laxatives. Mixtures containing a docusate salt and a contact laxative are of special concern since the docusate salt may enhance the absorption of the other agent in the mixture.

The following listing of available mixtures is provided for information only; it is not intended to be complete and, in certain instances, represents an unfortunate commentary on the motives that led to the formulation of these products. This listing does not signify a recommendation for use.

Agoral (Parke-Davis). Emulsion containing white phenolphthalein 200 mg and mineral oil 4.2 g/15 ml (nonprescription).
Dialose Plus (Stuart). Each capsule contains casanthranol 30 mg and docusate potassium 100 mg (nonprescription).
Dorbantyl (3M Personal Care). Each capsule contains danthron 25 mg and docusate sodium 50 mg; each Forte capsule contains danthron 50 mg and docusate sodium 100 mg (both nonprescription).
Doxidan (Hoechst-Roussel). Each capsule contains danthron 50 mg and docusate calcium 60 mg (nonprescription).
Haley's M-O (Winthrop-Breon). Emulsion containing magnesium hydroxide and mineral oil 25% (nonprescription).
Maltsupex (Wallace). Each tablet contains malt soup extract 750 mg and potassium 0.15 to 0.25 mEq; each 5 ml of liquid and 0.56 ounce of power contain malt soup extract 16 g and potassium 3.1 to 5.5 mEq (all forms nonprescription).
Peri-Colace (Mead Johnson). Each capsule contains casanthranol 30 mg and docusate sodium 100 mg; each 5 ml of syrup contains casanthranol 10 mg and docusate sodium 20 mg (alcohol 10%) (both forms nonprescription).
Senokap DSS (Purdue Frederick). Each capsule contains senna concentrate 163 mg and docusate sodium 50 mg.
Senokot S (Purdue Frederick). Each tablet contains senna concentrate 187 mg and docusate sodium 50 mg (nonprescription).
Unilax (Ascher). Each tablet contains danthron 75 mg and docusate sodium 150 mg (nonprescription).

Cited References

Laxative drug products for over-the-counter human use; tentative final monograph. *Federal Register* 50:2124-2158, (Jan 15), 1985.
Oral electrolyte solutions for colonic lavage before colonoscopy or barium enema. *Med Lett Drugs Ther* 27:39-40, 1985.
Donowitz M, et al: Effects of Senokot on rat intestinal electrolyte

transport: Evidence of Ca^{++} dependence. *Gastroenterology* 87:503-512, 1984.

Fingl E: Laxatives and cathartics, in Gilman AG, et al (eds): *The Pharmacological Basis of Therapeutics,* ed 6. New York, Macmillan, 1980, 1002-1012.

Girard CM: Comparison of Golytely lavage with standard diet/cathartic preparation for double contrast barium enema. *Am J Roentgenol* 142:1147-1149, 1984.

Godding EW: Bowel function and dysfunction: Prevention of constipation. *Pharmaceut J* 229-230, (Feb 25) 1984 A.

Godding EW: Bowel function and dysfunction: Rehabilitation of the constipated bowel; case histories. *Pharmaceut J* 198-200, (Feb 18) 1984 B.

Godding EW: Bowel function and dysfunction: Chemical laxatives. *Pharmaceut J* 168-169, (Feb 11) 1984 C.

Gullikson GW, et al: Effects of anionic laxatives on hamster small intestinal membrane structure and function: Relationship to surface activity. *Gastroenterology* 73:501-511, 1977.

Kallman H: Constipation in the elderly. *Am Fam Physician* 27:179-184, (Jan) 1983.

Klein H: Constipation and fecal impaction. *Med Clin North Am* 66:1135-1141, 1982.

Meisel JL, et al: Human rectal mucosa: Proctoscopic and morphological changes caused by laxatives. *Gastroenterology* 72:1274-1279, 1977.

Michael KA, et al: Whole bowel irrigation for mechanical colon cleansing. *Clin Pharmacy* 4:414-424, 1985.

Moriarity KJ, et al: Study on mechanism of action of dioctyl sodium sulphosuccinate in normal human jejunum. *Gastroenterology* 82:1134, 1982.

Sparberg M: Practical pointers for treating constipation. *Drug Ther* 14:97-105, (May) 1984.

Stephen AM, Cummings JH: Mechanism of action of dietary fibre in human colon. *Nature* 284:283-284, 1980.

Stratton JW, Mackeigan, JM: Treating constipation. *Am Fam Physician* 25:139-142, (June) 1982.

Tedesco FJ, et al: Laxative use in constipation. *Am J Gastroenterol* 80:303-309, 1985.

Zumoff B, Hellman L: Absorption of sodium from hypertonic sodium phosphate enema solutions. *Dis Col Rect* 21:440-443, 1978.

Agents Used in Disorders of the Liver, Biliary Tract, and Pancreas

55

DISORDERS OF THE LIVER

Portal Systemic Encephalopathy

Etiology: Portal systemic encephalopathy (PSE) is a metabolic disorder of the central nervous system that usually occurs as a complication of hepatic cirrhosis with shunting, but also may result from deficiency of urea cycle enzymes. It often is associated with varying degrees of impaired consciousness, which is presumed to result primarily from defective conversion of ammonia to urea. Hyperammonemia is caused by the entry of portal blood directly into the systemic circulation through collateral vessels that bypass the liver (eg, cirrhosis), through intrahepatic shunting (eg, acute hepatitis), or through surgical shunts. Some investigators believe that derangements in plasma amino acid patterns are also causal factors (Fischer, 1982). The branched-chain amino acids (valine, leucine, and isoleucine) are decreased and the aromatic amino acids (phenylalanine, tryptophan, and tyrosine) are increased in patients with cirrhosis and the initial stage of coma. However, neither the increased level of blood ammonia nor the decreased level of branched-chain amino acids correlates well with the severity of the encephalopathy.

The primary etiologic role of hyperammonemia in PSE has been challenged, because other neurotoxins produced by the action of gut bacteria on dietary protein are not removed by the liver and gain access to the brain (Jones, 1983). These neurotoxins include dimethyl sulfide and other mercaptans, gamma aminobutyric acid, phenol, false neurotransmitters such as octopamine, and short- and medium-chain fatty acids. Many of these substances may interact to produce a synergistic toxic effect in the brain.

Therapy: Current therapy is aimed at minimizing the contact time between colonic bacteria and protein to reduce the formation of ammonia and other neurotoxins. Sources of excess protein in the gastrointestinal tract (eg, hemorrhage) are treated or removed, dietary protein is decreased, dialysis is used to remove ammonia from the blood, and laxatives or antibiotics are administered to cleanse the bowel of bacteria. Laxatives and enemas increase the excretion of ammonia.

The primary drugs used to manage PSE are neomycin [Mycifradin], a poorly absorbed antibiotic that decreases bacterial production of ammonia, and lactulose [Cephulac], a synthetic disaccharide that may enhance ammonia uptake by bacteria and/or enhance its excretion. Lactulose is effective for acute as well as prolonged maintenance therapy; neomycin is useful for short-term management of severe disease. Neomycin may have a more rapid onset of action, but lactulose is less toxic and is preferred, especially in older patients and those with renal impairment or constipation. In clinical trials, a combination of lactulose and neomycin was not more effective than either drug alone (Crossley and Williams, 1984).

Neomycin is partially absorbed and can cause significant adverse effects, particularly in patients with impaired renal function. Metronidazole [Flagyl, Metryl], a safer antimicrobial agent, is being evaluated in clinical trials and may prove to be a useful alternative to neomycin. Unlike neomycin, metronidazole is effective against anaerobic bacteria (Crossley and Williams, 1984); adverse reactions are rare, but significant central nervous system effects may develop with prolonged use.

Investigationally, lactose, a precursor of lactulose, appears to be effective in PSE associated with lactase deficiency. Another investigational disaccharide, lactitol (beta galactoside sorbitol), is more palatable than lactulose and has been effective in clinical trials (Lanthier and Morgan, 1985).

In one study, short-term administration of oral zinc supplements appeared to benefit patients with PSE (Reding et al, 1984). Zinc probably acts by correcting a deficiency of this metal that compromises the conversion of ammonia to urea, but improvement may be only temporary.

Branched-chain amino acids may be effective in early or mild PSE and allow ingestion of larger amounts of protein (Egberts et al, 1985). However, oral administration may not improve brain function or enhance survival in most patients (*Lancet*, 1984; *Intern Med Alert*, 1985). Intravenous infusion may be useful but is impractical. An alpha keto analogue of leucine, alpha ketoisocaproate, or the ornithine salt of various keto analogues of branched-chain amino acids may improve symptoms in some patients (Crossley and Williams, 1984).

Drug Evaluations

LACTULOSE
[Cephulac]

ACTIONS. Lactulose, a poorly absorbed, synthetic disaccharide prepared from lactose, reduces blood ammonia levels. It is not metabolized in the upper intestinal tract and thus is not absorbed. Lactulose is degraded in the colon by intestinal bacteria into low-molecular-weight organic acids that decrease the pH of the colonic contents and have an osmotic laxative action. Acidification enhances the transport of blood ammonia to the colonic lumen where it is converted to ammonium ion, which is poorly absorbed; colonic transit time is accelerated by the laxative effect of the organic acids and the excretion of ammonium ion is increased. Lactulose also may allow colonic

bacteria to take up ammonia (Vince et al, 1978; Conn, 1978).

USES. Lactulose is used for the treatment of acute episodes and for long-term maintenance therapy in portal systemic encephalopathy (PSE); it also improves protein tolerance in patients with advanced hepatic cirrhosis (Conn et al, 1977; Atterbury et al, 1978). The frequency and severity of recurrences are reduced in approximately 75% of patients with PSE and an increase in protein intake and discontinuation of neomycin are usually possible. Improvement may be noted within one to three days, but maximal benefits may not be evident for 10 to 14 days.

For maximum efficacy, several bowel movements are required daily, but this may create a significant nursing problem and promote bed sores in nonambulatory (especially comatose) patients.

ADVERSE REACTIONS. Lactulose may cause transient abdominal distention and discomfort, flatulence, nausea, and vomiting. Excessive doses cause diarrhea.

DOSAGE AND PREPARATIONS.
Oral: Adults, for acute portal systemic encephalopathy, initially, 30 to 45 ml hourly; when laxation occurs, the frequency of administration may be reduced to three or four times daily. For maintenance, 30 to 45 ml three or four times daily. Dosage should be adjusted every one or two days to produce two or three soft stools daily. *Older children and adolescents,* 40 to 90 ml daily in two or three divided doses. If the initial dose causes diarrhea, subsequent amounts should be reduced.
Rectal: Adults, 300 ml is mixed with 700 ml of water or saline and given as a retention enema. The enema is retained for 30 to 60 minutes and administration may be repeated every four to six hours. Coma may be relieved within two hours after the first enema. Enemas should be reserved for adults in impending coma or the coma stage of encephalopathy and when the danger of aspiration exists.

Cephulac (Merrell Dow). Syrup 10 g/15 ml (<2.2 g galactose, <1.2 g lactose, and ≤1.2 g other sugars).

NEOMYCIN SULFATE
[Mycifradin Sulfate]

ACTIONS AND USES. When given orally, this poorly absorbed aminoglycoside reduces hyperammonemia in patients with portal systemic encephalopathy (PSE), presumably by destroying intestinal bacteria. This mechanism of action has been questioned, however, because neomycin is ineffective against anaerobic gut flora, which are the predominant bacteria generating ammonia and other neurotoxins.

Neomycin is effective for short-term management of severe PSE. It has a more rapid onset of action than lactulose, but the latter is less toxic and is preferred for long-term therapy.

ADVERSE REACTIONS AND PRECAUTIONS. Diarrhea and reversible malabsorption are the most common adverse effects. Superinfections may result from prolonged use. Ototoxicity or nephrotoxicity may occur in patients with inflammatory bowel disease or renal insufficiency.

DOSAGE AND PREPARATIONS.
Oral: Adults, initially, 4 to 12 g daily in divided doses for five to six days; for maintenance, 2 to 3 g daily.
  Generic. Tablets 500 mg.
  Mycifradin Sulfate (Upjohn). Solution (oral) 125 mg/5 ml and tablets 500 mg equivalent to 87.5 and 350 mg of base, respectively.

Portal Hypertension

Shunt surgery may control recurrent esophageal or gastric bleeding and reduce portal vein pressure in patients with hepatic cirrhosis. However, prophylactic shunt surgery is no longer recommended because it often produces hepatic encephalopathy and does not prolong survival significantly (Clark, 1982).

The preferred management of esophageal varices is injection of sclerosing substances, such as sodium morrhuate and sodium tetradecyl sulfate. Sclerotherapy, which may be required indefinitely in most patients, decreases the frequency of bleeding episodes and the number of transfusions required. It is not yet known if this procedure prolongs survival. Sclerotherapy may be useful prophylactically in patients with severe or moderate liver disease. Prophylactic therapy should be reserved for patients with recent bleeding from varices; benefits in patients who have never bled are unclear.

Sclerotherapy is more effective than intravenous infusion of vasopressin for treatment of acute variceal bleeding. Theoretically, some adverse cardiovascular effects of vasopressin may be avoided by simultaneous administration of nitroglycerin or nitroprusside.

Propranolol [Inderal] has been reported to prevent recurrent variceal bleeding in low-risk alcoholic patients with portal hypertension and cirrhosis (Lebrec et al, 1981), but the results of another well-controlled study conducted in patients with a variety of liver diseases showed the drug to be ineffective (Burroughs et al, 1983). Propranolol has little value in patients with cirrhosis and severe liver disease not related to alcoholism and its usefulness in high-risk surgical patients with ascites may be limited because it produces sodium retention in these patients. Propranolol also may be less useful in cirrhotic patients with significant alteration of clotting factors because it inhibits platelet aggregation. Until more data become available, this drug probably should be reserved for patients in controlled clinical studies or those who refuse other therapy (Reynolds, 1983).

Wilson's Disease and Primary Biliary Cirrhosis

Wilson's Disease: Abnormal hepatic deposition of copper with accumulation occurs in Wilson's disease. Penicillamine [Cuprimine, Depen] facilitates the renal transport of copper. This drug is effective orally and most treated patients have a normal life span. The amount of copper in the diet must be restricted to less than 2 mg/day to achieve a negative copper balance. The usual period required for improvement in results of hepatic function tests is 6 to 18 months.

Asymptomatic individuals homozygous for Wilson's disease also should receive penicillamine to prevent the development of neurologic or hepatic symptoms.

In an occasional patient, use of this drug is associated with a hypersensitivity reaction and dosage reduction or desensitization is required. A number of the adverse reactions reported in patients who receive penicillamine for autoimmune diseases, such as primary biliary cirrhosis or rheumatoid arthritis, occur less frequently in patients with Wilson's disease. However, prolonged therapy may be associated with a variety of undesirable effects, including proteinuria and nephrotic syndrome, which are usually reversible upon discontinuation of this drug.

Trientine (trien) [Cuprid], is a useful alternative in patients who cannot tolerate penicillamine. Like penicillamine, trientine produces a negative copper balance, improves symptoms, and is effective for prolonged therapy in Wilson's disease. In contrast to penicillamine, toxicity is low; iron deficiency anemia is the only adverse effect noted (Deiss, 1983). (See the evaluation in Chapter 80, Drugs Used in the Treatment of Poisoning.)

Zinc has been effective investigationally in Wilson's disease (Brewer et al, 1983). Oral zinc acetate produces a negative copper balance, probably by inducing the formation of an intestinal mucosal metallothionein that binds dietary and endogenous copper. Intestinal mucosal cells containing the copper-bound metallothionein are sloughed and removed with the feces. Since penicillamine produces zinc deficiency, body stores of zinc must be built up before zinc can inhibit copper absorption. For this reason, zinc acetate should be administered for at least two weeks before penicillamine is withdrawn. Zinc acetate rarely causes adverse reactions but occasionally irritates the gastric mucosa. Compliance may be a problem; five daily doses are required in contrast to two to four daily doses of penicillamine (Brewer et al, 1983). The effectiveness of long-term treatment with zinc in patients with Wilson's disease remains to be established. At present, zinc is recommended only for patients unable to tolerate penicillamine or for pregnant women; it should be avoided in acutely ill patients not previously treated with penicillamine.

Primary Biliary Cirrhosis: No satisfactory treatment exists for primary biliary cirrhosis. Drug therapy is supportive and is aimed at reducing symptoms and minimizing complications (Maddrey, 1984).

Cholestyramine resin [Questran] or colestipol [Colestid] relieves pruritus, which is often disabling in these patients. Large volume plasmapheresis relieves pruritus in the rare patient who does not respond to colestipol or cholestyramine. Antihistamines or phenobarbital also are occasionally useful.

Deficiencies of vitamins A, D, and K may occur in severely jaundiced patients with steatorrhea and malabsorption, and administration of these fat-soluble vitamins may be necessary. A low-fat diet supplemented with medium-chain triglycerides also is used to treat symptomatic steatorrhea. There is no effective treatment for osteoporosis, the major bone disorder observed in this disease. Although the administration of vitamin D or its derivatives may slow the progression of osteoporosis or reverse it in an occasional patient, no convincing evidence for efficacy is available.

Xanthomas and other manifestations of hyperlipidemia are occasionally relieved by prolonged treatment with cholestyramine. The iron deficiency anemia that often develops in patients with primary biliary cirrhosis can be treated with oral iron preparations.

The results of a number of well-controlled studies (Matloff et al, 1982; Dickson et al, 1985) indicate that, in contrast to previously published reports (Deering et al, 1977; Epstein et al, 1981), penicillamine may not relieve symptoms significantly or prolong survival in patients with primary biliary cirrhosis. Therefore, the use of this toxic agent must be considered questionable at this time.

Corticosteroids and azathioprine [Imuran] have no role in the treatment of primary biliary cirrhosis. Corticosteroids may aggravate osteoporosis and appear to have no effect on the course of the disease.

Drug Evaluation

PENICILLAMINE
[Cuprimine, Depen]

$$CH_3 - \underset{\underset{CH_3}{|}}{\overset{\overset{SH}{|}}{C}} - \underset{\underset{H}{|}}{\overset{\overset{NH_2}{|}}{C}} - \overset{\overset{O}{||}}{C}OH$$

ACTIONS AND USES. This synthetic sulfhydryl compound is a degradation product of penicillin but has no antibacterial activity. It combines with copper, iron, mercury, lead, and arsenic to form soluble complexes that are readily excreted by the kidneys.

Most patients with Wilson's disease who are treated with this orally effective agent have a normal life span. Penicillamine facilitates the renal transport of copper. In order to achieve a negative copper balance, the amount of copper in the diet must be restricted to less than 2 mg/day. Improvement in results of hepatic function tests usually requires 6 to 18 months of treatment. Severe neurologic damage is not always completely reversible. Prophylactic administration is recommended for individuals homozygous for Wilson's disease before clinical symptoms develop.

The results of controlled studies utilizing penicillamine for primary biliary cirrhosis are conflicting. Initial studies reported that penicillamine improved survival (Epstein et al, 1981), but neither symptoms nor survival improved significantly in two other studies (Matloff et al, 1982; Dickson et al, 1985). Copper overload in patients with primary biliary cirrhosis is not a principal factor in its development. Any activity of penicillamine in this disorder appears to result from its anti-inflammatory action rather than from its ability to chelate copper. The high incidence of adverse reactions requiring cessation of therapy and its questionable efficacy in this disease have led to the recommendation that penicillamine not be used for histologically advanced primary biliary cirrhosis (Maddry, 1984; Dickson et al, 1985).

ADVERSE REACTIONS. More adverse reactions occur in patients with primary biliary cirrhosis than in those with Wilson's disease. Drug withdrawal may be required because of intolerance. Adverse effects include skin rash, loss of taste, proteinuria, and anorexia. Serious adverse reactions include nephrotic syndrome, thrombocytopenia, and autoimmune disorders (systemic lupus erythematosus, Goodpasture's syndrome, peripheral neuropathy, polymyositis, myasthenia gravis, pemphigus). Most of these adverse reactions are reversible upon discontinuation of the drug.

The pharmacokinetics, other adverse effects, and precautions associated with the use of penicillamine are discussed in Chapter 31, Agents Used to Treat Urologic Disorders.

DOSAGE AND PREPARATIONS. Penicillamine should be given on an empty stomach between meals and at bedtime; the last dose should be given at least three hours after the evening meal. Dosage must be individualized and can be determined only by measuring the urinary excretion of copper. If the patient is on a low-copper diet and is using an oral cation exchange resin, negative copper balance will result if the urinary excretion of copper is 0.5 to 1 mg or more every 24 hours.

Oral: For Wilson's disease, *older children and adults*, initially, 125 or 250 mg daily, increased gradually over a four- to eight-week period as indicated by side effects and urinary copper excretion. The usual maintenance dose is 250 mg four times daily; however, if efficacy is not compromised, it is recommended that the total daily dose be limited to 500 to 750 mg to minimize untoward effects. *Infants over 6 months and young children*, a single daily dose of 250 mg dissolved in fruit juice.

For primary biliary cirrhosis (investigational indication), the same dosage as for Wilson's disease has been given.

Cuprimine (Merck Sharp & Dohme). Capsules 125 and 250 mg.
Depen (Wallace). Tablets 250 mg.

DISORDERS OF THE BILIARY TRACT

Composition of Bile Acids and Salts: The primary bile acids, cholic acid and chenodeoxycholic acid, are formed from cholesterol in the liver. Deoxycholic and lithocholic acids are produced by 7-dehydroxylation of cholic acid and chenodeoxycholic acid, respectively, by anaerobic intestinal bacteria. Ursodeoxycholic acid is formed from chenodeoxycholic acid by bacterial action in the large intestine and possibly also from the 7-keto derivative of chenodeoxycholic acid in the liver.

Bile acids do not occur as such, but rather as N-glycine or N-taurine conjugates. Conjugation increases their solubility, makes them more resistant to precipitation by calcium, and decreases passive intestinal absorption. Lithocholic acid is not only conjugated with glycine or taurine but also is sulfated at the 3 position. Sulfation decreases intestinal absorption, thus hastening elimination of this hepatotoxic bile acid.

Endogenous Actions of Bile: Bile serves in man as the unique excretory pathway for cholesterol, which is present in bile in the form of mixed micelles. Cholesterol is secreted into the intestine during digestion and a mixed micelle with a new composition is formed; this new aggregate contains predominantly fatty acids and monoglycerides formed by the action of lipase and colipase on dietary triglycerides.

Bile acids facilitate absorption by enhancing the diffusion of solubilized fat digestion products through the unstirred layer of water that coats the intestinal mucosa. Micellar solubilization of fat-soluble vitamins is essential for their absorption. The bile acids are reabsorbed mainly in the ileum by active transport and return to the liver, where they are extracted and re-excreted in bile. The bile acid pool (ie, the mass of bile acids in the enterohepatic circulation) circulates six to ten times a day. The only input of bile acids into the enterohepatic circulation is by synthesis from cholesterol; the only loss is by fecal excretion.

Many conditions interfere with the enterohepatic circulation of bile acids. The major disturbances are biliary obstruction, biliary fistula, ileal disease or resection, and bacterial overgrowth (eg, in the stagnant loop syndrome). These defects impair micelle formation, causing maldigestion of fat and steatorrhea.

Replacement Therapy

At present, no preparation of conjugated bile acids is satisfactory for replacement therapy. Commercial ox bile preparations do not provide an adequate amount of conjugated bile acids (about 4 to 8 g are secreted with each meal) and produce diarrhea (dihydroxy bile acids induce secretion of water and electrolytes by the colon). Thus, their use to treat vague symptoms attributable to deficiency of bile or intestinal malfunction does not appear to be justifiable and may cause undesirable side effects. However, successful replacement therapy with bile acids has been reported in one patient with an ileostomy and significant steatorrhea (Fordtran et al, 1982).

Synthetic dehydrocholic acid [Decholin] is metabolized to cholic acid (and hydroxy-oxo bile acids) in the liver. A hydrocholeretic effect has been reported, but controlled studies demonstrating the therapeutic utility of this agent is lacking.

Gallstone Dissolution Therapy

Bile acids play an important role in solubilizing cholesterol in bile. When their secretion is decreased or cholesterol secretion is increased, bile contains excess cholesterol that may precipitate from solution and form gallstones.

Cholelithiasis affects about 10% of the population of the United States (20% over age 40). The most common cause is probably overconsumption of cholesterol and calories; inade-

quate exercise may be contributory, and metabolic as well as genetic factors may also be important. The symptoms of active disease include biliary colic and jaundice if bile duct obstruction occurs, but the majority of patients remain asymptomatic. There is a question of whether therapy is required for the latter patients; many practitioners believe that treatment of asymptomatic patients is unwise (Hofmann, 1982; Ransohoff et al, 1983; Tangedahl, 1983; Tyor, 1983).

Drug Therapy: At present, chenodiol (chenodeoxycholic acid) [Chenix] and the investigational agent, ursodeoxycholic acid, are used for gallstone dissolution therapy in carefully selected patients. Symptoms may be rapidly relieved by these agents, but relief also occurs in many patients given a placebo. Relatively large doses of chenodiol (13 to 15 mg/kg/day) decrease cholesterol secretion into bile, thus desaturating bile and dissolving gallstones (Palmer and Carey, 1982). However, surgery is preferred for most patients when intervention is required.

Results of the National Cooperative Gallstone Study (NCGS) to determine drug efficacy were disappointing (Schoenfield et al, 1981). In this controlled, multicenter trial, more than 900 patients received chenodiol 375 or 750 mg/day for two years. The larger dose completely or partially dissolved gallstones in 27% of patients; the smaller amount was beneficial in only 14% of patients. The poor overall response resulted from the small doses employed. Lean patients responded better than heavy or obese patients. It is now clear that chenodiol is less effective in doses smaller than 13 mg/kg/day (Tangedahl et al, 1983).

In the NCGS, chenodiol increased serum cholesterol (particularly low density lipoproteins) by 10% and produced clinically significant intrahepatic cholestasis that required termination of therapy in 3% of patients receiving the larger dose (750 mg/day). In several patients, the lesions resembled those induced by lithocholic acid (the major metabolite of chenodiol), which has caused biliary tract inflammation, adenomas, or hepatomas in mice. Mild diarrhea also occurred but did not require suspension of treatment.

In a number of studies, ursodeoxycholic acid was as effective as chenodiol in dissolving cholesterol gallstones; moreover, response was more rapid in some patients and significantly fewer side effects (ie, liver dysfunction, diarrhea) occurred (Ward et al, 1984). When available, ursodeoxycholic acid will be the drug of choice for gallstone dissolution, although reports of calcification of gallstones acquired during treatment with this agent are disquieting.

Radiopaque or large calculi are relatively resistant to dissolution by either bile acid, as are cholesterol stones containing more than 4% calcium. Dissolution often occurs only until a pigment layer, a calcified shell, or an insoluble nidus is reached.

Overall, some dissolution occurs in 40% to 80% of appropriately selected patients within two years after treatment with either chenodiol or ursodeoxycholic acid; about one-half of these patients experience total dissolution of stones. Complete dissolution occurs more often in women, in patients with high normal serum cholesterol concentrations, in thin patients, and in those with cholesterol gallstones less than 15 mm in diameter or noncalcified radiolucent stones that are "floating" (ie, that float during oral cholecystography). Gallstones dissolve completely in over 80% of those with floating radiolucent stones when either bile acid is taken for up to two years. However, only 10% to 15% of patients have this type of stone. Patients receiving ursodeoxycholic acid or chenodiol must have a functioning gallbladder, no history of recurrent attacks of biliary colic, and stones within the gallbladder should not be pigmented or calcified (Ward et al, 1984). Pre-existing liver disease not related to gallstones is a contraindication to use of chenodeoxycholic acid; neither bile acid should be used in patients with laboratory evidence of hepatobiliary obstruction or cholestasis. Pregnant women or those likely to become pregnant should not be treated with chenodiol or ursodeoxycholic acid.

Dissolution requires three months to two years, depending on the size and composition of the stones, and is best assessed by oral cholecystography or ultrasound examination performed at six-month intervals. Nonvisualization is not an indication for discontinuing treatment unless dissolution can be confirmed on three sequential cholecystograms taken over a one-year period. Therapy should be continued for at least three months after apparent complete dissolution. Partial dissolution at six months is a good predictive factor for eventual complete dissolution in patients receiving oral chenodiol 15 mg/kg/day or ursodeoxycholic acid 8 to 10 mg/kg/day. Patients who do not respond to chenodiol after nine months or to ursodeoxycholic acid after six months probably will not improve after 24 months. Therapy should be discontinued if there is no significant decrease in stone size after 16 months (Tyor, 1983; Tangedahl, 1983). After two years of treatment with chenodiol, further therapy for two years in the doses used in the NCGS provided little additional benefit (Marks et al, 1984 A).

Following complete dissolution of gallstones with chenodiol, 25% to 75% of patients experience recurrences within five years. Retreatment is usually successful.

Available evidence does not support maintenance therapy with low-dose chenodiol or ursodeoxycholic acid after complete dissolution of gallstones. Low-dose prophylaxis with chenodiol 375 mg/kg/day did not prevent recurrence in patients whose gallstones were completely dissolved with this drug (Marks et al, 1984 B).

Combination therapy with ursodeoxycholic acid and chenodiol may have synergistic effects, because these agents act by different mechanisms, and their combined use is under investigation.

Criteria for Choice of Surgical or Medical Therapy: It has been recommended that chenodiol be reserved for patients who require treatment but refuse surgery or in whom surgery would be hazardous (Isselbacher, 1981). However, delaying surgery may increase operative morbidity and mortality in poor-risk patients (McSherry, 1981).

If gallstone dissolution therapy is considered, a staging of gallstone and gallbladder disease has been proposed to serve as a basis for selection of no therapy, medical (gallstone dissolution) therapy, or surgical therapy (Hofmann, 1982). Asymptomatic patients are divided into Stage I (supersaturated or lithogenic bile) and Stage II (crystallization detectable only by duodenal drainage). Patients in Stage I or II do not require therapy. In Stage III patients (uncomplicated radiolucent cholelithiasis with normal gallbladder function), medical or surgical therapy is recommended if intervention is appropriate. Gallstone dissolution therapy should be reserved for compliant patients with normal liver function tests. Surgery is recommended for patients in Stage IV (cholelithiasis with inflammation and gallbladder dysfunction) and Stage V (acute cholecystitis due to cystic duct obstruction by a gallstone).

The attainment of ideal body weight and a high-fiber diet are recommended to diminish stone formation whether medical or surgical therapy is elected.

Bile Duct Stones: Recurrent bile duct stones are usually composed of calcium bilirubinate and calcium soaps; they are resistant to dissolution by oral chenodiol or ursodeoxycholic acid. Contact dissolution with cholesterol solvents, such as monooctanoin [Moctanin], is only occasionally successful.

Retained bile duct stones are a significant problem after cholecystectomy or choledochotomy; those containing more than 40% cholesterol can be dissolved by contact dissolution using monooctanoin within one to four weeks. To obtain direct access to the stones, monooctanoin is administered through a T-tube, nasobiliary catheter, or percutaneous transhepatic catheter (Hofmann et al, 1981; Jarrett et al, 1981; Allen and Thistle, 1983; Tritapepe et al, 1984). Oral chenodiol or ursodeoxycholic acid also can be used, but complete dissolution usually requires six months to two years and these drugs are more expensive than monooctanoin.

The administration of methyl *tert*-butyl ether (MTBE) through a percutaneous transhepatic catheter has been used investigationally for contact dissolution of bile duct and gallbladder cholesterol stones in less than eight hours without serious adverse effects (Allen et al, 1985).

Drug Evaluations

CHENODIOL (Chenodeoxycholic Acid)
[Chenix]

ACTIONS AND USES. Chenodiol, a natural bile acid, decreases cholesterol saturation of bile by decreasing the secretion of cholesterol and perhaps by increasing the secretion of bile acids. Thus, it promotes the dissolution of radiolucent cholesterol gallstones in selected patients (Hofmann, 1982). Radiopaque gallstones (containing calcium) and some radiolucent calcium bilirubinate stones (containing pigment) are resistant to dissolution.

Chenodiol has a limited role in gallstone dissolution therapy. Considerable commitment by both the physician and patient is required for successful therapy. Up to one-third of patients do not complete the required duration of therapy (usually 24 months) (Tangedahl et al, 1983). The effectiveness of this agent and guidelines for its use are discussed in the Introduction to this section.

ADVERSE REACTIONS. Intermittent dose-related diarrhea is usually the only side effect. The dose should be reduced by one-half until the diarrhea abates and then increased gradually to the original level. It is rarely necessary to discontinue treatment because of diarrhea. Dyspepsia is uncommon and usually diminishes or disappears two to four weeks after initiation of therapy.

Significant abnormalities in the results of liver function tests may be noted in up to 10% of patients. A reversible increase in the serum transaminase level develops in some individuals. Therefore, serum transaminase levels should be measured before initiating treatment; at one-, three-, and six-month intervals during administration; and at six-month intervals thereafter. If levels are more than twice the upper limit of normal, an unrelated viral hepatitis should be excluded. Chenodiol should be discontinued if alkaline phosphatase or bilirubin levels are elevated markedly.

The major metabolite of chenodiol is lithocholic acid, which may cause portal tract inflammation in hypersensitive patients. Chenodiol increases the low density lipoprotein fraction of cholesterol by about 10%, which may be a risk factor for atherosclerosis (Albers et al, 1982). The high density lipoprotein fraction is unaffected.

PRECAUTIONS. Relative contraindications include inflammatory diseases of the bile duct or bowel, obstructive hepatobiliary diseases, acute cholecystitis, and acute or chronic hepatitis. Women of childbearing age should receive chenodiol only in conjunction with effective contraception, because safety during pregnancy has not been documented (FDA Pregnancy Category X). For the same reason, it is not advisable to use this drug in lactating mothers.

DRUG INTERACTIONS. Cholestyramine, colestipol, and aluminum-containing antacids bind chenodiol and decrease its absorption; therefore, simultaneous administration of these agents is not advised.

POISONING. No cases of overdosage have been reported; however, on a theoretical basis, it is recommended that gastric lavage be performed immediately with at least 1 L of a suspension of cholestyramine or charcoal (2 g/100 ml of water), followed by 50 ml of aluminum hydroxide suspension orally.

PHARMACOKINETICS. See the discussion of Composition of Bile Acids and Salts in the Introduction. In patients with normal liver function, the intestinal absorption and hepatic uptake of chenodeoxycholic acid are so rapid that only a slight increase in blood concentration occurs.

DOSAGE AND PREPARATIONS. Chenodiol should be taken with meals or milk since it dissolves more rapidly in intestinal chyme when bile and pancreatic juice are present.

Oral: Adults, initially, 500 mg/day should be given and the amount gradually increased after one or two weeks until an approximate dose of 15 mg/kg/day (1 g/day) in divided amounts is reached. Doses less than 13 mg/kg/day are less effective. Convenient doses based on a 250-mg tablet size appear in the following Table (adapted from Tangedahl, 1983):

Body Weight (kg)	Total Daily Dose (mg)	Number of Tablets	
		Morning	Evening
up to 60	750	1	2
up to 75	1,000	1	3
up to 90	1,250	2	3
up to 107	1,500	2	4
over 107	1,750	3	4

Investigationally, a single bedtime dose combined with a low-cholesterol diet almost doubles the rate of gallstone dissolution (Kupfer et al, 1982), thus reducing the duration and cost of therapy.

Chenix (Reid-Rowell). Tablets 250 mg.

URSODEOXYCHOLIC ACID

ACTIONS. This investigational drug is synthesized from chenodeoxycholic or cholic acid. The endogenous compound is formed from chenodeoxycholic acid (chenodiol) by colonic bacteria (Bachrach and Hofmann, 1982). Like chenodiol, ursodeoxycholic acid decreases the saturation index (ie, the bile concentration of cholesterol relative to bile acids), which results in dissolution of cholesterol from the surface of gallstones.

Unlike chenodiol, ursodeoxycholic acid does not efficiently solubilize cholesterol in micellar solution or increase the secretion of bile acids into bile. Instead it promotes the formation of a lecithin-cholesterol liquid layer at the surface of the stone (Fromm, 1984).

Ursodeoxycholic acid decreases the availability of cholesterol for secretion into the bile, perhaps by enhancing the formation of bile acids from cholesterol but apparently not by decreasing cholesterol synthesis. It also inhibits the absorption of cholesterol.

USES. Ursodeoxycholic acid is about as effective as chenodiol in dissolving radiolucent gallstones in carefully selected patients. This agent alone or in combination with chenodeoxycholic acid may become the therapy of choice for this use. Symptoms are usually relieved rapidly after use of ursodeoxycholic acid. As with chenodiol, radiopaque gallstones (containing calcium) and some radiolucent calcium bilirubinate stones (containing pigment) are resistant to therapy. The effectiveness of this agent and guidelines for its use are discussed in the Introduction to this section.

ADVERSE REACTIONS AND PRECAUTIONS. Dose-related diarrhea and hypersensitivity-related elevation of serum transaminase and alkaline phosphatase levels are observed rarely; the incidence and severity of these side effects are significantly less than with chenodiol. Hepatic damage has not occurred.

Calcification of the gallstone surface occurs during ursodeoxycholic acid therapy in about 10% of patients and may interfere with further dissolution. If significant calcification occurs or symptoms worsen, surgery is indicated. Ursodeoxycholic acid does not appear to alter serum cholesterol levels in patients with cholelithiasis.

The precautions, drug interactions, and treatment of poisoning are similar to those of chenodiol (see the evaluation).

PHARMACOKINETICS. Ursodeoxycholic acid is absorbed from the intestine and rapidly taken up by the liver, from which it is excreted into bile in the form of glycine and taurine conjugates. Like chenodiol, this agent is converted principally to lithocholic acid in the distal intestine by colonic bacteria. Because the portion of lithocholic acid that is absorbed is sulfated in the liver, this potentially hepatotoxic compound is detoxified. In patients with normal liver function, oral absorption and hepatic uptake occur so rapidly that only a small increase in blood concentration occurs.

Enterohepatic recirculation of ursodeoxycholyl conjugates is quite efficient. The half-life following oral administration is 3.5 to 5.8 days.

Ursodeoxycholic acid may enhance the hypolipidemic effects of clofibrate, further reducing serum triglyceride and serum bile acid levels.

DOSAGE AND PREPARATIONS. This drug should be taken with meals or milk since it dissolves more rapidly in intestinal chyme when bile and pancreatic juice are present.
Oral: Adults, 8 to 10 mg/kg/day twice daily (usually a 250-mg capsule administered in the morning and evening). Alternatively, a single nighttime dose may be given and is considered more efficacious by some authorities.
    (Investigational drug)

MONOOCTANOIN
[Moctanin]

ACTIONS AND USES. The major constituents of this semisynthetic vegetable oil are the mono- and diglycerides of octanoic and decanoic acids. The product is predominantly glyceryl 1-mono-octanoate.

Monooctanoin has been effective in up to two-thirds of patients with retained radiolucent biliary duct stones containing more than 40% cholesterol (Palmer and Hofmann, 1986). It is only occasionally effective in recurrent bile duct stones and is ineffective in pigment stones with little cholesterol. When a surgically removed gallstone is available, it should be tested for solubility in monooctanoin; a useful solvent for testing is methyl *tert*-butyl ether (Allen et al, 1985). Alternatively, the stones can be incubated in monooctanoin at body temperature with stirring. If analysis shows the stone to be other than cholesterol or if no dissolution is observed after 72 hours of incubation, monooctanoin therapy should not be instituted.

ADVERSE REACTIONS AND PRECAUTIONS. Infusion is usually well tolerated if the rate is slow (3 to 5 ml/hour). The perfusion pressure must be kept below 15 cm. Too rapid infusion often causes mild diarrhea, nausea, and abdominal pain (Steinhagen and Pertsemlidis, 1983; Allen and Thistle, 1983; Tritapepe et al, 1984). Minor irritation of the gastric and duodenal mucosa sometimes occurs but appears to be insignificant (Tritapepe et al, 1984). Use of this agent is contraindicated in patients with pre-existing liver disease.

DOSAGE AND PREPARATIONS. Monooctanoin is administered as a continuous perfusion through a catheter inserted directly into the common bile duct, generally via a T-tube or nasobiliary tube placed by endoscopy. *It is essential to utilize an overflow manometer, peristaltic pump (preferred), or similar measure to assure that perfusion pressure does not exceed 15 cm H_2O. The rate should not exceed 3 to 5 ml/hour at a pressure of 10 cm H_2O* to minimize gastrointestinal and/or biliary irritation. Administration may be interrupted during meals.

This agent must not be administered intravenously or intramuscularly. The solution should be warmed to 60 to 80 F prior to perfusion and its temperature should not fall below 65 F during administration.

The duration of perfusion is 7 to 21 days. If T-tube cholangiograms taken at intervals of three to four days do not show a decrease in the number or size of gallstones after seven days of treatment, continued therapy is unlikely to be successful.
    Moctanin (Ascot). Solution (sterile) in 120 ml containers.

DISORDERS OF THE PANCREAS

Optimum digestion of fat, carbohydrate, and protein depends upon the exocrine function of the pancreas (ie, secretion of lipase, amylase, trypsin, and chymotrypsin). Pancreatic secretion of bicarbonate also is necessary to protect these enzymes from denaturation by acid and pepsin. When pancreatic secretion is impaired by pancreatectomy, chronic relapsing pancreatitis, cystic fibrosis, or pancreatic duct obstruction caused by carcinoma or stricture, pancreatic enzyme replacement is necessary.

The duodenal pH in patients with chronic pancreatitis is often less than 5.0 late in the postprandial period. Glycine-conjugated bile acids may precipitate below pH 5.0, which reduces their availability and further impairs fat absorption. When the patient's history and physical examination are inconclusive for diagnosis, the secretin stimulation test is employed. This is probably the most commonly used direct method to determine the degree of impairment of pancreatic exocrine function. However, simpler indirect tests, such as the bentiromide or two-stage carbon 14-triolein test, have been devised for this assessment (Goff, 1981; Toskes, 1984).

Patients with severe pancreatic insufficiency manifested by high fecal fat excretion may have either a high or low rate of acid secretion. Those with a low rate of secretion respond well to enzyme replacement with conventional (plain) preparations. Those with a high rate of secretion may require enteric-coated preparations.

Replacement Therapy

Drug Selection: Pancreatic enzymes (lipase, protease, and amylase) are extracted from hog pancreas. Pancreatin and pancrelipase are effective for replacement therapy in diseases accompanied by a marked decrease in the secretion of these enzymes (eg, chronic pancreatitis, benign or malignant pancreatic tumors, cystic fibrosis, pancreatectomy). However, these enzymes should be used only after the diagnosis of exocrine pancreatic insufficiency has been confirmed. There is no rationale for their use in gastrointestinal disorders unrelated to pancreatic enzyme deficiency, as remedies for dyspepsia, or as "digestive aids."

Successful enzyme replacement therapy relieves symptoms of steatorrhea (diarrhea, abdominal fullness, or bloating and cramps) and prevents further weight loss or produces a gain in weight. Therapy can be assessed by comparing the 24-hour fat excretion in stool during therapy with a baseline measurement (Glendell and Cello, 1983).

Pancrelipase has largely replaced other pancreatic extracts used clinically. Some products are available in enteric-coated form to avoid destruction of the enzymes by gastric pepsin or inactivation by acid pH. However, the coating does not dissolve until the luminal pH is greater than 6.0, which may affect availability in the duodenum and upper jejunum where the enzyme is needed most. Enteric-coated microspheres are useful, but enteric-coated tablets containing pancreatin or pancrelipase have little clinical value (Graham, 1986).

The benefits obtained from enteric-coated microspheres and plain preparations usually are similar; in general, plain preparations are preferred because they contain more enzyme. However, the enteric-coated microspheres may be more beneficial in patients with high rates of acid secretion.

Lipase is irreversibly inactivated below pH 4.0. The use of adjuvants, such as antacids or histamine$_2$ blockers, to raise the pH of the intragastric contents has been employed in an attempt to improve the effectiveness of pancreatic enzymes in patients with relatively low rates of acid secretion as well as in those with relatively high acid output. However, patients with low rates of gastric acid secretion rarely require adjuvant therapy, for most respond adequately to the enzymes alone. The use of adjuvants in these patients will reduce the steatorrhea even further but the added improvement (although often statistically significant) is usually not clinically significant. In contrast, because patients with high rates of acid secretion will inactivate much of the enzyme in plain preparations, a good clinical response requires the use of adjuvants (and/or enteric-coated microspheres). Concomitant administration of sodium bicarbonate or aluminum hydroxide before or with a meal relieves steatorrhea more than the enzymes alone (Graham, 1982). Antacids containing calcium or magnesium do not reduce steatorrhea and may increase it in some patients. In addition, all antacids increase intragastric volume, which dilutes enzyme concentration and may decrease their effectiveness.

For children with cystic fibrosis, some physicians recommend adding pancreatic enzymes to applesauce, but this is inappropriate since the low pH immediately and irreversibly inactivates lipase.

Bile salts or proteolytic enzymes of plant origin (eg, proteolytic enzymes from *Carica papaya* [Papase]) are of no benefit in exocrine pancreatic insufficiency.

Adverse Reactions and Precautions: Although allergic reactions to the animal protein in enzyme preparations occur only rarely, allergic rhinitis and bronchospasm have resulted from sensitization induced by repeated inhalation of the powder. These enzymes should be used cautiously in patients sensitive to pork. Respiratory symptoms caused by inhalation of pancreatic powder may develop in the absence of sensitivity to ingested pork.

Large doses of pancreatic enzymes may produce diarrhea, nausea, abdominal cramps, or pain. A high-fiber diet may decrease the efficacy of oral pancreatic enzymes. In patients with diabetes, the value of a high-fiber diet must be weighed against the need to reduce steatorrhea (Dutta and Hlasko, 1985).

Dosage Requirements: Dosage should be individualized and is based on the activity of the lipase, protease, and amylase in each product rather than on the weight of the extract. Requirements depend upon the degree of maldigestion and malabsorption, the amount of fat in the diet, and the enzyme activity of each preparation. Enzyme tablets should be taken with every meal and snack for maximal effectiveness. Compliance is a problem, particularly in alcoholics.

Rarely, it may be necessary to reduce the dietary intake of fat. This is required usually only in patients with persistent watery diarrhea after steatorrhea has been reduced. In such patients, medium-chain triglycerides may be necessary to supply additional calories.

Preparations of much higher specific activity than those presently available are urgently needed to simplify and facilitate treatment.

Pain Relief in Chronic Pancreatitis

In investigational studies, oral pancreatic enzyme tablets have relieved recurrent abdominal pain in patients with chronic pancreatitis. This beneficial effect may result from feedback inhibition of pancreatic exocrine secretion. Pain is relieved much more effectively in patients with mild chronic or nonalcoholic pancreatitis than in those with severe pancreatic insufficiency (Isaksson and Ihse, 1983; Goldberg and Barkin, 1983; Toskes, 1983).

Drug Evaluations

PANCREATIN

Pancreatin preparations are derived from hog pancreas and contain varying amounts of amylase, proteases, lipases, and other constituents. In the FDA tentative final monograph on exocrine pancreatic insufficiency drug products, pancreatin preparations are classified as safe and effective (*Federal Register*, 1985). Preparations containing pancreatin have been largely supplanted clinically by pancrelipase preparations because of the latter's greater enzyme activity.

See the Introduction to this section for indications and precautions.

DOSAGE AND PREPARATIONS.

Oral: Adults, 4 to 18 g of extract (triple U.S.P. strength) daily in divided doses at mealtimes; an extra dose should be taken with any food eaten between meals. Administration at one- or two-hour intervals throughout the day or before and within an hour after meals also has been suggested, but no apparent advantage is gained from administration of the enzymes at any time other than when food is ingested, presumably because food acts as a buffer of gastric acidity and the gastric pH is highest during the digestive period. *Children*, initially, 300 to 600 mg with each meal. Dosage or frequency of administration may be increased to further reduce steatorrhea if nausea, vomiting, or diarrhea does not occur.

> **Pancreatin** (Lilly). Tablets (enteric-coated) containing pancreatin 1 g (lipase 2,000 U.S.P. units, protease 25,000 U.S.P. units, and amylase 25,000 U.S.P. units); tablets (plain) containing pancreatin 325 mg (lipase 650 U.S.P. units, protease 8,125 U.S.P. units, and amylase 8,125 U.S.P. units) (both forms nonprescription).

PANCRELIPASE

> [Cotazym, Cotazym-S, Festal II, Ilozyme, Pancrease, Viokase]

The action of pancrelipase, which is derived from hog pancreas, is qualitatively similar to that of other pancreatic enzyme preparations; however, its lipase activity is greater, permitting better control of steatorrhea. (At present, Ilozyme is the most potent product in terms of lipase activity.) Pancrelipase preparations contain much more enzyme activity than pancreatin preparations and have largely supplanted the latter. Pancrelipase also may be more acceptable to patients than pancreatin because of the smaller dosage required. The enteric-coated microspheres may be more useful than plain or enteric-coated products in patients with high rates of acid excretion. The plain tablets are preferred in other patients.

In the FDA tentative final monograph on exocrine pancreatic insufficiency drug products, pancrelipase preparations are classified as safe and effective (*Federal Register*, 1985).

See the Introduction to this section for indications and precautions. Caution is advised when administering pancrelipase to patients sensitive to pork. Pancrelipase is classified in FDA Pregnancy Category C.

DOSAGE AND PREPARATIONS.

Oral: Adults, 600 to 900 mg (one to three tablets or capsules) before each meal, 900 mg with meals, 600 mg within an hour after meals, and 300 mg with any food eaten between meals. *Children*, 300 to 600 mg taken in the same manner outlined for adults. In severe deficiency, 1 g every waking hour has been given.

> **Cotazym** (Organon). Each capsule (porcine) (plain, flavored) contains lipase 8,000 U.S.P. units, protease 30,000 U.S.P. units, amylase 30,000 U.S.P. units, and precipitated calcium carbonate 25 mg.
>
> **Cotazym-S** (Organon). Each capsule (porcine) (enteric-coated microspheres) contains lipase 5,000 U.S.P. units, protease 20,000 U.S.P. units, and amylase 20,000 U.S.P. units. (NOTE: Capsules should not be crushed or chewed.)
>
> **Festal II** (Hoechst-Roussel). Each tablet (enteric-coated) contains lipase 6,000 U.S.P. units, protease 20,000 U.S.P. units, and amylase 30,000 U.S.P. units (nonprescription).
>
> **Ilozyme** (Adria). Each tablet (porcine) contains lipase 11,000 U.S.P. units, protease 30,000 U.S.P. units, and amylase 30,000 U.S.P. units.
>
> **Pancrease** (McNeil). Each capsule (porcine) (enteric-coated microspheres) contains no less than lipase 4,000 U.S.P. units, protease 25,000 U.S.P. units, and amylase 20,000 U.S.P. units. (Note: Capsules should not be crushed or chewed.)
>
> **Viokase** (Robins). Each tablet (porcine) contains lipase 8,000 U.S.P. units, protease 30,000 U.S.P. units, and amylase 30,000 U.S.P. units; each 0.7 g of powder (porcine) contains lipase 16,800 U.S.P. units, protease 70,000 U.S.P. units, and amylase 70,000 U.S.P. units. (NOTE: The bad taste of the powder reduces compliance.)

MIXTURES

The following mixtures contain bile constituents and derivatives, enzymes, sedatives (eg, phenobarbital), antispasmodics, cellulase, and other ingredients; they are marketed for the treatment of many ill-defined gastrointestinal syndromes. There is no scientific rationale or evidence of efficacy to support the use of most of these mixtures and no established indications for ox bile, pepsin, and hydrochloric acid. Pancreatic enzymes are indicated only when an exocrine pancreatic deficiency has been demonstrated, in which case adequate quantities of the enzymes alone should be prescribed. When the other active ingredients of these mixtures are required, they should be prescribed separately rather than in combination with useless or inappropriate drugs. For these reasons, use of these mixtures cannot be justified. Examples of commonly used products are listed only for information.

> **Cholan HMB** (Pennwalt). Each tablet contains dehydrocholic acid 250 mg, phenobarbital 8 mg, and homatropine methylbromide 2.5 mg.
>
> **Cotazym-B** (Organon). Each tablet contains lipase 4,000 U.S.P. units, protease 15,000 U.S.P. units, amylase 15,000 U.S.P. units, mixed conjugated bile salts 65 mg, and cellulase 2 mg (nonprescription).
>
> **Donnazyme** (Robins). Each tablet contains pancreatin 300 mg

and bile salts 150 mg (in enteric-coated core) and hyoscyamine sulfate 0.0518 mg, atropine sulfate 0.0097 mg, scopolamine hydrobromide 0.0033 mg, phenobarbital 8.1 mg, and pepsin 150 mg (in outer layer).

Entozyme (Robins). Each tablet contains pepsin 250 mg (in outer layer) and pancreatin 300 mg and bile salts 150 mg (in enteric-coated core).

Festalan (Hoechst-Roussel). Each tablet contains lipase 6,000 U.S.P. units, protease 20,000 U.S.P. units, amylase 30,000 U.S.P. units, and atropine methylnitrate 1 mg (in outer layer).

Kutrase (Rorer). Each capsule contains lipase 75 mg, protease 6 mg, amylase 30 mg, hyoscyamine sulfate 0.0625 mg, and phenyl-toloxamine citrate 15 mg.

Cited References

Branched-chain amino acids in treatment of latent portosystemic encephalopathy. *Intern Med Alert* 30-31 (April 30), 1985.

Exocrine pancreatic insufficiency drug products for over-the-counter human use; tentative final monograph. *Federal Register* 50:46594-46600, 1985.

Hepatic encephalopathy today. *Lancet* 1:489-491, 1984.

Albers JJ, et al: National Cooperative Gallstone Study: Effect of chenodeoxycholic acid on lipoproteins and apolipoproteins. *Gastroenterology* 82:638-646, 1982.

Allen MJ, Thistle JL: Management of biliary duct stones. *Drug Ther (Hosp)* 8:17-24, (July) 1983.

Allen MJ, et al: Rapid dissolution of gallstones by methyl tert-butyl ether. *N Engl J Med* 312:217-220, 1985.

Atterbury CE, et al: Neomycin-sorbitol and lactulose in treatment of acute portal-systemic encephalopathy: Controlled, double-blind clinical trial. *Am J Digest Dis* 23:398-406, 1978.

Bachrach WH, Hofmann AF: Ursodeoxycholic acid in treatment of cholesterol cholelithiasis, parts I and II. *Digest Dis Sci* 27:737-761, 833-856, 1982.

Brewer GJ, et al: Oral zinc therapy for Wilson's disease. *Ann Intern Med* 99:314-320, 1983.

Burroughs AK, et al: Controlled trial of propranolol for prevention of recurrent variceal hemorrhage in patients with cirrhosis. *N Engl J Med* 309:1539-1542, 1983.

Clark ML: Portal hypertension, (editorial). *J R Soc Med* 75:761-764, 1982.

Conn HO: Lactulose: Drug in search of modus operandi. *Gastroenterology* 74:624-626, 1978.

Conn HO, et al: Comparison of lactulose and neomycin in treatment of chronic portal-systemic encephalopathy: Double-blind controlled trial. *Gastroenterology* 72:573-583, 1977.

Crossley JR, Williams R: Progress in treatment of chronic portosystemic encephalopathy. *Gut* 25:85-98, 1984.

Deering TB, et al: Effect of d-penicillamine on copper retention in patients with primary biliary cirrhosis. *Gastroenterology* 72:1208-1212, 1977.

Deiss A: Treatment of Wilson's disease, (editorial). *Ann Intern Med* 99:398-400, 1983.

Dickson ER, et al: Trial of D-penicillamine in advanced primary biliary cirrhosis. *N Engl J Med* 312:1011-1015, 1985.

Dutta S, Hlasko J: Dietary fiber in pancreatic disease: Effect of high fiber diet on fat malabsorption in pancreatic insufficiency and in vitro study of interaction of dietary fiber with pancreatic enzymes. *Am J Clin Nutr* 41:517-525, 1985.

Egberts E-H, et al: Branched chain amino acids in treatment of latent portosystemic encephalopathy: Double-blind placebo-controlled crossover study. *Gastroenterology* 88:887-895, 1985.

Epstein O, et al: D-penicillamine treatment improves survival in primary biliary cirrhosis. *Lancet* 1:1275-1277, 1981.

Fischer JE: Amino acids in hepatic coma. *Digest Dis Sci* 27:97-102, 1982.

Fordtran JS, et al: Ox bile treatment of severe steatorrhea in ileectomy patient. *Gastroenterology* 82:564-568, 1982.

Fromm H: Gallstone dissolution and cholesterol-bile acid-lipoprotein axis: Propitious effects of ursodeoxycholic acid. *Gastroenterology* 87:229-233, 1984.

Glendell JH, Cello JP: Chronic pancreatitis, in Sleisenger MH, Fordtran JS (eds): *Gastrointestinal Disease: Pathophysiology, Diagnosis, Management.* Philadelphia, WB Saunders, vol II, 1983, 1503-1505.

Goff JS: Pancreatic exocrine function testing. *West J Med* 135:368-375, 1981.

Goldberg H, Barkin JS: Treatment of chronic pancreatitis. *Compr Ther* 9:53-56, (Nov) 1983.

Graham DY: Pancreatic enzyme replacement: Effect of antacids or cimetidine. *Digest Dis Sci* 27:485-490, 1982.

Graham DY: Treatment of steatorrhea in chronic pancreatitis. *Hosp Pract* 21:125-129, (Jan 15) 1986.

Hofmann AF: Gallstone-dissolving drugs: New approach to old disease. *Drug Ther* 12:57-71, (Feb) 1982.

Hofmann AF, et al: Clinical experience with mono-octanoin for dissolution of bile duct stones: Uncontrolled multicenter trial. *Digest Dis Sci* 26:954-955, 1981.

Isaksson G, Ihse I: Pain reduction by oral pancreatic enzyme preparation in chronic pancreatitis. *Digest Dis Sci* 28:97-102, 1983.

Isselbacher KJ: Chenodiol for gallstones: Dissolution or disillusion? *Ann Intern Med* 95:377-379, 1981.

Jarrett LN, et al: Intraductal infusion of mono-octanoin: Experiences in 24 patients. *Lancet* 1:68-70, 1981.

Jones EA: Enigma of hepatic encephalopathy. *Postgrad Med J* 59(suppl 4):42-54, 1983.

Kupfer S, et al: Gallstone dissolution rate during chenic acid therapy. *Digest Dis Sci* 27:1025-1029, 1982.

Lanthier PL, Morgan MY: Lactitol in treatment of chronic hepatic encephalopathy: Open comparison with lactulose. *Gut* 26:415-420, 1985.

Lebrec D, et al: Propranolol for prevention of recurrent gastrointestinal bleeding in patients with cirrhosis: Controlled study. *N Engl J Med* 305:1371-1374, 1981.

Maddrey WC: Primary biliary cirrhosis. *Res Staff Physician* 30:30pc-38pc, 1984.

Marks JW, et al: Additional chenodiol therapy after partial dissolution of gallstones with two years of treatment. *Ann Intern Med* 100:383-384, 1984 A.

Marks JW, et al: Low-dose chenodiol to prevent gallstone recurrence after dissolution therapy. *Ann Intern Med* 100:376-381, 1984 B.

Matloff DS, et al: Prospective trial of D-penicillamine in primary biliary cirrhosis. *N Engl J Med* 306:319-326, 1982.

McSherry CK: National Cooperative Gallstone Study Report: Surgeon's perspective. *Ann Intern Med* 95:379-380, 1981.

Palmer RH, Carey MC: Optimistic view of National Cooperative Gallstone Study. *N Engl J Med* 306:1171-1174, 1982.

Palmer KR, Hofmann AF: Intraductal mono-octanoin for direct dissolution of bile duct stones: Experience in 343 patients. *Gut* 27:196-202, 1986.

Ransohoff DF, et al: Prophylactic cholecystectomy or expectant management for silent gallstones. *Ann Intern Med* 99:199-204, 1983.

Reding P, et al: Oral zinc supplementation improves hepatic encephalopathy: Results of randomized controlled trial. *Lancet* 2:493-495, 1984.

Reynolds TB: What to do about esophageal varices? *N Engl J Med* 309:1575-1577, 1983.

Schoenfield LJ, et al: Chenodiol (chenodeoxycholic acid) for dissolution of gallstones: National Cooperative Gallstone Study, controlled trial of efficacy. *Ann Intern Med* 95:257-282, 1981.

Steinhagen RM, Pertsemlidis D: Monooctanoin dissolution of retained biliary stones in high risk patients. *Gastroenterology* 78:756-760, 1983.

Tangedahl TN: Management of gallstones: New option of bile acid therapy. *Postgrad Med* 74:115-121, (Nov) 1983.

Tangedahl T, et al: Drug and treatment efficacy of chenodeoxycholic acid in 97 patients with cholelithiasis and increased surgical risk. *Digest Dis Sci* 28:545-551, 1983.

Toskes PP: Pancreatic extract does decrease abdominal pain in patients with chronic pancreatitis. *Gastroenterology* 84:1629, 1983.

Toskes PP: Bentiromide test for pancreatic exocrine insufficiency. *Pharmacotherapy* 4:74-80, 1984.

Tritapepe R, et al: Treatment of retained biliary stones with mono-octanoin: Report of 16 patients. *Am J Gastroenterol* 79:710-714, 1984.

Tyor MP: Selecting patients for gallstone-dissolving therapy. *Drug Ther* 13:237-252, (April) 1983.

Vince A, et al: Effect of lactulose on ammonia production in fecal incubation system. *Gastroenterology* 74:544-549, 1978.

Ward A, et al: Ursodeoxycholic acid: Review of its pharmacological properties and therapeutic efficacy. *Drugs* 27:95-131, 1984.

Dermatologic Preparations *56*

THERAPEUTIC AGENTS

    Anti-inflammatory Corticosteroids

    Corticosteroid-Antibiotic Mixtures

    Keratolytic Agents

    Antiacne Agents

    Antidandruff-Antiseborrheic Agents

    Antipsoriatic Agents

    Agents Affecting Pigmentation

    Topical Anesthetics and Antipruritics

    Cytotoxic Agents

    Agents Used in Skin Ulcers

    Agents Used to Stimulate Hair Growth

    Miscellaneous Agents

PROPHYLACTIC AGENTS

    Antiperspirants and Deodorants

    Sunscreens

VEHICLES

    Constituents

    Wet Dressings

    Lotions

    Gels

    Creams and Ointments

    Urea

    Propylene Glycol

    Pastes

    Soaps, Soap Substitutes, and Shampoos

    Baths and Body Oils

When a topical rather than a systemic preparation is selected to treat a cutaneous disorder, both the active ingredient(s) and the vehicle must be taken into account. The choice of active ingredient depends upon an accurate diagnosis; the choice of vehicle depends upon the character of the affected skin and site of the lesion. The dermatologic preparations discussed are divided into three main categories: (1) agents used therapeutically, (2) agents used prophylactically, and (3) vehicles.

In general, concentration or dose, vehicle, and container size are listed for prescription drugs but not for most OTC preparations. General guidelines for determining the amount of topical medication to apply once the concentration of active ingredient(s) and vehicle have been selected are presented in Table 1. Information on adverse reactions, contraindications, and precautions appear in the introduction for each therapeutic class.

THERAPEUTIC AGENTS

Anti-inflammatory Corticosteroids

Uses: Seborrheic dermatitis, atopic dermatitis, lichen simplex chronicus, nummular eczematous dermatitis, and pruritus ani generally respond to topical corticosteroids of low to medium potency (Robertson and Maibach, 1983; Bickers et al,

1984; Pollat, 1984). Phototoxic reactions and contact dermatitis due to allergens, irritant chemicals, dryness (inflammatory xerosis), and heat and moisture (intertrigo) also respond, particularly the nonweeping later phases. These drugs are useful in mild psoriasis of the face and body folds, but that affecting the palms, soles, elbows, and knees usually requires more potent topical steroids. The latter also are generally required for discoid lupus erythematosus, sarcoidosis, necrobiosis lipoidica diabeticorum, hypertrophic lichen planus, lichen striatus, familial benign pemphigus, and pretibial myxedema. If higher concentrations with occlusion are ineffective for hypertrophic lichen planus, psoriasis, and alopecia areata, intralesional injection may be necessary. The intralesional route is recommended for hypertrophic scars early in their development, keloids, granuloma annulare, acne cysts, prurigo nodularis, and chondrodermatitis nodularis helicus. Systemic corticosteroids may be required for acute, severe, allergic, contact dermatitis.

Hydrocortisone acetate [Orabase HCA] or triamcinolone acetonide [Kenalog in Orabase] dental paste may be useful adjunctively in nonherpetic oral inflammatory and ulcerative lesions.

Topical corticosteroids are contraindicated in varicella and vaccinia.

Actions: The mechanisms of action of the corticosteroids are related to vasoconstriction and suppression of membrane permeability, mitotic activity, the immune response, and re-

TABLE 1.
AMOUNT OF TOPICAL MEDICATION FOR TREATMENT*

Area Treated	Single Application (g)	Application Three Times Daily for		
		1 week	2 weeks g(oz)	4 weeks
Hands, head, face, anogenital area	2	45 (1.5)	90 (3)	180 (6)
One arm, anterior or posterior trunk	3	60 (2)	120 (4)	240 (8)
One leg	4	90 (3)	180 (6)	360 (12)
Entire body	30	630 (21) 1¼ (lb)		

The amounts recommended apply whether a lotion, cream, or ointment is presecribed (Lynfield and Schechter, 1984). Adapted from Arndt, 1983.

lease of inflammatory mediators. Vasoconstriction decreases extravasation of serum into the skin and inhibits swelling and discomfort. The lysosomal membrane-stabilizing effect inhibits the release of cytotoxic chemicals that cause pain and pruritus. Suppression of mitotic activity diminishes epidermal hyperplasia, but undesirable epidermal and dermal atrophy may result from excessive interference with these synthetic pathways. Corticosteroids suppress the immune response by interfering with lymphokine enhancement of the immune response, thus limiting migration of immune-effector substances to the site of inflammation. Suppression of phospholipase A diminishes the availability of the arachidonic acid necessary in the production of some mediators of inflammation.

Drug Selection: In addition to the disorder and its severity, selection of a corticosteroid depends primarily upon the drug's inherent potency, concentration, formulation, and method of application; the site of disease; the patient's age; and the expense.

The formulation and method of application affect the degree of absorption; selection also is influenced by the character of the lesions (wet or dry). See the section on Vehicles for a more detailed discussion. An occlusive wrap can increase absorption as much as tenfold.

Selected topical corticosteroids are grouped on the basis of potency in Table 2 (Cornell and Stoughton, 1984, 1985; Stoughton and Cornell, 1985). The most potent topical corticosteroids are generally fluorinated compounds. Although agents in this group may be effective when less potent corticosteroids are inadequate, the risk of adverse reactions also is increased. A more potent corticosteroid may be required for less permeable regions (eg, palms, soles, back) and for more recalcitrant disorders. A low-potency steroid may be adequate in permeable areas (eg, scalp, axilla, face, eyelids, neck, perineum, genitals). A less potent steroid also should be considered for maintenance therapy, particularly for chronic skin diseases. Hydrocortisone is a steroid of choice in responsive conditions because it is inexpensive and its application to extensive areas for prolonged periods is relatively safe.

Younger individuals, especially infants, and elderly patients with atrophic skin may be more susceptible to the effects of

TABLE 2.
POTENCY RANKING OF SOME COMMONLY USED TOPICAL CORTICOSTEROIDS[1,2]

HIGH POTENCY

I. Betamethasone dipropionate ointment 0.05%[3] (optimized vehicle)
   Diprolene ointment
   Clobetasol propionate ointment 0.05%[3]
   Temovate ointment

II. Amcinonide ointment 0.1%
   Cyclocort ointment
   Betamethasone dipropionate ointment 0.05%
   Diprosone ointment
   Desoximetasone cream 0.25%
   Topicort cream
   Desoximetasone gel 0.05%
   Topicort gel
   Desoximetasone ointment 0.25%
   Topicort ointment
   Diflorasone diacetate ointment 0.05%
   Florone ointment
   Maxiflor ointment
   Fluocinonide cream 0.05%
   Lidex cream
   Fluocinonide gel 0.05%
   Lidex gel
   Fluocinonide ointment 0.05%
   Lidex ointment
   Halcinonide cream 0.1%
   Halog cream

III. Betamethasone dipropionate cream 0.05%
   Diprosone cream
   Betamethasone valerate ointment 0.1%
   Valisone ointment
   Diflorasone diacetate cream 0.05%
   Florone cream
   Maxiflor cream
   Triamcinolone acetonide cream 0.5%
   Aristocort cream (HP)

INTERMEDIATE POTENCY

IV. Betamethasone benzoate ointment 0.025%
　　Benisone ointment
　Desoximetasone cream 0.05%
　　Topicort LP cream
　Fluocinolone acetonide cream 0.2%
　　Synalar cream (HP)
　Fluocinolone acetonide ointment 0.025%
　　Synalar ointment
　Flurandrenolide ointment 0.05%
　　Cordran ointment
　Hydrocortisone valerate ointment 0.2%[4]
　　Westcort ointment
　Triamcinolone acetonide ointment 0.1%
　　Aristocort ointment
　　Kenalog ointment

V. Betamethasone benzoate cream 0.025%
　　Benisone cream
　Betamethasone dipropionate lotion 0.02%
　　Diprosone lotion
　Betamethasone valerate cream 0.1%
　　Valisone cream
　Betamethasone valerate lotion 0.1%
　　Valisone lotion
　Fluocinolone acetonide cream 0.025%
　　Synalar cream
　Flurandrenolide cream 0.05%
　　Cordran cream
　Hydrocortisone butyrate cream 0.1%[4]
　　Locoid cream
　Hydrocortisone valerate cream 0.2%[4]
　　Westcort cream
　Triamcinolone acetonide cream 0.1%
　　Kenalog cream
　Triamcinolone acetonide lotion 0.1%
　　Kenalog lotion

LOW POTENCY

VI. Desonide cream 0.05%[4]
　　Tridesilon cream
　Fluocinolone acetonide solution 0.01%
　　Synalar solution

VII. Topical preparations of hydrocortisone,[4] dexamethasone, prednisolone,[4] and methylprednisolone[4]

[1]*Adapted from Cornell and Stoughton, 1984*
[2]*Group I is the most potent and potency descends with each group to group VII, which is least potent (I, II, III = high-potency steroids; IV, V = intermediate-potency steroids; VI, VII = low-potency steroids). There is no significant difference between agents within any given group; within each group, the generic names of the compounds are arranged alphabetically.*
HP = high potency, LP = low potency
[3]*Package insert specifies no more then 45 g weekly [Diprolene] and 50 g weekly [Temovate] for two weeks followed by a rest period; not used under occlusive dressings*
[4]*Nonfluorinated steroids*

topical corticosteroids. Careful monitoring and use of less potent agents usually are indicated.

Expense can be a significant factor. The prototype of this group (hydrocortisone) is available generically over-the-counter in 0.5% strength, and thus generally costs less than most trademarked, higher potency preparations. However, because more aggressive therapy with higher potency corticosteroids may lessen the duration of illness, the number of work days lost, and the incidence of noncompliance, relative expense is best determined by the physician for the individual patient.

Adverse Reactions and Precautions: Predictable adverse reactions to topical corticosteroids are related directly to inherent potency, concentration of drug dispersed, volume applied, skin condition, duration of use, site and area of application, and use of occlusive vehicles or wraps (Robertson and Maibach, 1983; Bickers et al, 1984; Pollat, 1984). Epidermal and dermal atrophy resulting in thinning of the skin, striae, telangiectasia, and senile-type purpura are most commonly seen in highly absorptive areas (ie, face, neck, axilla, perineum, genitals).

Less common local effects include rosacea-like dermatoses, perioral dermatitis, acne, folliculitis, and nonhealing leg ulcers. Hypopigmentation occurs, especially in blacks. Hypertrichosis is a side effect of the more potent corticosteroids. Ocular hypertension has been reported. Allergic contact dermatitis is rare and often is caused by the vehicle rather than the steroid. A comparison of the vehicles used in topical corticosteroid preparations is available (Tan et al, 1986). Superficial epidermal fissures that resemble erythema craquele rarely follow termination of prolonged occlusive therapy.

When the more potent steroids used for eczema and psoriasis are discontinued, rebound erythroderma or pustulation may develop on all body surfaces. Corticosteroids can mask or aggravate dermatophytoses, impetigo, or scabies (see the section on Corticosteroid-Antibiotic Mixtures).

Pregnancy and Lactation: If prolonged use of occlusive dressings and/or application on extensive areas are avoided, adverse effects during pregnancy or lactation do not occur. Excessive absorption of the more potent corticosteroids causes fetal abnormalities in animals but no well-controlled, adequate studies have been performed in pregnant women (FDA Pregnancy Category C).

Toxicity: Systemic toxicity is usually observed only when high-potency corticosteroids are applied to extensive areas under occlusive dressings for prolonged periods, especially in diseases that alter cutaneous permeability (eg, exfoliative erythroderma). Miliaria and bacterial and candidal infections are more common with use of occlusive dressings. Systemic toxicity is generally not a major concern except in children, especially those undergoing occlusive therapy, who may experience growth suppression even when relatively small amounts of steroid are absorbed systemically.

Systemic effects generally do not occur when the total weekly dose of a high-potency steroid does not exceed 30 g in adults or 10 g in children. If (1) the dose of high-potency steroid exceeds 50 g in adults or 30 g in children, (2) daily treatment is required for more than two weeks, or (3) liver function is impaired, and it is not possible to reduce the dose or dosage schedule (eg, alternate-day therapy) or substitute a less potent steroid (Parish et al, 1985), assessment of hypothalamic-pituitary-adrenal (HPA) function may be indicated. Individuals taking large total doses of high-potency corticosteroids, with or without occlusive dressings, should receive a supplemental systemic corticosteroid if surgery is necessary. For the signs and symptoms of systemic toxicity, see Chapter 61, Adrenal Corticosteroids in Nonendocrine Diseases.

Dosage and Preparations: Small amounts of the lotion, cream, or ointment should be rubbed gently on involved areas. Initially, application two to four times daily may be required. Once control is established, the frequency of application should be reduced to the minimum to avoid relapse. Application once or twice a day may be sufficient.

AMCINONIDE:
Cyclocort (Lederle). Cream and ointment 0.1% in 15, 30, and 60 g containers.
BETAMETHASONE:
Generic. Cream, ointment, and lotion 0.1%.
BETAMETHASONE BENZOATE:
Benisone (Rydelle). Cream, gel, and ointment 0.025% in 15 and 60 g containers; lotion 0.025% in 15 and 60 ml containers.
Uticort (Parke-Davis). Cream, gel, and ointment 0.025% in 15 and 60 g containers; lotion 0.025% in 15 and 60 ml containers.
BETAMETHASONE DIPROPIONATE:
Alphatrex (Savage). Cream and ointment 0.05% in 15 and 45 g containers.
Diprolene (Schering). Ointment 0.05% in 15 and 45 g containers. (NOTE: Diprolene has much higher potency than Diprosone.)
Diprosone (Schering). Aerosol 0.1% in 85 g containers; cream and ointment 0.05% in 15 and 45 g containers; lotion 0.05% in 20 and 60 ml containers.
BETAMETHASONE VALERATE:
Generic. Cream, ointment, and lotion 0.1%.
Betatrex (Savage). Cream and ointment 0.1% in 15 and 45 g containers; lotion 0.1% in 60 ml containers.
Beta-Val (Lemmon). Cream 0.1% in 15 and 45 g containers.
Valisone (Schering). Cream 0.01% in 15 and 60 g containers and 0.1% in 15, 45, 110, and 430 g containers; lotion 0.1% in 20 and 60 ml containers; ointment 0.1% in 15 and 45 g containers.
CLOBETASOL PROPIONATE:
Temovate (Glaxo). Cream and ointment 0.05%.
CLOCORTOLONE PIVALATE:
Cloderm (Ortho). Cream 0.1% in 15 and 45 g containers.
DESONIDE:
DesOwen (Owen). Cream 0.05% in 15 and 60 g containers.
Tridesilon (Miles). Cream and ointment 0.05% in 15 and 60 g containers.
DESOXIMETASONE:
Topicort (Hoechst-Roussel). Cream 0.25% in 15, 60, and 120 g containers and 0.05% (**Topicort LP**) in 15 and 60 g containers; gel 0.05% in 15 and 60 g containers; ointment 0.25% in 15 and 60 g containers.
DEXAMETHASONE:
Aeroseb-Dex (Herbert). Aerosol 0.01% in 60 g containers.
Decaderm (Merck Sharp & Dohme). Gel 0.1% in 30 g containers.
Decaspray (Merck Sharp & Dohme). Aerosol 0.04% in 25 g containers.
DEXAMETHASONE SODIUM PHOSPHATE:
Decadron Phosphate (Merck Sharp & Dohme). Cream 0.1% in 15 and 30 g containers.
DIFLORASONE DIACETATE:
Florone (Dermik). Cream and ointment 0.05% in 15, 30, and 60 g containers.
Maxiflor (Herbert). Cream and ointment 0.05% in 15, 30, and 60

g containers.
FLUOCINOLONE ACETONIDE:
Generic. Cream 0.01% and 0.025% in 15, 60, and 425 g containers; ointment 0.025% in 15, 30, and 60 g containers; solution 0.01% in 20 and 60 ml containers.
Fluonid (Herbert). Cream 0.01% and 0.025% in 15 and 60 g containers; ointment 0.025% in 15 and 60 g containers; solution 0.01% in 20 and 60 ml containers.
Synalar (Syntex). Cream 0.01% and 0.025% in 15, 30, 60, 120, and 425 g containers and 0.2% (**Synalar-HP**) in 12 g containers; ointment 0.025% in 15, 30, 60, 120, and 425 g containers; solution 0.01% in 20 and 60 ml containers.
Synemol (Syntex). Cream 0.025% in 15, 30, 60, and 120 g containers.
FLUOCINONIDE:
Lidex (Syntex). Cream and ointment 0.05% in 15, 30, 60, and 120 g containers; gel 0.05% in 15, 30, 60, and 120 g containers; solution 0.05% in 20 and 60 ml containers.
FLURANDRENOLIDE:
Generic. Lotion 0.05% in 15 and 60 ml containers.
Cordran (Dista). Cream and ointment 0.05% in 15, 30, 60, and 225 g containers and 0.025% in 30, 60, and 225 g containers; tape 4 mcg/cm² in 7.5 cm X 60 cm and 7.5 cm X 200 cm rolls; lotion 0.05% in 15 and 60 ml containers.
HALCINONIDE:
Halog (Squibb). Cream 0.025% in 15 and 60 g containers and 0.1% in 15, 30, 60, and 240 g containers; ointment 0.1% in 15, 30, 60, and 240 g containers; solution 0.1% in 20 and 60 ml containers.
HYDROCORTISONE:
Generic. Cream, lotion, and ointment.
Aeroseb-HC (Herbert). Aerosol 0.5% in 60 g containers.
Alphaderm (Norwich Eaton). Cream 1% in a stabilized carbamide (urea) delivery system in 30 and 100 g containers.
Cetacort (Owen). Lotion 0.25% in 120 ml containers; 0.5% and 1% in 60 ml containers.
Cort-Dome (Miles). Cream 0.25% in 30 and 120 g containers, 0.5% in 15 and 30 g containers, and 1% in 15 and 30 g containers; lotion 0.25% and 0.5% in 120 ml containers and 1% in 30 ml containers.
Cortril (Pfipharmecs). Ointment 1% in 15 g containers.
Dermacort (Rowell). Cream 1% in 454 g containers; lotion 0.5% in 120 ml containers (nonprescription) and 1% in 120 ml containers.
Hytone (Dermik). Cream 1% in 28.4 and 113.4 g containers and 2.5% in 28.4 and 56.7 g containers; ointment 0.5% in 28.4 g containers, 1% in 28.4 and 113.4 g containers, and 2.5% in 28.4 g containers; lotion 1% in 118.3 ml containers and 2.5% in 59 ml containers.
Nutracort (Owen). Cream 1% in 30, 60, and 120 g containers; lotion 0.25% and 0.5% in 120 ml containers and 1% in 60 and 120 ml containers.
Penecort (Herbert). Cream 1% in 30 and 60 g containers and 2.5% in 30 g containers; ointment 2.5% in 30 g containers; topical solution in 30 and 60 ml containers.
Synacort (Syntex). Cream 1% in 15, 30, and 60 g containers and 2.5% in 30 g containers.
HYDROCORTISONE ACETATE:
Cortef Acetate (Upjohn). Ointment 1% in 20 g containers.
Orabase HCA (Hoyt). Dental paste 0.5% in 5 g containers.
HYDROCORTISONE BUTYRATE:
Locoid (Owen). Cream and ointment 0.1% in 15 and 45 g containers.
HYDROCORTISONE VALERATE:
Westcort (Westwood). Cream 0.2% in 15, 45, 60, and 120 g containers; ointment 0.2% in 15, 45, and 60 g containers.
METHYLPREDNISOLONE ACETATE:
Medrol Acetate (Upjohn). Ointment 0.25% and 1% in 7.5 and 30 g containers.

TRIAMCINOLONE ACETONIDE:

Generic. Cream 0.025% and 0.1% in 15, 80, 240, and 454 g containers and 0.5% in 15 and 120 g containers; lotion 0.025% in 60 ml containers and 0.1% in 15 and 60 ml containers; ointment 0.025% and 0.1% in 15, 80, 120, and 240 g containers and 0.5% in 15 and 20 g containers.

Aristocort (Lederle). Cream 0.025% and 0.1% in 15, 60, and 240 g containers and 0.5% in 15 and 240 g containers; ointment 0.1% in 15, 60, and 240 g containers and 0.5% in 15 and 240 g containers.

Aristocort A (Lederle). Cream 0.025% in 15 and 60 g containers, 0.1% in 15, 60, and 240 g containers, and 0.5% in 15 and 240 g containers; ointment 0.1% in 15 and 60 g containers and 0.5% in 15 g containers.

Kenalog (Squibb). Cream 0.025% in 15, 80, and 240 g containers, 0.1% in 15, 60, 80, and 240 g containers, and 0.5% in 20 g containers; lotion 0.025% and 0.1% in 15 and 60 ml containers; ointment 0.025% in 15, 80, and 240 g containers, 0.1% in 15, 60, 80, and 240 g containers, and 0.5% in 20 g containers; aerosol 0.147 mg/g in 23 and 63 g containers.

Kenalog-H (Squibb). Cream 0.1% in 15 and 60 g containers.

Kenalog in Orabase (Squibb). Dental paste 0.1% in 5 g containers.

Triacet (Lemmon). Cream 0.025% and 0.1% in 15 and 80 g containers and 0.5% in 15 g containers.

Trymex (Savage). Cream 0.025% and 0.1% in 15, 80, and 454 g containers and 0.5% in 15 g containers; ointment 0.025% and 0.1% in 15 and 80 g containers.

Corticosteroid-Antibiotic Mixtures

When secondary pyoderma is superimposed on pre-existing dermatitis or when allergic inflammatory dermatitis (eg, eczema) develops in response to primary pyoderma, the concomitant use of a topical corticosteroid and antibiotic may be indicated. The criteria for selection of topical antibiotics and antifungal agents are presented in Chapter 74, Topical Anti-infective Agents: Drugs Used on Skin and Mucous Membranes. Criteria for selection of topical corticosteroids are presented in the preceding section on Anti-inflammatory Corticosteroids.

The use of combination products containing a topical corticosteroid and topical antibiotic or antifungal agent is controversial (Leyden and Kligman, 1978; Hodge, 1980). Those opposed argue that there is insufficient evidence that these mixtures are more effective than the steroid alone in secondary pyodermas and that such therapy may increase the risk of development of resistant organisms and allergic contact dermatitis (especially with neomycin). Those in favor point out that combination therapy significantly improves results when (1) therapy is initiated early; (2) is limited to one or two weeks' duration; (3) is avoided in patients with intertrigo, diaper dermatitis, and stasis dermatitis or skin ulcers to decrease the incidence of antibiotic sensitivity; and (4) is chosen on the basis of the area and probable organism involved (eg, neomycin for glabrous skin infections predominantly caused by *Staphylococcus aureus*).

A listing of representative mixtures follows. The following concentrations of antimicrobial agents are commonly present: neomycin sulfate 0.5%, polymyxin B sulfate 5,000 to 10,000 units/g, bacitracin 400 to 500 units/g, and nystatin 100,000 units/g.

AVAILABLE MIXTURES.

DEXAMETHASONE AND NEOMYCIN:

NeoDecadron (Merck Sharp & Dohme). Cream containing dexamethasone phosphate 0.1% and neomycin sulfate 0.5% in 15 and 30 g containers.

FLUOCINOLONE AND NEOMYCIN:

Neo-Synalar (Syntex). Cream containing fluocinolone acetonide 0.025% and neomycin sulfate 0.5% in 15, 30, and 60 g containers.

FLURANDRENOLIDE AND NEOMYCIN:

Cordran-N (Dista). Cream and ointment containing flurandrenolide 0.05% and neomycin sulfate 0.5% in 15, 30, and 60 g containers.

HYDROCORTISONE AND NEOMYCIN:

Generic. Ointment containing hydrocortisone 1% and neomycin 0.5%.

Neo-Cort-Dome (Miles). Cream containing hydrocortisone 0.5% and neomycin sulfate 0.5% in 15 g containers.

Neo-Cortef (Upjohn). Cream containing hydrocortisone acetate 1% and neomycin sulfate 0.5% in 20 g containers; ointment containing hydrocortisone acetate 0.5%, 1%, and 2.5% and neomycin sulfate 0.5% in 5 (1% and 2.5% concentrations only) and 20 g containers.

HYDROCORTISONE, NEOMYCIN, AND POLYMYXIN B:

Cortisporin (Burroughs Wellcome). Cream containing hydrocortisone acetate 0.5%, neomycin sulfate 0.5%, and polymyxin B 10,000 units in 7.5 g containers.

HYDROCORTISONE, NEOMYCIN, POLYMYXIN B, AND BACITRACIN ZINC:

Cortisporin (Burroughs Wellcome). Ointment containing hydrocortisone 1%, neomycin sulfate 0.5%, polymyxin B sulfate 5,000 units, and bacitracin zinc 400 units in 15 g containers.

METHYLPREDNISOLONE AND NEOMYCIN:

Neo-Medrol Acetate Topical (Upjohn). Topical containing methylprednisolone acetate 0.25% or 1% and neomycin sulfate 0.5% in 7.5 and 30 g containers.

PREDNISOLONE AND NEOMYCIN:

Neo-Delta-Cortef (Upjohn). Ointment containing prednisolone acetate 0.5% and neomycin sulfate 0.5% in 20 g containers.

TRIAMCINOLONE AND NYSTATIN:

Mycolog II (Squibb), *Mytrex F* (Savage). Cream and ointment containing triamcinolone acetonide 0.1% and nystatin 100,000 units in 15, 30, 60, and 120 (*Mycolog II* only) g containers.

Myco-Triacet II (Lemmon). Cream and ointment containing triamcinolone acetonide 0.1% and nystatin 100,000 units in 15, 30, and 60 (cream only) g containers.

Keratolytic Agents

Sulfur, resorcinol, and salicylic acid alter keratin and have weak antibacterial and antifungal activity. Keratolysis may be minimal (peeling) or result in extensive desquamation of the stratum corneum. Sulfur and resorcinol have a peeling effect at available therapeutic concentrations. Low concentrations of salicylic acid (3% to 6%) have a peeling action; concentrations exceeding 20% are keratolytic and are employed principally in the management of verrucae (warts), corns, and calluses. See the section on Antiviral Agents for Warts and Molluscum Contagiosum in Chapter 74, Topical Anti-infective Agents: Drugs Used on Skin and Mucous Membranes.

1006

SULFUR

RESORCINOL

Numerous nonprescription preparations contain sulfur or resorcinol in concentrations of 2% to 10%. Sulfur alone or with resorcinol is used for the topical treatment of acne vulgaris, dandruff, seborrheic dermatoses, superficial fungal infections, and diaper dermatoses. However, more potent and specific keratolytic, antifungal, and antibacterial agents are available for these conditions and are preferred.

Sulfur and/or resorcinol also have been combined with other active topical agents (eg, salicylic acid, coal tar products) in nonprescription preparations for psoriasis.

Nonprescription shampoos that contain salicylic acid 2% and sulfur 2% to 5% are available to treat seborrhea capitis. A preparation containing sulfur 3% and salicylic acid 6% in petrolatum is an alternative agent in erythrasma or superficial fungal infections.

Some physicians use sulfur 6% in petrolatum for scabies (and occasionally in pediculosis) in pregnant women, infants, and young children (see the section on Anti-infestation Agents in Chapter 74, Topical Anti-infective Agents: Drugs Used on Skin and Mucous Membranes).

PRECIPITATED SULFUR, U.S.P.:
Generic. Powder. Ointments containing sulfur 3% to 15% may be compounded by the pharmacist.
Sulfur Soap (Stiefel). Bar 10% precipitated sulfur.
RESORCINOL:
Available only as ingredient of mixtures.
SULFUR AND SALICYLIC ACID OR SODIUM SALICYLATE:
Fostex Medicated Cleansing Bar (Westwood), **Meted 2** (Rydelle), **pHisoDan Shampoo** (Winthrop-Breon), **SAStid** (Stiefel), **Sebulex** (Westwood), **Vanseb** (Herbert) (all forms nonprescription).

SALICYLIC ACID

USES. Salicylic acid 3% to 6% in an ointment base is useful in seborrheic dermatitis, acne, and psoriasis. The 6% concentration in petrolatum is used to thin or remove calluses. This concentration in a gel vehicle with propylene glycol 60% [Hydrisalic, Keralyt] is particularly effective when applied under occlusive dressings to treat ichthyosis but may cause irritation (see the evaluation on Propylene Glycol in the section on Vehicles).

Salicylic acid is used to treat superficial fungal infections, but more potent agents are available. A preparation containing benzoic acid 6% and salicylic acid 3% (Whitfield's ointment) is effective, but the antifungal effect is attributed to a keratolytic rather than fungistatic action. Keratolytic agents may be necessary initially when fungal infections in deeper layers are otherwise inaccessible to the more potent antifungal agents.

ADVERSE REACTIONS AND PRECAUTIONS. This drug is absorbed readily and is excreted slowly in the urine. Thus, salicylic acid should not be applied over large areas, in high concentrations, or for prolonged periods to extremities, in diabetics, or in patients with peripheral vascular disease, since acute inflammation and ulceration may occur after such use. This acid is not effective in a zinc oxide paste (eg, Lassar's Plain Zinc Paste) because it forms zinc salicylate, which is pharmacologically inactive.

Ointments or lotions containing salicylic acid are odorless and do not stain the skin.

DOSAGE AND PREPARATIONS.
Topical: To remove calluses, the ointment is applied at bedtime and washed off in the morning. An emery board or scalpel blade may be necessary to remove excessive callus.

The collodion solution is applied to corns; after drying, an adhesive moleskin is applied to the affected area for one to three days. The softened necrotic tissue is pared with a scalpel blade or scissors. Applications and parings are repeated as necessary.

SALICYLIC ACID, U.S.P.:
Generic. Powder.
SALICYLIC ACID COLLODION, U.S.P.
40% SALICYLIC ACID PLASTER, U.S.P.:
Numerous commercial products available. Selected concentrations (usually 5% to 17%) can be compounded by a pharmacist.
AVAILABLE MIXTURES.
Hydrisalic (Pedinol), **Keralyt** (Westwood). Gel containing salicylic acid 6% in a propylene glycol and alcohol vehicle in 30 g containers.
Saligel (Stiefel). Gel containing salicylic acid 5% with alcohol base 14% in 60 g containers.
Duofilm (Stiefel), **Salactic Film** (Pedinol). Flexible collodion containing salicylic acid 16.7% and lactic acid 16.7% in 15 ml containers.
Occlusal (GemDerm). Salicylic acid 17% with alcohol 20% in a polyacrylic vehicle in 15 ml containers.
BENZOIC AND SALICYLIC ACIDS OINTMENT:
Mixture available under the name Whitfield's Ointment in 30, 45, and 454 g containers (nonprescription).

Antiacne Agents

Acne vulgaris principally affects adolescents and young adults, who often are genetically predisposed. This disorder is caused by an exaggerated response to androgenic steroids (eg, testosterone, dehydroepiandrosterone, 17-hydroxyprogesterone) that results in an increase in the turnover of follicular cells, which are extremely cohesive (follicular retention hyperkeratosis), and an increase in sebum production. Since sebum serves as a substrate for lipase-producing *Propionibacterium acnes*, irritant free fatty acids are increased correspondingly. In addition, this bacterium releases at least two low-molecular-weight chemotactic factors that cause inflammation. The pilosebaceous follicles on the face, neck, chest, shoulders, and back are most commonly involved (Juhlin et al, 1980; Matsuoka, 1983; Shalita, 1984; Wilson, 1985).

Mild acne is characterized by oily skin and closed and open comedones; in moderate acne, papules, pustules, and inflammation are present. The primary lesions of severe acne vulgaris are nodules and inflammatory cysts that result in subsequent pitting or hypertrophic scars. Purulent abscesses are infrequent. An especially severe form of cystic or nodular acne is designated as acne conglobata or cystic acne.

Nondrug Therapy: Some acneiform eruptions are induced by industrial chemicals or drugs, especially corticosteroids, androgens, iodides, bromides, and androgenic progestins that are components of some oral contraceptives. If oral contraception is required, preparations with a higher ratio of estrogen to progestin should be chosen to minimize the androgenic effect of the progestin; progestin-only preparations should not be used. Efforts to limit or avoid these chemicals and drugs, as well as humid environments and occlusive cosmetic oils and greases, may be as important in the treatment of mild to moderate acne as drug therapy.

Dietary factors do not appear to be relevant in acne management. Gentle cleansing of affected areas two or three times daily minimizes surface oiliness, but scrubbing with or without abrasives may damage the delicate hair follicle openings through which sebum must flow.

Comedo extraction and chemosurgery, dermabrasion, or collagen injection may be useful in selected patients.

Drug Therapy: A number of objectives are beneficial in acne therapy (eg, reduction of sebum output and follicular retention hyperkeratosis, decreasing the number of *P. acnes* organisms, control of infection). The extent of follicular hyperkeratosis, occlusion, and inflammation determines therapy. Acne that is unresponsive to over-the-counter topical products, such as sulfur, resorcinol, salicylic acid, and benzoyl peroxide (2.5% to 5%) alone or in combination, requires a better program of compliance and physician instruction, as well as use of more potent medications, such as benzoyl peroxide 10%, tretinoin, and/or topical antibiotics. Severe, acute, inflammatory acne usually responds to systemic antibiotics given with topical agents initially; low-dose systemic or topical antibiotics can be used for maintenance (Stern et al, 1984 A). The sebostatic agent, isotretinoin, should be reserved for patients with severe cystic or nodular conglobate acne unresponsive to other therapy; *it is contraindicated during pregnancy.*

The use of estrogens or spironolactone in women for their antiandrogen action is investigational and should be reserved for individuals unresponsive to conventional therapy. The use of low-dose dexamethasone in patients with elevated androgen levels is investigational (Marynick et al, 1983).

Drug Selection: *Mild Acne.* Numerous nonprescription products of diverse formulation are available for mild acne, including bar soaps, soap-free cakes, liquid cleansers, lotions, gels, and creams. Abrasive particles (aluminum oxide, sodium tetraborate, polyethylene) are often included to remove surface debris, and alcohol or acetone is present to promote drying. Keratolytics added to promote peeling and comedolysis include sulfur, resorcinol, benzoyl peroxide, and salicylic acid. Hot compresses may be as effective as some nonprescription products.

Based on recommendations of an Advisory Panel on OTC Antimicrobial (II) Drug Products, the FDA has published a tentative final monograph on topical acne drug products (*Federal Register,* [Jan 15] 1985). Benzoyl peroxide, sulfur, and resorcinol with sulfur are considered to be safe and effective for the treatment of acne. Salicylic acid 0.5% to 2% is also safe and effective, but data are insufficient to determine the safety of concentrations above 2%. Astringents (aluminum and zinc salts), which promote drying, are classified as ineffective. Antiseptics, which are present in many formulations, are classified as unsafe and/or ineffective. The antimicrobial, povidone-iodine, is considered safe, but data are insufficient to permit its final classification as effective.

Moderate Acne. Useful topical drugs for inflammatory acne include benzoyl peroxide, tretinoin [Retin-A], and antibiotics.

Benzoyl peroxide lotions and creams are nonprescription products, but most gels are available only by prescription. Concentrations of 5% or 10% may be used in patients with mild to moderate acne who were previously untreated or inadequately treated. Both benzoyl peroxide and tretinoin are sometimes given for an additive effect: tretinoin for nighttime use and benzoyl peroxide for daytime use.

Topical clindamycin [Cleocin T], erythromycin [Akne-mycin, A/T/S, Erycette, EryDerm, Erymax, Staticin, T-Stat], meclocycline sulfosalicylate [Meclan], and tetracycline [Topicycline] also are useful in inflammatory acne. Although all of these topical antibiotics are widely used in the treatment of acne, few controlled comparative studies are available. Clindamycin was reported to be more effective than topical tetracycline in mild to moderate inflammatory facial acne, and the incidence and severity of adverse effects, such as burning, pruritus, erythema, or peeling, were similar (Padilla et al, 1981). Initial controlled short-term studies comparing 1.5% erythromycin to 1% clindamycin in moderate acne revealed little difference in efficacy and adverse reactions. Considerably more data are needed to establish the comparative efficacy of topical antibiotic preparations in the treatment of acne. Concern exists about this therapy, because antibiotic-resistant strains of bacteria may emerge at a more rapid rate (Eady et al, 1982).

Results of controlled studies showed topical clindamycin to be as efficacious as oral tetracycline 500 mg daily for inflammatory acne (Stoughton et al, 1980; Gratton et al, 1982). Based on the systemic side effects produced and pharmacokinetic data, topical absorption appears to be clinically insignificant; however, pseudomembranous colitis has been reported rarely after use of this route (Milstone et al, 1981; Rosen and Waisman, 1981). Therefore, patients with regional enteritis or ulcerative colitis should not receive topical clindamycin. No adequate, well-controlled, teratogenic studies are available; however, in reproductive studies in animals, the drug had no adverse effect. Clindamycin is present in human milk after systemic administration, but its presence after topical administration is unknown.

If inflammation is severe enough to warrant systemic antibiotic therapy, tetracycline is the drug of choice because of its effectiveness, low toxicity, and low cost. Oral doses of 250 mg four times daily may be required initially for severe inflammation. Optimum response generally requires 6 to 12 weeks, and 250 to 500 mg daily may be necessary for prolonged maintenance therapy. Alternatively, if tolerated, 500 mg twice daily or 1 g daily may be prescribed to improve compliance. Erythromycin is an acceptable alternative. Oral clindamycin 300 to 450 mg/day is equally effective; however, because pseudomembranous colitis occurs on occasion after oral administration, it should not be used orally for acne except in rare situations.

Cross resistance between topical clindamycin and erythromycin (but not oral or topical tetracycline) is usually present. Minocycline [Minocin] 50 to 200 mg daily orally is suggested if resistance develops to all three antibiotics. Administration once daily is adequate even during the acute inflammatory stage. A lack of interaction with food and more rapid alleviation of inflammation (Hubbell et al, 1982) are advantages of minocycline compared to tetracycline; the latter is less expensive, however.

Severe Acne. The treatment of severe, recalcitrant, cystic acne usually requires dermatologic consultation and more aggressive therapy. Larger doses of oral tetracycline (2 g/day), isotretinoin [Accutane], intralesional injection of corticosteroids, or hot compresses with sulfurated lime solution [Vleminckx] may be necessary. Oral estrogen therapy in women is rarely indicated since isotretinoin [Accutane] became available.

BENZOYL PEROXIDE

ACTIONS AND USES. Benzoyl peroxide is effective in acne vulgaris because of its keratolytic effect. Its bacteriostatic activity against *Propionibacterium acnes* may decrease the production of irritant free fatty acids in the follicle. However, some investigators dispute the relevance of free fatty acids in the pathogenesis of acne. Benzoyl peroxide is available in untinted or tinted vehicles in concentrations of 2.5% to 10%. Cream, lotion, and gel formulations are used for mild to moderate acne.

ADVERSE REACTIONS AND PRECAUTIONS. Benzoyl peroxide is absorbed to some extent after topical application to the forearm of primates. Benzoic acid is a major metabolite; however, it is cleared rapidly via the kidney and cumulation does not occur with therapeutic doses (Yeung et al, 1983). Systemic toxicity has not been reported in man. Some irritation must be accepted, since a dose-response relationship may exist between efficacy and irritation. Local irritation may be severe but is readily reversible and easily managed by reducing the frequency of use and dose.

Contact sensitivity is observed in 1% to 3% of patients under conditions of recommended use. Benzoyl peroxide should not be applied under an occlusive dressing, because it is a potent experimental contact sensitizer (delayed hypersensitivity), and a recent study in volunteers revealed that a reaction occurred in 70% of subjects after use of occlusive patches containing a 5% or 10% concentration. When sensitivity is suspected, patch tests may be performed with a freshly prepared 0.5% concentration in petrolatum.

DOSAGE AND PREPARATIONS. To avoid severe irritation, the patient should be instructed to limit the volume of material and the frequency of application initially and to increase the amount and duration of contact gradually as tolerance permits. The following is a conservative approach, assumes that the benzoyl peroxide can be washed off, and may be modified for individual patients.

Topical: The formulation is applied and left on the skin for 15 minutes the first evening. The length of exposure is increased by 15 minutes each evening thereafter until the preparation is tolerated for two hours. Benzoyl peroxide then may be left on overnight. An additional application may be necessary in the morning after sensitivity and response are determined. Contact with eyes, eyelids, and mucous membranes should be avoided. Gels containing acetone or alcohol tend to be more drying.

Liquid Cleanser:
Benzac W Wash (Owen) 5% and 10% in 120 ml containers; *Desquam-X Wash* (Westwood) 4% and 10% in 150 ml containers.
Fostex Wash (Westwood) 10% in 150 ml containers (nonprescription).

Gel (alcohol vehicle):
Generic 5% and 10% in 45 and 120 g containers; *Benzac 5, 10* (Owen) in 60 g containers; *5-, 10-Benzagel* (Dermik) in 45 and 90 g containers; *PanOxyl 5, 10* (Stiefel) in 60 and 120 g containers.

Gel (without alcohol):
Fostex 5% BPO (Westwood) in 20 g containers (nonprescription); *PanOxyl AQ 2.5%, 5%, 10%* (Stiefel) in 60 and 120 g containers; *Benzac W 2.5, 5, 10* (Owen) in 60 and 90 g containers; *Buf-Oxal 10* (3M) 10% in 60 ml containers (nonprescription); *Clear by Design* (Herbert) 2.5% in 45 and 90 g containers (nonprescription); *Desquam-X 5, 10* (Westwood), *Persa-Gel 5, 10* (Ortho), *Xerac BP 5, 10* (Person & Covey) in 45 and 90 g containers (nonprescription).

Cleansing Bar:
Fostex Cleansing Bar (Westwood) 10% (nonprescription); *PanOxyl Bar 5, 10* (Stiefel) (nonprescription).

Cream:
Clearasil (Vicks) 10% in 30 g containers; *Persadox* (paraben-free) 5%, *Persadox-HP* (Owen) 10% in 30 g containers (all forms nonprescription).

Lotion:
Generic 5% and 10% in 30 ml containers; *Benoxyl 5, 10* (Stiefel) in 30 and 60 ml containers; *Clearasil* (Vicks) 10% in 30 ml containers; *Loroxide* (Dermik) 5.5% in 25 g containers; *Oxy 5, 10* (Norcliff Thayer) 5% and 10% in 30 ml containers; *Persadox-HP* (Owen) 10% in 30 ml containers; *pHisoAc BP* (Winthrop-Breon) 10% in 30 g containers; *Vanoxide* (Dermik) 5% in 25 and 50 g containers (all forms nonprescription).

AVAILABLE MIXTURES.
Sulfoxyl (Stiefel). Lotion containing benzoyl peroxide 5% and sulfur 2% (Regular) or benzoyl peroxide 10% and sulfur 5% (Strong) in 30 ml containers.
Vanoxide-HC (Dermik). Lotion containing benzoyl peroxide 5% and hydrocortisone 0.5% in 25 and 50 ml containers.

CLINDAMYCIN PHOSPHATE
[Cleocin T]

ERYTHROMYCIN
[Akne-mycin, A/T/S, Erycette, EryDerm, Erymax, Staticin, T-Stat]

MECLOCYCLINE SULFOSALICYLATE
[Meclan]

TETRACYCLINE HYDROCHLORIDE
[Topicycline]

Topical antibiotic therapy is effective in the management of inflammatory acne vulgaris. For further discussion of topical, as well as systemic, antibiotic therapy for acne, see the introduction to this section.

DOSAGE AND PREPARATIONS.
Topical: The preparation is applied twice daily, morning and evening.

CLINDAMYCIN PHOSPHATE:
Cleocin T (Upjohn). Solution 1% in a 50% isopropyl alcohol and water vehicle in 30, 60, and 474 ml containers.
ERYTHROMYCIN:
Generic. Solution 1.5% and 2% in 60 ml containers.
Akne-mycin (Hermal). Ointment 2% in 25 g containers.
A/T/S (Hoechst Roussel). Solution 2% in a 66% alcohol vehicle in 60 ml containers.
Erycette (Ortho). Pledgets 2% in a 66% alcohol vehicle.
EryDerm (Abbott). Solution 2% in a 77% alcohol vehicle in 60 ml containers.
Erymax (Herbert). Solution 2% in a 66% alcohol vehicle in 120 ml containers.
Staticin (Westwood). Solution 1.5% in a 55% alcohol vehicle in 60 ml containers.
T-Stat (Westwood). Solution 2% in a 71% alcohol vehicle in 60 ml containers.
MECLOCYCLINE SULFOSALICYLATE:
Meclan (Ortho). Cream 1% in an aqueous (nonalcohol) vehicle in 20 and 45 g containers.
TETRACYCLINE HYDROCHLORIDE:
Topicycline (Norwich Eaton). Powder with diluent (n-decyl methyl sulfoxide, sodium bisulfite, and sucrose esters in 40% alcohol). Preparation must be reconstituted to make 70 ml of solution containing 2.2 mg/ml.
AVAILABLE MIXTURE.
Benzamycin (Dermik). Gel containing erythromycin 30 mg and benzoyl peroxide 50 mg/g (after reconstitution) in 23.3 g containers.

ISOTRETINOIN
[Accutane]

ACTIONS AND USES. ***Acne Conglobata or Cystic Acne:*** This *cis* configuration of retinoic (vitamin A) acid is very effective in acne conglobata, but it should be reserved for patients who do not respond to conventional therapy, including systemic antibiotics, because of its severe side effects.

Isotretinoin reduces sebaceous gland cell size, increases differentiation of pilosebaceous follicular cells, alters keratinization patterns, decreases sebum production, and decreases the growth of *Propionibacterium acnes* within the follicle. Its anti-inflammatory action is proposed to be due to inhibition of superoxide production and beta-glucuronidase release in neutrophils.

In early studies, lesions resistant to conventional therapy, including systemic antibiotics, cleared completely in most patients who received 1 to 2 mg/kg daily for four to five months (Rumsfield et al, 1983; Strauss et al, 1984; Ward et al, 1984). The recommended dose now is 0.5 to 1 mg/kg/day. A second course of therapy may be necessary for significant recurrences. However, an interim period of at least two months is suggested before beginning a second course because improvement usually continues after the first course is terminated.

Intensive clinical studies of isotretinoin continue. The following uses are investigational:

Disorders of Keratinization: More prolonged therapy may be required in some of the following disorders (DiGiovanna and Peck, 1983): Darier's disease, lamellar ichthyosis, keratosis palmaris et plantaris, erythrokeratoderma, keratoacanthoma, acantholytic dermatosis (Grover's disease), acne rosacea, pityriasis rubra pilaris, and premature sebaceous gland hyperplasia. Less than satisfactory responses were observed in patients with nevus comedonicus, x-linked ichthyosis, and Netherton's syndrome, which has worsened following therapy.

Hidradenitis Suppurativa and Mycosis Fungoides (Cutaneous T-cell Lymphoma): Limited case reports suggest that some patients respond to isotretinoin or etretinate. No comparative studies have been conducted and treatment must be considered palliative.

Gram-negative Folliculitis: Isotretinoin 0.5 to 1 mg/kg/day for five months is very effective in this condition and remissions are sustained (James and Leyden, 1985). An antibacterial action presumably is not responsible. *Staphylococcus aureus* nasal carriage develops in most patients, but colonization has not been a source of significant infection and can be minimized by applying antibiotic ointment to the anterior inner nares.

Basal and Squamous Cell Carcinomas: Although results of limited studies are encouraging, isotretinoin's definitive role has not been established.

Pustular Psoriasis: Although isotretinoin is effective in pustular psoriasis, another retinoid, etretinate, is much preferred.

ADVERSE REACTIONS AND PRECAUTIONS. Although almost all patients experience reversible cheilitis, discontinuation of therapy is seldom required. Xerosis and facial desquamation are common. Palmoplantar desquamation, pruritus, brittle nails, and alteration or loss of hair are uncommon at usual doses (0.5 to 1 mg/kg/day). Dryness of the mouth, nose, and eyes; epistaxis; conjunctivitis; and inflammation of the urethral meatus may be observed. Rarely, pyogenic granuloma-like acne lesions may develop (Exner et al, 1983).

Headaches and insomnia are observed in 10% and 5% of patients, respectively. Pseudotumor cerebri and/or papilledema were associated with the use of isotretinoin. Lens opacities in patients with keratinizing disorders may be related to long-term use of isotretinoin, especially with large doses (*FDA Drug Bull*, 1983; Fraunfelder et al, 1985). Isotretinoin has not been proved to cause regional enteritis, but it has been associated temporally with inflammatory bowel disease, including regional enteritis.

Transient elevations in the sedimentation rate and serum levels of alanine and aspartate transaminases are relatively common.

Triglyceride levels were elevated in approximately 25% of 500 patients; high density lipoproteins decreased in approximately 15% and cholesterol levels increased in about 7% of these patients. The changes were reversible and their significance has not been established (Colburn and Gibson, 1985). Monitoring for hyperlipidemia is recommended just before treatment is begun and weekly or biweekly thereafter until the lipid response is established. Peak lipid responses usually are evident after four weeks in men, but may not be observed for 12 weeks in women (Bershad et al, 1985). These elevations are related to isotretinoin blood concentration rather than dose, and individuals with high or borderline high serum lipids or those with pre-existing hypertriglyceridemia are most susceptible (Colburn and Gibson, 1985).

Exacerbation of arthritis or onset of arthralgias has been observed in 15% to 20% of patients with cystic acne.

Hyperuricemia, occasionally symptomatic (painful great toe), has been reported in nine patients (*FDA Drug Bull*, 1983). The condition responded to phenylbutazone, and these patients continued therapy with isotretinoin.

Skeletal hyperostosis occurred 6 to 12 months after larger than usual doses of isotretinoin (3 to 4 mg/kg/day) were given to patients with chronic disorders of keratinization and appeared to be drug induced. This effect often persisted after termination of therapy. Similar changes have also been reported in a few patients with acne given therapeutic doses.

A macular erythematous rash induced by isotretinoin has not been definitively ascribed to photosensitivity, but protection from the sun is recommended.

Individuals under treatment should not donate blood.

PREGNANCY. Isotretinoin is teratogenic; its placement in FDA Pregnancy Category X signifies that the risk of using this drug during pregnancy clearly outweighs the benefits and it is *contraindicated* during pregnancy. Congenital abnormalities include hydrocephalus, microcephaly, microtia, agenesis of the ear canals, conotruncal malformations, aortic arch atresia, ventricular septal defects, facial dysmorphism, microphthalmos, micrognathia, and cleft palate (*Morbid Mortal Week Rep*, [April 6] 1984; Lammer et al, 1985).

Women of childbearing potential should not receive isotretinoin until pregnancy is excluded and contraception should be used for at least one month before, during, and one month (many physicians prefer three months) following discontinuation of therapy. These patients should be counseled on the risk to the fetus if pregnancy occurs during treatment and on the desirability of continuing any such pregnancy.

Physicians are urged to report exposures in pregnant women to Roche by calling collect (201) 235-3021. Arrangements for analyses of abortuses can be made by contacting the Epidemiology Development Branch, Division of Drugs and Biologics Experience, FDA, Rockville, MD, 20852 or the Department of Environmental and Drug-Induced Pathology, Armed Forces Institute of Pathology, Washington, DC, 20306; telephone (202) 576-2434.

PHARMACOKINETICS. Maximum blood concentration occurs one to four hours after oral administration; the presence of food may double the amount absorbed. Isotretinoin is nearly 100% bound to plasma albumin at all therapeutic concentrations.

A major metabolite, 4-oxo-isotretinoin, is formed, then glucuronidated and excreted via the biliary tract. Enterohepatic circulation occurs in some individuals.

Isotretinoin has a mean harmonic elimination half-life of ten hours in patients with cystic acne, and this value did not change significantly following use of 40 mg twice daily for 25 days. The mean harmonic half-life of isotretinoin in patients with keratinizing disorders was about 16 hours, while that of its metabolite, 4-oxo-isotretinoin, was 29 hours (Brazzell et al, 1983). Negligible amounts are excreted in the urine (Khoo et al, 1982).

DOSAGE AND PREPARATIONS. Topical agents, such as benzoyl peroxide, sulfur, and tretinoin, should be discontinued before starting isotretinoin therapy, because they potentiate the drying effect of isotretinoin. Vitamin A supplements also should be discontinued.

Oral: For most *adults,* the initial dose should be 0.5 to 1 mg/kg given in two divided doses daily for 15 to 20 weeks. Patients whose disease is very severe or manifested primarily on the body instead of the face, as well as patients who weigh more than 70 kg, may require the maximum recommended dose of 2 mg/kg/day. Although lower doses (0.1 up to 0.5 mg/kg) may be effective and side effects are not remarkably different in frequency or severity than with larger doses, relapses are reported to be more common (Strauss et al, 1984).

If the total cyst count has been reduced by more than 70% before 15 to 20 weeks have elapsed, the drug may be discontinued. After two months without therapy and if warranted by significant recurrence or persistent severe cystic acne, a second course may be initiated.

Accutane (Roche). Capsules 10, 20, and 40 mg.

TRETINOIN
[Retin-A]

ACTIONS AND USES. This retinoid is an all *trans* configuration of retinoic acid (vitamin A acid) used topically to treat acne vulgaris. It also is effective in some disorders of keratinization (eg, lamellar ichthyosis, Darier's disease).

Tretinoin decreases cohesiveness of the follicular epithelial cells and increases epidermal cell mitosis and cell turnover. It has been suggested that increased turnover of follicular epithelium prevents blockage by keratinous plugs and extrudes existing microcomedones. Acne may be aggravated during the first six weeks of therapy, but good results are noted after three or four months in most patients. Tretinoin also thins the stratum corneum, which enhances the penetration of other antiacne agents.

ADVERSE REACTIONS AND PRECAUTIONS. Tretinoin is potentially irritating, particularly if used incorrectly. Within 48 hours, the skin may become red and begin to peel. Once-nightly application initially and avoidance of excessive sun or sunlamp exposure reduce irritation and help to determine individual tolerance to the drug.

Tretinoin should not be used on eczematous skin. Contact with the corners of the mouth, nose, eyes, or mucous membranes must be minimized. The patient should be instructed to avoid concomitant use of other keratolytic preparations (eg, sulfur, resorcinol, salicylic acid, benzoyl peroxide) and abrasive soaps except as directed by the physician. The number of face washings should be limited to two or three a day initially.

Commercially available formulations of tretinoin penetrate the skin but do not cause systemic toxicity. Contact sensitization has been noted only rarely. An appropriate patch test concentration (0.1% in petrolatum) can be obtained from the manufacturer.

DOSAGE AND PREPARATIONS.
Topical: The patient should be instructed to avoid concomitant use of keratolytic preparations (eg, sulfur, resorcinol, salicylic acid) and abrasive soaps except as directed by the physician. Initially, one application nightly to the entire area involved is usually sufficient. The preparation should be applied to dry skin, preferably 15 to 30 minutes after washing. The amount, frequency of application, and dosage form (tretinoin 0.01% gel and 0.05% cream are most frequently prescribed) should be individualized to minimize irritation while maintaining effective comedolytic action. The liquid preparation is generally more irritating.

>*Retin-A* (Ortho). Cream 0.05% and 0.1% in 20 and 45 (0.05% only) g containers; gel 0.01% and 0.025% in 15 and 45 g containers (alcohol 90%); liquid 0.05% in 28 ml containers (alcohol 55%).

Antidandruff-Antiseborrheic Agents

Dandruff and seborrheic dermatitis are associated with increased rates of maturation and proliferation of epidermal cells, although other characteristics of these disorders, such as type of scale, sebum retention, epidermal hyperplasia, dermal capillary proliferation, areas of involvement, and presence of inflammation, differ considerably.

Dandruff affects individuals who are at the upper limit of normal variation with respect to rate of turnover of epidermal cells. The excessive scaling (scurf) is most obvious on the scalp and is not accompanied by inflammation, alteration of sebum kinetics, pathologic change, or epidermal hyperplasia.

Seborrheic dermatitis is an inflammatory scaling disease of the scalp and face, especially the nasolabial folds; occasionally, the eyelids, upper middle anterior chest, and intertriginous areas also are involved. When sebum is retained, the scales become oily; epidermal hyperplasia and an abnormal number of parakeratotic cells are present. Pruritus is common.

Because corticosteroids decrease mitotic activity and epidermal cell proliferation, they are effective in the treatment of dandruff and seborrheic dermatitis; other effective agents are also presumed to have a cytostatic action. However, evidence based upon the investigational oral (Ford et al, 1984) and topical (Skinner et al, 1985) use of the antifungal agent, ketoconazole, suggests that the yeast, *Pityrosporum ovale*, may be involved in the pathogenesis of both dandruff and seborrhea. Thus, unlike the corticosteroids, the modest antifungal action of zinc pyrithione [Danex, DHS Zinc, Head and Shoulders, Sebulon, Zincon], selenium sulfide [Exsel, Selsun, Selsun Blue], and chloroxine [Capitrol] may be more relevant than their cytostatic action in these disorders. Sulfur and/or salicylic acid have weak, if any, antifungal action, and their role in these disorders may depend on their keratolytic action.

Although dandruff can be controlled by frequent application of bland shampoos (four to six washings per week), most individuals require medicated shampoos. Shampoos containing tar or sulfur and salicylic acid are beneficial, but zinc pyrithione or selenium sulfide are more effective and are required for resistant cases.

Chloroxine [Capitrol], a dichlorohydroxy quinoline, is a recently approved shampoo; when applied topically, it has antibacterial and antifungal activities against staphylococcal and *Pityrosporum* species, respectively. Topical pharmacokinetic data in humans are unavailable. The preparation should not be used on acutely inflamed (exudative) lesions, and discoloration of light-colored hair (eg, blond, grey, bleached) may occur.

Zinc pyrithione, selenium sulfide, and sulfur/salicylic acid shampoos are effective in seborrhea capitis. Seborrheic blepharitis usually responds to daily treatment of the eyelids and lashes with shampoos. Some physicians prefer sulfacetamide/corticosteroid preparations (see Chapter 20, Miscellaneous Ophthalmic Preparations). Low- or intermediate-potency topical corticosteroids may be indicated if involvement is widespread, particularly when inflammation is prominent (see the section on Anti-inflammatory Corticosteroids).

SELENIUM SULFIDE
[Exsel, Selsun, Selsun Blue]

ACTIONS AND USES. Selenium sulfide shampoos are effective in the treatment of dandruff and seborrhea capitis. This agent also is used to treat tinea versicolor (see the section on Antifungal Agents in Chapter 74, Topical Anti-infective Agents: Drugs Used on Skin and Mucous Membranes). The antidandruff and antiseborrheic effects are purported to result from cytostatic activity (*Federal Register*, [Dec 3] 1982) and substantivity (ie, residual adherence to the skin after shampoo and rinse), although the antifungal action may contribute to their usefulness as well (see the Introduction to this section).

Selenium sulfide is sporicidal for *Trichophyton tonsurans*, the causative agent of tinea capitis; use of the shampoo twice weekly is an effective adjunct to oral griseofulvin (Allen et al, 1982).

ADVERSE REACTIONS AND PRECAUTIONS. Little or no toxicity has been observed when selenium sulfide is applied as directed to normal skin and hair. The drug irritates conjunctival mucosa on contact and should not be applied to large areas of skin with marked dermatitic lesions because it may act as an irritant. The product should not be used when acute inflammation or exudation is present, because absorption may be increased. Allergic contact dermatitis has not been documented.

DOSAGE AND PREPARATIONS. For seborrhea capitis and dandruff, one or two teaspoonsful of the shampoo are applied and allowed to remain on the scalp for five to ten minutes before being rinsed off thoroughly. Alternatively, some physicians prefer two consecutive applications of shampoo and omit the time for retention. The preparation should be used once or twice weekly only. Contact with the eyes should be avoided.

    Generic. Lotion shampoo 1% (nonprescription) and 2.5%.
    Exsel (Herbert), *Selsun* (Abbott). Lotion shampoo 2.5% in 120 ml containers.
    Selsun Blue (Abbott). Lotion 1% in 120 and 240 ml containers (nonprescription).

ZINC PYRITHIONE

Zinc pyrithione shampoos are widely used nonprescription formulations that are effective in the treatment of dandruff, seborrhea capitis, and tinea versicolor.

Zinc pyrithione possesses cytostatic (*Federal Register*, [Dec 3] 1982) and antifungal actions. Its effectiveness in dandruff and seborrhea is purported to result from its cytostatic activity and substantivity (ie, residual adherence to the skin after shampoo and rinse), but the antifungal action may affect these disorders as well (see the Introduction). For its use in tinea versicolor, see Chapter 74.

These shampoos have no apparent toxicity when applied as directed to normal skin and hair.

DOSAGE AND PREPARATIONS. For dandruff and seborrhea, one or two teaspoonsful of shampoo are applied and allowed to remain on the scalp for up to five minutes before rinsing off thoroughly; the application is then repeated. Application once or twice weekly controls dandruff in many individuals. Contact with the eyes should be avoided.

    Available Trademarks.
    Danex (Herbert) 1%, *DHS Zinc* (Person & Covey) 2%, *Head and Shoulders* (Procter & Gamble) 2%, *Sebulon* (Westwood) 2%, *Zincon* (Lederle) 1% (all forms nonprescription).

Antipsoriatic Agents

Clinical variants of psoriasis (Farber and Nall, 1984 A; Lowe, 1985; Roenigk and Maibach, 1985 A and B) include the following entities:

Psoriasis vulgaris is a common chronic papulosquamous disease characterized by dry, thick, silver-white, adherent or flaky scale on red papules and sharply demarcated erythematous slightly raised plaques. Epidermal proliferation is intense, resulting in large numbers of parakeratotic cells and acanthosis. Nails and the skin of the scalp, elbows, knees, and sacral, intertriginous, and anogenital areas are the primary sites of involvement. The palms and soles may have eczematous or hyperkeratotic marginated plaques, or be involved with an acute onset of keratolysis-like lesions; nails are often pitted and dystrophic. A family history of psoriasis is common. Less severe cases of this form of psoriasis usually respond well to conventional drug therapy.

Psoriatic arthritis is not accepted by all dermatologists as a clinical variant; however, seronegative arthritis is present in 5% to 10% of patients, and it generally responds favorably to drug therapy.

Guttate psoriasis is characterized by spotty oval lesions 1 to 2 cm in diameter and is common in children and young adults following upper respiratory tract infection with beta-hemolytic streptococci. It is quite responsive to conventional therapy.

Pustular psoriasis is a severe disabling form of the disease characterized by sterile superficial pustules associated with the typical lesions of psoriasis vulgaris, psoriatic nail changes, and very painful fissuring of the skin. In its most severe form, acute generalized pustular psoriasis, the mucous membranes also are involved and leukocytosis, high fever, and prostration are present.

Both pustular psoriasis and *erythrodermic psoriasis*, a severe exfoliative disorder involving the entire skin surface, most often occur as rebound phenomena after withdrawal of systemic corticosteroids and are more resistant to conventional drug therapy.

Pathogenesis: Epidermal hyperproliferation appears to be related to abnormal metabolic pathways (ie, altered cyclic nucleotide metabolism, elevated polyamine-forming capacity, abnormal arachidonic acid transformations) (Lowe, 1983; Voorhees, 1983; Anderson, 1985). Streptococcal throat infections, drugs (eg, propranolol, lithium, indomethacin and possibly other nonsteroidal anti-inflammatory agents), emotional stress, and injury often trigger the onset of psoriasis (Farber and Nall, 1984 B).

Drug Therapy: The management of psoriasis depends principally on its severity (Lowe, 1983; Farber and Nall, 1984 A; Anderson, 1985).

Mild Psoriasis. Many patients with mild involvement can be managed with topical agents alone, usually intermediate- to high-potency corticosteroids, with or without occlusion. Some dermatologists recommend the concomitant use of phototherapy (erythemogenic doses of UVB light) if topical corticosteroids with occlusion therapy is not adequate.

If the thick hyperkeratotic scale and crusts cannot be removed by moist occlusive dressings, nonprescription formulations (ointment, gel, and shampoo) containing salicylic acid 5% to 6% alone or with propylene glycol, alcohol, sulfur, urea (in 10% to 20% ointment or cream), and/or tar are used for their keratolytic action.

Moderate Psoriasis. The cytostatic agents (ie, corticosteroids, tar, anthralin [Anthra-Derm, Drithocreme, Lasan]) are commonly used topically to restore a normal rate of epidermal cell proliferation and keratinization in moderately severe psoriasis.

Periodic use of UVB light and topical coal tar (Goeckerman regimen) or topical anthralin applied traditionally (Ingram regimen) (Ashton et al, 1983) or in a short-contact, high-concentration regimen (Farber and Nall, 1984 A; Lowe et al, 1984) is an alternative when coal tar or a low concentration of anthralin alone is inadequate. Suberythemogenic doses of UVB light plus coal tar appear to be as effective as erythemogenic doses of UVB light alone (Lowe, 1983; Menkes et al, 1985).

When treatment regimens become complex, management in psoriasis day-care centers is recommended (Farber and Nall, 1984 A) to optimize therapy and reduce cost by avoiding hospitalization.

Severe Psoriasis. When severe disabling psoriasis does not respond adequately to the above agents, two alternative drug therapies are often beneficial but may be associated with greater risk. The first employs the cytotoxic drug, methotrexate [Folex, Mexate]. The second utilizes the psoralen, methoxsalen [Oxsoralen], with ultraviolet type A light, which is termed photochemotherapy (PUVA therapy) (see the evaluation for a discussion of photochemotherapy). Relapses are common whether methotrexate or PUVA therapy is used.

Etretinate [Tegison], a retinoic acid derivative, is currently under investigation (Peck, 1982). Vitamin A regulates the proliferation and differentiation of epithelial cells and, with its naturally occurring derivative, retinol, is essential for vision. Epithelial metaplasia due to vitamin A deficiency resembles that occurring in a number of precancerous disorders. Since physiologic doses of vitamin A correct this type of metaplasia, it has been investigated for use in many tumors; however, the pharmacologic doses used investigationally were toxic. Consequently, many synthetic derivatives of vitamin A and related natural derivatives (collectively termed retinoids) were screened for antitumor activity (Elias and Williams, 1981; Peck, 1982; Bollag, 1983; Spielvogel et al, 1985), and were found to be moderately successful for certain superficial dermal and bladder tumors. Most importantly, other dermal actions of vitamin A (ie, inhibition of keratinization, antiinflammatory and immunostimulant effects, diminished sebaceous gland function) have been selectively attained, often with minimization of some serious toxic effects (Dicken, 1984; Goodman, 1984).

Clinically useful retinoids include tretinoin (trans retinoic acid) [Retin A] and isotretinoin (cis retinoic acid) [Accutane], which are used principally for acne and severe recalcitrant cystic acne, respectively, and the investigational agent, etretinate, which is principally used for severe psoriasis unresponsive to conventional therapy. Etretinate is reported to be especially effective in pustular and erythrodermic psoriasis (Mahrle et al, 1982; Ward et al, 1983; Dicken, 1984). Relapses are common on cessation of treatment, but most patients respond when etretinate therapy is resumed (Farber and Nall, 1984 A). Other retinoids, Ro 10-1670 (Geiger et al, 1984) and the especially potent arotinoid, Ro-13-6298 (Tsambaos and Orfanos, 1983), are under investigation for psoriasis.

A controlled study supports the efficacy of peritoneal dialysis in the treatment of psoriasis (Whittier et al, 1983); however, results are not always encouraging (Klemm-Mayer et al, 1984)

and the procedure should be considered experimental (Farber and Nall, 1984 A).

ANTHRALIN
[Anthra-Derm, Drithocreme, Lasan]

ACTIONS AND USES. Anthralin was developed as a synthetic substitute for chrysarobin in the treatment of psoriasis. It reduces epidermal cell DNA synthesis and mitotic activity of hyperplastic epidermis (Lowe and Breeding, 1981), thus restoring a normal rate of proliferation and keratinization in patients with moderately severe psoriasis. Anthralin is the most effective nonsteroidal topical agent for psoriasis (Ashton et al, 1983; Lowe et al, 1984). If necessary, it may be used with periodic erythemogenic ultraviolet phototherapy. However, frequent irritation, especially with concentrations above 0.1%, as well as the need for specialized care in a supervised setting, has limited the use of this therapy to dermatologists.

Compared to the conventional overnight 8-hour or 24-hour Ingram regimens, short-contact high-concentration regimens suitable for outpatient or day-care centers (Ashton et al, 1983; Lowe et al, 1984; Farber and Nall, 1984 A; Schaefer, 1985) cause less staining and irritation and are less expensive.

ADVERSE REACTIONS AND PRECAUTIONS. Significant percutaneous absorption of anthralin has not been observed. Irritation occurs frequently, especially with concentrations above 0.1%. Excessive erythema may occur on adjacent normal skin and may require reducing the frequency of application. Sensitivity reactions are rare.

Contact with the eyes may cause conjunctivitis. Anthralin may stain fabrics permanently and the hair and skin temporarily.

Anthralin should be applied only to quiescent or chronic patches of psoriasis; it should not be used on acute eruptions or excessively inflamed areas and should be used cautiously, if at all, on the face or intertriginous areas.

It has been suggested that anthralin may be contraindicated in patients with impaired renal function because of possible renal toxicity after percutaneous absorption, but renal or hepatic toxicity has not been substantiated. On the contrary, short-term toxicologic studies using paste and ointment forms indicate that concentrations up to 0.4% do not impair kidney or liver function.

Anthralin is classified in FDA Pregnancy Category C.

DOSAGE AND PREPARATIONS. When the response to anthralin has not been previously established, the 0.1% strength should be used initially and, if necessary, stronger concentrations then substituted. Anthralin may be used in two ways: the conventional overnight regimen and the short-contact regimen (investigational). In the overnight regimen, the ointment is applied without a dressing at bedtime and should remain on the lesions for 8 to 12 hours. Care must be taken to avoid staining of clothing and bed linens; either old clothing should be worn or the treated areas should be covered with suitable dressings. The next morning, the ointment is removed and a corticosteroid cream may be applied during the day to control or prevent irritation.

In the modified short-contact regimen (investigational), 0.1% anthralin ointment is applied initially, left on for 30 minutes, then washed off with soap and hot water. The concentration is increased by 0.5% to a maximum of 3% at three-day intervals; it is left on for 10 minutes providing no burning or irritation is observed (Lowe et al, 1984; Schaefer, 1985). Formulations containing more than 1% anthralin are unstable.

Salicylic acid 0.2% may be incorporated into anthralin ointments as a stabilizer, and the strength may be increased to 3% for a keratolytic action on thickened lesions on the soles.

Generic. Ointment 0.1%, 0.25%, 0.5%, and 1% in 45 g containers.

Anthra-Derm (Dermik). Ointment in petrolatum 0.1%, 0.25%, 0.5%, and 1% in 42.5 g containers.

Drithocreme (American Dermal). Cream 0.1%, 0.25%, 0.5%, and 1% (**Drithocreme HP**) in 50 g containers.

Lasan (Stiefel). Cream 0.1%, 0.2%, 0.4%, and 1% (**Lasan HP-1**) in 65 g containers; ointment 0.4% with salicylic acid in 60 g containers.

ETRETINATE
[Tegison]

ACTIONS AND USES. Etretinate is an aromatic retinoid developed in Europe that is undergoing clinical trials in the United States (Ward et al, 1983). It is effective in patients with common psoriasis and is especially useful in severe forms, such as generalized pustular, palmar and plantar pustular, and erythrodermic psoriasis (Mahrle et al, 1982; Wolska et al, 1983; Moy et al, 1985).

Other disorders of keratinization (eg, pityriasis rubra pilaris, Darier's disease, ichthyosis) also respond to etretinate. Lichen planus, keratoacanthoma, mycosis fungoides, and multiple warts in immunocompromised patients were reported to respond, but studies are limited. In other limited studies, etretinate was effective in some patients with precancerous lesions (eg, oral leukoplakia, actinic keratosis, xeroderma pigmentosum, arsenical keratosis, keratoacanthoma) and may be useful adjunctively in basal cell carcinoma and superficial epithelial tumors of the bladder wall.

Modest improvement of the arthritis present in 5% to 10% of patients with psoriasis has been reported. More studies are required to determine the definitive role of etretinate combined with PUVA, anthralin, tars, and topical corticosteroids, although synergism is evident (ie, reduced dose of each component elicited the same response).

Etretinate inhibits keratinization, proliferation, and differentiation of epithelial tissues and inhibits ornithine decarboxylase, which is essential for polyamine synthesis (Lowe et al, 1982 A). These actions are probably responsible in part for its efficacy in proliferative and hyperkeratotic skin disorders. The anti-inflammatory and immunomodulator actions are less defined, but etretinate inhibits the motility and migration of neutrophils and eosinophils into the epidermis, which reduces the antibody-dependent cell-mediated cytotoxicity of polymorphonuclear leukocytes (Ellis et al, 1985); stimulates cell-mediated cytotoxicity and T-killer cells; and suppresses the mitogenic response of lymphocytes.

ADVERSE REACTIONS AND PRECAUTIONS. Common side effects include dryness of the lips (cheilitis), mouth, and nose; epistaxis may result.

More serious side effects include loss of hair (22%), which has accounted for the majority of withdrawals from therapy; thinning and desquamation of the skin; exfoliation of the palms and soles; pseudotumor cerebri; and nail dystrophies.

Etretinate has not caused the hepatic changes associated with excessive vitamin A (Foged et al, 1984); however, hepatitis with eosinophilia presumed to result from hypersensitivity has developed. Dose-dependent elevations of SGPT and, to a lesser extent, alkaline phosphatase may resolve with continued therapy or on cessation of treatment. Skeletal hyperostosis has been reported in one patient receiving a low daily dose (Burge and Ryan, 1985). Effects on serum lipids are reported to be much less than those of isotretinoin (Vahlquist et al, 1985), but data are limited.

PREGNANCY. Like vitamin A and isotretinoin, etretinate is a potent teratogen (FDA Pregnancy Category X). Contraception should be practiced for one and preferably two months before and during therapy. Because the drug persists in the body for an extended period, the anticipated recommendation is to avoid pregnancy for two years following cessation of therapy.

PHARMACOKINETICS. Etretinate is administered orally; its bioavailability is approximately 40%. Milk is reported to enhance absorption. This drug is converted to an active, more water-soluble, retinoid metabolite, Ro 10-1670, which is also under investigation. Numerous inactive metabolites are found in the urine; however, about 75% of the dose is recovered from the feces.

The time to peak absorption varies from 2.5 to 6 hours. Etretinate is 98% bound to plasma proteins, principally albumin. The volumes of distribution of etretinate and its active metabolite are 150 L and 210 L, respectively. Steady-state concentrations range from 100 to 500 ng/ml.

Etretinate has a much longer elimination half-life (about 120 days) than its active metabolite, Ro 10-1670, and isotretinoin (8 to 10 hours). This slow terminal elimination phase probably results from accumulation in fatty tissue from which it is slowly released. Accumulation also may explain the prolonged remissions achieved with etretinate therapy. The lengthening of the elimination half-life with multiple dosing is probably due to lack of assay sensitivity at drug concentrations obtained after single-dose administration rather than to alterations in etretinate's pharmacokinetics (Lucek and Colburn, 1985).

DOSAGE AND PREPARATIONS. *See the warning in the Pregnancy section of this evaluation.*

Oral: Adults, for severe psoriasis, 0.75 mg to 1 mg/kg daily in divided amounts, depending on the patient's response (maximum, 75 mg daily). The dose may have to be reduced to 0.3 to 0.5 mg/kg daily in patients who are sensitive to the drug. Treatment is continued for two weeks after remission is observed or for a maximum of 16 weeks. Therapy is usually discontinued after four weeks if no response is evident.

Tegison (Roche).

(Investigational drug)

METHOTREXATE

METHOTREXATE SODIUM
[Folex, Mexate]

ACTIONS AND USES. Methotrexate, a cytotoxic agent, controls severe, recalcitrant, disabling psoriasis that does not respond adequately to corticosteroids, phototherapy, tar, and anthralin. Diagnosis must be established by dermatologic consultation prior to use of methotrexate.

Actively proliferating tissues (eg, epidermal hyperplasia associated with psoriasis and other disorders of keratinization) are sensitive to this dihydrofolate reductase and thymidylate synthesis inhibitor. Methotrexate also has been used to treat other proliferative and autoimmune disorders (eg, systemic lupus erythematosus, severe epidermolytic ichthyosis or keratoderma, pityriasis rubra pilaris, dermatomyositis, mycosis fungoides, Reiter's disease, bullous pemphigoid, and pemphigus vulgaris). Success has been variable.

Considerable expertise is required for patient selection and pretreatment evaluation (eg, liver biopsy); dosage schedules and post-treatment evaluations must be individualized and drug interactions must be considered. Guidelines for the use of methotrexate in refractory psoriasis have been published by the Psoriasis Task Force of the National Program for Dermatology (Roenigk et al, 1982; Roenigk and Maibach, 1983).

For other uses of this drug, see Chapter 64, Drugs Used in Cancer Chemotherapy.

ADVERSE REACTIONS AND PRECAUTIONS. The incidence and severity of adverse reactions are less when methotrexate is used for psoriasis than for neoplasms because of the lower doses required. However, hepatotoxicity is of concern when methotrexate is used for prolonged periods, even at lower doses.

The most common adverse reactions are nausea, malaise, and leukopenia. Chills, fever, fatigue, and dizziness are less common. The most common reason for discontinuing therapy is gastrointestinal side effects.

Methotrexate causes bone marrow depression; interstitial pneumonitis, hepatic cirrhosis and failure, immunosuppression, hemorrhagic enteritis, seizures, renal failure, and altered fertility occur less frequently.

Because methotrexate has caused congenital abnormalities and fetal death, it is not recommended for women of childbearing potential (FDA Pregnancy Category D).

Methotrexate must be used cautiously and only by physicians experienced in antimetabolite therapy. The patient should be informed fully of the risks involved and should remain under the close supervision of a physician during treatment with methotrexate.

See the evaluation on methotrexate in Chapter 64, Drugs Used in Cancer Chemotherapy, for a more detailed discussion of adverse reactions, precautions, and drug interactions.

PHARMACOKINETICS. Conventional oral doses are readily absorbed in most patients; peak serum levels are reached in one to two hours. One-half of the drug is reversibly bound to plasma proteins.

Methotrexate has a triphasic half-life. The first phase (alpha plasma elimination half-life, 0.75 hours) is due to tissue distribution; the second phase (beta elimination half-life, 3.5 to 4 hours) is due to renal clearance and biliary excretion; a slow terminal phase ranging from 10 to 27 hours is probably due to enterohepatic recycling.

About 10% of an administered dose is metabolized to 7-hydroxymethotrexate and is eliminated by the kidney. About 50% to 90% of methotrexate is excreted by the kidney within 24 hours. Clearance ranges from 0.63 to 2.62 ml/min/kg (Chen et al, 1984).

DOSAGE AND PREPARATIONS. Leucovorin is a specific antidote that can be life-saving in serious methotrexate overdosage.

A current, widely used schedule is based on knowledge of cell proliferation kinetics. Because the psoriatic cell completes its germinative cycle in 37 hours, once weekly all psoriatic cells will be targets for methotrexate. Two equally effective, commonly used schedules are: (1) a large oral, intravenous, or intramuscular dose given once weekly; or (2) three oral doses weekly given over a 36-hour period. Studies to date indicate that when a certain amount of drug is given in one dose, there are fewer toxic effects than when the same amount is dispensed in divided doses over five to seven days.

Oral, Intramuscular, Intravenous: *Adults,* dosage schedules cited below are for the average 70-kg adult. A test dose of 5 to 10 mg should be used initially to detect any idiosyncratic reaction.

(1) *Weekly single oral, intramuscular, or intravenous dose schedule*: (a) The usual range for oral administration is 7.5 to 25 mg/week; occasional patients require a maximum of 37.5 mg/week. It is recommended that the total be increased gradually (2.5 to 5 mg/week) with appropriate monitoring of the blood counts. (b) The usual range for intramuscular or rapid ("push") intravenous dosage is 7.5 to 50 mg/week; occasional patients require a maximum of 100 mg/week. Slow intravenous drip should never be used. As the total dose of methotrexate is gradually increased, blood counts should be monitored more carefully.

(2) *Divided oral dose schedule*: 2.5 to 5 mg at 12-hour intervals for three doses each week. Dosage may be increased gradually by 2.5 mg/week but total dose should not exceed 25 mg/week and blood counts should be monitored.

All schedules should be continually individualized, and the dosage should be reduced and rest periods increased to the greatest possible extent with any schedule.

The goal is not necessarily to achieve complete clearing of psoriasis, but rather to achieve adequate control with the minimum dosage and the longest rest period. The use of methotrexate may permit the return to conventional topical therapy, which should be encouraged.

METHOTREXATE:
Methotrexate (Lederle). Tablets 2.5 mg.

METHOTREXATE SODIUM:
(Strengths expressed in terms of the base)
Folex (Adria). Powder (lyophilized, preservative-free) in 25, 50, and 100 mg containers.
Methotrexate (Lederle). Powder (lyophilized, preservative-free) in 20, 50, and 100 mg containers; solution 2.5 and 25 mg/ml in 2 ml containers (alcohol 0.9%).
Methotrexate LPF (Lederle). Solution (preservative-free) 25 mg/ml in 2, 4, and 8 ml containers.
Mexate (Bristol). Powder (lyophilized, preservative-free) in 20, 50, 100, and 250 mg containers.

PHOTOCHEMOTHERAPY (PUVA THERAPY)

Long-wave ultraviolet radiation in the A range (320 to 400 nm), UVA, only produces erythema or pigmentation with long exposures, but concomitant use of a circulating photo-sensitizer (eg, a psoralen) markedly enhances the response. The development of oral psoralen with UVA photochemotherapy as a therapeutic tool has been reviewed (Fitzpatrick and Pathak, 1984). Photochemotherapy, originally termed PUVA therapy (*Psoralen* with *UVA* light), is used to treat severe psoriasis (Bickers et al, 1984; Farber and Nall, 1984 A). It is thought to act by forming psoralen-DNA photo adducts that interfere with the hyperproliferative epidermal cell turnover characteristic of psoriasis (Anderson and Voorhees, 1980). The psoralen, methoxsalen, is used orally with controlled exposures to UVA light to enhance inhibition of epidermal cells and avoid severe burns. Lesions usually clear after 12 to 18 therapy sessions usually given over four to six weeks. Photochemotherapy is used in patients with extensive, active disease who have not responded to conventional regimens (steroids, phototherapy, tars, and anthralins).

The factors that determine the frequency of maintenance therapy have been evaluated (Henseler et al, 1981; Stern and Melski, 1982; Melski and Stern, 1982).

Photochemotherapy appears to be effective in severe psoriasis, the early stages of mycosis fungoides (Powell et al, 1984), and vitiligo (Pathak et al, 1984). Uncontrolled studies support its use in alopecia areata, dyshidrotic or atopic eczema, polymorphic light eruption (Bickers, 1983), and persistent light reactivity.

ADVERSE REACTIONS. Acute adverse reactions to PUVA are pruritus, nausea, and painful erythema; however, potential toxic effects are of considerable concern. Occasionally, the stimulation of melanogenesis may lead to mottling and lentigenes. Hypopigmentation has been reported (Todes-Taylor et al, 1983).

Photochemotherapy increases the risk of premature aging of the skin and skin cancer in fair-skinned individuals with skin types I to III. The risk is increased nine- to twelvefold for squamous cell carcinomas of the skin (Farber et al, 1983; Stern et al, 1984 B) and twofold for basal cell carcinoma. Patients previously exposed to carcinogens (eg, prior irradiation, chemical carcinogens) may be more at risk (Morison et al, 1983; Roelandts, 1984; Stern et al, 1984 B).

A cataractogenic action has not been established conclusively in patients with proper eye protection (Marks, 1982).

PRECAUTIONS. Criteria for patient selection and dosing regimens are complex (Epstein et al, 1979; Henseler et al, 1981). Photochemotherapy should be performed only by dermatologists experienced in its use. The manufacturer of methoxsalen (Elder Pharmaceuticals, Inc) distributes information for physicians and patients.

The Committee on Drugs of the American Academy of Pediatrics recommends that under no circumstances should children with psoriasis receive such therapy unless it is administered by qualified specialists.

TARS

ACTIONS AND USES. Tar suppresses epidermal cell DNA synthesis and mitotic activity (Lowe et al, 1982 B; Lowe, 1983; Menkes et al, 1985) and restores a normal rate of proliferation.

Tars, most commonly coal tar, are used to treat chronic lichenified and papulosquamous eruptions (Hjorth and Jacobsen, 1983). Although they have been largely supplanted by topical corticosteroids in mild psoriasis, recalcitrant seborrheic dermatitis, atopic dermatitis, and lichen simplex chronicus, tars are beneficial in these disorders. Phototherapy with suberythemogenic or erythemogenic doses of UVB light following removal of tar may enhance the suppression of hyperplastic skin in proliferative disorders, and a number of dermatologists use this combination (Goeckerman regimen) for moderately severe psoriasis (Muller and Perry, 1984).

Nonprescription ointment and shampoo formulations containing tar, sulfur, and salicylic acid are used if an additional keratolytic action is desired to remove thick crusts.

Tars incorporated into lotions, creams, or ointments containing hydrocortisone 0.25% to 1% and iodoquinol (diiodohydroxyquin) 1% are promoted for the treatment of infected eczemas and atopic dermatitis. Controlled studies comparing this regimen to hydrocortisone or halogenated quinoline alone are not available.

ADVERSE REACTIONS. An important disadvantage of all tar preparations is their lack of uniformity. Tar formulations are irritating and cause smarting and burning. They may be photosensitizing, have an unpleasant odor, and frequently stain the skin and hair. Inappropriate or excessive use may aggravate lesions (particularly in guttate or pustular psoriasis) or cause folliculitis. However, the irritation caused by usual concentrations of coal tar is minimal and appears to be negligible in patients with psoriasis. Tars rarely cause allergic sensitization. Juniper tar, birch tar, and pine tar cause sensitization more often and have no advantage over coal tar. Systemic toxicity is not observed following topical administration.

Crude coal tar and its derivatives contain aromatic hydrocarbons and may have carcinogenic potential when used for prolonged periods (Zackheim, 1978). Considerable experience with the Goeckerman regimen reveals that the incidence of skin cancer is not appreciably increased in patients with psoriasis (Muller and Perry, 1984).

COAL TAR (liquor carbonis detergens), U.S.P.:
Generic. Solution 20%. This solution may contain an emulsifier,

polysorbate 80 [Tween 80], which forms a fine dispersion when 60 ml is added to the bath. The solution can be incorporated into creams or ointments (2% to 5%) or into tincture of green soap for a shampoo (10%).

Body Oil:
Balnetar (Westwood) 2.5%, *Lavatar* (Doak) 33.3%, *Neutrogena T/Derm* (Neutrogena) (nonprescription), *Polytar Bath* (Stiefel) 25% (nonprescription), *Zetar Emulsion* (Dermik) 30%.

Cream:
Fototar (Elder) 1.6%.

Gel:
Aquatar (Herbert) 2.5%, *Estar* (Westwood) 5%, *psoriGel* (Owen) 7.5% (nonprescription).

Lotion:
Doak Tar (Doak) 5% (nonprescription).

Ointment:
Medotar (Medco) 1% (nonprescription), *Unguentum Bossi* (Doak) 5%.

Paste:
Tarpaste (Doak) 5% (nonprescription).

Shampoo:
Doak Tar Shampoo (Doak) 3%, *Pentrax Tar* (Rydelle) 4%, *Polytar* (Stiefel) 1%, *T/Gel* (Neutrogena) 2%, *Zetar* (Dermik) 1% (all forms nonprescription).

Soap:
Packer's Pine Tar (Rydelle) 5.87%, *Polytar* (Stiefel) 1% (nonprescription).

AVAILABLE MIXTURES.
COAL TAR, SULFUR, AND SALICYLIC ACID:

Ointment:
Pragmatar (Menley & James) 4% with precipitated sulfur 3% and salicylic acid 3% (nonprescription).

Shampoo:
Sebutone (Westwood) 0.5% with salicylic acid 2% and sulfur 2% (nonprescription).
Vanseb-T (Herbert) 5% with salicylic acid 1% and sulfur 2% (nonprescription).

Scalp Conditioner:
T/Gel Scalp Solution (Neutrogena) 2% with salicylic acid 2%.

Agents Affecting Pigmentation

Hydroquinone [Eldoquin, Melanex], a skin bleaching agent, is applied topically to treat localized macules of *hyperpigmentation*, such as freckles, lentigenes, postinflammatory states, and melasma due to pregnancy or oral contraceptives.

Acquired localized disorders of *hypopigmentation* include vitiligo, which is characterized by loss of melanocytes, or depigmentation caused by inflammation following bullae, burns, infections, atrophy, or scarring of the skin. Congenital diffuse hypopigmentation and depigmentation (ie, albinism) are distinguished by the presence of melanocytes that lack tyrosinase, the enzyme that produces melanin.

Application of the psoralen compounds, trioxsalen and methoxsalen, with subsequent exposure to UVA light (photochemotherapy), may stimulate melanin synthesis and repigmentation except in albinism. Psoralens may be used orally in vitiligo involving less than 40% of the body surface. If the vitiliginous area is less than 50 to 60 cm², topical rather than oral administration can be considered. If more than 40% of the body surface is affected, it may be easier to lessen or destroy the pigmentation of nonvitiliginous areas with monobenzone.

HYDROQUINONE
[Eldoquin, Melanex]

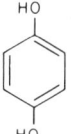

ACTIONS AND USES. The skin bleaching agent, hydroquinone, may decrease cutaneous hyperpigmentation when applied topically in various localized conditions, such as freckles, lentigenes, postinflammatory states, and melasma due to pregnancy or oral contraceptives. The decrease in hyperpigmentation may be permanent and may overshoot the desired color so that the lesion appears vitiliginous, but its effect is usually reversible. Since sunlight darkens the lesions and offsets the bleaching action of hydroquinone, some nonprescription preparations of hydroquinone 2% also contain sunscreens. A preparation containing an opaque sunscreen [Eldopaque, Eldopaque Forte] may be required to suppress the effect of sunlight on the lesion completely.

Hydroquinone acts by decreasing the proliferative and melanin synthesizing activity of melanocytes. It inhibits tyrosinase in melanocytes, which depresses melanin synthesis, melanin granule movement, and melanocyte growth. Hydroquinone is also toxic to melanocytes.

ADVERSE REACTIONS AND PRECAUTIONS. High concentrations of hydroquinone (4% to 10%) may cause ochronosis with continuous use. No other serious untoward effects have been reported. Tingling or burning on application with subsequent erythema and inflammation was reported in 8% and 32% of patients, respectively, when a 2% or 5% concentration of hydroquinone was used. Therapy need not be terminated if inflammation occurs, but topical hydrocortisone may be given to alleviate this reaction.

Allergic contact dermatitis occurs far less frequently than irritation; a 1% concentration of hydroquinone in petrolatum can be obtained from the manufacturer and is suitable for patch testing. Contact with the eyes should be avoided.

DOSAGE AND PREPARATIONS.
Topical: Adults and adolescents over 12 years, the preparation is applied to the involved areas twice daily for six to eight weeks. An opaque sunscreen also should be applied during the day on areas that cannot easily be protected from exposure to the sun to prevent recurrence of hyperpigmentation.

For especially resistant cases, a formula composed of hydroquinone 0.5% to 2% and tretinoin 0.1% in hydrophilic ointment or equal parts of alcohol and propylene glycol can be compounded and is applied twice daily for six weeks (Arndt, 1983; Pathak, 1984).
Eldoquin (Elder). Cream 2% (nonprescription) or 4% (**Forte**) in 15 and 30 g containers; lotion 2% in 15 g containers.
Melanex (Neutrogena). Solution 3% in 30 ml containers.
AVAILABLE MIXTURES.
HYDROQUINONE AND SUNSCREENS:
Eldopaque (Elder). Cream containing hydroquinone 2% (nonprescription) or 4% (Forte) in a talc opaque base in 15 and 30 g containers.

Porcelana with Sunscreen (Jeffry Martin). Cream 2% with octyl dimethyl PABA 2.5% in 120 g containers (nonprescription).
Solaquin (Elder). Cream containing hydroquinone 2% (nonprescription) or 4% (Forte) and ethyl dihydroxypropyl PABA 5%, dioxybenzone 3%, and oxybenzone in 30 g containers; gel containing hydroquinone 4% (Forte) and ethyl dihydroxypropyl PABA 5% and dioxybenzone 3% in 30 g containers.

METHOXSALEN
[Oxsoralen]

USES. Methoxsalen is administered to treat small vitiliginous lesions. The drug is applied topically to small macules ranging from 6 to 50 cm²; the area is subsequently exposed to sunlight or UVA radiation (320 to 400 nm). The general principles of therapy are similar to those of photochemotherapy (see the discussion on Photochemotherapy in the section on Antipsoriatic Agents). Oral administration is recommended for larger areas of involvement (up to 40% of the body surface). Topical or oral therapy should be supervised closely by the physician.

ADVERSE REACTIONS AND PRECAUTIONS. High concentrations of topical methoxsalen and overexposure to UVA radiation can cause photosensitivity reactions (severe erythema and blistering). Therefore, methoxsalen must be diluted to 1:10,000 or 1:1,000 and the duration of UVA radiation carefully controlled.

Gastric discomfort occasionally follows oral administration and is minimized by giving the drug with milk or meals. To protect the eyes and lips, blue-grey sunglasses (with side shields to prevent reflected radiation) opaque to UVA light and a light-screening lipstick should be used for 24 or preferably 48 hours after drug ingestion. A cataractogenic action has been established in animals, but this hazard can be avoided if proper sunglasses are used.

Methoxsalen is contraindicated in patients with hepatic insufficiency and diseases associated with photosensitivity (eg, porphyria, acute systemic lupus erythematosus, hydroa). Other photosensitizing drugs (eg, phenothiazines, tar) should not be given concomitantly. If overdose occurs, an emetic should be considered, and the patient should remain in a darkened room for eight hours or until cutaneous reactions subside.

PHARMACOKINETICS. In normal individuals, an oral dose of methoxsalen is almost completely absorbed (95%). Time to peak plasma concentration is two to three hours. The duration of photosensitizing action is about ten hours. Methoxsalen is metabolized in the liver and more than 90% of a single dose is excreted in the urine within 12 hours. Accumulation has not been observed in normal individuals.

DOSAGE AND PREPARATIONS.
Topical: For small vitiliginous lesions 6 to 50 cm², low concentrations are applied on alternate days to the affected area (50 to 200 mcg/in²). Many physicians begin with a 0.1% concentration because of the strong potential for blister formation. The surrounding normal skin is protected by an opaque sunscreen. After 30 to 45 minutes, the treated area is exposed to a long-wave ultraviolet radiation source for 30 to 60 seconds; the lesions are then washed with soap and water, and a broad spectrum or opaque sunscreen is applied. Direct sunlight should be avoided. Exposure is increased gradually but should not exceed one-half the minimal erythemal dose.
Oxsoralen (Elder). Lotion 1% in 30 ml containers.
Oxsoralen lotion should never be dispensed directly to the patient for home application.

Oral: *Adults and children over 12 years,* for repigmentation of idiopathic vitiligo (lesions generally larger than 6 cm² to a maximum of 40% of the body surface), 20 mg/day as a single dose 2 to 2.5 hours before exposure to ultraviolet radiation. Patients with brown or black skin can receive 40 mg/day (0.6 mg/kg). UVA exposure usually is limited to five minutes initially and gradually increased to 30 minutes if required. The risk of severe burn to the vitiliginous skin is considerable with methoxsalen. Sunlight exposure also must be limited (see the manufacturer's literature for suggested time limitations) and sunscreens, appropriate sunglasses, and light-screening lipstick must be employed for 24 to 48 hours after exposure to UVA radiation (see Precautions).
Oxsoralen (Elder). Capsules 10 mg.

MONOBENZONE
[Benoquin]

Monobenzone is the monobenzyl ether of hydroquinone. Its action is similar to that of hydroquinone except that extensive selective destruction of melanocytes also occurs. Monobenzone causes irreversible depigmentation and is used to remove the few remaining areas of normal pigmentation in patients with generalized vitiligo covering at least 60% of the body. Patient consent should be obtained for achieving total depigmentation.

ADVERSE REACTIONS AND PRECAUTIONS. The adverse effects are similar to those caused by hydroquinone, except that the incidence of sensitization is higher.

Monobenzone therapy is often difficult to manage and requires careful patient follow-up; bizarre patterns of hypopigmentation may occur at sites distant from the area of application. Alternative management programs should be considered before monobenzone is tried in the treatment of vitiligo, ie, continuous sunscreen protection, psoralen compounds, masking preparations (eg, Covermark Cream), staining type cosmetics (eg, Vitadye).

DOSAGE AND PREPARATIONS.
Topical: *Adults and adolescents over 12 years,* the preparation is applied to the involved areas twice daily for three to nine months. An opaque sunscreen also should be applied during the day on areas that cannot easily be protected from exposure to the sun to prevent recurrence of hyperpigmentation.
Benoquin (Elder). Ointment 20% in 37.5 g containers.

TRIOXSALEN
[Trisoralen]

USES. Trioxsalen, a psoralen derivative, increases tolerance to sunlight in sun-sensitive individuals. Tolerance of the skin to ultraviolet light is enhanced by increasing pigmentation and, possibly, by thickening of the stratum corneum; therefore, administration of trioxsalen must be followed in approximately two hours by exposure to sunlight or, in expert hands, to long-wave ultraviolet radiation (320 to 400 nm [UVA]). This regimen of trioxsalen and light exposure is potentially danger-ous to patients with fair skin who are more likely to develop keratoses and basal and squamous cell carcinomas.

ADVERSE REACTIONS. Extensive clinical experience with short-term administration indicates that trioxsalen has minimal toxicity. Gastric discomfort is noted occasionally but can be minimized by taking the medication with food.

See the discussion on Photochemotherapy in the section on Antipsoriatic Agents for discussion of the potential cataracto-genic and carcinogenic actions of the psoralens.

PRECAUTIONS. The psoralens are *not* sunscreens. Since photoprotection develops gradually during multiple treatments, patients are susceptible to sunburn during initial treatment periods. Therefore, the dosage and length of exposure to the sun must be controlled closely to prevent injury to the skin. To protect eyes and lips, blue-gray plastic sunglasses (with side shields) opaque to UVA light and a light-screening lipstick should be used during exposure and for at least 24 and preferably 48 hours following administration. If overdosage occurs, the patient should remain in a darkened room for eight hours or until cutaneous reactions subside.

Trioxsalen is contraindicated in patients with diseases asso-ciated with photosensitivity, such as porphyria (porphyria cutanea tarda and erythropoietic porphyria), discoid or sys-temic lupus erythematosus, and xeroderma pigmentosum. Other photosensitizing drugs (eg, phenothiazines) should not be given concomitantly.

DOSAGE AND PREPARATIONS. The potential for producing a severe burn is considerable; the package insert should be read before prescribing this medication.

Oral: Adults and children over 12 years, for increasing tolerance to sunlight, the daily dose usually should not exceed 20 mg, and the total dosage should not exceed 28 to 36 tablets (four tablets daily in divided doses taken three days weekly on alternate days). Graduated, measured, daily exposures to sunlight or ultraviolet radiation should occur two to three hours after ingestion of the tablets. See the manufacturer's literature for suggested time limitations of sun exposure and Precau-tions for eye and lip protection.

For large lesions of vitiligo (the potential for producing a severe burn is considerable; caution and consultation is ad-vised), 0.6 mg/kg daily is given two or three times a week two hours before exposure to 10 to 15 minutes of sunlight at 2 PM.

Exposure is increased by 5 to 10 minutes per treatment until a mild erythema develops 12 to 18 hours after exposure that becomes maximal at 48 hours. During exposure to solar radiation, the patient should be in the prone or supine position and should change position at half of the exposure time. If the desired result is not obtained after 60 minutes of exposure, the dose of trioxsalen is increased by 10-mg increments to a maximum of 80 mg daily. Repigmentation, especially on the face and neck, is usually evident after three to four months of treatment. Since few patients benefit from longer use, therapy should be discontinued if results are not significant after four months.

See the Precautions section for eye and lip protection.
Trisoralen (Elder). Tablets 5 mg.

Topical Anesthetics and Antipruritics

For moderately extensive dermatitic eruptions, an agent with anti-inflammatory activity in an appropriate vehicle or a local antipruritic agent in a lotion or cream formulation (eg, menthol 0.25% to 2%, phenol 0.5% to 1.5%, camphor 1% to 3%) usually relieves pruritus and/or pain and avoids the use of topical anesthetics.

Oral nonsedating H_1 antihistamines such as astemizole [Hismanal] (investigational) and terfenadine [Seldane] are effective only when pruritus is due to peripheral release of histamine (eg, wheal reactions of urticaria and dermogra-phism). The sedating H_1 histamine antagonists or certain other sedatives (eg, benzodiazepines) are required for more com-mon pruritic dermatoses (eg, eczema, psoriasis, lichen planus) in which pruritus is unrelated to peripheral histamine release (Krause and Shuster, 1983). See also Chapter 58, Histamine and Antihistamines.

Certain antihistamines have local anesthetic activity when applied to mucocutaneous and abraded cutaneous areas, but, because of the risk of allergic contact dermatitis, systemic rather than topical administration is advisable for pruritus.

Topical local anesthetics may be useful in selected disorders affecting mucous membranes, mucocutaneous junctions, and abraded inflamed skin (eg, aphthous stomatitis, oral or anogenital herpes simplex lesions) and for pain caused by cytotoxic therapy for anal and genital warts. They are rarely useful in nonspecific pruritus ani and vulvae and may be sensitizing.

Numerous nonprescription topical mixtures containing a local anesthetic (most commonly, benzocaine) and usually an antiseptic are available for sunburn but they often are ineffec-tive, probably because the concentration of anesthetic is too low and penetration is poor even in sunburned skin. At least a 10% concentration of benzocaine, and probably 20%, usually is necessary.

The selection of a topical local anesthetic is based on its availability in a suitable vehicle (ie, solution, viscous solution, jelly, cream, ointment), the patient's prior history of sensitiza-tion, and the desired duration of action. Dibucaine and dimeth-isoquin may have the longest duration of action (two to four hours). Most local anesthetics are available without prescrip-tion. In the following listing, they are divided into amide, ester, and miscellaneous (nonamide and nonester) categories for selection in cases of known sensitivity.

Rash, urticaria, edema, or other manifestations of allergy may develop during use of a topical local anesthetic, but these reactions are rare during short-term therapy. These drugs should be used cautiously in patients with allergies or a strong family history of allergy. See also Chapter 15, Local Anesthetics.

Rectal formulations containing local anesthetics are available for relief of symptoms associated with anorectal disorders (see Chapter 53, Agents Used in Disorders of the Lower Intestinal Tract).

AMIDE LOCAL ANESTHETICS.
DIBUCAINE:
Generic. Ointment 1% (nonprescription).
Nupercainal (CIBA). Cream 0.5% in 45 g containers; ointment 1% in 30 and 60 g containers (both forms nonprescription).
LIDOCAINE:
Generic. Ointment 5%.
Xylocaine (Astra). Ointment 2.5% in 35 g containers (nonprescription) and 5% in 3.5 and 35 g containers; solution 2% (viscous) in 100 and 450 ml containers; solution 4% in 50 ml containers; jelly 2% in 30 ml containers; oral spray 10% in 60 ml containers.

AMINOBENZOATE ESTER LOCAL ANESTHETICS.
BENZOCAINE:
Generic. Cream 5% (nonprescription).
Americaine (American Critical Care). Aerosol 20% in 20, 60, and 120 g containers (nonprescription); gel lubricant 20% in 30 g containers; ointment 20% in 30 g containers (nonprescription).
Rhulicaine (Rydelle). Aerosol 20% in 120 ml containers.
BUTAMBEN PICRATE:
Butesin Picrate (Abbott). Ointment 1% in 28.4 g containers (nonprescription).
TETRACAINE:
Pontocaine (Winthrop-Breon). Cream (as hydrochloride) 1%, ointment 0.5% in 30 g containers (both forms nonprescription); solution 2% in 30 and 118 ml containers.

NONAMIDE AND NONAMINOBENZOATE ESTER LOCAL ANESTHETICS.
BENZYL ALCOHOL:
Topic (Syntex). Gel 5% in 60 g containers (nonprescription).
DYCLONINE HYDROCHLORIDE:
Dyclone (Astra). Solution 0.5% and 1% in 30 ml containers.
PRAMOXINE HYDROCHLORIDE:
Tronolane (Abbott). Cream 1% in 30 and 90 g containers; suppositories 1% (both forms nonprescription).
Tronothane (Abbott). Cream 1% in 30 g containers (nonprescription).

Cytotoxic Agents

The cytotoxic agents, cantharidin and podophyllin, are used for certain types of warts (see the section on Antiviral Agents in Chapter 74, Topical Anti-infective Agents: Drugs Used on Skin and Mucous Membranes). Methotrexate is employed to treat psoriasis (see the section on Antipsoriatic Agents). Topical fluorouracil is used to treat actinic keratoses.

FLUOROURACIL
[Efudex, Fluoroplex]

ACTIONS AND USES. This cytotoxic drug is used topically to remove multiple premalignant actinic keratoses; curettage or cryotherapy is preferred for isolated lesions (Bennett et al, 1985). Fluorouracil is more effective for keratoses on the face, forehead, bald scalp, and ears. Concentrations of 1% to 2% often are adequate for the face and forehead; higher concentrations may produce severe inflammation in these areas. Some physicians apply an intermediate-potency, nonfluorinated, topical corticosteroid subsequently to reduce inflammation. Lesions on the hands and arms may require higher concentrations, longer treatment periods, or initial therapy with 0.05% tretinoin. Actinic keratoses may recur. Although the inflammatory response may be lessened by limiting the area of initial application, the ultimate effectiveness of treatment is related to the inflammatory response and duration of therapy.

Superficial basal cell carcinomas respond to fluorouracil, but a 5% concentration and a longer duration of therapy (usually a month) are required. For other uses of fluorouracil, see Chapter 64, Drugs Used in Cancer Chemotherapy.

The healing process may continue for one to two months after therapy is stopped; restoration of skin color and texture is usually satisfactory.

Fluorouracil acts selectively against atypical epidermal cells by inhibiting DNA and RNA synthesis. Even lesions that are not grossly visible respond; for this reason, fluorouracil should be applied to the entire affected area. The drug has less effect on normal epidermis unless occlusive dressings are used.

ADVERSE REACTIONS AND PRECAUTIONS. Pruritus and irritation are the most common adverse reactions. Intense burning pain is reported occasionally. Severe reactions can be avoided by careful selection and instruction of patients. Systemic reactions are uncommon after topical use. Before therapy is initiated, the patient should be informed that inflammation, prolonged discoloration of skin, and a burning sensation may develop.

If there is excessive inflammation on normal skin, treatment should be discontinued. Fluorouracil should be applied with care to sensitive areas (eg, around the eyes, nasolabial folds). Exposure to sunlight during and for one or two months following treatment should be minimized. Since allergic reactions occur, the final drug product may be utilized for diagnostic patch tests, and intradermal tests sometimes are required.

DOSAGE AND PREPARATIONS. Commercial preparations are available in a variety of concentrations and vehicles. Solutions in propylene glycol are more active than creams containing equivalent concentrations of the drug.
Topical: Fluorouracil is applied twice daily for two to four weeks until a maximal inflammatory response occurs; the

frequency of application may require adjustment in accordance with the intensity of the response.

If allergic reactions are not severe, the drug can be applied every three to seven days to maintain the therapeutic effect.

Efudex (Roche). Cream 5% in 25 g containers; solution 2% and 5% with propylene glycol in 10 ml containers.

Fluoroplex (Herbert). Cream 1% in 30 g containers; solution 1% with propylene glycol in 30 ml containers.

Agents Used in Skin Ulcers

Prevention is paramount in the management of skin ulcers. Supersoft support and placement of a patient in the 30° oblique position on either side are recommended to avoid decubitus ulcers (Seiler and Stähelin, 1985 A). A number of agents are available as adjuncts in the management of skin ulcers; general supportive care and treatment of complications (eg, stasis, trauma, infection) are necessary for optimal results (Friedman and Su, 1983; Parish and Witkowski, 1983; Roenigk, 1983, 1985; Seiler and Stähelin, 1985 B).

It is essential that patients, particularly the elderly who are most likely to develop stasis and decubitus ulcers, receive adequate hydration and nutrition; enteral supplementation or total parenteral nutrition may be necessary to resolve resistant ulcers. Bedrest to reduce tissue oxygen demands and frequent changes of position to alleviate pressure also are valuable. Restoration of vascular sufficiency to an involved extremity enhances wound healing; correction of anemia increases the efficiency of available circulation. Surgical curettage of eschar following use of topical viscous lidocaine may be helpful.

Transparent, occlusive, synthetic films (eg, Bioclusive, Op-Site, Tegaderm) that are permeable to oxygen and water vapor but impermeable to liquids and bacteria and hydrocolloid dressing [DuoDerm], which is not permeable to oxygen but does have absorptive capacity, may be indicated to minimize bacterial contamination, drying, and pain.

Skin grafting is necessary for lesions larger than 3 cm that have sufficient granulation tissue to support epithelial regeneration. Silver nitrate sticks or 10% solution may control excessive granulation tissue that interferes with epithelial regeneration.

An appropriate topical antiseptic or antibiotic should be used to inhibit bacterial growth. Silver sulfadiazine [Flint SSD, Silvadene], which is used principally for burns, has been recommended for treatment of chronic pressure ulcers instead of saline and povidone-iodine (Kucan et al, 1981). Although clinical experience suggests that resistance of gram-negative bacilli would be greater with silver sulfadiazine, this agent is especially effective against the gram-negative organism, *Pseudomonas aeruginosa* (Melotte et al, 1985). Any threatening invasive infection should be treated with systemic antibiotics in addition. Hyperglycemia, uremia, and edema also should be corrected.

The value of *topical debriding enzymes*, collagenase [Biozyme-C, Santyl], fibrinolysin with desoxyribonuclease [Elase], and sutilains [Travase], is controversial. These agents

degrade protein and thus aid in the removal of necrotic tissue, clotted blood, purulent exudates, or fibrinous accumulations resulting from burns, trauma, inflammation, infected wounds, or ulcers. By promoting wound cleansing, they facilitate healing, but some physicians question the findings of the limited data available.

Effective enzymatic action depends upon proper wound preparation prior to application (ie, adequate cleansing of the site to remove detritus, providing for subsequent drainage when necessary). Cross hatching of eschar may be necessary to ensure the enzyme's adequate contact with the wound. Insufficient action may result from improper storage of the enzyme, use of an inappropriate vehicle, or concomitant administration of agents that destroy or inhibit the enzyme (eg, heavy metals, some antiseptics, hexachlorophene). Failure also may result from drying of the substrate, persistence of foreign material or sequestra, and inaccessible location of pus, as in osteomyelitis of cancellous bone.

Dextranomer [Debrisan] is a hydrophilic cross-linked dextran polymer available as small beads (Heel et al, 1979). It is not a debriding agent, but rather a cleansing agent that acts by developing powerful suction forces that absorb wound secretions and products so that they will not interfere with wound healing. It should be used only during the wet exudative phase of healing; it is not effective in dry wounds.

COLLAGENASE

[Biozyme-C, Santyl]

ACTIONS AND USES. Collagenase is an enzyme derived from fermentation of *Clostridium histolyticum*. It is effective in managing dermal ulcers from various causes (eg, peripheral vascular disorders, pressure sores) and severe burns. Complete debridement usually occurs in 10 to 14 days; granulation, epithelialization, and healing follow.

Collagenase degrades denatured and undenatured collagen, whereas other proteolytic enzymes act only on denatured collagen. For this reason, it has been claimed that this enzyme produces better debridement by acting on collagen fibers at the wound edges, which anchor necrotic slough to the base. In vitro studies indicate that collagenase does not act on fat, keratin, fibrin, muscle, or collagen in newly formed granulation tissue.

Activity is optimal between pH 6.0 and 8.0; the enzyme is inactivated at pH 5.0 or lower and at pH 8.5 or higher, as well as at temperatures above 56 C. It also is inactivated by detergents, benzalkonium chloride, hexachlorophene, nitrofurazone, tincture of iodine, and heavy metals and substances containing them (eg, thimerosal, silver nitrate, aluminum acetate).

Several topical antibiotics (eg, bacitracin, neomycin, polymyxin B) do not interfere with the activity of collagenase and may be used if infection is present. Systemic antibiotics may be required for more severe infections.

ADVERSE REACTIONS AND PRECAUTIONS. Adverse reactions are uncommon; slight erythema may develop in surrounding tissue. Irritation may be prevented by applying a protectant (eg, zinc oxide paste, U.S.P. [Lassar's Plain Zinc Paste]) to the surrounding tissue. Enzymatic action can be stopped when desired by application of aluminum acetate solution, U.S.P. (Burow's solution).

DOSAGE AND PREPARATIONS.

Topical: The ointment is applied once daily or more frequently if the dressing becomes soiled. It may be applied directly to deep lesions; for shallow wounds, it can be applied to a sterile gauze pad placed over the wound. Prior to application, the lesion should be cleansed with hydrogen peroxide or Dakin's solution followed by normal saline; antiseptics that inactivate the enzyme should not be used. If such materials have been applied to the lesion, they must be removed completely by washing before collagenase is used. The ointment should be confined to the area of the lesion; surrounding healthy skin can be protected by covering with zinc oxide paste.

> **Biozyme-C** (Armour), **Santyl** (Knoll). Ointment 250 units/g in white petrolatum in 15 and 30 (**Santyl** only) g containers.

FIBRINOLYSIN WITH DESOXYRIBONUCLEASE COMBINED
[Elase]

This preparation contains fibrinolysin (plasmin) and desoxyribonuclease of bovine origin. Fibrinolysin acts on fibrin in blood clots and exudates and is used topically to remove necrotic debris and exudates from wounds, ulcers, and burns and to irrigate abscess cavities and sinus tracts.

Dermatitis, swelling, and erythema may occur. Precautions should be taken to prevent allergic reactions in patients with a history of sensitivity to mercury (from the preservative) or bovine products.

DOSAGE AND PREPARATIONS.

Topical: Adults and children, the ointment or solution is applied at least twice daily until optimal debridement is obtained.

> **Elase** (Parke-Davis). Ointment containing fibrinolysin 1 unit and desoxyribonuclease 666.6 units/g with thimerosal in a base containing liquid petrolatum and polyethylene in 10 and 30 g containers; powder (lyophilized, for solution) containing fibrinolysin 25 units (Loomis) and desoxyribonuclease 15,000 units (modified Christensen method) with thimerosal in 30 ml containers.

SUTILAINS
[Travase]

ACTIONS AND USES. Sutilains contains a proteolytic enzyme elaborated by *Bacillus subtilis*. The enzyme is most effective within a pH range of 6 to 6.8. It is virtually inactive on viable tissue but dissolves necrotic tissue. Sutilains is used to remove purulent exudate from skin surfaces in second- and third-degree burns. This agent also is used in the management of decubitus ulcers, traumatic and pyogenic wounds, and ulcers secondary to peripheral vascular disease.

ADVERSE REACTIONS AND PRECAUTIONS. Untoward effects are mild and consist of transient pain, paresthesia,

hemorrhage, and dermatitis. The enzyme should be discontinued if bleeding or dermatitis occurs. Systemic allergic reactions have been reported in man, and immunologic studies have shown that an antibody response may occur.

Detergents or antiseptics (eg, benzalkonium chloride, hexachlorophene, iodine, nitrofurazone) should not be used concomitantly because denaturation of the enzyme may occur. Sutilains should not come into contact with the eyes. If this occurs, the eyes should be rinsed with a copious amount of water (preferably sterile).

Use of sutilains is contraindicated in fungating neoplastic lesions; in necrotic areas where bone, tendon, fascia, or cartilage is exposed; or in wounds involving major body cavities or nerve tissue.

DOSAGE AND PREPARATIONS.

Topical: Adults and children, after cleansing and irrigating the wound area, the ointment is applied in a thin layer 1/4 to 1/2 inch beyond the area to be debrided and the site is covered with a loose wet dressing. A wet environment is important for enzymatic action. Application may be repeated three or four times daily. If there is no demonstrable debriding action within 24 to 48 hours, further application is unlikely to have an effect.

> **Travase** (Flint). Ointment (sterile) containing approximately 82,000 casein units of sutilains/g in a base containing white petrolatum and polyethylene in 14.2 g containers.

DEXTRANOMER
[Debrisan]

ACTIONS AND USES. Dextranomer is a hydrophilic polymer consisting of a three-dimensional network of cross-linked dextran chains. It is available as beads that are 0.1 to 0.3 mm in diameter or as a paste; each gram of beads absorbs 4 ml of fluid. Spaces within and between the beads generate suction forces of up to 200 mm Hg. Low-molecular-weight substances less than 1,000 daltons (eg, peptides) are absorbed into the beads, and high-molecular-weight substances (eg, proteins such as fibrin and its split products, wound detritus) are absorbed into the bead interspaces. Presumably this action creates a more favorable environment for wound healing (Heel et al, 1979). The role of dextranomer in wound management is as a cleansing agent.

Unlike debriding enzymes, dextranomer does not attack collagen or fibrin. It is suggested that large necrotic areas be debrided surgically or enzymatically prior to use of dextranomer. Dextranomer is indicated only for exudative ulcers and wounds.

ADVERSE REACTIONS AND PRECAUTIONS. Isolated cases of erythema, pain, subjective irritation, and bleeding have been reported, usually associated with dressing changes; these reactions rarely necessitate discontinuation of therapy. Spilling the beads on the floor can make the floor dangerously slippery.

DOSAGE AND PREPARATIONS.

Topical: For exudative lesions, the wound is filled with beads to a depth of at least 6 mm. (An area of ulceration 3 cm in diameter will require approximately 4 g of beads.) A light bandage is applied to hold the beads in place. Paste may be necessary for hard-to-reach areas or irregular surfaces. Dextranomer becomes greyish yellow when saturated and should then be removed by gentle irrigation, if possible; vigorous irrigation may be necessary, however. The frequency of dressing changes depends upon the degree of exudation from the wound; once or twice daily is usually necessary.

> **Debrisan** (Johnson & Johnson). Beads in 4, 25, 60, and 120 g containers; paste (sterile) in 10 g containers (both forms nonprescription).

Agents Used to Stimulate Hair Growth

Normal terminal scalp hair growth (anagen phase) is relatively steady over a three-year period, at which time the follicle enters a resting stage (telogen phase) for about three months. New growth then ensues and the old hair is pushed out of the follicle. Most follicles continue this cycle throughout life, but, in patients with pattern baldness, follicles in the areas of hair loss become progressively smaller, produce thinner and less pigmented indeterminate hair, then vellus hairs, and finally no hairs.

Minoxidil is a potent direct vasodilator used to treat hypertension (see Chapter 28, Antihypertensive Agents). This agent produces hypertrichosis and improves hereditary androgen-dependent alopecia (male or female pattern baldness) in a minority of patients. Topical use of this agent is being tested to stimulate hair growth in androgenetic (pattern) alopecia, as well as in alopecia areata (patchy baldness), alopecia totalis (total scalp baldness), and alopecia universalis (total body baldness) (Weiss and West, 1985). The latter three conditions, which are reported to have an autoimmune pathogenesis (Mitchell and Krull, 1984), have shown some response to the investigational immunostimulant, inosiplex [Isoprinosine] (Galbraith et al, 1984; Lowy et al, 1985).

MINOXIDIL
[Regaine]

ACTIONS AND USES. Minoxidil causes elongation of follicles in the area of alopecia (Headington and Novak, 1984); new follicles are not formed. Minoxidil has no endocrine action. Topical application causes a dose-dependent increase in dermal blood flow, which may contribute to hair regrowth. In alopecia areata, decreases in the perifollicular lymphocytic infiltrate and opening of previously closed dermal vessels occur in areas of regrowth.

Limited controlled studies utilizing topical minoxidil 1% to 3% twice daily for months have demonstrated good responses in about one-third of subjects (Fenton and Wilkinson, 1983, Weiss et al, 1984; De Villez, 1985; Olsen et al, 1985; Weiss and West, 1985). In alopecia areata, a 5% concentration appears to be most effective (Weiss et al, in press). Good to excellent responses are based not only on number of new hairs, but also on hair growth beyond the vellus stage, ie, cosmetically acceptable.

Onset of action is usually from one to two and one-half months, but may be longer in some patients. Responses have been most satisfactory in patients with smaller areas of baldness. Shorter duration of hair loss may favorably affect response in androgenetic alopecia (De Villez, 1985; Olsen et al, 1985), but it has no relevance in alopecia areata (Weiss et al, 1984; Weiss et al, in press). The beneficial effect ceases when use of minoxidil is discontinued.

ADVERSE REACTIONS AND PRECAUTIONS. A few cases of allergic contact dermatitis have been reported, but local reactions are minimal and treatment is well tolerated. Absorption appears to be minimal based on the observation that 1.6% to 3.9% of an applied dose was found in the urine (Franz, 1985); the few cardiovascular signs or symptoms reported during clinical trials were not thought to be drug related. However, because of variations in concentration and formulation of extemporaneous preparations, adverse events may not be predictable. Therefore, the FDA strongly recommends that topical formulations not be compounded from available oral tablets for this use (*FDA Drug Bull*, 1985).

> **Regaine** (Upjohn).
> (Investigational drug)

Miscellaneous Agents

COLLODION

This mixture of pyroxylin, ether, and alcohol forms a sticky, tenacious film that adheres to the skin upon drying. Flexible collodion also contains camphor 0.2% and castor oil 0.3% and is used as a protectant for fissures. Collodion may be used as a protectant from the irritating effects of tar in the treatment of psoriasis or salicylic acid in the treatment of corns, calluses, and warts. This mixture also is employed as a vehicle for salicylic and lactic acids.

> COLLODION, U.S.P.:
> **Generic.** Liquid in 120 and 474 ml containers.
> FLEXIBLE COLLODION, U.S.P.:
> **Generic.** Liquid in 120, 474, and 3,792 ml containers.

DAPSONE

SULFAPYRIDINE

$$H_2N \text{—} \langle \text{benzene ring} \rangle \text{—} SO_2NH \text{—} \langle \text{pyridine ring} \rangle$$

The sulfonamide, sulfapyridine, was once the treatment of choice for dermatitis herpetiformis but in large part has been replaced by the antileprosy sulfone, dapsone. This compound is relatively insoluble and is absorbed slowly following oral administration. The risk of crystalluria with sulfapyridine, unlike many of the newer sulfonamides, is high. The drug is quite toxic and would be considered obsolete except for its use as an alternative to dapsone for dermatitis herpetiformis.

Dermatitis herpetiformis is a chronic disease characterized by clusters of intensely pruritic papules, urticaria-like lesions, vesicles, and bullae on the extensor surfaces. A gluten-sensitive jejunopathy similar to that found in celiac disease is observed in so many of these patients that the jejunopathy and dermatitis are considered parts of the same disease complex. A gluten-free diet often reverses the generally asymptomatic jejunal abnormality, but strict adherence to the diet is required for months to reverse the skin lesions; some patients remain resistant and reversal is never achieved with diet alone (Katz et al, 1980). Dapsone usually controls the skin lesions rapidly, and adherence to a gluten-free diet usually allows dosage reduction or eventual discontinuation of drug therapy. Deposition of IgA in dermal papillae, HLA association, gluten sensitivity, and antireticulin antibodies suggest that the disease is an immunologic disorder. An immunosuppressive action of dapsone characterized by inhibition of cytotoxicity induced by the myeloperoxidase-peroxide-halide system supports that concept (Stendahl et al, 1978).

Since the bullous eruption of systemic lupus erythematosus resembles dermatitis herpetiformis histologically, dapsone has been tried in a small number of patients with this disease. In one study, response was rapid and satisfactory (Hall et al, 1982).

Usual daily doses of dapsone (100 to 200 mg) relieve acute dermatologic symptoms in one to three days, but slightly larger amounts (200 to 300 mg daily) can produce hemolysis, methemoglobinemia, or leukopenia in less than two weeks. Agranulocytosis is a rare complication. Weekly complete blood counts are recommended during the first month of therapy and every three to four months thereafter.

Less common side effects of dapsone include dose-related hepatitis and peripheral motor neuropathy that may be idiosyncratic and is usually manifested by weakness not always reversible on drug withdrawal. Reversible, severe hypoalbuminemia has been reported in two patients after 3 and 11 years of dapsone therapy for dermatitis herpetiformis.

See the evaluation on Dapsone in Chapter 75, Antimycobacterial Agents, for additional information on pharmacokinetics, adverse reactions, and precautions.

DOSAGE AND PREPARATIONS.

DAPSONE:

Oral: *Adults,* 50 mg three or four times daily.
   Generic. Tablets 25 and 100 mg.

SULFAPYRIDINE:

Oral: *Adults,* 500 mg to 1 g four times daily; up to 6 g daily has been used.
   Generic. Tablets 500 mg.

PLASTIC FILMS

Synthetic films (eg, polyvinylidene chloride, polyethylene) are widely used as occlusive dressings in dermatologic therapy. Occlusion prevents evaporation of perspiration and enhances penetration of certain medications (eg, adrenal corticosteroids) through the skin. Polyethylene film is a useful adjunct in the treatment of psoriasis, skin ulcers, some eczemas, and keratodermas.

Occlusion can cause folliculitis, overgrowth of *Candida*, and other conditions resulting from maceration and heat, especially during hot weather.

   Glad Wrap (Union Carbide). Also available in tubular form for occlusion of extremities.
   Similar Preparation.
   Saran Wrap (Dow). Vinylidene polymer plastic.

PROPHYLACTIC AGENTS

Antiperspirants and Deodorants

Undesirable body odor results from the action of bacteria on organic constituents of apocrine gland sweat. The more voluminous, watery eccrine sweat promotes this process by increasing wetness, which favors bacterial growth.

Two classes of nonprescription drugs diminish this phenomenon (*Federal Register*, [Aug 20] 1982). Topically applied *antiperspirants* reduce eccrine gland sweat by 20% to 60%, depending upon the agent and method of application; aerosols tend to be least effective. Aluminum chlorohydrate, aluminum zirconium chlorohydrate, aluminum chloride, or buffered aluminum sulfate are the principal active agents in over-the-counter antiperspirants. They probably interfere with the formation of sweat, partially occlude the ducts, and exert an antibacterial action that contributes to the deodorant effect.

Topically applied *antiseptics*, usually in the form of antimicrobial bar soaps, do not reduce sweating. Their antimicrobial deodorant action should be distinguished from the effect of masking fragrances in cosmetic preparations. The active ingredient is carbanilide, triclocarban, or triclosan. Representative bar soaps include Coast, Dial, Irish Spring, Jergens Clear Complexion Bar, Lifebuoy, Phase III, Safeguard, and Zest. (See the section on Antiseptics and Disinfectants in Chapter 74, Topical Anti-infective Agents: Drugs Used on Skin and Mucous Membranes.)

The most common adverse effects of antiperspirants are stinging, burning, itching, and irritation. Less common reactions include dermatitis and open ulceration. These preparations should be discontinued at the first sign of irritation, which usually disappears without further complications. Contact sensitization is rare; if patch testing is desirable, the manufacturer should be contacted for appropriate materials, for the final formulation may be inadequate for this purpose.

Certain deodorant drugs are taken orally to control ostomy odors. The FDA has recognized as safe and effective the nonprescription drugs, bismuth subgallate (200 to 400 mg up to four times daily) and chlorophyllin copper complex (100 to 200 mg daily), for this indication (*Federal Register*, [June 17] 1985).

OTC antiperspirant products are inadequate to treat severe hyperhidrosis of the palms, soles, and axillae. Prescription products containing aluminum chloride hexahydrate 6.25% [Xerac AC] or 20% [Drysol] in absolute ethyl alcohol appear to be effective in some patients when applied without occlusion; for greater effectiveness, the preparation is applied under plastic occlusive dressing to *dry* axillae at bedtime and is washed off in the morning. The number of treatments required depends upon the individual. Severe irritation occurs frequently. Glutaral 2% in a buffered solution (pH 7.5) [Cidex] is available without prescription and has an anhidrotic effect when applied to the palms and soles but not the axillae. It appears to act by occluding the sweat ducts (see the discussion on Aldehydes in the section on Antiseptics and Disinfectants in Chapter 74).

> **Drysol** (Person & Covey). Aluminum chloride hexahydrate 20% in anhydrous ethyl alcohol 93% in 35 ml containers.
>
> **Xerac AC** (Person & Covey). Aluminum chloride hexahydrate 6.25% in anhydrous ethyl alcohol 96% in 35 and 60 ml containers.

Sunscreens

Although sunlight is used therapeutically (phototherapy) in neonatal jaundice, psoriasis, and related papulosquamous disorders, it has many acute and chronic adverse effects on the skin. Fair-skinned individuals with normal skin require only 10 to 20 minutes of exposure to sunlight initially during spring or early summer to develop perceptible sunburn (minimal erythema dose, MED). Exposure times of 60 to 90 minutes can lead to an acute, painful sunburn reaction with blisters. Sun-sensitive individuals should minimize direct exposure to sunlight and should go outdoors only when solar irradiation is less intense and with as much protection from opaque clothing and accessories as possible. These individuals preferably should remain indoors between 10 AM and 4 PM, especially during the summer.

Sun Sensitivity: The variation in sun sensitivity and ability to produce pigment among individuals has led to the following classification of six skin types: (I) always burns, never tans; (II) burns easily, tans minimally; (III) burns moderately, tans gradually; (IV) burns minimally, tans well; (V) rarely burns, tans profusely; (VI) never burns, deeply pigmented.

Solar radiation includes ultraviolet (6%), visible (46%), and infra-red (48%) radiation. Ultraviolet radiation is divided into three categories (1) UVA or near ultraviolet, 320 to 400 nm; (2) UVB, 290 to 320 nm; (3) UVC, 200 to 290 nm.

Uncontrolled exposure to solar radiation causes sunburn, skin aging, actinic keratosis, and skin cancer (basal and squamous cell carcinomas). UVA radiation may enhance UVB-induced skin carcinogenesis and aging. UVB and UVA

radiation also stimulate melanin pigmentation (tanning reaction), but the latter produces tanning only in individuals with skin types III to VI. UVC radiation from the sun is filtered by the ozone layer in the stratosphere and does not reach the earth's surface. It is emitted by artificial sources and is a weak germicide. No appreciable tanning occurs with UVC radiation. However, the erythemogenic (sunburn) potential of UVC is greater than that of UVB, and UVB is 800 to 1,000 times more erythemogenic than UVA radiation. Sunscreens vary in their ability to block out UVA and UVB radiation.

Sunscreen Characteristics: Sunscreens help to prevent sunburn, actinic keratosis, and premature aging of the skin (solar elastosis). They are indicated especially in (1) individuals who burn easily (skin types I through III); (2) individuals hypersensitive to sunlight; (3) patients taking photosensitizing or phototoxic medications (eg, thiazides, phenothiazines, sulfonamides, sulfonylureas, psoralens, demeclocycline); (4) patients with photosensitivity caused by systemic lupus erythematosus or porphyria; (5) medical personnel and patients who may be exposed to ultraviolet bactericidal lamps; and (6) individuals traveling to equatorial areas.

Sunscreens are now labeled with a *sun protective factor (SPF)* that ranges from 2 to 15. This factor is defined as the ratio of the amount of ultraviolet energy required to produce a minimal erythema dose (MED) through the applied sunscreen product to the amount required to produce the same reaction without the sunscreen. Five product categories are based on SPF numbers: SPF 2-4, minimal protection from sunburn but permit suntanning; SPF 4-6, moderate protection but permit suntanning; SPF 6-8, extra protection from sunburn and permit limited suntanning; SPF 8-15, maximum protection from sunburn and permit limited suntanning; SPF over 15, most protection from sunburn and permit no suntanning. SPF usually is determined in human volunteers with skin types I through III under laboratory conditions using an ultraviolet emitting lamp to simulate solar radiation.

Chemical sunscreens include (UV absorption spectrum in parentheses) para-aminobenzoic acid (PABA) and its two esters (290 to 320), benzophenones (250 to 360), cinnamates (290 to 320), and salicylates (290 to 320). The FDA has approved about 25 chemicals for use as suncreens. Physical sunscreens (zinc oxide, talc, or titanium dioxide) scatter ultraviolet and visible radiation and thus are opaque to all wavelengths of light. They are effective and useful to protect selected areas of the body (eg, nose, cheeks, shoulders), but are cosmetically unappealing.

Sunscreen Selection: The effectiveness of sunscreen preparations depends on the absorption spectrum of the principal agent(s), concentration, and vehicle. Increasing the concentration increases protection, but the two are not directly proportional. Certain esters of para-aminobenzoic acid (PABA) are more substantive (ie, the ability of the preparation to resist removal during sweating and swimming) than PABA alone (Sayre et al, 1979; Pathak, 1982); however, the vehicle also affects substantivity (Kaidbey and Kligman, 1981; Pathak, 1982). In one extensive comparative study, MMM What-A-Tan, Sundown 8 and 15, SuperShade 15, PreSun 15, Elizabeth Arden 15, Piz Buin 12, Ti-Screen 15, and TOTAL Eclipse 15 exhibited excellent resistance to sweating and good resistance to water immersion (Pathak, 1982; Pathak et al, 1985).

Preparations containing less effective sunscreens or lower concentrations of effective agents are marketed for individuals who wish to acquire a tan while avoiding sunburn. These preparations are less suitable for individuals with skin types I and II.

Precautions: Contact sensitivity and photosensitivity occur in a few individuals with most chemical agents, but a nonsensitizing preparation usually can be found. Sparing use is recommended initially until lack of sensitization is assured. Individuals sensitive to benzocaine, procaine, para-phenylene diamine (hair dyes), and sulfanilamide probably should avoid formulations containing PABA and its esters; those sensitive to thiazides and other sulfa drugs should avoid PABA esters as well (Pathak, 1982). If patch and photopatch testing facilities are available, sensitivity to these agents may be determined definitively. This permits specific recommendations for individual patients and avoids mandating against all related chemicals (Mathias et al, 1978). Highly alcoholic vehicles should not be used on eczematous or otherwise inflamed skin.

Adjunctive Preparations: Baby oil or mineral oil (with or without iodine), lubricating creams or lotions, cocoa butter, coconut oil, and tanning butters also are available. These preparations provide no protection against sunburn and may induce miliaria and folliculitis; their sole virtue is that they minimize skin dryness.

A number of artificial tanning preparations (bronzers, body gels, face colors) are available to give the skin a tanned appearance without exposure to the sun; these preparations provide no protection against sunburn unless a sunscreen is incorporated in the formulation.

In some instances, aspirin, corticosteroids, and indomethacin are claimed to provide some degree of protection; however, these agents should not be used as systemic sunscreens.

Products: Laboratory methodology is not yet standardized, and the SPF's for the following preparations tend to overestimate the degree of protection (Pathak et al, 1985). The lettered designations in parentheses denote the active ingredient(s) and are listed to aid the physician when contact dermatitis is known or anticipated: (a) para-aminobenzoic acid, (b) esters of para-aminobenzoic acid (glyceryl, padimate O), (c) benzophenones, (d) cinnamates, (e) salicylates, (f) titanium dioxide, (g) zinc oxide, (h) red veterinary petrolatum, (i) anthranilates.

See the discussion of skin types under the section on Sun Sensitivity when selecting the following products with differing SPF ranges.

SPF RANGE 10-15 FOR SKIN TYPE I and II
Alo-Sun SPF 15 Sunblock Stick (Aloe Creme) (b,c); ***Alo-Sun Fashion Tan SPF 15 Sunblock Lotion*** (Aloe Creme) (b,c); ***Coppertone Waterproof Sunblock Lotion 15*** (Plough) (b,c); ***Coppertone Faces Lotion 15*** (Plough) (b,c); ***Coppertone Lipkote 15*** (Plough) (b,c); ***Elizabeth Arden 15*** (Elizabeth Arden) (b,c); ***MMM What-A-Tan*** (3 M) (b,c); ***Pabanol Lotion*** (Elder) (a); ***PreSun 15 Sunscreen Lotion*** (Westwood) (a,b); ***PreSun 15 Creamy Sunscreen Lotion*** (Westwood) (b,c); ***Solbar Plus 15 Sunscreen Cream*** (Person & Covey) (b,c); ***Solbar PabaFree 15*** (Person & Covey) (c); ***Solar Cream SPF 15*** (Doak) (a,f); ***Sundown Ultra 15 Sunscreen Lotion*** (Johnson & Johnson) (b,c); ***Super Shade Waterproof Sunblock 15 Lotion*** (Plough) (b,c);

Total Eclipse 15 Sunscreen Lotion (Dorsey) (b,c) (all forms nonprescription).

SPF RANGE 6-8 FOR SKIN TYPE III
A-Fil (Rydelle) (f,i); ***Coppertone Waterproof Sunscreen Lotion 6, 8*** (Plough) (b,c); ***Coppertone Noskote 8*** (Plough) (c,e); ***Coppertone Face Lotion 6*** (Plough) (b); ***Eclipse Original Sunscreen Gel, Lotion*** (Dorsey) (b); ***PreSun 8 Lotion, Creamy Lotion, Gel*** (Westwood) (a); ***RVPaque Ointment [10%]*** (Elder) (d,g,h); ***Shade Waterproof Sunscreen [6]*** (Plough) (b,c); ***Sundown Maximal 8 Sunscreen Lotion*** (Johnson & Johnson) (b,c); ***Sundown Extra [6] Sunscreen Lotion*** (Johnson & Johnson) (b,c).

SPF RANGE 4-6 FOR SKIN TYPE IV
Coppertone Lite Formula Suntan Lotion 4 (Plough) (e); ***Coppertone Waterproof Suntan Lotion 4*** (Plough) (b,c); ***Coppertone Face Lotion 4*** (Plough) (b); ***Maxafil 4-6*** (Johnson Wax) (d,i); ***Pabagel*** (Owen) (a); ***Partial Eclipse*** (Dorsey) (b); ***Shade Waterproof Sunscreen Lotion 4*** (Plough) (b,c); ***Solbar Cream*** (Person & Covey) (c); ***PreSun 4 Sunscreen Lotion*** (Westwood) (b); ***Sun Dare Creamy or Clear 4-6*** (Rydelle) (d); ***Sun Stick 4-6*** (Rydelle) (e).

SPF RANGE 2-4 FOR SKIN TYPE V and VI
Coppertone Suntan Oil 2 (Plough) (e); ***RVP Ointment*** (Elder) (h); ***Sundown Moderate [4] Sunscreen Lotion*** (Johnson & Johnson) (b).

VEHICLES

Dermatologic vehicles are designed to deliver topical medication in the most beneficial manner (McKay, 1983). They are used on occasion to enhance penetration of skin by active agents. They can be therapeutic in their own right when properly used. Their actions include skin cleansing, cooling, drying, lubrication, softening, hydration, and protection.

Criteria for selection of a vehicle include its drying, hydrating, or lubricating activity; the manner in which it holds, releases, or assists in the absorption of the active ingredients; and suitability for use on the area intended. Liquids (eg, lotions, solutions, shampoos, sprays) are convenient for application to hairy areas. Emulsified vanishing-type creams are most appropriate for use in body folds (intertriginous sites); if an ointment is used in such areas, it must be spread thinly to avoid maceration.

Constituents: The principal constituents of vehicles include liquids (water, alcohol, or organic solvents), powders, oils, and ointment bases; pharmaceutic aids often are present as additives.

Liquids have desirable properties in addition to their usefulness as vehicles. Water acts as a vehicle and as a hydrating agent in wet dressings, lotions, baths, creams, and some ointments. When applied as hot or cold compresses, water alters skin temperature and macerates the superficial layer of the skin. Alcohols are solvents and are used to cool the skin; depending upon the concentration, they may be antiseptic and astringent. Glycerin, a solvent and emollient in lotions, creams, and pastes, is miscible with water and alcohol. Propylene glycol is an excellent solvent and preservative; it has replaced glycerin as the vehicle for many topical therapeutic agents, cosmetics, and body and hand lotions. It is hygroscopic and has considerable moistening and softening actions. Subjective irritation (burning and stinging) may limit its use.

Powders increase evaporation, reduce friction and pruritus, and provide a cooling sensation. They are dusted on the skin or are present as a component of lotions and pastes. Examples of U.S.P. powders include zinc oxide, zinc stearate, magnesium stearate, talc, cornstarch, bentonite, titanium dioxide, and precipitated calcium carbonate.

Zinc oxide and talc (mainly hydrous magnesium silicate) are protective and absorb some water when applied as a paste in petrolatum. Zinc oxide mixed with a small amount of ferric oxide has a pink color; this mixture, calamine, is used in shake lotions. Although insoluble in water, bentonite (hydrated aluminum silicate) combines with water to form a gel; it improves the dispersion of zinc oxide and sulfur in oil-in-water mixtures. Titanium dioxide is opaque to both UVA and UVB radiation and is an ingredient of lotions or pastes used as sunscreens. Precipitated calcium carbonate is a fine white powder that is insoluble in alcohol and water; it gives a dry sensation and is more absorbent than talc. Talc alone is a lubricant but it may cause severe granulomatous reactions when applied to wounds.

Oils are liquid or semisolid hydrocarbons of mineral, vegetable, or animal origin. Vegetable and mineral oils are most widely used for topical therapy. Cottonseed, corn, castor, olive, and peanut oils are commonly incorporated in creams and lotions. Their emollient effect is similar, but odor, storage stability, and emulsifying capabilities differ.

Mineral oil is a mixture of high-molecular-weight hydrocarbons obtained from petroleum. It is used alone or as an ingredient in lotions, creams, or ointments and, unlike vegetable or animal oils, does not become rancid. Stabilizers (eg, tocopherol, butylhydroxytoluene) often are added. The United States Pharmacopeia requires that the stabilizer be identified on the label. Topically applied mineral oil is relatively free of untoward effects, except in acne-prone patients.

Like oils, *ointment bases* are used in various creams and ointments. They include semisolid vegetable and animal fats and waxes, petroleum hydrocarbons, and silicones.

Emulsifying agents are *pharmaceutic-aid additives* used in topical dermatologic products to provide stability and homogeneity for immiscible liquids. Glyceryl monostearate, polyethylene glycol derivatives (polyoxyl 40 stearate, polysorbate 80), and sodium lauryl sulfate are used as emulsifying agents in lotions, creams, and ointments that contain oily ingredients and water. Other additives include cetyl palmitate and related esters, which improve the consistency and appearance of creams; stearic acid and stearyl alcohol, which act as lubricants or emollients; silicones, which act as antifoaming agents; and methylcellulose and gum tragacanth, which are inert substances used as suspending agents in lotions, creams, ointments, and pastes. The parabens (methylparaben, propylparaben, and butylparaben), oxyquinoline sulfate, organic quaternary ammonium compounds, quaternium 15 [Dowicil 200], imidazolidinyl urea [Germall], parachlorometaxylenol, sorbic acid, benzyl alcohol, and chlorobutanol frequently are added as antimicrobial preservatives. Most of these agents are innocuous at the low concentrations present; however, the parabens rarely produce allergic contact dermatitis and sodium lauryl sulfate has the potential for producing irritation. Some additives increase the stratum corneum's permeability

not only to medicaments but to noxious agents and thus may directly or indirectly produce irritation.

Wet Dressings

Wet dressings are indicated for acute inflammation characterized by vesicular eruptions with exudation, oozing (weeping), and crusting. The soft, saturated, tepid dressings should be changed every 5 to 15 minutes for a period of 30 minutes to two hours, depending upon the severity of the inflammation. This process may be repeated three or four times daily.

Water is the most important ingredient in wet dressings. In addition to providing evaporative cooling, it is cleansing and helps to drain exudates; the vasoconstriction that results from cooling combats the first stage of an acute inflammatory response. These effects are lost if the wet dressing is occluded by wrapping or covering with plastic or rubber, and softening and maceration of the skin surface result. Aluminum acetate, potassium permanganate, copper and zinc sulfates, acetic acid, or silver nitrate may be added for their presumptive antibacterial or astringent action.

A 5% aluminum acetate solution, U.S.P. (Burow's solution), diluted 1:10 to 1:40, is commonly used as a wet dressing. Potassium permanganate 0.025% to 0.1% has astringent properties but stains the skin. *Tablets should be completely dissolved if placed in a tub of water, because they can produce cutaneous necrosis if the patient sits on them.* Silver nitrate solution 0.1% to 0.5% stains the skin but has more antibacterial activity than the other metal salts listed; however, it also permanently stains clothing and linens.

ALUMINUM ACETATE SOLUTION, U.S.P.
ALUMINUM CHLORIDE HEXAHYDRATE, N.F.
ALUMINUM SULFATE AND CALCIUM ACETATE:
Domeboro (Miles), **Bluboro** (Herbert). Powder (nonprescription).
POTASSIUM PERMANGANATE, U.S.P.
SILVER NITRATE, U.S.P.

Lotions

The term lotion (sometimes called "shake lotion") historically refers to a suspension of powder in a liquid medium (usually water) that requires shaking before application. The term recently has been extended to include commercial emulsions that are usually of thin, uniform consistency.

Lotions are used for subacute inflammatory lesions after the severe exudative phase has ceased. Their protective, drying, cooling effect is especially useful at intertriginous sites or in areas of widespread eruptions. A basic white shake lotion contains zinc oxide, talc, glycerin, and water. Calamine may be added for a flesh tint. Alcohol may be added (to a concentration of 15%) to enhance the drying effect.

Menthol 0.25% to 2%, phenol 0.5% to 1.5%, and camphor 1% to 3% have a weak antipruritic action; the latter two agents alter cutaneous nerve transmission, while menthol imparts a cooling sensation. See the evaluation on Phenol in the section on Antiseptics and Disinfectants in Chapter 74 for precautions.

Salicylic acid 1% to 2% and coal tar solution 3% to 10% may have an antipruritic action.

CALAMINE LOTION, U.S.P.

PHENOLATED CALAMINE LOTION, U.S.P.

MENTHOL LOTION WITH PHENOL:
Schamberg's Lotion (C & M Pharmacal) (nonprescription).

MENTHOL, CAMPHOR, AND PHENOL LOTION:
Sarna Lotion (Stiefel) (nonprescription).

MENTHOL, CAMPHOR, AND/OR CALAMINE:
Rhulicream, Rhuligel, Rhulispray (Rydelle) (nonprescription).

Gels

Gels used for topical preparations are transparent or opaque colloidal dispersions prepared in a solid or semisolid (jelly-like) state. Aqueous, acetone, alcohol, or propylene glycol gels of organic polymers, such as agar, gelatin, hydroxypropyl cellulose, carbomer methylcellulose, pectin, and polyethylene glycol, are primarily used. The gel liquifies on contact with skin and dries to a greaseless nonocclusive film.

The presence of large amounts of water and other solvents characterizes the subclass of gels known as jellies. Jellies are used as vehicles, particularly for application to mucous membranes, and as lubricants for surgical gloves, finger cots, catheters, and sexual intercourse.

A significant percentage of patients experience subjective irritation (burning, stinging) or drying after using gels.

Creams and Ointments

These semisolid preparations serve as vehicles for many drugs and are used alone for their emollient and protective properties. Creams and ointments are particularly suitable for the chronic inflammatory stage of skin diseases. Dry, scaling, thickened, pruritic, and lichenified lesions respond to their softening and lubricating properties. Creams and certain ointments hold or attract water to promote skin rehydration; other types of ointments repel water. Most ointments are sufficiently occlusive to promote the cutaneous absorption of drugs.

Creams and *emulsion ointment bases* consist of emulsions of oil (hydrophobic hydrocarbons, animal or vegetable fats, organic alcohols) and water. Oil-in-water (O/W) emulsions are less greasy and more easily removed (water-washable or vanishing creams) than water-in-oil (W/O) emulsions; however, the latter provide more lubrication and occlusion.

When the amount of oil exceeds that of water by a certain proportion, the emulsion changes from a pourable cream to a semisolid ointment. Although generally true, neither the official nor the manufacturers' designation of a product as a cream or ointment always correlates with O/W or W/O emulsification type, eg, Cold Cream, U.S.P. (W/O); Hydrophilic Ointment, U.S.P. (O/W).

Hydrophilic ointment contains white petrolatum, stearyl alcohol, sodium lauryl sulfate, and propylene glycol in water with preservatives. It is a good vehicle for water-soluble medica-

ments, has good esthetic properties, and imparts a pleasing sensation. Irritation has been noted, probably due to the emulsifier, sodium lauryl sulfate.

Cold cream, a water-in-mineral oil emulsion containing white wax, cetyl esters, wax, mineral oil, and sodium borate, is widely used. It lubricates and hydrates the skin and imparts a cooling sensation.

The remaining three classes of ointments contain essentially no water. Some are soluble in water or will attract and hold it; others are completely insoluble in water, hold little if any water, or may be water-repellent, depending upon the base used.

Water-absorbent ointment bases are mixtures of oleaginous materials and emulsifying agents. They are insoluble in water but absorb it and are difficult to wash off. These substances are water-in-oil emulsion ointment bases when hydrated. Examples include Hydrophilic Petrolatum, U.S.P., and Anhydrous Lanolin, U.S.P. The former is composed of white petrolatum, cholesterol, stearyl alcohol, and white wax; it is less greasy and more acceptable cosmetically than petrolatum. Anhydrous lanolin is an oleaginous substance obtained from sheep's wool; it contains less than 0.25% water but is capable of absorbing a considerable amount. It is an ingredient of commercial ointments and some bath oil preparations.

Oleaginous ointment bases are water-repellent and consist of hydrophobic hydrocarbons, hydrogenated vegetable fats, or siloxanes (silicones); some are synthetic mixtures with waxes. They are anhydrous, insoluble in water, and absorb little or no water. They are difficult to wash off, will not dry out, and generally change little during storage (although some fats may become rancid on aging). Oleaginous ointment bases are suitable for use alone or as a vehicle in patients who are sensitive to other bases and/or their ingredients (emulsifiers, stabilizers, preservatives).

Petrolatum, N.F., the most important agent of this group, is a purified mixture of high-molecular-weight hydrocarbons obtained from petroleum. This ointment is protective and emollient when applied to the skin and is an excellent base or vehicle for topical medicaments. It varies in color (off-white to light amber), composition, and consistency depending upon the petroleum source and manner of preparation. White Petrolatum, U.S.P., a bleached form of yellow petrolatum, is more esthetically pleasing and, therefore, is the form most commonly used. Yellow petrolatum is preferable for tar preparations because the bleaching agent in white petrolatum may inactivate tars. White Ointment, U.S.P., is white petrolatum with 5% white wax added. This preparation is firmer at room temperature than petrolatum.

Depending upon their degree of polymerization, silicones are available as liquid or semisolid preparations. The latter have the properties of other oleaginous ointment bases, except that they are considerably more water-repellent and have a low surface tension, which increases penetration into skin creases. Silicones are used as aqueous-barrier creams because they repel water and provide intimate coverage; however, they do not act as a barrier for organic compounds that may be contact irritants. The polydimethylsiloxanes (dimethicone) are stable, nonsensitizing, and nonirritating.

Water-soluble ointment bases (eg, polyethylene glycol ointment) are greaseless and anhydrous. They absorb water, are water soluble, and are good vehicles for the topical delivery of water-soluble drugs. The oil-in-water emulsion, Hydrophilic Ointment, U.S.P., is soluble in water and can be used similarly.

OIL-IN-WATER EMULSIONS:
Hydrophilic Ointment, U.S.P.
Acid Mantle Cream (Dorsey), *Cetaphil Lotion* (Owen), *Keri Lotion* (Westwood), *LactiCare Lotion* (Stiefel), *Lubriderm Cream* (Warner/Lambert), *Moisturel* (Westwood), *Nivea Cream* (Beiersdorf), *Nutraderm Cream* (Owen), *Purpose Dry Skin Cream* (Ortho), *Shepard's Skin Cream* (Dermik), *Sofenol-5* (C & M Pharmacal) (all forms nonprescription).

WATER-IN-OIL EMULSIONS:
Cold Cream, U.S.P.
Lanolin, U.S.P.
Eucerin (Beiersdorf), *Polysorb Hydrate* (Fougera), *Vaseline Petroleum Jelly* (Chesebrough Ponds) (nonprescription).

WATER-ABSORBENT OINTMENT BASES:
Hydrophilic Petrolatum, U.S.P.
Anhydrous Lanolin, U.S.P.
Aquaphor (Beiersdorf), *Unibase* (Parke-Davis), *Velvachol* (Owen) (nonprescription).

OLEAGINOUS (WATER-REPELLENT) OINTMENT BASES:
Petrolatum, N.F.
White Petrolatum, U.S.P.
White Ointment, U.S.P.
Dimethicone, U.S.P.

WATER-SOLUBLE OINTMENT BASE:
Polyethylene Glycol Ointment, U.S.P.

UREA

Urea, in a suitable cream or ointment vehicle, may soften the skin in ichthyotic and other dry, scaly conditions, such as psoriasis or atopic dermatitis. It disrupts the normal hydrogen bonding of keratinic proteins through its hydrating and keratolytic actions; this, in turn, promotes desquamation of the stratum corneum. It has not been established whether the antipruritic effect results from a direct action or from improvement of the skin condition.

Urea is used to accelerate cutaneous penetration of active ingredients; it increases hydrocortisone absorption twofold.

Subjective irritation (burning and stinging) may be noted with higher concentrations.

Generic. Crystals (bulk).
Aquacare (Herbert). Cream, lotion 2% and cream lotion 10% (*Aquacare*/*HP*).
Carmol-10 (Syntex). Lotion 10%.
Carmol-20 (Syntex). Cream 20%.
Nutraplus (Owen). Cream, lotion 10%.
(All forms nonprescription)

Available Mixture.
Carmol HC (Syntex). Cream containing urea 10% and hydrocortisone acetate 1% in 30 and 120 g containers.

PROPYLENE GLYCOL

Propylene glycol, a widely used vehicle in dermatologic formulations, is isotonic in 2% concentrations. Concentrations up to 70% alter keratin to hydrate and soften the skin and cause desquamation of scales, particularly when used under occlusive dressings.

Propylene glycol and other hydroalcoholic gels augment the keratolytic action of salicylic acid; this combination may be effective in ichthyosis. If the formulation contains 6% salicylic acid, no more than 20% of the body surface should be covered at any one time to prevent excessive absorption of salicylate.

Initially the preparation is applied nightly to wet skin (an occlusive dressing may be applied at bedtime) and the preparation is washed off in the morning. The frequency of application is reduced when improvement is noted. Subjective irritation (burning and stinging) occurs, particularly if the skin is damaged. Patients who cannot tolerate propylene glycol probably experience a special form of irritation but only rarely develop allergic contact dermatitis (Trancik and Maibach, 1982).

Available Mixtures.
Hydrisalic (Pedinol), *Keralyt* (Westwood). Gel containing salicylic acid 6% in a propylene glycol and alcohol vehicle in 30 g containers.
Lac-Hydrin (Westwood). Lotion containing lactic acid 12% and propylene glycol in 150 ml containers.

Pastes

Simple pastes are made by incorporating a finely divided powder into an ointment base. The resulting mixture protects the skin against external irritants and sunlight. The ointment base is usually petrolatum, and the powder is zinc oxide, talc, starch, bentonite, aluminum oxide, or titanium dioxide. Titanium dioxide has particularly good sunscreen properties. Coloring matter may be added to make the mixture cosmetically acceptable. A paste containing zinc oxide, starch, and white petrolatum in a 1:1:4 ratio, Zinc Oxide Paste, U.S.P. (Lassar's Plain Zinc Paste), is a commonly prescribed protective paste. Starch may act as substrate for some organisms. Pastes generally are poor vehicles for delivering active pharmacologic agents and for inhibiting water evaporation, but they adhere well and protect skin from friction caused by clothing and bandages. They are applied in subacute and chronic dermatoses, particularly in infants, but generally should be avoided in weeping lesions and hairy areas. Removal of pastes is facilitated by use of mineral or vegetable oil.

Soaps, Soap Substitutes, and Shampoos

Ordinary soaps are sodium or potassium salts of fatty acids. These anionic surfactants and cationic detergent cleansers emulsify fats, thereby promoting the removal of foreign particles from the skin. The pH of toilet bars varies in solution; some bar soaps are alkaline (pH 9.0 to 10.5) in solution, and superfatted bar soaps are at the lower end of this range. Neutral toilet bars contain synthetic surfactants and have a solution pH of 7.5 or slightly less. Badly irritated skin generally should not be exposed to soaps, detergents, or cleansers other than water.

Medicated soaps are widely available. Some abrasive soaps contain inert aluminum oxide, polyethylene, or sodium tetraborate decahydrate particles (see the section on Antiacne

Agents). Antimicrobial soaps contain antiseptics in sufficient concentration to be effective deodorants or useful as hand-washes for health care personnel, for preoperative preparation of the skin, or for surgical scrubs.

Shampoos are liquid soaps or detergents used to wash the hair and clean the scalp of scales. Most bar soaps can be used similarly. The detergent properties of special shampoos for use on dry, normal, or oily hair are different. Shampoos also are used as vehicles for applying medication to the scalp for dandruff, seborrheic dermatitis, or psoriasis.

NEUTRAL SOAPS OR SOAP SUBSTITUTES:
Acne-Aid Cleansing Bar (Stiefel), *Aveenobar* (Rydelle), *Caress* (Lever), *Dove* (Lever), *Drytergent* (C & M Pharmacal), *Lowila* (Westwood), *Oilatum Soap* (Stiefel), *pHisoDerm* (Winthrop-Breon), *Vel* (Colgate).

SUPERFATTED SOAPS:
Aveenobar Oilated (Rydelle), *Basis* (Beiersdorf), *Camay, Coast* (Procter & Gamble), *Irish Spring* (Colgate), *Nivea Creme Soap* (Beiersdorf), *Neutrogena* (Neutrogena), *Shield* (Lever).

Baths and Body Oils

Pruritus that accompanies acute dermatitis or extensive exanthematous lesions is often alleviated by immersion of the part or the entire body in water. Cooling diminishes pruritus safely and effectively. When baths are used to hydrate the skin, subsequent gentle drying is desirable, followed by use of an emollient to retard water evaporation.

Colloidal substances can be added to baths for their soothing and antipruritic activities. A paste made up of 2 cups of starch and 4 cups of cold water or colloidal oatmeal (Aveeno-bath Regular, Aveenobath Oilated) is added to a tub half-filled with water.

Occasionally it is desirable to add an oil to bath water. Since oils are insoluble in water, emulsifiers are often added to enhance dispersion and form a milky mixture of microglobules of oil-in-water. A fine film of oil remains on the skin after the bath. Since the addition of oils may make tubs slippery, body oils should be applied to wet skin after the bath in the elderly and children.

These products may be helpful in ichthyosis or pruritic and chronic eczematous dermatosis. Since these surfactant-treated oils impart a pleasing sensation to the skin, they are often used as emollients. Solutions of coal tar oils also are available for addition to baths; they are particularly useful for treating psoriasis.

MINERAL OIL AND LANOLIN OIL:
Alpha Keri (Westwood).

MINERAL OIL:
Domol (Miles), *Lubath* (Warner/Lambert).

SESAME SEED OIL:
Neutrogena Body Oil (Neutrogena).

Cited References

Adverse effects with isotretinoin. *FDA Drug Bull* 13:21-30, (Nov) 1983.

Antiperspirant drug products for over-the-counter human use; tentative final monograph. *Federal Register* 47:36492-36505, (Aug 20) 1982.

Deodorant drug products for internal use for over-the-counter human use; tentative final monograph; proposed rulemaking. *Federal Register* 50:25162-25167, (June 17) 1985.

Isotretinoin: Newly recognized human teratogen. *Morbid Mortal Week Rep* 33:171-173, (April 6) 1984.

OTC drug products for control of dandruff, seborrheic dermatitis, and psoriasis; establishment of monograph. *Federal Register* 47:54646-54684, (Dec 3) 1982.

Topical acne drug products for over-the-counter human use; tentative final monograph. *Federal Register* 50:2172-2182, (Jan 15) 1985.

Unapproved use of minoxidil. *FDA Drug Bull* 15:38, (Dec) 1985.

Allen HB, et al: Selenium sulfide: Adjunctive therapy for tinea capitis. *Pediatrics* 69:81-83, 1982.

Anderson TF: Psoriasis: New reasons for using time-honored empiric therapy. *Consultant* 39-55, (March 15) 1985.

Anderson TF, Voorhees JJ: Psoralen photochemotherapy of cutaneous disorders. *Annu Rev Pharmacol Toxicol* 20:235-257, 1980.

Arndt KA: *Manual of Dermatologic Therapeutics with Essentials of Diagnosis*, ed 3. Boston, Little, Brown and Company, 1983, 109-110.

Ashton RE, et al: Anthralin: Historical and current perspectives. *J Am Acad Dermatol* 9:173-192, 1983.

Bennett R, et al: Current management using 5-fluorouracil: 1985. *Cutis* 36:218-236, 1985.

Bershad S, et al: Changes in plasma lipids and lipoproteins during isotretinoin therapy for acne. *N Engl J Med* 313:981-985, 1985.

Bickers DR: Position paper: PUVA therapy. *J Am Acad Dermatol* 8:265-270, 1983.

Bickers DR, et al: Phototherapy and photochemotherapy, in Bickers DR, et al: *Clinical Pharmacology of Skin Disease*. New York, Churchill Livingstone, 1984, 200-216.

Bollag W: Development of retinoids in experimental and clinical oncology and dermatology. *J Am Acad Dermatol* 9:797-805, 1983.

Brazzell RK, et al: Pharmacokinetics of isotretinoin during repetitive dosing to patients. *Eur J Clin Pharmacol* 24:695-702, 1983.

Burge S, Ryan T: Diffuse hyperostosis associated with etretinate, (letter). *Lancet* 2:397-398, 1985.

Chen ML, et al: Specific HPLC assay to determine pharmacokinetics of methotrexate in patients. *Int J Clin Pharmacol Ther Toxicol* 22:1-6, 1984.

Colburn WA, Gibson DM: Isotretinoin kinetics after 80 to 320 mg oral doses. *Clin Pharmacol Ther* 37:411-414, 1985.

Cornell RC, Stoughton RB: Use of topical steroids in psoriasis. *Dermatol Clin* 2:397-409, 1984.

Cornell RC, Stoughton RB: Correlation of vasoconstrictor assay and clinical activity in psoriasis. *Arch Dermatol* 121:63-67, 1985.

De Villez RL: Topical minoxidil therapy in hereditary androgenetic alopecia. *Arch Dermatol* 121:197-202, 1985.

Dicken CH: Retinoids: Review. *J Am Acad Dermatol* 11:541-552, 1984.

DiGiovanna JJ, Peck GL: Oral synthetic retinoid treatment in children. *Pediatr Dermatol* 1:77-88, 1983.

Eady EA, et al: Use of antibiotics in acne therapy: Oral or topical administration? *J Antimicrob Chemother* 10:89-115, 1982.

Elias PM, Williams ML: Retinoids, cancer, and skin. *Arch Dermatol* 117:160-180, 1981.

Ellis CN, et al: Etretinate therapy for psoriasis: Reduction of antibody-dependent cell-mediated cytotoxicity of polymorphonuclear leukocytes. *Arch Dermatol* 121:877-880, 1985.

Epstein JH, et al: Current status of oral PUVA therapy for psoriasis. *J Am Acad Dermatol* 1:106-117, 1979.

Exner JH, et al: Pyogenic granuloma-like acne lesions during isotretinoin therapy. *Arch Dermatol* 119:808-811, 1983.

Farber EM, Nall L: Appraisal of measures to prevent and control psoriasis. *J Am Acad Dermatol* 10:511-517, 1984 A.

Farber EM, Nall L: Psoriasis: Review of recent advances in treatment. *Drugs* 28:324-346, 1984 B.

Farber EM, et al: Long-term risks of psoralen and UV-A therapy for psoriasis. *Arch Dermatol* 119:426-431, 1983.

Fenton DA, Wilkinson JD: Topical minoxidil in treatment of alopecia areata. *Br Med J* 287:1015-1017, 1983.

Fitzpatrick TB, Pathak MA: Research and development of oral psoralen and longwave radiation photochemotherapy: 2000 BC-1982 AD, in Pathak MA, Dunnick JK (eds): *Photobiologic, Toxicologic, and Pharmacologic Aspects of Psoralens*, (monograph 66). Bethesda, MD, USPHS, NIH, NCI, 1984, 3-11.

Foged E, et al: Histologic changes in liver during etretinate treatment. *J Am Acad Dermatol* 11:580-583, 1984.

Ford GP, et al: Response of seborrhoeic dermatitis to ketoconazole. *Br J Dermatol* 111:603-607, 1984.

Franz TJ: Percutaneous absorption of minoxidil in man. *Arch Dermatol* 121:203-206, 1985.

Fraunfelder FT, et al: Adverse ocular reactions possibly associated with isotretinoin. *Am J Ophthalmol* 100:534-537, 1985.

Friedman SJ, Su WPD: Management of leg ulcers. *Am Fam Physician* 27:219-226, (Feb) 1983.

Galbraith GMP, et al: Open-label trial of immunomodulation therapy with inosiplex (Isoprinosine) in patients with alopecia totalis and cell-mediated immunodeficiency. *J Am Acad Dermatol* 11:224-230, 1984.

Geiger EM, et al: Clinical evaluation of aromatic retinoid, RO 10-1670, in severe psoriasis. *Curr Ther Res* 35:735-740, 1984.

Goodman DS: Vitamin A and retinoids in health and disease. *N Engl J Med* 310:1023-1031, 1984.

Gratton D, et al: Topical clindamycin versus systemic tetracycline in treatment of acne. *J Am Acad Dermatol* 7:50-53, 1982.

Hall RP, et al: Bullous eruption of systemic lupus erythematosus: Dramatic response to dapsone therapy. *Ann Intern Med* 97:165-170, 1982.

Headington JT, Novak E: Clinical and histologic studies of male pattern baldness treated with topical minoxidil. *Curr Ther Res* 36:1098-1106, 1984.

Heel RC, et al: Dextranomer: Review of its general properties and therapeutic efficacy. *Drugs* 18:89-102, 1979.

Henseler T, et al: Oral 8-methoxypsoralen photochemotherapy of psoriasis: European PUVA study; cooperative study among 18 European centres. *Lancet* 1:853-857, 1981.

Hjorth N, Jacobsen M: Coal tar. *Semin Dermatol* 2:281-286, 1983.

Hodge L: Corticosteroid/antibiotic combinations: When should they be used? *Drugs* 19:380-382, 1980.

Hubbell CG, et al: Efficacy of minocycline compared with tetracycline in treatment of acne vulgaris. *Arch Dermatol* 118:989-992, 1982.

James WD, Leyden JJ: Treatment of gram-negative folliculitis with isotretinoin: Positive clinical and microbiologic response. *J Am Acad Dermatol* 12:319-324, 1985.

Juhlin L, et al (eds): Acne symposia. *Acta Derm Venereol* Suppl 89:1-95, 1980.

Kaidbey KH, Kligman AM: Appraisal of efficacy and substantivity of new high-potency sunscreens. *J Am Acad Dermatol* 4:566-570, 1981.

Katz SI, et al: Dermatitis herpetiformis: Skin and gut. *Ann Intern Med* 93:857-874, 1980.

Khoo K-C, et al: Pharmacokinetics of isotretinoin following single oral dose. *J Clin Pharmacol* 22:395-402, 1982.

Klemm-Mayer H, et al: Plasma exchange therapy in psoriasis. *Acta Derm Venereol (Stockh)* Suppl 113:142-144, 1984.

Krause L, Shuster S: Mechanism of action of antipruritic drugs. *Br Med J* 287:1199-1200, 1983.

Kucan JO, et al: Comparison of silver sulfadiazine, povidone-iodine, and physiological saline in treatment of chronic pressure ulcers. *J Am Geriatr Soc* 29:232-235, 1981.

Lammer EJ, et al: Retinoic acid embryopathy. *N Engl J Med* 313:837-841, 1985.

Leyden JJ, Kligman AM: Efficacy of steroid-antibiotic combinations. *Drug Ther* 8:114-120, (Feb) 1978.

Lowe NJ: Psoriasis therapy: Current perspective. *West J Med* 139:184-189, 1983.

Lowe NJ: *Practical Psoriasis Therapy.* Chicago, Year Book Medical Publishers, 1985.

Lowe NJ, Breeding J: Anthralin: Different concentration effects on epidermal cell DNA synthesis rates in mice and clinical responses in human psoriasis. *Arch Dermatol* 117:698-700, 1981.

Lowe NJ, et al: Etretinate therapy for psoriasis inhibits epidermal

ornithine decarboxylase. *J Am Acad Dermatol* 6:697-698, 1982 A.

Lowe NJ, et al: New coal tar extract and coal tar shampoos: Evaluation by epidermal cell DNA synthesis suppression assay. *Arch Dermatol* 118:487-489, 1982 B.

Lowe NJ, et al: Anthralin for psoriasis: Short-contact anthralin therapy compared with topical steroid and conventional anthralin. *J Am Acad Dermatol* 10:69-72, 1984.

Lowy M, et al: Clinical and immunologic response to Isoprinosine in alopecia areata and alopecia universalis: Association with auto-antibodies. *J Am Acad Dermatol* 12:78-84, 1985.

Lucek RW, Colburn WA: Clinical pharmacokinetics of retinoids. *Clin Pharmacokinet* 10:38-62, 1985.

Lynfield YL, Schechter S: Choosing and using a vehicle. *J Am Acad Dermatol* 10:56-59, 1984.

Mahrle G, et al: Oral treatment of keratinizing disorders of skin and mucous membranes with etretinate: Comparative study of 113 patients. *Arch Dermatol* 118:97-100, 1982.

Marks JM: Adverse effects of ultraviolet light therapy. *Adverse Drug React Bull* No 95:348-351, (Aug) 1982.

Marynick SP, et al: Androgen excess in cystic acne. *N Engl J Med* 308:981-986, 1983.

Mathias CGT, et al: Allergic contact photodermatitis to para-aminobenzoic acid. *Arch Dermatol* 114:1665-1666, 1978.

Matsuoka LY: Acne. *J Pediatr* 103:849-854, 1983.

McKay M: Topical dermatologic therapy. *Primary Care* 10:513-524, 1983.

Melotte P, et al: Efficacy of 1% silver sulfadiazine cream in treating bacteriological infection of leg ulcers. *Curr Ther Res* 37:197-202, 1985.

Melski JW, Stern RS: Annual rate of psoralen and ultraviolet-A treatment of psoriasis after initial clearing. *Arch Dermatol* 118:404-411, 1982.

Menkes A, et al: Psoriasis treatment with suberythemogenic ultraviolet B radiation and coal tar extract. *J Am Acad Dermatol* 12:21-25, 1985.

Milstone ER, et al: Pseudomembranous colitis after topical application of clindamycin. *Arch Dermatol* 117:154-155, 1981.

Mitchell AJ, Krull EA: Alopecia areata: Pathogenesis and treatment. *J Am Acad Dermatol* 11:763-775, 1984.

Morison WL, et al: Abnormal lymphocyte function following long-term PUVA therapy for psoriasis. *Br J Dermatol* 108:445-450, 1983.

Moy RL, et al: Isotretinoin vs etretinate therapy in generalized pustular and chronic psoriasis. *Arch Dermatol* 121:1297-1301, 1985.

Muller SA, Perry HO: Goeckerman treatment in psoriasis: Six decades of experience at Mayo Clinic. *Cutis* 34:265-269, 1984.

Olsen EA, et al: Topical minoxidil in early male pattern baldness. *J Am Acad Dermatol* 13:185-192, 1985.

Padilla RS, et al: Topical tetracycline hydrochloride vs topical clinda-mycin phosphate in treatment of acne: Comparative study. *Int J Dermatol* 20:445-448, 1981.

Parish LC, Witkowski JA: Decubitus ulcers: How to intervene effective-ly. *Drug Ther* 13:225-231, (May) 1983.

Parish LC, et al: Topical corticosteroids. *Int J Dermatol* 24:435-436, 1985.

Pathak MA: Sunscreens: Topical and systemic approaches for protec-tion of human skin against harmful effects of solar radiation. *J Am Acad Dermatol* 7:285-312, 1982.

Pathak MA, et al: Safety and effectiveness of 8-methoxypsoralen, 4,5′,8-trimethylpsoralen, and psoralen in vitiligo, in Pathak MA, Dunnick JK (eds): *Photobiologic, Toxicologic and Pharmacologic Aspects of Psoralens*, (monograph 66). Bethesda, MD, USPHS, NIH, NCI, 1984, 165-174.

Pathak MA, et al: Principles of photoprotection in sunburn and suntanning, and topical and systemic photo-protection in health and diseases: Sunscreens. *J Dermatol Surg Oncol* 11:575-579, 1985.

Peck GL: Retinoids: Therapeutic use in dermatology. *Drugs* 24:341-351, 1982.

Pollat PA (ed): Use and misuse of topical steroids. *Fam Med Rep* 2:173-179, (Summer/Fall) 1984.

Powell FC, et al: Treatment of parapsoriasis and mycosis fungoides:

Role of psoralen and long-wave ultraviolet light A (PUVA). *Mayo Clin Proc* 59:538-546, 1984.

Robertson DB, Maibach HI: Topical corticosteroids. *Semin Dermatol* 2:238-249, 1983.

Roelandts R: Mutagenicity and carcinogenicity of methoxsalen plus UV-A. *Arch Dermatol* 120:662-669, 1984.

Roenigk HH Jr: Medical and surgical management of leg ulcers. *Primary Care* 10:411-427, 1983.

Roenigk HH Jr: Leg ulcers, in Provost TT, Farmer ER: *Current Therapy in Dermatology, 1985-1986*. Philadelphia, BC Decker, 1985, 250-253.

Roenigk HH Jr, Maibach HI: Methotrexate. *Semin Dermatol* 2:231-237, 1983.

Roenigk HH Jr, Maibach HI: *Psoriasis*. New York, Marcel Dekker, 1985 A.

Roenigk HH Jr, Maibach HI (eds): Psoriasis. *Semin Dermatol* 4:271-326, 1985 B.

Roenigk HH Jr, et al: Methotrexate guidelines: Revised. *J Am Acad Dermatol* 6:145-155, 1982.

Rosen T, Waisman M: Topically administered clindamycin in treatment of acne vulgaris and other dermatologic disorders. *Pharmacotherapy* 1:201-205, 1981.

Rumsfield JA, et al: Isotretinoin in severe recalcitrant cystic acne: Review. *Drug Intell Clin Pharm* 17:329-333, 1983.

Sayre RM, et al: Performance of six sunscreen formulations on human skin: Comparison. *Arch Dermatol* 115:46-49, 1979.

Schaefer H: Short-contact therapy, (editorial). *Arch Dermatol* 121:1505-1509, 1985.

Seiler WO, Stähelin HB: Decubitus ulcers: Preventive techniques for elderly patients. *Geriatrics* 40:53-60, 1985 A.

Seiler WO, Stähelin HB: Decubitus ulcers: Treatment through five therapeutic principles. *Geriatrics* 40:30-44, 1985 B.

Shalita AR: New advances in treatment of acne. *Res Staff Physician* 30:75-82, (Jan) 1984.

Skinner RB Jr, et al: Double-blind treatment of seborrheic dermatitis with 2% ketoconazole cream. *J Am Acad Dermatol* 12:852-856, 1985.

Spielvogel RL, et al: Oral isotretinoin therapy for familial Muir-Torre syndrome. *J Am Acad Dermatol* 12:475-480, 1985.

Stendahl O, et al: Inhibition of polymorphonuclear leukocyte cytotoxicity by dapsone: Possible mechanism in treatment of dermatitis herpetiformis. *J Clin Invest* 61:214-220, 1978.

Stern RS, Melski JW: Long-term continuation of psoralen and ultraviolet-A treatment of psoriasis. *Arch Dermatol* 118:400-403, 1982.

Stern RS, et al: Topical versus systemic agent treatment for papulopustular acne: Cost-effectiveness analysis. *Arch Dermatol* 120:1571-1578, 1984 A.

Stern RS, et al: Cutaneous squamous-cell carcinoma in patients treated with PUVA. *N Engl J Med* 310:1156-1161, 1984 B.

Stoughton RB, Cornell RC: Topical corticosteroids in psoriasis, in Roenigk HH Jr, Maibach HI (eds): *Psoriasis*. New York, Marcel Dekker, 1985, 337-352.

Stoughton RB, et al: Double-blind comparison of topical 1% clindamycin phosphate (Cleocin) and oral tetracycline 500 mg/day in treatment of acne vulgaris. *Cutis* 26:424-429, 1980.

Strauss JS, et al: Isotretinoin therapy for acne: Results of multicenter dose-response study. *J Am Acad Dermatol* 10:490-496, 1984.

Tan PL, et al: Current topical corticosteroid preparations. *J Am Acad Dermatol* 14:79-93, 1986.

Todes-Taylor N, et al: Occurrence of vitiligo after psoralens and ultraviolet A therapy. *J Am Acad Dermatol* 9:526-532, 1983.

Trancik RJ, Maibach HI: Propylene glycol: Irritation or sensitization? *Contact Dermatitis* 8:185-189, 1982.

Tsambaos D, Orfanos CE: Antipsoriatic activity of new synthetic retinoid: Arotinoid RO 13-6298. *Arch Dermatol* 119:746-751, 1983.

Vahlquist C, et al: Sequential comparison of etretinate (Tigason) and isotretinoin (Roaccutane) with special regard to their effects on serum lipoproteins. *Br J Dermatol* 112:69-76, 1985.

Voorhees JJ: Leukotrienes and other lipoxygenase products in pathogenesis and therapy of psoriasis and other dermatoses, (editorial). *Arch Dermatol* 119:541-547, 1983.

Ward A, et al: Etretinate: Review of its pharmacological properties and therapeutic efficacy in psoriasis and other skin disorders. *Drugs* 26:9-43, 1983.

Ward A, et al: Isotretinoin: Review of its pharmacological properties and therapeutic efficacy in acne and other skin disorders. *Drugs* 28:6-37, 1984.

Weiss VC, West DP: Topical minoxidil therapy and hair regrowth, (editorial). *Arch Dermatol* 121:191-192, 1985.

Weiss VC, et al: Alopecia areata treated with topical minoxidil. *Arch Dermatol* 120:457-463, 1984.

Weiss VC, et al: Topical minoxidil dose response effect in alopecia areata. *Arch Dermatol*, (in press).

Whittier FC, et al: Peritoneal dialysis for psoriasis: Controlled study. *Ann Intern Med* 99:165-168, 1983.

Wilson DG (ed): Advances in management of acne in general practice and in hospital. *J R Soc Med* 78(suppl 10):1-31, 1985.

Wolska H, et al: Etretinate in severe psoriasis. *J Am Acad Dermatol* 9:883-889, 1983.

Yeung D, et al: Benzoyl peroxide: Percutaneous penetration and metabolic disposition. II. Effect of concentration. *J Am Acad Dermatol* 9:920-924, 1983.

Zackheim HS: Should therapeutic coal-tar preparations be available over-the-counter? (letter). *Arch Dermatol* 114:125-126, 1978.

Other Selected References

Handbook of Nonprescription Drugs, ed 7. Washington, DC, American Pharmaceutical Association, 1982.

Arndt KA: *Manual of Dermatologic Therapeutics with Essentials of Diagnosis*, ed 3. Boston, Little, Brown and Company, 1983.

Bickers DR, et al: *Clinical Pharmacology of Skin Disease*. New York, Churchill Livingstone, 1984, 1-321.

Fitzpatrick TB, et al (eds): *Dermatology in General Medicine*, ed 3. New York, McGraw-Hill, 1982.

Marzulli FN, Maibach HI (eds): *Dermatotoxicology*. New York, Hemisphere Press, 1983.

Moschella SL, Hurley HJ (eds): *Dermatology, Vol I & II*, ed 2. Philadelphia, WB Saunders, 1985.

Provost TT, Farmer ER: *Current Therapy in Dermatology, 1985-1986*. Philadelphia, BC Decker, 1985.

INTRODUCTION

ANTIGENS

ANTIBODIES

CELLS PARTICIPATING IN THE IMMUNE RESPONSE

CELL COLLABORATION IN THE IMMUNE RESPONSE

During the past 15 years, there has been a considerable increase in the understanding of the mechanisms involved in the activation and regulation of the immune system in humans. There has been a virtual explosion of technologic advances in cell hybridization and cloning, production of monoclonal antibodies, immunochemistry, immunogenetics, and recombinant DNA technology that has allowed extremely sophisticated approaches to understanding the immune response.

This chapter presents an overview of the immune response to provide background information to guide the physician's use of immunoreactive drugs. The reader is encouraged to seek further information on immunology, especially in those areas not covered in this chapter, by referring to the numerous immunologic textbooks that are available, such as those listed in the references.

Several features characterize the immune response. The cardinal feature is the specificity of the response in which the system can recognize very fine differences between closely related antigens. The normal immune system can distinguish between materials that are self or non-self (foreign); only rarely does the system react to constituent materials of the body (autoimmunity).

The immune system consists of a number of lymphoid organs (thymus, lymph nodes, spleen, and tonsils), aggregates of lymphoid tissue in nonlymphoid organs (eg, Peyer's patches in the gut), and lymphoid cells dispersed in the bone marrow, blood, and connective and epithelial tissues. The immune response involves the cooperative interaction between phagocytic cells, regulatory lymphocytes (T-helper and T-suppressor cells), effector lymphocytes (cytocidal T-cells, antibody-producing B-cells), and other effector cells (eg, mast cells). Antigen stimulation causes proliferation of both T- and B-lymphocytes in response to the production of growth factors (interleukin-2, B-cell growth factor). The immune system's memory allows subsequent exposure to the inciting antigen to evoke more rapid proliferation of affected lymphocytes and enhanced, earlier production of antibody. The immune response can be enhanced by substances such as adjuvants

and certain immunomodulators or depressed by other immunomodulators or even abrogated by the induction of tolerance (see Chapter 63, Immunomodulators). A subset of T-lymphocytes, T-suppressor (Ts) cells, serves a normal regulatory function in inhibiting antibody production and the activity of effector T-lymphocytes, while other regulatory lymphocytes, the T-helper (Th) cells, assist in promoting these same functions. Finally, the immune response is controlled by genes of the major histocompatibility complex, which determine the ability to respond to an antigen. Deletion of an immune response (Ir) gene can lead to an immunodeficiency disease in any of the arms of the immune system.

Thus, the immune system is an intricate network capable of exerting multiple effects varying from protection against an invading pathogen or destruction of cancer cells to an attack upon normal constituent cells of the body.

ANTIGENS

The term, antigen, has been operationally defined as a substance capable of stimulating the production of antibody that will react with the inducing substance in a specific and demonstrable manner. However, this definition is incomplete since antigens also may provoke a cellular response, such as delayed hypersensitivity and tolerance. In a broader sense, antigens are substances capable of inducing an immune response that includes lymphoid cell proliferation and synthesis of recognition molecules (antibodies or cellular receptors) that can be shown to combine specifically with the inducing antigen. The term, *immunogen*, may be preferred, for it may better convey the concept of a substance giving rise to an immune response.

Antigens comprise a structurally diverse group consisting of proteins, polysaccharides, lipids, and nucleic acids. Their molecular weight varies from less than a thousand to several million daltons. Although a molecular size threshold for immunogenicity has not been established, in general the larger the molecule, the greater its immunogenicity. This has been attributed to the increased chemical complexity of larger molecules and, consequently, the increased likelihood of the presence of different antigenic determinants (epitopes). (An epitope is the smallest antigen structural unit that is recognized by antibody; the antigenic pattern is the largest structure recognized by a given antibody population.) Four general types of antigens are recognized: (1) haptens, (2) natural immunogens, (3) artificial immunogens obtained by modification of natural ones, and (4) synthetic immunogens, such as amino acid polymers composed of one, two, or three different amino acids.

Haptens are small molecules that are capable of combining with antibody molecules but are unable to stimulate an immune response unless they are coupled to a carrier immunogenic molecule. The carrier molecule is usually a protein or synthetic polypeptide. An example of a hapten is 2,4-dinitrophenol (DNP), which when conjugated to bovine gamma globulin is capable of inducing antibodies against itself when injected into a suitable animal, such as a rabbit.

To be immunogenic, a hapten need not be linked covalently to the carrier; several highly immunogenic haptens are bound to the carrier by charge interactions. Many immunologic drug reactions are due to the fact that the offending drug behaves as a hapten by binding to host protein; an example is the binding of penicillin to serum protein, which then stimulates an immune response to penicillin. Upon subsequent exposure to the same molecule, a hypersensitivity reaction occurs. In many contact hypersensitivities (poison ivy, oak and sumac, metals, etc), the sensitizing antigen is a hapten that becomes conjugated to skin protein. Injection of a hapten-protein conjugate produces antibodies with different specificities: those directed toward the hapten, those directed toward the carrier protein, and, occasionally, those directed to the region of contact between the hapten and the carrier protein ("anti-link" antibodies).

Several factors determine the immunogenicity of a molecule. These factors include foreignness, chemical composition and complexity, genetic constitution of the responding animal, dose and route of administration, immunization schedule, use of adjuvants, and the availability and functional status of helper T-lymphocytes, which recognize determinants on the antigen. Foreignness of the antigen is of major importance for the host species. Substances that are most foreign are most likely to stimulate a strong immune response since a larger number of distinct epitopes would be recognized. The occurrence of autoimmunity indicates that lymphocytes bearing receptors for self-antigens, as well as those with receptors for foreign antigens, are present in the host.

The nature of the antigen has an important influence on the method of immunization employed. Particulate antigens —bacteria, viruses, erythrocytes—readily elicit an antibody response after intravenous or intracutaneous administration at many different doses. In contrast, many soluble proteins and carbohydrates require more intense immunization and adjuvants may be necessary to enhance the response. In general, conditions that favor increased phagocytosis of antigen or increase the inflammatory response enhance immunogenicity.

Most antigens require T-lymphocyte participation before an antibody or cell-mediated response can be produced. These are referred to as T-dependent (thymus dependent) antigens and include heterologous serum proteins and erythrocytes and synthetic polypeptides of L-amino acids. T-independent antigens do not require direct T-cell participation to produce an antibody and appear to stimulate B-lymphocytes (antibody-producing cells) directly. These antigens include endotoxin, lipopolysaccharides (LPS), pneumococcal polysaccharides, and certain synthetic antigens, such as polyvinyl pyrrolidone and polymers of D-amino acids. Many T-independent antigens have a characteristic structure consisting of repeating units and are degraded slowly. The antibody response to T-independent antigens is principally or exclusively of the IgM class and shows poor immunological memory. Moreover, these antigens are often polyclonal activators of B-lymphocytes, ie, they nonspecifically stimulate large numbers of B-cells to multiply and differentiate into antibody-producing cells. LPS is such a B-cell mitogen: large doses stimulate the proliferation and differentiation of many sets of B-cells that produce the types of antibody that they were genetically committed to produce regardless of the nature of the stimulus. However, at limiting doses, LPS binds preferentially to B-cells possessing specific receptors and, consequently, the antibody produced is primarily anti-LPS.

Ultimately, injected protein antigen is catabolized by the usual pathways and eliminated as amino acids or small peptides.

ANTIBODIES

Antibodies are immunoglobulin glycoproteins that combine specifically with antigens. Most of these proteins migrate as gamma globulins during electrophoresis. All immunoglobulins have a common structure consisting of two light (L) polypeptide chains and two heavy (H) polypeptide chains arranged as shown in the Figure. Five classes of human immunoglobulin have been identified: IgG, IgA, IgM, IgD, and IgE. These classes are distinguished on the basis of the structure of their H chain known, respectively, as γ, α, μ, δ, and ϵ. There are only two types of L chains, kappa (κ) and lambda (λ). These

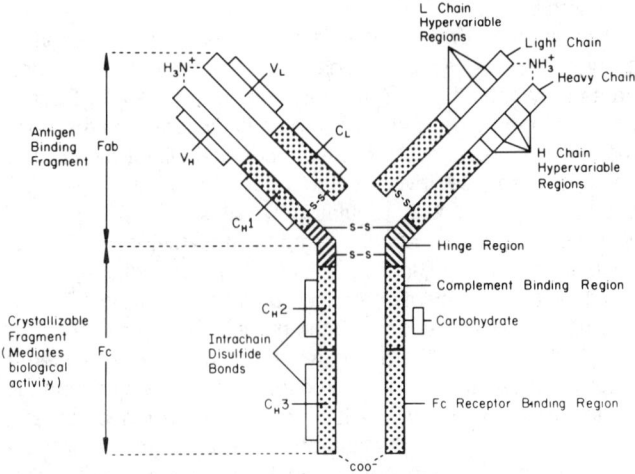

Schematic representation of the human IgG molecule

are bound to the heavy chains through disulfide (S-S) linkages; the H chains are bound to each other through two S-S bridges.

Most of our knowledge concerning immunoglobulin structure and function comes from studies on IgG. The proteolytic enzyme, papain, splits the IgG molecule at the hinge region into three fragments, two of the fragments are similar and bind antigen (fragment antigen binding or Fab). The Fab portion consists of both light chains and their neighboring H chain linked through S-S bridges. The third portion does not combine with antigen but is readily crystalizable and hence is known as the Fc fragment. The Fc portion contains the regions responsible for binding to cells, fixing complement, and traversing the placenta. The Fc fragment accounts for approximately one-third of the IgG molecule, and the Fab fragment for approximately two-thirds.

Both L and H chains contain regions at the carboxy terminus in which the amino acid sequences are identical and hence are referred to as the *constant* or "C" region (C_L or C_H, respectively), and the amino terminus contains a region in which the sequence is variable and thus is known as the variable or V region (V_L or V_H, respectively). The C_H segment consists of three approximately equal regions referred to as C_H1, C_H2, and C_H3. The C_H1 portion is separated from the other C_H portions by the hinge region. Intrachain disulfide bonds are present in both the V and C regions of the IgG molecule. Carbohydrate is bound to the C_H2 region, which also binds complement.

Some positions in the V region show great variability in sequence composition and are known as *hypervariable* regions. There are three hypervariable regions in the V_L segment and four in the V_H segment. The residues between hypervariable regions are known as "framework" residues. The V_H and V_L regions contain the antigen-binding cleft within the Fab portion of the antibody molecule. Further, the folding of the V_H and V_L regions brings the hypervariable regions into close proximity forming a structure complementary to an epitope. The framework residues serve to maintain the hypervariable regions in appropriate alignment in the antigen-binding site. Changes in the hypervariable regions are responsible for the great number of specific antigen-binding sites necessary to handle the vast diversity of antigen determinants.

IgG is the principal immunoglobulin in human serum. This monomer is the predominant antibody type found after antigenic challenge. The fetus does not produce IgG, but this immunoglobulin readily crosses the placenta and maternal IgG can be found in the fetus and newborn. There are four subclasses of IgG based on differences in the heavy chains —$\gamma1$, $\gamma2$, $\gamma3$, $\gamma4$. All four subclasses are proportionally represented in the antibody response to some antigens; however, certain antigens may induce primarily one of the subclasses. Antibodies to carbohydrates tend to be IgG_2, while anti-DNA antibodies are primarily IgG_1 and IgG_3. IgG_3 has the lowest synthetic and highest catabolic rate and the shortest serum half-life of any of the subclasses. Various biological and physical properties of IgG are shown in Tables 1 and 2.

IgA exists as a monomer and as a dimer. It is the main immunoglobulin in secretions, where it exists as a dimer. The dimer is held together by a polypeptide-joining chain (J-chain) and disulfide bridges. In addition, the dimer in secretions (saliva, tears, intestinal fluid) contains a polypeptide chain called the secretory component (SC) or piece. The SC appears to protect dimeric IgA from proteolytic digestion by gastrointestinal enzymes. It is produced by local serous-type secretory epithelial cells and is present on the surface membrane of these cells; this has led to speculation that SC may be a receptor for dimeric IgA. Passage through or between these cells allows the SC piece to be added, and its addition to dimeric IgA is thought to allow the molecules to cross the mucosal epithelium by exocytosis (reverse pinocytosis). Thus, the production of secretory IgA is considered unusual because it involves the cooperation of two different types of cells, antibody-secreting plasma cells and serous epithelial cells. There are two subclasses of IgA, IgA_1 and IgA_2, based on differences in the heavy α chain. The IgA_2 molecules are further subclassified based on genetic markers into two subcategories A2m(1) and A2m(2).

IgM is the largest immunoglobulin (molecular weight, 890,000) and is a pentamer consisting of five identical subunits that contain two κ or λ light chains and two heavy μ chains. The five monomeric subunits are held together in a circle by S-S bonds between the heavy chains. In addition, IgM contains a J chain similar to that in dimeric IgA, which aids in holding the molecule together. IgM is highly efficient in fixing complement and is much more effective than IgG in agglutinating erythrocytes and bacteria and in bactericidal reactions. Monomeric IgM is present on the surfaces of B-cells where it is thought to act as an antigen receptor. After an initial lag phase, IgM is the first antibody to appear following the primary antigen dose. It usually reaches a peak at seven days. At this time, IgG antibody is detected and generally reaches maximal titers in 10 to 14 days. During the period in which IgG titers are rising, IgM titers fall and little can be detected four to five weeks after the primary antigen dose. In the secondary response (anamnestic or booster response), both IgM and IgG titers rise exponentially, but only the IgG response is significantly greater and longer lasting; IgM titers are the same as or only slightly higher than in the primary response. IgM-producing cells become poor memory cells, and a second antigen challenge does not produce a typical anamnestic response. Thus, the presence of IgM is useful in establishing whether an infection is of recent origin. There is evidence that IgG- or IgA-bearing lymphocytes develop sequentially from IgM- or IgM/IgD-bearing precursor lymphocytes.

IgD is a monomer consisting of two Δ heavy chains and two κ or two λ light chains. It is a minor component of serum immunoglobulins, and the rate of synthesis is approximately 100 times less than that of IgG. IgD also has a high catabolic rate and its plasma half-life is only three days. IgD does not fix complement or sensitize skin. Most umbilical cord and adult B-cells have IgD on their surface and it has been suggested that IgD may be an early antigen cell receptor.

IgE is a large monomer (molecular weight, 185,000) consisting of two heavy ϵ chains and two κ or λ light chains. Its serum concentration is very low and it has the shortest plasma half-life, the lowest rate of synthesis, and the highest catabolic rate of all the immunoglobulin classes. IgE plays a cardinal role in immediate hypersensitivity. It binds strongly through its Fc portion to receptors on mast cells and basophils. Antigen

TABLE 1.
PROPERTIES OF THE FOUR HUMAN IgG SUBCLASSES

Property	IgG_1	IgG_2	IgG_3	IgG_4
Percent total IgG	65-70	23-28	4-8	3-4
Placental transfer	+	+	+	+
Complement fixation (C_{1q})	+	+	+	−
IgE blocking	−	−	−	+
Heterologous skin fixation	+	−	+	−
Binding to Fc receptors on:				
neutrophils	+	+	+	+
monocytes	+	−	+	−
Antibody-dependent cytotoxic cells	+	+	+	−
Bacterial antibodies	+	+	+	+
Rh antibodies	+	−	+	−
Blood group A antibodies	+	+	+	+
Factor VIII antibodies	−	−	−	+
DNA antibodies	+	−	+	−

(allergen) then interacts with two adjacent IgE molecules to form an antigen bridge. This causes local membrane changes that result in the release of mediators (histamine, slow reacting substance of anaphylaxis, and eosinophilic chemotactic factor) that trigger immediate hypersensitivity reactions. Levels of allergen-specific IgE are elevated in atopic individuals. It has been speculated that IgE may have a protective role against parasites, but no conclusive data has been presented.

Immunoglobulin molecules themselves are antigenic, which can be demonstrated by injecting them into different animal species or into individuals of the same species with a different genetic background. Three different types of antigenic determinants have been demonstrated on immunoglobulins: *isotypic, allotypic,* and *idiotypic.*

Isotypic determinants occur on all heavy and light chains. For example, antiserum directed toward the isotypic determinants of the γ heavy chain of human IgG will recognize all normal human IgG molecules.

Allotypic determinants are antigenic determinants present on heavy and light chains of only certain individuals and are inherited according to Mendelian laws. Allotypic determinants have been demonstrated on the γ heavy chain of IgG, the α heavy chain of IgA, the μ heavy chain of IgM, and the κ and λ light chains. About 20 allotypic determinants (called Gm markers) have been found on the γ heavy chains, chiefly on the Fc portion. κ light chains contain a set of three allotypic markers referred to as Inv 1, Inv 2, and Inv 3. Each IgG subclass has its own allotypic markers that are controlled by codominant alleles.

Idiotypic determinants are localized on the variable portion of light and heavy chains and arise as a result of the unique configuration of the amino acid sequences constituting the antigen combining site of an antibody. Idiotypic determinants may be located on either the V_H or V_L chain, but generally both polypeptide chains contribute to their formation. There are two functional categories of these determinants: those that are related to the antigen-combining site and those that are not (called framework determinants).

Anti-idiotypic antibodies directed toward the antigen-combining site have a three-dimensional structure resembling the inciting antigen, ie, they are an "internal image" of the antigen. They are considered to be an important mechanism for controlling the immune response and form the basis for a network theory of regulating the immune response (Jerne, 1974). In this theory, the immune system is viewed as a network of V domains based on the interactions between idiotypes and anti-idiotypes. Idiotypes on antibody molecules and lymphocyte antigen receptors are the chief components of this network. Prior to antigen administration, the system is in a state of dynamic equilibrium mediated by idiotype/anti-idiotype interactions. The administration of antigen disturbs this equilibrium and specific antibody is produced. Idiotypic determinants on the antibody molecule induce the synthesis of anti-idiotypic antibodies in the same individual. The latter inhibit the proliferation of clones of B-cells and T-cells initially stimulated by antigen, thus terminating the initial immune response.

There are many reports in the literature that support the concept of idiotypic networks regulating the immune response. For example, following booster immunization with tetanus toxoid, anti-idiotype-bearing cells have been detected, as has as auto-anti-idiotypic antibody; the latter was found to inhibit the synthesis of tetanus toxoid antibody (Geha, 1983).

Since anti-idiotypic antibody directed to the antigen combining site of the antibody molecule forms the internal image of the antigen, it is possible to utilize this category of anti-idiotypic antibody for antigen mimicry. Such an antibody should produce the same type of antibody engendered by the injection of antigen. This is the theoretical basis for the use of anti-idiotypic

TABLE 2.
PROPERTIES OF THE FIVE CLASSES OF HUMAN ANTIBODIES

Property	IgG	IgA	IgM	IgD	IgE
Molecular weight	160,000	170,000-340,000	890,000	170,000-200,000	185,000
Serum concentration (mg%)	1,250	280	120	0.3-30	0.002-0.2
Plasma half-life (days)	23	6	5	3	2
Percent carbohydrate	3	8	12	12	12
Heavy chain	γ	α	μ	δ	ϵ
Heavy chain subgroup	$\gamma1, \gamma2, \gamma3, \gamma4$	α_1, α_2	μ_1, μ_2	—	—
Light chain	κ or λ	κ or λ	κ or λ	κ or λ	κ or λ
J chain	None	+ (dimeric) − (monomeric)	+	None	None
Found in	serum, amniotic fluid	serum, secretions, colostrum, saliva, tears, GI tract	serum	serum	serum
Placental transfer	+	−	−	−	−
Complement fixing	+	−	+	−	−
Beneficial activities	Toxin neutralizing, agglutinating, opsonizing, bacteriolytic with complement	Toxin neutralizing, agglutinating, ?opsonizing	Toxin neutralizing, agglutinating, bacteriolytic with complement, antigen receptor on B lymphocytes	Antigen receptor on B lymphocytes	Mediate changes in vascular permeability
Injurious activities	Antigen-antibody complexes can cause tissue injury, eg, Arthus reaction, serum sickness	?	Antigen-antibody complexes can cause tissue injury, eg, Arthus reaction, serum sickness	?	Local and systemic immediate hypersensitivity or anaphylactic reactions

antibody as a mimic antigen for a vaccine; it is an alternative means of inducing immunity without ever exposing the host to the antigens of an infectious agent. Several investigational anti-idiotypic vaccines have been produced; for example, poliovirus neutralizing antibody has been induced in mice using monoclonal anti-idiotypic antibody (Uytdehaag and Osterhaus, 1985). Studies are in progress to develop an anti-idiotypic vaccine for HTLV-III, the etiologic agent of the acquired immunodeficiency syndrome (AIDS).

CELLS PARTICIPATING IN THE IMMUNE RESPONSE

A number of different types of cells participate in the immune response. Lymphocytes are the major group. These cells have receptor molecules on their surface that enable them to recognize and bind antigen. After interaction with antigen, the lymphocytes are activated and carry out various effector functions. Other cells that also play important roles in the immune response include monocytes, macrophages, poly-

morphonuclear leukocytes, and granulocytes. These cells carry out crucial effector functions such as phagocytosis, increasing vascular permeability, and/or processing antigen during immune induction. Polymorphonuclear leukocytes, eosinophils, basophils, and mast cells take part in the antibody-mediated inflammatory response. Phagocytic monocytes participate both as auxiliary cells during immune induction and as effector cells in cell-mediated immune reactions.

The lymphocytes are in a highly dynamic state and about 50% recirculate in blood and lymph. The remainder are the principal cells of lymphoid tissues (thymus, lymph nodes, and spleen) or are important constituents of certain nonlymphoid tissues (eg, the respiratory and gastrointestinal tract), thus forming a diffuse lymphoid component. In mammals, the primary lymphoid organ is the thymus where antigen-independent differentiation of lymphocytes takes place, (ie, where mature T- and B-cells are generated from stem cells). The lymph nodes and spleen are secondary lymphoid organs in which mature B- and T-cells and phagocytes (antigen-trapping cells) are found in large numbers; in these organs, antigen is concentrated, cell division is antigen driven, and specific immune responses are generated.

TABLE 3.
SURFACE ANTIGENS ASSOCIATED WITH HUMAN T CELL DIFFERENTIATION AND FUNCTION

Antigens*	Molecular Weight	Percent Positive		Comments
		Thymocytes	Peripheral T Cells	
T11	55,000	95	100	Associated with sheep red blood cell rosette receptor
T10	37,000	95	5	Present on early stem cells, some B cells, activated peripheral T cells
T9	190,000	10	0	Transferrin receptor, present on activated T cells
T8	32,000 43,000	80	35	Present on cytotoxic/suppressor cells
T6	44,000	70	0	Equivalent to murine TL antigen
T4	60,000	75	65	Present on helper/inducer T cells
T3	20,000 23,000 26,000	20	100	Associated with the T cell receptor for antigen
T1	67,000	95	100	Equivalent to murine Thy 1 antigen

*Identified with monoclonal antibodies
Adapted from Stobo, 1984

There are two major categories of lymphocytes: B-cells (referring to the avian bursa of Fabricus or bone marrow in mammals) and T-cells (referring to the thymus). B-cells are the precursors of antibody-forming cells (plasma cells) and are derived from bone marrow stem cells by an antigen-independent maturation process in the bone marrow. T-cells are derived from the thymus also by an antigen-independent maturation process and are responsible for various cell-mediated reactions and important regulatory functions.

In the thymus, maturation of T-cells is marked by the appearance of cell surface antigens (T-antigens) that enable the cells to respond to an antigen, ie, they become immuno-competent (see Table 3). Thymic hormones play an important role in the T-cell maturation process (see Chapter 63, Immuno-modulators). Another important marker of T-cell differentiation is the enzyme, terminal deoxynucleotidyl transferase, which adds mononucleotides to DNA segments in the absence of template and is considered to be important for the generation of immunologic diversity. It is found in prothymocytes, immature thymocytes, and some bone marrow cells but is absent in mature T-cells. After maturation in the thymus, the lymphocytes enter the bloodstream and migrate to the peripheral lymphoid system (ie, lymph nodes, spleen, Peyer's patches, tonsils, appendix). There is evidence to suggest that the "homing in" of lymphocytes to lymphoid tissues is guided by specific antigens ("homing" antigens) present on lymphocytes.

In secondary lymphoid organs, B- and T-lymphocytes and phagocytic cells (macrophages) are compartmentalized. In the lymph node, for example, T-lymphocytes are found principally in the paracortical areas, whereas B-lymphocytes are found in and around germinal centers in the cortex. Plasma cells occur principally in the medulla, whereas macrophages are distribut-ed throughout the node. Lymphocytes enter the lymph node via afferent lymphatics, move through the sinuses, and leave via efferent lymphatics. More than 50 times as many lymphocytes leave the node as enter it. Less than 5% of the lymphocytes are derived from precursors in the lymph node; the majority come from the bloodstream, thus underscoring the importance of lymphocyte recirculation. Most recirculating lymphocytes are long-lived T-cells, but a few B-cells also come from the bloodstream. Most of the B-cells in the node are found in the germinal centers of the peripheral cortex.

Lymphocyte circulation consists of three major types. The first is the seeding of stem cells from the fetal liver or bone marrow to primary lymphoid organs, followed by distribution of differentiated cells to the peripheral lymphoid system. Recirculation of lymphocytes from blood to lymph to blood is the second type. This occurs very rapidly and does not involve cell proliferation. Average transit times for long-lived T-cells is about 0.6 hours in the blood, 5 to 6 hours in the spleen, and 15 to 20 hours in the lymph nodes. The transit time for B-lymphocytes is longer, (eg, 30 hours in lymph nodes). Cortico-steroids markedly alter lymphocyte traffic and thus produce a leukopenia (see Chapter 63).

B-Lymphocytes: B-lymphocytes produce immunoglobulin and have this class of molecule on their cell surface; they constitute 5% to 15% of peripheral blood lymphocytes. Most B-cells have both monomeric IgM and IgD on the cell surface; about 25% have only IgM or IgD, and only 1% have IgG or IgA. These surface immunoglobulins act as antigen receptors: B-cells bearing these specific antigen receptors are present prior to antigen challenge. These cells are committed to the synthesis of uniquely specific antibodies and develop during normal cell differentiation. Antigen binds to cells bearing specific receptors for it. Antigen binding to the receptors stimulates specific lymphocytic clones to proliferate and further differentiate into plasma cells and long-lived memory cells. The plasma cell is the end stage of the antigen-driven differentiation process and does not divide. It actively secretes more than 90% of the immunoglobulin molecules it synthesizes, but very little of these molecules are found on its membrane. The plasma cell has a half-life of only two or three days.

Immunologic responses by B-cells usually require cooperative interaction with T-cells. However, a certain class of antigens, called thymus (T)-independent antigens, may stimulate a restricted response by acting directly on B-cells and does not require collaboration between T-cells and B-cells.

Immature B-cells have membrane-bound IgM and, as they develop, express IgD also. Following antigen stimulation, there is often a switch in the heavy chain isotype expressed, which may be sequential (from IgM to IgG_3 to IgG_1, etc) or direct (from IgM to any other heavy chain isotype). Evidence suggests that the latter is most common. The mechanism underlying isotype switching is not clear. These changes are also seen in the plasma cells that develop from B-cells.

T-Lymphocytes: The two major categories of T-cells are effector T-lymphocytes and regulatory T-lymphocytes. Effector T-lymphocytes are responsible for cell-mediated immune reactions, such as delayed hypersensitivity reactions, allograft rejection, graft-versus-host reactions, and the elimination of tumor cells and virus-infected cells. Cytotoxic T-lymphocytes ("killer" cells) have the capacity to kill other cells and express the T_8 phenotype. Effector cells involved in delayed hypersensitivity carry the T_4 phenotype (see Table 4). Regulatory T-lymphocytes modulate the immune response by amplification (helper cells) or suppression (suppressor cells) of B-lymphocytes or other T-lymphocytes (eg, cytotoxic T-cells). T-helper cells carry the T_4 antigen and aid immunoglobulin synthesis by B-cells and cytotoxic activity by other T-cells. A subset of this group, T-inducer cells, also carries the T_4 antigen and induces the activity of suppressor T-cells. T-suppressor cells carry the T_8 antigen and decrease the immune response of both B- and T-cells and suppress the T-helper cell response. T-helper and T-suppressor cells interact in complex ways to modulate the immune response by secreting regulatory proteins (lymphokines) or by direct contact with the participating cells.

T-cells do not recognize free circulating antigen and respond only to antigen on a cell surface. T-cell antigen receptors only recognize antigen in conjunction with autologous antigens of the major histocompatibility complex (MHC). T_4 cells require MHC class II molecules, whereas T_8 cells require MHC class I molecules. For an immune response to occur, the antigen receptor on a T-cell must simultaneously recognize the antigen and the MHC molecule. This phenomenon is known as MHC restriction.

The receptor for antigen on T-cells consists of five distinct proteins known as the T_3 complex. This complex is present on all mature peripheral T cells and on medullary thymocytes. Monoclonal antibodies to T_3 inhibit antigen-induced proliferation of all T-lymphocytes. The antigen recognizing portion of this complex contains two glycosylated polypeptide chains, α and β, which are linked by disulfide bonds to form a heterodimer. Both the α and β chains contain constant and variable portions that are analogous to those on immunoglobulin molecules. Most evidence suggests that T cells recognize both foreign antigen and MHC molecules with a single receptor rather than having a separate receptor for each. Studies using haptens have demonstrated that T- and B-cells recognize different parts of an antigen.

Null Cells: A small proportion of lymphocytes bear neither T- nor B-cell surface markers and have been called "null" cells. Most of these cells have complement (C_3) receptors and Fc receptors. They appear to represent different types of lymphocyte cell lines that are probably in some stage of differentiation. There are two categories of such cells: (1) K (killer) cells that carry out antibody-dependent cell-mediated cytotoxic reactions, and (2) NK (natural killer) cells whose cytotoxic activity does not require previous sensitization or antibody. A proportion of K cells produce immunoglobulins when placed in culture, suggesting a B-cell lineage. The origin of NK cells is not known, but it has been suggested that they may be of T-cell lineage. Most of the NK activity has been

TABLE 4.
PHENOTYPIC AND FUNCTIONAL HETEROGENEITY AMONG PERIPHERAL BLOOD T CELLS

Function	T Cell Phenotype	
	T1, T3, T4, T11	T1, T3, T8, T11
Effector cells for delayed hypersensitivity	+	−
Effector cells for cytotoxicity	−	+
Help for immunoglobulin synthesis	+	−
Help for cytotoxicity	+	−
Supressor for immunoglobulin synthesis and delayed hypersensitivity	−	+
Inducer of suppressor	+	−

From Stites DP, et al (eds): Basic & Clinical Immunology, *ed 5. Los Altos, CA, Lange Medical Publications, 1984, 71. (Reprinted with permission)*

associated with large granular lymphocytes. Both K and NK cells play important roles in defense against infectious diseases.

CELL COLLABORATION IN THE IMMUNE RESPONSE

It is now known that the collaboration of several different cell types and their products is required for an immune response. This is illustrated most clearly by the production of antibody as a consequence of challenge with a T-cell dependent antigen (most antigens are T-cell dependent).

First, phagocytic cells take up the offending antigen (such as a virus) by endocytosis, catabolize the proteins, and then display the "processed" antigen on their cell surface. The phagocytes involved usually are macrophages, but monocytes, Langerhans cells of the skin, dendritic cells, keratinocytes, and brain astrocytes can serve as antigen processing and presenting cells. The macrophage not only processes the antigen and presents it on its surface to T-cells, but also secretes the monokine, interleukin-1 (IL-1). According to one proposed model (Bendtzen, 1983), a precursor T-cell population (T-pre) reacts with the presented antigen and the appropriate MHC class protein on the surface of the macrophage. Contact with these antigens and stimulation by IL-1 causes the T-pre cells to develop surface receptors for IL-2, a T-cell growth factor. In addition, antigen presentation together with IL-1 induces T-helper cells to elaborate IL-2, which interacts with the IL-2 receptor to trigger T-cell proliferation. T-pre cells develop into helper, suppressor, or cytotoxic cells. Proliferation of these cells continues as long as they possess IL-2 receptors and IL-2 is available. Some activated T-cells become memory cells.

T-helper cells also secrete another lymphokine, gamma interferon. This substance enhances the synthesis of MHC class I and II molecules on cells, thus increasing the efficacy of antigen presentation to T-cells (see Chapter 63). In addition, gamma interferon enhances the activity of NK cells and other cytocidal cells. Antigen-activated T-cells secrete yet another lymphokine, IL-3, an important regulator of hematopoiesis, which promotes T-stem cell maturation and enhances mast cell growth.

The B-lymphocytes are also activated by antigen and lymphokines. One lymphokine, human B-cell growth factor (BCGF), is produced by T-lymphocytes and is involved in the proliferation of activated B-lymphocytes (Maizel et al, 1983). BCGF has been purified and demonstrated to be distinct from IL-2 (Mehta et al, 1985). There is some evidence that IL-2 can sustain proliferation of B-cells and that activated B-lymphocytes carry functional IL-2 receptors (see Chapter 63). Once activated, B-cells proliferate and some differentiate into antibody-secreting plasma cells, while others become memory cells. Because B- and T-memory cells are present, a second challenge of antigen results in interaction with many more antigen-sensitive T- and B-cells, and much more antibody is produced in a much shorter period of time (anamnestic response).

The immune response is terminated by the activities of T-suppressor cells. These cells are important not only in controlling antibody production, but also because they play a major role in preventing autoimmune disease.

Cited References

Bendtzen K: Biological properties of interleukins. *Allergy* 38:219-226, 1983.

Geha RS: Presence of circulating anti-idiotype-bearing cells after booster immunization with tetanus toxoid (TT) and inhibition of anti-TT antibody synthesis by auto-anti-idiotypic antibody. *J Immunol* 130:1634-1639, 1983.

Jerne NK: Towards network theory of immune system. *Ann Immunol (Inst Pasteur)* 125C:373-389, 1974.

Maizel A, et al: Proliferation of human B lymphocytes mediated by a soluble factor. *Fed Proc* 42:2753-2756, 1983.

Mehta SR, et al: Purification of human B cell growth factor. *J Immunol* 135:3298-3302, 1985.

Stobo JD: Lymphocytes, in Stites DP, et al (eds): *Basic & Clinical Immunology*, ed 5. Los Altos, CA, Lange Medical Publications, 1984, 569-585.

Uytdehaag FGCM, Osterhaus ADME: Induction of neutralizing antibody in mice against poliovirus type II with monoclonal anti-idiotypic antibody. *J Immunol* 134:1225-1229, 1985.

Other Selected References

Bach J-F (ed): *Immunology*, ed 2. New York, John Wiley & Sons, 1982.

Barrett JT: *Textbook of Immunology: An Introduction to Immunochemistry and Immunobiology*, ed 4. St Louis, CV Mosby, 1983.

Myrvik QN, Weiser RS: *Fundamentals of Immunology*, ed 2. Philadelphia, Lea & Febiger, 1984.

Stites DP, et al (eds): *Basic & Clinical Immunology*, ed 5. Los Altos, CA, Lange Medical Publications, 1984.

Histamine and Antihistamines *58*

HISTAMINE

Histamine is a low-molecular-weight amine that is stored in tissue mast cells and circulating basophils throughout the body. Release of histamine results from antigen-antibody reactions or exposure to various substances, including drugs, chemicals, dyes, foods, alkaloids, and venoms. (See Chapter 57, The Immune Response.)

Histamine interacts with specific receptors in various target tissues. Receptors are subdivided into histamine 1 (H_1) and histamine 2 (H_2) receptors. The action of histamine on cells of different tissues depends upon the function of the cell and the ratio of H_1:H_2 receptors.

Activation of H_1 receptors contracts smooth muscle and increases vascular permeability and mucus secretion; some of these effects may be mediated through increased intracellular cyclic guanosine monophosphate (cGMP). In the central nervous system, histamine probably serves as a neurotransmitter.

Activation of H_2 receptors primarily causes gastric acid secretion, but vascular dilation with cutaneous flushing also occurs. Histamine stimulates secretion of gastric acid within the gastric mucosa, increasing the concentration of cyclic adenosine monophosphate (cAMP) and decreasing the levels of cGMP; H_2 antihistamines block these actions. A reciprocal relationship may exist in the lung where bronchial smooth muscle is constricted following stimulation of H_1 receptors by histamine but is relaxed following stimulation of H_2 receptors by H_2 receptor agonists. See Chapter 52, Agents Used in Disorders of the Upper Gastrointestinal Tract, for further discussion of H_2 antihistamines.

The principal action of histamine on smooth muscle occurs in the lung, where it may contribute to the bronchoconstriction of asthma; significant effects also occur in intestinal smooth muscle. Important clinical effects of histamine include: (1) Vasodilation of small blood vessels and increased capillary permeability; when large amounts enter the circulation rapidly, vasodilation may be severe enough to cause vascular shock. (2) Mediation of the wheal and flare component of the triple response in skin; histamine often is used as a positive control during skin testing for allergic conditions. (3) Production of pruritus in allergic urticaria and angioedema.

Histamine is occasionally used as an H_2 agonist to stimulate secretion of stomach acids in the diagnosis of pernicious anemia, atrophic gastritis, and gastric carcinoma. Other H_2 receptor agonists (the investigational agents, dimaprit and impromidine) are much more selective in their action on gastric secretion.

ANTIHISTAMINES

The antihistamines discussed in this chapter are H_1 receptor blocking agents, which are among the most widely used drugs. Like histamine, H_1 antagonists contain a substituted ethylamine moiety, but, unlike histamine, most H_1 antagonists have other groupings in place of the primary amino structure and single aromatic ring. Antihistamines are classified according to these other groupings as amino alkyl ethers (diphenhydramine, carbinoxamine, clemastine), ethylenediamines (pyrilamine, tripelennamine), alkylamines (brompheniramine, chlorpheniramine, dexchlorpheniramine, triprolidine), and phenothiazines (methdilazine, promethazine, trimeprazine). There are several miscellaneous agents with widely varying added groupings (azatadine, cyproheptadine, diphenylpyraline, hydroxyzine, phenindamine). (See Tables 1 and 2.)

Traditional antihistamines cause sedation, impair coordination, and have other effects on the central nervous system. Newer agents (terfenadine and the investigational agents, astemizole, acrivastine, and mequitazine) do not cross the blood-brain barrier in appreciable amounts and are nonsedating in most patients.

The potency and adverse effects of the H_1 receptor blocking

TABLE 1.
ACTIONS OF STRUCTURAL GROUPS OF TRADITIONAL ANTIHISTAMINES

Class	Antihistaminic Activity	Sedative Effects	Anticholinergic Activity	Antiemetic Effects	Gastrointestinal Side Effects	Duration of Action
AMINO ALKYL ETHERS (Ethanolamines)	+ to ++	+ to +++	+++	++ to +++	+	4 to 6 hours
ETHYLENEDIAMINES	+ to ++	+ to ++	—	—	+++	4 to 6 hours
ALKYLAMINES (Propylamines)	++ to +++	+ to ++	++	—	+	4 to 25 hours
PHENOTHIAZINES	+ to +++	+++	+++	++++	—	4 to 24 hours

Adapted from Ziment I, 1978.

agents vary. When one antihistamine must be substituted for another because of ineffectiveness or tolerance, it is advisable to select the succeeding drug from a different chemical group. Administration of a single dose of a long-acting traditional antihistamine in the evening may relieve symptoms without producing sedation or other adverse effects in patients whose symptoms are prominent in the morning (Drouin, 1985). Nonsedating antihistamines are the drugs of choice for patients who cannot tolerate the central nervous system effects of the traditional antihistamines.

Actions and Uses

Antihistamines probably act by competing reversibly for histamine receptor sites on cells, thus preventing the actions of histamine on target organs. These agents also may inhibit the release of histamine and other inflammatory mediators from mast cells and basophils (Togias et al, 1986). Antihistamines do not reverse effects that have already occurred, and thus are more effective in preventing rather than treating symptoms of allergy and anaphylaxis. Antihistamines prevent the vasodilation, increased capillary permeability, tissue edema, and pruritus that occur in urticaria and angioedema; they also are of value in preventing rhinorrhea of upper respiratory allergy. Usual doses of the traditional antihistamines do not inhibit the smooth muscle contraction that causes bronchospasm in asthmatics; however, they do inhibit histamine-mediated bronchoconstriction in histamine challenge tests.

Although many symptoms of allergic disease can be prevented or ameliorated by antihistamines, relief is often incomplete, probably because other mediator substances not affected by antihistamines are released with histamine. Antihistamines usually relieve only symptoms that are histamine-mediated. In addition, limitations on dosage may make it difficult to achieve concentrations at receptor sites large enough to compete with histamine. Antihistamines often control mild allergic symptoms of recent onset but are less helpful for chronic illness and are least effective in severe disorders, such as anaphylaxis. Since antihistamines are best utilized for prevention rather than treatment, oral administration usually is recommended.

Upper Respiratory Disorders: Antihistamines relieve mild symptoms of allergic rhinitis (sneezing, rhinorrhea, and pruritus of the nose, eyes, and throat) of recent onset but are less effective when not given on a regular basis or when the symptoms are pronounced or prolonged. These agents do not relieve nasal congestion. Seasonal allergic rhinitis (hay fever) is more responsive to antihistamine therapy than the nonseasonal chronic form. These drugs are less likely to be helpful in vasomotor rhinitis and their value in infectious rhinitis is limited. Symptomatic relief sometimes experienced by patients with vasomotor or infectious rhinitis can be attributed to the drying effect on nasal mucosa caused by the anticholinergic action of some antihistamines.

The nonsedating antihistamines appear to be as effective as the traditional antihistamines in these allergic conditions (Sorkin and Heel, 1985; Richards et al, 1984). However, in some studies, terfenadine in recommended doses was reported to be less effective than traditional antihistamines or astemizole (investigational agent) for hay fever. In patients with seasonal allergic rhinitis, terfenadine has a more rapid onset of action (one to three hours) than astemizole (one to six days) (Girard et al, 1985; Sussman and Kobric, 1985) and may be more useful when rapid relief is required. Astemizole may be more useful for prophylaxis.

Lower Respiratory Disorders: Although the H_1 antihistamines prevent the bronchospasm caused by inhalation of histamine, they are much less effective in bronchospasm caused by other chemical mediators (eg, prostaglandins, leukotrienes, acetylcholine). Certain H_1 antagonists (eg, hydroxyzine) may have a slight bronchodilating effect. At best, these antihistamines offer mild protection against bronchospasm. In patients with both hay fever and asthma, the traditional antihistamines can be used to treat hay fever symptoms since it is no longer believed that the anticholinergic drying actions of some of these agents aggravate asthma.

The efficacy of antihistamines in the common cold and other respiratory infections has been reviewed (West et al, 1975). Current evidence indicates that none of these agents prevents colds or significantly shortens the duration of infection, although mild symptomatic relief has been reported in some patients. Despite this lack of substantial effectiveness, antihistamines are common ingredients of cold remedies (see Chapter 21, Decongestant, Cough, and Cold Preparations).

Dermatologic Conditions: Acute urticaria and infantile eczema, particularly the pruritic component, often are alleviated by oral antihistamines. Chronic urticaria responds to hydroxyzine or another sedating antihistamine but also appears to improve with prolonged administration of nonsedating antihistamines. In one study, terfenadine was reported to be less effective than azatadine for chronic urticaria (Drouin, 1985). The simultaneous use of an H₁ and H₂ antagonist may be more effective in chronic urticaria than either drug alone. The relatively long half-lives of hydroxyzine and terfenadine permit administration once or twice daily and increase their usefulness.

Antihistamines also prevent physical urticaria such as that produced by cold or exercise. The pruritus of atopic or contact dermatitis may be relieved by sedative antihistamines as a result of their central nervous system depressant actions. In patients with severe pruritus, the dual effects of sedation and histamine receptor blockade can be particularly helpful, especially if these drugs are used at bedtime.

Some patients with angioedema respond to antihistamines, but epinephrine should be used for severe angioedema, especially in life-threatening situations (anaphylaxis) with laryngeal involvement (see the section on Treatment of Anaphylactic Shock in Chapter 62, Agents for Active and Passive Immunity).

Antihistamines are sometimes used topically to treat allergic conjunctivitis, allergic dermatitis, pruritus caused by insect stings, and similar conditions. However, local application for long periods may cause sensitization. Accordingly, oral administration is preferred.

Hypersensitivity Phenomena: Antihistamines aid in the treatment of urticaria and pruritus associated with anaphylaxis and other allergic reactions (eg, penicillin sensitivity; food allergies; wasp, yellow jacket, and hornet stings; acute reactions to drugs and allergen injections). However, these drugs are ineffective in combating servere symptoms of hypersensitivity resulting in anaphylaxis (eg, hypotension, upper respiratory obstruction due to laryngeal edema) because mediators other than histamine may be involved.

Epinephrine is the agent of choice for anaphylaxis and other allergic emergencies (see Chapter 62), but antihistamines can be used as adjuncts to control secondary effects on skin and mucosa.

Transfusion Reactions: Antihistamines may ameliorate histamine-induced flushing, urticaria, and pruritus associated with mild transfusion reactions not caused by incompatibility or pyrogens, but these agents do not prevent such reactions. Antihistamines should not be given routinely to patients receiving blood but may be administered prophylactically to those with a history of transfusion reactions. They should never be added to blood being transfused.

Miscellaneous Uses: The sedative effect of the traditional antihistamines is the basis for their use, particularly hydroxyzine and promethazine, for preoperative medication (see Chapter 17, Adjuncts to Anesthesia).

The traditional antihistamines are the principal components of most over-the-counter sleep aids. The amount of antihistamine permitted in each dose is generally limited and tolerance to the sedative effect develops quickly. Nevertheless, several fatalities from overdosage have been reported with use of these products. (See also Chapter 5, Drugs Used for Anxiety and Sleep Disorders.)

Antihistamines may help to prevent allergic reactions to contrast media. Diphenhydramine has been employed most commonly, usually in conjunction with corticosteroids; when indicated, they are given parenterally before the intravenous administration of contrast media. The addition of ephedrine may further reduce allergic reactions (Greenberger et al, 1985).

The piperazine antihistamines (buclizine [Bucladin-S], cyclizine [Marezine], and meclizine [Antivert, Bonine]) and the amino alkyl ether, dimenhydrinate [Dramamine], are used principally for motion sickness (see Chapter 14, Drugs Used in Vertigo and Vomiting). Some antihistamines are used in parkinsonism (see Chapter 11, Drugs Used in Extrapyramidal Movement Disorders).

For information on specific antihistamines, see Table 2.

Adverse Reactions

Therapeutic doses of traditional H₁ antagonists cause adverse effects that are rarely serious and often disappear after a few days of continued usage. However, there is marked variation in tolerance among individuals.

The most common adverse effect of the traditional antihistamines is sedation. Daytime drowsiness may be a problem, especially while driving or operating machinery; most patients become tolerant to sedation within a few days or a few weeks. Administration of traditional antihistamines with relatively long serum half-lives (eg, chlorpheniramine, brompheniramine, hydroxyzine) as a single dose at bedtime may prevent or decrease daytime sedation in adults (Drouin, 1985). Patients should be warned that simultaneous ingestion of alcohol or other central nervous system depressants increases somnolence. Other untoward effects include dizziness, lassitude, incoordination, fatigue, tinnitus, and diplopia. Paradoxically, euphoria, nervousness, irritability, insomnia, tremors, and increased tendency toward convulsions also may occur, especially in children.

In therapeutic doses, nonsedating antihistamines produce few adverse effects. Unlike their traditional counterparts, these drugs rarely produce drowsiness and do not potentiate that caused by alcohol, diazepam, or other central nervous system depressants. These nonsedating agents also do not impair psychomotor performance. In large doses, mequitazine (investigational agent) is more likely than terfenadine or astemizole (investigational agent) to cause sedation and other signs of central nervous depression (Nicholson and Stone, 1983).

The next most common side effects of traditional antihistamines include gastrointestinal symptoms, such as loss of appetite, nausea, vomiting, abdominal discomfort, constipation, or diarrhea. The use of the nonsedating agent, astemizole, for longer than two weeks may increase appetite and cause weight gain (Wilson and Hillas, 1982).

Many traditional antihistamines have anticholinergic actions that are manifested in about 3% of patients as dryness of the mouth, throat, and nasal airway; tightness of the chest; palpitations; headache; and prostatism (urinary retention) or

TABLE 2.
ANTIHISTAMINES

Drug	Usual Dosage	Preparations	Comment
AMINO ALKYL ETHERS Diphenhydramine Hydrochloride	*Oral: Adults,* 25-50 mg 3 or 4 times daily. *Children under 12 years,* 5 mg/kg in 4 divided doses over a 24-hour period. *Intravenous (preferred), Intramuscular (deep): Adults,* 10-50 mg (maximum, 400 mg daily). *Children,* 5 mg/kg daily in 4 divided doses (maximum, 300 mg daily). *Topical:* Cream or lotion applied as needed to affected area.	*Generic.* Capsules, elixir, syrup, and solution *Benadryl* (Parke-Davis). Capsules 25 and 50 mg; elixir 12.5 mg/5 ml; solution (for injection) 10 mg/ml in 10 and 30 ml containers and 50 mg/ml in 1 and 10 ml containers; cream 2% in 30 and 60 g containers (nonprescription) *Caladryl* (Parke-Davis). Cream 1% in 15 and 45 g containers (nonprescription); lotion 1 % in 30, 75, and 180 ml containers (nonprescription)	Most widely used antihistamine for parenteral administration in treatment of anaphylactic and other allergic reactions. May be given with epinephrine but is not a substitute for it. Incidence of drowsiness high. Diphenhydramine and other antihistamines applied topically may cause sensitization (contact dermatitis). Drug should not be used in premature and newborn infants. Drug should not be used with ototoxic antibiotics, as the ototoxicity may be masked.
Carbinoxamine Maleate	*Oral: Adults,* 12-32 mg daily in divided doses. *Children,* 0.2 mg/kg 3 or 4 times daily.	*Clistin* (McNeil). Tablets 4 mg.	Lowest incidence of drowsiness of the amino alkyl ethers. Anticholinergic effect comparatively weak.
Clemastine Fumarate	*Oral: Adults,* 1.34-2.68 mg 2 to 3 times daily (maximum, 8.04 mg daily).	*Tavist* (Sandoz). Tablets 1.34 and 2.68 mg	Drowsiness is the most frequent side effect, but the incidence of central sedative effects is generally low. Anticholinergic effect very weak.
ETHYLENEDIAMINES Tripelennamine Citrate	*Oral:* (Doses expressed in terms of hydrochloride salt.) *Adults,* 25-50 mg every 4 to 6 hours. *Children,* 5 mg/kg/24 hours divided into 4 to 6 doses.	*PBZ* (Geigy). Elixir 37.5 mg (equivalent to 25 mg hydrochloride)/5 ml; tablets 25 and 50 mg	Incidence of sedation lower than with diphenhydramine. Dizziness common.
Tripelennamine Hydrochloride	*Oral: Adults,* 25-50 mg every 4 to 6 hours (tablets) or 100 mg 2 or 3 times daily (timed-release form). *Children,* 5 mg/kg/24 hours in 4 to 6 divided doses (tablets) or, for *children over 5 years,* 50 mg 2 or 3 times daily (timed-release form). *Topical:* Cream applied as needed.	*Generic.* Tablets, powder, cream *PBZ* (Geigy). Cream 2% in 30 g containers *PBZ-SR* (Geigy). Tablets (timed-release) 100 mg	
Pyrilamine Maleate	*Oral: Adults,* 75-100 mg daily in 3 or 4 divided doses. *Children,* information is inadequate to establish dose.	*Generic.* Tablets	Incidence of drowsiness low.

(Continued on next page)

Drug	Usual Dosage	Preparations	Comment
ALKYLAMINES Chlorpheniramine Maleate	*Oral: Adults,* 2-4 mg 3 or 4 times daily (tablets, syrup) or 8 mg 1 to 3 times daily or 12 mg 1 or 2 times daily (timed-release form). *Children under 12 years,* 0.35 mg/kg daily divided into 4 doses; *7 years and older,* 8 mg every 12 hours (timed-release form). *Intramuscular, Intravenous, Subcutaneous: Adults,* 5-40 mg (intravenous injection should be made over period of 1 minute). *Subcutaneous: Children under 12 years,* 0.35 mg/kg daily divided into 4 doses.	*Generic.* Capsules (plain, timed-release),* tablets, solution, syrup *Chlor-Trimeton* (Schering). Syrup 2 mg/5 ml (nonprescription); tablets 4 mg (nonprescription); tablets (timed-release) 8 (nonprescription) and 12 mg; solution (for injection) 10 mg/ml in 1 ml containers. *Teldrin* (Menley & James). Capsules (timed-release) 8 and 12 mg (nonprescription)	Drowsiness most common reaction, but overall incidence low. Common ingredient in cold remedies.
Brompheniramine Maleate	*Oral: Adults,* 4 mg every 4 to 6 hours (maximum, 24 mg daily) (tablets, elixir) or 8-12 mg 2 or 3 times daily (timed-release form). *Children 6 to 12 years,* 2 mg every 4 to 6 hours (maximum, 12 mg daily) (tablets, elixir) or 8-12 mg every 12 hours (timed-release form); *2 to 6 years,* 1 mg every 4 to 6 hours (maximum, 6 mg daily) (elixir). *Intramuscular, Intravenous, Subcutaneous: Adults,* 5-20 mg every 6 to 12 hours (maximum, 40 mg daily). *Children under 12 years,* 0.5 mg/kg daily divided into 3 or 4 doses.	*Generic.* Elixir, tablets (plain, timed-release), solution *Dimetane* (Robins). Elixir 2 mg/5 ml (nonprescription); tablets 4 mg (nonprescription); tablets (timed-release) 8 (nonprescription) and 12 mg. *Dimetane-Ten* (Robins). Solution (for injection) 10 mg/ml in 1 ml containers	Most common reaction is drowsiness, but overall incidence low.
Dexchlorpheniramine Maleate	*Oral: Adults,* 1 or 2 mg 3 or 4 times daily (tablets, syrup) or 4 or 6 mg 2 times daily, and, for resistant cases, 8 mg 2 times daily or 6 mg 3 times daily (timed-release form). *Children under 12 years,* 0.15 mg/kg daily divided into 4 doses.	*Generic.* Syrup, tablets (plain, timed-release) *Polaramine* (Schering). Syrup 2 mg/5 ml; tablets 2 mg; tablets (timed-release) 4 and 6 mg	Incidence of reactions low; most common reaction is drowsiness.
Triprolidine Hydrochloride	*Oral: Adults,* 2.5 mg 3 or 4 times daily. *Children over 6 years,* 1.25 mg 3 or 4 times daily; *under 6 years,* (syrup) 0.3-0.6 mg 3 or 4 times daily, depending on age.	*Generic.* Syrup, tablets *Actidil* (Burroughs Wellcome). Syrup 1.25 mg/5 ml; tablets 2.5 mg (nonprescription).	Incidence of reactions low; most common reaction is drowsiness.

(Continued on next page)

TABLE 2. ANTIHISTAMINES (continued)

Drug	Usual Dosage	Preparations	Comment
PHENOTHIAZINES Methdilazine Methdilazine Hydrochloride	*Oral: Adults*, 16-32 mg daily divided into 2 to 4 doses. *Children over 3 years*, 4 mg 2 to 4 times daily.	*Tacaryl* (Westwood). Tablets (chewable) 3.6 mg (equivalent to 4 mg of hydrochloride) *Tacaryl [hydrochloride]* (Westwood). Syrup 4 mg/5 ml; tablets 8 mg	Used primarily as antipruritic. Drowsiness less prominent than with other phenothiazines used as antihistamines. Most serious adverse reactions of other phenothiazines not reported with methdilazine.
Promethazine Hydrochloride	*Oral: Adults*, 25 mg at bedtime or 12.5 mg 4 times daily. *Children*, 25 mg at bedtime or 6.25-12.5 mg 3 times daily. *Rectal, Intramuscular, Intravenous: Adults*, 25 mg repeated in 2 hours if necessary. *Intramuscular: Children*, no more than one-half adult dose.	*Generic.* Tablets, solution, syrup *Phenergan* (Wyeth). Syrup 6.25 and 25 mg/5 ml; tablets 12.5, 25, and 50 mg; suppositories 12.5, 25, and 50 mg; solution (for injection) 25 and 50 mg/ml in 1 ml containers	Pronounced sedative effect limits use in many ambulatory patients. All precautions applicable to phenothiazines should be observed (see Chapter 6). Photosensitization is contraindication to further use.
Trimeprazine Tartrate	*Oral: Adults*, 10 mg daily divided into 4 doses (tablets, syrup) or 2 doses (timed-release form). *Children 6 months to 3 years*, 3.75 mg daily divided into 3 doses; *3 to 12 years*, 7.5 mg daily divided into 3 doses.	*Temaril* (Smith Kline & French). Capsules (timed-release) 5 mg; syrup 2.5 mg/5 ml; tablets 2.5 mg	Used primarily as antipruritic. Drowsiness most common reaction. All precautions applicable to phenothiazines should be observed (see Chapter 6).
MISCELLANEOUS Azatadine Maleate	*Oral: Adults*, 1-2 mg twice daily. *Children*, dosage has not been established.	*Optimine* (Schering). Tablets 1 mg	Chemically similar to cyproheptadine. Drowsiness most common side effect.
Cyproheptadine Hydrochloride	*Oral: Adults*, 4-20 mg daily in divided doses. Dosage must be individualized and should not exceed 0.5 mg/kg daily. *Children 2 to 6 years*, 2 mg 2 or 3 times daily (maximum, 12 mg daily); *7 to 14 years*, 4 mg 2 or 3 times daily (maximum, 16 mg daily).	*Generic.* Syrup, tablets *Periactin* (Merck Sharp & Dohme). Syrup 2 mg/5 ml; tablets 4 mg	Used to relieve pruritus. Reported to be especially useful in cold urticaria. Drowsiness most common reaction. Drug should not be used in premature and newborn infants.
Diphenylpyraline Hydrochloride	*Oral: Adults*, 5 mg every 12 hours (maximum, 10 mg daily) *Children over 6 years*, 5 mg every 24 hours. *Children 2 to 6 years*, not recommended.	*Hispril* (Smith Kline & French). Capsules (timed-release)* 5 mg	General antihistamine with mild sedative effect.
Hydroxyzine Hydrochloride Hydroxyzine Pamoate	*Oral: Adults*, initially, 25 mg 3 times daily, increased if necessary to 100 mg 4 times daily. *Children under 6 years*, 50 mg daily divided into 3-4 doses; *over 6 years*, 50-100 mg daily divided into 3-4 doses.	*Generic.* Solution, syrup, tablets (hydrochloride); capsules (pamoate). *Atarax [hydrochloride]* (Roerig). Syrup 10 mg/5 ml; tablets 10, 25, 50 and 100 mg *Vistaril [pamoate]* (Pfizer). Capsules 25, 50 and 100 mg; suspension (oral) equivalent to 25 mg hydrochloride/5 ml	This piperazine is agent of choice in chronic urticaria and many dermatologic allergies. Drowsiness most common reaction. Contraindicated during early pregnancy.

(Continued on next page)

Drug	Usual Dosage	Preparations	Comment
Phenindamine Tartrate	*Oral: Adults,* 25 mg 4 times daily. *Children 6 to 12 years,* 12.5 mg 4 times daily; *under 6 years,* dosage not established.	*Nolahist* (Carnrick). Tablets 25 mg (nonprescription)	May cause drowsiness. Excitation can occur, particularly in children.
NONSEDATING AGENTS Terfenadine	*Oral: Adults and children 12 years or over,* 60 mg twice daily. *Children 6 to 12 years,* 30 to 60 mg twice daily adjusted according to weight; *3 to 5 years,* 15 mg twice daily (Sorkin and Heel, 1984).	*Seldane* (Merrell Dow). Tablets 60 mg	Rapid onset of action (1 to 3 hours). Sedation, impaired coordination, and other signs of CNS depression do not occur. Neither efficacy nor adverse reactions are increased by giving large doses (2 to 3 times the therapeutic amount).
Astemizole (Investigational)	*Oral: Adults and children over 12 years,* 10 mg once daily taken on an empty stomach. In patients with severe symptoms, 30 mg daily as a single dose for up to 8 days, then 10 mg daily. *Children 6 to 12 years,* dosage is halved; *less than 6 years,* 0.2 mg/kg in suspension form (Richards et al, 1984).	*Hismanal* (Janssen).	Slow onset of action (1 to 6 days); thus, most useful for prophylaxis. Sedation, impaired coordination, and other signs of CNS depression do not occur.
Acrivastine (Investigational)	*Oral: Adults and children over 12 years,* 4 mg 3 or 4 times daily or 8 mg 2 times daily (Cohen et al, 1985).	—(Burroughs Wellcome).	Rapid onset of action (1 to 2 hours). Tachyphylaxis does not occur with chronic administration. Sedation, impaired coordination, and other signs of CNS depression are markedly reduced compared to traditional antihistamines.

*Bioavailability of drug in timed-release form may be neither uniform nor reliable.

dysuria. The incidence of these effects is less in patients receiving the nonsedating antihistamines. Monoamine oxidase inhibitors prolong and intensify the anticholinergic effects of antihistamines.

Any of the usual manifestations of drug allergy may develop when antihistamines are given orally. More commonly, allergic dermatitis occurs after topical application of an antihistamine. Leukopenia and agranulocytosis occur rarely.

Although the traditional antihistamines have a relatively large margin of safety, their widespread use makes acute poisoning common. The central nervous system effects of the drugs, especially their central anticholinergic effects, are most likely to cause difficulty (eg, toxic psychosis).

Precautions

Since antihistamines inhibit the cutaneous histamine response, they should be withdrawn before skin testing for allergies is undertaken. Compliance can be verified by documenting suppression of the histamine-mediated wheal and flare reaction. Antihistamines should not be given prophylactically to patients receiving allergen injections.

There are no clear guidelines for safe use of antihistamines in pregnant women.

Pharmacokinetics

The clinical pharmacokinetics of antihistamines have been reviewed (Paton and Webster, 1985).

Of the traditional antihistamines, only brompheniramine, chlorpheniramine, promethazine, hydroxyzine, and diphenhydramine have been studied extensively. These drugs appear to be metabolized by the liver and thus may accumulate in patients with severe hepatic disease. They and their metabolites are excreted chiefly by the kidneys. The elimination half-lives of these drugs are: diphenhydramine, about 4 hours; promethazine, 10 to 14 hours; chlorpheniramine, 14 to 25 hours; and brompheniramine, about 25 hours. Total body clearances in adults range from 5 to 12 ml/kg/min and apparent volumes of distribution are large (more than 4 L/kg).

Following oral administration of most traditional agents, effects appear within 15 to 30 minutes, are maximal within one hour, and persist for four to six hours. Some antihistamines have a considerably longer duration of action (see Table 1). In single-dose studies, the serum half-lives of chlorpheniramine, brompheniramine, and hydroxyzine exceeded 20 hours in adults; therefore, administration of these drugs once or twice daily may be possible if the results are applicable to chronic administration (Drouin, 1985). The serum half-lives of these drugs are shorter in children and administration two or three times daily may be required. Intramuscular or intravenous injection produces a more prompt action, but rapid intravenous administration may cause hypotension.

Although bioequivalence has been demonstrated for some timed-release preparations (see Table 2), others may be less effective than conventional dosage forms.

Extensive pharmacokinetic data are available for the non-sedating antihistamines, terfenadine (Sorkin and Heel, 1985) and astemizole (Richards et al, 1984). Neither drug appears to cross the blood-brain barrier.

Terfenadine is well absorbed and peak concentrations occur one to two hours after an oral dose. This drug is extensively and rapidly metabolized, primarily to two major metabolites, and is well distributed in the tissues. More than 98% of a dose is bound to plasma proteins, which contributes to the difficulty in crossing the blood-brain barrier. Terfenadine is eliminated by fecal (60%) and urinary (40%) excretion. The elimination half-life is relatively long in healthy adults (16 to 23 hours) (Sorkin and Heel, 1985).

After oral administration of astemizole, peak plasma levels occur in one to four hours. Concomitant ingestion of food significantly decreases its bioavailability. Astemizole undergoes extensive first-pass metabolism in the liver to several active and inactive metabolites, and it is well distributed in the tissues. In human volunteers, the drug was 96% bound to plasma proteins. Astemizole and its metabolites are excreted slowly following a single oral dose; 54% to 73% of the dose is recovered in the feces within 14 days. The apparent elimination half-life of unchanged drug and metabolites is 18 to 20 days.

Mixtures

Many fixed-ratio mixtures containing an antihistamine with other agents, most commonly adrenergic nasal decongestants and analgesics, are marketed for the treatment of allergies and upper respiratory infections. The combination of more than one ingredient in an individual dosage form can be recommended for convenience only. It is unlikely that all of the drugs in the mixture are provided in the exact dose needed by the individual patient. Thus, a combination may produce sedation in one patient and overstimulation in another. However, they are popular with physicians and patients and are convenient and generally safe.

For a listing of commonly prescribed mixtures containing antihistamines, see Chapter 21, Decongestant, Cough, and Cold Preparations.

Cited References

Drouin MA: H₁ antihistamines: Perspective on use of conventional and new agents. *Ann Allergy* 55:747-752, 1985.

Girard JP, et al: Double-blind comparison of astemizole, terfenadine and placebo in hay fever with special regard to onset of action. *J Int Med Res* 13:102-108, 1985.

Greenberger PA, et al: Prophylaxis against repeated radiocontrast media reactions in 857 cases: Adverse experience with cimetidine and safety of β-adrenergic antagonists. *Arch Intern Med* 145:2197-2200, 1985.

Nicholson AN, Stone BM: H₁-antagonist mequitazine: Studies on performance and visual function. *Eur J Clin Pharmacol* 25:563-566, 1983.

Paton DM, Webster DR: Clinical pharmacokinetics of H₁-receptor antagonists (antihistamines). *Clin Pharmacokinet* 10:477-497, 1985.

Richards DM, et al: Astemizole: Review of its pharmacodynamic properties and therapeutic efficacy. *Drugs* 28:38-61, 1984.

Sorkin EM, Heel RC: Terfenadine: Review of its pharmacodynamic properties and therapeutic efficacy. *Drugs* 29:34-56, 1985.

Sussman GL, Kobric M: Treatment of seasonal allergic rhinitis with astemizole, non-sedating antihistamine: Results of open, multicenter clinical trial. *Todays' Therapeutic Trends* 2:11-19, 1985.

Togias AG, et al: Demonstration of inhibition of mediator release from human mast cells by azatadine base: In vivo and in vitro evaluation. *JAMA* 255:225-229, 1986.

West S, et al: Review of antihistamines and common cold. *Pediatrics* 56:100-107, 1975.

Wilson JD, Hillas JL: Astemizole: New long-acting antihistamine in treatment of seasonal allergic rhinitis. *Clin Allergy* 12:131-140, 1982.

Ziment I: *Respiratory Pharmacology and Therapeutics.* Philadelphia, WB Saunders, 1978.

Antiarthritic Drugs

The drugs discussed in this chapter are used to treat rheumatoid arthritis, juvenile arthritis, ankylosing spondylitis, psoriatic arthritis, Reiter's syndrome, osteoarthritis (degenerative joint disease), and fibrositic disorders. They include nonsteroidal anti-inflammatory drugs, analgesics, gold compounds, penicillamine, antimalarial drugs, corticosteroids, and cytotoxic agents.

There are many types of arthritis, and more than one form may occur in the same patient. Therefore, an accurate diagnosis is important for proper management, including drug selection. Arthritic diseases are characterized by inflammation and tissue damage at joints. The pathogenesis is incompletely understood, although the immune response plays a prominent role in producing both inflammation and local tissue damage.

The inflammatory process is mediated by a variety of endogenous chemicals, including immunologic factors; those that precipitate the inflammatory cascade can be categorized as vasoactive substances, chemotactic factors, and agents causing cell and tissue damage (Rodnan et al, 1983). Among the vasoactive substances are histamine, serotonin, protein constituents of the complement system, bradykinin, and prostaglandins. Prostaglandin levels are increased in the synovial fluid of patients with rheumatoid arthritis and osteoarthritis, and prostaglandin E_2 has been shown to degrade articular cartilage. Furthermore, all effective nonsteroidal anti-inflammatory drugs inhibit prostaglandin synthesis, thereby reducing the concentration of prostaglandins, as well as that of other products of the synthetic pathway (eg, thromboxane A_2). However, these drugs do not affect the lipoxygenase pathway and thus do not affect the production of leukotrienes.

Tissue damage results from the complex interplay of humoral and cellular immune responses. Antigen-antibody complex-es accumulate in synovial tissues and activate the complement system with engagement of the cellular immune response. This cellular response is characterized by release of lysosomal enzymes, prostaglandins, and free oxygen radicals, which contribute to tissue damage and the inflammatory process. It is believed that remission-inducing (disease-modifying) drugs partially suppress the immune response. Remission-inducing antiarthritic drugs include the gold compounds, the antimalarials, penicillamine, and cytotoxic agents. Because the precise nature of the etiologic stimulus is not known, understanding of their mechanism of action is limited.

Although the following discussion is limited to drug therapy, it should be recognized that mechanical problems seldom respond to drugs alone and that other measures must be employed (ie, physical therapy, exercise, surgery, adaptive devices). Furthermore, the impact of the disease on all aspects of the patient's life must be assessed with the help of a social worker, occupational therapist, vocational rehabilitation specialist, and sometimes a psychiatrist. Patient education and understanding of the disease and its management, including expectations from drug therapy, are important in achieving therapeutic success.

DISEASES AND THERAPY

Rheumatoid Arthritis

This inflammatory disease occurs in about 1% of the adult population and is two and one-half times more common in women than in men. The incidence peaks in the fourth and fifth decades, but rheumatoid arthritis can appear anytime from childhood to old age. Rheumatoid arthritis is usually bimodal in age pattern of onset, either in the 20's to 30's or again with equal incidence of onset in postmenopausal females. The incidence of disease for both sexes may equalize after age 60.

Symptoms: Rheumatoid arthritis is a systemic disorder characterized primarily by inflammation of the synovium with destruction of cartilage and bone. Early manifestations include fatigue, weight loss, anorexia, and general malaise. The major clinical manifestations are diffuse and prolonged morning stiffness; pain on motion; tenderness and/or swelling of multiple joints, usually symmetrical; subcutaneous nodules; and typical roentgenographic changes. Extra-articular complications, such as anemia, vasculitis, scleritis, pleurisy, pericarditis, and peripheral neuropathy, also may develop.

Therapy: The primary aims in the treatment of rheumatoid arthritis are to reduce pain and inflammation, maintain joint mobility, and prevent deformity. Gold compounds, including oral gold, and cyclophosphamide [Cytoxan, Neosar] suppress the destructive course of the disease. Penicillamine [Cuprimine, Depen], chloroquine [Aralen], and hydroxychloroquine [Plaquenil] also may have this effect but data are not yet available to support this assumption. The nonsteroidal anti-inflammatory drugs provide symptomatic relief but whether they alter the course of disease remains an active area of investigation.

Proper management, including drug selection, is determined by the severity or stage of disease. The effectiveness of therapy is difficult to evaluate because spontaneous remissions and exacerbations occur in almost all patients. However, few remissions are complete and there is a tendency toward gradual progression of the disease. Appropriate treatment requires long-term therapy and the cooperation and motivation of the patient.

In the early stages of disease, a basic conservative program achieves the desired goals in most patients; this includes rest periods, appropriate exercise and physical therapy, adequate nutrition, avoidance of extremes in climate, attention to emotional and psychological factors, and use of a salicylate or another nonsteroidal anti-inflammatory drug. The patient's status must be re-evaluated periodically and treatment modified accordingly.

Salicylates are the preferred anti-inflammatory drugs for initial therapy because they are least expensive and rapidly effective. However, doses larger than those required for analgesia must be given to reduce inflammation. Although the latter action is most important in arthritis, the analgesic effect of salicylates may enhance their therapeutic value. A dosage that controls symptoms without producing unacceptable side effects should be prescribed, and full therapeutic amounts should be taken regularly for as long as synovitis is present. The dosage must be individualized because of differences in body weight and variations in the pharmacokinetics of salicylates among individuals. Serum salicylate concentrations are used to establish the dose; the most satisfactory anti-inflammatory concentration is 15 to 30 mg/dl. Pain and stiffness are alleviated in more than 90% of patients; objective improvement also can be documented. However, additional therapy is required in more than one-half of these patients.

Aspirin often is the initial drug of choice and is the least expensive nonsteroidal anti-inflammatory drug. However, this agent can be toxic to the gastrointestinal tract; several studies have shown that, of all the nonsteroidal anti-inflammatory drugs, aspirin has the greatest propensity to produce erosions in the stomach (Roth, 1984; Hart and Huskisson, 1984). Some rheumatologists believe that toxicity and the complexities of aspirin's pharmacokinetics make it undesirable for the long-term treatment of rheumatoid arthritis, especially since newer nonsteroidal anti-inflammatory drugs are available that are both safer and more convenient to use (O'Brien, 1983).

When prolonged use of large doses of regular aspirin cannot be tolerated because of gastric irritation, nonacetylated alternatives (eg, salsalate, choline salicylate) or enteric-coated or matrix-release aspirin or rectal suppository formulations may be tried. All preparations produce similar salicylate blood levels. The enteric-coated preparations cause fewer gastric lesions than uncoated or buffered aspirin, and other salicylates (choline magnesium trisalicylate, magnesium salicylate, salsalate) may cause fewer gastrointestinal side effects than aspirin. Newer nonacetylated salicylates, such as choline magnesium trisalicylate and salsalate, offer the additional advantage of administration twice daily (Roth, 1983).

Alternatively, one of the newer nonsteroidal analgesic/anti-inflammatory agents (ie, diflunisal [Dolobid], fenoprofen [Nalfon], ibuprofen [Motrin, Rufen], ketoprofen [Orudis], naproxen [Anaprox, Naprosyn], piroxicam [Feldene], sulindac [Clinoril], tolmetin [Tolectin], meclofenamate [Meclomen]) may be tried in patients who cannot tolerate or do not respond to aspirin. Like aspirin, these agents have anti-inflammatory, analgesic, and antipyretic actions. They appear to be as effective as aspirin in rheumatoid arthritis, and equieffective doses generally produce fewer gastrointestinal reactions and less gastrointestinal bleeding; nevertheless, they should be used very cautiously in patients with a history of peptic ulcer or upper gastrointestinal bleeding. Enteric-coated preparations may be of benefit in these patients. Less common but potentially more serious adverse reactions (eg, hepatic toxicity, fluid retention and edema, renal dysfunction, hypersensitivity reactions) should be kept in mind when these drugs are considered for long-term therapy. Particular toxicities appear to be unique to different chemical classes of drugs. Thus, bone marrow toxicity is related to pyrazolones, central nervous system and gastrointestinal toxicity to indolacetic acid derivatives, gastric toxicity to oxicams, and anaphylactoid hypersensitivity to pyrrole acetic acid derivatives (tolmetin). Preference for one drug over another varies among patients and physicians (Wasner et al, 1981). Many new nonsteroidal anti-inflammatory drugs are being evaluated, but whether any of these will have advantages over currently available drugs remains to be determined.

Different drugs and dosages should be tried to determine the optimum regimen for each individual. It should be kept in mind that adequate doses must be given for sufficient periods (two to four weeks) to evaluate efficacy before another drug is substituted (Scherbel and Wilke, 1981). If the first nonsteroidal anti-inflammatory drug fails, one or two more should be tried. The concurrent use of aspirin and other nonsteroidal anti-inflammatory drugs may produce drug interactions (see the evaluations) and usually is not recommended, although additive effects may result from some combinations.

Indomethacin [Indocin], an older nonsteroidal anti-inflammatory drug, is effective in moderate to severe rheumatoid arthritis, including acute exacerbations of chronic disease, but it is used more commonly in osteoarthritis and ankylosing spondylitis. Small doses should be given initially and the amount increased gradually to the level of tolerance (see the evaluation).

Opioid analgesics may relieve severe articular pain, but drugs with high abuse potential should not be used routinely. However, those with low abuse potential (eg, an agonist-antagonist) may be useful if the pain is severe.

If the symptoms of active rheumatoid arthritis fail to improve adequately after a sufficient trial with the basic conservative program (including nonsteroidal anti-inflammatory agents) and if the disease is progressing and involves multiple joints, consideration should be given to adding a so-called remission-inducing drug to the regimen (O'Duffy and Luthra, 1984; Roth, 1984). Opinions vary on which drug should be used first, but generally a gold compound, penicillamine, or hydroxychloroquine has the most favorable benefit/risk ratio. Some rheumatologists administer a parenteral gold compound (aurothioglucose [Solganal], gold sodium thiomalate [Myochrysine]) first because there has been more experience with these drugs. Some advocate their use early during the course of disease when there is active inflammation, but others prefer to postpone administration until more conservative therapy has been tried. In either case, patients should be informed of the potential adverse effects of gold therapy; that frequent, repeated injections are required over a long period; and that beneficial effects may not be observed for 10 to 24 weeks after initiation of therapy. If significant improvement is observed and therapy is tolerated, maintenance injections should be continued for several years and, possibly, indefinitely.

An orally effective gold compound, auranofin [Ridaura], is now available. Beneficial effects and the frequency of side effects appear to be comparable to those of injectable gold, but adverse reactions may be less severe (Chaffman et al, 1984). Thus, this oral preparation may be preferable to parenteral forms (see the evaluation).

Results of controlled studies have established the effectiveness of penicillamine in rheumatoid arthritis. It is an alternative to gold and is given orally. Penicillamine appears to be as effective as gold compounds or the immunosuppressive agent, azathioprine, and some rheumatologists prefer to give it before using gold compounds. Penicillamine is reserved for patients with severe, progressive disease that does not respond adequately to standard drug therapy. With current dosage regimens, the prevalence of adverse reactions appears to be lower than in early trials using larger doses. Nevertheless, patients must be monitored carefully. Because beneficial effects may not be observed for two to three months or more, anti-inflammatory drugs should be continued. Penicillamine is not effective in ankylosing spondylitis and other HLA-B27-associated arthropathies.

The antimalarial agents, chloroquine and hydroxychloroquine, partially suppress disease in 70% of patients with rheumatoid arthritis. The potential for visual impairment has limited their use, but they are the least hazardous remission-inducing drugs. The size of the dose appears to be the most important factor in development of retinal toxicity, and small doses can be given for long periods (eg, hydroxychloroquine 200 mg for two to three years) without toxic effects. Ocular reactions occur rarely when appropriate doses are prescribed (prevalence less than 1%) and are reversible (Mackenzie, 1981). Ophthalmologic examinations should be performed every six months. Retinal damage may appear or progress even after the drug is discontinued when excessive daily doses have been used. Chloroquine and hydroxychloroquine must be given for at least three to six months before maximum beneficial effects are noted. If a low-dose schedule is not effective after a trial of at least six months, agents in another class should be substituted.

Systemic corticosteroids usually improve functional capacity, relieve pain, and control inflammation, although joint destruction may continue. However, their usefulness is limited by their numerous adverse effects. Therefore, systemic use of these drugs should be reserved for patients with moderately severe, rapidly progressing rheumatoid arthritis that does not respond to other antirheumatic agents, for those threatened with severe disability or unemployability, for those with significant systemic involvement, and for patients with later onset of disease (over 60 years of age). They also may be used on a short-term basis during initiation of gold or penicillamine therapy (Bennett, 1979), but the difficulty of withdrawing the steroid must be considered. Prednisone and prednisolone are most commonly used systemically. The minimum dosage that improves symptoms and signs should be used; the initial dose should be low and increased (up to 7.5 mg prednisone or equivalent) if necessary for extra-articular manifestations. Complete relief is not sought; therefore, amelioration of disability may be the major indication for these agents unless extra-articular signs are present.

When only one or two joints are affected or present a major problem, pain can be relieved for long periods by injecting long-acting corticosteroids intra-articularly. Synovitis can be controlled for weeks to months when long-acting preparations are used. The prevalence of rapid joint damage is usually less than 1%. Dose and frequency of injections must be individualized; the smallest dose should be administered as infrequently as possible to provide relief. It is suggested that injection into a single joint should not be repeated more than three times yearly.

Certain cytotoxic agents have been effective in patients with severe disease. Azathioprine [Imuran], cyclophosphamide [Cytoxan], and methotrexate [Folex, Mexate] have been studied most extensively in rheumatoid arthritis. Although controlled trials have shown that cyclophosphamide may be very beneficial in selected patients, it appears to be more toxic than azathioprine or methotrexate. Its use is therefore limited by its serious adverse effects, including bone marrow suppression, increased infections, mucous membrane lesions, cystitis, and possibly increased incidence of neoplastic disease.

Small doses of azathioprine (1.5 mg/kg/day) given for up to three years were effective in some cases of severe recalcitrant rheumatoid arthritis. The low-dosage regimen reduced the risk of serious adverse reactions, including oncogenesis (Van Wanghe and Dequeker, 1982).

The weekly administration of methotrexate 7.5 to 10 mg orally or by injection as a single dose or every 12 hours for three doses also has been effective in refractory rheumatoid arthritis (Thompson et al, 1984; Willkens and Watson, 1982; Ward, 1984; Weinblatt et al, 1985). One study (Thompson et al, 1984) indicated that methotrexate may have a more rapid onset of therapeutic effect than other remission-inducing agents. The risk/benefit ratio of low-dose methotrexate for rheumatoid arthritis requires further study, especially the long-term risks of hepatic cirrhosis and neoplasms, which are substantially reduced by low-dose pulse therapy. It is now felt that methotrexate is not oncogenic as are other cytotoxic agents (Willkens, 1985).

Another regimen utilized small doses of cyclophosphamide, azathioprine, and hydroxychloroquine for severe refractory rheumatoid arthritis. In an open trial, the disease was suppressed at least partially in 14 of 17 patients within 16 months and complete remission occurred in five patients (McCarty and Carrera, 1982). These results require verification by controlled clinical trials. Such combined therapy of these potentially toxic agents is considered investigational for severe resistant cases by experienced research workers.

The benefit/risk ratio of drugs that affect the immune mechanism should be considered carefully for each patient. Controlled trials are required to determine the effects of prolonged use of cytotoxic agents and immunosuppressives in rheumatoid arthritis. Because of their many serious adverse reactions, these agents should be reserved for patients with advanced disease who fail to respond to more conventional management. (See also Chapter 63, Immunomodulators, and Chapter 64, Drugs Used in Cancer Chemotherapy.)

In summary, pharmacologic management of rheumatoid arthritis can be thought of as based on three separate groupings: nonsteroidal anti-inflammatory drugs (including salicylates), corticosteroids, and remission-inducing drugs (slow-acting antirheumatic drugs).

Juvenile Arthritis

Symptoms: This disease has three main onset subtypes: (1) systemic (acute febrile or Still's disease), (2) pauciarticular (four or fewer joints affected), and (3) polyarticular (five or more joints affected). The subtype is determined by manifestations during the first six months of disease and varies with respect to age at onset, sex, number and distribution of joints affected, results of serologic tests, extra-articular manifestations, and prognosis. For appropriate therapy, juvenile arthritis must be differentiated (usually by exclusion) from several other diseases with similar manifestations commonly seen in children (eg, rheumatic fever, ankylosing spondylitis, septic arthritis, trauma, malignancy).

During the first ten years of disease, chronic iridocyclitis develops in about one-fourth of patients with the early onset pauciarticular type and a positive test for antinuclear factor.

Since iridocyclitis is frequently asymptomatic at onset and may be detected only by slit-lamp examination, children with this type of juvenile arthritis should be examined at least every six months so that therapy can be instituted when necessary. Mydriatics and corticosteroids (local and systemic) prevent further complications and loss of vision.

Myocarditis is a rare but particularly hazardous manifestation of systemic onset juvenile arthritis and may lead to cardiac enlargement and heart failure. Joint involvement in this type is variable.

The prognosis is good for most children with juvenile arthritis. Overall, more than 75% have remissions without joint damage. However, severe destructive arthritis occurs in more than 50% of patients with polyarticular disease who have a positive test for rheumatoid factor. Severe arthritis develops in only about 10% to 15% of children in the polyarticular, seronegative group and in about 20% of those in the systemic (acute febrile) group. Polyarticular disease usually begins in late childhood and resembles severe adult-onset rheumatoid arthritis. The arthritis is only rarely severe in those with the pauciarticular type. However, more severe polyarticular disease develops in later years in some children with the pauciarticular subset. The incidence of HLA-B27 is high (75%) and serologic tests for antinuclear antibodies and rheumatoid factor are negative in patients who develop pauciarticular disease during late childhood. There is some evidence that these patients, who are primarily teenage boys, are likely to develop spondylitis or sacroiliitis with increasing duration of disease.

Therapy: Drug therapy for juvenile arthritis is only one part of total management, which includes a home program of supportive measures performed by parents and regular follow-up care by the physician. Treatment is most effective when initiated early. Aspirin is preferred initially, regardless of the onset subtype. Beneficial effects may not appear for one to two weeks and significant changes may not be observed for several months. Aspirin should be administered for at least six months after articular signs and symptoms have subsided. The drug then may be discontinued gradually, but should be reinstituted if symptoms recur.

Since tinnitus, the usual sign of aspirin toxicity, may be difficult to determine in young children, serum salicylate concentrations should be monitored to establish optimal dosage. Lethargy and episodic hyperpnea are early signs of toxicity; if these occur, aspirin should be discontinued until the signs abate and resumed in a slightly smaller dose. Gastrointestinal disturbances are uncommon in children but, if they occur, other preparations (eg, enteric-coated aspirin, choline salicylate) can be tried. Serum salicylate concentrations of 20 to 30 mg/dl are generally safe and effective. Because transaminase levels usually increase with prolonged administration, they should be monitored frequently during dosage adjustment and every two to three months thereafter. Hepatotoxicity may be dose related and occurs more frequently when serum salicylate levels exceed 25 mg/dl (Calabro, 1981).

As in adult rheumatoid arthritis, a newer nonsteroidal anti-inflammatory agent may be tried when aspirin is not tolerated; however, children's doses have been established only for tolmetin. Because of the potentially serious adverse reactions of indomethacin and phenylbutazone, these drugs should be avoided in children under 14 years.

If polyarticular disease progresses and no improvement is noted after four to six months of nonsteroidal anti-inflammatory therapy, gold compounds may be added to the regimen. Gold therapy is of considerable value in many children, although its effects may not be apparent for several months. The initial dose usually is 0.2 mg/kg, and is increased after one week by 0.5 mg/kg. If no adverse reactions (skin rash, oral ulcers, leukopenia, or proteinuria) occur, 1 mg/kg may be given in the third week (Nelson, 1982) and this amount usually is administered weekly for about 20 weeks. Toxic effects are similar to those in adults; patients should be observed closely and appropriate laboratory tests should be performed prior to each injection (see the evaluations on Gold Compounds). Studies employing oral gold are being performed in patients with juvenile arthritis. Preliminary results show that the efficacy and frequency of side effects are similar to those reported in adults.

Penicillamine was about as effective as gold in a few studies but, because of potential toxicity, it should be used only under carefully controlled conditions.

Antimalarial agents also are useful for children, and some clinicians prefer to employ them before gold compounds; however, care must be taken to calculate the dosage correctly, based on lean body weight, as in adults. The children's dose is the same as that for adults: 4 mg/kg/day of chloroquine and 6.4 mg/kg/day of hydroxychloroquine.

Oral corticosteroids should not be administered routinely because of their serious adverse reactions and the problems associated with withdrawal. They should be reserved for seriously ill children with polyarticular disease who do not respond to aspirin and other anti-inflammatory drugs (eg, tolmetin), and therapy should be limited to a few months (Baum, 1983). Alternate-day therapy may be useful for some patients. Systemic corticosteroids are recommended in children with myocarditis. Intra-articular injection may be useful but no more than three or four injections should be made into the same joint each year to prevent cartilage damage. Topical corticosteroids are essential in the treatment of chronic iridocyclitis; rarely, local injection or systemic administration is needed when topical application does not control inflammation.

Ankylosing Spondylitis

Symptoms: This form of arthritis differs in many respects from rheumatoid arthritis (Calin, 1979) and is characterized by involvement of the sacroiliac joints, the spinal apophyseal joints, and the paravertebral soft tissues. The peripheral joints, usually only the hips and shoulders, also are affected in about 30% of patients. Ankylosing spondylitis occurs most often in the second or third decade of life. Onset is usually insidious with primary symptoms of back pain and early morning stiffness. Symptoms tend to progress and the disease becomes chronic. This disorder also may affect other body systems; uveitis occurs in about 25% of patients and pulmo-

nary disease may mimic tuberculosis in the upper lung fields (Calin, 1979).

The HLA-B27 antigen has been found in about 95% of patients with ankylosing spondylitis. This antigen also is found in a large percentage of patients with other rheumatic diseases in which spondylitis occurs (Reiter's syndrome, psoriatic arthritis). The use of HLA-B27 as a diagnostic aid is controversial and few rheumatologists use it in this fashion.

Early recognition and initiation of appropriate therapy are important for successful treatment of ankylosing spondylitis. Although progression of the disease may not be modified by any available therapy, relief of pain and inflammation and maintenance of function usually are possible. Spontaneous remissions and exacerbations occur, and the prognosis generally is good.

Therapy: The mainstay of treatment is a daily exercise regimen to maintain spinal mobility and muscle strength. Nonsteroidal anti-inflammatory drugs aid in this goal by minimizing pain and stiffness.

Although aspirin may be effective for mild attacks, it usually does not relieve severe pain. Indomethacin is considered the drug of choice. Some newer nonsteroidal anti-inflammatory drugs (eg, piroxicam, sulindac) also are effective and may be better tolerated than indomethacin. Piroxicam may improve compliance because it is given once daily (Tannenbaum et al, 1984). Phenylbutazone also may provide symptomatic relief but, because of its potential to produce severe blood dyscrasias, it should be used only after other drugs have failed (see the evaluation).

Systemic corticosteroids are rarely needed unless iridocyclitis or vasculitis occurs and these compounds should be avoided, if possible. Gold compounds are not effective and the antimalarials and penicillamine have not been studied adequately in this condition.

Psoriatic Arthritis

Symptoms: This arthropathy occurs in about 7% of patients with psoriasis. Onset is insidious and asymmetric inflammation involving only a few joints is common. In approximately 80% of patients, peripheral joints are affected primarily. The distal interphalangeal joints of fingers and toes are involved most frequently. Sacroiliitis and spondylitis also are common; patients with HLA-B27 antigen have a higher risk of developing these disorders. Psoriasis also has been associated with HLA-B13 and BW17; BW38 has been associated with peripheral joint disease (Calin, 1979).

Therapy: The psoriasis as well as the arthritis must be treated (see Chapter 56, Dermatologic Preparations). Prognosis for psoriatic arthritis is good, for this disease generally is not severe or disabling (Vasey et al, 1982). Remissions of peripheral arthritis sometimes parallel those of the skin disease.

In general, treatment of arthritic symptoms is similar to that for rheumatoid arthritis. Aspirin is not as effective as in rheumatoid arthritis but it may be helpful in mild cases. Indomethacin controls pain and increases the range of spinal motion. A newer nonsteroidal anti-inflammatory drug may be substituted when there is no response to the older drugs. Antimalarial drugs may be effective, although exacerbation of skin disease may be severe if the patient is allergic (Kuflik, 1980). Gold compounds are beneficial in some patients. Systemic corticosteroids may improve both the skin and joint disease, but the dosage required usually is so large that adverse reactions result and withdrawal of steroids may exacerbate psoriasis; thus, they have virtually no role in the treatment of this condition. Methotrexate 2.5 to 5 mg every 12 hours for three doses weekly has been effective. Because of its potential toxicity (especially involving the liver and bone marrow), it should be reserved for progressive disease unresponsive to more conventional drugs and administered only by physicians experienced in its use. Also, during initial use, a complete blood count and liver function tests should be obtained every one to four weeks and eventually no less often than every two months (Vasey et al, 1982).

Reiter's Syndrome

Symptoms: This disease occurs primarily in young adult males. The etiology is unknown, but two epidemiologic forms are recognized: the epidemic form that follows dysentery and the endemic or venereal form that presumably follows sexual contact. The genitourinary, ocular, skeletal, and mucocutaneous systems are affected. Reiter's syndrome may be self-limiting but can become chronic and produce disability. There are many similarities between this syndrome and psoriatic arthritis. The HLA-B27 antigen is present in about 80% of patients with Reiter's syndrome and its determination may aid in diagnosis.

Therapy: There is no specific treatment for Reiter's syndrome. Anti-inflammatory drugs suppress pain, but the musculoskeletal symptoms are less responsive. Aspirin does not appear to be as effective as other nonsteroidal anti-inflammatory drugs. Indomethacin should be considered in the selection of an initial agent. A newer nonsteroidal anti-inflammatory drug may be tried as an alternative. Phenylbutazone also is effective but the potential for serious adverse reactions must be considered. Systemic corticosteroids should be avoided because they are usually less effective, although intra-articular injection of a long-acting steroid is useful when one or two joints cause major problems. Cytotoxic therapy may be indicated in patients with chronic severe disease (Calin, 1979). Oral methotrexate 7.5 to 10 mg weekly and azathioprine 1 to 2.5 mg/kg/day are beneficial in some patients resistant to other therapies (Gerber, 1984).

Osteoarthritis

Symptoms: This disease has been referred to as degenerative joint disease and traditionally has been regarded as noninflammatory and a part of the aging process. However, it is now generally agreed that an inflammatory component exists; hence, the term, osteoarthritis, appears to be appropriate. The exact pathogenesis is unknown, although the disorder is characterized by narrowing of joints with degeneration of articular cartilage and proliferative changes at the joint margins. As in rheumatoid arthritis, the initial inflammatory episode may be caused by various factors (eg, trauma, infection, metabolic disorder, prolonged joint inflammation). Several years may elapse between the provocative event and the appearance of disease, during which time there are few if any symptoms of osteoarthritis (Ehrlich, 1979; Huskisson, 1979). Episodes of secondary inflammation occur infrequently, and the inflammatory component is much less marked than in rheumatoid arthritis.

Osteoarthritis is common in middle-aged and elderly individuals, but it is not necessarily a part of the aging process. It is not considered to be a systemic disease and can be localized at a particular joint. Weight-bearing joints (knee and hip) are most commonly affected; the spine is involved less frequently. Finger joint involvement is limited to the distal interphalangeal joints (Heberden's nodes) and the proximal interphalangeal joints (Bouchard's nodes). The carpometacarpal joint in the thumb often is involved. Symptoms are referable to the joint involved, and the most common is pain that becomes worse with use of the joint. Pain at night is common; stiffness in the morning and after sitting also occurs often, but does not last as long as in rheumatoid arthritis.

Therapy: Measures to reduce strain on weight-bearing joints, physical therapy (including the application of heat or cold to reduce pain), appropriate exercise and rest, and drug therapy are all important in the management of osteoarthritis. Since inflammation contributes to symptoms, nonsteroidal anti-inflammatory agents are more effective than simple analgesics because of their combined activity. Aspirin taken regularly in adequate doses is the usual initial agent; however, the newer nonsteroidal anti-inflammatory drugs (eg, diflunisal, fenoprofen, ibuprofen, ketoprofen, naproxen, sulindac, tolmetin) may be better tolerated, especially by older patients who are more likely to have osteoarthritis (Ehrlich, 1979; Calabro, 1983) (see the evaluations). If pain is not relieved by one of these agents, indomethacin may be used. Indomethacin has been particularly effective in osteoarthritis involving the hip, hands, knees, and shoulders. Other analgesics (eg, acetaminophen, codeine) are sometimes used either alone or in addition to the anti-inflammatory drugs, but drugs with abuse potential should be avoided if possible.

Systemic corticosteroids are not indicated in this condition and may cause serious adverse effects. Intra-articular injection of long-acting preparations is less beneficial than in rheumatoid arthritis; the injections may relieve synovitis temporarily but may not prevent or reduce cartilage degeneration. However, these agents may be used to relieve symptoms in a contracted joint in order to permit institution of physical therapy to restore function. Surgical procedures utilizing total joint replacement are preferred when the joint deteriorates to instability.

NONSTEROIDAL ANTI-INFLAMMATORY AGENTS

These drugs (aspirin and nonacetylated salicylates, diflunisal [Dolobid], fenoprofen [Nalfon], ibuprofen [Motrin, Rufen], ketoprofen [Orudis], naproxen [Anaprox, Naprosyn], piroxicam [Feldene], sulindac [Clinoril], tolmetin [Tolectin], meclofenamate [Meclomen], indomethacin, and phenylbutazone) are used primarily for their anti-inflammatory and analgesic activities in the treatment of chronic arthritic conditions and certain soft tissue disorders associated with pain and inflammation. They are effective in rheumatoid arthritis, juvenile arthritis, ankylosing spondylitis, Reiter's syndrome, psoriatic arthritis, osteoarthritis, and acute gouty arthritis (see Table). Some of these drugs also are used to relieve pain (see Chapter 4, General Analgesics) and headache (see Chapter 13, Drugs Used to Treat Migraine and Other Headaches).

Mechanism of Action: Nonsteroidal anti- inflammatory drugs block the synthesis of prostaglandins by inhibiting cyclo-oxygenase, which converts arachidonic acid to cyclic endoperoxides, precursors of prostaglandins.

Prostaglandin E_2 and PGI_2 (prostacyclin) are potent vasodilators that increase vascular permeability, thus promoting inflammatory reactions. It has been suggested that the therapeutic effects, as well as the adverse reactions, of nonsteroidal anti-inflammatory drugs are related primarily to inhibition of the synthesis of these prostaglandins (Robinson, 1983). However, since stable prostaglandins are both pro- and anti-inflammatory (Weissman, 1985), further definition of the mechanism of action is needed.

Other possible mechanisms include modulation of T-cell function, inhibition of chemotaxis of inflammatory cells, stabilization of lysosomal membranes, and decreased release of superoxide radicals or increased scavenging of these compounds at the site of inflammation (Bhalla and Simon, 1984).

Pharmacokinetics: All nonsteroidal anti- inflammatory drugs are absorbed rapidly after oral administration. When taken with food, the rate and sometimes the extent of absorption are decreased. The onset of analgesic effects generally occurs within one hour and time to peak serum concentration ranges from 0.5 to 5 hours (Porter, 1984). The antirheumatic action may not be apparent for one to two weeks and time to peak effect varies from one to four weeks.

Plasma concentrations of all of the nonsteroidal anti-inflammatory drugs except aspirin and naproxen correlate poorly with therapeutic efficacy. Plasma salicylate concentrations of 20 to 30 mg/dl correlate well with anti-inflammatory activity.

Except for salicylates, these drugs are tightly bound to plasma proteins, especially albumin. This extensive binding increases the likelihood of drug interactions with concomitant administration of anticoagulants or oral hypoglycemic agents, which also are extensively bound to plasma proteins.

The liver is the major site for metabolism of the nonsteroidal anti-inflammatory drugs. The major pathway for excretion is the kidney, although significant amounts of most of these drugs are excreted in the feces.

The elimination half-lives vary greatly; the longest is that of piroxicam, which ranges from 37 to 86 hours (Lipman, 1982; Porter, 1984). The frequency of administration necessary to achieve anti-inflammatory activity can affect compliance. For example, studies have demonstrated that compliance is poor (40% to 57.5%) in arthritic patients treated with multiple doses of nonsteroidal anti-inflammatory drugs. Some of the newer

nonsteroidal anti-inflammatory drugs and timed-release forms of the older drugs require less frequent administration. Piroxicam is unique in this respect since it requires administration only once daily. Choline magnesium trisalicylate can be given once or twice daily, and naproxen and sulindac can be given twice daily. Diflunisal also may be administered twice daily, although it is more useful in osteoarthritis and other painful states than in rheumatoid arthritis (Bhalla and Simon, 1984). The timed-release preparation of indomethacin sustains therapeutic drug concentrations for up to 12 hours. Aspirin can sometimes be given two or three times daily, especially in timed-release preparations.

Adverse Reactions: The use of the nonsteroidal anti-inflammatory drugs has been associated with a broad spectrum of adverse reactions. The prolonged administration of large doses of these drugs, as in rheumatic disease, enhances the probability and potential severity of reactions. Indeed, the nonsteroidal anti-inflammatory drugs account for approximately one-third of all adverse reactions reported to the Food and Drug Administration. Although this can be construed only as a direct measure of rate of reporting resulting from their widespread use rather than rate of occurrence, it does emphasize the importance of careful patient monitoring, especially in the elderly.

The most frequent or severe adverse reactions are dermatologic, gastrointestinal, renal, hepatic, hematologic, and immunologic in nature. Although all nonsteroidal anti-inflammatory drugs have been associated with such reactions, there are differences that often provide the basis for drug selection.

Central nervous system reactions have been observed with all the nonsteroidal anti-inflammatory drugs and include dizziness, lightheadedness, drowsiness, headache, and confusion. Indomethacin, diflunisal, fenoprofen, and piroxicam are most likely to produce such effects (Rainsford, 1984). Indomethacin causes headache in more than 10% of patients. Behavioral disturbances, such as depersonalization and depression, have been reported occasionally with this drug.

Dermatologic reactions also are common with the use of nonsteroidal anti-inflammatory drugs. Cited frequencies vary (Rainsford, 1984; Stern and Bigby, 1984); however, tolmetin, sulindac, and piroxicam commonly cause dermatologic reactions. Urticaria, exanthema, photosensitivity, and pruritus are reported most often. Toxic epidermal necrolysis and erythema multiforme have occurred. Rarely, skin rash may presage an anaphylactic reaction, which has been noted in a very small percentage of patients taking aspirin and in smaller percentages taking other nonsteroidal drugs.

Gastrointestinal disturbances are the most common side effects of these drugs. Such reactions include nausea, vomiting, dyspepsia, epigastric pain, diarrhea, constipation, bleeding, and ulceration with bleeding. A majority of the ulcers occurring in treated arthritic patients are gastric; in contrast, in the general population, only one-twentieth of ulcers are gastric (Silvoso et al, 1979; Caruso et al, 1980). Fatalities from gastrointestinal bleeding or hemorrhage with ulceration have been reported.

Aspirin, piroxicam, and indomethacin frequently produce gastrointestinal toxicity, including life-threatening reactions. A

Drug	Chemical Class	Uses*	Initial Drug or Drug of Choice	Number of Daily Doses
Aspirin	Salicylate	RA, OA, JA,	RA, OA, JA	3–4
Diflunisal	Salicylate	RA, OA		2
Fenoprofen	Propionic acid derivative	RA, OA, AS, PA, RS		3–4
Ibuprofen	Propionic acid derivative	RA, OA, AS, PA, RS		3–4
Indomethacin	Pyrrole acetic acid derivative	RA, OA, AS, PA, RS	AS, RS	2–3
Ketoprofen	Propionic acid derivative	RA, OA		3–4
Meclofenamate	Anthranilic acid derivative	RA, OA		3–4
Naproxen	Propionic acid derivative	RA, OA, JA, AS, PA, RS		2
Phenylbutazone	Pyrazolon	AS, RS, RA		3–4
Piroxicam	Oxicam	RA, OA, AS		1–2
Nonacetylated Salicylates Choline, magnesium or sodium salicylate	Salicylate	RA, OA, JA, AS, PA, RS	RA, OA	varies with preparation
Choline magnesium trisalicylate				
Salsalate				
Sulindac	Pyrrole acetic acid derivative	RA, OA, AS, PA, RS		2
Tolmetin	Pyrrole acetic acid derivative	RA, OA, JA, AS, PA, RS		3–4

*Rheumatoid arthritis (RA), osteoarthritis (OA), juvenile arthritis (JA), ankylosing spondylitis (AS), psoriatic arthritis (PA), Reiter's syndrome (RS)

particularly high incidence of diarrhea has been associated with use of meclofenamate. The nonacetylated salicylates, naproxen, and ibuprofen appear to be less damaging to the gastrointestinal system than the other nonsteroidal compounds. The gastrointestinal toxicity of sulindac is due to systemic blockade of prostaglandins rather than toxicity, since this is a prodrug requiring conversion by the liver to the active metabolite. Such molecular manipulation has not spared the drug the toxicity of other nonsteroidal anti-inflammatory drugs, however.

The effects of nonsteroidal anti-inflammatory drugs on *renal function* are mediated by inhibition of prostaglandin synthesis. In normal individuals, prostaglandins do not appear to affect renal function (Robinson, 1983). Thus, nonsteroidal anti-inflammatory drug therapy should not pose an excessive risk in such patients. Indeed, an epidemiologic study (Fox and Jick, 1984) indicated that the association of these drugs with renal toxicity was "rare." However, caution is warranted in patients at risk of compromised renal function, in whom prostaglandins are important in maintaining renal blood flow. Factors that

Potential Serious Adverse Reactions	Interaction with Anticoagulants	Relative Contraindications
GI, Hypersensitivity, Hearing loss	Definite	Upper GI disease, hypersensitivity to aspirin, bleeding disorders, renal dysfunction, liver dysfunction, pregnancy
GI	Possible	Upper GI disease, hypersensitivity to aspirin, renal dysfunction, pregnancy
GI, Renal	Possible	Upper GI disease, hypersensitivity to aspirin, renal dysfunction, pregnancy
GI	Unlikely	Upper GI disease, hypersensitivity to aspirin, renal dysfunction
GI, Edema	Possible	Upper GI disease, hypersensitivity to aspirin, renal dysfunction, cardiac disease, hypertension, proctitis, rectal bleeding, pregnancy, nursing
GI	Possible	Upper GI disease, hypersensitivity to aspirin, renal dysfunction
GI	Definite	Upper GI disease, hypersensitivity to aspirin, renal dysfunction, pregnancy
GI	Unlikely	Upper GI disease, hypersensitivity to aspirin, renal dysfunction
Hematologic, GI, Edema	Definite	Upper GI disease, bleeding disorders, hepatic dysfunction, renal or cardiac disease, drug allergy, pancreatitis, parotitis, stomatitis, temporal arteritis, polymyalgia rheumatica, pregnancy, nursing, children
GI	Possible	Upper GI disease, hypersensitivity to aspirin, renal dysfunction, cardiac disease, hypertension, pregnancy
GI	Possible	Upper GI disease, hypersensitivity to nonacetylated salicylates, renal dysfunction, pregnancy
GI	Unlikely	Upper GI disease, hypersensitivity to aspirin, renal dysfunction, pregnancy
GI	Unlikely	Upper GI disease, hypersensitivity to aspirin, renal dysfunction, bleeding disorders, pregnancy

predispose patients to drug-induced renal insufficiency include advanced age, renal dysfunction, atherosclerosis, hepatic cirrhosis, concurrent diuretic therapy, and acute gouty arthritis (Robinson, 1983; Blackshear et al, 1985).

Renal reactions induced by nonsteroidal anti-inflammatory drugs are manifested as renal insufficiency, nephrotic syndrome with interstitial nephritis, hyperkalemia, hyponatremia, and papillary necrosis. Renal insufficiency has been estimated to occur in 20% of predisposed patients (see above). Nephrotic syndrome with interstitial nephritis is rare but has been reported with increasing frequency in recent years, especially with use of fenoprofen (O'Brien, 1983). These renal complications improve if the offending agent is discontinued early.

All nonsteroidal anti-inflammatory drugs can impair renal function in patients at risk. Fenoprofen is most commonly associated with such adverse effects. Indomethacin and phenylbutazone have produced significant edema, especially in the extremities. It has been suggested that sulindac may have a renal-sparing effect (Bunning and Barth, 1982). That the renal-sparing effect of sulindac might result from its failure to inhibit renal prostaglandin synthesis has not been borne out (Svendsen et al, 1984). In one study, renal prostaglandin synthesis was inhibited in nine of ten patients with rheumatoid arthritis and congestive heart failure who received sulindac 400 mg daily. This effect was reversed after four weeks, suggesting the need for further study.

Hepatic dysfunction caused by nonsteroidal anti-inflammatory drugs occurs occasionally and usually is mild. Drug-related abnormalities in liver function tests (elevated levels of transaminase, alkaline phosphatase, and total bilirubin) are not uncommon, but irreversible hepatic damage is rare (Paulus, 1982). Abnormal results of liver function tests have been produced most frequently by aspirin, especially in patients with juvenile rheumatoid arthritis and systemic lupus erythematosus (Robinson, 1983). Serious hepatic effects have been reported rarely for almost all nonsteroidal anti-inflammatory drugs. Predisposing factors include advanced age, impaired renal function, large doses, and prolonged therapy (Paulus, 1982).

Serious *hematologic reactions* are rare. All of these agents inhibit platelet aggregation, but only aspirin's effect is irreversible. Aplastic anemia, agranulocytosis, and related blood dyscrasias have been reported rarely. Phenylbutazone has the greatest propensity to produce these potentially fatal reactions; the mortality rate is estimated to be 2.2/100,000 patients (Hart and Huskisson, 1984).

Hypersensitivity reactions generally are manifested by dermatologic effects or by difficulty in breathing. Aspirin causes anaphylactic reactions characterized by bronchospasm and dyspnea, sweating, sudden weakness, fainting, and collapse. Estimates of the incidence of these side effects vary between 0.001% and 0.02% of the general population (Rainsford, 1984). Generally, cross-sensitivity to other nonsteroidal anti-inflammatory drugs and the yellow food dye, tartrazine, occurs. Asthma, hay fever, and nasal polyps are predictive of a predisposition to these allergic reactions.

Miscellaneous side effects reported with the nonsteroidal anti-inflammatory drugs include tinnitus, hearing loss, blurred vision, taste dysfunction, tachycardia, palpitations, and esophageal stricture. See evaluations for more specific information.

Precautions: Considering the widespread utilization of nonsteroidal anti-inflammatory drugs and the chronic conditions for which they are used, this class of drugs is relatively safe. Awareness of adverse reactions and adherence to precautions minimize the potential for many adverse effects.

Ingestion with milk or food or after meals can reduce gastrointestinal discomfort. When the patient has a history of or active peptic ulcer, the benefits of a nonsteroidal drug must be weighed carefully against the risks. Naproxen, ibuprofen, and the nonacetylated salicylates are less toxic to the gastrointestinal tract than other nonsteroidal anti-inflammatory drugs.

Patients with atherosclerosis, hepatic cirrhosis (especially if ascites is present), or renal insufficiency and those receiving diuretic therapy concurrently require close monitoring. Additionally, the elderly usually have reduced renal function and should be monitored. In patients at risk, the BUN and creatinine levels should be determined at the initiation of therapy and the tests should be repeated at regular intervals during prolonged therapy (Bhalla and Simon, 1984). Proteinuria, hematuria, and cells and casts in the urine are important early signals of compromised renal function (Roth, 1984). Consideration should be given to reducing the dose in patients at risk.

Precautions should be taken to avoid hepatic toxicity (Paulus, 1982). The SGPT appears to be the most sensitive indicator of liver function. Patients with signs or symptoms suggesting liver impairment should be evaluated further. If abnormal test results persist or worsen or if signs and symptoms of liver disease develop, the drug should be discontinued.

Because the nonsteroidal anti-inflammatory drugs impair platelet aggregation and prolong bleeding time, they should be used cautiously in patients with bleeding disorders. The presence of a bleeding disorder is a relative contraindication to the use of aspirin. Furthermore, aspirin should be discontinued several days prior to surgery; other nonsteroidal drugs need not be stopped until 24 to 48 hours before surgery (Bhalla and Simon, 1984). Serious consideration should be given to the potential for severe hematologic reactions, especially in the elderly, when use of phenylbutazone is being considered.

The occurrence of a hypersensitivity reaction to a nonsteroidal anti-inflammatory drug is a contraindication to subsequent use, and it is likely that patients sensitive to one nonsteroidal agent will be sensitive to others. Patients with nasal polyps, asthma, urticaria, or hay fever should be given these drugs only with great care and only when absolutely necessary (Bhalla and Simon, 1984).

Tinnitus and hearing loss require reduction of the dose of any nonsteroidal anti-inflammatory drug.

Chronic administration of aspirin during pregnancy may be associated with prolonged gestation, longer labor, greater blood loss at delivery, and antepartum and postpartum hemorrhage. In addition, premature closure of patent ductus arteriosus may occur with the use of indomethacin and probably other nonsteroidal anti-inflammatory drugs (Thurnau, 1983). Thus, nonsteroidal anti-inflammatory drugs should be discontinued during pregnancy, if possible. If their use is essential, the lowest effective dose should be utilized and treatment should be discontinued several days (aspirin) or one to two days before delivery. Use of this class of drugs in nursing mothers should be avoided.

Drug Interactions: Concomitant administration of nonsteroidal anti-inflammatory drugs and anticoagulants can produce significant adverse effects. The actions of anticoagulants may be enhanced by their displacement from plasma protein binding sites, increased prothrombin times, or inhibition of metabolism. Thus, the concurrent administration of aspirin, phenylbutazone (Verbeeck et al, 1983), or indomethacin should be avoided. Ibuprofen, naproxen, tolmetin, and sulindac can be used with anticoagulants if appropriate precautions are taken, including measurement of prothrombin time daily for the first five days of combined therapy (Rodnan et al, 1983).

The hypoglycemic effect of the sulfonylureas may be enhanced by coadministration of salicylates or phenylbutazone. Displacement from plasma protein binding sites and inhibition of renal tubular secretion are the postulated mechanisms with salicylates. Displacement from binding sites and inhibition of degradative metabolism may account for the interaction with phenylbutazone. Moderate to large doses of these drugs should be given cautiously to patients receiving oral hypoglycemic agents.

Antacids may alter the absorption and sometimes the disposition of a nonsteroidal anti-inflammatory drug. Aspirin prolongs the half-life of penicillin G, increases the activity of methotrexate, and inhibits the uricosuric effect of sulfinpyrazone [Anturane]. Indomethacin inhibits the diuretic effect of furosemide [Lasix].

The use of two nonsteroidal anti-inflammatory drugs together confers no additional benefit over the use of an individual agent. Exceptions may include the addition of small doses of salicylates to a longer acting nonsteroidal agent for additional analgesic activity (Roth, 1984) and the use of one drug for daytime treatment and another at bedtime to relieve morning pain and stiffness.

The coadministration of ketoprofen with methotrexate has been reported to prolong and increase serum methotrexate concentrations (Thyss et al, 1986). In three of four patients observed with such increased concentrations, severe methotrexate toxicity resulted in death. It remains to be determined whether these interactions of ketoprofen and methotrexate also occur with other nonsteroidal anti-inflammatory drugs.

Drug Evaluations

SALICYLATES

USES. The salicylates have a long history of efficacy in relieving pain and stiffness and improving routine task performance in arthropathies. Of the salicylates, aspirin is the drug of choice in active rheumatoid arthritis, juvenile arthritis, and osteoarthritis. It is not as effective in ankylosing spondylitis, Reiter's syndrome, or psoriatic arthritis.

Aspirin is used primarily for its anti-inflammatory effect in rheumatoid arthritis and must be administered in maximally tolerated doses; smaller doses may be adequate in osteoarthritis. If it cannot be tolerated because of gastrointestinal disturbances, enteric-coated preparations, the suppository form, or another salicylate may be tried. Comparative data are limited, although it has been shown that blood salicylate levels are comparable for the different preparations. If salicylates are not tolerated or effective, another nonsteroidal agent should be tried.

ADVERSE REACTIONS, PRECAUTIONS, AND INTERACTIONS. Gastrointestinal disturbances are the most common adverse reactions. Nausea, vomiting, and gastric distress occur in 10% to 30% of patients receiving large doses of aspirin; taking the drug with food decreases the likelihood of such reactions. Occult bleeding occurs in about 70% of patients receiving plain or buffered aspirin; 2 to 6 ml of blood may be lost daily, but losses of up to 10 ml daily may occur and result in iron deficiency anemia. There appears to be no correlation between the incidence of gastric distress and occult bleeding. Blood loss is not decreased by the simultaneous ingestion of food. Nonacetylated salicylates, such as choline salicylate, choline magnesium trisalicylate, and salsalate (salicylsalicylic acid), cause less gastrointestinal bleeding with comparable blood levels than plain or buffered aspirin. The prevalence of gastric ulcers and erosions is lower with nonacetylated salicylates and possibly enteric-coated and matrix-release preparations than with uncoated or buffered aspirin. Thus, these preparations may be preferred for long-term use (Roth, 1984).

The incidence of peptic ulcer is increased in patients with rheumatoid arthritis who take aspirin for prolonged periods, and this drug may activate ulcer and precipitate massive hemorrhage. Therefore, an active ulcer is a relative contraindication to administration of aspirin; a nonacetylated salicylate may be safer. The risk of gastric ulceration is increased when alcohol and aspirin are taken concomitantly.

Tinnitus and hearing loss are the most common initial signs of toxicity (salicylism) in adults and may be used to determine the maximal acceptable daily dose. However, they are not a reliable indication of toxicity in some elderly patients, who may not develop tinnitus even with large doses, or in children. Signs of overdosage in children include hyperventilation with acidosis, increased metabolic rate, and disturbances in carbohydrate and lipid metabolism; the earliest symptoms may be lethargy and episodic hyperpnea. When initiating therapy, the dosage for children and elderly patients should be increased gradually and cautiously, and these patients should be observed closely for early signs of ototoxicity.

A very small percentage of patients are hypersensitive to aspirin and may develop rash or an asthmatic-type anaphylactic reaction, which can be life-threatening. The incidence of these reactions is highest in those with asthma, hay fever, or nasal polyps. Hypersensitive patients should avoid aspirin or aspirin-containing products, as well as preparations containing the yellow dye, tartrazine, because of cross sensitivity. Some patients sensitive to aspirin also are sensitive to other nonsteroidal anti-inflammatory agents that inhibit prostaglandin synthesis; however, asthmatic-type reactions have not been associated with sodium or magnesium salicylates.

Large doses of salicylates prolong prothrombin time, but this effect is clinically insignificant. Since aspirin (but not sodium salicylate or other nonacetylated salicylates) inhibits platelet aggregation irreversibly and prolongs bleeding time, it should be avoided in patients receiving heparin or coumarin anticoagulants and in those with severe liver disease or bleeding disorders (eg, hemophilia). Abnormal results of liver function studies are common in children with juvenile arthritis receiving prolonged aspirin therapy and in adults with systemic lupus erythematosus. Hepatic effects are reversible upon discontinuation of the drug.

Aspirin temporarily decreases renal function, most commonly in patients with renal disease. The uricosuric effect of probenecid and sulfinpyrazone is diminished by the salicylates. Since the renal clearance of salicylates is increased by corticosteroids, toxicity may occur when corticosteroids are discontinued in patients receiving large doses of salicylates concomitantly. The use of aspirin with another nonsteroidal anti-inflammatory drug may produce a drug interaction (see evaluations).

Patients on a sodium-restricted diet should not be given sodium salicylate. Individuals with renal insufficiency may develop hypermagnesemia after use of magnesium salicylate. Salsalate is the "pure" salicylate. Its double salicylate moiety only uncouples in the alkaline medium of the bowel. Thus, it bypasses a potentially troubled upper gastrointestinal tract and qualifies as the only prodrug of the salicylate series (Roth, 1985).

For additional information on adverse reactions and interactions, see Chapter 4, General Analgesics.

PHARMACOKINETICS. The pharmacokinetics of salicylates are complex. The half-life increases with dosage so that an increase in dose may produce a disproportionate increase in plasma drug levels. There is considerable individual variation in metabolism (Levy, 1979). See also Chapter 4.

DOSAGE AND PREPARATIONS. The dose should be individualized and adjusted to the amount that produces an adequate anti-inflammatory effect. Blood salicylate levels and therapeutic effect do not correlate well with dose, but a plasma concentration greater than 15 mg/dl is usually required for efficacy; levels above 30 mg/dl are frequently toxic. If there is any uncertainty about the adequacy of dosage, toxicity, or patient compliance, plasma salicylate concentrations should be determined.

Oral, Rectal: *Adults,* for rheumatoid arthritis, 3.6 to 5.4 g of aspirin or the equivalent salicylate daily in divided doses. For osteoarthritis, doses usually can be reduced. For juvenile arthritis of pauciarticular or polyarticular onset, *children weighing 25 kg or less,* up to 120 mg/kg daily; *children weighing more than 25 kg,* 2.4 to 3.6 g daily. Those with systemic (acute febrile) onset may require larger doses. Since these doses may be toxic, it is usually advisable to start with two-thirds of the anticipated optimal dose and increase this amount gradually to the maximally tolerated dose.

Administration with meals reduces gastrointestinal disturbances. Milk or a small meal at bedtime delays absorption and prolongs the therapeutic effect to allay morning stiffness. Alternatively, a larger dose may be given at bedtime or enteric-coated preparations may be used.

ASPIRIN:
NOTE: Because most manufacturers express dosage sizes of aspirin in grains rather than milligrams, the grain sizes with approximate milligram equivalents are given.
Generic. Tablets 5, 7 1/2, and 10 gr (325, 500, and 650 mg); tablets (buffered) 5 gr (325 mg); tablets (enteric-coated) 5 and 10 gr (325 and 650 mg); suppositories 1, 2, 3, 5, 10, and 20 gr (60, 130, 195, 325, and 650 mg and 1.2 g) (all forms nonprescription).
Available Trademarks.
Arthritis Pain Formula (Whitehall). Tablets 487.5 mg with calcium carbonate, magnesium oxide, and magnesium carbonate (nonprescription).
Ascriptin (Rorer). Tablets 325 mg with magnesium and aluminum hydroxide 75 mg or 150 mg (*Ascriptin A/D*) (nonprescription).
Bufferin (Bristol-Myers). Tablets 324 mg with magnesium carbonate 97.2 mg and aluminum glycinate 48.6 mg (nonprescription).
Cama (Dorsey). Tablets 500 mg with magnesium oxide 150 mg and aluminum hydroxide 150 mg (nonprescription).
Easprin (Parke-Davis). Tablets (enteric-coated) 975 mg.
Ecotrin (Menley & James). Tablets (enteric-coated) 325 and 500 mg (nonprescription).

Measurin (Winthrop-Breon). Tablets (timed-release) 650 mg (nonprescription).
Zorprin (Boots). Tablets (timed-release) 800 mg.
SODIUM SALICYLATE:
Generic. Tablets (plain, enteric-coated) 325 and 650 mg (nonprescription).
CHOLINE SALICYLATE:
Arthropan (Purdue Frederick). Each 5 ml of liquid is equivalent in salicylate content to 650 mg of aspirin (nonprescription).
CHOLINE MAGNESIUM TRISALICYLATE:
Trilisate (Purdue Frederick). Each tablet contains choline salicylate 293, 440, or 587 mg and magnesium salicylate 362, 544, or 725 mg to provide 500, 750, or 1,000 mg of salicylate; each 5 ml of liquid contains choline salicylate 293 mg and magnesium salicylate 362 mg to provide 500 mg of salicylate.
MAGNESIUM SALICYLATE:
Magan (Adria). Tablets 545 mg.
Mobidin (Ascher). Tablets 600 mg.
SALSALATE (Salicylsalicylic Acid):
Disalcid (Riker). Capsules 500 mg; tablets 500 and 750 mg.

DIFLUNISAL
[Dolobid]

ACTIONS AND USES. Diflunisal is a fluoridated salicylic acid derivative. Like aspirin, it has analgesic, anti-inflammatory, and antipyretic activities and inhibits prostaglandin synthesis. This peripherally acting, nonopioid analgesic has a long duration of action.

Diflunisal is effective in the symptomatic treatment of osteoarthritis and rheumatoid arthritis. Comparative studies showed that diflunisal 500 to 750 mg daily was as effective as aspirin 2 to 3 g, ibuprofen 800 mg to 1.2 g (Umbenhauer, 1983), and the timed-release preparation of indomethacin (Gordin et al, 1984).

For other uses, see Chapter 4, General Analgesics.

ADVERSE REACTIONS AND PRECAUTIONS. Diflunisal is generally well tolerated. In clinical trials, the overall incidence of gastrointestinal reactions, dizziness, edema, and tinnitus was lower than with aspirin. Gastrointestinal disturbances are most common; the incidence of nausea, pain, dyspepsia, and diarrhea is 3% to 9%. Fecal blood loss was significantly lower than with aspirin in one clinical study (Rider, 1983). However, peptic ulcer and bleeding have been reported. Diflunisal inhibits platelet function to a lesser degree than aspirin and the inhibition is reversible. Acute renal failure and Stevens-Johnson syndrome have been reported. Cross sensitivity may occur in patients sensitive to aspirin.

Other adverse reactions are similar to those of the nonsteroidal anti-inflammatory drugs in general. Diflunisal is classified in FDA Pregnancy Category C.

For additional uses, adverse reactions, and precautions, see the Introduction and Chapter 4, General Analgesics.

OVERDOSE. Overdose (more than 15 g) has resulted in hyperventilation, tachycardia, sweating, and cardiopulmonary arrest. When used alone, the lowest dose of diflunisal at which a death has been reported was 15 g. In a mixed-drug overdose, ingestion of 7.5 g of diflunisal resulted in death. Gastric lavage and general supportive care should be provided. The effectiveness of forced diuresis or forced alkaline diuresis has not been established (Court and Volans, 1984).

DRUG INTERACTIONS. Diflunisal displaces anticoagulants from plasma protein binding sites, resulting in prolonged prothrombin time. Concurrent administration of diflunisal and indomethacin has been associated with fatal gastrointestinal hemorrhage; therefore, these two drugs should not be given together. Diflunisal decreases the hyperuricemic effect of furosemide and hydrochlorothiazide. Diflunisal has no effect on the diuretic activity of furosemide, but it significantly increased levels of hydrochlorothiazide. Concomitant administration of aluminum hydroxide reduces the extent of absorption of diflunisal. Diflunisal increases the plasma concentration of acetaminophen.

PHARMACOKINETICS. Diflunisal is rapidly absorbed after oral administration with peak plasma concentrations occurring one to three hours after ingestion (Verbeeck et al, 1983; Davies, 1983). Diflunisal exhibits dose-dependent kinetics; the elimination half-life ranges from 5 to 20 hours. Ingestion every 12 hours produces steady-state plasma levels within three to nine days.

DOSAGE AND PREPARATIONS.

Oral: *Adults,* for osteoarthritis, 500 mg to 1 g daily in two divided doses. Dosage may be increased or decreased according to the patient's response. Maintenance doses should not exceed 1.5 g daily. For rheumatoid arthritis, 1 g daily in two divided doses has been used in clinical trials.

   Dolobid (Merck Sharp & Dohme). Tablets 250 and 500 mg.

FENOPROFEN CALCIUM
  [Nalfon]

ACTIONS AND USES. Like aspirin, this phenylpropionic acid derivative has anti-inflammatory, analgesic, and antipyretic properties and inhibits prostaglandin synthesis, but the influence of this action on clinical effects is not known.

Fenoprofen is effective as initial therapy or as an alternative to aspirin in rheumatoid arthritis and osteoarthritis. Results of comparative studies in patients with rheumatoid arthritis indicated that fenoprofen 2.4 g daily was approximately equivalent to aspirin 3.9 g daily and, in one study, was superior to sulindac 400 mg (Durance et al, 1979).

In osteoarthritis, the benefit of fenoprofen 1.2 to 1.8 g daily was similar to that obtained with aspirin 2 to 3 g, and 2 g of fenoprofen and was comparable to 300 mg of phenylbutazone. Fenoprofen 1.2 g was more efficacious than sulindac 400 mg in one study (Thompson et al, 1979).

Fenoprofen relieved symptoms in a few patients with anky-losing spondylitis, but additional studies are needed to establish its comparative efficacy in this condition. Fenoprofen may prove useful as alternative therapy in psoriatic arthritis and Reiter's syndrome.

ADVERSE REACTIONS AND PRECAUTIONS. The most common adverse reactions are gastrointestinal disturbances (eg, dyspepsia, constipation, nausea, vomiting). These reactions occur less frequently with fenoprofen than with aspirin. The amount of gastrointestinal bleeding also is less than with aspirin. However, since a few cases of ulceration have been observed, fenoprofen should be used with caution in patients with a history of peptic ulcer.

Central nervous system reactions include drowsiness, dizziness, headache, nervousness, and confusion. Pruritus, rash, sweating, palpitations, tremor, tinnitus, blurred vision, and decreased hearing, as well as sensitivity to the drug, have been reported.

Fenoprofen has produced nephrotic syndrome with interstitial nephritis. Periodic renal function tests should be performed in patients at risk.

Elevations of serum transaminase, lactic dehydrogenase, and alkaline phosphatase levels have been observed in some patients. Fenoprofen reduces platelet aggregation and adhesiveness and increases bleeding time. Thrombocytopenia, agranulocytosis, and aplastic anemia have been reported rarely. Therefore, this drug should be used very cautiously in patients with bleeding disorders and in those receiving anticoagulants.

Because of the potential for cross sensitivity, fenoprofen should not be given to patients who experience symptoms of asthma, rhinitis, or urticaria when given aspirin and other nonsteroidal anti-inflammatory drugs.

This drug is classified in FDA Pregnancy Category B.

OVERDOSE. Overdosage (0.3 to 3 g in children, 2 to 15 g in adults) with fenoprofen is rare and symptoms usually are mild. Manifestations include hypotension, tachycardia, and difficulty in breathing. Two cases of severe toxicity have been reported. Gastric lavage, activated charcoal, and a cathartic produced a favorable response in one patient. In the other, hypothermia, coma, and respiratory depression culminated in fatal cardiac arrest (Court and Volans, 1984).

DRUG INTERACTIONS. Fenoprofen may displace anticoagulants or oral hypoglycemic agents from plasma binding sites, thus increasing their activity. If concurrent use is necessary, patients should be observed closely. Aspirin enhances the metabolic clearance of fenoprofen, thus reducing plasma concentrations of the drug.

PHARMACOKINETICS. Fenoprofen is rapidly absorbed after oral administration, and peak plasma levels occur within 90 minutes. The plasma half-life is about 160 minutes and does not appear to be dose dependent. Absorption and availability are not affected by the concomitant administration of an antacid (aluminum and magnesium hydroxides).

Fenoprofen is metabolized and excreted almost exclusively in the urine in conjugated form. The drug is highly bound to plasma protein and may displace other protein-bound drugs from their binding sites, resulting in drug interactions.

DOSAGE AND PREPARATIONS.

Oral: Adults, for rheumatoid arthritis or osteoarthritis, 300 to 600 mg three or four times daily. Total daily dosage should not exceed 3.2 g. After a satisfactory response is obtained, the dose is adjusted to the patient's needs. If gastrointestinal reactions occur, fenoprofen may be given with meals or milk. Dosage for *children* has not been established.

    Nalfon (Dista). Capsules 200 and 300 mg; tablets 600 mg (strengths expressed in terms of the base).

IBUPROFEN
[Motrin, Rufen]

ACTIONS AND USES. Ibuprofen is a phenylpropionic acid derivative with analgesic, anti-inflammatory, and antipyretic actions. Like aspirin and other nonsteroidal anti-inflammatory drugs, it inhibits prostaglandin synthesis. Ibuprofen is effective for the symptomatic treatment of rheumatoid arthritis and osteoarthritis and has been reported to be useful in ankylosing spondylitis and psoriatic arthritis. It also may be useful as an alternative agent in Reiter's syndrome.

In rheumatoid arthritis, ibuprofen is as effective as aspirin, piroxicam, indomethacin, and tolmetin. Ibuprofen may be administered with maintenance doses of gold salts for additional symptomatic relief; it also may be given with corticosteroids.

In osteoarthritis, therapeutic doses of ibuprofen are as effective as aspirin, aspirin and acetaminophen, sulindac, and indomethacin.

ADVERSE REACTIONS AND PRECAUTIONS. The overall incidence of adverse reactions is low, and ibuprofen appears to be one of the better tolerated nonsteroidal anti-inflammatory drugs. The most common reactions are nausea and vomiting; diarrhea, constipation, heartburn, and epigastric pain occur less frequently. In studies designed to measure gastrointestinal bleeding, patients receiving ibuprofen for as long as one year experienced less gastrointestinal bleeding than those receiving aspirin. Nevertheless, severe, sometimes fatal, gastrointestinal bleeding has occurred, but a cause-and-effect relationship has not been established. Thus, those with an active ulcer or a history of such ulcers should be monitored carefully when taking ibuprofen.

Central nervous system reactions reported occasionally include dizziness, lightheadedness, and headache. Maculopapular, erythematous, or urticarial rashes and generalized pruritus also have occurred.

Toxic amblyopia, characterized by reduced visual acuity and difficulty in color discrimination, has been observed in a few patients. Although a definite cause-and-effect relationship was not established, the symptoms disappeared after ibuprofen was discontinued. Ophthalmologic examination of numerous patients did not reveal similar visual disturbances. Nevertheless, patients receiving ibuprofen should have a complete ophthalmologic examination if they experience any visual disturbances.

Meaningful (three times the upper limit of normal) elevations of serum transaminases (SGPT or SGOT) occurred in less than 1% of patients in controlled clinical trials. Severe hepatic reactions, including jaundice and fatal hepatitis, have been reported. Hyperuricemia also has occurred sporadically.

Fluid retention and edema have been reported; therefore, ibuprofen should be used with caution in patients with a history of cardiac decompensation. Acute renal failure has been reported in patients with significantly compromised renal function. Thus, the drug should be used cautiously in patients with impaired renal function and careful monitoring is necessary.

Ibuprofen inhibits platelet aggregation less than aspirin or indomethacin. A slight, probably clinically insignificant, decrease in hemoglobin and hematocrit values has been observed. Lymphopenia, agranulocytosis, and hemolytic anemia have been reported rarely.

Since cross sensitivity may occur, ibuprofen should not be used in patients known to be hypersensitive to aspirin or other nonsteroidal anti-inflammatory drugs and in those with nasal polyps, angioedema, and bronchospastic reactions to aspirin. Hypersensitivity reactions (eg, fever, rash, nausea, vomiting, abdominal pain, hypotension) and increased serum transaminase levels have been reported in several patients with systemic lupus erythematosus receiving ibuprofen.

There is no evidence that ibuprofen has any teratogenic effect in rabbits and rats. However, since this agent was found in the fetal circulation of animals after administration to the mothers during late pregnancy, it appears to cross the placenta. This drug is classified in FDA Pregnancy Category B. Ibuprofen was not detectable in the breast milk of mothers taking 2 g daily (Townsend et al, 1984).

OVERDOSE. More than 100 cases of overdosage have been reported; the estimated intake varied from 1.2 g in children to 16 g in an adult. Symptoms included dizziness, nystagmus, apnea, unconsciousness, and hypotension. All patients recovered with no apparent sequelae. Since no specific antidote is known, standard supportive treatment should be instituted: The stomach should be emptied by induced vomiting or lavage, and urine output should be maintained to ensure excretion of the drug.

DRUG INTERACTIONS. Measurements of clotting function were not affected when doses up to 2.4 g/day of ibuprofen were given to patients receiving warfarin sodium, but larger amounts may displace warfarin from protein binding sites. Ibuprofen may be one of the safer nonsteroidal anti-inflammatory drugs for concurrent use with anticoagulants (Hansten, 1983).

The concomitant administration of single doses of ibuprofen and aspirin had no effect on the availability or elimination of either drug; however, multiple doses of these drugs decreased the blood levels of ibuprofen.

PHARMACOKINETICS. Ibuprofen is rapidly absorbed following oral administration, and peak plasma concentrations occur in one to two hours. When the drug is taken immediately after meals, absorption is delayed but the total amount absorbed is not decreased. The drug is highly bound (99%) to plasma protein. There is no evidence of drug accumulation. Ibuprofen is rapidly eliminated from plasma; the half-life after single or multiple doses is 1.8 to 2.6 hours. This agent is rapidly metabolized by hydroxylation and carboxylation and is excreted in the urine almost exclusively as four inactive metabolites. Excretion is essentially complete within 24 hours.

DOSAGE AND PREPARATIONS.

Oral: Adults, for rheumatoid arthritis and osteoarthritis, including flareups of chronic disease, 1.2 to 3.2 g daily in divided doses. Because of the variability in response, the optimal dose for each patient must be determined individually. Daily dosage should not exceed 3.2 g. The dosage for osteoarthritis may be smaller than that for rheumatoid arthritis. There is insufficient experience with this drug in *children under 14 years* to establish a dose.

    Rufen (Boots), **Generic**. Tablets 400 and 600 mg.
    Motrin (Upjohn). Tablets 300, 400, 600, and 800 mg.

INDOMETHACIN
[Indocin]

ACTIONS AND USES. Indomethacin is a nonsteroidal anti-inflammatory compound of the indole group with analgesic and antipyretic effects. Like aspirin and other nonsteroidal anti-inflammatory drugs, indomethacin inhibits prostaglandin synthesis; other actions (eg, interference with migration of leukocytes, inhibition of phosphodiesterase) may contribute to its anti-inflammatory effect.

Because of its potential to cause severe adverse effects, this agent is not recommended as a simple analgesic or antipyretic. Indomethacin is the drug of choice in the treatment of ankylosing spondylitis and should be considered for initial use in Reiter's syndrome. It also is useful as an anti-inflammatory agent in moderate to severe rheumatoid arthritis and osteoarthritis, particularly of the hands, hips, knees, and shoulders. It may be useful as an alternative agent in the treatment of psoriatic arthritis. The timed-release formulation is comparable to the other formulations in patient tolerance and efficacy and it offers the advantage of once- or twice-daily dosing (Yeh, 1982).

Indomethacin is used to treat attacks of acute gouty arthritis (see Chapter 60, Agents Used in Gout and Hyperuricemia), but the timed-release preparation should not be used for this indication. Indomethacin is effective in bursitis, tendinitis, and traumatic synovitis.

ADVERSE REACTIONS. Gastrointestinal disturbances (nausea, vomiting, abdominal distress, indigestion, epigastric burning, constipation, diarrhea) have been observed in 3% to 9% of patients and may be lessened by giving the drug with food. Less common, but more significant, effects are single or multiple ulcerations of the esophagus, stomach, duodenum, or small intestine; perforation and hemorrhage, sometimes fatal, have been reported. Occult bleeding with secondary anemia may occur in the absence of an ulcer. Other gastrointestinal reactions are anorexia, stomatitis, gastritis, and perforation of pre-existing sigmoid lesions; ulcerative colitis and regional enteritis occur rarely.

The timed-release preparation causes the same frequency of gastrointestinal and other side effects as comparable doses of the immediate-release preparation (Rhymer et al, 1982).

Central nervous system effects (headaches, vertigo, dizziness, somnolence, depression, and fatigue) are common. Headaches occur in more than 10% of patients and are usually severe in the morning; if they persist, treatment should be discontinued. Convulsions, peripheral neuropathy, lightheadedness, syncope, confusion, coma, and behavioral disturbances, such as depersonalization, also have been reported occasionally.

Ocular complications (corneal deposits and retinal disturbances) have been observed after prolonged use of indomethacin. A thorough ophthalmologic examination is required if blurred vision develops. Tinnitus occurs commonly, but deafness is infrequent.

Leukopenia, hemolytic or aplastic anemia, purpura, bone marrow depression, agranulocytosis, and thrombocytopenia are observed rarely during therapy with indomethacin.

Fatalities caused by hepatitis with jaundice have been reported. As with other nonsteroidal anti-inflammatory drugs, liver function tests may be abnormal. If abnormalities persist or worsen or if clinical manifestations of liver disease develop, the drug should be discontinued.

Dermatologic and hypersensitivity reactions (pruritus, urticaria, rash, erythema nodosum, angioedema, angiitis, alopecia, dyspnea, acute respiratory distress, and a rapid fall in blood pressure resembling shock) also may occur.

Indomethacin rarely has caused acute renal failure, but renal dysfunction usually was reversible when the drug was discontinued. Renal function should be assessed periodically in patients with chronic renal disease.

PRECAUTIONS AND CONTRAINDICATIONS. Indomethacin is contraindicated in pregnant women, nursing mothers, infants, and children 14 years of age and under, since safe conditions for use in these patients have not been established. The drug also is contraindicated in patients with active gastrointestinal lesions or a history of recurrent gastrointestinal lesions. Indomethacin should be used with caution in the elderly and in those with epilepsy, parkinsonism, or emotional or psychiatric problems, since it may aggravate these conditions.

OVERDOSE. Overdose (75 to 175 mg in children, 175 to 1,500 mg in adults) is manifested by drowsiness, gastric irritation, nausea, headache, and tinnitus. Sixty-one percent of patients remained asymptomatic after taking up to 2.5 g (Court and Volans, 1984).

DRUG INTERACTIONS. Like aspirin and other nonsteroidal anti-inflammatory agents, indomethacin inhibits platelet aggregation. This effect appears to be related to dose and plasma concentration and is of shorter duration than that produced by aspirin. Indomethacin should be used very cautiously in patients with coagulation defects. If concomitant administration of indomethacin and an anticoagulant is necessary, the patient should be observed for alterations in prothrombin time and the dose of anticoagulant adjusted accordingly.

The administration of aspirin with indomethacin has been reported to decrease the blood level of indomethacin, but other studies have not confirmed this interaction. The concurrent use of these drugs does not generally produce a better therapeutic effect except when a large dose of indomethacin (50 to 100 mg) is given at night in conjunction with aspirin during the day. The significant gastric toxicity of aspirin and indomethacin individually and the potentially serious additive toxicity of the combination should be considered, however.

The plasma levels of indomethacin may be increased by the concomitant administration of probenecid; thus, lower doses of indomethacin may be used in patients receiving both drugs.

Since indomethacin has been reported to reduce the natriuretic and antihypertensive effects of furosemide, patients receiving both drugs should be observed carefully for interactions. The combination of triamterene and indomethacin impaired renal function in healthy subjects (Favre et al, 1982).

Blunting of the antihypertensive effect of beta-blocking agents by nonsteroidal anti-inflammatory drugs, including indomethacin, has been reported. Therefore, when using beta-blocking agents to treat hypertension, patients should be observed carefully to confirm that the desired therapeutic effect is being obtained.

The concomitant administration of indomethacin and lithium caused a clinically relevant increase in lithium plasma concentrations and produced delirium in one patient (Herschberg and Sierles, 1983).

PHARMACOKINETICS. Indomethacin is rapidly and almost completely absorbed after oral administration. About 90% of a dose is bound to plasma proteins. Indomethacin is metabolized in the liver by demethylation, deacetylation, and glucuronide conjugation; the metabolites and unchanged drug are excreted in the bile and urine. About 60% of the dose is recovered in the urine and 33% in the feces.

Absorption is slower when the drug is taken with meals but the extent of absorption is not affected. The half-life of indomethacin is 5 to 10 hours (Helleberg, 1981) but there is marked inter- and intraindividual variation (Verbeeck et al, 1983). This variation is due to extensive enterohepatic recycling through excretion of the glucuronide metabolite in the bile followed by reabsorption of indomethacin after hydrolysis (Yeh, 1982).

Rectal administration reduces times to peak plasma concentration but also decreases peak concentrations. Bioavailability studies on the timed-release preparation (containing 75 mg of the drug, of which 25 mg is released immediately) showed a statistically significant reduction (55%) in peak plasma concentration and significantly less variation in plasma concentrations.

DOSAGE AND PREPARATIONS.
Oral: For ankylosing spondylitis, osteoarthritis, and rheuma-

toid arthritis, *adults,* initially, 25 mg two or three times daily. If well tolerated, the daily dose may be increased by 25 or 50 mg at weekly intervals until a maximum of 150 to 200 mg daily is reached. Some patients may respond in four to six days while others require up to one month of therapy. In acute exacerbations, it may be necessary to increase the daily dose by 25 or 50 mg. After the acute phase is controlled, the daily dose should be reduced until the smallest effective dose is given or the drug can be discontinued.

For painful shoulder (bursitis, tendinitis), 25 mg three or four times daily, usually for 7 to 14 days. After the signs and symptoms of inflammation have been controlled for several days, the drug should be discontinued.

The timed-release preparation [Indocin SR] can be taken once daily to sustain plasma concentrations comparable to those obtained with 25 mg three times a day. In addition, one timed-release capsule taken in the morning and one in the evening were as effective as the conventional 50-mg capsule taken three times a day.

Generic. Capsules 25 and 50 mg.
Indocin (Merck Sharp & Dohme). Capsules 25 and 50 mg; capsules (timed-release) 75 mg (*Indocin SR*).

KETOPROFEN
[Orudis]

ACTIONS AND USES. Ketoprofen is a propionic acid derivative with analgesic, anti-inflammatory, and antipyretic actions. It is effective for the treatment of rheumatoid arthritis and osteoarthritis. As with other nonsteroidal anti-inflammatory drugs, the therapeutic effects of ketoprofen are thought to be mediated, at least in part, by inhibition of prostaglandin synthesis.

ADVERSE REACTIONS AND PRECAUTIONS. The most common adverse reactions are dyspepsia, nausea, vomiting, abdominal pain, headache, dizziness, tinnitus, visual disturbance, rash, and impairment of renal function. Peptic ulceration and gastrointestinal bleeding have been noted in less than 1% of individuals taking ketoprofen. Patients with an active ulcer or a history of gastrointestinal problems who receive ketoprofen should be closely monitored.

Interstitial nephritis and nephrotic syndrome have been associated infrequently with the use of ketoprofen. As with other nonsteroidal anti-inflammatory drugs, ketoprofen may precipitate renal failure, especially in patients with impaired renal function, heart failure, or liver dysfunction; in individuals taking diuretics; and in the elderly. Renal effects are reversible when ketoprofen is discontinued.

Peripheral edema has been observed in approximately 2% of patients taking ketoprofen. Thus, the drug should be used cautiously in patients with fluid retention, hypertension, or heart failure.

Hepatic dysfunction, including serious hepatic reactions

such as jaundice, has been observed in less than 1% of patients taking ketoprofen. Thus, patients with signs or symptoms suggesting hepatic dysfunction and abnormal results of liver function tests should be evaluated for more severe hepatic reactions.

Hypocoagulability, agranulocytosis, anemia, hemolysis, purpura, and thrombocytopenia have been associated with use of ketoprofen. Hemoglobin values should be determined frequently in patients with initial hemoglobin values of 10 g/dl or less who require long-term therapy.

Ketoprofen is contraindicated in hypersensitive patients. Since cross sensitivity may occur, ketoprofen should not be used in patients known to be hypersensitive to aspirin or other nonsteroidal anti-inflammatory drugs.

Studies in rats and rabbits failed to demonstrate any teratogenic effect. However, since studies in animals don't always predict the occurrence of teratogenicity in man, ketoprofen should be used only when the risk justifies the benefit. This drug is classified in FDA Pregnancy Category B. Data on the concentration of ketoprofen in human breast milk are not available, but this drug is not recommended for use in nursing mothers.

OVERDOSE. Only mild symptoms have been observed in the 20 patients who received an overdose of ketoprofen. Vomiting and drowsiness were most prominent in four of these patients. One individual ingested 5 g without sequelae. Since no specific antidote is known, standard supportive measures should be instituted. The stomach should be emptied by induced vomiting or lavage. The drug is dialyzable; therefore, hemodialysis may be useful to remove circulating drug.

DRUG INTERACTIONS. The concomitant administration of ketoprofen and aspirin decreased the protein binding and increased the clearance of ketoprofen from plasma. Although the clinical significance of this interaction has not been established, these two drugs should not be used together.

Patients taking diuretics are at greater risk of developing renal failure, and the addition of ketoprofen to diuretic therapy increases the risk. In patients taking hydrochlorothiazide and ketoprofen, urinary potassium and chloride excretion was reduced compared to hydrochlorothiazide alone.

The concomitant administration of ketoprofen and methotrexate has resulted in severe methotrexate toxicity, including death (Thyss et al, 1986).

PHARMACOKINETICS. Ketoprofen is rapidly absorbed following oral administration; peak plasma concentrations occur in 0.5 to 2 hours. When ketoprofen is taken immediately after meals, its absorption is delayed but the total amount absorbed is not affected. The drug is highly bound (99%) to plasma protein.

The mean elimination half-life is five hours in the normal geriatric population and three hours in younger individuals. About 60% of the drug is excreted in urine primarily as the glucuronide metabolite. Enterohepatic circulation may account for the other 40% absorbed.

DOSAGE AND PREPARATIONS.
Oral: Adults, for rheumatoid arthritis and osteoarthritis, initially, 75 mg three times daily or 50 mg four times daily. Minor side

effects may be relieved by using a lower dose, which may still have an adequate therapeutic effect. If the drug is well tolerated but not maximally effective, the dose may be increased to a maximum of 300 mg daily.

Elderly patients and those with impaired renal function, the dose should be reduced by one-half to one-third.

Orudis (Wyeth). Capsules 50 and 75 mg.

MECLOFENAMATE SODIUM MONOHYDRATE
[Meclomen]

ACTIONS AND USES. This halogenated anthranilic acid derivative is related chemically to the analgesic, mefenamic acid. Both compounds have analgesic, anti-inflammatory, and antipyretic activities, but meclofenamate had a more potent anti-inflammatory effect in animal studies. Like aspirin and other nonsteroidal anti-inflammatory drugs, meclofenamate inhibits prostaglandin synthesis. It also competes for binding at prostaglandin receptor sites. These actions probably have a significant influence on its clinical effects.

In several controlled studies, meclofenamate was effective in the symptomatic treatment of rheumatoid arthritis and osteoarthritis. Meclofenamate 300 mg/day was as effective as aspirin 3.6 g/day in rheumatoid arthritis; in osteoarthritis of the hip or knee, meclofenamate 200 to 300 mg/day was as effective as indomethacin 100 to 150 mg/day (Dresner, 1978). In one study, meclofenamate or aspirin was administered to patients with rheumatoid arthritis who were receiving gold compounds or corticosteroids; results indicated that meclofenamate was as effective as aspirin.

Meclofenamate has been used for one to three years. Although its effectiveness was maintained during this period, approximately 25% of patients discontinued therapy because of adverse reactions (Preston, 1978).

ADVERSE REACTIONS AND PRECAUTIONS. Gastrointestinal reactions were reported most frequently. Diarrhea occurred in 10% to 33% of patients and was severe enough to require discontinuation of treatment in about 4%. This adverse reaction is most likely to occur early in therapy, and is reversible when the dose is reduced or the drug is discontinued.

Nausea with or without vomiting occurred in about 10% and abdominal pain in about 7% of patients. Less common gastrointestinal reactions include pyrosis and flatulence. Symptoms usually can be controlled by reducing the dose or temporarily discontinuing therapy. Gastric or duodenal ulcers were reported occasionally (incidence, 0.9% in double-blind and long-term studies), usually in patients with a history of ulcers; thus, the drug should be used with caution in such patients. Fecal blood loss with meclofenamate 300 or 400 mg/day was less than with aspirin 3.6 g/day.

The incidence of central nervous system reactions, such as headache and dizziness, was less than with indomethacin. The incidence of rashes of various types was about the same as with aspirin (4%).

The hematocrit, hemoglobin, and erythrocyte count decreased in about 10% of patients, but discontinuation of the drug was rarely required. Low white cell counts were observed rarely. The relationship between these changes and administration of the drug is not understood. If anemia is suspected in patients on long-term therapy, hemoglobin and hematocrit values should be determined. In contrast to aspirin, meclofenamate did not prolong bleeding time or reduce collagen-induced platelet aggregation after repeated administration.

Increased serum alkaline phosphatase, transaminase (SGOT, SGPT), creatinine, and blood urea nitrogen levels occurred occasionally but usually returned to normal even when administration of the drug was continued.

Meclofenamate should not be used during pregnancy because there is no experience with its use in pregnant women. Some fetotoxicity, but no major teratogenicity, was observed in animals.

OVERDOSE. Overdose may produce central nervous system stimulation marked by agitation and generalized seizures. Renal toxicity, manifested by oliguria, anuria, or azotemia, may follow. Management includes emesis or lavage and instillation of activated charcoal into the stomach. General supportive measures also should be utilized.

DRUG INTERACTIONS. When meclofenamate was administered to patients already receiving warfarin sodium, the dose of warfarin had to be reduced. Therefore, prothrombin time should be monitored during simultaneous use.

The concomitant administration of aspirin and meclofenamate decreased the plasma level of the latter drug, but the plasma salicylate concentration was not affected. Meclofenamate did not affect the uricosuric action of sulfinpyrazone when the two drugs were given together.

PHARMACOKINETICS. Following a single oral dose, peak plasma concentrations occur in one-half to one hour. When taken with food, absorption is delayed, but the total amount absorbed is not altered. The absorption of meclofenamate was not affected by the concurrent administration of a magnesium-aluminum hydroxide antacid. Meclofenamate is highly bound (99%) to plasma proteins. The plasma half-life following a single dose is two hours; the half-life after multiple doses for four days is 3.3 hours. The drug does not accumulate in the body. It is metabolized to a hydroxymethyl derivative (25%), which also has anti-inflammatory activity, and a carboxy derivative (6%); both metabolites are excreted as glucuronide conjugates. A small amount of drug is excreted unchanged. Approximately two-thirds of the dose is excreted in the urine and one-third in the feces.

DOSAGE AND PREPARATIONS. Dosage should be individualized on the basis of each patient's needs and response. A low dose should be given initially and increased as necessary. *Oral: Adults,* for rheumatoid arthritis and osteoarthritis, 200 to 400 mg daily in three or four equal doses. The drug may be taken with meals or milk. After a satisfactory response is obtained, the dosage should be adjusted as necessary. If a severe adverse reaction occurs, the drug should be discontinued. A dosage for *children* has not been established.

Meclomen (Parke-Davis). Capsules 50 and 100 mg of meclofenamic acid in the form of meclofenamate sodium monohydrate.

NAPROXEN
[Naprosyn]

NAPROXEN SODIUM
[Anaprox]

ACTIONS AND USES. Naproxen is chemically related to the phenylpropionic acid group of drugs. It has analgesic, anti-inflammatory, and antipyretic actions and, like other nonsteroidal anti-inflammatory drugs, also inhibits prostaglandin synthesis. This drug is effective in the symptomatic treatment of rheumatoid arthritis, juvenile arthritis, ankylosing spondylitis, osteoarthritis, and acute gouty arthritis. It also may be useful as an alternative agent in the treatment of psoriatic arthritis and Reiter's syndrome.

Comparative studies in patients with rheumatoid arthritis showed that naproxen 500 mg daily was as efficacious as aspirin 3.6 to 4.8 g. Studies comparing naproxen to other nonsteroidal anti-inflammatory drugs have indicated that naproxen is equally or more effective than ibuprofen, fenoprofen, or indomethacin in this disorder. The drug's steroid-sparing effect was demonstrated in a limited number of patients who were also receiving a corticosteroid for rheumatoid arthritis and, when naproxen was given to patients receiving gold therapy, it enhanced the therapeutic effect. Naproxen was as effective as aspirin, indomethacin, or sulindac in patients with osteoarthritis.

ADVERSE REACTIONS AND PRECAUTIONS. Naproxen is one of the better tolerated nonsteroidal anti-inflammatory drugs. The most common adverse reactions are gastrointestinal disturbances (eg, heartburn, dyspepsia, abdominal pain, constipation, diarrhea). The gastric mucosa is less severely affected in short-term studies of normal volunteers and less gastrointestinal bleeding has been observed than with aspirin; however, bleeding occasionally is severe and ulceration has been reported. Controlled studies with endoscopy in rheumatoid arthritis have indicated gastropathy and ulcer progression. Therefore, this drug should be used with caution in patients with a history of peptic ulcer.

Like aspirin, naproxen inhibits platelet aggregation and prolongs bleeding time; however, this effect is reversible upon discontinuation of naproxen.

Central nervous system effects reported occasionally are headache, drowsiness, and dizziness or vertigo. Other adverse reactions occurring occasionally include pruritus, rash, urticaria, sweating, tinnitus, edema, and visual and hearing disturbances. As with other prostaglandin inhibitors, glomerular nephritis, interstitial nephritis, and nephrotic syndrome have been reported with naproxen. Since the drug is eliminated largely by the kidney, it should be used with caution in patients with impaired renal function. Pulmonary infiltration with eosinophils has been reported, and this complication should be considered when pulmonary involvement is a component of the underlying disease.

Naproxen readily crosses the placenta following oral administration to pregnant women and is excreted in the milk of lactating women. Thus, this drug should not be used during pregnancy or lactation. This drug is classified in FDA Pregnancy Category B.

OVERDOSE. Overdose with naproxen usually causes only mild to moderate symptoms. The most severe reaction reported was a seizure in a patient who ingested 35 g.

DRUG INTERACTIONS. Naproxen is highly bound to plasma protein (99%) and may displace other albumin-bound drugs from their binding sites. Therefore, patients receiving such drugs (eg, oral anticoagulants, sulfonylureas, hydantoins) should be observed for interactions. The concomitant administration of probenecid increases the plasma concentration and half-life of naproxen. The rate of absorption is decreased slightly by magnesium and aluminum hydroxide and is increased by sodium bicarbonate.

PHARMACOKINETICS. Naproxen is rapidly absorbed after oral administration; the peak plasma concentration occurs within two to four hours. Absorption is not significantly delayed by the presence of food. Naproxen is highly bound (99%) to plasma proteins at plasma concentrations between 23 and 40 mcg/ml. The drug is metabolized by demethylation and subsequent glucuronide conjugation. The elimination half-life is 12 to 15 hours and excretion occurs largely in the urine.

DOSAGE AND PREPARATIONS.
Oral: *Adults,* for rheumatoid arthritis and osteoarthritis, 500 to 750 mg daily divided into two doses (morning and evening). The dose may be increased or decreased during long-term use, depending upon the patient's response. The effects of doses exceeding 1 g have not been studied.

NAPROXEN:
Naprosyn (Syntex). Tablets 250, 375, and 500 mg.
NAPROXEN SODIUM:
Anaprox (Syntex). Tablets equivalent to 250 mg base.

PHENYLBUTAZONE
[Azolid, Butazolidin]

ACTIONS AND USES. Phenylbutazone has anti-inflammatory, antipyretic, and analgesic activities. It is especially effective in the treatment of ankylosing spondylitis and acute gouty arthritis. It also is effective in rheumatoid arthritis and Reiter's syndrome.

Phenylbutazone poses a significant risk of blood dyscrasia that counterbalances the benefits of its potent anti-inflammatory activity. As a general rule, phenylbutazone should be prescribed only after other nonsteroidal anti-inflammatory drugs have failed and when the severity of symptoms warrants the risk of a blood disorder.

ADVERSE REACTIONS AND PRECAUTIONS. The most serious adverse reactions associated with phenylbutazone are blood dyscrasias. Leukopenia, agranulocytosis, and aplastic anemia occur infrequently. The fatality rate from such effects has been estimated to be 2.2/100,000 patients (Hart and Huskisson, 1984). These adverse reactions may occur shortly after initiation of therapy or after prolonged treatment. Hematologic toxicity may develop abruptly or gradually and may become apparent days or weeks after cessation of therapy. In patients older than 60 years, especially women, phenylbutazone should be restricted to short-term use (one week maximum) if possible. Blood counts, including platelet determinations, should be performed regularly during prolonged treatment, but these tests cannot be depended upon to predict the blood dyscrasia. Therefore, patients should be advised to discontinue the drug and notify their physician immediately if fever, sore throat, or stomatitis develops.

Rashes, water retention and edema, and gastrointestinal disturbances ranging from mild irritation to ulceration occur and can be serious (eg, toxic epidermal necrolysis, gastrointestinal hemorrhage). Other adverse reactions include jaundice, hepatitis, purpura, and hematuria.

A careful medical history and complete physical and laboratory examinations (including blood count and urinalysis) should be performed prior to initiation of therapy with phenylbutazone. These tests should be repeated at regular intervals. Patients should be warned not to exceed the recommended dose and to discontinue the drug and report to the physician when fever, sore throat, oral lesions, dyspepsia, epigastric pain, unusual bleeding or bruising, black or tarry stools, symptoms of anemia, skin rashes, significant weight gain, or edema occurs. If long-term treatment is needed, the lowest effective dose should be used and patients should be informed of the risks.

Phenylbutazone is contraindicated in children under 14 years and in senile patients. It also is contraindicated in individuals with gastrointestinal lesions or a history of recurrent lesions; in those with renal, hepatic, or cardiovascular disease; and in patients with a history of blood dyscrasias or drug allergy. Phenylbutazone also is contraindicated in patients with pancreatitis, parotitis, stomatitis, temporal arteritis, and polymyalgia rheumatica. This drug should be used with extreme caution, if at all, in patients with borderline or overt congestive heart failure because it may produce severe fluid retention.

OVERDOSE. Mild poisoning with phenylbutazone has been associated with nausea, abdominal pain, and drowsiness. In more severe cases, hyperpyrexia, electrolyte disturbances, and cardiovascular and pulmonary complications can lead to renal failure, hepatic complications, ECG abnormalities, and blood dyscrasias. In all cases of overdose, gastric lavage and activated charcoal should be administered immediately (Court and Volans, 1984).

DRUG INTERACTIONS. Since phenylbutazone may prolong the prothrombin time in patients receiving coumarin anticoagulants concomitantly, combined use should be avoided. Phenylbutazone may increase the hypoglycemic effect of insulin and the oral hypoglycemic agents. It also reduces iodine uptake by the thyroid.

PHARMACOKINETICS. Phenylbutazone is rapidly and completely absorbed following oral administration. Peak plasma concentrations occur within 2.5 ± 1.4 hours, and the drug is highly bound to plasma protein. The major metabolite of phenylbutazone is the active form, oxyphenbutazone, which undergoes glucuronidation and is excreted mainly in the urine. The elimination half-life of phenylbutazone is 84 ± 23 hours and there is large inter- and intraindividual variation.

DOSAGE AND PREPARATIONS.
Oral: Adults, for ankylosing spondylitis, 300 mg daily in three or four equally divided doses. A one-week trial period is considered adequate to determine response. If a favorable response does not occur, the drug should be discontinued. The maintenance dose should not exceed 300 mg daily. If symptoms can be controlled with a maintenance dose of 100 to 200 mg daily, the drug may be given for longer periods under careful and close supervision. In patients 60 years and older, phenylbutazone should be restricted to short-term treatment periods only (if possible, maximum of one week).
  Azolid (USV), *Butazolidin* (Geigy), *Generic.* Capsules and tablets 100 mg.

PIROXICAM
[Feldene]

ACTIONS. Piroxicam differs chemically from other nonsteroidal anti-inflammatory drugs but has similar anti-inflammatory, analgesic, and antipyretic activities. Like other nonsteroidal anti-inflammatory drugs, piroxicam inhibits prostaglandin synthesis by blocking cyclo-oxygenase; it has no effect on lipoxygenase. The drug also inhibits chemotaxis, release of lysosomal enzymes, and neutrophil aggregation. Piroxicam has been reported to have a greater effect than other nonsteroidal anti-inflammatory drugs in inhibiting rheumatoid factor production and increasing phytohemagglutinin response and the percentage of suppressor T-cells in peripheral blood (Goodwin et al, 1983). The significance of these effects on its anti-inflammatory and antiarthritic actions is not clear.

USES. In controlled clinical studies, this agent was effective in the symptomatic treatment of rheumatoid arthritis and osteoarthritis. It also appears to be useful in ankylosing spondylitis and acute gouty arthritis, but additional studies are needed to establish comparative effectiveness and dosages in these conditions. Piroxicam can be administered once daily.

In studies on patients with rheumatoid arthritis, piroxicam 20 mg daily was as effective as aspirin 4.7 g daily in relieving signs and symptoms and was at least as effective as indomethacin, ibuprofen, naproxen, and sulindac.

In patients with osteoarthritis, piroxicam 20 mg/day relieved pain and improved joint movement as well as aspirin 3.9 g/day or, in a limited number of patients, indomethacin 75 mg/day (Turner, 1982; Dessain, 1982).

In a limited number of studies, piroxicam was reported to relieve pain in acute musculoskeletal disorders (eg, bursitis, tendinitis), after postpartum episiotomy, postoperatively, and after dental procedures, fractures, or trauma. However, comparative efficacy and analgesic doses have not been established.

ADVERSE REACTIONS AND PRECAUTIONS. Gastrointestinal reactions occurred in about 20% of patients. Epigastric distress and nausea were noted most frequently; abdominal discomfort, constipation, diarrhea, and flatulence also were reported. Peptic ulcer developed in about 1% of patients, and the incidence of gastric irritation and ulcer increased with doses greater than 20 mg daily. Perforation of ulcers and severe gastrointestinal bleeding resulting in death have occurred. Thus, piroxicam should be used with extreme caution in patients with a history of upper gastrointestinal disease.

Since hemoglobin and hematocrit levels were decreased in some patients, these values should be determined if anemia develops. Like aspirin, piroxicam inhibits platelet aggregation and prolongs bleeding time. Aplastic anemia has been associated with piroxicam therapy.

Peripheral edema has occurred in about 2% of patients receiving piroxicam. Congestive heart failure (five cases) and myocardial infarction also have been reported (Fowler and Arnold, 1983). Thus, piroxicam should be used very cautiously in patients with impaired cardiac function, hypertension, reduced renal function of the elderly, or other conditions predisposing to fluid retention.

Elevation of BUN levels (reversible), acute renal failure, and hyperkalemia have occurred. Because piroxicam is excreted primarily by the kidney, it should be used cautiously in patients with impaired renal function.

Severe dermatologic reactions (eg, exfoliative dermatitis, fatal pemphigus vulgaris) have been reported rarely. Other adverse reactions observed occasionally include rash, pruritus, dizziness, somnolence, and headache.

Cross sensitivity with aspirin and other prostaglandin inhibitors may occur; therefore, piroxicam is contraindicated in patients with a history of nasal polyps and angioedema or bronchospasm induced by aspirin or other anti-inflammatory drugs.

OVERDOSE. Sixteen cases of poisoning have been reported; 13 patients had no symptoms after ingesting 300 to 400 mg. Two patients experienced dizziness and blurred vision after 200 to 300 mg. One patient who ingested 600 mg became comatose but recovered fully.

DRUG INTERACTIONS. Aspirin and piroxicam should not be

used concomitantly. Piroxicam is highly bound to plasma proteins and may displace other albumin-bound drugs from binding sites. Therefore, patients receiving oral anticoagulants, sulfonylureas, or hydantoins should be monitored carefully. The concomitant administration of lithium and piroxicam increased lithium plasma concentrations.

PHARMACOKINETICS. Following oral administration, piroxicam is rapidly absorbed; peak plasma levels occur in three to five hours. With repeated daily doses of 20 mg, steady-state plasma levels of 3 to 5 mcg/ml are attained in 7 to 12 days. Plasma levels of piroxicam are not affected by the administration of antacids.

Concentration of the drug in synovial fluid is about 40% of that in plasma. The apparent volume of distribution ranges from 0.12 to 0.14 L/kg, and mean half-life is about 50 hours (range, 30 to 86 hours). The drug is extensively bound (99%) to plasma proteins. Piroxicam is metabolized predominantly by hydroxylation and subsequent conjugation with glucuronic acid. It is excreted primarily in the urine; a small amount is excreted in the feces, and about 2% to 5% is excreted unchanged.

DOSAGE AND PREPARATIONS.

Oral: Adults, for rheumatoid arthritis and osteoarthritis, 20 mg daily as a single dose or in divided doses; the incidence of gastrointestinal reactions is likely to increase with larger doses. Assessment of the drug's efficacy should be delayed for about two weeks to allow time for attainment of steady-state plasma levels. The dosage for *children* has not been established.

Feldene (Pfizer). Capsules 10 and 20 mg.

SULINDAC
[Clinoril]

ACTIONS AND USES. Sulindac is a substituted indene analogue of indomethacin and has similar anti-inflammatory, analgesic, and antipyretic properties. It is as effective as aspirin in rheumatoid arthritis and osteoarthritis and appears to be comparable to phenylbutazone in ankylosing spondylitis. Sulindac may be useful as an alternative agent in the treatment of psoriatic arthritis or Reiter's syndrome.

ADVERSE REACTIONS AND PRECAUTIONS. The most common reactions are abdominal pain, dyspepsia, nausea, constipation, and diarrhea. The incidence of gastrointestinal disturbances generally is lower than with aspirin and is about the same as with ibuprofen. Sulindac causes less gastrointes-

tinal bleeding than aspirin; however, peptic ulceration and gastrointestinal bleeding have been reported rarely. Therefore, sulindac should be used cautiously in patients with a history of gastrointestinal disease and should not be prescribed for those with active gastrointestinal bleeding.

Central nervous system effects include dizziness, drowsiness, and headache; the incidence of these effects is about the same as with aspirin and ibuprofen but less than with indomethacin. Other common adverse reactions are rash, pruritus, edema, and tinnitus.

Like aspirin and other nonsteroidal anti-inflammatory drugs, sulindac inhibits platelet aggregation and prolongs bleeding time. Therefore, it should be used cautiously in patients with bleeding disorders.

Acute renal failure has been reported with sulindac, although this drug affects renal function less than other nonsteroidal anti-inflammatory drugs in patients with chronic glomerular disease. Nevertheless, the drug should be used cautiously in patients with impaired renal function, and the dose should be reduced if necessary.

As with other nonsteroidal anti-inflammatory drugs, results of liver function tests may be abnormal; hepatitis, jaundice, or both have occurred. If abnormal test results persist or worsen or clinical signs and symptoms of liver disease develop, the drug should be discontinued.

Other serious reactions associated with sulindac include toxic epidermal necrolysis, Stevens-Johnson syndrome, and pancreatitis. As with other nonsteroidal anti-inflammatory agents, hypersensitivity reactions have occurred. Pregnant and nursing women should avoid the use of sulindac.

OVERDOSE. Few cases of overdose with sulindac have been reported and symptoms have not been serious.

DRUG INTERACTIONS. Although sulindac and its sulfide metabolite are highly bound to plasma protein, no clinically significant interaction with oral anticoagulants or oral hypoglycemic agents has been reported in normal patients. Plasma levels of the active sulfide were depressed by the concomitant administration of aspirin but not acetaminophen or propoxyphene.

PHARMACOKINETICS. About 90% of a dose is absorbed rapidly following oral administration, and the drug's disposition is complex. The parent drug (sulfoxide) is inactive but is reduced reversibly to the sulfide (active metabolite) and oxidized irreversibly to the sulfone (inactive metabolite). Sulindac, sulfone, and their conjugates are excreted primarily in the urine; less than 1% of a dose appears in the urine as the sulfide metabolite. The sulfide, which is responsible for the biological activities of the parent drug, is eliminated slowly from plasma (half-life, about 16 hours). Results of studies in animals have indicated that sulindac and its metabolites are excreted in the bile to varying degrees; thus, they may be reabsorbed unchanged, biotransformed, or excreted.

DOSAGE AND PREPARATIONS.

Oral: For *adults* with rheumatoid arthritis, osteoarthritis, and ankylosing spondylitis, the usual initial dose is 150 mg twice daily with food. Patients with rheumatoid arthritis usually require 200 mg twice daily. The dosage should be adjusted according to the patient's response. Doses above 400 mg/day are not recommended. Dosage for *children* has not been established.

Clinoril (Merck Sharp & Dohme). Tablets 150 and 200 mg.

TOLMETIN SODIUM
[Tolectin]

ACTIONS AND USES. Tolmetin alleviates symptoms of rheumatoid arthritis, and its effectiveness has been maintained with long-term use (two years). In patients with rheumatoid arthritis, tolmetin was as effective as aspirin, indomethacin, ibuprofen, and phenylbutazone. Patients receiving corticosteroid or gold therapy experienced greater relief when tolmetin was added to the regimen. Concomitant administration of tolmetin and acetaminophen relieves symptoms more than tolmetin alone, but the combination of tolmetin and aspirin provided no advantage over use of the individual drugs.

This agent also is as effective as aspirin in juvenile arthritis. Its effectiveness in osteoarthritis is similar to that of aspirin, ibuprofen, and indomethacin. In a limited number of studies, tolmetin was comparable to indomethacin in ankylosing spondylitis. In addition, it has been reported to reduce pain in nonarticular and traumatic painful conditions, but data are insufficient to establish its usefulness conclusively. Tolmetin may be useful as an alternative agent in the treatment of psoriatic arthritis and Reiter's syndrome.

Like other nonsteroidal anti-inflammatory agents, tolmetin inhibits prostaglandin synthetase in vitro and enhances deficient T-cell function. However, the significance of these actions is not precisely understood.

ADVERSE REACTIONS AND PRECAUTIONS. The most frequently reported adverse reactions are gastrointestinal disturbances; however, they occur less frequently than with aspirin. Epigastric distress (heartburn, dyspepsia, and abdominal pain) is most common; other reactions include nausea, vomiting, and constipation. Gastrointestinal bleeding is reported occasionally, but usual doses of tolmetin cause less occult gastrointestinal bleeding than with aspirin. In clinical studies, peptic ulcer occurred in approximately 2% of patients, but many of these had a history of peptic ulcer disease. Therefore, it is advisable to use tolmetin cautiously in patients with such a history.

Central nervous system reactions include headache, dizziness, lightheadedness, nervousness, and drowsiness. These effects occurred less frequently than with indomethacin. Other reactions observed occasionally are rash or urticaria, pruritus, tinnitus, and mild edema related to sodium retention.

Tolmetin decreases platelet adhesiveness and increases bleeding time; thus, it should not be used in patients with bleeding disorders. Unlike aspirin, this drug has a minimal effect on platelet aggregation. Because of the potential for cross sensitivity with aspirin and other nonsteroidal anti-inflammatory drugs, tolmetin should not be given to patients who experience symptoms of asthma, rhinitis, or urticaria when given aspirin.

As with other nonsteroidal anti-inflammatory drugs, nephrotic syndrome has been reported with tolmetin. Patients with impaired renal function should be monitored carefully and the dose may need to be reduced, since the drug is eliminated by the kidney.

Since tolmetin causes pseudoproteinuria in tests involving acid precipitation, other methods for detecting proteinuria should be used in patients receiving this drug.

Tolmetin is a chemical analogue of zomepirac, which was associated with a substantial number of cases of anaphylaxis, some of which were fatal. The incidence of anaphylaxis with tolmetin has been higher than with other nonsteroidal anti-inflammatory agents.

OVERDOSE. No serious side effects have occurred in patients reported to have taken an overdose of tolmetin.

DRUG INTERACTIONS. Tolmetin does not affect the anticoagulant activity of warfarin or the hypoglycemic effect of insulin or sulfonylureas.

PHARMACOKINETICS. Tolmetin is rapidly and completely absorbed after oral administration; peak plasma concentrations occur in 30 to 60 minutes. Absorption is not significantly affected by the short- or long-term administration of an antacid mixture of magnesium and aluminum hydroxides. The drug is highly bound (99%) to plasma protein. It undergoes biotransformation by oxidation of its aromatic methyl group, and 70% of the dose is recovered in the urine as this oxidized metabolite (Verbeeck et al, 1983). The elimination half-life is one to three hours.

DOSAGE AND PREPARATIONS.
Oral: Adults, for rheumatoid arthritis, initially, 400 mg three times daily. After a therapeutic response is achieved, the dose is adjusted to the patient's needs; 600 mg to 1.8 g daily is optimal for most patients. For osteoarthritis, 600 mg to 1.6 g daily usually is adequate. *Children over 2 years,* 20 mg/kg daily in divided doses initially; for maintenance, 15 to 30 mg/kg daily.

Tolectin (McNeil). Capsules (**Tolectin DS**) 400 mg; tablets 200 mg (strengths expressed in terms of base).

REMISSION-INDUCING DRUGS

The remission-inducing drugs include dissimilar chemical agents of varying but significant toxicity. Functional improvement rather than complete remission in rheumatoid arthritis is the characteristic outcome with use of these drugs.

Antimalarials appear to be the least toxic remission-inducing drugs at appropriate low doses but also are the least effective in rheumatoid arthritis. They may be selectively useful in sun-sensitive systemic lupus erythematosus, however. Oral gold may be less toxic but is less effective than parenteral gold therapy. Penicillamine, methotrexate, and azathioprine also may be administered. Corticosteroids are not yet regarded as remission-inducing drugs. Opinion is divided on which of these drugs should be used alternatively under which particular circumstances in rheumatoid arthritis. It is agreed, however, that these agents should be administered only by those trained and experienced in the use of such toxic agents in more advanced stages of rheumatoid and related disease progression.

These drugs vary widely in their mechanisms of action and adverse reactions (see the following evaluations). A general discussion of methotrexate may be found in Chapter 64, Drugs Used in Cancer Chemotherapy.

Antimalarial Agents

CHLOROQUINE PHOSPHATE

HYDROXYCHLOROQUINE SULFATE
[Plaquenil Sulfate]

ACTIONS AND USES. The 4-aminoquinoline compounds, chloroquine and hydroxychloroquine, have similar actions, but hydroxychloroquine is prescribed more commonly to treat rheumatoid arthritis, usually as second-line therapy. These drugs also are employed in juvenile arthritis, lupus erythematosus, and other inflammatory connective tissue diseases. Their value is limited by toxicity and the variable beneficial effects obtained; 70% of patients with rheumatoid arthritis experience moderate relief of symptoms. Because clinical improvement is slow, a three- to six-month trial is necessary to obtain maximal benefits and the recommended dosage must not be exceeded.

ADVERSE REACTIONS AND PRECAUTIONS. Ocular toxicity is the only serious complication noted; all other side effects are reversible. Retinopathy appears to be dose related; the risk is greater with larger doses, even when given for short periods, than with small doses administered over a prolonged period. Serious retinal changes occur infrequently (incidence less than 1%). Progressive impairment of vision and eventual blindness, even after the drug is discontinued, have been reported after daily doses of 0.75 to 1 g of chloroquine, but have not been observed following use of small doses. The retinopathy, which

starts in the area of the macula, appears to affect pigmentation; increased granularity and edema of the retina are the earliest findings. Regular ophthalmologic examinations (eg, visual acuity, visual fields, color testing, retinal and corneal biomicroscopy) should be performed prior to initiating therapy and every six months during therapy. The drug should be discontinued at the first sign of change in the ocular fundus.

Other adverse reactions include mild headache, gastrointestinal disturbances (diarrhea, nausea, abdominal cramps), rash, and neuropsychiatric effects (eg, emotional changes). Acute intermittent porphyria and neuromyopathy also may occur. The skin lesions of psoriasis may be aggravated and exfoliative dermatitis has been reported rarely; therefore, the antimalarial agents should be used in patients with psoriatic arthritis only after they have been informed of the possible consequences. Patients with G6PD deficiency should be observed closely for hemolytic anemia. Discontinuation of therapy because of side effects is necessary in approximately 3% to 7% of patients.

After acute overdosage, toxic symptoms may be noted within 30 minutes and death may occur. Children are especially sensitive to these drugs; therefore, patients should be warned to keep the drug out of their reach.

PHARMACOKINETICS. Antimalarial drugs are readily absorbed from the gastrointestinal tract. The plasma half-life during prolonged therapy is six to seven days. The drugs are deposited in tissues (eg, lungs, kidney, eyes), and 50% is excreted in one week. Because 3% to 5% of the drug in tissue is more firmly bound, complete excretion may take months or even years after therapy is discontinued.

DOSAGE AND PREPARATIONS.
CHLOROQUINE PHOSPHATE:
Oral: Adults, a maximum of 250 mg once daily with the evening meal or at bedtime. Dosage should be calculated on the basis of ideal body weight and should not exceed 4 mg/kg/day. This dose has been shown to maintain stable plasma levels within the therapeutic range.
Generic. Tablets 250 mg.
HYDROXYCHLOROQUINE SULFATE:
Oral: Adults, 200 mg once or twice daily with meals. Dosage should be calculated on the basis of ideal body weight and should not exceed 6.4 mg/kg/day.
Plaquenil Sulfate (Winthrop-Breon). Tablets 200 mg (equivalent to 155 mg of base).

Gold Compounds

AUROTHIOGLUCOSE
[Solganal]

GOLD SODIUM THIOMALATE
[Myochrysine]

$$CH_2CO^-Na^+$$
$$|$$
$$AuSCHCO^-Na^+ \cdot H_2O$$

ACTIONS AND USES. Active adult and juvenile arthritis are the principal indications for these agents, but beneficial effects also have been obtained in some patients with psoriatic arthritis. Although their exact mechanism of action is not known, the gold compounds exert an anti-inflammatory effect in these disorders and, unlike most antiarthritic drugs, may alter the course of the disease. They should be considered in the treatment of rheumatoid arthritis that progresses despite adherence to a conservative program of salicylates or other nonsteroidal anti-inflammatory drugs, rest, and physical therapy for several months. Therapy should be initiated before irreversible changes have occurred in the involved joints. The concomitant use of a nonsteroidal anti-inflammatory agent is necessary unless complete remission of arthritis has occurred. The gold compounds appear to be equally effective, but there is some evidence that aurothioglucose is less toxic (Lawrence, 1976), although the injections are more painful.

ADVERSE REACTIONS AND PRECAUTIONS. The usefulness of chrysotherapy is limited by toxicity. Dermatitis (ranging from erythema to exfoliative dermatitis) and lesions of the mucous membranes (stomatitis and, more rarely, proctitis and vaginitis) are common and may be serious. Pruritus may signify the early development of a skin reaction. When a pruritic skin lesion of uncertain etiology appears, gold therapy must be discontinued immediately, for another dose may produce a much more severe reaction.

Hematologic reactions (eg, eosinophilia, leukopenia, thrombocytopenia, hypoplastic or aplastic anemia) are rare; some fatalities have occurred. Effects on the kidney range from proteinuria to the nephrotic syndrome or glomerulitis with hematuria, and symptoms usually disappear with early recognition and discontinuation of the drug.

Hepatitis, cholestatic jaundice, severe enterocolitis, interstitial lung disease, and encephalopathy have developed rarely.

Anaphylactoid or "nitritoid-type" reactions (eg, flushing, syncope, dizziness, sweating), as well as nausea, vomiting, and weakness may occur with the thiomalate preparation, but they are probably caused by the vehicle rather than the gold. Substituting aurothioglucose usually alleviates these symptoms.

Some patients experience a transient flare within 24 hours after the injection. It is thought that these patients eventually respond well to gold therapy. In a few patients, this reaction is so severe that prednisone must be given for a few days to control it.

Toxic effects may be observed after the first injection, during the course of therapy, or several months after chrysotherapy has been discontinued. Their incidence and severity appear to depend upon dosage; severe effects are most common after a cumulative dosage of 400 to 800 mg has been administered. Since these reactions are unpredictable, patients should be questioned about symptoms of toxicity (eg, rash, purple blotches, pruritus, stomatitis, metallic taste) prior to each injection. A complete blood count, including platelet estimation, should be performed before the first treatment to serve as a baseline value and should be repeated before every second injection throughout the period of treatment. Qualitative urine protein estimates should be performed before each injection. If toxicity develops, gold therapy should be discontinued immediately. Treatment with topical or systemic corticosteroids may be necessary, and the chelating agent, dimercaprol [BAL in Oil], may be used to increase the excretion of gold.

Gold compounds should be used with extreme caution in patients with impaired renal or hepatic function, blood disorders, rash, or marked hypertension. They are contraindicated in patients with severe debilitation, systemic lupus erythematosus, or previous signs of gold toxicity. They are seldom needed during pregnancy but, if their use is contemplated, the benefit/risk ratio should be considered (FDA Pregnancy Category C). Diabetes mellitus or congestive heart failure should be under control before initiating gold therapy.

DOSAGE AND PREPARATIONS.
Intramuscular (gluteal): Adults, initially, single weekly injections of 10 mg the first week, 25 mg the second week, and 25 or 50 mg the third week and each week thereafter until a total dose of 800 mg to 1 g has been administered. If there is no response after 1 g has been given, the patient may be considered unresponsive and the drug discontinued, or the dose may be increased by 10 mg every one to four weeks (maximum, 100 mg in a single injection). If the patient has improved and no toxic effects have developed, dosage may be reduced. If the clinical course remains stable, 25 to 50 mg may be given every two to three weeks and then at monthly intervals.

Comparative studies have demonstrated that 10 or 25 mg is as effective as the usual 50-mg dose and that the response is not related to serum level of gold (Sharp et al, 1977). A remission after one year of maintenance therapy had been considered an indication for complete withdrawal of the drug, but many rheumatologists now feel that gold therapy probably should be continued indefinitely on a reduced dosage schedule. If relapse occurs when the interval between doses is increased or the drug is discontinued, the former schedule should be reinstituted.

For juvenile arthritis, recommendations vary; a usual dose for *children* is 1 mg/kg weekly for 20 weeks and the same dose at two- to four-week intervals thereafter for as long as therapy is beneficial and there are no signs of toxicity. Single doses for children and all but the largest adolescents should not exceed 50 mg.

AUROTHIOGLUCOSE:
Solganal (Schering). Suspension (sterile) 50 mg/ml in sesame oil with aluminum monostearate 2% and propylparaben 1 mg/ml in 10 ml containers.

GOLD SODIUM THIOMALATE:
Myochrysine (Merck Sharp & Dohme). Solution (sterile, aqueous) 10 and 25 mg/ml with benzyl alcohol 0.5% in 1 ml containers and 50 mg/ml with benzyl alcohol 0.5% in 1 and 10 ml containers.

AURANOFIN
[Ridaura]

ACTIONS AND USES. Auranofin differs chemically and in some pharmacologic actions from the older gold compounds (Walz et al, 1982 A). Unlike the latter preparations, which must be given parenterally, auranofin is effective when administered orally for rheumatoid arthritis. Like the other gold compounds, auranofin modifies the disease process and may induce remissions. Thus, it is a useful alternative and may be preferred to parenteral gold compounds for chrysotherapy of rheumatoid arthritis.

Auranofin decreases morning stiffness and the number of painful and swollen joints and increases grip strength. In addition, a decrease in weakness, fatigue, and progressive weight loss was reported by some patients. A reduction in erythrocyte sedimentation rate and rheumatoid factor paralleled the clinical response to auranofin.

In comparative studies, clinical improvements produced by auranofin were comparable to those produced by gold sodium thiomalate. However, fewer patients discontinued auranofin than the parenteral gold compound during the study (Gottlieb, 1980).

Like other gold compounds, auranofin has an immunomodulator action, although some of these effects differ from those of gold sodium thiomalate. The mechanism of these actions and their exact relationship to the therapeutic effects of auranofin in rheumatoid arthritis are not known (Walz et al, 1982 B).

ADVERSE REACTIONS AND PRECAUTIONS. The most frequent adverse reactions to auranofin are gastrointestinal disturbances (changes in bowel habits, loose stools, diarrhea). They generally occur within the first three months of therapy and are usually transient. If they persist, reduction of the dosage may improve symptoms. Diarrhea was reported in about 50% of patients; other gastrointestinal reactions include abdominal pain, nausea, dyspepsia, and anorexia. Skin reactions (eg, pruritus, rash) are mild and occur in about 30% of patients. Alopecia and conjunctivitis have been reported in 2% and 10% of patients, respectively.

Proteinuria was reported in about 4% of patients, but required discontinuation of therapy in only 0.7%. Abnormal results of liver function tests occurred in 0.4% of patients in U.S. studies. Anemia, leukopenia, eosinophilia, and thrombocytopenia developed infrequently and were reversible upon discontinuation of the drug.

Auranofin is contraindicated in patients with a history of gold-induced anaphylactic reactions, necrotizing enterocolitis, pulmonary fibrosis, exfoliative dermatitis, bone marrow aplasia, or other severe hematologic disorders.

PHARMACOKINETICS. Following oral administration of a single dose (6 mg), peak plasma levels occurred in 1.5 to 2.5 hours; approximately 25% of the dose was absorbed. With repeated daily doses, little day-to-day variation occurred in blood gold levels once steady state was achieved. The mean levels after three and six months of therapy (6 mg/day) were approximately the same: 0.62 ± 0.19 mcg/ml and 0.68 ± 0.45 mcg/ml, respectively. Blood gold levels following auranofin administration were about one-third of those reported with parenteral gold compounds, although the serum half-life of the latter was shorter. The gold from auranofin appeared to be more rapidly and completely excreted.

A major portion of the blood gold content was found to be associated with the cellular elements. After six months of administration (3 mg twice daily), the mean plasma terminal half-life was 17 to 25.5 days and the mean total body terminal half-life was 80.8 days. About 85% of the recoverable gold is excreted in the feces and 15% in the urine. Approximately 100% of a single dose of Au[195]-labeled auranofin was excreted over six months. (See reviews by Gottlieb, 1982; Blocka et al, 1982.)

DOSAGE AND PREPARATIONS.
Oral: The optimal therapeutic dose appears to be 6 mg/day given in one or two doses. Smaller doses can be used if this amount is not tolerated. Blood gold levels are dose related, but there appears to be no correlation between blood levels and therapeutic efficacy. Larger dosages (9 mg/day) caused a greater incidence of gastrointestinal adverse reactions but have been tolerated by some patients.
　Ridaura (Smith Kline & French). Capsules 3 mg.

Other Drugs

PENICILLAMINE
[Cuprimine, Depen]

ACTIONS AND USES. Comparative studies indicate that penicillamine, a chelating drug, may be as effective as gold compounds or azathioprine in rheumatoid arthritis. It is also beneficial in many patients with seropositive or seronegative juvenile polyarthritis (Ansell and Hall, 1981). This drug is not useful in ankylosing spondylitis, psoriatic arthritis, or other HLA-B27 associated diseases.

The mechanism of action is not known, but penicillamine has immunosuppressive activity and appears to affect immune complex levels, possibly by exerting an effect on T-cells. Many of this drug's effects are similar to those of the gold compounds.

Because it may cause serious adverse reactions, penicillamine should be reserved for patients with severe, active disease that has not responded adequately to more conservative drug therapy. Physicians who prescribe it should be familiar with its action and patients should be supervised closely.

ADVERSE REACTIONS AND PRECAUTIONS. The incidence of adverse reactions is high and may be related to the large doses used in early studies. Some effects are related to the rate of dosage increase and may be prevented by titrating the dose carefully.

The most common adverse reactions are pruritus, rash, anorexia, epigastric pain, nausea, vomiting, or occasional diarrhea and an alteration in taste that may be transient. Serious reactions involving the hematologic system (thrombocytopenia, leukopenia, agranulocytosis, and aplastic anemia) and renal system (proteinuria, hypoalbuminemia, nephrotic syndrome) have been observed. Proteinuria and/or hematuria may develop during therapy and may be warning signs of membranous glomerulopathy, which can progress to a nephrotic syndrome. Close observation of these patients is essential. In some patients, proteinuria disappears with continued therapy; in others, penicillamine must be discontinued. When proteinuria or hematuria develops, the physician must ascertain whether it is drug-induced or is unrelated to penicillamine therapy. Other serious reactions reported occasionally are lupus-like disease, pemphigus, Goodpasture's syndrome, myasthenia gravis, obliterative bronchiolitis, and polymyositis.

Blood and urine tests should be performed periodically, and complete blood cell counts, including platelets, must be obtained at two-week intervals during the first six months of treatment and monthly thereafter. Blood urea nitrogen and creatinine levels should be monitored occasionally. Patients over 65 years appear to have a greater risk of developing hematologic toxicity. If urinary protein excretion is greater than 1 g/24 hours, the drug should be discontinued or the dose reduced. Reduction of dosage corrects proteinuria in some patients after several months. Penicillamine must be discontinued if significant hypoalbuminemia, nephrotic syndrome, hematuria, drug fever, or other symptoms of toxicity develop.

PHARMACOKINETICS. Penicillamine is rapidly absorbed from the intestine after oral administration; the peak plasma concentration usually occurs in about 130 minutes. Metabolism is complex; five forms appear in plasma and the percentage of each urinary metabolite varies somewhat with the disease being treated. Plasma elimination half-life is 60.7 $\pm$ 8.2 minutes. Urinary excretion is 21.2% $\pm$ 2.3% within 24 hours; 50% of an oral dose is excreted in the feces, but the metabolites have not been identified (Perrett, 1981; Wiesner et al, 1981).

DOSAGE AND PREPARATIONS. The dose must be individualized on the basis of the clinical response and adverse reactions. Because of the long latent period of the clinical response, changes in dosage should not be made at intervals of less than two to three months. Other medication, except gold, antimalarial agents, cytotoxic drugs, and phenylbutazone, should be continued when penicillamine is given. After clinical improvement is observed, the other drugs can be withdrawn gradually. Penicillamine should be given on an empty stomach (about one hour before meals) to ensure maximum absorption.

Oral: Adults, initially, 125 mg/day as a single dose; the amount may be increased by increments of 125 mg/day at two- to three-month intervals to 500 mg/day. No further increase should be made until the patient's response can be assessed (Rodnan et al, 1983). If no adverse reactions occur and the therapeutic effect is incomplete, up to 750 mg/day may be tried. *Children,* initially 5 mg/kg/day; the dosage may be increased to 10 to 15 mg/kg/day after two months if no effect is seen with the lower amounts (Baum, 1983).

Children, the dosage should start at 5 mg/kg/day after two months if no effect is seen at the lower doses (Baum, 1983).

Cuprimine (Merck Sharp & Dohme). Capsules 125 and 250 mg.
Depen (Wallace). Tablets 250 mg.

AZATHIOPRINE
[Imuran]

USES. This immunosuppressive agent is effective in rheumatoid arthritis; however, because of potential toxic effects, use of azathioprine should be limited to severe, active, progressive disease that does not respond to conventional management, including other drug therapy. Other agents should be continued when azathioprine is given, with the exception of slow-acting drugs (gold, antimalarials, penicillamine), because the effects of combined use of the latter drugs with azathioprine have not been determined. Azathioprine is about as effective as gold, penicillamine, or cyclophosphamide. It appears to have a slower onset than penicillamine and to be less toxic than cyclophosphamide (Bunch and O'Duffy, 1980).

ACTIONS. Azathioprine, an imidazolyl derivative of mercaptopurine, is rapidly metabolized to the latter, which is also active and accounts for most of the effects of this compound. The exact mechanism of the immunosuppressant and anti-inflammatory actions of azathioprine in rheumatoid arthritis is not known.

ADVERSE REACTIONS AND PRECAUTIONS. The incidence of adverse reactions is less when azathioprine is given for rheumatoid arthritis than when it is used as an immunosuppressant in renal homotransplantation. Hematologic reactions (leukopenia, thrombocytopenia, anemia) occur most frequently (incidence, 28%). These are dose related and usually are mild, but leukopenia is occasionally pronounced and severe. Severe bone marrow depression occurs infrequently. Therefore, complete blood counts, including platelets, should be performed periodically during therapy (eg, weekly during the first month, twice monthly during the second and third months, and monthly thereafter). If there is a rapid fall, a persistent low leukocyte count, or other evidence of bone marrow depression, the dose should be reduced or the drug discontinued.

Although serious infections are a potential hazard of immunosuppressant therapy, the incidence of infections has not increased in patients receiving azathioprine for rheumatoid arthritis.

Gastrointestinal disturbances usually are mild and occur soon after treatment is begun; nausea and vomiting have been reported in about 12% of patients with rheumatoid arthritis. Hepatotoxicity is uncommon (incidence, less than 1%), but it may be severe; the effects generally are reversible after discontinuation of the drug.

An increase in lymphoma, reticulum cell sarcoma, and other neoplasms has been noted in renal transplant patients receiving azathioprine. Although the risk of malignancies is less in patients with rheumatoid arthritis, acute myelogenous leukemia, non-Hodgkin's lymphoma, and solid tumors have been reported in these patients.

Azathioprine is teratogenic in animals and, since it crosses the placenta in man, the drug should not be used during pregnancy.

If azathioprine is given with allopurinol, the dose should be reduced to about one-third or one-fourth the usual amount because the inhibition of xanthine oxidase by allopurinol reduces the conversion of mercaptopurine to its major inactive metabolite, 6-thiouric acid. Since this metabolite is excreted in the urine, the dose of azathioprine also should be reduced in patients with renal dysfunction.

For other uses, adverse reactions, and precautions, see Chapter 63, Immunomodulators.

DOSAGE AND PREPARATIONS.

Oral: Adults, initially, about 1 mg/kg (50 to 100 mg) as a single dose or in two divided doses daily. This may be increased after six to eight weeks by 0.5 mg/kg/day at four-week intervals to a maximum of 2.5 mg/kg/day. A therapeutic response may not be observed for six to eight weeks; thus, at least 12 weeks should be allowed to determine whether the patient is refractory to treatment. If the response is satisfactory and there are no toxic effects, the drug may be continued for long-term therapy, but the smallest effective maintenance dose should be used and the patient should be monitored carefully.

Imuran (Burroughs Wellcome). Tablets 50 mg.

ADRENAL CORTICOSTEROIDS

Of the systemic corticosteroids, prednisone and prednisolone are most commonly used in rheumatic disorders and are equally effective when given orally. Others, preferably those with little mineralocorticoid activity, also may be administered in equivalent doses, although their greater potency may make dosage adjustment difficult. The dose should be reduced gradually at frequent intervals, when possible, and the corticosteroid can be withdrawn gradually in many patients. Others require small maintenance doses in order to perform their jobs or household duties or to take care of themselves. The adjunctive use of a nonsteroidal anti-inflammatory agent may permit use of smaller doses of the steroid.

For equivalency and adverse reactions, see Chapter 61, Adrenal Corticosteroids in Nonendocrine Diseases.

Intra-articular injection of a long-acting corticosteroid (eg, prednisolone tebutate [Hydeltra-T.B.A.], betamethasone sodium phosphate and acetate [Celestone Soluspan], triamcinolone acetonide [Kenalog], triamcinolone hexacetonide [Aristospan], methylprednisolone acetate [depMedalone, Depo-Medrol]) temporarily relieves pain when only a few joints are markedly affected. Effects last several weeks to months, depending upon the preparation used. Several rheumatologists have reported that triamcinolone preparations are the most potent and have the longest duration of action (Gray et al, 1981). See Chapter 61 for suitable preparations and doses.

Corticotropin can be used in selected hospitalized patients for flareups of rheumatoid arthritis (Roth, 1980).

DOSAGE AND PREPARATIONS.

PREDNISONE, PREDNISOLONE:

Oral: Adults, for rheumatoid arthritis, the daily dose should not exceed 7.5 mg prednisone equivalents or 5 mg equivalents in postmenopausal women (Roth, 1984). The amount should be adjusted at three- to seven-day intervals, depending upon response, to the maintenance level. Discontinuation of therapy should be gradual with dosage reductions of 1 mg/month (Bhalla and Simon, 1984).

For *children,* small doses (as little as 2 to 3 mg/day) sometimes improve juvenile polyarticular arthritis with severe inflammation that is unresponsive to other medications (Baum, 1983). If possible, 1-mg tablets should be given in divided doses during the day. Alternate-day therapy is preferred and can be utilized if symptoms are controlled satisfactorily during the day on which no medication is given.

For preparations, see Chapter 61.

Cited References

Ansell BM, Hall MA: Penicillamine in chronic arthritis of childhood. *J Rheumatol* 8(suppl 7):112-115, 1981.

Baum J: Pharmacologic treatment of juvenile arthritis. *Compr Ther* 9:8-13, (Sept) 1983.

Bennett RM: Management of rheumatoid arthritis. *Compr Ther* 5:23-35, (Aug) 1979.

Bhalla AK, Simon LS: Clinical evaluation of antiarthritic agents. *Compr Ther* 10:40-50, (Aug) 1984.

Blackshear JL, et al: Renal complications of nonsteroidal anti-inflammatory drugs: Identification and monitoring of those at risk. *Semin Arthritis Rheum* 14:163-175, 1985.

Blocka K, et al: Single dose pharmacokinetics of auranofin in rheumatoid arthritis. *J Rheumatol* 9(suppl 8):110-119, 1982.

Bunch TW, O'Duffy JD: Disease-modifying drugs for progressive rheumatoid arthritis. *Mayo Clin Proc* 55:161-179, 1980.

Bunning RD, Barth WF: Sulindac: Potentially renal-sparing nonsteroidal anti-inflammatory drug. *JAMA* 248:2864-2867, 1982.

Calabro JJ: Management of juvenile rheumatoid arthritis. *Compr Ther* 7:30-36, (Feb) 1981.

Calabro JJ: Relieving ache of osteoarthritis. *Emerg Med* 15:110-157, (Feb 28) 1983.

Calin A: Ankylosing spondylitis and other seronegative spondylarthritides. *Compr Ther* 5:41-47, (Aug) 1979.

Caruso I, et al: Gastroscopic evaluation of anti-inflammatory agents. *Br Med J* 280:75-78, 1980.

Chaffman M, et al: Auranofin: Preliminary review of its pharmacological properties and therapeutic use in rheumatoid arthritis. *Drugs* 27:378-424, 1984.

Court H, Volans GN: Poisoning after overdose with non-steroidal anti-inflammatory drugs. *Adv Drug React Acc Pois Rev* 3:1-21, 1984.

Davies RO: Review of animal and clinical pharmacology of diflunisal. *Pharmacotherapy* 3(suppl 1):9S-22S, 1983.

Dessain P: Efficacy and toleration of piroxicam in general practice: Multicenter study of osteoarthritis, in *Advances in Arthritis Therapy: An International Review of Piroxicam.* Postgraduate Medicine:Custom Communications, April, 1982.

Dresner AJ: Multicenter studies with sodium meclofenamate (Meclomen) in the United States and Canada. *Curr Ther Res* 23(suppl):90-106, (April) 1978.

Durance RA, et al: Multicentre comparative analgesic study of fenoprofen and sulindac in rheumatoid arthritis. *Curr Ther Res* 26:791-798, 1979.

Ehrlich GE: Pathogenesis and treatment of osteoarthritis. *Compr Ther* 5:36-40, (Aug) 1979.

Favre L, et al: Reversible acute renal failure from combined triamterene and indomethacin: Study in healthy subjects. *Ann Intern Med* 96:317-320, 1982.

Fowler RW, Arnold KG: Non-steroidal analgesic and anti-inflammatory agents, (letter). *Br Med J* 287:835, 1983.

Fox DA, Jick H: Nonsteroidal anti-inflammatory drugs and renal disease. *JAMA* 251:1299-1300, 1984.

Gerber RC: Diagnosis and management of Reiter's syndrome. *Compr Ther* 10:51-57, (Aug) 1984.

Goodwin JS, et al: Administration of nonsteroidal anti-inflammatory agents in patients with rheumatoid arthritis: Effects on indexes of cellular immune status and serum rheumatoid factor levels. *JAMA* 250: 2485-2488, 1983.

Gordin A, et al: Comparison of slow-release indomethacin and diflunisal in patients with arthrosis. *Curr Med Res Opin* 9:275-279, 1984.

Gottlieb NL: Comparative metabolism, efficacy, and toxicity of oral and parenteral gold compounds. *Rheumatologie* 32:245-246, 1980.

Gottlieb NL: Comparative pharmacokinetics of parenteral and oral gold compounds. *J Rheumatol* 9(suppl 8):99-109, 1982.

Gray RG, et al: Local corticosteroid injection treatment in rheumatic disorders. *Semin Arthritis Rheum* 10:231-254, 1981.

Hansten PD: Nonsteroidal anti-inflammatory drugs and oral anticoagulants. *Drug Interact Newslett* 3:49-53, (Nov) 1983.

Hart FD, Huskisson EC: Non-steroidal anti-inflammatory drugs: Current status and rational therapeutic use. *Drugs* 27:232-255, 1984.

Helleberg L: Clinical pharmacokinetics of indomethacin. *Clin Pharmacokinet* 6:245-258, 1981.

Herschberg SN, Sierles FS: Indomethacin-induced lithium toxicity. *Am Fam Physician* 28:155-157, (Aug) 1983.

Huskisson EC: Osteoarthritis: Changing concepts in pathogenesis and treatment. *Postgrad Med* 65:97-104, (March) 1979.

Kuflik EG: Effect of antimalarial drugs on psoriasis. *Cutis* 26:153-155, 1980.

Lawrence JS: Comparative toxicity of gold preparations in treatment of rheumatoid arthritis. *Ann Rheum Dis* 35:171-173, 1976.

Levy G: Pharmacokinetics of salicylate in man. *Drug Metab Rev* 9:3-19, 1979.

Levy G, Giacomini KM: Rational aspirin dosage regimens. *Clin Pharmacol Ther* 23:247-252, 1978.

Lipman AG: Anti-inflammatories: Overview of subtle differences. *Mod Med* 227-228, (Sept) 1982.

Mackenzie AH: Ocular safety of huge cumulative antimalarial dosage, (abstract). *Arthritis Rheum* 24(suppl):70S, (April) 1981.

McCarty DJ, Carrera GF: Intractable rheumatoid arthritis: Treatment with combined cyclophosphamide, azathioprine, and hydroxychloroquine. *JAMA* 248:1718-1723, 1982.

Nelson AM: Juvenile rheumatoid arthritis: Drug therapy plan and look at prognosis. *Mod Med* 187-196, (Nov) 1982.

Nuki G: Non-steroidal analgesic and anti-inflammatory agents. *Br Med J* 287:39-43, 1983.

O'Brien WM: Pharmacology of nonsteroidal anti-inflammatory drugs: Practical review for clinicians. *Am J Med* 75:32-39, 1983.

O'Duffy JD, Luthra HS: Current status of disease-modifying drugs in progressive rheumatoid arthritis. *Drugs* 27:373-377, 1984.

Paulus HE: FDA arthritis advisory committee meeting. *Arthritis Rheum* 25:1124-1125, 1982.

Perrett D: Metabolism and pharmacology of D-penicillamine in man. *J Rheumatol* 8(suppl 7):41-50, 1981.

Porter RS: Factors determining efficacy of NSAIDs. *Drug Intell Clin Pharm* 18:42-51, 1984.

Preston SN: Safety of sodium meclofenamate (Meclomen). *Curr Ther Res* 23(suppl):107-112, (April) 1978.

Rainsford K: Side-effects of anti-inflammatory/analgesic drugs: Epidemiology and gastrointestinal tract. *TIPS* 156-159, (April) 1984.

Rhymer AR, et al: Double-blind trial comparing indomethacin sustained release capsules (Indocid-R) with indomethacin capsules in patients with rheumatoid arthritis. *Rheumatol Rehabil* 21:101-106, 1982.

Rider JA: Comparison of fecal blood loss after use of aspirin and diflunisal. *Pharmacotherapy* 3(suppl 1):61S-64S, 1983.

Robinson DR: Prostaglandins and mechanism of action of anti-inflammatory drugs. *Am J Med* 75:26-31, 1983.

Rodnan GP, et al (eds): *Primer on the Rheumatic Diseases,* ed 8. Atlanta, GA, Arthritis Foundation, 1983.

Roth SH: Corticosteroid therapy, in: *New Directions in Arthritis Therapy.* Littleton, MA, PSG Publishing Company, 1980.

Roth SH: Emerging new arthritis drugs: Clinician's opinion. *Postgrad Med* 73:125-134, (March) 1983.

Roth SH: Arthritis and rheumatism: Old questions, new answers. *Compr Ther* 10:58-64, (Aug) 1984.

Roth SH: Salicylates, in Roth SH (ed): *Rheumatic Therapeutics.* New York, McGraw-Hill, 1985.

Scherbel AL, Wilke WS: New nonsteroidal anti-inflammatory drugs. *Geriatrics* 10:67-75, (Oct) 1981.

Sharp JT, et al: Comparison of two dosage schedules of gold salts in treatment of rheumatoid arthritis. *Arthritis Rheum* 20:1179-1187, 1977.

Silvoso GR, et al: Incidence of gastric lesions in patients with rheumatic disease on chronic aspirin therapy. *Ann Intern Med* 91:517-520, 1979.

Stern RS, Bigby M: Expanded profile of cutaneous reactions to nonsteroidal anti-inflammatory drugs: Reports to specialty-based system for spontaneous reporting of adverse reactions to drugs. *JAMA* 252:1433-1437, 1984.

Svendsen UG, et al: Renal excretion of prostaglandins and changes in plasma renin during treatment with either sulindac or naproxen in patients with rheumatoid arthritis and thiazide treated heart failure. *J Rheumatol* 11:779-782, 1984.

Tannenbaum H, et al: Double blind multicenter trial comparing piroxicam and indomethacin in ankylosing spondylitis with long-term follow-up. *Curr Ther Res* 36:426-435, 1984.

Thompson M, et al: Comparative clinical study of fenoprofen and sulindac in osteoarthritis. *Curr Ther Res* 26:779-790, 1979.

Thompson RN, et al: Controlled two-centre trial of parenteral methotrexate therapy for refractory rheumatoid arthritis. *J Rheumatol* 11:760-763, 1984.

Thurnau GR: Rheumatoid arthritis. *Clin Obstet Gynecol* 26:558-578, 1983.

Thyss A, et al: Clinical and pharmacokinetic evidence of life-threatening interaction between methotrexate and ketoprofen. *Lancet* 1:256-258, 1986.

Townsend RJ, et al: Excretion of ibuprofen into breast milk. *Am J Obstet Gynecol* 149:184-186, 1984.

Turner R: Review of management of rheumatoid arthritis with piroxicam, in *Advances in Arthritis Therapy: An International Review of Piroxicam.* Postgraduate Medicine:Custom Communications, April, 1982.

Umbenhauer ER: Diflunisal in treatment of pain of osteoarthritis: Summary of clinical studies. *Pharmacotherapy* 3(suppl 1):55S-60S, 1983.

Van Wanghe P, Dequeker J: Compliance and long-term effect of azathioprine in 65 rheumatoid arthritis cases. *Ann Rheum Dis* 41(suppl):40-43, 1982.

Vasey FB, et al: Clinical aspects of psoriatic arthritis. *Compr Ther* 8:34-39, (April) 1982.

Verbeeck RK, et al: Clinical pharmacokinetics of non-steroidal anti-inflammatory drugs. *Clin Pharmacokinet* 8:297-331, 1983.

Walz DT, et al: Comparative pharmacology and biological effects of different gold compounds. *J Rheumatol* 9(suppl 8):54-60, 1982 A.

Walz DT, et al: Mechanisms of action of auranofin: Effects on human immune response. *J Rheumatol* 9(suppl 8):32-36, 1982 B.

Ward JR: Prospective randomized controlled trial of low dose pulse methotrexate in rheumatoid arthritis, (abstract). *Arthritis Rheum* 27(suppl):540, 1984.

Wasner C, et al: Nonsteroidal anti-inflammatory agents in rheumatoid arthritis and ankylosing spondylitis. *JAMA* 246:2168-2172, 1981.

Weinblatt ME, et al: Efficacy of low-dose methotrexate in rheumatoid arthritis. *N Engl J Med* 312:818-822, 1985.

Weissman G: Mechanisms of inflammation. SEAPAL Meeting, Bangkok, Jan 1985.

Wiesner RH, et al: Pharmacokinetics of D-penicillamine in man. *J Rheumatol* 8(suppl 7):51-55, 1981.

Willkens RF: Immunomodulating agents, in Roth SH (ed): *Rheumatic Therapeutics*. New York, McGraw-Hill, 1985.

Willkens RF, Watson MA: Methotrexate: Perspective of use in treatment of rheumatic diseases. *J Lab Clin Med* 100:314-321, 1982.

Yeh KC: Indomethacin and indomethacin sustained release: Comparison of their pharmacokinetic profiles. *Semin Arthritis Rheum* 12(suppl 1):136-141, 1982.

Agents Used in Gout and Hyperuricemia

60

Gout is characterized biochemically by hyperuricemia and clinically by episodes of severe, acute arthritis. The untreated disease may develop through four stages: (1) asymptomatic hyperuricemia, which infrequently progresses to acute gout; (2) acute gouty arthritis, which is usually monoarticular but may be polyarticular; (3) asymptomatic intercritical (interval) period; and (4) chronic tophaceous gout (30% to 40% of patients with gout develop tophi). If the disease is diagnosed early and appropriate therapy is employed promptly, gout usually can be arrested and complications of gout (eg, destructive joint lesions, renal disease) can be prevented.

The hyperuricemia that underlies the clinical manifestations of acute gouty arthritis commonly is classified as primary or secondary. Primary hyperuricemia may result from overproduction of uric acid, decreased renal excretion of uric acid, or both. The precise mechanism of uric acid overproduction is undefined in most cases. A deficiency of hypoxanthine-guanine-phosphoribosyl transferase or increased activity of phosphoribosyl-pyrophosphate synthetase may lead to elevated levels of 5-phosphoribosyl-1-pyrophosphate, which drives the synthesis of uric acid (Rodnan et al, 1983).

Impaired renal clearance of uric acid is much more common than overproduction. In many patients with gout, the renal capacity to excrete uric acid is defective. This capacity depends upon the integrity of a four-component model of filtration, reabsorption, secretion, and postsecretory reabsorption. Decreased tubular secretion or enhanced tubular reabsorption are the most likely mechanisms in primary hyperuricemia.

Secondary hyperuricemia develops during the course of another disease or is the consequence of some external precipitating event (eg, drug therapy). Like primary hyperuricemia, the underlying causes of secondary hyperuricemia are the overproduction and/or decreased renal excretion of uric acid. For example, in patients with myeloproliferative disorders, increased bone marrow activity results in increased production and turnover of both cells and nucleic acids, which lead to elevated blood concentrations of uric acid. Renal elimination of uric acid may be compromised by diuretic therapy or chronic ingestion of alcohol, which also may lead to elevated blood concentrations.

Symptoms of acute gout usually develop at serum uric acid concentrations above 7 mg/dl in males and 6 mg/dl in females as measured by the uricase method. These concentrations characteristically promote deposition of monosodium urate crystals in synovial fluid, which eventually causes an acute inflammatory attack. Although the precise mechanism is not known, events responsible for an attack include leukocytic phagocytosis of crystals, activation of the kallikrein and complement systems, disruption of lysosomes within the leukocytes, and subsequent disruption of whole cells with release of lysosomal enzymes into the synovial fluid (Kelley, 1983).

Many disorders are associated with hyperuricemia and the symptoms of acute gout may resemble those of several other types of arthritis; thus, a precise differential diagnosis is necessary for proper treatment. Demonstration of monosodium urate crystals in synovial fluid leukocytes or tophi is diagnostic of gout. In addition, the combination of hyperuricemia, monoarticular arthritis that resolves with an intercritical period, and a prompt response to colchicine usually differentiates gout from similar conditions (Holmes, 1981). For a more complete discussion of the diagnosis of acute gouty arthritis developed by the American Rheumatism Association, see Wallace et al, 1977. For details and procedures of diagnosis, see reviews (eg, Kelley, 1983) and specialized texts (eg, Talbott and Yu, 1976; Wyngaarden and Kelley, 1976).

Drug Therapy

The principal objectives of the treatment of gout are: (1) to terminate the inflammatory process of an acute attack, and (2) to reduce hyperuricemia in order to prevent formation of urate deposits and recurrent attacks and to promote the resolution of tophi in tophaceous gout. It should be noted that there is some disagreement on the necessity of reducing hyperuricemia in all patients with gout. In high-risk patients with secondary hyperuricemia, particularly those with neoplasm-related hyperuricemia who are receiving antineoplastic agents, reduction of hyperuricemia may be necessary to avoid obstructive uropathy.

Colchicine and the nonsteroidal anti-inflammatory drugs, especially indomethacin [Indocin], are most commonly used to treat attacks of acute gouty arthritis. Drugs employed to reduce hyperuricemia are probenecid [Benemid, SK-Probenecid] and sulfinpyrazone [Anturane], which increase the renal excretion of uric acid, and allopurinol [Lopurin, Zyloprim], which decreases the formation of uric acid. These agents should not be used to treat acute attacks because they are ineffective and may exacerbate or precipitate an acute attack.

Acute Gouty Arthritis: Drug selection depends upon the physician's or patient's experience with a certain drug. Medication is most effective when given early during an acute attack, and patients should be advised to take the drug at the first signs of an impending acute attack.

Colchicine and indomethacin are the preferred agents for the treatment of acute gouty arthritis. Colchicine is the drug most frequently employed for an initial attack because the relative specificity of its therapeutic effect in gout contributes to the establishment of the diagnosis.

Indomethacin is preferred for subsequent attacks because it has demonstrated efficacy and because it causes fewer gastrointestinal disturbances than colchicine. Several newer nonsteroidal anti-inflammatory drugs (fenoprofen [Nalfon], ibuprofen [Motrin, Rufen], naproxen [Anaprox, Naprosyn], piroxicam [Feldene], and sulindac [Clinoril]) also are effective. Because

of its adverse reactions, including blood dyscrasias, phenylbutazone [Azolid, Butazolidin] should be reserved for patients with a history of severe treatment-resistant attacks that have responded favorably to the drug in the past. Phenylbutazone should be used only after therapeutic measures, including other nonsteroidal anti-inflammatory drugs, have been unsatisfactory and should be used for no longer than five to seven days.

Intramuscular or intravenous administration of corticotropin (ACTH) or oral or intra-articular injection of a corticosteroid rarely is necessary in very severe acute attacks or in patients who fail to respond to the other anti-inflammatory agents. Colchicine should be given with and after discontinuation of corticotropin or steroids to prevent rebound attacks.

Intercritical (Interval) Period: Proper management of patients with gout during the intercritical (asymptomatic) period includes drug therapy, attention to diet for control of body weight and excess intake of purines, and avoidance of precipitating factors. Many patients do well during the intercritical phase without drug therapy. This discussion is limited to a consideration of appropriate drug therapy.

Small daily doses of colchicine (one or two tablets) are used to prevent recurrent acute attacks. Some clinicians do not initiate prophylactic therapy unless two or three attacks occur within a one-year period. If symptoms of an impending acute attack occur during prophylactic therapy, the dose of colchicine should be increased. An attack usually can be aborted with a few tablets (Talbott, 1980).

After the inflammation of an acute attack has subsided, the administration of drugs that decrease the serum uric acid level (allopurinol, probenecid, sulfinpyrazone) should be considered to avoid the other physiologic manifestations of gout. Opinions vary regarding the time in the treatment program when antihyperuricemic therapy, if indicated, should be started. Most clinicians prefer to withhold these drugs after only one attack if hyperuricemia is mild and renal function is normal; others believe that hyperuricemia severe enough to produce one acute attack should be treated (Wyngaarden and Kelley, 1976). Serum urate levels should not be reduced suddenly, because the rapid mobilization of urate from body pools may precipitate an acute attack.

Since uricosuric agents and allopurinol may precipitate an attack of acute gouty arthritis during the initial treatment, small doses should be used initially and the amount increased gradually.

The choice between allopurinol or a uricosuric is based on the production and, thus, excretion of uric acid. Patients consuming a normal diet who have normal renal function and in whom the 24-hour urinary uric acid excretion is less than 800 mg should be treated with a uricosuric. When uric acid excretion is persistently above 800 mg, overproduction of uric acid can be presumed and the patient should be treated with allopurinol. Allopurinol also is preferred in patients with renal insufficiency or nephrolithiasis and tophi. The objective of treatment in these patients is to maintain normal serum and urinary uric acid levels.

Regardless of which drug is used to treat hyperuricemia, serum urate levels should be measured regularly to determine the efficacy of treatment. To help avoid urate renal calculi during uricosuric therapy, a large flow of alkaline urine (pH 6.0 to 6.5) should be maintained by increasing fluid intake and administering sodium bicarbonate and/or acetazolamide. Renal function should be assessed periodically (eg, monthly) during this therapy.

Tophaceous Gout: The objective of treatment in tophaceous gout is to decrease the serum uric acid concentration to less than 7 mg/dl in males and 6 mg/dl in females, thereby allowing tophi to be reduced in size without precipitating crystals in the kidneys or joints. Because allopurinol reduces the load of uric acid excreted by the kidney and because the amount of uric acid that is mobilized from tophi is phenomenally high, this drug is preferred. In the rare patient with adequate renal function who is not controlled by a single medication, allopurinol may be used with probenecid. Such combination therapy does not necessitate changing either drugs' dosage and usually lowers serum urate concentration (Kelley, 1983).

Secondary Hyperuricemia: Secondary hyperuricemia may result from excessive production and/or decreased renal excretion of uric acid. Overproduction occurs in various myeloproliferative disorders, such as polycythemia vera, myeloid metaplasia, leukemia, or lymphoma, as well as during the treatment of these diseases with drugs that cause a breakdown of cellular nucleic acid. Patients with these diseases should be given allopurinol prior to treatment with cytotoxic drugs (see the evaluation on Allopurinol for precautions). Decreased renal excretion of uric acid occurs in such conditions as lead nephropathy, glycogen storage disease, and sickle cell disease; the endogenous production of uric acid also is increased in the latter two conditions.

Several drugs, including salicylates in low doses, pyrazinamide, niacin, ethambutol [Myambutol], and alcohol, may increase the serum uric acid level. Hyperuricemia often is induced by diuretics that are widely used to treat hypertension, but the routine use of drugs to reduce serum uric acid in these patients is unnecessary. Antihypertensive therapy should be the primary treatment in patients with both gout and hypertension, since studies suggest that renal disease is a more common complication of uncontrolled hypertension than uncontrolled hyperuricemia. If the serum urate level exceeds 10 mg/dl in females and 13 mg/dl in males, hyperuricemia should be treated with a uricosuric agent (Simkin, 1979) and colchicine should be given concomitantly during the early months of therapy to prevent attacks of acute gout (see Chapter 29, Diuretics).

Asymptomatic Hyperuricemia: The advisability of treating asymptomatic hyperuricemia is controversial. The risk of developing gouty arthritis and nephropathy is proportional to the degree of hyperuricemia. Mild hyperuricemia with no clinical manifestations of gout need not be treated. Treatment should be instituted if symptoms of gout develop; if there is a family history of gout, nephrolithiasis, or renal failure; or if there is marked overproduction of uric acid as indicated by the daily urinary excretion of more than 1 g with rigid purine restriction (Kelley, 1983).

Pseudogout: Pseudogout is a term used to describe deposition of calcium pyrophosphate in joint cartilage. Clinically, it resembles acute gouty arthritis and is characterized by acute inflammation and pain in one or more joints that lasts several days or more. It is thought to result from an inflammatory response to calcium pyrophosphate crystals in the synovial fluid similar to that seen in patients with acute gout due to accumulation of urate crystals. The magnitude of this inflammatory response is generally much less than that seen in acute gouty arthritis.

The newer nonsteroidal anti-inflammatory drugs are effective in relieving inflammation and pain. When large joints are affected acutely, thorough aspiration alone or with injection of corticosteroids may be beneficial. Colchicine can be useful when administered intravenously in usual therapeutic doses; oral administration generally is less effective (Rodnan et al, 1983).

Drug Evaluations

DRUGS USED IN ACUTE GOUTY ARTHRITIS

COLCHICINE

ACTIONS. The beneficial effects of colchicine in acute gout are attributable to its anti-inflammatory action, but other inflammatory diseases are affected only slightly. Colchicine has several biological actions, but their exact relationship to its clinical effect in gout has not been demonstrated conclusively (Dallaverde et al, 1982).

USES. Colchicine reduces inflammation and relieves pain in acute gouty arthritis. It is preferred by some clinicians for the initial attack. Therapy should begin at the first sign of an attack and continue until symptoms subside, gastrointestinal distress develops, or the maximal dose is given. This drug may be administered orally or intravenously. The oral route is not used as frequently as in the past because of gastrointestinal disturbances and the availability of other drugs. If oral administration is contraindicated, the drug may be given intravenously, but care must be taken to prevent extravasation, which causes sloughing of skin and subcutaneous tissues. Some clinicians prefer this route because it produces a more rapid response and avoids gastrointestinal disturbances. Relief of pain and inflammation usually occurs within 24 to 48 hours after oral therapy and 6 to 12 hours after intravenous injection, but several days may elapse before swelling subsides completely. It may be difficult to obtain prompt relief with nontoxic doses if there is delay in treatment or inconsistency in the dosage schedule.

Use of small doses of colchicine during the intercritical period may prevent acute attacks or diminish their severity and facilitate treatment. Colchicine also is given to prevent attacks of acute gouty arthritis that may be precipitated during the initial months of treatment with uricosurics or allopurinol, but this combined therapy should be individualized. Colchicine should be given until all visible or radiographically demonstrated tophi are dissolved. In the absence of tophi, it is advisable to continue therapy for one year. The dosage should be adjusted to provide maximal freedom from acute attacks without adverse reactions. Patients receiving colchicine prophylaxis sometimes respond to small therapeutic doses, thus terminating an acute attack without unpleasant reactions.

Intravenous colchicine may be used to control acute attacks of pseudogout (Tabatabai and Cummings, 1980; Spilberg et al, 1980).

When taken prophylactically, colchicine may prevent the episodic attacks of painful serositis characteristic of familial Mediterranean fever and may improve the symptoms of amyloidosis (Ravid et al, 1977). Alternatively, short courses of colchicine taken at the very onset of symptoms may abort attacks in some patients. Results of one study indicated that the drug increases survival in patients with primary amyloidosis (Rubinow et al, 1981).

Colchicine has been reported to be effective in the treatment of Paget's disease of bone (Theodors et al, 1981), dermatitis herpetiformis (Silvers et al, 1980), acute febrile neutrophilic dermatosis (Suehisa et al, 1983), erythema nodosum leprosum (Sarojini and Mshana, 1983), and idiopathic thrombocytopenic purpura resistant to standard treatment (Strother et al, 1984).

ADVERSE REACTIONS AND PRECAUTIONS. When given orally, colchicine causes gastrointestinal reactions in about 80% of patients, especially when maximal doses are used. These include nausea and vomiting or abdominal pain, as well as the so-called therapeutic endpoint of diarrhea. The warning provided by gastrointestinal intolerance tends to protect the patient from toxic doses. As soon as symptoms of intolerance occur, administration should be discontinued, irrespective of the status of joint symptoms. Drugs to control vomiting and diarrhea may be given when indicated. Gastrointestinal distress does not develop after intravenous administration of therapeutic amounts, but extravasation produces inflammation and necrosis of the skin and soft tissues.

More severe reactions have been reported rarely and generally have been associated with overdosage (therapeutic or suicidal), liver disease, delayed excretion caused by kidney damage, and especially with combinations of these factors. These reactions have included bone marrow depression with leukopenia and thrombocytopenia, purpura, peripheral neuritis, myopathy, anuria, alopecia, hepatocellular failure, hypersensitivity reactions, and hemorrhagic colitis. Disseminated intravascular coagulation is a frequent manifestation of severe colchicine toxicity; it appears within 48 hours and often is fatal. Treatment of toxicity is symptomatic and supportive.

Colchicine should be given with special caution to debilitated patients and to those with hepatic, renal, cardiovascular, or gastrointestinal disease. Intravenous administration is contraindicated in patients with leukopenia or severe hepatic or renal disease. Colchicine is classified as an FDA Pregnancy Category D substance.

PHARMACOKINETICS. Following oral administration of 2 mg, a mean peak plasma level of 2.2 ng/ml was reached after two hours; however, absorption was variable. Following intravenous injection of a 1-mg bolus in normal subjects, the mean elimination half-life was 65 ± 15 minutes and total clearance was 601 ± 155 ml/min. Volume of distribution was 49.5 ± 9.5 L. Colchicine levels declined biexponentially, fitting a two-compartment open-body model. The drug is concentrated in peripheral leukocytes and small but significant amounts are excreted in urine. The metabolism of colchicine is not completely known (Halkin et al, 1980).

DOSAGE AND PREPARATIONS.

Oral: For acute attacks, *adults,* 0.5 or 0.6 mg (one tablet) is administered hourly; alternatively, 1 or 1.2 mg (two tablets) may be given initially, followed by 0.5 or 0.6 mg every two hours until articular symptoms subside or gastrointestinal distress occurs. A maximum dose of 6 mg may be administered, but most patients cannot tolerate this amount. For prophylaxis, the dosage depends upon the sensitivity of the patient to gastrointestinal reactions. Usually 0.5 to 1 mg daily is given (Yu, 1982); 0.5 mg should be given every two hours if symptoms of an impending attack occur.

Generic. Tablets 0.5 and 0.6 mg.

Intravenous: For acute attacks, *adults,* 2 mg initially, followed by one or two additional doses of 1 mg each at six-hour intervals if needed. When given promptly, one or two infusions usually terminate an attack. Some clinicians recommend a single dose of 2 mg rather than repeated administration of smaller amounts, which increases the risk of extravasation and tissue necrosis. The total dose for one course of treatment should not exceed 4 mg. To minimize sclerosis of the vein, the contents of the 2-ml vial should be diluted to 20 ml with sterile normal sodium chloride injection and administered slowly over no less than five minutes. Solutions containing a bacteriostatic agent or 5% dextrose should not be used; any solution containing a precipitate should be discarded.

Generic. Solution 0.5 mg/ml in 2 ml containers.

Anti-inflammatory Drugs

ADRENAL CORTICOSTEROIDS

CORTICOTROPIN (ACTH)
[Acthar, Cortrophin Gel, Cortrophin-Zinc]

Although rarely needed, corticotropin or systemic corticosteroids may be effective in unusually severe acute attacks or in patients who do not respond to other anti-inflammatory drugs. Some clinicians believe that the use of corticotropin is not justified and a steroid is preferable (Simkin, 1979). These agents should not be administered for more than a few days and should not be given to treat chronic gout. To prevent rebound attacks, colchicine 0.6 mg two or three times daily should be given with and for seven days after discontinuation of corticotropin or steroids.

If the acute attack is limited to a single joint, a corticosteroid injected intra-articularly usually relieves pain. Oral anti-inflammatory drugs should be given concomitantly.

For adverse reactions and precautions, see Chapter 61, Adrenal Corticosteroids in Nonendocrine Diseases, and Chapter 42, Agents Related to Anterior Pituitary and Hypothalamic Function.

DOSAGE AND PREPARATIONS.
CORTICOTROPIN:
Intramuscular: Adults, 40 to 80 units every six to eight hours for two to three days; the dose then is reduced gradually until the medication can be withdrawn completely.
Intravenous: Adults, 40 to 80 units diluted in 250 to 500 ml of normal saline administered by intravenous drip.

> Available generically and as *ACTH*. Gel (repository) 40 and 80 units/ml in 5 ml containers; powder 40 and 80 units.
> *Acthar* (Armour). Powder (sterile, lyophilized) 25 and 40 units; gel (repository) 40 and 80 units/ml in 1 and 5 ml containers (*H.P. Acthar Gel*).
> *Cortrophin Gel* (Organon). Gel (repository) 40 and 80 units/ml in 5 ml containers.
> *Cortrophin-Zinc* (Organon). Suspension (repository, for intramuscular use only) 40 units with 2 mg of zinc/ml in 5 ml containers.
> **Additional Trademarks.**
> *Cortigel-40, -80* (Savage), *Cotropic Gel 40, 80* (Reid-Provident).

ADRENAL CORTICOSTEROIDS:
The doses vary greatly depending upon the individual preparation, but oral doses of 20 to 30 mg daily of prednisone and intra-articular injection of 8 to 40 mg of prednisolone tebutate or 2 to 20 mg of triamcinolone hexacetonide, depending on size of joint, are suggested (Simkin, 1979; Talbott, 1980; Holmes, 1981).

See Chapter 61 for preparations.

INDOMETHACIN
[Indocin]

USES. Indomethacin's anti-inflammatory properties are useful in the short-term treatment of attacks of acute gouty arthritis, and indomethacin is the drug of choice when the diagnosis is well established. Efficacy is comparable to that of colchicine. Indomethacin also may be beneficial in acute pseudogout.

ADVERSE REACTIONS AND PRECAUTIONS. The adverse reactions produced by indomethacin, some of which may be serious, generally are dose and time dependent. Gastrointestinal effects (nausea, vomiting, dyspepsia, diarrhea, abdominal pain, constipation) or central nervous system effects (dizziness, headache, tinnitus, vertigo, somnolence, depression, and fatigue) are most common.

Indomethacin should not be given to patients with an active ulcer, a history of recurrent gastrointestinal lesions, nasal polyps associated with angioedema, or a history of bronchospastic reaction to aspirin or other nonsteroidal anti-inflammatory drugs. The drug should be used cautiously in the elderly, since the incidence of adverse reactions appears to be higher in these patients.

When indomethacin is administered with probenecid, the tubular secretion of indomethacin is inhibited and the plasma concentration is increased; thus, a smaller dose of indomethacin may be satisfactory. Indomethacin also may interact with aspirin, lithium, and furosemide. See also Chapter 59, Antiarthritic Drugs.

DOSAGE AND PREPARATIONS.
Oral: For attacks of acute gout, *adults,* initially, 50 mg, followed by 25 mg three or four times daily until symptoms subside. Pain usually is relieved within two to four hours, tenderness and heat in 24 to 36 hours, and swelling gradually disappears, usually in three to five days. The dose is then reduced rapidly to cessation of therapy. Indomethacin should be taken with food, immediately after meals, or with antacids to reduce gastrointestinal irritation.
Rectal: Adults, 25 to 50 mg two to four times daily. Pediatric dose has not been established.

> *Generic.* Capsules 25 and 50 mg.
> *Indocin* (Merck Sharp & Dohme). Capsules 25 and 50 mg; suppositories 50 mg.

PHENYLBUTAZONE
[Azolid, Butazolidin]

ACTIONS AND USES. Phenylbutazone has proven effectiveness in attacks of acute gouty arthritis due to its anti-inflammatory and analgesic actions. Phenylbutazone should be used only in treatment-resistant patients with a history of positive response to the drug. Because of its potential to cause adverse reactions, especially with long-term use, phenylbutazone should not be used prophylactically or in the treatment of chronic gout.

ADVERSE REACTIONS AND PRECAUTIONS. Phenylbutazone may produce serious adverse reactions, particularly hematologic effects, even with short-term use. Thus, the patient should be supervised carefully during treatment and therapy should be discontinued immediately if any serious reactions occur. This drug is classified in FDA Pregnancy Category C. (For other adverse reactions and precautions, see Chapter 59, Antiarthritic Drugs.)

DOSAGE AND PREPARATIONS.
Oral: For acute attacks, *adults,* initially, 200 mg, followed by 100 mg four times daily for two to three days with gradual reduction of the dose over the next few days. Articular inflammation usually subsides within four days and therapy should not be continued for more than five to seven days.

> *Azolid* (USV), *Butazolidin* (Geigy), *Generic.* Capsules and tablets 100 mg.

Newer Nonsteroidal Anti-inflammatory Drugs

FENOPROFEN CALCIUM

IBUPROFEN

NAPROXEN

SULINDAC

These nonsteroidal anti-inflammatory drugs were developed primarily to treat arthritis but, because of their anti-inflammatory and analgesic actions, are also useful in acute gout. Although only sulindac and naproxen are labeled for use in gout, results of clinical studies have demonstrated that the others are also effective. There is insufficient evidence to indicate that any of these drugs is superior to the others as the initial agent in an acute attack. However, any of them may be tried as substitutes for colchicine (Baum, 1978; Talbott, 1980), especially if the diagnosis has been confirmed.

These nonsteroidal anti-inflammatory agents also are alternatives to colchicine for prophylaxis prior to and during initial therapy with allopurinol or uricosurics. They may be effective as nonspecific therapy in acute pseudogout.

For a discussion of adverse reactions, precautions, and interactions, see Chapter 59, Antiarthritic Drugs.

DOSAGE AND PREPARATIONS.

FENOPROFEN CALCIUM:

Oral: For acute attacks, dosage has not been established; in the investigational studies, 800 mg was given every six hours for three to eight days, depending upon response.

IBUPROFEN:

Oral: For acute attacks, dosage has not been established; in investigational studies, 800 mg was given every eight hours initially, reduced to 400 mg every six hours for 24 to 72 hours after symptoms subsided.

NAPROXEN:

Oral: For acute attacks, initially, 750 mg, followed by 250 mg every eight hours until the attack subsides.

SULINDAC:

Oral: For acute attacks, *adults,* 200 mg twice a day. The dose can be reduced after a satisfactory response has occurred; seven days of therapy are usually sufficient.

For preparations, see Chapter 59.

DRUGS USED FOR TOPHACEOUS GOUT AND OTHER HYPERURICEMIAS

ALLOPURINOL

[Lopurin, Zyloprim]

USES. Allopurinol is the preferred drug in the treatment of chronic tophaceous gout; it reduces serum urate levels, usually within a few days to two weeks. Prolonged treatment inhibits the formation of tophi and mobilizes stored urates, which causes a gradual regression in the size of tophi already formed. Allopurinol is especially useful in patients with chronic gout complicated by renal insufficiency or uric acid renal calculi, although careful titration of dose is important.

This drug is used to treat hyperuricemia associated with excessive production of uric acid (urinary uric acid excretion more than 800 mg/24 hours). This often occurs in patients with polycythemia vera, myeloid metaplasia, leukemia, or lymphoma, as well as during the treatment of these conditions with cytotoxic agents that break down cellular nucleic acids, which leads to acute uric acid nephropathy. Patients with these disorders should receive allopurinol prior to cytotoxic drug therapy. In patients with the Lesch-Nyhan syndrome, allopurinol controls blood uric acid levels and prevents nephropathy, tophi, and arthritis but has no effect on the neurologic and behavioral manifestations.

Like the uricosurics, allopurinol may increase the frequency of attacks of acute gouty arthritis during the early stages of treatment; therefore, colchicine or a nonsteroidal anti-inflammatory drug should be given prophylactically during the initial months of therapy (see the evaluation on Colchicine), and patients should receive appropriate treatment if acute attacks occur. Attacks usually diminish in number and severity after several months of treatment with allopurinol.

ACTIONS. Unlike uricosuric agents, allopurinol decreases the renal excretion of uric acid and its action is not antagonized by salicylates.

Allopurinol decreases the production of uric acid by inhibiting xanthine oxidase, which converts hypoxanthine to xanthine and xanthine to uric acid; plasma and urine concentrations of uric acid are thus reduced. Allopurinol also inhibits de novo purine synthesis through a feedback mechanism. This action requires the presence of hypoxanthine-guanine phosphoribosyltransferase. Children with Lesch-Nyhan syndrome, who lack this enzyme, and the few adults with a partial deficiency do not benefit from this effect.

Allopurinol is itself metabolized by xanthine oxidase to oxipurinol, which also inhibits xanthine oxidase. Oxipurinol has a considerably longer plasma half-life than allopurinol, thus accounting for the latter's long duration of action, which permits administration of allopurinol once daily.

ADVERSE REACTIONS AND PRECAUTIONS. Allopurinol is tolerated well by most patients (McInnes et al, 1981). However, a toxic syndrome associated with hypersensitivity has been reported (Hande et al, 1984). Manifestations include a diffuse, erythematous, desquamating, skin rash; fever; hepatic dysfunction; eosinophilia; and renal dysfunction. Of the 78 reported cases of severe allopurinol toxic syndrome, 16 have resulted in death.

Most patients who developed this syndrome took 200 to 400 mg daily for two to four weeks and had renal insufficiency. The causative factor may be allopurinol's active metabolite, oxipurinol, since its long half-life is prolonged further in patients with impaired renal function. In a study of six cases (Hande et al,

1984), the serum oxipurinol half-life was related inversely to renal creatinine clearance. Because of the increased potential for toxicity, allopurinol should be avoided or doses reduced in patients with renal insufficiency (see Dosage and Preparations).

Of the 78 cases reported, 52 patients were being treated for asymptomatic hyperuricemia. Thus, the incidence of toxicity could be reduced by avoiding use of this drug in patients with asymptomatic hyperuricemia and by reducing the dose in patients with renal insufficiency. If a rash and/or fever develop, allopurinol should be discontinued. Some patients recover spontaneously after drug withdrawal, while others require steroids or hemodialysis.

The long-term administration of allopurinol has been associated with cataracts in a few patients (Fraunfelder et al, 1982; Lerman et al, 1982, 1984); however, a causal relationship has not been established. Patients receiving allopurinol should undergo periodic ophthalmologic examinations and, if lens opacity is present, the drug should be discontinued.

Reactions that occur occasionally include nausea, vomiting, diarrhea, abdominal discomfort, drowsiness, headache, and a metallic taste. Rare reactions for which a causal relationship has not been established include peripheral neuritis, precipitation of peptic ulcer or increase in ulcer symptoms, tachycardia, pancreatitis, pyelonephritis, increased blood urea nitrogen levels, anemia, retinopathy, and macular degeneration. One death associated with bone marrow depression has been reported.

Hepatic effects ranging from altered liver function (increased serum levels of alkaline phosphatase and transaminases) to hepatitis, which may be part of a generalized hypersensitivity reaction, have been reported frequently. Granulomatous hepatitis has been reported rarely. If anorexia, weight loss, or pruritus develops in patients taking allopurinol, liver function should be evaluated.

Xanthine renal calculus formation occurs rarely, even in patients with Lesch-Nyhan syndrome.

Allopurinol is relatively contraindicated in patients with liver disease and bone marrow suppression.

Studies in animals have shown that allopurinol has no teratogenic effects. However, there is no information on the effects of xanthine oxidase inhibition on the human fetus, and the potential benefits should be weighed against the possible risk to the fetus before allopurinol is used in pregnant women or women of childbearing age.

DRUG INTERACTIONS. Because allopurinol inhibits the oxidation of mercaptopurine, the dose of the latter must be reduced to one-third or one-fourth of the usual amount when both drugs are given concomitantly. Since mercaptopurine is a metabolite of azathioprine, similar precautions should be observed when using the latter drug. Allopurinol also appears to increase the toxicity of other cytotoxic agents (eg, cyclophosphamide). Anemia, nausea, pain, pruritus, and tremors have developed in patients receiving allopurinol and vidarabine. Thus, caution is advised when these two drugs are administered concomitantly (Friedman and Grasela, 1981).

The incidence of rash after administration of ampicillin is unusually high in patients receiving allopurinol concomitantly. Allopurinol should be discontinued promptly when rash occurs,

since this reaction may become serious if treatment is continued.

Allopurinol inhibits hepatic drug metabolizing enzymes; thus, drugs metabolized by these enzymes (eg, coumarin derivatives) should be given in lower doses.

PHARMACOKINETICS. Following a single oral dose of 300 mg, about 80% of the dose is absorbed. Peak serum concentrations of 1.4 ± 0.23 ng/ml are reached in one to two hours; oxipurinol, the major metabolite, attains a peak concentration of 5.20 ± 0.65 ng/ml in 5.2 to 6.5 hours. The half-life of allopurinol is 1.3 ± 0.1 hours and that of oxipurinol is 21.2 ± 0.4 hours (Chang et al, 1981). Most of the oxipurinol is excreted unchanged by the kidney.

DOSAGE AND PREPARATIONS. Dosage should be individualized to obtain the desired serum urate level (7 mg/dl or less in males and 6 mg/dl or less in females) as determined by frequent measurements. Allopurinol is better tolerated if taken after meals.

Oral: *Adults,* dosage must be individualized. Initially, 100 mg/day, increased at weekly intervals by 100 mg until the serum uric acid level is normal or near normal. An effective range for most patients with normal renal function is 200 to 300 mg daily. The maintenance dosage should be reduced in patients with renal insufficiency. Frequent follow-up examinations of serum urate and renal function help to establish the minimal effective dose that maintains the serum urate level below 7 mg/dl (males) or 6 mg/dl (females).

For secondary hyperuricemias, the optimal dose is the smallest amount necessary to maintain serum uric acid levels within the normal range. *Adults,* 100 to 200 mg daily is the minimum effective dose (maximum, 800 mg); *children 6 to 10 years with malignancies,* 300 mg daily; *under 6 years,* 150 mg daily.

Lopurin (Boots), **Zyloprim** (Burroughs Wellcome), **Generic.** Tablets 100 and 300 mg.

Rectal: Extemporaneous rectal suppositories have been prepared from tablets for use in patients unable to take oral medications; however, absorption of the drug in suppository form was poor and erratic. Although clinical efficacy, as determined by the decrease in serum uric acid level, has been reported, additional studies are needed to confirm these results. Therefore, this route does not appear to be an effective alternative to oral administration (Chang et al, 1981).

PROBENECID
[Benemid, SK-Probenecid]

ACTIONS AND USES. The uricosuric effect of probenecid is attributed to inhibition of the tubular reabsorption of filtered urate. This effective uricosuric agent is used to prevent or reduce the joint changes and tophi that occur in chronic gout; it is chosen primarily for patients with normal renal function whose 24-hour urinary uric acid excretion is less than 800 mg. Probenecid usually has no significant uricosuric activity when the glomerular filtration rate is less than 30 ml/min, and thus is not always effective in patients with chronic renal insufficiency. It has been used in patients with renal impairment, but an increase in dosage may be required. This drug is not indicated in acute attacks of gouty arthritis.

Since acute attacks of gout may occur during the initial months of therapy, colchicine or a nonsteroidal anti-inflammatory drug should be given concomitantly during this period. (See the evaluation on Colchicine.)

Probenecid also is used to increase the blood levels and prolong the antibacterial action of penicillin preparations by blocking their renal tubular secretion. It has been shown to prolong the half-life of dyphylline (see Chapter 22, Drugs Used in Bronchial Disorders).

ADVERSE REACTIONS AND PRECAUTIONS. Probenecid is well tolerated by most patients. Gastrointestinal reactions (anorexia, nausea, vomiting), headache, hypersensitivity reactions (including anaphylaxis, dermatitis, pruritus, and fever), urinary frequency, anemia, dizziness, and flushing have occurred. Hemolytic anemia, which may be related to G6PD deficiency; aplastic anemia; nephrotic syndrome; and hepatic necrosis have been reported rarely.

Initially, a large volume (2 to 3 L/day) of urine should be maintained to minimize urate precipitation in the urinary tract. Probenecid is contraindicated in patients with a history of renal calculi, especially uric acid stones, because it may aggravate or precipitate this condition. The drug also should not be used in patients whose glomerular filtration rate is less than 50% of normal.

DRUG INTERACTIONS. Salicylates diminish the effect of probenecid and should not be used concomitantly. Probenecid inhibits the renal transport of sulfinpyrazone, sulfonylureas, indomethacin, penicillin, aminosalicylic acid, sulfonamides (mostly as inactive conjugates), pantothenic acid, iodomethamate and related iodinated organic acids, aminohippuric acid, 17-ketosteroids, phenolsulfonphthalein, and sulfobromophthalein. The dosage of these agents should be modified when they are administered with probenecid. The drug has been reported to increase plasma levels of rifampin and methotrexate.

Since probenecid increases the renal excretion of oxipurinol, inhibition of xanthine oxidase is reduced when probenecid is given with allopurinol. However, in tophaceous gout, it can be given with allopurinol for more rapid dissolution of tophi. When probenecid was given with sulindac, the plasma levels of sulindac and its sulfone metabolite were increased, but the plasma sulfide levels were only slightly affected. Probenecid slows the clearance of naproxen by inhibiting hepatic metabolism; thus, concomitant use of these drugs results in higher plasma levels of naproxen (Runkel et al, 1978).

PHARMACOKINETICS. Probenecid is readily absorbed following oral administration. Peak plasma concentrations are observed three to four hours after a 0.5-g dose. Mean elimination half-life was 4.2 hours after the 0.5-g dose. With larger doses, saturable probenecid elimination kinetics were observed, which suggests that the drug may accumulate upon repeated administration. Probenecid is metabolized by side chain oxidation and glucuronidation. It is excreted in urine principally as the acylglucuronides and oxidized metabolites. Little probenecid is excreted unchanged in urine (Selen et al, 1982).

DOSAGE AND PREPARATIONS.
Oral: Dosage should be individualized to obtain the desired serum urate level. *Adults,* 250 mg one or two times daily for one week or more depending on response; the amount is then increased slowly to the minimum dose necessary to maintain normal serum urate levels. Usually 1 g/day is sufficient, but some patients may require 1.5 g/day or more.

Benemid (Merck Sharp & Dohme), **SK-Probenecid** (Smith Kline & French), **Generic**. Tablets 500 mg.

SULFINPYRAZONE
[Anturane]

ACTIONS AND USES. Sulfinpyrazone is a congener of phenylbutazone, but it lacks the latter's anti-inflammatory, analgesic, and sodium-retaining properties. This effective uricosuric agent is used to treat tophaceous gout and hyperuricemia during the intercritical period. It is more potent than probenecid on a weight basis and is chosen primarily for patients with normal renal function whose 24-hour urinary uric acid excretion is less than 800 mg. It is of no immediate value in acute attacks of gouty arthritis.

Because acute attacks of gout may increase in frequency or severity during the initial months of therapy with sulfinpyrazone, colchicine or a nonsteroidal anti-inflammatory drug should be given concomitantly during this period. (See the evaluation on Colchicine.)

Since sulfinpyrazone inhibits platelet function, it has been studied as an antithrombotic agent (Margulies et al, 1980).

ADVERSE REACTIONS AND PRECAUTIONS. The most frequently reported adverse reactions are abdominal pain and nausea. Since reactivation or exacerbation of peptic ulcer also has been reported, sulfinpyrazone should be used cautiously in patients with a history of ulcer and is contraindicated in those with active peptic ulcer. Rash is uncommon; anemia, leukopenia, agranulocytosis, and thrombocytopenia have occurred rarely.

An adequate fluid intake and alkalization of the urine should be maintained to minimize the renal deposition of urate during therapy until the serum urate level is within the normal range. The drug should be used with caution in patients with impaired renal function or a history of renal calculi, especially uric acid stones, because of the possibility of aggravating or precipitating the condition. Sulfinpyrazone should not be used when the glomerular filtration rate is less than 50% of normal. Patients with significant renal impairment should have periodic evaluations of their renal function. Sulfinpyrazone is contraindicated in patients with a history of blood dyscrasias.

DRUG INTERACTIONS. Like probenecid, sulfinpyrazone reduces the renal tubular excretion of aminohippuric acid, phenolsulfonphthalein, and salicylic acid; therefore, diagnostic procedures based upon measurement of these substances are invalidated by therapy with sulfinpyrazone. Salicylates diminish the effect of sulfinpyrazone and should not be used concomitantly.

Like phenylbutazone, sulfinpyrazone may potentiate the actions of insulin and oral hypoglycemic agents; therefore, it should be used with caution in patients receiving these drugs. Because of its chemical relationship to phenylbutazone and the similarity of some adverse effects, sulfinpyrazone should be used cautiously, if at all, in patients known to be sensitive to phenylbutazone; however, serious reactions are less common than with phenylbutazone. Sulfinpyrazone has no effect on sodium reabsorption.

PHARMACOKINETICS. Sulfinpyrazone is rapidly and completely absorbed following oral administration. Peak blood levels occur in about one hour and the half-life is one to three hours. It is highly bound to plasma protein. Most of the drug is excreted unchanged in urine; the remainder is metabolized to the parahydroxyl analogue, which also has uricosuric activity.

DOSAGE AND PREPARATIONS.
Oral: Adults, 100 to 200 mg two times daily given with meals or with milk. The dose is increased gradually over a one-week period until the dosage required to control blood urate levels is reached, usually 200 to 400 mg. The dose then may be reduced to the minimal effective level.

Anturane (CIBA), *Generic.* Capsules 200 mg; tablets 100 mg.

Mixture

PROBENECID AND COLCHICINE
[ColBENEMID]

This mixture of probenecid and colchicine is designed to facilitate maintenance therapy of chronic gout, but its usefulness is limited because the amount of each ingredient cannot be individualized. If the usual dosage of probenecid were used, this mixture would provide a greater amount of colchicine than needed by many patients and less than that needed by some.

For adverse reactions and precautions, see the evaluations on Colchicine and Probenecid.

DOSAGE AND PREPARATIONS. The dosage is based upon the patient's requirement for the individual ingredients, provided that these have been established individually and are consistent with the ratio present in this preparation. (See the evaluations on Probenecid and Colchicine.)

ColBENEMID (Merck Sharp & Dohme), *Generic.* Each tablet contains probenecid 500 mg and colchicine 0.5 mg.

Cited References

Baum J: Modern concepts in treatment of gout. *Drug Ther* 8:76-81, (May) 1978.

Chang S-L, et al: Bioavailability of allopurinol oral and rectal dosage forms. *Am J Hosp Pharm* 38:365-368, 1981.

Dallaverde E, et al: Mechanism of action of colchicine. V. Neutrophil adherence and phagocytosis in patients with acute gout treated with colchicine. *J Pharmacol Exp Ther* 223:197-202, 1982.

Fraunfelder FT, et al: Cataracts associated with allopurinol therapy. *Am J Ophthalmol* 94:137-140, 1982.

Friedman HM, Grasela T: Adenine arabinoside and allopurinol: Possible adverse drug interaction, (letter). *N Engl J Med* 304:423, 1981.

Halkin H, et al: Colchicine kinetics in patients with familial Mediterranean fever. *Clin Pharmacol Ther* 28:82-87, 1980.

Hande KR, et al: Severe allopurinol toxicity: Description and guidelines for prevention in patients with renal insufficiency. *Am J Med* 76:47-56, 1984.

Holmes EW Jr: Rational approach to gout. *Drug Ther* 11:117-124, (Feb) 1981.

Kelley WN: Gout and other disorders of purine metabolism, in Petersdorf RG, et al (eds): *Harrison's Principles of Internal Medicine,* ed 10. New York, McGraw-Hill, 1983, 517-524.

Lerman S, et al: Allopurinol therapy and cataractogenesis in humans. *Am J Ophthalmol* 94:141-146, 1982.

Lerman S, et al: Further studies on allopurinol therapy and human cataractogenesis. *Am J Ophthalmol* 97:205-209, 1984.

Margulies EH, et al: Sulfinpyrazone: Review of its pharmacological properties and therapeutic use. *Drugs* 20:179-197, 1980.

McInnes GT, et al: Acute adverse reactions attributed to allopurinol in hospitalised patients. *Ann Rheum Dis* 40:245-249, 1981.

Ravid M, et al: Prolonged colchicine treatment in four patients with amyloidosis. *Ann Intern Med* 87:568-570, 1977.

Rodnan GP, et al (eds): Gout, in: *Primer on the Rheumatic Diseases,* ed 8. Atlanta, GA, Arthritis Foundation, 1983, 120-128.

Rubinow AS, et al: Colchicine therapy in amyloidosis: Preliminary report. *Arthritis Rheum* 24(suppl):124, (April) 1981.

Runkel R, et al: Naproxen-probenecid interaction. *Clin Pharmacol Ther* 24:706-713, 1978.

Sarojini PA, Mshana RN: Use of colchicine in management of erythema nodosum leprosum (ENL), (letter). *Lepr Rev* 54:151-156, 1983.

Selen A, et al: Pharmacokinetics of probenecid following oral doses in human volunteers. *J Pharmaceut Sci* 71:1238-1242, 1982.

Silvers DN, et al: Treatment of dermatitis herpetiformis with colchicine. *Arch Dermatol* 116:1373-1374, 1980.

Simkin PA: Management of gout. *Ann Intern Med* 90:812-816, 1979.

Spilberg I, et al: Colchicine and pseudogout. *Arthritis Rheum* 23:1062-1063, 1980.

Strother SV, et al: Colchicine therapy for refractory idiopathic thrombocytopenic purpura. *Arch Intern Med* 144:2198-2200, 1984.

Suehisa S, et al: Colchicine in treatment of acute febrile neutrophilic dermatosis (Sweet's syndrome). *Br J Dermatol* 108:99-101, 1983.

Tabatabai MR, Cummings NA: Intravenous colchicine in treatment of acute pseudogout. *Arthritis Rheum* 23:370-374, 1980.

Talbott JH: Gouty arthritis: Disease for all ages. *Geriatrics* 35:69-78, (May) 1980.

Talbott JR, Yu TF: *Gout and Uric Acid Metabolism.* New York, Stratton Intercontinental, 1976.

Theodors A, et al: Colchicine in treatment of Paget disease of bone: New therapeutic approach. *Clin Ther* 3:365-373, 1981.

Wallace SL, et al: Preliminary criteria for classification of acute arthritis of primary gout. *Arthritis Rheum* 20:895-900, 1977.

Wyngaarden JB, Kelley WN: *Gout and Hyperuricemia.* New York, Grune & Stratton, 1976.

Yu TF: Efficacy of colchicine prophylaxis in articular gout: Reappraisal after 20 years. *Semin Arthritis Rheum* 12:256-264, 1982.

Other Selected References

Boss GR, Seegmiller JE: Hyperuricemia and gout: Classification, complications and management. *N Engl J Med* 300:1459-1468, 1979.

Fox IH, Kelley WN: Management of gout. *JAMA* 242:361-364, 1979.

Gordon GV, Schumacher HR: Management of gout. *Am Fam Physi-*

cian 19:91-97, (Jan) 1979.

Klinenberg JR: Hyperuricemia and gout. *Med Clin North Am* 61:299-312, 1977.

Klinenberg JR: Role of kidneys in pathogenesis of gout. *Postgrad Med* 63:145-150, (May) 1978.

Scott JT: Long-term management of gout and hyperuricaemia. *Br Med J* 281:1164-1166, 1980.

Talbott JH: Treating gout: Successful methods of prevention and control. *Postgrad Med* 63:175-180, (May) 1978.

Wallace SL: Colchicine. *Semin Arthritis Rheum* 3:369-381, 1974.

Wedeen RP: Hyperuricemia and gouty nephropathy: Persisting controversy. *Drug Ther* 11:45-52, (Oct) 1981.

Yu TF: Nephrolithiasis in patients with gout. *Postgrad Med* 63:164-170, (May) 1978.

Adrenal Corticosteroids in Nonendocrine Diseases

61

ACTIONS

INDICATIONS

ADVERSE REACTIONS

PRECAUTIONS

WITHDRAWAL FROM THERAPY

ALTERNATE-DAY THERAPY

DRUG SELECTION

PREPARATIONS

Corticosteroids with predominantly glucocorticoid activity are used to treat a wide variety of nonendocrine diseases. Efficacy is related to their anti-inflammatory and immunomodulating actions, which are not associated with physiologic concentrations of hormones but become apparent only when pharmacologic doses are administered. Patients receiving systemic corticosteroids for nonendocrine disorders are at risk of developing adverse effects, such as cushingoid features, increased susceptibility to infection, and suppression of the hypothalamic-pituitary-adrenal (HPA) axis. Therefore, the expected benefits must be weighed against the possible adverse effects before initiating therapy. Guidelines for the judicious use of corticosteroids include the following:

(1) The presence of a steroid-responsive condition must be ascertained initially.

(2) Corticosteroid therapy should be initiated only after less toxic therapy has been ineffective.

(3) Dosage should be based on the severity of the disease; the smallest amount that controls a specific symptom or sign should be used. The purpose of therapy is to achieve an acceptable degree of palliation; complete remission is usually not an appropriate therapeutic goal.

(4) Dosage, frequency of administration, duration of therapy, and corticosteroid preparations influence the therapeutic response and the frequency of adverse reactions. Systemic administration of a single large dose (ie, 1 to 2 mg/kg of prednisone or equivalent) is virtually without ill effects and may decrease morbidity; this justifies the use of such therapy in life-threatening emergencies when the diagnosis is only tentative. Generally, the severity of adverse reactions increases

with the duration of therapy and size of the dose and is directly related to the degree of immunosuppressive anti-inflammatory effect.

(5) When possible, the corticosteroid should be administered locally to concentrate therapeutic effects on the diseased tissue and minimize adverse effects.

(6) To avoid adrenal crisis before HPA axis responsiveness returns after prolonged therapy, pharmacologic doses of glucocorticoids must be reduced gradually over weeks to months except in unusual circumstances. In some cases, adrenal responsiveness to corticotropin (ACTH) should be tested (see the evaluation on Cosyntropin in Chapter 42, Agents Related to Anterior Pituitary and Hypothalamic Function).

(7) When possible, once the underlying disease is in remission, alternate-day therapy should be used to minimize adverse effects.

ACTIONS

At the molecular level, glucocorticoids act by passively entering a target cell and rapidly binding to intracellular cytoplasmic steroid receptors. After the steroid-receptor complexes undergo conformational changes termed "activation," they have a high affinity for nuclei and DNA. They bind to acceptor sites in the nuclear chromatin, altering the levels of specific mRNAs. Consequently, there are changes in the rates of synthesis of protein translated from these hormone-regulated mRNAs, which, in turn, mediate the response to glucocorticoids.

Glucocorticoids act at multiple sites. They do not block the interaction of antibodies with sensitized lymphocytes or the release of histamine or kinins that is initiated by this process. Rather, they block the multiple tissue responses to these stimuli. Glucocorticoids prevent the initiation of the cascade of reactions leading to the production of certain prostaglandins and leukotrienes by inducing the production and release of a protein (macrocortin, lipomodulin) that inhibits phospholipase A_2, an enzyme that releases free arachidonic acid from membrane phospholipids. At high tissue concentrations, they may stabilize lysosomal enzymes, thus preventing the spillage of hydrolytic enzymes. Glucocorticoids increase the number of beta-agonist receptors on cell membranes. They help to maintain capillary integrity and interfere with the movement of immune complexes across basement membranes. Glucocorticoids maintain vascular tone, possibly by potentiating the action of vasoconstrictors.

Glucocorticoids exert a broad range of effects on circulating leukocytes. They produce lymphocytopenia, which lasts for about 24 hours (see Table 1). The decrease in circulating lymphocytes in man is due to redistribution rather than lysis of lymphocytes as occurs in "corticosteroid-sensitive" animals, such as the mouse, rat, and rabbit (Fauci et al, 1976). Circulating neutrophils increase because mature neutrophils are released from the bone marrow and movement from the blood to other tissues decreases. Other circulating leukocytes decrease after glucocorticoid administration.

Corticosteroids also alter the function of monocytes, macrophages, and T-lymphocytes. During an antigen-antibody interaction, migration inhibitory factor (MIF) is released from lymphocytes and interleukin-1 (IL-1) is released from macrophages. MIF inhibits the mobility of macrophages, causing accumulation in the surrounding area. Glucocorticoids prevent the macrophage reaction to MIF and inhibit phagocytosis and digestion of antigens. Interleukin-1 stimulates T cells to synthesize and release interleukin-2 (IL-2), which binds to antigenically stimulated receptors located on the membranes of certain T cells and cause the T cells to replicate. Glucocorticoids inhibit IL-1 and IL-2 production and inhibit the T-lymphocyte-mediated proliferation of lymphocytes that normally follows exposure to mitogens and antigens. The antigenically stimulated receptors are unaffected, however, and the cells will proliferate if exogenous IL-2 is added to the culture medium.

By inhibiting the inflammatory process at the cellular level, glucocorticoids decrease its clinical manifestations (eg, heat, redness, tenderness), but the underlying disorder is unaffected.

INDICATIONS

In this chapter, only those indications not discussed elsewhere in the book are reviewed.

Allergic Disorders: Glucocorticoids promptly relieve symptoms in many allergic states, including bronchial asthma; nonseasonal allergic rhinitis; seasonal allergic rhinitis (hay fever, pollinosis); reactions to drugs, serum, and transfusions; and allergic dermatoses. They are generally reserved for control of acute episodes and are not a substitute for other medication (eg, beta-adrenergic agonists for asthma, antihistamines for hay fever) or avoidance of allergens. In relatively minor conditions, prednisone 60 mg (or equivalent) is given for two or three days and the amount is then reduced by 10 mg daily until therapy is discontinued. In emergencies (eg, status asthmaticus, anaphylactic reactions), steroids should be employed only as adjuncts to epinephrine, cardiorespiratory support, and, in status asthmaticus, a beta-adrenergic agonist and aminophylline. (See also Chapter 22, Drugs Used in Bronchial Disorders, and Chapter 62, Agents for Active and Passive Immunity.)

Cerebral Edema: Glucocorticoids are most effective when edema is of the vasogenic type, such as that caused by brain tumors, especially metastases and glioblastomas; they are somewhat less effective in edema caused by astrocytomas and meningiomas. Edema resulting from brain abscesses responds to glucocorticoid therapy; that produced by closed head injury is least responsive. There is doubt about the benefit of glucocorticoids in ischemic brain edema; these agents appear to have a deleterious effect in patients with malaria (Warrell et al, 1982).

The role of glucocorticoids in the treatment of severe head injury remains controversial. In animal studies, functional recovery improved in dogs and cats receiving massive doses (ie, methylprednisolone 15 to 30 mg/kg, dexamethasone 3 to 6 mg/kg) within one hour of induced spinal cord injury (Braughler and Hall, 1985); smaller doses or delay of therapy was ineffective. However, in clinical studies, glucocorticoids lack

TABLE 1.
GLUCOCORTICOID-INDUCED SHIFTS IN CIRCULATING LEUKOCYTES

Leukocyte Population	Absolute Number of Cells in Circulation	Relative Proportion of Cells	Time to Peak Effect (Hours)	Time to Recovery (Hours)
Neutrophils	⇈	⇈	4–6	24
Eosinophils	⇊	⇊	4–8	72
Basophils	⇊	⇊	8	72
Monocytes	⇊	⇊	4–6	24
Lymphocytes	⇊	↓	4–6	24
T-lymphocytes	⇊	⇊	4–6	24
B-lymphocytes	↓	↑	4–6	24

Adapted from Cupps and Fauci, 1982

beneficial activity and are detrimental in some instances. For example, in one study, patients receiving "large" doses of methylprednisolone (a bolus of 1 g intravenously, repeated daily for ten days) fared worse than patients receiving "standard" doses (a bolus of 100 mg intravenously, repeated daily for ten days) (Bracken et al, 1984). Further studies are needed to determine the role of glucocorticoids in head trauma.

These steroids have been used for brain edema associated with stroke, but opinion is divided on their efficacy. They also are sometimes used with mannitol to treat brain edema associated with Reye's syndrome.

Collagen Disorders: Generally, steroids are most beneficial when large doses (1 to 2 mg/kg of prednisone or the equivalent) are given during acute exacerbations; the effectiveness of long-term maintenance therapy varies. Some manifestations of *systemic lupus erythematosus* may be controlled by glucocorticoids. Topical preparations are used if dermatologic symptoms predominate, and systemic therapy is appropriate when nephritis, central nervous system disturbances, and hematologic complications, such as hemolytic anemia or thrombocytopenia, are present. Symptoms and serologic values (eg, serum complement, anti-DNA antibodies) may aid in determining the minimum dosage that improves survival rates (Urman and Rothfield, 1977).

Short-term use of large doses (1 to 2 mg/kg of prednisone or the equivalent) may be required for remission, particularly when the central nervous system is involved. Fewer exacerbations occur if the dose is reduced gradually at the rate of 10% of the daily dose per week after the patient's condition stabilizes (Yount et al, 1975). If serum complement levels rise and then decrease as the dose is reduced, the amount should be increased and the rate of reduction slowed. "Pulse" dosing with methylprednisolone (1 g/day for three days) has been tried in severe disease, and studies evaluating efficacy continue. The combination of an immunosuppressive agent, such as azathioprine [Imuran] or cyclophosphamide [Cytoxan], with a glucocorticoid appears to be more beneficial than either type of agent alone in slowing the progression of renal failure in patients with lupus nephritis (Carette et al, 1983).

Polymyositis and *dermatomyositis* are treated initially with large doses of glucocorticoids (1 to 2 mg/kg of prednisone daily for two to three months); the amount can be decreased gradually after the initial response. Six months often are required before the dose can be reduced to 7.5 to 10 mg daily. More abrupt reduction of the dose may cause recurrence of weakness and an increase in plasma creatine phosphokinase. Maintenance therapy may be required for years and more than 50% of patients require steroids indefinitely. Most patients who discontinue glucocorticoid therapy do so within three years after diagnosis. Immunosuppressive agents (eg, azathioprine, antilymphocytic globulin, methotrexate) have been used as adjuncts in selected patients with dermatomyositis not controlled by steroids alone.

Steroids relieve the signs of *polyarteritis nodosa* (systemic necrotizing vasculitis) and may improve the five-year survival rate, which is about 15% without treatment. Therapy is initiated with prednisone 40 to 60 mg daily; the dose is then reduced to the lowest effective amount for maintenance. When glucocorticoids alone are used in polyarteritis nodosa, the five-year

survival rate exceeds 50%. A major complication of systemic necrotizing vasculitis is bowel infarction; when glucocorticoids are used alone, the signs and symptoms of ischemic bowel frequently are masked. The addition of a cytotoxic drug improves the response in some patients. The combination may be advisable when there are life-threatening complications, renal involvement, or no sign of remission after two to three months of steroid therapy (Armstrong and Conn, 1981). Hypertension must be controlled but is not a contraindication to steroid therapy. Residual hypertension is common in those who survive.

Polymyalgia rheumatica occurs in older patients (usually over 60 years) and is improved by glucocorticoid therapy to suppress symptoms and maintain the erythrocyte sedimentation rate below 30 mm/hour (Behn et al, 1983). Small doses (eg, prednisone 10 to 20 mg daily) are used initially and the amount can be reduced by 1 mg/month in patients taking 10 mg daily or less. The incidence of *temporal arteritis* (giant cell arteritis) is high in patients with polymyalgia rheumatica who generally require larger doses to control the disease (initial dose, prednisone 20 mg or more daily). Because of the high risk of temporal arteritis, some practitioners favor treating all patients who have polymyalgia rheumatica with steroids.

Mixed connective tissue disease (MCTD) responds well to glucocorticoids. Most symptoms can be controlled with alternate-day therapy and steroids often can be discontinued eventually. Differential diagnosis of MCTD and systemic scleroderma is essential, however, because glucocorticoids do not improve the vascular lesions or fibrosis produced by the latter disorder.

Hematologic Disorders: Idiopathic and acquired *autoimmune hemolytic anemia* may respond to glucocorticoids, which are sometimes the sole therapeutic agents utilized. Glucocorticoids do not reduce hemolysis in transfusion reactions, although they may lessen drug-induced hemolysis. In *erythroblastopenia* (pure erythrocyte aplasia, congenital hypoplastic anemia, Blackfan-Diamond syndrome), small maintenance doses given on alternate days may eliminate dependence on transfusion and may be the treatment of choice.

Rarely, glucocorticoids produce remissions of variable length in *aplastic anemia*. They may be useful when a suitable donor for bone marrow transplantation is not available and in patients with less severe disease. Following immunosuppression and pending the availability of a suitable donor, androgens and anabolic steroids also may be utilized (see Chapter 38, Androgens and Anabolic Steroids).

Although their effectiveness has not been proved in controlled trials, glucocorticoids generally are recommended as initial therapy for *idiopathic thrombocytopenic purpura* (ITP). ITP is considered an autoimmune disease, and antibodies (most commonly IgG) have been found adhering to platelets in up to 90% of patients. Glucocorticoids are thought to act by inhibiting the phagocytosis of antibody-associated platelets, thus increasing platelet life span. Doses of 1 to 1.5 mg/kg of prednisone or the equivalent produce remission in 40% to 60% of patients (Rote and Lau, 1985; Burns and Saleem, 1983). Splenectomy should be considered for those who do not respond adequately after two to six months of therapy. It is unclear whether glucocorticoids reduce the risk of life-threatening intracranial hemorrhage. Long-term steroid therapy has no role in the treatment of ITP.

The treatment of ITP during pregnancy usually is conservative. Many pregnant women with moderate disease do not require treatment, but those with severe ITP do. Most clinicians prescribe the lowest dose of glucocorticoid that increases the platelet count and returns the bleeding time to normal (Kelton, 1983). Infants of mothers with ITP are at risk for thrombocytopenia. Steroid therapy during pregnancy may protect the fetus, but generalizations cannot be made concerning its effectiveness in controlling the fetal platelet count. If the neonatal platelet count drops below 50,000 to 75,000 platelets/mm³, prednisone 1 to 2 mg/kg/day, exchange transfusions, and immune globulin should be considered (Rote and Lau, 1985).

Hepatic Diseases: The effectiveness and safety of glucocorticoids in the treatment of liver disease depend upon the form involved and the condition of the patient. These agents are used in the initial therapy of *subacute hepatic necrosis* (prednisolone 60 to 100 mg/day) and autoimmune *chronic active hepatitis* (prednisone 20 to 60 mg/day). Medication traditionally is withdrawn gradually when there are signs of maximal improvement; if relapse occurs, more prolonged therapy is required. However, recent data show that not all patients with chronic active hepatitis who initially responded to steroids will respond to these drugs again if relapse occurs. Therefore, some experts suggest life-long maintenance steroid therapy (ie, prednisone 5 to 15 mg/day) for selected patients with chronic active hepatitis. Concomitant administration of azathioprine sometimes allows reduction of the glucocorticoid dose.

Patients with hepatitis B surface antigens who have chronic active hepatitis should *not* receive glucocorticoid therapy, because remission is delayed, complications occur more frequently, and the mortality rate is higher.

In *alcoholic hepatitis*, the beneficial effects of glucocorticoid therapy are probably limited to seriously ill patients with encephalopathy, in whom survival rates are enhanced. These agents may be used in *sarcoidosis* when acute inflammatory changes coexist with functional abnormalities as demonstrated by liver biopsy. Glucocorticoids also may be effective in other types of hepatic granulomata except those due to infections or neoplasms.

Glucocorticoids may be beneficial in drug-induced hepatic disorders, but controlled studies are lacking. Whether these agents are effective in biliary cirrhosis or infectious mononucleosis has not been demonstrated adequately. They are *not* indicated for the treatment of acute viral hepatitis or inactive postnecrotic cirrhosis.

Renal Disease: In patients less than 16 years of age, the most common subtype of idiopathic *nephrotic syndrome* is minimal change nephrosis, which generally responds to glucocorticoids. The initial dosage is prednisone 1 to 1.5 mg/kg/day or the equivalent. Both daily and alternate-day administration have been utilized; 80% to 90% of children respond within four to eight weeks, although a three-month course is usual. Two-thirds of those who respond never experience relapse or do so no more than once yearly; courses of glucocorticoids may be repeated in the latter. The remaining responsive

patients relapse two to four times yearly and may require more prolonged therapy, preferably on an alternate-day schedule. The addition of an alkylating agent (cyclophosphamide [Cytoxan] or chlorambucil [Leukeran]) to the regimen may maintain remission in children with frequent relapses; these drugs also may be used in steroid-resistant patients. Alkylating agents should be administered only when necessary because of their side effects (Martinez-Maldonado and Garcia, 1981).

Adults with nephrotic syndrome may respond to alternate-day prednisone therapy, depending upon the subtype present; in decreasing order of responsiveness these are: minimal change nephrosis, membranous nephropathy, diffuse proliferative nephritis, and focal sclerosis (Bolton et al, 1977).

The following regimens, alternated monthly for six months, were reported to relieve proteinuria and preserve renal function in adults with idiopathic membranous nephropathy: intravenous methylprednisolone 1 g daily for 3 days, followed by either oral methylprednisolone 0.4 mg/kg/day or prednisone 0.5 mg/kg/day for 27 days, then oral chlorambucil 0.2 mg/kg/day for 30 days (Ponticelli et al, 1984).

Respiratory Disorders: Glucocorticoids have palliative effects in *pulmonary sarcoidosis* but apparently have little influence on the development of pulmonary fibrosis or the eventual outcome of the disease. They generally are reserved for patients in whom functioning of a vital extrapulmonary organ is impaired and those with stage 2 or 3 pulmonary sarcoidosis. Patients with a differential count of pretreatment bronchoalveolar lavage (BAL) specimens containing greater than 35% lymphocytes are more likely to respond favorably than patients with BAL lymphocytes less than 35% (Hollinger et al, 1985). Therapy is initiated with prednisone 30 to 40 mg (or 40 to 60 mg on alternate days) for six to eight weeks; the dose then is reduced to the lowest effective amount.

The *respiratory distress syndrome* (RDS) is a significant cause of death in premature neonates. Antenatal administration of glucocorticoids reduces the incidence, severity, and mortality rate. Treatment appears to be more effective in female infants. These agents may induce enzymes that accelerate the production of lung surfactant by type 2 pneumonocytes. Administration of steroids after RDS has developed does not enhance survival, because there is a latent period (up to several days) before enzyme induction occurs.

Glucocorticoids have been of significant benefit in pregnancies of 26 to 34 weeks when delivery occurred at least 24 hours after initiating treatment. In pregnancies of this length, the patient may be treated if the lecithin/sphingomyelin ratio is less than 2 or if amniotic fluid analysis is unavailable. No definite effect has been noted during pregnancies with longer gestation periods. Effectiveness appears to be maximal if delivery occurs 24 to 48 hours after administration of steroid, and the effect is lost after seven days. Therefore, some physicians recommend a second course of therapy after one week if indications persist. During premature labor, a uterine relaxant (eg, ritodrine) is administered with the glucocorticoid to delay labor. Premature rupture of the membranes does not accelerate fetal pulmonary maturation.

In the most commonly used regimen, betamethasone sodium phosphate [Celestone Soluspan] 12 mg is injected intramuscularly twice at 24-hour intervals. It has been suggested that betamethasone is preferable to hydrocortisone, prednisone, or prednisolone because the maternal:fetal ratio is lower, thus allowing administration of a relatively smaller effective dose. Other clinicians suggest that intravenous hydrocortisone acts earlier than intramuscular betamethasone and is preferred when rapid action is necessary. In various trials utilizing hydrocortisone, the equivalent doses were larger than with betamethasone, however. Dexamethasone also has been beneficial. Methylprednisolone is less effective than betamethasone.

In pregnancies complicated by severe pre-eclampsia, the number of fetal deaths increased after glucocorticoid therapy, and neonatal hypoglycemia was observed. Apgar scores and onset of lactation were unaffected. Although the neonatal cortisol level was suppressed for several days, adrenal insufficiency was not reported. In some studies, the incidence of maternal infection increased, particularly when there was premature rupture of membranes.

Prophylactic administration of glucocorticoids for RDS is not indicated in women with severe pre-eclampsia or when immediate delivery is required for maternal or neonatal survival (ie, maternal infection, fetal distress, abruptio placentae, placenta previa).

Prenatal administration of glucocorticoids to animal fetuses retarded somatic growth and compromised central nervous system development. The dose and duration of administration exceeded those used in humans. When 12 mg betamethasone is administered to women prenatally, fetal blood levels of glucocorticoid are similar to those observed during stress. The steroid is cleared from the fetal circulation within three days. In children observed for four years after prophylactic steroid treatment for RDS, no significant alterations in growth or development have been observed. The possibility that a long latent period or a rare adverse effect may be identified eventually cannot be ignored, however, and monitoring of these children must continue before this form of therapy can be accepted unequivocally. For reviews and discussion of the issues involved in prevention of RDS with glucocorticoids, see Ballard and Ballard, 1979; Ballard et al, 1979; Shields and Resnik, 1979; and *Drug Ther Bull*, 1980.

Shock: Although glucocorticoids are commonly used to treat shock, they are clearly indicated only for that produced by adrenocortical insufficiency (addisonian shock) and probably for septic shock, but there is no universal agreement on their effectiveness for the latter. Although clinical evidence is limited and equivocal, glucocorticoids appear to be ineffective in cardiogenic, hypovolemic, or traumatic shock. However, they may be useful in any type of shock if the patient has relative adrenal insufficiency.

The mechanisms by which corticosteroids act in septic shock are not completely understood, but probably involve effects on cellular and subcellular membranes with consequent effects on cellular metabolism. Steroids improve tissue perfusion; preserve capillary endothelial integrity; and stabilize lysosomal membranes.

Massive doses of steroids are beneficial in patients with chills, high fever, confusion, lethargy, reduced blood pressure, and tachypnea with respiratory alkalosis who are likely to develop septic shock (Sheagren, 1981). In addition, corticosteroids appear to reverse septic shock when administered shortly after diagnosis. When these drugs are given before irreversible damage has occurred, they increase survival. They do not, however, appear to affect overall mortality in patients with severe, late septic shock (Sprung et al, 1984). Massive doses (30 mg/kg of methylprednisolone or 3 to 6 mg/kg of dexamethasone intravenously) are employed and may be repeated every four to six hours for two or three doses. Most experts prefer methylprednisolone to dexamethasone because the former has a shorter duration of action and penetrates cellular compartments more rapidly. These doses produce very high plasma concentrations (eg, 1 mg/ml of methylprednisolone) that inhibit complement-induced polymorphonuclear leukocyte aggregation. When steroid therapy is of brief duration (five days or less), the hypothalamic-pituitary-adrenal axis is suppressed for up to five days after completion of therapy (Streck and Lockwood, 1979).

ADVERSE REACTIONS

Corticosteroids have many potential adverse effects that are often extensions of their pharmacologic actions. The incidence of adverse reactions correlates with the dose, frequency and route of administration, duration of therapy, age and condition of the patient, and underlying disease.

Gastrointestinal Reactions: Glucocorticoids decrease the protection provided by the gastric mucus barrier, interfere with tissue repair, and, in some patients, increase gastric acid and pepsinogen production. There is no universal agreement on whether steroids per se are responsible for the peptic ulcers encountered during therapy. However, glucocorticoid therapy may mask the symptoms of peptic ulcer so that perforation or hemorrhage occurs without antecedent pain; therefore, periodic examination of the stools for occult blood is suggested.

Data from 71 controlled trials in which more than 5,000 patients randomly received either systemic corticosteroids (or ACTH) or nonsteroid therapy showed that peptic ulcer disease occurred in 1.8% of 3,064 steroid-treated patients and in 0.8% of 2,897 control subjects (relative risk, 2.3) (Messer et al, 1983). The relative risk of gastrointestinal hemorrhage in steroid-treated patients was 1.5.

When separate analyses were performed for double-blind studies, studies using only oral steroids, studies using only parenteral steroids, and studies excluding patients with a history of ulcer, a similar relative risk was found. The incidence of ulcers varied directly with the dose of steroids.

These findings appear to conflict with those of Conn and Blitzer (1976); the latter pooled data from 50 controlled studies and reported that there was no statistical relationship (ie, p <0.05) between steroid use and peptic ulcer disease. However, their study did suggest an association, and there was an increased relative risk of 1.7 overall for patients taking steroids, which is similar to that reported by Messer et al (1983). Thus, there is no conflict between the findings of the two studies.

More recent data show that corticosteroids caused peptic ulcers in only 1 in 100 patients (0.8/100 controls had ulcers, 1.8/100 treated patients had ulcers), an increase of 1 patient per 100. Therefore, antiulcer drugs should not be prescribed routinely for patients receiving corticosteroids. Instead, therapy to prevent ulcers should be used only when other medications that increase the risk of peptic ulcer disease (eg, nonsteroidal anti-inflammatory drugs) are taken concomitantly.

If an ulcer occurs, the corticosteroid should be discontinued slowly (using the method described), unless it is life-saving, and antiulcer therapy should be given (Spiro, 1983). See Chapter 52, Agents Used in Disorders of the Upper Gastrointestinal Tract, for antiulcer therapy.

Edema: Since glucocorticoids with little or no mineralocorticoid activity are now available, electrolyte imbalance is observed less frequently. Edema is best treated by restricting dietary sodium at the inception of therapy. If edema occurs, sodium intake should be reduced sharply; if it persists, the patient should receive a glucocorticoid with less mineralocorticoid activity. However, caution is required if large doses of any corticosteroid are given for prolonged periods to patients with cardiovascular or severe renal disease, for even slight fluid retention may be dangerous.

Hypokalemia: Severe hypokalemia may cause asthenia, paralysis, or arrhythmias that may proceed to cardiac arrest. The incidence of hypokalemia is related to the mineralocorticoid activity of a specific glucocorticoid and can be avoided in most patients by restricting dietary sodium, consuming foods rich in potassium (eg, bananas), supplementing the diet with oral potassium, and using a steroid with minimal mineralocorticoid activity. Concurrent use of potassium-wasting diuretics (eg, thiazides) may exacerbate potassium loss. See also Chapter 46, Replenishers and Regulators of Water and Electrolytes.

Osteoporosis: This common but infrequently recognized adverse effect is associated with long-term use of glucocorticoids. The morphologic findings are bone loss in areas with a high content of trabecular bone, such as the ribs and vertebrae, and enlargement of the marrow cavity. Fractures are most common in these bones. Glucocorticoids appear to decrease bone formation directly through suppression of osteoblastic formation. They also act indirectly by inhibiting calcium absorption from the gastrointestinal tract and reabsorption from the renal tubules; hypocalcemia results and increases the plasma parathyroid hormone concentration, which ultimately increases bone resorption (Baylink, 1983).

A number of early studies assessed the occurrence of steroid-induced osteoporosis in patients with rheumatoid arthritis, in whom the incidence of generalized osteoporosis is high regardless of whether glucocorticoids are used in therapy. However, steroid-induced bone loss and osteoporosis have recently been shown to occur in patients with asthma, a condition not normally associated with osteoporosis (Adinoff and Hollister, 1983; Rüegsegger et al, 1983).

The amount of bone loss is related to the dose and duration of steroid therapy. Doses as low as prednisone 5 mg daily (or equivalent) or 25 mg every other day result in demonstrable bone loss within one year in a significant number of patients.

Patients should be monitored with bone densitometry if available, and those at risk for osteoporosis should receive vitamin D 50,000 IU twice weekly or calcifediol 40 to 60 mcg daily and elemental calcium 1.5 g daily for prophylaxis. Treatment of osteoporosis is discussed in Chapter 49, Agents Affecting Calcium Metabolism.

Osteonecrosis: Corticosteroid-induced osteonecrosis most commonly affects the femoral head but also may involve the head of the humerus, femoral condyles, tibial plateau, talus, and capitulum. A number of mechanisms have been suggested, including fat embolism, hypercoagulability, increased intraosseous pressure, and swelling of fat cells, but none have been proven. The first symptoms (joint pain and stiffness) are often noted 12 to 24 months after first exposure. Techniques recommended for early diagnosis are bone marrow pressure recordings and intraosseous venography (Nixon, 1984).

Osteonecrosis is most commonly associated with prolonged corticosteroid therapy, but it also has occurred following brief high-dose treatment (McCluskey and Gutteridge, 1982; Sambrook et al, 1984; Taylor, 1984). Current data suggest that large doses are a factor leading to osteonecrosis in predisposed patients (Zizic et al, 1985).

Negative Nitrogen Balance: Negative nitrogen balance results from the excessive breakdown of protein by glucocorticoids; this may be modified somewhat by administration of anabolic agents and a high-protein diet. However, there is no evidence that anabolic agents protect tissues from atrophy and osteoporosis.

Carbohydrate and Lipid Metabolism: Glucocorticoids elevate plasma glucose concentrations 10% to 20% by increasing gluconeogenesis and decreasing cellular sensitivity to insulin. They aggravate diabetes, but ketosis generally is not a problem and diabetes can be controlled by modifying the diet or adjusting the dose of hypoglycemic agents. Glucocorticoids also can make latent diabetes chemically apparent. However, patients with normal pancreatic insulin production and response are not affected. Serum triglyceride concentrations may become elevated.

Central Nervous System Effects: Large doses of glucocorticoids cause behavioral and personality changes usually manifested by euphoria. Other signs include insomnia, increased appetite, nervousness, irritability, and hyperkinesia. Psychotic episodes, including manic-depressive and paranoid states and acute toxic psychoses, have been reported occasionally. Symptoms may occur within days to two weeks after initiating therapy or may develop in a subsequent course of therapy. They may disappear partly or completely upon dosage reduction. It has been suggested that tricyclic antidepressants have a deleterious effect on steroid-induced psychoses.

Patients sometimes become psychologically dependent on these drugs. Glucocorticoid abuse also has been reported when patients took the drug for an inappropriate indication. Pre-existing psychiatric illness does not appear to increase the risk of mental problems during steroid therapy. However, this history may influence the character of the emotional manifestation. In some instances, it may be impossible to determine whether psychiatric symptoms are caused by steroid therapy or the underlying condition (eg, systemic lupus erythematosus) (Ling et al, 1981).

Growth Suppression: Because growth is suppressed in children receiving long-term, daily, divided-dose glucocorticoid therapy, use of such regimens in children should be restricted to the most urgent indications. Alternate-day therapy with a short-acting agent (see Table 2) usually avoids or minimizes growth suppression. When daily administration is required, a short-acting steroid taken as a single dose at 7 to 8 AM minimizes growth suppression and is preferred over multiple daily doses.

Myopathy: Pharmacologic doses of corticosteroids cause protein catabolism and can lead to myopathy. This disorder develops slowly and the weakness primarily involves the proximal musculature of the upper and lower extremities. Myopathy responds to a reduction in dosage, and recovery occurs slowly over a period of months. Myopathy is most often associated with use of 9α-fluorinated steroids, such as triamcinolone; it rarely occurs in patients receiving less than 30 mg daily of prednisone or the equivalent. It has been suggested that myopathy may be reversed by physical exercise, but further studies are needed to verify this (Horber et al, 1985).

Ocular Effects: Systemic administration and ocular application of glucocorticoids occasionally elevate intraocular pressure by decreasing outflow facility (open-angle glaucoma). The tendency to develop these symptoms is inherited in a recessive autosomal pattern and occurs most frequently in patients with primary open-angle glaucoma and their relatives, especially homozygous individuals. An exaggerated intraocular pressure response is also common among diabetics and myopes. Glucocorticoid therapy may be continued if topical agents control the ocular hypertension. (See Chapter 20, Miscellaneous Ophthalmic Preparations.)

Posterior subcapsular cataracts (PSCC) are common in patients receiving prolonged systemic or topical glucocorticoid therapy. There is disagreement on whether PSCC is associated with dose, duration of therapy, or the patient's age. Some experts think that patients receiving prednisone 10 mg daily (or the equivalent) or less or those treated for less than six months to one year are unlikely to develop PSCC. In contrast, others believe that the most important factor in PSCC may be individual susceptibility rather than extent of exposure. Children (especially those treated for rheumatoid arthritis) are affected more often than adults.

Miscellaneous Reactions: Acne, hirsutism, menstrual disorders, facial rounding, thin and shiny skin, supraclavicular fat pads, weight gain due to increased appetite, headache, pseudotumor cerebri, hypertension, impotence, hyperhidrosis, flushing, vertigo, chronic pancreatitis, intestinal perforation, hepatomegaly, hyperlipidemia, and acceleration of atherosclerosis have been reported with glucocorticoid therapy.

PRECAUTIONS

Pharmacologic doses of glucocorticoids may suppress the signs and symptoms of disease that are required for diagnosis through their anti-inflammatory and anti-immunologic actions. Perforation of a peptic ulcer may occur with minimal discomfort. Septicemia may progress without fever, probably due to the corticosteroid's effect on hypothalamic temperature control or suppression of pyrogen production.

The degradation of glucocorticoids is increased markedly in patients with hyperthyroidism. Pharmacologic doses have been given empirically to some patients with thyrotoxic crises (thyroid storm) because the compensatory increase in adrenal secretion may be inadequate in this condition. Glucocorticoid action is enhanced in patients with hypothyroidism or hepatic damage.

Infection and Other Stress: Resistance to infection is decreased during prolonged treatment with pharmacologic doses of glucocorticoids, for the same mechanisms that prevent the destruction of tissue by inflammation also may increase vulnerability to infectious agents. The patient is predisposed to all types of infection (bacterial, viral, fungal, parasitic) and susceptibility is often increased by the underlying disease (eg, systemic lupus erythematosus, leukemia). Fewer infections may occur when the dosage interval is increased (as in alternate-day therapy) so that immunologic defenses remain intact.

Reactivation of quiescent tuberculosis in patients receiving glucocorticoids is well documented. Since skin sensitivity to tuberculin is usually lost during treatment with moderate to large daily doses of glucocorticoids (about 20 mg of prednisone or the equivalent daily), tuberculin skin testing is recommended for all patients before initiating long-term, daily, high-dose therapy. (Patients on alternate-day therapy may not be affected.) Those with positive skin tests may be candidates for appropriate chemotherapy. There are insufficient data to recommend isoniazid chemoprophylaxis for patients treated with low doses of glucocorticoids (less than 10 mg of prednisone daily) (see Chapter 75, Antimycobacterial Agents).

Large doses of steroids also diminish or inhibit the positive reaction to histoplasmin skin tests and suppress the reaction to patch tests for allergy.

Host defenses are impaired in patients receiving large doses of glucocorticoids, and this increases susceptibility to fungal infections, especially candidiasis. The incidence and severity of bacterial and viral infections also are increased. Since glucocorticoids tend to mask symptoms, intercurrent infections may become severe before their presence is recognized. Glucocorticoids are especially hazardous when herpes simplex keratitis is present. Early recognition and institution of appropriate treatment are the only safeguards against these serious complications.

The body requires greater than normal amounts of glucocorticoids under conditions of stress, including infectious illnesses. Individuals with normal adrenal function secrete larger amounts of corticosteroids during the early phase of most infections. Those dependent on exogenous steroids (whether for replacement or nonendocrine indications) require larger doses during stress since they are unable to secrete adequate additional amounts of endogenous hormone. When infection occurs in patients treated for a prolonged period with pharmacologic doses of glucocorticoids, a dilemma occurs: Administering the larger doses needed for the nonspecific, stress-related functions of glucocorticoids may further compromise resistance to infection. For mild illness, if the maintenance dose is low, the usual solution is to double the normal dose. In patients already receiving doses exceeding the amount produced endogenously under maximum stress (approximately 60 mg or more of prednisone or the equivalent daily), probably no additional steroid is necessary for mild illness. All patients should be treated concomitantly with an appropriate antimicrobial agent.

Normal adults may secrete 250 to 300 mg of cortisol daily in response to major stress (eg, trauma, surgery). When patients taking pharmacologic doses of glucocorticoids undergo such stress, the suppressed pituitary secretes insufficient ACTH and the adrenal glands may be unable to secrete the extra hormone required. Additional exogenous corticosteroid is given in the dosage and for the duration appropriate for the severity of the stress. For example, for major surgery, hydrocortisone 100 mg intravenously every six hours is given on the day of surgery and the dose is reduced by 20% to 30% daily for three days; for minor surgery, a similar regimen is administered for one day. For procedures such as colonoscopy or dental extractions, hydrocortisone 100 mg may be given with preoperative medications, followed by 20 mg orally that evening (Collins and Byyny, 1980).

Hypothalamic-Pituitary-Adrenal Axis Suppression: Administration of exogenous glucocorticoids will result in some degree of suppression (through negative feedback of glucocorticoid) of the hypothalamic-pituitary-adrenal (HPA) axis. The suppression generally is proportional to the size of the dose, relative glucocorticoid activity, biological half-life, and, most importantly, duration of therapy. Prolonged therapy produces adrenal atrophy and inhibits pituitary function (which requires more time for recovery). If patients have been receiving pharmacologic doses for more than one month, it may be assumed that they are unable to secrete normal amounts of hormone or to respond to stress by increasing secretion. However, there is wide individual variation in the dose and duration of treatment required to produce HPA suppression. Significant adrenal suppression may occur within one week after large doses of a glucocorticoid are given. In general, however, less than 5 mg of prednisone daily or the equivalent causes little suppression. Divided doses (three or four daily) are more suppressive than single daily doses, and doses administered before bedtime are more suppressive than those given earlier in the day.

The same precautions exercised by patients receiving adrenal replacement therapy, such as carrying a steroid identification card and bracelet and keeping emergency supplies of medication, also apply to those receiving large doses of these hormones for nonendocrine conditions. (See also the section on Precautions in Chapter 37, Agents Used to Treat Adrenal Dysfunction.)

Pregnancy and Lactation: The placenta has extensive 11-beta-ol-dehydrogenase activity, an enzyme that metabolizes glucocorticoids to their inactive 11-ketosteroid counterparts. Studies using perfused human placenta showed that cortisol, prednisolone, prednisone, and dexamethasone all were extensively metabolized before crossing the placenta and entering the fetus. Thus, there appears to be no significant advantage of one preparation over the others in raising fetal circulatory concentrations of glucocorticoids (Levitz et al, 1978).

When very large pharmacologic doses must be used for prolonged periods during pregnancy, fetal adrenal hypoplasia may occur. The state of neonatal adrenal function must be assessed and replacement therapy provided if necessary. When steroids are discontinued, normal adrenal function is recovered eventually.

These drugs are classified in FDA Pregnancy Category C.

Corticosteroids are found in the breast milk of lactating women receiving systemic therapy. However, it is probably safe for a lactating mother to nurse her infant if she is taking small doses.

Drug Interactions: The metabolism of corticosteroids is increased by drugs that induce certain hepatic metabolizing enzymes (eg, phenobarbital, phenytoin [Dilantin], rifampin [Rifadin, Rimactane]). If one of these agents is given concomitantly, an increase in the maintenance dose of corticosteroid may be necessary.

Methylprednisolone clearance was reduced in asthmatic patients also taking troleandomycin [Tao]. This may result in either therapeutic enhancement of steroid activity or cushingoid side effects, and the dosage of steroid may require reduction (Szefler et al, 1980). This effect also occurs with concomitant administration of erythromycin.

Estrogen increases levels of corticosteroid-binding globulin, thereby increasing the bound (inactive) fraction; however, this effect is balanced by decreased metabolism, which prolongs the half-life of the steroid. When therapy with estrogens or estrogen-containing preparations is initiated, a reduction in corticosteroid dose may be required, and increased amounts may be needed when estrogen treatment is terminated.

Large doses of intravenous methylprednisolone increased plasma cyclosporine concentrations in renal transplant patients. The dose of cyclosporine may need to be reduced when glucocorticoid therapy is initiated (Klintmalm and Säwe, 1984).

Corticosteroids have a hyperglycemic effect and may increase the requirement for hypoglycemic drugs. The potassium balance should be monitored in patients taking corticosteroids (especially those with a significant mineralocorticoid activity), particularly when amphotericin B and thiazide or loop diuretics are taken concurrently, for such combinations can cause potassium depletion. Corticosteroid administration is associated with greater clearance of salicylates and decreased effectiveness of anticoagulants, and the dosage of these drugs may require adjustment when steroid therapy is initiated or discontinued.

Effects on Laboratory Tests: Corticosteroids may increase the blood level of glucose, sometimes resulting in diabetes mellitus and glycosuria. This reflects not only elevated blood glucose but a lowered renal threshold for glucose. Potent glucocorticoids (eg, dexamethasone) decrease urinary levels of 17-ketosteroids and 17-hydroxysteroids due to the negative feedback effect on secretion of endogenous hormones.

WITHDRAWAL FROM THERAPY

Several patterns of response to steroid withdrawal have been described (Dixon and Christy, 1980). These include HPA suppression with or without symptoms, exacerbation of the disease being treated, and physical or psychological dependence with otherwise normal function.

The length of time and the rate of dosage reduction necessary for withdrawal from pharmacologic steroid therapy depend on the degree of HPA suppression (related to dose and duration of therapy) and the response of the underlying disease. A variety of schedules have been suggested (Byyny, 1976; Fass, 1979; Collins and Byyny, 1980; Chamberlain and Meyer, 1981).

Glucocorticoids given in large doses for one to three days probably suppress HPA function only temporarily and they can be withdrawn suddenly or gradually over one week. After one month or more of treatment, dosage reduction usually begins by administering a single dose in the morning to minimize adrenal suppression. The dose may be reduced by 2.5 to 5 mg of prednisone or the equivalent every three to seven days until 5 mg/day is given. At this time, hydrocortisone 20 mg daily is substituted and the dose is reduced by 2.5 mg at weekly intervals to reach a daily dose of 10 mg (see Table 3). Alternatively, the dose may be reduced by 25% weekly until 10 mg/day of prednisone or the equivalent is given. This amount is administered on alternate days and finally discontinued. The maximum rate of dosage reduction is limited by the patient's response; too rapid withdrawal may exacerbate symptoms of the underlying disease or lead to withdrawal symptoms.

Short- or intermediate-acting agents (see Table 2), such as hydrocortisone or prednisone, should be employed, since long-acting agents, such as betamethasone or dexamethasone, offer no therapeutic advantage but cause more prolonged adrenal suppression. The adrenal gland begins to regain the ability to respond to corticotropin stimulation at daily doses of 5 to 7.5 mg of prednisone or the equivalent.

The entire process of recovery of HPA axis function occurs in stages and may be rapid or may require one year or more for completion. Children tend to recover function more quickly than adults (Chamberlain and Meyer, 1981). During the first phase of recovery, plasma ACTH levels normalize, followed by secretion of normal basal levels of cortisol. This is usually achieved within several months and indicates recovery of adrenal responsiveness to corticotropin and resumption of the cortisol feedback mechanism. This stage of recovery is indicated by a morning (before taking the morning dose of corticosteroid, or on the morning of no medication when using alternate-day therapy) plasma cortisol level greater than 10 mcg/dl. In the second phase, normal corticotropin and cortisol secretory responses to stressful stimuli return. This can be demonstrated in patients with normal morning cortisol levels by a normal response to an ACTH stimulation test (see Table 3 and Chapter 42, Agents Related to Anterior Pituitary and Hypothalamic Function). A few patients with normal responses to ACTH stimulation tests have been reported to have an abnormal serum cortisol response to insulin tolerance tests, which may indicate acute adrenal insufficiency (Borst et al, 1982). Because extended suppression is possible, those who received systemic glucocorticoid therapy during the previous year should be given appropriate doses of steroids during stress unless recovery of the HPA axis has been confirmed by appropriate tests.

Corticotropin injections should not be used to accelerate recovery from adrenal atrophy because further HPA suppression occurs even though adrenal secretion is stimulated.

In addition to HPA suppression, withdrawal of glucocorticoid therapy may be accompanied by malaise, fever, myalgia, arthralgia, fatigue, and restlessness. This syndrome may be mistaken for an exacerbation of the underlying disease, particularly in patients with rheumatoid arthritis. Gradual reduction of the dose and treatment with nonsteroidal anti-inflammatory drugs minimizes these problems.

Some patients become psychologically dependent on glucocorticoids (Flavin et al, 1983), particularly those given repeated courses of therapy for recurring symptoms (eg, those with asthma or certain dermatologic conditions). Dependence also may occur when the underlying disease is inactive. Since euphoria and rapid relief occur when glucocorticoid therapy is initiated, it may be difficult to convince the patient to accept repeated attempts to withdraw medication with its attendant discomforts.

ALTERNATE-DAY THERAPY

Glucocorticoid therapy may be initiated with a single daily dose or multiple daily doses. After symptoms are controlled by daily therapy, most chronic diseases respond to alternate-day administration of intermediate-acting glucocorticoids (prednisone, prednisolone, methylprednisolone). The advantages are less suppression of the HPA axis, convenience that may enhance compliance, and a lower incidence of adverse effects. For example, when pharmacologic doses of glucocorticoids are given daily to children, the rate of growth is decreased; however, normal growth patterns are maintained with alternate-day therapy. Alternate-day therapy produces less inhibition of intestinal calcium absorption and results in less bone loss.

There are many methods of transferring patients from daily to alternate-day therapy. One effective approach has been to reduce the daily dose to prednisone 40 to 50 mg (or the equivalent dose of an intermediate-acting agent) (Kehrl and Fauci, 1983). Then, the daily dose on the day designated as "on" is doubled to 80 to 100 mg. The dose on the "off" day is decreased gradually by 5 to 10 mg. Tapering is continued until the dose on the "off" day is 20 mg, at which point the dose is reduced by 2.5 mg until the patient receives no steroid on the "off" day. If remission is maintained, the dose on the "on" day is reduced to the least amount that controls symptoms. If a relapse occurs, the dose on the "on" day is increased sufficiently to reinduce remission.

The most common reasons for failure of transfer from daily to alternate-day therapy are too rapid conversion and inadequate dose on the "on" day. Although not all patients can be adequately controlled, the benefits of alternate-day therapy justify trial in most patients receiving prolonged glucocorticoid therapy.

With the alternate-day regimen, the steroid is administered every other morning between 7 and 8 AM. This simulates the natural circadian rhythm of glucocorticoid secretion (early

TABLE 2.
GLUCOCORTICOID PROPERTIES AND ROUTES OF ADMINISTRATION

Drug	Effect*			Half-life (hours)	
	Onset	Peak (hours)	Duration+	Plasma	Biological
SHORT-ACTING					
Cortisone				0.5	8–12
Acetate					
Oral	Rapid	2	1.25–1.5 days		
IM	Slow	20–48			
Hydrocortisone				1.5–2	8–12
Oral		1	1.25–1.5 days		
IM		4–8			
Rectal (retention enema)	3–5 days				
Acetate					
IA, IS, IB, IL, ST		24–48	3–28 days		
Rectal (foam)	5–7 days				
Cypionate					
Oral	Slower than tablet	1–2			
Sodium Phosphate					
IV	Rapid				
IM	Rapid	1			
Sodium Succinate					
IV	Rapid				
IM	Rapid	1	Variable		
INTERMEDIATE-ACTING					
Methylprednisolone				3.0	18–36
Oral		1–2	1.25–1.5 days		
Acetate					
IM	Slow (6–48 hours)	4–8 days	7–28 days		
IA, IL, ST	Very slow	7 days	7–35 days		
Sodium Succinate					
IV	Rapid				
IM	Rapid				
Prednisolone				2.1–3.5	18–36
Oral		1–2	1.25–1.5 days		
Acetate					
IM	Slow				
Acetate/Sodium Phosphate					
IM			Up to 28 days		
IB, IS, IA, ST			3–28 days		
Sodium Phosphate					
IV	Rapid	1			
IM	Rapid	1			
IA, IL, ST			3–21 days		
Tebutate					
IA, IL, ST	Slow (1–2 days)		7–21 days		

(Continued on next page)

Drug	Effect*			Half-life (hours)	
	Onset	Peak (hours)	Duration+	Plasma	Biological
Prednisone				3.4–3.8	18–36
Oral		1–2	1.25–1.5 days		
Triamcinolone				2–>5	18–36
Oral		1–2	2.25 days		
Acetonide					
IM	Slow (24–48 hours)		7–30 days		
IB, IA, IS, IL, ST			7–30 days		
Diacetate					
Oral		1–2			
IM	Slow		4–28 days		
IL			7–14 days		
IA, IS, ST			7–40 days		
Hexacetonide					
IA, IL			21–28 days		
LONG-ACTING					
Betamethasone				3–5	36–54
Oral		1–2	3.25 days		
Sodium Phosphate					
IV	Rapid				
IM	Rapid				
Acetate/Sodium Phosphate					
IM	1–3 hours		7 days		
IA, IS			7–14 days		
IL, ST			7 days		
Dexamethasone				3–4.5	36–54
Oral		1–2	2.75 days		
Acetate					
IM		8	6 days		
IA, ST, IL			7–21 days		
Sodium Phosphate					
IV	Rapid				
IM	Rapid				
IA, IS, IL, ST			3–21 days		
Paramethasone				3–4.5	36–54
Acetate					
Oral		1–2	2 days		

Adapted from USP Dispensing Information. *Rockville, MD, The United States Pharmacopeial Convention, Inc, vol. I, 1986.*

Abbreviations: *IA* = intra-articular   *IB* = intrabursal   *IL* = intralesional   *IM* = intramuscular
    IS = intrasynovial   *IV* = intravenous   *SC* = subcutaneous   *ST* = soft tissue

*Actual onset, peak, and duration of action depend upon route and site of administration, solubility of dosage form, dose administered, and condition being treated.
+Duration of action is based on biological half-life.

TABLE 3.
PROTOCOL FOR GLUCOCORTICOID WITHDRAWAL[1]

Step	Interval	Observation	Result	Glucocorticoid and Dose
I	Variable	Underlying disease present	Worsening of underlying disease	Variable; gradually decrease dose to hydrocortisone 20 mg/day or equivalent
			Symptoms and signs of steroid withdrawal	Increase dose if disease worsens; continue if disease is quiescent; increase dose for stress
II	4 weeks	8 AM plasma cortisol	Plasma cortisol: When <10 mcg/100 ml	Begin hydrocortisone 20 mg/day; decrease by 2.5 mg/day once/week to 10 mg each morning and continue this dosage; increase dose for stress
			When >10 mcg/100 ml	Stop hydrocortisone; supplement dose for stress
III	4 weeks—Indefinite	8 AM 250 mcg IM cosyntropin[2] test	When plasma cortisol increased by <6 mcg/100 ml or maximum <20 mcg/100 ml (or both)	Supplement dose for stress
IV	4 weeks—Indefinite	8 AM 250 mcg IM cosyntropin[2] test	When plasma cortisol increased by >6 mcg/100 ml or maximum >20 mcg/100 ml	Stop supplementation for stress
V	Indefinite	Routine	———	As indicated

[1]See text for discussion.
[2]Synthetic (1 to 24 amino acids) corticotropin (ACTH)
Adapted from Byyny, 1976

morning peak, evening nadir) and produces less suppression of the hypothalamic-pituitary-adrenal axis. Ideally, the level of *exogenous* hormone is high on the morning of treatment and that of *endogenous* hormone is normal on the morning that medication is withheld, for the HPA axis is not suppressed on that day.

Alternate-day therapy is preferred for maintenance whenever feasible. This regimen is reported to be particularly effective in asthma, systemic lupus erythematosus, uveitis, and nephrotic syndrome. Alternate-day therapy may not be adequate in severe conditions, such as renal transplantation or certain hematologic and malignant disorders. Some patients, especially those with rheumatoid arthritis and adults with ulcerative colitis, may become symptomatic or experience an exacerbation on the day that the glucocorticoid is withheld. If symptoms persist despite an increase in dose, a single morning dose is preferred to a more suppressive daily divided-dose schedule.

DRUG SELECTION

Localized therapy is generally preferred because it minimizes adverse effects. It should be noted, however, that local or topical administration of large doses can have systemic effects. When systemic administration is required, the oral route is preferred for the ease in regulation of dose and the variety of regimens.

Prednisone is the usual preparation of choice for oral administration, because it has the longest history of usage and is reliable, readily available, and inexpensive. Prednisone is metabolized to the active metabolite, prednisolone, by the liver. This conversion was thought to be impeded in patients with acute liver disease, and it was suggested that prednisolone may be preferred in this situation. However, further studies show that the conversion of prednisone to prednisolone is not impaired significantly in patients with liver disease (Uribe et al, 1982). Thus, there appears to be little real advantage in using one preparation over another in patients with liver disease or hypoalbuminemia from other causes (Pickup, 1979).

Prednisone has slight but significant mineralocorticoid activity. In patients with hypertension, congestive heart failure, or other conditions in which salt retention is a problem, a preparation with even less mineralocorticoid activity may be chosen (see Table 4). This is particularly important when unusually large doses must be prescribed.

Cortisone and hydrocortisone have the most mineralocorticoid activity among the available glucocorticoids. Systemic administration should be limited to short-term use, for prolonged administration of pharmacologic doses may result in

TABLE 4.
GLUCOCORTICOID PROPERTIES

	Glucocorticoid Potency	Equivalent Dose (mg)	Mineralocorticoid Potency
SHORT-ACTING			
Hydrocortisone	1	20.0	2+
Cortisone	0.8	25.0	2+
INTERMEDIATE-ACTING			
Meprednisone	4–5	4.0	0
Methylprednisolone	5	4.0	0
Prednisolone	4	5.0	1+
Prednisone	4	5.0	1
Triamcinolone	5	4.0	0
LONG-ACTING			
Betamethasone	25–30	0.60	0
Dexamethasone	25–30	0.75	0
Paramethasone	10	2.0	0

For preparations, see listing at end of chapter. For topical preparations, see Chapters 20, Miscellaneous Ophthalmic Agents; 22, Drugs Used in Bronchial Disorders; 56, Dermatologic Preparations; 58, Agents Used in Disorders of the Lower Intestinal Tract; and 73, Topical Anti-infective Agents: Otic and Ophthalmic Preparations.

sodium and water retention, hypertension, and hypokalemia; sodium restriction and potassium supplementation may be necessary.

Dexamethasone has minimal mineralocorticoid activity and is commonly chosen to treat vasogenic cerebral edema. Mild diuresis with sodium loss may occur in patients who had been receiving other glucocorticoids.

Triamcinolone often produces a mild diuresis with sodium loss during the first days of treatment whether or not the patient is frankly edematous; conversely, edema may occur in patients with a decreased glomerular filtration rate. Certain adverse reactions are unique to triamcinolone; myopathy is encountered more frequently, and this agent tends to cause anorexia (with resultant weight loss) rather than stimulation of appetite, and sedation and depression rather than euphoria.

PREPARATIONS

Numerous synthetic corticosteroids have been developed by modifying the chemical structure of hydrocortisone (cortisol, Compound F) (see the Figure). The analogues thus produced may differ from the parent compound in half-life, potency, and sodium-retaining activity. Prednisone and prednisolone were produced by introducing a double bond between carbon atoms 1 and 2 (Δ-1 analogues) of cortisone and hydrocortisone, respectively; this increased glucocorticoid activity while decreasing mineralocorticoid effects. Other

synthetic preparations have either glucocorticoid (dexamethasone, betamethasone) or mineralocorticoid (desoxycorticosterone) activity almost exclusively; most have been synthesized primarily for their glucocorticoid effects and are widely used in nonendocrine diseases.

When considering the therapeutic efficacy of the corticosteroids, it is important to remember that separation of glucocorticoid and mineralocorticoid activity is incomplete. Some agents that are considered to be primarily glucocorticoids (eg, hydrocortisone, cortisone, prednisone, prednisolone) possess variable mineralocorticoid activity as well and, therefore, cause sodium retention and potassium depletion when used in pharmacologic amounts.

The plasma half-lives of the synthetic glucocorticoids are variable and often are considerably longer than that of hydrocortisone. The tissue half-lives determine biological effectiveness. Although they generally correlate with plasma half-lives, the relationship is not linear: tissue half-lives always exceed plasma half-lives. The relative potency is a measure of anti-inflammatory and HPA suppressive activities. However, the degree and duration of HPA suppression caused by the long-acting glucocorticoids, betamethasone and dexamethasone, are greater than would be predicted on the basis of their plasma half-lives and relative potencies. Table 2 lists the properties of glucocorticoids currently marketed in the United States.

Glucocorticoids may be administered by a number of routes, depending upon the nature of the disease and the condition of

GLUCOCORTICOID STRUCTURES

	$C_1 - C_2$	C_6	C_9	C_{11}	C_{16}
Short-acting					
Cortisone	single bond	—H	---H	=O	—H
Hydrocortisone	single bond	—H	---H	◀OH	—H
Intermediate-acting					
Methylprednisolone	double bond	---CH₃	---H	◀OH	—H
Prednisolone	double bond	—H	---H	◀OH	—H
Prednisone	double bond	—H	---H	=O	—H
Triamcinolone	double bond	—H	---F	◀OH	---OH
Long-acting					
Betamethasone	double bond	—H	---F	◀OH	——CH₃
Dexamethasone	double bond	—H	---F	◀OH	---CH₃
Paramethasone	double bond	---F	---H	◀OH	---CH₃

the patient. The intravenous route is preferred in emergencies, and the intramuscular route may be utilized temporarily when oral medication cannot be taken, but the oral route is used whenever possible. Depot preparations may be injected intra-articularly (eg, in rheumatoid arthritis), extra-articularly (eg, in bursitis, tenosynovitis, localized noninfectious tissue inflammatory disorders), and intralesionally (eg, keloids, psoriasis). Rectal preparations are employed in inflammatory bowel conditions (see Chapter 53, Agents Used in Disorders of the Lower Intestinal Tract) and topical preparations are used for dermatologic disorders (see Chapter 56, Dermatologic Preparations).

PREPARATIONS. For specific routes employed, see Table 2.

BETAMETHASONE:
Celestone (Schering). Syrup 0.6 mg/5 ml (alcohol 1%); tablets 0.6 mg.

BETAMETHASONE SODIUM PHOSPHATE:
Celestone Phosphate (Schering), **Generic.** Solution 4 mg/ml in 5 ml containers.

BETAMETHASONE ACETATE AND BETAMETHASONE SODIUM PHOSPHATE:
Celestone Soluspan (Schering). Each ml of suspension contains betamethasone acetate 3 mg and betamethasone sodium phosphate 3 mg in 5 ml containers.

CORTISONE ACETATE:
Generic. Suspension 25 mg/ml in 10 and 20 ml containers and 50 mg/ml in 10 ml containers; tablets 5, 10, and 25 mg.
Cortone Acetate (Merck Sharp & Dohme). Suspension 25 mg/ml in 20 ml containers and 50 mg/ml in 10 ml containers; tablets 25 mg.

DEXAMETHASONE:
Generic. Elixir 0.5 mg/5 ml; solution (oral) 0.5 mg/5 ml (alcohol-free) and 0.5 mg/0.5 ml (alcohol 10%); tablets 0.25, 0.5, 0.75, 1, 1.5, 2, 4, and 6 mg.
Decadron (Merck Sharp & Dohme). Elixir 0.5 mg/5 ml (alcohol 5%); tablets 0.25, 0.5, 0.75, 1.5, 4, and 6 mg.
Dexone (Rowell), **Hexadrol** (Organon). Tablets 0.5, 0.75, and 1.5 mg.

DEXAMETHASONE ACETATE:
Dalalone D.P. (Forest). Suspension (repository) 16 mg/ml in 1 and 5 ml containers (not for intralesional use).
Dalalone L.A. (Forest), **Decaject-L.A.** (Mayrand), **Generic.** Suspension (repository) 8 mg/ml in 5 ml containers.
Decadron-LA (Merck Sharp & Dohme). Suspension (repository) 8 mg/ml in 1 and 5 ml containers.

DEXAMETHASONE SODIUM PHOSPHATE:
Generic. Solution 4 mg/ml in 1, 5, 10, and 30 ml containers, 10 mg/ml in 1 and 10 ml containers, and 24 mg/ml in 5 and 10 ml containers (for intravenous use only).
Dalalone (Forest). Solution 4 mg/ml in 5 ml containers.
Decadron Phosphate (Merck Sharp & Dohme). Solution 4 mg/ml in 1, 2.5, 5, and 25 ml containers and 24 mg/ml in 5 and 10 ml containers (for intravenous use only).
Hexadrol Phosphate (Organon). Solution 4 mg/ml in 1 and 5 ml containers, 10 mg/ml in 1 and 10 ml containers, and 20 mg/ml in 5 ml containers (intravenous or intramuscular use only).

Available Mixture:
Decadron Phosphate with Xylocaine (Merck Sharp & Dohme). Each milliliter of solution contains dexamethasone sodium phosphate 4 mg and lidocaine hydrochloride 10 mg in 5 ml containers.

HYDROCORTISONE:
Generic. Suspension 25 and 50 mg/ml in 10 ml containers.
Cortef (Upjohn). Suspension 50 mg/ml in 5 ml containers; tablets 5, 10, and 20 mg.
Hydrocortone (Merck Sharp & Dohme). Tablets 10 and 20 mg.

HYDROCORTISONE ACETATE:
Generic. Suspension 25 and 50 mg/ml in 5 and 10 ml containers.
Hydrocortone Acetate (Merck Sharp & Dohme). Suspension 25 and 50 mg/ml in 5 ml containers.

HYDROCORTISONE CYPIONATE:
Cortef (Upjohn). Suspension 10 mg/5 ml.

HYDROCORTISONE SODIUM PHOSPHATE:
Hydrocortone Phosphate (Merck Sharp & Dohme). Solution 50 mg/ml in 2 and 10 ml containers.

HYDROCORTISONE SODIUM SUCCINATE:
A-hydroCort (Abbott), **Solu-Cortef** (Upjohn), **Generic.** Powder 100, 250, and 500 mg and 1 g.

METHYLPREDNISOLONE:
Generic. Tablets 4 mg.
Medrol (Upjohn). Tablets 2, 4, 8, 16, 24, and 32 mg.

METHYLPREDNISOLONE ACETATE:
Generic. Suspension 20 mg/ml in 10 ml containers, 40 mg/ml in 1, 5, and 10 ml containers, and 80 mg/ml in 1 and 5 ml containers.
depMedalone (Forest). Suspension 40 and 80 mg/ml in 5 ml containers.
Depo-Medrol (Upjohn). Suspension 20 mg/ml in 5 ml containers, 40 mg/ml in 1, 5, and 10 ml containers, and 80 mg/ml in 1 and 5 ml containers.

METHYLPREDNISOLONE SODIUM SUCCINATE:
Solu-Medrol (Upjohn), **Generic.** Powder 40, 125, and 500 mg and 1 g.

PARAMETHASONE ACETATE:
Haldrone (Lilly). Tablets 1 and 2 mg.

PREDNISOLONE:
Delta-Cortef (Upjohn), **Sterane** (Pfipharmecs), **Generic.** Tablets 5 mg.
Prelone (Muro). Syrup 15 mg/5 ml (alcohol 5%).

PREDNISOLONE ACETATE:
Generic. Suspension 25 and 50 mg/ml in 10 and 30 ml containers and 100 mg/ml in 10 ml containers.
Savacort-50 (Savage). Suspension 50 mg/ml in 10 ml containers.
PREDNISOLONE ACETATE AND PREDNISOLONE SODIUM PHOSPHATE:
Durapred (Reid-Provident), *Generic.* Each ml of suspension contains prednisolone acetate 80 mg and prednisolone sodium phosphate 20 mg in 10 ml containers.
PREDNISOLONE SODIUM PHOSPHATE:
Generic. Solution 20 mg/ml in 10 ml containers.
Hydeltrasol (Merck Sharp & Dohme). Solution 20 mg/ml in 2 and 5 ml containers.
PREDNISOLONE TEBUTATE:
Generic. Suspension 20 mg/ml in 10 ml containers.
Hydeltra-T.B.A. (Merck Sharp & Dohme). Suspension 20 mg/ml in 1 and 5 ml containers.
PREDNISONE:
Generic. Solution oral 5 mg/5 ml (alcohol 5%); tablets 1, 2.5, 5, 10, 20, 25, and 50 mg.
Deltasone (Upjohn). Tablets 2.5, 5, 10, 20, and 50 mg.
Meticorten (Schering). Tablets 1 mg.
Orisone (Rowell). Tablets 1, 5, 10, 20, and 50 mg.
SK-Prednisone (Smith Kline & French). Tablets 5 mg.
TRIAMCINOLONE:
Generic. Tablets 4 mg.
Aristocort (Lederle). Tablets 1, 2, 4, 8, and 16 mg.
Kenacort (Squibb). Tablets 4 and 8 mg.
TRIAMCINOLONE ACETONIDE:
Generic. Suspension 40 mg/ml in 1 and 5 ml containers.
Kenalog (Squibb). Suspension 10 mg/ml in 5 ml containers and 40 mg/ml in 1, 5, and 10 ml containers.
TRIAMCINOLONE DIACETATE:
Generic. Suspension 40 mg/ml in 1, 5, and 10 ml containers.
Aristocort Diacetate (Lederle). Syrup 2 mg/5 ml; suspension 25 and 40 mg/ml in 5 ml containers.
Kenacort Diacetate (Squibb). Syrup 4 mg/5 ml.
TRIAMCINOLONE HEXACETONIDE:
Aristospan (Lederle). Suspension 5 mg/ml in 5 ml containers (intralesional) and 20 mg/ml in 1 and 5 ml containers (intra-articular).

Cited References

Corticosteroids can prevent neonatal respiratory distress syndrome. *Drug Ther Bull* 18:101-102, 1980.

Adinoff AD, Hollister JR: Steroid-induced fractures and bone loss in patients with asthma. *N Engl J Med* 309:265-268, 1983.

Armstrong SD, Conn DL: Diagnosis and management of polyarteritis nodosa. *Compr Ther* 7:37-44, (Feb) 1981.

Ballard PL, Ballard RA: Corticosteroids and respiratory distress syndrome: Status 1979. *Pediatrics* 63:163-165, 1979.

Ballard RA, et al: Prenatal administration of betamethasone for prevention of respiratory distress syndrome. *J Pediatr* 94:97-101, 1979.

Baylink DJ: Glucocorticoid-induced osteoporosis, (editorial). *N Engl J Med* 309:306-308, 1983.

Behn AR, et al: Polymyalgia rheumatica and corticosteroids: How much for how long? *Ann Rheum Dis* 42:374-378, 1983.

Bolton WK, et al: Therapy of idiopathic nephrotic syndrome with alternate day steroids. *Am J Med* 62:60-70, 1977.

Borst GC, et al: Discordant cortisol response to exogenous ACTH and insulin-induced hypoglycemia in patients with pituitary disease. *N Engl J Med* 306:1462-1464, 1982.

Bracken MB, et al: Efficacy of methylprednisolone in acute spinal cord injury. *JAMA* 251:45-52, 1984.

Braughler JM, Hall ED: Current application of "high-dose" steroid therapy for CNS injury: Pharmacological perspective. *J Neurosurg* 62:806-810, 1985.

Burns TR, Saleem A: Idiopathic thrombocytopenic purpura. *Am J Med* 75:1001-1007, 1983.

Byyny RL: Withdrawal from glucocorticoid therapy. *N Engl J Med* 295:30-32, 1976.

Carette S, et al: Controlled studies of oral immunosuppressive drugs in lupus nephritis. *Ann Intern Med* 99:1-8, 1983.

Chamberlain P, Meyer WJ III: Management of pituitary-adrenal suppression secondary to corticosteroid therapy. *Pediatrics* 67:245-251, 1981.

Collins TR, Byyny RL: Clinical use of glucocorticoids. *Compr Ther* 6:63-72, (Nov) 1980.

Conn HO, Blitzer BL: Nonassociation of adrenocorticosteroid therapy and peptic ulcer. *N Engl J Med* 294:473-479, 1976.

Cupps TR, Fauci AS: Corticosteroid-mediated immunoregulation in man. *Immunol Rev* 65:133-155, 1982.

Dixon RB, Christy NP: On various forms of corticosteroid withdrawal syndrome. *Am J Med* 68:224-230, 1980.

Fass B: Glucocorticoid therapy for nonendocrine disorders: Withdrawal and "coverage." *Pediatr Clin North Am* 26:251-256, 1979.

Fauci AS, et al: Glucocorticosteroid therapy: Mechanisms of action and clinical considerations. *Ann Intern Med* 84:304-315, 1976.

Flavin DK, et al: Corticosteroid abuse: Unusual manifestation of drug dependence. *Mayo Clin Proc* 58:764-766, 1983.

Hollinger WM, et al: Prediction of therapeutic response in steroid-treated pulmonary sarcoidosis: Evaluation of clinical parameters, bronchoalveolar lavage, gallium-67 lung scanning, and serum angiotensin-converting enzyme levels. *Am Rev Respir Dis* 132:65-69, 1985.

Horber FF, et al: Evidence that prednisone-induced myopathy is reversed by physical training. *J Clin Endocrinol Metab* 61:83-88, 1985.

Kehrl JH, Fauci AS: Clinical use of glucocorticoids. *Ann Allergy* 50:2-8, 1983.

Kelton JG: Management of pregnant patient with idiopathic thrombocytopenic purpura. *Ann Intern Med* 99:796-800, 1983.

Klintmalm G, Säwe J: High dose methylprednisolone increases plasma cyclosporin levels in renal transplant recipients, (letter). *Lancet* 1:731, 1984.

Levitz M, et al: Transfer and metabolism of corticosteroids in perfused human placenta. *Am J Obstet Gynecol* 132:363-366, 1978.

Ling MHM, et al: Side effects of corticosteroid therapy: Psychiatric aspects. *Arch Gen Psychiatry* 38:471-477, 1981.

Martinez-Maldonado M, Garcia A: Practical approach to nephrotic syndrome. *Drug Ther* 11:79-91, (March) 1981.

McCluskey J, Gutteridge DH: Avascular necrosis of bone after high doses of dexamethasone during neurosurgery. *Br Med J* 284:333-334, 1982.

Messer J, et al: Association of adrenocorticosteroid therapy and peptic ulcer disease. *N Engl J Med* 309:21-24, 1983.

Nixon JE: Early diagnosis and treatment of steroid induced avascular necrosis of bone. *Br Med J* 288:741-744, 1984.

Pickup ME: Clinical pharmacokinetics of prednisone and prednisolone. *Clin Pharmacokinet* 4:111-128, 1979.

Ponticelli C, et al: Controlled trial of methylprednisolone and chlorambucil in idiopathic membranous nephropathy. *N Engl J Med* 310:946-950, 1984.

Rote NS, Lau RJ: Immunologic thrombocytopenic purpura. *Clin Obstet Gynecol* 28:84-100, 1985.

Rüegsegger P, et al: Corticosteroid-induced bone loss: Longitudinal study of alternate day therapy in patients with bronchial asthma using quantitative computed tomography. *Eur J Clin Pharmacol* 25:615-620, 1983.

Sambrook PN, et al: Osteonecrosis after high dosage, short term corticosteroid therapy. *J Rheumatol* 11:514-516, 1984.

Sheagren JN: Septic shock and corticosteroids, (editorial). *N Engl J Med* 305:456-458, 1981.

Shields JR, Resnik R: Fetal lung maturation and antenatal use of glucocorticoids to prevent respiratory distress syndrome. *Obstet Gynecol Surv* 34:343-363, 1979.

Spiro HM: Is the steroid ulcer a myth? (editorial). *N Engl J Med* 309:45-47, 1983.

Sprung CL, et al: Effects of high-dose corticosteroids in patients with septic shock. *N Engl J Med* 311:1137-1143, 1984.

Streck WF, Lockwood DH: Pituitary adrenal recovery following short-term suppression with corticosteroids. *Am J Med* 66:910-914, 1979.

Szefler SJ, et al: Effect of troleandomycin on methylprednisolone elimination. *J Allergy Clin Immunol* 66:447-451, 1980.

Taylor LJ: Multifocal avascular necrosis after short-term high-dose steroid therapy: Report of three cases. *J Bone Joint Surg* 66-B:431-433, 1984.

Uribe M, et al: Comparative serum prednisone and prednisolone concentrations following administration to patients with chronic active liver disease. *Clin Pharmacokinet* 7:452-459, 1982.

Urman JD, Rothfield NF: Corticosteroid treatment in systemic lupus erythematosus: Survival studies. *JAMA* 238:2272-2276, 1977.

Warrell DA, et al: Dexamethasone proves deleterious in cerebral malaria: Double-blind trial in 100 comatose patients. *N Engl J Med* 306:313-319, 1982.

Yount WJ, et al: Corticosteroid therapy of collagen vascular disorders, in Azarnoff DL (ed): *Steroid Therapy*. Philadelphia, WB Saunders, 1975, 269-286.

Zizic TM, et al: Corticosteroid therapy associated with ischemic necrosis of bone in systemic lupus erythematosus. *Am J Med* 79:596-604, 1985.

Agents for Active and Passive Immunity

62

Immunization is an inclusive term denoting the process of inducing immunity or providing it artificially through administration of a vaccine or antiserum. Active immunization is induced by natural infection or by a vaccine or toxoid that causes the recipient to produce specific antibodies and antitoxins. The immunologic response responsible for protection is unknown for some vaccines (eg, BCG) but may be due in part to cell-mediated immunity. In the case of BCG, empiric observations of protection following vaccine administration have served as a guide. Passive immunization is the provision of temporary immunity through administration of preformed antibodies produced in another individual by natural infection or active immunization. Three types of agents are employed for passive immunization: pooled human immune globulin, specific immune globulin, and antitoxin.

The ultimate goal of most immunization programs is the eradication of communicable diseases through the use of vaccines and antiserums. For example, an effective worldwide immunization program with smallpox vaccine has eradicated the natural disease. Immunization also may have the immediate goal of preventing specific diseases in selected individuals and groups.

Attainment of a high proportion of immune individuals in a community is the most effective means of preventing communicable disease. Universal immunization is an important part of good health care and should be pursued actively through routine and intensive programs to ensure that all children and other susceptible persons are immunized. In the United States, universal immunization with diphtheria/tetanus/pertussis, poliovirus, haemophilus influenzae type b, and measles/mumps/rubella vaccines has been recommended.

The Immunization Practices Advisory Committee (ACIP) of the United States Public Health Service regularly updates information on vaccines and antiserums and periodically revises recommendations for their use. ACIP advisories and recommendations are published in the widely circulated *Morbidity and Mortality Weekly Report* and the pertinent articles are routinely reported in the *Journal of the American Medical*

Association. Physicians should consult these publications for updated information on vaccines and antiserums. The American Academy of Pediatrics and the American College of Physicians also publish recommendations for the use of vaccines. The physician should also consult the manufacturer's package insert.

VACCINES AND TOXOIDS

Vaccines are suspensions of living or killed microorganisms (bacteria, viruses) or components thereof employed to induce active immunity. Certain vaccines (diphtheria/tetanus/pertussis, measles/mumps/rubella, poliomyelitis, and haemophilus influenzae type b) are used routinely for pediatric immunization, while others (eg, hepatitis B, rabies, influenza, meningococcal, pneumococcal, BCG, plague, anthrax, typhoid, cholera, yellow fever) are indicated primarily for those at special risk. Most vaccines are intended for use in normal, healthy individuals, although they may be safe and effective in persons with diseases or conditions not adversely affected by them.

Vaccines are used prophylactically, usually before exposure to infectious disease but may be used in individuals previously exposed to a specific disease. The following are examples. Pre-exposure rabies immunization is given only to selected individuals at high risk (eg, veterinarians, animal handlers), but rabies vaccine is administered routinely after contact with the virus, usually through an animal bite. Measles vaccine given within five days after exposure prevents disease in 68% of household contacts. This is thought to be due to the shorter incubation period for vaccine measles (seven days) compared to natural measles (11 days).

VIRAL VACCINES. These are composed of live attenuated viruses (eg, measles, mumps, rubella vaccines, oral poliovirus vaccine), inactivated nonliving whole viruses (eg, influenza vaccine, rabies vaccine), or antigenic components of the virus particle (eg, influenza "split-virus" vaccine, hepatitis B vaccine) and may contain a single agent (eg, measles, hepatitis B) or a combination (eg, measles/mumps/rubella).

In normal recipients, vaccines containing live, attenuated microorganisms produce a mild or subclinical infection that results in active immunity. Replication of the virus in the vaccines is essential to the induction of immunity. Most vaccines containing live, attenuated viruses require only a single administration to provide long-term protection. However, three doses of live oral poliovirus vaccine are recommended to ensure immunity to all three serotypes. In addition to systemic protection, oral poliovirus vaccine also appears to stimulate local immunity by inducing IgA at the portal of entry.

Inactivated vaccines must contain a sufficient antigenic mass to induce the desired immune response, since the organisms in these preparations cannot replicate in the host. Repeated administration is usually necessary to induce long lasting immunity. The primary immunization schedule usually consists of two to three doses, with booster doses to maintain immunity.

BACTERIAL VACCINES. These are prepared from whole bacteria (eg, pertussis vaccine) or from purified capsular polysaccharides of certain bacteria (eg, pneumococcal vaccine, meningococcal vaccine, haemophilus influenzae type B vaccine). Except for BCG and live oral typhoid vaccine, bacterial vaccines are composed of nonliving agents. The live attenuated bacterial vaccines act in a manner analogous to that described for live virus vaccines.

Bacterial vaccines stimulate the production of various antibodies. Those antibodies that appear to play a protective role are directed against antigens on the surface of a bacterial cell (eg, polysaccharide antigens). Coating of these bacterial antigens with antibodies renders the organisms more susceptible to phagocytosis (opsonins), to lysis by complement (lytic antibodies), or to aggregation (antisurface antigen antibodies) and subsequent phagocytosis.

Inactivated bacterial vaccines are usually given in two or three doses, except for polysaccharide vaccines, which provide years of protection after a single dose.

TOXOIDS. Toxoids are modified bacterial exotoxins that have been neutralized by treatment with formaldehyde. They retain the ability to stimulate the production of antibodies that combine with toxin. The two agents used clinically are tetanus and diphtheria toxoids. Both are available as single agents or as combinations with or without pertussis vaccine.

COMPONENTS OF VACCINES AND TOXOIDS. Physicians should be familiar with the major constituents of vaccines and toxoids, since they may cause adverse effects (eg, hypersensitivity reactions).

Immunizing Antigen(s): In some preparations (eg, hepatitis B surface antigen, tetanus toxoid), this is a single, well-defined material, while in others (eg, pertussis vaccine, live virus vaccines), it is complex and poorly defined.

Suspending Fluid: This may be simple (sterile water or saline) or complex (eg, tissue culture fluid). Small amounts of proteins and other material derived from the biological system or medium of preparation (eg, egg protein, serum protein, cell culture antigens) may be included.

Preservatives, Stabilizers, Antibiotics: Mercurials, glycine, and certain antibiotics are present to prevent bacterial growth or stabilize the antigen. These materials occasionally cause hypersensitivity reactions in certain individuals.

Adjuvants: Certain vaccines contain an aluminum compound to intensify the immune response and to aid in retention of the antigen at the depot site, which prolongs the stimulant effect. Adjuvants are employed in vaccines containing inactivated microorganisms or their products (eg, toxoids, hepatitis B vaccine). Vaccines containing adjuvants should not be injected subcutaneously or intracutaneously, since local irritation, inflammation, granuloma, or necrosis may follow. They should be injected deep into muscle masses.

ANTISERUMS AND IMMUNE GLOBULINS

These substances are used both prophylactically and therapeutically to provide temporary immunity against infectious agents, microbial exotoxins, and snake and insect venoms. Antiserums provide protection by the passive transfer of antibodies produced in another individual by natural infection (eg, hepatitis B immune globulin) or active immunization with a known immunogen (eg, rabies antiserum, human or equine). The protection afforded may be specific, as with diphtheria antitoxin, or general, as with human immune globulin (gamma globulin).

Antiserums are commonly used when (1) no vaccine is available and use of antibody prevents or modifies the disease (eg, hepatitis A); (2) protection is needed immediately and there is insufficient time to stimulate the patient's own antibodies through active immunization (eg, hepatitis B, rabies prophylaxis, certain exposures to measles); (3) a specific microbial toxin (eg, botulism) is best managed by administration of antibody; (4) clinical disease is present and an antibody is known to neutralize the effect of the unfixed toxin (eg, diphtheria, tetanus, snake or spider envenomation); or (5) the patient has diminished or absent capacity to produce antibodies (eg, immunosuppression caused by cancer chemotherapy or radiation treatment; immunodeficiency disease).

Antiserums for clinical use are of human or equine origin. Serious hypersensitivity reactions (serum sickness, anaphylaxis) occur much more often with equine antiserums. In addition, antibodies from heterologous species, such as those in equine antiserums, disappear from the blood rapidly; often none remain after seven to ten days. In contrast, the half-life of human antiserums is approximately four weeks.

Immune globulin is a sterile serum protein solution (15% to 18%) containing antibodies from human blood. It is derived from pooled human serum and consists primarily of immunoglobulin G (95% IgG); small amounts of other immunoglobulins (IgM, IgA) and serum proteins also are present. Immune globulin contains antibodies in proportion to those in the population from which it was derived, and large numbers of donors are employed to ensure that adequate amounts of desired antibodies (eg, measles, hepatitis) are included.

Specific immune globulins are obtained from plasma donors preselected for high titers of the desired antibody (eg, hepatitis B, varicella-zoster, rabies, vaccinia, tetanus). Some preparations are obtained from individuals hyperimmunized with a specific vaccine (eg, vaccinia, tetanus, rabies), while others are obtained from pooled plasma drawn from subjects with naturally high antibody titers to a specific antigen (eg, varicella-zoster, hepatitis B). In all other respects, specific immune globulin preparations conform to the description of immune globulin.

Antitoxins are antibodies directed against a toxin (eg, microbial exotoxin, snake or spider venom) that combine specifically with it to neutralize toxicity. Antitoxins for human use are principally of equine origin (antivenins; diphtheria, botulism, and tetanus antitoxins), but tetanus antitoxin of human origin (tetanus immune globulin) is available.

Antivenins are antitoxins directed against the venom of a snake (eg, North American coral snake) or insect (black widow spider). All antivenins for human use are of equine origin and are used only after envenomation has occurred.

Antiserums and immune globulin preparations contain antibodies that combine with antigenic sites on the infectious organism or toxin, resulting in anti-invasive, neutralizing, or antitoxic activity. Passive immunization with these materials results in protection of short duration (one to three months). Protective antiviral (neutralizing) antibodies inhibit adsorption, penetration, and normal uncoating of the virus. Since antibodies do not penetrate the intact cell, they act only on extracellular viruses. Antitoxins combine avidly with specific toxins. Once combined with antibody, the toxin's action is inhibited and it is said to be neutralized; however, antitoxin cannot affect fixed toxin or reverse its prior effect.

ADVERSE REACTIONS

VACCINES. Adverse reactions have been reported for all vaccines. These are usually local and transient but may be systemic and immediate or delayed. Local inflammatory reactions at the site of injection are most common. Systemic reactions (eg, fever, rash, hypersensitivity) occur infrequently but most subside within 48 hours; they usually can be managed with symptomatic treatment only. The following four types of adverse reactions have been encountered with vaccines.

Mild Local Reactions: These effects are the most common and occur after use of most vaccines. A local inflammatory reaction (eg, erythema, tenderness) develops at the site of injection. Induration is seen less often.

Severe Local Reactions: This type of reaction is most commonly encountered with certain live vaccines, such as smallpox and BCG, which produce a lesion at the injection site that leaves a scar. With BCG vaccine, severe ulceration and keloidal scars may result.

Mild Systemic Reactions: Following vaccination, transient fever, malaise, or mild headache may occur, but usually these reactions subside within 48 hours and require symptomatic treatment only.

Severe, Nonallergic Systemic Reactions: These reactions are rare, may be of a "toxic" nature, and may be characterized by a severe febrile response, severe headache, febrile or nonfebrile convulsions, or postimmunization encephalomyelitis. Examples include the systemic reactions that develop occasionally in children after pertussis vaccination; reactions to vaccination or booster doses of typhoid, cholera, or plague vaccine; and the rare instances of paralytic poliomyelitis that develop after administration of live oral poliovirus vaccine.

Hypersensitivity Reactions: Sensitivity reactions occur very rarely. Allergic reactions are thought to be due to the following vaccine constituents: (1) Trace amounts of egg protein in influenza and yellow fever vaccines. (2) Antibiotic(s) in the vaccines; for example, measles/mumps/rubella vaccine contains a small amount of neomycin and some individuals allergic to neomycin may experience a delayed-type of local reaction (erythematous, pruritic papule) 48 to 72 hours after injection of the vaccine. (3) Some component of the infectious agent itself or one of its products. Rarely, urticarial reactions have been observed in individuals receiving tetanus or diphtheria toxoids and these are thought to be hypersensitivity reactions to the immunogens themselves.

ANTISERUMS AND IMMUNE GLOBULINS. Adverse reactions to antiserums are much more common than to vaccines or immune globulins. Serious hypersensitivity reactions occur with much greater frequency with use of antiserums of equine origin than to those of human origin. Serious reactions to human immune globulins are uncommon, although anaphylaxis and systemic collapse have been reported. The most common reaction is discomfort on administration. Organic mercurials (eg, thimerosal) are used as preservatives in these products and may accumulate in patients given immune globulins over a prolonged period. However, only one instance of proven mercury sensitivity has been reported.

Animal serums pose a special risk because of sensitivity reactions. Three types of reactions occur: (1) Anaphylactic reactions develop seconds to minutes after injection and consist of urticaria, dyspnea, cyanosis, and shock. (See following discussion.) (2) Serum sickness consisting of rash, urticaria, arthritis, adenopathy, and fever occurs hours or days after injection. It is more common in persons who received prior serum injections or large doses and may be managed with salicylates, antihistamines, ephedrine, or corticosteroids. (3) Acute febrile reactions are usually mild and may be treated with salicylates. Rarely, these reactions may result in death due to hyperpyrexia.

ANAPHYLACTIC SHOCK. Anaphylaxis is an acute systemic manifestation of immediate hypersensitivity and is often life-threatening. Release of mediators (eg, histamine, leukotrienes, prostaglandins) by mast cells and basophils is responsible for the many complex and varied reactions. Upper airway obstruction and circulatory collapse are the most serious manifestations and can be fatal in minutes. Laryngeal edema followed by hypotension, bronchospasm, and arrhythmias are the most common life-threatening complications. In the vast majority of patients, pruritic urticaria develops and is considered to be the hallmark of anaphylaxis, although severe episodes can occur in its absence. Generalized reactions are rare and occur primarily when vaccines containing egg protein are used; systemic reactions to equine globulins are more common.

Therapy is aimed at preventing or reversing complications and includes administration of epinephrine, immediate attention to the airway, cardiac monitoring, and establishing intravenous access. Immediate attention to the upper airway is imperative, for most fatal reactions involve obstruction at this site. Hypoxia should be treated by establishing a patent airway and administering oxygen. Endotracheal intubation may be necessary and tracheostomy may be indicated in the presence of laryngeal edema.

The usual treatment for vascular shock (eg, maintaining body temperature, elevating the lower extremities) also may be needed. For severe cardiovascular collapse, it may be necessary to administer epinephrine directly into the heart and to initiate cardiopulmonary resuscitation. Intravenous fluids should be administered and intravenous infusion of norepinephrine [Levophed] may be required to support blood pressure (adults, 2 to 8 ml of solution added to 500 ml of 5% dextrose injection and given at a rate adjusted to maintain satisfactory blood pressure).

Epinephrine 1:1,000 is the primary drug used in anaphylaxis because of its combined alpha- and beta-adrenergic agonist properties. The alpha component increases peripheral resistance and decreases urticaria. The beta component increases cyclic adenosine monophosphate (cAMP) levels to inhibit further release of mediators, relax bronchial smooth muscle, and increase cardiac rate and contractility. The dosages in Table 1 should be given at the earliest sign of anaphylaxis.

Antihistamines (eg, diphenhydramine) are usually considered part of the standard treatment of anaphylactic reactions but play no role in immediate treatment, for they do not reverse effects already produced by histamine. Antihistamines act by competitively inhibiting histamine at receptor sites but have no effect on SRS-A and, thus, bronchospasm is not reversed. However, these agents reverse such cutaneous manifestations as pruritus and thus may be used adjunctively. For reactions that have been reversed by epinephrine therapy, diphenhydramine can be given orally, but it should be given parenterally for life-threatening episodes.

Patients who develop severe wheezing without vascular shock should be treated initially with epinephrine, which may be followed by use of theophylline or a sympathomimetic bronchodilator (see Chapter 22, Drugs Used in Bronchial Disorders).

Since corticosteroids neither prevent nor reverse anaphylactic symptoms, they are not useful in emergencies but are often given to shorten the course of the reaction. Those who advocate their use in refractory cases (when hypotension or bronchospasm is present) believe that corticosteroids may decrease the duration or severity of symptoms in prolonged reactions. Steroids may prevent the effects of (1) some mediators (prostaglandins, leukotrienes) that are not preformed but are released after antigen stimulation and may have extended effects, and (2) circulating antigen that may

TABLE 1.
TREATMENT OF ANAPHYLACTIC SHOCK

Route	Dosage	
	Adults	Children
Initial (repeated every 5 min): Subcutaneous (preferred), Intramuscular (epinephrine 1:1,000)	0.5 ml	0.01 ml/kg (maximum 0.3 ml)
Inadequate response to intramuscular or subcutaneous administration: Intravenous (epinephrine 1:10,000)*	0.25 to 0.5 ml at 15-min intervals	0.01 ml/kg every 5 to 15 min, as needed

*Solution diluted 1:10,000 by adding 1 ml of 1:1,000 solution to syringe containing 9 ml of physiologic saline injection. A ready-made 1:10,000 solution can be obtained from several manufacturers.

persist and cause a recurrence of symptoms. However, clinical studies do not conclusively support the use of steroids in anaphylaxis or determine an agent of choice.

Hypotensive patients who do not respond to repeated doses of epinephrine, intravenous fluids, and antihistamines may be treated with pressor agents. Although the agent of choice is controversial, some investigators prefer dopamine (Lucke and Thomas, 1983; Fath and Cerra, 1984).

Acidosis may result from hypoxia and decreased cardiac output; treatment with sodium bicarbonate has been recommended (Fath and Cerra, 1984).

For a more detailed discussion on anaphylaxis and its treatment, see Lucke and Thomas, 1983, and Fath and Cerra, 1984.

PRECAUTIONS

The physician should be aware of the following general recommendations and precautions when administering a vaccine, immune globulin, or serum of animal origin.

Any difficulties encountered in the practical use of immunizing agents should be reported by telephone *and* in writing to the manufacturer or through local and state health departments to one of the following:

Immunization Division of the Centers for Disease Control, Department of Health and Human Services, Atlanta, GA 30333; telephone: day (404) 329-1880, night (404) 329-2888

Food and Drug Administration, through the Drug Experience Report (FD 1639) available from the Division of Drug Epidemiology and Drug Experience, HFD-210, FDA, 5600 Fishers Lane, Rockville, MD 20857 and reproduced in this book (see back cover).

VACCINES. When feasible, live virus vaccines not administered on the same day should be given at least one month apart because of the possibility of viral interference. Some vaccines contain preservatives (eg, thimerosal) or trace amounts of antibiotics (eg, neomycin) to which some patients may be hypersensitive. However, no currently recommended vaccine contains penicillin or a derivative.

Immunosuppressed patients, such as those with leukemia, lymphoma, or generalized malignancy, generally should not receive live virus vaccines, for virus replication may be enhanced in these patients. Live vaccine should not be administered to patients undergoing immunosuppressive therapy until three months after all such therapy has been discontinued. Because immunodeficient patients may not have an adequate response to vaccination, it is advisable to determine antibody levels or use another appropriate immunologic parameter to assess the efficacy of immunization and to guide future management. Oral poliovirus vaccine should not be given to a member of a household in which there is a family history of immunodeficiency until the immune competence of the recipient and other family members is known. Vaccine virus excreted by the recipient may be communicated to an immunodeficient person and complications may result.

Immunization is generally contraindicated in patients with progressive neurologic disorders, but those with stable neuro-logic disorders may be vaccinated. Persons with severe febrile illnesses should not be immunized until they have recovered.

Except for poliovirus and yellow fever vaccines, live virus vaccines are not recommended for pregnant women or those likely to become pregnant within three months of vaccination. When a vaccine must be given during pregnancy, it is prudent to wait until the second or third trimester, and then only when there is substantial risk of exposure to the wild virus. Inactivated poliovirus vaccine is preferred for adults when there is sufficient time to complete the series.

Live virus vaccines should not be given within three months of administration of human immune globulin, since antibodies present in the latter may inhibit virus replication and the desired immune response.

IMMUNE GLOBULINS. Immune globulin should be given only for diseases in which its efficacy has been established.

Since immune globulin preparations may contain trace amounts of IgA, patients selectively deficient for IgA may develop antibody to it and subsequently react to immune globulins, serum plasma, or whole blood. Normal individuals may develop antibodies to genetic types of IgG that differ from their own.

Aggregates of IgG may form on standing and rarely cause systemic reactions (eg, anaphylaxis) after administration of immune globulins.

Isoimmunization is a possibility in immunocompetent individuals given immune globulin.

ANIMAL SERUMS. Because of their potential for causing serious hypersensitivity reactions, animal serums should be used only when other forms of therapy or prophylaxis (eg, human immune globulin) are not available. Before using any animal serum, a careful inquiry should be made into the prospective recipient's history of hypersensitivity and appropriate tests for hypersensitivity (scratch, eye, or intracutaneous skin test) should be performed. (See following discussion.)

No serum should be injected or any test for hypersensitivity performed unless there is a syringe containing 0.5 ml of 1:1,000 aqueous epinephrine (maximum initial dose) within immediate reach.

TESTS FOR HYPERSENSITIVITY. Antigens in vaccines and antiserums may cause hypersensitivity reactions. Certain constituents of vaccines (eg, egg protein, antibiotics) may cause allergic reactions and sensitive individuals should not receive vaccines at all, since they are principally used for prophylaxis.

An intracutaneous skin test preceded by a scratch or eye (conjunctival) test must be performed before injection of any animal serum, regardless of whether or not the patient has ever received the serum species. For any of the following sensitivity tests, the concomitant use of antihistamines may invalidate the testing procedure. Epinephrine should always be available during testing, desensitization, or administration.

Conjunctival Test: One drop of a 1:10 dilution of the test serum in isotonic sodium chloride solution is instilled into one conjunctival sac. One drop of isotonic sodium chloride solution is instilled into the other to serve as a control. A positive test is manifested by lacrimation and conjunctival injection in 10 to 30 minutes.

Scratch Test: One drop of a 1:100 dilution of the test serum in saline is applied to a superficial scratch on the skin (eg, on the distal forearm). A positive reaction consists of erythema and wheal formation at the site. As a control, a similar test using saline only is performed at a distant site (eg, the other forearm).

Intradermal Test: This test is performed only if the conjunctival or scratch test is negative. FOR INDIVIDUALS WITH NO KNOWN ALLERGIES, 0.1 ml of a 1:100 dilution of the serum in saline is injected. As a control, the saline diluent only is injected at a distant site. A positive reaction consists of wheal formation in 10 to 30 minutes. IN PERSONS WITH A HISTORY OF ALLERGY, the test dose is reduced to 0.05 ml of a 1:1,000 dilution.

The physician is cautioned that intradermal skin tests have resulted in fatalities but eye and scratch tests have not. *Skin tests should never be performed unless a syringe containing 0.5 ml of epinephrine 1:1,000 (maximum initial dose) is within immediate reach.*

A negative eye or skin test is *not* an absolute guarantee that sensitivity is absent, but only indicates that sensitivity is probably lacking.

Desensitization for Serum Reactions: If a test for hypersensitivity is positive or if there is a history of allergy in a patient whose need for animal serum is imperative, it is still possible to proceed with passive immunization. In such instances, the following desensitization procedure may increase the patient's tolerance to the foreign protein. However, it is dangerous to assume that true desensitization occurs.

The following doses are injected every 15 minutes if they can be tolerated without local or systemic reaction: (1) 0.05 ml of 1:20 dilution subcutaneously; (2) 0.1 ml of 1:10 dilution subcutaneously; (3) 0.3 ml of 1:10 dilution subcutaneously; (4) 0.1 ml undiluted serum subcutaneously; (5) 0.2 ml undiluted serum intramuscularly; (6) 0.5 ml undiluted serum intramuscularly; and (7) the remaining therapeutic dose intramuscularly. It is recommended that a written record of pulse, blood pressure, and respiration taken before each succeeding injection should be maintained.

ROUTE, SITE, AND TECHNIQUE OF IMMUNIZATION

Each immunobiologic agent has a recommended route of administration based upon prior clinical trials and experience. To avoid untoward local or systemic effects and to ensure optimal efficacy, the practitioner should not deviate from the recommended route.

Injectable immunobiologics should be given in an area with minimal opportunity for local, neural, vascular, or tissue injury. Usually, *subcutaneous injections* are administered into the thigh of infants and the deltoid area of older children and adults. *Intradermal injections* are generally given on the volar surface of the forearm, except for human diploid cell rabies vaccine, which is given in the deltoid area to avoid severe reactions. At the present time, the preferred sites for *intramuscular injection* are the anterolateral aspect of the upper thigh for children under 3 years and the deltoid muscle of the upper arm for older children and adults. However, for children, the site should be determined individually based on the volume of material to be injected and the size of the muscle mass.

Under most circumstances, the upper, outer aspect of the buttocks should not be used for routine immunizations. In those rare instances when this site must be used (eg, for administration of large volumes of immune globulin), the upper outer mass of the gluteus maximus away from the central region of the buttocks should be selected to avoid injury to the sciatic nerve.

A sterile disposable syringe and needle should be used for each injection to minimize contamination. If different vaccines are given at the same time, each injection should be in a different site.

Most widely used vaccines are both safe and effective when given simultaneously. This is practical in certain circumstances: imminent exposure to several infectious diseases, preparation for foreign travel or uncertainty of patient return, and integration with other health care activities (eg, well-infant visits).

Inactivated vaccines may be given at the same time at different injection sites. However, vaccines commonly associated with adverse reactions (eg, cholera, typhoid, plague) should be given on separate occasions.

Most live virus vaccines may be administered on the same day. In children, antibody responses to oral poliovirus vaccine given with measles/mumps/rubella vaccine are comparable to those realized when these vaccines are given on separate occasions. However, data suggest that the antibody response to a live virus vaccine administered within one month after another live virus vaccine may be diminished. Therefore, it is usually recommended that live virus vaccines not given on the same day be spaced at least one month apart.

In general, an inactivated vaccine and a live virus vaccine may be given simultaneously at separate sites with no more than the usual precautions that apply for the individual vaccines.

IMMUNIZATION SCHEDULES

As a general rule, vaccines are recommended for the youngest age group at risk and capable of responding to vaccination. The objective of most routine immunization programs is not only to protect the individual, but to control and eventually eliminate infectious disease in a community through the development of high levels of immunity.

Schedules for routine primary active immunization against diphtheria, tetanus, pertussis (whooping cough), poliomyelitis, measles, rubella, mumps, and haemophilus influenzae type B have been developed by the U.S. Public Health Services Advisory Committee on Immunization Practices and the Committee on Infectious Diseases of the American Academy of Pediatrics (see Tables 2, 3, and 4). Their recommendations for the scheduling of immunizations are based upon the following factors: Vaccines that every normal infant and child should receive, optimal and practical ages for immunization, efficacy and tolerance of combinations of vaccines, current epidemiology of the diseases, possibility of the integration of vaccinations with other health care activities (well-infant visits), and other practical aspects of administration.

IMMUNIZATION RECORDS. Every physician should maintain a permanent record of the immunization history of each patient so that information can be updated regularly and those in need of immunization can be identified easily and recalled.

Whatever system of recording is used, it is recommended that the following data be included: Date of administration, vaccine or other biologic administered, manufacturer, lot number, expiration date, site and route of administration, unexpected or unusual adverse reactions.

Permanent, comprehensive immunization records also should be maintained by the parent. In addition, immunization records (containing at least immunization dates) should be kept by institutions, such as schools and day care centers. Since persons frequently relocate, it is recommended that personal immunization records be maintained by all individuals.

PEDIATRIC IMMUNIZATIONS. The recommendations in Tables 2, 3, and 4 are influenced by: (1) the risks of the disease for specific age groups; (2) the risk of complications; (3) the ability of an age group to respond to a vaccine; and (4) the possible presence of maternal antibody, which could interfere with the expected immune response.

Recent data suggest that patients with a history of convulsions are more likely to experience seizures following pertussis vaccination. Thus, it is recommended that immunization with DTP or DT vaccines be deferred until the first birthday in infants and young children in whom seizures have occurred or who develop seizures before completion of the four-dose primary series until it can be determined that there is no evolving neurologic disorder. Infants and children with stable neurologic conditions or a family history of convulsions may be vaccinated (Immunization Practices Advisory Committee, 1985 A).

A decision on whether to proceed with DTP immunization usually can be made within a few months and should be made at no later than 1 year of age for infants who have received less than three doses. A minimum of three doses at intervals of at least four weeks is necessary for adequate immunity.

ADULT IMMUNIZATIONS. Immunization programs are usually proposed for children to achieve long-term universal immunity in a population. Despite these efforts, a portion of the adolescent and adult population remains susceptible to one or more common communicable diseases, and these individuals may be candidates for certain routine pediatric vaccines.

Diphtheria: Specific adult immunization programs are not considered necessary for diphtheria, for this disease is rare (occasional outbreaks occur in susceptible migrant workers and their families). However, it has been estimated that immunity to the disease is lacking in nearly one-half of the adult population. For this reason, the divalent toxoid, Td, rather than monovalent tetanus toxoid has been recommended for routine use.

Tetanus: Most adults over 50 years are inadequately immunized against tetanus. If the primary vaccination series has

TABLE 2. RECOMMENDED SCHEDULE FOR ACTIVE IMMUNIZATION OF NORMAL INFANTS AND CHILDREN*

Recommended Age	Vaccine(s)	Comments
2 mo	DTP,[1] OPV[2]	Can be initiated earlier in areas of high endemicity
4 mo	DTP, OPV	2-mo interval desired for OPV to avoid interference
6 mo	DTP (OPV)	OPV optional for areas where polio might be imported (e.g., some areas of Southwest United States)
15 mo	Measles, Mumps, Rubella (MMR)[3]	MMR preferred
18 mo	DTP, OPV	Consider as part of primary series—DTP essential
24 mo	Hib[4]	
4–6 yr[5]	DTP, OPV	
14–16 yr	Td[6]	Repeat every 10 years for lifetime

[1]*DTP—Diphtheria and tetanus toxoids with pertussis vaccine.*
[2]*OPV—Oral, attenuated poliovirus vaccine contains poliovirus types 1, 2, and 3.*
[3]*MMR—Live measles, mumps, and rubella viruses in a combined vaccine (see text for discussion of single vaccines).*
[4]*Haemophilus influenzae type B polysaccharide vaccine.*
[5]*Up to the seventh birthday.*
[6]*Td—Adult tetanus toxoid (full dose) and diphtheria toxoid (reduced dose) in combination.*
For all products used, consult manufacturers' brochure for instructions for storage, handling, and administration.
Biologics prepared by different manufacturers may vary, and those of the same manufacturer may change from time to time. The package insert should be followed for a specific product.
*Adapted from American Academy of Pediatrics, Report of the Committee on Infectious Diseases, 1982.

been completed, a booster dose of tetanus toxoid (preferably Td) should be given every 10 years. A single booster should restore protection when more than 10 years have elapsed since the last dose. It should be noted that tetanus organisms have a worldwide distribution, the mortality for untreated tetanus is 40%, and only those who are specifically immunized are protected.

Pertussis: Pertussis (whooping cough) is rare in adults and usually is not serious. Thus, immunization of this age group is

TABLE 3.
RECOMMENDED IMMUNIZATION SCHEDULES FOR INFANTS AND CHILDREN
NOT INITIALLY IMMUNIZED AT USUAL RECOMMENDED TIMES IN EARLY INFANCY

Timing	Recommended Schedules				Comments
	Preferred Schedule	Alternatives			
		#1	#2	#3	
First Visit	DTP #1, OPV #1, Tuberculin test (PPD)	MMR, PPD	DTP #1, OPV #1, PPD	DTP#1, OPV#1, MMR, PPD	MMR should be given no younger than 15 mo. old.
1 month after first visit	MMR	DTP #1, OPV #1	MMR, DTP #2	DTP #2	—
2 months after first visit	DTP #2, OPV #2	—	DTP #3, OPV #2	DTP #3, OPV #2	—
3 months after first visit	(DTP #3)	DTP #2, OPV #2	—	—	In preferred schedule, DTP #3 can be given if OPV #3 is not to be given until 10–16 months.
4 months after first visit	DTP #3, (OPV #3)	—	(OPV #3)	(OPV #3)	OPV #3 optional for areas for likely importation of polio (e.g., some southwestern states).
5 months after first visit	—	DTP #3 (OPV #3)	—	—	(Same as 4 months)
10–16 months after last dose	DTP #4, OPV # 3 or OPV #4	DTP #4, OPV #3 or OPV #4	DTP #4, OPV #3 or OPV #4	DTP #4, OPV #3 or OPV #4	—
24 months	Hib	—	—	—	—
Preschool	DTP #5, OPV #4 or OPV #5	DTP #5, OPV #4 or OPV #5	DTP #5, OPV #4 or OPV #5	DTP #5, OPV #4 or OPV #5	Preschool dose not necessary if DTP #4 or #5 given after fourth birthday.
14–16 yr old	Td	Td	Td	Td	Repeat every 10 years

Alternative #1 can be used in those more than 15 months old if measles is occurring in the community.

Alternative #2 allows for more rapid DTP immunization.

Alternative #3 should be reserved for those whose access to medical care is compromised by poor compliance.

DTP = Diphtheria and tetanus toxoids with pertussis vaccine.

OPV = Oral, attenuated poliovirus vaccine contains types 1, 2, and 3.

Tuberculin test = Mantoux (intradermal PPD) preferred. Frequency of tests depends on local epidemiology. The Committee recommends annual or biennial testing unless local circumstances dictate less frequent or no testing.

MMR = Live measles, mumps, and rubella viruses in a combined vaccine (see text for discussion of single vaccines).

Hib = Haemophilus influenzae type B polysaccharide vaccine

Td = Adult tetanus toxoid (full dose) and diphtheria toxoid (reduced dose) in combination.

For all products used, consult manufacturer's brochure for instructions for storage, handling, and administration. Biologics prepared by different manufacturers may vary, and those of the same manufacturer may change from time to time. The package insert should be followed for a specific product.

Adapted from American Academy of Pediatrics, Report of the Committee on Infectious Diseases, 1982.

not necessary. Pertussis vaccine is not generally given after the seventh birthday because of the mild nature of the disease in adults and the occurrence of adverse reactions to the vaccine.

Poliomyelitis: Routine poliovirus vaccination of adults residing in the U.S. is not recommended. Most adults are already immune and the risk of exposure is very small. However, adults at increased risk of exposure include (1) travelers to areas where poliomyelitis is prevalent; (2) members of population groups with disease caused by poliovirus; (3) certain laboratory personnel working with virulent polioviruses; (4) health care workers in frequent contact with poliomyelitis patients; and (5) unimmunized or inadequately immunized parents or other adults residing in the same household as children to be given live oral poliovirus vaccine. (Susceptible adult contacts are at slight risk of infection resulting from fecal excretion of revertant viruses.) Adults who are household contacts of children to be given oral poliovirus vaccine should follow the most appropriate schedule as outlined below before the vaccine is administered to the child.

TABLE 4.
RECOMMENDED IMMUNIZATION SCHEDULE FOR PERSONS 7 YEARS OF AGE OR OLDER

Timing	Vaccine(s)	Comments
First visit	Td #1[1], OPV #1[2], and MMR[3]	OPV not routinely administered to those 18 years of age or older
2 months after first Td, OPV	Td #2, OPV #2	—
6–12 months after second Td, OPV	Td #3, OPV #3	OPV #3 may be given as soon as 6 weeks after OPV #2
10 years after Td #3	Td	Repeat every 10 years throughout life

[1]*Td-Tetanus and diphtheria toxoids (adult type) are used after the seventh birthday. The DTP doses given to children under 7 who remain incompletely immunized at age 7 or older should be counted as prior exposure to tetanus and diphtheria toxoids (eg, a child who previously received 2 doses of DTP needs only 1 dose of Td to complete a primary series).*

[2]*OPV-Oral, attenuated poliovirus vaccine contains poliovirus types 1, 2, and 3. When polio vaccine is to be given to individuals 18 years of older, IPV is preferred.*

[3]*MMR-Live measles, mumps, and rubella viruses in a combined vaccine. Persons born before 1956 can generally be considered immune to measles and mumps and need not be immunized. Rubella vaccine may be given to persons of any age, particularly to women of childbearing age. MMR may be used since administration of vaccine to persons already immune is not deleterious.*

Adapted from Immunization Practices Advisory Committee, 1983.

For adults at increased risk of exposure to poliovirus, the following recommendations are based on the immune status of the individual:

A. *Unvaccinated or uncertain immune status*: Primary vaccination with inactivated poliovirus vaccine. If time does not permit administration of at least three doses, the following schedules are recommended: (1) Less than eight weeks, but more than four: Two doses of inactivated vaccine at least four weeks apart. (2) Less than four weeks: A single dose of live oral poliovirus vaccine. In both instances, the remaining doses of vaccine should be given later at the recommended interval if the person remains at increased risk.

B. *Incompletely immunized*: Adults who have received less than a full course of either the oral or inactivated vaccine should be given the remaining doses of the respective vaccine regardless of the interval since the last dose.

C. *Completion of a primary course of either poliovirus vaccine*: Those who have completed a primary course of oral poliovirus vaccine may be given another dose of the same vaccine. Those who have completed a primary course of inactivated poliovirus vaccine may be given a dose of either the oral or inactivated vaccine.

Measles: A significant proportion of young adults appears to be susceptible to measles, for they escaped immunization programs and natural exposure was reduced because of "herd" immunity. Epidemics of measles have occurred in older teenagers, college students, and young adults. Measles in adults is often more severe than in children.

Serologic surveys have shown that virtually all persons born before 1956 are immune. However, a significant proportion of persons born since 1956 may be susceptible. It has been suggested, therefore, that all nonimmune persons born since 1956 be immunized. Recipients of the earlier, inactivated measles vaccine may not be protected from natural measles infection and the disease may be more serious in these individuals. These persons should be vaccinated with the current live virus vaccine. In addition, any person who was immunized prematurely (eg, before the first birthday), received immune globulin within three months prior to the live vaccine, or received improperly handled vaccine should be reimmunized.

Mumps: In postpubertal persons, mumps may produce significant discomfort (eg, orchitis, oophoritis); orchitis occurs in up to 20% of postpubertal males, but sterility is rare. Meningoencephalitis occurs occasionally, but permanent sequelae are rare. Mumps vaccine may be given to susceptible adults. Immune globulin does not prevent mumps.

Rubella: The primary objective of immunization against rubella in childhood is to prevent infection in pregnant women, because transplacental transfer of the virus to the fetus may cause serious congenital abnormalities. Despite widespread immunization of children, it is estimated that 15% to 20% of women of childbearing age are susceptible to rubella. All females of childbearing age should be given rubella vaccine unless serologic testing reveals that they are immune or were vaccinated previously. Pregnant females should be excluded because of the potential risk to the fetus. Vaccinees are advised not to become pregnant for three months after vaccination and are encouraged to use some form of birth control during this period.

Although the value of immune globulin has not been established in proven or presumably susceptible pregnant women exposed to rubella, patients should receive the preparation when therapeutic abortion is not performed. It is also recommended that susceptible mothers be vaccinated in the immediate postpartum period.

Studies have shown that 15% to 20% of young adult males are susceptible to rubella. Since these individuals may spread the virus to pregnant women, they also should be vaccinated.

IMMUNIZATIONS FOR TRAVELERS

Requirements and recommendations for specific immunizations and health practices for travel to various countries change yearly. The best source of up-to-date information is *Health Information for International Travel*, which is published annually by the Centers for Disease Control and can be obtained from the Superintendent of Documents, U.S. Government Printing Office, Washington, DC 20402.

Infants less than 6 months are usually exempt from requirements for certain vaccines, but they should receive the usual pediatric immunizations at the recommended intervals.

In the following discussion, immunizations are divided into three convenient groups: (1) Prerequisite for entry into a country or area, (2) commonly recommended, and (3) occasionally recommended.

Immunizations Required for Entry

Yellow Fever: Presently, this disease occurs only in Africa and South America. Vaccination is required in some African countries for entering travelers; other countries require vaccination only for those entering from areas considered to harbor the virus. The vaccine is usually recommended for all persons over 6 months of age who travel in areas where the disease is occurring. Pregnant women and infants under 6 months should be considered for vaccination if travel to a high-risk area is anticipated and cannot be postponed. Protection is effective for 10 years. The vaccine must be administered at an approved Yellow Fever Vaccination Center (consult state or local health departments).

Studies indicate that antibody titers of both yellow fever and cholera are reduced if the vaccines are given simultaneously or within three weeks of each other.

Cholera: Vaccination is not required for travel to most countries, but some countries require cholera vaccination for all travelers or for those coming from an endemic area. In the United States, cholera is exceedingly rare. Cholera vaccines have limited effectiveness. Although booster doses enhance protection, only one dose is necessary to meet international requirements and is valid for six months.

Immunizations Commonly Recommended

Typhoid Fever: Immunization is recommended for travelers to areas where typhoid fever and poor sanitation exist. The killed vaccine is about 70% effective but often causes local reaction at the injection site of one to two days' duration, fever, malaise, and headache. Protection lasts four to six months.

A live oral typhoid vaccine (Ty21a) is available in some countries and may soon be available in the U.S. It is essentially nonreactogenic and was more than 90% effective in one field trial.

Hepatitis A: This disease occurs worldwide and is spread by the fecal-oral route. Immune globulin is recommended for travelers to developing countries who will tour areas with primitive sanitation. It should be given close to the time of departure. All active immunizations should be completed before immune globulin is given (at least two weeks between the administration of the last dose of vaccine and the injection of immune globulin).

Poliomyelitis: Vaccination is usually recommended for non-immune or inadequately immunized travelers to areas where poliomyelitis is prevalent and sanitation is poor. Depending upon immune status and history, either the killed or live poliovirus vaccine may be employed.

Tetanus: Tetanus immunization is recommended for everyone at home or traveling abroad. A booster injection combined with diphtheria toxoid should be given every 10 years to those who have completed the primary series.

Immunizations Occasionally Recommended

Diphtheria: The bacteria causing diphtheria are distributed throughout the world. Travelers at high risk of infection are those in contact with children of poorer areas in underdeveloped nations. In spite of immunization programs, many adults are susceptible. A tetanus/diphtheria toxoid (Td) booster injection is recommended every 10 years for those who have completed the primary series.

Rabies: Vaccination with rabies vaccine is recommended only for travelers anticipating contact with animals or prolonged residence in areas where exposure to rabies is a constant threat.

Plague: Vaccination is not recommended unless there is a substantial risk of infection. Immunization is generally recommended only for travelers who expect to have contact with rodents, rabbits, or fleas in areas where plague is enzootic (eg, Southeast Asia, Africa, South America).

Hepatitis B: Although not ordinarily recommended for travelers, the vaccine should be considered for certain individuals going to areas where the disease is highly endemic (eg, Southeast Asia, sub-Saharan Africa). Health care personnel whose work requires handling of body fluids and individuals expecting to have sexual contact with persons at risk are candidates for the vaccine. In order to complete the full immunization series, vaccination should begin six months in advance of the anticipated travel date.

Measles: Many adolescents and young adults are susceptible to measles and measles in adults is often more serious than in children. Traveling may place these individuals at increased risk of exposure. It is suggested that anyone born after 1956 who has not been vaccinated and does not have physician-documented history of infection should consider receiving measles vaccine before traveling.

Meningococcal Polysaccharide Vaccine: Immunization is not usually recommended for adults, but travelers to countries where meningococcal disease is epidemic (eg, sub-Saharan Africa from Mauritania to Ethiopia) are candidates for the vaccine.

ROUTINE IMMUNIZING AGENTS

Diphtheria

Diphtheria is primarily a disease of childhood, but it may occur in all age groups. Since the use of immunization on a large scale, diphtheria has become rare but localized outbreaks are reported occasionally. The disease is caused by invasion of the skin or upper respiratory tract by *Corynebacterium diphtheriae*, which produces toxins that cause systemic manifestations, including peripheral neuropathy and myocarditis.

Active immunization is achieved with the use of diphtheria toxoid, a preparation of formaldehyde-inactivated toxins of *C. diphtheriae*. It is usually given in combination with tetanus toxoid and pertussis vaccine (DTP) for primary immunization of infants and young children. In addition, diphtheria toxoid is available in combination with tetanus toxoid without pertussis vaccine in a pediatric preparation (DT) or an adult preparation (Td).

Diphtheria antitoxin also may be useful for prophylaxis in exposed, nonimmunized, susceptible individuals who are not under close surveillance. Most commonly, however, it is used with appropriate antibiotic therapy to treat clinical diphtheria. The most important aspect of treatment is to give a large dose of antitoxin at the earliest possible moment. The dose depends on the severity and duration of the clinical disease and is substantially increased if the diphtheritic membrane is extensive or the illness is prolonged (see the evaluation). The antitoxin probably is of no value for cutaneous lesions.

DIPHTHERIA AND TETANUS TOXOIDS AND PERTUSSIS VACCINE ADSORBED (DTP)

This combination of diphtheria and tetanus toxoids with pertussis vaccine is the recommended preparation for routine primary immunization and recall (booster) injections in children under 7 years.

The combined triple antigens are not recommended for use on or after the seventh birthday. There are two reasons for this recommendation: (1) Both the incidence and severity of disease decrease with age and the vaccine may cause undesirable adverse reactions, and (2) the diphtheria component is present in a high dose that is not recommended for individuals over 7 years. Tetanus and diphtheria toxoids, adult type (Td), may be used for primary immunization of older patients (7 years or more); diphtheria and tetanus toxoids, pediatric type (DT), may be used in younger children when pertussis vaccine is contraindicated.

ADVERSE REACTIONS AND PRECAUTIONS. The most common untoward effects include transient fever and tenderness, erythema, and induration at the site of injection. Systemic reactions, such as drowsiness, fretfulness, vomiting, and anorexia, are also common. Persistent crying or a transient shock-like episode has occurred less frequently. Reactions involving the central nervous system are rare but may develop after any DTP injection in a course. Manifestations include convulsions, uncontrollable screaming, or encephalopathy, which may lead to permanent defects. It has been calculated that DTP vaccine carries an attributable risk of serious neurologic reaction of 1/110,000 doses; the risk of neurologic damage that persists for one year has been estimated at 1/310,000 doses (*Br Med J*, 1981). Because data suggest that infants and young children with a history of convulsions are more likely to develop seizures after pertussis immunization, it has been recommended that immunization with any vaccine containing pertussis be deferred in these patients until it can be determined that there is no evolving neurologic disorder (Immunization Practices Advisory Committee, 1984 A, 1985 A) (see also Immunization Schedules).

The vaccine is contraindicated in patients with acute febrile respiratory disease or fever over 100 F and in those undergoing immunosuppressive therapy. Absolute contraindications include the occurrence of the following adverse events after DTP or monovalent pertussis vaccination: (1) allergic hypersensitivity; (2) fever of 105 F or higher within 48 hours; (3) collapse or shock-like state within 48 hours; (4) persistent, inconsolable crying lasting three hours or more or an unusual, high-pitched cry occurring within 48 hours; (5) convulsion(s) with or without fever occurring within three days; (6) encephalopathy occurring within seven days, including severe alterations in consciousness with generalized or focal neurologic signs (Immunization Practices Advisory Committee, 1985 A).

An ad hoc panel of the American Medical Association has published a report on pertussis vaccine injury, including severe irreversible and reversible reactions, likely duration and sequelae, and clinical criteria for attribution (AMA Ad Hoc Panel on Pertussis Vaccine Injury, 1985).

DOSAGE.

Intramuscular: Children 2 months to the seventh birthday, initially, 0.5 ml, followed by two more doses at four- to eight-week intervals. A reinforcing fourth dose is given about one year after the third and a booster dose is given when the child is 4 to 6 years old. This booster dose is not necessary if the fourth dose in the primary series was given on or after the fourth birthday. DTP should not be used after the seventh birthday.

Each 0.5 ml of DTP contains 4 protective units of pertussis antigen. A total of at least 12 units is recommended; more than 70% of immunized individuals will be protected from pertussis after this amount is administered.

(See the manufacturer's recommendations for volume dose of preparation used.)

Manufacturers: Lederle (**Tri-Immunol**), Connaught.

DIPHTHERIA AND TETANUS TOXOIDS ADSORBED (Pediatric) (DT)

Diphtheria and tetanus toxoids pediatric (DT) may be used for primary immunization and recall injections in children up to 7 years of age when pertussis vaccine must be given separately or omitted. It should not be used in older individuals.

Following the initial injection of DT vaccine, the serum antibody titer rises to a low level, peaks after one to two months, and then subsides if no further vaccine is given. The titer rises rapidly after subsequent injections, reaches a peak 10 to 15 days later, and gradually declines thereafter. After the primary immunization series has been completed, booster doses establish protective serum levels within five to seven days that may last for several years.

ADVERSE REACTIONS AND PRECAUTIONS. As with other routine immunization procedures, use of combined diphtheria and tetanus toxoids should be deferred in the presence of active infection or febrile acute respiratory tract disease. A history of a neurologic or severe hypersensitivity reaction following a previous dose is a contraindication to further use of DT toxoids. Erythema, induration, and tenderness at the injection site develop in some patients. Systemic reactions, such as fever, drowsiness, fretfulness, vomiting, anorexia, and persistent crying, are sometimes observed. Neurologic complications following tetanus toxoid administration have been reported rarely.

DOSAGE.

Intramuscular: Children less than 12 months, three 0.5-ml injections administered at different sites at four-week intervals, followed by a fourth dose 6 to 12 months later. *Children over 12 months,* two doses four weeks apart, followed by a third dose 6 to 12 months later (Immunization Practices Advisory Committee, 1984 A). A booster dose is given when the child is 4 to 6 years old, but it is not necessary if the fourth dose in the primary series was given on or after the fourth birthday.

Manufacturers: Lederle, Sclavo, Squibb/Connaught, Wyeth.

TETANUS AND DIPHTHERIA TOXOIDS ADSORBED FOR ADULT USE (Td)

Tetanus and diphtheria toxoids adsorbed for adult use (Td) is used for primary immunization or recall (booster) injections in adults and children 7 years and older. This preparation contains the same amount of tetanus toxoid as DTP but only one-sixth to one-twelfth of the diphtheria toxoid contained in pediatric preparations. It is preferred to tetanus toxoid alone in wound management (see Table 5).

Serum antibody responses are similar to those seen with the pediatric vaccine. High levels of immunity to diphtheria are reached in recipients after primary immunization. These levels can be maintained by booster immunization at ten-year intervals with a low dose of toxoid.

ADVERSE REACTIONS. Reactions to Td are usually mild in patients under 20 years. They include erythema, induration, and tenderness at the site of injection; fever and malaise also may occur. Booster injections may produce severe reactions to either component. These are most likely to occur in persons who have received large numbers of booster doses. Neurologic complications following tetanus toxoid administration have been reported rarely.

DOSAGE.

Intramuscular: Adults and children 7 years and older, two injections of 0.5 ml with an interval of four to six weeks between injections. A reinforcing dose to complete basic immunization is given 6 to 12 months later and every ten years thereafter.

Manufacturers: Lederle, Sclavo, Squibb/Connaught, Wyeth.

DIPHTHERIA TOXOID ADSORBED (Pediatric)

This monovalent vaccine is a sterile suspension of diphtheria toxoid adsorbed onto aluminum hydroxide. It is used for active immunization of children under 6 years of age in whom tetanus toxoid and/or pertussis vaccine is contraindicated. For those over 6 years, products containing diphtheria toxoid for adult immunization (Td) are employed.

ADVERSE REACTIONS AND PRECAUTIONS. Mild local reactions (redness, tenderness, and induration at the injection site) have been observed. Systemic reactions include transient fever, malaise, flushing, generalized urticaria or pruritus, tachycardia, and hypotension. These effects are especially likely to occur in patients who have received a large number of booster injections.

The vaccine should not be used to treat active diphtheria infections. Immunization should be deferred in the presence of acute or active infection. A diminished antibody response may occur in patients undergoing immunosuppressive therapy and, therefore, primary diphtheria immunization should be deferred until such treatment is terminated. If immunization is attempted during such treatment, an additional dose should be given one month after immunosuppressive therapy has ceased. Postponement of immunization is recommended in patients with a history of central nervous system disorders or convulsions until the situation is clarified. The vaccine should not be given intracutaneously.

DOSAGE.

Intramuscular: Children less than 6 years, two injections of 0.5 ml given six to eight weeks apart. A third 0.5-ml dose is given approximately one year later.

Manufacturer: Sclavo.

DIPHTHERIA ANTITOXIN

This antitoxin is a sterile solution of enzyme-treated antibodies obtained from the serum of horses immunized with diphtheria toxoid alone or in conjunction with diphtheria toxin. It is used to treat active cases of diphtheria, and a few experts believe it should be considered for prophylaxis in exposed, nonimmunized, susceptible individuals who are not under close surveillance. For active cases, antitoxin should be administered on the basis of a clinical diagnosis of diphtheria without waiting for bacteriologic confirmation. Appropriate antimicrobial therapy (eg, penicillin, erythromycin) helps eliminate bacteria from the infected sites but is of no value against the toxin. Active immunization with diphtheria toxoid, using a different site, should be initiated at the same time that diphtheria antitoxin is given, because recovery from the disease does not necessarily confer immunity.

ADVERSE REACTIONS AND PRECAUTIONS. Serum sickness (urticaria, fever, pruritus, malaise, arthralgia) may occur in 7 to 14 days. The incidence of serum sickness caused by the currently available enzyme-treated serum is about 5%. The extent and severity of reactions depend on the amount of horse serum administered, the hypersensitivity of the patient, and the history of previous serum injections. Before injecting diphtheria antitoxin, it is essential to determine whether the patient has received a previous injection of animal serum or has a history of asthma or allergy. A skin or conjunctival test for sensitivity should be performed in all patients (see the Introduction).

DOSAGE. The entire dose required should be given at one time if possible. Enough antitoxin must be administered to neutralize all the circulating toxin and any that may continue to be produced; usually one-half is given intravenously and one-half intramuscularly.

Intramuscular: Adults and children, all asymptomatic, nonimmunized contacts of patients with diphtheria should receive prompt prophylaxis through immunization with diphtheria toxoid, appropriate antimicrobial therapy, and continued surveillance for seven days. Patients not being monitored also should be given diphtheria antitoxin as follows:

If sensitivity tests are negative or desensitization has been completed, the patient is given 2,000 to 10,000 units of antitoxin, depending on the length of time since exposure, extent of exposure, and condition of the patient.

For treatment, dosage depends upon the site, severity, and duration of infection. Suggested ranges for *adults and children* are: pharyngeal or laryngeal disease of 48 hours' duration, 20,000 to 40,000 units; nasopharyngeal lesions, 40,000 to 60,000 units; extensive disease of three or more days' duration, 80,000 to 120,000 units.

Intravenous (slow infusion): Adults and children, for treatment only, same as intramuscular dose.

Manufacturers: Sclavo, Squibb/Connaught.

Tetanus

Tetanus is not communicable; it results from the introduction of *Clostridium tetani,* a spore-forming anaerobic bacillus, into an area of injury. Under certain local tissue conditions (eg, low oxygen tension), the spore is converted to the vegetative form, which produces an exotoxin, tetanospasmin, which acts on the nervous system. Although tetanus is rare in the United States, the mortality rate is approximately 50%. Most cases of clinical disease occur in adults who have not received the primary immunization series or the necessary boosters to maintain adequate immunity. Fortunately, the disease is completely preventable by adequate immunization.

Since there is no natural immunity to tetanus, prophylaxis must be achieved by immunization: actively with tetanus toxoid, passively with tetanus immune globulin, or both. To provide adequate protection, it is important (1) that all children receive the recommended primary immunizations; (2) that booster injections be given every ten years; (3) that a history of immunizations be obtained from adult patients and booster injections be given as necessary; and (4) that an injured patient receive appropriate treatment of wounds and tetanus prophylaxis when indicated.

Primary immunization schedules are given in Tables 2, 3, and 4. Schedules for the use of prophylactic agents in wound management are given in Table 5.

Prophylaxis: Since complete primary immunization with tetanus toxoid protects for ten years or more, boosters are required only every ten years in those who have completed the primary series, unless the wound is "tetanus prone" (eg, deep puncture). It is necessary to determine whether a patient completed primary immunization and, if not, how many doses

were given. Primary immunization should be completed in patients who received fewer than the recommended doses, including those given as part of wound management.

The preparation of choice for tetanus immunization in persons 7 years and older is Td (tetanus and diphtheria toxoids adsorbed, for adult use). Many adults are susceptible to diphtheria and simultaneous administration of diphtheria toxoid will enhance protection against this disease.

For children less than 7 years, the products employed are diphtheria and tetanus toxoids and pertussis vaccine adsorbed (DTP) or diphtheria and tetanus toxoids adsorbed (for pediatric use) (DT) if pertussis vaccine is contraindicated.

TABLE 5.
GUIDE TO TETANUS PROPHYLAXIS IN ROUTINE WOUND MANAGEMENT[1]

History of adsorbed tetanus toxoid (doses)	Clean, minor wounds		All other wounds[2]	
	Td[3]	TIG	Td[3]	TIG
Unknown or <3	Yes	No	Yes	Yes
>3[4]	No[5]	No	No[6]	No

[1]Adapted from Immunization Practices Advisory Committee, 1985 A.

[2]Such as, but not limited to, wounds contaminated with dirt, feces, soil, and saliva; puncture wounds; avulsions; and wounds from missiles, crushing, burns, and frostbite.

[3]For children under 7 years, DTP (DT if pertussis vaccine is contraindicated) is preferred to tetanus toxoid alone. For persons 7 years old and older, Td is preferred to tetanus toxoid alone.

[4]If only three doses of fluid toxoid have been received, a fourth dose of toxoid, preferably adsorbed toxoid, should be given.

[5]Yes if more than five years since last dose (More frequent boosters are not needed and can accentuate side effects.)

Clinical Tetanus: Treatment of clinical tetanus includes injection of tetanus immune globulin (human). This preparation is preferred to the older equine antitoxin, which may cause hypersensitivity reactions. The antitoxin neutralizes circulating toxin but does not affect that attached to the neuromuscular endplate. Other measures include appropriate wound management with debridement if necessary; administration of antibiotics (penicillin or tetracycline), sedatives, and muscle relaxants; and other supportive therapy (eg, quiet environment).

TETANUS TOXOID

TETANUS TOXOID ADSORBED

Tetanus toxoid is a sterile preparation of inactivated toxin of *Clostridium tetani.* It is available in fluid or adsorbed form; *the latter is preferred* because it usually induces higher antitoxin titers and a longer duration of protection.

An immunizing course of tetanus toxoid is highly effective, produces few adverse reactions, and provides long-lasting protection against tetanus. This agent usually is given with diphtheria toxoid and pertussis vaccine (DTP) for primary immunization of infants and children under 7 years of age. For primary immunization of adults and children 7 years and older, Td (tetanus and diphtheria toxoids adsorbed for adult use) is preferred to tetanus toxoid alone to provide a booster immunization of diphtheria. For children under 7 years in whom the pertussis component is contraindicated, DT is recommended. (See these evaluations.)

Tetanus toxoid in combination with diphtheria toxoid (as Td or DT) also is used prophylactically for wound management in patients who are not completely immunized. Considerations in treatment are the condition of the wound and whether to use tetanus toxoid alone for active immunization or to use tetanus immune globulin in addition for passive immunization. (See Table 5.)

At least three injections of tetanus toxoid are needed to induce sufficient levels of neutralizing antibody. Immunity lasts up to ten years in 95% of vaccinees and a blood level equal to or greater than 0.01 IU tetanus antitoxin will be maintained.

ADVERSE REACTIONS AND PRECAUTIONS. Adverse reactions occur infrequently and include erythema, induration, and tenderness at the site of injection; fever, malaise, and neurologic complications are rare. The incidence of adverse reactions may be higher in persons over 25 years of age. High antibody levels following too frequent booster doses of tetanus toxoid have been associated with hypersensitivity reactions. (See also the evaluations on the combinations of tetanus toxoid with diphtheria toxoid and pertussis vaccine.)

DOSAGE.

Intramuscular: The adsorbed form is preferred to the fluid preparation. Tetanus toxoid adsorbed, for *adults and children* not previously immunized, three injections of 0.5-ml; the second injection is given four to six weeks after the first and the third injection is given one year after the second. A booster dose is given every ten years.

Manufacturers: Lederle, Sclavo, Squibb/Connaught, Wyeth.

TETANUS IMMUNE GLOBULIN (TIG)

Tetanus immune globulin is a sterile solution of globulins obtained from the plasma of adults hyperimmunized with tetanus toxoid. It is indicated in the prophylaxis and treatment of persons with wounds potentially contaminated by *Clostridium tetani* and is preferred to tetanus antitoxin of equine origin for passive immunization.

Passive immunization is indicated for individuals with tetanus-prone wounds who have never been actively immunized with Tetanus toxoid; whose immune status is uncertain and cannot be established conclusively; whose last recall (booster) dose or last dose of the basic immunization series was more than ten years prior to injury; or whose wound has been unattended for more than 24 hours.

TIG induces longer lasting protective levels of circulating antitoxin with considerably lower doses than either the equine or bovine antitoxin. It has a half-life of approximately four weeks and appreciable serum levels are maintained for up to 14 weeks. It supplements, but does not replace, antibiotic therapy for management of wounds. Active immunization with tetanus toxoid should be initiated concomitantly using a different injection site and different syringe.

ADVERSE REACTIONS. Because tetanus immune globulin is of human origin, it is relatively free from the risk of hypersensitivity reactions. As with other gamma globulin preparations, pain and erythema may occur at the site of injection.

DOSAGE. Tetanus immune globulin should be given intramuscularly only.

Intramuscular: For prophylaxis, *adults and children*, 250 to 500 units by deep intramuscular injection. (Tetanus toxoid adsorbed may be given concurrently in a separate syringe and at a different site.) If threat of tetanus infection persists, the dose may be repeated at four-week intervals.

For treatment, therapy usually is employed only when prior immunization is incomplete. An optimum therapeutic dose has not been established but the following amounts are recommended: *Adults*, 3,000 to 6,000 units; *children*, a single dose of 500 to 3,000 units. Part of the dose may be placed in the wound area (Academy of Pediatrics, 1982).

Available Trademarks.
Homo-Tet (Savage), **Hu-Tet** (Hyland), **Hyper-Tet** (Cutter), **Tetanus Immune Globulin** (Wyeth).

TETANUS ANTITOXIN EQUINE

Tetanus antitoxin is a sterile solution of concentrated antibody proteins obtained from the blood of horses hyperimmunized with tetanus toxin or toxoid. It is one component of therapy in patients with clinical tetanus. It also may be used prophylactically in nonimmunized patients with tetanus-prone wounds; however, because of the risk of hypersensitivity reactions, tetanus antitoxin should be used only when tetanus immune globulin (human) is not available.

Appropriate tests for sensitivity to equine serum should precede the use of tetanus antitoxin (see the Introduction). Epinephrine 1:1,000 should be available for prompt treatment of severe reactions.

When given for prophylaxis, tetanus antitoxin should be administered intramuscularly to lessen the severity of reactions, which range from pain at the site of injection to serum sickness (arthralgia, urticaria, fever, malaise) and anaphylactic shock. For therapy, the intravenous route is employed to neutralize circulating tetanus toxin rapidly. Active immunization with tetanus toxoid should be initiated at the same time that tetanus antitoxin is given using a different injection site and a different syringe.

DOSAGE.

Intramuscular: Adults and children, for prophylaxis, 1,500 to 5,000 units, depending upon body weight (<30 kg, 1,500 units; >30 kg, 3,000 to 5,000 units).

Intravenous: Adults and children, for treatment, 50,000 to 100,000 units. Part of the dose is given intravenously and the rest is given intramuscularly.

Manufacturer: Sclavo.

Pertussis

Pertussis is a highly communicable disease caused by the bacterium, *Bordetella pertussis.* About 80% of clinical cases occur during the first five years of life, and most deaths occur in infants less than 1 year; fatalities are rare in older patients. Therefore, vaccination early in life is strongly recommended, preferably as part of the routine primary immunization program (see Tables 2, 3, and 4). Although the immunology of the infection and the specific immune mechanisms of vaccination are not well understood, the widespread use of pertussis vaccine during the past 35 years has markedly reduced the morbidity and mortality from the disease.

PERTUSSIS VACCINE ADSORBED

Pertussis vaccine adsorbed is a preparation of whole killed bacteria. It is a sterile suspension of killed *Bordetella pertussis* in saline solution containing aluminum phosphate and thimerosal. Research is in progress to determine the specific antigenic components so that an improved vaccine, free of irrelevant material, can be prepared.

Pertussis vaccine adsorbed is used when immunization with the monovalent vaccine is preferred. It also may be used as a booster during outbreaks of pertussis. Pertussis vaccine appears to be more effective in protecting against clinical pertussis than against subclinical infection with *Bordetella pertussis.* Short-lived protection may be mediated through secretory IgA in respiratory epithelium.

This vaccine is usually administered with diphtheria and tetanus toxoids as DTP (see that evaluation). Monovalent pertussis vaccine is rarely indicated. Since the incidence and mortality of pertussis decrease with age, while local and systemic reactions to the vaccine increase, pertussis immunization is not generally recommended for those over 7 years.

ADVERSE REACTIONS AND PRECAUTIONS. Convulsions in infants following use of DTP have been reported; therefore, no vaccine containing the pertussis antigen should be administered without an evaluation in any child who has previously had a DTP-associated convulsion. Rare, severe encephalopathic reactions also have been described. If pertussis vaccine does induce such reactions, the incidence is clearly lower than that of similar effects produced by the disease.

Common adverse reactions include induration, local tenderness, fever, and malaise. Formation of sterile abscesses is rare. (See also evaluation of DTP vaccine and other individual components.)

DOSAGE.

Intramuscular: Children 2 months to 6 years, three injections of 0.5 ml each given four to eight weeks apart. Booster doses of 0.5 ml each should be given at 2 and 5 years of age. Recall injections after intimate exposure may be given to children up to 7 years. *Adults,* 0.25-ml booster may be given to medical personnel exposed during pertussis epidemics, as well as to adolescents at risk.

The total human immunizing dose of three 0.5-ml injections contains 12 protective units of pertussis vaccine. Monovalent pertussis vaccine may be obtained from the Biologic Products Division, Michigan Department of Health, PO Box 30035, Lansing, MI 48909.

Measles

Prior to the development of an effective vaccine, measles was a common childhood disease sometimes associated with pneumonia, acute encephalitis, subacute sclerosing panencephalitis, and death. Since the use of live attenuated measles virus vaccine, morbidity and mortality have decreased markedly. However, when immunization efforts have lapsed, there has been a resurgence of cases. At present, programs are under way to eliminate measles from the United States.

Measles vaccination may be accomplished with the individual measles virus vaccine or with a combination product containing measles with rubella or measles with mumps and rubella. The last is more commonly used for routine immunization programs because it requires only a single injection and provides earlier protection against the specific diseases.

MEASLES VIRUS VACCINE LIVE

This vaccine is a bacteriologically sterile preparation containing a highly attenuated strain of measles (rubeola) virus grown in chick embryo cell cultures. A noncommunicable, mild measles virus infection develops in susceptible individuals and results in the production of protective antibodies. The vaccine is highly immunogenic and a seroconversion rate of 90% to 95% is expected. Little or no virus is excreted and secondary spread to contacts is not a problem.

Vaccine-induced antibody levels may decline over time but protection appears to be permanent. Vaccine failure may be due to thermal inactivation of the live virus or to pre-existing neutralizing antibodies, either of which may inhibit viral replication and the subsequent development of host immunity. The simultaneous administration of immune globulin to reduce adverse reactions is not recommended, since this may interfere with the immunogenicity of the vaccine.

Immunization with live measles vaccine is recommended for all children at or after 15 months of age when transplacental passive immunity has dissipated. It may be given as early as 6 months of age in high-risk situations, such as an outbreak of measles in an institution or community. In such instances, immunization should be repeated after 15 months of age. In addition, because of the possibility of inadequate immunity, live measles vaccine should be given to children who received the vaccine for any reason prior to 12 months of age or who received the older inactivated measles virus vaccine. Most adults are immune to measles, but vaccination may be advisable for high school and college students during an epidemic or for adults in isolated communities where measles is not endemic.

ADVERSE REACTIONS AND PRECAUTIONS. There are usually no reactions to the vaccine, but moderate fever, rash, or both occur occasionally and convulsions associated with high fever rarely. Other central nervous system effects observed rarely include encephalitis and encephalopathy, but the risk of these reactions is less than with natural measles. Although subacute sclerosing panencephalitis has been reported in children who received the vaccine, it is clear that measles vaccination offers good protection against this late complication of the disease.

Anaphylactic reactions rarely have been reported after administration of measles vaccine, which is prepared in chick embryo cell culture, to persons with known allergy to egg protein (Herman et al, 1983). A procedure for desensitization of children with positive skin tests to both egg albumin and vaccine has been described (Herman et al, 1983).

Exposure to measles is not a contraindication to vaccination. If the vaccine is given within 72 hours after exposure to measles, protection may be provided. Immune globulin may be used to modify measles in a susceptible person (see that evaluation) but should not be used concurrently with the vaccine.

The vaccine should not be administered to pregnant females and pregnancy should be avoided for three months following vaccination (FDA Pregnancy Category C).

DOSAGE.
Subcutaneous: *Children 15 months or older,* a single dose of 0.5 ml of reconstituted vaccine is injected, preferably into the outer aspect of the upper arm. It is essential that only the diluent supplied with the vaccine be used for reconstitution.

Available Trademark.
Attenuvax (Merck Sharp & Dohme).

Mumps

Mumps occurs primarily in children 5 to 15 years of age and is reported in about twice as many males as females because it is more apt to be overt or recognized in the former. It is a relatively benign, self-limiting disease. The principal clinical manifestation, parotitis, may be unpleasant or debilitating, although many infections are asymptomatic. Orchitis occurs in up to 20% of postpubertal males, but sterility is rare. Meningoencephalitis occurs occasionally, but permanent sequelae are also rare. Deafness may result from infection. Since the introduction of live mumps virus vaccine in 1967, the incidence of clinical mumps and morbidity due to complications have declined markedly.

MUMPS VIRUS VACCINE LIVE

Live mumps virus vaccine is a suspension of the Jeryl Lynn strain of virus grown in chick embryo culture. It produces a subclinical, noncommunicable infection and provides active immunity in over 90% of persons following a single subcutaneous injection. Levels of circulating antibodies are significantly lower than following natural infection, but are adequate to provide protection for many years, probably for life. Vaccine failures may be due to virus inactivation during storage or to pre-existing neutralizing antibody.

Immunization is recommended for all children at any age after 12 months. It is not recommended for children under 12 months since retention of maternal neutralizing antibodies may interfere with the immune response. The vaccine is of particular value in susceptible individuals approaching puberty, adolescents, and adults. It is not necessary, however, to test for susceptibility before vaccination.

Mumps vaccine may be given alone or in combination with rubella or with live measles and rubella virus vaccines; this triple combination is commonly used in routine immunization programs and is the vaccine of choice. (Mumps and measles combined vaccine is not marketed in the United States.)

Mumps vaccine may not provide protection when given after exposure to the disease. Immune globulin does not provide postexposure prophylaxis; thus, its use is not recommended.

ADVERSE REACTIONS AND PRECAUTIONS. Mumps vaccine produces very few adverse reactions. Fever or tenderness at the site of injection has been reported. Parotitis has occurred occasionally. Allergic reactions are uncommon and usually are mild and brief. Manifestations of central nervous system involvement are very rare. There is no evidence that mumps vaccine produces diabetes.

The vaccine should not be used during pregnancy, in patients with hypogammaglobulinemia or dysgammaglobulinemia, in those receiving immunosuppressive therapy (eg, corticosteroids, irradiation, antineoplastic agents), in those with severe febrile illness, or in those with blood dyscrasias, leukemia, lymphomas, or malignant neoplasms affecting the bone marrow or lymphoid system. It should not be given for three months after administration of immune serum globulin. There is no evidence to preclude its use in persons with allergies to eggs, chickens, or feathers that are not anaphylactic in nature.

DOSAGE.
Subcutaneous: *Adults and children 12 months or older,* the total volume (0.5 ml) of reconstituted vaccine is administered. The reconstituted vaccine retains potency for eight hours at 2 to 8 C in the dark; it should be discarded if not used within that period. Only the diluent supplied should be used for reconstitution.

Available Trademark.
Mumpsvax (Merck Sharp & Dohme).

Rubella

The primary objective of immunization against rubella is to prevent infection in pregnant women because transplacental transfer of the virus to the fetus may cause serious congenital abnormalities. Rubella in children generally is benign and self-limiting, but this age group may be a major source of infection for pregnant women.

Following the introduction of live attenuated rubella virus vaccines, the number of cases of rubella and congenital rubella syndrome decreased; also, the anticipated periodic epidemics of rubella have not occurred.

Immunization recommendations include: (1) All children between the ages of 12 months to puberty should receive rubella vaccine, preferably in combination with measles and mumps vaccines, as part of their routine immunization program. (2) School records should be audited annually to permit identification and vaccination of children before puberty. (3) All females of childbearing age should receive rubella vaccine unless they were previously vaccinated or serologic testing reveals that they are immune. Females in this age group should be asked if they are pregnant and excluded from immunization with rubella if they are. The theoretical risks should be explained to these individuals and they should understand that pregnancy must be avoided for three months after immunization. (4) Susceptible mothers should be vaccinated in the immediate postpartum period before discharge from the hospital. (5) All other children, adolescents, and adults (especially women) who are considered to be susceptible should be vaccinated if there are no contraindications.

RUBELLA VIRUS VACCINE LIVE

Live rubella virus vaccine is a suspension of attenuated rubella virus derived from the Wistar Institute RA 27/3 strain grown in human diploid cell (WI-38) culture. The vaccine produces a mild infection in susceptible persons resulting in the production of protective antibodies. Excretion of small amounts of live virus from the nose or throat occurs in most vaccinees 7 to 28 days after vaccination. Nevertheless, contact spread is not known to occur. Thus, there is no hazard for susceptible pregnant females exposed to vaccinated children.

Antibody response induced by this vaccine resembles natural rubella more closely than that produced by the earlier vaccines. Rubella antibody levels are detectable in over 95% of patients within four to six weeks following vaccination and persist for as long as 16 years, suggesting active immunity of long duration. Antibody levels may decline over time. Reinfection following exposure to wild rubella virus, as evidenced by increased antibody levels without viremia or disease, occurs in a small number of vaccinees. However, over 90% of vaccinees are protected against both clinical rubella and viremia for at least 15 years and probably for life.

ADVERSE REACTIONS AND PRECAUTIONS. Adverse reactions include fever; rash, induration, erythema, and tenderness at the site of injection; and regional adenopathy. Transient arthritis, arthralgia, and polyneuritis may occur within two months after immunization. Up to 3% of children have been reported to experience arthralgia, but arthritis was rare in these patients. In contrast, 12% to 20% of women vaccinees experience arthralgias. Encephalitis also has been reported very rarely but a causal association has not been demonstrated. The incidence of untoward reactions seems to increase with age and is probably higher in females.

Rubella virus vaccine is contraindicated in pregnant women. Vaccination should be avoided in patients with blood dyscrasias, leukemia, lymphomas, generalized malignancy, active untreated tuberculosis, or immunodeficiencies and in those receiving immunosuppressive therapy (corticosteroids, antineoplastic drugs, or irradiation). Vaccination should be postponed during a febrile illness. If, however, a pregnant woman is inadvertently given the vaccine, experience to date indicates that the risk of vaccine-associated malformations is negligible.

Rubella vaccine should not be given routinely within three months after receiving plasma, blood transfusion, or immune globulin therapy.

DOSAGE.

Subcutaneous: *Adults and children 12 months or older,* the total volume of reconstituted vaccine is injected, preferably into the outer aspect of the upper arm. It should not be given intravenously or intranasally.

The vaccine should be refrigerated and protected from light. It must remain refrigerated after reconstitution and should be discarded if not used within eight hours. Only the diluent supplied should be used to reconstitute the vaccine.

Available Trademark.
Meruvax II (Merck Sharp & Dohme).

MEASLES, MUMPS, AND RUBELLA VIRUS VACCINE LIVE (MMR)

Live measles, mumps, and rubella virus vaccine is a suspension of the same attenuated viruses present in the monovalent vaccines. It is indicated for simultaneous routine immunization of children 15 months of age or older and may be used in adolescents and adults who have not been vaccinated against or experienced any or all of the natural infections. Clinical studies have shown that the vaccine produces antibody levels comparable to those obtained with the use of each monovalent vaccine given at properly spaced intervals. Persistence of immunity is similar to that observed with the live, attenuated monovalent vaccines.

Adverse reactions and precautions generally are the same as those associated with the monovalent vaccines (see the evaluations). The vaccine is usually well tolerated, but malaise, mild fever, and regional lymphadenopathy occur occasionally.

DOSAGE.

Subcutaneous: *Children 12 months of age or older,* the total volume of reconstituted vaccine (0.5 ml) is injected into the outer aspect of the upper arm.

Available Trademark.
M-M-R II (Merck Sharp & Dohme).

MEASLES AND RUBELLA VIRUS VACCINE LIVE

Live measles and rubella virus vaccine is a suspension of the same attenuated viruses present in equivalent monovalent vaccines. Available evidence indicates that it produces a serologic response equivalent to that induced by the individual measles and rubella vaccines. It is used for simultaneous immunization against measles and rubella in children from 15 months of age to puberty and in adults.

Adverse reactions and precautions are the same as those associated with the monovalent vaccines (see the evaluations).

DOSAGE.
Subcutaneous: *Adults and children 12 months of age or older,* the total volume of the reconstituted vaccine is injected into the outer aspect of the upper arm.

> Available Trademark.
> **M-R-VAX II** (Merck Sharp & Dohme).

RUBELLA AND MUMPS VIRUS VACCINE LIVE

Live rubella and mumps virus vaccine is a suspension of the same attenuated viruses present in equivalent monovalent vaccines. The vaccine is used for the simultaneous routine immunization of children 12 months of age to puberty who have been vaccinated against measles or experienced the natural disease but who have no history of immunizing exposure to rubella and mumps viruses. The vaccine produces antibody levels comparable to those stimulated by the monovalent vaccines given separately; the degree of protection against natural disease is also comparable.

Contraindications, precautions, and adverse reactions are the same as those associated with the monovalent vaccines (see the evaluations).

DOSAGE.
Subcutaneous: *Children 12 months of age to puberty,* the total volume of reconstituted vaccine (0.5 ml) is injected into the outer aspect of the upper arm. The reconstituted vaccine should be stored at 2 to 8 C and discarded if not used within eight hours.

> Available Trademark.
> **Biavax II** (Merck Sharp & Dohme).

Poliomyelitis

The virtual elimination of poliomyelitis from the United States by the use of vaccines is one of the most important medical achievements in recent years. Although the risk of poliomyelitis in the United States is very small, epidemics could occur if the immunity of the population is not maintained by immunizing all children beginning in the first year of life. Subclinical infection with wild strains is no longer a significant natural means of establishing or maintaining immunity and thus universal vaccination of infants and children is increasingly important.

Oral poliovirus vaccine (OPV) and inactivated poliovirus vaccine (IPV) are available in the United States. The oral vaccine is the agent of choice for routine immunization of children. For unimmunized adults at risk, primary immunization with IPV is recommended. If protection is needed in less than four weeks, a single dose of OPV is recommended, followed by IPV if the person remains at increased risk.

POLIOVIRUS VACCINE INACTIVATED (IPV)

This vaccine contains the three serotypes of poliovirus propagated in monkey kidney cell culture and rendered noninfectious by formalin treatment. Properly prepared killed vaccines do not spread virus to contacts or cause poliomyelitis. IPV is safe for use in immunodeficient patients and their household contacts, but the immune response may be inadequate in the immunodeficient. Nevertheless, the vaccine may be administered to these patients in an attempt to provide some degree of protection.

IPV was used extensively in the United States until the early sixties and considerably decreased the incidence of poliomyelitis. Epidemiologic studies show that IPV diminished the spread of wild poliovirus in vaccinated communities. However, some vaccinated individuals have developed abortive infections with both wild and attenuated vaccine viruses and have excreted these strains in their feces. IPV is used in several small European countries and, in Sweden where it has been used exclusively, it has essentially eradicated poliomyelitis.

Following primary immunization, seroconversions occur in over 95% of vaccinees. After an initial decline during the year following vaccination, circulating antibodies remain stable and may persist for as long as 12 years.

The vaccine may be given to susceptible adults at risk of exposure by reason of travel. Physicians may administer a primary series of vaccinations to such persons or, when constrained by time, at least two doses one month apart.

Primary immunization consists of four doses for persons of all ages. As with OPV, the primary schedule for children is usually integrated with DTP vaccination (see Table 2). No serious adverse effects have been reported.

DOSAGE.
PRIMARY IMMUNIZATION:
Subcutaneous: *Infants,* immunization should be started at the initial visit (6 to 12 weeks of age). Three doses of 1 ml each are administered into the subcutaneous tissue near the insertion of the deltoid muscle at intervals of four to eight weeks; a fourth 1-ml dose is given 6 to 12 months after the third dose. *Older children and adults at increased risk of exposure who are unvaccinated* are given the same regimen. *Adults with incomplete primary immunization* may complete the series regardless of the interval since the last dose.
REINFORCING (BOOSTER) IMMUNIZATION:
Children who have received four primary immunization doses should be given a booster dose of 1 ml prior to entering school. Additional doses may be given every five years thereafter. *Adults over 18 years* at increased risk of exposure who have completed primary immunization may be given a 1-ml booster dose.

> *Manufacturer:* Squibb/Connaught.

POLIOVIRUS VACCINE LIVE ORAL TRIVALENT (OPV)

This vaccine contains attenuated poliovirus types I, II, and III and stimulates production of mucosal antibodies in the digestive tract as well as circulating antibodies. Oral poliovirus vaccine is the agent of choice for prevention of paralytic poliomyelitis. It is easily administered and long-lasting immunity is achieved quickly.

In susceptible individuals, the type-specific, serum-neutralizing antibody titer begins to increase about one week after ingestion and reaches a peak about three weeks later. A primary series produces an immune response to each of the three virus types in over 95% of recipients.

Other viruses in the intestinal tract (eg, enteroviruses) may interfere with the replication of vaccine virus, thus interfering with the development of immunity. In areas where enterovirus infections are common (tropical and subtropical regions), this may be a problem. In addition, an inhibitory substance in the alimentary tract of some infants living in tropical areas may prevent the multiplication of vaccine virus in the intestine and thus reduce the number of successful immunizations. Vaccine success rates in tropical areas have been as low as 50% compared to the 95% response rate characteristic of U.S. programs.

OPV is recommended routinely for all infants and children who do not have immune deficiency diseases or altered immune states and do not live with persons having these disorders.

Initial vaccination is not recommended prior to 6 weeks of age because of persistence of maternal antibodies. However, in certain tropical areas where poliomyelitis is endemic, it may be advisable to start immunization as early as 3 days of age.

Routine immunization of adults living in the continental United States is unnecessary because most are immune, exposure to wild virus is unlikely, and there may be a slightly greater risk of vaccine-associated paralysis in adults than in children. However, any nonimmunized adult who might be exposed to poliovirus by traveling to epidemic or endemic areas should receive OPV or IPV (see Immunization Schedules). If there is not sufficient time for at least two doses of IPV, one dose of the oral vaccine is preferred.

ADVERSE REACTIONS AND PRECAUTIONS. OPV rarely has been associated with paralytic disease. Most authorities believe that a causal relationship exists between the development of paralytic poliomyelitis in certain recipients and their close contacts (contact within two months after administration) and the reversion to greater neurovirulence of vaccine progeny. However, the risk of vaccine-associated paralysis is extremely small for recipients and their close contacts (1 in approximately 3.2 million doses), especially when weighed against the benefits.

Tonsillectomy, adenoidectomy, and pregnancy are not contraindications to the use of vaccine when immunization is required, as during an epidemic. The vaccine should not be administered if the patient has diarrhea. Immunization is contraindicated when the immune state of the recipient may be altered, as in those with dysgammaglobulinemia, lymphoma, leukemia, and generalized malignancies, as well as in patients receiving therapeutic regimens that may impair cellular immunity (eg, corticosteroids, antineoplastic agents, immunosuppressive agents, irradiation). OPV should not be given to a member of a household in which there is a history of immunodeficiency until the immune status of the recipient and other children in the family is determined to be normal. It also is prudent to recommend that vaccine recipients avoid close household-type contact with all immunosuppressed persons for at least six to eight weeks.

DOSAGE. This vaccine is never administered by injection.

Oral: Each dose of trivalent poliovirus vaccine contains approximately 800,000 tissue culture infective doses (TCID$_{50}$) of Type I virus, 100,000 of Type II, and 500,000 of Type III. For primary immunization, three doses are administered.

Infants, the primary series of three doses is usually administered at 2, 4, and approximately 18 months of age (American Academy of Pediatrics, 1982). Some authorities prefer to administer the third dose at age 6 months to those who live in or travel to endemic areas.

Children, adolescents, and adults, two doses administered not less than six and preferably eight weeks apart; the third dose is given 12 months later. Children who have completed primary immunization should be given a single additional dose of vaccine prior to entering elementary school. *Children and adults who have completed primary immunization and are at increased risk* by virtue of contact, travel, or occupation may be given a single additional dose.

Available Trademark.
Orimune (Lederle).

Haemophilus influenzae Type b Infections

Haemophilus influenzae type b (Hib) is a principal cause of serious systemic bacterial disease in children and is the most common cause of bacterial meningitis in the United States. Approximately 12,000 cases of Hib meningitis occur yearly, primarily in children under 5 years, and virtually all cases are caused by type b strains. The mortality rate ranges from 5% to 10% and neurologic sequelae develop in 25% to 35% of survivors. Other diseases caused by Hib include epiglottitis, pneumonia, septic arthritis, cellulitis, osteomyelitis, pericarditis, and sepsis. Although *H. influenzae* is a major cause of otitis media, only 5% to 10% of cases are produced by type b strains; the majority of cases are caused by nonencapsulated (nontypeable) strains.

In the United States, the cumulative risk of systemic Hib disease during the first five years of life is estimated to be 1 in 200. Of those children who develop Hib disease, rates are highest between age 6 and 12 months; 35% to 40% of systemic Hib disease occurs in children over 18 months and approximately 25% occurs in children over 24 months. Groups at increased risk are Native Americans, blacks, persons in lower socioeconomic classes, and patients with asplenia, sickle cell disease, Hodgkin's disease, or antibody immunodeficiency syndromes. In addition, children who attend day care centers may have a substantially increased risk of Hib disease (Redmond and Pichichero, 1984).

HAEMOPHILUS b POLYSACCHARIDE VACCINE

Haemophilus b polysaccharide vaccine is derived from the purified polysaccharide capsule of *Haemophilus influenzae* type b (Hib); it is a linear copolymer of ribose-ribitol-phosphate. The vaccine contains 25 mcg of purified polysaccharide in each 0.5-ml dose.

In vitro, antibodies to the Hib polysaccharide antigen mediate complement-dependent bacteriolysis and opsonization; in vivo, they protect animals from experimental infection. As with other polysaccharide vaccines (T-independent antigens), response depends on age: response is poor in infants but improves by age 18 months. Ninety percent of children 24 months or older exhibit a significant antibody response. Studies in Finland indicated that the vaccine reduced the rate of bacteremic Hib disease by 90% in children age 18 months to 5 years; the vaccine was not effective in younger children (Peltola et al, 1984). (See also the evaluation on Haemophilus influenzae Type B Polysaccharide-Diphtheria Toxoid Conjugate Vaccine in the section on Investigational Agents.)

Hib polysaccharide vaccine is recommended for all children 24 months to 6 years of age to protect against diseases caused by *H. influenzae* type b. Immunization may be considered at 18 months, especially for those in high-risk groups (see introduction above). It is anticipated that protection will last at least 1.5 to 3.5 years and routine revaccination is not recommended, although high-risk patients may require a second dose within 18 months of the first to ensure adequate protection. The vaccine is not recommended for children under 18 months.

Data are inadequate to make recommendations for older children and adults at increased risk of Hib disease.

ADVERSE REACTIONS. Current preparations appear to cause few reactions. Mild local and febrile reactions are uncommon; less than 1% of recipients experience fever (101.3 F).

DOSAGE.

Subcutaneous: *Children 24 months to 6 years*, 0.5 ml of reconstituted vaccine.

Available Trademarks.
b-CAPSA I (Mead Johnson), **Hib-Imune** (Lederle), **HibVax** (Connaught).

Viral Hepatitis

Three clinically similar diseases are included under this term, but each is etiologically and epidemiologically distinct: (1) hepatitis A ("infectious" hepatitis), (2) hepatitis B ("serum" hepatitis), and (3) non-A, non-B hepatitis. Delta hepatitis virus (sometimes called hepatitis D virus) is a defective RNA-containing virus that produces infection only in the presence of active hepatitis B virus (HBV) infection. Since delta virus depends on HBV replication for growth, prevention of HBV infection in susceptible persons also prevents delta infection. Vaccine is available only for hepatitis B.

Hepatitis A: Immune globulin is effective for prophylaxis against hepatitis A, especially when given early, and is recommended for travelers to high-risk areas for hepatitis A. It is not indicated in patients with clinical manifestations of the disease or in those exposed more than two weeks previously. Both intravenous and intramuscular preparations are currently available.

Hepatitis B: HBV infection is fairly uncommon in the general population of the United States but is highly prevalent in certain risk groups. The lifetime risk varies from about 5% for the general population to nearly 100% for the highest risk groups (see Table 6). About 200,000 persons are infected with HBV each year in the United States and 25% subsequently develop jaundice. Between 6% and 10% of infected young adults become carriers and 25% of these develop chronic active hepatitis. (A carrier has been defined as a person who is HBsAg-positive on at least two occasions six months apart.) There are 500,000 to 1,000,000 carriers in the United States and the number is thought to be more than 200 million worldwide. The carrier state may lead to chronic liver disease, including massive hepatic necrosis, chronic active hepatitis, cirrhosis, and hepatocellular carcinoma. The disease is highly endemic in China, Southeast Asia, sub-Saharan Africa, most Pacific islands, and the Amazon basin. Thus, the development of the inactivated HBV vaccine meets an urgent need.

After infection with hepatitis B virus (HBV), a significant number of patients develop chronic persistent, chronic active, or chronic active hepatitis with cirrhosis. The five-year survival rates have been estimated as 97% for patients with chronic persistent hepatitis, 86% for those with chronic active hepatitis, and 55% for individuals with chronic active hepatitis with cirrhosis (Weissberg et al, 1984). There is no treatment for chronic active hepatitis. However, hepatitis B can be prevented through vaccination and administration of hepatitis B immune globulin (HBIG).

Postexposure prophylaxis to prevent infection with HBV should be considered in the following situations: perinatal exposure of a neonate born to a mother known to be positive for hepatitis B surface antigen (HBsAg), accidental exposure (percutaneous or permucosal) to HBsAg-positive blood, and sexual exposure to an HBsAg-positive person.

Studies have demonstrated that a combination of hepatitis B vaccine and HBIG prevents chronic HBV infection in approximately 90% of infants born to HBsAg-positive mothers. Because of these findings, it has been recommended that the vaccine/immune globulin combination also be used for prophylaxis after acute exposure to HBsAg-positive blood. This combination should provide long-lasting immunity and may prevent HBV disease after exposure. The value of HBV vaccine for postexposure prophylaxis following a single sexual contact with an HBsAg-positive person is unknown and, therefore, it is not routinely used; HBIG alone is recommended for susceptible persons with a single sexual contact (Immunization Practices Advisory Committee, 1985 B).

The principal objective of postexposure prophylaxis of neonates is to prevent the establishment of an HBV carrier state. Approximately 80% to 90% of infants born to HBsAg- and HBeAg-positive mothers become infected with HBV and about 90% of infected infants become chronic HBV carriers. Approximately 25% of these carriers die of cirrhosis or primary hepatocellular carcinoma. If the mother is HBsAg-positive but HBeAg-negative or if anti-HBe is present, transmission of HBV to the infant occurs in less than 25% and 12% of cases, respectively. In such cases, transmission rarely leads to chronic infection, but severe acute disease, including fatal fulminating hepatitis in the neonate, has been observed. Therefore, prophylaxis of all infants born to HBsAg-positive mothers, regardless of HBeAg status, is recommended.

TABLE 6.
EXPECTED HEPATITIS B VIRUS (HBV) PREVALENCE IN VARIOUS POPULATION GROUPS

	Prevalence of Serologic Markers of HBV Infection	
	HBsAg* ————— % —————	All Markers
HIGH-RISK GROUPS		
Immigrants/refugees from areas of high HBV endemicity	13	70–85
Clients in institutions for the mentally retarded	10–20	35–80
Users of illicit parenteral drugs	7	60–80
Homosexually active males	6	35–80
Household contacts of HBV carriers	3–6	30–60
Patients of hemodialysis units	3–10	20–80
INTERMEDIATE-RISK GROUPS		
Prisoners (male)	1–8	10–80
Staff of institutions for the mentally retarded	1	10–25
Health-care workers (frequent blood contact)	1–2	15–30
LOW-RISK GROUPS		
Health-care workers (no or infrequent blood contact)	0.3	3–10
Healthy adults (first-time volunteer blood donors)	0.3	3–5

*HBsAg = hepatitis B surface antigen.
Adapted from Immunization Practices Advisory Committee, 1985 B.

It is very important that prenatal HBsAg screening be performed on all pregnant women in high-risk groups (see Table 7). They should be tested routinely for HBsAg during prenatal visits. If this is not done, screening should be performed at the time of delivery or immediately thereafter, for the efficacy of HBIG decreases markedly if treatment is delayed longer than 48 hours after delivery. If a positive test is not determined until after delivery and a venous sample from the infant is HBsAg-negative, prophylactic therapy should still be given.

TABLE 7.
WOMEN FOR WHOM PRENATAL HBsAg SCREENING IS RECOMMENDED

1. Women of Asian, Pacific Island, or Alaskan Eskimo descent, whether immigrant or U.S. born
2. Women born in Haiti or sub-Saharan Africa.
3. Women with histories of:
   a. Acute or chronic liver disease.
   b. Work or treatment in a hemodialysis unit.
   c. Work or residence in an institution for the mentally retarded.
   d. Rejection as a blood donor.
   e. Blood transfusion on repeated occasions.
   f. Frequent occupational exposure to blood in medico-dental settings.
   g. Household contact with an HBV carrier or hemodialysis patient.
   h. Multiple episodes of venereal disease.
   i. Percutaneous use of illicit drugs.

From Immunization Practices Advisory Committee, 1985 B.

HBIG preferably should be given within 12 hours and the first dose of HBV vaccine administered within seven days of birth (see Table 8). An HBsAg test at six months is recommended; a positive test indicates therapeutic failure and the third dose of vaccine need not be given. In order to monitor the success of treatment, the infant's blood should be tested at 12 to 15 months for HBsAg and anti-HBs. Immunization with HBV vaccine should not postpone other pediatric vaccinations. Similarly, administration of HBIG at birth should not interfere with the DTP or poliovirus vaccine usually administered at 2 months of age.

For susceptible persons who have had sexual contact with an HBsAg-positive partner and those who continue to have such contact with a person who has acute disease before becoming HBsAg-negative, a single dose of HBIG is recommended. A second dose should be given for heterosexual exposures if the index patient remains HBsAg-positive three months after detection. Regular sexual partners of known HBV carriers or index patients who remain HBsAg-positive for six months should receive HBV vaccine. The vaccine is recommended for all susceptible homosexual men.

Several factors that must be considered before instituting prophylaxis following permucosal exposure to blood known or suspected of being HBsAg-positive are (1) the vaccination status of the exposed person, (2) the source of the blood, and (3) the HBsAg status of the source. Table 9 summarizes the recommendations for HBV prophylaxis after percutaneous, ocular, or mucous membrane exposure. HBV vaccination is recommended for any exposure in previously unvaccinated individuals and should be initiated within seven days of exposure. For passive immunization, HBIG should be given as soon as possible, preferably within 24 hours, as its usefulness

TABLE 8.
HEPATITIS B VIRUS POSTEXPOSURE RECOMMENDATIONS

	HBIG		Vaccine	
Exposure	Dose	Recommended Timing	Dose	Recommended Timing
Perinatal	0.5 ml IM	Within 12 hours of birth	0.5 ml (10 mcg) IM	Within 12 hours of birth*; repeat at 1 and 6 months
Sexual	0.06 ml/kg IM	Single dose within 14 days of sexual contact	+	—

*The first dose can be given the same time as the HBIG dose but at a different site.
+Vaccine is recommended for homosexual men and for regular sexual contacts of HBV carriers and is optional in initial treatment of heterosexual contacts of persons with acute HBV.
From Immunization Practices Advisory Committee, 1985 B.

seven days or more after exposure is not known. If HBIG is not available, an equivalent dose of immune globulin may be substituted. No treatment is necessary for vaccinated individuals with adequate levels of anti-HBs. For individuals with known exposure to HBsAg-positive materials whose antibody levels are inadequate, a dose of HBIG should be administered and a vaccine booster given at a different site. If the status of the source is unknown but there is a high risk that it is HBsAg-positive, additional prophylaxis is necessary only if the exposed individual is known to be unresponsive to vaccine. In such cases, the source should be tested for HBsAg and, if positive, the exposed patient should receive a dose of HBIG immediately and a booster dose of HBV vaccine. As the risk of HBV infection is minimal for vaccinated persons exposed to a low-risk or unknown source of HBsAg, no specific treatment is indicated.

Non-A, Non-B Hepatitis: No specific vaccine or antiserum is currently available for non-A, non-B hepatitis.

HEPATITIS B VACCINE INACTIVATED

This vaccine is a noninfectious formalin-inactivated preparation derived from the surface antigen (HBsAg) of hepatitis B virus. HBsAg is harvested and purified from HBsAg-positive blood donated by carriers of hepatitis B virus. Each ml of HBV vaccine contains 20 mcg of HBsAg protein and is formulated in an alum adjuvant. It is initially purified by ultracentrifugation. This is then followed by a three-step inactivation process involving 8 M urea, pepsin at pH 2.0, and 1:4,000 formalin. The procedure inactivates HBV and representative viruses from all known groups, including retroviruses. There is no evidence that acquired immunodeficiency syndrome (AIDS) can be transmitted by this product.

Hepatitis B vaccine is indicated for immunization against infection caused by all known B virus subtypes. Vaccination is recommended for persons over 3 months of age at increased risk of infection, such as populations with a high incidence of

TABLE 9.
RECOMMENDATIONS FOR HEPATITIS B PROPHYLAXIS FOLLOWING PERCUTANEOUS EXPOSURE

	Exposed Person	
Source	Unvaccinated	Vaccinated
HBsAG-positive	1. HBIG × 1 immediately* 2. Initiate HB vaccine+ series.	1. Test exposed person for anti-HBs. 2. If inadequate antibody, HBIG (× 1) immediately plus HB vaccine booster dose.
Known source High-risk HBsAg-positive	1. Initiate HB vaccine series 1. 2. Test source for HBsAg. If positive, HBIG × 1.	1. Test source for HBsAg only if exposed is vaccine nonresponder; if source is HBsAg-positive, give HBIG × 1 immediately plus HB vaccine booster dose.
Low-risk HBsAg-positive	Initiate HB vaccine series.	Nothing required.
Unknown source	Initiate HB vaccine series.	Nothing required.

*HBIG dose 0.06 ml/kg IM.
+HB vaccine dose 20 mcg IM for adults; 10 mg IM for infants or children under 10 years of age. First dose within 1 week; second and third doses, 1 and 6 months later.
From Immunization Practices Advisory Committee, 1985 B.

disease (eg, Alaskan Eskimos, Indochinese and Haitian refugees), health care personnel, hematology and hemodialysis patients and staff, patients and staff of institutions for the mentally retarded, morticians and embalmers, blood bank and fractionation workers, recipients of blood clotting factor concentrates, homosexual males, household and sexual contacts of HBV carriers, prostitutes, heterosexually active persons with multiple sexual partners, illicit drug users, prisoners, and international travelers who will be in highly endemic areas for more than six months (see Table 6).

The three-dose regimen stimulates production of neutralizing antibodies in 85% to 96% of vaccinees, and immunity probably lasts five years; a single booster injection then may be necessary to maintain immunity. However, in hemodialysis patients, immunogenicity and efficacy are much lower than in normal adults and the duration of protection in these patients is unknown. The immunologic response of infants and children to a course of three 10-mcg doses has been excellent. A suboptimal response may follow injection into the buttock, for injections into this site may inadvertently be deposited in fat where the vaccine is less well mobilized.

Adverse effects are mainly local, mild, and transitory. Slight tenderness at the injection site is most common (10% of adults and 4% of children). Pregnancy is not a contraindication to use of the vaccine.

DOSAGE.
Intramuscular: *Children birth to 10 years*, a series of three 0.5-ml (10 mcg) injections, the second given one month after the first, and the third six months later. *Adults and children over 10 years*, a series of three 1-ml (20 mcg) injections, the second given one month after the first, and the third six months later. The deltoid muscle is the preferred site in adults. *Dialysis and immunocompromised patients*, a series of three 2-ml (20 mcg/ml) doses (for each 2-ml dose, two 1-ml injections are given at different sites), the second given one month after the first, and the third six months later.

Available Trademark.
Heptavax-B (Merck Sharp & Dohme).

HEPATITIS B IMMUNE GLOBULIN (HBIG)

This sterile solution of immune globulin is prepared from the pooled plasma of donors with high titers of antibody to hepatitis B surface antigen (anti-HBsAg).

HBIG is indicated for postexposure prophylaxis following parenteral exposure (eg, accidental "needle-stick," direct mucous membrane contact [accidental splash]) or oral ingestion (pipetting accident) of HBsAg-positive materials, such as blood, plasma, or serum. It is also indicated for infants born to HBsAg-positive mothers (especially those who also are HBeAg-positive), since these infants are at risk of acquiring hepatitis B infection. Susceptible persons who are sexual contacts of HBsAg-positive individuals also are candidates for the antiserum. This product is of no value in the treatment of fulminant acute or chronic active hepatitis B. (See also introduction to this section.)

Adverse reactions include local pain and tenderness at the injection site, urticaria, and angioedema.

DOSAGE.
Intramuscular: For *adults and children*, 0.06 ml/kg; the usual adult dose is 3 to 5 ml administered as soon as possible (within seven days) after exposure and repeated in 28 to 30 days.

For *newborn infants,* the usual dose is 0.5 ml given as soon after birth as possible and no later than 24 hours. Doses of 0.5 ml should be repeated at three and six months.

Intravenous administration should be avoided.

Available Trademarks.
H-BIG (Abbott), ***Hep-B-Gammagee*** (Merck Sharp & Dohme), ***HyperHep*** (Cutter).

Influenza

INFLUENZA VIRUS VACCINE

This polyvalent vaccine is prepared from types A and B influenza viruses grown in embryonated chicken eggs. It is available as an inactivated "whole virus" or "split virus" product. In addition to its use in adults, split virus vaccine only is recommended for children less than 13 years because it causes fewer side effects than the whole virus vaccine. Formulations are reviewed regularly and changed when necessary to include strains that are anticipated to be prevalent in the community.

Annual vaccination is the single most important measure in controlling infection and is recommended for the following groups in order of priority (Immunization Practices Advisory Committee, 1984 C):

(1) Adults and children with chronic cardiovascular or pulmonary disorders that required medical attention during the preceding year. Also, residents of nursing homes and other chronic care facilities.

(2) Medical personnel, including physicians, who have extensive contact with high-risk patients.

(3) Individuals over 65 years old. Also, adults and children with chronic metabolic diseases (including diabetes mellitus), renal disease, anemia, impaired immunologic function, or asthma that required hospitalization or other medical attention during the preceding year.

In addition, the vaccine may be used by any person wishing to decrease the probability of acquiring influenza. For influenza control programs in institutions, it is recommended that no less than 80% of residents be vaccinated.

The vaccine induces production of antibodies to the H (hemagglutinin) and N (neuraminidase) antigens of each of the virus strains contained in the vaccine. Antibodies to the H antigen are associated with virus neutralization, while N antibodies are associated with amelioration of the severity of the disease. Efficacy varies from 0% to 90%, depending upon the antigenic match between the vaccine strains and the prevalent infecting virus strain.

The potency of these vaccines is high and protective levels of antibody can be expected in young adults within four weeks. The elderly, the very young, and patients with certain chronic diseases may develop lower antibody titers. In these patients, the vaccine may be less effective in preventing infection and involvement of the upper respiratory tract than in reducing the incidence and severity of lower respiratory tract involvement or other complications. In one study conducted on residents of nursing homes, influenza immunization was reported to attenuate infection; unvaccinated persons were more likely to develop pneumonia, be hospitalized, and/or die of influenza-like illness (Patriarca et al, 1985).

ADVERSE REACTIONS AND PRECAUTIONS. Currently available purified vaccines are well tolerated. Split virus vaccines appear to cause fewer adverse effects than whole virus vaccines. Fever, malaise, myalgia, and other systemic symptoms are less common in adults than in children. Reactions may appear within 6 to 12 hours and disappear within one to two days. Allergic reactions are rare because current vaccines contain very small quantities of egg protein.

The vaccine may be given to pregnant women, although it is prudent to wait until the second or third trimester.

DOSAGE. See the manufacturer's literature. Recommendations for vaccine composition and administration are widely publicized each year.

Available Trademarks.
Fluogen (Parke-Davis), *Fluzone* (Squibb/Connaught), *Influenza Virus Vaccine Trivalent, Types A and B* (Wyeth).

Pneumococcal Pneumonia

PNEUMOCOCCAL POLYSACCHARIDE VACCINE

The incidence of serious pneumococcal disease remains high. Pneumococcal pneumonia occurs in all age groups; the incidence gradually increases in adults over 40 years and increases twofold in those over 60 years. Despite antibiotic therapy, death occurs in approximately 20% of patients with bacteremic pneumococcal pneumonia and 30% of patients with meningitis. Mortality is highest in patients with certain underlying medical conditions and older persons; in high-risk patients, mortality may be as high as 40% for those with bacteremic disease and 55% for those with meningitis. Prophylaxis with pneumococcal vaccines may reduce mortality and morbidity.

The current formulation of polyvalent vaccine contains purified capsular polysaccharides from 23 of the most common pneumococcal types frequently associated with disease in adults and children (see manufacturers' package insert). These 23 types cause about 87% of bacteremic pneumococcal disease in the United States. Each 0.5-ml dose of vaccine contains 25 mcg of the purified capsular material from each type dissolved in isotonic saline solution with 0.25% phenol [Pneumovax] or 0.01% thimerosal [Pnu-Imune] as preservative.

Immunization with pneumococcal polysaccharide vaccines should be considered for those in the following special groups: (1) adults over 65; (2) persons over 2 years with certain chronic diseases associated with increased risk of pneumococcal disease, such as chronic cardiac, pulmonary, hepatic, and renal disease; Hodgkin's disease; multiple myeloma; cirrhosis; alcoholism; cerebrospinal fluid leaks; and metabolic diseases such as diabetes mellitus; (3) persons over 2 years with chronic conditions that may be complicated by pneumococcal disease, such as sickle cell anemia or other causes of

functional or anatomic splenic dysfunction (eg, splenectomy); or (4) those who are immunocompromised.

Recurrent pneumococcal otitis media or sinusitis in children is not an indication for vaccination. The vaccine should be given at least two weeks before elective splenectomy. The interval between vaccine administration and the initiation of immunosuppressive therapy should be as long as possible. Influenza vaccine may be given simultaneously with pneumococcal vaccine if different injection sites and different syringes are used.

The duration of protection provided by pneumococcal vaccine is unknown. Antibody levels are detectable five years after immunization. Revaccination is not recommended in adults previously vaccinated with any polyvalent pneumococcal vaccine, since local reactions (Arthus type) may be more frequent and severe. Children less than 2 years of age have an unsatisfactory antibody response.

Only a few studies have utilized pneumococcal vaccine in children. One study employed octavalent vaccine in patients 2 to 25 years old with sickle cell disease or asplenia; the occurrence of bacteremic pneumococcal disease was reduced significantly (Ammann et al, 1977).

In a study on a tetradecavalent pneumococcal vaccine, the efficacy ranged between 60% and 80% in persons over 60 years with no underlying illness (Broome et al, 1980) but was lower in patients with cirrhosis or renal failure (Immunization Practices Advisory Committee, 1984 D). In a case-control study utilizing 90 patients with systemic evidence of pneumococcal infection and matched controls, vaccine efficacy was 0% for severely immunocompromised patients, 70% for patients 55 years or older, and 77% for patients at moderately increased risk of pneumococcal infections (Shapiro and Clemens, 1984).

Using serotype distribution in unvaccinated and vaccinated groups as a basis of comparison, the overall efficacy of a pneumococcal vaccine containing 14 virus strains was estimated to be 64% and did not appear to differ significantly with age; in persons over 65 years, with or without underlying illness, efficacy was reported to be 61%. These findings led the authors to recommend the use of pneumococcal vaccine in selected populations (Bolan et al, 1986). This view was supported by results of a study that showed that vaccination against pneumococcal pneumonia was cost-effective and that benefits would be enhanced if the vaccine were more widely used (Sisk and Riegelman, 1986). In a position paper, the Health and Public Policy Committee of the American College of Physicians (1986) concluded that physicians were underusing the pneumococcal vaccine in patients who could clearly be expected to benefit from it.

Although the foregoing studies suggest that pneumococcal vaccine confers substantial protection against systemic pneumococcal infections, additional studies are needed to validate these findings with the 23-valent vaccine before definitive statements can be made concerning efficacy in the elderly and others at increased risk of serious pneumococcal disease.

ADVERSE REACTIONS AND PRECAUTIONS. Serious adverse effects to pneumococcal vaccines are rare. The most common reactions are local erythema and tenderness at the injection site, which usually subside within one to two days; local induration is noted less frequently. Fever may occur. Anaphylactic reactions have been reported rarely. The vaccine is contraindicated in those with febrile respiratory illness or active infection, children under 2 years, and during pregnancy.

DOSAGE.

Subcutaneous, Intramuscular: A single 0.5-ml dose. Intravenous inoculation should be avoided.

> Available Trademarks.
> **Pneumovax 23** (Merck Sharp & Dohme), **Pnu-Imune 23** (Lederle).

Rabies

Pre-exposure Immunization: Pre-exposure immunization is considered for persons at high risk of exposure to rabies virus (eg, veterinarians, animal handlers, certain laboratory workers, persons spending one month or more in countries where rabies is a constant threat, spelunkers) and those whose vocation or avocation brings them into contact with potentially rabid domestic or wild animal species. Pre-exposure prophylaxis is given to (1) protect against inapparent exposure to rabies, (2) protect persons when postexposure therapy might be delayed, and (3) simplify postexposure therapy by eliminating the need for immune globulin and decreasing the number of required doses of vaccine. It should be noted that pre-exposure immunization does not eliminate the need for postexposure prophylaxis following exposure; it only reduces the extent of the needed regimen.

For pre-exposure immunization, 1 ml of human diploid cell rabies vaccine (HDCV) is given on days 0, 7, and 21 or 28. Booster doses are administered at six-month to two-year intervals (see Table 10).

Although clinical rabies is rare in the United States, many persons receive prophylactic treatment because of possible exposure. Although dog and cat bites are the principal reasons for treatment, rabies in domestic animals has decreased considerably since the widespread use of veterinary vaccines. However, rabies in wildlife has become more widespread in recent years and wild animals now constitute the most important source of infection for both humans and domestic animals. In the United States, only Hawaii has remained free of rabies.

Appropriate management depends upon the risk of infection and the efficacy and risk of prophylactic treatment. Carnivorous animals (especially skunks, foxes, coyotes, raccoons, and bobcats) and bats are more likely to be infective than other animals. Bites of rabbits, squirrels, chipmunks, rats, and mice rarely, if ever, call for rabies prophylaxis; rabies is rare in rodents and no human rabies has resulted from a rodent bite. Properly immunized domestic animals are not likely to develop rabies. In doubtful or unusual cases, the local health authority should be consulted. Even in areas where rabies is enzootic, if adequate data indicate that infection is not present in the particular species, the local authority may recommend that no specific rabies immunoprophylaxis be given.

Postexposure Immunization: The management of patients exposed to possibly rabid animals should follow the guidelines given in Table 11. It is more likely that an animal is rabid if the attack is unprovoked. (Bites following attempts to handle or feed an apparently healthy animal should generally be regarded as provoked.) Nonbite exposure to rabies virus, such as contact with potentially infectious material from a rabid animal or an infectious aerosol (eg, in bat caves), also is possible. Thus, each case must be evaluated individually. Dogs and cats should be isolated and observed by a veterinarian for ten days after the bite. If no clinical signs of rabies develop during this period, it can be considered that no exposure to rabies occurred. However, if the animal is killed or dies, the head should be sent to the local health authorities for confirmatory diagnosis.

As part of the postexposure prophylactic treatment, all bite wounds, as well as scratches and skin abrasions exposed to licks of animals, should be immediately and thoroughly flushed with copious amounts of soap and water. If available, 20% tincture of green soap should be used; subsequent use of 70% alcohol may increase the efficacy of local treatment. If debridement is necessary, the wound area may be infiltrated with a local anesthetic. If possible, bite wounds should not be sutured immediately. Antibiotics may be given and appropriate tetanus prophylaxis initiated if indicated.

Postexposure prophylaxis should be initiated as soon as possible after exposure. Two types of immunoprophylactic agents are employed: (1) human diploid cell rabies vaccine (HDCV), which is used to induce active immunity but requires seven to ten days for a measurable antibody response, and (2) immune globulins, which are used to provide rapid protection for a short time (half-life, about 21 days). Two immune globulin products that are employed are: Rabies immune globulin (RIG) prepared from the plasma of donors hyperimmunized with rabies vaccine, and equine antirabies serum (ARS) obtained from horses immunized against fixed rabies virus. Both products are effective; however, ARS causes serum sickness in over 40% of adult recipients. Adverse effects are rare with RIG and, therefore, it is the product of choice.

Postexposure antirabies immunization for both bite and nonbite exposures usually includes administration of both immune globulin (preferably RIG) and vaccine. The exception is a person who has been previously immunized with a rabies vaccine and has recently been documented as having an adequate rabies antibody titer. Such persons should receive only the vaccine (two doses three days apart), for administration of antibody in these circumstances could interfere with the expected anamnestic response. The first dose of HDCV should be given as soon as possible after exposure of a previously immunized person. The Immunization Practices Advisory Committee (1984 B) recommends that additional doses be given on days 3, 7, 14, and 28. (WHO recommends a sixth dose at 90 days.) RIG is administered only at the beginning of prophylaxis to provide passive immunity until the patient starts to produce his own antibodies. If RIG administration is delayed for some reason, it may be given up to the eighth day after the first dose of vaccine; it is not indicated after this time as it can be presumed that an antibody response to the vaccine has occurred. If ARS must be used,

TABLE 10.
PRE-EXPOSURE RABIES IMMUNIZATION

Criteria for Pre-exposure Immunization			
Risk Category	Nature of Risk	Typical Populations	Pre-exposure Regimen
Continuous	Virus present continuously, often in high concentrations. Aerosol, mucous membrane, bite, or nonbite exposure possible. Specific exposures may go unrecognized.	Rabies research lab workers[1] Rabies biologics production workers	Primary pre-exposure immunization course[2] Serology every 6 months Booster immunization when antibody titer falls below acceptable level
Frequent	Exposure usually episodic, with source recognized, but exposure may also be unrecognized. Aerosol, mucous membrane, bite, or nonbite exposure.	Rabies diagnostic lab workers[1], spelunkers, veterinarians, and animal control and wildlife workers in rabies epizootic areas	Primary pre-exposure immunization course Booster immunization or serology every 2 years[3]
Infrequent (greater than population-at-large)	Exposure nearly always episodic with source recognized. Mucous membrane, bite, or nonbite exposure.	Veterinarians and animal control and wildlife workers in areas of low rabies endemicity. Certain travelers to foreign rabies epizootic areas. Veterinary students	Primary pre-exposure immunization course Booster immunization or serology
Rare (population-at-large)	Exposure always episodic, mucous membrane, or bite with source recognized	U.S. population-at-large, including individuals in rabies epizootic areas	No pre-exposure immunization

[1]Judgment of relative risk and extra monitoring of immunization status of laboratory workers is the responsibility of the laboratory supervisor.

[2]Pre-exposure immunization consists of three doses of HDCV 1 ml IM (ie, deltoid area) one each on days 0, 7, and 28. Administration of routine booster doses of vaccine depends on exposure risk category as noted above. Pre-exposure immunization of immunosuppressed persons is not recommended.

[3]Pre-exposure booster immunization consists of one dose of HDCV 1 ml/dose IM (deltoid area). Acceptable antibody level is 1:5 titer (complete inhibition in RFFIT at 1:5 dilution). Boost if titer falls below 1:5.

Adapted from Immunization Practices Advisory Committee, 1984 B.

the recommended dose is 40 IU/kg (about 18 IU/1b). If possible, up to one-half the dose of RIG should be used to infiltrate the wound. Neither RIG nor ARS should be given at the same site as the rabies vaccine.

If the immune status of a previously vaccinated person who did not receive the recommended HDCV regimen is not known, the full primary postexposure regimen (RIG plus five doses of HDCV) may be necessary. However, if antibody is present in a serum sample collected prior to vaccine administration, treatment may be discontinued after two doses of HDCV. (See Table 12.)

HUMAN DIPLOID CELL RABIES VACCINE (HDCV)

This inactivated virus vaccine is prepared from fixed rabies virus grown in human diploid cell cultures (WI-38 or MRC-5).

Pre-exposure prophylaxis provides the basis for a rapid anamnestic response to booster doses of the vaccine. HDCV is indicated for persons at high risk of exposure to rabies, including physicians and others who treat rabid patients, veterinarians, certain laboratory workers, animal handlers, spelunkers, and others who may be exposed to rabid animals or spend time in regions where animal rabies occurs. Vaccination is recommended for children living in or visiting countries where exposure to rabies is a constant threat. (Children are generally more at risk than adults.)

The vaccine is used in postexposure treatment to provide active immunity. Previously immunized individuals may experience a rapid anamnestic response. It is strongly recommended that passive immunization with human rabies immune globulin be initiated simultaneously with the rabies vaccine. Persons with recently documented adequate rabies antibody titer may be protected by administration of the vaccine only (see also Table 10).

The antibody response requires seven to ten days to develop, but persists for as long as a year or more. Seroconversion has been observed after only one dose, but multiple doses are required to reach 100%. Booster doses at two-year intervals are necessary to maintain adequate antibody titers. In persons working with live rabies virus or involved in vaccine production, rabies antibody titers should be measured every six months and boosters given as needed to maintain adequate antibody levels.

ADVERSE REACTIONS AND PRECAUTIONS. Reactions are

TABLE 11.
RABIES POSTEXPOSURE PROPHYLAXIS GUIDE

Animal species	Condition of animal at time of attack	Treatment of exposed person[1]
DOMESTIC Dog and cat	Healthy and available for 10 days of observation	None, unless animal develops rabies[2]
	Rabid or suspected rabid	RIG[3] and HDCV
	Unknown (escaped)	Consult public health officials. If treatment is indicated, give RIG[3] and HDCV
WILD Skunk, bat, fox, coyote, raccoon, bobcat, and other carnivores	Regard as rabid unless proven negative by laboratory tests[4]	RIG[3] and HDCV
OTHER Livestock, rodents, and lagomorphs (rabbits and hares)	Consider individually. Local and state public health officials should be consulted on questions about the need for rabies prophylaxis. Bites of squirrels, hamsters, guinea pigs, gerbils, chipmunks, rats, mice, other rodents, rabbits, and hares almost never call for antirabies prophylaxis.	

The above recommendations are only a guide. In applying them, take into account the animal species involved, the circumstances of the bite or other exposure, the vaccination status of the animal, and presence of rabies in the region. Local or state public health officials should be consulted if questions arise about the need for rabies prophylaxis.
[1]*All bites and wounds should immediately be thoroughly cleansed with soap and water. If antirabies treatment is indicated, both rabies immune globulin (RIG) and human diploid cell rabies vaccine (HDCV) should be given as soon as possible, regardless of the interval from exposure. Local reactions to vaccines are common and do not contraindicate continuing treatment. Discontinue vaccine if fluorescent antibody tests of the animal are negative.*
[2]*During the usual holding period of 10 days, begin treatment with RIG and HDCV at first sign of rabies in a dog or cat that has bitten someone. The symptomatic animal should be killed immediately and tested.*
[3]*If RIG is not available, use antirabies serum, equine (ARS). Do not use more than the recommended dosage.*
[4]*The animal should be killed and tested as soon as possible. Holding for observation is not recommended.*
Adapted from Immunization Practices Advisory Committee, 1984 B.

principally mild local (incidence 25%) or systemic effects (incidence 20%). The vaccine is considerably less reactogenic than the earlier vaccines.

An immune complex-like reaction has been reported. The reaction occurs 2 to 21 days postinjection; symptoms include generalized urticaria, arthralgia, arthritis, angioedema, nausea, vomiting, fever, and malaise. It occurs in up to 6% of persons receiving booster doses, but is much less frequent in those given primary immunization. In none of the reported cases has the reaction been life-threatening. Persons who experience these reactions should not receive further doses of HDCV unless they are likely to have been exposed and have inadequate rabies antibody titers.

Corticosteroids, antineoplastic drugs, and immunosuppressive agents may interfere with the development of active immunity and predispose the exposed patient to active rabies. Unless these agents are essential, they should be discontinued during postexposure vaccine therapy. Serum antibody levels should be measured in these patients and rabies immune globulin should be given.

Once treatment with rabies vaccine has been initiated, it should not be interrupted because of local or mild systemic

TABLE 12.
POSTEXPOSURE RABIES IMMUNIZATION*

Persons not previously immunized:	RIG, 20 IU/kg body weight, one-half infiltrated at bite site (if possible), remainder IM; 5 doses of HDCV, 1 ml IM (ie, deltoid area), one each on days 0, 3, 7, 14 and 28
Persons previously immunized+:	Two doses of HDCV, 1 ml IM (ie deltoid area), one each on days 0 and 3. RIG should not be administered.

All postexposure treatment should begin with immediate thorough cleansing of all wounds with soap and water.
+*Pre-exposure immunization with HDCV, prior postexposure prophylaxis with HDCV, or persons previously immunized with any other type of rabies vaccine and a documented history of positive antibody response to the prior vaccination.*
Adapted from Immunization Practices Advisory Committee, 1984 B.

reactions. These can usually be managed with anti-inflammatory and antipyretic agents. Serious systemic anaphylactic or neuroparalytic reactions are rare and must be evaluated carefully; assistance may be sought from state health departments or the Centers for Disease Control. Such serious reactions should be reported to state health departments or the CDC (404) 329-3095 during working hours; (404) 329-2888 at other times.

Pregnancy is not a contraindication to postexposure prophylaxis and, if there is substantial risk, pre-exposure prophylaxis may be indicated.

DRUG INTERACTION. In a randomized, controlled clinical trial, chloroquine 300 mg per week significantly reduced the mean antibody response to immunization with intradermal HDCV rabies vaccine (Pappaioanou et al, 1986).

DOSAGE.
Intramuscular: Adults and children, for pre-exposure immunoprophylaxis, 1 ml is injected into the deltoid area on days 0, 7, and 21 or 28. Booster immunization, *adults and children*, individuals at risk should have a serum antibody test every two years to determine if revaccination is necessary. If antibody levels are inadequate, a single 1-ml dose may be given in the deltoid area and the level measured again in two to three weeks.

For postexposure immunization, see Table 10.

Available Trademark.
Imovax (Merieux).

RABIES IMMUNE GLOBULIN (RIG)

RIG is a sterile solution of antirabies immunoglobulin prepared by cold ethanol fractionation of plasma from donors hyperimmunized with the rabies vaccine. The globulin solution is stabilized with glycine and contains thimerosal as a preservative. The product is standardized to contain an average of 150 IU/ml.

RIG is indicated for all persons with known or suspected exposure to rabies virus and is given in conjunction with rabies vaccine. However, individuals previously immunized with rabies vaccine and a documented positive antibody response should be given only the vaccine. Repeated doses of RIG should not be administered once rabies vaccine has been injected, for this could prevent full development of active immunity.

DOSAGE.
Intramuscular: 20 IU/kg; one-half of the material should be infiltrated around the wound if feasible. RIG is used as soon as possible after a suspected exposure to rabies and always in conjunction with rabies vaccine (see Immunization Schedules also).

Available Trademarks.
Hyperab (Cutter), *Imogam* (Merieux).

ANTIRABIES SERUM EQUINE (ARS)

This sterile solution of refined and concentrated globulins contains rabies antibodies from the blood of horses immunized against fixed rabies virus. The content of neutralizing antibody is standardized to contain 1,000 IU/vial (125 IU/ml) and the volume in each vial is adjusted by the manufacturer on the basis of the antibody potency in each lot. At the present time, a 1,000-IU vial contains approximately 5 ml.

Hyperimmune equine serum is used only when human rabies immune globulin (RIG) is unavailable. RIG is preferred because ARS has a considerably higher risk of adverse reactions. Serum sickness occurs in over 40% of adults; the incidence is lower in children. ARS is always used in conjunction with rabies vaccine and is usually administered only once to provide protective antibodies until the patient responds to vaccination. As with all equine serums, tests for sensitivity and desensitization procedures should be performed prior to use (see the Introduction). ARS should not be administered intravenously because of the potential for serious reactions.

DOSAGE.
Intramuscular: Adults and children, 40 IU/kg; up to one-half of the total dose should be infiltrated around the wound. A course of rabies vaccine also should be initiated immediately (see Table 10).

Manufacturer: Sclavo.

VACCINES USED UNDER SPECIAL CIRCUMSTANCES

ANTHRAX VACCINE, ADSORBED

Anthrax vaccine consists of a culture filtrate containing a protective antigen that is elaborated during the microaerophilic growth in a chemically defined medium of an avirulent, nonencapsulated strain of *Bacillus anthracis*. This vaccine is recommended for laboratory personnel who work with *B. anthracis*; individuals who work with imported animal hides, furs, bonemeal, wool, hair (especially goat hair), and bristles; and veterinarians who may encounter anthrax-infected animals or carcasses. The vaccine is recommended only for adults 18 to 65 years since studies to date have been conducted only in this age group.

The basic immunization series consists of six subcutaneous injections. Immunity can be maintained by booster injections at one-year intervals. The vaccine is approximately 90% effective.

Adverse reactions are usually mild and local. Approximately 94% of those receiving the basic series of immunizations and 87% of those given the booster series experience no reaction. A moderate local reaction may develop in individuals with a history of anthrax infection; this history may be considered a contraindication.

DOSAGE.
Subcutaneous: Adults 18 to 65 years of age, for primary immunization, the initial series consists of three 0.5-ml doses at two-week intervals followed by three additional 0.5-ml injections at six-month intervals beginning six months after the first dose of the initial series.

For booster immunization, *adults under 65 years*, 0.5 ml given at yearly intervals to maintain immunity.

The vaccine is available through the Centers for Disease Control, Host Factors Division (404) 329-3356 Monday through Friday 8 a.m. to 4:30 p.m. Eastern time.

BCG VACCINE

BCG vaccine is a standardized preparation of a living BCG (Bacillus Calmette-Guerin) strain used for active immunization against tuberculosis. BCG is an attenuated strain of bovine tubercle bacillus (*Mycobacterium bovis*). The Danish 1077 substrain is used to produce the Glaxo vaccine, while a substrain of the Pasteur Institute strain is used in the vaccine marketed by Antigen International, Inc. All BCG vaccines are presumed to be derived from the original strain, but they may vary in immunogenicity and efficacy. Data on these vaccines have been obtained primarily from other countries and do not necessarily pertain to the vaccine available in the United States. Efficacy of current vaccines has not been clearly established.

BCG vaccine is not recommended for routine immunization but should be reserved for persons with a negative reaction to a tuberculin skin test who are repeatedly exposed to untreated or inadequately treated patients with sputum-positive pulmonary tuberculosis. The vaccine is also suggested for members of well-defined groups with excessive rates of new infections and inadequate control over therapeutic regimens.

In normal tuberculin-negative recipients, proper intradermal injection of vaccine results in localized skin infection. A lesion appears within seven to ten days, reaches a maximum diameter of about 8 mm after five weeks, then gradually regresses to form a scar in approximately three months. A successful "take" is characterized by conversion to tuberculin-positivity that should be confirmed by tuberculin testing two to three months after vaccination. If the test is negative, vaccination should be repeated.

BCG vaccine also has been used as an adjuvant to enhance antibody formation (see Chapter 63, Immunomodulators) and to treat certain types of localized cancer (see Chapter 64, Drugs Used in Cancer Chemotherapy).

ADVERSE REACTIONS AND PRECAUTIONS. The frequency and severity of adverse reactions vary with the BCG substrain employed. The Danish 1077 substrain is reported to cause fewer untoward reactions than other BCG strains. Lymphadenitis (incidence, 10%), local ulceration that may become severe and persistent, ulcers resulting from autoinoculation, granulomas, and transient urticaria of the limbs and trunk may occur. Keloidal scars and, rarely, lupus reactions of the skin develop in some individuals. Osteomyelitis occurs more frequently in neonates than in adults (adults, 1/1,000,000 vaccinees; neonates, 5/100,000 vaccinees). Isolated cases of disseminated BCG infection and death have been reported (1 to 10/10,000,000 vaccinees), principally in children with an impaired immune response.

BCG vaccine is *contraindicated* in tuberculin-positive individuals, those recently given smallpox vaccinations, and burn patients. It should not be given to pregnant women or patients with extensive skin infections. It is also contraindicated in patients with cellular or combined immunodeficiencies and in those receiving immunosuppressive agents, including corticosteroids.

BCG vaccine is not effective in patients taking isoniazid, rifampin, streptomycin, or other drugs that inhibit the growth of the organism. Successful vaccination permanently converts individuals to tuberculin-positivity and thus negates the diagnostic utility of the tuberculin test.

DOSAGE. BCG vaccine should be protected from light and kept in the refrigerator during long-term storage (<10 C).

Intradermal: Adults with negative tuberculin skin tests who are at risk from continued exposure to active disease may be given the freshly reconstituted vaccine. See the manufacturers' instructions for further information on dosage and administration.

Manufacturers: Glaxo, University of Illinois (marketed by Antigen International, Inc).

CHOLERA VACCINE

This combined bacterial vaccine consists of the Ogawa and Inaba strains of *Vibrio cholerae*, inactivated by phenol and suspended in a saline solution containing 0.5% phenol as a preservative. Many public health officials feel that killed whole cell cholera vaccines are minimally effective and do not prevent disease transmission. Protective immunity develops in only 25% to 50% of recipients and lasts a short time. The low level of immunity begins to recede in three to six months. Consequently, a booster dose should be administered every six months as long as there is risk of exposure. Use of the vaccine in community immunization programs is of limited value in controlling a cholera outbreak.

The U.S. Public Health Service does not require cholera vaccination for entry into the United States from infected areas, and the World Health Organization no longer recommends routine vaccination for travel to or from infected areas. Nevertheless, some countries in Asia, the Middle East, and Africa still require evidence of cholera vaccination for entry. The vaccine is not recommended for infants under 6 months of age.

Malaise, fever, and induration and erythema may occur at the site of injection. The vaccine is contraindicated in individuals who experienced a serious reaction to previous injections.

DOSAGE.

Intramuscular, Subcutaneous: Primary immunization consists of two doses given one week to one month apart; booster doses of identical size are advised at six-month intervals as long as there is risk of exposure. The amounts given in each dose are: *adults and children over 10 years*, 0.5 ml; *children 5 to 10 years*, 0.3 ml; and *6 months through 4 years*, 0.2 ml.

Intradermal: For *adults and children over 5 years*, two doses of 0.2 ml given one week to one month apart for primary immunization; booster doses of 0.2 ml are given at six-month intervals if necessary.

A single dose (primary or booster) by any of the foregoing

routes within six months of travel will satisfy international health regulations where immunization with cholera vaccine is required.

Manufacturers: Lederle, Wyeth.

MENINGOCOCCAL POLYSACCHARIDE VACCINES

Outbreaks of meningococcal infections occur in closed populations of infants, children, and military recruits and there is a high incidence of secondary cases among household contacts. Despite antimicrobial therapy, the case-fatality rate is about 10% for meningococcal meningitis and 20% for meningococcemia. Meningococcal disease is most common in the pediatric age group, especially infants 6 to 12 months of age. The causative organism, *Neisseria meningitidis,* has at least seven serogroups based upon differing capsular polysaccharides. Groups B, C, and W-135 cause 85% to 95% of meningococcal infections in the United States. Groups A, C, Y, and W-135 polysaccharide antigens are quite immunogenic, but serogroup B, which causes 50% to 55% of all cases, does not readily induce antibody production. Although serogroup A is responsible for only a few cases in the United States, it is the most frequent cause of epidemics in other countries. Certain chronic conditions (asplenia, complement deficiency) appear to predispose to severe meningococcal infections. Military recruits were once considered to be at very high risk for meningococcal disease, particularly group C, but routine use of an A/C vaccine has greatly reduced the incidence of the disease.

Routine immunization with meningococcal polysaccharide vaccines is not recommended, but should be considered for individuals with terminal complement component deficiencies, those with anatomic or functional asplenia, travelers to countries where meningococcal disease is epidemic, and military recruits.

The vaccine available for civilian and military use in the United States is quadrivalent and contains serogroups A, C, Y, and W-135. It contains 50 mcg of each of the purified capsular polysaccharides. Clinical studies have demonstrated the immunogenicity and efficacy of the A and C components in military recruits. However, children under 2 years respond poorly to the A/C vaccine as they do to other polysaccharide vaccines. The Y and W-135 components have been shown to be immunogenic in adults and children over 2 years of age. It is thought that the clinical protection induced by the quadrivalent vaccine persists for at least three years, although antibody titers to the A and C components diminish markedly during this time, especially in young children.

ADVERSE REACTIONS AND PRECAUTIONS. Adverse reactions are more common in children than adults and include erythema, induration, malaise, low-grade fever, and axillary adenopathy.

Meningococcal polysaccharide vaccines should not be used in pregnant women because effects on the fetus are unknown. However, the vaccine has been given to pregnant women in Brazil with no reported adverse effects.

DOSAGE.
A/C/Y/W-135 QUADRIVALENT VACCINE:
Subcutaneous: *Adults and children over 2 years,* 0.5 ml as a single injection. Booster injections may be indicated for children first vaccinated when less than 4 years of age who remain at high risk.

Available Trademark.
Menomune (Squibb/Connaught)

PLAGUE VACCINE

Plague vaccine is prepared from *Yersinia pestis* grown on artificial media, killed with formaldehyde, and preserved with 0.5% phenol. Its use is recommended for all laboratory and field personnel working with *Y. pestis,* those engaged in aerosol experimentation, and field personnel working in enzootic areas. In addition, vaccination should be considered for laboratory personnel working with *Y. pestis* or infected rodents, those whose work brings them into frequent contact with wild rodents in plague enzootic areas (eg, southwestern United States), and those residing in enzootic or epidemic areas where avoidance of rodents and fleas is not possible.

It is generally believed that immunization greatly increases the chance of recovery from bubonic plague, but the degree of protection against the pneumonic form is unknown. Plague vaccine should not be relied upon as a principal preventive measure. Control of rodents and their ectoparasites is most effective.

ADVERSE REACTIONS. Adverse reactions include local erythema and induration, malaise, mild lymphadenopathy, hyperpyrexia, and, occasionally, headache. Booster injections increase the incidence and severity of adverse reactions. Sensitivity reactions (urticaria, asthma) are rare.

DOSAGE.
Intramuscular: *Adults and children over 10 years,* for primary vaccination, one 1-ml dose, followed in four weeks by a second dose of 0.2 ml. A third injection of 0.2 ml six months after the first injection completes the primary series. If essential, an accelerated schedule of three doses of 0.5 ml each at weekly intervals may be given; however, the efficacy of this schedule has not been determined. Booster injections of 0.1 to 0.2 ml every six months are recommended for individuals who remain at risk. After three such doses, boosters at one- to two-year intervals should provide the needed protection. *Children under 10 years* receive the same series at the same intervals, but at a reduced dosage as follows: *Infants 1 year or less,* first dose 0.2 ml, second and third doses 0.04 ml, booster dose 0.02 to 0.04 ml; *1 to 4 years,* first dose 0.4 ml, second and third doses 0.08 ml, booster dose 0.04 to 0.08 ml; *5 to 10 years,* first dose 0.6 ml, second and third doses 0.12 ml, booster dose 0.06 to 0.12 ml.

Manufacturer: Cutter.

SMALLPOX VACCINE

In 1980, the World Health Organization declared the world free of smallpox in the natural state, which attested to the highly effective worldwide immunization programs. All but four of the 160 member states of WHO have officially discontinued routine smallpox vaccination. International Certificates of Vaccination are no longer required of travelers. In the United States, general distribution of the vaccine to the civilian population was discontinued in May, 1983, in an attempt to end its misuse in diseases such as warts and herpes. The only currently recommended nonmilitary use of the vaccine is for laboratory personnel who work with the virus or a closely related orthopox virus and those involved in vaccine production.

Vaccinia immune globulin is available through the Centers for Disease Control to treat the clinical complications of smallpox vaccination in certain individuals.

Smallpox vaccine is a live virus vaccine prepared from vaccinia virus-infected calf lymph and contains traces of antibiotics used during processing (polymyxin B sulfate, dihydrostreptomycin sulfate, chlortetracycline hydrochloride, and neomycin sulfate).

Smallpox vaccination is indicated only for laboratory workers directly involved with smallpox or closely related orthopox viruses (eg, monkeypox, vaccinia) and for military personnel.

The virus multiplies at the site of inoculation and produces a local skin lesion that subsequently resolves. These events elicit the production of virus-neutralizing antibodies and active immunity to smallpox. The inoculation site should be inspected six to eight days after vaccination. Interpretation of the response is as follows:

Primary Vaccination: A typical Jennerian vesicle forms after successful vaccination. If none is found, vaccination should be repeated using vaccine from a different lot until a successful result is obtained.

Upon revaccination, two responses are defined by the WHO Expert Committee on Smallpox:

Major Reaction: The reaction is vesicular, pustular, or consists of an area of definite palpable induration or congestion. It is surrounded by a lesion that may be a crust or an ulcer. This reaction indicates that virus multiplication has probably taken place and that revaccination is successful.

Equivocal Reaction: This is any reaction other than a major reaction; it may indicate residual immunity sufficient to suppress virus multiplication or may represent an allergic reaction to the vaccine. Revaccination should be repeated with vaccine from another lot if an equivocal reaction is observed.

Immunity lasts at least three years. Revaccination is recommended at three-year intervals.

ADVERSE REACTIONS AND PRECAUTIONS. Complications may follow either primary (see Table 13) or booster inoculations. The risk of adverse effects after revaccination is extremely low but complications have occurred, especially in patients with underlying disease, in those receiving immunosuppressive therapy, or in subjects who have not been vaccinated for many years. The latter may respond as primary vaccinees.

Smallpox vaccine is *contraindicated* in individuals with eczema, other skin conditions, wounds, or burns and in household contacts of such individuals; patients receiving radiation therapy, corticotropin (ACTH), antimetabolites, corticosteroids, or immunosuppressive drugs; people with known or suspected disorders of gamma globulin synthesis; individuals with leukemia, lymphomas, other reticuloendothelial malignancies, or other malignant neoplasms affecting the bone marrow or lymphatic systems; and pregnant women.

Any vaccine remaining at the vaccination site should be removed with clean dry gauze or cotton. These, as well as other vaccination materials, should be sterilized before disposal.

Smallpox vaccine should not be used to treat warts or prevent recurrent herpes infections.

SOURCE. At present, smallpox vaccine is no longer available in the United States for use in the general public. The Department of Defense has a policy of immunizing personnel on active or reserve duty and in the National Guard. At the present time, the Centers for Disease Control is the only source of smallpox vaccine for civilians. Physician requests for the vaccine should be sent to: Drug Immunobiologic and Vaccine Service, Center for Infectious Diseases, Building 1, Room 1259, Centers for Disease Control, Atlanta, GA 30333 (404) 329-3356.

VACCINIA IMMUNE GLOBULIN

Vaccinia immune globulin (VIG) is a solution of immunoglobulins prepared from the serum of persons recently immunized with vaccinia virus. VIG is used to treat the clinical complica-

TABLE 13.
COMPLICATION RATES PER MILLION PRIMARY SMALLPOX VACCINATIONS IN THE UNITED STATES BY AGE AND DIAGNOSIS

	Age of Vaccinee (years)			
	1	1–4	5–19	20+
Death (from all complications)	5	0.5	0.5	Unknown
Postvaccinal Encephalitis	6	2	2.5	4
Vaccinia Necrosum	1	0.5	1	7
Eczema Vaccinatum	14	44	35	30
Generalized Vaccinia	394	233	140	212
Accidental Infection	507	577	371	606
Erythematous Urticarial Reactions	Unkown	9,600	Unknown	Unknown

From Lane and Millar, 1971.

tions (eczema vaccinatum, vaccinia necrosum, ocular vaccinia, generalized vaccinia) of smallpox vaccination. It is also used prophylactically following exposure to smallpox and for the prevention and modification of vaccinia infection. VIG is of no benefit in patients with postvaccinal encephalitis. This immune globulin should be administered as soon as possible after the onset of symptoms. Doses may be large and should be given over 24 to 36 hours. More detailed information may be obtained from the Centers for Disease Control, International Health Program Office (404) 329-3526.

DOSAGE.

Intramuscular: Adults and children, for smallpox exposure, 0.3 ml/kg administered within 24 hours of exposure into the buttock or anterolateral aspect of the thigh. Doses over 10 ml should be divided and injected at two or more sites. Simultaneous vaccination or revaccination for smallpox should be conducted.

For prevention or modification of vaccinia infection, *adults and children*, 0.3 ml/kg should be given as soon as possible after exposure. Doses over 10 ml should be injected at two or more sites.

For treatment of postvaccinal complications, *adults and children*, 0.6 ml/kg administered as soon as possible after symptoms appear. Doses over 10 ml should be injected at two or more sites. The dose may be repeated, depending on severity of symptoms and response to treatment.

> Vaccinia immune globulin is an investigational drug available through the Center for Infectious Diseases, Centers for Disease Control. Emergency requests from physicians for the antiserum should be made to (404) 329-3145 Monday through Friday, 8 am to 4:30 pm Eastern time or (404) 329-2888 at all other times.

TYPHOID VACCINE

Typhoid vaccine is a sterile saline suspension of phenol and heat-killed typhoid bacilli (*Salmonella typhi*) of a strain (Ty-2) selected for high antigenicity. The vaccine contains 0.5% phenol as a preservative. The current inactivated vaccine is approximately 70% effective against infectious doses commonly found in contaminated water and milk, but it may not protect against large doses, such as those present in heavily contaminated foods.

The administration of the vaccine is followed by the production of agglutinins and bactericidal antibodies, which eliminate bacteria from the blood. However, intracellular bacteria inaccessible to these antibodies may multiply and produce endotoxins that have injurious effects even in the presence of circulating antibodies. Fecal carriage load of typhoid bacilli is not reduced by circulating antibodies.

Immunity wanes with time, and booster doses should be given every three years to those who are continuously at risk. Although a natural infection increases resistance, second attacks of typhoid have occurred.

Routine immunization is not indicated in the United States but is recommended for persons with intimate exposure to a known carrier in the household or those traveling to areas where typhoid fever is endemic. Flood conditions are not an indication for immunization.

ADVERSE REACTIONS AND PRECAUTIONS. Adverse reactions to typhoid vaccine include local erythema, tenderness at the site of injection, malaise, myalgia, headache, and fever. The reactions usually begin within 24 hours of administration and persist for one or two days. The vaccine is contraindicated in the presence of acute respiratory illness or other active infections, in immunocompromised patients, or in those who have previously experienced an allergic reaction to the vaccine. Safety of the vaccine during pregnancy has not been established and its use should be individualized to reflect actual need. The vaccine should be used with caution in patients with a severe febrile illness or a history of febrile convulsions following vaccine administration (especially children).

DOSAGE.

Subcutaneous: Adults and children over 10 years, two 0.5-ml doses four or more weeks apart or, if insufficient time exists, three 0.5-ml doses at weekly intervals, but this schedule may be less effective. *Children 6 months to 10 years,* two 0.25-ml doses four or more weeks apart or three doses at weekly intervals. If there is continued or repeated exposure, a booster dose should be given at least every three years; *adults and children over 10 years* should receive 0.5 ml, and *children under 10 years,* 0.25 ml.

Manufacturer: Wyeth.

YELLOW FEVER VACCINE

This live, attenuated virus vaccine is prepared from the 17D strain grown in chicken embryos. When the vaccine is administered subcutaneously, infection develops, followed by low-grade viremia in three to nine days. Most virus multiplication is then thought to occur in the lymph nodes, spleen, and bone marrow. Immunity develops by the seventh day and lasts for ten years or more. Revaccination is required after ten years by countries that require a vaccination certificate.

Yellow fever vaccine must meet standards established by the World Health Organization and must be administered at WHO-approved centers located in most cities in the United States; information on specific locations may be obtained from city or county public health officers and the Public Health Service.

Vaccination is recommended for persons 6 months of age or older traveling to or living in countries in which yellow fever is endemic (currently parts of Africa and South America). It is recommended for persons traveling outside urban areas of countries where yellow fever is endemic, for the areas of yellow fever activity often exceed the officially reported infected zones. Pregnant women and infants under 6 months should be considered for immunization if travel in high-risk areas is absolutely necessary and exposure to mosquitos cannot be avoided. Vaccination is also recommended for laboratory personnel who might be exposed to the virulent yellow fever virus.

A certificate of vaccination against yellow fever is required by certain countries in which the disease is endemic. Since requirements may change, all travelers should seek current information from health departments.

Available evidence suggests that yellow fever vaccine may be administered concomitantly with other live virus vaccines without impairment of antibody response or increase in adverse effects. If not given concurrently, four weeks should elapse between administration of live virus vaccines. Simultaneous administration of cholera and yellow fever vaccines reduces the antibody levels to both vaccines. When possible, these agents should be given at a minimal interval of three weeks. If not possible, it is recommended that they be given simultaneously.

ADVERSE REACTIONS AND PRECAUTIONS. Adverse reactions are generally mild and consist of headache, myalgia, or low-grade fever in 2% to 5% of vaccinees. The vaccine is contraindicated in individuals highly sensitive to eggs; those with febrile illnesses or dysgammaglobulinemia; or those receiving corticosteroid, antineoplastic, or immunosuppressive drugs. It is prudent to avoid vaccinating pregnant women. If the sole reason for vaccinating a pregnant woman or an individual with known allergy is to satisfy international travel requirements, physicians should make efforts to obtain a waiver.

DOSAGE.

Subcutaneous: *Adults and children over 6 months,* 0.5 ml of reconstituted vaccine. International regulations do not require revaccination more frequently than every ten years.

Available Trademark.
YF-Vax (Squibb/Connaught).

OTHER IMMUNE GLOBULINS

IMMUNE GLOBULIN (IG)

Immune globulin (formerly immune serum globulin) is a sterile solution of immunoglobulin, primarily IgG, containing 16.5% ± 1.5% protein that is prepared by cold ethanol precipitation of pooled human plasma. Only plasma units nonreactive for hepatitis B surface antigen (HBsAg) are employed. IG contains glycerin and the preservative, thimerosal.

IG preparations consist of a pool of antibodies that neutralize or otherwise modify the activity of the agents (eg, measles virus) to which their specificities are directed and, hence, protect the host. These protective antibodies to common infectious agents are characteristic of the donor population from which the IG preparations are made. Thus, different lots of IG vary in specific antibody titer.

IG contains all four immunoglobulin subclasses and all of the known IgG genetic groups. Although 95% of the preparation is IgG, traces of IgA, IgM, and other serum proteins are present. Patients with isolated IgA deficiency may develop antibodies to any IgA-containing preparation and, on future exposure to products containing IgA, may develop an anaphylactic reaction. IG aggregates in vitro and, therefore, intravenous use is contraindicated as it may cause severe, even fatal, reactions.

USES. **Hepatitis:** Immune globulin contains antibodies to both the hepatitis A virus and the hepatitis B surface antigen (anti-HBs). Studies have shown that IG is protective if given before exposure or during the incubation period of hepatitis A. It is not indicated in patients with clinical manifestations of the disease or in those exposed more than two weeks previously. It is recommended for travelers to countries where there is a significant risk of infection with hepatitis A. It is also recommended for postexposure prophylaxis against hepatitis A, household and sexual contacts of infected patients, and individuals at risk during outbreaks of hepatitis A in day care centers, schools, institutions for custodial care, and hospitals. When there is a common source of exposure, such as an infected food handler, IG prophylaxis may be considered if immune globulin can be administered within two weeks of exposure.

Radioimmunoassays have shown that IG contains an anti-HBs titer of at least 1:100, while HBIG has a titer of 1:100,000. Therefore, it has been recommended that IG be used as an alternative to HBIG, when the latter is not available, for postexposure prophylaxis following percutaneous (needlestick or bite), ocular (eye splash), or permucosal exposure to HBsAg-positive material. IG should be administered as soon as possible after exposure (within seven days) and repeated 25 to 30 days later.

IG also has been suggested for prophylaxis after percutaneous exposure to blood from patients with non-A, non-B hepatitis.

Measles: IG is indicated to prevent or modify measles (rubeola) in susceptible persons exposed less than six days previously, especially household contacts of measles patients (particularly infants under 1 year) for whom the risk of complications is high. Children with generalized malignancy, immune deficiency disease, or those receiving immunosuppressive therapy who are exposed to measles should receive IG immediately.

Immunoglobulin Deficiency: IG is used prophylactically in patients with immunoglobulin (IgG) deficiency to prevent serious infection. It may not prevent infections in the respiratory or gastrointestinal tract or other secretory tissues. Prophylactic use, especially against encapsulated bacteria, is effective in Bruton-type, sex-linked, congenital agammaglobulinemia, agammaglobulinemia with thymoma, and acquired agammaglobulinemia.

Varicella: If varicella-zoster immune globulin is unavailable, IG may be used to modify varicella virus infection in immunocompromised individuals. However, lots differ in antibody titer to varicella-zoster virus and results vary accordingly.

Rubella: Some studies have indicated that the use of IG in exposed, susceptible women may lessen the likelihood of infection and fetal damage. However, the routine use of IG for prophylaxis in early pregnancy is of dubious value and cannot be justified.

ADVERSE REACTIONS AND PRECAUTIONS. Adverse reactions consist of local pain, tenderness at the injection site, urticaria (occasional), and angioedema. IG must not be administered intravenously. Because of the possibility of systemic reactions, epinephrine should be immediately available to treat acute allergic symptoms.

DOSAGE.

Intramuscular: For hepatitis A postexposure prophylaxis (household or close personal contacts of infected individuals), *adults and children,* 0.02 ml/kg as soon as possible after

TABLE 14.
INDICATIONS AND GUIDELINES FOR USE OF VARICELLA-ZOSTER IMMUNE GLOBULIN (VZIG) FOR PROPHYLAXIS OF CHICKENPOX (VARICELLA)

I. Exposure criteria for which VZIG is indicated (patients must meet both criteria)
   1. One of the following types of exposure to chickenpox or zoster patient(s):
      a. Continuous household contact
      b. Playmate contact (>1 hour play indoors)
      c. Hospital contact (in same 2- to 4- bed room or adjacent beds in a large ward or prolonged face-to-face contact with an infectious staff member or patient)
      d. Newborn contact (newborn of mother who had onset of chickenpox ≤5 days before delivery or within 48 hours after delivery, regardless of prior administration of VZIG to the mother)
   2. Exposure occurred ≤96 hours prior to contemplated administration of VZIG

II. Persons for whom VZIG is indicated (all four criteria should be met)
   1. Susceptible to varicella-zoster infection
   2. Significant exposure (see I above)
   3. Age <15 years; administration to immunocompromised adolescents and adults and other older patients on an *individual* basis
   4. One of the following underlying illnesses or conditions:
      a. Leukemia or lymphoma
      b. Congenital or acquired immunodeficiency
      c. Immunosuppressive treatment
      d. Newborn of mother who had onset of chickenpox <5 days before delivery or within 48 hours after delivery
      e. Premature infant (≥28 weeks' gestation born to a mother with a negative history of chickenpox)
      f. Premature infant (<28 weeks' gestation or birthweight ≤1 kg) regardless of maternal history

Adapted from Immunization Practices Advisory Committee, 1984 E.

exposure. The use of IG two weeks after exposure or after onset of symptoms is not indicated.

For travel in areas where hepatitis A is common (preexposure prophylaxis), *adults and children*, 0.02 ml/kg for less than two-month length of stay; 0.06 ml/kg repeated every five months for longer visits. For postexposure prophylaxis, 0.02 ml/kg (Immunization Practices Advisory Committee, 1985 B).

For measles prophylaxis or modification of infections in exposed susceptible *adults and children*, 0.25 ml/kg (maximum, 15 ml) administered less than six days following exposure. No more than 5 ml should be injected at any one site. *Children with leukemia, lymphoma, loss of cell-mediated immunity, or immunosuppression*, 0.5 ml/kg.

For prophylaxis in *adults and children* with immunoglobulin deficiency, initially, 1.32 ml/kg, followed by 0.66 ml/kg every three to four weeks. Frequency of administration should be determined by clinical response (absent or infrequent infections).

   Available Trademarks.
   Gammar (Armour), **Gammastan** (Cutter), **Immuglobin** (Savage), **Immune Serum Globulin** (Hyland, Wyeth).

IMMUNE GLOBULIN INTRAVENOUS (IGIV)

Intravenous immune globulin is a sterile solution of plasma proteins containing IgG antibodies from pooled human plasma. Only plasma units nonreactive for hepatitis B surface antigen are used. It is prepared for intravenous use either by treatment with pepsin at acid pH [Sandoglobulin] or reduction with dithiothreitol and alkylation with iodoacetamide [Gamimune]. The preparation contains no less than 90% immunoglobulin consisting of all the IgG subclasses and trace amounts of IgA and IgM. IGIV is used in place of intramuscular immune globulin preparations when an immediate increase in circulating immunoglobulin levels is required or when intramuscular injections are contraindicated.

IGIV is indicated to treat immunodeficiency disease, such as agammaglobulinemia, hypogammaglobulinemia, and combined immunodeficiency. It has been used in acute idiopathic thrombocytopenic purpura (ITP) and, in patients less than 13 years old, has been as effective as steroids in increasing the platelet count (Imbach et al, 1981). Its use in older patients has not been studied in prospectively controlled clinical trials. Studies suggest that IGIV also may be useful in chronic ITP in children and adults (Bussel et al, 1983; Abe et al, 1983; Newland et al, 1983; Carroll et al, 1984; Oral et al, 1984; Warrier and Lusher, 1984). The mechanism of action in ITP has not been elucidated but may include blockade of Fc receptors.

IGIV has also been used investigationally for other autoimmune diseases, such as myasthenia gravis (Ippoliti et al, 1984) and Kawasaki disease (Furusho et al, 1984). Preliminary studies suggest that large doses of IGIV may suppress the spontaneous inhibitor of factor VIII (antihemophiliac factor) found in certain patients (Sultan et al, 1984; Zimmermann et al, 1985).

Approximately six days after intravenous administration, IGIV is evenly distributed in the intra- and extravascular compartments. It has an intravascular half-life of about three weeks. As with physiologic IgG, IGIV may cross the placenta, but only during the final weeks of pregnancy. It should be used during pregnancy only if clearly indicated.

ADVERSE REACTIONS AND PRECAUTIONS. Immune globulin is *contraindicated* in patients known to have experienced an anaphylactic reaction or severe systemic response to immune serum globulin (human) and in individuals with selective IgA deficiencies or class specific anti-IgA. A precipitous fall in blood pressure and signs and symptoms of anaphylaxis have been observed in some patients. These events appear to be related to infusion rate, which should be carefully controlled and monitored. IGIV should be given only intravenously (the intramuscular route has not been evaluated) through a separate line and *not* mixed with other fluids or medications.

Inflammatory reactions due to antigen overload occur in less than 1% of patients with normal immune functions. If the initial infusion rate exceeds 1 ml/minute, adverse reactions (eg, flushing, chills, wheezing, malaise, dizziness) develop in approximately 10% of patients. Rarely, anaphylactic reactions occur in patients previously sensitized to antigens in the preparation.

DOSAGE.

GAMIMUNE:

Intravenous: For prophylaxis in immunodeficiency syndromes, *adults and children*, 100 mg/kg (2 ml/kg) at a rate of 0.01 to 0.02 ml/kg/min for 30 minutes. If there is no discomfort, the rate may be increased up to to 0.04 ml/kg/min. If side effects occur, the rate should be reduced or the infusion interrupted until symptoms subside. The infusion may then be resumed at a rate that is tolerated by the patient.

Immune globulin may be administered once a month. If the clinical response is inadequate or the level of IgG achieved in the circulation is insufficient, the dose may be increased to 200 mg/kg (4 ml/kg) or the infusion may be given more than once a month.

SANDOGLOBULIN:

Intravenous: For prophylaxis in immunodeficiency syndromes, *adults and children*, 200 mg/kg once monthly. If the clinical response or the level of serum IgG is insufficient, the dose may be increased to 300 mg/kg or the infusion may be repeated more frequently. The initial infusion must be given as a 3% solution at a rate of 0.5 to 1 ml/min. After 15 to 30 minutes, the infusion rate may be increased. If, after the first dose, large doses must be administered repeatedly, a 6% solution may be given at an initial infusion rate of 1 to 1.5 ml/min.

For treatment of idiopathic thrombocytopenic purpura, 400 mg/kg on five consecutive days.

Available Trademarks.
Gamimune (Cutter), *Sandoglobulin* (Sandoz).

VARICELLA-ZOSTER IMMUNE GLOBULIN (HUMAN) (VZIG)

VZIG is a sterile 16% to 18% solution of the globulin fraction of human plasma of which not less than 99% is IgG; trace amounts of IgA and IgM also are present. VZIG is derived from plasma selected for high titers of varicella-zoster antibodies. Only plasma units nonreactive for hepatitis B surface antigen are employed. The plasma pools are fractionated by cold ethanol precipitation of the proteins and the final product contains 100 to 180 mg/ml of protein.

VZIG is not the same as zoster immune globulin (ZIG), although the terms have been used synonymously. The two preparations are derived from different donor populations: ZIG was derived from the serum of convalescent zoster patients, whereas VZIG is derived from the plasma of healthy adults. VZIG has replaced ZIG commercially.

VZIG is intended for passive immunization of selected, susceptible individuals (eg, immunocompromised children) at high risk of varicella-associated complications following significant exposure to the virus (see Table 14). Effectiveness is maximum when treatment is initiated as soon as possible after exposure; VZIG has not been evaluated for efficacy beyond 96 hours after initial exposure.

There is no evidence that VZIG modifies established varicella-zoster infections. Its principal use in pregnancy is to prevent complications of varicella in susceptible women rather than to prevent intrauterine infection.

The decision to administer VZIG should be evaluated on an individual basis; most adults are probably immune. Postexposure administration of VZIG may ameliorate and not prevent clinical illness, in which case varicella may still be contagious. The incubation period for varicella infection in immunocompromised patients may be prolonged an additional 14 to 18 days and healthy individuals who receive VZIG should be considered contagious for 10 to 28 days following exposure or until all lesions have healed.

VZIG should never be administered intravenously.

Since licensure, VZIG has been produced by the Massachusetts Public Health Biologic Laboratories, which distributes the preparation in its own state. It is distributed elsewhere by the American Red Cross Services-Northeast Region through regional blood centers. The Centers for Disease Control ([404] 329-3753) maintains a listing of telephone numbers of these distribution centers and continues to provide consultation regarding the indications for VZIG.

DOSAGE.

Intramuscular: *Adults*, 125 units/10 kg (see table below). Each 125 units (2.5 ml) must be injected into a different site. [Data do not exist from which a calculation of the most appropriate dose for adults can be made. The ACIP states that a dose of 625 units is probably sufficient for healthy adults, but larger doses may be necessary in immunocompromised patients (Immunization Practices Advisory Committee 1984 E).]

Body Weight (kg)	Units	Vials	Injection Sites
0–10	125	1	1
10.1 to 20	250	2	2
20.1 to 30	375	3	3
30.1 to 40	500	4	4
Over 40	625	5	5

It has been recommended that postexposure prophylaxis with VZIG be repeated at three-week intervals in persons with continued or repeated exposure to varicella until such risk is no longer present unless there is laboratory evidence of adequate immunity at the time of re-exposure (Immunization Practices Advisory Committee, 1984 E).

EQUINE ANTISERUMS

BOTULISM ANTITOXIN TRIVALENT

Botulism antitoxin is a refined, concentrated preparation of globulins obtained from horses immunized with botulinus toxins types A, B, and E and modified by enzymatic digestion. It may be administered by intramuscular or intravenous injection.

Botulism antitoxin neutralizes the toxin produced by *Clostridium botulinum* in persons who have ingested contaminated foods or acquired toxin through other means ("wound" botulism, infant botulism due to colonization of the gastrointestinal tract). It is most effective when given early.

The outcome of treatment depends largely on the interval between the onset of symptoms and the time when the peak of the injected antitoxin is reached. The incubation period for botulism is usually 12 to 48 hours after ingestion of contaminated food. Experimental data on the amount of circulating antitoxin needed to counteract botulinus toxin poisoning in humans is lacking. Since death may result from untreated botulism, it is important to administer the antitoxin as soon as possible to symptomatic patients. The level and duration of circulating antibody titer depend upon the dose and route of administration.

Since the amount or type of botulinus toxin ingested is not usually known, the entire contents of one vial of trivalent antitoxin should be given intravenously. In addition, to provide a reservoir from which additional antitoxin may be absorbed, the contents of another vial may be given by intramuscular injection. If the signs and symptoms worsen, additional doses may be indicated at two to four hours. Management of botulism also should include elimination of toxin by induced vomiting or gastric lavage, rapid purgation, high enemas, and optimum respiratory care.

ADVERSE REACTIONS AND PRECAUTIONS. Adverse effects are those of any equine globulin preparation, especially hypersensitivity reactions. About 9% of patients experience an allergic reaction.

The antitoxin should never be administered without conducting appropriate sensitivity tests. Patients who appear to be sensitive to equine serum should first be desensitized and the antitoxin should then be administered over several hours until the total dose has been given.

Aminoglycosides may potentiate the neurotoxins of *C. botulinum* and should not be used.

DOSAGE AND PREPARATIONS.

Intravenous, Intramuscular: For symptomatic botulism, *adults,* initially, *after sensitivity testing,* one vial intravenously and one vial intramuscularly. After four hours if signs and symptoms worsen, one vial intravenously; another vial may be given intravenously after 12 to 24 hours.

For prophylaxis after ingestion of *C. botulinum*-contaminated food, one-fifth to one vial, *intramuscularly.* If symptoms appear, additional antitoxin should be administered.

Botulism Antitoxin Trivalent is supplied in vials of 7 to 10 ml containing the following amounts of antitoxin: Type A, 7,500 IU; Type B, 5,500 IU; Type E, 8,500 IU. It may be obtained from the Centers for Disease Control, Atlanta, GA 30333. The Centers' telephone numbers are: (404) 329-3753; off-duty hours (404) 329-2888.

ANTIVENINS

Snakebites

It has been estimated that about 8,000 people are bitten by snakes annually but only 12 to 15 of these bites are fatal. Pit vipers (rattlesnakes, cottonmouths [water moccasins], and copperheads) are responsible for most of the bites in the United States. Rattlesnake bites are the most serious, followed by those of cottonmouth and copperhead. Copperhead envenomation usually does not cause major systemic injury.

Envenomation does not necessarily occur after snakebite; about one of five pit viper bites is "dry," ie, not associated with injection of venom. Furthermore, the amount of venom injected with each bite varies. Although they rarely bite people, are small with short fangs, and often do not inject much venom, coral snake bites can be dangerous and symptoms may not appear for many hours. Coral snake venom is chiefly paralytic (neurotoxic) in action and, customarily, only minimal to moderate tissue reaction and pain occur at the site of the bite. The adult LD_{100} has been estimated to be 4 to 5 mg of the dried venom. Under laboratory conditions, bites of the coral snake (*M. f. fulvius*) have yielded 1 to 28 mg of venom, depending upon the size of the snake.

Polyvalent crotalidae antivenin and North American coral snake antivenin neutralize the venoms of certain poisonous snakes indigenous to the United States. Venoms of snakes found outside the United States usually require other antivenins. The Oklahoma Poison Information Center ([405] 271-5454) in cooperation with the Oklahoma City Zoo maintains an Antivenin Index (Rappolt et al, 1978) and can provide information on the availability of snake antivenins; it also maintains a snakebite consultation service for physicians. The physician also is encouraged to consult the literature (eg, Russell, 1983) and manufacturers of antivenin preparations for recommended methods of management of venomous snakebite and precautions regarding the use of antivenin.

Antivenins are prepared by injecting horses with venoms to induce the production of antibodies. Their use carries the risk inherent in the injection of foreign protein; thus, it is important to observe the criteria for use of these agents carefully.

Since there is some risk of sensitization or reaction to antivenin, careful evaluation of the patient's condition should precede the decision to begin treatment. Signs and symptoms of envenomation include fang marks, swelling, and edema that develop within 20 minutes and pain, which is not always severe. Systemic signs and symptoms include weakness, syncope, paresthesia, and hypotension; blurred vision and ecchymoses are less common. Treatment with antivenin should be initiated as soon as the diagnosis is established.

The antivenins are diluted in normal saline and usually

administered intravenously. Small amounts may be given intramuscularly, but these agents should never be injected into the fingers or toes. Adequate dosage is critical and prompt administration is essential. Children may require larger doses than adults.

In addition to antivenins, management of envenomation should include appropriate antitetanus therapy and adequate supportive management.

ANTIVENIN (CROTALIDAE) POLYVALENT

Antivenin (Crotalidae) polyvalent is an antiserum prepared from refined and concentrated serum globulins obtained from horses immunized against the venoms of the pit vipers, *Crotalus adamanteus* (eastern diamond rattlesnake), *C. atrox* (western diamond rattlesnake), *C. durissus terrificus* (tropical rattlesnake, Cascabel), and *Bothrops atrox* (fer-de-lance).

This antivenin is indicated only to treat envenomation due to bites of the specified crotalids (pit vipers): rattlesnakes (*Crotalus, Sistrurus*); copperhead and cottonmouth moccasins (*Agkistrodon*), including *A. halys* of Korea and Japan; fer-de-lance and other species of *Bothrops*; tropical rattler (*Crotalus durissus* and similar species); Cantil (*A. bilineatus*); and bushmaster (*Lachesis mutus*) of Central and South America.

The severity of envenomation should be estimated as soon as possible before administration of antivenin. The amount of the first dose is based on this estimate (none, minimal, moderate, or severe). (See Dosage and Preparations.)

The antivenin is most effective when given within four hours of the bite, less effective after eight hours, and of questionable value after 12 hours. Nevertheless, in severe poisonings, antivenin therapy should be given even 24 hours after the snakebite.

ADVERSE REACTIONS AND PRECAUTIONS. The principal adverse effect is hypersensitivity to the equine serum proteins in the preparation. Since severe envenomation can be fatal, this risk must be weighed carefully against the risk of withholding antivenin. A procedure has been described for use in severely envenomated patients with positive sensitivity tests (see Wingert and Wainschel, 1975).

DOSAGE AND PREPARATIONS. Lyophilized preparations are active for at least five years; they are readily soluble in water for injection and should be reconstituted immediately prior to administration. For intravenous use, a 1:1 or 1:10 dilution is made of antivenin reconstituted in sodium chloride or 5% dextrose injection. The initial 5 to 10 ml should be infused over a three- to five-minute period. If no signs of a systemic reaction appear, intravenous infusion may be continued at the maximum rate. The intravenous route usually is preferred and is mandatory in the case of shock. Maximum blood levels of antivenin are not reached until eight or more hours after intramuscular administration.

Intravenous: Adults and children, initial dosage is based upon the extent of envenomation. Envenomation by large snakes in children or small adults requires larger doses of antivenin. The amount administered to a child is not based on weight. For minimum envenomation, 20 to 40 ml; moderate envenomation, 50 to 90 ml; severe envenomation, 100 to 150 ml or more. The need for additional antivenin must be based on the clinical response to the initial dose and continuing assessment of the patient's condition. If warranted, an additional 10 to 50 ml may be administered.

See the manufacturer's literature for more detailed dosage information.

Antivenin (Crotalidae) Polyvalent (Equine Origin) (Wyeth). Lyophilized preparation with 10 ml of bacteriostatic water for injection.

NORTH AMERICAN CORAL SNAKE ANTIVENIN

This is a refined, concentrated, and lyophilized preparation of serum globulins obtained from the fractionated blood of horses immunized with the venom of the eastern coral snake (*Micrurus fulvius fulvius*). This antivenin neutralizes venom of *M. f. tenere* (Texas coral snake) but *not* that of *Micruroides euryxanthus* (Arizona or Sonoran coral snake). Each 10-ml vial contains sufficient material to neutralize approximately 250 mouse LD_{50} or about 2 mg of *M. f. fulvius* venom.

Severe and even fatal envenomation from a coral snakebite may occur without significant tissue reaction. Death from respiratory paralysis has occurred within four hours. Some patients require ten or more vials to neutralize the venom dose injected by the snake.

The intravenous route is preferred and antivenin should be given as soon as possible and before signs and symptoms occur. If signs and symptoms are already present when the patient is first seen, antivenin should be given promptly. The rate of infusion is determined by the severity of signs and symptoms and tolerance to the antivenin.

With vigorous treatment and careful observation, patients with complete respiratory paralysis have recovered, indicating that this effect is reversible. The use of morphine or other narcotics that depress respiration is *contraindicated*. Sedatives should be used with extreme caution.

DOSAGE. Appropriate history and testing should be conducted prior to administration, since this antivenin is prepared from horse serum. In the event of sensitivity (if the history is positive and either the skin or conjunctival test is strongly positive), administration is contraindicated in all but acute emergencies. *Constant attendance and observation of the patient are mandatory during administration of antivenin.*

Intravenous: Adults and children, an intravenous drip of 250 to 500 ml sodium chloride injection is begun and the contents of three to five vials of antivenin (30 to 50 ml) are administered directly into the intravenous tubing or added to the reservoir bottle. In either case, the first 1 to 2 ml should be injected over a three- to five-minute period with careful observation of the patient for anaphylactic reaction. If no evidence of sensitivity appears, the infusion may be continued at an appropriate rate until the equivalent of 30 to 50 ml of undiluted antivenin in 250 to 500 ml sodium chloride injection has been given (30 minutes in previously healthy adults). Additional antivenin may be given if required.

Manufacturer: Wyeth.

Arthropod Bites

Biting or stinging insects possess venoms that contain deleterious substances. Unlike snakebite, the volume of toxin injected by insects and most spiders and scorpions usually is too small to cause serious problems except in hypersensitive individuals. In these individuals, insect stings cause anaphylactic shock and prophylactic hyposensitization is essential for management.

Spider bites and scorpion stings cause injury by envenomation and are, therefore, the only arthropod-caused injuries currently amenable to treatment with antivenin. The only spider antivenin readily available is black widow spider antivenin.

The venom of the Arizona bark scorpion contains several potent components that act at the neuromuscular junction and also may affect the sympathetic nervous system. Symptoms include marked restlessness, especially in children; hypertonicity; pharyngeal spasms; drooling; fecal and urinary incontinence; hyperthermia; and sometimes paralysis. Beta-adrenergic blocking agents have been suggested for tachycardia and hypertension. Many patients are unable to locate the site of the sting, since most scorpion venoms produce minimal local reaction. An antivenin against the Arizona bark scorpion produced from goat serum is available in Arizona only. For the most part, treatment is symptomatic and most stings do not require medical care.

Like scorpion venom, the lethal fraction of black widow spider venom is a protein that causes destabilization of cell membranes and degranulation of nerve terminals resulting in the release of neurotransmitters. Central and peripheral nervous system excitement, autonomic activity, muscle spasm, vasoconstriction, and hypertension result from envenomation.

BLACK WIDOW SPIDER ANTIVENIN

Black widow spider antivenin is prepared from the serum of horses immunized against the venom of the black widow spider (*Lactrodectus mactans*). Each vial contains not less than 6,000 antivenin units (1 unit of antivenin will neutralize one murine lethal dose of venom).

The earliest possible use of antivenin is recommended for greatest effectiveness. If possible, the patient should be hospitalized. Supportive therapy may include warm baths, intravenous methocarbamol or 10% calcium gluconate solution to control myalgia, and diazepam to lessen extreme restlessness. Morphine may be required for pain, but since the spider venom is a neurotoxin and may cause respiratory paralysis, caution should be employed when considering the use of morphine or a barbiturate. Corticosteroids also have been used with varying results. No apparent benefit is gained by local treatment (eg, tourniquets, incision, suction).

The antivenin is indicated *only* for the treatment of envenomation due to the bite of the black widow spider. In individuals between age 16 and 60, antivenin use may be deferred and treatment with muscle relaxants considered.

A test for hypersensitivity to horse serum should be performed prior to use of this preparation (see the Introduction).

DOSAGE AND PREPARATIONS.

Intramuscular (anterolateral thigh): Adults and children, the entire contents of one container (2.5 ml restored serum) is administered. One dose usually relieves symptoms in one to three hours; a second dose may be needed.

Intravenous: This is the preferred route in severe cases, in children under 12 years, or in those in shock. The contents of the container is diluted in 10 to 50 ml of saline and administered over a 15-minute period.

Antivenin (Lactrodectus mactans) (Equine Origin) (Merck Sharp & Dohme). Powder (for suspension) containing not less than 6,000 Antivenin Units with 2.5 ml of sterile water for injection.

INVESTIGATIONAL AGENTS

Vaccines

HAEMOPHILUS INFLUENZAE TYPE b POLYSACCHARIDE-DIPHTHERIA TOXOID CONJUGATE VACCINE (PRP-D)

The incidence of *H. influenzae* type b (Hib) disease is highest in infants under 18 months of age and peaks between age 6 to 12 months. Unfortunately, Hib polysaccharide vaccine is not effective in the most susceptible age group, apparently because of the T-cell independent nature of this vaccine. In an effort to enhance immunogenicity, the polysaccharide (PRP) vaccine has been conjugated with diphtheria toxoid in the hope that such a conjugate would behave as a T-dependent antigen.

The vaccine is prepared by conjugating diphtheria toxoid with adipic acid dihydrazide and covalently coupling it to cyanogen bromide activated polysaccharide antigen (PRP). The conjugated vaccine (PRP-D) is then purified by chromatography.

In animals, PRP-D functions as a T-cell dependent antigen and induces booster responses and a switch from IgM to IgG production.

A study conducted in adults reported that, one month after intramuscular injection of PRP-D, the concentration of IgG and IgM antibodies to the PRP antigen increased approximately three times over that observed with the PRP vaccine alone. Also, there was a 12.4-fold increase in IgG antibody to diphtheria toxoid in PRP-D recipients, but no increase was noted in individuals given only PRP vaccine (Lepow et al, 1984). These results were confirmed in a second study conducted in adults (Granoff et al, 1984). Moreover, the latter study demonstrated that there was no further increase in anti-PRP antibodies after a second injection given one month after the first, there was a progressive decline in antibody, and there was no statistical difference between groups given the PRP-D or PRP vaccine after 12 months.

Encouraging results were reported in a study conducted in infants 9 to 15 months of age (Lepow et al, 1985). After the initial dose, 97% given the PRP-D vaccine versus 44% given PRP alone demonstrated a greater than twofold increase in anti-PRP antibody. Moreover, levels of antibody in the PRP-D group were 27 times greater than those in the PRP group. In infants 9 to 11 months of age, the IgM response was greater than the IgG response; in those older than 11 months, the IgG response was greater. A booster effect was observed in most infants after a second dose of the conjugated vaccine; this did not occur with the PRP vaccine alone. In addition, the conjugated vaccine significantly increased diphtheria antitoxin levels, but no booster effect to diphtheria toxin was observed after a second dose.

In all studies, adverse effects to the conjugated vaccine have been minimal, consisting principally of mild local reactions. The data suggest that, in infants, the conjugated vaccine behaves as a T-dependent antigen, induces a booster response to PRP, and is associated with an IgM-IgG class switch after a second dose (Lepow et al, 1985).

RECOMBINANT YEAST DNA HEPATITIS B VACCINE

Production of a human hepatitis B vaccine from the plasma of HBV carriers is restricted by the supply of infected plasma. Also, stringent and highly technical procedures must be performed to purify the immunizing antigen (HBsAg) and to inactivate any infectious agents present in plasma. These procedures are effective but are costly and time consuming. To meet the worldwide need for a hepatitis B vaccine, other means of preparation have been investigated. A promising alternative is the use of recombinant DNA technology for in vitro synthesis of HBsAg. In 1982, the synthesis and assembly of HBsAg particles in the yeast, *Saccharomyces cerevisiae*, were accomplished (Valenzuela et al, 1982) with construction of an autonomously replicating plasmid that contained the HBsAg-coding sequences linked to the yeast alcohol dehydrogenase I promoter. The recombinant synthesized and accumulated particulate antigens specifically reacting with HBsAg antibodies. These particles were found to be approximately 20 nm in size and resembled those used in the preparation of the plasma vaccine.

A vaccine has been formulated from the virus antigen produced in yeast cells by adsorption onto alum adjuvant. Chimpanzees immunized with this vaccine were protected from subsequent challenge with virulent virus (McAleer et al, 1984). The vaccine was given intramuscularly at 0, 1, and 6 months to healthy, low-risk, seronegative adults (Scolnick et al, 1984). By three months, 80% to 100% of vaccinees were antibody positive; one month after the last dose, large boosts in antibody titer were observed. Mild soreness at the injection site was the most common complaint; no serious adverse effects were observed.

The recombinant hepatitis B vaccine (10 mcg/dose) was compared to the plasma vaccine (20 mcg/dose) in a study on 30 healthy, seronegative, young adults given the vaccines intramuscularly at 0, 1, and 6 months. One month after the last dose, the results for the two groups were similar in seroconversion rates and anti-HBs titers. However, in the group receiving recombinant vaccine, the immune response appeared to develop more slowly (Jilg et al, 1984). In a similar study conducted in military recruits given equal doses (10 mcg/dose) of recombinant and plasma vaccine, antibody levels in the first three months were similar for the two groups; however, after the last dose of vaccine, levels were significantly lower in the group receiving recombinant vaccine (Papaevangelou et al, 1985). A third study involving 107 seronegative health professionals revealed essentially the same immune response in individuals given 5 or 10 mcg of recombinant vaccine compared to a group given 20 mcg of plasma vaccine (Davidson and Krugman, 1985).

ROTAVIRUS VACCINE LIVE ORAL ATTENUATED

Approximately 50% of hospital admissions for acute diarrhea in children and 20% to 40% of all acute diarrheas in developing countries are due to rotavirus infections. Generally, acute diarrheas associated with rotaviruses are more severe than cases not associated with this group of agents. It has been estimated that worldwide about one million deaths in children are associated with rotavirus diarrhea. Thus, there has been considerable interest in developing a vaccine to prevent rotavirus infection.

One promising approach is use of an attenuated bovine rotavirus to induce cross protection against human rotaviruses, since both bovine and human strains share a common group antigen. The Nebraska strain of bovine rotavirus is related antigenically to human rotavirus strains of subgroup 1. An attenuated derivative of this strain, RIT 4237, grows well in monkey kidney cell cultures and has been used investigationally. Immunization with the RIT 4237 strain protected piglets against human rotavirus strains of subgroup 2 and 3 (Zissis et al, 1983).

A preliminary study was conducted in adults and children to assess the immunogenicity and safety of the RIT 4237 vaccine. In adults, many of whom were initially seropositive, the vaccine was safe (ie, did not produce clinical symptoms) and a booster response occurred in 2 of 20 subjects. Seroconversion occurred after a single oral dose in up to 88% of children who were initially seronegative and a booster response was observed in at least 25% of initially seropositive children (Vesikari et al, 1983).

A randomized, double-blind, placebo-controlled trial was conducted with RIT 4237 vaccine in children during a human subgroup 2 rotavirus outbreak to assess the vaccine's ability to protect against natural infection. Infants 8 to 11 months were given a single oral dose of vaccine or placebo and observed clinically and serologically for five months. No adverse effects attributable to the vaccine were observed and the protection rate was calculated to be 88% (Vesikari et al, 1984 A).

Seroconversion rates in infants receiving a single oral dose of the RIT 4237 vaccine were enhanced by giving the vaccine after the ingestion of milk to neutralize gastric acid destruction of the vaccine virus (Vesikari et al, 1984 B).

It remains to be established whether the RIT 4237 vaccine can protect against all rotavirus subgroups and how long vaccine-induced protection will last.

TYPHOID VACCINE LIVE ORAL

The protection afforded by parenterally administered killed typhoid vaccines is inadequate against large numbers of organisms and adverse reactions are common. In addition, the relative importance of humoral immunity to typhoid has been questioned and it has been suggested that local defense mechanisms at the intestinal mucosa are the dominant immune determinants.

Oral vaccines have stimulated local immunity in other diseases and, in general, have been nonreactogenic. A live oral typhoid vaccine has been produced and may be the first of a series of similarly conceived mutant bacterial vaccines. This consists of a mutant strain (Ty 21a) of *Salmonella typhi* that lacks the enzyme, uridine diphosphate (UDP)-galactose-4-epimerase, and contains greatly reduced levels of two other enzymes involved in galactose metabolism (Germanier and Fürer, 1975). Consequently, immunogenic lipopolysaccharides that act as antigens are synthesized in amounts insufficient to maintain cell wall integrity. More importantly, galactose-1-phosphate and UDP-galactose accumulate. These events result in bacterial lysis. Thus, the vaccine is quite antigenic but the organism has limited viability in man due to its autodestructive nature. The Ty 21a mutant is stable and reversion to wild type has not been observed in laboratory or field trials.

In the first clinical trial of the Ty 21a vaccine, it was 87% effective in protecting vaccinees challenged with virulent typhoid bacilli five to nine weeks after immunization (Gilman et al, 1977). Excretion of *S. typhi* Ty 21a was not observed after the third day, there was no evidence of reversion to the wild type, and significantly fewer virulent *S. typhi* bacilli (emanating from the challenge dose) were excreted in the feces. Three-year results of field trials in an endemic area indicated a protection rate of 95% (Wahdan et al, 1982). Fecal IgA antibodies to *S. typhi* antigens were observed in volunteers 25 days after vaccine administration; however, these antibodies were not present at 24 months. It has been suggested that IgA does not remain in the enteric tract for long periods if the specific antigens do not persist there (Cancellieri and Fara, 1985).

Subsequent trials conducted in a highly endemic area of Chile showed varying levels of efficacy (0% to 70%), perhaps related to the formulation used to protect the vaccine from gastric acid. Studies on vaccine formulation are continuing.

Adverse reactions observed with live oral typhoid vaccine are minimal and include vomiting, nausea, abdominal pain, and fever.

> This investigational vaccine is made by the Swiss Serum and Vaccine Institute in Bern, Switzerland, and is licensed in Switzerland and in several European and South American countries. A license application has been submitted in the United States.

VARICELLA-ZOSTER VACCINE LIVE ATTENUATED

Although a number of live varicella vaccines have been developed, the attenuated vaccine derived from the Oka strain has been most widely tested and is considered to be the leading candidate for development. The Oka strain was originally isolated in 1974 in Japan from a child with varicella. It was attenuated by passage at 34 C on human embryo fibroblasts, followed by passages at 37 C in cell cultures of guinea pig embryo cells and human diploid (WI-38) cells. Studies performed in Japan on normal and immunocompromised children and children with leukemia in remission or with solid tumors demonstrated that the vaccine was well tolerated, immunogenic, and protective against natural varicella infection.

A double-blind, placebo-controlled trial of attenuated Oka vaccine was conducted on 956 children 1 to 14 years old with a negative history of varicella. The vaccine was well tolerated and produced few adverse reactions in the 468 children who received it, and there was no clinical evidence of viral spread. Seroconversion was observed in 94% of vaccinated children. During a nine-month surveillance period, no vaccinated child developed varicella, whereas 39 cases occurred in placebo recipients; thus, within the limits of the study, the vaccine appeared to be 100% effective (Weibel et al, 1984).

The safety and efficacy of Oka vaccine has also been investigated in children with leukemia in remission. In a study involving 191 children (mean age 6 years), there was serologic evidence of immunogenicity after one dose in about 80% of recipients and after two doses in more than 90%. The major adverse effect was a mild rash, which occurred in 36% of recipients after the first dose and in 14% after the second dose. Those with rash were more likely to transmit vaccine virus to others. The vaccine was considered to be about 80% effective in preventing clinical varicella in these leukemic children and completely effective in preventing severe varicella (Gershon et al, 1984).

Zoster has occurred rarely in recipients of live varicella vaccine. Only two cases of zoster were found in 4,000 or more recipients of the attenuated Oka vaccine in Japan. In the United States, one case of vaccine-induced zoster occurred in a child with acute lymphocytic leukemia nearly two years after administration of the vaccine (Williams et al, 1985). Fortunately, both the vaccine virus and strains isolated from vaccinated patients with malignancies who developed either varicella or zoster are as susceptible to acyclovir as wild type viruses (Shiraki et al, 1984).

Immune Globulin

CYTOMEGALOVIRUS IMMUNE GLOBULIN

Cytomegalovirus (CMV) infection is a significant hazard for recipients of renal, bone marrow, or cardiac allografts. It is the major viral pathogen encountered in renal transplant recipients. Current therapy with antiviral agents, such as vidarabine and acyclovir, in immunosuppressed patients has not been successful. Attempts at active immunization with CMV vaccine have also been disappointing. Another approach being evaluated is passive immunization with specific antibody. A method was devised to extract CMV immune globulin from selected normal donor blood and concentrate specific antibody about twentyfold (Zaia et al, 1979). A CMV immune globulin preparation suitable for intravenous administration has also been prepared; it was found to be safe and to raise CMV serum antibody titers significantly (Snydman et al, 1984).

In one study, CMV immune globulin given intramuscularly significantly reduced the number of infections in seronegative marrow transplant recipients who did not receive granulocyte transfusions compared to untreated controls. However, no protection was observed in patients who received granulocytes from seropositive donors, presumably because exogenous antibody was not effective against intracellular virus in the donor preparations (Meyers et al, 1983). Seven renal transplant recipients with severe CMV infection were treated with anti-CMV antibody; six received fractionated hyperimmune anti-CMV immune globulin. The immune globulin preparation was administered both intraperitoneally and by slow subcutaneous infusion. Five patients had complete and sustained responses within one day of antibody therapy. No adverse reactions were observed (Nicholls et al, 1983).

These studies suggest that CMV immune globulin may prevent CMV disease in transplant patients. It also may be useful in other groups, such as newborn infants and patients exposed to large quantities of leukocytes during whole blood transfusions. Passive immunization with CMV immune globulin circumvents the theoretical problem posed by the oncogenic potential of CMV vaccine, and, therefore, may be the preferred immunization procedure.

Cited References

Pertussis vaccine. *Br Med J* 282:1563-1564, 1981.

Abe T, et al: Clinical effect of intravenous immunoglobulin in chronic idiopathic thrombocytopenic purpura. *Blut* 47:69-75, 1983.

American Academy of Pediatrics: *Report of the Committee on Infectious Diseases*, ed 19. Evanston, IL, American Academy of Pediatrics, 1982.

AMA Ad Hoc Panel on Pertussis Vaccine Injury: Pertussis vaccine injury. *JAMA* 254:3083-3084, 1985.

Ammann AJ, et al: Polyvalent pneumococcal-polysaccharide immunization of patients with sickle-cell anemia and patients with splenectomy. *N Engl J Med* 297:897-900, 1977.

Bolan G, et al: Pneumococcal vaccine efficacy in selected populations in the United States. *Ann Intern Med* 104:1-6, 1986.

Broome CV, et al: Pneumococcal disease after pneumococcal vaccination: Alternative method to estimate efficacy of pneumococcal vaccine. *N Engl J Med* 303:549-552, 1980.

Bussel JB, et al: Intravenous gammaglobulin for chronic idiopathic thrombocytopenic purpura. *Blood* 62:480-486, 1983.

Cancellieri V, Fara GM: Demonstration of specific IgA in human feces after immunization with live Ty 21a *Salmonella typhi* vaccine. *J Infect Dis* 151:482-484, 1985.

Carroll RR, et al: Intravenous immunoglobulin administration in treatment of severe chronic immune thrombocytopenic purpura. *Am J Med* 76:181-186, 1984.

Davidson M, Krugman S: Immunogenicity of recombinant yeast hepatitis B vaccine. *Lancet* 1:108-109, 1985.

Fath JJ, Cerra FB: Therapy of anaphylactic shock. *Drug Intell Clin Pharm* 18:14-21, 1984.

Furusho K, et al: High-dose intravenous gammaglobulin for Kawasaki disease. *Lancet* 2:1055-1058, 1984.

Germanier R, Fürer E: Isolation and characterization of Gal E mutant Ty 21a of *Salmonella typhi*: Candidate strain for live, oral typhoid vaccine. *J Infect Dis* 131:553-558, 1975.

Gershon AA, et al: Live attenuated varicella vaccine: Efficacy for children with leukemia in remission. *JAMA* 252:355-362, 1984.

Gilman RH, et al: Evaluation of UDP-glucose-4-epimeraseless mutant of *Salmonella typhi* as live oral vaccine. *J Infect Dis* 136:717-723, 1977.

Granoff DM, et al: Immunogenicity of *Haemophilus influenzae* type b polysaccharide-diphtheria toxoid conjugate vaccine in adults. *J Pediatr* 105:22-27, 1984.

Health and Public Policy Committee, American College of Physicians: Pneumococcal vaccine. *Ann Intern Med* 104:118-120, 1986.

Herman JJ, et al: Allergic reactions to measles (rubeola) vaccine in patients hypersensitive to egg protein. *J Pediatr* 102:196-198, 1983.

Imbach P, et al: High dose intravenous gammaglobulin for idiopathic thrombocytopenic purpura in childhood. *Lancet* 2:1228, 1981.

Immunization Practices Advisory Committee: Inactivated hepatitis B virus vaccine. *Ann Intern Med* 97:379-383, 1982.

Immunization Practices Advisory Committee (ACIP): General recommendations on immunization. *Morbid Mortal Week Rep* 32:1-17, 1983.

Immunization Practices Advisory Committee (ACIP): Supplementary statement of contraindications to receipt of pertussis vaccine. *Morbid Mortal Week Rep* 33:169-171, 1984 A.

Immunization Practices Advisory Committee (ACIP): Rabies prevention—United States, 1984. *Morbid Mortal Week Rep* 33:393-402, 408, 1984 B.

Immunization Practices Advisory Committee (ACIP): Prevention and control of influenza. *Morbid Mortal Week Rep* 33:253-266, 1984 C.

Immunization Practices Advisory Committee (ACIP): Update: Pneumococcal polysaccharide vaccine usage—United States. *Morbid Mortal Week Rep* 33:273-281, 1984 D.

Immunization Practices Advisory Committee (ACIP): Varicella-zoster immune globulin for prevention of chickenpox. *Morbid Mortal Week Rep* 33:84-100, 1984 E.

Immunization Practices Advisory Committee (ACIP): Diphtheria, tetanus, and pertussis: Guidelines for vaccine prophylaxis and other preventive measures. *Morbid Mortal Week Rep* 34:405-426, 1985 A.

Immunization Practices Advisory Committee (ACIP): Recommendations for protection against viral hepatitis. *Morbid Mortal Week Rep* 34:313-335, 1985 B.

Ippoliti G, et al: High-dose intravenous gammaglobulin for myasthenia gravis, (letter). *Lancet* 2:809-810, 1984.

Jilg W, et al: Clinical evaluation of recombinant hepatitis B vaccine. *Lancet* 2:1174-1175, 1984.

Lane JM, Miller JD: Risks of smallpox vaccination complications in the United States. *Am J Epidemiol* 93:238-240, 1971.

Lepow ML, et al: Safety and immunogenicity of *Haemophilus influenzae* type b polysaccharide-diphtheria toxoid conjugate vaccine in adults. *J Infect Dis* 150:402-406, 1984.

Lepow ML, et al: Safety and immunogenicity of *Haemophilus influenzae* type b polysaccharide-diphtheria conjugate vaccine in infants 9 to 15 months of age. *J Pediatr* 106:185-189, 1985.

Lucke WC, Thomas H Jr: Anaphylaxis: Pathophysiology, clinical presentations and treatment. *J Emerg Med* 1:83-95, 1983.

McAleer WJ, et al: Human hepatitis B vaccine from recombinant yeast. *Nature* 307:178-180, 1984.

Meyers JD, et al: Prevention of cytomegalovirus infection by cytomegalovirus immune globulin after marrow transplantation. *Ann Intern Med* 98:442-446, 1983.

Newland AC, et al: High-dose intravenous IgG in adults with autoimmune thrombocytopenia. *Lancet* 1:84-87, 1983.

Nicholls AJ, et al: Hyperimmune immunoglobulin for cytomegalovirus infections, (letter). *Lancet* 1:532-533, 1983.

Oral A, et al: Intravenous gamma globulin in treatment of chronic idiopathic thrombocytopenic purpura in adults. *Am J Med* 76:187-192, 1984.

Papaevangelou G, et al: Immunogenicity of recombinant hepatitis B vaccine, (letter). *Lancet* 1:455-456, 1985.

Pappaioanou M, et al: Antibody response to preexposure human diploid-cell rabies vaccine given concurrently with chloroquine. *N Engl J Med* 314:280-284, 1986.

Patriarca PA. et al: Efficacy of influenza vaccine in nursing homes: Reduction in illness and complications during influenzae A (H3N2) epidemic. *JAMA* 253:1136-1139, 1985.

Peltola H, et al: Prevention of *Haemophilus influenzae* type b bacteremic infections with the capsular polysaccharide vaccine. *N Engl J Med* 310:1561-1566, 1984.

Rappolt RT, et al: Medical toxicologist's notebook: Snakebite treatment and international antivenin index. *Clin Toxicol* 13:409-438, 1978.

Redmond SR, Pichichero ME: *Haemophilus influenzae* type b disease: Epidemiologic study with special reference to day-care centers. *JAMA* 252:2581-2584, 1984.

Russell FE: *Snake Venom Poisoning*. Great Neck, NY, Scholium International, 1983.

Scolnick EM, et al: Clinical evaluation in healthy adults of hepatitis B vaccine made by recombinant DNA. *JAMA* 251:2812-2815, 1984.

Shapiro ED, Clemens JD: Controlled evaluation of protective efficacy of pneumococcal vaccine for patients at high risk of serious pneumococcal infections. *Ann Intern Med* 101:325-330, 1984.

Shiraki K, et al: Susceptibility to acyclovir of Oka-strain varicella vaccine and vaccine-derived viruses isolated from immunocompromised patients, (letter). *J Infect Dis* 150:306-307, 1984.

Sisk JE, Riegelman RK: Cost effectiveness of vaccination against pneumococcal pneumonia: Update. *Ann Intern Med* 104:79-86, 1986.

Snydman DR, et al: Pilot trial of novel cytomegalovirus immune globulin in renal transplant recipients. *Transplantation* 38:553-557, 1984.

Sultan Y, et al: Anti-idiotypic suppression of autoantibodies to factor VIII (antihaemophilic factor) by high-dose intravenous gamma-globulin. *Lancet* 2:765-768, 1984.

Valenzuela P, et al: Synthesis and assembly of hepatitis B virus surface antigen particles in yeast. *Nature* 298:347-350, 1982.

Vesikari T, et al: Immunogenicity and safety of live oral attenuated bovine rotavirus vaccine strain RIT 4237 in adults and young children. *Lancet* 2:807-811, 1983.

Vesikari T, et al: Protection of infants against rotavirus diarrhoea by RIT 4237 attenuated bovine rotavirus strain vaccine. *Lancet* 1:977-981, 1984 A.

Vesikari T, et al: Increased "take" rate of oral rotavirus vaccine in infants after milk feeding, (letter). *Lancet* 2:700, 1984 B.

Wahdan MH, et al: Controlled field trial of live *Salmonella typhi* strain Ty 21a oral vaccine against typhoid: Three-year results. *J Infect Dis* 145:292-295, 1982.

Warrier I, Lusher JM: Intravenous gamma globulin treatment for chronic idiopathic thrombocytopenic purpura in children. *Am J Med* 76:193-198, 1984.

Weibel RE, et al: Live attenuated varicella virus vaccine: Efficacy trial in healthy children. *N Engl J Med* 310:1409-1415, 1984.

Weissberg JI, et al: Survival in chronic hepatitis B: Analysis of 379 patients. *Ann Intern Med* 101:613-616, 1984.

Williams DL, et al: Herpes zoster following varicella vaccine in child with acute lymphocytic leukemia. *J Pediatr* 106:259-261, 1985.

Wingert WA, Wainschel J: Diagnosis and management of envenomation by poisonous snakes. *South Med J* 68:1015-1026, 1975.

Zaia JA, et al: Cytomegalovirus immune globulin: Production from selected normal donor blood. *Transplantation* 27:66-67, 1979.

Zimmerman R, et al: Intravenous IgG for patients with spontaneous inhibitor to factor VIII, (letter). *Lancet* 1:273-274, 1985.

Zissis G, et al: Protection studies in colostrum-derived piglets of bovine rotavirus vaccine candidate using human rotavirus strains for challenge. *J Infect Dis* 148:1061-1068, 1983.

Other Selected References

Venomous bites and stings. *J Toxicol Clin Toxicol* 21:417-560, 1983-1984.

Committee on Immunization, American College of Physicians: *Guide for Adult Immunization*. Philadelphia, American College of Physicians, 1985.

Lerner RA, et al (eds): *Vaccines 85: Molecular and Chemical Basis of Resistance to Parasitic, Bacterial, and Viral Diseases*. New York, Cold Spring Harbor Laboratory, 1985.

Immunomodulators

Immunomodulators adjust the immune response to a desired level of activity through the processes of immunosuppression (eg, corticosteroids, cytotoxic drugs, antiserums), induction of tolerance (desensitization), or immunopotentiation (eg, immune globulin replacement therapy).

Exposure to foreign antigen elicits a complex response in which the immune system plays a major role. The sequence of events comprising the immune response can be divided into five stages: (1) uptake and processing of antigen; (2) transfer of information and triggering of effector cells of the immune system; (3) proliferation, differentiation, and maturation of involved lymphocytes; (4) synthesis and release of mediator substances and antibodies; and (5) responses to mediators, antibodies, and effector cells.

It is theoretically possible to regulate the immune response at each of these levels, but most currently used drugs are cytotoxic compounds that were originally tested for use in cancer chemotherapy and act by interfering with production of involved lymphocytes (stage 3).

Immunosuppression: The immune response can be suppressed by producing tolerance to a specific antigen. Immunologic tolerance is defined as failure of the immune system to respond to a specific antigen after prior exposure to that antigen and is thought to be due to either elimination of responding lymphocyte clones or inhibition of the immune system by regulatory mechanisms. It is possible to produce tolerance to both cell-mediated and humoral immune responses. The nature of the antigen, the amount, and the route of administration influence the degree of tolerance. In general, the greater the immunocompetence of the organism, the more difficult it is to induce tolerance. Nevertheless, irradiation or administration of antilymphocyte globulin followed by exposure to antigen may produce tolerance to specific antigens.

Specific IgE antibody can be suppressed in the allergic patient by repeated administration of specific antigen; the technique produces a "tolerance" to this antigen, which has been referred to as allergic immunotherapy. It is not known to what extent this "tolerance" is due to suppression of IgE formation or, more likely, to induction of IgG molecules that compete with IgE for the allergen. Desensitization to insect venom, for example, is an important immunotherapeutic measure for sensitive individuals who may respond to bee stings with anaphylaxis.

Injection of antibodies produced elsewhere and passively transferred can inhibit or suppress specific antibody production by a negative feedback mechanism or by masking the antigen with the exogenous antiserum. Thus, if anti-Rh_o antibody is given to an Rh-negative mother at the time of delivery of her Rh-positive child, sensitization and anti-Rh_o antibody production can be avoided.

Immunosuppressive agents inhibit immune responses. Their action is usually nonspecific, but some agents have a degree of specificity. For example, antilymphocyte serum suppresses T-lymphocyte activity more than B-lymphocyte activity, and cyclosporine [Sandimmune] inhibits the T-helper/inducer subset without affecting expression of the preformed T-suppressor/cytotoxic subset or B-lymphocyte function. Some nonspecific suppressants, such as methotrexate [Folex, Mexate], are cell cycle specific; others, like cyclophosphamide [Cytoxan, Neosar], are not specific for any phase of the cell cycle. The cellular responses to these agents vary widely. The immunosuppressive action of all nonspecific drugs is obtained only at doses close to toxic levels. (For detailed information about immunosuppressants in cancer chemotherapy, see Chapter 64.)

Corticosteroid therapy is the mainstay in the treatment of many immune diseases. Corticosteroids and cyclosporine have a wider margin of safety than the cytotoxic drugs. Combination therapy with a corticosteroid and the immunosuppressants, azathioprine [Imuran] and cyclosporine, is used to suppress allograft rejection.

The cytotoxic drugs, cyclophosphamide, chlorambucil [Leukeran], and methotrexate, are effective antineoplastic agents, especially when used in a large dose, pulsed regimen: The larger doses enhance neoplastic cytotoxicity and pulsed therapy permits recovery of the immune response. Conversely, smaller doses of these drugs are effective in conventional regimens to maintain immunosuppression with minimal toxicity. In view of their considerable potential toxicity, antineoplastic drugs usually are reserved for autoimmune, immune complex, or granulomatous diseases and vasculitides that do not respond adequately to corticosteroid therapy.

Two factors that determine a cytotoxic drug's ability to reduce a population of immunoreactive cells are the cell cycle specificity of the agent and the proliferative status of the target cell. The former refers to the phase of the mitotic cycle in which the drug exerts its effect; the latter refers to the phase of the mitotic cycle of the target cells. Cytotoxic agents can be classified as: (1) *Phase-specific drugs*, which are toxic only during a specific phase of the mitotic cycle. Examples include azathioprine, cytarabine, mercaptopurine, and methotrexate, all of which are primarily S phase (stage of DNA synthesis) inhibitors. (2) *Cycle-specific drugs* (eg, cyclophosphamide), which affect both intermitotic and cycling cells, although there is preferential toxicity for proliferating cells. (3) *Cycle-nonspecific drugs* (eg, mechlorethamine), which are toxic to both intermitotic and proliferating cells.

Prior to antigen challenge, lymphocytes are predominantly in the intermitotic phase; after contact with antigen, they actively proliferate. Cycle-nonspecific drugs are most inhibitory when given just prior to antigen challenge. Phase-specific drugs are only active when cells are replicating (after antigen challenge). Cycle-specific drugs are effective before and after antigen challenge. (See Table 1.)

Suppression of Allograft Rejection: The most common rejection response to a histoincompatible kidney, marrow, liver, or heart graft is the development of cytotoxic T-lymphocytes. Monocytes and B-lymphocytes also play a role; the latter are

TABLE 1.
SUMMARY OF USES OF CYTOTOXIC IMMUNOSUPPRESSIVE DRUGS

DISORDERS IN WHICH CYTOTOXIC DRUGS ARE PROBABLY CLINICALLY BENEFICIAL:

Rheumatoid arthritis
Systemic lupus erythematosus
Lipoid nephrosis
Wegener's granulomatosis
Chronic active hepatitis
Inflammatory bowel disease
Autoimmune hemolytic anemia
Immune thrombocytopenia
Circulating anticoagulants
Systemic necrotizing vasculitis
Goodpasture's syndrome

Adapted from Webb and Winkelstein, 1984.

especially prominent during accelerated or "white graft" rejection. Corticosteroids are indispensable to attenuate rejection episodes. Lymphocyte immune globulin seems to be useful in allotransplantation because it markedly suppresses T-lymphocyte mediated immune responses.

The immunosuppressive agent, cyclosporine, has shown great promise in suppressing allograft rejection. This potent drug prolonged the survival of allografts and even xenografts in laboratory animals. Heart, lung, kidney, pancreas, liver, skin, muscle, nerve cells, bone marrow, small intestine, cornea, islets of Langerhans, ovaries, and fallopian tubes have been transplanted successfully in cyclosporine-treated animals. In man, cyclosporine has greatly improved the success of transplantation and is the drug of choice for maintenance of heart and liver allografts. However, in kidney transplants from living, related donors, some clinicians have been quite satisfied with graft and patient survival in those receiving azathioprine and steroids.

Cyclosporine selectively suppresses T-lymphocyte functions without producing myelosuppression. In vitro, the growth of bone marrow-derived myeloid, erythroid, or B-lymphocyte cell lines is not inhibited. Cyclosporine suppresses primary and, to a lesser degree, secondary antibody responses to T-cell-*dependent* antigens and is a potent inhibitor of delayed hypersensitivity. B-lymphocyte responses to T-cell-independent antigens or similar activators are not affected. This agent depletes medullary thymocytes and splenic T-lymphocytes. The number and function of T-helper/inducer lymphocytes are impaired selectively; cyclosporine reversibly inhibits the initial macrophage T-lymphocyte activation and impairs the production of interleukin-2, a growth factor essential for T-cell proliferation and differentiation into cytotoxic T-cells. The drug acts principally during the G0-G1 phase of the T-cell cycle and thus does not inhibit mature, proliferating T-cells. The inhibition of antibody production to T-cell-dependent antigens is a consequence of impaired T-helper cell function, which is required for B-cell growth and differentiation. There is a relative sparing of T-suppressor cells, for the production of suppressor cell-inducing lymphokines by T-helper cells does not seem to be inhibited; thus, there may be a selective expansion of T-suppressor cell populations. Suppressor cells appear to be important in maintaining an unresponsive state to allografts. The function of human natural killer (NK) cells does not seem to be affected by therapeutic concentrations of cyclosporine.

For optimal suppression of T-cell function, cyclosporine must be present in the early phase of the immune response; maximum suppression occurs during the first 24 hours of antigen stimulation. The critical period is during induction of the immune response against the allograft, since T-cells already primed by antigen are resistant to cyclosporine. (For reviews of cyclosporine, see Cohen et al, 1984; Bendtzen, 1984; and Ptachcinski et al, 1985 A.)

For a discussion of the serious adverse effects that limit use of cyclosporine, see the evaluation.

Immunologic Augmentation: It is possible to reconstitute a deficient immune system by transplanting bone marrow and thymus tissue, but these techniques are not in widespread clinical use. Immune globulin also augments the immune response. Transfer factor, a dialyzable extract of immune lymphocytes, has been investigated as a method of transferring cell-mediated immunity in humans. (See the evaluation in the section on Miscellaneous Investigational Agents.)

Some agents amplify the production of antibodies. These adjuvants are administered with antigen to increase the immune response to that antigen. Aluminum phosphate is an example of a specific immunostimulant of this type; when added to tetanus toxoid, this mineral salt markedly enhances the ability of the toxoid to stimulate antibody production. Other methods employed experimentally in animals to enhance antibody production include (1) use of antigen with water-in-oil emulsions containing killed mycobacteria (complete Freund's adjuvant) or without mycobacteria (incomplete Freund's adjuvant), and (2) use of synthetic polynucleotides and bacterial endotoxins.

The exact mechanisms of action of these techniques are obscure, but some facts are apparent. Mineral salts provoke granulomas at the site of injection, which stimulates macrophage activity and slows antigen absorption. Freund's adjuvant markedly slows antigen absorption and increases dispersal while stimulating T-cell activity. Endotoxins stimulate DNA synthesis in B-lymphocytes. Cellular actions of the adjuvants are being investigated.

Immunologic Replacement: There is currently no synthetic drug to treat immunodeficiency diseases, but various forms of immunotherapy are available and some may even have a curative effect on the underlying disease. Marrow transplant has been beneficial in marrow failure and other immunodeficiencies. Thymic hormones have been administered in an attempt to stimulate the immune system in very young and very old patients. The usefulness of bone marrow or thymus transplantation is limited by the availability of appropriate donors. Nevertheless, they do offer a therapeutic avenue of approach.

When there is a deficiency in the immune system, replacement with immune globulin (gamma globulin) sometimes has been helpful. Immune globulin is derived from human plasma and contains most of the antibodies found in whole blood. The preparation consists primarily of IgG with lesser amounts of IgM. Since IgA, found mostly in mucosal surfaces, is not present in significant amounts in these preparations, immune globulin cannot be used for IgA deficiency. It is administered most commonly for the prevention of measles and hepatitis A and for replacement therapy in agammaglobulinemia. Its recommended use for the treatment of immunodeficient conditions is shown in Table 2. Specific immune globulin is preferred for prophylaxis after exposure (see Chapter 62, Agents for Active and Passive Immunity).

Interleukin-2, interferon, and transfer factor, which are products of the immune system, show some promise for stimulating immunity. The anthelmintic, levamisole (investigational drug), appears to improve the function of an intact but depressed immune system, but no effect has been demonstrated on the normal system.

Plasmapheresis: In recent years, plasmapheresis has been used to manage immunopathologic diseases, such as myasthenia gravis, some types of hepatitis, and rheumatic, autoimmune, and immune complex diseases. The clinical usefulness of this technique has been demonstrated in a limited number of conditions, including myasthenia gravis, Goodpasture's syndrome, and thrombotic thrombocytopenia purpura. Its usefulness in systemic lupus erythematosus is quite controversial.

In plasmapheresis, dialysis equipment can remove 6 to 8 L of plasma in two to four hours and exchange this with reconstituted plasma, albumin, or purified plasma protein fraction. Theoretically, plasmapheresis will remove specific autoantibodies; nonspecific inflammatory mediators, such as complement or fibrinogen; and immune complexes. However, the technique is costly, there are no prospective controlled

TABLE 2.
TREATMENT OF IMMUNODEFICIENCY WITH IMMUNE GLOBULIN (GAMMA GLOBULIN)

B-CELL DISORDERS (intramuscular or intravenous preparations may be used)

   Acquired hypogammaglobulinemia
   Secondary hypogammaglobulinemia when associated with infection
   X-linked hypogammaglobulinemia

   Do NOT use in selective IgA deficiency.

T-CELL DISORDERS (intramuscular or intravenous preparations may be used)

   Use only when an antibody response has been demonstrated to be absent (intravenous preparation may be given).

   Wiskott-Aldrich syndrome (intramuscular preparation is not recommended)

PHAGOCYTIC DISORDERS

   Not recommended

COMPLEMENT DISORDERS

   Not recommended

Adapted from Ammann, 1984.

studies, and the side effects are unknown. Thus, plasmapheresis is considered an investigational technique. (See Chapter 35, Blood, Blood Components, and Blood Substitutes.)

ADVERSE REACTIONS AND PRECAUTIONS

Reactions peculiar to each drug are discussed in the evaluations, but certain general statements can be made. Suppression of bone marrow by cytotoxic agents inhibits the function of phagocytes, neutrophils, and, to a lesser degree, monocytes. Suppression of these final effector cells increases the risk of overwhelming infection. The more subtle forms of a drug's ability to inhibit immunoinflammatory responses emerge clinically as infection with unusual pathogens, such as *Pneumocystis carinii, Listeria monocytogenes,* cytomegalovirus, or *Toxoplasma gondii*. More common is gram-negative bacteremia or *Streptococcus pneumoniae* infection.

Although the risk of infection in a compromised host is well appreciated, the risk of neoplasia in patients undergoing immunomodulator therapy is less clear but of great importance. The incidence of neoplasia is higher in patients with renal and heart transplants. This may represent a complex situation involving multiple immunosuppressive agents and the stimulatory presence of a foreign graft. Data exist concerning the emergence of tumors in patients treated with low-dose, immunosuppressive, cytotoxic therapy. Reports of highly malignant lymphomas predominate, but solid tumors in young patients also have been described. The confounding variable is that the diseases being treated cause abnormal immune responses and, on that basis alone, are associated with a high risk of neoplasia.

Alkylating agents produce oligospermia and sometimes permanent azoospermia. To assure future childbearing potential, males should be informed that cryogenic storage of spermatozoa prior to the initiation of therapy is available.

The use of any immunomodulator entails both theoretical and actual risks to the patient. The risk/benefit ratio should be determined and informed consent should be obtained.

Drug Evaluations

ANTI-INFLAMMATORY AGENTS

GLUCOCORTICOIDS

ACTIONS. Corticosteroids have broad effects on both immune and inflammatory processes. Human lymphocytes are relatively resistant to lysis by corticosteroids and effects are not based on the cytotoxicity of these agents. Upon immune activation, however, human lymphocytes become more sensitive and lysis of antigen-activated lymphocytes may occur in the presence of glucocorticoids during treatment for graft rejection. There is evidence that proliferating lymphocytes are sensitive to steroids, but become resistant after reaching the effector stage. Except at extremely high doses, the cytotoxic process is not inhibited by corticosteroids unless they are added during the early sensitization phase of cytotoxic cells.

Normal human lymphocytes, monocytes, neutrophils, and eosinophils contain specific glucocorticoid receptors. Although heterogeneity of receptors has been reported for different lymphocyte populations, a functional significance for this variability has not been established, except in preliminary studies suggesting that production of lymphokines, such as interleukin-2 (IL-2) and macrophage mitogenic factor, may be receptor-mediated.

Corticosteroids markedly alter lymphocyte traffic and induce peripheral blood lymphopenia. Lymphocytopenia is more pronounced for T-cells; it does not appear to result from selective depression of T-subsets (Schuyler et al, 1984), but rather from redirection of normal lymphocyte traffic. B-cells are less affected. B-cells have been reported to metabolize cortisol more rapidly than T-cells, which suggests a mechanism for their increased resistance (Klein et al, 1980). Lymphocytes tend to sequester within lymph nodes and bone marrow, but total body lymphocyte mass is probably not decreased. The rapid sequestration of lymphocytes in the extravascular pool probably protects allografts from invasion by cytotoxic T-lymphocytes.

Although other circulating leukocytes decrease in number or remain relatively unchanged, the number and proportion of neutrophils increase temporarily. This increase has been attributed to release of mature neutrophils from the bone marrow coupled with decreased egress from the blood. The latter accounts for failure of neutrophils and leukocytes to accumulate at inflamed sites.

Production of IL-1 by monocytes and IL-2 by lymphocytes is suppressed by glucocorticoids. There is also evidence that corticosteroids render IL-2-producing T-cells unresponsive to IL-1. The bactericidal activity of monocytes is reduced substantially in patients receiving glucocorticoids; delayed skin test reactivity also is reduced. T-lymphocyte responses to mitogens and antigens are suppressed by these agents. Suppressor cells that spontaneously appear in vivo also are inhibited by glucocorticoids, although studies have indicated that suppressor cells are resistant in vitro. Serum IgG, IgA, and, to a lesser degree, IgM are suppressed by glucocorticoids; maximal suppression occurs two to four weeks after administration. Serum IgE levels appear to be minimally affected, but late-phase components of immediate hypersensitivity are altered. Thus, some B-cell responses are affected but it is not known whether the effect is direct or mediated through some other component of the immune system.

Glucocorticoids do not inhibit the release of histamine or protect against histamine shock.

See also Chapter 61, Adrenal Corticosteroids in Nonendocrine Diseases.

USES. A wide variety of immunologically mediated diseases have been treated with glucocorticoids: connective tissue diseases (eg, systemic lupus erythematosus, rheumatoid arthritis), severe asthma, vasculitides, granulomatous diseases, autoimmune hemolytic anemia, and organ transplant rejection. Chronic disease may require prolonged use of suppressive doses and careful consideration must be given to the selection of a therapeutic regimen. Choice will depend on the severity of the disorder, the anticipated dose and duration of therapy, presence of factors predisposing to complications, and alternative modes of therapy to reduce glucocorticoid requirements. In most patients, a shorter acting drug, eg, prednisone, is preferred since it can be used in a manner that closely resembles the diurnal cortisol cycle.

ADVERSE REACTIONS AND PRECAUTIONS. See Chapter 61.

DOSAGE AND PREPARATIONS.

Oral, Parenteral: Prednisone 1 to 2 mg/kg (or the equivalent) provides tissue and serum concentrations with lymphoid, neutrophil, and monocyte effects. Doses higher than 2 mg/kg probably do not increase the therapeutic effect but do increase drug-related morbidity.

A common regimen employs a single morning dose of prednisone. The lowest dose should be given in the least toxic interval that is sufficient to control the disease. However, for active diseases, a dose sufficient to produce remission should be employed (eg, 1 mg/kg/day of prednisone in up to three divided doses). The dose is then adjusted until the lowest effective amount is determined; the patient then can be converted to alternate-day therapy until the drug can be discontinued.

In acute necrotizing inflammatory states, morning administration or divided daily doses are preferred to an alternate-day regimen when starting therapy. Once the disease or inflammatory condition is relatively stable, persistent attempts should be made to give the steroid on alternate days, since this reduces most adverse effects.

Many schedules have been tried. A popular one is calculating the alternate-day dose as double the daily dosage. The dose also can be reduced gradually on alternate days. When severe drug reactions occur or erythema multiforme syndromes involving mucous membranes are being treated, intravenous administration is preferred because severe gastrointestinal mucosal loss may impair absorption.

For preparations, see Chapters 37 and 61.

NONSTEROIDAL ANTI-INFLAMMATORY AGENTS

ACTIONS. Salicylates suppress inflammation nonspecifically by inhibiting prostaglandin synthesis. However, under certain circumstances, as in individuals sensitive to aspirin, salicylates may actually enhance the release of prostaglandins. They also reduce adhesion of neutrophils to vascular endothelium, alter platelet aggregation, enhance fibrinolysis, and inhibit the activation of kallikrein. Salicylates have a mild immunosuppressive action.

Phenylbutazone [Azolid, Butazolidin] and indomethacin [Indocin] also inhibit prostaglandin synthetase, which interferes with prostaglandin synthesis. They may produce abnormalities in neutrophils that cause defective chemotaxis (phenylbutazone) and reduce platelet aggregation, but usual immunologic parameters are not affected. Changes in the immune response are probably caused by suppression of inflammation. However, unlike glucocorticoids, the anti-inflammatory action of phenylbutazone and indomethacin is nonspecific and does not

increase the propensity to infections, probably because these drugs do not interfere with superoxide production.

For further information, see Chapter 59, Antiarthritic Drugs.

CYTOTOXIC DRUGS

Immunosuppression can be achieved by agents that kill immunologically competent cells. These agents, like those used for cancer chemotherapy, are not selectively toxic for lymphocytes but are capable of killing any cell that can replicate. The activity of cytotoxic drugs may depend upon the phase of the mitotic cycle in which the drug exerts its effect (see the Introduction). Cytotoxic drugs inhibit both B-cell and T-cell responses, but they do not inhibit all immune responses equally. The primary immune response is more readily inhibited than a secondary one; drugs that are effective in an unsensitized situation may have little or no effect in a sensitized system.

Cytotoxic drugs are often used to treat autoimmune disorders. Their generalized cytotoxicity is a hazard, particularly to rapidly dividing cells of the bone marrow.

The undesired effects of cytotoxic immunosuppressive drugs include bone marrow suppression with neutropenia, thrombocytopenia, and anemia; gastrointestinal disturbances; sterility; infections resulting from generalized suppression of immune responses; and increased risk of malignancies, especially lymphoma.

AZATHIOPRINE
[Imuran]

AZATHIOPRINE SODIUM
[Imuran]

ACTIONS AND USES. Azathioprine is a derivative of mercaptopurine, to which it is converted rapidly after administration, and has similar biological activity. Mercaptopurine is an S-phase specific compound that acts by competitive enzyme inhibition to inhibit purine biosynthesis and thus decreases the rate of cell replication (see the evaluation on Mercaptopurine in Chapter 64, Drugs Used in Cancer Chemotherapy). Azathioprine suppresses T-cell more than B-cell activity; it has limited anti-inflammatory properties. Clinically, the number of mononuclear and granulocytic cells available for migration to an area of inflammation is decreased. It also inhibits the proliferation of promyelocytes within bone marrow, thus decreasing the number of circulating monocytes available to become macrophages in the peripheral blood.

Azathioprine exerts its maximum immunosuppressive effect when given immediately after immunologic challenge (induction phase). When given prior to antigen challenge (preinduction phase), it may augment antibody response in specific immunoglobulin classes. Azathioprine is not effective when given in the effector phase (proliferation and maturation phases). Therefore, the compound has no effect on established graft rejections or secondary responses.

Azathioprine has been used extensively in allotransplantation procedures; it also has been administered in systemic lupus erythematosus, rheumatoid arthritis, polymyositis, Crohn's disease, and other collagen, vascular, and systemic inflammatory states. It is at least as effective as the alkylating agents and is less toxic. Usual daily doses do not have pronounced effects on immunologic responses per se. A clinical response is not noted for two to four weeks.

ADVERSE REACTIONS AND PRECAUTIONS. The frequency and severity of adverse effects depend on the dose and duration of administration and on any underlying disease or concomitant therapy. Toxic effects on the gastrointestinal tract and hematologic systems are most common. In addition, the risk of secondary infection and neoplasia is increased. The incidence of hematologic toxicity, neoplasia, and infection is significantly higher in renal homotransplantation than in rheumatoid arthritis (eg, infection rate is 50 to 60 times higher in renal transplant patients). The high incidence of toxicity following renal transplantation may be due to the accumulation of metabolites normally eliminated by the kidney.

Bone marrow depression is uncommon with conventional doses of azathioprine, but is a possibility with larger doses. Hematologic toxicity is usually limited to mild leukopenia and thrombocytopenia. A limited number of cases of acute idiosyncratic aplastic anemia has occurred shortly after initiation of therapy or suddenly during a previously stable course.

Nausea, vomiting, and gastrointestinal discomfort are common during the first few months of azathioprine therapy and usually respond to dosage adjustment. Enzyme changes characteristic of hepatocellular necrosis and cholestasis may occur relatively early (one or two weeks) but also extremely late (years) during treatment and usually require discontinuing the drug. If administration must be continued, close observation is essential, since deaths from hepatic decompensation have occurred. Pancreatitis and hypersensitivity-type interstitial pneumonitis have been reported occasionally.

Other uncommon adverse effects are skin rash, alopecia, fever, arthralgia, steatorrhea, and negative nitrogen balance.

Since severe leukopenia and/or thrombocytopenia may develop in patients receiving azathioprine, complete blood and platelet counts should be performed at regular intervals. Prompt reduction in dosage or withdrawal of the drug may be necessary if there is evidence of serious bone marrow depression.

Azathioprine is carcinogenic in animals and is associated with increased risk of neoplasia in transplant patients. There may be a prohibitive risk of neoplasia in patients with rheumatoid arthritis who have been treated with alkylating agents.

Azathioprine is mutagenic and teratogenic in laboratory animals and transplacental transmission of drug and metabolites has been reported in man. Therefore, risk versus benefit should be assessed carefully before administering azathioprine to pregnant patients and, whenever possible, its use should be avoided. It is not recommended for treating arthritis in pregnant women.

DRUG INTERACTIONS. Because allopurinol inhibits xanthine oxidase, the enzyme required for 6-mercaptopurine metabolism, the dose of azathioprine should be reduced to one-third or one-fourth the usual maintenance amount in patients taking this drug concomitantly. Drugs known to induce (phenytoin, phenobarbital, rifampin) or inhibit (ketoconazole, erythromycin) hepatic microsomal enzymes may alter the clearance of azathioprine.

PHARMACOKINETICS. Oral azathioprine is efficiently absorbed. After oral administration of 35-S-azathioprine, maximum serum radioactivity occurs at one to two hours and the half-life is five hours (decay rate for all 35-S-containing metabolites).

Azathioprine is cleaved in vivo to mercaptopurine, which is then catabolized to various oxidized and methylated derivatives, including 6-thiouric acid, the major metabolite. The latter is formed after oxidation of mercaptopurine by xanthine oxidase in the liver. About 10% of azathioprine is cleaved between the sulfur and purine ring to form 1-methyl-4-nitro-5-thioimidazole. Proportions of metabolites differ in individual patients, which may account for variability in drug effects.

Azathioprine is mainly eliminated by metabolic degradation. Small amounts of unchanged drug and mercaptopurine are eliminated by the kidney. Following oral administration, no azathioprine or mercaptopurine is detectable in the urine after eight hours.

Mercaptopurine derived from the metabolism of azathioprine is widely distributed in body tissues, but only a small percentage enters the cerebrospinal fluid. About 30% of both azathioprine and mercaptopurine is bound to serum protein. Usual doses of azathioprine produce low blood levels (less than 1 mcg/ml) of both the foregoing compounds and both quickly leave the circulation. Neither the magnitude nor the duration of the clinical response can be predicted from the blood levels, since these correlate with thiopurine nucleotide levels in tissues rather than in blood. The effects of azathioprine may persist long after clearance is complete.

DOSAGE AND PREPARATIONS. Azathioprine is a potent immunosuppressive agent and should be used under the direction of a physician familiar with the risk associated with this type of therapy. The patient should be evaluated carefully and monitored adequately during treatment.

Oral, Intravenous: For allotransplantation, initially, 3 to 5 mg/kg/day as a single dose beginning on the day of transplant. For maintenance, 1 to 3 mg/kg/day. Intravenous administration is used in patients who are unable to tolerate oral medication; the oral form is substituted as soon as possible.

AZATHIOPRINE:
Imuran (Burroughs Wellcome). Tablets 50 mg.
AZATHIOPRINE SODIUM:
Imuran (Burroughs Wellcome). Powder (lyophilized, sterile) equivalent to azathioprine 100 mg.

CHLORAMBUCIL
[Leukeran]

This bifunctional alkylating agent has not been used extensively for immunosuppression in the United States. Behcet's syndrome, systemic lupus erythematosus, and Wegener's granulomatosis have been reported to respond to low doses of chlorambucil. In one controlled trial, a chlorambucil/methylprednisolone regimen was reported to be effective for the treatment of idiopathic membranous nephropathy (Ponticelli et al, 1984).

Chlorambucil is a slow-acting nitrogen mustard that is cell cycle nonspecific but has a marked lympholytic effect. The induction time for an immunologic effect is longer than for cyclophosphamide, but serious hematologic depression appears to occur less frequently and urinary excretion is not impaired. Chlorambucil is a very potent alkylator and is carcinogenic in humans. It can produce infertility and is probably mutagenic and teratogenic in humans (Pregnancy Category D). It should not be used as an immunosuppressive agent except in life-threatening disease.

See also Chapter 64, Drugs Used in Cancer Chemotherapy, for a more detailed discussion.

DOSAGE AND PREPARATIONS.
Oral: 0.05 to 0.1 mg/kg daily.
   Leukeran (Burroughs Wellcome). Tablets 2 mg.

CYCLOPHOSPHAMIDE
[Cytoxan, Neosar]

ACTIONS AND USES. Cyclophosphamide is an alkylating agent of the cyclic mustard group. It is a prodrug that requires metabolic activation by liver enzymes before it can alkylate cellular substances. It has greater effect on the B-cell lymphocytes than on the T-cell lymphocytes. A possible mechanism of immunosuppression is direct cytotoxicity on immunocompetent lymphocytes, especially those that have undergone antigenic differentiation and division. Cyclophosphamide inhibits an established immune response, which usually is present in patients considered to be candidates for immunomodulatory therapy.

Cyclophosphamide can be given orally and intravenously. It does not cause severe tissue necrosis after inadvertent subcutaneous injection. Oral administration for 7 to 14 days is required before a clinically detectable immunomodulatory effect occurs.

Beneficial effects are most apparent in patients with Wegener's granulomatosis (in which cyclophosphamide is the drug of choice), in selected patients with severe rheumatoid arthritis, in children with nephrotic syndrome who do not respond to steroids or who relapse if steroids are discontinued, and in patients with autoimmune blood disorders, such as idiopathic thrombocytopenic purpura. Its effectiveness in other diseases, such as systemic lupus erythematosus and progressive multiple sclerosis, is being investigated. It has been used prophylactically in patients undergoing bone marrow transplantation.

ADVERSE REACTIONS AND PRECAUTIONS. Cyclophosphamide produces the same adverse effects as other cytotoxic agents, including reversible alopecia, nausea, and vomiting. Life-threatening reactions include bone marrow suppression, acute hemorrhagic cystitis, bladder telangiectasia, and abnormal urinary cytology. Adverse reactions involving the bladder can be minimized by increasing the fluid intake and emptying the bladder prior to sleep. Long-term use is associated with bladder fibrosis and carcinoma. Impaired urinary excretion has been reported with large doses only. Cyclophosphamide should be discontinued if hematuria occurs. Massive urinary bleeding may require supravesicular diversion. Acute myopericarditis, which can be fatal, may occur following large doses of cyclophosphamide given prior to bone marrow transplantation.

When cyclophosphamide therapy is selected for use in young patients, the probability of drug-induced infertility must be considered. Ovulation is inhibited and permanently impaired in 30% to 50% of women after continuous low-dose therapy; aspermia is common after three to six months of therapy. The teratogenic potential of cyclophosphamide appears to be low, but contraception should be encouraged during treatment (FDA Pregnancy Category C).

For other indications, adverse reactions, and dosages, see Chapter 64, Drugs Used in Cancer Chemotherapy.
   Cytoxan (Bristol-Myers). Powder 100, 200, and 500 mg and 1 and 2 g; tablets 25 and 50 mg.
   Neosar (Adria). Powder 100, 200, and 500 mg.

METHOTREXATE

METHOTREXATE SODIUM
[Folex, Mexate]

ACTIONS AND USES. Methotrexate is a phase-specific compound that acts by inhibiting folate metabolism. It has a marked affinity for dihydrofolic reductase, the enzyme required for thymidine and DNA synthesis.

This folic acid analogue has been administered for immunosuppression in organ transplant recipients. Many clinical transplant groups have used a 17-dose, 102-day methotrexate regimen for graft-versus-host disease (GVHD) in bone marrow recipients. A four-dose regimen (10 mg/M[2]/day on posttransplant days 1, 3, 6, and 11 only) is reported to be as effective as the 102-day regimen in preventing both acute and chronic GVHD (Smith et al, 1985).

Methotrexate has been beneficial in the treatment of severe psoriasis refractory to other therapy (see Chapter 56, Dermatologic Preparations). The drug is also used in patients with polymyositis or dermatomyositis. Methotrexate has been added to the regimens of patients with inflammatory muscle disease when no clinical response occurred after three to six months of therapy with prednisone 1 mg/kg.

ADVERSE REACTIONS AND PRECAUTIONS. The most common adverse effects are ulcerative stomatitis, leukopenia, nausea, and abdominal distress. Other side effects include marked myelosuppression with anemia, leukopenia, and thrombocytopenia. Pulmonary fibrosis also has developed.

Methotrexate may be hepatotoxic, especially when large doses or prolonged therapy is employed. Since early signs of hepatotoxicity may be absent, hepatic function tests should be performed both prior to and during therapy. Concomitant use of other hepatotoxic drugs (including alcohol) should be avoided. An intermittent dosage schedule appears to be less toxic than a continuous one.

Methotrexate has been reported to act as an abortifacient and has caused congenital abnormalities. Therefore, it is not recommended for women of childbearing potential (FDA Pregnancy Category D).

See Chapter 64, Drugs Used in Cancer Chemotherapy, for a more detailed discussion.

DOSAGE AND PREPARATIONS.
Intravenous: 25 to 50 mg is given weekly until a clinical or enzyme response occurs; the same amount is then given monthly.
Oral, Intramuscular, Intravenous: For severe psoriasis, see Chapter 56.

METHOTREXATE:
Methotrexate (Lederle). Tablets 2.5 mg.
METHOTREXATE SODIUM:
(Strengths expressed in terms of the base)
Folex (Adria). Powder (lyophilized) 25, 50, 100, and 250 mg.
Methotrexate (Lederle). Solution 2.5 mg/ml in 2 ml containers and 25 mg/ml in 2, 4, and 8 ml containers; powder (cryodesiccated) 20, 50, and 100 mg.
Mexate (Bristol). Powder (lyophilized) 20, 50, 100, and 250 mg.

T-LYMPHOCYTE SUPPRESSANT

CYCLOSPORINE
[Sandimmune]

ACTIONS AND USES. Cyclosporine is a metabolite produced by the fungus, *Tolypocladium inflatum Gams*. The active ingredient is a cyclic polypeptide consisting of 11 amino acids. The drug selectively inhibits T-helper cell function while allowing expansion of T-suppressor cells. The introduction of cyclosporine has substantially improved the success of transplantation.

The antilymphocyte effects of cyclosporine are described in the Introduction. The exact molecular mechanism of action is unclear. The drug inhibits the production of IL-2, but it is less clear whether the expression of IL-2 receptors is also inhibited. There is some indirect evidence that it may interfere with the function of IL-1, a macrophage-derived T-cell activator. Release of IL-3, a product of activated T-cells involved in mast cell growth and hemopoiesis, does not appear to be inhibited. In vitro, the synthesis of gamma interferon by human thymocytes and T-lymphocytes is inhibited by cyclosporine (Reem et al, 1983).

This potent immunosuppressant is indicated to prevent organ rejection in kidney, liver, and heart allogeneic transplants. The manufacturer's package insert states that it always should be used with adrenal corticosteroids. However, some transplant centers do not use corticosteroids except to treat existing rejection.

Although the manufacturer does not recommend the use of cyclosporine with nonsteroidal immunosuppressive drugs, some transplant centers have employed an investigational immunosuppressive regimen consisting of low-dose cyclosporine, azathioprine, and prednisone in renal transplant recipients; no increase in the incidence of infections or lymphomas has been noted (Fries et al, 1985; Illner et al, 1985; Slapak et al, 1985).

Cyclosporine may be used to prevent chronic rejection in patients previously treated with other immunosuppressants. It is the drug of choice for maintenance of kidney, liver, heart, and heart-lung allografts. One-year kidney transplant survivals have increased from approximately 50% (for conventional therapy) to about 75%; hospitalization time has decreased and patient survival has increased significantly (95% to 98% after one year). Survival of liver transplants has improved from about 30% to more than 70% after one year. One-year survival rates for heart transplants have increased to more than 60%.

Investigationally, cyclosporine has been used to treat established GVHD in bone marrow transplant patients and to prevent bone marrow transplant rejection. When used alone, it has had no advantage over conventional immunosuppressive measures in segmental pancreatic allograft recipients. However, a significant reduction in the incidence of GVHD occurred in marrow transplant patients who received both methotrexate and cyclosporine compared to those who received cyclosporine alone (33% and 54%, respectively). In addition, the actuarial survival rates for the two groups at 1.5 years were 80% and 55%, respectively (Storb et al, 1986).

Cyclosporine is being investigated for a number of autoimmune diseases. Of great interest are reports that insulin-dependent diabetes mellitus (IDDM) may be prevented or alleviated if treated immediately after diagnosis (Stiller et al, 1984; Mandrup-Poulsen et al, 1985; Assan et al, 1985). Other autoimmune diseases in which cyclosporine has been investigated include uveitis, Grave's ophthalmopathy, biliary cirrhosis, severe psoriasis, systemic lupus erythematosus, myasthenia gravis, multiple sclerosis, aplastic anemia, dermatomyositis, polymyositis, Crohn's disease, pure red cell aplasia, pemphigus, rheumatoid arthritis, and ulcerative colitis.

Cyclosporine also has been effective in the treatment of schistosomiasis, malaria, and *Coccidioides immitis* infections in experimental animals (Bueding et al, 1981; Nickell et al, 1982; Kirkland and Fierer, 1983).

ADVERSE REACTIONS. The principal adverse effects of cyclosporine are renal dysfunction, thromboembolism, neurotoxicity, hepatotoxicity, and hypertension; other effects include hirsutism and gingival hyperplasia.

Nephrotoxicity (incidence 25% to 38%) is the most frequent and important toxic effect of cyclosporine. In renal transplant patients, a major difficulty is differentiating nephrotoxicity from acute rejection episodes. The diagnosis of such toxicity is generally one of exclusion. This adverse event has been defined as an increase in serum creatinine levels of more than 25% over several days that is reversed by decreasing the dose of cyclosporine. In patients with acute renal allograft rejection, there is a sudden increase in serum creatinine associated with fever, graft tenderness, and decreased urine output and renal blood flow, and cellular infiltrate is observable on biopsy (Ptachcinski et al, 1985 A). The mechanism by which cyclosporine exerts its nephrotoxic effects is unknown. Histologic studies reveal glomerular thromboses, severe tubular damage, and giant mitochondria; fine needle biopsies reveal deposits of the drug.

In a retrospective study on 90 recipients of cadaveric kidney allografts who were treated with cyclosporine, 17 thromboembolic complications occurred in 13 patients. Increased concentrations of factor VIII C, fibrinogen, antithrombin III, and protein C were found in treated patients, and adenosine-5'-diphosphate-induced platelet aggregation was enhanced (Vanrenterghen et al, 1985). However, in a subsequent report, no increase in deep vein thrombosis could be associated with use of cyclosporine (Bergentz et al, 1985). The clinical impression of some investigators is that thromboembolic complications are not a common problem in patients receiving cyclosporine; however, they have been common in renal transplant patients treated with azathioprine and prednisolone (Zazgornik et al, 1985).

Neurotoxic effects associated with cyclosporine include hallucinations (Noll and Kulkarni, 1984), generalized epileptic seizures (Shah et al, 1984), and convulsions (Powell-Jackson et al, 1984; Beaman et al, 1985). Limb paresthesias have developed in approximately 50% and fine distal upper extremity tremor in 20% of patients receiving the drug. Seizures have been reported and tend to occur within the first month of treatment. Some seizures appear to be due to profound hypomagnesemia and renal magnesium wasting (Thompson et al, 1984; June et al, 1985). Adequate magnesium replacement has resolved seizures and prevented recurrences (Thompson et al, 1984).

Hepatotoxicity (incidence 4% to 7%) also has been seen in patients given cyclosporine. This is accompanied by an increase in both direct and total bilirubin concentrations; serum transaminases and alkaline phosphatase are increased in approximately 50% of patients with hyperbilirubinemia. A

reduction in cyclosporine dosage rapidly reverses the hepatotoxic effects.

Initially, there was concern over reports of lymphomas in cyclosporine-treated patients. Subsequent studies, however, revealed that the incidence of lymphoproliferative disease was no greater in treated patients than in other immunosuppressed patients.

Rarely, patients have developed a hypersensitivity reaction to intravenous cyclosporine, but no reactions have occurred with subsequent oral administration.

PRECAUTIONS. Therapeutic levels may be difficult to achieve in patients with malabsorption. Oral absorption is erratic and blood levels should be monitored. Subsequent dosage adjustments may be required to avoid toxicity due to overdose or organ rejection due to low drug levels.

Hypertension is a common adverse effect of cyclosporine and some patients may require antihypertensive therapy.

Renal and liver function tests should be performed regularly during therapy. Blood urea nitrogen levels may be elevated during therapy; this may be related to steroid therapy. In renal transplant patients, this does not necessarily indicate rejection and each patient must be evaluated individually before any dosage adjustment is made. Persistently high levels of BUN and creatinine that do not respond to adjustment in dosage may suggest that other immunosuppressive therapy should be considered. However, in addition to dose adjustment, other procedures, such as biopsy, renal flow scan, or ultrasound, are indicated prior to changing immunosuppressive therapy.

If there are signs of chronic unremitting rejection, it is preferable to remove the transplanted kidney rather than to increase dosage to a high level in an attempt to inhibit the rejection. Cyclosporine has not been proven effective in reversing established graft rejection. However, large doses may be indicated in some patients because of the highly variable pharmacokinetics of cyclosporine.

Monitoring of blood or plasma concentrations of cyclosporine has been recommended as a means of limiting toxicity while ensuring sufficient immunosuppression. However, no consensus appears to have been reached regarding assay, specimen, frequency of testing, or therapeutic range. Blood and serum concentrations of cyclosporine have been measured by radioimmunoassay and high performance liquid chromatography. The proposed range of therapeutic drug concentration depends on which assay is employed (Ptachcinski et al, 1985 A). The problems of blood level monitoring have been reviewed (Burkle, 1985; Cohen et al, 1984).

Large oral doses of cyclosporine are embryotoxic and fetotoxic in rats and rabbits. This drug should be used during pregnancy only if the potential benefit justifies the potential risk to the fetus (FDA Pregnancy Category C). Successful pregnancies in patients receiving cyclosporine have been reported. Cyclosporine is excreted in human milk; therefore, nursing should be avoided.

INTERACTIONS. Synergistic effects may occur when cyclosporine is used with other nephrotoxic drugs (eg, amphotericin B, aminoglycoside antibiotics, melphalan, trimethoprim).

Drugs that affect the mixed-function oxidase system can

alter the metabolism of cyclosporine. Ketoconazole and erythromycin inhibit microsomal enzyme function and have been reported to increase trough concentrations of cyclosporine. Enzyme inducers, such as phenytoin, phenobarbital, and rifampin, increase cyclosporine clearance. Thus, patients taking drugs known to affect microsomal enzyme functions should be monitored closely to determine if alterations in dose or dosing interval are necessary.

Large doses of methylprednisolone have been reported to increase plasma cyclosporine levels in renal transplant recipients and the metabolic clearance of prednisolone has been decreased by cyclosporine. These reports have been reviewed by Burkle, 1985.

PHARMACOKINETICS. Absorption of cyclosporine from the gastrointestinal tract is incomplete and variable. Although kinetics are highly variable, the manufacturer reported peak blood and plasma concentrations (Cmax) in approximately 3.5 hours; Cmax is about 1 ng/ml/mg of dose for plasma and 1.4 to 2.7 ng/ml/mg of dose for blood (for low to high doses). Compared to intravenous infusion, the absolute bioavailability of the oral solution is about 30%. Administration of cyclosporine with food has been reported to increase peak and trough blood concentrations, as well as the area under the blood concentration versus time curve (mean increase, 60%) (Ptachcinski et al, 1985 B). Malabsorption of oral cyclosporine is a common problem in patients following orthotopic liver transplantation.

The volume of distribution of cyclosporine ranges from less than 1 to 13 L/kg. Most of the drug is distributed outside the blood volume. Distribution is concentration-dependent in blood; 33% to 47% is in plasma, 4% to 9% in leukocytes, 5% to 12% in granulocytes, and 41% to 58% in erythrocytes. Uptake by leukocytes and erythrocytes becomes saturated at high concentrations. Approximately 90% is bound to plasma proteins, primarily lipoproteins. The volume of distribution varies from 4 to 13 L/kg.

Cyclosporine is extensively metabolized but there is no major metabolic pathway. Only 0.1% of a dose is excreted as unchanged drug in the urine; 15 metabolites have been characterized in human urine. The cytochrome P-450 liver enzyme systems are responsible for metabolism. The rate of cyclosporine clearance is low to intermediate and is highly variable. The rate appears to be higher in the late evening and morning, which indicates that trough levels should be determined at the same time each day.

Disposition of the drug from blood is biphasic with a terminal half-life ranging from 10 to 27 hours. Cyclosporine is eliminated primarily in the bile, and only 6% of a dose is excreted in the urine.

DOSAGE AND PREPARATIONS.

Intravenous, Oral: The dose should be determined carefully for each patient. The absorption of cyclosporine is erratic; therefore, cyclosporine blood concentrations should be monitored frequently and the dosage adjusted accordingly. Cyclosporine is routinely administered with adrenal corticosteroids; its use with other immunosuppressive agents is investigational.

Different transplant centers have employed different protocols. Some centers have not administered cyclosporine to renal transplant patients until after postoperative diuresis. For further information, see the manufacturer's package insert.

Sandimmune (Sandoz). Solution (intravenous) 50 mg/ml in 5 ml containers (alcohol 32.9%); solution (oral) 100 mg/ml (alcohol 12.5%).

AGENT FOR REPLACEMENT THERAPY

IMMUNE GLOBULIN

Immune globulin (gamma globulin, immune serum globulin) is derived from human plasma and contains most of the antibodies found in whole blood. The preparation consists primarily of IgG with lesser amounts of IgM. Since IgA, found mostly on mucosal surfaces, is not present in significant amounts in the preparation, immune globulin cannot be used for IgA deficiency.

Immune globulin is used most commonly for the prevention of measles and hepatitis A and for replacement therapy in congenital and acquired hypogammaglobulinemia. It is also used prophylactically when hepatitis B and varicella-zoster immune globulin are not available. Both intramuscular and intravenous formulations have been used to treat B-cell and T-cell disorders (see Table 1). For prophylaxis, the intramuscular preparation has been used principally. An advantage of the intravenous preparation is that large amounts of immune globulin can be administered. An intravenous formulation of immune globulin (IGIV) has been used to treat patients with idiopathic thrombocytopenic purpura. IGIV also has been used investigationally to treat various autoimmune diseases.

Frequently recurring upper respiratory infection in children should not be treated with immune globulin unless an immunodeficiency has been demonstrated. When interpreting blood levels in children, close attention must be paid to age-adjusted standards.

See also Table 2; Chapter 35, Blood, Blood Components, and Blood Substitutes; and Chapter 62, Agents for Active and Passive Immunity.

AGENT FOR ERYTHROBLASTOSIS FETALIS

Rh₀(D) IMMUNE GLOBULIN
[Gamulin Rh, HypRho-D, RhoGAM]

Rh₀D IMMUNE GLOBULIN (Microdose)
[HypRho-D Mini Dose, MICRhoGAM, Mini-Gamulin Rh]

Rh₀(D) immune globulin (RhIG) is a sterile, concentrated solution of immune globulin. It is prepared by cold alcohol fractionation of human plasma obtained from donors immunized to produce high levels of Rh₀(D) antibodies. Only plasma units nonreactive in tests for hepatitis B surface antigen are used.

ACTIONS AND USES. RhIG is indicated to prevent Rh

hemolytic disease of the newborn (erythroblastosis fetalis). It is administered to the $Rh_o(D)$-negative, D^u-negative mother within 72 hours after the birth of an $Rh_o(D)$-positive or D^u-positive infant when the following criteria are met: (1) The mother is $Rh_o(D)$- and D^u-negative and is not already sensitized to the $Rh_o(D)$ factor; (2) The infant is $Rh_o(D)$-positive or D^u-positive and has a negative direct Coombs' test due to anti-$Rh_o(D)$. (A positive direct Coombs' test may be caused by antibodies other than anti-$Rh_o(D)$; although therapy with RhIG is not contraindicated, the cause should be investigated.) If the fetal Rh status cannot be determined, it should be presumed to be Rh-positive.

RhIG is indicated for all nonimmunized $Rh_o(D)$-negative, D^u-negative women after abortion or ectopic pregnancy (unless the fetus or the father is shown to be Rh-negative), following amniocentesis or other abdominal trauma that allows fetal cells to enter the maternal circulation, and following transfusion in an $Rh_o(D)$-negative or D^u-negative premenopausal female with $Rh_o(D)$-positive or D^u-positive red blood cells or blood components prepared from blood containing such cells.

The routine use of RhIG during the 28th week of gestation in all Rh-negative women is favored by a large number of medical centers surveyed by the Committee on Obstetrics, Maternal and Fetal Medicine of the American College of Obstetricians and Gynecologists (Nichols, 1984).

RhIG acts by suppressing the specific immune response of Rh-negative individuals to Rh-positive red blood cells. Exposure to these red blood cells may result from pregnancy, abortion, delivery, amniocentesis, or transfusion. Prevention of sensitization to the $Rh_o(D)$ factor in pregnant $Rh_o(D)$-negative women prevents hemolytic disease of the newborn. Injection of RhIG suppresses the antibody response and the formation of anti-$Rh_o(D)$. Although the mechanism of action is unclear, it has been proposed that binding of passive antibody to circulating antigen prevents stimulation of antigen-sensitive cells and subsequent production of anti-$Rh_o(D)$.

Primary immunization occurs most often during labor and delivery in about 15% of the women at risk. Rh_o immunoprophylaxis fails to prevent sensitization in 10% to 15% of the women at risk. Reasons for these therapeutic failures may include previous undetected or overlooked Rh-positive pregnancies or transfusions or the administration of an inadequate dose of RhIG. The most frequent cause of apparent failure of postpartum prophylaxis is probably Rh immunization early during pregnancy.

The administration of RhIG within 72 hours of delivery of a full-term infant reduces the incidence of Rh isoimmunization as a result of pregnancy from 12% to 13% to 1% to 2%. The incidence of isoimmunization can be further reduced to less than 0.1% by administering the product in two doses, one at 28 weeks gestation and another following delivery. Protection against isoimmunization is decreased when the Rh antibody is administered more than 72 hours following delivery.

ADVERSE REACTIONS AND PRECAUTIONS. Adverse reactions are infrequent, mild, and generally confined to the site of injection. Slight elevations of temperature have been reported following injection. Other adverse effects are the same as those encountered with similar human immune globulin preparations (see Chapter 62, Agents for Active and Passive Immunity).

RhIG is contraindicated in Rh-positive patients and in Rh-negative patients who have already developed Rh antibodies. It must not be administered intravenously or given to the neonate. A broad spectrum compatibility test capable of detecting "incomplete" antibodies should be performed to determine if the patient already has been sensitized to the $Rh_o(D)$ factor.

DOSAGE AND PREPARATIONS. RhIG should be stored at 2 to 8 C but not frozen.

STANDARD PREPARATION:

Intramuscular: Postpartum, prophylaxis, miscarriage, abortion, ectopic pregnancy, *adults*, the entire content of one vial is administered. This is sufficient to suppress the immunizing potential of 15 ml of red blood cells or approximately 30 ml of whole blood. RhIG should be administered within 72 hours of the fetomaternal hemorrhage.

Transfusion accident, one vial will suppress the immune response to 15 ml of Rh-positive red blood cells. To calculate the volume of red blood cells in whole blood transfusions, the total volume of blood transfused is multiplied by the hematocrit of the donor; alternatively, the volume may be approximated by multiplying the total volume by 0.45.

    Generic. Unit-dose containers.

    Gamulin Rh (Armour), *HypRho-D* (Cutter), *RhoGAM* (Ortho). Packages containing a single dose.

MICRODOSE PREPARATION:

Intramuscular: This preparation contains approximately one-sixth the $Rh_o(D)$ antibody present in the standard preparation and is indicated only for $Rh_o(D)$-negative women undergoing abortion or miscarriage up to 12 weeks gestation, unless the father is Rh negative. *Adults,* one vial is usually sufficient and should be administered within 72 hours of the termination of pregnancy.

    HypRho-D Mini Dose (Cutter), *MICRhoGAM* (Ortho), *Mini-Gamulin Rh* (Armour). Single (microdose) containers.

IMMUNOSUPPRESSIVE ANTISERUM

LYMPHOCYTE IMMUNE GLOBULIN (Antithymocyte Globulin [Equine])
    [Atgam]

ACTIONS. Lymphocyte immune globulin is obtained from serum IgG of horses immunized with human T-cell lymphocytes. This preparation is a selective immunosuppressant that reduces the number of circulating, thymus-dependent lymphocytes (T-cells) that are partly responsible for graft rejection; it has little effect on B-cells and is not associated with severe lymphopenia. Activity may vary from lot to lot due to imprecise methods of measuring potency. Since it is usually administered with other immunosuppressants, such as corticosteroids and antimetabolites, the patient's response to the equine globulin is minimal and the incidence of hypersensitivity reactions is reduced.

USES. Lymphocyte immune globulin has been used primarily

to minimize allograft rejection in renal transplant patients. When it is administered at the time of rejection, resolution of the acute episode is enhanced. Efficacy and safety have not been demonstrated in renal transplant patients not receiving other immunosuppressive therapy concomitantly.

Lymphocyte immune globulin also is indicated for the treatment of moderate to severe aplastic anemia in patients who are unsuitable for bone marrow transplantation and may induce partial to complete hematologic remission when given with a regimen of supportive care. It has not been useful in patients who are suitable candidates for bone marrow transplantation or in patients with aplastic anemia secondary to neoplastic disease, storage disease, myelofibrosis, or Fanconi's syndrome or in patients exposed to myelotoxic agents or radiation. Lymphocyte immune globulin has been used investigationally in patients with T-cell malignancies or GVHD.

ADVERSE REACTIONS AND PRECAUTIONS. Common adverse effects (incidence 10% to 50%) include chills, fever, leukopenia, thrombocytopenia, and dermatologic reactions (rash, pruritus, urticaria, wheal and flare). Other reactions (incidence 1% to 5%) include arthralgia, chest or back pain, headache, nausea and/or vomiting, diarrhea, peripheral thrombophlebitis, stomatitis, dyspnea, hypotension, night sweats, and pain at the infusion site. Rarely (incidence less than 1%) anaphylaxis, serum sickness, tachycardia, laryngospasm, pulmonary edema, herpes simplex virus reactivation, local and systemic infections, or myalgias may occur.

Since lymphocyte immune globulin is of equine origin, the usual precautions should be observed (see Chapter 62, Agents for Active and Passive Immunity). Caution should be exercised when giving repeated doses of this preparation, and patients should be observed for signs of allergy. A skin test for sensitivity to equine serum is recommended prior to the first infusion. A systemic reaction, such as generalized rash, tachycardia, dyspnea, hypotension, or anaphylaxis, precludes further administration. Some previously masked reactions to the antiserum (hypersensitivity) may appear if doses of other immunosuppressants given concomitantly are reduced. Patients should be monitored carefully for leukopenia and thrombocytopenia, especially when the antiserum is used with corticosteroids, antimetabolites, or other immunosuppressive agents. Treatment should be discontinued if severe, unremitting thrombocytopenia or leukopenia develops. This antiserum is *contraindicated* in patients who previously experienced a severe systemic reaction to lymphocyte immune globulin or any equine immunoglobulin preparation.

Administration during pregnancy is not recommended. The antiserum has not been tested in pregnant or lactating women.

The patient should be observed carefully for signs of concurrent infection and treated promptly if infection develops.

DOSAGE AND PREPARATIONS. This agent is not well standardized and the dosage varies. The maximum tolerated dose has not been determined. The following dosages are examples of immunosuppressive regimens that have been employed. Lymphocyte immune globulin is used with other immunosuppressive agents. The manufacturer's instructions for pretesting and infusion procedures should be followed careful-

ly. Dilution of the product in dextrose or acidic solutions is not recommended. A dose should not be infused in less than four hours.

Intravenous: Renal allograft recipients, *adults,* 10 to 30 mg/kg daily; *children,* 5 to 25 mg/kg (experience with children is limited).

To delay rejection, *adults,* 15 mg/kg daily for 14 days, then every other day for 14 days for a total of 21 doses in 28 days. The first dose should be administered 24 hours before or after transplant.

For treatment of rejection, *adults,* the first dose is administered after diagnosis of the first rejection episode. The recommended dose is 10 to 15 mg/kg daily for 14 days. Additional alternate-day therapy up to a total of 21 doses may be given.

Aplastic anemia, *adults,* 10 to 20 mg/kg daily for 8 to 14 days. Additional alternate-day therapy up to a total of 21 doses may be administered. Since thrombocytopenia has been associated with this product, patients with aplastic anemia may need prophylactic platelet transfusions.

Atgam (Upjohn). Each milliliter of solution contains equine gamma globulin 50 mg stabilized in 0.3 molar glycine to a pH of about 6.8.

VENOM ALLERGENS FOR IMMUNOTHERAPY

The sting of the bee, wasp, hornet, or yellow-jacket poses a serious hazard for sensitive individuals who may respond to a second exposure with anaphylaxis. Anaphylactic shock caused by insect sting is no less hazardous than that caused by other allergens. There is much clinical experience to indicate that immunotherapeutic injections of protein extracts from *Hymenoptera* can produce a refractory state. However, for treatment of acute anaphylaxis, epinephrine is the drug of choice (see Chapter 62, Agents for Active and Passive Immunity).

For many years, hyposensitization therapy against the sting of *Hymenoptera* employed a whole body extract. Results of most recent investigations indicate that whole body extracts are ineffective or less effective than extracts from pure venom or venom sacs only. Whole body extracts have been withdrawn from the market by order of the Food and Drug Administration.

The diagnosis of insect hypersensitivity depends upon history, physical examination when possible, and determination of IgE antibody against *Hymenoptera* protein through skin or radioallergosorbent (RAST) testing. Skin testing was reported to be more sensitive than RAST in one study (Small et al, 1983). Individuals who experienced a severe systemic reaction involving airways or hypotension and a positive skin test are the only candidates for routine immunotherapy (Lichtenstein et al, 1979). It has been suggested that the only unequivocal criteria for immunotherapy are a history of a life-threatening reaction and a positive skin test to an insect venom (Ewan, 1985). Patients who experienced severe local reactions with a positive skin or RAST test should be considered for immunotherapy only if the reactions are incapacitating or there is clear progression of symptoms following repeated stings.

Neither the degree of reactivity to skin testing nor the level of response to RAST testing correlates with the degree of sensitivity to insect sting. There is a very narrow range between the diagnostic and irritant concentrations of the skin test antigens. Some individuals, particularly children, lose their sensitivity after several years without exposure. However, immunotherapy stimulates the production not only of protective IgG-blocking antibodies but also of IgE antibodies, which may tend to maintain the sensitivity. In some patients, protection does not appear to be related to IgG antibodies, which raises the possibility that other mechanisms may be involved during immunotherapy, such as stimulation of antigen-specific T-suppressor cells.

The degree of protection achieved with either venom or whole body extract is not clear. No endpoint has been established; the prevailing view appears to be that a minimum of three years' therapy is necessary.

ADVERSE REACTIONS AND PRECAUTIONS. Because severe systemic reactions may occur, *Hymenoptera* venom preparations should be given only by a physician experienced in administering allergens and/or after allergy consultation. In highly sensitive individuals, even the small dose used for skin tests may precipitate an anaphylactic reaction.

An anaphylactic reaction is always possible with use of any immunotherapeutic agent. For that reason, a tourniquet, epinephrine, and agents to treat shock and bronchospasm should be available. In addition, patients should remain in the office under close observation for one hour after an injection (see Chapter 62, Agents for Active and Passive Immunity).

Extensive local reactions can occur from skin tests or hyposensitization procedures (incidence, about 60% of patients undergoing hyposensitization). Systemic reactions have been noted in about 16% of adults receiving hyposensitization therapy. These may occur while increasing the dosage or after a maintenance dose. Symptoms include any of the following: pruritus, urticaria, sneezing, nasal discharge, hoarseness, coughing, wheezing, tachycardia, gastrointestinal discomfort and nausea, neck or chest pain, sweating, or lacrimation. Systemic reactions commonly occur shortly after injection; however, a serum sickness-like reaction manifested by fever, malaise, joint pain, and myalgia can appear up to 48 hours following injection. Local and systemic reactions are less common in children.

Because of the risks, the patient should be fully informed and kept under constant supervision. All patients receiving venom immunotherapy should be instructed in emergency self-injection procedures with subcutaneous epinephrine. An emergency insect sting treatment kit [Ana-Kit] containing prepackaged doses of epinephrine and antihistamines and instructions for use is available commercially. This kit should be prescribed for patients at risk from insect sting anaphylaxis and should be readily available at all times of possible exposure. Patients should be instructed by the physician regarding the proper use of the ANA kit.

Because antihistamines may interfere with skin test responses they should not be taken for 72 hours prior to skin testing. Safety during pregnancy has not been established. The benefit/risk ratio must be evaluated carefully because of the risk of serious systemic reactions.

ADMINISTRATION. The regimens for hyposensitization vary according to the recommendation of the manufacturer. Recommended dosage schedules may have to be adjusted for highly sensitive patients. A prick test followed by an intradermal test is recommended for diagnostic skin testing. The subcutaneous route is preferred for immunotherapy injections. It is important to include a negative control with diluent and a positive control with histamine to interpret the significance of the wheal and erythema reaction if it occurs. The product information sheet should be consulted for recommended diluent, dilutions, and interpretation of the skin test response.

Albay (Hollister-Stier). Diagnostic kits, maintenance kits, and bulk vials are available. Each vacuum-sealed bulk vial contains venom protein 550 mcg. When reconstituted with 5.5 ml of the appropriate diluent (50% glycerin, normal saline, or Hollister-Stier albumin-saline diluent), each vial contains 100 mcg/ml of an individual venom protein (honeybee, yellow jacket, yellow hornet, white-faced hornet, wasp, and mixed vespid). The manufacturer's recommendation for reconstitution should be followed closely.

Pharmalgen (Pharmacia). The diagnostic kit contains one vial each of 100 mcg of honey bee, yellow jacket, yellow hornet, white-faced hornet, and wasp venoms. The Venom Starter Kit is designed for new patient start-up therapy; it contains five vials of four different color-coded concentrations and is available for honey bee, yellow jacket, wasp and mixed vespids only. Treatment kits containing 6 x 100 mcg are available for all venoms included in the Diagnostic Kit as well as for mixed vespid (6 x 300 mcg). Multiple dose vials containing 1,000 mcg are available for honey bee, yellow jacket, and wasp, and one containing 3,000 mcg is available for mixed vespids. All products are supplied freeze dried; the appropriate diluent is available separately. When refrigerated, all freeze-dried preparations are stable for three years. Solutions containing 100 mcg/ml are stable for one year. Lower concentrations are stable for shorter periods.

MISCELLANEOUS INVESTIGATIONAL AGENTS

BCG VACCINE

ACTIONS AND USES. BCG is an attenuated strain of *Mycobacterium bovis*. It has been used in the past to induce immunity against tuberculosis but results have been variable. More recently, this agent has been administered as a nonspecific stimulator of the immune system in patients with cancer. Success in the treatment of tumors with BCG is most likely when the neoplasm is small and localized, the patient has a normally functioning immune system, there is close contact between BCG and tumor cells, and a sufficient number of viable organisms is administered.

BCG appears to act principally by nonspecifically stimulating the reticuloendothelial system. It is not known whether this is a primary effect or secondary to T-cell activation and lymphokine production. This agent activates natural killer cells and enhances the production of hematopoietic stem cells. BCG has been reported to cross-react with melanoma, leukemic, and hepatoma cells, which could explain reports of specific effects on these types of tumors. Macrophages affected by BCG become more active killer cells and more efficiently clear antigen and immune complexes and recruit other cells involved in the destruction of cancer cells. Under certain circumstances, BCG enhances tumor growth, apparently due to formation of immune complexes (BCG/anti-BCG) that block the cytotoxic action of lymphocytes and stimulation of antigen-specific T-suppressor cells.

BCG has been used investigationally in the treatment of malignant melanoma, acute lymphocytic leukemia, acute and chronic myelogenous leukemia, lymphomas, breast cancer, head and neck tumors, and cancer of the bladder, lung, or colon. In most of these clinical trials, effectiveness has been equivocal and few controlled trials have been performed. Efficacy was greatest in cutaneous melanoma, in which it was injected intralesionally (Morton et al, 1970), and in transitional cell carcinoma of the bladder, in which it was administered intravesically (Netto and Lemos, 1984; Brosman, 1985; Lamm, 1985; Kelley et al, 1985). BCG was reported to be ineffective in preventing recurrent genital herpes (Douglas et al, 1985).

To prevent disseminated BCG infection, BCG should not be given to immunosuppressed or immunodeficient patients. (See also Chapter 62, Agents for Active and Passive Immunity, and Chapter 64, Drugs Used in Cancer Chemotherapy.)

CORYNEBACTERIUM PARVUM (CP)

This suspension contains *Corynebacterium parvum*, a gram-positive bacterium, that has been heat-killed and formaldehyde-inactivated. It appears to be active only when given by injection.

CP is a nonspecific immunostimulant that is thought to activate macrophages to augment phagocytosis and cytotoxic activity. Its action may involve C_3 receptors; nonimmunologic mechanisms also may contribute to the antitumor action. Paradoxically, CP depresses T-cell function. In laboratory animals, CP inhibits growth and metastasis of various tumors; activity is greatest after intralesional injection. In man, intralesional injection has led to regression of cutaneous metastases of malignant melanoma. In many clinical trials, benefits have been negligible, except in the limited area of control of malignant effusions.

Many patients develop very high fever (up to 40.5 C), headache, nausea, and vomiting. Other adverse effects include peripheral vasoconstriction and hypertension.

INTERFERONS

ACTIONS. Initially, it was thought that only a single type of interferon existed. The material was characterized as a broad spectrum, antiviral, species-specific glycoprotein produced by all nucleated animal cells, which acted by inducing a refractory state to virus infection. It is now known that there are three major classes of interferons (alpha, beta, and gamma) having broad biological activities. These properties include inhibition of DNA synthesis, cell multiplication, antibody synthesis, delayed hypersensitivity, graft-versus-host disease (GVHD), and tumor growth. On the other hand, interferons enhance the activity of cytolytic T-cells and natural killer cells, the expression of HLA antigens and β_2-microglobulin on lymphocytes, HLA and tumor-associated antigens on cancer cells, and tumoricidal and phagocytic activity of macrophages. When small doses are given after antigen stimulation, antibody production and GVHD are enhanced.

All three types of interferon enhance the expression of HLA class I antigens, but gamma interferon appears to be the most potent inducer. Expression of class II HLA molecules (Ia or immunoassociated antigens) is associated only with gamma interferon. The effect of gamma interferon on expression of the two classes of Ia molecules, DR and DC, differs in that DC expression is increased two- to threefold more than DR expression (Ameglio et al, 1983). Ia expression on cells is required for proper antigen presentation to T-lymphocytes, and gamma interferon plays an important role in its regulation. All three classes enhance the production of IL-1. There is general agreement that gamma interferon is most potent in terms of antiproliferative and, especially, immunomodulating activity.

USES. Preclinical studies with animal interferons demonstrated that these agents had significant antiviral and antineoplastic activity in vivo. Clinical trials of human interferons as antiviral agents were initiated in the early 1960s and many trials are still in progress. More recently, interferons have been used therapeutically in a wide variety of malignancies. Early studies employed interferon from fibroblast cell cultures. This subsequently was replaced by interferon from human buffy coat cells of pooled blood from normal donors stimulated by Sendai virus. Both materials consisted of less than 1% interferon but did demonstrate some antiviral and antineoplastic activity in humans. Most recently, all three interferon types have been produced by recombinant DNA (rDNA) technology, which yields large quantities of interferon of high purity. The latter are now being studied in a number of clinical trials. The efficacy and adverse reactions observed with rDNA interferon have been similar to those obtained with cell culture materials. The majority of clinical studies utilizing rDNA human interferon to date have employed interferon alpha-2, the first form available in large quantities. The most successful results with alpha interferon have been obtained in hairy cell leukemia. Few studies have been reported with beta or gamma interferon prepared by rDNA technology (see also Chapter 64, Drugs Used in Cancer Chemotherapy, and Chapter 79, Antiviral Agents).

NOTE: The alpha form of interferon became available for treatment of hairy cell leukemia after this chapter was prepared. See the manufacturers' literature.

INTERLEUKIN-2

Interleukin-2 (IL-2), a lymphokine produced by activated helper T-lymphocytes, induces the proliferation of T-cells and promotes the differentiation of lymphocytes into cytotoxic cells. IL-2 also induces the production of gamma interferon and activates natural killer (NK) cells and other lymphokine-activated killer (LAK) cells. Activation of killer cells appears to be due to the induction of gamma interferon, which mediates the enhanced killing (Kawase et al, 1983; Weigent et al, 1983; Ortaldo et al, 1984; Itoh et al, 1985).

IL-2 has been cloned in bacteria through recombinant DNA technology, thus allowing the production of large amounts. No functional difference was observed between native and recombinant IL-2 in supporting the growth of IL-2-dependent cell lines, enhancing the generation of cytolytic cells in vitro, or generating LAK cells from lymphocyte preparations (Rosenberg et al, 1984). Studies with natural and recombinant materials have suggested that IL-2 can sustain proliferation but not differentiation of B-cells, that activated B-lymphocytes carry functional IL-2 receptors at their surface, and that IL-2 appears to increase the production of IL-1 (Jacques and Soulillou, 1985).

In vitro studies on animal and human cells have shown that T-cell responses are potentiated and restored. Since sufficient quantities of IL-2 have only recently become available, only a few clinical studies have been completed.

Lymphocytes from patients with acquired immunodeficiency syndrome produce significantly less IL-2 than cells from healthy controls and have a greatly decreased proliferative response to mitogen induction; addition of IL-2 to lymphocyte cultures from AIDS patients partially or fully restored this response in approximately 50% of treated cultures. However, clinical trials of IL-2 in AIDS patients did not affect the outcome of the disease. In one uncontrolled study, xenogeneic IL-2 with high biologic activity injected intralesionally caused significant tumor regression in five of six patients with bladder cancer (Pizza et al, 1984). Adoptive immunotherapy employing LAK cells and repeated injections of recombinant IL-2 was reported to be highly effective in reducing the numbers and size of established pulmonary sarcoma metastases in mice (Mulé et al, 1984). Preliminary results of this regimen in patients with cancer (subcutaneous metastatic melanoma, advanced rectal cancer) appear to be encouraging (*F-D-C Reports*, 1985).

INOSIPLEX (Inosine Pranobex, Methisoprinol)
[Isoprinosine]

Inosiplex has been studied as an antiviral agent for over a decade. Currently, it is being widely investigated because of its reported immunopotentiating properties. The mechanism of action is unknown. In vitro, inosiplex increased the T-cell proliferative response to mitogens and antigens, natural killer (NK) cell activity, and macrophage activity. The enhanced activities may be mediated through augmentation of IL-1 and IL-2 production. In vitro, cells from patients with depressed immunity showed significant improvement when exposed to inosiplex. For example, mitogen-induced lymphocyte proliferation, NK cell activity, neutrophil chemotaxis, and IL-2 production were restored to normal or near normal levels in cells collected from aging humans (Tsang et al, 1985). However, improvements in cell-mediated immunity in laboratory tests have been much easier to demonstrate than improvements in the clinical status of treated patients (see also Chapter 79, Antiviral Agents).
Isoprinosine (Newport).

LEVAMISOLE
[Ergamisol]

Levamisole, the levo-isomer of tetramisole and an established anthelmintic drug, was first reported to be an immunostimulant in 1972. Since then, it has been investigated in a large variety of disease states.

ACTIONS. The mechanism of action of levamisole is not completely understood. Depending upon the dose and time of administration, it either augments or depresses immune responses; it usually acts as an immunopotentiator. Immunopotentiation generally requires the simultaneous administration of a primary stimulus, such as antigen. Levamisole has been referred to as an "immunonormalizing" agent since a normal immune system is not stimulated. T-cell function is enhanced more than B-cell function. Delayed hypersensitivity reactions have been restored or increased in the elderly and in patients with malignant and nonmalignant diseases.

The drug appears to act directly on lymphocytes, macrophages, and granulocytes to modify their proliferation, mobility, and secretion. The maturation and proliferation of T-cells are enhanced, but NK or K cells do not appear to be affected. Some investigators consider the principal action of levamisole to be facilitation of monocyte chemotaxis; the drug also enhances monocyte phagocytosis. Defective Fc receptor activity of neutrophils has been restored (Patrone et al, 1985; Luzi et al, 1983).

USES. In clinical trials, levamisole's effects on cancer and a number of autoimmune disorders have been inconsistent. It has been reported to stabilize remission in breast, lung, head and neck, and stage IV gastric cancer; in leukemia; and in multiple myeloma. However, it also was reported to be ineffective or only slightly effective in breast cancer (Klefström et al, 1985; Kay et al, 1983), ovarian cancer (Khoo et al, 1984), and acute nonlymphocytic leukemia (Van Sloten et al, 1983). In patients with rheumatoid arthritis, levamisole was comparable to penicillamine in effectiveness. Efficacy also has been claimed in herpesvirus and bacterial infections (chronic brucellosis, leprosy, and staphylococcal infection), erythema multiforme, lupus erythematosus, and aphthous stomatitis. No effect was observed on amyotrophic lateral sclerosis, idiopathic nephrotic syndrome, or measles.

ADVERSE REACTIONS. The most severe adverse effects of levamisole are dermatitis and agranulocytosis (especially in individuals with HLA B27). The latter resolves on drug withdrawal. Other effects include a flu-like malaise, metallic taste, nausea and vomiting, and nervousness.
Ergamisol (Janssen).

MURAMYL DIPEPTIDE

Because BCG immunotherapy occasionally causes severe adverse effects, attempts have been made to use subfractions of the bacterium in the hope of reducing these complications. Muramyl dipeptide (MDP) is the smallest active component of the mycobacterial cell wall and retains the immunoadjuvant activity of BCG. This water-soluble fragment is administered orally. A large number of MDP analogues have been prepared and the parent compound and derivatives have been studied extensively as adjuvants for immunization.

In animals, MDP induces tumoricidal and bactericidal activities of macrophages and increases the secretion of monokines. When incorporated into oil with antigen, it augments the development of both cellular and humoral immunity. In vitro studies have shown that T-cell function and B-cell proliferation are enhanced.

Data on the activity of MDP in man are limited. In vitro, MDP encapsulated in liposomes enhanced the tumoricidal activity of human monocytes; a significantly smaller amount was required if MDP was incorporated into liposomes (Sone et al, 1984). Liposomes containing a derivative, muramyl tripeptide, have been reported to protect mice from fatal herpes simplex type 2 infection (Koff et al, 1985). When administered intraperitoneally, MDP inhibited the ascitic growth of four of five thymoma cell lines in mice (Phillips et al, 1983).

MUROMONAB CD3 (Murine Monoclonal Antibody, Anti-CD3, Human T-Cell Inhibitor)
[Orthoclone OKT3]

Muromonab CD3 is a monoclonal antibody to the T3 (CD3) antigen of human T-lymphocytes (Kung et al, 1979; Van Wauwe et al, 1980). The T3 molecule is associated with the antigen recognition site of T-cells and is essential for signal transduction (Chang et al, 1981). The monoclonal antibody is purified IgG_{2a} and contains two heavy chains of about 50,000 daltons and two light chains of approximately 25,000 daltons.

ACTIONS AND USES. Muromonab CD3 is used to reverse acute allograft rejection in renal transplant patients. It reverses graft rejection by blocking the function and generation of cytotoxic T-lymphocytes responsible for renal inflammation and destruction during acute renal rejection. Circulating T-lymphocytes bearing the T3 antigen are removed from the circulation within minutes following intravenous administration of muromonab CD3. Complement is not involved in this reaction and removal probably results from phagocytic activity of the reticuloendothelial system that follows opsonization by the monoclonal antibody.

In an early study, established renal allograft rejection episodes in eight patients were reversed within two to seven days by muromonab CD3 despite continued reduction of the steroid dosages employed (Cosimi et al, 1981). Similar success was encountered in a second study that also involved a small number of patients. In the latter study, production of human antimurine antibodies was observed, which suggested that administration of muromonab CD3 may be limited to a single short course in each patient (Burton et al, 1982). In a prospective, randomized, multicenter trial involving 123 patients undergoing acute rejection of cadaveric renal transplants, muromonab CD3 was reported to reverse 94% of the rejections compared to a 75% reversal rate obtained with conventional steroid treatment. The superior reversal rate with muromonab CD3 was reflected in improved one-year graft survival of 62% for the muromonab CD3 treated group versus 45% for the steroid-treated group (Ortho Multicenter Transplant Study Group, 1985).

Investigationally, muromonab CD3 is being used to treat rejection of other organ transplants, such as liver and heart.

ADVERSE REACTIONS AND PRECAUTIONS. Determinations of adverse reactions have been obtained primarily from patients who were simultaneously receiving low-dose immunosuppressive therapy, principally azathioprine and corticosteroids. A high incidence of adverse effects (pyrexia, chills, and dyspnea) has been observed following the first dose of this monoclonal antibody. Because severe pulmonary edema has been observed in approximately 2% of patients, it is recommended that muromonab CD3 not be given to hypervolemic patients and that all patients be closely supervised after administration of the first dose.

Patients treated with muromonab CD3 experience adverse reactions in addition to those caused by renal rejection only during the first two days of treatment. The majority of patients then experience pyrexia (90%) and chills (59%). Other adverse effects include chest pain (14%), dyspnea (21%), wheezing (13%), nausea (19%), vomiting (19%), diarrhea (14%), tremor (13%), headache (11%), and tachycardia (10%). The incidence of infections has not been significantly different from that seen with conventional immunosuppressive therapy.

Muromonab CD3 should not be given to patients who are hypersensitive to this product. Antibodies (IgM, IgG, and IgE) to muromonab CD3 have been observed during and following its use. One report of anaphylaxis and two possible cases of serum sickness have been associated with these antibodies.

Therapy should be conducted in facilities equipped and staffed with adequate laboratory and supportive medical resources. The product should not be administered to patients whose temperature exceeds 100 F; antipyretics may be used to reduce the temperature.

The safety and efficacy of muromonab CD3 in children have not been established, but patients as young as 2 years have received the drug with no unusual effects.

Muromonab CD3 should be given to pregnant women only if clearly needed (FDA Pregnancy Category C).

PHARMACOKINETICS. Following treatment with 5 mg/day for 14 days, mean serum trough levels increased during the first three days and then averaged 0.9 mcg/ml on days 3 to 14. The levels attained during therapy have been shown to block T-cell effector functions in vitro.

DOSAGE AND PREPARATIONS.
Intravenous: Adults, for the treatment of acute renal failure, 5 mg/day by intravenous push for 10 to 14 days using a low protein-binding (0.2 or 0.22) micron filter. Conventional immunosuppressive therapy given concomitantly should be decreased during the administration of this product. The manufacturer should be consulted for further information.

Orthoclone OKT3 (Ortho Pharmaceutical). Solution (sterile, buffered) 1 mg/ml in 5 ml containers.

THYMIC HORMONES

The epithelium of the thymus gland synthesizes many hormone-like factors that appear to play a major role in the regulation and differentiation of T-lymphocytes. Several active factors have been isolated from the thymus, including thymosin fraction 5 (TF-5), thymosin α-1, thymopoietin (TP), thymic humoral factor (THF), serum thymic factor (facteur thymique serique, FTS), and thymostimulin (TS). These thymic hormones are involved in the maturation of T-cell precursors and promote the differentiation and proliferation of mature T-cells. Blood levels are highest in childhood, decline during the third or fourth decade, and are low in elderly people. Levels are undetectable in patients with complete DiGeorge syndrome who lack the thymus. Because of the low levels in the elderly, thymic hormones have been evaluated in this group to enhance immune responsiveness.

Thymosin fraction 5 is an extract of calf thymus and contains over 20 peptides with molecular weights ranging from 2 to 15,000 daltons. TF-5 varies from lot-to-lot and may contain toxic contaminants. Although it is generally nonreactogenic in humans, hypersensitivity reactions to bovine antigens have been reported.

TF-5 induces the expression of antigens associated with maturation on precursor T-cells, stimulates terminal deoxynucleotidyl transferase (TdT, a DNA polymerase present only in prothymocytes and hence a marker for immature cells), and enhances the production of IL-2. TF-5 also augments the functions of both T-helper (Th) and T-suppressor (Ts) cells and, accordingly, either increases or decreases cytotoxic T-cell activity (Smalley et al, 1984). It does not appear to affect NK cell activity. In experimental models, TF-5 had some antitumor effects but, in human phase I studies, no significant reproducible modification of biologic response could be demonstrated (Smalley et al, 1984).

In phase II studies, TF-5 failed to produce any objective responses in patients with metastatic renal carcinoma (Dimitrov et al, 1985). However, in vitro, TF-5 was reported to enhance antitetanus antibody synthesis in cells collected from elderly patients; this effect was not noted in young patients (Ershler et al, 1984). Because of the variable responses obtained, the isolation, purification, and characterization of individual polypeptides in TF-5 have been given priority over further clinical testing of this material.

Thymosin α-1 (Tα₁) is a polypeptide found in TF-5; its gene has been cloned and it also has been synthesized. This peptide contains 28 amino acids and has a molecular weight of 3,100 daltons. Tα₁ enhances several T-cell functions in vitro, including the synthesis of migration inhibitory factor, the proliferative response to T-cell mitogens (but not alloantigens), Th cell activity, and antibody synthesis in secondary responses to T-dependent antigens. It also induces the expression of T-cell surface antigens and TdT at considerably lower doses than TF-5. While Tα₁ appears to augment the development of cytotoxic T-cells, it does not appear to activate NK cells. The maturation of T-precursor cells in vivo is induced by Tα₁ at significantly lower doses than TF-5. In animal models, it has demonstrated some efficacy in preventing experimental and spontaneous metastases (Smalley et al, 1984). Tα₁ enhanced both Th and Ts cell activity in old but not young mice; enhancement of Th cells predominated (Frasca et al, 1985).

In phase I clinical trials in a small group of patients, an indication of antitumor response and biological modification was reported following Tα₁ therapy in patients with a small tumor burden who had received local radiation therapy; how-

ever, no objective antitumor responses were reported (Smalley et al, 1984).

Thymopoietin is a pure polypeptide (molecular weight, 5,260) obtained from human thymus extract. Thymopoietin pentapeptide (TP5) has been synthesized and found to have the same biologic activity as the whole native molecule. TP5 appears to be related to the active site on the native molecule. In vivo, it has a half-life of 30 minutes.

In a small clinical study, TP5 was reported to induce clinical and immunologic improvement in three of three infants with DiGeorge syndrome and in three of six patients with T-cell defect (Aiuti et al, 1983 A). In a placebo-controlled, double-blind, randomized study, TP5 improved many clinical features of rheumatoid arthritis (Malaise et al, 1985). In a preliminary study on AIDS patients with lymphadenopathy, treatment improved blastogenic responses, restored delayed hypersensitivity, and produced some subjective improvement in constitutional symptoms (Clumeck et al, 1984).

Thymic humoral factor (THF) is isolated from calf thymus by dialysis and may be similar to thymosin fraction 5. It increases the production of T-lymphocytes in animals and man and leads to T-cell differentiation and maturation. In seven renal allograft patients undergoing acute rejection episodes, all of whom had a striking decrease in suppressor T-cells, in vitro incubation of lymphocytes with THF increased the number of Ts cells from very low levels to normal or above (Shohat et al, 1983).

Serum thymic factor (FTS), a nonapeptide produced by the thymus, has been synthesized. It modulates NK cell activity in mice; it increases activity but decreases the abnormally high level of NK activity in thymectomized mice. In vitro studies on human cells have shown that low concentrations increased and high concentrations decreased NK activity. In one limited clinical trial, FTS was found to increase NK activity in two of four cancer patients with low pretreatment NK values, but decreased NK activity in two of four patients with normal or elevated pretreatment NK values (Dokhelar et al, 1983).

Thymostimulin (TS) is another extract of calf thymus that has been found to enhance T-cell proliferation and differentiation. In one study involving 21 immunodeficient patients with recurrent herpes simplex labialis, a significant reduction in the number and severity of recurrences was observed that persisted for at least three months. In in vitro studies on lymphocytes, lymphoproliferative responses and NK cell activity were elevated (Aiuti et al, 1983 B).

The use of thymic hormones to treat human disease requires further clinical studies. The extent to which a thymic deficiency may contribute to the pathogenesis of any disease is important in defining the probable efficacy of thymic hormones. Studies employing purified materials derived from recombinant DNA technology or from chemical synthesis should not only identify the specific active factors and clarify their potential clinical role, but eliminate the lot-to-lot variation in thymic extracts that has made the determination of appropriate dosage a significant problem.

DIALYZABLE TRANSFER FACTOR

Dialyzable leukocyte extracts (DLE) are obtained from leukocytes lysed by alternate freezing and thawing. The original material described by Lawrence in 1955 was a crude preparation consisting of at least 60 distinct moieties. DLE are capable of transferring delayed skin hypersensitivity from a positive specific donor to a negative recipient. The antigen-specific activity in DLE is currently designated as dialyzable transfer factor (TFd). The precise chemical nature of TFd is unknown, but it has a molecular weight of 1,100 to 1,600 daltons, is stable at body temperature, and is resistant to the action of trypsin. It appears to be a small nucleopeptide containing both RNA and protein, but not DNA.

The mechanism of action of TFd has not been determined, but it may act on uncommitted stem cells to induce specificity for an antigen or group of antigens. It also has been suggested that TFd may assist in recruiting specific antigen-sensitive cells. It does not appear to affect humoral immunity.

The capacity of TFd to transfer antigen-specific immunity combined with its low toxicity has served as an impetus for a number of different clinical trials on patients with myriad conditions. Most consistent clinical success has been encountered in patients with chronic mucocutaneous candidiasis and the Wiskott-Aldrich syndrome. Results in disseminated coccidioidomycosis and other disseminated fungal infections also have been promising. TFd has been used to treat patients with immunodeficiency diseases and a variety of infectious and parasitic diseases. Although striking results have been reported for disseminated vaccinia, measles, pneumonia, congenital herpes zoster, and cytomegalovirus infection, there have been no controlled studies. Chronic cutaneous leishmaniasis also has been very responsive. No definite conclusions have been reached concerning the usefulness of TFd in cancer because only a few patients have been treated and no controlled trials have been performed. A significant problem has been the selection of appropriate leukocyte donors with cell-mediated immunity to the tumor in question.

Cited References

Lymphokine activated killer cell and interleukin-2 studies. *F-D-C Reports* (May 20) 1985.

Aiuti F, et al: Thymopoietin pentapeptide treatment of primary immunodeficiencies. *Lancet* 1:551-554, 1983 A.

Aiuti F, et al: Placebo-controlled trial of thymic hormone treatment of recurrent herpes simplex labialis infection in immunodeficient hosts. *Int J Clin Pharmacol Ther Toxicol* 21:81-86, 1983 B.

Ameglio F, et al: Differential effects of gamma interferon on expression of HLA class II molecules controlled by DR and DC loci. *Infect Immun* 42:122-125, 1983.

Ammann AJ: Immunodeficiency diseases, in Stites DP, et al (eds): *Basic & Clinical Immunology*, ed 5. Los Altos, CA, Lange Medical Publications, 1984, 384-422.

Assan R, et al: Metabolic and immunological effects of cyclosporin in recently diagnosed type 1 diabetes mellitus. *Lancet* 1:67-71, 1985.

Beaman M, et al: Convulsions associated with cyclosporin A in renal transplant recipients. *Br Med J* 290:139-140, 1985.

Bendtzen K: Ciclosporin (cyclosporin A): Prototype of new generation of immunosuppressive drugs. *Allergy* 39:565-571, 1984.

Bergentz SE, et al: Venous thrombosis and cyclosporin. *Lancet* 2:101-102, 1985.

Brosman SA: Use of bacillus Calmette-Guerin in therapy of bladder carcinoma in situ. *J Urol* 134:36-39, 1985.

Bueding E, et al: Antischistosomal effects of cyclosporin A. *Agents Actions* 11:380-383, 1981.

Burkle WS: Cyclosporine pharmacokinetics and blood level monitoring. *Drug Intell Clin Pharm* 19:101-105, 1985.

Burton RC, et al: Monoclonal antibodies to human T cell subsets: Use for immunologic monitoring and immunosuppression in renal transplantation. *J Clin Immunol* 2(suppl):142S-147S, (July) 1982.

Chang TW, et al: Does OKT3 monoclonal antibody react with an antigen-recognition structure on human T cells? *Proc Natl Acad Sci USA* 78:1805-1808, 1981.

Clumeck N, et al: Preliminary results on clinical and immunological effects of thymopentin in AIDS. *Int J Clin Pharm Res* 4:459-463, 1984.

Cohen DJ, et al: Cyclosporine: New immunosuppressive agent for organ transplantation. *Ann Intern Med* 101:667-682, 1984.

Cosimi AB, et al: Treatment of acute renal allograft rejection with OKT3 monoclonal antibody. *Transplantation* 32:535-539, 1981.

Dimitrov NV, et al: Phase II study of thymosin fraction 5 in treatment of metastatic renal cell carcinoma. *Cancer Treat Rep* 69:137-138, 1985.

Dokhelar M-C, et al: Effect of synthetic thymic factor (facteur thymique serique) on natural killer cell activity in humans. *Int J Immunopharm* 5:277-282, 1983.

Douglas JM, et al: Ineffectiveness and toxicity of BCG vaccine for prevention of recurrent genital herpes. *Antimicrob Agents Chemother* 27:203-206, 1985.

Ershler WB, et al: Specific antibody synthesis in vitro: II. Age-associated thymosin enhancement of antitetanus antibody synthesis. *Immunopharmacology* 8:69-77, 1984.

Ewan PW: Allergy to insect stings: Review. *J R Soc Med* 78:234-239, 1985.

Frasca D, et al: Enhancement of helper and suppressor T cell activities by thymosin α_1 injection in old mice. *Immunopharmacology* 10:41-49, 1985.

Fries D, et al: Prospective study of triple association: Cyclosporine, corticosteroids, and azathioprine in immunologically high-risk renal transplant. *Transplant Proc* 27:1231-1234, 1985.

Hurd ER: Immunosuppressive and anti-inflammatory properties of cyclophosphamide, azathioprine and methotrexate. *Arthritis Rheum* 16:84-88, 1973.

Illner W-D, et al: Cyclosporine in combination with azathioprine and steroids in cadaveric renal transplant. *Transplant Proc* 27:1181-1184, 1985.

Itoh K, et al: Generation of activated killer (AK) cells by recombinant interleukin 2 (rIL 2) in collaboration with interferon-γ (IFN-γ). *J Immunol* 134:3124-3129, 1985.

Jacques Y, Soulillou J-P: Third French workshop on interleukin-2: Joint report. *Lymphokine Res* 4:159-167, 1985.

June CH, et al: Profound hypomagnesemia and renal magnesium wasting associated with use of cyclosporine for marrow transplantation. *Transplantation* 39:620-624, 1985.

Kawase I, et al: Interleukin 2 induces γ-interferon production: Participation of macrophages and NK-like cells. *J Immunol* 131:288-292, 1983.

Kay RG, et al: Levamisole in primary breast cancer: Controlled study in conjunction with L-phenylalanine mustard. *Cancer* 51:1992-1997, 1983.

Kelley DR, et al: Intravesical bacillus Calmette-Guerin therapy for superficial bladder cancer: Effect of bacillus Calmette-Guerin viability on treatment results. *J Urol* 134:48-53, 1985.

Khoo SK, et al: Levamisole as adjuvant to chemotherapy of ovarian cancer: Results of randomized trial and 4-year follow-up. *Cancer* 54:986-990, 1984.

Kirkland TN, Fierer J: Cyclosporin A inhibits *Coccidioides immitis* in vitro and in vivo. *Antimicrob Agents Chemother* 24:921-924, 1983.

Klefström P, et al: Levamisole in treatment of stage II breast cancer: Five-year follow-up of randomized double-blind study. *Cancer* 55:2753-2757, 1985.

Klein A, et al: Difference between human B and T lymphocytes regarding their capacity to metabolize cortisol. *J Steroid Biochem* 13:517-520, 1980.

Koff WC, et al: Protection of mice against fatal herpes simplex type 2 infection by liposomes containing muramyl tripeptide. *Science* 228:495-497, 1985.

Kung PC, et al: Monoclonal antibodies defining distinctive human T cell surface antigens. *Science* 206:347-349, 1979.

Lamm DL: Bacillus Calmette-Guerin immunotherapy for bladder cancer. *J Urol* 134:40-47, 1985.

Lichtenstein LM, et al: Insect allergy: State of the art. *J Allergy Clin Immunol* 64:5-12, 1979.

Luzi G, et al: Levamisole therapy: Clinical and immunological evaluation in herpetic keratitis. *Int J Immunopharm* 5:197-199, 1983.

Malaise MG, et al: Treatment of active rheumatoid arthritis with slow intravenous injections of thymopentin: Double-blind placebo-controlled randomized study. *Lancet* 1:832-836, 1985.

Mandrup-Poulsen T, et al: Disappearance and reappearance of islet cell cytoplasmic antibodies in cyclosporin-treated insulin-dependent diabetics. *Lancet* 1:599-602, 1985.

Morton DL, et al: Immunological factors which influence response to immunotherapy in malignant melanoma. *Surgery* 68:158-164, 1970.

Mulé JJ, et al: Adoptive immunotherapy of established pulmonary metastases with LAK cells and recombinant interleukin-2. *Science* 225:1487-1489, 1984.

Netto RG Jr, Lemos GC: Bacillus Calmette-Guerin immunotherapy of infiltrating bladder cancer. *J Urol* 132:675-677, 1984.

Nichols EE: Routine antepartum Rh immune globulin administration. *JAMA* 252:2763, 1984.

Nickell SP, et al: Inhibition by cyclosporin A of rodent malaria in vivo and human malaria in vitro. *Infect Immun* 37:1093-1100, 1982.

Noll RB, Kulkarni R: Complex visual hallucinations and cyclosporine. *Arch Neurol* 41:329-330, 1984.

Ortaldo JR, et al: Effects of natural and recombinant IL 2 on regulation of IFN γ production and natural killer activity: Lack of involvement of TAC antigen for these immunoregulatory effects. *J Immunol* 133:779-783, 1984.

Ortho Multicenter Transplant Study Group: Randomized clinical trial of OKT3 monoclonal antibody for acute rejection of cadaveric renal transplants. *N Engl J Med* 313:337-342, 1985.

Patrone F, et al: Restoration of defective EA$_G$-rosetting capacity of cancer patient neutrophils by levamisole. *Cancer* 55:1668-1672, 1985.

Phillips NC, et al: Modulation of murine lymphoma growth by MDP, MDP(D-D) and cyclophosphamide: 1. Inhibition of growth in vivo. *Int J Immunopharm* 5:219-227, 1983.

Pizza G, et al: Tumour regression after intralesional injection of interleukin 2 (IL-2) in bladder cancer: Preliminary report. *Int J Cancer* 34:359-367, 1984.

Ponticelli C, et al: Controlled trial of methylprednisolone and chlorambucil in idiopathic membranous nephropathy. *N Engl J Med* 310:946-950, 1984.

Powell-Jackson PR, et al: Adult respiratory distress syndrome and convulsions associated with administration of cyclosporine in liver transplant recipients. *Transplantation* 38:341-343, 1984.

Ptachcinski RJ, et al: Cyclosporine. *Drug Intell Clin Pharm* 19:90-100, 1985 A.

Ptachcinski RJ, et al: Effect of food on cyclosporine absorption. *Transplantation* 40:174-176, 1985 B.

Reem GH, et al: Gamma interferon synthesis by human thymocytes and T lymphocytes inhibited by cyclosporin A. *Science* 221:63-65, 1983.

Rosenberg SA, et al: Biological activity of recombinant human interleukin-2 produced in *Escherichia coli. Science* 223:1412-1415, 1984.

Schuyler RM, et al: Prednisone and T-cell subpopulations. *Arch Intern Med* 144:973-975, 1984.

Shah D, et al: Generalised epileptic fits in renal transplant recipients given cyclosporin A. *Br Med J* 289:1347-1348, 1984.

Shohat B, et al: In vitro induction of T suppressor lymphocytes in recipients of renal allografts by THF, a thymic hormone. *Transplantation* 35:68-71, 1983.

Slapak M, et al: Use of low-dose cyclosporine in combination with azathioprine and steroids in renal transplantation. *Transplant Proc* 27:1222-1226, 1985.

Small P, et al: Venom immunotherapy: Critical evaluation of in vitro techniques. *Ann Allergy* 50:256-259, 1983.

Smalley RV, et al: Thymosins: Preclinical and clinical studies with fraction V and alpha-I. *Cancer Treat Rev* 11:69-84, 1984.

Smith BR, et al: Efficacy of short course (four doses) of methotrexate following bone marrow transplantation for prevention of graft-versus-host disease. *Transplantation* 39:326-329, 1985.

Sone S, et al: Potentiating effect of muramyl dipeptide and its lipophilic analog encapsulated in liposomes on tumour cell killing by human monocytes. *J Immunol* 132:2105-2110, 1984.

Stiller CR, et al: Effects of cyclosporine immunosuppression in insulin-dependent diabetes mellitus of recent onset. *Science* 223:1362-1367, 1984.

Storb R, et al: Methotrexate and cyclosporine compared with cyclosporine alone for prophylaxis of acute graft versus host disease after marrow transplantation for leukemia. *N Engl J Med* 314:729-735, 1986.

Thompson CB, et al: Association between cyclosporin neurotoxicity and hypomagnesaemia. *Lancet* 2:1116-1120, 1984.

Tsang KY, et al: In vitro restoration of immune response in aging humans by isoprinosine. *Int J Immunopharm* 7:199-206, 1985.

Vanrenterghen Y, et al: Thromboembolic complications and haemostatic changes in cyclosporin-treated cadaveric kidney allograft recipients. *Lancet* 1:999-1002, 1985.

Van Sloten K, et al: Evaluation of levamisole as adjuvant to chemotherapy for treatment of ANLL. *Cancer* 51:1576-1580, 1983.

Van Wauwe JP, et al: OKT3: Monoclonal antihuman T lymphocyte antibody with potent mitogenic properties. *J Immunol* 124:2708-2713, 1980.

Webb DR, Winkelstein A: Immunosuppression, immunopotentiation, and anti-inflammatory drugs, in Stites DP, et al (eds): *Basic & Clinical Immunology,* ed 5. Los Altos, CA, Lange Medical Publications, 1984, 271-287.

Weigent DA, et al: Interleukin 2 enhances natural killer cell activity through induction of gamma interferon. *Infect Immun* 41:992-997, 1983.

Zazgornik J, et al: Venous thrombosis and cyclosporin, (letter). *Lancet* 2:102, 1985.

Drugs Used in Cancer Chemotherapy

64

In the past half century, since the reduction of death rates due to infectious diseases, cancer has emerged as one of the leading causes of death in industrial societies. In the United States, cancer ranks second to heart disease in overall mortality and is the leading cause of death in women age 30 to 54 and in children age 3 to 14 (Carter et al, 1982). Although great efforts have been made in cancer research and major developments have occurred in molecular and cellular biology, many fundamental questions remain unanswered and the etiology and pathogenesis of the basic neoplastic process are still unknown.

All cancers are malignant tumors characterized by an unlimited growth potential and an ability to expand locally by invasion of surrounding tissues and systemically by metastasis to distant sites. However, depending on the organ system and cell type involved, each form of cancer has a unique natural history, pattern of spread, and response to therapy. Therefore, the physician engaged in the treatment of cancer is faced with not one but a multiplicity of diseases. When additional factors, such as extent of disease (eg, size of primary tumor, status of lymph nodes, presence of metastasis) and patient characteristics, are considered for each case, it becomes apparent that the treatment of cancer is sufficiently complex to present a considerable challenge even to the experienced oncologist.

The most important decision to be made in developing a treatment plan for the patient with cancer is to determine whether the goal is cure or palliation (eg, increased survival time, alleviation of symptoms, maintenance of close to normal function). When cure is considered possible, therapy must be appropriate and aggressive. The underlying principle of curative cancer therapy is the removal or eradication of the last neoplastic cell, since it appears that a single clonogenic malignant cell is capable of multiplying and eventually killing the host by the volume of its progeny (Skipper et al, 1964). Palliative therapy should provide benefits to the patient that outweigh the risks of treatment and ranges from aggressive chemotherapy, such as that employed for acute leukemias in adults, to no treatment at all.

Three major therapeutic modalities are currently employed in cancer treatment: surgery, radiation therapy, and chemotherapy (including hormones). Surgery and/or radiation usually are the initial treatment modalities for most solid cancers, particularly when cure is anticipated. However, surgical extirpation or irradiation of malignant tissue only eliminates localized and regional disease. At present, only one-third of patients are cured with surgery or radiation therapy alone; in the remaining patients, the tumor is already disseminated at the time of diagnosis and local therapy is ineffective (Martin, 1981).

Anticancer drugs can be effective in systemic neoplastic

disease. Chemotherapy traditionally has been the primary treatment modality in hematologic malignancies (eg, leukemias, lymphomas) and choriocarcinoma. Increased understanding of the pharmacology and mechanisms of action of several antineoplastic agents has led to rational application of these drugs, often in combination (combination chemotherapy). Such chemotherapy has resulted in five-year survival rates approaching 50% or better in disseminated Hodgkin's disease, acute lymphocytic leukemia in children, Burkitt's lymphoma, and choriocarcinoma. The five-year survival rates for some forms of disseminated non-Hodgkin's lymphoma also have been increased (Krakoff, 1981).

In the past, chemotherapy was used only secondarily to treat solid tumors unresponsive to surgery and radiation therapy. Although antineoplastic drugs are still widely used for palliation of certain disseminated cancers, greater emphasis is being placed on optimal chemotherapy for primary treatment with curative intent. Nonseminomatous testicular carcinomas, a class of rapidly growing tumors, are particularly sensitive to antineoplastic drugs and approximately 70% of disseminated testicular cancers can be cured by combination chemotherapy alone following orchiectomy (Einhorn, 1981). Chemotherapy combined with surgery and/or irradiation, termed adjuvant chemotherapy, has increased survival rates for a number of solid tumors. Although the greatest success has been achieved with relatively uncommon solid tumors in children (eg, Wilms' tumor, Ewing's sarcoma, embryonal rhabdomyosarcoma), survival also has been prolonged in other cancers (eg, osteogenic sarcoma, breast cancer) (Martin, 1981).

This chapter has been divided into four sections: basic principles of cancer chemotherapy; antineoplastic drug selection, including combination chemotherapy, adjuvant chemotherapy, and a brief overview of current chemotherapy for a number of human cancers; toxicities associated with the use of antineoplastic agents; and evaluations of individual antineoplastic drugs, including investigational agents.

PRINCIPLES OF CANCER CHEMOTHERAPY

The goal of cancer chemotherapy is to achieve selective toxicity against malignant tumor cells and to spare normal host cells. Selective toxicity of the degree associated with bacterial chemotherapy has not been possible in chemotherapy of cancers, however, because the differences between normal and malignant cells are much more subtle. With few exceptions, antineoplastic agents suppress proliferating cells, and toxicity to dividing normal cells (eg, bone marrow, gastrointestinal and germinal epithelia, hair follicles, lymphoid organs) is a routine consequence of cancer chemotherapy. Thus, successful treatment depends upon killing malignant tumor cells with doses that allow recovery of normal proliferating cells. Although many successes in cancer chemotherapy have been the result of empiricism, rationales for drug treatment based on tumor determinants, particularly cell kinetics, and pharmacologic and host factors have clearly evolved. For more detailed discussions, see Pratt and Ruddon, 1979; Carter et al, 1981; Carter and Livingston, 1982 A; DeVita, 1985; Mihich and Creaven, 1982; Skipper and Schabel, 1982; Steel, 1982; and Zubrod, 1982.

Tumor Determinants

Growth Fraction, Gompertzian Growth Curves: Rapidly growing cancers (eg, certain leukemias and lymphomas, choriocarcinoma, testicular cancer) are more susceptible to killing by antineoplastic agents than slower growing cancers (eg, nonsmall cell lung, colon, breast). A major determinant of the time it takes a malignant tumor to double its volume, ie, the mass doubling time, is its growth fraction, which is defined as the percentage of viable cells in active cell division. Actively dividing tumor cells usually are most sensitive to cytotoxic anticancer drugs. Certain normal tissues (eg, bone marrow, gastrointestinal mucosa, hair follicles) with high growth fractions also are susceptible to these drugs. Thus, the difference in growth fractions between tumor and normal cell populations is a very important factor in determining the outcome of chemotherapy. When active drugs are given in the proper schedule, tumors with a high growth fraction can be treated successfully with acceptable toxicity to normal tissues. This usually is not the case for tumors with low growth fractions, however.

Based on experimental tumor models, the growth curves of most cancers follow a Gompertzian function, ie, growth at every instant is exponential but with a growth constant that simultaneously is exponentially slowing. Thus, the doubling time increases as the tumor volume increases and is probably due to depletion of nutrients resulting in both increased cell loss and, more importantly, decreased growth fraction. Because it is estimated that a tumor must be 1 cm in diameter and contain approximately 1×10^9 cells to be diagnosed clinically, it is believed that many human cancers, particularly solid tumors, are approaching the plateau phase of the Gompertzian growth curve when they are diagnosed. Thus, the effectiveness of chemotherapy is further diminished by the smaller growth fractions associated with the relatively large tumors present at initial diagnosis.

The model implies that smaller tumors are more sensitive to chemotherapy and has provided a rationale for the treatment approaches now employed clinically. One approach is to remove large tumor volumes by surgery or irradiation (debulking) in the hope that the remaining cells will be stimulated into active division and, therefore, be susceptible to chemotherapy. This has been termed recruitment. Another approach (adjuvant chemotherapy) is to treat certain high-risk patients who have apparently local or regional disease with chemotherapy shortly after removing the primary tumor by surgery or irradiation. Because it is common for metastases to develop eventually after surgery or irradiation alone, adjuvant chemotherapy is initiated when metastases are small (micrometastases) and presumed to have large growth fractions.

Tumor Burden, Cell-kill Hypothesis: In addition to a decreased growth fraction, a large tumor burden imposes additional problems for effective chemotherapy: therapeutic concentrations of drug may not be able to penetrate large tumors, metastases are more likely to have occurred, greater heterogeneity within the tumor cell population increases the potential for drug resistance, and there are more tumor cells that must be killed. The last point deserves particular attention. Based on animal tumor models, it has been shown that antineoplastic drugs kill tumor cells by first-order kinetics, ie, a given dose of drug kills a constant fraction, rather than a constant number, of tumor cells. In other words, the same dose that can reduce the tumor burden from 1×10^{12} to 1×10^9 cells would be required to lower the number from 1×10^9 to 1×10^6 cells. Furthermore, it has been shown that one remaining viable tumor cell has the ability to repopulate and eventually kill the host.

The clinical implication of this cytokinetic data is that successful chemotherapy is most likely when the tumor burden is low. Also, since the dose-response curves for most antineoplastic drugs are quite steep, the use of maximally tolerated doses with optimal scheduling is recommended to obtain the highest log kill of tumor cells compatible with recovery of normal proliferating cells. Even when other reasons for treatment failure are disregarded, cure of cancer by chemotherapy cannot be accomplished if tumor cells repopulate more quickly than normal cells.

Presently, quantitative cytokinetic data on human cancers are considerably less accurate than those on experimental tumors. Estimation of total tumor burden, particularly for solid tumors, can be subject to considerable error. This is also true for estimates of cell-kill (eg, by measuring numbers of remaining leukemia cells or the decrease in size of a solid tumor) and rate of tumor cell repopulation (eg, by determining time to recurrence). Heterogeneity within tumor cell populations increases the imprecision. Furthermore, although the steep dose-response relationships observed for most anticancer drugs in experimental systems, which are the basis for the use of high-dose intermittent treatment scheduling, appear to hold true for human cancers, some exceptions have been observed. Thus, it is difficult to determine optimal dose, interval, and duration of treatment clinically. Although past knowledge should be utilized, certain assumptions and empiric decisions are often necessary.

Antineoplastic Agents and the Cell Cycle: To understand why only certain cells in a tumor are susceptible to drugs and how different drugs act, the phases of the cell cycle must be considered. All actively dividing cells pass through certain phases from one mitosis to the next. The first part of the interphase after completion of cell division is called the G_1 phase; during this phase, DNA synthesis is absent but RNA and protein synthesis continue normally. In late G_1, there is a burst of RNA synthesis and the S phase begins, during which cellular DNA is replicated. After completion of the S phase, a cell enters the G_2 period. During this phase, the cell is tetraploid, ie, it contains twice the DNA content, and it continues to synthesize RNA and protein. In mitosis (M phase), RNA and protein synthesis diminish abruptly while genetic material is segregated into daughter cells. After completion of mitosis, a cell may re-enter the G_1 phase and continue to proliferate, or the cell may enter a resting state, usually termed the G_0 phase. Some resting cells lose their ability to proliferate and are

irreversibly out of cycle. Other resting cells retain the potential to produce an unlimited line of descendants and are the so-called clonogenic or stem cells. The sensitivity of actively dividing cells to cytotoxic antineoplastic agents and the importance of a large growth fraction to the success of chemotherapy have been discussed. Resting clonogenic cells are also very important because they are most likely to survive chemotherapy and are necessary for the recovery of proliferating normal tissues; however, they also can repopulate the tumor, resulting in disease recurrence. Thus, the persistence of resting clonogenic tumor cells is a likely cause of chemotherapeutic failures.

A number of antineoplastic drugs are effective primarily during a specific part of the cell cycle and are classified as cell-cycle phase specific drugs. For example, cytarabine and hydroxyurea are S phase specific, ie, they exert their cytotoxic effects only on dividing cells in the S phase of the cell cycle. Other drugs, such as methotrexate and mercaptopurine, are also S phase specific, but their effects are considered to be self-limiting because they have other inhibitory actions that slow the entry of cells into the S phase. The mitotic spindle inhibitors, vincristine and vinblastine, are M phase specific drugs. Phase specific anticancer drugs are effective only against actively dividing cells. Furthermore, cytotoxic concentrations of phase specific drugs must be maintained long enough to expose a sufficient number of tumor cells during the sensitive phase.

The remaining antineoplastic drugs usually are considered to be cycle phase nonspecific and include alkylating agents, most antitumor antibiotics, cisplatin, and procarbazine. Distinctions are more relative than absolute, however, and many cycle phase nonspecific agents are more effective against proliferating cells and those in a specific phase of the cell cycle. For example, if alkylated DNA of a resting clonogenic tumor cell is repaired prior to entry of the cell into the DNA replicative cycle, that cell will be unaffected by the alkylating agent.

In animal tumor models, effective chemotherapeutic regimens have been developed on the basis of known cell cycle specificities of various antineoplastic agents. For example, when mice bearing L1210 leukemia cells were given vinblastine followed by cytarabine 16 hours later, therapeutic effectiveness was enhanced markedly (Vadlamudi and Goldin, 1971). Enhanced activity was not observed when the drugs were given at the same time. The explanation for these observations was that vinblastine arrested cells in M phase resulting in a synchronized cell population. About 16 hours later, essentially all of the cells entered the S phase and were sensitive to the effects of cytarabine. Thus, sequencing and timing of this two-drug combination were critical to its enhanced effectiveness. Clinical application of this approach requires a tumor with a large growth fraction. In addition, concomitant synchronization of normal proliferating cells (eg, bone marrow) should be avoided to obtain a selective antitumor effect.

Resistance: The presence of drug-resistant tumor cells is another important factor in the success or failure of cancer chemotherapy. A mathematical model has been developed

(Goldie and Coldman, 1979) for drug resistance in tumor cell populations, in which the likelihood of finding a single cell with resistance to a specific drug is related to both population size and frequency of mutation. Antineoplastic agents exert a positive selective pressure on tumor cell populations; replication of drug-resistant clones can result in drug-resistant tumors and therapeutic failures.

Some of the mechanisms identified are decreased cellular uptake or enhanced efflux (many drugs), increased target enzyme or altered affinity for target enzyme (methotrexate), decreased activation of drug (mercaptopurine and fluorouracil), increased deactivation of drug (cytarabine), increased DNA repair (alkylating agents), and increased utilization of salvage pathways for purine and pyrimidine biosynthesis (antimetabolites). In addition, tumor cells may develop pleiotropic drug resistance. After exposure to a single drug, cells may become cross-resistant to a number of structurally unrelated compounds with different mechanisms of action. It appears that resistant cells have impaired ability to accumulate and retain drug. A high-molecular-weight "P-glycoprotein" appears to be a phenotypic marker for this form of drug resistance. Reversal of this process has been reported using calcium channel blocking agents and calmodulin inhibitors.

To avoid drug resistance, combinations of drugs having different mechanisms of action that are individually effective in the specific tumor are employed and therapy is initiated when the tumor burden is small (see the section on Combination Chemotherapy).

Pharmacologic Determinants

The effectiveness of an antineoplastic agent is related directly to its pharmacologic disposition in the patient. Tumoricidal concentrations must reach the tumor cells and remain there for a sufficient time to kill the tumor cells. As with other drug classes, basic principles of pharmacology apply to anticancer drugs. The attainment of therapeutic concentrations inside the tumor cell depends upon absorption (eg, for oral preparations), plasma protein binding, distribution to various organs, rates of excretion (eg, renal, biliary) and metabolic transformation, and a drug's ability to penetrate into the (solid) tumor and cross individual tumor cell membranes. The following examples illustrate the importance of these factors.

Cyclophosphamide is a prodrug that must be metabolized by the hepatic mixed-function oxidase system before active drug can be generated. Mechlorethamine, dactinomycin, daunorubicin, and doxorubicin are very reactive chemically and must be administered intravenously to obtain a systemic effect and avoid local tissue necrosis. Cytarabine has an extremely short serum half-life (eg, 12 minutes for the initial phase) due to rapid inactivation by cytidine deaminase, particularly in the liver. Thus, this drug must be administered by continuous intravenous infusion to maintain effective concentrations. At present, the use of continuous infusions of a variety of chemotherapeutic agents is being investigated (Vogelzang, 1984).

Nitrosoureas and procarbazine are among the few antineo-plastic drugs that cross the blood-brain barrier in sufficient concentrations to be useful in brain tumors. High dose methotrexate and cytosine arabinoside also may provide adequate central nervous system levels. When most other antineoplastic agents are used systemically, the central nervous system can provide a pharmacologic sanctuary for tumor cells that can lead to relapse. It is for this reason that, in addition to systemic therapy, intrathecal methotrexate and CNS radiation therapy are given prophylactically to prevent central nervous system relapses in acute lymphocytic leukemia in children.

For tumors confined to the pleural or peritoneal cavities, intracavitary chemotherapy may allow high local concentrations of drug with acceptable systemic levels (Markman, 1985). Low blood flow to parts of large (ischemic) tumors often prevents adequate drug penetration to all tumor cells in the mass.

Finally, a sufficient concentration of most drugs must cross the individual tumor cell membrane to reach the site of action inside the cell. If the permeability barrier is too formidable, the drug will not be effective. Large doses of methotrexate are necessary to attain effective concentrations in osteogenic sarcoma cells, in part because of poor transport across the sarcoma cell membrane. Usually, such amounts would be prohibitively toxic to normal cells (eg, bone marrow). However, the subsequent administration of leucovorin (N^5N^{10}-formyl-tetrahydrofolate), which enters normal and malignant cells via a carrier-mediated transport mechanism, bypasses the methotrexate inhibition of dihydrofolate reductase in normal cells and "rescues" them from the cytotoxic antimetabolite. Thus, differences in membrane transport have been exploited to a therapeutic advantage, although the clinical efficacy of this approach remains controversial (see the evaluation on Methotrexate).

The attainment of selectively tumoricidal concentrations of an antineoplastic drug requires consideration of additional, complicating factors. As discussed earlier, not all tumor cells are susceptible to a cytotoxic anticancer drug at any given time (eg, only S phase cells are sensitive to cytarabine) and a certain percentage of dividing normal cells are likely to be killed. Furthermore, both tumor and normal cell growth kinetics will be perturbed by drug administration and subsequent drug sensitivities may be altered. Thus, dosage schedules must be optimized to yield a maximum tumor cell kill with minimum lethality to normal cells.

Host Determinants

A number of host factors also influence the response to cancer chemotherapy. Among the most important is the overall performance status (eg, Karnofsky Scale) of the patient. Generally, individuals who appear normal, are not complaining, and show no evidence of disease (eg, performance score of 100) are likely to have the best response to chemotherapy. As disease symptoms increase and the ability to function normally decreases, the prognosis for successful therapy diminishes. Patients who are disabled and require special care and assistance (eg, performance score of 40 or less) are less likely to improve significantly with chemotherapy.

Thus, for most cancers, patients who are diagnosed early have a greater chance for prolonged survival and possible cure.

The patient's immune status, particularly cell-mediated immunity, is another important correlate of response to chemotherapy. Immunocompetent individuals respond to chemotherapy more favorably than immunocompromised patients. The determination of immune status is complicated because the neoplastic disease produces immunologic defects, and most antineoplastic drugs are immunosuppressive due to their antiproliferative effect on blood cell-forming tissues. Generally, maintenance of immunocompetence has been accomplished most often by using intensive, intermittent, chemotherapy regimens in which time is allowed for recovery of these normal tissues.

Patients who have not received prior radiation or chemotherapy almost invariably show a better response than previously treated patients. Prior treatment usually decreases tolerance to the myelosuppressive effects of antineoplastic agents and the immune status is more likely to be compromised. As a result, the first attempt at therapy should be with maximal tolerated doses and optimal scheduling, particularly when cure is anticipated. Supportive measures, including platelet and granulocyte replacement transfusions, antimicrobial chemotherapy, hyperalimentation, and allopurinol administration to prevent uric acid-induced renal disease may increase the likelihood of success.

Other patient characteristics that influence the response to chemotherapy include age, sex, race, organ function, and the presence of other diseases. For example, the functional status of organs involved in drug elimination or particularly susceptible to drug toxicity must be considered. The dosages of methotrexate and doxorubicin may have to be reduced in patients with impaired renal or hepatic function, respectively, because these drugs are eliminated primarily by these organs. Similarly, doxorubicin, bleomycin, and cisplatin must be administered with caution or avoided in patients with pre-existing cardiac, pulmonary, or renal disease, respectively, because of their direct toxic effects on these organs.

ANTINEOPLASTIC DRUG SELECTION

A large number of antineoplastic agents are currently available for use in various cancers. The individual drugs are listed in Table 1 according to class, and important properties of each drug are summarized. Some antineoplastic drugs (eg, cyclophosphamide [Cytoxan, Neosar], methotrexate [Folex, Mexate], vincristine [Oncovin], doxorubicin [Adriamycin]) have broad spectrums of activity and are used in the treatment of many hematologic and solid cancers. In contrast, the use of other drugs is limited due to tissue-specific toxicity (eg, mitotane [Lysodren] for adrenocortical tissue, streptozocin [Zanosar] for beta cells of the islets of Langerhans) or undesirable toxicologic (eg, plicamycin [Mithracin]) or pharmacologic (eg, mechlorethamine [Mustargen]) properties.

A primary determinant of antineoplastic drug selection clinically is the sensitivity of a particular cancer to the various drugs. General knowledge of tumor sensitivities has primarily been obtained empirically in clinical trials. Although a reasonably reliable prediction can be made, individual tumors may not respond, resulting in chemotherapeutic failure. Analogous to susceptibility testing in bacteria, specific chemosensitivity tests for an individual patient's tumors would be highly desirable in cancer chemotherapy. Unfortunately, although several methods of in vitro chemosensitivity testing (Carney, 1984) have been developed, these techniques remain experimental. One exception is the estrogen receptor (ER) assay in advanced breast cancer. Patients with ER-negative tumors are not likely to respond to hormonal therapy and such patients are initially treated with chemotherapy. Patients with ER-positive tumors receive hormonal therapy, although the presence of estrogen receptors accurately predicts response in only about 60% of the cases. Recent studies suggest that concomitant measurement of tumor progesterone receptors may improve the predictive capability (McGuire, 1982).

Certain cancers, particularly those with a high growth fraction, are quite sensitive to chemotherapy. These include acute leukemias, lymphomas, many pediatric solid tumors, nonseminomatous testicular cancer, and small cell lung, ovarian, and breast carcinomas. Patients, even those with a poorer performance status, who have these types of cancers usually should be treated because of the possibility of a complete response leading to prolonged survival and, in some cases, cure. Consistent with the principles outlined in the preceding section, the first attempt at therapy should aim for maximal effectiveness, even if it is likely to be the most toxic. Drugs should be used in the largest possible doses to ensure an optimal tumor cell kill and should be administered by the routes and in the schedules designed to provide optimal selective toxicity to the tumors.

Many solid cancers, including renal, pancreatic, colorectal, and non-small cell lung carcinomas and melanomas remain relatively refractory to chemotherapy. For patients with these types of cancers, other factors (eg, performance status, age, extent of disease, expected drug-induced toxicity) must be considered before initiating chemotherapy. If chemotherapy is elected, participation in a therapeutic research protocol is the best approach.

Currently preferred regimens for various human cancers are listed in Table 2. The purpose of this list is to provide an overview of the role of chemotherapy in the treatment of different neoplastic diseases and to give the reader some knowledge of what drugs and drug combinations are being used. Because the ideal drug treatment protocol has not been clearly defined for any cancer, preferred drugs or combinations of drugs are likely to change as clinical trials identify more effective regimens. New developments in clinical cancer chemotherapy are being evaluated annually by leading medical oncologists (Marsoni and Wittes, 1984). Thus, some or many of the preferences listed in Table 2 are likely to become obsolete with time.

Combination Chemotherapy

Significant remissions or cures with single-agent chemotherapy have been obtained only for choriocarcinoma and Burkitt's lymphoma. In all other cancers for which chemotherapy has

TABLE 1.
SPECIFIC AGENTS USED IN CANCER CHEMOTHERAPY[1]

Drug	Cell Cycle Specificity	Route of Administration	Elimination
ALKYLATING AGENTS			
Nitrogen Mustards			
Chlorambucil [Leukeran]	Phase nonspecific	Oral	Metabolic
Cyclophosphamide CTX; [Cytoxan, Neosar]	Phase nonspecific	Intravenous, oral	Metabolic
Mechlorethamine Hydrochloride HN$_2$, Nitrogen Mustard; [Mustargen]	Phase nonspecific but M and G$_1$ most sensitive	Intravenous, intracavitary, topical	Metabolic
Melphalan L-PAM, Phenylalanine Mustard; [Alkeran]	Phase nonspecific	Oral	Metabolic
Aziridine Derivative			
Thiotepa	Phase nonspecific	Intravenous, intracavitary, intravesical, intrathecal	Metabolic
Alkyl Sulfonate			
Busulfan [Myleran]	Phase nonspecific	Oral	Metabolic
Nitrosoureas			
Carmustine BCNU; [BiCNU]	Phase nonspecific	Intravenous, topical	Metabolic
Lomustine CCNU; [CeeNU]	Phase nonspecific	Oral	Metabolic
Streptozocin Streptozotocin; [Zanosar]	Phase nonspecific but S phase most sensitive	Intravenous	Metabolic and renal
Triazene			
Dacarbazine DIC, DTIC; [DTIC-Dome]	Phase nonspecific	Intravenous	Metabolic
ANTIMETABOLITES			
Folic Acid Analogue			
Methotrexate and Methotrexate Sodium MTX, Amethopterin; [Folex, Methotrexate, Mexate]	S-phase specific but self-limiting	Intravenous, intramuscular, oral, intrathecal	Renal and liver
Pyrimidine Analogues			
Cytarabine Ara C, Cytosine Arabinoside; [Cytosar-U]	S-phase specific	Intravenous, subcutaneous, intrathecal	Metabolic

Major Toxicity[1]		
Acute	**Delayed**	**Indications**
Mild nausea and vomiting	*Bone marrow depression* (leukopenia, thrombocytopenia, anemia)	Chronic lymphocytic leukemia; Hodgkin's and non-Hodgkin's lymphomas; choriocarcinoma; testicular cancer; ovarian carcinoma
Nausea and vomiting	*Bone marrow depression* (leukopenia, thrombocytopenia); alopecia; hemorrhagic cystitis	Acute and chronic lymphocytic leukemias; Hodgkin's, non-Hodgkin's, and Burkitt's lymphomas; multiple myeloma; choriocarcinoma; testicular cancer; breast, lung, ovarian, endometrial, and cervical carcinomas; Ewing's and soft tissue sarcomas; rhabdomyosarcoma; neuroblastoma
Nausea and vomiting; local irritant	*Bone marrow depression* (leukopenia, thrombocytopenia)	Hodgkin's and non-Hodgkin's lymphomas, cutaneous T cell lymphomas
Mild nausea and vomiting	*Bone marrow depression* (leukopenia, thrombocytopenia, anemia)	Multiple myeloma; breast and ovarian carcinomas; melanoma
Mild nausea and vomiting; local pain	*Bone marrow depression* (leukopenia, thrombocytopenia, anemia)	Hodgkin's disease; breast and ovarian carcinomas; bladder (intravesically)
Mild nausea and vomiting	*Bone marrow depression* (leukopenia, thrombocytopenia, anemia); pulmonary fibrosis; hyperpigmentation of skin	Chronic myelogenous leukemia
Nausea and vomiting; local pain	*Bone marrow depression* (delayed leukopenia and thrombocytopenia; myelosuppression is cumulative); pulmonary fibrosis; renal and hepatic toxicity	Brain tumors; Hodgkin's and non-Hodgkin's lymphomas; multiple myeloma; gastric and colorectal carcinomas; melanoma
Nausea and vomiting	*Bone marrow depression* (delayed leukopenia, thrombocytopenia, anemia; myelosuppression is cumulative); alopecia; renal and hepatic toxicity	Brain tumors; Hodgkin's and non-Hodgkin's lymphomas; lung and colorectal carcinomas, melanoma
Nausea and vomiting; local pain	*Renal toxicity* (common); bone marrow depression (uncommon and usually mild); hepatotoxicity; hyperglycemia	Islet cell carcinoma, malignant carcinoid; pancreatic carcinoma; Hodgkin's disease
Nausea and vomiting; local pain	*Bone marrow depression* (leukopenia, thrombocytopenia); flu-like syndrome	Hodgkin's disease; melanoma; soft tissue sarcomas; neuroblastoma
Mild nausea and vomiting; diarrhea; acute hypersensitivity reactions	*Bone marrow depression* (leukopenia, anemia, thrombocytopenia); oral and gastrointestinal ulceration; renal tubular necrosis; hepatic fibrosis; pneumonitis; osteoporosis	Choriocarcinoma; acute lymphocytic leukemia; non-Hodgkin's lymphomas; osteogenic sarcoma; rhabdomyosarcoma; testicular cancer; head and neck, breast, lung, cervical, ovarian, and bladder carcinomas; medulloblastoma
Nausea and vomiting; fever; anaphylaxis (hypersensitivity)	*Bone marrow depression* (leukopenia, thrombocytopenia, anemia, megaloblastosis); stomatitis, hepatic dysfunction	Acute myelogenous leukemia; acute lymphocytic leukemia; non-Hodgkin's lymphomas

(Continued on next page)

TABLE 1 (continued)

Drug	Cell Cycle Specificity	Route of Administration	Elimination
Floxuridine [FUDR]	Phase nonspecific but acts on proliferating cells (cycle specific)	Intra-arterial	Metabolic
Fluorouracil 5-FU; [Adrucil, Fluorouracil]	Phase nonspecific but acts on proliferating cells (cycle specific)	Intravenous	Metabolic
Purine Analogues Mercaptopurine 6-MP; [Purinethol]	S-phase specific but self-limiting	Oral	Metabolic
Thioguanine 6-TG	S-phase specific	Oral, intravenous	Metabolic
NATURAL PRODUCTS **Antibiotics** Bleomycin Sulfate [Blenoxane]	Most active in G_2; also active in late G_1, early S, and M phases	Intravenous, intramuscular, subcutaneous	Renal and metabolic
Dactinomycin Actinomycin D; [Cosmegen]	Cycle nonspecific	Intravenous, isolation-perfusion	Biliary and renal
Daunorubicin Hydrochloride [Cerubidine]	Cycle nonspecific, but S phase most sensitive	Intravenous	Metabolic and biliary
Doxorubicin Hydrochloride [Adriamycin]	Cycle nonspecific but S phase most sensitive	Intravenous	Metabolic and biliary
Mitomycin [Mutamycin]	Cycle nonspecific but late G_1 and early S phases most sensitive	Intravenous	Metabolic
Plicamycin [Mithracin]	Cycle nonspecific; S phase probably most sensitive	Intravenous	Metabolic
Plant Alkaloids Vinblastine Sulfate VLB; [Velban]	M-phase specific	Intravenous	Metabolic and biliary

Major Toxicity[1]

Acute	Delayed	Indications
Nausea and vomiting; diarrhea	*Bone marrow depression* (leukopenia, thrombocytopenia, anemia); *oral and gastrointestinal ulceration;* alopecia; hyperpigmentation; dermatitis; cerebellar ataxia; hepatotoxicity	Carcinomas of the gastrointestinal tract
Nausea and vomiting; diarrhea	*Bone marrow depression* (leukopenia, thrombocytopenia, anemia); *oral and gastrointestinal ulceration;* alopecia; hyperpigmentation; dermatitis; cerebellar ataxia	Breast, colorectal, gastric, pancreatic, esophageal, hepatocellular, ovarian, endometrial, cervical, prostate, bladder, and head and neck carcinomas
Nausea, vomiting, and diarrhea (can be dose-limiting with bolus injection)	*Bone marrow depression* (particularly leukopenia; also thrombocytopenia, anemia); hepatotoxicity	Acute myelogenous leukemia
Occasional nausea and vomiting	*Bone marrow depression* (leukopenia, thrombocytopenia, anemia); cholestasis	Acute myelogenous leukemia; chronic myelogenous leukemia; acute lymphocytic leukemia
Mild nausea and vomiting (uncommon); fever; anaphylaxis and other hypersensitivity reactions	*Pneumonitis and pulmonary fibrosis;* cutaneous reactions; stomatitis; alopecia	Hodgkin's and non-Hodgkin's lymphomas; testicular cancer; squamous cell carcinomas (eg, head and neck, cervix, esophagus)
Nausea and vomiting; diarrhea; local irritant	*Bone marrow depression* (leukopenia, thrombocytopenia, anemia); *oral and gastrointestinal mucositis;* alopecia	Choriocarcinoma; Wilms' tumor; Ewing's, osteogenic, and soft tissue sarcomas; rhabdomyosarcoma; testicular cancer
Nausea and vomiting, diarrhea; red urine (not hematuria); local irritant; transient EKG changes	*Bone marrow depression* (leukopenia, thrombocytopenia, anemia); cardiac toxicity including irreversible congestive heart failure (total cumulative dose should not exceed 550 mg/M^2); alopecia; stomatitis; fever and chills.	Acute myelogenous leukemia; acute lymphocytic leukemia; neuroblastoma
Nausea and vomiting; diarrhea; red urine (not hematuria); local irritant; transient EKG changes	*Bone marrow depression* (leukopenia, thrombocytopenia, anemia); cardiac toxicity including irreversible congestive heart failure (total cumulative dose should not exeed 550 mg/M^2); alopecia; stomatitis; fever and chills	Acute myelogenous and acute lymphocytic leukemias; Hodgkin's and non-Hodgkin's lymphomas; multiple myeloma; testicular cancer; breast, lung, gastric, pancreatic, hepatocellular, bladder, prostatic, ovarian, endometrial, cervical, head and neck, and thyroid carcinomas; osteogenic, Ewing's, and soft tissue sarcomas; rhabdomyosarcoma; Wilms' tumor; neuroblastoma.
Nausea and vomiting; local irritant	*Bone marrow depression* (cumulative leukopenia, thrombocytopenia; also anemia); alopecia; stomatitis; renal toxicity; pulmonary toxicity	Gastric, colorectal, pancreatic, esophageal, lung, breast, cervical, and bladder carcinomas
Nausea and vomiting; diarrhea	*Bone marrow depression* (thrombocytopenia most marked; also, leukopenia and anemia); coagulation defects resulting in *hemorrhagic diathesis* (can occur in the absence of thrombocytopenia); hepatotoxicity; hypocalcemia; CNS toxicity; skin rashes and fever; renal toxicity	Testicular cancer
Nausea and vomiting; local irritant	*Bone marrow depression* (primarily leukopenia); mucositis; alopecia; neurologic toxicity as for vincristine but much less common	Hodgkin's and non-Hodgkin's lymphomas; testicular cancer; choriocarcinoma; breast carcinoma

(Continued on next page)

TABLE 1 (continued)

Drug	Cell Cycle Specificity	Route of Administration	Elimination
Vincristine Sulfate VCR; [Oncovin]	M-phase specific	Intravenous	Metabolic and biliary
Etoposide VP-16, VP-16213; [VePesid]	Appears to act primarily in G_2 phase; possibly in late S or M phases as well	Intravenous, oral	Liver and renal
Enzyme Asparaginase [Elspar]	Postmitotic G_1-phase specific	Intravenous, intramuscular	Metabolic

MISCELLANEOUS DRUGS

Heavy Metal Complex Cisplatin Cis-platin, CPDD; [Platinol]	Phase nonspecific but G_1 may be most sensitive	Intravenous	Primarily renal
Substituted Urea Hydroxurea [Hydrea]	S-phase specific	Oral	Primarily renal
Methyl Hydrazine Derivative Procarbazine Hydrochloride [Matulane]	Phase nonspecific	Oral	Metabolic
Adrenocortical Suppressant Mitotane o_1p-DDD; [Lysodren]	Phase nonspecific	Oral	Metabolic

HORMONES[2] AND ANTAGONISTS

	Classification		
Prednisone	Adrenal corticosteroid	Oral	Metabolic
Diethylstilbestrol DES	Estrogen	Oral	Metabolic
Ethinyl Estradiol	Estrogen	Oral	Metabolic
Testosterone Propionate	Androgen	Intramuscular	Metabolic

Major Toxicity[1]		
Acute	**Delayed**	**Indications**
Local irritant	*Neurologic toxicity* including peripheral neuropathy (eg, areflexia, muscular weakness, peripheral neuritis), paralytic ileus, cranial nerve palsies; alopecia; mild bone marrow depression	Acute and chronic lymphocytic leukemias; acute myelogenous leukemia; Hodgkin's and non-Hodgkin's lymphomas; small cell lung and breast carcinomas; Ewing's and soft tissue sarcomas; rhabdomyosarcoma; Wilms' tumor; neuroblastoma
Mild nausea and vomiting; orthostatic hypotension with rapid infusion	*Bone marrow depression* (primarily leukopenia; also thrombocytopenia, anemia); alopecia; peripheral neuropathy	Testicular cancer, lung carcinoma (particularly small cell); choriocarcinoma; acute myelogenous leukemia; non-Hodgkin's lymphomas
Nausea and vomiting; fever; chills; hypersensitivity reactions including anaphylaxis	Cerebral dysfunction (eg. disorientation, coma, seizures); acute hemorrhagic pancreatitis; coagulation defects; hepatic dysfunction	Acute lymphocytic leukemia
Nausea and vomiting (often severe and prolonged); fever; hypersensitivity reactions including anaphylaxis	*Nephrotoxicity including renal failure;* ototoxicity including hearing loss; bone marrow depression (leukopenia, thrombocytopenia, anemia); peripheral neuropathy; hypomagnesemia and hypocalcemia	Testicular cancer; ovarian, cervical, bladder, head and neck, non-small cell lung, and esophageal carcinomas; osteogenic sarcoma
Mild nausea and vomiting	*Bone marrow depression* (leukopenia, thrombocytopenia, anemia, megaloblastosis)	Chronic myelogenous leukemia
Nausea and vomiting	*Bone marrow depression* (leukopenia, thrombocytopenia, anemia; myelosuppression may be delayed); stomatitis; neurologic toxicity (CNS depression, peripheral neuropathy, myalgia, arthralgia); dermatitis; pneumonitis	Hodgkin's and non-Hodgkin's lymphomas; brain tumors; small cell lung carcinoma
Nausea and vomiting; diarrhea	Neurologic toxicity (mental depression, visual disturbances); dermatitis	Adrenocortical carcinoma
None	Hyperadrenocorticism; adverse reactions expected with corticosteroids, including sodium retention (edema, hypertension), glucose intolerance, accumulation of fat on face and trunk, osteoporosis, psychoses and euphoria, loss of skin collagen, increased susceptibility to infection, weight gain, growth retardation in children.	Acute and chronic lymphocytic leukemias; Hodgkin's and non-Hodgkin's lymphomas; multiple myeloma; breast carcinoma
Occasional nausea	Fluid retention; hypercalcemia; feminization, uterine bleeding; increased frequency of vascular accidents (especially at high doses); vaginal carcinoma in offspring of pregnant women given drug.	Prostatic and breast carcinomas (postmenopausal women)
None	Fluid retention; hypercalcemia; feminization; uterine bleeding; increased frequency of vascular accidents (especially at high doses).	Prostatic and breast carcinomas (postmenopausal women)
None	Fluid retention; masculinization; hypercalcemia.	Breast carcinoma

(Continued on next page)

TABLE 1 (continued)

Drug	Cell Cycle Specificity	Route of Administration	Elimination
Fluoxymesterone	Androgen	Oral	Metabolic
Leuprolide [Lupron]	LHRH agonist	Subcutaneous	Metabolic
Testolactone [Teslac]	Androgen	Oral	Metabolic
Hydroxyprogesterone Caproate	Progestin	Intramuscular	Metabolic
Medroxyprogesterone Acetate	Progestin	Oral, intramuscular	Metabolic
Megestrol Acetate	Progestin	Oral	Metabolic
Estramustine Phosphate Sodium [Emcyt]	Estradiol mustard	Oral	Metabolic
Tamoxifen Citrate [Nolvadex]	Antiestrogen	Oral	Metabolic
Aminoglutethimide [Cytadren]	Adrenal corticosteroid synthesis inhibitor	Oral	Metabolic, renal

[1]Usual dose-limiting toxicity is italicized.
[2]Individual hormone preparations listed are the ones most commonly employed in cancer chemotherapy.

had a major impact on prolonging survival, combinations of drugs have proven superior to single agents (see Table 2).

Circumvention of drug resistance may be an important reason for the greater success of combination chemotherapy over single agents. As discussed earlier, selection of de novo resistant cell lines from a heterogeneous tumor population can result in drug resistance. In addition, many antineoplastic agents are mutagenic and may directly produce a drug-resistant line. Pleiotropic drug resistance also may develop. However, when combination chemotherapy utilizing two or more noncross-resistant drugs is employed, therapeutic failure due to emergence of drug resistance is less likely.

Another major reason for the greater success of combination chemotherapy is that each drug can provide a maximal tumor cell kill within the range of toxicity tolerated by the host. If the drugs have minimal overlapping toxicities, optimal antitumor doses of each agent can be given. Thus, the total tumor cytoreduction will be much greater with an effective drug combination than with any single agent (Blum et al, 1982; DeVita, 1985).

Although some effective drug combinations have been designed entirely on the basis of biochemical or cytokinetic principles, most successful combination chemotherapy regimens used clinically have been derived empirically. The following guidelines are usually employed when choosing drugs for combination chemotherapy. (1) Drugs that are active against the tumor when used alone should be selected. If available, drugs that produce some fraction of complete responses are preferred to those that produce only partial responses. (2) The drugs included should have different

mechanisms of action to minimize the possibility of drug resistance. (3) Drugs selected should have minimally overlapping toxicities to allow the administration of full or nearly full doses of each active agent to result in a greater tumor cell kill. (4) The individual drugs should be optimally scheduled and the combination given at consistent intervals. Usually, the interval selected between cycles is the narrowest possible to allow recovery of the most sensitive normal target tissue, which usually is the bone marrow (Pratt and Ruddon, 1979; Blum et al, 1982; Carter and Livingston, 1982 A; DeVita, 1985).

An excellent example of the principles discussed above is the MOPP regimen used to treat advanced Hodgkin's disease. The drugs and dosage schedules employed in this combination are: mechlorethamine [Mustargen] 6 mg/M[2] intravenously on days one and eight; vincristine [Oncovin] 1.4 mg/M[2] intravenously on days one and eight; procarbazine [Matulane] 100 mg/M[2] orally on days one to fourteen; and prednisone 40 mg/M[2] orally on days one to fourteen (cycles one and four only). The cycle is repeated every four weeks for a minimum of six cycles or as many cycles as needed for complete remission, plus two additional cycles to consolidate the remission (DeVita et al, 1985).

When used alone, each of the drugs in the MOPP regimen is active in Hodgkin's disease but produces complete remissions in only a small percentage of patients. The individual drugs have different mechanisms: Mechlorethamine is an alkylating agent that cross links DNA; vincristine is an M-phase specific mitotic inhibitor that disrupts microtubules; procarbazine inhibits DNA and RNA synthesis (mechanism unknown); and prednisone is lympholytic via a steroid receptor mechanism.

Major Toxicity[1]

Acute	Delayed	Indications
None	Fluid retention; masculinization including hirsutism and painful clitoral hypertrophy; cholestatic jaundice; hypercalcemia	Breast carcinoma
	Disease flare; hot flashes; gynecomastia; loss of libido	Breast carcinoma; prostate carcinoma
None	Fluid retention; masculinization (usually minimal); hypercalcemia	Breast carcinoma
Local pain	Fluid retention (mild); hypercalcemia, cholestatic jaundice	Endometrial carcinoma
Local pain (injectable)	Fluid retention (mild), hypercalcemia	Breast and endometrial carcinomas
None	Fluid retention (mild); hypercalcemia	Breast and endometrial carcinomas
Nausea and vomiting; diarrhea	Fluid retention, gynecomastia; abnormal liver function tests	Prostatic carcinoma
Mild nausea and vomiting; hot flashes; transient increased bone or tumor pain	Vaginal bleeding; skin rashes; transient leukopenia and thrombocytopenia; hypercalcemia; pruritus vulvae; headache; retinopathy and corneal opacities with high-dose, long-term use	Breast carcinoma
Lethargy; ataxia; skin rash; orthostatic dizziness; fever; nausea	Masculinization; hypothyroidism; bone marrow depression	Breast carcinoma

In addition to the evaluations, the reader is referred to Pratt and Ruddon, 1979, pp 64–272, Med Lett Drugs Ther, 1980; Carter et al, 1981, pp 53-126; Krakoff, 1981; Schepartz et al, 1981; Carter and Livingston, 1982 B; Chabner and Myers, 1985; and Balis et al, 1983.

Although the dose-limiting toxicities of both mechlorethamine and procarbazine are bone marrow depression and, therefore, overlap, vincristine (dose-limiting neurotoxicity) and prednisone do not depress the bone marrow. Thus, the criteria of individually active drugs, different mechanisms of action, and nonoverlapping toxicities to allow maximally tolerated doses of each drug are essentially satisfied in the MOPP regimen. Furthermore, the scheduling of cycles four weeks apart accommodates the recovery time for bone marrow. Approximately 80% of patients go into complete remission and many more than 50% remain free of disease for more than ten years and are considered as cures. More recent data suggest that alternating treatment with MOPP and ABVD (see Table 2) may further increase the cure rate to greater than 80% for patients with stage IV Hodgkin's disease (Bonadonna and Santoro, 1982).

Combination chemotherapy has significantly prolonged survival, with some probable cures, in acute lymphocytic leukemia, certain non-Hodgkin's lymphomas, and testicular cancer (see Table 2). It should be noted that bone marrow-sparing agents (eg, vincristine, bleomycin [Blenoxane], cisplatin [Platinol], asparaginase [Elspar], prednisone) are included in each of these regimens.

In other cancers, particularly those that show good responses to a number of individual drugs, combination chemotherapy has clearly been superior to single-agent chemotherapy and now is employed routinely. Examples include small cell carcinoma of the lung, acute myelogenous leukemia, and breast carcinoma. In contrast, for many cancers that are only marginally sensitive to presently available drugs (eg, colorectal and renal carcinomas, melanoma), drug combinations have not significantly improved survival over single agents and may cause greater toxicity. Thus, combination chemotherapy usually is not recommended for these neoplastic diseases except in experimental protocols (see Table 2 and the references for more detailed information).

Adjuvant Chemotherapy

For many solid tumors, cures can be obtained with surgery or radiation therapy alone if the cancer is localized at the time of treatment. However, a high percentage of patients with apparently localized disease harbor undetectable metastases (micrometastases). Eventual relapse is likely in these patients and cure of late, macrometastatic disease with chemotherapy is rare. As a result of this problem, adjuvant systemic chemotherapy is being employed; cytotoxic therapy is initiated immediately after local surgery and/or radiation therapy to eradicate the micrometastases presumed to be present. Chemotherapy is presumed to be most effective immediately after cytoreductive surgery when the total micrometastatic body burden is smallest, and this has been the case in a number of animal model systems (Martin, 1981).

Clinically, encouraging results with adjuvant chemotherapy have been reported for a number of cancers, particularly pediatric cancers (eg, Wilms' tumor, rhabdomyosarcoma, Ewing's sarcoma), osteogenic sarcoma, and breast carcinoma. However, there is considerable controversy regarding interpretation of the various data, and adjuvant chemotherapy

TABLE 2.
CLINICAL RESPONSE TO CHEMOTHERAPEUTIC DRUGS

Type of Cancer	Drugs Currently Preferred	Alternative or Secondary Drugs	Other Drugs With Reported Activity
RESPONSIVE CANCERS (PROLONGED SURVIVAL AND PROBABLY SOME CURES)			
Choriocarcinoma			
Low Risk	Methotrexate	Dactinomycin, vinblastine, chlorambucil	Etoposide
High Risk	Methotrexate + dactinomycin + chlorambucil (MAC)	Methotrexate + dactinomycin + cyclophosphamide	
Burkitt's lymphoma	Cyclophosphamide + vincristine + methotrexate + doxorubicin + prednisone	Carmustine	Cytarabine
Hodgkin's disease	Mechlorethamine + vincristine + procarbazine + prednisone (MOPP)	Doxorubicin + bleomycin + vinblastine + dacarbazine (ABVD) *or* Carmustine + vinblastine + cyclophosphamide +procarbazine + prednisone (BCVPP)	Lomustine, carmustine, chlorambucil, thiotepa, altretamine[2] Streptozocin
Wilms' tumor	Dactinomycin + vincristine	Doxorubicin	
Embryonal rhabdo-myosarcoma	Vincristine + dactinomycin + cyclophosphamide (VAC)	Doxorubicin	Thiotepa, methotrexate
Acute lymphocytic leukemia of childhood	*Induction:* Vincristine + prednisone *Prophylaxis of CNS disease:* Intrathecal methotrexate and/or cranial irradiation *Maintenance:* Methotrexate + mercaptopurine	Vincristine + prednisone + daunorubicin *or* *Vincristine* + prednisone + asparaginase	Doxorubicin, cyclophosphamide mercaptopurine, cytarabine, thioguanine
Non-Hodgkin's Lymphomas Rapidly growing types (eg, diffuse histiocytic lymphoma)	Bleomycin + doxorubicin + cyclophosphamide + methotrexate + dexamethasone (M-BACOD) *or* Cyclophosphamide + doxorubicin + vincristine + prednisone (CHOP) *or* Bleomycin + doxorubicin + cyclophosphamide + vincristine + prednisone (BACOP) *or* Cyclophosphamide + vincristine + methotrexate (high dose with leucovorin rescue) + cytarabine (COMLA)	Combination of agents not previously utilized	Mechlorethamine, chlorambucil, vinblastine, procarbazine, carmustine, lomustine, cytarabine, altretamine,[2] etoposide[2]
Testicular cancer (nonseminomatous)	Cisplatin + vinblastine + bleomycin (PVB) *or* Vinblastine + dactinomycin + bleomycin + cisplatin + cyclophosphamide (VAB-VI)	Cisplatin + etoposide ± bleomycin (salvage therapy for patients not cured by PVB regimen)	Doxorubicin, chlorambucil, plicamycin, methotrexate

(Continued on next page)

Type of Cancer	Drugs Currently Preferred	Alternative or Secondary Drugs	Other Drugs With Reported Activity
Ewing's sarcoma	Vincristine + dactinomycin + cyclophosphamide (VAC)	Doxorubicin	Methotrexate (high dose wth leucovorin rescue)

MODERATELY RESPONSIVE CANCERS (PALLIATION AND PROBABLE PROLONGATION OF LIFE)

Type of Cancer	Drugs Currently Preferred	Alternative or Secondary Drugs	Other Drugs With Reported Activity
Acute myelogenous leukemia	*Induction:* Daunorubicin + cytarabine ± thioguanine	Doxorubicin + cytarabine ± thioguanine *or* *Doxorubicin* + cytarabine + vincristine + prednisolone	Azacitidine,[2] amsacrine,[2] high-dose cytarabine
	Maintenance: Investigational status; intensive sequential therapy with rotating drug combinations may prolong remission durations (Weinstein et al, 1980; Rai et al, 1981).		
Chronic myelogenous leukemia	*Chronic phase:* Busulfan	Hydroxyurea	Dibromomannitol,[2] mercaptopurine

	Blast crisis
	  Myeloblastic: Same regimens as for acute myelogenous leukemia (see above)
	  Lymphoblastic: Vincristine + prednisone		

Chronic lymphocytic leukemia	Chlorambucil + prednisone	Cyclophosphamide *or* Cyclophosphamide + vincristine + prednisone (COP)	
Multiple myeloma	Melphalan (or cyclophosphamide) + prednisone	Many combination regimens under study (see Woodruff, 1981)	Carmustine, doxorubicin, vincristine, chlorambucil, interferon[2]
Non-Hodgkin's Lymphomas Indolent types (eg, most nodular lymphomas)	Cyclophosphamide + vincristine + prednisone (CVP) *or* Chlorambucil *or* Cyclophosphamide	*Doxorubicin* + bleomycin + prednisone (ABP)	Mechlorethamine, vinblastine, procarbazine, carmustine, lomustine, altretamine,[2] etoposide[2], interferon[2]
Breast Carcinoma Adjuvant therapy[4]	Cyclophosphamide + methotrexate + fluorouracil *or* Cyclophosphamide + doxorubicin + fluorouracil (CAF)	Various protocols under investigation	
Advanced disease	*Hormones:* Oophorectomy (premenopausal); tamoxifen (postmenopausal)	Aminoglutethimide (plus replacement hydrocortisone)	Androgens, estrogens, progestins, corticosteroids
	Chemotherapy: Cyclophosphamide + methotrexate + fluorouracil (CMF) ± prednisone (CMFP) ± vincristine (CMFVP) *or* Cyclophosphamide + fluorouracil + prednisone (CFP) *or* Fluorouracil + doxorubicin + cyclophosphamide (FAC)	Doxorubicin + cyclophosphamide (AC) *or* Doxorubicin + vincristine (AV) *or* Regimen composed of other active drugs not used in primary therapy	Melphalan, vinblastine, thiotepa, mitomycin, vindesine,[2] leuprolide
Small cell carcinoma of lung	Doxorubicin + cyclophosphamide + vincristine *or* Cyclophosphamide + lomustine + methotrexate	Regimens composed of other active drugs not used, including etoposide	Procarbazine, altretamine,[2] cisplatin

(Continued on next page)

TABLE 2 (continued)

Type of Cancer	Drugs Currently Preferred	Alternative or Secondary Drugs	Other Drugs With Reported Activity
MODERATELY RESPONSIVE CANCERS (continued)			
Ovarian carcinoma	Combination including melphalan (or cyclophosphamide) + doxorubicin + cisplatin *or* Altretamine (hexamethymelamine)[2] + cyclophosphamide + methotrexate + fluorouracil (Hexa-CAF)	Doxorubicin or cisplatin or altretamine[2] depending on primary treatment	Chlorambucil, thiotepa, progestins
Islet cell carcinoma	Streptozocin + fluorouracil	Other streptozocin combinations under study	Dacarbazine
Prostate carcinoma	Diethylstilbestrol Leuprolide	Doxorubicin or cyclophosphamide or cisplatin or estramustine	Fluorouracil, ethinyl estradiol
Endometrial carcinoma	Progestin (eg, megestrol, hydroxyprogesterone, medroxyprogesterone)	Doxorubicin	Fluorouracil, cyclophosphamide
Osteogenic sarcoma	Doxorubicin *or* Methotrexate (high dose with leucovorin rescue)	Drug not used for primary treatment	Cisplatin, melphalan, mitomycin
Neuroblastoma, Advanced disease	Cyclophosphamide + vincristine + dacarbazine ± dosorubicin	Doxorubicin if not used in primary regimen	Daunorubicin, vinblastine, prednisone
PARTIALLY TO MINIMALLY RESPONSIVE CANCERS (POSSIBLE PALLIATION; MINIMAL TO NO INCREASE IN SURVIVAL)			
Adrenocortical carcinoma	Mitotane		
Bladder (also renal pelvis and ureters) transitional cell carcinoma	Cisplatin	Doxorubicin	Cyclophosphamide, fluorouracil, methotrexate, mitomycin
Bronchogenic carcinoma (non-small cell)	None (investigational area)	Doxorubicin; cyclophosphamide; cisplatin	Methotrexate, mitomycin, lomustine, vindesine,[2] etoposide, ifosfamide[2]
Cervical carcinoma	Cisplatin *or* Mitomycin	Bleomycin	Methotrexate, fluorouracil, vincristine, cyclophosphamide, doxorubicin, altretamine[2]
Colorectal carcinoma	Fluorouracil	Mitomycin *or* Semustine[2]	Carmustine, lomustine, tegafur[2]
Esophageal carcinoma	Cisplatin + fluorouracil		Bleomycin, mitomycin, vindesine,[2] methotrexate
Gastric carcinoma	Fluorouracil *or* Fluorouracil + doxorubicin + mitomycin (FAM)	Many combination regimens under study (see Macdonald et al, 1985	Carmustine, semustine.[2] tegafur,[2] cisplatin
Head and neck carcinoma	Methotrexate *or* Cisplatin *or* Cisplatin + bleomycin *or* Cisplatin + fluorouracil	Single agent or combination not utilized as primary therapy	Fluorouracil, cyclophosphamide, doxorubicin, vinblastine
Hepatocellular carcinoma	None (investigational)		Fluorouracil, doxorubicin
Melanoma	Dacarbazine	Nitrosourea (eg. carmustine, lomustine, semustine[2])	Interferon[2]

(Continued on next page)

Type of Cancer	Drugs Currently Preferred	Alternative or Secondary Drugs	Other Drugs With Reported Activity
Pancreatic carcinoma	None (investigational)	Various single agents and combinations under study (Sindelar et al, 1985)	Fluorouracil, doxorubicin, mitomycin, streptozocin, semustine[2]
Renal cell carcinoma	None (investigational)		Vinblastine Interferon[2]
Soft tissue sarcoma (adult)	Doxorubicin *or* Doxorubicin + dacarbazine (ADIC) *or* Cyclophosphamide + vincristine + doxorubicin + dacarbazine (CYVADIC)	Other combinations under investigation (see Bramwell and Pinedo, 1982)	Dactinomycin, methotrexate
Thyroid carcinoma	Doxorubicin		
Malignant Glioma	Carmustine *or* Lomustine	Procarbazine	Semustine,[2] etoposide

[1]*For many types of cancer listed, treatment routinely includes surgery and/or radiation therapy in addition to chemotherapy. The reader should refer to the listed (and other) references for detailed recommendations on the treatment of the various individual cancers as well as for specific dosage schedules of the currently preferred drug regimens.*
[2]*Investigational drug*

for most cancers should be considered investigational. A major problem in evaluating the effectiveness of adjuvant chemotherapy regimens is the prolonged follow-up time required for reliable statistical analysis (Carter and Glatstein, 1982 B).

Selection of appropriate drugs for adjuvant chemotherapy is based primarily on their effectiveness against advanced cancer. In general, adjuvant chemotherapy has been more successful against chemosensitive (eg, breast carcinoma) than chemoinsensitive (eg, colorectal carcinoma) cancers. Combinations of drugs usually are more effective than single agents and high-dose, intermittent courses of therapy are preferred. This presents another problem, however. Since a significant number of patients may remain disease-free with surgery or radiotherapy alone, the added risk of drug toxicity (and, in some cases, the induction of secondary malignancies, such as leukemia) must be weighed carefully against the potential benefit. This latter point emphasizes the importance of identifying high-risk recurrence groups who should receive adjuvant chemotherapy (Pratt and Ruddon, 1979; Martin, 1981; Carter and Glatstein, 1982 B; DeVita, 1985).

A brief discussion of adjuvant chemotherapy in breast cancer will illustrate some of these principles and problems. The prevalence of this disease in American women (100,000 new cases annually) and the propensity of this tumor to metastasize early have made it a prime candidate for adjuvant chemotherapy studies. Tumor status of axillary lymph nodes is considered to be the best prognostic indicator for recurrence with apparently localized breast cancer, and about one-half of all women with breast cancer have involved nodes. The ten-year relapse rates are 24%, 65%, and 86% for zero, one to three, and four or more positive nodes, respectively. Presently, it is recommended that all patients with positive nodes receive adjuvant chemotherapy and patients with negative nodes not be treated (National Institutes of Health Consensus-

Development Statement, 1980). Although this represents a very logical separation of high- and low-risk recurrence groups, some patients experience prolonged disease-free intervals after local therapy alone, and about 25% of negative node patients may benefit from adjuvant chemotherapy. The inclusion of additional prognostic factors (eg, ER status) may refine the definition of the high-risk recurrence group.

In the early 1970s, two large randomized prospective trials were designed to compare surgery alone to adjuvant chemotherapy with either melphalan (L-PAM) [Alkeran] or the combination of cyclophosphamide, methotrexate, and fluorouracil [Adrucil] (CMF) in women with positive lymph nodes. Both the single agent and the combination were previously shown to be active in disseminated breast cancer with overall response rates of approximately 20% and 50%, respectively. After eight years of follow-up, melphalan was shown to benefit only premenopausal women with fewer than four positive nodes (Harris et al, 1985). As in advanced breast cancer, the CMF combination appeared to be more active as an adjuvant and is one of the currently recommended adjuvant chemotherapy regimens for breast cancer.

Although breast cancer studies are at the forefront of the adjuvant chemotherapy strategy, even they leave certain questions unanswered. (1) Are these five- and ten-year relapse-free survivors cured or will late relapses develop? (2) Will overall survival continue to be (statistically) significantly greater in the treated group? (3) Would benefits have occurred in postmenopausal women if full doses of chemotherapy had been utilized? In addition, one must consider chronic toxicity or secondary malignancies in the treated patients. For example, are CMF-treated patients likely to develop hepatic fibrosis (eg, due to methotrexate) or acute leukemias? This could be a serious problem for newer protocols containing drugs such as doxorubicin, cisplatin, and bleomycin. In summary, adjuvant chemotherapy offers considerable promise for improvement of cure rates in a number of solid cancers, but well-designed and lengthy clinical trials will be necessary.

TOXICITY OF ANTINEOPLASTIC DRUGS

Because of the lack of readily exploitable biochemical differences between cancer and normal cells, the cytotoxic nature of most antineoplastic drugs, and the necessity for optimum dosing for the best response, most anticancer drugs have low therapeutic indices and produce cytotoxic effects in normal cells. The major acute and delayed toxicities of the various drugs are listed in Table 1 and discussed in the evaluations.

Myelosuppression: Bone marrow suppression is most significant in terms of morbidity and mortality caused by antineoplastic drugs and is the usual dose-limiting toxicity. Only the hormones, vincristine, bleomycin, asparaginase, and cisplatin have other major dose-limiting toxicities, which makes them desirable components of combination chemotherapy regimens (Mihich and Creaven, 1982).

Generally, leukopenia is more severe than thrombocytopenia, and anemia is less common. This is because the half-lives (and, thus, the doubling times of precursor marrow cells) of granulocytes (six hours) and platelets (five to seven days) are considerably shorter than red blood cells (about 120 days) and, therefore, they are more susceptible to the cytotoxicity of the drugs. Different types of agents produce different patterns of myelosuppression. Phase-specific agents that act only on proliferating cells (eg, methotrexate, vinblastine [Velban], the antipurines, and the antipyrimidines) usually produce a rapid granulocytopenia with a rapid recovery. In contrast, certain cycle nonspecific agents cause more prolonged bone marrow depression characterized by slow recovery and cumulative effects. Busulfan [Myleran], mitomycin [Mutamycin], and, in particular, the chloroethyl nitrosoureas (carmustine [BiCNU], lomustine [CeeNU], semustine [investigational]) can cause severe thrombocytopenia three to five weeks after drug administration. Other agents (eg, phase nonspecific but with a preference for proliferating cells) usually show an intermediate pattern. The effect on the platelet count may be more or less pronounced than the effect on the granulocyte count, and the kinetics to maximum depression (nadir) may differ. For example, cyclophosphamide and etoposide [VePesid] primarily affect granulocytes and rarely produce thrombocytopenia; the opposite is seen with plicamycin (mithramycin). Bone marrow depression is delayed with the nitrosoureas, with the nadir for thrombocytopenia (28 days) appearing about a week prior to the nadir for granulocytopenia (35 days).

Although the severity of bone marrow depression also varies among the antineoplastic drugs, it also depends on dose and patient factors, including age, nutritional status, marrow reserve, and prior radiation or chemotherapy (Hoagland, 1982; Mihich and Creaven, 1982).

Patients receiving myelosuppressive drugs must have careful monitoring of blood counts during and after therapy. Dosage reductions are often necessary when the white blood cell and platelet counts fail to return to adequate levels prior to the next course of therapy. The major consequences of granulocytopenia and thrombocytopenia are infection and bleeding, respectively. Supportive measures, including antibiotics, platelet and white cell transfusions, and protected environments, may be required (Hoagland, 1982).

Cytotoxicity to Other Proliferating Cells: Other proliferating normal tissues that are most susceptible to the cytotoxic effects of the antineoplastic drugs are the gastrointestinal and germinal epithelium, hair follicles, and lymphoid organs.

Gastrointestinal mucositis, most commonly stomatitis, can occur with a number of drugs. Severe mucositis with possible ulceration is observed most commonly with methotrexate, the fluorinated pyrimidines (eg, fluorouracil), dactinomycin [Cosmegen], doxorubicin, bleomycin, and vinblastine, and it may be dose limiting (Mitchell and Schein, 1982). A number of drugs cause partial or complete hair loss. In particular, cyclophosphamide and doxorubicin cause severe alopecia (see Dunagin, 1982). A variety of antineoplastic drugs, particularly the alkylating agents, depress spermatogenesis and can cause sterility.

Most antineoplastic drugs suppress cellular and humoral immunity. Immunosuppression often does not persist for long periods after treatment is discontinued and is less of a problem when intermittent scheduling is employed. However, cell-mediated immunity appears to be an important defense mechanism against the tumor and the immunocompromised patient is more susceptible to infection.

Immediate Side Effects: Most antineoplastic drugs have acute and delayed effects that can be both frequent and severe. Among the immediate side effects, nausea and vomiting are caused by most antineoplastic agents. Mechlorethamine, cisplatin, streptozocin, dacarbazine [DTIC-Dome], and azacytidine (investigational) cause vomiting, often severe, in essentially all patients. The sensory and stimulatory input underlying chemotherapy-induced vomiting is complex and in part is mediated through the chemoreceptor trigger zone (CTZ) in the brain. For this reason, combinations of antiemetics (eg, phenothiazines, butyrophenones, metoclopramide [Reglan], dronabinol [Marinol], dexamethasone, lorazepam [Ativan]) are utilized to provide the most effective control (Fortner et al, 1985). See Chapter 14, Drugs Used in Vertigo and Vomiting.

Local tissue necrosis due to drug extravasation is common. Doxorubicin, daunorubicin, dactinomycin, mechlorethamine, plicamycin, streptozocin, vincristine, vinblastine, and mitomycin are local irritants; therefore, these drugs must be administered intravenously with care to avoid extravasation (Dunagin, 1982).

Toxicity to Individual Organs: Important toxicities to individual organs and the antineoplastic drugs most frequently implicated are as follows:

Skin—Bleomycin (very common and includes hyperpigmentation, induration, erythema, vesicles, bullae) and busulfan (hyperpigmentation).

Lung—Bleomycin (usual dose-limiting toxicity; most often pneumonitis, but fatal pulmonary fibrosis can occur), busulfan and chloroethyl nitrosoureas (pulmonary fibrosis), mitomycin

C (pneumonitis, fibrosis), and methotrexate (pneumonitis).

Heart—Doxorubicin and daunorubicin (cumulative toxicity limits total dose to 550 mg/M²; ranges from transient EKG changes to cardiomyopathy with irreversible congestive heart failure).

Liver—Mercaptopurine, thioguanine, and sex steroids (cholestatic jaundice), asparaginase (fatty metamorphosis), nitrosoureas (hepatitis), and methotrexate (fibrosis and cirrhosis with prolonged use).

Pancreas—Asparaginase (hyperglycemia, hemorrhagic pancreatitis) and streptozocin (hyperglycemia).

Bladder—Cyclophosphamide (sterile hemorrhagic cystitis).

Kidney—Cisplatin (usual dose-limiting toxicity; acute renal tubular necrosis), streptozocin (usual dose-limiting toxicity; ranges from proteinuria to renal tubular atrophy), chloroethyl nitrosoureas and mitomycin (delayed onset nephrotoxicity that can progress to renal failure), high-dose methotrexate (renal tubular necrosis), and, indirectly, many cytotoxic drugs (hyperuricemic nephropathy due to large purine breakdown from tumor subsequent to cell killing).

Blood Coagulation—Plicamycin (hemorrhagic diathesis) and asparaginase (decreased clotting factors, reduced fibrinolytic activity).

Nervous System—Vincristine (usual dose-limiting toxicity; peripheral neuropathy ranging from decreased Achilles tendon reflex to areflexia; constipation due to autonomic dysfunction; and ptosis and diplopia due to cranial nerve palsies), asparaginase (cerebral dysfunction ranging from lethargy and confusion to severe depression and coma), fluorinated pyrimidines (cerebellar ataxia), procarbazine (altered consciousness, peripheral neuropathy), cisplatin (ototoxicity), intrathecal methotrexate (acute meningeal irritation, progressive meningoencephalopathy), and prednisone (manic psychosis or depression, altered sleep patterns) (Glatstein and Carter, 1982; Livingston 1982).

Hypersensitivity Reactions: Hypersensitivity reactions may be common and severe. Type I reactions characterized by urticaria, angioedema, and anaphylaxis are most commonly observed with asparaginase (1% mortality) followed by cisplatin and intravenous melphalan. Bleomycin-induced hyperpyrexia is quite common in lymphoma patients. Hypersensitivity reactions have been reported less frequently for methotrexate, doxorubicin, daunorubicin, cyclophosphamide, oral melphalan, and procarbazine (Weiss, 1982).

Mutagenicity, Teratogenicity, and Carcinogenicity: Many commonly employed antineoplastic drugs are mutagenic as well as teratogenic and some, including procarbazine and the alkylating agents, are carcinogenic in animals. The frequency of secondary malignancies, particularly acute leukemia, in patients treated for Hodgkin's disease, multiple myeloma, ovarian cancer, and possibly some other cancers is increased. The risk of secondary malignancies, which may not appear for many years after chemotherapy, must be considered in weighing benefits versus risks for any new therapy. This is particularly true for adjuvant chemotherapy in which improved survival must be balanced against the side effects of the drugs (Kyle, 1982).

Drug Evaluations

ALKYLATING AGENTS

The major types of clinically useful alkylating agents are the nitrogen mustards (chlorambucil [Leukeran], cyclophosphamide [Cytoxan, Neosar], mechlorethamine [Mustargen], melphalan [Alkeran]), the aziridine (thiotepa), the alkyl sulfonate (busulfan [Myleran]), the nitrosoureas (carmustine [BiCNU], lomustine [CeeNU]), and the triazene (dacarbazine [DTIC-Dome]).

The alkylating agents are cell cycle phase nonspecific in that they kill both resting and dividing cells, although most of these drugs are more active against proliferating cells.

These highly reactive drugs produce positively charged carbonium ion intermediates that readily form covalent bonds with a number of nucleophilic (negatively charged) cellular substances, such as phosphate, amino, sulfhydryl, hydroxyl, carboxyl, and imidazole groups. A particularly important reaction of the nitrogen mustards is alkylation of the 7-nitrogen of guanine in DNA; this can lead to chain scission, depurination, miscoding, and, in the case of bifunctional alkylating agents, cross-linking between two DNA strands, preventing replication. Although other reactions occur, the alkylation of DNA may be most destructive to the cell.

Toxicity of the alkylating agents is related to the drugs' cytotoxic effects. The normal tissues most affected are those with a rapid growth rate: the bone marrow, gastrointestinal and germinal epithelia, hair follicles, and lymphoid tissue. Bone marrow depression is the usual dose-limiting toxicity. Nausea and vomiting also are associated with most of these agents, particularly after intravenous administration.

Although the alkylating agents possess cytotoxic, mutagenic, and carcinogenic potential, they vary greatly in pharmacokinetic properties, lipid solubility, chemical reactivity, and membrane transport properties and are not uniformly cross-resistant. For example, cyclophosphamide and the nitrosoureas do not show cross resistance in the treatment of lymphomas. Thus, a consideration of the individual agents is necessary in order to understand their unique properties and optimal clinical usage.

Nitrogen Mustards

CHLORAMBUCIL
[Leukeran]

ACTIONS AND USES. This aromatic derivative of mechlorethamine is the slowest acting, least toxic nitrogen mustard in clinical use. It is cell cycle nonspecific and has a marked lympholytic effect.

Chlorambucil is a drug of choice in the palliative treatment of chronic lymphocytic leukemia. It is also effective in Hodgkin's disease, non-Hodgkin's lymphomas, multiple myeloma, and primary (Waldenstrom's) macroglobulinemia.

This agent has shown activity against carcinoma of the ovary, testicular cancer, and choriocarcinoma. In addition, it has been used to treat vasculitis as a complication of rheumatoid arthritis and autoimmune hemolytic anemias associated with cold agglutinins.

ADVERSE REACTIONS AND PRECAUTIONS. Hematologic toxicity is most prominent. Myelosuppression is usually moderate, gradual, and reversible. Leukopenia develops after the third week of treatment and continues for up to ten days after the last dose. Subsequently, the leukocyte count usually returns to normal rapidly. The dosage should be decreased if leukocyte or platelet counts fall below normal values and the drug should be discontinued if depression is severe.

Chlorambucil-related gastrointestinal, dermatologic, pulmonary, or hepatic toxicity is seldom encountered with usual therapeutic doses. Azoospermia in adult males, sterility in prepubertal and pubertal males, and amenorrhea have been reported. This drug is classified in FDA Pregnancy Category D. An increased incidence of secondary acute myelogenous leukemia has been associated with long-term use of chlorambucil.

In addition to blood counts, serum uric acid levels should be monitored frequently to detect hyperuricemia that could lead to renal failure.

PHARMACOKINETICS. Chlorambucil is well absorbed after oral administration. The plasma half-life is about 1.5 hours. The drug is metabolized rapidly to phenylacetic acid mustard and very little is excreted in the urine as unchanged drug.

DOSAGE AND PREPARATIONS.
Oral: For chronic lymphocytic leukemia and Hodgkin's or non-Hodgkin's lymphomas, 1 to 3 mg/M^2 daily as a single dose. Dosage adjustments are based on blood count.

An alternative schedule for the treatment of chronic lymphocytic leukemia is 15 to 20 mg/M^2 given as a single dose; the dose is repeated every two weeks and increased by 4 mg/M^2 until leukocytosis is controlled or toxicity is observed.

Leukeran (Burroughs Wellcome). Tablets 2 mg.

CYCLOPHOSPHAMIDE
[Cytoxan, Neosar]

$$ClCH_2CH_2 \overset{O}{\underset{N-P}{\nearrow}} \overset{O}{\underset{N}{\diagdown}} \cdot H_2O$$

ACTIONS AND USES. Cyclophosphamide is the most widely used alkylating agent and can be administered orally or intravenously. This cyclic phosphamide ester of mechlorethamine is cell cycle phase nonspecific. Cyclophosphamide itself does not have alkylating activity and is not a vesicant, but is a prodrug that must be metabolically activated in the liver by the microsomal cytochrome P450 mixed-function oxidase system before it can alkylate cellular constituents (see below). It is currently believed that phosphoramide mustard and nitrogen mustard, potent alkylating agents, are the active cytotoxic metabolites.

There are many indications for cyclophosphamide in the treatment of both hematologic and solid cancers. When given intravenously in large doses as a single agent, it has produced cures in some patients with Burkitt's lymphoma. In combination with other antineoplastic agents, it is a drug of choice in the treatment of non-Hodgkin's lymphomas (both indolent and aggressive histologic types), multiple myeloma, breast and small cell lung carcinomas, soft tissue sarcomas, and pediatric solid tumors, such as embryonal rhabdomyosarcoma, Ewing's sarcoma, and neuroblastoma (see Table 2). It is used in chronic lymphocytic leukemia and testicular and ovarian cancers and shows activity in acute lymphocytic leukemia, Hodgkin's disease, choriocarcinoma, and endometrial, cervical, prostatic, bladder, head and neck, and non-small cell lung carcinomas.

Cyclophosphamide has a marked immunosuppressive action and has been used in rheumatoid arthritis, nephrotic syndrome in children, and Wegener's granulomatosis. It is also administered before bone marrow transplantation to produce immunosuppression.

DRUG INTERACTIONS. Since this drug is activated in the liver, its metabolism can be affected by drugs that induce (eg, phenobarbital) or inhibit (eg, allopurinol) enzymes of the mixed-function oxidase system. Although the half-life of cyclophosphamide is altered by such drugs, its antitumor activity and therapeutic index do not change. In addition, cyclophosphamide can induce the microsomal enzymes responsible for its own metabolism.

ADVERSE REACTIONS AND PRECAUTIONS. A variety of toxic effects have been observed. Among the acute side effects, gastrointestinal disturbances, especially nausea and vomiting, are common. They usually begin six or more hours after administration and last about four hours.

The usual dose-limiting toxicity is bone marrow depression. The major effect is on leukocytes and thrombocytopenia is probably less severe than with other alkylating agents. The nadir of leukopenia usually occurs within one to two weeks after the start of administration, and recovery usually takes about ten days after the last dose. Blood counts must be monitored and the dosage reduced as necessary.

More than 50% of patients receiving intensive or prolonged therapy with cyclophosphamide experience alopecia, which is usually reversible.

A relatively common and potentially dose-limiting toxic effect is sterile hemorrhagic cystitis, which can result from a high concentration of active metabolites (eg, acrolein) in the bladder. This is ameliorated by ample fluid intake and frequent voiding. Instillation of thiol compounds into the bladder or systemic administration of N-acetylcysteine or sodium 2-mercapto-ethane sulfonate (MESNA) may reduce toxicity. Bladder fibrosis and carcinoma have been reported after long-term use of cyclophosphamide.

Other toxic effects are liver dysfunction, hyperpigmentation, oral ulceration, amenorrhea, azoospermia, irreversible pulmonary fibrosis, and water retention resulting from direct effects on the renal tubule. After use of very large single doses of cyclophosphamide, myocarditis and congestive heart failure developed and the cardiotoxic effect of doxorubicin was potentiated. Secondary malignancies also have been reported.

This drug is classified in FDA Pregnancy Category C.

PHARMACOKINETICS. Cyclophosphamide is well absorbed orally and peak plasma levels appear about one hour after oral use. It also is administered intravenously. This drug is metabolized in the liver to the inactive metabolite, 4-hydroxycyclophosphamide, which is in equilibrium with the acyclic tautomer, aldophosphamide. Although these metabolites are primarily oxidized further to additional inactive metabolites, some aldophosphamide is converted to phosphoramide mustard and nitrogen mustard, which are highly cytotoxic, and acrolein. It is believed that the active alkylating metabolites are generated in the tumor cells themselves, and cyclophosphamide is not toxic to normal liver cells.

The plasma half-life of cyclophosphamide is four to six hours; 50% to 70% is excreted in the urine in 48 hours, two-thirds as metabolites and one-third as parent drug. Active metabolites may accumulate in patients with severe renal impairment and a reduction in dosage may be required.

DOSAGE AND PREPARATIONS.

Intravenous: For patients with no hematologic deficiency, 500 mg to 1.5 g/M^2 is administered approximately at two- to four-week intervals. The dose is reduced, usually by one-third to one-half, in patients with impaired bone marrow function. Alternative dosage schedules are frequently used.

> *Cytoxan* (Bristol Myers). Powder (crystalline) 100, 200, and 500 mg and 1 and 2 g.
> *Neosar* (Adria). Powder (crystalline) 100, 200, and 500 mg.
> Use of benzyl alcohol-preserved diluents should be avoided.

Oral: When cyclophosphamide is given daily, the dose must be individualized for each patient. Doses of 60 to 120 mg/M^2 are used. Titration may be required after careful assessment of myelosuppression. Cyclophosphamide is best tolerated when given during or after meals.

> *Cytoxan* (Bristol Myers). Tablets 25 and 50 mg.

MECHLORETHAMINE HYDROCHLORIDE
[Mustargen]

$$\begin{array}{c} ClCH_2CH_2 \\ \diagdown \\ ^+NHCH_3 \quad Cl^- \\ \diagup \\ ClCH_2CH_2 \end{array}$$

ACTIONS AND USES. Mechlorethamine was the first alkylating agent used clinically. The major indication for this bifunctional alkylating agent is in disseminated Hodgkin's disease as part of the MOPP regimen (see the section on Combination Chemotherapy). It is also active in other lymphomas. Mechlorethamine may be useful in chronic myelocytic or lymphocytic leukemias, polycythemia vera, and cutaneous T cell lymphomas (mycosis fungoides and Sézary syndrome). Malignant pleural effusions may be palliated by intracavitary instillation. Topical mechlorethamine has been effective in patients with plaque stage cutaneous T cell lymphomas.

Major drawbacks to use of this drug are its chemical instability and strong vesicant action.

ADVERSE REACTIONS AND PRECAUTIONS. The most common immediate adverse reactions are nausea and vomiting, which are direct central nervous system effects. Vomiting may be severe, but usually stops within eight hours; nausea may persist for 24 hours. These reactions usually can be controlled by premedication with a sedative and an antiemetic. Anorexia, weakness, and diarrhea also may occur.

The most serious and usual dose-limiting toxic effect is bone marrow depression. Lymphopenia is usually apparent within 24 hours. The nadir of granulocytopenia and thrombocytopenia usually occurs within 7 to 21 days after drug administration. Hematologic recovery is usually adequate after four weeks, and rebound hyperplasia may be present from the fifth to seventh week.

Other toxic effects are maculopapular skin eruptions, alopecia, hearing loss and tinnitus, vertigo, jaundice, menstrual irregularities, impaired spermatogenesis, and total germinal aplasia. Hyperuricemia may develop, particularly in lymphoma patients. Adequate fluid intake should be instituted prior to drug treatment to prevent uric acid nephropathy, or allopurinol should be given. Various chromosomal abnormalities have been reported after mechlorethamine therapy; this drug is teratogenic, mutagenic, and carcinogenic.

Mechlorethamine is a potent vesicant. Thrombosis and thrombophlebitis may result from direct contact of the drug with the intima of the injected vein. Extravasation into subcutaneous tissue can cause severe, brawny induration and slough may result. If extravasation occurs, the area should be infiltrated with sterile isotonic sodium thiosulfate solution (1/6 molar), and an ice compress should be applied intermittently for 6 to 12 hours. Local corticosteroid injections may be of benefit.

Allergic hypersensitivity reactions are common after topical application and often require desensitization.

PHARMACOKINETICS. Mechlorethamine is highly reactive chemically and is hydrolized rapidly after intravenous injection; 90% disappears from blood in a few minutes. The drug penetrates cells through an active transport mechanism shared with the physiologic amine, choline. Excretion is via the urine, where approximately 50% appears in metabolized form in 24 hours. Less than 0.01% of unchanged drug is recovered in the urine.

DOSAGE AND PREPARATIONS. This agent has a marked vesicant action and is usually injected into the tubing of a freely flowing intravenous infusion. The compound undergoes rapid chemical transformation and decomposes on standing; thus, it must be prepared immediately before administration. The use of surgical gloves is advised during preparation.

Intravenous: For disseminated Hodgkin's disease and other lymphomas, 6 mg/M^2 on days one and eight as a component of the MOPP regimen; the course is repeated every 28 days. (See the section on Combination Chemotherapy.) An alternative schedule is 10 to 15 mg/M^2 repeated at four- to six-week intervals.

Intracavitary: For malignant pleural effusions, 10 to 15 mg/M^2. See the manufacturer's literature for more specific data.

Topical: The solution is prepared by dissolving 10 mg mechlorethamine in 50 to 60 ml of tap water. More dilute preparations are often necessary.

> *Mustargen* (Merck Sharp & Dohme). Powder (crystalline) 10 mg with sodium chloride q.s. 100 mg.

MELPHALAN
[Alkeran]

ACTIONS AND USES. This phenylalanine derivative of nitrogen mustard is cell cycle nonspecific. Like chlorambucil, melphalan contains an aromatic ring. The electron-withdrawing effect of the ring moiety decreases the rate of reactivity of the drug and, therefore, allows time for absorption and distribution after oral administration before alkylation occurs.

Melphalan is given orally and is an agent of choice in the palliative treatment of multiple myeloma. Cross resistance with cyclophosphamide is not typical. It is active in breast carcinoma and has been studied extensively as an adjuvant in the treatment of stage II breast carcinoma (see the section on Adjuvant Chemotherapy). Ovarian carcinoma also has responded to this agent. Melphalan has been used for arterial infusion of extremities affected by malignant melanoma. Although activity against testicular seminoma has been reported, the drug is not used clinically for this disease.

The agent is almost insoluble in water and only slightly soluble in alcohol. A parenteral preparation is available for investigational use only.

ADVERSE REACTIONS. Melphalan produces dose-limiting bone marrow depression that results in leukopenia, thrombocytopenia, and anemia. Blood counts must be monitored and the dosage reduced as necessary.

Nausea and vomiting have occurred after large doses of melphalan. Although its safety during pregnancy has not been evaluated, melphalan is potentially teratogenic and should not be used during this period unless absolutely necessary. Secondary acute myelogenous leukemia has been observed.

PHARMACOKINETICS. Absorption is variable after oral administration. Plasma levels can be measured to assure adequate bioavailability. Between 20% and 50% is excreted in the stool. The plasma half-life of parent drug appears to range between one and two hours, but most of an administered dose is chemically altered and metabolites persist in the body. Melphalan enters cells by an amino acid transport system. Less than 15% is excreted by the kidneys in the unchanged form. However, the drug should be used cautiously in patients with severe renal insufficiency, and dosage adjustments must be considered.

DOSAGE AND PREPARATIONS.
Oral: 6 to 8 mg/M^2 for four consecutive days every six weeks. The dosage is usually adjusted to produce a mild leukopenia (total leukocyte count, 3,000 to 3,500/microliter) for optimal results.

Alkeran (Burroughs Wellcome). Tablets 2 mg.

Aziridine
THIOTEPA

ACTIONS AND USES. Thiotepa is a cell cycle nonspecific trifunctional alkylating agent. This drug has been employed in the palliative management of carcinoma of the breast and ovary, although other agents are currently preferred. It has limited usefulness in lymphomas. Intracavitary instillation may control pleural or peritoneal effusions. Intravesical instillation is sometimes useful in superficial papillary carcinomas of the urinary bladder. Thiotepa has also been utilized in carcinomatous meningitis.

ADVERSE REACTIONS AND PRECAUTIONS. Thiotepa may produce nausea, anorexia, and headache, but the incidence is less than with mechlorethamine. It has a dose-limiting toxic effect on the bone marrow. Initial effects on the bone marrow may not become evident for 5 to 30 days (median, 15 days). As with other alkylating agents, the white blood cell and platelet counts are reliable guides.

Amenorrhea and impaired spermatogenesis have been observed. Thiotepa is teratogenic and, therefore, is contraindicated during the first trimester of pregnancy. The drug is also mutagenic and carcinogenic.

PHARMACOKINETICS. Thiotepa is unstable in acid and poorly absorbed from the gastrointestinal tract. It has a plasma half-life of 2 to 3 hours. It is not a vesicant and can be administered by direct intravenous injection, intracavitary or intravesical administration, or injection directly into a tumor site. Approximately 85% is excreted in the urine in 24 hours, primarily as metabolites. Patients with renal failure require reduced doses.

DOSAGE AND PREPARATIONS. Dosage must be individualized. The clinical response to thiotepa may be slow and too frequent administration can cause bone marrow depression.
Intravenous: 6 mg/M^2 daily for five days every four weeks if results of blood counts are acceptable.
Intravesical: For bladder instillation, 60 mg in 30 to 60 ml of distilled water is instilled into the bladder by catheter and retained for two hours. The patient may be repositioned every 15 minutes for maximum contact. Treatment is repeated at one- to four-week intervals.
Intrathecal: Doses from 1 to 10 mg/M^2 have been given at a concentration of 1 mg/ml in sterile water for injection.

Thiotepa (Lederle). Powder (sterile) 15 mg.

Alkyl Sulfonate

BUSULFAN
[Myleran]

$$CH_3SO_2O(CH_2)_4OSO_2CH_3$$

ACTIONS AND USES. The cytotoxic action of this cell cycle nonspecific bifunctional alkylating agent primarily affects granulocytes and, to some extent, platelets. Busulfan is the drug of choice in the palliative treatment of chronic myelogenous leukemia. It also may be useful in the myeloproliferative syndromes, polycythemia vera and myelofibrosis with myeloid metaplasia.

ADVERSE REACTIONS AND PRECAUTIONS. Toxic effects primarily affect the hematopoietic system, and leukopenia is usually dose limiting. The reduction in white blood cell count begins after about ten days of therapy and continues for two weeks after discontinuation of the drug. Busulfan can cause bone marrow hypoplasia, and peripheral leukopenia and thrombocytopenia may be prolonged (months). Thrombocytopenia may persist after leukocyte counts have returned to normal. The most likely cause of pancytopenia is failure to reduce or discontinue dosage as the blood counts decrease. Therefore, blood cell counts should be performed frequently. Busulfan should be employed with extreme caution in patients with a compromised marrow reserve (eg, because of prior cytotoxic therapy).

Hyperpigmentation may develop during prolonged therapy and may be part of an addisonian wasting syndrome manifested by asthenia, hypotension, nausea, vomiting, and weight loss. Usually there is no objective evidence of adrenal hypofunction.

Delayed effects, such as cataract, ovarian fibrosis, amenorrhea, testicular atrophy, aspermia, and gynecomastia, may occur. A rare and potentially fatal complication is the "busulfan lung" syndrome manifested by persistent cough and progressive dyspnea caused by intra-alveolar exudation of fibrin with subsequent organization. This may occur one to ten years after treatment is begun and usually results in fibrosis and death. Large doses of corticosteroids may be beneficial in the treatment of this disorder, but their use remains controversial.

Serum uric acid levels should be monitored frequently; hyperuricemia, which may result in nephropathy and acute renal failure, can be treated by hydration, alkalization of the urine, and administration of allopurinol.

This drug is classified in FDA Pregnancy Category D.

PHARMACOKINETICS. Busulfan is well absorbed after oral administration. It is cleared from the blood in two to three minutes; 10% to 50% is excreted within 24 hours as metabolites, primarily methanesulfonic acid.

DOSAGE AND PREPARATIONS.
Oral: For chronic intermittent therapy of chronic myelogenous leukemia, 2 to 6 mg/M² daily until the white blood count decreases to 10,000/microliter; treatment is discontinued until the white blood count increases to 50,000/microliter and then is resumed as before. For chronic continuous therapy, 2 to 6 mg/M² daily until the white blood count decreases to 10,000 to 20,000/microliter; the dose then is reduced as necessary (usually to 2 mg daily) to maintain the white blood count at this level.

Myleran (Burroughs Wellcome). Tablets 2 mg.

Nitrosoureas

The nitrosoureas most frequently used to treat cancer are the chloroethyl derivatives, carmustine, lomustine, and, investigationally, semustine. These nitrosoureas are unstable and decompose to alkylating and carbamoylating intermediates in aqueous media. Although a number of cellular constituents can be alkylated and carbamoylation of the ε-amino group of lysines is common, it appears that inhibition of DNA synthesis due to DNA alkylation is the lethal effect.

Nitrosoureas are absorbed rapidly from the gastrointestinal tract. They are metabolized rapidly and parent drugs quickly disappear from plasma. Metabolites, many inactive, have longer half-lives due to plasma protein binding and enterohepatic circulation. Most nitrosoureas undergo considerable biotransformation and are excreted in the urine as metabolites; only a small fraction is excreted as parent drug.

In contrast to other antineoplastic drugs, the nitrosoureas are quite lipid soluble and cross the blood-brain barrier. Thus, they are useful in central nervous system malignancies.

Delayed, dose-dependent, and cumulative depression of the hematopoietic system is the major adverse reaction. Bone marrow suppression appears to be more pronounced than with the classic (eg, nitrogen mustard) alkylating agents. Maximal depression of platelets and leukocytes occurs after three to five and four to six weeks of therapy, respectively, and usually last for one to two weeks. Severe nausea and vomiting also may be encountered.

Streptozocin, a glycosylated nitrosourea, differs from the chloroethylnitrosoureas in a number of its properties. In particular, the sugar moiety facilitates the uptake of this drug by pancreatic islet cells and significantly reduces bone marrow toxicity (see the evaluation).

CARMUSTINE (BCNU)
[BiCNU]

$$\underset{ClCH_2CH_2N - C - NHCH_2CH_2Cl}{\overset{NO\ \ O}{|\ \ ||}}$$

ACTIONS AND USES. Carmustine (bischloroethyl nitrosourea) alkylates DNA and, because it contains two chloroethyl groups, can cross link DNA, which is probably its most important action. Carmustine also alkylates RNA and proteins and carbamoylates amino acids, primarily the ε-amino group in lysine residues, in proteins. It is cell cycle phase nonspecific.

Since carmustine is highly lipid soluble with a relative lack of ionization at physiologic pH, it readily crosses the blood-brain barrier and is often a drug of choice in malignant tumors of the central nervous system. This drug is also active in multiple myeloma (in combination with prednisone), Hodgkin's disease, and non-Hodgkin's lymphomas. In lymphomas, it is used as secondary therapy in combination with other drugs when patients relapse or do not respond to primary therapy. Carmustine also has been used in melanoma, gastric and colorectal adenocarcinoma, and hepatoma. A topical solution has been used to treat cutaneous T cell lymphomas.

ADVERSE REACTIONS AND PRECAUTIONS. Bone marrow suppression is the usual dose-limiting toxicity. It is delayed in onset with platelet nadirs occurring four to five weeks and leukocyte nadirs five to six weeks after therapy is begun. Thrombocytopenia is usually more severe than leukopenia, but both may be dose limiting. Complete blood counts should be performed frequently for at least six weeks after each dose. Carmustine should not be given more often than every six weeks. Since the effect on the bone marrow is cumulative, dosage adjustments must be made on the basis of blood counts obtained after the prior dose.

Nausea and vomiting are noted frequently and are dose related. They occur within two hours and usually last four to six hours. Prior administration of antiemetics may control vomiting. Dose-related pulmonary toxicity has been observed often; the frequency is related to the total cumulative dose of carmustine. Symptoms include a hacking cough, dyspnea, or acute respiratory distress; deaths have been reported. Delayed-onset nephrotoxicity, including renal failure, has been reported with the nitrosoureas. Large doses have produced reversible hepatotoxicity in a small percentage of patients; this is manifested by increased transaminase, alkaline phosphatase, and bilirubin levels. There have been isolated reports of optic neuritis. The nitrosoureas are mutagenic, teratogenic, and carcinogenic. Accidental skin contact with the reconstituted drug has caused transient hyperpigmentation.

PHARMACOKINETICS. Carmustine is rapidly absorbed orally, but only intravenous preparations are available. Tissue uptake and metabolism occur rapidly; the elimination half-life of parent drug from serum is approximately 15 minutes. Metabolites are excreted primarily by the kidney. The drug readily enters the cerebrospinal fluid.

DOSAGE AND PREPARATIONS. Carmustine is dissolved in 3 ml of the sterile diluent supplied and then 27 ml of sterile water for injection is added aseptically. The resulting solution contains carmustine 3.3 mg/ml and may be diluted further with sodium chloride injection or 5% dextrose for injection.

Intravenous: As a single agent in previously untreated patients, 200 mg/M^2 is infused over a one- to two-hour period every six weeks. (More rapid infusion may produce intense pain and burning at the injection site.) This may be given as a single dose or 100 mg/M^2 may be given on two successive days. The dose should be reduced when carmustine is used with other myelosuppressive agents or in patients with impaired bone marrow function. Subsequent dosage is determined by the hematologic response to the preceding dose. The course should not be repeated until circulating blood elements have returned to acceptable levels (platelet count more than 100,000/microliter; leukocyte count more than 4,000/microliter); these levels usually are observed within six weeks.

Topical: Concentrations of 0.5 to 3 mg/ml in an aqueous solution with 30% alcohol has been used topically to treat plaque stage cutaneous T cell lymphoma.

  BiCNU (Bristol-Myers). Powder (lyophilized) 100 mg with 3 ml of sterile diluent (anhydrous ethyl alcohol).

LOMUSTINE (CCNU)
[CeeNU]

ACTIONS AND USES. This cyclohexylchloroethyl nitrosourea probably acts as an alkylating agent but, like other nitrosoureas, it may inhibit several key enzymatic processes. Although lomustine contains only a single alkylating function, it has been shown to produce interstrand cross links in DNA. Like carmustine, it also has carbamoylating activity. The drug is cell cycle phase nonspecific.

Because of its high lipid solubility and relative lack of ionization at physiologic pH, lomustine readily crosses the blood-brain barrier and is sometimes used to treat malignant tumors of the central nervous system. Lomustine also has been employed in combination regimens in small cell lung cancer (see Table 2). Activity has been reported in melanoma, Hodgkin's and non-Hodgkin's lymphomas, and breast, non-small cell lung, and colorectal carcinomas.

ADVERSE REACTIONS AND PRECAUTIONS. The most serious toxic effect is bone marrow suppression, which is delayed, dose related, dose limiting, and cumulative. Thrombocytopenia develops about four weeks and leukopenia about six weeks after a dose of lomustine; both persist for one to two weeks. Complete blood counts should be performed frequently for at least six weeks after each dose. Lomustine should not be given more often than every six weeks. Since the effect on the bone marrow is cumulative, dosage adjustments must be made on the basis of blood counts obtained after the prior dose.

Gastrointestinal disturbances (nausea and vomiting) occur two to six hours after administration and last less than 24 hours. Vomiting can be severe, but prior administration of antiemetics can decrease the frequency and duration. Other reactions include stomatitis, alopecia, anemia, and hepatotoxicity manifested by transient, reversible elevation of liver function tests. Neurologic reactions, such as disorientation, lethargy, ataxia, and dysarthria, have been noted but their relationship to medication is unclear. Delayed-onset nephrotoxicity, including renal failure, has been reported with the nitrosoureas. The nitrosoureas are teratogenic, mutagenic, and carcinogenic.

PHARMACOKINETICS. Lomustine is rapidly and completely absorbed after oral administration. Parent drug disappears rapidly from plasma. The plasma half-life of metabolites is 16 to 48 hours; 50% of the metabolized drug is excreted in the urine during the first 12 hours. Cerebrospinal fluid levels are 50% of plasma levels.

DOSAGE AND PREPARATIONS.
Oral: Adults and children, 130 mg/M^2 as a single dose every six weeks. In patients with impaired bone marrow function, the dose should be reduced to 100 mg/M^2 every six weeks. The

dose also must be reduced when lomustine is used with other myelosuppressive drugs. Blood counts should be monitored weekly and the dose should not be repeated before six weeks; circulating blood elements should return to acceptable levels (platelet count more than 100,000/microliter; leukocyte count more than 4,000/microliter). Lomustine should be taken on an empty stomach and alcohol should be avoided on the day of ingestion.

> **CeeNU** (Bristol-Myers). Capsules 10, 40, and 100 mg and dose pack containing two 100 mg, 40 mg, and 10 mg capsules each (stable for at least two years when stored at room temperature in tightly closed containers).

STREPTOZOCIN
[Zanosar]

ACTIONS. Streptozocin (1-methyl nitrosourea glucosamine) is an antibiotic originally derived from *Streptomyces achromogenes*. Although it is a nitrosourea, the glucose moiety confers properties that make this drug quite different from the chloroethyl nitrosoureas. It has alkylating activity and can cross link DNA, but this activity is weaker than with other nitrosoureas. It also inhibits precursor incorporation into DNA. Streptozocin is phase nonspecific, but cells in the S phase are most sensitive.

USES. Streptozocin is taken up selectively by pancreatic islet cells and is cytotoxic to malignant islet cell tumors. Thus, the principal therapeutic use of streptozocin has been in metastatic islet cell tumors (including insulin-secreting and noninsulin-secreting beta cell and nonbeta cell). Significant tumor regression (35% response rate) and a return to a normoglycemic state have occurred. Combination regimens containing streptozocin are currently under study; a regimen consisting of streptozocin plus fluorouracil was shown to be superior to single agent therapy (Moertel et al, 1980). The drug is also effective in patients with malignant carcinoid tumors; those of small bowel origin are most responsive. Streptozocin is either inactive or has equivocal status in other cancers. It may be of some value in combination regimens for pancreatic carcinoma and in secondary regimens for Hodgkin's disease.

ADVERSE REACTIONS AND PRECAUTIONS. Renal dysfunction is the major dose-limiting toxicity and occurs in 28% to 73% of patients. The drug is toxic to both renal tubules and glomeruli. Symptoms include renal tubular acidosis (eg, glycosuria, aminoaciduria, acetonuria), proteinuria, and azotemia. Nephrotoxicity can occur with a single dose; however, it is more common with repeated doses and develops in most patients receiving prolonged treatment. Renal function must be monitored continually in all patients. Mild abnormalities are often reversible upon discontinuation of drug, but irreversible damage will occur if treatment is continued. Patients with pre-existing renal dysfunction should not receive streptozocin. Urinary output should be maintained during and after treatment to ensure maximum dilution of the drug while it is passing through the kidney.

The other major adverse effects of streptozocin are nausea and vomiting. Vomiting occurs in almost all patients one to four hours after administration and can be severe and protracted. Phenothiazine antiemetics do not alleviate symptoms.

Hematologic toxicity is encountered only rarely, which makes this drug potentially useful for combination regimens. Glucose intolerance is usually inconsequential. Abnormal liver function tests are common and hepatotoxicity occasionally is severe. Streptozocin may cause a burning sensation upon administration. Miscellaneous untoward effects include fever and eosinophilia.

This drug is classified in FDA Pregnancy Category C.

PHARMACOKINETICS. Streptozocin is not orally active. After intravenous administration, it is rapidly cleared from plasma and is undetectable after three hours. The initial half-life of parent drug is 5 to 15 minutes, and the terminal half-life is 35 minutes. Metabolites are detected in plasma for up to 24 hours. The drug concentrates in certain tissues; the liver and kidneys contain the highest levels, and pancreas also concentrates streptozocin. Parent drug and metabolites are eliminated rapidly by the kidney; 60% to 70% of a dose is recovered in urine within four hours. Only 10% to 20% of an excreted dose is parent drug. Dosage reduction is required in patients with renal insufficiency.

DOSAGE AND PREPARATIONS.
Intravenous: 1 to 1.5 g/M² weekly; alternatively, 500 mg/M² daily for five days every six weeks.

> **Zanosar** (Upjohn). Powder (sterile) 1 g. (Refrigerate and protect from light.)

Triazene

DACARBAZINE
[DTIC-Dome]

ACTIONS AND USES. Dacarbazine was originally considered to be an antimetabolite, acting as an inhibitor of purine synthesis, and to interact with sulfhydryl groups in proteins. However, after metabolic activation in the liver, it has demonstrated alkylating activity, which is now believed to be the most important action. The drug inhibits RNA and protein synthesis more markedly than DNA synthesis. It is cell cycle nonspecific.

Dacarbazine is used in the palliative treatment of metastatic melanoma, but the overall response rate is only about 20% for this chemoinsensitive cancer. It is a component of the ABVD regimen, which is an alternative to MOPP in the treatment of advanced Hodgkin's disease (see Table 2). It also is a component of combination regimens used to treat soft tissue sarcomas and neuroblastoma. Dacarbazine is active in islet cell cancer.

ADVERSE REACTIONS. Myelosuppression is usually dose limiting and primarily affects leukocytes and platelets. This effect is somewhat delayed compared to classic nitrogen mustards. Leukopenia generally is reported after 10 days of therapy and thrombocytopenia after 10 to 15 days, but both effects may appear two to four weeks after the last dose.

Nausea and vomiting usually occur within one to three hours after administration and vomiting can last for up to 12 hours. These effects occur in about 90% of patients and may be severe. Prior administration of phenothiazines may not be effective. Rarely, intractable nausea and vomiting have necessitated discontinuance of therapy. Most patients develop tolerance and these symptoms subside after one to two days of treatment.

An "influenza-like" syndrome consisting of fever, myalgia, and malaise has been described with dacarbazine. Other untoward effects are pain at the infusion site, facial flushing, paresthesia, alopecia, and elevation of hepatic enzyme levels. Hepatic necrosis has been reported. Dacarbazine is teratogenic and carcinogenic in animals (FDA Pregnancy Category C). Anaphylaxis occurs rarely.

PHARMACOKINETICS. Since oral absorption is incomplete and highly variable, dacarbazine is administered only intravenously. It is metabolized in the liver first by N-demethylation to a monomethyl form and then to amino imidazole carboxamide (AIC) and diazomethane. The active carbonium ion is formed from diazomethane. Dacarbazine has a biphasic plasma decay with half-lives of 19 minutes and 5 hours. It is rapidly excreted by renal tubular secretion. About 40% is eliminated unchanged within six hours; the major metabolite in urine is AIC.

DOSAGE AND PREPARATIONS.
Intravenous: 250 mg/M²/day for five days every three to four weeks has been used for solid tumors.

For Hodgkin's disease, as part of the ABVD combination, 375 mg/M²/day on days one and fifteen and repeated every four weeks.

DTIC-Dome (Miles). Powder (sterile) 100 and 200 mg.

ANTIMETABOLITES

These compounds are chemically similar to naturally occurring metabolites, but they differ enough to interfere with normal metabolic pathways. Antimetabolites used in cancer chemotherapy interfere with important enzymatic reactions in the synthesis of nucleic acids, purines, pyrimidines, and their precursors. They also may be incorporated into nucleic acids in place of the corresponding normal nucleotides, which alter important cellular functions.

Folic acid, pyrimidine, and purine analogues act primarily during the DNA synthesizing phase of the cell cycle (S phase). Some act exclusively in S phase (eg, cytarabine) and others (eg, methotrexate, mercaptopurine) act both in S phase and prior to S phase and thus are self-limiting because they prevent entry of cells into the DNA synthesizing phase. The fluorinated pyrimidines appear to be exceptions; although they act preferentially on cycling cells, they are not phase specific.

Folic Acid Analogue

METHOTREXATE

METHOTREXATE SODIUM
[Folex, Mexate]

ACTIONS. Methotrexate is the 4-amino, N^{10}-methyl analogue of folic acid. It competitively inhibits mammalian dihydrofolate reductase, the enzyme that reduces dihydrofolic acid (FH_2) to tetrahydrofolic acid (FH_4). FH_4 is converted to various coenzymes required for one-carbon transfer reactions involved in the synthesis of thymidylate, purines, methionine, and glycine. Thus, inhibition of dihydrofolate reductase by methotrexate can lead to inhibition of DNA, RNA, and protein synthesis. Most studies suggest that the primary action is inhibition of thymidylate synthesis in which the requirements for FH_4 are stoichiometric with thymidine monophosphate production. The drug also has a weak, direct inhibitory effect on thymidylate synthetase. However, cytotoxicity is more efficient at higher drug levels, presumably because increased cell killing is enhanced by antipurine effects. Methotrexate is cell cycle-specific for the S phase, but it is self-limiting because of other effects on RNA and protein synthesis that slow the entry of cells into the S phase.

The block of dihydrofolate reductase can be bypassed clinically by use of leucovorin calcium (citrovorum factor). This "rescue" agent allows for recovery of normal tissue and thus permit use of larger doses of methotrexate (see section on Principles of Cancer Chemotherapy). In addition, thymidine, which restores intracellular pools of thymidine triphosphate, and carboxypeptidase G_1, an enzyme that hydrolyzes and inactivates methotrexate, have been used as rescue measures in clinical trials.

USES. Methotrexate, either alone or in combination depending on the risk factors, has been very effective in women with choriocarcinoma and related trophoblastic tumors; cures have been reported in most cases.

Although methotrexate induces complete remissions in acute lymphocytic leukemia of childhood, it is of more value for maintenance therapy and is an agent of choice in combination with mercaptopurine. Furthermore, intrathecal methotrexate and cranial irradiation are administered routinely to patients with acute lymphocytic leukemia to prevent meningeal metastases.

Methotrexate is a component of combination regimens used

to treat non-Hodgkin's and Burkitt's lymphomas and breast and ovarian carcinomas (see Table 2).

Large doses of methotrexate with leucovorin rescue have been used in osteogenic sarcoma, head and neck cancer, bronchogenic carcinoma, lymphomas, and leukemias. The value of this approach is questionable, however, because superior efficacy has not been demonstrated in a well-controlled clinical trial. Some experts contend that high-dose methotrexate with leucovorin rescue offers no advantages over conventional doses of methotrexate and is cumbersome and cost ineffective.

Methotrexate is a primary agent in the treatment of cutaneous T cell lymphomas and medulloblastoma. It has shown activity in testicular cancer, bladder and cervical carcinoma, soft tissue sarcomas, and embryonal rhabdomyosarcoma. Methotrexate also has been used in severe psoriasis and, investigationally, in severe rheumatoid arthritis (see Chapter 56, Dermatologic Preparations, and Chapter 59, Antiarthritic Drugs, respectively).

Resistance to methotrexate may develop as a result of increased dehydrofolate activity secondary to gene amplification or defective transport into malignant cells.

ADVERSE REACTIONS AND PRECAUTIONS. Toxicity to proliferating tissues most often involves the gastrointestinal tract, bone marrow, and oral mucosa. Stomatitis is common and is an indication for interruption of therapy, as is diarrhea. Hemorrhagic enteritis and intestinal perforation can occur if therapy is continued after diarrhea develops.

Myelosuppression (eg, leukopenia, thrombocytopenia, anemia) is the usual dose-limiting toxicity. Following a bolus dose or short-term infusion, the nadir usually appears between 5 and 14 days and recovery is rapid. More prolonged and severe toxicity has been observed in patients receiving higher doses and in those with poorer performance status or compromised bone marrow, liver, or renal function. Leucovorin may be used to rescue the bone marrow from the myelosuppressive effects of methotrexate if it is given within 42 hours of methotrexate. It is only partially effective when given later.

Since methotrexate is excreted principally by the kidneys, its use in patients with impaired renal function may increase toxicity. Therefore, renal function should be monitored prior to and during therapy. In addition, large doses have been associated with direct toxicity to the kidney, presumably due to precipitation of drug in the renal tubules. Adequate hydration and alkalization of the urine (using sodium bicarbonate or acetazolamide) enhance excretion of methotrexate.

Hepatic dysfunction has been observed after short- and long-term use. Acute reversible elevations in hepatic enzyme levels are often seen with high-dose therapy. Prolonged use may lead to fibrosis and occasionally cirrhosis. Liver function should be monitored.

Alopecia and dermatitis have been reported, and osteoporosis is observed occasionally in children on long-term maintenance therapy. An acute reversible pneumonitis of unknown etiology may develop, especially with intermittent therapy. It is characterized by fever, cough, shortness of breath, peripheral eosinophilia, and patchy pulmonary infiltrates. Acute hypersensitivity (eg, urticaria, wheezing, hypotension) has occurred

rarely. Central nervous system toxicity has been observed when methotrexate was given intrathecally, usually when central nervous system irradiation therapy also was administered.

This drug has been reported to be an abortifacient and should not be used during the first trimester of pregnancy. Because of possible teratogenic effects, it is recommended that a period of time (eg, six months) elapse between the end of therapy and conception in both males and females (FDA Pregnancy Category D).

DRUG INTERACTIONS. Vinca alkaloids, daunorubicin, and cytarabine increase the cellular uptake of methotrexate, while penicillin, hydroxyurea, mercaptopurine, neomycin, kanamycin, corticosteroids, bleomycin, and asparaginase decrease cellular uptake.

Methotrexate may be displaced from plasma albumin by sulfonamides, salicylates, tetracyclines, chloramphenicol, and phenytoin. In addition, salicylates and probenecid may compete with methotrexate for renal tubular secretion. Caution should be used if these drugs are given concomitantly.

Although vincristine interferes with efflux of methotrexate from cells, the therapeutic effect is not enhanced. Asparaginase may attenuate methotrexate toxicity by inhibiting protein synthesis. A synergistic effect has been reported when methotrexate was administered before fluorouracil. Accumulation of intracellular phosphoribosylpyrophosphate as a result of methotrexate treatment enhances the formation of fluorouracil nucleotides, which enhances cell killing.

PHARMACOKINETICS. Methotrexate can be given orally and conventional doses (eg, less than 25 mg/M^2) are readily absorbed; absorption is erratic at higher doses. Peak plasma levels are attained in one to four hours. The drug also is administered intravenously and intramuscularly. The peak plasma level is reached within one-half to two hours after intramuscular injection. The initial plasma half-life is two to four hours after parenteral administration; the elimination half-life is 8 to 15 hours after parenteral use and 8 to 10 hours after oral use.

Drug concentration and duration of cell exposure are critical determinants of cytotoxicity. One-half of the drug is bound to plasma proteins; 50% to 90% is excreted unchanged in the urine within 24 hours by glomerular filtration and active tubular secretion. Dose modifications are required in patients with renal insufficiency, and monitoring of plasma levels is indicated.

Methotrexate enters and exits cells by carrier-mediated active transport systems shared by the physiologic reduced folates. Intracellular storage is in the form of polyglutamate conjugates, which may be important determinants of the duration and site of drug action. The drug accumulates in the liver and kidney. The terminal elimination of methotrexate is very slow, for it persists in the liver and kidney for weeks.

Methotrexate does not enter the cerebrospinal fluid in therapeutic concentrations (except at high intravenous dose levels, ie, more than 1 g/M^2) and intrathecal administration is necessary. Third spaces (eg, pleural effusions, ascites) may act as drug depots and require evacuation prior to methotrexate administration.

DOSAGE AND PREPARATIONS.

Oral: 2.5 to 5 mg daily.

> METHOTREXATE:
> **Methotrexate** (Lederle). Tablets 2.5 mg.

Intramuscular, Intravenous: 25 mg/M^2 once or twice weekly. Dose modifications are based on toxicity. When used with cyclophosphamide and fluorouracil in breast carcinoma, 40 mg/M^2 intravenously on days one and eight every 28 days.

High-dose Intravenous: 1.5 g/M^2 with rescue every three weeks.

Intrathecal: 5 to 10 mg/M^2 (maximum, 12 mg in 10 ml Eliot's B solution) every two to five days until the cell count of cerebrospinal fluid returns to normal.

> METHOTREXATE SODIUM:
> (Strengths expressed in terms of the base.)
> **Methotrexate** (Lederle). Liquid (for injection) 2.5 mg/ml in 2 ml containers and 25 mg/ml in 2, 4, and 8 ml containers; powder (cryodesiccated) 20, 50, and 100 mg.
> **Folex** (Adria). Powder (lyophilized) 25, 50, and 100 mg.
> **Mexate** (Bristol-Myers). Powder (lyophilized) 20, 50, 100, and 250 mg.

Pyrimidine Analogues

CYTARABINE (Cytosine Arabinoside)
[Cytosar-U]

ACTIONS. This synthetic nucleoside differs from the normal nucleosides, cytidine and deoxycytidine, in that the sugar moiety is arabinose rather than ribose or deoxyribose. Cytarabine is converted sequentially by deoxycytidine kinase, dCMP kinase, and nucleoside diphosphate kinase to the triphosphate derivative, arabinofuranosylcytosine triphosphate (ara-CTP), which is the active metabolite. Ara-CTP interferes with DNA synthesis by inhibiting DNA polymerase and is incorporated into DNA, causing additional defects in chain termination. The effects are exerted during the S phase.

USES. The primary indication for cytarabine is acute myelogenous leukemia in combination with doxorubicin or daunorubicin and thioguanine. It also is used in the blastic crisis phase of chronic myelogenous leukemia, as secondary treatment of acute lymphocytic leukemia, and in combination regimens for non-Hodgkins's lymphomas. The drug can be administered intrathecally for meningeal leukemia.

Resistance to cytarabine may result from impaired cellular uptake, decreased activation secondary to decreased kinase activity, or enhanced metabolism from increased deaminase activity. High-dose cytarabine has been effective in overcoming drug resistance. Recently, low-dose cytarabine has been employed for myelodysplastic syndromes. It is not clear wheth-er the predominant effect is cytotoxicity or differentiation in these disorders.

ADVERSE REACTIONS AND PRECAUTIONS. The major dose-limiting toxic effect of cytarabine is bone marrow depression, which is dependent on the dose and schedule. It is characterized by leukopenia, thrombocytopenia, reticulocytopenia, and megaloblastosis. The leukopenia is caused primarily by granulocyte depression, and circulating lymphocytes are only minimally affected. The white blood cell depression has a biphasic course following continuous infusion for five days or rapid injections. There is an initial decrease in the first 24 hours with the nadir occurring on days seven to nine, followed by a brief increase that peaks around the twelfth day. Subsequently, a second and deeper fall reaches a nadir between days 15 to 24, with a rapid rise to above baseline in the next ten days. Platelet depression is noticeable at five days with the nadir occurring between days 12 to 15. Thereafter, a rapid rise to above baseline occurs in the next ten days. Frequent blood counts and bone marrow examinations are required.

Nausea and vomiting occur frequently, particularly after rapid intravenous infusion. Stomatitis, thrombophlebitis, hepatic dysfunction, fever, and, rarely, anaphylaxis also have been reported. Hyperuricemia secondary to rapid lysis of neoplastic cells may occur. Cytarabine is a potent immunosuppressant. It has been shown to be teratogenic in animals (FDA Pregnancy Category C). Because cytarabine is metabolized primarily in the liver, patients with impaired hepatic function may require a reduction in dosage.

Side effects of high-dose cytarabine regimens include conjunctival pain and photophobia (modified with steroid eyedrops), midline cerebellar dysfunction, and peripheral neuropathy. Intrathecal cytarabine may cause central nervous system toxicity.

PHARMACOKINETICS. Cytarabine is rapidly metabolized and less than 20% is absorbed after oral administration. Thus, it is given intravenously. The drug is deaminated rapidly, primarily in the liver, to uracil arabinoside, an inactive metabolite, and disappears from the blood in two phases, an initial fast phase with a half-life of 12 minutes and a second phase of approximately two hours. Eighty percent is excreted in the urine in 24 hours, 90% as uracil arabinoside and less than 10% as unchanged drug. A carrier mediated mechanism is responsible for cellular uptake.

Cerebrospinal fluid levels approach 40% to 50% of the plasma concentration after a two-hour intravenous infusion. Because of the low levels of deaminase in the cerebrospinal fluid, little conversion to uracil arabinoside occurs there.

With-high dose cytarabine regimens, peak plasma levels are approximately 100 times those observed with conventional doses.

DOSAGE AND PREPARATIONS. For induction therapy, patients should be hospitalized in a facility with adequate laboratory and supportive resources. In many treatment protocols, cytarabine is used in combination with other cytotoxic drugs.

Intravenous: For continuous intravenous infusion, 100 to 200 mg/M^2/24 hours. Generally, five- to seven-day infusions are given in conjunction with an anthracycline and thioguanine. If there is no response, the course is repeated; if remission does not occur after the second course, another therapeutic regimen should be substituted.

High-dose Intravenous: 3 g/M^2 infused over a one-hour period every 12 hours for a total of 12 doses.

Subcutaneous: For maintenance therapy in acute leukemia, 50 mg/M^2 weekly.

Low-dose Subcutaneous: 20 mg/M^2/day for 7 to 21 days.

Intrathecal: 50 to 100 mg in 10 ml of saline given one to three times weekly.

    Cytosar-U (Upjohn). Powder (sterile, cryodesiccated) 100 and 500 mg with diluent.

FLUOROURACIL (5 FU)
[Adrucil]

ACTIONS. This fluorinated pyrimidine was developed as a potential antineoplastic agent because of the observation that certain tumor cells utilized the normal pyrimidine base, uracil, for biosynthesis of DNA more effectively than did nontumor cells. Fluorouracil must be converted in vivo to the deoxynucleotide, 5-fluoro-2'-deoxyuridine 5'-monophosphate (FdUMP), which is the active metabolite. In animal tumor models, conversion of fluorouracil to FdUMP correlates well with tumor sensitivity, but this relationship has not been clearly established in human cancer. FdUMP inhibits thymidylate synthetase, which catalizes methylation of deoxyuridylic acid (dUMP) to thymidylic acid (dTMP), thereby preventing DNA synthesis. Although inhibition of thymidylate synthetase is generally accepted as the primary action, fluorouracil also is converted to the nucleotide, fluorouridine monophosphate (FUMP), which is readily incorporated into RNA and inhibits RNA processing and function. Fluorouracil is more toxic to proliferating than to nonproliferating cells, but there is no clear-cut cell cycle phase specificity. Resistance to fluorouracil could result from deletion of enzymes required for its activation or from an increase in thymidylate synthetase activity.

USES. The usefulness of fluorouracil is confined to solid tumors. It is used extensively in the palliative treatment of disseminated colorectal and breast carcinomas; when used alone, response rates are only about 20% and 30%, respectively. When given as a component of the CMF (and PF) regimen, fluorouracil is an agent of choice in adjuvant chemotherapy of breast cancer (see the section on Adjuvant Chemotherapy). A superior combination regimen has not yet been found for colorectal carcinoma.

This drug also is a component of the FAM combination used in the palliative treatment of gastric adenocarcinoma (see Table 2). Other responsive tumors are carcinomas of the ovary (eg, Hexa-CAF regimen), bladder, uterine cervix, endometrium, prostate, head and neck, pancreas, and esophagus and hepatoma.

ADVERSE REACTIONS AND PRECAUTIONS. The major toxic effects of fluorouracil occur in the gastrointestinal and hematopoietic systems. Anorexia, nausea, and vomiting are common. Stomatitis, esophagopharyngitis, and diarrhea are indications for interruption of therapy because severe ulceration of the oropharynx and bowel may develop. Gastrointestinal toxicity is usually dose limiting when the drug is given by intravenous infusion. In contrast, leukopenia is the usual dose-limiting toxicity after bolus intravenous administration. The nadir of the white blood cell count commonly occurs between day 7 and 14 after the first dose. Thrombocytopenia is much less prominent and may be observed between days 7 and 17. Monitoring of blood counts is necessary.

Other adverse effects are alopecia, dermatitis, and hyperpigmentation. Acute and chronic conjunctivitis have been seen. Reversible cerebellar ataxia occurs in 1% of patients, is probably dose related, and may occur at any time during therapy (usually after several months). Cerebellar signs may persist for several weeks after discontinuing the drug. Myocardial ischemia has been noted rarely with fluorouracil infusions. This drug is teratogenic in animals and may be carcinogenic.

The dose of fluorouracil should be decreased in patients with impaired hepatic function (eg, extensive liver metastases), and the drug should be used with caution in patients with poor nutritional status.

The use of intermittent intravenous infusions daily for four or five days markedly decreases hematologic toxicity. However, results of clinical studies do not indicate whether rapid injections or infusions are a superior treatment method. Prolonged infusions of fluorouracil have been associated with a hand-foot syndrome associated with pain, erythema, and desquamation.

DRUG INTERACTIONS. Pretreatment with methotrexate increases the formation of 5-fluorouracil nucleotide by increasing the intracellular content of phosphoribosylpyrophosphate. Allopurinol also may alter the effect of fluorouracil and its metabolite, oxypurinol, inhibits orotic acid phosphoribosyl transferase, which decreases toxicity and possibly improves the therapeutic index. Thymidine and other nucleosides enhance the incorporation of fluorouracil into RNA, and thymidine may delay the breakdown of fluorouracil by dihydrouracil dehydrogenase. However, these combinations have not improved clinical results.

PHARMACOKINETICS. Because of erratic absorption, fluorouracil is not routinely administered orally (an oral preparation is available in Europe). It is usually given intravenously. This drug also has been administered intra-arterially for direct delivery to the tumor (eg, hepatic artery for liver metastases) and by direct injection into effusions in body cavities (eg, in ovarian cancer). The plasma half-life after intravenous administration is 7.5 to 10 minutes and no unchanged drug is detectable after three hours. Intracellular drug levels persist much longer.

Fluorouracil is metabolized extensively in the liver; 60% to 80% is excreted as respiratory carbon dioxide in 8 to 12 hours and 15% is eliminated unchanged in urine within six hours. The drug enters effusions and the cerebrospinal fluid. Assays for fluorouracil in plasma are available.

DOSAGE AND PREPARATIONS.

Intravenous: Various regimens have been used. In one, a

loading dose of 400 to 500 mg/M² is given once daily for four successive days (maximum single daily dose, 800 mg); if no toxicity is observed, this is followed by a weekly maintenance dose. Some investigators repeat the loading dose regimen every four to five weeks.

With continuous infusion, 1 g/M² is administered daily for five days with acceptable toxicity and is repeated every three to four weeks. Dosage adjustments must be made if hematologic or gastrointestinal side effects develop.

Intra-arterial (Hepatic): 800 mg/M²/day for 14 to 21 days by continuous infusion.

   Adrucil (Adria), *Fluorouracil* (Roche). Solution 50 mg/ml in 10 ml containers.

TOPICAL FLUOROURACIL
   [Efudex]

ACTIONS AND USES. Topical preparations containing 2% or 5% fluorouracil are used to treat multiple actinic (solar) keratoses on the head and neck. The 5% concentration is used on keratoses in other areas and is useful in superficial basal cell carcinomas when conventional methods are impractical (eg, in patients with multiple lesions or difficult treatment sites). The diagnosis should be established before treatment is begun, since this method has not been proved effective in other types of basal cell carcinomas. If the lesions are isolated and easily accessible, conventional techniques are preferred because of their higher success rate. For a description of the mechanism of action, see the preceding evaluation on Fluorouracil. See also Chapter 56, Dermatologic Preparations.

ADVERSE REACTIONS AND PRECAUTIONS. The most frequently encountered local reactions are pain, pruritus, hyperpigmentation, and burning at the site of application. Other local reactions include dermatitis, scarring, soreness, tenderness, suppuration, scaling, and swelling. Use of an occlusive dressing may increase the incidence of inflammatory reactions in adjacent normal skin. A porous gauze dressing may be applied for cosmetic reasons without increasing the frequency of reactions. Patients should be informed that the treated areas may be unsightly during therapy and for several weeks thereafter. A topical corticosteroid cream may hasten the involution of severe inflammation following cessation of therapy.

Insomnia, stomatitis, irritability, medicinal taste, photosensitivity, lacrimation, and telangiectasia have been reported, although a causal relationship is remote. Laboratory abnormalities reported are leukocytosis, thrombocytopenia, toxic granulation, and eosinophilia. The safety of topical fluorouracil during pregnancy has not been established.

Topical fluorouracil is contraindicated in patients with known hypersensitivity to any of the components in the formulations. Prolonged exposure to ultraviolet rays during therapy should be avoided, for this may intensify the severity of reactions.

If fluorouracil is applied with the fingers, the hands should be washed immediately thereafter. It should be applied with care near the eyes, nose, and mouth.

Unresponsive solar keratoses should undergo biopsy to confirm the diagnosis, and follow-up biopsy of superficial basal cell carcinomas should be performed as indicated.

DOSAGE AND PREPARATIONS.
Topical: The response to application occurs in the following sequence: erythema, vesiculation, erosion, ulceration, necrosis, and epithelialization.

For actinic or solar keratosis, the cream or solution is applied twice daily in an amount sufficient to cover the lesions. Treatment is continued until the inflammatory response reaches the erosion, necrosis, and ulceration stage (usually for two to four weeks). Complete healing commonly occurs one to two months after cessation of therapy.

For superficial basal cell carcinoma, the 5% concentration is applied twice daily in an amount sufficient to cover the lesions. Treatment should be continued for at least three to six weeks and may be required for as long as 10 or 12 weeks. As in any neoplastic condition, the patient should be followed for a reasonable period to determine if a cure has been obtained.

   Efudex (Roche). Cream 5% in 25 g containers; solution 2% and 5% in 10 ml containers.

FLOXURIDINE
   [FUDR]

ACTIONS AND USES. Rationale for the use of floxuridine, the deoxyriboside derivative of fluorouracil, is based upon its distinctive metabolism, which depends upon the mode and rate of administration. Following intravenous or rapid intra-arterial injection, floxuridine is rapidly metabolized to fluorouracil and has the same efficacy and adverse effects. However, when floxuridine is given by slow, continuous, intra-arterial infusion, it is converted by a nucleoside kinase to the active agent, floxuridine monophosphate (FdUMP), which inhibits thymidylate synthetase and thus blocks DNA synthesis. With this method of administration, the dose can be reduced because floxuridine is pharmacologically more active than with bolus injection. Floxuridine has less effect on RNA than fluorouracil.

Although intra-arterial floxuridine has been used for palliation in certain malignancies (eg, carcinoma of the rectum, colon, and gastrointestinal tract and liver metastases from these sites), it does not appear to offer any advantages over intravenous fluorouracil. Furthermore, no controlled study has shown superior results with intra-arterial administration, which is both hazardous and expensive. When administered into the hepatic artery, the drug is metabolized immediately by the liver, with 95% removed on the first pass.

ADVERSE REACTIONS AND PRECAUTIONS. Local adverse reactions (eg, mucositis, localized erythema) are more prominent than systemic reactions after intra-arterial injection. Severe, possibly fatal sclerosing cholangitis and/or hepatitis has been observed after hepatic artery infusion and this method should be used cautiously in patients with hepatic dysfunction.

Systemic reactions are similar to those seen with fluorouracil. The most common are nausea, vomiting, diarrhea, stomatitis, and enteritis. Other adverse effects include anorexia, cramps, duodenal ulcer, gastritis, glossitis, pharyngitis, and dermatologic reactions (alopecia, dermatitis, pruritus, rash, ulceration). Anemia and leukopenia also occur. Elevated alkaline phosphatase, serum transaminase, serum bilirubin, and lactic dehydrogenase values have been noted. Acute and delayed central nervous system toxicity is manifested by ataxia, blurred vision, depression, nystagmus, vertigo, and lethargy. Complications of regional arterial infusion (eg, arterial aneurysm; ischemia and thrombosis; bleeding, leaking, and infection at the catheter site; thrombophlebitis) may occur.

Because of its toxicity and low therapeutic index, floxuridine should be given under the supervision of a physician experienced not only in cancer chemotherapy, but in the technique of intra-arterial infusion. Ambulatory patients must be hospitalized during the first course of treatment and should be informed about toxic manifestations. White blood cell and platelet counts should be performed regularly.

As with fluorouracil, floxuridine should be discontinued immediately when any of the following signs and symptoms appear: stomatitis, esophagopharyngitis, gastrointestinal ulceration and bleeding, diarrhea (five or more loose stools daily), intractable vomiting, leukocyte count less than 3,500/microliter or a rapidly decreasing count, thrombocytopenia with a platelet count less than 100,000/microliter, or hemorrhage from any site. Use of floxuridine is hazardous in patients with poor nutritional status or bone marrow depression, and it should be avoided in pregnant women, particularly during the first trimester, because of its potential teratogenicity.

DOSAGE AND PREPARATIONS.

Intra-arterial: The specialized nature of this technique requires the combined skills of a surgeon and oncologist. *Adults,* with the patient under general anesthesia, the catheter is inserted into the artery supplying the tumor and sutured to the vessel wall. An infusion pump is used to administer 5 to 20 mg/M²/24/hr continuously for 14 to 21 days. Infusion is continued until a local toxic reaction (eg, cutaneous erythema, mucositis) or systemic toxicity is noted. The infusion is stopped until the reaction subsides; additional courses then are given for as long as the response continues. Adequate courses of therapy have varied from one month to several years.

FUDR (Roche). Powder (sterile) 500 mg.

Purine Analogues

MERCAPTOPURINE
[Purinethol]

ACTIONS. Mercaptopurine, the thio analogue of hypoxanthine, is a prodrug that must be converted to 6-mercaptopurine-ribose-phosphate (6-MPRP), intracellularly by hypoxanthine-guanine phosphoribosyl transferase (HGPRT). This has been termed lethal synthesis. 6-MPRP interferes with purine biosynthesis both by feedback inhibition of the first step (phosphoribosylpyrophosphate amidotransferase) in purine biosynthesis and by blocking the conversion of inosinic acid to adenylic acid or guanylic acid. Triphosphorylated nucleotide metabolites are incorporated into DNA, and this may also be involved in the cytotoxic effects of the drug.

Mercaptopurine is cell cycle specific for the S phase but is self-limiting. Biochemical resistance can result from absence of the activating enzyme (HGPRT) or by increased concentration of a degrading enzyme, a membrane bound alkaline phosphatase.

USES. When used alone, mercaptopurine induces complete remission in approximately 25% of children and 10% of adults with acute lymphocytic leukemia. However, much better results are obtained with combination regimens (see Table 2). The major role of mercaptopurine in acute lymphocytic leukemia is in maintenance therapy, most often in combination with methotrexate. When administered after a prednisone/vincristine-induced remission, the incidence of prolonged complete bone marrow remissions approaches 80% in children.

Mercaptopurine is marginally effective in acute myelogenous leukemia in adults; complete remissions of short duration occur in less than 20% of patients. It is not a primary drug in this type of leukemia. Similarly, in the early phase of chronic myelogenous leukemia, the drug controls the disease in 30% to 50% of adults, but busulfan is the drug of choice for initial therapy.

ADVERSE REACTIONS AND PRECAUTIONS. The usual dose-limiting toxicity of mercaptopurine is bone marrow depression, including leukopenia, thrombocytopenia, and anemia. It is usually gradual in onset and may persist for several days after cessation of administration. Myelosuppression can be delayed and leukocyte counts should be performed weekly; mercaptopurine should be discontinued if an abnormal reduction occurs. The leukocyte count is used to establish a maintenance dose.

Anorexia, nausea, and vomiting occur in about 25% of adult patients and are usually mild. Oral and gastrointestinal ulcerations are much less common than with methotrexate and fluorouracil. Hepatic dysfunction is seen in about one-third of adults; it is less common in children. Cholestatic jaundice is most prominent but is usually reversible on cessation of therapy. Smaller doses are recommended in patients with impaired hepatic or renal function to avoid accumulation.

Since mercaptopurine is metabolized by xanthine oxidase to 6-thiouric acid, the dose should be reduced to 25% to 33% of the usual amount if allopurinol, a xanthine oxidase inhibitor, is used concomitantly for hyperuricemia. In the presence of allopurinol, 6-thioxanthine, an intermediate oxidation product, becomes the predominant metabolite eliminated.

Mercaptopurine is embryotoxic in animals and should be avoided during the first trimester of pregnancy. It produces chromosomal aberrations and is mutagenic and potentially carcinogenic. The drug is an immunosuppressant.

PHARMACOKINETICS. This agent is incompletely and erratically absorbed after oral administration (average, 20% to 50% of the administered dose). Peak plasma levels are attained in two hours; after eight hours, no drug is detectable. Mercaptopurine and its active nucleotide are metabolized extensively to a number of products in the liver; 50% of the drug and its metabolites are excreted in the urine in 24 hours. Mercaptopurine is about 20% bound to plasma proteins. Although it is widely distributed in body tissues, only a small percentage enters the cerebrospinal fluid after usual doses.

DOSAGE AND PREPARATIONS. The dosage varies from patient to patient and titration is necessary to obtain maximum effectiveness with acceptable toxicity. The following dosages are frequently employed. Modifications may be necessary when mercaptopurine is combined with other cytotoxic drugs.
Oral: For induction of remission, *adults and children over 5 years,* 100 mg/M^2 daily. If clinical improvement does not occur and leukocytes are not depressed within four weeks, the dose may be increased cautiously to a maximum of 200 mg/M^2 daily. The total daily dose may be given at one time and is calculated to the closest multiple of 25 mg. Alternatively, 500 to 700 mg/M^2/day is given for five days in combination with other drugs.

For maintenance therapy in *children* with acute lymphocytic leukemia in remission, 50 mg/M^2 daily as a single dose, usually in combination other drugs (most frequently with methotrexate). Administration may be continued for a prolonged period.

Therapy should be discontinued at the first sign of profound or rapid reductions in the leukocyte or platelet count; it may be reinstituted at one-half the previous dosage after toxic manifestations disappear.

Purinethol (Burroughs Wellcome). Tablets 50 mg.

THIOGUANINE

ACTIONS. Thioguanine, the thio analogue of guanine, is a prodrug that is converted to 6-thioguanine-ribose-phosphate (6-TGRP), an active metabolite, by the same pathway used by mercaptopurine. 6-TGRP is a feedback inhibitor of the initial (amidotransferase) step in purine biosynthesis. This metabolite also blocks the conversions of inosinic acid to guanylic acid (GMP) and of GMP to GDP. Thioguanine also is converted to the deoxynucleoside triphosphate, which can be incorporated into tumor cell DNA. Although some investigators believe that this is the major mechanism of cytotoxicity, the relative importance of the various sites of action remain to be elucidated. Thioguanine is cell cycle specific for the S phase. Tumor cells resistant to mercaptopurine usually exhibit cross resistance to thioguanine.

USES. The use of thioguanine is essentially confined to patients with acute leukemias. The combination of thioguanine and cytarabine induces complete responses in approximately 50% of adults with acute myelogenous leukemia. The rate is usually higher when cytarabine is combined with an anthracycline. Thioguanine is often employed as a third drug in these regimens. This drug also is active in the blast crisis of chronic myelogenous leukemia and in acute lymphocytic leukemia.

ADVERSE REACTIONS AND PRECAUTIONS. The usual dose-limiting toxicity of thioguanine is bone marrow depression resulting in leukopenia, thrombocytopenia, and anemia. Hemoglobin levels and white blood cell and platelet counts should be determined weekly or more frequently during remission induction therapy for acute leukemia. Thioguanine should be discontinued if leukocyte or platelet counts decrease suddenly. Therapy may be reinstituted when the cell counts return to normal levels.

Occasionally, nausea, vomiting, anorexia, and stomatitis may develop, especially if large doses are used. Gastrointestinal side effects are usually less severe with thioguanine than with mercaptopurine. Hepatic dysfunction, usually cholestatic jaundice, may occur. Lower doses may be required in patients with impaired hepatic or renal function. Hyperuricemia may develop as a consequence of tumor cell lysis; dosage does not require adjustment when allopurinol is given concomitantly. Thioguanine is potentially mutagenic and carcinogenic. It should not be given during the first trimester of pregnancy because of its potential teratogenic effects. It is immunosuppressive.

PHARMACOKINETICS. Thioguanine is incompletely absorbed when given orally, averaging about 30% of an administered dose. The elimination half-life of the parent drug is 1.5 hours, but peak plasma levels of metabolites are reached in six to eight hours. Between 24% and 46% is excreted in the urine as metabolites within 24 hours. Thioguanine also can be administered intravenously. It is cleared rapidly from plasma; more than 80% of a dose is excreted within 24 hours. Although thioguanine crosses the blood-brain barrier in animals after use of large doses, very little enters the cerebrospinal fluid of humans after usual clinical doses are employed.

Thioguanine and its active metabolites are extensively inactivated in the liver, primarily by methylation; 6-methylthioguanine is a major metabolite. Thioguanine is not extensively deaminated and only a small amount is converted to thiouric acid by xanthine oxidase. Thus, the dose of thioguanine does not require reduction in the presence of allopurinol.

DOSAGE AND PREPARATIONS. The dosage varies from patient to patient and titration is necessary to obtain maximum effectiveness with acceptable toxicity. The following dosages are frequently employed.
Oral: Adults and children, 80 mg/M^2 daily. If there is no response after four weeks, the amount may be increased cautiously to 120 mg/M^2 daily. If no clinical or laboratory evidence of improvement is observed, another class of drugs should be substituted. The total daily dose may be given at one time and is usually calculated to the closest multiple of 20 mg.

For induction of remission in acute myelogenous leukemia,

in combination with daunorubicin and cytarabine, *adults and children,* 100 mg/M² every 12 hours on days one through seven.

Thioguanine (Burroughs Wellcome). Tablets 40 mg.

ANTITUMOR ANTIBIOTICS

Like other antibiotics, these drugs are produced by microbial fermentation. The clinically useful antitumor antibiotics consist of the anthracyclines (daunorubicin, doxorubicin), dactinomycin, plicamycin (mithramycin), mitomycin, and bleomycin. These drugs either bind to or react with cellular DNA to exert their cytotoxic effect. The anthracyclines and dactinomycin are intercalating agents. Plicamycin also binds DNA noncovalently but is not an intercalating agent. Mitomycin covalently binds DNA, and bleomycin causes DNA strand scission. Because antitumor antibiotics are poorly absorbed by the gastrointestinal tract, they are usually administered intravenously.

BLEOMYCIN SULFATE
[Blenoxane]

(Main Component: Bleomycin A₂, in which R is (CH₃)₂S⁺CH₂ CH₂ CH₂—)

ACTIONS. The bleomycins are a family of complex glycopeptides extracted from a strain of *Streptomyces verticillus.* The bleomycin used clinically is a mixture consisting predominantly of bleomycin A_2 and B_2. This drug produces its cytotoxic effect by inhibiting DNA synthesis, primarily by generating free radicals that cause single- and double-strand scissions in the DNA molecule.

Bleomycin appears to exhibit some degree of cell cycle phase specificity. It is most active during the G_2 phase and has some activity in the late G_1, early S, and M phases.

USES. Bleomycin is useful in the treatment of testicular cancer and malignant lymphomas. It has some activity against squamous cell carcinomas of the head and neck region (eg, buccal mucosa, tongue, tonsil, pharynx), uterine cervix, and esophagus. This antibiotic has been administered intravesically to treat recurrent superficial bladder tumors.

Because it lacks significant myelosuppressive activity, bleomycin has been used extensively with other drugs (see Table 2 and the section on Combination Chemotherapy). The combination of bleomycin, vinblastine, and cisplatin is very effective in disseminated seminomatous and nonseminomatous testicular cancer and produces a high percentage of long-term

disease-free survivors who are probably cured of disease. In Hodgkin's disease, bleomycin has been added to the MOPP regimen; the combination of doxorubicin, bleomycin, vinblastine, and dacarbazine (ABVD) is an effective alternative to MOPP. Complete responses with long-term disease-free survival also have been observed in many patients with non-Hodgkin's lymphoma who received regimens containing bleomycin (eg, BACOP). The combination of bleomycin, mitomycin, and vincristine is active in the treatment of carcinoma of the cervix, but there are few complete responses and remissions are of short duration.

ADVERSE REACTIONS AND PRECAUTIONS. The usual dose-limiting toxic effect of bleomycin is pulmonary fibrosis, which occurs in approximately 10% of patients. The incidence and severity of pulmonary toxicity are related to the patient's age, the total dose, and the concomitant use of other agents. Patients older than 70 years or those receiving a total dose of more than 400 units are at greater risk. Radiation to the thorax probably increases the risk.

The development of pulmonary toxicity is usually delayed and may occur four to ten weeks after initiation of therapy. The radiographic appearance is typical of interstitial pneumonitis that may progress to pulmonary fibrosis. Rales, rhonchi, and, occasionally, pleural friction rubs usually precede radiographic changes. The lesions are found most frequently in the lower lobes and subpleural areas and consist of a fibrinous exudate, atypical proliferation of alveolar cells, hyaline membranes, interstitial and intra-alveolar fibrosis, and squamous metaplasia of the distal air spaces. Pulmonary function tests are not necessarily predictive. The most sensitive method for early detection of pulmonary toxicity may be serial determination of carbon monoxide diffusion capacity. The drug should be discontinued immediately if lung reaction is detected.

The incidence of hypersensitivity reactions ranging from chills and fever to anaphylaxis is high (20% to 50% of patients). Severe reactions are most common in lymphoma patients and test doses are recommended. Mucocutaneous changes (eg, alopecia; hyperpigmentation; pruritic erythema; hyperkeratosis; desquamation of hands, feet, and pressure areas; edema; mucositis) also occur frequently. Neither clinically significant myelosuppression nor immunosuppression has been reported.

The safety of bleomycin during pregnancy or lactation is unknown.

PHARMACOKINETICS. Bleomycin is inactive orally. When administered parenterally, it is distributed rapidly throughout the body. The highest concentrations appear in the skin, lung, kidney, peritoneum, and lymph nodes. However, bleomycin does not enter the cerebrospinal fluid. This drug is rapidly inactivated in all normal tissues except skin and lung. The plasma elimination half-life is about 2 to 4 hours; 45% to 70% is recovered in urine as active drug. Drug clearance is decreased and the plasma half-life is prolonged in patients with impaired renal function; dosage modifications are required.

DOSAGE AND PREPARATIONS. One mg has been defined as one unit of activity. For intramuscular or subcutaneous use, the contents of the ampul are dissolved in 1 to 5 ml of sterile water for injection, sodium chloride injection, or 5% dextrose injection. For intravenous use, the contents of the ampul are dissolved in 5 ml or more of sodium chloride injection or 5% dextrose injection and administered slowly over ten minutes.

Intramuscular, Intravenous, Subcutaneous: For squamous cell carcinomas, lymphomas, and testicular carcinoma, 10 to 20 units/M^2 once or twice weekly (to a total dose of 300 to 400 units). Because anaphylactic reactions may occur, patients with lymphomas should receive 2 units or less as the initial dose. If no acute reaction is observed, the regular dosage schedule may be used.

Intracavitary: After thoracostomy tube drainage, 15 to 240 units diluted in 100 ml of normal saline has been administered into the pleural space.

    Blenoxane (Bristol-Myers). Powder (sterile) 15 units.

DACTINOMYCIN (Actinomycin D)
[Cosmegen]

ACTIONS. This antitumor antibiotic, derived from *Streptomyces parvullus*, forms a stable complex with DNA and inhibits DNA-dependent RNA synthesis and, at higher concentrations, DNA synthesis. Dactinomycin also causes single strand DNA breaks. This drug is cell cycle nonspecific.

USES. Dactinomycin is effective in gestational choriocarcinoma. Effective therapy of Wilms' tumor requires multiple treatment modalities, including surgery, radiation therapy, and combination chemotherapy with dactinomycin and vincristine. Dactinomycin also is active in testicular tumors, embryonal rhabdomyosarcoma, Ewing's sarcoma, osteosarcoma, and other sarcomas.

ADVERSE REACTIONS AND PRECAUTIONS. The usual dose-limiting toxicity is bone marrow depression, usually leukopenia and thrombocytopenia. The nadir usually occurs between one and two weeks after a course of therapy. Thrombocytopenia is often seen first; leukopenia may be dose limiting. Blood counts should be monitored carefully. Dactinomycin should be given cautiously to those with renal or liver disease or impaired bone marrow function.

    Anorexia, nausea, and vomiting usually occur within a few hours after administration and may be ameliorated by antiemetics (eg, phenothiazines) given prior to therapy. Abdominal pain and diarrhea may occur. Stomatitis, cheilitis, glossitis, and proctitis are common and may be dose limiting. Oral and gastrointestinal ulcerations may develop.

    Dermatologic reactions include alopecia and acneiform eruption. Cutaneous erythema, desquamation, and hyperpigmentation also may occur, especially in previously irradiated areas. Dactinomycin potentiates the effects of ionizing radiation. Anaphylactic reactions have been reported.

    This drug is locally irritating and can cause cellulitis if extravasation occurs. Teratogenic and carcinogenic effects have been observed in animals (FDA Pregnancy Category C). Dactinomycin is immunosuppressive.

PHARMACOKINETICS. Dactinomycin is poorly absorbed orally and is administered intravenously. The drug is cleared rapidly from plasma by tissue uptake and DNA binding. It does not enter the cerebrospinal fluid. Dactinomycin has a long tissue and plasma half-life (36 hours) due to slow release from tissue stores. It is metabolized minimally and about 30% of a dose is excreted in bile and urine over seven days.

DOSAGE AND PREPARATIONS.

Intravenous: The usual dose is 0.4 to 0.6 mg/M^2 daily for a maximum of five days. In both adults and children, a second course may be administered after at least three weeks have elapsed, provided all signs of toxicity have disappeared. Dactinomycin is administered through a running intravenous infusion.

Isolation Perfusion Technique: The dosage schedules and technique vary; the literature should be consulted for details. In general, the following doses are suggested: 0.15 to 0.2 mg/M^2 for lower extremity or pelvis; 0.1 to 0.15 mg/M^2 for upper extremity. After bone marrow function has recovered (three to four weeks), the course is repeated.

    Cosmegen (Merck Sharp & Dohme). Powder (lyophilized) 0.5 mg with mannitol 20 mg.

DAUNORUBICIN HYDROCHLORIDE
[Cerubidine]

ACTIONS. Daunorubicin, an anthracycline antibiotic isolated from *Streptomyces peucetius*, forms a stable complex with DNA and inhibits DNA-dependent DNA and RNA synthesis. DNA damage also may result from free radical formation. In addition, anthracyclines may react directly with cell membranes to alter function. Daunorubicin is cycle nonspecific, but activity is greatest during the S phase. Tumor cell cross resistance is observed between daunorubicin and doxorubicin.

USES. The major indications for daunorubicin, in combination with other active drugs, are acute myelogenous and lymphocytic leukemias (see Table 2). The combination of cytarabine and daunorubicin (with or without thioguanine) is the treatment of choice for induction of remission in acute myelogenous leukemias. Complete response rates exceeding 60% are observed routinely with the two-drug combination. Daunorubicin is also active in neuroblastoma.

ADVERSE REACTIONS AND PRECAUTIONS. Myelosuppression is the usual dose-limiting toxicity. Leukopenia is usually more significant than thrombocytopenia, but severe aplasia may develop. The nadir for leukopenia generally occurs between 10 and 14 days, and recovery is gradual over the next one or two weeks. Monitoring of blood counts is essential.

Nausea and vomiting are usually mild but can be severe. Stomatitis also occurs; it typically begins as a burning sensation with erythema of the oral mucosa leading to ulceration in two or three days. Alopecia develops in about 80% of patients; it often has a sudden onset after three to four weeks of therapy but is usually reversible. Febrile reactions also may occur occasionally.

Cardiotoxicity is the major delayed adverse effect of daunorubicin. An acute syndrome characterized by transient, reversible changes in the electrocardiogram (eg, tachycardia, extrasystoles, ST-T wave alterations) may occur hours to days after a dose and is not related to the total dose. A cumulative, dose-dependent cardiomyopathy also may develop and sometimes leads to congestive heart failure that may not respond to treatment. Cardiotoxicity may be mediated by free radical formation. Cardiotoxicity may occur one to six months after treatment is discontinued. The risk of congestive heart failure increases when the total cumulative dose exceeds 550 mg/M² (maximum recommended dose). The total dose of daunorubicin should be limited to 400 mg/M² when radiation therapy to the mediastinum was administered previously. Also, the dosage should be modified if previous or concomitant cardiotoxic drug therapy is employed. Daunorubicin should be used with great caution in patients with significant heart disease.

Severe local tissue necrosis and sloughing may develop if extravasation occurs. Daunorubicin causes transient red discoloration of the urine that is of no clinical significance. The drug is mutagenic, carcinogenic, and teratogenic.

Dosage reductions may be necessary in patients with impaired hepatic function.

PHARMACOKINETICS. Daunorubicin is poorly absorbed orally. Plasma clearance is biphasic after intravenous administration with a first half-life of 45 minutes, indicating uptake by tissues, and an elimination half-life of 24 to 55 hours. The drug is metabolized rapidly in the liver and is distributed to the tissues as unchanged drug, a major active metabolite (daunorubicinol), and other metabolites. It is excreted slowly in the urine, mainly as metabolites, with 25% excreted in the first five days; there also is significant (eg, 40%) biliary excretion. Daunorubicin does not enter cerebrospinal fluid.

DOSAGE AND PREPARATIONS.
Intravenous: 30 to 60 mg/M² daily for three days, repeated at three- to six-week intervals. The drug is administered through a running intravenous line.
> **Cerubidine** (Wyeth). Powder (sterile, lyophilized) equivalent to 20 mg of base with mannitol 100 mg.

DOXORUBICIN HYDROCHLORIDE
[Adriamycin]

ACTIONS. Doxorubicin, an anthracycline antibiotic isolated from *Streptomyces peucetius*, is very similar in structure to daunorubicin. Doxorubicin inhibits DNA-dependent synthesis of DNA and RNA due to intercalation between base pairs of DNA. Damage to DNA also may be mediated by free radical formation. In addition, anthracyclines may react directly with cell membranes to alter function. The agent is cell cycle nonspecific but activity is greatest during the S phase. Tumor cell cross resistance is observed between doxorubicin and daunorubicin.

USES. Doxorubicin is one of the most effective antineoplastic agents and has been useful, most often in combination regimens, in acute lymphocytic and acute myelogenous leukemia; Hodgkin's disease and non-Hodgkin's lymphoma; sarcomas (Ewing's, osteogenic, rhabdomyosarcoma, and soft tissue); neuroblastoma; Wilms' tumor; carcinomas of the breast, lung, stomach, pancreas, bladder, prostate, ovary, endometrium, cervix, testes, and thyroid; squamous cell carcinoma of the head and neck; and hepatoma (see Table 2).

ADVERSE REACTIONS AND PRECAUTIONS. Toxicity affects the hematopoietic, cardiac, dermatologic, and gastrointestinal systems. Leukopenia is the usual dose-limiting toxicity, with the nadir occurring 10 to 15 days after initial administration. Blood counts usually return to normal levels approximately 21 days after administration. Thrombocytopenia and anemia follow a similar pattern but are of smaller magnitude. Blood counts must be monitored carefully.

Both acute and cumulative dose-dependent cardiotoxicity may occur. Acute effects may develop within a few minutes after a single intravenous dose and may persist for two weeks. They consist of electrocardiographic changes, such as sinus tachycardia, voltage reduction, flattening of the T-wave, depression of the S-T segment, and arrhythmias. Such changes are usually transient and reversible. Suspension of doxorubicin therapy should take into consideration the patient's overall status. The second type of cardiotoxicity is a delayed, cumulative, dose-dependent cardiomyopathy that may occur during or up to several weeks after completion of treatment. Doxorubicin must be discontinued when congestive heart failure secondary to diffuse cardiomyopathy develops. The total dose should not exceed 550 mg/M², since the risk of congestive heart failure increases markedly with larger amounts. This drug should not be given to patients with significantly impaired cardiac function. If it is used in patients who have received mediastinal irradiation, the total dose should not exceed 400 mg/M², because the risk of cardiotoxicity is increased in these patients. Other reported risk factors for doxorubicin-induced cardiomyopathy are hypertensive heart disease and concomitant administration of certain antineoplastic drugs (eg, high-dose cyclophosphamide). Cardiotoxicity may be mediated by free radical formation. Continuous infusion or weekly doxorubicin appears to be less cardiotoxic.

Alopecia is seen in about 80% of patients, and regrowth of hair is usually complete two to five months after cessation of therapy. Doxorubicin also may cause a recurrence of radiation-induced skin reactions and exacerbates tissue changes due to irradiation in mucous membranes and the liver.

Nausea and vomiting are common and usually moderate; diarrhea occurs occasionally. Mucositis (eg, stomatitis, esophagitis) may be severe with ulceration. Fever, chills, and urticaria have been observed and anaphylaxis may occur.

The urine may become red after administration of the red-colored doxorubicin, but the discoloration is transient and of no clinical significance.

Erythematous streaking and/or hives along the vein proximal to the site of injection may be observed. Extravasation causes severe tissue necrosis and sloughing; thus, great care in administration is needed.

Doxorubicin and related compounds are mutagenic, carcinogenic, and teratogenic in animals.

Dosage reductions are necessary in patients with impaired hepatic function.

PHARMACOKINETICS. Doxorubicin is poorly absorbed orally and is administered intravenously. Injection is followed by an initial rapid plasma clearance and significant tissue binding. The plasma decay curve of unaltered doxorubicin is triphasic with half-lives of 12 minutes, 3.3 hours, and 30 hours. Hepatic metabolism is rapid and several metabolites exist in plasma; the major metabolite is doxorubinol. Slow release from tissue binding sites prolongs the duration of drug and metabolites in plasma. After seven days, 40% to 50% of a dose is eliminated in bile, 50% as unchanged drug and 23% as active metabolite (adriamycinol). Only 5% to 10% is excreted in the urine.

DOSAGE AND PREPARATIONS.

Intravenous: 60 to 75 mg/M^2 given as a single dose every three weeks; alternatively, 20 mg/M^2 repeated every week. The drug is administered slowly by direct intravenous administration into the side arm of a freely running intravenous line. If daunorubicin has been given previously, the total cumulative dose of the two drugs should not exceed 500 mg/M^2.

Adriamycin (Adria). Powder (cryodesiccated) 10, 20, and 50 mg with 50, 100, and 250 mg of lactose, respectively.

MITOMYCIN
[Mutamycin]

ACTIONS. Mitomycin is isolated from *Streptomyces caespitosus*. After activation by intracellular reductases, the drug functions as a bifunctional alkylating agent. Cytotoxicity is probably due to the inhibition of DNA synthesis that results from cross linking of DNA. At high concentrations, RNA and protein synthesis also are inhibited. Mitomycin also can participate in free radical reactions. It is cell cycle nonspecific but appears to be most active in the late G_1 and early S phases.

USES. Mitomycin is used in the palliative treatment of various solid tumors. It is part of the FAM regimen used in gastric carcinoma (see Table 2). Other indications are non-small cell lung, cervical, colorectal, breast, bladder, pancreatic, and esophageal carcinomas.

ADVERSE REACTIONS AND PRECAUTIONS. The most significant toxic effect is dose-limiting myelosuppression, which is delayed and unpredictable. After a single dose of 20 mg/M^2, the average time to nadir is three and one-half weeks for leukopenia and four weeks for thrombocytopenia. Leukopenia persists for one to two weeks and thrombocytopenia for two to three weeks. The blood count recovers in about 75% of patients within eight weeks but does not return to within normal limits in the remaining 25%. There also is a cumulative effect and more profound and more prolonged myelosuppression is noted in subsequent courses.

Other adverse reactions include nausea, vomiting, anorexia, and stomatitis. Alopecia and skin rashes are seen frequently.

Renal toxicity, in the form of glomerular sclerosis, has been observed after several months of therapy. It does not appear to be dose related, and is manifested by increased levels of BUN and serum creatinine and often severe hypertension. Abnormal liver function tests also have been reported. Severe pulmonary toxicity may occur. Other rare manifestations of toxicity include fever, drowsiness, and diarrhea.

Cardiomyopathy has been reported in patients receiving doxorubicin and mitomycin. The toxicity is thought to result from a synergistic effect of these agents mediated through free radicals.

With multiple courses of mitomycin, a thrombotic microangiopathy resembling the hemolytic uremic syndrome has been seen.

Extravasation causes severe cellulitis and ulceration.

Mitomycin is teratogenic and carcinogenic in animals.

PHARMACOKINETICS. Mitomycin is not absorbed orally. It is cleared rapidly from plasma after intravenous administration (half-life, 10 to 17 minutes and a β half-life of 50 to 60 minutes). The agent is widely distributed throughout body tissues, except the central nervous system, and is metabolized rapidly, primarily in the liver. Only 10% is excreted unchanged in the urine. Urinary excretion increases with increasing dose, however, due to saturation of metabolic pathways.

DOSAGE AND PREPARATIONS.

Intravenous: 10 to 20 mg/M^2 every six to eight weeks administered through a running intravenous line.

Because of cumulative myelosuppression, patients must be re-evaluated after each course. Subsequent doses are adjusted on the basis of the nadir of myelosuppression from the previous dose and should not be administered until the leukocyte count has returned to 3,000 and the platelet count to

75,000. Doses greater than 20 mg/M^2 are more toxic but not more effective. The dose must be reduced appropriately when this drug is used with other myelosuppressive agents.

Mutamycin (Bristol-Myers). Powder 5 and 20 mg.

PLICAMYCIN (Mithramycin)
[Mithracin]

ACTIONS. This chromomycin antibiotic is produced by *Streptomyces plicatus*. It binds tightly to, but does not intercalate, DNA to inhibit nucleic acid synthesis. RNA synthesis is more severely affected than DNA synthesis. It is cell cycle nonspecific with some S phase specificity. Plicamycin also affects calcium metabolism, probably by suppressing osteoclastic bone resorption.

USES. The only indication for plicamycin is embryonal cell carcinoma of the testes. Since it exhibits considerable toxicity and other effective drugs (eg, cisplatin, bleomycin, vinblastine) are available, plicamycin is now a secondary drug for testicular cancer. Lower doses of plicamycin have been effective in severe hypercalcemia unresponsive to conventional therapy (see Chapter 49, Agents Affecting Calcium Metabolism).

ADVERSE REACTIONS AND PRECAUTIONS. The most important toxic effect associated with plicamycin is a dose-related bleeding syndrome that usually begins with an episode of epistaxis. Severe coagulation defects resulting in hemorrhagic diathesis and even death due to uncontrolled gastrointestinal hemorrhage have been reported. This syndrome is manifested by thrombocytopenia, prolonged prothrombin time, and depressed clotting factors II, V, VII, and X. The drug should be administered only to hospitalized patients and those who can be observed carefully with frequent monitoring of platelet count and prothrombin time during and after therapy. Leukopenia occurs less frequently.

Most patients experience anorexia, nausea, and vomiting, which may begin one to two hours after initiation of therapy and persist for 12 to 24 hours. The prior use of antiemetics may be helpful. Diarrhea and stomatitis occur occasionally. Other adverse effects are fever, facial edema, hyperpigmentation, acneiform rashes, drowsiness, lethargy, malaise, headache, and depression.

Abnormal results of liver and renal function tests have been observed and the serum calcium level is often decreased. Before each dose, the lactic dehydrogenase and blood urea nitrogen levels, prothrombin time, and platelet count must be monitored. Plicamycin is contraindicated in patients with coagulation disorders or thrombocytopenia. It should be used with

extreme caution in those with impaired liver and kidney function.

PHARMACOKINETICS. Plicamycin has minimal activity after oral administration and is usually given by intravenous infusion. It is excreted rapidly in the urine, 25% within 2 hours and 40% after 15 hours. Cerebrospinal fluid levels are comparable to those in the blood at four to six hours.

DOSAGE AND PREPARATIONS.

Intravenous: 1.75 mg/M^2 every two days for up to eight doses. This schedule is less toxic than daily administration. The dose is diluted in 1,000 ml of 5% dextrose in water or normal saline and infused over four to six hours. Extravasation can cause local irritation and cellulitis.

For the dosage used in hypercalcemia, see Chapter 49.

Mithracin (Miles). Powder (cryodesiccated) 2.5 mg with mannitol 100 mg and sufficient disodium phosphate to adjust to pH 7.

VINCA ALKALOIDS

Vinca alkaloids are derived from the periwinkle plant (*Vinca rosea*) and are mitotic inhibitors. They act by complexing with tubulin, the protein component of microtubules, and the mitotic spindle, thus interfering with the assembly of microtubules and interrupting cell division in metaphase. They are M phase specific. Since microtubules are also involved in other cellular processes (eg, axonal transport, secretory functions), the vinca alkaloids may affect these functions as well. For example, they inhibit the secretion of some hormones (eg, glucose-induced insulin release, TSH-mediated thyroid hormone secretions) and proteins.

Although vincristine and vinblastine have similar chemical structures and mechanisms of action, there are important differences in antitumor activity and dose-limiting toxicities. Also, patients who become resistant to one often respond to the other, which probably reflects differences in dosages rather than a true lack of cross-resistance.

Because the gastrointestinal absorption of vincristine and vinblastine is unpredictable, these drugs are given intravenously. They are highly irritating to tissue, however, and special precautions must be taken to avoid extravasation. Although the pharmacokinetics of the vinca alkaloids has not been delineated clearly, both drugs show triphasic elimination, primarily by biliary excretion and metabolism. Very little (3% to 8%) of either drug is recovered in the urine. The presently available pharmacologic data fail to explain the important clinical differences between vincristine and vinblastine. However, it has been suggested that the greater neurotoxicity of vincristine may be due, in part, to its longer elimination half-life, which prolongs contact with nerve tissue containing high concentrations of tubulin (Nelson, 1982).

Resistance to the vinca alkaloids may result from mutations in the tubulin protein, which affects drug binding, and decreased uptake and increased capacity for drug efflux. This latter phenomenon may account for concomitant resistance to anthracyclines and actinomycin D (ie, pleiotropic drug resistance).

A related compound, vindesine, is discussed in the section on Investigational Agents.

VINBLASTINE SULFATE
[Velban]

ACTIONS. Vinblastine is the sulfate salt of a dimeric alkaloid derived from the periwinkle plant, *Vinca rosea*. It binds to tubulin and prevents the assembly of the microtubular components of the mitotic spindle, leading to metaphase arrest.

USES. Vinblastine, in combination with cisplatin and bleomycin, is an agent of choice in disseminated nonseminomatous testicular cancer. Most patients treated with this regimen achieve long-term disease-free survival. This drug is a component of the ABVD regimen, an effective alternative to MOPP, in the treatment of advanced Hodgkin's disease (see Table 2). Vinblastine is active in non-Hodgkin's lymphomas, choriocarcinoma, breast carcinoma, neuroblastoma, head and neck cancer, mycosis fungoides, Kaposi's sarcoma, and histiocytosis X (Letterer-Siwe disease).

ADVERSE REACTIONS AND PRECAUTIONS. Dose-limiting leukopenia is the most common toxic effect of vinblastine, with the nadir occurring within five to ten days; recovery is observed within 7 to 14 days. With larger doses, the white blood cell count may not return to normal levels for three weeks. Thrombocytopenia and anemia are uncommon.

Neurotoxic effects have been reported in 5% to 20% of patients and include paresthesias, loss of deep tendon reflexes, peripheral neuritis, mental depression, headache, and convulsions.

Nausea and vomiting are common but usually can be controlled by antiemetic agents. Other gastrointestinal effects are stomatitis, glossitis, constipation, and adynamic ileus. Raynaud's phenomenon has recently been reported with use of vinblastine and/or bleomycin in testicular cancer.

Alopecia is reversible. Extravasation can cause phlebitis and severe cellulitis. Local injection of hyaluronidase and application of moderate heat help to disperse the drug, minimize discomfort, and avoid cellulitis.

Caution is necessary when vinblastine is used during pregnancy, and animal studies suggest that teratogenic effects may occur.

PHARMACOKINETICS. Vinblastine is poorly absorbed when given orally. After intravenous administration, there is a triphasic plasma clearance (first half-life, 0.06 hours; second half-life, 1.6 hours; third half-life, 25 hours). Approximately 80% of the drug is bound to plasma proteins. Vinblastine is excreted primarily in bile; 30% is excreted in stool as metabolites over the first three days, and 21% is excreted in the urine.

DOSAGE AND PREPARATIONS. Vinblastine should be given no more frequently than once every seven days. Dosage is based on body surface area and weekly white blood cell counts and should be decreased in the presence of liver disease.

Intravenous: 4 to 8 mg/M^2 weekly. In combination with cisplatin and bleomycin for testicular cancer, 0.2 mg/kg every three weeks for four courses.

Velban (Lilly). Powder (lyophilized, sterile) 10 mg.

VINCRISTINE SULFATE
[Oncovin]

ACTIONS. Vincristine is the sulfate salt of a dimeric alkaloid derived from the periwinkle plant, *Vinca rosea*. It is M phase specific and blocks mitosis with metaphase arrest by binding to tubulin and inhibiting the assembly of microtubules.

USES. Vincristine is active in a number of neoplastic diseases, including leukemias, lymphomas, sarcomas, and some carcinomas. Because it lacks dose-limiting myelosuppressive activity (see below), this drug is used extensively in combination regimens (see Table 2 and the section on Combination Chemotherapy).

When vincristine is combined with prednisone, complete remissions are induced in up to 90% of children with acute lymphocytic leukemia. The further addition of asparaginase or daunorubicin prolongs disease-free remissions. Vincristine also is very effective in combination regimens used to treat malignant lymphomas, including Hodgkin's, non-Hodgkin's, and Burkitt's lymphomas. For example, the combination of mechlorethamine, vincristine, procarbazine, and prednisone (MOPP regimen) is the treatment of choice in advanced

Hodgkin's disease and a high percentage of patients are cured. Combination regimens containing vincristine also are treatments of choice in Ewing's sarcoma, neuroblastoma, embryonal rhabdomyosarcoma, Wilms' tumor, soft tissue sarcomas, and small cell lung carcinoma (see Table 2). Vincristine also is active in acute myelogenous leukemia, chronic lymphocytic leukemia, multiple myeloma, and breast and cervical carcinomas.

ADVERSE REACTIONS. In contrast to vinblastine, vincristine does not produce serious bone marrow depression, which makes it particularly useful in combination with myelosuppressive agents. Leukopenia may develop but there is no effect on red blood cells or platelets.

Neurologic toxicity, particularly peripheral neuropathy, is usually dose limiting and is caused by vincristine binding to tubulin in neurotubules. Mild sensory neuropathy is common but does not require discontinuance of drug. Loss of the Achilles tendon reflex is usually the first sign of peripheral neuropathy. More serious manifestations include paresthesias (occasionally severe), loss of deep tendon reflexes, ataxia, foot drop, slapping gait, and muscle wasting. The primary muscle groups involved are the dorsiflexors of the hands and wrists and the extensors of the feet.

In addition to peripheral nerve dysfunction, disorders of the autonomic nervous system also may occur. Constipation and abdominal pain develop frequently and usually respond to enemas and laxatives, but, if severe, they may be dose limiting. Cranial nerve deficits (ptosis, diplopia, abducens nerve palsy, and vocal cord paralysis) also have been reported.

Nausea and vomiting are rare. Alopecia is observed in more than 20% of patients. Vincristine is a local irritant, and extravasation can cause phlebitis and severe cellulitis. This drug has been shown to promote release of antidiuretic hormone, which rarely has caused hyponatremia. Liver impairment increases toxicity.

PHARMACOKINETICS. Vincristine is poorly absorbed orally. After intravenous use, the plasma elimination is triphasic with half-lives of 0.08, 2.3, and 85 hours. The drug is incompletely metabolized by the liver and elimination is primarily via the bile; approximately 70% of a dose is excreted in the feces and about 12% is eliminated in the urine. Obstruction of liver outflow may require careful adjustment of dosage. Vincristine does not penetrate the central nervous system.

DOSAGE AND PREPARATIONS.
Intravenous: Adults, 1.4 mg/M^2 once weekly (maximum dose, 2 mg/M^2). *Children older than 1 year,* 2 mg/M^2 once weekly. *Children less than 10 kg or with body surface area less than 1 M^2,* 0.05 mg/kg once weekly to avoid excessive neurotoxicity. The therapeutic effect does not appear to be dose related, and toxic reactions increase significantly without increased benefit with larger doses. The drug is administered through a running intravenous line or is injected with care to prevent extravasation. The dose should be reduced in patients with liver disease. Vincristine should not be given intrathecally since this causes fatal ascending paralysis.

Oncovin (Lilly). Solution 1 mg/ml in 1, 2, and 5 ml containers.

MISCELLANEOUS AGENTS

ASPARAGINASE
[Elspar]

ACTIONS. Asparaginase is an enzyme derived from cultures of either *Escherichia coli* or *Erwinia carotovora.* (Elspar is derived from *E. coli.*) It catalyzes the hydrolysis of the amino acid, asparagine, to aspartic acid and ammonia, thus depleting the amount of asparagine available to tumor cells. Unlike normal cells, certain leukemic cells appear to lack asparagine synthetase and cannot convert aspartic acid to asparagine. Thus, they depend upon an exogenous source of asparagine. The asparagine-depleting action interferes with the synthesis of protein and subsequently DNA and RNA in tumor cells. Asparaginase probably is cell cycle-specific for the postmitotic G$_1$ phase.

Asparaginase was originally considered to be an antitumor agent that exploited a unique biochemical difference between normal and neoplastic cells. However, it is now known that many normal tissues are sensitive to asparaginase and various toxic effects can result. In addition, it has become apparent that human leukemic cells can quickly become resistant due to the emergence of strains that either induce asparagine synthetase or produce a mutated form of the enzyme. This drug is usually used in combination regimens.

USES. Asparaginase is indicated only in acute lymphocytic leukemia, most often combined with other chemotherapeutic agents (eg, prednisone and vincristine) to induce remissions in children.

ADVERSE REACTIONS AND PRECAUTIONS. The usefulness of asparaginase is limited by toxic effects. Major toxicities can be divided into those caused by immunologic sensitization to a foreign protein and those resulting from decreased protein synthesis.

Despite its immunosuppressive properties, hypersensitivity reactions ranging from urticaria to anaphylactic shock occur in approximately 10% to 15% of patients receiving asparaginase. They can develop during the initial course but are more frequently seen when the drug is readministered. The incidence of hypersensitivity reactions is increased when the interval between doses is seven days or longer. Allergic reactions are not completely predictable on the basis of an intradermal skin test. Physicians should be aware of the potential for anaphylactic shock and appropriate supportive measures should be readily available. Intravenous epinephrine usually terminates hypersensitivity reactions. Since there is no apparent cross reactivity between the *Escherichia coli* and *Erwinia carotovora* enzymes, patients sensitized to the *E. coli* enzyme may be treated with the *Erwinia* enzyme.

Neurotoxic reactions are observed primarily in adults. Approximately 25% of patients exhibit a decreased level of consciousness ranging from confusion to coma. Seizures or focal neurologic signs are rare. Although blood ammonia levels are increased, this does not appear to correlate with central nervous system toxicity, which is currently believed to be caused by decreased levels of asparagine and glutamine or inhibition of protein synthesis in the brain.

Inhibition of protein synthesis also may cause hypoalbuminemia resulting in peripheral edema and decreased circulating insulin resulting in hyperglycemia. In addition, decreased protein synthesis causes hypofibrinogenemia and decreases other clotting factors, particularly V, VII, VIII, and IX. However, severe bleeding is uncommon. Paradoxically, thrombosis may occur due to depletion of factors required for fibrinolysis. Reduction of circulating platelets also has occurred.

Pancreatitis has been observed in less than 15% of patients but may progress to severe hemorrhagic pancreatitis. Hepatotoxicity, with abnormal results of liver function tests, occurs in 50% to 75% of patients, and fatty metamorphosis of the liver has been observed. Azotemia, usually prerenal, occurs frequently. Acute renal shutdown and fatal renal insufficiency have been reported during treatment. Fatal hyperthermia also has been observed.

Approximately two-thirds of patients receiving asparaginase experience immediate side effects including nausea, vomiting, chills, and fever.

Myelosuppression is rare and usually not severe, although marked leukopenia has been reported.

PHARMACOKINETICS. Asparaginase is administered either intravenously or intramuscularly; peak blood levels are 50% lower after intramuscular injection. Plasma concentrations are proportional to the dose. The plasma half-life ranges from 8 to 30 hours and varies among preparations and individuals but is usually stable in a single individual. In patients who develop hypersensitivity to the enzyme, the half-life is shortened. This is probably due to a binding antibody that causes more rapid plasma clearance.

Little of the drug is distributed out of the vascular compartment, because of its large molecular size and highly ionized state in the body. Eventually, levels in lymph fluid approach 25% of the plasma concentrations. Very little drug is found in bile, urine, and cerebrospinal fluid. The inactivation of asparaginase is presumed to be due to serum proteases and the immune and reticuloendothelial systems.

DOSAGE AND PREPARATIONS. When administered intravenously, asparaginase should be injected into the tubing of a running infusion of sodium chloride injection or 5% dextrose in water over a period of at least 30 minutes. Because allergic reactions may occur, an intradermal skin test should be performed prior to initial administration and when the drug is readministered after a week or more has elapsed between courses. However, negative results do not preclude the possibility of an allergic reaction.

Intravenous: Children, when used following therapy with prednisone and vincristine, 1,000 IU/kg/day for 10 successive days beginning on day 22 of the treatment period. The administration of asparaginase with or immediately before a course of vincristine and prednisone may increase toxicity.

Intramuscular: Adults and children, in a combination induction regimen with prednisone and vincristine, 6,000 IU/M² on days 4, 7, 10, 13, 16, 19, 22, 25, and 28.

   Elspar (Merck Sharp & Dohme). Lyophilized plug or powder containing 10,000 IU with 80 mg of mannitol in 10 ml containers.

For reconstitution, 5 ml of sterile water for injection or sodium chloride injection is added. The solution may be used within an eight-hour period following reconstitution if it remains clear.

CISPLATIN (CPDD)
[Platinol]

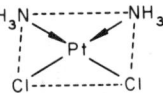

ACTIONS. Cisplatin is a heavy metal coordination complex containing a central atom of platinum surrounded by two chloride atoms and two ammonia molecules in the cis position. Its biochemical properties are similar to those of bifunctional alkylating agents; it produces interstrand and intrastrand cross links in DNA and is apparently cell cycle nonspecific.

USES. Cisplatin is indicated in the treatment of metastatic testicular and ovarian cancers and is one of the most active drugs against testicular tumors. An effective combination for patients with disseminated seminomatous and nonseminomatous testicular cancer includes cisplatin, bleomycin, and vinblastine. Long-term survival and probable cures occur in about 70% of patients. In metastatic ovarian carcinoma, the combination of cisplatin, doxorubicin, and an alkylating agent (eg, cyclophosphamide) has produced encouraging results. Patients with bladder and cervical carcinoma and head and neck cancer also have responded to this agent. Activity in osteogenic sarcoma and non-small cell lung, esophageal, and gastric carcinomas has been reported.

ADVERSE REACTIONS AND PRECAUTIONS. The most frequent and serious toxicity produced by cisplatin is impaired renal function due to a direct toxic effect on renal tubules. This is manifested by elevations in BUN, creatinine, and serum uric acid levels and/or decreased creatinine clearance. Nephrotoxicity is first noted during the second week of therapy after the initial dose and is dose related and cumulative. Renal function must return to normal before another dose of cisplatin can be given. Intravenous infusion, hydration, and diuretics have been used to reduce nephrotoxicity. Other nephrotoxic drugs (eg, aminoglycosides) should be avoided in patients receiving cisplatin.

Other major dose-related manifestations of toxicity are myelosuppression, nausea and vomiting, ototoxicity, and neurotoxicity. Myelosuppression occurs in 25% to 30% of patients treated with cisplatin and is most pronounced with larger doses (more than 50 mg/M²). The nadirs in circulating platelet and leukocyte counts occur between days 18 and 23 (range, 7.5 to 45), and most patients recover by day 39 (range, 13 to 62). Decreased hemoglobin levels of more than 2 g Hb/dl parallel the occurrence of leukopenia and thrombocytopenia.

Nausea and vomiting occur in almost all patients treated with cisplatin and are occasionally so severe that the drug must be discontinued. These reactions usually begin within one to four hours after treatment and last up to 24 hours. Nausea and anorexia may persist for up to one week after treatment. Large intravenous doses of metoclopramide [Reglan] alleviate emesis (Gralla et al, 1981).

Ototoxicity, manifested by tinnitus and/or hearing loss in the high frequency range (4,000 to 8,000 Hz), has been observed in up to 31% of patients treated with a single dose of 50 mg/M² of cisplatin. Ototoxic effects may be more severe in children. Hearing loss may be unilateral or bilateral and tends to become more severe with repeated doses. The ability to hear normal conversational tones may be decreased occasionally. Audiometry should be performed prior to and during cisplatin therapy.

Neurotoxicity, usually characterized by peripheral neuropathies, may be irreversible. Loss of taste and seizures also have been reported.

Decreased levels of serum calcium, magnesium, potassium, and sodium have been observed in patients receiving cisplatin. These effects may be related to the intravenous infusion of large volumes of fluid. In many cases, decreased levels of electrolytes may persist for several weeks and are due to inappropriate electrolyte excretion resulting from renal tubular damage.

In patients previously treated with cisplatin, anaphylactoid reactions (facial edema, wheezing, tachycardia, and hypotension) have been observed within a few minutes after readministration.

Cisplatin is mutagenic, teratogenic, and probably carcinogenic.

PHARMACOKINETICS. Cisplatin is administered intravenously. The plasma disappearance curve is biphasic with half-lives of 25 to 49 minutes and 58 to 73 hours, respectively. More than 90% of the drug present during the second phase is bound to plasma proteins. Elimination occurs primarily via the kidney. Although up to 30% is excreted in the urine during the first 24 hours, only 25% to 45% is recovered from urine after five days. Very little drug is found in feces. Significant tissue binding occurs, particularly in the liver, kidney, intestine, and testes, and the drug persists in the body for prolonged periods. Little cisplatin appears to enter the cerebrospinal fluid.

DOSAGE AND PREPARATIONS.

Intravenous: When given as a single agent, 60 to 120 mg/M² once every three to four weeks.

When combined with vinblastine and bleomycin in the treatment of testicular cancer, 20 mg/M² daily for five days (days one to five) is administered every three weeks for four courses.

Pretreatment hydration with 1 to 2 L of 5% dextrose in 0.5% normal saline infused for 8 to 12 hours is recommended. Adequate hydration and urinary output must be maintained during the following 24 hours. Mannitol with or without furosemide is often administered concomitantly to ensure adequate diuresis. The course should not be repeated until the serum creatinine level is below 1.5 mg/dl and/or the BUN level is below 25 mg/dl and circulating blood elements are at an acceptable level (platelet count more than 100,000/microliter, leukocyte count more than 4,000/microliter). Subsequent doses also should be withheld until an audiometric analysis indicates that auditory acuity is within normal limits.

Trials using large doses of cisplatin (40 mg/M² daily for five days) with hypertonic saline diuresis are in progress.

Platinol (Bristol-Myers). Powder (lyophilized) 10 and 50 mg.

ETOPOSIDE (VP-16-213)
[VePesid]

ACTIONS. Etoposide is a semisynthetic glycosidic derivative of podophyllotoxin (extract of the mandrake plant). However, it is not a spindle poison and does not produce metaphase arrest. It arrests cells in the late S or G₂ phase, but the mechanism is unclear.

USES. Etoposide exhibits considerable activity in small cell lung carcinoma (average response rate, 40%) and is being actively investigated as a component of combination regimens in this disease. It is active in advanced nonseminomatous testicular cancer and is an agent of choice in combinations used to salvage patients not cured by the standard PVB regimen (see Table 2). Etoposide is also active in choriocarcinoma, acute myelogenous leukemia, non-Hodgkin's lymphomas, and childhood solid tumors, and exhibits some activity in non-small cell lung cancer and breast cancer.

ADVERSE REACTIONS AND PRECAUTIONS. Hematologic toxicity, predominantly leukopenia, is most frequently dose limiting. White blood cell count nadirs occur between 8 and 14 days and recovery occurs by days 16 to 21. Nausea and vomiting are usually mild. Hypotension can occur following intravenous push injection and this drug should be given by infusion only. Alopecia is relatively common. Fever, chills, and palpitations have been reported. Peripheral neuropathy, which may be cumulative with that caused by other neurotoxins (eg, vinca alkaloids, cisplatin), also has been observed. This drug is classified in FDA Pregnancy Category D.

PHARMACOKINETICS. Etoposide has been given orally as a drinking ampul and about 20% to 80% of a dose is absorbed from the gastrointestinal tract. It is also given intravenously. The drug is extensively bound (94%) to plasma proteins. The plasma decay is biphasic with half-lives of 2 and 5 hours. About 45% of a dose is recovered in the urine after 72 hours, approximately two-thirds as unchanged drug. Despite the lipophilicity of etoposide, cerebrospinal fluid levels are generally below 10% of plasma concentrations in most patients. The dose of etoposide should be reduced in patients with severe hepatic dysfunction.

DOSAGE AND PREPARATIONS.

Intravenous: 50 to 100 mg/M² is infused daily for five days. Alternatively, 100 mg/M²/day is given on days one, three, and five every three to four weeks in combination with other drugs. Etoposide must not be given by rapid intravenous injection because orthostatic hypotension may occur from the pharmaceutical solvent system.

VePesid (Bristol-Myers). Solution 20 mg/ml in 2.5 and 5 ml containers.

HYDROXYUREA
[Hydrea]

$$\begin{array}{c} NH_2 \\ | \\ C=O \\ | \\ NHOH \end{array}$$

ACTIONS. Hydroxyurea blocks DNA synthesis by inhibiting ribonucleoside diphosphate reductase, an enzyme that catalyzes the conversion of ribonucleoside diphosphates to deoxyribonucleoside diphosphates. This drug is S phase specific.

USES. Hydroxyurea is most commonly employed in the palliative treatment of chronic myelogenous leukemia.

ADVERSE REACTIONS AND PRECAUTIONS. Myelosuppression (leukopenia, thrombocytopenia, anemia, megaloblastosis) is most prominent and dose limiting, but recovery is usually rapid when hydroxyurea is discontinued. Anorexia, nausea, and vomiting are uncommon and stomatitis is rare. Dermatologic reactions (maculopapular rash, pruritus, and alopecia) are mild and reversible. Less common are central nervous system disturbances (headache, dizziness, disorientation, hallucinations, convulsions). Impairment of renal function with hyperuricemia, uric acid calculi, and elevated BUN levels has been reported.

Blood, bone marrow, renal, and hepatic function should be evaluated prior to and at weekly intervals during therapy. Hydroxyurea should be discontinued if the white blood cell count falls below 2,500/microliter or the platelet count below 100,000/microliter. Administration may be resumed when blood counts return to satisfactory levels. Anemia can be corrected by blood transfusions without discontinuing hydroxyurea. Because hydroxyurea is excreted primarily by the kidneys, it must be used with caution in patients with impaired renal function. Since this drug has caused teratogenic effects in experimental animals, it should not be used in women of childbearing age.

PHARMACOKINETICS. Hydroxyurea is readily absorbed from the gastrointestinal tract after oral administration. Peak plasma levels are reached in about two hours; within 24 hours, the plasma concentration is essentially zero. The drug is eliminated primarily by the kidney and 80% of an oral dose is recovered in urine within 12 hours.

DOSAGE AND PREPARATIONS.
Oral: 1,000 mg/M² daily. Titration is often required. The dose should be decreased in patients with impaired marrow or renal function.

Hydrea (Squibb). Capsules 500 mg.

MITOTANE
[Lysodren]

ACTIONS. Chemically, mitotane (o, p'-DDD) is similar to the insecticides, DDD and DDT. In toxicology studies in dogs, mitotane produced necrosis and atrophy of the adrenal cortex, particularly the zona fasciculata and zona reticularis. Although it is selectively toxic to adrenal cortical cells, the precise mechanism of action is unknown.

USES. Mitotane is indicated in the palliative treatment of both functional and nonfunctional inoperable carcinoma of the adrenal cortex. The tumor mass is reduced significantly in 34% to 54% of patients, and the mean duration of response is about ten months.

Mitotane rapidly decreases the level of corticosteroids and their metabolites in blood and urine. This response is useful for adjusting the dose and monitoring the course of hyperadrenocorticism (Cushing's syndrome) due to adrenal tumor or hyperplasia.

ADVERSE REACTIONS AND PRECAUTIONS. Gastrointestinal disturbances (anorexia, nausea, vomiting, and diarrhea) occur in 80% of patients and are usually dose limiting. About 40% of patients experience central nervous system side effects (lethargy and somnolence, 25%; dizziness or vertigo, 15%). About 15% of patients develop dermatitis. Less frequent adverse effects are visual disturbances (eg, blurred vision, diplopia, lens opacities, retinopathy), albuminuria, hemorrhagic cystitis, flushing, hyperpyrexia, orthostatic hypotension, and hypertension. Hypersensitivity to mitotane has been reported and is a contraindication to use.

PHARMACOKINETICS. Approximately 40% of an oral dose is absorbed from the gastrointestinal tract; the remaining 60% is recovered unchanged in feces. Daily doses of 5 to 15 g produce blood concentrations of 10 to 90 mcg/ml of unchanged drug and 30 to 50 mcg/ml of a metabolite. Plasma concentrations of mitotane are measurable for six to nine weeks after discontinuation of therapy. Although the drug is found in all tissues, fat is the primary site of storage. Approximately 25% of an oral or parenteral dose can be recovered in urine as a water-soluble metabolite.

DOSAGE AND PREPARATIONS.
Oral: Initially, 8 to 10 g is given in three or four divided doses daily. The dose is increased gradually to the maximum tolerated amount. This may vary from 2 to 16 g but is usually 8 to 10 g daily. If adverse reactions occur, the dose is reduced until the maximal tolerated amount is determined. Therapy should be supervised by a physician familiar with the use of mitotane, and patients should be hospitalized until a maintenance dose is established. Treatment should be continued as long as clinical benefit is apparent. If no improvement is observed after three months of therapy with the maximal tolerated dose, the drug should be discontinued.

Lysodren (Bristol-Myers). Tablets 500 mg.

PROCARBAZINE HYDROCHLORIDE
[Matulane]

ACTIONS. The mechanism of action of this methylhydrazine derivative is uncertain, but conversion to active metabolites appears to be necessary. The inhibition of DNA, RNA, and subsequent protein synthesis occurs. The methylation and/or alkylation of nucleic acids are possible mechanisms. Aberrant transmethylation of purine bases and transfer RNA also has been observed. Auto-oxidation of procarbazine to hydrogen peroxide and hydroxy radicals produces effects resembling those of ionizing radiation, but these oxidation products do not appear to be the critical cytotoxic intermediates. Procarbazine is cell cycle nonspecific.

USES. The primary use of procarbazine is in advanced Hodgkin's disease in combination with mechlorethamine, vincristine, and prednisone (MOPP regimen). This regimen produces in a high percentage of long-term disease-free survivors (see the section on Combination Chemotherapy). Procarbazine also is effective in primary and metastatic brain tumors, small cell bronchogenic carcinoma, and non-Hodgkin's lymphomas.

ADVERSE REACTIONS AND PRECAUTIONS. Bone marrow depression and gastrointestinal disturbances are the primary toxic manifestations. Leukopenia and thrombocytopenia are usually dose limiting and may be delayed for several weeks after the start of treatment. Like other hydrazine derivatives, procarbazine also may cause hemolysis. Nausea and vomiting occur frequently and may be dose limiting, but tolerance usually develops with continued administration. Stomatitis, dysphagia, and diarrhea are less common.

Neurologic reactions (eg, lethargy, drowsiness, depression, peripheral neuropathy with paresthesia, nystagmus, ataxia) have been noted in 10% to 20% of patients. Other untoward effects include myalgia, arthralgia, orthostatic hypotension, dermatitis, pruritus, hyperpigmentation, and alopecia. The drug is immunosuppressive and a potent mutagen. It is teratogenic and carcinogenic in animals.

DRUG INTERACTIONS. The effects of central nervous system depressants (eg, barbiturates, phenothiazines, narcotics) may be enhanced. This appears to be due to a procarbazine-induced decrease in cytochrome P-450 levels, which decreases the metabolism of these drugs. Its hypnotic effect may be additive with that of other drugs. A disulfiram-like reaction may occur when alcohol is ingested concomitantly. Since procarbazine inhibits monoamine oxidase, sympathomimetics, tricyclic antidepressants, and beverages or foods with a high tyramine content (eg, bananas, ripe cheese, red wine, yogurt) should be avoided.

PHARMACOKINETICS. Procarbazine is rapidly and completely absorbed following oral administration. The drug initially concentrates in the liver and kidney and readily crosses the blood-brain barrier. The plasma half-life of parent drug is approximately 10 minutes. It is rapidly converted, primarily in liver microsomes and also in erythrocytes, to azo procarbazine, which is metabolized further to active and inactive metabolites. Approximately 45% to 70% of a dose is excreted in the urine during the first 24 hours as metabolites, particularly the inactive N-isopropylterephthalamic acid derivative. About 30% of the N-methyl group appears in respiratory CO_2.

DOSAGE AND PREPARATIONS.

Oral: Initially, 100 mg/M² is given daily; the dose is increased over a one-week period to 150 to 200 mg/M². This amount is maintained for three weeks and then reduced to 100 mg/M² daily until toxicity develops. The dose should be decreased in patients with hepatic, renal, or bone marrow dysfunction.

As a component of the MOPP regimen, 100 mg/M² is given daily for 14 days every four weeks.

Matulane (Roche). Capsules equivalent to 50 mg of the base.

SODIUM PHOSPHATE P 32

USES. Sodium phosphate P 32 is a β-emitting radioactive isotope used principally to treat the proliferative phase of polycythemia vera. When administered orally or intravenously, it is taken up by tissues with high phosphate turnover, including neoplastic and bone marrow cells. It inhibits proliferation of bone marrow cells and thus reduces the erythrocyte count, packed red blood cell volume, and hypervolemia associated with this myeloproliferative disorder. Following an appropriate dose, a latent period of one to three months is succeeded by a smooth progression into complete hematologic remission lasting six months to several years. A second dose of sodium phosphate P 32 may be required within the initial six months for satisfactory remission, and phlebotomies often are performed to maintain the hematocrit at normal levels during the induction period.

This isotope also may be useful for palliative treatment in the early phase of chronic myelogenous leukemia.

ADVERSE REACTIONS AND PRECAUTIONS. Although usual doses rarely cause radiation sickness, dosage should be individualized to ensure minimal radiation exposure to the patient and laboratory personnel. Excessive amounts can cause leukopenia, thrombocytopenia, and anemia. Periodic blood cell counts should be performed. This agent is contraindicated when the leukocyte count is less than 5,000/microliter or the platelet count less than 150,000/microliter. There is evidence that sodium phosphate P 32 is leukemogenic in patients with polycythemia vera, but the incidence appears to be lower than with chlorambucil. Presently, the benefits of sodium phosphate P 32 appear to outweigh the risks of acute leukemia, particularly in patients over age 40, but further studies are required.

This agent is classifed in FDA Pregnancy Category C.

Treatment with sodium phosphate P 32 is restricted to physicians licensed by the Nuclear Regulatory Commission.

DOSAGE AND PREPARATIONS.

Oral: For polycythemia vera, initially, 6 millicuries.

Intravenous: For polycythemia vera, 2.3 millicuries/M², depending upon the initial erythrocyte, leukocyte, and platelet counts and the patient's body surface area. Phlebotomy may be performed adjunctively.

Generic (Mallinckrodt). Solution 0.67 millicuries/ml in 10 ml containers (5 millicuries radioactivity/container).

HORMONES AND ANTAGONISTS

Hormone-sensitive tumors may be hormone-dependent, hormone-responsive, or both. A hormone-dependent tumor regresses on removal of the hormonal stimulus. This has been accomplished by ablative surgery, as in oophorectomy for the initial treatment of premenopausal women with estrogen receptor-positive, advanced breast cancer. Orchiectomy is often the treatment of choice for men with advanced prostate cancer. Preventing hormonal stimulation of hormone-dependent tumors with drugs has been accomplished only in breast cancer. Tamoxifen, an antiestrogen, and aminoglutethimide, an inhibitor of adrenal corticosteroid synthesis, prevent estrogen stimulation of breast cancer cells. Presently, tamoxifen is a treatment of choice in pre- and postmenopausal women with estrogen receptor-positive, advanced breast cancer.

Hormone-responsive tumors regress when pharmacologic amounts of hormones are administered regardless of whether previous signs of hormone sensitivity were observed. The major hormone-responsive cancers include carcinomas of the breast, prostate, and endometrium; lymphomas; and certain leukemias. Hormonal substances that inhibit the growth of certain human tumors are steroids and include estrogens, progestins, androgens, and adrenal corticosteroids. Each of these classes of steroids has been used in advanced breast carcinoma. Estrogens are drugs of choice in advanced prostatic carcinoma. Progestins are drugs of choice in advanced endometrial carcinoma and have shown activity in ovarian cancer. The effects of the various steroids are palliative except for the cytotoxic effect of glucocorticoids (eg, prednisone) on lymphoid cells. Glucocorticoids are routinely employed in combination chemotherapy regimens to treat lymphomas and certain leukemias, often with curative intent. Examples include the MOPP regimen for Hodgkin's disease, the CHOP and BACOP regimens for histiocytic lymphomas, and remission induction regimens for acute lymphocytic leukemia (see Table 2).

The precise mechanisms of action of the steroid hormones are not completely understood. In some cancers (eg, breast, lymphoid, probably endometrial), the effectiveness of therapy depends upon the presence of specific steroid receptor proteins in the cytoplasm of tumor cells and, in some cases (eg, glucocorticoid action on lymphoblasts), binding of the hormone to the receptor appears to be required. The absence or loss of specific hormone receptor proteins can be correlated with a lack of antineoplastic effects. For example, estrogen receptor-negative breast tumors usually do not respond to hormonal therapy (see the section on Antineoplastic Drug Selection). See Section VI, Endocrine and Metabolic Agents, for a comprehensive discussion of steroid hormones.

ADRENAL CORTICOSTEROIDS

ACTIONS. The precise mode of action of the adrenal corticosteroids (glucocorticoids) is unknown, but they must bind to specific membrane at cytoplasmic receptor proteins in tumor cells to exert their antitumor effect. Many cells are targets for the adrenal corticosteroids and physiologic effects vary widely. In lymphoid tissues, glucocorticoids induce cell death. They interfere with lymphoid proliferation and cause dissolution of lymphocytes and regression of lymphatic tissue. It has been suggested that the effects result from a decrease in utilization of energy due to glucose deprivation.

USES. Because of their cytotoxic effect on lymphoid tissues, the major indications for adrenal corticosteroids are acute and chronic lymphocytic leukemia, Hodgkin's disease, and non-Hodgkin's lymphomas. They are also used in multiple myeloma and breast carcinoma. Adrenal corticosteroids are not myelosuppressive and usually are given in combination with other chemotherapeutic agents (see Table 2).

Adrenal corticosteroids also are given to treat certain complications of cancer, particularly hypercalcemia in steroid-responsive tumors and brain edema associated with intracranial metastases. They also are used in conjunction with radiation therapy to reduce edema in critical areas (eg, superior mediastinum, brain, spinal cord). The corticosteroids may produce temporary symptomatic improvement in critically ill patients by suppressing fever, sweating, and pain and by restoring appetite, lost weight, strength, and a sense of well-being.

ADVERSE REACTIONS AND PRECAUTIONS. Long-term therapy can cause cushingoid features with accumulation of fat on the trunk and face. Metabolic effects include sodium retention, which may result in edema, heart failure, and hypertension; potassium loss, which may produce muscle weakness; and decreased glucose tolerance, which may result in glycosuria and overt diabetes mellitus. Loss of skin collagen can result in paper thin skin and cutaneous striae. Proximal myopathy, osteoporosis, and vertebral compression fractures can develop. Peptic ulcerations may occur. Pituitary-adrenal suppression and retardation or interruption of growth have been observed in children. Euphoria is common and some patients may develop psychoses.

Caution should be exercised in patients receiving long-term steroid therapy, since they are more susceptible to severe infections, and sudden withdrawal of medication or development of stress may result in acute adrenocortical insufficiency. To minimize the complications of corticosteroid therapy, an attempt should be made to reduce the dosage.

For a more detailed discussion on adrenal corticosteroids, see Chapter 61, Adrenal Corticosteroids in Nonendocrine Diseases.

DOSAGE AND PREPARATIONS.
PREDNISONE:
Oral: 10 to 100 mg daily.

In combination with vincristine (with or without daunorubicin or asparaginase) for induction of remission in acute lymphocytic leukemia, 40 mg/M^2 daily in divided doses for four to six weeks.

As a component of the MOPP regimen in advanced Hodgkin's disease, 40 mg/M^2 daily on days 1 through 14 (cycles one and four only).

As a component of the CVP regimen in non-Hodgkin's lymphomas (indolent-behaving histologies), 100 mg/M^2 daily on days one through five every four weeks.

As a component of the CHOP regimen in non-Hodgkin's lymphoma (aggressive histologies), 100 mg/M^2 daily on days one through five every three weeks.

As part of the BACOP regimen in non-Hodgkin's lymphoma

(aggressive histologies), 60 mg/M² daily on days 15 through 28 every four weeks.

DEXAMETHASONE, DEXAMETHASONE SODIUM PHOSPHATE: *Oral, Intramuscular, Intravenous:* To reduce cerebral edema, 4 to 16 mg daily in divided doses.

For preparations, see Chapter 61.

ESTROGENS

USES. Estrogens are used in the palliative management of estrogen receptor-positive metastatic breast carcinoma in postmenopausal women, although the antiestrogen, tamoxifen, is now the primary therapy for these patients. Estrogens also are used in the palliative treatment of advanced carcinoma of the prostate.

In breast carcinoma, estrogen induces objective tumor responses in 50% to 60% of patients with estrogen receptor-positive tumors. Positive responses are confined primarily to metastatic disease in soft tissues and bone and last about 12 to 14 months. Tumor regression may not be apparent for several weeks, and therapy must be continued for 8 to 12 weeks before effectiveness can be evaluated. If the response is favorable, therapy should be continued until there is evidence of disease progression. Occasionally, the tumor may again regress when estrogen is withdrawn.

Disseminated prostatic carcinoma can be palliated by orchiectomy or estrogen therapy in about 75% of cases. Successful treatment is manifested almost immediately by reduced bone pain and decreased acid phosphatase levels.

ADVERSE REACTIONS AND PRECAUTIONS. When estrogens are used to treat breast carcinoma, adverse effects include edema, nausea, anorexia, altered libido, breast tenderness, abdominal cramps, dizziness, irritability, and urinary frequency. Fluid retention may be severe, especially in patients with cardiovascular disease. Pigmentation of nipples and areola occurs in almost all patients.

Occasionally, bone pain and the neoplastic process are exacerbated. Hypercalcemia is a potentially fatal complication. Estrogens should be discontinued and appropriate treatment for hypercalcemia must be instituted. However, hypercalcemia may indicate the likelihood of a favorable antitumor response later and, unless the tumor is progressing rapidly by objective measures, treatment should be resumed after the hypercalcemia resolves.

Since the liver inactivates estrogens, toxic effects tend to be more severe in the presence of hepatic damage. Rarely, cholestatic jaundice may occur.

Urinary incontinence when coughing or straining is a frequent complaint of older women. Postmenopausal patients should be warned that uterine bleeding often occurs with prolonged high-dose estrogen therapy or upon withdrawal of estrogen. Vaginal carcinoma has been reported rarely in the offspring of women who used diethylstilbestrol during pregnancy.

When estrogens are used for prostatic carcinoma, gynecomastia and impotence are expected adverse effects. Fluid retention may be hazardous and should be treated appropriately. The risk of cardiovascular complications increases with larger doses. Diethylstilbestrol diphosphate can cause pruritus and burning pain in the anogenital region or at metastatic sites during or after administration. These effects may be ameliorated by slowing the rate of intravenous infusion and administering antihistamines or sedatives simultaneously. Hypophosphatemia secondary to renal excretion may occur.

DOSAGE AND PREPARATIONS.

CHLOROTRIANISENE:
Oral: For prostatic carcinoma, 12 to 25 mg daily.

CONJUGATED ESTROGENS:
Oral: For breast carcinoma, 10 mg three times daily; for prostatic carcinoma, 3.75 to 7.5 mg daily.

DIETHYLSTILBESTROL (DES):
Oral: For breast carcinoma, 5 mg three times daily (range, 5 to 15 mg daily); for prostatic carcinoma, 1 to 3 mg daily.

DIETHYLSTILBESTROL DIPHOSPHATE:
Intravenous: For prostatic carcinoma, 500 mg dissolved in 300 ml of saline or 5% dextrose on the first day; 1 g in 300 ml of saline or dextrose is then given daily for five days or more, depending upon the response of the patient. The infusion should be administered slowly (20 to 30 drops/min) during the first 10 to 15 minutes and then the rate of flow adjusted so that the entire amount is given within one hour. Following the first intensive course of therapy, 250 to 500 mg may be administered in a similar manner once or twice weekly, or oral maintenance therapy may be instituted.
Oral: For prostatic carcinoma, 50 mg three times daily, increased to 200 mg or more if necessary.

ESTERIFIED ESTROGENS:
Oral: For breast carcinoma, 10 mg three times daily; for prostatic carcinoma, 1.25 mg or more three times daily.

ETHINYL ESTRADIOL:
Oral: For breast carcinoma, 0.5 to 1 mg three times daily; for prostatic carcinoma, 0.15 to 0.3 mg daily.

POLYESTRADIOL PHOSPHATE:
Intramuscular (deep): For prostatic carcinoma, initially, 40 mg every two to four weeks or less frequently. If the response is not satisfactory, up to 80 mg may be given.

See Chapter 39 for preparations.

ANDROGENS

USES. Androgens are used in the palliative management of estrogen receptor-positive, disseminated breast carcinoma in postmenopausal women, although the antiestrogen, tamoxifen, is now the primary therapy for these patients. Androgens induce objective responses in 50% to 60% of patients with estrogen receptor-positive tumors. Responses generally last 12 to 14 months. Soft tissue metastases are most responsive, followed by osseous lesions; metastases to viscera are least responsive. As with estrogens, several weeks may elapse before a response to androgen therapy is evident (see the preceding evaluation on Estrogens).

Testolactone is relatively inert hormonally, produces less masculinization, and induces a tumor remission rate similar to that observed with other androgens. The prototype parenteral androgen preparations, testosterone propionate and enanthate, although as effective as other androgens, are now rarely used because of their marked virilizing effect. Fluoxymesterone and dromostanolone are less virilizing than testosterone.

ADVERSE REACTIONS AND PRECAUTIONS. Adverse effects include fluid retention, hypercalcemia, masculinization (clitoral enlargement, hirsutism, deepening of the voice, increased libido, acne), alopecia, and erythrocythemia. Cholestatic jaundice has been noted with oral therapy, and hepatocellular neoplasms have rarely been associated with long-term therapy. Rarely, exacerbation of the malignant process may occur.

Androgens are contraindicated in patients with cardiorenal disease or hypercalcemia and in pregnant women or nursing mothers. If hypercalcemia develops, the androgen should be discontinued immediately and appropriate corrective measures instituted (eg, forced hydration, diuretics, adrenal corticosteroids, oral phosphate therapy, plicamycin).

DOSAGE AND PREPARATIONS.
DROMOSTANOLONE PROPIONATE:
Intramuscular: 100 mg three times weekly.
   Drolban (Lilly). Solution 50 mg/ml in 10 ml containers.
FLUOXYMESTERONE:
Oral: 15 to 30 mg daily in divided doses.
   See Chapter 38, Androgens and Anabolic Steroids, for preparations.
METHYLTESTOSTERONE:
Oral: 200 mg in divided doses.
Buccal: 100 mg daily in divided doses.
   See Chapter 38 for preparations.
TESTOLACTONE:
Oral: 250 mg four times daily.
   Teslac (Squibb). Tablets 50 mg.
TESTOSTERONE ENANTHATE, TESTOSTERONE PROPIONATE:
Intramuscular: 100 mg three times weekly.
   See Chapter 38 for preparations.

PROGESTINS

USES. Progestins are the hormones of choice for the palliative management of disseminated endometrial carcinoma. Response rates average 33%, and well differentiated tumors respond more frequently. The response depends on the presence of progesterone receptors in the tumor. Positive responders have prolonged survival (eg, about two years for responders versus six months for nonresponders) (Perez et al, 1985). Treatment is continued until the disease recurs. Progestins also have shown some activity in breast and ovarian cancer. They appear to be as effective as tamoxifen for the treatment of estrogen receptor-positive postmenopausal breast cancer. They are inactive in renal cancer despite a report to the contrary.

ADVERSE REACTIONS AND PRECAUTIONS. Adverse reactions are usually minimal; anorexia, fluid retention, and pain at the site of injection may occur. Hypercalcemia develops occasionally if there are osseous metastases.

DOSAGE AND PREPARATIONS.
HYDROXYPROGESTERONE CAPROATE:
Intramuscular: 1 g twice weekly.

See Chapter 39, Estrogens, Progestins, and Other Agents Used to Treat Gynecologic Conditions, for preparations.
MEDROXYPROGESTERONE ACETATE:
Intramuscular: Initially, 400 mg to 1 g weekly; for maintenance, 400 mg monthly.
   See Chapter 39 for preparations.
MEGESTROL ACETATE:
Oral: For breast carcinoma, 160 mg/day in four divided doses. For endometrial carcinoma, 40 to 320 mg daily in divided doses.

   See Chapter 39 for preparations.

ESTRAMUSTINE PHOSPHATE SODIUM
   [Emcyt]

ACTIONS. Estramustine phosphate is composed of nitrogen mustard, a bifunctional alkylating agent, linked chemically to estradiol. Its precise mechanism of action is unknown; the liberation of nornitrogen mustard into the blood appears to be minimal and the agent is not myelosuppressive. Some patients with prostatic cancer refractory to estrogen therapy respond to estramustine. Thus, the drug appears to act in tumor cells by more than one mechanism.

USES. Estramustine is indicated for the palliative management of patients with advanced prostatic carcinoma. A wide range of response rates have been reported; the rates are generally higher in previously untreated patients, but estramustine does not appear to be more effective than estrogen alone. Response rates in patients previously treated with hormones are usually about 25%, although some have been higher. Durations of response also are variable (3 to 36 months). Since some patients who have become refractory to estrogen therapy respond to estramustine, its major indication would appear to be in this group of patients (Carter et al, 1981).

ADVERSE REACTIONS AND PRECAUTIONS. The adverse effects associated with estramustine are primarily due to the estrogenic component. Gynecomastia is most common. Fluid retention is relatively common and the drug should be used with caution in patients with cardiovascular disease. An increased risk of vascular accidents is associated with estrogen therapy, particularly when large doses are used. Hypercalcemia, although uncommon, is serious. Minor gastrointestinal upset, nausea, and diarrhea occasionally are observed. Altered liver function tests (eg, LDH and/or SGOT) are common, and caution should be exercised when administering this drug to patients with hepatic impairment. This drug is potentially mutagenic, carcinogenic, and teratogenic.

PHARMACOKINETICS. Estramustine is well absorbed after oral administration. The drug is rapidly dephosphorylated and the predominant metabolite in blood is estromustine (17-keto analogue of estramustine) with lesser amounts of estramustine. Peak concentrations of estromustine (1 mcg/ml) are reached two to three hours following a dose of 7.5 mg/kg. Elimination from plasma appears to be multiphasic; the half-life of the terminal phase is about 20 hours. In addition to estromustine and estramustine, estrone and estradiol are biotransformation products of estramustine phosphate. Excretion via the biliary route appears most likely.

DOSAGE AND PREPARATIONS.

Oral: Doses range from 1 to 10 capsules daily in three or four divided doses. Although responses (eg, decreased bone pain) have been seen after two weeks, patients should be treated for 30 to 90 days before evaluating therapy. Treatment should be continued until evidence of disease progression is observed.

　　Emcyt (Roche). Capsules equivalent to 140 mg estramustine phosphate (sodium 12.5 mg/capsule). (Refrigerate; protect from light.)

TAMOXIFEN CITRATE
[Nolvadex]

ACTIONS. Tamoxifen is a nonsteroidal antiestrogenic agent. The antiestrogenic effects appear to be related to the drug's ability to compete with estradiol for binding to estrogen receptors (eg, in breast cancer cells). Tamoxifen forms a stable complex with the estrogen receptor that is translocated to the nucleus, but the tamoxifen-receptor complex does not stimulate RNA and protein synthesis. Furthermore, cytoplasmic estrogen receptor content is depleted in the presence of drug.

USES. Tamoxifen is currently the drug of choice for the palliative treatment of advanced breast cancer in pre- and postmenopausal women with estrogen receptor-positive tumors.

Overall response rates in postmenopausal women with advanced ER-positive breast cancer average about 60% with durations of response ranging from 4 to more than 40 months (median, 8 months). Soft tissue and osseous lesions respond better than visceral disease. Previous hormonal therapy with or without previous cytotoxic treatment does not preclude a response to tamoxifen. Also, some patients who responded to antiestrogen treatment and then relapsed have benefited from further hormonal therapy. Currently, studies are being performed to assess the value of tamoxifen in various combination regimens for adjuvant chemotherapy and as the sole adjuvant agent in postmenopausal women.

ADVERSE REACTIONS AND PRECAUTIONS. Adverse effects of tamoxifen occur less frequently and are significantly milder than with androgens or estrogens. No life-threatening adverse reactions were reported in more than 1,000 patients, and less than 3% could not tolerate tamoxifen. Those who temporarily withdrew from therapy or required dosage reduction because of side effects were able to tolerate reduced dosage or resume therapy.

The most common reactions were nausea or vomiting and hot flashes, which occurred in 10% to 20% of patients. The platelet count decreased temporarily but hemorrhage did not result; leukopenia was transient, even with continued therapy. Increased tumor and bone pain occurred. Vaginal bleeding or discharge, menstrual irregularities, and skin rash were reported less frequently. Other uncommon untoward effects were hypercalcemia (osseous lesions), peripheral edema, anorexia, pruritus vulvae, depression, dizziness, lightheadedness, and headache. Abnormal results of liver function tests have been reported rarely. Tamoxifen is carcinogenic and interferes with reproductive function in animals. There is no evidence that tamoxifen is carcinogenic in man.

Four cases of retinal and corneal damage occurred following use of very large doses in phase I studies (120 to 160 mg twice daily for more than 17 months). This is equivalent to 20 to 30 years of therapy at recommended dosage levels.

PHARMACOKINETICS. Data on the pharmacokinetics of tamoxifen have been established, in part, by radioisotope studies in women. Peak plasma levels occur at four to seven hours and only 20% to 30% is present as parent drug. There is an initial half-life of 7 to 14 hours with secondary peaks at four or more days. Radioactivity is excreted slowly in the feces and only a small amount is detectable in the urine. Most of a single dose is eliminated in conjugated form; less than 30% is excreted in hydroxylated or unchanged form. Tamoxifen apparently undergoes enterohepatic circulation.

DOSAGE AND PREPARATIONS.

Oral: 10 to 20 mg twice daily. If there is no response in one month, the dosage should be increased to 20 mg twice daily.

　　Nolvadex (Stuart). Tablets equivalent to 10 mg of the base. (Protect from heat and light.)

AMINOGLUTETHIMIDE
[Cytadren]

Aminoglutethimide is currently under investigation for the treatment of breast cancer.

ACTIONS. Aminoglutethimide inhibits the enzymatic conversion of cholesterol to delta[5]-pregnenolone, the first step in adrenal corticosteroid biosynthesis, thereby reducing the synthesis of glucocorticoids, mineralocorticoids, and other steroids. In addition, it inhibits the aromatase enzyme that converts androstenedione to estrone and estradiol in extradrenal tissues. Because the adrenal gland is the principal source of estrogens in postmenopausal and oophorectomized women, this dual inhibitory action lowers plasma estrogen levels to the same extent as surgical adrenalectomy.

USES. Aminoglutethimide plus replacement hydrocortisone (to prevent reflex ACTH hypersecretion from overcoming adrenal inhibition) has been shown to be as effective as surgical adrenalectomy in the treatment of postmenopausal women with estrogen receptor-positive advanced breast carcinoma (Santen et al, 1981). Thus, "medical adrenalectomy" appears to be a preferred alternative to surgery and its associated high morbidity and occasional mortality. Overall response rates are approximately 50% in women with ER-positive tumors. Durations of response average 30 months in complete responders and 14 months in partial responders. Responses occur primarily in soft tissue (47%) and bone (35%) metastases (Santen et al, 1982).

In a randomized crossover trial comparing tamoxifen to aminoglutethimide plus hydrocortisone, response rates and durations were approximately the same. Because of its lower potential for toxicity and greater experience with its use, tamoxifen should be considered the drug of choice in postmenopausal women with ER-positive advanced breast cancer, but aminoglutethimide plus hydrocortisone is an alternative choice for patients who fail or relapse with tamoxifen.

Aminoglutethimide is also useful in suppressing adrenal function in some patients with Cushing's syndrome (see Chapter 37, Agents Used to Treat Adrenal Dysfunction).

ADVERSE REACTIONS AND PRECAUTIONS. Aminoglutethimide causes acute soporific side effects; 40% of patients experience lethargy and 10% have ataxia. Tolerance usually develops to these adverse effects after four to six weeks, presumably due to induction of drug metabolizing enzymes. Morbilliform skin rash and nausea and anorexia are also common side effects, but they usually disappear after one to two weeks of therapy. Orthostatic hypotension characterized by dizziness and weakness occurs in about 10% of patients and mineralocorticoid supplements may be required. Headache, tachycardia, myalgia, fever, vomiting, and pruritus have been reported. Masculinization and hirsutism can occur in women and precocious sexual development in boys. Goiters with mild hypothyroidism have been observed with long-term use because the drug blocks iodination of tyrosine. Hematologic abnormalities (eg, leukopenia, thrombocytopenia, pancytopenia, agranulocytosis) have been reported. Elevations in liver enzymes (eg, SGOT, alkaline phosphatase) occur. The drug is a teratogen in animals and is classified in FDA Pregnancy Category D. Since aminoglutethimide accelerates the metabolism of dexamethasone, it should not be used in glucocorticoid replacement therapy.

PHARMACOKINETICS. Aminoglutethimide is absorbed by the gastrointestinal tract after oral administration. Between 20% and 25% is bound to plasma proteins. Prior to previous drug exposure, the plasma half-life is 13 hours; after one to two weeks of drug administration, the half-life decreases to seven hours. This is presumed to be due to induction of drug metabolizing enzymes, although the mechanisms are unclear. Four metabolites have been identified, of which aceto-aminoglutethimide is most prominent. After oral administration, 50% of a dose is excreted in the urine unchanged and 20% to 50% is excreted as aceto-aminoglutethimide.

DOSAGE AND PREPARATIONS.

Oral: For breast carcinoma, 250 mg twice daily for two weeks, increased to 250 mg four times daily thereafter. This schedule reduces soporific symptoms and allows induction of an increased rate of drug metabolism. Hydrocortisone is given concomitantly in large doses (60 mg at bedtime, 20 mg in the morning and at 5 PM for a total of 100 mg daily) for the initial two weeks to reduce the severity of skin rash; thereafter, the dose is reduced to 40 mg daily (20 mg at bedtime, 10 mg in the morning, and 10 mg at 5 PM).

For the dosage schedule in Cushing's syndrome, see Chapter 37.

Cytadren (CIBA). Tablets 250 mg.

LEUPROLIDE
[Lupron]

H — 5 — OxoPro — His — Trp — Ser — Tyr — D — Leu — Leu — Arg — Pro — NHEt   ·   CH$_3$COOH

The growth and function of prostate cells and of prostatic tumor cells are stimulated by dihydrotestosterone, which is formed within the prostate gland by the conversion of testosterone. Reducing the amount of testosterone available for conversion is an effective means of treating prostate cancer. This can be achieved by orchiectomy or the administration of exogenous estrogens, such as diethylstilbestrol (DES). Although orchiectomy has been advocated as first-line treatment for prostatic cancer, the psychological effects can be damaging. Treatment with DES has been associated with major thromboembolic morbidity and mortality. Thus, in selected patients, leuprolide offers an important alternative to estrogens and orchiectomy in the initial management of prostatic cancer.

ACTIONS. Leuprolide acetate, a nonapeptide, is a synthetic analogue of luteinizing hormone-releasing hormone (LH-RH), a decapeptide; and has greater potency than the natural hormone. Like other potent agonists, a D-amino acid is substituted in the sixth position and the N-terminus is modified by substitution of an ethylanide moiety for glycine. Agonist analogue peptides with differing amino acid sequences have been found to have paradoxical effects on the pituitary, which results in initial stimulation, but subsequent inhibition of the release of follicle-stimulating hormone (FSH) and luteinizing hormone (LH). This decreases testicular and ovarian steroidogenesis.

The hypothalamic-pituitary-testicular (HPT) axis controls testosterone production. The hypothalamus produces LH-RH which is then transported to the pituitary gland where it stimulates the production of (LH and FSH). LH stimulates the production of testosterone in the testes.

Leuprolide acts as a potent inhibitor of gonadotropin secretion when therapeutic doses are given continuously. Initial doses increase LH and FSH, resulting in transient increases in testosterone and dihydrotestosterone in males and estrone and estradiol in premenopausal females. Prolonged administration has the paradoxical effect of down regulating LH and FSH receptors in the pituitary gland, decreasing testosterone to castration levels in males, and reducing estrogens to postmenopausal levels in premenopausal females. The decreases are observed within two to four weeks after initiation of treatment. Castrate levels of testosterone have been observed in patients treated for up to three years. The ultimate effect of leuprolide is the inhibition of testicular steroidogenesis by interference with 17-hydroxylase and 17,20-desmolase activity. When the analogue is discontinued, gonadotropins and androgens levels return to normal.

Leuprolide does not affect adrenal androgen production or alter serum prolactin or cortisol levels.

USES. Leuprolide is indicated for the palliative treatment of advanced prostatic cancer when orchiectomy or estrogen is not indicated or is unacceptable to the patient.

DES and leuprolide were compared in a randomized controlled trial involving 199 previously untreated patients with prostatic cancer. Both drugs suppressed testosterone and dihydroxytestosterone and decreased acid phosphatase to comparable levels. An objective response was seen in 86% of those in the leuprolide group and in 85% of those in the DES group. One-year survival rates were 87% in patients receiving leuprolide and 78% in patients receiving DES (Leuprolide Study Group, 1984).

Leuprolide appears to be much less effective in patients previously treated with orchiectomy or DES. In one multicenter trial, 19 of 47 previously untreated patients (40%) had partial (18/47) or complete (1/47) response to leuprolide, whereas 0/26 patients who had undergone orchiectomy and only 1/21 patients previously treated with hormone demonstrated an objective response (Smith et al, 1985).

Investigationally, leuprolide has displayed some activity in the treatment of breast cancer (Harvey et al, 1985).

ADVERSE REACTIONS. Initial stimulation of gonadotropin release and sex steroid production may cause disease flare-up during the first weeks of therapy. Between 3% and 10% of patients complain of increased bone pain, but this usually declines with subsequent treatment. A few patients may have a transient elevation in BUN levels. Exacerbations of signs and symptoms is a concern in patients with vertebral metastases and/or urinary obstruction, for this may lead to neurologic problems or increased obstruction.

Hot flashes are common (incidence 41% to 51%) but decrease in frequency and severity over time. Gynecomastia, nausea and vomiting, edema, and thrombophlebitis are infrequent complications. Impotence and loss of libido may occur as with DES. Patients receiving DES were reported to experience more frequent gynecomastia, nausea and vomiting, edema, and thromboembolism than those receiving leuprolide; however hot flashes were reported more often in those in the leuprolide group (Leuprolide Study Group, 1984).

PRECAUTIONS. Patients with metastatic vertebral lesions and/or urinary tract obstruction should be monitored during the first few weeks of therapy. Such patients may not be able to tolerate the worsening of symptoms that may occur during this period due to the initial increase in circulating testosterone levels.

Serum levels of testosterone and acid phosphatase should be monitored. Castration levels of testosterone are usually reached in two to four weeks and acid phosphatase levels decrease to values near baseline by the fourth week.

PHARMACOKINETICS. The plasma half-life of leuprolide is about three hours. The drug is not active when given orally. The metabolism, distribution, and excretion of leuprolide in man has not been reported.

DOSAGE AND PREPARATIONS.
Subcutaneous: *Adults*, 1 mg as a single daily injection.
   Lupron (TAP Pharmaceuticals). Solution 1 mg/0.2 ml in 2.8 ml containers.

INVESTIGATIONAL DRUGS

Anthracycline Analogues

A large number of anthracycline analogues are now undergoing clinical evaluation. Structural differences account for variations in the toxicity profiles of these drugs, while significant experimental anticancer activity is maintained.

ACLARUBICIN (Aclacinomycin A; ACM-A)

Aclarubicin, isolated from *Streptomyces galidaeus*, inhibits RNA polymerase more than DNA polymerase and is thought to have a different mechanism of action from that of doxorubicin.

Aclarubicin has demonstrated activity in breast, lung, gastric, and ovarian cancer and is effective in non-Hodgkin's lymphomas.

Aclarubicin can cause myelosuppression, nausea, vomiting, liver damage, and phlebitis. It appears to be less cardiotoxic than doxorubicin. Alopecia is unusual.

DOSAGE AND PREPARATIONS.
Intravenous: 100 mg/M² every three weeks.
   Aclarubicin (Bristol-Myers).

4'-DEOXYDOXORUBICIN (DxDx)

ACTIONS. 4'-deoxydoxorubicin, a derivative of doxorubicin, differs from the parent compound only in the reduction of the 4' position on the glycosamine moiety. Its postulated mechanism of action is the same as that for other anthracycline compounds, but 4'-deoxydoxorubicin causes greater stabilization of the DNA helix against heat denaturation and is more active against DNA polymerase.

USES. 4'-deoxydoxorubicin is expected to have a spectrum of activity similar to that of doxorubicin. In animal models, 4'deoxydoxorubicin was not totally cross resistant with doxorubicin. However, it is anticipated that 4'-deoxydoxorubicin will be significantly less active against tumors previously exposed to the parent compound.

ADVERSE REACTIONS AND PRECAUTIONS. Side effects include myelosuppression, nausea and vomiting, alopecia, and superficial phlebitis with an urticarial eruption along the injected vein. In animal toxicology studies, myocardial damage was not seen, and cardiotoxicity was not observed in phase I clinical trials. However, cardiac damage that is probably attributable to 4'-deoxydoxorubicin has been described recently.

PHARMACOKINETICS. 4'-deoxydoxorubicin can be administered orally or intravenously. The plasma decay curve after intravenous use is multiphasic with half-lives of 4 to 6 minutes and 66 hours. The aglygone metabolite is detected only for the first hour and the largest degradation product is deoxyadriamycinol. Excretion is primarily through the biliary system.

DOSAGE.
Intravenous, Oral: 30 to 40 mg/M² every three weeks.

MENOGARIL (7-OMEN)

ACTIONS AND USES. Menogaril is a semisynthetic derivative of the anthracycline antibiotic, nogalamycin. Analogues of nogalamycin differ from other anthracyclines by the attachment of a sugar to the D ring rather than to the A ring. Menogaril appears to differ substantially from doxorubicin in its mechanism of action; it binds only weakly to DNA and does not inhibit RNA polymerase activity.

It is anticipated that menogaril will have a spectrum of activity similar to that of doxorubicin. However, preclinical studies suggest that menogaril is six times less potent.

ADVERSE REACTIONS AND PRECAUTIONS. Menogaril has produced leukopenia, local cutaneous reactions, diarrhea, and radiation recall. A relative platelet-sparing effect has been observed. Menogaril is cardiotoxic. Hepatic, renal, and pulmonary toxicities have occurred in animals.

PHARMACOKINETICS. Menogaril can be administered orally or intravenously. Orally, menogaril has a bioavailability of approximately 30%. As with other anthracycline derivatives, plasma clearance is multiphasic. Excretion is primarily through the biliary system; less than 10% is excreted in the urine.

DOSAGE.
Intravenous: 200 mg/M² every three to four weeks.

MITOXANTRONE HYDROCHLORIDE
(Dihydroxyanthracenedione; Novantrone)

ACTIONS AND USES. This substituted alkylaminoanthraquinone, like all aminoanthraquinones, is a potent inhibitor of DNA and RNA synthesis in vitro and binds strongly to DNA. However, not all of these derivatives have antitumor effects, and antitumor activity may be due to some mechanism other than, or in addition to, those discussed above. A number of bis (substituted aminoalkylamino) anthraquinones have been shown to be intercalating agents and mitoxantrone probably acts by intercalating base pairs of the DNA double helix.

Mitoxantrone is expected to have a spectrum of activity similar to that of doxorubicin.

ADVERSE REACTIONS AND PRECAUTIONS. The amino sugar moiety is thought to be responsible for the cardiotoxicity of the anthracyclines. Substitution of select amino- or alkylamino-substituted side chains may eliminate this side effect. In addition to its potential for cardiotoxicity, mitoxantrone can cause myelosuppression, nausea and vomiting, phlebitis, and renal and hepatic toxicity. Extravasation can cause tissue necrosis and sloughing.

PHARMACOKINETICS. Mitoxantrone is administered intravenously. The drug disappears from plasma in a biphasic pattern with an elimination half-life of 20 to 36 hours. Most of the compound is excreted in the biliary system; only 10% is excreted in the urine.

DOSAGE AND PREPARATIONS.
Intravenous: 14 mg/M² every three weeks.
    Mitoxantrone Hydrochloride (Lederle).

Cisplatin Analogues

Several analogues of cisplatin are now undergoing clinical evaluation. The new analogues have been developed with the hope that antitumor activity will equal that of cisplatin while gastrointestinal and renal toxicity will be less.

CARBOPLATIN (CBDCA)

Carboplatin is a substituted malonato complex of platinum in the II oxidation state. It is anticipated that carboplatin will have a spectrum of activity similar to that of cisplatin.

ADVERSE REACTIONS. Carboplatin is less nephrotoxic and ototoxic than cisplatin. Nausea and vomiting are usually mild. Myelosuppression is the dose-limiting toxicity; thrombocytopenia is most pronounced.

PHARMACOKINETICS. CBDCA is only 6% to 8% protein bound (cisplatin is 95% to 99% protein bound) and therefore has a more rapid elimination half-life (t1/2 β is 3 to 7.2 hours). Peak plasma levels are dose dependent.

DOSAGE AND PREPARATIONS.
Intravenous: 400 mg/M² every 28 days.
    Carboplatin (Bristol-Myers).

CHIP (Cis-dichloro-trans dihydroxy-bis-isopropylamine platinum I.L.V.)

This cisplatin analogue is a heavy metal coordination complex containing a central atom of platinum. It has a mechanism of action similar to that of the parent compound and produces inter- and intrastrand cross-links in DNA. CHIP apparently is cell cycle nonspecific.

It is anticipated that CHIP will have a spectrum of activity similar to that of cisplatin.

ADVERSE REACTIONS AND PRECAUTIONS. CHIP is less nephrotoxic and ototoxic than cisplatin. Nausea and vomiting are common and hypersensitivity reactions have been observed. Thrombocytopenia is often dose limiting.

PHARMACOKINETICS. CHIP has biphasic plasma decay with half-lives of approximately 0.4 to 2.2 hours and 58 to 103 hours. Urinary excretion of platinum has ranged from 15% to 61% of dose at 24 hour and 16.5% to 63% at 48 hours.

DOSAGE.
Intravenous: 275 mg/M² every 28 days.

Polyamine Synthesis Inhibitors

Polyamines have been implicated in cell growth and division and their inhibition may retard neoplastic growth.

DIFLUOROMETHYLORNITHINE (DFMO)

ACTIONS AND USES. Difluoromethylornithine irreversibly inhibits ornithine decarboxylase and thus inhibits polyamine biosynthesis in mammalian cells.

In vitro studies utilizing rodent tumor cell lines have demonstrated cytostatic activity. In vitro tests and studies in mice have demonstrated that this drug has activity against human small cell lung cancer lines. To date, however, difluoromethylornithine has not been effective alone in clinical trials. It appears that its antitumor effect can be potentiated by nitrosoureas and interferon.

For the investigational use of difluoromethylornithine in the treatment of pneumocystis pneumonia, see Chapter 77, Antiprotozoal Agents.

ADVERSE REACTIONS AND PRECAUTIONS. Myelosuppression is typically the dose-limiting side effect; thrombocytopenia may be pronounced. Nausea and vomiting are not significant. Anorexia and fatigue occur frequently. Diarrhea is common and often requires dose modification. Reversible ototoxicity has been observed.

PHARMACOKINETICS. Difluoromethylornithine has a plasma half-life of three to four hours after an oral dose.

DOSAGE.
Oral: 2.25 g/M² daily in divided doses every six hours.

METHYL-GLYOXALBIS-GUANYLHYDRAZONE (MGBG)

ACTIONS AND USES. MGBG selectively inhibits the synthesis of spermidine from putrescine by blocking S-adenosyl methionine decarboxylase. Spermidine reverses most of the toxic effects of MGBG.

Therapeutic responses have been observed in acute myelocytic leukemia and non-Hodgkin's lymphomas. The drug also has demonstrated activity in solid tumors.

ADVERSE REACTIONS AND PRECAUTIONS. Side effects include mucositis, cutaneous lesions, phlebitis, ulceration after extravasation, alopecia, nausea and vomiting, delayed hypoglycemia, peripheral neuropathy, vasculitis, and hypotension after rapid infusion.

PHARMACOKINETICS. There is a biphasic drug elimination. An initial rapid half-life is followed by prolonged terminal elimination. The compound is not extensively metabolized. Approximately 60% of an intravenous dose is excreted primarily as unchanged drug in the urine; less than 20% appears in the feces.

DOSAGE.
Intravenous: 500 to 700 mg/M² every week.

Miscellaneous Investigational Drugs

ALTRETAMINE (Hexamethylmelamine)

ACTIONS. The structure of this synthetic agent resembles that of triethylenemelamine, an alkylating agent. The precise mechanism of action of altretamine is unknown, however. Although it is metabolized to intermediates with alkylating activity, this drug is not consistently cross resistant with the classic alkylating agents. Altretamine inhibits the incorporation of precursors into DNA and RNA in vitro.

USES. Altretamine is active in ovarian, small cell lung, cervical, and breast carcinoma and in malignant lymphomas. When used alone, objective response rates of approximately 30% have been reported in ovarian and small cell bronchogenic carcinomas. Altretamine is a component of the Hexa-CAF regimen used in ovarian carcinoma (see Table 2) and is under investigation as a component in other combination therapy.

ADVERSE REACTIONS AND PRECAUTIONS. Nausea and vomiting are common (50% to 70% of patients) and may be severe; they usually increase with subsequent doses and require discontinuation of therapy after two to three weeks. Moderate, reversible leukopenia and thrombocytopenia have occurred occasionally; nevertheless, this drug is a good candidate for inclusion in combination regimens. With repeated courses, peripheral neuropathy has been reported; two cases were irreversible. Other adverse reactions include numbness, paresthesia, depression, confusion, drowsiness, and hallucinations.

PHARMACOKINETICS. Altretamine is absorbed following oral administration. It is metabolized rapidly in the liver. Metabolites are excreted in urine and 62% is recovered within 24 hours. The plasma half-life of parent drug ranges from 4.7 to 10.2 hours.

DOSAGE.
Oral: 240 to 320 mg/M² daily in four divided doses for 21 days.

AMINOTHIADIAZOLE (A-TDA)

Aminothiadiazole appears to act by blocking the polymerization of adenosine monophosphate and guanasine monophosphate, which leads to increased synthesis of uric acid, xanthine, and hypoxanthine. Allopurinol partially blocks uric acid formation without affecting toxicity or activity. Nicotinamide antagonizes the antitumor activity of aminothiadiazole.

Preclinical studies suggest that aminothiadiazole has some activity in rodent and human tumors.

Mucositis is the dose-limiting toxicity. Rash is common. Uric acid is elevated in most patients despite use of allopurinol, but symptoms do not occur. Hematologic toxicity is unusual.

DOSAGE.
Intravenous: 125 to 150 mg/M² weekly. Simultaneous administration of allopurinol 300 mg daily is required.

AMSACRINE (m-AMSA)
[Amsidyl]

ACTIONS. Amsacrine is a synthetic aminoacridine that exerts its cytotoxic effect by intercalating DNA and inhibiting DNA synthesis. The drug is probably cell cycle nonspecific, but cells in G₂ and S phases are more sensitive.

USES. The primary use of this drug is for induction of remission in acute leukemia in adults who have relapsed or are refractory to conventional therapy. Amsacrine has induced complete remissions in 10% to 20% of patients with acute myelogenous leukemia refractory to both cytarabine and anthracyclines. Remission durations have been short, however. Amsacrine also has modest activity in acute lymphocytic leukemia and non-Hodgkin's lymphoma.

ADVERSE REACTIONS AND PRECAUTIONS. Leukopenia develops in almost all patients and is the usual dose-limiting toxicity. Nadirs occur around day 12 and recovery occurs between days 25 and 28. Other reported adverse reactions include mild nausea and vomiting, mucositis, seizures, local tissue irritation, and possible cardiotoxicity, which may be additive to that of the anthracyclines.

PHARMACOKINETICS. The terminal half-life after intravenous administration ranges from 7 to 17.4 hours. Amsacrine is metabolized in the liver and excreted via the bile. Patients with hepatic dysfunction require dosage adjustments.

DOSAGE AND PREPARATIONS.
Intravenous: For induction of remission in acute leukemia, 120 to 200 mg/M² daily for five days.
Amsidyl (Parke-Davis).

AZACITIDINE (5-Azacytidine; Ladakamycin)
[Mylosar]

ACTIONS AND USES. This antimetabolite, an analogue of cytidine, is rapidly phosphorylated and incorporated into both RNA and DNA. By disrupting the translation of nucleic acid sequences into protein, protein synthesis is inhibited. Moreover, azacitidine affects de novo pyrimidine synthesis by inhibiting orotidylic acid decarboxylase. It is cell cycle specific for the S phase.

The major indication for azacitidine is acute myelogenous leukemia refractory to conventional therapy.

ADVERSE REACTIONS AND PRECAUTIONS. Dose-limiting toxicity is usually hematologic, and is manifested by leukopenia, thrombocytopenia, and anemia. Nausea and vomiting are common and may be severe and prolonged. Symptoms are ameliorated by prolonged or continuous infusion. Antiemetics appear to be most helpful if taken 24 to 48 hours before therapy is begun. Other toxic effects are diarrhea, neuromuscular disturbances, fever, hepatotoxicity, hypotension, and skin rash.

PHARMACOKINETICS. Azacitidine is metabolized rapidly, initially by deamination; 70% to 90% of a dose is recovered in urine within 24 hours.

DOSAGE AND PREPARATIONS.
Intravenous: 50 to 400 mg/M² given by continuous infusion for five days. Preparations must be formulated every 6 to 12 hours because the drug is unstable in aqueous solutions.
Mylosar (Upjohn).

AZIRIDINYLBENZOQUINONE (AZQ)

The exact mechanism of action is unknown, but the chemical structure suggests that this drug may have an alkylating activity. In preclinical studies, aziridinylbenzoquinone was reported to exert some action on rodent and human tumors. Its ability to penetrate the central nervous system has resulted in clinical trials in patients with brain tumors.

Myelosuppression is the dose-limiting toxicity. Anorexia, diarrhea, weight loss, and mild elevations in the results of liver function tests have been noted occasionally.

DOSAGE.
Intravenous: 40 mg/M² every three weeks.

FLUDARABINE PHOSPHATE (2 Fluoro-ara-AMP)

ACTIONS AND USES. Fludarabine is the 2-fluoro, 5'-phosphate derivative of 9-β-D-arabinofuranosyladenine (Ara-A). It is resistant to deamination by adenosine deaminase. Its metabolite, 2-fluoro-ara-ATP, inhibits DNA polymerase.

Preclinical studies suggest that fludarabine has activity against rodent and human tumors. In Phase I clinical trials, non-Hodgkin's lymphomas were responsive.

ADVERSE REACTIONS AND PRECAUTIONS. Myelosuppression is dose limiting; leukopenia is most pronounced. Neurotoxic effects (eg, lethargy, somnolence) are common. Nausea and vomiting, stomatitis, and renal insufficiency also have been noted.

PHARMACOKINETICS. Fludarabine is metabolized rapidly to 2-fluoro-ara-A. The metabolite has a triexponential decay curve with half-lives of 5.42 minutes, 1.4 hours, and 10.2 hours. Total body clearance appears to be related to creatinine clearance.

DOSAGE.
Intravenous: 18 mg/M² for five days every four weeks.

HOMOHARRINGTONINE

ACTIONS AND USES. Homoharringtonine and its congener, harringtonine, are cephalotoxine alkaloids derived from evergreen trees in China. Homoharringtonine inhibits protein synthesis and thus the synthesis of DNA and RNA. There is also evidence that the drug induces a dose-dependent differentiation with a loss of proliferative activity.

Preclinical studies suggest that homoharringtonine has some activity in rodent and human tumors. Responses in acute myelocytic leukemia have been observed in preliminary clinical trials.

ADVERSE REACTIONS AND PRECAUTIONS. Bolus injections have been associated with severe, sometimes irreversible hypotension. Other significant side effects include arrhythmias (ameliorated by prolonged infusion), myelosuppression, fluid retention, hyperglycemia, diarrhea, nausea, alopecia, neuralgias, and mucositis.

PHARMACOKINETICS. Homoharringtonine has a biphasic terminal plasma half-life of 14.4 hours.

DOSAGE.
Intravenous: 3.25 to 4 mg/M² by continuous infusion daily for five days every four weeks.

INTERFERONS

ACTIONS. Interferon refers to a family of glycoproteins that are defined biologically by their ability to inhibit viral replication. Presently, three types of human interferons, designated HuIFN-α (leukocyte), HuIFN-β (fibroblast), and HuIFN-γ (T lymphocyte), are known (see Chapter 79, Antiviral Agents, and Chapter 63, Immunomodulators, for a more detailed discussion). The mechanisms by which interferons influence tumor growth are poorly understood. Direct inhibition of tumor cell growth, alteration of tumor cell surface properties, and immunomodulation of host defense mechanisms (eg, activation of natural killer [NK] cells) have been postulated.

USES. A number of clinical trials have been performed. Antitumor responses were reported in breast and renal cell cancer, osteogenic sarcoma, non-Hodgkin's lymphomas, multiple myeloma, chronic myelogenous leukemia, hairy cell leukemia, Kaposi's sarcoma, and cutaneous T cell lymphomas.

ADVERSE REACTIONS AND PRECAUTIONS. Side effects of interferons include fever, chills, myalgias, headache, fatigue, reversible leukopenia and thrombocytopenia (usually hypoplastic, although immune-mediated suppression may occur),

and transient elevations of liver enzymes. Significant nephrotoxicity is uncommon. Arrhythmias have been reported. Large doses have caused somnolence and seizures. Patients may develop antibodies against interferon.

DOSAGE.
Interferons can be administered intravenously, intramuscularly, or subcutaneously. Dosage depends on the preparation and route of administration.

NOTE: The alpha form of interferon became available for treatment of hairy cell leukemia after this chapter was prepared. See the manufacturers' literature.

IFOSFAMIDE (Noxamide)
[Ifex]

ACTIONS AND USES. This structural analogue of cyclophosphamide must be activated by the microsomal enzyme system of the liver. Its reactive metabolites are capable of covalent binding to protein and DNA.

Activity has been observed in non-small cell lung cancer, Hodgkin's and non-Hodgkin's lymphomas, breast cancer, ovarian cancer, testicular cancer, and acute and chronic leukemias. The spectrum of activity is similar to that of cyclophosphamide.

ADVERSE REACTIONS AND PRECAUTIONS. Ifosfamide is less myelosuppressive than cyclophosphamide. Nausea and vomiting are common. Large doses may cause lethargy and confusion. Local reactions, transient elevations of hepatic enzymes, and alopecia have occurred. The most serious side effect is hemorrhagic cystitis due to excretion of alkylating metabolites. Vigorous hydration and acetylcysteine and/or ascorbic acid have been employed to prevent this complication.

PHARMACOKINETICS. Ifosfamide is metabolized more slowly than cyclophosphamide. The plasma half-life is approximately 15 hours after a bolus dose.

DOSAGE AND PREPARATIONS.
Intravenous: 1.8 g/M² daily for five days every three weeks.
Ifex (Mead Johnson).

ISOTRETINOIN (13-cis-retinoic acid)
[Accutane]

ACTIONS AND USES. Vitamin A and its analogues (retinoids) are essential for epithelial cell differentiation. Deficiency of vitamin A promotes tissue metaplasia and neoplasia in various animal and organ culture models. Isotretinoin is a geometic isomer of retinoic acid.

In animal models, retinoids have been shown to delay the appearance, retard the growth, and cause regression of cancers of the skin; respiratory, urinary, and gastrointestinal tracts; pancreas; stomach; cervix; and mammary gland. Retinoids have been effective in benign dermatologic conditions (eg, severe acne) and in the treatment of basal cell carcinomas and cutaneous T cell lymphomas. Clinical trials evaluating the role of isotretinoin as a chemopreventive agent are in progress.

See also Chapter 56, Dermatologic Preparations.

ADVERSE REACTIONS AND PRECAUTIONS. Dry skin and mucous membranes are common. Exfoliation and increased susceptibility to sunburn may occur. The most frequent adverse reaction is cheilitis. Conjunctivitis is less common. Corneal opacities also have been reported. Nonspecific gastrointestinal and musculoskeletal disorders are frequent. Pseudotumor cerebri have developed.

Laboratory abnormalities include altered serum lipids with elevated plasma triglyceride levels and a mild to moderate decrease in high density lipoprotein levels. Cholesterol may be minimally elevated during treatment. These lipid abnormalities are reversible with cessation of therapy. Mild myelosuppression may be seen. Transient increases in liver enzymes are noted.

Isotretinoin is teratogenic and should not be given to pregnant women (FDA Pregnancy Category X). Patients sensitive to parabens should not receive isotretinoin, for they are used as preservatives in the formulation. See also Chapter 56.

DOSAGE AND PREPARATIONS.
Oral: 40 mg/M^2 daily.
   Accutane (Roche). Capsules 10, 20, and 40 mg.
   (Investigational indication)

N-METHYLFORMAMIDE (N-MF)

ACTIONS AND USES. N-methylformamide belongs to a class of polar-planar compounds that induce differentiation of specific cells in vitro. Both murine virus-infected erythroleukemia cells and human promyelocytic leukemia cells (HLGO) differentiate in the presence of N-methylformamide. It is thought that polar compounds act by changing the conformation of DNA or a DNA-protein complex, which alters transcription of the genes that regulate cellular differentiation.

Preclinical studies suggest that N-methylformamide has some activity in certain rodent and human tumors. Phase II clinical trials are in progress.

ADVERSE REACTIONS AND PRECAUTIONS. Anorexia, nausea, and vomiting are common side effects. Reversible hepatotoxicity has been observed.

DOSAGE.
Intravenous: 800 mg/M^2/day for five days every four weeks. Glass syringes or glass containers should be used.

An oral preparation also has been used.

MITOLACTOL (Dibromodulcitol)

$$
\begin{array}{c}
CH_2Br \\
| \\
H-C-OH \\
| \\
HO-C-H \\
| \\
HO-C-H \\
| \\
H-C-OH \\
| \\
CH_2Br
\end{array}
$$

ACTIONS AND USES. Mitolactol, a halogenated sugar alcohol, appears to act as an alkylating agent, although all of the drug's actions cannot be explained on this basis.

Clinical activity has been reported in acute and chronic leukemias, Hodgkin's and non-Hodgkin's lymphomas, breast cancer, lung cancer, and melanoma.

ADVERSE REACTIONS AND PRECAUTIONS. Mitolactol is myelosuppressive and produces leukopenia and thrombocytopenia. Nausea and vomiting are mild. Pulmonary and hepatic complications have been noted rarely.

PHARMACOKINETICS. After oral administration, blood levels are observed in 15 minutes. The parent molecule is rapidly hydrolyzed in plasma to various epoxides and debrominated derivatives, including monobromodulcitol. Renal excretion is the primary route of elimination for mitolactol and its metabolites.

DOSAGE.
Oral: 130 mg/M^2 daily.

PCNU (1-C2-chloroethyl)-3-(2,6-dioxo-3-piperidyl)-1-nitrosourea)

This nitrosourea analogue has high lipid solubility and alkylating activity and low carbamoylating activity. Its primary mechanism of action is DNA alkylation. Preclinical studies suggest that PCNU has some activity in rodent and human tumors.

Myelosuppression is dose limiting (less prolonged than with other nitrosoureas). Renal, pulmonary, and hepatic toxicity are rare.

DOSAGE.
Intravenous: 90 mg/M^2 every six weeks. Glass syringes should be used.

PENTOSTATIN (2′Deoxycoformycin)
[Potentiator]

ACTIONS AND USES. Pentostatin is a potent inhibitor of adenosine deaminase that binds tightly to the enzyme. Inhibition of adenosine deaminase leads to an accumulation of deoxy-adenosine triphosphate (dATP) and appears to inhibit cell proliferation. Lymphoid cells are particularly sensitive to this effect.

Pentostatin has shown activity in acute and chronic lymphocytic leukemia, non-Hodgkin's lymphomas, cutaneous T cell lymphomas, and hairy cell leukemia.

ADVERSE REACTIONS AND PRECAUTIONS. Toxicity has included myelosuppression (lymphopenia may be pronounced), conjunctivitis, and panserositis. Central nervous system side effects are frequent and range from lethargy to coma. Renal toxicity includes hyperuricemia; pulmonary toxicity also developed. Immune suppression with reactivation of herpes zoster infection is common.

DOSAGE AND PREPARATIONS.
Intravenous: 5 mg/M^2 for three days every four weeks.
   Potentiator (Parke-Davis).

RAZOXANE

ACTIONS AND USES. This bis-dioxopiperazine compound inhibits proliferating cells in the G$_2$-M phase of the cell cycle. The precise mechanism of action remains to be elucidated, but razoxane inhibits DNA synthesis. Significant activity has been reported in leukemia and non-Hodgkin's lymphomas.

ADVERSE REACTIONS AND PRECAUTIONS. Leukopenia is the principal toxic effect. Nausea and vomiting are common and usually mild. Alopecia, dermatitis, and a flu-like syndrome have been reported. The drug is immunosuppressive, radiosensitizing, and teratogenic.

PHARMACOKINETICS. Bioavailability is erratic. The plasma half-life is approximately 3.5 hours. The drug is extensively metabolized and appears to be excreted by the kidneys and biliary system (with possible significant enterohepatic recirculation).

DOSAGE.
Oral: 3 g/M^2 in divided doses every six hours for one day/week for six weeks.

SEMUSTINE (Methyl CCNU)

ACTIONS. Semustine, a chloroethyl nitrosourea, probably acts as an alkylating agent. Although this drug contains only one alkylating function, it produces interstrand cross links in DNA. Like other nitrosoureas, semustine may inhibit several key enzymatic processes and also has carbamoylating activity. This drug is cell cycle nonspecific.

USES. Therapeutic responses have been observed in patients with brain tumors; gastric, colorectal, and pancreatic adenocarcinomas; Hodgkin's disease; non-Hodgkin's lymphomas; and malignant melanoma. Although the response rates of gastrointestinal malignancies (eg, stomach, colon, pancreas) are low, semustine is being investigated as a component of various combination regimens in these diseases.

ADVERSE REACTIONS AND PRECAUTIONS. Nausea and vomiting occur four to six hours after administration and last six to eight hours. Vomiting can be severe; prior administration of antiemetics decreases the frequency and duration.

The dose-limiting toxicity is bone marrow suppression with delayed leukopenia (nadir of white blood cell count occurs six weeks after administration) and thrombocytopenia (nadir occurs after about four weeks). This myelosuppression is cumulative. Anemia is less apparent. Blood counts must be performed frequently for at least six weeks following each dose. Subsequent doses should not be given for at least six weeks, and adjustments must be made on the basis of the nadir from the prior dose. Secondary leukemias have been reported.

Delayed nephrotoxicity, including renal failure, has been reported frequently, particularly in children. Nephrotoxicity appears to be related to the total cumulative dose. In one study, five of six children receiving total doses greater than 1,500 mg/M^2 developed renal damage (Harmon et al, 1979). Approximately 25% of adults receiving doses in excess of 1.4 g/M^2 developed renal abnormalities. Individuals who received a lower total dose were unaffected (Micetich et al, 1981). Renal function must be monitored continually. If renal function tests (eg, BUN, creatinine clearance, serum creatinine) are abnormal, semustine should be discontinued. This drug should not be administered with other nephrotoxic drugs.

Other adverse effects include alopecia, pulmonary fibrosis (with prolonged use), and abnormal liver function tests. The drug is teratogenic, mutagenic, and carcinogenic.

PHARMACOKINETICS. Semustine is rapidly absorbed from the gastrointestinal tract following oral administration, and the parent drug rapidly disappears from plasma. The plasma half-lives of major metabolites are long (eg, chloroethyl moiety, 36 hours; cyclohexyl moiety, 72 hours); these metabolites are eliminated via the kidney. Like other chloroethyl nitrosoureas, semustine readily crosses the blood-brain barrier.

DOSAGE.
Oral: 200 mg/M^2 as a single dose every six weeks.

SPIROGERMANIUM (NSC)
[Spiro 32]

ACTIONS AND USES. Spirogermanium is an azaspirane that incorporates germanium into the heterocyclic ring structure. It inhibits protein synthesis with secondary depression of RNA and DNA synthesis.

Preclinical studies suggest this drug's activity in rodent and human tumors. In preliminary clinical trials, breast cancer, ovarian cancer, and non-Hodgkin's lymphoma have been responsive.

ADVERSE REACTIONS AND PRECAUTIONS. Neurotoxicity is dose limiting and includes lethargy, fatigue, transient vertigo, ataxia, euphoria, diplopia, seizures, and paresthesias. Neurologic side effects are reversible, and slow infusion diminishes these complications. Transient elevations of hepatic enzymes have been noted. Renal toxicity is uncommon.

PHARMACOKINETICS. Following intravenous injection, most of the drug attaches to cellular elements; trace amounts remain in the serum bound to protein. There is a biphasic decay curve with half-lives of 10 to 20 minutes and 60 to 200 minutes.

DOSAGE AND PREPARATIONS.

Intravenous: 200 to 300 mg/M^2 twice weekly.
 Spiro 32 (Unimed).

TEGAFUR (Ftorafur)

ACTIONS. This pyrimidine antimetabolite is structurally similar to floxuridine [FUDR] and appears to be converted slowly to fluorouracil in vivo. Thus, it probably acts as an inhibitor of thymidylate synthetase.

USES. The clinical and experimental antitumor activity of tegafur is similar to that of fluorouracil; greatest activity is seen in gastric, colorectal, and breast carcinoma. The drug appears to offer no therapeutic advantages over fluorouracil but has a number of toxicologic disadvantages.

ADVERSE REACTIONS AND PRECAUTIONS. The dose-limiting toxicity of tegafur is different from that of fluorouracil. The drug is minimally myelosuppressive. However, it produces considerable diarrhea, cramps, vomiting, and mucositis, which is most often dose limiting. Also, it is more neurotoxic than fluorouracil. Common manifestations are altered mental status and cerebellar ataxia.

PHARMACOKINETICS. Tegafur is reliably absorbed after oral administration but is more frequently given by the intravenous route in this country. The parent compound has a prolonged plasma half-life of 6 to 16 hours and is eliminated by conversion to hydroxylated metabolites. Tegafur readily penetrates into the central nervous system.

DOSAGE AND PREPARATIONS.

Intravenous, Oral: 1 to 1.5 g/M^2 daily in courses of 14 to 21 days, repeated every 28 days.
 Tegafur (Mead Johnson).

TENIPOSIDE (VM-26)

Teniposide, a semisynthetic podophyllotoxin, arrests cells in the late S or G_2 phase, but the mechanism is unclear.

Teniposide has significant activity in Hodgkin's and non-Hodgkin's lymphoma. Responses also have been seen in lymphocytic leukemia in children.

Myelosuppression is the typical dose-limiting toxicity. Hypotension has occurred after rapid intravenous injection. Anaphylactic reactions have been reported, and chemical phlebitis is not uncommon.

Teniposide is extensively bound to serum proteins (about 99%). Plasma clearance is biphasic with a terminal half-life of 8 to 24 hours. The drug is extensively metabolized.

DOSAGE AND PREPARATIONS.

Intravenous: 50 mg/M^2 daily for five days every four weeks.
 Teniposide (Bristol-Myers).

VINDESINE SULFATE
 [Eldisine]

ACTIONS AND USES. This synthetic derivative of vinblastine produces mitotic arrest by disrupting the assembly of microtubules.

Vindesine has been active in a variety of cancers, including acute lymphoblastic leukemia, Hodgkin's and non-Hodgkin's lymphomas, breast carcinoma, malignant melanoma, and non-small cell lung cancer.

ADVERSE REACTIONS AND PRECAUTIONS. Like vinblastine, the usual dose-limiting toxicity of vindesine is myelosuppression, with neutropenia predominating over thrombocytopenia. Neurotoxicity is usually less severe than that caused by vincristine but may be dose limiting. Paresthesias, muscle weakness, and loss of deep tendon reflexes occur frequently. Cumulative neurotoxicity precludes the use of vindesine with other vinca alkaloids. Gastrointestinal symptoms include nausea, vomiting, and diarrhea. Alopecia ranges from mild to total hair loss. Dermatitis, stomatitis, fever, and myalgias are less common. Vindesine is a tissue irritant.

PHARMACOKINETICS. Vindesine appears to resemble other vinca alkaloids in its pharmacokinetic and pharmacologic behavior. Elimination from the blood is triphasic after intravenous administration; the half-lives are 0.04, 0.9, and 24 hours.

DOSAGE AND PREPARATIONS. Each 5-mg ampul is reconstituted with 5 ml of the diluent provided. When refrigerated the solution is stable for four weeks.

Intravenous: Administration is by slow push into the tubing of a free-flowing intravenous line. The most common dose employed is 3 to 4 mg/M^2 every week.

Eldisine (Lilly).

ZOLADEX

This analogue of gonadotropin-releasing hormone has substitutions for the L-amino acid glycine in positions six and ten. Zoladex is 50 to 100 times more potent and the duration of action is longer than that of the natural peptide. Zoladex is effective in the treatment of prostate and breast cancer.

Initial stimulation of gonadotropin release and sex steroid production may cause a disease flare during the first weeks of therapy. Hot flashes are common. Gynecomastia, nausea and vomiting, edema, and thrombophlebitis are infrequent complications. Loss of libido may occur.

DOSAGE.

Subcutaneous: 3.6 mg every four weeks.

Zoladex depot is supplied as a totally biodegradable, lactic-glycolic acid copolymer impregnated with 3.6 mg zoladex in a disposable syringe device mounted on a −16 gauge hypodermic needle.

Cited References

Cancer chemotherapy. *Med Lett Drugs Ther* 22:101-106, 1980.

Blum RH, et al: Principles of dose, schedule, and combination chemotherapy, in Holland JF, Frei E III (eds): *Cancer Medicine*, ed 2. Philadelphia, Lea & Febiger, 1982, 730-752.

Bonadonna G, Santoro A: ABVD chemotherapy in treatment of Hodgkin's disease. *Cancer Treat Rev* 9:21-35, 1982.

Bramwell VHC, Pinedo HM: Treatment of metastatic bone and soft-tissue sarcomas, in Carter SK, et al (eds): *Principles of Cancer Treatment*. New York, McGraw-Hill, 1982, 718-733.

Carney DN, Winkler CW: In vitro assays of chemotherapeutic sensitivity, in De Vita VT Jr, et al (eds): *Important Advances in Oncology*. Philadelphia, JB Lippincott, 1985.

Carter SK, Glatstein E: Neuroblastoma, in Carter SK, et al (eds): *Principles of Cancer Treatment*. New York, McGraw-Hill, 1982 A, 869-872.

Carter SK, Glatstein E: Principles of combined-modality treatment involving chemotherapy (adjuvant chemotherapy), in Carter SK, et al (eds): *Principles of Cancer Treatment*. New York, McGraw-Hill, 1982 B, 281-287.

Carter SK, Livingston RB: Principles of cancer chemotherapy, in Carter SK, et al (eds): *Principles of Cancer Treatment*. New York, McGraw-Hill, 1982 A, 95-110.

Carter SK, Livingston RB: Drugs available to treat cancer, in Carter SK, et al (eds): *Principles of Cancer Treatment*. New York, McGraw-Hill, 1982 B, 111-145.

Carter SK, Rubens RD: Management of locally advanced and disseminated breast cancer. *Lancet* 2:795-797, 1981.

Carter SK, et al: *Chemotherapy of Cancer*, ed 2. New York, John Wiley & Sons, 1981.

Carter SK, et al: Introduction: Cancer treatment and clinical research in perspective, in Carter SK, et al (eds): *Principles of Cancer Treatment*. New York, McGraw-Hill, 1982, 3-13.

Chabner BA, Myers CE: Clinical pharmacology of cancer chemotherapy, in DeVita VT Jr, et al (eds): *Cancer, Principles and Practice of Oncology*. Philadelphia, JB Lippincott, 1985, 287-328.

DeVita VT Jr: Principles of chemotherapy, in DeVita VT Jr, et al (eds): *Cancer, Principles and Practice of Oncology*. Philadelphia, JB Lippincott Co, 1985, 257-286.

DeVita VT Jr, et al: Hodgkin's disease and non-Hodgkin's lymphomas, in DeVita VT Jr, et al (eds): *Cancer, Principles and Practice of Oncology*. Philadelphia, JB Lippincott, 1985, 1623-1710.

Dunagin WG: Clinical toxicity of chemotherapeutic agents: Dermatologic toxicity. *Semin Oncol* 9:14-22, 1982.

Einhorn LH: Testicular cancer as model for curable neoplasm: Richard and Hinda Rosenthal Foundation Award Lecture. *Cancer Res* 41:3275-3280, 1981.

Glatstein E, Carter SK: Chronic toxicity of cancer treatment, in Carter SK, et al (eds): *Principles of Cancer Treatment*. New York, McGraw-Hill, 1982, 221-232.

Goldie JH, Coldman AJ: Mathematical model for relating the drug sensitivity of tumors to their spontaneous mutation rate. *Cancer Treat Rep* 63:1727-1733, 1979.

Gralla RJ, et al: Antiemetic efficacy of high-dose metoclopramide: Randomized trials with placebo and prochlorperazine in patients with chemotherapy-induced nausea and vomiting. *N Engl J Med* 305:905-909, 1981.

Harmon WE, et al: Chronic renal failure in children treated with methyl CCNU. *N Engl J Med* 300:1200-1203, 1979.

Harris JR, et al: Cancer of breast, in DeVita VT Jr, et al (eds): *Cancer, Principles and Practice of Oncology*. Philadelphia, JB Lippincott, 1985, 1119-1173.

Harvey HA, et al: Medical castration produced by the GnRH analog, Leuprolide, to treat metastatic breast cancer. *J Clin Oncol* 3:1068-1072, 1985.

Hoagland HC: Hematologic complications of cancer chemotherapy. *Semin Oncol* 9:95-102, 1982.

Krakoff IH: Cancer chemotherapeutic agents. *Ca* 31:130-140, 1981.

Kyle RA: Second malignancies associated with chemotherapeutic agents. *Semin Oncol* 9:131-142, 1982.

Leuprolide Study Group: Leuprolide versus diethylstilbestrol for metastatic prostate cancer. *N Engl J Med* 311:1281-1286, 1984.

Livingston RB: Management of acute toxicity of chemotherapeutic agents, in Carter SK, et al (eds): *Principles of Cancer Treatment*. New York, McGraw-Hill, 1982, 206-211.

Macdonald JS, et al: Cancer of stomach, in DeVita VT Jr, et al (eds): *Cancer, Principles and Practice of Oncology*. Philadelphia, JB Lippincott, 1985, 659-690.

Markman M: Intracavitary chemotherapy for malignant disease confined to body cavities. *West J Med* 142:364-368, 1985.

Marsoni S, Wittes R: Clinical development of anticancer agents: National Cancer Institute perspective. *Cancer Treat Rep* 68:77-85, 1984.

Martin DS: Scientific basis for adjuvant chemotherapy. *Cancer Treat Rev* 8:169-189, 1981.

McGuire WL: Hormone receptors and hormonal treatment of breast cancer, in Carter SK, et al (eds): *Principles of Cancer Treatment*. New York, McGraw-Hill, 1982, 352-357.

Micetich KC, et al: Nephrotoxicity of semustine (methyl-CCNU) in patients with malignant melanoma receiving adjuvant chemotherapy. *Am J Med* 71:967-972, 1981.

Mihich E, Creaven PJ: Principles of pharmacology and toxicology, in Holland JF, Frei E III (eds): *Cancer Medicine*, ed 2. Philadelphia, Lea & Febiger, 1982, 685-715.

Mitchell EP, Schein PS: Gastrointestinal toxicity of chemotherapeutic agents. *Semin Oncol* 9:52-64, 1982.

Moertel CG, et al: Streptozocin alone compared with streptozocin plus fluorouracil in treatment of advanced islet-cell carcinoma. *N Engl J Med* 303:1189-1194, 1980.

National Institutes of Health Consensus-Development Panel: Adjuvant chemotherapy of breast cancer. *N Engl J Med* 303:831-832, 1980.

Nelson RL: Comparative clinical pharmacology and pharmacokinetics of vindesine, vincristine, and vinblastine in human patients with cancer. *Med Pediatr Oncol* 10:115-127, 1982.

Perez CA, et al: Gynecologic tumors, in DeVita VT Jr, et al (eds): *Cancer, Principles and Practice of Oncology*. Philadelphia, JB Lippincott, 1985, 1013-1082.

Pratt WB, Ruddon RW: *The Anticancer Drugs*. New York, Oxford University Press, 1979.

Rai KR, et al: Treatment of acute myelocytic leukemia: Study by Cancer and Leukemia Group B. *Blood* 58:1203-1212, 1981.

Santen RJ, et al: Randomized trial comparing surgical adrenalectomy with aminoglutethimide plus hydrocortisone in women with advanced breast cancer. *N Engl J Med* 305:545-551, 1981.

Santen RJ, et al: Aminoglutethimide as treatment of postmenopausal women with advanced breast carcinoma. *Ann Intern Med* 96:94-101, 1982.

Schepartz SA, et al: New approaches in cancer chemotherapy. *Pharm Times* 47:84-96, 1981.

Sindelar WF, et al: Cancer of pancreas, in DeVita VT Jr, et al: *Cancer, Principles and Practice of Oncology*. Philadelphia, JB Lippincott, 1985, 691-740.

Skipper HE, Schabel FM Jr: Quantitative and cytokinetic studies in experimental tumor systems, in Holland JF, Frei E III (eds): *Cancer Medicine*, ed 2. Philadelphia, Lea & Febiger, 1982, 663-685.

Skipper HE, et al: Experimental evaluation of potential anticancer agents. XIII. On the criteria and kinetics associated with "curability" of experimental leukemia. *Cancer Chemother Rep* 35:1-111, 1964.

Smith JA Jr, et al: Clinical effects of gonadotropin-releasing hormone analogue in metastatic carcinoma of prostate. *Urology* 25:106-114, 1985.

Steel GG: Cytokinetics of neoplasia, in Holland JF, Frei E III (eds): *Cancer Medicine*, ed 2. Philadelphia, Lea & Febiger, 1982, 177-189.

Stiehm ER, et al: Interferon: Immunobiology and clinical significance. *Ann Intern Med* 96:80-93, 1982.

Vadlamudi S, Goldin A: Influence of mitotic cycle inhibitors on antileukemic activity of cytosine arabinoside (NSC-63878) in mice bearing leukemia L1210. *Cancer Chemother Rep* 55:547-555, 1971.

Vogelzang NJ: Continuous infusion chemotherapy: Critical review. *J Clin Oncol* 2:1289-1304, 1984.

Weinstein HJ, et al: Treatment of acute myelogenous leukemia in children and adults. *N Engl J Med* 303:473-478, 1980.

Weiss RB: Hypersensitivity reactions to cancer chemotherapy. *Semin Oncol* 9:5-13, 1982.

Woodruff R: Treatment of multiple myeloma. *Cancer Treat Rev* 8:225-270, 1981.

Zubrod CG: Principles of chemotherapy (introduction), in Holland JF, Frei E III (eds): *Cancer Medicine*, ed 2. Philadelphia, Lea & Febiger, 1982, 627-632.

Other Selected References

Balis FM, et al: Clinical pharmacokinetics and commonly used anticancer drugs. *Clin Pharmacokinet* 8:202-232, 1983.

Carter SK, et al (eds): *Principles of Cancer Treatment*. New York, McGraw-Hill, 1982.

DeVita VT Jr, et al (eds): *Cancer, Principles and Practice of Oncology*. Philadelphia, JB Lippincott, 1985.

Dorr RT, Fritz WL: *Cancer Chemotherapy Handbook*. New York, Elsevier, 1980.

Holland JF, Frei E III (eds): *Cancer Medicine*, ed 2. Philadelphia, Lea & Febiger, 1982.

Antimicrobial Therapy and Chemoprophylaxis of Infectious Diseases

65

INTRODUCTION

PRINCIPLES OF ANTIMICROBIAL DRUG SELECTION

Diagnosis

Organism Resistance

Patient Response Variation

Outpatient Versus Inpatient Drug Treatment

Cost

OTHER PRINCIPLES OF THERAPY FOR ACTIVE INFECTIOUS DISEASE

Relief of Obstruction, Drainage, Surgery, Debridement, and Foreign Body Removal

Supportive Care

Monitoring of Patient Response

TABLE 1: ANTIMICROBIAL DRUG SELECTION FOR COMMON INFECTIOUS DISEASES

TABLE 2: TREATMENT OF SEXUALLY TRANSMITTED DISEASES (STD)

TABLE 3: ANTIMICROBIAL CHEMOPROPHYLAXIS FOR AMBULATORY PATIENTS

TABLE 4: ANTIMICROBIAL CHEMOPROPHYLAXIS FOR SURGICAL PATIENTS

Antimicrobial drugs are used extensively by physicians, and the list of clinically useful agents grows increasingly longer. The large number of active antimicrobial drugs offers the patient with an infection a greater chance for cure with less drug-related toxicity and provides alternative choices despite the continuing emergence of drug-resistant pathogenic organisms. For the prescribing physician, however, appropriate drug selection has become increasingly difficult.

The primary goal of this chapter is to present an overview of information and guidelines for antimicrobial drug selection for the treatment of active infections as well as for chemoprophylaxis. In addition, the various principles of active infectious disease therapy are briefly reviewed.

Tables are employed to provide rapid access to specific information on drug selection for a given clinical situation. Table 1 lists the common infectious diseases, organisms most often responsible, and preferred and alternative antimicrobial agents for specific and/or empiric (presumptive) therapy. Table 2 provides more detailed guidelines for the treatment of sexually transmitted diseases (STD). Tables 3 and 4 list specific antimicrobial chemoprophylactic regimens for ambulatory and surgical prophylaxis, respectively.

Principles of Antimicrobial Drug Selection

Selection of the most appropriate antimicrobial drug for the treatment of an infection is based on several criteria. First, a determination of the primary focus of infection and the possible organism(s) involved can establish a presumptive or definitive *diagnosis*. The most effective classes of antimicrobial agents then can be identified. The possibility of *organism resistance* to any of these drugs must be considered in order to determine which drugs can successfully eradicate the organism. *Patient response variation*, ie, predicting the response of an individual patient to both the organism and the proposed therapy, also aids the physician in determining the most effective, least toxic agents for treatment. Additional criteria required to identify the actual drug(s) of choice for a particular patient include *outpatient versus inpatient management* and *cost*.

Diagnosis: The most probable organism(s) causing an infection often can be determined by the available clinical evidence, including the known or suspected etiology and the primary focus of infection. A reasonably reliable prediction is possible if the infection is associated with trauma, burns, drug addiction, sexual activity, contaminated intimate-contact devices (eg, urethral or intravenous catheter, prosthetic implants), recent hospitalization, prior infection or antibiotic use, and if the primary focus of infection is localized in the meninges, skin, cardiovascular system, upper or lower respiratory system, urinary tract, bone, joints, gastrointestinal tract, reproductive system, or above or below the diaphragm.

A Gram stain of an *adequate* specimen is a simple, rapid, and inexpensive method that can be particularly helpful in diagnosis when done by someone skilled in this technique. Although not always cost effective, culture and susceptibility tests yield the most accurate information and are especially important when the infection is probably due to organisms that vary in their susceptibility to first-choice drugs, eg, gram-negative bacilli. It is important to obtain appropriate specimens for cultures of body fluids, exudates, and blood before starting antimicrobial therapy. Anaerobic cultures should be obtained when anaerobic infections are considered.

Table 1 lists common infectious diseases by organ system(s) involvement, and the most probable organism(s) responsible. The usual first-choice and alternative antimicrobial regimens for specific and/or empiric (presumptive) therapy are shown.

Organism Resistance: Although a number of organisms continue to be predictably susceptible to selected antimicrobial agents (eg, susceptibility of *Treponema pallidum*, *Streptococcus pyogenes*, and *Neisseria meningitidis* to penicillin G), the development of clinically important resistant organisms is common because of the selective pressures applied by antimicrobial drug usage. Organism resistance occurs both through plasmid transfer, either by conjugation or transduction, and from chromosomal mutations. Both the rate of emergence and extent of resistance can vary between organisms and from drug to drug. When resistance to a drug is not absolute, the administration of larger dosages of drug that do not cause serious adverse effects may be adequate for clinical cure. In contrast, combinations of antimicrobial drugs are necessary for the effective treatment of tuberculosis to avoid the rapid development of highly resistant strains of *Mycobacterium tuberculosis* that readily appear when single drugs are used.

Antimicrobial susceptibility testing is necessary whenever there is doubt about the susceptibility of a given organism. For bacteria such as *Staphylococcus aureus* and various facultative and aerobic gram-negative bacilli, to which resistance is common, susceptibility testing is particularly important.

Patterns of antimicrobial susceptibility can vary from one geographic area to another, among different hospitals within a given area, and between community-acquired and hospital-acquired infections. A current, locally generated antibiotic susceptibility profile for selected organisms is a good source for establishing the probable type and degree of resistance.

Patient Response Variation: In addition to the virulence of the organism, the severity of an infection is determined by the genetic constitution, age, and health of the patient. Individuals at the extremes of age, those with inadequate humoral and cellular defense mechanisms, and/or those with associated disorders (especially hypovolemia, hypoxemia, and/or acidosis) are most susceptible. An immunologically incompetent patient with a malignancy who is receiving radiation and cytotoxic drugs is the classic example used to define the high-risk individual with an infection. Using bactericidal rather than bacteriostatic agents when both are available or using a combination of antibiotics rather than a single drug may be required in high-risk individuals.

In the drug selection process, pharmacokinetic factors that affect the patient's response to the proposed antibiotic(s) must be considered in order to achieve an effective drug concentration at the site of infection. Selection based on parenteral rather than oral absorption may be indicated. Distribution characteristics also may determine the drug of choice. This is of particular importance for infections in the cerebrospinal fluid. Small lipophilic molecules, such as chloramphenicol, isoniazid, metronidazole, rifampin, sulfonamides, and trimethoprim, penetrate into cerebrospinal fluid better than highly charged or larger molecular weight molecules, such as aminoglycosides, amphotericin B, first and most second generation cephalosporins, clindamycin, and polymyxins. Ampicillin, piperacillin, ethambutol, flucytosine, methicillin, nafcillin, penicillin G, vancomycin, and the third generation cephalosporins achieve adequate therapeutic levels when the meninges are inflamed. If an agent that exhibits poor cerebrospinal fluid penetration must be used, however, lumbar intrathecal or intraventricular (through a shunt) administration may be necessary. Trimethoprim, usually administered in combination with sulfamethoxazole, doxycycline, and erythromycin (for gram-positive bacteria only) may have to be considered in chronic prostatic infections because of their better penetration into noninflamed prostatic tissue. The remaining two pharmacokinetic parameters, drug metabolism and elimination, must be considered for patients with impaired hepatic or renal function. For example, dosage adjustments must be made for the aminoglycosides in patients with renal insufficiency to avoid severe toxicity, especially ototoxicity and nephrotoxicity.

Additional factors that may eliminate an effective agent from consideration include (1) a reliable history of an allergic reaction to the antibiotic (eg, urticaria, angioedema, wheezing, anaphylaxis); (2) potential adverse interactions (eg, avoiding additive nephrotoxicity, ototoxicity, or hepatotoxicity) when other drugs are being given for associated illnesses; and (3) predictable adverse reactions that are unacceptable in certain patients (eg, use of tetracyclines in pregnant women or young children).

Outpatient Versus Inpatient Drug Treatment: These drug treatment modes are distinguished primarily by the severity of the infection and the anticipated compliance with therapy. Among efficacious alternatives, low toxicity and ease of administration (usually by the oral route) are the most important factors in drug selection for outpatients; using drugs that require less frequent administration may improve compliance. In contrast, drug efficacy and the rapid attainment of inhibitory, preferably bactericidal, concentrations at the site of infection are primary considerations in hospitalized patients with life-threatening infections, even when very toxic drugs must be administered. Empiric therapy with parenteral (usually intravenous) antimicrobial agents frequently is required in these patients before results of culture and susceptibility tests are available.

Drug selection is usually more difficult for inpatients than for ambulatory patients because (1) the patient is more severely affected; (2) nosocomial infections are often associated with uncommon or resistant organisms; (3) the patient is at higher risk for both the organism involved and the drug selected; and (4) associated illnesses often are present.

The following core-group of antibiotics is widely used for systemic antimicrobial therapy in ambulatory patients: the penicillins (especially penicillin V, benzathine penicillin G, ampicillin, amoxicillin, and the orally effective penicillinase-resistant penicillins, cloxacillin and dicloxacillin), erythromycin, sulfisoxazole, tetracyclines, oral cephalosporins, trimethoprim, and the drug combinations trimethoprim/sulfamethoxazole [Bactrim, Septra] and erythromycin/sulfisoxazole [Pediazole]. These drugs are effective when employed appropriately and have a good record of safety. (See Table 1 and other chapters in this section for specific indications.)

Cost: The impact of drug cost continues to be widely discussed. Although the physician's primary responsibility is to select the antimicrobial agent that is most likely to effect a complete cure in the shortest time, alternative preparations of the same antibiotic are often available. The selection of an appropriate, equally effective, but less expensive preparation may ensure compliance in selected patients. The physician is encouraged to seek unbiased sources of information that compare the cost of equally effective preparations. Such sources include the Pharmacy and Therapeutics Committee in local hospitals and antibiotic audit cost-effectiveness reviews in the literature (providing regional costs are consonant with those listed). Potentially effective mechanisms to decrease antibiotic drug costs within hospitals include the use of competitive bidding for similar antimicrobials (eg, antipseudomonal penicillins, third generation cephalosporins, aminoglycosides), and to use (equally effective) drugs that require less frequent administration.

Other Principles of Therapy for Active Infectious Diseases

If the preferred antimicrobial agent has been selected on the basis of the preceding criteria, treatment with that drug in an appropriate dosage should produce a concentration of antimicrobial agent at the site of infection that is adequate to eradicate the causative organism. In addition, optimum therapy will also require that the following general principles be given equal consideration.

Relief of Obstruction, Drainage, Surgery, Debridement, and Foreign Body Removal: Relief of gastrointestinal or ureteral obstruction; incision and adequate drainage of furuncles, abscesses, and wound infections; surgical repair of a ruptured colon or removal of an infected gallbladder; as well as debridement of animal and human bite wounds when indicated are necessary to achieve an optimum effect from any antimicrobial agent. In many cases, mechanical correction is the primary indication for a successful clinical outcome.

A foreign body, including intimate-contact medical devices (eg, catheters of all types regardless of location, intrauterine devices, prostheses, pacemakers) that must remain in place should always be considered potential sources of infection in a diagnostic work-up. Successful antimicrobial treatment of an infection associated with a foreign body usually requires the latter's removal.

Supportive Care: Mild to moderate hypovolemia, electrolyte imbalances, and/or acidosis should be corrected in order to improve the overall management of the patient. Adequate supportive care may help to prevent therapeutic failure in moderate to severe infections. Life-threatening septic shock and other types of cardiovascular depression may require additional aggressive therapy with dopamine, digitalis, and/or corticosteroids. Management of increased intracranial pressure is another vital aspect of the supportive care of a patient with an infectious disease (ie, meningitis). Diphtheria antitoxin and tetanus immune globulin (human) also should be administered when indicated.

Monitoring of Patient Response: Monitoring of patient response to antimicrobial therapy is essential to determine the efficacy of treatment and whether a change in drug therapy is indicated. The frequency of monitoring patient response to therapy is related directly to the severity of the infection.

Measurements of clinical variables, such as resolution of fever, leukocytosis, and other signs of inflammation, and disappearance of the causative organism from post-treatment cultures, are primary methods of determining response to therapy. When a potentially toxic antimicrobial agent (eg, aminoglycoside) is administered for a prolonged period, monitoring of serum drug concentrations during therapy usually is desirable. Similarly, when a prolonged serum bactericidal effect is necessary to cure an infection (eg, infective endocarditis), measurement of serum bactericidal titers during therapy frequently is done to assess the adequacy of treatment, although this is controversial.

Therapeutic failure or an adverse event demands an individualized analysis of possible etiologies in order to distinguish between the two. Therapeutic failures commonly occur because of (1) inadequate concentration and/or duration of the antimicrobial agent at the site of infection; (2) prior or developing organism resistance to the drug(s) selected; (3) concomitant development of an unrelated infection or superinfection that is unresponsive to the drug selected; (4) failure to correct an aggravating factor that limits the effectiveness of the antibiotic (eg, failure to drain an abscess, remove a foreign implant, or correct the cause of compromised humoral or cellular immunity); (5) laboratory error resulting in inadequate therapy; or (6) noncompliance by an ambulatory patient.

The appearance of an adverse event most probably is related to (1) an adverse drug reaction or drug interaction; or

(2) signs or symptoms resulting from the concomitant onset of an associated illness.

Other mechanisms also may produce therapeutic failure or adverse events. However, the diligent physician who reviews the mechanisms listed above for cause and makes appropriate changes will prevent adverse outcomes for many of the infections being treated.

TABLE 1. ANTIMICROBIAL DRUG SELECTION FOR COMMON INFECTIOUS DISEASES

The purpose of this Table is to present synopses of antimicrobial drug therapy recommendations for common infectious diseases. Drug selection guidelines presented in the Table represent a consensus based on an evaluation of the current medical literature and the opinions of expert consultants in infectious diseases.

Unless stated otherwise, common causative organisms and appropriate antimicrobial drug selection will be for community-acquired infections in normal (eg, immunocompetent) hosts. When included, hospital-acquired (nosocomial) infections or infections in compromised hosts (eg, neutropenic, diabetic, alcoholic) will be indicated as such.

Depending on the location of the infection, antimicrobial drug selection may be for (1) specific therapy following identification of the causative organism; (2) therapy based primarily on the results of a Gram stain; and/or (3) initial empiric therapy pending the results of cultures or clinical response. Drug selection at these different levels will be considered, when appropriate, for each infection.

The content of this Table is limited by the constraints of space. Therefore, it is not possible to provide a detailed discussion of antimicrobial drug therapy or to include all possible drug regimens for each infectious disease. The reader is encouraged to consult the cited references for additional information. The antimicrobial agents, including dosage information, are discussed in other chapters within this section.

The following are recommended general references on infectious disease therapy:

(1) **Textbooks**: Mandell et al, 1979, 1984; Kagan, 1980; Yoshikawa et al, 1980; Braude, 1981, 1986; Feigin and Cherry, 1981; Hoeprich, 1983; Kass and Platt, 1983; McCracken and Nelson, 1983; Reese and Douglas, 1983, 1986; Remington and Klein, 1983; Holmes et al, 1984; Ristuccia and Cunha, 1984; (2) **Pocketbooks and Manuals**: Eisenberg et al, 1980; Fairbanks, 1980; *American Academy of Pediatrics Redbook*, 1982; Conte and Barriere, 1984; Gardner and Provine, 1984; The Medical Letter, 1984, 1986; Nelson, 1985; Sanford, 1985, 1986; (3) **Reviews**: Cunha, 1982; Neu, 1982; Fekety, 1983, 1984, 1985; McHenry and Weinstein, 1983; Speck and Blumer, 1983; Wilkowske and Hermans, 1983; *Med Lett Drugs Ther*, 1984, 1986.

NOTE: In this Table, when the preferred drug therapy is a penicillin derivative, but the patient is allergic to this class of antibiotics, the first nonpenicillin drug (or combination) listed usually becomes the preferred drug therapy. However, skin testing and desensitization may be indicated for certain serious infections (eg, infective endocarditis). Cephalosporins should not be administered to patients who have experienced an immediate-type hypersensitivity reaction to penicillins (see Chapters 66, Penicillins, and 67, Cephalosporins and Related Agents, respectively, for the names of specific penicillin and cephalosporin analogues).

SKIN INFECTIONS

Impetigo, Nonbullous

The primary causative organism is *Streptococcus pyogenes* (group A, beta hemolytic, gram-positive cocci). Frequently, mixtures of *S. pyogenes* and *Staphylococcus aureus* (gram-positive cocci) are isolated from lesions, but the staphylococci traditionally have been considered to be secondary invaders.

Systemic (usually oral) antimicrobial drug therapy is indicated and usually is EMPIRIC based on the clinical presentation. Presently, there is some controversy on the most appropriate drug selection for nonbullous impetigo. Traditionally, therapy has been directed only against *S. pyogenes* even when *S. aureus* also is present, because the staphylococci have been assumed to be secondary colonizers. However, a number of experts now believe that *S. aureus* also can be pathogenic and they recommend antimicrobial drugs that are active against both *S. pyogenes* and penicillinase-producing *S. aureus*. Debridement and cleansing of lesions also are indicated.

Selected references: Dillon, 1980; Melish, 1981 A; Witkowski and Parish, 1982; Schachner et al, 1983; Aly and Maibach, 1984; Conte and Barriere, 1984; Swartz, 1984; Nelson, 1985; Sanford, 1985; Magnussen, 1986. See also Chapter 74, Topical Anti-Infective Agents: Drugs Used on Skin and Mucous Membranes.

EMPIRIC THERAPY

(A) *Streptococcus pyogenes* only

PREFERRED THERAPY:
Penicillin V potassium
ALTERNATIVE THERAPY:
Erythromycin; Penicillin G Benzathine (IM)
REMARKS:
(1) Duration of therapy with oral antibiotics is 10 days. A single intramuscular injection of penicillin G benzathine is equally effective and is preferred when patient compliance is a likely problem.
(2) Penicillin V potassium usually is preferred to penicillin G (orally, for 10 days) because it is more acid-stable, provides greater and more reliable bioavailability, and can be taken with meals.
(3) Of the agents listed, only erythromycin is active against penicillinase-producing strains of *S. aureus*. However, in recent experience, between 5% and 10% of these strains derived from skin infections have been erythromycin-resistant.

(B) *Streptococcus pyogenes* and *Staphylococcus aureus* (penicillinase-producing)

PREFERRED THERAPY:
Cloxacillin (or Dicloxacillin)
ALTERNATIVE THERAPY:

Erythromycin; Oral cephalosporin (cephalexin, cephradine); Clindamycin
REMARKS:
(1) Cloxacillin and dicloxacillin generally are preferred to oxacillin and nafcillin for oral administration because they are better and more reliably absorbed.

Impetigo, Bullous

The causative organism is *Staphylococcus aureus* (usually group II, phage type 71). Bullae represent an exfoliative reaction of the epidermis to an exotoxin (exfoliatin) elaborated by this strain of *S. aureus*.

Systemic (usually oral) antimicrobial drug therapy is indicated and usually is EMPIRIC based on the clinical presentation. Debridement and cleansing of lesions also are indicated.

Selected references: Dillon, 1980; Melish, 1981 A; Witkowski and Parish, 1982; Schachner et al, 1983; Aly and Maibach, 1984; Swartz, 1984; Nelson, 1985; Magnussen, 1986. See also Chapter 74: Topical Anti-Infective Agents, Drugs Used on Skin and Mucous Membranes.

EMPIRIC THERAPY
(*Staphylococcus aureus* [penicillinase-producing])

PREFERRED THERAPY:
Cloxacillin (or Dicloxacillin)
ALTERNATIVE THERAPY:
Erythromycin; Oral cephalosporin (cephalexin, cephradine); Clindamycin

REMARKS:
(1) Cloxacillin and dicloxacillin generally are preferred to oxacillin and nafcillin for oral administration because they are better and more reliably absorbed.

Staphylococcal Scalded Skin Syndrome

The staphylococcal scalded skin syndrome usually occurs in neonates and young children and is a potentially severe disease caused by the exfoliative toxin of *Staphylococcus aureus* (usually phage group II).

Parenteral antimicrobial drug therapy is indicated initially and usually is EMPIRIC based on the clinical presentation and skin biopsy. Supportive therapy (eg, fluid and electrolyte replacement) also is indicated.

Selected references: Melish, 1981 B; Swartz, 1984; Nelson, 1985.

EMPIRIC THERAPY
(*Staphylococcus aureus* [penicillinase-producing])

PREFERRED THERAPY:
Nafcillin OR Oxacillin
ALTERNATIVE THERAPY:
Cefazolin, Cephalothin, or Cephapirin; Vancomycin; Clindamycin
REMARKS:
(1) Methicillin is not recommended (except in newborns) because it is associated with a higher incidence of interstitial nephritis.
(2) If methicillin-resistant strains of *S. aureus* are suspected, substitute vancomycin for the antistaphylococcal penicillin.

Folliculitis, Furunculosis, and Carbuncles

The vast majority of these infections are caused by *Staphylococcus aureus* (gram-positive cocci).

Most cases of folliculitis and mild furunculosis can be controlled by local measures (eg, warm soaks to encourage spontaneous drainage). Carbuncles and furuncles with surrounding cellulitis and/or fever, or if located in the midfacial area, require systemic (usually oral) antibiotic therapy. Drug selection is usually EMPIRIC (based on the clinical presentation) or based on Gram stain. Drainage of these large, fluctuant cutaneous abscesses (except possibly on lips and nose) also is indicated.

Selected references: Melish, 1981 C; Witkowski and Parish, 1982; Aly and Maibach, 1984; Conte and Barriere, 1984; Swartz, 1984; Magnussen, 1986. See also Chapter 74, Topical Anti-Infective Agents: Drugs Used on Skin and Mucous Membranes.

EMPIRIC THERAPY
(*Staphylococcus aureus* [penicillinase-producing])

PREFERRED THERAPY:
Cloxacillin OR Dicloxacillin
ALTERNATIVE THERAPY:
Erythromycin; Oral cephalosporin (cephalexin; cephradine); Clindamycin
REMARKS:
(1) Cloxacillin and dicloxacillin generally are preferred to oxacillin and nafcillin for oral administration because they are better and more reliably absorbed.
(2) Recurrent furunculosis is a problem in certain patients and is associated with persistent colonization of the anterior nares by coagulase-positive *S. aureus*. In addition to careful skin cleansing, care of clothing, and care of dressings, application of topical antibiotics (eg, neomycin, bacitracin) to nasal vestibules may prevent recurrences. Rifampin (adults, orally 600 mg daily for 10 days) has been shown to eradicate these organisms from most nasal carriers for up to 12 weeks (Wheat et al, 1983). This agent, given in combination with an antistaphylococcal penicillin to prevent the emergence of rifampin-resistant *S. aureus*, may be useful in managing recurrent furunculosis in those patients in whom other measures have failed.

Whirlpool Folliculitis

A folliculitis caused by *Pseudomonas aeruginosa* is associated with improperly maintained whirlpools, hot tubs, and swimming pools. The disease is usually self-limiting (Gustafson et al, 1983; see also Chapter 74, Topical Anti-Infective Agents: Drugs Used on Skin and Mucous Membranes).

Ecthyma

The primary causative organism is *Streptococcus pyogenes* (group A, beta hemolytic, gram-positive cocci).

Systemic (usually oral) antimicrobial drug therapy is indicated and usually is EMPIRIC based on the clinical presentation. Debridement and cleansing of lesions also are indicated.

Selected references: Witkowski and Parish, 1982; Aly and Maibach, 1984; Swartz, 1984. See also Chapter 74, Topical

Anti-Infective Agents: Drugs Used on Skin and Mucous Membranes.

EMPIRIC THERAPY
(*Streptococcus pyogenes*)

PREFERRED THERAPY:
Penicillin V potassium
ALTERNATIVE THERAPY:
Erythromycin
REMARKS:
(1) Penicillin V potassium usually is preferred to penicillin G (oral) because it is more acid-stable, provides greater and more reliable bioavailability, and can be taken with meals.

Erysipelas

The primary causative organism is *Streptococcus pyogenes* (group A, beta hemolytic, gram-positive cocci).

Systemic antimicrobial drug therapy is necessary and usually is EMPIRIC based on the clinical presentation. Oral or parenteral administration may be indicated initially, depending on the severity of the infection.

Selected references: Melish, 1981 C; Witkowski and Parish, 1982; Aly and Maibach, 1984; Conte and Barriere, 1984; Swartz, 1984; Nelson, 1985; Magnussen, 1986. See also Chapter 74, Topical Anti-Infective Agents: Drugs Used on Skin and Mucous Membranes.

EMPIRIC THERAPY
(*Streptococcus pyogenes*)

PREFERRED THERAPY:
Penicillin V potassium (oral) OR **Penicillin G Procaine (IM)** OR **Penicillin G (IV)** depending on severity
ALTERNATIVE THERAPY:
Erythromycin (oral); Cephalosporin (oral cephalexin, cephradine; parenteral cefazolin, cephalothin, cephapirin)
REMARKS:
(1) Penicillin V potassium usually is preferred to penicillin G (oral) because it is more acid-stable, provides greater and more reliable bioavailability, and can be taken with meals.

Cellulitis

The vast majority of these infections are caused by *Streptococcus pyogenes* (group A, beta hemolytic, gram-positive cocci) and *Staphylococcus aureus*. *Haemophilus influenzae* type b is a common cause of cellulitis in children less than 5 years, but is a rare pathogen in adults. It most commonly occurs as a unilateral infection of the cheek (buccal or facial cellulitis), has a blue-red to purple-red color, and is not associated with a primary portal of entry (eg, cut, laceration, insect bite). Enteric gram-negative bacilli (eg, *Escherichia coli*, *Klebsiella, Enterobacter*) are occasional pathogens, usually in patients with complicating factors (eg, immunosuppression, diabetes mellitus).

Systemic antimicrobial drug therapy is necessary and usually is EMPIRIC based on the clinical presentation. Oral or parenteral administration may be indicated initially, depending on the severity of the infection. Some experts recommend needle aspiration of the leading edge of the cellulitis to obtain material for Gram stain and culture, but the yield is usually low. Blood cultures may be positive when there is associated bacteremia.

Selected references: Melish, 1981 C; Witkowski and Parish, 1982; Carter and Feldman, 1983; Aly and Maibach, 1984; Swartz, 1984; Nelson, 1985; Sanford, 1985; Hook et al, 1986; Magnussen, 1986. See also Chapter 74, Topical Anti-Infective Agents: Drugs Used on Skin and Mucous Membranes.

EMPIRIC THERAPY

(A) Cellulitis (Majority of Cases)
(*Streptococcus pyogenes* and *Staphylococcus aureus* [penicillinase-producing])

PREFERRED THERAPY:
Cloxacillin (or Dicloxacillin) (oral)
OR
Nafcillin (or Oxacillin) (parenteral) depending on severity
ALTERNATIVE THERAPY:
Erythromycin (oral); Cephalosporin (oral cephalexin, cephradine; parenteral cefazolin, cephalothin, cephapirin); Vancomycin (parenteral); Clindamycin (oral or parenteral)
REMARKS:
(1) Cloxacillin and dicloxacillin generally are preferred to oxacillin and nafcillin for oral administration because they are better and more reliably absorbed.
(2) Most experts do not recommend methicillin because of an increased risk of interstitial nephritis.
(3) Penicillin G parenterally or penicillin V potassium orally should be substituted for antistaphylococcal penicillins if *Streptococcus pyogenes* is shown to be the causative organism or susceptibility of *S. aureus* strain is proven.
(4) For methicillin-resistant strains of *S. aureus*, vancomycin is the drug of choice.

(B) Facial cellulitis in children less than 5 years
(*Haemophilus influenzae* type b, *Staphylococcus aureus*, and *Streptococcus pyogenes*)

PREFERRED THERAPY:
Cefuroxime
OR
Nafcillin (or Oxacillin) *plus* **Chloramphenicol**
ALTERNATIVE THERAPY:
Cefotaxime; Ceftizoxime; Ceftriaxone
REMARKS:
(1) Switch to most effective drug regimen after culture and susceptibility test results are available.
(2) Cefuroxime, despite less clinical experience, appears to be superior to cefamandole for this indication. Cefuroxime has increased stability to *H. influenzae* TEM-1 beta lactamase, a longer half-life, and a better adverse reaction profile and most importantly, has not been associated with "breakthrough" *H. influenzae* type b meningitis, presumably because it can penetrate into cerebrospinal fluid more effectively than cefamandole (see Nelson, 1983). Cefamandole is NOT recommended as an initial therapy for children less than 5 years because of its poor penetration into the cerebrospinal fluid.
(3) The above regimens also are recommended empirically in children less than 5 years with periorbital cellulitis or with cellulitis in other sites when accompanied by high fever or significant toxicity, evidence of infection elsewhere (eg, meningitis), or if the lesion has a blue-red to purple-red discoloration.

Erythrasma

The causative organism is *Corynebacterium minutissimum*. Local treatment may be sufficient for mild cases. Systemic (usually oral) antimicrobial drug therapy is indicated for persistent and/or widespread disease.

Selected references: Duncan, 1983; Aly and Maibach, 1984; Swartz, 1984. See also Chapter 74, Topical Anti-Infective Agents: Drugs Used on Skin and Mucous Membranes.

SPECIFIC THERAPY
Corynebacterium minutissimum
(gram-positive bacilli)

> PREFERRED THERAPY:
> **Erythromycin**

Superficial Fungal Infections

Dermatophytic infections (tinea capitis, tinea corporis, tinea cruris, tinea pedis, and tinea unguium) are caused by species of *Trichophyton, Epidermophyton,* and *Microsporum*. Mucocutaneous mycotic infections include only candidiasis, which is caused by *Candida albicans*. For treatment guidelines, see Chapter 74, Topical Anti-Infective Agents: Drugs Used on Skin and Mucous Membranes.

Scabies

The causative organism is the itch mite, *Sarcoptes scabiel*. For treatment guidelines, see Chapter 74, Topical Anti-Infective Agents: Drugs Used on Skin and Mucous Membranes.

Pediculosis

Pediculosis in man is caused by three types of lice: *Phthirus pubis* (crab louse), *Pediculus humanus* (body louse), and *Pediculus capitis* (head louse). For treatment guidelines, see Chapter 74, Topical Anti-Infective Agents: Drugs Used on Skin and Mucous Membranes.

Acne Vulgaris

Acne vulgaris, a chronic inflammatory disease of the sebaceous glands, is believed to be associated with the bacterium *Propionibacterium (Corynebacterium) acnes*. For treatment guidelines, see Chapter 56, Dermatologic Preparations.

Cold Sores (Labial Herpes)

The causative organism is herpes simplex virus. Antiviral therapy in the normal host currently is investigational and specific recommendations are NOT available. For additional discussion, see Chapter 79, Antiviral Agents.

Shingles (Varicella-Zoster)

The causative organism is varicella-zoster virus. Antiviral therapy in the normal host currently is investigational and specific recommendations are NOT available. For additional discussion, see Chapter 79, Antiviral Agents.

Decubitus Ulcers, with Sepsis

Causative organisms include *Staphylococcus aureus* (gram-positive cocci); streptococci (gram-positive cocci), including *S. pyogenes* and enterococci; aerobic gram-negative bacilli, including Enterobacteriaceae and *Pseudomonas aeruginosa*; and anaerobic bacteria, including *Bacteroides fragilis* (gram-negative bacilli), gram-positive cocci, and clostridia (gram-positive bacilli).

Antimicrobial drug therapy (parenteral) initially is EMPIRIC pending results of blood cultures. Broad spectrum antibacterial coverage against both aerobic bacteria (enteric gram-negative bacilli, *S. aureus*, non-group D streptococci) and anaerobic bacteria, especially *B. fragilis*, is necessary. Some experts also recommend coverage against enterococci (*S. faecalis*). Local (eg, pressure relief, debridement of necrotic tissue) and supportive (eg, nutritional replenishment) therapy also are indicated.

Selected references: Conte and Barriere, 1984; Cooney and Reuler, 1984; Sanford, 1985; Magnussen, 1986. See also Chapter 74, Topical Anti-Infective Agents: Drugs Used on Skin and Mucous Membranes.

EMPIRIC THERAPY
(Gram-negative enteric bacilli [Enterobacteriaceae]; *Pseudomonas aeruginosa*; *Bacteroides fragilis* and other anaerobic bacteria [eg, *Peptococcus, Peptostreptococcus*, clostridia]; *Staphylococcus aureus*; non-group D streptococci [eg, *S. pyogenes*]; *Streptococcus faecalis* [group D; enterococci])

> PREFERRED THERAPY:
> **Clindamycin *plus* Aminoglycoside (gentamicin, tobramycin, amikacin, netilmicin) *with or without* Penicillin G (or Ampicillin)**
> ALTERNATIVE THERAPY:
> **Chloramphenicol *plus* Aminoglycoside**
> REMARKS:
> (1) The above regimens were obtained from literature sources. However, many additional regimens were considered reasonable alternatives by our consultants. Regimens suggested by at least two or more consultants include: Metronidazole *plus* aminoglycoside *with or without* penicillin G (or ampicillin); cefoxitin *with or without* aminoglycoside; mezlocillin (or piperacillin) *plus* aminoglycoside; cefazolin *plus* mezlocillin (or piperacillin); nafcillin (or oxacillin) *plus* mezlocillin (or piperacillin); imipenem/cilastatin alone.
> (2) Switch to most effective drug regimen after culture and susceptibility test results are available.

Burns, Infected (Sepsis)

The most common causative organisms are gram-negative bacilli, including *Escherichia coli, Klebsiella, Enterobacter, Proteus, Providencia, Serratia marcescens,* and *Pseudomonas aeruginosa*. Frequently, these are hospital-acquired (nosocomial) pathogens that may be resistant to conventional antibiotics. *Staphylococcus aureus* also is an important cause of infection in burn patients. Methicillin-resistant strains may be prevalent in some hospitals.

Systemic (parenteral) antimicrobial drug therapy is indicated for infected burns and, ultimately, drug selection should be specific based on culture and susceptibility data. When the causative organism is unknown, EMPIRIC therapy, as outlined below, is indicated initially. Appropriate local (eg, debridement) and supportive (eg, nutritional replenishment) treatment measures also are required. This includes the topical application of antimicrobial agents (silver sulfadiazine, mafenide acetate) to control infection within the essentially avascular burn eschar (see Chapter 74, Topical Anti-Infective Agents: Drugs Used on Skin and Mucous Membranes).

Selected references: Burke, 1979; Demling, 1983, 1985; Conte and Barriere, 1984; Sanford, 1985.

EMPIRIC THERAPY
(Gram-negative bacilli [as listed above];
Staphylococcus aureus)

> PREFERRED THERAPY:
> **Nafcillin (or Oxacillin)** *plus* **Aminoglycoside (gentamicin, tobramycin, amikacin, netilmicin)**
> OR
> **Antipseudomonal Penicillin (carbenicillin, ticarcillin, mezlocillin, piperacillin, azlocillin)** *plus* **Aminoglycoside**
> ALTERNATIVE THERAPY:
> **Cephalosporin** *plus* **Aminoglycoside; Vancomycin** *plus* **Aminoglycoside**
> REMARKS:
> (1) Definitive guidelines for empiric therapy are not available. Each of the above combination regimens has been suggested by various infectious disease experts. An antistaphylococcal agent (nafcillin or oxacillin; cefazolin, cephalothin, or cephapirin; vancomycin) plus an aminoglycoside provides optimum activity against *S. aureus* and adequate coverage against most gram-negative bacilli. Vancomycin is required for methicillin-resistant *S. aureus* strains. Combining an antipseudomonal penicillin with an aminoglycoside provides optimum activity against *P. aeruginosa* and increased coverage against other gram-negative bacilli but may be inadequate for staphylococcal infections. A second or third generation cephalosporin plus an aminoglycoside also increases coverage against gram-negative bacilli and may be adequate for *S. aureus*. Ceftazidime is the preferred cephalosporin for *P. aeruginosa*. The regimen selected for the individual patient should depend on the particular clinical situation and the likelihood of specific pathogens being involved (eg, organism(s) isolated from recent culture; organism(s) that are currently prevalent in the burn unit). Furthermore, the particular aminoglycoside, cephalosporin, antistaphylococcal agent, and/or antipseudomonal penicillin used for empiric therapy should be selected on the basis of locally generated antibiotic susceptibility profiles.
> (2) Switch to most effective drug regimen after culture and susceptibility test results are available.

CENTRAL NERVOUS SYSTEM INFECTIONS

Meningitis, Bacterial

The most common causative organisms vary with patient age and are usually subdivided according to the following three age groups:

(1) OLDER CHILDREN AND ADULTS: The most frequently encountered pathogens are *Streptococcus pneumoniae* (pneumococcus) and *Neisseria meningitidis* (meningococcus); the incidence of meningitis due to *Escherichia coli* and other Enterobacteriaceae increases in adults over 60 years;

(2) CHILDREN 1 MONTH TO 6 YEARS: The most common causative organism is *Haemophilus influenzae* type b; *N. meningitidis* and *S. pneumoniae* also are encountered;

(3) NEONATES LESS THAN 1 MONTH: The predominant organisms are group B streptococci *(Streptococcus agalactiae)*, *E. coli* and other gram-negative enteric bacilli, and *Listeria monocytogenes*; streptococci other than group B also may be encountered.

Antimicrobial drug therapy of bacterial meningitis can be either SPECIFIC (ie, when the causative organism is known or highly suspected based on results of a Gram stain or a rapid diagnostic test such as counter-immunoelectrophoresis [CIE] or latex agglutination) or EMPIRIC (ie, when the bacterial etiology is unknown, but the institution of effective antimicrobial drug therapy is mandatory). Parenteral, preferably intravenous, antimicrobial drug administration is necessary.

Selected references: Bell, 1981; Parker, 1981; Neu, 1982; Pfenninger et al, 1982; Rahal and Simberkoff, 1982; Report from a Swedish Study Group, 1982; Del Rio et al, 1983; McCracken and Nelson, 1983; Nelson, 1983; Steele and Bradsher, 1983; Barriere and Flaherty, 1984; Congeni, 1984; McCracken et al, 1984; McGee and Kaiser, 1984; *Med Lett Drugs Ther*, 1984, 1986; Schaad et al, 1984; Barson et al, 1985; Bryan et al, 1985; Jacobs et al, 1985; Naqvi et al, 1985; Steele, 1985; Cherubin and Eng, 1986; Van Voris and Roberts, 1986; Whitby and Finch, 1986.

SPECIFIC THERAPY

Streptococcus pneumoniae
(gram-positive cocci)

> PREFERRED THERAPY:
> **Penicillin G**
> ALTERNATIVE THERAPY:
> **Chloramphenicol; Cefuroxime; Cefotaxime; Ceftizoxime; Ceftriaxone**
> REMARKS:
> (1) Susceptibility testing (via oxacillin disc or MIC) is recommended because penicillin G-insensitive and penicillin G-resistant strains have been reported. Chloramphenicol may be effective against insensitive strains; vancomycin is active in vitro against totally resistant strains (Tweardy et al, 1983).
> (2) Chloramphenicol is bactericidal for *S. pneumoniae*.

Neisseria meningitidis
(gram-negative cocci)

> PREFERRED THERAPY:
> **Penicillin G**
> ALTERNATIVE THERAPY:
> **Chloramphenicol; Cefuroxime; Cefotaxime; Ceftizoxime; Ceftriaxone; Ceftazidime**
> REMARKS:
> (1) Penicillin G is not effective for prophylaxis of the meningococcal carrier state; rifampin is the drug of choice (see Table 3, Antimicrobial Chemoprophylaxis for Ambulatory Patients).
> (2) Chloramphenicol is a bactericidal antibiotic for *N. meningitidis*.

Haemophilus influenzae (type b)
(gram-negative bacilli)

PREFERRED THERAPY:
Ampicillin *plus* Chloramphenicol initially
ALTERNATIVE THERAPY:
Chloramphenicol alone; Cefotaxime; Cefuroxime; Ceftizoxime; Ceftriaxone; Ceftazidime
REMARKS:
(1) Beta lactamase-producing strains are resistant to ampicillin and rare strains are resistant to chloramphenicol (some are resistant to both antibiotics). Therefore, combined treatment is recommended until susceptibility is determined. Ampicillin usually is preferred for sensitive strains.
(2) Chloramphenicol is a bactericidal antibiotic for *H. influenzae*.
(3) Ampicillin is not effective for prophylaxis of the *H. influenzae* (type b) carrier state; rifampin is the drug of choice (see Table 3, Antimicrobial Chemoprophylaxis for Ambulatory Patients).

Streptococcus agalactiae (group B)
(gram-positive cocci)

PREFERRED THERAPY:
Penicillin G OR Ampicillin
ALTERNATIVE THERAPY:
See Remarks
REMARKS:
(1) Alternative antimicrobial therapy to the penicillins has not been studied.
(2) Penicillin-tolerant strains are occasionally encountered. Combination therapy with ampicillin (or penicillin G) *plus* an aminoglycoside (eg, gentamicin) is recommended (McCracken, 1983).

Escherichia coli and other aerobic gram-negative enteric bacilli

PREFERRED THERAPY:
Cefotaxime OR Ceftizoxime OR Ceftriaxone OR Ceftazidime
ALTERNATIVE THERAPY:
Aminoglycoside (gentamicin, tobramycin, amikacin, netilmicin) *with or without* Ampicillin; Chloramphenicol
REMARKS:
(1) Susceptibility testing is recommended.
(2) Presently, cefotaxime is the only listed third generation cephalosporin that is labeled for this indication. However, most of our consultants recommended the inclusion of ceftizoxime, ceftriaxone, and ceftazidime as suitable alternatives. Although moxalactam is labeled for aerobic gram-negative enteric bacillary meningitis, most of our consultants do not recommend this third generation cephalosporin because of serious bleeding disorders associated with its use (see also Chapter 67, Cephalosporins and Related Agents).
(3) Cefotaxime, ceftizoxime, ceftriaxone, and moxalactam are NOT recommended if *Pseudomonas aeruginosa* is a likely causative organism; only ceftazidime is active against this organism (see below).
(4) Aminoglycoside also may be given by lumbar intrathecal or intraventricular administration. Some of our consultants questioned the efficacy of these approaches.
(5) Chloramphenicol frequently is NOT bactericidal for gram-negative enteric bacilli in the central nervous system and high failure rates have been reported.
(6) Intravenous trimethoprim/sulfamethoxazole may be a useful alternative for gram-negative bacilli that are resistant to third generation cephalosporins (eg, *Acinetobacter calcoaceticus*, *Pseudomonas cepacia*, or *Flavobacterium meningosepticum*) (Levitz and Quintiliani, 1984). This combination is not active against *P. aeruginosa*, however.

Pseudomonas aeruginosa
(gram-negative bacilli)

PREFERRED THERAPY:
Antipseudomonal penicillin (carbenicillin, ticarcillin, mezlocillin, piperacillin, azlocillin) *plus* Aminoglycoside (gentamicin, tobramycin, amikacin, netilmicin)
ALTERNATIVE THERAPY:
Ceftazidime *plus* Aminoglycoside
REMARKS:
(1) Aminoglycoside is administered parenterally and intrathecally, either intralumbarly or intraventricularly through an Ommaya reservoir.
(2) Ceftazidime alone also has been effective in the treatment of *P. aeruginosa* meningitis in a limited number of patients (Fong and Tomkins, 1985). Because development of resistance is a concern, however, the authors recommended using a concomitant parenteral aminoglycoside for the first week of treatment.

Listeria monocytogenes
(gram-positive bacilli)

PREFERRED THERAPY:
Ampicillin *with or without* Aminoglycoside (gentamicin, tobramycin, amikacin, netilmicin)
ALTERNATIVE THERAPY:
Penicillin G *with or without* Aminoglycoside
REMARKS:
(1) Combination regimen is synergistic in vitro. Most consultants recommended combination therapy for *L. monocytogenes* meningitis.
(2) Aminoglycoside also may be given by lumbar intrathecal or intraventricular administration. Some of our consultants questioned the efficacy of these approaches.
(3) Trimethoprim/sulfamethoxazole may be a useful alternative in the penicillin-allergic patient (Levitz and Quintiliani, 1984).

EMPIRIC THERAPY
Empiric therapy of bacterial meningitis is based upon the patient's age for reasons presented above.

Adults (less than 60 years)
(*Streptococcus pneumoniae* and *Neisseria meningitidis*)

PREFERRED THERAPY:
Penicillin G
ALTERNATIVE THERAPY:
Chloramphenicol
REMARKS:
(1) Some penicillin G-insensitive or penicillin G-resistant *S. pneumoniae* have been reported (see earlier Remark).
(2) Because of the increasing incidence of *Haemophilus influenzae* (type b) meningitis in young adults and in some geographical areas, some experts substitute ampicillin for penicillin G, or use combination therapy with a penicillin plus chloramphenicol, or use a third generation cephalosporin, such as cefotaxime or ceftriaxone, that is active against all three organisms.
(3) In older adults (greater than 60 years), additional causative organisms (eg, *Escherichia coli*) should be considered and antimicrobial therapy directed accordingly (eg, cefotaxime, ceftriaxone).

Infants and children (1 month to 6 years)
(*Haemophilus influenzae* type b, *Neisseria meningitidis*, and *Streptococcus pneumoniae*)

PREFERRED THERAPY:
Ampicillin *plus* Chloramphenicol
ALTERNATIVE THERAPY:
Chloramphenicol alone; Cefuroxime; Cefotaxime; Ceftriaxone
REMARKS:
(1) Switch to most effective drug regimen after susceptibility test results are available.
(2) Some pediatric infectious disease consultants recommended that empiric coverage continue to include *H. influenzae* in children older than six years (eg, up to 12 years) because this organism causes bacterial meningitis in these older children.
(3) In infants between 1 and 3 months, group B streptococci also may be causative. Because ampicillin and chloramphenicol are antagonistic in vitro against this pathogen, most pediatric infectious disease experts recommended ampicillin *plus* cefotaxime (or ceftriaxone or cefuroxime) for empiric therapy of bacterial meningitis in this age group (see Nelson, 1985; Siegel, 1985).

Neonates (less than 1 month)
(*Streptococcus agalactiae* [group B], *Escherichia coli* and other gram-negative enteric bacilli, *Listeria monocytogenes*, and other streptococci)

PREFERRED THERAPY:
Ampicillin *plus* Aminoglycoside (gentamicin, tobramycin, amikacin, netilmicin)
ALTERNATIVE THERAPY:
Ampicillin *plus* Cefotaxime OR Ampicillin *plus* Ceftriaxone
REMARKS:
(1) Penicillin G may be substituted for ampicillin in these combination regimens.
(2) Some pediatric infectious disease consultants suggested that ampicillin *plus* moxalactam is another effective alternative regimen for this indication.
(3) No additional benefit from lumbar intrathecal or intraventricular administration of aminoglycoside has been shown in neonates and these routes are not recommended (McCracken, 1981).
(4) Switch to most effective drug regimen after susceptibility test results are available.

EAR INFECTIONS

Otitis Media, Acute

Acute otitis media is a very common infection in infants and children, particularly those under 3 years.

The most common causative organisms in all age groups are *Streptococcus pneumoniae* (pneumococcus) and *Haemophilus influenzae* (usually nontypable strains). Other pathogens include *Branhamella (Neisseria) catarrhalis*, *Streptococcus pyogenes* (group A, beta hemolytic), and, rarely, *Staphylococcus aureus*. The importance of *B. catarrhalis* as a pathogen appears to be increasing (Wald, 1984). In neonates up to 6 weeks, particularly those in nursery intensive care units, gram-negative enteric bacilli (eg, *Escherichia coli*) and *S. aureus* may cause up to 20% of cases.

Antimicrobial drug therapy (oral) in ADULTS, CHILDREN, and INFANTS is usually EMPIRIC and should be effective against the two most likely pathogens, *S. pneumoniae* and *H. influenzae*. In NEONATES, many experts recommend initial

treatment to be the same as for neonatal sepsis pending isolation of the causative organism (see Sepsis, Neonatal).

Selected references: Paradise, 1980; Schwartz and Schwartz, 1980; *Med Lett Drugs Ther*, 1981; Klein and Bluestone, 1982; McCracken, 1984.

EMPIRIC THERAPY
Adults, Children, and Infants (greater than 6 weeks)
(*Streptococcus pneumoniae* and *Haemophilus influenzae* [usually nontypable strains])

PREFERRED THERAPY:
Amoxicillin
ALTERNATIVE THERAPY:
Erythromycin *plus* Sulfisoxazole OR Trimethoprim/Sulfamethoxazole OR Cefaclor OR Amoxicillin/Potassium Clavulanate [Augmentin]
REMARKS:
(1) Although ampicillin is a cost-effective alternative, amoxicillin usually is preferred because it is better absorbed, requires fewer doses per day, can be taken with meals, and may cause less diarrhea. Other aminopenicillins (eg, bacampicillin, cyclacillin) do not appear to offer any important advantages over amoxicillin.
(2) All alternative regimens should be effective for infections caused by amoxicillin-resistant (beta lactamase-producing) strains of *H. influenzae*. Such strains are prevalent (eg, up to 40%) in some geographic areas. The majority of *B. catarrhalis* strains also produce beta lactamase.
(3) An alternative regimen (except Augmentin) should be used in patients allergic to penicillin. However, cefaclor should not be used in patients who have experienced an immediate-type hypersensitivity reaction to penicillin.
(4) Some consultants suggested doxycycline as a possible alternative in penicillin-allergic adults. This drug should not be given to pregnant women or children under 8 years.

External Otitis

External otitis is a common inflammatory condition involving the skin of the external auditory canal. When there is a breakdown in the natural defenses, inflammation and secondary infection may ensue. The most common causative bacteria are *Pseudomonas aeruginosa*, *Escherichia coli*, *Staphylococcus aureus*, streptococci, or species of *Proteus*.

EMPIRIC THERAPY
PREFERRED THERAPY:
Topical (otic) neomycin *plus* polymyxin B (or colistin)
ALTERNATIVE THERAPY:
Topical (otic) acetic acid
REMARKS:
(1) Cleansing the ear canal is the most important part of therapy.
(2) Topical (otic) chloramphenicol is indicated only if the causative organism is proven to be susceptible.

EYE INFECTIONS

Conjunctivitis, Bacterial

The most common causative organisms in purulent bacterial conjunctivitis in adults, children, and infants (excluding neonates) are *Staphylococcus aureus*, *Streptococcus pneumo-*

niae, *Staphylococcus epidermidis, Haemophilus influenzae,*
and *Moraxella lacunata* (commonly isolated with *S. aureus*).
Nonpurulent conjunctivitis is commonly caused by viruses,
allergens, or chemical irritants.

EMPIRIC THERAPY
Adults, Children and Infants (Excluding Neonates)

PREFERRED THERAPY:
**Topical (ophthalmic) neomycin-bacitracin-polymyxin B.
Gramicidin may be substituted for bacitracin.**
ALTERNATIVE THERAPY:
Topical (ophthalmic) sulfacetamide
REMARKS:
(1) Topical (ophthalmic) gentamicin, tobramycin, chloramphenicol, tetracycline, or erythromycin is indicated if the causative organism is proven to be susceptible.

Ophthalmia Neonatorum

The most common causative organisms of infectious conjunctivitis during the first ten to twenty days of life are *Chlamydia trachomatis* (onset, 5 to 20 days), *Neisseria gonorrhoeae* (onset, 2 to 5 days), and *Staphylococcus aureus* (onset, variable). *Haemophilus influenzae* and *Streptococcus pneumoniae* also may be causative. Appropriate Gram stain and culture of exudate and diagnostic test for chlamydia (eg, culture, direct fluorescent antibody or Giemsa stained conjunctival scrapings) are necessary to determine the causative organism.

Inclusion conjunctivitis due to *C. trachomatis* and gonococcal ophthalmia are sexually transmitted diseases and treatment guidelines can be found in Table 2, Treatment of Sexually Transmitted Diseases (STD). Antimicrobial drug selection for ophthalmia neonatorum caused by *S. aureus* is shown below.

Ophthalmology consultation should be obtained promptly for patients with ophthalmia neonatorum.

Selected references: McCracken and Nelson, 1983; *Morbid Mortal Week Rep*, 1985; Nelson, 1985 A; Riley and Baker, 1986.

SPECIFIC THERAPY

Chlamydia trachomatis
REMARKS:
(1) See Table 2 for treatment guidelines.

Neisseria gonorrhoeae
(gram-negative cocci)
REMARKS:
(1) See Table 2 for treatment guidelines.

Staphylococcus aureus
(gram-positive cocci)

SERIOUS INFECTIONS

PREFERRED THERAPY:
Oxacillin (or Methicillin) (parenteral) *with or without* Neomycin (topical ophthalmic)

REMARKS:
(1) Nafcillin is not recommended for neonates by some experts because of its erratic pharmacokinetics, particularly in jaundiced infants; methicillin rarely is nephrotoxic in neonates (Nelson, 1985 B).
(2) Penicillin G should be substituted for antistaphylococcal penicillins if susceptibility is proven.
(3) For methicillin-resistant strains of *S. aureus*, vancomycin is the drug of choice.

MINOR INFECTIONS

PREFERRED THERAPY:
Neomycin (topical ophthalmic) only
ALTERNATIVE THERAPY:
Bacitracin (topical ophthalmic)
REMARKS:
(1) Systemic antimicrobial therapy is not required for minor infections.

UPPER RESPIRATORY TRACT INFECTIONS

Rhinitis, Acute

Acute rhinitis (common cold) is the most common upper respiratory tract infection. However, the etiology is viral and antimicrobial drug therapy is either NOT effective or practical.

Pharyngitis/Tonsillitis, Acute

The majority of these infections are caused by viruses for which antimicrobial drug therapy is NOT effective.

The most common cause of acute bacterial pharyngitis is the group A, beta hemolytic streptococcus (*Streptococcus pyogenes*). Streptococcal pharyngitis ("strep throat"), including scarlet fever, is most common in children between 5 and 15 years and is diagnosed by throat culture or by newer rapid diagnostic tests. Prevention of rheumatic fever is a primary treatment goal.

Less frequent, but important, causes of acute bacterial pharyngitis include *Neisseria gonorrhoeae* and *Corynebacterium diphtheriae*. Gonococcal pharyngitis is a sexually transmitted disease and treatment guidelines can be found in Table 2, Treatment of Sexually Transmitted Diseases (STD). Diphtheria is relatively rare in the United States today, but it is a potentially life-threatening disease.

Selected references: Levy et al, 1983; Shulman, 1984; Shulman et al, 1984; Gerber and Markowitz, 1985; *Morbid Mortal Week Rep*, 1985; Nelson, 1985; Hall and Douglas, 1986.

SPECIFIC THERAPY

Streptococcus pyogenes (group A, beta hemolytic)
(gram-positive cocci)

PREFERRED THERAPY:
Penicillin V potassium (orally, for 10 days) OR penicillin G benzathine (intramuscularly, single dose)
ALTERNATIVE THERAPY:
Erythromycin (orally, for 10 days)

REMARKS:
(1) Penicillin V potassium usually is preferred to penicillin G (orally, for 10 days) because it is more acid stable, provides greater and more reliable bioavailability, and can be taken with meals.
(2) Recently, it has been reported that early penicillin treatment of streptococcal pharyngitis can rapidly relieve symptoms in children (Nelson, 1984; Krober et al, 1985; Randolph et al, 1985), suggesting that initiation of drug therapy before the results of throat culture are available may be beneficial. However, this issue is controversial (see Smith, 1984; Fulginiti, 1985). The availability of new rapid diagnostic tests for group A streptococci that are fairly sensitive and highly specific may make earlier diagnosis and, therefore, immediate initiation of specific therapy possible (*Med Lett Drugs Ther*, 1985).

Neisseria gonorrhoeae
(gram-negative cocci)
REMARKS:
(1) See Table 2 for treatment guidelines.

Corynebacterium diphtheriae
(gram-positive bacilli)

PREFERRED THERAPY:
Antitoxin *plus* Penicillin G
ALTERNATIVE THERAPY:
Antitoxin *plus* Erythromycin
REMARKS:
(1) Antitoxin is necessary to neutralize toxin produced by *C. diphtheriae*; antimicrobial therapy eradicates the organism and prevents spread.

Laryngitis, Acute

Acute laryngitis is caused by viruses for which antimicrobial drug therapy is NOT effective.

Laryngotracheitis, Acute

Acute laryngotracheitis (viral croup) usually occurs in children under 3 years. It is caused by viruses for which antimicrobial drug therapy is NOT effective. (NOTE: Bacterial tracheitis is a relatively rare syndrome that mimics viral croup. Causative organisms include *Staphylococcus aureus*, group A β-hemolytic streptococci and *Haemophilus influenzae* type b. Empiric therapy with intravenous antibiotics should be rapidly initiated. Nafcillin plus chloramphenicol OR Cefuroxime OR Third generation cephalosporin [eg, cefotaxime] are possible regimens.)

Epiglottitis, Acute

Acute epiglottitis is seen most frequently in children between 2 and 7 years, but may occur at any age. The causative organism usually is *Haemophilus influenzae* (type b).
This rapidly progressive and potentially fatal disease should be considered a medical emergency. MAINTENANCE OF AN ADEQUATE AIRWAY IS OF PRIMARY IMPORTANCE. Antimicrobial drug therapy (parenteral) is initially EMPIRIC pending the results of cultures and susceptibility tests.

Selected references: Zack, 1983; Nelson, 1985; Hall and Douglas, 1986.

EMPIRIC THERAPY
Children
(*Haemophilus influenzae* [type b])

PREFERRED THERAPY:
Ampicillin *plus* Chloramphenicol
ALTERNATIVE THERAPY:
Chloramphenicol alone; Cefotaxime; Ceftizoxime; Ceftriaxone; Ceftazidime; Cefuroxime
REMARKS:
(1) Beta lactamase-producing strains of *H. influenzae* (type b) are resistant to ampicillin and rare strains are resistant to chloramphenicol. Therefore, combined treatment is recommended until susceptibility is determined. Ampicillin usually is preferred for susceptible strains.
(2) Clinical experience with third generation cephalosporins (eg, cefotaxime) and cefuroxime is more limited, but these cephalosporin derivatives are highly active against *H. influenzae* in vitro, including beta lactamase-producing strains.
(3) Antimicrobial drug therapy of adults with acute epiglottitis appears to be the same as for children (see Cohen, 1984).

Sinusitis, Acute

The most common causative organisms in both adults and children are *Streptococcus pneumoniae* (pneumococcus) and *Haemophilus influenzae* (usually nontypable strains). *Branhamella (Neisseria) catarrhalis* (more common in children), *Streptococcus pyogenes* (group A, beta hemolytic), alpha hemolytic streptococci, and *Staphylococcus aureus* are isolated much less frequently.
Antimicrobial drug therapy (usually oral) in ADULTS AND CHILDREN is usually EMPIRIC and should be effective against the two most likely pathogens, *S. pneumoniae* and *H. influenzae*.

Selected references: Gwaltney et al, 1981; Gwaltney, 1983; Levy et al, 1983; Wald, 1983; Bluestone, 1985; Hall and Douglas, 1986.

EMPIRIC THERAPY
Adults and Children
(*Streptococcus pneumoniae* and *Haemophilus influenzae* [usually nontypable strains])

PREFERRED THERAPY:
Amoxicillin
ALTERNATIVE THERAPY:
Trimethoprim/Sulfamethoxazole OR **Cefaclor** OR **Erythromycin *plus* Sulfisoxazole** OR **Amoxicillin/Potassium Clavulanate [Augmentin]**
REMARKS:
(1) Although ampicillin is a cost-effective alternative, amoxicillin usually is preferred because it is better absorbed, requires fewer doses per day, can be taken with meals, and may cause less diarrhea. Other aminopenicillins (eg, bacampicillin) do not appear to offer any important advantages over amoxicillin.
(2) All alternative regimens should be effective for infections caused by amoxicillin-resistant (beta lactamase-producing) strains of *H. influenzae*. Such strains are prevalent (eg, up to 40%) in some geographic areas. The majority of *B. catarrhalis* strains also produce beta-lactamase.

(3) An alternative regimen (except Augmentin) should be used in penicillin-allergic patients. However, cefaclor should not be used in patients who have had an immediate-type hypersensitivity reaction to penicillin.

(4) Some consultants suggested doxycycline as a possible alternative in penicillin-allergic adults. This drug should not be given to pregnant women or children under 8 years.

(5) Prolonged sinus infection in inadequately treated or untreated patients can lead to chronic sinusitis, which is characterized by irreversible damage to the sinus mucous membrane. Anaerobic bacteria (*Bacteroides*, gram-positive anaerobic cocci, *Fusobacterium*) are the predominant organisms isolated (Frederick and Braude, 1974; Brook, 1981). Patients with chronic sinusitis should be referred to an otorhinolaryngologist. Surgical procedures to facilitate drainage may be necessary. Antimicrobial therapy may be useful for acute exacerbations.

(6) Some cases of sinusitis may be severe and parenteral antimicrobial therapy is required.

Influenza

Influenza is caused by influenza A or B virus. Conventional antibiotics are NOT effective for viral infections. Amantadine, if administered within 48 hours of onset of symptoms, is effective against influenza A infection; it also is effective for prophylaxis (see Chapter 79, Antiviral Agents).

LOWER RESPIRATORY TRACT INFECTIONS

Bronchitis, Acute and Bronchiolitis

Acute bronchitis is caused primarily by viruses for which antimicrobial drug therapy is NOT effective. *Mycoplasma pneumoniae* is occasionally the causative organism. Drug selection for this organism is listed below.

Bronchiolitis usually occurs in infants between 2 and 8 months. It is caused by viruses for which antimicrobial drug therapy is NOT effective.

Selected references: Gwaltney, 1984; Hall and Hall, 1984; *Med Lett Drugs Ther*, 1984, 1986.

SPECIFIC THERAPY
Mycoplasma pneumoniae

PREFERRED THERAPY:
Erythromycin OR **Tetracycline**
REMARKS:
(1) Tetracyclines should not be given to pregnant women or children under 8 years.

Acute Exacerbations of Chronic Bronchitis

Streptococcus pneumoniae (pneumococcus) and *Haemophilus influenzae* are the two bacterial species most frequently isolated from the sputum of patients with acute exacerbations of chronic bronchitis. Respiratory viruses and, to a lesser extent, *Mycoplasma pneumoniae* also have been associated with acute exacerbation. An unequivocal causative role of these organisms in acute exacerbations of chronic bronchitis remains to be determined, however.

The effectiveness of short-term antimicrobial drug therapy for acute exacerbations of chronic bronchitis is difficult to assess based on the available data and this area remains controversial. Many infectious disease experts recommend antimicrobial drug therapy (usually oral) directed against *S. pneumoniae* and *H. influenzae* (and possibly *M. pneumoniae*) in patients with increased cough and purulent sputum production, but without evidence of pneumonia. Treatment is continued or altered as indicated by patient response and/or results of sputum culture.

Selected references: Tager and Speizer, 1975; Fedson and Rusthoven, 1979; Nicotra et al, 1982; Smialowicz, 1982; Van Scoy, 1983; Hurst, 1984; Reynolds, 1984; Hall and Douglas, 1986.

EMPIRIC THERAPY
Adults

(*Streptococcus pneumoniae* and *Haemophilus influenzae* [and possibly *Mycoplasma pneumoniae*])

PREFERRED THERAPY:
Amoxicillin OR **Tetracycline (or Doxycycline)**
ALTERNATIVE THERAPY:
Trimethoprim/Sulfamethoxazole; Cefaclor; Amoxicillin/ Potassium Clavulanate [Augmentin]
REMARKS:
(1) Although ampicillin is a cost-effective alternative, amoxicillin usually is preferred because it is better absorbed, requires fewer doses per day, can be taken with meals, and may cause less diarrhea. Other aminopenicillins (eg, bacampicillin) do not appear to offer any important advantages over amoxicillin.

(2) Trimethoprim/sulfamethoxazole, cefaclor, and Augmentin should be effective for infections caused by amoxicillin-resistant (beta lactamase-producing) strains of *H. influenzae*. Such strains are prevalent (eg, up to 40%) in some geographic areas.

(3) Of the drugs listed, tetracycline (or doxycycline) is the only effective drug against *M. pneumoniae*. However, it is the least active drug against *S. pneumoniae* and *H. influenzae* and one of the alternative drugs may be required for tetracycline-resistant strains of these organisms. (Note: Some consultants prefer doxycycline to tetracycline because it is more active in vitro and exhibits better penetration into bronchial secretions.)

(4) Amoxicillin and Augmentin should not be used in penicillin-allergic patients; cefaclor should not be used in patients who have had an immediate-type hypersensitivity reaction to penicillin.

(5) Tetracyclines should not be given to pregnant women or children under 8 years.

Pertussis (Whooping Cough)

Selected references: *American Academy of Pediatrics Redbook*, 1982; Conte and Barriere, 1984; Geller, 1984; *Med Lett Drugs Ther*, 1984, 1986; Wilkins and Wehrle, 1984.

SPECIFIC THERAPY
Bordetella pertussis
(gram-negative bacilli)

PREFERRED THERAPY:
Erythromycin
ALTERNATIVE THERAPY:
Trimethoprim/Sulfamethoxazole; Tetracycline
REMARKS:
(1) Antimicrobial agents only reduce infectivity by eliminating *B. pertussis* carriage. There is not convincing evidence that they

affect the course of the disease syndrome, which is caused by a toxin. Supportive care is essential. Corticosteroids significantly alter the severity and duration of pertussis and may be indicated.

(2) Erythromycin orally (adults, 500 mg four times daily; children, 50 mg/kg daily in four divided doses) for 14 days appears to be the most effective regimen. (Note: A retrospective analysis of the literature suggests that erythromycin estolate has been more effective than erythromycin ethylsuccinate or erythromycin stearate in eliminating B. pertussis carriage, presumably due to better penetration of the estolate into respiratory secretions [Bass, 1985].) Less clinical experience has been obtained with the alternative antimicrobial agents.

(3) Ampicillin is active against B. pertussis in vitro, but does not reduce communicability or modify the clinical course. Pertussis Immune Globulin (Human) is of no value.

(4) Tetracyclines should not be given to pregnant women or children under 8 years.

Pneumonia

The most common causative organisms of community-acquired pneumonia in otherwise normal hosts are Streptococcus pneumoniae (acute bacterial [typical] pneumonia), viruses (viral pneumonias), and Mycoplasma pneumoniae (atypical pneumonia syndrome). Relative incidences are related to patient age as follows:

(1) ADULTS GREATER THAN 40 YEARS, S. pneumoniae;

(2) ADULTS LESS THAN 40 YEARS AND CHILDREN GREATER THAN 5 YEARS, M. pneumoniae;

(3) INFANTS AND CHILDREN LESS THAN 5 YEARS (EXCEPT NEWBORNS), viruses.

Acute bacterial pneumonias are much more common in debilitated elderly patients and persons with predisposing conditions. Although S. pneumoniae is usually the most common causative organism, other bacteria are also important pathogens in these patients. Common predisposing conditions and probable causative bacteria are as follows:

(1) CHRONIC OBSTRUCTIVE PULMONARY DISEASE: S. pneumoniae and Haemophilus influenzae;

(2) CHRONIC ALCOHOLISM: S. pneumoniae, anaerobic bacteria (aspiration pneumonia), H. influenzae, Klebsiella pneumoniae, Staphylococcus aureus, and Mycobacterium tuberculosis (tuberculosis);

(3) POSTINFLUENZA BACTERIAL PNEUMONIA: S. pneumoniae, S. aureus, and H. influenzae;

(4) ELDERLY NURSING HOME PATIENTS: S. pneumoniae, S. aureus, K. pneumoniae (and other gram-negative bacilli), and H. influenzae;

(5) PATIENTS WITH MENTAL OBTUNDATION, SWALLOWING PROBLEMS, ESOPHAGEAL DISORDERS, SEIZURE DISORDERS, AND POOR DENTAL HYGIENE: Anaerobic bacteria (aspiration pneumonia);

(6) CYSTIC FIBROSIS: Pseudomonas aeruginosa and S. aureus;

(7) IMMUNOCOMPROMISED HOSTS: Multiple etiologies, including gram-negative bacilli (eg, Escherichia coli, K. pneumoniae, P. aeruginosa), S. aureus, and other bacteria, as well as viral (eg, cytomegalovirus), fungal (eg, Aspergillus), and protozoal (eg, Pneumocystis carinii) pathogens. The likely spectrum of causative organisms will vary, depending on the cause of the immunodeficiency (eg, S. aureus, aerobic gram-negative bacilli, and Aspergillus are likely pathogens in neutropenic patients).

Additional causative organisms of atypical pneumonia syndromes include Legionella pneumophila, Chlamydia trachomatis, C. psittaci, and Coxiella burnetii. L. pneumophila, a gram-negative bacillus, is the etiologic agent in Legionnaires' disease. It can cause pneumonia in normal hosts and is a particularly important pathogen in elderly patients with predisposing conditions. The incidence of nonepidemic community-acquired pneumonia due to L. pneumophila has increased and is quite common in some reported series. C. trachomatis is a common cause of afebrile pneumonia in infants between 2 and 15 weeks of age who have acquired this sexually transmitted organism from mothers with genital infections. Ornithosis (C. psittaci) and Q fever (C. burnetii, a rickettsial organism) are relatively rare atypical pneumonias associated with exposure to birds and farm animals, respectively.

Ideally, antimicrobial drug selection for a patient with pneumonia should be based on the isolation of a specific causative organism from a site not usually colonized (eg, blood, pleural fluid, respiratory tract). However, this may be impossible or impractical in many cases. Thus, antimicrobial drug therapy of community-acquired pneumonia usually is initiated with varying degrees of empiricism based on a number of factors. These include: (1) an adequate history (eg, age, smoking and drinking habits, underlying diseases and predisposing conditions, immune status, recent exposure to specific pathogens, and occupational, travel, and animal exposure history); (2) the clinical presentation (eg, onset, fever, nature of cough, sputum, and pleuritic pain); and the results of (3) physical examination; (4) chest x-ray (eg, location of infiltrates, presence of consolidation, effusion, cavitation); (5) clinical laboratory tests (eg, white blood cell count); and, of particular importance, (6) Gram stain of a reliable sputum specimen (less than 10 squamous epithelial cells and greater than 25 polymorphonuclear leukocytes per low power field).

SPECIFIC THERAPY, as outlined below, can be employed when the causative organism is known or highly suspected based on the results of Gram stain and/or these other factors. When the specific etiologic agent is unknown and other factors make the diagnosis equivocal, the institution of rational EMPIRIC THERAPY usually is necessary.

Selected references: Brunton et al, 1982; Kannangara and LeFrock, 1982 A and B; Neu, 1982; Pennington, 1982; Francke, 1983; Long, 1983; Perlino, 1983; Rosenberg and LeFrock, 1983; Smith 1983; Van Scoy, 1983; Weinstein and Fields, 1983; Conte and Barriere, 1984; Donowitz and Mandell, 1984; Gleckman and Roth, 1984; Med Lett Drugs Ther, 1984, 1986; Nelson, 1985; Sanford, 1985; Teele, 1985; Betts and Reese, 1986.

SPECIFIC THERAPY (ACUTE BACTERIAL PNEUMONIA)

Streptococcus pneumoniae
(gram-positive cocci)

PREFERRED THERAPY:
Penicillin G (IV) OR **Penicillin G Procaine (IM)** OR **Penicillin V**

potassium (oral) depending on severity
ALTERNATIVE THERAPY:
Erythromycin; First Generation Cephalosporin (cefazolin, cephalothin, cephapirin, cephradine)
REMARKS:
(1) Rare strains of *S. pneumoniae* are totally resistant to penicillin G; these strains are susceptible to vancomycin.

Haemophilus influenzae
(gram-negative bacilli)

PREFERRED THERAPY:
Ampicillin *plus* Chloramphenicol initially
ALTERNATIVE THERAPY:
Chloramphenicol alone; Cefuroxime; Cefotaxime; Ceftizoxime; Ceftriaxone; Ceftazidime; Trimethoprim/Sulfamethoxazole
REMARKS:
(1) Beta lactamase-producing strains are resistant to ampicillin and rare strains are resistant to chloramphenicol. Therefore, combined treatment is recommended until susceptibility is determined. Ampicillin usually is preferred for sensitive strains.
(2) All alternative regimens should be effective against ampicillin-resistant strains of *H. influenzae*. Although clinical experience is more limited, many experts prefer cefuroxime or a third generation cephalosporin to chloramphenicol for these resistant strains or when susceptibility is unknown.
(3) Cefamandole is NOT recommended. Its activity against β-lactamase-producing *H. influenzae* is unreliable and it exhibits poor penetration into cerebrospinal fluid.

Staphylococcus aureus
(gram-positive cocci)

PREFERRED THERAPY:
Nafcillin OR Oxacillin
ALTERNATIVE THERAPY:
First Generation Cephalosporin (cefazolin, cephalothin, cephapirin, cephradine); Vancomycin
REMARKS:
(1) Most experts do not recommend methicillin in adults because of an increased risk of interstitial nephritis.
(2) Penicillin G should be substituted for antistaphylococcal penicillins if susceptibility is proven.
(3) For methicillin-resistant strains of *S. aureus*, vancomycin is the drug of choice.

Klebsiella pneumoniae and other gram-negative enteric bacilli

PREFERRED THERAPY:
Cefotaxime; Ceftizoxime; Ceftriaxone; Ceftazidime
ALTERNATIVE THERAPY:
First Generation Cephalosporin (cefazolin, cephalothin, cephapirin, cephradine) *plus* Aminoglycoside (gentamicin, tobramycin, amikacin, netilmicin)
REMARKS:
(1)Susceptibility testing is recommended.
(2) Increased nephrotoxicity has been observed when cephalothin is combined with an aminoglycoside. This has not been reported for other cephalosporins.

Pseudomonas aeruginosa
(gram-negative bacilli)

PREFERRED THERAPY:
Antipseudomonal Penicillin (carbenicillin, ticarcillin, mezlocillin, piperacillin, azlocillin) *plus* Aminoglycoside (gentamicin, tobramycin, amikacin, netilmicin)
ALTERNATIVE THERAPY:
Ceftazidime (or Cefoperazone) *plus* Aminoglycoside (gentamicin, tobramycin, amikacin, netilmicin)
REMARKS:
(1) Most experts recommend combination therapy for systemic infections caused by *P. aeruginosa*.

Anaerobic bacteria from oropharyngeal flora, including *Peptococcus, Peptostreptococcus, Fusobacterium*, and *Bacteroides* (aspiration pneumonia)

PREFERRED THERAPY:
Penicillin G
ALTERNATIVE THERAPY:
Clindamycin
REMARKS:
(1) Penicillin G-resistant strains of *Bacteroides* species (eg, *B. melaninogenicus*) have been increasing. Clindamycin is preferred for these organisms.

Mycobacterium tuberculosis
(acid fast bacilli)
REMARKS:
(1) See Chapter 75, Antimycobacterial Agents, for treatment guidelines.

SPECIFIC THERAPY (ATYPICAL PNEUMONIA SYNDROMES)

Mycoplasma pneumoniae

PREFERRED THERAPY:
Erythromycin OR Tetracycline
REMARKS:
(1) Tetracyclines should not be given to pregnant women or children under 8 years.

Legionella pneumophila
(gram-negative bacillus)

PREFERRED THERAPY:
Erythromycin *with or without* Rifampin
REMARKS:
(1) In those patients who fail to respond to erythromycin alone, who are critically ill, or who have severe underlying disease, rifampin can be added to erythromycin therapy. Rifampin should not be used alone, however, due to the rapid emergence of resistant organisms.

Chlamydia trachomatis (chlamydial pneumonia in infants)
REMARKS:
(1) See Table 2, Treatment of Sexually Transmitted Diseases (STD), for treatment guidelines.

Chlamydia psittaci (ornithosis; psittacosis)

PREFERRED THERAPY:
Tetracycline
ALTERNATIVE THERAPY:
Chloramphenicol
REMARKS:
(1) Tetracyclines should not be given to pregnant women or children under 8 years.

Coxiella burnetii (rickettsial organism responsible for Q fever)

PREFERRED THERAPY:
Tetracycline
ALTERNATIVE THERAPY:
Chloramphenicol
REMARKS:
(1) Tetracyclines should not be given to pregnant women or children under 8 years.

EMPIRIC THERAPY

Guidelines for empiric therapy of community-acquired pneumonia based on patient age and the presence of predisposing conditions (if any) are presented. However, it must be emphasized that no single regimen can cover all possible pathogens and antimicrobial drug selection for any given patient should take into consideration all relevant factors (see above).

Adults (no predisposing condition)

(*Streptococcus pneumoniae* and *Mycoplasma pneumoniae* are most likely; *Legionella pneumophila* is less common.)

PREFERRED THERAPY:
Erythromycin
REMARKS:
(1) If *L. pneumophila* is the likely causative organism, a larger dose of erythromycin is necessary.

Adults (chronic lung disease; alcoholism; postinfluenza pneumonia; debilitated elderly patients)

(*Streptococcus pneumoniae, Haemophilus influenzae, Staphylococcus aureus, Klebsiella pneumoniae*, oropharyngeal anaerobic bacteria, and *Legionella pneumophila*)

PREFERRED THERAPY:
Second Generation Cephalosporin (cefuroxime, cefoxitin, cefamandole) alone
OR
First Generation Cephalosporin (cefazolin, cephalothin, cephapirin, cephradine) *plus* Aminoglycoside (gentamicin, tobramycin, amikacin, netilmicin)
OR
Second Generation Cephalosporin (cefuroxime, cefoxitin, cefamandole) *plus* Aminoglycoside (gentamicin, tobramycin, amikacin, netilmicin)
REMARKS:
(1) Each of the above regimens has been suggested as preferred therapy by different experts. Selection of a particular regimen should depend on the individual clinical setting (eg, a second generation cephalosporin alone may be adequate for most patients with mild to moderate pneumonia). Some consultants also suggested ampicillin *plus* an aminoglycoside *with or without* nafcillin (or oxacillin) as an alternative regimen to those listed in order to provide better coverage against anaerobic bacteria.
(2) None of the above regimens is effective against *L. pneumophila*. Some experts recommend the addition of erythromycin to cover this pathogen.
(3) Third generation cephalosporins, especially cefotaxime, ceftizoxime, and ceftriaxone, should be effective against all of the above pathogens (except *L. pneumophila*). However, they generally are not recommended empirically for community-acquired pneumonias because these infections are not likely to be caused by multiple-drug-resistant gram-negative bacilli and third generation cephalosporins are very expensive and associated with the potential for emergence of resistant organisms.

(4) Switch to most effective drug regimen after susceptibility test results are available.

Children (greater than 5 years)

(*Mycoplasma pneumoniae* is most likely; *Streptococcus pneumoniae* is less common. Viruses also may cause pneumonia in this age group, but antimicrobial drug therapy is NOT effective.)

PREFERRED THERAPY:
Erythromycin

Infants and Children (less than 5 years; except newborns)

(Viruses are the most common causes of pneumonia in this age group, but antimicrobial drug therapy is NOT effective. *Streptococcus pneumoniae* and *Haemophilus influenzae* type b are the common bacterial causes and antimicrobial drug therapy should be directed against these pathogens when they are suspected.)

PREFERRED THERAPY:
Cefuroxime
OR
Ampicillin *plus* Chloramphenicol
ALTERNATIVE THERAPY:
Chloramphenicol alone; Cefotaxime; Ceftizoxime; Ceftriaxone
REMARKS:
(1) Switch to most effective drug regimen after susceptibility test results are available.
(2) Cefuroxime, despite less clinical experience, appears to be superior to cefamandole for this indication. Cefuroxime has increased stability to *H. influenzae* TEM-1 beta lactamase, a longer half-life, and a better adverse reaction profile and, most importantly, has not been associated with "breakthrough" *H. influenzae* type b meningitis, presumably because it can penetrate into cerebrospinal fluid more effectively than cefamandole (see Nelson, 1983). Cefamandole is NOT recommended as an initial therapy for children less than five years because of its poor penetration into cerebrospinal fluid.
(3) Some consultants recommended nafcillin (or oxacillin) *plus* chloramphenicol in the severely ill child to increase coverage against *Staphylococcus aureus*.
(4) For children who are well enough to be treated as outpatients, oral amoxicillin (alternative, erythromycin *plus* sulfisoxazole) is preferred.
(5) *Chlamydia trachomatis* may cause up to one-third of cases of pneumonia in infants between one and six months. If clinical suspicion of *C. trachomatis* is high, erythromycin should be added to the regimen. Infants in this age group who are treated as outpatients should receive erythromycin *plus* sulfisoxazole.

Neonates

REMARKS:
(1) Intrapartum bacterial pneumonia most frequently is caused by *Streptococcus agalactiae* (group B) and gram-negative enteric bacilli (eg, *Escherichia coli*). Initial antimicrobial drug therapy is the same as for neonatal sepsis pending isolation of the causative organism (see Sepsis, Neonatal).
(2) Afebrile pneumonia due to *Chlamydia trachomatis* is seen in neonates between 2 and 15 weeks; this sexually transmitted pathogen is acquired from infected mothers. See Table 2, Treatment of Sexually Transmitted Diseases (STD), for treatment guidelines. See also Infants and Children (Less Than 5 Years; Except Newborns) above for additional remarks.

INFECTIONS OF THE CARDIOVASCULAR SYSTEM

Endocarditis, Infective

Streptococci and staphylococci are the major causes of infective endocarditis, accounting for approximately 70% and 20% of cases, respectively. Bacterial endocarditis caused by streptococci usually occurs in patients with underlying heart disease and follows a subacute course. Viridans streptococci (eg, *S. sanguis, S. mutans, S. milleri, S. mitior*) cause about 40% of cases; enterococci (eg, *S. faecalis*) cause about 10% of cases; and nonhemolytic, microaerophilic, anaerobic, or nonenterococcal group D (eg, *S. bovis*) streptococci cause the remaining 20% of cases. *Staphylococcus aureus* (coagulase-positive) is the major cause of acute bacterial endocarditis. This pathogen can infect normal as well as diseased heart valves.

Prosthetic valve endocarditis is an infrequent but serious complication of cardiac valve replacement. *Staphylococcus epidermidis* (coagulase-negative) and *S. aureus* are common pathogens in both early onset (less than two months) and late onset (greater than two months) prosthetic valve endocarditis. Aerobic gram-negative bacilli (common), diphtheroids, fungi, and streptococci are other causes of early onset disease; streptococci are common causative organisms of late onset disease.

S. aureus (50%), streptococci (20%), including enterococci, gram-negative bacilli (20%), particularly *Pseudomonas aeruginosa*, and fungi (10%), primarily *Candida*, are the causative organisms of infective endocarditis in narcotic addicts.

The causative organism of infective endocarditis usually can be isolated from blood cultures, and antimicrobial drug therapy should be SPECIFIC and bactericidal for the offending pathogen. In patients with acute infective endocarditis, EMPIRIC therapy should be employed until the results of blood cultures are known. EMPIRIC therapy usually is unnecessary for subacute forms of the disease. Surgical removal of the infected valve also may be required; this is common in prosthetic valve endocarditis.

Host defense mechanisms play a minimal role in the control of infective endocarditis, and cure is dependent on the administration of adequate dosages (ie, prolonged, high-dose, parenteral administration) of *bactericidal* antibiotics. The usefulness of monitoring serum bactericidal activity is controversial (Scheld and Sande, 1984; Wolfson and Swartz, 1985). Achieving a peak serum bactericidal titer, ie, the killing activity of the patient's serum obtained at the anticipated peak serum antibiotic concentration, of at least 1:8 has been considered a desirable goal. However, a retrospective review of 17 studies failed to confirm any correlation between serum bactericidal activity and therapeutic success (Coleman et al, 1982). In a multicenter collaborative evaluation of a standardized serum bactericidal test, peak serum bactericidal titers of ≥64 mcg/ml and trough titers ≥ 32 mcg/ml were associated with bacteriologic cure; adjustment of antibiotic dosages to achieve these titers was recommended to provide optimal therapy of infective endocarditis (Weinstein et al, 1985). However, limitations of this study have been noted (Mellors et al, 1986; Weinstein et al, 1986).

Selected references: Sande and Scheld, 1980; Geraci and Wilson, 1982; Thompson, 1982; Van Scoy, 1982; Wilkowske, 1982; Wilson et al, 1982 A, B and C; Hoeprich and Durack, 1983; Gnann and Cobbs, 1984; Scheld and Sande, 1984; Nelson, 1985; Brandriss, 1986.

SPECIFIC THERAPY

Penicillin-sensitive streptococci (minimum inhibitory concentration [MIC] <0.2 mcg/ml), including most viridans streptococci and S̄. bovis (nonenterococcal group D) (gram-positive cocci)

PREFERRED THERAPY:
Penicillin G *with or without* Streptomycin
ALTERNATIVE THERAPY:
Cefazolin, Cephalothin, Cephapirin, or Cephradine; Vancomycin
REMARKS:
(1) The optimum preferred regimen has not been clearly identified and some controversy exists among experts. The following three regimens are suggested with advantages and disadvantages:
(a) Aqueous penicillin G (adults, 10-20 million U/day IV in divided doses every three to four hours) or penicillin G procaine (adults, 1.2 million U every six hours IM) for two weeks *plus* streptomycin (adults with normal renal function, 7.5 mg/kg [not to exceed 0.5 g] every 12 hours IM) for two weeks is considered by many to be the most cost-effective regimen for patients with native valve endocarditis who are less than 65 years without renal impairment, eighth nerve defects, or serious complications. However, other experts still prefer to treat penicillin-sensitive streptococcal endocarditis for four weeks.
(b) Aqueous penicillin G (adults, 10-20 million U/day IV in divided doses every three to four hours; children, 150,000 units/kg/day IV in divided doses every four to six hours) for four weeks is preferred in patients with relative contraindications to the use of streptomycin, including age greater than 65 years, renal impairment, or eighth nerve deficits. This is the preferred regimen of many experts for the majority of patients.
(c) Aqueous penicillin G (adults, 10-20 million U/day IV in divided doses every three to four hours; children, 150,000 units/kg/day IV in divided doses every four to six hours) for four weeks *plus* streptomycin (adults with normal renal function, 7.5 mg/kg [not to exceed 0.5 g] every 12 hours IM; children with normal renal function, 30 mg/kg/day IM in divided doses every 12 hours) for the initial two weeks is preferred for patients with complicated disease (eg, central nervous system involvement, shock, prosthetic valve). Some experts consider this the preferred regimen for all patients who can tolerate streptomycin.
(2) Some of our consultants would substitute gentamicin (adults with normal renal function, 1 mg/kg IM or IV every eight hours; children with normal renal function, 6 mg/kg/day IM or IV in divided doses every eight hours) for streptomycin in the above regimens.
(3) For viridans streptococcal strains that are relatively resistant to penicillin G (MIC >0.2 mcg/ml), high-dose penicillin G (IV) for four weeks *plus* streptomycin (IM) or gentamicin (IM or IV) for four weeks is recommended (see Specific Therapy of Enterococcal Endocarditis below).
(4) For patients who are potentially allergic to penicillin G, appropriate skin testing for penicillin allergy is recommended before selection of alternative therapy. Four weeks of intravenous cefazolin, cephalothin, cephapirin, or cephradine can be used in penicillin-allergic patients who are not allergic to cephalosporins. All others should receive four weeks of intravenous vancomycin.

Enterococci (Streptococcus faecalis, Streptococcus faecium, Streptococcus durans) and other penicillin-resistant streptococci (MIC >0.2 mcg/ml)
(gram-positive cocci)

PREFERRED THERAPY:
Penicillin G plus **Gentamicin**
OR
Penicillin G plus **Streptomycin**
ALTERNATIVE THERAPY:
Vancomycin plus **Gentamicin**
OR
Vancomycin plus **Streptomycin**
REMARKS:
(1) Adult dosages are penicillin G 20 million U/day IV in divided doses every three to four hours (higher dose if necessary); streptomycin 7.5 mg/kg (not to exceed 0.5 g) IM every 12 hours in patients with normal renal function; gentamicin 1 mg/kg IM or IV every 8 hours in patients with normal renal function; and vancomycin 7.5 mg/kg (not to exceed 0.5 g) IV every 6 hours in patients with normal renal function. Duration of therapy is four to six weeks. Patients with symptoms of enterococcal endocarditis for more than three months or those with mitral valve infections should be treated for six weeks; patients without these high-risk factors can be treated for four weeks (Wilson et al, 1984).
(2) Synergistic antimicrobial combinations are required for bactericidal activity and cure of enterococcal endocarditis.
(3) Streptomycin usually is preferred for susceptible strains of enterococci; gentamicin is recommended if the organism is resistant (ie, MIC >2000 mcg/ml) to streptomycin. Because 40% of enterococcal strains are resistant to streptomycin, gentamicin should be used when susceptibility testing cannot be performed. Tobramycin generally should not be substituted for gentamicin or streptomycin.
(4) Ampicillin is two- to four-fold more active than penicillin G against enterococci in vitro, but the clinical relevance, if any, is uncertain. Some experts prefer ampicillin (adults, 12 g/day) over penicillin G, however.
(5) Pediatric preferred therapy: Ampicillin (150 mg/kg/day IV or IM in 4 to 6 divided doses for 30 days) plus gentamicin (children with normal renal function, 6 mg/kg/day IV or IM in 3 divided doses during first 10 to 14 days). Alternative therapy: Penicillin G (250,000 units/kg/day in 4 to 6 divided doses) plus streptomycin (children with normal renal function, 20 to 30 mg/kg/day IM in 2 divided doses) for 30 days; OR Vancomycin (children with normal renal function, 40 mg/kg/day IV in 4 divided doses) with or without an aminoglycoside.
(6) For patients who are potentially allergic to penicillin G, appropriate skin testing for penicillin allergy is recommended. Some experts recommend desensitization procedures in patients with positive skin tests. The alternative regimen of vancomycin plus an aminoglycoside should be effective, but nephrotoxicity and ototoxicity may be additive and careful monitoring of renal and eighth nerve function is necessary. (Note: Vancomycin probably should not be used alone because of its lack of bactericidal activity in vitro and its poor performance in experimental enterococcal endocarditis.)

Staphylococcus aureus (methicillin-sensitive)
(gram-positive cocci)

PREFERRED THERAPY:
Nafcillin OR **Oxacillin**
ALTERNATIVE THERAPY:
Vancomycin; Cephalothin, Cefazolin, Cephapirin, or Cephradine
REMARKS:
(1) Adult dosages are nafcillin 12 g/day IV; oxacillin 12 g/day IV; cephalothin 12 g/day IV; cefazolin 6-8 g/day IV; cephapirin 12 g/day IV; vancomycin 7.5 mg/kg (not to exceed 0.5 g) IV every six hours in patients with normal renal function. Duration of therapy is four to six weeks.
(2) Pediatric dosages: Nafcillin 150 mg/kg/day IV in 4 divided doses for 42 days; OR Vancomycin 40 mg/kg/day IV in 4 divided doses in patients with normal renal function. Efficacy of cephalosporins in pediatric cases is not established.
(3) Most experts do not recommend the use of methicillin in adults and children because of an increased risk of interstitial nephritis.
(4) Penicillin G (adults, 20 million U/day IV) may be substituted for antistaphylococcal penicillins if susceptibility is proven.
(5) The role of combination chemotherapy with an antistaphylococcal penicillin plus gentamicin (patients with normal renal function: adults, 1 mg/kg IM or IV every eight hours; children, 6 mg/kg/day in 3 divided doses) in S. aureus endocarditis remains controversial. This combination exhibits synergistic activity against S. aureus in vitro and has greater bactericidal activity than an antistaphylococcal penicillin alone in a rabbit endocarditis model. In humans, nafcillin plus gentamicin accelerated the clearance of bacteremia compared to nafcillin alone, but did not alter the cure rate, morbidity, or mortality (Korzeniowski et al, 1982). These data led to the suggestion that combination therapy could be used for the initial three to five days of therapy; after clearance of bacteremia, the aminoglycoside (and its associated toxicity) could be discontinued. Some experts recommend combination therapy in severely ill patients, patients who respond poorly to single drug therapy, or for endocarditis caused by tolerant strains of S. aureus (ie, when the minimum bactericidal concentration [MBC] is much greater than the MIC). Rifampin also has been added to an antistaphylococcal penicillin if bacteremia fails to clear with a single agent, or for possible abscesses, or for secondary staphylococcal meningitis. Its use is investigational.
(6) For patients who are potentially allergic to penicillin, appropriate skin testing for penicillin allergy is recommended before selection of alternative therapy. Patients who are allergic to penicillins may be treated with intravenously administered vancomycin (see dosage suggested above). First generation cephalosporins, including cephalothin, cefazolin, cephapirin, and cephradine can be used in patients who are allergic to penicillin but not to cephalosporins.

Staphylococcus aureus (methicillin-resistant)
(gram-positive cocci)

PREFERRED THERAPY:
Vancomycin
REMARKS:
(1) For patients with normal renal function: Adults, 7.5 mg/kg (not to exceed 0.5 g) IV every six hours; children, 40 mg/kg/day IV in four divided doses.
(2) Alternatively, patients may be treated with intravenous trimethoprim/sulfamethoxazole (20 mg/kg trimethoprim component daily in four equally divided doses).
(3) Methicillin-resistant S. aureus should also be considered cephalosporin-resistant, but this may not be reliably demonstrated by routine in vitro susceptibility tests.

Staphylococcus epidermidis
(gram-positive cocci)

PREFERRED THERAPY:
Vancomycin plus **Rifampin** plus **Gentamicin**
REMARKS:
(1) Adult dosages are: Vancomycin 7.5 mg/kg (not to exceed 0.5 g) IV every six hours in patients with normal renal function; and rifampin 300 mg orally every eight hours. Duration of therapy is six weeks. The adult dosage of gentamicin is 1 mg/kg IM or IV every eight hours in patients with normal renal function for the initial 14 days of therapy.

(2) Pediatric dosages: Vancomycin 40 mg/kg/day IV in 4 divided doses in patients with normal renal function; rifampin 10 to 20 mg/kg/day orally in 2 divided doses; and gentamicin 6 mg/kg/day IV in 3 divided doses in patients with normal renal function.

(3) *S. epidermidis* should be considered methicillin-resistant and cephalosporin-resistant until proven otherwise. The preferred therapy listed above appears to be the best based on a prospective study (see Karchmer et al, 1984). Previously, it was shown that cure rates of patients treated with vancomycin were increased by the addition of rifampin or gentamicin (Karchmer et al, 1983). However, the development of rifampin-resistant *S. epidermidis* with treatment failure has been reported in patients receiving only vancomycin plus rifampin therapy for prosthetic valve endocarditis (Karchmer et al, 1983 and 1984; Chamovitz et al, 1985). When gentamicin is added to the regimen, the emergence of rifampin resistance is significantly decreased (Karchmer et al, 1984). Any *S. epidermidis* strains isolated after initiation of rifampin-containing regimens should be tested for rifampin susceptibility.

(4) Resistance of *S. epidermidis* to methicillin or cephalosporins may not be apparent by routine in vitro susceptibility testing (Lowy and Hammer, 1983; Karchmer et al, 1983; Thornsberry, 1984). Thus, the use of β-lactam antibiotics to treat *S. epidermidis* prosthetic valve endocarditis has resulted in a high failure rate (Karchmer et al, 1983).

(5) *S. epidermidis* usually infects prosthetic heart valves; surgical removal of the affected valve frequently is necessary.

EMPIRIC THERAPY

Empiric antimicrobial drug therapy of acute infective endocarditis is recommended prior to isolation of the causative organism from blood culture.

Acute Infective Endocarditis - Natural Valve

(*Staphylococcus aureus* and *Streptococcus faecalis* [enterococcus]; also *Streptococcus pyogenes* [group A, β hemolytic], *Streptococcus pneumoniae* [pneumococcus], *Neisseria* species, and, occasionally, *Haemophilus* species)

PREFERRED THERAPY:
Nafcillin (or Oxacillin) *plus* Gentamicin *plus* Penicillin G (or Ampicillin)
ALTERNATIVE THERAPY:
Vancomycin *plus* Gentamicin
REMARKS:
(1) Guidelines for therapy are controversial and not all of our consultants agreed with the regimens listed above. When methicillin-resistant staphylococci are potential causative organisms, empiric therapy with vancomycin plus gentamicin is preferred.

(2) Adult dosages are: nafcillin 12 g/day IV; oxacillin 12 g/day IV; gentamicin 1 mg/kg IM or IV every 8 hours in patients with normal renal function; penicillin G 20 million U/day IV; ampicillin 12 g/day IV; and vancomycin 7.5 mg/kg (not to exceed 0.5 g) IV every 6 hours in patients with normal renal function.

(3) Pediatric dosages are: nafcillin 150 mg/kg/day IV in 4 divided doses; gentamicin 6 mg/kg/day IV in 3 divided doses in patients with normal renal function; penicillin G 100 to 200 mg/kg/day IV in 4 divided doses; ampicillin 200 mg/kg/day IV in 3 divided doses; and vancomycin 40 mg/kg/day IV in 4 divided doses in patients with normal renal function.

(4) Switch to most effective drug regimen after culture and susceptibility test results are available. (Note: Routine susceptibility testing for methicillin-resistant staphylococci may be unreliable [Thornsberry, 1984].)

Acute Infective Endocarditis - Prosthetic Valve

(*Staphylococcus epidermidis* [methicillin-resistant strains], *Staphylococcus aureus*, corynebacteria, gram-negative bacilli, streptococci)

PREFERRED THERAPY:
Vancomycin *plus* Gentamicin *plus* Rifampin
REMARKS:
(1) Guidelines for therapy are controversial and not all of our consultants agreed with the regimen listed above.

(2) Adult dosages are: vancomycin 7.5 mg/kg (not to exceed 0.5 g) IV every 6 hours in patients with normal renal function; gentamicin 1 mg/kg IM or IV every 8 hours in patients with normal renal function; and rifampin orally 300 to 600 mg every 12 hours or 300 mg every eight hours.

(3) Pediatric dosages are: Vancomycin 40 mg/kg/day IV in 4 divided doses in patients with normal renal function; gentamicin 6 mg/kg/day IV in 3 divided doses in patients with normal renal function; rifampin 10 to 20 mg/kg/day orally in 2 divided doses.

(4) Switch to most effective drug regimen after culture and susceptibility test results are available. (Note: Routine susceptibility testing for methicillin-resistant staphylococci may be unreliable [Thornsberry, 1984].)

GASTROINTESTINAL AND INTRA-ABDOMINAL INFECTIONS

Infectious Gastroenteritis/Infectious Diarrhea

Infectious gastroenteritis/infectious diarrhea can be caused by viruses, bacteria, and protozoa.

Rotavirus and Norwalk virus are the most common viral etiologies of infectious gastroenteritis. Infants between 6 and 24 months are most frequently affected by rotavirus. Norwalk virus tends to occur in epidemics and usually affects school-age children, adolescents, and adults. Antimicrobial drug therapy is NOT effective for viral infections. Therapy is primarily supportive and consists of correction of dehydration and electrolyte imbalance.

Infectious gastroenteritis/infectious diarrhea caused by bacteria usually is subdivided into three categories:

(1) Acute food poisoning can be caused by ingestion of a preformed enterotoxin. *Staphylococcus aureus* (gram-positive cocci), *Bacillus cereus* (gram-positive bacilli), and *Clostridium perfringens* (anaerobic gram-positive bacilli) are the common bacterial pathogens. Disease is frequently self-limited. Supportive therapy (replacement of fluids and electrolytes) may be necessary, but antimicrobial drug therapy is not indicated.

Although botulism (*Clostridium botulinum*) is a type of acute food poisoning, it is a life-threatening disease characterized by blockade of neuromuscular transmission that is caused by a preformed neurotoxin. Ventilatory support and specific antitoxin are indicated.

(2) Acute secretory diarrheas, characterized by watery diarrhea without fecal leukocytes, are caused by enterotoxins elaborated by causative bacteria. Enterotoxigenic strains of *Escherichia coli* and *Vibrio cholerae* are the major pathogens. Acute secretory diarrheas are common in underdeveloped countries; enterotoxigenic *E. coli* is the most common cause of travelers' diarrhea.

Supportive therapy (replacement of fluids and electrolytes) and SPECIFIC antimicrobial drug therapy are indicated in the treatment of cholera. Correction of dehydration and electrolyte imbalance also may be necessary in diarrhea caused by enterotoxigenic *E. coli*, but the role of antimicrobial drug therapy is presently unclear. Limited studies suggest that such therapy may decrease the severity and duration of the illness.

(3) Invasive bacteria or those that produce a cytotoxic toxin can cause bloody diarrhea with other constitutional symptoms (eg, fever). Major pathogens include *Shigella* species (eg, *S. flexneri*, *S. sonnei*), *Salmonella* species (eg, *S. enteritidis*), *Campylobacter jejuni*, invasive strains of *Escherichia coli*, *Yersinia enterocolitica*, *Vibrio parahaemolyticus*, and *Aeromonas hydrophila*.

When necessary, supportive therapy (replacement of fluids and electrolytes) is indicated for diarrhea caused by any of these pathogens. SPECIFIC antimicrobial drug therapy is recommended for *Shigella* infections. The role of antimicrobial drug therapy for infections caused by the other pathogens is less clear. Acute diarrheal illnesses are often mild and self-limited and antimicrobial drugs are unnecessary in these cases. When diarrhea is severe and protracted or there is associated bacteremia, SPECIFIC antimicrobial drug therapy usually is recommended.

Giardia lamblia (giardiasis), *Entamoeba histolytica* (amebiasis), and *Cryptosporidium* are the major protozoal etiologies of infectious diarrhea. Treatment guidelines can be found in Chapter 77, Antiprotozoal Agents.

Selected references: Black, 1982; San Joaquin and Marks, 1982; Blaser, 1983; Fekety, 1983; Pickering, 1983; Satterwhite and DuPont, 1983; Conte and Barriere, 1984 A; *Med Lett Drugs Ther*, 1984, 1986; George et al, 1985; Hruska, 1986. See also Chapter 53, Agents Used in Disorders of the Lower Intestinal Tract.

SPECIFIC THERAPY

(A) Supportive therapy (replacement of fluids and electrolytes) plus specific antimicrobial drug therapy is recommended for infectious gastroenteritis/infectious diarrhea caused by the following:

Shigella species
(gram-negative bacilli)

PREFERRED THERAPY:
Trimethoprim/Sulfamethoxazole
ALTERNATIVE THERAPY:
Ampicillin; Tetracycline; Nalidixic Acid
REMARKS:
(1) Antibiotics are indicated because they shorten the duration of illness and decrease the relapse rate.
(2) Ampicillin-resistant strains are common; this drug frequently is preferred when susceptibility is proven.
(3) Amoxicillin should not be substituted for ampicillin for *Shigella* infections.
(4) Tetracyclines should not be given to pregnant women or children under 8 years.

Vibrio cholerae (cholera)
(gram-negative bacilli)

PREFERRED THERAPY:
Tetracycline
ALTERNATIVE THERAPY:
Trimethoprim/Sulfamethoxazole; Furazolidone; Chloramphenicol
REMARKS:
(1) Antibiotics are indicated because they reduce the duration and volume of diarrhea.
(2) Tetracyclines should not be given to pregnant women or children under 8 years.

Giardia lamblia (giardiasis)
(protozoan)
REMARKS:
(1) See Chapter 77, Antiprotozoal Agents, for treatment guidelines.

Entamoeba histolytica (amebiasis)
(protozoan)
REMARKS:
(1) See Chapter 77, Antiprotozoal Agents, for treatment guidelines.

(B) Infectious gastroenteritis/infectious diarrhea caused by the following pathogens frequently is self-limiting, and supportive therapy (replacement of fluids and electrolytes) ALONE is adequate. When diarrhea is severe or protracted or there is associated bacteremia, SPECIFIC antimicrobial drug therapy also is recommended.

Salmonella species (nontyphoidal)
(gram-negative bacilli)
REMARKS:
(1) Gastroenteritis is self-limited and requires supportive therapy only. Antibiotics may prolong the carrier state. When systemic illness (eg, bacteremia) is present, treat with antimicrobial agents as for typhoid fever (see Typhoid Fever below).
(2) Some pediatric infectious disease consultants consider treatment with antimicrobials appropriate for younger children (eg, under one year).

Campylobacter jejuni
(gram-negative bacilli)

PREFERRED THERAPY:
Erythromycin
ALTERNATIVE THERAPY:
Tetracycline; Gentamicin; Chloramphenicol
REMARKS:
(1) Definitive treatment guidelines are lacking. Erythromycin shortens duration of shedding of *C. jejuni* from feces, but its effect on the clinical course of gastroenteritis is less clear. Some erythromycin-resistant strains have been reported. Some experts prefer gentamicin or chloramphenicol for patients with sepsis.
(2) Tetracyclines should not be given to pregnant women or children less than 8 years.
(3) Trimethoprim/sulfamethoxazole usually is NOT effective against *C. jejuni*.

Escherichia coli (invasive strains)
(gram-negative bacilli)

REMARKS:

(1) The role of antimicrobial drug therapy is unclear. Some experts recommend trimethoprim/sulfamethoxazole (alternative, ampicillin) as for *Shigella*. Laboratory confirmation of invasive *E. coli* infection is not generally available.

Yersinia enterocolitica
(gram-negative bacilli)

REMARKS:

(1) Most cases of gastroenteritis appear to resolve spontaneously. The role of antimicrobial drug therapy is unknown. Trimethoprim/sulfamethoxazole, aminoglycosides (eg, gentamicin), tetracycline, and chloramphenicol are active.

Vibrio parahaemolyticus
(gram-negative bacilli)

REMARKS:

(1) Most cases of gastroenteritis appear to resolve spontaneously. The role of antimicrobial drug therapy is unknown. Tetracycline is active.

Aeromonas hydrophila
(gram-negative bacilli)

REMARK:

(1) The role of antimicrobial drug therapy is unknown. Trimethoprim/sulfamethoxazole and tetracycline appear to be active.

Escherichia coli (enterotoxigenic strains)
(gram-negative bacilli)

REMARKS:

(1) Most cases of gastroenteritis appear to resolve spontaneously. The role of antimicrobial drug therapy is unclear, although limited studies suggest that trimethoprim/sulfamethoxazole (alternative, trimethoprim) decreases the severity and duration of illness (see Travelers' Diarrhea below). Laboratory confirmation of enterotoxigenic *E. coli* infection is not generally available.

Travelers' Diarrhea

Infectious diarrhea occurs in as many as 50% of United States travelers to underdeveloped regions (eg, Mexico, South America, Africa, Southern and Southeast Asia). Enterotoxigenic *Escherichia coli* is the causative organism in approximately 50% of the cases. *Shigella* (15%), *Salmonella* (10%), *Giardia* (4%), and *Campylobacter* (3%) are other important pathogens.

Presently, guidelines for the prevention and treatment of travelers' diarrhea are not definitive. All experts agree that awareness and avoidance of possible sources of contamination is of primary importance. The role of antimicrobial prophylaxis is controversial, but the current consensus is that the risks outweigh the benefits for most (if not all) travelers (DuPont et al, 1985; *Med Lett Drugs Ther*, 1985; National Institutes of Health Consensus Development Conference, 1985; see also Table 3, Antimicrobial Chemoprophylaxis for Ambulatory Patients).

Treatment of travelers' diarrhea frequently is unnecessary because most cases are mild and self-limited. Maintenance of fluid and electrolyte balance is of primary importance, al-though most individuals do not develop serious dehydration. Antimotility agents (eg, loperamide, diphenoxylate with atropine [Lomotil]) or bismuth subsalicylate [Pepto-Bismol] may help relieve symptoms in milder cases (DuPont et al, 1985; NIH Consensus Development Conference, 1985; see also Chapter 53, Agents Used in Disorders of the Lower Intestinal Tract). A prospective, randomized, double-blind, placebo-controlled study suggests that early (within 48 hours of onset of illness) EMPIRIC antimicrobial drug treatment (as outlined below) of travelers' diarrhea can decrease the severity and duration of the illness in most patients (DuPont et al, 1982). Such therapy is indicated in patients with moderate to severe symptoms (three or more loose stools in an eight-hour period with nausea, vomiting, abdominal cramps, fever, or blood in the stools [NIH Consensus Development Conference, 1985]). Travelers who have persistent diarrhea with serious fluid loss, fever, and blood or mucus in the stools should seek medical attention.

It is recommended that travelers to areas of high risk obtain an antimotility drug (or bismuth subsalicylate) and an antimicrobial agent prior to their trip in order to avoid buying over-the-counter drugs abroad with potentially dangerous ingredients (NIH Consensus Development Conference, 1985).

Selected references: Gorbach, 1982; Satterwhite and DuPont, 1983; Weiss, 1983; DuPont et al, 1985; NIH Consensus Development Conference, 1985; Johnson et al, 1986.

EMPIRIC THERAPY
(Enterotoxigenic *Escherichia coli* and *Shigella* species)

PREFERRED THERAPY:
Trimethoprim/Sulfamethoxazole
ALTERNATIVE THERAPY:
Trimethoprim
REMARKS:

(1) Dosages are trimethoprim 160 mg/sulfamethoxazole 800 mg twice daily for five days; trimethoprim 200 mg twice daily for five days. Treatment for three days appears to be equally effective and is the duration of therapy recommended by the NIH Consensus Development Conference (1985).

(2) Both regimens were more effective than placebo for infections caused by culture-proven enterotoxigenic *E. coli* or *Shigella* and when diarrhea was not associated with a detectable pathogen.

(3) Five percent of patients receiving trimethoprim/sulfamethoxazole and 8% of patients receiving trimethoprim were treatment failures. Such cases may be due to *Campylobacter* or *Giardia* and appropriate investigation is recommended.

(4) Preliminary evidence suggests that doxycycline (100 mg twice daily) also is effective for the treatment of travelers' diarrhea (NIH Consensus Development Conference, 1985).

Antibiotic-Associated Pseudomembranous Colitis

The most important cause of antibiotic-associated pseudomembranous colitis is *Clostridium difficile* which secretes cytotoxins.

General treatment measures include discontinuation of the causative antimicrobial agent when possible and supportive therapy (replacement of fluids and electrolytes). When necessary, SPECIFIC antimicrobial therapy directed against *C. difficile* is recommended. See also Chapter 68, Macrolides and Lincosamides.

Selected references: Bartlett, 1981; Chang, 1981; Gotz and Rand, 1982; Tedesco, 1982; Fekety, 1983.

SPECIFIC THERAPY

Clostridium difficile
(gram-positive bacilli)

PREFERRED THERAPY:
Vancomycin (oral)
ALTERNATIVE THERAPY:
Metronidazole (oral); Bacitracin (oral); Cholestyramine resin
REMARKS:
(1) A major disadvantage of vancomycin is its high cost. Most experts agree that the usual adult dosage of 500 mg four times per day (5 to 10 days) can be reduced to 125 mg four times per day (5-10 days) in most patients with no decrease in efficacy; this has been demonstrated in a randomized clinical trial (Fekety et al, 1984). Thus, cost of therapy with this agent can be decreased fourfold.
(2) A prospective, randomized study has suggested that metronidazole (adults, 250 mg four times daily) is a cost-effective alternative to vancomycin (Teasley et al, 1983). Greater clinical experience with this agent appears to be necessary before it can be recommended routinely for all patients. However, it appears to be an effective and less expensive alternative to vancomycin for mild to moderate cases. Metronidazole has been reported to induce C. difficile pseudomembranous colitis in a few patients.
(3) Between 10% and 20% of patients relapse after initial successful treatment with vancomycin or metronidazole. Antimicrobial drug-resistant strains of C. difficile are not causative, however, because retreatment of these patients with vancomycin or metronidazole frequently is successful. Persistent fecal carriage of C. difficile after treatment is an important risk factor for relapse.
(4) Cholestyramine resin acts by neutralizing C. difficile toxins. The efficacy of this agent has been variable depending on the institution. It should be used only in mild cases of antibiotic-associated pseudomembranous colitis. Because the resin also binds vancomycin, simultaneous use should be avoided.
(5) Experience with bacitracin is very limited. In a prospective, randomized study, bacitracin (adults, 20,000 units four times daily) was significantly less effective than vancomycin (adults, 125 mg four times daily) in clearing C. difficile from the stools, although resolution of symptoms and incidence of relapses were similar in each treatment group (Young et al, 1985).

Typhoid Fever

Typhoid fever is caused by *Salmonella typhi*. SPECIFIC antimicrobial drug therapy should be directed against this organism.

Selected references: Hornick, 1983; Satterwhite and DuPont, 1983; Conte and Barriere, 1984 B; *Med Lett Drugs Ther*, 1984, 1986; Hruska, 1986.

SPECIFIC THERAPY

Salmonella typhi
(gram-negative bacilli)

PREFERRED THERAPY:
Chloramphenicol
ALTERNATIVE THERAPY:
Ampicillin (or Amoxicillin); Trimethoprim/Sulfamethoxazole

REMARKS:
(1) Chloramphenicol-resistant strains of *S. typhi* have been reported in Mexico and Southeast Asia.
(2) Chloramphenicol is not effective in the treatment of the chronic carrier state. Ampicillin (alternative, amoxicillin) has been effective in patients without gallbladder disease. Cholecystectomy is recommended for patients with gallbladder disease.

Hepatitis, Infectious

The major causes of infectious hepatitis are hepatitis A, hepatitis B, and non-A, non-B hepatitis viruses. Antimicrobial drug therapy is NOT effective for these viral infections.

Cholecystitis, Acute

Acute cholecystitis usually results when the cystic duct becomes obstructed by gallstones; secondary bacterial infection occurs in about 50% to 70% of cases. *Escherichia coli*; other gram-negative enteric bacilli, such as *Klebsiella*, *Enterobacter*, and *Proteus* species; and nonhemolytic streptococci, including enterococci, are causative organisms. Anaerobic bacteria, including *Bacteroides fragilis* and clostridia, also may be involved, particularly in the elderly. When anaerobic bacteria are present, they frequently are part of polymicrobial infections containing mixtures of anaerobic bacteria and aerobic gram-negative enteric bacilli.

Surgery is the primary treatment of gallstone-associated cholecystitis, but the timing of surgery is controversial. Because most cases of acute cholecystitis resolve spontaneously, some surgeons recommend waiting two to three months after the inflammation has subsided. Others advocate immediate surgery. Antimicrobial drug therapy (parenteral) of acute cholecystitis should be regarded as adjunctive to surgery (ie, to prevent spread of infection and to sterilize the bloodstream of any associated bacteremia). Drug selection usually is EMPIRIC pending the results of blood cultures and/or biliary operative culture data. Antibiotics usually do not eradicate local infection within the biliary tree because penetration of the drugs into bile is inadequate in the presence of obstruction.

Selected references: Swenson, 1979; Conte and Barriere, 1984 B; Levison and Pontzer, 1984; Hruska, 1986.

EMPIRIC THERAPY
(*Escherichia coli* and other enteric gram-negative bacilli [*Klebsiella, Enterobacter, Proteus* species]; *Streptococcus faecalis* [group D; enterococcus]; possible anaerobic bacteria [*Bacteroides fragilis*, clostridia])

PREFERRED THERAPY:
Ampicillin *plus* Aminoglycoside (gentamicin, tobramycin, amikacin, netilmicin)
ALTERNATIVE THERAPY:
See Remarks.
REMARKS:
(1) The combination of cefoxitin *plus* aminoglycoside (gentamicin, tobramycin, amikacin, netilmicin) is recommended by one expert (Sanford, 1985). This regimen would provide adequate coverage against enteric gram-negative bacilli and anaerobic bacteria, including *B. fragilis*, but may be inadequate against enterococci.

(2) For mild infections, single-agent therapy usually is considered adequate. First generation cephalosporins (eg, cefazolin) and ampicillin are most frequently recommended. Cefoxitin, a second generation cephalosporin, also is a reasonable agent, especially in the older patient who may have an anaerobic infection.

(3) For life-threatening clinical situations, including perforation with peritonitis or obstructive suppurative cholangitis, immediate surgery and antibiotic regimens (eg, clindamycin [or metronidazole] *plus* aminoglycoside *with or without* ampicillin [or penicillin G]), as recommended for peritonitis, are usually necessary (see Peritonitis Secondary to Bowel Perforation below).

Peritonitis Secondary to Bowel Perforation

These infections are typically polymicrobial and contain a mixture of aerobic and anaerobic bacteria that originate from the microbial flora of the large bowel. Among the aerobic bacteria, *Escherichia coli*, other gram-negative enteric bacilli (eg, *Klebsiella, Proteus*), and streptococci, particularly enterococci (*Streptococcus faecalis*), are the major causative organisms. *Bacteroides fragilis* is a very common and particularly important anaerobic pathogen. Other common anaerobic bacteria include gram-positive cocci (*Peptostreptococcus* and *Peptococcus*) and clostridia.

The primary treatment of peritonitis secondary to bowel perforation is prompt surgical intervention to correct the intra-abdominal disease processes or injuries that caused the infection or to provide drainage of purulent materials. Supportive therapy (eg, fluid and electrolyte repletion) also is necessary. Antimicrobial therapy is indicated as an adjunct to control bacteremia, prevent the formation of metastatic foci of infection, reduce suppurative complications after bacterial contamination, and prevent local spread of existing infection.

Antimicrobial drug therapy (parenteral) of peritonitis secondary to bowel perforation initially is EMPIRIC pending results of cultures obtained from blood and peritoneal fluid. Broad spectrum antibacterial coverage against both enteric gram-negative bacilli (the aerobic component) and anaerobic bacteria, especially *B. fragilis*, is necessary. Whether enterococci also should be routinely covered is somewhat controversial; some experts recommend such coverage in more severely ill patients.

Selected references: Levison, 1979; Gorbach and McGowan, 1981; Tally, 1981; Fekety, 1982; Conte and Barriere, 1984 B; Levison and Pontzer, 1984; Finegold et al, 1985; DiPiro et al, 1986; Hruska, 1986.

EMPIRIC THERAPY

(*Escherichia coli* and other gram-negative enteric bacilli [eg, *Klebsiella, Proteus* species]; *Bacteroides fragilis* and other anaerobic bacteria [eg, *Peptococcus, Peptostreptococcus*]; optional, *Streptococcus faecalis* [group D; enterococcus])

PREFERRED THERAPY:
Clindamycin *plus* Aminoglycoside (gentamicin, tobramycin, amikacin, netilmicin) *with or without* Ampicillin (or Penicillin G)
OR

Metronidazole *plus* Aminoglycoside *with or without* Ampicillin (or Penicillin G)
OR
Cefoxitin alone (see Remarks)
ALTERNATIVE THERAPY:
Chloramphenicol *plus* Aminoglycoside
OR
Antipseudomonal Penicillin (carbenicillin, ticarcillin, mezlocillin, piperacillin, azlocillin) *plus* Aminoglycoside
OR
Cefoxitin *plus* Aminoglycoside *with or without* Ampicillin (or Penicillin G)
OR
Imipenem/cilastatin alone (see Remarks)
REMARKS:
(1) Switch to most effective drug regimen after susceptibility test results are available.
(2) For severely ill patients, a two-drug regimen containing an aminoglycoside plus an agent with excellent activity against anaerobic bacteria, including *B. fragilis*, is indicated. The above list of recommended regimens is based on the current literature and consensus opinion among consultants. Many experts feel that ampicillin (or penicillin G) should be added to the regimen (ie, triple antibiotic therapy) to increase coverage against enterococci, but this is controversial.
(3) Choice of aminoglycoside depends on local susceptibility patterns. Metronidazole, chloramphenicol, and clindamycin are most active against *B. fragilis*, but some strains are resistant to clindamycin (Tally et al, 1985). Hematologic toxicity is associated with chloramphenicol.
(4) Cefoxitin is active against most anaerobic bacteria, including *B. fragilis*, and a number of enteric gram-negative bacilli. When used alone, this agent was shown to be as effective as clindamycin *plus* aminoglycoside for community-acquired intra-abdominal infections in a controlled clinical study (Tally et al, 1981). Some experts prefer cefoxitin alone for community-acquired infections in mild to moderately ill patients. It should be noted, however, that up to 20% of *B. fragilis* strains may be resistant to cefoxitin in some geographic locations (Tally et al, 1985).
(5) Various third generation cephalosporins, including moxalactam, cefotaxime, and ceftizoxime, also have been effective for secondary peritonitis when used alone. Each of these antibiotics has excellent activity against aerobic gram-negative enteric bacilli. Moxalactam has activity in vitro against *B. fragilis* comparable to cefoxitin, but serious bleeding has been associated with its use and, generally, it is not recommended. The other third generation cephalosporins are less active against *B. fragilis* and they do not appear to offer any advantages over cefoxitin when used alone. Some consultants suggested the combination of a third generation cephalosporin (eg, cefotaxime) *plus* an antianaerobic agent (eg, clindamycin) for patients at increased risk for aminoglycoside toxicity (eg, impaired renal function).
(6) Some consultants prefer the newer, extended spectrum penicillins (eg, piperacillin, mezlocillin) to the carboxypenicillins (ticarcillin, carbenicillin) because they are more active against enterococci and *B. fragilis*. These agents should not be used alone because they are susceptible to β-lactamases and resistant bacterial strains are relatively common.
(7) Imipenem, a recently approved β-lactamase stable carbapenem antibiotic, has the broadest antimicrobial spectrum of currently available β-lactam antibiotics, that includes aerobic gram-negative bacilli (including *P. aeruginosa*), gram-positive cocci (including enterococci), and anaerobic bacteria (including *B. fragilis*). Although clinical experience is limited, this agent looks promising for empiric monotherapy of polymicrobial infections such as secondary peritonitis (Solomkin et al, 1985). Imipenem is administered in a 1:1 fixed ratio combination with cilastatin, which is a specific inhibitor of dehydropeptidase-I, a renal enzyme that inactivates imipenem (see Chapter 67, Cephalosporins and Related Agents).

URINARY TRACT INFECTIONS

Pyelonephritis, Acute

Acute pyelonephritis, a particularly important illness in young children, women of childbearing age, and the elderly, is characterized by fever, chills, flank pain, and costovertebral angle tenderness, often associated with dysuria, urgency, and frequency. The syndrome is accompanied by pyuria and $>10^5$ bacteria/ml of urine.

Escherichia coli is responsible for approximately 90% of initial infections that are community-acquired. *Proteus mirabilis*, *Klebsiella pneumoniae*, *Enterobacter* species and *Streptococcus faecalis* (group D, enterococci) are occasional causative organisms. These latter pathogens and other gram-negative bacilli, including indole-positive *Proteus* (*Morganella morganii*, *Providencia rettgeri*, *Proteus vulgaris*), *Serratia marcescens*, and *Pseudomonas aeruginosa* are more frequently encountered in patients who have had repeated courses of antimicrobial therapy for recurrent infections, those who have undergone frequent instrumentation because of structural abnormalities of the urinary tract, and individuals with hospital-acquired (nosocomial) infections.

Although ultimate antimicrobial drug selection for acute pyelonephritis should be SPECIFIC and based on urine culture and susceptibility data, EMPIRIC therapy, frequently based on Gram stain of urine, is indicated initially. Customarily, patients with acute symptomatic infection require hospitalization and parenteral antimicrobial drug therapy. This includes bacteremic patients, toxic patients, older patients, and patients with underlying disease. Mildly ill, nonbacteremic patients with initial attacks can sometimes be treated as outpatients with oral antimicrobial drugs.

Selected references: Cunha, 1981; *Med Lett Drugs Ther*, 1981; Carson, 1982; Fang et al, 1982; Abraham et al, 1983; Gleckman, 1983; Conte and Barriere, 1984; Sobel and Kaye, 1984; Valenti and Reese, 1986.

EMPIRIC THERAPY

(If possible, a Gram stain of urine should be obtained to aid in appropriate antimicrobial drug selection.)

Inpatient Therapy
(*Escherichia coli* most likely in initial, community-acquired infection; other gram-negative bacilli; *Streptococcus faecalis* [group D; gram-positive enterococcus])

PREFERRED THERAPY:
Aminoglycoside (gentamicin, tobramycin, amikacin, netilmicin) plus Ampicillin (parenteral)
ALTERNATIVE THERAPY:
Parenteral First Generation Cephalosporin (cefazolin, cephalothin, cephapirin) plus Aminoglycoside; Trimethoprim/Sulfamethoxazole (parenteral); Third Generation Cephalosporin (cefotaxime, ceftizoxime, ceftriaxone, ceftazidime, cefoperazone)
REMARKS:
(1) Parenteral ampicillin should no longer be used alone, even for community-acquired infections in patients without previous episodes, due to organism resistance in 20% to 30% of cases.
(2) If Gram stain of urine shows gram-positive cocci in chains, indicating enterococci, ampicillin should be used.
(3) Third generation cephalosporins may be preferred in patients with renal impairment, especially when multiple-resistant gram-negative bacilli are possible causative organisms (eg, hospital-acquired infection). However, none of these agents is active against enterococci. Only ceftazidime and cefoperazone have activity against *Pseudomonas aeruginosa*.
(4) Switch to most effective, least toxic, and least expensive drug regimen after susceptibility test results are available.
(5) Most patients with acute pyelonephritis become afebrile by 48 hours after initiating therapy with appropriate antimicrobial agents. Continuing fever beyond 48 hours requires further investigation (eg, for urinary obstruction or intrarenal or perinephric abscess).
(6) Parenteral therapy is usually given for at least 24-48 hours after patient becomes afebrile. Then switch to oral therapy. Total duration of therapy is usually 14 days. If relapse occurs, a more prolonged course of therapy for six weeks is indicated; evaluation for underlying urinary tract abnormalities also is recommended.
(7) In males with acute pyelonephritis, continuation of antimicrobial therapy for at least six weeks is recommended because at least one-half of these patients have prostatic infection and shorter courses of therapy will lead to recurrences.
(8) In infants and children, followup urine cultures are particularly important after an episode of acute pyelonephritis as these individuals are potentially at risk of renal scars or failure of normal growth of the infected kidney.

Outpatient Therapy
(*Escherichia coli* most likely in initial, community-acquired infection; other gram-negative bacilli; *Streptococcus faecalis* [group D; gram-positive enterococcus])

PREFERRED THERAPY:
Trimethoprim/Sulfamethoxazole (oral)
ALTERNATIVE THERAPY:
Cephalosporin (oral)
REMARKS:
(1) If Gram stain of urine shows gram-positive cocci in chains, indicating enterococci, ampicillin should be used.
(2) Switch to most effective, least toxic, and least expensive drug regimen after susceptibility test results are available.
(3) Duration of therapy is usually 14 days. If relapse occurs, a more prolonged course of therapy for six weeks is indicated; evaluation for underlying urinary tract abnormalities also is recommended.

Cystitis, Acute

Acute cystitis is particularly common in women of childbearing or middle age. Symptoms of dysuria, frequency, urgency, and suprapubic pain accompanied by pyuria and $>10^5$ bacteria/ml of urine have been the traditional criteria used to define this superficial bladder infection. Two important points require emphasis, however. First, it is now apparent that a significant proportion ($>30\%$) of women with symptoms restricted to the lower urinary tract have silent renal infection (subclinical pyelonephritis). These patients generally require more prolonged antimicrobial drug therapy, as discussed below in this section. Second, a large percentage of women with clinical cystitis (symptoms of dysuria, frequency, and urgency accompanied by pyuria) have a "negative" or "low-count" urine culture (<10⁵ bacteria/ml). Traditionally, these women have been said to suffer from the "acute urethral syndrome," meaning infection localized to the urethra. However, it now is clear that many of these women have infection of both the urethra and bladder, with urine colony counts <10⁵ bacteria/ml (Stamm et al, 1980, 1981, 1982). These data suggest that the standard criteria for significant bacteriuria (>10⁵ bacteria/ml) may require downward adjustment in a symptomatic woman. Antimicrobial drug therapy of these patients is considered in the section on the Acute Urethral Syndrome below.

Escherichia coli is by far the most common causative organism of acute cystitis acquired in the community. *Staphylococcus saprophyticus* appears to be the second most frequent cause, particularly in younger women. The growth of "coagulase-negative staphylococci" in pure culture from the urine may represent infection with *S. saprophyticus* and should not be dismissed as a contaminant. Other gram-negative bacilli (for specific organisms, see section on Pyelonephritis, Acute above) and *Streptococcus faecalis* (group D, enterococci) are infrequent pathogens in initial episodes of community-acquired lower urinary tract infections.

Antimicrobial drug therapy (oral) of initial episodes of community-acquired acute cystitis is initially EMPIRIC. For adult women who are not pregnant, who have no apparent renal parenchymal involvement, who do not have findings suggesting subclinical pyelonephritis (underlying urinary tract disease, diabetes mellitus or other conditions or therapies producing an immunocompromised state, a history of urinary infections in childhood, documented relapses in the past, or recent acute pyelonephritis), whose symptoms are recent (less than seven days), and who are available for follow-up, most experts now recommend a single dose of an appropriate antimicrobial agent. Conventional, multiple-dose antimicrobial therapy for 7 to 14 days is recommended for all other patients, including women with possible upper urinary tract infection (subclinical pyelonephritis), pregnant women, males, and children. Most experts recommend urologic evaluation in men and children because of the increased probability of underlying urinary tract abnormalities in these patients.

Selected references: Cunha, 1981; Kunin, 1981; *Med Lett Drugs Ther*, 1981; Schaeffer et al, 1981; Carson, 1982; Fang et al, 1982; Stamm, 1982 A; Abraham et al, 1983; Farrar, 1983; Gleckman, 1983; Komaroff, 1984, 1986; Sobel and Kaye, 1984; Carlson and Mulley, 1985; Valenti and Reese, 1986.

EMPIRIC THERAPY

Single-dose therapy

(Recommended only for adult women who are not pregnant, have no apparent renal parenchymal involvement, have no evidence of subclinical pyelonephritis, have recent symptoms [<7 days], and are available for follow up. *Escherichia coli* is most likely causative organism; *Staphylococcus saprophyticus*; other gram-negative bacilli)

PREFERRED THERAPY:
Trimethoprim/Sulfamethoxazole (160 mg/800 mg [one "double-strength" tablet] or 320 mg/1600 mg [two "double-strength" tablets])

ALTERNATIVE THERAPY:
Sulfisoxazole (1 or 2 g); Trimethoprim (400 mg); Tetracycline (2.5 g); Amoxicillin (3 g)

REMARKS:
(1) Advantages of single-dose therapy are increased compliance, decreased adverse drug reactions, lower cost, and decreased likelihood of emergence of resistant bacterial strains.
(2) Trimethoprim/sulfamethoxazole was preferred by most of our consultants.
(3) Most experts do not obtain a urine culture at the initial visit. It is recommended that a urine culture be obtained one week after single-dose therapy as evidence of cure or to identify relapse. Patients who fail to respond to single-dose therapy or who relapse (usually within 36 to 96 hours) are considered to have silent renal infection, although rapid reinfection from the perineum also may occur. (Note: Some experts consider response to single-dose therapy as a localization test to distinguish upper from lower urinary tract infection.) These patients are cultured and started on conventional multiple-dose antimicrobial drug therapy for 10-14 days (see below). Follow-up is essential. Early relapse requires more prolonged course of therapy for six weeks; evaluation for underlying urinary tract abnormalities also is recommended in these patients.
(4) Some reports have suggested that trimethoprim/sulfamethoxazole is superior to amoxicillin for this indication (Carlson and Mulley, 1985; Hooton et al, 1985). Some consultants feel that amoxicillin or sulfonamides alone should not be used empirically unless resistance to these drugs is known to be low (eg, less than 10%) within a given community.
(5) Parenteral aminoglycosides also have been effective as single-dose therapy; however, oral cephalosporins have NOT been effective.

Conventional (multiple-dose) therapy (7-14 days)

(Recommended for all patients except women who qualify for single-dose therapy [see above]. *Escherichia coli* is most likely causative organism; other gram-negative bacilli; *Staphylococcus saprophyticus*; *Streptococcus faecalis* [group D; enterococcus])

PREFERRED THERAPY:
Sulfisoxazole (or Sulfamethoxazole) OR Ampicillin (or Amoxicillin) OR Trimethoprim/Sulfamethoxazole OR Nitrofurantoin OR Cinoxacin

ALTERNATIVE THERAPY:
Trimethoprim; Tetracycline; Oral Cephalosporin (cephalexin, cephradine)

REMARKS:
(1) Sulfisoxazole (or sulfamethoxazole) is preferred by many experts because it is the least expensive regimen. However, sulfonamide resistance is prevalent in many communities. Some consultants do not recommend its use empirically unless resistance is known to be low (eg, less than 10% of isolates). Sulfonamides should not be used in pregnant women near term or in newborns.
(2) Because resistance to ampicillin and amoxicillin is prevalent in many communities, some consultants do not recommend their use empirically unless resistance is known to be low (eg, less than 10% of isolates).
(3) Tetracyclines should not be used in pregnant women or children under 8 years. Trimethoprim should not be used in pregnant women.
(4) The urinary tract analgesic, phenazopyridine, may provide symptomatic relief of dysuria and urethral irritation during the initial 24-48 hours. It should be discontinued after 48 hours.
(5) If relapse occurs, suggesting silent renal infection, a more

prolonged course of therapy for six weeks is indicated; evaluation for underlying urinary tract abnormalities also is recommended.

Asymptomatic Bacteriuria

Patients with asymptomatic bacteriuria have significant bacteriuria (ie, $>10^5$ bacteria/ml of urine) but do not have clinical symptoms of urinary tract infection. Antimicrobial drug therapy is recommended for pregnant women (who have a 40% chance of developing pyelonephritis), diabetics, other immunocompromised patients, and children. Because asymptomatic bacteriuria of childhood can be a manifestation of underlying structural abnormality, it is recommended that children receive a urological evaluation, including cultures. Choice of drugs in children is dependent on culture results (tetracyclines contraindicated in children under 8 years). Pregnant women can be given conventional multiple-dose therapy as for acute cystitis (see Cystitis, Acute above). Tetracyclines, trimethoprim, and sulfonamides (near term only) should not be administered to pregnant women.

Whether treatment of asymptomatic bacteriuria in nonpregnant, otherwise healthy, ambulatory adults would be beneficial remains to be determined.

Selected references: *Med Lett Drugs Ther*, 1981; Fang et al, 1982; Farrar, 1983; Sobel and Kaye, 1984; Valenti and Reese, 1986.

Acute Urethral Syndrome

Women with the acute urethral syndrome have symptoms of acute cystitis (ie, dysuria, frequency, urgency), but do not have significant bacteriuria as defined by traditional criteria (ie, $>10^5$ bacteria/ml). Based on the work of Stamm et al (1980, 1981, 1982), women with the acute urethral syndrome can be subdivided into three categories. Patients with pyuria (≥ 8 leukocytes/ml of unspun urine) and between 10^2 and 10^5 bacteria (primarily *Escherichia coli*; also, *Staphylococcus saprophyticus*) per ml of urine essentially are considered to have acute bacterial urethrocystitis, ie, bacterial infection of both the urethra and bladder. Those with pyuria and sterile urine cultures usually are infected with *Chlamydia trachomatis* and have a sexually transmitted disease. (NOTE: *Neisseria gonorrhoeae* and Herpes simplex virus also may cause the acute urethral syndrome.) Women in either of the above categories are said to have the "dysuria-pyuria" syndrome. Patients with no pyuria and a sterile urine culture have no demonstrable infection. (NOTE: Vaginitis must always be considered in the differential diagnosis.)

Antimicrobial drug therapy (oral) is indicated for women with symptoms of dysuria, frequency, or urgency who also have pyuria (ie, patients who have the "dysuria-pyuria" syndrome), but not for women who lack pyuria and bacteria in their urine. Two approaches to treatment currently are being recommended. EMPIRIC antimicrobial therapy to cover all potential pathogens (ie, *Escherichia coli*, *Staphylococcus saprophyticus*, *Chlamydia trachomatis*, *Neisseria gonorrhoeae*) is recommended by some experts. The other, usually preferred, approach is first to differentiate probable coliform (or staphylo-

coccal) infection from chlamydial (or gonococcal) infection using clinical, epidemiologic, and (rapidly available) laboratory data and then treat the patient with a more SPECIFIC, albeit still EMPIRIC, antimicrobial drug regimen. Criteria that suggest coliform (or staphylococcal) infection include abrupt onset of symptoms (<4 days), hematuria, suprapubic pain, previous urinary tract infection, and no recent change in sexual partner. Criteria that suggest chlamydial (or gonococcal) infection include gradual onset of symptoms, >7-day history of symptoms, no hematuria, no suprapubic pain, and recent change in sexual partners. Cervical Gram stain and culture for *N. gonorrhoeae* and rapid immunologic diagnostic testing for *C. trachomatis* may allow for SPECIFIC therapy directed against either of these sexually transmitted pathogens. Treatment guidelines for gonococcal and chlamydial infections and for the acute urethral syndrome caused by these sexually transmitted pathogens can be found in Table 2, Treatment of Sexually Transmitted Diseases (STD).

Selected references: Cunha, 1981; Fang et al, 1982; Stamm, 1982 B; Abraham et al, 1983; Komaroff, 1984, 1986; Sobel and Kaye, 1984; *Morbid Mortal Week Rep*, 1985; Valenti and Reese, 1986.

EMPIRIC THERAPY

(A) Usually effective against all potential pathogens, including *Escherichia coli*, *Staphylococcus saprophyticus*, *Chlamydia trachomatis*, *Neisseria gonorrhoeae*

PREFERRED THERAPY:
Doxycycline
REMARKS:
(1) Dosage is 100 mg twice daily for 10 days (Stamm et al, 1981).
(2) Tetracycline is less expensive than doxycycline and should be an effective alternative.
(3) In vitro, resistance to tetracyclines is not uncommon among *E. coli* (up to 30%) and is increasing among gonococci.
(4) Tetracyclines should not be administered to pregnant women or children under 8 years.

(B) Presumed bacterial infection of bladder/urethra; therapy directed against *Escherichia coli*, *Staphylococcus saprophyticus*
REMARKS:
(1) Treat as for acute cystitis with single-dose therapy (preferred, if appropriate) or conventional (multiple-dose) therapy (7-14 days). See section entitled Cystitis, Acute above for specific recommendations.

(C) Presumed sexually transmitted infection; therapy directed against *Chlamydia trachomatis* and/or *Neisseria gonorrhoeae*
REMARKS:
(1) See Table 2 for treatment guidelines.

Recurrent Urinary Tract Infections

Recurrent episodes of urinary tract infection can be either due to *relapse* or *reinfection*.

Relapse refers to a recurrence of infection after treatment by the same organism that caused the initial infection. They usually occur within two weeks after completion of a course of therapy. Relapse usually indicates the presence of renal involvement, structural abnormality of the urinary tract (eg, calculi), or, in males, chronic prostatitis. Patients with relapsing urinary tract infections require thorough urologic evaluation to identify surgically correctable abnormalities. If no urological defect is found and the patient has failed to respond to a conventional two-week course of therapy, which suggests a deep-seated tissue infection of the kidney, a longer six-week course of therapy is indicated (see sections above entitled Pyelonephritis, Acute and Cystitis, Acute for specific antimicrobial regimens). Males with chronic bacterial prostatitis also require prolonged courses of appropriate antimicrobial therapy (see section below entitled Prostatitis, Chronic).

Reinfections are due to introduction of a new organism (from the fecal-perineal flora) that is different from the one previously treated. They account for more than 80% of recurrent urinary tract infections in women and girls and usually involve only the lower urinary tract. Most reinfections occur within weeks to months of the preceding urinary tract infection. If episodes of reinfection are infrequent, each episode can be treated as a separate infection with single-dose or conventional therapy as outlined in the section above entitled Cystitis, Acute. If reinfections are frequent (eg, three or more episodes per year), long-term antimicrobial prophylaxis may be indicated. See Table 3, Antimicrobial Chemoprophylaxis for Ambulatory Patients, for guidelines.

Selected references: *Med Lett Drugs Ther*, 1981; Fang et al, 1982; Farrar, 1983; Sobel and Kaye, 1984; Valenti and Reese, 1986.

Urethritis

Urethritis in sexually active males is usually caused by *Neisseria gonorrhoeae* (uncomplicated gonorrhea) or *Chlamydia trachomatis* (nonspecific [non-gonococcal] urethritis). See Table 2, Treatment of Sexually Transmitted Diseases (STD), for treatment guidelines for these sexually transmitted infections.

Prostatitis, Acute

Escherichia coli is the causative organism in the majority ($\geq$80%) of cases of acute bacterial prostatitis. Other gram-negative bacilli, including *Klebsiella, Proteus, Enterobacter*, and *Pseudomonas* (rare), and *Streptococcus faecalis* (group D, enterococci) are occasional causative organisms.

Antimicrobial drug therapy of acute prostatitis initially is EMPIRIC pending results of urine cultures and susceptibility tests.

Selected references: Meares, 1979; Cunha, 1981; Farrar, 1983; Sobel and Kaye, 1984; Orland et al, 1985; Valenti and Reese, 1986.

EMPIRIC THERAPY
(*Escherichia coli* most likely; other enteric gram-negative bacilli; *Streptococcus faecalis* [group D, gram-positive enterococcus])

PREFERRED THERAPY:
Trimethoprim/Sulfamethoxazole (oral)
OR
Aminoglycoside (gentamicin, tobramycin, amikacin, netilmicin) *plus* Ampicillin (parenteral)
ALTERNATIVE THERAPY:
Trimethoprim alone
REMARKS:
(1) Although many antibacterial agents appear to penetrate the inflamed prostate adequately, many experts prefer trimethoprim/sulfamethoxazole because of the good penetration of trimethoprim into prostatic tissue. If the causative organism is susceptible and clinical response is favorable, many experts will continue trimethoprim/sulfamethoxazole (160 mg/800 mg twice daily) for 30 days in an attempt to prevent the development of chronic prostatitis.
(2) Parenteral therapy with an aminoglycoside *plus* ampicillin may be preferred initially in patients with pronounced systemic symptoms. When the patient becomes afebrile, appropriate oral therapy, based on urine culture and susceptibility testing, is recommended for 30 days.

Prostatitis, Chronic

Chronic bacterial prostatitis is the most common cause of relapsing urinary tract infections in males. *Escherichia coli* is the causative organism in the majority of cases. Other gram-negative bacilli, including *Klebsiella, Proteus, Enterobacter*, and *Pseudomonas* (rare), and *Streptococcus faecalis* (group D, enterococci) are occasional causative organisms. Nonbacterial prostatitis is quite similar to chronic bacterial prostatitis, but an infectious etiology is presently unclear. *Chlamydia trachomatis* and *Ureaplasma urealyticum* have been suggested to be causative in some cases.

Diagnosis of chronic bacterial prostatitis is by prostatic localization test, which shows significantly higher bacterial counts in fluid expressed by prostatic massage or urine voided after massage when compared to urine cultured prior to prostatic massage. Antimicrobial drug therapy (oral) is initiated if bacteria are cultured. Drug selection is limited, however, because few antimicrobial agents adequately penetrate into prostatic fluid.

Selected references: Meares, 1979; Cunha, 1981; Carson, 1982; Farrar, 1983; Sobel and Kaye, 1984; Orland et al, 1985; Valenti and Reese, 1986.

EMPIRIC THERAPY
(*Escherichia coli* most likely; other enteric gram-negative bacilli; *Streptococcus faecalis* [group D, gram-positive enterococcus])

PREFERRED THERAPY:
Trimethoprim/Sulfamethoxazole
ALTERNATIVE THERAPY:
Trimethoprim alone
REMARKS:
(1) Most experts prefer trimethoprim/sulfamethoxazole because of the good penetration of trimethoprim into prostatic fluid. If the

causative organism is susceptible, most experts will administer trimethoprim/sulfamethoxazole (160 mg/800 mg twice daily) for 12 weeks.

(2) Despite prolonged therapy, a significant number of failures will result. Urologic evaluation and surgical resection may be indicated in these patients. Alternatively, some experts initiate long-term suppressive therapy with trimethoprim/sulfamethoxazole (80 mg/400 mg daily) to control symptoms and protect against recurrent urinary tract infections.

(3) Carbenicillin indanyl has been used by some experts as alternative therapy of chronic bacterial prostatitis (see Orland et al, 1985). Rifampin *plus* trimethoprim is a proposed regimen but clinical data are very limited (see Sobel and Kaye, 1984).

(4) Doxycycline and erythromycin have been suggested in cases of nonbacterial prostatitis in which *Chlamydia trachomatis* or *Ureaplasma urealyticum* are potential causative organisms.

INFECTIONS OF THE MALE REPRODUCTIVE TRACT

Genital Ulcers

Causative organisms include Herpes simplex virus, *Treponema pallidum* (syphilis), *Haemophilus ducreyi* (chancroid), *Calymmatobacterium granulomatis* (granuloma inguinale), and LGV serotypes of *Chlamydia trachomatis* (lymphogranuloma venereum). These are sexually transmitted infections. For treatment guidelines, see Table 2, Treatment of Sexually Transmitted Diseases (STD). See also Chapter 79, Antiviral Agents, for treatment guidelines to genital herpes infections.

Epididymo-orchitis, Acute

Acute epididymo-orchitis has two forms. A sexually transmitted form usually occurs in men under 35 years, is associated with urethritis, and is caused by *Chlamydia trachomatis* and/or *Neisseria gonorrhoeae*. Nonsexually transmitted epididymo-orchitis usually occurs in men over 35 years, is associated with midstream pyuria and bacteriuria, and is usually caused by *Escherichia coli*; other Enterobacteriaceae and *Pseudomonas aeruginosa* are occasional pathogens. (NOTE: Mumps and Coxsackie (pleurodynia) should be considered in the infectious differential diagnosis of epididymo-orchitis. Tuberculosis also may cause epididymitis.)

Antimicrobial drug therapy of nonsexually transmitted acute epididymo-orchitis is initially EMPIRIC pending results of urine cultures and susceptibility tests. For treatment of sexually transmitted acute epididymo-orchitis, see Table 2, Treatment of Sexually Transmitted Diseases (STD).

Selected references: Pong, 1983; Berger, 1984; *Morbid Mortal Week Rep*, 1985; Sanford, 1985.

EMPIRIC THERAPY

Nonsexually Transmitted Epididymo-orchitis
(*Escherichia coli* is most frequent pathogen; other Enterobacteriaceae)

PREFERRED THERAPY:
Trimethoprim/Sulfamethoxazole

ALTERNATIVE THERAPY:
Ampicillin (or Amoxicillin); Sulfisoxazole (or sulfamethoxazole); Tetracycline; Trimethoprim alone
REMARKS:
(1) For patients with fever, leukocytosis, severe pain and swelling, and a toxic clinical presentation, initial parenteral therapy with an aminoglycoside (gentamicin, tobramycin, amikacin, netilmicin) frequently is preferred. Third generation cephalosporins (eg, cefotaxime) are alternatives for the severely ill patient.

(2) Switch to most effective, least toxic, and least expensive drug regimen after susceptibility test results are available.

(3) Urologic evaluation is indicated.

(4) In prepubertal males, epididymitis is usually caused by coliforms or *Staphylococcus aureus*. Preferred empiric therapy: Nafcillin *plus* Aminoglycoside (Nelson, 1985).

Sexually Transmitted Epididymo-orchitis
(*Chlamydia trachomatis* and/or *Neisseria gonorrhoeae*)
REMARKS:
(1) See Table 2 for treatment guidelines.

INFECTIONS OF THE FEMALE REPRODUCTIVE TRACT

Vaginitis

The major causative organisms of infectious vaginitis are *Candida albicans* (candidiasis), *Trichomonas vaginalis* (trichomoniasis), several species of vaginal bacteria (including anaerobic bacteria) that interact to produce the syndrome called bacterial vaginosis (formerly nonspecific vaginitis), and Herpes simplex virus. Sexual transmission is believed to play a limited role in candidiasis. In contrast, trichomoniasis, bacterial vaginosis, and genital herpes are sexually transmitted diseases.

Antimicrobial drug therapy of infectious vaginitis is SPECIFIC for the causative organism. Drug selection for vaginal candidiasis is outlined below. For treatment guidelines for trichomoniasis and bacterial vaginosis, see Table 2, Treatment of Sexually Transmitted Diseases (STD). Treatment of genital herpes infections is discussed in Chapter 79, Antiviral Agents.

Selected references: Gibbs, 1983; *Morbid Mortal Week Rep*, 1985; Sanford, 1985; Penn, 1986.

SPECIFIC THERAPY

Candida albicans (candidiasis)
(fungus)

PREFERRED THERAPY:
Miconazole (intravaginal) OR Clotrimazole (intravaginal)
ALTERNATIVE THERAPY:
Nystatin (intravaginal)
REMARKS:
(1) Larger intravaginal doses and a shorter duration of therapy for miconazole (200 mg/day for three days) and clotrimazole (500 mg as a single dose) appear to be as effective as traditional dosage regimens for these agents. For nystatin, a longer treatment period (14 days) may be required. For a detailed discussion, see Chapter 74, Topical Anti-Infective Agents: Drugs Used on Skin and Mucous Membranes.

Trichomonas vaginalis (trichomoniasis)

(protozoan)

REMARKS:

(1) See Table 2 for treatment guidelines.

Bacterial vaginosis caused by the interaction of several species of vaginal bacteria (including anaerobic bacteria)

REMARKS:

(1) See Table 2 for treatment guidelines.

Herpes simplex virus (genital herpes)

REMARKS:

(1) See Chapter 79, Antiviral Agents, for treatment guidelines.

Cervicitis

Major causative organisms include *Neisseria gonorrhoeae, Chlamydia trachomatis,* and Herpes simplex virus. These are sexually transmitted infections. For treatment guidelines, see Table 2, Treatment of Sexually Transmitted Diseases (STD). See also Chapter 79, Antiviral Agents, for treatment guidelines for genital herpes infection.

Pelvic Inflammatory Disease (PID)

Important causative organisms include *Neisseria gonorrhoeae, Chlamydia trachomatis,* anaerobic bacteria (eg, *Bacteroides,* gram-positive cocci), facultative gram-negative bacilli (eg, *Escherichia coli*), and *Mycoplasma hominis.* Treatment guidelines for pelvic inflammatory disease are outlined in Table 2, Treatment of Sexually Transmitted Diseases (STD). See also the review by Burnakis and Hildebrandt, 1986.

BONE AND JOINT INFECTIONS

Septic Arthritis

The most common causative organisms of septic arthritis vary with patient age and are usually subdivided according to the following five age groups:

(1) NEONATES AND YOUNG INFANTS LESS THAN 2 MONTHS: The predominant organisms are *Staphylococcus aureus,* group B streptococci (*Streptococcus agalactiae*), and gram-negative enteric bacilli (eg, *Escherichia coli*) (NOTE: *Neisseria gonorrhoeae* from an infected mother also may be causative);

(2) CHILDREN 2 MONTHS TO 4 YEARS: *Haemophilus influenzae* (more common under 2 years), *S. aureus* (less common under 2 years), and streptococci (eg, *S. pyogenes, S. pneumoniae*) are the common causative organisms;

(3) CHILDREN 5 TO 15 YEARS: *S. aureus* and streptococci are the major pathogens;

(4) SEXUALLY ACTIVE ADOLESCENTS AND ADULTS (USUALLY BETWEEN 15 AND 40 YEARS): *Neisseria gonorrhoeae* causes most cases; *S. aureus* and streptococci are less common;

(5) OLDER ADULTS (>40 YEARS): *S. aureus* is the predominant pathogen; streptococci, gram-negative bacilli (often associated with predisposing conditions), and *N. gonorrhoeae* are less common causative organisms.

Although ultimate antimicrobial drug selection for septic arthritis should be SPECIFIC and based on culture (synovial fluid, blood, other sites as indicated) and susceptibility data, EMPIRIC therapy is indicated initially. As outlined below, initial drug selection is based on the age of the patient and results of synovial fluid Gram stain, when available. Parenteral antibiotics are recommended. Adequate removal of purulent joint fluid (eg, needle aspiration, open drainage) also is required.

Selected references: Syriopoulou and Smith, 1981; Neu, 1982; Aronoff and Scoles, 1983; McCracken and Nelson, 1983; Conte and Barriere, 1984; LeFrock and Kannangara, 1984; *Med Lett Drugs Ther,* 1984, 1986; Smith, 1984; Goldenberg and Reed, 1985; *Morbid Mortal Week Rep,* 1985; Nelson, 1985 A; Sanford, 1985 A; Roberts and Mock, 1986.

EMPIRIC THERAPY (BASED ON INITIAL GRAM STAIN)

Neonates and Young Infants (Less Than 2 Months)

(A) Gram-positive cocci

(*Staphylococcus aureus; Streptococcus agalactiae* [group B])

PREFERRED THERAPY:

Oxacillin OR Methicillin

ALTERNATIVE THERAPY:

Cefazolin or Cephalothin

REMARKS:

(1) In contrast to older children and adults, nafcillin is not recommended in neonates by some experts because of erratic pharmacokinetics, particularly in jaundiced infants; methicillin rarely is nephrotoxic in neonates (Nelson, 1985 B).

(2) Penicillin G should be substituted for antistaphylococcal penicillins if susceptibility of *S. aureus* strain is proven.

(3) For methicillin-resistant strains of *S. aureus,* vancomycin is the drug of choice.

(4) For infections caused by group B streptococci, penicillin G or ampicillin is preferred. Some experts would add either of these agents to the antistaphylococcal penicillin prior to culture and susceptibility test results to improve coverage against group B streptococci.

(B) Gram-negative bacilli

(*Escherichia coli* and other gram-negative enteric bacilli)

PREFERRED THERAPY:

Aminoglycoside (gentamicin, tobramycin, amikacin, netilmicin)

ALTERNATIVE THERAPY:

Cefotaxime; Ceftriaxone; Ceftazidime

REMARKS:

(1) Switch to most effective drug regimen after susceptibility test results are available.

(2) Cefotaxime and ceftriaxone are NOT recommended if *Pseudomonas aeruginosa* is a likely pathogen. Ceftazidime *plus* an aminoglycoside OR an antipseudomonal penicillin (carbenicillin, ticarcillin, piperacillin, azlocillin, mezlocillin) *plus* an aminoglycoside are alternative regimens for *P. aeruginosa* infections.

Infants and Young Children (2 months to 4 years)

(A) Gram-positive cocci

(*Staphylococcus aureus*; streptococci [*S. pyogenes; S. pneumoniae*])

PREFERRED THERAPY:
Nafcillin OR Oxacillin
ALTERNATIVE THERAPY:
Cefazolin, Cephalothin, or Cephapirin; Vancomycin; Clindamycin
REMARKS:
(1) Most experts do not recommend methicillin because of an increased risk of interstitial nephritis.
(2) Penicillin G should be substituted for antistaphylococcal penicillins if susceptibility of *S. aureus* strain is proven.
(3) For methicillin-resistant strains of *S. aureus*, vancomycin is the drug of choice.
(4) For infections caused by streptococci, penicillin G is preferred.

(B) Gram-negative coccobacilli

(*Haemophilus influenzae*)

PREFERRED THERAPY:
Ampicillin *plus* Chloramphenicol initially
ALTERNATIVE THERAPY:
Chloramphenicol alone; Cefuroxime; Cefotaxime; Ceftizoxime; Ceftriaxone; Ceftazidime; Trimethoprim/Sulfamethoxazole
REMARKS:
(1) Beta lactamase-producing strains of *H. influenzae* are resistant to ampicillin and rare strains are resistant to chloramphenicol. Therefore, combined treatment is recommended until susceptibility is determined. Ampicillin usually is preferred for sensitive strains.
(2) All alternative regimens should be effective against ampicillin-resistant strains of *H. influenzae*. Although clinical experience is more limited, some experts prefer cefuroxime or a third generation cephalosporin to chloramphenicol for these resistant strains or when susceptibility is unknown.
(3) Cefamandole is NOT recommended as an initial therapy for children less than five years because of its poor penetration into cerebrospinal fluid.

Children (5 To 15 Years)

(A) Gram-positive cocci

(*Staphylococcus aureus*; streptococci [*S. pyogenes; S. pneumoniae*])
REMARKS:
(1) See Infants and Young Children (2 Months to 4 Years) above for drug selection recommendations and remarks.

Sexually Active Adolescents and Adults (usually between 15 and 40 years)

(A) Gram-negative cocci

(*Neisseria gonorrhoeae*)
REMARKS:
(1) See Table 2, Treatment of Sexually Transmitted Diseases (STD), for treatment guidelines.

(B) Gram-positive cocci

(*Staphylococcus aureus*; streptococci [*S. pyogenes; S. pneumoniae*])

REMARKS:
(1) See Infants and Young Children (2 Months to 4 Years) above for drug selection recommendations and remarks.

Older Adults (Greater Than 40 Years)

(A) Gram-positive cocci

(*Staphylococcus aureus*; streptococci [*S. pyogenes; S. pneumoniae*])
REMARKS:
(1) See Infants and Young Children (2 Months to 4 Years) above for drug selection recommendations and remarks.

(B) Gram-negative cocci

(*Neisseria gonorrhoeae*)
REMARKS:
(1) See Table 2, Treatment of Sexually Transmitted Diseases (STD), for treatment guidelines.

(C) Gram-negative bacilli

(Enterobacteriaceae; *Pseudomonas aeruginosa*)

PREFERRED THERAPY:
Antipseudomonal Penicillin (carbenicillin, ticarcillin, mezlocillin, piperacillin, azlocillin) *plus* Aminoglycoside (gentamicin, tobramycin, amikacin, netilmicin)
ALTERNATIVE THERAPY:
Third Generation Cephalosporin (ceftazidime, cefoperazone, cefotaxime, ceftizoxime; ceftriaxone) *with or without* Aminoglycoside
REMARKS:
(1) Septic arthritis caused by gram-negative bacilli is more common in patients with predisposing risk factors (eg, prior noninfectious joint disease, immunosuppression, narcotic use, underlying chronic debilitating disease). Most experts recommend that coverage include *P. aeruginosa*.
(2) Most experts recommend combination therapy for systemic infections in which *P. aeruginosa* is a probable causative organism.
(3) Third generation cephalosporins alone are NOT recommended for *P. aeruginosa* infections. Among these agents, ceftazidime is the most active against this pathogen. It is the preferred cephalosporin if *P. aeruginosa* is suspected.
(4) Switch to most effective drug regimen after susceptibility test results are available.

EMPIRIC THERAPY (NO ORGANISMS SEEN ON GRAM STAIN)

Neonates and Young Infants (Less Than 2 Months)
(*Staphylococcus aureus*; *Streptococcus agalactiae* [group B]; *Escherichia coli* and other gram-negative enteric bacilli)

PREFERRED THERAPY:
Oxacillin (or Methicillin) *plus* Aminoglycoside (gentamicin, tobramycin, amikacin, netilmicin)
ALTERNATIVE THERAPY:
Cefazolin (or Cephalothin) *plus* Aminoglycoside
OR
Oxacillin (or Methicillin) *plus* Cefotaxime (or Ceftriaxone or Ceftazidime)
REMARKS:
(1) Switch to most effective drug regimen after susceptibility test results are available.
(2) In contrast to older children and adults, nafcillin is not

recommended in neonates by some experts because of erratic pharmacokinetics, particularly in jaundiced infants; methicillin rarely is nephrotoxic in neonates (Nelson, 1985 B).

(3) If methicillin-resistant strains of *S. aureus* are suspected, substitute vancomycin for the antistaphylococcal penicillin.

(4) Some experts would add penicillin G or ampicillin to the above regimens to improve coverage against group B streptococci.

Infants and Young Children (2 Months To 4 Years)

(*Haemophilus influenzae*; *Staphylococcus aureus*; streptococci [*S. pyogenes*; *S. pneumoniae*])

PREFERRED THERAPY:
Cefuroxime
OR
Nafcillin (or Oxacillin) *plus* **Chloramphenicol**
ALTERNATIVE THERAPY:
Cefotaxime; Ceftizoxime; Ceftriaxone
REMARKS:

(1) Switch to most effective drug regimen after susceptibility test results are available.

(2) Because ampicillin-resistant strains of *H. influenzae* are common in most geographic areas, alternative agents (eg, cefuroxime, chloramphenicol) are preferred until susceptibility test results are known.

(3) Most experts do not recommend methicillin because of an increased risk of interstitial nephritis.

(4) Cefuroxime, despite less clinical experience, appears to be superior to cefamandole for this indication. Cefuroxime has increased stability to *H. influenzae* TEM-1 beta lactamase, a longer half-life, and a better adverse reaction profile and, most importantly, has not been associated with "breakthrough" *H. influenzae* type b meningitis, presumably because it can penetrate into cerebrospinal fluid more effectively than cefamandole (see Nelson, 1983). Cefamandole is NOT recommended as an initial therapy for children less than five years because of its poor penetration into cerebrospinal fluid.

(5) If methicillin-resistant strains of *S. aureus* are suspected, vancomycin should be used in combination with agents active against *H. influenzae*.

(6) Cefotaxime, ceftizoxime, and ceftriaxone have less antistaphylococcal activity than antistaphylococcal penicillins and cefuroxime. Some experts recommend adding a second antibiotic (eg, nafcillin, vancomycin) for optimal antistaphylococcal activity pending results of susceptibility tests.

(7) Because septic arthritis caused by *H. influenzae* usually occurs in infants between 2 months and 2 years, some experts use age 2 years, rather than 4 years, as the cutoff for coverage against this pathogen. In contrast, others recommend regimens containing activity against *H. influenzae* in children up to 6 years.

Children (5 to 15 Years)

(*Staphylococcus aureus*; streptococci [*S. pyogenes*, *S. pneumoniae*])

PREFERRED THERAPY:
Nafcillin OR **Oxacillin**
ALTERNATIVE THERAPY:
Cefazolin, Cephalothin, or Cephapirin; Vancomycin; Clindamycin
REMARKS:

(1) Switch to most effective drug regimen after susceptibility test results are available. Use penicillin G if organism is susceptible.

(2) Most experts do not recommend methicillin because of an increased risk of interstitial nephritis.

(3) If methicillin-resistant strains of *S. aureus* are suspected, substitute vancomycin for the antistaphylococcal penicillin.

(4) Some experts recommend the addition of an aminoglycoside

(gentamicin, tobramycin, amikacin, netilmicin) or third generation cephalosporin (ceftazidime, cefotaxime, ceftizoxime, ceftriaxone) to include coverage against gram-negative bacilli in patients with predisposing risk factors (eg, prior noninfectious joint disease, immunosuppression, narcotic use, underlying chronic debilitating disease).

Sexually Active Adolescents and Adults (usually between 15 and 40 years)

(Unless the clinical presentation suggests alternative etiologies, *Neisseria gonorrhoeae* is the most likely causative organism in young healthy adults).

REMARKS:

(1) See Table 2, Treatment of Sexually Transmitted Diseases (STD), for treatment guidelines.

(2) Some experts recommend the addition of nafcillin (or oxacillin) to provide adequate coverage against *Staphylococcus aureus*.

Older Adults (Greater Than 40 Years)

(*Staphylococcus aureus* most common; streptococci [*S. pyogenes*; *S. pneumoniae*])

REMARKS:

(1) See Children (5 to 15 Years) above for drug selection recommendations and remarks.

Osteomyelitis, Acute

Acute hematogenous osteomyelitis can occur in all age groups, but is most common in children under 16 years. Microbial etiology is related to age and the presence of associated risk factors. In NEONATES AND YOUNG INFANTS (<3 MONTHS), group B streptococci (*Streptococcus agalactiae*), *Staphylococcus aureus*, and gram-negative enteric bacilli (eg, *Escherichia coli*) are all important causative organisms. In CHILDREN (>3 MONTHS) AND ADULTS, *Staphylococcus aureus* is, by far, the major causative organism. Streptococci, especially *S. pyogenes*, also cause this infection in children and occasionally in adults. In contrast to septic arthritis (see previous section entitled Septic Arthritis), *Haemophilus influenzae* is a relatively rare cause of osteomyelitis in infants and children under 6 years. Gram-negative bacilli (eg, Enterobacteriaceae, *Pseudomonas aeruginosa*) are more likely to cause osteomyelitis in high-risk patients, including intravenous drug abusers, hemodialysis patients, diabetics, and patients with underlying debilitating diseases (eg, alcoholism, malignancy). Acute osteomyelitis is a particularly common infection in CHILDREN AND ADULTS WITH ASSOCIATED HEMOGLOBINOPATHY (SICKLE CELL DISEASE); *Salmonella* species are major causative organisms in these patients.

Although ultimate antimicrobial drug selection for acute osteomyelitis should be specific and based on culture (blood, aspirates of subperiosteal pus or intraosseous lesions) and susceptibility data, EMPIRIC therapy is indicated initially. As outlined below, initial drug selection is based on the age of the patient. High-dose parenteral antibiotics are recommended.

Selected references: Kaplan, 1982; Prober, 1982; Aronoff and Scoles, 1983; Brooks and Pons, 1983; McCracken and Nelson, 1983; Conte and Barriere, 1984; Zack, 1984; Nelson, 1985 A; Sanford, 1985 B; Chapman, 1986.

EMPIRIC THERAPY

Neonates and Young Infants (Less Than 3 Months)
(*Streptococcus agalactiae* [group B]; *Staphylococcus aureus*; *Escherichia coli* and other gram-negative enteric bacilli)

PREFERRED THERAPY:
Oxacillin (or Methicillin) *plus* **Aminoglycoside (gentamicin, tobramycin, amikacin, netilmicin)**
ALTERNATIVE THERAPY:
Cefazolin (or Cephalothin) *plus* **Aminoglycoside**
OR
Oxacillin (or Methicillin) *plus* **Cefotaxime (or Ceftriaxone or Ceftazidime)**
REMARKS:
(1) Switch to most effective drug regimen after susceptibility test results are available.
(2) In contrast to older children and adults, nafcillin is not recommended in neonates by some experts because of erratic pharmacokinetics, particularly in jaundiced infants; methicillin rarely is nephrotoxic in neonates (Nelson, 1985 B).
(3) If methicillin-resistant strains of *S. aureus* are suspected, substitute vancomycin for the antistaphylococcal penicillin.
(4) Cefotaxime and ceftriaxone are NOT recommended if *Pseudomonas aeruginosa* is a likely pathogen. Ceftazidime *plus* an aminoglycoside OR an antipseudomonal penicillin (carbenicillin, ticarcillin, piperacillin, azlocillin, mezlocillin) *plus* an aminoglycoside are alternative regimens for *P. aeruginosa* infections.
(5) Some experts would add penicillin G or ampicillin to the above regimens to improve coverage against group B streptococci.
(6) Duration of therapy is usually four to six weeks.

Children (Greater Than 3 Months) and Adults
(*Staphylococcus aureus*)

PREFERRED THERAPY:
Nafcillin OR Oxacillin
ALTERNATIVE THERAPY:
Cefazolin, Cephalothin, or Cephapirin; Vancomycin; Clindamycin
REMARKS:
(1) Switch to most effective drug regimen after susceptibility test results are available. Use penicillin G if organism is susceptible.
(2) Most experts do not recommend methicillin because of an increased risk of interstitial nephritis.
(3) If methicillin-resistant strains of *S. aureus* are suspected, substitute vancomycin for the antistaphylococcal penicillin.
(4) Although *H. influenzae* is an infrequent pathogen in osteomyelitis, some experts recommend that initial, empiric coverage include this pathogen in children under 6 years. Cefuroxime alone (Nelson, 1983) or the addition of chloramphenicol, a third generation cephalosporin (cefotaxime, ceftizoxime, ceftriaxone, ceftazidime), or ampicillin (usually not recommended initially because of the prevalence of resistant strains of *H. influenzae*) to the antistaphylococcal penicillin are alternative regimens for these patients.
(5) Some experts recommend the addition of an aminoglycoside (gentamicin, tobramycin, amikacin, netilmicin) or, alternatively, a third generation cephalosporin (ceftazidime, cefoperazone, cefotaxime, ceftizoxime, ceftriaxone) to include coverage against gram-negative bacilli in patients with predisposing risk factors (intravenous drug users, hemodialysis patients, diabetics, and patients with underlying debilitating diseases).
(6) Duration of therapy is usually four to six weeks. Traditionally, parenteral antibiotics have been used throughout the course of therapy. To decrease cost and the potential complications associated with long-term parenteral administration, a switch to oral antibiotics during the course of therapy may be indicated in selected patients (eg, children with *S. aureus* or streptococcal osteomyelitis in the absence of complicating risk factors) provided that certain criteria are fulfilled: (1) isolation of a bacterial pathogen that is sensitive to an oral agent; (2) administration of the drug in a fashion that ensures peak serum bactericidal titers greater than 1:8 and trough titers greater than 1:2 (monitoring serum bactericidal titers throughout course of therapy is essential); (3) clinical improvement during the first 5-7 days of intravenous antibiotics; and (4) patient compliance must be assured (usually by hospitalization).

Children and Adults with Associated Hemoglobinopathy (Sickle Cell Disease)
(*Staphylococcus aureus*; *Salmonella*; other coliform bacteria)

PREFERRED THERAPY:
Nafcillin (or Oxacillin) *plus* **Ampicillin**
ALTERNATIVE THERAPY:
Nafcillin (or Oxacillin) *plus* **Chloramphenicol; Cefazolin (or Cephalothin or Cephapirin)** *plus* **Chloramphenicol**
REMARKS:
(1) Switch to most effective drug regimen after susceptibility test results are available.
(2) Most experts do not recommend methicillin because of an increased risk of interstitial nephritis.
(3) If methicillin-resistant strains of *S. aureus* are suspected, substitute vancomycin for the antistaphylococcal penicillin.
(4) Duration of therapy is usually four to six weeks.

BACTEREMIAS AND SEPSIS

Sepsis of Unknown Etiology

In many cases of sepsis, the probable causative organism can be determined from a suspected source of primary infection prior to blood culture results (for specific examples, see the other sections of this Table). After adequate clinical evaluation, if no primary source of infection responsible for bacteremia can be identified and blood culture results are not yet available, EMPIRIC antimicrobial drug therapy (parenteral) to cover the more likely pathogens should be initiated. In NONCOMPROMISED ADULTS AND CHILDREN GREATER THAN 5 YEARS, coverage should include gram-negative bacilli, especially *Escherichia coli* and *Klebsiella pneumoniae*, and gram-positive cocci, including *Staphylococcus aureus*, *Streptococcus pneumoniae*, and other streptococci. In NONCOMPROMISED INFANTS AND CHILDREN LESS THAN 5 YEARS (EXCEPT NEWBORNS), coverage should include *Streptococcus pneumoniae* and other streptococci, *Haemophilus influenzae*, and *Neisseria meningitidis*; some experts also recommend coverage against *Staphylococcus aureus*. For treatment of sepsis in NEONATES, see the following section entitled Sepsis, Neonatal.

Selected references: Cherry, 1983; Ellner, 1983; Nelson, 1983; *Med Lett Drugs Ther*, 1984, 1986; Sanford, 1985; Foltzer and Reese, 1986.

EMPIRIC THERAPY

Noncompromised Adults and Children (greater than 5 years)

(Gram-negative bacilli [eg, *Escherichia coli, Klebsiella pneumoniae*]; *Staphylococcus aureus; Streptococcus pneumoniae*; other streptococci)

PREFERRED THERAPY:
Nafcillin (or Oxacillin) *plus* **Aminoglycoside (gentamicin, tobramycin, amikacin, netilmicin)**
OR
First Generation Cephalosporin (cefazolin, cephalothin, cephapirin, cephradine) *plus* **Aminoglycoside (gentamicin, tobramycin, amikacin, netilmicin)**
ALTERNATIVE THERAPY:
Cefotaxime; Ceftizoxime; Ceftriaxone; Ceftazidime; Cefoperazone; Imipenem/cilastatin
REMARKS:
(1) Some experts would add ampicillin (or penicillin G) to provide adequate coverage against enterococci (eg, *Streptococcus faecalis*), *Neisseria*, and *Haemophilus influenzae*.
(2) If methicillin-resistant *Staphylococcus aureus* are suspected, substitute vancomycin for the penicillinase-resistant penicillin or the cephalosporin.
(3) If anaerobic infection with *Bacteroides fragilis* is possible (eg, suspected intra-abdominal focus), clindamycin, metronidazole, or other anti-*B. fragilis* drug should be added.
(4) Selection of the particular aminoglycoside should be based on locally generated antibiotic susceptibility profiles.
(5) Most experts do not recommend methicillin in adults because of an increased risk of interstitial nephritis.
(6) Less clinical experience has been obtained with third generation cephalosporins (cefotaxime, ceftizoxime, ceftriaxone, ceftazidime, cefoperazone). They may be preferred to aminoglycosides for suspected gram-negative sepsis when meningitis (not cefoperazone) or renal failure may be present. Disadvantages include poor antipseudomonal activity (except ceftazidime), potential for the emergence of resistant bacterial strains, and high cost.
(7) Imipenem, a recently approved carbapenem antibiotic, has the broadest antimicrobial spectrum of currently available β-lactam antibiotics and it is resistant to most β-lactamases. Although clinical experience is limited, this agent may be useful for empiric monotherapy of community-acquired bacteremia in nonimmunocompromised adults and children. Imipenem is administered in a 1:1 fixed ratio combination with cilastatin, which is a specific inhibitor of dehydropeptidase-I, a renal enzyme that inactivates imipenem (see Chapter 67, Cephalosporins and Related Agents).
(8) Switch to most effective drug regimen after blood culture and susceptibility test results are available.

Noncompromised Infants and Children (less than 5 years, excluding newborns)

(*Streptococcus pneumoniae, Haemophilus influenzae, Neisseria meningitidis*, other streptococci; some experts also recommend coverage against *Staphylococcus aureus*)

PREFERRED THERAPY:
Nafcillin (or Oxacillin) *plus* **Chloramphenicol**
OR
Cefuroxime
OR
Ampicillin *plus* **Chloramphenicol**

ALTERNATIVE THERAPY:
Cefotaxime; Ceftizoxime; Ceftriaxone

REMARKS:
(1) Each of the above regimens has been recommended by various experts.
(2) Chloramphenicol, cefuroxime, cefotaxime, ceftizoxime, and ceftriaxone are active against beta lactamase-producing *H. influenzae*, which are prevalent in most geographical areas.
(3) The regimen of ampicillin *plus* chloramphenicol may be inadequate for infections caused by *S. aureus*.
(4) Most experts do not recommend methicillin because of an increased risk of interstitial nephritis.
(5) Cefuroxime, despite less clinical experience, appears to be superior to cefamandole for this indication. Cefuroxime has increased stability to *H. influenzae* TEM-1 beta lactamase, a longer half-life, a better adverse reaction profile, and, most importantly, has not been associated with "breakthrough" *H. influenzae* type b meningitis, presumably because it can penetrate into cerebrospinal fluid more effectively than cefamandole (Nelson, 1983). Cefamandole is NOT recommended as an initial therapy for children less than five years because of its poor penetration into the cerebrospinal fluid.
(6) In infants between 1 and 3 months, group B streptococci also may be causative. Many pediatric infectious disease experts recommend ampicillin *plus* cefotaxime (or ceftriaxone or cefuroxime) for empiric therapy in this age group.
(7) Switch to most effective drug regimen after blood culture and susceptibility test results are available.

Sepsis, Neonatal

The most common causative organisms are *Escherichia coli* and group B streptococci (*Streptococcus agalactiae*). Other causative organisms include *Listeria monocytogenes, Klebsiella-Enterobacter* species, *Proteus* species, group D streptococci (enterococci and *S. bovis*), and non-group D, alpha-hemolytic streptococci. After 5 days of age, nosocomial infections caused by *Staphylococcus aureus* and multiply-resistant gram-negative enteric bacilli also are a possibility.

Initial antimicrobial drug therapy (parenteral) of neonatal sepsis is EMPIRIC pending the results of blood cultures and susceptibility tests.

Selected references: Harris and Polin, 1983; Klein et al, 1983; McCracken and Nelson, 1983; Nelson, 1985; Steinhoff, 1986.

EMPIRIC THERAPY (NEONATES LESS THAN 1 MONTH)

(*Streptococcus agalactiae* [group B] and other streptococci, including enterococci; *Escherichia coli* and other gram-negative enteric bacilli; *Listeria monocytogenes*)

PREFERRED THERAPY:
Ampicillin *plus* **Aminoglycoside (gentamicin, tobramycin, amikacin, netilmicin)**
ALTERNATIVE THERAPY:
Ampicillin *plus* **Cefotaxime**
OR
Ampicillin *plus* **Ceftriaxone**
REMARKS:
(1) Penicillin G may be substituted for ampicillin in these combination regimens.
(2) Selection of the particular aminoglycoside should be based on locally generated antibiotic susceptibility profiles.

(3) If *S. aureus* is a suspected pathogen, a penicillinase-resistant penicillin (oxacillin or methicillin) can be added to the regimen.

(4) Switch to most effective drug regimen after blood culture and susceptibility test results are available.

(5) The rapid emergence of resistant strains of certain gram-negative bacilli (eg, *Enterobacter cloacae*) to third generation cephalosporins has caused concern among some neonatologists about the widespread use of these agents as part of routine, initial empiric regimens in the closed environments of neonatal intensive care units (Bryan et al, 1985; McCracken, 1985).

Fever in the Patient with Neutropenia (<500 Granulocytes/mm³)

Febrile neutropenic patients frequently will have a bacteremia. The most common causative organisms are gram-negative bacilli, particularly *Escherichia coli, Klebsiella* species, and *Pseudomonas aeruginosa*. Gram-positive cocci, particularly *Staphylococcus aureus* and *Staphylococcus epidermidis* (the incidence of infection with this pathogen is high in certain cancer centers), and *Candida* also are relatively common pathogens.

Antimicrobial drug therapy prior to blood culture results is essential. In the absence of a primary focus of infection, EMPIRIC therapy to cover the most common pathogens is initiated. Optimal doses of parenteral broad spectrum, bactericidal antibiotics in synergistic combinations should be selected.

Selected references: Wade, 1982; Drusano and Schimpff, 1983; Klastersky, 1983; *Med Lett Drugs Ther*, 1984, 1986; Pizzo, 1984; Mayer and DeTorres, 1985; Sanford, 1985; Foltzer and Reese, 1986.

EMPIRIC THERAPY
(*Escherichia coli, Klebsiella* species, and *Pseudomonas aeruginosa*; see Remarks)

PREFERRED THERAPY:
Aminoglycoside (gentamicin, tobramycin, amikacin, netilmicin) *plus* **Antipseudomonal Penicillin (carbenicillin, ticarcillin, piperacillin, azlocillin, mezlocillin)**

ALTERNATIVE THERAPY:
Aminoglycoside (gentamicin, tobramycin, amikacin, netilmicin) *plus* **Third Generation Cephalosporin (ceftazidime, cefoperazone, cefotaxime, ceftizoxime; ceftriaxone)**

REMARKS:
(1) Selection of the particular aminoglycoside should be based on locally generated antibiotic susceptibility profiles. Amikacin should be used when gentamicin- and tobramycin-resistant strains are prevalent.

(2) Some experts use a triple drug regimen that also includes a first generation cephalosporin (eg, cefazolin) or a penicillinase-resistant penicillin (eg, nafcillin), but presently available data fail to show any clear advantages for a three-drug combination when compared to recommended two-drug regimens. However, when *S. aureus* is a suspected pathogen, the addition of a first generation cephalosporin or a penicillinase-resistant penicillin (eg, nafcillin) to the regimen is recommended.

(3) Methicillin-resistant *Staphylococcus epidermidis* is a common cause of fever in the neutropenic patient in some cancer centers. Vancomycin is required to treat infections caused by this pathogen (see Wade et al, 1982).

(4) Use of ceftazidime alone or in combination with an antistaphylococcal drug (eg, nafcillin, vancomycin) for febrile neutropenic patients appears promising. However, additional data are necessary before specific recommendations can be made (see also Chapter 67, Cephalosporins and Related Agents).

(5) Switch to most effective drug regimen after blood culture and susceptibility test results are available. (Note: In patients with persistent granulocytopenia, continuation of a broad-spectrum combination of antibiotics appears to have some prophylactic value and is preferable.)

(5) If fever responds to therapy, but neutropenia (<500 granulocytes/mm³) persists, continued administration of the empiric antibiotic regimen is recommended.

(6) Persistent fever and granulocytopenia in the absence of documented bacterial infection (ie, negative culture) suggest possible fungal infection by *Candida*; addition of amphotericin B to the regimen should be considered.

Toxic Shock Syndrome

Toxic shock syndrome is an acute, febrile exanthematous illness characterized by the involvement of multiple organ systems and subsequent desquamation. It occurs primarily in young menstruating females who use tampons. The exact cause of toxic shock syndrome is still uncertain, but it is believed to be due to exotoxin produced by *Staphylococcus aureus* colonizing the vagina. This syndrome also may occur in patients with other *S. aureus* infections (eg, post-operative wound infection).

Antimicrobial drug therapy does not appear to play an important role in treating the acute phase of toxic shock syndrome. Supportive measures (eg, maintenance of adequate blood pressure) are of primary importance. Antibiotics (parenteral) are useful in preventing recurrences of the syndrome.

Selected references: *Morbid Mortal Week Rep*, 1983; Wager, 1983; Wiesenthal, 1983; Foltzer and Reese, 1986.

SPECIFIC THERAPY

PREFERRED THERAPY:
Nafcillin OR **Oxacillin**
ALTERNATIVE THERAPY:
First Generation Cephalosporin (eg, cefazolin)
REMARKS:
(1) Most experts do not recommend methicillin in adults because of an increased risk of interstitial nephritis.
(2) Vancomycin can be used in patients allergic to penicillins and cephalosporins.

MISCELLANEOUS INFECTIONS

SPECIFIC antimicrobial drug therapy for miscellaneous bacterial, actinomycetic, rickettsial, and spirochetal infections is outlined below. Treatment guidelines for fungal, protozoal, helminthic, and viral infections are discussed in Chapters 76, Antifungal Agents for Systemic Mycoses; 77, Antiprotozoal Agents; 78, Anthelmintics; and 79, Antiviral Agents, respectively.

Anthrax

Selected references: Conte and Barriere, 1984; *Med Lett Drugs Ther*, 1984, 1986; Nelson, 1985 A.

Bacillus anthracis
(gram-positive, spore-forming bacilli)

> PREFERRED THERAPY:
> **Penicillin G**
> ALTERNATIVE THERAPY:
> **Erythromycin; Tetracycline**
> REMARKS:
> (1) Tetracyclines should not be used in pregnant women or children less than 8 years.

Clostridial Myonecrosis (Gas Gangrene)

Selected references: Bornstein, 1981; *Med Lett Drugs Ther*, 1984, 1986; Nelson, 1985 A and B; Sanford, 1985 A.

Clostridium perfringens common; also C. novyi, C. septicum
(gram-positive bacilli)

> PREFERRED THERAPY:
> **Penicillin G**
> ALTERNATIVE THERAPY:
> **Chloramphenicol; Clindamycin; Metronidazole; Tetracycline**
> REMARKS:
> (1) High-dose, intravenous penicillin G (approximately 20 million units per day) is indicated.
> (2) Emergency surgical debridement is of primary importance. Hyperbaric oxygen therapy frequently is used. Antitoxin is no longer recommended.
> (3) Tetracyclines should not be used in pregnant women or children less than 8 years.

Erysipeloid

The predominant form is an acute, localized cellulitis caused by *Erysipelothrix rhusiopathiae*. Infection usually occurs in the finger or hand following an abrasion, scratch, or puncture wound while handling organic material (eg, raw fish or poultry) containing the organism. Erysipeloid is an occupational disease of fishermen, butchers, and others handling raw fish or poultry. Rarely, the organism causes bacteremia and endocarditis.

Selected references: Conte and Barriere, 1984; Magnussen, 1986.

Erysipelothrix rhusiopathiae
(gram-positive bacilli)

> PREFERRED THERAPY:
> **Penicillin G**
> ALTERNATIVE THERAPY:
> **Erythromycin**

Listeria monocytogenes Infections

Selected references: Conte and Barriere, 1984; *Med Lett Drugs Ther*, 1984, 1986; Nelson, 1985 A; Sanford, 1985 B.

Listeria monocytogenes
(gram-positive bacilli)

> PREFERRED THERAPY:
> **Ampicillin (or Penicillin G) *with or without* Aminoglycoside (gentamicin, tobramycin, amikacin, netilmicin)**
> ALTERNATIVE THERAPY:
> **Trimethoprim/Sulfamethoxazole; Tetracycline; Chloramphenicol; Erythromycin**
> REMARKS:
> (1) Combination regimen is synergistic in vitro. It is recommended for serious infections (sepsis, endocarditis, meningitis).

Tetanus

Tetanus is manifested by tonic muscle spasms and hyperreflexia that are caused by an exotoxin produced by the sporulated form of *Clostridium tetani*. Treatment includes administration of human hyperimmune globulin to neutralize the toxin, supportive care, and the administration of antimicrobial drug therapy, as outlined below.

Selected references: Band and Bennett, 1983; *Med Lett Drugs Ther*, 1984, 1986; Nelson, 1985 A and B; Magnussen, 1986. Guidelines for the prevention of tetanus can be found in Chapter 62, Agents for Active and Passive Immunity.

Clostridium tetani
(gram-positive, spore-forming bacilli)

> PREFERRED THERAPY:
> **Penicillin G**
> ALTERNATIVE THERAPY:
> **Tetracycline**
> REMARKS:
> (1) Avoid intramuscular injections.
> (2) Tetracyclines should not be used in pregnant women or children less than 8 years.

Brucellosis

Selected references: Conte and Barriere, 1984; *Med Lett Drugs Ther*, 1984, 1986; Nelson, 1985 A and B; Sanford, 1985 B.

Brucella
(gram-negative bacilli)

> PREFERRED THERAPY:
> **Tetracycline *with or without* Streptomycin**
> ALTERNATIVE THERAPY:
> **Chloramphenicol *with or without* Streptomycin; Trimethoprim/Sulfamethoxazole**
> REMARKS:
> (1) Combination regimens are recommended for severe infections.

(2) Trimethoprim/sulfamethoxazole *plus* rifampin or tetracycline *plus* rifampin are other alternative regimens, but clinical experience is limited.

(3) Tetracyclines should not be used in pregnant women or children less than 8 years.

Glanders

Selected references: *Med Lett Drugs Ther*, 1984, 1986; Nelson, 1985 A.

Pseudomonas mallei
(gram-negative bacilli)

PREFERRED THERAPY:
Tetracycline *plus* Streptomycin
ALTERNATIVE THERAPY:
Chloramphenicol *plus* Streptomycin
REMARKS:
(1) Tetracyclines should not be used in pregnant women or children less than 8 years.

Melioidosis

Selected references: Sanford, 1979; Thin, 1981; Conte and Barriere, 1984; *Med Lett Drugs Ther*, 1984, 1986; Nelson, 1985 A and B; Sanford, 1985 B.

Pseudomonas pseudomallei
(gram-negative bacilli)

PREFERRED THERAPY:
Trimethoprim/Sulfamethoxazole
OR
Tetracycline *with or without* Chloramphenicol
ALTERNATIVE THERAPY:
Chloramphenicol *plus* Kanamycin, Gentamicin, or Tobramycin; Sulfonamide
REMARKS:
(1) Combination regimens are recommended for severe infections.
(2) Tetracyclines should not be used in pregnant women or children less than 8 years.

Pasteurella multocida Infections

Pasteurella multocida is the most common causative organism of infections resulting from dog and cat bites or scratches.

Selected references: Goscienski, 1983; *Med Lett Drugs Ther*, 1984, 1986; Nelson, 1985 A; Sanford, 1985 B; Magnussen, 1986.

Pasteurella multocida
(gram-negative coccobacilli)

PREFERRED THERAPY:
Penicillin G
ALTERNATIVE THERAPY:
Tetracycline; Cephalosporin; Chloramphenicol
REMARKS:
(1)Tetracyclines should not be used in pregnant women or children less than 8 years.

Plague

Selected references: Conte and Barriere, 1984; *Med Lett Drugs Ther*, 1984, 1986; Nelson, 1985 A; Sanford, 1985 B.

Yersinia pestis
(gram-negative bacilli)

PREFERRED THERAPY:
Streptomycin
ALTERNATIVE THERAPY:
Tetracycline; Chloramphenicol; Gentamicin; Trimethoprim/Sulfamethoxazole
REMARKS:
(1) Some experts recommend a combination regimen containing streptomycin *plus* tetracycline.
(2) Tetracyclines should not be used in pregnant women or children less than 8 years.

Pseudomonas cepacia Infections

Selected references: *Med Lett Drugs Ther*, 1984, 1986; Nelson, 1985 A; Sanford, 1985 B.

Pseudomonas cepacia
(gram-negative bacilli)

PREFERRED THERAPY:
Trimethoprim/Sulfamethoxazole
ALTERNATIVE THERAPY:
Chloramphenicol; Ceftazidime

Rat Bite Fever

Causative organisms are *Spirillum minus* and *Streptobacillus moniliformis* (Haverhill Fever). Antimicrobial drug selection is the same for either organism.

Selected references: Conte and Barriere, 1984; *Med Lett Drugs Ther*, 1984, 1986; Nelson, 1985 A.

Spirillum minus
(gram-negative bacilli)

PREFERRED THERAPY:
Penicillin G
ALTERNATIVE THERAPY:
Tetracycline; Streptomycin
REMARKS:
(1) Tetracyclines should not be used in pregnant women or children less than 8 years.

Streptobacillus moniliformis
(gram-negative bacilli)

PREFERRED THERAPY:
Penicillin G
ALTERNATIVE THERAPY:
Tetracycline; Streptomycin
REMARKS:
(1) Tetracyclines should not be used in pregnant women or children less than 8 years.

Tularemia

Selected references: Hornick, 1983; Conte and Barriere, 1984; *Med Lett Drugs Ther*, 1984, 1986; Nelson, 1985 A and B; Sanford, 1985 B.

Francisella tularensis
(gram-negative coccobacilli)

PREFERRED THERAPY:
Streptomycin
ALTERNATIVE THERAPY:
Gentamicin, Tobramycin, or Amikacin; Tetracycline; Chloramphenicol
REMARKS:
(1) Tetracycline and chloramphenicol are less effective alternatives and relapses have occurred due to persistence of *F. tularensis*.
(2) Tetracyclines should not be used in pregnant women or children less than 8 years.

Vincent's Infection

Selected references: Attebery, 1981; *Med Lett Drugs Ther*, 1984, 1986; Nelson, 1985 A; Sanford, 1985 A.

Leptotrichia buccalis
(gram-negative bacilli)

PREFERRED THERAPY:
Penicillin G
ALTERNATIVE THERAPY:
Tetracycline; Erythromycin; Clindamycin
REMARKS:
(1) Tetracyclines should not be used in pregnant women or children less than 8 years.

Leprosy

The causative organism is *Mycobacterium leprae* (acid fast bacilli). See Chapter 75, Antimycobacterial Agents, for treatment guidelines.

Atypical Mycobacterial Infections

Causative organisms include *Mycobacterium kansasii, M. avium-intracellulare-scrofulaceum* complex, *M. fortuitum*, and *M. marinum*. See Chapter 75, Antimycobacterial Agents, for treatment guidelines.

Actinomycosis

Selected references: Conte and Barriere, 1984; *Med Lett Drugs Ther*, 1984, 1986; Nelson, 1985 A and B; Sanford, 1985 B and C; Gold and Kinderlehrer, 1986.

Actinomyces israelii
(anaerobic, gram-positive, branching, filamentous bacteria)

PREFERRED THERAPY:

Penicillin G
ALTERNATIVE THERAPY:
Tetracycline; Clindamycin; Erythromycin
REMARKS:
(1) High-dose, intravenous penicillin G (10 to 20 million units daily) for the initial four to six weeks, followed by oral penicillin V for 6 to 12 months often is recommended for deep-seated cervicofacial infections. Surgical debridement and drainage frequently are necessary.
(2) Tetracyclines should not be used in pregnant women or children less than 8 years.

Nocardiosis

Selected references: Hoeprich, 1983; Conte and Barriere, 1984; *Med Lett Drugs Ther*, 1984, 1986; Nelson, 1985 A and B; Sanford, 1985 B and C; Gold and Kinderlehrer, 1986.

Nocardia asteroides
(aerobic, gram-positive, branching, filamentous bacteria)

PREFERRED THERAPY:
Sulfonamide (trisulfapyrimidines, sulfadiazine, sulfisoxazole)
ALTERNATIVE THERAPY:
Trimethoprim/Sulfamethoxazole; Minocycline; Ampicillin *plus* Erythromycin; Amikacin; Cycloserine
REMARKS:
(1) Optimum treatment guidelines presently are unclear. Some experts prefer trimethoprim/sulfamethoxazole over a sulfonamide alone (see Smego et al, 1983).
(2) Prolonged therapy for 6 to 12 months usually is recommended. Surgical excision or drainage frequently is necessary.

Rickettsial Infections

This group of diseases is caused by rickettsiae (obligate, intracellular, pleomorphic bacteria). All are characterized by fever, headache, rash (except Q fever), influenza-like symptoms, and prostration. Diseases with worldwide or at least United States distribution include Q fever (*Coxiella burnetii*), rickettsialpox (*Rickettsia akari*), Rocky Mountain spotted fever (*R. rickettsii*), epidemic or Brill-Zinsser typhus (*R. prowazekii*), and endemic or murine typhus (*R. mooseri*). Antimicrobial drug therapy is the same for all rickettsial infections.

Selected references: Eisenberg et al, 1980; *Med Lett Drugs Ther*, 1984, 1986; Nelson, 1985 A and B; Sanford, 1985 B.

Rickettsia

PREFERRED THERAPY:
Tetracycline
ALTERNATIVE THERAPY:
Chloramphenicol
REMARKS:
(1) Tetracyclines should not be used in pregnant women or children less than 8 years.

Leptospirosis

Selected references: Conte and Barriere, 1984; McClain et al, 1984; *Med Lett Drugs Ther*, 1984, 1986; Nelson, 1985 A and B; Sanford, 1985 A.

Leptospira species
(spirochete)

PREFERRED THERAPY:
Penicillin G OR **Doxycycline** OR **Tetracycline**
REMARKS:
(1) Therapy early in the course of illness (within four days of onset) appears to favorably affect the signs and symptoms of leptospirosis.
(2) Tetracyclines should not be used in pregnant women or children less than 8 years.

Lyme Disease

Lyme disease is caused by *Borrelia burgdorferi,* a spirochete that is transmitted by *Ixodes* ticks. The disease is characterized initially by a distinctive skin lesion, erythema chronicum migrans, often accompanied by nonspecific constitutional symptoms, including fever, headache, myalgias, and arthralgias. Arthritic, neurologic, or cardiac complications may develop in some patients weeks to months after the initial lesion.

Early treatment of Lyme disease with appropriate antimicrobial agents has been shown to shorten the duration of erythema chronicum migrans and to prevent or ameliorate late complications of the disease.

Selected references: Benach et al, 1983; Meyerhoff, 1983; Steere et al, 1983 A, B and C; Bruhn, 1984; *Med Lett Drugs Ther*, 1984, 1986; *Morbid Mortal Week Rep*, 1984; Nelson, 1985 B.

Borrelia burgdorferi
(spirochete)

PREFERRED THERAPY:
Tetracycline
ALTERNATIVE THERAPY:
Penicillin G; Penicillin V; Erythromycin
REMARKS:
(1)Tetracycline and penicillin V were more effective than erythromycin in resolving erythema chronicum migrans and associated symptoms in a prospective, randomized study (Steere et al, 1983 B). Tetracycline appeared to be more effective in preventing the late complications of Lyme disease.
(2) Tetracyclines should not be used in pregnant women or children less than 8 years.
(3) Intravenous penicillin G (20 million units daily for 10 days) was shown to be effective in the treatment of meningitis associated with Lyme disease in a small number of patients (Steere et al, 1983 D). This regimen also was effective in 11 of 20 patients with Lyme arthritis (Steere et al, 1985). However, the optimal antimicrobial drug treatment of arthritis and other complications of this disease (eg, cardiac conduction abnormalities) presently is unresolved.

Relapsing Fever

Selected references: Southern, 1983; *Med Lett Drugs Ther*, 1984, 1986; Nelson, 1985 A; Sanford, 1985 A and B.

Borrelia recurrentis and other *Borrelia* species
(spirochete)

PREFERRED THERAPY:
Tetracycline
ALTERNATIVE THERAPY:
Chloramphenicol; Erythromycin; Penicillin G
REMARKS:
(1) Tetracyclines should not be used in pregnant women or children under 8 years.

Syphilis

Syphilis is caused by *Treponema pallidum* (spirochete). See Table 2, Treatment of Sexually Transmitted Diseases (STD), for treatment guidelines for this sexually transmitted infection.

Yaws

Selected references: *Med Lett Drugs Ther*, 1984, 1986; Nelson, 1985 A.

Treponema pertenue
(spirochete)

PREFERRED THERAPY:
Penicillin G
ALTERNATIVE THERAPY:
Tetracycline
REMARKS:
(1) Tetracyclines should not be used in pregnant women or children less than 8 years.

TABLE 2. TREATMENT OF SEXUALLY TRANSMITTED DISEASES (STD)

Sexually transmitted diseases (STD) are among the more common infections in the United States and have become a major public health problem. The well-known venereal diseases, gonorrhea and syphilis, continue to be two of the most common reportable infectious diseases. In addition, the spectrum of diseases known to be sexually transmitted has enlarged considerably, especially among homosexual or bisexual males. Presently, more than 20 etiologic agents that are associated with a variety of STD-related syndromes have been identified.

Guidelines for the selection of appropriate antimicrobial drugs in the treatment of a number of sexually transmitted diseases, ie, infections in which sexual contact is the primary or an important mechanism of transmission, are presented. Most of the recommendations are consistent with 1985 treatment guidelines proposed by the Centers for Disease Control (*Morbid Mortal Week Rep*, 1985 A).

CHLAMYDIA TRACHOMATIS INFECTIONS

Infections caused by *Chlamydia trachomatis* are the most prevalent sexually transmitted diseases in the United States today. The importance of serious complications (eg, pelvic inflammatory disease, infertility) related to chlamydial infections has been established. Diagnosis and treatment of these infections frequently are based on the clinical syndrome since chlamydial cultures often are unavailable. Recently developed direct fluorescent antibody [Microtrak] and enzyme-linked immunoassay [Chlamydiazyme] techniques can also be used to diagnose chlamydial genital infections. The following guidelines are for treatment of *laboratory-proven* infections caused by *C. trachomatis* (other than lymphogranuloma venereum [LGV] strains). For approaches to the treatment of common chlamydia-associated syndromes when laboratory confirmation is not available, see the section of this Table entitled, Common STD-Associated Syndromes. See also *Morbid Mortal Week Rep*, 1985 B.

Uncomplicated Urethral, Endocervical, or Rectal Infection in Adults (Confirmed Infection)

RECOMMENDED REGIMEN(S):
Tetracycline Hydrochloride: Orally, 500 mg four times daily for seven days;
OR
Doxycycline: Orally, 100 mg twice daily for seven days.
ALTERNATIVE REGIMEN(S):
(for patients in whom tetracyclines are contraindicated or not tolerated)
Erythromycin base or stearate: Orally, 500 mg four times daily for seven days;
OR
Erythromycin ethylsuccinate: Orally, 800 mg four times daily for seven days.
REMARKS:
(1) Sulfonamides also are active against *C. trachomatis*. Although optimal dosages of sulfonamides for chlamydial infection have not been defined, sulfamethoxazole, orally, 1 g twice daily for 10 days is probably effective.
(2) Persons exposed to *C. trachomatis* (sexual partners) should be examined for STD and treated with one of the above regimens.
(3) When taken as directed, the tetracycline and erythromycin regimens listed above are highly effective (>95% cure rates). Therefore, posttreatment *C. trachomatis* test-of-cure cultures may be omitted if laboratory resources are limited. Test-of-cure cultures may not become positive until three to six weeks after treatment. When they are positive, patients should be retreated with one of the above regimens and any interim sex partners should be treated.
(4) Pregnant women with laboratory-proven *C. trachomatis* infections and/or those whose sexual partners have nongonococcal urethritis should be treated with one of the above erythromycin regimens. For women who cannot tolerate these regimens, one-half the daily dose (250 mg base or stearate; 400 mg ethylsuccinate) four times daily for at least 14 days should be used. The optimal dose and duration of antibiotic therapy for pregnant women has not been established. There are no completely studied alternative regimens for women who are allergic to erythromycin or those who cannot tolerate this antibiotic. Proven treatment failures should be retreated with erythromycin in either of the dosage schedules outlined above. Simultaneous treatment of the male partner(s) with tetracycline or doxycycline is an important component of the therapeutic regimen. Pregnant women at particular risk for chlamydial infections should undergo diagnostic testing for *C. trachomatis* if possible at their first prenatal visit and during the third trimester. Important risk factors include the following: unmarried, age less than 20 years, residence in a socially disadvantaged community (eg, inner city) and the presence of other sexually transmitted diseases.

Neonatal Conjunctivitis and Pneumonia (Confirmed Infection)

Conjunctivitis

RECOMMENDED REGIMEN:
Erythromycin syrup: Orally, 50 mg/kg/day divided into four doses for two weeks.
REMARKS:
(1) Appropriate tests to rule out *Neisseria gonorrhoeae* as the cause should be done.
(2) The diagnosis of chlamydial conjunctivitis can be established by culture, direct fluorescent antibody, or Giemsa-stained conjunctival scrapings.
(3) There is no indication that topical therapy provides additional benefit.
(4) If inclusion conjunctivitis recurs after stopping therapy, erythromycin treatment should be reinstituted for an additional one to two weeks.

Pneumonia

RECOMMENDED REGIMEN:
Erythromycin syrup: Orally, 50 mg/kg/day divided into four doses for two weeks.
REMARKS:
(1) The optimal duration for therapy has not been established.
(2) Parents of newborn infants with chlamydial infection (conjunctivitis or pneumonia) should be treated with one of the recommended regimens for chlamydial infection.

GONOCOCCAL INFECTIONS

These guidelines, as proposed by the Centers for Disease Control, take into account the following observations: (1) the high frequency of coexisting chlamydial and gonococcal infections; (2) the increased recognition of serious complications of chlamydial and gonococcal infections; (3) the difficulty in diagnosing chlamydial infections; (4) the increasing incidence of infections due to both penicillinase-producing *Neisseria gonorrhoeae* (PPNG) and chromosomal-mediated *N. gonorrhoeae* (CMRNG); (5) reports of the emergence of tetracycline-resistant gonococci in some geographic areas; and (6) the availability of new antimicrobials (eg, new cephalosporins) that appear to be effective in treating gonococcal infections. Regimens have been recommended based on the general criteria of efficacy, safety, ease of administration, and cost.

Because of the changing pattern of antimicrobial resistance, periodic testing for antimicrobial susceptibility of a sample of *N. gonorrhoeae* isolates and all isolates associated with treatment failures should be an integral part of gonorrhea control programs.

Uncomplicated Urethral, Endocervical, or Rectal Infection in Adults

RECOMMENDED REGIMEN(S):
Amoxicillin/Ampicillin: Orally, amoxicillin 3 g or ampicillin 3.5 g, either with probenecid 1 g;
OR

Aqueous Procaine Penicillin G: Intramuscularly, 4.8 million units injected at two sites, with probenecid 1 g orally.
OR
Ceftriaxone: Intramuscularly, 250 mg without probenecid.

Followed By

Tetracycline Hydrochloride: Orally, 500 mg four times daily for seven days;
OR
Doxycycline: Orally, 100 mg twice daily for seven days.
OR
For patients in whom tetracyclines are contraindicated or not tolerated, erythromycin base or stearate, orally, 500 mg four times daily for seven days or erythromycin ethylsuccinate, orally, 800 mg four times daily for seven days.
REMARKS:
(1) The order of presentation does not indicate preference, but aqueous procaine penicillin G may be less desirable because of associated pain and toxicity.
(2) An important concern in the treatment of gonorrhea is coexisting chlamydial infection, documented in up to 45% of women with gonorrhea when adequate chlamydial cultures were performed. Only tetracycline (or doxycycline) is active against both gonococcal and chlamydial infections, but the increasing emergence of tetracycline-resistant *N. gonorrhoeae* strains argues against its use as a first-line drug for gonorrhea (Jaffe et al, 1981; Faruki et al, 1985; Rice et al, 1985; *Morbid Mortal Week Rep*, 1985 C; Hook and Holmes, 1985). Concern also exists about the problem of patient compliance with multiple-day tetracycline/doxycycline regimens for gonococcal infections and the low cure rate of only 90% reported for women with gonococcal infections given tetracycline alone (Stamm et al, 1984). To address these concerns, administration of a single-dose penicillin or cephalosporin regimen for gonorrhea is recommended just prior to a tetracycline or doxycycline regimen.
(3) The advantages of the combined regimen are: (a) it provides adequate single-dose treatment for gonorrhea; (b) it is effective against chlamydial infections; and (c) it is effective against pharyngeal gonococcal infections. Disadvantages are: (a) the requirement for a multiple-day, multiple-dose regimen for treatment of chlamydial infection; (b) the risk of secondary vulvovaginal candidiasis in women probably is enhanced; (c) test-of-cure culture for gonorrhea must be delayed until three or four days after the completion of dual therapy; (d) unknown potential for selection of resistant strains of *C. trachomatis* if compliance is poor; and (e) unknown potential for masking *C. trachomatis* infections in those who only partially comply with treatment.
(4) In women with rectal infection, any of the above regimens are effective. However, ampicillin/amoxicillin and tetracycline/doxycycline are not effective for rectal gonococcal infections in men. Thus, homosexual men with rectal gonococcal infection should be treated with ceftriaxone, 250 mg intramuscularly (preferred), or aqueous procaine penicillin G, 4.8 million units intramuscularly injected at two sites, plus probenecid, 1 g orally (see Remark 1). For those allergic to penicillins and cephalosporins, use spectinomycin, 2 g intramuscularly. These regimens provide adequate treatment for urethral and rectal gonococcal infection, but spectinomycin is not recommended for the treatment of pharyngeal gonococcal infection. Homosexual men are less likely than heterosexual men to have coexistent chlamydial infections; therefore, routine additional tetracycline or doxycycline treatment is not recommended.
(5) Either the amoxicillin/ampicillin or ceftriaxone regimen is recommended for pregnant women with uncomplicated gonorrhea. Aqueous procaine penicillin G also is effective, but is less desirable because of associated pain and toxicity. Follow-up therapy with one of the erythromycin regimens is necessary to treat coexisting chlamydial infection. Tetracycline or doxycycline should not be used in pregnant women because of potential

adverse effects for the fetus. All pregnant women should have endocervical cultures for *N. gonorrhoeae* at the first prenatal visit. A second culture for gonococci and a test for *C. trachomatis* late in the third trimester should be done on women at high risk of sexually transmitted diseases.
(6) The tetracycline or doxycycline regimen is recommended for penicillin- and cephalosporin-allergic patients, except for men with anorectal gonorrhea or pregnant women. A single intramuscular injection of spectinomycin 2 g is recommended in these individuals and in those penicillin- and cephalosporin-allergic patients who cannot tolerate tetracyclines. Some infectious disease experts now prefer spectinomycin as the primary alternative for all penicillin- and cephalosporin-allergic patients (Hook and Holmes, 1985; see also Remark 2 above).
(7) All the above recommended regimens (except spectinomycin alone) should cure incubating syphilis (seronegative, without clinical signs of syphilis). All patients with gonorrhea should have a serologic test for syphilis which, if present, should be treated with additional therapy appropriate for the stage of syphilis (see the section entitled Syphilis).
(8) Patients with proven or suspected penicillinase-producing *N. gonorrhoeae* (PPNG) infection or those in whom gonorrhea persists after treatment with a recommended regimen should receive a single intramuscular injection of either spectinomycin 2 g or ceftriaxone 250 mg. Tetracycline, doxycycline, or erythromycin should be added to treat coexisting chlamydial infection. To treat pharyngeal gonococcal infection due to PPNG, administer ceftriaxone 250 mg intramuscularly or nine tablets of trimethoprim/sulfamethoxazole (80 mg/400 mg) as a single daily dose for five days.
(9) Chromosomally mediated (beta-lactamase negative) resistant *N. gonorrhoeae* (CMRNG) have been reported in the United States. Spectinomycin or ceftriaxone (dosage regimens as above) should be effective against these strains (*Morbid Mortal Week Rep*, 1984).
(10) Women and heterosexual men exposed to gonorrhea (sexual partners) should be examined, cultured, and treated prophylactically with an appropriate recommended regimen which covers both gonococcal and chlamydial infections. Homosexual men exposed to gonorrhea should be examined, cultured, and treated for gonorrhea.
(11) Follow-up cultures should be obtained from the infected site(s) three to seven days after completion of treatment. In addition, rectal cultures should be obtained from all women treated for gonorrhea.
(12) Although a number of the beta-lactamase-stable second and third generation cephalosporins are effective in uncomplicated gonorrhea, ceftriaxone has become the preferred agent. This long-acting ($t_{1/2} = 8$ hours) third generation cephalosporin has outstanding in vitro activity against *N. gonorrhoeae*, including PPNG and CMRNG strains. Administered intramuscularly as a single 250 mg dose, it has been highly effective in uncomplicated gonorrhea in adults, including urethral, endocervical, anorectal, and pharyngeal forms of this infection (Handsfield and Murphy, 1983; Judson et al, 1983, 1985; Collier et al, 1984; see also Chapter 67, Cephalosporins and Related Agents).
(13) Although benzathine penicillin G is effective in the treatment of syphilis, it has no place in the treatment of gonorrhea. Penicillins and cephalosporins *not recommended* for the treatment of gonorrhea include: benzathine penicillin G, oral penicillin G, penicillin V, cloxacillin, dicloxacillin, cephradine, cephalothin, cephapirin, cefazolin, cephalexin, cefadroxil, and cefaclor.

Disseminated Gonococcal Infection in Adults (Arthritis-Dermatitis Syndrome)

RECOMMENDED REGIMEN(S):
Aqueous Crystalline Penicillin G: Intravenously, 10 million units per day for at least three days, followed by amoxicillin

500 mg (or ampicillin 500 mg) orally four times daily to complete at least seven days of antibiotic treatment;
OR
Amoxicillin/Ampicillin: Orally, amoxicillin 3 g (or ampicillin 3.5 g), each with probenecid 1 g, followed by amoxicillin 500 mg (or ampicillin 500 mg) four times daily for at least seven days;
OR
Cefoxitin: Intravenously, 1 g four times daily for at least seven days;
OR
Cefotaxime: Intravenously, 500 mg four times daily for at least seven days;
OR
Ceftriaxone: Intravenously, 1 g once daily for seven days.
REMARKS:
(1) Except for homosexual men, patients treated with one of the above regimens should be given an additional seven days of tetracycline, doxycycline, or erythromycin, as outlined in the previous section, for possible coexistent chlamydial infection.
(2) Patients allergic to penicillins and cephalosporins may be treated with tetracycline hydrochloride, orally, 500 mg four times daily for at least seven days OR doxycycline, orally, 100 mg twice daily for at least seven days.
(3) For disseminated infections caused by PPNG, the cefoxitin, cefotaxime, or ceftriaxone regimen is recommended.
(4) Hospitalization is recommended, especially for patients who cannot reliably comply with treatment, have uncertain diagnoses, have purulent joint effusions, or have other complications. Attempts should be made to exclude endocarditis or meningitis.
(5) Although open drainage of joints other than the hip is not indicated, repeated aspiration may be necessary. Intra-articular injection of antibiotics is contraindicated.
(6) Meningitis and endocarditis caused by *N. gonorrhoeae* require high-dose intravenous penicillin therapy. Optimal duration of therapy is unknown, but most authorities treat patients with gonococcal meningitis for 10 to 14 days and gonococcal endocarditis for one month. Therapy of penicillin-allergic patients must be individualized. Treatment of PPNG- or CMRNG-related meningitis or endocarditis should be undertaken in consultation with an expert.

Gonococcal Ophthalmia in Adults

RECOMMENDED REGIMEN:
Aqueous Crystalline Penicillin G: Intravenously, 10 million units daily for five days.
REMARKS:
(1) For PPNG infections, use one of the following for five days: cefoxitin 1 g or cefotaxime 500 mg, intravenously, each given four times daily, or ceftriaxone, intramuscularly, 1 g once daily.
(2) Patients should be hospitalized. Irrigation of the eyes with saline or buffered ophthalmic solutions may be useful adjunctive therapy to eliminate discharge. All patients must have careful ophthalmologic assessment for ocular complications.
(3) Topical antibiotic preparations alone are not sufficient and are unnecessary when appropriate systemic antibiotic therapy is given.

Neonatal Gonococcal Infections

No apparent illness, but born to mother with gonococcal infection

RECOMMENDED REGIMEN:
Aqueous Crystalline Penicillin G: Intramuscularly or intravenously, 50,000 units (full-term infants) or 20,000 units (low-birth-weight infants) as a single injection.

REMARKS:
(1) The infant born to a mother with untreated gonorrhea is at high risk of infection and requires treatment.
(2) Topical prophylaxis for neonatal ophthalmia is not adequate treatment for infections at other sites.
(3) Clinical illness requires additional treatment as outlined below.

Gonococcal ophthalmia

RECOMMENDED REGIMEN:
Aqueous Crystalline Penicillin G: Intravenously, 100,000 units/kg/day in four divided doses for seven days.
REMARKS:
(1) Cefotaxime or gentamicin in doses appropriate for neonates is preferred for PPNG infections.
(2) Patients should be hospitalized and isolated for 24 hours after initiation of treatment. Irrigation of the eyes with saline or buffered ophthalmic solutions may be useful adjunctive therapy to eliminate discharge. Topical antibiotics should not be given.
(3) Both parents must be treated.
(4) Simultaneous ophthalmic infection with *C. trachomatis* has been reported and should be considered in patients who do not respond satisfactorily.

Bacteremia and arthritis

RECOMMENDED REGIMEN:
Aqueous Crystalline Penicillin G: Intravenously, 100,000 units/kg/day in four divided doses for at least seven days.
REMARK:
(1) For penicillin-resistant strains, experience is limited and should be decided in consultation with an expert. Cefotaxime, cefoxitin, or ceftriaxone may be useful.

Meningitis

RECOMMENDED REGIMEN:
Aqueous Crystalline Penicillin G: Intravenously, 100,000 units/kg/day in four divided doses for at least ten days.
REMARK:
(1) For penicillin-resistant strains, experience is limited and should be decided in consultation with an expert. Cefotaxime or ceftriaxone may be useful.

Gonococcal Infections in Older children

Uncomplicated gonorrhea in children <45 kg

RECOMMENDED REGIMEN(S):
Amoxicillin: Orally, 50 mg/kg plus probenecid 25 mg/kg (maximum, 1 g);
OR
Ceftriaxone: Intramuscularly, 125 mg.
REMARKS:
(1) Children weighing≥45 kg should receive adult regimens (see Uncomplicated Urethral, Endocervical, or Rectal Infection in Adults).
(2) Ceftriaxone should be used for proctitis and pharyngitis.
(3) Children who are allergic to penicillins and cephalosporins should receive spectinomycin intramuscularly, 40 mg/kg as a single dose. Children over 8 years may be given tetracycline hydrochloride (orally, 40 mg/kg/day in four divided doses for five days).
(4) Children with PPNG infection should receive spectinomycin in appropriate doses. Ceftriaxone may be useful, but data are unavailable.

(5) All patients should have follow-up cultures, and the source of infection should be identified, examined, and treated. Child abuse should be carefully considered and evaluated.

(6) Patients should be evaluated for coinfection with *C. trachomatis*.

Complicated gonorrhea

REMARKS:

The alternative regimens used in adults (see Disseminated Gonococcal Infection in Adults [Arthritis-Dermatitis Syndrome]) may be used in appropriate pediatric dosages (tetracyclines should not be used in children under 8 years).

COMMON STD-ASSOCIATED SYNDROMES

Several, often serious, clinical syndromes are associated with STD. Some are more clearly defined than others. The following guidelines outline approaches to the initial treatment of these conditions when complete bacteriologic evaluation is not possible or while awaiting the results of specific laboratory tests.

Nongonococcal Urethritis (NGU)

The most common causative organisms are *Chlamydia trachomatis* or *Ureaplasma urealyticum*.

RECOMMENDED REGIMEN(S):
Tetracycline Hydrochloride: Orally, 500 mg four times daily for seven days;
OR
Doxycycline: Orally, 100 mg twice daily for seven days.
REMARKS:
(1) For patients in whom tetracyclines are contraindicated or not tolerated, erythromycin base or stearate, orally, 500 mg four times daily for seven days or erythromycin ethylsuccinate, orally, 800 mg four times daily for seven days is recommended.
(2) Sexual partners of patients with NGU should be examined for STD and treated with an appropriate recommended regimen.
(3) Patients should be advised to return if symptoms persist or recur.

Acute Pelvic Inflammatory Disease (PID)

Acute pelvic inflammatory disease (PID) includes endometritis, salpingitis, parametritis, and peritonitis and refers to an acute clinical syndrome attributed to the ascending spread of microorganisms, unrelated to pregnancy or surgery, from the vagina and endocervix to the endometrium, fallopian tubes, and/or contiguous structures.

Causative organisms include *Neisseria gonorrhoeae*, *Chlamydia trachomatis*, anaerobic bacteria (eg, *Bacteroides*; gram-positive cocci), facultative gram-negative bacilli (eg, *Escherichia coli*), *Mycoplasma hominis*, and rarely *Actinomyces israelii*. The treatment of choice is not established and no single agent is active against the entire spectrum of pathogens.

The following are examples of combination regimens with broad activity against major pathogens in PID. The regimens have been subdivided into those used for inpatient treatment and those employed in ambulatory patients. Hospitalization is indicated when (1) the diagnosis is uncertain; (2) surgical emergencies, such as appendicitis and ectopic pregnancy, cannot be excluded; (3) a pelvic abscess is suspected; (4) severe illness precludes outpatient management; (5) the patient is pregnant; (6) the patient is a prepubertal child; (7) the patient is unable to follow or tolerate an outpatient regimen; (8) the patient has failed to respond to outpatient therapy; or (9) clinical follow-up within 72 hours following the start of antibiotic treatment cannot be arranged. Many experts recommend hospitalization for all patients with PID.

Inpatient Treatment

RECOMMENDED REGIMEN(S):
(A) Doxycycline: Intravenously, 100 mg twice daily;
Plus
Cefoxitin: Intravenously, 2 g four times daily.
Continue drugs intravenously for at least four days and at least 48 hours after patient improves. Then continue doxycycline 100 mg, orally, twice daily to complete 10 to 14 days of total therapy.
REMARKS:
(1) This regimen theoretically provides optimal coverage for *N. gonorrhoeae*, including PPNG, and *C. trachomatis*. It may not provide optimal treatment for anaerobes, pelvic mass, or PID associated with an intrauterine device (IUD).

(B) Clindamycin: Intravenously, 600 mg four times daily;
Plus
Gentamicin (or tobramycin): Intravenously, 2 mg/kg initially, followed by 1.5 mg/kg three times daily in patients with normal renal function.
Continue drugs intravenously for at least four days and at least 48 hours after patient improves. Then continue clindamycin 450 mg, orally, four times daily to complete 10 to 14 days of total therapy.
REMARKS:
(1) This regimen provides optimal activity against anaerobes and facultative gram-negative rods, and limited clinical data (Wasserheit et al, 1986) suggest adequate activity against *C. trachomatis* and *N. gonorrhoeae*. Amikacin may be substituted when gentamicin- or tobramycin-resistant strains of aerobic gram-negative bacilli are known or suspected to be present.

Ambulatory Treatment

RECOMMENDED REGIMEN(S):
Cefoxitin: Intramuscularly, 2 g; OR Amoxicillin: Orally, 3 g; OR Ampicillin: Orally, 3.5 g; OR Aqueous Procaine Penicillin G: Intramuscularly, 4.8 million units at two sites (each along with probenecid 1 g orally); OR Ceftriaxone: Intramuscularly, 250 mg.

Followed By

Doxycycline: Orally, 100 mg twice daily for 10 to 14 days.
REMARKS:
(1) Treatment with penicillins or cephalosporins alone is not recommended.
(2) Cefoxitin or ceftriaxone plus doxycycline provides activity against *N. gonorrhoeae*, including PPNG, and *C. trachomatis*. The other combinations are not effective against PPNG.
(3) Although tetracycline hydrochloride (orally, 500 mg four times daily) can be substituted for doxycycline, it is less active against

certain anaerobes and requires more frequent dosing; both represent drawbacks in treatment of PID.

(4) Outpatients should be re-evaluated after 48 to 72 hours for response.

(5) Sexual partners of patients with PID should be examined for STD and promptly treated with a regimen effective against uncomplicated gonococcal and chlamydial infections.

(6) Single doses of penicillin or cephalosporin antibiotic followed by oral tetracycline may not provide sustained activity against many strains of chromosomally mediated resistant *N. gonorrhoeae* or the facultative or anaerobic organisms involved in PID. No data are available on the therapy of PID caused by CMRNG. These patients should be followed in consultation with an expert.

Acute Epididymo-orchitis

Acute epididymo-orchitis has two forms: a sexually transmitted form usually associated with urethritis and commonly caused by *Chlamydia trachomatis* and/or *Neisseria gonorrhoeae*, and a nonsexually transmitted form associated with urinary tract infections caused by Enterobacteriaceae or *Pseudomonas*. Urine should be examined by Gram stain and culture to exclude bacteriuria in all patients, including those with urethritis. Testicular torsion is a surgical emergency that should be considered in all cases.

Sexually transmitted epididymo-orchitis occurs primarily in young adults (eg, <35 years) and is associated with the presence of urethritis, absence of underlying genitourinary pathology, and absence of gram-negative rods on Gram stain of urine. Recommended treatment for this form of epididymo-orchitis is outlined below. For drug selection for nonsexually transmitted acute epididymo-orchitis, see Table 1, Antimicrobial Drug Selection for Common Infectious Diseases.

Sexually transmitted epididymo-orchitis

RECOMMENDED REGIMEN(S):
Amoxicillin: Orally, 3 g; OR Ampicillin: Orally, 3.5 g; OR Aqueous Procaine Penicillin G: Intramuscularly, 4.8 million units at two sites (each along with probenecid 1 g orally); OR Spectinomycin: Intramuscularly, 2 g; OR Ceftriaxone: Intramuscularly, 250 mg.

Followed By

Tetracycline Hydrochloride: Orally, 500 mg four times daily for ten days; OR Doxycycline: Orally, 100 mg twice daily for ten days.
REMARKS:
(1) For patients in whom tetracyclines are contraindicated or not tolerated, erythromycin base or stearate, orally, 500 mg four times daily for seven days or erythromycin ethylsuccinate, orally, 800 mg four times daily for seven days is recommended.
(2) For epididymitis caused by PPNG, clinical experience is limited, but a 10-day course of therapy with oral trimethoprim/sulfamethoxazole or parenteral ceftriaxone, cefotaxime, cefoxitin, or spectinomycin may be used.
(3) Bed rest and scrotal elevation are recommended until fever and local inflammation subside. Failure to improve within three days requires re-evaluation.
(4) Sexual partners of patients with sexually transmitted acute epididymo-orchitis should be examined for STD and promptly treated with a regimen effective against uncomplicated gonococcal and chlamydial infection.

Bacterial Vaginosis

Vaginal discharge associated with bacterial vaginosis is a common syndrome associated with sexual activity in women.

Vaginal discharge associated with bacterial vaginosis is nonirritating, malodorous, thin, and homogeneous white. The vaginal pH is elevated (>4.5), and there is elaboration of malodorous amines (fishy odor) from the discharge fluid after alkalization with 10% potassium hydroxide. Microscopic examination of vaginal fluid typically reveals small, gram-negative coccobacillary organisms associated with epithelial cells (clue cells). It is now believed that several species of vaginal bacteria interact to produce the syndrome. Cultures for *Gardnerella vaginalis* are not useful and are not recommended for the diagnosis of this syndrome.

RECOMMENDED REGIMEN:
Metronidazole: Orally, 500 mg twice daily for seven days is an effective treatment.
REMARKS:
(1) Alternative regimen is ampicillin (or amoxicillin) orally, 500 mg four times daily for seven days. This regimen is less effective, but may be used for pregnant women or patients for whom metronidazole is contraindicated.
(2) Treatment of asymptomatic carriers of *G. vaginalis* is not recommended.
(3) Treatment of male sexual partners does not reduce the risk of recurrence of bacterial vaginosis in the index case.

Mucopurulent Cervicitis

The presence of mucopurulent endocervical exudate often reflects cervicitis due to chlamydial or gonococcal infection. Criteria for the presumptive diagnosis of mucopurulent cervicitis include: (1) mucopurulent secretion from the endocervix which may appear yellow or green when viewed on a white cotton-tipped swab (positive swab test); (2) >10 polymorphonuclear leukocytes per microscopic oil immersion field (x 1,000) in a Gram-stained smear of endocervical secretions; and (3) cervicitis, determined by cervical friability (bleeding when the first swab culture is taken) and/or by erythema or edema within a zone of cervical ectopy. For treatment of mucopurulent cervicitis, see the following remarks.
REMARKS:
(1) If *N. gonorrhoeae* is found on Gram stain or culture of endocervical or urethral discharge, treatment should be given as recommended for uncomplicated gonorrhea in adults (see section entitled Gonococcal Infections: Uncomplicated Urethral, Endocervical, or Rectal Infection in Adults).
(2) If *N. gonorrhoeae* is not found and/or chlamydial infection is proven or suspected, treatment should be given as recommended for chlamydial infection in adults (see section entitled *Chlamydia Trachomatis* Infections: Uncomplicated Urethral, Endocervical, or Rectal Infection in Adults [Confirmed Infection]).
(3) Male sexual partners of women with mucopurulent cervicitis attributed to gonococcal or chlamydial infection should be evaluated for STD and treated with the same regimen as their sex partners.

Acute Urethral Syndrome (Dysuria-Pyuria Syndrome)

The acute urethral syndrome is a common syndrome that may be associated with STD in women. Description and treatment of the acute urethral syndrome are discussed primarily in Table 1, Antimicrobial Drug Selection for Common Infectious Diseases. For drug selection when the sexually transmitted pathogens, *Chlamydia trachomatis* and/or *Neisseria gonorrhoeae*, are the suspected causative organisms, see the following remarks.

REMARKS:

(1) If *N. gonorrhoeae* is found on Gram stain or culture of endocervix, urethra, or urine, treatment should be given as recommended for uncomplicated gonorrhea in adults (see section entitled Gonococcal Infections: Uncomplicated Urethral, Endocervical, or Rectal Infection in Adults).

(2) If *N. gonorrhoeae* is not found and/or chlamydial infection is proven or suspected, treatment should be given as recommended for chlamydial infection in adults (see section entitled *Chlamydia Trachomatis* Infections: Uncomplicated Urethral, Endocervical, or Rectal Infection in Adults [Confirmed Infection]).

(3) Male sexual partners of women with sexually transmitted acute urethral syndrome attributed to gonococcal or chlamydial infection should be evaluated for STD and treated as recommended for contacts exposed to gonorrhea or chlamydial infection.

Vulvovaginal Candidiasis

REMARKS:

(1) This common vaginal infection generally is not considered a sexually transmitted disease. For drug selection and treatment guidelines, refer to Table 1, Antimicrobial Drug Selection for Common Infectious Diseases, and Chapter 74, Topical Anti-infective Agents: Drugs Used on Skin and Mucous Membranes.

TRICHOMONIASIS

This vaginal infection is caused by *Trichomonas vaginalis*. Antimicrobial drug therapy should be active against this organism.

RECOMMENDED REGIMEN:
Metronidazole: Orally, 2 g in a single dose.
REMARKS:

(1) Alternative regimen: Metronidazole, orally, 250 mg three times daily for seven days.

(2) Asymptomatic women with trichomoniasis should be treated as for symptomatic women.

(3) Male sexual partners of women with trichomoniasis should be treated with metronidazole, orally, 2 g, as a single dose, and examined for coexistent STD.

(4) Tests to determine cure should be sought whenever possible. Resistance of *Trichomonas vaginalis* to metronidazole has been observed but is rare. Patients who fail treatment should be retreated with the same regimen. Persistent failures should be managed in consultation with an expert. Metronidazole, orally, 2 g daily for three days has been successful in patients infected with *T. vaginalis* strains mildly resistant to metronidazole, but experience with this regimen is limited.

(5) Metronidazole is contraindicated during the first trimester of pregnancy and should be avoided throughout pregnancy. Clotrimazole 100 mg intravaginally at bedtime for seven days may

produce symptomatic improvement and some cures. Other local treatments may be used for symptomatic relief, but have low cure rates.

(6) Lactating women may be treated with metronidazole, orally, 2 g, in a single dose. Although no adverse reactions in nursing infants have been reported, breast-feeding is not recommended for at least 24 hours after therapy.

(7) Infants with symptomatic trichomoniasis or persistent urogenital trichomonal colonization beyond the fourth week of life can be treated with metronidazole 10 to 30 mg/kg daily for five to eight days.

(8) Children (prepubertal) with trichomonal infection should be treated with metronidazole, orally, 15 mg/kg daily divided into three doses for seven to ten days. Child abuse should be carefully considered and evaluated.

GENITAL HERPES SIMPLEX VIRUS INFECTIONS

Genital herpes infection is caused by Herpes simplex virus; it may be chronic and recurrent and there is no known cure. For treatment guidelines, see Chapter 79, Antiviral Agents.

GENITAL AND ANAL WARTS (CONDYLOMATA ACUMINATA)

The treatment of genital and anal warts has not been well studied. No treatment is completely satisfactory. Genital and anal warts are caused by human papilloma virus (HPV) and have recently been linked to the development of squamous cell genital cancers. For these reasons, atypical or persistent warts should be biopsied. A Papanicolaou smear is recommended for all women with genital warts. Women with cervical warts should not be treated until the results of the Pap smear are available to guide therapy. Although podophyllin is widely used in the treatment of genital and anal warts, some experts feel that cryotherapy, when available, may be preferable.

External Genital/Perianal Warts

RECOMMENDED REGIMENS:
Cryotherapy, eg, liquid nitrogen or carbon dioxide (dry ice)
OR
Podophyllin: 10% in compound tincture of benzoin. Apply carefully to each wart, avoiding normal tissue. Wash off thoroughly in one to four hours. Some consultants use a longer period, but this must be individualized after patient tolerance and compliance have been established. Repeat once or twice weekly. If warts do not regress after four applications, alternative treatments are indicated.
REMARKS:

(1) Podophyllin should not be used during pregnancy.

(2) Alternative therapies: Electrosurgery; surgical removal.

(3) Women with external genital warts often have coexistent vaginal or cervical warts. At a minimum, a Pap smear is indicated for detection of cervical warts or other cytologic abnormalities. Colposcopy in consultation with an expert should be considered.

Vaginal/Cervical Warts

Vaginal/cervical warts are often found only by Pap smear or colposcopy. Women with vaginal/cervical warts should be examined by an experienced colposcopist. Treatment of vaginal/cervical warts is complicated and should be carried out in consultation with an expert. Current therapies include:

Cryotherapy
Fluorouracil
REMARKS:
(1) Podophyllin 10% in compound tincture of benzoin may be used for vaginal warts only if great care is taken to ensure that the treated area is dried before removing the speculum. Because podophyllin is absorbed and is toxic, use of large amounts should be avoided. Podophyllin is *not recommended* for cervical warts.

Urethral/Meatal Warts

RECOMMENDED REGIMEN:
Podophyllin: 10% in compound tincture of benzoin may be used for accessible meatal warts. Great care should be taken to ensure that the treated area is dried before contact with normal mucosa is allowed. Podophyllin must be thoroughly washed off after one to four hours. Treatment should be undertaken in consultation with an expert. Access to urethroscopy is important for management. Podophyllin should not be used for urethral warts (see Remarks below).
REMARKS:
(1) Alternative therapy: Cryotherapy (eg, liquid nitrogen, solid carbon dioxide).
(2) Urethral Warts: Intraurethral warts should be suspected in men with recurrent meatal warts. Urethroscopy is necessary to diagnose this condition. Intraurethral 5% fluorouracil or thiotepa may be effective in this condition, but neither has been adequately evaluated. Podophyllin should not be used.

Anal Warts

RECOMMENDED REGIMENS:
Cryotherapy (eg, liquid nitrogen, solid carbon dioxide) may be used to treat anal warts accessible to anoscope.
OR
Podophyllin: 10% in compound tincture of benzoin may be used to treat anal warts accessible to anoscope. Extreme care must be taken to avoid exposure of normal mucosa to podophyllin. Allow the treated area to dry before removal of the anoscope. Podophyllin must be washed off after one to four hours. Many consultants avoid the use of podophyllin for anal warts.
REMARKS:
(1) Alternative therapy: Electrocautery.
(2) Patients with extensive anal warts should be referred for proctologic evaluation.

Oral Warts

Oral warts should be treated with:

Cryotherapy (eg, liquid nitrogen, solid carbon dioxide)
Electrosurgery
Surgical removal
REMARK:
(1) Podophyllin is contraindicated for oral warts.

SYPHILIS

Antimicrobial therapy should be directed against the causative organism, *Treponema pallidum*. Parenteral penicillin G is the drug of choice in the nonallergic patient for the treatment of all stages of syphilis. The preparation(s) used (ie, benzathine, aqueous procaine, or aqueous crystalline penicillin G), and the dose and length of treatment depend on the stage of disease.

Early Syphilis

Primary, secondary, or latent syphilis of less than one year's duration

RECOMMENDED REGIMEN:
Benzathine Penicillin G: Intramuscularly, 2.4 million units in a single dose.
REMARKS:
(1) Penicillin-allergic patients should receive tetracycline hydrochloride, orally, 500 mg four times daily for 15 days. Although this regimen appears to be effective, optimal patient compliance may be difficult to achieve.
(2) Penicillin-allergic patients who cannot tolerate tetracycline should have their allergy confirmed. If confirmed, these patients should receive erythromycin, orally, 500 mg four times daily for 15 days only if compliance and serologic follow-up can be assured. Otherwise, the patient should be referred to an expert.
(3) Post-treatment quantitative nontreponemal tests are recommended at 3, 6, and 12 months. Cerebrospinal fluid examination is recommended at the last visit for patients who received regimens other than penicillin.
(4) Retreatment: The possibility of reinfection should always be considered when retreating patients with early syphilis. A CSF examination should be performed before retreatment unless reinfection and a diagnosis of early syphilis can be established. Retreatment should be considered when: (a) Clinical signs or symptoms of syphilis persist or recur; (b) there is a fourfold increase in the titer of a nontreponemal test; or (c) an initially high-titer nontreponemal test fails to decrease fourfold within a year. Patients should be retreated with the schedules recommended for syphilis of more than one year's duration. In general, only one retreatment course is indicated because patients may maintain stable, low titers of nontreponemal tests or have irreversible anatomical damage.
(5) Persons exposed to infectious syphilis within the previous three months and other persons at high risk should be tested for syphilis and treated as for early syphilis.

Syphilis of More Than One Year's Duration (Except Neurosyphilis)

Syphilis of more than one year's duration, including latent, cardiovascular, or late benign syphilis, but not neurosyphilis

RECOMMENDED REGIMEN:
Benzathine Penicillin G: Intramuscularly, 2.4 million units weekly for three successive weeks (7.2 million units total).
REMARKS:
(1) The optimal treatment schedules for syphilis of greater than one year's duration have been less well established than schedules for early syphilis. In general, syphilis of longer duration requires more prolonged therapy.
(2) Penicillin-allergic patients should receive tetracycline hydrochloride, orally, 500 mg four times daily for 30 days. The efficacy of this regimen is not documented by published clinical data and patient compliance may be difficult to achieve. Cerebrospinal fluid examinations should be performed prior to therapy to exclude asymptomatic neurosyphilis.
(3) Penicillin-allergic patients who cannot tolerate tetracycline

should have their allergy confirmed. If confirmed, these patients should receive erythromycin, orally, 500 mg four times daily for 30 days only if compliance and serologic follow-up can be assured. Otherwise, the patient should be hospitalized and managed by an expert. Cerebrospinal fluid examinations should be performed prior to therapy to exclude asymptomatic neurosyphilis.

(4) Cerebrospinal fluid examination is desirable for all patients with syphilis of more than one year's duration to exclude asymptomatic neurosyphilis.

(5) Post-treatment quantitative nontreponemal tests are recommended at 3, 6, 12, and 24 months. Cerebrospinal fluid examination is recommended at the last visit for patients who received regimens other than penicillin.

(6) Therapy is recommended for established cardiovascular syphilis, although antibiotics may not reverse the pathology associated with this disease.

Neurosyphilis

Published studies show that a total dose of 6 to 9 million units of penicillin G over a three- to four-week period results in a satisfactory clinical response in approximately 90% of patients with neurosyphilis. Regimens employing benzathine penicillin G in standard doses or procaine penicillin G in doses under 2.4 million units daily do not consistently provide treponemicidal levels of penicillin G in CSF, and several case reports document the failure of such regimens to cure neurosyphilis.

RECOMMENDED REGIMENS:
Aqueous Crystalline Penicillin G: Intravenously, 2 to 4 million units every four hours for ten days, followed by benzathine penicillin G, intramuscularly, 2.4 million units weekly for three successive weeks;
OR
Aqueous Procaine Penicillin G: Intramuscularly, 2.4 million units daily, plus probenecid 500 mg orally four times daily, both drugs for ten days, followed by benzathine penicillin G, intramuscularly, 2.4 million units weekly for three successive weeks;
OR
Benzathine Penicillin G: Intramuscularly, 2.4 million units weekly for three successive weeks.

REMARKS:
(1) These regimens are considered potentially effective, but none has been adequately studied. Benzathine penicillin G, used alone, should be reserved for patients who are unlikely to comply with the other regimens.

(2) Penicillin-allergic patients should have their allergy confirmed and be referred to an expert.

(3) Cerebrospinal fluid examination should be performed in patients with clinical symptoms or signs consistent with neurosyphilis.

(4) Post-treatment serologic tests at periodic intervals, clinical evaluations every six months, and cerebrospinal fluid examinations repeated for at least three years are recommended.

Syphilis in Pregnancy

All pregnant women should have a nontreponemal serologic test for syphilis, such as the VDRL or RPR test, at the first prenatal visit. Refer to CDC guidelines (*Morbid Mortal Week Rep*, 1985 A) for subsequent tests in high-risk or seroreactive patients.

RECOMMENDED REGIMEN(S):
Penicillin: Pregnant women who are not allergic to penicillin should receive the appropriate preparations and dosage schedules for the stage of syphilis as recommended for nonpregnant patients. (See Early Syphilis, Syphilis of More Than One Year's Duration [Except Neurosyphilis], and Neurosyphilis.)

REMARKS:
(1) Treatment failures have been reported with benzathine penicillin G regimens in pregnant women (Mascola et al, 1984).

(2) The treatment of choice for penicillin-allergic pregnant women is controversial. The CDC guidelines state: "Patients at all stages of pregnancy who have documented allergy to penicillins: (1) If compliance and serologic follow-up can be assured, administer erythromycin in dosage schedules appropriate for the stage of syphilis as recommended for the treatment of nonpregnant patients. Infants born to mothers treated during pregnancy with erythromycin for early syphilis should be treated with penicillin. (2) If compliance and serologic follow-up cannot be assured, the patient should be hospitalized and managed in consultation with an expert. Tetracycline is not recommended in pregnant women because of potential adverse effects on the fetus."

(3) Pregnant women who have been treated for early syphilis should have monthly quantitative nontreponemal serologic tests for the remainder of the current pregnancy. Women who show a fourfold rise in titer should be retreated. Treated women who do not show a fourfold decrease in titer in a three-month period should be retreated. After delivery, follow-up is as outlined for nonpregnant patients.

Congenital Syphilis

Congenital syphilis may occur if the mother has syphilis during pregnancy. If the mother has received adequate penicillin treatment during pregnancy, the risk to the infant is small. However, all infants should be examined carefully at birth, at 1 month, and every 3 months for the first 15 months, and then every 6 months until nontreponemal serologic tests are negative or stable at low titer. If a serologic test is positive at 3 months, the infant should be treated for congenital syphilis.

Infected infants are frequently asymptomatic at birth and may be seronegative if the maternal infection occurred late in gestation. Infants should be treated at birth if maternal treatment was inadequate or unknown, did not include penicillin, or if adequate follow-up of the infant cannot be assured.

Infants with congenital syphilis should have a CSF examination before treatment to provide a baseline for follow-up. Regardless of CSF results, children should be treated with a regimen effective for neurosyphilis.

Symptomatic infants or asymptomatic infants

RECOMMENDED REGIMENS:
Aqueous Crystalline Penicillin G: Intramuscularly or intravenously, 25,000 units/kg twice daily for at least ten days;
OR
Aqueous Procaine Penicillin G: Intramuscularly, 50,000 units/kg daily for at least ten days.

REMARKS:
(1) In asymptomatic infants whose mothers were treated adequately with a penicillin regimen during pregnancy, treatment is not necessary if follow-up can be assured. In asymptomatic infants whose follow-up cannot be assured, many consultants choose to treat the infant with benzathine penicillin G 50,000 units/kg intramuscularly in a single dose. It is recognized that data

on the efficacy of this regimen in congenital neurosyphilis are lacking. Therefore, if neurosyphilis cannot be excluded, the aqueous crystalline penicillin G or procaine penicillin G regimens are recommended. Only penicillin regimens are recommended for neonatal congenital syphilis.

(2) After the neonatal period, penicillin therapy for congenital syphilis should be with the same dosages used for neonatal congenital syphilis. For larger children, the total dose of penicillin need not exceed the dosage used in adult syphilis of more than one year's duration.

(3) Post-treatment quantitative nontreponemal tests are recommended at 3, 6, and 12 months.

CHANCROID

Chancroid is a form of genital ulcers caused by *Haemophilus ducreyi*. The diagnosis is best made by isolation of *H. ducreyi* from ulcers and/or lymph nodes. The susceptibility of *H. ducreyi* to antimicrobial agents differs among geographic regions and this should be taken into account when selecting therapy.

RECOMMENDED REGIMENS:
Erythromycin: Orally, 500 mg four times daily for seven days;
OR
Ceftriaxone: Intramuscularly, 250 mg as a single dose.
(Note: Not evaluated in the United States but probably effective [see Taylor et al, 1985].)
ALTERNATIVE REGIMENS:
Trimethoprim/sulfamethoxazole: Orally, one double-strength tablet (160/800 mg) twice daily for at least seven days.
(Note: The susceptibility of *H. ducreyi* to this combination of antimicrobial agents varies widely; use should be limited to areas where favorable susceptibility patterns have been established.)
OR
Trimethoprim/sulfamethoxazole: Orally, four double-strength tablets (160/800 mg) in a single dose.
(Note: Recommended only in areas where *H. ducreyi* susceptibility to these antimicrobials has been established. Not evaluated in the United States.)
OR
Amoxicillin (500 mg) plus clavulanic acid (125 mg) three times daily for seven days.
(Note: Not evaluated in the United States.)
REMARKS:
(1) Successfully treated ulcers are almost invariably clinically improved by seven days after institution of therapy. If they are not, use of an alternative regimen should be considered.
(2) Clinical resolution of lymph nodes is slower than that of ulcers and may require aspiration, even during successful therapy. Fluctuant lymph nodes should be aspirated through healthy adjacent normal skin. Incision and drainage or excision of nodes delay healing and are contraindicated. Apply compresses to ulcers to remove necrotic material.
(3) Sexual partners should be treated with a recommended regimen.
(4) Antimicrobial susceptibility testing should be done on *H. ducreyi* isolated from patients who fail to respond to the recommended therapies.

LYMPHOGRANULOMA VENEREUM

Genital, inguinal, or anorectal infection due to a LGV serotype of *Chlamydia trachomatis*.

RECOMMENDED REGIMEN:
Tetracycline Hydrochloride: Orally, 500 mg four times daily for at least two weeks.
REMARKS:
(1) Although evaluated less extensively, alternative regimens are: Doxycycline, orally, 100 mg twice daily for at least two weeks; or Erythromycin, orally, 500 mg four times daily for at least two weeks; or
Sulfamethoxazole, orally, 1 g twice daily for at least two weeks. Other sulfonamides can be used in equivalent dosage.
(2) Fluctuant lymph nodes should be aspirated as needed through healthy adjacent normal skin. Incision and drainage or excision of nodes delay healing and are contraindicated. Late sequelae, such as stricture and/or fistula, may require surgical intervention.
(3) Sex partners of patients with LGV should be treated with one of the recommended regimens.

GRANULOMA INGUINALE (DONOVANOSIS)

Granuloma inguinale is a form of genital ulcers caused by *Calymmatobacterium granulomatis* and antimicrobial drug therapy should be active against this organism.

Selected references: Felman and Nikitas, 1981; Hart, 1979, 1984; Lynch, 1982.

RECOMMENDED REGIMEN:
Tetracycline: Orally, 500 mg four times daily for three weeks or until there is complete healing of all lesions.
REMARKS:
(1) For treatment failures or patients who are allergic to or cannot tolerate tetracyclines, gentamicin and chloramphenicol are alternative antibiotics.
(2) A variant of chancroid mimics granuloma inguinale and accounts for most cases clinically diagnosed as granuloma inguinale in the Atlanta, GA area. Minocycline and erythromycin appear to be effective (Kraus et al, 1982; Werman et al, 1983).

SCABIES

This skin infection is caused by the itch mite, *Sarcoptes scabiei*. For treatment guidelines, see Chapter 74, Topical Anti-infective Agents: Drugs Used on Skin and Mucous Membranes.

PEDICULOSIS PUBIS

This infection is caused by *Phthirus pubis* (crab louse), which primarily infests the pubic region. For treatment guidelines, see Chapter 74, Topical Anti-infective Agents: Drugs Used On Skin And Mucous Membranes.

ENTERIC INFECTIONS

Enteric infections can be sexually transmitted and are primarily observed in homosexual or bisexual men due to sexual practices that frequently involve anal-oral contact. Common causative organisms include *Campylobacter jejuni*, *Shigella* species, nontyphoidal *Salmonella* species, *Entamoeba histolytica*, and *Giardia lamblia*. Treatment of sexually transmitted enteric infections should be based on etiologic diagnosis. Symptomatic individuals; asymptomatic, infected individuals for whom anal-oral contact is a sexual practice; and persons whose work or social situation is associated with a likelihood of transmission (eg, food handlers, hospital workers, day-care center employees) are recommended for treatment, and sexual partners at risk for fecal-oral transmission should be evaluated.

For drug selection for infections caused by *Campylobacter jejuni*, *Shigella*, and nontyphoidal *Salmonella* species, see Table 1, Antimicrobial Drug Selection for Common Infectious Diseases. Treatment of amebiasis and giardiasis are discussed in Chapter 77, Antiprotozoal Agents.

VIRAL HEPATITIS

No specific therapy is available for the various types of acute viral hepatitis whether sexually transmitted or not. For recommendations for protection against viral hepatitis, see *Morbid Mortal Week Rep*, 1985 D; see also Chapter 62, Agents for Active and Passive Immunity.

ACQUIRED IMMUNODEFICIENCY SYNDROME

Acquired immunodeficiency syndrome (AIDS) is a sexually transmissible infection caused by a retrovirus presently known as human T-cell lymphotropic virus type III/lymphadenopathy-associated virus (HTLV-III/LAV). Presently, the only available control measure is primary prevention of sexually transmitted HTLV-III/LAV infection. No interventions have been demonstrated to eradicate or alter the course of HTLV-III/LAV infection (secondary prevention) or to rehabilitate persons with overt AIDS (tertiary prevention). At present, there is no established treatment available to reverse the immune dysfunction of AIDS. Experimental studies to evaluate the efficacy of immunomodulatory agents and compounds active against HTLV-III/LAV are in progress. Treatment for many of the infections and neoplastic complications of AIDS has been successful (Armstrong et al, 1985; Drake et al, 1985; Frederick et al, 1985; Furio and Wordell, 1985; Gelman et al, 1985; Small et al, 1985; Volberding et al, 1985), but requires consultation with specialists in infectious diseases, oncology, or dermatology.

PREVENTION OF OPHTHALMIA NEONATORUM

Instillation of a prophylactic agent into the eyes of all newborn infants is recommended as required by laws in most states. None of the presently recommended approaches for prophylaxis against gonococcal and chlamydial ophthalmia neonatorum is completely effective.

RECOMMENDED REGIMEN(S):
Erythromycin (0.5%) ophthalmic ointment OR **tetracycline (1%) ophthalmic ointment** OR **silver nitrate (1%) solution immediately postpartum and never later than one hour after birth. Drugs are given in a single application into each conjunctival sac with no rinsing of the eyes. Single-use tubes or ampuls are preferred to multiple-use tubes.**
REMARKS:
(1) Silver nitrate is effective in preventing gonococcal infections, but does not prevent chlamydial disease and frequently causes chemical conjunctivitis.
(2) Erythromycin is effective in preventing both gonococcal and chlamydial ophthalmia and does not cause chemical conjunctivitis, but the topical use of this drug does not prevent nasopharyngeal carriage of *C. trachomatis* or chlamydial pneumonia. Furthermore, erythromycin prophylaxis is considerably more expensive than silver nitrate prophylaxis.
(3) Tetracycline ointment has not been as extensively evaluated as has erythromycin, but it appears to be as effective.
(4) Efficacy of tetracycline and erythromycin in the prevention of gonococcal ophthalmia due to penicillinase-producing *N. gonorrhoeae* (PPNG) is unknown.
(5) Bacitracin is not recommended.

TABLE 3. ANTIMICROBIAL CHEMOPROPHYLAXIS FOR AMBULATORY PATIENTS

The purpose of antimicrobial chemoprophylaxis is to prevent the development of symptomatic infection or to prevent the spread of disease. This is accomplished by administering an antimicrobial agent before, during, or shortly after exposure to an infectious agent. Whether chemoprophylaxis is justified depends on a number of factors, including: (1) the likelihood that the patient will develop symptomatic infection if chemoprophylaxis is not used; (2) the severity of the disease to be prevented; (3) the effectiveness of nonspecific host defenses; (4) the efficacy of the drug in preventing the infection; (5) the acceptability of the drug, based on its adverse reaction potential; (6) the duration of exposure to the infectious agent; (7) the likelihood and consequences of promoting resistance to the drug(s) used; and (8) the cost and availability of the prophylactic regimen (Flynn and Hoeprich, 1983).

Chemoprophylaxis is most often successful when it is directed against a specific pathogenic microorganism that is highly susceptible to the antimicrobial agent and remains sensitive throughout the period of prophylaxis. The use of penicillin G benzathine to prevent recurrent attacks of rheumatic fever by group A, beta hemolytic streptococci is an example of chemoprophylaxis directed against a specific pathogen. Prevention of infections at particular body sites by a range of pathogens is more difficult, but can be successfully achieved if the period of risk is defined and brief, if the expected pathogens have predictable antimicrobial susceptibility, and if the site is accessible to the drug. The use of trimethoprim/sulfamethoxazole to prevent recurrent urinary tract infections is an example of this type of chemoprophylaxis. Chemoprophylaxis to prevent secondary infections by any or all microorganisms in patients who are ill with other diseases generally has been unsuccessful. However, short-term chemoprophylaxis with trimethoprim/sulfamethoxazole has been reported to reduce the frequency of bacterial infection in severely neutropenic patients (see Walsh and Schimpff, 1983).

Situations in which antimicrobial chemoprophylaxis of nonsurgical infections in ambulatory patients is of proven, or probable, benefit are discussed below with guidelines for antimicrobial agents of choice, dosages, and durations of prophylaxis. See Table 4 for antimicrobial chemoprophylaxis for surgical patients. Immunoprophylaxis of infectious diseases is discussed in Chapter 62, Agents for Active and Passive Immunity.

General references: Mills and Jawetz, 1982; Scheifele, 1982; Wilson, 1983; Brachman, 1984; Sande and Mandell, 1985.

Prevention of Bacterial Endocarditis

Antimicrobial chemoprophylaxis of bacterial endocarditis in patients with (1) prosthetic heart valves, (2) most forms of congenital heart disease (excluding uncomplicated secundum atrial septal defect), (3) surgically constructed systemic-pulmonary shunts, (4) rheumatic or other acquired valvular heart disease, (5) hypertrophic cardiomyopathy (IHSS), (6) previous history of bacterial endocarditis, and (7) mitral valve prolapse with insufficiency (see NOTE below) is recommended prior to all dental and various other invasive procedures of the upper respiratory, genitourinary, or lower gastrointestinal tract that may be associated with transitory bacteremia. Prophylaxis should be effective against viridans streptococci (from oral or respiratory foci) or enterococci (from genitourinary or lower gastrointestinal foci), the likely causative organisms of infective endocarditis. Although the effectiveness of specific regimens has not been documented in controlled clinical studies, the recommendations of the American Heart Association (AHA) Committee on the Prevention of Rheumatic Fever and Bacterial Endocarditis (Shulman et al, 1984) are most widely accepted. These guidelines are outlined below. Similar recommendations have been proposed by others (for example, see *Med Lett Drugs Ther*, 1984, 1986; Durack, 1984; Keys, 1982; Report of a Working Party of the British Society for Antimicrobial Chemotherapy, 1982).

NOTE: Definitive data to provide guidance in management of patients with mitral valve prolapse are particularly limited. In general, such patients are clearly at low risk of development of endocarditis, but the risk-benefit ratio of prophylaxis in mitral valve prolapse is uncertain (Shulman et al, 1984). For additional information on this controversial issue, see Bor and Himmelstein, 1984; Clemens and Ransohoff, 1984; Durack, 1984; Baddour and Bisno, 1986; Chadwick and Shulman, 1986; Kaye, 1986.

A. Prophylaxis for dental procedures (including cleaning) and surgery or instrumentation of the upper respiratory tract (risk of bacteremia with various procedures is discussed in Everett and Hirschmann, 1977; LeFrock and Molavi, 1982; and Shulman et al, 1984)

PROPHYLACTIC REGIMEN(S)

STANDARD ORAL PENICILLIN-CONTAINING REGIMEN:
Penicillin V (*adults*, 2 g; *children less than 27 kg*, 1 g) one hour before procedure, then (*adults*, 1 g; *children*, 500 mg) six hours later.

REMARKS:
(1) This is the preferred regimen for most patients.
(2) Penicillin V is the preferred form of oral penicillin because it is relatively resistant to gastric acid.
(3) For patients unable to take oral antibiotics prior to a procedure, aqueous penicillin G (*adults*, 2 million units; *children*, 50,000 units/kg) IV or IM 30 to 60 minutes before procedure, then (*adults*, 1 million units; *children*, 25,000 units/kg) six hours later may be substituted.
(4) In unusual circumstances or in the case of delayed healing, it may be necessary to provide additional doses of antibiotics even though bacteremia rarely persists longer than 15 minutes after procedure.

STANDARD ORAL REGIMEN FOR PATIENTS ALLERGIC TO PENICILLIN:
Erythromycin (*adults*, 1 g; *children*, 20 mg/kg) one hour before procedure, then (*adults*, 500 mg; *children*, 10 mg/kg) six hours later.

REMARKS:
(1) For patients unable to tolerate oral erythromycin, changing to a different erythromycin preparation may be beneficial. Otherwise, an oral cephalosporin (1 g one hour before procedure, then 500 mg six hours later) may be·useful. However, data are lacking to allow specific recommendation of this latter regimen.

SPECIAL PARENTERAL PENICILLIN-CONTAINING REGIMEN:
Ampicillin (*adults*, 1 to 2 g; *children*, 50 mg/kg) IM or IV *plus* gentamicin (*adults*, 1.5 mg/kg; *children*, 2 mg/kg) IM or IV one-half hour before procedure, followed by oral penicillin V (*adults*, 1 g; *children*, 500 mg) six hours later. Alternatively, the parenteral regimen may be repeated once eight hours later.

REMARKS:
(1) An oral regimen is safer and is preferred in most patients. Parenteral regimens are recommended when maximal protection is desired, especially for patients with prosthetic valves or surgically constructed systemic-pulmonary shunts, or those who have had endocarditis previously. For patients receiving continuous oral penicillin for rheumatic fever prophylaxis, oral erythromycin is appropriate unless other high-risk circumstances exist. See Shulman et al, 1984 for additional discussion.

SPECIAL PARENTERAL REGIMEN FOR PATIENTS ALLERGIC TO PENICILLIN:
Vancomycin (*adults*, 1 g; *children*, 20 mg/kg) IV *slowly* over one hour starting one hour prior to procedure. Because of the long half-life of vancomycin, a repeat dose should not be necessary.

B. Prophylaxis for genitourinary tract or gastrointestinal tract surgery or instrumentation (risk of bacteremia with various procedures is discussed in Everett and Hirschmann, 1977; LeFrock and Molavi, 1982; Shulman et al, 1984)

PROPHYLACTIC REGIMEN(S)

STANDARD PARENTERAL PENICILLIN-CONTAINING REGIMEN:
Ampicillin (*adults*, 2 g; *children*, 50 mg/kg) IM or IV *plus* gentamicin (*adults*, 1.5 mg/kg; *children*, 2 mg/kg) IM or IV one-half to one hour before procedure. This regimen may be repeated once eight hours later.

REMARKS:
(1) This is the preferred regimen for most patients who require parenteral therapy.
(2) In patients with compromised renal function, it may be necessary to modify or omit the second dose of gentamicin.

SPECIAL PARENTERAL REGIMEN FOR PATIENTS ALLERGIC TO PENICILLIN:

Vancomycin (*adults*, 1 g; *children*, 20 mg/kg) given IV *slowly over one hour plus* gentamicin (*adults*, 1.5 mg/kg; *children*, 2 mg/kg) IM or IV one hour before procedure. This regimen may be repeated once 8 to 12 hours later.

REMARK:

(1) In patients with compromised renal function, it may be necessary to modify or omit the second dose of each drug.

SPECIAL ORAL PENICILLIN-CONTAINING REGIMEN:

Amoxicillin (*adults*, 3 g, *children*, 50 mg/kg) one hour before procedure, then (*adults,* 1.5 g, *children*, 25 mg/kg) six hours later.

REMARK:

(1) This oral regimen may be substituted for minor or repetitive procedures in low-risk patients.

Prevention of Recurrent Attacks of Rheumatic Fever (Secondary Prevention)

The recommendations of the American Heart Association's (AHA) Committee on Rheumatic Fever and Infective Endocarditis of the Council on Cardiovascular Disease in the Young (Shulman et al, 1984) are generally accepted.

Prevention of recurrent rheumatic fever depends upon continuous prophylaxis with antimicrobial agents effective against group A, beta hemolytic streptococci *(Streptococcus pyogenes)*. Prophylaxis is recommended for patients who have a well-documented history of rheumatic fever or Sydenham's chorea and those who show definite evidence of rheumatic heart disease. Recommended regimens are listed below.

The most effective protection from rheumatic recurrences is afforded by long-term continuous chemoprophylaxis, possibly for life. It is known, however, that risk of recurrence decreases with the age of the patient and as the time interval since the most recent attack increases. Furthermore, patients without rheumatic heart disease are at less risk for recurrence than those with cardiac involvement. Thus, physicians may wish to make exceptions to maintaining prophylaxis indefinitely, especially in older patients, on an individual basis. The AHA committee has recommended that the decision on duration of prophylaxis in each individual patient take into account the risk of acquiring a streptococcal infection, the anticipated recurrence rate per infection, and the consequences of recurrence. Adults with a high risk of exposure to streptococcal infection include parents of young children, teachers, physicians, nurses, allied medical personnel, military personnel, other individuals living in crowded situations, and members of lower socioeconomic classes. Individuals with high recurrence rates per infection are those with rheumatic heart disease, those with an attack of rheumatic fever in the preceding five years, and those with multiple previous attacks.

PROPHYLACTIC REGIMEN(S)

PREFERRED REGIMEN:

Penicillin G benzathine, intramuscularly, 1.2 million units every four weeks.

REMARKS:

(1) This is the most effective method of secondary prevention.

(2) Recommended for patients at high risk for recurrence, particularly those with rheumatic heart disease.

(3) Disadvantages are inconvenience and the pain of intramuscular injection.

ALTERNATIVE (ORAL) REGIMENS:

Sulfadiazine, orally, 1 g once daily for patients >60 lbs or 500 mg once daily for patients <60 lbs.

OR

Penicillin V, orally, 125 or 250 mg twice daily

REMARKS:

(1) Efficacy of oral regimens are similar, but they are less than intramuscular penicillin G benzathine. Thus, the oral regimens are most appropriate for patients with a lower risk of recurrence (eg, late adolescent or young adult who has not had rheumatic attack in preceding five years).

(2) Success depends on long-term patient compliance.

(3) Sulfisoxazole (1 g once daily) is probably an effective alternative to sulfadiazine, although comparative data are not available.

(4) Penicillin V is preferred to penicillin G because it is more acid-stable.

(5) Erythromycin, orally, 250 mg twice daily is recommended in patients allergic to both penicillins and sulfonamides.

Prevention of Tuberculosis

Recommendations for chemoprophylaxis of tuberculosis can be found in Chapter 75, Antimycobacterial Agents.

Prevention of Meningococcal Disease

Antimicrobial chemoprophylaxis is recommended for household (including index case) and other intimate contacts of patients with meningococcal disease. In addition to household contacts, persons at highest risk include nursery school or day-care center contacts (ie, young children), other very close day-to-day contacts who are exposed to the patient's oral secretions either through kissing or sharing of food or beverages, and medical personnel who perform mouth-to-mouth resuscitation on the patient. These contacts may receive antimicrobial prophylaxis as soon as possible, preferably within 24 hours of diagnosis of the primary case. Prophylaxis is not indicated for casual school or work contacts or for routine contacts of the hospitalized patient. Prophylactic regimens should eliminate nasopharyngeal carriage of *Neisseria meningitidis*.

Selected references: *Med Lett Drugs Ther*, 1981; *American Academy of Pediatrics Redbook*, 1982; Shapiro, 1982; Feder, 1983.

PROPHYLACTIC REGIMEN(S)

PREFERRED REGIMEN:

Rifampin (Oral: *Adults*, 600 mg twice daily; *children 1 month to 12 years*, 10 mg/kg twice daily; *newborns less than 1 month*, 5 mg/kg twice daily) for two days.

REMARKS:

(1) Rifampin should not be used in pregnant women.

(2) Sulfonamides are preferred only if the meningococcal isolate is known to be susceptible. Sulfadiazine (Oral: *Adults*, 1 g twice daily; *children 1 to 12 years*, 500 mg twice daily; *infants 2 months to 1 year,* 500 mg once daily) OR sulfisoxazole (Oral: *Adults*, 1 g twice daily; *children 1 to 6 years*, 500 mg twice daily; *infants 2 months to 1 year*, 250 mg twice daily) for two days are effective regimens. Sulfonamides should not be used in pregnant women at term or in newborn infants less than 2 months.

(3) Although minocycline (100 mg twice daily for five days) is an effective alternative in adults, it generally is not recommended because it causes frequent vestibular side effects. Tetracyclines should not be used in pregnant women or children less than 8 years.

(4) Penicillin G and chloramphenicol, preferred drugs in the treatment of meningococcal meningitis, are not useful for chemoprophylaxis because they fail to eliminate nasopharyngeal carriage of *N. meningitidis*.

(5) Presently available meningococcal polysaccharide vaccines are not substitutes for chemoprophylaxis since an antibody response is not seen for five days to two weeks following vaccine administration. Presently available vaccines are only effective against meningococcal disease caused by serogroups A, C, Y, and W-135, which cause 50% of cases of meningococcal disease. Group C vaccine is not effective in children less than 2 years. For uses of meningococcal vaccines, see *Morbid Mortal Week Rep*, 1985 and Chapter 62, Agents for Active and Passive Immunity.

Prevention of *Haemophilus influenzae* Type b Disease

An increased risk of secondary invasive *Haemophilus influenzae* type b disease exists among household contacts less than 4 years. Day care center contacts less than 4 years also may be at increased risk, but the magnitude of this is unclear at the present time. Rifampin (20 mg/kg/day for four days) effectively eliminates the oropharyngeal carrier state in 95% of treated individuals. In a single, controlled clinical trial, this regimen was shown to prevent secondary *H. influenzae* type b disease (Band et al, 1984). This study has been criticized for flaws in design and conclusions, however, (Osterholm and Murphy, 1984).

Based on the above information, the Committee on Infectious Diseases of the American Academy of Pediatrics has issued revised recommendations for antimicrobial chemoprophylaxis of invasive *H. influenzae* type b disease (Committee on Infectious Diseases, 1984). These replace previous recommendations by this committee (*American Academy of Pediatrics Redbook*, 1982) that generated considerable controversy among infectious disease experts (for references see Daum et al, 1982; Fulginiti, 1982; Nelson, 1982; Shapiro, 1982; Murphy et al, 1983; Siegel, 1984).

The revised recommendations are as follows:

(1) Family members of the index case and parents of other close contacts (eg, from day care centers) should be informed of the increased risk of disease and the need for prompt medical evaluation of any febrile illnesses.

(2) Rifampin prophylaxis is indicated for all household contacts (children and adults) in households where there are children (other than index case) less than 49 months of age. A household contact is an individual residing in the residence of the index patient or a nonresident who spent four or more hours with the index patient for five of the seven days preceding hospital admission of the index patient. Prophylaxis should be initiated as soon as possible because 54% of secondary cases occur during the first week after hospitalization of the index patient.

(3) The index case should also receive prophylaxis after completion of therapy for the primary infection and before returning to the household.

(4) The management of day care centers and nursery school contact groups should be individualized. Supervisory personnel and parents should be educated to encourage prompt medical evaluation of febrile episodes in attendees. Definitive recommendations regarding administration of rifampin prophylaxis in day care centers cannot be made at this time because (a) the risk of secondary disease in centers with a single case is uncertain; (b) the efficacy of rifampin in day care centers is unknown; and (c) the logistical problems of cost and responsibility to coordinate chemoprophylaxis programs in day care centers are substantial. The advisability of rifampin prophylaxis in centers where a single case has occurred is controversial. However, most experts advise administering rifampin to all infants and supervisory personnel when two or more cases of invasive *H. influenzae* type b disease have occurred among attendees within 60 days. Strict and prompt compliance by attendees and supervisory personnel would be required for rifampin prophylaxis to be successful.

(5) Prophylaxis is not recommended for pregnant women who are contacts of the index patient because the effects of rifampin on the fetus are unknown.

PROPHYLACTIC REGIMEN(S)

PREFERRED REGIMEN:
Rifampin (Oral: *Adults and children*, 20 mg/kg once daily [maximum dose, 600 mg daily] for four days).
REMARKS:
(1) The dose for very young infants is not established. Some reduce the dose of rifampin to 10 mg/kg per dose in infants less than one month.
(2) Rifampin is not commercially available as an oral suspension. For patients unable to swallow rifampin capsules, preweighed rifampin powder mixed with a small amount of applesauce immediately prior to administration may be given. A rifampin suspension (1% in simple syrup), if used, should be freshly prepared and shaken vigorously prior to administration. Rifampin stains soft contact lenses.
(3) Ampicillin and chloramphenicol, preferred drugs in the treatment of *H. influenzae* type b disease, are not useful for chemoprophylaxis because they fail to eliminate oropharyngeal carriage of the organism.
(4) An *H. influenzae* type b polysaccharide vaccine is now licensed for use in the United States. A single dose is recommended for all children at 24 months of age. Children at high risk, such as day care center attendees, may be vaccinated at 18 months, but immunity may not be complete. Unfortunately, the vaccine does not protect children below this age in whom the incidence of invasive disease is highest (see *Morbid Mortal Week Rep*, 1985). This capsular polysaccharide vaccine has been shown to be safe and effective in children older than 18 months in a large-scale trial in Finland, but does not elicit adequate antibody responses in children less than 18 months (Peltola et al, 1984). For additional discussion see Chapter 62, Agents for Active and Passive Immunity.

Prevention of Pneumococcal Infection in Splenectomized Patients

Anatomic or functionally asplenic patients (eg, those with sickle cell disease), particularly children, are susceptible to overwhelming infection with encapsulated bacteria, including *Streptococcus pneumoniae*, *Haemophilus influenzae*, and *Neisseria meningitidis*. Antimicrobial chemoprophylaxis directed against *S. pneumoniae* traditionally has been recommended for children and adolescents after splenectomy or diagnosis of chronic splenic dysfunction. Whether to use similar chemoprophylaxis in adult patients is less clear.

Selected references: *Med Lett Drugs Ther*, 1977; *American Academy of Pediatrics Redbook*, 1982; Reese and Betts, 1986.

PROPHYLACTIC REGIMEN(S)

PREFERRED REGIMEN:
Penicillin V (Oral: *Children*, 125 mg twice daily; *adults*, 250 mg twice daily)
REMARKS:
(1) Some experts recommend use of ampicillin (25 to 50 mg/kg/day) or amoxicillin (20 mg/kg/day) for children less than five years of age to include coverage against *H. influenzae*.
(2) Penicillin G benzathine (intramuscularly, 1.2 million units every four weeks) also has been suggested for this indication (see Sanford, 1985).
(3) Duration of prophylaxis in children usually has ranged from two to four years.
(4) Splenectomized or sickle cell disease patients older than 2 years also should receive pneumococcal 23-valent polysaccharide vaccine (*Morbid Mortal Week Rep*, 1984). Immunization with quadrivalent (A, C, Y, W-135) meningococcal vaccine also is recommended (*Morbid Mortal Week Rep*, 1985 A). Splenectomized or sickle cell disease patients older than 18 months also should receive Haemophilus b Polysaccharide vaccine, although only limited data on immunogenicity and clinical efficacy in this group are available (*Morbid Mortal Week Rep*, 1985 B). See Chapter 62, Agents for Active and Passive Immunity, for additional discussion.

Prevention of Recurrent Bacterial Urinary Tract Infections (Reinfections) in Women

Young to middle-aged nonpregnant women with three or more recurrent episodes of new infection (reinfection) per year are candidates for long-term antimicrobial chemoprophylaxis. There should be no history of prior urological surgery, renal calculi, or known genitourinary tract abnormality.

Selected references: Stamm, et al, 1980, 1981, 1982; *Med Lett Drugs Ther*, 1981; Ronald and Harding, 1981; Fang et al, 1982; Farrar, 1983; Valenti and Reese, 1986.

PROPHYLACTIC REGIMEN(S)

PREFERRED REGIMEN:
Trimethoprim (40 mg)/sulfamethoxazole (200 mg), ie, one-half of a regular strength tablet, orally, at bedtime three times per week on Sunday, Wednesday, and Friday (a daily regimen also is effective).
ALTERNATIVE REGIMENS:
Nitrofurantoin, 50 mg (or nitrofurantoin macrocrystals, 100 mg), orally, once daily at bedtime
OR
Trimethoprim, 50 to 100 mg, orally, once daily at bedtime.
REMARKS:
(1) Duration of prophylaxis generally is six months. If recurrence

of infection then occurs within three months, prophylaxis frequently is reinstituted for two years.
(2) Trimethoprim/sulfamethoxazole penetrates vaginal secretions very well and effectively eradicates Enterobacteriaceae from the fecal reservoir and prevents perineal colonization. Emergence of resistant bacterial strains has not been a problem. Serious adverse reactions have been rare.
(3) In one study, serious adverse reactions (eg, pulmonary toxicity) were reported with long-term nitrofurantoin administration (Holmberg et al, 1980).
(4) Whether the use of trimethoprim alone will lead to more rapid emergence of trimethoprim-resistant bacterial strains than the combination is still unresolved. Many experts prefer to reserve trimethoprim alone for patients who are allergic to sulfonamides.
(5) Long-term, low dose cinoxacin (500 mg once daily at bedtime) also has been effective for the prevention of recurrent urinary tract infections (Landes, 1980). Some urological consultants like this agent because it has not been associated with plasmid-mediated, transferable resistance.
(6) Prior to beginning chemoprophylaxis, any acute urinary tract infection should be treated with appropriate antimicrobial agents and a sterile urine culture should be obtained (usually two weeks after treatment).
(7) A screening intravenous pyelogram (IVP) is no longer considered necessary for the majority of women who are candidates for long-term chemoprophylaxis. An exception is relapsing urinary tract infections due to urease-producing bacteria (eg, *Proteus*), where infected urinary calculi must be considered.
(8) Recurrences of urinary tract infection in some women appear to correlate temporally with sexual intercourse. For such patients, a single prophylactic dose of an appropriate antimicrobial agent taken immediately after intercourse appears to prevent active infections. Despite less clinical experience, this approach may be an acceptable alternative to long-term chemoprophylaxis for selected women.
(9) Another strategy for managing recurrent urinary tract infections is to prescribe antimicrobial drugs for susceptible women to keep at home and self-administer when symptoms arise. Intermittent self-therapy with single-dose trimethoprim (320 mg)/sulfamethoxazole (1,600 mg) was shown to be efficacious and economical in selected women (eg, those in whom the symptomatic episode was most likely acute cystitis rather than urethritis or vaginitis; those with ability to accurately self-diagnose acute cystitis) (Wong et al, 1985).

Prevention of *Chlamydia trachomatis* Infections, Gonococcal Infections, and Syphilis in Sexual Contacts

Guidelines for the prevention of these infections in sexual contacts can be found in Table 2, Treatment of Sexually Transmitted Diseases (STD).

Prevention of Ophthalmia Neonatorum

Guidelines for the prevention of ophthalmia neonatorum can be found in Table 2, Treatment of Sexually Transmitted Diseases (STD).

Prevention of Malaria

Recommendations for chemoprophylaxis of malaria can be found in Chapter 77, Antiprotozoal Agents.

Prevention of Influenza A Infection

Recommendations for chemoprophylaxis of influenza A infection with amantadine can be found in Chapter 79, Antiviral Agents. Immunoprophylaxis with influenza vaccine is discussed in Chapter 62, Agents for Active and Passive Immunity.

Prevention of Pertussis in Exposed Persons

Exposure to pertussis can result in clinical disease in both immunized and unimmunized contacts. Thus, antimicrobial chemoprophylaxis is recommended for household and other close contacts.

Selected references: *American Academy of Pediatrics Redbook*, 1982; Feder, 1983.

PROPHYLACTIC REGIMEN(S)

PREFERRED REGIMEN:
Erythromycin, orally 50 mg/kg/day (maximum, 1,500 mg), divided into three or four doses for 14 days.
REMARKS:
(1) Erythromycin has been shown to eliminate carriage of *Bordetella pertussis*, but efficacy in preventing disease is not fully established. (Note: A retrospective analysis of the literature suggests that erythromycin estolate has been more effective than erythromycin ethylsuccinate or erythromycin stearate in eliminating *B. pertussis* carriage, presumably due to better penetration of the estolate into respiratory secretions [Bass, 1985].)
(2) Trimethoprim/sulfamethoxazole is recommended by some experts, but its value is less well established.
(3) Previously immunized close contacts less than 7 years of age should also receive a booster dose of vaccine, preferably as DTP, unless they have received a booster dose within the previous six months.
(4) Contacts not previously immunized should receive erythromycin for ten days after the contact is broken; if it is not possible to break the contact, they should be treated for the duration of the cough in the index patient, or until the patient has received seven days of treatment with erythromycin.

Prevention of Recurrent Acute Otitis Media

Antimicrobial chemoprophylaxis has decreased the number of recurrent episodes of acute otitis media in children in various studies, but conclusive evidence that the advantages outweigh the disadvantages for this management option are lacking. Furthermore, the indications for prophylaxis, the most effective drugs, and the optimum duration of prophylaxis have not been clearly established. Although more definitive clinical studies are necessary, many infectious disease experts currently recommend antimicrobial chemoprophylaxis (as outlined below) as a reasonable approach in children with at least three episodes of acute otitis media in the previous six months or four episodes in one year.

Selected references: Paradise, 1981; Klein and Bluestone, 1982; *Med Lett Drugs Ther*, 1983.

PROPHYLACTIC REGIMEN(S)

PREFERRED REGIMEN:
Sulfisoxazole, orally, 50 mg/kg once daily at bedtime.
ALTERNATIVE REGIMENS:
Amoxicillin, orally, 20 mg/kg once daily at bedtime
OR
Trimethoprim (4 mg/kg)/sulfamethoxazole(20 mg/kg), orally, once daily at bedtime.
REMARKS:
(1) Duration of prophylaxis is for about six months or during the winter and spring when the incidence of respiratory tract infections is high.
(2) Sulfisoxazole is generally preferred because of proven effectiveness, safety, and low cost.
(3) If episodes of acute otitis media occur during prophylaxis, an alternative regimen should be used for treatment.
(4) If episodes of acute otitis media recur after conclusion of prophylaxis, reinstitution of chemoprophylaxis or myringotomy with insertion of tympanostomy tubes are alternative management options.
(5) Hazards of antimicrobial chemoprophylaxis include potential for adverse drug reactions and emergence of resistant bacterial strains.
(6) Because chemoprophylaxis potentially could alleviate symptoms of acute otitis media without eliminating middle ear effusion, monthly evaluation of patients for middle ear effusion is recommended.

Prevention of Travelers' Diarrhea

Although effective chemoprophylactic regimens (as outlined below) are available, antimicrobial agents are *not recommended* for the prevention of travelers' diarrhea because the risks associated with widespread administration of these agents outweigh the benefits of preventing an illness that usually is mild and self-limiting. These risks include the potential for: (1) serious adverse drug reactions; (2) the development of superinfections; and (3) the emergence of widespread bacterial resistance to the antimicrobial agents being used (NIH Consensus Development Conference, 1985). For most travelers, awareness and avoidance of possible sources of microbial contamination are of primary importance. If diarrhea develops, supportive therapy (replacement of fluids and electrolytes) may be indicated. Early treatment with trimethoprim/ sulfamethoxazole (or trimethoprim alone) has been shown to decrease the severity of diarrhea caused by enterotoxigenic *Escherichia coli* and *Shigella*, the most common pathogens in travelers' diarrhea (DuPont et al, 1982); doxycycline also appears to be effective (NIH Consensus Development Conference, 1985). Antimotility agents (eg, loperamide) or bismuth subsalicylate may be useful for mild cases. Thus, early treatment of travelers' diarrhea is a preferable alternative to prophylaxis (NIH Consensus Development Conference, 1985). See also Table 1 for more detailed discussion.

For trips of short duration (two weeks or less) to areas with high incidences of diarrhea, chemoprophylaxis has been considered a reasonable approach by some infectious disease experts for certain groups of travelers including (1) persons on important business trips; (2) military personnel on short stay; (3) individuals with increased susceptibility to infectious diarrhea (achlorhydria, known gastric resection, use of cimetidine-like drugs or antacids, or presence of dysgammaglobuline-mia); and (4) persons at greater risk for complications from dehydration or underlying disease (diuretic/digitalis therapy or history of diverticulitis) (see DuPont et al, 1985). However, the NIH Consensus Development Conference (1985) found no basis for employing antimicrobial chemoprophylaxis in these select groups of travelers and, therefore, it is not recommended. The conference report does contain a statement that some travelers may wish to consult with their physician and may elect to use prophylactic antimicrobial agents for travel under special circumstances, once the risks and benefits are clearly understood.

Selected references: Sack et al, 1978, 1979; DuPont et al, 1980, 1983, 1985; Gorbach, 1982; *Med Lett Drugs Ther*, 1983, 1985; Satterwhite and DuPont, 1983; Weiss, 1983; Siegel, 1984; NIH Consensus Development Conference, 1985.

PROPHYLACTIC REGIMEN(S)

PREFERRED REGIMEN:

Trimethoprim (160 mg)/sulfamethoxazole (800 mg), ie, one double-strength tablet, orally, once daily beginning on day of travel and continuing until two days after return home.

REMARKS:

(1) This is probably the most effective chemoprophylactic regimen currently available because it prevents travelers' diarrhea caused by either enterotoxigenic *E. coli* or *Shigella*.

(2) Generally well tolerated, but skin rashes (3%) have been observed. Sulfonamides rarely cause severe skin (eg, Stevens-Johnson syndrome) or hematologic (eg, hemolytic and aplastic anemias) adverse reactions.

(3) Trimethoprim alone (200 mg once daily) was less effective than the combination, but may be useful in patients who are allergic to sulfonamides.

ALTERNATIVE REGIMENS:

Doxycycline, orally, 200 mg on day of travel, followed by 100 mg once daily, continuing until two days after return home OR

Pepto-Bismol, orally, 60 ml (containing 1.05 g bismuth subsalicylate) four times daily beginning on day of travel and continuing until two days after return home.

REMARKS:

(1) Doxycycline is effective only against susceptible strains of enterotoxigenic *E. coli*. Some strains of this organism, as well as most *Shigella* and *Salmonella*, are resistant.

(2) Drug-induced gastrointestinal upset, including diarrhea, and photosensitivity reactions are important side effects of tetracyclines. Also tetracyclines should not be administered to pregnant women or children less than 8 years.

(3) The large volumes of Pepto-Bismol used in controlled studies are an inconvenience for most travelers. A laboratory study by Graham et al (1983) suggests that bismuth subsalicylate (600-mg doses) in nonliquid form also is effective in preventing travelers' diarrhea. In a recent field trial involving U.S. students in Mexico, two bismuth subsalicylate tablets (263 mg/tablet) four times daily for three weeks provided a 66% protection rate against travelers' diarrhea when compared to placebo (diarrhea incidences, 13% [drug] versus 38% [placebo]) (DuPont et al, 1986).

(4) The salicylate contained in 240 ml of Pepto-Bismol is equivalent to eight 5-grain aspirin tablets. This regimen should not be used in patients allergic to salicylates, those taking large daily doses of aspirin for arthritis, or individuals receiving oral anticoagulants, uricosurics, or methotrexate (*Med Lett Drugs Ther*, 1980).

(5) The bismuth subsalicylate contained in a 60-ml dose of Pepto-Bismol significantly decreased the bioavailability of doxycycline, 200 mg orally (Ericsson et al, 1982). Thus, the two agents should not be taken together to prevent travelers' diarrhea.

TABLE 4. ANTIMICROBIAL CHEMOPROPHYLAXIS FOR SURGICAL PATIENTS

The purpose of antimicrobial chemoprophylaxis for surgical patients is to reduce the risk of postoperative wound infection. The benefit of prophylaxis for each surgical procedure must be weighed against the potential risks to both the patient and the environment, including adverse drug reactions, superinfections, and the emergence of antibiotic-resistant bacterial strains, and the monetary cost of antimicrobial administration.

Surgical procedures are classified into four categories according to the expected risk of postoperative infection: *clean, clean-contaminated, contaminated*, and *dirty*. Generally, prophylaxis should be limited to patients at high risk of postoperative infection, ie, those undergoing clean-contaminated or contaminated surgery, or those in whom the development of an infection might be associated with a catastrophic end result, such as patients undergoing clean surgical procedures involving the insertion of prostheses. Dirty surgery implies that infection already exists and the use of antimicrobial agents in such procedures usually is considered treatment rather than prophylaxis.

The timing and duration of antimicrobial administration are important for effective surgical prophylaxis. An adequate concentration of a drug that is active against the likely pathogens must be present in vulnerable tissues during the procedure, which is the time of maximal contamination. Thus, for most surgical procedures, antimicrobial prophylaxis should begin just prior to the operation. Usually, a single parenteral (usually intravenous) dose administered shortly before the first surgical incision (usually at induction of anesthesia) provides sufficient tissue concentrations of antimicrobial agent throughout the procedure. Additional doses given either earlier or later usually are unnecessary. A second dose frequently is administered postoperatively, however, but prophylaxis for more than 24 hours is not indicated. When the surgical procedure is prolonged, an additional dose of antimicrobial agent, intraoperatively, may be required to maintain adequate tissue concentrations.

Guidelines for antimicrobial chemoprophylaxis of those surgical procedures for which prophylaxis is justified, based on controlled clinical trials, are presented below. However, it should be emphasized that definitive recommendations remain to be established, pending the results of future studies.

Selected references: Hirschmann and Inui, 1980; DiPiro et al, 1981, 1983; Hirschmann, 1981; Lennard and Dellinger, 1981; *Med Lett Drugs Ther*, 1981, 1985; Nichols, 1981, 1984; Flynn and Hoeprich, 1983; Guglielmo et al, 1983; Polk et al, 1983; Burnakis, 1984; Conte and Barriere, 1984; Conte et al, 1984; Gilbert, 1984; Sanford, 1985; Reese and Betts, 1986.

ABDOMINAL SURGERY

Elective Biliary Tract Surgery (Clean-Contaminated)

INDICATIONS:

Prophylaxis is recommended only for high-risk patients, including those over 70 years, or patients with jaundice, acute cholecystitis, or common duct stones.

POTENTIAL PATHOGENS:
Gram-negative enteric bacilli (*Escherichia coli, Klebsiella*), *Streptococcus faecalis* (group D; enterococcus), and *Clostridium perfringens* (less than 20% of cases)

RECOMMENDED REGIMEN:
Cefazolin[1] (*adults*, 1 g IV at induction of anesthesia)

ALTERNATIVE REGIMEN:
Ampicillin (*adults*, 1 g IV at induction of anesthesia) *plus* gentamicin (or tobramycin) (*adults*, 1.5 mg/kg IV at induction of anesthesia)

REMARKS:
(1) Ampicillin alone also appears to be an effective alternative (Levi et al, 1984). Some consultants suggest adding gentamicin only for seriously ill patients, those requiring prophylaxis for endocarditis (see Table 3, Antimicrobial Chemoprophylaxis for Ambulatory Patients), and for immunocompromised patients.
(2) Trimethoprim (160 mg)/sulfamethoxazole (800 mg) IV at induction of anesthesia appears to be an effective alternative.

Gastroduodenal Surgery (Clean-Contaminated)

INDICATIONS:
Prophylaxis is recommended only for high-risk patients with decreased gastric acidity or motility. This includes patients with gastric ulcer, gastric malignancy, obstructing or bleeding duodenal ulcer, and achlorhydria or those receiving chronic cimetidine therapy. Prophylaxis is not recommended for patients with routine, nonobstructing duodenal ulcer.

POTENTIAL PATHOGENS:
Mixed oropharyngeal flora (eg, aerobic and anaerobic streptococci); gram-negative bacilli; and *Staphylococcus aureus*

RECOMMENDED REGIMEN:
Cefazolin[1] (*adults*, 1 g IV at induction of anesthesia)

Elective Colorectal Surgery (Clean-Contaminated)

INDICATIONS:
Current consensus is that all patients undergoing elective procedures should receive mechanical bowel preparation and prophylactic antimicrobial agents orally. Parenteral antimicrobial prophylactic regimens should be used in emergency procedures or in patients with bowel obstruction (see REMARKS).

POTENTIAL PATHOGENS:
Gram-negative enteric bacilli (eg, *Escherichia coli*); anaerobic bacteria (especially *Bacteroides fragilis*); and rarely *Streptococcus faecalis* (group D; enterococcus)

RECOMMENDED REGIMEN (ORAL):
Neomycin *plus* erythromycin base (orally, 1 g of each at 1 PM, 2 PM, and 11 PM on the day prior to surgery [surgery at 8 AM])

ALTERNATIVE REGIMENS (PARENTERAL):
Cefoxitin (*adults*, 2 g IV at induction of anesthesia)
OR
Clindamycin (*adults*, 600 mg IV at induction of anesthesia) (or metronidazole, *adults*, 1 g IV infused over 30 to 60 minutes prior to induction of anesthesia) *plus* gentamicin (or tobramycin) (*adults*, 1.5 mg/kg IV at induction of anesthesia)

REMARKS:
(1) Whether an oral or an appropriate parenteral regimen is better, or both together are better than either alone, remains to be determined (*Med Lett Drugs Ther*, 1985). Some consultants suggested combined oral and parenteral agents in certain situations (eg, fistulas, partial bowel obstruction, colostomy closures) where contact of the oral antimicrobials throughout the bowel cannot be assured.

(2) For prolonged operations (eg, greater than four hours), a second intraoperative dose of cefoxitin is indicated because of its short elimination half-life.
(3) Various third generation cephalosporins have been shown to be effective for prophylaxis of elective colorectal surgery, but whether they offer any advantages over cefoxitin remains to be established by comparative, controlled clinical trials.

Colorectal Surgery (Dirty)

INDICATIONS:
Surgery for penetrating abdominal trauma, colon perforation, appendiceal abscess or perforation, or ruptured viscus often is followed by postoperative infection. Current consensus is that empiric antimicrobial treatment, rather than prophylaxis, is indicated (see REMARKS).

POTENTIAL PATHOGENS:
Gram-negative enteric bacilli (eg, *Escherichia coli*); anaerobic bacteria (especially *Bacteroides fragilis*); and *Streptococcus faecalis* (group D; enterococcus)

RECOMMENDED REGIMENS:
Clindamycin (*adults*, 600 mg IV immediately and then every six hours for 5 to 10 days) *plus* gentamicin (or tobramycin) (*adults*, 1.5 mg/kg IM or IV immediately and then every eight hours for 5 to 10 days)
OR
Cefoxitin (*adults*, 2 g IV immediately and then every six hours for 5 to 10 days) *with or without* gentamicin (or tobramycin) (*adults*, 1.5 mg/kg IM or IV immediately and then every eight hours for 5 to 10 days)

REMARKS:
(1) Some experts also add ampicillin (or penicillin G) to the regimen to cover enterococci (eg, *S. faecalis*).
(2) An alternative dosing schedule for clindamycin is 900 mg IV every eight hours.
(3) Established intra-abdominal infections (peritonitis or abscess) can be avoided in patients with bacterial contamination of the abdomen secondary to penetrating abdominal trauma if prompt surgical intervention and administration of appropriate antimicrobial agents are performed. In these patients, cefoxitin alone appears to be as effective as combination regimens containing clindamycin plus an aminoglycoside in preventing infections after penetrating abdominal injuries (Hofstetter et al, 1984; Nichols et al, 1984; Jones et al, 1985). Furthermore, when antimicrobial agents are given as soon as possible after injury, it appears that shorter courses (eg, 24 to 48 hours) are as effective in preventing infections as traditional 5 to 7 day durations of therapy (Stone et al, 1979; Oreskovich et al, 1982; Hofstetter et al, 1984; Jones et al, 1985; Dellinger et al, 1986; see also DiPiro et al, 1986).
(4) See also the discussion on Peritonitis Secondary to Bowel Perforation in Table 1, Antimicrobial Drug Selection for Common Infectious Diseases.

CARDIOVASCULAR SURGERY

Cardiac Surgery (Clean)

INDICATIONS:
Prophylaxis is recommended when a prosthetic heart valve is inserted to decrease the risk of prosthetic valve endocarditis, a frequently fatal infection. The usefulness of prophylaxis in coronary artery bypass graft surgery remains unestablished, although some experts feel it is justified. Prophylaxis usually is not recommended for pacemaker insertion or cardiac catheterization.

POTENTIAL PATHOGENS:
Staphylococcus aureus; S. epidermidis; diphtheroids; gram-negative enteric bacilli; and rarely fungi

RECOMMENDED REGIMEN:

Cefazolin[1] (**adults, 2 g IV at induction of anesthesia**)

ALTERNATIVE REGIMEN:

Vancomycin (adults, 1 g IV infused over 60 minutes prior to induction of anesthesia)

REMARKS:

(1) For prolonged operations (greater than four hours), a second intraoperative dose of cefazolin is recommended.

(2) Some surgeons prefer to continue prophylaxis for an additional 48 to 72 hours until vascular monitoring catheters are removed.

(3) Cefazolin (or another parenteral first generation cephalosporin) usually is preferred to penicillinase-resistant penicillins (nafcillin, oxacillin) because it is more active against *S. epidermidis*.

(4) In hospitals with a high incidence of methicillin-resistant staphylococcal strains, vancomycin is the likely drug of choice.

Peripheral Vascular Surgery (Clean)

INDICATIONS:

Prophylaxis is recommended for arterial reconstructive surgery of the abdominal aorta and vascular operations on the lower leg involving a groin incision. Generally, prophylaxis is probably justified for any vascular procedure in which a prosthesis is inserted. It usually is not recommended for brachial or carotid arterial surgery if a prosthesis is not involved; the incidence of infection is low and there are no data on the effectiveness of prophylaxis.

POTENTIAL PATHOGENS:

Staphylococcus aureus; S. epidermidis; and gram-negative enteric bacilli

RECOMMENDED REGIMEN:

Cefazolin[1] (**adults, 1 g IV at induction of anesthesia**)

REMARK:

(1) Vancomycin (dosage as above for Cardiac Surgery) is alternative agent.

OBSTETRIC-GYNECOLOGIC SURGERY

Hysterectomy (Clean-Contaminated)

INDICATIONS:

Prophylaxis is recommended for vaginal hysterectomy. The role of antimicrobial prophylaxis in abdominal hysterectomy is less clear, although some clinical trials have shown significantly decreased rates of postoperative wound infection. Thus, prophylaxis for abdominal hysterectomy is probably a reasonable option.

POTENTIAL PATHOGENS:

Escherichia coli and other Enterobacteriaceae; anaerobic bacteria (eg, gram-positive cocci, *Bacteroides*); *Streptococcus faecalis* (group D; enterococcus); and *S. agalactiae* (group B)

RECOMMENDED REGIMEN:

Cefazolin[1] (**adults, 1 g IV at induction of anesthesia**)

REMARKS:

(1) Cefoxitin, other second and third generation cephalosporins, extended spectrum penicillins, and metronidazole have been shown to be effective for prophylaxis of vaginal hysterectomy, but whether any of these antimicrobial agents offers any advantages over cefazolin remains to be established by comparative, controlled clinical trials (see also the Footnote).

Cesarean Section (Clean-Contaminated)

INDICATIONS:

Prophylaxis appears to be useful in reducing postoperative infectious complications (eg, endometritis) in certain high-risk women. This includes patients in labor or with ruptured membranes, or those who require internal fetal monitoring. The usefulness of prophylaxis in routine vaginal deliveries is not established.

POTENTIAL PATHOGENS:

Escherichia coli and other Enterobacteriaceae; anaerobic bacteria (eg, gram-positive cocci, *Bacteroides*); *Streptococcus faecalis* (group D; enterococcus); and *S. agalactiae* (group B)

RECOMMENDED REGIMEN:

Cefazolin[1] (**adults, 1 g IV after cord clamping**)

REMARKS:

(1) Cefoxitin, other second and third generation cephalosporins, and extended spectrum penicillins have been shown to be effective for prophylaxis of cesarean section, but whether any of these antimicrobial agents offers any advantages over cefazolin remains to be established by comparative, controlled clinical trials (see also the Footnote).

(2) To avoid delivery of the antibiotic to the fetus, the first dose for prophylaxis should be administered after the cord is clamped.

ORTHOPEDIC SURGERY

Orthopedic Surgery (Clean)

INDICATIONS:

Prophylaxis decreases postoperative infection following total hip replacement, a potentially disastrous complication, and is recommended. Prophylaxis also appears to be justified for other artificial joint insertions and is recommended for hip fracture operations in which fixation is achieved with a nail, plate, or a prosthetic femoral head. Other clean orthopedic surgery not involving the insertion of a prosthesis usually does not require prophylactic antimicrobial drugs; the incidence of infection is low and the effectiveness of prophylaxis is unproven.

POTENTIAL PATHOGENS:

Staphylococcus aureus; S. epidermidis; and other skin flora

RECOMMENDED REGIMEN:

Cefazolin[1] (**adults, 1 g IV at induction of anesthesia**)

ALTERNATIVE REGIMENS:

Nafcillin (or oxacillin) (adults, 1 g IV at induction of anesthesia)

OR

Vancomycin (adults, 1 g IV infused over 60 minutes prior to induction of anesthesia)

REMARKS:

(1) Cefazolin (or another first generation cephalosporin) usually is preferred to penicillinase-resistant penicillins (nafcillin, oxacillin) because it is more active against *S. epidermidis*.

(2) In hospitals with a high incidence of methicillin-resistant staphylococcal strains, vancomycin is the likely drug of choice.

Compound Fracture (Dirty)

INDICATIONS:

Infection is likely and empiric antimicrobial treatment, rather than prophylaxis, is indicated.

POTENTIAL PATHOGENS:

Staphylococcus aureus; Streptococcus pyogenes (group A, beta hemolytic); and clostridia

RECOMMENDED REGIMENS:

Cefazolin[1] (**adults, 1 g IM or IV immediately and then every eight hours for 5 to 10 days**)

OR

Nafcillin (or oxacillin) (adults, 1 g IV immediately and then every four hours for 5 to 10 days)

ALTERNATIVE REGIMENS:
Vancomycin (*adults*, 7.5 mg/kg IV, infused over a 60-minute period, immediately and then every eight hours for 5 to 10 days)
OR
Clindamycin (*adults*, 600 mg IV immediately and then every six hours for 5 to 10 days)
REMARKS:
(1) Some experts would add penicillin G for better coverage against clostridia.
(2) Nafcillin (or oxacillin) is preferred to methicillin because the latter is associated with a higher incidence of interstitial nephritis.

OTOLARYNGOLOGIC SURGERY

Head and Neck Surgery (Contaminated)

INDICATIONS:
Prophylaxis is recommended for surgical procedures requiring an incision that enters the oral cavity or pharynx (eg, as in surgery for laryngeal and pharyngeal carcinomas).
POTENTIAL PATHOGENS:
Mixture of oropharyngeal aerobic bacteria (eg, *Staphylococcus aureus*, streptococci, gram-negative bacilli [eg, *Klebsiella*]) and anaerobic bacteria (eg, peptococci, peptostreptococci, *Bacteroides* [seldom *B. fragilis*])
RECOMMENDED REGIMENS:
Cefazolin[1] (*adults*, 1 g IV at induction of anesthesia)
OR
Clindamycin (*adults*, 300 to 600 mg IV at induction of anesthesia) *plus* gentamicin (or tobramycin) (*adults*, 1.5 mg/kg IV at induction of anesthesia)
REMARKS:
(1) Although most experts recommend cefazolin, the results of a double blind, randomized clinical trial suggested that clindamicin *plus* gentamicin was significantly more effective in prophylaxis (Johnson et al, 1984). The dosage of cefazolin was 500 mg every eight hours in this study, however.

FOOTNOTE
1. Cephalothin and cephapirin are alternatives to cefazolin. However, cefazolin usually is preferred because it has the following advantages: (1) a longer serum half-life; (2) higher tissue levels (for equivalent weight of drug); and (3) less pain with IM injection. Based on current data, there is no advantage to using second or third generation cephalosporins in this situation.

REFERENCES

Introduction

Eliopoulos GM, Moellering RC Jr: Principles of antibiotic therapy. *Med Clin North Am* 66:3-15, 1982.

McHenry MC, Weinstein AJ: Antimicrobial drugs and infections in ambulatory patients: Some problems and perspectives. *Med Clin North Am* 67:3-16, 1983.

Moellering RC Jr: Principles of anti-infective therapy, in Mandell GL, et al (eds): *Principles and Practice of Infectious Diseases*, ed 2. New York, John Wiley & Sons, 1984, 153-164.

Reese RE, Betts RF: Antibiotic use, in Reese RE, Douglas RG Jr (eds): *A Practical Approach to Infectious Diseases*, ed 2. Boston, Little, Brown and Company, 1986, 559-679.

Sande MA, Mandell GL: Antimicrobial agents: General considerations, in Gilman AG, et al (eds): *The Pharmacological Basis of Therapeutics*, ed 7. New York, Macmillan, 1985, 1066-1094.

Wilkowske CJ, Hermans PE: General principles of antimicrobial therapy. *Mayo Clin Proc* 58:6-13, 1983.

Table 1: Antimicrobial Drug Selection for Common Infectious Diseases

INTRODUCTION

(A) Textbooks

Braude AI (ed): *Medical Microbiology and Infectious Diseases*, eds 1 and 2. Philadelphia, WB Saunders, 1981, 1986.

Feigin RD, Cherry JD (eds): *Textbook of Pediatric Infectious Diseases*. Philadelphia, WB Saunders, 1981, vols I and II.

Hoeprich PD (ed): *Infectious Diseases*, ed 3. Philadelphia, Harper & Row, 1983.

Holmes KK, et al (ed): *Sexually Transmitted Diseases*. New York, McGraw-Hill, 1984.

Kagan BM (ed): *Antimicrobial Therapy*, ed 3. Philadelphia, WB Saunders, 1980.

Kass EH, Platt R (eds): *Current Therapy in Infectious Disease, 1983-1984*. Philadelphia, BC Decker, 1983.

Mandell GL, et al (eds): *Principles and Practice of Infectious Diseases*, eds 1 and 2. New York, John Wiley & Sons, 1979, 1984.

McCracken GH Jr, Nelson JD: *Antimicrobial Therapy for Newborns*, ed 2. New York, Grune & Stratton, 1983.

Reese RE, Douglas RG Jr (eds): *A Practical Approach to Infectious Diseases*, eds 1 and 2. Boston, Little, Brown and Company, 1983, 1986.

Remington JS, Klein JO (ed): *Infectious Diseases of the Fetus and Newborn*, ed 2. Philadelphia, WB Saunders, 1983.

Ristuccia AM, Cunha B (eds): *Antimicrobial Therapy*. New York, Raven Press, 1984.

Yoshikawa TT, et al (eds): *Infectious Diseases: Diagnosis and Management*. Boston, Houghton Mifflin, 1980.

(B) Pocketbooks and Manuals

Report of the Committee on Infectious Diseases: *American Academy of Pediatrics Redbook*, ed 19. Evanston, IL, American Academy of Pediatrics, 1982.

Conte JE Jr, Barriere SL: *Manual of Antibiotics and Infectious Diseases*, ed 5. Philadelphia, Lea & Febiger, 1984.

Eisenberg MS, et al: *Manual of Antimicrobial Therapy and Infectious Diseases*. Philadelphia, WB Saunders, 1980.

Fairbanks DNF: *Pocket Guide to Antimicrobial Therapy in Otolaryngology*. Washington, DC, American Council of Otolaryngology —Head and Neck Surgery, 1980.

Gardner P, Provine HT: *Manual of Acute Bacterial Infections*. Boston, Little, Brown and Company, 1984.

The Medical Letter: *Handbook of Antimicrobial Therapy*. New Rochelle, NY, The Medical Letter, Inc, 1984, 1986.

Nelson JD: *Pocketbook of Pediatric Antimicrobial Therapy*, ed 6. Baltimore, Williams & Wilkins, 1985.

Sanford JP: *Guide to Antimicrobial Therapy, 1985*. West Bethesda, MD, private publication, 1985.

Sanford JP: *Guide to Antimicrobial Therapy, 1986*. West Bethesda, MD, private publication, 1986.

(C) Reviews

The choice of antimicrobial drugs. *Med Lett Drugs Ther* 26:19-26, 1984; 28:33-40, 1986.

Cunha BA (ed): Symposium on antimicrobial therapy. *Med Clin North Am* 66:1-316, 1982 (26 articles).

Fekety R (ed): *Reviews of Infectious Diseases, 1983*. Orlando, Grune & Stratton, 1983.

Fekety R (ed): *Reviews of Infectious Diseases, 1984*. Orlando, Grune & Stratton, 1984.

Fekety R (ed): *Reviews of Infectious Diseases, 1985*. Orlando, Grune & Stratton, 1985.

McHenry MC, Weinstein AJ (eds): Symposium on infections in office practice. *Med Clin North Am* 67:1-261, 1983 (14 articles).

Neu HC: Clinical uses of cephalosporins. *Lancet* 2:252-255, 1982.

Speck WT, Blumer JL (eds): Symposium on anti-infective therapy, Parts I and II. *Pediatr Clin North Am* 30:1-240, 241-416, 1983 (29 articles).

Wilkowske CJ, Hermans PE: General principles of antimicrobial therapy. *Mayo Clin Proc* 58:6-13, 1983.

SKIN INFECTIONS

Aly R, Maibach HI: Pyodermas: Avoiding the empiric approach: Parts I and II. *Fam Med Rep* 2:17-24, 25-32, (Winter/Spring) 1984.

Burke JF: Burns, in Mandell GL, et al (eds): *Principles and Practice of Infectious Diseases.* New York, John Wiley & Sons, 1979, vol 1, 838-843.

Carter S, Feldman WE: Etiology and treatment of facial cellulitis in pediatric patients. *Pediatr Infect Dis* 2:222-224, 1983.

Conte JE Jr, Barriere SL: *Manual of Antibiotics and Infectious Diseases,* ed 5. Philadelphia, Lea & Febiger, 1984, 105.

Cooney TG, Reuler JB: Pressure sores. *West J Med* 140:622-624, 1984.

Demling RH: Infections following burns, in Hoeprich PD (ed): *Infectious Diseases,* ed 3. Philadelphia, Harper & Row, 1983, 1348-1351.

Demling RH: Burns. *N Engl J Med* 313:1389-1398, 1985.

Dillon HC Jr: Topical and systemic therapy for pyodermas. *Int J Dermatol* 19:443-451, 1980.

Duncan WC: Erythrasma and trichomycosis axillaris, in Hoeprich PD (ed): *Infectious Diseases,* ed 3. Philadelphia, Harper & Row, 1983, 933-936.

Gustafson TL, et al: Pseudomonas folliculitis: Outbreak and review. *Rev Infect Dis* 5:1-8, 1983.

Hook EW III, et al: Microbiologic evaluation of cutaneous cellulitis in adults. *Arch Intern Med* 146:295-297, 1986.

Magnussen CR: Skin and soft tissue infections, in Reese RE, Douglas RG Jr (eds): *A Practical Approach to Infectious Diseases,* ed 2. Boston, Little, Brown and Company, 1986, 99-122.

Melish ME: Impetigo, in Braude AI (ed): *Medical Microbiology and Infectious Diseases.* Philadelphia, WB Saunders, 1981 A, 1553-1557.

Melish ME: Staphylococcal scalded skin syndrome, in Braude AI (ed): *Medical Microbiology and Infectious Diseases.* Philadelphia, WB Saunders, 1981 B, 1563-1567.

Melish ME: Pyogenic skin infections, in Braude AI (ed): *Medical Microbiology and Infectious Diseases.* Philadelphia, WB Saunders, 1981 C, 1557-1563.

Nelson JD: *1985 Pocketbook of Pediatric Antimicrobial Therapy,* ed 6. Baltimore, Williams & Wilkins, 1985, 22-23.

Nelson JD: Cefuroxime: Cephalosporin with unique applicability to pediatric practice. *Pediatr Infect Dis* 2:394-396, 1983.

Sanford JP: *Guide to Antimicrobial Therapy, 1985.* West Bethesda, MD, private publication, 1985, 27-30.

Schachner L, et al: Therapeutic update of superficial skin infections. *Pediatr Clin North Am* 30:397-404, 1983.

Swartz MN: Cellulitis and superficial infections, in Mandell GL, et al (eds): *Principles and Practice of Infectious Diseases,* ed 2. New York, John Wiley & Sons, 1984, 598-609.

Wheat LJ, et al: Long-term studies of effect of rifampin on nasal carriage of coagulase-positive staphylococci. *Rev Infect Dis* 5(suppl 3):S459-S462, (July-Aug) 1983.

Witkowski JA, Parish LC: Bacterial skin infections: Management of common streptococcal and staphylococcal lesions. *Postgrad Med* 72:166-185, (Oct) 1982.

CENTRAL NERVOUS SYSTEM INFECTIONS

The choice of antimicrobial drugs. *Med Lett Drugs Ther* 26:19-26, 1984; 28:33-40, 1986.

Barriere SL, Flaherty JF: Third generation cephalosporins: Critical evaluation. *Clin Pharm* 3:351-373, 1984.

Barson WJ, et al: Prospective comparative trial of ceftriaxone vs conventional therapy for treatment of bacterial meningitis in children. *Pediatr Infect Dis* 4:362-368, 1985.

Bell WE: Treatment of bacterial infections of central nervous system. *Ann Neurol* 9:313-327, 1981.

Bryan JP, et al: Comparison of ceftriaxone and ampicillin plus chloramphenicol for therapy of acute bacterial meningitis. *Antimicrob Agents Chemother* 20:361-368, 1985.

Cherubin CE, Eng RHK: Experience with use of cefotaxime in treatment of bacterial meningitis. *Am J Med* 80:398-404, 1986.

Congeni BL: Comparison of ceftriaxone and traditional therapy of bacterial meningitis. *Antimicrob Agents Chemother* 25:40-44, 1984.

Del Rio M, et al: Ceftriaxone versus ampicillin and chloramphenicol for treatment of bacterial meningitis in children. *Lancet* 1:1241-1244, 1983.

Fong IW, Tomkins KB: Review of *Pseudomonas aeruginosa* meningitis with special emphasis on treatment with ceftazidime. *Rev Infect Dis* 7:604-612, 1985.

Jacobs RF, et al: Prospective randomized comparison of cefotaxime vs ampicillin and chloramphenicol for bacterial meningitis in children. *J Pediatr* 107:129-133, 1985.

Levitz RE, Quintiliani R: Trimethoprim-sulfamethoxazole for bacterial meningitis. *Ann Intern Med* 100:881-890, 1984.

McCracken GH Jr: Perinatal bacterial diseases, in Feigin RD, Cherry JD (eds): *Textbook of Pediatric Infectious Diseases.* Philadelphia, WB Saunders, 1981, vol I, 747-768.

McCracken GH Jr: New concepts in management of infants and children with meningitis. *Pediatr Infect Dis* 2:551-555, 1983.

McCracken GH Jr, Nelson JD: *Antimicrobial Therapy for Newborns,* ed 2. New York, Grune & Stratton, 1983, 119-127.

McCracken GH Jr, et al: Moxalactam therapy for neonatal meningitis due to gram-negative enteric bacilli: Prospective controlled evaluation. *JAMA* 252:1427-1432, 1984.

McGee ZA, Kaiser AB: Acute meningitis, in Mandell GL, et al (eds): *Principles and Practice of Infectious Diseases,* ed 2. New York, John Wiley & Sons, 1984, 560-573.

Naqvi SH, et al: Cefotaxime therapy of neonatal gram-negative bacillary meningitis. *Pediatr Infect Dis* 4:499-502, 1985.

Nelson JD: Cefuroxime: Cephalosporin with unique applicability to pediatric practice. *Pediatr Infect Dis* 2:394-396, 1983.

Nelson JD: *1985 Pocketbook of Pediatric Antimicrobial Therapy,* ed 6. Baltimore, Williams & Wilkins, 1985, 38-39.

Neu HC: New beta-lactamase-stable cephalosporins. *Ann Intern Med* 97:408-419, 1982.

Parker RH: Diagnosis and treatment of bacterial meningitis. *Drug Ther (Hosp)* 6:33-42, (Aug) 1981.

Pfenninger J, et al: Cefuroxime in bacterial meningitis. *Arch Dis Child* 57:539-543, 1982.

Rahal JJ, Simberkoff MS: Host defense and antimicrobial therapy in adult gram-negative bacillary meningitis. *Ann Intern Med* 96:468-474, 1982.

Report from a Swedish Study Group: Cefuroxime versus ampicillin and chloramphenicol for treatment of bacterial meningitis. *Lancet* 1:295-298, 1982.

Schaad UB, et al: Extended experience with cefuroxime therapy of childhood bacterial meningitis. *Pediatr Infect Dis* 3:410-416, 1984.

Siegel J: Prevention and treatment of group B streptococcal infections. *Pediatr Infect Dis* 4(suppl):S33-S36, 1985.

Steele RW: Ceftriaxone: Increasing half-life and activity of third generation cephalosporins. *Pediatr Infect Dis* 4:188-191, 1985.

Steele RW, Bradsher RW: Comparison of ceftriaxone with standard therapy for bacterial meningitis. *J Pediatr* 103:138-141, 1983.

Tweardy DJ, et al: Susceptibility of penicillin-resistant pneumococci to eighteen antimicrobials: Implications for treatment of meningitis. *J Antimicrob Chemother* 12:133-139, 1983.

Van Voris LP, Roberts NJ Jr: Central nervous system infections, in

Reese RE, Douglas RG Jr (eds): *A Practical Approach to Infectious Diseases*, ed 2. Boston, Little, Brown and Company, 1986, 123-155.

Whitby M, Finch R: Bacterial meningitis: Rational selection and use of antibacterial drugs. *Drugs* 31:266-278, 1986.

EAR INFECTIONS

Antimicrobial agents for acute otitis media. *Med Lett Drugs Ther* 23:93-95, 1981.

Klein JO, Bluestone CD: Acute otitis media. *Pediatr Infect Dis* 1:66-73, 1982.

McCracken GH Jr: Antimicrobial therapy for acute otitis media. *Pediatr Infect Dis* 3:383-386, 1984.

Paradise JL: Otitis media in infants and children. *Pediatrics* 65:917-943, 1980.

Schwartz RH, Schwartz DM: Acute otitis media: Diagnosis and drug therapy. *Drugs* 19:107-118, 1980.

Wald ER: Changing trends in microbiology of otitis media with effusion. *Pediatr Infect Dis* 3:380-383, 1984.

EYE INFECTIONS

1985 STD treatment guidelines. *Morbid Mortal Week Rep* 34(suppl):75S-108S, 1985.

McCracken GH Jr, Nelson JD: *Antimicrobial Therapy for Newborns*, ed 2. New York, Grune & Stratton, 1983, 152-156.

Nelson JD: *1985 Pocketbook of Pediatric Antimicrobial Therapy*, ed 6. Baltimore, Williams & Wilkins, 1985 A, 13.

Nelson JD: *1985 Pocketbook of Pediatric Antimicrobial Therapy*, ed 6. Baltimore, Williams & Wilkins, 1985 B, 7-8.

Riley GJ, Baker AS: Eye infections, in Reese RE, Douglas RG Jr (eds): *A Practical Approach to Infectious Diseases*, ed 2. Boston, Little, Brown and Company, 1986, 156-173.

UPPER RESPIRATORY TRACT INFECTIONS

Rapid office diagnostic tests for streptococcal pharyngitis. *Med Lett Drugs Ther* 27:49-51, 1985.

1985 STD treatment guidelines. *Morbid Mortal Week Rep* 34(suppl):75S-108S, 1985.

Bluestone CD (ed): Diagnosis and management of sinusitis in children. *Pediatr Infect Dis* 4(suppl):S49-S81, 1985 (9 papers).

Brook I: Bacteriologic features of chronic sinusitis in children. *JAMA* 246:967-969, 1981.

Cohen EL: Epiglottitis in adult: Recognizing and treating acute case. *Postgrad Med* 75:309-311, (March) 1984.

Frederick J, Braude AI: Anaerobic infection of paranasal sinuses. *N Engl J Med* 290:135-137, 1974.

Fulginiti VA: Still more on streptococcal pharyngitis: Important disease with yet unresolved clinical issues, (editorial). *JAMA* 253:1302, 1985.

Gerber MA, Markowitz M: Management of streptococcal pharyngitis reconsidered. *Pediatr Infect Dis* 4:518-526, 1985.

Gwaltney JM: Acute sinusitis in adults. *Am J Otolaryngol* 4:422-423, 1983.

Gwaltney JM, et al: Etiology and antimicrobial treatment of acute sinusitis. *Otol Rhinol Laryngol* 90:68-71, 1981.

Hall CB, Douglas RG Jr: Infections of upper respiratory tract, trachea, and bronchi, in Reese RE, Douglas RG Jr (eds): *A Practical Approach to Infectious Diseases*, ed 2. Boston, Little, Brown and Company, 1986, 174-201.

Krober MS, et al: Streptococcal pharyngitis: Placebo-controlled double-blind evaluation of clinical response to penicillin therapy. *JAMA* 253:1271-1274, 1985.

Levy ML, et al: Infections of upper respiratory tract. *Med Clin North Am* 67:153-171, 1983.

Nelson JD: Effect of penicillin therapy on symptoms and signs of streptococcal pharyngitis. *Pediatr Infect Dis* 3:10-13, 1984.

Nelson JD: *1985 Pocketbook of Pediatric Antimicrobial Therapy*, ed 6. Baltimore, Williams & Wilkins, 1985, 28.

Randolph MF, et al: Effect of antibiotic therapy on clinical course of streptococcal pharyngitis. *J Pediatr* 106:870-875, 1985.

Shulman ST: Decline of rheumatic fever: What impact on our management of pharyngitis? *Am J Dis Child* 138:426-427, 1984.

Shulman ST, et al: Prevention of rheumatic fever: Statement for health professionals by the Committee on Rheumatic Fever and Infective Endocarditis of the Council on Cardiovascular Disease in the Young. *Circulation* 70:1118A-1122A, 1984.

Smith AL: Does penicillin improve symptoms of strep throat? *Pediatr Alert* 9:17-18, 1984.

Wald ER: Acute sinusitis in children. *Pediatr Infect Dis* 2:61-68, (March) 1983.

Zack BG: Managing croup and epiglottitis: Clinical challenge. *Drug Ther (Hosp)* 8:74-87, (Feb) 1983.

LOWER RESPIRATORY TRACT INFECTIONS

Report of the Committee on Infectious Diseases. *American Academy of Pediatrics Redbook*, ed 19. Evanston, IL, American Academy of Pediatrics, 1982, 198-202.

The choice of antimicrobial drugs. *Med Lett Drugs Ther* 26:19-26, 1984; 28:33-40, 1986.

Bass JW: Pertussis: Current status of prevention and treatment. *Pediatr Infect Dis* 4:614-619, 1985.

Betts RF, Reese RE: Lower respiratory tract infections (including tuberculosis), in Reese RE, Douglas RG Jr (eds): *A Practical Approach to Infectious Diseases*, ed 2. Boston, Little, Brown and Company, 1986, 202-257.

Brunton JL, et al: Diagnosis and treatment of pneumonia. *Compr Ther* 8:8-18, (Sept) 1982.

Conte JE Jr, Barriere SL: *Manual of Antibiotics and Infectious Diseases*, ed 5. Philadelphia, Lea & Febiger, 1984, 102-104, 121-123, 124-131.

Donowitz GR, Mandell GL: Acute pneumonia, in Mandell GL, et al (eds): *Principles and Practice of Infectious Diseases*, ed 2. New York, John Wiley & Sons, 1984, 394-404.

Fedson DS, Rusthoven J: Acute lower respiratory disease. *Prim Care* 6:13-41, 1979.

Francke E: Legionnaires' disease: Clinical and pathologic features and current management. *Postgrad Med* 73:347-354, (Feb) 1983.

Geller RJ: Pertussis syndrome: Persistent problem. *Pediatr Infect Dis* 3:182-186, 1984.

Gleckman RA, Roth RM: Community-acquired bacterial pneumonia in the elderly. *Pharmacotherapy* 4:81-88, 1984.

Gwaltney JM Jr: Acute bronchitis, in Mandell GL, et al (eds): *Principles and Practice of Infectious Diseases*, ed 2. New York, John Wiley & Sons, 1984, 385-387.

Hall CB, Douglas RG Jr: Infections of upper respiratory tract, trachea, and bronchi, in Reese RE, Douglas RG Jr (eds): *A Practical Approach to Infectious Diseases*, ed 2. Boston, Little, Brown and Company, 1986, 174-201.

Hall CB, Hall WJ: Bronchiolitis, in Mandell GL, et al (eds): *Principles and Practice of Infectious Diseases*, ed 2. New York, John Wiley & Sons, 1984, 390-394.

Hurst DJ: Comparison of cefaclor and tetracycline in treatment of bacterial bronchitis. *Clin Therapeut* 6:163-169, 1984.

Kannangara DW, LeFrock JL: Solving etiologic puzzle of pneumonia. *Drug Ther (Hosp)* 7:35-45, (Dec) 1982 A.

Kannangara DW, LeFrock JL: Targeting pneumonia therapy. *Drug Ther (Hosp)* 7:49-58, (Dec) 1982 B.

Long SS: Treatment of acute pneumonia in infants and children. *Pediatr Clin North Am* 30:297-321, 1983.

Nelson JD: Cefuroxime: Cephalosporin with unique applicability to pediatric practice. *Pediatr Infect Dis* 2:394-396, 1983.

Nelson JD: *1985 Pocketbook of Pediatric Antimicrobial Therapy*, ed 6. Baltimore, Williams & Wilkins, 1985, 28-32.

Neu HC: New beta-lactamase-stable cephalosporins. *Ann Intern Med* 97:408-419, 1982.

Nicotra MB, et al: Antibiotic therapy of acute exacerbations of chronic bronchitis: Controlled study using tetracycline. *Ann Intern Med* 97:18-21, 1982.

Pennington JE: Treating pneumonia: Thirteen keys to avoiding costly errors. *Mod Med* 50:66-80, (Jan) 1982.

Perlino CA: Anaerobic pulmonary infections. *Compr Ther* 9:15-20, (May) 1983.

Reynolds HY: Chronic bronchitis and acute infectious exacerbations, in Mandell GL, et al (eds): *Principles and Practice of Infectious Diseases*, ed 2. New York, John Wiley & Sons, 1984, 387-390.

Rosenberg M, LeFrock JL: Choosing antibiotic therapy for pneumonia. *Am Fam Physician* 28:246-251, (Nov) 1983.

Sanford JP: *Guide to Antimicrobial Therapy*, 1985. West Bethesda, MD, private publication, 1985, 21-25.

Smialowicz CR: Clinical and bacteriological evaluation of cefaclor and tetracycline in acute episodes of bacterial bronchitis. *Clin Therapeut* 5:113-119, 1982.

Smith CB: *Mycoplasma pneumoniae* infections: Diagnosis and therapy. *Drug Ther* 13:89-102, (June) 1983.

Tager I, Speizer FE: Role of infection in chronic bronchitis. *N Engl J Med* 292: 563-571, 1975.

Teele D: Pneumonia: Antimicrobial therapy for infants and children. *Pediatr Infect Dis* 4:330-335, 1985.

Van Scoy RE: Office management of lower respiratory infections in adults. *Med Clin North Am* 67:173-186, 1983.

Weinstein L, Fields B (eds): *Seminars in Infectious Disease: Pneumonias*. New York, Thieme-Stratton, vol V, 1983.

Wilkins J, Wehrle PF: Bordetella species (including whooping cough), in Mandell GL, et al (eds): *Principles and Practice of Infectious Diseases*, ed 2. New York, John Wiley & Sons, 1984, 1301-1305.

INFECTIONS OF THE CARDIOVASCULAR SYSTEM

Brandriss MW: Cardiac infections, in Reese RE, Douglas RG Jr (eds): *A Practical Approach to Infectious Diseases*, ed 2. Boston, Little, Brown and Company, 1986, 258-283.

Chamovitz B, et al: Prosthetic valve endocarditis caused by *Staphylococcus epidermidis*: Development of rifampin resistance during vancomycin and rifampin therapy. *JAMA* 253:2867-2868, 1985.

Coleman DL, et al: Association between serum inhibitory and bactericidal concentrations and therapeutic outcome in bacterial endocarditis. *Am J Med* 73:260-267, 1982.

Geraci JE, Wilson WR: Endocarditis due to gram-negative bacteria: Report of 56 cases. *Mayo Clin Proc* 57:145-148, 1982.

Gnann JW Jr, Cobbs CG: Infections of prosthetic valves and intravascular devices, in Mandell GL, et al (eds): *Principles and Practice of Infectious Diseases*, ed 2. New York, John Wiley & Sons, 1984, 530-539.

Hoeprich PD, Durack DT: Infective endocarditis, in Hoeprich PD (ed): *Infectious Diseases*, ed 3. Philadelphia, Harper & Row, 1983, 1171-1187.

Karchmer AW, et al: *Staphylococcus epidermidis* causing prosthetic valve endocarditis: Microbiologic and clinical observations as guides to therapy. *Ann Intern Med* 98:447-455, 1983.

Karchmer AW, et al: Methicillin-resistant *Staphylococcus epidermidis* (SE) prosthetic valve (PV) endocarditis (E): Therapeutic trial, (abstract 476). *24th Interscience Conference on Antimicrobial Agents and Chemotherapy*. Washington, DC, Oct 8-10, 1984.

Korzeniowski O, et al: Combination antimicrobial therapy for *Staphylococcus aureus* endocarditis in patients addicted to parenteral drugs and in nonaddicts: Prospective study. *Ann Intern Med* 97:496-503, 1982.

Lowy FD, Hammer SM: *Staphylococcus epidermidis* infections. *Ann Intern Med* 99:834-839, 1983.

Mellors JW, et al: Value of serum bactericidal test in management of patients with bacterial endocarditis. *Eur J Clin Microbiol* 5:67-70, 1986.

Nelson JD: *1985 Pocketbook of Pediatric Antimicrobial Therapy*, ed 6. Baltimore, Williams & Wilkins, 1985, 22-42.

Sande MA, Scheld WM: Combination antibiotic therapy of bacterial endocarditis. *Ann Intern Med* 92:390-395, 1980.

Scheld WM, Sande MA: Endocarditis and intravascular infections, in Mandell GL, et al (eds): *Principles and Practice of Infectious Diseases*, ed 2. New York, John Wiley & Sons, 1984, 504-530.

Thompson RL: Staphylococcal infective endocarditis. *Mayo Clin Proc* 57:106-114, 1982.

Thornsberry C: Methicillin-resistant (heteroresistant) staphylococci. *Antimicrob Newslett* 1:43-47, 1984.

Van Scoy RE: Culture-negative endocarditis. *Mayo Clin Proc* 57:149-154, 1982.

Weinstein MP, et al: Multicenter collaborative evaluation of standardized serum bactericidal test as prognostic indicator in infective endocarditis. *Am J Med* 78:262-269, 1985.

Weinstein MP, et al: Current status of serum bactericidal test as monitor of therapeutic efficacy in serious infections. *Antimicrob Newslett* 3:9-14, 1986.

Wilkowske CJ: Enterococcal endocarditis. *Mayo Clin Proc* 57:101-105, 1982.

Wilson WR, et al: General considerations in diagnosis and treatment of infective endocarditis. *Mayo Clin Proc* 57:81-85, 1982 A.

Wilson WR, et al: Treatment of penicillin-sensitive streptococcal infective endocarditis. *Mayo Clin Proc* 57:95-100, 1982 B.

Wilson WR, et al: Prosthetic valve endocarditis. *Mayo Clin Proc* 57:155-161, 1982 C.

Wilson WR, et al: Treatment of streptomycin-susceptible and streptomycin-resistant enterococcal endocarditis. *Ann Intern Med* 100:816-823, 1984.

Wolfson JS, Swartz MN: Serum bactericidal activity as monitor of antibiotic therapy. *N Engl J Med* 312:968-975. 1985.

GASTROINTESTINAL AND INTRA-ABDOMINAL INFECTIONS

The choice of antimicrobial drugs. *Med Lett Drugs Ther* 26:19-26, 1984; 28:33-40, 1986.

Immunizations and chemoprophylaxis for travelers. *Med Lett Drugs Ther* 27:33-36, 1985.

Bartlett JG: Antibiotic-associated pseudomembranous colitis. *Hosp Pract* 16:85-95, (Dec) 1981.

Black RE: Prophylaxis and therapy of secretory diarrhea. *Med Clin North Am* 66:611-621, 1982.

Blaser MJ: Current approach to acute diarrheal illnesses. *Drug Ther* 13:114-123, (Feb) 1983.

Chang TW: Antimicrobial-associated diarrhea and enterocolitis. *Drug Ther (Hosp)* 6:71-78, (May) 1981.

Conte JE Jr, Barriere SL: *Manual of Antibiotics and Infectious Diseases*, ed 5. Philadelphia, Lea & Febiger, 1984 A, 115-116.

Conte JE Jr, Barriere SL: *Manual of Antibiotics and Infectious Diseases*, ed 5. Philadelphia, Lea & Febiger, 1984 B, 100, 117-118.

DiPiro JT, et al: Current concepts in clinical therapeutics: Intra-abdominal infections. *Clin Pharm* 5:34-50, 1986.

DuPont HL, et al: Treatment of travelers' diarrhea with trimethoprim/sulfamethoxazole and with trimethoprim alone. *N Engl J Med* 307:841-844, 1982.

DuPont HL, et al: Chemotherapy and chemoprophylaxis of travelers' diarrhea, (editorial). *Ann Intern Med* 102:260-261, 1985.

Fekety R: Clinical importance of anaerobic infections. *Drug Ther (Hosp)* 7:47-58, (Oct) 1982.

Fekety R: Recent advances in management of bacterial diarrhea. *Rev Infect Dis* 5:246-257, 1983.

Fekety R, et al: Comparative efficacy of low vs. high dose oral vancomycin (125 mg or 500 mg four times per day) in treatment of adults with antibiotic associated *Clostridium difficile* colitis, (abstract 818). *24th Interscience Conference on Antimicrobial Agents and Chemotherapy*. Washington DC, Oct 8-10, 1984.

Finegold SM, et al: Anaerobic infections (parts I and II). *DM* 31:1-77, 1-97, 1985.

George WL, et al: *Aeromonas*-related diarrhea in adults. *Arch Intern Med* 145:2207-2211, 1985.

Gorbach SL: Travelers' diarrhea. *N Engl J Med* 307:881-883, 1982.

Gorbach SL, McGowan K: Comparative clinical trials in treatment of intra-abdominal sepsis. *J Antimicrob Chemother* 8(suppl D):95-104, 1981.

Gotz VP, Rand KH: Medical management of antimicrobial-associated diarrhea and colitis. *Pharmacotherapy* 2:100-109, 1982.

Hornick RB: Typhoid fever, in Hoeprich PD (ed): *Infectious Diseases*, ed 3. Philadelphia, Harper & Row, 1983, 662-668.

Hruska JF: Gastrointestinal and intra-abdominal infections, in Reese RE, Douglas RG Jr (eds): *A Practical Approach to Infectious Diseases*, ed 2. Boston, Little, Brown and Company, 1986, 284-326.

Johnson PC, et al: Comparison of loperamide with bismuth subsalicylate for treatment of acute travelers' diarrhea. *JAMA* 255:757-760, 1986.

Levison ME: Peritonitis and intra-abdominal abscess, in Mandell GL, et al (eds): *Principles and Practice of Infectious Diseases*. New York, John Wiley & Sons, 1979, vol 1, 609-643.

Levison ME, Pontzer RE: Peritonitis and other intra-abdominal infections, in Mandell GL, et al (eds): *Principles and Practice of Infectious Diseases*, ed 2. New York, John Wiley & Sons, 1984, 476-503.

National Institutes of Health Consensus Development Conference: Travelers' diarrhea. *JAMA* 253:2700-2704, 1985.

Pickering LK: Antimicrobial therapy of gastrointestinal infections. *Pediatr Clin North Am* 30:373-388, 1983.

Sanford JP: *Guide to Antimicrobial Therapy, 1985*. West Bethesda, MD, private publication, 1985, 11.

San Joaquin VH, Marks MI: New agents in diarrhea. *Pediatr Infect Dis* 1:53-65, 1982.

Satterwhite TK, DuPont HL: Infectious diarrhea in office practice. *Med Clin North Am* 67:203-220, 1983.

Solomkin JS, et al: Randomized trial of imipenem/cilastatin versus gentamicin and clindamycin in mixed flora infections. *Am J Med* 78(suppl 6A):85-91, 1985.

Swenson RM: Cholecystitis and cholangitis, in Mandell GL, et al (eds): *Principles and Practice of Infectious Diseases*. New York, John Wiley & Sons, 1979, vol 1, 644-649.

Tally FP: Therapeutic approaches to anaerobic infection. *Hosp Pract* 16:117-132, 1981.

Tally FP, et al: Randomized comparison of cefoxitin with or without amikacin and clindamycin plus amikacin in surgical sepsis. *Ann Surg* 193:318-323, 1981.

Tally FP, et al: Nationwide study of susceptibility of *Bacteroides fragilis* group in the United States. *Antimicrob Agents Chemother* 28:675-677, 1985.

Teasley DG, et al: Prospective randomised trial of metronidazole versus vancomycin for *Clostridium difficile*-associated diarrhoea and colitis. *Lancet* 2:1043-1046, 1983.

Tedesco FJ: Pseudomembranous colitis: Pathogenesis and therapy. *Med Clin North Am* 66:655-664, 1982.

Weiss BD: Traveler's diarrhea: Update 1983. *Am Fam Physician* 27:193-195, (April) 1983.

Young GP, et al: Antibiotic-associated colitis due to *Clostridium difficile*: Double-blind comparison of vancomycin with bacitracin. *Gastroenterology* 89:1038-1045, 1985.

URINARY TRACT INFECTIONS

1985 STD treatment guidelines. *Morbid Mortal Week Rep* 34(suppl):75S-108S, 1985.

Treatment of urinary tract infections. *Med Lett Drugs Ther* 23:69-70, 1981.

Abraham E, et al: Cystitis and pyelonephritis. *Ann Emerg Med* 12:228-234, 1983.

Carlson KJ, Mulley AG: Management of acute dysuria: Decision-analysis model of alternative strategies. *Ann Intern Med* 102:244-249, 1985.

Carson CC: How to treat urinary tract infections. *Drug Ther* 12:72-78, (Nov) 1982.

Conte JE Jr, Barriere SL: *Manual of Antibiotics and Infectious Diseases*, ed 5. Philadelphia, Lea & Febiger, 1984, 101, 119-120.

Cunha BA: Urinary tract infections: Part 1, Pathophysiology and diagnostic approach; Part 2, Therapeutic approach. *Postgrad Med* 70:141-145, 149-157, (Dec) 1981.

Fang LST, et al: Clinical management of urinary tract infection. *Pharmacotherapy* 2:91-99, 1982.

Farrar WE Jr: Infections of urinary tract. *Med Clin North Am* 67:187-201, 1983.

Gleckman RA: Urinary tract infection in women: New perspectives on office management. *Postgrad Med* 73:277-282, (May) 1983.

Hooton TM, et al: Single-dose therapy for cystitis in women: Comparison of trimethoprim/sulfamethoxazole, amoxicillin, and cyclacillin. *JAMA* 253:387-390, 1985.

Komaroff AL: Acute dysuria in women. *N Engl J Med* 310:368-375, 1984.

Komaroff AL: Urinalysis and urine culture in women with dysuria. *Ann Intern Med* 104:212-218, 1986.

Kunin CM: Duration of treatment of urinary tract infections. *Am J Med* 71:849-854, 1981.

Meares EM Jr: Prostatitis. *Ann Rev Med* 30:279-288, 1979.

Orland SM, et al: Prostatitis, prostatosis, and prostatodynia. *Urology* 25:439-459, 1985.

Schaeffer AJ, et al: Comparison of cinoxacin and trimethoprim/sulfamethoxazole in treatment of urinary tract infections. *J Urol* 125:825-827, 1981.

Sobel JD, Kaye D: Urinary tract infections, in Mandell GL, et al (eds): *Principles and Practice of Infectious Diseases*, ed 2. New York, John Wiley & Sons, 1984, 426-452.

Stamm WE: Recent developments in diagnosis and treatment of urinary tract infections. *West J Med* 137:213-220, 1982 A.

Stamm WE: Management of acute urethral syndrome. *Drug Ther* 12:155-164, (June) 1982 B.

Stamm WE, et al: Causes of acute urethral syndrome. *N Engl J Med* 303:409-415, 1980.

Stamm WE, et al: Treatment of acute urethral syndrome. *N Engl J Med* 304:956-958, 1981.

Stamm WE, et al: Diagnosis of coliform infection in acutely dysuric women. *N Engl J Med* 307:463-468, 1982.

Valenti WM, Reese RE: Genitourinary tract infections, in Reese RE, Douglas RG Jr (eds): *A Practical Approach to Infectious Diseases*, ed 2. Boston, Little, Brown and Company, 1986, 327-358.

INFECTIONS OF THE MALE REPRODUCTIVE TRACT

1985 STD treatment guidelines. *Morbid Mortal Week Rep* 34(suppl):75S-108S, 1985.

Berger RE: Epididymitis, in Holmes KK, et al (eds): *Sexually Transmitted Diseases*. New York, McGraw-Hill, 1984, 650-662.

Nelson JD: *1985 Pocketbook of Pediatric Antimicrobial Therapy*, ed 6. Baltimore, Williams & Wilkins, 1985, 22-42.

Pong RS: Epididymitis, in Conn HF (ed): *Current Therapy, 1983*. Philadelphia, WB Saunders, 1983, 516-517.

Sanford JP: *Guide to Antimicrobial Therapy, 1985*. West Bethesda, MD, private publication, 1985, 13-17.

INFECTIONS OF THE FEMALE REPRODUCTIVE TRACT

1985 STD treatment guidelines. *Morbid Mortal Week Rep* 34(suppl):75S-108S, 1985.

Burnakis TG, Hildebrandt NB: Pelvic inflammatory disease: Review with emphasis on antimicrobial therapy. *Rev Infect Dis* 8:86-116, 1986.

Gibbs RS: Sexually transmitted diseases in the female. *Med Clin North Am* 67:221-234, 1983.

Penn RL: Gynecological and obstetrical infections, in Reese RE, Douglas RG Jr (eds): *A Practical Approach to Infectious Diseases*, ed 2. Boston, Little, Brown and Company, 1986, 385-421.

Sanford JP: *Guide to Antimicrobial Therapy, 1985*. West Bethesda, MD, private publication, 1985, 13-17.

BONE AND JOINT INFECTIONS

The choice of antimicrobial drugs. *Med Lett Drugs Ther* 26:19-26, 1984; 28:33-40, 1986.

1985 STD treatment guidelines. *Morbid Mortal Week Rep* 34(suppl):75S-108S, 1985.

Aronoff SC, Scoles PV: Treatment of childhood skeletal infections. *Pediatr Clin North Am* 30:271-280, 1983.

Brooks GF, Pons VG: Osteomyelitis, in Hoeprich PD (ed): *Infectious Diseases*, ed 3. Philadelphia, Harper & Row, 1983, 1318-1330.

Chapman SW: Osteomyelitis, in Reese RE, Douglas RG Jr (eds): *A Practical Approach to Infectious Diseases*, ed 2. Boston, Little, Brown and Company, 1986, 440-462.

Conte JE Jr, Barriere SL: *Manual of Antibiotics and Infectious Diseases*, ed 5. Philadelphia, Lea & Febiger, 1984, 94, 110-111.

Goldenberg DL, Reed JI: Bacterial arthritis. *N Engl J Med* 312:764-771, 1985.

Kaplan SL: Osteomyelitis in children. *Compr Ther* 8:69-75, (Oct) 1982.

LeFrock JL, Kannangara DW: Treatment of infectious arthritis. *Am Fam Physician* 30:252-257, (Sept) 1984.

McCracken GH Jr, Nelson JD: *Antimicrobial Therapy for Newborns*, ed 2. New York, Grune & Stratton, 1983, 172-176.

Nelson JD: Cefuroxime: Cephalosporin with unique applicability to pediatric practice. *Pediatr Infect Dis* 2:394-396, 1983.

Nelson JD: *1985 Pocketbook of Pediatric Antimicrobial Therapy*, ed 6. Baltimore, Williams & Wilkins, 1985 A, 15, 24-25.

Nelson JD: *1985 Pocketbook of Pediatric Antimicrobial Therapy*, ed 6. Baltimore, Williams & Wilkins, 1985 B, 7-8.

Neu HC: Clinical uses of cephalosporins. *Lancet* 2:252-255, 1982.

Prober CG: Oral antibiotic therapy for bone and joint infections. *Pediatr Infect Dis* 1:8-10, 1982.

Roberts NJ Jr, Mock DJ: Joint infections, in Reese RE, Douglas RG Jr (eds): *A Practical Approach to Infectious Diseases*, ed 2. Boston, Little, Brown and Company, 1986, 422-439.

Sanford JP: *Guide to Antimicrobial Therapy, 1985*. West Bethesda, MD, private publication, 1985 A, 19.

Sanford JP: *Guide to Antimicrobial Therapy, 1985*. West Bethesda, MD, private publication, 1985 B, 4.

Smith JW: Infectious arthritis, in Mandell GL, et al (eds): *Principles and Practice of Infectious Diseases*, ed 2. New York, John Wiley & Sons, 1984, 697-704.

Syriopoulou VP, Smith AL: Osteomyelitis and septic arthritis, in Feigin RD, Cherry JD (eds): *Textbook of Pediatric Infectious Diseases*. Philadelphia, WB Saunders, 1981, vol I, 550-568.

Zack BG: Acute hematogenous osteomyelitis: Challenge to clinical acumen. *Postgrad Med* 75:103-111, (Feb) 1984.

BACTEREMIAS AND SEPSIS

The choice of antimicrobial drugs. *Med Lett Drugs Ther* 26:19-26, 1984; 28:33-40, 1986.

Update: Toxic-shock syndrome: United States. *Morbid Mortal Week Rep* 32:398-399, 1983.

Bryan CS, et al: Gentamicin vs cefotaxime for therapy of neonatal sepsis: Relationship to drug resistance. *Am J Dis Child* 139:1086-1089, 1985.

Cherry JD: Selection of antimicrobial agents for initial treatment of suspected septicemia in infants and children. *Rev Infect Dis* 5(suppl):S32-S39, 1983.

Drusano GL, Schimpff SC: Granulocytopenic cancer patient: When and how to initiate empiric antimicrobial therapy. *Drug Ther (Hosp)* 8:25-32, (Feb) 1983.

Ellner JJ: Septic shock. *Pediatr Clin North Am* 30:365-371, 1983.

Foltzer MA, Reese RE: Bacteremias and sepsis, in Reese RE, Douglas RG Jr (eds): *A Practical Approach to Infectious Diseases*, ed 2. Boston, Little, Brown and Company, 1986, 47-74.

Harris MC, Polin RA: Neonatal septicemia. *Pediatr Clin North Am* 30:243-258, 1983.

Klastersky J: Empiric treatment of infections in neutropenic patients with cancer. *Rev Infect Dis* 5(suppl):S21-S31, 1983.

Klein JO, et al: Selection of antimicrobial agents for treatment of neonatal sepsis. *Rev Infect Dis* 5(suppl):S55-S64, 1983.

Mayer KH, DeTorres OH: Current guidelines on use of antibacterial drugs in patients with malignancies. *Drugs* 29:262-279, 1985.

McCracken GH Jr: Use of third-generation cephalosporins for treatment of neonatal infections, (editorial). *Am J Dis Child* 134:1079-1080, 1985.

McCracken GH Jr, Nelson JD: *Antimicrobial Therapy for Newborns*, ed 2. New York, Grune & Stratton, 1983, 119-127.

Nelson JD: Cefuroxime: Cephalosporin with unique applicability to pediatric practice. *Pediatr Infect Dis* 2:394-396, 1983.

Nelson JD: *1985 Pocketbook of Pediatric Antimicrobial Therapy*, ed 6. Baltimore, Williams & Wilkins, 1985, 12-18.

Pizzo PA: Empiric therapy and prevention of infection in immunocompromised host, in Mandell GL, et al (eds): *Principles and Practice of Infectious Diseases*, ed 2. New York, John Wiley & Sons, 1984, 1680-1688.

Sanford JP: *Guide to Antimicrobial Therapy, 1985*. West Bethesda, MD, private publication, 1985, 30-31.

Steinhoff MC: Neonatal sepsis and infections, in Reese RE, Douglas RG Jr (eds): *A Practical Approach to Infectious Diseases*, ed 2. Boston, Little, Brown and Company, 1986, 75-98.

Wade JC: Principles of empiric antibiotic usage in febrile patients with granulocytopenia. *J Antimicrob Chemother* 9(suppl A):215-222, 1982.

Wade JC, et al: *Staphylococcus epidermidis*: Increasing cause of infection in patients with granulocytopenia. *Ann Intern Med* 97:503-508, 1982.

Wager GP: Toxic shock syndrome: Review. *Am J Obstet Gynecol* 146:93-102, 1983.

Wiesenthal AM: Toxic shock syndrome: Update. *Drug Ther* 13:109-120, (June) 1983.

MISCELLANEOUS INFECTIONS

The choice of antimicrobial drugs. *Med Lett Drugs Ther* 26:19-26, 1984; 28:33-40, 1986.

Update: Lyme disease: United States. *Morbid Mortal Week Rep* 33:268-270, 1984.

Attebery HR: Vincent's infection, in Braude AI (ed): *Medical Microbiology and Infectious Diseases*. Philadelphia, WB Saunders, 1981, 823-825.

Band JD, Bennett JV: Tetanus, in Hoeprich PD (ed): *Infectious Diseases*, ed 3. Philadelphia, Harper & Row, 1983, 1107-1114.

Benach JL, et al: Spirochetes isolated from the blood of two patients with Lyme disease. *N Engl J Med* 308:740-742, 1983.

Bornstein DL: Clostridial myonecrosis, in Braude AI (ed): *Medical Microbiology and Infectious Diseases*. Philadelphia, WB Saunders, 1981, 1775-1782.

Bruhn FW: Lyme disease. *Am J Dis Child* 138:467-470, 1984.

Conte JE Jr, Barriere SL: *Manual of Antibiotics and Infectious Diseases*, ed 5. Philadelphia, Lea & Febiger, 1984, 124-131.

Eisenberg MS, et al: *Manual of Antimicrobial Therapy and Infectious Diseases*. Philadelphia, WB Saunders, 1980, 180-182.

Gold JWM, Kinderlehrer DA: Fungal infections, in Reese RE, Douglas RG Jr (eds): *A Practical Approach to Infectious Diseases*, ed 2. Boston, Little, Brown and Company, 1986, 474-513.

Goscienski PJ: Zoonoses. *Pediatr Infect Dis* 2:69-81, 1983.

Hoeprich PD: Nocardiosis, in Hoeprich PD (ed): *Infectious Diseases*, ed 3. Philadelphia, Harper & Row, 1983, 419-427.

Hornick RB: Tularemia, in Hoeprich PD: *Infectious Diseases*, ed 3. Philadelphia, Harper & Row, 1983, 1220-1226.

Magnussen CR: Skin and soft-tissue infections, in Reese RE, Douglas RG Jr (eds): *A Practical Approach to Infectious Diseases*, ed 2. Boston, Little, Brown and Company, 1986, 99-122.

McClain JB, et al: Doxycycline therapy for leptospirosis. *Ann Intern Med* 100:696-698, 1984.

Meyerhoff J: Lyme disease. *Am J Med* 75:663-670, 1983.

Nelson JD: *1985 Pocketbook of Pediatric Antimicrobial Therapy*, ed 6. Baltimore, Williams & Wilkins, 1985 A, 44-51.

Nelson JD: *1985 Pocketbook of Pediatric Antimicrobial Therapy*, ed 6. Baltimore, Williams & Wilkins, 1985 B, 22-42.

Sanford JP: *Pseudomonas* species (including melioidosis and glanders), in Mandell GL, et al (eds): *Principles and Practice of*

Douglas RG Jr (eds): *A Practical Approach to Infectious Diseases,*, ed 2. Boston, Little, Brown and Company, 1986, 327-358.

Wong ES, et al: Management of recurrent urinary tract infections with patient-administered single-dose therapy. *Ann Intern Med* 102:302-307, 1985.

PREVENTION OF PERTUSSIS IN EXPOSED PERSONS

Report of the Committee on Infectious Diseases: *American Academy of Pediatrics Redbook*, ed 19. Evanston, IL, American Academy of Pediatrics, 1982, 198-202.

Bass JW: Pertussis: Current status of prevention and treatment. *Pediatr Infect Dis* 4:614-619, 1985.

Feder HM Jr: Chemoprophylaxis in ambulatory pediatrics. *Pediatr Infect Dis* 2:251-257, 1983.

PREVENTION OF RECURRENT ACUTE OTITIS MEDIA

Chemoprophylaxis for recurrent acute otitis media. *Med Lett Drugs Ther* 25:102-103, 1983.

Klein JO, Bluestone CD: Acute otitis media. *Pediatr Infect Dis* 1:66-73, 1982.

Paradise JL: Antimicrobial prophylaxis for recurrent acute otitis media. *Ann Otol Rhinol Laryngol* 90(suppl 84):53-57, 1981.

PREVENTION OF TRAVELERS' DIARRHEA

Immunization and chemoprophylaxis for travelers. *Med Lett Drugs Ther* 27:33-36, 1985.

Immunization and chemoprophylaxis for travelers: Travelers' diarrhea. *Med Lett Drugs Ther* 25:39-40, 1983.

Salicylate in Pepto-Bismol. *Med Lett Drugs Ther* 22:63, 1980.

DuPont HL, et al: Prevention of travelers' diarrhea (emporiatric enteritis): Prophylactic administration of subsalicylate bismuth. *JAMA* 243:237-241, 1980.

DuPont HL, et al: Treatment of travelers' diarrhea with trimethoprim/sulfamethoxazole and with trimethoprim alone. *N Engl J Med* 307:841-844, 1982.

DuPont HL, et al: Prevention of travelers' diarrhea with trimethoprim/sulfamethoxazole and trimethoprim alone. *Gastroenterology* 84:75-80, 1983.

DuPont HL, et al: Chemotherapy and chemoprophylaxis of travelers' diarrhea. *Ann Intern Med* 102:260-261, 1985.

DuPont HL, et al: Prevention of travelers' diarrhea by tablet formulation of bismuth subsalicylate, (abstract). *Gastroenterology* 90:1401, 1986.

Ericsson CD, et al: Influence of subsalicylate bismuth on absorption of doxycycline. *JAMA* 247:2266-2267, 1982.

Gorbach SL: Travelers' diarrhea. *N Engl J Med* 307:881-883, 1982.

Graham DY, et al: Double-blind comparison of bismuth subsalicylate and placebo in prevention and treatment of enterotoxigenic *Escherichia coli*-induced diarrhea in volunteers. *Gastroenterology* 85:1017-1022, 1983.

National Institutes of Health Consensus Development Conference: Travelers' diarrhea. *JAMA* 253:2700-2704, 1985.

Sack DA, et al: Prophylactic doxycycline for travelers' diarrhea: Results of prospective double-blind study of Peace Corps volunteers in Kenya. *N Engl J Med* 298:758-763, 1978.

Sack RB, et al: Prophylactic doxycycline for travelers' diarrhea: Results of prospective double-blind study of Peace Corps volunteers in Morocco. *Gastroenterology* 76:1368-1373, 1979.

Satterwhite TK, DuPont HL: Infectious diarrhea in office practice. *Med Clin North Am* 67:203-220, 1983.

Siegel JD: Prophylactic antibiotics. *Pediatr Infect Dis* 3:537-541, 1984.

Weiss BD: Traveler's diarrhea: Update 1983. *Am Fam Physician* 27:193-195, (April) 1983.

Table 4: Antimicrobial Chemoprophylaxis for Surgical Patients

Antimicrobial prophylaxis for surgery. *Med Lett Drugs Ther* 23:77-80, 1981; 27:105-108, 1985.

Burnakis TG: Surgical antimicrobial prophylaxis: Principles and guidelines. *Pharmacotherapy* 4:248-271, 1984.

Conte JE Jr, Barriere SL: *Manual of Antibiotics and Infectious Diseases*, ed 5. Philadelphia, Lea & Febiger, 1984, 145-149.

Conte JE Jr, et al: *Antibiotic Prophylaxis in Surgery: Comprehensive Review*. Philadelphia, JB Lippincott, 1984.

Dellinger EP, et al: Efficacy of short-course antibiotic prophylaxis after penetrating intestinal injury: Prospective randomized trial. *Arch Surg* 121:23-30, 1986.

DiPiro JT, et al: Antimicrobial prophylaxis in surgery: Parts I and II. *Am J Hosp Pharm* 38:320-334, 487-494, 1981.

DiPiro JT, et al: Prophylactic use of antimicrobials in surgery. *Curr Probl Surg* 20:69-132, 1983.

DiPiro JT, et al: Current concepts in clinical therapeutics: Intra-abdominal infections. *Clin Pharm* 5:34-50, 1986.

Flynn NM, Hoeprich PD: Chemoprophylaxis of infectious diseases, in Hoeprich PD (ed): *Infectious Diseases*, ed 3. Philadelphia, Harper & Row, 1983, 238-254.

Gilbert DN: Current status of antibiotic prophylaxis in surgical patients. *Bull NY Acad Med* 60:340-357, 1984.

Guglielmo BJ, et al: Antibiotic prophylaxis in surgical procedures: Critical analysis of the literature. *Arch Surg* 118:943-955, 1983.

Hirschmann JV: Rational antibiotic prophylaxis. *Hosp Pract* 16:105-123, (Nov) 1981.

Hirschmann JV, Inui TS: Antimicrobial prophylaxis: Critique of recent trials. *Rev Infect Dis* 2:1-23, 1980.

Hofstetter SR, et al: Prospective comparison of two regimens of prophylactic antibiotics in abdominal trauma: Cefoxitin versus triple drug. *J Trauma* 24:307-310, 1984.

Johnson JT, et al: Antimicrobial prophylaxis for contaminated head and neck surgery. *Laryngoscope* 94:46-51, 1984.

Jones RC, et al: Evaluation of antibiotic therapy following penetrating abdominal trauma. *Ann Surg* 201:576-585, 1985.

Lennard ES, Dellinger EP: Prophylactic antibiotics in surgery: Rationale for family physician. *J Fam Pract* 12:461-467, 1981.

Levi JU, et al: Ampicillin versus cefamandole in biliary tract surgery: Prospective, randomized clinical and bacteriological study. *Am Surg* 50:412-417, 1984.

Nichols RL: Use of prophylactic antibiotics in surgical practice. *Am J Med* 70:686-692, 1981.

Nichols RL: Postoperative infections and antimicrobial prophylaxis, in Mandell GL, et al (eds): *Principles and Practice of Infectious Diseases*, ed 2. New York, John Wiley & Sons, 1984, 1637-1644.

Nichols RL, et al: Risk of infection after penetrating abdominal trauma. *N Engl J Med* 311:1065-1070, 1984.

Oreskovich MR, et al: Duration of preventive antibiotic administration for penetrating abdominal trauma. *Arch Surg* 117:200-205, 1982.

Polk HC Jr, et al: Guidelines for prevention of surgical wound infection. *Arch Surg* 118:1213-1217, 1983.

Reese RE, Betts RF: Antibiotic use, in Reese RE, Douglas RG Jr (eds): *A Practical Approach to Infectious Diseases*, ed 2. Boston, Little, Brown and Company, 1986, 559-679.

Sanford JP: *Guide to Antimicrobial Therapy 1985*. West Bethesda, MD, private publication, 1985, 80-84.

Stone HH, et al: Prophylactic and preventive antibiotic therapy: Timing, duration and economics. *Ann Surg* 189:691-699, 1979.

A unique combination of high efficacy and relatively low toxicity, even in immature infants (Eichenwald and Mc-Cracken, 1978), makes the penicillins one of the most commonly prescribed and generally useful groups of antibiotics.

Chemistry, Source, and Classification

All penicillins contain a common nucleus (6-aminopenicillanic acid) composed of a thiazolidine ring (A) and a β-lactam ring (B) connected to a side chain (R_3) (see Figure 1). The penicillin nucleus, including an intact β-lactam ring, is necessary for biological activity, but the side chain primarily determines antibacterial spectrum, sensitivity to acid and β-lactamases, and pharmacokinetic properties. The natural penicillin, penicillin G, is extracted from cultures of *Penicillium chrysogenum.* Semisynthetic penicillins are prepared by incorporating specific precursors in mold cultures, by chemically modifying a natural penicillin, or by adding side chains to 6-aminopenicillanic acid. The last method is most frequently employed (see Mandell and Sande, 1980).

Presently, 20 penicillin derivatives are marketed in the United States. These can be classified according to antimicro-bial spectrum into the following subclasses: natural penicillins, penicillinase-resistant (antistaphylococcal) penicillins, amino-penicillins, antipseudomonal penicillins, and amidino penicil-lins (see Figure 1). There are significant differences among penicillin subclasses, particularly with regard to uses. Differences among members of a given subclass frequently are of a pharmacologic nature, although one compound in a group may be more active than another. For detailed discussion, see the following sections in this Introduction and the evaluations.

Mechanism of Action

In the presence of penicillin, the cell walls of sensitive bacteria develop abnormally, which ultimately results in the death of the organism. Penicillins exert their bactericidal effect on actively dividing cells and have little or no effect on intracellular organisms, dormant bacteria, or organisms that lack cell walls (eg, eukaryotic cells).

The rigid structure of the bacterial cell wall is due to peptidoglycan, a mucopeptide made up of linear polysaccha-ride chains cross linked by peptide bonds. Bacterial cell wall synthesis is a complex process that involves at least 30 enzymes; it is usually subdivided into three stages. In the first stage, cell wall precursor (UDP-acetylmuramyl-pentapeptide) is synthesized and accumulates in the cytoplasm of the bacterial cell. Cycloserine [Seromycin], an antibiotic occasionally used to treat tuberculosis, inhibits precursor formation. In the second stage, the UDP-acetylmuramyl-pentapeptide binds to phospholipid in the cell membrane and is then linked to UDP-N-acetylglucosamine with release of uridine nucleotides. This disaccharide pentapeptide undergoes further modification (eg, the addition of five glycine residues in *Staphylococcus aureus*) and finally is linked to pre-existing portions of the cell wall, resulting in a linear peptidoglycan polymer. Vancomycin [Vancocin] and bacitracin inhibit different steps in this second stage. The third stage occurs outside the cell membrane and involves the cross linking of linear peptidoglycan polymers via peptide bonds, thus completing formation of the tough outer envelope of the bacterial cell. Traditionally, the β-lactam antibiotics, including the penicillins and cephalosporins, have been considered to be inhibitors of this terminal cross linking step, ie, inhibitors of transpeptidation (Tipper and Wright, 1979; see also Pratt, 1977).

The above explanation now appears to be oversimplified, however, and the penicillins' actual mechanism of action is not completely understood. In *S. aureus*, bactericidal concentrations inhibit the transpeptidase enzyme that catalyzes the cross-linking reaction. Although it is believed to be important, this effect probably does not completely explain the bactericidal action of penicillin. In gram-positive species, cell wall lysis also seems to depend upon the ability of penicillin to decrease the availability of an inhibitor of bacterial murein hydrolase, a cell wall autolytic enzyme whose normal function is unclear. In the presence of penicillin, this uninhibited autolysin destroys the structural integrity of the cell wall (Tomasz, 1979; see also Pratt, 1977). Thus, the penicillins may increase breakdown of the cell wall as well as inhibit synthesis.

A number of penicillin-binding proteins (PBPs) that are associated with bacterial cell membranes have been identified and isolated from both gram-positive and gram-negative bacteria. These proteins are believed to be enzymes (eg, transpeptidases, carboxypeptidases) that are involved in bacterial cell wall division, wall elongation, septum formation, and the maintenance of cell shape. Each bacterial species has a unique set of PBPs that are numbered in order of decreasing molecular weight. The PBPs of gram-negative and gram-positive bacteria differ extensively, but PBPs of some gram-negative bacteria appear to have similarities. Based primarily on studies done with *Escherichia coli*, the critical PBPs of gram-negative bacteria are PBP1, which consists of PBPs 1A and 1Bs; PBP2; and PBP3. Most penicillins and cephalosporins bind to PBP1 and/or PBP3, which cause bacterial cell lysis and the production of long filamentous forms, respectively. In contrast, amdinocillin binds to PBP2 and produces ovoid cells. The PBPs that are critical in gram-positive bacteria are PBP1, PBP2, and PBP4. Activity of penicillins (eg, penicillin G) against streptococci and staphylococci correlates with binding to essential PBPs in these species. In summary, the selective affinity patterns of β-lactam antibiotics for PBPs of different bacterial species vary with the agent and provide the basis for

the distinctive structural or physiologic effects caused by the antimicrobial agent (see Spratt, 1980; Neu, 1982 A, 1983 A, 1984 A; Tomasz, 1982).

Other factors also affect the antibacterial activity of β-lactam antibiotics. These include the stability of the antibiotic to various β-lactamases produced by gram-positive and gram-negative bacteria and the ability of a drug to penetrate the outer membrane of gram-negative bacteria (see also the section on Resistance).

Antimicrobial Spectrum

Natural Penicillins: Penicillin G (benzylpenicillin) is the penicillin of choice for infections caused by susceptible gram-positive cocci, including *Streptococcus pyogenes* (group A), *S. agalactiae* (group B), nonenterococcal group D streptococci (eg, *S. bovis*), viridans streptococci, *S. pneumoniae* (rare strains are resistant), anaerobic streptococci (*Peptostreptococcus*), *Peptococcus*, and microaerophilic streptococci. Enterococci (eg, *S. faecalis*) are less susceptible than other streptococci, but penicillin G is useful in enterococcal infections, particularly endocarditis (in combination with gentamicin or streptomycin; see Uses section). Most strains of *Staphylococcus aureus* produce β lactamase and are resistant. However, penicillin G is preferred for non-β lactamase-producing *S. aureus* that are shown to be susceptible.

Susceptible gram-positive bacilli include *Bacillus anthracis*, most strains of *Corynebacterium diphtheriae*, *Listeria monocytogenes*, *Erysipelothrix rhusiopathiae*, most clostridia (eg, *Cl. perfringens*, *Cl. tetani*), and *Eubacterium*.

Penicillin G is a drug of choice for susceptible gram-negative cocci, including *Neisseria meningitidis* and *N. gonorrhoeae*. Penicillinase-producing *N. gonorrhoeae* (PPNG) are resistant, however. The number of reported PPNG infections among civilians doubled (from 3,000 to 6,000 cases) in the United States for the first nine months of 1985 when compared to 1984; significant outbreaks occurred in Florida, New York city, and Los Angeles (*Morbid Mortal Week Rep,* 1986). In some countries (eg, Philippines), PPNG infections are very common (see Handsfield, 1982). More recently, an increasing number of high-level, chromosomally mediated (β lactamase-negative), resistant *N. gonorrhoeae* (CMRNG) have been reported in the United States (*Morbid Mortal Week Rep*, 1984; Faruki et al, 1985; Hook and Holmes, 1985; Rice et al, 1985). *Veillonella*, anaerobic gram-negative cocci, are susceptible to penicillin G.

Susceptible gram-negative bacilli include *Streptobacillus moniliformis*, *Pasteurella multocida*, *Leptotrichia buccalis*, and *Spirillum minor*. Although many strains of *Haemophilus influenzae* are susceptible in vitro, an aminopenicillin (eg, ampicillin, amoxicillin) is generally preferred clinically for infections due to this organism. β lactamase-producing *H. influenzae* are resistant. Among gram-negative anaerobic bacilli, most *Fusobacterium* and oropharyngeal strains of *Bacteroides* are susceptible. However, some strains of *B. melaninogenicus* are resistant. The *B. fragilis* group are usually resistant. Most other gram-negative bacilli are resistant to penicillin G,

FIGURE 1. CHEMICAL STRUCTURES OF PENICILLINS

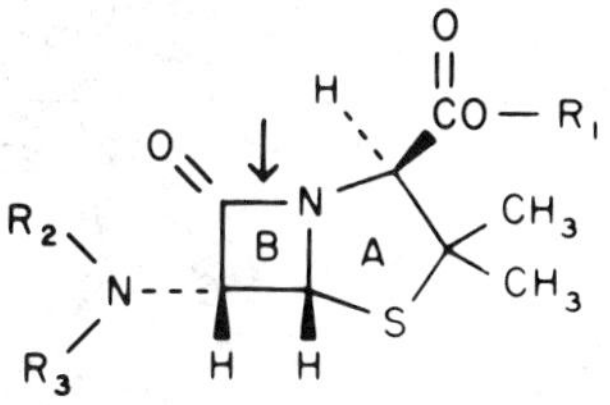

Penicillin Nucleus[1]

Generic Name	R_1	R_2	R_3
NATURAL PENICILLINS			
Penicillin G[2]	H	H	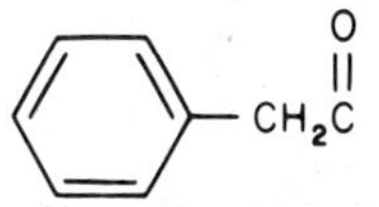
Penicillin V	H	H	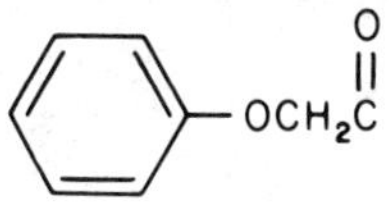
PENICILLINASE–RESISTANT PENICILLINS			
Methicillin	H	H	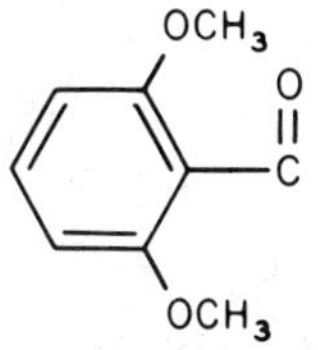
Nafcillin	H	H	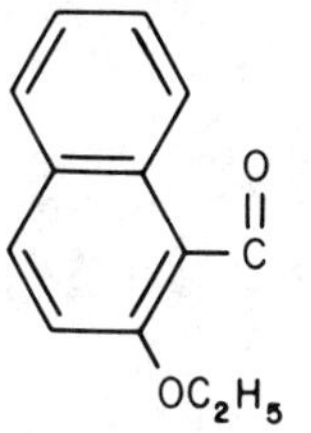
ISOXAZOLYL PENICILLINS			
Oxacillin	H	H	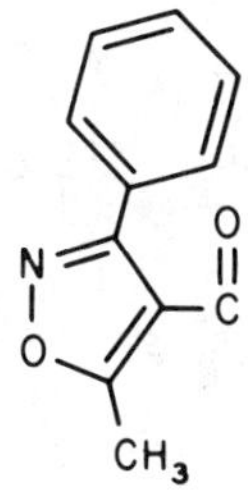
Cloxacillin	H	H	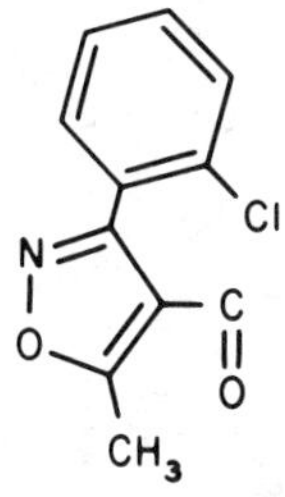

[1]For 6-aminopenicillanic acid, $R_1 = R_2 = R_3 = H$; A = thiazolidine ring; B = β-lactam ring. The arrow is the site of β-lactamase attack. [2]Penicillin G procaine (not shown) is a stable aqueous suspension of a poorly water-soluble (0.4%) crystalline salt that contains equimolar amounts of procaine and penicillin G, the active drug. Penicillin G benzathine (not shown) is a stable aqueous suspension of a very poorly water-soluble (0.02%) salt that contains one mole of an ammonium base and two moles of penicillin G, the active drug.

FIGURE 1. CHEMICAL STRUCTURES OF PENICILLINS (continued)

Generic Name	R₁	R₂	R₃
Dicloxacillin	H	H	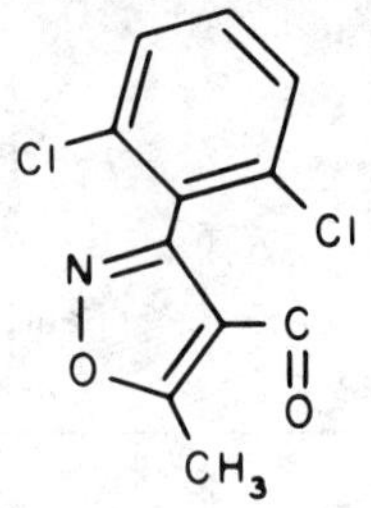

AMINOPENICILLINS

Ampicillin	H	H	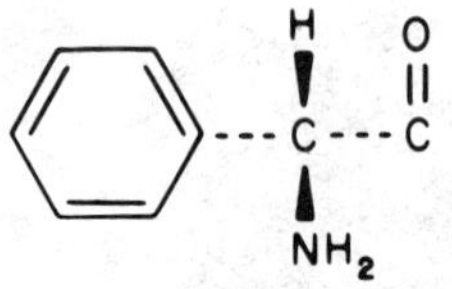
Amoxicillin	H	H	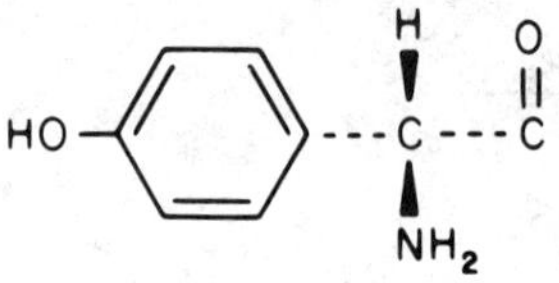
Bacampicillin	CH₃ O / CHO–COCH₂CH₃	H	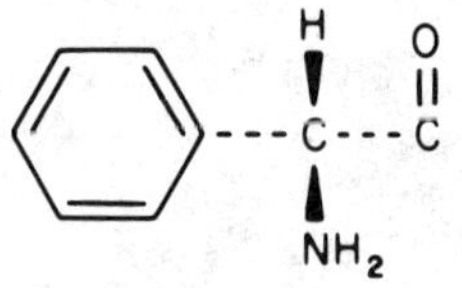
Cyclacillin	H	H	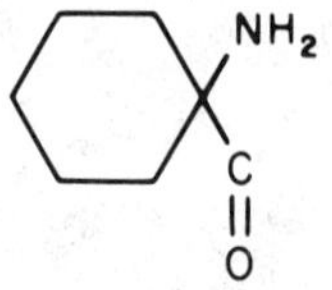

ANTIPSEUDOMONAL PENICILLINS

CARBOXYPENICILLINS

Carbenicillin	H	H	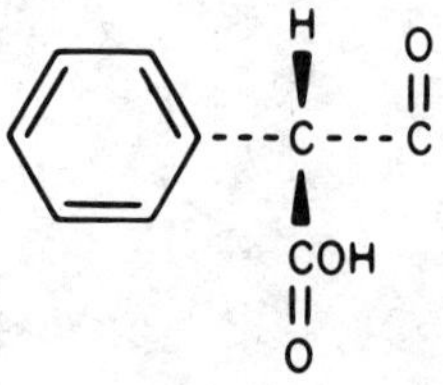
Carbenicillin Indanyl	H	H	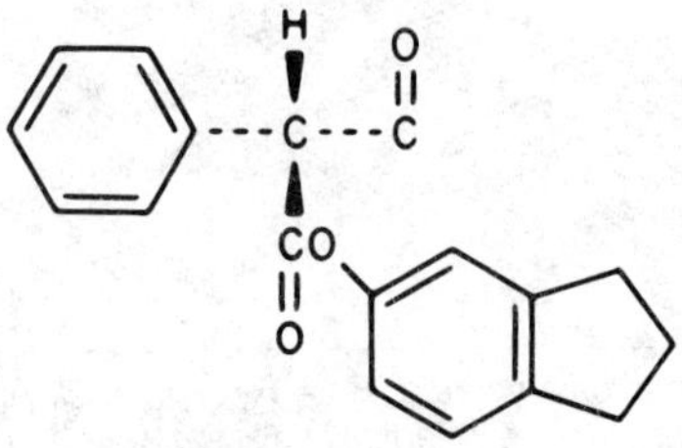

(Continued on next page)

FIGURE 1. CHEMICAL STRUCTURES OF PENICILLINS (continued)

Generic Name	R₁	R₂	R₃

Generic Name R_1 R_2 R_3

Ticarcillin   H   H

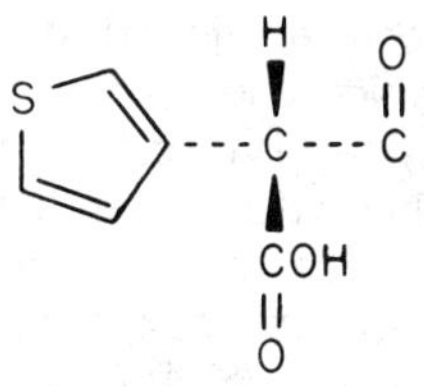

ACYLUREIDOPENICILLINS

Azlocillin   H   H

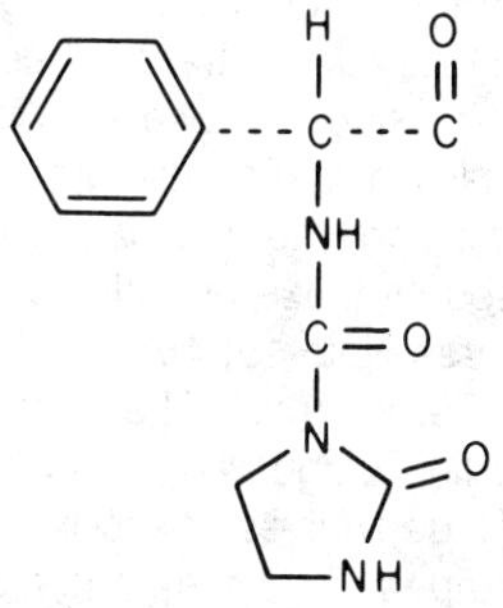

Mezlocillin   H   H

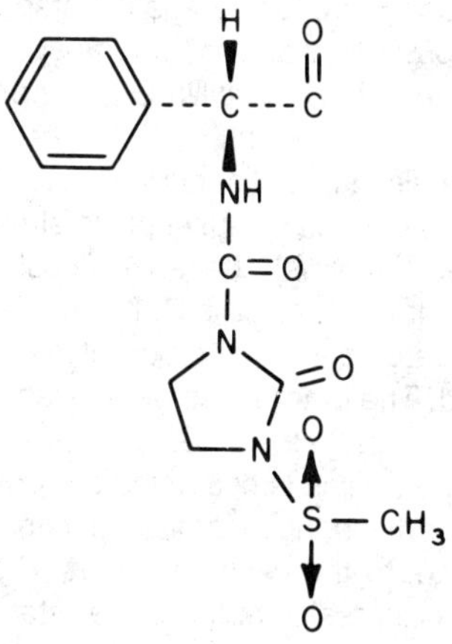

PIPERAZINE PENICILLIN

Piperacillin   H   H

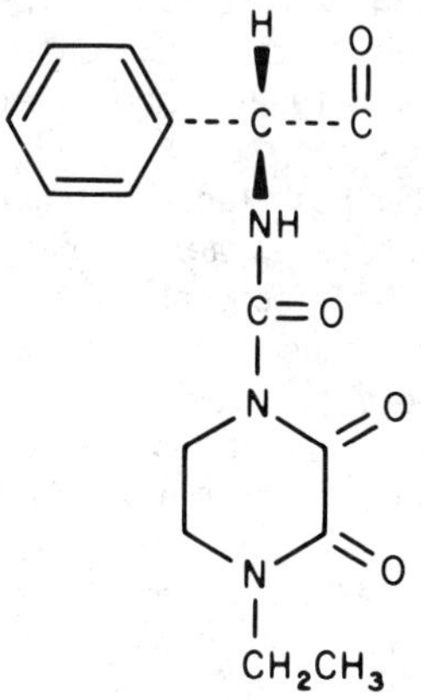

AMIDINO PENICILLIN

Amdinocillin   H

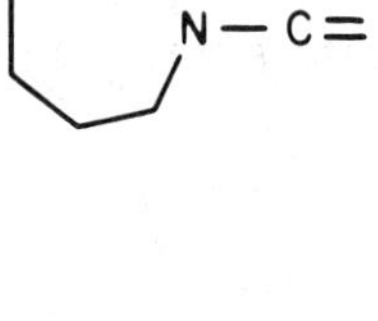

including important clinical pathogens, such as the Enterobacteriaceae and *Pseudomonas aeruginosa*.

Actinomyces israelii are susceptible to penicillin G, but *Nocardia* are resistant. Spirochetes, including *Treponema pallidum*, *T. pertenue*, *Leptospira*, and *Borrelia burgdorferi*, the causative organism of Lyme disease, are susceptible. Mycobacteria, mycoplasma, chlamydia, rickettsia, fungi, amebae, plasmodia, and viruses are resistant to all penicillins.

The in vitro activity of penicillin V (phenoxymethyl penicillin) [Ledercillin VK, PenVee K, Uticillin VK, V-Cillin K, Veetids] against most gram-positive bacteria is comparable to that of penicillin G. It frequently is preferred for infections (eg, streptococcal pharyngitis) requiring oral administration (see also the Uses and Pharmacokinetics sections). However, this derivative is less active than penicillin G against gram-negative bacteria, particularly *Neisseria* and *Haemophilus*, and it is not indicated for infections caused by these organisms.

For additional discussion, see Neu, 1984 A.

Penicillinase-Resistant Penicillins: The penicillinase-resistant penicillins (methicillin [Staphcillin], nafcillin [Nafcil, Unipen]) and the isoxazolyl derivatives, oxacillin [Bactocill, Prostaphlin], cloxacillin [Cloxapen, Tegopen], and dicloxacillin [Dycill, Dynapen, Pathocil]), are active against staphylococci, including β lactamase-producing strains, and most streptococci, but they are less potent than penicillin G. Enterococci (eg, *Streptococcus faecalis*) are resistant.

Currently, these semisynthetic penicillins are drugs of choice only for infections caused by susceptible staphylococci (eg, *S. aureus*, *S. epidermidis*), because most of these organisms are now resistant to penicillin G. If bacterial susceptibility studies demonstrate sensitivity to penicillin G, this form should be administered. The emergence of resistant strains of *S. aureus* and, to a greater extent, *S. epidermidis* to the penicillinase-resistant penicillins is becoming a problem in the United States, particularly in nosocomial infections. These strains also are resistant to the cephalosporins. Problems in identifying these methicillin-resistant (heteroresistant) staphylococci using standard in vitro susceptibility tests are well known (see Thornsberry, 1984; *Med Lett Drugs Ther*, 1986). Vancomycin is the drug of choice against these organisms. For additional discussion, see Neu, 1982 B, and Molavi and Le Frock, 1984.

Although some gram-positive bacilli (eg, *Clostridium perfringens*, *Corynebacterium diphtheriae*, *Listeria monocytogenes*) are susceptible in vitro, antistaphylococcal penicillins are not used clinically for infections caused by these organisms. Gram-negative bacteria generally are resistant.

Aminopenicillins: Another group of semisynthetic penicillins, the aminopenicillins, include ampicillin [Amcill, Omnipen, Polycillin, Principen], amoxicillin [Amoxil, Larotid, Polymox, Trimox], bacampicillin [Spectrobid], and cyclacillin [Cyclapen-W]. With few exceptions, the antibacterial spectra of the aminopenicillins are comparable. The in vitro potencies of ampicillin, which can be administered as the parent drug or generated from the hydrolysis of the prodrug, bacampicillin, and amoxicillin are similar. Cyclacillin is less active on a weight basis.

The gram-positive antibacterial spectrum of the aminopenicillins is similar to that of penicillin G, but these drugs are more active against *Streptococcus faecalis* (enterococcus) and *Listeria monocytogenes*. Because the aminopenicillins are sensitive to β lactamases, most staphylococci are resistant. The gram-negative cocci, *Neisseria meningitidis* and *N. gonorrhoeae* (except PPNG and CMRNG), are susceptible to the aminopenicillins.

Most strains of *Haemophilus influenzae* are susceptible, but resistant β lactamase-producing strains are continually emerging. In contrast to penicillin G, several aerobic gram-negative enteric bacilli are susceptible to the aminopenicillins, including strains of *Escherichia coli*, *Proteus mirabilis*, *Salmonella*, and *Shigella* (amoxicillin is less active than ampicillin against *Shigella* and is not used clinically). However, resistant β lactamase-producing strains of these organisms are present, which has significantly diminished the usefulness of the aminopenicillins for infections caused by these bacteria in some locations (see also the Uses section). Other Enterobacteriaceae (eg, *Klebsiella*, *Enterobacter*, *Serratia*, indole-positive *Proteus*, *Providencia*), *Pseudomonas aeruginosa*, and *Acinetobacter* are resistant to the aminopenicillins. Among gram-negative anaerobic bacteria, *Fusobacterium* and oropharyngeal strains of *Bacteroides* are usually susceptible, but the *B. fragilis* group are resistant. Ampicillin is active against *Gardnerella* (*Haemophilus*) *vaginalis*.

For additional discussion, see Wright and Wilkowske, 1983; Neu, 1984 A; and Sahm et al, 1985.

Antipseudomonal Penicillins: The antipseudomonal penicillins are semisynthetic derivatives that include the carboxypenicillins, carbenicillin [Geocillin, Pyopen], ticarcillin [Ticar], and carbenicillin indanyl [Geocillin], an ester of carbenicillin for oral administration; the acylureidopenicillins, azlocillin [Azlin] and mezlocillin [Mezlin]; and the piperazine penicillin, piperacillin [Pipracil]. Like the aminopenicillins, all antipseudomonal penicillins are susceptible to destruction by β lactamases elaborated by gram-positive and gram-negative bacteria.

Antipseudomonal penicillins have a broader spectrum of activity against gram-negative bacilli when compared to ampicillin. Non-β lactamase-producing strains of *Haemophilus influenzae* are susceptible. Among the Enterobacteriaceae, many strains of *Escherichia coli*, *Proteus mirabilis*, *Salmonella*, *Shigella*, *Enterobacter*, *Citrobacter*, and indole-positive *Proteus* (*Providencia rettgeri*, *Morganella morganii*, *Proteus vulgaris*) are susceptible to all of these analogues. Generally, mezlocillin and piperacillin are slightly more potent than azlocillin, ticarcillin, and carbenicillin for most of these organisms. Furthermore, mezlocillin, piperacillin, and, to a lesser extent, azlocillin, are active against some *Klebsiella* and *Serratia* strains. Most *Serratia* and essentially all *Klebsiella* are resistant to carbenicillin and ticarcillin.

The antipseudomonal penicillins are active against many strains of *Pseudomonas aeruginosa*, which accounts for their major clinical advantage over earlier penicillins (eg, ampicillin, penicillin G). In vitro, the order of decreasing potency for the various antipseudomonal penicillins against *P. aeruginosa* is piperacillin ≥ azlocillin > mezlocillin = ticarcillin > carbenicillin. Whether this is of clinical significance is presently unresolved. Many strains of *Acinetobacter* also are susceptible to the antipseudomonal penicillins.

Among gram-negative anaerobic bacteria, *Fusobacterium*

and *Bacteroides*, including many strains of *B. fragilis*, are susceptible.

The number of strains of gram-negative bacilli that are resistant to the antipseudomonal penicillins is quite large, however, and the emergence of resistant β lactamase-producing strains is relatively common. Thus, it is usually necessary to test for susceptibility before instituting therapy with these agents, especially when they are used alone. Furthermore, combination therapy with an antipseudomonal penicillin plus an aminoglycoside is strongly recommended for systemic *P. aeruginosa* infections (see also the Uses section).

Mezlocillin, piperacillin, and azlocillin are comparable to ampicillin in activity against gram-positive bacteria and gram-negative cocci. Carbenicillin and ticarcillin generally are less potent against these organisms and have poor activity against enterococci (eg, *Streptococcus faecalis*). β lactamase-producing strains of staphylococci are resistant to all of the antipseudomonal penicillins.

For additional discussion, see Eliopoulos and Moellering, 1982; Neu, 1982 C, 1983 B, 1984 A; Parry and Pancoast, 1984; Norris, 1985; and Sahm et al, 1985.

Amidino Penicillins: Amdinocillin [Coactin], known as mecillinam outside the United States, has a spectrum of activity that differs from other penicillins. This agent is active against many enteric gram-negative bacilli, including *Escherichia coli*, *Klebsiella pneumoniae*, *Enterobacter* species, *Citrobacter* species, *Salmonella enteritidis* species and *S. typhi*, and *Shigella* species. Some *Proteus mirabilis* and *Serratia marcescens* strains also are susceptible. The diarrheal pathogens, *Campylobacter jejuni*, *Yersinia enterocolitica*, and *Aeromonas hydrophila*, are highly susceptible to amdinocillin. However, this agent is not reliably active against most gram-positive bacteria, *Haemophilus influenzae*, indole-positive *Proteus*, *Pseudomonas aeruginosa* and other nonfermenting gram-negative bacilli, or anaerobic organisms (eg, the *Bacteroides fragilis* group) (see Neu, 1983 A, 1985; *Med Lett Drugs Ther*, 1985 A; Sahm et al, 1985).

The basis for this unique spectrum of antibacterial activity is the affinity of amdinocillin for PBP2 of gram-negative bacteria, a penicillin-binding protein that causes bacterial cells to be converted to osmotically stable round forms. Other penicillins (and cephalosporins) bind mostly to PBP1 and/or PBP3 of gram-negative bacteria. Amdinocillin does not bind to PBPs of gram-positive bacteria (see also the section on Mechanism of Action).

The unusual mode of action of amdinocillin suggested that combining this agent with conventional penicillins or cephalosporins might result in a synergistic interaction. This has been observed in vitro with a number of enteric gram-negative bacilli. However, synergistic activity has only occurred with approximately 50% of bacterial isolates and is not predictable for any particular species. Thus, the clinical usefulness of such combinations remains uncertain (see Neu, 1983 A, 1985; Cleeland and Squires, 1983; Farrar, 1984; *Med Lett Drugs Ther*, 1985 A).

Amdinocillin is susceptible to β lactamase inactivation, but is more resistant than ampicillin to the common plasmid-mediated TEM-1 β lactamase (Neu, 1985; see also the section on Resistance).

Resistance

Mechanisms of resistance to penicillin antibiotics include: (1) inactivation by bacterial β lactamases; (2) decreased permeability of the bacterial cell to the penicillin, which prohibits the antibiotic from reaching the appropriate binding proteins; (3) alterations in penicillin-binding proteins(s) that prevent binding to the penicillin; and (4) tolerance. Clinically, the most important mechanism of acquired resistance is the production of inactivating enzymes (ie, β lactamases) by staphylococci and gram-negative bacteria. β lactamases cleave the β-lactam ring of the penicillin nucleus resulting in the formation of inactive penicilloic acid derivatives (see Figure 1).

Staphylococcal β lactamases are encoded by plasmids that can be transferred from one bacterium to another by transduction. These enzymes can be induced and are secreted extracellularly. They are considered to be true penicillinases because they inactivate penicillin molecules, but not cephalosporins. Methicillin, nafcillin, and the isoxazolyl derivatives (oxacillin, cloxacillin, and dicloxacillin) are resistant to staphylococcal penicillinases and are preferred for staphylococcal infections. Methicillin-resistant staphylococci are being encountered clinically. The mechanism is related to failure to bind penicillin-binding proteins.

Genetic information for the various β lactamases produced by gram-negative bacteria can be either chromosomal- or plasmid-mediated. These enzymes may be either constitutive or inducible and are located in the periplasmic space between the inner and outer membranes of the bacterial cell. Some β lactamases of gram-negative bacteria are specific for either penicillins or cephalosporins, but others can hydrolyze both molecules. Also, differences in β lactamase stability among various penicillins account for some of the differences in in vitro activities against some gram-negative bacteria.

The cell walls of gram-negative bacteria are covered by a lipopolysaccharide-containing outer membrane. Some penicillins (eg, the penicillinase-resistant penicillins) are unable to penetrate through the porin protein channels of this outer membrane. Therefore, gram-negative bacteria are naturally resistant to these agents. In addition, some gram-negative bacteria, including *Neisseria gonorrhoeae*, *Serratia*, *Enterobacter*, and *Pseudomonas*, have acquired resistance to ampicillin and/or antipseudomonal penicillins due to changes in their cell envelopes that have decreased permeability to the antibiotic.

Clinically, resistance due to altered penicillin-binding proteins (PBPs) appears to be relatively uncommon. In addition to methicillin-resistant *Staphylococcus aureus* and *S. epidermidis* (see above), highly resistant South African strains of *Streptococcus pneumoniae* have PBPs with reduced binding affinities for penicillins. Resistance due to altered PBPs also has been demonstrated in *Streptococcus faecalis*, *Neisseria gonorrhoeae*, and *Haemophilus influenzae*.

Tolerance to penicillins has been reported primarily in gram-positive bacteria, such as *Staphylococcus aureus*, *Streptococcus sanguis*, and *Streptococcus pneumoniae*. Penicillin-tolerant strains are resistant to the lethal action of a normally bactericidal penicillin. In vitro, tolerant strains are suggested initially by large differences between the minimal inhibitory concentration (MIC), which is usually within the normal range, and the minimal bactericidal concentration (MBC), which is much higher; confirmation of tolerance requires follow-up time-kill studies and more detailed microbiologic studies using genetically and physiologically homogeneous cultures of the isolate. The mechanistic basis of tolerance is not completely understood. Many of these strains appear to have a suppressed murein hydrolase (autolytic enzyme) activity that prevents their lysis, although other mechanisms also may be involved (Handwerger and Tomasz, 1985).

For additional discussion, see Hamilton-Miller, 1982; Neu, 1982 A, 1984 A.

Uses

Penicillins are bactericidal antibiotics with a high therapeutic to toxic ratio; they are frequently drugs of choice for infections caused by susceptible organisms in nonallergic patients.

Penicillin G is preferred for infections caused by most frequently encountered gram-positive bacteria (except staphylococci and, in some situations, enterococci) and gram-negative cocci. It also is the drug of choice for infections caused by certain gram-negative bacilli, actinomycetes, and spirochetes (see Reese and Betts, 1983; Wright and Wilkowske, 1983; Neu, 1984 A).

Procaine penicillin G and benzathine penicillin G are repository forms that provide tissue depots from which drug is absorbed over hours (procaine penicillin G) or days (benzathine penicillin G). Administered intramuscularly, these preparations are indicated for certain infections when prolonged therapeutic blood levels are achievable and the frequent dosing requirements of aqueous penicillin G (due to its short half-life) are undesirable. In particular, procaine penicillin G frequently is preferred in certain forms of gonorrhea, and benzathine penicillin G is used in the treatment of syphilis and streptococcal pharyngitis. When high, sustained levels of antibiotic are required, however, parenteral aqueous penicillin G should be used (see Reese and Betts, 1983; Wright and Wilkowske, 1983; Neu, 1984 A).

Penicillin V is more acid stable than penicillin G and equivalent oral doses produce higher blood levels. Furthermore, the absorption of this phenoxymethyl derivative is not affected by the presence of food in the gastrointestinal tract. Thus, penicillin V is frequently preferred to penicillin G when oral administration is indicated (eg, streptococcal pharyngitis), although larger oral doses of buffered penicillin G are equally effective (see Reese and Betts, 1983; Wright and Wilkowske, 1983; Neu, 1984 A; see also the section on Pharmacokinetics).

The penicillinase-resistant penicillins offer no therapeutic advantages over penicillin G except in staphylococcal infections, in which the majority of strains are now resistant to penicillin G. Thus, these agents are drugs of choice for staphylococcal infections. The penicillinase-resistant penicillins differ mainly in their pharmacologic properties (see the section on Pharmacokinetics). Parenteral nafcillin, oxacillin, and methicillin are alternative choices for serious staphylococcal infections. In adults, methicillin has been associated with interstitial nephritis most frequently and the other agents are often preferred. Oral dicloxacillin, cloxacillin, and, less frequently, oxacillin are alternative choices for mild to moderate infections. When methicillin-resistant strains of *Staphylococcus aureus* (or *S. epidermidis*) are known or suspected to be present, vancomycin is required (see Neu, 1982 B; Molavi and Le Frock, 1984; see also Chapter 72, Miscellaneous Antibacterial Agents).

Aminopenicillins usually are drugs of choice for infections caused by enterococci (penicillin G often is preferred in enterococcal endocarditis, however) and susceptible *Haemophilus influenzae* and Enterobacteriaceae, particularly *Proteus mirabilis* and community-acquired *Escherichia coli*. Ampicillin, the prototype of this group, is often the agent of choice against susceptible organisms because it is less expensive than the other aminopenicillins and is the only agent of this class available for parenteral administration in the United States. Amoxicillin may be preferred for oral use, however, because it is absorbed more rapidly and completely and equivalent doses produce higher serum levels than ampicillin. Furthermore, absorption of amoxicillin is not affected by the presence of food, and diarrhea appears to occur less often, particularly in young children. Higher serum levels also may be achieved by using bacampicillin, a proampicillin. Generally, bacampicillin and cyclacillin do not offer significant clinical advantages over amoxicillin, and they are more expensive (see Neu, 1979, 1984 A; Scheife and Neu, 1982; McCracken, 1983; Reese and Betts, 1983; see also the section on Pharmacokinetics).

Despite their broad antibacterial spectra, the parenteral antipseudomonal penicillins (carbenicillin, ticarcillin, azlocillin, mezlocillin, piperacillin) are currently drugs of choice only for infections caused by *Pseudomonas aeruginosa* or susceptible aerobic gram-negative bacilli that are resistant to other penicillins and cephalosporins. Systemic pseudomonal infections are usually serious and difficult to eradicate; they frequently are of nosocomial origin and affect compromised hosts (eg, neutropenic cancer patients, cystic fibrosis patients); and they may be associated with the emergence of resistant bacterial strains, particularly when treated with an antipseudomonal penicillin alone. Thus, most infectious disease experts recommend that systemic *P. aeruginosa* infections virtually always be treated with an antipseudomonal penicillin plus an aminoglycoside (gentamicin [Garamycin, Jenamicin], tobramycin [Nebcin], amikacin [Amikin], netilmicin [Netromycin]. Such combinations often have demonstrated antibacterial synergism against *P. aeruginosa*. Also, the rate of emergence of resistant organisms should be decreased with combination therapy. Antipseudomonal penicillins and aminoglycosides should not be mixed together physically, however, because they inactivate one another (see Drug Interactions section; see also Chapter 70, Aminoglycosides).

The descending order of in vitro activity of the antipseudomonal penicillins against *P. aeruginosa* is piperacillin $\geq$ azlocillin > mezlocillin = ticarcillin > carbenicillin. The clinical significance of this in vitro data is undetermined. However, most physicians have preferred ticarcillin over carbenicillin for infections caused by *P. aeruginosa* because it can be given in lower dosages, resulting in decreased sodium load and other adverse effects to the patient. Whether the newer agents, piperacillin, mezlocillin, or azlocillin, will offer significant clinical advantages over ticarcillin is presently unresolved. Piperacillin, azlocillin, and mezlocillin contain less sodium per gram than ticarcillin and carbenicillin, which is an advantage in patients who must severely restrict sodium intake. Differences in drug acquisition costs may be an important factor in selecting an antipseudomonal penicillin for general use in a given hospital (see *Med Lett Drugs Ther*, 1981, 1982 A and B; Eliopoulos and Moellering, 1982; Neu, 1982 C; Wright and Wilkowske, 1983; Drusano et al, 1984; Parry and Pancoast, 1984).

Carbenicillin indanyl sodium is an oral antipseudomonal penicillin that is used only for urinary tract infections, including chronic bacterial prostatitis. The blood levels obtained with this analogue are not high enough to be effective systemically.

Parenterally administered amdinocillin, either alone or in combination with other β-lactam antibiotics, has been shown to be effective for complicated and uncomplicated urinary tract infections caused by susceptible Enterobacteriaceae, primarily *Escherichia coli*, *Klebsiella*, and *Enterobacter* (Demos and Green, 1983; Cox, 1983; Ward et al, 1983; King et al, 1983; Rotstein and Farrar, 1983; see also the review by Neu, 1985). However, it is presently unknown whether this antibiotic offers any clinical advantages over other agents (eg, penicillins, cephalosporins, trimethoprim/sulfamethoxazole [Bactrim, Septra]). Furthermore, although combinations of amdinocillin and various other β-lactam agents exhibit synergy against a number of enteric gram-negative bacilli in vitro, these data cannot easily be extrapolated to clinical effectiveness. Clinical experience with amdinocillin for infections outside the urinary tract is very limited. Thus, the current role of this agent in infectious disease therapy appears to be small (Farrar, 1984; *Med Lett Drugs Ther*, 1985 A; Neu, 1985).

Specific infections for which the penicillins are the preferred (or alternative) drugs are summarized below according to site of infection. For additional discussion, see Chapter 65, Antimicrobial Therapy and Chemoprophylaxis of Infectious Diseases.

Skin: Pyodermas are caused by *Staphylococcus aureus* (eg, folliculitis, furuncles, carbuncles, bullous impetigo) or *Streptococcus pyogenes* (eg, erysipelas, ecthyma, nonbullous impetigo) and frequently require systemic antibiotics. Penicillinase-resistant penicillins are drugs of choice for staphylococcal pyodermas; penicillin G or penicillin V is preferred for streptococcal pyodermas.

Intravenous penicillin G is the drug of choice for gas gangrene due to *Clostridium perfringens,* although surgical debridement is most important for this infection.

Infections following burns frequently are caused by *Pseudomonas aeruginosa*. An antipseudomonal penicillin combined with an aminoglycoside is preferred therapy.

Central Nervous System: Aqueous penicillin G administered intravenously is the drug of choice in bacterial meningitis caused by susceptible strains of *Neisseria meningitidis* or *Streptococcus pneumoniae* (rare strains are resistant). Since meningitis in adults under age 60 is infrequently caused by

Haemophilus influenzae (usually type b) or other gram-negative bacilli, large doses of penicillin G often are preferred in these patients even before the results of culture and susceptibility tests are available. In patients over 60 years, the incidence of meningitis caused by penicillin G-resistant, aerobic gram-negative enteric bacilli (eg, *Escherichia coli*) is increasing. The third generation cephalosporins (eg, cefotaxime [Claforan]) are now the drugs of choice in proven aerobic gram-negative enteric bacillary meningitis (see Landesman et al, 1981; Rahal and Simberkoff, 1982; see also Chapter 67, Cephalosporins and Related Agents).

Large doses of intravenous ampicillin are effective against susceptible strains of *Haemophilus influenzae*, and this aminopenicillin is a drug of first choice in infants and children with meningitis caused by these organisms. Because ampicillin-resistant (β lactamase-producing) strains of *H. influenzae* have been reported in most areas of the United States, it is currently recommended that chloramphenicol [Chloromycetin, Mychel] 100 mg/kg/day be given intravenously with ampicillin for initial treatment before the results of culture and sensitivity tests are known. If only ampicillin-sensitive organisms are cultured from the cerebrospinal fluid, chloramphenicol can be discontinued. Cefuroxime [Zinacef] and third generation cephalosporins (eg, cefotaxime, ceftriaxone [Rocephin]) also are effective in *H. influenzae* meningitis, including disease caused by β lactamase-producing strains; some experts now prefer these agents for initial treatment (see also Chapter 67).

In infants less than 1 month of age, causative organisms of bacterial meningitis include *Streptococcus agalactiae* (group B), *Escherichia coli* and other coliforms, *Listeria monocytogenes,* and other streptococci. Ampicillin (or penicillin G) in combination with an aminoglycoside is the preferred empiric therapy for meningitis in this age group; ampicillin plus cefotaxime is an alternative regimen. Ampicillin (or penicillin G) are primary agents for group B streptococcal and *L. monocytogenes* infections.

Intravenous penicillin G may be indicated for anaerobic infections of the central nervous system (eg, brain abscess), depending on the probable causative organism(s) (most anaerobic bacteria above the diaphragm are susceptible). Alternative antibiotics include chloramphenicol and metronidazole [Flagyl I.V., Flagyl I.V. RTU, Flagyl]. The latter drug is particularly effective against the *Bacteroides fragilis* group.

Intravenously administered aqueous crystalline penicillin G is a drug of choice for neurosyphilis (*Treponema pallidum*) and gonococcal meningitis (*Neisseria gonorrhoeae*); see Chapter 65, Table 2, for a detailed discussion.

Ear: The most common causative organisms of acute otitis media are *Streptococcus pneumoniae* and *Haemophilus influenzae*. Amoxicillin (or ampicillin) is the drug of choice for this infection. However, the incidence of amoxicillin-resistant *H. influenzae* is increasing. Erythromycin plus a sulfonamide, trimethoprim/sulfamethoxazole, cefaclor [Ceclor], and amoxicillin/potassium clavulanate [Augmentin] are effective alternatives for these resistant strains. Augmentin combines amoxicillin with a β-lactamase inhibitor to restore activity against various β lactamase-producing bacteria (see Mixtures of Penicillins with Clavulanic Acid [β Lactamase Inhibitor]).

Upper Respiratory Tract: Acute sinusitis is caused by the same organisms that cause acute otitis media. Amoxicillin (or ampicillin) is a drug of choice.

Oral penicillin V (ten-day course of therapy) or intramuscular benzathine penicillin G (single injection) is the preferred drug for pharyngitis due to *Streptococcus pyogenes* (group A, β hemolytic). Treatment of streptococcal pharyngitis with penicillin decreases the risk of acute rheumatic fever.

Penicillin G is a drug of choice for Vincent's gingivitis and frequently is preferred for periodontal infections caused by anaerobic bacteria in the oral cavity. Penicillin V may be used in mild infections.

Penicillin G procaine is among the preferred drugs for gonococcal pharyngitis caused by susceptible strains of *Neisseria gonorrhoeae*. However, ampicillin (or amoxicillin) has not been adequate for this form of gonorrhea. When infection is caused by penicillin-resistant *N. gonorrhoeae* (eg, PPNG), intramuscular ceftriaxone and oral trimethoprim/sulfamethoxazole appear to be effective (see Chapter 65, Table 2, for a detailed discussion).

Specific antitoxin plus antibiotic therapy with penicillin G (or erythromycin) is required to treat diphtheria caused by *Corynebacterium diphtheriae*. Penicillin G can be used to eliminate the carrier state, although many infectious disease experts prefer erythromycin.

Epiglottitis is a life-threatening infection caused by *Haemophilus influenzae* type b. Intravenous ampicillin (for known susceptible strains) or chloramphenicol is the drug of choice for this infection; combined therapy is recommended initially until susceptibility is determined. Third generation cephalosporins, used alone, also are effective. Maintaining an airway is of critical importance in acute epiglottitis.

Lower Respiratory Tract: The most common causative bacterial organism of community-acquired, acute, typical pneumonia in a normal host is *Streptococcus pneumoniae*. Penicillin G is the drug of choice for this infection and procaine penicillin G is usually adequate in uncomplicated cases.

In infants and young children, *Haemophilus influenzae* may be the causative organism of pneumonia. Parenteral ampicillin is the drug of choice for susceptible organisms; chloramphenicol, cefuroxime, third generation cephalosporins (eg, cefotaxime), or trimethoprim/sulfamethoxazole should be effective against ampicillin-resistant *H. influenzae*.

Penicillin G is traditionally preferred for bronchopulmonary infections caused by anaerobic bacteria (eg, aspiration pneumonia). The major penicillin G-resistant anaerobic pathogen, *Bacteroides fragilis,* is not a frequent cause of infections above the diaphragm. Penicillin G-resistant (β lactamase-producing) strains of *B. melaninogenicus*, a common anaerobic pathogen in the respiratory tract, are increasing, however. Clindamycin [Cleocin] usually is an effective alternative for these infections (see Chapter 68, Macrolides and Lincosamides).

Nosocomial pneumonias are most frequently caused by gram-negative bacilli. When *P. aeruginosa* is the infectious agent, an antipseudomonal penicillin in combination with an aminoglycoside is recommended. When *Staphylococcus aureus* is the documented cause of pneumonia, a penicillinase-resistant penicillin is frequently preferred.

It should be emphasized that penicillins are not active against the organisms that cause atypical pneumonias (eg, *Mycoplasma pneumoniae, Chlamydia, Legionella pneumophila*). Erythromycin (or tetracycline [except for *Legionella*]) is preferred for atypical pneumonias.

Heart: The most common causative organisms of infective endocarditis are streptococci, principally viridans streptococci (eg, *S. sanguis, S. mutans, S. milleri, S. mitior*), but also frequently enterococci (eg, *S. faecalis*). Viridans streptococci usually are highly sensitive to penicillin G, and this agent (with or without streptomycin) is primarily employed. Enterococcal endocarditis is optimally treated with combination therapy. Traditionally, penicillin G (or ampicillin) plus streptomycin has been the preferred regimen because antibacterial synergism is observed. A number of enterococcal strains are now highly resistant to streptomycin, however. The substitution of gentamicin for streptomycin in the combination usually is effective in these cases (see also Chapter 70, Aminoglycosides).

Acute bacterial endocarditis is most frequently caused by *Staphylococcus aureus*. A penicillinase-resistant penicillin (with or without gentamicin) is preferred for susceptible strains. For methicillin-resistant *S. aureus*, vancomycin is required. *S. epidermidis*, which is often methicillin-resistant, is a common cause of prosthetic valve endocarditis. Vancomycin plus rifampin [Rifadin, Rimactane] plus gentamicin currently appears to be the preferred regimen (Karchmer et al, 1984), but exact guidelines remain to be established. When a prosthetic heart valve is involved, surgical removal is usually required.

For rare cases of endocarditis due to *Pseudomonas aeruginosa* (eg, in intravenous drug abusers), an antipseudomonal penicillin plus an aminoglycoside is recommended; surgery is required if the infection is on the left side of the heart.

Gastrointestinal Tract: Ampicillin in combination with an aminoglycoside frequently is used for empiric therapy of biliary tract infections. Causative organisms of these infections include *Escherichia coli* and other Enterobacteriaceae and the gram-positive enterococci.

Ampicillin (but not amoxicillin) may be effective in gastroenteritis caused by susceptible *Shigella* strains. However, the number of ampicillin-resistant shigellae is considerable and trimethoprim/sulfamethoxazole is now the therapy of choice for shigellosis. No antibiotics are recommended for simple gastroenteritis due to *Salmonella*. However, ampicillin, amoxicillin, and trimethoprim/sulfamethoxazole are alternatives to chloramphenicol for systemic infections (eg, bacteremia, enteric fever syndrome including typhoid fever) caused by *Salmonella* species, including *S. typhi*; these agents often are effective against chloramphenicol-resistant strains. Ampicillin (6 g daily for one to three months) has eliminated the typhoid carrier state in patients without gallstones.

Peritonitis following bowel perforation is usually caused by a mixture of pathogens, including aerobic gram-negative bacilli; anaerobic bacteria, particularly the *Bacteroides fragilis* group; and enterococci. The antipseudomonal penicillins in combination with an aminoglycoside (to eradicate aerobic gram-negative bacilli) have been effective since these penicillins have significant activity against the *B. fragilis* group. However, clindamycin and metronidazole are current drugs of choice for the *B. fragilis* group and are more frequently used in combination with an aminoglycoside to treat these mixed infections; penicillin G or ampicillin also may be added. Cefoxitin alone also has been effective in peritonitis (ie, mild to moderate illness and when the infection is community-acquired).

Urinary Tract: *Escherichia coli* causes more than 90% of initial urinary tract infections. Other coliform organisms and enterococci less frequently cause these infections. In addition, *Staphylococcus saprophyticus* also causes some cases of acute bacterial cystitis, particularly in younger women.

For mild (nonbacteremic) cases of acute pyelonephritis in ambulatory patients, oral ampicillin or amoxicillin may be effective, but resistance to these aminopenicillins among community-acquired *E. coli* has become a problem in many geographic locations. Oral trimethoprim/sulfamethoxazole often is a preferred alternative. For more severe cases, parenteral ampicillin in combination with an aminoglycoside frequently is recommended until results of cultures and susceptibility tests are available.

Presently, single-dose antimicrobial therapy is preferred for initial attacks of acute bacterial cystitis in females who are not pregnant, have no renal parenchymal involvement, have no evidence of subclinical pyelonephritis, and are available for follow-up. A single 3-g dose of oral amoxicillin is an alternative to trimethoprim/sulfamethoxazole (preferred) for this indication. Other effective agents include sulfisoxazole [Gantrisin], trimethoprim alone [Proloprim, Trimpex], tetracycline, or an aminoglycoside. For all other patients, traditional therapy for 7 to 14 days is recommended. Drugs of choice include trimethoprim/sulfamethoxazole, sulfisoxazole, ampicillin, amoxicillin, nitrofurantoin, and cinoxacin. Penicillins are not generally used for prophylaxis of recurrent urinary tract infections or empiric treatment of the acute urethral syndrome.

The causative organisms and treatment of acute prostatitis in males are similar to those for acute pyelonephritis. However, the aminopenicillins are not indicated for chronic bacterial prostatitis. Prolonged therapy with trimethoprim/sulfamethoxazole (alternative, trimethoprim alone) is preferred in chronic prostatitis, which is often difficult to eradicate. Oral carbenicillin indanyl also may be useful.

For the role of penicillins in the treatment of urethritis, see the section below on sexually transmitted diseases and Chapter 65, Table 2.

Female Reproductive Tract: Acute pelvic inflammatory disease frequently is caused by a mixture of pathogens, including *Neisseria gonorrhoeae*, *Chlamydia trachomatis*, anaerobic bacteria (eg, *Bacteroides*, gram-positive cocci), facultative gram-negative bacilli (eg, *Escherichia coli*), *Actinomyces israelii*, and *Mycoplasma hominis*. The drug or combination of drugs employed depends on the most likely causative organism(s) and the severity of the infection. Currently, other antimicrobials are preferred to penicillins for inpatient regimens, but single-dose ampicillin (or amoxicillin) or penicillin G procaine may be recommended in ambulatory patients (milder cases) when penicillin-sensitive *N. gonorrhoeae* is the probable pathogen. Follow-up therapy with oral doxycycline frequently is recommended to cover potential coexisting *C. trachomatis* infection adequately (see Chapter 65, Table 2, for a detailed discussion).

Bacterial vaginosis, a syndrome that has been associated with *Gardnerella* (*Haemophilus*) *vaginalis*, is now believed to be caused by the interaction of several species of vaginal bacteria, including anaerobes. This syndrome can be treated effectively with oral ampicillin. However, metronidazole is the current drug of choice. Penicillins are not indicated in other forms of vaginitis.

For the role of penicillins in the treatment of cervicitis, see the section below on sexually transmitted diseases and Chapter 65, Table 2.

Male Reproductive Tract: Epididymo-orchitis in males under 35 years frequently is a sexually transmitted form caused by *Neisseria gonorrhoeae* and/or *Chlamydia trachomatis*. Ampicillin (or amoxicillin) or penicillin G procaine is effective in acute epididymo-orchitis due to *N. gonorrhoeae*, but the increasing frequency of *C. trachomatis* as the causative organism has made follow-up therapy with tetracycline (or doxycycline [Vibramycin]) the recommendation of the Centers for Disease Control (see Chapter 65, Table 2, for a detailed discussion). In males over age 35, *E. coli* and other coliforms are the most likely causative organisms of acute epididymo-orchitis. Although choice of therapy depends on the severity of the disease, trimethoprim/sulfamethoxazole and ampicillin (or amoxicillin) are among the preferred drugs.

Bone and Joint: *Staphylococcus aureus* and, to a lesser extent, streptococci (eg, *S. pyogenes*, *S. pneumoniae*) are the most common causes of septic arthritis in adults over age 40 and children under 15 years. A parenteral penicillinase-resistant penicillin (eg, nafcillin, oxacillin) is the drug of choice when the Gram stain reveals that a gram-positive coccus is the causative organism; it also should be given when no organism is seen on Gram stain. *Haemophilus influenzae* is an important pathogen for this disease in children between 2 months and 4 years. Parenteral ampicillin is preferred for susceptible strains of this organism. In patients between the ages of 15 and 40, *Neisseria gonorrhoeae* is the most likely cause of septic arthritis. For the role of penicillins in treatment, see the section below on sexually transmitted diseases; see also Chapter 65, Table 2.

The most likely causative organism of acute hematogenous osteomyelitis is *S. aureus,* and a parenteral penicillinase-resistant penicillin is the drug of choice. Gram-negative bacilli also may cause this infection in newborn infants, and combined therapy with a penicillinase-resistant penicillin and an aminoglycoside is indicated in these patients.

Sepsis: Parenterally administered penicillins frequently are preferred to treat sepsis caused by susceptible pathogens (eg, penicillin G for *Streptococcus pneumoniae*; nafcillin, oxacillin, or methicillin for *Staphylococcus aureus*). They also may be used in combination regimens for empiric therapy before the etiologic agent has been identified. For example, a penicillinase-resistant penicillin (alternative, first generation cephalosporin) plus an aminoglycoside often is recommended for sepsis of unknown etiology in nonimmunocompromised adults and older children; ampicillin plus an aminoglycoside is a regimen of choice in neonatal sepsis; and an antipseudomonal penicillin plus an aminoglycoside is usually preferred in febrile neutropenic patients.

Other Infections: The penicillins, particularly penicillin G, play a role in the treatment of certain infectious diseases that involve more than one organ system. Penicillin G is the preferred drug in actinomycosis (*Actinomyces israelii*), anthrax (*Bacillus anthracis*), and, in combination with tetanus immune globulin (human), tetanus (*Clostridium tetani*). Penicillin G and its repository forms (procaine or benzathine penicillin G) are preferred drugs in syphilis; penicillin G and the aminopenicillins are used to treat disseminated gonorrhea (see the section below on sexually transmitted diseases; see also Chapter 65, Table 2). Parenteral penicillinase-resistant penicillins are given to patients with the toxic shock syndrome. Antimicrobial drugs do not appear to play an important role in the treatment of the acute phase of this disease; supportive measures (eg, maintenance of adequate blood pressure) are of primary importance. Antibiotics are useful in preventing recurrences of the syndrome.

Penicillin G is the preferred antibiotic for various other infections, including erysipeloid (*Erysipelothrix rhusiopathiae*), rat bite fever (*Spirillum minor*), *Pasteurella multocida* infections, yaws (*Treponema pertenue*), and arthritis and meningitis associated with Lyme disease. Penicillin G (or penicillin V) is an alternative to tetracycline in early Lyme disease. Penicillin G is an alternative to doxycycline for leptospirosis.

Sexually Transmitted Diseases: Penicillin G and its repository forms are drugs of choice for all stages of syphilis in the nonallergic patient. In adults, benzathine penicillin G is preferred in early syphilis; syphilis of more than one year's duration (except neurosyphilis); and for persons exposed to infectious syphilis (contacts). For neurosyphilis, aqueous crystalline penicillin G (intravenous) or penicillin G procaine (intramuscular) followed by penicillin G benzathine is recommended. Symptomatic congenital syphilis is treated with aqueous crystalline penicillin G or penicillin G procaine; asymptomatic infants (with normal cerebrospinal fluid) who are at increased risk also should be treated. For detailed treatment guidelines, see Chapter 65, Table 2.

Penicillins are drugs of choice or among the preferred alternatives for all forms of gonorrhea in the nonallergic patient. However, penicillins are not effective against penicillinase-producing *N. gonorrhoeae* (PPNG) or chromosomal-mediated resistant *N. gonorrhoeae* (CMRNG) strains or for coexisting *Chlamydia trachomatis* infection, which has been documented in up to 45% of gonorrhea patients for whom adequate chlamydial cultures are done (*Morbid Mortal Week Rep*, 1985 A). In adults with uncomplicated gonococcal infection or sexual contacts, large single doses of intramuscular penicillin G procaine (active in urogenital, anorectal, and pharyngeal forms) or oral amoxicillin or ampicillin (not active in anorectal [in men] or pharyngeal forms) are among the preferred alternatives. Single-dose ceftriaxone also is a drug of choice for all forms of uncomplicated gonorrhea; this third generation cephalosporin also is active against PPNG and CMRNG strains. Because coexisting chlamydial infection is a primary concern, most authorities recommend seven days of additional therapy with tetracycline or doxycycline (*Morbid Mortal Week Rep*, 1985 A and B; *Med Lett Drugs Ther*, 1984 A; Hook and Holmes, 1985). Intravenous aqueous crystalline penicillin G usually is preferred for gonococcal arthritis (oral amoxicillin and ampicillin are among the alternatives), endocarditis, meningitis, and ophthalmia in adults and for all types of neonatal gonococcal infections. For detailed treatment guidelines, see Chapter 65, Table 2.

Prophylaxis: Penicillins also have played an important role in prophylaxis. Monthly injections of benzathine penicillin G (preferred) or twice daily administration of oral penicillin V are recommended to prevent recurrent attacks of rheumatic fever (secondary prevention) in patients with a well documented history of rheumatic fever and those who show definite evidence of rheumatic heart disease. The optimal duration of continuous antimicrobial prophylaxis remains unsettled. Although it has been suggested that prophylaxis should be continued for life, the necessity for such prolonged prophylaxis has not been firmly established. See Chapter 65, Table 3, or the American Heart Association Committee Report on Prevention of Rheumatic Fever for a more detailed discussion (Shulman et al, 1984 A).

Prophylaxis of bacterial endocarditis in patients with (1) prosthetic heart valves, (2) most forms of congenital heart disease, (3) surgically constructed systemic-pulmonary shunts, (4) rheumatic or other acquired valvular heart disease, (5) hypertrophic cardiomyopathy (IHSS), (6) previous history of bacterial endocarditis, or (7) mitral valve prolapse with insufficiency is recommended prior to all dental and various other invasive procedures of the upper respiratory, genitourinary, or lower gastrointestinal tract that may be associated with transitory bacteremia. Because viridans streptococci (from oral or upper respiratory foci) or enterococci (from lower gastrointestinal or genitourinary foci) are likely causative organisms of infective endocarditis, penicillins are primary antibiotics in prophylactic regimens for nonallergic individuals. Specific regimens, as recommended by the American Heart Association's Committee on the Prevention of Rheumatic Fever and Bacterial Endocarditis, are listed in Chapter 65, Table 3. For additional information, see the committee's report (Shulman et al, 1984 B).

Monthly injections of benzathine penicillin G or twice daily administration of oral penicillin V (for two to four years in children) can be used for the prophylaxis of pneumococcal infection in splenectomized patients. Some experts prefer amoxicillin in children under five years to include coverage against *Haemophilus influenzae*. Immunization with pneumococcal 23-valent polysaccharide vaccine can serve as an adjunct for protection against pneumococcal infection. Quadrivalent meningococcal vaccine and Haemophilus b polysaccharide vaccine also should be considered in splenectomized patients. For detailed discussion, see Chapter 65, Table 3.

Oral amoxicillin, once daily for about six months, is an alternative to sulfisoxazole for the prevention of recurrent acute otitis media (see Chapter 65, Table 3).

For the role of penicillins in the prophylaxis of sexual contacts of gonorrhea or syphilis patients, see the section above on sexually transmitted diseases and Chapter 65, Table 2.

Parenteral penicillinase-resistant penicillins are alternatives to cefazolin for antimicrobial prophylaxis of certain surgical procedures (eg, total hip replacement). For detailed discussion, see Chapter 65, Table 4.

Adverse Reactions and Precautions

Hypersensitivity Reactions: The major adverse effects of the penicillins are hypersensitivity reactions that range in severity from skin rashes to immediate anaphylaxis. The incidence of hypersensitivity to the penicillins has been estimated to be between 1% and 10%. Among the antimicrobials, this group of drugs causes the largest number of allergic reactions, which may reflect wide use of the penicillins rather than specific potential for sensitization. Topical application or exposure to dust or aerosol containing a penicillin once was the most common source of hypersensitization. Today, parenteral and oral preparations probably are chiefly responsible, although an individual who has never received a penicillin may develop a reaction through previous exposure to normal environmental sources of penicillium molds or penicillins (eg, in milk).

Once a hypersensitivity reaction occurs to any penicillin, it should be assumed that the patient will react to all other drugs in the class. Also, about 5% to 10% of penicillin-allergic patients are sensitive to cephalosporins, and individuals who have experienced an immediate-type hypersensitivity reaction to penicillins should not receive cephalosporins (see Chapter 67, Cephalosporins and Related Agents). The occurrence of an untoward reaction to penicillin does not necessarily imply repetition of the effect on subsequent exposures, however. Allergic reactivity can be lost or the reaction may not have been hypersensitive in nature (see below).

Penicillin and its metabolites are low-molecular-weight haptens that must bind to carrier molecules (eg, host protein, cell membranes) to be immunogenic. Most of the penicillin bound to tissue protein (about 95%) is in the penicilloyl form and this is called the major antigenic determinant. Other metabolites (eg, penicilloate, penilloate, penicilloyl-amine) and native penicillin itself, also may be bound to tissue (about 5%) and are collectively called minor antigenic determinants. The terms major and minor refer only to the quantity of hapten available and not to their immunologic importance.

Penicillins may cause hypersensitivity reactions by any one of four immune mechanisms:

Type I reactions are mediated by IgE antibodies, which fix to the surface of tissue mast cells, causing release of vasoactive compounds (eg, histamine). Manifestations include urticaria, angioedema, and anaphylaxis, as well as rhinitis, asthma, and laryngeal edema. Reactions may be accompanied by fever. Severe anaphylaxis, hypotension, and death are rare, however. It is estimated that only 0.02% of courses of penicillin treatment are associated with a severe IgE-mediated allergic response, but the mortality rate in affected patients is about 10%.

Type I responses often are immediate (within one hour after administration), but accelerated urticaria and other reactions may be observed 1 to 72 hours after the drug is given. These reactions usually resolve within 48 hours after the drug is stopped but may persist for several days.

Both the major and minor antigenic determinants can cause IgE-mediated hypersensitivity reactions. However, minor determinants are the major cause of anaphylactic reactions. Type I reactions are the adverse effects most likely to be reported and, like all undesirable responses to penicillins, may occur after oral or parenteral administration. Severe anaphylaxis is more prevalent after parenteral injection (Patterson and Anderson, 1982).

Although early reports suggested that allergic reactions to penicillin, especially anaphylaxis, are more common in atopic patients, more recent studies showed that these reactions occur no more often in atopic individuals than in the rest of the population. An individual should not be denied penicillin on the basis of other allergic manifestations when there is no history or clear-cut evidence of hypersensitivity to penicillin. Nevertheless, it would seem prudent to evaluate such individuals more thoroughly for penicillin allergy than those with no history of allergic phenomena.

Type II reactions are caused by cytotoxic antibodies of the IgG class. Penicillin, most likely the penicilloyl determinant, acts as a hapten on the cell surface and reacts with antipenicillin antibodies, resulting in the activation of complement and the eventual destruction of the cell. Hemolytic anemia is mediated by this mechanism.

Type III reactions involve the formation of immune complexes of IgG or IgM antibodies and penicillin antigens, most likely the penicilloyl determinant. These complexes are deposited in tissue spaces or on cells of the skin, kidneys, or other organs. There is complement fixation. Polymorphonuclear leukocytes are attracted by the immune reactant, and an inflammatory response occurs. Serum sickness is caused by this mechanism.

Type IV reactions are classified as delayed (72 hours or more following administration of the drug) and are mediated by T-lymphocytes that react with tissue-bound drug. Contact dermatitis is an example of a type IV reaction.

Some adverse reactions to penicillins are categorized as idiopathic. Although abnormal immune responses have been reported, specific immune mechanisms have not been identified. These include maculopapular drug eruptions, interstitial nephritis, drug fever, and eosinophilia. Exfoliative dermatitis and the Stevens-Johnson syndrome are rare adverse reactions that appear to be allergic in nature.

Hypersensitivity-type rashes may occur following the administration of any penicillin but, at least in the case of ampicillin, the vast majority do not appear to be allergic in nature. These mildly pruritic maculopapular eruptions usually occur within 1 to 28 days, are not associated with positive skin tests, and resolve whether or not ampicillin administration is continued. Such rashes are particularly common in patients with viral infections, such as infectious mononucleosis, and with concomitant allopurinol therapy (see the section on Drug Interactions and Interference with Laboratory Tests). They do not preclude the future use of a penicillin.

In order to minimize the risk of penicillin hypersensitivity reactions, a careful history should be taken with regard to previous allergic reactions. For most patients with a positive history, an alternative, noncross-reacting antimicrobial agent usually can be selected. When an effective alternative is not available, skin testing can help to identify patients at high risk of developing an IgE-mediated (eg, immediate) reaction (see below). If an allergic reaction does occur, epinephrine (subcutaneous or intramuscular for mild reactions and intravenous for more serious reactions) will usually abort the reaction and can be lifesaving in severe anaphylactic reactions. (See the discussion on Treatment of Anaphylactic Shock in Chapter 62, Agents for Active and Passive Immunity.) Accelerated and late urticaria may be treated with antihistamines. Maculopapular rashes are self-limiting, but antihistamines relieve pruritus.

For more detailed discussion, see Van Arsdel, 1981; Condemi, 1983; Saxon, 1983; Sher, 1983; Sogn, 1984.

Tests for Hypersensitivity. The earliest tests for penicillin hypersensitivity utilized intradermal injection of a small amount of penicillin G. This procedure is unreliable and dangerous, since even a small amount of penicillin can cause severe reactions or death in sensitive individuals.

Preparations that more accurately predict reactions to the penicillins are available. One of these, benzylpenicilloyl-polylysine (BPO-PL) [Pre-Pen], is a major antigenic determinant of benzylpenicillin; a concentration of 6×10^{-5} M is used. The second preparation is a benzylpenicillin minor determinant mixture (BP-MDM) containing penicillin breakdown products (eg, penilloates, sodium benzyl penicilloylate), prepared by the method of Levine and Redmond (1969), and used in a concentration of 2×10^{-2} M. The minor determinants must be freshly prepared, since they are unstable and no satisfactory technique has been developed to market them. Both major and minor determinants possess a greater margin of safety than penicillin G itself. Nevertheless, prick tests should be performed prior to intradermal injection because the risk of anaphylaxis is greater when a larger amount is injected.

BPO-PL and BP-MDM used as a combined testing procedure probably predict 95% or more of penicillin IgE-mediated hypersensitivity reactions. In one study of 86 adults and 167 children (Warrington et al, 1978), it was found that, of 169 patients with negative skin tests, only two children exhibited mild reactions when challenged with penicillin, an incidence of 1.2%. The same study showed that, when BPO-PL was used alone, up to 31% of allergic patients had false-negative tests for hypersensitivity. Also, reactivity to BP-MDM is more often associated with severe anaphylactic reactions than reactivity to BPO-PL (Levine and Redmond, 1969). Skin tests do not predict non-IgE hypersensitivity reactions, such as serum sickness, hemolytic anemia, contact dermatitis, maculopapular rashes, or interstitial nephritis.

Other Adverse Reactions: The penicillins per se are relatively nontoxic in man. Most reactions are caused by the irritant effects of excessive concentration or reactions to a related molecule (eg, procaine toxicity from injection of procaine penicillin G). Pain and sterile inflammation may occur at the site of intramuscular injection, and phlebitis or thrombophlebitis is sometimes seen when these drugs are given intravenously. Pyrosis, anorexia, nausea, vomiting, and mild to severe diarrhea may result from irritation of the gastrointestinal tract, especially with oral administration. Ampicillin has been associated with diarrhea most frequently.

The most serious consequences of the irritant properties of the penicillins involve the nervous system. Accidental injection into a peripheral nerve causes pain and dysfunction of that part of the body innervated by the nerve. This effect usually is slowly reversible. High concentrations of penicillin in the central nervous system may cause arachnoiditis, convulsions, or fatal encephalopathy. For example, convulsions may follow intravenous injection of a large dose of penicillin G (eg, more than 20 million units in adults), especially in epileptics, infants, or other susceptible individuals (eg, patients with renal insufficiency).

Immediate-type reactions to the procaine component of penicillin G procaine may occur in some individuals, particularly when a large single dose is administered in the treatment of gonorrhea (4.8 million units). These reactions may be manifested by mental disturbances, including anxiety, confusion, agitation, depression, weakness, seizures, hallucinations, combativeness, and expressed fear of impending death. Reactions occur in 1 of 500 patients and are transient, lasting 15 to 30 minutes.

Nephropathy, an allergic reaction manifested as interstitial nephritis, has been reported. The clinical syndrome is characterized by fever, macular rash, eosinophilia, proteinuria, hematuria, leukocyturia, and eosinophiluria; ultimately, the reaction can progress to acute renal failure. Interstitial nephritis occurs most often with methicillin but may be caused by any of the penicillins. Patients usually recover when the drug is discontinued, but fatalities have been reported. Hemorrhagic cystitis also has been reported rarely with methicillin (for additional discussion see the evaluation).

Rapid administration of massive intravenous doses of penicillin G potassium (1.7 mEq of potassium/million units) may produce hyperkalemia, arrhythmias, and cardiac arrest, particularly in patients with impaired renal function.

The administration of large intravenous doses of any penicillin, particularly carbenicillin and ticarcillin, can produce hypokalemia due to the large amount of nonreabsorbable anion in the distal renal tubules. Excessive sodium intake also can be a problem with carbenicillin and ticarcillin, both disodium salts, in patients with impaired sodium excretion mechanisms (eg, those with pre-existing cardiac, renal, or hepatic disease).

Hematologic toxicity occurs rarely following administration of the penicillins. Neutropenia has been observed after use of all penicillins, particularly with large doses, and is reversible after discontinuation of therapy. Coombs'-positive hemolytic anemia is rare. High concentrations of all penicillins, particularly carbenicillin and ticarcillin, bind adenosine diphosphate receptors in platelets and prevent normal platelet aggregation. This can result in prolongation of the bleeding time. However, clinically significant bleeding occurs infrequently.

Transient increases in liver enzymes (eg, serum glutamic-oxaloacetic transaminase [SGOT]) have been reported occasionally for a number of penicillins (eg, nafcillin, isoxazolyl penicillins, aminopenicillins, antipseudomonal penicillins). Symptoms of hepatitis have rarely been associated with these elevated enzyme levels in patients receiving oxacillin.

Penicillins alter the bacterial flora in certain areas of the body (eg, intestinal tract, respiratory tract) by eliminating sensitive micro-organisms. This usually is of little clinical significance, and re-establishment of the normal microflora occurs after therapy. However, serious superinfections with resistant organisms (eg, *Klebsiella, Pseudomonas, Candida*) may follow long-term therapy with any penicillin; this may be more likely with broad spectrum analogues.

Antibiotic-associated pseudomembranous colitis (AAPMC) due to *Clostridium difficile* may develop during or after penicillin therapy. Ampicillin has been one of the more frequently implicated antibiotics in this disorder. This potentially life-threatening adverse effect requires prompt discontinuation of the offending antibiotic, maintenance of fluid and electrolyte balance, and possible therapy with oral vancomycin (see also Chapters 68, Macrolides and Lincosamides, and 72, Miscellaneous Antibacterial Agents).

Generally, penicillins have proven to be the safest antibiotics for use during pregnancy. Although less information is available concerning the safety of the newer semisynthetic penicillin derivatives during pregnancy, there is no evidence that these agents will be teratogenic (see Chow and Jewesson, 1985). The penicillins are classified in FDA Pregnancy Category B.

For additional discussion of adverse reactions and precautions, see Barza, 1977; Neu, 1979, 1982 B and C, 1984 A; Scheife and Neu, 1982; Wright and Wilkowske, 1983; and Drusano et al, 1984.

Drug Interactions and Interference with Laboratory Tests

The antipseudomonal penicillins (carbenicillin, ticarcillin, mezlocillin, azlocillin, piperacillin), which usually are given in large doses, have been shown to inactivate aminoglycosides, particularly gentamicin and tobramycin, when mixed together in intravenous solutions. This practice should be avoided. Furthermore, in patients with renal failure, in vivo antagonism has been observed and may be clinically significant. Serum aminoglycoside concentrations should be monitored in such patients and the dosage adjusted accordingly (Mangini, 1984; Hansten, 1985 A). For a more detailed discussion, see Chapter 70, Aminoglycosides.

Theoretically, bacteriostatic antibiotics that inhibit protein synthesis (eg, chloramphenicol, tetracyclines, erythromycin, clindamycin) could interfere with the bactericidal effect of penicillins. However, the clinical significance is not known and such combinations are recommended under certain circumstances (eg, chloramphenicol plus ampicillin for empiric therapy of *Haemophilus influenzae* meningitis). When such combinations are considered necessary, it is recommended that adequate amounts of each drug be administered and, if possible, the penicillin should be given a few hours or more before the bacteriostatic antibiotic (see Hansten, 1985 A).

Elevated serum methotrexate levels have been reported in a patient receiving large doses (30 g daily) of carbenicillin concomitantly. An enhanced methotrexate effect may be observed (see Hansten, 1985 A).

Isolated cases of breakthrough bleeding and pregnancy have been reported in women receiving oral contraceptives and antibiotics, including ampicillin. The clinical significance is unknown, but the addition of other forms of contraception appears warranted when a course of ampicillin (or other antimicrobial) therapy is initiated in a woman on oral contraceptives (see Back et al, 1981; Hansten and Horn, 1985; see also Chapter 40, Contraceptive Agents).

Oral neomycin has been shown to decrease the gastrointestinal absorption of penicillin V, presumably due to the production of a malabsorption syndrome. Although this has not been demonstrated for other penicillins, it is recommended that parenteral penicillins be used when patients are receiving oral neomycin (Hansten, 1985 A).

Either allopurinol or hyperuricemia appears to predispose patients receiving ampicillin to rashes (Jick and Porter, 1981). No special precautions appear to be necessary, however (Hansten, 1985 A).

The bioavailability of atenolol [Tenormin] was reported to be decreased by concurrent administration of oral ampicillin in six healthy volunteers; exercise tachycardia was significantly higher than after atenolol alone (Schäfer-Korting, 1983). Although additional data are required, it should be recognized that an altered response to atenolol may occur if ampicillin therapy is started or stopped (Hansten, 1985 B).

Warfarin resistance, demonstrated by decreased prothrombin time, was observed in one patient receiving high-dose intravenous nafcillin therapy. The warfarin half-life was markedly reduced when the patient received nafcillin. Both the prothrombin time and warfarin half-life gradually returned to expected values after discontinuation of nafcillin (Qureshi et al, 1984). Although confirmation of this report is necessary, an altered response to warfarin is a possibility if nafcillin therapy is initiated or discontinued (Hansten, 1984).

Large doses of some penicillins (eg, penicillin G, nafcillin, azlocillin, mezlocillin) have been associated with false-positive reactions for urinary protein (pseudoproteinuria) when certain methods have been employed (eg, sulfosalicylic acid and boiling test, acetic acid test, biuret reaction, nitric acid test). This should be distinguished from the true proteinuria that may follow the use of methicillin, oxacillin, and perhaps other penicillins.

Pharmacokinetics

The claims that one penicillin is clinically superior to another based on in vitro sensitivity are questionable, because such tests do not take into account factors such as stability in gastric acid, rates of absorption and excretion, degree of protein binding, diffusion into abscesses or body cavities, and minimal effective blood and tissue concentrations.

Absorption: There are marked differences in oral absorption of the penicillins (see Table 1). Oral preparations of penicillin G are susceptible to destruction by gastric acid and are absorbed erratically and incompletely. To obtain comparable blood concentrations, the oral dose of penicillin G must be four to five times greater than the intramuscular dose. Because the oral absorption of penicillin G also is decreased in the presence of food, this penicillin must be given one hour before or two hours after meals to ensure adequate blood levels.

Penicillin V potassium is less susceptible to acid destruction

TABLE 1.
CLASSIFICATION OF THE PENICILLINS
WITH SOME PHARMACOKINETIC DATA[1]

Class and Generic Name	Trade Name(s)	Route(s) of Administration	Oral Absorption (%)
NATURAL PENICILLINS			
Penicillin G	Many (see evaluation)	Oral Intramuscular Intravenous	20–30
Penicillin V	Many (see evaluation)	Oral	60
PENICILLINASE-RESISTANT (ANTISTAPHYLOCOCCAL) PENICILLINS			
Methicillin	Staphcillin	Intramuscular Intravenous	None
Nafcillin	Nafcil Unipen Nallpen	Oral Intramuscular Intravenous	Erratic (10-20)
Isoxazolyl Penicillins			
Oxacillin	Bactocill Prostaphlin	Oral Intramuscular Intravenous	30
Cloxacillin	Cloxapen Tegopen	Oral	50
Dicloxacillin	Dycill Dynapen Pathocil	Oral	50
AMINOPENICILLINS			
Ampicillin	Many (see evaluation)	Oral Intramuscular Intravenous	40
Amoxicillin	Amoxil Larotid Polymox Trimox	Oral	75–90
Bacampicillin[2]	Spectrobid	Oral	~95
Cyclacillin	Cyclapen-W	Oral	~95
ANTIPSEUDOMONAL PENICILLINS			
Carboxypenicillins			
Carbenicillin	Geopen Pyopen	Intramuscular Intravenous	None
Carbenicillin Indanyl[2]	Geocillin	Oral	30
Ticarcillin	Ticar	Intramuscular Intravenous	None
Acylureidopenicillins			
Azlocillin	Azlin	Intravenous Intramuscular	None
Mezlocillin	Mezlin	Intramuscular Intravenous	None
Piperazine Penicillin			
Piperacillin	Pipracil	Intramuscular Intravenous	None

Protein Bound (%)	Metabolized (%)	Urinary Recovery (%)	Approximate Half-life (hours)	Volume of Distribution (L/kg)
50–60	20	20 (oral) 60–90 (parenteral)	0.5	~0.2
80	55	29–37	0.5–1	~0.2
35–40	10	80	0.5	0.43±0.1
87–90	60	30	0.5	0.1–0.3
90–93	45–50	30–50	0.5	~0.2
93–95	20	30–50	0.5	0.1
95–97	10	60	0.5–0.7	0.09±0.02
17–20	10	40–45 (oral) 90 (parenteral)	1	0.17–0.31
17–20	10	50–70	1	0.25–0.42
17–20	10	75	1	0.32±0.11
20	15–17	80	0.5–0.75	---
50–60	2	85–95	1.1	0.18
50–60	2	30	1.1	0.18
50–60	10–15	75–85	1.2	0.22
20–40	<10	50–70	0.8–1	~0.2
16–42	<10	45–70	0.8–1.2	~0.2
16–22	---	60–80	1–1.3	~0.2

(Continued on next page)

Class and Generic Name	Trade Name(s)	Route(s) of Administration	Oral Absorption (%)
AMIDINO PENICILLIN			
Amdinocillin	Coactin	Intramuscular Intravenous	None

[1]*Pharmacokinetic data were obtained from the following references: Barza, 1977; Neu, 1979, 1982 B and C, 1984 A, 1985; Med Lett Drugs Ther, 1981, 1982 A and B; Eliopoulos and Moellering, 1982; Fortner et al, 1982; McCloskey et al, 1982; Scheife and Neu, 1982; McCracken, 1983; Wright and Wilkowske, 1983; Drusano et al, 1984; Molavi and LeFrock, 1984; Parry and Pancoast, 1984.*
[2]*These penicillins are prodrugs; after oral absorption, bacampicillin is hydrolyzed to ampicillin, and carbenicillin indanyl is hydrolyzed to carbenicillin.*

than penicillin G and, when given with meals, produces blood levels almost as high as those obtained when the drug is taken on an empty stomach. Comparable doses of penicillin V produce blood levels that are two- to fivefold higher than those obtained with penicillin G. Thus, penicillin V is frequently preferred for oral administration.

Methicillin is not used orally because of susceptibility to gastric acid. The other penicillinase-resistant penicillins are resistant to gastric acid, but their absorption is incomplete (see Table 1). Also, nafcillin and, to a lesser extent, oxacillin are absorbed more erratically than cloxacillin and dicloxacillin. The oral use of nafcillin is not recommended. The absorption of all penicillinase-resistant penicillins is impeded by food in the stomach.

The aminopenicillins are resistant to gastric acid. However, amoxicillin and bacampicillin, which is hydrolized to ampicillin, are better absorbed than ampicillin, particularly in the presence of food. Amoxicillin is frequently the preferred aminopenicillin for oral use because its bioavailability is superior to that of ampicillin.

The antipseudomonal penicillins (eg, carbenicillin, ticarcillin, azlocillin, mezlocillin, piperacillin) are acid-labile and are not absorbed orally. However, carbenicillin indanyl sodium, an ester derivative, is adequately absorbed to yield antibacterial concentrations in urine and it is used for certain urinary tract infections.

Amdinocillin is not absorbed following oral administration and must be administered parenterally.

Transient high blood concentrations of penicillin G can be produced by injecting an aqueous solution intravenously or intramuscularly every three to six hours. However, intramuscular administration is irritating and painful. When large doses (eg, 10 million units or more daily) are required, penicillin G must be given intravenously. High tissue levels can be obtained after continuous or intermittent intravenous infusion. Intrathecal injection should never be used because of the irritant effect of even small doses on the central nervous system.

When more sustained effects are desired, less soluble repository preparations may be given intramuscularly for infections caused by susceptible micro-organisms. Penicillin G procaine can be given every 6 to 12 hours or even once daily, depending upon the infection and the dose needed. Penicillin G benzathine provides detectable blood levels for as long as four weeks after a single intramuscular injection. However,

because the blood levels produced are low, this form of penicillin is effective against only very susceptible organisms such as *Treponema pallidum* (see also the Uses section).

Penicillin preparations for topical use are no longer marketed in the United States, since hypersensitization is a frequent complication.

Distribution: Plasma protein binding of the penicillins varies widely (see Table 1). Only the free drug has antibacterial activity. However, the protein-penicillin complex dissociates readily and, as free drug is withdrawn from plasma, additional penicillin is unbound from protein stores.

The penicillins are well distributed to most areas of the body, including lung, liver, kidney, muscle, bone, and placenta. High concentrations are achieved in urine. Most of these agents, especially ampicillin, amoxicillin, nafcillin, piperacillin, mezlocillin, and azlocillin, are present in the bile in concentrations well above the minimal inhibitory levels for most sensitive organisms and are reabsorbed from the intestine. In the presence of inflammation, concentrations achieved in synovial, pericardial, pleural, and peritoneal fluids and the middle ear are sufficient to inhibit most bacteria. Diffusion into cerebrospinal fluid, the eye, and the prostate is poor, even when very large doses are given, unless inflammation is present.

Penicillins cross the placenta. Compounds with low protein binding may produce fetal serum concentrations equivalent to those in the maternal serum 30 to 60 minutes after injection. Highly protein-bound penicillins achieve only low concentrations in both the fetal serum and the amniotic fluid.

Elimination: Most penicillins are excreted rapidly in the urine, primarily as unchanged drug. Active renal tubular secretion is the predominant mechanism; probenecid delays excretion. The rate of elimination is decreased in newborns because of reduced renal function. Only nafcillin is excreted primarily by the liver; 60% of a dose is metabolized. Penicillin V and oxacillin also are metabolized significantly. Other penicillins are metabolized to a minor degree. Biliary excretion of penicillins does occur, but probably is important only for nafcillin, mezlocillin, azlocillin, and piperacillin.

The dosage of some penicillins should be adjusted if renal function is impaired. Creatinine clearance rates of 30 to 50 ml/min require dosage modification of carbenicillin and ticarcillin; rates of 10 ml/min or less require that the dosage of all penicillins, except the isoxazolyl compounds (oxacillin, cloxacillin, dicloxacillin) and nafcillin, be reduced or given at longer intervals (see the evaluations).

Protein Bound (%)	Metabolized (%)	Urinary Recovery (%)	Approximate Half-life (hours)	Volume of Distribution (L/kg)
5–10	---	75–90	0.8–1	---

Drug Evaluations

NATURAL PENICILLINS

PENICILLIN G

Penicillin G is a naturally derived (from *Penicillium chrysogenum*) antibiotic for oral and parenteral use.

MECHANISM OF ACTION, ANTIMICROBIAL SPECTRUM, AND RESISTANCE. Penicillin G inhibits cell wall formation in susceptible bacteria and usually is bactericidal.

This antibiotic is active in vitro against most gram-positive bacteria (except β lactamase-producing staphylococci), gram-negative cocci, and anaerobic bacteria (except the *Bacteroides fragilis* group). Spirochetes and certain gram-negative bacilli also are susceptible. However, the Enterobacteriaceae and *Pseudomonas aeruginosa* are resistant.

Penicillin G is hydrolized by β lactamases produced by various bacteria, including *Staphylococcus aureus*, *Neisseria gonorrhoeae*, and *Haemophilus influenzae*, and is not active against these strains.

For a detailed discussion of the mechanism of action, antimicrobial spectrum, and resistance properties of the penicillins, see the Introduction.

USES. Penicillin G has a high therapeutic/toxic ratio and its cost to the patient is relatively low. It is frequently the drug of choice for infections caused by susceptible organisms in nonallergic patients. Infections for which penicillin G is a preferred drug include group A beta hemolytic streptococcal infections (eg, pyodermas, pharyngitis), pneumococcal pneumonia and meningitis, meningococcal meningitis, gonococcal infections, syphilis, penicillin-sensitive streptococcal (eg, viridans streptococci, *S. bovis*) endocarditis, enterococcal endocarditis (in combination with streptomycin or gentamicin), anaerobic infections above the diaphragm, and other less common infections, such as anthrax, clostridial myonecrosis (gas gangrene), diphtheria (as adjunct to antitoxin), tetanus (as adjunct to human hyperimmune globulin), erysipeloid, *Pasteurella multocida* infections, rat bite fever, actinomycosis, leptospirosis, yaws, and meningitis and arthritis associated with Lyme disease. For detailed discussions, see the Introduction; see also Chapter 65, Antimicrobial Therapy and Chemoprophylaxis of Infectious Diseases.

Penicillin G is available in oral and parenteral form and as repository salts. Drug selection usually depends on the severity of the infection being treated. Since oral preparations are absorbed erratically and penicillin G is destroyed by gastric acid, this route should be used only for mild or stabilized infections and long-term prophylaxis. The drug should be taken one hour before or two hours after a meal. Penicillin V generally is preferred for oral administration because it results in more reliable bioavailability and can be administered with food (see the evaluation).

Aqueous crystalline penicillin G, available as the potassium (usually preferred) or sodium salt, is administered intramuscularly or intravenously to produce high serum concentrations rapidly. When large doses are indicated for severe infections (eg, pneumococcal meningitis, enterococcal endocarditis, gas gangrene), the intravenous route should be used.

Because aqueous crystalline penicillin G is rapidly eliminated from the body by renal tubular secretion (eg, half-life, 30 minutes in patients with normal renal function), frequent dosing is necessary. The concomitant administration of probenecid will prolong the half-life of penicillin G by competitive inhibition of active tubular secretion.

Penicillin G procaine and penicillin G benzathine are poorly soluble repository forms of penicillin G that are administered intramuscularly. They provide tissue depots from which active drug can be absorbed over a period of hours (penicillin G procaine) or days (penicillin G benzathine). Thus, they are useful for certain infections caused by sensitive organisms when prolonged therapeutic blood levels are desirable (and achievable) but the frequent dosing requirements of aqueous crystalline penicillin G can be avoided. Uses of procaine penicillin G include uncomplicated gonococcal infections, some cases (eg, uncomplicated) of pneumococcal pneumonia, moderately severe group A β hemolytic streptococcal infections (eg, skin, soft tissue), penicillin-sensitive streptococcal endocarditis (combined with streptomycin), and other less common infections. Penicillin G benzathine is used in streptococcal pharyngitis, syphilis, and for the secondary prophylaxis of rheumatic fever.

For additional discussion, see the Introduction; see also Chapter 65.

ADVERSE REACTIONS AND PRECAUTIONS. Hypersensitivity reactions are the most common adverse effects of penicillin G (see the Introduction), and this drug should be avoided in patients known to be allergic to penicillins. An alternative antibacterial agent, selected on the basis of organism susceptibility and the type and severity of infection involved, should be given to patients with a history of penicillin allergy. Examples include (1) erythromycin for pharyngitis due to *Streptococcus pyogenes* or pneumonia due to *Streptococcus pneumoniae;* (2) first generation cephalosporins (eg, cefazolin, cephalothin, cephapirin) for certain serious streptococcal (eg, endocarditis due to viridans streptococci) and most staphylococcal infections; (3) clindamycin for anaerobic infections and some staphylococcal infections; (4) chloramphenicol for meningitis due to *S. pneumoniae* and *Neisseria meningitidis;* (5) tetracyclines for gonorrhea and syphilis; and (6) vancomycin for enterococcal endocarditis. Because cross-sensitivity between penicillins and cephalosporins exists in some individuals, patients with immediate-type hypersensitivity reactions to penicillin should not receive cephalosporins.

When a hypersensitivity reaction to penicillin G occurs, the drug should be discontinued immediately and appropriate ameliorative treatment given if necessary (see the Introduction). In most instances, discontinuation of penicillin G is sufficient. If further treatment is necessary, another antibacterial agent should be substituted based on the criteria listed above.

High-dose therapy in neonates or in patients with renal disease or rapid intravenous administration of more than 20 million units daily may produce convulsions; intravenous doses larger than this have been used to treat endocarditis caused by sensitive organisms, but this is rarely necessary. Intrathecal administration is not justified.

For a detailed discussion of the adverse reactions and precautions, see the Introduction.

In addition to the standard adverse reactions associated with penicillin G, the procaine component of penicillin G procaine has been associated with immediate, but transient, mental disturbances after injection of large single doses (eg, 4.8 million units). The Jarisch-Herxheimer reaction has been reported in patients treated for syphilis with penicillin G benzathine.

DRUG INTERACTIONS AND INTERFERENCE WITH LABORATORY TESTS. See the Introduction.

PHARMACOKINETICS. Penicillin G can be administered orally, intramuscularly, and intravenously. Oral preparations are susceptible to destruction by gastric acid and are absorbed erratically and incompletely; usually, between 20% and 30% of an oral dose is absorbed, primarily in the duodenum. Following a dose of 500 mg (800,000 units) in fasting adults, peak serum levels of total drug range between 1.5 and 2.5 mcg/ml after 30 to 60 minutes; peak levels of free drug are between 0.6 and 1 mcg/ml. Absorption in neonates and the elderly is greater because gastric pH is higher. The presence of food in the gastrointestinal tract decreases absorption; penicillin G should be administered either one hour before or two to three hours after a meal.

Peak serum levels are attained approximately 15 to 30 minutes after intramuscular injection and immediately after intravenous administration of aqueous crystalline penicillin G. Levels usually are about four- to fivefold higher than those following oral administration. For example, a 625-mg (1,000,000 units) intravenous dose of aqueous crystalline penicillin G results in a total peak serum level of about 10 mcg/ml.

About 60% of circulating penicillin G is bound to plasma protein, primarily albumin. The volume of distribution approximates that of the extracellular fluid volume, ie, 0.2 L/kg. The drug readily distributes to many tissues (eg, muscle, lung, liver, kidney, bone) and body fluids (eg, interstitial, synovial, pericardial, peritoneal, pleural). High concentrations are achieved in bile and urine. Penetration into cerebrospinal fluid, the aqueous humor, and the prostate is poor in the absence of inflammation, but therapeutic concentrations can be achieved for susceptible organisms in the presence of inflammation. Penicillin G crosses the placenta.

Penicillin G is rapidly eliminated. Following parenteral administration, between 60% and 90% of a dose is excreted in the urine within one hour, primarily by renal tubular secretion. Excretion is delayed by probenecid. Additionally, a small percentage of drug is eliminated via the bile, and up to 20% is metabolized to inactive penicilloic acid derivatives. The beta phase elimination half-life is approximately 0.5 hours in patients with normal renal function. The half-life is prolonged in patients with renal impairment (eg, 6 to 10 hours in anuric patients) and dosage adjustments are necessary. Because of incompletely developed renal function in young infants and deteriorating renal function in the elderly, the half-life of penicillin G is longer in these patients.

The elimination of oral penicillin G is the same as for the parenteral form. However, only about 20% of a dose is recovered from urine as unchanged drug because of limited gastrointestinal absorption. Most unabsorbed penicillin G is inactivated by bacteria in the colon; the amount of unchanged drug in feces is low.

Penicillin G Procaine: This repository form of penicillin G slowly releases active drug from the tissue depot at the site of intramuscular injection. A plateau-type of peak serum level (eg, approximately 3 mcg/ml after a 750-mg [1.2 million units] dose) is reached after one to three hours and falls slowly over 15 to 20 hours. Usually 60% to 90% of a dose is excreted in the urine within 24 to 36 hours, but drug may be detected in serum five to seven days after injection. Although penicillin G procaine does not result in the rapid, high serum concentrations that can be achieved with an equivalent parenteral dose of aqueous crystalline penicillin G, it provides a more prolonged therapeutic serum level for certain susceptible microorganisms (see the Uses section and the Introduction). Thus, a longer, more convenient dosing interval can be used.

Penicillin G Benzathine: This repository form of penicillin G very slowly releases active drug from the tissue depot at the site of intramuscular injection. The result is a low peak serum level (eg, 0.1 mcg/ml 24 hours after a 750-mg [1,200,000 units] dose), but a very flat serum concentration versus time curve. Serum levels of penicillin G are detectable for up to 30 days. These prolonged, low serum levels are therapeutically effective for certain infections caused by highly susceptible microorganisms (eg, syphilis due to *Treponema pallidum*, pharyngitis due to *Streptococcus pyogenes*) and obviate the need for more frequent dosing intervals (see the Uses section and the Introduction).

DOSAGE AND PREPARATIONS. To convert units of penicillin G to milligrams, 1 unit is equivalent to 0.6 mcg.

PENICILLIN G POTASSIUM:

Oral: A dose is administered one hour before or two hours after meals. *Adults and children over 12 years*, 1.6 to 3.2 million units daily in divided doses four times daily (The Medical Letter, 1984); *children under 12 years*, 40,000 to 80,000 units/kg daily in divided doses every six to eight hours (Nelson, 1985 A).

> **Generic.** Powder (for oral solution) 250,000 and 400,000 units/5 ml; powder (for oral suspension) 250,000 and 400,000 units/5 ml; tablets 200,000, 250,000, 400,000, 500,000, 800,000, and 1,000,000 units; tablets (buffered) 200,000, 250,000, and 400,000 units.
>
> **Pentids, Pentids 400, Pentids 800** (Squibb). Powder (for syrup, buffered) 200,000 and 400,000 units/5 ml; tablets (buffered) 200,000, 400,000, and 800,000 units.
>
> **Additional Trademarks.**
>
> **Pfizerpen G** (Pfipharmecs), **SK-Penicillin G** (Smith Kline & French).

PENICILLIN G SODIUM, POTASSIUM:

Intramuscular, Intravenous: Total daily dosage and route of administration depend on the type and severity of infection. For example, high-dose intravenous penicillin G is used in meningitis (eg, pneumococcal, meningococcal), some forms of endocarditis (eg, enterococcal) and severe clostridial infections.

Adults, 1.2 to 24 million units daily (The Medical Letter, 1984). Daily dosage can be given intermittently in equally divided doses at four (range, two to six)-hour intervals or by constant intravenous infusion. Large doses (10 to 20 million units daily) should be given intravenously.

Children, 100,000 to 250,000 units/kg daily in divided doses every four hours (Nelson, 1985 A).

Infants over 7 days and weighing more than 2 kg, 100,000 units/kg daily in divided doses every six hours; for meningitis, 200,000 units/kg daily in divided doses every six hours; *over 7 days and weighing less than 2 kg,* 75,000 units/kg daily in divided doses every eight hours; for meningitis, 150,000 units/kg daily in divided doses every eight hours; *under 7 days and weighing more than 2 kg,* 50,000 units/kg daily in divided doses every 8 hours; for meningitis, 150,000 units/kg daily in divided doses every eight hours; *under 7 days and weighing less than 2 kg,* 50,000 units/kg daily in divided doses every 12 hours; for meningitis, 100,000 units/kg daily in divided doses every 12 hours (Nelson, 1985 B).

For dosage guidelines in gonococcal infections and syphilis, see Chapter 65, Table 2.

> PENICILLIN G (AQUEOUS) POTASSIUM:
> **Generic.** Powder (sterile) 200,000, 500,000, and 1, 5, 10, and 20 million units; powder (buffered) 1 and 5 million units.
>
> PENICILLIN G (AQUEOUS) SODIUM:
> **Generic.** Powder (sterile) 5 million units.

PROCAINE PENICILLIN G:

Intramuscular: Adults and children, 600,000 to 1.2 million units daily in one or two doses depending upon the condition being treated. Ten days to two weeks of therapy is usually sufficient. *Newborn infants,* 50,000 units/kg once daily.

Certain patients with infective endocarditis caused by penicillin-sensitive streptococci (eg, most viridans streptococci, *S. bovis*) have been successfully treated with procaine penicillin G 1.2 million units four times daily for two to four weeks plus streptomycin 500 mg twice daily for the initial two weeks (see Chapter 65, Table 1).

For dosage guidelines in the treatment of gonorrhea and syphilis, see Chapter 65, Table 2.

> **Generic.** Suspension (sterile) 300,000 units/ml in 10 ml containers.
>
> **Crysticillin 300 A.S.** (Squibb), **Duracillin A.S.** (Lilly). Suspension (sterile, aqueous) 300,000 units/ml in 10 ml containers.
>
> **Crysticillin 600 A.S.** (Squibb). Suspension (sterile, aqueous) 500,000 units/ml in 12 ml containers.
>
> **Pfizerpen-AS** (Pfipharmecs). Suspension (aqueous) 300,000 units/ml in 10 ml containers.
>
> **Wycillin** (Wyeth). Suspension (sterile, aqueous) 600,000 units/ml in 1, 2, and 4 ml containers.

BENZATHINE PENICILLIN G:

Intramuscular: Adults, 1.2 million units in a single dose; *older children,* a single injection of 900,000 units; *infants and children weighing less than 27.3 kg,* a single dose of 50,000 units/kg.

For dosage guidelines in the treatment of syphilis, see Chapter 65, Table 2.

For dosage guidelines in the prophylaxis of rheumatic fever, see Chapter 65, Table 3.

> **Bicillin L-A** (Wyeth). Suspension (sterile) 300,000 units/ml in 10 ml containers, 600,000 units/ml in 1, 2, and 4 ml containers.
>
> **Permapen** (Pfipharmecs). Suspension (aqueous) 600,000 units/ml in 2 ml containers.

Oral: Although an oral preparation of benzathine penicillin G is available, it has no recommended indications and dosages are not presented.

> **Bicillin** (Wyeth). Tablets 200,000 units.

COMBINATIONS OF PENICILLIN G:

Combinations of procaine penicillin G and benzathine penicillin G are marketed for the convenience of physicians who believe that they may be helpful in situations requiring both immediate and long-term effects when the patient cannot conveniently return for care. In general, however, it is preferable to administer penicillins as single-entity preparations for specific indications. Thus, dosage recommendations are not given.

> **Bicillin C-R** (Wyeth). Suspension (aqueous) containing benzathine penicillin G and procaine penicillin G 150,000 units/ml each in 10 ml containers or 300,000 units/ml each in 1, 2, and 4 ml containers.
>
> **Bicillin C-R 900/300** (Wyeth). Suspension (aqueous) containing benzathine penicillin G 900,000 units and procaine penicillin G 300,000 units/2 ml in 2 ml containers.

PENICILLIN V

POTASSIUM PENICILLIN V

[Ledercillin VK, Pen-Vee K, SK-Penicillin VK, V-Cillin K, Veetids]

Penicillin V (phenoxymethyl penicillin) is a semisynthetic derivative for oral use.

MECHANISM OF ACTION, ANTIMICROBIAL SPECTRUM, AND RESISTANCE. The activity of penicillin V against most gram-positive bacteria is comparable to that of penicillin G. However, this semisynthetic derivative is less active against gram-negative micro-organisms (eg, *Neisseria, Haemophilus*).

Penicillin V is sensitive to β lactamases and β lactamase-producing strains of various bacteria (eg, most staphylococci) are resistant.

For a detailed discussion of the mechanism of action, antimicrobial spectrum, and resistance properties of the penicillins, see the Introduction.

USES. Penicillin V usually is preferred to penicillin G when oral administration is indicated because it is more reliably absorbed and can be administered with food (see Pharmacokinetics below). Major uses of penicillin V include group A β-hemolytic streptococcal pharyngitis (10-day course), mild streptococcal pyodermas, mild respiratory tract infections caused by *Streptococcus pneumoniae*, secondary prophylaxis of rheumatic fever (penicillin G benzathine preferred), and oral prophylaxis of infective endocarditis in certain high-risk patients prior to dental procedures or upper respiratory tract surgery or instrumentation.

For a more detailed discussion, see the Introduction; see also Chapter 65, Antimicrobial Therapy and Chemoprophylaxis of Infectious Diseases.

ADVERSE REACTIONS AND PRECAUTIONS. Hypersensitivity reactions are the most common adverse effects. For a discussion of these and other adverse reactions, see the Introduction.

DRUG INTERACTIONS AND INTERFERENCE WITH LABORATORY TESTS. See the Introduction.

PHARMACOKINETICS. In contrast to penicillin G, penicillin V is stable in gastric acid. Approximately 60% of an orally administered dose is absorbed from the gastrointestinal tract, primarily from the duodenum. Following a dose of 500 mg (800,000 units), peak serum levels of total drug range from 3 to 5 mcg/ml after 30 to 60 minutes; peak levels of free drug are about 0.8 mcg/ml. Unlike penicillin G, the presence of food in the gastrointestinal tract does not decrease absorption appreciably. The potassium salt of penicillin V is better absorbed than other salts.

Because penicillin V produces total serum levels that are two- to fivefold higher than comparable doses of penicillin G and because it exhibits less individual variability in absorption, it often is preferred for oral administration. However, larger doses of oral penicillin G should produce comparable therapeutic results. When higher serum levels are required (eg, for more serious infections), parenteral penicillin G is indicated.

Like other penicillins, penicillin V primarily distributes into the extracellular fluid volume and is eliminated rapidly by renal tubular secretion. The half-life is 30 to 60 minutes; probenecid delays elimination. Approximately 55% of a dose of penicillin V is metabolized to penicilloic acid derivatives, however. For additional discussion, see the Introduction.

DOSAGE AND PREPARATIONS.
Oral: Adults, 125 to 500 mg four times daily. In the presence of severe renal impairment (creatinine clearance, 10 ml/min or less), the dose probably should not exceed 250 mg every six hours. *Children,* 25 to 50 mg/kg daily in divided doses every six to eight hours. The duration of treatment for streptococcal pharyngitis should be ten days.

For dosage guidelines in the prophylaxis of bacterial endocarditis in high-risk patients prior to dental procedures or surgery or instrumentation of the upper respiratory tract and for the prophylaxis of rheumatic fever, see Chapter 65, Table 3.

PENICILLIN V:
Generic. Powder for oral solution (plain, buffered) and oral suspension 125 and 250 mg/5 ml; tablets 125, 250, and 500 mg.
POTASSIUM PENICILLIN V:
Generic. Powder for oral solution 125 and 250 mg/5 ml; tablets 250 and 500 mg.
Ledercillin VK (Lederle), **SK-Penicillin VK** (Smith Kline & French), **Veetids** (Squibb). Powder for oral solution 125 and 250 mg/5 ml; tablets 250 and 500 mg.
Pen-Vee K (Wyeth), **V-Cillin K** (Lilly). Powder for oral solution 125 and 250 mg/5 ml; tablets 125, 250, and 500 mg.

Additional Trademarks.
Beepen-VK (Beecham), **Betapen-VK** (Bristol), **Pfizerpen VK** (Pfipharmecs), **Repen-VK** (Reid-Provident), **Robicillin VK** (Robins), **Uticillin VK** (Upjohn).

PENICILLINASE-RESISTANT (ANTISTAPHYLOCOCCAL) PENICILLINS

METHICILLIN SODIUM
[Staphcillin]

Methicillin sodium is a water-soluble, penicillinase-resistant semisynthetic salt for parenteral use.

MECHANISM OF ACTION, ANTIMICROBIAL SPECTRUM, AND RESISTANCE. Methicillin is active against most *Staphylococcus aureus*, including β lactamase-producing strains. Many strains of *S. epidermidis* also are sensitive. Because most staphylococci produce β lactamase and are resistant to penicillin G, the penicillinase-resistant penicillins are primary drugs for infections caused by these pathogens (see Uses). Most streptococci, including *S. pyogenes, S. pneumoniae*, and viridans streptococci, also are susceptible to the antistaphylococcal penicillins. However, penicillin G is more potent against streptococci and is preferred clinically. Enterococci are resistant to methicillin. Gram-negative bacteria generally are resistant.

In recent years, methicillin-resistant strains of *Staphylococcus aureus* have been increasing in the United States. The Centers for Disease Control has determined that the proportion of methicillin-resistant isolates in hospitals doubled (from 2.4% to 4.9%) between 1975 and 1980. These resistant strains also occur in the community. Methicillin resistance is even more common among strains of *S. epidermidis*, which is a primary pathogen in infections associated with prosthetic devices and other foreign bodies. Staphylococcal resistance to methicillin is due to decreased affinity of the drug for penicillin-binding proteins (PBPs) present in these resistant strains. Such strains also are resistant to the other penicillinase-resistant penicillins and to the cephalosporins, although this may not be reliably demonstrated by routine in vitro antimicrobial susceptibility tests. Presently, vancomycin is the drug of choice for infections caused by these pathogens (see Lowy and Hammer, 1983; Neu, 1984 B; Sheagren, 1984; Thornsberry, 1984).

For additional discussion of the mechanism of action, antimicrobial spectrum, and resistance properties of the penicillins, see the Introduction.

USES. Penicillinase-resistant (antistaphylococcal) penicillins are recommended only for infections known or suspected to be caused by penicillinase-producing staphylococci. Since most strains of *S. aureus* are now resistant to penicillin G, antistaphylococcal penicillins are usually drugs of choice for most *S. aureus* infections. Penicillin G is preferred when susceptibility is confirmed. Methicillin-resistant *S. aureus* are increasing, however, and may represent a significant proportion of staphylococcal strains in some hospitals. Vancomycin is required for these organisms.

Parenteral penicillinase-resistant penicillins are used for serious *S. aureus* infections, such as bacteremias, endocarditis, meningitis, osteomyelitis, septic arthritis, pneumonia, empyema, severe pyodermas, and renal abscess. Nafcillin and oxacillin usually are preferred to methicillin in adults because of the association of interstitial nephritis with the latter agent (see Adverse Reactions and Precautions). Methicillin is used in neonates, however, because interstitial nephritis is rare in this age group. For additional discussion, see the Introduction; Chapter 65, Antimicrobial Therapy and Chemoprophylaxis of Infectious Diseases; and the evaluations of Nafcillin and Oxacillin; see also Neu, 1982 B; Molavi and LeFrock, 1984; and Sheagren, 1984.

Parenteral penicillinase-resistant penicillins also are preferred for susceptible *S. epidermidis* infections. However, methicillin-resistant strains of this pathogen are common. Thus, vancomycin appears to be the antibiotic of choice for empiric therapy of *S. epidermidis* infections pending the availability of accurate susceptibility data (Lowy and Hammer, 1983; Thornsberry, 1984; see also Chapters 65 and 72, Miscellaneous Antibacterial Agents).

ADVERSE REACTIONS AND PRECAUTIONS. Methicillin generally is well tolerated; untoward effects are usually mild and most commonly consist of allergic reactions typical of all penicillins (see the Introduction).

Interstitial nephritis has been associated with use of methicillin more frequently than with other antistaphylococcal penicillins. The incidence appears to be greater in males than in females. Methicillin-induced nephrotoxicity may develop at any age (but is uncommon in neonates) and is not dose-related. The disease begins 2 to 37 days (mean, 15 days) after initiation of therapy and is characterized by fever, rash, eosinophilia, hematuria, proteinuria, leukocyturia, and eosinophiluria. Ultimately, the reaction can progress to renal failure. Biopsy of the kidney routinely shows an interstitial infiltrate of mononuclear and eosinophilic cells with tubular damage, but no glomerular lesions. In most cases, renal function returns to normal when the drug is discontinued. The mechanism is unknown, but interstitial nephritis may be a hypersensitivity reaction because of the lack of a dose relationship, the presence of rash and eosinophilia, the renal pathology, and

the occurrence of cross-sensitivity in some patients when another penicillin was substituted (Ditlove et al, 1977).

Hemorrhagic cystitis has been reported with methicillin and is most likely to occur in patients with low urine output given large doses. The mechanism is unknown.

DRUG INTERACTIONS AND INTERFERENCE WITH LABORATORY TESTS. See the Introduction.

PHARMACOKINETICS. Methicillin is labile in gastric acid and is not absorbed following oral administration. Thus, it must be administered parenterally. Peak serum levels of 12 to 17 mcg/ml are attained 30 to 60 minutes after intramuscular injection of 1 g. After an intravenous dose of 1 g, peak serum levels range between 20 and 40 mcg/ml.

Between 35% and 40% of circulating methicillin is bound to plasma protein, primarily albumin. Methicillin exhibits the lowest plasma protein binding among the antistaphylococcal penicillins. Like other penicillins, this drug primarily distributes into the extracellular fluid volume.

Methicillin is rapidly eliminated primarily by renal tubular secretion; probenecid delays excretion. Approximately 80% of a dose is recovered as unchanged drug in the urine; less than 10% is metabolized. The half-life in patients with normal renal function is approximately 30 minutes. The half-life is prolonged in patients with renal impairment (eg, about 4 hours in anuric patients) and dosage adjustments are necessary. For additional discussion, see the Introduction.

DOSAGE AND PREPARATIONS. Methicillin can be administered by intramuscular injection (solution containing 500 mg/ml), direct intravenous injection (solution containing 20 mg/ml at the rate of 10 ml/minute), or by continuous intravenous drip. See the manufacturer's instructions for the appropriate dilution of the drug, a list of compatible diluents and intravenous solutions, and stability of methicillin in these solutions. When used in conjunction with other drugs, methicillin should not be physically mixed with the other agent(s).

Intramuscular, Intravenous: Adults, 4 to 12 g daily in equally divided doses every four to six hours (The Medical Letter, 1984). In those with severe renal impairment (creatinine clearance, 10 ml/min or less), the dose of methicillin probably should not exceed 2 g every twelve hours (The Medical Letter, 1984).

Children, 100 to 200 mg/kg daily in equally divided doses every four to six hours (The Medical Letter, 1984).

Infants over 7 days and weighing more than 2 kg, 100 mg/kg daily in divided doses every six hours; for meningitis, 200 mg/kg daily in divided doses every six hours; *infants over 7 days and weighing less than 2 kg,* 75 mg/kg daily in divided doses every eight hours; for meningitis, 150 mg/kg daily in divided doses every eight hours; *infants under 7 days and weighing more than 2 kg,* 75 mg/kg daily in divided doses every eight hours; for meningitis, 150 mg/kg daily in divided doses every eight hours; *infants under 7 days and weighing less than 2 kg,* 50 mg/kg daily in divided doses every 12 hours; for meningitis, 100 mg/kg daily in divided doses every 12 hours (Nelson, 1985 B).

Staphcillin (Bristol). Powder (buffered) 1, 4, 6, and 10 g (900 mg methicillin base with 3 mEq sodium/g).

NAFCILLIN SODIUM
[Nafcil, Nallpen, Unipen]

This semisynthetic penicillin is highly resistant to staphylococcal β lactamases and is usually administered parenterally. It is stable in gastric acid, but is absorbed more erratically after oral administration than most other penicillinase-resistant penicillins (eg, dicloxacillin, cloxacillin); therefore, the oral route is not recommended.

MECHANISM OF ACTION, ANTIMICROBIAL SPECTRUM, AND RESISTANCE. The mechanism of action, antimicrobial spectrum, and resistance properties are the same as for methicillin (see that evaluation and the Introduction). On a weight basis, nafcillin is more potent than methicillin in vitro against susceptible bacteria.

USES. The indications for parenteral nafcillin are the same as those for methicillin with the primary use being serious infections caused by *Staphylococcus aureus* (see the evaluation on Methicillin). Nafcillin (or oxacillin) usually is preferred to methicillin in adults and older children because of the association of interstitial nephritis with the latter agent. However, nafcillin usually is not recommended in neonates or patients with hepatic disease. Nafcillin pharmacokinetics in the newborn are erratic, especially in those with jaundice.

For additional discussion, see the Introduction; Chapter 65, Antimicrobial Therapy and Chemoprophylaxis of Infectious Diseases; and the evaluations on Methicillin and Oxacillin. See also Neu, 1982 B; Molavi and LeFrock, 1984; and Sheagren, 1984.

ADVERSE REACTIONS AND PRECAUTIONS. Nafcillin generally is well tolerated; untoward effects are usually mild and most commonly consist of allergic reactions typical of all penicillins (see the Introduction). Neutropenia, which is immediately reversible on discontinuation of the drug, has been reported in 10% to 20% of patients receiving 150 to 200 mg/kg daily for 10 to 14 days or longer (Conte and Barriere, 1984).

DRUG INTERACTIONS AND INTERFERENCE WITH LABORATORY TESTS. See the Introduction.

PHARMACOKINETICS. Although nafcillin is available for oral administration, absorption is usually low (10% to 20% of a dose) and erratic. Thus, this antistaphylococcal penicillin primarily is administered parenterally. Peak serum levels of 5 to 8 mcg/ml are attained 60 minutes after intramuscular injection of 500 mg. After an intravenous dose of 15 mg/kg, peak serum levels range between 20 and 40 mcg/ml.

Between 87% and 90% of circulating nafcillin is bound to plasma protein, primarily albumin. Nafcillin exhibits significantly greater plasma protein binding than methicillin, but is less protein bound than the isoxazolyl derivatives. Like other penicillins, nafcillin primarily distributes into the extracellular fluid volume. Concentrations achieved in bile in the absence of obstruction are higher than for other antistaphylococcal penicillins. Penetration into cerebrospinal fluid is adequate in the presence of inflammation (see Molavi and LeFrock, 1984).

Unlike other penicillins, nafcillin is primarily excreted by the liver and, to a lesser extent, by the kidney. In patients with normal renal and liver function, approximately 60% of a dose is metabolized in the liver, about 10% is eliminated unchanged in bile, and approximately 30% is recovered in urine. The beta phase elimination half-life is about 30 minutes; it is increased minimally (to 80 minutes) in anuric patients. Thus, dosage adjustments are not required in these patients. However, dosage adjustments are necessary if there also is coexisting hepatic dysfunction. For additional discussion, see the Introduction.

DOSAGE AND PREPARATIONS.
Oral: Serum levels of nafcillin after oral administration are low and unpredictable, and this route is not recommended. The following dosages are included only for completeness. Nafcillin should be administered at least one hour before or two hours after meals. *Adults,* 2 to 4 g daily in equally divided doses every six hours; *children,* 50 to 100 mg/kg daily in four divided doses every six hours.
Strengths expressed in terms of the base:
Unipen (Wyeth). Capsules (buffered) 250 mg; powder for oral solution 250 mg/5 ml; tablets (buffered) 500 mg.
Intramuscular, Intravenous: Nafcillin can be administered by intramuscular injection (solution containing 250 mg/ml), direct intravenous injection (required amount of drug diluted in 15 to 30 ml and injected over 5 to 10 minutes), or by continuous intravenous drip. See the manufacturers' instructions for the appropriate dilution of the drug, a list of compatible diluents and intravenous solutions, and stability of nafcillin in these solutions. When used in conjunction with other drugs, nafcillin should not be physically mixed with the other agent(s).

Adults, 2 to 9 g daily in equally divided doses every four to six hours; up to 12 g daily can be given for severe infections (The Medical Letter, 1984). *Children,* 100 to 200 mg/kg daily in equally divided doses every four to six hours (The Medical Letter, 1984). Although nafcillin generally is not recommended for newborn infants, the following dosage guidelines are presented: *infants over 7 days and weighing more than 2 kg,* 75 mg/kg daily in divided doses every six hours; *infants over 7 days and weighing less than 2 kg,* 75 mg/kg daily in divided doses every eight hours; *infants under 7 days and weighing more than 2 kg,* 50 mg/kg daily in divided doses every eight hours; *infants under 7 days and weighing less than 2 kg,* 50 mg/kg daily in divided doses every 12 hours (Nelson, 1985 B).

Dosage adjustments are not required in patients with impaired renal function.
Strengths expressed in terms of the base:
Nafcil (Bristol), *Nallpen* (Beecham). Powder (buffered) 500 mg and 1, 2, and 10 g (sodium, 2.9 mEq/g).
Unipen (Wyeth). Powder (buffered) 500 mg and 1, 1.5, 2, 4, and 10 g (sodium, 2.9 mEq/g).

OXACILLIN SODIUM
[Bactocill, Prostaphlin]

Oxacillin is a semisynthetic, penicillinase-resistant penicillin for parenteral or oral use. This isoxazolyl derivative is chemically related to cloxacillin and dicloxacillin.

MECHANISM OF ACTION, ANTIMICROBIAL SPECTRUM, AND RESISTANCE. The mechanism of action, antimicrobial spectrum, and resistance properties are the same as for methicillin (see that evaluation and the Introduction). On a weight basis, oxacillin is more potent than methicillin in vitro against susceptible bacteria.

USES. The indications for parenteral oxacillin are the same as those for methicillin, with the primary use being serious infections caused by *Staphylococcus aureus* (see the evaluation on Methicillin). Oxacillin (or nafcillin) usually is preferred to methicillin in adults and older children because of the association of interstitial nephritis with the latter agent. Oral oxacillin is an alternative to dicloxacillin and cloxacillin for the treatment of mild to moderate *S. aureus* infections of the skin and soft tissues, respiratory and genitourinary tracts, and joints.

For additional discussion, see the Introduction; Chapter 65, Antimicrobial Therapy and Chemoprophylaxis of Infectious Diseases; and the evaluations on Methicillin, Nafcillin, Cloxacillin, and Dicloxacillin. See also Neu, 1982 B; Molavi and LeFrock, 1984; and Sheagren, 1984.

ADVERSE REACTIONS AND PRECAUTIONS. Oxacillin is generally well tolerated; untoward effects are usually mild and most commonly consist of allergic reactions typical of all penicillins (see the Introduction). Elevations in hepatic enzymes (eg, SGOT) have been reported more frequently with oxacillin than other antistaphylococcal penicillins. Reversible cholestatic hepatitis also has occurred. Abnormal results of liver function tests are reversible when the drug is discontinued (see Neu, 1982 B).

DRUG INTERACTIONS AND INTERFERENCE WITH LABORATORY TESTS. See the Introduction.

PHARMACOKINETICS. Oxacillin can be administered orally, intramuscularly, and intravenously. Although oxacillin is stable in gastric acid, only about 30% of an oral dose is absorbed by the gastrointestinal tract. Following administration of 500 mg to fasting individuals, total peak serum levels of 4 to 6 mcg/ml are attained in about one hour; peak levels of free drug are approximately 0.6 mcg/ml. Although peak serum levels of total (ie, bound and unbound) oxacillin are lower than with equivalent doses of cloxacillin and dicloxacillin, the levels of free drug are similar for all three derivatives due to differences in plasma protein binding. The presence of food decreases the absorption of oxacillin and this drug should be administered on an empty stomach, preferably one hour before or two hours after meals.

Following intramuscular injection of 500 mg, peak serum levels of 14 to 16 mcg/ml are achieved after 30 to 60 minutes. A peak serum level of approximately 40 mcg/ml is obtained after a 1-g intravenous dose.

Between 90% and 93% of circulating oxacillin is bound to plasma protein, but it is the least bound of the isoxazolyl penicillin derivatives (see evaluations of Cloxacillin and Dicloxacillin). Like other penicillins, oxacillin primarily distributes into the extracellular fluid volume.

Oxacillin is rapidly eliminated, primarily by renal tubular secretion; probenecid delays excretion. Between 30% and 50% is recovered from urine as unchanged drug. Oxacillin is metabolized to a greater extent than other isoxazolyl penicillins; between 45% and 50% of a dose is metabolized. The beta phase elimination half-life in patients with normal renal function

is approximately 30 minutes. The half-life is increased minimally (to 30 to 60 minutes) in anuric patients and dosage adjustments are not required in these patients. For additional discussion, see the Introduction.

DOSAGE AND PREPARATIONS.

Oral: Oxacillin should be taken at least one hour before or two hours after meals. *Adults and children weighing more than 40 kg,* 500 mg to 1 g every four to six hours; *less than 40 kg,* 50 to 100 mg/kg daily in divided doses every six hours.

> Strengths expressed in terms of the base:
> **Bactocill** (Beecham). Capsules 250 and 500 mg.
> **Prostaphlin** (Bristol). Capsules 250 and 500 mg; powder for oral solution 250 mg/5 ml.

Intramuscular, Intravenous: Oxacillin can be administered by intramuscular injection (solution containing 250 mg/1.5 ml), direct intravenous injection (solution containing $\leq$ 100 mg/ml and injected slowly to avoid vein irritation), or by continuous intravenous drip. See the manufacturers' instructions for the appropriate dilution of the drug, a list of compatible diluents and intravenous solutions, and stability of oxacillin in these solutions. When used in conjunction with other drugs, oxacillin should not be physically mixed with the other agent(s).

Adults, 2 to 12 g daily in equally divided doses every four to six hours; maximum daily dose is 12 g (The Medical Letter, 1984). *Children,* 100 to 200 mg/kg daily in equally divided doses every four to six hours (The Medical Letter, 1984). *Infants over 7 days and weighing more than 2 kg,* 150 mg/kg daily in divided doses every six hours; *infants over 7 days and weighing less than 2 kg,* 100 mg/kg daily in divided doses every eight hours; *infants under 7 days and weighing more than 2 kg,* 75 mg/kg daily in divided doses every eight hours; *infants under 7 days and weighing less than 2 kg,* 50 mg/kg daily in divided doses every 12 hours (Nelson, 1985 B).

Dosage adjustments are not required in patients with renal impairment.

> Strengths expressed in terms of the base:
> **Bactocill** (Beecham). Powder 500 mg and 1, 2, 4, and 10 g (sodium, 2.8 mEq/g).
> **Prostaphlin** (Bristol). Powder 250 and 500 mg and 1, 2, 4, and 10 g (sodium, 2.8 mEq/g).

CLOXACILLIN SODIUM
[Cloxapen, Tegopen]

Cloxacillin is a semisynthetic, penicillinase-resistant penicillin for oral use. This isoxazolyl derivative is chemically related to oxacillin and dicloxacillin.

MECHANISM OF ACTION, ANTIMICROBIAL SPECTRUM, AND RESISTANCE. The mechanism of action, antimicrobial spectrum, and resistance properties are the same as for methicillin (see that evaluation and the Introduction). On a weight basis, cloxacillin is more potent than methicillin in vitro against susceptible bacteria.

USES. Orally administered cloxacillin (or dicloxacillin) is a preferred drug for the treatment of mild to moderate *Staphylococcus aureus* infections of the skin and soft tissue (the most common use), respiratory and genitourinary tracts, and joints. For more severe infections, a parenteral penicillinase-resistant penicillin should be used initially (see evaluations of Methicillin, Nafcillin, and Oxacillin).

For additional discussion, see the Introduction; Chapter 65, Antimicrobial Therapy and Chemoprophylaxis of Infectious Diseases; and the evaluation of Dicloxacillin. See also Neu, 1982 B; Molavi and LeFrock, 1984; and Sheagren, 1984.

ADVERSE REACTIONS AND PRECAUTIONS. Cloxacillin generally is well tolerated; untoward effects are usually mild and most commonly consist of gastrointestinal disturbances or allergic reactions typical of all penicillins (see the Introduction).

DRUG INTERACTIONS AND INTERFERENCE WITH LABORATORY TESTS. See the Introduction.

PHARMACOKINETICS. Cloxacillin is stable in gastric acid and about 50% of an oral dose is absorbed by the gastrointestinal tract. Following administration of 500 mg to fasting individuals, total peak serum levels of approximately 10 mcg/ml are attained in about one hour; peak levels of free drug are 0.6 mcg/ml. Although peak serum levels of total (ie, bound and unbound) cloxacillin are lower than with equivalent doses of dicloxacillin, the levels of free drug are similar due to differences in plasma protein binding. The presence of food decreases the absorption of cloxacillin and this drug should be administered on an empty stomach, preferably one hour before or two hours after meals.

Between 93% and 95% of circulating cloxacillin is bound to plasma protein. Among the isoxazolyl penicillins, cloxacillin is less bound than dicloxacillin but more bound than oxacillin (see the evaluations). Like other penicillins, cloxacillin primarily distributes into the extracellular fluid volume.

Cloxacillin is rapidly eliminated, primarily by renal tubular secretion; probenecid delays excretion. Between 30% and 50% is recovered from urine as unchanged drug; approximately 20% is metabolized. The beta phase elimination half-life in patients with normal renal function is approximately 30 minutes. The half-life is not significantly increased in anuric patients and dosage adjustments are not required in these patients. For additional discussion, see the Introduction.

DOSAGE AND PREPARATIONS.
Oral: Cloxacillin should be taken at least one hour before or two hours after meals. *Adults and children weighing 20 kg or more*, 500 mg to 1 g every six hours (250 mg every six hours is recommended by the manufacturer for mild to moderate upper respiratory tract infections or localized skin and soft tissue infections). *Children weighing less than 20 kg,* 50 to 100 mg/kg daily in four equal doses every six hours.

A parenteral penicillinase-resistant penicillin (eg, nafcillin, oxacillin) should be used initially for serious staphylococcal infections.

Strengths expressed in terms of the base:
Generic. Capsules 200, 250, and 500 mg; powder for oral solution 125 mg/5 ml.
Cloxapen (Beecham). Capsules 250 and 500 mg.
Tegopen (Bristol). Capsules 250 and 500 mg; powder for oral solution 125 mg/5 ml.

DICLOXACILLIN SODIUM
[Dycill, Dynapen, Pathocil]

Dicloxacillin is a semisynthetic, penicillinase-resistant penicillin for oral use. This isoxazolyl derivative is chemically related to cloxacillin and oxacillin.

MECHANISM OF ACTION, ANTIMICROBIAL SPECTRUM, AND RESISTANCE. The mechanism of action, antimicrobial spectrum, and resistance properties are the same as for methicillin (see that evaluation and the Introduction). On a weight basis, dicloxacillin is more potent than methicillin in vitro against susceptible bacteria.

USES. Orally administered dicloxacillin (or cloxacillin) is a preferred drug for the treatment of mild to moderate *Staphylococcus aureus* infections of the skin and soft tissues (the most common use), respiratory and genitourinary tracts, and joints. For more severe infections, a parenteral penicillinase-resistant penicillin should be used initially (see evaluations of Methicillin, Nafcillin, and Oxacillin).

For additional discussion, see the Introduction; Chapter 65, Antimicrobial Therapy and Chemoprophylaxis of Infectious Diseases; and the evaluation of Cloxacillin. See also Neu, 1982 B; Molavi and LeFrock, 1984; and Sheagren, 1984.

ADVERSE REACTIONS AND PRECAUTIONS. Dicloxacillin generally is well tolerated; untoward effects are usually mild and most commonly consist of gastrointestinal disturbances or allergic reactions typical of all penicillins (see the Introduction).

DRUG INTERACTIONS AND INTERFERENCE WITH LABORATORY TESTS. See the Introduction.

PHARMACOKINETICS. Dicloxacillin is stable in gastric acid, and about 50% of an oral dose is absorbed by the gastrointestinal tract. Following administration of 500 mg to fasting individuals, total peak serum levels of approximately 15 mcg/ml are attained in about one hour; peak levels of free drug are 0.6 mcg/ml. Although peak serum levels of total (ie, bound and unbound) dicloxacillin are higher than with equivalent doses of cloxacillin, the levels of free drug are similar due to differences in plasma protein binding. The presence of food decreases the absorption of dicloxacillin and this drug should be administered on an empty stomach, preferably one hour before or two hours after meals.

Between 95% and 97% of circulating dicloxacillin is bound to plasma protein and it is the most highly protein bound isoxazolyl penicillin (see the evaluations of Oxacillin and Cloxacillin). Like other penicillins, dicloxacillin primarily distributes into the extracellular fluid volume.

Dicloxacillin is rapidly eliminated, primarily by renal tubular secretion; probenecid delays excretion. Approximately 60% is recovered from urine as unchanged drug; about 10% is metabolized. The beta phase elimination half-life in patients with normal renal function ranges from 30 to 42 minutes. The half-life is not significantly increased in anuric patients and dosage adjustments are not required in these patients. For additional discussion, see the Introduction.

DOSAGE AND PREPARATIONS.
Oral: Dicloxacillin should be taken at least one hour before or two hours after meals. *Adults and children weighing 40 kg or more*, 1 to 2 g daily in equally divided doses every six hours; the maximum daily dose is 4 g (The Medical Letter, 1984) (125 mg every six hours is recommended by the manufacturer for mild to moderate upper respiratory tract infections or localized

skin and soft tissue infections). *Children weighing less than 40 kg*, 12.5 to 25 mg/kg daily in equally divided doses every six hours (The Medical Letter, 1984).

A parenteral penicillinase-resistant penicillin (eg, nafcillin, oxacillin) should be used initially for serious staphylococcal infections.

Strengths expressed in terms of the base:

Dycill (Beecham), *Generic.* Capsules 250 and 500 mg.
Dynapen (Bristol). Capsules 125, 250, and 500 mg; powder for oral suspension 62.5 mg/5 ml.
Pathocil (Wyeth). Capsules 250 and 500 mg; powder for oral suspension 62.5 mg/5 ml.

AMINOPENICILLINS

AMPICILLIN
[Amcill, Omnipen, Polycillin, Principen]

AMPICILLIN SODIUM
[Omnipen-N, Polycillin-N]

Ampicillin is a semisynthetic penicillin for oral and parenteral use.

MECHANISM OF ACTION, ANTIMICROBIAL SPECTRUM, AND RESISTANCE. Ampicillin inhibits cell wall formation in susceptible bacteria and usually is bactericidal.

Like penicillin G, ampicillin is active in vitro against most gram-positive bacteria (except β lactamase-producing staphylococci), gram-negative cocci, and anaerobic bacteria (except the *Bacteroides fragilis* group). This aminopenicillin has a broader antimicrobial spectrum than penicillin G, however, and is active against certain aerobic gram-negative bacilli, including *Haemophilus influenzae, Escherichia coli, Proteus mirabilis, Salmonella* species, and *Shigella* species.

Ampicillin is hydrolyzed by β lactamases produced by various bacteria, including *Staphylococcus aureus, Neisseria gonorrhoeae, Haemophilus influenzae*, and various Enterobacteriaceae (eg, *E. coli, Salmonella, Shigella*), and is not active against these strains.

For a detailed discussion of the mechanism of action, antimicrobial spectrum, and resistance properties of the penicillins, see the Introduction.

USES. Ampicillin is bactericidal, has a high therapeutic to toxic ratio, can be administered parenterally as well as orally, and is of relatively low cost to the patient. Thus, it frequently is a preferred drug for infections caused by susceptible organisms in nonallergic patients, although it usually should not be substituted for penicillin G when the latter drug is equally effective. Many experts prefer amoxicillin over ampicillin for oral administration because gastrointestinal absorption of amoxicillin is greater, resulting in higher serum concentrations; the presence of food does not interfere with its absorption; and amoxicillin appears to cause less diarrhea. Other aminopenicillins (bacampicillin, cyclacillin) do not appear to offer any significant advantages over these two drugs and they are more expensive (see the evaluations).

Infections for which ampicillin is the preferred or alternative drug include acute bacterial cystitis (usually caused by a susceptible *E. coli*); other urinary tract infections (eg, acute pyelonephritis, acute prostatitis, acute epididymo-orchitis) caused by susceptible bacteria; uncomplicated gonorrhea (not effective for pharyngitis, anorectal infections in men, or PPNG infections); disseminated gonorrhea; bacterial vaginosis caused by the interaction of several species of vaginal bacteria; meningitis, epiglottitis, pneumonia, and skin infections (eg, facial cellulitis) caused by susceptible *H. influenzae*; acute otitis media; acute sinusitis; shigellosis (many strains of *Shigella* are resistant); and *Salmonella* infections (eg, bacteremia, enteric fever but not simple gastroenteritis) caused by susceptible strains.

Ampicillin also is employed frequently in combination with another antibiotic for: (1) empiric therapy before organism susceptibility to ampicillin is known (eg, ampicillin plus chloramphenicol for *H. influenzae* meningitis); (2) empiric therapy when one (or more) of a number of possible causative organisms may be involved (eg, ampicillin plus an aminoglycoside for meningitis or bacteremia in the newborn, biliary tract infections, acute pyelonephritis); and (3) for antibacterial synergism (eg, ampicillin [alternative, penicillin G] plus gentamicin [alternative streptomycin] for enterococcal endocarditis). Ampicillin plus gentamicin is the standard parenteral regimen for prophylaxis of endocarditis in certain high-risk patients prior to genitourinary or lower gastrointestinal tract surgery or instrumentation.

For a more detailed discussion, see the Introduction; see also Chapter 65, Antimicrobial Therapy and Chemoprophylaxis of Infectious Diseases.

ADVERSE REACTIONS AND PRECAUTIONS. Ampicillin is usually well tolerated. Adverse reactions are generally mild and consist most often of skin rashes or diarrhea. The incidence of diarrhea has been reported to be as great as 11% in adults and 20% in children, although these figures may be high. Diarrhea usually is not severe enough to require discontinuing the drug. However, antibiotic-associated pseudomembranous colitis (AAPMC) caused by *Clostridium difficile* may occur during ampicillin therapy. Although this adverse effect is relatively rare, ampicillin has been one of the more frequently implicated antibiotics. This potentially life-threatening adverse effect requires prompt discontinuation of ampicillin, maintenance of fluid and electrolyte balance, and possible therapy with oral vancomycin (see also Chapter 68, Macrolides and Lincosamides, and Chapter 72, Miscellaneous Antibacterial Agents).

Skin rashes develop more often with ampicillin (incidence, 3% to 9%) and other aminopenicillins than with penicillin G. Only a small percentage (eg, approximately 1% to 5%) of these rashes are truly allergic (eg, urticarial) in nature and require discontinuing the antibiotic. This incidence presumably is about the same as with other penicillins. However, the majority of skin rashes caused by the aminopenicillins are characteristically diffuse, nonurticarial, maculopapular rashes that usually appear seven to ten days after initiation of therapy, will almost always subside despite continued therapy, and are rarely dangerous. The mechanism that underlies the rash is not clear, but many feel that it is primarily a toxic phenomenon rather than an immunologic reaction. It is clearly not an IgE-mediated hypersensitivity reaction. The incidence of this type of rash is particularly high in patients with viral infections, most notably infectious mononucleosis (70% to 90%), or lymphatic leukemia (90%) and in those receiving concurrent allopurinol therapy (15% to 22%). These rashes are not contraindications to the use of ampicillin or other penicillins, nor should they be considered an indication that the patient is allergic to penicillin.

Other adverse reactions, both allergic and nonallergic, that are typical of all penicillins can occur with ampicillin. For a detailed discussion, see the Introduction.

DRUG INTERACTIONS AND INTERFERENCE WITH LABORATORY TESTS. See the Introduction.

PHARMACOKINETICS. Ampicillin can be administered orally, intramuscularly, and intravenously. Although it is stable in gastric acid, only about 30% to 50% of an oral dose is absorbed by the gastrointestinal tract. Following a 500-mg dose to fasting individuals, peak serum levels of 2.5 to 5 mcg/ml are attained in one to two hours. The presence of food in the gastrointestinal tract decreases absorption. Many experts prefer amoxicillin to ampicillin for oral administration because its absorption is superior and unaffected by the presence of food (see the evaluation). Following intramuscular injection of 500 mg of ampicillin, peak serum levels of approximately 8 mcg/ml are achieved within one hour. A peak serum level of approximately 40 mcg/ml is obtained after a 1-g intravenous dose.

Approximately 20% of circulating ampicillin is bound to plasma protein. Like other penicillins, ampicillin primarily distributes into the extracellular fluid volume. High concentrations are achieved in bile and urine. Penetration into cerebrospinal fluid is adequate in the presence of inflammation.

Ampicillin is rapidly eliminated, primarily by renal tubular secretion; probenecid delays excretion. Urinary recovery of unchanged drug is approximately 90% after parenteral administration and 40% (due to incomplete absorption) after oral administration. Only about 10% of a dose is metabolized. The beta phase elimination half-life is approximately one hour in patients with normal renal function. The half-life is prolonged in patients with renal impairment (eg, 8 to 12 hours in anuric patients) and dosage adjustments are necessary. For additional discussion, see the Introduction.

DOSAGE AND PREPARATIONS.

AMPICILLIN (TRIHYDRATE OR ANHYDROUS):

Oral: Ampicillin preferably is given one hour before or two hours after meals. *Adults*, 2 to 4 g daily in equally divided doses every six hours; *children,* 50 to 100 mg/kg daily in equally divided doses every six hours (The Medical Letter, 1984).

For dosage recommendations in gonorrhea, see Chapter 65, Table 2.

Strengths expressed in terms of the base:
Generic. Capsules 250 and 500 mg; powder for oral suspension 125 and 250 mg/5 ml.
Omnipen (Wyeth). Capsules (anhydrous) 250 and 500 mg; powder for oral suspension (trihydrate) 100 mg/ml (pediatric), 125, 250, and 500 mg/5 ml.
Amcill (Parke-Davis), **Polycillin** (Bristol). Capsules (trihydrate) 250 and 500 mg; powder for oral suspension (trihydrate) 100 mg/ml (pediatric), 125, 250, and 500 (**Polycillin** only) mg/5 ml.

Principen (Squibb). Capsules (trihydrate) 250 and 500 mg; powder for oral suspension (trihydrate) 125 and 250 mg/5 ml.
Additional Trademarks.
Pfizerpen-A (Pfipharmecs), **SK-Ampicillin** (Smith Kline & French), **Supen** (Reid-Provident), **Totacillin** (Beecham).
AVAILABLE MIXTURES.
Polycillin-PRB (Bristol), **Generic.** Powder for oral suspension containing ampicillin (trihydrate) 3.5 g and probenecid 1 g.
Principen W/Probenecid (Squibb). Capsules containing ampicillin (trihydrate) 3.5 g and probenecid 1 g/nine capsule package.

AMPICILLIN SODIUM:

Intravenous, Intramuscular: Ampicillin can be administered by intramuscular injection, direct intravenous injection, or intravenous drip. The intravenous route generally is preferred. See the manufacturers' literature for the appropriate dilution of the drug, a list of compatible diluents and intravenous solutions, and stability of ampicillin in those solutions.

Adults, 2 to 12 g daily in equally divided doses every six hours; the maximum daily dose in equally divided doses every four hours should be used for meningitis (The Medical Letter, 1984). *Children*, 100 to 200 mg/kg daily in equally divided doses every six hours; for meningitis in children caused by ampicillin-sensitive *H. influenzae* type b, up to 400 mg/kg daily in equally divided doses every four hours is recommended (The Medical Letter, 1984).

Infants over 7 days and weighing more than 2 kg, 100 mg/kg daily in divided doses every six hours; for meningitis, 200 mg/kg daily in divided doses every six hours; *infants over 7 days and weighing less than 2 kg*, 75 mg/kg daily in divided doses every eight hours; for meningitis, 150 mg/kg daily in divided doses every eight hours; *infants under 7 days and weighing more than 2 kg*, 75 mg/kg daily in divided doses every eight hours; for meningitis, 150 mg/kg daily in divided doses every eight hours; *infants under 7 days and weighing less than 2 kg*, 50 mg/kg daily in divided doses every 12 hours; for meningitis, 100 mg/kg daily in divided doses every 12 hours (Nelson, 1985 B).

In the presence of severe renal impairment (creatinine clearance, 10 ml/min or less), the dosage interval should be increased to 12 hours (The Medical Letter, 1984).

For dosage recommendations in the prophylaxis of infective endocarditis, see Chapter 65, Table 3.

Strengths expressed in terms of the base:
Generic. Powder 500 mg.
Omnipen-N (Wyeth), **Polycillin-N** (Bristol). Powder 125, 250, and 500 mg and 1, 2, and 10 g.
Additional Trademarks.
SK-Ampicillin-N (Smith Kline & French), **Totacillin-N** (Beecham).

AMOXICILLIN TRIHYDRATE
[Amoxil, Larotid, Polymox, Trimox]

Amoxicillin is a semisynthetic aminopenicillin for oral use.

MECHANISM OF ACTION, ANTIMICROBIAL SPECTRUM, AND RESISTANCE. The in vitro antimicrobial spectrum of amoxicillin is essentially identical to that of ampicillin (see the evaluation). However, amoxicillin has somewhat less activity against *Shigella* species and, combined with its better absorption, is not useful clinically for the gastrointestinal infections caused by this pathogen.

Amoxicillin is hydrolyzed by β lactamases produced by various bacteria, including *Staphylococcus aureus, Neisseria gonorrhoeae, Haemophilus influenzae*, and various Enterobacteriaceae (eg, *Escherichia coli, Salmonella*) and is not active against these strains.

For a detailed discussion of the mechanism of action, antimicrobial spectrum, and resistance properties of the penicillins, see the Introduction.

USES. Infections for which amoxicillin is the preferred or alternative drug include acute otitis media and acute sinusitis (except when caused by β lactamase-producing *H. influenzae*) acute bacterial cystitis (usually caused by susceptible *E. coli*), other urinary tract infections caused by susceptible bacteria, uncomplicated gonorrhea (not effective for pharyngitis, anorectal infections in men, or PPNG infections), disseminated gonorrhea, and susceptible *Salmonella* infections (eg, enteric fever but not for simple gastroenteritis). For a more detailed discussion, see the Introduction and Chapter 65, Antimicrobial Therapy and Chemoprophylaxis of Infectious Diseases.

Many infectious disease experts prefer amoxicillin to ampicillin for infections requiring oral administration because amoxicillin is more completely absorbed from the gastrointestinal tract (better bioavailability), food does not interfere with its absorption, and it appears to cause less diarrhea than ampicillin, particularly in children. Other aminopenicillins (bacampicillin, cyclacillin) do not appear to offer any significant advantage over amoxicillin and they are more expensive (see the Introduction and the evaluations. See also Neu, 1979, 1984 A; McCracken, 1983; Reese and Betts, 1983).

ADVERSE REACTIONS AND PRECAUTIONS. Adverse reactions to amoxicillin are similar to those seen with ampicillin. However, diarrhea occurs less frequently with amoxicillin, particularly in children (see the evaluation of Ampicillin and the Introduction; see also Neu, 1979).

DRUG INTERACTIONS AND INTERFERENCE WITH LABORATORY TESTS. See the Introduction.

PHARMACOKINETICS. Amoxicillin is stable in gastric acid and between 75% and 90% of an oral dose is absorbed from the gastrointestinal tract. Following a dose of 500 mg, peak serum levels range from 6 to 8 mcg/ml after one to two hours. The presence of food in the gastrointestinal tract does not decrease absorption appreciably. Because amoxicillin is more completely absorbed than ampicillin and, in contrast to the latter drug, absorption is not appreciably affected by the presence of food, many experts prefer this aminopenicillin for oral administration.

Approximately 20% of circulating amoxicillin is bound to plasma protein. Like other penicillins, amoxicillin primarily distributes into the extracellular fluid volume. High concentrations are achieved in bile and urine.

Amoxicillin is rapidly eliminated, primarily by renal tubular secretion; probenecid delays excretion. Between 50% and 70% of a dose is recovered from urine as unchanged drug; approximately 10% is metabolized. The beta phase elimination half-life in patients with normal renal function is approximately one hour. The half-life is prolonged in patients with renal impairment (eg, 8 to 16 hours in anuric patients) and dosage adjustments are necessary. For additional discussion, see the Introduction.

DOSAGE AND PREPARATIONS.
Oral: Adults and children weighing more than 20 kg, 750 mg to 1.5 g daily (doses as large as 1 g every four hours have been used in some adults); *less than 20 kg*, 20 to 40 mg/kg daily. These amounts are administered at eight-hour intervals. The larger doses are used in more severe infections. In the presence of severe renal impairment (creatinine clearance, 10 ml/min or less), the adult dose probably should not exceed 500 mg every 12 hours.

For dosage recommendations in gonorrhea, see Chapter 65, Table 2.

Generic. Capsules 250 and 500 mg; powder for oral suspension 125 and 250 mg/5 ml.

Amoxil (Beecham), **Larotid** (Roche), **Polymox** (Bristol). Capsules 250 and 500 mg; powder for oral suspension 50 mg/ml (pediatric) and 125 and 250 mg/5 ml; tablets (chewable) 125 and 250 mg (**Amoxil** only).

Trimox (Squibb). Capsules 250 and 500 mg; powder for oral suspension 125 and 250 mg/5 ml.

Additional Trademarks.
Sumox (Reid-Provident), **Utimox** (Parke-Davis), **Wymox** (Wyeth).

BACAMPICILLIN HYDROCHLORIDE
[Spectrobid]

Bacampicillin is the 1-ethoxycarbonyloxyethyl ester of ampicillin. This prodrug has little antibacterial action itself but is rapidly and completely converted to ampicillin in vivo by hydrolytic cleavage of the ester moiety from the ampicillin base.

MECHANISM OF ACTION, ANTIMICROBIAL SPECTRUM, AND RESISTANCE. The antibacterial spectrum of bacampicillin is identical to that of ampicillin, since it is hydrolyzed to ampicillin (see the Introduction and the evaluation).

USES. The uses of bacampicillin are very similar to those of oral ampicillin or amoxicillin. Major indications are acute otitis media and acute sinusitis (except when caused by β lactamase-producing *Haemophilus influenzae*), acute bacterial cystitis (usually caused by susceptible strains of *Escherichia coli*), other urinary tract infections caused by susceptible bacteria, and uncomplicated gonorrhea. Bacampicillin does not appear to offer any significant clinical advantages over amoxicillin for routine use and it is more expensive (see the Introduction and the evaluation of Amoxicillin; see also Scheife and Neu, 1982; McCracken, 1983).

ADVERSE REACTIONS AND PRECAUTIONS. Adverse reactions to bacampicillin are similar to those seen with ampicillin. However, diarrhea occurs less frequently with bacampicillin, presumably due to more complete absorption (see the evaluation of Ampicillin and the Introduction; see also Scheife and Neu, 1982).

DRUG INTERACTIONS AND INTERFERENCE WITH LABORATORY TESTS. See the Introduction.

PHARMACOKINETICS. Bacampicillin is stable in gastric acid. It is rapidly and almost completely (95%) absorbed from the gastrointestinal tract following oral administration. During the process of absorption, bacampicillin is hydrolyzed to ampicillin, the active drug; approximately 1.4 mg of bacampicillin is equivalent to 1 mg of ampicillin. Following 400 mg, 800 mg, and 1,600 mg doses of bacampicillin, average peak serum ampicillin concentrations of 7.9, 12.9, and 20.1 mcg/ml, respectively, are attained in 45 to 60 minutes. These are considerably higher than those obtained for equivalent doses of ampicillin because of the superior absorption of the prodrug. In contrast to ampicillin, the presence of food in the gastrointestinal tract does not decrease the absorption of bacampicillin.

The distribution and elimination of bacampicillin-derived ampicillin are essentially identical to that observed after administration of the parent compound. Approximately 75% of a dose is recovered from urine as unchanged drug within eight hours. (See the evaluation on Ampicillin and the Introduction; see also Neu, 1981.)

DOSAGE AND PREPARATIONS. The interval between doses recommended by the manufacturer is longer than that for ampicillin or amoxicillin. This so-called "pulse-dosing" appears to produce equally effective results but offers no clear-cut advantage over more frequent administration of ampicillin or amoxicillin and this drug is considerably more expensive.

Oral: Adults, 800 mg to 1.6 g daily in equally divided doses every 12 hours; *children*, 25 to 50 mg/kg daily in equally divided doses every 12 hours. In the presence of severe renal impairment (creatinine clearance, 10 ml/min or less), the adult dose probably should not exceed 800 mg every 24 hours (Norris and Mandell, 1985).

For uncomplicated gonorrhea, adults 1.6 g plus probenecid 1 g as a single oral dose.

> **Spectrobid** (Roerig). Tablets 400 mg (equivalent to 280 mg ampicillin); powder for oral suspension 125 mg/5 ml (equivalent to 87.5 mg ampicillin).

CYCLACILLIN
[Cyclapen-W]

Cyclacillin is an aminopenicillin that is chemically related to ampicillin. It is administered orally.

MECHANISM OF ACTION, ANTIMICROBIAL SPECTRUM, AND RESISTANCE. The in vitro antimicrobial spectrum of cyclacillin is similar to that of ampicillin and amoxicillin. However, on a weight basis, cyclacillin is less active than these other aminopenicillins. Cyclacillin is inactivated by β lactamase-producing bacterial strains. See the evaluations of Ampicillin and Amoxicillin and the Introduction.

USES. The uses of cyclacillin are very similar to those of oral ampicillin and amoxicillin. Major indications are acute otitis media and acute sinusitis (except when caused by β lactamase-producing *Haemophilus influenzae*) and uncomplicated urinary tract infections (cystitis) caused by susceptible *Escherichia coli* and *Proteus mirabilis*. However, cyclacillin does not appear to offer any significant clinical advantages over amoxicillin and it is more expensive (see the Introduction and the evaluation of Amoxicillin).

ADVERSE REACTIONS AND PRECAUTIONS. Adverse reactions to cyclacillin are similar to those seen with ampicillin. However, diarrhea occurs less frequently with cyclacillin, presumably due to more complete absorption (see the evaluation of Ampicillin and the Introduction).

DRUG INTERACTIONS AND INTERFERENCE WITH LABORATORY TESTS. See the Introduction.

PHARMACOKINETICS. Cyclacillin is stable in gastric acid and it is rapidly and almost completely (95%) absorbed from the gastrointestinal tract following oral administration. Following a dose of 500 mg, peak serum levels of 11 to 12 mcg/ml are achieved in 40 to 60 minutes. The effect of food on absorption is not known. Although peak serum levels of cyclacillin are higher and appear earlier than those obtained for a comparable (ie, 500 mg) dose of ampicillin, cyclacillin is less active than ampicillin in vitro for most pathogens and is eliminated more rapidly; serum cyclacillin concentrations are lower than those of ampicillin after three hours (see below). Consequently, no differences in clinical efficacy have been reported. See also the evaluation of Ampicillin and the Introduction.

About 20% of circulating cyclacillin is bound to plasma proteins and it penetrates into most tissues and body fluids. Cyclacillin is rapidly eliminated, primarily by renal tubular secretion; probenecid delays excretion. Between 65% and 70% of a dose is recovered from urine as unchanged drug within six hours. Approximately 15% is metabolized to a penicilloic acid metabolite. The half-life in patients with normal renal function is 30 to 40 minutes. The half-life is prolonged in patients with renal impairment and dosage adjustments are necessary.

DOSAGE AND PREPARATIONS.

Oral: Adults, 1 to 2 g daily in equally divided doses every six hours; *children*, 50 to 100 mg/kg daily in equally divided doses every six hours (The Medical Letter, 1984).

For patients with reduced renal function, the dosage interval should be increased to 12 to 24 hours when creatinine clearance is 50 to 10 ml/min and to 24 hours when it is less than 10 ml/min (The Medical Letter, 1984).

> **Cyclapen-W** (Wyeth). Tablets 250 and 500 mg; powder for oral suspension 125 and 250 mg/5 ml.

ANTIPSEUDOMONAL PENICILLINS

CARBENICILLIN DISODIUM
[Geopen, Pyopen]

CARBENICILLIN INDANYL SODIUM
[Geocillin]

Carbenicillin disodium is a semisynthetic carboxypenicillin. It is labile in gastric acid and must be administered parenterally for systemic infections. Carbenicillin indanyl sodium, an ester of carbenicillin, can be given orally for urinary tract infections. Once absorbed, the indanyl ester is rapidly hydrolyzed to carbenicillin, the active drug.

MECHANISM OF ACTION, ANTIMICROBIAL SPECTRUM,

AND RESISTANCE. Carbenicillin inhibits cell wall formation in susceptible bacteria and usually is bactericidal.

Carbenicillin is active against most gram-positive bacteria and gram-negative cocci. In general, its activity against these bacteria is considerably less than that of penicillin G or ampicillin, however, and this antipseudomonal penicillin offers no clinical advantages. Enterococci (eg, *Streptococcus faecalis*) and β lactamase-producing staphylococci are resistant to carbenicillin.

Carbenicillin's spectrum of activity against aerobic gram-negative bacilli is expanded when compared to ampicillin. Among the Enterobacteriaceae, many strains of *Enterobacter* and indole-positive *Proteus* (*Providencia rettgeri, Morganella morganii, Proteus vulgaris*) are susceptible as are *Escherichia coli, Proteus mirabilis, Salmonella*, and *Shigella*. Most *Serratia* and essentially all *Klebsiella* are resistant, however. Carbenicillin also is active against many strains of *Pseudomonas aeruginosa*, which accounts for its major clinical advantage over earlier penicillins (eg, ampicillin, penicillin G). Many strains of *Acinetobacter* also are sensitive. Among the anaerobes, *Fusobacterium* and *Bacteroides*, including many strains of *B. fragilis*, are susceptible.

Carbenicillin is inactivated by β lactamases. The number of carbenicillin-resistant strains of gram-negative bacilli is quite large and the emergence of resistant β lactamase-producing strains is relatively common. Thus, it is usually necessary to do susceptibility testing before instituting therapy with this agent, especially when it is used alone. Furthermore, combination therapy with an antipseudomonal penicillin plus an aminoglycoside generally is recommended for systemic *P. aeruginosa* infections (see Uses).

For a detailed discussion of the mechanism of action, antimicrobial spectrum, and resistance properties of the penicillins, see the Introduction.

USES. Despite its broad antimicrobial spectrum, the only primary clinical indication for carbenicillin is suspected or proven systemic *P. aeruginosa* infection. These include infections of the skin and soft tissue (eg, infected burns), central nervous system (eg, postneurosurgical meningitis), ear (eg, malignant otitis externa), lower respiratory tract (eg, nosocomial pneumonias, especially in immunocompromised hosts and cystic fibrosis patients), heart (eg, endocarditis, particularly in intravenous drug abusers), urinary tract (eg, recurrent infections), and blood (eg, bacteremia in immunocompromised hosts) and for empiric therapy in febrile neutropenic patients.

Systemic pseudomonal infections usually are serious and difficult to eradicate; frequently are of nosocomial origin and affect compromised hosts (eg, neutropenic cancer patients, cystic fibrosis patients); and may be associated with the emergence of resistant bacterial strains, particularly when an antipseudomonal penicillin is given alone. Thus, most infectious disease experts recommend that systemic *P. aeruginosa* infections virtually always be treated with an antipseudomonal penicillin plus an aminoglycoside (gentamicin, tobramycin, amikacin, netilmicin). Such combinations have demonstrated antibacterial synergisms against *P. aeruginosa*. Also, the rate of emergence of resistant organisms should be decreased with combination therapy. Antipseudomonal penicillins and amino-

glycosides should not be mixed together physically, however, because they inactivate one another (see Drug Interactions and the Introduction; see also Chapter 70, Aminoglycosides).

The descending order of in vitro activity of the antipseudomonal penicillins against *P. aeruginosa* is piperacillin ≥ azlocillin > mezlocillin = ticarcillin > carbenicillin. The clinical significance of this in vitro data is undetermined. However, most physicians prefer ticarcillin to carbenicillin for infections caused by *P. aeruginosa* because it can be given in lower dosages, resulting in decreased sodium load and other adverse effects (eg, hypokalemia, abnormal coagulation) to the patient. Whether the newer agents, piperacillin, mezlocillin, or azlocillin, will offer significant clinical advantages over ticarcillin is presently unresolved (see the evaluations and the Introduction). Differences in drug acquisition costs may be an important factor in selecting an antipseudomonal penicillin for general use in a given hospital.

Antipseudomonal penicillins exhibit antibacterial activity against most anaerobic bacteria, including many strains of *Bacteroides fragilis*. Thus, they have been combined with an aminoglycoside for mixed aerobic-anaerobic intra-abdominal or gynecologic pelvic infections, but other antibiotics active against the *B. fragilis* group, such as clindamycin, metronidazole, chloramphenicol, and cefoxitin, usually are preferred.

Antipseudomonal penicillins also may be indicated for systemic infections caused by other susceptible aerobic gram-negative bacilli (eg, *Enterobacter*, indole-positive *Proteus, Providencia, Acinetobacter, Escherichia coli*) that are resistant to other penicillins and cephalosporins.

Despite carbenicillin's broad antibacterial spectrum, resistant bacteria are fairly common and resistance has developed during therapy. Thus, this drug should not be used alone for empiric therapy of suspected infections.

In general, antipseudomonal penicillins should not be used when narrower spectrum, less expensive antibiotics (eg, penicillin G, ampicillin) are as effective and of no greater toxicity.

Oral carbenicillin indanyl is hydrolyzed in the body to carbenicillin, the active metabolite. Although plasma concentrations are low, the active drug is rapidly excreted in the urine and is useful in the treatment of urinary tract infections caused by susceptible gram-negative bacilli, particularly *Pseudomonas aeruginosa, Enterobacter*, and *Proteus* species. Carbenicillin indanyl also has been used in chronic prostatitis due to susceptible bacteria (eg, *Escherichia coli*).

For a more detailed discussion, see the Introduction; see also Chapter 65, Antimicrobial Therapy and Chemoprophylaxis of Infectious Diseases.

ADVERSE REACTIONS AND PRECAUTIONS. Carbenicillin is relatively well tolerated, but any of the adverse reactions associated with the use of penicillins may occur with this derivative (see the Introduction).

A variety of hypersensitivity reactions (eg, rashes, urticaria, fever) have been reported, although anaphylactic reactions are uncommon.

Gastrointestinal disturbances are infrequent, but pseudomembraneous colitis caused by *Clostridium difficile* has occurred. However, the incidence is less than with ampicillin (see that evaluation).

Various hematologic abnormalities have occurred with carbenicillin and are more common after prolonged, high-dose, parenteral administration. As with several other penicillins, neutropenia and eosinophilia have been reported. Carbenicillin is the penicillin derivative most frequently associated with abnormal blood clotting. In high concentrations, this antibiotic can bind to adenosine diphosphate receptors in platelets and prevent normal platelet aggregation, thus prolonging the bleeding time. This is a dose-related phenomenon. Although clinically significant bleeding occurs infrequently, it is more likely in patients with underlying renal dysfunction.

The large intravenous doses of carbenicillin usually used in clinical practice can cause electrolyte disorders. Hypokalemia has occurred due to the large amount of nonreabsorbable anion present in the distal renal tubules. Large doses of this disodium salt may contribute significantly to the sodium load in patients with impaired sodium excretion mechanisms (eg, those with renal, cardiac, or hepatic disease). Each gram of carbenicillin contains 4.7 mEq of sodium.

As with other penicillins given in large intravenous doses, convulsions can occur if serum levels are excessive (eg, in patients with renal failure in whom dosage adjustments are not made). Local pain at the site of intramuscular injection and phlebitis following intravenous administration have been reported. Elevated serum transaminase (SGOT, SGPT) levels have been observed; these are reversible. Interstitial nephritis has been reported rarely. Clinically significant superinfections have occurred.

For additional discussion, see the Introduction; see also Neu, 1982 C.

DRUG INTERACTIONS AND INTERFERENCE WITH LABORATORY TESTS. Carbenicillin and other antipseudomonal penicillins can inactivate aminoglycosides, particularly gentamicin and tobramycin. Therefore, these antibiotics should not be mixed together prior to administration. Furthermore, in patients with renal failure, in vivo antagonism has been observed. Serum aminoglycoside concentrations should be monitored in such patients and the dosage adjusted accordingly (Mangini, 1984; Hansten, 1985 A; see also Chapter 70, Aminoglycosides).

For a discussion of other drug interactions involving the penicillins, see the Introduction.

PHARMACOKINETICS. Carbenicillin is labile in gastric acid and is not absorbed following oral administration. Thus, it must be administered parenterally. Peak serum levels between 20 mcg/ml and 30 mcg/ml are attained about one hour after intramuscular injection of 1 g. Intravenous infusion at a rate of 1 g/hr results in average serum concentrations of 150 mcg/ml. Peak serum concentrations of up to 500 mcg/ml can be achieved following the rapid (15 to 30 minutes) intravenous administration of 5 g.

About 50% of circulating carbenicillin is bound to plasma protein. Like other penicillins, carbenicillin primarily distributes into the extracellular fluid volume.

Carbenicillin is rapidly eliminated, primarily by renal tubular secretion; probenecid delays excretion. Approximately 95% of a dose is recovered as unchanged drug in urine, 75% to 85%

within the first nine hours; less than 5% is metabolized. The half-life in patients with normal renal function is about one hour. The half-life is prolonged in patients with renal impairment (eg, 13 to 16 hours in anuric patients) and dosage adjustments are necessary.

In contrast to carbenicillin, carbenicillin indanyl is stable in gastric acid. After oral administration, approximately 30% of a dose is absorbed from the gastrointestinal tract and rapidly hydrolyzed to carbenicillin, the active drug. Peak serum levels of about 10 mcg/ml are attained approximately one hour after administration of two tablets (equivalent to 764 mg of carbenicillin). These levels are inadequate for systemic infections and this drug is indicated only for urinary tract infections (see Uses).

For additional discussion, see the Introduction.

DOSAGE AND PREPARATIONS. The following dosages are recommended for infections caused by *Pseudomonas aeruginosa*. Consult the manufacturers' literature for dosage recommendations for infections caused by other pathogens.

CARBENICILLIN DISODIUM:

Intramuscular: This route is used primarily for uncomplicated urinary tract infections. No more than 2 g should be injected at one time. Intravenous therapy in higher doses should be used for serious urinary tract and systemic infections.

Adults, for uncomplicated urinary tract infections, 4 to 8 g daily in divided doses every six hours; *children*, for urinary tract infections, 50 to 200 mg/kg daily in divided doses every four to six hours.

Intravenous: This is the preferred route for serious urinary tract and systemic infections. Carbenicillin disodium can be administered by slow injection or by intermittent or continuous infusion. See the manufacturer's literature for the appropriate dilution of the drug, a list of compatible diluents and intravenous solutions, and stability of carbenicillin in these solutions.

For urinary tract infections, *adults*, uncomplicated infections, 4 to 8 g daily in divided doses every six hours; for serious infections, 200 mg/kg daily by continuous or intermittent infusion; *children*, 50 to 200 mg/kg daily in divided doses every four to six hours.

For severe systemic infections (eg, septicemia, respiratory or soft tissue infections), *adults*, 400 to 500 mg/kg daily (30 to 40 g daily) in divided doses every four to six hours or by continuous infusion; *children*, 400 to 500 mg/kg daily in divided doses every four to six hours or by continuous infusion (up to 600 mg/kg daily can be administered [The Medical Letter, 1984]); *infants weighing more than 2 kg and ≤ 3 days*, 100 mg/kg initially, then 300 mg/kg daily in divided doses every six hours; *infants weighing more than 2 kg and over 3 days*, 400 mg/kg daily in divided doses every six hours; *infants weighing less than 2 kg and ≤ 7 days*, 100 mg/kg initially, then 225 mg/kg daily in divided doses every eight hours; *infants weighing less than 2 kg and over 7 days*, 400 mg/kg daily in divided doses every six hours.

For infections other than urinary tract infections complicated by renal insufficiency (creatinine clearance, <5 ml/min), *adults*, 2 g every 8 to 12 hours; during peritoneal dialysis, 2 g every six hours; during hemodialysis, 2 g every four hours.

Clinical data are insufficient to recommend a dose for *children with impaired renal function.*

Geopen (Pfipharmecs). Powder (sterile) 1, 2, and 5 g containers (intravenous and intramuscular) and 5, 10 and 30 g containers (intravenous only) (sodium, 4.7 mEq/g).

Pyopen (Beecham). Powder (sterile) in 1, 2, and 5 g containers (intravenous and intramuscular) and 2, 5, 10, and 20 g containers (intravenous) (sodium, 5.3 mEq/g).

CARBENICILLIN INDANYL SODIUM:

Oral: For urinary tract infections in *adults,* one to two tablets four times daily. Clinical data are insufficient to recommend a dose for *children.* (See also the manufacturer's literature.)

This drug should be avoided in patients with severe renal impairment (creatinine clearance, 10 ml/min or less).

Geocillin (Roerig). Tablets equivalent to 382 mg of carbenicillin.

TICARCILLIN DISODIUM
[Ticar]

Ticarcillin disodium is a semisynthetic carboxypenicillin that is closely related to carbenicillin. Since it is not absorbed orally, it must be given either intravenously or intramuscularly.

MECHANISM OF ACTION, ANTIMICROBIAL SPECTRUM, AND RESISTANCE. The antibacterial spectrum of ticarcillin is the same as that of carbenicillin (see that evaluation) except that ticarcillin is two- to fourfold more active in vitro against *Pseudomonas aeruginosa* (Eickhoff and Ehret, 1976). Some strains of *P. aeruginosa* develop resistance fairly rapidly. Like carbenicillin, ticarcillin is active in vitro against the *Bacteroides fragilis* group (Roy et al, 1977; Henderson et al, 1977), and clinical studies (Webb et al, 1978, and others) indicate that it is useful in anaerobic infections caused by this organism.

Ticarcillin is inactivated by β lactamase-producing organisms. As with carbenicillin, the number of ticarcillin-resistant strains is quite large for many bacteria and susceptibility testing is usually necessary before institution of therapy, especially when ticarcillin is used alone.

For a detailed discussion of the mechanism of action, antimicrobial spectrum, and resistance properties of the penicillins, see the Introduction.

USES. The indications for ticarcillin are similar to those for carbenicillin with the primary use being suspected or proven infections caused by *P. aeruginosa* (see the evaluation on Carbenicillin). It may be used in bacterial septicemia, skin and soft tissue infections, respiratory tract infections, and genitourinary tract infections.

Like carbenicillin, the combination of ticarcillin with an aminoglycoside usually results in antibacterial synergism against *P. aeruginosa* and combination therapy is recommended for systemic infections caused by this pathogen. Ticarcillin frequently is preferred to carbenicillin for *P. aeruginosa* infections. Because of its greater in vitro activity, ticarcillin can be given in lower dosages, resulting in decreased sodium load and other adverse effects (eg, hypokalemia, abnormal coagulation) to the patient. The combination of ticarcillin plus an aminoglycoside has been successful for many *P. aeruginosa* infections. Whether the newer antipseudomonal penicillins, piperacillin, mezlocillin, or azlocillin, will

offer significant clinical advantages over ticarcillin is presently unresolved (see the evaluations and the Introduction). As with carbenicillin, ticarcillin and aminoglycosides should not be mixed together (see Drug Interactions and the Introduction; see also Chapter 70, Aminoglycosides).

For a more detailed discussion of the uses of antipseudomonal penicillins, see the evaluation of Carbenicillin and the Introduction; see also Chapter 65, Antimicrobial Therapy and Chemoprophylaxis of Infectious Diseases.

ADVERSE REACTIONS AND PRECAUTIONS. Adverse reactions to ticarcillin are similar to those seen with carbenicillin. These include various hypersensitivity reactions, dose-related inhibition of platelet aggregation with the potential for bleeding, and hypokalemia. For a more detailed discussion of these and other adverse reactions, see the evaluation of Carbenicillin and the Introduction; see also Neu, 1982 C.

Each gram of ticarcillin disodium contains 5.2 mEq of sodium and large doses may contribute significantly to the salt load in patients with impaired sodium excretion mechanisms (eg, those with renal, cardiac, or liver disease). At usual therapeutic doses, the actual sodium content administered is less than with carbenicillin, but more than with the newer antipseudomonal penicillins (eg, azlocillin, mezlocillin, piperacillin), which are monosodium salts (see the evaluations).

DRUG INTERACTIONS AND INTERFERENCE WITH LABORATORY TESTS. Ticarcillin and other antipseudomonal penicillins can inactivate aminoglycosides, particularly gentamicin and tobramycin. Therefore, these antibiotics should not be mixed together prior to administration. Furthermore, in patients with renal failure, in vivo antagonism has been observed. Serum aminoglycoside concentrations should be monitored in such patients and the dosage adjusted accordingly (Mangini, 1984; Hansten, 1985 A; see also Chapter 70, Aminoglycosides).

For a discussion of other drug interactions involving the penicillins, see the Introduction.

PHARMACOKINETICS. Ticarcillin is labile in gastric acid and is not absorbed following oral administration. Thus, it must be administered parenterally. Peak serum levels between 20 mcg/ml and 30 mcg/ml are attained about one hour after a 1 g intramuscular injection. Rapid intravenous injection of 5 g produces serum concentrations greater than 300 mcg/ml after 15 minutes.

Between 50% and 60% of circulating ticarcillin is bound to plasma protein. Like other penicillins, ticarcillin primarily distributes into the extracellular fluid volume.

Ticarcillin is rapidly eliminated, primarily by renal tubular secretion; probenecid delays excretion. Between 75% and 85% of a dose is recovered as unchanged drug in the urine; 10% to 15% is metabolized to penicilloic acid derivatives. The half-life in patients with normal renal function is about 1.2 hours. The half-life is prolonged in patients with renal impairment (eg, about 15 hours in anuric patients) and dosage adjustments are necessary. For additional discussion, see the Introduction.

DOSAGE AND PREPARATIONS.

Intramuscular: This route is used primarily for uncomplicated urinary tract infections. No more than 2 g should be injected at one time. Intravenous therapy in higher doses should be used for serious urinary tract and systemic infections.

For uncomplicated urinary tract infections, *adults,* 4 g daily in divided doses every six hours; *children weighing less than 40 kg,* 50 to 100 mg/kg daily in divided doses every six to eight hours.

Intravenous: This is the preferred route for serious urinary tract and systemic infections. Ticarcillin disodium can be administered by slow injection or by intermittent or continuous infusion. See the manufacturer's literature for the appropriate dilution of the drug, a list of compatible diluents and intravenous solutions, and stability of ticarcillin in these solutions.

For severe systemic infections (eg, septicemia, respiratory tract, skin and soft tissue, intra-abdominal, and female pelvic and genital tract infections), *adults,* 200 to 300 mg/kg daily in divided doses every three, four, or six hours; *children weighing less than 40 kg,* 200 to 300 mg/kg/day in divided doses every four or six hours (the daily dose should not exceed that used for adults); *infants weighing more than 2 kg and ≤ 7 days,* 225 mg/kg daily in divided doses every eight hours; *infants weighing more than 2 kg and over 7 days,* 300 mg/kg daily in divided doses every eight hours; *infants weighing less than 2 kg and ≤ 7 days,* 150 mg/kg daily in divided doses every 12 hours; *infants weighing less than 2 kg and over 7 days,* 225 mg/kg daily in divided doses every eight hours.

For uncomplicated urinary tract infections, *adults,* 4 g daily in divided doses every six hours; *children weighing less than 40 kg,* 50 to 100 mg/kg/day in divided doses every six to eight hours.

For urinary tract infections with complications, *adults and children,* 150 to 200 mg/kg/day in divided doses every four to six hours.

The following schedule is used for *adults and children weighing more than 40 kg* with renal insufficiency (see also the manufacturer's literature): An initial loading dose of 3 g followed by:

Creatinine Clearance (ml/min)	Dosage
>60	3 g every 4 hours
60–30	2 g every 4 hours
30–10	2 g every 8 hours
<10	2 g every 12 hours (or 1 g intramuscularly every 6 hours)
<10 (with hepatic dysfunction)	2 g every 24 hours (or 1 g intramuscularly every 12 hours)
Patients on peritoneal dialysis	3 g every 12 hours
Patients on hemodialysis	2 g every 12 hours supplemented with 3 g after each dialysis

Ticar (Beecham). Powder 1, 3, 6, and 20 g (equivalent to base) (sodium, 5.2 mEq/g).

AZLOCILLIN SODIUM
[Azlin]

Azlocillin is a broad spectrum, semisynthetic penicillin for parenteral use; it is not absorbed when given orally. Chemically, it is an acylureidopenicillin and is related to mezlocillin.

MECHANISM OF ACTION, ANTIMICROBIAL SPECTRUM, AND RESISTANCE. The antibacterial spectrum of azlocillin is very similar to that of mezlocillin (see that evaluation). However, there are some differences. In particular, azlocillin is considerably less active than mezlocillin against *Klebsiella* but is more active against *Pseudomonas aeruginosa* (Fu and Neu, 1978 A). As with mezlocillin, an inoculum effect of some strains of this organism to azlocillin has been observed in vitro, but the clinical significance of this observation has not been determined.

Azlocillin is sensitive to β lactamases. Like the other antipseudomonal penicillins, a large percentage of strains of gram-negative bacilli may be resistant to azlocillin. Therefore, this antibiotic should not be used alone until results of susceptibility tests are known.

For a detailed discussion of the mechanism of action, antimicrobial spectrum, and resistance properties of the penicillins, see the Introduction.

USES. The indications for azlocillin are similar to those for carbenicillin and ticarcillin with the primary use being suspected or proven infections caused by *P. aeruginosa* (see the evaluation on Carbenicillin). It may be used in lower respiratory, urinary tract, skin structure, and bone and joint infections and bacterial septicemia. In vitro, azlocillin combined with an aminoglycoside (eg, gentamicin, tobramycin, amikacin) often produced a synergistic effect against *P. aeruginosa* (Neu and Fu, 1978 A). As with carbenicillin and ticarcillin, such a combination is recommended in *P. aeruginosa* infections or in empiric therapy of severe infections. Since aminoglycosides are inactivated by azlocillin when they are mixed in solution (Pickering and Rutherford, 1981), these drugs should be administered separately.

Clinical experience with azlocillin is more limited than with carbenicillin or ticarcillin in the United States. Presently, it is unclear whether this analogue provides significant advantages over these older penicillins, at least in terms of improved cure rates. Despite azlocillin's broad antibacterial spectrum, resistant bacteria are fairly common and resistance has developed during therapy. Thus, this drug should not be used alone for empiric therapy.

For a more detailed discussion of the uses of antipseudomonal penicillins, see the evaluation of Carbenicillin and the Introduction; see also Chapter 65, Antimicrobial Therapy and Chemoprophylaxis of Infectious Diseases.

ADVERSE REACTIONS AND PRECAUTIONS. Azlocillin is generally well tolerated. Minor gastrointestinal disturbances and skin rashes appear to be the most common side effects. Other adverse effects (eg, hypersensitivity reactions, thrombophlebitis, leukopenia and eosinophilia, platelet dysfunction, elevated hepatic enzyme levels, central nervous system irritation, hypokalemia) that are typical of the antipseudomonal penicillins either have been reported or are likely to occur with azlocillin (see the evaluation of Carbenicillin and the Introduction; see also Parry, 1983). Whether the incidence of certain adverse reactions, such as hypokalemia or platelet dysfunction, will be less with azlocillin compared to carbenicillin and ticarcillin remains to be determined.

Each gram of azlocillin monosodium contains 2.17 mEq (49.8 mg) of sodium and large doses may contribute significantly to the sodium load in patients with impaired sodium excretion mechanisms (eg, those with renal, cardiac, or liver disease). However, therapeutic doses of azlocillin contain less sodium than the disodium salts, ticarcillin or carbenicillin, a possible advantage in these patients (see the evaluations of Ticarcillin and Carbenicillin).

DRUG INTERACTIONS AND INTERFERENCE WITH LABORATORY TESTS. Azlocillin and other antipseudomonal penicillins can inactivate aminoglycosides, particularly gentamicin and tobramycin (Pickering and Rutherford, 1981). Therefore, these antibiotics should not be mixed together prior to administration. Furthermore, in patients with renal failure, in vivo antagonism has been observed. Serum aminoglycoside concentrations should be monitored in such patients and the dosage adjusted accordingly (Mangini, 1984; Hansten, 1985 A; see also Chapter 70, Aminoglycosides).

For a discussion of other drug interactions involving the penicillins, see the Introduction.

PHARMACOKINETICS. Azlocillin is labile in gastric acid and is not absorbed following oral administration. Thus, it must be administered parenterally. Mean serum levels observed five minutes after rapid intravenous injection (5 to 10 minutes) of 2 g and 5 g were 239 mcg/ml and 527 mcg/ml, respectively. Immediately after intravenous infusion (30 minutes) of 2 or 3 g, average serum levels of 165 mcg/ml and 214 mcg/ml, respectively, were measured. Serum levels are not proportional to dose.

Between 20% and 40% of circulating azlocillin is bound to plasma protein. Like other penicillins, azlocillin primarily distributes into the extracellular fluid volume. High concentrations are achieved in bile and urine.

Azlocillin is rapidly eliminated, primarily by renal tubular secretion; probenecid delays excretion. Between 50% and 70% of a dose is recovered as unchanged drug in the urine within 24 hours; less than 10% is metabolized to penicilloic acid derivatives. The half-life in patients with normal renal function is about one hour and is dose-dependent, ie, it increases somewhat with larger doses. The half-life is prolonged in patients with renal impairment and dosage adjustments are necessary in those with moderate to severe insufficiency. For additional discussion, see the Introduction; see also Bergan, 1983.

DOSAGE AND PREPARATIONS.

Intravenous (slow injection over a five-minute period or longer or by intermittent infusion over a 30-minute period): For uncomplicated urinary tract infections, *adults,* 2 g every six hours (100 to 125 mg/kg daily). For complicated urinary tract infections, *adults,* 3 g every six hours (150 to 200 mg/kg daily).

For severe lower respiratory tract, skin and skin structure, and bone and joint infections or septicemia, *adults,* 3 g every four hours or 4 g every six hours (225 to 300 mg/kg daily).

For life-threatening infections, dosage may be increased to 4 g every four hours (maximum, 24 g daily). The usual duration of therapy is 10 to 14 days but may be longer for some infections.

The following schedule is suggested for serious systemic infections in *adults with impaired renal function* (creatinine clearance, ≤ 30 ml/min): 2 g every 8 hours if creatinine clearance is 10 to 30 ml/min and 3 g every 12 hours if creatinine clearance is <10 ml/min. For patients undergoing hemodialysis for renal failure, 3 g should be given after each dialysis and then every 12 hours. (See the manufacturer's literature for additional information.)

Experience with azlocillin in children and infants is limited; the drug is not recommended for neonates. In *children with acute exacerbation of cystic fibrosis,* 75 mg/kg every four hours (450 mg/kg daily); total dosage should not exceed 24 g daily. The drug may be infused over a 30-minute period.

> *Azlin* (Miles). Powder (sterile) 2, 3, and 4 g (equivalent to base) or (for infusion) 2, 3, and 4 g (equivalent to base) (sodium, 2.17 mEq/g).

MEZLOCILLIN SODIUM
[Mezlin]

Mezlocillin sodium is a broad spectrum, semisynthetic penicillin for parenteral use; it is not absorbed when given orally. Chemically, it is an acylureidopenicillin and is related to azlocillin.

MECHANISM OF ACTION, ANTIMICROBIAL SPECTRUM, AND RESISTANCE. Among the currently available penicillins, mezlocillin exhibits one of the broadest spectrums of activity, including organisms susceptible to both ampicillin and carbenicillin (see the evaluations). However, like these other penicillins, mezlocillin also is sensitive to β lactamases.

In vitro, mezlocillin is less active than penicillin G against *Streptococcus pneumoniae* and is comparable to ampicillin against *S. faecalis.* Penicillinase-producing staphylococci are resistant, however. Most strains of *Haemophilus influenzae* and *Neisseria gonorrhoeae* are sensitive. Mezlocillin is more active than either ampicillin or carbenicillin against *Escherichia coli, Klebsiella, Enterobacter, Citrobacter, Acinetobacter, Serratia, Pseudomonas aeruginosa,* and the *Bacteroides fragilis* group. However, as with carbenicillin and ticarcillin, a large percentage of strains of gram-negative bacilli may be resistant to mezlocillin (Fu and Neu, 1978 A). Consequently, the drug should not be used alone until results of susceptibility tests are known.

Mezlocillin's activity against *P. aeruginosa* is about equal to that of ticarcillin but less than that of piperacillin and azlocillin; some ticarcillin- and carbenicillin-resistant organisms have exhibited susceptibility to mezlocillin. Some strains of *P. aeruginosa* have developed resistance fairly rapidly, however. In one study, an inoculum effect of some strains of this organism to mezlocillin appeared to be greater than that previously observed with either ticarcillin or carbenicillin (Fu and Neu, 1978 A), but the clinical significance of this observation has not been determined.

For a detailed discussion of the mechanism of action, antimicrobial spectrum, and resistance properties of the penicillins, see the Introduction.

USES. The indications for mezlocillin are similar to those for carbenicillin and ticarcillin with the primary use being suspected or proven infections caused by *P. aeruginosa* (see the evaluation on Carbenicillin). It may be used in bacterial septicemia and skin and soft tissue, intra-abdominal, gynecologic, and urinary and lower respiratory tract infections. Although mezlocillin is effective in uncomplicated gonorrhea, other drugs are preferred (see Table 2 in Chapter 65).

In vitro, mezlocillin combined with an aminoglycoside (eg, gentamicin, tobramycin, amikacin) often produced a synergistic effect against a number of susceptible organisms, including *P. aeruginosa* (Neu and Fu, 1978 A; Schassan et al, 1978). As with carbenicillin and ticarcillin, such a combination is recommended in *P. aeruginosa* infections or in empiric therapy of severe infections. Since aminoglycosides are inactivated by mezlocillin when they are mixed together in solution (Pickering and Rutherford, 1981), these drugs should be administered separately.

Clinical experience with mezlocillin is more limited than with carbenicillin or ticarcillin in the United States. Presently, it is unclear whether this analogue provides significant advantages over these older penicillins, at least in terms of improved cure rates. Despite mezlocillin's broad antibacterial spectrum, resistant bacteria are fairly common and resistance has developed during therapy. Thus, this drug should not be used alone for empiric therapy of suspected infections.

For a more detailed discussion of the uses of antipseudomonal penicillins, see the evaluation of Carbenicillin and the Introduction; see also Chapter 65, Antimicrobial Therapy and Chemoprophylaxis of Infectious Diseases.

ADVERSE REACTIONS AND PRECAUTIONS. Mezlocillin is generally well tolerated. The most common side effects have been skin rashes and minor gastrointestinal disturbances (incidence, 2% to 3%). Other adverse effects (eg, hypersensitivity reactions, thrombophlebitis, leukopenia and eosinophilia, platelet dysfunction, elevated hepatic enzyme levels, central nervous system irritation, hypokalemia) that are typical of the antipseudomonal penicillins either have been reported or are likely to occur with mezlocillin (see the evaluation of Carbenicillin and the Introduction; see also Parry and Neu, 1982).

Studies in normal volunteers have shown that the effect of mezlocillin on platelet function was less than that of carbenicillin (Copelan et al, 1983; Ballard et al, 1984) or ticarcillin (Somani et al, 1983), which suggests that the risk of a clinical bleeding disorder may be less with mezlocillin. Whether the incidence of other adverse reactions such as hypokalemia will be less with mezlocillin compared to these older antipseudomonal penicillins remains to be determined.

Each gram of mezlocillin monosodium contains 1.85 mEq (42.6 mg) of sodium and large doses may contribute significantly to the sodium load in patients with impaired sodium excretion mechanisms (eg, those with renal, cardiac, or liver disease). However, therapeutic doses of mezlocillin contain less sodium than the disodium salts, ticarcillin or carbenicillin, a possible advantage in these patients (see the evaluations Ticarcillin and Carbenicillin).

DRUG INTERACTIONS AND INTERFERENCE WITH LABORATORY TESTS. Mezlocillin and other antipseudomonal penicillins can inactivate aminoglycosides, particularly gentamicin and tobramycin (Pickering and Rutherford, 1981). Therefore, these antibiotics should not be mixed together prior to administration. Furthermore, in patients with renal failure, in vivo antagonism has been observed. Serum aminoglycoside concentrations should be monitored in such patients and dosage adjusted accordingly (Mangini, 1984; Hansten, 1985 A; see also Chapter 70, Aminoglycosides).

For a discussion of other drug interactions involving the penicillins, see the Introduction.

PHARMACOKINETICS. Mezlocillin is labile in gastric acid and is not absorbed following oral administration. Thus, it must be administered parenterally. After intramuscular injection of 1 g, a peak serum level of about 15 mcg/ml is achieved in approximately 45 minutes. Mean serum levels observed five minutes after rapid intravenous injection (five minutes) of 2 g and 5 g were 253 mcg/ml and 411 mcg/ml, respectively. Immediately after intravenous infusion (30 minutes) of 3 g, an average serum level of 263 mcg/ml was measured. Serum levels are not proportional to dose.

Between 16% and 42% of circulating mezlocillin is bound to plasma protein. Like other penicillins, mezlocillin primarily distributes into the extracellular fluid volume. High concentrations are achieved in bile and urine.

Mezlocillin is rapidly eliminated, primarily by renal tubular secretion; probenecid delays excretion. Between 45% and 70% of a dose is recovered as unchanged drug in the urine; less than 10% is metabolized to penicilloic acid derivatives. Up to 26% of a dose may be excreted in the bile. The half-life in patients with normal renal function is about one hour and is dose-dependent, ie, it increases somewhat with larger doses, suggesting that saturable extrarenal mechanisms are also involved (Bergan, 1978). The half-life is prolonged in patients with renal impairment and dosage adjustments are necessary in those with moderate to severe insufficiency. For additional discussion, see the Introduction.

DOSAGE AND PREPARATIONS.
Intramuscular: For uncomplicated urinary tract infections, *adults,* 1.5 to 2 g every six hours (100 to 125 mg/kg daily).

For uncomplicated gonorrhea, *adults,* 1 to 2 g as a single dose one-half hour after the administration of probenecid 1 g orally.

No more than 2 g should be injected at one time.
Intravenous (direct injection over a three to five-minute period or by intermittent infusion over a 30-minute period): For uncomplicated urinary tract infections, *adults,* 1.5 to 2 g every six hours (100 to 125 mg/kg daily). For severe urinary tract infections, *adults,* 3 g every six hours (150 to 200 mg/kg daily).

For severe lower respiratory tract, intra-abdominal, gynecologic, and skin and skin structure infections or septicemia, *adults*, 4 g every six hours or 3 g every four hours (225 to 300 mg/kg daily).

For life-threatening infections, dosage may be increased to 4 g every four hours (maximum, 24 g daily). The usual duration of therapy is 7 to 10 days but may be longer for some infections.

The following schedule is suggested for serious systemic infections in *adults with impaired renal function* (creatinine clearance, ≤ 30 ml/min): 3 g every eight hours if creatinine clearance is 10 to 30 ml/min and 2 g every eight hours if creatinine clearance is <10 ml/min. For life-threatening infections, the same doses may be administered every six hours. Patients on hemodialysis for renal failure should be given 3 to 4 g after each dialysis and then every 12 hours. Patients on peritoneal dialysis should be given 3 g every 12 hours. (See the manufacturer's literature for additional information.)

Experience with mezlocillin in *children and infants* is limited. The following dosage schedules are recommended by the manufacturer for serious infections: *Infants and children 1 month to 12 years*, 50 mg/kg every four hours; *newborn infants 1 week to 1 month and weighing more than 2 kg*, 75 mg/kg every six hours; *1 week to 1 month and weighing less than 2 kg*, 75 mg/kg every eight hours; *less than 1 week*, 75 mg/kg every 12 hours.

   Mezlin (Miles). Powder (sterile) 1, 2, 3, and 4 g (equivalent to base) or (for infusion) 2, 3, and 4 g (equivalent to base) (sodium, 1.85 mEq/g).

PIPERACILLIN SODIUM
[Pipracil]

Piperacillin is a broad spectrum, semisynthetic penicillin for parenteral use; it is not absorbed when given orally.

SPECTRUM OF ACTIVITY. Piperacillin and mezlocillin have essentially identical antibacterial spectra and, in vitro, the potencies of these extended spectrum penicillins are comparable for most susceptible bacteria, including *Escherichia coli, Klebsiella, Enterobacter, Proteus mirabilis,* indole-positive *Proteus, Citrobacter, Acinetobacter, Serratia, Providencia, Salmonella, Shigella,* streptococci (including *S. faecalis),* and the *Bacteroides fragilis* group (Fu and Neu, 1978 B). (See also the evaluation on Mezlocillin.) Piperacillin is more active in vitro than all other penicillins against *Pseudomonas aeruginosa,* and its potency is similar to that of gentamicin (Fu and Neu, 1978 B; Winston et al, 1978). This drug has been shown to be active against a number of bacterial strains that are resistant to other penicillins (eg, ticarcillin, carbenicillin). Piperacillin is sensitive to β lactamases, however, and organisms that produce these inactivating enzymes (eg, most staphylococci) are resistant. As with other broad spectrum β lactamase-sensitive penicillins, a number of strains of various gram-negative bacilli are resistant to piperacillin and acquired drug resistance can be expected to be a problem with this antibiotic. Consequently, piperacillin should not be used alone until results of susceptibility tests are known.

Like mezlocillin, an inoculum effect and large differences between minimal inhibitory concentrations (MIC) and minimal bactericidal concentrations (MBC) have been observed in vitro with *P. aeruginosa.*

For a detailed discussion of the mechanism of action, antimicrobial spectrum, and resistance properties of the penicillins, see the Introduction.

USES. The indications for piperacillin are similar to those for carbenicillin, ticarcillin, mezlocillin, and azlocillin with the primary use being suspected or proven infections caused by *P. aeruginosa* (see the evaluation on Carbenicillin). It may be used in bacterial septicemia and skin and soft tissue, intra-abdominal, gynecologic, bone and joint, and urinary and lower respiratory tract infections (Winston et al, 1980; Pancoast et al, 1981). Although piperacillin is effective in uncomplicated gonorrhea, other drugs are preferred (see Table 2 in Chapter 65).

In vitro, piperacillin combined with an aminoglycoside (eg, gentamicin, tobramycin, amikacin) often produces a synergistic effect against a number of susceptible organisms, including *P. aeruginosa* (Fu and Neu, 1978 B; Winston et al, 1978). As with carbenicillin, ticarcillin, mezlocillin, and azlocillin, such a combination is recommended in *P. aeruginosa* infections or in empiric therapy of severe infections, particularly in immunocompromised patients. Combination therapy also is recommended to decrease the emergence of piperacillin-resistant organisms, which have appeared when piperacillin was used alone (Winston et al, 1980; Simon et al, 1980). In a small, randomized, double-blind comparison of empiric antibiotic therapy for febrile, granulocytopenic cancer patients, piperacillin plus amikacin was similar to ticarcillin plus amikacin in both efficacy and toxicity. The emergence of resistant organisms was less in patients who received piperacillin plus amikacin, however (Wade et al, 1981). Aminoglycosides are inactivated by piperacillin when the two drugs are mixed together (Pickering and Rutherford, 1981). Therefore, they should be administered separately.

Like mezlocillin, clinical experience with piperacillin is more limited than with carbenicillin or ticarcillin in the United States. Presently, it is unclear whether this analogue provides significant advantages over these older penicillins, at least in terms of improved cure rates. Despite piperacillin's broad antibacterial spectrum, resistant bacteria are fairly common and resistance has developed during therapy. Thus, this drug should not be used alone for empiric therapy of suspected infections.

For a more detailed discussion of the uses of antipseudomonal penicillins, see the evaluation of Carbenicillin and the Introduction; see also Chapter 65, Antimicrobial Therapy and Chemoprophylaxis of Infectious Diseases.

ADVERSE REACTIONS AND PRECAUTIONS. Piperacillin is generally well tolerated. The most common side effects have been thrombophlebitis (4%), diarrhea (3%), and skin rashes (2%). Other adverse reactions (eg, hypersensitivity reactions, leukopenia and eosinophilia, platelet dysfunction, elevated hepatic enzyme levels, central nervous system irritation, hypokalemia) that are typical of the antipseudomonal penicillins either have been reported or are likely to occur with piperacillin (see the evaluation of Carbenicillin and the Introduction; see also Fortner et al, 1982; Holmes et al, 1984).

Based on a study in normal volunteers, the effect of piperacillin on platelet function may be less than that of carbenicillin or ticarcillin at equivalent dosages (Gentry et al, 1981). Whether the incidence of other adverse reactions, such as hypokalemia, will be less with piperacillin compared to these older antipseudomonal penicillins remains to be determined. A high incidence of fever has been reported in patients with cystic fibrosis who received piperacillin (Stead et al, 1984).

Each gram of piperacillin monosodium contains 1.85 mEq (42.5 mg) of sodium, and large doses may contribute significantly to the sodium load in patients with impaired sodium excretion mechanisms (eg, those with renal, cardiac, or liver disease). However, therapeutic doses of piperacillin contain less sodium than the disodium salts, ticarcillin or carbenicillin, a possible advantage in these patients (see the evaluations of Ticarcillin and Carbenicillin).

DRUG INTERACTIONS AND INTERFERENCE WITH LABORATORY TESTS. Piperacillin and other antipseudomonal penicillins can inactivate aminoglycosides, particularly gentamicin and tobramycin (Pickering and Rutherford, 1981). Therefore, these antibiotics should not be mixed together prior to administration. Furthermore, in patients with renal failure, in vivo antagonism has been observed. Serum aminoglycoside concentrations should be monitored in such patients and dosage adjusted accordingly (Mangini, 1984; Hansten, 1985 A; see also Chapter 70, Aminoglycosides).

For a discussion of other drug interactions involving the penicillins, see the Introduction.

PHARMACOKINETICS. Piperacillin is labile in gastric acid and is not absorbed following oral administration. Thus, it must be administered parenterally. After intramuscular injection of 2 g, a peak serum level of about 36 mcg/ml is achieved in approximately 30 minutes. Mean serum levels observed immediately after rapid intravenous injection (two to three minutes) of 2 g and 4 g were 305 mcg/ml and 412 mcg/ml, respectively. Immediately after intravenous infusion (30 minutes) of 4 g or 6 g, average serum levels of 244 mcg/ml and 353 mcg/ml, respectively, were measured. Serum levels are not proportional to dose.

Between 16% and 22% of circulating piperacillin is bound to plasma proteins. Like other penicillins, piperacillin primarily distributes into the extracellular fluid volume. High concentrations are achieved in bile and urine.

Piperacillin is rapidly eliminated, primarily by renal tubular secretion; probenecid delays excretion. Between 60% and 80% of a dose is recovered as unchanged drug in the urine within 24 hours. Up to 25% of an administered dose may be excreted in the bile. The half-life in patients with normal renal function is about one hour and is dose-dependent, ie, it increases somewhat with larger doses. The half-life is prolonged in patients with renal impairment and dosage adjustments are necessary in those with moderate to severe insufficiency. For additional discussion, see the Introduction.

DOSAGE AND PREPARATIONS.
Intramuscular: For uncomplicated urinary tract infections and

most community-acquired pneumonia, *adults,* 6 to 8 g (100 to 125 mg/kg) daily in equally divided doses every 6 to 12 hours.

For uncomplicated gonorrhea, *adults,* 2 g as a single dose one-half hour after the administration of probenecid 1 g orally.

No more than 2 g should be injected at one time.

Intravenous (by direct injection over a three- to five-minute period or by intermittent infusion over a 20- to 30-minute period): For uncomplicated urinary tract infections and most community-acquired pneumonia, *adults,* 6 to 8 g (100 to 125 mg/kg) daily in equally divided doses every 6 to 12 hours.

For complicated urinary tract infections, *adults,* 8 to 16 g (125 to 200 mg/kg) daily in equally divided doses every six to eight hours.

For severe lower respiratory tract, intra-abdominal, gynecologic, skin and soft tissue infections or septicemia, *adults,* 12 to 18 g (200 to 300 mg/kg) daily in equally divided doses every four to six hours.

The maximum daily dose for adults is usually 24 g/day. The usual duration of therapy is 7 to 10 days but may be longer for some infections.

The following schedule is suggested for serious systemic infections *in adults with impaired renal function* (creatinine clearance, <40 ml/min): 4 g every eight hours if creatinine clearance is 20 to 40 ml/min and 4 g every 12 hours if creatinine clearance is <20 ml/min. Patients on hemodialysis for renal failure should be given 2 g every eight hours and 1 g after each dialysis. (See the manufacturer's literature for additional information.)

Dosage labeling for piperacillin for *children under 12 years* has not been approved. Most infectious disease experts suggest 200 to 300 mg/kg daily in divided doses every four to six hours for serious systemic infections (The Medical Letter, 1984; Nelson, 1985 A).

Pipracil (Lederle). Powder (sterile) 2, 3, and 4 g (equivalent to base) or (for infusion) 2, 3, and 4 g (equivalent to base) (sodium 1.85 mEq/g).

AMIDINO PENICILLIN

AMDINOCILLIN
[Coactin]

Amdinocillin is a semisynthetic penicillin for parenteral use. It is not absorbed when given orally.

MECHANISM OF ACTION, ANTIMICROBIAL SPECTRUM, AND RESISTANCE. Unlike other penicillins and cephalosporins, amdinocillin binds preferentially to penicillin binding protein 2 (PBP2) of gram-negative bacteria to produce osmotically stable round forms. It does not bind to PBPs of gram-positive bacteria (Neu, 1983 A, 1985).

Amdinocillin is active against many enteric gram-negative bacilli, including *Escherichia coli, Klebsiella pneumoniae, Enterobacter species, Citrobacter* species, *Salmonella enteritidis* species and *Salmonella typhi,* and *Shigella* species. Some *Proteus mirabilis* and *Serratia marcescens* strains also are susceptible. The diarrheal pathogens, *Campylobacter jejuni, Yersinia enterocolitica,* and *Aeromonas hydrophila,* are highly susceptible to amdinocillin. However, this agent is not reliably active against most gram-positive bacteria, *Haemophilus influenzae*, indole-positive *Proteus, Pseudomonas aeruginosa* and other nonfermenting gram-negative bacilli, or anaerobic bacteria (eg, the *Bacteroides fragilis* group) (see Neu, 1983 A, 1985; *Med Lett Drugs Ther*, 1985 A; Sahm et al, 1985).

Amdinocillin acts synergistically with other penicillins and cephalosporins in vitro to inhibit some strains of enteric gram-negative bacilli. However, there seems to be no way to predict which strains will respond in this manner. Thus, the clinical utility of such combinations remains uncertain (see Neu, 1983 A, 1985; Cleeland and Squires, 1983; Farrar, 1984; *Med Lett Drugs Ther*, 1985 A).

Amdinocillin is susceptible to inactivation by β lactamases but is more resistant than ampicillin to the common plasmid-mediated TEM-1 β lactamase (Neu, 1985; see also the section on Resistance). For additional discussion, see the Introduction.

USES. Parenterally administered amdinocillin, either alone or in combination with other β-lactam antibiotics, has been shown to be effective for complicated and uncomplicated urinary tract infections caused by susceptible Enterobacteriaceae, primarily *Escherichia coli, Klebsiella*, and *Enterobacter* (Demos and Green, 1983; Cox, 1983; Ward et al, 1983; King et al, 1983; Rotstein and Farrar, 1983; see also the review by Neu, 1985). However, it is not presently known whether this antibiotic offers any clinical advantages over other agents (eg, other penicillins, cephalosporins, trimethoprim/sulfamethoxazole). Furthermore, although combinations of amdinocillin and various other β-lactam agents exhibit synergy against a number of enteric gram-negative bacilli in vitro, these data cannot easily be extrapolated to clinical effectiveness. Clinical experience with amdinocillin for infections outside the urinary tract is very limited. Thus, the current role of this agent in infectious disease therapy appears to be small (Farrar, 1984; *Med Lett Drugs Ther*, 1985 A; Neu, 1985; see also the Introduction).

ADVERSE REACTIONS AND PRECAUTIONS. Amdinocillin is generally well tolerated. The most frequently reported adverse reactions occur in about 5% of patients and include eosinophilia, thrombocytosis, and elevations in serum aspartate aminotransferase (SGOT) and alkaline phosphatase. Adverse reactions reported in about 1% of patients include skin rashes, thrombophlebitis, diarrhea and nausea, dizziness, and anemia, neutropenia, and leukopenia. Pruritus and/or urticaria, pain at the injection site, vomiting, drowsiness and lethargy, elevated blood pressure, vaginitis, thrombocytopenia, and elevations in serum alanine aminotransferase (SGPT) have been reported rarely. Nephritis and seizures have not yet been reported, but amdinocillin has the potential to produce any of the hypersensitivity reactions or other adverse effects that have occurred with penicillins (see the Introduction). Patients allergic to any penicillin should be considered allergic to amdinocillin.

DRUG INTERACTIONS AND INTERFERENCE WITH LABORATORY TESTS. See the Introduction.

PHARMACOKINETICS. Amdinocillin is not absorbed following oral administration. Thus, it must be administered parenterally.

After intramuscular injection of 10 mg/kg, a peak serum concentration of 26 mcg/ml was achieved in approximately 30 minutes. Following intravenous infusion of 10 mg/kg over 15 minutes, the average peak serum level was 61 mcg/ml (range, 34 to 80 mcg/ml).

Between 5% and 10% of circulating amdinocillin is bound to plasma protein. Like other penicillins, amdinocillin primarily distributes into the extracellular fluid volume. High concentrations are achieved in urine.

Amdinocillin is rapidly eliminated, primarily by renal tubular secretion; probenecid delays excretion. Between 75% and 90% of a dose is recovered as unchanged drug in the urine. Amdinocillin is metabolized minimally. The half-life in patients with normal renal function is between 50 and 60 minutes. It is prolonged slightly (3.3 hours) in patients with severe renal insufficiency (creatinine clearance less than 10 ml/minute). Simultaneous infusion of amdinocillin and cephalothin did not alter the pharmacokinetic properties of either drug (Gambertoglio et al, 1983).

For additional discussion, see the Introduction; see also Neu, 1985, and the manufacturer's literature.

DOSAGE AND PREPARATIONS.
Intramuscular, Intravenous: Adults, 10 mg/kg every four to six hours.

In *adults* with moderate to severe renal impairment (creatinine clearance less than 30 ml/min), the dosage should be limited to 10 mg/kg every six to eight hours.

For additional discussion, see the manufacturer's literature.
Coactin (Roche). Powder 500 mg and 1 g.

MIXTURES OF PENICILLINS WITH CLAVULANIC ACID (β LACTAMASE INHIBITOR)

Clavulanic acid is a β lactam isolated from *Streptomyces clavuligerus* (Figure 2). It has only weak antibacterial properties of its own, but is a potent inhibitor of many bacterial β lactamases.

FIGURE 2. CHEMICAL STRUCTURE OF CLAVULANIC ACID

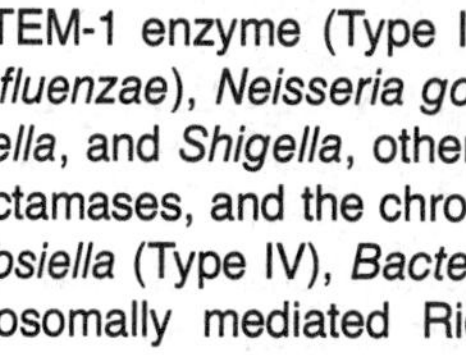

Clavulanic acid inhibits the plasmid-mediated exoenzymes from staphylococci and the gram-negative β lactamases of the Richmond Types II, III, IV, and V. These include the common plasmid-mediated TEM-1 enzyme (Type III) present in *Haemophilus* (eg, *H. influenzae*), *Neisseria gonorrhoeae*, *Escherichia coli, Salmonella*, and *Shigella*, other plasmid-mediated gram-negative β lactamases, and the chromosomally mediated enzymes of *Klebsiella* (Type IV), *Bacteroides fragilis*, and *Legionella*. Chromosomally mediated Richmond Type I β lactamases that are present in *Enterobacter, Serratia, Morganella, Citrobacter, Pseudomonas*, and *Acinetobacter* are not inhibited by clavulanic acid (see Table 2; see also

1330

TABLE 2.
INHIBITION OF BETA-LACTAMASES BY CLAVULANIC ACID

Beta-lactamases	Name	Organism	Inhibition by Clavulanic Acid
Plasmid		*Staphylococcus aureus*	Yes
Plasmid	TEM-1	*Escherichia coli* *Haemophilus* *Neisseria gonorrhoeae* *Salmonella* *Shigella*	Yes
Plasmid	TEM-2	*E. coli*	Yes
Plasmid	SHV-1	*Klebsiella*	Yes
Plasmid	OXA 1, 2, 3	*E. coli*	Variable
Plasmid	PSE 1, 2, 3	*Pseudomonas*	Variable
Chromosomal	Type Ia*	*Enterobacter* *Morganella* *Citrobacter* *Serratia*	No
Chromosomal	Type Id*	*Pseudomonas*	No
Chromosomal	Type IV, K1*	*Klebsiella*	Yes
Chromosomal		*Bacteroides*	Yes
Chromosomal		*Legionella*	Yes

*Richmond-Sykes classification (Richmond and Sykes, 1973)
Adapted from Neu, 1984 C

Reading and Cole, 1977; Neu and Fu, 1978 B; Wise et al, 1978; Neu, 1984 C).

The mechanism of inhibition by clavulanic acid depends on the particular β lactamase. Although reversible inhibition is seen, clavulanic acid frequently acts as a suicide inactivator, which, after forming an acylenzyme intermediate, irreversibly inactivates the enzyme (Bush and Sykes, 1983; Neu, 1984 C).

Clinically, clavulanic acid is being used in fixed-ratio combinations with β-lactam antibiotics that alone are susceptible to β-lactamase inactivation. Presently, amoxicillin/potassium clavulanate [Augmentin] and ticarcillin/potassium clavulanate [Timentin] are marketed in the United States. The rationale for these combinations is that clavulanic acid irreversibly binds β lactamases and protects the β lactam antibiotic from inactivation by β lactamase-producing bacteria. Thus, the useful antibacterial spectrum of the β-lactam agent is extended to include these bacterial strains.

AMOXICILLIN/POTASSIUM CLAVULANATE
[Augmentin]

The combination of amoxicillin trihydrate, an aminopenicillin, and potassium clavulanate, a β-lactamase inhibitor, is marketed in 2:1 and 4:1 fixed-ratio dosage forms for oral administration.

MECHANISM OF ACTION, ANTIMICROBIAL SPECTRUM, AND RESISTANCE. Amoxicillin alone is active in vitro against a wide variety of gram-positive and gram-negative bacteria, including group A and other streptococci, pneumococci, enterococci, many anaerobic bacteria, *Neisseria meningitidis*, many strains of *Salmonella*, and nonβ lactamase-producing strains of staphylococci, gonococci, *Haemophilus influenzae*, and *Branhamella catarrhalis*. At levels achievable in urine, many strains of *Escherichia coli* and *Proteus mirabilis* will be susceptible (see the evaluation and the Introduction). The addition of clavulanic acid does not alter the susceptibility of amoxicillin-sensitive strains and extends the in vitro activity of amoxicillin to include, at achievable serum concentrations, β lactamase-producing strains of *H. influenzae, H. ducreyi, Neisseria gonorrhoeae, Staphylococcus aureus* (but not methicillin-resistant strains), and *B. catarrhalis*. At achievable urine concentrations, many β lactamase-producing strains of *E. coli, Klebsiella, Proteus,* and *Citrobacter diversus* will be susceptible. *Bacteroides fragilis* and *Legionella pneumophila* also are sensitive in vitro to amoxicillin/potassium clavulanate. The combination is not active against *Pseudomonas aeruginosa* and *Serratia* and many strains of *Enterobacter, Morganella,* and *Providencia* are resistant (see *Med Lett Drugs Ther*, 1984 B; Neu, 1984 C; Weber et al, 1984; Smith and LeFrock, 1985).

For a discussion of the mechanism of action of clavulanic acid, see above; for a discussion of the mechanism of action of amoxicillin, see the Introduction.

USES. Amoxicillin/potassium clavulanate appears to be an effective alternative to erythromycin/sulfisoxazole, trimethoprim/sulfamethoxazole, and cefaclor for the treatment of acute otitis media and acute sinusitis caused by amoxicillin-resistant *H. influenzae* and *B. catarrhalis* (see *Med Lett Drugs Ther*, 1984 B; Weber et al, 1984; Smith and LeFrock, 1985). In one study, this combination was superior to cefaclor for acute otitis media in children, although the incidence of side effects, particularly mild diarrhea, was greater with amoxicillin/potassium clavulanate (Odio et al, 1985).

Amoxicillin/potassium clavulanate appears to be effective oral therapy for mild to moderate lower respiratory tract infections caused by β lactamase-producing *H. influenzae* and *B. catarrhalis* (Wallace et al, 1985; for others, see Weber et al, 1984). Further comparative evaluation of this combination with other therapies is necessary before its role in lower respiratory tract infections can be clearly defined.

Many studies have demonstrated the effectiveness of amoxicillin/potassium clavulanate in primary and recurrent urinary tract infections caused by susceptible *E. coli* and other bacteria, including many strains resistant to amoxicillin alone (Iravani and Richard, 1982; Brumfitt and Hamilton-Miller, 1984; for others, see Weber et al, 1984; Smith and LeFrock, 1985). This combination appears to be suitable for the treatment of complicated and recurrent urinary tract infections caused by susceptible pathogens (see Weber et al, 1984). Also, because of the increasing emergence of community-acquired *E. coli* resistant to amoxicillin alone, amoxicillin/potassium clavulanate may become important in the treatment of uncomplicated urinary tract infections. However, further studies are needed to evaluate the relative efficacy of this combination compared to other antimicrobial agents (eg, trimethoprim/sulfamethoxazole) in urinary tract infections. In one small study, amoxicillin/potassium clavulanate was at least as effective as trimethoprim/sulfamethoxazole following a seven-day course of therapy (Fancourt et al, 1984).

Amoxicillin/potassium clavulanate has been effective in skin and soft tissue infections caused by susceptible pathogens, including β lactamase-producing *S. aureus* (see Weber et al, 1984; Smith and LeFrock, 1985). However, any advantages over currently recommended agents (eg, oral penicillinase-resistant penicillins) remain to be determined.

Amoxicillin/potassium clavulanate was effective in chancroid caused by β lactamase-producing *H. ducreyi* (Fast et al, 1982). Clinical studies are very limited, however, and erythromycin, ceftriaxone, or trimethoprim/sulfamethoxazole currently is preferred. Although single large doses of amoxicillin (3 g)/potassium clavulanate (125 to 500 mg) were effective in some cases of uncomplicated gonorrhea caused by penicillinase-producing *N. gonorrhoeae* (PPNG), failures have been reported (DeKoning et al, 1981; Lawrence and Shanson, 1983; Munday et al, 1985). A number of effective parenteral antibiotics (eg, spectinomycin, ceftriaxone, cefoxitin, cefotaxime) already are available for these infections.

Amoxicillin/potassium clavulanate may be useful in human and animal bite wounds (Goldstein et al, 1984; see also *Med Lett Drugs Ther*, 1984 B).

ADVERSE REACTIONS AND PRECAUTIONS. Amoxicillin/potassium clavulanate generally is well tolerated; less than 3% of patients discontinued therapy because of side effects. The most frequently reported adverse reactions were diarrhea/loose stools (9%), nausea (3%), skin rashes and urticaria (3%), vomiting (1%), and vaginitis (1%). Diarrhea appears to be more frequent with amoxicillin/potassium clavulanate than with amoxicillin alone (see *Med Lett Drugs Ther*, 1984 B; Weber et al, 1984; Smith and LeFrock, 1985). It is more common with larger doses of clavulanic acid (eg, 250 mg or more).

Less frequently reported adverse reactions include abdominal discomfort, flatulence, headache, dizziness, and moderate increases in serum transaminase (SGOT, SGPT) concentrations. Two cases of pseudomembraneous colitis have been reported.

Amoxicillin/potassium clavulanate has the potential to produce any of the hypersensitivity reactions or other adverse effects associated with amoxicillin therapy alone (see the evaluation and the Introduction). Patients allergic to any penicillin should be considered allergic to amoxicillin/potassium clavulanate.

This drug is classified in FDA Pregnancy Category B.

DRUG INTERACTIONS AND INTERFERENCE WITH LABORATORY TESTS. See the Introduction.

PHARMACOKINETICS. Amoxicillin/potassium clavulanate is stable in gastric acid and is well absorbed from the gastrointestinal tract following oral administration; absorption is not affected by food, milk, or antacids. Peak serum concentrations of 4.4 and 7.6 mcg/ml of amoxicillin and 2.3 mcg/ml of clavulanic acid occur one to two hours after doses of amoxicillin (250 mg)/potassium clavulanate (125 mg) (one Augmentin '250' tablet) and amoxicillin (500 mg)/potassium clavulanate (125 mg) (one Augmentin '500' tablet), respectively. The amoxicillin serum concentrations achieved with the combination are comparable to those observed with amoxicillin alone (see the evaluation).

About 20% of circulating amoxicillin and 30% of clavulanic acid are bound to plasma protein. Both agents primarily distribute into the extracellular fluid volume. High concentrations are achieved in urine. Adequate concentrations of both drugs are found in bile, pleural and peritoneal fluid, and middle ear fluid. Both agents penetrate poorly into sputum, and concentrations in cerebrospinal fluid are very low in the absence of inflammation. Both amoxicillin and clavulanic acid cross the placenta.

Both amoxicillin and clavulanic acid are excreted by the kidneys. Probenecid delays excretion of amoxicillin, but not of clavulanic acid. Approximately 50% to 70% of amoxicillin, and 25% to 40% of clavulanic acid are recovered as unchanged drugs in the urine after six hours. Clavulanic acid appears to undergo considerable metabolism. The elimination half-lives of amoxicillin and clavulanic acid are about 1.3 hours and 1 hour, respectively. Elimination of both drugs is prolonged in patients with impaired renal function; dosage adjustments are made for the amoxicillin component.

For additional discussion, see Weber et al, 1984, Smith and LeFrock, 1985, and the manufacturer's literature; see also the evaluation of Amoxicillin.

DOSAGE AND PREPARATIONS.

Oral: *Adults and children weighing more than 40 kg*, the usual dose is amoxicillin 250 mg/potassium clavulanate 125 mg (one Augmentin '250' tablet) every eight hours; for more severe infections and infections of the respiratory tract, amoxicillin 500 mg/potassium clavulanate 125 mg (one Augmentin '500' tablet) every eight hours (*NOTE:* Since both Augmentin '250' and '500' tablets contain the same amount of clavulanic acid, ie, 125 mg as the potassium salt, two Augmentin '250' tablets are not equivalent to one Augmentin '500' tablet).

Children weighing less than 40 kg, the usual dose is 20 mg/kg daily (based on the amoxicillin component) in divided doses every eight hours; for otitis media, sinusitis, lower respiratory infections, and other more severe infections, 40 mg/kg daily (based on the amoxicillin component) in divided doses every eight hours.

Augmentin '250', '500' Tablets (Beecham). Tablets containing 250 or 500 mg amoxicillin (as trihydrate) and 125 mg clavulanic acid (as potassium; potassium, 0.63 mEq/tablet); **Augmentin '125', '250' for Oral Suspension** (Beecham). Powder for oral suspension containing 125 or 250 mg amoxicillin and 31.25 or 62.5 mg clavulanic acid (as potassium salt)/5 ml (potassium, 0.16 or 0.32 mEq/5 ml); **Augmentin '125', '250' Chewable Tablets** (Beecham). Chewable tablets containing 125 or 250 mg amoxicillin (as trihydrate) and 31.25 or 62.5 mg clavulanic acid (as potassium; potassium, 0.16 or 0.32 mEq/tablet).

TICARCILLIN DISODIUM/POTASSIUM CLAVULANATE
[Timentin]

The combination of ticarcillin disodium, a carboxypenicillin, and potassium clavulanate, a β-lactamase inhibitor, is marketed in a 30:1 fixed-ratio dosage form for parenteral administration.

MECHANISM OF ACTION, ANTIMICROBIAL SPECTRUM, AND RESISTANCE.

Ticarcillin alone is a broad spectrum antipseudomonal penicillin that is active in vitro against most gram-positive bacteria (except enterococci and β lactamase-producing staphylococci), gram-negative cocci, and, when compared to ampicillin, an expanded spectrum of gram-negative bacilli, including *Escherichia coli*, *Proteus mirabilis*, indole-positive *Proteus* (*Providencia rettgeri*, *Morganella morganii*, *Proteus vulgaris*), *Enterobacter*, *Pseudomonas aeruginosa*, *Acinetobacter*, and the *Bacteroides fragilis* group. However, β lactamase-producing strains of these gram-negative bacilli can inactivate ticarcillin and are relatively common (see the evaluation and the Introduction).

The addition of clavulanic acid does not alter the susceptibility of ticarcillin-sensitive strains and extends the in vitro activity of ticarcillin to include, at achievable serum concentrations, β lactamase-producing strains of many Enterobacteriaceae, including *Escherichia coli*, *Klebsiella pneumoniae* and *K. oxytosa*, *Citrobacter diversus* and *C. amaloneticus*, *Proteus vulgaris*, *Providencia rettgeri* and *P. stuartii*, and some strains of *Serratia marcescens* and *Enterobacter*; the *Bacteroides fragilis* group; *Haemophilus* species; *Neisseria* species; and staphylococci (except methicillin-resistant strains). However, the in vitro susceptibilies of *Pseudomonas aeruginosa*, *Acineto-*

bacter calcoaceticus, and a number of *Serratia marcescens* and *Enterobacter* strains are not enhanced by the presence of clavulanic acid at concentrations expected in serum. Thus, these organisms should be considered resistant to ticarcillin/potassium clavulanate if they are resistant to ticarcillin alone (Barry et al, 1984; Clarke and Zemcov, 1984; Fuchs et al, 1984; see also *Med Lett Drugs Ther*, 1985 B).

For a discussion of the mechanism of action of clavulanic acid, see above; for a discussion of the mechanism of action of ticarcillin, see the Introduction.

USES. Ticarcillin/potassium clavulanate is indicated for serious lower respiratory tract, urinary tract, bone and joint, and skin and soft tissue infections, and septicemia caused by susceptible β lactamase-producing strains of various gram-negative bacilli and *Staphylococcus aureus* or by ticarcillin-susceptible organisms. Because of its broad antibacterial spectrum against gram-positive and gram-negative bacteria, including many β lactamase-producing strains, this combination is being promoted for the treatment of mixed infections and for presumptive therapy prior to the identification of the causative organisms (see the manufacturer's literature). Clinical experience with ticarcillin/potassium clavulanate is limited, however, and published results of prospective, randomized, double-blind, comparative clinical trials with conventional antimicrobial therapies generally are unavailable. Thus, it is difficult to identify specific clinical situations in which this combination would be preferred to other agents. Its expanded spectrum of activity against β lactamase-producing strains of various Enterobacteriaceae (eg, *Escherichia coli*, *Klebsiella*), the *Bacteroides fragilis* group, and *Staphylococcus aureus* appear to be advantages when compared to ticarcillin alone. On the other hand, attainable serum concentrations of clavulanic acid do not enhance the susceptibility of *Pseudomonas aeruginosa* to ticarcillin. Thus, as with ticarcillin alone, ticarcillin/potassium clavulanate should be combined with an aminoglycoside for systemic *P. aeruginosa* infections. Such combination therapy also is recommended empirically for febrile neutropenic patients (see the evaluations of Ticarcillin and Carbenicillin and the Introduction). See also *Med Lett Drugs Ther*, 1985 B.

ADVERSE REACTIONS AND PRECAUTIONS. Ticarcillin/potassium clavulanate generally is well tolerated and adverse reactions are similar to those seen with ticarcillin alone. These may include hypersensitivity reactions (eg, skin rash), central nervous system disturbances (eg, headache), gastrointestinal disturbances (eg, nausea, diarrhea), hematologic abnormalities (eg, platelet dysfunction with potential for bleeding), and electrolyte disturbances (eg, hypokalemia) (see the evaluations on Ticarcillin and Carbenicillin and the Introduction). Patients allergic to any penicillin should be considered allergic to ticarcillin/potassium clavulanate.

This drug is classified in FDA Pregnancy Category B.

DRUG INTERACTIONS AND INTERFERENCE WITH LABORATORY TESTS. As with ticarcillin alone, the mixing of ticarcillin/potassium clavulanate with an aminoglycoside in parenteral solutions prior to administration can inactivate the aminoglycoside. In vivo antagonism in patients with renal failure also can occur (see the evaluation on Ticarcillin and

Chapter 70, Aminoglycosides).

For a discussion of other drug interactions involving the penicillins, see the Introduction.

PHARMACOKINETICS. After intravenous infusion (30 minutes) of ticarcillin (3 g)/potassium clavulanate (100 mg) (Timentin 3.1 g formulation), peak serum concentrations of both drugs were attained immediately after completion of the infusion. Ticarcillin serum concentrations were similar to those produced by an equivalent dose of ticarcillin alone (mean peak serum concentration, 330 mcg/ml). The corresponding mean peak serum concentration of clavulanic acid was 8 mcg/ml (manufacturer's literature).

About 45% of circulating ticarcillin and 9% of clavulanic acid are bound to plasma proteins. Both agents primarily distribute into the extracellular fluid volume. High concentrations are achieved in the urine.

Both ticarcillin and clavulanic acid are excreted by the kidneys. Probenecid delays excretion of ticarcillin, but not of clavulanic acid. Approximately 60% to 70% of ticarcillin and 35% to 45% of clavulanic acid are recovered as unchanged drugs in the urine after six hours. Clavulanic acid appears to undergo considerable metabolism. The elimination half-lives of ticarcillin and clavulanic acid in normal volunteers are about 1.1 hours. Elimination of both drugs is prolonged in patients with impaired renal function; dosage adjustments are made for the ticarcillin component.

For additional discussion, see the manufacturer's literature; see also the evaluation of Ticarcillin.

DOSAGE AND PREPARATIONS.

Intravenous: Ticarcillin/potassium clavulanate should be administered by intermittent infusion over 30 minutes. See the manufacturer's literature for the appropriate dilution of the drug, a list of compatible diluents and intravenous solutions, and stability of ticarcillin/potassium clavulanate in these solutions. The manufacturer's dosage recommendations are as follows:

For systemic and urinary tract infections for *average (60 kg) adults*, ticarcillin 3 g/potassium clavulanate 100 mg, ie, 3.1 g Timentin, every four to six hours; for *patients weighing less than 60 kg*, 200 to 300 mg/kg daily (based on the ticarcillin component) in divided doses every four to six hours. For *infants and children under 12*, dosages have not been established.

In *adults with renal insufficiency*, an initial loading dose of 3.1 g should be followed by doses based on creatinine clearance and type of dialysis as indicated below:

Creatinine Clearance (ml/min)	Dosage
>60	3.1 g every 4 hours
60–30	2 g every 4 hours
30–10	2 g every 8 hours
<10	2 g every 12 hours
<10 (with hepatic dysfunction)	2 g every 24 hours
Patients on peritoneal dialysis	3.1 g every 12 hours
Patients on hemodialysis	2 g every 12 hours supplemented with 3.1 g after each dialysis

Half-life of ticarcillin in patients with renal failure, about 13 hours

Timentin (Beecham). Powder (sterile) containing 3 g ticarcillin (as disodium salt) and 100 mg clavulanic acid (as potassium salt) in 3.1 g containers (sodium, 4.75 mEq/g).

Cited References

Mezlocillin sodium (Mezlin). *Med Lett Drugs Ther* 23:110-111, 1981.

Piperacillin sodium (Pipracil). *Med Lett Drugs Ther* 24:48-49, 1982 A.

Azlocillin sodium (Azlin). *Med Lett Drugs Ther* 24:113-114, 1982 B.

Treatment of sexually transmitted disease. *Med Lett Drugs Ther* 26:5-10, 1984 A.

Amoxicillin-clavulanic acid (Augmentin). *Med Lett Drugs Ther* 26:99-100, 1984 B.

Amdinocillin. *Med Lett Drugs Ther* 27:30-32, 1985 A.

Ticarcillin-clavulanic acid (Timentin). *Med Lett Drugs Ther* 27:69-70, 1985 B.

Antimicrobial susceptibility tests. *Med Lett Drugs Ther* 28:2-4, 1986.

Chromosomally mediated resistant *Neisseria gonorrhoeae*—United States. *Morbid Mortal Week Rep* 33:408-410, 1984.

1985 STD treatment guidelines. *Morbid Mortal Week Rep* 34:75S-108S, 1985 A.

Chlamydia trachomatis infections: Policy guidelines for prevention and control. *Morbid Mortal Week Rep* 34:53S-74S, 1985 B.

Penicillinase-producing *Neisseria gonorrhoeae*—United States, Florida. *Morbid Mortal Week Rep* 35:12-14, 1986.

Back DJ, et al: Interindividual variation and drug interactions with hormonal steroid contraceptives. *Drugs* 21:46-61, 1981.

Ballard JO, et al: Comparison of effects of mezlocillin, carbenicillin, and placebo on normal hemostasis. *Antimicrob Agents Chemother* 25:153-156, 1984.

Barry AL, et al: In vitro activity of ticarcillin plus clavulanic acid against bacteria isolated in three centers. *Eur J Clin Microbiol* 3:203-206, 1984.

Barza M: Antimicrobial spectrum, pharmacology, and therapeutic use of antibiotics: Part 2. Penicillins. *Am J Hosp Pharm* 74:57-67, 1977.

Bergan T: Pharmacokinetics of mezlocillin in healthy volunteers. *Antimicrob Agents Chemother* 14:801-806, 1978.

Bergan T: Review of pharmacokinetics and dose dependency of azlocillin in normal subjects and patients with renal insufficiency. *J Antimicrob Chemother* 11(suppl B):101-114, 1983.

Brumfitt W, Hamilton-Miller JMT: Amoxicillin plus clavulanic acid in treatment of recurrent urinary tract infections. *Antimicrob Agents Chemother* 25:276-278, 1984.

Bush K, Sykes RB: β-lactamase inhibitors in perspective. *J Antimicrob Chemother* 11:97-107, 1983.

Chow AW, Jewesson PJ: Pharmacokinetics and safety of antimicrobial agents during pregnancy. *Rev Infect Dis* 7:287-313, 1985.

Clarke AM, Zemcov SJV: Clavulanic acid in combination with ticarcillin: In vitro comparison with other β-lactams. *J Antimicrob Chemother* 13:121-128, 1984.

Cleeland A, Squires E: Enhanced activity of beta-lactam antibiotics with amdinocillin in vitro and in vivo. *Am J Med* 75(suppl 2A):21-29, (Aug 29) 1983.

Condemi JJ: Allergy to penicillin and other antibiotics, in Reese RE, Douglas RG (eds): *A Practical Approach to Infectious Diseases*. Boston, Little, Brown and Company, 1983, 163-180.

Conte JE, Barriere SL: *Manual of Antibiotics and Infectious Diseases*, ed 5. Philadelphia, Lea & Febiger, 1984, 63-64.

Copelan EA, et al: Comparison of effects of mezlocillin and carbenicillin on haemostasis in volunteers. *J Antimicrob Chemother* 11(suppl C):43-49, 1983.

Cox CE: Parenteral amdinocillin for treatment of complicated urinary tract infections. *Am J Med* 75(suppl 2A):82-84, (Aug 29) 1983.

DeKoning GAJ, et al: Combination of clavulanic acid and amoxicillin (Augmentin) in treatment of patients infected with penicillinase producing gonococci, (letter). *J Antimicrob Chemother* 8:81-82, 1981.

Demos CH, Green E: Review of clinical experience with amdinocillin monotherapy and comparative studies. *Am J Med* 75(suppl 2A):72-81, (Aug 29) 1983.

Ditlove J, et al: Methicillin nephritis. *Medicine* 56:483-491, 1977.

Drusano GL, et al: Acylampicillins: Mezlocillin, piperacillin, and azlocillin. *Rev Infect Dis* 6:13-32, 1984.

Eichenwald HF, McCracken GH Jr: Antimicrobial therapy in infants and children: Part I. Review of antimicrobial agents. *J Pediatr* 93:337-356, 1978.

Eickhoff TC, Ehret JM: Comparative activity in vitro of ticarcillin BL-P1654 and carbenicillin. *Antimicrob Agents Chemother* 10:241-244, 1976.

Eliopoulos GM, Moellering RC Jr: Azlocillin, mezlocillin, and piperacillin: New broad-spectrum penicillins. *Ann Intern Med* 97:755-760, 1982.

Fancourt GJ, et al: Augmentin (amoxycillin-clavulanic acid) compared with co-trimoxazole in urinary tract infections. *Br Med J* 289:82-83, 1984.

Farrar WE: Amdinocillin, (editorial). *Ann Intern Med* 101:389-390, 1984.

Faruki H, et al: Community-based outbreak of infection with penicillin-resistant *Neisseria gonorrhoeae* not producing penicillinase (chromosomally mediated resistance). *N Engl J Med* 313:607-611, 1985.

Fast MV, et al: Treatment of chancroid by clavulanic acid with amoxycillin in patients with β-lactamase-positive *Haemophilus ducreyi* infection. *Lancet* 2:509-511, 1982.

Fortner CL, et al: Piperacillin sodium: Antibacterial spectrum, pharmacokinetics, clinical efficacy, and adverse reactions. *Pharmacotherapy* 2:287-299, 1982.

Fu KP, Neu HC: Azlocillin and mezlocillin: New ureido penicillins. *Antimicrob Agents Chemother* 13:930-938, 1978 A.

Fu KP, Neu HC: Piperacillin: New penicillin active against many bacteria resistant to other penicillins. *Antimicrob Agents Chemother* 13:358-367, 1978 B.

Fuchs PC, et al: In vitro activity of ticarcillin plus clavulanic acid against 632 clinical isolates. *Antimicrob Agents Chemother* 25:392-394, 1984.

Gambertoglio JG, et al: Amdinocillin pharmacokinetics: Simultaneous administration with cephalothin and cerebrospinal fluid penetration. *Am J Med* 75(suppl 2A):54-59, (Aug 29) 1983.

Gentry LO, et al: Effects of sodium piperacillin on platelet function in normal volunteers. *Antimicrob Agents Chemother* 19:532-533, 1981.

Goldstein EJ, et al: Animal and human bite wounds: Comparative study, Augmentin versus penicillin ± dicloxacillin. *Postgrad Med J* 76 (suppl): 105-110, 1984

Hamilton-Miller JMT: β-lactamases and their clinical significance. *J Antimicrob Chemother* 9(suppl B):11-19, 1982.

Handsfield HH: PPNG infections: Current status and guidelines for therapy. *Drug Ther* 12:118-124, (July) 1982.

Handwerger S, Tomasz A: Antibiotic tolerance among clinical isolates of bacteria. *Rev Infect Dis* 7:368-386, 1985.

Hansten PD: Warfarin and nafcillin. *Drug Interact Newslett* 4:24, 1984.

Hansten PD: *Drug Interactions*, ed 5. Philadelphia, Lea & Febiger, 1985 A, 194-260.

Hansten PD: *Drug Interactions*, ed 5. Philadelphia, Lea & Febiger, 1985 B, 23.

Hansten PD, Horn JR: Inhibition of oral contraceptive efficacy. *Drug Interact Newslett* 5:7-10, 1985.

Henderson DK, et al: Comparative susceptibility of anaerobic bacteria to ticarcillin, cefoxitin, metronidazole, and related antimicrobial agents. *Antimicrob Agents Chemother* 11:679-682, 1977.

Holmes B, et al: Piperacillin: Review of its antibacterial activity, pharmacokinetic properties, and therapeutic uses. *Drugs* 28:375-425, 1984.

Hook EW III, Holmes KK: Gonococcal infections. *Ann Intern Med* 102:229-243, 1985.

Iravani A, Richard GA: Treatment of urinary tract infections with combination of amoxicillin and clavulanic acid. *Antimicrob Agents Chemother* 22:672-677, 1982.

Jick H, Porter JB: Potentiation of ampicillin skin reactions by allopurinol or hyperuricemia. *J Clin Pharmacol* 21:456-458, 1981.

Karchmer AW, et al: Methicillin-resistant *Staphylococcus epidermidis* (SE) prosthetic valve (PV) endocarditis (E): Therapeutic trial, (abstract 476). *24th Interscience Conference on Antimicrobial Agents and Chemotherapy.* Washington, DC, Oct 8-10, 1984.

King JW, et al: Systemic infections treated with amdinocillin in combination with other beta-lactam antibiotics. *Am J Med* 75(suppl 2A):90-95, (Aug 29) 1983.

Landesman SH, et al: Past and current roles of cephalosporin antibiotics in treatment of meningitis: Emphasis on use in gram-negative bacillary meningitis. *Am J Med* 71:693-703, 1981.

Lawrence AG, Shanson DC: Augmentin for treatment of penicillinase-producing *Neisseria gonorrhoeae*, (abstract 473). *23rd Interscience Conference on Antimicrobial Agents and Chemotherapy.* Las Vegas, NV, Oct 24-26, 1983.

Levine BB, Redmond AP: Minor haptenic determinant-specific reagins of penicillin hypersensitivity in man. *Int Arch Allergy Appl Immunol* 35:445-455, 1969.

Lowy FD, Hammer SM: *Staphylococcus epidermidis* infections. *Ann Intern Med* 99:824-839, 1983.

Mandell GL, Sande MA: Antimicrobial agents: Penicillins and cephalosporins, in Gilman AG, et al (eds): *The Pharmacological Basis of Therapeutics*, ed 6. New York, Macmillan, 1980, 1126-1261.

Mangini RJ (ed): *Drug Interaction Facts*. St Louis, JB Lippincott, 1984, 14.

McCloskey RV, et al: Microbiology, pharmacology, and clinical use of mezlocillin sodium. *Pharmacotherapy* 2:300-312, 1982.

McCracken GH Jr: Comparative evaluation of aminopenicillins for oral use. *Pediatr Infect Dis* 2:317-329, 1983.

The Medical Letter: *Handbook of Antimicrobial Therapy.* New Rochelle, NY, The Medical Letter, Inc, 1984, 38-47.

Molavi A, LeFrock JL: Antistaphylococcal penicillins, in Ristuccia AM, Cunha BA (eds): *Antimicrobial Therapy.* New York, Raven Press, 1984, 183-195.

Munday PE, et al: Treatment of gonorrhea with clavulanate-potentiated amoxicillin (Augmentin). *Sex Transm Dis* 12:163-165, 1985.

Nelson JD: *1985 Pocketbook of Pediatric Antimicrobial Therapy*, ed 6. Baltimore, Williams & Wilkins, 1985 A, 64-75.

Nelson JD: *1985 Pocketbook of Pediatric Antimicrobial Therapy*, ed 6. Baltimore, Williams & Wilkins, 1985 B, 20-21.

Neu HC: Amoxicillin. *Ann Intern Med* 90:356-360, 1979.

Neu HC: Pharmacokinetics of bacampicillin. *Rev Infect Dis* 3:110-116, 1981.

Neu HC: Penicillins: New insights into their mechanisms of activity and clinical use. *Bull NY Acad Sci* 58:681-695, 1982 A.

Neu HC: Antistaphylococcal penicillins. *Med Clin North Am* 66:51-60, 1982 B.

Neu HC: Carbenicillin and ticarcillin. *Med Clin North Am* 66:61-77, 1982 C.

Neu HC: Penicillin-binding proteins and role of amdinocillin in causing bacterial cell death. *Am J Med* 75(suppl 2A):9-20, (Aug 29) 1983 A.

Neu HC: Structure-activity relations of new β-lactam compounds and in vitro activity against common bacteria. *Rev Infect Dis* 5(suppl 2):S319-S336, 1983 B.

Neu HC: Penicillins, in Mandell GL, et al (eds): *Principles and Practice of Infectious Diseases*, ed 2. New York, John Wiley & Sons, 1984 A, 166-180.

Neu HC: Treatment of methicillin-resistant staphylococcus infections. *Antimicrob Newslett* 1:47-48, 1984 B.

Neu HC: Other beta-lactam antibiotics, in Mandell GL, et al (eds): *Principles and Practice of Infectious Diseases*, ed 2. New York, John Wiley & Sons, 1984 C, 187-192.

Neu HC: Amdinocillin: Novel penicillin: Antimicrobial activity, pharmacology and clinical use. *Pharmacotherapy* 5:1-10, 1985.

Neu HC, Fu KP: Synergy of azlocillin and mezlocillin combined with aminoglycoside antibiotics and cephalosporins. *Antimicrob Agents Chemother* 13:813-819, 1978 A.

Neu HC, Fu KP: Clavulanic acid, novel inhibitor of β-lactamases. *Antimicrob Agents Chemother* 14:650-665, 1978 B.

Norris SM: Penicillins with antipseudomonal activity. *Infect Control* 6:165-168, 1985.

Norris SM, Mandell GL: Tables of antimicrobial agent pharmacology, in Mandell GL, et al, (eds): *Anti-Infective Therapy*. New York, John Wiley & Sons, 1985, 428-503.

Odio CM, et al: Comparative treatment trial of Augmentin versus cefaclor for acute otitis media with effusion. *Pediatrics* 75:819-826, 1985.

Pancoast S, et al: Clinical evaluation of piperacillin therapy for infection. *Arch Intern Med* 141:1447-1450, 1981.

Parry MF: Tolerance and safety of azlocillin. *J Antimicrob Chemother* 11(suppl B):223-228, 1983.

Parry MF, Neu HC: Safety and tolerance of mezlocillin. *J Antimicrob Chemother* 9(suppl A):273-280, 1982.

Parry MF, Pancoast SJ: Antipseudomonal penicillins, in Ristuccia AM, Cunha BA (eds): *Antimicrobial Therapy*. New York, Raven Press, 1984, 197-207.

Patterson R, Anderson J: Allergic reactions to drugs and biologic agents. *JAMA* 248:2637-2645, 1982.

Pickering LK, Rutherford I: Effect of concentration and time upon inactivation of tobramycin, gentamicin, netilmicin, and amikacin by azlocillin, carbenicillin, mecillinam, mezlocillin, and piperacillin. *J Pharmacol Exp Ther* 217:345-349, 1981.

Pratt WB: *Chemotherapy of Infection*. New York, Oxford University Press, 1977, 22-84.

Qureshi GD, et al: Warfarin resistance with nafcillin therapy. *Ann Intern Med* 100:527-529, 1984.

Rahal JJ, Simberkoff MS: Host defense and antimicrobial therapy in adult gram-negative bacillary meningitis. *Ann Intern Med* 96:468-474, 1982.

Reading C, Cole M: Clavulanic acid: Beta-lactamase-inhibiting beta-lactam from *Streptomyces clavuligerus*. *Antimicrob Agents Chemother* 11:852-857, 1977.

Reese RE, Betts RF: Antibiotic use, in Reese RE, Douglas RG (eds): *A Practical Approach to Infectious Diseases*. Boston, Little, Brown and Company, 1983, 51-162.

Rice RJ, et al: Changing trends in gonococcal antibiotic resistance in the United States, 1983-1984. *CDC Surveill Summ* 33:11SS-15SS, 1985.

Richmond MM, Sykes RB: β-lactamases of gram-negative bacteria and their possible physiological role. *Adv Microb Physiol* 9:31-88, 1973.

Rotstein C, Farrar WE Jr: Amdinocillin in combination with beta-lactam antibiotics for treatment of serious gram-negative infections. *Am J Med* 75(suppl 2A):96-99, (Aug 29) 1983.

Roy I, et al: In vitro activity of ticarcillin against anaerobic bacteria compared with that of carbenicillin and penicillin. *Antimicrob Agents Chemother* 11:258-261, 1977.

Sahm DF, et al: β-lactam antibiotics: Extended spectrum penicillins. *Antimicrob Newslett* 2:14-16, 1985.

Saxon A: Immediate hypersensitivity reactions to β-lactam antibiotics. *Rev Infect Dis* 5(suppl 2):S368-S379, 1983.

Schäfer-Korting M, et al: Atenolol interaction with aspirin, allopurinol, and ampicillin. *Clin Pharmacol Ther* 33:283-288, 1983.

Schassan HH, et al: Mezlocillin: New acyl ureidopenicillin. *Chemotherapy* 24:134-142, 1978.

Scheife RT, Neu HC: Bacampicillin hydrochloride: Chemistry, pharmacology, and clinical use. *Pharmacotherapy* 2:313-321, 1982.

Sheagren JN: *Staphylococcus aureus*: Persistent pathogen, parts 1 and 2. *N Engl J Med* 310:1368-1373, 1437-1442, 1984.

Sher TH: Penicillin hypersensitivity: Review. *Pediatr Clin North Am* 30:161-176, 1983.

Shulman ST, et al: Prevention of rheumatic fever: Statement for health professionals by Committee on Rheumatic Fever and Infective Endocarditis of Council on Cardiovascular Disease in the Young. *Circulation* 70:1118A-1122A, 1984 A.

Shulman ST, et al: Prevention of bacterial endocarditis: Statement for health professionals by Committee on Rheumatic Fever and Infective Endocarditis of Council on Cardiovascular Disease in the Young. *Circulation* 70:1123A-1127A, 1984 B.

Simon GI, et al: Clinical trial of piperacillin with acquisition of resistance by *Pseudomonas* and clinical relapse. *Antimicrob Agents Chemother* 18:167-170, 1980.

Smith BR, LeFrock JL: Amoxicillin-potassium clavulanate: Novel β-lactamase inhibitor. *Drug Intell Clin Pharm* 19:415-420, 1985.

Sogn DD: Penicillin allergy. *J Allergy Clin Immunol* 74:589-593, 1984.

Somani P, et al: Effects of mezlocillin, ticarcillin, and placebo on blood coagulation and bleeding time in normal volunteers. *J Antimicrob Chemother* 11(suppl C):33-41, 1983.

Spratt BG: Biochemical and genetical approaches to the mechanism of action of penicillin. *Philos Trans R Soc Lond (Biol)* 289:273-283, 1980.

Stead RJ, et al: Adverse reactions to piperacillin in cystic fibrosis. *Lancet* 1:857-858, 1984.

Thornsberry C: Methicillin-resistant (heteroresistant) staphylococci. *Antimicrob Newslett* 1:43-47, (June) 1984.

Tipper DJ, Wright A: Structure and biosynthesis of bacterial cell walls, in Sokatch JR, Ornstein LA (eds): *The Bacteria*. New York, Academic Press, 1979, vol 7, 291-426.

Tomasz A: Mechanism of irreversible antimicrobial effects of penicillins: How beta-lactam antibiotics kill and lyse bacteria. *Ann Rev Microbiol* 33:113-137, 1979.

Tomasz A: Penicillin-binding proteins in bacteria. *Ann Intern Med* 96:502-504, 1982.

Van Arsdel PP Jr: Drug allergy: Update. *Med Clin North Am* 65:1087-1103, 1981.

Wade JC, et al: Piperacillin or ticarcillin plus amikacin: Double-blind prospective comparison of empiric antibiotic therapy for febrile granulocytopenic cancer patients. *Am J Med* 71:983-990, 1981.

Wallace RJ Jr, et al: Amoxicillin-clavulanic acid in treatment of lower respiratory tract infections caused by β-lactamase-positive *Haemophilus influenzae* and *Branhamella catarrhalis*. *Antimicrob Agents Chemother* 27:912-915, 1985.

Ward TT, et al: Combination amdinocillin and cefoxitin therapy of multiply-resistant *Serratia marcescens* urinary tract infections. *Am J Med* 75(suppl 2A):85-89, (Aug 29) 1983.

Warrington RJ, et al: Diagnosis of penicillin allergy by skin testing: Manitoba experience. *Can Med Assoc J* 118:787-791, 1978.

Webb D, et al: Ticarcillin disodium in anaerobic infections. *Arch Intern Med* 138:1618-1620, 1978.

Weber DJ, et al: Amoxicillin and potassium clavulanate, an antibiotic combination: Mechanism of action, pharmacokinetics, antimicrobial spectrum, clinical efficacy, and adverse effects. *Pharmacotherapy* 4:122-136, 1984.

Winston DJ, et al: In vitro studies of piperacillin, new semisynthetic penicillin. *Antimicrob Agents Chemother* 13:944-960, 1978.

Winston DJ, et al: Piperacillin therapy for serious bacterial infections. *Am J Med* 69:255-261, 1980.

Wise R, et al: In vitro study of clavulanic acid in combination with penicillin, amoxicillin, and carbenicillin. *Antimicrob Agents Chemother* 13:389-393, 1978.

Wright AJ, Wilkowske CJ: Penicillins. *Mayo Clin Proc* 58:21-32, 1983.

Other Selected References

Barza M, Weinstein L: Pharmacokinetics of penicillins in man. *Clin Pharmacokinet* 1:297-308, 1976.

Bergan T: Penicillins, in Schonfeld H (ed): *Antibiotics and Chemotherapy*. Basel, S. Karger, 1978, vol 25, 1-122.

Brogden RN, et al: Amoxycillin: Review of its antibacterial and pharmacokinetic properties and therapeutic use. *Drugs* 9:88-140, 1975.

Craig WA, Kirby WMM (eds): Pulse dosing of antimicrobial drugs with special reference to bacampicillin. *Rev Infect Dis* 3:1-177, 1981 (23 papers).

Jackson D, Phillips I (eds): From penicillin to piperacillin. *J Antimicrob Chemother* 9(suppl B):1-101, 1982 (10 papers).

Klein JD (ed): Use of extended-spectrum penicillins for selected serious infections in infants and children, (symposium). *J Pediatr* 106:1021-1056, 1985 (5 papers).

Leigh DA, et al (eds): Timentin—ticarcillin plus clavulanic acid: Laboratory and clinical perspective. *J Antimicrob Chemother*

17 (suppl C):1–244, 1986 (30 papers).

Moellering RC Jr, et al (eds): International review of amdinocillin: New beta-lactam antibiotic. *Am J Med* 75(suppl 2A):1-138, (Aug 29) 1983 (22 papers).

Nelson JD, McCracken GH Jr: Mezlocillin and related antibiotics. *Pediatr Infect Dis* 1:42-43, 1982.

Neu HC (ed): Beta-lactamase inhibition: Therapeutic advances. *Am J Med* 79(suppl 5B):1-196, 1985 (39 papers).

Neu HC, Wise R (eds): Mezlocillin. *J Antimicrob Chemother* 9(suppl A):1-299, 1982 (46 papers).

Neu HC, et al (eds): Azlocillin: Antipseudomonas penicillin. *J Antimicrob Chemother* 11(suppl B):1-239, 1983 (28 papers).

Neu HC, et al (eds): Mezlocillin: Broad spectrum penicillin: Update. *J Antimicrob Chemother* 11(suppl C):1-108, 1983 (14 papers).

Prince AS, Neu HC: New penicillins and their use in pediatrics. *Pediatr Clin North Am* 30:3-16, 1983.

Cephalosporins and Related Agents

Since the introduction of cephalothin [Keflin, Seffin] for clinical use in the early 1960s, the cephalosporins have become a widely used and rapidly expanding class of antibiotics. Presently, 16 cephalosporins and 2 chemically related antibiotics, cefoxitin [Mefoxin], a cephamycin, and moxalactam [Moxam], an oxa-β-lactam, are being marketed in the United States. Undoubtedly, additional cephalosporin derivatives will be approved for use in the future.

CHEMISTRY AND CLASSIFICATION

Like the penicillins, cephalosporins contain a β-lactam ring that is necessary for antimicrobial activity. However, the penicillins are derivatives of 6-aminopenicillanic acid (6-APA) (see Chapter 66, Penicillins), whereas the parent nucleus of the cephalosporins is 7-aminocephalosporanic acid (7-ACA) (see Figure 1). This compound is derived from cephalosporin C, which is a fermentation product of *Cephalosporium acremonium*.

7-Aminocephalosporanic acid is composed of a dihydrothiazine ring (A) and a β-lactam ring (B), and it is resistant to penicillinases, such as those produced by staphylococci. This nucleus has been modified with different side chains to create a whole family of cephalosporin antibiotics (see Figure 1). Modifications (R_1) at position 7 of the β-lactam ring are associated with changes in antibacterial activity and stability to β-lactamases. Substitutions (R_2) at position 3 of the dihydrothiazine ring affect metabolism and pharmacokinetic properties of the drugs to a greater extent than antibacterial activity.

The cephamycins are related chemically to cephalosporin C, differing primarily in that they possess a 7-α-methoxy group (R_3), which enhances stability to certain β-lactamases. Cefoxitin is derived from cephamycin C, which is elaborated by *Streptomyces lactamdurans*.

Moxalactam has a dihydro-oxazine ring instead of the dihydrothiazine ring common to the cephalosporins and cephamycins. Therefore, technically it is not a penicillin, cephalosporin, or cephamycin but is related to all three. It also is a totally synthetic compound.

For additional discussion of chemistry, see Neu, 1982 A, 1983, 1985 A; Garzone et al, 1983 A; Barriere and Flaherty, 1984; Mandell, 1984; Norris, 1984 A; Quintiliani et al, 1984; and Fried and Hinthorn, 1985.

It is convenient to classify the cephalosporins and related agents as first, second, or third generation compounds based on their activity against gram-negative bacteria. The first generation cephalosporins were the initial agents developed and they have a narrower gram-negative antibacterial spectrum than the compounds developed later. However, first generation analogues generally are more active against gram-positive bacteria than second and third generation cephalosporins. First generation cephalosporins currently marketed in the United States include cephalothin, cefazolin [Ancef, Kefzol], and cephapirin [Cefadyl] for parenteral use only; cephalexin [Keflex] and cefadroxil [Duricef, Ultracef] for oral use only; and cephradine [Anspor, Velosef], which can be administered orally or parenterally.

The available second generation cephalosporins are cefamandole [Mandol], cefoxitin, cefuroxime [Zinacef], cefonicid [Monocid], and ceforanide [Precef] for parenteral use; and cefaclor [Ceclor] for oral administration. Although there are differences among individual agents, second generation cephalosporins generally are more active against gram-negative bacteria than first generation analogues. Cefoxitin and cefuroxime are more resistant to certain gram-negative bacterial β-lactamases than most other compounds.

The third generation cephalosporins are even more active and have a still broader in vitro spectrum of activity against gram-negative bacteria, including organisms resistant to earlier generation cephalosporins. They also show increased stability to β-lactamases produced by many gram-negative bacteria. The third generation cephalosporins generally are less active than first generation analogues against gram-positive bacteria, however. Currently, parenteral cefotaxime [Claforan], ceftizoxime [Cefizox], ceftriaxone [Rocephin], moxalactam, cefoperazone [Cefobid], and ceftazidime [Fortaz, Tazicef, Tazidime] are available in the United States. Ceftazidime and cefoperazone are more active against *Pseudomonas aeruginosa* than the other available third generation cephalosporins (see Antimicrobial Spectrum). Cefmenoxime [Cefmax] and cefsulodin [Cefomonil] are investigational. The latter agent has a much narrower antibacterial spectrum than other third generation cephalosporins but a greater specificity for *P. aeruginosa*.

For additional discussion, see Neu, 1982 A; Bertino and Speck, 1983; Garzone et al, 1983 A; *Med Lett Drugs Ther*, 1983 A; Thompson and Wright, 1983; Barriere and Flaherty, 1984; Mandell, 1984; Norris, 1984 A; Quintiliani et al, 1984; Fried and Hinthorn, 1985; Tartaglione and Polk, 1985.

MECHANISM OF ACTION

The cephalosporins are primarily bactericidal antibiotics with a mechanism of action very similar to that of the penicillins. These β-lactam antibiotics inhibit the third and final stage of bacterial cell wall formation by preferentially binding to one or more penicillin binding proteins (PBPs) that are located beneath the cell walls of susceptible bacteria. Thus, the intrinsic activity of a cephalosporin against a particular bacterial strain depends, in part, on its binding affinity to these protein receptor molecules. For example, first generation cephalosporins exhibit greater affinity for essential PBPs of staphylococci than third generation derivatives. Conversely, third generation cephalosporins usually have greater affinity for critical PBPs of the Enterobacteriaceae. Other factors also affect the antibacterial activity of β-lactam antibiotics. These include the stability of the antibiotic to various β-lactamases produced by gram-positive and gram-negative bacteria and the ability of a drug to penetrate the outer membrane of gram-negative bacteria (see also the section on Resistance). For a detailed discussion on the mechanism of action of β-lactam antibiotics, see Chapter 66, Penicillins; see also Neu, 1982 B, 1985 A.

ANTIMICROBIAL SPECTRUM

First Generation Cephalosporins: All of these agents have similar antibacterial spectra that include most gram-positive and some gram-negative bacteria.

The first generation cephalosporins have the highest degree of activity in vitro against gram-positive bacteria. They are active against most staphylococci, including penicillinase-producing *S. aureus*. However, methicillin-resistant staphylococci should be considered resistant to all cephalosporins, although in vitro resistance is not always readily demonstrated. Most streptococci, including *S. pyogenes* (group A, β-hemolytic), *S. agalactiae* (group B), viridans streptococci, anaerobic streptococci, and *S. pneumoniae* are susceptible. Enterococci (eg, *S. faecalis*) and penicillin-resistant *S. pneumoniae* are resistant to all cephalosporins, however. There do not appear to be major differences in activity between the various parenteral first generation cephalosporins against gram-positive cocci, although cephalothin may be slightly more active against staphylococci. The parenteral agents generally are more active than oral cephalosporins in vitro against aerobic gram-positive cocci.

Susceptible gram-positive bacilli include certain clostridia (eg, *Clostridium perfringens*) and *Corynebacterium diphtheriae*. *Listeria monocytogenes* should be considered resistant to all cephalosporins.

The clinically relevant spectrum of first generation cephalosporins against gram-negative bacteria is limited to *Escherichia coli*, *Klebsiella*, and *Proteus mirabilis*. Cefazolin generally is more active than cephalothin. Variable percentages of strains of these three species are resistant to the first generation cephalosporins, however; these are more common in hospital-acquired infections. These resistant strains may be susceptible to second and particularly third generation cephalosporins (see below).

Although in vitro susceptibility to first generation cephalosporins has been demonstrated for many strains of *Salmonella*, *Shigella*, *Haemophilus influenzae*, and the gram-negative cocci, *Neisseria gonorrhoeae* and *N. meningitidis*, clinical usefulness is minimal. Indole-positive *Proteus*, *Providencia*,

FIGURE 1.   CHEMICAL STRUCTURES OF CEPHALOSPORINS

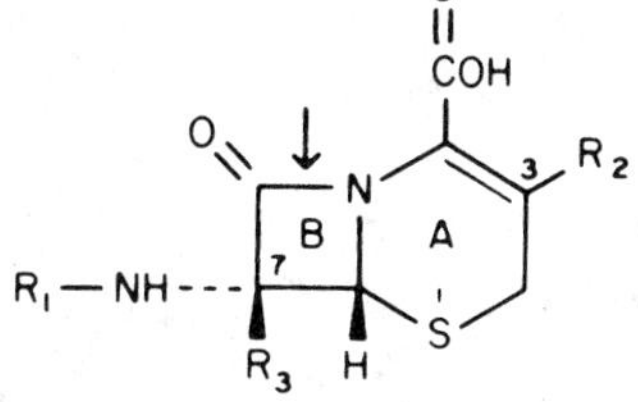

Cephalosporin Nucleus[1]

Generic Name (Trade Name)	R₁	R₂	R₃
First Generation			
Cephalothin (Keflin, Seffin)	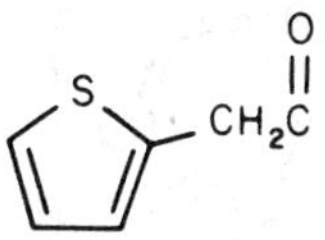 (thienyl)$CH_2C(=O)$	$CH_2OCCH_3(=O)$	H
Cefazolin (Ancef, Kefzol)	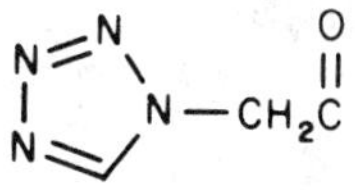 (tetrazolyl)$CH_2C(=O)$	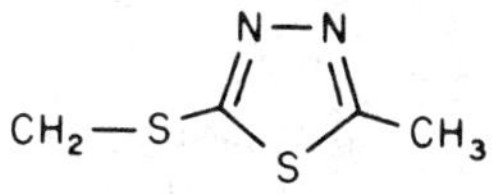 CH_2–S–(thiadiazolyl)–CH_3	H
Cephapirin (Cefadyl)	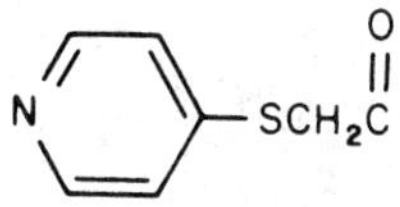 (pyridyl)$SCH_2C(=O)$	$CH_2OCCH_3(=O)$	H
Cephradine (Anspor, Velosef)	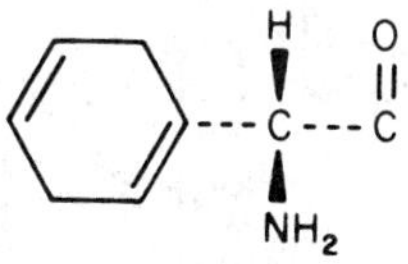 (cyclohexadienyl)$CH(NH_2)C(=O)$	CH_3	H
Cephalexin (Keflex)	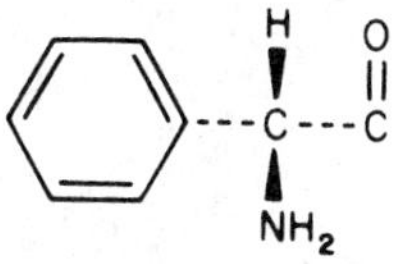 (phenyl)$CH(NH_2)C(=O)$	CH_3	H
Cefadroxil (Duricef, Ultracef)	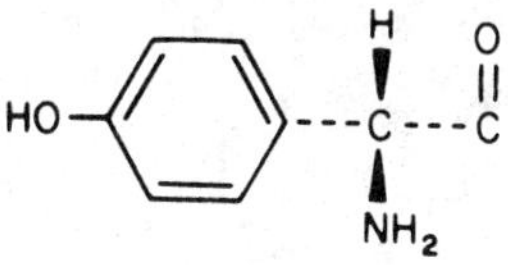 HO–(phenyl)$CH(NH_2)C(=O)$	CH_3	H
Second Generation			
Cefamandole Nafate (Mandol)	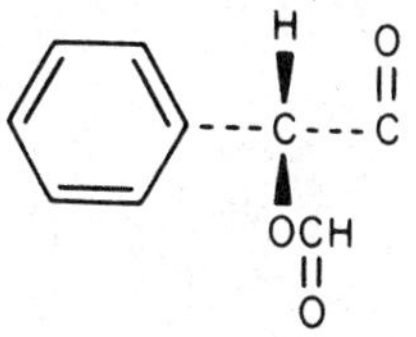 (phenyl)$CH(OCH=O)C(=O)$	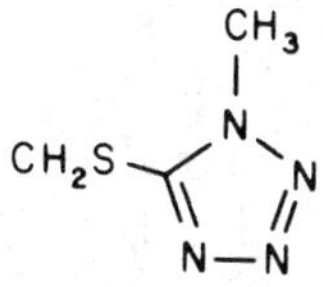 CH_2S–(methyltetrazolyl)	H
Cefoxitin (Mefoxin)	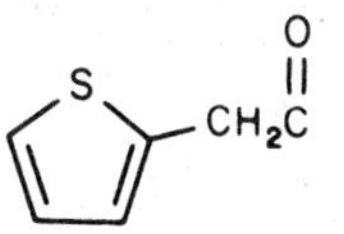 (thienyl)$CH_2C(=O)$	$CH_2OCNH_2(=O)$	OCH_3

(Continued on next page)

FIGURE 1 (continued)

Generic Name (Trade Name)	R₁	R₂	R₃
Cefuroxime (Zinacef)	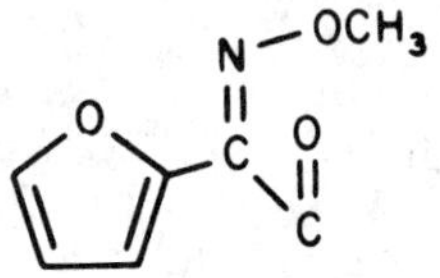	CH_2OCNH_2 (O)	H
Cefonicid (Monocid)	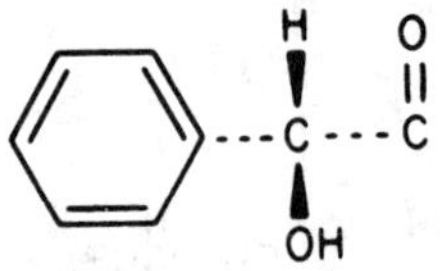	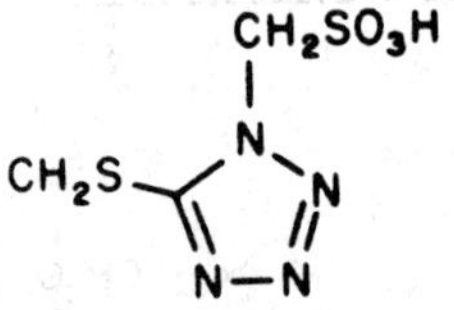 CH_2SO_3H / tetrazole / CH_3S	H
Ceforanide (Precef)	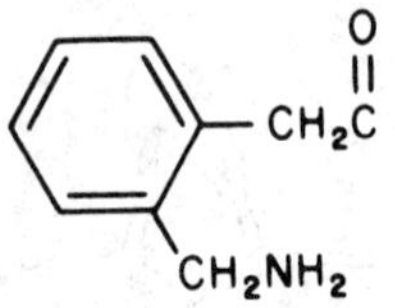	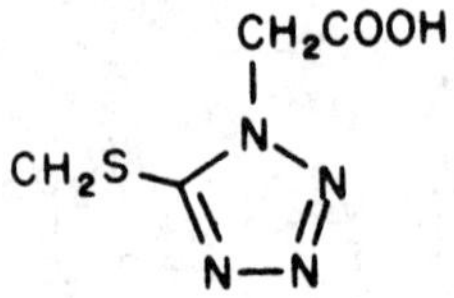 CH_2COOH / tetrazole / CH_3S	H
Cefaclor (Ceclor)	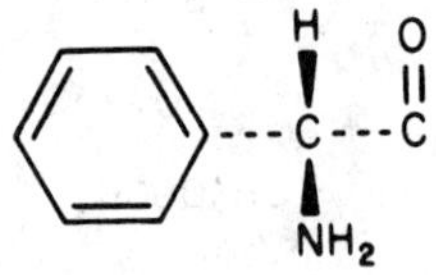	Cl	H
Third Generation			
Cefotaxime (Claforan)	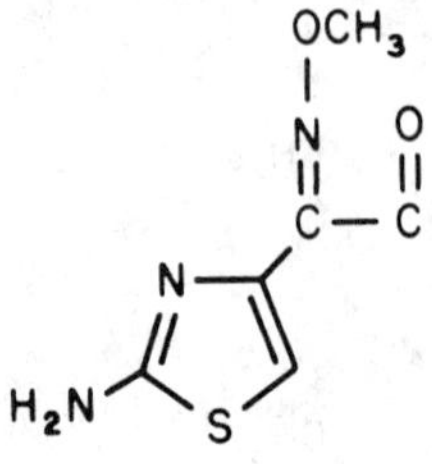	CH_2OCCH_3 (O)	H
Ceftizoxime (Cefizox)	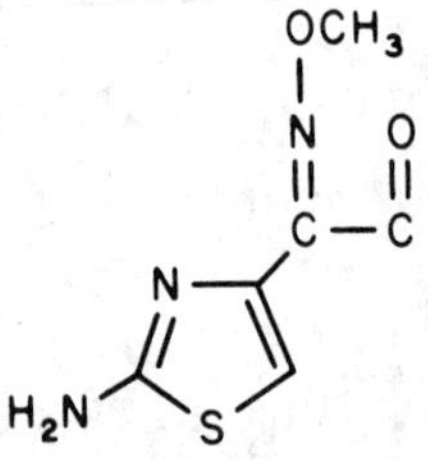	H	H
Ceftriaxone (Rocephin)	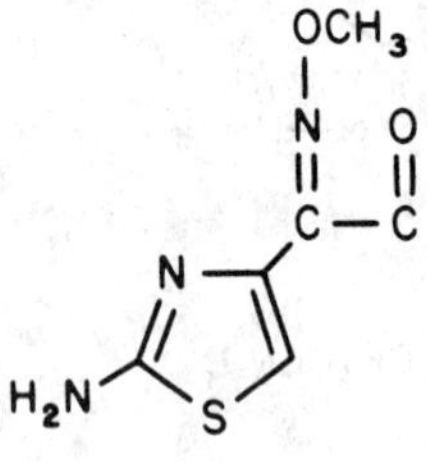	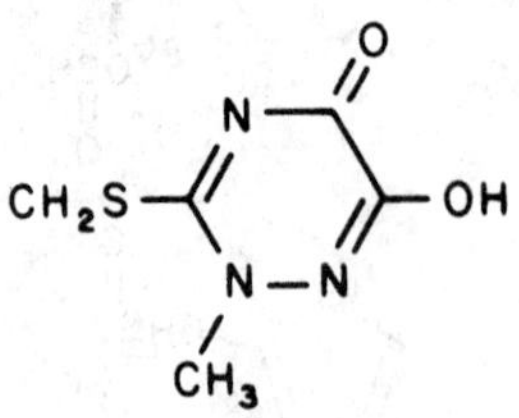 CH_3S / triazinone / CH_3	H

FIGURE 1 (continued)

Generic Name (Trade Name)	R_1	R_2	R_3
Cefmenoxime[2] (Cefmax)	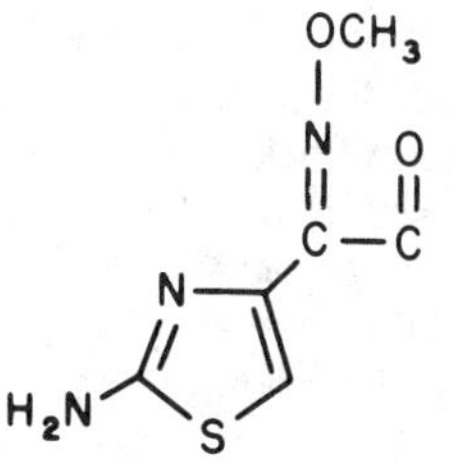	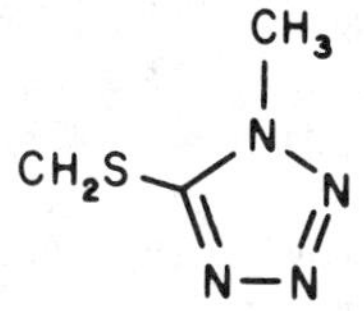	H
Ceftazidime (Fortaz, Tazidime, Tazicef)	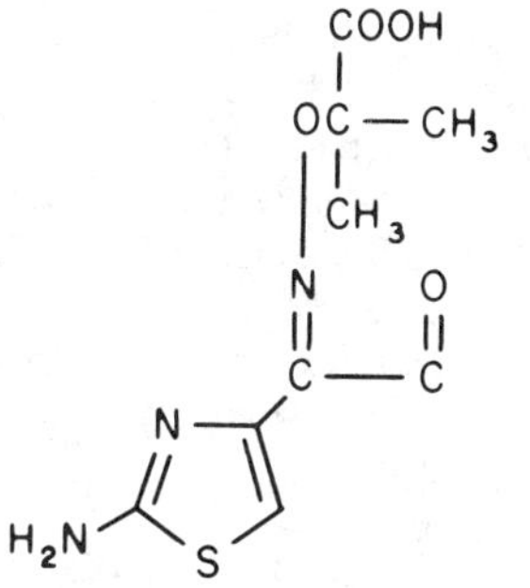	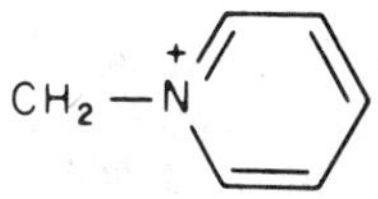	H
Cefoperazone (Cefobid)	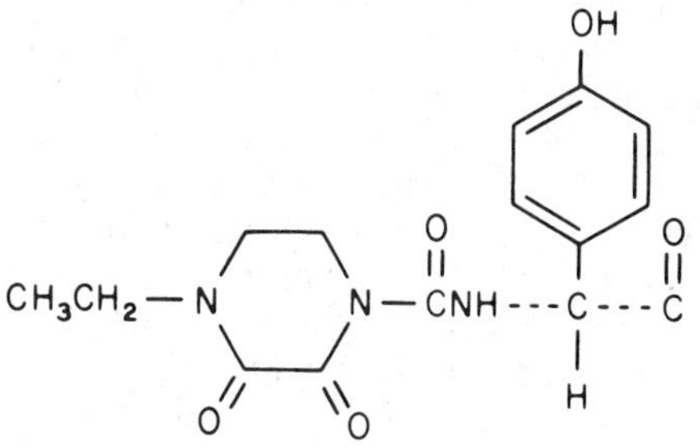	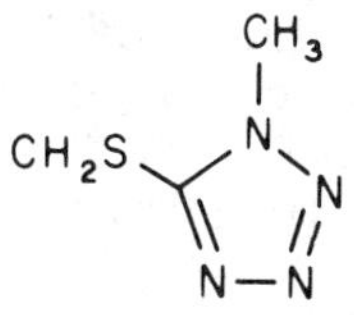	H
Moxalactam[3] (Moxam)	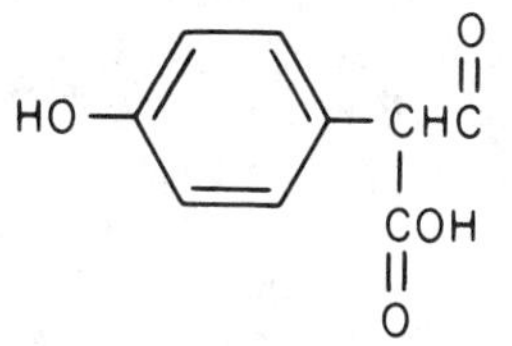	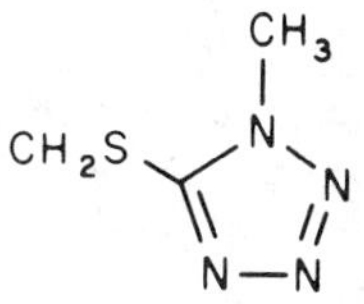	OCH_3
Cefsulodin[2] (Cefomonil)	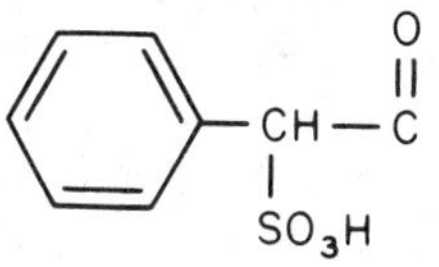	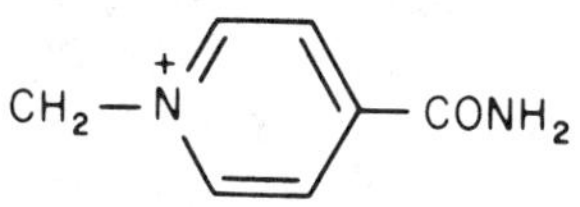	H

[1]For 7-aminocephalosporanic acid (7-ACA), $R_1 = R_3 = H$ and $R_2 = CH_2OCCH_3$; A = dihydrothiazine ring; B = beta-lactam ring. The arrow is the site of beta-lactamase attack.
[2]Investigational drug
[3]Moxalactam is actually an oxy-cephem antimicrobial; it has an oxygen atom instead of sulfur in position one of ring A (see the Cephalosporin Nucleus).

Enterobacter, Serratia, Citrobacter, Pseudomonas, Acinetobacter, and the *Bacteroides fragilis* group are resistant. *Legionella pneumophila* should be considered resistant to the cephalosporins.

For additional discussion, see Bertino and Speck, 1983; Garzone et al, 1983 B; Jones and Preston, 1983; *Med Lett Drugs Ther*, 1983 A; Thompson and Wright, 1983; Mandell, 1984; Norris, 1984 B; Quintiliani et al, 1984; Fried and Hinthorn, 1985; Sahm et al, 1985 A.

Second Generation Cephalosporins: These antibiotics have enhanced activity against a greater variety of gram-negative bacteria when compared to first generation cephalosporins. The second generation agents also differ among themselves with regard to their activities against various bacteria.

Second generation cephalosporins are active against most staphylococci, including penicillinase-producing *S. aureus*, *Streptococcus pyogenes*, *S. pneumoniae*, *S. agalactiae*, viridans streptococci, and gram-positive anaerobes (eg, *Peptococcus*, *Peptostreptococcus*, clostridia). As with first generation agents, enterococci (eg, *S. faecalis*), methicillin-resistant staphylococci, penicillin-resistant pneumococci, and *Listeria monocytogenes* are resistant.

The activity of parenteral second generation cephalosporins against most streptococci and pneumococci is comparable to or slightly less than that observed with parenteral first generation agents. On the other hand, activity of the second generation derivatives against staphylococci is quite variable. The most active agents are cefamandole and cefuroxime, which are slightly less active than first generation agents. Cefoxitin and the newer second generation cephalosporins with longer half-lives, cefonicid and ceforanide, have inferior activity against staphylococci. Oral cefaclor has comparable activity in vitro to cephalexin against gram-positive cocci. In general, second generation cephalosporins offer no clinical advantages over first generation derivatives for infections caused by gram-positive bacteria.

Neisseria gonorrhoeae and *N. meningitidis*, gram-negative cocci, are susceptible to the second generation cephalosporins. Of particular clinical relevance are (1) the high degree of activity of cefoxitin for *N. gonorrhoeae*, including penicillinase-producing strains (PPNG), and (2) the good activity of cefuroxime against the meningococcus, because this is the only second generation cephalosporin that adequately penetrates into cerebrospinal fluid (see the discussion on Uses and Pharmacokinetics).

The second generation cephalosporins are considerably more active against *Haemophilus influenzae* than the first generation antibiotics and also are active against many ampicillin-resistant strains. Among the parenteral second generation agents, cefuroxime appears to be the most useful clinically. When compared to cefamandole, it has increased stability to β-lactamases (eg, plasmid-mediated TEM-1) produced by *H. influenzae*. More important, its ability to achieve therapeutic concentrations in cerebrospinal fluid against this common meningeal pathogen is a distinct advantage over other second generation cephalosporins (see Uses and Pharmacokinetics). Oral cefaclor is more active than cephalexin against *H. influenzae* and is useful in otitis media (see Uses).

Among the Enterobacteriaceae, second generation cephalosporins are more active than first generation agents against *Escherichia coli*, *Klebsiella*, and *Proteus mirabilis*, including strains resistant to first generation drugs. All have good activity against *Citrobacter diversus*. For other Enterobacteriaceae, the activity often varies with the second generation agent being considered. Cefamandole, cefuroxime, cefonicid, and ceforanide are most similar and are active against many isolates of *C. freundii*, *Enterobacter* species, and the indole-positive *Proteae*; they are not active against *Serratia* species. In contrast, cefoxitin is less active against *C. freundii* and *Enterobacter* species but is more active against indole-positive *Proteae*, especially *Proteus vulgaris*, and it is active against some *Serratia* species. Strains resistant to second generation cephalosporins are relatively common among some species of Enterobacteriaceae. The third generation cephalosporins clearly have superior activity against most Enterobacteriaceae (see below).

Cefoxitin has the best activity of any currently available cephalosporin against the *Bacteroides fragilis* group because it is not usually hydrolyzed by β-lactamases produced by these gram-negative anaerobic bacilli. Most other anaerobic bacteria, except some *Clostridium* species and a few *Fusobacterium*, also are susceptible to cefoxitin. Thus, this second generation cephalosporin is clinically useful in pelvic and intra-abdominal infections in which *B. fragilis* is a common pathogen (see Uses).

Second generation cephalosporins are not active against *Pseudomonas aeruginosa* or *Acinetobacter*.

For additional discussion, see Barriere and Mills, 1982; Muytjens and van der Ros-van de Repe, 1982; Bertino and Speck, 1983; Garzone et al, 1983 B; Gold and Rodriguez, 1983; *Med Lett Drugs Ther*, 1983 A; Smith and LeFrock, 1983; Thompson and Wright, 1983; Dudley et al, 1984; Mandell, 1984; Norris, 1984 B; Pontzer and Kaye, 1984; Quintiliani et al, 1984; Fried and Hinthorn, 1985; Sahm et al, 1985 A; Sanders et al, 1985; Tartaglione and Polk, 1985.

Third Generation Cephalosporins: These antibiotics generally have increased potency and a wider spectrum of activity against clinically important gram-negative bacteria when compared to first and second generation cephalosporins. Comparative in vitro activities of the third generation cephalosporins are summarized in Table 1.

Although the third generation cephalosporins are active against most staphylococci, including penicillinase-producing strains, they are considerably less potent than first generation agents (eg, cephalothin, cefazolin). Moxalactam and ceftazidime are the least active third generation cephalosporins against *S. aureus* and coagulase-negative staphylococci. Methicillin-resistant staphylococci are resistant to all of these agents. Cefotaxime, ceftizoxime, ceftriaxone, and cefmenoxime (investigational) have excellent activity against *Streptococcus pyogenes*, *S. agalactiae*, and *S. pneumoniae*. Ceftazidime, cefoperazone, and, in particular, moxalactam are less active against streptococci and pneumococci. Enterococci (eg, *S. faecalis*) and penicillin-resistant pneumococci are resistant to all of these agents, as are *Listeria monocytogenes*. In general, third generation cephalosporins offer no clinical advantages over first generation derivatives for infections (other than meningitis) caused by gram-positive bacteria.

Currently available third generation cephalosporins are highly active against *Neisseria gonorrhoeae*, including penicillinase-producing strains (PPNG); ceftriaxone and cefotaxime are used clinically for infections caused by these organisms (see Uses). *N. meningitidis* also is very susceptible to these agents.

Third generation cephalosporins show excellent activity against many aerobic gram-negative bacilli, including *Haemophilus influenzae* and most of the Enterobacteriaceae (eg, *Escherichia coli, Klebsiella, Enterobacter, Proteus, Morganella, Providencia, Citrobacter, Serratia, Salmonella, Shigella*) including strains resistant to earlier generation cephalosporins, penicillins, and aminoglycosides. This activity is related to the agents' excellent β-lactamase stability and high affinity for penicillin binding proteins. Third generation cephalosporins offer distinct clinical advantages over earlier generation cephalosporins against these aerobic gram-negative bacilli. In general, *Enterobacter* species, *Citrobacter freundii, Serratia marcescens*, and *Providencia* species are less susceptible to the third generation agents than other Enterobacteriaceae, but there is a fair amount of variability among published reports. Cefoperazone generally is less active than other third generation cephalosporins against Enterobacteriaceae. This drug is more susceptible to certain β-lactamases (eg, TEM-1, TEM-2), and β-lactamase-producing strains of *E. coli* and *Klebsiella* that are susceptible to other third generation cephalosporins, have been resistant to cefoperazone.

The activity of third generation cephalosporins against *Pseudomonas aeruginosa* is variable. Ceftazidime has the greatest activity, including some strains that are resistant to aminoglycosides and antipseudomonal penicillins. Cefoperazone and cefsulodin (investigational) also have good activity against *P. aeruginosa*; the other agents are considerably less active. Cefsulodin is unique in that it is only active against *P. aeruginosa* and some *S. aureus*; other bacteria (eg, Enterobacteriaceae) are resistant. Other than ceftazidime, third generation cephalosporins generally are not very active against *Acinetobacter* species.

Although third generation cephalosporins are active against anaerobic streptococci, some clostridia (not *C. difficile*), fusobacteria, actinomycetes, and most *Bacteroides*, they generally are inferior to the penicillins. Against the *B. fragilis* group, only moxalactam has activity comparable to that of cefoxitin; the other third generation agents have inferior activity against this pathogen.

For additional discussion, see Bodey et al, 1981; Beam, 1982, 1985; Funk and Strausbaugh, 1982; Muytjens and van der Ros-van de Repe, 1982; Neu, 1982 A; Bertino and Speck, 1983; Carmine et al, 1983 A and B; Fass, 1983; Garzone et al, 1983 B; *Med Lett Drugs Ther*, 1983 A; Barriere and Flaherty, 1984; Mandell, 1984; Neu and Scully, 1984; Quintiliani et al, 1984; Richards et al, 1984; Stamm, 1984; Fried and Hinthorn, 1985; Gentry, 1985; Norris, 1985; Richards and Brogden, 1985; Richards and Heel, 1985; Sahm et al, 1985 B; Thornsberry, 1985.

RESISTANCE

Mechanisms of resistance to cephalosporins include: (1) inactivation by bacterial β-lactamases (see Figure 1); (2) decreased permeability of the bacterial cell to the cephalosporin, which prohibits the antibiotic from reaching the appropriate binding proteins; and, (3) alterations in penicillin binding protein(s) that prevent binding to the cephalosporin. Clinically, β-lactamase inactivation and, to a lesser extent, altered permeability are most important in gram-negative bacteria. Decreased affinity for penicillin binding proteins occurs with some gram-positive bacteria, but it is not a common cause of clinical resistance to cephalosporins among gram-negative bacteria.

A number of β-lactamases have been identified. The enzymes produced by *Staphylococcus aureus* are considered to be true penicillinases because they inactivate penicillin molecules but not cephalosporins. Thus, all cephalosporins are active against penicillinase-producing *S. aureus*. The decreased activities of newer generation cephalosporins against staphylococci appear to be due to decreased affinities for penicillin binding proteins rather than increased susceptibilities to β-lactamases. Methicillin-resistant staphylococci are resistant to cephalosporins; this is due to alterations in penicillin binding proteins. The lack of activity of cephalosporins against penicillin-resistant pneumococci and enterococci also is related to failure to bind critical penicillin binding proteins in these bacteria.

The β-lactamases of gram-negative bacteria fall into five broad enzyme classes (Richmond and Sykes, 1973; Sykes, 1982). These enzymes can be chromosomal- or plasmid-mediated, constitutive or inducible, and are strategically located in the periplasmic space between the inner and outer membranes of the bacterial cell. Some of these enzymes preferentially inactivate either penicillins or cephalosporins, while others work equally well on both classes of drugs. First generation cephalosporins are susceptible to many β-lactamases produced by gram-negative bacteria. This accounts, in part, for their more limited antibacterial spectrum and the development of strains resistant to their antibacterial effect (see Mandell, 1984). Second generation cephalosporins, particularly cefoxitin and cefuroxime, and most third generation derivatives have been chemically engineered to be considerably more stable to β-lactamase degradation. Thus, in addition to greater intrinsic antibacterial activity, newer generations of cephalosporins are less likely to be inactivated by β-lactamases (see Neu, 1982 C; Sykes and Bush, 1983).

Variable susceptibility to different β-lactamases is still evident with the newer cephalosporins, however. For example, some strains of *E. coli* and *Klebsiella* are resistant to cefoperazone because this drug remains susceptible to certain β-lactamases (eg, TEM-1, TEM-2) that may be produced by these bacteria (Sykes and Bush, 1983). Differences in susceptibility of *B. fragilis* and *P. aeruginosa* to the various analogues can be explained in part by differences in susceptibilities of the various drugs to β-lactamases elaborated by these organisms (Sykes and Bush, 1983). With increased use of the newer cephalosporins, it is likely that strains resistant to all of these drugs will emerge to some extent. For example, strains of

TABLE 1.
COMPARATIVE IN VITRO ACTIVITY OF SEVEN THIRD GENERATION CEPHALOSPORINS[1,2]

Organism	Cefotaxime	Ceftizoxime	Ceftriaxone
Staphylococcus aureus	++	++	++
Staphylococcus epidermidis	++	+/++	+/++
Streptococcus, Group A	+++	++++	++++
Streptococcus, Group B	++++	++++	++++
Streptococcus pneumoniae	+++/++++	+++	+++/++++
Haemophilus influenzae[4]	++++	++++	++++
Neisseria gonorrhoeae[4]	++++	++++	++++
Neisseria meningitidis	++++	++++	++++
Escherichia coli	+++/++++	+++	+++/++++
Klebsiella pneumoniae	+++/++++	+++/++++	+++
Enterobacter aerogenes	++/+++	++	+++
Enterobacter cloacae	+/++	+/++	+/++
Citrobacter freundii	+/++	++	++
Citrobacter diversus	+++	+++	+++
Serratia marcescens	++	++/+++	++
Proteus mirabilis	++++	++++	++++
Morganella morganii	++	+++	++++
Providencia stuartii	++/+++	++	++
Pseudomonas aeruginosa[5]	R(64)	R(64)	R(64)

[1]Adapted from Barriere and Flaherty, 1984. Data for ceftazidime obtained from Bodey et al, 1981; Muytjens and van der Ros-van de Repe, 1982; Fass, 1983; Neu, 1983; Richards and Brogden, 1985; and Thornsberry, 1985. This table was generated from published reports of in vitro susceptibilities from a variety of geographic areas. However, susceptibilities to these drugs may differ markedly in a given institution from data in the table.

[2]Legend: ++++ = MIC_{90} ≤0.1 mcg/ml (highly susceptible); +++ = MIC_{90} 0.2-1 mcg/ml (very susceptible); ++ = MIC_{90} 2-8 mcg/ml (susceptible); + = MIC_{90} 16-32 mcg/ml (moderately susceptible); R = MIC_{90} >32 mcg/ml (resistant)

[3]Investigational drug

[4]Includes penicillinase-producing strains

[5]MIC_{90} in parentheses

resistant *P. aeruginosa* and *Serratia marcescens* have already appeared due to permeability mechanisms (see Sanders, 1985).

Of increasing concern is the rapid development of resistance to β-lactamase stable, third generation cephalosporins by certain nonfastidious gram-negative bacilli, particularly species of *Enterobacter*, *Serratia*, and *Pseudomonas*. Therapeutic failures and relapses have been reported. The mechanism involves induction or derepression of Type I chromosomal β-lactamases that appear to bind (but not hydrolyze) these antibiotics with high affinity and render them inactive. Furthermore, routine antimicrobial susceptibility test procedures may fail to detect these strains (see Sanders, 1983, 1984; Sanders and Sanders, 1983, 1985).

The above discussion emphasizes the importance of maintaining locally generated antibiotic susceptibility profiles and of performing appropriate in vitro susceptibility tests when using the cephalosporins (see Amsterdam, 1984; Sanders, 1984; Sahm et al, 1985 A and B).

USES

The cephalosporins are broad spectrum bactericidal antibiotics with a high therapeutic/toxic ratio. They are effective in a wide variety of infections and are used frequently. However, first and second generation analogues usually have not been regarded as antibiotics of first choice for the treatment of most infections because of the availability of equally effective and less expensive alternatives. The third generation cephalosporins will likely become primary drugs for some infections, but additional clinical investigation is required to demonstrate that they are as reliable as the already proven therapeutic agents. A problem with these newer agents also is their relatively high

Cefmenoxime[3]	Ceftazidime	Cefoperazone	Moxalactam
++	+	++	+
++	R/+	++	R/+
++++	+++	+++	++
++++	+++	+++	++
++++	+++	+++/++++	++/+++
++++	+++/++++	+++	++++
++++	+++/++++	++++	++++
++++	++++	++++	++++
+++/++++	+++	+/++	+++
+++/++++	+++	+/++	+++
+++	++/+++	+/++	++/+++
++	+/++	+/++	++/+++
++	++	+	++
+++	+++	+++	+++
++	+++	+/++	++
++++	++++	+++	+++
+++	++	++	+++
++	++	+	++
R(64)	++(8)	+(32)	+(32)

cost to the patient. As the number of cephalosporins continues to expand, drug selection among the available agents will become more difficult.

For additional discussion, see Chapter 65, Antimicrobial Therapy and Chemoprophylaxis of Infectious Diseases; see also Neu, 1982 A and D; Brooks and Barriere, 1983; Garzone et al, 1983 B; *Med Lett Drugs Ther*, 1983 A; Barriere and Flaherty, 1984; Mandell, 1984; Norris, 1984 B, 1985; Smith, 1984; Eichenwald, 1985; Fried and Hinthorn, 1985; Sanders et al, 1985; Tartaglione and Polk, 1985.

Parenteral First Generation Cephalosporins: Antimicrobial chemoprophylaxis during certain surgical procedures effectively reduces the risk of postoperative wound infection. Parenteral first generation cephalosporins frequently are preferred for prophylaxis during many of these procedures, including prosthetic heart valve insertion, reconstructive surgery of the abdominal aorta, total hip replacement, gastroduodenal and biliary tract surgery in high-risk patients, vaginal and abdominal hysterectomy, cesarean section in high-risk patients, head and neck surgery requiring an incision that enters the oral cavity or pharynx, and pulmonary resection. Cefazolin usually is preferred over other first generation analogues because it produces higher serum concentrations and has a longer elimination half-life (see Pharmacokinetics). Usually, a single dose administered shortly before the first surgical incision (eg, intravenously at induction of anesthesia) provides sufficient tissue concentrations of cefazolin throughout the procedure. Additional doses given either earlier or later usually are unnecessary; continuation of prophylaxis for more than 24 hours after surgery is not indicated. For a more detailed discussion, see Chapter 65, Table 4; see also DiPiro et al, 1981, 1983; Lennard and Dellinger, 1981; *Med Lett Drugs Ther*, 1981, 1985 C; Guglielmo et al, 1983; Burnakis, 1984; Conte et al, 1984; Gilbert, 1984. Although a number of second and third generation cephalosporins have been shown to be effective as prophylactic agents for various surgical procedures (see Tartaglione and Polk, 1985; Barriere and Flaherty, 1984), there is no evidence, based on controlled, comparative clinical studies, that these newer cephalosporins offer any advantages over first generation cephalosporins. Thus, at present, none are indicated over available therapy (*Med Lett Drugs Ther*, 1983 A, 1985 C; DiPiro et al, 1983, 1984; Rapp and Blue, 1985).

Parenterally administered first generation cephalosporins (cephalothin, cefazolin, cephapirin, cephradine) are rarely drugs of choice for the treatment of bacterial infections. They may be used in serious infections caused by gram-positive cocci (except enterococci), *Klebsiella pneumoniae, Escherichia coli*, or *Proteus mirabilis*, based on the results of susceptibility tests. These include infections of the lower respiratory tract, skin, soft tissues, bone, joints, heart, and urinary tract and bacteremias. They are not effective in meningitis. First generation cephalosporins may be combined with an aminoglycoside for serious *Klebsiella* infections (eg, pneumonia) or to provide broad spectrum empiric coverage for severe community-acquired infections (eg, pneumonia, sepsis) in nonimmunocompromised patients.

First generation cephalosporins often are the preferred alternatives to antistaphylococcal penicillins or penicillin G for serious staphylococcal and/or streptococcal (except enterococcal) infections when the patient is allergic to penicillins. Cephalosporins should not be administered to patients who experienced an immediate-type hypersensitivity reaction to a penicillin, however (see Adverse Reactions and Precautions; see also Chapter 66, Penicillins). These infections include severe pyodermas, staphylococcal pneumonia, pneumococcal pneumonia (erythromycin is often preferred), septic arthritis, osteomyelitis, and endocarditis caused by viridans streptococci and *Staphylococcus aureus* (not methicillin-resistant strains).

When a cephalosporin is used for a gram-positive infection, first generation derivatives are recommended because they have the best activity against gram-positive bacteria and they are less expensive than newer cephalosporins. Cefazolin usually is the preferred parenteral first generation cephalosporin because of its better pharmacokinetic properties (see above and Pharmacokinetics); also, it is less painful than cephalothin and cephapirin when administered intramuscularly.

For additional discussion, see Chapter 65, Table 1; see also Neu, 1982 D; *Med Lett Drugs Ther*, 1983 A; Mandell, 1984; Fried and Hinthorn, 1985.

Parenteral Second Generation Cephalosporins: Clinical uses of second generation cephalosporins must differentiate the two patterns of antibacterial activity included in this generation: that of cefoxitin and that of the other second generation derivatives (see Antimicrobial Spectrum).

Cefoxitin is suitable for treating intra-abdominal infections that result from breaches in the intestinal mucosa. Such infections usually are caused by mixtures of aerobic gram-negative enteric bacilli and anaerobic bacteria, including the *Bacteroides fragilis* group. For community-acquired infections, cefoxitin alone has been shown to be as effective as the traditional therapy of clindamycin [Cleocin] plus gentamicin [Garamycin] (Tally et al, 1981; Nichols et al, 1984). It frequently is the preferred drug in mild to moderately ill patients with community acquired infections. For more severely ill patients and/or for intra-abdominal infections of nosocomial origin, an aminoglycoside should be included (see Chapter 65, Table 1; see also Neu, 1982 D; LeFrock et al, 1984 A; Fried and Hinthorn, 1985; Sanders et al, 1985). Other anti-*B. fragilis* drugs include clindamycin, metronidazole [Flagyl, Metryl], chloramphenicol [Chloromycetin, Mychel], and the antipseudomonal penicillins.

Gynecologic pelvic infections (eg, acute pelvic inflammatory disease, endometritis, pelvic cellulitis) can be caused by a variety of bacterial pathogens and frequently are caused by more than one organism. Etiologic agents include members of the normal vaginal microflora, such as facultative gram-negative bacilli (eg, *Escherichia coli*) and anaerobic bacteria (eg, *Bacteroides* [*B. bivius, B. disiens*, and, less frequently, *B. fragilis*], gram-positive cocci), and the sexually transmitted pathogens, *Neisseria gonorrhoeae* and *Chlamydia trachomatis*. Depending on the clinical situation and likely causative organisms, cefoxitin, alone or in combination, may be the preferred drug (see Neu, 1982 D; LeFrock et al, 1984 B; Sanders et al, 1985). It is active against *N. gonorrhoeae*, including penicillinase-producing strains (PPNG); many gram-negative bacilli; and most anaerobic bacteria, including *B. fragilis*. Combination with doxycycline [Vibramycin] will expand coverage to include *C. trachomatis*; this combined regimen is recommended by the Centers for Disease Control for acute pelvic inflammatory diseases likely to be caused by sexually transmitted pathogens (*Morbid Mortal Week Rep*, 1985). Combination of cefoxitin with an aminoglycoside will expand coverage against aerobic gram-negative bacilli, but may not be adequate against *C. trachomatis*. An alternative to cefoxitin-containing regimens is clindamycin plus an aminoglycoside, which provides good coverage against anaerobic bacteria and aerobic gram-negative bacilli, but may not be adequate against *N. gonorrhoeae* or *C. trachomatis*. For additional discussion, see Chapter 65, Table 2.

Cefoxitin alone also has been effective in mixed aerobic-anaerobic skin and soft tissue infections (Sanders et al, 1985). It is an alternative to ceftriaxone, a long-acting third generation cephalosporin, for disseminated gonococcal infections caused by PPNG. Although it is an effective alternative to spectinomycin [Trobicin] for uncomplicated gonorrhea caused by PPNG, ceftriaxone is now the preferred cephalosporin (*Morbid Mortal Week Rep*, 1985). Depending on the results of susceptibility tests, cefoxitin may be used in serious lower respiratory tract, urinary tract, bone, joint, skin, and soft tissue infections or bacteremias, provided that equally effective, less toxic, and less expensive alternatives are not available. Because of its greater activity against the *B. fragilis* group when compared to first generation cephalosporins, cefoxitin is used to prevent infections after colorectal surgery in patients who cannot take the oral neomycin/erythromycin combination (due to emergency operations or intestinal obstruction) (see Chapter 65, Table 4).

Cefamandole and the newer second generation cephalosporins, cefuroxime, ceforanide, and cefonicid, have similar antibacterial spectra (see Antimicrobial Spectrum). Any of these agents may be used to treat infections of the lower respiratory tract, urinary tract, skin and skin structures, bone, and joints or bacteremias caused by susceptible bacteria, provided that equally effective, less toxic, and less expensive alternatives are not available. All of these agents have been approved for perioperative prophylaxis during certain surgical procedures (Tartaglione and Polk, 1985), but none have been shown to offer any advantages over first generation cephalosporins (DiPiro et al, 1984; Rapp and Blue, 1985). Presently, it would appear that only one of these agents needs to be included in the hospital formulary. Based on the current evidence, cefuroxime appears to be the preferred drug, particularly if the hospital treats pediatric patients.

Cefuroxime resembles cefamandole and, despite more limited clinical experience, appears to offer a number of advantages. These include increased stability to certain β-lactamases (eg, TEM-1 of *Haemophilus influenzae*); a longer half-life (1.3 hours versus 0.6 to 0.8 hours), which permits a longer dosing interval; and the absence of hypoprothrombinemia and a disulfiram-like reaction as adverse effects (see Antimicrobial Spectrum, Resistance, Pharmacokinetics, and Adverse Reactions and Precautions). In particular, cefuroxime, unlike cefamandole, can achieve adequate concentrations in cerebrospinal fluid and thus is effective in meningitis caused by the common meningeal pathogens, *H. influenzae* (including β-lactamase-producing strains), *Neisseria meningitidis*, and *Streptococcus pneumoniae* (Pfenninger et al, 1982; Report from a Swedish Study Group, 1982; see also Pharmacokinetics). Furthermore, the "breakthrough" meningitis that has been reported with the use of cefamandole has not yet been observed with cefuroxime (see Gold and Rodriguez, 1983; Nelson, 1983; Smith and LeFrock, 1983; *Med Lett Drugs Ther*, 1984 A; Eichenwald, 1985; Sanders et al, 1985). Thus, cefuroxime has become a preferred drug among many pediatric infectious disease experts for single-agent empiric therapy of community-acquired bacterial pneumonia, suppurative bone and joint infections, and buccal and orbital cellulitis in infants and young children between 2 months and 4 years because it provides adequate coverage against the likely causative organisms (ie, *Staphylococcus aureus*, streptococci, pneumococci, and *H. influenzae*). Furthermore, cefuroxime appears to be an effective single-agent alternative to ampicillin plus chloramphenicol for initial therapy of meningitis in infants and young children (see Nelson, 1983; Eichenwald, 1985; see also Chapter 65, Table 1). Certain third generation cephalosporins (eg, ceftriaxone, cefotaxime) also appear to be useful for this latter indication (see discussion below). Cefuroxime is active against *Neisseria gonorrhoeae*, including PPNG strains, and is suggested by the Centers for Disease Control for those rare cases of acute pelvic inflammatory disease that occur in prepubertal females (*Morbid Mortal Week Rep*, 1985).

When compared to cefuroxime or cefamandole, the elimination half-lives of cefonicid (t½, 4.5 hours) and ceforanide (t½, 3 hours) are longer, which permit dosage intervals of 24 and 12 hours, respectively (Barriere and Mills, 1982; Dudley et al,

1984; Pontzer and Kaye, 1984; Tartaglione and Polk, 1985; see also Pharmacokinetics). Thus, these agents have the potential to reduce the cost of drug therapy. However, both ceforanide and cefonicid have considerably less activity in vitro than cefuroxime or cefamandole against *Staphylococcus aureus*. Failures with cefonicid in the treatment of staphylococcal infections have been reported (see Dudley et al, 1984; Pontzer and Kaye, 1984; Tartaglione and Polk, 1985). Ceforanide also has inferior activity against *Haemophilus influenzae* (Barriere and Mills, 1982; *Med Lett Drugs Ther*, 1984 B; Tartaglione and Polk, 1985). Unlike cefuroxime, neither cefonicid or ceforanide adequately penetrates into cerebrospinal fluid to be useful in meningitis (Tartaglione and Polk, 1985). Presently, clinical experience with cefonicid, particularly in serious infections, is very limited (Jacob and Layne, 1984), and any role for this agent in infectious disease therapy or surgical prophylaxis will depend on the results of further clinical studies (*Med Lett Drugs Ther*, 1984 C). Ceforanide does not appear to offer any advantages over cefuroxime or cefonicid and its clinical usefulness probably will be limited (*Med Lett Drugs Ther*, 1984 B).

Parenteral Third Generation Cephalosporins: In contrast to first and most second generation cephalosporins, the available third generation cephalosporins (except cefoperazone) show considerable promise in certain types of meningitis. Cefotaxime and moxalactam have produced excellent results in gram-negative enteric bacillary meningitis, particularly against *Escherichia coli*, *Klebsiella*, and *Proteus* (Landesman et al, 1981; Cherubin et al, 1982; Rahal, 1982; Rahal and Simberkoff, 1982). Because of high failure rates with chloramphenicol and the difficulties associated with intrathecal aminoglycoside administration, these third generation cephalosporins have become drugs of choice for meningitis known to be caused by gram-negative enteric bacilli (see Chapter 65, Table 1; see also Corrado et al, 1982; Rahal and Simberkoff, 1982; *Med Lett Drugs Ther*, 1983 A; Barriere and Flaherty, 1984; Mandell, 1984; Fried and Hinthorn, 1985). Although clinical experience is very limited, ceftizoxime, ceftriaxone, and ceftazidime also appear promising for this indication. Ceftazidime appears to be the most useful third generation cephalosporin for meningitis caused by *Pseudomonas aeruginosa* (Fong and Tomkins, 1985). Presently, ceftazidime plus an aminoglycoside should be considered an alternative regimen to an antipseudomonal penicillin plus an aminoglycoside for this indication; the aminoglycoside is administered intravenously and intrathecally (or intraventricularly). Although ceftazidime alone has been effective in a limited number of cases of *P. aeruginosa* meningitis (Fong and Tomkins, 1985), additional clinical studies are necessary before it can be recommended as monotherapy for this very serious infection.

All of the above third generation cephalosporins also have been very effective against meningitis caused by *Haemophilus influenzae* (including β-lactamase-producing strains), a frequent causative organism in young children. Presently, ampicillin and chloramphenicol are preferred; however, some infectious disease consultants now favor cefuroxime, cefotaxime, or ceftriaxone for initial treatment of *H. influenzae* type b meningitis. Penicillin G remains the drug of choice for pneumococcal and meningococcal meningitis; chloramphenicol is an alternative. Ceftriaxone and cefotaxime have excellent activity in vitro against all three of these common meningeal pathogens, and they have been shown to be as effective as ampicillin plus chloramphenicol for the empiric therapy of meningitis in infants and young children (Del Rio et al, 1983; Steele and Bradsher, 1983; Congeni, 1984; Barson et al, 1985; Bryan et al, 1985; Jacobs et al, 1985). A twice daily dosage schedule was adequate for the long-acting ceftriaxone; in one study (Bryan et al, 1985), once daily administration was effective. Thus, these third generation cephalosporins and the second generation derivative cefuroxime (see above) should be considered as effective single-agent alternatives to ampicillin plus chloramphenicol for pediatric meningitis (see Chapter 65, Table 1).

Neonatal meningitis is caused by *Streptococcus agalactiae* (group B) and other streptococci, *Escherichia coli* and other gram-negative enteric bacilli, and *Listeria monocytogenes*. The currently recommended empiric therapy for neonatal meningitis is ampicillin plus an aminoglycoside, but ampicillin plus a third generation cephalosporin (cefotaxime, moxalactam, or ceftriaxone) is an effective alternative regimen (see Chapter 65, Table 1; see also McCracken et al, 1984; Eichenwald, 1985; Naqvi et al, 1985). Third generation cephalosporins should not be used alone for this indication because none are active against *L. monocytogenes* or enterococci and some agents, such as moxalactam, lack adequate activity against group B streptococci (see Neu, 1982 A and D; Barriere and Flaherty, 1984; see also Antimicrobial Spectrum).

All third generation cephalosporins are highly active against *Neisseria gonorrhoeae*, including penicillinase-producing strains (PPNG) (see Antimicrobial Spectrum). In particular, the long-acting ceftriaxone ($t_{1/2}$, 8 hours), administered intramuscularly in a single 250-mg dose, has been shown to be very effective in uncomplicated gonorrhea in adults, including urethral, cervical, anorectal, and pharyngeal forms of this infection (Handsfield and Murphy, 1983; Judson et al, 1983, 1985; Collier et al, 1984). Presently, it is among the preferred drugs (alternatives: amoxicillin, ampicillin, penicillin G procaine) for uncomplicated gonococcal infections, including PPNG and chromosomal-mediated resistant *N. gonorrhoeae* (CMRNG) infections (*Morbid Mortal Week Rep*, 1985). Although cephalosporins are likely to cure incubating syphilis, they are not active against *Chlamydia trachomatis* and concomitant therapy with a tetracycline is recommended for coexisting chlamydial infections (*Morbid Mortal Week Rep*, 1985). Intravenous ceftriaxone, cefotaxime, and cefoxitin (see above) are alternatives to intravenous penicillin G or oral amoxicillin (or ampicillin) for disseminated gonococcal infections; these cephalosporins are recommended for PPNG infections. A single 250-mg intramuscular dose of ceftriaxone is a treatment of choice (alternative, oral erythromycin for seven days) for chancroid caused by *Haemophilus ducreyi* (*Morbid Mortal Week Rep*, 1985). For a more detailed discussion, see Chapter 65, Table 2.

The third generation cephalosporins have been effective, frequently as empiric monotherapy, in a wide variety of serious gram-negative bacillary infections outside the central nervous system. These include lower respiratory tract, complicated urinary tract, intra-abdominal, gynecologic, skin and skin structure, bone, and joint infections and bacteremias; these infections often are of nosocomial origin (see Neu, 1982 D; Barriere and Flaherty, 1984; Smith, 1984; see also Other Selected References for symposia publications on the individual agents). However, the exact role of third generation cephalosporins in these infections and optimal drug selection among the available third generation derivatives remain to be clarified. The decision to use a third generation cephalosporin should depend, in part, on the particular clinical situation and locally generated antibiotic susceptibility profiles. In general, less expensive, narrower spectrum, first (or second) generation cephalosporins should be used when they are equally effective. First generation cephalosporins clearly are preferable for known gram-positive bacterial infections and for surgical prophylaxis (see Neu, 1982 D; *Med Lett Drugs Ther*, 1983 A; DiPiro et al, 1984; Mandell, 1984; Fried and Hinthorn, 1985).

The following represent some of the more likely uses of third generation cephalosporins in serious gram-negative bacillary infections, based on current clinical experience: (1) When bacteria that are known to be multiply-resistant to other, less expensive antibiotics (eg, penicillins, older cephalosporins), but are susceptible to a third generation cephalosporin, the latter is indicated. (2) When equally effective, third generation cephalosporins are usually preferred to aminoglycosides because of the ototoxicity and nephrotoxicity associated with the latter agents. This is especially important in patients at increased risk for aminoglycoside toxicity (see Chapter 70, Aminoglycosides) or those requiring prolonged therapy (eg, osteomyelitis). (3) The high in vitro activity of third generation cephalosporins against most gram-negative bacilli may make these agents more desirable than less expensive alternatives for certain severe infections, such as pneumonia caused by *Klebsiella pneumoniae* (see Neu, 1982 D; Barriere and Flaherty, 1984; Mandell, 1984; Smith, 1984; Fried and Hinthorn, 1985).

Monotherapy with a third generation cephalosporin, as an alternative to antimicrobial combination therapy that frequently includes an aminoglycoside, for broad spectrum empiric treatment of serious infections (eg, pneumonia, septicemia) or to treat infections of polymicrobial origin (eg, intra-abdominal, pelvic) appears promising (Oblinger et al, 1982; Mandell et al, 1983; Stone et al, 1983; Warren et al, 1983; Smith et al, 1984; see also Neu, 1982 D; Barriere and Flaherty, 1984; Smith, 1984; Moellering, 1985 A; and Chapter 65, Table 1). However, additional comparative studies are necessary before definitive recommendations can be made. An important consideration for empiric therapy of nosocomial infections is the incidence of *Pseudomonas aeruginosa* in a particular hospital. Of the available third generation cephalosporins, ceftazidime is the most active agent against this organism. When used alone, ceftazidime has been as effective as standard combination therapy (eg, antipseudomonal penicillin plus aminoglycoside) for nosocomial sepsis (Rapp et al, 1984; Cone et al, 1985; Young, 1985), acute pulmonary exacerbations of cystic fibrosis (Mastella et al, 1983; Gold et al, 1985), and for initial therapy of febrile neutropenic patients (see Smith, 1984; Pizzo et al, 1985). However, ceftazidime-resistant strains of *P. aeruginosa* have been isolated and monotherapy with this agent for serious *P. aeruginosa* infections and for initial therapy of febrile neutropenic patients requires further study (see the evaluation).

Selecting a particular third generation cephalosporin for routine use is somewhat difficult because they rarely have been compared directly for clinical efficacy and toxicity. Guidelines for drug selection usually are based on noncomparative clinical studies, in vitro antimicrobial activity, pharmacokinetics, adverse reaction profiles, and cost. Relative advantages and disadvantages of the currently available third generation cephalosporins are listed in Table 2. As discussed above, when *P. aeruginosa* is a probable causative organism, ceftazidime is the preferred third generation cephalosporin. Cefoperazone is an alternative, but it has inferior activity against most strains of this organism. When *P. aeruginosa* is not under consideration, ceftriaxone, ceftizoxime, and cefotaxime have advantages over moxalactam, which has unacceptable hematologic toxicity, and cefoperazone, which also has been associated with hematologic side effects, has poorer activity against many Enterobacteriaceae, is not recommended for meningitis, and is not labeled for use in children, infants, and neonates. Ceftriaxone, ceftizoxime, and cefotaxime have

good activity against most gram-positive bacteria, excellent activity against most gram-negative bacteria, and good adverse reaction profiles that are similar to first and most second generation cephalosporins. These three agents differ primarily in pharmacokinetic properties and in the amount of clinical experience. The primary advantage of cefotaxime is lengthy clinical experience, particularly in gram-negative enteric bacillary meningitis. However, current consensus recommends that it be administered every four to six hours for serious infections, although some experts argue that an 8 hour dosage interval is adequate because of the more prolonged half-life (about 1.6 hours) of desacetylcefotaxime, its active metabolite (see the evaluation). Ceftizoxime is essentially identical to cefotaxime, but it has a longer half-life and can be administered every eight hours for serious infections. It is not labeled for use in gram-negative enteric bacillary meningitis or in infants less than six months. Ceftriaxone has the longest half-life ($t_{1/2}$, 8 hours) among third generation cephalosporins and can be administered once daily for most serious infections and twice daily for meningitis. If competitively priced and no new serious adverse reactions are found with this agent, it may become the preferred third generation cephalosporin. See also Antimicrobial Spectrum, Adverse Reactions and Precautions, Pharmacokinetics, and the evaluations.

TABLE 2.
ADVANTAGES AND DISADVANTAGES OF THE THIRD GENERATION CEPHALOSPORINS[1]

Drug	Advantages	Disadvantages
Cefotaxime [Claforan]	1. Greater clinical experience 2. Good overall activity against gram-positive and gram-negative bacteria 3. Proven efficacy in gram-negative enteric bacillary meningitis. Also is labeled for use in *Haemophilus influenzae*, *Neisseria meningitidis*, and *Streptococcus pneumoniae* meningitis. 4. Good adverse reaction profile—like first generation cephalosporins 5. Labeled for use in children, infants, and neonates	1. Requires four- to six-hour dosing interval for serious infections (see text); eight-hour interval for less serious infections. 2. Poor activity against *Pseudomonas aeruginosa*; fair activity against *Bacteroides fragilis* 3. Expensive—average wholesale price, $10.81/g[2]
Ceftizoxime [Cefizox]	1. Good overall activity against gram-positive and gram-negative bacteria 2. Eight-hour dosing interval for serious infections; 12-hour interval for less serious infections 3. Good adverse reaction profile—like first generation cephalosporins	1. Poor activity against *Pseudomonas aeruginosa*; fair activity against *Bacteroides fragilis* 2. Not labeled for use in gram-negative enteric bacillary meningitis (labeled only for *Haemophilus influenzae* meningitis) 3. Not labeled for use in infants less than 6 months 4. Expensive—average wholesale price, $11.18/g[2]
Ceftriaxone [Rocephin]	1. Good overall activity against gram-positive and gram-negative bacteria 2. 24-hour dosing interval for most serious infections; 12-hour interval for meningitis 3. Good adverse reaction profile—like first generation cephalosporins 4. Labeled for use in *Haemophilus influenzae*, *Neisseria meningitidis*, and *Streptococcus pneumoniae* meningitis 5. Labeled for use in children, infants, and neonates	1. Poor activity against *Pseudomonas aeruginosa*; fair/poor activity against *Bacteroides fragilis* 2. Not labeled for use in gram-negative enteric bacillary meningitis 3. Expensive—average wholesale price, $27.54/g[2]

(Continued on next page)

TABLE 2.
ADVANTAGES AND DISADVANTAGES OF THE THIRD GENERATION CEPHALOSPORINS[1] (continued)

Drug	Advantages	Disadvantages
Ceftazidime [Fortaz, Tazicef, Tazidime]	1. Good activity against *Pseudomonas aeruginosa* 2. Eight-hour dosing interval for serious infections; 12-hour interval for less serious infections 3. Good adverse reaction profile—like first generation cephalosporins 4. Labeled for use in children, infants, and neonates	1. Less active against gram-positive bacteria, particularly staphylococci 2. Poor activity against *Bacteroides fragilis* 3. Not labeled for use in gram-negative enteric bacillary meningitis (labeled for *Haemophilus influenzae* and *Neisseria meningitidis* meningitis; some success in *Pseudomonas aeruginosa* meningitis has been noted) 4. Expensive—average wholesale price, 11.02/g[2,3]
Cefoperazone [Cefobid]	1. Greater clinical experience 2. Eight-hour dosing interval for serious infections; 12-hour interval for less serious infections 3. Fair activity against *Pseudomonas aeruginosa*	1. Lower beta-lactamase stability and, therefore, less active against most gram-negative bacteria (eg, Enterobacteriaceae) 2. Fair/poor activity against *Bacteroides fragilis* 3. Hypoprothrombinemia and bleeding episodes (uncommon) 4. Ethanol intolerance 5. Not labeled for use in meningitis 6. Not labeled for use in children, infants, and neonates 7. Expensive—average wholesale price, $11.28/g[2]
Moxalactam [Moxam]	1. Greater clinical experience 2. Eight-hour dosing interval for serious infections; 12-hour interval for less serious infections 3. Proven efficacy in gram-negative enteric bacillary meningitis 4. Good activity against *Bacteroides fragilis* 5. Labeled for use in children, infants, and neonates	1. Less active against gram-positive bacteria 2. Hypoprothrombinemia, suppression of platelet function, and bleeding episodes (relatively common and fatalities have occurred) 3. Ethanol intolerance 4. Enterococcal superinfections 5. Poor activity against *Pseudomonas aeruginosa* 6. Expensive—average wholesale price, $10.68/g[2]

[1] None of the third generation cephalosporins is active against enterococci, methicillin-resistant staphylococci, penicillin-resistant pneumococci, Listeria monocytogenes, or Clostridium difficile.
[2] Average wholesale prices obtained from 1985 Drug Topics Redbook (Oradell, NJ, Medical Economics Co, 1985) and monthly updates through October, 1985. Actual hospital pharmacy cost and price charged to patient will vary among institutions.
[3] Average wholesale price shown is for Fortaz; prices of Tazicef and Tazidime were not available when this table was prepared. Because ceftazidime is being marketed by three manufacturers, hospital pharmacies may be able to reduce their acquisition cost through competitive bidding.

Oral Cephalosporins: Cephalexin, cephradine, cefadroxil, and cefaclor are rarely drugs of choice for bacterial infections, but these expensive oral antibiotics may be indicated in mild to moderate infections of the respiratory tract, urinary tract, skin and skin structures, and bone caused by susceptible organisms when preferred agents are ineffective or cannot be tolerated. Likely indications for first generation derivatives (cephalexin, cephradine, cefadroxil) include urinary tract infections when the causative organism is resistant to preferred and less expensive drugs (eg, sulfonamides, ampicillin, trimethoprim/sulfamethoxazole [Bactrim, Septra]) and minor staphylococcal pyodermas in patients with non-IgE-mediated (ie, nonimmediate) hypersensitivity reactions to penicillins. Cefaclor, a second generation cephalosporin, is more active than the other agents against *Haemophilus influenzae* and is active against many amoxicillin-resistant *H. influenzae* and *Branhamella catarrhalis* strains. This agent is an alternative to erythromycin/sulfisoxazole [Pediazole], trimethoprim/sulfamethoxazole, and amoxicillin/potassium clavulanate [Augmentin] for acute otitis media and acute sinusitis caused by these amoxicillin-resistant organisms. For additional discussion of oral cephalosporins, see Chapter 65, Table 1; see also Neu, 1982 D; Reese and Betts, 1983; Rehm and McHenry, 1983; Norris, 1984 B; Eichenwald, 1985; and Gordon, 1985.

Sequential parenteral-oral cephalosporin therapy for suppurative bone and joint infections in infants and children has been successfully employed. However, large doses of oral cephalosporins usually are required, organism susceptibility must be known, and careful monitoring for compliance and serum bactericidal activity is required (see Nelson et al, 1982; Eichenwald, 1985).

ADVERSE REACTIONS AND PRECAUTIONS

Hypersensitivity Reactions: Cephalosporins generally are well tolerated. Hypersensitivity reactions are the most common systemic adverse effects. The majority of these are maculopapular skin rashes that usually occur after several days of therapy. Rashes frequently are accompanied by fever and eosinophilia. Immediate-type, IgE-mediated reactions, including urticaria, bronchospasm, and anaphylaxis, are uncommon with the cephalosporins. Immune-mediated leukopenia, thrombocytopenia, and anemia have been reported rarely and are reversible with discontinuation of treatment. Direct and indirect positive Coombs' tests are relatively common with large doses, but hemolytic anemia is rare and usually mild. A serum sickness reaction, characterized by skin rash with polyarthritis and, frequently, fever, has been associated most often with cefaclor (Murray et al, 1980; Ackley and Felsher, 1981; Leng and Anderson, 1985; Levine, 1985).

Although the chemical structures of cephalosporins and penicillins are similar (see Chemistry and Classification; see also Chapter 66, Penicillins), cross-hypersensitivity between these two groups of antibiotics is low. Clinically, probably less than 5% of individuals with a history of penicillin allergy, including those with a history of IgE-mediated reactions, also are allergic to cephalosporins (Saxon, 1983; Quintiliani et al, 1984). Therefore, it generally is considered safe to administer a cephalosporin to a patient with a history of a non-IgE-mediated hypersensitivity reaction (eg, maculopapular skin rash) to penicillins. However, the current consensus is that cephalosporins should not be used in individuals who experienced immediate hypersensitivity reactions (eg, urticaria, angioedema, bronchospasm, anaphylaxis) to penicillins because the consequences of these adverse reactions could be catastrophic (Quintiliani et al, 1984).

Hematologic Reactions: Bleeding has been reported with cefamandole, cefoperazone, and, particularly, moxalactam. A total of 2.5% of clinical trial patients treated for four or more days with moxalactam experienced a bleeding event, most of which were serious (manufacturer's literature). Each of these cephalosporins contains a methylthiotetrazole side chain that has been associated with hypoprothrombinemia in some patients, particularly elderly debilitated individuals, those with severe renal insufficiency, and malnourished patients receiving total parenteral nutrition. The prolongation of prothrombin time appears to result from interference with hepatic vitamin K metabolism by the methylthiotetrazole side chain of these cephalosporins (Andrassy et al, 1985), but eradication of vitamin K-producing intestinal microorganisms also may be involved (Bang and Kammer, 1983). Administration of vitamin K reverses the hypoprothrombinemia. In some patients, prophylactic vitamin K administration may be desirable when using these three cephalosporins; vitamin K (adults, 10 mg per week) is now recommended in all patients receiving moxalactam (see the evaluation).

Moxalactam also has prolonged the bleeding time and caused bleeding diathesis in some patients because of dose-dependent inhibition of platelet function (Weitekamp and Aber, 1983). This is not reversible by vitamin K. In adults with normal renal function, doses exceeding 4 g per day for more than three days may result in platelet dysfunction. Patients with reduced renal function are particularly susceptible. Bleeding time should be monitored in patients requiring more than 4 g of moxalactam per day and who are treated for more than three days. All patients with renal dysfunction should have appropriate dosage adjustments and should be monitored periodically with bleeding times. If the bleeding time becomes unduly prolonged, moxalactam should be discontinued (see evaluation). Because of the coagulopathy associated with moxalactam use, other third generation cephalosporins usually are preferred (see Uses).

Gastrointestinal Reactions: Gastrointestinal disturbances associated with cephalosporins include pyrosis, anorexia, nausea, vomiting, and diarrhea. Cefoperazone may cause more diarrhea than other cephalosporins, perhaps because of greater biliary excretion (Carlberg et al, 1982; Mulligan et al, 1982). Rarely, antibiotic-associated pseudomembranous colitis (AAPMC) due to *Clostridium difficile* occurs with the cephalosporins. If this potentially life-threatening adverse effect develops, the drug should be discontinued, supportive measures should be initiated to maintain normal fluid and electrolyte balance, and, if necessary, treatment with oral vancomycin (alternative, metronidazole) should be instituted (see Chapter 68, Macrolides and Lincosamides, and Chapter 72, Miscellaneous Antibacterial Agents).

Renal and Hepatic Reactions: Cephalosporins may temporarily increase blood urea nitrogen (BUN) levels, but generally they are not considered to be nephrotoxic at usually recommended doses. However, cephalothin rarely has caused more serious nephrotoxicity (tubular necrosis), especially when given in large doses or to patients with pre-existing renal impairment. Additive nephrotoxicity has been reported when cephalothin and an aminoglycoside were administered concomitantly (see Drug Interactions and Interference with Laboratory Tests). Some signs of hepatic dysfunction, manifested by transient increases in serum transaminase (SGOT, SGPT) and alkaline phosphatase concentrations, also have been noted following administration of the cephalosporins. Reversible cholestatic jaundice has been reported rarely.

Miscellaneous Reactions: Cephalosporins are irritants and can cause pain at the site of intramuscular injection or thrombophlebitis after intravenous administration. Among first generation cephalosporins, cefazolin is less irritating than cephalothin, cephapirin, and cephradine and is preferred for intramuscular use. Phlebitis usually can be prevented by alternating veins or by slow injection of a solution diluted with sodium chloride or dextrose injection. Intrathecal injection of cephalosporins is not recommended, because animal studies and limited clinical observations indicate that this route may be neurotoxic; nystagmus, hallucinations, and convulsions have been observed.

Cephalosporins may cause clinically significant superinfections. *Pseudomonas, Candida*, and enterococci (particularly with third generation derivatives like moxalactam) are likely causative organisms. If superinfection occurs, appropriate measures should be undertaken.

The risk to the fetus when the cephalosporins are administered to pregnant women has not been fully assessed but, as with the penicillins, there is no evidence of teratogenicity in man (see Chow and Jewesson, 1985). All cephalosporins except moxalactam are in FDA Pregnancy Category B; moxalactam is in Category C.

For additional discussion of adverse reactions and precautions, see *Med Lett Drug Ther*, 1983 A; Barriere and Flaherty, 1984; Mandell, 1984; Quintiliani et al, 1984; Smith, 1984; Fried and Hinthorn, 1985; Tartaglione and Polk, 1985; Norrby, 1986.

DRUG INTERACTIONS AND INTERFERENCE WITH LABORATORY TESTS

An increase in nephrotoxicity has been observed in patients receiving an aminoglycoside plus cephalothin (Wade et al, 1978; for others, see Luft, 1982; Mangini, 1984 A; and Hansten, 1985). This appears to be most likely in patients with pre-existing renal disease. Except for cephaloridine (no longer marketed), there is no evidence that other cephalosporins also potentiate aminoglycoside nephrotoxicity (see Mangini, 1984 A). Current recommendations are to administer aminoglycoside-cephalosporin combinations with caution, particularly in patients with pre-existing renal disease (Hansten, 1985). Avoidance of cephalothin in these patients should be considered.

Cephalothin also may increase the nephrotoxic effects of colistimethate and renal function should be monitored. The availability of alternative antibiotics probably makes use of this combination unnecessary (Mangini, 1984 B; Hansten, 1985).

Acute alcohol intolerance, ie, a disulfiram-like reaction, has been attributed to certain cephalosporins containing a methylthiotetrazole side chain. Facial flushing, nausea, headache, sweating, tachycardia, and, infrequently, hypotensive episodes have been reported in patients who imbibed alcohol while receiving cefamandole, cefoperazone, moxalactam, or the investigational drug, cefmenoxime (Neu and Prince, 1980; Portier et al, 1980; Kannangara et al, 1984; for others, see Witt and Witt, 1983; Mangini, 1984 C; Hansten, 1985; Stockley, 1985). Symptoms usually occur within 30 minutes of alcohol ingestion and last for several minutes to several hours. The exact incidence of this reaction is not known. Methylthiotetrazole-containing cephalosporins increased acetaldehyde concentrations in animals when ethanol was administered (Buening et al, 1981), and although not completely understood, acetaldehyde accumulation is presumed to be the cause of this reaction in humans. It is recommended that alcoholic beverages or ethanol-containing pharmaceuticals be avoided in patients receiving cefamandole, cefoperazone, moxalactam, or cefmenoxime and for two to three days after antibiotic treatment is discontinued (Hansten, 1985).

A false-positive reaction for glucose in the urine may occur when Benedict's or Fehling's solution or Clinitest tablets are employed. Cephalosporins apparently do not interfere with results obtained from enzyme-based tests, such as Tes-Tape or Clinistix.

High concentrations of cefoxitin, ceforanide, or cephalothin may interfere with measurement of creatinine levels by the Jaffe reaction and produce false results (see Guay et al, 1983). Serum samples from cefoxitin-treated patients should not be analyzed for creatinine if withdrawn within two hours of drug administration.

PHARMACOKINETICS

Some pharmacokinetic values for the cephalosporins are shown in Table 3.

Oral Cephalosporins: Cephalexin, cephradine, and cefadroxil (first generation cephalosporins) and cefaclor (second generation cephalosporin) are stable in gastric acid and can be administered orally. All are well absorbed from the gastrointestinal tract and similar peak serum concentrations are attained with comparable doses (eg, approximately 15 mcg/ml after a dose of 500 mg). Except for cefadroxil, the presence of food decreases the rate of absorption in adults, but the extent of absorption (ie, the area under the serum concentration time curve [AUC]) is unchanged (see Nightingale et al, 1980; Norris, 1984 B; Fried and Hinthorn, 1985). In infants and children, the ingestion of milk was reported to decrease the bioavailability of cephalexin and cephradine, but not cefadroxil or cefaclor (Ginsburg, 1982).

All of the oral cephalosporins bind poorly to plasma proteins. Although these agents distribute to a wide variety of tissues and body fluids, they do not achieve therapeutic concentrations in the cerebrospinal fluid, even in the presence of inflammation.

Oral cephalosporins are eliminated by the kidneys, primarily by renal tubular secretion, and are recovered as unchanged drugs in the urine. Excretion is delayed by probenecid. The elimination half-lives of cephalexin, cephradine, and cefaclor are similar (about 50 minutes). However, the elimination half-life of cefadroxil is more prolonged (about 90 minutes), allowing a longer dosing interval. Dosage reductions are required when cephalexin, cephradine, or cefadroxil are used in patients with impaired renal function. Cefaclor, however, is unstable in biological fluids and does not accumulate in these patients.

See also Table 3 and the evaluations. For additional discussion, see Nightingale et al, 1975, 1980; Rehm and McHenry, 1983; Norris, 1984 B; Quintiliani et al, 1984; and Fried and Hinthorn, 1985.

Parenteral First Generation Cephalosporins: These agents can be administered intravenously or intramuscularly. Cefazolin is preferred to cephalothin, cephapirin, and cephradine for intramuscular administration because it causes less pain at the site of injection. At equivalent doses, cefazolin achieves peak serum concentrations significantly higher than those obtained with other first generation cephalosporins. This is due, in part, to the higher plasma protein binding and lower volume of distribution observed with cefazolin.

Parenteral first generation cephalosporins distribute to a wide variety of tissues (eg, myocardium, bone, gallbladder) and body fluids (eg, pericardial, pleural, synovial, bile, urine). However, they fail to achieve therapeutic concentrations in the cerebrospinal fluid, even in the presence of inflammation.

All parenterally administered first generation cephalosporins are eliminated by the kidneys. However, the mechanisms and rates of elimination differ among the four agents. Both cephalothin and cephapirin are partially metabolized to considerably less active desacetyl metabolites. Parent drugs plus metabolites are rapidly eliminated by renal tubular secretion. Cephradine also is rapidly eliminated by renal tubular secretion, but it is not metabolized. The half-lives of cephalothin, cephapirin, and cephradine are under one hour. In contrast, cefazolin is eliminated more slowly ($t_{1/2}$, 1.8 hours) by glomerular filtration and renal tubular secretion. Because of its higher and more prolonged serum concentrations, cefazolin usually can be given in lower doses and less frequently than other parenteral first generation cephalosporins and, thus, often is preferred (see Uses). The half-lives of all of these analogues are prolonged in patients with renal impairment and dosage adjustments are required.

See also Table 3 and the evaluations. For additional discussion, see Nightingale et al, 1975, 1980; Quintiliani and Nightingale, 1978; Norris, 1984 B; Quintiliani et al, 1984; and Fried and Hinthorn, 1985.

Parenteral Second Generation Cephalosporins: These agents can be administered intravenously or intramuscularly. At equivalent dosages, peak serum concentrations vary among the individual agents. In general, cefonicid achieves the highest peak serum concentration followed by ceforanide, cefuroxime, and the older derivatives, cefoxitin and cefamandole. Plasma protein binding also varies; cefonicid is the most highly bound (greater than 95%) and cefuroxime is the least bound (33%) second generation cephalosporin.

All of these agents distribute to a wide variety of tissues and body fluids, including pleural and synovial fluids, sputum, bone, bile, and urine. However, cefuroxime is the only second generation cephalosporin that achieves therapeutic concentrations in the cerebrospinal fluid of patients with meningitis (see Gold and Rodriguez, 1983; see also Uses).

All parenteral second generation cephalosporins are excreted as unchanged drugs via the kidneys by glomerular filtration and renal tubular secretion. They are not metabolized. These agents differ in their rates of elimination, however. The half-lives of the newer derivatives, particularly cefonicid ($t_{1/2}$, 3.5 to 4.5 hours) and ceforanide ($t_{1/2}$, 2.7 to 3 hours), are considerably longer than those of cefoxitin and cefamandole ($t_{1/2}$, less than one hour). The half-life of cefuroxime is 1.3 to 1.7 hours. The half-lives of all of these agents are prolonged in patients with renal impairment and dosage adjustments are necessary.

Longer dosing intervals can be employed with cefonicid (24 hours), ceforanide (12 hours), and cefuroxime (eight hours) when compared to cefoxitin and cefamandole (four to six hours). The pharmacokinetics of these newer second generation cephalosporins, particularly cefonicid, have the potential to reduce the cost of cephalosporin therapy. However, equal or improved efficacy (without added toxicity) of these newer agents must be clearly established by comparative clinical trials before they can be recommended over established therapies (see Uses).

See also Table 3 and the evaluations. For additional discussion, see Barriere and Mills, 1982; Gold and Rodriguez, 1983; Smith and LeFrock, 1983; Dudley et al, 1984; Norris, 1984 B;

Pontzer and Kaye, 1984; Fried and Hinthorn, 1985; Sanders et al, 1985; and Tartaglione and Polk, 1985.

Parenteral Third Generation Cephalosporins: All presently available third generation cephalosporins are poorly absorbed orally and must be administered intravenously or intramuscularly. At equivalent doses, peak serum concentrations vary among the individual agents. In general, ceftriaxone and cefoperazone achieve the highest peak serum concentrations. This is due, in part, to their higher plasma protein binding and lower volumes of distribution.

Third generation cephalosporins distribute to a wide variety of tissues (eg, myocardium, myometrium, bone, gallbladder) and body fluids (eg, synovial, pleural, peritoneal, pericardial). Adequate biliary concentrations are achieved with all of these agents, and very high concentrations are observed with cefoperazone and ceftriaxone. Urinary concentrations achieved with all third generation cephalosporins are far in excess of minimum inhibitory concentrations for susceptible organisms.

In contrast to first and second generation cephalosporins (except cefuroxime), the third generation agents are able to penetrate inflamed meninges to achieve therapeutic cerebrospinal fluid concentrations for a number of pathogens, including *Escherichia coli* and other gram-negative enteric bacilli, *Haemophilus influenzae, Neisseria meningitidis,* and, for some analogues, *Streptococcus pneumoniae.* Except for cefoperazone, for which cerebrospinal fluid penetration has been more variable, the third generation cephalosporins are promising agents for meningitis (see Uses).

The third generation cephalosporins exhibit considerable differences in elimination routes and half-lives. Cefotaxime is the only third generation agent that undergoes metabolism. This compound is partially metabolized by hepatic esterases to desacetylcefotaxime, which is four- to eightfold less active than the parent compound. Cefotaxime and its metabolite are eliminated primarily by renal tubular secretion; probenecid delays excretion. Cefotaxime has the shortest half-life (one hour) among third generation cephalosporins and, therefore, must be administered the most frequently (eg, every six hours for serious infections). Because cefotaxime has an important nonrenal route of elimination, little parent drug accumulates in individuals with renal impairment. However, elimination of the desacetyl metabolite is prolonged and dosage reductions are recommended when the creatinine clearance is less than 20 ml/min.

Ceftizoxime, ceftazidime, and moxalactam are excreted as unchanged drugs by the kidneys. Ceftizoxime ($t_{1/2}$, 1.4 to 1.8 hours) is eliminated by glomerular filtration and renal tubular secretion; probenecid delays excretion. In contrast, ceftazidime ($t_{1/2}$, 1.8 hours) and moxalactam ($t_{1/2}$, 2 to 2.3 hours) are eliminated by glomerular filtration, and probenecid does not affect their rates of excretion. The intermediate elimination half-lives of these three agents allows them to be administered every eight hours for serious infections. The half-lives of ceftizoxime, ceftazidime, and moxalactam are substantially longer in individuals with renal impairment and dosage reductions are necessary to avoid drug accumulation.

Ceftriaxone is eliminated as unchanged drug both via the renal (about 60%, by glomerular filtration) and biliary (about

TABLE 3.
PHARMACOKINETIC VALUES FOR THE CEPHALOSPORINS[1]

Generic Name	Trade Name(s)	Route(s) of Administration	Plasma Protein Bound (%)	Volume of Distribution (L/kg)
FIRST GENERATION				
Cephalothin	Keflin, Seffin	Intravenous Intramuscular	70	0.26±0.11
Cefazolin	Ancef, Kefzol	Intravenous Intramuscular	85	0.12±0.03
Cephapirin	Cefadyl	Intravenous Intramuscular	45-50	0.13±0.05
Cephradine	Anspor, Velosef	Oral Intravenous Intramuscular	10-20	0.25±0.01
Cephalexin	Keflex	Oral	10-15	0.26±0.03
Cefadroxil	Duricef, Ultracef	Oral	15-20	0.31
SECOND GENERATION				
Cefamandole	Mandol	Intravenous Intramuscular	70-80	0.16±0.05
Cefoxitin	Mefoxin	Intravenous Intramuscular	70-80	0.13-0.22
Cefuroxime	Zinacef	Intravenous Intramuscular	33	0.19±0.04
Ceforanide	Precef	Intravenous Intramuscular	80	0.16-0.19
Cefonicid	Monocid	Intravenous Intramuscular	95-98	0.11
Cefaclor	Ceclor	Oral	25	0.24-0.36

Metabolized (%)	Urinary Recovery (%)	Approximate Half-Life (hours)	Effect of Probenecid	References
20-30	70-80(50)[2]	0.5-0.9	+	Nightingale et al, 1975, 1980; Bennett et al, 1983; Norris, 1984 B; Benet and Sheiner, 1985
None	95	1.8	+	Nightingale et al, 1975, 1980; Quintiliani and Nightingale, 1978; Bennett et al, 1983; Norris, 1984 B; Benet and Sheiner, 1985
40	90(50)[2]	0.6-0.8	+	Nightingale et al, 1975, 1980; Bennett et al, 1983; Norris, 1984 B; Benet and Sheiner, 1985
None	90	0.8	+	Nightingale et al, 1975, 1980; Bennett et al, 1983; Norris, 1984 B; Benet and Sheiner, 1985.
None	90	0.9	+	Nightingale et al, 1975, 1980; Bennett et al, 1983; Rehm and McHenry, 1983; Norris, 1984 B; Benet and Sheiner, 1985
None	90	1.4	+	Nightingale et al, 1980; Bennett et al, 1983; Rehm and McHenry, 1983; Norris, 1984 B
None	80-95	0.6-1	+	Nightingale et al, 1980; Norris, 1984 B; Benet and Sheiner, 1985; Sanders et al, 1985; Tartaglione and Polk, 1985
<2	80-95	0.7-1	+	Nightingale et al, 1980; Bennett et al, 1983; Norris, 1984 B; Sanders et al, 1985; Tartaglione and Polk, 1985
None	90-95	1.3-1.7	+	Gold and Rodriquez, 1983; Smith and LeFrock, 1983; Norris, 1984 B; Benet and Sheiner, 1985; Tartaglione and Polk, 1985
None	90	2.7-3.0	−	Barriere and Mills, 1982; Bennett et al, 1983; Norris, 1984 B; Tartaglione and Polk, 1985
None	90	3.5-4.5	+	Dudley et al, 1984; Norris, 1984 B; Pontzer and Kaye, 1984; Benet and Sheiner, 1985; Tartaglione and Polk, 1985
None	60-85	0.6-0.9	+	Nightingale et al, 1980; Bennett et al, 1983; Rehm and McHenry. 1983; Norris, 1984 B

(Continued on next page)

TABLE 3.
PHARMACOKINETIC VALUES FOR THE CEPHALOSPORINS[1] (continued)

Generic Name	Trade Name(s)	Route(s) of Administration	Plasma Protein Bound (%)	Volume of Distribution (L/kg)
THIRD GENERATION				
Cefotaxime	Claforan	Intravenous Intramuscular	38	0.25-0.39
Ceftizoxime	Cefizox	Intravenous Intramuscular	30	0.35-0.40
Ceftriaxone	Rocephin	Intravenous Intramuscular	83-96	0.12-0.14
Cefmenoxime[5]	Cefmax	Intravenous Intramuscular	77	0.23
Ceftazidime	Fortaz, Tazicef, Tazidime	Intravenous Intramuscular	17	0.21-0.28
Cefoperazone	Cefobid	Intravenous Intramuscular	87-93	0.14-0.20
Moxalactam	Moxam	Intravenous Intramuscular	50	0.25-0.40
Cefsulodin[5]	Cefomonil	Intravenous Intramuscular	15-30	0.22-0.31

[1]The pharmacokinetic values shown in this Table represent average or most frequently reported values from the literature. In some cases, however, there is considerable variation among different laboratories.
[2]Number in parentheses represents percentage of dose excreted in the urine as unchanged drug.
[3]The half-life of desacetylcefotaxime is 1.5 to 1.6 hours.
[4]Although the primary route of excretion is renal, about 40% of a dose is eliminated unchanged in the bile. Dosage reductions are not necessary in patients with severe renal dysfunction.
[5]Investigational drug in the United States
[6]Unlike other cephalosporins, the primary route of excretion is biliary (70% as unchanged drug). Dosage reductions are not necessary in patients with severe renal dysfunction.

Metabolized (%)	Urinary Recovery (%)	Approximate Half-Life (hours)	Effect of Probenecid	References
30-50	85(50-60)[2]	1-1.1[3]	+	LeFrock et al, 1982; Neu, 1982 A; Carmine et al, 1983 A; Garzone et al, 1983 A; Barriere and Flaherty, 1984; Balant et al, 1985; Benet and Sheiner, 1985
None	80-90	1.4-1.8	+	Neu, 1982 A; Bennett et al, 1983; Garzone et al, 1983 A; Barriere and Flaherty, 1984; Balant et al, 1985; Richards and Heel, 1985
None	40-65[4]	6-9	−	Neu, 1982 A; Bennett et al, 1983; Garzone et al, 1983 A; Barriere and Flaherty, 1984; Patel and Kaplan, 1984; Richards et al, 1984; Balant et al, 1985; Beam, 1985
?	75-80	1	+	Neu, 1982 A; Bennett et al, 1983; Barriere and Flaherty, 1984
None	75-90	1.8	−	Neu, 1982 A; Garzone et al, 1983 A; Smith, 1984; Balant et al, 1985; Benet and Sheiner, 1985; Gentry, 1985; Richards and Brogden, 1985
None	25[6]	1.9-2.1	−	Funk and Strausbaugh, 1982; Neu, 1982 A; Bennett et al, 1983; Garzone et al, 1983 A; Barriere and Flaherty, 1984; Balant et al, 1985
None	70-94	2-2.3	−	Fitzpatrick and Standiford, 1982; Neu, 1982 A; Bennett et al, 1983; Carmine et al, 1983 B; Garzone et al, 1983 A: Barriere and Flaherty, 1984; Balant et al 1985
?	50-70	1.6-1.9	−	Neu, 1982 A; Bennett et al, 1983; Smith, 1984; Balant et al, 1985

40%) routes. It has the longest elimination half-life (six to nine hours) of any third generation cephalosporin and can be administered once daily for serious infections outside the central nervous system. Thus, it is a particularly attractive agent because of the potential for cost savings. It also may be useful for home intravenous antibiotic therapy. The elimination half-life of ceftriaxone is only minimally increased in patients with severe renal impairment and dosage reductions are unnecessary. Accumulation does occur in patients with severe combined renal and hepatic failure and dosage modifications are required.

Cefoperazone is the only cephalosporin eliminated primarily unchanged in bile (about 70%); about 25% of a dose is recovered in the urine. This third generation cephalosporin has an intermediate elimination half-life (1.9 to 2.1 hours); most infectious disease experts recommend an eight-hour dosing interval for serious infections. Accumulation of cefoperazone does not occur in patients with end-stage renal disease and the half-life is only increased two- to fourfold in the presence of hepatic disease. However, substantial accumulation occurs in patients with combined renal and hepatic failure and dosage reductions are necessary.

See also Table 3 and the evaluations. For additional discussion, see Neu, 1982 A; Garzone et al, 1983 A; Barriere and Flaherty, 1984; Smith, 1984; Balant et al, 1985; and Noble and Barza, 1985.

Drug Evaluations

PARENTERAL FIRST GENERATION CEPHALOSPORINS

CEPHALOTHIN SODIUM
[Keflin, Seffin]

MECHANISM OF ACTION, ANTIMICROBIAL SPECTRUM, AND RESISTANCE. The mechanism of action, antimicrobial spectrum, and resistance properties are essentially the same as for cefazolin (see that evaluation and the Introduction). Cephalothin is highly resistant to staphylococcal β-lactamases.

USES. Cephalothin has the same indications as cefazolin, but the latter drug frequently is preferred because it achieves higher serum concentrations, has a longer elimination half-life, and causes less pain on intramuscular injection (see the evaluation on Cefazolin Sodium and the Introduction).

ADVERSE REACTIONS AND PRECAUTIONS. See the Introduction. Nephrotoxicity (renal tubular necrosis) has been reported rarely with cephalothin, usually when large doses were given or after administration to patients with renal impairment.

DRUG INTERACTIONS AND INTERFERENCE WITH LABORATORY TESTS. Cephalothin plus an aminoglycoside can increase nephrotoxicity, particularly in patients with pre-existing renal disease. For additional discussion, see the Introduction.

PHARMACOKINETICS. Because of pain on intramuscular injection, cephalothin usually is administered intravenously. Peak serum concentrations of 30 to 60 mcg/ml are obtained after an intravenous dose of 1 g.

Approximately 70% of circulating cephalothin is bound to plasma protein. The volume of distribution is 0.26 ± 0.11 L/kg. The drug enters many tissues and body fluids, but it fails to achieve therapeutic concentrations in cerebrospinal fluid even in the presence of inflammation. Cephalothin crosses the placenta.

Up to 30% of cephalothin is metabolized to the less active desacetyl metabolite. Parent drug and metabolite are excreted by the kidneys, primarily by renal tubular secretion; probenecid delays excretion. The elimination half-life ranges from 30 to 55 minutes. The half-life is prolonged in patients with renal impairment and dosage adjustments are required.

DOSAGE AND PREPARATIONS. Cephalothin can be administered intravenously (preferred) or by intramuscular injection deep into a large muscle mass to minimize pain and induration. Intravenous administration can be by slow injection or by intermittent or continuous infusion. See the manufacturer's instructions for the appropriate dilution of the drug, compatible diluents and intravenous solutions, and stability of cephalothin in these solutions.

Intravenous, Intramuscular (deep): Adults, 2 to 12 g daily in equally divided doses every four to six hours (The Medical Letter, 1984). The usual dosage is 500 mg to 1 g every four to six hours, depending on the severity of the infection and the susceptibility of the causative organism. In severe, life-threatening infections, doses up to 2 g every four hours may be required.

Infants and children, 75 to 125 mg/kg daily in equally divided doses every four to six hours (The Medical Letter, 1984; Nelson, 1985 A). The manufacturer recommends a dosage range of 80 to 160 mg/kg daily in divided doses.

Newborns over 7 days and weighing more than 2 kg, intravenously, 80 mg/kg daily in divided doses every six hours; *newborns over 7 days and weighing less than 2 kg,* intravenously, 60 mg/kg daily in divided doses every eight hours; *newborns 0 to 7 days and weighing more than 2 kg,* intravenously, 60 mg/kg daily in divided doses every eight hours; *newborns 0 to 7 days and weighing less than 2 kg,* intravenously, 40 mg/kg daily in divided doses every 12 hours (Nelson, 1985 B).

Patients with impaired renal function require modification in doses and/or frequency of administration depending on the degree of impairment, severity of the infection, and susceptibility of the causative organism. Various dosage recommendations for these patients have been proposed. For *adults with impaired renal function,* the manufacturer of Keflin recommends an intravenous loading dose of 1 to 2 g and maximum maintenance dosages as shown in the following table.

Alternative dosage recommendations for *adults with impaired renal function* are 500 mg to 2 g every six hours for creatinine clearance of 80 to 50 ml/min; every eight hours for

Renal Function	Maximum Adult Maintenance Dosage
Mild Impairment (Ccr = 80-50 ml/min)	2.5 g every 6 hours
Moderate Impairment (Ccr = 50-25 ml/min)	1.5 g every 6 hours
Severe Impairment (Ccr = 25-10 ml/min)	1 g every 6 hours
Marked Impairment (Ccr = 10-2 ml/min)	0.5 g every 6 hours
Essentially No Function (Ccr <2 ml/min)	0.5 g every 8 hours when dialysis is not being performed

From manufacturer's literature

creatinine clearance of 50 to 10 ml/min; every 12 hours for creatinine clearance less than 10 ml/min (The Medical Letter, 1984). A supplemental dose should be given after hemodialysis (Norris and Mandell, 1985).

Generic. Solution 1 and 2 g (equivalent to base) in 0.9% sodium chloride or 5% dextrose in 50 ml containers.
Keflin (Lilly). Powder 1, 2, 4, and 20 g (equivalent to base) (sodium 2.8 mEq/g).
Seffin (Glaxo). Powder 1, 2, and 10 g (equivalent to base).

CEFAZOLIN SODIUM
[Ancef, Kefzol]

MECHANISM OF ACTION, ANTIMICROBIAL SPECTRUM, AND RESISTANCE. The clinically relevant antimicrobial spectra of first generation cephalosporins are the same. These agents have excellent activity against most gram-positive bacteria, including nonpenicillinase- and penicillinase-producing staphylococci, streptococci (except enterococci), and many anaerobic bacteria. In general, they are more active than second or third generation cephalosporins against gram-positive bacteria. Gram-negative activity of first generation cephalosporins essentially is limited to *Escherichia coli, Klebsiella,* and *Proteus mirabilis.* Cefazolin generally is more active than cephalothin. However, all first generation agents are less active than second and, particularly, third generation cephalosporins against these gram-negative species.

For additional discussion of the mechanism of action, antimicrobial spectrum, and resistance properties of the cephalosporins, see the Introduction.

USES. Parenteral first generation cephalosporins frequently are drugs of choice for prophylaxis during certain cardiovascular, orthopedic, gastroduodenal, biliary tract, obstetric-gynecologic, head and neck, and thoracic surgical procedures. Cefazolin usually is preferred to other first generation cephalosporins because it has superior pharmacokinetic properties (ie, higher plasma protein binding, lower volume of distribution, and slower rate of elimination) that result in higher and more sustained serum concentrations (see the Introduction; see also Chapter 65, Antimicrobial Therapy and Chemoprophylaxis of Infectious Diseases, Table 4).

Parenterally administered first generation cephalosporins are rarely drugs of choice for the treatment of bacterial infections. However, they may be used to treat serious lower respiratory tract, skin, soft tissue, bone, joint, heart, or urinary tract infections and bacteremias, based on the results of susceptibility tests. They are not effective in meningitis. Frequently, they are preferred for serious staphylococcal and/or streptococcal (except enterococcal) infections (eg, pneumonia, septic arthritis, osteomyelitis, endocarditis) in patients who are allergic to penicillins. However, they should not be used in patients who have experienced an immediate-type (IgE-mediated) hypersensitivity reaction to a penicillin. First generation cephalosporins may be given with an aminoglycoside for *Klebsiella* pneumonia and for severe infections before the results of culture studies are known. Because of its pharmacokinetic advantages, cefazolin often is preferred to other first generation cephalosporins for these indications (see the Introduction; see also Chapter 65, Table 1).

ADVERSE REACTIONS AND PRECAUTIONS. See the Introduction. Cefazolin causes less pain on intramuscular injection than other first generation cephalosporins.

DRUG INTERACTIONS AND INTERFERENCE WITH LABORATORY TESTS. See the Introduction.

PHARMACOKINETICS. Cefazolin is administered intramuscularly or intravenously. Peak serum concentrations of approximately 65 mcg/ml and 185 mcg/ml are achieved after intramuscular and intravenous doses of 1 g, respectively. The higher serum concentrations obtained with cefazolin compared to cephalothin, cephapirin, and cephradine are due, in part, to higher plasma protein binding and a smaller volume of distribution (see the Introduction and these evaluations).

Approximately 85% of circulating cefazolin is bound to plasma protein. The volume of distribution is 0.12 ± 0.03 L/kg. The drug enters many tissues (eg, myocardium, bone, gallbladder) and body fluids (eg, pericardial, pleural, synovial). Adequate concentrations are achieved in bile and high concentrations are obtained in urine. However, cefazolin fails to achieve therapeutic concentrations in cerebrospinal fluid even in the presence of inflammation. Cefazolin crosses the placenta.

Up to 95% of a dose is excreted in the urine as unchanged drug by glomerular filtration and renal tubular secretion. Cefazolin is not metabolized. The elimination half-life is approximately 1.8 hours, which is considerably longer than that of cephalothin, cephapirin, and cephradine (see the Introduction and the evaluations). The half-life is prolonged in patients with renal impairment and dosage adjustments are required.

DOSAGE AND PREPARATIONS. Cefazolin can be administered intramuscularly by injection into a large muscle mass or intravenously by direct injection or by intermittent or continuous infusion. Pain is uncommon after intramuscular injection. See the manufacturer's instructions for the appropriate dilution of the drug, compatible diluents and intravenous solutions, and stability of cefazolin in these solutions.

Intramuscular, Intravenous: *Adults,* 1 to 6 g daily in equally divided doses every six to eight hours (The Medical Letter, 1984). The usual dosage for mild infections caused by susceptible gram-positive cocci, 250 to 500 mg every eight hours; for moderate to severe infections, 500 mg to 1 g every six to eight hours; for severe, life-threatening infections (eg, endocarditis, septicemia), 1 to 1.5 g every six hours. For acute uncomplicated urinary tract infections, 1 g every 12 hours is probably adequate. For dosage recommendations in perioperative prophylaxis, see Chapter 65, Table 4.

Children and infants over 1 month, 25 to 100 mg/kg daily in equally divided doses every six to eight hours (The Medical Letter, 1984). The usual dosage for mild to moderately severe infections is 25 to 50 mg/kg daily in divided doses every six to eight hours. For severe infections, 100 mg/kg daily may be required.

Newborns over 7 days and weighing more than 2 kg, 60 mg/kg daily in divided doses every eight hours; *newborns over 7 days and weighing less than 2 kg*, 40 mg/kg daily in divided doses every 12 hours; *newborns 0 to 7 days*, 40 mg/kg daily in divided doses every 12 hours (Nelson, 1985 B).

Patients with impaired renal function require modification in doses and/or frequency of administration depending on the degree of impairment, severity of the infection, and susceptibility of the causative organism. Various dosage recommendations for these patients have been proposed. For *adults with impaired renal function*, the manufacturers of Ancef and Kefzol recommend an initial loading dose appropriate to the severity of the infection and maintenance dosages as follows:

Creatinine clearance of 55 ml/min or greater or serum creatinine of 1.5 mg/dl or less, full therapeutic doses; creatinine clearance of 35 to 54 ml/min or serum creatinine of 1.6 to 3 mg/dl, full therapeutic doses with dosage interval restricted to at least eight hours; creatinine clearance of 11 to 34 ml/min or serum creatinine of 3.1 to 4.5 mg/dl, one-half the usual dose every 12 hours; creatinine clearance of 10 ml/min or less or serum creatinine of 4.6 mg/dl or greater, one-half the usual dose every 18 to 24 hours (manufacturers' product information brochure).

Alternative dosage recommendations for *adults with impaired renal function* are 0.5 to 1.5 g every 8 hours for creatinine clearance of 80 to 50 ml/min; 0.5 to 1 g every 8 to 12 hours for creatinine clearance of 50 to 10 ml/min; 0.5 to 1 g every 24 hours for creatinine clearance less than 10 ml/min (The Medical Letter, 1984). A supplemental dose of 0.25 to 0.5 g should be given after hemodialysis (Norris and Mandell, 1985).

In *children with impaired renal function*, a usual therapeutic dose can be given as a loading dose, followed by maintenance doses according to the following schedule: creatinine clearance 70 to 40 ml/min, 60% of the usual daily dose in equally divided doses every 12 hours; 40 to 20 ml/min, 25% of usual daily dose in equally divided doses every 12 hours; 20 to 5 ml/min, 10% of normal daily dose every 24 hours. See the manufacturers' literature for further information.

Strengths expressed in terms of base.
Ancef (Smith Kline & French). Powder (lyophilized, sterile) 250 and 500 mg and 1, 5, and 10 g (sodium 2 mEq/g); solution (sterile) 500 mg and 1 g in 5% dextrose in 50 ml containers.
Kefzol (Lilly). Powder (sterile) 250 and 500 mg and 1 and 10 g (sodium 2.1 mEq/g).

CEPHAPIRIN SODIUM
[Cefadyl]

MECHANISM OF ACTION, ANTIMICROBIAL SPECTRUM, AND RESISTANCE. The mechanism of action, antimicrobial spectrum, and resistance properties are essentially the same as for cefazolin (see that evaluation and the Introduction).

USES. Cephapirin has the same indications as cefazolin, but the latter drug frequently is preferred because it achieves higher serum concentrations, has a longer elimination half-life, and causes less pain on intramuscular injection (see the evaluation on Cefazolin Sodium and the Introduction).

ADVERSE REACTIONS AND PRECAUTIONS. See the Introduction.

DRUG INTERACTIONS AND INTERFERENCE WITH LABORATORY TESTS. See the Introduction.

PHARMACOKINETICS. The pharmacokinetics of cephapirin are similar to those of cephalothin. Because of pain on intramuscular injection, cephapirin usually is administered intravenously. Peak serum concentrations of 40 to 70 mcg/ml are obtained after an intravenous dose of 1 g.

Between 45% and 50% of circulating cephapirin is bound to plasma proteins. The volume of distribution is 0.13 ± 0.05 L/kg. The drug enters many tissues and body fluids, but it fails to achieve therapeutic concentrations in cerebrospinal fluid even in the presence of inflammation. Cephapirin crosses the placenta.

Up to 40% of cephapirin is metabolized to the less active desacetyl metabolite. Parent drug and metabolite are excreted by the kidneys, primarily by renal tubular secretion; probenecid delays excretion. The elimination half-life ranges from 35 to 50 minutes. The half-life is prolonged in patients with renal impairment and dosage adjustments are required.

DOSAGE AND PREPARATIONS. Cephapirin can be administered intravenously (preferred) or by intramuscular injection deep into a large muscle mass to minimize pain and induration. Intravenous administration can be by slow injection or by intermittent or continuous infusion. See the manufacturer's instructions for the appropriate dilution of the drug, compatible diluents and intravenous solutions, and stability of cephapirin in these solutions.

Intravenous, Intramuscular (deep): Adults, 2 to 12 g daily in equally divided doses every four to six hours (The Medical Letter, 1984). The usual dosage is 500 mg to 1 g every four to six hours, depending on the severity of the infection and the susceptibility of the causative organism. In severe, life-threatening infections, doses up to 2 g every four hours may be required.

Children and infants over 3 months, 40 to 80 mg/kg in equally divided doses every six hours (Nelson, 1985 A). Cephapirin has not been extensively studied in infants under three months and dosage guidelines are unavailable.

Patients with impaired renal function require modification in dose and/or frequency of administration depending on the degree of impairment, severity of the infection, and susceptibility of the causative organism. Various dosage recommendations for these patients have been proposed. For *adults with reduced renal function* (moderately severe oliguria or serum creatinine greater than 5 mg/dl), the manufacturer recommends a dose of 7.5 to 15 mg/kg every 12 hours. Patients with severely reduced renal function who are undergoing hemodialysis should receive 7.5 to 15 mg/kg just before dialysis and every 12 hours thereafter.

Alternative dosage recommendations for *adults with impaired renal function*, 500 mg to 2 g every six hours for creatinine clearance of 80 to 50 ml/min; every eight hours for creatinine clearance of 50 to 10 ml/min; every 12 hours for creatinine clearance less than 10 ml/min (The Medical Letter, 1984). A supplemental dose of 7.5 to 15 mg/kg should be given just before hemodialysis (Norris and Mandell, 1985).

> *Cefadyl* (Bristol). Powder (sterile) 500 mg and 1, 2, 4, and 20 g (equivalent to base) (sodium 2.36 mEq/g).

CEPHRADINE
[Anspor, Velosef]

Cephradine can be administered orally and parenterally. The evaluation is included under Oral Cephalosporins (see below).

PARENTERAL SECOND GENERATION CEPHALOSPORINS

CEFAMANDOLE NAFATE
[Mandol]

MECHANISM OF ACTION, ANTIMICROBIAL SPECTRUM, AND RESISTANCE. Cefamandole has a broader antibacterial spectrum against aerobic gram-negative bacilli than the first generation cephalosporins. Among the Enterobacteriaceae, it often has greater activity against *Escherichia coli*, *Klebsiella*, and *Proteus mirabilis*, including cephalothin-resistant strains; its spectrum also includes some indole-positive *Proteus*, *Citrobacter*, and *Enterobacter* strains. Cefamandole-resistant strains of Enterobacteriaceae occur and are relatively common for some species. Third generation cephalosporins clearly have superior activity against most Enterobacteriaceae. Cefamandole is not active against the nonfermenting gram-negative bacilli, *Pseudomonas aeruginosa* and *Acinetobacter* species. Activity against the *Bacteroides fragilis* group, gram-negative anaerobic bacilli, is poor (see the Introduction).

Compared to first generation cephalosporins, cefamandole has enhanced in vitro activity against *Haemophilus influenzae*, including many ampicillin-resistant strains. However, it is less active than ampicillin against ampicillin-sensitive *H. influenzae*. Furthermore, possible tolerance of *H. influenzae* isolates, ineffective killing, and an inoculum effect have been observed with cefamandole (see Sanders et al, 1985). Third generation cephalosporins and cefuroxime are more reliably active against *H. influenzae* when compared to cefamandole (see the evaluations and the Introduction).

Cefamandole is active against most gram-positive bacteria, including nonpenicillinase- and penicillinase-producing staphylococci, streptococci (except enterococci), and anaerobic bacteria. Although its potency against gram-positive bacteria is comparable to or only slightly less than first generation cephalosporins, cefamandole offers no advantages for known gram-positive infections.

Cefamandole is active in vitro against *Neisseria meningitidis* and many *N. gonorrhoeae* strains but is not used clinically in these infections.

For additional discussion of the mechanism of action, antimicrobial spectrum, and resistance properties of the cephalosporins, see the Introduction.

USES. Cefamandole is rarely the drug of choice for the treatment of bacterial infections. It may be used to treat infections of the lower respiratory tract, urinary tract, skin and skin structures, bone, and joints or bacteremias caused by susceptible bacteria, provided that equally effective, less toxic, and less expensive alternatives are unavailable. For example, this second generation cephalosporin may be indicated as a replacement for an aminoglycoside to treat infections caused by gram-negative bacilli (eg, *E. coli*, *Klebsiella*, *Proteus*) when susceptibility to cefamandole is known. Although this drug has been used as an alternative to ampicillin or chloramphenicol for serious infections (eg, pneumonia) caused by *H. influenzae*, some failures have been reported (see Sanders et al, 1985). Also, cefamandole is not effective in meningitis. The third generation cephalosporins and cefuroxime are better alternatives for *H. influenzae* infections. They are more reliably active against β-lactamase-producing strains and are useful in meningitis (see the evaluations and the Introduction).

Cefamandole is active against *S. pneumoniae*, *H. influenzae*, *S. aureus*, *K. pneumoniae*, and oropharyngeal anaerobes and has been used empirically, either alone or with an aminoglycoside to treat community-acquired pneumonia in adults with certain predisposing factors (eg, chronic lung disease, alcoholism, postinfluenza bacterial pneumonia, debilitated elderly patients). Cefuroxime or third generation cephalosporins may be preferred, however. None of the cephalosporins is active against *Legionella pneumophila* or other organisms (eg, *Mycoplasma pneumoniae*) causing atypical pneumonias.

Cefamandole is active against group A, β-hemolytic streptococci, *S. aureus*, pneumococci, and *H. influenzae* and has been used as single-agent empiric therapy in young children (2 months to 4 years) with pneumonia, bone and joint infections, or buccal and orbital cellulitis. However cefamandole does not penetrate adequately into cerebrospinal fluid and "breakthrough" meningitis, especially with *H. influenzae* type b, has been reported (see Nelson, 1983; Eichenwald, 1985; Sanders et al, 1985). Cefuroxime is preferred for these pediatric infections (see the evaluation and the Introduction).

Cefamandole does not appear to offer any advantages over first generation cephalosporins against known gram-positive bacterial infections or for surgical prophylaxis (see the Introduction; see also Chapter 65, Antimicrobial Therapy and Chemoprophylaxis of Infectious Diseases, Table 4).

ADVERSE REACTIONS AND PRECAUTIONS. Hypersensitivity reactions (eg, maculopapular rash, fever, eosinophilia, urticaria) and other adverse effects associated with cephalosporins have been observed with cefamandole (see the Introduction). In addition, this second generation derivative contains a methylthiotetrazole side chain and has been associated with hypoprothrombinemia and, occasionally, bleeding. Elderly debilitated patients, individuals with severe renal insufficien-

Renal Function	Less Severe Infections (Adult Maintenance Dosage)	Life-threatening Infections (Maximum Adult Maintenance Dosage)
Mild Impairment (Ccr = 80-50 ml/min)	0.75-1.5 g every 6 hours	1.5 g every 4 hours or 2 g every 6 hours
Moderate Impairment (Ccr = 50-25 ml/min)	0.75-1.5 g every 8 hours	1.5 g every 6 hours or 2 g every 8 hours
Severe Impairment (Ccr = 25-10 ml/min)	0.5-1 g every 8 hours	1 g every 6 hours or 1.25 g every 8 hours
Marked Impairment (Ccr = 10-2 ml/min)	0.5-0.75 g every 12 hours	0.67 g every 8 hours or 1 g every 12 hours
Essentially No Function (Ccr <2 ml/min)	0.25-0.5 g every 12 hours	0.5 g every 8 hours or 0.75 g every 12 hours

From manufacturer's literature

cy, and malnourished patients receiving total parenteral nutrition are at highest risk. Vitamin K reverses the hypoprothrombinemia, and prophylactic administration may be desirable in some patients (see the Introduction).

DRUG INTERACTIONS AND INTERFERENCE WITH LABORATORY TESTS. Methylthiotetrazole-containing cephalosporins have been associated with a disulfiram-like reaction. For additional discussion, see the Introduction.

PHARMACOKINETICS. Cefamandole is administered intramuscularly or intravenously. Peak serum concentrations of 20 to 36 mcg/ml (after 30 to 120 minutes) and 88 to 139 mcg/ml (after 10 minutes) are obtained after intramuscular and intravenous doses of 1 g, respectively.

Between 70% and 80% of circulating cefamandole is bound to plasma protein. The volume of distribution is 0.16 ± 0.05 L/kg. This drug enters many tissues (eg, myocardium, bone, gallbladder) and body fluids (eg, pleural, synovial). High concentrations are obtained in bile and urine. However, it fails to achieve therapeutic concentrations in cerebrospinal fluid even in the presence of inflammation. Cefamandole crosses the placenta.

Approximately 85% of a dose is excreted by the kidneys (glomerular filtration and renal tubular secretion) as unchanged drug over an eight-hour period; excretion is delayed by probenecid. Cefamandole is not metabolized. The elimination half-life is 35 to 60 minutes. The half-life is prolonged in patients with renal impairment and dosage adjustments are required.

DOSAGE AND PREPARATIONS. Cefamandole can be administered by intramuscular injection into a large muscle mass or intravenously by direct injection or intermittent or continuous infusion. See the manufacturer's instructions for the appropriate dilution of the drug, compatible diluents and intravenous solutions, and stability of cefamandole in these solutions.

Intravenous, Intramuscular (deep): Adults, 1.5 to 12 g daily in equally divided doses every four to eight hours (The Medical Letter, 1984). The usual dosage range is 500 mg to 1 g every four to eight hours, depending on the severity of the infection and the susceptibility of the causative organism. For severe, life-threatening infections, up to 2 g every four hours may be required.

Children and infants over 1 month, 50 to 150 mg/kg daily in equally divided doses every four to eight hours (The Medical Letter, 1984). For most infections, 50 to 100 mg/kg daily in equally divided doses every four to eight hours has been effective. In severe infections, up to 150 mg/kg daily (not to exceed the maximum adult dose) may be given.

Patients with impaired renal function require modification in doses and/or frequency of administration depending on the degree of impairment, severity of the infection, and susceptibility of the causative organism. Various dosage recommendations for these patients have been proposed. In *adults with impaired renal function*, the manufacturer recommends an initial loading dose of 1 to 2 g and maintenance dosages as shown in the table (see above).

Alternative dosage recommendations for *adults with impaired renal function* are 1 to 2 g every six hours for creatinine clearance of 80 to 50 ml/min; 1 to 2 g every eight hours for creatinine clearance of 50 to 10 ml min; 0.5 to 1 g every 12 hours for creatinine clearance less than 10 ml/min (The Medical Letter, 1984).

Mandol (Lilly). Powder (sterile) 500 mg and 1, 2, and 10 g (equivalent to base) (sodium 3.3 mEq/g).

CEFOXITIN SODIUM
[Mefoxin]

Cefoxitin, a β-lactam antibiotic closely related to the cephalosporins, is technically classified as a cephamycin. It is derived from cephamycin C, which is produced by *Streptomyces lactamdurans*.

MECHANISM OF ACTION, ANTIMICROBIAL SPECTRUM, AND RESISTANCE. The presence of a 7-α-methoxyl group (see Figure 1) provides cefoxitin with a high degree of resistance to β-lactamases. This antibiotic has a broader antibacterial spectrum against gram-negative bacteria than first generation cephalosporins. Among the Enterobacteriaceae, it is more active against *Escherichia coli*, *Klebsiella*, and *Proteus mirabilis*, including cephalothin-resistant strains; its spectrum also includes indole-positive *Proteus* species, especially *P. vulgaris*; *Providencia* species; and some strains of *Serratia marcescens*. It is less active than cefamandole against *Enterobacter* species, however. The nonfermenting gram-negative bacilli, *Pseudomonas aeruginosa* and *Acinetobacter* species, are resistant.

Cefoxitin is the most active cephalosporin against the *Bacteroides fragilis* group because it is resistant to β-lactamases produced by these anaerobic gram-negative bacilli. Usually between 85% and 95% of *B. fragilis* clinical isolates are susceptible, depending on the institution (*Med Lett Drugs Ther*, 1984 D). Other anaerobic bacteria, except some *Clostridium* species (other than *C. perfringens*) and a few *Fusobacterium* strains, also are susceptible.

Cefoxitin has good activity against *Neisseria gonorrhoeae*, including penicillinase-producing strains (PPNG) and is useful clinically in these infections. Although this antibiotic is active against *N. meningitidis* and *H. influenzae*, including β-lactamase-producing strains, it usually is not used for infections caused by these bacteria.

Although cefoxitin is active against most gram-positive bacteria, including nonpenicillinase- and penicillinase-producing staphylococci and streptococci (except enterococci), it is less potent than first generation cephalosporins, particularly against staphylococci. It offers no advantages over these earlier generation cephalosporins for gram-positive infections.

For additional discussion of the mechanism of action, antimicrobial spectrum, and resistance properties of the cephalosporins, see the Introduction.

USES. Cefoxitin is useful in the treatment of intra-abdominal infections, such as peritonitis secondary to bowel perforation. These are frequently polymicrobial infections caused by mixtures of aerobic gram-negative enteric bacilli (eg, *Escherichia coli*) and anaerobic bacteria, including the *Bacteroides fragilis* group. Initial therapy usually is empiric and broad spectrum antimicrobial coverage is indicated. Cefoxitin alone appears to be as effective as clindamycin plus an aminoglycoside for mild to moderately ill patients with community-acquired intra-abdominal infection (Tally et al, 1981; Nichols et al, 1984) and frequently is the preferred drug in such situations. For more severely ill patients and/or for nosocomial infections, combination therapy with an anti-*B. fragilis* agent (eg, metronidazole, clindamycin, chloramphenicol, cefoxitin) plus an aminoglycoside is indicated (see the Introduction and Chapter 65, Antimicrobial Therapy and Chemoprophylaxis of Infectious Diseases, Table 1).

Gynecologic pelvic infections (eg, pelvic inflammatory disease, endometritis, pelvic cellulitis) also are typically mixed infections involving aerobic and anaerobic bacteria and cefoxitin has a role in therapy. For pelvic inflammatory disease in sexually active women, cefoxitin plus doxycycline is a preferred regimen of the Centers for Disease Control (*Morbid Mortal Week Rep*, 1985). In such patients, cefoxitin provides antimicrobial coverage against *Neisseria gonorrhoeae*, including PPNG strains; many gram-negative bacilli; and most anaerobic bacteria, including the *B. fragilis* group. Doxycycline expands the spectrum to include *Chlamydia trachomatis* (see the Introduction and Chapter 65, Table 2).

Cefoxitin has been useful in the treatment of uncomplicated and disseminated gonococcal infections caused by PPNG strains. However, the more highly active third generation agent, ceftriaxone, is now the preferred cephalosporin (*Morbid Mortal Week Rep*, 1985; see also Chapter 65, Table 2).

Because of its greater activity against the *B. fragilis* group when compared to first generation cephalosporins, cefoxitin usually is the preferred parenteral antibiotic for prophylaxis in colorectal surgical procedures (see the Introduction and Chapter 65, Table 4).

Depending on the results of susceptibility tests, cefoxitin may be used in serious lower respiratory tract, urinary tract, bone, joint, skin, and soft tissue infections or bacteremias, provided that equally effective, less toxic, and less expensive alternatives are unavailable.

ADVERSE REACTIONS AND PRECAUTIONS. These are the same as for first generation cephalosporins. Hypoprothrombinemia and bleeding have not been reported (see the Introduction).

DRUG INTERACTIONS AND INTERFERENCE WITH LABORATORY TESTS. See the Introduction. High serum concentrations of cefoxitin may interfere with measurement of creatinine by the Jaffe method. Serum samples withdrawn within two hours of cefoxitin administration should not be assayed for serum creatinine concentrations.

PHARMACOKINETICS. Cefoxitin is administered intramuscularly or intravenously. Peak serum concentrations of 20 to 25 mcg/ml (after 20 to 30 minutes) and 56 to 110 mcg/ml (after 5 minutes) are obtained after intramuscular and intravenous doses of 1 g, respectively.

Between 70% and 80% of circulating cefoxitin is bound to plasma protein. The volume of distribution ranges from 0.13 to 0.22 L/kg. The antibiotic reaches therapeutic levels in a number of tissues and body fluids, including myometrium; pleural and synovial fluids; bile; and urine. However, it fails to achieve therapeutic concentrations in cerebrospinal fluid even in the presence of inflammation. Cefoxitin crosses the placenta.

Approximately 85% of a dose is excreted by the kidneys (glomerular filtration and renal tubular secretion) as unchanged drug over a six-hour period. Excretion is delayed by probenecid and cefoxitin is minimally metabolized. The elimination half-life is approximately 40 to 60 minutes. The half-life is prolonged in patients with renal impairment and dosage adjustments are required.

DOSAGE AND PREPARATIONS. Cefoxitin can be administered by intramuscular injection deep into a large muscle mass or intravenously by direct injection or by intermittent or continuous infusion. Large doses should be given only by the intravenous route because of the large volumes or high concentrations required. See the manufacturer's instructions for the appropriate dilution of the drug, compatible diluents and intravenous solutions, and stability of cefoxitin in these solutions.

Intravenous, Intramuscular (deep): Adults, 3 to 12 g daily in equally divided doses every four to eight hours (The Medical Letter, 1984). The usual dosages for mild uncomplicated infections are 1 g every six to eight hours intravenously or intramuscularly (total daily dosage, 3 to 4 g); for moderate or severe infections, 1 g every four hours or 2 g every six to eight hours intravenously (total daily dosage, 6 to 8 g); for life-threatening infections, 2 g every four hours or 3 g every six hours intravenously (total daily dosage, 12 g). For uncomplicated gonorrhea (including PPNG), 2 g intramuscularly with probenecid, 1 g orally, given at the same time or up to 30 minutes before cefoxitin. For disseminated gonococcal infection, gonococcal ophthalmia, and pelvic inflammatory disease, see Chapter 65, Table 2. For perioperative prophylaxis in colorectal surgical procedures, see Chapter 65, Table 4.

Infants over 3 months and children, 80 to 160 mg/kg daily divided into four to six equal doses. The maximum daily dosage is 12 g.

Patients with impaired renal function require modification in doses and/or frequency of administration depending on the degree of impairment, severity of the infection, and susceptibility of the causative organism. Various dosage recommendations for these patients have been proposed. For *adults with impaired renal function*, the manufacturer recommends an initial loading dose of 1 to 2 g and maintenance dosages as follows:

Renal Function	Adult Maintenance Dosage
Mild Impairment (Ccr = 50-30 ml/min)	1-2 g every 8-12 hours
Moderate Impairment (Ccr = 29-10 ml/min)	1-2 g every 12-24 hours
Severe Impairment (Ccr = 9-5 ml/min)	0.5-1 g every 12-24 hours
Essentially No Function (Ccr <5 ml/min)	0.5-1 g every 24-48 hours

From manufacturer's literature

In patients undergoing hemodialysis, a loading dose of 1 to 2 g can be given after each hemodialysis session, followed by a maintenance dose as indicated above.

Alternative dosage recommendations for *adults with impaired renal function* are 1 to 2 g every eight hours for creatinine clearance of 80 to 50 ml/min; 1 to 2 g every 12 hours for creatinine clearance of 50 to 10 ml/min; 0.5 to 1 g every 12 to 24 hours for creatinine clearance less than 10 ml/min (The Medical Letter, 1984). A supplemental dose of 1 to 2 g should be given after hemodialysis (Norris and Mandell, 1985).

Mefoxin (Merck Sharp & Dohme). Powder (sterile) 1, 2, and 10 g (equivalent to base) (sodium 2.3 mEq/g); solution 1 and 2 g (equivalent to base) in 5% dextrose in 50 ml containers.

CEFUROXIME SODIUM
[Zinacef]

MECHANISM OF ACTION, ANTIMICROBIAL SPECTRUM, AND RESISTANCE. Cefuroxime has good activity against most staphylococci, including β-lactamase-producing strains. However, the antistaphylococcal activity of this second generation cephalosporin is less than that of cephalothin. Cefuroxime has excellent activity against streptococci, including *S. pyogenes* (group A, β-hemolytic), *S. agalactiae* (group B), *S.*

pneumoniae, viridans streptococci, and anaerobic streptococci (*Peptostreptococcus*). However, enterococci are resistant. Gram-positive anaerobes, including *Peptococcus* and many clostridia, are usually susceptible. In general, despite its excellent activity against gram-positive bacteria, cefuroxime does not appear to offer any clinical advantages over first generation cephalosporins for infections (other than meningitis) known to be caused by these organisms.

The gram-negative cocci, *Neisseria meningitidis* and *N. gonorrhoeae*, including β-lactamase-producing strains (PPNG), are very susceptible. Cefuroxime is more active than first generation cephalosporins against *Haemophilus influenzae*, including ampicillin-resistant strains. It exhibits excellent stability to β-lactamases produced by this gram-negative bacillus. *Branhamella catarrhalis*, including β-lactamase-positive strains, also are susceptible.

Among the Enterobacteriaceae, cefuroxime is more active than first generation cephalosporins against *Escherichia coli*, *Klebsiella*, and *Proteus mirabilis*, including some cephalothin-resistant strains, and its spectrum also includes most *Citrobacter* and some *Enterobacter* and indole-positive *Proteus* strains. However, third generation cephalosporins clearly have superior activity against most Enterobacteriaceae. Cefuroxime is not active against the nonfermenting gram-negative bacilli, *Pseudomonas aeruginosa* and *Acinetobacter* species. The *Bacteroides fragilis* group (gram-negative anaerobic bacilli) usually are resistant.

In summary, the antimicrobial spectrum of cefuroxime is similar to that of cefamandole (see the evaluation). However, cefuroxime has increased resistance to certain β-lactamases (eg, TEM-1) of various gram-negative bacteria (eg, *Haemophilus influenzae*, *Neisseria gonorrhoeae*), a potential clinical advantage for infections caused by these bacterial strains (see Gold and Rodriguez, 1983; Nelson, 1983; Smith and LeFrock, 1983).

For additional discussion of the mechanism of action, antimicrobial spectrum, and resistance properties of the cephalosporins, see the Introduction.

USES. Cefuroxime has become a preferred drug for single-agent empiric therapy of serious community-acquired bacterial pneumonia, suppurative bone and joint infections, or buccal and orbital cellulitis in infants and young children between 2 months and 4 years. This drug provides adequate coverage against the likely causative organisms, *Haemophilus influenzae* (including β-lactamase-producing strains), pneumococci, *Streptococcus pyogenes*, and *Staphylococcus aureus*. Furthermore, unlike cefamandole, "breakthrough" meningitis has not been reported with cefuroxime (see Gold and Rodriguez, 1983; Nelson, 1983; Smith and Lefrock, 1983; *Med Lett Drugs Ther*, 1984 A; Eichenwald, 1985; Sanders et al, 1985). This is because cefuroxime can achieve adequate concentrations in cerebrospinal fluid to be effective in meningitis caused by the common meningeal pathogens, *H. influenzae*, *S. pneumoniae*, and *Neisseria meningitidis* (Pfenninger et al, 1982; Report from a Swedish Study Group, 1982). Presently, it appears to be a promising single-agent alternative to ampicillin plus chloramphenicol for initial treatment of meningitis in infants and young children (see Nelson, 1983; Eichenwald, 1985; see also the Introduction and Chapter 65, Antimicrobial Therapy and Chemoprophylaxis of Infectious Diseases, Table 1).

Other indications for cefuroxime appear to be similar to those for cefamandole (see the evaluation). Despite more limited clinical experience, cefuroxime appears to offer a number of advantages over this older cephalosporin, including increased β-lactamase stability (eg, TEM-1 of *H. influenzae*), more reliable cerebrospinal fluid penetration, a longer elimination half-life, and the absence of hypoprothrombinemia and a disulfiram-like reaction as adverse effects (see the Introduction).

ADVERSE REACTIONS AND PRECAUTIONS. These are the same as for first generation cephalosporins. Hypoprothrombinemia and bleeding have not been reported (see the Introduction).

DRUG INTERACTIONS AND INTERFERENCE WITH LABORATORY TESTS. See the Introduction. A disulfiram-like reaction has not been reported.

PHARMACOKINETICS. Cefuroxime is administered intramuscularly or intravenously. The peak serum concentration obtained after intramuscular injection of 0.75 g was approximately 27 mcg/ml after 45 minutes (range, 15 to 60 minutes). Following intravenous doses of 0.75 and 1.5 g, serum concentrations were approximately 50 and 100 mcg/ml, respectively, at 15 minutes.

Approximately 33% of circulating cefuroxime is bound to plasma protein. The volume of distribution approximates that of the extracellular fluid, ie, 0.2 L/kg. The antibiotic reaches therapeutic levels in a number of tissues (interstitial fluids) and body fluids, including pleural and synovial fluids, sputum, bile, bone, and urine. Unlike first and other second generation cephalosporins, cefuroxime penetrates the inflamed meninges and achieves cerebrospinal fluid concentrations that are adequate for the treatment of bacterial meningitis caused by susceptible organisms (eg, *S. pneumoniae, H. influenzae, N. meningitidis*). Cefuroxime crosses the placenta.

More than 90% of a dose of cefuroxime is excreted in the urine as unchanged drug within 24 hours; it is not metabolized. Elimination appears to be by renal tubular secretion and glomerular filtration and is delayed by probenecid. The elimination half-life is approximately 1.3 to 1.7 hours, which is longer than that of cefamandole (0.6 to 1 hour). The half-life is prolonged in patients with renal impairment and dosage adjustments are required when the creatinine clearance falls below 20 ml/min. The half-life in infants less than 1 week ranges from 3.5 to 5.5 hours.

DOSAGE AND PREPARATIONS. Cefuroxime can be administered by intramuscular injection deep into a large muscle mass or intravenously by direct injection or by intermittent or continuous infusion. See the manufacturer's instructions for the appropriate dilution of the drug, compatible diluents and intravenous solutions, and stability of cefuroxime in these solutions.

Intravenous, Intramuscular (deep): Adults, 2.25 to 9 g daily in equally divided doses every eight hours (The Medical Letter, 1984). The usual dosages for uncomplicated urinary tract infections, skin and skin structure infections, disseminated gonococcal infections, and uncomplicated pneumonia are 750 mg every eight hours; for severe or complicated infections, 1.5

g every eight hours. In life-threatening infections or infections due to less susceptible organisms, 1.5 g every six hours may be required. In bacterial meningitis, the dose should not exceed 3 g every eight hours. For uncomplicated gonococcal infections, 1.5 g intramuscularly given as a single dose at two different sites together with probenecid, 1 g orally.

Infants and children over 3 months, 50 to 100 mg/kg daily in equally divided doses every six to eight hours. The higher dosage (not to exceed the maximum adult dosage) should be used for the more severe or serious infections. For bacterial meningitis, 200 to 240 mg/kg daily in equally divided doses every six to eight hours.

Modification of dosage is unnecessary in patients with creatinine clearances above 20 ml/min. The manufacturer recommends that *adults* with creatinine clearances of 20 to 10 ml/min receive 750 mg every 12 hours and those with creatinine clearances less than 10 ml/min receive 750 mg every 24 hours. In *children* with impaired renal function, the manufacturer recommends that the frequency of administration be modified as for adults. In patients undergoing hemodialysis, a supplemental dose of cefuroxime should be given after each dialysis period.

> *Zinacef* (Glaxo). Powder (sterile) 750 mg and 1.5 g (equivalent to base) (sodium 2.4 mEq/g).
> **Additional Trademark:**
> *Kefurox* (Lilly).

CEFONICID SODIUM
[Monocid]

Cefonicid is a semisynthetic second generation cephalosporin that is structurally similar to cefamandole (see Figure 1).

MECHANISM OF ACTION, ANTIMICROBIAL SPECTRUM, AND RESISTANCE. The mechanism of action, antimicrobial spectrum, and resistance properties of cefonicid are similar to those of cefamandole. Like cefamandole, the in vitro activity of cefonicid against aerobic gram-negative bacteria generally is superior to that of first generation cephalosporins, but inferior to that of third generation cephalosporins. Cefonicid is usually active against *Escherichia coli, Proteus mirabilis, Klebsiella, Citrobacter diversus*, and *Neisseria meningitidis*. It also has good activity against *N. gonorrhoeae* and *Haemophilus influenzae*, including β-lactamase-producing strains. Its activity against *Enterobacter* species and *C. freundii* is variable. *Serratia marcescens, Providencia, Pseudomonas aeruginosa, Acinetobacter*, and the *Bacteroides fragilis* group (gram-negative anaerobic bacilli) are usually resistant.

Most gram-positive cocci, including nonpenicillinase- and penicillinase-producing *Staphylococcus aureus* and streptococci (except enterococci), are susceptible in vitro. However, the activity of cefonicid against those organisms, especially staphylococci, is less than that of first generation cephalosporins, cefamandole, and cefuroxime. The activity against *S. aureus* is decreased in the presence of serum, which appears to result from the high binding of cefonicid to plasma proteins (see Pharmacokinetics).

For additional discussion, see *Med Lett Drugs Ther*, 1984 C; Dudley et al, 1984; Pontzer and Kaye, 1984; Tartaglione and

Creatinine Clearance (ml/min/1.73 M²)	Mild to Moderate Infections (Adult Maintenance Dosage)	Severe Infections (Adult Maintenance Dosage)
79-60	10 mg/kg every 24 hours	25 mg/kg every 24 hours
59-40	8 mg/kg every 24 hours	20 mg/kg every 24 hours
39-20	4 mg/kg every 24 hours	15 mg/kg every 24 hours
19-10	4 mg/kg every 48 hours	15 mg/kg every 48 hours
9-5	4 mg/kg every 3-5 days	15 mg/kg every 3-5 days
<5	3 mg/kg every 3-5 days	4 mg/kg every 3-5 days

NOTE: It is not necessary to administer additional dosage following dialysis.
From manufacturer's literature

Polk, 1985; see also the Introduction and the evaluations of Cefamandole Nafate and Cefuroxime Sodium.

USES. Cefonicid has the longest elimination half-life (3.5 to 4.5 hours) among currently available first and second generation cephalosporins and, administered once daily, has been shown to be effective in urinary tract, lower respiratory tract, skin and skin structure, bone, and joint infections caused by susceptible bacteria (see Jacob and Layne, 1984). Because of its once daily dosing interval, cefonicid has the potential to be less expensive than other cephalosporins and may be useful in outpatient therapy (see Kunkel and Iannini, 1984). However, current clinical experience with this long-acting second generation cephalosporin, particularly in serious infections, is very limited and randomized, double-blinded, comparative clinical trials with established therapies generally are unavailable (see *Med Lett Drugs Ther*, 1984 C; Dudley et al, 1984; Pontzer and Kaye, 1984; Tartaglione and Polk, 1985). Thus, its role in infectious disease therapy is largely undefined.

There is concern over the efficacy of cefonicid in *Staphylococcus aureus* infections because this agent was ineffective in three of four patients with *S. aureus* endocarditis (Chambers et al, 1984) and, in one study (Lea et al, 1982), cefonicid was shown to be less effective than cefazolin for skin and soft tissue infections caused by this pathogen. Cefonicid is not recommended for the treatment of bacterial meningitis (see *Med Lett Drugs Ther*, 1984 C). When administered as a single 1-g dose, it has been less than adequate for anorectal or pharyngeal gonococcal infections (Handsfield and Murphy, 1985). Although single-dose (1 g) cefonicid has been shown to be effective as perioperative prophylaxis in various surgical procedures, including biliary tract surgery, vaginal and abdominal hysterectomy, cesarean section, colorectal surgery, and prosthetic arthroplasty (see Jacob and Layne, 1984), no advantages over currently recommended cephalosporins (usually cefazolin) have been shown in controlled clinical trials (see DiPiro et al, 1984; *Med Lett Drugs Ther*, 1984 C; Rapp and Blue, 1985; see also Chapter 65, Antimicrobial Therapy and Chemoprophylaxis of Infectious Diseases, Table 4). For additional discussion, see the Introduction.

ADVERSE REACTIONS AND PRECAUTIONS. Cefonicid generally has been well tolerated and most adverse reactions (eg, hypersensitivity reactions, pain on intramuscular injection, gastrointestinal disturbances, mild reversible laboratory abnormalities) are similar to those of first generation cephalosporins (see the Introduction). A "flu-like syndrome" developed in 3 of 15 patients receiving the drug for more than 2 weeks (Kunkel and Iannini, 1984). Although cefonicid contains a methylthiotetrazole side chain, it has not been associated with hypoprothrombinemia or a disulfiram-like reaction. The absence of these side effects may be related to the presence of a methylsulfonic acid group on the methylthiotetrazole side chain rather than the methyl group present in cefamandole, cefoperazone, and moxalactam (see Pontzer and Kaye, 1984; see also the Introduction and Figure 1).

DRUG INTERACTIONS AND INTERFERENCE WITH LABORATORY TESTS. See the Introduction. A disulfiram-like reaction has not been reported (see the above discussion).

PHARMACOKINETICS. Cefonicid is administered intramuscularly or intravenously. Peak serum concentrations of 98 mcg/ml (after one to two hours) and 221 mcg/ml (after five minutes) are obtained after intramuscular and intravenous doses of 1 g, respectively.

Greater than 95% of circulating cefonicid is bound to plasma protein. The volume of distribution is approximately 0.11 L/kg. Therapeutic levels are achieved in a number of tissues (eg, bone, gallbladder wall, uterus) and body fluids (eg, sputum, wound fluid, pleural and pericardial fluids, bile). High concentrations are obtained in urine. However, therapeutic concentrations are not achieved in cerebrospinal fluid even in the presence of inflammation. Cefonicid crosses the placenta.

More than 90% of a dose is excreted by the kidneys (renal tubular secretion and glomerular filtration) as unchanged drug within 24 hours. Excretion is delayed by probenecid. Cefonicid is not metabolized. The elimination half-life is approximately 3.5 to 4.5 hours. The half-life is prolonged in patients with renal impairment and dosage adjustments are required.

DOSAGE AND PREPARATIONS. Cefonicid can be administered by intramuscular injection deep into a large muscle mass or intravenously by direct injection or infusion. See the manufacturer's instructions for the appropriate dilution of the drug, compatible diluents and intravenous solutions, and stability of cefonicid in these solutions.

Intramuscular (deep), Intravenous: Adults, 500 mg to 2 g once daily. The usual dosages for uncomplicated urinary tract infections are 500 mg once daily; for mild to moderate infections, 1 g once daily; for severe or life-threatening infections, 2 g once daily. With a dosage of 2 g intramuscularly once daily, one-half of the dose is given in different large muscle masses.

Dosage recommendations for *children* currently are unavailable.

Patients with impaired renal function require modification in doses and/or frequency of administration depending on the degree of impairment, severity of the infection, and susceptibility of the causative organisms. For *adults with impaired renal function*, the manufacturer recommends an initial loading dose of 7.5 mg kg, intramuscularly or intravenously, followed by maintenance dosages as shown in the table on previous page.

> **Monocid** (Smith Kline & French). Powder (sterile) 500 mg and 1 and 10 g (equivalent to base) (sodium 3.7 mEq/g).

CEFORANIDE
[Precef]

Ceforanide is a semisynthetic second generation cephalosporin that is structurally similar to cefamandole (see Figure 1).

MECHANISM OF ACTION, ANTIMICROBIAL SPECTRUM, AND RESISTANCE. The mechanism of action, antimicrobial spectrum, and resistance properties of ceforanide are similar to those of cefamandole. Like cefamandole, the in vitro activity of ceforanide against members of the Enterobacteriaceae family generally is superior to that of first generation cephalosporins but inferior to that of third generation cephalosporins. Ceforanide is usually active against *Escherichia coli, Klebsiella, Proteus mirabilis,* and *Citrobacter diversus,* including some cephalothin-resistant strains. Activity against indole-positive *Proteus* species and *Enterobacter* species is variable; *Serratia marcescens* are resistant. The nonfermenting gram-negative bacilli, *Pseudomonas aeruginosa* and *Acinetobacter,* are resistant. The *Bacteroides fragilis* group, anaerobic gram-negative bacilli, also are resistant.

Neisseria meningitidis, N. gonorrhoeae, and *Haemophilus influenzae,* including β-lactamase-producing strains, usually are susceptible in vitro. However, ceforanide is considerably less active than cefuroxime, cefamandole, or cefonicid against *H. influenzae.*

Most gram-positive cocci, including nonpenicillinase- and penicillinase-producing *Staphylococcus aureus* and streptococci (except enterococci), are susceptible in vitro. However, the activity of ceforanide against these organisms, particularly staphylococci, is less than that of first generation cephalosporins, cefamandole, and cefuroxime.

For additional discussion, see Barriere and Mills, 1982; Garzone et al, 1983 B; *Med Lett Drugs Ther,* 1984 B; and Tartaglione and Polk, 1985. See also the Introduction and the evaluations on Cefamandole Nafate, Cefuroxime Sodium, and Cefonicid Sodium.

USES. Ceforanide has a longer elimination half-life (2.7 to 3 hours) than currently available first and second generation cephalosporins (except cefonicid) and, administered twice daily, has been shown to be effective in urinary tract, community-acquired lower respiratory tract, skin and skin structure, bone, and joint infections caused by susceptible bacteria (see Barriere and Mills, 1982; LeFrock et al, 1984 C; Tartaglione and Polk, 1985). In one study, ceforanide failed to eradicate *H. influenzae* from the sputum of patients with pneumonia, although clinical outcomes were successful (Wallace et al, 1981); in addition, one infant treated with ceforanide

for periorbital cellulitis caused by *H. influenzae* type b relapsed with bacteremia one week after therapy was stopped (Thirumoorthi et al, 1983).

Ceforanide 1 to 2 g every 12 hours intramuscularly also has been shown to be effective for right-sided endocarditis caused by *S. aureus* and nonenterococcal streptococci in intravenous drug abusers. However, serum bactericidal titers for ceforanide against *S. aureus* were inferior to those seen with antistaphylococcal penicillins (eg, nafcillin) or first generation cephalosporins (Cooper et al, 1981; Greenman et al, 1984).

Ceforanide fails to achieve therapeutically effective concentrations in cerebrospinal fluid and is not useful in bacterial meningitis.

Presently, clinical experience with ceforanide is very limited and randomized, double-blinded comparative clinical trials with established therapies generally are unavailable (Barriere and Mills, 1982; *Med Lett Drugs Ther,* 1984 B; Tartaglione and Polk, 1985). Thus, its role in infectious disease therapy is largely undefined. Ceforanide does not appear to offer any advantages over first generation cephalosporins for infections caused by gram-positive bacteria or for perioperative prophylaxis and is inferior to cefuroxime and third generation cephalosporins for *H. influenzae* infections (see *Med Lett Drugs Ther,* 1984 B; Tartaglione and Polk, 1985; see also the Introduction and the evaluations).

ADVERSE REACTIONS AND PRECAUTIONS. Ceforanide generally has been well tolerated and the majority of adverse reactions (eg, hypersensitivity reactions, gastrointestinal disturbances, mild reversible laboratory abnormalities) are similar to those reported with first generation cephalosporins (see the Introduction). Although ceforanide contains a methylthiotetrazole side chain, it has not been associated with hypoprothrombinemia or a disulfiram-like reaction. The absence of these side effects may be related to the presence of a carboxymethyl group on the methylthiotetrazole side chain rather than the methyl group present in cefamandole, cefoperazone, and moxalactam (see Barriere and Mills, 1982, and Tartaglione and Polk, 1985. See also the Introduction and Figure 1).

DRUG INTERACTIONS AND INTERFERENCE WITH LABORATORY TESTS. See the Introduction. A disulfiram-like reaction has not been reported (see the above discussion).

PHARMACOKINETICS. Ceforanide is administered intramuscularly or intravenously. Peak serum concentrations of approximately 70 mcg/ml (after one hour) and 125 mcg/ml (after a 30-minute infusion) are obtained after intramuscular and intravenous doses of 1 g, respectively.

About 80% of circulating ceforanide is bound to plasma protein. The volume of distribution ranges from 0.16 to 0.19 L/kg. The antibiotic reaches therapeutic levels in a number of tissues (eg, bone, gallbladder, myocardium) and body fluids (eg, pericardial and synovial fluids, bile). High concentrations are obtained in urine. However, therapeutic concentrations are not achieved in cerebrospinal fluid even in the presence of inflammation. Ceforanide crosses the placenta.

More than 90% of a dose is excreted as unchanged drug via the kidneys, primarily by glomerular filtration. Probenecid does not delay excretion. Ceforanide is not metabolized. The elimination half-life is approximately 2.7 to 3 hours. The half-life is prolonged in patients with renal impairment and dosage adjustments are required.

DOSAGE AND PREPARATIONS. Ceforanide can be administered by intramuscular injection deep into a large muscle mass or intravenously by direct injection or infusion. See the manufacturer's instructions for the appropriate dilution of the drug, compatible diluents and intravenous solutions, and stability of ceforanide in these solutions.

Intramuscular (deep), Intravenous: *Adults,* 1 to 2 g daily in equally divided doses every 12 hours; *children,* 20 to 40 mg/kg daily in equally divided doses every 12 hours.

Patients with impaired renal function require modification in doses and/or frequency of administration depending on the degree of impairment, severity of the infection, and susceptibility of the causative organism. The manufacturer recommends a 12-hour dosing interval when creatinine clearance is 60 ml/min/1.73 M^2 or greater; a 24-hour dosing interval when creatinine clearance is between 59 and 20 ml/min/1.73 M^2; a 48-hour dosing interval when creatinine clearance is between 19 and 5 ml/min/1.73 M^2; and a 48- to 72-hour dosing interval when creatinine clearance is less than 5 ml/min/1.73 M^2. Patients on hemodialysis should receive a supplemental dose (adults, 0.5 to 1 g) after each hemodialysis session (Norris and Mandell, 1985).

Precef (Bristol). Powder (sterile) 500 mg and 1 g (equivalent to base).

PARENTERAL THIRD GENERATION CEPHALOSPORINS

CEFOTAXIME SODIUM
[Claforan]

Cefotaxime is one of several third generation cephalosporins that contain an aminothiazolyl-acetyl side chain with an α-*syn*-methoximino group at the 7-position of the β-lactam ring (see Figure 1). The aminothiazolyl side chain enhances antibacterial activity, particularly against Enterobacteriaceae, and the methoximino group imparts stability against hydrolysis by many β-lactamases (see Neu, 1982 A). Cefotaxime was the first cephalosporin of the third generation to be marketed in the United States.

MECHANISM OF ACTION, ANTIMICROBIAL SPECTRUM, AND RESISTANCE. Cefotaxime has increased potency and a wider spectrum of activity against clinically important gram-negative bacteria when compared to first and second generation cephalosporins. This drug has excellent activity against *Neisseria meningitidis, N. gonorrhoeae, Haemophilus influenzae,* and most of the Enterobacteriaceae (eg, *Escherichia coli, Klebsiella, Enterobacter, Proteus, Morganella, Providencia, Citrobacter, Serratia, Salmonella, Shigella*), including strains that are resistant to earlier generation cephalosporins, penicillins, and aminoglycosides. This activity is related to cefotaxime's excellent β-lactamase stability and high affinity for penicillin binding proteins in these gram-negative bacteria. The nonfermenting gram-negative bacilli, *Pseudomonas aerugino-*

sa and *Acinetobacter,* generally are resistant, however. Cefotaxime has only fair activity against the *Bacteroides fragilis* group, anaerobic gram-negative bacilli.

Among gram-positive bacteria, cefotaxime has excellent activity against *Streptococcus pyogenes, S. agalactiae,* and *S. pneumoniae* and good activity against nonpenicillinase- and penicillinase-producing staphylococci. However, this agent offers no clinical advantages over first generation cephalosporins for infections (other than meningitis) that are known to be caused by gram-positive bacteria. Enterococci, methicillin-resistant staphylococci, penicillin-resistant pneumococci, and *Listeria monocytogenes* are resistant to all cephalosporins.

Although cefotaxime is stable to the hydrolytic activity of most β-lactamases, resistance to this third generation cephalosporin can occur among certain nonfastidious gram-negative bacilli, particularly *Enterobacter, Serratia,* and *Pseudomonas* species, via the induction of Type I chromosomal β-lactamases that appear to tightly bind and, therefore, inactivate the drug.

In vivo, cefotaxime is partially metabolized to 3-desacetylcefotaxime, an active, β-lactamase-stable metabolite. The antibacterial activity of desacetylcefotaxime is four- to eightfold less than that of cefotaxime, but this metabolite is more active than cefazolin, cefamandole, and cefoxitin against most aerobic gram-negative bacteria. Studies in vitro suggest that cefotaxime and desacetylcefotaxime act synergistically against a number of bacterial strains (see Jones et al, 1982; Neu, 1982 E; Chin and Neu, 1984).

For additional discussion of the mechanism of action, antimicrobial spectrum, and resistance properties of the cephalosporins, see the Introduction.

USES. Cefotaxime is useful in the treatment of certain types of bacterial meningitis and, among third generation cephalosporins, clinical experience is probably greatest with this agent. It is a preferred drug for meningitis caused by susceptible gram-negative enteric bacilli (eg, *Escherichia coli, Klebsiella, Proteus*). However, it should not be considered adequate single-drug therapy for meningitis caused by *Pseudomonas aeruginosa.* Cefotaxime (and most third generation cephalosporins) is effective in meningitis caused by *Haemophilus influenzae,* including β-lactamase-producing strains. Presently, it is an alternative to ampicillin plus chloramphenicol for this indication. Cefotaxime is active against the common causative organisms (*H. influenzae, Neisseria meningitidis, Streptococcus pneumoniae*) of meningitis in infants and young children and is an effective single-agent alternative to ampicillin plus chloramphenicol for the empiric therapy of meningitis in this age group. The combination of ampicillin plus cefotaxime is an alternative to ampicillin plus an aminoglycoside for initial therapy of neonatal meningitis. For additional discussion, see the Introduction; see also Chapter 65, Antimicrobial Therapy and Chemoprophylaxis of Infectious Diseases, Table 1.

Cefotaxime has been effective, frequently as empiric monotherapy, in a wide variety of serious gram-negative bacillary infections outside the central nervous system. These include lower respiratory tract, complicated urinary tract, intra-abdominal, gynecologic, skin and skin structure, bone, and joint infections and bacteremias. These frequently are of nosocomial origin and are caused by bacterial strains that are resistant to penicillins, older cephalosporins, and aminoglycosides. However, the exact role of cefotaxime (or other third generation cephalosporins) in the treatment of these infections remains to be determined. It would appear to be particularly useful (1) for infections caused by susceptible gram-negative bacilli that exhibit multiple resistance to other, less expensive antimicrobial agents; (2) as an effective alternative to a more toxic aminoglycoside, particularly in patients at high risk for aminoglycoside toxicity or when prolonged therapy is required (eg, for osteomyelitis); and (3) for certain serious infections, such as *Klebsiella* pneumonia, for which a third generation cephalosporin is the most active agent. Cefotaxime alone eventually may replace combination regimens that contain an aminoglycoside for initial treatment of seriously ill patients with infections of undetermined etiology, but when gram-negative aerobic bacilli are suspected pathogens. However, additional clinical studies are necessary before specific recommendations can be made. Cefotaxime should not be used alone when *P. aeruginosa* is a likely causative organism.

Cefotaxime (or other third generation cephalosporins) should not be used when less expensive, narrower spectrum, first (or second) generation cephalosporins are equally effective (eg, for known gram-positive infections, perioperative prophylaxis). For additional discussion, see the Introduction and Chapter 65, Table 1.

Cefotaxime has been useful in the treatment of uncomplicated and disseminated gonococcal infections caused by PPNG strains. However, the more active third generation agent, ceftriaxone, is now the preferred cephalosporin for these infections (*Morbid Mortal Week Rep*, 1985; see also Chapter 65, Table 2).

ADVERSE REACTIONS AND PRECAUTIONS. These are the same as for first generation cephalosporins. Hypoprothrombinemia and bleeding have not been reported (see the Introduction).

DRUG INTERACTIONS AND INTERFERENCE WITH LABORATORY TESTS. See the Introduction. A disulfiram-like reaction has not been reported.

PHARMACOKINETICS. Cefotaxime is administered intramuscularly or intravenously. Peak serum concentrations obtained after intramuscular or intravenous injections of 1 g are 20 mcg/ml (after 30 minutes) and 100 mcg/ml, respectively. Following intravenous infusion of 1 g over a 30-minute period, peak serum levels of 40 to 45 mcg/ml are achieved.

About 38% of circulating cefotaxime is bound to plasma protein. Volumes of distribution ranging from 0.25 to 0.39 L/kg have been reported. Cefotaxime has been shown to distribute into a variety of tissues and body fluids, including synovial, pericardial, pleural, and peritoneal fluids; bile; and urine. It enters cerebrospinal fluid in the presence of inflammation and achieves therapeutic concentrations for a number of pathogens. This antibiotic crosses the placenta.

Up to 50% of a dose is metabolized to desacetylcefotaxime, which has some antimicrobial activity, and other unknown, inactive metabolites. Parent drug and metabolites are excreted via the kidneys by renal tubular secretion and glomerular filtration; probenecid delays excretion. Between 50% and 60%

of a dose is recovered as unchanged drug in the urine; 15% to 25% is recovered as desacetylcefotaxime. The elimination half-life of cefotaxime is about one hour; the half-life of desacetylcefotaxime is 1.6 hours. Little parent drug accumulates in patients with impaired renal function. However, elimination of the desacetyl metabolite is prolonged and dosage reduction is recommended when the creatinine clearance is less than 20 ml/min.

DOSAGE AND PREPARATIONS. Cefotaxime can be administered by intramuscular injection deep into a large muscle mass or intravenously by direct injection or by intermittent or continuous infusion. See the manufacturer's instructions for the appropriate dilution of the drug, compatible diluents and intravenous solutions, and stability of cefotaxime in these solutions.

Intravenous, Intramuscular (deep): Adults, 2 to 12 g daily in equally divided doses every four to six hours (The Medical Letter, 1984). The usual dosage for moderate to severe infections is 1 to 2 g every six hours; for life-threatening infections, up to 2 g is given every four hours (Reese and Betts, 1983). Some infectious disease experts and the manufacturer recommend 1 to 2 g every six to eight hours for moderate to severe infections. The manufacturer recommends 1 g every 12 hours for uncomplicated urinary tract infections. For uncomplicated gonorrhea (including PPNG), 1 g intramuscularly as a single dose without probenecid. For disseminated gonococcal infections or gonococcal ophthalmia, see Chapter 65, Table 2.

Infants over 1 month and children, 100 to 200 mg/kg daily in equally divided doses every four to six hours (The Medical Letter, 1984). The larger dosage is recommended for meningitis. *Neonates over 7 days*, 150 mg/kg daily in divided doses every eight hours; *neonates 0 to 7 days*, 100 mg/kg daily in divided doses every 12 hours (The Medical Letter, 1984; Nelson, 1985 B).

Patients with impaired renal function require modification in doses and/or frequency of administration depending on the degree of impairment, severity of the infection, and susceptibility of the causative organism. Various dosage recommendations for these patients have been proposed. The manufacturer recommends that the dose of cefotaxime be halved when creatinine clearance is less than 20 ml/min/1.73 M². Alternative dosage recommendations for patients with impaired renal function are to increase the dosage interval to 6 to 12 hours for creatinine clearance of 50 to 10 ml/min and to 12 hours for creatinine clearance less than 10 ml/min (The Medical Letter, 1984). A supplemental dose equal to 50% of the maintenance dose should be given after hemodialysis (Norris and Mandell, 1985).

Claforan (Hoechst-Roussel). Powder (sterile) 1, 2, and 10 g (equivalent to base) (sodium 2.2 mEq/g).

CEFTIZOXIME SODIUM
[Cefizox]

Ceftizoxime is an aminothiazolyl *syn*-methoximino cephalosporin that is structurally very similar to cefotaxime (see Figure 1).

Renal Function	Creatinine Clearance (ml/min)	Less Severe Infections (Adult Maintenance Dosage)	Life-threatening Infections (Adult Maintenance Dosage)
Mild Impairment	79-50	500 mg every 8 hours	0.75-1.5 g every 8 hours
Moderate to Severe Impairment	49-5	250-500 mg every 12 hours	0.5-1 g every 12 hours
Dialysis Patients	4-0	500 mg every 48 hours or 250 mg every 24 hours	0.5-1 g every 48 hours or 0.5 g every 24 hours

From manufacturer's literature

MECHANISM OF ACTION, ANTIMICROBIAL SPECTRUM, AND RESISTANCE. The mechanism of action, antimicrobial spectrum, and resistance properties are essentially the same as for cefotaxime (see that evaluation and the Introduction; see also Barriere and Flaherty, 1984; Neu, 1984 A; Richards and Heel, 1985).

USES. Ceftizoxime has been effective, frequently as empiric monotherapy, in a wide variety of serious gram-negative bacillary infections, including lower respiratory tract, complicated urinary tract, intra-abdominal, gynecologic, skin and skin structure, bone, and joint infections and bacteremias. These frequently are of nosocomial origin and are caused by bacterial strains that are resistant to penicillins, older cephalosporins, and aminoglycosides. This drug is not recommended as sole therapy for *Pseudomonas aeruginosa* infections, however (see Parks et al, 1982; Barriere and Flaherty, 1984; Neu, 1984 A; Richards and Heel, 1985). The exact role of ceftizoxime in the treatment of these infections remains to be determined, but it appears to have indications very similar to those of cefotaxime (see that evaluation; see also the Introduction and Chapter 65, Antimicrobial Therapy and Chemoprophylaxis of Infectious Diseases, Table 1).

The elimination half-life of ceftizoxime (1.4 to 1.8 hours) is longer than that of cefotaxime (about one hour). Thus, it has the advantage of a more prolonged dosage interval. However, clinical experience with ceftizoxime, particularly for meningitis, is more limited than with cefotaxime. Although ceftizoxime has approved labeling for meningitis caused by *Haemophilus influenzae* and looks promising for other forms of bacterial meningitis (Overturf et al, 1984), additional clinical studies are necessary before conclusions can be made on its usefulness.

ADVERSE REACTIONS AND PRECAUTIONS. These are the same as for first generation cephalosporins. Hypoprothrombinemia and bleeding have not been reported (see the Introduction).

DRUG INTERACTIONS AND INTERFERENCE WITH LABORATORY TESTS. See the Introduction. A disulfiram-like reaction has not been reported.

PHARMACOKINETICS. Ceftizoxime is administered intramuscularly or intravenously. The peak serum concentration obtained after intramuscular injection of 1 g was 39 mcg/ml (after 60 minutes). Following intravenous infusion of 1 g over a 30-minute period, serum levels of 80 to 90 mcg/ml were achieved.

Approximately 30% of circulating ceftizoxime is bound to plasma proteins. Volumes of distribution ranging from 0.35 to 0.40 L/kg have been reported. Ceftizoxime has been shown to distribute into a variety of tissues and body fluids, including pleural, ascitic, prostatic, surgical wound, and peritoneal fluids; bile; urine; saliva; aqueous humor; heart; gallbladder; bone; and biliary, peritoneal, prostatic, and uterine tissues. Ceftizoxime enters cerebrospinal fluid in the presence of inflammation. This antibiotic crosses the placenta and is found in breast milk.

Up to 90% of a dose is excreted in the urine as unchanged drug by renal tubular secretion and glomerular filtration; excretion is delayed by probenecid. Ceftizoxime is not metabolized. The elimination half-life is approximately 1.4 to 1.8 hours. The half-life is prolonged in patients with renal impairment and dosage adjustments are required.

DOSAGE AND PREPARATIONS. Ceftizoxime can be administered by intramuscular injection deep into a large muscle mass or intravenously by direct injection or by intermittent or continuous infusion. See the manufacturer's instructions for the appropriate dilution of the drug, compatible diluents and intravenous solutions, and stability of ceftizoxime in these solutions.

Intravenous, Intramuscular (deep): Adults, 2 to 12 g daily in equally divided doses every eight to 12 hours (The Medical Letter, 1984). The usual dosages are as follows: for moderate infections outside the urinary tract, 1 g every 8 to 12 hours intramuscularly or intravenously; for severe or refractory infections, 1 g every 8 hours or 2 g every 8 to 12 hours intramuscularly or intravenously; for life-threatening infections, 3 to 4 g every 8 hours intravenously (up to 2 g every 4 hours has been given). For uncomplicated urinary tract infections, the manufacturer recommends 500 mg every 12 hours (a higher dosage is recommended for urinary tract infections caused by *Pseudomonas aeruginosa*). For uncomplicated gonorrhea (including PPNG), 1 g intramuscularly as a single dose without probenecid. When 2 g is administered intramuscularly, one-half of the dose is given in different large muscle masses.

Children 6 months or older, 150 to 200 mg/kg daily in equally divided doses every six to eight hours (not to exceed the maximum daily dosage for adults). Dosage guidelines for infants less than six months have not been established.

Patients with impaired renal function require modification in doses and/or frequency of administration depending on the degree of impairment, severity of the infection, and susceptibility of the causative organism. In *adults with impaired renal function*, the manufacturer recommends an initial loading dose of 500 mg to 1 g intramuscularly or intravenously and maintenance dosages as shown in the table (see above):

No additional supplemental dosing is required following hemodialysis. However, the dosage schedule should be timed so that the dose (according to the table on previous page) is given at the end of the dialysis session.

Cefizox (Smith, Kline & French). Powder (sterile) 1 and 2 g (equivalent to base) (sodium 2.6 mEq/g); solution 1 and 2 g in 5% dextrose in 50 ml containers.

CEFTRIAXONE SODIUM
[Rocephin]

Ceftriaxone is an aminothiazolyl *syn*-methoximino cephalosporin that is structurally similar to cefotaxime and ceftizoxime (see Figure 1).

MECHANISM OF ACTION, ANTIMICROBIAL SPECTRUM, AND RESISTANCE. The mechanism of action, antimicrobial spectrum, and resistance properties are essentially the same as for cefotaxime (see that evaluation and the Introduction; see also Barriere and Flaherty, 1984; Cleeland and Squires, 1984; Richards et al, 1984; Beam, 1985).

USES. Ceftriaxone has outstanding activity against *Neisseria gonorrhoeae*, including penicillinase-producing strains (PPNG) and chromosomal-mediated resistant *N. gonorrhoeae* (CMRNG). A single intramuscular 250-mg dose of this long-acting third generation cephalosporin has been highly effective in uncomplicated gonorrhea in adults, including urethral, endocervical, anorectal, and pharyngeal forms of this infection (Handsfield and Murphy, 1983; Judson et al, 1983 and 1985; Collier et al, 1984). Presently, it is among the preferred drugs (alternatives: ampicillin, amoxicillin, penicillin G procaine) for all uncomplicated gonococcal infections and is a drug of choice for proctitis in men, pharyngitis, and PPNG and CMRNG infections (*Morbid Mortal Week Rep*, 1985). Because cephalosporins are not active against *Chlamydia trachomatis*, follow-up therapy with a tetracycline for seven days is recommended for coexisting chlamydial infections. Ceftriaxone 1 g intravenously once daily for seven days also is useful in disseminated gonococcal infections and is a preferred drug for PPNG infections (*Morbid Mortal Week Rep*, 1985). A single intramuscular 250-mg dose of ceftriaxone, was highly effective in the treatment of chancroid (Taylor et al, 1985); it is a preferred drug (alternative, erythromycin) for this infection caused by *Haemophilus ducreyi* (*Morbid Mortal Week Rep*, 1985). For additional discussion, see the Introduction and Chapter 65, Antimicrobial Therapy and Chemoprophylaxis of Infectious Diseases, Table 2.

Ceftriaxone is highly active against the common causative organisms (*Haemophilus influenzae*, *Neisseria meningitidis*, *Streptococcus pneumoniae*) of meningitis in infants and young children and it has been shown to be an effective single-agent alternative to ampicillin plus chloramphenicol for the empiric therapy of meningitis in this age group (Del Rio et al, 1983; Steele and Bradsher, 1983; Congeni, 1984; Barson et al, 1985; Bryan et al, 1985). This agent also looks promising for gram-negative enteric bacillary meningitis (eg, *Escherichia coli*, *Klebsiella*) and, in combination with ampicillin, for neonatal meningitis; however, additional clinical studies are necessary before conclusions can be made on its usefulness. It is not active against *Listeria monocytogenes*, enterococci, or *Pseudomonas aeruginosa*. For additional discussion, see the Introduction and Chapter 65, Table 1.

Ceftriaxone has been effective, frequently as empiric monotherapy, in a wide variety of serious gram-negative bacillary infections, including lower respiratory tract, complicated urinary tract, intra-abdominal, gynecologic, skin and skin structure, bone, and joint infections and bacteremias. These frequently are of nosocomial origin and are caused by bacterial strains that are resistant to penicillins, older cephalosporins, and aminoglycosides. This drug is not recommended as sole therapy of *Pseudomonas aeruginosa* infections, however (see Barriere and Flaherty, 1984; McClosky, 1984; Richards et al, 1984; Beam, 1985). The exact role of ceftriaxone in the treatment of these infections remains to be determined, but the indications appear to be very similar to those of cefotaxime (see that evaluation, the Introduction, and Chapter 65, Table 1).

The major advantage of ceftriaxone is a long elimination half-life (six to nine hours) that permits administration once daily for most infections. Thus, the potential to reduce the cost of antimicrobial therapy and, for certain infections, to administer parenteral antibiotics in an outpatient setting may be realized with ceftriaxone. However, clinical experience with this agent is more limited than with cefotaxime.

Although single-dose ceftriaxone has been shown to be effective as perioperative prophylaxis for various surgical procedures (see Beam, 1985), no advantages over currently recommended cephalosporins, usually cefazolin, have been shown in controlled clinical trials (see DiPiro et al, 1984; Barriere, 1985; Polk, 1985; see also the Introduction and Chapter 65, Table 4).

ADVERSE REACTIONS AND PRECAUTIONS. Ceftriaxone generally has been well tolerated and most adverse reactions (eg, skin rashes and other hypersensitivity reactions, diarrhea and other gastrointestinal disturbances, mild reversible laboratory abnormalities) are similar to those reported for first generation cephalosporins (see the Introduction). Hypoprothrombinemia is very rare and bleeding has not been reported. Although ceftriaxone does not possess the methylthiotetrazole side chain that has been associated with coagulopathy, the manufacturer suggests that monitoring of prothrombin time, with supplemental vitamin K, may be reasonable in patients with impaired vitamin K synthesis or low vitamin K stores (eg, chronic hepatic disease, malnutrition). Because of its broad antimicrobial spectrum and high biliary excretion, ceftriaxone markedly alters colonic flora, but diarrhea has been reported in only 3% to 6% of patients and the incidence of superinfections with resistant organisms does not appear to be greater than with other third generation cephalosporins (see Barriere and Flaherty, 1984; Moskovitz, 1984; Oakes et al, 1984; Richards et al, 1984; Beam, 1985; Noble and Barza, 1985).

DRUG INTERACTIONS AND INTERFERENCE WITH LABORATORY TESTS. See the Introduction. Although ceftriaxone does not contain a methylthiotetrazole side chain, a disulfiram-like reaction has been reported in one patient (Moskovitz, 1984). It has been suggested by one of our consultants that the methylthiotriazine group at the 3-position of ceftriaxone may have structural similarities to the methylthiotetrazole side chain of cefamandole, cefoperazone, and moxalactam (see Figure 1).

PHARMACOKINETICS. Ceftriaxone is administered intramuscularly or intravenously. A peak serum concentration of 40 to 45 mcg/ml is obtained between two and three hours after intramuscular injection of 500 mg. Following intravenous infusion of 1 g over a 30-minute period, a serum concentration of approximately 150 mcg/ml is achieved.

Between 83% and 96% of circulating ceftriaxone is bound to plasma protein. Protein binding is concentration-dependent; the free ceftriaxone fraction increases from 4% to 17% over the serum concentration range of 5 mcg/ml to 300 mcg/ml. The apparent volume of distribution of (total) ceftriaxone is 0.12 to 0.14 L/kg. Ceftriaxone distributes to a wide variety of tissues (eg, myometrium, gallbladder wall, bone) and body fluids (eg, synovial, pleural, peritoneal). Large concentrations are present in bile and urine. Ceftriaxone enters the cerebrospinal fluid in the presence of inflammation and achieves therapeutic concentrations for a number of pathogens. This antibiotic crosses the placenta.

Ceftriaxone is eliminated by both renal (glomerular filtration) and biliary routes. It is not metabolized. Between 40% and 65% of a dose is recovered from urine as unchanged drug; the remainder is secreted into bile and ultimately is found in the feces as microbiologically inactive compounds. The elimination half-life is between six and nine hours in healthy volunteers. Elimination is prolonged only slightly in patients with severe renal impairment and dosage adjustments are unnecessary. The effect of hepatic dysfunction on elimination also is minimal. However, accumulation occurs in those with combined renal and hepatic impairment and dosage reductions are required.

DOSAGE AND PREPARATIONS. Ceftriaxone can be administered by intramuscular injection deep into a large muscle mass or intravenously by intermittent infusion. See the manufacturer's instructions for the appropriate dilution of the drug, compatible diluents and intravenous solutions, and stability of ceftriaxone in those solutions.

Intramuscular (deep), Intravenous: Adults, the usual dosage is 1 to 2 g once daily (or in equally divided doses every 12 hours) depending on the type and severity of the infection (*Med Lett Drugs Ther*, 1985 A; manufacturer's literature). The total daily dose should not exceed 4 g. For uncomplicated gonococcal infections, 250 mg intramuscularly as a single dose. *Infants and children*, for serious infections other than meningitis, 50 to 75 mg/kg daily (maximum of 2 g per day) in equally divided doses every 12 hours; for meningitis, 100 mg/kg daily (maximum of 4 g per day) in divided doses every 12 hours, with or without a loading dose of 75 mg/kg (*Med Lett Drugs Ther*, 1985 A; manufacturer's literature).

Dosage adjustments are unnecessary in patients with impaired renal or hepatic function. However, the manufacturer recommends monitoring of serum concentrations in patients with severe renal impairment (eg, dialysis patients) and in those with combined renal and hepatic dysfunction.

Rocephin (Roche). Powder (sterile) 250 and 500 mg and 1, 2, and 10 g (equivalent to base) (sodium 3.6 mEq/g).

CEFTAZIDIME
[Fortaz, Tazicef, Tazidime]

Ceftazidime is an aminothiazolyl cephalosporin similar to cefotaxime, ceftizoxime, and ceftriaxone. However, it differs from these agents because it contains a 2-carboxy-2-oxypropane imino group rather than a methoximino group, which the others have (see Figure 1). The carboxy side chain of ceftazidime reduces its activity against gram-positive cocci but increases its activity against *Pseudomonas aeruginosa* (see Neu, 1982 A).

Ceftazidime is being marketed by three manufacturers in the United States, which should allow hospital pharmacies to reduce their acquisition cost through competitive bidding.

MECHANISM OF ACTION, ANTIMICROBIAL SPECTRUM, AND RESISTANCE. Ceftazidime is a broad spectrum β-lactamase-stable third generation cephalosporin. Like other aminothiazolyl cephalosporins (eg, cefotaxime) and moxalactam, it has excellent activity against a variety of gram-negative bacteria, including *Neisseria meningitidis, N. gonorrhoeae, Haemophilus influenzae*, and most Enterobacteriaceae (eg, *Escherichia coli, Klebsiella, Enterobacter, Proteus, Morganella, Providencia, Citrobacter, Serratia, Salmonella, Shigella*). Strains of these gram-negative bacteria that are resistant to earlier generation cephalosporins, penicillins, and aminoglycosides frequently are susceptible.

The primary advantage of ceftazidime when compared to other currently available third generation cephalosporins is its good activity against *Pseudomonas aeruginosa*. It is superior to cefoperazone and, in most instances, is more active in vitro than aminoglycosides, carbenicillin, ticarcillin, azlocillin, and piperacillin against *P. aeruginosa*, including strains that are resistant to these other antibiotics. Ceftazidime also is active against many strains of other nonfermenting gram-negative bacilli, including other *Pseudomonas* species (eg, *P. cepacia*) and *Acinetobacter*.

Among gram-positive bacteria, ceftazidime is generally active in vitro against nonpenicillinase- and penicillinase-producing *Staphylococcus aureus*, but it is less potent than cefotaxime, ceftizoxime, and ceftriaxone and is considerably less active than first generation cephalosporins. Activity against coagulase-negative staphylococci (eg, *S. epidermidis*) is marginal and many strains are resistant. As with all cephalosporins, methicillin-resistant staphylococci are resistant. Most streptococci (except enterococci) are susceptible to ceftazidime, but it is less potent than cefotaxime, ceftizoxime, ceftriaxone, and the first generation cephalosporins. Penicillin-resistant pneumococci and *Listeria monocytogenes* are resistant to ceftazidime and all other cephalosporins.

Overall, the activity of ceftazidime against anaerobic bacteria is fair, but it has poor activity against the *Bacteroides fragilis* group. Clostridia (other than *C. perfringens*) usually are resistant.

Although ceftazidime is stable to the hydrolytic activity of most β-lactamases, resistance has emerged during therapy with this antibiotic, particularly among *Pseudomonas* and *Enterobacter* species (see Sanders and Sanders, 1985).

For additional discussion of the mechanism of action, antimicrobial spectrum, and resistance properties of ceftazidime, see the Introduction; see also Smith, 1984; Gentry, 1985; and Richards and Brogden, 1985.

USES. Ceftazidime has been effective, frequently as empiric monotherapy, in a wide variety of serious infections caused by *Pseudomonas aeruginosa* and other aerobic gram-negative bacilli. These include lower respiratory tract, complicated urinary tract, skin and soft tissue, bone, and joint infections and bacteremias. These are frequently of nosocomial origin and are caused by bacterial strains that are resistant to penicillins, other cephalosporins, and aminoglycosides (see Smith, 1984; Gentry, 1985; *Med Lett Drugs Ther*, 1985 B; Richards and Brogden, 1985). Thus, ceftazidime appears to be a useful agent for hospital-acquired gram-negative infections and would be preferred to other third generation cephalosporins when *P. aeruginosa* is a potential causative organism. Although this agent has been used to treat intra-abdominal and gynecologic infections (see Smith, 1984), its usefulness as a single agent in these situations must be questioned because of its lack of efficacy against many strains of *Bacteroides fragilis* (see Gleckman, 1985; Moellering, 1985 B; Richards and Brogden, 1985). For additional discussion, see the Introduction.

Ceftazidime appears to be the most useful third generation cephalosporin for meningitis caused by *P. aeruginosa* (Fong and Tomkins, 1985). Presently, it should be considered an alternative to an antipseudomonal penicillin for combination therapy with an aminoglycoside (intravenous and intrathecal administration). Although ceftazidime alone also has been effective in a limited number of cases of *P. aeruginosa* meningitis (Fong and Tompkins, 1985), additional clinical studies are necessary before it can be recommended as monotherapy for this very serious infection. Ceftazidime also appears to be promising for meningitis caused by gram-negative enteric bacilli, such as *Escherichia coli*, *Klebsiella*, and *Proteus* (see Norrby, 1985), but experience with cefotaxime and moxalactam is greater. In one study, ceftazidime was as effective as ampicillin plus chloramphenicol for meningitis in infants and children from 1 month to 15 years; causative organisms were primarily *Haemophilus influenzae*, *Neisseria meningitidis*, and *Streptococcus pneumoniae* (Rodriguez et al, 1985). However, cefuroxime, cefotaxime, and ceftriaxone have been studied more extensively. For additional discussion, see the Introduction and the evaluations; see also Chapter 65, Antimicrobial Therapy and Chemoprophylaxis of Infectious Diseases, Table 1.

Ceftazidime may be particularly useful in patients whose underlying conditions predispose them to infections with *P. aeruginosa*. Used alone, ceftazidime has produced clinical improvement in some patients with acute pulmonary exacerbations of cystic fibrosis (Mastella et al, 1983; Blumer et al, 1985; Gold et al, 1985) and was as effective as ticarcillin plus tobramycin in a randomized, controlled trial (Gold et al, 1985). Although short-term reductions in sputum colony counts of *P. aeruginosa* were observed, ceftazidime failed to produce long-term *P. aeruginosa* eradication. This is consistent with results obtained with other antipseudomonal antibiotics. The response to ceftazidime was less satisfactory in cystic fibrosis patients with lower respiratory tract infections caused by *P. cepacia* (Gold et al, 1985).

Because of its good activity against *P. aeruginosa*, ceftazidime also has been used alone and in combination with other agents for presumptive and definitive therapy of bacterial infections in neutropenic patients. Some published studies suggest that ceftazidime monotherapy may be as effective as standard combination regimens (eg, antipseudomonal penicillin plus aminoglycoside) for initial therapy of febrile neutropenic patients (de Pauw et al, 1983; Morgan et al, 1983; Reilly et al, 1983; Pizzo et al, 1984; see also Smith, 1984; Pizzo et al, 1985). However, in some studies, "breakthrough" infections with gram-positive bacteria have been frequent, prompting some investigators to recommend the addition of an agent (eg, nafcillin, vancomycin) with good gram-positive activity for primary coverage in neutropenic patients (Darbyshire et al, 1983; Fainstein et al, 1983; Ramphal et al, 1983). In summary, the use of ceftazidime monotherapy in this setting may provide potential cost advantages over traditional combination therapy and would enable the clinician to avoid the nephrotoxicity that occurs in certain patients receiving aminoglycosides. However, ceftazidime's relative lack of activity against gram-positive bacteria, particularly staphylococci, and the reports of emergence of resistance during therapy of *Pseudomonas* infections (Sanders and Sanders, 1985) must make one cautious in contemplating its use as a single agent in neutropenic patients; further data attesting to its efficacy in this setting are needed (Gleckman, 1985; Moellering, 1985 B; Richards and Brogden, 1985; Yost and Ramphal, 1985).

As with other third generation cephalosporins, ceftazidime is not indicated for infections that can be effectively treated (or prevented) with less expensive, narrower spectrum, first (or second) generation cephalosporins. In particular, it offers no advantages over first generation cephalosporins for known gram-positive infections or for perioperative prophylaxis (see the Introduction).

ADVERSE REACTIONS AND PRECAUTIONS. These are the same as for first generation cephalosporins. Hypoprothrombinemia and bleeding have not been reported (see the Introduction; see also Smith, 1984; Gentry, 1985; Richards and Brogden, 1985).

DRUG INTERACTIONS AND INTERFERENCE WITH LABORATORY TESTS. See the Introduction. A disulfiram-like reaction has not been reported.

PHARMACOKINETICS. Ceftazidime is administered intravenously or intramuscularly. Peak serum concentrations obtained after intramuscular and bolus intravenous injections of 1 g are 39 mcg/ml (after 60 minutes) and 107 to 119 mcg/ml, respectively. Following intravenous infusion of 1 g over a 30-minute period, peak serum levels of about 70 mcg/ml are achieved.

Approximately 17% of circulating ceftazidime is bound to plasma protein. Apparent volumes of distribution ranging from 0.21 to 0.28 L/kg have been reported. Ceftazidime has been shown to distribute into a variety of tissues (eg, gallbladder wall, myometrium, bone) and body fluids (eg, peritoneal, pleural, and synovial fluids; bile). High concentrations are obtained in urine. Ceftazidime enters the cerebrospinal fluid in the presence of inflammation and achieves therapeutic concentrations for a number of pathogens. This antibiotic crosses the placenta.

Between 80% and 90% of a dose is excreted in the urine as unchanged drug within 24 hours by glomerular filtration without renal tubular secretion. Probenecid has no effect on elimination. Ceftazidime is not metabolized. The elimination half-life is approximately 1.8 hours. The half-life is prolonged in patients with renal impairment and dosage adjustments are required.

DOSAGE AND PREPARATIONS. Ceftazidime can be administered by intramuscular injection deep into a large muscle mass or intravenously by direct injection or by intermittent or continuous infusion. See the manufacturer's instructions for the appropriate dilution of the drug, compatible diluents and intravenous solutions, and stability of ceftazidime in these solutions.

Intramuscular (deep), Intravenous: *Adults*, the usual dosage for moderately severe infections is 1 to 2 g intravenously every 8 to 12 hours; for serious or life-threatening infections such as meningitis or fever in a granulocytopenic patient, the maximum dosage of 2 g every eight hours should be used (*Med Lett Drugs Ther*, 1985 B).

The following dosages are recommended by the manufacturer for specific indications: uncomplicated urinary tract infections, 250 mg intravenously or intramuscularly every 12 hours; bone and joint infections, 2 g intravenously every 12 hours; complicated urinary tract infections, 500 mg intravenously or intramuscularly every eight to 12 hours; uncomplicated pneumonia and mild skin and skin structure infections, 500 mg to 1 g intravenously or intramuscularly every 8 hours; serious gynecologic and intra-abdominal infections, 2 g intravenously every eight hours; meningitis, 2 g intravenously every eight hours; very severe life-threatening infections, especially in immunocompromised patients, 2 g intravenously every eight hours; pseudomonal pulmonary infections in patients with cystic fibrosis and normal renal function, 30 to 50 mg/kg intravenously every eight hours (maximum, 6 g daily).

Infants and children from 1 month to 12 years, 30 to 50 mg/kg intravenously every eight hours (maximum, 6 g daily) (*Med Lett Drugs Ther*, 1985 B; manufacturer's literature). The higher dosage (50 mg/kg every eight hours) is recommended for immunocompromised children or children with cystic fibrosis or meningitis.

Neonates 1 to 4 weeks, 30 mg/kg intravenously every eight hours; *neonates 0 to 7 days*, 30 mg/kg intravenously every 12 hours; the dose should be increased to 50 mg/kg for neonatal meningitis (*Med Lett Drugs Ther*, 1985 B). (NOTE: The manufacturer recommends a dosage of 30 mg/kg intravenously every 12 hours for neonates 0 to 4 weeks).

Patients with impaired renal function require modification in doses and/or frequency of administration depending on the degree of impairment, severity of the infection, and susceptibility of the causative organism. In *adults with impaired renal function*, the manufacturer recommends an initial loading dose of 1 g and maintenance dosages as follows:

Creatinine Clearance (ml/min)	Adult Maintenance Dosage
50-31	1 g every 12 hours
30-16	1 g every 24 hours
15-6	500 mg every 24 hours
<5	500 mg every 48 hours

From manufacturer's literature

For patients with severe infections who would normally receive 6 g daily were it not for renal insufficiency, the unit dose given in the table above may be increased 50% or the dosing frequency increased appropriately. In adults undergoing hemodialysis, a loading dose of 1 g is recommended,

followed by 1 g after each dialysis period.

Ceftazidime can also be used in patients undergoing intraperitoneal dialysis and continuous ambulatory peritoneal dialysis. In adults, a loading dose of 1 g is given, followed by 500 mg every 24 hours. In addition to intravenous use, ceftazidime can be incorporated in dialysis fluid at a concentration of 250 mg/2 L of dialysis fluid (manufacturer's literature).

Fortaz (Glaxo). Powder (sterile) 500 mg and 1, 2, and 6 g (equivalent to anhydrous ceftazidime) (sodium 2.3 mEq/g)
Tazicef (Smith Kline & French). Powder (sterile) 1 and 2 g (equivalent to ceftazidime activity) (sodium 2.3 mEq/g).
Tazidime (Lilly). Powder (sterile) 500 mg and 1 and 2 g (equivalent to ceftazidime activity) (sodium 2.3 mEq/g).

CEFOPERAZONE SODIUM
[Cefobid]

This semisynthetic cephalosporin differs structurally from other third generation cephalosporins (see Figure 1). Similar to piperacillin, cefoperazone contains a piperazine side chain at position 7 of the cephalosporin nucleus. This enhances its antipseudomonal activity but decreases its stability to certain β-lactamases. Like cefamandole and moxalactam, cefoperazone contains a methylthiotetrazole side chain at position 3 that increases antibacterial activity and helps to prevent metabolism of the drug but also is associated with certain adverse effects (see Neu, 1983).

MECHANISM OF ACTION, ANTIMICROBIAL SPECTRUM, AND RESISTANCE. Similar to other third generation cephalosporins, cefoperazone has increased potency and a wider spectrum of activity against clinically important gram-negative bacteria when compared to first and second generation cephalosporins. This drug has excellent activity against *Neisseria meningitidis*, *N. gonorrhoeae*, and *Haemophilus influenzae*, including β-lactamase-producing strains of these species. Cefoperazone also is highly active against most Enterobacteriaceae (eg, *Escherichia coli*, *Klebsiella*, *Enterobacter*, *Proteus*, *Morganella*, *Providencia*, *Citrobacter*, *Serratia*, *Salmonella*, *Shigella*), but other third generation cephalosporins generally are superior. Cefoperazone is more susceptible to certain β-lactamases (eg, TEM-1, TEM-2), and β-lactamase-producing organisms, including strains of *E. coli* and *Klebsiella*, that are susceptible to other third generation cephalosporins occasionally will be resistant to cefoperazone (Sykes and Bush, 1983). Cefoperazone has better activity against *Pseudomonas aeruginosa* than other currently available third generation cephalosporins with the exception of ceftazidime. The activity of cefoperazone against *Acinetobacter*, nonfermenting gram-negative bacilli, is poor. Although most anaerobic bacteria are susceptible, many *Bacteroides fragilis* strains are resistant.

Among gram-positive bacteria, cefoperazone has good activity against nonpenicillinase- and penicillinase-producing staphylococci and most streptococci (except enterococci). However, as with other third generation cephalosporins, this agent offers no clinical advantages over first generation cephalosporins for infections that are known to be caused by gram-positive bacteria.

Cefoperazone has been reported to be a poorer inducer of Type I β-lactamases of certain gram-negative bacilli (eg,

Enterobacter cloacae) when compared to other third generation cephalosporins (Minami et al, 1980; Sykes and Bonner, 1985). Whether this is an advantage clinically is unknown.

For additional discussion on the mechanism of action, antimicrobial spectrum, and resistance properties of cefoperazone, see the Introduction; see also Funk and Strausbaugh, 1982; Barriere and Flaherty, 1984; Smith, 1984.

USES. Cefoperazone has been effective, frequently as empiric monotherapy, in a wide variety of serious gram-negative bacillary infections outside the central nervous system. These include lower respiratory tract, complicated urinary tract, intra-abdominal, gynecologic, skin and skin structure, bone, and joint infections and bacteremias. These infections often are of nosocomial origin and are caused by bacterial strains that are resistant to penicillins, older cephalosporins, and aminoglycosides (see Funk and Strausbaugh, 1982; Warren et al, 1983; Barriere and Flaherty, 1984; Cohen et al, 1984).

The exact role of cefoperazone in the treatment of serious gram-negative bacillary infections remains to be determined, however. This agent has better activity than cefotaxime, ceftizoxime, ceftriaxone, and moxalactam against *Pseudomonas aeruginosa*. However, most infectious disease experts do not recommend cefoperazone as sole therapy for serious systemic *P. aeruginosa* infections (see *Med Lett Drugs Ther*, 1983 B; Barriere and Flaherty, 1984; Quintiliani et al, 1984). Furthermore, ceftazidime has better activity than cefoperazone against this gram-negative organism and now appears to be the preferred third generation cephalosporin for infections known or presumed to be caused by *P. aeruginosa* (see the evaluation and the Introduction).

Cefoperazone has inferior activity in vitro against most Enterobacteriaceae and, with the exception of moxalactam, has been associated with more undesirable adverse reactions (eg, hypoprothrombinemia, bleeding) than other third generation cephalosporins. Also, it exhibits variable penetration into cerebrospinal fluid and it is not indicated for meningitis. Thus, the apparent disadvantages of cefoperazone appear to outweigh its advantages when compared to other available third generation cephalosporins. However, well-controlled clinical trials comparing cefoperazone to the other agents are generally unavailable. For additional discussion, see the Introduction.

As with other third generation cephalosporins, cefoperazone is not indicated for infections that can be effectively treated (or prevented) with less expensive, narrower spectrum first (or second) generation cephalosporins. In particular, it offers no advantages over first generation cephalosporins for known gram-positive infections or for perioperative prophylaxis (see the Introduction).

ADVERSE REACTIONS AND PRECAUTIONS. Hypersensitivity reactions (eg, maculopapular rash, fever, eosinophilia) and other adverse effects associated with cephalosporins have been observed with cefoperazone (see the Introduction). Because of its broad antimicrobial spectrum and high biliary excretion, cefoperazone markedly alters colonic flora (Alestig et al, 1983; see also Barriere and Flaherty, 1984; Noble and Barza, 1985). Diarrhea was reported frequently in some studies (Carlberg et al, 1982; Mulligan et al, 1982; Mastella et al, 1983; see also Barriere and Flaherty, 1984) but not in others (Cohen et al, 1984). Superinfections with resistant organisms occur, but the incidence does not appear to be

greater than with other third generation cephalosporins (see Barriere and Flaherty, 1984; Noble and Barza, 1985).

Cefoperazone contains a methylthiotetrazole side chain and has been associated with hypoprothrombinemia and, occasionally, bleeding. Elderly debilitated patients, individuals with severe renal insufficiency, and malnourished patients receiving total parenteral nutrition are at highest risk. Vitamin K reverses the hypoprothrombinemia, and prophylactic administration may be desirable in some patients (see the Introduction).

DRUG INTERACTIONS AND INTERFERENCE WITH LABORATORY TESTS. Methylthiotetrazole-containing cephalosporins also have been associated with a disulfiram-like reaction. For additional discussion, see the Introduction.

PHARMACOKINETICS. Cefoperazone is administered intramuscularly or intravenously. Peak serum concentrations obtained after intramuscular and intravenous injections of 1 g are 65 to 74 mcg/ml (after one hour) and 200 mcg/ml (within 15 minutes), respectively. Following intravenous infusion of 1 g over a 15-minute period, a serum level of 153 mcg/ml is achieved.

Between 87% and 93% of circulating cefoperazone is bound to plasma proteins. Volumes of distribution ranging from 0.14 to 0.20 L/kg have been reported. The drug penetrates into most body fluids and tissues; highest concentrations occur in bile. Antibacterial concentrations can be achieved in the cerebrospinal fluid when the meninges are inflamed. However, penetration into cerebrospinal fluid has been variable and cefoperazone is not used to treat meningitis. The drug crosses the placenta.

Approximately 70% of a dose is eliminated in the bile as unchanged drug. About 30% is eliminated in the urine (glomerular filtration). The serum half-life ranges from 1.9 to 2.1 hours and is not prolonged in patients with renal impairment. In patients with hepatic dysfunction, the serum half-life is prolonged two- to fourfold and there is a compensatory increase in urinary excretion. Cefoperazone accumulates in patients with combined renal and hepatic failure and dosage adjustments are necessary.

DOSAGE AND PREPARATIONS. Cefoperazone can be administered by intramuscular injection deep into a large muscle mass or intravenously by intermittent or continuous infusion. See the manufacturer's instructions for the appropriate dilution of the drug, compatible diluents and intravenous solutions, and stability of cefoperazone in these solutions.

Intramuscular (deep), Intravenous: *Adults*, 2 to 4 g daily in equally divided doses every 12 hours is the usual dosage recommended by the manufacturer. In severe infections or infections caused by less sensitive organisms, the manufacturer states that the dose and/or frequency of administration may be increased. Patients have been successfully treated with a total daily dosage of 6 to 12 g divided into two, three or four administrations ranging from 1.5 to 4 g per dose. Most infectious disease experts recommend a dosing interval of every eight hours (or even every six hours) for serious or life-threatening infections (Garzone et al, 1983 A; The Medical Letter, 1984; Fried and Hinthorn, 1985; Noble and Barza, 1985).

Children, 100 to 150 mg/kg daily in divided doses every 8 to 12 hours has been recommended (Nelson, 1985 A). However there is no approved labeling for use in children.

The dosage usually does not require adjustment in patients with severely impaired renal function. A total daily dosage above 4 g generally is unnecessary in those with hepatic disease and/or biliary obstruction. If higher dosages are used, serum concentrations should be monitored. In patients with both hepatic dysfunction and significant renal disease, dosage should not exceed 1 to 2 g daily and serum concentrations should be monitored.

> **Cefobid** (Roerig). Powder (sterile) in 1 and 2 g containers (equivalent to base) (sodium 1.5 mEq/g).

MOXALACTAM DISODIUM
[Moxam]

This broad spectrum, β-lactam antibiotic differs from the other third generation cephalosporins in that it is an oxa-β-lactam (1-oxa-cephalosporin) in which the sulfur of the dihydrothiazine ring is replaced by an oxygen to form a dihydro-oxazine ring (see Figure 1). It is a totally synthetic molecule and it is administered only parenterally.

MECHANISM OF ACTION, ANTIMICROBIAL SPECTRUM, AND RESISTANCE. As with the aminothiazolyl cephalosporins (eg, cefotaxime), moxalactam has increased potency and β-lactamase stability and a wider spectrum of activity against clinically important gram-negative bacteria when compared to first or second generation cephalosporins. This drug has excellent activity against *Neisseria meningitidis, N. gonorrhoeae, Haemophilus influenzae*, and most Enterobacteriaceae (eg, *Escherichia coli, Klebsiella, Enterobacter, Proteus, Morganella, Providencia, Citrobacter, Serratia, Salmonella, Shigella*), including strains that are resistant to earlier generation cephalosporins, penicillins, and aminoglycosides. Moxalactam is the only third generation cephalosporin with reasonably good activity against the *Bacteroides fragilis* group; it is comparable to cefoxitin against these gram-negative anaerobic bacilli. The nonfermenting gram-negative bacilli, *Pseudomonas aeruginosa* and *Acinetobacter*, generally are resistant, however.

Although moxalactam is active against nonpenicillinase- and penicillinase-producing staphylococci and most streptococci (except enterococci), it is inferior to other third generation cephalosporins against these gram-positive bacteria.

For additional discussion of the mechanism of action, antimicrobial spectrum, and resistance properties of moxalactam, see the Introduction; see also Fitzpatrick and Standiford, 1982; Carmine et al, 1983 B; Barriere and Flaherty, 1984.

USES. Substantial clinical experience has been obtained with moxalactam. This drug has been effective in the treatment of meningitis caused by gram-negative enteric bacilli (eg, *E. coli, Klebsiella, Proteus*) and *H. influenzae*. Moxalactam has been effective, frequently as empiric monotherapy, in a wide variety of serious gram-negative bacillary infections outside the central nervous system, including lower respiratory tract, complicated urinary tract, intra-abdominal, gynecologic, skin and skin structure, bone, and joint infections and bacteremias. These frequently are of nosocomial origin and are caused by bacterial strains that are resistant to penicillins, older cephalosporins, and aminoglycosides.

Unfortunately, moxalactam has been associated with serious bleeding episodes, including fatalities, in a number of patients. With the availability of an increasing number of comparably effective and less toxic third generation cephalosporins, the usefulness of moxalactam has diminished greatly. For additional discussion, see the Introduction; see also Barriere and Flaherty, 1984.

ADVERSE REACTIONS AND PRECAUTIONS. All of the adverse reactions common to the cephalosporins (eg, skin rash, other hypersensitivity reactions, gastrointestinal disturbances) may occur with moxalactam (see the Introduction).

Clinically, bleeding has been a particularly common and serious problem with moxalactam. It has been reported that 2.5% of clinical trial patients receiving this antibiotic for four days or longer suffered a bleeding event, most of which were serious (manufacturer's literature). Numerous case reports of moxalactam-associated coagulopathy, including some fatalities, have appeared in the literature (Holt et al, 1981; Pakter et al, 1982; Jones and Kimbrough, 1983; Lee et al, 1983; MacLennan et al, 1983; Panwalker and Rosenfeld, 1983; Slonaker and Luper, 1983; Weitekamp and Aber, 1983; Au and Geiger, 1984; Bach, 1984; Brandstetter et al, 1984; Conly et al, 1984; Meisel, 1984).

Moxalactam affects hemostasis via three mechanisms: hypoprothrombinemia, platelet dysfunction, and, very rarely, immune-mediated thrombocytopenia. Like cefamandole and cefoperazone, moxalactam contains a methylthiotetrazole side chain and has caused hypoprothrombinemia and bleeding in certain patients, particularly elderly, debilitated patients, those individuals with severe renal insufficiency, and malnourished patients receiving total parenteral nutrition. Prothrombin times should be monitored; if they become prolonged, vitamin K should be given. Because vitamin K can prevent the hypoprothrombinemia, it is now recommended that vitamin K (adults, 10 mg per week) be administered prophylactically to all patients receiving moxalactam (manufacturer's literature).

Moxalactam also has caused prolonged bleeding time and bleeding diathesis in some patients by inhibiting platelet function; this is dose dependent and not reversible by vitamin K (Weitekamp and Aber, 1983; Weitekamp et al, 1985). In adults with normal renal function, doses greater than 4 g per day for more than three days may result in platelet dysfunction (manufacturer's literature), although lower dosages also have been implicated (Bach, 1984). Patients with reduced renal function are particularly susceptible. The manufacturer recommends that the bleeding time be monitored in patients requiring more than 4 g of moxalactam per day and who are treated for more than three days. All patients with renal dysfunction should have appropriate dosage adjustments and should be monitored periodically with bleeding times. If the bleeding time becomes unduly prolonged, moxalactam should be discontinued. If hemorrhage should occur by this mechanism, the drug should be discontinued and appropriate supportive measures (eg, administration of fresh frozen plasma, packed red cells, platelet concentrates) should be undertaken. Substitution of moxalactam with another beta lactam antibiotic that also can cause platelet dysfunction (eg, carbenicillin) should be with caution.

Superinfections with enterococci have been reported more

Creatinine Clearance (ml/min/1.73 M²)	Renal Function	Life-threatening Infections (Maximum Adult Maintenance Dosage)	Less Severe Infections (Adult Maintenance Dosage)
>80	Normal	4 g every 8 hours	0.5-2 g every 8-12 hours
50-80	Mild Impairment	3 g every 8 hours	0.5-1 g every 8 hours
25-50	Moderate Impairment	2 g every 8 hours or 3 g every 12 hours	0.25-1 g every 12 hours
2-25	Severe Impairment	1 g every 8 hours or 1.25 g every 12 hours	0.25-0.5 g every 8 hours
<2	0	1 g every 24 hours	0.25-0.5 g every 12 hours

From manufacturer's literature

frequently with moxalactam than with other third generation cephalosporins. This may be associated with moxalactam's very poor activity against these organisms (see Jones and Thornsberry, 1985).

DRUG INTERACTIONS AND INTERFERENCE WITH LABORATORY TESTS. Similar to other methylthiotetrazole-containing cephalosporins, moxalactam has been associated with a disulfiram-like reaction. For additional discussion, see the Introduction.

Concomitant use of "high-dose" heparin (more than 20,000 units/day), oral anticoagulants, and other drugs that affect hemostasis (eg, aspirin) are factors that may increase the risk of bleeding during therapy with moxalactam.

PHARMACOKINETICS. Moxalactam is administered intramuscularly or intravenously. Peak serum concentrations after intramuscular and intravenous injections of 1 g are 23 to 52 mcg/ml (after one to two hours) and 95 to 120 mcg/ml, respectively. Following intravenous infusion of 1 g over 30 minutes, a serum level of 60 to 70 mcg/ml is achieved.

Approximately 50% of circulating moxalactam is bound to plasma proteins. Volumes of distribution ranging from 0.25 to 0.40 L/kg have been reported. Moxalactam has been shown to distribute into a variety of tissues and body fluids, including pleural, interstitial, peritoneal, and synovial fluids; bile; urine; aqueous humor; bronchial secretions; bone; prostatic tissue; and atrial appendage. Moxalactam enters the cerebrospinal fluid in the presence of inflammation and achieves therapeutic concentrations for a number of pathogens. This antibiotic crosses the placenta and is found in breast milk.

Up to 90% of a dose of moxalactam is excreted in the urine as unchanged drug within 24 hours; it is not metabolized. The primary mechanism of elimination is by glomerular filtration and probenecid has little effect on excretion. The serum half-life ranges from 2 to 2.3 hours. The half-life is prolonged in patients with renal impairment and dosage adjustments are required.

DOSAGE AND PREPARATIONS. Moxalactam can be administered by intramuscular injection deep into a large muscle mass or intravenously by direct injection or by intermittent or continuous infusion. See the manufacturer's instructions for the appropriate dilution of the drug, compatible diluents and intravenous solutions, and stability of moxalactam in these solutions.

It is recommended that patients who receive moxalactam be given 10 mg of vitamin K per week prophylactically. Bleeding times should be monitored in patients who receive more than 4 g moxalactam per day for more than three days. All patients with significantly reduced renal impairment should have appropriate dosage reduction (see below) and bleeding times should be monitored periodically.

Intramuscular (deep), Intravenous: Adults, 1 to 12 g daily in equally divided doses every 8 to 12 hours (Norris and Mandell, 1985). Most infectious disease experts recommend 2 g every eight hours for serious infections (Fitzpatrick and Standiford, 1982; Reese and Betts, 1983; Fried and Hinthorn, 1985; Noble and Barza, 1985). For life-threatening infections (eg, meningitis) or infections caused by less susceptible organisms, up to 4 g every eight hours may be needed. (NOTE: The manufacturer states that the usual daily dosage is 2 to 4 g administered every 8 to 12 hours and that most mild to moderate infections can be expected to respond to 500 mg to 2 g every 12 hours. The manufacturer's recommendations for specific infections are as follows: mild skin and skin structure infections and uncomplicated pneumonia, 500 mg every eight hours; mild, uncomplicated urinary tract infections, 250 mg every 12 hours; urinary tract infections that are more difficult to treat, 500 mg every 12 hours; serious urinary tract infections, 500 mg every eight hours; life-threatening infections or infections caused by less susceptible organisms, up to 4 g every eight hours.)

Children, 150 to 200 mg/kg daily in equally divided doses every six to eight hours; *infants 1 month to 1 year*, 200 mg/kg daily in equally divided doses every six hours; *neonates 1 to 4 weeks*, 150 mg/kg daily in equally divided doses every eight hours; *neonates 0 to 7 days*, 100 mg/kg daily in equally divided doses every 12 hours. In pediatric gram-negative meningitis, an initial loading dose of 100 mg/kg is recommended by the manufacturer. The maximum daily dosage recommended by the manufacturer for serious infections is 200 mg/kg (not to exceed 12 g).

Patients with impaired renal function require modification in doses and/or frequency of administration depending on the degree of impairment, severity of the infection, and susceptibility of the causative organism. In *adults with impaired renal function*, the manufacturer recommends an initial loading dose of 1 to 2 g and maintenance dosages as shown in the table (see above).

The serum half-life of moxalactam during hemodialysis ranges from two to five hours. Maintenance doses should be repeated following regular hemodialysis.

Moxam (Lilly). Powder (sterile) 1, 2, and 10 g (equivalent to base).

NOTE: *The following evaluation was added after this chapter was completed.*

CEFOTETAN DISODIUM
[Cefotan]

Cefotetan is a cephamycin antibiotic derived semisynthetically from oganomycin G, which is produced by *Streptomyces oganonensis*. Like cefoxitin and moxalactam, it contains a 7α-methoxy substitution on the basic cephalosporin nucleus that enhances its stability to most β-lactamases. Cefotetan generally is classified as a third generation cephalosporin because it is more active than first and second generation cephalosporins against gram-negative bacteria. However, many experts would consider it a second generation agent (see Ward and Richards, 1985).

MECHANISM OF ACTION, ANTIMICROBIAL SPECTRUM, AND RESISTANCE. The mechanism of action of cefotetan is the same as for other cephalosporins (see the Introduction).

In general, cefotetan has increased potency and a broader antimicrobial spectrum against gram-negative bacteria than first and second generation cephalosporins. Among the Enterobacteriaceae, it has excellent activity against *Escherichia coli*, *Klebsiella* species, *Proteus mirabilis*, and *Proteus vulgaris* with most strains susceptible in vitro at concentrations less than 1 mcg/ml. Other *Proteus* species, *Providencia* and *Morganella* species, and *Salmonella* and *Shigella* species are susceptible at concentrations less than 8 mcg/ml. Activity against *Enterobacter*, *Serratia*, and *Citrobacter* species is variable and, generally, cefotetan is less active than other third generation cephalosporins against these species.

Cefotetan is active against *Haemophilus influenzae* and *Neisseria gonorrhoeae*, including β-lactamase-producing strains. However, its potency (MIC_{90}, 1 to 4 mcg/ml) is comparable to that of the second generation cephalosporins (eg, cefoxitin, cefamandole) and is considerably less than other third generation cephalosporins. Cefotetan is active against *Neisseria meningitidis*.

The nonfermenting gram-negative bacilli, *Pseudomonas aeruginosa* and *Acinetobacter* species, are resistant to cefotetan.

Cefotetan has only modest activity against most gram-positive cocci (MIC_{90} = 2 to 16 mcg/ml), including nonpenicillinase- and penicillinase-producing staphylococci and most streptococci. It is similar to moxalactam in activity against these species, but is less active than cefotaxime, ceftizoxime, and ceftriaxone. In general, third generation cephalosporins offer no advantages over first generation derivatives (eg, cefazolin) for known gram-positive bacterial infec-

tions. None of the cephalosporins are active against enterococci (eg, *Streptococcus faecalis*), methicillin-resistant staphylococci, penicillin G-resistant pneumococci, and *Listeria monocytogenes*.

Cefotetan exhibits modest in vitro activity against anaerobic bacteria. *Bacteroides* (including the *B. fragilis* group), *Clostridium,* and *Fusobacterium* species usually are more susceptible to cefotetan, cefoxitin, and moxalactam than cephalosporins lacking the 7α-methoxy substitution, but activity varies considerably among different institutions. Like cefoxitin, cefotetan is less active than clindamycin, metronidazole, chloramphenicol, and imipenem against the clinically important *Bacteroides* (eg, *B. fragilis*) species. Most anaerobic gram-positive cocci are susceptible to cefotetan.

Like other 7α-methoxy cephalosporins, cefotetan is resistant to most β-lactamases, although it is hydrolyzed by certain β-lactamases from *Pseudomonas aeruginosa* and *Enterobacter cloacae*. Resistant strains of *Bacteroides fragilis*, *Serratia liquifaciens*, and *Citrobacter freundii* also have been reported.

For additional discussion, see Ward and Richards, 1985.

USES. Cefotetan has been shown to be effective in intra-abdominal, obstetric and gynecologic, skin and soft tissue, complicated urinary tract, and lower respiratory tract infections caused by susceptible bacteria. Studies are too limited to establish efficacy in bacteremias and sepsis, gonorrhea, meningitis, and infections in immunocompromised patients (see Ward and Richards, 1985).

In general, clinical experience with cefotetan is very limited and randomized, double-blinded comparative trials with established therapies are unavailable. Thus, any role for this agent in infectious disease therapy remains largely undefined. It would appear that the most likely indications for cefotetan would be similar to those for cefoxitin and include intra-abdominal and obstetric-gynecologic infections. These are frequently polymicrobial, involving both aerobic gram-negative bacilli and anaerobic bacteria (including the *B. fragilis* group). When compared to cefoxitin, cefotetan has an expanded spectrum of activity against aerobic gram-negative bacilli and a longer elimination half-life (about 3.5 hours), which allows it to be administered twice daily. However, like cefamandole, cefoperazone, and moxalactam, cefotetan contains a methylthiotetrazole side chain that has been associated with hypoprothrombinemia and bleeding. Thus, it remains to be established by additional, comparative clinical trials whether cefotetan offers advantages over cefoxitin for these infections. It should be emphasized that up to 20% of *B. fragilis* strains are resistant to these cephalosporins in some institutions and they probably should not be used alone for severely ill patients with intra-abdominal infections (see Antimicrobial Spectrum, Adverse Reactions and Precautions, and Pharmacokinetics, the evaluation of cefoxitin, and the Introduction; see also Chapter 65, Antimicrobial Therapy and Chemoprophylaxis of Infectious Diseases, Tables 1 and 2).

Although cefotetan has been shown to be effective as perioperative prophylaxis in various surgical procedures, including biliary tract surgery, vaginal and abdominal hysterectomy, cesarean section, and colorectal surgery (see Ward and Richards, 1985), no advantages over currently recommended cephalosporins (usually cefazolin) have been shown in controlled clinical trials. For additional discussion, see the Introduction and Chapter 65, Table 4.

ADVERSE REACTIONS AND PRECAUTIONS. Cefotetan generally has been well tolerated in clinical trial patients and the adverse reaction profile has been similar to other cephalosporins. Hypersensitivity reactions (eg, rash, pruritus, fever), gastrointestinal disturbances (eg, diarrhea, nausea, vomiting), local reactions (eg, phlebitis, local pain), and minor hematologic (eg, eosinophilia, leukopenia) and hepatic (eg, elevated SGOT, SGPT, alkaline phosphatase) laboratory abnormalities have been reported most frequently (Ward and Richards, 1985; manufacturer's literature; see also the Introduction). Cefotetan is classified in FDA Pregnancy Category B.

Cefotetan contains a methylthiotetrazole side chain, but hypoprothrombinemic bleeding problems have not yet been reported clinically (see Ward and Richards, 1985). However, the potential for prolongation of prothrombin time with bleeding should be considered. Elderly debilitated patients, individuals with severe renal insufficiency, and malnourished patients receiving total parenteral nutrition are at highest risk. Prothrombin times should be monitored in patients at risk and exogenous vitamin K administered as indicated (see the Introduction).

DRUG INTERACTIONS AND INTERFERENCE WITH LABORATORY TESTS. Methylthiotetrazole-containing cephalosporins have been associated with a disulfiram-like reaction, but this has not yet been reported for cefotetan (see Ward and Richards, 1985). However, the potential for this interaction should be considered. For additional discussion of this and other drug interactions, see the Introduction.

PHARMACOKINETICS. Cefotetan is not absorbed following oral administration and must be administered intramuscularly or intravenously. Bioavailability after intramuscular injection is 100%. Peak serum concentrations obtained after intramuscular and bolus intravenous injections of 1 g are 50 to 80 mcg/ml (after one to two hours) and 140 to 250 mcg/ml, respectively. Following intravenous infusion of 1 g over a 30-minute period, peak serum levels of approximately 160 mcg/ml are achieved.

Approximately 88% of circulating cefotetan is bound to plasma protein. Apparent volumes of distribution ranging from 8 to 13 L have been reported, indicating distribution to the extracellular water space. Cefotetan has been shown to distribute into a variety of tissues and body fluids, including skin, muscle, fat, myometrium, endometrium, cervix, ovary, kidney, ureter, bladder, maxillary sinus mucosa, tonsil, bile, peritoneal fluid, umbilical cord serum, and amniotic fluid. High concentrations are obtained in urine. Penetration into cerebrospinal fluid appears to be low, but data are very limited.

Cefotetan is eliminated by the renal route. Between 51% and 81% of a dose is recovered as unchanged drug in the urine over a 24-hour period. The drug does not appear to be metabolized. The elimination half-life in adults with normal renal function ranges from 3 to 4.4 hours. In pediatric subjects, a slightly shorter half-life (range, 1.85 to 3.5 hours) usually is observed; in newborn infants with urinary tract infections, a longer half-life of 5.4 hours has been reported. The elimination half-life is prolonged in patients with impaired renal function and dosage adjustments are necessary.

For additional discussion, see Ward and Richards, 1985 and the manufacturer's literature.

DOSAGE AND PREPARATIONS. Cefotetan can be administered by intramuscular injection deep into a large muscle mass or intravenously by direct injection or by intermittent infusion. See the manufacturer's instructions for the appropriate dilution of the drug, compatible diluents and intravenous solutions, and stability of cefotetan in these solutions.

Intramuscular (deep), Intravenous: Adults, 1 to 6 g daily in equally divided doses every 12 hours is the dosage range recommended by the manufacturer. The usual adult dosage is 1 or 2 g every 12 hours. The following general guidelines for dosage of cefotetan according to type of infection have been recommended by the manufacturer: urinary tract, 500 mg every 12 hours or 1 to 2 g every 24 hours or 1 to 2 g every 12 hours; other sites, 1 to 2 g every 12 hours; severe, 2 g every 12 hours (intravenous); life-threatening, 3 g every 12 hours (intravenous). The maximum daily dosage should not exceed 6 g.

Patients with impaired renal function require modification in doses and/or frequency of administration depending on the degree of impairment, severity of the infection, and susceptibility of the causative organism. For *adults with impaired renal function*, the manufacturer recommends: for creatinine clearance of >30 ml/min, the usual recommended dose every 12 hours; for creatinine clearance of 10 to 30 ml/min, the usual recommended dose every 24 hours; for creatinine clearance of <10 ml/min, the usual recommended dose every 48 hours. Alternatively, the dosing interval may remain constant at 12 hour intervals, but the dose reduced to one-half the usual recommended dose for patients with creatinine clearance of 10 to 30 ml/min, and one-quarter of the usual recommended dose for patients with creatinine clearance of <10 ml/min. For patients undergoing intermittent hemodialysis, one-quarter of the usual recommended dose should be given every 24 hours on days between dialysis and one-half the usual recommended dose on the day of dialysis.

Pediatric dosage guidelines are presently unavailable.

Cefotan (Stuart). Powder (sterile) 1 and 2 g (equivalent to base) (sodium 5.5 mEq/g).

ORAL CEPHALOSPORINS

CEPHALEXIN MONOHYDRATE
[Keflex]

MECHANISM OF ACTION, ANTIMICROBIAL SPECTRUM, AND RESISTANCE. The clinically relevant antibacterial spectrum of cephalexin is similar to that of other first generation cephalosporins. It is active against most gram-positive bacteria, including nonpenicillinase- and penicillinase-producing staphylococci, streptococci (except enterococci), and many anaerobic bacteria. The in vitro potency against gram-positive cocci generally is less than that of parenteral first generation cephalosporins (eg, cephalothin, cefazolin). The gram-negative antibacterial activity of first generation cephalosporins essentially is limited to *Escherichia coli, Klebsiella,* and

Proteus mirabilis. Cephalexin is not very active against *Haemophilus influenzae*.

For additional discussion of the mechanism of action, antimicrobial spectrum, and resistance properties of the cephalosporins, see the Introduction.

USES. Cephalexin is rarely the drug of choice for bacterial infections. It may be indicated in mild to moderate infections of the respiratory tract, urinary tract, skin and skin structures, and bone caused by susceptible organisms when preferred agents are ineffective or cannot be tolerated. It often is among the alternatives for penicillins in patients who exhibit hypersensitivity reactions (other than the immediate type) to penicillins. For example, cephalexin is a likely alternative to antistaphylococcal penicillins in certain staphylococcal pyodermas. Although it could be used in streptococcal infections (eg, pharyngitis), erythromycin is usually the preferred alternative to penicillin G. Cephalexin usually is not recommended in upper respiratory tract infections or otitis media in which *H. influenzae* is an important pathogen; cefaclor may be useful for this organism, however (see that evaluation). Cephalexin may be useful for urinary tract infections when the causative organism is resistant to currently preferred drugs (eg, sulfisoxazole, ampicillin, trimethoprim/sulfamethoxazole) but sensitive to cephalexin.

A consistent problem with the oral cephalosporins has been their relatively high cost to the patient, a factor the physician should take into consideration when alternative, less expensive, but equally effective antibacterial drugs are available.

For additional discussion, see the Introduction; see also Chapter 65, Antimicrobial Therapy and Chemoprophylaxis of Infectious Diseases, Table 1.

ADVERSE REACTIONS AND PRECAUTIONS. Cephalexin generally is well tolerated. Gastrointestinal disturbances (eg, diarrhea) and hypersensitivity reactions (eg, skin rash) are most common. For detailed discussion, see the Introduction.

DRUG INTERACTIONS AND INTERFERENCE WITH LABORATORY TESTS. See the Introduction.

PHARMACOKINETICS. Cephalexin is stable to gastric acid and is well absorbed following oral administration. Following doses of 250 mg, 500 mg, and 1 g, average peak serum concentrations of approximately 9, 18, and 32 mcg/ml, respectively, were obtained at one hour. Although food delays absorption, the total amount of drug absorbed is not affected.

Cephalexin is only 10% to 15% bound to plasma protein. The volume of distribution is 0.26 ± 0.03 L/kg. The drug enters most tissues and body fluids, but fails to achieve therapeutic concentrations in cerebrospinal fluid even in the presence of inflammation. Cephalexin crosses the placenta.

Approximately 90% of a dose is excreted as unchanged drug in the urine within eight hours, primarily by renal tubular secretion. Excretion is delayed by probenecid. The elimination half-life is approximately 50 minutes. The half-life is prolonged in patients with renal impairment and dosage adjustments are required.

DOSAGE AND PREPARATIONS.
Oral: Adults, 1 to 4 g daily in equally divided doses every six hours (maximum, 4 g daily in divided doses). If more than 4 g is needed, a parenteral cephalosporin should be substituted.

Children, 25 to 50 mg/kg daily in equally divided doses every six hours; for severe infections, this dosage may be doubled.

Patients with impaired renal function require modifications in doses and/or frequency of administration depending on the degree of impairment, severity of the infection, and susceptibility of the causative organism. Various dosage recommendations for these patients have been proposed. One recommendation is to increase the dosing interval to 8 to 12 hours when creatinine clearance is between 50 and 10 ml/min and to 24 to 48 hours when creatinine clearance is less than 10 ml/min (The Medical Letter, 1984).

Keflex (Dista). Capsules 250 and 500 mg; drops (pediatric) 100 mg/ml (after reconstitution); suspension 125 and 250 mg/5 ml (after reconstitution); tablets 1 g.

CEPHRADINE
[Anspor, Velosef]

Cephradine is the only cephalosporin currently available in the United States that can be administered both orally and parenterally. Structurally, it is a close congener of cephalexin (see Figure 1).

MECHANISM OF ACTION, ANTIMICROBIAL SPECTRUM, AND RESISTANCE. The mechanism of action, antimicrobial spectrum, and resistance properties are essentially the same as for cephalexin (see that evaluation and the Introduction).

USES. Oral cephradine has the same indications as cephalexin (see that evaluation and the Introduction). Intramuscular or intravenous cephradine has the same indications as cefazolin, but the latter drug frequently is preferred because it achieves higher serum concentrations, has a longer elimination half-life, and causes less pain on intramuscular injection (see the evaluation of Cefazolin Sodium and the Introduction).

ADVERSE REACTIONS AND PRECAUTIONS. Cephradine generally is well tolerated. Gastrointestinal disturbances (eg, diarrhea) and hypersensitivity reactions (eg, skin rash) are most common. For detailed discussion, see the Introduction.

DRUG INTERACTIONS AND INTERFERENCE WITH LABORATORY TESTS. See the Introduction.

PHARMACOKINETICS. Cephradine is stable in gastric acid and is well absorbed when given orally. Following doses of 250 mg, 500 mg, and 1 g, average peak serum concentrations of approximately 9, 17, and 24 mcg/ml, respectively, were obtained within one hour. Although food delays absorption, the total amount of drug absorbed is not affected.

Cephradine also can be administered intramuscularly and intravenously. Peak serum concentrations after intramuscular injection (eg, 5.8 to 6.3 mcg/ml after a 500-mg dose) are actually lower than those obtained by the oral route, but total drug absorbed is the same. Cephradine is absorbed more slowly and serum concentrations are lower in women than in men after injection into the gluteus maximus. A single intravenous dose of 1 g cephradine results in an average peak serum level of 86 mcg/ml after five minutes.

Cephradine is only 10% to 20% bound to plasma protein. The volume of distribution is 0.25 ± 0.01 L/kg. The drug enters most tissues and body fluids, but therapeutic concentrations are not achieved in cerebrospinal fluid even in the presence of inflammation. Cephradine crosses the placenta.

Approximately 90% of a dose is excreted as unchanged drug in the urine within six hours, primarily by renal tubular secretion. Excretion is delayed by probenecid. The serum half-life is approximately 50 minutes. It is prolonged in patients with renal impairment and dosage adjustments are required.

DOSAGE AND PREPARATIONS. Cephradine can be administered orally, intramuscularly deep into a large muscle mass, or intravenously by direct injection or by intermittent or continuous infusion. See the manufacturer's instructions for the appropriate dilution of the drug, compatible diluents and intravenous solutions, and stability of cephradine in these solutions.

Oral: Adults, 1 to 4 g daily in equally divided doses every six hours; *children over 9 months*, 25 to 50 mg/kg daily in equally divided doses every six hours (The Medical Letter, 1984). The maximum daily dosage should not exceed 4 g.

Patients with impaired renal function require modification in doses and/or frequency of administration depending on the degree of impairment, severity of the infection, and susceptibility of the causative organism. Various dosage recommendations for these patients have been proposed. For *adults with impaired renal function*, the manufacturers recommend 500 mg every 6 hours when creatinine clearance is greater than 20 ml/min; 250 mg every 6 hours when creatinine clearance is between 20 and 5 ml/min; and 250 mg every 12 hours when creatinine clearance is less than 5 ml/min. If the patient is on chronic, intermittent hemodialysis, 250 mg should be given at the start of dialysis and 250 mg at 12 hours and 36 to 48 hours after the start of dialysis. Children may require dosage modification proportional to their weight and the severity of infection.

   Anspor (Smith Kline & French), *Velosef* (Squibb). Capsules 250 and 500 mg; suspension 125 and 250 mg/5 ml.

Intravenous, Intramuscular (deep): Adults, 2 to 8 g daily in equally divided doses every four to six hours (The Medical Letter, 1984). The usual daily dosage is 500 mg to 1 g every six hours. In severe infections, up to 8 g daily may be given in divided doses every four to six hours. *Children over 1 year*, 50 to 100 mg/kg daily in equally divided doses every six hours (The Medical Letter, 1984; Nelson, 1985 A).

Patients with impaired renal function require modification in doses and/or frequency of administration depending on the degree of impairment, severity of the infection, and susceptibility of the causative organism. Various dosage recommendations for these patients have been proposed. In *adults with impaired renal function*, the manufacturer recommends an initial loading dose of 750 mg intravenously and maintenance doses of 500 mg intravenously at the time intervals listed below:

Creatinine Clearance	Dosage Interval
>20 ml/min	6-12 hours
15-19 ml/min	12-24 hours
10-14 ml/min	24-40 hours
5-9 ml/min	40-50 hours
<5 ml/min	50-70 hours

From manufacturer's literature

Further modification of the dosage schedule may be necessary in children.

   Velosef (Squibb). Powder (sterile) 250 and 500 mg and 1 g (intramuscular or intravenous) and 2 and 4 g (intravenous only) (sodium 6 mEq/g).

   Velosef for Infusion (Squibb). Powder (sterile, sodium-free) 2 g (intravenous infusion).

CEFADROXIL
[Duricef, Ultracef]

This orally administered first generation cephalosporin is structurally similar to cephalexin (see Figure 1).

MECHANISM OF ACTION, ANTIMICROBIAL SPECTRUM, AND RESISTANCE. The mechanism of action, antimicrobial spectrum, and resistance properties of cefadroxil are essentially the same as for cephalexin (see that evaluation and the Introduction).

USES. Cefadroxil has the same indications as cephalexin (see that evaluation and the Introduction). Elimination of cefadroxil is more prolonged, however, and the longer dosing interval may increase patient compliance.

ADVERSE REACTIONS AND PRECAUTIONS. Cefadroxil generally is well tolerated. Gastrointestinal disturbances (eg, diarrhea) and hypersensitivity reactions (eg, skin rash) are most common. For detailed discussion, see the Introduction.

DRUG INTERACTIONS AND INTERFERENCE WITH LABORATORY TESTS. See the Introduction.

PHARMACOKINETICS. Cefadroxil is stable in gastric acid and is well absorbed following oral administration. Following single doses of 500 mg and 1 g, average peak serum concentrations of approximately 16 and 28 mcg/ml, respectively, were obtained at 1.5 to 2 hours. Absorption does not appear to be affected by the presence of food.

Cefadroxil is only 15% to 20% bound to plasma protein. The apparent volume of distribution is 0.31 L/kg. The drug enters most tissues and body fluids, but therapeutic concentrations are not achieved in cerebrospinal fluid even in the presence of inflammation. Cefadroxil crosses the placenta.

More than 90% of a dose is excreted as unchanged drug in the urine within 24 hours by renal tubular secretion and glomerular filtration. Excretion is delayed by probenecid. The serum half-life of approximately 1.4 hours is somewhat longer than that of cephalexin or cephradine. The half-life is prolonged in patients with renal impairment and dosage adjustments are required.

DOSAGE AND PREPARATIONS.

Oral: Adults, 1 to 2 g daily in equally divided doses every 12 hours or once every 24 hours (*Med Lett Drugs Ther*, 1983 A). The usual dosages recommended by the manufacturer are: for uncomplicated lower urinary tract infections, ie, cystitis, 1 to 2 g daily in a single dose or in divided doses every 12 hours; for all other urinary tract infections, 2 g daily in divided doses every 12 hours; for skin and skin structure infections, 1 g daily as a single dose or in divided doses every 12 hours; for group A, β-hemolytic streptococcal pharyngitis or tonsillitis, 1 g daily in divided doses every 12 hours for 10 days.

Children, 30 mg/kg daily in divided doses every 12 hours. (The Medical Letter, 1984; Nelson, 1985 A).

In patients with impaired renal function, doses and/or frequency of administration must be modified depending on the degree of renal impairment, severity of the infection, and susceptibility of the causative organism. In *adults with renal impairment*, the manufacturers suggest a loading dose of 1 g followed by administration of 500 mg at the following intervals: Mild to moderate impairment (Ccr 50 to 25 ml/min), every 12 hours; moderate to severe impairment (Ccr 25 to 10 ml/min), every 24 hours; severe impairment to essentially no function (Ccr 10 to 0 ml/min), every 36 hours. Patients with a creatinine clearance value of more than 50 ml/min may be considered to have normal renal function for therapeutic purposes.

> *Duricef* (Mead Johnson). Capsules 500 mg; tablets 1 g; suspension 125, 250, and 500 mg/5 ml.
> *Ultracef* (Bristol). Capsules 500 mg; tablets 1 g; suspension 125 and 250 mg/5 ml.

CEFACLOR
[Ceclor]

This orally administered second generation cephalosporin is structurally similar to cephalexin (see Figure 1).

MECHANISM OF ACTION, ANTIMICROBIAL SPECTRUM, AND RESISTANCE. Cefaclor has an in vitro antibacterial spectrum similar to that of the oral first generation cephalosporins, except that it generally is more active against gram-negative bacilli. In particular, it is more active than cephalexin against *Haemophilus influenzae*, including ampicillin-resistant strains; some *H. influenzae* strains are resistant to cefaclor, however (see the evaluation on Cephalexin Monohydrate and the Introduction).

USES. Cefaclor is rarely the drug of choice for the treatment of bacterial infections. It is used primarily in the treatment of acute otitis media and acute sinusitis caused by strains of *H. influenzae* or *Branhamella catarrhalis* that are resistant to amoxicillin, the usual drug of choice. Cefaclor is an alternative to erythromycin/sulfisoxazole, trimethoprim/sulfamethoxazole, and amoxicillin/potassium clavulanate for infections caused by these resistant strains and usually is preferred in patients who are allergic to sulfonamides. For additional discussion, see the Introduction and Chapter 65, Antimicrobial Therapy and Chemoprophylaxis of Infectious Diseases, Table 1.

Similar to oral first generation cephalosporins, cefaclor may be indicated in other mild to moderate infections of the respiratory tract, urinary tract, or skin and skin structures caused by susceptible organisms when preferred agents are ineffective or cannot be tolerated (see the evaluation on Cephalexin Monohydrate and the Introduction).

ADVERSE REACTIONS AND PRECAUTIONS. Cefaclor generally is well tolerated. Gastrointestinal disturbances and hypersensitivity reactions are most common. Serum sickness-like reactions have been reported more frequently with cefaclor than with other cephalosporins (Murray et al, 1980; Ackley and Felsher, 1981; Leng and Anderson, 1985; Levine, 1985). In a large comparative study, the incidences of serum sickness, erythema multiforme, and urticaria were significantly greater in infants and children receiving cefaclor than in those given amoxicillin (Levine, 1985).

For detailed discussion of the adverse reactions and precautions associated with cephalosporin use, see the Introduction.

DRUG INTERACTIONS AND INTERFERENCE WITH LABORATORY TESTS. See the Introduction.

PHARMACOKINETICS. Cefaclor is stable in gastric acid and is well absorbed following oral administration. Following administration of 250 mg, 500 mg, and 1 g doses to fasting subjects, average peak serum levels of approximately 7, 13, and 23 mcg/ml, respectively, were obtained in 30 to 60 minutes. Although the presence of food delays absorption and decreases the peak level by 25% to 50%, the total amount of drug absorbed is not affected.

Cefaclor is only 25% bound to plasma protein. The apparent volume of distribution ranges between 0.24 and 0.36 L/kg. The drug enters most tissues and body fluids, but therapeutic concentrations are not achieved in cerebrospinal fluid even in the presence of inflammation. Cefaclor crosses the placenta.

Between 60% and 85% of a dose is excreted as unchanged drug in the urine within eight hours, primarily by renal tubular secretion. Excretion is delayed by probenecid. The serum half-life ranges from 0.6 to 0.9 hours in patients with normal renal function and is only slightly prolonged in individuals with renal impairment. In those with no renal function, the half-life of cefaclor is 2.3 to 2.8 hours. The drug does not accumulate in such patients because it is unstable in biological fluids.

DOSAGE AND PREPARATIONS.
Oral: Adults, 750 mg to 1.5 g daily in equally divided doses every eight hours (The Medical Letter, 1984). The usual dosage is 250 mg every eight hours; for severe infections or those caused by less susceptible organisms, 500 mg every eight hours. The maximum daily dosage recommended by the manufacturer is 4 g.

Children and infants over 1 month, 20 to 40 mg/kg daily in equally divided doses every eight hours (The Medical Letter, 1984). For otitis media, severe infections, or those caused by less susceptible organisms, the larger dosage (40 mg/kg/day) is recommended. The maximum daily dosage is 1 g.

In patients with impaired renal function, cefaclor usually can be administered without modification of the usual dosage. For patients on hemodialysis, a supplemental dose should be administered after each dialysis session (Norris and Mandell, 1985).

> *Ceclor* (Lilly). Capsules 250 and 500 mg; powder (for oral suspension) 125 and 250 mg/5 ml.

RELATED BETA LACTAM AGENTS

IMIPENEM/CILASTATIN SODIUM
[Primaxin]

Imipenem

Cilastatin

Imipenem is the chemically stable N-formimidoyl derivative of thienamycin, an antibiotic isolated from *Streptomyces cattleya*. It is the first of a new class of β-lactam antibiotics called *carbapenems*. The carbapenems have the 4:5 fused ring lactam of the penicillins with the substitution of carbon for sulfur and the presence of unsaturation in the five-member ring (see Birnbaum et al, 1985; see also Chapter 66, Penicillins). Imipenem has the broadest antibacterial spectrum of any β-lactam antibiotic presently available.

When given alone, imipenem is extensively metabolized by dehydropeptidase-1, a dipeptidase enzyme located in the brush border of proximal renal tubular cells, and very low concentrations of active drug are obtained in the urine. Thus, imipenem is administered in a 1:1 fixed-ratio combination with cilastatin, a specific inhibitor of dehydropeptidase-1. By preventing the metabolism of imipenem, cilastatin significantly increases urinary recovery of active drug. Furthermore, it decreases the renal toxicity (acute tubular necrosis) of imipenem that occurs in experimental animals when the antibiotic is administered alone (see Barza, 1985; Birnbaum et al, 1985).

MECHANISM OF ACTION, ANTIMICROBIAL SPECTRUM, AND RESISTANCE. Imipenem has potent activity against most clinically important species of bacteria, including isolates that are resistant to other antibiotics. It is an inhibitor of bacterial cell wall formation and is rapidly bactericidal against most bacteria that it inhibits. Imipenem exerts its antibacterial effect by binding to critical penicillin binding proteins (PBPs) of susceptible gram-positive and gram-negative bacteria. Unlike the cephalosporins and most penicillins, this antibiotic preferentially binds to PBP-2 of aerobic gram-negative bacilli to produce round cells; it also strongly inhibits PBP-1 resulting in a rapidly lethal effect. Other factors that contribute to the excellent activity of imipenem are its good penetration through the outer membrane of gram-negative bacteria and its marked stability to attack by both plasmid- and chromosomal-mediated β-lactamases of most bacterial species, including strains resistant to other antibiotics (Barza, 1985; Jones, 1985; Kropp et al, 1985; Neu, 1985 B).

Imipenem has excellent activity against most gram-positive bacteria. It is very active against nonpenicillinase- and penicillinase-producing strains of *Staphylococcus aureus* and coagulase-negative staphylococci. Activity against methicillin-resistant staphylococci is variable, however, and many strains are resistant. *Streptococcus pneumoniae* and beta-hemolytic streptococci (eg, *S. pyogenes*) are highly susceptible. Imipenem also is active against penicillin-resistant pneumococci, although the minimal inhibitory concentrations are higher. In contrast to the cephalosporins, *Streptococcus faecalis* (group D enterococci) are inhibited in vitro by imipenem. However, *S. faecium* usually are resistant. This drug also is active in vitro against *Listeria monocytogenes*.

Imipenem is extremely active against most species of gram-negative aerobic bacteria. *Neisseria meningitidis*, *N. gonorrhoeae*, and *Haemophilus influenzae*, including β-lactamase-producing strains of these species, are highly susceptible. The drug is comparable in activity to the most potent third generation cephalosporins against most Enterobacteriaceae (eg, *Escherichia coli*, *Klebsiella*, *Enterobacter*, *Proteus*, *Morganella*, *Providencia*, *Citrobacter*, *Serratia*, *Salmonella*, *Shigella*), including strains that are resistant to antipseudomonal penicillins, aminoglycosides, and third generation cephalosporins. Imipenem has potency similar to that of ceftazidime against *Pseudomonas aeruginosa* and is very active against *Acinetobacter*. However, *Pseudomonas maltophilia* and *P. cepacia* are resistant.

Imipenem is the most active β-lactam antibiotic against clinically important species of anaerobic bacteria (eg, *Bacteroides*, *Fusobacterium*, *Veillonella*, *Peptococcus*, *Peptostreptococcus*, most clostridia), including the *Bacteroides fragilis* group. Its potency is comparable to that of clindamycin and metronidazole. However, *Clostridium difficile*, the cause of pseudomembranous colitis, is only moderately susceptible.

Imipenem also is active in vitro against various other bacteria including *Campylobacter jejuni*, *Yersinia enterocolitica*, *Aeromonas hydrophila*, *Actinomyces* species, *Nocardia asteroides*, and *Legionella*, but it is not known if the drug will be clinically useful for infections caused by these organisms.

For most bacteria, the minimum bactericidal concentration (MBC) of imipenem is similar to the minimum inhibitory concentration (MIC). However, the MBC may be much higher than the MIC for *Streptococcus faecalis* (enterococci), methicillin-resistant strains of *Staphylococcus aureus* and *S. epidermidis*, *Listeria monocytogenes*, and some strains of *Pseudomonas aeruginosa*. The combination of imipenem plus an aminoglycoside frequently is synergistic in vitro against *S. faecalis*, *S. aureus*, and *L. monocytogenes* organisms that show a difference between inhibition and killing, although the clinical significance is unclear. In one study (Indrelie et al, 1984), the synergistic activity in vitro against enterococci of imipenem plus an aminoglycoside was significantly less than for penicillin G plus an aminoglycoside. Against *P. aeruginosa* and the Enterobacteriaceae, in vitro synergism with imipenem and an aminoglycoside has been infrequent in most reported studies.

Unlike many β-lactam antibiotics, the effect of increasing inoculum concentration on imipenem susceptibility is minimal for most bacteria.

Because of its marked stability to practically all known β-lactamases, resistance to imipenem by this mechanism is very rare. The drug is hydrolyzed by a β-lactamase from *Pseudomonas maltophilia*, and two strains of *Bacteroides fragilis* were reported to have β-lactamases that inactivate imipenem.

Imipenem is a good inducer of Type I β-lactamases present in certain gram-negative bacilli, such as *Enterobacter cloacae* and *Pseudomonas aeruginosa*. In contrast to the decreased antibacterial activity that results when cephamycins or amino-thiazolyl cephalosporins induce β-lactamases, the strains with increased β-lactamase are not resistant to imipenem. However, they are resistant to cephalosporins and penicillins. These properties may account for both the general lack of cross-resistance of imipenem with other β-lactam antibiotics as well as the in vitro antagonism frequently observed when imipenem is combined with another β-lactam agent.

Occasional strains of *Serratia marcescens* and *Enterobacter cloacae* are resistant to imipenem. The mechanisms are unclear but may be related to decreased permeability. Imipenem-resistant strains of *Pseudomonas aeruginosa* have emerged during therapy. These strains may be susceptible to other antipseudomonal antibiotics (eg, antipseudomonal penicillins, third generation cephalosporins, aminoglycosides).

For additional discussion of the mechanism of action, antimicrobial spectrum, and resistance properties of imipenem, see Barza, 1985; Jones, 1985; Kropp et al, 1985; Neu, 1985 B.

USES. Imipenem/cilastatin has been effective, frequently as empiric monotherapy, in a wide variety of serious infections caused by gram-positive cocci, aerobic gram-negative bacilli, and anaerobic bacteria; many of these infections were of nosocomial origin and were caused by bacterial strains that were resistant to other antibiotics (see Barza, 1985; Wang et al, 1985). These include lower respiratory tract infections (Acar, 1985; Salata et al, 1985), intra-abdominal infections (Kager and Nord, 1985; Solomkin et al, 1985), obstetric and gynecologic infections (Berkeley et al, 1985; Sweet, 1985), complicated urinary tract infections (Cox and Corrado, 1985; Sheehan and Ronald, 1985), skin and soft tissue infections (Fass et al, 1985; Marier, 1985), osteomyelitis (MacGregor and Gentry, 1985), endocarditis primarily caused by *Staphylococcus aureus* (Dickinson et al, 1985; Donabedian and Freimer, 1985), and bacteremias (Eron, 1985). In randomized, comparative clinical trials, imipenem/cilastatin has compared favorably to moxalactam (Eron et al, 1983; Calandra et al, 1984), cefotaxime (Baumgartner and Glauser, 1983; Diaz-Mitoma et al, 1985), and the combination of clindamycin plus gentamicin (Report from a Scandinavian Study Group, 1984; Guerra et al, 1985; Solomkin et al, 1985) for the treatment of serious infections.

The exact role of imipenem/cilastatin in infectious disease therapy has not yet been defined. However, this new drug may be particularly useful in the treatment of infections caused by mixtures of bacteria for which a combination of antibiotics, often including an aminoglycoside, would otherwise be necessary. Examples include pulmonary, intra-abdominal, and soft tissue infections. The good activity of imipenem/cilastatin against the *Bacteroides fragilis* group and enterococci when compared to third generation cephalosporins appears to make it preferable for the treatment of mixed intra-abdominal infections (see Barza, 1985; Neu, 1985 C). Because resistant strains of *Pseudomonas aeruginosa* frequently have emerged during therapy with imipenem/cilastatin (Acar, 1985; Eron, 1985; Iannini et al, 1985; Marier, 1985; Salata et al, 1985; Trumbore et al, 1985), its use alone for serious infections caused by this pathogen probably should be avoided (Barza, 1985). The role of imipenem/cilastatin in the treatment of meningitis; febrile, neutropenic cancer patients; and enterococcal endocarditis remains to be established (Barza, 1985).

ADVERSE REACTIONS AND PRECAUTIONS. Based on a review of 2,516 clinical trial patients, imipenem/cilastatin (dosage range, 1 to 4 g of each component daily) generally has been well tolerated and its adverse reaction profile resembles that of most other β-lactam antibiotics (Calandra et al, 1985).

Hypersensitivity reactions were observed in 2.7% of patients and included drug fever, pruritus, urticaria, and other rashes; anaphylactic reactions were not reported. However, the incidence of allergic reactions to imipenem/cilastatin could actually be higher because all patients with a history of serious allergy to β-lactam antibiotics were excluded from clinical trials. Of 12 patients with a history of nonanaphylactic hypersensitivity reactions to penicillins, imipenem/cilastatin produced allergic manifestations in two patients.

The most common clinical adverse reactions to imipenem/cilastatin were those involving the gastrointestinal tract. Drug-related nausea and vomiting were observed in 1.3% and 0.9% of patients, respectively. In some patients, a syndrome characterized by nausea and vomiting and accompanied by hypotension, dizziness, and sweating has been associated with rapid intravenous infusion of imipenem/cilastatin. However, this syndrome is unpredictable in that slowing the rate of infusion does not always solve the problem. In such cases, the drug may have to be discontinued.

Diarrhea occurred in about 3.3% of patients who received imipenem/cilastatin. *Clostridium difficile* or its toxin was reported in 0.76% of patients and actual pseudomembranous colitis, diagnosed by colonoscopy, occurred in four patients (0.16%).

Local adverse reactions at the site of infusion, usually phlebitis/thrombophlebitis, were considered to be drug related in about 2% of patients.

Seizures were reported in about 1% of patients receiving imipenem/cilastatin, but were considered drug-related in only seven patients (0.3%). Most patients who experienced seizures were elderly, had predisposing factors (eg, head injury, intracranial neoplasm, prior history of convulsions, alcoholism) and were severely ill at the time of treatment. Furthermore, most of these patients had renal insufficiency and may have received a relatively high dose of drug. Seizures seemed to respond to a reduction in dosage or discontinuation of imipenem/cilastatin therapy, and to treatment with diphenylhydantoin or benzodiazepines. Whether imipenem/cilastatin is more epileptogenic than other β-lactam antibiotics is unknown. Caution is recommended in patients at increased risk for convulsions (eg, epileptics). Dosages of imipenem/cilastatin greater than 2 g daily are not recommended in patients with renal insufficiency (Barza, 1985).

Imipenem/cilastatin has not been associated with nephrotoxicity or coagulopathies.

Among severely ill patients, the incidences of colonization with resistant bacteria and fungi were 3.2% and 8%, respectively. The incidence of actual superinfections were 2.8% for bacteria, usually *Pseudomonas aeruginosa* or *P. maltophilia*, and 1.5% for *Candida*.

Laboratory abnormalities associated with the use of imipenem/cilastatin appear to be relatively mild and reversible. Most common were transient elevations in liver function values, including aspartate aminotransferase (1.1%), alanine aminotransferase (1.2%), and alkaline phosphatase (0.8%). Eosinophilia and positive direct Coombs' test results have been observed. However, hemolytic anemia has not occurred. Reversible neutropenia, thrombocytopenia, and hypoprothrombinemia have been reported rarely. Thrombocytosis was observed in 15 patients (0.6%).

Despite its broad antimicrobial spectrum, the impact of imipenem/cilastatin on the fecal flora has been modest. This probably is due to the limited biliary secretion of this drug (Nord et al, 1985; Wexler and Finegold, 1985).

Use of imipenim/cilastatin in pregnant women has not been established. It is classified in FDA Pregnancy Category C.

PHARMACOKINETICS. When imipenem is administered alone by the intravenous route, the levels excreted in the urine are low and variable (6% to 38% of the dose) between subjects because of renal inactivation. Thus, this new carbapenem antibiotic is coadministered with an equal amount of cilastatin, a dehydropeptidase-1 inhibitor.

Neither imipenem nor cilastatin is appreciably absorbed following oral administration and, therefore, must be given by a parenteral route. Mean plasma concentrations after a 30-minute intravenous infusion of 1 g of each drug were 52 and 65 mcg/ml, respectively. Six hours later, these values had fallen to 1 mcg or less per milliliter.

Approximately 20% of circulating imipenem is bound to plasma protein. The drug is well distributed into most tissues and body fluids. In patients with meningitis, cerebrospinal fluid concentrations ranged between 0.5 and 11 mcg/ml following administration of 1 g every six hours for four doses (Modai et al, 1984), suggesting that this agent may be useful for bacterial meningitis. Concentrations of imipenem in bile generally are low due to limited biliary excretion. Urinary concentrations are high. No data are available regarding drug concentrations in milk, placenta, or fetal tissue.

When coadministered with cilastatin, about 70% of a dose of imipenem is excreted as unchanged drug in urine; both glomerular filtration and renal tubular secretion are involved. The remainder is eliminated non-renally, primarily by metabolic inactivation. Approximately 75% of cilastatin also is recov-

ered as unchanged drug in urine. The remainder appears to be metabolized and 12% of a dose is recovered in urine as N-acetyl cilastatin, the major metabolite. Less than 1% of imipenem or cilastatin is excreted in the feces. The elimination half-lives of both imipenem and cilastatin are about one hour in patients with normal renal function. In patients with renal failure, the half-life of imipenem increases to 3.5 to 4 hours and the half-life of cilastatin increases to 16 hours; dosage adjustments are necessary. Both drugs are substantially removed by hemodialysis; the half-lives are 2.5 hours for imipenem and 3.8 hours for cilastatin. Supplemental dosing after hemodialysis is necessary.

For additional discussion, see Barza, 1985; Drusano and Standiford, 1985; Gibson et al, 1985; Rogers et al, 1985.

DOSAGE AND PREPARATIONS. The dosages listed refer to the amount of imipenem to be administered; an equal amount of cilastatin will also be present in the solution. The drug is infused intravenously over 20 to 60 minutes, depending on the dose. See the manufacturer's instructions for the appropriate dilution of the drug, compatible diluents and intravenous solutions, and the stability of imipenem/cilastatin in these solutions.

Intravenous: Adults, 2 g daily in equally divided doses every six hours is expected to be the usual dosage. Up to 4 g daily may be given for life-threatening infections or for infections caused by less susceptible organisms (Barza, 1985).

The following dosing schedule for adults with normal renal function is recommended by the manufacturer:

Type or Severity of Infection	Gram-positive Organisms Anaerobes Highly Susceptible Gram-negative Organisms	Other Gram-negative Organisms
Mild	250 mg q6h	500 mg q6h
Moderate	500 mg q8h–500 mg q6h	500 mg q6h–1 g q8h
Severe, life-threatening	500 mg q6h	1 g q8h–1 g q6h
Uncomplicated urinary tract infection	250 mg q6h	250 mg q6h
Complicated urinary tract infection	500 mg q6h	500 mg q6h

(Maximum daily dosage not to exceed 50 mg/kg/day or 4 g/day, whichever is lower.)
From manufacturer's literature

For *adults with impaired renal function*, the following dosages (based on a body weight of 70 kg) have been recommended by the manufacturer:

Creatinine Clearance (ml/min/ 1.73 m²)	Renal Function	Less Severe Infections or Presence of Highly Susceptible Organisms	Life Threatening Infections— Maximum Dosage
30-70	Mild impairment	500 mg q8h	500 mg q6h
20-30	Moderate impairment	500 mg q12h	500 mg q8h
5-20	Severe to marked impairment	250 mg q12h	500 mg q12h
0-5	None, but on hemodialysis	250 mg q12h	500 mg q12h

From manufacturer's literature

A supplemental dose of imipenem/cilastatin should be given after each hemodialysis session unless the next dose is scheduled within four hours.

Primaxin (Merck, Sharp & Dohme). Powder (sterile) 250 and 500 mg (equivalent to imipenem component).

AZTREONAM
[Azactam]

Aztreonam is the first of a new class of β-lactam antimicrobial agents called *monobactams* to be investigated for clinical use. Unlike the penicillins, cephalosporins, and carbapenems, which have fused double-ring nuclei, the monobactams are monocyclic β-lactam agents containing 3-aminomonobactamic acid as the basic nucleus (see following Figure 2).

The first monobactams to be discovered were naturally occurring compounds isolated from bacteria (eg, *Gluconobacter, Acetobacter, Chromobacterium*), but they exhibited poor antibacterial properties. In contrast, aztreonam is a totally synthetic monobactam that has been chemically engineered (principally by the addition of an aminothiazole oxime side chain with an added carboxylic acid group at the 3-position and an α-methyl group at the 4-position) to have potent activity against aerobic gram-negative bacteria, including *Pseudomonas aeruginosa*, and excellent stability to β-lactamases (Sykes and Bonner, 1985; see also Chapter 66, Penicillins; Figure 1; and the evaluation on Imipenem/Cilastatin Sodium).

MECHANISM OF ACTION, ANTIMICROBIAL SPECTRUM, AND RESISTANCE. Similar to other classes of β-lactam antibiotics, aztreonam is an inhibitor of bacterial cell wall formation. This antimicrobial agent readily traverses the outer membrane barrier of aerobic gram-negative bacteria and has a high affinity for penicillin binding protein 3 (PBP-3). This interaction causes filamentation of bacteria, inhibition of cell division, and, ultimately, cell death. Bactericidal concentrations of aztreonam are closely associated with inhibitory concentrations. In contrast to its effect on aerobic gram-negative bacteria, aztreonam fails to bind appreciably to essential PBPs of gram-positive or anaerobic bacteria.

Aztreonam exhibits a narrow spectrum of antimicrobial activity in that it is active solely against aerobic gram-negative bacteria. *Neisseria meningitidis, N. gonorrhoeae,* and *Haemophilus influenzae,* including β-lactamase-producing strains of these species, are highly susceptible. Aztreonam has potency comparable to that of third generation cephalosporins against most Enterobacteriaceae (eg, *Escherichia coli, Klebsiella, Enterobacter, Proteus, Morganella, Providencia, Citrobacter, Serratia, Salmonella, Shigella*), including strains that are resistant to penicillins, older cephalosporins, and aminoglycosides. Aztreonam also is active against most strains of *Pseudomonas aeruginosa,* including strains that are resistant to other antipseudomonal antibiotics (eg, antipseudomonal penicillins, aminoglycosides). Its potency against this organism is similar to that of ceftazidime. Aztreonam has poor activity against other *Pseudomonas* species, however, and is not active against *Acinetobacter*.

As can be expected from its poor interaction with PBPs of gram-positive bacteria and anaerobes, aztreonam is inactive against these organisms.

Like most third generation cephalosporins, aztreonam possesses a high degree of resistance to enzymatic hydrolysis by most common plasmid- and chromosomal-mediated β-lactamases. However, as with these other agents, resistance to aztreonam can occur among certain nonfastidious gram-negative bacilli, particularly *Enterobacter, Serratia,* and *Pseudomonas,* due to inducible Type I chromosomal β-lactamases that appear to tightly bind and, therefore, inactivate (nonhydrolytic) the drug. Aztreonam has been reported to be a poor inducer of Type I β-lactamases of certain gram-negative bacilli (eg, *Enterobacter cloacae, Proteus*) when compared to cefoxitin and some third generation cephalosporins (see Sykes and Bonner, 1985), but the clinical significance of this observation remains to be determined.

The effect of increasing inoculum concentration on aztreonam susceptibility generally is small for most susceptible bacteria. Unlike the aminoglycosides, the activity of aztreonam is not decreased in an anaerobic or acidic environment.

The narrow spectrum of aztreonam will encourage use of

the drug in combination with other antibiotics to expand antimicrobial coverage during empiric therapy or for mixed infections. The in vitro activities of nafcillin, cloxacillin, erythromycin, or vancomycin against gram-positive bacteria and of clindamycin or metronidazole against various anaerobic bacteria were not inhibited by combination with aztreonam. Additive or indifferent responses usually were observed. When aztreonam was combined with gentamicin, tobramycin, or amikacin, synergistic activity against a high percentage of strains of *P. aeruginosa* has been reported (see Sykes and Bonner, 1985).

For additional discussion of the mechanism of action, antimicrobial spectrum, and resistance properties of aztreonam, see Neu, 1984 B; Guay and Koskoletos, 1985; Hopefl, 1985; Sykes and Bonner, 1985.

USES. Aztreonam has been effective in serious gram-negative aerobic bacillary infections; many of these were of nosocomial origin and were caused by bacterial strains that were resistant to other antibiotics (Giamarellou et al, 1984; Greenberg et al, 1984; Torres and Ramírez-Ronda, 1984; Childs, 1985; Pastorek et al, 1985; Pribyl et al, 1985; Scully and Neu, 1985; Simons and Lee, 1985; see also Guay and Koskoletos, 1985; Henry and Bendush, 1985). These include complicated urinary tract, lower respiratory tract, skin and skin structure, obstetric and gynecologic, intra-abdominal, and bone and joint infections and bacteremias. When necessary, aztreonam was combined with another antimicrobial agent (eg, antistaphylococcal penicillin, vancomycin, clindamycin, metronidazole) to expand the antimicrobial spectrum for mixed infections or empiric therapy.

Presently, clinical experience with aztreonam is limited and its ultimate role in infectious disease therapy is unclear. The antimicrobial activity of this monobactam is very similar to that of the aminoglycosides. In a limited number of randomized, controlled clinical trials, aztreonam was shown to be more effective than tobramycin for nosocomial gram-negative pneumonias (Schentag et al, 1985) and as effective as gentamicin for serious gram-negative urinary tract infections (Sattler et al, 1984). The combination of aztreonam plus clindamycin was similar in efficacy to tobramycin plus clindamycin for serious lower respiratory tract infections caused by aerobic gram-negative bacilli (Rodriguez et al, 1985) and to gentamicin plus clindamycin for endometritis after cesarean section (Gibbs et al, 1985). Thus, aztreonam appears to be a potentially less toxic alternative to the aminoglycosides for serious gram-negative bacillary infections, particularly in patients at high risk for aminoglycoside toxicity and for those requiring prolonged therapy. However, additional studies comparing aztreonam to aminoglycosides as well as to third generation cephalosporins, particularly ceftazidime, and imipenem/cilastatin are necessary before making definite conclusions (see Guay and Koskoletos, 1985; Neu, 1985 D; see also Chapter 70, Aminoglycosides, the Introduction, and these evaluations). The role of aztreonam in gram-negative bacillary meningitis and in febrile neutropenic patients remains to be established (Neu, 1985 D).

ADVERSE REACTIONS AND PRECAUTIONS. Based on a review of 2,117 clinical trial patients, aztreonam generally has been well tolerated and its adverse reaction profile resembles that of most other β-lactam antibiotics (Henry and Bendush, 1985).

Pain and phlebitis at the intravenous injection site was the most frequent adverse effect, occurring in 2.4% of patients. Mild gastrointestinal upset was observed in less than 2% of patients; nausea (0.8%) and diarrhea (0.7%) were most common. Only one case of *Clostridium difficile*-associated diarrhea was reported; the patient had received prior antibiotics.

Rash occurred in 1.5% of patients treated with aztreonam. Of 134 patients with a history of allergy to penicillin and/or cephalosporins, only one developed a possible IgE-mediated urticarial rash. The potential for immunological cross-reactivity between aztreonam and the penicillin and cephalosporin classes of antibiotics has been investigated. Studies in rabbits have demonstrated negligible cross-reactivity between antiaztreonam and antibenzylpenicillin and anticephalothin antibodies (Adkinson et al, 1984; Saxon et al, 1985). Studies in humans showed that none of 41 patients with documented IgE-reactive skin tests to various penicillin determinants concurrently demonstrated reproducible reactivity to any aztreonam reagents (Saxon et al, 1984, 1985). Although caution is warranted, these results indicate that there is very little cross-reactivity between the monobactam, aztreonam, and other β-lactam antibiotics.

Aztreonam has not been associated with nephrotoxicity, neurotoxicity, or coagulopathies.

Superinfections were reported in 9.7% of patients receiving aztreonam; about 40% of these required specific therapy. The most frequently encountered pathogens were enterococci (Henry and Bendush, 1985). Enterococcal colonization or superinfection in the urinary tract of patients receiving aztreonam has been observed frequently in some clinical studies (Chandrasekar et al, 1984; Sattler et al, 1984).

Laboratory abnormalities associated with the use of aztreonam appear to be relatively mild and reversible. Transient elevations in serum concentrations of hepatic transaminases (SGOT, SGPT) were most frequently reported; the average incidence was 4% for all clinical trial patients (Henry and Bendush, 1985), but was as high as 36% in one study (Greenberg et al, 1984).

The impact of aztreonam on the fecal flora is primarily directed against facultative gram-negative bacilli (eg, Enterobacteriaceae) with lesser effects on strict anaerobic bacteria (Jones et al, 1984; de Vries-Hospers et al, 1984).

DRUG INTERACTIONS. Concurrent administration of aztreonam with cephradine, clindamycin, gentamicin, metronidazole, or nafcillin in 48 healthy male volunteers resulted in no clinically significant pharmacokinetic drug interactions (Creasey et al, 1984).

PHARMACOKINETICS. Aztreonam is not absorbed following oral administration and must be administered intramuscularly or intravenously. Bioavailability after intramuscular injection is 100%. Peak serum concentrations obtained after intramuscular and bolus intravenous injections of 1 g are 46 mcg/ml (after 60 minutes) and 125 mcg/ml, respectively. Following intravenous infusion of 1 g over a 30-minute period, peak serum levels of 164 mcg/ml are achieved.

Approximately 56% of circulating aztreonam is bound to plasma protein. Apparent volumes of distribution ranging from 0.11 to 0.18 L/kg have been reported, indicating distribution to the extracellular water space. Aztreonam has been shown to distribute into a variety of tissues and body fluids, including synovial and blister fluids, bronchial secretions, bone, and bile. High concentrations are obtained in urine. Aztreonam has been shown to penetrate the uninflamed prostate (Madsen et al, 1984) and uninflamed or inflamed meninges (Duma et al, 1984) to achieve concentrations that are likely to be higher than the minimal inhibitory concentrations for most Enterobacteriaceae. Concentrations attained in cerebrospinal fluid of patients with inflamed meninges were, on the average, fourfold greater than those obtained in the absence of inflammation. Aztreonam crosses the placenta.

About 65% to 70% of a dose of aztreonam is excreted in the urine as unchanged drug by glomerular filtration and tubular secretion; probenecid delays excretion. About 7% of a dose is metabolized and the metabolite is also eliminated in urine. Only 1% of a dose is recovered as unchanged drug in feces. The elimination half-life of aztreonam in adults with normal renal function is 1.7 hours (range 1.6 to 2.1 hours). A similar half-life is observed in pediatric patients over 1 month; in newborns, the half-life ranges from 2.5 hours in those weighing more than 2.5 kg to 5.7 hours in those weighing less than 2.5 kg (Stutman et al, 1984).

In patients with impaired renal function, the elimination half-life of aztreonam is prolonged (eg, to six hours in renal failure) and dosage adjustments are necessary. About 50% of the drug is removed during hemodialysis and supplemental dosing is required. Total body clearance of aztreonam decreases by 20% to 25% in patients with alcoholic cirrhosis and dosage adjustments may be necessary (eg, when therapy is prolonged).

For additional discussion of pharmacokinetics, see Swabb et al, 1981, 1983; Scully et al, 1983; Guay and Koskoletos, 1985; Swabb, 1985.

DOSAGE AND PREPARATIONS.

Intramuscular, Intravenous: *Adults,* 1 to 8 g daily in divided doses every six to 12 hours has been the dosage range used in study protocols (see Guay and Koskoletos, 1985). Dosages most frequently used in clinical trials for moderate to severe infections are 1 g every eight to 12 hours; for severe or life-threatening infections, 2 g every six to eight hours (see Hopefl, 1985).

For *adults with impaired renal function,* the following dosage guidelines have been suggested (Fillastre et al, 1985): Following a normal loading dose, administer maintenance doses equal to 50% (creatinine clearance, 80 to 30 ml/min), 33% (creatinine clearance, 29 to 10 ml/min), or 25% (creatinine clearance, <10 ml/min) of the normal dose at regular dosage intervals. Alternatively, administer the normal dose at two times (creatinine clearance, 80 to 30 ml/min), three times (creatinine clearance, 29 to 10 ml/min), or four times (creatinine clearance, <10 ml/min) the normal dosage interval. Patients requiring hemodialysis should, in addition, receive half their maintenance dose after each dialysis session.

Azactam (Squibb).
(Investigational drug)

Cited References

Antimicrobial prophylaxis for surgery. *Med Lett Drugs Ther* 23:77-80, 1981.

Choice of cephalosporins. *Med Lett Drugs Ther* 25:57-60, 1983 A.

Cefoperazone sodium (Cefobid). *Med Lett Drugs Ther* 25:29-30, 1983 B.

Cefuroxime sodium (Zinacef). *Med Lett Drugs Ther* 26:15-16, 1984 A.

Ceforanide (Precef). *Med Lett Drugs Ther* 26:91-92, 1984 B.

Cefonicid sodium (Monocid). *Med Lett Drugs Ther* 26:71-72, 1984 C.

Drugs for anaerobic infections. *Med Lett Drugs Ther* 26:87-89, 1984 D.

Ceftriaxone sodium (Rocephin). *Med Lett Drugs Ther* 27:37-39, 1985 A.

Ceftazidime (Fortaz). *Med Lett Drugs Ther* 27:85-87, 1985 B.

Antimicrobial prophylaxis for surgery. *Med Lett Drugs Ther* 27:105-108, 1985 C.

1985 STD treatment guidelines. *Morbid Mortal Week Rep* 34(suppl):75S-108S, 1985.

Acar JF: Therapy for lower respiratory tract infection with imipenem/cilastatin: Review of worldwide experience. *Rev Infect Dis* 7(suppl 3):S513-S517, 1985.

Ackley AM Jr, Felsher J: Adverse reactions to cefaclor. *South Med J* 74:1550, 1981.

Adkinson NF Jr, et al: Immunology of monobactam aztreonam. *Antimicrob Agents Chemother* 25:93-97, 1984.

Alestig K, et al: Effect of cefoperazone on faecal flora. *J Antimicrob Chemother* 12:163-167, 1983.

Amsterdam D: Editorial comment. *Antimicrob Newslett* 1:32-33, 1984.

Andrassy K, et al: Hypoprothrombinemia caused by cephalosporins. *J Antimicrob Chemother* 12:133-136, 1985.

Au JP, Geiger GS: Thrombocytopenia associated with moxalactam administration. *Drug Intell Clin Pharm* 18:140-143, 1984.

Bach MC: Prolonged bleeding time associated with 'low-dose' moxalactam therapy, (letter). *JAMA* 251:3082, 1984.

Balant L, et al: Clinical pharmacokinetics of third generation cephalosporins. *Clin Pharmacokinet* 10:101-143, 1985.

Bang NU, Kammer RB: Hematologic complications associated with β-lactam antibiotics. *Rev Infect Dis* 5(suppl 2):S380-S393, 1983.

Barriere SL: Ceftriaxone: Beta-lactamase-stable, broad-spectrum cephalosporin with extended half-life, (commentary). *Pharmacotherapy* 5:252-253, 1985.

Barriere SL, Flaherty JF: Third generation cephalosporins: Critical evaluation. *Clin Pharm* 3:351-373, 1984.

Barriere SL, Mills J: Ceforanide: Antibacterial activity, pharmacology, and clinical efficacy. *Pharmacotherapy* 2:322-327, 1982.

Barson WJ, et al: Prospective comparative trial of ceftriaxone vs conventional therapy for treatment of bacterial meningitis in children. *Pediatr Infect Dis* 4:362-368, 1985.

Barza M: Imipenem: First of new class of beta-lactam antibiotics. *Ann Intern Med* 103:552-560, 1985.

Baumgartner JD, Glauser MP: Comparative study of imipenem in severe infections. *J Antimicrob Chemother* 12(suppl D):141-148, 1983.

Beam TR Jr: Third generation cephalosporins, parts I and II. *Ration Drug Ther* 16:1-6 (June), 1-5 (July), 1982.

Beam TR Jr: Ceftriaxone: Beta-lactamase-stable, broad spectrum cephalosporin with extended half-life. *Pharmacotherapy* 5:237-253, 1985.

Benet LZ, Sheiner LB: Design and optimization of dosage regimens. Pharmacokinetic data, in Gilman AG, et al (eds): *The Pharmacological Basis of Therapeutics*, ed 7. New York, MacMillan, 1985, 1663-1733.

Bennett WM, et al: Drug prescribing in renal failure: Dosing guidelines for adults. *Am J Kidney Dis* 3:155-193, 1983.

Berkeley AS, et al: Imipenem/cilastatin in treatment of obstetric and gynecologic infections. *Am J Med* 78(suppl 6A):79-84, 1985.

Bertino JS Jr, Speck WT: Cephalosporin antibiotics. *Pediatr Clin North Am* 30:17-26, 1983.

Birnbaum J, et al: Carbapenems, new class of beta-lactam antibiotics: Discovery and development of imipenem/cilastatin. *Am J Med* 78(suppl 6A):3-21, 1985.

Blumer JL, et al: Ceftazidime therapy in patients with cystic fibrosis and multiply-drug-resistant *Pseudomonas*. *Am J Med* 79(suppl 2A):37-46, 1985.

Bodey GP, et al: Comparative in vitro study of new cephalosporins. *Antimicrob Agents Chemother* 20:226-230, 1981.

Brandstetter RD, et al: Moxalactam disodium-induced pulmonary hemorrhage. *Chest* 86:644-645, 1984.

Brooks GF, Barriere SL: Clinical use of new beta-lactam drugs: Practical considerations for physicians, microbiology laboratories, pharmacists, and formulary committees. *Ann Intern Med* 98:530-535, 1983.

Bryan JP, et al: Comparison of ceftriaxone and ampicillin plus chloramphenicol for therapy of acute bacterial meningitis. *Antimicrob Agents Chemother* 28:361-368, 1985.

Buening MK, et al: Disulfiram-like reaction to β-lactams, (letter). *JAMA* 245:2027-2028, 1981.

Burnakis TG: Surgical antimicrobial prophylaxis: Principles and guidelines. *Pharmacotherapy* 4:248-271, 1984.

Calandra GB, et al: Multiclinic randomized study of comparative efficacy, safety and tolerance of imipenem/cilastatin and moxalactam. *Eur J Clin Microbiol* 3:478-487, 1984.

Calandra GB, et al: Review of adverse experiences and tolerability in first 2,516 patients treated with imipenem/cilastatin. *Am J Med* 78(suppl 6A):73-78, 1985.

Carlberg H, et al: Intestinal side effects of cefoperazone. *J Antimicrob Chemother* 10:483-487, 1982.

Carmine AA, et al: Cefotaxime: Review of its antimicrobial activity, pharmacological properties and therapeutic use. *Drugs* 25:223-289, 1983 A.

Carmine AA, et al: Moxalactam (latamoxef): Review of its antibacterial activity, pharmacokinetic properties, and therapeutic use. *Drugs* 26:279-333, 1982 B.

Chambers HF, et al: Failure of once-daily regimen of cefonicid for treatment of endocarditis due to *Staphylococcus aureus*. *Rev Infect Dis* 6(suppl 4):S870-S874, 1984.

Chandrasekar PH, et al: Enterococcal superinfection and colonization with aztreonam therapy. *Antimicrob Agents Chemother* 26:280-282, 1984.

Cherubin CE, et al: Treatment of gram-negative bacillary meningitis: Role of new cephalosporin antibiotics. *Rev Infect Dis* 4(suppl):S453-S464, 1982.

Childs SJ: Aztreonam in treatment of urinary tract infection. *Am J Med* 78(suppl 2A):44-46, 1985.

Chin N, Neu HC: Cefotaxime and desacetylcefotaxime: Example of advantageous antimicrobial metabolism. *Diagn Microbiol Infect Dis* 2:21S-31S, 1984.

Chow AW, Jewesson PJ: Pharmacokinetics and safety of antimicrobial agents during pregnancy. *Rev Infect Dis* 7:287-313, 1985.

Cleeland R, Squires E: Antimicrobial activity of ceftriaxone: Review. *Am J Med* 77(suppl 4C):3-11, 1984.

Cohen MS, et al: Multicenter clinical trial of cefoperazone sodium in the United States. *Am J Med* 77(suppl 1B):35-41, 1984.

Collier AC, et al: Comparative study of ceftriaxone and spectinomycin in the treatment of uncomplicated gonorrhea in women. *Am J Med* 77(suppl 4C):68-72, 1984.

Cone LA, et al: Ceftazidime versus tobramycin-ticarcillin in treatment of pneumonia and bacteremia. *Antimicrob Agents Chemother* 28:33-36, 1985.

Congeni BL: Comparison of ceftriaxone and traditional therapy of bacterial meningitis. *Antimicrob Agents Chemother* 25:40-44, 1984.

Conly JM, et al: Hyperprothrombinemia in febrile, neutropenic patients with cancer: Association with antimicrobial suppression of intestinal microflora. *J Infect Dis* 150:202-212, 1984.

Conte JE Jr, et al: *Antibiotic Prophylaxis in Surgery: Comprehensive Review*. Philadelphia, JB Lippincott, 1984.

Cooper RH, et al: Evaluation of ceforanide as treatment for staphylococcal and streptococcal endocarditis. *Antimicrob Agents Chemother* 19:256-259, 1981.

Corrado ML, et al: Designing appropriate therapy in treatment of gram-negative bacillary meningitis. *JAMA* 248:71-74, 1982.

Cox CE, Corrado ML: Safety and efficacy of imipenem/cilastatin in treatment of complicated urinary tract infections. *Am J Med* 78(suppl 6A):92-94, 1985.

Creasey WA, et al: Pharmacokinetic interaction of aztreonam with other antibiotics. *J Clin Pharmacol* 24:174-180, 1984.

Darbyshire PJ, et al: Ceftazidime in treatment of febrile immunosuppressed children. *J Antimicrob Chemother* 12(suppl 2A):357-360, 1983.

Del Rio M, et al: Ceftriaxone versus ampicillin and chloramphenicol for treatment of bacterial meningitis in children. *Lancet* 1:1241-1244, 1983.

dePauw BE, et al: Randomized study of ceftazidime versus gentamicin plus cefotaxime for infections in severe granulocytopenic patients. *J Antimicrob Chemother* 12(suppl A):93-99, 1983.

de Vries-Hospers HG, et al: Selective decontamination of digestive tract with aztreonam: Study of 10 health volunteers. *J Infect Dis* 150:636-642, 1984.

Diaz-Mitoma F, et al: Prospective, randomized comparison of imipenem/cilastatin and cefotaxime for treatment of lung, soft tissue, and renal infections. *Rev Infect Dis* 7(suppl 3):S452-S457, 1985.

Dickinson G, et al: Efficacy of imipenem/cilastatin in endocarditis. *Am J Med* 78(suppl 6A):117-121, 1985.

DiPiro JT, et al: Antimicrobial prophylaxis in surgery, parts 1 and 2. *Am J Hosp Pharm* 38:320-334, 487-494, 1981.

DiPiro JT, et al: Prophylactic use of antimicrobials in surgery. *Curr Probl Surg* 20:69-132, 1983.

DiPiro JT, et al: Prophylactic parenteral cephalosporins in surgery: Are newer agents better? *JAMA* 252:3277-3279, 1984.

Donabedian H, Freimer EN: Pathogenesis and treatment of endocarditis. *Am J Med* 78(suppl 6A):127-133, 1985.

Drusano GL, Standiford HC: Pharmacokinetic profile of imipenem/cilastatin in normal volunteers. *Am J Med* 78(suppl 6A):47-53, 1985.

Dudley MN, et al: Review of cefonicid, long-acting cephalosporin. *Clin Pharm* 3:23-32, 1984.

Duma RJ, et al: Penetration of aztreonam into cerebrospinal fluid of patients with and without inflamed meninges. *Antimicrob Agents Chemother* 26:730-733, 1984.

Eichenwald HF: Antimicrobial therapy in infants and children: Update 1976-1985. Part I. *J Pediatr* 107:161-168, 1985.

Eron LJ: Imipenem/cilastatin therapy of bacteremia. *Am J Med* 78(suppl 6A):95-99, 1985.

Eron LJ, et al: Imipenem versus moxalactam in treatment of serious infections. *Antimicrob Agents Chemother* 24:841-846, 1983.

Fainstein V, et al: Randomized study of ceftazidime compared to ceftazidime and tobramycin for treatment of infections in cancer patients. *J Antimicrob Chemother* 12(suppl A):101-110, 1983.

Fass RJ: Comparative in vitro activities of third-generation cephalosporins. *Arch Intern Med* 143:1743-1745, 1983.

Fass RJ, et al: Treatment of skin and soft tissue infections with imipenem/cilastatin *Am J Med* 78(suppl 6A):110-112, 1985.

Fillastre JP, et al: Pharmacokinetics of aztreonam in patients with chronic renal failure. *Clin Pharmacokinet* 10:91-100, 1985.

Fitzpatrick BJ, Standiford HC: Comparative evaluation of moxalactam: Antimicrobial activity, pharmacokinetics, adverse reactions, and clinical efficacy. *Pharmacotherapy* 2:197-212, 1982.

Fong IW, Tomkins KB: Review of *Pseudomonas aeruginosa* meningitis with special emphasis on treatment with ceftazidime. *Rev Infect Dis* 7:604-612, 1985.

Fried JS, Hinthorn DR: Cephalosporins. *DM* 31:1-60, (July) 1985.

Funk EA, Strausbaugh LJ: Antimicrobial activity, pharmacokinetics, adverse reactions, and therapeutic indications of cefoperazone. *Pharmacotherapy* 2:185-196, 1982.

Garzone P, et al: Third-generation and investigational cephalosporins: I. Structure-activity relationships and pharmacokinetic review. *Drug Intell Clin Pharm* 17:507-515, 1983 A.

Garzone P, et al: Third-generation and investigational cephalosporins: II. Microbiologic review and clinical summaries. *Drug Intell Clin Pharm* 17:615-622, 1983 B.

Gentry LO: Antimicrobial activity, pharmacokinetics, therapeutic indications, and adverse reactions of ceftazidime. *Pharmacotherapy* 5:254-267, 1985.

Giamarellou H, et al: Evaluation of aztreonam in difficult-to-treat infections with prolonged posttreatment followup. *Antimicrob*

Agents Chemother 26:245-249, 1984.

Gibbs RS, et al: Aztreonam versus gentamicin, each with clindamycin, in treatment of endometritis. *Obstet Gynecol* 65:825-829, 1985.

Gibson TP, et al: Imipenem/cilastatin: Pharmacokinetic profile in renal insufficiency. *Am J Med* 78(suppl 6A):54-61, 1985.

Gilbert DN: Current status of antibiotic prophylaxis in surgical patients. *Bull NY Acad Med* 60:340-357, 1984.

Ginsburg CM: Comparative pharmacokinetics of cefadroxil, cefaclor, cephalexin, and cephradine in infants and children. *J Antimicrob Chemother* 10(suppl B):27-31, 1982.

Gleckman RA: Antimicrobial activity, pharmacokinetics, therapeutic indications, and adverse reactions of ceftazidime, (commentary). *Pharmacotherapy* 5:265-266, 1985.

Gold B, Rodriguez WJ: Cefuroxime: Mechanisms of action, antimicrobial activity, pharmacokinetics, clinical applications, adverse reactions and therapeutic indications. *Pharmacotherapy* 3:82-100, 1983.

Gold R, et al: Controlled trial of ceftazidime vs ticarcillin and tobramycin in treatment of acute respiratory exacerbations in patients with cystic fibrosis. *Pediatr Infect Dis* 4:172-177, 1985.

Gordon RC: Sorting out the cephems: Role of new cephalosporins in pediatric therapeutics. *Pediatr Ann* 14:278-287, 1985.

Greenberg RN, et al: Treatment of serious gram-negative infections with aztreonam. *J Infect Dis* 150:623-630, 1984.

Greenman RL, et al: Twice-daily intramuscular ceforanide therapy of *Staphylococcus aureus* endocarditis in parenteral drug abusers. *Antimicrob Agents Chemother* 25:16-19, 1984.

Guay DRP, Koskoletos C: Aztreonam, new monobactam antimicrobial. *Clin Pharm* 4:516-526, 1985.

Guay DRP, et al: Interference of selected second- and third-generation cephalosporins with creatinine determination. *Am J Hosp Pharm* 40:435-438, 1983.

Guerra JG, et al: Imipenem/cilastatin vs gentamicin/clindamycin for treatment of moderate to severe infections in hospitalized patients. *Rev Infect Dis* 7(suppl 3):S463-S470, 1985.

Guglielmo BJ, et al: Antibiotic prophylaxis in surgical procedures: Critical analysis of the literature. *Arch Surg* 118:943-955, 1983.

Handsfield HH, Murphy VL: Comparative study of ceftriaxone and spectinomycin for treatment of uncomplicated gonorrhoea in men. *Lancet* 2:67-70, 1983.

Handsfield HH, Murphy VL: Treatment of uncomplicated gonorrhea in women with single-dose cefonicid. *Sex Transm Dis* 12:90-92, 1985.

Hansten PD: *Drug Interactions*, ed 5. Philadelphia, Lea & Febiger, 1985, 194-260.

Henry SA, Bendush CB: Aztreonam: Worldwide overview of treatment of patients with gram-negative infections. *Am J Med* 78(suppl 2A):57-64, 1985.

Holt RJ, et al: Hypoprothrombinemia associated with moxalactam treatment of septic sternoclavicular arthritis due to *Citrobacter diversus*. *Drug Intell Clin Pharm* 15:288-289, 1981.

Hopefl AW: Aztreonam: Overview. *Drug Intell Clin Pharm* 19:171-175, 1985.

Iannini PB, et al: Imipenem/cilastatin: General experience in community hospital. *Am J Med* 78(suppl 6A):122-126, 1985.

Indrelie JA, et al: Synergy of imipenem or penicillin G and aminoglycosides against enterococci isolated from patients with infective endocarditis. *Antimicrob Agents Chemother* 26:909-912, 1984.

Jacob LS, Layne P: Cefonicid: Overview of clinical studies in United States. *Rev Infect Dis* 6(suppl 4):S791-S802, 1984.

Jacobs RF, et al: Prospective randomized comparison of cefotaxime vs ampicillin and chloramphenicol for bacterial meningitis in children. *J Pediatr* 107:129-133, 1985.

Jones PG, et al: Effect of aztreonam on throat and stool flora of cancer patients. *Antimicrob Agents Chemother* 26:941-943, 1984.

Jones RN: Review of in vitro spectrum of activity of imipenem. *Am J Med* 78(suppl 6A):22-32, 1985.

Jones RN, et al: Antimicrobial activity of desacetylcefotaxime alone and in combination with cefotaxime: Evidence of synergy. *Rev Infect Dis* 4(suppl):S366-S373, 1982.

Jones RN, Preston DA: Antimicrobial activity of cephalexin against old and new pathogens. *Postgrad Med J* 59(suppl 5):9-15, 1983.

Jones RN, Thornsberry C: Gram-positive superinfections: Consequence of modern β-lactam chemotherapy. *Antimicrob Newslett* 2:17-24, 1985.

Jones SR, Kimbrough RC III: Moxalactam and hemorrhage, (letter). *Ann Intern Med* 99:126, 1983.

Judson FN, et al: Comparative study of ceftriaxone and aqueous procaine penicillin G in treatment of uncomplicated gonorrhea in women. *Antimicrob Agents Chemother* 23:218-220, 1983.

Judson FN, et al: Comparative study of ceftriaxone and spectinomycin for treatment of pharyngeal and anorectal gonorrhea. *JAMA* 253:1417-1419, 1985.

Kager L, Nord CE: Imipenem/cilastatin in treatment of intra-abdominal infections: Review of worldwide experience. *Rev Infect Dis* 7(suppl 3):S518-S521, 1985.

Kannangara DW, et al: Disulfiram-like reactions with newer cephalosporins: Cefmenoxime. *Am J Med Sci* 287:45-47, 1984.

Kropp H, et al: Antibacterial activity of imipenem: First thienamycin antibiotic. *Rev Infect Dis* 7(suppl 3):S389-S410, 1985.

Kunkel MJ, Iannini PB: Cefonicid in once-daily regimen for treatment of osteomyelitis in ambulatory setting. *Rev Infect Dis* 6(suppl 4):S865-S869, 1984.

Landesman SH, et al: Past and current roles for cephalosporin antibiotics in treatment of meningitis: Emphasis on use in gram-negative bacillary meningitis. *Am J Med* 71:693-703, 1981.

Lea AS, et al: Comparative trial of cefonicid vs cefazolin for treatment of skin and soft tissue infections caused by gram-positive cocci, (abstract 794). *23rd Interscience Conference on Antimicrobial Agents and Chemotherapy*. Miami Beach, Oct 4-6, 1982.

Lee S, et al: Coagulopathy associated with moxalactam, (letter). *JAMA* 249:2019-2020, 1983.

LeFrock JL, et al: Mechanism of action, antimicrobial activity, pharmacology, adverse effects, and clinical efficacy of cefotaxime. *Pharmacotherapy* 2:174-184, 1982.

LeFrock JL, et al: Nonprophylactic role of cephalosporins in surgery. *Bull NY Acad Med* 60:394-402, 1984 A.

LeFrock JL, et al: Nonprophylactic role of cephalosporins in obstetrics and gynecology. *Bull NY Acad Med* 60:416-425, 1984 B.

Le Frock JL, et al: In vitro and clinical evaluation of ceforanide. *Am J Med Sci* 287:21-25, 1984 C.

Leng M, Anderson PO: Serum sickness with cefaclor. *Drug Intell Clin Pharm* 19:186-187, 1985.

Lennard ES, Dellinger EP: Prophylactic antibiotics in surgery: Rationale for family physician. *J Fam Pract* 12:461-467, 1981.

Levine LR: Quantitative comparison of adverse reactions to cefaclor vs amoxicillin in surveillance study. *Pediatr Infect Dis* 4:358-361, 1985.

Luft FC: Cephalosporin and aminoglycoside interactions: Clinical and toxicologic implications, in Whelton A, Neu HC (eds): *The Aminoglycosides: Microbiology, Clinical Use, and Toxicology*. New York, Marcel Dekker, 1982, 387-399.

MacGregor RR, Gentry LO: Imipenem/cilastatin in treatment of osteomyelitis. *Am J Med* 78(suppl 6A):100-103, 1985.

MacLennan FM, et al: Severe depletion of vitamin-K-dependent clotting factors during postoperative latamoxef therapy, (letter). *Lancet* 1:1215, 1983.

Madsen PO, et al: Aztreonam concentrations in human prostatic tissue. *Antimicrob Agents Chemother* 26:20-21, 1984.

Mandell GL: Cephalosporins, in Mandell GL, et al (eds): *Principles and Practice of Infectious Diseases*, ed 2. New York, John Wiley & Sons, 1984, 180-187.

Mandell LA, et al: Multicentre prospective randomized trial comparing ceftazidime with cefazolin/tobramycin in treatment of hospitalized patients with nonpneumococcal pneumonia. *J Antimicrob Chemother* 12(suppl A):9-20, 1983.

Mangini RJ (ed): *Drug Interaction Facts*. St Louis, JB Lippincott, 1984 A, 12.

Mangini RJ (ed): *Drug Interaction Facts*. St Louis, JB Lippincott, 1984 B, 455.

Mangini RJ (ed): *Drug Interaction Facts*. St Louis, JB Lippincott, 1984 C, 245.

Marier RL: Role of imipenem/cilastatin in treatment of soft tissue infections. *Am J Med* 78(suppl 6A):140-144, 1985.

Mastella G, et al: Alternative antibiotics for treatment of pseudomonas infections in cystic fibrosis. *J Antimicrob Chemother* 12(suppl A):297-311, 1983.

McClosky RV: Clinical and bacteriologic efficacy of ceftriaxone in the United States. *Am J Med* 77(suppl 4C):97-103, 1984.

McCracken GH Jr, et al: Moxalactam therapy for neonatal meningitis due to gram-negative enteric bacilli: Prospective controlled evaluation. *JAMA* 252:1427-1432, 1984.

The Medical Letter: *Handbook of Antimicrobial Therapy.* New Rochelle, NY, The Medical Letter, Inc, 1984, 38-47.

Meisel S: Severe bleeding diathesis associated with moxalactam administration. *Drug Intell Clin Pharm* 18:721-722, 1984.

Minami S, et al: Induction of β-lactamase by various β-lactam antibiotics in *Enterobacter cloacae. Antimicrob Agents Chemother* 18:382-385, 1980.

Modai J, et al: Imipenem penetration into cerebrospinal fluid of patients with bacterial meningitis, (abstract 601). *24th Interscience Conference on Antimicrobial Agents and Chemotherapy.* Washington, DC, Oct 8-10, 1984.

Moellering RC Jr: Can third-generation cephalosporins eliminate need for antimicrobial combinations? *Am J Med* 79(suppl 2A):104-109, 1985 A.

Moellering RC Jr: Ceftazidime: New broad spectrum cephalosporin. *Pediatr Infect Dis* 4:390-393, 1985 B.

Morgan G, et al: Ceftazidime as single agent in management of children with fever and neutropenia. *J Antimicrob Chemother* 12(suppl A):347-351, 1983.

Moskovitz BL: Clinical adverse effects during ceftriaxone therapy. *Am J Med* 77(suppl 4C):84-88, 1984.

Mulligan ME, et al: Impact of cefoperazone therapy on fecal flora. *Antimicrob Agents Chemother* 22:226-230, 1982.

Murray DL, et al: Cefaclor: Cluster of adverse reactions, (letter). *N Engl J Med* 303:1003, 1980.

Muytjens HL, van der Ros-van de Repe J: Comparative activities of 13 β-lactam antibiotics. *Antimicrob Agents Chemother* 21:925-934, 1982.

Naqvi SH, et al: Cefotaxime therapy of neonatal gram-negative bacillary meningitis. *Pediatr Infect Dis* 4:499-502, 1985.

Nelson JD: Cefuroxime: Cephalosporin with unique applicability to pediatric practice. *Pediatr Infect Dis* 2:394-396, 1983.

Nelson JD: *1985 Pocketbook of Pediatric Antimicrobial Therapy*, ed 6. Baltimore, Williams & Wilkins, 1985 A, 64-75.

Nelson JD: *1985 Pocketbook of Pediatric Antimicrobial Therapy*, ed 6. Baltimore, Williams & Wilkins, 1985 B, 20-21.

Nelson JD, et al: Benefits and risks of sequential parenteral-oral cephalosporin therapy for suppurative bone and joint infections. *J Pediatr Orthoped* 2:255-262, 1982.

Neu HC: New beta-lactamase-stable cephalosporins. *Ann Intern Med* 97:408-419, 1982 A.

Neu HC: Factors that affect *in vitro* activity of cephalosporin antibiotics. *J Antimicrob Chemother* 10(suppl C):11-23, 1982 B.

Neu HC: In vitro activity, human pharmacology, and clinical effectiveness of new β-lactam antibiotics. *Ann Rev Pharmacol Toxicol* 22:599-642, 1982 C.

Neu HC: Clinical uses of cephalosporins. *Lancet* 2:252-255, 1982 D.

Neu HC: Antibacterial activity of desacetylcefotaxime alone and in combination with cefotaxime. *Rev Infect Dis* 4(suppl):S374-S378, 1982 E.

Neu HC: Structure-activity relations of new β-lactam compounds and in vitro activity against common bacteria. *Rev Infect Dis* 5(suppl 2):S319-S337, 1983.

Neu HC: Ceftizoxime: β-lactamase-stable, broad-spectrum cephalosporin: Pharmacokinetics, adverse effects, and clinical use. *Pharmacotherapy* 4:47-60, 1984 A.

Neu HC: Other beta-lactam antibiotics, in Mandell GL, et al (eds): *Principles and Practice of Infectious Diseases*, ed 2. New York, John Wiley & Sons, 1984, 187-193, 1984 B.

Neu HC: Relation of structural properties of beta-lactam antibiotics and antibacterial activity. *Am J Med* 79(suppl 2A):2-13, 1985 A.

Neu HC: Carbapenems: Special properties contributing to their activity. *Am J Med* 78(suppl 6A):33-40, 1985 B.

Neu HC: Summary of imipenem/cilastatin symposium. *Am J Med* 78(suppl 6A):165-167, 1985 C.

Neu HC: Current state of infectious diseases: Potential areas of directed therapy with aztreonam. *Am J Med* 78(suppl 2A):77-80, 1985 D.

Neu HC, Prince AS: Interaction between moxalactam and alcohol, (letter). *Lancet* 1:1422, 1980.

Neu HC, Scully BE: Activity of cefsulodin and other agents against *Pseudomonas aeruginosa. Rev Infect Dis* 6(suppl 3):S667-S677, 1984.

Nichols RL, et al: Risk of infection after penetrating abdominal trauma. *N Engl J Med* 311:1065-1070, 1984.

Nightingale CH, et al: Pharmacokinetics and clinical use of cephalosporin antibiotics. *J Pharm Sci* 64:1899-1927, 1975.

Nightingale CH, et al: Cephalosporins, in Evans WE, et al (eds): *Applied Pharmacokinetics: Principles of Therapeutic Drug Monitoring.* San Francisco, Applied Therapeutics, 1980, 240-274.

Noble JT, Barza M: Pharmacokinetic properties of newer cephalosporins: Valid basis for drug selection? *Drugs* 30:175-181, 1985.

Nord CE, et al: Effect of imipenem/cilastatin on colonic microflora. *Rev Infect Dis* 7(suppl 3):S432-S434, 1985.

Norrby SR: Role of cephalosporins in treatment of bacterial meningitis in adults: Overview with special emphasis on ceftazidime. *Am J Med* 79(suppl 2A):56-61, 1985.

Norrby SR: Adverse reactions and interactions with newer cephalosporin and cephamycin antibiotics. *Med Toxicol* 1:32-46, 1986.

Norris SM: Cephalosporin antibiotic agents. I. Considered as a group. *Infect Control* 5:493-496, 1984 A.

Norris SM: Cephalosporin antibiotic agents. II. First- and second-generation agents. *Infect Control* 5:577-582, 1984 B.

Norris SM: Cephalosporin antibiotic agents. III. Third generation cephalosporins. *Infect Control* 6:78-83, 1985.

Norris SM, Mandell GL: Tables of antimicrobial agent pharmacology, in Mandell GL, et al (eds): *Anti-Infective Therapy.* New York, John Wiley & Sons, 1985, 428-503.

Oakes M, et al: Abnormal laboratory test values during ceftriaxone therapy. *Am J Med* 77(suppl 4C):89-96, 1984.

Oblinger MJ, et al: Moxalactam therapy vs standard antimicrobial therapy for selected serious infections. *Rev Infect Dis* 4(suppl):S639-S649, 1982.

Overturf GD, et al: Treatment of bacterial meningitis with ceftizoxime. *Antimicrob Agents Chemother* 25:258-262, 1984.

Pakter RL, et al: Coagulopathy associated with use of moxalactam. *JAMA* 248:1100, 1982.

Panwalker AP, Rosenfeld J: Hemorrhage, diarrhea, and superinfection associated with use of moxalactam, (letter). *J Infect Dis* 147:171-172, 1983.

Parks D, et al: Ceftizoxime: Clinical evaluation of efficacy and safety in the U.S.A. *J Antimicrob Chemother* 10(suppl C):327-338, 1982.

Pastorek JG II, et al: Aztreonam plus clindamycin as therapy for pelvic infections in women. *Am J Med* 78(suppl 2A):47-50, 1985.

Patel IH, Kaplan SA: Pharmacokinetic profile of ceftriaxone in man. *Am J Med* 77(suppl 4C):17-25, 1984.

Pfenninger J, et al: Cefuroxime in bacterial meningitis. *Arch Dis Child* 57:539-543, 1982.

Pizzo P, et al: Monotherapy vs combination antibiotics for initial empiric management of febrile (F+) granulocytopenic (G+) cancer patients (Pts), (abstract 380). *24th Interscience Conference on Antimicrobial Agents and Chemotherapy.* Washington, DC, Oct 8-10, 1984.

Pizzo PA, et al: New beta-lactam antibiotics in granulocytopenic patients: New options and new questions. *Am J Med* 79(suppl 2A):75-82, 1985.

Polk R: Ceftriaxone: Beta-lactamase-stable, broad-spectrum cephalosporin with an extended half-life, (commentary). *Pharmacotherapy* 5:251-252, 1985.

Pontzer RE, Kaye D: Cefonicid: Long-acting, second-generation cephalosporin: Antimicrobial activity, pharmacokinetics, clinical efficacy, and adverse effects. *Pharmacotherapy* 4:325-333, 1984.

Portier H, et al: Interaction between cephalosporins and alcohol, (letter). *Lancet* 2:263, 1980.

Pribyl C, et al: Aztreonam in treatment of serious orthopedic infections. *Am J Med* 78(suppl 2A):51-56, 1985.

Quintiliani R, Nightingale CH: Cefazolin. *Ann Intern Med* 89(part I):650-656, 1978.

Quintiliani R, et al: Cephalosporins: Overview, in Ristuccia AM, Cunha BA (eds): *Antimicrobial Therapy*. New York, Raven Press, 1984, 289-303.

Rahal JJ Jr: Moxalactam therapy for gram-negative bacillary meningitis. *Rev Infect Dis* 4(suppl):S606-S609, 1982.

Rahal JJ, Simberkoff MS: Host defense and antimicrobial therapy in adult gram-negative bacillary meningitis. *Ann Intern Med* 96:468-474, 1982.

Ramphal R, et al: Early results of comparative trial of ceftazidime versus cephalothin, carbenicillin and gentamicin in treatment of febrile granulocytopenic patients. *J Antimicrob Chemother* 12(suppl A):81-88, 1983.

Rapp RP, Blue D: Role of extended half-life second generation cephalosporins in surgical prophylaxis. *Drug Intell Clin Pharm* 19:214-215, 1985.

Rapp RP, et al: Ceftazidime versus tobramycin/ticarcillin in treating hospital acquired pneumonia and bacteremia. *Pharmacotherapy* 4:211-215, 1984.

Reese RE, Betts RF: Antibiotic use, in Reese RE, Douglas RG (eds): *A Practical Approach to Infectious Diseases*. Boston, Little Brown & Co, 1983, 51-162.

Rehm SJ, McHenry MC: Oral antimicrobial drugs. *Med Clin North Am* 67:57-98, 1983.

Reilly JT, et al: Ceftazidime compared to tobramycin and ticarcillin in immunocompromised haematological patients. *J Antimicrob Chemother* 12(suppl A):89-92, 1983.

Report from a Scandinavian Study Group: Imipenem/cilastatin versus gentamicin/clindamycin for treatment of serious bacterial infections. *Lancet* 1:868-871, 1984.

Report from a Swedish Study Group: Cefuroxime versus ampicillin and chloramphenicol for treatment of bacterial meningitis. *Lancet* 1:295-298, 1982.

Richards DM, Brogden RN: Ceftazidime: Review of its antibacterial activity, pharmacokinetic properties, and therapeutic use. *Drugs* 29:105-161, 1985.

Richards DM, Heel RC: Ceftizoxime: Review of its antibacterial activity, pharmacokinetic properties, and therapeutic use. *Drugs* 29:281-329, 1985.

Richards DM, et al: Ceftriaxone: Review of its antibacterial activity, pharmacological properties and therapeutic use. *Drugs* 27:469-527, 1984.

Richmond MH, Sykes RG: β-lactamases of gram-negative bacteria and their possible physiological role. *Rev Microb Physiol* 9:31-88, 1973.

Rodriguez JR, et al: Efficacy and safety of aztreonam-clindamycin versus tobramycin-clindamycin in treatment of lower respiratory tract infections caused by aerobic gram-negative bacilli. *Antimicrob Agents Chemother* 27:246-251, 1985.

Rodriguez WJ, et al: Ceftazidime in treatment of meningitis in infants and children over one month of age. *Am J Med* 79(suppl 2A):52-55, 1985.

Rogers JD, et al: Pharmacokinetics of imipenem and cilastatin in volunteers. *Rev Infect Dis* 7(suppl 3):S435-S446, 1985.

Sahm DF, et al: β-lactam antibiotics: First- and second-generation cephalosporins. *Antimicrob Newslett* 2:25-28, 1985 A.

Sahm DF, et al: β-lactam antibiotics: Third-generation cephalosporins and other newer β-lactams. *Antimicrob Newslett* 2:33-40, 1985 B.

Salata RA, et al: Pneumonia treated with imipenem/cilastatin. *Am J Med* 78(suppl 6A):104-109, 1985.

Sanders CC: Novel resistance selected by new expanded-spectrum cephalosporins: Concern. *J Infect Dis* 147:585-589, 1983.

Sanders CC: Failure to detect resistance in antimicrobial susceptibility tests: "Very major" error of increasing concern. *Antimicrob Newslett* 1:27-31, 1984.

Sanders CC, Sanders WE Jr: Emergence of resistance during therapy with newer β-lactam antibiotics: Role of inducible β-lactamases and implications for the future. *Rev Infect Dis* 5:639-648, 1983.

Sanders CC, Sanders WE Jr: Microbial resistance to newer generation β-lactam antibiotics: Clinical and laboratory implications. *J Infect Dis* 151:399-406, 1985.

Sanders CV, et al: Cefamandole and cefoxitin. *Ann Intern Med* 103:70-78, 1985.

Sattler FR, et al: Aztreonam compared with gentamicin for treatment of serious urinary tract infections. *Lancet* 1:1315-1318, 1984.

Saxon A: Immediate hypersensitivity reactions to β-lactam antibiotics. *Rev Infect Dis* 5(suppl 2):S368-S379, 1983.

Saxon A, et al: Lack of cross-reactivity between aztreonam, a monobactam antibiotic, and penicillin in penicillin-allergic subjects. *J Infect Dis* 149:16-22, 1984.

Saxon A, et al: Investigation into immunologic cross-reactivity of aztreonam with other beta lactam antibiotics. *Am J Med* 78(suppl 2A):19-26, 1985.

Schentag JJ, et al: Treatment with aztreonam or tobramycin in critical care patients with nosocomial gram-negative pneumonia. *Am J Med* 78(suppl 2A):34-41, 1985.

Scully BE, Neu HC: Use of aztreonam in treatment of serious infections due to multiresistant gram-negative organisms, including *Pseudomonas aeruginosa*. *Am J Med* 78:251-261, 1985.

Scully BE, et al: Pharmacology of aztreonam after intravenous infusion. *Antimicrob Agents Chemother* 24:18-22, 1983.

Sheehan GJ, Ronald AR: Imipenem in urinary tract infections. *Curr Ther Res* 37:1141-1151, 1985.

Simons WJ, Lee TJ: Treatment of gram-negative infections with aztreonam. *Am J Med* 78(suppl 2A):27-30, 1985.

Slonaker CE, Luper WE: Moxalactam-associated platelet dysfunction, (letter). *JAMA* 250:729-730, 1983.

Smith BR: Cefsulodin and ceftazidime, two antipseudomonal cephalosporins. *Clin Pharm* 3:373-385, 1984.

Smith BR, LeFrock JL: Cefuroxime: Antimicrobial activity, pharmacology, and clinical efficacy. *Therapeut Drug Monitor* 5:149-160, 1983.

Smith CR, et al: Cefotaxime compared with nafcillin plus tobramycin for serious bacterial infections: Randomized, double-blind trial. *Ann Intern Med* 101:469-477, 1984.

Solomkin JS, et al: Randomized trial of imipenem/cilastatin versus gentamicin and clindamycin in mixed flora infections. *Am J Med* 78(suppl 6A):85-91, 1985.

Stamm JM: Cefmenoxime: In vitro activity. *Am J Med* 77(suppl 6A):1-3, 1984.

Steele RW, Bradsher RW: Comparison of ceftriaxone with standard therapy for bacterial meningitis. *J Pediatr* 103:138-141, 1983.

Stockley IH: Disulfiram-type reaction with some cephalosporins. *Pharmaceut J* 234:239-240, 1985.

Stone HH, et al: Third-generation cephalosporins for polymicrobial surgical sepsis. *Arch Surg* 118:193-200, 1983.

Stutman HR, et al: Single-dose pharmacokinetics of aztreonam in pediatric patients. *Antimicrob Agents Chemother* 26:196-199, 1984.

Swabb EA: Review of clinical pharmacology of monobactam antibiotic aztreonam. *Am J Med* 78(suppl 2A):11-18, 1985.

Swabb EA, et al: Pharmacokinetics of monobactam SQ 26,776 after single intravenous doses in healthy subjects. *J Antimicrob Chemother* 8(suppl E):131-140, 1981.

Swabb EA, et al: Metabolism and pharmacokinetics of aztreonam in healthy subjects. *Antimicrob Agents Chemother* 24:394-400, 1983.

Sweet RL: Imipenem/cilastatin in treatment of obstetric and gynecologic infections: Review of worldwide experience. *Rev Infect Dis* 7(suppl 3):S522-S527, 1985.

Sykes RB: Classification and terminology of enzymes that hydrolyze β-lactam antibiotics. *J Infect Dis* 145:762-765, 1982.

Sykes RB, Bonner DP: Aztreonam: First monobactam. *Am J Med* 78(suppl 2A):2-10, 1985.

Sykes RB, Bush K: Interaction of new cephalosporins with β-lactamases and β-lactamase-producing gram-negative bacilli. *Rev Infect Dis* 5(suppl 2):S356-S367, 1983.

Tally FP, et al: Randomized comparison of cefoxitin with or without amikacin and clindamycin plus amikacin in surgical sepsis. *Ann Surg* 193:318-323, 1981.

Tartaglione TA, Polk RE: Review of new second-generation cephalosporins: Cefonicid, ceforanide, and cefuroxime. *Drug Intell Clin Pharm* 19:188-198, 1985.

Taylor DN, et al: Comparative study of ceftriaxone and trimethoprim/sulfamethoxazole for treatment of chancroid in Thailand. *J Infect Dis* 152:1002-1006, 1985.

Thirumoorthi MC, et al: Efficacy and safety of ceforanide in treatment of childhood infections. *Pediatr Infect Dis* 2:377-380, 1983.

Thompson RL, Wright AJ: Cephalosporin antibiotics. *Mayo Clin Proc* 58:79-87, 1983.

Thornsberry C: Review of in vitro activity of third-generation cephalosporins and other newer beta-lactam antibiotics against clinically important bacteria. *Am J Med* 79(suppl 2A):14-20, 1985.

Torres A, Ramírez-Ronda CH: Aztreonam in treatment of serious gram-negative infections. *Curr Ther Res* 36:875-881, 1984.

Trumbore D, et al: Multicenter study of clinical efficacy of imipenem/cilastatin for treatment of serious infections. *Rev Infect Dis* 7(suppl 3):S476-S481, 1985.

Wade JC, et al: Cephalothin plus aminoglycoside is more nephrotoxic than methicillin plus an aminoglycoside. *Lancet* 2:604-606, 1978.

Wallace RJ, et al: Ceforanide and cefazolin therapy of pneumonia: Comparative clinical trial. *Antimicrob Agents Chemother* 20:648-652, 1981.

Wang C, et al: Efficacy and safety of imipenem/cilastatin: Review of worldwide clinical experience. *Rev Infect Dis* 7(suppl 3):S528-S536, 1985.

Ward A, Richards DM: Cefotetan: Review of its antibacterial activity, pharmacokinetic properties and therapeutic use. *Drugs* 30:382-426, 1985.

Warren JW, et al: Randomized, controlled trial of cefoperazone vs cefamandole-tobramycin in treatment of putative, severe infections with gram-negative bacilli. *Rev Infect Dis* 5(suppl):S173-S180, 1983.

Weitekamp MR, Aber RC: Prolonged bleeding times and bleeding diathesis associated with moxalactam administration. *JAMA* 249:69-71, 1983.

Weitekamp MR, et al: Effects of latamoxef, cefotaxime, and cefoperazone on platelet function and coagulation in normal volunteers. *J Antimicrob Chemother* 16:95-101, 1985.

Wexler HM, Finegold SM: Impact of imipenem/cilastatin therapy on normal fecal flora. *Am J Med* 78(suppl 6A):41-46, 1985.

Witt LG, Witt LD: Cephalosporins and ethanol. *Drug Interact Newslett* 3:27-30, 1983.

Yost RL, Ramphal R: Ceftazidime review. *Drug Intell Clin Pharm* 19:509-513, 1985.

Young LS: Ceftazidime in treatment of nosocomial sepsis. *Am J Med* 79(suppl 2A):89-95, 1985.

Other Selected References

Cefamandole and cefoxitin. *Med Lett Drugs Ther* 21:13-15, 1979.

Cefmenoxime: New broad-spectrum antibiotic. *Am J Med* 77(suppl 6A):1-59, 1984 (14 papers).

Cefotaxime sodium (Claforan). *Med Lett Drugs Ther* 23:61-62, 1981.

Ceftizoxime sodium (Cefizox). *Med Lett Drugs Ther* 25:109-110, 1983.

Current and future directions in use of antimicrobial agents. *Bull NY Acad Med* 60:313-446, 1984 (13 papers).

Imipenem-cilastatin sodium (Primaxin). *Med Lett Drugs Ther* 28:29-31, 1986.

Moxalactam disodium (Moxam) *Med Lett Drugs Ther* 24:13-14, 1982.

Two new oral cephalosporins. *Med Lett Drugs Ther* 21:85-87, 1979.

Acar JF, Neu HC: Gram-negative aerobic bacterial infections: Focus on directed therapy, with special reference to aztreonam. *Rev Infect Dis* 7(suppl 4):S537-S843, 1985 (42 papers).

Brogden RN, Heel RC: Aztreonam: Review of its antibacterial activity, pharmacokinetic properties, and therapeutic use. *Drugs* 31:96-130, 1986.

Brogden RN, et al: Cefoxitin: Review of its antibacterial activity, pharmacological properties and therapeutic use. *Drugs* 17:1-37, 1979.

Brogden RN, et al: Cefoperazone: Review of in vitro antimicrobial activity, pharmacological properties and therapeutic efficacy. *Drugs* 22:423-460, 1981.

Cherubin CE, et al (eds): Current status of cefotaxime sodium: New cephalosporin. *Rev Infect Dis* 4(suppl):S281-S488, 1982 (27 papers).

Conte JE Jr (ed): Clinical and economic impact of cefonicid. *Rev Infect Dis* 6(suppl 4):S777-S937, 1984 (24 papers).

Cunha BA, Ristuccia AM: Third generation cephalosporins. *Med Clin North Am* 66:283-291, 1982.

Farber BF, Moellering RC Jr: New cephalosporins. *Drug Ther* 12:51-59, (May) 1982.

Finegold SM, Kirby WMM (eds): Changing patterns of hospital infections: Implications for therapy. *Am J Med* 77(suppl 1B):1-41, 1984 (6 papers).

Geddes AM, Stille W (eds): Imipenem: First thienamycin antibiotic. *Rev Infect Dis* 7(suppl 3):S353-S536, 1985 (24 papers).

Geddes AM, et al (eds): Cefotaxime: New cephalosporin antibiotic. *J Antimicrob Chemother* 6(suppl A):1-303, 1980 (55 papers).

Gleckman R: Third-generation cephalosporins: Plea for restraint, (editorial). *JAMA* 142:1267-1268, 1982.

Hoffbrand BI, Kory M (eds): Cephalexin: Twelve years of clinical and laboratory experience. *Postgrad Med J* 59(suppl 5):1-56, 1983 (9 papers).

Jones RN, et al (eds): Workshop on five years of clinical experience with cefotaxime (with special references to gram-positive infections). *Infection* 13(suppl 1):S1-S162, 1985 (32 papers).

Klein JO, Neu HC (eds): Empiric therapy of bacterial infections: Evaluation of cefoperazone. *Rev Infect Dis* 5(suppl 1):S1-S209, 1983 (22 papers).

Lambert HP, et al (eds): Ceftazidime in clinical practice. *J Antimicrob Chemother* 12(suppl A):1-414, 1983 (63 papers).

Lyon JA: Cefoperazone (Cefobid, Pfizer). *Drug Intell Clin Pharm* 17:7-11, 1983.

Lyon JA: Imipenem/cilastatin: First carbapenem antibiotic. *Drug Intell Clin Pharm* 19:894-899, 1985.

Lüthy R, et al (eds): Perspective of imipenem. *J Antimicrob Chemother* 12(suppl D):1-156, 1983 (13 papers).

Mandell GL, Sande MA: Cephalosporins, in Gilman AG, et al (eds): *The Pharmacological Basis of Therapeutics*, ed 7. New York, Macmillan, 1985, 1137-1149.

Moellering RC Jr (ed): Clinical significance of newer beta-lactam antibiotics: Focus on cefuroxime. *Therapeutics Today Series*. New York, ADIS Press, 1983, vol 3, 1-126 (13 papers).

Moellering RC Jr (ed): Ceftriaxone: Long-acting cephalosporin. *Am J Med* 77(suppl 4C):1-118, 1984 (21 papers).

Moellering RC Jr (ed): Symposium on ceftriaxone: Long-acting cephalosporin. *Am J Surg* 148(suppl 4A):1-43, 1984 (10 papers).

Moellering RC Jr, Young LS (eds): Moxalactam international symposium. *Rev Infect Dis* 4(suppl):S489-S726, 1982 (38 papers).

Nahata MC, Barson WJ: Ceftriaxone: Third generation cephalosporin. *Drug Intell Clin Pharm* 19:900-906, 1985.

Neu HC (ed): Aztreonam: Monocyclic beta-lactam antibiotic. *Am J Med* 78(suppl 2A):1-80, 1985 (14 papers).

Neu HC (ed): Advances in cephalosporin therapy: Beyond the third generation. *Am J Med* 79(suppl 2A):1-118, 1985 (19 papers).

Neu HC, Phillips I (eds): Cefotaxime. *J Antimicrob Chemother* 14(suppl B):1-344, 1984 (50 papers).

Neu HC, et al (eds): Ceftizoxime, broad-spectrum β-lactamase stable cephalosporin. *J Antimicrob Chemother* 10(suppl C):1-355, 1982 (46 papers).

Phillips I, Wise R (eds): Role of cefadroxil in oral antibiotic therapy. *J Antimicrob Chemother* 10(suppl B):1-162, 1982 (24 papers).

Phillips I, et al (eds): Cefotetan: New cephamycin. *J Antimicrob Chemother* 11(suppl A):1-239, 1983 (32 papers).

Polk RE: Moxalactam (Moxam, Eli Lilly). *Drug Intell Clin Pharm* 16:104-114, 1982.

Quintiliani R (ed): Symposium on cefotetan. *Am J Obstet Gynecol* 154:945-963, 1986 (4 papers).

Quintiliani R, et al: First and second generation cephalosporins. *Med Clin North Am* 66:183-197, 1982.

Remington JS (ed): Carbapenems: New class of antibiotics. *Am J Med* 78(suppl 6A):1-167, 1985 (25 papers).

Sykes RB, Phillips I (eds): Aztreonam, synthetic monobactam. *J Antimicrob Chemother* 8(suppl E):1-148, 1981 (17 papers).

Williams JD, Casewell MW (eds): Ceftazidime. *J Antimicrob Chemother* 8(suppl B):1-358, 1981 (61 papers).

Young LS: *Pseudomonas aeruginosa*: Biology, immunology, and therapy: Cefsulodin symposium. *Rev Infect Dis* 6(suppl 3):S603-S776, 1984 (20 papers).

Macrolides and Lincosamides

MACROLIDES

Erythromycin and troleandomycin [TAO], derived from strains of *Streptomyces erythreus* and *S. antibioticus*, respectively, are the only macrolide antibiotics presently marketed in the United States. Chemically, these drugs contain a macrocyclic lactone ring to which sugars are attached (see Figure 1). Erythromycin is of major clinical importance. This antibiotic has some primary indications and frequently is the preferred alternative to penicillin G for a number of infections in penicillin-allergic individuals. It is considered to be among the safest antibiotics in use today (Steigbigel, 1984). Troleandomycin is an obsolete drug of little use in the treatment of infectious diseases. Therefore, the discussion in this section will focus primarily on erythromycin.

Mechanism of Action: Erythromycin inhibits bacterial protein synthesis by binding to the 50S ribosomal subunit, which prevents elongation of the peptide chain; other macrolides act similarly. Erythromycin does not bind to mammalian 80S ribosomes; this accounts in part for its selective toxicity (Mao et al, 1970). Competition experiments indicate that the binding sites for the macrolides overlap those for chloramphenicol and the lincosamides but are not identical to them. The binding of one of these antibiotics to the ribosome may inhibit the reaction of the other (see Pratt, 1977). There are no clinical indications for the concurrent use of these antibiotics.

Erythromycin may be bacteriostatic or bactericidal depending on the concentration of drug, organism susceptibility, the growth rate, and the size of the inoculum. Bacterial killing is favored by higher antibiotic concentrations, lower bacterial density, and rapid growth. The antibacterial activity of erythromycin increases progressively over the pH range 5.5 to 8.5 for

FIGURE 1. CHEMICAL STRUCTURES OF MACROLIDES

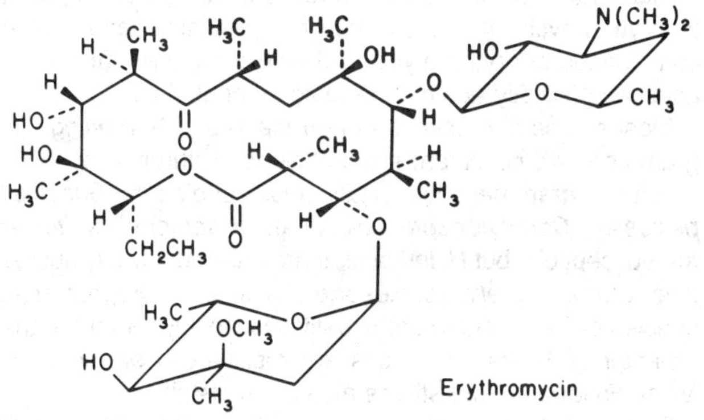

Erythromycin

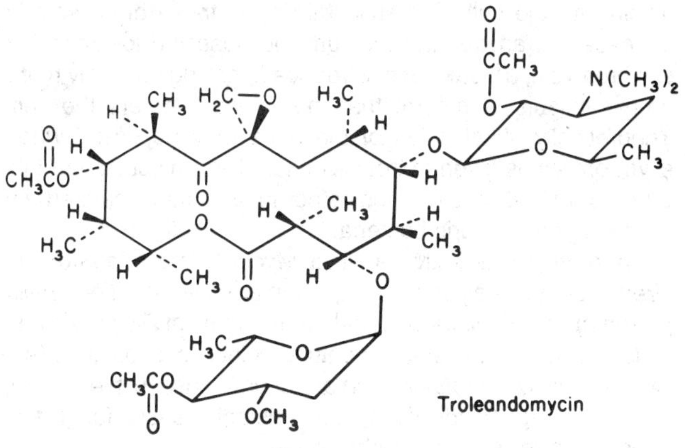

Troleandomycin

both gram-positive and gram-negative bacteria (see Steigbigel, 1984; Washington and Wilson, 1985).

Antimicrobial Spectrum: Erythromycin has a relatively broad spectrum and is active in vitro against most gram-positive and some gram-negative bacteria, actinomycetes, mycoplasmas, spirochetes, chlamydiae, rickettsiae, and certain atypical mycobacteria (Nicholas, 1977; Gribble and Chow, 1982; Steigbigel, 1984; Washington and Wilson, 1985).

Among gram-positive cocci, *Streptococcus pyogenes* (group A, beta-hemolytic streptococci) and *S. pneumoniae* are highly susceptible to erythromycin, although occasional strains (eg, about 5% of group A streptococci) are resistant in the United States (see Steigbigel, 1984). Erythromycin also is active against most viridans and anaerobic streptococci. It is inhibitory against a number of strains of *S. faecalis* (group D enterococci). Most *Staphylococcus aureus* and *S. epidermidis* are susceptible. Some strains of *S. aureus*, particularly in hospitals, are resistant or rapidly develop resistance during therapy. Approximately 12% of *S. aureus* strains causing nosocomial infections were resistant to erythromycin in the years 1980 to 1983 (see Washington and Wilson, 1985).

Susceptible gram-positive bacilli include *Bacillus anthracis, Clostridium tetani, Corynebacterium diphtheriae* (occasional strains are resistant), *C. minutissimum,* and *Listeria monocytogenes.* Many strains of *Clostridium perfringens* are only moderately susceptible. Erythromycin is active against *Actinomyces israelii. Nocardia asteroides* has variable susceptibility to erythromycin alone, but may be quite susceptible to the combination of erythromycin and ampicillin, which appears to act synergistically against the majority of strains.

Most strains of *Neisseria gonorrhoeae* and *N. meningitidis,* gram-negative cocci, are susceptible to erythromycin.

Among gram-negative bacilli, most strains of *Bordetella pertussis, Campylobacter jejuni,* and *Haemophilus ducreyi* are susceptible, but *H. influenzae* are only moderately susceptible. Some *Brucella* species are susceptible. Oropharyngeal species of *Bacteroides* are usually susceptible, but more than one-half of *B. fragilis* strains are resistant to erythromycin. Many *Fusobacterium* strains also are resistant.

The majority of aerobic gram-negative bacilli, including the Enterobacteriaceae (eg, *Escherichia coli*) are resistant to erythromycin. This is because the cell envelopes of most gram-negative bacilli prevent the passive diffusion of erythromycin into the cell. The susceptibility of these organisms is increased in an alkaline medium, because the ionization of erythromycin, a weak base, is reduced, making relatively more drug available in a form that more readily enters the cell. Theoretically, alkalization of the urine may be useful when erythromycin is given to treat a urinary tract infection, but this drug is rarely, if ever, indicated in infections caused by gram-negative enteric bacteria.

Erythromycin is active against *Mycoplasma pneumoniae, Ureaplasma urealyticum, Treponema pallidum, Legionella pneumophila, L. micdadei,* and many strains of *Rickettsia* and *Chlamydia.* Some strains of nontuberculous mycobacteria (eg, *M. kansasii, M. scrofulaceum*) are usually susceptible in vitro, but others (eg, *M. fortuitum*) are resistant. Yeasts, fungi, and viruses are resistant to erythromycin.

Troleandomycin is less active and has no clinical advantage over erythromycin.

Resistance: Various mechanisms of resistance to erythromycin have been reported. One mechanism involves an alteration in a protein component of the bacterial 50S ribosomal subunit resulting in decreased binding affinity for erythromycin (and often to other macrolides and lincosamides). This one-step, high-level resistance is due to a chromosomal mutation and has been demonstrated in *Bacillus subtilis, Streptococcus pyogenes, Escherichia coli,* and probably *Staphylococcus aureus.*

Decreased binding of erythromycin (and often other macrolides and lincosamides) to its target site also can result from an alteration in the 23S RNA component of the 50S ribosomal subunit by methylation of adenine. This occurs in *S. aureus* and probably *S. pyogenes* and *Streptococcus faecalis.* This resistance appears to be mediated by a plasmid that contains a gene for an RNA methylase. It can be constitutive or inducible. The latter has been observed in *S. aureus* (Weisblum et al, 1971). RNA methylase is induced when the concentration of erythromycin is too low to inhibit protein synthesis. Thus, when organisms are exposed to low concentrations of erythromycin (about 10^{-8} M), they become resistant to all macrolides and lincosamides. In contrast, if the organism is initially exposed to high concentrations of erythromycin (greater than 10^{-7} M), staphylococcal growth is inhibited and induced resistance is blocked because protein synthesis is inhibited. This has been termed "dissociated resistance" (see Steigbigel, 1984).

Another mechanism of resistance, decreased permeability of the cell wall to erythromycin, is exhibited by the Enterobacteriaceae (see also Antimicrobial Spectrum).

Uses: Erythromycin is the preferred or alternative therapy for a number of indications as outlined below. For additional discussion, see Chapter 65, Antimicrobial Therapy and Chemoprophylaxis of Infectious Diseases.

Erythromycin is the drug of choice for the treatment of atypical pneumonia caused by *Mycoplasma pneumoniae.* This antibiotic reduces the duration of illness and accelerates radiologic clearing of pulmonary infiltrates. Tetracycline is an effective alternative in nonpregnant adults.

Because erythromycin also is an effective alternative to penicillin G for pneumococcal pneumonia (see below), this antibiotic frequently is preferred for empiric therapy of mild to moderate cases of community-acquired pneumonia in older children and younger adults without predisposing conditions. *M. pneumoniae* and *Streptococcus pneumoniae* are the most common causes of pneumonia in this population (see also Table 1 in Chapter 65).

Erythromycin is the drug of choice in pneumonia caused by *Legionella pneumophila* (Legionnaires' disease), but the usual daily dose (2 g orally) may be inadequate for cure (Sanford, 1979). It has been suggested that intravenous injection of 2 to 4 g daily is more likely to be effective, although organisms may persist despite therapy and radiographic evidence of resolution often requires many weeks. Rifampin frequently is added to the regimen for severely ill patients or for those who do not respond satisfactorily to erythromycin alone. Erythromycin also is effective for infections caused by *L. micdadei* (Pittsburgh pneumonia agent).

A 14-day course of erythromycin is recommended for patients with pertussis. Although antimicrobial therapy does not affect the course of this disease, which is caused by a toxin, erythromycin eliminates *B. pertussis* carriage in the nasopharynx and, therefore, reduces infectivity. This antibiotic also is administered prophylactically to exposed persons, although proof of efficacy is not fully established (Report of the Committee on Infectious Diseases, 1982).

Patients with acute diphtheria, including some who have failed to respond to penicillin, have been treated successfully with erythromycin and diphtheria antitoxin. The antibiotic eradicates the causative organism and prevents spread. Erythromycin is preferred for treating carriers of this disease.

Chlamydia trachomatis infections in infants (eg, pneumonia, conjunctivitis) and children (eg, urethritis, cervicitis secondary to sexual abuse) are primary indications for the use of erythromycin. This antibiotic appears to be as effective as the tetracyclines for chlamydial infections, and it is safer in children under 8 years in whom tetracyclines cause mottling and staining of teeth. Erythromycin also is the drug of choice for chlamydial infections (eg, cervicitis, pelvic inflammatory disease) in pregnant women, in whom tetracyclines are contraindicated (see also Table 2 in Chapter 65).

Erythromycin is considered to be the drug of choice for gastroenteritis caused by *Campylobacter jejuni,* but definitive treatment guidelines are lacking. Although erythromycin shortened the duration of shedding of *C. jejuni* from feces, it failed to alter the clinical course of gastroenteritis when therapy was begun four or more days after the onset of symptoms (Anders et al, 1982; Mandal et al, 1984). It appears that mild cases of *C. jejuni* gastroenteritis are self-limited and erythromycin should be reserved for severe illness or when transmission of the organism must be prevented. Some strains of *C. jejuni* are resistant to erythromycin.

The combination of erythromycin base and neomycin has reduced the number of infections associated with elective colorectal surgery. This oral combination is the preferred prophylactic regimen for this type of surgery (see also Table 4 in Chapter 65).

Erythromycin is the drug of choice in erythrasma, a superficial skin infection caused by *Corynebacterium minutissimum.*

Erythromycin is routinely employed as an alternative to penicillin G in patients who cannot tolerate penicillins (eg, usually due to hypersensitivity). As a penicillin G alternative, erythromycin is used in the treatment of pharyngitis, scarlet fever, impetigo, cellulitis, and erysipelas caused by group A *Streptococcus pyogenes.* Pneumonia and bronchitis caused by *S. pneumoniae* also respond favorably (see Table 1 in Chapter 65). It also is an alternative to penicillin G in the prophylaxis of recurrences of rheumatic fever in patients who have a history or demonstrable sequelae of rheumatic fever but are allergic to penicillin. Sulfadiazine may be preferred, however. Prophylactic therapy with erythromycin to prevent endocarditis is indicated in certain penicillin-allergic patients with cardiac abnormalities prior to dental procedures or instrumentation of the upper airway (see Table 3 in Chapter 65).

Acute otitis media due to *S. pneumoniae* or *S. pyogenes* usually responds to erythromycin, but a penicillin (usually amoxicillin or ampicillin) continues to be the drug of choice. In acute otitis media caused by *H. influenzae,* the concentration of erythromycin achieved in the middle ear may be insufficient to eradicate the organism. The combination of erythromycin and a sulfonamide usually is more effective than erythromycin alone in children with otitis media caused by *H. influenzae.* This combination is useful when the patient is allergic to penicillins or when amoxicillin (or ampicillin)-resistant strains of *H. influenzae* are encountered. A fixed-ratio combination product containing erythromycin ethylsuccinate and sulfisoxazole acetyl [Pediazole] is available (see Chapter 71, Sulfonamides and Trimethoprim). Trimethoprim/sulfamethoxazole [Bactrim, Septra], cefaclor [Ceclor], and amoxicillin/potassium clavulanate [Augmentin] are other alternatives for this indication (see Table 1 in Chapter 65).

Erythromycin may be used in patients with relatively minor staphylococcal infections (eg, bullous impetigo, carbuncles) caused by penicillin G-susceptible or penicillin G-resistant strains. It is not a drug of first choice for severe staphylococcal infections, however, since it is usually bacteriostatic against this organism. Furthermore, the emergence of appreciable numbers of resistant strains of *S. aureus* limits the use of erythromycin. The availability of penicillinase-resistant penicillins (eg, nafcillin [Nafcil, Unipen], oxacillin [Bactocill, Prostaphlin], dicloxacillin [Dycill, Dynapen]) and the cephalosporins (eg, cefazolin [Ancef, Kefzol], cephalothin [Keflin], cephradine [Anspor, Velosef]) has reduced the need to use the erythromycins in serious staphylococcal infections.

Erythromycin is an alternative to penicillin G in the treatment of anthrax. Although it is not a preferred alternative, erythromycin may be used instead of penicillin G to treat gas gangrene, but debridement remains the most essential therapeutic procedure; erythromycin also rapidly eradicates *C. tetani* from wounds. Erythromycin has been employed as an alternative to penicillin G in the treatment of Vincent's gingivitis, erysipeloid, actinomycosis, *Listeria* infections, and certain anaerobic infections above the diaphragm. It may be combined with ampicillin to treat *Nocardia* infections.

This antibiotic may be used as an alternative to penicillin G for early and late syphilis, although tetracycline is the current preferred alternative in penicillin-allergic patients. Erythromycin is the drug of choice in penicillin-allergic pregnant women with syphilis. Congenital syphilis has occurred in offspring, however (Fenton and Light, 1976; Fiumara, 1983). Syphilitic patients who are treated with erythromycin must be followed carefully to assure eradication of the organism. Erythromycin also has been used as an alternative drug in disseminated gonorrhea (arthritis-dermatitis syndrome). Although tetracyclines are the preferred antibiotics for *C. trachomatis* infections (eg, urethritis, cervicitis, proctitis, pelvic inflammatory disease, lymphogranuloma venereum) in nonpregnant adults, erythromycin is an effective alternative. Erythromycin may be preferred for urethritis caused by *Ureaplasma urealyticum.* It is a drug of choice in chancroid (alternative, ceftriaxone). See also Table 2 in Chapter 65 and *Morbid Mortal Week Rep,* 1985, for additional discussion.

For use of erythromycin in eye infections and acne vulgaris, see Chapters 73, Topical Anti-infective Agents: Otic and Ophthalmic Preparations, and 56, Dermatologic Preparations, respectively.

Troleandomycin offers no advantages over erythromycin in the treatment of infectious diseases and is not recommended. It is used occasionally in severe asthma in combination with methylprednisolone (see the evaluation and Chapter 22, Drugs Used in Bronchial Disorders).

Adverse Reactions and Precautions: Erythromycin is one of the safest antimicrobial agents and seldom causes serious adverse reactions.

Gastrointestinal irritation, including epigastric distress, nausea, vomiting, and diarrhea, is the most common adverse effect produced by erythromycin and usually is associated with oral administration. Irritation is dose related and gastrointestinal intolerance is more common and severe with larger doses (eg, 2 g or more daily). Some brands of enteric-coated tablets and the ester derivatives (eg, ethylsuccinate, estolate) may be taken with food to minimize these untoward effects.

Hypersensitivity reactions, such as skin rashes, drug fever, and eosinophilia, have occurred occasionally; serious reactions (eg, anaphylaxis, interstitial nephritis) are rare.

The most serious toxic effect of erythromycin is a characteristic syndrome of cholestatic hepatitis. Erythromycin estolate has been associated with hepatotoxicity most often (see Nicholas, 1977; Gribble and Chow, 1982; Steigbigel, 1984; Washington and Wilson, 1985). Other erythromycins, most notably the ethylsuccinate ester, also have been associated with hepatic dysfunction but, in contrast to the estolate, only a few cases have been reported (Viteri et al, 1979; Zafrani et al, 1979; Sullivan et al, 1980; Hosker and Jewell, 1983; Inman and Rawson, 1983; Phillips, 1983; Diehl et al, 1984; Patel and Schneider, 1984). Patients 12 years of age or older appear to be most susceptible.

Hepatotoxicity typically begins after ten days of therapy, but occurs most frequently and rapidly (within two to three days) in patients who previously received erythromycin estolate. Symptoms consist of nausea, vomiting, and upper right quadrant pain, followed by jaundice, fever, and changes in hepatic function tests suggesting cholestatic hepatitis. These may be accompanied by rash, leukocytosis, and eosinophilia. The syndrome appears to be a hypersensitivity reaction because it may rapidly return upon rechallenge. It is reversible when the antibiotic is discontinued and no deaths have been reported.

Despite the relative rarity of this adverse effect, erythromycin estolate should be used with caution, particularly in adults. Other forms of erythromycin are preferred in patients with a history of liver disease, in those with pre-existing liver disease, or in those suspected of having impaired liver function.

Sensorineural hearing loss, although extremely rare, has been associated with use of large doses (Nicholas, 1977) or renal failure (Bennett et al, 1980) and has occurred more frequently in older patients (Haydon et al, 1984). It develops within a few hours to several days and is manifested as marked bilateral hearing loss that gradually reverses on discontinuation of the drug.

Suprainfections, including pseudomembranous colitis caused by *Clostridium difficile,* have been reported with erythromycin.

Thrombophlebitis occurs with intravenous administration. This can be minimized by slow infusion of more dilute solutions. Intramuscular administration of erythromycin is not recommended because injection is extremely painful.

Safety during pregnancy is not established, but congenital defects have not been reported despite widespread use. Erythromycin estolate has been associated with elevated serum glutamic oxaloacetic transaminase (SGOT) concentrations in about 10% of pregnant women (McCormack et al, 1977). This ester probably should not be used in pregnant women.

Troleandomycin may cause hepatic changes (eg, jaundice, hyperbilirubinemia, abnormal results of liver function tests) if administered for two weeks or longer. These effects are usually reversible if the drug is discontinued promptly. The most common adverse effects are hypersensitivity reactions, nausea, vomiting, diarrhea, anal burning, and headache. Anaphylactic reactions also have occurred. Because of its potential toxicity, troleandomycin is contraindicated in conditions requiring long-term therapy (eg, acne), in patients with hepatic disease or dysfunction, and in those sensitive to the drug.

Drug Interactions: Erythromycin can reduce clearance and increase serum theophylline levels in some patients, particularly those receiving large doses of the methylated xanthine. The mechanism appears to be inhibition of hepatic metabolism of theophylline by erythromycin. Because the potential for theophylline toxicity (eg, nausea, vomiting, cardiovascular instability, seizures) is increased, patients should be carefully monitored. Measurement of theophylline plasma concentrations is recommended (see Hansten, 1983 A; Ludden, 1985).

Plasma levels of carbamazepine [Tegretol] also can be elevated by erythromycin, leading to carbamazepine toxicity (eg, nausea, vomiting, drowsiness, nystagmus, ataxia). Close clinical monitoring of patients receiving these two drugs concurrently is recommended (see Hansten, 1983 B; Vajda and Bladin, 1984; Carranco et al, 1985; Ludden, 1985). Concomitant administration of erythromycin and warfarin [Coumadin, Panwarfin] can result in prolongation of prothrombin time with possible hemorrhage. Monitoring of prothrombin time is necessary when these drugs are given together (see Schwartz et al, 1983; Husserl, 1983; Sato et al, 1984; Hansten and Horn, 1985; Ludden, 1985). Similar to troleandomycin (see the evaluation), the elimination of methylprednisolone is reduced by erythromycin (LaForce et al, 1983; see Ludden, 1985). Although less well studied than the theophylline-erythromycin interaction, the mechanism for the interaction of erythromycin with each of the above three drugs also appears to be inhibition of hepatic drug metabolism by erythromycin (see Ludden, 1985).

Troleandomycin is a more potent inhibitor of microsomal drug metabolism than erythromycin and all of the above interactions also can occur with this agent (see Ludden, 1985).

Approximately 10% of patients convert substantial amounts of digoxin to inactive metabolites in the gastrointestinal tract. Certain antimicrobial agents, including erythromycin, have been shown to alter gut microbial flora and prevent the inactivation of digoxin. Thus, marked increases in serum digoxin levels can occur in these individuals. The effects of this interaction can persist for several months (Lindenbaum et al,

1981). Careful clinical monitoring of patients receiving these drugs is recommended (Doherty, 1981).

Acute ergot toxicity (eg, peripheral vasospasm) has been reported when erythromycin was administered to a patient receiving ergotamine tartrate [Ergomar, Ergostat] (Francis et al, 1984). This also has been reported for troleandomycin (see Ludden, 1985). The mechanism is unknown. Careful clinical monitoring for symptoms of ergot toxicity is recommended when ergot alkaloids and macrolides are given concurrently.

Erythromycin, primarily a bacteriostatic antibiotic, presumably may interfere with the action of bactericidal agents such as the penicillins. However, the clinical significance is unknown. Such a combination should be used only when it has been demonstrated to be beneficial.

Parenteral dosage forms of the erythromycins may be physically and/or chemically incompatible with solutions containing vitamin B complex, ascorbic acid, cephalothin, tetracycline, colistin [Coly-Mycin S], chloramphenicol, heparin, metaraminol [Aramine], and phenytoin [Dilantin].

Interference with Laboratory Tests: Erythromycin may cause false-positive elevations in SGOT concentrations when determined by colorimetric methods. This must be distinguished from drug-induced hepatotoxicity (see above). Erythromycin also may falsely elevate urinary catecholamine and 17-hydroxycorticosteroid levels.

Pharmacokinetics: The only form of erythromycin known to be biologically active in vivo is the free base. When given orally, however, erythromycin base is inactivated by gastric acid, resulting in decreased gastrointestinal absorption (Nicholas, 1977). Thus, a large number of derivatives and formulations have been prepared to optimize stability and absorption. Shielding the erythromycin base from acid degradation in the stomach by providing either a protective film coating [Erythromycin Base Filmtab] or enteric coating (ie, E-Mycin, ERYC, Ery-Tab, Ilotycin, Robimycin, RP-Mycin) has been one approach. Chemical modification of the erythromycin molecule itself to decrease acid inactivation is the other method. This has been accomplished by preparing the stearate salt (ie, Erypar, Erythrocin Stearate, Ethril, Pfizer-E, SK-Erythromycin, Wyamycin S), the ethylsuccinate ester (ie, E.E.S., E-Mycin E, EryPed, Pediamycin, Wyamycin E) or the lauryl sulfate salt of the propionyl ester, termed the estolate [Ilosone]. The ester and ester salt of erythromycin are tasteless and form stable suspensions in water; they usually are preferred in young children.

Peak serum levels obtained after administration of single doses of various erythromycin preparations appear in the Table. Peak serum levels are affected by several factors, including the chemical structure, the coating, the number of doses, and if the subject is fasting. There is considerable variation among subjects and from study to study.

Erythromycin base is absorbed intact. The nature of the coating applied to erythromycin base tablets affects both the time course and total amount of absorption. Absorption of film-coated erythromycin base tends to be erratic and administration under fasting conditions is required. Although erratic absorption of some enteric-coated tablets has been reported, other preparations provide excellent bioavailability in the fasting and nonfasting states with both single- and multiple-dose regimens (Fraser, 1980; also see Gribble and Chow, 1982).

Erythromycin stearate is absorbed as the base after dissociation in the duodenum. Erythromycin stearate also is acid labile and bioavailability is decreased significantly when this derivative is taken with food. Also, higher serum levels are achieved when the stearate is taken with large (eg, 250 ml) as opposed to small (eg, 20 ml) volumes of water in fasting individuals (Welling et al, 1978).

Erythromycin estolate is acid stable. It is absorbed as the propionyl ester and subsequently hydrolyzed to the free base. The absorption of the estolate is not affected by food. Total serum levels of erythromycin (bioactive erythromycin base plus bioinactive erythromycin propionate) are at least three to four times greater following absorption of the estolate than the base or stearate. However, only 20% to 30% of the circulating drug represents the bioactive base; the remainder is unchanged propionyl ester (Bechtol et al, 1976). Thus, the actual concentrations of base achieved are similar to those obtained when other oral preparations are taken in the fasting state. For example, studies (DiSanto et al, 1980) comparing enteric-coated tablets of erythromycin base and capsules containing erythromycin estolate revealed essentially no difference in the plasma concentrations of bioactive erythromycin.

Erythromycin ethylsuccinate is absorbed directly as the inactive ester. Although the extent of in vivo hydrolysis of this derivative to free base (about 55%) is greater than for the estolate, the actual serum levels of bioactive free base are less because less total drug is absorbed. Because of the high therapeutic/toxic ratio for the erythromycins, the larger dose of the ethylsuccinate ester that is required usually does not cause increased toxicity. However, in one controlled trial comparing erythromycin ethylsuccinate (25 mg/kg twice daily) to erythromycin estolate (15 mg/kg twice daily) for group A streptococcal pharyngitis in children, bacteriologic failure rates and gastrointestinal intolerance were significantly higher in the group receiving the ethylsuccinate ester (Ginsburg et al, 1984). Food does not affect the absorption of the ethylsuccinate ester and some studies suggest that food can enhance absorption (Fraser, 1980; also see Gribble and Chow, 1982).

When oral erythromycin preparations are administered in the correct dose and with proper timing in relation to food intake, it appears that no one type of preparation offers a significant therapeutic advantage, at least in mild to moderate infections caused by susceptible organisms (see Gribble and Chow, 1982; *Federal Register*, 1982; Steigbigel, 1984). Erythromycin estolate usually is not recommended for adults because of the increased risk of cholestatic hepatitis (see Adverse Reactions and Precautions). In children, however, this derivative rarely causes hepatitis and some pediatric infectious disease experts prefer the estolate over the ethylsuccinate because of better bioavailability (Ginsburg et al, 1976, 1982, 1984; *Med Lett Drugs Ther*, 1985). When high blood levels are required (eg, for serious infections), the glucceptate and lactobionate salts may be given intravenously.

Erythromycin passes readily into most tissues and body fluids (including prostatic fluid) and is distributed throughout total body water. The volume of distribution is 0.72 ± 0.20 L/kg, and the drug is 70% to 75% protein bound. Useful therapeutic concentrations cannot be attained in cerebrospinal fluid, except for extremely susceptible organisms, even in the presence of inflammation. This agent crosses the placenta, but

PEAK SERUM LEVELS OF ERYTHROMYCIN IN ADULTS[a]

Preparation	Dose (mg)	Route	Peak Serum Level	
			Hours After Dose	mcg/ml
Base	250	Oral	4	0.3-1.0[b]
	500			0.3-1.9
Stearate	250 (fasting)	Oral	3	0.2-1.3
	500 (fasting)		3	0.4-1.8
	500 (after food)		3	0.1-0.4[c]
Ethylsuccinate	500	Oral	0.5-2.5	1.5[d] (0.6[e])
Estolate	250	Oral	2-4	1.4-1.7[d]
	500		3.5-4	4.2[d] (1.1[e])
Lactobionate	200	Intravenous	Immediately	3-4
	500		1	9.9
Gluceptate	250	Intravenous	Immediately	3.5-10.7
	1000		1	9.9

[a]From Steigbigel NH: Erythromycin, lincomycin, and clindamycin, in Mandell GL, et al (eds): Principles and Practice of Infectious Diseases, ed 2. New York, John Wiley & Sons, 1984, 226. (Reprinted with permission)
[b]Somewhat higher levels reported with some enteric-coated preparations after repeated doses (MacDonald et al, 1977; DiSanto and Chodos, 1981).
[c]Recent studies note higher levels (to 2.8 mcg/ml) with dose taken during a meal (Malmborg, 1979).
[d]Total drug (inactive ester and free base)
[e]Free base

fetal blood levels are no higher than 10% (usually closer to 2%) of those present in the maternal circulation.

Erythromycin is concentrated in the liver and high concentrations are excreted into the bile in the absence of obstruction. Some of the absorbed drug is demethylated in the liver. A considerable portion of an oral dose is eliminated in the feces, resulting largely from biliary excretion, but some represents unabsorbed drug. Only 2% to 5% of an oral dose and 12% to 15% of an intravenous dose is eliminated in the urine.

The reported half-life of erythromycin varies from one to more than three hours in normal individuals (Bennett et al, 1980; Benet and Sheiner, 1980). The half-life is increased to approximately five hours in anuric patients. There is no need, therefore, to adjust dosage in patients with renal insufficiency. Erythromycin is not removed by peritoneal dialysis or hemodialysis.

Because erythromycin is excreted primarily by the liver, caution should be exercised in patients with impaired hepatic function. The estolate ester is not recommended in such patients (see Adverse Reactions and Precautions).

Drug Evaluations

ERYTHROMYCIN

[film-coated: Erythromycin Base Filmtabs; enteric-coated: E-Mycin, ERYC, Ery-Tab, Ilotycin, Robimycin, RP-Mycin]

ERYTHROMYCIN ESTOLATE
[Ilosone]

ERYTHROMYCIN ETHYLSUCCINATE
[E.E.S., E-Mycin E, EryPed, Pediamycin, Wyamycin E]

ERYTHROMYCIN GLUCEPTATE
[Ilotycin Gluceptate]

ERYTHROMYCIN LACTOBIONATE
[Erythrocin Lactobionate-IV]

ERYTHROMYCIN STEARATE
[Erypar, Erythrocin Stearate, Ethril, Pfizer-E, SK-Erythromycin, Wyamycin S]

All erythromycins (base, salt, esters) have the same spectrum of antibacterial activity and uses; adverse reactions also are similar, except that erythromycin estolate has a greater propensity to cause hepatotoxicity. See the introductory section on Macrolides for a detailed discussion.

DOSAGE AND PREPARATIONS. All doses and strengths are expressed in terms of the base. For group A streptococcal infections, therapy should be continued for at least ten days. *Oral:* (Base) *Adults,* 250 to 500 mg every six hours. Alternative schedules for the lower dosage are 333 mg every eight hours (*E-Mycin* and *Ery-Tab* only) or 500 mg every 12 hours.

See the manufacturers' labeling to determine whether a specific preparation should be administered with or without food.

(Estolate) *Adults*, 250 to 500 mg every six hours. Alternative schedule for the lower dosage is 500 mg every 12 hours.

(Ethylsuccinate) *Adults,* 400 to 800 mg four times daily. Alternative schedules for the lower dosage are 600 mg every eight hours or 800 mg every 12 hours.

(Stearate) *Adults,* 250 to 500 mg every six hours. Alternative schedule for the lower dosage is 500 mg every 12 hours. Preferably, the drug is given on an empty stomach. See the manufacturers' recommendations for specific preparations.

(All forms) For severe infections in *adults,* up to 4 g may be given daily in divided doses. These larger doses (eg, 4 g daily) are necessary for the treatment of known or suspected *Legionella* infections. *Children,* 30 to 50 mg/kg daily in four divided doses; for severe infections, the dose may be doubled.

For prophylaxis of rheumatic fever or infective endocarditis, see Chapter 65, Antimicrobial Therapy and Chemoprophylaxis of Infectious Diseases, Table 3.

For treatment of sexually transmitted diseases, including chlamydial infections, chancroid, and syphilis, see Chapter 65, Table 2.

For prophylaxis of elective colorectal surgery, see Chapter 65, Table 4.

ERYTHROMYCIN:
Generic. Powder; tablets (plain, enteric-coated) 250 and 500 mg.
Erythromycin Base Filmtab (Abbott). Tablets (film-coated) 250 and 500 mg.
E-Mycin (Upjohn). Tablets (enteric-coated) 250 and 333 mg.
ERYC (Parke-Davis). Capsules 250 mg (enteric-coated pellets).
Ery-Tab (Abbott). Tablets (enteric-coated) 250, 333, and 500 mg.
Ilotycin (Dista), *Robimycin* (Robins), *RP-Mycin* (Reid-Provident). Tablets (enteric-coated) 250 mg.

ERYTHROMYCIN ESTOLATE:
Generic. Capsules, tablets 250 mg; suspension 125 and 250 mg/5 ml.
Ilosone (Dista). Capsules 125 and 250 mg; drops 100 mg/ml; suspension 125 and 250 mg/5 ml; tablets (chewable) 125 and 250 mg; tablets 500 mg.

ERYTHROMYCIN ETHYLSUCCINATE:
Generic. Granules, powder for suspension 200 mg/5 ml after reconstitution; suspension 200 and 400 mg/5 ml; tablets 400 mg.
E.E.S. (Abbott). Powder for oral suspension 100 mg/2.5 ml after reconstitution; granules for oral suspension 200 mg/5 ml after reconstitution; suspension 200 and 400 mg/5 ml; tablets (chewable) 200 mg, (film-coated) 400 mg.
E-Mycin E (Upjohn), *Wyamycin E* (Wyeth). Suspension 200 and 400 mg/5 ml.
EryPed (Abbott). Powder for oral suspension 400 mg/5 ml after reconstitution.
Pediamycin (Ross). Powder for oral suspension 100 mg/2.5 ml after reconstitution; granules for oral suspension 200 mg/5 ml after reconstitution; suspension 200 and 400 mg/5 ml.

ERYTHROMYCIN STEARATE:
Generic. Tablets (film-coated) 250 and 500 mg, (enteric-coated) 250 mg.
Erypar (Parke-Davis), *Erythrocin Stearate Filmtab* (Abbott), *Ethril* (Squibb), *SK-Erythromycin* (Smith Kline & French), *Wyamycin S* (Wyeth). Tablets (film-coated) 250 and 500 mg.
Pfizer-E (Pfipharmecs). Tablets (film-coated) 250 mg.

Intravenous: For severe infections, *adults,* 1 to 4 g daily; *children*, 15 to 50 mg/kg daily (maximum, 4 g daily) (Norris and Mandell, 1985). The larger doses (eg, 4 g daily) are necessary for known or suspected *Legionella* infections.

Continuous infusion is preferable, but administration in divided doses at intervals not greater than every six hours also is effective. Because of the irritating properties of erythromycin, intravenous push is not acceptable. For instructions on the preparation of intravenous solutions and drug administration, consult the manufacturers' literature.

An oral dosage form should be substituted as soon as possible.

ERYTHROMYCIN GLUCEPTATE:
Ilotycin Gluceptate (Dista). Powder 250 and 500 mg and 1 g.
ERYTHROMYCIN LACTOBIONATE:
Generic, Erythrocin Lactobionate-IV (Abbott). Powder (sterile, lyophilized) 500 mg and 1 g.

TROLEANDOMYCIN
[TAO]

Use of troleandomycin for infectious diseases is seldom indicated because much more effective and potentially less toxic agents are available. For antibacterial spectrum, adverse reactions and precautions, and interactions, see the introductory section on Macrolides.

The oral combination of troleandomycin plus methylprednisolone is used occasionally as a last resort in patients with severe asthma who are not adequately controlled by high doses of the steroid alone. Troleandomycin is a steroid-sparing agent that decreases the clearance and increases the plasma levels of methylprednisolone, presumably by inhibiting hepatic microsomal drug metabolism (see Ludden, 1985). See also Chapter 22, Drugs Used in Bronchial Disorders, for additional discussion.

DOSAGE AND PREPARATIONS.
Oral: Adults, 250 to 500 mg four times daily; *children,* 6.6 to 11 mg/kg every six hours. For group A streptococcal infections, therapy should be continued for at least ten days.

For severe asthma, see Chapter 22.
TAO (Roerig). Capsules equivalent to 250 mg of oleandomycin.

LINCOSAMIDES

The lincosamides include lincomycin [Lincocin], an antibacterial agent produced by *Streptomyces lincolnensis* var. *lincolnensis*, and its semisynthetic derivative, clindamycin [Cleocin]. These drugs contain an amino acid linked to an amino sugar. Clindamycin (7-chloro-7-deoxylincomycin) differs chemically from lincomycin by the substitution of a chlorine atom for a hydroxyl group on the parent molecule (see Figure 2). With this slight molecular modification, clindamycin has increased antibacterial potency and is better absorbed from the gastrointestinal tract after oral administration (McGehee et al, 1968). Thus, it is the preferred lincosamide for clinical use and the discussion in this section will focus primarily on clindamycin.

Mechanism of Action: Clindamycin and lincomycin inhibit bacterial protein synthesis by binding to the 50S ribosomal subunit and probably prevent elongation of the peptide chain by interfering with peptidyl transfer (see Davis, 1980). Compe-

FIGURE 2. CHEMICAL STRUCTURES OF LINCOSAMIDES

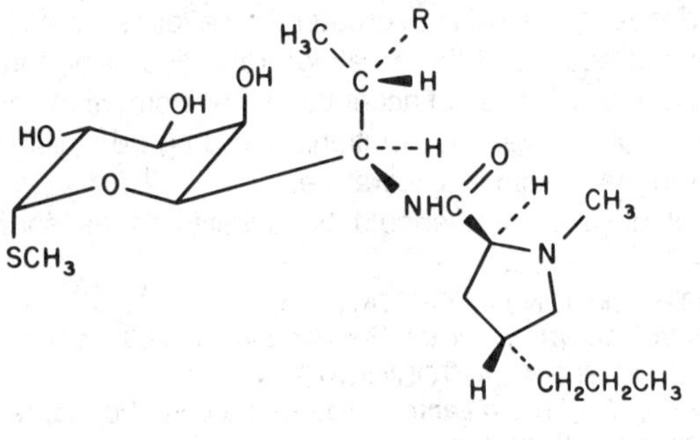

GENERIC NAME	R
Lincomycin	OH
Clindamycin	Cl

tition experiments have demonstrated that the clindamycin ribosomal binding site overlaps those for chloramphenicol and erythromycin, but they are not identical (see Pratt, 1977). There are no clinical indications for the concurrent use of these antibiotics.

The lincosamides are primarily bacteriostatic. However, depending on the antibiotic concentration, the organism's susceptibility, and the size of the inoculum, bactericidal activity has been demonstrated against some organisms (eg, *Streptococcus pneumoniae, S. pyogenes, Bacteroides fragilis*).

Antimicrobial Spectrum: The lincosamides are active against most gram-positive and anaerobic gram-negative bacteria; clindamycin is more potent than lincomycin.

Clindamycin resembles erythromycin in its activity in vitro against various streptococci, including *S. pneumoniae, S. pyogenes,* and viridans streptococci. However, *S. faecalis* is resistant. It also is active against *Staphylococcus aureus,* although some resistant strains have been reported. *Corynebacterium diphtheriae* are susceptible.

Anaerobic organisms susceptible to clindamycin in vitro include *Bacteroides* species (including the *B. fragilis* group [from 3% to 7% of strains are resistant (Tally et al, 1985)]), *Fusobacterium, Propionibacterium, Eubacterium, Bifidobacterium, Peptococcus* (about 10% are resistant), *Peptostreptococcus* and *Veillonella* species, microaerophilic streptococci, clostridia (most *C. perfringens* [*welchii*] and *C. tetani* are susceptible, but *C. sporogenes* and *C. tertium* often are resistant), and several *Actinomyces* species.

Although most strains of *Mycoplasma pneumoniae* are susceptible, other antibiotics (eg, erythromycin, tetracycline) are preferred. Most aerobic gram-negative bacteria (eg, the Enterobacteriaceae, *Haemophilus influenzae, Neisseria meningitidis*) are resistant to the lincosamides. Most *Nocardia* species are resistant. Yeasts, fungi, and viruses also are resistant.

Resistance: Acquired resistance to clindamycin has been observed for gram-positive cocci and the *Bacteroides fragilis* group.

Occasional clinical isolates of clindamycin-resistant *Streptococcus pneumoniae, S. pyogenes*, and viridans streptococci have been reported; these strains also are resistant to lincomycin and usually to erythromycin.

Strains of *Staphylococcus aureus* also may become resistant to clindamycin. In vitro, staphylococcal resistance usually develops in a slow, stepwise manner, but can occur more rapidly in strains that are already resistant to erythromycin. Clinical isolates of clindamycin-resistant staphylococci frequently are resistant to erythromycin. Cross-resistance between clindamycin and lincomycin is complete for staphylococci. Mechanisms appear to involve alterations in the 50S ribosomal binding site or in the 23S RNA component of the 50S subunit (see Steigbigel, 1984; see also the section on Macrolides).

Resistance of *B. fragilis* to clindamycin in the United States during 1981, 1982, and 1983 was assessed in a multicenter study. The average rate of resistance was 6%, 3%, and 7%, respectively, but this ranged from 0 to 17% in various institutions (Tally et al, 1985). High-level, plasmid-mediated, transferable clindamycin resistance has been demonstrated; resistance to erythromycin also is carried on these genes (Tally et al, 1979, 1983). Clinically, clindamycin-resistant *B. fragilis* strains have been shown to cause severe infections (Yee et al, 1982). Because antimicrobial resistance can be a problem with this organism, antimicrobial susceptibility testing should be performed.

Uses: Clindamycin is preferred to lincomycin for all indications because it has greater antibacterial potency and is better absorbed after oral administration (see Antimicrobial Spectrum and Pharmacokinetics). The number of indications for clindamycin is limited, however, because of the potential for life-threatening antibiotic-associated pseudomembranous colitis and the availability of equally effective, less toxic alternatives.

Clindamycin often is effective in anaerobic infections. It has been widely used and usually is considered a drug of choice for intra-abdominal sepsis (eg, peritonitis secondary to bowel perforation) and nonvenereal gynecologic pelvic infections (eg, pelvic or tubo-ovarian abscess, endometritis). These infections usually involve penicillin G-resistant anaerobic bacteria, particularly the *Bacteroides fragilis* group (the most common group of anaerobic pathogens in intra-abdominal sepsis) or *B. bivius* (a common genital tract pathogen). These infections usually are polymicrobial and are caused by a mixture of aerobic gram-negative bacilli (eg, Enterobacteriaceae) as well as anaerobic bacteria, and an aminoglycoside is combined with clindamycin to eradicate the aerobic organisms. Metronidazole [Flagyl, Metryl], chloramphenicol, and, depending on local susceptibility patterns, cefoxitin [Mefoxin] and the antipseudomonal penicillins (eg, piperacillin [Pipracil]) also are effective against penicillin G-resistant anaerobes, particularly the *B. fragilis* group, and are alternatives to clindamycin for these infections (see Finegold et al, 1975, 1985; Tally, 1981; Bartlett, 1982; Fekety, 1982; *Med Lett Drugs Ther*, 1984; DiPiro et al, 1986; see also Chapter 65, Antimicrobial Therapy and Chemoprophylaxis of Infectious Diseases, Tables 1 and 2). Cefoxitin alone may be adequate for certain community-acquired intra-abdominal infections (Tally et al, 1981).

Certain serious soft tissue infections, such as infected decubitus ulcers with sepsis, frequently are associated with anaerobic bacteria, including the *B. fragilis* group, as well as coliforms. Clindamycin, usually in combination regimens, is a preferred drug for the anaerobic pathogens. This drug is not suitable for central nervous system infections (eg, brain abscess) caused by anaerobic bacteria because of poor penetration of the blood-brain barrier. Chloramphenicol and metronidazole are preferred for penicillin G-resistant anaerobes (eg, the *B. fragilis* group) in the central nervous system. Clindamycin also has been disappointing in anaerobic bacterial endocarditis. When members of the *B. fragilis* group are causative, metronidazole is the drug of choice because of its consistent bactericidal activity against this organism (see Chapter 72, Miscellaneous Antibacterial Agents).

For anaerobic infections above the diaphragm, including orodental infections, aspiration pneumonia, and lung abscess, penicillin G traditionally has been the preferred antibiotic. Clindamycin is an effective alternative in penicillin-allergic patients and for bronchopulmonary infections that fail to respond to penicillin G. The role of clindamycin in serious bronchopulmonary infections may become more prominent, however. Penicillin G-resistant strains of *Bacteroides melaninogenicus*, a common anaerobic pathogen in the respiratory tract, are increasing and, although relatively uncommon, members of the *B. fragilis* group cause some bronchopulmonary infections (see Tally, 1981; Bartlett, 1982; *Med Lett Drugs Ther*, 1984). In a prospective, randomized, controlled, clinical trial comparing clindamycin to penicillin G for the treatment of community-acquired putrid lung abscess, clindamycin was superior (Levison et al, 1983); however, some flaws in this study have been noted (Bartlett and Gorbach, 1983).

Clindamycin has been used as an alternative to penicillin G in infections caused by *Clostridium perfringens* and *Actinomyces israelii*.

Clindamycin may be indicated as an alternative antibiotic for infections caused by susceptible gram-positive cocci, usually *Staphylococcus aureus*, in patients who are allergic to both penicillins and cephalosporins. These include skin and soft tissue infections, septic arthritis, and osteomyelitis. Clindamycin penetrates bone very well and has been a useful alternative in osteomyelitis, although some experts prefer vancomycin [Vancocin], a bactericidal drug, in patients who are allergic to the beta lactams. Because clindamycin is unreliably bactericidal against *S. aureus* and because of the potential for the emergence of resistant strains, it usually is not recommended for deep-seated or life-threatening *S. aureus* infections (eg, endocarditis, sepsis). For most mild staphylococcal skin infections (eg, pyodermas), group A streptococcal infections (eg, pyodermas, pharyngitis), and pneumococcal infections (eg, acute sinusitis, acute otitis media, pneumonia) in penicillin-allergic patients, erythromycin usually is preferred to clindamycin because it is less toxic. See Chapter 65, Table 1, for additional discussion.

Clindamycin has been effective in certain surgical prophylactic regimens, particularly in combination with an aminoglycoside in 'dirty' colorectal and urologic surgical procedures (see Chapter 65, Table 4).

Topical clindamycin [Cleocin T] has been effective in the treatment of acne (see Chapter 56, Dermatologic Preparations).

Antibiotic-Associated Pseudomembranous Colitis (AAPMC): Lincomycin and clindamycin are usually well tolerated. A common adverse effect is diarrhea; the incidence associated with clindamycin therapy has been reported to be as low as 2% and as high as 21% (mean, about 8%). The lincosamides are capable of causing antibiotic-associated pseudomembranous colitis (AAPMC) that can be fatal. AAPMC has been estimated to occur in less than 0.01% to more than 10% of patients (Tedesco, 1977; Swartzberg et al, 1977; Gurwith et al, 1977; Lusk et al, 1977; Neu et al, 1977); this variable incidence may reflect different diagnostic methods and the variable epidemiology of *Clostridium difficile*. Essentially all antibiotics can cause diarrhea, however, including AAPMC. Those most frequently associated with AAPMC are ampicillin, the lincosamides, and the cephalosporins (see Fekety, 1978; Bartlett, 1981; Chang, 1981). Thus, the following discussion of AAPMC applies to other antibiotics in addition to the lincosamides.

Older individuals, particularly those with chronic, debilitating diseases, are at greater risk of developing AAPMC. The incidence is unrelated to the route of administration, total dosage, duration of therapy, or underlying disease.

The most frequently observed clinical features of AAPMC are watery diarrhea, crampy abdominal pain, fever, and leukocytosis. Mucus and blood in the stools also may be observed. Sigmoidoscopic examination often shows plaque-like lesions (pseudomembranes) on the colonic or rectal mucosa. Histologically, the pseudomembrane is composed of polymorphonuclear leukocytes, chronic inflammatory cells, fibrin, and epithelial debris (Tedesco, 1982 A).

The majority of patients present with watery diarrhea between the fourth and ninth days of therapy. However, 25% to 40% of patients develop diarrhea and AAPMC from two to as long as ten weeks after completion of therapy. Diarrhea that develops during antibiotic administration usually is self-limiting and ceases 4 to 14 days after the medication is discontinued. The disorder is usually more protracted (two to four weeks' duration) and debilitating in patients who continue to receive antibiotic therapy in spite of diarrhea, or in those who initially develop diarrhea after the course of antibiotic therapy has been completed (see Tedesco, 1982 A).

The syndrome has been studied in detail using Syrian hamsters as an animal model (Rifkin et al, 1977, 1978 A; Lusk et al, 1978). In the hamster, AAPMC is caused by an enterotoxin produced by *Clostridium difficile*, and passive immunization with *C. sordellii* antitoxin protects against AAPMC after administration of clindamycin. A heat-labile toxin has been demonstrated in the feces of patients with AAPMC induced by clindamycin and ampicillin (Larson and Price, 1977; Larson et al, 1977; Rifkin et al, 1978 B; Bartlett et al, 1978), and enterotoxigenic strains of *C. difficile* usually can be identified (Fekety, 1978; Tedesco et al, 1978).

AAPMC should be suspected in any patient who develops diarrhea during or up to four weeks after therapy with these agents. Although sigmoidoscopy may be sufficient to visualize colonic changes in the majority of cases, the etiologic diagnosis of *C. difficile*-induced pseudomembranous colitis requires demonstration of the *C. difficile* toxin by tissue culture assay or with newer, more rapid immunologic methods (eg, enzyme-linked immunosorbent assay [ELISA]) (see Chang, 1981; Tedesco, 1982 A).

Once AAPMC has been diagnosed, the offending antibiotic should be discontinued and procedures initiated to restore and maintain normal fluid and electrolyte balance. If diarrhea continues or if it begins after antimicrobials have been stopped, additional treatment is necessary. Specific therapy aimed at either eradication of the C. difficile organism or removal of the toxin is now available (see Tedesco, 1982 A; Gotz and Rand, 1982). Oral vancomycin (125 to 500 mg every six hours for 5 to 10 days in adults with normal renal function) is considered the antibiotic of choice (see Table 1 in Chapter 65, Antimicrobial Therapy and Chemoprophylaxis of Infectious Diseases, and Chapter 72, Miscellaneous Antibacterial Agents). Responses are usually prompt and impressive; diarrhea, fever, and abdominal cramps usually subside in two to four days and toxin levels in stool samples decline gradually over three to seven days. Oral metronidazole (250 mg four times daily or 500 mg three times daily [see Chapter 72]), bacitracin (25,000 units four times daily [see Chapter 72]), and cholestyramine [Questran] (or colestipol [Colestid]) anion exchange resin (4 g of either resin three times daily) also have been shown to be useful in treating AAPMC. Like vancomycin, metronidazole and bacitracin eradicate the C. difficile organism, but there is less experience with these antibiotics. Metronidazole was shown to be as effective as vancomycin in a prospective, randomized trial (Teasley et al, 1983) and may become a less costly alternative in some patients. In a few cases, metronidazole has caused AAPMC, however. Cholestyramine (or colestipol) binds and neutralizes the toxin. Because the resin also binds vancomycin, simultaneous use should be avoided. Success rates have been variable with cholestyramine and it appears to be more effective for mild AAPMC. Occasionally, additional aggressive supportive treatment also may be necessary, particularly in elderly patients.

Relapses of AAPMC have been observed in 10% to 20% of patients after initial successful treatment with vancomycin, metronidazole, or bacitracin. Persistent fecal carriage of C. difficile after treatment is an important risk factor. Most patients respond to a repeat course of vancomycin or metronidazole and experience only one relapse. However, some individuals suffer multiple relapses. Optimum treatment guidelines for recurrent AAPMC are unknown, but a tapering dose of vancomycin in conjunction with cholestipol resin has been used successfully in a few patients (Tedesco, 1982 B).

Although steroids have been used systemically, there is little evidence that they are beneficial in AAPMC. Antiperistaltic drugs, such as loperamide and the antidiarrheal mixture, diphenoxylate with atropine [Lomotil], are not recommended for the treatment of AAPMC. Their effectiveness is questionable, they may prevent clearance of the toxin from the stool, and toxic megacolon has been associated with their use in AAPMC.

Although AAPMC is not unique to the lincosamides, is relatively uncommon, and is treatable, physicians should prescribe lincosamides only when clearly indicated, and they should be alert to the potential for this adverse reaction.

Other Adverse Reactions and Precautions: In addition to diarrhea, other reported adverse effects of the lincosamides on the gastrointestinal tract include nausea and vomiting.

Hypersensitivity reactions have occurred with both clindamycin and lincomycin. Generalized, mild to moderate, morbilliform-like skin rashes are relatively common. Pruritus, maculopapular rash, and urticaria also have been observed. Severe hypersensitivity reactions, such as erythema multiforme and anaphylaxis, have been reported rarely with these antibiotics.

Transient leukopenia and eosinophilia have been reported. In addition, agranulocytosis and thrombocytopenia rarely have been associated with use of the lincosamides. These effects are reversible following withdrawal of the drugs.

Transitory changes in liver function tests have occurred after administration of lincomycin and clindamycin. More serious hepatotoxicity, including jaundice, has been reported rarely.

A medicinal taste experienced during infusions of 600 mg or more of clindamycin is probably due to the high concentrations of drug in saliva.

Hypotension, electrocardiographic changes, and, rarely, cardiac arrest have been associated with the rapid administration of large intravenous doses of lincomycin. Cardiac arrest also has been reported in a patient after 600 mg of undiluted clindamycin was injected over several minutes into a central intravenous line (Aucoin et al, 1982).

The safety of these drugs during pregnancy has not been established, although no harmful effects have been observed in several hundred pregnant women who have taken lincomycin or clindamycin during all stages of pregnancy.

Although pain, induration, and sterile abscesses after intramuscular administration and thrombophlebitis after intravenous administration have been reported, local irritative reactions are uncommon and these drugs are generally well tolerated after parenteral administration.

Drug Interactions: Clindamycin and lincomycin have a slight neuromuscular blocking effect and may enhance the action of other neuromuscular blocking drugs. A solution of clindamycin phosphate is chemically incompatible with ampicillin, phenytoin, barbiturates, aminophylline, calcium gluconate, and magnesium sulfate (Steigbigel, 1984).

Pharmacokinetics: Essentially all (90%) of an oral dose of clindamycin hydrochloride is absorbed, and mean peak plasma concentrations of 2.5 and 3.6 mcg/ml have been attained 45 to 60 minutes after ingestion of 150 and 300 mg, respectively, in adults. Clindamycin palmitate also is absorbed rapidly and efficiently after oral administration, but serum levels are slightly lower. Food interferes with the absorption of oral lincomycin, but the absorption of clindamycin preparations does not appear to be appreciably retarded.

After intravenous administration, biologically inactive clindamycin phosphate is rapidly converted to active clindamycin. In healthy adults, peak serum levels of active drug were 7, 10, 11, and 14 mcg/ml after infusions of 300 mg (over 10 minutes), 600 mg (over 20 minutes), 900 mg (over 30 minutes), and 1.2 g (over 45 minutes), respectively. After intramuscular administration, peak levels of clindamycin are reached after three hours in adults and after one hour in children. With both oral and parenteral preparations of clindamycin, peak serum concentrations increase linearly (but not proportionally) with increases in dosage.

Clindamycin is approximately 90% protein bound. The volume of distribution is 93.6 ± 0.2 L (Benet and Sheiner, 1980). It is widely distributed throughout the body and penetrates well into various tissues and body fluids, including saliva, sputum, respiratory tissue, pleural fluid, bile, liver, gallbladder, appendix, soft tissues, prostate, semen, and bones and joints (see LeFrock et al, 1982). However, effective concentrations are not attained in the cerebrospinal fluid, even when meninges are inflamed. Clindamycin readily crosses the placenta. This drug is actively transported into polymorphonuclear leukocytes and macrophages and achieves relatively high concentrations in experimental abscesses (see Steigbigel, 1984).

Clindamycin is primarily metabolized in the liver to bioactive and inactive metabolites. N-demethyl clindamycin (more active than parent drug) and clindamycin sulfoxide (less active) are the major bioactive metabolites. Metabolites are excreted in the urine and bile. Only 10% of an administered dose is excreted unchanged in the urine.

The elimination half-life of clindamycin is approximately three hours in normal individuals and is only slightly increased in patients with markedly reduced renal or hepatic function. Therefore, little or no dosage modification is needed for patients with mild to moderate renal or hepatic impairment. Dosage reduction is recommended in patients with combined severe renal and hepatic disease. Hemodialysis and peritoneal dialysis do not remove clindamycin from the serum.

For a description of the clinical pharmacology of lincomycin, see Fass, 1980.

Drug Evaluations

CLINDAMYCIN HYDROCHLORIDE
[Cleocin Hydrochloride]

CLINDAMYCIN PALMITATE HYDROCHLORIDE
[Cleocin Pediatric]

CLINDAMYCIN PHOSPHATE
[Cleocin Phosphate]

Clindamycin is a semisynthetic derivative of lincomycin that is more potent and better absorbed than the parent compound. Thus, it is the preferred lincosamide for all indications. For antimicrobial spectrum, uses, pharmacokinetics, adverse reactions and precautions, and interactions, see the introduction on Lincosamides.

DOSAGE AND PREPARATIONS. For group A streptococcal infections, treatment should be continued for at least ten days. *Oral:* (Hydrochloride) *Adults,* for serious infections, 150 to 300 mg every six hours; for more severe infections, 300 to 450 mg every six hours. *Children,* for serious infections, 8 to 16 mg/kg daily in three or four divided doses; for more severe infections, 16 to 20 mg/kg daily in three or four divided doses.

(Palmitate Hydrochloride) *Adults and children weighing more than 10 kg*, for serious infections, 8 to 12 mg/kg daily in three or four divided doses; for severe infections, 13 to 16 mg/kg daily in three or four divided doses; for more severe infections, 17 to 25 mg/kg daily in three or four divided doses. *Children weighing 10 kg or less,* 37.5 mg three times daily is the minimum recommended dose.

CLINDAMYCIN HYDROCHLORIDE:
Cleocin Hydrochloride (Upjohn). Capsules 75 and 150 mg (equivalent to base).
CLINDAMYCIN PALMITATE HYDROCHLORIDE:
Cleocin Pediatric (Upjohn). Granules for suspension 75 mg/5 ml (equivalent to base).

Intramuscular: Intramuscular injection of more than 600 mg at a single site is frequently painful and is not recommended. Oral therapy should be substituted as soon as possible. *Adults,* for serious infections with aerobic gram-positive cocci and more sensitive anaerobes, 600 mg to 1.2 g daily in two, three, or four equally divided doses. For more severe infections, particularly those caused by *Bacteroides fragilis, Peptococcus,* or *Clostridium* (other than *C. perfringens*), 1.2 to 2.7 g daily in two, three, or four equally divided doses. *Children over 1 month,* for serious infections, 15 to 25 mg/kg (alternative, 350 mg/M²) daily in three or four equally divided doses; for more severe infections, 25 to 40 mg/kg (alternative, 450 mg/M²) daily in three or four equally divided doses (minimum, 300 mg daily).

Intravenous: Oral therapy should be substituted as soon as possible. *Adults,* for serious infections with aerobic gram-positive cocci and more sensitive anaerobes, 600 mg to 1.2 g daily in two, three, or four equally divided doses; for more severe infections, particularly those caused by *B. fragilis, Peptococcus,* or *Clostridium* (other than *C. perfringens*), 1.2 to 2.7 g daily in two, three, or four equally divided doses; for life-threatening infections, as much as 4.8 g daily has been given. Alternatively, the initial dose may be administered as a single rapid infusion, followed by continuous infusion (see manufacturer's recommendations). *Children over 1 month,* for serious infections, 15 to 25 mg/kg (alternative, 350 mg/M²) daily in three or four equally divided doses; for more severe infections, 25 to 40 mg/kg (alternative, 450 mg/M²) daily (minimum, 300 mg).

Clindamycin phosphate should *not* be injected intravenously undiluted as a bolus. It should be diluted with an appropriate solution for injection to a concentration of not more than 12 mg/ml and infused at a rate of not more than 30 mg/min. See manufacturer's recommendations for appropriate infusion rates.

CLINDAMYCIN PHOSPHATE:
Cleocin Phosphate (Upjohn). Solution (sterile) 150 mg/ml in 2, 4, and 6 ml containers (equivalent to base).

LINCOMYCIN HYDROCHLORIDE MONOHYDRATE
[Lincocin]

Lincomycin offers no therapeutic advantages over clindamycin. Consequently, it has become obsolete.

For antimicrobial spectrum, adverse reactions, and precautions, see the introduction on Lincosamides.

DOSAGE AND PREPARATIONS. For group A streptococcal infections, therapy should be continued for at least ten days.

Oral: *Adults,* for serious infections, 500 mg three times daily; for more severe infections, 500 mg four times daily; *children and infants over 1 month,* for serious infections, 30 mg/kg daily in three or four divided doses; for more severe infections, 60 mg/kg daily in three or four divided doses.

Lincocin (Upjohn). Capsules 250 (pediatric) and 500 mg (equivalent to base).

Intramuscular: *Adults,* for serious infections, 600 mg every 24 hours; for more severe infections, 600 mg every 12 hours or more often; *children and infants over 1 month,* for serious infections, 10 mg/kg every 24 hours; for more severe infections, 10 mg/kg every 12 hours or more often.

Intravenous: *Adults,* for serious infections, 600 mg to 1 g every 8 to 12 hours; dosage may be increased to a maximum of 8 g daily for more severe infections. *Children and infants over 1 month,* 10 to 20 mg/kg daily (depending on the severity of the infection) in two or three divided doses.

Lincomycin should *not* be injected intravenously undiluted as a bolus because cardiopulmonary arrest has occurred with rapid intravenous administration of large doses. The drug should be diluted with an appropriate solution for intravenous injection to a concentration of not more than 1 g/100 ml and infused slowly over a period of not less than one hour (see manufacturer's recommendations).

Lincocin (Upjohn). Solution (sterile) 300 mg/ml in 2 and 10 ml containers (equivalent to base).

Cited References

Drugs for anaerobic infections. *Med Lett Drugs Ther* 26:87-89, 1984.

Erythromycin estolate: Withdrawal of proposal to revoke provisions for certification of tablets and capsules; response to petition; labeling. *Federal Register* 47:22547-22568, (May 25) 1982.

Oral erythromycins. *Med Lett Drugs Ther* 27:1-3, 1985.

1985 STD treatment guidelines. *Morbid Mortal Week Rep* 34(suppl):S75-S108, 1985.

Anders BJ, et al: Double-blind placebo-controlled trial of erythromycin for treatment of *Campylobacter* enteritis. *Lancet* 1:131-132, 1982.

Aucoin P, et al: Clindamycin-induced cardiac arrest. *South Med J* 75:768, 1982.

Bartlett JG: Antibiotic-associated pseudomembranous colitis. *Hosp Pract* 16:85-95, (Dec) 1981.

Bartlett JG: Anti-anaerobic antibacterial agents. *Lancet* 2:478-481, 1982.

Bartlett JG, Gorbach SL: Penicillin or clindamycin for primary lung abscess? *Ann Intern Med* 98:546-548, 1983.

Bartlett JG, et al: Antibiotic-associated pseudomembranous colitis due to toxin-producing clostridia. *N Engl J Med* 298:531-534, 1978.

Bechtol LD, et al: Erythromycin esters: Comparative in vivo hydrolysis and bioavailability. *Curr Ther Res* 20:610-622, 1976.

Benet LZ, Sheiner LB: Design and optimization of dosage regimens: Pharmacokinetic data, in Gilman AG, et al (eds): *The Pharmacological Basis of Therapeutics,* ed 6. New York, Macmillan, 1980, 1675-1737.

Bennett WM, et al: Drug therapy in renal failure: Dosing guidelines for adults. I. Antimicrobial agents, analgesics. *Ann Intern Med* 93:62-89, 1980.

Carranco E, et al: Carbamazepine toxicity induced by concurrent erythromycin therapy. *Arch Neurol* 42:187-188, 1985.

Chang T-W: Antimicrobial-associated diarrhea and enterocolitis. *Drug Ther (Hosp)* 6:71-78, (May) 1981.

Davis BD: Protein synthesis, in Davis BD, et al (eds): *Microbiology,* ed 3. Hagerstown, MD, Harper & Row, 1980, 229-255.

Diehl AM, et al: Cholestatic hepatitis from erythromycin ethylsuccinate: Report of two cases. *Am J Med* 76:931-934, 1984.

DiPiro JT, et al: Current concepts in clinical therapeutics: Intra-abdominal infections. *Clin Pharm* 5:34-50, 1986.

DiSanto AR, Chodos DJ: Influence of study design in assessing food effects on absorption of erythromycin base and erythromycin stearate. *Antimicrob Agents Chemother* 20:190-196, 1981.

DiSanto AR, et al: Comparative bioavailability evaluation of erythromycin base and its salts and esters. I. Erythromycin estolate capsules versus enteric-coated erythromycin base tablets. *J Clin Pharmacol* 20:437-443, 1980.

Doherty JE: Digoxin-antibiotic drug interaction, (editorial). *N Engl J Med* 305:827-828, 1981.

Fass RJ: Lincomycin and clindamycin, in Kagan BM (ed): *Antimicrobial Therapy,* ed 3. Philadelphia, WB Saunders, 1980, 97-116.

Fekety R: Antibiotic-associated pseudomembranous colitis. *Clin Microbiol Newslett* (preview issue) Oct 1978.

Fekety R: Clinical importance of anaerobic infections. *Drug Ther (Hosp)* 7:47-58, (Oct) 1982.

Fenton LJ, Light IJ: Congenital syphilis after maternal treatment with erythromycin. *Obstet Gynecol* 47:492-494, 1976.

Finegold SM, et al: Management of anaerobic infections. *Ann Intern Med* 83:375-389, 1975.

Finegold SM, et al: Anaerobic infections. *DM* 31:Part I, 1-77; Part II, 1-97, (Oct; Nov) 1985.

Fiumara NJ: Therapy guidelines for sexually transmitted diseases, (letter). *J Am Acad Dermatol* 9:600-601, 1983.

Francis H, et al: Severe vascular spasm due to erythromycin-ergotamine interaction. *Clin Rheumatol* 3:243-246, 1984.

Fraser DG: Selection of oral erythromycin product. *Am J Hosp Pharm* 37:1199-1205, 1980.

Ginsburg CM, et al: Concentrations of erythromycin in serum and tonsil: Comparison of estolate and ethylsuccinate suspensions. *J Pediatr* 89:1011-1013, 1976.

Ginsburg CM, et al: Management of group A streptococcal pharyngitis: Randomized controlled study of twice-daily erythromycin ethylsuccinate versus erythromycin estolate. *Pediatr Infect Dis* 1:384-387, 1982.

Ginsburg CM, et al: Erythromycin therapy for group A streptococcal pharyngitis: Results of comparative study of estolate and ethylsuccinate formulations. *Am J Dis Child* 138:536-539, 1984.

Gotz VP, Rand KH: Medical management of antimicrobial-associated diarrhea and colitis. *Pharmacotherapy* 2:100-109, 1982.

Gribble MJ, Chow AW: Erythromycin. *Med Clin North Am* 66:79-89, 1982.

Gurwith MJ, et al: Diarrhea associated with clindamycin and ampicillin therapy: Preliminary results of cooperative study. *J Infect Dis* 135(suppl):104-110, 1977.

Hansten PD: Erythromycin-theophylline: Updated. *Drug Interact Newslett* 3:13-15, 1983 A.

Hansten PD: Carbamazepine and erythromycin. *Drug Interact Newslett* 3:39-40, 1983 B.

Hansten PD, Horn JR: Erythromycin and warfarin. *Drug Interact Newslett* 5:37-40, 1985.

Haydon RC, et al: Erythromycin ototoxicity: Analysis and conclusions based on 22 case reports. *Otolaryngol Head Neck Surg* 92:678-684, 1984.

Hosker JP, Jewell DP: Transient, selective factor X deficiency and acute liver failure following chest infection treated with erythromycin. *Postgrad Med J* 59:514-515, 1983.

Husserl FE: Erythromycin-warfarin interaction, (letter). *Arch Intern Med* 143:1831, 1836, 1983.

Inman WHW, Rawson NS: Erythromycin estolate and jaundice. *Br Med J* 286:1954-1955, 1983.

LaForce CF, et al: Inhibition of methylprednisolone elimination in presence of erythromycin therapy. *J Allergy Clin Immunol* 72:34-39, 1983.

Larson HE, Price AB: Pseudomembranous colitis: Presence of clostridial toxin. *Lancet* 2:1312-1314, 1977.

Larson HE: Undescribed toxin in pseudomembranous colitis. *Br Med J* 1:1246-1248, 1977.

LeFrock JL, et al: Clindamycin. *Med Clin North Am* 66:103-120, 1982.

Levison ME, et al: Clindamycin compared with penicillin for treatment of anaerobic lung abscess. *Ann Intern Med* 98:466-471, 1983.

Lindenbaum J, et al: Inactivation of digoxin by gut flora: Reversal by antibiotic therapy. *N Engl J Med* 305:789-794, 1981.

Ludden TM: Pharmacokinetic interactions of macrolide antibiotics. *Clin Pharmacokinet* 10:63-79, 1985.

Lusk RH, et al: Gastrointestinal side effects of clindamycin and ampicillin therapy. *J Infect Dis* 135(suppl):111-119, 1977.

Lusk RH, et al: Clindamycin-induced enterocolitis in hamsters. *J Infect Dis* 137:464-475, 1978.

Malmborg A-S: Effect of food on absorption of erythromycin: Study of two derivatives, the stearate and the base. *J Antimicrob Chemother* 5:591-599, 1979.

Mandal BK, et al: Double-blind placebo-controlled trial of erythromycin in treatment of clinical *Campylobacter* infection. *J Antimicrob Chemother* 13:619-623, 1984.

Mao JCH, et al: Biochemical basis for selective toxicity of erythromycin. *Biochem Pharmacol* 19:391-399, 1970.

McCormack WM, et al: Hepatotoxicity of erythromycin estolate during pregnancy. *Antimicrob Agents Chemother* 12:630-635, 1977.

McDonald PJ, et al: Studies on absorption of newly developed enteric-coated erythromycin base. *J Clin Pharmacol* 17:601-606, 1977.

McGehee RF Jr, et al: Comparative studies of antibacterial activity in vitro and absorption and excretion of lincomycin and clindamycin. *Am J Med Sci* 256:279-292, 1968.

Neu HC, et al: Incidence of diarrhea and colitis associated with clindamycin therapy. *J Infect Dis* 135(suppl):120-125, 1977.

Nicholas P: Erythromycin: Clinical review. I. Clinical pharmacology. *NY State J Med* 77:2088-2094, 1977.

Norris SM, Mandell GL: Tables of antimicrobial agent pharmacology, in Mandell GL, et al (eds): *Anti-Infective Therapy*. New York, John Wiley & Sons, 1985, 470-471.

Patel J, Schneider R: Hepatotoxic reaction to erythromycin ethylsuccinate. *South Med J* 77:1343-1349, 1984.

Phillips KG: Hepatotoxicity of erythromycin ethylsuccinate in child, (letter). *Can Med Assoc J* 129:411-412, 1983.

Pratt WB: *Chemotherapy of Infection*. New York, Oxford University Press, 1977, 142-149.

Report of the Committee on Infectious Diseases: *American Academy of Pediatrics Redbook*, ed 19. Evanston, IL, American Academy of Pediatrics, 1982, 198-202.

Rifkin GD, et al: Antibiotic-induced colitis: Implication of toxin neutralized by *Clostridium sordellii* antitoxin. *Lancet* 2:1103-1106, 1977.

Rifkin GD, et al: Gastrointestinal and systemic toxicity of fecal extracts from hamsters with clindamycin-induced colitis. *Gastroenterology* 74:52-57, 1978 A.

Rifkin GD, et al: Neutralization by *Clostridium sordellii* antitoxin of toxins implicated in clindamycin-induced cecitis in hamster. *Gastroenterology* 75:422-424, 1978 B.

Sanford JP: Legionnaires' disease: First thousand days. *N Engl J Med* 300:654-656, 1979.

Sato RI, et al: Warfarin interaction with erythromycin. *Arch Intern Med* 144:2413-2414, 1984.

Schwartz J, et al: Interaction between warfarin and erythromycin. *South Med J* 76:91-93, 1983.

Steigbigel NH: Erythromycin, lincomycin, and clindamycin, in Mandell GL, et al (eds): *Principles and Practice of Infectious Diseases,* ed 2. New York, John Wiley & Sons, 1984, 224-231.

Sullivan D, et al: Erythromycin ethylsuccinate hepatotoxicity. *JAMA* 243:1074, 1980.

Swartzberg JE, et al: Clinical study of gastrointestinal complications associated with clindamycin therapy. *J Infect Dis* 135(suppl):99-103, 1977.

Tally FP: Therapeutic approaches to anaerobic infections. *Hosp Pract* 16:117-132 (Dec) 1981.

Tally FP, et al: Plasmid-mediated, transferable resistance to clindamycin and erythromycin in *Bacteroides fragilis*. *J Infect Dis* 139:83-88, 1979.

Tally FP, et al: Randomized comparison of cefoxitin with or without amikacin and clindamycin plus amikacin in surgical sepsis. *Ann Surg* 193:318-323, 1981.

Tally FP, et al: Susceptibility of *Bacteroides fragilis* group in United States in 1981. *Antimicrob Agents Chemother* 23:536-540, 1983.

Tally FP, et al: Nationwide study of susceptibility of *Bacteroides fragilis* group in United States. *Antimicrob Agents Chemother* 28:675-677, 1985.

Teasley DG, et al: Prospective randomized trial of metronidazole versus vancomycin for *Clostridium difficile*-associated diarrhoea and colitis. *Lancet* 2:1043-1046, 1983.

Tedesco FJ: Clindamycin and colitis: Review. *J Infect Dis* 135(suppl):95-98, 1977.

Tedesco FJ: Pseudomembranous colitis: Pathogenesis and therapy. *Med Clin North Am* 66:655-664, 1982 A.

Tedesco FJ: Treatment of recurrent antibiotic-associated pseudomembranous colitis. *Am J Gastroenterol* 77:220-221, 1982 B.

Tedesco FJ, et al: Oral vancomycin for antibiotic-associated pseudomembranous colitis. *Lancet* 2:226-228, 1978.

Vajda FJE, Bladin PF: Carbamazepine-erythromycin base interaction, (letter). *Med J Aust* 1:81, 1984.

Viteri AL, et al: Erythromycin ethylsuccinate-induced cholestasis. *Gastroenterology* 76:1007-1008, 1979.

Washington JA II, Wilson WR: Erythromycin: Microbial and clinical perspective after 30 years of clinical use, parts 1 and 2. *Mayo Clin Proc* 60:189-203, 271-278, 1985.

Weisblum B, et al: Erythromycin-inducible resistance in *Staphylococcus aureus*: Requirements for induction. *J Bacteriol* 106:835-847, 1971.

Welling PG, et al: Bioavailability of erythromycin stearate: Influence of food and fluid volume. *J Pharm Sci* 67:764-766, 1978.

Yee MH, et al: Clinical significance of clindamycin-resistant *Bacteroides fragilis*. *JAMA* 248:1860-1863, 1982.

Zafrani ES, et al: Cholestatic and hepatocellular injury associated with erythromycin esters: Report of nine cases. *Digest Dis Sci* 24:385-396, 1979.

Other Selected References

Erythromycin symposium. *Scott Med J* 22(suppl 1):349-407, 1977.

Derrick CW Jr, Reilly KM: Erythromycin, lincomycin, and clindamycin. *Pediatr Clin North Am* 30:63-69, 1983.

Ginsburg CM: Macrolides: Erythromycin, troleandomycin, and josamycin, in Kagan BM (ed): *Antimicrobial Therapy*, ed 3. Philadelphia, WB Saunders, 1980, 84-97.

Kucers A: Chloramphenicol, erythromycin, vancomycin, tetracycline. *Lancet* 2:425-429, 1982.

Nelson JD (Chairman): Evolving role of erythromycin in medicine: Proceedings of symposium. *Pediatr Infect Dis* 5:118-176, 1986.

Nicholas P: Erythromycin: Clinical review. II. Therapeutic uses. *NY State J Med* 77:2243-2246, 1977.

TETRACYCLINES

Source, Chemistry, and Classification

The tetracycline antibiotics were discovered as the result of a systematic screening of soil samples collected from many parts of the world for antibiotic-producing microorganisms. The first tetracycline to be introduced was chlortetracycline in 1948. Presently, six tetracycline analogues are marketed in the United States. Tetracycline, oxytetracycline [Terramycin], and demeclocycline [Declomycin] are naturally derived compounds from various species of *Streptomyces*. Methacycline [Rondomycin] and doxycycline [Vibramycin] are derived semi-synthetically from oxytetracycline, and minocycline [Minocin] is prepared by chemical modification of tetracycline.

All tetracyclines contain a hydronaphthacene nucleus consisting of four fused rings. Differences among the various analogues are determined by different substitutions on the basic structure (Figure).

The tetracyclines are broad spectrum antimicrobial agents. In general, patterns of microbial susceptibility and resistance to the tetracyclines are similar, but there are some differences in the degree of activity among the various analogues. The

CHEMICAL STRUCTURES OF TETRACYCLINES

Generic Name	R_1	R_2	R_3	R_4
SHORT-ACTING				
Tetracycline	H	OH	CH_3	H
Oxytetracycline	H	OH	CH_3	OH
INTERMEDIATE-ACTING				
Demeclocycline	Cl	OH	H	H
Methacycline	H	$=CH_2$		OH
LONG-ACTING				
Doxycycline	H	H	CH_3	OH
Minocycline	$N(CH_3)_2$	H	H	H

newer tetracyclines, minocycline and doxycycline, are more active than the parent compound against some organisms. The tetracyclines differ considerably in their pharmacology, and these antibiotics are usually subdivided into short- (tetracycline, oxytetracycline), intermediate- (demeclocycline, methacycline), and long-acting (doxycycline, minocycline) analogues.

Mechanism of Action

Tetracyclines interfere with protein synthesis by blocking the attachment of aminoacyl transfer RNA to the acceptor site on the messenger RNA-ribosome complex (Pratt, 1977). Binding of antibiotic occurs primarily at the bacterial 30S ribosomal subunit. Tetracyclines also can inhibit mammalian protein synthesis in cell-free systems. Their selective toxicity for bacteria appears to depend, in part, on energy-dependent uptake of antibiotic by bacterial, but not mammalian, cells. This results in a greater accumulation of tetracyclines by bacterial cells. However, active transport does not account for the high sensitivity of various intracellular microorganisms (eg, rickettsia, chlamydia) to tetracyclines, and other factors appear to be involved.

Tetracyclines are usually bacteriostatic at blood levels achieved clinically.

Antimicrobial Spectrum

Tetracyclines are effective in vitro against a great variety of bacteria, including gram-positive, gram-negative, aerobic, and anaerobic organisms. In addition, they are active against spirochetes, mycoplasmas, rickettsiae, chlamydiae, and some protozoa (Siegel, 1978, part II; Ory, 1980; Cunha et al, 1982; Standiford, 1984).

Among gram-positive cocci, most strains of *Streptococcus pneumoniae* are susceptible to the tetracyclines. A number of strains of *S. pyogenes* (group A), *S. agalactiae* (group B), viridans streptococci, and anaerobic streptococci also are susceptible. However, the tetracyclines usually are not used to treat streptococcal infections because many strains are resistant and more effective drugs (eg, penicillin G, erythromycin, cephalosporins) are available. Essentially all strains of *S. faecalis* (group D, enterococcus) are resistant. Many strains of *Staphylococcus aureus* are resistant to the tetracyclines, although minocycline has greater antistaphylococcal activity than other analogues.

Tetracyclines are active against a number of gram-positive bacilli including *Bacillus anthracis*, *Erysipelothrix rhusiopathiae*, *Clostridium tetani*, and *Listeria monocytogenes*. These antibiotics are alternatives to the penicillins in infections caused by these organisms.

Most *Neisseria gonorrhoeae* (gram-negative cocci) are susceptible, but there has been an increasing emergence of tetracycline-resistant strains in the United States (Jaffe et al, 1981; Faruki et al, 1985; Hook and Holmes, 1985; *Morbid Mortal Week Rep*, 1985 A; Rice et al, 1985). The Centers for Disease Control no longer recommends tetracyclines as first-line drugs for gonococcal infections (*Morbid Mortal Week Rep*, 1985 B; see also Uses). *N. meningitidis* are susceptible to the tetracyclines, particularly minocycline. However, the usefulness of this drug in meningococcal prophylaxis is limited by an unacceptably high incidence of vestibular side effects.

Tetracyclines are active against and are among the preferred antibiotics in infections caused by a number of gram-negative bacilli including *Brucella*, *Pseudomonas mallei*, *P. pseudomallei*, *Vibrio cholerae*, and *Calymmatobacterium granulomatis*. They also are active against *Francisella tularensis*, *Campylobacter jejuni*, *Haemophilus ducreyi* (a number of strains have become resistant), *Yersinia pestis*, *Y. enterocolitica*, *Pasteurella multocida*, *Spirillum minor*, *Leptotrichia buccalis*, *Bordetella pertussis*, and *Acinetobacter*.

Among gram-negative anaerobes, *Fusobacterium* and a number of *Bacteroides* strains are susceptible. Resistant strains of the *B. fragilis* group are common for most tetracycline analogues, however. Doxycycline is the most active analogue against the *B. fragilis* group, but other drugs (eg, clindamycin [Cleocin], metronidazole [Flagyl, Metryl]) generally are preferred for infections caused by this pathogen.

Tetracyclines are active against some strains of *H. influenzae*, *Shigella*, and community-acquired *Escherichia coli*. However, many strains of Enterobacteriaceae (eg, *E. coli*, *Klebsiella*, *Enterobacter*, indole-positive *Proteus*) are resistant. *Pseudomonas aeruginosa* are almost uniformly resistant.

Tetracyclines are among the agents of choice in infections caused by *Mycoplasma pneumoniae* and *Ureaplasma urealyticum*. They are the drugs of choice for chlamydial (eg, *C. trachomatis*, *C. psittaci*) and rickettsial (eg, *R. akari*, *R. rickettsii*, *R. prowazekii*, *R. mooseri*, *Coxiella burnetii*) infections. Among the spirochetes, tetracyclines are active against *Borrelia recurrentis*, *B. burgdorferi* (cause of Lyme disease), *Treponema pallidum*, and *T. pertenue*. They are alternatives to penicillin G for infections caused by *Actinomyces israelii*, and minocycline is active against *Nocardia asteroides*. Doxycycline is active against *Legionella pneumophila*, although erythromycin (with or without rifampin [Rifadin, Rimactane]) is the drug of choice. The atypical mycobacteria, *M. fortuitum* and *M. marinum*, are susceptible to doxycycline and minocycline, respectively.

High concentrations of tetracyclines are active against the protozoans, *Entamoeba histolytica*, *Dientamoeba fragilis*, *Balantidium coli*, and certain strains of *Plasmodium falciparum*.

Resistance

Several species of bacteria have become increasingly resistant to the tetracyclines (Siegel, 1978, part I). Many Enterobacteriaceae (eg, *Shigella*, *E. coli*) and most *P. aeruginosa* are resistant. Many strains of staphylococci, streptococci, and *Bacteroides* are no longer susceptible. Even some strains of pneumococci and *N. gonorrhoeae* have become resistant to the tetracyclines.

Resistance may occur through several mechanisms. Strains of mutant *E. coli* with tetracycline-resistant ribosomes have been isolated in the laboratory, and there is evidence that some bacteria may be induced to synthesize enzymes that degrade the antibiotic. The primary mechanism of resistance, however, is decreased uptake of tetracyclines by the bacterial cell due to alterations in the energy-dependent transport process. Resistance to one tetracycline usually implies resistance to all, except for minocycline's activity against *S. aureus* and doxycycline's activity against *B. fragilis.*

Resistance can be passed from one organism to another by transfer of small plasmids (circular, self-replicating, extrachromosomal DNA) called R-factors that contain genetic information for the development of resistance. An R-factor often induces resistance to several antibiotics simultaneously. *E. coli* have been shown to acquire resistance by conjugation, that is, by the direct passage of genetic material between bacteria. Staphylococci may transfer resistance when a bacteriophage (a virus capable of infecting bacteria) carries the plasmid into the cell.

Uses

Tetracyclines are the preferred or alternative drugs for a number of infectious diseases as outlined below. Tetracycline, the least expensive analogue, generally is preferred and is administered orally when possible. For additional discussion, see Chapter 65, Antimicrobial Therapy and Chemoprophylaxis of Infectious Diseases.

Tetracyclines are drugs of choice in brucellosis (often combined with streptomycin), cholera, relapsing fever, melioidosis (combined with chloramphenicol in seriously ill patients), glanders (combined with streptomycin), leptospirosis, early stages of Lyme disease (Steere et al, 1983), *Mycoplasma pneumoniae* infections (erythromycin is preferred by some physicians), and rickettsial infections (ie, Rocky Mountain spotted fever, typhus fever, Q fever, rickettsialpox). Some physicians prefer chloramphenicol for rickettsial infections.

Tetracyclines are preferred drugs for chlamydial infections (ie, nongonococcal urethritis, pelvic inflammatory disease, epididymitis, lymphogranuloma venereum, psittacosis, trachoma, inclusion conjunctivitis, keratoconjunctivitis). They are drugs of choice for various other venereal diseases, including granuloma inguinale and urethritis due to *Ureaplasma urealyticum* (some physicians prefer erythromycin). They may be effective against chancroid, but a number of strains of *H. ducreyi* are now resistant and erythromycin, ceftriaxone [Rocephin], or trimethoprim/sulfamethoxazole [Bactrim, Septra] usually is preferred. Because of the increasing emergence of resistant *Neisseria gonorrhoeae* strains (see Antimicrobial Spectrum), tetracyclines are now alternatives to penicillin or ceftriaxone for gonorrhea (eg, urethritis, cervicitis, proctitis [not effective in men], pelvic inflammatory disease, epididymitis, pharyngitis, septic arthritis, bacteremia). Although penicillin G is still the drug of choice for syphilis, tetracycline is an alternative. Likewise, tetracycline is an alternative to penicillin for prophylaxis in sexual contacts of patients with gonorrhea or syphilis. Tetracycline, in contrast to penicillin, also will be active in nongonococcal urethritis (eg, due to *C. trachomatis*). See *Morbid Mortal Week Rep*, 1985 B, and Table 2 in Chapter 65

for detailed discussions on the treatment of chlamydial infections, gonorrhea, syphilis, and other sexually transmitted diseases.

Other diseases for which tetracyclines provide effective therapy and may be suitable alternatives include actinomycosis, tularemia, anthrax, yaws, plague, *Pasteurella multocida* infections, gastroenteritis caused by *Yersinia enterocolitica* and *Campylobacter jejuni,* Vincent's angina, Whipple's disease, tetanus, rat bite fever, tropical sprue, and certain *Listeria* infections. Tetracyclines can be effective in the treatment of acute, uncomplicated lower urinary tract infections (cystitis); other useful antimicrobial agents include trimethoprim/sulfamethoxazole, sulfisoxazole [Gantrisin], ampicillin, and nitrofurantoin [Furadantin, Macrodantin]).

Atypical pneumonias caused by *Chlamydia, Coxiella, Francisella, Mycoplasma,* and *Legionella* have become difficult diagnostic and therapeutic problems. If *Legionella pneumophila* is the most likely causative organism, erythromycin is the drug of choice. However, for other cases of atypical pneumonia in which the diagnosis is uncertain, tetracyclines are active against most of the potential causative organisms.

Although the role of infection in the pathogenesis of acute exacerbations of chronic bronchitis has yet to be clarified, it has been customary to prescribe antibiotics. The tetracyclines are one class of antibiotics that have been used for this indication. Amoxicillin, trimethoprim/sulfamethoxazole, and cefaclor [Ceclor] are alternatives.

The efficacy of tetracycline in acne is well documented (Ad Hoc Committee on Use of Antibiotics in Dermatology, 1975), and it is the drug of first choice when systemic therapy is required for chronic, severe, inflammatory lesions refractory to topical therapy alone. See Chapter 56, Dermatologic Preparations, for a more detailed discussion of acne treatment.

Tetracyclines also have been used in acute intestinal amebiasis (*Entamoeba histolytica*), balantidiasis, dientamoebiasis, in combination with parenteral quinine for malaria caused by chloroquine-resistant strains of *Plasmodium falciparum* (alternative, simultaneous use of sulfonamide and pyrimethamine), and bacillary dysentery caused by susceptible strains of *Shigella*. See Chapter 77, Antiprotozoal Agents, for additional discussion.

Doxycycline is the preferred tetracycline for certain infections. Because doxycycline has a high degree of activity against pneumococci, group A streptococci, and *Haemophilus influenzae* and excellent penetration into respiratory secretions, some consider this agent to be the tetracycline of choice for acute exacerbations of chronic bronchitis (Cunha et al, 1982).

Chronic prostatitis is a difficult therapeutic problem because few active drugs can achieve therapeutic concentrations in noninflamed prostatic tissue. Gram-negative bacteria, particularly *E. coli,* cause the majority of cases and trimethoprim/sulfamethoxazole is the therapy of choice; carbenicillin indanyl also is used. Because of its relatively high lipid solubility, doxycycline also penetrates the noninflamed prostate and may be effective, especially when *C. trachomatis* is a possible pathogen (Cunha, 1981; Cunha et al, 1982).

Doxycycline is often the drug of choice for the empiric

treatment of the acute urethral syndrome (symptoms characteristic of cystitis, but less than 100,000 organisms/ml of urine) because the most likely causative organisms (*E. coli, Staphylococcus saprophyticus*, and chlamydia) are usually susceptible (Stamm et al, 1981). Conventional tetracycline also should be effective for this indication, however.

Organisms that cause acute pelvic inflammatory disease include *N. gonorrhoeae, C. trachomatis*, anaerobic bacteria (eg, *Bacteroides*, gram-positive cocci), facultative gram-negative bacilli (eg, *E. coli*), *Actinomyces israelii*, and *Mycoplasma hominis*, and treatment regimens are designed to cover a broad range of pathogens. A tetracycline usually is included and doxycycline is the recommended analogue (*Morbid Mortal Week Rep*, 1985 B; see also Table 2 in Chapter 65). It has better activity against most anaerobes, including *B. fragilis*, than conventional tetracycline and certain pharmacokinetic advantages (see Pharmacokinetics). Also, when intravenous administration is necessary, doxycycline is better tolerated than tetracycline.

Doxycycline has been shown to prevent travelers' diarrhea caused by enterotoxigenic *E. coli* (Sack et al, 1978, 1979). Prophylaxis generally is not recommended, however, because of the potential for adverse drug reactions (eg, photosensitivity) and the emergence of resistant bacterial strains (National Institutes of Health Consensus Development Conference, 1985; see also Table 3 in Chapter 65). Despite limited clinical experience, doxycycline appears to be an effective alternative to trimethoprim/sulfamethoxazole in the treatment of more severe cases of travelers' diarrhea (National Institutes of Health Consensus Development Conference, 1985).

Doxycycline (combined with amikacin) is a preferred regimen for *Mycobacterium fortuitum* infections.

In general, doxycycline offers a number of pharmacologic advantages over conventional tetracycline, including better gastrointestinal absorption resulting in the need for smaller doses, a longer half-life that permits longer intervals between doses, increased lipid solubility leading to higher tissue levels, and a mechanism of elimination that is independent of renal function and causes less diarrhea (see Pharmacokinetics). However, doxycycline is considerably more expensive than tetracycline, an important consideration in drug selection for those infections in which the two analogues are equally effective. Thus, tetracycline remains the preferred analogue for most infections. Doxycycline is the recommended tetracycline derivative for patients with impaired renal function.

Minocycline is more active than the other tetracyclines against *Nocardia asteroides* and is an alternative drug in nocardiosis. This antibiotic also is effective in *Mycobacterium marinum* infections. The good activity of minocycline against *Neisseria meningitidis* has led to its use in the prophylaxis of the meningococcal carrier state. However, the high incidence of vestibular toxicity has limited its usefulness in this and other infections (see Adverse Reactions and Precautions).

Adverse Reactions and Precautions

Gastrointestinal: The tetracyclines produce varying degrees of gastrointestinal irritation in some patients. These effects are more common after oral administration. Anorexia, pyrosis, nausea, vomiting, flatulence, and diarrhea are most common. They are usually dose related and occur in about 10% of patients receiving 2 g or more of tetracycline or its equivalent daily, and their incidence increases after prolonged administration. These reactions usually are not disabling but may become severe enough to require discontinuation or interruption of therapy. The presence of food may ameliorate the irritating effects of oral tetracyclines on the upper gastrointestinal tract. However, food decreases the absorption of some analogues (eg, tetracycline) more than others (eg, doxycycline) (see Pharmacokinetics).

When diarrhea is severe or persistent, it is important to determine whether it is due to nonspecific irritation, suprainfection of the bowel by staphylococci, or pseudomembranous colitis caused by overgrowth of *Clostridium difficile*. The latter conditions can be life-threatening and are more likely to occur in elderly, debilitated patients. Management must be prompt and requires immediate cessation of tetracycline administration. Fluid and electrolyte replacement, other supportive therapy, and treatment with oral vancomycin [Vancocin] (alternatives: metronidazole, cholestyramine [Questran]) may be necessary. Poorly absorbed tetracyclines (eg, tetracycline hydrochloride) are more likely to cause diarrhea and alter the enteric flora than well absorbed analogues (eg, doxycycline).

Esophageal ulceration with retrosternal pain that is intensified by swallowing has been reported after ingestion of tetracycline and doxycycline, usually when capsules were taken without water at bedtime.

Other undesirable gastrointestinal reactions include dryness of the mouth, stomatitis sometimes associated with vesiculo-papular oral lesions, glossitis and black hairy tongue, pharyngitis, hoarseness, dysphagia, and proctitis. Most of these reactions result from suppression of normal enteric flora with overgrowth of resistant organisms. Inflammatory lesions caused by candidal overgrowth of the oral, vulvovaginal, and perianal regions also may be seen.

Renal: All tetracyclines can produce negative nitrogen balance and increase blood urea nitrogen (BUN) levels, presumably by inhibiting protein synthesis in host cells. This is generally of no clinical importance when usual doses are given to patients with normal renal function, but tetracyclines may exacerbate renal dysfunction (eg, increase azotemia, hyperphosphatemia, acidosis) in patients with impaired renal function.

Tetracyclines other than doxycycline should not be used in patients with renal dysfunction. Unlike the other analogues, doxycycline is excreted by the gastrointestinal tract under these circumstances; its half-life will remain unchanged and it will not accumulate in the serum of patients with renal insufficiency (see also Pharmacokinetics).

Demeclocycline causes nephrogenic diabetes insipidus characterized by polyuria, polydipsia, and weakness in some patients. The syndrome is reversible upon discontinuation of the antibiotic. This effect has been utilized therapeutically to reverse the chronic syndrome of inappropriate secretion of antidiuretic hormone (SIADH) (Forrest et al, 1978; see also Chapter 30, Agents Affecting Water Homeostasis).

Degradation products in outdated tetracycline preparations have produced a Fanconi-like syndrome. Albuminuria, glycosuria, aminoaciduria, hypophosphatemia, hypokalemia, and renal tubular acidosis are manifestations of this condition. Such formulations are no longer available and it is unlikely that this complication will recur. The use of outdated tetracyclines also has been associated with a systemic lupus erythematosus-like syndrome. As with any drug, outdated preparations should not be used.

Hepatic: The tetracyclines may cause liver damage that is sometimes associated with pancreatitis, particularly when large doses (2 g or more of tetracycline daily) are administered intravenously. The damage is detectable by liver function studies. Diffuse, fine, vacuolar, fatty metamorphosis of the liver has been demonstrated histologically (Timbrell, 1983). Patients with pre-existing hepatic or renal insufficiency, those suffering from malnutrition, or individuals receiving other hepatotoxic drugs are at increased risk. Hepatotoxicity is a particular hazard to pregnant or postpartum women with pyelonephritis or other renal dysfunction. A number of deaths have been reported, most of them occurring when doses of tetracycline greater than 1 g daily were given intravenously. Therefore, tetracyclines should not be administered to pregnant women unless there are no therapeutic alternatives.

Bones and Teeth: Tetracyclines are deposited in developing bones and teeth where they can chelate with calcium to form a tetracycline-calcium orthophosphate complex. Bone growth is depressed temporarily in the fetus and in young children. The danger is greatest from midpregnancy to 3 years of age, but it may continue to age 7 and possibly longer. The incidence is influenced more by the total quantity of tetracycline ingested by mother or child than by the duration of treatment.

Tetracyclines can interfere with the development of deciduous teeth when administered antepartum or in children up to 4 to 6 months and of permanent teeth when administered to children between age 4 to 6 months and 6 years or older. Permanent discoloration of teeth ranging from gray-brown to yellow can result, and enamel hypoplasia has been reported. The degree of discoloration correlates with the total quantity of antibiotic administered and increases with repeated courses.

Because of these adverse effects, tetracyclines should not be used during the last half of pregnancy or in children under 8 years (see statement of Committee on Drugs, American Academy of Pediatrics, 1975) unless there are compelling reasons to do so. Some infectious disease experts consider it reasonable to administer a single course of tetracycline to a young child with a known serious infection (eg, Rocky Mountain spotted fever) when alternative therapy (eg, chloramphenicol) is potentially more toxic. Doxycycline and oxytetracycline may produce less tooth discoloration than other analogues.

Nervous System: Vestibular toxicity is unique to minocycline. This very lipid-soluble tetracycline analogue appears to concentrate in lipid-laden cells of the vestibular apparatus to produce vertigo. Symptoms of lightheadedness, loss of balance, dizziness, nausea, and tinnitus usually begin two to three days after therapy is initiated and occur in a high percentage of patients (eg, up to 70% receiving the drug for meningococcal prophylaxis). This adverse effect is more common in women than in men. Although vestibular toxicity is reversible after discontinuation of the drug, it has limited the use of minocycline. Patients receiving this analogue should be advised of this adverse effect and cautioned about driving a motor vehicle or operating machinery if they experience central nervous system side effects.

The tetracyclines can cause a rare condition known as pseudotumor cerebri. Tense bulging of the fontanelles caused by increased intracranial pressure occurs in infants and meningeal irritation with papilledema is observed in adults. Except for the elevated pressure, the spinal fluid is normal and the diagnosis, chiefly one of exclusion, may require careful neurologic appraisal. When the antibiotic is discontinued, spinal fluid pressure returns to normal over a period of days or weeks.

Photosensitivity: Reactions upon exposure to the sun or other sources of ultraviolet light have been noted occasionally. Sensitivity is produced by all analogues but is most common after use of demeclocycline. Usual manifestations are exaggerated sunburn and marked erythema; rarely, bullae develop in exposed areas of the body. Photosensitivity is reversible over a period of days or weeks. A few cases of papular eruption have been reported, and onycholysis occurs in about 25% of those affected. Patients likely to be exposed to direct sunlight or ultraviolet light should be advised that an exaggerated sunburn reaction can occur with tetracyclines.

Hypersensitivity: Hypersensitivity reactions most often involve the skin, although they are generally infrequent. Urticaria, angioedema, exfoliative dermatitis, idiopathic nonthrombocytopenic purpura, and exacerbations of systemic lupus erythematosus have been reported. Anaphylaxis has been reported rarely. Patients who are allergic to any of the tetracyclines should not receive these drugs.

Hematologic: Tetracyclines have been shown to depress plasma prothrombin activity. Patients receiving anticoagulant therapy may require a reduction in the dosage of anticoagulant.

Hemolytic anemia, thrombocytopenia, neutropenia, and eosinophilia have occurred rarely with tetracyclines.

Miscellaneous: Tetracyclines can cause thrombophlebitis after intravenous administration. This is more likely to occur with short-acting analogues (tetracycline, oxytetracycline) than long-acting derivatives (doxycycline, minocycline). Intramuscular injection of tetracycline or oxytetracycline is extremely painful and this route of administration is not recommended.

When given for prolonged periods, tetracyclines have been reported to produce brown-black discoloration of the thyroid gland. However, no abnormalities in thyroid function are known to occur.

Pigmentation of the skin, nails, and mucous membranes has been reported, most frequently after use of minocycline. This analogue also has been associated with tooth discoloration in young adults treated for acne (Poliak et al, 1985).

Drug Interactions

Divalent or trivalent cations (eg, Mg^{++}, Fe^{++}, Zn^{++}, Al^{+++}, Ca^{+++}) can chelate tetracyclines. Thus, tetracyclines should not be administered with milk or milk products, antacids, vitamin and mineral preparations, or cathartics containing divalent or trivalent cations because insoluble complexes form, resulting in decreased and erratic absorption of the antibiotic (see also Pharmacokinetics).

Tetracyclines are primarily bacteriostatic and may interfere with the bactericidal action of penicillins. Generally, concomitant administration is not recommended. When such combinations are considered necessary, it is recommended that adequate amounts of each drug be administered and, if possible, the penicillin should be given a few hours or longer before the tetracycline.

Concomitant administration of tetracyclines and methoxyflurane [Penthrane] has caused serious renal toxicity and deaths have been reported. These drugs should not be used together.

The half-life of doxycycline may be decreased by concurrent administration of carbamazepine [Tegretol], phenytoin [Dilantin], or barbiturates, which increase the hepatic metabolism of this antibiotic.

The bismuth subsalicylate contained in a 60-ml dose of Pepto-Bismol significantly decreased the bioavailability of oral doxycycline 200 mg (Ericsson et al, 1982). Thus, the two agents should not be taken together to prevent travelers' diarrhea.

Tetracyclines can increase plasma prothrombin time and, despite minimal clinical evidence, could potentiate the effects of coumarin-type anticoagulants. Reduction of the anticoagulant dose may be necessary.

Concurrent administration of tetracyclines and diuretics can increase blood urea nitrogen (BUN) concentrations. However, the clinical significance is uncertain and no special precautions appear to be necessary.

Sodium bicarbonate and cimetidine [Tagamet] have been reported to decrease the absorption of the tetracyclines, but the clinical significance is unclear.

Approximately 10% of patients convert substantial amounts of digoxin to inactive metabolites in the gastrointestinal tract. Certain antimicrobial agents, including tetracycline, have been shown to alter gut microbial flora and prevent the inactivation of digoxin. Thus, marked increases in serum digoxin levels can occur in these individuals. The effects of this interaction can persist for several months (Lindenbaum et al, 1981). Careful clinical monitoring of patients is recommended (Doherty, 1981).

Isolated cases of breakthrough bleeding and pregnancy have been reported in women receiving oral contraceptives and antibiotics, including tetracyclines. The clinical significance is unknown, but the addition of other forms of contraception appears warranted when a course of tetracycline therapy is initiated in a woman on oral contraceptives (see Back et al, 1981; Hansten and Horn, 1985; see also Chapter 40, Contraceptive Agents).

Oxytetracycline has been reported to enhance the hypoglycemic effect of insulin in a few patients, and insulin requirements may be reduced (Hansten, 1979).

Pharmacokinetics

Some pharmacokinetic properties of the tetracyclines are compared in the Table.

Routes of Administration: Tetracyclines usually are given orally, the preferred route of administration. Tetracycline hydrochloride, oxytetracycline hydrochloride, doxycycline hyclate, and minocycline hydrochloride also can be administered intravenously. This route is employed initially in those with severe infections or malabsorption syndromes and in critically ill or comatose patients. Rapid intravenous injection (less than five minutes) should be avoided. The long-acting analogues (doxycycline, minocycline) usually are less irritating to the vein than the short-acting derivatives (tetracycline, oxytetracycline), and thus are less likely to cause thrombophlebitis. Intramuscular injection of tetracycline or oxytetracycline also can be employed but is extremely painful, even when the preparation contains a local anesthetic and is injected into a large muscle mass. Furthermore, the serum concentrations attained tend to be low, even with maximum doses. Thus, intramuscular administration is not recommended.

Absorption: The short-acting (tetracycline and oxytetracycline) and intermediate-acting (demeclocycline and methacycline) tetracyclines are adequately but incompletely absorbed from the gastrointestinal tract; absorption is decreased in the presence of food. The long-acting analogues, doxycycline and minocycline, are more completely absorbed, and absorption appears to be affected only slightly by the presence of food. The primary site of absorption for the tetracyclines is the proximal small intestine.

Tetracyclines form insoluble complexes in the gut with calcium, magnesium, zinc, iron, aluminum, and other bivalent and trivalent cations. Therefore, the presence of milk and milk products, vitamin and mineral preparations, or cathartics and antacids containing metal salts may result in decreased and erratic absorption. In contrast, achlorhydria does not appear to interfere with the gastrointestinal absorption of these drugs (see Cunha et al, 1982).

Peak serum concentrations generally are attained one to three hours after oral administration and correlate with the degree of absorption of the various analogues. A 500-mg dose of tetracycline hydrochloride results in a peak serum concentration of 4 mcg/ml, highest of the short- (or intermediate-) acting analogues. Doxycycline and minocycline, given in single 200-mg doses, achieve serum concentrations of approximately 2.5 mcg/ml.

After intravenous administration of tetracycline hydrochloride 500 mg, serum concentrations are approximately 8 mcg/ml at 30 minutes and decrease to 2 to 3 mcg/ml by five hours. Intravenous injection of the usual 200-mg loading dose of doxycycline or minocycline produces serum concentrations of approximately 4 mcg/ml after 30 minutes. Once tissue distribution of the long-acting analogues occurs, levels are almost identical to the concentrations achieved orally.

Distribution: The tetracyclines are bound to plasma proteins to varying degrees. Although values reported in the literature are quite variable, the intermediate- and long-acting analogues usually exhibit greater plasma protein binding.

The apparent volume of distribution for most tetracyclines is greater than that of extracellular body water, which indicates sequestration in tissues, most likely the liver. Minocycline and doxycycline have the smallest volumes of distribution.

PHARMACOKINETIC VALUES FOR THE TETRACYCLINES[1]

Antibiotic	Oral Dose Absorbed (%)	Half-life (hours)	Renal Clearance[2] (ml/min/1.73m²)	Urinary Recovery (%)	Apparent Volume of Distribution[2] (liters)	Protein Binding[3] (%)
SHORT-ACTING						
Oxytetracycline	58	9	99	70	128	35
Tetracycline	77	8	74	60	108	65
INTERMEDIATE-ACTING						
Methacycline	58	14	31	60	79	90
Demeclocycline	66	12	35	39	121	91
LONG-ACTING						
Doxycycline	93	18	20	42	50	93
Minocycline	95	16	9	6	60	76

[1]From Standiford HC: Tetracyclines and chloramphenicol, in Mandell GL, et al (eds): Principles and Practice of Infectious Diseases, ed 2. New York, John Wiley & Sons, 1984, 209. Reprinted by permission.
[2]Following single dose intravenous administration.
[3]Ultrafiltration technique

As a group, tetracyclines penetrate variably into many different body fluids and tissues including bile, liver, lung, kidney, prostate, urine, cerebrospinal fluid, brain, sputum, and bone. The highest concentrations are found in bile and are 5 to 20 times those in the serum. Concentrations of conventional tetracycline in the cerebrospinal fluid are approximately 10% to 20% of those in the serum. Tetracyclines have an affinity for rapidly growing or metabolizing tissue and tend to localize in the liver and new bone and teeth, particularly before birth and during the first three years of life. The tetracyclines cross the placenta and appear in the milk of lactating women.

The tetracyclines differ markedly in their lipid solubility, which correlates directly with tissue penetration. Since doxycycline and minocycline are considerably more lipid soluble than the shorter acting tetracyclines, they penetrate into tissues and secretions more efficiently. For example, doxycycline has excellent penetration into endometrial, myometrial, prostatic, and renal tissues. This may explain, in part, its efficacy in the treatment of pelvic inflammatory disease, chronic prostatitis, and chronic pyelonephritis. Similarly, therapeutic concentrations of minocycline are achieved in saliva and tears to eradicate the meningococcal carrier state. Unfortunately, the high lipid solubility of minocycline also appears to result in its concentration in the lipid-laden cells of the vestibular apparatus leading to the vestibular toxicity that is unique to this analogue.

Elimination: The tetracyclines usually are classified on the basis of their duration of action (see the Table). Although these drugs undergo enterohepatic circulation and are, in part, recoverable in the feces, their half-lives are determined primarily by the rates of excretion by the kidneys. Tetracycline and oxytetracycline are eliminated rapidly by glomerular filtration as unchanged drugs and thus have the shortest half-lives. Demeclocycline and methacycline are intermediate. The half-lives of all of these drugs are prolonged significantly in patients with renal insufficiency.

Minocycline has a low renal clearance and less than 10% of a dose is recovered unchanged in urine. The drug undergoes enterohepatic circulation and may be metabolized to a considerable extent. Its high lipid solubility causes it to be retained in fatty tissues. The half-life of this drug is prolonged in patients with renal insufficiency but not in those with hepatic failure.

The elimination of doxycycline, the longest acting tetracycline, differs from the other analogues and is independent of both renal and hepatic function. This drug is excreted in the feces, largely as an inactive chelated product. Thus, the dose does not require modification in patients with renal or hepatic insufficiency. Furthermore, the inactive product has relatively less impact on the intestinal microflora resulting in a lower incidence of irritative diarrhea and candidal overgrowth.

Doxycycline offers a number of pharmacologic advantages over conventional tetracycline, including better gastrointestinal absorption resulting in the need for smaller doses, a longer half-life that permits longer intervals between doses, increased lipid solubility leading to higher tissue levels, and a mechanism of elimination that is independent of renal function and causes less diarrhea. However, when the two analogues are equally effective (see the section on Uses), the considerably lower cost of tetracycline should be an important consideration in drug selection.

Drug Evaluations

SHORT-ACTING TETRACYCLINES

TETRACYCLINE
[Achromycin V, SK-Tetracycline, Sumycin]

TETRACYCLINE HYDROCHLORIDE
[Achromycin, Achromycin V, Cyclopar, Panmycin, Robitet, Sumycin, Tetracyn]

Tetracycline is the most widely used drug in its class. The low cost of this analogue compared to that of the other agents is frequently an important consideration in drug selection.

See the Introduction for a complete discussion of the actions, antimicrobial spectrum, uses, pharmacokinetics, adverse reactions and precautions, and drug interactions of tetracycline.

DOSAGE AND PREPARATIONS. Tetracyclines should not be used in pregnant or nursing women or children under 8 years unless there are compelling reasons to do so. This agent should not be used in patients with impaired renal function.

Oral: Therapy should be continued for at least 24 to 48 hours after signs and symptoms have subsided. Tetracycline should be given one hour before or two hours after meals (see Pharmacokinetics). *Adults,* 250 to 500 mg every six hours; the larger dose should be reserved for severe infections. *Children over 8 years,* 25 to 50 mg/kg daily in four divided doses.

For the treatment of brucellosis, 500 mg four times daily for three weeks with streptomycin, intramuscularly, 1 g twice daily the first week and once daily the second week.

For treatment of sexually transmitted diseases, including chlamydial and gonococcal infections and syphilis, see Table 2 in Chapter 65, Antimicrobial Therapy and Chemoprophylaxis of Infectious Diseases.

For treatment of acne, see Chapter 56, Dermatologic Preparations.

TETRACYCLINE:
(Strengths expressed in terms of the hydrochloride salt.)
Generic. Suspension and syrup 125 mg/5 ml.
Achromycin V (Lederle). Suspension 125 mg/5 ml.
SK-Tetracycline (Smith Kline & French). Syrup 125 mg/5 ml (alcohol 1%).
Sumycin (Squibb). Syrup (buffered with potassium metaphosphate) 125 mg/5 ml.
TETRACYCLINE HYDROCHLORIDE:
Generic. Capsules 250 and 500 mg; tablets 250 mg.
Achromycin V (Lederle), *Cyclopar* (Parke-Davis), *Robitet* (Robins), *Tetracyn* (Pfipharmecs). Capsules 250 and 500 mg.
Panmycin (Upjohn). Capsules 250 mg.
Sumycin (Squibb). Capsules, tablets 250 and 500 mg.

Intravenous: Intravenous therapy is indicated only when oral therapy is inadequate or not tolerated. Oral therapy should be substituted as soon as possible. *Adults,* 250 to 500 mg at 12-hour intervals (maximum, 500 mg every six hours). *Children over 8 years,* 12 mg/kg daily in divided doses every 12 hours; 10 to 20 mg/kg daily may be given, depending on the severity of the infection.

The contents of the vial should be diluted before administration (see the manufacturer's literature) and injected at a rate not exceeding 2 mg/min (normally a two-hour infusion).

TETRACYCLINE HYDROCHLORIDE:
Achromycin IV (Lederle). Powder (sterile) 250 and 500 mg with ascorbic acid 625 mg or 1.25 g.

Intramuscular: This route generally is not recommended and should be used only when oral or intravenous therapy is not feasible, because injection can be extremely painful. The solution should be injected deep into a large muscle mass such as gluteal muscle.

Adults and children over 8 years weighing more than 40 kg, 250 mg once every 24 hours or 300 mg in divided doses at 8-to 12-hour intervals. *Children over 8 years weighing less than 40 kg,* 15 to 25 mg/kg daily to a maximum of 250 mg in a single daily injection or in divided doses at 8- to 12-hour intervals.

TETRACYCLINE HYDROCHLORIDE:
Achromycin IM (Lederle). Powder (sterile) 100 mg and 250 mg with procaine hydrochloride 40 mg, magnesium chloride 46.84 mg, and ascorbic acid 250 or 275 mg, respectively.

OXYTETRACYCLINE
[Terramycin]

OXYTETRACYCLINE HYDROCHLORIDE
[Terramycin]

The actions, antimicrobial spectrum, indications, pharmacokinetics, adverse reactions and precautions, and interactions of oxytetracycline are similar to those of tetracycline (see the Introduction). However, the cost of oxytetracycline is considerably greater than that of tetracycline.

DOSAGE AND PREPARATIONS. Tetracyclines should not be used in pregnant or nursing women or children under 8 years unless there are compelling reasons to do so. Oxytetracycline should not be used in patients with impaired renal function.

Oral: Therapy should be continued for at least 24 to 48 hours after signs and symptoms have subsided. Oxytetracycline should be given one hour before or two hours after meals (see Pharmacokinetics). *Adults,* 1 to 2 g daily in four equally divided doses, depending upon the severity of the infection. (Note: For Terramycin film-coated tablets only, the manufacturer recommends 500 mg initially, then 250 mg every six hours, as the usual average dosage. A total of 2 to 4 g/day may be indicated in severe infections.) *Children over 8 years,* 25 to 50 mg/kg daily in four equally divided doses.

OXYTETRACYCLINE:
Terramycin (Pfipharmecs). Tablets (film-coated) 250 mg.
OXYTETRACYCLINE HYDROCHLORIDE:
Generic. Capsules 250 mg.
Terramycin (Pfipharmecs). Capsules equivalent to 250 mg of base.

Intravenous: Intravenous therapy is indicated only when oral therapy is inadequate or not tolerated. Oral therapy should be substituted as soon as possible. *Adults,* 500 mg to 1 g daily divided into two doses at 12-hour intervals. *Children over 8 years,* 12 mg/kg daily in divided doses every 12 hours; 10 to 20 mg/kg daily in two divided doses may be given, depending on the severity of the infection.

To prepare the solution, 250 mg is dissolved in 10 ml of sterile water for injection and then diluted to a final volume of 100 ml with 5% dextrose or sodium chloride injection.

OXYTETRACYCLINE HYDROCHLORIDE:
Terramycin IV (Pfipharmecs). Powder 250 and 500 mg with ascorbic acid.

Intramuscular: This route generally is not recommended and should be used only when oral or intravenous therapy is not feasible, because injection can be extremely painful. The solution should be injected deep into a large muscle mass such as gluteal muscle.

Adults, 250 mg once every 24 hours or 300 mg in divided

doses at 8- to 12-hour intervals, depending upon the severity of illness; *children over 8 years*, 15 to 25 mg/kg daily to a maximum of 250 mg in a single daily injection or in divided doses at 8- to 12-hour intervals.

OXYTETRACYCLINE:

Terramycin (Pfipharmecs). Solution 50 mg/ml with 2% lidocaine in 2 and 10 ml containers and 125 mg/ml with 2% lidocaine in 2 ml containers.

INTERMEDIATE-ACTING TETRACYCLINES

DEMECLOCYCLINE HYDROCHLORIDE
[Declomycin]

The actions, antimicrobial spectrum, indications, and adverse effects of demeclocycline are comparable to those of tetracycline, but its half-life (12 hours) is somewhat longer (see the Introduction). Therefore, longer intervals between doses may be employed. The cost of demeclocycline is considerably greater than that of tetracycline, however.

Demeclocycline is the tetracycline most frequently associated with photosensitivity reactions at therapeutic dosage levels. Also, this analogue has been implicated in a few cases of nephrogenic diabetes insipidus, all of which were reversible within four weeks after medication was discontinued. This side effect has been utilized therapeutically to reverse the chronic syndrome of inappropriate secretion of antidiuretic hormone (SIADH) (see Chapter 30, Agents Affecting Water Homeostasis).

DOSAGE AND PREPARATIONS. Tetracyclines should not be used in pregnant or nursing women or children under 8 years unless there are compelling reasons to do so. Demeclocycline should not be used in patients with impaired renal function. *Oral:* Therapy should be continued for at least 24 to 48 hours after signs and symptoms have subsided. Demeclocycline should be given one hour before or two hours after meals (see Pharmacokinetics). *Adults,* 600 mg daily in two or four divided doses; *children over 8 years*, 6 to 12 mg/kg daily, depending on the severity of the infection, in two or four divided doses.

Declomycin (Lederle). Capsules 150 mg; tablets 150 and 300 mg.

METHACYCLINE HYDROCHLORIDE
[Rondomycin]

Methacycline is an analogue of oxytetracycline. Its actions, antimicrobial spectrum, indications, and adverse effects are similar to those of tetracycline, but its half-life (14 hours) is somewhat longer (see the Introduction). The cost of methacycline is considerably greater than that of tetracycline.

DOSAGE AND PREPARATIONS. Tetracyclines should not be used in pregnant or nursing women or children under 8 years unless there are compelling reasons to do so. Methacycline should not be used in patients with impaired renal function. *Oral:* Therapy should be continued for at least 24 to 48 hours after signs and symptoms have subsided. Methacycline should be given one hour before or two hours after meals (see

Pharmacokinetics). *Adults,* 600 mg daily in two or four divided doses; *children over 8 years*, 6 to 12 mg/kg daily, depending on the severity of the infection, in two or four divided doses.

Rondomycin (Wallace). Capsules 150 and 300 mg (equivalent to 140 mg and 280 mg of base, respectively).

LONG-ACTING TETRACYCLINES

DOXYCYCLINE CALCIUM
[Vibramycin]

DOXYCYCLINE HYCLATE
[Doryx, SK-Doxycycline Hyclate, Vibramycin]

DOXYCYCLINE MONOHYDRATE
[Vibramycin]

Doxycycline, a synthetic analogue of oxytetracycline, provides certain pharmacokinetic advantages over tetracycline and is more active against some organisms. Thus, it is the analogue of choice for certain indications (eg, pelvic inflammatory disease) and in patients with impaired renal function (see the Introduction). However, doxycycline is considerably more expensive than tetracycline. For those indications in which any member of this class of antibiotics would be equally effective, tetracycline usually is preferred because of cost considerations.

See the Introduction for a complete discussion of the actions, antimicrobial spectrum, uses, pharmacokinetics, adverse reactions and precautions, and drug interactions of doxycycline.

DOSAGE AND PREPARATIONS. Tetracyclines should not be used in pregnant or nursing women or children under 8 years unless there are compelling reasons to do so. *Oral:* Therapy should be continued for at least 24 to 48 hours after signs and symptoms have subsided. If gastric irritation occurs, doxycycline can be administered with food. The absorption of this agent is not markedly affected by the presence of food. The manufacturer recommends that doxycycline not be given just prior to bedtime; an upright position should be maintained after administration.

Adults and children over 8 years weighing 45 kg or more, 200 mg on the first day of treatment divided into two doses at 12-hour intervals, followed by 100 mg daily as a single dose or in two doses every 12 hours or, for more severe infections, 100 mg every 12 hours. *Children over 8 years weighing less than 45 kg*, 4.4 mg/kg on the first day of treatment divided into two doses at 12-hour intervals, followed by 2.2 mg/kg daily as a single dose or in two doses every 12 hours; for more severe infections, 2.2 mg/kg is given every 12 hours. In *patients with renal impairment*, doxycycline in recommended doses does not accumulate excessively.

For treatment of sexually transmitted diseases, including pelvic inflammatory disease (PID) and other chlamydial and gonococcal infections, see Table 2 in Chapter 65, Antimicrobial Therapy and Chemoprophylaxis of Infectious Diseases.

For the prophylaxis of travelers' diarrhea, 200 mg on the day of travel, followed by 100 mg once daily, continuing until two days after return home (Sack et al, 1978, 1979; Satterwhite and DuPont, 1983); prophylaxis generally is not recommended, however (see Uses). For treatment of travelers' diarrhea, 100 mg every 12 hours for three to five days (National Institutes of Health Consensus Development Conference, 1985) (investigational use).

DOXYCYCLINE CALCIUM:
Vibramycin (Pfizer). Syrup equivalent to 50 mg of base/5 ml.
DOXYCYCLINE HYCLATE:
Generic. Capsules 50 and 100 mg; tablets 100 mg.
Doryx (Parke-Davis). Capsules equivalent to 100 mg of base.
SK-Doxycycline Hyclate (Smith Kline & French), **Vibramycin** (Pfizer). Capsules equivalent to 50 and 100 mg of base; tablets [**Vibra-Tabs**] equivalent to 100 mg of base.
DOXYCYCLINE MONOHYDRATE:
Vibramycin (Pfizer). Powder for oral suspension equivalent to 25 mg of base/5 ml after reconstitution.

Intravenous: Intravenous therapy is indicated only when oral therapy is inadequate or not tolerated. Oral therapy should be substituted as soon as possible. The duration of intravenous infusion may vary with the dose (100 to 200 mg/day), but is usually one to four hours. A recommended minimum infusion time for 100 mg of a 0.5 mg/ml solution is one hour. The therapeutic antibacterial serum activity usually persists for 24 hours following use of the recommended dosage. See the manufacturer's literature for instructions on the preparation of solution for intravenous administration.

Adults and children over 8 years weighing 45 kg or more, 200 mg on the first day of treatment given in one or two infusions, followed by 100 to 200 mg daily (depending upon the severity of infection) in one or two infusions. *Children over 8 years weighing less than 45 kg,* 4.4 mg/kg on the first day of treatment given in one or two infusions, followed by 2.2 mg/kg to 4.4 mg/kg daily (depending upon the severity of infection) in one or two infusions. In *patients with renal impairment,* doxycycline in recommended doses does not accumulate excessively.

For the treatment of pelvic inflammatory disease (PID), see Table 2 in Chapter 65.

DOXYCYCLINE HYCLATE:
Vibramycin IV (Pfizer). Powder (sterile) equivalent to 100 or 200 mg of base with ascorbic acid 480 or 960 mg, respectively.

MINOCYCLINE HYDROCHLORIDE
[Minocin]

The clinical use of minocycline is limited by the vestibular toxicity that is unique to this tetracycline analogue. Also, it is considerably more expensive than tetracycline. See the Introduction for a complete discussion of the actions, antimicrobial spectrum, uses, pharmacokinetics, adverse reactions and precautions, and drug interactions of minocycline.

DOSAGE AND PREPARATIONS. Tetracyclines should not be used in pregnant or nursing women or children under 8 years unless there are compelling reasons to do so. Minocycline should not be used in patients with impaired renal function.

Oral: Therapy should be continued for at least 24 to 48 hours after signs and symptoms have subsided. If gastric irritation occurs, minocycline can be administered with food. The absorption of this agent is not markedly affected by the presence of food. *Adults,* 200 mg initially, followed by 100 mg every 12 hours (alternatively, 50 mg every six hours). *Children over 8 years,* 4 mg/kg initially, followed by 2 mg/kg every 12 hours.

For meningococcal prophylaxis, *adults,* 100 mg every 12 hours for five days. However, this regimen is associated with a high incidence of vestibular toxicity (see Table 3 in Chapter 65).

For *Mycobacterium marinum* infections, optimal dosage has not been established; 100 mg twice daily for six to eight weeks has been effective in a limited number of patients.

MINOCYCLINE HYDROCHLORIDE:
Minocin (Lederle). Capsules and tablets equivalent to 50 and 100 mg of base; oral suspension equivalent to 50 mg of base/5 ml (alcohol 5%).

Intravenous: Intravenous therapy is indicated only when oral therapy is inadequate or not tolerated. Oral therapy should be substituted as soon as possible. *Adults,* 200 mg initially, followed by 100 mg every 12 hours (maximum, 400 mg daily). *Children over 8 years,* 4 mg/kg initially, followed by 2 mg/kg every 12 hours.

The drug should be diluted before administration (see the manufacturer's literature).

MINOCYCLINE HYDROCHLORIDE:
Minocin IV (Lederle). Powder (sterile) 100 mg.

MIXTURES

Only two fixed-ratio combinations containing a tetracycline and other agents presently are available for systemic use. Proof of efficacy is lacking for both products and there is no justification for their use. They are evaluated briefly only for the sake of completeness.

UROBIOTIC

This product contains a tetracycline, a sulfonamide, and a urinary analgesic and is promoted for the treatment of urinary tract infections, although tetracyclines are not primary drugs for this indication. Since there is no recognized advantage for the fixed-ratio combination (eg, no synergism has been demonstrated between tetracyclines and sulfonamides), the use of either agent alone is preferred.

Because proof of efficacy is lacking, no dosage recommendation is made.

Urobiotic-250 (Roerig). Each capsule contains oxytetracycline hydrochloride equivalent to oxytetracycline 250 mg, sulfamethizole 250 mg, and phenazopyridine hydrochloride 50 mg.

MYSTECLIN-F

This mixture contains tetracycline and amphotericin B, an antifungal agent, and is promoted for the prevention of candidal overgrowth in patients receiving tetracycline therapy.

However, the rationale for the use of this fixed-ratio combination is weak. Intestinal candidiasis does not occur frequently, and there is no clinical evidence that the routine prophylactic administration of this antifungal agent reduces its incidence. It is preferable to prescribe antifungal drugs separately to treat intestinal candidiasis when clinically indicated.

Because proof of efficacy is lacking, no dosage recommendation is made.

Mysteclin-F (Squibb). Each capsule contains tetracycline hydrochloride 250 mg and amphotericin B 50 mg; each 5 ml of syrup contains tetracycline hydrochloride 125 mg and amphotericin B 25 mg. Preparations buffered with potassium metaphosphate.

CHLORAMPHENICOL

CHLORAMPHENICOL
[Chloromycetin, Mychel]

CHLORAMPHENICOL PALMITATE
[Chloromycetin Palmitate]

CHLORAMPHENICOL SODIUM SUCCINATE
[Chloromycetin Sodium Succinate, Mychel-S]

Chloramphenicol is a broad spectrum antibiotic that was originally derived from *Streptomyces venezuelae* but is now prepared synthetically. The potential of this drug to cause fatal aplastic anemia has limited its usefulness to the treatment of serious infections in which the location of the infection or the susceptibility of the causative organism limits or prevents the use of less toxic agents. In particular, chloramphenicol often is preferred for the treatment of typhoid fever caused by *Salmonella typhi*, meningitis caused by ampicillin-resistant *Haemophilus influenzae*, and susceptible anaerobic bacterial infections, including brain abscess and intra-abdominal sepsis (see Uses).

MECHANISM OF ACTION. Chloramphenicol acts by inhibiting bacterial protein synthesis. This antibiotic reversibly binds to the 50S subunit of the bacterial 70S ribosome and prevents the attachment of the amino acid-containing end of the aminoacyl-tRNA to the acceptor site on the ribosome. Thus, the amino acid substrate cannot interact with the enzyme, peptidyl transferase, and peptide bond formation does not occur (Pratt, 1977). Chloramphenicol usually is bacteriostatic but can be bactericidal against common meningeal pathogens (*H. influenzae, Neisseria meningitidis, Streptococcus pneumoniae*) at therapeutic concentrations (Rahal and Simberkoff, 1979).

Mammalian mitochondria contain 70S ribosomes with physical and chemical characteristics similar to those found in bacterial cells. Many of the adverse effects of chloramphenicol, including dose-dependent bone marrow depression and the gray syndrome, appear to result from inhibition of protein synthesis in host mitochondria (see also Adverse Reactions and Precautions).

ANTIMICROBIAL SPECTRUM. Chloramphenicol is active in vitro against a great variety of bacteria, including gram-positive, gram-negative, aerobic, and anaerobic organisms. In addition, this antibiotic is effective against rickettsiae, chlamydiae, spirochetes, and mycoplasmas (Standiford, 1984).

Among gram-positive cocci, *Streptococcus pneumoniae, S. pyogenes, S. agalactiae*, and viridans streptococci are usually susceptible. Enterococci (eg, *S. faecalis*) are variably susceptible. Most strains of *Staphylococcus aureus* are susceptible, but this varies with local utilization patterns. *Peptococcus* and *Peptostreptococcus*, anaerobic gram-positive cocci, are susceptible.

Susceptible gram-positive bacilli include *Bacillus* species, *Listeria monocytogenes, Corynebacterium diphtheriae*, clostridia (including *C. perfringens*), and *Eubacterium*.

Most strains of *Neisseria meningitidis* and *N. gonorrhoeae*, gram-negative cocci, are susceptible. *Veillonella* species, obligate anaerobes, also are susceptible.

Among gram-negative bacilli, *H. influenzae* are usually susceptible. Chloramphenicol also is active against *Brucella* species, *Bordetella pertussis, Pasteurella multocida, Pseudomonas pseudomallei, P. mallei, P. cepacia, Yersinia pestis, Vibrio cholerae, Francisella tularensis, Campylobacter jejuni*, and anaerobic gram-negative rods, including the *Bacteroides fragilis* group, other *Bacteroides* species, and *Fusobacterium*. Response of the Enterobacteriaceae is variable; many organisms that were originally susceptible are now resistant. Salmonellae, including *S. typhi*, are generally susceptible in the United States, although imported strains (eg, from Mexico, India, Vietnam) may be highly resistant. The drug is active against most strains of *Shigella, Escherichia coli, Klebsiella pneumoniae*, and *Proteus mirabilis*. However, most strains of *Serratia, Enterobacter, Providencia*, and *Proteus rettgeri* are resistant. *Pseudomonas aeruginosa* are resistant.

Rickettsiae (*R. akari, R. rickettsii, R. prowazekii, R. mooseri, Coxiella burnetii*), chlamydiae (*C. trachomatis, C. psittaci*), mycoplasmas, and treponemes are usually susceptible.

RESISTANCE. Chloramphenicol resistance among most gram-negative bacilli is due to drug inactivation by an acetyltransferase that is R-factor mediated. Resistance in gram-positive bacteria appears to develop by a similar mechanism, but is less well understood. *P. aeruginosa* and some strains of *Proteus* and *Klebsiella* become resistant through a nonenzymatic mechanism involving an inducible change in permeability that blocks the entry of chloramphenicol into the bacterial cell.

USES. Chloramphenicol has a relatively low therapeutic:toxic ratio and rarely has caused fatal aplastic anemia (see Adverse Reactions and Precautions). This antibiotic should not be used to treat trivial infections, indications for which there are equally effective and less toxic alternatives, or as a prophylactic agent. However, chloramphenicol has somewhat unique properties of lipid solubility with good penetration into cerebrospinal fluid (see Pharmacokinetics) and is active against a number of important microbial pathogens, including some that are not readily treated by alternative drugs (see Antimicrobial Spectrum). Thus, chloramphenicol is recommended for well defined indications in seriously ill patients, as outlined below, when the location of the infection or the susceptibility of the causative organism limits or prevents the use of less toxic agents. For additional discussion, see Chapter 65, Antimicrobial Therapy and Chemoprophylaxis of Infectious Diseases.

Chloramphenicol generally is regarded as the drug of choice for the treatment of acute typhoid fever. Resistant strains of *S. typhi* have not become a serious problem in the United States, although they have appeared in other countries (eg, Mexico, India, Vietnam). Ampicillin, amoxicillin, and trimethoprim/sulfamethoxazole are alternatives for the treatment of typhoid fever, including chloramphenicol-resistant strains. Relapses respond to retreatment with chloramphenicol, but this compound is not effective in typhoid carriers, who should be treated with ampicillin or amoxicillin (if the strain is sensitive to either of these drugs), trimethoprim/sulfamethoxazole, or, if cholecystitis or cholelithiasis is present, by cholecystectomy. Approximately 10% of patients become postinfective carriers following administration of chloramphenicol, whereas ampicillin or amoxicillin may essentially eliminate the carrier state.

For severe salmonellosis (eg, bacteremia, invasive disease) caused by nontyphoidal *Salmonella* species, chloramphenicol, ampicillin, amoxicillin, and trimethoprim/sulfamethoxazole are alternative regimens. Drug selection often depends on antimicrobial resistance patterns in a particular geographic location. It is emphasized that antimicrobial drugs are not recommended for gastroenteritis caused by *Salmonella*, which is usually self-limited. Antimicrobial therapy may not shorten the duration of illness and may prolong the convalescent carrier state.

Chloramphenicol readily penetrates the blood-brain barrier (see Pharmacokinetics) and often is preferred for infections of the central nervous system caused by susceptible organisms. This antibiotic is bactericidal in vitro against most strains of the common meningeal pathogens, *Haemophilus influenzae* (type b), *N. meningitidis*, and *S. pneumoniae*. Presently, chloramphenicol is the drug of choice for meningitis caused by ampicillin-resistant strains of *H. influenzae*; third generation cephalosporins and cefuroxine [Zinacef] are effective alternatives (see discussion below; see also Chapter 65, Table 1, and Chapter 67, Cephalosporins and Related Agents). Because of the increasing prevalence of these strains, it is recommended that both ampicillin and chloramphenicol be administered initially to patients (eg, infants and children) with suspected *H. influenzae* meningitis before the results of susceptibility tests are known. Meningitis caused by *N. meningitidis* or *S. pneumoniae* (including penicillin-insensitive strains) usually responds to chloramphenicol, and this antibiotic is the preferred treatment in patients who are allergic to penicillin G. Although chloramphenicol-resistant strains of *H. influenzae*, *N. meningitidis*, and *S. pneumoniae* have been reported in the United States, their incidence remains rare. Most authorities now consider chloramphenicol to be an inappropriate drug for gram-negative enteric bacillary meningitis involving susceptible strains of Enterobacteriaceae, presumably due to its lack of bactericidal activity; third generation cephalosporins (eg, cefotaxime [Claforan]) are preferred (Rahal and Simberkoff, 1982; Barriere and Flaherty, 1984; see also Chapter 65, Table 1, and Chapter 67).

Chloramphenicol is frequently preferred for anaerobic infections in the central nervous system (eg, brain abscess). Penicillin G and metronidazole are alternatives. When *Bacteroides fragilis* is the likely causative organism, either metronidazole or chloramphenicol should be used because this gram-negative anaerobic bacillus usually is resistant to penicillin G. For empiric therapy of pyogenic brain abscesses, combination therapy with penicillin G plus chloramphenicol (or metronidazole) frequently is employed.

In addition to meningitis, *H. influenzae* frequently causes other serious infections, particularly in infants and young children. These include acute epiglottitis, pneumonia, facial cellulitis, and septic arthritis. Because of the prevalence of ampicillin-resistant strains of *H. influenzae* in most geographic locations, it has become necessary to use alternative antimicrobial agents for these infections, at least for empiric therapy (ie, before culture and susceptibility test results are available). Many infectious disease experts currently prefer chloramphenicol, often in combination with ampicillin, for these infections. Newer cephalosporins, including cefuroxime, a second generation agent, and most of the third generation analogues (eg, cefotaxime, ceftizoxime [Cefizox], ceftriaxone [Rocephin]), also are highly effective for ampicillin-resistant *H. influenzae* infections, including meningitis, and may eventually replace chloramphenicol for certain indications (see Neu, 1982; Nelson, 1983; also see Table 1 in Chapter 65, Antimicrobial Therapy and Chemoprophylaxis of Infectious Diseases; and Chapter 67, Cephalosporins and Related Compounds).

Most anaerobic bacteria are susceptible to chloramphenicol, including virtually all strains of the *B. fragilis* group (which are resistant to most penicillins and cephalosporins) and clostridia (which are relatively resistant to most cephalosporins and may be resistant to clindamycin). Anaerobic infections above the diaphragm, such as orodental infections, aspiration pneumonia, and lung abscess, involve anaerobic bacteria that are usually susceptible to penicillin G. However, some experts prefer clindamycin for these infections when they are serious and fulminant or fail to respond to penicillin G. For serious anaerobic infections below the diaphragm (eg, intra-abdominal abscess, peritonitis secondary to bowel perforation), *B. fragilis* usually is an important pathogen, and clindamycin, metronidazole, and chloramphenicol often are considered to be drugs of choice for infections caused by this organism. Cefoxitin [Mefoxin] and the antipseudomonal penicillins (eg, ticarcillin, piperacillin) also are useful against the *B. fragilis* group. Because intra-abdominal infections are usually caused by mixtures of anaerobes and aerobic gram-negative bacilli, an aminoglycoside is usually added to cover the aerobic organisms (see Fekety, 1982; Chapter 68, Macrolides and Lincosamides; and Chapter 72, Miscellaneous Antibacterial Agents).

Chloramphenicol is as effective as the tetracyclines in Rocky Mountain spotted fever, Q fever, and other rickettsial infections. It can be used when the tetracyclines are contraindicated (eg, in pregnant women, infants and children under 8 years; in hypersensitive patients; when parenteral antibiotics are necessary because of severe illness).

Chloramphenicol frequently is combined with a tetracycline for the treatment of severe melioidosis. This antibiotic is an effective alternative in glanders (with streptomycin), brucellosis (with or without streptomycin), plague, certain chlamydial infections (eg, psittacosis), relapsing fever, *Pseudomonas cepacia* infections, tularemia, *Pasteurella multocida* infections, and gas gangrene.

Chloramphenicol is effective in certain ocular and otic infections (see Chapter 73, Topical Anti-infective Agents: Otic and Ophthalmic Preparations).

ADVERSE REACTIONS AND PRECAUTIONS. **Hematologic:** The most important adverse effects of chloramphenicol are on the hematopoietic system and can be subdivided into two types of bone marrow depression. The first type is characterized by anemia (with or without thrombocytopenia and leukopenia), reticulocytopenia, and increased levels of serum iron. There is increased cellularity of bone marrow with cytoplasmic vacuolization and maturation arrest of erythroid and myeloid precursors. This form of bone marrow depression is common, occurs during therapy, and is dose related. It is more likely to occur in patients receiving large doses (eg, 4 g or more per day) or prolonged therapy and in those with impaired hepatic function. It frequently is associated with serum levels greater than 25 mcg/ml. This type of bone marrow depression is not a prodrome to aplastic anemia (see below) and is reversible within one to three weeks after the drug is discontinued. The mechanism appears to be related to inhibition of host mitochondrial protein synthesis.

The second, more serious type of bone marrow depression is aplastic anemia. This is not dose related and typically occurs weeks to months after the drug has been discontinued. It is characterized by peripheral pancytopenia and hypoplastic or aplastic bone marrow. The prognosis is very poor, since the anemia usually is irreversible. The incidence of aplastic anemia has been estimated to be 1 in 25,000 to 1 in 40,000 courses of therapy. It is believed to be an idiosyncratic reaction of unknown mechanism. It has been suggested that the nitrated benzene radical of chloramphenicol, or one of its metabolites, may cause irreversible marrow toxicity in genetically predisposed individuals (Yunis et al, 1980). Interestingly, thiamphenicol, an analogue of chloramphenicol used in Europe and Japan, has the nitro group on the benzene ring replaced by a methysulfone and it has not been associated with aplastic anemia (see Standiford, 1984).

There is debate as to whether oral chloramphenicol is more likely to cause aplastic anemia than other routes. Although the incidence following intravenous administration is extremely low, some cases have been reported (Domart et al, 1961; Grilliat et al, 1966; Restrepo and Zambrano, 1968; Wallerstein et al, 1969; Daum et al, 1979; Plaut and Best, 1982; Alavi, 1983). It also has been observed after topical ophthalmic administration (Rosenthal and Blackman, 1965; Carpenter, 1975; Abrams et al, 1980; Fraunfelder et al, 1982; Fraunfelder and Bagby, 1983). Thus, it must be assumed that this serious

adverse effect can occur when chloramphenicol is administered by *any* route.

Chloramphenicol also may precipitate hemolytic anemia in patients with the Mediterranean form of glucose-6-phosphate dehydrogenase (G6PD) deficiency; individuals with milder type A G6PD deficiency (usually blacks) usually are not affected.

Since dose-related bone marrow depression can occur in any patient and is reversible, serial blood monitoring should be conducted in all patients receiving chloramphenicol. Complete blood counts and differential reticulocyte counts should be measured frequently (eg, every two to three days) to permit early detection of bone marrow depression. Serum iron levels also may be monitored. The drug should be discontinued or, at the least, the dosage should be reduced when there is evidence of bone marrow depression (eg, white blood cell count less than 3,000/mm³ [Bartlett, 1982]). Unfortunately, routine hemograms cannot predict the occurrence of aplastic anemia.

When possible, prolonged or repeated courses of chloramphenicol or concomitant administration with other drugs that depress the bone marrow should be avoided.

Gray Syndrome: The "gray syndrome" refers to a potentially fatal adverse effect that has occurred with excessive dosage. This syndrome generally is associated with serum chloramphenicol concentrations greater than 40 mcg/ml, which can inhibit host mitochondrial electron transport in the liver, myocardium, and skeletal muscle (see Bartlett, 1982; Ambrose, 1984; Shalit and Marks, 1984). It is manifested initially by vomiting, tachypnea, abdominal distention, cyanosis, green stools, lethargy, and an ashen color. It can progress to vasomotor collapse and death, which commonly occurs within two days of initial symptoms. The gray syndrome is most common in neonates (usually less than 2 weeks), particularly premature infants, who receive excessive amounts of the drug. This is because such patients have inadequate glucuronyl transferase activity combined with decreased renal excretion of unconjugated chloramphenicol. If chloramphenicol must be administered to premature infants and neonates, the dosage should be reduced (see Dosage and Preparations) and antibiotic serum concentrations should be monitored. Although this syndrome has been termed the "gray baby syndrome," it can also occur in older children and adults with excessive serum levels of the drug (eg, from overdosage, in patients with hepatic dysfunction).

Chloramphenicol crosses the placenta and is excreted in breast milk. Therefore, it should be avoided, if possible, in pregnant women, particularly those near term or in labor, or breast-feeding mothers.

Neurologic: Neurologic complications are usually associated with prolonged chloramphenicol therapy and include optic neuritis, peripheral neuritis, mental confusion, and delirium. Visual loss associated with optic neuritis may not be completely reversible. Vision should be monitored in selected patients (eg, those on long-term therapy) because of the risk of optic neuritis. Patients should be requested to report any visual loss promptly.

Gastrointestinal: Nausea, vomiting, glossitis, unpleasant taste, stomatitis, and diarrhea have been reported. Although bacterial or fungal suprainfections can occur, antibiotic-associated pseudomembranous colitis due to *Clostridium difficile* is uncommon.

Hypersensitivity: Rashes, urticaria, angioedema, and anaphylaxis have been observed, but are uncommon. Herxheimer-like reactions have been reported during treatment of typhoid fever.

DRUG INTERACTIONS. Chloramphenicol can prolong the half-lives and increase the serum concentrations of phenytoin, tolbutamide, chlorpropamide, dicumarol, and possibly other drugs by inhibiting their metabolism by hepatic microsomal enzymes. Increased toxicity and deaths have been reported. Conversely, phenobarbital, phenytoin, and rifampin (Prober, 1985) have been reported to decrease the serum concentration of chloramphenicol, presumably because of hepatic enzyme induction. Monitoring of chloramphenicol serum concentrations is recommended during concomitant administration with other drugs that may affect its pharmacokinetics.

Chloramphenicol may delay the response of anemias to iron, folic acid, or vitamin B_{12}. This antibiotic may interfere with the anamnestic response to tetanus toxoid. Concomitant administration of chloramphenicol and active immunizing agents probably should be avoided.

Antagonism of penicillin's bactericidal effect by chloramphenicol has been demonstrated in vitro and in animal studies. However, the clinical significance is unclear. This combination should be used only when such treatment has been demonstrated to be beneficial.

PHARMACOKINETICS. Three preparations of chloramphenicol are available for systemic use: chloramphenicol base in capsules for oral use; chloramphenicol palmitate, a tasteless ester, in suspension for oral use; and chloramphenicol succinate, a soluble ester, for intravenous administration. The palmitate and succinate esters are prodrugs that require hydrolysis to liberate biologically active chloramphenicol.

Absorption: Chloramphenicol base is readily absorbed from the gastrointestinal tract; bioavailability ranging from 76% to 93% has been reported. Peak plasma concentrations have been observed between 0.5 and 6 hours, and occur between 0.5 and 2 hours with products having fast dissolution and deaggregation rates (see Ambrose, 1984). After a single 1-g dose, a mean peak plasma concentration of 11.2 mcg/ml was reported at one hour. Multiple dosing at six-hour intervals resulted in somewhat higher plasma concentrations on the second day (18.4 mcg/ml after the fifth dose) with no subsequent increases (manufacturer's literature).

Chloramphenicol palmitate must be hydrolyzed by pancreatic esterases in the small intestine to active chloramphenicol base, which is subsequently absorbed. Bioavailability of chloramphenicol is approximately 80% when administered as the palmitate ester and peak plasma concentrations usually occur two to three hours after administration (see Ambrose, 1984). The absorption of chloramphenicol after oral administration of the palmitate ester has been reported to be incomplete, prolonged, and erratic in premature and term newborns (Shankaran and Kauffman, 1984).

After intravenous administration, circulating chloramphenicol succinate must be hydrolyzed to free chloramphenicol, the active drug; this probably occurs in the liver, kidney, and lung. Initially, it was believed that metabolic conversion of the succinate ester to free chloramphenicol was rapid and complete, but this is not the case. The rate and extent of hydrolysis of chloramphenicol succinate are variable and incomplete and, on the average, about 30% of a dose is eliminated as unhydrolyzed ester in the urine in both adults and children. In addition, there is wide interpatient variability in the amount of succinate ester that is excreted in urine. Thus, the mean 70% bioavailability of free chloramphenicol following intravenous administration of chloramphenicol succinate is actually lower than that obtained following oral administration. More importantly, bioavailability after intravenous administration is quite variable among patients, especially in newborns, infants, and young children (see Kauffman et al, 1981 A and B; Smith and Weber, 1983; Ambrose, 1984; Kramer et al, 1984; Shalit and Marks, 1984). In newborns (eg, less than 1 month), both the hydrolysis and renal excretion of chloramphenicol succinate appear to be considerably reduced when compared to other age groups (see Ambrose, 1984; Shalit and Marks, 1984).

Distribution: Between 50% and 60% of circulating chloramphenicol is bound to plasma protein. Reported mean values for the apparent volume of distribution range from 0.6 to 1 L/kg (see Ambrose, 1984). The drug has good lipid solubility and readily penetrates most tissues and body fluids. This includes the cerebrospinal fluid where levels approximately one-half the corresponding plasma level can be achieved with or without meningitis. Levels in brain tissue are higher than those in plasma. Therapeutic concentrations are achieved in synovial, pleural, and ascitic fluid. Good penetration into the aqueous and vitreous humors is also observed. Chloramphenicol readily crosses the placenta and can be found in breast milk. Only small amounts of active chloramphenicol are recovered from bile (see Ambrose, 1984; Standiford, 1984).

Metabolism and Excretion: Chloramphenicol is eliminated primarily by metabolism to inactive products. In patients with normal hepatic function, approximately 90% of chloramphenicol is conjugated to the glucuronide in the liver. The inactive conjugate subsequently is excreted by the kidneys. Minor metabolites also have been identified. Only about 5% to 15% is excreted by glomerular filtration as active, unchanged chloramphenicol in urine. The mean elimination half-life is approximately four hours in adults and children (see Ambrose, 1984).

The metabolism and excretion of chloramphenicol are diminished in young children, particularly in neonates and premature infants in whom hepatic (eg, glucuronyl transferase system) and renal function are not fully developed. Mean elimination half-lives of chloramphenicol have been reported to be about nine hours in neonates from 1 week to 2 months and 12 hours in those less than 1 week of age; there is substantial individual variation (see Smith and Weber, 1983; Ambrose, 1984).

Patients with hepatic dysfunction (eg, cirrhosis) conjugate active chloramphenicol at a slower rate, resulting in a prolonged elimination half-life and accumulation in serum. Dosage reductions are necessary.

With impaired renal function, there is a delay in the excretion of the glucuronide conjugate, but this metabolite is biologically inactive and apparently nontoxic. After oral administration, the elimination half-life of chloramphenicol is unchanged and serum accumulation of the active and potentially toxic free drug does not occur. Chloramphenicol bioavailability in patients with renal dysfunction may be greater after intravenous infusion, however, because less succinate ester will be excreted in urine (see Ambrose, 1984). Neither peritoneal nor hemodialysis alters serum levels sufficiently to require dosage alterations.

Monitoring Chloramphenicol Serum Concentrations: In general, peak serum chloramphenicol concentrations of 10 to 20 mcg/ml and trough concentrations of 5 to 10 mcg/ml are desirable for most infections. This drug has a low therapeutic:toxic ratio, and dose-dependent bone marrow depression has been associated with peak serum concentrations greater than 25 mcg/ml and trough concentrations greater than 10 mcg/ml (see Ambrose, 1984; see also the section on Adverse Reactions and Precautions). Therefore, sequential monitoring of peak and trough serum chloramphenicol concentrations is indicated to ensure efficacy and prevent toxicity (see Bartlett, 1982; Smith and Weber, 1983; Ambrose, 1984; Shalit and Marks, 1984). This is particularly important for pediatric patients in whom wide variations in chloramphenicol metabolism and excretion have been reported. Dosage requirements may vary threefold in children of the same age. Even greater variation is observed in newborn and young infants, making serum monitoring imperative in this age group (Friedman et al, 1979; Kauffman et al, 1981 A; Tuomanen et al, 1981; Yogev et al, 1981). Monitoring of serum chloramphenicol concentrations is also very important in individuals with hepatic dysfunction, those with renal impairment who are given the succinate ester intravenously, and patients receiving concomitant therapy with other drugs (eg, phenytoin, phenobarbital, rifampin) that can alter chloramphenicol pharmacokinetics (see Drug Interactions) (see Bartlett, 1982; Smith and Weber, 1983; Ambrose, 1984; Shalit and Marks, 1984). Currently, enzymatic and high pressure liquid chromatographic (HPLC) methods are preferred for monitoring because they have good sensitivity, specificity, and reproducibility (Bartlett, 1982; Ambrose, 1984; Shalit and Marks, 1984).

DOSAGE AND PREPARATIONS. Current dosage recommendations for oral chloramphenicol base or palmitate or for intravenous chloramphenicol sodium succinate are the same, despite some differences in bioavailability among these preparations (see Pharmacokinetics). The intravenous route is recommended initially in the treatment of most serious infections. Oral therapy may be substituted when conditions warrant. Intramuscular administration generally is not recommended because delayed absorption results in substantially lower serum concentrations and therapeutic failures have been reported.

In general, peak chloramphenicol serum concentrations of 10 to 20 mcg/ml and trough concentrations of 5 to 10 mcg/ml are desirable for most infections. Sequential monitoring of peak and trough chloramphenicol serum concentrations is recommended because of the low therapeutic:toxic ratio of this antibiotic and the wide interpatient variation in chloramphenicol pharmacokinetics that has been observed. This is of particular importance in pediatric patients, especially newborns and premature infants, patients with hepatic dysfunction, and those receiving concomitant therapy with other drugs that can alter chloramphenicol pharmacokinetics (see Pharmacokinetics and Drug Interactions).

Oral, Intravenous: *Adults*, 50 mg/kg daily in divided doses every six hours for most indications (eg, typhoid fever, rickettsial infections); 100 mg/kg daily in divided doses every six hours for meningitis and brain abscess (see Standiford, 1984). Ideally, serum concentrations of chloramphenicol should be monitored periodically (see above).

Children, 50 to 75 mg/kg daily in divided doses every six hours for most indications; 75 to 100 mg/kg daily in divided doses every six hours for meningitis (Nelson, 1985 A). Ideally, serum concentrations of chloramphenicol should be monitored periodically (see above).

Neonates over 7 days weighing more than 2 kg, 50 mg/kg daily in divided doses every 12 hours; *neonates from birth to 7 days weighing more than 2 kg,* 25 mg/kg once daily; *neonates under 2 kg,* 25 mg/kg once daily (Nelson, 1985 B). Serum concentrations of chloramphenicol should be monitored periodically (see above).

In *patients with impaired hepatic function*, dosage reductions may be necessary. Clear guidelines are not available and, ideally, serum levels should be monitored. In *adults*, an initial loading dose of 1 g followed by 500 mg every six hours has been suggested (see Standiford, 1984).

CHLORAMPHENICOL:
Generic. Capsules 250 and 500 mg.
Chloromycetin (Parke-Davis), **Mychel** (Rachelle). Capsules 250 mg.

CHLORAMPHENICOL PALMITATE:
Chloromycetin Palmitate (Parke-Davis). Suspension (oral) equivalent to chloramphenicol 150 mg/5 ml.

CHLORAMPHENICOL SODIUM SUCCINATE:
Chloromycetin Sodium Succinate (Parke-Davis), **Mychel-S** (Rachelle), **Generic.** Powder (for injection) 1 g (equivalent to 100 mg of chloramphenicol/ml when reconstituted [see manufacturer's instructions]).

Cited References

Tetracycline-resistant *Neisseria gonorrhoeae*—Georgia, Pennsylvania, New Hampshire. *Morbid Mortal Week Rep* 34:563-570, 1985 A.

1985 STD treatment guidelines. *Morbid Mortal Week Rep* 34(suppl):75S-108S, 1985 B.

Abrams SM, et al: Marrow aplasia following topical application of chloramphenicol eye ointment. *Arch Intern Med* 140:576-577, 1980.

Ad Hoc Committee on Use of Antibiotics in Dermatology, American Academy of Dermatology: Systemic antibiotics for treatment of acne vulgaris: Efficacy and safety. *Arch Dermatol* 111:1630-1636, 1975.

Alavi JB: Aplastic anemia associated with intravenous chloramphenicol. *Am J Hematol* 15:375-379, 1983.

Ambrose PJ: Clinical pharmacokinetics of chloramphenicol and chloramphenicol succinate. *Clin Pharmacokinet* 9:222-238, 1984.

Back DJ, et al: Interindividual variation and drug interactions with hormonal steroid contraceptives. *Drugs* 21:46-61, 1981.

Barriere SL, Flaherty JF: Third generation cephalosporins: Critical evaluation. *Clin Pharm* 3:351-373, 1984.

Bartlett JG: Chloramphenicol. *Med Clin North Am* 66:91-102, 1982.

Carpenter G: Chloramphenicol eye-drops and marrow aplasia. *Lancet* 2:326-327, 1975.

Committee on Drugs, American Academy of Pediatrics: Requiem for tetracyclines. *Pediatrics* 55:142-143, 1975.

Cunha BA: Urinary tract infections: 2. Therapeutic approach. *Postgrad Med* 70:149-157, (Dec) 1981.

Cunha BA, et al: Tetracyclines. *Med Clin North Am* 66:293-302, 1982.

Daum RS, et al: Fatal aplastic anemia following apparent 'dose-related' chloramphenicol toxicity. *J Pediatr* 94:403-406, 1979.

Doherty JE: Digoxin-antibiotic drug interaction. *N Engl J Med* 305:827-828, 1981.

Domart A, et al: Aplasie médullaire mortelle aprés administration de chloramphénicol par voie intra-musculaire chez duex adultes. *Sem Hop Paris* 37:2256-2258, 1961.

Ericsson CD, et al: Influence of subsalicylate bismuth on absorption of doxycycline. *JAMA* 247:2266-2267, 1982.

Faruki H, et al: Community-based outbreak of infection with penicillin-resistant *Neisseria gonorrhoeae* not producing penicillinase (chromosomally-mediated resistance). *N Engl J Med* 313:607-611, 1985.

Fekety R: Clinical importance of anaerobic infections. *Drug Ther (Hosp)* 7:47-48, (Oct) 1982.

Forrest JN Jr, et al: Superiority of demeclocycline over lithium in treatment of chronic syndrome of inappropriate secretion of antidiuretic hormone. *N Engl J Med* 298:173-177, 1978.

Fraunfelder FT, Bagby GC Jr: Ocular chloramphenicol and aplastic anemia, (letter). *N Engl J Med* 307:1536, 1983.

Fraunfelder FT, et al: Fatal aplastic anemia following topical administration of ophthalmic chloramphenicol. *Am J Ophthalmol* 93:356-360, 1982.

Friedman CA, et al: Chloramphenicol disposition in infants and children. *J Pediatr* 95:1071-1077, 1979.

Grilliat JP, et al: Cytopenié mortelle aprés therapeutique par hemisuccinate de chloramphenicol. *Ann Med Nancy* 5:754-762, 1966.

Hansten PD: Antidiabetic drug interactions. *Drug Interactions*, ed 4. Philadelphia, Lea & Febiger, 1979, 104.

Hansten PD, Horn JR: Initiation of oral contraceptive efficacy. *Drug Interact Newslett* 5:7-10, 1985.

Hook EW III, Holmes KK: Gonococcal infections. *Ann Intern Med* 102:229-243, 1985.

Jaffe HW, et al: Infections due to penicillinase-producing *Neisseria gonorrhoeae* in the United States: 1976-1980. *J Infect Dis* 144:191-197, 1981.

Kauffman RE, et al: Pharmacokinetics of chloramphenicol and chloramphenicol succinate in infants and children. *J Pediatr* 98:315-320, 1981 A.

Kauffman RE, et al: Relative bioavailability of intravenous chloramphenicol succinate and oral chloramphenicol palmitate in infants and children. *J Pediatr* 99:963-967, 1981 B.

Kramer WG, et al: Comparative bioavailability of intravenous and oral chloramphenicol in adults. *J Clin Pharmacol* 24:181-186, 1984.

Lindenbaum J, et al: Inactivation of digoxin by gut flora: Reversal by antibiotic therapy. *N Engl J Med* 305:789-794, 1981.

National Institutes of Health Consensus Development Conference: Travelers' diarrhea. *JAMA* 253:2700-2704, 1985.

Nelson JD: Cefuroxime: Cephalosporin with unique applicability to pediatric practice. *Pediatr Infect Dis* 2:394-396, 1983.

Nelson JD: *1985 Pocketbook of Pediatric Antimicrobial Therapy*, ed 6. Baltimore, Williams & Wilkins, 1985 A, 64-75.

Nelson JD: *1985 Pocketbook of Pediatric Antimicrobial Therapy*, ed 6. Baltimore, Williams & Wilkins, 1985 B, 20-21.

Neu HC: New beta-lactamase-stable cephalosporins. *Ann Intern Med* 97:408-419, 1982.

Ory EM: Tetracyclines, in Kagan BM (ed): *Antimicrobial Therapy*, ed 3. Philadelphia, WB Saunders, 1980, 117-126.

Plaut ME, Best WR: Aplastic anemia after parenteral chloramphenicol: Warning renewed, (letter). *N Engl J Med* 306:1486, 1982.

Poliak SC, et al: Minocycline-associated tooth discoloration in young adults. *JAMA* 254:2930-2932, 1985.

Pratt WB: *Chemotherapy of Infection*. New York, Oxford University Press, 1977, 127-175.

Prober CG: Effect of rifampin on chloramphenicol levels, (letter). *N Engl J Med* 312:788-789, 1985.

Rahal JJ Jr, Simberkoff MS: Bactericidal and bacteriostatic action of chloramphenicol against meningeal pathogens. *Antimicrob Agents Chemother* 16:13-18, 1979.

Rahal JJ Jr, Simberkoff MS: Host defense and antimicrobial therapy in adult gram-negative bacillary meningitis. *Ann Intern Med* 96:468-474, 1982.

Restrepo A, Zambrano F: Anemia aplastica tardia secundaria a cloranfenicol. Descripcion de diez casos. *Antioquia Medica* 18:593-606, 1968.

Rice RJ, et al: Changing trends in gonococcal antibiotic resistance in the United States, 1983-1984. *CDC Surveill Summ* 33:11SS-15SS, 1985.

Rosenthal RL, Blackman A: Bone-marrow hypoplasia following use of chloramphenicol eyedrops. *JAMA* 191:148-149, 1965.

Sack DA, et al: Prophylactic doxycycline for travelers' diarrhea: Results of prospective double-blind study of Peace Corps volunteers in Kenya. *N Engl J Med* 298:758-763, 1978.

Sack RB, et al: Prophylactic doxycycline for travelers' diarrhea: Results of prospective double-blind study of Peace Corps volunteers in Morocco. *Gastroenterology* 76:1368-1373, 1979.

Satterwhite TK, DuPont HL: Infectious diarrhea in office practice. *Med Clin North Am* 67:203-220, 1983.

Shalit I, Marks MI: Chloramphenicol in the 1980s. *Drugs* 28:281-291, 1984.

Shankaran S, Kauffman RE: Use of chloramphenicol palmitate in neonates. *J Pediatr* 105:113-116, 1984.

Siegel D: Tetracyclines: New look at old antibiotic: I. Clinical pharmacology, mechanism of action, and untoward effects. II. Clinical use. *NY State J Med* 78:950-956, 1115-1120, 1978.

Smith AL, Weber A: Pharmacology of chloramphenicol. *Pediatr Clin North Am* 30:209-236, 1983.

Stamm WE, et al: Treatment of acute urethral syndrome. *N Engl J Med* 304:956-958, 1981.

Standiford HC: Tetracyclines and chloramphenicol, in Mandell GL, et al (eds): *Principles and Practice of Infectious Diseases*, ed 2. New York, John Wiley & Sons, 1984, 206-216.

Steere AC, et al: Treatment of early manifestations of Lyme disease. *Ann Intern Med* 99:22-26, 1983.

Timbrell JA: Drug hepatotoxicity. *Br J Clin Pharmacol* 15:3-14, 1983.

Tuomanen EI, et al: Oral chloramphenicol in treatment of *Haemophilus influenzae* meningitis. *J Pediatr* 99:968-974, 1981.

Wallerstein RO, et al: Statewide study of chloramphenicol therapy and fatal aplastic anemia. *JAMA* 208:2045-2050, 1969.

Yogev R, et al: Pharmacokinetic comparison of intravenous and oral chloramphenicol in patients with *Haemophilus influenzae* meningitis. *Pediatrics* 67:656-660, 1981.

Yunis AA, et al: Nitroso-chloramphenicol: Possible mediator in chloramphenicol-induced aplastic anemia. *J Lab Clin Med* 96:36-46, 1980.

Other Selected References

Barza M, Schiefe RT: Antimicrobial spectrum, pharmacology and therapeutic use of antibiotics: Part 1. Tetracyclines. *Am J Hosp Pharm* 34:49-57, 1977.

Kucers A: Chloramphenicol, erythromycin, vancomycin, tetracyclines. *Lancet* 2:425-429, 1982.

Meissner HC, Smith AL: Current status of chloramphenicol. *Pediatrics* 64:348-356, 1979.

Reese RE, Betts RF: Antibiotic use, in Reese RE, Douglas RG Jr (eds): *A Practical Approach to Infectious Diseases*. Boston, Little, Brown and Company, 1983, 123-127, 137-141.

Ristuccia AM: Chloramphenicol: Clinical pharmacology in pediatrics. *Therapeut Drug Monitor* 7:159-167, 1985.

Aminoglycosides

The aminoglycoside antibiotics were discovered as the result of a systematic screening of soil actinomycetes for the elaboration of antimicrobial substances. Streptomycin, the first clinically useful aminoglycoside, was isolated in 1944.

Presently, nine aminoglycoside antibiotics are approved for use in the United States. Streptomycin, neomycin [Mycifradin, Neobiotic], kanamycin [Kantrex, Klebcil], tobramycin [Nebcin], and paromomycin [Humatin] are natural compounds derived from various species of *Streptomyces*; gentamicin [Garamycin] and sisomicin [Siseptin] are obtained from species of *Micromonospora*. Amikacin [Amikin] and netilmicin [Netromycin] are semisynthetic aminoglycosides produced by chemical modification of kanamycin and sisomicin, respectively. Sisomicin is not currently marketed in the United States.

In general, aminoglycosides have similar antibacterial spectra and pharmacokinetic properties, and their potential toxicities affect the same organ systems. However, subtle and important differences do exist.

Chemistry

The aminoglycosides are more appropriately designated aminoglycosidic aminocyclitols. These agents all contain a six-membered aminocyclitol ring (aglycone) to which are attached a variety of amino-containing and nonamino-containing sugars by glycosidic linkages. The aminocyclitol ring of streptomycin is streptidine. The other aminoglycosides have 2-deoxystreptamine as the aglycone in a centrally located position.

The 2-deoxystreptamine subclass can be further subdivided into aminoglycoside families based on the number and types of sugars attached to the aminocyclitol ring. The neomycin family, which includes neomycin and paromomycin, has three sugars (two amino hexoses and one nonamino pentose) attached to 2-deoxystreptamine. The kanamycin (kanamycin, tobramycin, amikacin) and gentamicin (gentamicin, sisomicin, netilmicin) families have only two amino hexoses attached to this central aglycone. These latter two families differ in the type of 3-amino hexose found in the C ring position; for the kanamycin family it is kanosamine and for the gentamicin family it is garosamine. Variations within families of aminoglycosides result from differences in side chains on the amino sugars and, in the case of amikacin and netilmicin, on the aglycone. The chemical structures of the aminoglycosides are shown in the Figure.

Mechanism of Action

Under aerobic conditions, the aminoglycosides are bactericidal, but their exact mechanism of action is unknown. These antibiotics must be actively transported into susceptible bacteria. Based on studies done primarily with streptomycin, the aminoglycosides bind to the bacterial 30S ribosomal subunit to produce a nonfunctional 70S initiation complex that, in turn, results in the inhibition of bacterial cell protein synthesis and misreading of the genetic code (Pratt, 1977; Tanaka, 1982; Moellering, 1983; Lietman, 1984). The 2-deoxystreptamine-containing aminoglycosides also bind to the 30S subunit, inhibit protein synthesis, and cause incorrect reading of the genetic code. However, they appear to have different interactions with this subunit when compared to streptomycin. These analogues also have been shown to bind to the 50S subunit. For example, the binding of amikacin to the 50S subunit is competitively inhibited by neomycin and gentamicin (Benveniste and Davies, 1973). Thus, there is evidence of selective affinities for 30S and 50S binding sites among the 2-deoxystreptamine-containing aminoglycosides (Pratt, 1977; Tanaka, 1982; Moellering, 1983; Lietman, 1984).

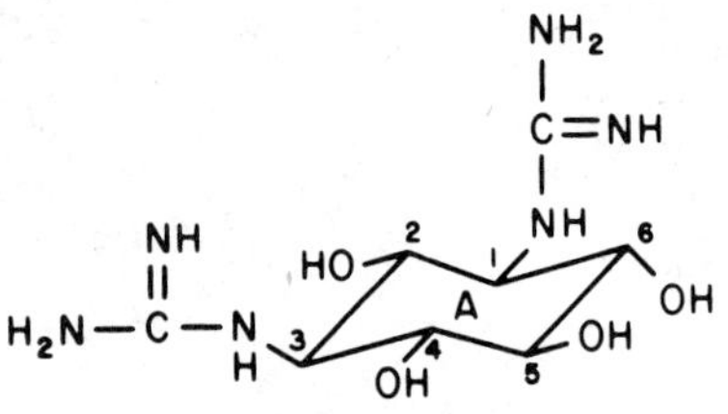

STREPTIDINE

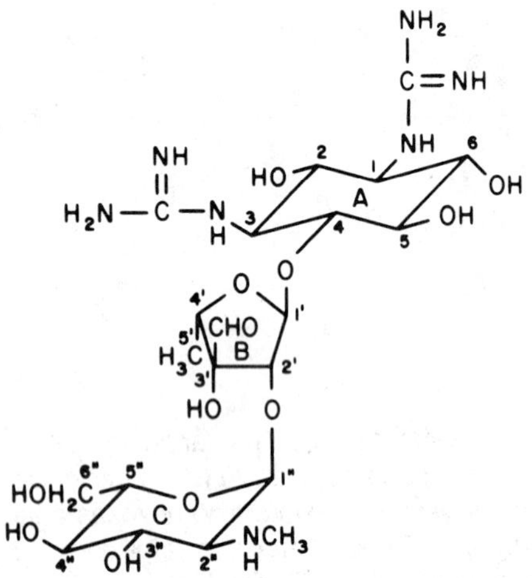

STREPTOMYCIN

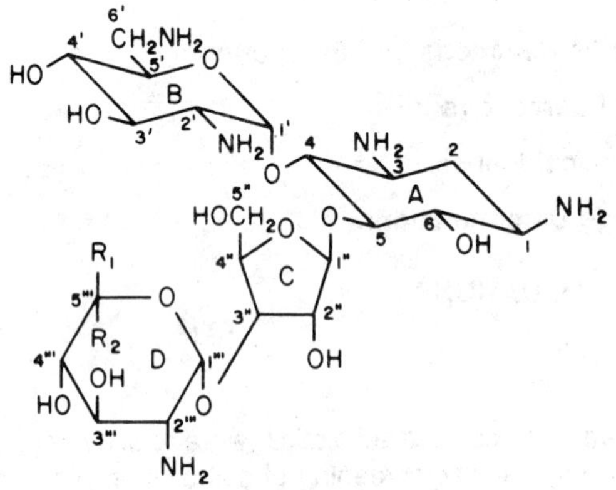

NEOMYCIN[1]

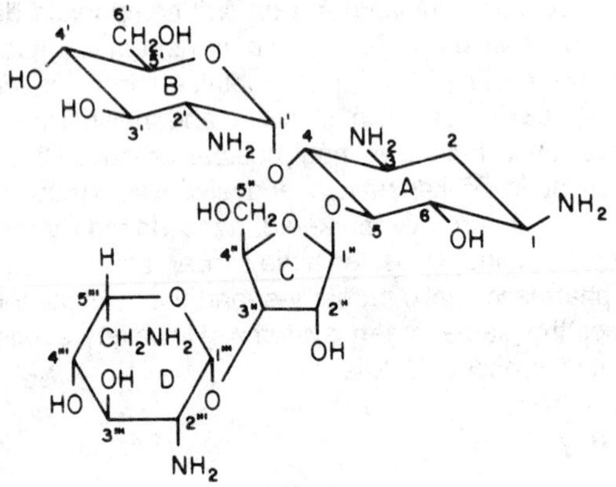

PAROMOMYCIN

[1]Commercially available preparations of gentamicin, neomycin, and kanamycin are actually mixtures. Gentamicin contains approximately equal amounts of gentamicin C_1 ($R_1 = R_2 = CH_3$), C_2 ($R_1 = CH_3$; $R_2 = H$), and C_{1A} ($R_1 = R_2 = H$). Neomycin contains approximately equal amounts of neomycin B ($R_1 = H$; $R_2 = CH_2NH_2$) and C ($R_1 = CH_2NH_2$; $R_2 = H$). Kanamycin is primarily kanamycin A (structure shown) with less than 5% kanamycin B (not shown).

THE AMINOGLYCOSIDES

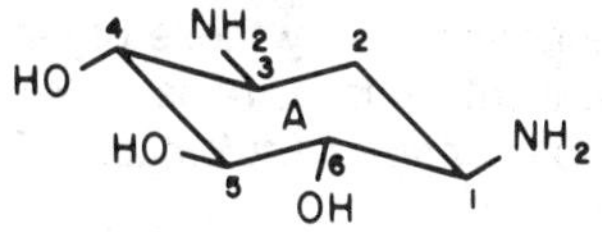

2-DEOXYSTREPTAMINE

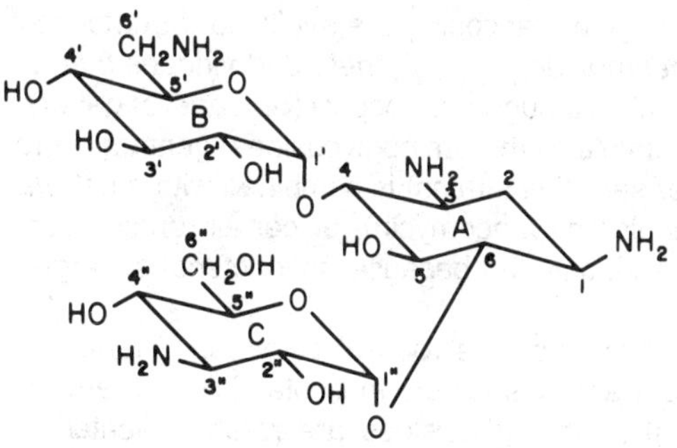

KANAMYCIN[1]

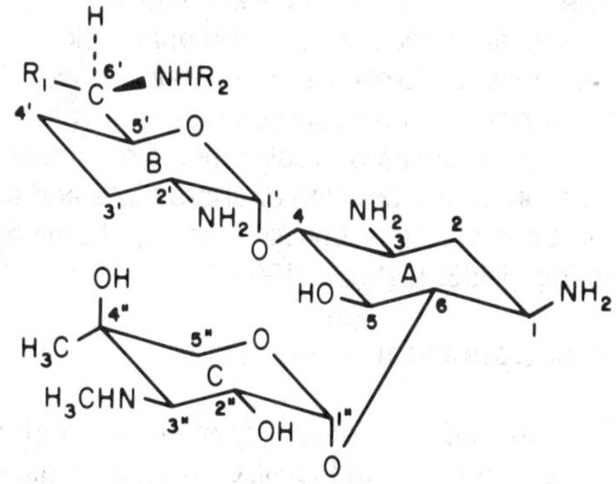

GENTAMICIN[1]

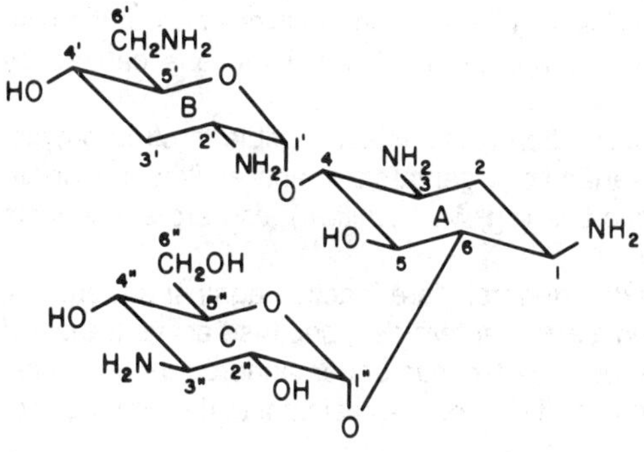

TOBRAMYCIN

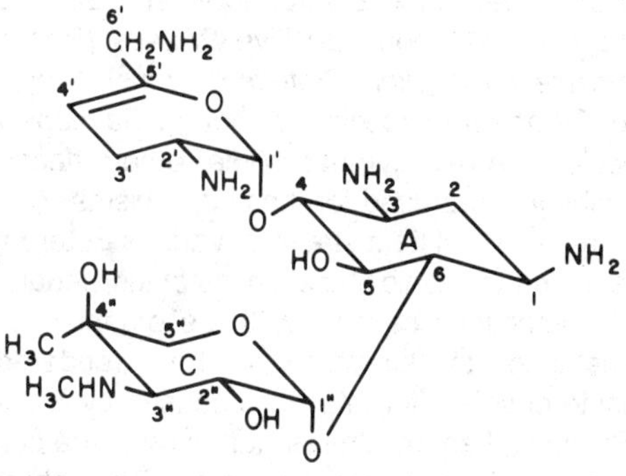

SISOMICIN

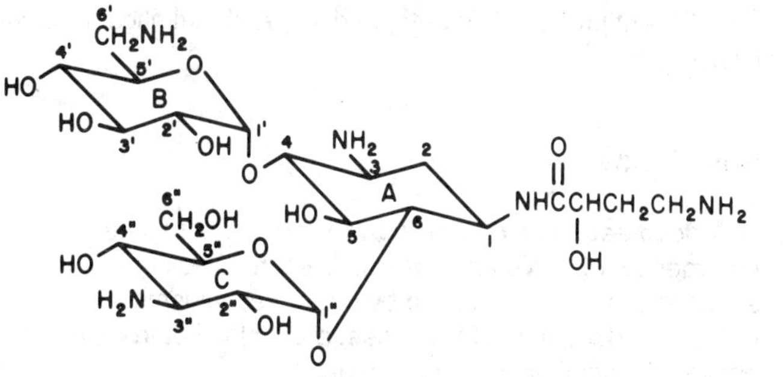

AMIKACIN

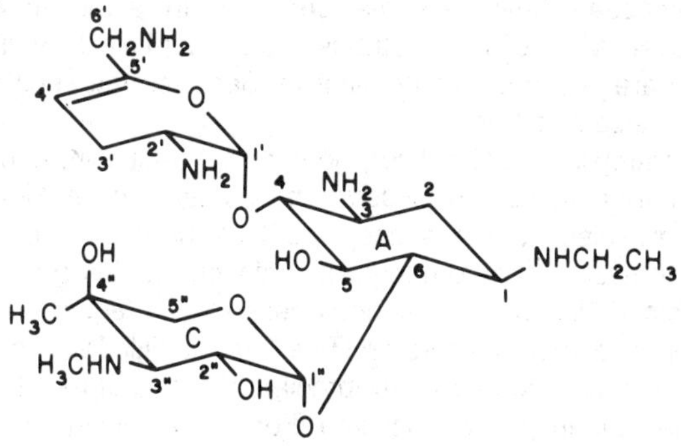

NETILMICIN

It is still not known why the aminoglycosides are bactericidal, while other antibiotics that impair protein synthesis (eg, chloramphenicol, tetracyclines) are usually only bacteriostatic. Bacterial cell death does not appear to correlate with the production of faulty proteins due to misreading of the genetic code. The lethal effect of the aminoglycosides may result from their high affinity for the 30S subunit that leads to essentially irreversible binding (Pratt, 1977; Moellering, 1983), but other mechanisms (eg, an effect on bacterial membranes) also may be involved (Hancock, 1981; Tanaka, 1982; Lietman, 1984).

The active transport of aminoglycosides across bacterial cell membranes is inhibited by divalent cations (eg, Ca^{++}, Mg^{++}), hyperosmolarity, reduced pH, and anaerobiosis. Thus, the activity of these antibiotics is markedly reduced in the anaerobic environment of an abscess or in hyperosmolar acidic urine. The interactions with calcium and magnesium are particularly relevant to the creation of appropriate and consistent media for the in vitro susceptibility testing of aminoglycosides (Moellering, 1983; Lietman, 1984).

Antimicrobial Spectrum

The major useful spectrum of activity of the aminoglycoside antibiotics includes aerobic and facultative gram-negative bacilli and *Staphylococcus aureus* (see Korzeniowski and Hook, 1979; Moellering, 1983).

Enterobacteriaceae that are usually susceptible include *Escherichia coli, Klebsiella, Enterobacter* and *Serratia* species, *Proteus mirabilis*, indole-positive *Proteus (Providencia rettgeri, Morganella morganii, Proteus vulgaris), Providencia stuartii,* and *Citrobacter* species. Although *Salmonella* and *Shigella* species are usually susceptible, other effective and less toxic antibiotics are used for these organisms.

The emergence of resistant strains of various Enterobacteriaceae has affected the clinical usefulness of individual aminoglycosides for infections caused by these organisms. Widespread resistance to streptomycin has rendered this aminoglycoside obsolete for infections caused by Enterobacteriaceae. Similarly, kanamycin-resistant strains are common, particularly in hospitals. Presently, gentamicin, tobramycin, amikacin, and netilmicin have sufficient activity against Enterobacteriaceae to be recommended clinically for systemic infections. Gentamicin- and tobramycin-resistant strains of Enterobacteriaceae have become prevalent in some hospitals, however. Most of these strains are susceptible to amikacin; many are susceptible to netilmicin. See also the sections on Resistance and Uses.

Tobramycin (most active), gentamicin, amikacin, and netilmicin are active against *Pseudomonas aeruginosa*. However, this organism is not susceptible to kanamycin, neomycin, streptomycin, or paromomycin. Aminoglycosides are usually combined with an antipseudomonal penicillin (eg, carbenicillin [Geopen, Pyopen], ticarcillin [Ticar], mezlocillin [Mezlin], azlocillin [Azlin], piperacillin [Pipracil]) or an antipseudomonal cephalosporin (eg, ceftazidime [Fortaz, Tazidime], cefoperazone [Cefobid]) for serious systemic infections caused by *P. aeruginosa*.

Other susceptible aerobic gram-negative bacilli include *Acinetobacter* and *Haemophilus* species. Aminoglycosides generally are not used to treat *Haemophilus* infections, however, because more effective, less toxic antibiotics are available.

Streptomycin is active against *Brucella, Francisella tularensis, Yersinia pestis, Pseudomonas mallei,* and *Spirillum minor* and is useful for infections caused by these organisms (see Uses section and evaluation). Some strains of *Haemophilus ducreyi* and *Calymmatobacterium granulomatis* also are susceptible.

Among gram-positive cocci, only staphylococci (eg, *S. aureus*) are inhibited by the aminoglycosides. However, these antibiotics have seldom been used as sole agents in serious staphylococcal infections, because less toxic antibiotics (eg, penicillinase-resistant penicillins, cephalosporins, clindamycin [Cleocin], vancomycin [Vancocin]) are available. Streptococci, including *S. pneumoniae, S. pyogenes,* and viridans streptococci are resistant. Although enterococci (*S. faecalis*) generally are not susceptible to the aminoglycosides, gentamicin (or streptomycin for sensitive strains) is combined with a cell wall inhibitor (eg, penicillin, vancomycin) for certain enterococcal infections (eg, endocarditis) because antibacterial synergism is observed.

Although the gram-positive rods of *Bacillus, Listeria,* and *Corynebacterium* are susceptible to gentamicin, tobramycin, and amikacin, the aminoglycosides are rarely indicated for infections caused by these organisms. Ampicillin plus an aminoglycoside frequently is synergistic in vitro against *L. monocytogenes,* however.

Neisseria gonorrhoeae and *N. meningitidis* (gram-negative cocci) are susceptible to some aminoglycosides, but these drugs generally are not used to treat infections caused by these organisms.

Mycobacterium tuberculosis is susceptible to streptomycin (most active), kanamycin, gentamicin, and amikacin. Certain atypical mycobacteria (eg, *M. fortuitum*) also are susceptible to amikacin.

Aminoglycosides generally are inactive against anaerobes, including clostridia and *Bacteroides*, because active transport of these drugs does not occur under anaerobic conditions. Rickettsiae, fungi, and viruses are resistant to the aminoglycosides.

Entamoeba histolytica, the causative organism of amebiasis, and various tapeworms, including *Taenia saginata, T. solium, Dipylidium caninum, Diphyllobothrium latum,* and *Hymenolepis nana,* are susceptible to paromomycin (see Chapters 77, Antiprotozoal Agents, and 78, Anthelmintics, respectively).

Resistance

Widespread use of aminoglycosides has resulted in the emergence of resistant strains. Bacterial resistance to the aminoglycosides is achieved by three mechanisms: (1) alteration of the ribosome, (2) decreased antibiotic uptake, and (3) enzymatic inactivation of the drugs.

Clinically, the third mechanism is the most common and important type of resistance. Inactivation occurs when extrachromosomal genes (plasmids), transmitted by bacterial conjugation or other mechanisms, cause the production of enzymes that modify the aminoglycosides by acetylation of specific amino groups or phosphorylation or adenylylation of specific hydroxyl groups (Benveniste and Davies, 1973; Courvalin and Carlier, 1981; Mitsuhashi and Kawabe, 1982; Phillips, 1982; Davies, 1983; Moellering, 1983; Hare and Miller, 1984; Lietman, 1984). Current evidence indicates that the modified antibiotic is unable to bind to ribosomal target sites. This, in turn, is thought to interfere with the aminoglycoside transport mechanism and prevents further uptake of active drug into the bacterial cell (Davies and Smith, 1978; Dickie et al, 1978; Davies, 1983; Moellering, 1983).

Several acetyltransferases (AAC), phosphotransferases (APH), and adenylyltransferases (ANT) have been identified; some are widely distributed among bacterial species, whereas others are more limited. Each has a characteristic spectrum of activity against different aminoglycosides, depending on the presence or absence of the group on which it acts or its inaccessibility resulting from the protective effects of other substituents in the molecule (Table 1). Furthermore, isoenzymes that have slightly different substrate profiles have been identified for a number of these modifying enzymes. Thus, many different patterns of aminoglycoside cross-resistance can emerge as the result of the overlapping substrate specificities exhibited by these modifying enzymes (Mitsuhashi and Kawabe, 1982; Phillips, 1982; Davies, 1983; Hare and Miller, 1984; Lietman, 1984).

The prevalence of individual aminoglycoside-inactivating enzymes varies widely both with respect to geographic location and time. Therefore, different patterns of aminoglycoside resistance exist among countries; among hospitals in any country, state, or city; and even among wards within a hospital (Lietman, 1984). For the United States in general, streptomy-

cin is clinically obsolete for infections caused by the Enterobacteriaceae and the usefulness of kanamycin against these organisms is limited because of the widespread prevalence of modifying enyzmes that are active against these aminoglycoside analogues. In one major study (Hare and Miller, 1984), the incidence of resistance mechanisms that affect gentamicin, tobramycin, amikacin, or netilmicin was compared. ANT (2"), AAC (3), and AAC (6') were the most prevalent aminoglycoside-inactivating enzymes found among clinical isolates of gram-negative bacilli in this country. Each of these enzymes is active against gentamicin and tobramycin and cross-resistance between these two aminoglycosides is common. However, some gentamicin-resistant *Pseudomonas* remain susceptible to tobramycin. Gentamicin-resistant strains that produce acetyltransferases also usually are resistant to netilmicin, but Enterobacteriaceae that produce adenylyltransferases are usually susceptible to the latter drug because it is not inactivated by these enzymes. Organisms resistant to both gentamicin and tobramycin often are sensitive to amikacin, which is not susceptible to most aminoglycoside-inactivating enzymes (see Table 1). This discussion emphasizes the importance of maintaining locally generated antibiotic susceptibility profiles and of performing susceptibility tests when using aminoglycosides.

Gram-negative bacilli that are resistant to amikacin frequently are resistant to all aminoglycosides; strains of *E. coli*, *Pseudomonas*, *Enterobacter*, and *Serratia* have been isolated that are resistant to all aminoglycosides. The mechanism is nonenzymatic and results from decreased uptake of antibiotic by the bacterial cell (Moellering, 1983). Despite increased clinical use, resistance to amikacin has not appeared to increase in some institutions (Price et al, 1981; Moody et al,

TABLE 1.
CLASSES OF AMINOGLYCOSIDE-MODIFYING ENZYMES[1]

Enzyme	Substrate	Source
PHOSPHOTRANSFERASES (APH)		
APH (3')[2]	KM, NM, PM[3]	Enterobacteriaceae, *Pseudomonas*, staphylococci, *Streptococcus faecalis*
APH (2")	GM, KM, TM, NTL (+/−)	Staphylococci, *Streptococcus faecalis*
APH (3")	SM	Enterobacteriaceae, *Pseudomonas*, staphylococci, *Streptococcus faecalis*
APH (6)	SM	*Pseudomonas*
ADENYLYLTRANSFERASES (ANT or AAD)		
ANT (3")	SM	Enterobacteriaceae, *Pseudomonas*
ANT (6)	SM	Staphylococci
ANT (2")	GM, KM, TM	Enterobacteriaceae, *Pseudomonas*
ANT (4')	KM, NM, PM, TM, AK	Staphylococci
ACETYLTRANSFERASES (AAC)		
AAC (3)[2]	GM, TM, KM, NM, PM, NTL	Enterobacteriaceae, *Pseudomonas*
AAC (6')[2]	KM, NM, GM[4], TM, NTL, AK (variable)	Enterobacteriaceae, *Pseudomonas*, staphylococci, *Streptococcus faecalis*
AAC (2')	GM, TM, NTL, NM, PM	*Providencia stuartii, Proteus rettgeri*

[1]*Adapted from reviews by Mitsuhashi and Kawabe, 1982: Phillips, 1982; Davies, 1983; and Hare and Miller, 1984.*
[2]*Substrate profiles vary with isozymic form of the enzyme.*
[3]*Abbreviations are: AK = amikacin; GM = gentamicin; KM = kanamycin; NM = neomycin; NTL = netilmicin; PM = paromomycin; SM = streptomycin; TM = tobramycin*
[4]*Gentamicins C_{1A} and C_2 are modified, but gentamicin C_1 is not modified by this enzyme.*

1982; Betts et al, 1984; Gerding and Larson, 1985). However, this observation is not universal (Levine et al, 1985), and the occurrence of amikacin resistance requires continued surveillance.

Chromosomal mutations that alter the 30S ribosomal subunit binding site can result in a rapid, single-step resistance to streptomycin. Clinically, this type of resistance appears to be important for *Mycobacterium tuberculosis* and enterococci, but not for gram-negative bacilli. Although ribosomal resistance to 2-deoxystreptamine-containing aminoglycosides has been demonstrated, it is generally uncommon and not of much clinical importance (Moellering, 1983; Lietman, 1984).

Uses

Aminoglycosides must be administered parenterally for systemic infections. Gentamicin, tobramycin, amikacin, netilmicin, kanamycin, and streptomycin are the currently available parenteral aminoglycosides. These agents are indicated in severe, complicated infections caused by susceptible organisms. Because of their ototoxic and nephrotoxic potential, these antibiotics should not be used in trivial infections or in those that can be eradicated with less toxic antibacterial agents.

Parenteral Aminoglycosides for Serious Aerobic Gram-negative Bacillary Infections: The primary use of parenteral aminoglycosides, either alone or in combination regimens, is for the treatment of serious infections caused by aerobic gram-negative bacilli, principally the Enterobacteriaceae and *Pseudomonas aeruginosa*. These include bacteremias; intraabdominal infections (eg, peritonitis secondary to bowel perforation, nonvenereal pelvic inflammatory disease); skin and soft tissue infections (eg, infected burns with sepsis, necrotizing fasciitis); lower respiratory tract infections (eg, nosocomial pneumonia); bone and joint infections (eg, osteomyelitis, septic arthritis); complicated urinary tract infections (eg, acute pyelonephritis); and meningitis (intrathecal administration required except in newborns) (see Neu, 1982 A; see also Chapter 65, Antimicrobial Therapy and Chemoprophylaxis of Infectious Diseases). Gentamicin, tobramycin, amikacin, netilmicin, or kanamycin may be used for these infections when the susceptibility of the causative organism is known. Generally, widespread resistance of the Enterobacteriaceae to streptomycin has rendered this drug obsolete for common gram-negative bacterial infections.

Empiric therapy with an aminoglycoside frequently is necessary for a presumed gram-negative bacillary infection before the identification and susceptibility of the causative organism are known. Under these circumstances, drug selection should depend on a number of factors, including the incidence of aminoglycoside resistance at a given hospital based on current locally generated antibiotic susceptibility profiles for selected organisms, the severity and type of infection (community acquired or nosocomial), possible differences in drug toxicity, the ability to monitor aminoglycoside serum concentrations, and the cost of antibiotic therapy (Reese and Betts, 1983). Presently, there is considerable controversy as to whether any one aminoglycoside offers significant advantages over the other analogues to warrant being the drug of choice. A major reason for this problem is lack of well designed, controlled clinical trials comparing aminoglycosides (Smith and Lietman, 1982). The following discussion considers some of the advantages and disadvantages of each agent with regard to the above factors. Ultimately, each hospital must comparatively evaluate the aminoglycosides relative to their institution's requirements before selecting a particular agent for the hospital formulary.

Gentamicin, tobramycin, amikacin, and netilmicin usually are considered when selecting an aminoglycoside for general use. Kanamycin is not active against *Pseudomonas aeruginosa* and resistance to this agent among the Enterobacteriaceae is widespread in many hospitals. Thus kanamycin has no advantages over the other aminoglycosides in serious gram-negative bacillary infections.

Presently, gentamicin and tobramycin are the aminoglycosides most frequently selected for general use. Either agent is an appropriate drug of choice for infections that are likely to be caused by susceptible organisms. The patent for gentamicin has expired and it is considerably less expensive than tobramycin, amikacin, or netilmicin. In a cost-conscious environment, this is an important consideration when all other factors are equal.

Tobramycin is more potent in vitro against *P. aeruginosa*, including some gentamicin-resistant strains, and frequently is preferred, often in combination with an antipseudomonal penicillin, for infections likely to be caused by this organism (eg, infection in the neutropenic patient). Conclusive proof that tobramycin is clinically superior to gentamicin against *P. aeruginosa* has not been shown, however (Young et al, 1981; Lietman, 1984).

Some infectious disease experts have recommended tobramycin over gentamicin for all infections likely to be caused by susceptible organisms because tobramycin has been reported to be less nephrotoxic (based on serum creatinine determinations) than gentamicin (Smith et al, 1980; and others [see reviews by Rozek, 1984; Whelton, 1985]). Although this result was not confirmed by others (Fong et al, 1981; and others [see reviews by Rozek, 1984; Whelton, 1985]) and the design of the study by Smith et al, (1980) has been criticized (De Torres, 1981; Ristuccia and Cunha, 1982), consensus opinion based on all of the available evidence does suggest that tobramycin is probably less nephrotoxic than gentamicin. However, nephrotoxicity associated with aminoglycoside therapy usually is mild and reversible, and it seldom requires additional hospitalization or dialysis. When the data from the study by Smith et al (1980) were subjected to decision analysis to evaluate the relative cost-effectiveness of gentamicin and tobramycin, it was concluded that the former agent was more cost-effective despite its greater nephrotoxic potential (Holloway et al, 1984). Furthermore, it has been shown that when gentamicin serum concentrations are carefully monitored and dosages are calculated by an individualized pharmacokinetic method (Sawchuck and Zaske, 1976; Sawchuck et al, 1977), the nephrotoxicity observed with gentamicin is minimal (Zaske et al, 1980, 1981, 1982 A, B, and C). In summary, the use of tobramycin over gentamicin for all patients does not appear to be warranted. Tobramycin may be preterable in patients at increased risk for nephrotoxicity, such as the elderly and those requiring prolonged therapy (see Moore et al, 1984 A; Whelton, 1985; see also section on Adverse Reactions and Precautions), particularly when individualized dosing methods are not employed.

Other than the above, data that clearly show differences in toxicity (eg, nephrotoxicity, ototoxicity) among the four major aminoglycosides (ie, gentamicin, tobramycin, amikacin, netilmicin) in humans are presently unavailable. In animal studies, netilmicin has been shown to be less ototoxic and nephrotoxic than gentamicin, tobramycin, and amikacin (Szot and Tabachnick, 1980). These differences generally have not been demonstrated unequivocally in humans (*Med Lett Drugs Ther*, 1983; Craig et al, 1983; Guay, 1983), although a retrospective review of aminoglycoside toxicity from clinical studies published between 1975 and 1982 suggests that netilmicin may be less ototoxic than the other aminoglycosides (Kahlmeter and Dahlager, 1984). In one multicenter, controlled clinical trial, the combination of netilmicin plus ticarcillin was reported to be significantly less ototoxic than tobramycin plus ticarcillin (Lerner et al, 1983). However, confirmation of these results and additional clinical experience with this aminoglycoside are necessary before it can be recommended over other analogues (see *Med Lett Drugs Ther*, 1983; Craig et al, 1983; Guay, 1983). As discussed above, netilmicin is considerably more expensive than gentamicin.

Cross-resistance between gentamicin and tobramycin is common, and resistance to these two aminoglycosides is becoming more widespread, particularly in nosocomial infections. Amikacin usually is effective in infections caused by organisms (eg, strains of Enterobacteriaceae, *P. aeruginosa*) that are resistant to gentamicin and tobramycin because it is less susceptible to aminoglycoside-inactivating enzymes (see section on Resistance). Thus, amikacin should be the drug of choice for empiric therapy of infections caused by aerobic gram-negative bacilli in hospitals where gentamicin- and tobramycin-resistant strains are common. Furthermore, even in hospitals without a major resistance problem, when there is concern about gentamicin- and tobramycin-resistant gram-negative bacilli in a particular clinical situation (eg, severe nosocomial infection in a patient who is immunosuppressed, on prior antibiotics, or in the intensive care unit), amikacin frequently is recommended for initial therapy before the results of susceptibility tests are known. Netilmicin also is active against some gentamicin- and tobramycin-resistant strains of various Enterobacteriaceae. However, it does not appear to offer any advantages in spectrum of activity over amikacin and clinical experience with this agent is more limited (see *Med Lett Drugs Ther*, 1983; Craig et al, 1983; Guay, 1983). Presently, netilmicin is less expensive than amikacin (based on average wholesale prices obtained from *1985 Drug Topics Redbook* [Oradell, NJ, Medical Economics Co, 1985] and monthly updates through January, 1986) and this may be a consideration in some hospitals.

The selection of amikacin as the aminoglycoside of choice for general use presently is a controversial issue. Many infectious disease experts have recommended that this antibi-

otic be reserved for situations in which gentamicin or tobramycin resistance is a problem. The rationale is that extensive use of amikacin will result in the unnecessary emergence of amikacin-resistant bacterial strains. However, there is no evidence that restriction of amikacin has delayed the emergence of resistance to this drug (Levin, 1981; Reese and Betts, 1983; Davies, 1983; Lietman, 1984). Furthermore, in some hospitals where amikacin has become the primary aminoglycoside, resistance to this agent has not increased (Price et al, 1981; Moody et al, 1982; Betts et al, 1984; Gerding and Larson, 1985). In addition to its lower resistance potential, some infectious disease experts prefer amikacin over gentamicin (or tobramycin) for general use because of a better pharmacokinetic profile, including more reliable predictability of adequate, nontoxic, peak serum concentrations, a higher therapeutic ratio, and a longer dosing interval, and decreased susceptibility to inactivation by beta-lactam antibiotics (Levin, 1981; Ristuccia and Cunha, 1982, 1985; Holm et al, 1983; see also the section on Drug Interactions and the evaluations). The clinical significance of these factors is unclear, however (Levin, 1981), and others have reported wide interpatient variation in amikacin pharmacokinetics similar to gentamicin and tobramycin (see Mangione and Schentag, 1980; Zaske, 1980; Finley et al, 1982; Bauer and Blouin, 1983). As discussed above, amikacin is considerably more expensive than gentamicin, an important consideration for hospitals where gentamicin resistance is not a problem.

Specific Uses of Streptomycin: Streptomycin frequently is the preferred drug in the treatment of tularemia, plague, severe brucellosis (in combination with a tetracycline or chloramphenicol), and glanders (in combination with a tetracycline or chloramphenicol). See also Chapter 65, Antimicrobial Therapy and Chemoprophylaxis of Infectious Diseases, Table 1.

Streptomycin, used only in combination regimens to prevent the emergence of resistant strains, is now a second-line drug in the treatment of tuberculosis. Kanamycin also is used rarely for this disease. Guidelines for the treatment and prophylaxis of tuberculosis are discussed in Chapter 75, Antimycobacterial Agents.

Streptomycin has been used in granuloma inguinale and chancroid, but other antimicrobial drugs (tetracycline for granuloma inguinale and erythromycin, ceftriaxone [Rocephin], or trimethoprim/sulfamethoxazole for chancroid) are preferred (see Chapter 65, Table 2).

For the use of streptomycin in the treatment of infective endocarditis, see the following section, Antibiotic Combinations, and the evaluation.

Uses of Oral Aminoglycosides: Gastrointestinal absorption of orally administered aminoglycosides is negligible in patients with normal renal function and an intact gastrointestinal tract (see section on Pharmacokinetics). Some analogues have been used by the oral route for their local effects in the gastrointestinal tract.

Neomycin, kanamycin, and paromomycin have been used to suppress the bacterial flora of the bowel as a prophylactic measure before elective colorectal surgery. Presently, oral neomycin plus erythromycin base is a regimen of choice for this indication (see Chapter 65, Table 4).

Neomycin is used as an adjunct in the treatment of hepatic coma because it decreases the number of ammonia-forming bacteria in the intestinal tract. For additional discussion, see Chapter 55, Agents Used in Disorders of the Liver, Biliary Tract, and Pancreas.

Neomycin reduces the absorption of cholesterol by precipitating it from micellar solution and has been used in patients with type IIa hyperlipoproteinemia. It should be reserved for patients who have failed to respond to conventional therapy and who have a high risk of ischemic heart disease. For additional discussion, see Chapter 50, Agents Used to Treat Hyperlipidemia.

Paromomycin, usually in combination with iodoquinol [Yodoxin], is an alternative to metronidazole [Flagyl, Metryl] alone (preferred) in the treatment of mild to moderately severe intestinal amebiasis. This aminoglycoside is not effective in extraintestinal amebiasis. For additional discussion, see Chapter 77, Antiprotozoal Agents.

Paromomycin is an alternative to niclosamide [Niclocide] (preferred) in the treatment of tapeworm infections. For additional discussion, see Chapter 78, Anthelmintics.

Uses of Topical Aminoglycosides: The administration of neomycin as a peritoneal or pleural irrigant after surgery is of questionable value and may be dangerous, since a sufficient amount of drug can be absorbed to cause serious ototoxicity and nephrotoxicity (Davia et al, 1970; Masur et al, 1976; Weinstein et al, 1977) or neuromuscular blockade, particularly when used with muscle relaxants.

Neomycin [Myciguent] is most commonly used topically for infections of the eye, ear, and skin, frequently as a component of an antibiotic mixture. Topical ophthalmic preparations of gentamicin [Garamycin, Genoptic] and tobramycin [Tobrex] are used in conjunctivitis caused by susceptible gram-negative bacilli. Although a dermatologic preparation of gentamicin [Garamycin] is available for topical application, such use is *not recommended* because selection of gentamicin-resistant strains occurs very rapidly; widespread resistance has been reported in burn units where topical gentamicin was used. Additional information on the use of the aminoglycosides in infectious diseases of the eye, ear, and skin can be found in Chapters 73, Topical Anti-infective Agents: Otic and Ophthalmic Preparations, and 74, Topical Anti-infective Agents: Drugs Used on Skin and Mucous Membranes.

Antibiotic Combinations

Aminoglycosides frequently are combined with another antibiotic to treat certain infections. The reasons for employing combination therapy are: (1) to obtain a synergistic antibacterial effect, (2) to prevent the emergence of antibiotic-resistant bacteria, and (3) to expand the antimicrobial spectrum (see Rahal, 1978). The following combinations are often employed clinically (see also Chapter 65, Antimicrobial Therapy and Chemoprophylaxis of Infectious Diseases):

(1) An antipseudomonal penicillin (carbenicillin, ticarcillin, mezlocillin, piperacillin, azlocillin) is frequently combined with an aminoglycoside (gentamicin, tobramycin, amikacin, netilmicin) for serious infections caused by Pseudomonas aerugino-

sa because of their synergistic antibacterial effect against this organism. For example, carbenicillin and gentamicin or tobramycin were synergistic against more than 80% of *P. aeruginosa* isolates tested (Kluge et al, 1974). In addition, the emergence of resistant organisms is decreased when such combinations are used. Antipseudomonal penicillins and aminoglycosides should not be mixed together physically, however, because they covalently interact (1:1 molar ratio) and this results in a loss of aminoglycoside activity. Inactivation also has been observed in vivo in patients with severe renal disease despite separate administration of the drugs. Amikacin is less susceptible to inactivation by antipseudomonal penicillins than gentamicin or tobramycin (Holt et al, 1976; Pickering and Rutherford, 1981; Blair et al, 1982; Glew and Pavuk, 1983; Lietman, 1984; see also the section on Drug Interactions).

(2) An antipseudomonal aminoglycoside (gentamicin, tobramycin, amikacin, netilmicin) in combination with an antipseudomonal penicillin and/or a cephalosporin are used routinely for initial empiric therapy in febrile leukopenic immunocompromised patients. Expanded antibacterial coverage with synergistic combinations of bactericidal antibiotics is recommended in such patients to avoid potentially disastrous outcomes. Because of problems with gentamicin and tobramycin resistance, amikacin often is the preferred aminoglycoside for this indication.

(3) Penicillin G or ampicillin in combination with streptomycin (for susceptible strains) or gentamicin has a synergistic action against many enterococci (eg, *Streptococcus faecalis*). Such combinations are employed to treat enterococcal endocarditis for which effective bactericidal activity is necessary. Similarly, streptomycin and penicillin G are more rapidly bactericidal against viridans streptococci, although penicillin G alone is very active against this organism. The combination of an aminoglycoside with vancomycin also is synergistic against most streptococci, including enterococci. Because additive ototoxicity and nephrotoxicity may occur (see the section on Drug Interactions), this combination should be administered only when it is necessary (eg, for enterococcal endocarditis in patients allergic to penicillin).

(4) A penicillinase-resistant penicillin (or vancomycin) plus an aminoglycoside often is synergistic against *Staphylococcus aureus*; however, the clinical indications for such combination therapy remain to be clarified.

(5) Gentamicin, tobramycin, amikacin, or netilmicin may be combined with a cephalosporin in serious *Klebsiella* infections or as empiric therapy for nosocomial pneumonia. Although cephalosporin/aminoglycoside combinations exhibit synergistic activity, some controversy exists concerning their use because increased nephrotoxicity has been seen with cephalothin/aminoglycoside combinations (Wade et al, 1978; see also the section on Drug Interactions).

(6) Gentamicin, tobramycin, amikacin, or netilmicin often is used in combination with a drug effective against the *Bacteroides fragilis* group (eg, clindamycin, metronidazole, chloramphenicol, cefoxitin [Mefoxin], antipseudomonal penicillin) to treat abdominal or pelvic sepsis or prophylactically prior to "dirty" colorectal or urologic surgery.

(7) Gentamicin, tobramycin, amikacin, or netilmicin may be

used with another antibiotic in other empiric therapy when an expanded antimicrobial spectrum is desirable (eg, with ampicillin for neonatal meningitis or biliary tract infections).

(8) Oral neomycin plus erythromycin base is a regimen of choice for prophylaxis of elective colorectal surgery.

Some combinations of an aminoglycoside and a nonaminoglycoside antibiotic are antagonistic. In vitro tests and studies in animals have shown that chloramphenicol and tetracycline antagonize the actions of streptomycin in infections caused by streptococci and *Klebsiella*. Similarly, chloramphenicol antagonizes the action of gentamicin in *P. mirabilis* infections in neutropenic mice or in mice with meningitis.

Adverse Reactions and Precautions

The aminoglycosides have a low therapeutic/toxic ratio when compared to most other antibiotics used systemically. In particular, they have the potential to produce irreversible ototoxicity. They also are nephrotoxic and neurotoxic. Parenteral administration of neomycin and paromomycin should be avoided because of the extreme toxicity associated with these analogues.

Ototoxicity: All aminoglycosides have the potential to produce irreversible ototoxicity; both the hearing (cochlear) and equilibrium (vestibular) functions may be affected. These antibiotics are toxic initially to the hair cells and then to the supporting cells of the neuroepithelium and secretory tissues of the vestibular and cochlear apparatuses of the inner ear. Cellular damage appears to be related to the accumulation and slow elimination of aminoglycosides from the perilymph and endolymph that bathe the relevant target cells. Toxicity is frequently irreversible and is cumulative (eg, with prolonged or repeated courses of therapy) because the cells of the cochlear and vestibular apparatuses cannot regenerate once they have been destroyed (Bendush, 1982; Lietman, 1984; Whelton, 1985).

Clinical manifestations of auditory toxicity include tinnitus, a feeling of "fullness" in the ears, or any degree of hearing loss from temporary inability to detect certain (usually high frequency) tones to total, irreversible deafness. The hearing loss is usually bilateral, although unilateral hearing loss has been reported. If they occur, tinnitus or a feeling of "fullness" in the ear may be an early sign of ototoxicity, and patients should be instructed to report such sensations as soon as they occur. However, these symptoms frequently are not reliable premonitors of auditory toxicity (Lietman, 1984). By the time hearing loss can be detected by inability of the patient to react to normal conversational tones, considerable permanent damage may have occurred. Audiograms should be considered for certain high-risk patients including those with renal failure and those receiving prolonged therapy (ten days or longer). However, it may not be possible to obtain reliable audiograms in critically ill patients. Auditory testing is not routinely performed in patients without associated risk factors.

Symptoms of vestibular toxicity include nausea, vomiting, vertigo, dizziness, and an unsteady gait with nystagmus. These are difficult to evaluate in ill patients. Laboratory measurement of vestibular function by electronystagmography is not obtained in most patients receiving aminoglycosides.

Ototoxicity is dose related and is associated with excessive aminoglycoside serum concentrations. It is more likely to occur with prolonged (more than ten days) or repeated courses of aminoglycoside therapy. Ototoxicity also can occur after discontinuation of drug. Inappropriately high dosing in patients with impaired renal function, dehydrated individuals, the elderly, or the obese increases the risk of ototoxicity. Other reported risk factors include the presence of bacteremia, fever, liver dysfunction, the ratio of serum urea nitrogen to serum creatinine as a measure of hypovolemia, and concurrent administration of other ototoxic drugs, such as ethacrynic acid [Edecrin] (see Bendush, 1982; Ackerman et al, 1984; Lietman, 1984; Moore et al, 1984 B; Whelton, 1985; see also the section on Drug Interactions). Aminoglycoside serum concentrations should be carefully monitored and adjusted in these high-risk patients (see section on Dosage Determinations).

Some aminoglycosides (eg, neomycin, kanamycin, amikacin) impair auditory acuity most frequently, while others (eg, streptomycin, gentamicin) primarily affect vestibular function. Tobramycin appears to affect both functions almost equally (see Bendush, 1982). However, all aminoglycosides will cause both hearing loss and equilibrium imbalance if a high concentration is maintained in the inner ear for a sufficient period.

The incidence of aminoglycoside ototoxicity reported in the literature ranges from 2% to 24%; this wide variation presumably is due to differences in patient populations, the criteria used to determine ototoxicity, and whether serum concentrations were optimally controlled (see Ackerman et al, 1984). In a series of well-controlled, prospective clinical trials done at Johns Hopkins, the incidence of auditory or vestibular toxicity with gentamicin, tobramycin, and amikacin has been estimated to occur in 3% to 5% of patients based on audiometric or electronystagmographic testing, respectively; clinically detectable hearing loss or vestibular dysfunction occurred in about 0.5% of patients (see Lietman, 1984). Clinically detectable ototoxicity has not been observed with gentamicin or tobramycin in a large number of patients when dosages were calculated by an individualized pharmacokinetic method (Zaske et al, 1980, 1981, 1982 A, B, and C; Cipolle et al, 1980).

Clinically, the ototoxic potentials of the important systemically administered agents (gentamicin, tobramycin, amikacin) do not appear to differ significantly (see Lietman, 1984), although one report suggests that tobramycin is less vestibulotoxic than gentamicin (Fee, 1983). In animal studies, netilmicin has been shown to be less ototoxic than gentamicin, tobramycin, and amikacin (Szot and Tabachnick, 1980). These differences generally have not been demonstrated unequivocally in humans (*Med Lett Drugs Ther*, 1983; Craig et al, 1983; Guay, 1983), although a retrospective review of aminoglycoside toxicity from clinical studies published between 1975 and 1982 suggests that netilmicin may be less ototoxic than the other aminoglycosides (Kahlmeter, and Dahlager, 1984). In one multicenter controlled clinical trial, netilmicin (plus ticarcillin) was reported to be significantly less ototoxic than tobramycin (plus ticarcillin) (Lerner et al, 1983). However, a definitive statement on relative ototoxicity requires additional clinical evaluation (see also Uses).

Nephrotoxicity: All aminoglycosides are nephrotoxic to proximal renal tubules. These antibiotics are actively reabsorbed by proximal renal tubular cells where they accumulate and are retained for prolonged periods. Concentrations of aminoglycosides in renal cortex are 5- to 50-fold higher than plasma concentrations. The morphologic effects of aminoglycosides on proximal renal tubular cells consist of cellular swelling and the appearance of cytoplasmic vacuoles and myeloid bodies within lysosomes. Eventually, tubular necrosis can occur. Glomerular filtration subsequently is decreased, but glomerular lesions have not yet been observed in humans. The mechanism for reduced glomerular filtration presently is unclear (see Lietman and Smith, 1983; Lietman, 1984; Whelton, 1985).

Clinically, the earliest effects of aminoglycoside-induced nephrotoxicity begin to appear within one to two days and include proteinuria caused by increased excretion of β_2-microglobulin and several renal tubular enzymes (alanine aminopeptidase, β-D-glucosaminidase, alkaline phosphatase). Urinary casts that result from sloughing of proximal renal tubules also appear. Although these early effects are the most sensitive indicators of renal tubular dysfunction, most infectious disease experts consider them to be too sensitive and nonspecific to be clinically useful. Clinical nephrotoxicity usually is defined by elevations in serum creatinine (alternative, blood urea nitrogen [BUN]) (Lietman and Smith, 1983; Lietman, 1984; Whelton, 1985). For example, one group (Lietman and Smith, 1983) defines nephrotoxicity as an increase in serum creatinine levels of ≥ 0.5 mg/dl if the initial serum creatinine level is <3 mg/dl, or an increase of ≥ 1 mg/dl if the initial serum creatinine level is >3 mg/dl. Elevations in serum creatinine reflect reductions in glomerular filtration rate. This usually occurs only after several days (eg, five to seven days) of aminoglycoside therapy.

The severity of aminoglycoside nephrotoxicity can range from trivial effects on proximal renal tubules to life-threatening acute tubular necrosis. A syndrome of hypokalemia, hypocalcemia, and hypomagnesemia has been reported rarely. Fortunately, nephrotoxicity usually is mild when aminoglycoside dosage is adjusted carefully for changing glomerular function. Furthermore, it is usually, if not always, reversible with drug discontinuation because proximal renal tubular cells, unlike the hair cells of the inner ear, readily regenerate. Aminoglycoside nephrotoxicity usually is nonoliguric (Lietman and Smith, 1983; Lietman, 1984; Whelton, 1985). Nephrotoxicity should not be a deterrent to the use of these antibiotics in therapeutically effective doses. Nevertheless, aminoglycosides should be used for clear indications in seriously ill patients, and serum creatinine and BUN levels should be measured routinely.

Nephrotoxicity is dose related and is more likely to occur with prolonged (more than ten days) or repeated courses of aminoglycoside therapy. It frequently has been associated with elevated serum aminoglycoside trough concentrations (>2 mcg/ml for gentamicin or tobramycin; >4 mcg/ml for netilmicin; >10 mcg/ml for amikacin). However, it is unclear whether this is a true cause-and-effect relationship or simply reflects an already diminished glomerular filtration rate. Inappropriately high dosing in patients with impaired renal function, dehydrated individuals, the elderly, and the obese increases the risk of nephrotoxicity. Other reported risk factors for aminoglycoside nephrotoxicity include the presence of hypotension, liver dysfunction, female sex, a high initial creatinine clearance, and concurrent administration of other nephrotoxic agents. Potent diuretics (eg, furosemide [Lasix]) can increase the risk of nephrotoxicity if volume depletion is not corrected (see Lietman and Smith, 1983; Ackerman et al, 1984; Lietman, 1984; Moore et al, 1984 A; Whelton, 1985). Aminoglycoside serum concentrations should be carefully monitored and adjusted in these high-risk patients (see section on Dosage Determinations).

The incidence of aminoglycoside nephrotoxicity has been reported to range from 1% to 25% or greater in various clinical trials (see Whelton, 1985). The considerable variability among studies is presumably because of differences in the definition of nephrotoxicity, clinical protocols, methodologies, patient populations, the aminoglycoside employed, dosage regimens, and method of determining aminoglycoside dosing (eg, individualized, nomogram).

A number of clinical studies have been undertaken to identify differences in the inherent nephrotoxic potentials of the important systemically administered aminoglycosides (gentamicin, tobramycin, amikacin, netilmicin) (for reviews, see Rozek, 1984; Whelton, 1985). In most cases, data that convincingly show differences in nephrotoxicity are unavailable. Present evidence does suggest that tobramycin probably is less nephrotoxic than gentamicin and this has caused considerable controversy in drug selection between these analogues (see Uses). Although netilmicin has been shown to be less nephrotoxic than gentamicin, tobramycin, and amikacin in animal studies (Szot and Tabachnak, 1980), these differences generally have not been demonstrated unequivocally in humans (*Med Lett Drugs Ther*, 1983; Craig et al, 1983; Guay, 1983).

Neuromuscular Blockade: The aminoglycosides rarely cause neuromuscular blockade that can lead to progressive flaccid paralysis and potentially fatal respiratory arrest. This adverse effect is associated with very high concentrations of aminoglycoside at the neuromuscular junction. The risk is greatest with intraperitoneal or intrapleural instillation of large doses or after rapid (bolus) intravenous administration, but a curare-like paralysis also has been seen rarely following intravenous infusion, intramuscular injection, or even oral administration. Blockade is most common in patients already compromised by other drugs (eg, general anesthetics, neuromuscular blocking agents [see section on Drug Interactions]), diseases (eg, myasthenia gravis), or conditions (eg, hypocalcemia) that affect neuromuscular transmission. Blockade usually can be counteracted by the prompt administration of calcium gluconate; response to cholinesterase inhibitors, such as neostigmine [Prostigmin], has been variable.

Hypersensitivity: Hypersensitivity reactions have been observed occasionally following use of aminoglycosides. Rashes, pruritus, urticaria, and, rarely, exfoliative dermatitis have been reported. Drug fever, hypotension, and anaphylactic shock also have been associated with aminoglycoside use. Patients who are allergic to aminoglycosides should not receive these drugs.

Topical application of neomycin frequently has resulted in sensitization to the drug (see Chapter 74, Topical Anti-infective Agents: Drugs Used on Skin and Mucous Membranes).

Miscellaneous Adverse Reactions: Gastrointestinal side effects are usually mild. Nausea, vomiting, stomatitis, and diarrhea have been reported. Suprainfection caused by non-susceptible organisms has occurred, but pseudomembranous colitis due to *Clostridium difficile* is extremely rare (or does not occur) with aminoglycosides. A malabsorption syndrome may occur after prolonged oral administration.

Blood dyscrasias, including anemia, eosinophilia, neutropenia, thrombocytopenia (including purpura), and agranulocytosis have been reported rarely. Aplastic anemia has been reported very rarely with streptomycin.

Headache, lethargy, paresthesias, tremor, peripheral neuritis, arthralgia, and, rarely, convulsions have been reported.

Increased SGOT, SGPT, LDH, and unbound serum bilirubin levels, possibly drug-related, sometimes develop.

Pain at the site of intramuscular injection also has been noted.

Although there is no conclusive evidence that the aminoglycosides are teratogenic, ototoxic, or nephrotoxic in the fetus, it must be assumed that these effects are possible. Aminoglycosides should be given to pregnant women only when life-threatening infections do not respond to other antibiotics.

Drug Interactions

Aminoglycosides and various penicillin derivatives chemically interact in a 1:1 molar ratio by forming a covalent bond between an amino group on the aminoglycoside and a carboxyl group from a broken beta-lactam ring. However, for this reaction to proceed efficiently, a high molar ratio of penicillin to aminoglycoside is required. Thus, only the aminoglycoside activity is measurably lost (see Lietman, 1984). Clinically, the antipseudomonal penicillins (carbenicillin, ticarcillin, mezlocillin, azlocillin, piperacillin), which usually are given in large doses, have been shown to inactivate aminoglycosides, particularly gentamicin and tobramycin, when mixed together in intravenous solutions prior to administration. This practice should be avoided. When these antibiotics are administered separately, loss of aminoglycoside activity in vivo is unlikely in patients with normal renal function. However, in vivo antagonism has been reported in patients with renal failure (see Mangini, 1984; Hansten, 1985 A); this may be clinically significant. Amikacin appears to be less susceptible than gentamicin or tobramycin to inactivation by antipseudomonal penicillins both in vitro (Holt et al, 1976; Pickering and Rutherford, 1981; Glew and Pavuk, 1983) and in patients with renal failure (Blair et al, 1982). Netilmicin also has been reported to be less susceptible to inactivation by antipseudomonal penicillins in vitro (Pickering and Rutherford, 1981). Current recommendations are that serum concentrations of any aminoglycoside should be monitored and dosage adjusted accordingly in patients with renal failure who receive these drugs in combination with antipseudomonal penicillins (Mangini, 1984; Hansten, 1985 A). Serum specimens containing aminoglycoside-penicillin combinations should be tested immediately or frozen before antibiotic assay (Pickering and Rutherford, 1981).

The ototoxicity produced by ethacrynic acid can be additive with aminoglycoside ototoxicity. The drugs should be used together with extreme caution (Hansten, 1985 A). Whether additive ototoxicity also occurs with the other loop diuretics (furosemide, bumetanide [Bumex]) presently is an unresolved issue. The combination of furosemide (or bumetanide) and an aminoglycoside has been shown to be more toxic to the cochlea than the aminoglycoside alone in animal studies. However, enhanced toxicity of these combinations in humans is not supported by existing data (see Guglielmo, 1984). In a retrospective analysis of three prospective, controlled, randomized, double-blind clinical trials evaluating nephrotoxicity and auditory toxicity of gentamicin, tobramycin, and amikacin, the concurrent administration of furosemide did not increase the incidence of aminoglycoside ototoxicity (or nephrotoxicity) (Smith and Lietman, 1983). Until more information is available, it is suggested that physicians closely follow aminoglycoside serum concentrations and monitor for signs of nephrotoxicity and ototoxicity in patients receiving furosemide (or bumetanide) concurrently with an aminoglycoside (Guglielmo, 1984). Also, it should be emphasized that appropriate monitoring of the patient's hydration status is particularly important when potent diuretics are administered with aminoglycosides. Excessive administration of any of these diuretics may potentiate both the nephrotoxicity and ototoxicity of the aminoglycosides by decreasing extracellular fluid volume and thus increasing serum levels of antibiotic (see Whelton, 1985; see also section on Adverse Reactions and Precautions).

Skeletal muscle relaxants (eg, succinylcholine [Anectine, Quelicin, Sucostrin], tubocurarine) produce neuromuscular blockade that can be potentiated by the aminoglycosides and cause respiratory paralysis. They should be given concomitantly only with extreme caution. Calcium or anticholinesterase agents may counteract the blockade (see Hansten, 1985 A; see also the section on Adverse Reactions and Precautions).

Additive or synergistic nephrotoxicity has been observed when aminoglycosides are administered concurrently with certain other nephrotoxic agents. This has been documented for methoxyflurane [Penthrane] and aminoglycosides should not be given to patients who recently received this anesthetic unless absolutely necessary (Hansten, 1985 A). Administration of aminoglycosides with amphotericin B [Fungizone] (Churchill and Seely, 1977), vancomycin (Farber and Moellering, 1983; Odio et al, 1984), cisplatin [Platinol] (Dentino et al, 1978), cyclosporine [Sandimmune] (Hansten, 1984), or intravenous indomethacin [Indocin IV] (given for closure of patent ductus arteriosus in neonates) (Zarfin et al, 1985) also can result in increased nephrotoxicity. When administration of one of these combination regimens is necessary, close monitoring of renal function is essential.

An increase in nephrotoxicity has been observed in patients receiving an aminoglycoside plus cephalothin [Keflin] (Wade et al, 1978; for others, see Luft, 1982; Mangini, 1984, and Hansten, 1985 A). This appears to be most likely in patients with pre-existing renal disease. Except for cephaloridine (no longer on the market), there is no evidence that other cephalosporins also potentiate aminoglycoside nephrotoxicity (see Mangini, 1984). Current recommendations are to administer aminoglycoside-cephalosporin combinations with caution, particularly in patients with pre-existing renal disease (Hansten,

1985 A). Avoidance of cephalothin in these patients should be considered.

It has been suggested that the symptoms of aminoglycoside ototoxicity can be masked by dimenhydrinate [Dramamine]. Although clinical examples are lacking, the possibility should be anticipated (Hansten, 1985 A).

For information on incompatibility between parenteral aminoglycosides and other drugs or substances in intravenous solutions, see Trissel, 1983.

Orally administered neomycin or kanamycin may potentiate the action of coumarin anticoagulants by reducing bacterial vitamin K production in the large intestine and/or by decreasing vitamin K absorption. Dietary vitamin K deficiency is an additional predisposing factor. More careful monitoring of prothrombin time is recommended in patients receiving concomitant oral neomycin (or kanamycin) and coumarin anticoagulants (Hansten, 1985 B). Oral neomycin also appears to inhibit the gastrointestinal absorption of digoxin. Serum digoxin levels should be monitored when concomitant oral neomycin administration is necessary (Hansten, 1985 A).

Pharmacokinetics

Absorption: The aminoglycosides are highly polar polycations at the pH of the small intestine and are poorly absorbed from the intact gastrointestinal tract. Following oral administration, serum concentrations are too low to be therapeutic for systemic infections. Nevertheless, ingestion of quantities sufficient to reduce bacterial flora in the bowel or to treat hepatic coma may produce detectable serum levels, especially in patients with renal failure. Aminoglycosides penetrate poorly through intact skin, but considerable absorption may occur following topical application to large denuded or burned areas. Variable amounts are absorbed during irrigation of closed body cavities or infected wounds.

Aminoglycosides must be given intramuscularly or intravenously for systemic infections. After intramuscular injection, almost 100% of the dose is absorbed, and peak serum concentrations usually are attained after approximately 60 minutes (range, 30 to 90 minutes). The concentrations are similar to those attained 30 minutes after completion of an intravenous infusion of an equal dose over a 30-minute period. Average peak serum concentrations for gentamicin (1.5 mg/kg), tobramycin (1.5 mg/kg), amikacin (7.5 mg/kg), netilmicin (2 mg/kg), and kanamycin (7.5 mg/kg) are 4 to 8, 4 to 8, 15 to 25, 7, and 20 to 25 mcg/ml, respectively. However, wide interpatient variations in peak serum concentrations have been reported after standard doses of aminoglycosides (Cipolle et al, 1980; Zaske, 1980; Zaske et al, 1980, 1981, 1982 B and C).

Distribution: The aminoglycosides are bound weakly to serum proteins; streptomycin is approximately 35% bound and the other aminoglycosides are less than 10% bound. The aminoglycosides distribute mainly to extracellular fluids; the volume of distribution using a two-compartment model is between 0.2 and 0.3 L/kg (Korzeniowski and Hook, 1979), although considerable interpatient variation has been reported (Cipolle et al, 1980; Zaske, 1980; Zaske et al, 1980, 1981,

1982 B and C). Various factors can affect the volume of distribution. For example, the presence of edema or ascites increases the volume of distribution and decreases serum levels. The reverse usually is true in obese patients. These drugs distribute poorly into adipose tissue and dosage adjustment may be required in obese individuals.

Aminoglycoside concentrations in body tissues and fluids are lower than corresponding serum levels except in the urine and kidney where these drugs become tightly bound to renal cortical tissue (see Neu, 1982 B; Ristuccia and Cunha, 1982; and Lietman, 1984). Penetration into cerebrospinal fluid is inadequate for antibacterial action in adults, even in the presence of inflammation; lumbar intrathecal or intraventricular injection is necessary. However, therapeutic levels may be achieved in cerebrospinal fluid of neonates with meningitis after intravenous administration (see McCracken, 1981). Antibacterial levels cannot be attained in the vitreous humor of the eye and are not attained consistently in the aqueous humor. Direct instillation by intravitreal or subconjunctival injection, respectively, is necessary to treat infections in these spaces. Biliary concentrations usually are variable and lower than serum levels. Concentrations approximating 25% to 50% of serum levels are achieved in bronchial, pleural, pericardial, peritoneal, and synovial fluids. These drugs readily enter the perilymph of the inner ear and concentrations found in this space correlate with ototoxicity. The aminoglycosides also cross the placenta (Weinstein et al, 1976), and effects upon the fetus or newborn infant must be considered if an aminoglycoside is administered during pregnancy. They should be given to pregnant women only when life-threatening infections do not respond to other antibiotics.

Excretion: The aminoglycosides are eliminated almost entirely unchanged by glomerular filtration. Although some proximal tubular reabsorption may occur (see section on Adverse Reactions and Precautions), these drugs are not metabolized. More than 90% of a dose is recovered in urine as unchanged drug within 24 hours.

In adults and infants more than 6 months old with normal renal function, the elimination (beta) half-life of the aminoglycosides is two to three hours, although considerable interpatient variation has been reported (Cipolle et al, 1980; Zaske, 1980; Zaske et al, 1980, 1981, 1982 B and C). In infants less than 1 week old, particularly those born prematurely or of low birth weight (less than 2 kg), the half-life may be 8 to 11 hours. The half-life in neonates with a birth weight exceeding 2 kg is approximately five hours. The half-life usually is decreased in febrile patients. Since aminoglycosides are excreted by the kidney, a very sharp increase in elimination half-life is observed with decreases in renal function (eg, up to thirty to fortyfold in uremic patients). Dosage adjustment is necessary in such patients to avoid the serious toxicities of the aminoglycosides (see the sections on Adverse Reactions and Precautions and Dosage Determinations). The aminoglycosides can be removed by hemodialysis and peritoneal dialysis.

During administration of the first three to five doses of an aminoglycoside, plasma clearance exceeds renal excretion by 10% to 20%. Thereafter, an equilibrium is maintained. The initial lag phase represents saturation of binding sites in tissues (eg, concentration in renal cortex). The half-life of tissue-bound aminoglycoside is long (eg, 30 to 700 hours) and these drugs can be recovered in the urine for 20 days or longer after discontinuation of therapy.

Dosage Determinations

The following factors apply to parenterally administered aminoglycosides:

(1) The aminoglycosides have a narrow therapeutic:toxic ratio, ie, there is a narrow range between serum concentrations that are therapeutically effective and those that are toxic.

(2) A number of studies have shown that adequate peak serum aminoglycoside concentrations are associated with desired therapeutic response (Noone et al, 1974; Zaske et al, 1982 A; Moore et al, 1984 C and D; see also Burton et al, 1985) and that subinhibitory serum aminoglycoside concentrations can result in treatment failures (Jackson and Riff, 1971; Anderson et al, 1976; see also Burton et al, 1985). For example, mortality from gram-negative bacteremia was significantly less in patients who had peak serum gentamicin, tobramycin, or amikacin concentrations greater than 5, 5, or 20 mcg/ml, respectively (Moore et al, 1984 C). Similarly, successful outcome in gram-negative pneumonia was significantly greater in patients who had peak serum gentamicin, tobramycin, or amikacin concentrations equal to or greater than 7, 7, or 28 mcg/ml, respectively (Moore et al, 1984 D). The higher serum concentrations required for pneumonia probably reflect poor penetration of aminoglycosides into bronchial secretions and other local factors (eg, decreased pH of sputum, presence of pus).

(3) A correlation between excessive serum aminoglycoside concentrations, particularly when they are maintained throughout the course of therapy, and the toxicity (ototoxicity, nephrotoxicity) caused by these agents also is accepted by most infectious disease experts (for reviews, see Zaske, 1980; Wenk et al, 1984; Burton et al, 1985). For gentamicin, tobramycin, amikacin, kanamycin, and netilmicin, peak concentrations greater than 12, 12, 35, 35, or 16 mcg/ml, respectively, and trough concentrations greater than 2, 2, 10, 10, or 4 mcg/ml, respectively, are associated with an increased probability of ototoxicity and nephrotoxicity.

(4) In contrast to the good correlation between serum aminoglycoside concentrations and efficacy (or toxicity), the relationship between standard doses of aminoglycosides and the serum drug concentrations that are attained is generally poor. Wide variations in aminoglycoside pharmacokinetics, particularly in volumes of distribution and elimination rates, exist among patients. This is true not only for patients with known risk factors (eg, renal failure, dehydration), but also for individuals with normal renal function (Cipolle et al, 1980; Mangione and Schentag, 1980; Zaske, 1980; Zaske et al, 1980, 1981, 1982 B and C; Ackerman et al, 1984; for others, see Burton et al, 1985). Thus, standard aminoglycoside dosage regimens may have substantial error for individual patients.

Because of the above, serum concentrations of aminoglycosides should be monitored when feasible to assure adequate therapeutic levels and to avoid potentially toxic concentrations.

This is particularly important in seriously ill or poorly responding patients and for those individuals who are likely to require dosage adjustments. This includes (1) patients with pre-existing renal disease; (2) patients with rapidly changing renal function or fluid status; (3) elderly patients; (4) obese patients; (5) patients with sepsis; (6) febrile patients who may have supranormal renal clearance; (7) patients with altered or changing volumes of distribution due to diseases such as cirrhosis (ascites) or heart failure (edema); (8) burn patients; (9) cystic fibrosis patients; (10) patients receiving other drugs that can affect aminoglycoside serum concentrations (eg, antipseudomonal penicillins that can inactivate aminoglycosides in vivo in patients with renal dysfunction; potent diuretics); (11) azotemic patients on dialysis (aminoglycosides are dialyzable molecules); and (12) neonates.

Guidelines for peak and trough serum aminoglycoside concentrations have been established to help the clinician obtain a favorable therapeutic outcome with a minimum risk of toxicity. The desired peak concentrations are 6 to 10 mcg/ml for gentamicin, tobramycin, and netilmicin and 20 to 30 mcg/ml for amikacin. The desired trough concentrations are 1 to 2 mcg/ml for gentamicin, tobramycin, and netilmicin and 4 to 8 mcg/ml for amikacin. Within these guidelines, higher trough and peak concentrations should be selected for patients with more severe infections (eg, gram-negative pneumonia) or infections with less susceptible isolates (Ackerman et al, 1984). Peak concentrations should be obtained approximately 30 minutes after completion of a 30- to 60-minute intravenous infusion or one hour after an intramuscular injection. Trough concentrations should be obtained within 15 minutes of the next dose under steady-state conditions (see Haas and Collins, 1982, and Ristuccia and Cunha, 1982). Serum concentration data can be used optimally when the exact times for beginning and ending an intravenous infusion (or the time of an intramuscular injection) and the exact times for obtaining serum samples have been noted. A number of fast and reliable assay methods for aminoglycosides currently are available (see Wenk et al, 1984).

Individualization of aminoglycoside dosage regimens with serum concentrations can be accomplished either by utilizing pharmacokinetic principles (Sawchuk and Zaske, 1976; Sawchuk et al, 1977) or by the trial and error method. When available, pharmacokinetic based dosing appears to be superior. In this method, three timed serum concentrations are obtained over two to three half-lives, preferably during the first dosing interval. The serum concentration-time data are then used to determine drug pharmacokinetic parameters, ie, volume of distribution and elimination rate constant, for the individual patient. After the physician has determined the desired peak and trough concentrations, the pharmacokinetic parameters are used to calculate the patient's dose and dosage interval. Equations and programs for computers and programmable calculators are available to "fit" the serum concentration-time data, calculate pharmacokinetic parameters, and determine the patient's dosage regimen. As deemed appropriate, serum concentrations should be monitored periodically throughout the course of therapy and necessary dosage adjustments made to control serum concentrations.

The Sawchuk-Zaske individualized pharmacokinetic dosing

method has been evaluated extensively with gentamicin (Zaske et al, 1982 B) in burn (Zaske et al, 1982 A), surgical (Zaske et al, 1980), gynecologic (Zaske et al, 1981), and elderly (Zaske et al, 1982 C) patients. It also has been tested in a limited number of patients given tobramycin (Cipolle et al, 1980) or amikacin (Zaske, 1980). In all of these studies, wide interpatient variation in pharmacokinetic parameters was observed and dosage requirements both below and above "standard" regimens were necessary to achieve desired peak and trough serum concentrations. Measured peak and trough serum concentrations obtained with this pharmacokinetic dosing method were in close agreement with predicted values. Furthermore, the incidence of nephrotoxicity was less than 2% and ototoxicity was not observed clinically. In burn patients, survival was significantly increased in patients receiving individualized dosages of gentamicin when compared to those given standard dosage regimens (Zaske et al, 1982 A), and pharmacokinetic based dosing was determined to be cost-effective in these patients (Bootman et al, 1979).

When pharmacokinetic based dosing is not available, individualization of aminoglycoside dosage regimens with serum concentrations can be done by the trial-and-error method. Peaks and troughs can be measured in a patient and doses and dosage intervals can then be adjusted using empirical judgments in order to achieve acceptable peak and trough serum concentrations. For example, once the initial dosage regimen has been selected, peak and trough serum concentrations should be determined after the steady state level has been achieved (four to five drug half-lives). In critically ill patients, a peak concentration also should be determined after the loading dose to ensure that it is within the desired therapeutic range. A trough concentration usually is obtained around the fifth to seventh day and intermittently thereafter as an indication of drug accumulation (NOTE: Some experts recommend monitoring both peak and trough concentrations beginning on the second or third day). Patients who are likely to need dosage adjustments during therapy (eg, due to changes in volume of distribution or renal function) will require more intensive monitoring (see Haas and Collins, 1982).

The trial-and-error method is useful when the patient is at steady state and the clinician is skilled in using the data. Otherwise, many dosage errors can occur because important data, such as the dose, time of infusion, and time of sample collection, frequently are obtained in an uncontrolled manner. Also, the trial-and-error method usually requires more time than the pharmacokinetic based dosing method for optimal adjustment of dosage (Zaske, 1980; Ackerman et al, 1984).

A number of nomograms also are available to help determine the appropriate dosage of aminoglycosides both in patients with normal renal function and in those with various degrees of renal impairment. Unfortunately, these predictive algorithms generally are based on the invalid assumptions of a constant volume of distribution for all patients and that creatinine clearance (or serum creatinine) has a high degree of correlation with aminoglycoside clearance (Zaske, 1980). Thus, there can be substantial variation in serum concentrations achieved with the use of these nomograms when compared to predicted values (Lesar et al, 1982; for others, see Burton et al, 1985). Nomograms do provide acceptable initial

dosage guidelines, however, and are valuable in initiating treatment, but further dosage adjustment should depend on measured peak and trough serum concentrations (Zaske, 1980; Ackerman et al, 1984).

When serum aminoglycoside concentrations cannot be measured, however, dosage guidelines based on predictive nomograms can be used. The method of Sarubbi and Hull (1978), which is applicable to gentamicin, tobramycin, amikacin, kanamycin, and netilmicin, generally is preferred. This method utilizes estimates of renal function, lean body weight, age, and sex to predict required dosage regimens. The method allows the physician to select a different dose or dosing interval for varying degrees of renal function and severity of infection. The procedure is as follows:

An appropriate loading dose, expressed in mg/kg of ideal body weight, is selected from the dosing chart (Table 2) to attain a peak serum concentration (mcg/ml) in the expected range. The aminoglycoside antibiotics are poorly distributed in adipose tissue. Therefore, the loading dose is calculated using the lean (or ideal) body weight of the patient in order to avoid abnormally elevated serum concentrations in obese patients. Ideal (nonobese) body weight is calculated as follows:

Male Ideal Weight = 50 kg + 2.3 kg for every inch over 5 feet

Female Ideal Weight = 45.5 kg + 2.3 kg for every inch over 5 feet

Maintenance dosage is based on the weight-corrected creatinine clearance [C(c)cr] of the patient. This value can be calculated for males and females as follows:

$$C(c)cr \ male = \frac{140 - age}{serum \ creatinine}$$

$$C(c)cr \ female = 0.85 \times C(c)cr \ male$$

The maintenance dose is then calculated as a percentage of the loading dose according to the corrected clearance determination and can be administered every 8, 12, or 24 hours as shown on the dosage chart (Table 2). The interval between doses should be extended to 12 or 24 hours as C(c)cr declines (eg, less than 50% to 60% of the loading dose) in order to avoid drug accumulation and unnecessarily elevated trough serum concentrations.

Drug Evaluations

GENTAMICIN SULFATE
[Garamycin]

Gentamicin is a mixture of three closely related antibacterial substances (gentamicins C_1, C_2, and C_{1A}) obtained from cultures of *Micromonospora purpurea*.

MECHANISM OF ACTION, ANTIMICROBIAL SPECTRUM, AND RESISTANCE. Gentamicin primarily is active against aerobic gram-negative bacilli, including the Enterobacteria-

TABLE 2.
AMINOGLYCOSIDE DOSING CHART

1. Select Loading Dose in mg/kg (IDEAL WEIGHT) to provide peak serum concentrations in range listed below for desired aminoglycoside.

Aminoglycoside	Usual Loading Dose	Expected Peak Serum Concentrations
Tobramycin Gentamicin	1.5 to 2 mg/kg	4 to 10 mcg/ml
Amikacin Kanamycin	5 to 7.5 mg/kg	15 to 30 mcg/ml
Netilmicin	1.3 to 3.25 mg/kg*	4 to 12 mcg/ml*

2. Select Maintenance Dose (as percentage of chosen loading dose) to continue peak serum concentrations indicated above according to desired dosing interval and the patient's corrected creatinine clearance.

Percentage of Loading Dose Required for Dosage Interval Selected

C(c)cr (ml/min)	Half-life** (hours)	8 hours	12 hours	24 hours
90	3.1	84%	—	—
80	3.4	80	91%	—
70	3.9	76	88	—
60	4.5	71	84	—
50	5.3	65	79	—
40	6.5	57	72	92%
30	8.4	48	63	86
25	9.9	43	57	81
20	11.9	37	50	75
17	13.6	33	46	70
15	15.1	31	42	67
12	17.9	27	37	61
10***	20.4	24	34	56
7	25.9	19	28	47
5	31.5	16	23	41
2	46.8	11	16	30
0	69.3	8	11	21

*Values for netilmicin were taken from the manufacturer's literature.

**Alternatively, one-half of the chosen loading dose may be given at an interval approximately equal to the estimated half-life.

***Dosing for patients with C(c)cr <10 ml/min should be assisted by measured serum levels.

From Sarubbi FA Jr, Hull JH. Amikacin serum concentrations: Prediction of levels and dosage guidelines. Ann Intern Med 89:612-618, 1978.

ceae (eg, *Escherichia coli*) and *Pseudomonas aeruginosa*. It also is active against *Staphylococcus aureus*.

In vitro, the potency of gentamicin is similar to that of tobramycin for most bacterial species; it is somewhat more potent on a weight basis than amikacin and kanamycin. Gentamicin generally is more active in vitro than tobramycin against *Serratia*, but is less active against *P. aeruginosa*.

Gentamicin-resistant strains of Enterobacteriaceae and *P.*

aeruginosa are prevalent in some hospitals; cross-resistance with tobramycin is common. Many of these strains are susceptible to amikacin, which is resistant to most aminoglycoside-inactivating enzymes.

For a detailed discussion on the mechanism of action, antimicrobial spectrum, and resistance properties of the aminoglycosides, see the Introduction.

USES. Gentamicin is administered parenterally and is used to treat serious infections caused by aerobic gram-negative bacilli (eg, a number of the Enterobacteriaceae, *P. aeruginosa*). These include lower respiratory tract, intra-abdominal, soft tissue, bone or joint, wound, and complicated urinary tract infections; bacteremias; and meningitis.

Gentamicin often is the preferred aminoglycoside for general use in hospitals where bacterial resistance to this agent is not a problem (based on locally generated antimicrobial susceptibility profiles). Its major advantage over tobramycin, amikacin, and netilmicin is lower cost (due to the expiration of its patent). The empiric use of gentamicin (or tobramycin) is not justified in hospitals where gentamicin resistance is common, and amikacin is the aminoglycoside of choice. For a detailed discussion of aminoglycoside drug selection for aerobic gram-negative bacillary infections, see the Introduction.

The combination of gentamicin plus penicillin G (or ampicillin) exhibits synergistic activity against enterococci (eg, *Streptococcus faecalis*) and this frequently is the regimen of choice for the treatment of enterococcal endocarditis. Streptomycin often is preferred to gentamicin for streptomycin-susceptible strains of enterococci (see Chapter 65, Antimicrobial Therapy and Chemoprophylaxis of Infectious Diseases, Table 1; see also the evaluation on Streptomycin Sulfate).

Gentamicin is now the preferred aminoglycoside for the prophylaxis of endocarditis. It is administered with ampicillin as the standard parenteral regimen for high-risk patients (eg, those with prosthetic heart valves, most forms of congenital heart disease, rheumatic or other acquired valvular heart disease, hypertrophic cardiomyopathy [IHSS], mitral valve prolapse with insufficiency) prior to genitourinary or gastrointestinal tract surgery and instrumentation. This parenteral combination regimen also is indicated for patients in whom maximal protection is desired (eg, for patients with prosthetic heart valves) prior to dental procedures and upper respiratory tract surgical procedures (Shulman et al, 1984; see also Chapter 65, Table 3).

For other uses of gentamicin, either alone or in combination, see the Introduction.

ADVERSE REACTIONS AND PRECAUTIONS. Gentamicin has the potential to produce irreversible ototoxicity; both the hearing (cochlear) and equilibrium (vestibular) functions may be affected. Nephrotoxicity that usually is mild and reversible and, rarely, neuromuscular blockade are other potentially serious adverse reactions of gentamicin. For a detailed discussion, see the Introduction. This drug is classified in FDA Pregnancy Category C.

DRUG INTERACTIONS. Gentamicin appears to be more readily inactivated by antipseudomonal penicillins (eg, carbenicillin, ticarcillin) than amikacin both in vitro (Holt et al, 1976; Glew and Pavuk, 1983) and in vivo in patients with renal failure

(Blair et al, 1982). For a detailed discussion of this and other drug interactions, see the Introduction.

PHARMACOKINETICS. The pharmacokinetics of the parenterally administered aminoglycosides are similar, including an extracellular volume of distribution, poor penetration into cerebrospinal fluid, and elimination as unchanged drug by glomerular filtration. However, wide interpatient variation in aminoglycoside pharmacokinetics has been reported (see the Introduction).

DOSAGE AND PREPARATIONS. The following are standard dosages for gentamicin. However, monitoring of aminoglycoside serum concentrations and individualization of dosage regimens, preferably based on pharmacokinetic principles (Sawchuk-Zaske method), is recommended, particularly for seriously ill or poorly responding patients and for other high-risk individuals in whom dosage adjustments are likely to be necessary (eg, the elderly, neonates, patients with impaired renal function or changing volumes of distribution). Predictive nomograms (eg, Sarubbi-Hull) may provide acceptable dosage guidelines for initiation of treatment. For detailed discussion, see the Introduction.

For gentamicin, prolonged peak serum concentrations exceeding 12 mcg/ml and rising trough serum levels greater than 2 mcg/ml should be avoided (see the Introduction).

Intramuscular, Intravenous: When given intravenously, gentamicin can be diluted in 5% dextrose or isotonic sodium chloride injection and administered over approximately 30 minutes. The total duration of therapy by either route generally should not exceed ten days.

Patients with normal renal function: Adults, 3 to 5 mg/kg daily in three equally divided doses every eight hours. The larger dose is used only for life-threatening infections. *Children,* 6 to 7.5 mg/kg daily in three equally divided doses every eight hours. *Infants 1 week or older,* 7.5 mg/kg daily in three equally divided doses every eight hours. *Premature or full-term neonates less than 1 week,* 5 mg/kg daily in two divided doses every 12 hours.

For dosages for the treatment and prophylaxis of infective endocarditis, see Chapter 65, Antimicrobial Therapy and Chemoprophylaxis of Infectious Diseases, Tables 1 and 3, respectively.

Patients with impaired renal function: Dosage modification is indicated. Whenever possible, gentamicin serum concentrations should be monitored to help determine dosage (see above and the Introduction). If these measurements are unavailable or unreliable, gentamicin may be given to *adults* according to the dosing chart proposed by Sarubbi and Hull (see the Introduction).

Patients undergoing hemodialysis: Adults, for most infections, 1 to 1.7 mg/kg (depending upon the severity of infection) at the end of each six-hour dialysis period. *Children,* 2 mg/kg at the end of each six-hour dialysis period. Gentamicin serum levels must be measured in patients undergoing dialysis.

Garamycin (Schering), **Generic.** Solution (sterile) 10 mg/ml (pediatric) in 2 ml containers and 40 mg/ml in 2 and 20 ml containers (strengths expressed in terms of the base).

Additional Trademark.
Jenamicin (Hauck).

Intrathecal: Direct administration of "preservative-free" gentamicin preparation into the cerebrospinal fluid is intended as adjunctive therapy in patients with central nervous system infections. Although dosage depends upon factors such as age and weight of the patient, site of injection, degree of obstruction to cerebrospinal fluid flow, the amount of cerebrospinal fluid estimated to be present, and concomitant treatment with intramuscular or intravenous gentamicin, generally recommended dosages are, *adults,* 4 to 8 mg once daily; *children and infants 3 months and older,* 1 to 2 mg once daily.

Garamycin Intrathecal (Schering). Solution (sterile, preservative-free) 2 mg/ml in 2 ml containers.

TOBRAMYCIN SULFATE
[Nebcin]

This water-soluble aminoglycoside is derived from *Streptomyces tenebrarius*.

MECHANISM OF ACTION, ANTIMICROBIAL SPECTRUM, AND RESISTANCE. Tobramycin primarily is active against aerobic gram-negative bacilli, including the Enterobacteriaceae (eg, *Escherichia coli*) and *Pseudomonas aeruginosa*. On a weight basis, it is two to five times more active in vitro than gentamicin against *P. aeruginosa*. Strains of *P. aeruginosa* that are moderately resistant to gentamicin are usually sensitive to tobramycin. When there is a high degree of resistance to gentamicin, however, the organisms also will be resistant to tobramycin. This drug is usually less active in vitro than gentamicin against *Serratia marcescens*.

Cross-resistance between tobramycin and gentamicin is common and resistant strains of aerobic gram-negative bacilli are prevalent in some hospitals. Many of these strains are susceptible to amikacin, which is resistant to most aminoglycoside-inactivating enzymes.

Most gram-positive organisms except *Staphylococcus aureus* are resistant to tobramycin. In contrast to gentamicin, this drug has poor activity in combination with penicillin G (or ampicillin) against some enterococci (essentially all strains of *Streptococcus faecium* are highly resistant).

For a detailed discussion on the mechanism of action, antimicrobial spectrum, and resistance properties of the aminoglycosides, see the Introduction.

USES. Tobramycin is administered parenterally to treat serious infections caused by aerobic gram-negative bacilli (eg, a number of the Enterobacteriaceae, *P. aeruginosa*). These include lower respiratory tract, intra-abdominal, soft tissue, bone or joint, wound, and complicated urinary tract infections; bacteremias; and meningitis.

Tobramycin frequently is the aminoglycoside of choice for infections caused by *P. aeruginosa* because of its greater in vitro activity against this organism. However, superior clinical efficacy is unproven. It usually is given in combination with an antipseudomonal penicillin for severe, systemic *P. aeruginosa* infections (see the Introduction).

Some infectious disease experts have preferred the more costly tobramycin to gentamicin as the aminoglycoside for general use in hospitals where resistance is not a problem because it appears to be less nephrotoxic. However, this does not appear to be warranted when all of the available data are evaluated. For a detailed discussion of aminoglycoside drug selection, see the Introduction.

Amikacin is the aminoglycoside of choice in hospitals where gentamicin and tobramycin resistance is a problem (see the Introduction).

ADVERSE REACTIONS AND PRECAUTIONS. Tobramycin has the potential to produce irreversible ototoxicity; both hearing (cochlear) and equilibrium (vestibular) functions may be affected. Nephrotoxicity that usually is mild and reversible and, rarely, neuromuscular blockade are other potentially serious adverse reactions of tobramycin. For a detailed discussion, see the Introduction. This drug is classified in FDA Pregnancy Category D.

DRUG INTERACTIONS. Tobramycin appears to be more readily inactivated by antipseudomonal penicillins (eg, carbenicillin, ticarcillin) than amikacin based on in vitro studies (Holt et al, 1976; Glew and Pavuk, 1983). For a detailed discussion of this and other drug interactions, see the Introduction.

PHARMACOKINETICS. The pharmacokinetics of the parenterally administered aminoglycosides are similar, including an extracellular volume of distribution, poor penetration into cerebrospinal fluid, and elimination as unchanged drug by glomerular filtration. However, wide interpatient variation in aminoglycoside pharmacokinetics has been reported (see the Introduction).

DOSAGE AND PREPARATIONS. The following are standard dosages for tobramycin. However, monitoring of aminoglycoside serum concentrations and individualization of dosage regimens, preferably based on pharmacokinetic principles (Sawchuk-Zaske method), is recommended, particularly for seriously ill or poorly responding patients and for other high-risk individuals in whom dosage adjustments are likely to be necessary (eg, the elderly, neonates, patients with impaired renal function or changing volumes of distribution). Predictive nomograms (eg, Sarubbi-Hull) may provide acceptable dosage guidelines for initiation of treatment. For detailed discussion, see the Introduction.

For tobramycin, prolonged peak serum concentrations exceeding 12 mcg/ml and rising trough serum levels greater than 2 mcg/ml should be avoided (see the Introduction).

Intramuscular, Intravenous: When given intravenously, tobramycin can be diluted in 5% dextrose or isotonic sodium chloride injection and administered over approximately 30 minutes. The total duration of therapy by either route generally should not exceed ten days.

Patients with normal renal function: Adults, 3 to 5 mg/kg daily in three equally divided doses every eight hours. The larger dose is used only for life-threatening infections. *Children*, 6 to 7.5 mg/kg daily in three equally divided doses every eight hours. *Premature or full-term neonates 1 week of age or less*, up to 4 mg/kg daily in two divided doses every 12 hours.

Patients with impaired renal function: Dosage modification is indicated. Whenever possible, tobramycin serum concentrations should be monitored to help determine dosage (see above and the Introduction). If these measurements are unavailable or unreliable, tobramycin may be given to *adults* according to the dosing chart proposed by Sarubbi and Hull (see the Introduction).

Nebcin (Lilly). Solution (sterile) 10 mg/ml (pediatric) in 2 ml containers and 40 mg/ml in 1.5 and 2 ml containers; powder 1.2 g (strengths expressed in terms of the base).

AMIKACIN SULFATE
[Amikin]

Amikacin, the first semisynthetic aminoglycoside to be marketed, is a water-soluble acylated derivative of kanamycin A. This chemical modification protects susceptible hydroxyl and amino groups from aminoglycoside-inactivating enzymes, thus making amikacin resistant to most of the enzymes that inactivate kanamycin, gentamicin, tobramycin, and netilmicin.

MECHANISM OF ACTION, ANTIMICROBIAL SPECTRUM, AND RESISTANCE. Amikacin primarily is active against aerobic gram-negative bacilli, including the Enterobacteriaceae (eg, *Escherichia coli*) and *Pseudomonas aeruginosa*. It also is active against *Staphylococcus aureus*, *Mycobacterium tuberculosis*, and certain atypical mycobacteria (eg, *M. fortuitum*).

In vitro, amikacin is somewhat less potent on a weight basis than either gentamicin or tobramycin. However, this is not clinically significant because amikacin also is less toxic on a weight basis and larger doses can be administered.

Amikacin is susceptible to only two of the known aminoglycoside-inactivating enzymes, the acetyltransferase, AAC 6′, and the adenylylating enzyme, ANT 4′ (see Table 1 in the Introduction). Therefore, it is active against many gentamicin- and tobramycin-resistant strains of aerobic gram-negative bacilli. Bacterial strains that are resistant to amikacin usually have a defective aminoglycoside transport mechanism. These mutants exhibit cross-resistance to all other aminoglycosides.

For a detailed discussion on the mechanism of action, antimicrobial spectrum, and resistance properties of the aminoglycosides, see the Introduction.

USES. Amikacin is used parenterally to treat serious infections caused by susceptible aerobic gram-negative bacilli (eg, a number of the Enterobacteriaceae, *P. aeruginosa*). Such infections include bacteremias and intra-abdominal, soft tissue (including burns), bone or joint, lower respiratory tract, and complicated urinary tract infections.

The major advantage of amikacin is its superior resistance profile (see previous section and the Introduction). Thus, amikacin is the aminoglycoside of choice for infections caused by aerobic gram-negative bacilli that are known or suspected to be resistant to other aminoglycosides. It should be the aminoglycoside for general use in hospitals where resistance to gentamicin and tobramycin is known to be high. Furthermore, even in hospitals without a major resistance problem, when there is concern about gentamicin- and tobramycin-resistant gram-negative bacilli in a particular clinical situation (eg, severe nosocomial infection in a patient who is immunosuppressed, on prior antibiotics, or in the intensive care or burn unit), amikacin frequently is recommended for initial therapy before the results of susceptibility tests are known.

Since amikacin is the only currently available aminoglycoside effective against many gentamicin- and tobramycin-resistant organisms, many infectious disease experts have felt that its use should be restricted to minimize the emergence of additional resistant strains. However, there is no evidence that such restriction has delayed the emergence of resistance to amikacin (Levin, 1981; Reese and Betts, 1983; Davies, 1983; Lietman, 1984). Furthermore, encouraging reports from hospitals that rely on amikacin as the primary aminoglycoside suggest that resistance to amikacin does not increase despite more widespread use (see Levin, 1981; Price et al, 1981; Moody et al, 1982; Betts et al, 1984; Gerding and Larson, 1985). Nevertheless, general use of amikacin in hospitals without a gentamicin (or tobramycin) resistance problem remains a controversial issue. Amikacin is considerably more expensive than gentamicin, an important consideration in a cost-conscious environment. For a detailed discussion of aminoglycoside drug selection, see the Introduction.

ADVERSE REACTIONS AND PRECAUTIONS. Amikacin has the potential to produce irreversible ototoxicity; both the hearing (cochlear) and equilibrium (vestibular) functions may be affected. Nephrotoxicity that usually is mild and reversible and, rarely, neuromuscular blockade are other potentially serious adverse reactions of amikacin. Based on the available comparative studies, toxicity caused by amikacin in humans does not appear to be significantly different in incidence or severity from that caused by gentamicin or tobramycin. For a detailed discussion, see the Introduction.

DRUG INTERACTIONS. When compared to gentamicin and tobramycin, amikacin is less susceptible to inactivation by antipseudomonal penicillins (eg, carbenicillin, ticarcillin) both in vitro (Holt et al, 1976; Glew and Pavuk, 1983) and in vivo in patients with renal failure (Blair et al, 1982). Amikacin may have clinical advantages in patients with renal failure who require concurrent therapy with an antipseudomonal penicillin. For a detailed discussion of this and other drug interactions, see the Introduction.

PHARMACOKINETICS. The pharmacokinetics of the parenterally administered aminoglycosides are similar, including an extracellular volume of distribution, poor penetration into cerebrospinal fluid, and elimination as unchanged drug by glomerular filtration (see the Introduction).

Although it has been suggested that amikacin pharmacokinetics are more predictable than those of gentamicin and tobramycin (see Levin, 1981; Ristuccia and Cunha, 1982, 1985; Holm et al, 1983; see also the Introduction), wide interpatient variation in amikacin pharmacokinetics has been reported (see Mangione and Schentag, 1980; Zaske, 1980; Finley et al, 1982; Bauer and Blouin, 1983). Thus, as with other aminoglycosides, monitoring of serum concentrations with individualization of dosage, preferably based on pharmacokinetic principles (Sawchuk-Zaske method), is recommended for amikacin (see section below and the Introduction). Theoretically, amikacin may achieve a higher therapeutic ratio against those bacterial strains with minimum inhibitory concentrations (MICs) that are similar for gentamicin, tobramycin, and amikacin because higher serum concentrations of amikacin can be achieved (Dyas et al, 1983).

DOSAGE AND PREPARATIONS. The following are standard dosages for amikacin. However, monitoring of aminoglycoside serum concentrations and individualization of dosage regimens, preferably based on pharmacokinetic principles (Sawchuk-Zaske method), is recommended, particularly for seriously ill or poorly responding patients and for other high-risk individuals in whom dosage adjustments are likely to be necessary (eg, the elderly, neonates, patients with impaired renal function or changing volumes of distribution). Predictive nomograms (eg, Sarubbi-Hull) may provide acceptable dosage guidelines for initiation of treatment. For detailed discussion, see the Introduction.

For amikacin, prolonged peak serum concentrations exceeding 35 mcg/ml and rising trough serum levels greater than 10 mcg/ml should be avoided (Meyer, 1981; see also the Introduction).

Intramuscular, Intravenous: When given intravenously, amikacin can be diluted in 5% dextrose or isotonic sodium chloride injection and should be infused over a 30- to 60-minute period in adults and a one- to two-hour period in infants.

Uncomplicated infections caused by susceptible organisms usually respond in 24 to 48 hours. If a response is not observed in three to five days, bacterial sensitivity should be redetermined and therapy re-evaluated. For both adults and children, except in unusual circumstances, the duration of therapy should not exceed ten days.

Patients with normal renal function: Adults, children, and older infants, 15 mg/kg daily in equally divided doses at 8- or 12-hour intervals. The total daily dose for adults in the heavier weight classes should not exceed 1.5 g. When indicated for uncomplicated urinary tract infections in adults, 250 mg twice daily is frequently sufficient. *Neonates* should be given a loading dose of 10 mg/kg, followed by 7.5 mg/kg every 12 hours.

Patients with impaired renal function: Dosage modification is indicated. Whenever possible, amikacin serum concentrations should be monitored to help determine dosage (see above and the Introduction). If these measurements are unavailable or unreliable, amikacin may be given to *adults* according to the dosing chart proposed by Sarubbi and Hull (see the Introduction).

Amikin (Bristol). Solution (sterile) 50 mg/ml in 2 ml containers and 250 mg/ml in 2 and 4 ml containers.

NETILMICIN
[Netromycin]

Netilmicin, a semisynthetic aminoglycoside, is the 1-N-ethyl derivative of sisomicin.

MECHANISM OF ACTION, ANTIMICROBIAL SPECTRUM, AND RESISTANCE. Netilmicin primarily is active against aerobic gram-negative bacilli, including the Enterobacteriaceae (eg, *Escherichia coli*) and *Pseudomonas aeruginosa*. It also is active against *Staphylococcus aureus*. In general, the in vitro potency of netilmicin is similar to that of gentamicin and tobramycin. However, netilmicin is less active against *Pseudomonas aeruginosa* than these aminoglycosides. The clinical significance of this difference is unknown (*Med Lett Drugs Ther*, 1983; Craig et al, 1983; Guay, 1983).

Netilmicin is susceptible to fewer aminoglycoside-inactivating enzymes than gentamicin and tobramycin (see Table 1 in the Introduction), and some gram-negative bacilli that are resistant to these latter agents will be susceptible to netilmicin. However, most of these strains are sensitive to amikacin as well, and amikacin also is active against most netilmicin-resistant strains of these bacteria. Thus, netilmicin does not appear to offer any advantages in spectrum of activity over amikacin for the treatment of gentamicin- or tobramycin-resistant organisms (*Med Lett Drugs Ther*, 1983; Craig et al, 1983; Guay, 1983).

For a detailed discussion on the mechanism of action, antimicrobial spectrum, and resistance properties of the aminoglycosides, see the Introduction.

USES. Netilmicin is given parenterally to treat serious infections caused by aerobic gram-negative bacilli (eg, a number of Enterobacteriaceae, *P. aeruginosa*). These include bacteremias and lower respiratory tract, intra-abdominal, soft tissue, bone or joint, wound, and complicated urinary tract infections.

The clinical role of netilmicin, the most recently approved aminoglycoside, presently is unresolved. In clinical situations in which gentamicin- or tobramycin-resistant bacterial strains are unlikely, the therapeutic efficacy of netilmicin appears to be no greater than that of these older analogues. Gentamicin is considerably less expensive than netilmicin. When gentamicin (or tobramycin) resistance is a problem, the drug of choice for empiric therapy is amikacin because it is the least susceptible aminoglycoside to enzymatic inactivation. However, netilmicin is an effective alternative for susceptible bacterial isolates and presently is less expensive than amikacin (see the Introduction). It appears that the use of netilmicin will remain somewhat limited unless it can be shown in well-controlled clinical trials to be significantly less ototoxic (or nephrotoxic) in humans when compared to the other currently available aminoglycosides (*Med Lett Drugs Ther*, 1983; Craig et al, 1983; Guay, 1983; see also the following section and the Introduction).

ADVERSE REACTIONS AND PRECAUTIONS. Netilmicin has the potential to produce irreversible ototoxicity; both hearing (cochlear) and equilibrium (vestibular) functions may be affected. Nephrotoxicity that usually is mild and reversible and, rarely, neuromuscular blockade are other potentially serious adverse reactions of netilmicin.

In animal studies, netilmicin has been shown to be less ototoxic and nephrotoxic than gentamicin and tobramycin (Szot and Tabachnick, 1980). These differences generally have not been demonstrated unequivocally in humans (*Med Lett Drugs Ther*, 1983; Craig et al, 1983; Guay, 1983), although a retrospective review of aminoglycoside toxicity from clinical studies published between 1975 and 1982 suggests that netilmicin may be less ototoxic than the other aminoglycosides (Kahlmeter and Dahlager, 1984). In one multicenter, controlled clinical trial, the combination of netilmicin plus ticarcillin was reported to be significantly less ototoxic than tobramycin plus ticarcillin (Lerner et al, 1983). If further studies confirm that the incidence of ototoxicity is significantly lower with netilmicin, its role in therapy, particularly in patients at increased risk for ototoxicity, will be enhanced.

For a detailed discussion of aminoglycoside adverse reactions and precautions, see the Introduction. This drug is classified in FDA Pregnancy Category D.

DRUG INTERACTIONS. When compared to gentamicin and tobramycin, netilmicin was reported to be less susceptible to inactivation by antipseudomonal penicillins (eg, carbenicillin, ticarcillin) in vitro (Pickering and Rutherford, 1981). For a detailed discussion of this and other drug interactions, see the Introduction.

PHARMACOKINETICS. The pharmacokinetics of the parenterally administered aminoglycosides are similar, including an extracellular volume of distribution, poor penetration into cerebrospinal fluid, and elimination as unchanged drug by glomerular filtration. However, wide interpatient variations in aminoglycoside pharmacokinetics have been reported (see the Introduction).

DOSAGE AND PREPARATIONS. The following are standard dosages for netilmicin cited in the manufacturer's literature. However, monitoring of aminoglycoside serum concentrations and individualization of dosage regimens, preferably based on pharmacokinetic principles (Sawchuk-Zaske method), is recommended, particularly for seriously ill or poorly responding patients and for other high-risk individuals in whom dosage adjustments are likely to be necessary (eg, the elderly, neonates, patients with impaired renal function or changing volumes of distribution). Predictive nomograms (eg, Sarubbi-Hull) may provide acceptable dosage guidelines for initiation of treatment. For detailed discussion, see the Introduction.

For netilmicin, prolonged peak serum concentrations exceeding 16 mcg/ml and rising trough serum levels greater than 4 mcg/ml should be avoided (manufacturer's literature; see also the Introduction).

Intramuscular, Intravenous: When given intravenously in *adults*, a single dose of netilmicin injection may be diluted in 50 to 200 ml of various parenteral solutions (see manufacturer's literature for a list of compatible parenteral solutions). In infants and children, the volume of diluent is decreased according to the fluid requirements of the patient. The solution may be infused over a period of 30 minutes to two hours.

The duration of therapy with netilmicin usually ranges from 7 to 14 days.

Patients with normal renal function: Adults with serious systemic infections, 4 to 6.5 mg/kg daily in equally divided doses every 8 to 12 hours. *Adults with complicated urinary tract infections*, 3 to 4 mg/kg daily in equally divided doses every 12 hours. *Infants and children (6 weeks through 12 years)*, 5.5 to 8 mg/kg daily in equally divided doses every 8 to 12 hours. *Neonates (less than 6 weeks)*, 4 to 6.5 mg/kg daily in equally divided doses every 12 hours.

Patients with impaired renal function: Dosage modification is indicated. Whenever possible, netilmicin serum concentrations should be monitored to help determine dosage (see above and the Introduction). If these measurements are unavailable or unreliable, netilmicin may be given to *adults* according to the dosing chart proposed by Sarubbi and Hull (see the Introduction).

Netromycin (Schering). Solution (sterile) 10 (neonatal) and 25 mg/ml (pediatric) in 2 ml containers and 100 mg/ml in 1.5 ml containers.

KANAMYCIN SULFATE
[Kantrex, Klebcil]

Kanamycin is derived from *Streptomyces kanamyceticus*. It is a mixture of kanamycins A (more than 95%) and B (less than 5%).

MECHANISM OF ACTION, ANTIMICROBIAL SPECTRUM, AND RESISTANCE. Kanamycin is active against aerobic gram-negative bacilli, principally members of the Enterobacteriaceae (eg, *Escherichia coli*). Unlike gentamicin, tobramycin, amikacin, and netilmicin, it is not active against *Pseudomonas aeruginosa*. Strains of *Mycobacterium tuberculosis* and *Staphylococcus aureus* frequently are sensitive to kanamycin.

Kanamycin is susceptible to a number of aminoglycoside-inactivating enzymes (see Table 1 in the Introduction) and kanamycin-resistant bacterial strains are prevalent in many geographic locations.

For a detailed discussion on the mechanism of action, antimicrobial spectrum, and resistance properties of the aminoglycosides, see the Introduction.

USES. Parenterally administered kanamycin may still be used to treat serious infections caused by susceptible aerobic gram-negative bacilli, primarily Enterobacteriaceae. These include bacteremias and lower respiratory tract, intra-abdominal, soft tissue, bone and joint, and complicated urinary tract infections. However, bacterial resistance to kanamycin is common and other aminoglycosides (gentamicin, tobramycin, amikacin, netilmicin) are usually preferred for systemic use. Also, kanamycin is not effective against infections caused by *P. aeruginosa*. For a detailed discussion of aminoglycoside drug selection, see the Introduction.

Kanamycin is used in combination therapy for active treatment of tuberculosis only if susceptibility studies indicate its value over other primary and secondary antituberculous drugs. Since this is relatively uncommon, kanamycin is rarely used in tuberculosis therapy. See Chapter 75, Antimycobacterial Agents, for treatment guidelines for tuberculosis.

Oral kanamycin is used to suppress the bacterial flora of the bowel as a prophylactic measure before elective colorectal surgery. Kanamycin, administered orally, also has been used as an adjunct in the treatment of hepatic coma because it decreases the number of ammonia-forming bacteria in the intestinal tract. See also Chapter 55, Agents Used in Disorders of the Liver, Biliary Tract, and Pancreas.

ADVERSE REACTIONS AND PRECAUTIONS. Kanamycin has the potential to produce irreversible ototoxicity. Both the hearing (cochlear) and equilibrium (vestibular) functions may be affected, but this aminoglycoside usually has been associated with auditory toxicity (Bendush, 1982). Nephrotoxicity that usually is mild and reversible and, rarely, neuromuscular blockade are other potentially serious adverse reactions of kanamycin. For a detailed discussion, see the Introduction.

Although intestinal absorption is poor, caution must be exercised when this drug is given orally to patients with renal insufficiency, since toxic levels may result. As with neomycin, a malabsorption syndrome may occur after prolonged oral use.

DRUG INTERACTIONS. See the Introduction.

PHARMACOKINETICS. The pharmacokinetics of the parenterally administered aminoglycosides are similar, including an extracellular volume of distribution, poor penetration into cerebrospinal fluid, and elimination as unchanged drug by glomerular filtration. However, wide interpatient variation in aminoglycoside pharmacokinetics has been reported (see the Introduction).

DOSAGE AND PREPARATIONS. The following are standard dosages for kanamycin. However, monitoring of aminoglycoside serum concentrations and individualization of dosage regimens, preferably based on pharmacokinetic principles (Sawchuk-Zaske method), is recommended, particularly for seriously ill or poorly responding patients and for other high-risk individuals in whom dosage adjustments are likely to be necessary (eg, the elderly, neonates, patients with impaired renal function or changing volumes of distribution). Predictive nomograms (eg, Sarubbi-Hull) may provide acceptable dosage guidelines for initiation of treatment. For detailed discussion, see the Introduction.

For kanamycin, prolonged peak serum concentrations exceeding 35 mcg/ml and rising trough serum levels greater than 10 mcg/ml should be avoided (see the Introduction).

Intramuscular, Intravenous: When the intravenous route must be used, the drug should be diluted to 2.5 to 5 mg/ml in normal sodium chloride injection or 5% dextrose injection and the appropriate dose infused slowly over a 30- to 60-minute period. Duration of therapy with parenteral kanamycin generally should not exceed ten days.

Adults, children, and older infants with normal renal function, 15 mg/kg daily in two equally divided doses every 12 hours (occasionally, an eight-hour interval is used). The maximum daily dose in adults is 1.5 g. *Neonates up to 1 week with normal renal function who weigh less than 2 kg,* 15 mg/kg daily in two equally divided doses every 12 hours. *Neonates up to 1 week with normal renal function who weigh more than 2 kg,* 20 mg/kg daily in two equally divided doses every 12 hours.

Patients with impaired renal function: Dosage modification is indicated and should be determined on the basis of serum concentrations (see above and the Introduction). If this cannot be done, the dosing chart proposed by Sarubbi and Hull can be used for *adults* (see the Introduction).

Kantrex (Bristol), **Klebcil** (Beecham), **Generic.** Solution (sterile) 37.5 (pediatric) and 250 mg/ml in 2 ml containers and 333 mg/ml in 3 ml containers (strengths expressed in terms of the base).

Oral (not for systemic effects): *Adults,* as an adjunct in extended therapy of hepatic coma, 8 to 12 g daily in divided doses. *Adults,* as an adjunct in short-term mechanical cleansing of the large bowel, 1 g every hour for four hours, followed by 1 g every six hours for 36 to 72 hours. *Infants and children,* for suppression of bowel flora, 150 to 250 mg/kg daily in divided doses every hour to every six hours (Nelson, 1985).

Kantrex (Bristol). Capsules equivalent to 500 mg of base.

STREPTOMYCIN SULFATE

Streptomycin, derived from *Streptomyces griseus*, is bactericidal against a variety of aerobic gram-negative bacilli and certain mycobacteria. This drug is not commonly used today, however, since more effective aminoglycosides (ie, gentamicin, tobramycin, amikacin, netilmicin) are available and other equally effective and safer antituberculosis agents (eg, isoniazid, rifampin, ethambutol) are preferred.

MECHANISM OF ACTION, ANTIMICROBIAL SPECTRUM, AND RESISTANCE. Streptomycin is active against *Brucella, Francisella tularensis, Yersinia pestis, Pseudomonas mallei, Spirillum minor, Calymmatobacterium granulomatis, Haemophilus ducreyi,* and *Mycobacterium tuberculosis.* Although this drug has a broad spectrum of activity in vitro against common aerobic gram-negative bacilli (eg, Enterobacteriaceae), the widespread emergence of resistant strains has rendered it clinically obsolete for infections caused by these organisms.

Naturally resistant organisms include *Pseudomonas aeruginosa,* most gram-positive organisms, anaerobic bacteria, rickettsiae, fungi, and viruses.

For a detailed discussion on the mechanism of action, antimicrobial spectrum, and resistance properties of the aminoglycosides, see the Introduction.

USES. Streptomycin frequently is the preferred drug in the treatment of tularemia, plague, severe brucellosis (in combination with a tetracycline or chloramphenicol), and glanders (in combination with a tetracycline or chloramphenicol). It is an alternative agent in rat bite fever. See also the Introduction and Chapter 65, Antimicrobial Therapy and Chemoprophylaxis of Infectious Diseases, Table 1. It also has been used in granuloma inguinale and chancroid, but other drugs currently are preferred (see Chapter 65, Table 2). In plague, streptomycin is so rapidly bactericidal that it occasionally precipitates a Herxheimer-like reaction, which can be fatal.

This antibiotic has been used for years with large doses of penicillin G (or ampicillin) to treat enterococcal endocarditis because the combination is synergistic against susceptible enterococci (see the Introduction). However, 40% to 50% of enterococcal strains are now almost totally resistant to streptomycin in vitro (eg, minimal inhibitory concentration, >2,000 mcg/ml) and the combination is not synergistic against these organisms. The combination of gentamicin and penicillin G (or ampicillin) is usually effective against streptomycin-resistant enterococci. Combinations of streptomycin and penicillin G are still commonly used for endocarditis caused by viridans streptococci, which usually is sensitive both in vitro and in vivo. See also Chapter 65, Table 1.

Streptomycin currently is a second-line drug in the treatment of tuberculosis. It is used in combination therapy for retreatment of tuberculosis. Streptomycin is most commonly used when organism resistance precludes the use of isoniazid and/or rifampin, and/or parenteral management is desirable. See Chapter 75, Antimycobacterial Agents, for treatment guidelines for tuberculosis.

ADVERSE REACTIONS AND PRECAUTIONS. Streptomycin has the potential to produce irreversible ototoxicity. Both the hearing (cochlear) and equilibrium (vestibular) functions may be affected, but this aminoglycoside more frequently has been associated with vestibular toxicity (Bendush, 1982). Other neurologic toxicities associated with the use of streptomycin include peripheral and optic neuritis and neuromuscular blockade.

Nephrotoxicity appears to occur less commonly with streptomycin than with the other aminoglycosides.

Streptomycin causes hypersensitivity reactions ranging from skin rashes (fairly common) to exfoliative dermatitis and anaphylactic shock. Hematopoietic reactions (neutropenia and, rarely, agranulocytosis, aplastic anemia, or thrombocytopenic purpura) have been reported.

Administration of streptomycin to pregnant women has been reported to affect eighth cranial nerve function in the fetus (Conway and Birt, 1965). Streptomycin should not be given with other ototoxic drugs because effects may be additive.

Streptomycin is usually administered intramuscularly. Injection should be deep into the muscle since pain and sterile abscesses have developed with more superficial injection. The intrapleural or intrathecal route is rarely, if ever, employed. The latter route has produced radiculitis, transverse myelitis, arachnoiditis, nerve root pain, and even paraplegia.

The topical application of streptomycin is contraindicated because of the high risk of sensitization and rapidly developing bacterial resistance.

For a detailed discussion of aminoglycoside adverse reactions and precautions, see the Introduction.

DRUG INTERACTIONS. See the Introduction.

PHARMACOKINETICS. Peak serum levels of 15 to 20 mcg/ml (0.5 g) or 30 to 40 mcg/ml (1 g) are reached approximately 30 minutes after intramuscular injection. These levels should not be exceeded. Streptomycin exhibits the greatest degree of protein binding of the aminoglycosides (35%). As with other aminoglycosides, streptomycin distributes into the extracellular fluid volume and is eliminated as unchanged drug by glomerular filtration. Between 30% and 90% of a dose may be recovered in the urine during the first 24 hours after injection. For a detailed discussion of aminoglycoside pharmacokinetics, see the Introduction.

DOSAGE AND PREPARATIONS. All doses are expressed in terms of the base and are for patients with normal renal function. Dosage for patients with renal impairment must be based upon creatinine clearance and decreased in direct proportion to the degree of dysfunction.

Intramuscular: Adults, 15 to 25 mg/kg daily in two divided doses for seven to ten days and 1 g daily thereafter; *children,* 20 to 40 mg/kg daily in two divided doses; *premature and newborn infants,* 10 to 20 mg/kg daily in two divided doses.

For tularemia, an accepted dosage for *adults* is 2 g daily in divided doses every 12 hours; for plague, 2 g daily in divided doses every 12 hours; and for brucellosis, 1 g daily in divided doses every 12 hours together with tetracycline (Lietman, 1984).

For tuberculosis, see Chapter 75, Antimycobacterial Agents. For infective endocarditis due to penicillin-sensitive streptococci (eg, viridans streptococci), see Chapter 65, Antimicrobial Therapy and Chemoprophylaxis of Infectious Diseases, Table 1. For enterococcal endocarditis caused by streptomycin-susceptible enterococci, see Chapter 65, Table 1.

    Generic. Powder (for solution) 1 and 5 g; solution 400 mg/ml in 2.5 and 12.5 ml containers and 500 mg/ml in 10 ml containers (strengths expressed in terms of the base).

NEOMYCIN SULFATE
    [Mycifradin Sulfate, Neobiotic]

Neomycin, derived from *Streptomyces fradiae*, is the most toxic aminoglycoside antibiotic and should not be administered parenterally for systemic infections. Its therapeutic application is limited primarily to topical and oral administration for local antibacterial effects.

MECHANISM OF ACTION, ANTIMICROBIAL SPECTRUM, AND RESISTANCE. In vitro, neomycin is active against many aerobic gram-negative bacilli, principally members of the Enterobacteriaceae (eg, *Escherichia coli*). *Pseudomonas aeruginosa* are resistant, however. Many strains of *Staphylococcus aureus* are sensitive, but most other gram-positive bacteria are resistant. Other resistant organisms include anaerobic bacteria, rickettsiae, fungi, and viruses.

For a detailed discussion on the mechanism of action, antimicrobial spectrum, and resistance properties of the aminoglycosides, see the Introduction.

USES. Oral neomycin, in combination with erythromycin base, is frequently the preferred regimen for prophylaxis in elective colorectal surgery (see the Introduction and Chapter 65, Antimicrobial Therapy and Chemoprophylaxis of Infectious Diseases, Table 4). Neomycin can be used orally as an adjunct in the treatment of hepatic coma, since the drug reduces the number of ammonia-producing bacteria in the intestinal tract (see the Introduction and Chapter 55, Agents Used in Disorders of the Liver, Biliary Tract, and Pancreas). Oral neomycin also is used in type IIa hyperlipoproteinemia (see the Introduction and Chapter 50, Agents Used to Treat Hyperlipidemia). Neomycin has been administered orally in an attempt to control diarrhea caused by enteropathogenic *E. coli*, but evidence demonstrating its effectiveness is lacking.

Neomycin is most commonly used topically to treat infections of the eye, ear, and skin, frequently as a component of an antibiotic mixture. For these indications, see Chapters 73, Topical Anti-infective Agents: Otic and Ophthalmic Preparations, and 74, Topical Anti-infective Agents: Drugs Used on Skin and Mucous Membranes.

Parenteral administration of neomycin for systemic infections should be avoided because of serious ototoxicity and nephrotoxicity.

The value of this drug as a peritoneal or pleural irrigant is questionable and absorption may be sufficient to cause serious toxicity.

ADVERSE REACTIONS AND PRECAUTIONS. Although only small amounts of neomycin are absorbed following oral administration, this antibiotic may accumulate, particularly in patients with renal impairment, and cause toxicity (Ward and Rounthwaite, 1978). Diarrhea, superinfections, and a malabsorption syndrome (particularly with prolonged use) are the most common adverse reactions following oral administration.

Although parenteral preparations of neomycin are still marketed, their use is universally condemned since safer, equally effective antibiotics are available. When given parenterally, neomycin is highly ototoxic and nephrotoxic; these effects are dose related. Nephrotoxicity may be reversible, but ototoxicity that involves the cochlear portion of the inner ear is usually irreversible and may progress insidiously after the drug is discontinued. Intraperitoneal or intravenous use has caused apnea.

Neomycin should not be administered with other drugs that are potentially ototoxic or nephrotoxic, since effects may be additive.

Topical application of neomycin frequently has resulted in sensitization.

DRUG INTERACTIONS. See the Introduction.

PHARMACOKINETICS. Neomycin is minimally absorbed from the gastrointestinal tract following oral administration. Unabsorbed neomycin is excreted unchanged in the feces. Any drug that is absorbed will be excreted via the kidneys (glomerular filtration) as unchanged drug.

DOSAGE AND PREPARATIONS.
Oral: For prophylaxis in patients undergoing elective intestinal or colorectal surgery, *adults*, neomycin plus erythromycin base (1 g of each at 1 PM, 2 PM, and 11 PM on the day prior to surgery [surgery at 8 AM], accompanied by mechanical bowel preparation). No postoperative dose is necessary. See also Chapter 65, Table 4.

For dosages for hepatic coma and type IIa hyperlipoproteinemia, see Chapters 55, Agents Used in Disorders of the Liver, Biliary Tract, and Pancreas, and 50, Agents Used to Treat Hyperlipidemia, respectively.

For diarrhea caused by enteropathogenic *E. coli* (proof of efficacy is lacking), *adults,* 50 mg/kg daily in four divided doses; *newborn and premature infants,* 10 to 50 mg/kg daily in four divided doses; *older infants and children,* 50 to 100 mg/kg daily in four divided doses.

    Mycifradin Sulfate (Upjohn). Solution 125 mg/5 ml and tablets 500 mg equivalent to 87.5 and 350 mg of base, respectively.
    Neobiotic (Pfipharmecs), *Generic.* Tablets 500 mg.

Topical: For detailed information on dosages and preparations for topical application to the eye, ear, and skin, see Chapters 73, Topical Anti-infective Agents: Otic and Ophthalmic Preparations, and 74, Topical Anti-infective Agents: Drugs Used on Skin and Mucous Membranes.

Intramuscular: The parenteral administration of neomycin is not recommended and no useful dosage regimen is recognized.

    Generic. Powder (sterile) 500 mg.
    Mycifradin Sulfate (Upjohn). Powder (sterile) 500 mg (equivalent to 350 mg of base).

PAROMOMYCIN SULFATE
    [Humatin]

Paromomycin, an aminoglycoside antibiotic derived from *Streptomyces rimosus*, has antibacterial, amebicidal, and anthelmintic properties. It is administered only orally for local effects in the intestinal lumen.

MECHANISM OF ACTION, ANTIMICROBIAL SPECTRUM, AND RESISTANCE. Paromomycin is active against many aerobic gram-negative bacilli, principally members of the Enterobacteriaceae (eg, *Escherichia coli*). *Pseudomonas aeruginosa* are resistant, however. Many strains of *Staphylococcus aureus* are susceptible, but most other gram-positive bacteria are resistant.

Entamoeba histolytica, the causative organism of amebiasis, and various tapeworms, including *Taenia saginata*, *T. solium*, *Diphyllobothrium latum*, *Dipylidium caninum*, and *Hymenolepis nana*, are susceptible to paromomycin.

For a detailed discussion on the mechanism of action, antimicrobial spectrum, and resistance properties of the aminoglycosides, see the Introduction.

USES. Paromomycin is administered only orally for local effects in the intestinal lumen and is used as a secondary drug for the following: Prophylaxis of elective colorectal surgery (neomycin plus erythromycin base are preferred); adjunct in the treatment of hepatic coma (neomycin is preferred); generally used with other drugs (eg, iodoquinol) as an alternative to metronidazole alone (preferred) in the treatment of asymptomatic or mild to moderate symptomatic intestinal amebiasis (paromomycin is not effective in extraintestinal amebiasis) (see also Chapter 77, Antiprotozoal Agents); as an alternative to niclosamide (preferred) in the treatment of intestinal tapeworm infection (see also Chapter 78, Anthelmintics).

ADVERSE REACTIONS. Paromomycin may cause nausea, abdominal cramps, and diarrhea, particularly when doses exceed 3 g daily. Overgrowth of nonsusceptible organisms and a malabsorption syndrome may occur after prolonged administration.

Paromomycin should be used cautiously in patients with ulcerative lesions of the intestinal tract because it may be absorbed in such patients and cause nephrotoxicity.

DRUG INTERACTIONS. See the Introduction.

PHARMACOKINETICS. Paromomycin is minimally absorbed from the gastrointestinal tract following oral administration. It is primarily eliminated in the feces as unchanged drug.

DOSAGE AND PREPARATIONS. Paromomycin may be better tolerated if taken with meals.

Oral: For hepatic coma, *adults*, 4 g daily in divided doses at regular intervals for five to six days.

For dosages for intestinal amebiasis and intestinal tapeworm infections, see Chapters 77, Antiprotozoal Agents, and 78, Anthelmintics, respectively.

Humatin (Parke-Davis). Capsules 250 mg.

Cited References

Netilmicin sulfate (Netromycin). *Med Lett Drugs Ther* 25:65-67, 1983.

Ackerman BH, et al: Aminoglycoside therapy: Improving patient response and safety. *Postgrad Med* 75:177-185, (Feb) 1984.

Anderson ET, et al: Simultaneous antibiotic levels in "breakthrough" gram-negative rod bacteremia. *Am J Med* 61:493-497, 1976.

Bauer LA, Blouin RA: Influence of age on amikacin pharmacokinetics in patients without renal disease: Comparison with gentamicin and tobramycin. *Eur J Clin Pharmacol* 24:639-642, 1983.

Bendush CL: Ototoxicity: Clinical considerations and comparative information, in Whelton A, Neu HC (eds): *The Aminoglycosides: Microbiology, Clinical Use, and Toxicology*. New York, Marcel Dekker, 1982, 453-486.

Benveniste R, Davies J: Mechanisms of antibiotic resistance in bacteria. *Annu Rev Biochem* 42:471-506, 1973.

Betts RF, et al: Five-year surveillance of aminoglycoside usage in university hospital. *Ann Intern Med* 100:219-222, 1984.

Blair DC, et al: Inactivation of amikacin and gentamicin by carbenicillin in patients with end-stage renal failure. *Antimicrob Agents Chemother* 22:376-379, 1982.

Bootman JL, et al: Individualizing gentamicin dosage regimens in burn patients with gram-negative septicemia: Cost-benefit analysis. *J Pharmaceut Sci* 68:267-272, 1979.

Burton ME, et al: Comparison of drug dosing methods. *Clin Pharmacokinet* 10:1-37, 1985.

Churchill DN, Seely J: Nephrotoxicity associated with combined gentamicin-amphotericin B therapy. *Nephron* 19:176-181, 1977.

Cipolle RJ, et al: Systematically individualizing tobramycin dosage regimens. *J Clin Pharmacol* 20:570-580, 1980.

Conway N, Birt BD: Streptomycin in pregnancy: Effect on foetal ear. *Br Med J* 2:260-263, 1965.

Courvalin P, Carlier C: Resistance towards aminoglycoside-aminocyclitol antibiotics in bacteria. *J Antimicrob Chemother* 8(suppl A):57-69, 1981.

Craig WA, et al: Netilmicin sulfate: Comparative evaluation of antimicrobial activity, pharmacokinetics, adverse reactions, and clinical efficacy. *Pharmacotherapy* 3:305-315, 1983.

Davia JE, et al: Uremia, deafness, and paralysis due to irrigating antibiotic solutions. *Arch Intern Med* 125:136-139, 1970.

Davies JE: Resistance to aminoglycosides: Mechanisms and frequency. *Rev Infect Dis* 5(suppl):S261-S267, 1983.

Davies J, Smith DI: Plasmid-determined resistance to antimicrobial agents. *Annu Rev Microbiol* 32:469-518, 1978.

Dentino M, et al: Long term effect of cis-diamminedichloride platinum (CDDP) on renal function and structure in man. *Cancer* 41:1274-1281, 1978.

DeTorres OH: Closer look at aminoglycosides. *Clin Ther* 3:399-412, 1981.

Dickie P, et al: Effect of enzymatic adenylylation on dihydrostreptomycin accumulation in *Escherichia coli* carrying an R-factor: Model explaining aminoglycoside resistance by inactivating mechanisms. *Antimicrob Agents Chemother* 14:569-580, 1978.

Dyas A, et al: Reproducibility study of pharmacokinetics of amikacin, gentamicin, and tobramycin: Three-way crossover study. *J Antimicrob Chemother* 12:371-376, 1983.

Farber BF, Moellering RC Jr: Retrospective study of toxicity of preparations of vancomycin from 1974 to 1981. *Antimicrob Agents Chemother* 23:138-141, 1983.

Fee WE Jr: Gentamicin and tobramycin: Comparison of ototoxicity. *Rev Infect Dis* 5(suppl 2):S304-S313, 1983.

Finley RS, et al: Comparison of standard versus pharmacokinetically adjusted amikacin dosing in granulocytopenic cancer patients. *Antimicrob Agents Chemother* 22:193-197, 1982.

Fong IW, et al: Comparative toxicity of gentamicin versus tobramycin: Randomized prospective study. *J Antimicrob Chemother* 7:81-88, 1981.

Gerding DN, Larson TA: Aminoglycoside resistance in gram-negative bacilli during increased amikacin use: Comparison of experience in 14 United States hospitals with experience in the Minneapolis Veterans Administration Medical Center. *Am J Med* 79(suppl 1A):1-7, 1985.

Glew RH, Pavuk RA: Stability of gentamicin, tobramycin, and amikacin in combination with four β-lactam antibiotics. *Antimicrob Agents Chemother* 24:474-477, 1983.

Guay DRP: Netilmicin (Netromycin, Schering-Plough). *Drug Intell Clin Pharm* 17:83-91, 1983.

Guglielmo RB: Furosemide-aminoglycoside interaction. *Drug Interact Newslett* 4:34-35, 1984.

Haas EJ, Collins GE: Guidelines for aminoglycoside dosing. *Drug Ther (Hosp)* 7:57-66, (June) 1982.

Hancock REW: Aminoglycoside uptake and mode of action—with

special reference to streptomycin and gentamicin: I. Antagonists and mutants. II. Effects of aminoglycosides on cells. *J Antimicrob Chemother* 8:249-276, 429-445, 1981.

Hansten PD: Cyclosporine interactions. *Drug Interact Newslett* 41:29-31, 1984.

Hansten PD: *Drug Interactions*, ed 5. Philadelphia, Lea & Febiger, 1985 A, 194-199.

Hansten PD: *Drug Interactions*, ed 5. Philadelphia, Lea & Febiger, 1985 B, 67-68.

Hare RS, Miller GH: Mechanisms of aminoglycoside resistance. *Antimicrob Newslett* 1:77-84, 1984.

Holloway JJ, et al: Comparative cost effectiveness of gentamicin and tobramycin. *Ann Intern Med* 101:764-769, 1984.

Holm SE, et al: Prospective, randomized study of amikacin and gentamicin in serious infections with focus on efficacy, toxicity and duration of serum levels above the MIC. *J Antimicrob Chemother* 12:393-402, 1983.

Holt HA, et al: Interactions between aminoglycoside antibiotics and carbenicillin or ticarcillin. *Infection* 4:107-109, 1976.

Jackson GG, Riff LJ: *Pseudomonas* bacteremia: Pharmacologic and other bases for failure of treatment with gentamicin. *J Infect Dis* 124(suppl):S185-S191, 1971.

Kahlmeter G, Dahlager JI: Aminoglycoside toxicity: Review of clinical studies published between 1975 and 1982. *J Antimicrob Chemother* 13(suppl A):9-22, 1984.

Kluge RM, et al: Carbenicillin-gentamicin combination against *Pseudomonas aeruginosa*: Correlation with gentamicin sensitivity. *Ann Intern Med* 81:584-587, 1974.

Korzeniowski OM, Hook EW: Aminocyclitols: Aminoglycosides and spectinomycin, in Mandell GL, et al (eds): *Principles and Practice of Infectious Diseases*. New York, John Wiley & Sons, 1979, 249-273.

Lerner AM, et al: Randomised, controlled trial of comparative efficacy, auditory toxicity, and nephrotoxicity of tobramycin and netilmicin. *Lancet* 1:1123-1126, 1983.

Lesar TS, et al: Gentamicin dosing errors with four commonly used nomograms. *JAMA* 248:1190-1193, 1982.

Levin S: Antibiotics of choice in suspected serious sepsis. *J Antimicrob Chemother* 8(suppl A):133-142, 1981.

Levine JF, et al: Amikacin-resistant gram-negative bacilli: Correlation of occurrence with amikacin use. *J Infect Dis* 151:295-300, 1985.

Lietman PS: Aminoglycosides and spectinomycin: Aminocyclitols, in Mandell GL, et al (eds): *Principles and Practice of Infectious Diseases*, ed 2. New York, John Wiley & Sons, 1984, 192-206.

Lietman PS, Smith CR: Aminoglycoside nephrotoxicity in humans. *Rev Infect Dis* 5(suppl 2):S284-S293, 1983.

Luft FC: Cephalosporin and aminoglycoside interactions: Clinical and toxicologic implications, in Whelton A, Neu HC (eds): *The Aminoglycosides: Microbiology, Clinical Use, and Toxicology*. New York, Marcel Dekker, 1982, 387-399.

Mangini RJ (ed): *Drug Interaction Facts*. St Louis, JB Lippincott, 1984, 12-14.

Mangione A, Schentag JJ: Therapeutic monitoring of aminoglycoside antibiotics: Approach. *Therapeut Drug Monitor* 2:159-167, 1980.

Masur H, et al: Neomycin toxicity revisited. *Arch Surg* 111:822-825, 1976.

McCracken GH Jr: Perinatal bacterial diseases, in Feigin RD, Cherry JD (eds): *Textbook of Pediatric Infectious Diseases*. Philadelphia, WB Saunders, 1981, vol 1, 747-768.

Meyer RD: Amikacin: Drugs five years later. *Ann Intern Med* 95:328-332, 1981.

Mitsuhashi S, Kawabe H: Aminoglycoside antibiotic resistance in bacteria, in Whelton A, Neu HC (eds): *The Aminoglycosides: Microbiology, Clinical Use, and Toxicology*. New York, Marcel Dekker, 1982, 97-122.

Moellering RC Jr: In vitro antibacterial activity of aminoglycoside antibiotics. *Rev Infect Dis* 5(suppl 2):S212-S232, 1983.

Moody MM, et al: Long-term amikacin use: Effects on aminoglycoside susceptibility patterns of gram-negative bacilli. *JAMA* 248:1199-1202, 1982.

Moore RD, et al: Risk factors for nephrotoxicity in patients treated with aminoglycosides. *Ann Intern Med* 100:352-357, 1984 A.

Moore RD, et al: Risk factors for development of auditory toxicity in patients receiving aminoglycosides. *J Infect Dis* 149:23-30, 1984 B.

Moore RD, et al: Association of aminoglycoside plasma levels with mortality in patients with gram-negative bacteremia. *J Infect Dis* 149:443-448, 1984 C.

Moore RD, et al: Association of aminoglycoside plasma levels with therapeutic outcome in gram-negative pneumonia. *Am J Med* 77:657-662, 1984 D.

Nelson JD: *1985 Pocketbook of Pediatric Antimicrobial Therapy*, ed 6. Baltimore, Williams & Wilkins, 1985, 70.

Neu HC: Clinical use of aminoglycosides, in Whelton A, Neu HC (eds): *The Aminoglycosides: Microbiology, Clinical Use, and Toxicology*. New York, Marcel Dekker, 1982 A, 611-628.

Neu HC: Pharmacology of aminoglycosides, in Whelton A, Neu HC (eds): *The Aminoglycosides: Microbiology, Clinical Use, and Toxicology*. New York, Marcel Dekker, 1982 B, 125-142.

Noone P, et al: Experience in monitoring gentamicin therapy during treatment of serious gram-negative sepsis. *Br Med J* 1:477-481, 1974.

Odio C, et al: Nephrotoxicity associated with vancomycin-aminoglycoside therapy in four children. *J Pediatr* 105:491-493, 1984.

Phillips I: Aminoglycosides. *Lancet* 2:311-315, 1982.

Pickering LK, Rutherford I: Effect of concentration and time upon inactivation of tobramycin, gentamicin, netilmicin, and amikacin by azlocillin, carbenicillin, mecillinam, mezlocillin, and piperacillin. *J Pharmacol Exp Ther* 217:345-349, 1981.

Pratt WB: *Chemotherapy of Infection*. New York, Oxford University Press, 1977, 85-126.

Price KE, et al: Epidemiological studies of aminoglycoside resistance in U.S.A. *J Antimicrob Chemother* 8(suppl A):89-105, 1981.

Rahal JJ Jr: Antibiotic combinations: Clinical relevance of synergy and antagonism. *Medicine* 57:179-195, 1978.

Reese RE, Betts RF: Antibiotic use: Aminoglycosides, in Reese RE, Douglas RG Jr (eds): *A Practical Approach to Infectious Diseases*. Boston, Little, Brown and Company, 1983, 106-118.

Ristuccia AM, Cunha BA: Aminoglycosides. *Med Clin North Am* 66:303-312, 1982.

Ristuccia AM, Cunha BA: Review: Overview of amikacin. *Therapeut Drug Monitor* 7:12-25, 1985.

Rozek JL: Aminoglycoside antibiotics. *Antimicrob Newslett* 1:51-56, 1984.

Sarubbi FA Jr, Hull JH: Amikacin serum concentrations: Prediction of levels and dosage guidelines. *Ann Intern Med* 89:612-618, 1978.

Sawchuk RJ, Zaske DE: Pharmacokinetics of dosing regimens which utilize multiple intravenous infusions: Gentamicin in burn patients. *J Pharmacokinet Biopharm* 4:183-195, 1976.

Sawchuk RJ, et al: Kinetic model for gentamicin dosing with use of individual patient parameters. *Clin Pharmacol Ther* 21:362-369, 1977.

Shulman ST, et al: Prevention of bacterial endocarditis: Statement for Health Professionals by the Committee on Rheumatic Fever and Infective Endocarditis of the Council on Cardiovascular Disease in the Young. *Circulation* 70:1123A-1127A, 1984.

Smith CR, Lietman PS: Comparative clinical trials of aminoglycosides, in Whelton A, Neu HC (eds): *The Aminoglycosides: Microbiology, Clinical Use, and Toxicology*. New York, Marcel Dekker, 1982, 497-509.

Smith CR, Lietman PS: Effect of furosemide on aminoglycoside-induced nephrotoxicity and auditory toxicity in humans. *Antimicrob Agents Chemother* 23:133-137, 1983.

Smith CR, et al: Double-blind comparison of nephrotoxicity and auditory toxicity of gentamicin and tobramycin. *N Engl J Med* 302:1106-1109, 1980.

Szot RJ, Tabachnick IIA: Animal studies with netilmicin. *Clin Trials J* 17:318-337, 1980.

Tanaka N: Mechanism of action of aminoglycoside antibiotics, in Umezawa H, Hooper IR (eds): *Handbook of Experimental Pharmacology*. New York, Springer-Verlag, 1982, vol 62, 221-266.

Trissel LA: *Handbook on Injectable Drugs*, ed 3. Washington, DC, American Society of Hospital Pharmacists, 1983.

Wade JC, et al: Cephalothin plus an aminoglycoside is more nephrotoxic than methicillin plus an aminoglycoside. *Lancet* 2:604-606, 1978.

Ward KM, Rounthwaite FJ: Neomycin ototoxicity. *Ann Otol Rhinol Laryngol* 87:211-215, 1978.

Weinstein AJ, et al: Placental transfer of clindamycin and gentamicin in term pregnancy. *Am J Obstet Gynecol* 124:688-691, 1976.

Weinstein AJ, et al: Systemic absorption of neomycin irrigating solution. *JAMA* 238:152-153, 1977.

Wenk M, et al: Serum level monitoring of antibacterial drugs: Review. *Clin Pharmacokinet* 9:475-492, 1984.

Whelton A: Therapeutic initiatives for avoidance of aminoglycoside toxicity. *J Clin Pharmacol* 25:67-81, 1985.

Young LS, et al: Aminoglycosides in treatment of bacteraemic infections in immunocompromised host. *J Antimicrob Chemother* 8(suppl A):121-132, 1981.

Zarfin Y, et al: Possible indomethacin-aminoglycoside interaction in preterm infants. *J Pediatr* 106:511-513, 1985.

Zaske DE: Aminoglycosides: Counterpoint discussion, in Evans WE, et al (eds): *Applied Pharmacokinetics: Principles of Therapeutic Drug Monitoring*. San Francisco, Applied Therapeutics, 1980, 210-239.

Zaske DE, et al: Gentamicin dosage requirements: Wide interpatient variations in 242 surgery patients with normal renal function. *Surgery* 87:164-169, 1980.

Zaske DE, et al: Increased gentamicin dosage requirements: Rapid elimination in 249 gynecology patients. *Am J Obstet Gynecol* 139:896-900, 1981.

Zaske DE, et al: Increased burn patient survival with individualized dosages of gentamicin. *Surgery* 91:142-149, 1982 A.

Zaske DE, et al: Gentamicin pharmacokinetics in 1,640 patients: Method for control of serum concentrations. *Antimicrob Agents Chemother* 21:407-411, 1982 B.

Zaske DE, et al: Wide interpatient variations in gentamicin dose requirements for geriatric patients. *JAMA* 248:3122-3126, 1982 C.

Other Selected References

Advances in aminoglycoside therapy: Amikacin. *J Infect Dis* 134(suppl):242-460, (Nov) 1976.

Symposium on amikacin. *Am J Med* 62:863-966, 1977.

Blumer JL, Reed MD: Clinical pharmacology of aminoglycoside antibiotics in pediatrics. *Pediatr Clin North Am* 30:195-208, 1983.

Burkle WS: Comparative evaluation of aminoglycoside antibiotics for systemic use. *Drug Intell Clin Pharm* 15:847-862, 1981.

Finland M, Neu HC (eds): Tobramycin, symposium. *J Infect Dis* 134(suppl):1-234, 1976.

Gerding DN (ed): Role of aminoglycosides as first-line therapy in multiple clinical settings. *Am J Med* 79(suppl 1A):1-76, 1985 (11 articles).

Gilbert DN, Sanford JP (eds): Clinical perspective of antibiotic therapy: Aminoglycosides vs broad-spectrum β-lactams. *Rev Infect Dis* 5(suppl 2):S211-S316, 1983 (11 articles).

Meyers BR: Aminoglycosides, in Kagan BM (ed): *Antimicrobial Therapy*, ed 3. Philadelphia, WB Saunders, 1980, 56-76.

Noone P: Sisomicin, netilmicin, and dibekacin: Review of their antibacterial activity and therapeutic use. *Drugs* 27:548-578, 1984.

Sande MA, Mandell GL: Antimicrobial agents: Aminoglycosides, in Gilman AG, et al (eds): *The Pharmacological Basis of Therapeutics*, ed 6. New York, Macmillan, 1980, 1162-1180.

Solberg CO, et al (eds): Netilmicin. *J Antimicrob Chemother* 13(suppl A):1-83, 1984 (10 articles).

Whelton A, Neu HC (eds): *The Aminoglycosides: Microbiology, Clinical Use, and Toxicology*. New York, Marcel Dekker, 1982.

SULFONAMIDES

Introduction

History, Chemistry, and Scope of Discussion

Mechanism of Action

Antimicrobial Spectrum

Resistance

Uses

Adverse Reactions and Precautions

Drug Interactions and Interference with Laboratory Tests

Pharmacokinetics

Drug Evaluations

Short-acting Sulfonamides

Intermediate-acting Sulfonamide

Mixtures

Mixture Containing Only Sulfonamides

Mixtures Containing a Sulfonamide and Another Drug

DIHYDROFOLATE REDUCTASE INHIBITORS

Trimethoprim

Mixture: Trimethoprim/Sulfamethoxazole

SULFONAMIDES

History, Chemistry, and Scope of Discussion

The modern antimicrobial chemotherapeutic era began in the early 1930's when Prontosil, a chemical developed by the German dye industry, was shown to combat streptococcal infection in mice after metabolism to para-aminobenzene sulfonamide (sulfanilamide), an antibacterial compound.

Sulfanilamide is similar in structure to para-aminobenzoic acid (PABA), a precursor required by bacteria for folic acid synthesis (Figure 1). The clinically useful sulfonamides are synthetically derived from sulfanilamide. Most derivatives contain a free para-amino group, which is necessary for antibacterial activity, and heterocyclic aromatic substitutions on the sulfonamide group (Figure 1). Such modifications of the basic sulfanilamide molecule result in increased antibacterial activity. The nature of these substitutions also determines other pharmacologic properties of the drug, such as absorption, solubility, and gastrointestinal tolerance.

Although many sulfonamides have been tested for clinical usefulness, only five derivatives currently are marketed in the United States as single-entity drugs for systemic use. These include the short-acting sulfonamides, sulfisoxazole [Gantrisin], sulfacytine [Renoquid], sulfamethizole [Thiosulfil], and sulfadiazine, and the intermediate-acting analogue, sulfamethoxazole [Gantanol]. The structures of these derivatives are shown in Figure 1. Long-acting sulfonamides (eg, sulfamethoxypyridazine, sulfameter) are no longer available as single agents because they have been associated with severe hypersensitivity reactions, such as the Stevens-Johnson syndrome.

This section is limited to a discussion of the above single-entity preparations and systemic fixed-ratio mixtures containing more than one sulfonamide or a sulfonamide and another drug (see the discussion on Mixtures).

For information on sulfonamides limited to use in the gastrointestinal tract (eg, sulfasalazine), eye (eg, sulfacetamide), or skin (eg, mafenide, silver sulfadiazine), see Chapters 53, Agents Used in Disorders of the Lower Intestinal Tract; 73, Topical Anti-infective Agents: Otic and Ophthalmic Preparations; and 74, Topical Anti-infective Agents: Drugs Used on Skin and Mucous Membranes, respectively.

Mechanism of Action

Bacteria require tetrahydrofolic acid, a derivative of folic acid, as a cofactor in the synthesis of thymidine, purines, and, ultimately, DNA. Most bacterial cells are impermeable to folic acid and must synthesize it from para-aminobenzoic acid (PABA). The sulfonamides are structural analogues of PABA and competitively inhibit the synthesis of dihydropteroic acid, the immediate precursor of dihydrofolic acid, from PABA and pteridine (see Figure 2). Mammalian cells are unaffected by this inhibition because they require preformed folic acid and cannot synthesize it.

The sulfonamides are primarily bacteriostatic at therapeutic concentrations. However, it has been shown that when bacteria are grown in media containing purines and amino acids but a low concentration of thymine, exposure to sulfonamides can be bactericidal because of "thymineless death." This bactericidal effect has been demonstrated in human blood and urine (Then and Angehrn, 1973 A and B; Pratt, 1977).

Sulfonamide-induced inhibition of bacterial cell growth can be reversed in vitro by adding certain agents (eg, thymidine, purines, methionine, serine) to the growth medium. This may be of clinical importance, since pus may contain many of these substances as the result of cell breakdown, and their presence may inhibit the effectiveness of these drugs in purulent infections. Also, when in vitro sensitivity is being determined, it is

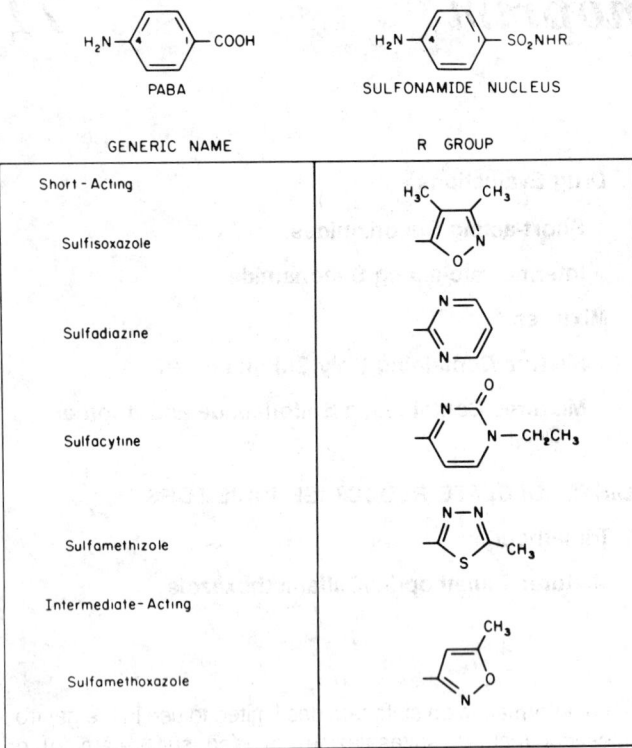

Figure 1. Chemical structures of para-aminobenzoic acid (PABA) and sulfonamides for systemic use.

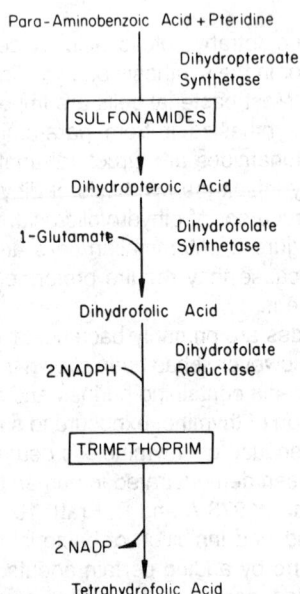

Figure 2. Pathway for the synthesis of tetrahydrofolic acid in bacteria and the sites of inhibition by the sulfonamides and trimethoprim. From Wormser GP, Keusch GT: Trimethoprim-sulfamethoxazole in the United States. Ann Intern Med 91:420-429, 1979. (Reprinted with permission)

essential that the culture medium be free of PABA, since trace amounts of this compound may interfere with results.

Antimicrobial Spectrum

The sulfonamides are active against both gram-positive and gram-negative bacteria. Their in vitro spectrum includes *Streptococcus pyogenes*, *S. pneumoniae*, some strains of *Bacillus anthracis* and *Corynebacterium diphtheriae*, *Haemophilus influenzae*, *H. ducreyi*, *Brucella*, *Pseudomonas pseudomallei*, *Vibrio cholerae*, *Yersinia pestis*, and *Calymmatobacterium granulomatis*. *Chlamydia trachomatis*, *Actinomyces*, *Nocardia* species (*N. asteroides* is highly sensitive), and the protozoans, *Plasmodium falciparum* and *Toxoplasma gondii*, are susceptible (Mandell and Sande, 1980).

Although *Neisseria gonorrhoeae* and *N. meningitidis* were susceptible in the past, the majority of strains are now resistant. Similarly, most strains of *Shigella sonnei* and *S. flexneri* are now resistant (Mandell and Sande, 1980).

Escherichia coli usually are susceptible to sulfonamides when present in the urinary tract, particularly if the organism is community-acquired and the infection has not been treated previously. *Klebsiella* species, *Proteus mirabilis*, and *Serratia marcescens* vary in their in vitro susceptibility. *Enterobacter aerogenes*, *Pseudomonas aeruginosa*, and most *Proteus* species occasionally are susceptible in vitro, but diseases caused by these bacteria seldom respond to sulfonamides. Resistant organisms include *Francisella tularensis*, *Leptospira*, *Bordetella pertussis*, *Borrelia*, *Mycobacterium tuberculosis*, *M. leprae*, *Treponema pallidum*, rickettsiae, amebae, fungi, and viruses (Mandell and Sande, 1980).

Resistance

Many bacteria become highly resistant to the sulfonamides during therapy. Resistance can be chromosomally mediated or transferred by R-factors. The latter method frequently is seen with Enterobacteriaceae. The mechanisms of resistance include (1) overproduction of PABA; (2) a decreased affinity of dihydropteroate synthetase for the sulfonamide; (3) a decreased permeability of the bacterium to the drug; and (4) increased inactivation of the drug. Cross-resistance between sulfonamides is usual.

Acquired resistance to the sulfonamides is widespread and severely limits their clinical usefulness. For example, significant resistance among gonococci, meningococci, staphylococci, streptococci, and shigellae has rendered the sulfonamides clinically obsolete in treating infections caused by these bacteria.

Uses

Urinary Tract Infections: The sulfonamides were once a mainstay in the treatment of infectious diseases, but their importance has diminished as bacterial resistance has increased and more effective antibiotics have been developed.

Nevertheless, because of their established effectiveness, low cost, and the relative lack of toxicity of the newer compounds, sulfonamides are among the drugs of choice for acute, uncomplicated urinary tract infections (ie, cystitis) caused by susceptible bacterial strains, particularly *E. coli* (the causative organism in about 90% of initial infections). Ampicillin [Amcill, Omnipen, Polycillin, Principen], amoxicillin [Amoxil, Larotid, Polymox, Trimox], trimethoprim/sulfamethoxazole [Bactrim, Septra], and nitrofurantoin [Furadantin, Macrodantin] are effective alternatives. Sulfonamides often are effective in the treatment of asymptomatic bacteriuria in pregnant women, but they should not be administered near term because of possible adverse effects on the neonate (see section on Adverse Reactions and Precautions).

Sulfonamides should not be used to treat acute pyelonephritis; parenteral antibiotics (eg, an aminoglycoside) frequently are required for this infection. The use of sulfonamides for the prophylaxis of recurrent urinary tract infections also is not recommended. However, trimethoprim/sulfamethoxazole (also trimethoprim alone, nitrofurantoin) often is preferred for this indication (see the section on Dihydrofolate Reductase Inhibitors). For a more detailed discussion of antimicrobial drug selection for urinary tract infections, see Chapter 65, Antimicrobial Therapy and Chemoprophylaxis of Infectious Diseases.

For greatest effectiveness in urinary tract infections, use of a sulfonamide that is excreted in high concentration (largely in the active rather than the acetylated form), is reasonably soluble in acidic urine, and maintains adequate levels in the blood and tissues during the period of maximum excretion is desirable. The short-acting drugs that most nearly meet these criteria are sulfisoxazole, sulfamethizole, and sulfacytine; sulfisoxazole frequently is preferred because it is the least expensive derivative. In addition to traditional multiple-dose therapy, sulfisoxazole has been shown to be effective as single-dose (2 g) therapy of initial attacks of cystitis in nonpregnant women without renal involvement.

The intermediate-acting analogue, sulfamethoxazole (alone or combined with trimethoprim), also is used in uncomplicated urinary tract infections. This derivative can be administered less frequently than sulfisoxazole (twice versus four times per day), but it is somewhat less soluble in urine. The combination of sulfamethoxazole/trimethoprim often is preferred over a single sulfonamide (see the section on Dihydrofolate Reductase Inhibitors).

Nocardiosis: Sulfonamides, including sulfadiazine, sulfisoxazole, trisulfapyrimidines, and sulfamethoxazole, traditionally have been preferred drugs for nocardiosis. Trimethoprim/sulfamethoxazole, minocycline [Minocin], and ampicillin plus erythromycin are alternative therapies for *N. asteroides* infections.

Miscellaneous Bacterial Infections: Although not the drugs of choice, certain sulfonamides, including sulfisoxazole and sulfamethoxazole, can be used to treat chlamydial pneumonia in infants, lymphogranuloma venereum, chancroid, and melioidosis.

Respiratory Tract Infections and Acute Otitis Media: Certain respiratory tract infections (eg, acute sinusitis) and otitis media caused by susceptible streptococci, pneumococci,

or *Haemophilus influenzae* may respond to the sulfonamides, but other antimicrobial agents currently are preferred. However, sulfamethoxazole/trimethoprim frequently is employed in these infections (see the section on Dihydrofolate Reductase Inhibitors). Sulfonamides also may be combined with erythromycin (or penicillin) to treat otitis media caused by amoxicillin-resistant strains of *H. influenzae*. A fixed-ratio combination containing sulfisoxazole acetyl and erythromycin ethylsuccinate [Pediazole] is widely used for this infection and in penicillin-allergic patients with acute otitis media (see the section on Mixtures).

Antimicrobial Chemoprophylaxis: Sulfadiazine (or sulfisoxazole) is recommended for the prophylaxis of rheumatic fever in penicillin-allergic patients. Erythromycin is an alternative. Sulfonamides should *not* be used in the treatment of established streptococcal pharyngitis because they fail to eradicate the causative organism, and late sequelae (eg, rheumatic fever, glomerulonephritis) may develop.

Rifampin [Rifadin, Rimactane] is the drug of choice for prophylaxis of meningococcal meningitis in household or other close contacts. Sulfadiazine (or sulfisoxazole) can be used only if the susceptibility of the organism to this agent is known. Sulfonamides are no longer used to treat meningococcal meningitis because of the prevalence of resistant strains of *Neisseria meningitidis*.

Sulfisoxazole is commonly used for the chemoprophylaxis of recurrent otitis media, although conclusive evidence that the advantages outweigh the disadvantages for this management option is lacking.

Protozoal Infections: Sulfonamides also are used in various protozoal infections. Sulfadoxine, a long-acting derivative available only with pyrimethamine in a fixed-ratio combination [Fansidar] in the United States, and sulfadiazine may be used adjunctively in combination with pyrimethamine in malaria caused by chloroquine-resistant strains of *Plasmodium falciparum*. Sulfadiazine with pyrimethamine, the primary agent, is useful in toxoplasmosis due to *Toxoplasma gondii*. *Pneumocystis carinii* infections may be treated with trimethoprim/sulfamethoxazole (see the section on Dihydrofolate Reductase Inhibitors). For additional discussion on the treatment of these protozoal infections, see Chapter 77, Antiprotozoal Agents.

Adverse Reactions and Precautions

The sulfonamides are capable of producing a wide variety of adverse reactions that affect a number of organ systems, including the blood and bone marrow, skin, kidney, liver, and nervous system.

Cutaneous and Mucocutaneous: Hypersensitivity reactions affecting the skin and mucous membranes include urticaria and maculopapular rashes that are often accompanied by pruritus and fever. More serious dermatologic reactions (eg, exfoliative dermatitis, toxic epidermal necrolysis, erythema nodosum) occur less frequently. The sulfonamides rarely may provoke erythema multiforme and its severe form, Stevens-Johnson syndrome, especially in children. This syndrome involves both the skin and mucous membranes and is fatal in up to 25% of patients (Araujo and Flowers, 1984). Therefore, sulfonamide therapy should be discontinued in patients who develop a skin rash and the illness re-evaluated.

Photosensitivity reactions also have occurred with the use of sulfonamides. Patients should be cautioned that an exaggerated sunburn reaction after exposure to the sun is possible during sulfonamide therapy.

Hematologic: The incidence of blood dyscrasias is low, but they can be extremely serious and deaths have occurred. Sulfonamides may cause agranulocytosis, hemolytic or aplastic (rare) anemia, leukopenia, thrombocytopenia, hypoprothrombinemia, and eosinophilia. Hemolytic anemia has been observed in patients with and without deficiency of erythrocytic glucose-6-phosphate dehydrogenase (G6PD). This hazard should be borne in mind if there is a family history of G6PD deficiency, which is most common in blacks and Mediterranean ethnic groups.

Blood studies performed at regular intervals are necessary during prolonged therapy with any sulfonamide, since they detect the milder leukopenias. Clinical signs, such as sore throat, fever, pallor, purpura, or jaundice, may be early indications of serious blood disorders and blood counts should be performed.

Hypersensitivity Reactions: In addition to hypersensitivity reactions involving the skin and blood, sulfonamides may cause drug fever, a serum sickness-like syndrome, urticaria, anaphylaxis, polyarteritis nodosa, and systemic lupus erythematosus. An allergic reaction to one sulfonamide precludes the later use of another derivative.

Renal: Older, less soluble sulfonamides, including sulfadiazine, frequently caused crystalluria in the kidney, renal calices and pelvis, ureters, or bladder that resulted in hematuria, irritation, and obstruction. This complication was minimized by maintenance of a high urine flow and alkalization of the urine to increase solubility of the drug. The risk of crystalluria has diminished markedly with the use of more soluble sulfonamides (eg, sulfisoxazole). However, since these agents are excreted primarily by the kidneys, an adequate urine volume must be maintained. Before sulfonamide therapy is begun, urinary output should be 1,000 to 1,500 ml/day for individuals with normal renal function and appropriate hydration (eg, maintenance of an adequate fluid intake) should be continued throughout the treatment period. Because the sulfonamides are more soluble in alkaline urine, efforts to alkalize the urine (eg, with sodium bicarbonate) may be desirable in some patients.

Sulfonamides infrequently cause toxic nephrosis with oliguria and anuria but without evidence of crystalluria. Tubular necrosis or necrotizing angiitis are the pathologic manifestations of this adverse effect.

Sulfonamides must be used cautiously in patients with impaired renal function. Frequent urinalyses with microscopic examination are advisable in patients receiving sulfonamides.

Hepatic: Hepatitis with focal or diffuse necrosis and cholestatic jaundice may occur. The conjugation of sulfonamides is reduced in patients with impaired liver function, and toxic reactions may follow usual therapeutic doses.

Neurologic: Reactions involving the central nervous system include headache, lethargy, dizziness, and mental depression. Peripheral neuritis, psychoses, ataxia, vertigo, tinnitus, and convulsions have been reported rarely.

Gastrointestinal: Anorexia, nausea, vomiting, and diarrhea are common side effects of sulfonamide therapy.

Metabolic Effects: Sulfonamides cross the placenta and are excreted into breast milk. Since they compete with bilirubin for albumin binding, high levels of free bilirubin can cause kernicterus in infants born to mothers who take sulfonamides near term and in nursing neonates whose mothers are taking sulfonamides. The use of sulfonamides in pregnant women near term or in nursing mothers is inadvisable. In addition, sulfonamides should not be given to infants less than 2 months of age.

Miscellaneous Reactions: Sulfonamides have been reported to produce goiters.

Local irritation has been reported with sulfonamides that are administered by injection.

Drug Interactions and Interference With Laboratory Tests

Sulfonamides may displace certain drugs from plasma albumin and/or inhibit their biotransformation, thus potentiating their pharmacologic effect. For example, hypoglycemia has been reported after antibacterial sulfonamides were given to a few patients receiving tolbutamide [Orinase, SK-Tolbutamide] or chlorpropamide [Diabinese]; for this reason, these agents should be given cautiously to patients receiving any oral hypoglycemic agent. Sulfonamides also should be used cautiously with coumarin anticoagulants, methotrexate, and phenytoin [Dilantin], since they have been reported to enhance the action of these agents. Conversely, sulfonamides may be displaced from plasma protein binding sites by other drugs (eg, phenylbutazone [Azolid, Butazolidin], salicylates, probenecid [Benemid, SK-Probenecid]), resulting in increased sulfonamide activity.

Sulfamethizole [Thiosulfil] and sulfathiazole have formed insoluble precipitates with formaldehyde in the urine; therefore, concomitant administration of sulfonamides (especially the less soluble analogues) with methenamine compounds (eg, methenamine mandelate [Mandelamine]) should be avoided.

PABA-containing compounds and local anesthetics derived from PABA (eg, procaine [Novocain]) may directly inhibit the activity of sulfonamides.

Sulfonamides have been reported to produce false-positive Benedict's tests for urine glucose and false-positive sulfosalicylic acid tests for urine proteins. Sulfisoxazole has been reported to interfere with the Urobilistix test for urinary urobilinogen.

Pharmacokinetics

Routes of Administration: The sulfonamides usually are given orally. When parenteral administration is indicated, sulfisoxazole diolamine may be given subcutaneously or intravenously. Sulfadiazine sodium also may be administered intravenously. When the intravenous route is used, the drug must be well diluted and injected slowly to avoid extravasation. The alkaline sodium salts are too irritating to be given intramuscularly or subcutaneously.

Absorption: Following oral administration, the systemic sulfonamides are readily absorbed from the gastrointestinal tract, primarily from the small intestine. Estimates of therapeutically effective serum concentrations for most infections vary between 60 and 150 mcg/ml of free (ie, unconjugated, unbound) sulfonamide. Because the sulfonamides are concentrated in the urine, however, the serum levels necessary in the treatment of urinary tract infections may be lower than those needed for systemic infections. The serum levels of sulfacytine and sulfamethizole are too low to treat systemic infections outside the urinary tract because of rapid elimination of these drugs.

Distribution: All sulfonamides are reversibly bound to plasma proteins in varying degrees. These drugs are widely distributed throughout the body; concentrations approaching 80% of serum levels may be attained in pleural, synovial, peritoneal, and cerebrospinal fluids. Sulfonamides readily cross the placenta and are present in fetal blood and amniotic fluid. Blood and tissue levels are related to the degrees of protein binding and lipid solubilities of the various analogues.

Metabolism: Sulfonamides are metabolized to varying extents in the liver by acetylation or conjugation with glucuronic acid. Either process may alter solubility of the drug in urine, the major route of excretion. Acetylated metabolites and many conjugates are inactive.

Elimination: Both active unchanged sulfonamides and their metabolites are excreted by the kidneys. Excretion is primarily by glomerular filtration, although tubular reabsorption and active tubular secretion may play a role. The half-lives of sulfonamides are dependent on the rates of renal excretion. Generally, urinary excretion is more rapid for sulfonamides with low pKa values (eg, sulfisoxazole). Alkalization of the urine increases solubility and enhances urinary excretion.

The sulfonamides can be classified according to their duration of action in the body as short-, intermediate-, or long-acting. The long-acting sulfonamides are no longer marketed as single agents in the United States, however, because they have been associated with hypersensitivity reactions, such as the Stevens-Johnson syndrome.

Short-acting Sulfonamides: Sulfisoxazole, sulfamethizole, and sulfacytine are short-acting sulfonamides with half-lives of four to seven hours. Sulfamethizole and sulfacytine are eliminated primarily as unchanged drugs that are readily soluble in urine. Sulfisoxazole is eliminated as acetylated (30%) and free drug; both forms are readily soluble in urine.

Although sulfadiazine also is classified as short-acting, its half-life is 17 hours. It is partially acetylated. In contrast to other systemic sulfonamides, urinary solubility is a problem with sulfadiazine and the patient must be kept well hydrated (maintain urine volume of at least 1,500 ml/day in adults) to avoid crystalluria (see Adverse Reactions and Precautions).

Other short-acting sulfonamides (eg, sulfamerazine, sulfamethazine) are relatively insoluble or weakly anti-infective and are rarely used except in combination with other drugs. Sulfamerazine and sulfamethazine are combined with sulfadiazine in a short-acting mixture known as trisulfapyrimidines (see the section on Mixtures).

Intermediate-acting Sulfonamide: Sulfamethoxazole is an intermediate-acting sulfonamide with a half-life that ranges between 10 and 12 hours. It is partially acetylated. Although sulfamethoxazole requires less frequent administration than sulfisoxazole (twice versus four times daily), its acetylated metabolite is less soluble in urine. Thus, the risk of crystalluria is somewhat greater and the patient should be adequately hydrated (maintain urine volume of at least 1,500 ml/day in adults).

Drug Evaluations

Short-acting Sulfonamides

SULFACYTINE
[Renoquid]

MECHANISM OF ACTION, ANTIMICROBIAL SPECTRUM, AND RESISTANCE. See the Introduction.

USES. Sulfacytine is used only to treat acute, uncomplicated urinary tract infections caused by susceptible bacteria. However, sulfisoxazole is usually preferred to this sulfonamide. Because of rapid renal excretion, the plasma levels of sulfacytine are low and the drug is not used for systemic infections outside of the urinary tract.

ADVERSE REACTIONS AND PRECAUTIONS, DRUG INTERACTIONS, AND INTERFERENCE WITH LABORATORY TESTS. See the Introduction.

PHARMACOKINETICS. Sulfacytine is absorbed rapidly following oral administration. The half-life is approximately four hours, and the drug is 86% bound to serum proteins. More than 90% of a given dose is excreted by the kidneys, almost entirely in the free, active form. Sulfacytine is highly soluble in urine within the normal acidic pH range.

DOSAGE AND PREPARATIONS.
Oral: Adults, 500 mg initially, followed by 250 mg four times daily for up to ten days. *Children under 14 years* probably should not receive sulfacytine, since experience in children is lacking.
   Renoquid (Glenwood). Tablets 250 mg.

SULFADIAZINE

SULFADIAZINE SODIUM

MECHANISM OF ACTION, ANTIMICROBIAL SPECTRUM, AND RESISTANCE. See the Introduction.

USES. Sulfadiazine is a preferred drug for nocardiosis. Trisulfapyrimidines and sulfisoxazole are other sulfonamides that are used in this disease. Although sulfadiazine may be administered in the treatment of urinary tract infections, it is no longer a recommended sulfonamide because large doses and alkalization of the urine are necessary. The more soluble analogues (eg, sulfisoxazole) should be given for this indication. Sulfadiazine (or sulfisoxazole) is indicated for the prophylaxis of rheumatic fever in penicillin-allergic patients. Erythromycin is an alternative. The use of sulfadiazine for the prophylaxis of meningococcal meningitis in household or other close contacts should be restricted to cases in which the causative organism is known to be susceptible. Rifampin is the current drug of choice for this prophylactic indication.

Sulfadiazine may be a preferred sulfonamide in certain other susceptible systemic infections (eg, in combination with pyrimethamine for toxoplasmosis or for prophylaxis of malaria in which chloroquine-resistant strains of *Plasmodium falciparum* are common).

ADVERSE REACTIONS AND PRECAUTIONS. Sulfadiazine is less soluble in the urine than other currently available sulfonamides (eg, sulfisoxazole). Thus, the risk of crystalluria is greater. Patients receiving sulfadiazine must be kept well hydrated in order to maintain an adequate urinary volume (at least 1,500 ml daily in adults). Alkalization of the urine (eg, with sodium bicarbonate) increases urinary solubility.

For other adverse reactions and precautions, see the Introduction.

DRUG INTERACTIONS AND INTERFERENCE WITH LABORATORY TESTS. See the Introduction.

PHARMACOKINETICS. Orally administered sulfadiazine is rapidly absorbed and peak serum levels are attained within three to six hours after a single dose. About 45% of circulating sulfadiazine is bound to plasma proteins. The drug is widely distributed in body fluids and tissues, and therapeutic concentrations are attained in the cerebrospinal fluid. Between 15% and 40% of a dose is acetylated; both acetylated and unchanged drug are excreted by the kidney. The half-life is 17 hours.

DOSAGE AND PREPARATIONS. The blood level should be maintained at 100 to 150 mcg/ml.
Oral: Adults, 2 to 4 g initially, then 1 g every four to six hours. *Children and infants over 2 months,* 75 mg/kg initially, then 150 mg/kg daily in four to six divided doses. The total daily dose should not exceed 6 g. Duration of therapy for nocardiosis is four to six months or longer.

For prophylaxis of rheumatic fever, 500 mg once daily for patients under 27 kg and 1 g daily for those over 27 kg.

For prophylaxis of meningococcal disease (only if the *Neisseria meningitidis* isolate is known to be susceptible), *adults,* 1 g twice daily for two days; *children 1 to 12 years,* 500 mg twice daily for two days; *infants 2 months to 1 year,* 500 mg once daily for two days.

For dosage in toxoplasmosis, see Chapter 77, Antiprotozoal Agents.

SULFADIAZINE:
Generic. Tablets 500 mg.

Intravenous: Parenteral administration is not recommended and is rarely used. The sodium salt is highly alkaline and irritating. When parenteral administration is necessary, the drug may be given intravenously after it is well diluted with isotonic sodium chloride injection. Intrathecal, subcutaneous, or intramuscular administration is contraindicated.

Adults, initially, 100 mg/kg up to a total of 5 g, then 30 to 50 mg/kg every six to eight hours. *Children over 2 months,* 50 mg/kg initially, then 100 mg/kg daily in four divided doses. Oral therapy should be substituted as soon as possible.

SULFADIAZINE SODIUM:
Generic. Powder.

SULFAMETHIZOLE
[Thiosulfil]

MECHANISM OF ACTION, ANTIMICROBIAL SPECTRUM, AND RESISTANCE. See the Introduction.

USES. Sulfamethizole is used only to treat acute, uncomplicated urinary tract infections caused by susceptible bacteria. However, sulfisoxazole is usually preferred to this sulfonamide. Because of rapid renal excretion, the plasma levels of sulfamethizole are low and the drug is not used for systemic infections outside of the urinary tract.

ADVERSE REACTIONS AND PRECAUTIONS, DRUG INTERACTIONS, AND INTERFERENCE WITH LABORATORY TESTS. See the Introduction.

PHARMACOKINETICS. Sulfamethizole is readily absorbed following oral administration and is rapidly eliminated by renal excretion (80% of a dose is recovered in urine within eight hours). Approximately 90% of a dose is excreted in the active unchanged form, which is readily soluble in urine within the normal acidic pH range.

DOSAGE AND PREPARATIONS.
Oral: Adults, 500 mg to 1 g three or four times daily. *Children and infants over 2 months,* 30 to 45 mg/kg daily in four divided doses.

Thiosulfil Forte (Ayerst). Tablets 500 mg.

SULFISOXAZOLE
[Gantrisin]

SULFISOXAZOLE ACETYL
[Gantrisin]

SULFISOXAZOLE DIOLAMINE
[Gantrisin]

MECHANISM OF ACTION, ANTIMICROBIAL SPECTRUM, AND RESISTANCE. See the Introduction.

USES. Sulfisoxazole is a preferred sulfonamide for the treatment of acute, uncomplicated urinary tract infections; it is as effective as the other analogues and is less expensive. In addition to traditional multiple-dose therapy, a single 2-g dose of sulfisoxazole has been shown to be effective in treating initial attacks of cystitis in women who are not pregnant and who have no renal parenchymal involvement (see the Introduction).

Sulfisoxazole frequently is the preferred sulfonamide for susceptible systemic infections. Because of problems with amoxicillin-resistant strains of *Haemophilus influenzae,* sulfisoxazole, in combination with a penicillin or erythromycin, is often used to treat otitis media caused by such strains. This sulfonamide frequently is used for prophylaxis of recurrent otitis media. It is an alternative to sulfadiazine and trisulfapyrimidines in nocardiosis. Although it is not the drug of choice, sulfisoxazole has been used in chancroid, lymphogranuloma venereum, chlamydial pneumonia in infants, and melioidosis and for prophylaxis of rheumatic fever and meningococcal disease.

ADVERSE REACTIONS AND PRECAUTIONS, DRUG INTERACTIONS, AND INTERFERENCE WITH LABORATORY TESTS. See the Introduction.

PHARMACOKINETICS. Sulfisoxazole is absorbed rapidly and completely from the gastrointestinal tract following oral administration. Sulfisoxazole acetyl is a tasteless soluble derivative for oral use that usually is preferred by children. It is converted to sulfisoxazole in the intestine and, therefore, absorption of active drug is delayed with this preparation. Sulfisoxazole diolamine also is soluble and, since it causes minimal tissue irritation, is administered intravenously or subcutaneously. Oral administration of sulfisoxazole is preferred, however.

Sulfisoxazole is 90% bound to plasma proteins. The volume of distribution (0.15 L/kg) approximates that of the extracellular fluid. The drug readily distributes to most tissues and body fluids, including pleural, synovial, peritoneal, and cerebrospinal fluids, and crosses the placenta.

About 30% of a dose of sulfisoxazole is acetylated, and both the free and acetylated drug are rapidly eliminated by the kidneys. The half-life ranges from five to six hours, and about 95% of a dose is recovered from the urine within 24 hours. Both the free and acetylated forms are highly soluble in urine within the normal acidic pH range.

DOSAGE AND PREPARATIONS. All concentrations are expressed in terms of the base.
Oral: Adults, 2 to 4 g initially, then 4 to 8 g daily in four to six divided doses. *Children over 2 months,* 75 mg/kg initially, then 150 mg/kg daily in divided doses every four hours (maximum, 6 g daily). The dosage of the concentrated, timed-release preparation (***Lipo Gantrisin***) is: *Adults,* 4 to 5 g every 12 hours; *children over 2 months,* initially, 60 to 75 mg/kg, then 120 to 150 mg/kg daily in two divided doses (maximum, 6 g daily).

For single-dose therapy of initial attacks of acute uncomplicated lower urinary tract infections (ie, cystitis) in *adult women who are not pregnant and have no renal involvement,* 2 g in a single dose.

For dosages for prophylaxis of rheumatic fever, meningococcal disease, or recurrent otitis media, see Chapter 65, Antimicrobial Therapy and Chemoprophylaxis of Infectious Diseases, Table 3.
SULFISOXAZOLE:
Gantrisin (Roche), ***Generic.*** Tablets 500 mg.

SULFISOXAZOLE ACETYL:
Gantrisin (Roche). Suspension (pediatric) 500 mg/5 ml; syrup 500 mg/5 ml; liquid (timed-release) 1 g/5 ml (***Lipo Gantrisin***).
Intravenous, Subcutaneous: *Adults and children over 2 months,* 50 mg/kg initially, then 100 mg/kg daily in four (intravenous) or three (subcutaneous) divided doses.
SULFISOXAZOLE DIOLAMINE:
Gantrisin (Roche). Solution 400 mg/ml in 5 ml containers.
(NOTE: Gantrisin injectable was discontinued after this chapter was completed.)

Intermediate-acting Sulfonamide

SULFAMETHOXAZOLE
[Gantanol]

MECHANISM OF ACTION, ANTIMICROBIAL SPECTRUM, AND RESISTANCE. See the Introduction.

USES. The indications for this intermediate-acting sulfonamide are the same as for sulfisoxazole and include lower urinary tract and certain systemic infections caused by susceptible organisms. Because sulfamethoxazole is eliminated more slowly than sulfisoxazole, it requires less frequent administration, which may help with compliance. However, the acetylated metabolite of sulfamethoxazole is less soluble in urine and the risk of crystalluria is greater. During therapy, maintenance of an adequate urinary output (at least 1,500 ml daily in adults) by ensuring adequate fluid intake is important, but alkalization of the urine usually is unnecessary. See the evaluation on Sulfisoxazole and the Introduction.

Sulfamethoxazole also is marketed with trimethoprim as a fixed-ratio combination for oral and parenteral use (see the evaluation on this mixture).

ADVERSE REACTIONS AND PRECAUTIONS, DRUG INTERACTIONS, AND INTERFERENCE WITH LABORATORY TESTS. See the Introduction.

PHARMACOKINETICS. Sulfamethoxazole is completely absorbed following oral administration, although it is absorbed more slowly than sulfisoxazole. It is 70% bound to plasma proteins. The volume of distribution (0.21 L/kg) approximates that of the extracellular fluid. The drug readily distributes to most tissues and body fluids, including pleural, synovial, peritoneal, and cerebrospinal fluids, and crosses the placenta.

Sulfamethoxazole is partially acetylated; both free and acetylated drug are eliminated by the kidneys, primarily by glomerular filtration. The half-life ranges from 10 to 12 hours, which is longer than the half-life of sulfisoxazole. As discussed above, acetylated sulfamethoxazole is less soluble than acetylated sulfisoxazole in the urine.

DOSAGE AND PREPARATIONS.
Oral: Adults, 2 g initially, then 1 g two or, for severe infections, three times daily. *Children over 2 months,* initially, 50 to 60 mg/kg then one-half of this amount every 12 hours (maximum, 75 mg/kg/24 hours).
Generic. Tablets 500 mg and 1 g.
Gantanol (Roche). Suspension 500 mg/5 ml; tablets 500 mg and 1 g (***Gantanol DS***).

MIXTURES

Mixture Containing Only Sulfonamides

The rationale for combining several sulfonamides in a single preparation for systemic use is that the solubilities of the sulfonamides are independent of each other but their therapeutic effects are additive. Use of combination therapy thereby decreases the risk of crystalluria. Trisulfapyrimidines is the only such mixture still marketed. The availability of newer single-entity agents (eg, sulfisoxazole) that are more soluble in urine has made combined sulfonamide preparations essentially obsolete for systemic indications.

TRISULFAPYRIMIDINES
[Terfonyl]

This combination contains equal amounts of sulfadiazine, sulfamerazine, and sulfamethazine. It appears to produce somewhat higher total blood levels of sulfonamide than equal doses of sulfadiazine alone, but the effectiveness remains the same. The incidence of crystalluria (but not of other untoward effects) is reduced with trisulfapyrimidines when compared to larger doses of the individual components. However, newer sulfonamides (eg, sulfisoxazole) are considerably more soluble than trisulfapyrimidines and are usually preferred.

For actions, antimicrobial spectrum, indications, adverse reactions and precautions, and drug interactions, see the Introduction.

DOSAGE AND PREPARATIONS.
Oral: Adults, 3 to 4 g initially, then 1 g every six hours. *Children and infants over 2 months,* 75 mg/kg initially, then 150 mg/kg daily in four to six divided doses.
  Terfonyl (Squibb), **Generic.** Suspension 500 mg/5 ml; tablets 500 mg.

Mixtures Containing a Sulfonamide and Another Drug

Fixed-ratio combinations containing a sulfonamide and phenazopyridine, a urinary tract analgesic, or a sulfonamide and another antimicrobial agent presently are available for systemic use. See the evaluations for discussions. See the section on Dihydrofolate Reductase Inhibitors for the evaluation on Trimethoprim/Sulfamethoxazole.

SULFONAMIDES AND PHENAZOPYRIDINE

Phenazopyridine, a urinary tract analgesic, is combined with sulfonamides (eg, sulfisoxazole, sulfamethizole, sulfamethoxazole) in fixed-ratio preparations promoted for the treatment of urinary tract infections. Since phenazopyridine may relieve such symptoms as pain, burning, urgency, and frequency, its concomitant use with a sulfonamide may be beneficial. However, this analgesic preferably should be given separately rather than in a fixed-ratio combination product so that it can be eliminated from the regimen as soon as symptoms are controlled. Phenazopyridine therapy should not be continued beyond the first 48 hours in urinary tract infections because efficacy has not been demonstrated after this time (*Federal Register*, 1983).

Some sulfonamide/phenazopyridine preparations also contain a tetracycline; these are not recommended (see Chapter 69, Tetracyclines and Chloramphenicol).

DOSAGE AND PREPARATIONS.
Oral: Dosage is the same as that for the sulfonamide without phenazopyridine (see the appropriate evaluation). Treatment with the fixed-ratio combination products should not exceed two days. The sulfonamide should be given alone after this period.
  Azo Gantanol (Roche). Each tablet contains sulfamethoxazole 500 mg and phenazopyridine hydrochloride 100 mg.
  Azo Gantrisin (Roche). Each tablet contains sulfisoxazole 500 mg and phenazopyridine hydrochloride 50 mg.
  Thiosulfil-A (Ayerst). Each tablet contains sulfamethizole 250 or 500 mg (**Thiosulfil-A Forte**) and phenazopyridine hydrochloride 50 mg.
Because proof of efficacy is lacking, the following product is not recommended:
  Urobiotic-250 (Roerig). Each capsule contains sulfamethizole 250 mg, oxytetracycline hydrochloride equivalent to oxytetracycline 250 mg, and phenazopyridine hydrochloride 50 mg.

ERYTHROMYCIN ETHYLSUCCINATE AND SULFISOXAZOLE ACETYL
[Pediazole]

This fixed-ratio combination is used to treat acute otitis media and also may be effective in acute bacterial sinusitis. The most likely causative organisms of these infections are *Streptococcus pneumoniae* and *Haemophilus influenzae*. Amoxicillin (or ampicillin) traditionally has been preferred, but the increasing emergence of resistant strains of *H. influenzae* is becoming a major problem in some areas. The alternative therapies for patients in whom amoxicillin-resistant *H. influenzae* is a possibility or who cannot tolerate penicillins are erythromycin (to cover *S. pneumoniae*) plus a sulfonamide (to cover *H. influenzae*), trimethoprim/sulfamethoxazole, and cefaclor [Ceclor]. The latter drug is inappropriate in patients who exhibit an immediate-type hypersensitivity reaction to penicillin, however.

There is no antibacterial advantage (eg, no synergistic action) when erythromycin and sulfisoxazole are combined in a fixed-ratio preparation; administration of the two agents independently should be as effective. However, the fixed-ratio combination is more convenient to administer, a possible advantage in young children with acute otitis media.

The actions, pharmacokinetics, and adverse effects associated with Pediazole are the same as those expected from equivalent doses of the individual agents (see the evaluation on Sulfisoxazole in this chapter and on Erythromycin in Chapter 68, Macrolides and Lincosamides).

DOSAGE AND PREPARATIONS.
Oral: Children over 2 months may be given the drug every six

hours for ten days according to the following schedule suggested by the manufacturer: *Less than 8 kg*, dosage is adjusted according to body weight; *8 kg*, 2.5 ml; *16 kg*, 5 ml; *24 kg*, 7.5 ml; and *more than 45 kg*, 10 ml. These doses are administered every six hours.

> **Pediazole** (Ross). Granules for reconstitution in 100, 150, and 200 ml containers. Reconstituted suspension contains erythromycin ethylsuccinate equivalent to 200 mg erythromycin activity and sulfisoxazole acetyl equivalent to 600 mg sulfisoxazole/5 ml.

DIHYDROFOLATE REDUCTASE INHIBITORS

Trimethoprim, a 2,4-diaminopyrimidine, is the prototype of a group of nonsulfonamide drugs that inhibit dihydrofolate reductases of bacterial (also protozoal) but not mammalian cells, thus preventing the formation of tetrahydrofolic acid. This ability to selectively inhibit an enzyme that is essential to the growth of certain bacteria results in antibacterial activity with limited toxicity to the host. Furthermore, the combination of trimethoprim with a sulfonamide (eg, sulfamethoxazole) results in a synergistic antibacterial effect due to the sequential blockade of two steps in the same biosynthetic pathway (see Figure 2 in the Introduction and the evaluation on Trimethoprim/Sulfamethoxazole).

TRIMETHOPRIM
[Proloprim, Trimpex]

MECHANISM OF ACTION. Trimethoprim competitively inhibits the conversion of dihydrofolic acid to tetrahydrofolic acid by blocking the action of bacterial dihydrofolate reductase (see Figure 2 in the Introduction). Trimethoprim is about 50,000 times more active against bacterial dihydrofolate reductase than against the human enzyme. Lack of tetrahydrofolic acid prevents the one-carbon transfer reactions necessary for the synthesis of certain amino acids (eg, glycine, methionine), purines, and thymidine and, ultimately, DNA, RNA, and protein. Since thymidine biosynthesis by thymidylate synthetase requires stoichiometric amounts of tetrahydrofolic acid, this is believed to be the critical reaction that is prevented by trimethoprim. Trimethoprim may be bacteriostatic or bactericidal depending on the growth conditions. Because pus contains thymine and thymidine, the action of trimethoprim may be inhibited in necrotic wounds containing pus and other cellular debris.

ANTIMICROBIAL SPECTRUM. Trimethoprim is active in vitro against many gram-positive cocci, including *Staphylococcus aureus*, *S. saprophyticus*, *Streptococcus pyogenes*, *S. pneumoniae*, viridans streptococci, and *S. faecalis*. Some gram-positive bacilli, such as *Corynebacterium diphtheriae* and *Listeria monocytogenes*, also are susceptible. *Clostridium perfringens* and most anaerobes are resistant, however.

The gram-negative cocci, *Neisseria meningitidis* and *N. gonorrhoeae*, show a variable response, but many strains are resistant.

The majority of clinically important aerobic gram-negative bacilli, including *Escherichia coli*, *Klebsiella*, *Enterobacter*, *Proteus mirabilis*, *Serratia marcescens*, *Salmonella*, *Shigella*, and *Haemophilus influenzae*, are susceptible. *Pseudomonas aeruginosa*, *Bacteroides*, and other anaerobes are resistant, however.

Nocardia asteroides is variably susceptible. Trimethoprim is active against certain pathogenic protozoa (eg, *Pneumocystis carinii*), *Toxoplasma* species, and plasmodia that cause malaria.

Treponema pallidum and *Mycobacterium tuberculosis* are resistant. Trimethoprim is not effective against fungi or viruses.

RESISTANCE. Several mechanisms may confer resistance to trimethoprim. Thymine- or thymidine-dependent bacterial mutants are intrinsically resistant to trimethoprim because they lack thymidylate synthetase and, thus, depend on exogenous thymine and thymidine for growth (Brumfitt and Hamilton-Miller, 1980). Fortunately, such organisms appear to cause disease only rarely in man (Maskell et al, 1978). Organisms may develop resistance to trimethoprim by altering the nature of dihydrofolate reductase (eg, increased levels of enzyme and/or decreased affinity for trimethoprim) or by decreasing permeability of the bacteria to the drug. An enzyme that destroys trimethoprim is not elaborated.

Acquired resistance to trimethoprim can be mediated by both chromosomal and plasmid mechanisms (see Rubin and Swartz, 1980; Brogden et al, 1982). Among the Enterobacteriaceae, a high-level resistance to trimethoprim that results from the production of a trimethoprim-resistant dihydrofolate reductase is increasing and may be of particular clinical importance. This type of resistance is mediated by transferable plasmids or by transposons (Acar and Goldstein, 1982; Towner, 1982; Brumfitt et al, 1983).

Considerable controversy has revolved around whether trimethoprim alone is more likely to cause the development of resistant bacterial strains than the combination of trimethoprim and sulfamethoxazole. The combination was originally marketed in preference to trimethoprim alone because of the drugs' synergistic action and because it was believed that the exclusive use of the combination would prevent the emergence of organisms resistant to either agent. Although considerable clinical work has been conducted to test the latter premise, the controversy has not been completely resolved. In Finland, where trimethoprim alone has been used to treat urinary tract infections for over ten years, widespread resistance to this drug has not emerged (Kasanen and Sundquist, 1982). Similar results were reported in London (Brumfitt et al, 1983). However, an increase in trimethoprim-resistant but sulfonamide-sensitive clinical isolates of Enterobacteriaceae in Nottingham has been reported (Towner, 1982). To date, significant resistance has not developed to either the combination or to trimethoprim alone in the United States. In summary, although there is no strong evidence that there will be a more rapid increase in resistance to trimethoprim as the result of its use alone, additional clinical experience with trimethoprim alone and continued surveillance of resistance patterns is necessary before more definitive recommendations can be made (see the evaluation on Trimethoprim/Sulfamethoxazole; also, see Rubin and Swartz, 1980; Friesen et al, 1981; Brogden et al, 1982; Reeves, 1982; Smith and Sensakovic, 1982).

USES. Trimethoprim alone is labeled only for the initial treatment of acute, uncomplicated urinary tract infections (eg, cystitis) caused by susceptible organisms, particularly *E. coli*, *P. mirabilis*, *K. pneumoniae*, *Enterobacter* species, and *S. saprophyticus*. Urinary concentrations of the drug greatly exceed those required to inhibit sensitive pathogens, and trimethoprim appears to be as effective as trimethoprim/ sulfamethoxazole for initial episodes of acute, uncomplicated urinary tract infections (see Brogden et al, 1982). However, a sulfonamide, ampicillin, or amoxicillin frequently is preferred for this infection when caused by a susceptible organism (see Table 1 in Chapter 65, Antimicrobial Therapy and Chemoprophylaxis of Infectious Diseases).

A single daily dose of trimethoprim also is effective for the prophylaxis of recurrent urinary tract infections in women. Presently, however, trimethoprim/sulfamethoxazole is preferred for this indication (see this evaluation and Chapter 65, Table 3).

Trimethoprim, a relatively lipophilic compound, is one of the few antibacterial agents that adequately penetrates into the uninflamed prostate gland. Therefore, it is useful in the treatment of chronic bacterial prostatitis, an infection that is difficult to cure. Presently, trimethoprim/sulfamethoxazole is the regimen of choice for this infection and trimethoprim is used in sulfonamide-allergic patients. Some infectious disease experts believe that trimethoprim alone should be the preferred agent for chronic prostatitis, however, because sulfamethoxazole fails to achieve therapeutic concentrations in the uninflamed prostate (Friesen et al, 1981; Reeves, 1982). See also the evaluation on Trimethoprim/Sulfamethoxazole and Chapter 65, Table 1.

Trimethoprim appears to be an effective alternative to trimethoprim/sulfamethoxazole in certain patients (eg, sulfonamide-allergic) both for the treatment and prophylaxis of travelers' diarrhea (DuPont et al, 1982, 1983; see also Chapter 65, Tables 1 and 3).

It has been suggested that trimethoprim alone also may be useful in other infections (eg, otitis media, upper and lower respiratory tract infections, typhoid fever). However, the available clinical evidence is very limited and additional studies are necessary. For treatment of *Pneumocystis carinii* pneumonitis, only the combination of trimethoprim/sulfamethoxazole should be employed (see the evaluation).

A primary advantage of trimethoprim over trimethoprim/ sulfamethoxazole is the likelihood of fewer adverse effects when compared to sulfonamides. Also, trimethoprim can be given to patients with impaired renal function or to those who cannot tolerate sulfonamides (Kunin et al, 1978). However, the fear of increasing the emergence of trimethoprim-resistant organisms when the drug is used alone, particularly with prolonged use or in hospital environments, is a potential problem that remains controversial (see the preceding section on Resistance).

ADVERSE REACTIONS AND PRECAUTIONS. Trimethoprim generally is well tolerated. The overall frequency of side effects with this drug alone has been less than for trimethoprim/ sulfamethoxazole when these regimens have been compared in the treatment of urinary tract infections (see Brogden et al, 1982).

The most common adverse effects are pruritus and skin rash. Maculopapular and morbilliform rashes have been reported most often, but exfoliative dermatitis also has been observed. Gastrointestinal reactions also are common and include epigastric distress, nausea, vomiting, and glossitis. Hematologic reactions, including thrombocytopenia, leukopenia, neutropenia, megaloblastic anemia, and methemoglobinemia, are rare and occur most often when large doses and/or prolonged therapy are used or when the drug is administered to patients with folate deficiencies. Fever and elevated levels of serum transaminases, bilirubin, blood urea nitrogen, and serum creatinine have been noted.

Trimethoprim should be used with caution in patients with possible folate deficiency (eg, alcoholics, debilitated patients, pregnant women, patients receiving phenytoin, patients with malabsorption syndromes). Folinic acid can be administered concomitantly to prevent the antifolate effects of trimethoprim without decreasing its antibacterial efficacy.

Caution is recommended in patients with impaired renal or hepatic function. Dosage reductions are necessary when creatinine clearance is between 15 and 30 ml/minute. The use of trimethoprim in patients with a creatinine clearance below 15 ml/min is not recommended.

Since trimethoprim is a folate antagonist, it might be expected to cause teratogenic effects. Fetal malformations have occurred in rats given large doses, but have not yet been reported clinically. Nevertheless, because of the lack of published data on use of the drug in pregnant women and because folate levels are probably marginal during pregnancy, trimethoprim is generally contraindicated in pregnant women or should be used only when the potential benefit justifies the potential risk to the fetus (FDA Pregnancy Category C). Caution should be exercised when trimethoprim is administered to nursing mothers since it is excreted in human milk and may interfere with folate metabolism in the nursing infant. Infants younger than 2 months should not be given the drug since its safety has not been established in this age group.

PHARMACOKINETICS. Trimethoprim is absorbed rapidly and completely from the gastrointestinal tract. Peak serum concentrations are attained one to four hours after oral administration. Mean peak serum levels of approximately 1 mcg/ml can be attained after an initial dose of 100 mg.

Trimethoprim is not highly protein bound; levels of 40% to 70% have been reported (Bennett et al, 1980). It is widely distributed in the body and the volume of distribution is 1.8 ± 0.2 L/kg (Benet and Sheiner, 1980). This compound is relatively lipophilic and diffuses well into tissues and body fluids (Brumfitt and Hamilton-Miller, 1980; Friesen et al, 1981; Brogden et al, 1982). Concentrations equal to or greater than serum levels occur in prostate tissue and fluid, saliva, sputum, bronchial and vaginal secretions, and cerebrospinal and synovial fluids. Therapeutic concentrations also can be achieved in bile, seminal fluid, bone tissue, and aqueous humor. Trimethoprim readily crosses the placenta.

The kidneys are the main organs of excretion through glomerular filtration and tubular secretion. The half-life in patients with normal renal function is 11 ± 1.4 hours (Benet and Sheiner, 1980); the half-life is prolonged in those with severe renal impairment. After oral administration, 50% to 60% of a dose is recovered in the urine within 24 hours; about 80% is unchanged drug and the remainder is inactive oxidized or hydroxylated metabolites. Urinary concentrations of trimethoprim are considerably higher than serum levels. After a single oral dose of 100 mg, urine concentrations ranged from 30 to 160 mcg/ml during the first four hours and declined to between 18 and 91 mcg/ml from 8 to 24 hours.

DOSAGE AND PREPARATIONS.

Oral: For acute, uncomplicated urinary tract infections, *adults and children over 12 years*, 100 mg every 12 hours or 200 mg every 24 hours, each for ten days. The use of trimethoprim in patients with creatinine clearance of less than 15 ml/min is not recommended. When creatinine clearance is between 15 and 30 ml/min, a dose of 50 mg every 12 hours should be employed.

For prophylaxis of recurrent urinary tract infections in women, *adults*, 50 to 100 mg once daily at bedtime. Duration of prophylaxis generally is for six months.

For chronic prostatitis (eg, in sulfonamide-allergic patients), *adults*, 200 mg twice daily for 12 weeks.

For the treatment of travelers' diarrhea, *adults*, 200 mg twice daily for five days (DuPont et al, 1982). For the prophylaxis of travelers' diarrhea, *adults*, 200 mg once daily beginning on day of travel and continuing two days after return home (DuPont et al, 1983; Satterwhite and DuPont, 1983).

Proloprim (Burroughs Wellcome). Tablets 100 and 200 mg.
Trimpex (Roche), **Generic.** Tablets 100 mg.

Mixture

TRIMETHOPRIM/SULFAMETHOXAZOLE
[Bactrim, Septra]

MECHANISM OF ACTION. Trimethoprim/sulfamethoxazole inhibits sequential steps in the synthesis of tetrahydrofolic acid, an essential metabolic cofactor in the bacterial synthesis of purines, thymidine, glycine, and methionine. Sulfonamides, including sulfamethoxazole, are structural analogues of PABA and block the synthesis of dihydropteroic acid, the immediate precursor of dihydrofolic acid, from PABA and pteridine. Trimethoprim subsequently acts to inhibit the reduction of dihydrofolic acid to the metabolically active tetrahydrofolic acid by the enzyme, dihydrofolate reductase (see Figure 2 in the Introduction). The most important consequence of this sequential enzymatic inhibition appears to be the interruption of thymidine synthesis.

Combining the two antimetabolites has the following theoretical advantages. Antibacterial synergism is observed in vitro, ie, most bacteria are considerably more susceptible to the combination than to either of the agents used alone.

Whereas the individual drugs are primarily bacteriostatic at therapeutic concentrations, the combination is usually bactericidal. The concomitant use of the two drugs also should reduce the rate of emergence of resistant bacterial strains.

Since mammalian cells do not produce folic acid, the sulfamethoxazole-induced inhibition of folic acid synthesis does not take place in man. Also, the affinity of trimethoprim for bacterial dihydrofolate reductase is about 50,000 times greater than for the human enzyme. Thus, a high therapeutic/toxic ratio is obtained with trimethoprim/sulfamethoxazole.

ANTIMICROBIAL SPECTRUM. Among aerobic gram-negative enteric bacteria, *Escherichia coli, Proteus mirabilis, Salmonella* (including *S. typhi*), *Shigella,* and *Citrobacter* are very susceptible. Indole-positive *Proteus, Serratia marcescens, Klebsiella pneumoniae, Enterobacter,* and *Providencia stuartii* are moderately susceptible.

Other gram-negative bacilli that are very susceptible to trimethoprim/sulfamethoxazole include *Haemophilus influenzae, Vibrio cholerae,* and *Yersinia pestis. Acinetobacter, Bordetella pertussis, Brucella, Gardnerella (Haemophilus) vaginalis, H. ducreyi, Pseudomonas pseudomallei, P. cepacia,* and *Yersinia enterocolitica* also are susceptible. *Bacteroides* and *Fusobacterium,* gram-negative anaerobes, are usually resistant. *Pseudomonas aeruginosa* is resistant.

Most strains of *Neisseria meningitidis* and *N. gonorrhoeae,* gram-negative cocci, are susceptible.

Most gram-positive bacteria are susceptible to trimethoprim/sulfamethoxazole in vitro, but there are only limited clinical data regarding treatment of systemic infections caused by these organisms. *Staphylococcus aureus* (including many methicillin-resistant strains), *Streptococcus pneumoniae,* and *S. pyogenes* are susceptible in vitro, although resistant strains of *S. pneumoniae* have been reported. The response of *S. faecalis* is variable.

Nocardia, Chlamydia trachomatis, and *Pneumocystis carinii* are susceptible. *Mycobacterium marinum* is susceptible, but other mycobacteria are resistant. *Treponema pallidum* is resistant.

The maximum synergistic interaction between trimethoprim and sulfamethoxazole is observed when the microorganism is susceptible to both drugs. However, synergistic activity also has been observed when organisms are sulfamethoxazole-resistant and trimethoprim-susceptible or moderately trimethoprim-resistant. Intrinsic susceptibility to trimethoprim is a major factor in determining the efficacy of the combination.

RESISTANCE. The frequency of development of bacterial resistance to trimethoprim/sulfamethoxazole is considered to be lower than it is to either of the agents alone. Resistance to trimethoprim has received the most attention. Major mechanisms include increased levels of dihydrofolate reductase and production of an altered dihydrofolate reductase with a decreased binding affinity for trimethoprim. Decreased permeability of the bacterial cell to trimethoprim has been reported rarely (eg, for *Pseudomonas aeruginosa*). In gram-negative bacteria (eg, Enterobacteriaceae), resistance frequently is associated with the presence of R-factors that can be transferred to susceptible organisms by conjugation. Resistance to trimethoprim also may be chromosomally mediated or carried on transposons (see also the evaluation on Trimethoprim). For mechanisms of resistance to sulfonamides, see the Introduction.

Presently, controversy exists concerning whether there is, in fact, less development of resistance to trimethoprim/sulfamethoxazole than to trimethoprim alone. Some infectious disease experts have suggested that the latter agent used alone may be just as effective but less toxic than the combination for certain infections (eg, acute urinary tract and upper respiratory tract infections, otitis media, prostatitis). Additional clinical experience with trimethoprim alone and continued surveillance of resistance patterns are necessary before more definitive recommendations can be made (see the evaluation on Trimethoprim; also, see Rubin and Swartz, 1980; Friesen et al, 1981; Brogden et al, 1982; Reeves, 1982; Smith and Sensakovic, 1982).

USES. Trimethoprim/sulfamethoxazole is a preferred or alternative antimicrobial regimen for a number of infectious diseases as outlined below. For additional discussion, see Chapter 65, Antimicrobial Therapy and Chemoprophylaxis of Infectious Diseases.

Urinary Tract Infections: This combination is recommended for the treatment of upper or lower urinary tract infections due to susceptible strains of *Escherichia coli, Klebsiella, Enterobacter, Proteus mirabilis, P. vulgaris,* and *Morganella morganii.* Intravenous administration is preferred for severe infections.

For conventional (multiple-dose) treatment (7 to 14 days) of initial episodes of uncomplicated urinary tract infections, effective single-agent therapy (eg, with sulfisoxazole or ampicillin) may be preferred to trimethoprim/sulfamethoxazole, depending upon resistance patterns of urinary isolates. However, this combination has been shown to be particularly useful in single-dose treatment of initial attacks of acute cystitis in nonpregnant women with no renal parenchymal involvement and who are available for follow-up. The recommended dose for adults is trimethoprim 160 mg/sulfamethoxazole 800 mg (ie, one double-strength tablet). Amoxicillin 3 g or sulfisoxazole 2 g are alternatives.

Trimethoprim (40 mg)/sulfamethoxazole (200 mg), ie, one-half regular-strength tablet, at bedtime three times per week on Sunday, Wednesday, and Friday is preferred for the long-term (eg, six months or longer) prophylaxis of recurrent urinary tract infections in selected women. Once daily nitrofurantoin or trimethoprim alone is an alternative.

Trimethoprim/sulfamethoxazole is the therapy of choice for acute and chronic prostatitis. Chronic prostatitis requires a prolonged course of therapy (eg, adults, trimethoprim 160 mg/sulfamethoxazole 800 mg [ie, one double-strength tablet] twice daily for 12 weeks). Trimethoprim alone and carbenicillin indanyl are alternatives for chronic prostatitis.

Respiratory Tract Infections: Trimethoprim/sulfamethoxazole is useful for the treatment of acute otitis media and acute sinusitis caused by susceptible strains of *Streptococcus pneumoniae* and *Haemophilus influenzae* when there are advantages over amoxicillin, the usual drug of choice (eg, in penicillin-allergic patients, presence of amoxicillin-resistant *H. influenzae* strain). This combination

also has been used as an alternative to sulfisoxazole or ampicillin for long-term (eg, six months) prophylaxis of recurrent otitis media in selected children.

Trimethoprim/sulfamethoxazole is recommended for acute exacerbations of chronic bronchitis caused by susceptible strains of *S. pneumoniae* and *H. influenzae* when there are advantages over single agents (eg, amoxicillin, tetracycline). Based on currently available data, however, the effectiveness of antimicrobial drug therapy for this indication is uncertain.

Although not the therapy of choice, trimethoprim/sulfamethoxazole can be effective in pneumonias caused by sensitive *H. influenzae* or other gram-negative bacteria. Intravenous administration should be used in seriously ill patients.

Trimethoprim/sulfamethoxazole is an alternative to erythromycin for the elimination of *B. pertussis* carriage in patients with pertussis.

Trimethoprim/sulfamethoxazole is *not* recommended for pharyngitis due to *Streptococcus pyogenes* because failures have been reported.

Gastrointestinal Infections: Trimethoprim/sulfamethoxazole is the regimen of choice for shigellosis caused by susceptible strains of *Shigella flexneri* and *S. sonnei.* Antibacterial agents shorten the duration of illness and decrease the relapse rate in this disease.

Antibacterial agents are not useful for simple gastroenteritis caused by *Salmonella.* However, they are indicated for typhoid fever (*S. typhi*) or for systemic infections (eg, bacteremia) caused by other species of *Salmonella.* Presently, trimethoprim/sulfamethoxazole is an alternative to chloramphenicol and ampicillin for these infections. The combination also may be effective in eliminating chronic *Salmonella* carriage.

Travelers' diarrhea is most frequently caused by enterotoxigenic strains of *Escherichia coli* (about 50% of cases); *Shigella* (15%) and other enteric pathogens are less common causes of this disease. Trimethoprim/sulfamethoxazole has been shown to be effective in the treatment of travelers' diarrhea (DuPont et al, 1982) and presently is recommended for more severe cases (National Institutes of Health Consensus Development Conference, 1985). This combination also is effective for the prophylaxis of travelers' diarrhea (DuPont et al, 1983). Prophylaxis generally is not recommended, however, because of the potential for adverse drug reactions and the emergence of resistant bacterial strains (National Institutes of Health Consensus Development Conference, 1985; see also Table 3 in Chapter 65).

Trimethoprim/sulfamethoxazole is an alternative to tetracycline in cholera.

Sexually Transmitted Diseases: Although most strains of *Neisseria gonorrhoeae* are susceptible to trimethoprim/sulfamethoxazole, single-dose regimens of other drugs (eg, amoxicillin, ampicillin, ceftriaxone [Rocephin], penicillin G procaine, spectinomycin [Trobicin]) usually are preferred for uncomplicated gonococcal infections. Larger oral doses of trimethoprim/sulfamethoxazole (ie, a single daily dose of nine regular strength [80 mg/400 mg] tablets for five days) appear to be particularly useful in pharyngeal gonococcal infections caused by penicillinase-producing *N. gonorrhoeae* (PPNG) strains because spectinomycin is not effective in this form of the disease. However, a single 250-mg dose of ceftriaxone, intramuscularly, also is effective and may be preferred (see *Morbid Mortal Week Rep*, 1985, and Chapter 65, Table 2).

Trimethoprim/sulfamethoxazole is an alternative to erythromycin or ceftriaxone (preferred regimens) in chancroid. Although chlamydial infections and granuloma inguinale may respond to this combination, tetracyclines are preferred. This preparation is not active in syphilis.

Trimethoprim/sulfamethoxazole has been used as an alternative to metronidazole or ampicillin for bacterial vaginosis (formerly called nonspecific vaginitis), but published clinical data are lacking.

Other Infections: Trimethoprim/sulfamethoxazole is a therapy of choice for melioidosis (tetracycline with or without chloramphenicol is preferred by some clinicians) and *Pseudomonas cepacia* infections. This combination also may be an effective alternative for nocardiosis (sulfonamides, eg, sulfadiazine, trisulfapyrimidines, are usually preferred); brucellosis (tetracycline with or without streptomycin is preferred); and infections caused by *Mycobacterium marinum* (minocycline is preferred).

Trimethoprim/sulfamethoxazole may be useful in serious infections, including meningitis, osteomyelitis, bacteremia, and endocarditis, caused by susceptible gram-negative bacteria when other antibacterial agents are ineffective or not tolerated. This combination may be an effective alternative to ampicillin (or penicillin G) with or without an aminoglycoside for the treatment of meningitis caused by *Listeria monocytogenes* (Levitz and Quintiliani, 1984). In a double-blind, randomized, prospective study, intravenous trimethoprim/sulfamethoxazole (640/3,200 mg daily) was shown to be as effective as vancomycin in the treatment of serious methicillin-resistant *Staphylococcus aureus* infections, including bacteremias, endocarditis, septic arthritis, and osteomyelitis (Markowitz et al, 1983). Currently, each of these indications is considered investigational.

Pneumocystis carinii Pneumonia: This opportunistic protozoal infection frequently occurs in immunocompromised patients. High-dose oral or intravenous trimethoprim/sulfamethoxazole is considered to be the therapy of choice for this disease in children and adults with cancer or organ transplants because it is at least as effective but less toxic than the available alternative, pentamidine isethionate [Pentam 300] (Hughes et al, 1978; Winston et al, 1980; Sattler and Remington, 1981; Hughes, 1982; Young, 1982; Siegel et al, 1984). This combination also is effective in the prevention of *P. carinii* pneumonia (Hughes et al, 1977), and prophylaxis may be indicated in selected patients (eg, children with acute lymphocytic leukemia who are at high risk for this infection).

P. carinii pneumonia also is one of the most common opportunistic infections in patients with acquired immunodeficiency syndrome (AIDS). Although trimethoprim/sulfamethoxazole has been shown to be effective against *P. carinii* infections in some AIDS patients, its use has been associated with a high incidence of adverse reactions (see the section on Adverse Reactions and Precautions; see also Jaffe et al, 1983; Mitsuyasu et al, 1983; Gordin et al, 1984; Kovacs

et al, 1984; *Med Lett Drugs Ther*, 1985). Thus, it is not clear at the present time whether trimethoprim/sulfamethoxazole or pentamidine isethionate is preferred for *P. carinii* pneumonia in AIDS patients. Usually, these patients receive one regimen initially and the alternative regimen is substituted if there is poor response or a significant adverse reaction. For additional discussion, see Chapter 77, Antiprotozoal Agents.

Prophylaxis in Neutropenic Patients: Trimethoprim/sulfamethoxazole has been reported to be effective in reducing the incidence of gram-negative rod bacteremia in neutropenic patients, usually those with acute leukemias, in a number of clinical studies (Gurwith et al, 1979; Dekker et al, 1981; Kauffman et al, 1983; Wade et al, 1983; Riben et al, 1983; Estey et al, 1984). Some studies have failed to show a benefit from prophylaxis, however (Gaya et al, 1980; Henry et al, 1984; Kramer et al, 1984). Also, infections with trimethoprim/sulfamethoxazole-resistant organisms and prolongation of neutropenia in patients treated with this antimicrobial combination have been reported (Dekker et al, 1981; Wade et al, 1983; Woods et al, 1984). The role of trimethoprim/sulfamethoxazole in the prophylaxis of gram-negative bacillary infection in neutropenic cancer patients remains investigational and additional clinical trials are indicated.

ADVERSE REACTIONS AND PRECAUTIONS. Trimethoprim/sulfamethoxazole usually is well tolerated by adults (Lawson and Paice, 1982; Wormser et al, 1982) and children (Gutman, 1984); however, severe, including fatal, adverse reactions have been reported rarely (*FDA Drug Bull*, 1984). Any adverse effect reported with the use of sulfonamides or trimethoprim may occur following administration of the combination (see the Introduction and the evaluation on Trimethoprim).

Skin rashes are among the most common adverse effects caused by trimethoprim/sulfamethoxazole and are most often due to hypersensitivity to the sulfonamide component. These are usually mild, diffuse, maculopapular rashes that are reversible upon discontinuation of the drug. Serious skin reactions, including toxic epidermal necrolysis, erythema multiforme, exfoliative dermatitis, and the Stevens-Johnson syndrome, have occurred rarely.

Sulfonamides have caused leukopenia, thrombocytopenia, eosinophilia, agranulocytosis, bone marrow aplasia, and hemolytic anemia (both related to hypersensitivity and to G6PD deficiency). Some of these are hypersensitivity reactions. Because blood dyscrasias have been reported, blood tests should be performed at regular intervals during prolonged therapy. Although such tests detect the milder leukopenias, the sudden appearance of sore throat, fever, pallor, purpura, or jaundice may be an indication of a serious blood disorder and blood counts should be obtained.

Increased incidences of hematologic abnormalities, most commonly a transient and reversible neutropenia, in children receiving oral or intravenous trimethoprim/sulfamethoxazole have been reported by some investigators (Ardati et al, 1979; Asmar et al, 1981; see also Worsmer et al, 1982). However, it is unclear whether many of these observed hematologic abnormalities were actual adverse reactions caused by trimethoprim/sulfamethoxazole or were due to some other cause, such as an underlying viral illness (see Gutman, 1984; Feldman et al, 1985).

In addition to hypersensitivity reactions involving the skin and blood, trimethoprim/sulfamethoxazole has been associated with chills, drug fever, allergic vasculitis, a lupus erythematosus-like syndrome, and anaphylaxis. The sulfonamide component probably is the causative drug. Patients who are allergic to either component of the combination should not be given trimethoprim/sulfamethoxazole.

Trimethoprim has caused megaloblastosis due to its folate-depleting effect. This is uncommon and usually occurs in patients prone to folate deficiency including alcoholics, debilitated patients, pregnant women, patients receiving phenytoin, and patients with malabsorption syndromes. The administration of folinic acid reverses or prevents the adverse effect without affecting antimicrobial effectiveness.

Trimethoprim/sulfamethoxazole has caused mild reversible increases in serum creatinine levels. Interstitial nephritis is an uncommon, reversible adverse effect more frequently seen in patients with renal disease. Crystalluria can occur; therefore, patients taking this medication should maintain an adequate fluid intake. The dosage should be reduced in patients with impaired renal function. Liver damage (eg, inflammation, cholestatic jaundice) develops rarely.

Upper gastrointestinal irritation, manifested by anorexia, nausea, and vomiting, is common. Glossitis and stomatitis also have occurred. Diarrhea is relatively rare. Trimethoprim/sulfamethoxazole causes minimal change in the composition of the anaerobic fecal flora.

Headache, depression, hallucinations, and neuritis have occurred and are probably caused by the sulfonamide. Trimethoprim/sulfamethoxazole has been reported to cause aseptic meningitis in isolated patients (Kremer et al, 1983; Derbes, 1984).

Sulfonamides are similar chemically to some goitrogens and oral hypoglycemic agents. Goiters and hypoglycemia have occurred rarely.

This combination should not be used during pregnancy unless the potential benefits outweigh the risks (FDA Pregnancy Category C). Because of the risk of kernicterus, it should not be given to pregnant women at term, nursing mothers, or infants less than 2 months. Use of trimethoprim/sulfamethoxazole should be restricted in all patients considered to have marginal or reduced levels of folates, such as pregnant women, alcoholics, or malnourished individuals.

Pain and irritation have been reported infrequently following intravenous administration.

A high incidence (up to 80%) of adverse reactions to trimethoprim/sulfamethoxazole occurs in AIDS patients receiving this combination for the treatment or prophylaxis of *P. carinii* pneumonia (Jaffe et al, 1983; Mitsuyasu et al, 1983; Gordin et al, 1984; Kovacs et al, 1984). These adverse reactions are characterized by recurrent fever, maculopapular skin rash, and peripheral cytopenias (eg, neutropenia, thrombocytopenia). These are believed to be hypersensitivity reactions because they recur with drug rechallenge. Discontinuation of trimethoprim/sulfamethoxazole therapy frequently is necessary in these patients. Case reports on two AIDS patients suggest that administration of diphenhydramine (intravenous) with or without epinephrine (subcutaneous) may control these hypersensitivity reactions and allow continued therapy with trimethoprim/sulfamethoxazole (Gibbons and Lindauer, 1985).

DRUG INTERACTIONS. Trimethoprim/sulfamethoxazole may potentiate the anticoagulant effect of warfarin. Prothrombin time should be monitored. Trimethoprim/sulfamethoxazole can displace certain drugs from plasma protein binding sites. In particular, the combination has been shown to potentiate the hypoglycemic effect of oral hypoglycemic drugs and the bone marrow depressant effect of methotrexate. The half-life of phenytoin is prolonged. Sulfamethoxazole can be displaced from plasma protein binding sites by certain acidic drugs including phenylbutazone, dicumarol, and salicylic acid. Thrombocytopenia has occurred more frequently when sulfonamides and thiazide diuretics were administered concomitantly. Hyponatremia has been reported with concomitant trimethoprim and diuretic administration (Eastell and Edmonds, 1984).

PHARMACOKINETICS. Although the pharmacokinetics of trimethoprim and sulfamethoxazole are not identical, they are sufficiently similar that the administration of the fixed-ratio combination is rational in this regard.

Both trimethoprim and sulfamethoxazole are well absorbed from the upper intestinal tract. When administered in the standard 1:5 ratio tablet containing 80 mg of trimethoprim and 400 mg of sulfamethoxazole, peak plasma concentrations (of free drugs) of approximately 1 mcg/ml trimethoprim and 20 mcg/ml sulfamethoxazole are achieved in one to four hours. In vitro, the 1:20 ratio appears to provide optimum synergy against a number of bacterial species.

Trimethoprim/sulfamethoxazole also can be administered intravenously for more severe infections. Following repeated intravenous administration of 160 mg trimethoprim and 800 mg sulfamethoxazole every eight hours, the steady-state peak and trough plasma concentrations were 8.8 and 5.6 and 106 and 71 mcg/ml for trimethoprim and sulfamethoxazole, respectively.

Approximately 44% of trimethoprim and 70% of sulfamethoxazole are bound to plasma proteins. The volume of distribution of trimethoprim (1.8 L/kg) is considerably greater than that of sulfamethoxazole (0.21 L/kg). Because of the lipophilic properties of trimethoprim, it reaches considerably higher concentrations in various tissues and fluids when compared to sulfamethoxazole. These include prostatic fluid and tissue, vaginal secretions, middle ear fluid, cerebrospinal fluid, sputum, pleural effusions, lung tissue, bile, and aqueous humor. Because of differences in distribution between the two drugs, the 1:20 plasma ratio between trimethoprim and sulfamethoxazole is not obtained in these other body tissues and fluids. However, synergism occurs at other ratios. Trimethoprim/sulfamethoxazole crosses the placenta and is excreted in breast milk.

Both trimethoprim and sulfamethoxazole are eliminated primarily by the kidneys; both glomerular filtration and tubular secretion are involved. Approximately 50% to 60% of a dose of trimethoprim is recovered in the urine within 24 hours, 80% of which appears as unchanged drug; the remainder is excreted as inactive metabolites. In contrast, only about 20% to 30% of sulfamethoxazole is excreted into urine as active drug; acetylated and glucuronide-conjugated metabolites make up the rest. Although the urinary concentrations of both bioactive trimethoprim and sulfamethoxazole are greater than the serum levels, the ratio of trimethoprim to sulfamethoxazole in the typically acidic urine of most patients is about 1:1. In an alkaline urine, the trimethoprim:sulfamethoxazole ratio will decrease.

The half-lives of trimethoprim and sulfamethoxazole are about 9 to 11 hours and 10 to 12 hours, respectively. In those with renal failure, trimethoprim/sulfamethoxazole can accumulate if the dosage is not reduced. Therapeutic levels of trimethoprim (but not sulfamethoxazole) usually can be achieved in the urine of patients with severe renal insufficiency. Trimethoprim and nonacetylated sulfamethoxazole can be removed by hemodialysis, although metabolites of sulfamethoxazole can accumulate and cause crystalluria.

DOSAGE AND PREPARATIONS.

Oral: The following dosages are for patients with normal renal function: *Adults,* for urinary tract infections, one double strength (DS) tablet, two regular strength tablets, or four teaspoonsful (20 ml) of suspension every 12 hours for 10 to 14 days. For shigellosis, the same dosage is administered for five days. For acute exacerbations of chronic bronchitis, the same dosage is administered for 14 days. For the treatment of travelers' diarrhea, the same dosage is administered for five days (DuPont et al, 1982). For prophylaxis of travelers' diarrhea, one DS tablet or two regular strength tablets once daily beginning on day of travel and continuing two days after return home (DuPont et al, 1983; Satterwhite and DuPont, 1983). See the Uses section for dosages in single-dose treatment of initial attacks of acute cystitis in women; prophylaxis of recurrent urinary tract infections in women; chronic prostatitis; and pharyngeal gonococcal infections caused by PPNG.

Children, for urinary tract infections or acute otitis media, 8 mg/kg of trimethoprim and 40 mg/kg of sulfamethoxazole daily in two divided doses every 12 hours for 10 days. The same dose can be given for five days to treat shigellosis. The following table may be used as a guideline in *children 2 months or older:*

Weight		Dose (every 12 hours)	
lb	kg	teaspoonsful	tablets*
22	10	1 (5 ml)	1/2
44	20	2 (10 ml)	1
66	30	3 (15 ml)	1 1/2
88	40	4 (20 ml)	2
			(or 1 *DS* tablet)

*regular strength

The oral preparation is contraindicated in *infants under 2 months.*

For severe infections, the daily amount may be increased by one-half and given in three divided doses.

The dosage for treatment of *Pneumocystis carinii* pneumonitis is 20 mg/kg of trimethoprim and 100 mg/kg of sulfamethoxazole daily in equally divided doses every six hours for 14 days. The following table can be used as a guideline in *children:*

Weight		Dose (every 6 hours)	
lb	kg	teaspoonsful	tablets*
18	8	1 (5 ml)	1/2
35	16	2 (10 ml)	1
53	24	3 (15 ml)	1 1/2
70	32	4 (20 ml)	2
			(or 1 *DS* tablet)

*regular strength

For prophylaxis of *P. carinii* infection, 5 mg/kg of trimethoprim and 25 mg/kg of sulfamethoxazole daily (Hughes, 1982; Wormser et al, 1982).

For patients with impaired renal function, it is recommended that the usual dose be given if creatinine clearance is >30 ml/min; that the dose be reduced to one-half the usual amount if creatinine clearance is between 15 and 30 ml/min; and that the combination not be used if creatinine clearance is <15 ml/min. All patients should maintain an adequate urine volume to prevent crystalluria.

> **Bactrim** (Roche), **Septra** (Burroughs Wellcome), **Generic.** Each 5 ml of suspension contains sulfamethoxazole 200 mg and trimethoprim 40 mg; each tablet contains sulfamethoxazole 400 mg and trimethoprim 80 mg; each double-strength tablet contains sulfamethoxazole 800 mg and trimethoprim 160 mg (**Bactrim-DS, Septra-DS**).

Intravenous: *Adults and children over 2 months with normal renal function,* for severe urinary tract infections and shigellosis, 8 to 10 mg/kg daily (based on the trimethoprim component) in two to four equally divided doses at intervals of 6, 8, or 12 hours for up to 14 days for severe urinary tract infections or five days for shigellosis.

For *P. carinii* pneumonitis, 15 to 20 mg/kg daily (based on the trimethoprim component) in three or four equally divided doses at six- or eight-hour intervals for up to 14 days.

The intravenous preparation is contraindicated in *infants under 2 months.*

For patients with impaired renal function, it is recommended that the usual dose be given if creatinine clearance is >30 ml/min; that the dose be reduced to one-half the usual amount if creatinine clearance is between 15 and 30 ml/min; and that the combination not be used if creatinine clearance is <15 ml/min. All patients should maintain an adequate urine volume to prevent crystalluria.

> **Bactrim I.V.** (Roche). Solution (sterile) containing trimethoprim 16 mg/ml and sulfamethoxazole 80 mg/ml in 5, 10, and 30 ml containers.
> **Septra I.V.** (Burroughs Wellcome). Solution (sterile) containing trimethoprim 16 mg/ml and sulfamethoxazole 80 mg/ml in 5, 10, and 20 ml containers.

Cited References

Human drugs; combination drug containing sulfamethoxazole and phenazopyridine hydrochloride and related combination drugs;

drug efficacy study implementation; conditions for approval and marketing phenazopyridine-containing drug products; labeling requirements. *Federal Register* 48:34516-34519, 1983.

Pentamidine for *Pneumocystis carinii* pneumonia. *Med Lett Drugs Ther* 27:6-7, 1985.

Serious adverse reactions with sulfonamides. *FDA Drug Bull* 14:5-6, 1984.

1985 STD treatment guidelines. *Morbid Mortal Week Rep* 34(suppl):75S-108S, 1985.

Acar JF, Goldstein FW: Genetic aspects and epidemiologic implications of resistance to trimethoprim. *Rev Infect Dis* 4:270-275, 1982.

Araujo OE, Flowers FP: Stevens-Johnson syndrome. *J Emerg Med* 2:129-135, 1984.

Ardati KO, et al: Intravenous trimethoprim/sulfamethoxazole in treatment of serious infections in children. *J Pediatr* 95:801-806, 1979.

Asmar BI, et al: Hematologic abnormalities after oral trimethoprim/sulfamethoxazole therapy in children. *Am J Dis Child* 135:1100-1103, 1981.

Benet LZ, Sheiner LB: Design and optimization of dosage regimens: Pharmacokinetic data, in Gilman AG, et al (eds): *The Pharmacological Basis of Therapeutics,* ed 6. New York, Macmillan, l980, 1734.

Bennett WM, et al: Drug therapy in renal failure: Dosing guidelines for adults. I. Antimicrobial agents, analgesics. *Ann Intern Med* 93:62-69, 1980.

Brogden RN, et al: Trimethoprim: Review of its antibacterial activity, pharmacokinetics and therapeutic use in urinary tract infections. *Drugs* 23:405-430, 1982.

Brumfitt W, Hamilton-Miller JMT: Trimethoprim. *Br J Hosp Med* 23:283-288, 1980.

Brumfitt W, et al: Evidence for slowing in trimethoprim resistance during 1981: Comparison with earlier years. *J Antimicrob Chemother* 11:503-509, 1983.

Dekker AW, et al: Prevention of infection by trimethoprim-sulfamethoxazole plus amphotericin B in patients with acute nonlymphocytic leukemia. *Ann Intern Med* 95:555-559, 1981.

Derbes SJ: Trimethoprim-induced aseptic meningitis. *JAMA* 252:2865-2866, 1984.

DuPont HL, et al: Treatment of travelers' diarrhea with trimethoprim-sulfamethoxazole and with trimethoprim alone. *N Engl J Med* 307:841-844, 1982.

DuPont HL, et al: Prevention of travelers' diarrhea with trimethoprim-sulfamethoxazole and trimethoprim alone. *Gastroenterology* 84:75-80, 1983.

Eastell R, Edmonds CJ: Hyponatremia associated with trimethoprim and a diuretic. *Br Med J* 289:1658-1659, 1984.

Estey E, et al: Infection prophylaxis in acute leukemia: Comparative effectiveness of sulfamethoxazole and trimethoprim, ketoconazole, and combination of the two. *Arch Intern Med* 144:1562-1568, 1984.

Feldman S, et al: Similar hematologic changes in children receiving trimethoprim/sulfamethoxazole or amoxicillin for otitis media. *J Pediatr* 106:995-1000, 1985.

Friesen WT, et al: Trimethoprim: Clinical use and pharmacokinetics. *Drug Intell Clin Pharm* 15:325-330, 1981.

Gaya H, et al: Double-blind placebo controlled trial of prophylactic trimethoprim and sulfamethoxazole (TMP-SMX) for prevention of infection in granulocytopenic patients, (abstract 331). *20th Interscience Conference on Antimicrobial Agents and Chemotherapy.* New Orleans, Sept 22-24, 1980.

Gibbons RB, Lindauer JA: Successful treatment of *Pneumocystis carinii* pneumonia with trimethoprim/sulfamethoxazole in hypersensitive AIDS patients, (letter). *JAMA* 253:1259-1260, 1985.

Gordin FM, et al: Adverse reactions to trimethoprim-sulfamethoxazole in patients with acquired immunodeficiency syndrome. *Ann Intern Med* 100:495-499, 1984.

Gurwith MJ, et al: Prospective controlled investigation of prophylactic trimethoprim/sulfamethoxazole in hospitalized granulocytopenic patients. *Am J Med* 66:248-256, 1979.

Gutman LT: Use of trimethoprim-sulfamethoxazole in children: Review of adverse reactions and indications. *Pediatr Infect Dis* 3:349-357, 1984.

Henry SA, et al: Oral trimethoprim/sulfamethoxazole in attempt to prevent infection after induction chemotherapy for acute leukemia. *Am J Med* 77:663-666, 1984.

Hughes WT: Trimethoprim-sulfamethoxazole therapy for *Pneumocystis carinii* pneumonitis in children. *Rev Infect Dis* 4:602-607, 1982.

Hughes WT, et al: Successful chemoprophylaxis for *Pneumocystis carinii* pneumonitis. *N Engl J Med* 297:1419-1426, 1977.

Hughes WT, et al: Comparison of pentamidine isethionate and trimethoprim-sulfamethoxazole in treatment of *Pneumocystis carinii* pneumonia. *J Pediatr* 92:285-291, 1978.

Jaffe HS, et al: Complications of co-trimoxazole in treatment of AIDS-associated *Pneumocystis carinii* pneumonia in homosexual men. *Lancet* 2:1109-1111, 1983.

Kasanen A, Sundquist H: Trimethoprim alone in treatment of urinary tract infections: Eight years of experience in Finland. *Rev Infect Dis* 4:358-365, 1982.

Kauffman CA, et al: Trimethoprim/sulfamethoxazole prophylaxis in neutropenic patients: Reduction of infections and effect on bacterial and fungal flora. *Am J Med* 74:599-607, 1983.

Kovacs JA, et al: *Pneumocystis carinii* pneumonia: Comparison between patients with acquired immunodeficiency syndrome and patients with other immunodeficiencies. *Ann Intern Med* 100:663-671, 1984.

Kramer BS, et al: Prophylaxis of fever and infection in adult cancer patients: Placebo-controlled trial of oral trimethoprim-sulfamethoxazole plus erythromycin. *Cancer* 53:329-335, 1984.

Kremer I, et al: Aseptic meningitis as adverse effect of co-trimoxazole, (letter). *N Engl J Med* 308:1481, 1983.

Kunin CM, et al: Trimethoprim therapy for urinary tract infection. *JAMA* 239:2588-2590, 1978.

Lawson DH, Paice BJ: Adverse reactions to trimethoprim-sulfamethoxazole. *Rev Infect Dis* 4:429-433, 1982.

Levitz RE, Quintiliani R: Trimethoprim-sulfamethoxazole for bacterial meningitis. *Ann Intern Med* 100:881-890, 1984.

Mandell GL, Sande MA: Antimicrobial agents: Sulfonamides, trimethoprim-sulfamethoxazole, and urinary tract antiseptics, in Gilman AG, et al (eds): *The Pharmacological Basis of Therapeutics,* ed 6. New York, MacMillan, 1980, 1106-1125.

Markowitz N, et al: Comparative efficacy and toxicity of trimethoprim-sulfamethoxazole (TS) versus vancomycin (V) in therapy of serious *S. aureus* (Sa) infections, (abstract 638). *23rd Interscience Conference on Antimicrobial Agents and Chemotherapy.* Las Vegas, Oct 24-26, 1983.

Maskell R, et al: Human infections with thymine-requiring bacteria. *J Med Microbiol* 11:33-45, 1978.

Mitsuyasu R, et al: Cutaneous reaction to trimethoprim-sulfamethoxazole in patients with AIDS and Kaposi's sarcoma, (letter). *N Engl J Med* 308:1535-1536, 1983.

National Institutes of Health Consensus Development Conference: Travelers' diarrhea. *JAMA* 253:2700-2704, 1985.

Pratt WB: *Chemotherapy of Infection.* New York, Oxford University Press, 1977, 176-202.

Reeves D: Sulfonamides and trimethoprim. *Lancet* 2:370-373, 1982.

Riben PD, et al: Reduction in mortality from gram-negative sepsis in neutropenic patients receiving trimethoprim/sulfamethoxazole therapy. *Cancer* 51:1587-1592, 1983.

Rubin RH, Swartz MN: Trimethoprim-sulfamethoxazole. *N Engl J Med* 303:426-432, 1980.

Satterwhite TK, DuPont HL: Infectious diarrhea in office practice. *Med Clin North Am* 67:203-220, 1983.

Sattler FR, Remington JS: Intravenous trimethoprim-sulfamethoxazole therapy for *Pneumocystis carinii* pneumonia. *Am J Med* 70:1215-1221, 1981.

Siegel SE, et al: Treatment of *Pneumocystis carinii* pneumonitis: Comparative trial of sulfamethoxazole-trimethoprim versus pentamidine in pediatric patients with cancer; Report from the Childrens Cancer Study Group. *Am J Dis Child* 138:1051-1054, 1984.

Smith LG, Sensakovic J: Trimethoprim-sulfamethoxazole. *Med Clin North Am* 66:143-156, 1982.

Then R, Angehrn P: Sulfonamide-induced "thymineless death" in *Escherichia coli. J Gen Microbiol* 76:255-263, 1973 A.

Then R, Angehrn P: Nature of bactericidal action of sulfonamides and trimethoprim, alone and in combination. *J Infect Dis* 128(suppl):S498-S501, 1973 B.

Towner KJ: Resistance to trimethoprim among urinary tract isolates in United Kingdom. *Rev Infect Dis* 4:456-460, 1982.

Wade JC, et al: Selective antimicrobial modulations as prophylaxis against infection during granulocytopenia: Trimethoprim-sulfamethoxazole versus nalidixic acid. *J Infect Dis* 147:624-634, 1983.

Winston DJ, et al: Trimethoprim-sulfamethoxazole for treatment of *Pneumocystis carinii* pneumonia. *Ann Intern Med* 92:762-769, 1980.

Woods WG, et al: Myelosuppression associated with co-trimoxazole as prophylactic antibiotic in maintenance phase of childhood acute lymphocytic leukemia. *J Pediatr* 105:639-644, 1984.

Wormser GP, et al: Co-trimoxazole (trimethoprim-sulfamethoxazole): Updated review of its antibacterial activity and clinical efficacy. *Drugs* 24:459-518, 1982.

Young LS: Trimethoprim-sulfamethoxazole in treatment of adults with pneumonia due to *Pneumocystis carinii. Rev Infect Dis* 4:608-613, 1982.

Other Selected References

Trimethoprim. *Med Lett Drugs Ther* 22:69-70, 1980.

Finland M, et al (eds): Trimethoprim-sulfamethoxazole revisited. *Rev Infect Dis* 4:185-618, 1980 (56 papers).

Gleckman R, et al: Intravenous sulfamethoxazole-trimethoprim: Pharmacokinetics, therapeutic indications, and adverse reactions. *Pharmacotherapy* 1:206-211, 1981.

Hughes WT: Trimethoprim/sulfamethoxazole. *Pediatr Clin North Am* 30:27-30, 1983.

Reese RE, Betts RF: Antibiotic use: Sulfonamides and trimethoprim-sulfamethoxazole; trimethoprim, in Reese RE, Douglas RG Jr (eds): *Practical Approach to Infectious Diseases.* Boston, Little, Brown and Company, 1983, 127-135.

Zinner SH, Mayer KH: Sulfonamides and trimethoprim, in Mandell GL, et al (eds): *Principles and Practice of Infectious Diseases,* ed 2. New York, John Wiley & Sons, 1984, 237-244.

Miscellaneous Antibacterial Agents

VANCOMYCIN

RIFAMPIN

METRONIDAZOLE

SPECTINOMYCIN

POLYMYXINS

BACITRACIN

URINARY TRACT ANTISEPTICS

INVESTIGATIONAL QUINOLONES

VANCOMYCIN HYDROCHLORIDE
[Vancocin]

Vancomycin is a glycopeptide antibiotic derived from *Streptomyces orientalis*. This drug was introduced in the late 1950s because of its efficacy against penicillin-resistant staphylococci, but was largely replaced by the less toxic antistaphylococcal penicillins and cephalosporins in the 1960s. A resurgence in the use of vancomycin has occurred in recent years, primarily because of the increase in methicillin-resistant staphylococcal infections and because of the recognition of *Clostridium difficile* as the major cause of antibiotic-associated pseudomembranous colitis.

MECHANISM OF ACTION. Vancomycin inhibits the biosynthesis of peptidoglycan polymers during bacterial cell wall formation. The drug also injures protoplasts by altering their cytoplasmic membranes. It usually is bactericidal for multiplying organisms.

ANTIMICROBIAL SPECTRUM. Vancomycin is primarily active against gram-positive bacteria. It is one of the most potent antibiotics against *Staphylococcus aureus* and *S. epidermidis*, including methicillin- and cephalothin-resistant strains. The minimal inhibitory concentration (MIC) for most strains is less than or equal to 5 mcg/ml. Although the minimal bactericidal concentration (MBC) usually is similar to the MIC, some strains of staphylococci may be tolerant to the bactericidal effect of vancomycin. These strains appear to be deficient in autolysins that are necessary to kill the bacterial cell.

Streptococcus pyogenes and *S. pneumoniae* (including penicillin G-resistant strains) are highly susceptible. Vancomycin usually inhibits the growth of viridans streptococci, *S. bovis*, *S. agalactiae* (group B), and enterococci (eg, *S. faecalis*) at concentrations attainable in vivo, but may not be bactericidal against some strains of these species. This is particularly true for enterococci. Antibacterial synergism against this organism is usually obtained when vancomycin is combined with an aminoglycoside, particularly gentamicin or streptomycin. Anaerobic or microaerophilic streptococci are usually susceptible.

Vancomycin-sensitive gram-positive bacilli include clostridia (including *C. difficile*), *Bacillus anthracis*, and *Corynebacterium diphtheriae*. *Flavobacterium meningosepticum* is susceptible at concentrations between 16 and 25 mcg/ml, but other gram-negative bacilli, mycobacteria, *Bacteroides*, and fungi are resistant.

RESISTANCE. Bacterial resistance rarely develops during therapy. Since vancomycin is chemically unrelated to other antibiotics, cross-resistance with other antibiotics does not occur.

USES. Intravenous vancomycin should be restricted to serious infections caused by susceptible staphylococci or other gram-positive bacteria when other antibiotics are ineffective or not tolerated.

Vancomycin is the drug of choice for methicillin-resistant staphylococcal infections, including bacteremia, endocarditis, osteomyelitis, pneumonia, soft tissue infections, and meningitis. Intrathecal administration may be required to treat meningitis.

Prosthetic valve endocarditis frequently is caused by methicillin-resistant *Staphylococcus epidermidis*. Vancomycin, alone or in combination with rifampin and/or gentamicin, is the drug of choice for this indication.

Vancomycin is recommended for serious staphylococcal infections in patients who cannot receive (eg, due to hypersensitivity) or have failed to respond to penicillins and cephalosporins.

Vancomycin, in combination with gentamicin or streptomycin, is the drug of choice for enterococcal endocarditis in penicillin-allergic patients. Although vancomycin can be used to treat endocarditis caused by viridans streptococci in penicillin-allergic patients, first generation cephalosporins (eg, cefazolin, cephalothin, cephapirin) usually are preferred (unless there also is cephalosporin hypersensitivity).

Intravenous vancomycin is useful for prophylaxis of infective endocarditis in high-risk patients who are allergic to penicillin and are undergoing dental or certain other surgical procedures.

Vancomycin is an alternative to first generation cephalosporins or antistaphylococcal penicillins for prophylaxis during certain surgical procedures (eg, cardiac valve replacement, total hip replacement) in patients allergic to penicillins and cephalosporins.

Vancomycin is poorly absorbed by the gastrointestinal tract, and oral vancomycin is the drug of choice for antibiotic-associated pseudomembranous colitis (AAPMC) caused by *Clostridium difficile*.

See also Chapter 65, Antimicrobial Therapy and Chemoprophylaxis of Infectious Diseases.

ADVERSE REACTIONS AND PRECAUTIONS. In general, the purified preparations of vancomycin now available are well tolerated when properly administered. Frequent reports of adverse reactions with early preparations appear to have been caused by impurities. In addition, there is now a better awareness of the hazards of rapid intravenous administration.

Phlebitis at the site of infusion is the most common problem associated with vancomycin administration, and may be avoided by frequently changing the site of infusion.

Fever, chills, and a histamine-like reaction characterized by flushing; tingling; pruritus; tachycardia; an erythematous macular rash involving the face, neck, upper trunk, back and arms; and systemic arterial hypotension (the "red neck syndrome") can occur with too rapid intravenous administration of vancomycin. Profound hypotension and, rarely, cardiac arrest have been reported after inadvertent bolus injection. Slow intravenous infusion of vancomycin over 60 minutes in a large volume of fluid reduces the incidence of these symptoms and this is the recommended method of administration.

It appears that the frequency of infusion-related anaphylactoid reactions increases with concomitant administration of anesthetic agents (Miller and Tausk, 1977; Waters and Rosenberg, 1981; Odio et al, 1984; Slight et al, 1985). The manufacturer suggests that these events may be reduced by administering vancomycin as a 60-minute infusion prior to anesthetic induction.

Ototoxicity is the most serious adverse effect of vancomycin. It is manifested by auditory nerve damage and hearing loss. Ototoxicity is infrequent at serum concentrations below 30 mcg/ml, but is common at levels of 80 mcg/ml or more. Large doses, prolonged therapy, advanced age, and impaired renal function increase the risk. Concomitant or sequential use of other ototoxic or nephrotoxic agents also increases the risk.

Dose-dependent nephrotoxicity was relatively common with earlier preparations of vancomycin, but occurs less frequently and is reversible when presently available preparations are administered appropriately. In one study, the concomitant administration of vancomycin and an aminoglycoside resulted in significantly elevated serum creatinine concentrations in 35% of patients (Farber and Moellering, 1983).

Other adverse effects include skin rash in 3% to 5% of patients, reversible neutropenia (2%), and eosinophilia. Nausea and an unpleasant taste have been reported with oral administration.

Renal function should be monitored frequently in patients receiving intravenous vancomycin. Caution should be exercised in patients over 60 years, those with pre-existing renal or otic disease, and when certain other drugs (eg, aminoglycosides) are administered concurrently. Measurement of vancomycin serum concentrations is recommended in high-risk patients. Serial audiograms are recommended for certain high-risk patients, including those with renal failure or on prolonged therapy.

DRUG INTERACTIONS. Vancomycin is incompatible in intravenous solution with heparin, chloramphenicol, methicillin, and adrenal corticosteroids.

PHARMACOKINETICS. Vancomycin is poorly absorbed from the gastrointestinal tract after oral administration, although high concentrations are attained in stools. Intramuscular injection causes severe pain and is not recommended. Therefore, vancomycin must be given intravenously to treat systemic infections. Intermittent infusion over at least 60 minutes is preferred, since rapid infusion may cause alarming erythematous or urticarial reactions that primarily involve the upper part of the body (the "red neck syndrome").

Following slow intravenous infusion of 1 g, peak levels of 20 to 50 mcg/ml and trough levels of 5 to 10 mcg/ml are observed. Between 10% and 55% of circulating vancomycin is bound to plasma proteins. The volume of distribution is 0.47 to 0.84 L/kg. Adequate levels of drug appear in most body fluids (eg, pleural, ascitic, pericardial, synovial). Low levels are found in bile, however. In patients with normal renal function, high concentrations are attained in urine. The drug does not penetrate the uninflamed meninges, but therapeutic levels may be attained in cerebrospinal fluid in the presence of meningitis. Intrathecal administration may be necessary in some patients, however. Information on vancomycin concentrations in human tissues is not available.

Vancomycin is eliminated by the kidneys, primarily by glomerular filtration; 80% to 90% of a dose appears in the urine as unchanged drug within 24 hours. The usual elimination half-life in adults with normal renal function ranges from 5 to 11 hours (mean, 6 hours). Elimination half-lives are 5.9 to 9.8 hours in newborns, 4.1 hours in older infants, and 2.2 to 3 hours in children. In anuric patients, the half-life may be prolonged to eight or nine days. Dosage reductions are necessary in patients with renal insufficiency.

DOSAGE AND PREPARATIONS. Reconstituted solutions are stable for 96 hours (intravenous) or one week (oral) if refrigerated.

Intravenous: Vials containing 500 mg should be diluted with 100 to 200 ml of 0.9% sodium chloride injection or 5% dextrose in sterile water for injection and administered slowly by intermittent infusion over a period of at least 60 minutes to reduce the risk of thrombophlebitis and hypotension. Continuous infusion should be used only when intermittent infusion is not feasible. In *adults of average size with normal renal function*, the usual dosage is 2 g daily given in two or four divided doses. Some patients may require higher dosages, which should be determined by measurement of serum concentrations. In *children and infants older than 1 month with normal renal function*, the usual dosage is 40 mg/kg daily given in four divided doses. Larger doses (eg, 60 mg/kg daily in four divided doses) may be required in patients with central nervous system infections and, if there is no response to intravenous therapy after 48 hours, intrathecal administration of 3 to 5 mg may be required (see McHenry and Gavan, 1983). In *infants from 8 days to 1 month with normal renal function*, the manufacturer suggests an initial dose of 15 mg/kg followed by 10 mg/kg every eight hours. In *infants from 0 to 7 days with normal renal function*, the manufacturer suggests an initial dose of 15 mg/kg followed by 10 mg/kg every 12 hours.

Patients with impaired renal function must receive reduced dosages. Monitoring of peak and trough vancomycin serum concentrations to achieve peak concentrations no higher than 30 to 40 mcg/ml (usually 20 to 25 mcg/ml is desired) and trough concentrations between 5 and 10 mcg/ml is recommended. Other methods also are available for administration of vancomycin to patients with impaired renal function. In one method, following a loading dose of 15 mg/kg in adults, the daily maintenance dose in milligrams is 150 plus 15 times the creatinine clearance (Ccr) in milliliters per minute (see Chapter 2, Drug Response Variation and Dosing Information for calculation of Ccr). This produces a vancomycin steady-state serum concentration of 20 mcg/ml. Another method is to give 1 g to adults every 36 hours when the serum creatinine concentration is between 1.5 and 5 mg/dl and 1 g every 10 to 14 days when the serum creatinine concentration is greater than 5 mg/dl. Still another approach is to use a published nomogram that is designed to yield vancomycin steady-state serum concentrations of 15 mcg/ml (Moellering et al, 1981). However, each of these methods provides only an estimation of the optimal dose in such patients. If administration of the drug is to be continued beyond two to three days, the serum concentrations should be measured to adjust dosage in the individual patient. Hemodialysis does not remove vancomycin; peritoneal dialysis may decrease serum concentrations modestly.

See Table 3 in Chapter 65, Antimicrobial Therapy and Chemoprophylaxis of Infectious Diseases, for dosage in chemoprophylaxis of infective endocarditis.

Vancocin (Lilly). Powder equivalent to 500 mg of base.
Oral: Adults, an aqueous solution containing 125 to 500 mg may be given every six hours. The lower dose is probably effective for most cases of pseudomembranous colitis caused by *C. difficile* (Fekety et al, 1984; see also Table 1 in Chapter 65, Antimicrobial Therapy and Chemoprophylaxis of Infectious Diseases). *Children*, 50 mg/kg daily in divided doses every six hours.

Vancocin (Lilly). Powder equivalent to 1 or 10 g of base.

RIFAMPIN
[Rifadin, Rimactane]

Rifampin, a semisynthetic derivative of rifamycin B, is a primary drug in the treatment of tuberculosis (see Chapter 75, Antimycobacterial Agents). Until recently, use of rifampin in nontuberculous infections generally was not recommended because of the potential for rapid emergence of resistant bacterial strains. However, the use of this antibiotic has been gradually broadening.

MECHANISM OF ACTION. Rifampin binds to the β subunit of bacterial DNA-dependent RNA polymerase and blocks initiation of RNA synthesis in susceptible bacteria. The drug is bactericidal.

ANTIMICROBIAL SPECTRUM. Rifampin is the most potent available antibiotic against *Staphylococcus aureus* and *S. epidermidis*, including methicillin-resistant strains. The minimal inhibitory concentration (MIC) for most strains is less than 0.015 mcg/ml (Thornsberry et al, 1983). Some strains of methicillin-resistant *S. epidermidis* also are resistant to rifampin, however.

Most streptococci, including *S. pyogenes* (group A), *S. pneumoniae, S. agalactiae* (group B), and viridans streptococci, are susceptible. The drug is somewhat less active against enterococci (*S. faecalis*).

Other sensitive bacteria include *Listeria monocytogenes, Clostridium difficile,* most other anaerobes (including the *B. fragilis* group), *Neisseria gonorrhoeae, N. meningitidis, Haemophilus influenzae,* and *Legionella pneumophila.* In vitro, rifampin is considerably more potent than erythromycin against *L. pneumophila. Chlamydia trachomatis* and *C. psittaci* are also sensitive. Rifampin is active against *Mycobacterium tuberculosis* and certain atypical mycobacteria. Most aerobic, gram-negative bacilli (eg, *Escherichia coli, Klebsiella, Proteus, Pseudomonas*) are resistant.

RESISTANCE. High-level resistance to rifampin develops rapidly due to mutations that alter the β subunit of RNA polymerase. Cross-resistance with other antimicrobial agents generally does not occur. Because of the rapid emergehce of resistance, *rifampin should not be used alone to treat established infections.*

USES. Rifampin is a first-line drug in the treatment of tuberculosis. For a discussion of its role in this and other mycobacterial infections, see Chapter 75, Antimycobacterial Agents.

Rifampin eliminates nasopharyngeal carriage of *Neisseria meningitidis* and currently is the preferred drug for chemoprophylaxis of close contacts of patients with meningococcal meningitis. Similarly, this drug also eliminates oropharyngeal carriage of *Haemophilus influenzae* type b and is recommended by the American Academy of Pediatrics to prevent secondary *H. influenzae* type b disease (Committee on Infectious Diseases, American Academy of Pediatrics, 1984; see also Table 3 in Chapter 65, Antimicrobial Therapy and Chemoprophylaxis of Infectious Diseases). Rifampin is not indicated for the treatment of meningitis caused by either of these pathogens, however. Short-term prophylaxis of meningitis is the only indication for rifampin monotherapy.

Although still considered investigational, rifampin, always in combination with one or more other antibiotics, is being used in a variety of staphylococcal infections for which treatment with more conventional drugs has been less than satisfactory. Most experts recommend that rifampin be given with vancomycin to treat prosthetic valve endocarditis caused by methicillin-resistant strains of *S. epidermidis.* In a retrospective study, the combination of vancomycin plus rifampin produced higher serum bactericidal titers in eight patients and appeared to improve the clinical outcome compared to vancomycin alone (Karchmer et al, 1983).

The combined use of rifampin plus a penicillinase-resistant penicillin (eg, nafcillin) or vancomycin may be useful in *S. aureus* endocarditis complicated by metastatic abscesses or in patients who fail to respond to single-agent therapy. Clinical data are minimal, however.

Based on limited clinical data, the combination of rifampin and nafcillin or vancomycin may improve response rates in chronic staphylococcal osteomyelitis.

The addition of rifampin to a penicillinase-resistant penicillin or vancomycin may be appropriate in the treatment of other serious staphylococcal infections that fail to respond to single-agent therapy, although, here too, use of such combinations must be considered investigational.

Rifampin can eradicate nasal carriage of staphylococci (Wheat et al, 1983) and the combination of rifampin and an oral antistaphylococcal penicillin (to prevent emergence of resistance to rifampin) may be useful in some patients with recurrent furunculosis.

The use of rifampin with erythromycin generally is indicated in the treatment of *L. pneumophila* infections that fail to respond to erythromycin alone. Some experts recommend combination therapy for all severe infections caused by this pathogen.

Rifampin can kill susceptible intracellular bacteria. It has been shown to eradicate staphylococci present in neutrophils of patients with chronic granulomatous disease and may be useful in this disease. Its role in diseases such as brucellosis presently is unclear.

ADVERSE REACTIONS AND PRECAUTIONS. Rifampin has caused very few adverse reactions when used for short-term prophylaxis of meningitis. Red discoloration of the urine is common and permanent staining of soft contact lenses has been reported.

Adverse reactions and precautions associated with chronic daily and/or intermittent rifampin therapy are discussed in Chapter 75, Antimycobacterial Agents.

DRUG INTERACTIONS. See Chapter 75.

PHARMACOKINETICS. Rifampin is well absorbed from the gastrointestinal tract after oral administration. Elimination is primarily via the biliary route following desacetylation (to active metabolite) in the liver. Rifampin is highly lipid soluble and exhibits excellent penetration into most tissues and body fluid compartments, including hidden recesses, such as cerebrospinal fluid, abscesses, and leukocytes. See Chapter 75 for a detailed discussion of pharmacokinetics.

DOSAGE AND PREPARATIONS.
Oral: Adults, 600 mg daily as a single dose or divided into two doses; in life-threatening infections (eg, prosthetic valve endocarditis), a maximum daily dose of 1.2 g may be given. *Children,* 10 to 20 mg/kg daily.

For prophylaxis of meningococcal disease, *adults,* 600 mg twice daily for two days; *children 1 month to 12 years,* 10 mg/kg twice daily for two days; *newborns less than 1 month,* 5 mg/kg twice daily for two days.

For prophylaxis of *H. influenzae* type b disease, *adults and children,* 20 mg/kg once daily (maximum, 600 mg daily) for four days. For young infants, dosage has not been established. Some experts administer 10 mg/kg once daily for four days to *infants less than 1 month.*

Rifadin (Merrell Dow). Capsules 150 and 300 mg.
Rimactane (CIBA). Capsules 300 mg.

METRONIDAZOLE
[Flagyl, Flagyl I.V. RTU, Metryl]

METRONIDAZOLE HYDROCHLORIDE
[Flagyl I.V.]

$$O_2N \underset{N}{\overset{N-CH_2CH_2OH}{\bigtriangleup}} CH_3$$

Metronidazole, a synthetic 5-nitroimidazole, exhibits selective activity against virtually all obligate anaerobic microorganisms, including bacteria and protozoa. The effectiveness of oral metronidazole in trichomonal vaginitis, amebiasis, and giardiasis is well established (see Chapter 77, Antiprotozoal Agents). The role of this antimicrobial agent (oral and intravenous formulations) in anaerobic bacterial infections is evaluated in the following discussion.

MECHANISM OF ACTION. The selective action of metronidazole against anaerobic bacteria is due to the preferential reduction of the 5'-nitro group of the parent drug by these organisms, presumably by a ferredoxin-like system. An anaerobic environment is required for reduction to proceed. The short-lived active intermediate products formed subsequently interact with bacterial DNA and perhaps other macromolecules. Although the precise mechanism of action is unknown, double strand scissions in DNA probably are produced. Metronidazole is not activated by, and therefore fails to inhibit, most aerobic and facultative organisms.

Unlike other drugs, metronidazole is consistently bactericidal to susceptible anaerobic bacteria.

ANTIMICROBIAL SPECTRUM. Clinically important susceptible anaerobic bacteria include *Bacteroides, Fusobacterium, Clostridium* (including *C. difficile*), *Peptococcus,* and *Peptostreptococcus.* Of particular importance is the essentially uniform susceptibility of the commonly encountered *Bacteroides fragilis* group, anaerobic gram-negative bacilli that often are resistant to other antibacterial agents. Only one-fourth of the strains of *Actinomyces* and *Arachnia,* the causative agents of actinomycosis, are susceptible and most strains of other nonsporing, gram-positive, anaerobic rods (these seldom cause infection) are resistant to metronidazole. Except for *Gardnerella* (*Haemophilus*) *vaginalis* and *Campylobacter fetus,* facultative anaerobes, microaerophilic bacteria, and obligate aerobes usually are not susceptible.

RESISTANCE. Acquired resistance is rare. Since metronidazole is not related chemically to other drugs used in anaerobic bacterial infections, cross-resistance does not occur.

USES. Anaerobic bacterial infections that respond to metronidazole include brain abscess, intra-abdominal and pelvic infections, osteomyelitis, septic arthritis, and endocarditis. In contrast, anaerobic infections of the lower respiratory tract (eg, aspiration pneumonia, lung abscess, empyema) have not responded consistently (presumably because of the concomitant presence of non-anaerobic organisms) and the drug of choice remains penicillin G (or clindamycin). Many foci infected with anaerobic bacteria also are infected by aerobic pathogens that are not susceptible to metronidazole. These mixed infections usually must be treated with metronidazole and other drugs (eg, an aminoglycoside) to eradicate the aerobic bacteria.

In those anaerobic infections for which metronidazole has been shown to be effective, it is the drug of first choice in the rare case of endocarditis caused by penicillin-resistant *Bacteroides* species, most commonly *B. fragilis*. The consistent bactericidal effect of metronidazole against this organism makes it particularly useful in this disease. Although chloramphenicol may still be preferred by some infectious disease experts for anaerobic infections of the central nervous system (eg, subdural empyema, brain abscess), metronidazole is a most effective drug due to its excellent penetration into the central nervous system, its consistent bactericidal activity, and its success in clinical trials. Metronidazole appears to be as effective as clindamycin (or other drugs active against *B. fragilis*) in intra-abdominal, pelvic, skin, and soft tissue infections and is considered a good choice for infections caused by organisms, particularly *B. fragilis*, that are resistant to other drugs.

In addition to antimicrobial drug therapy, surgical debridement of necrotic tissue and drainage of abscesses are important for the successful treatment of anaerobic infections.

The efficacy of metronidazole in surgical prophylactic regimens, particularly in patients undergoing colon or gynecologic surgery, has been established by well-controlled clinical trials in other countries. Although the drug is widely used for this purpose in Europe, there is less experience with metronidazole for surgical prophylaxis in the United States. In this country, it presently is labeled for prophylaxis in elective colorectal surgery.

Oral metronidazole is the preferred drug to treat bacterial vaginosis (formerly called nonspecific vaginitis), a syndrome now believed to be caused by the interaction of several species of vaginal bacteria, including anaerobes.

Oral metronidazole has been shown to effectively treat antibiotic-associated colitis (AAC) caused by *Clostridium difficile* (Teasley et al, 1983). However, current consensus is that oral vancomycin remains the drug of choice despite its higher cost (see that evaluation and Chapters 65, Antimicrobial Therapy and Chemoprophylaxis of Infectious Diseases [Table 1], and 68, Macrolides and Lincosamides). Metronidazole also may be effective when used intravenously to treat AAC in patients who cannot take oral therapy.

For the use of metronidazole in trichomoniasis, amebiasis, and giardiasis, see Chapter 77, Antiprotozoal Agents.

Metronidazole is being used investigationally for the treatment of Crohn's disease (see Chapter 53, Agents Used in Disorders of the Lower Intestinal Tract).

ADVERSE REACTIONS AND PRECAUTIONS. Metronidazole is generally well tolerated. The most common adverse effects are minor gastrointestinal disturbances (eg, nausea, epigastric distress, anorexia). Vomiting and diarrhea are less common. Isolated cases of pseudomembranous colitis caused by *C. difficile* have been reported. Other untoward effects include dryness of the mouth, unpleasant metallic taste, maculopapular rash, urticaria, urethral and vaginal burning, darkening of the urine, headache, dizziness, fever, and thrombophlebitis after intravenous infusion.

The most serious adverse effects involve the central nervous system and include convulsions and peripheral neuropathy, which is characterized mainly by numbness or paresthesia of an extremity. These effects are rare unless large doses or prolonged therapy is employed. If abnormal neurologic symptoms are observed, the drug must be discontinued immediately. Metronidazole should be used cautiously in individuals with a history of seizures or other central nervous system disorders.

Reversible neutropenia occurs in less than 1% of patients receiving metronidazole. Total and differential leukocyte counts are recommended before and after therapy.

Isolated cases of metronidazole-induced pancreatitis (Plotnick et al, 1985) and gynecomastia (Fagan et al, 1985) have been reported.

Because metronidazole is metabolized slowly in patients with hepatic disease, the drug may accumulate in plasma, particularly if there is also renal impairment. Therefore, the dosage should be reduced in these patients.

Metabolites of metronidazole excreted in the urine in man have been shown to be mutagenic in in vitro bacterial systems, but there is no evidence of mutagenicity in mammalian cells. The drug is carcinogenic in mice and possibly in rats, but not in hamsters, when large doses are administered for very prolonged periods. In at least one study, treated rats survived longer than controls; this may have contributed to the increased incidence of tumors. Although there is no evidence that the incidence of cancer is increased in humans exposed to metronidazole, the data presently available are sufficient only to exclude a large risk of cancer because of the long latent period associated with chemical carcinogenesis.

Metronidazole crosses the placenta and is excreted in breast milk. Although the drug has not been shown to be teratogenic in animals or man, benefits and risks should be weighed carefully before it is given to pregnant women or nursing mothers. Generally, it is not recommended during pregnancy, particularly during the first trimester. It is classified in FDA Pregnancy Category B.

Metronidazole has been reported to lower serum cholesterol and triglyceride levels (Davis et al, 1983). The mechanism and clinical significance are unknown.

DRUG INTERACTIONS AND INTERFERENCE WITH LABORATORY TESTS. Metronidazole inhibits the metabolism of warfarin and other coumarins, which potentiates their anticoagulant effect. Therefore, concomitant use should be avoided or the dosage of the anticoagulant should be reduced to maintain the desired prothrombin time.

Metronidazole has caused an intolerance to alcohol similar to that produced by disulfiram. Although not all patients exhibit a reaction, individuals receiving metronidazole should be advised not to drink alcohol because abdominal cramps, nausea, vomiting, headaches, and flushing may occur. This drug should never be administered concomitantly with disulfiram.

Cimetidine prolongs the plasma clearance of metronidazole, presumably by inhibiting metabolic enzymes (Gugler and Jensen, 1983); toxic concentrations of metronidazole may be produced. Drugs that induce microsomal liver enzymes (eg, phenobarbital) may accelerate the elimination of metronidazole, resulting in reduced plasma concentrations.

Metronidazole may interfere with certain types of determinations of serum chemistry values, such as aspartate aminotransferase (AST, SGOT), alanine aminotransferase (ALT, SGPT), lactate dehydrogenase (LDH), triglycerides, and hexokinase glucose. Values of zero may be observed. All of the assays in which interference has been reported involve enzymatic coupling of the assay to oxidation-reduction of nicotine adenine dinucleotide. Interference is due to the similarity in absorbance peaks of NADH (340 nm) and metronidazole (322 nm) at pH 7.

PHARMACOKINETICS. Metronidazole is well absorbed following oral administration. Peak plasma concentrations occur one to two hours after administration and are proportional to the dose (eg, oral administration of 250, 500, and 2,000 mg produced peak plasma levels of 6, 12, and 40 mcg/ml, respectively). Absorption is not significantly affected by food, although the time to peak plasma concentrations is increased. Metronidazole is variably absorbed when administered rectally (suppository).

Intravenous infusion is recommended initially for serious anaerobic bacterial infections. Plasma concentrations also are proportional to dose with this method of administration. Using a standard intravenous dosage regimen (15 mg/kg loading dose, followed by 7.5 mg/kg every six hours), peak and trough steady-state plasma concentrations average 25 and 18 mcg/ml, respectively.

Plasma concentrations of metronidazole are similar during the elimination phase after equivalent intravenous and oral doses.

Less than 20% of circulating metronidazole is bound to plasma proteins. The drug is widely distributed throughout all body tissues, and the volume of distribution is 0.8 L/kg.

Bactericidal concentrations are achieved in vaginal secretions, seminal fluid, saliva, empyema fluid, hepatic abscesses, pelvic tissues (eg, myometrium), bone, and bile. Metronidazole penetrates well into cerebrospinal fluid, including brain abscesses. It crosses the placenta and appears in breast milk.

Metronidazole is metabolized primarily in the liver; the major metabolites are 1-(2-hydroxyethyl)-2-hydroxymethyl-5-nitroimidazole, 2-methyl-5-nitroimidazole-1-yl-acetic acid, and glucuronide conjugates.

Metronidazole and its metabolites are eliminated primarily in the urine (60% to 80% of the dose); 6% to 15% is excreted in the feces. Less than 20% of a dose is excreted as unchanged drug.

The normal half-life of metronidazole is approximately eight hours. In patients with impaired hepatic function, the plasma clearance of metronidazole is decreased, and a dosage adjustment is likely to be necessary. Although the half-life of parent metronidazole is not increased in patients with renal failure, dosage adjustment may be required in some patients with renal insufficiency because of the retention of biologically active metabolites (eg, 1-(2-hydroxyethyl)-2-hydroxymethyl-5-nitroimidazole). Metronidazole and its metabolites are rapidly removed from serum by hemodialysis.

DOSAGE AND PREPARATIONS. The intravenous route is recommended initially in the treatment of most serious anaerobic bacterial infections. Oral therapy may be substituted when conditions warrant.

Intravenous: Metronidazole hydrochloride [Flagyl I.V.] or metronidazole intravenous solution [Flagyl I.V. RTU] must be administered slowly, either as a continuous or intermittent infusion. Metronidazole hydrochloride cannot be administered by direct intravenous injection (intravenous bolus) because of its low pH (0.5 to 2.0) after reconstitution. The reconstituted drug should be diluted further with intravenous fluid to a concentration not exceeding 8 mg/ml, neutralized to pH 6.0 to 7.0 with sodium bicarbonate, and administered by intravenous infusion. Metronidazole intravenous solution [Flagyl I.V. RTU] is a ready-to-use isotonic solution that does not require dilution or buffering before infusion.

Adults, for anaerobic infections, a loading dose of 15 mg/kg is infused over one hour, followed by maintenance doses of 7.5 mg/kg infused over a one-hour period every six to eight hours (maximum, 4 g/24-hour period). Accumulation may occur if treatment is prolonged and the dosage may have to be reduced, particularly in patients with hepatic insufficiency. The usual duration of therapy is 7 to 14 days but may be longer for some infections (eg, joints, bone, endocardium).

METRONIDAZOLE:
Flagyl I.V. RTU (Searle). Solution (sterile) 5 mg/ml in 100 ml containers.
METRONIDAZOLE HYDROCHLORIDE:
Flagyl I.V. (Searle). Powder (sterile, lyophilized) equivalent to 500 mg of base.

Oral: Adults, for anaerobic infections, 7.5 mg/kg every six hours.

For bacterial vaginosis, *adults,* 500 mg twice daily for seven days.

For pseudomembranous colitis caused by *C. difficile, adults,* 500 mg three times daily for 7 to 15 days; alternative dosage, 250 mg four times daily for 10 days.

For dosages in trichomoniasis, amebiasis, and giardiasis, see Chapter 77, Antiprotozoal Agents.

METRONIDAZOLE:
Flagyl (Searle), *Metryl* (Lemmon). Tablets 250 and 500 mg.
Additional Trademark.
Satric (Savage).

SPECTINOMYCIN HYDROCHLORIDE
[Trobicin]

Spectinomycin is an aminocyclitol antibiotic produced by a strain of *Streptomyces spectabilis*. It differs structurally and biologically from the aminoglycosides.

MECHANISM OF ACTION. Spectinomycin interacts with the bacterial 30S ribosomal subunit to inhibit protein synthesis, but the mechanism is unknown. It does not cause misreading of polyribonucleotides as do the aminoglycosides. It is usually bacteriostatic, but appears to be bactericidal for some pathogens, including *Neisseria gonorrhoeae*.

ANTIMICROBIAL SPECTRUM. Spectinomycin is active against most strains of *Neisseria gonorrhoeae*, including penicillinase-producing strains (PPNG) and chromosomal-mediated resistant *N. gonorrhoeae* (CMRNG). Although a number of other gram-positive and gram-negative bacteria are susceptible, the presence of naturally resistant strains and the rapid emergence of acquired resistance to this antibiotic has limited its usefulness to gonococcal infections. *Chlamydia trachomatis* and *Treponema pallidum*, other common pathogens of sexually transmitted diseases, are resistant. Some strains of *Ureaplasma urealyticum* are susceptible.

RESISTANCE. Spectinomycin-resistant strains of gonococci can be selected in vitro. Resistance can be relative or absolute, and both plasmid-mediated enzyme inactivations and chromosomal mutations that alter the 30S ribosome have been observed. Although relatively uncommon, spectinomycin-resistant clinical isolates have been reported, including a few strains that also produced penicillinase (Ashford et al, 1981; *Morbid Mortal Week Rep*, 1983). Thus far, clinically resistant strains appear to be the result of chromosomal mutations.

USES. Spectinomycin is used primarily to treat uncomplicated anogenital gonorrhea (urethritis and proctitis in men, cervicitis and proctitis in women) when the causative organism is susceptible and the primary drugs (amoxicillin, ampicillin, aqueous procaine penicillin G, ceftriaxone) are ineffective or cannot be tolerated (eg, due to hypersensitivity). The following recommendations for its use are based on the current treatment guidelines for sexually transmitted diseases as proposed by the Centers for Disease Control (*Morbid Mortal Week Rep*, 1985 A; see also Table 2 in Chapter 65, Antimicrobial Therapy and Chemoprophylaxis of Infectious Diseases).

Although penicillinase-producing *N. gonorrhoeae* (PPNG) accounted for only about 0.4% of all reported gonococcal infections in the United States in 1982, the incidence of these strains was increasing rapidly. Outbreaks of PPNG infections have been reported from several areas within the United

States; in some countries (eg, Philippines), PPNG infections are very common (see Jaffe et al, 1981; Handsfield, 1982; *Morbid Mortal Week Rep*, 1984 A, 1986). More recently, an increasing number of high level, chromosomally-mediated (β-lactamase-negative), penicillin-resistant *N. gonorrhoeae* (CMRNG) have been reported in the United States (*Morbid Mortal Week Rep*, 1984 B; Faruki et al, 1985; Hook and Holmes, 1985; Rice et al, 1985). Presently, single intramuscular injections of spectinomycin 2 g or ceftriaxone 250 mg are the drug regimens of choice for uncomplicated gonococcal infections caused by PPNG or CMRNG strains. Also, either of these antibiotics should be used in patients in whom gonorrhea persists after treatment with a penicillin regimen because a PPNG or CMRNG infection is a possibility. Spectinomycin should be used for these infections in patients who are allergic to cephalosporins.

Spectinomycin is not indicated in uncomplicated gonorrhea due to strains that are sensitive to a primary agent and when the patient can tolerate the preferred drug. Presently, tetracycline is recommended by the CDC for most patients who are allergic to penicillins and cephalosporins. However, tetracycline should not be used in pregnant women or children under 8 years. Furthermore, it is not effective against anorectal gonococcal infections in men. Such infections are common in homosexual men. Thus, spectinomycin is a drug of first choice in pregnant women, children under 8 years, and homosexual men with uncomplicated gonorrhea who are allergic to penicillins and cephalosporins, and it may be used instead of tetracycline in other patients if the latter drug is ineffective or not tolerated. Because of the increasing emergence of tetracycline-resistant *N. gonorrhoeae* strains (Jaffe et al, 1981; Faruki et al, 1985; Rice et al, 1985; *Morbid Mortal Week Rep*, 1985 B; Hook and Holmes, 1985), some infectious disease experts now prefer spectinomycin as the primary alternative for all penicillin- and cephalosporin-allergic patients with uncomplicated anogenital gonorrhea (Hook and Holmes, 1985).

Spectinomycin should not be used to treat pharyngeal gonococcal infections, since it fails to eradicate the infection in more than 50% of patients. The ceftriaxone regimen or trimethoprim/sulfamethoxazole (orally, nine regular-strength tablets [80 mg/400 mg] once daily for five days) is preferred for pharyngeal infections caused by PPNG. Spectinomycin is not effective in syphilis or nongonococcal urethritis caused by *Chlamydia trachomatis*. Because of the high frequency of coexisting chlamydial and gonococcal infections, the CDC recommends that spectinomycin be followed by a seven-day course of tetracycline or doxycycline (alternative, erythromycin) to treat coexisting chlamydial infection in most patients (except homosexual men).

Presently, spectinomycin is not listed in the CDC guidelines as a preferred drug for disseminated gonococcal infections caused by PPNG strains (cefoxitin, cefotaxime, and ceftriaxone are recommended) or in penicillin- and cephalosporin-allergic individuals (tetracycline and doxycycline are recommended). However, spectinomycin is an effective alternative for disseminated gonococcal infections and is preferred in some clinical situations (eg, in penicillin- and cephalosporin-allergic pregnant women) (see Mills and Brooks, 1984).

ADVERSE REACTIONS AND PRECAUTIONS. Adverse effects occur infrequently and include pain at the site of injection, nausea, vomiting, abdominal cramps, chills, fever, insomnia, pruritus, urticaria, and oliguria. A case of systemic anaphylaxis has been reported (Bender et al, 1983). Unlike the aminoglycosides, spectinomycin does not appear to cause cochlear, vestibular, or renal toxicity.

Results of laboratory tests may be abnormal following multiple doses; decreased hemoglobin, hematocrit, and creatinine clearance and elevated alkaline phosphatase, blood urea nitrogen (BUN), and serum glutamic pyruvic transaminase (SGPT) levels have been reported.

Although the safety of spectinomycin during pregnancy has not been established, this drug does not appear to be teratogenic. Therefore, it may be appropriate for use in pregnant women who are allergic to other antigonococcal drugs or who fail to respond to other treatment. Spectinomycin has been used to treat gonorrhea in prepubertal children.

Because spectinomycin does not eliminate incubating syphilis, serologic tests for syphilis should be performed at the time of treatment with spectinomycin and again in two to three months.

PHARMACOKINETICS. Spectinomycin is rapidly and completely absorbed following intramuscular injection. Mean peak serum concentrations of 100 mcg/ml are achieved one hour after administration of 2 g; at eight hours, mean serum concentrations are 15 mcg/ml. The drug is weakly bound to plasma proteins. It is concentrated in the urine where levels of 1,000 to 2,000 mcg/ml can be attained. Penetration into saliva is poor, which accounts for the poor efficacy in pharyngeal gonorrhea. The elimination half-life is one to three hours in individuals with normal renal function. It is increased in patients with renal impairment. Approximately 80% of the dose is excreted in the urine as unchanged drug and in a biologically active form.

DOSAGE AND PREPARATIONS.
Intramuscular: For uncomplicated gonorrhea, *adults,* 2 g as a single dose; this dose also is indicated for retreatment after other antibiotic therapy has failed. For patients living in areas where antibiotic resistance is known to be prevalent, 4 g is preferred and should be divided between two gluteal sites. *Children under 45 kg,* 40 mg/kg as a single dose (*Morbid Mortal Week Rep,* 1985 A).

For disseminated gonococcal infection, *adults,* 2 g twice a day for three days (Mills and Brooks, 1984).

> *Trobicin* (Upjohn). Powder (sterile, for solution) 2 and 4 g with 3.2 and 6.2 ml of diluent, respectively (contains 400 mg/ml when reconstituted).

POLYMYXINS

The polymyxins are a group of related polypeptides elaborated by strains of *Bacillus polymyxa.* Only polymyxin B [Aerosporin] and E (colistin [Coly-Mycin S]) have a sufficient margin of safety to be useful therapeutically. Colistimethate sodium [Coly-Mycin M], a sulfomethyl derivative of colistin, is the parenteral form of polymyxin E.

MECHANISM OF ACTION. The polymyxins are cationic surface-active compounds at physiologic pH. They exert their antibiotic effect by interacting with phospholipid components in the cytoplasmic membranes of susceptible bacteria and, therefore, disrupt the osmotic integrity of the cell membrane. The precise biochemical mechanism is unclear, however. They are bactericidal.

ANTIMICROBIAL SPECTRUM. Polymyxins are active against a number of aerobic gram-negative bacilli. In particular, they exhibit excellent activity against *Pseudomonas aeruginosa.* Other organisms that are usually susceptible include *Escherichia coli, Klebsiella pneumoniae, Enterobacter, Salmonella, Shigella, Haemophilus, Bordetella, Pasteurella,* and *Vibrio. Proteus, Providencia,* and *Serratia marcescens* are usually resistant. Polymyxins are not active against *Neisseria,* gram-positive bacteria, most obligate anaerobes, or fungi.

RESISTANCE. Acquired bacterial resistance develops slowly, and the overall efficacy of the polymyxins has remained fairly constant. Resistant bacteria usually have cell walls that prevent access of the drug to the cytoplasmic membrane. Cross-resistance is observed between polymyxin B and colistin, but not with other classes of antibiotics.

USES. Indications for parenteral polymyxin B or colistimethate sodium are extremely limited; they are not drugs of choice for any infection. Their primary use is in serious infections (eg, bacteremia, urinary tract) caused by strains of *P. aeruginosa* (or other aerobic gram-negative bacilli) that are resistant to other drugs (eg, aminoglycosides, antipseudomonal penicillins), or when patients with these infections cannot tolerate or are allergic to the preferred drugs. Intrathecal administration is necessary when polymyxin B is used in meningitis.

Aerosolized polymyxin B has been used to treat respiratory infections due to *Pseudomonas* in patients with cystic fibrosis or bronchiectasis and to prevent *Pseudomonas* infections in respiratory intensive care units. The effectiveness of this approach is limited, however, because pneumonias due to resistant organisms frequently develop.

Polymyxin B, in combination with neomycin, has been used as a bladder irrigant to prevent urinary tract infections in patients with indwelling catheters.

Oral colistin sulfate has been used in infants and children to treat diarrhea caused by enteropathogenic *E. coli.*

Polymyxin B is most commonly used topically for infections of the eye, ear, and skin, frequently as a component of an antibiotic mixture (see Chapters 73, Topical Anti-infective Agents: Otic and Ophthalmic Preparations, and 74, Topical Anti-infective Agents: Drugs Used on Skin and Mucous Membranes). Colistin sulfate also has been used topically for certain infections of the ear.

ADVERSE REACTIONS AND PRECAUTIONS. Parenteral polymyxins can cause serious nephrotoxicity and neurotoxicity. These adverse reactions have significantly limited the usefulness of these antibiotics as systemic agents.

Dose-dependent nephrotoxicity is a common and serious adverse effect. At usual therapeutic doses, approximately 20% of patients experience some degree of nephrotoxicity. This is usually manifested by elevated blood urea nitrogen (BUN) and elevated serum creatinine. Mild nephrotoxicity is usually reversible after the drug is discontinued, but some patients develop renal failure and acute tubular necrosis. This is more likely to occur with large doses or prolonged therapy and appears to be due to cumulative binding of polymyxins to renal tubular epithelium. Patients with pre-existing renal disease or receiving other nephrotoxic drugs (eg, aminoglycosides) are at increased risk.

Renal function should be monitored frequently when polymyxins are given. Polymyxins should be administered cautiously to patients with impaired renal function and dosage adjustments are necessary.

Neurotoxicity also is a common and serious adverse effect of the polymyxins. Transient neurologic disturbances, including dizziness, vertigo, ataxia, slurred speech, blurred vision, drowsiness, confusion, circumoral paresthesias, and numbness of the extremities, have been observed following parenteral administration. These adverse reactions are dose related and disappear soon after the drugs have been discontinued. However, larger doses can cause neuromuscular blockade and respiratory arrest. Neuromuscular blockade is not reversed by neostigmine, but may respond to calcium gluconate. Neurotoxicity is most likely to occur in patients with impaired renal function or pre-existing neuromuscular disease (eg, myasthenia gravis). Patients receiving neuromuscular blocking drugs (eg, tubocurarine), other potentially neurotoxic drugs (eg, aminoglycosides), an anesthetic with prominent muscle relaxant properties (eg, enflurane), or parenteral magnesium, quinidine, or quinine are at increased risk.

Respiratory arrest has been reported following administration of polymyxins as irrigants into serous cavities (eg, peritoneum) or as aerosols.

Allergic reactions are rare, but urticaria and shock due to histamine release have occurred with too rapid intravenous infusion.

Polymyxin B causes pain at the site of intramuscular injection and this route of administration is not recommended. When intramuscular injection of polymyxin B is necessary, the inclusion of a local anesthetic may decrease the pain.

DRUG INTERACTIONS. The concomitant use of polymyxins with other nephrotoxic drugs (eg, aminoglycosides) should be avoided, if possible, because nephrotoxicity may be additive.

Drugs that may impair neuromuscular transmission also should not be given with polymyxins, if possible, because respiratory arrest may occur. Such drugs include the neuromuscular blocking agents (eg, tubocurarine), aminoglycosides, anesthetics with prominent muscle relaxant properties (eg, enflurane), and parenteral quinidine, quinine, or magnesium.

PHARMACOKINETICS. Polymyxins are not absorbed from the gastrointestinal tract following oral administration except in neonates. Polymyxin B is usually given intravenously, but intrathecal administration is required to treat meningitis. The intramuscular route is not recommended. Intravenous infusion of polymyxin B (25,000 units/kg) yields peak serum concentrations of about 5 mcg/ml.

Colistimethate sodium can be administered intravenously or intramuscularly, and it is preferred to polymyxin B when intramuscular administration is desired. Following intramuscular injection, peak serum levels of 5 to 6 mcg/ml are achieved after about two hours. Colistimethate sodium is partially metabolized in the body to the more active colistin.

Colistin sulfate is used orally for a local antibacterial effect.

Polymyxins do not pass readily into cerebrospinal fluid or other body compartments (eg, pleural, synovial, brain tissue), but they cross the placenta. High concentrations are achieved in urine. Plasma protein binding may be as high as 75%. Effectiveness is reduced in the presence of pus or other organic material.

Polymyxins are excreted renally, primarily by glomerular filtration. The plasma half-lives of polymyxin B and colistimethate sodium are 6 to 7 hours and 2 to 4.5 hours, respectively, in patients with normal renal function.

DOSAGE AND PREPARATIONS.
POLYMYXIN B SULFATE:
Intravenous: *Adults and children with normal renal function,* 1.5 to 2.5 mg (15,000 to 25,000 units)/kg daily. The total daily dose generally should not exceed 2.5 mg (25,000 units)/kg, although *infants* usually tolerate up to 4 mg (40,000 units)/kg daily if needed. Dextrose injection 5% may be used as a vehicle and one-half of the daily dose should be given by continuous intravenous drip every 12 hours. To avoid widespread neuromuscular blockade, this drug should not be injected rapidly as a single bolus.

Intramuscular: This route is not recommended routinely because marked pain occurs at the site of injection. A 1% procaine hydrochloride solution in sodium chloride may be used as a vehicle to help reduce the pain. Otherwise, water for injection or sodium chloride solution for injection may be used as a vehicle.

Adults and children with normal renal function, 2.5 to 3 mg (25,000 to 30,000 units)/kg daily in divided doses every four to six hours. *Infants* may tolerate up to 4 mg (40,000 units)/kg daily, and *premature or newborn infants* with *P. aeruginosa* infections may be given 4.5 mg (45,000 units)/kg of polymyxin B sulfate daily.

Intrathecal: For *P. aeruginosa* meningitis, *adults and children over 2 years with normal renal function,* 5 mg (50,000 units) once daily for three to four days, followed by 5 mg (50,000 units) once every other day; *children under 2 years with normal renal function,* 2 mg (20,000 units) once daily for three to four days, or 2.5 mg (25,000 units) once every other day. These amounts are given for at least two weeks after cultures of the cerebrospinal fluid become negative and the sugar content has returned to normal.

In *patients with impaired renal function,* the parenteral dosage of polymyxin B should be reduced in proportion to the degree of renal impairment as determined by measurement of creatinine clearance or blood creatinine levels. The following guidelines may be used (Fekety, 1984):

Creatinine Clearance (Ccr)	Daily Dosage
Normal or ≥80% of normal	2.5-3 mg/kg
80% to ≥30% of normal	First day: 2.5 mg/kg Daily thereafter: 1-1.5 mg/kg
<30% of normal	First day: 2.5 mg/kg Every 2-3 days thereafter: 1-1.5 mg/kg
With Anuria	First day: 2.5 mg/kg Every 5-7 days thereafter: 1 mg/kg

Aerosporin (Burroughs Wellcome), *Generic*.
Powder (sterile) 500,000 units equivalent to 50 mg of polymyxin B sulfate.

Topical: See Chapters 73, Topical Anti-infective Agents: Otic and Ophthalmic Preparations, and 74, Topical Anti-infective Agents: Drugs Used on Skin and Mucous Membranes.

COLISTIMETHATE SODIUM:

Intramuscular, Intravenous: The intravenous dose should be administered slowly by intravenous drip. *Adults and children with normal renal function,* 2.5 to 5 mg/kg daily in divided doses every 8 or 12 hours (maximum, 300 mg daily). *Adults with impaired renal function,* following an initial dose of 2.5 to 5 mg/kg, the dosage should be modified according to the following schedule (see the manufacturer's literature for further information):

	RENAL IMPAIRMENT		
	Mild	Moderate	Marked
Serum Creatinine (mg/dl)	1.3-1.5	1.6-2.5	2.6-4.0
Daily Dose (mg/kg)	2.5-3.8	2.5	1.5
Dosage Interval (hours)	12	12-24	36

Coly-Mycin M (Parke-Davis). Powder (sterile, lyophilized) equivalent to 150 mg base.

COLISTIN SULFATE:

Oral: Infants and children, 5 to 15 mg/kg daily in three divided doses.

Coly-Mycin S (Parke-Davis). Powder for oral suspension equivalent to 300 mg of base, providing the equivalent of 25 mg of base/5 ml when suspended in 37 ml of distilled water.

BACITRACIN

Bacitracin is a mixture of polypeptide antibiotics produced by a strain of *Bacillus subtilis*.

MECHANISM OF ACTION. Bacitracin inhibits the formation of the linear peptidoglycan chains that are major components of the bacterial cell wall. It is bactericidal.

ANTIMICROBIAL SPECTRUM. Most gram-positive bacteria, including staphylococci, streptococci, and *Clostridium difficile*, are susceptible to bacitracin. Although this agent is active against *Neisseria* and *Haemophilus influenzae*, most gram-negative bacteria are resistant.

RESISTANCE. Acquired bacterial resistance to bacitracin is rare.

USES. Indications for systemic (intramuscular) bacitracin are extremely limited due to its nephrotoxicity and the availability of more effective drugs. It may be used as a drug of last resort in infants with serious staphylococcal infections (eg, pneumonia) resistant to all other antibiotics. Similarly, bacitracin has been administered intrathecally for the rare case of staphylococcal meningitis that does not respond to other therapy.

Bacitracin is only negligibly absorbed from the gastrointestinal tract. In limited studies, oral bacitracin has been effective in pseudomembranous colitis caused by *Clostridium difficile*, although relapses may occur (investigational use). Presently, the drug of choice is oral vancomycin, and metronidazole is an effective alternative (see the evaluations and Chapters 65, Antimicrobial Therapy and Chemoprophylaxis of Infectious Diseases [Table 1], and 68, Macrolides and Lincosamides).

Bacitracin is most commonly used topically for infections of the eye and skin caused by susceptible gram-positive bacteria (eg, staphylococci, streptococci). Frequently, it is combined with other antibiotics (eg, neomycin, polymyxin B) to increase the antibacterial spectrum. See Chapters 73, Topical Anti-infective Agents: Otic and Ophthalmic Preparations, and 74, Topical Anti-infective Agents: Drugs Used on Skin and Mucous Membranes, for additional discussion.

ADVERSE REACTIONS AND PRECAUTIONS. *Bacitracin is highly nephrotoxic and systemic administration should be avoided, if possible.* Glomerular and tubular necrosis have occurred after systemic use. Renal function should be monitored if the drug must be used systemically.

Intramuscular injection of bacitracin is quite painful.

PHARMACOKINETICS. Bacitracin is not absorbed from the gastrointestinal tract following oral administration. If systemic administration is necessary, the drug is injected intramuscularly. Absorption of the antibiotic is rapid and complete after intramuscular injection; peak blood concentrations are reached in one to two hours.

Distribution is relatively widespread after parenteral administration. However, only traces are found in the cerebrospinal fluid unless the meninges are inflamed.

Bactericidal plasma concentrations may be present for four to six hours after a single intramuscular dose. The drug is eliminated slowly by glomerular filtration; the quantity recovered in the urine varies from 10% to 40% in the first 24 hours.

DOSAGE AND PREPARATIONS.

Intramuscular: When parenteral administration is essential, the following amounts may be given: *Infants weighing less than 2.5 kg,* 900 units/kg daily in two or three divided doses. *Infants over 2.5 kg,* 1,000 units/kg daily in two or three divided doses.

Generic. Powder (for injection) 10,000 and 50,000 units.

Oral: For pseudomembranous colitis caused by *C. difficile,* *adults,* 25,000 units four times daily for seven to ten days (investigational use; oral form not available commercially). *Topical:* See Chapters 73 and 74.

URINARY TRACT ANTISEPTICS

Nitrofurantoin [Furadantin (microcrystalline), Macrodantin (macrocrystalline)], nalidixic acid [NegGram], cinoxacin [Cinobac], and methenamine [Hiprex, Mandelamine, Urex] are used only to treat and/or prevent urinary tract infections. These agents are active against common urinary tract pathogens and, since they are concentrated in the urine, have been classified as urinary tract antiseptics.

NITROFURANTOIN
[Furadantin (microcrystalline), Macrodantin (macrocrystalline)]

MECHANISM OF ACTION. The mechanism of action of this synthetic nitrofuran compound is unclear. There is evidence that nitrofurantoin inhibits a variety of enzyme systems in bacteria, and it has been postulated that it interferes with the early stages of bacterial carbohydrate metabolism by inhibiting acetyl coenzyme A.

ANTIMICROBIAL SPECTRUM. Nitrofurantoin is active against a wide spectrum of common urinary tract pathogens. Bacteria with a minimum inhibitory concentration (MIC) of less than or equal to 32 mcg/ml of drug are considered sensitive.

Most strains of *Escherichia coli*, a gram-negative coliform responsible for about 90% of initial urinary tract infections, are susceptible. About two-thirds of the strains of other coliforms, but only one-third of *Klebsiella-Enterobacter* strains, are sensitive. Most *Proteus* and *Serratia* species are moderately to completely resistant. *Pseudomonas aeruginosa* and other *Pseudomonas* species are resistant.

Staphylococcus aureus, S. saprophyticus, and *Streptococcus faecalis* (enterococci), gram-positive cocci that can cause urinary tract infections, are susceptible to nitrofurantoin.

Although in vitro susceptibility of *Salmonella, Shigella, Neisseria, Streptococcus pyogenes, S. pneumoniae, Corynebacterium,* and many anaerobes has been shown, nitrofurantoin is of little importance clinically for infections caused by these organisms.

For additional discussion, see Mayrer and Andriole, 1982; Andriole, 1984.

RESISTANCE. Sensitive bacteria do not readily develop resistance to nitrofurantoin during therapy.

USES. Nitrofurantoin is one of a number of alternative antibac-

terial agents (eg, trimethoprim/sulfamethoxazole, sulfisoxazole, ampicillin, amoxicillin, cinoxacin) recommended for the treatment of uncomplicated lower urinary tract infections (eg, cystitis) caused by susceptible bacteria.

Nitrofurantoin also is one of the recommended drugs (trimethoprim/sulfamethoxazole and trimethoprim alone are others) for the prophylaxis of recurrent lower urinary tract infections.

Although nitrofurantoin may be active in upper urinary tract infections, other agents usually are preferred. Nitrofurantoin is not useful for infections outside the urinary tract.

For additional discussion on the treatment and prophylaxis of urinary tract infections, see Chapter 65, Antimicrobial Therapy and Chemoprophylaxis of Infectious Diseases.

ADVERSE REACTIONS AND PRECAUTIONS. The overall incidence of adverse effects is relatively high (10% or more). Gastrointestinal irritation is most common. Symptoms include anorexia, nausea, and vomiting; diarrhea and abdominal pain occur less frequently. Gastrointestinal intolerance is less frequent with the macrocrystalline preparation. Administration of the drug with food or milk may control these side effects. Superinfection is rare.

Acute, subacute, and chronic pulmonary reactions have occurred. Acute pneumonitis was reported frequently in one Swedish study (Holmberg et al, 1980), but the incidence of this adverse reaction in other countries appears to be quite low (see D'Arcy, 1985). Acute pneumonitis is manifested by sudden onset of fever, chills, cough, chest pain, dyspnea, pulmonary infiltration with consolidation or pleural effusion on x-ray, and eosinophilia. The elderly are more likely to be affected. The reaction usually occurs during the first week of therapy, is reversible on discontinuation of treatment, and may respond to a corticosteroid. It is believed to be a hypersensitivity reaction because it quickly recurs with drug rechallenge. In subacute pneumonitis, symptoms are more insidious, fever and eosinophilia are less common, and symptoms resolve more slowly. Chronic pulmonary reactions are rare and usually occur in patients on prolonged therapy (eg, more than six months). Common findings are malaise, dyspnea on exertion, cough, and altered pulmonary function. Diffuse interstitial pneumonitis and/or fibrosis are common. The severity and reversibility of the chronic pulmonary reaction usually correlate with the duration of therapy after symptoms first appear. Permanent impairment of pulmonary function may occur and fatalities have been reported. This chronic reaction also is considered to be allergic in origin.

If any of these pulmonary reactions occur, nitrofurantoin should be discontinued and appropriate treatment should be instituted. Patients on long-term therapy should be monitored.

Other types of hypersensitivity reactions occur less frequently but may be severe. Rash and urticaria are most common, but chills and fever are sometimes seen. Hepatotoxicity, manifested as hepatitis, including chronic active hepatitis, and cholestatic jaundice, develops rarely. Arthralgia, angioedema, a lupus erythematosus-like syndrome, and anaphylaxis also have been reported.

Headache, drowsiness, dizziness, nystagmus that is readily reversible, and peripheral polyneuropathy have been reported. The peripheral neuritis, an ascending sensorimotor neuropathy, may be progressive and is one of the most serious adverse effects of nitrofurantoin. It is more common in patients with renal failure or in elderly patients receiving prolonged therapy. Anemia, diabetes, electrolyte imbalance, vitamin B deficiency, and debilitating disease are other predisposing conditions for this adverse reaction.

Leukopenia, granulocytopenia, eosinophilia, and megaloblastic anemia have been reported. Acute hemolytic anemia may occur in individuals with glucose-6-phosphate dehydrogenase (G6PD) deficiency (eg, 10% of blacks have this defect). A similar reaction may occur in infants with premature red cell enzyme systems (glutathione instability). Therefore, nitrofurantoin should not be administered to patients with G6PD deficiency, to infants less than 1 month, or to pregnant women at term because of the possibility of hemolytic anemia.

Large doses of nitrofurantoin depress spermatogenesis through a direct action on seminiferous tubules. Usual therapeutic doses do not appear to have this effect.

DRUG INTERACTIONS. Nitrofurantoin interferes with the urinary antimicrobial action of nalidixic and oxolinic acids; the drugs should not be given concomitantly.

PHARMACOKINETICS. Nitrofurantoin is administered orally, and it is rapidly and completely absorbed from the gastrointestinal tract. Both a microcrystalline [Furadantin] and a macrocrystalline [Macrodantin] form are available. The larger macrocrystals dissolve more slowly in the intestine and this form is more slowly absorbed than the microcrystalline formulation. This appears to result in a lower incidence of gastrointestinal intolerance, although the therapeutic efficacies of the two formulations are the same.

The presence of food in the intestine decreases the rate of absorption but appears to increase bioavailability. The duration of therapeutic urinary concentrations is prolonged by about two hours when the drug is administered with food.

Serum concentrations of nitrofurantoin are low (less than 2 mcg/ml) when usual doses are given, and the drug does not accumulate in the serum of patients with normal renal function. Therapeutic concentrations are not achieved in most body tissues. Although nitrofurantoin crosses the blood-brain barrier and the placenta, it does so to a very small extent. About 60% of a dose is reversibly bound to plasma proteins.

The serum half-life is approximately 20 minutes in patients with normal renal function. About two-thirds of a dose is rapidly metabolized in all body tissues, especially the liver. The remaining one-third is rapidly excreted into the urine by glomerular filtration and tubular secretion in a therapeutically active, unchanged form; an average dose of nitrofurantoin yields a urine concentration of approximately 200 (range, 50 to 250) mcg/ml in patients with normal renal function. In an acid urine, nitrofurantoin, a weak acid, is partially reabsorbed in the un-ionized form, resulting in lower urinary concentrations. However, the urine should not be alkalized to increase drug levels because antibacterial activity is significantly diminished at the higher pH.

Recovery of nitrofurantoin from urine is linearly related to creatinine clearance. If creatinine clearance is less than 40 ml/min, urinary concentrations of nitrofurantoin are inadequate

and blood levels of the drug are elevated, which increases the danger of toxicity. Therefore, nitrofurantoin should not be administered to patients with significantly diminished renal function.

For additional discussion, see Mayrer and Andriole, 1982; Andriole, 1984.

DOSAGE AND PREPARATIONS.
Oral: *Adults,* 50 to 100 mg three or four times daily. Most uncomplicated urinary tract infections caused by susceptible bacteria in patients with normal renal function are adequately treated with 50 mg three times daily. *Children,* 5 to 7 mg/kg every 24 hours in four divided doses.

For prophylaxis of frequently recurring urinary tract infections in *adults,* 50 to 100 mg at bedtime may be adequate; in *children,* doses as low as 1 mg/kg daily, given in a single or in two divided doses, may be adequate.

NITROFURANTOIN:
Generic (microcrystalline). Capsules, tablets 50 and 100 mg.
Furadantin (microcrystalline) (Norwich Eaton). Suspension 25 mg/5 ml; tablets 50 and 100 mg.
Macrodantin (macrocrystalline) (Norwich Eaton). Capsules 25, 50, and 100 mg.

NALIDIXIC ACID
[NegGram]

MECHANISM OF ACTION. Nalidixic acid binds to the A subunit of bacterial DNA gyrase, an enzyme responsible for the supercoiling of DNA (Gellert et al, 1977). This interaction leads to inhibition of bacterial DNA replication.

ANTIMICROBIAL SPECTRUM. Nalidixic acid is active against most Enterobacteriaceae that are common urinary tract pathogens (bacteria with minimum inhibitory concentrations [MICs] of less than or equal to 16 mcg/ml are considered sensitive). In particular, most strains of *Escherichia coli,* the causative organism of about 90% of initial urinary tract infections, are susceptible. Most strains of *Proteus, Klebsiella,* and *Enterobacter* also are sensitive. *Pseudomonas* species and gram-positive bacteria, including staphylococci and enterococci, are resistant to nalidixic acid.

Some nonurinary tract pathogens, including *Brucella* and some strains of *Salmonella* and *Shigella,* are susceptible to nalidixic acid.

For additional discussion, see Mayrer and Andriole, 1982; Andriole, 1984.

RESISTANCE. Although resistance to nalidixic acid does not appear to be transferable, the emergence of resistant bacteria by other mechanisms does occur and has caused problems clinically. Cross-resistance with cinoxacin is common.

USES. Nalidixic acid is effective orally for the treatment of uncomplicated lower urinary tract infections (eg, cystitis) caused by susceptible bacteria. However, other drugs (eg, trimethoprim/sulfamethoxazole, sulfisoxazole, ampicillin, amoxicillin, nitrofurantoin, cinoxacin) are more frequently preferred.

Nalidixic acid also has been used in the prophylaxis of recurrent lower urinary tract infections. However, trimethoprim/sulfamethoxazole, trimethoprim alone, or nitrofurantoin is preferred for prophylaxis.

This drug is not useful for upper urinary tract infections or for infections outside the urinary tract.

For additional discussion on the treatment and prophylaxis of urinary tract infections, see Chapter 65, Antimicrobial Therapy and Chemoprophylaxis of Infectious Diseases.

ADVERSE REACTIONS AND PRECAUTIONS. The incidence of untoward effects associated with nalidixic acid is low. The most common reactions are nausea, vomiting, rash, and urticaria. Diarrhea, abdominal pain, fever, eosinophilia, and photosensitivity occur occasionally. Patients taking this drug should be warned against excessive exposure to sunlight. Superinfection with fungal organisms has not been noted.

Hemolytic anemia has been reported; patients with glucose-6-phosphate dehydrogenase (G6PD) deficiency seem to be most susceptible. Leukopenia and thrombocytopenia also have developed. Cholestasis is rare.

Visual disturbances sometimes occur after administration of nalidixic acid. These include blurred vision, diplopia, photophobia, altered color perception, and abnormal accommodation. Symptoms disappear when therapy is discontinued.

Neurologic side effects include headache, malaise, drowsiness, dizziness, weakness, vertigo, and visual disturbances (see above). These adverse effects are reversible when nalidixic acid is discontinued. Occasionally, toxic psychoses and convulsions have occurred with large doses, particularly in young children or in patients with predisposing factors (eg, epilepsy, parkinsonism, mental instability, cerebral arteriosclerosis). In infants, nalidixic acid has caused increased intracranial pressure, resulting in papilledema and bulging fontanelles.

Nalidixic acid should not be administered to patients with a history of seizure disorders and should be used with caution in patients with severe renal or hepatic insufficiency.

This drug should not be given to pregnant women during the first trimester; no adverse effects to the fetus have been reported during the second or third trimesters. Its use is contraindicated in nursing mothers and in infants under 3 months. Nalidixic acid is not recommended for prepubertal children, for studies have shown that erosion of weight-bearing joints occurs in immature animals.

DRUG INTERACTIONS AND INTERFERENCE WITH LABORATORY TESTS. Nitrofurantoin interferes with the therapeutic effects of nalidixic acid and the two drugs should not be administered concomitantly. Nalidixic acid may potentiate the effects of oral anticoagulants (eg, warfarin, dicumarol) by displacing them from serum albumin binding sites.

The glucuronide conjugates of nalidixic acid may react with Benedict's solution or Clinitest tablets to give a false-positive reaction for urine glucose. This does not occur when Clinistix or Tes-Tape strips are used.

PHARMACOKINETICS. Nalidixic acid is almost completely absorbed from the gastrointestinal tract following oral administration.

Two hours after an oral dose of 1 g, plasma levels of 20 to 50 mcg/ml are attained; two-thirds represents nalidixic acid (93% plasma protein bound) and one-third is hydroxynalidixic acid (68% plasma protein bound), which is an active metabolite. The drug does not accumulate in tissues; only the kidney has levels higher than plasma. Therapeutically active concentrations of drug are not achieved in body sites other than the urine.

Nalidixic acid is rapidly excreted into urine; 85% represents an inactive conjugate and most of the remainder is hydroxynalidixic acid. Urine concentrations of hydroxynalidixic acid are 25 to 250 mcg/ml after a single 0.5- to 1-g dose and range from 100 to 500 mcg/ml with continued administration. Most sensitive bacteria are inhibited by less than or equal to 16 mcg/ml.

Although nalidixic acid and its metabolites are excreted almost exclusively by the kidney, effective therapeutic levels can be achieved in patients with moderate to advanced renal failure. Furthermore, active metabolites do not accumulate in azotemic patients even after prolonged therapy. However, the inactive conjugate may accumulate and, despite the fact that toxicity has not been reported, the drug probably should not be given to individuals with advanced renal or hepatic disease; conjugation of the drug may be impaired in the latter.

For additional discussion, see Mayrer and Andriole, 1982; Andriole, 1984.

DOSAGE AND PREPARATIONS.
Oral: Adults, 4 g daily in four divided doses for one week is usually sufficient to treat uncomplicated lower urinary tract infections.

NegGram (Winthrop-Breon). Suspension 250 mg/5 ml; tablets 250 and 500 mg and 1 g.

CINOXACIN
[Cinobac]

MECHANISM OF ACTION, ANTIMICROBIAL SPECTRUM, AND RESISTANCE. The antimicrobial properties of cinoxacin are comparable to those of nalidixic acid, to which it is related chemically (see that evaluation). Cross-resistance is seen between the two drugs. Plasmid (R-factor)-mediated resistance has not been reported for cinoxacin.

USES. Cinoxacin is effective orally for the treatment of uncomplicated lower urinary tract infections (eg, cystitis) caused by susceptible bacteria. It is one of a number of alternative antibacterial agents (eg, trimethoprim/sulfamethoxazole, sulfisoxazole, ampicillin, amoxicillin, nitrofurantoin) for this indication. This agent also appears to be effective in the prophylaxis of recurrent lower urinary tract infections. However, trimethoprim/sulfamethoxazole, trimethoprim alone, and nitrofurantoin have been more extensively evaluated and are currently recommended by the majority of our consultants. Cinoxacin is not indicated for infections outside the urinary tract. For additional discussion on the treatment and prophylaxis of urinary tract infections, see Chapter 65, Antimicrobial Therapy and Chemoprophylaxis of Infectious Diseases.

When compared to nalidixic acid, cinoxacin appears to have the advantages of a longer dosage interval, fewer adverse reactions, and a lower propensity to induce bacterial resistance during clinical use, but clinical experience with this agent is more limited (Guay, 1982; Sisca et al, 1983).

ADVERSE REACTIONS AND PRECAUTIONS. Cinoxacin is usually well tolerated; the overall incidence of adverse effects is reported to be about 5% (Sisca et al, 1983; Burt, 1984). The most common adverse reactions are nausea, vomiting, hypersensitivity reactions (pruritus, rash, urticaria, edema), dizziness, and headache. Other central nervous system effects include restlessness, insomnia, a tingling sensation, photophobia, and tinnitus. Although seizures have not been observed with cinoxacin, they have been reported rarely for chemically related drugs (eg, nalidixic acid). The drug also has caused anorexia, abdominal cramps, diarrhea, and perineal burning. Visual disturbances (eg, blurred vision) have been attributed to this agent. In general, the frequency and severity of adverse reactions appear to be less for cinoxacin than for nalidixic acid (Guay, 1982; Sisca et al, 1983).

Hematology and blood chemistry appear to be largely unaltered by cinoxacin, although hematocrit (hemoglobin) levels were reduced and eosinophilia has occurred. No overt renal or hepatic abnormalities have developed despite some modification of SGOT, SGPT, BUN, serum creatinine, and alkaline phosphatase values.

Because cinoxacin is excreted primarily by the kidney, the dosage should be reduced in patients with impaired renal function and the drug should not be given to anuric patients.

No teratogenic effects have been reported in man or animals, but no well-controlled studies have been performed in pregnant women. Therefore, cinoxacin should not be used during pregnancy or lactation (FDA Pregnancy Category B). The drug should not be given to prepuberal children since, like nalidixic acid, it causes erosion of weight-bearing joints in immature animals.

PHARMACOKINETICS. Cinoxacin is rapidly and almost completely absorbed from the gastrointestinal tract following oral administration. Although the presence of food delays absorption and lowers peak serum concentrations, the total amount absorbed is not decreased.

Mean peak serum concentrations of 15 mcg/ml are attained approximately two hours after ingestion of 500 mg. Between 60% and 70% of the drug is bound to plasma protein. Therapeutically active concentrations of drug are not achieved in body fluids other than the urine.

The serum half-life of cinoxacin is 1.5 hours. The drug is concentrated in the urine. Mechanisms include glomerular filtration and tubular secretion. More than 95% of a dose is excreted in the first 24 hours; 50% to 55% is unaltered drug and the remainder is inactive metabolites. A dose of 500 mg produces average urine concentrations of 250 to 300 mcg/ml within four hours. The half-life of cinoxacin is increased in patients with impaired renal function.

For additional discussion see Guay, 1982; Sisca et al, 1983.

DOSAGE AND PREPARATIONS.

Oral: Adults, 1 g daily in two or four divided doses given at equal intervals for 7 to 14 days. In the presence of renal impairment, the schedule given in the table can be used:*

Creatinine Clearance (ml/min/1.73 M²)	Renal Function	Dosage
>80	Normal	500 mg every 12 hours
80-50	Mild Impairment	250 mg every 8 hours
50-20	Moderate Impairment	250 mg every 12 hours
<20	Marked Impairment	250 mg every 24 hours

*From manufacturer's literature

Cinobac (Dista). Capsules 250 and 500 mg.

METHENAMINE

METHENAMINE HIPPURATE
[Hiprex, Urex]

METHENAMINE MANDELATE
[Mandelamine]

MECHANISM OF ACTION. Methenamine itself does not exert an antibacterial effect. In an acid medium, this tertiary amine is hydrolyzed to formaldehyde, the active degradation product. Formaldehyde appears to kill bacteria by denaturing proteins.

Adequate urinary acidification (pH less than or equal to 5.5) and adequate time for hydrolysis to occur in urine (about two hours) are necessary for methenamine to exert its antibacterial effect. The concomitant administration of various weak acids, such as hippuric acid (methenamine hippurate), mandelic acid (methenamine mandelate), ascorbic acid, ammonium chloride, and those contained in certain foods (eg, cranberries), is frequently recommended to further lower urinary pH. Also, hippuric and mandelic acids have weak bacteriostatic activities that are independent of formaldehyde generation. The contribution of these weak acids to the bactericidal effect of methenamine is questionable, however.

For additional discussion, see Mayrer and Andriole, 1982; Andriole, 1984.

ANTIMICROBIAL SPECTRUM. Virtually all bacteria and fungi are susceptible to formaldehyde (at approximately 20 mcg/ml). However, certain urease-positive bacteria (eg, *Proteus*) can convert urea to ammonium hydroxide, which can prevent the conversion of methenamine to formaldehyde.

RESISTANCE. Resistance to formaldehyde does not develop; thus, methenamine-resistant organisms are unknown.

USES. Methenamine is used for prophylaxis of recurrent urinary tract infections, but other drugs (eg, trimethoprim/sulfamethoxazole, trimethoprim alone, nitrofurantoin) are preferred. However, when residual urine is present (eg, prostatism, neurogenic bladder), methenamine is an excellent drug for long-term prophylaxis because there is sufficient time to generate formaldehyde in bladder urine and no formaldehyde-resistant organisms are known.

Methenamine is not recommended for treatment of acute urinary tract infections.

For additional discussion on the treatment and prophylaxis of urinary tract infections, see Chapter 65, Antimicrobial Therapy and Chemoprophylaxis of Infectious Diseases.

ADVERSE REACTIONS AND PRECAUTIONS. Methenamine and its salts are relatively safe and usually well tolerated. Gastrointestinal irritation and nausea have occurred, presumably caused by the generation of formaldehyde, an irritant, in the acid milieu of the stomach. The use of enteric-coated tablets may decrease these irritant effects. Similarly, bladder irritation, characterized by dysuria, frequency, and hematuria, has been reported. Large doses can cause acute inflammation of the urinary tract, which necessitates discontinuation of therapy and administration of an alkalizing salt (eg, sodium bicarbonate). Skin rashes have occurred.

Because ammonia is generated during methenamine hydrolysis, this drug should not be administered to patients with hepatic insufficiency.

Methenamine base is not contraindicated in the presence of renal insufficiency, and azotemic patients readily convert urinary methenamine to formaldehyde. However, the salts of methenamine are contraindicated in dehydrated patients and in those with severe renal disease. When the urinary output is decreased severely, methenamine salts may precipitate and cause crystalluria. Methenamine salts also should be avoided in patients with gout, since they may precipitate urate crystals in the urine.

The pH of the urine should be monitored to assure that an acidic medium is present for the hydrolysis of methenamine to formaldehyde. Patients should be instructed to avoid ingesting substances that could increase urinary pH (eg, citrus fruits, milk and milk products, antacids containing sodium carbonate or bicarbonate). Likewise, the ingestion of copious amounts of fluid may be counterproductive because the increased diuresis may increase urinary pH and dilute urinary formaldehyde concentrations to subinhibitory levels. Protein-rich diets with liberal amounts of cranberries, plums, prunes, and, possibly, the ingestion of acidifying agents (eg, ascorbic acid, ammonium chloride) are often recommended to maintain an acid urine. The value of these acidifying agents at the usual amounts ingested is questionable, however. The contributions of mandelic acid and hippuric acid to the antibacterial effect of methenamine, when administered in the commercially available acid salt forms, are probably negligible.

For additional discussion, see Mayrer and Andriole, 1982; Andriole, 1984.

DRUG INTERACTIONS. Drugs that increase urinary pH (eg, acetazolamide, sodium bicarbonate) prevent the hydrolysis of methenamine to formaldehyde. Methenamine should not be given to patients receiving these drugs.

The concomitant administration of sulfamethizole or sulfathiazole with methenamine has resulted in crystalluria. Methenamine should not be used with sulfonamides.

PHARMACOKINETICS. Methenamine and its salts are absorbed rapidly from the gastrointestinal tract following oral administration. Between 10% and 30% of a dose may be hydrolyzed in the gastric acid of the stomach. Enteric-coated preparations decrease formaldehyde generation in the stomach.

Methenamine is distributed throughout total body water, including red blood cells; cerebrospinal, synovial, and pericardial fluids; and aqueous and vitreous humors. However, the drug has no antibacterial activity in these fluids because formaldehyde is not generated at physiologic pH.

Over 90% of methenamine is excreted in the urine within 24 hours; up to 20% of this is hydrolyzed to free formaldehyde. The transit time through the kidney is too brief for adequate formaldehyde generation; thus, activity is limited to the bladder. At pH 5.0 to 5.5, about two hours are required to generate bactericidal levels of formaldehyde, which can be maintained for up to six hours or until the patient voids. The intake of copious amounts of fluids with methenamine may increase diuresis and urine pH and dilute the formaldehyde concentration to subinhibitory levels (see Mayrer and Andriole, 1982).

DOSAGE AND PREPARATIONS.

METHENAMINE, METHENAMINE MANDELATE:

Oral: Adults, 1 g four times daily after each meal and at bedtime; *children under 6 years,* 50 mg/kg daily divided into three doses; *children 6 to 12 years,* 500 mg four times daily.

METHENAMINE:
Generic. Tablets 500 mg; bulk (granules).

METHENAMINE MANDELATE:
Generic. Suspension 500 mg/5 ml; tablets (plain) 500 mg and 1 g; tablets (enteric-coated) 250 and 500 mg and 1 g.
Mandelamine (Parke-Davis). Granules 500 mg and 1 g; suspension 250 and 500 (Forte) mg/5 ml; tablets (plain, enteric-coated) 500 mg and 1 g.

METHENAMINE HIPPURATE:

Oral: Adults and children over 12 years, 1 g twice daily; *children 6 to 12 years,* 500 mg to 1 g twice daily.
Hiprex (Merrell Dow), *Urex* (Riker). Tablets 1 g.

PHENAZOPYRIDINE HYDROCHLORIDE
[Pyridium]

ACTIONS AND USES. Phenazopyridine is *not* a urinary tract antiseptic. However, it is excreted in the urine where it has an analgesic effect on the urinary tract mucosa. Thus, it is used to relieve pain, burning, urgency, and frequency of urination associated with irritation of the lower urinary tract. These symptoms can result from infection (eg, cystitis), trauma, surgery, catheterization, and endoscopy. Because this drug provides only symptomatic relief, prompt appropriate treatment of the cause of the pain must be instituted. Phenazopyridine should be discontinued when symptoms are controlled. It should not be continued beyond the first 48 hours in urinary tract infections because efficacy has not been demonstrated after this time period (Federal Register, 1983).

Many fixed-ratio combinations containing antibacterial agents and phenazopyridine are available, but separate drug administration is preferred.

ADVERSE REACTIONS AND PRECAUTIONS. The principal adverse reactions are gastrointestinal disturbances, which occur occasionally. A yellowish tinge to the skin or sclerae may indicate accumulation due to impaired renal excretion; therapy should be discontinued. A few cases of hemolytic anemia and hepatic toxicity have been reported, usually at overdose levels. Overdosage or prolonged use in patients with diminished renal function may produce methemoglobinemia. The use of phenazopyridine is contraindicated in patients with renal insufficiency or severe hepatitis. The drug is an azo dye and colors the urine red or orange; clothing is likely to be stained, and the stain is difficult to remove from fabric.

Long-term administration of phenazopyridine has induced neoplasia in rats and mice. Although no association between phenazopyridine and human cancer has been reported, adequate epidemiologic studies have not been conducted (Federal Register, 1983).

PHARMACOKINETICS. Following oral administration, approximately 90% of the dose is eliminated in the urine within 24 hours, about 40% as unchanged drug and 50% as aniline and its metabolites, mainly p-aminophenol and N-acetyl-p-aminophenol (acetaminophen).

DOSAGE AND PREPARATIONS.
Oral: *Adults,* 200 mg three times daily after meals; *children 6 to 12 years,* 100 mg three times daily after meals.
Pyridium (Parke-Davis), *Generic.* Tablets 100 and 200 mg.

INVESTIGATIONAL QUINOLONES

A group of synthetic quinolone derivatives (6-fluoro-7-piperazino-4-quinolones), which are related chemically to nalidixic acid, are being investigated as antibacterial agents for urinary tract and other infections. Derivatives include norfloxacin [Noroxin], ciprofloxacin, enoxacin, ofloxacin, pefloxacin, and amifloxacin. The new quinolones are more active than nalidixic acid against gram-negative urinary tract pathogens (eg, *Escherichia coli* and other Enterobacteriaceae). In addition, they have an expanded antibacterial spectrum that includes *Pseudomonas aeruginosa* and gram-positive bacteria (eg, staphylococci, enterococci). All of these agents can be administered orally and parenteral formulations are being investigated for some (eg, ciprofloxacin). Norfloxacin is the most extensively studied of these new quinolone derivatives

and an evaluation of this agent, based on the available, albeit limited, clinical data, is presented.

For a general review of the fluoroquinolones, see Wolfson and Hooper, 1985, and Hooper and Wolfson, 1985; for a review of norfloxacin, see Holmes et al, 1985.

NORFLOXACIN
[Noroxin]

MECHANISM OF ACTION. Norfloxacin is a bacterial DNA gyrase inhibitor (Crumplin et al, 1984). Thus, it appears to act via the same mechanism as nalidixic acid. It is usually bactericidal for susceptible bacteria (see Holmes et al, 1985).

ANTIMICROBIAL SPECTRUM. Norfloxacin is highly active against most Enterobacteriaceae that are urinary tract pathogens. *Escherichia coli* (the causative organism in over 90% of initial urinary tract infections), *Klebsiella, Enterobacter, Proteus mirabilis, Morganella morganii, Proteus vulgaris, Providencia, Citrobacter,* and *Serratia* are susceptible. Some strains of *Providencia* and *Serratia* are less sensitive, however. Norfloxacin is 10- to 100-fold more active than nalidixic acid against these pathogens (Neu and Labthavikul, 1982; Norrby and Jonsson, 1983; Newsom, 1984; see also Holmes et al, 1985; Wolfson and Hooper, 1985).

The antimicrobial spectrum of norfloxacin is broader than that of nalidixic acid. In particular, this agent is active against *Pseudomonas aeruginosa,* including strains that are resistant to other antibacterial agents (Forward et al, 1983; see also Holmes et al, 1985). Other *Pseudomonas* (eg, *P. maltophilia*) and *Acinetobacter* appear to be less sensitive.

Norfloxacin is highly active in vitro against most enteric pathogens, including *Shigella, Salmonella,* enterotoxigenic *E. coli, Yersinia enterocolitica, Aeromonas hydrophila, Vibrio parahaemolyticus,* and *Campylobacter jejuni. Clostridium difficile* are resistant (Carlson et al, 1983; see also Holmes et al, 1985).

Haemophilus influenzae (gram-negative coccobacilli) and the gram-negative cocci, *Neisseria meningitidis* and *N. gonorrhoeae,* including beta lactamase-producing strains (PPNG), are highly susceptible (Newsom, 1984; see also Holmes et al, 1985).

In contrast to nalidixic acid, norfloxacin is active against most gram-positive bacteria, although inhibitory concentrations generally are higher than for gram-negative bacteria. Susceptible gram-positive bacteria include staphylococci (eg, *S. aureus,* including methicillin-resistant strains; *S. epidermidis; S. saprophyticus,* a common urinary pathogen), streptococci (eg, *S. pyogenes; S. pneumoniae; S. agalactiae; S. faecalis,* a common urinary pathogen) and *Listeria* (Neu and Labthavikul, 1982; Newsom, 1984; see also Holmes et al, 1985; Wolfson and Hooper, 1985).

In general, norfloxacin has demonstrated poor activity against anaerobic bacteria (see Holmes et al, 1985).

In vitro activities of newer quinolones, including enoxacin, ciprofloxacin, ofloxacin, and amifloxacin, have been compared with norfloxacin in published studies (for review, see Wolfson and Hooper, 1985). Enoxacin, amifloxacin, and norfloxacin show comparable activity against most bacteria, although amifloxacin is more active against *Acinetobacter* (Chin and Neu, 1983; John and Twitty, 1984). Ofloxacin is more active than norfloxacin against *Acinetobacter, Gardnerella vaginalis*, and most gram-positive bacteria (Wise et al, 1984). These two agents show similar activity against other bacteria. Ciprofloxacin is the most potent quinolone tested; it is 2- to 32-fold more active than norfloxacin, depending on the bacterial strain (Fass, 1983; Barry et al, 1984; Chin and Neu, 1984). It has activity in vitro against *Chlamydia trachomatis* (Heessen and Muytjens, 1984).

The activity of norfloxacin (and other quinolones) is unaffected by the presence of serum, but is decreased in an acidic urine. Factors in addition to pH appear to be involved. Although the clinical significance of this phenomenon is not completely clear, concentrations of drug achieved in urine appear to be more than sufficient for most urinary pathogens (Newsom, 1984; see also Holmes et al, 1985). The in vitro activity of norfloxacin (and other quinolones) is little affected by inoculum size or the type of medium (see Holmes et al, 1985).

RESISTANCE. Whether acquired resistance to norfloxacin and the other new quinolones will become a major problem clinically, as is the case for nalidixic acid, remains to be determined. The frequency of appearance of organisms resistant to norfloxacin has been reported to be less than to nalidixic acid (Duckworth and Williams, 1984). Although gradual, stepwise decreases in susceptibility to the newer quinolones have been produced in vitro by serial passage of gram-negative bacilli through subinhibitory concentrations of these agents, the increases in minimal inhibitory concentrations (MICs) were not sufficient to be of clinical significance in urinary tract infections. Whether resistance would be clinically important in systemic infections is unknown. All of the quinolone derivatives exhibited cross-resistance (Barry and Jones, 1984). Plasmid-mediated, transferable resistance has not been reported for the quinolones (see Wolfson and Hooper, 1985).

USES. Clinical experience with norfloxacin is limited and virtually all of the published studies have been for the treatment of urinary tract infections. This agent compared favorably with trimethoprim/sulfamethoxazole in the treatment of acute uncomplicated urinary tract infections in women in two comparative trials (Haase et al, 1984; Watt et al, 1984). Norfloxacin has been effective in the treatment of complicated urinary tract infections in small groups of elderly or hospitalized patients (Panichi et al, 1983; Leigh et al, 1984; Leigh and Emmanuel, 1984). A number of these infections were caused by *Pseudomonas aeruginosa* and other multiresistant pathogens. Although additional clinical trials are necessary, norfloxacin appears to be potentially useful as an orally administered antibacterial agent for urinary tract infections caused by *P. aeruginosa* and other multiple drug-resistant gram-negative bacilli.

Oral norfloxacin (two 600-mg doses separated by an interval of four hours) was shown to be as effective as intramuscular spectinomycin in the treatment of acute gonococcal urethritis in males. Many of these infections were caused by penicillinase-producing *N. gonorrhoeae* (PPNG) (Crider et al,

1984). Further clinical study of this oral quinolone in penicillin-resistant gonococcal infections appears warranted.

For additional discussion, see Holmes et al, 1985; Hooper and Wolfson, 1985.

ADVERSE REACTIONS AND PRECAUTIONS. Norfloxacin generally has been well tolerated based on the clinical studies currently published. The most common adverse reactions are gastrointestinal irritation (3% to 4%), including nausea, vomiting, and anorexia; minor central nervous system side effects (less than 2%), including headache, dizziness, drowsiness, and photophobia; and hypersensitivity reactions (less than 1%), usually skin rash. Serious neurologic reactions (eg, psychoses, convulsions) that have occurred occasionally with nalidixic acid have not been reported with norfloxacin.

Crystalluria has been reported when large doses of norfloxacin (1.2 to 1.6 g) were given to normal volunteers (Swanson et al, 1983). This has not been observed at lower doses.

For additional discussion, see Holmes et al, 1985.

PHARMACOKINETICS. Norfloxacin is absorbed from the gastrointestinal tract following oral administration; oral bioavailability has been estimated to be approximately 70% (see Holmes et al, 1985). Peak serum concentrations are attained in one to two hours and have been reported to be 0.75, 1.58, 2.41, 3.15, and 3.87 mcg/ml with doses of 200, 400, 800, 1,200, and 1,600 mg, respectively (Swanson et al, 1983). Approximately 14% of circulating drug is bound to plasma proteins.

Information on distribution of norfloxacin into various tissues and body fluids is limited. High concentrations are achieved in urine; they peak in one to two hours and have been reported to be 200, 478, 697, 992, and 1,045 mcg/ml with doses of 200, 400, 800, 1,200, and 1,600 mg, respectively. Norfloxacin also has been detected in bile (Wise, 1984) and noninflamed prostatic tissue (Bologna et al, 1983).

The metabolism and excretion of norfloxacin are not completely understood. Approximately 30% of a dose is recovered as unchanged drug in urine. The mechanism of elimination appears to be renal tubular secretion. The elimination half-life is 3.5 hours in individuals with normal renal function and increases to 7.7 hours when the creatinine clearance falls below 10 ml/min. Norfloxacin also is metabolized and six metabolites have been identified. The fate of these metabolites is unclear (Wise, 1984), but urinary excretion of metabolites accounts for less than 10% of an administered dose (see Holmes et al, 1985).

DOSAGE AND PREPARATIONS.

Oral: The most frequently used dosage for *adults with urinary tract infections* is 800 mg daily in equally divided doses every 12 hours. Dosage reductions are recommended in patients with moderate to severe renal impairment, ie, when creatinine clearance is 30 ml/min or less. A dosage of 400 mg once daily is recommended when creatinine clearance is between 30 and 10 ml/min. No data on dosing intervals or safety are available for patients with creatinine clearances of less than 10 ml/min.

For *uncomplicated gonococcal urethritis in adult males*, two 600-mg doses separated by a four-hour interval was effective (Crider et al, 1984).

Noroxin (Merck Sharp & Dohme).
(Investigational drug)

Cited References

Human drugs; combination drug containing sulfamethoxazole and phenazopyridine hydrochloride and related combination drugs; drug efficacy study implementation; conditions for approval and marketing phenazopyridine-containing drug products; labelling requirement. *Federal Register* 48:34516-34519, 1983.

Spectinomycin-resistant penicillinase-producing *Neisseria gonorrhoeae*. *Morbid Mortal Week Rep* 32:51-52, 1983.

Gonorrhea—United States, 1983. *Morbid Mortal Week Rep* 33:361-363, 1984 A.

Chromosomally mediated resistant *Neisseria gonorrhoeae*—United States. *Morbid Mortal Week Rep* 33:408-410, 1984 B.

1985 STD treatment guidelines. *Morbid Mortal Week Rep* 34(suppl):75S-108S, 1985 A.

Tetracycline-resistant *Neisseria gonorrhoeae*—Georgia, Pennsylvania, New Hampshire. *Morbid Mortal Week Rep* 34:563-570, 1985 B.

Penicillinase-producing *Neisseria gonorrhoeae*—United States, Florida. *Morbid Mortal Week Rep* 35:12-14, 1986.

Andriole VT: Urinary tract agents: Quinolones, nitrofurantoin, and methenamine, in Mandell GL, et al (eds): *Principles and Practice of Infectious Diseases*, ed 2. New York, John Wiley & Sons, 1984, 244-253.

Ashford WA, et al: Spectinomycin-resistant penicillinase-producing *Neisseria gonorrhoeae*. *Lancet* 2:1035-1037, 1981.

Barry AL, Jones RN: Cross-resistance among cinoxacin, ciprofloxacin, DJ-6783, enoxacin, nalidixic acid, norfloxacin, and oxolinic acid after in vitro selection of resistant population. *Antimicrob Agents Chemother* 25:775-777, 1984.

Barry AL, et al: Antibacterial activities of ciprofloxacin, norfloxacin, oxolinic acid, cinoxacin, and nalidixic acid. *Antimicrob Agents Chemother* 25:633-637, 1984.

Bender BS, et al: Systemic anaphylaxis caused by parenteral spectinomycin. *South Med J* 76:1456-1457, 1983.

Bologna M, et al: Bactericidal intraprostatic concentrations of norfloxacin, (letter). *Lancet* 2:280, 1983.

Burt RAP: Review of adverse reactions associated with cinoxacin and other drugs used to treat urinary tract infections. *Urology* 23:101-107, 1984.

Carlson JR, et al: Comparative in vitro activities of ten antimicrobial agents against bacterial enteropathogens. *Antimicrob Agents Chemother* 24:509-513, 1983.

Chin N, Neu HC: In vitro activity of enoxacin, a quinolone carboxylic acid, compared with those of norfloxacin, new β-lactams, aminoglycosides, and trimethoprim. *Antimicrob Agents Chemother* 24:754-763, 1983.

Chin N, Neu HC: Ciprofloxacin, quinolone carboxylic acid compound active against aerobic and anaerobic bacteria. *Antimicrob Agents Chemother* 25:319-326, 1984.

Committee on Infectious Diseases, American Academy of Pediatrics: Revision of recommendation for use of rifampin prophylaxis of contacts of patients with *Haemophilus influenzae* infection. *Pediatrics* 74:301-302, 1984.

Crider SR, et al: Treatment of penicillin-resistant *Neisseria gonorrhoeae* with oral norfloxacin. *N Engl J Med* 311:137-140, 1984.

Crumplin GC, et al: Investigations into mechanism of action of antibacterial agent norfloxacin. *J Antimicrob Chemother* 13(suppl B):9-23, 1984.

D'Arcy PF: Nitrofurantoin. *Drug Intell Clin Pharm* 19:540-547, 1985.

Davis JL, et al: Metronidazole lowers serum lipids. *Ann Intern Med* 99:43-44, 1983.

Duckworth GJ, Williams JD: Frequency of appearance of resistant variants to norfloxacin and nalidixic acid. *J Antimicrob Chemother* 13(suppl B):33-38, 1984.

Fagan TC, et al: Metronidazole-induced gynecomastia. *JAMA* 254:3217, 1985.

Farber BF, Moellering RC Jr: Retrospective study of toxicity of preparations of vancomycin from 1974 to 1981. *Antimicrob Agents Chemother* 23:138-141, 1983.

Faruki H, et al: Community-based outbreak of infection with penicillin-resistant *Neisseria gonorrhoeae* not producing penicillinase (chromosomally mediated resistance). *N Engl J Med* 313:607-611, 1985.

Fass RJ: In vitro activity of ciprofloxacin (Bay o 9867). *Antimicrob Agents Chemother* 24:568-574, 1983.

Fekety R: Polymyxins, in Mandell GL, et al (eds): *Principles and Practice of Infectious Diseases*, ed 2. New York, John Wiley & Sons, 1984, 235-237.

Fekety R, et al: Comparative efficacy of low vs high dose oral vancomycin (125 or 500 mg four times per day) in treatment of adults with antibiotic associated *Clostridium difficile* colitis, (abstract 818). *24th Interscience Conference on Antimicrobial Agents and Chemotherapy*. Washington, DC, Oct 8-10, 1984.

Forward KR, et al: Comparative activities of norfloxacin and fifteen other antipseudomonal agents against gentamicin-susceptible and -resistant *Pseudomonas aeruginosa* strains. *Antimicrob Agents Chemother* 24:602-604, 1983.

Gellert M, et al: Nalidixic acid resistance: Second genetic character involved in DNA gyrase activity. *Proc Natl Acad Sci USA* 74:4772-4776, 1977.

Guay DRP: New drug evaluations: Cinoxacin. *Drug Intell Clin Pharm* 16:916-921, 1982.

Gugler R, Jensen JC: Interaction between cimetidine and metronidazole, (letter). *N Engl J Med* 309:1518-1519, 1983.

Haase DA, et al: Comparative trial of norfloxacin and trimethoprim-sulfamethoxazole in the treatment of women with localized, acute, symptomatic urinary tract infections and antimicrobial effect on periurethral and fecal microflora. *Antimicrob Agents Chemother* 26:481-484, 1984.

Handsfield HH: PPNG infections: Current status and guidelines for therapy. *Drug Ther* 12:118-124, (July) 1982.

Heessen FWA, Muytjens HL: In vitro activities of ciprofloxacin, norfloxacin, pipemidic acid, cinoxacin, and nalidixic acid against *Chlamydia trachomatis*. *Antimicrob Agents Chemother* 25:123-124, 1984.

Holmberg L, et al: Adverse reactions to nitrofurantoin: Analysis of 921 reports. *Am J Med* 69:733-738, 1980.

Holmes B, et al: Norfloxacin: Review of its antibacterial activity, pharmacokinetic properties, and therapeutic use. *Drugs* 30:482-513, 1985.

Hook EW III, Holmes KK: Gonococcal infections. *Ann Intern Med* 102:229-243, 1985.

Hooper DC, Wolfson JS: Fluoroquinolones: Pharmacology, clinical uses, and toxicities in humans. *Antimicrob Agents Chemother* 28:716-721, 1985.

Jaffe HW, et al: Infections due to penicillinase-producing *Neisseria gonorrhoeae* in the United States: 1976-1980. *J Infect Dis* 144:191-197, 1981.

John JF Jr, Twitty JA: Amifloxacin activity against well-defined gentamicin-resistant, gram-negative bacteria. *Antimicrob Agents Chemother* 26:781-784, 1984.

Karchmer AW, et al: *Staphylococcus epidermidis* causing prosthetic valve endocarditis: Microbiologic and clinical observations as guides to therapy. *Ann Intern Med* 98:447-455, 1983.

Leigh DA, Emmanuel FXS: Treatment of *Pseudomonas aeruginosa* urinary tract infections with norfloxacin. *J Antimicrob Chemother* 13(suppl B):85-88, 1984.

Leigh DA, et al: Comparative study using norfloxacin and amoxycillin in treatment of complicated urinary tract infections in geriatric patients. *J Antimicrob Chemother* 13(suppl B):79-83, 1984.

Mayrer AR, Andriole VT: Urinary tract antiseptics. *Med Clin North Am* 66:199-208, 1982.

McHenry MC, Gavan TL: Vancomycin. *Pediatr Clin North Am* 30:31-47, 1983.

Miller R, Tausk HC: Anaphylactoid reaction to vancomycin during anesthesia: Case report. *Anesth Analg* 56:870-872, 1977.

Mills J, Brooks GF: Disseminated gonococcal infection, in Holmes KK, et al (eds): *Sexually Transmitted Diseases.* New York, McGraw-Hill, 1984, 229-237.

Moellering RC Jr, et al: Vancomycin therapy in patients with impaired renal function: Nomogram for dosage. *Ann Intern Med* 94:343-346, 1981.

Neu HC, Labthavikul P: In vitro activity of norfloxacin, a quinolone-carboxylic acid, compared with that of β-lactams, aminoglycosides, and trimethoprim. *Antimicrob Agents Chemother* 22:23-27, 1982.

Newsom SWB: Antimicrobial spectrum of norfloxacin. *J Antimicrob Chemother* 13(suppl B):25-31, 1984.

Norrby SR, Jonsson M: Antibacterial activity of norfloxacin. *Antimicrob Agents Chemother* 23:15-18, 1983.

Odio C, et al: Adverse reactions to vancomycin used as prophylaxis for CSF shunt procedures. *Am J Dis Child* 138:17-19, 1984.

Panichi G, et al: Norfloxacin (MK-0366) treatment of urinary tract infections in hospitalized patients. *J Antimicrob Chemother* 11:589-592, 1983.

Plotnick BH, et al: Metronidazole-induced pancreatitis. *Ann Intern Med* 103:891-892, 1985.

Rice RJ, et al: Changing trends in gonococcal antibiotic resistance in the United States, 1983-1984. *CDC Surveill Summ* 33:11SS-15SS, 1985.

Sisca TS, et al: Cinoxacin: Review of its pharmacological properties and therapeutic efficacy in treatment of urinary tract infections. *Drugs* 25:544-569, 1983.

Slight PH, et al: Trial of vancomycin for prophylaxis of infections after neurosurgical shunts, (letter). *N Engl J Med* 312:921, 1985.

Swanson BN, et al: Norfloxacin disposition after sequentially increasing oral doses. *Antimicrob Agents Chemother* 23:284-288, 1983.

Teasley DG, et al: Prospective randomized trial of metronidazole versus vancomycin for *Clostridium difficile*-associated diarrhoea and colitis. *Lancet* 2:1043-1046, 1983.

Thornsberry C, et al: Rifampin: Spectrum of antibacterial activity. *Rev Infect Dis* 5(suppl 3):S412-S417, 1983.

Waters BG, Rosenberg M: Vancomycin-induced hypotension. *Oral Surg* 52:239-240, 1981.

Watt B, et al: Norfloxacin versus cotrimoxazole in treatment of uncomplicated urinary tract infection: Multicenter trial. *J Antimicrob Chemother* 13(suppl B):89-94, 1984.

Wheat LJ, et al: Long-term studies of effect of rifampin on nasal carriage of coagulase-positive staphylococci. *Rev Infect Dis* 5(suppl 3):S459-S462, 1983.

Wise R: Norfloxacin: Review of pharmacology and tissue penetration. *J Antimicrob Chemother* 13(suppl B):59-64, 1984.

Wise R, et al: In vitro activity of enoxacin (CI-919), a new quinoline derivative, compared with that of other antimicrobial agents. *J Antimicrob Chemother* 13:237-244, 1984.

Wolfson JS, Hooper DC: Fluoroquinolones: Structures, mechanisms of action and resistance, and spectra of activity in vitro. *Antimicrob Agents Chemother* 28:581-586, 1985.

Other Selected References

Metronidazole hydrochloride (Flagyl I.V.). *Med Lett Drugs Ther* 23:13-14, 1981.

Edson RS, Rosenblatt JE: Parenteral metronidazole therapy of serious anaerobic infection. *Drug Ther* 12:229-232, (April) 1982.

Farr B, Mandell GL: Rifampin, in Mandell GL, et al (eds): *Principles and Practice of Infectious Diseases,* ed 2. New York, John Wiley & Sons, 1984, 216-220.

Fekety R: Vancomycin, in Mandell GL, et al (eds): *Principles and Practice of Infectious Diseases,* ed 2. New York, John Wiley & Sons, 1984, 232-235.

Holloway WJ: Spectinomycin. *Med Clin North Am* 66:169-173, 1982.

Horton J, Pankey GA: Polymyxin B, colistin, and sodium colistimethate. *Med Clin North Am* 66:135-142, 1982.

Kapusnik JE, et al: Use of rifampin in staphylococcal infections: Review. *J Antimicrob Chemother* 13(suppl C):61-66, 1984.

Leigh DA, Wise R (eds): Norfloxacin: New quinolone for urinary infections. *J Antimicrob Chemother* 13(suppl B):1-142, 1984 (17 papers).

Sande MA (ed): Use of rifampin in treatment of nontuberculous infections. *Rev Infect Dis* 5(suppl 3):S399-S632, 1983 (42 papers).

Schaad UB, et al: Clinical pharmacology and efficacy of vancomycin in pediatric patients. *J Pediatr* 96:119-126, 1980.

Stranz MH, Bradley WE: Metronidazole (Flagyl IV, Searle). *Drug Intell Clin Pharm* 15:838-846, 1981.

Tally FP, Sullivan CE: Metronidazole: In vitro activity, pharmacology and efficacy in anaerobic bacterial infections. *Pharmacotherapy* 1:28-38, 1981.

Wise RI, Kory M (eds): Reassessments of vancomycin: Potentially useful antibiotic. *Rev Infect Dis* 3(suppl):S199-S300, 1981 (16 papers).

Wise R, Reeves D (eds): Vancomycin therapy. *J Antimicrob Chemother* 14(suppl D):1-109, 1984 (14 papers).

Topical Anti-Infective Agents: Otic and Ophthalmic Preparations

The products discussed in this chapter are those applied locally in the external ear canal to treat external otitis and impacted cerumen and those applied topically in the eye to treat infections of the lids, conjunctiva, or cornea.

OTIC INFECTIONS

External Otitis

External otitis is an inflammatory condition involving the skin of the external auditory canal. Common causative factors are trauma from attempts at cleaning or other manipulation by the patient, environmental factors (eg, high temperature and humidity), accumulation of cerumen, and frequent exposure to water (swimmers' ear). The normal pH of the ear canal is slightly acidic (4.0-5.0); breakdown of this acid mantle with subsequent elevation of the pH into the alkaline range allows pathogenic organisms to overwhelm the normal flora and cause infection. The most common infecting bacterium is *Pseudomonas aeruginosa; Staphylococcus aureus* and species of *Proteus* also are common bacterial pathogens. *Candida* and *Aspergillus* are the most common causes of otomycosis. A primary viral eruption also occurs. Infections may be localized (furuncle) or diffuse, deep or superficial, and may involve any part of the external ear.

The signs and symptoms of external otitis vary according to etiologic agent, chronicity, extension, and specific location and include pruritus, pain, tenderness, erythema, edema, hearing loss, ulceration, granulation tissue, and odoriferous discharge.

A feeling of fullness and some reversible hearing loss may result from filling of the ear canals with debris and pus. Tinnitus even may be present if the ear drum is directly or indirectly involved.

The management of external otitis requires removal of purulent secretions, cerumen, foreign bodies, polyps, and granulation tissue, preferably under microscopic guidance. The offending organism should be identified whenever possible, and appropriate medications prescribed as indicated.

Drugs for instillation into the ear usually are dissolved or suspended in a liquid vehicle. They must come in contact with the infected area to be effective. Medicated creams or ointments may be used for dry, crusted lesions, and powder is used frequently for its desiccant properties. See Chapter 56, Dermatologic Preparations, for a listing of topical anti-infective preparations and corticosteroid-antibiotic mixtures.

For mild pruritus, a weak corticosteroid cream applied with a cotton-tipped applicator will provide relief. See Chapter 56 for a listing of topical corticosteroid preparations. When the ear canal is swollen, weeping, and inflamed, an aluminum acetate solution is effective; it has anti-inflammatory, antipruritic, and astringent properties and is nonsensitizing. A steroid cream also may be used for pruritus in the cavum concha and outer portion of the canal. It may be applied with the fingertips or carefully with a cotton applicator.

To relieve the pain that usually accompanies acute external otitis or otitis media when the tympanic membrane is intact, local anesthetics, usually benzocaine or lidocaine, have been applied topically in the ear canal. However, since their absorption from the skin or tympanic membrane is extremely poor

TABLE 1.
TOPICAL OTIC ANALGESIC AGENTS

Preparation	Analgesics	Other Ingredients	Container Size
Americaine Solution (American Critical Care)	Benzocaine 20%	Benzethonium chloride 0.1%, glycerin 1%	15 ml
Auralgan Otic Solution (Ayerst)	Benzocaine 1.4% Antipyrine 5.4%	Glycerin, oxyquinolone sulfate	15 ml
Tympagesic Solution (Adria)	Benzocaine 5% Antipyrine 5%	Phenylephrine hydrochloride 0.25%, propylene glycol	13 ml

and depends partially upon the preparation, the effectiveness of local anesthetics is unpredictable. Benzocaine also may cause hypersensitivity reactions and macerate the keratin layer of skin, obscuring important clinical signs and making diagnosis and monitoring of progress difficult. Therefore, systemic analgesics (eg, codeine, aspirin and codeine) are usually preferred. (See Table 1 for topical otic analgesic preparations.)

DRUG SELECTION. Antibacterial and antifungal agents are used empirically to treat external ear infections.

Antibacterial Agents: Several single-entity topical antibacterial preparations are commercially available for bacterial infections of the external ear and appear to be effective. See Table 2, Anti-infective Agents for Topical Otic Therapy, for dosage and preparations.

Topical otic preparations used to treat external otitis usually contain more than one antibacterial agent (see Table 3). The proposed rationale for these mixtures is that they have a wide antibacterial spectrum that includes both gram-positive and gram-negative organisms. Such fixed-ratio mixtures for topical use have reasonable therapeutic value but may cause the adverse reactions associated with each ingredient. Topical preparations containing neomycin and polymyxin B or colistin (polymyxin E) are often considered drugs of choice for empiric therapy of acute external otitis (Fairbanks, 1980 A and B; Cody et al, 1981). An alternative is aqueous acetic acid solution 2% to 5%, which is active against most pathogens causing external otitis, particularly *Pseudomonas*. Chloramphenicol and gentamicin ophthalmic drops are generally reserved for patients refractory to less toxic therapy.

Preparations that contain a corticosteroid in addition to an antibacterial agent may be useful when external otitis is complicated by severe inflammation or allergic dermatitis. There is no evidence that the corticosteroid enhances the efficacy of the antibiotics, however. Preparations containing a corticosteroid are contraindicated in patients with herpes simplex, vaccinia, and varicella. See Table 3 for preparations. For further information on actions and adverse reactions of adrenal corticosteroids, see Chapter 20, Miscellaneous Ophthalmic Preparations, and Chapter 61, Adrenal Corticosteroids in Nonendocrine Diseases.

Systemic antibiotics are rarely needed to treat external otitis. Their use should be limited to those occasions when there is a positive identification of the pathogen and resolution with topical medication seems delayed. The vast majority of cases of acute otitis externa are caused by gram-negative bacteria or by fungus. The empiric use of antibiotics should be discouraged.

Patients who do not respond to the usual treatment, especially diabetics or the elderly, should be observed more closely, for they may develop malignant or necrotizing otitis externa caused by *Pseudomonas aeruginosa*. It begins in the soft tissues of the external auditory canal, progresses to involve the cartilage and perichondrium of the canal, and eventually leads to osteitis of the temporal bone and base of the skull. If the patient is not hospitalized and given intravenous antipseudomonal antibiotics (eg, tobramycin [Nebcin], ticarcillin [Ticar]), complications such as facial nerve palsy, multiple cranial nerve palsies, osteomyelitis, and intracranial infection may result. Even with the improved therapy, the overall mortality rate exceeds 15%.

Acetic acid solutions (2% to 5%) have antibacterial and antifungal activity, particularly against *Pseudomonas aeruginosa, Candida,* and *Aspergillus.* They reduce swelling and relieve other signs and symptoms of external otitis. Acetic acid solution is well tolerated, nonsensitizing, and does not produce resistant organisms. It does, however, have an unpleasant vinegar-like odor and can be very painful when applied to the middle ear through a tympanostomy tube or a perforation. If irritation or symptoms of sensitivity to the vehicle occur, the medication should be discontinued.

Chloramphenicol has a broad spectrum of activity against many organisms; strains of *Staphylococcus aureus, Escherichia coli,* and *Proteus* species are susceptible. It is useful topically to treat resistant superficial infections of the external auditory canal caused by these organisms. Signs of local irritation have been reported in patients sensitive to this preparation. If these occur, chloramphenicol should be discontinued. It should be kept in mind that blood dyscrasias have been associated with systemic use of this drug and have been reported after prolonged therapy with a topical ophthalmic preparation. For further information on antibacterial activity and adverse reactions, see Chapter 69, Tetracyclines and Chloramphenicol.

Neomycin, an aminoglycoside antibiotic, is effective against *Escherichia, Enterobacter aerogenes,* and most species of

TABLE 2.
ANTI-INFECTIVE AGENTS FOR TOPICAL OTIC THERAPY

Preparation	Concentration	Other Ingredients	Dosage	Container Size
ANTIBACTERIAL AGENTS Acetic Acid				
VoSol Otic Solution (Wallace), Generic	2%	Propylene glycol diacetate 3%	*Adults and children*, (VoSol Otic Solution) initially, when possible a cotton wick is saturated, inserted into the ear canal, and kept moist for 24 hours; the wick is then	15 and 30 ml
Otic Domeboro Solution (Miles)	2%	Aluminum acetate (modified Burow's solution)	removed and five drops are instilled directly into the ear canal three or four times daily. (Otic Domeboro Solution) Four to six drops are instilled every two or three hours.	60 ml
Chloramphenicol Chloromycetin Otic (Parke-Davis)	0.5%	Propylene glycol	*Adults and children*, two or three drops are instilled three times daily.	15 ml
ANTIBACTERIAL AGENTS WITH CORTICOSTEROID*	---	---	*Solutions and Suspensions Adults*, four drops; *children*, three drops. The preparation is instilled three or four times daily or may be applied on a wick and inserted into the ear canal. The wick should be kept moist and changed every 24 hours. *Creams and Ointments Adults and children*, a liberal amount is applied to affected area two to four times daily.	---
ANTIFUNGAL AGENTS Acetic Acid	(See Vosol Otic Solution)	---	---	---
Amphotericin B Fungizone Lotion (Squibb)	3%	Propylene glycol	*Adults and children*, a liberal amount is applied to lesions two to four times daily. Duration of therapy depends on patient response.	30 ml
Clotrimazole Lotrimin (Schering)	1%	Polyethylene glycol	*Adults and children*, three or four drops instilled three times daily with weekly or biweekly cleaning of the ear canal.	10 and 30 ml
m-Cresyl Acetate Cresylate Solution (Rescei)	25%	Propylene glycol, isopropanol 25%, chlorobutanol 1%, benzyl alcohol 1%, castor oil 5%	*Adults and children*, two to four drops as required.	15 ml

*See Table 3 for composition and preparations of topical otic solutions and suspensions.
See Chapter 56, Dermatologic Preparations, for composition and preparations of topical creams and ointments.

Klebsiella, Salmonella, Shigella, and *Proteus;* many strains of *Staphylococcus aureus* also are sensitive. It has only weak activity against many strains of *Pseudomonas,* which is the most common bacterial isolate in external otitis. Therefore, topical preparations containing neomycin also contain polymyxin B or colistin, which have antipseudomonal activity, and hydrocortisone. Such preparations are indicated in the treatment of external otitis caused by susceptible organisms.

TABLE 3.
MIXTURES FOR TOPICAL OTIC THERAPY[1]

Preparation[2]	Anti-infective Agent	Corticosteroid	Other Ingredients	Container Size
Coly-Mycin S Otic with Neomycin and Hydrocortisone Suspension (Parke-Davis)	Colistin sulfate (equivalent to 3 mg base), neomycin sulfate (equivalent to 3.3 mg base)/ml	Hydrocortisone acetate 1%	Thonzonium bromide 0.05%, acetic acid, thimerosal 0.002%, polysorbate 80	5 and 10 ml
Cortisporin Otic Solution[3] (Burroughs Wellcome)	Neomycin sulfate (equivalent to 3.5 mg base), polymyxin B sulfate 10,000 units/ml	Hydrocortisone 1%	Cupric sulfate, glycerin, propylene glycol, potassium metabisulfite 0.1%	10 ml
Cortisporin Otic Suspension[3] (Burroughs Wellcome)	Neomycin sulfate (equivalent to 3.5 mg base), polymyxin B sulfate 10,000 units/ml	Hydrocortisone 1%	Cetyl alcohol, propylene glycol, polysorbate 80, thimerosal 0.01%	10 ml
Otic Tridesilon Solution (Miles)	Acetic acid 2%	Desonide 0.05%	Propylene glycol	10 ml
Otobiotic Solution (Schering)	Polymyxin B sulfate 10,000 units/ml	Hydrocortisone 0.5%	Propylene glycol	15 ml
Otocort Solution (Lemmon)	Neomycin sulfate (equivalent to 3.5 mg base), polymyxin B sulfate 10,000 units/ml	Hydrocortisone 1%	Propylene glycol, glycerin, potassium metabisulfite	10 ml
Pyocidin-Otic Solution (Berlex)	Polymyxin B sulfate 10,000 units/ml	Hydrocortisone 0.5%	Propylene glycol	10 ml
VoSol HC Otic Solution (Wallace)	Acetic acid 2%	Hydrocortisone 1%	Propylene glycol diacetate, benzethonium chloride 0.02%	10 ml

[1]See Chapter 56, Dermatologic Preparations, for composition and preparations of topical creams and ointments.
[2]See Table 2 for dosage.
[3]See manufacturers' literature for choice between solution and suspension.

Neomycin is a topical sensitizer, and cutaneous hypersensitivity reactions may result from its use in the ear. The reported prevalence of hypersensitivity to topical neomycin 20% (commercially available otic preparations generally contain neomycin 0.33% to 0.5%) has ranged from 3.7% to 60% in individuals with contact dermatitis or chronic dermatoses. However, the prevalence is only about 1% when neomycin is used on undamaged skin for no more than seven days (Prystowsky et al, 1979). If irritation or sensitivity develops, neomycin should be discontinued. The physician must always be alert for these reactions, since they frequently mimic the disease being treated. Such reactions usually can be recognized because the inflammatory process spreads to the tragus, antitragus, and lobule of the ear and the infection worsens rather than improves with continued treatment. Cross sensitization can occur between neomycin and other aminoglycosides and may prevent the subsequent use of these antibacterial agents.

Aminoglycosides are ototoxic when given systemically and ototoxicity has been demonstrated in laboratory animals after *topical* application of gentamicin and neomycin to the round window membrane and middle ear. Although this effect has not been demonstrated in man, the theoretical possibility of ototoxicity should be considered when aminoglycoside otic preparations are prescribed in patients with perforated tympanic membranes or tympanostomy tubes. For further information on antibacterial activity and adverse reactions, see Chapter 70, Aminoglycosides.

Polymyxin B and *colistin* (polymyxin E) are effective against *Pseudomonas aeruginosa, Escherichia,* and some other gram-negative organisms that commonly infect the ear. They lack ototoxic properties and therefore are particularly useful in patients with perforated ear drums or tubes. However, they are not active against other organisms that often cause external otitis, such as *Proteus* or gram-positive bacteria. A polymyxin is commonly included in otic mixtures that are indicated for external otitis caused by susceptible organisms. Adverse reactions are uncommon, but treatment should be discontinued if irritation or sensitivity occurs.

Antifungal Agents: Most fungi, particularly those infecting superficial layers of skin, require a warm, moist, dark area and dead tissue for growth. Mycotic infections also may follow the use of certain antibiotics (eg, aminoglycosides) or prolonged topical application of corticosteroids.

Otomycoses are characterized by the cotton-like appearance of the surface in different colors, pruritus, and desquamation. The white, black, brown, or bluish color identifies the different families of fungi. The precise nature of the fungus may be determined by culture on appropriate media or appearance on a potassium hydroxide-treated slide. *Candida* and *Aspergillus* most often cause otomycosis.

Most important in the management of fungal infections is meticulous, gentle cleansing of the skin of the ear canal; keratolytic agents also may be helpful. After cleansing, an antifungal preparation is instilled or applied to the skin of the ear canal. Treatment should continue for one or two weeks after disappearance of all clinical symptoms and evidence of the disease because fungal infections often recur. When there is a mixed infection of fungus and bacteria, a preparation containing both antifungal and antibacterial agents is useful.

Amphotericin B [Fungizone] is the most effective topical antifungal agent; it is active against a variety of fungi, particularly *Candida*. Other antifungal agents present in some preparations include acetic acid, cresyl acetate, and parachlorometaxylenol. *Clotrimazole* [Lotrimin] drops are very effective in the local treatment of refractory fungal external otitis. Propylene glycol is dehydrating to fungi, and this ingredient enhances the effectiveness of antifungal agents. In addition, the low pH of some otic preparations provides an unsuitable medium for growth of many fungi.

See Table 2, Anti-infective Agents for Topical Otic Therapy.

Cerumen-Softening and Cerumenolytic Agents

Cerumen (ear wax) is produced by the apocrine and sebaceous glands in the outer one-third of the external ear canal. It is hydrophobic and probably bacteriostatic and fungistatic; thus, the wax provides a protective coating for the external auditory canal. The type of wax produced is genetically determined. Those in western countries produce moist cerumen while those in eastern countries produce dry cerumen. Normally, the canal is self-cleaning, but the physiologic mechanism for removing cerumen occasionally becomes inefficient and excessive amounts accumulate. The most frequent causes of breakdown of this mechanism are misguided attempts to remove wax by the patient, narrow tortuous ear canals, or excessive hair growth in the ear. The self-cleaning mechanism of the ear canal is less effective in clearing dry cerumen than

moist cerumen. Occlusion of the ear canal by a large mass of cerumen can produce significant conductive hearing loss and predispose to the development of external otitis.

Patients who have chronic difficulty with hard, but not impacted, cerumen should instill light mineral oil (baby oil) or glycerin into the ear canal occasionally to soften the cerumen and promote normal removal.

Professional cleaning may be needed occasionally to remove wax and epithelial debris. This can be performed painlessly and efficiently. Some otologists advise their patients to fill the canal with mineral oil, which is inexpensive and nonallergenic, and plug the ear at night with cotton, which is removed in the morning. This oil treatment is initiated three nights before the office visit for professional cleaning and may be continued for one to three days. In addition to softening the debris, oil separates the dead skin from the living surface, permitting almost the entire mass to be removed gently with a –5 or –7 French suction tube. Thus, rapid removal of wax and debris with a minimum of discomfort and instrumentation is possible. Use of an ear bulb syringe to irrigate the canal gently with water at body temperature or normal saline may facilitate removal of the cerumen. A solution of carbamide peroxide in glycerin [Debrox] also may aid in the removal of excessive or hardened cerumen. Glycerin softens the wax and the effervescent oxygen released from peroxide loosens tissue debris. The ear canal should be be dried thoroughly after treatment, either chemically (eg, 70% isopropyl alcohol, 2% acetic acid solution [VōSol Otic]) or by blowing air into the ear with an ear bulb syringe or hair dryer to prevent maceration of the skin.

If external otitis is present in addition to impacted cerumen, it should be treated as discussed above. The instillation of an antibiotic-steroid preparation to reduce inflammation also may aid in softening the wax.

If impacted cerumen causes little or no inflammation, removal under direct visualization with a ring curette, wire loop, or another suitable instrument is preferable to irrigation. Extreme care should be taken not to traumatize the canal, since this portion of the ear is very sensitive to instrumentation. If the wax cannot be removed mechanically, a wax-softening or, rarely, a cerumenolytic agent may be used, followed by irrigation. A solution of triethanolamine polypeptide oleate-condensate in propylene glycol [Cerumenex] is promoted as a cerumenolytic agent. However, results of clinical studies comparing its efficacy to that of other preparations are conflicting. This solution must be used with extreme care since it causes severe contact dermatitis in some patients.

See Table 4, Topical Cerumenolytic Agents, for preparations. These are listed for information only; their superiority to other similar preparations is not implied.

OCULAR INFECTIONS

Bacteria are implicated as causative pathogens in most eye infections; viruses are the next most frequent and fungi are the least common pathogens (Pavan-Langston, 1983). Nonspecialists usually can manage many superficial infections of the eyelids and conjunctiva, but more severe infections, those that

TABLE 4.
TOPICAL CERUMENOLYTIC AGENTS

Preparation	Cerumenolytic Agents	Other Ingredients	Container Size
Cerumenex Drops (Purdue Frederick)	Triethanolamine polypeptide oleate-condensate 10%	Propylene glycol, chlorobutanol 0.5%	6 and 12 ml
Debrox Drops* (Marion)	Carbamide peroxide 6.5%	Anhydrous glycerin	15 and 30 ml

Nonprescription

respond poorly to therapy, or those that involve other parts of the eye usually require treatment by an ophthalmologist.

Cultures and scrapings are recommended to assist in the diagnosis of infections more serious than routine blepharoconjunctivitis. Bacteria normally present on the eyelids must be considered when interpreting the results of culture or sensitivity tests.

ROUTES OF ADMINISTRATION. Anti-infective agents are applied topically as drops to treat conjunctival and corneal infections and as ointment to treat conjunctival or eyelid infections. Topical therapy is often adequate for superficial infections of these structures. Ointments provide more prolonged contact than solutions but may interfere with vision when used in the daytime and may decrease the bioavailability of a second topically applied drug.

Anterior subconjunctival injection of certain drugs is employed occasionally in conjunction with topical application to deliver additional antibiotic to the cornea and anterior chamber of the eye. Anterior (subconjunctival) and posterior (retrobulbar) sub-Tenon's injections are used to treat infections of the vitreous and retina. These routes are employed by ophthalmologists to treat serious infections for which topical and systemic therapy may be insufficient. Drugs that cause toxic effects when given systemically may be used by these routes with less risk of general adverse reactions. Subconjunctival and retrobulbar injections are often quite painful but may be repeated every 12 to 24 hours at different sites, depending upon the disease and its severity.

Systemic antibiotics are given with local therapy to treat some forms of severe conjunctivitis, endophthalmitis, and infections of the soft tissue of the lids, ocular adnexa, and orbit. Systemic antibiotics are used in gonococcal conjunctivitis and keratitis. Systemic therapy and periocular injections do not produce therapeutic antibiotic levels in the vitreous for most bacterial infections.

Systemically administered ampicillin, dicloxacillin, chloramphenicol, cephalothin, and minocycline provide potentially therapeutic levels in the cornea, iris, sclera, choroid, retina, and aqueous of the normal eye when given in adequate doses. Many other agents that do not readily penetrate the normal eye will enter the inflamed eye; these include penicillin G, methicillin, nafcillin, oxacillin, erythromycin, aminoglycosides, polymyxins, and flucytosine. Tetracycline, streptomycin, and amphotericin B penetrate the eye poorly when given systemically and are of limited usefulness when administered by this route.

For endophthalmitis, most ophthalmologists inject antibiotics directly into the vitreous humor to obtain a high intraocular concentration. Since the interior of the eye cannot tolerate high concentrations of most drugs, the dose must be chosen carefully to provide an effective concentration that is not toxic to the retina or other ocular structures. The injectable form should be used because topical products contain preservatives that are toxic to the retina and corneal endothelium.

Antibacterial, antifungal, and antiviral agents that are used topically to treat ocular infections are discussed below. Concentrations for topical use may be found in Tables 5 to 7 and commercially available topical preparations are listed in Tables 8 and 9. See the appropriate chapters in Section XI for antimicrobial spectrum, adverse reactions, and preparations of systemically administered anti-infectives.

Bacterial Conjunctivitis and Blepharitis

Bacterial blepharitis is often persistent and difficult to treat. It commonly produces chronically red lid margins, often in association with seborrhea. The most common causative organism is *Staphylococcus aureus*. Therapy consists of frequent lid scrubs with baby shampoo, and topical bacitracin or erythromycin. If the condition is resistant to topical therapy, systemic therapy with erythromycin, tetracycline, or dicloxacillin may alleviate the infection (Barza and Baum, 1983).

For further information on drug selection, see discussion on Antibacterial Agents.

Acute bacterial conjunctivitis is a relatively common infection caused by a variety of organisms that induces a purulent or mucopurulent conjunctival discharge, eyelid edema, a foreign body sensation, and sticking shut of the lids on awakening. *Neisseria gonorrhoeae* and *N. meningitidis* produce a characteristic "hyperpurulent" discharge with aching pain, tenderness, chemosis, and marked lymphadenopathy on the involved side. Pseudomembranes, an uncommon sign in acute bacterial conjunctivitis, suggest infection by *Streptococcus pyogenes* or adenovirus. Most acute conjunctivitis is nonpurulent, however, and is commonly caused by viruses (especially adenovirus), allergens, and chemical irritants.

Staphylococcus aureus, S. epidermidis, Streptococcus pneumoniae, Haemophilus influenzae, and *Moraxella lacunata* are the most common causative pathogens in adults, children, and infants (excluding neonates). *Pseudomonas aeruginosa* has become a more common etiologic agent with the increased use of contact lenses. It is potentially the most harmful organism because it releases enzymes that rapidly digest the cornea and cause rapid progression of disease.

Treatment of acute bacterial conjunctivitis generally includes instillation of topical antibacterial agents, such as bacitracin, gentamicin, erythromycin, and sulfacetamide. These topical anti-infectives are effective in the great majority of patients with typical bacterial conjunctivitis. Combinations such as neomycin-bacitracin-polymyxin B, bacitracin-polymyxin B, or gramicidin-neomycin-polymyxin B can be prescribed with reasonable confidence for minor infections.

In corneal infections, fortified or concentrated antibacterial eyedrops are instilled every 15 to 30 minutes. In conjunctival infections, commercially available drops are instilled every four hours or more frequently. Antibacterial ointments are applied in the conjunctival sac three or four times daily or as nighttime medication in association with daytime administration of drops.

Conjunctivitis caused by *Staphylococcus aureus* tends to be chronic; therefore, bacitracin ointment should be applied at bedtime for one month after all signs of infection have disappeared.

Any patient with infectious conjunctivitis that persists for longer than two weeks and is worsening or spreading to the cornea should be referred immediately to an ophthalmologist. Corticosteroids should be avoided when treating infectious conjunctivitis, for they cause immunologic incompetence and increase the severity of bacterial, viral, and fungal infections.

Inclusion conjunctivitis, also known as inclusion blennorrhea in the newborn, is caused by *Chlamydia trachomatis* and is becoming increasingly common, presumably because of changes in sexual customs. It is acquired by the newborn during passage through the infected cervix. Papillary conjunctivitis, lacrimation, lid swelling, diffuse infiltration, chemosis, and mucopurulent discharge develop after an incubation period of 5 to 14 days. The Centers for Disease Control guidelines for treating culture-proven neonatal inclusion conjunctivitis recommend systemic erythromycin 50 mg/kg/day divided into four doses for at least two weeks. Parents of infected neonates also should be treated.

In adults, *Chlamydia* cause inclusion conjunctivitis and trachoma. Both infections may be treated with topical tetracycline or erythromycin ointment applied five times daily for three weeks with oral tetracycline 1 to 1.5 g daily. Doxycycline [Vibramycin] may be the preferred tetracycline because it is administered only twice daily. Oral erythromycin should be substituted for tetracycline in children under 8 years.

For *prophylaxis against neonatal conjunctivitis,* topical application of silver nitrate (Credé prophylaxis) is legally required in many states. One drop of a 1% solution (preferably packaged in wax ampuls) is instilled in the conjunctival sac of each eye immediately after delivery. It should not be rinsed from the eyes. Concentrations greater than 1% should not be used. Silver nitrate prophylaxis has greatly reduced the incidence of gonococcal conjunctivitis in the newborn, but it may cause local irritation and is not effective against *Chlamydia trachomatis*, the most common cause of neonatal conjunctivitis today.

Some states permit a specific topical antibiotic to be used for prophylaxis instead of silver nitrate. Erythromycin or tetracycline ointment is recommended by the Centers for Disease Control as an acceptable alternative. Erythromycin is effective against chlamydial conjunctivitis but not against nasopharyngeal chlamydial infections or subsequent pneumonia. Its efficacy against gonococcal neonatal conjunctivitis has not been studied in a high-risk population (Hammerschlag et al, 1980). Tetracycline may be less effective than erythromycin for prophylaxis of neonatal chlamydial conjunctivitis (Hammerschlag et al, 1980; Rettig et al, 1981). Tetracycline also may be less effective than silver nitrate for prophylaxis of neonatal gonococcal conjunctivitis (Stenson et al, 1981).

Bacterial Keratitis and Endophthalmitis

The signs and symptoms of *bacterial corneal ulcers* include pain, foreign body sensation, photophobia, distinct epithelial ulceration covered with mucopurulent exudate, focal stromal infiltration and ulceration, and iridocyclitis. The severity depends upon the infecting organism, the patient's condition, and the period elapsed prior to treatment. Predisposing factors include ocular trauma, corneal disorders, and previous administration of corticosteroid therapy (Musch et al, 1983).

The most common causative pathogens in bacterial keratitis are, in approximately decreasing order of frequency, *Staphylococcus aureus, Pseudomonas aeruginosa, Streptococcus pneumoniae, Klebsiella pneumoniae, Moraxella*, and the Enterobacteriaceae (*Escherichia coli, Proteus, Citrobacter, Enterobacter*, and *Serratia*).

The management of suppurative microbial keratitis requires an accurate diagnosis, appropriate antimicrobial therapy modified in accordance with the clinical condition and laboratory findings, and termination of therapy when feasible. A management algorithm has been developed that bases initial therapy on the interpretation of corneal smears, assessment of severity, and clinical impression (Jones, 1981). Initially, antibiotics are applied topically as drops every 15 to 30 minutes for the first 24 to 48 hours. Gentamicin ophthalmic drops are very useful (generally in combination with a cephalosporin) in the treatment of susceptible bacterial corneal ulcers and should be fortified (eg, by adding 2 ml of the parenteral form of gentamicin [40 mg/ml] to the 5-ml ophthalmic dropper bottle). Subconjunctival injections may be required when compliance is questionable, or in infants and young children who cry and thus the topical antibiotics are diluted and the drops are squeezed out of the eye. (See Table 5 for concentrations of the principal antibiotics.)

Serious corneal infections may cause permanent scarring or perforate the eye with loss of vision.

Endophthalmitis is a rare but devastating ocular complication of surgery or penetrating eye trauma. It involves the uveal tract, vitreous body, and retina and produces eye pain, loss of vision, conjunctival and ciliary injection, chemosis, lid swelling, corneal edema, hypopyon, and decreased or absent red reflex on ophthalmoscopic examination. The major causative bacteria are *Staphylococcus aureus, S. epidermidis, Streptococcus, Pseudomonas*, and *Proteus*.

Prompt and aggressive management with subconjunctival,

TABLE 5.
ANTIBACTERIAL AGENTS FOR OPHTHALMIC THERAPY*

| Drug | Concentration | | Daily Dosage Subconjunctival |
	Solution or Suspension	Ointment	
Amikacin	10 mg/ml	—	75–100 mg
Ampicillin	—	—	50–250 mg
Bacitracin	10,000 units/ml**	400–500 units/g	10,000 units
Carbenicillin	4 mg/ml	—	100 mg
Cefazolin	—	—	50–100 mg
Cephalothin	—	—	25–50 mg
Chloramphenicol	5 mg/ml	10 mg/g	50–100 mg
Clindamycin	—	—	15–40 mg
Colistin	5–10 mg/ml	—	15–20 mg
Erythromycin	5–10 mg/ml	5 mg/g	100 mg
Gentamicin	3–10 mg/ml	3 mg/g	20–40 mg
Methicillin	—	—	100–200 mg
Neomycin	2.5–5 mg/ml	5 mg/g	0.25–0.5 mg
Penicillin G	10,000–100,000 units/ml	—	500,000–1,000,000 units
Polymyxin B	10,000–20,000 units/ml	5,000–10,000 units/g	25,000 units
Sulfacetamide	100–300 mg/ml	100–300 mg/g	—
Tetracycline	10 mg/ml	10 mg/g	—
Tobramycin	3–10 mg/ml	3 mg/g	10–40 mg
Vancomycin	50 mg/ml	—	25 mg

*See Table 8 for preparations.
**See also Ellis, 1981; Pettit, 1976; Grayson, 1979; Jones, 1980; Henkind and Walsh, 1985.

intravitreal, and systemic antibacterial agents with subconjunctival injection and oral administration of corticosteroids is needed to minimize loss of vision (Forster et al, 1980). Topical antibacterial agents are of little value in initial treatment because the infection is in the uvea, vitreous, and retina.

DRUG SELECTION. Most superficial bacterial infections can be controlled by an appropriate topical antibiotic or antibiotic combination product. Except for self-limited or minor infections, identification of the causative organism by culture and smears should be attempted. Treatment should be delayed until the culture specimens have been collected.

Sulfacetamide sodium, bacitracin, gramicidin, neomycin, polymyxin B, and colistin are rarely administered systemically and are available commercially for topical use as single-entity preparations or in mixtures. Commercial ophthalmic preparations containing erythromycin, chloramphenicol, gentamicin, tobramycin, tetracycline, chlortetracycline, and sulfisoxazole also are available. Neomycin appears to be the most allergenic of these drugs.

Sulfacetamide sodium [Ak-Sulf, Bleph-10, Cetamide, Sulamyd, Vasosulf] is effective against some gram-positive and gram-negative organisms. It is bacteriostatic, not bactericidal, and many organisms are resistant. Sulfacetamide may be useful for mild acute bacterial conjunctivitis, such as that caused by *Haemophilus aegyptius*, *Streptococcus pneumoniae*, and many strains of *Staphylococcus aureus*. It is also commonly used to treat chronic blepharitis and conjunctivitis, but its efficacy in these conditions is questionable.

The antibacterial spectrum of *bacitracin* [Baciguent] is similar to that of penicillin G. It is preferred to penicillin for topical treatment of superficial staphylococcal and streptococcal infections because few strains of organisms are resistant, allergic reactions occur less frequently, and future sensitization to penicillin is avoided. *Gramicidin* is similar in activity to bacitracin, but is available only in combination products.

Neomycin is bactericidal and active against many gram-positive and gram-negative organisms, including *Proteus*. It produces sensitization (or toxicity) more readily than other topical antibiotics, particularly if given for longer than five to six days. In sensitized individuals, allergic conjunctivitis may worsen signs and symptoms, causing the unwary physician to intensify therapy instead of discontinuing the drug.

Polymyxin B [Aerosporin] and *colistin* [Coly-Mycin S] are bactericidal against most gram-negative organisms, including *Pseudomonas aeruginosa*, *Escherichia coli*, *Klebsiella pneumoniae*, and *Enterobacter aerogenes*. They are not effective against *Proteus* or gram-positive organisms. The minimal effective concentration of polymyxin B is 10,000 units/ml (*Federal Register*, 1980). Organisms resistant to polymyxin B are often resistant to colistin.

Combinations containing bacitracin (or gramicidin), neomycin, and polymyxin B (eg, Mycitracin, Neosporin) are widely used in ocular therapy because of their broad spectrum of activity.

Erythromycin [Ilotycin] is well tolerated and is effective against many gram-positive organisms, including *Streptococcus pneumoniae* and *S. pyogenes*. Staphylococci occasionally are resistant to this antibiotic at the beginning of therapy;

however, many strains become resistant during long-term therapy. Silver nitrate is ineffective in preventing neonatal chlamydial conjunctivitis. Erythromycin is effective against chlamydial conjunctivitis but not against nasopharyngeal chlamydial infections or subsequent pneumonia. (See the discussion on prophylaxis against neonatal conjunctivitis.)

Chloramphenicol [Chloroptic, Econochlor, Ophthochlor] is a broad spectrum antibiotic that is often used topically to treat acute conjunctivitis caused by *Haemophilus* and *Moraxella*. Topical chloramphenicol rarely causes sensitization. Fifteen cases of significant blood dyscrasias or aplastic anemia have been reported during or several months after continuous or intermittent use of chloramphenicol eyedrops or ointment (Fraunfelder and Meyer, 1985). Its use should be restricted to infections resistant to all other antibiotics (Baum, 1980).

The aminoglycosides, *gentamicin* [Garamycin, Genoptic] and *tobramycin* [Tobrex], are active against a wide variety of gram-negative and gram-positive organisms. These agents are particularly useful because of their significant activity against *Pseudomonas, Proteus, Klebsiella, E. coli,* and staphylococci. Since occasional strains of *Pseudomonas* are resistant, polymyxin B or colistin may be considered as additional therapy for pseudomonal conjunctivitis.

In addition to these commercial preparations, eyedrops may be formulated by diluting parenteral antibiotics with balanced salt solution or artificial tears and adjusting for isotonicity. The solubility and stability of antibiotics prepared in this manner may vary (Osborn et al, 1976). Since the stability of these solutions is not assured, they should be prepared just prior to application. Most solutions are stable for a week.

A number of products contain a fixed-dose combination of a corticosteroid and an antibacterial agent, and these are used by some ophthalmologists to treat conditions in which both may be required. These mixtures should *not* be used to treat conjunctivitis or blepharitis of unknown origin. For further discussion, see Chapter 20, Miscellaneous Ophthalmic Preparations.

See Table 8 for single-entity preparations and Table 9 for fixed-dose combinations.

Fungal Infections

Fungal infections of the eye occur most commonly in warm climates after injury or surgery or when host resistance is decreased. The increased incidence of oculomycosis observed in recent years has been attributed to the widespread use of corticosteroids and, possibly, broad spectrum antibiotics.

Over 100 varieties of fungi have been identified as ocular pathogens. The fungi most frequently cultured from mycotic corneal ulcers are *Aspergillus* (usually *A. fumigatus*), *Fusarium solani, Candida albicans, Cephalosporium,* and *Curvularia*.

DRUG SELECTION. Most antifungal agents penetrate the eye poorly when applied topically. Natamycin is the only

TABLE 6.
ANTIFUNGAL AGENTS FOR TOPICAL OPHTHALMIC THERAPY*

Drug	Concentration	Dosage
Amphotericin B	0.5–1.5 mg/ml (suspension)	One drop every half hour and then every hour.
Miconazole	10 mg/ml (solution)	Initially, one drop every hour day and night for 4–10 days, followed by one drop every hour during the day for 2–4 weeks, then one drop six times daily for 3–7 weeks.
Natamycin	50 mg/ml** (suspension)	For fungal keratitis, initially one drop is instilled every hour during the day and every 2 hours at night. After 3–4 days, the frequency of administration may be reduced to one drop 6–8 times daily. Therapy should be continued for 14–21 days. For fungal blepharitis and conjunctivitis, an initial dose of 4–6 daily applications may be sufficient.
Nystatin	25,000 units/ml (suspension)	Initially, one drop every 15 minutes. Alternatively, the powder may be dusted onto the lesion.
	100,000 units/g (dermatologic ointment)	Ointment is applied 4 times daily.

*See Table 8 for preparations.
**Available in this concentration as ophthalmic products.

TABLE 7.
ANTIVIRAL AGENTS FOR TOPICAL OPHTHALMIC THERAPY*

Drug	Concentration	Dosage
Idoxuridine	1 mg/ml (0.1% solution)	One drop every hour during the day and every 2 hours at night. Alternatively, 1 drop every minute for 5 instillations, repeated every 4 hours. When healing appears to be complete, treatment should be continued for 3-5 days at a dose of 1 drop every 2 hours during the day and every 4 hours at night. Therapy generally should not be continued for more than 21 days.
	5 mg/g (0.5% ointment)	Ointment is applied 4-5 times daily or as nighttime medication. Treatment should be continued for 3-5 days after healing appears to be complete. Therapy generally should not be continued for more than 21 days.
Trifluridine	10 mg/ml (1% solution)	Initially, 1 drop every 2 hours while awake (maximum, 9 drops daily). When healing appears to be complete, treatment should be continued for 7 days at a dosage of 1 drop every 4 hours while awake (minimum, 5 drops daily). Therapy generally should not be continued for more than 21 days.
Vidarabine	30 mg/g (3% ointment)	One-half inch applied 5 times daily at 3-hour intervals. When healing appears to be complete, treatment should be continued for 7 days at a reduced dosage (eg, twice daily). Therapy generally should not be continued for more than 21 days.
Acyclovir**	30 mg/g (3% ointment)	One-half inch applied 5 times daily at 3- to 4- hour intervals and continued for at least 3 days after complete healing. Therapy generally should not be continued for more than 21 days.

*See Table 8 for preparations.
**Investigational use

antifungal drug available in the United States as a topical ophthalmic product. Dilute solutions or suspensions of some systemic antifungal drugs, such as nystatin, amphotericin B, and miconazole, also have been used for topical therapy. The subconjunctival route also has been employed, but some antifungal agents are very irritating when given by this route.

Amphotericin B [Fungizone] has significant activity against various fungi, particularly Candida, Coccidioides, Cryptococcus, Histoplasma, Blastomyces, and Sporotrichum. When administered systemically, intraocular penetration is poor and large doses must be used, thereby increasing the risk of hepatic and renal toxicity. However, a very dilute solution (ie, 0.05% to 0.15%) may be applied topically to treat keratomycoses caused by susceptible organisms and is considered by some experts to be the drug of choice. Strong concentrations cause severe local irritation and should be avoided.

Natamycin (pimaricin) [Natacyn] is a well tolerated topical agent that is effective in a variety of keratomycoses caused by Fusarium and Cephalosporium species. Because of its broad spectrum of activity, natamycin was the drug of choice for topical antifungal therapy. It penetrates the cornea poorly and is ineffective against deep forms of fungal keratitis. Allergic reactions have been reported rarely.

Nystatin [Mycostatin, Nilstat] is used topically to treat external ocular infections caused by Candida or Aspergillus. It is of little or no value in other fungal infections.

Miconazole may be useful topically to treat corneal infections caused by Candida and Aspergillus and is reported to penetrate the eye relatively well. The intravenous preparation (miconazole [Monistat I.V.]) has been employed for this purpose, but it may cause superficial punctate keratitis with prolonged topical use (Foster, 1981).

Flucytosine [Ancobon] is a relatively nontoxic antifungal agent that is administered orally. It has not been used widely in ophthalmology but appears to be useful in ocular infections caused by Candida albicans or Cryptococcus neoformans. Because resistant strains may develop, concomitant administration of amphotericin B has been recommended. Flucytosine has been used topically (product not available commercially) in a 1% to 1.5% concentration to treat ocular fungal infections.

See Table 6 for topical dosage. See also Jones, 1980, and Henkind and Walsh, 1985.

Viral Infections

Primary ocular herpes simplex infection is characterized by follicular conjunctivitis and vesicular lesions of the eyelids, which may be accompanied by punctate keratitis. Recurrent infection is generally manifested by epithelial keratitis, usually in the form of dendritic ulceration or, less commonly, as geographic or ameboid ulcers. Stromal keratitis and uveitis develop in 10% to 20% of patients.

TABLE 8.
TOPICAL OPHTHALMIC ANTI-INFECTIVE PREPARATIONS (SINGLE-ENTITY)

Preparation	Preservatives	Container Size
ANTIBACTERIAL AGENTS		
Bacitracin		
*Ointment 500 units/g**		
Baciguent (Upjohn)	Chlorobutanol 0.65%	3.5 g
Chloramphenicol		
Ointment 1%		
Chloromycetin (Parke-Davis)	Preservative free	3.5 g
Chloroptic S.O.P. (Allergan)	Chlorobutanol 0.5%	3.5 g
Econochlor (Alcon)	Preservative free	3.5 g
Solution 0.5%		
Chloroptic (Allergan)	Chlorobutanol 0.5%	7.5 ml
Econochlor (Alcon)	Thimerosal 0.01%	2.5 and 15 ml
Ophthochlor (Parke-Davis)	Preservative free	15 ml
Chlortetracycline		
Ointment 1%		
Aureomycin (Lederle)	Preservative free	3.75 g
Erythromycin		
Ointment 0.5%		
Ilotycin (Dista)	Preservative free	3.75 g
Gentamicin		
*Ointment 0.3%**		
Garamycin (Schering)	Methylparaben, propylparaben	3.75 g
Genoptic S.O.P. (Allergan)	Methylparaben, propylparaben	3.5 g
Solution 0.3%		
Garamycin (Schering)	Benzalkonium chloride	5 ml
Genoptic (Allergan)	Benzalkonium chloride	5 ml
Polymyxin B		
*Sterile Powder**		
Aerosporin (Burroughs Wellcome)	Preservative Free	500,000 units/vial
Silver Nitrate		
Solution 1%		
Generic		Single-dose ampuls
Sulfacetamide Sodium		
*Ointment 10%**		
Cetamide (Alcon)	Methylparaben, propylparaben	3.5 g
Sulamyd (Schering)	Benzalkonium chloride, methylparaben, propylparaben	3.5 g
*Solution 10%**		
Ak-Sulf (Akorn)	Chlorobutanol 0.2%, methylparaben, propylparaben, sodium thiosulfate 0.2%	15 ml
Bleph-10 Liquifilm (Alcon)	EDTA, sodium thiosulfate, thimerosal 0.005%	5 and 15 ml
Sulamyd (Schering)	Methylparaben, propylparaben	5 ml
*Solution 15%**		
Isopto-Cetamide (Alcon)	Methylparaben, propylparaben, sodium thiosulfite 0.3%	5 and 15 ml
Vasosulf** (CooperVision)	Methylparaben, propylparaben, sodium thiosulfate	5 and 15 ml

(Continued on next page)

TABLE 8.
TOPICAL OPHTHALMIC ANTI-INFECTIVE PREPARATIONS (SINGLE-ENTITY) (continued)

Preparation	Preservatives	Container Size
ANTIBACTERIAL AGENTS (continued)		
Sulfisoxazole Diolamine		
Ointment 4%		
Gantrisin (Roche)	Phenylmercuric acid 1:50,000	3.5 g
Solution 4%		
Gantrisin (Roche)	Phenylmercuric acid 1:100,000	15 ml
Tetracycline Hydrochloride		
Ointment 1%		
Achromycin (Lederle)	Preservative free	3.75 g
Suspension 1%		
Achromycin (Lederle)	Preservative free	0.5 and 4 ml
Tobramycin		
Ointment 0.3%		
Tobrex (Alcon)	Chlorobutanol 0.5%	3.5 g
Solution 0.3%		
Tobrex (Alcon)	Benzalkonium chloride 0.01%	5 ml
ANTIFUNGAL AGENT		
Natamycin		
Suspension 5%		
Natacyn (Alcon)	Benzalkonium chloride 0.02%	15 ml
ANTIVIRAL AGENTS		
Idoxuridine		
Ointment 0.5%		
Stoxil (Smith Kline & French)	Preservative free	4 g
Solution 0.1%		
Dendrid (Alcon)	EDTA, benzalkonium chloride 0.01%	15 ml
Herplex (Allergan)	Benzalkonium chloride, EDTA	15 ml
Stoxil (Smith Kline & French)	Thimerosal 1:50,000	15 ml
Trifluridine		
Solution 10 mg/ml		
Viroptic (Burroughs Wellcome)	Thimerosal 0.001%	7.5 ml
Vidarabine		
Ointment 3%		
Vira-A (Parke-Davis)	Preservative free	3.5 g

*Available generically
**With phenylephrine hydrochloride 0.125%

Epithelial disease has been treated successfully by mechanical debridement, but current therapy utilizes a topical antiviral agent with or without debridement. Corticosteroids are contraindicated in patients with epithelial viral infections because they allow the infection to spread; dense corneal scarring and loss of vision may result.

Most forms of stromal keratitis and uveitis are believed to be caused by immune mechanisms and may respond to topical corticosteroids. However, concomitant administration of an antiviral agent is usually advisable because the steroid may enhance virus growth.

DRUG SELECTION. Three antiviral agents are available in the United States for topical ophthalmic use: idoxuridine (IDU) [Dendrid, Herplex, Stoxil], vidarabine [Vira-A], and trifluridine [Viroptic]. These agents interfere with viral synthesis of DNA and are effective topically in herpes simplex infections of the conjunctiva and cornea.

In uncomplicated dendritic keratitis, the antiviral drugs are similar in efficacy, but trifluridine may be more effective than vidarabine against ameboid ulcers (Coster et al, 1979). Idoxuridine and trifluridine also have been used to treat vaccinia infections of the eye. There appears to be no cross sensitivity or cross resistance among these drugs, and patients allergic or resistant to one may benefit from treatment with another.

Antiviral agents are of no established value in treating stromal keratitis and uveitis; however, trifluridine is more likely

TABLE 9.
ANTIBACTERIAL MIXTURES FOR TOPICAL OPHTHALMIC THERAPY

Preparation	Antibacterial Agents	Preservatives	Container Size
Chloromyxin (Parke-Davis)	Chloramphenicol 10 mg and polymyxin B sulfate 10,000 units/g	Preservative free	3.5 g
Mycitracin Ophthalmic Ointment (Upjohn)	Bacitracin 500 units, neomycin sulfate 5 mg (equivalent to 3.5 mg base), and polymyxin B sulfate 5,000 units/g	Chlorobutanol 0.5%	3.5 g
Neosporin Ophthalmic Ointment (Burroughs Wellcome)	Bacitracin zinc 400 units, neomycin sulfate 5 mg (equivelant to 3.5 mg base), and polymyxin B sulfate 10,000 units/g	Preservative free	3.5 g
Neosporin Ophthalmic Solution (Burroughs Wellcome)	Gramicidin 0.025 mg, neomycin sulfate 2.5 mg (equivelant to 1.75 mg base), and polymyxin B sulfate 10,000 units/ml	Thimerosal 0.001%	10 ml
Polysporin Ophthalmic Ointment (Burroughs Wellcome)	Bacitracin zinc 500 units and polymyxin B sulfate 10,000 units/g	Preservative free	3.5 g
Statrol Ophthalmic Ointment (Alcon)	Neomycin sulfate 5 mg (equivalent to 3.5 mg base) and polymyxin B sulfate 10,000 units/g	Methylparaben, propylparaben	3.5 g
Statrol Ophthalmic Solution (Alcon)	Neomycin sulfate 5 mg (equivalent to 3.5 mg base) and polymyxin B sulfate 16,250 units/ml	Benzalkonium chloride	5 ml
Terramycin Ophthalmic Ointment (Pfipharmecs)	Oxytetracycline hydrochloride 5 mg and polymyxin B sulfate 10,000 units/g	Preservative free	3.5 g

to penetrate the cornea and may prove to be beneficial in these conditions.

Acyclovir [Zovirax] is an antiviral preparation used investigationally to treat ocular viral infections. It selectively inhibits viral DNA synthesis, penetrates the eye well, is minimally metabolized, and appears to be well tolerated. In comparative studies, acyclovir was as effective as idoxuridine, vidarabine, and trifluridine or more effective than idoxuridine and vidarabine in treating dendritic keratitis (Falcon, 1983; Richards et al, 1983). Initial reports suggest that acyclovir may be beneficial in treating geographic and stromal herpetic keratitis (Pavan-Langston et al, 1978; Klauber and Ottovay, 1982); however, further studies involving a larger number of patients are required to confirm these findings.

Idoxuridine, vidarabine, and trifluridine may cause local irritation (toxic and/or allergic), photophobia, edema of the eyelids and cornea, punctal occlusion, and superficial punctate keratopathy. The risk of corneal toxicity is increased by prolonged treatment or administration to patients with dry-eye syndromes. In theory, antiviral drugs might interfere with epithelial regeneration and inhibit stromal healing, and irreversible conjunctival cicatrization has been reported following long-term (more than one year) administration of idoxuridine (Lass et al, 1983). For reactions caused by acyclovir, see Chapter 79, Antiviral Agents.

See Table 7 for dosage and Table 8 for preparations.

Cited References

Oligosaccharide, peptide, and certain other antibiotic drugs. *Federal Register* 45:57735-57737, 1980.

Barza M, Baum J: Ocular infections. *Med Clin North Am* 67:131-152, 1983.

Baum J: Antibiotic use in ophthalmology, in Duane TD (ed): *Clinical Ophthalmology*. Hagerstown, MD, Harper & Row, 1980, vol 4, 1-20.

Cody DTR, et al: *Diseases of the Ear, Nose, and Throat: A Guide to Diagnosis and Management.* Chicago, Year Book Medical Publishers, 1981.

Coster DJ, et al: Treatment of amoeboid herpetic ulcers with adenine arabinoside or trifluorothymidine. *Br J Ophthalmol* 63:418-421, 1979.

Ellis PP: *Ocular Therapeutics and Pharmacology,* ed 6. St Louis, CV Mosby, 1981.

Fairbanks DNF: *Pocket Guide to Antimicrobial Therapy in Otolaryngology.* Washington, DC, American Council of Otolaryngology-Head and Neck Surgery, 1980 A.

Fairbanks DNF: Otic topical agents. *Otolaryngol Head Neck Surg* 88:327-331, 1980 B.

Falcon MG: Herpes simplex virus infections of eye and their management with acyclovir. *J Antimicrob Chemother* 12(suppl B):39-43, 1983.

Forster RK, et al: Management of infectious endophthalmitis. *Ophthalmology* 87:313-318, 1980.

Foster CS: Miconazole therapy for keratomycosis. *Am J Ophthalmol* 91:622-629, 1981.

Fraunfelder FT, Meyer SM: Side effects of drugs, in Reinecke RD (ed): *Ophthalmology Annual.* Norwalk, CT, Appleton-Century-Crofts, 1985, vol 1, 179-191.

Grayson M: *Diseases of the Cornea.* St Louis, CV Mosby, 1979.

Hammerschlag MR, et al: Erythromycin ointment for ocular prophylaxis of neonatal chlamydial infection. *JAMA* 244:2291-2293, 1980.

Henkind P, Walsh JB: Pharmaceuticals in ophthalmology. 3. Antimicrobial therapy, in: *Physicians' Desk Reference for Ophthalmology,* ed 13. Oradell, NJ, Medical Economics, 1985, 4-8.

Jones DB: Ocular infections, in Kagan BM (ed): *Antimicrobial Therapy.* Philadelphia, WB Saunders, 1980.

Jones DB: Decision-making in management of microbial keratitis. *Ophthalmology* 88:814-820, 1981.

Klauber A, Ottovay E: Acyclovir and idoxuridine treatment of herpes simplex keratitis: Double-blind clinical study. *Acta Ophthalmol* 60:838-844, 1982.

Lass JH, et al: Idoxuridine-induced conjunctival cicatrization. *Arch Ophthalmol* 101:747-750, 1983.

Musch DC, et al: Demographic and predisposing factors in corneal ulceration. *Arch Ophthalmol* 101:1545-1548, 1983.

Osborn E, et al: Stability of ten antibiotics in artificial tear solutions. *Am J Ophthalmol* 82:775-780, 1976.

Pavan-Langston D: Diagnosis and therapy of common eye infections: Bacterial, viral, fungal. *Compr Ther* 9:33-42, (May) 1983.

Pavan-Langston D, et al: Acyclic antimetabolite therapy of experimental herpes simplex keratitis. *Am J Ophthalmol* 86:618-623, 1978.

Pettit TH: Management of bacterial corneal ulcers, in Leopold IH, Burns RP (eds): *Symposium on Ocular Therapy.* New York, John Wiley & Sons, 1976, vol 8, 57-65.

Prystowsky SD, et al: Allergic contact sensitivity to nickel, neomycin, ethylenediamine, and benzocaine: Relationships between age, sex, history of exposure, and reactivity to standard patch tests and use tests in general population. *Arch Dermatol* 115:959-962, 1979.

Rettig PJ, et al: Postnatal prophylaxis of chlamydial conjunctivitis, (letter). *JAMA* 246:2321-2322, 1981.

Richards DM, et al: Acyclovir: Review of its pharmacodynamic properties and therapeutic efficacy. *Drugs* 26:378-438, 1983.

Stenson S, et al: Conjunctivitis in newborn: Observations on incidence, cause, and prophylaxis. *Ann Ophthalmol* 13:329-334, 1981.

Topical Anti-Infective Agents: Drugs Used on Skin and Mucous Membranes

74

TOPICAL ANTIBIOTICS

CHEMOTHERAPEUTIC AGENTS FOR BURNS

ANTIFUNGAL AGENTS FOR DERMATOPHYTIC AND
SUPERFICIAL CANDIDAL INFECTIONS

ANTIVIRAL AGENTS FOR WARTS AND MOLLUSCUM
CONTAGIOSUM

ANTI-INFESTATION AGENTS

Scabies

Pediculosis

ANTISEPTICS AND DISINFECTANTS

TOPICAL ANTIBIOTICS

Skin infections (pyodermas) caused by bacteria are classified as primary or secondary. Group A beta-hemolytic *Streptococcus* (*S. pyogenes*) and *Staphylococcus aureus* are the most common causative organisms (Witkowski and Parish, 1982; Aly and Maibach, 1984). Gram-negative pathogens are much less common etiologic agents, but they may cause certain secondary pyodermas (eg, infected burns, infected dermal stasis ulcers in the elderly).

Folliculitis, furuncles, carbuncles, and bullous impetigo are typical primary staphylococcal pyodermas; nonbullous facial impetigo usually is caused by staphylococci or mixed streptococci and staphylococci. Most cases of nonbullous impetigo, ecthyma, erysipelas, and cellulitis are caused by group A (group B in the newborn) beta-hemolytic streptococci.

Secondary pyodermas may appear in conjunction with skin disorders, such as insect, animal, or human bites; burns; other dermatoses; and fungal or viral infections. The most common serious secondary pyodermas are observed in patients with second- or third-degree burns, dermal stasis ulcers, eczematous dermatitis, or intertrigo and in debilitated or immunocompromised patients.

The general management and topical antibiotic therapy for uncomplicated bacterial pyodermas are presented in this section. For information on pyodermas associated with specific conditions, see the discussion on burn therapy in this chapter and on wound management in Chapter 56, Dermatologic Preparations. For fungal pyodermas, see the discussion on Antifungal Agents for Dermatophytic and Superficial Candidal Infections in this chapter.

Management: Warm moist compresses or soaks for wound cleansing, debridement, and promotion of drainage are useful adjuncts to drug therapy in pyodermas. Surgical incision and drainage or excision may be necessary for selected furuncles and carbuncles.

Topical antibiotics may be effective in some primary and secondary pyodermas, especially those superimposed on chronic dermatitis. When used adjunctively with systemic antibiotics, topical agents help to reduce contagion.

Topical antibiotic therapy and local cleansing may be sufficient for limited uncomplicated superficial folliculitis, limited impetigo, and ecthyma, especially when the patient or family members are able to perform gentle debridement of the thick crusts prior to application of the topical antibiotic (Leyden and Kligman, 1978).

Furuncles, carbuncles, or abscesses with surrounding cellulitis and causing fever or recurrent lesions usually require a systemic antibiotic. Systemic administration also is usually preferred for extensive streptococcal skin infections (Witkowski and Parish, 1982; Aly and Maibach, 1984).

When systemic administration is necessary, a penicillinase-resistant penicillin is often employed for staphylococcal pyodermas, although erythromycin is preferred by many pediatricians and dermatologists because it is safe and sensitization is uncommon. Penicillin is the drug of choice for streptococcal pyodermas; erythromycin is an alternate in patients allergic to penicillin. Infections caused by resistant organisms (eg, methicillin-resistant staphylococci, *H. influenzae*), by multiple organisms (eg, mixed anaerobic/aerobic gram-positive/gram-negative flora in infected dermal ulcers in diabetics), or infections in noncompliant patients may require use of vancomycin, ampicillin, a cephalosporin, clindamycin, or metronidazole. For systemic therapy of skin infections caused by other organisms, see Table 1 in Chapter 65, Antimicrobial Therapy and Chemoprophylaxis of Infectious Diseases.

Drug Selection: Since culturing of skin infections is often inappropriate and multiple organisms often are present, mixtures of poorly absorbed topical antibiotics are used frequently to improve the spectrum of antibacterial activity. However, a Gram stain of the lesion may aid in drug selection. The poorly absorbed topical antibiotics that are seldom used systemically (bacitracin, gramicidin, neomycin, and polymyxin B) are especially useful in limited pyodermas. Neomycin has the broadest spectrum of activity and is particularly effective against staphylococci. Streptococci and other gram-positive organisms are especially susceptible to bacitracin and also to gramicidin. Many gram-negative organisms, except *Proteus* and *Serratia*, are susceptible to polymyxin B.

Because topical antibiotics can promote resistance by selecting out mutants (Lacey, 1984), some dermatologists recommend that no antibiotic that is used systemically be employed in a topical preparation. Other authorities feel that the development of resistant strains does not appear to be a major problem in outpatient use. Topical antibiotics that are also given systemically (except for clioquinol [iodochlorhydroxyquin]) include the following drugs.

Tetracycline ointment [Achromycin], chlortetracycline ointment [Aureomycin], and oxytetracycline (available only in combination with polymyxin B [Terramycin]) in ointment and powder form have a broad spectrum of activity and are available without prescription as first-aid antibiotics.

Gentamicin cream or ointment [Garamycin] has a more limited spectrum of activity and is available only on prescription. Gentamicin is useful occasionally for *Pseudomonas* infections unresponsive to poorly absorbed topical antibiotics (eg, limited infection in burns or stasis ulcers).

Clioquinol (iodochlorhydroxyquin) [Vioform] is not an antibiotic; it has limited antibacterial and antifungal activity. Single-entity nonprescription preparations are available in cream and ointment forms. It also is used occasionally in combination with a corticosteroid [Racet, Vioform-Hydrocortisone] in localized bacterial infections and dermatophytoses associated with certain inflammatory skin conditions. Topical clioquinol's benefit-risk ratio currently is being questioned (see the section on Antifungal Agents for Dermatophytic and Superficial Candidal Infections).

Special formulations of erythromycin [A/T/S, EryDerm, Erymax, Erycette, Staticin], tetracycline [Topicycline, T-Stat], meclocycline sulfosalicylate [Meclan], and clindamycin [Cleocin T] are used exclusively to suppress *Propionibacterium acnes*, which is presumed to reduce the inflammatory response to fatty acids produced by *P. acnes*. These preparations are not used for pyodermas (see the section on Agents Used in Acne Vulgaris in Chapter 56, Dermatologic Preparations).

Drug Evaluations

BACITRACIN
[Baciguent]

ACTIONS AND USES. This polypeptide antibiotic is rarely used systemically. Topical preparations contain bacitracin alone or the zinc salt in combination with other poorly absorbed antibiotics and/or corticosteroids.

Bacitracin is bactericidal against gram-positive organisms, including the most common skin pathogens, staphylococci and streptococci. It is inactive against most gram-negative organisms, including *Pseudomonas*. Acquired bacterial resistance is rare.

Topical bacitracin is beneficial in primary pyodermas (eg, superficial folliculitis, limited ecthyma, impetigo) and limited secondary pyodermas not caused by gram-negative organisms. It is used with systemic antibiotics in more extensive gram-positive pyodermas to control infection, promote healing, and reduce contagion locally.

ADVERSE REACTIONS AND PRECAUTIONS. Hypersensitivity reactions, usually manifested as allergic dermatitis or conjunctivitis, may be severe but are rare when bacitracin is applied topically (Fisher, 1983). Bacitracin is not absorbed significantly from the skin; therefore, it may be used during pregnancy or lactation.

DOSAGE AND PREPARATIONS.
Topical: Adults and children, the ointment is applied to lesions three or four times daily and at bedtime.
> *Generic.* Ointment 500 units/g in 1.5, 15, 30, 120, and 454 g containers (nonprescription).
> *Baciguent* (Upjohn). Ointment 500 units/g in 15, 30, and 120 g containers (nonprescription).

NEOMYCIN SULFATE
[Myciguent]

ACTIONS AND USES. This broad spectrum aminoglycoside antibacterial agent is too toxic for parenteral use and is very poorly absorbed orally. Therefore, neomycin is used topically on the skin alone or in combination with other poorly absorbed antibiotics and/or corticosteroids.

Neomycin may be beneficial when used alone in limited primary pyodermas (superficial folliculitis, ecthyma, impetigo) and limited secondary pyodermas (eg, infectious eczematoid dermatitis, infected dermal ulcers, intertrigo). Infections caused by staphylococci are most responsive. Systemic antibiotics are preferred by most physicians for more extensive pyodermas, but neomycin may be useful with systemic antibiotic therapy to control infection, promote healing, and reduce contagion locally.

ADVERSE REACTIONS AND PRECAUTIONS. In one investigational study, hypersensitivity to topical neomycin 20% (a 3.5% concentration is available commercially) occurred in 3.7% to 60% of individuals with contact dermatitis or chronically damaged skin (eg, stasis dermatitis). However, the incidence was only about 1% after application to undamaged skin if treatment was limited to seven days. Cross sensitivity with other aminoglycoside antibiotics may occur. Results of the patch test utilizing 20% neomycin in petrolatum should be determined at 48 and 96 hours.

Neomycin is not absorbed significantly from the skin; therefore, it may be used during pregnancy or lactation.

DOSAGE AND PREPARATIONS.

Topical: An appropriate preparation is applied one or two times daily.

> *Generic.* Ointment 5 mg/g in 15 and 30 g containers (nonprescription).

> *Myciguent* (Upjohn). Cream 5 mg (equivalent to 3.5 mg of base)/g in 15 g containers; ointment 5 mg (equivalent to 3.5 mg of base)/g in 15, 30, and 120 g containers (nonprescription).

POLYMYXIN B SULFATE

ACTIONS AND USES. This cationic surface-active polypeptide antibiotic is rarely used systemically. Polymyxin B is not available as a single-entity preparation for topical application because its spectrum of action is limited to gram-negative organisms, including *Pseudomonas*, that are less commonly involved in pyodermas. It is combined with other poorly absorbed antibiotics and/or corticosteroids to treat limited primary pyodermas (superficial folliculitis, ecthyma, and impetigo) and secondary pyodermas; such preparations also may be used with systemic antibiotics in more extensive pyodermas to control infection, promote healing, and reduce contagion locally. Bacterial resistance to polymyxin B develops slowly.

ADVERSE REACTIONS AND PRECAUTIONS. Although rare, hypersensitivity is the most common adverse reaction to topical polymyxin B (Fisher, 1983). Polymyxin is not absorbed significantly from the skin; therefore, it may be used during pregnancy or lactation.

PREPARATIONS. Single-entity preparations are not available. See following listing for mixtures.

MIXTURES.

> BACITRACIN AND POLYMYXIN B:
> *Polysporin* (Burroughs Wellcome). Powder, aerosol, and ointment, *Generic.* Ointment (all forms nonprescription).
> BACITRACIN, POLYMYXIN B, AND NEOMYCIN:
> *Mycitracin* (Upjohn), *Neo-Polycin* (Merrell Dow), *Neosporin* (Burroughs Wellcome), *Generic.* Ointment (nonprescription).
> NEOMYCIN AND GRAMICIDIN:
> *Spectrocin* (Squibb). Ointment (nonprescription).
> NEOMYCIN AND POLYMYXIN B:
> *Neosporin Cream* (Burroughs Wellcome). Cream (nonprescription).
> OXYTETRACYCLINE AND POLYMYXIN B:
> *Terramycin* (Pfipharmecs). Ointment and powder (both forms nonprescription).

CHEMOTHERAPEUTIC AGENTS FOR BURNS

Burns are classified on the basis of severity (ie, superficial partial thickness, deep partial thickness, full thickness); extent (percentage of body surface area); etiology (ie, thermal,

electrical, chemical); and area of involvement (eg, inhalation, perineal, facial). The infected burn wound represents a unique therapeutic problem (Moleski, 1978; Pegg, 1982). Since blood supply to the injured skin is usually compromised, topical administration is necessary to distribute the antimicrobial compound at the involved site.

The principal gram-positive bacteria isolated from infected burn wounds are staphylococci (predominant) and beta-hemolytic streptococci. The most common gram-negative organisms are *Pseudomonas aeruginosa* and *Escherichia coli*; *Klebsiella, Enterobacter, Proteus, Providencia,* and *Serratia* also may be causative organisms. Fungi, especially *Candida albicans*, are present in 10% to 15% of infected burns.

Management: Nondrug procedures (eg, avoiding bacterial contamination; debridement under strict aseptic conditions; avoidance of ointments and alcohol-based, scented, deodorant soaps to minimize irritation and sensitization; fluid and electrolyte replacement; metabolic and nutritional management [Jacoby, 1984; Molnar and Burke, 1984] when indicated) are usually adequate for the general management of burns (Moylan, 1983). When necessary, pain medications and tetanus prophylaxis are indicated. Oxygen may be necessary to support respiratory function.

Prophylactic topical antibiotic therapy is controversial. Many clinicians do not recommend topical antibiotics when sepsis is not a threat, because wound maceration may be encouraged and the danger of contamination during application is increased. Other clinicians feel that topical antibiotics are indicated for prophylaxis, especially when burns increase the risk of infection, as in (1) burns of the hands, feet, or perineum; (2) burns in poor-risk patients (eg, elderly, children, diabetics, alcoholics, patients with congestive heart failure, those receiving corticosteroid therapy); (3) burns complicated by fractures or soft tissue injury; (4) electrical burns; (5) inhalation burns; (6) partial-thickness burns of more than 15% (adults) or 10% (children) or full-thickness burns over more than 2% to 3% of the body surface area. Many physicians recommend topical antibacterial agents for heavily colonized but not obviously infected burns and most physicians recommend them for infected burns. However, some physicians do not employ them for even severely infected burns if adequate facilities are available for daily debridement under aseptic conditions.

If bacteremia is present or anticipated, systemic antibiotic therapy may be necessary. Early wound closure may be associated with lower rates of infection and mortality (Wolfe et al, 1983; Demling, 1985).

Drug Selection for Topical Application (MacMillan, 1980; Pegg, 1982): Silver sulfadiazine [Flint SSD, Silvadene], mafenide [Sulfamylon], povidone-iodine, nitrofurazone [Furacin], silver nitrate, and gentamicin [Garamycin] are available for the prevention and treatment of infected burns. Silver sulfadiazine is widely used for severe extensive burns. It does not penetrate the eschar as well as mafenide, but it does not produce the often severe pain on application or the occasional acid-base disturbances that are characteristic of the latter drug. Although nitrofurazone is bactericidal for many gram-positive and gram-negative organisms present in surface infections, strains of *Pseudomonas* often are not susceptible. Povidone-iodine may cause mild pain on application and it does not penetrate eschar as well as silver sulfadiazine, mafenide and nitrofurazone; it is effective against *Candida*, as is silver sulfadiazine.

Gentamicin is recommended only when the causative organism is *Pseudomonas* or other sensitive gram-negative species resistant to silver sulfadiazine and mafenide. Although silver nitrate solution is economical and effective, the frequent applications required to minimize drying, pain on application, staining, and occasional acid-base disturbances have limited its use.

Drug Evaluations

SILVER SULFADIAZINE
[Flint SSD, Silvadene]

ACTIONS AND USES. This topical sulfonamide is the drug of choice to treat infected burn wounds and grafts and to prevent burn wound infections in selected patients at high risk. It is effective against a wide variety of gram-positive and gram-negative organisms, including *Pseudomonas*, and also *Candida*. The antibacterial action does not appear to be entirely attributable to the sulfonamide content; silver also has bacteriostatic properties (Fox, 1983).

ADVERSE REACTIONS AND PRECAUTIONS. Silver sulfadiazine does not cause electrolyte disturbances, even after prolonged contact with the burned area. Application is usually painless, unlike that of mafenide, although approximately 2.5% of patients experience rash, pruritus, or a burning sensation.

Significant quantities of sulfadiazine can be absorbed following prolonged treatment of extensive burns. Accordingly, all adverse reactions attributable to systemic sulfonamides, except hypersensitivity, may occur (see Chapter 71, Sulfonamides and Trimethoprim). Monitoring of serum levels during prolonged treatment is not necessary except, possibly, in patients with impaired renal or hepatic function.

Safe use of silver sulfadiazine during pregnancy has not been established but in view of the hazards of sepsis with severe burns (greater than 20%), the use of silver sulfadiazine in such patients must be determined individually. If possible, it should not be used at term or in premature infants or newborns during the first month of life to avoid kernicterus.

There is no evidence that silver sulfadiazine has contact sensitizing potential. It is not contraindicated for patients with a history of sulfonamide sensitivity (Degreef and Dooms-Goossens, 1985).

DOSAGE AND PREPARATIONS.
Topical: Following cleansing and debridement of the wound, the cream is applied with a sterile gloved hand to a thickness of 1 to 3 mm. All interstices and crevices of the irregular burn surface should be covered with cream. Because of the drug's

low solubility, the antimicrobial action persists for many hours; thus, once-daily application is usually adequate, although some patients may require twice-daily application. Silver sulfadiazine should be applied more frequently to burned areas from which the cream might be removed by movement of the patient. Therapy is continued until satisfactory healing has occurred or the burn site is ready for grafting.

Although dressings are unnecessary, a layer of fine mesh gauze covered with a roller bandage will help ensure contact of the drug with the wound and is more comfortable than no dressing to most patients.

Silver sulfadiazine softens eschar but, by decreasing local bacterial action, it decreases its autolysis. Therefore, hydrotherapy and debridement should be performed daily for removal of eschar, especially in patients with full-thickness burns.
> *Flint SSD* (Flint). Cream (water-miscible) 10 mg/g in 50 and 400 g containers.
> *Silvadene* (Marion). Cream (water-miscible) 10 mg/g in 20, 50, 400, and 1,000 g containers.

MAFENIDE ACETATE
[Sulfamylon]

ACTIONS AND USES. Mafenide is not a true sulfonamide chemically but has essentially the same antibacterial spectrum as silver sulfadiazine and is particularly effective against susceptible strains of *Pseudomonas aeruginosa*. The action of mafenide, unlike that of most sulfonamides, is not inhibited by pus and body fluids. It is highly soluble and diffuses into and through eschar. It may be the drug of choice if thick eschar is present (eg, electrical burns). Because of the pain produced on application and its potential for adverse reactions, some authorities do not use mafenide for established infections. It is used principally as a less preferred alternative to silver sulfadiazine to prevent infection in selected high-risk patients with heavily colonized burns.

ADVERSE REACTIONS AND PRECAUTIONS. Unlike silver sulfadiazine, mafenide causes pain that can be severe at the site of application. Allergic skin reactions and acid-base disturbances (hyperchloremic metabolic acidosis with tachypnea and hyperventilation) also may develop. The acid-base disturbances result from the inhibition of carbonic anhydrase by mafenide and its principal metabolite.

DOSAGE AND PREPARATIONS.
Topical: Following cleansing and debridement of the wound, the cream is applied with a sterile gloved hand to a thickness of 1 mm two or three times daily. It should be applied more frequently to burned areas from which the cream might be removed by movement of the patient. Therapy is continued until satisfactory healing has occurred or until the burn site is ready for grafting. Dressings can be applied over the cream, although this is unnecessary. Because the drug's antibacterial activity delays separation of eschar, daily hydrotherapy and mechanical debridement are advisable, especially in patients with full-thickness burns.

Sulfamylon (Winthrop-Breon). Cream (water-miscible) equivalent to 85 mg of base/g in 56.7, 113.4, and 411 g containers.

NITROFURAZONE
[Furacin]

Nitrofurazone, a synthetic nitrofuran, is bactericidal for many gram-positive and gram-negative organisms. However, strains of *Pseudomonas* are often not susceptible, which has restricted use of this drug to the treatment of limited infected burns. Silver sulfadiazine is preferred.

Allergic contact dermatitis has been reported (the overall rate is about 1.1%); hypersensitivity is more common on damaged skin. Under normal conditions of topical use, significant amounts of nitrofurazone are not absorbed into the systemic circulation.

DOSAGE AND PREPARATIONS.
Topical: Once-daily application is usually adequate. Therapy is continued until satisfactory healing has occurred.

Generic. Ointment (soluble dressing) 0.2% in 30 and 454 g containers; solution 0.2% in 474 and 3,792 ml containers.

Furacin (Norwich Eaton). Cream (water-miscible) 0.2% in 14 and 28 g containers; ointment (soluble dressing) 0.2% in 28, 56, 135, 368, and 454 g containers.

POVIDONE-IODINE
[Acu-dyne, Betadine, Efodine, Pharmadine, Polydine]

ACTIONS AND USES. Povidone-iodine, an iodophor, is a complex of iodine and the nonsurfactant polymer, polyvinyl-pyrrolidone. The iodophor complex releases free iodine gradually and in low concentration and has a broad antimicrobial spectrum. Rapid development of resistant bacterial strains does not appear to be a problem.

Povidone-iodine is used to prevent and treat burn sepsis. However, silver sulfadiazine or mafenide is generally preferred for most burn infections, especially moderately extensive partial- and full-thickness burns.

Povidone-iodine does not penetrate eschar as well as silver sulfadiazine and mafenide.

ADVERSE REACTIONS AND PRECAUTIONS. Mild pain may occur on application to burns. Povidone-iodine is less irritating and less toxic than aqueous and alcoholic solutions of elemental iodine. Although the frequency of hypersensitivity reactions varies, sensitization appears to be uncommon (Lachapelle, 1984).

Under normal conditions of use in burns of less than 15% to 20% of body surface area, povidone-iodine is not significantly absorbed into the systemic circulation. Systemic absorption of iodine may occur if the burned area is extensive (Zellner and Bugyi, 1985). The blood iodine concentration peaks in two to three days, and the value returns to normal about one week after discontinuation of povidone-iodine. No clinically significant adverse reactions related to blood iodine concentrations were noted.

DOSAGE AND PREPARATIONS.
Topical: See manufacturers' recommendations.
(All forms nonprescription)

Generic. Ointment in 1.5, 30, and 454 g containers; solution in 120, 240, and 474 and 3,792 ml containers.

ACU-dyne (Acme United). Ointment in 1.2, 2.7, and 454 g containers.

Betadine (Purdue-Frederick). Aerosol spray in 90 ml containers; aerosol foam (Helafoam solution) in 250 g containers; ointment in 0.94, 3.8, 30, and 454 g containers; solution in 15, 30, 240, 474, 948, and 3,792 ml containers; concentrate (for whirlpool) in 3,792 ml containers.

Efodine (Fougera). Ointment in 0.94, 30, and 454 g containers.

Pharmadine (Sherwood). Ointment in 1, 1.5, 30, and 454 g containers; solution in 15, 120, 240, 474, 948, and 3,792 ml containers; solution (for whirlpool) in 3,792 ml containers.

Polydine (Century). Ointment in 30, 120, and 454 g containers; solution in 30, 120, 240, 474, and 3,792 ml containers.

ANTIFUNGAL AGENTS FOR DERMATOPHYTIC AND SUPERFICIAL CANDIDAL INFECTIONS

For therapeutic purposes, the mycoses may be classified as superficial, deep, or systemic. This section describes the antifungal agents used for superficial mycoses. Those used for deep and systemic mycoses and chronic mucocutaneous candidiasis are discussed in Chapter 76, Antifungal Agents for Systemic Mycoses.

The common use of nonprescription antifungal products prior to consultation of a physician is an important consideration in the treatment of superficial mycoses. In such instances, the physician initially should confirm the diagnosis and, if correct, should determine that the nonprescription medication (often as potent as some prescription preparations) has been used properly before another antifungal agent is substituted. Because of the importance of this consideration, the prescription status of the antifungal agents used to treat superficial dermatophytic and candidal infections is noted where appropriate in the following discussion, as well as in the Table and evaluations.

DERMATOPHYTOSIS. Dermatophytic infections, the most common superficial mycoses, involve the skin, hair, and nails and are caused by species of *Epidermophyton*, *Trichophyton*, and *Microsporum*. They are usually treated with topical agents. Resistant fungi or involvement of the hair or nails usually require the prolonged (months) oral administration of griseofulvin or ketoconazole [Nizoral] (investigational use).

Drug Selection: For *mild to moderate tinea infections*, miconazole, a broad spectrum imidazole, is effective when applied for 14 to 28 days, depending on the extent and site of involvement; it is available over-the-counter [Micatin]. Limited clinical studies suggest that tioconazole is equally effective (East, 1983; Clissold and Heel, 1986). This agent also has fungicidal action on *Candida*, as well as the fungistatic action typical of other imidazoles that may prove advantageous

THERAPY FOR SUPERFICIAL MYCOSES

Drug	Route of Administration	Preparations	Body Perineum Foot Hand	Scalp Nails Beard	Tinea Versicolor	Skin	Mouth	Vagina
			Site of Dermatophytic (Tinea) Infection			Site of Candidal Infection		
Ciclopirox olamine			+		+	+		
Loprox	Topical	Cream						
Griseofulvin[1]			+[2]	+[3]				
Generic	Oral	Capsules						
Fulvicin U/F, P/G	Oral	Tablets						
Grisactin Ultra								
Gris-PEG								
Grifulvin V	Oral	Suspension, tablets						
Grisactin	Oral	Capsules, tablets						
Haloprogin			+		+	+		
Halotex	Topical	Cream, solution						
Clioquinol			+					
Vioform*	Topical	Cream, ointment						
Selenium sulfide					+			
Exsel, Selsun	Topical	Lotion						
Tolnaftate			+		+			
Aftate*	Topical	Aerosol powder, gel, powder, liquid aerosol, liquid spray						
Tinactin*	Topical	Aerosol powder, cream, liquid aerosol, powder, solution						
Zeasorb-AF	Topical	Powder	+		+			
Compound Undecylenic Acid			+					
Generic*	Topical	Ointment						
Desenex*	Topical	Aerosol powder, ointment, powder, solution, foam, soap						
Pyrithione zinc					+			
Danex*, DHS-Zinc*, Head and Shoulders*, Zincon*	Topical	Shampoo						
IMIDAZOLES								
Butoconazole								
Femstat	Intravaginal	Cream						+
Clotrimazole								
Lotrimin, Mycelex	Topical	Cream, solution	+		+	+		
Mycelex Troche	Oral	Troches					+	
Gyne-Lotrimin	Intravaginal	Cream, tablets						+
Mycelex G	Intravaginal	Cream, tablets						+
Econazole								
Spectazole	Topical	Cream	+		+	+		
Ketoconazole			+[4]	+[4]	+[4]	+[4]	+[4]	+[4]
Nizoral	Oral	Tablets						

(Continued on next page)

Drug	Route of Administration	Preparations	Body Perineum Foot Hand	Scalp Nails Beard	Tinea Versicolor	Skin	Mouth	Vagina
Miconazole nitrate								
Micatin*	Topical	Cream, powder, aerosol powder, liquid aerosol	+	+		+		
Monistat-Derm	Topical	Cream, lotion	+	+		+		
Monistat 7	Intravaginal	Cream, suppositories						
Monistat 3	Intravaginal	Suppositories						+
POLYENE ANTIBIOTICS								
Amphotericin B						+		
Fungizone	Topical	Cream, lotion, ointment						
Nystatin								
Generic	Oral (nonabsorbed)	Tablets					+	
	Intravaginal	Tablets						+
	Topical	Cream				+		
Mycostatin	Oral (nonabsorbed)	Drops, tablets					+	
	Intravaginal	Tablets						+
	Topical	Cream, ointment, powder				+		+
Nilstat	Oral (nonabsorbed)	Tablets					+	
	Intravaginal	Tablets						+
	Topical	Cream, ointment, powder				+		
O-V Statin	Oral (nonabsorbed)	Tablets					+	
	Intravaginal	Tablets						+

Site of Dermatophytic (Tinea) Infection — columns: Body Perineum Foot Hand | Scalp Nails Beard | Tinea Versicolor.
Site of Candidal Infection — columns: Skin | Mouth | Vagina.

*Nonprescription (Miconazole is also available on prescription.)

[1]The preparations of griseofulvin listed are not interchangeable; dosage recommendations are based on differences in absorption based principally on particle size and formulation.

[2]Griseofulvin is not recommended for trivial dermatophytic infections that usually respond to topical therapy alone.

[3]Topical therapy can be considered for mild involvement of these sites. Generally, oral griseofulvin is the drug of choice for moderate to severe infection.

[4]Investigational uses for tinea and candidal cutaneous and acute mucocutaneous infections; however, ketoconazole is the drug of choice for chronic mucocutaneous candidiasis.

(Beggs and Polman, 1985) but is not yet marketed in the United States.

Other nonprescription drugs for the treatment of mild, superficial tinea infections of the trunk, groin, pelvis, or soles include tolnaftate [Aftate, Tinactin, Zeasorb-AF] and compound undecylenic acid [Desenex]. Controlled clinical trials support the effectiveness of tolnaftate in athlete's foot, jock itch, and ringworm and compound undecylenic acid in athlete's foot.

Any antifungal effect of salicylic acid observed clinically is attributed to its keratolytic effect. This agent may be sufficient for superficial mild infections and also may be useful to make infections in deeper layers accessible to more potent antifungal agents.

In addition to its limited antibacterial activity, clioquinol (iodochlorhydroxyquin) [Vioform] has antifungal activity; it is available as a single-entity preparation for the treatment of limited bacterial and dermatophytic infections, but there is concern about its topical absorption (see the evaluation).

Triacetin [Enzactin] is used topically in limited superficial fungal infections. Its antifungal action may be partly due to alteration of pH and the keratolytic action of acetic acid, which is released slowly from triacetin by esterases in fungi, skin, and serum.

One controlled study showed that cyclohexanol (combined with thymol or triacetin) was effective in tinea pedis but comparative studies are unavailable.

Carbol-fuchsin solution (Castellani's Paint) is still used on occasion to treat chronic intertrigo of the toes but causes stinging and staining. More effective agents are available.

Haloprogin [Halotex] is effective against tinea and may be considered when over-the-counter medications are inadequate.

Moderately severe infections usually respond to topical clotrimazole [Lotrimin, Mycelex], econazole [Spectazole], or miconazole [Monistat-Derm]. All of these imidazoles, as well as the more recently approved imidazole, sulconazole [Sulcosyn], appear to be about equally effective when used under comparable conditions of patient selection and compliance.

In limited controlled studies, the spectrum of activity and efficacy of ciclopirox [Loprox], a hydroxypyridone, in tinea infections are comparable to those of the imidazoles. In tinea pedis and versicolor, ciclopirox produced a more rapid and complete clinical response than clotrimazole (Kligman et al, 1985; Cullen et al, 1985).

Oral griseofulvin is absorbed systemically and is not recommended for trivial tinea infections that usually are relieved by topical therapy alone. However, *moderate to severe tinea infections* of the palms, soles, and fingernails usually require griseofulvin but administration must be continued for months. This is the drug of choice for tinea barbae and tinea capitis when the causative organism is *Trichophyton tonsurans*, *Microsporum audouini*, or *M. canis* (Laude et al, 1982; Krowchuk et al, 1983; Rudolph, 1985). Topical agents may help control the infection during the eradication period. A systemic corticosteroid also may be necessary if kerions are present. At least one month but often three to six months of therapy is required for clinical cure. Ketoconazole is being evaluated for use in severe dermatophytic infections when griseofulvin is contraindicated.

Tinea versicolor is caused by the pathogenic hyphal form (*Pityrosporum furfur*) of the lipophilic yeast, *Pityrosporum orbiculare*, which resides on normal skin. Selenium sulfide suspension [Exsel, Selsun], an antidandruff remedy, is effective when applied to affected areas for 15 to 30 minutes daily for 7 to 14 days. Sodium thiosulfate 25% with salicylic acid 1% [Tinver] also is effective when applied to affected areas twice a day for several weeks. Acrisorcin [Akrinol] is useful, but residual soap on the skin inactivates the drug and mutagenic effects have been observed in submammalian species. The clinical significance of these findings has not been established, but long-term carcinogenicity studies are under way. Other prescription drugs that clear tinea versicolor when used for an adequate length of time include ciclopirox, haloprogin, clotrimazole, and econazole. Although oral ketoconazole is effective, its use for this infection remains investigational because less toxic agents are available. Griseofulvin is ineffective.

Nonprescription drugs used in tinea versicolor include an antidandruff drug, zinc pyrithione shampoo [Danex, DHS-Zinc, Head and Shoulders, Zincon] (applied for five minutes daily for 14 days), tolnaftate, and miconazole.

SUPERFICIAL CANDIDIASIS. *Candida albicans* most often causes disease, but *C. parapsilosis* and *C. pseudotropicalis* also have been implicated. The common acute form of mucocutaneous candidiasis usually affects moist skin or mucous membranes (eg, orocutaneous [perleche]; oropharyngeal [thrush]; esophageal; perianal, vulvovaginal, intertriginous areas). Patients with certain forms of cancer, acquired or congenital immunodeficiency syndrome, poor nutrition, severe burns, diabetes mellitus, or hepatic and/or renal failure and those known to abuse narcotics, undergoing peritoneal dialysis, and receiving adrenal corticosteroids, antineoplastic drugs, oral contraceptives, or broad spectrum antibacterial agents are predisposed to candidiasis of intertriginous areas and mucous membranes. Pregnancy or use of oral contraceptives predisposes to candidal vulvovaginitis.

Chronic mucocutaneous candidiasis is uncommon and also most often develops in immunocompromised or debilitated patients. The skin, scalp, nails, and mucous membranes are extensively involved and a systemic antifungal agent is usually required; topical agents may be used adjunctively.

Drug Selection: *Cutaneous candidiasis* responds to topical preparations of the polyene antibiotics, amphotericin B [Fungizone] and nystatin [Mycostatin, Nilstat]; haloprogin [Halotex]; ciclopirox [Loprox]; and the imidazoles (clotrimazole [Lotrimin, Mycelex], econazole [Spectazole], and miconazole [Micatin, Monistat-Derm]). Oral ketoconazole [Nizoral] is effective (investigational indication), but its use should be restricted to severe cutaneous candidiasis associated with chronic mucocutaneous candidiasis, for which it is the drug of choice. Topical antifungal therapy may be required in addition. Intravenous amphotericin B is effective for chronic mucocutaneous candidiasis; however, the relapse rate is very high when the drug is stopped, and prolonged administration can cause serious adverse reactions (see also Chapter 76, Antifungal Agents for Systemic Mycoses). Candidiasis limited to the skin does not respond to topical undecylenic acid, topical tolnaftate, or oral griseofulvin. Clioquinol (iodochlorhydroxyquin) has only limited antifungal activity.

Vaginal preparations of nystatin [Mycostatin, Nilstat, Nystex, O-V Statin], clotrimazole [Gyne-Lotrimin, Mycelex-G, Mycelex-G-500], and miconazole [Monistat 3, Monistat 7] are available to treat *vaginal candidiasis*. Nystatin may be as effective as the imidazoles, but a longer treatment period (14 days) may be required for clinical cure. Larger doses of miconazole or clotrimazole used for a shorter duration appear to be as effective as traditional regimens (eg, miconazole [Monistat 3] 200 mg/day for three days versus 100 mg/day for seven days [Monistat 7]; clotrimazole 500 mg as a single dose versus 200 mg/day for three days) (Hughes and Kriedman, 1984; Fleury et al, 1985).

When used as a vaginal cream in a dose of 100 mg/day for three days, a recently approved imidazole, butoconazole [Femstat] also is reported to be as effective as miconazole 100 mg/day for seven days (Bradbeer et al, 1985).

Oral ketoconazole has been used investigationally in vaginal candidiasis. However, in view of its greater potential for serious systemic adverse reactions, its use should be restricted to patients with chronic recurrent severe infections that do not respond to conventional topical therapy (Sobel, 1985).

Management of predisposing factors (eg, treatment of concurrent polymicrobial vaginitis, avoidance of tight-fitting synthetic underwear, short courses of topical estrogen for atrophic vaginitis in postmenopausal women) will improve the chances for therapeutic success with any systemic or topical antifungal agent (Meech et al, 1985).

Drug Evaluations

CICLOPIROX OLAMINE
[Loprox]

ACTIONS AND USES. This antifungal agent, a hydroxypyridone, is chemically unrelated to the broad spectrum imidazoles. Its action is attributed to inhibition of uptake of precursors of macromolecular synthesis from the medium (Sakurai et al, 1978).

Limited controlled studies suggest that ciclopirox is as effective as clotrimazole in the treatment of cutaneous candidal and dermatophytic infections, including tinea versicolor (Cullen et al, 1985; Jue et al, 1985; Kligman et al, 1985). Its final role in tinea capitis, tinea barbae, and moderately severe tinea infections of the palms, soles, or nails remains to be determined.

ADVERSE REACTIONS AND PRECAUTIONS. Side effects are reported to be infrequent and minor (eg, pruritus, burning). The drug appears to be nonsensitizing. Systemic toxicity has not been reported following topical application.

Safety and effectiveness in children less than 10 years have not been established.

PREGNANCY AND LACTATION. Reproduction studies in mice, rats, rabbits, and monkeys utilizing various routes of administration and doses ten or more times the topical human dose have had no effect on fertility or the fetus. However, no adequate or well-controlled studies have been performed in pregnant women. This drug is classified in FDA Pregnancy Category B.

It is not known whether ciclopirox is excreted in human milk, but, because many drugs are, caution should be exercised when ciclopirox is administered to nursing women.

PHARMACOKINETICS. Tagged studies of ciclopirox in polyethylene glycol 400 showed that an average of 1.3% of the dose was absorbed when the cream was applied to 750 cm^2 on the back and was followed by six hours of occlusion. Of the amount absorbed, the biologic half-life was 1.7 hours and excretion occurred via the kidney.

DOSAGE AND PREPARATIONS.
Topical: The preparation is applied to the affected area twice daily. The use of occlusive wrappings or dressings is not recommended. Although improvement may be noted in one week, clinical cure usually requires a minimum of two to four weeks, depending on the site and extent of involvement.

Loprox (Hoechst-Roussel). Cream 1% in 15, 30, and 90 g containers.

CLIOQUINOL (Iodochlorhydroxyquin)
[Vioform]

ACTIONS AND USES. Clioquinol, an 8-hydroxyquinolone related to iodoquinol, has limited topical antibacterial and antifungal activity. It is effective orally, but the oral preparation has been withdrawn from the United States market because it has an appreciable toxic potential for producing subacute myelo-optic neuropathy (SMON).

Clioquinol is available as a single-entity nonprescription agent and in mixtures for topical application in the treatment of limited fungal infections of the skin, such as tinea pedis (athlete's foot), and limited primary and secondary bacterial pyodermas (eg, superficial folliculitis, uncomplicated impetigo, infected dermal ulcers, infectious eczematoid dermatitis, intertrigo). It is not used topically on the eye or mucous membranes.

Recent studies on the topical absorption of clioquinol have raised serious concerns about the risk/benefit ratio of this agent (Ezzedeen et al, 1984). In one study, following application to intact adult human skin for twelve hours, topical absorption was rapid and extensive. The drug was detectable in the blood at two hours, reached a stable blood concentration by four hours, and an average of 40% ± 6.5% of the dose was absorbed (Stohs et al, 1984).

ADVERSE REACTIONS AND PRECAUTIONS. Irritation and hypersensitivity reactions occur only rarely, but patients who are hypersensitive to iodine should not receive this medication.

The hydroxy group of clioquinol interacts with the ferric chloride test for phenylketonuria to yield a false-positive result if the compound is present on the diaper or in the urine. Clioquinol stains hair and fabrics.

DOSAGE AND PREPARATIONS.
Topical: An appropriate preparation is applied to the affected area two or three times a day.

Generic. Cream 3% in 30 and 454 g containers; ointment 3% in 30, 60, and 454 g containers (both forms nonprescription).

Vioform (CIBA). Cream, ointment 3% in 30 g containers (nonprescription).

AVAILABLE MIXTURES.

HYDROCORTISONE AND CLIOQUINOL or IODOQUINOL (diiodohydroxyquin):

Generic. Cream and ointment containing hydrocortisone 0.5% or 1% and clioquinol 3%.

Racet (Lemmon). Cream containing hydrocortisone 0.5% and clioquinol 3% in 15 and 30 g containers or hydrocortisone 1% and clioquinol 3% in 15 g containers.

Vioform-Hydrocortisone (CIBA). Cream containing hydrocortisone 0.5% and clioquinol 3% in 15 and 30 g containers or hydrocortisone 1% and clioquinol 3% in 5 and 20 g containers;

lotion containing hydrocortisone 1% and clioquinol 3% in 15 ml containers; ointment containing hydrocortisone 0.5% and clioquinol 3% in 30 g containers; ointment containing hydrocortisone 1% and clioquinol 3% in 20 g containers.
Vytone (Dermik). Cream containing hydrocortisone 0.5% or 1% and iodoquinol 1% in 28.3 g containers.

GRISEOFULVIN

[*Microcrystalline:* Fulvicin-U/F, Grifulvin V, Grisactin;
[*Ultramicrocrystalline:* Fulvicin P/G, Grisactin Ultra, Gris-PEG]

ACTIONS. Griseofulvin is derived from a species of *Penicillium*. Its fungicidal effect is limited to actively growing organisms, since one of the major cellular effects of griseofulvin is to inhibit fungal mitosis by binding to intracellular microtubular protein.

USES. Griseofulvin is effective orally for dermatophytic (tinea) infections except tinea versicolor. It is not recommended routinely for trivial fungal infections that usually respond to a topical agent alone and is ineffective for bacterial or candidal infections.

Griseofulvin is the drug of choice for tinea barbae and tinea capitis caused by *Tricophyton tonsurans*, *Microsporum audouini*, or *M. canis* (Laude et al, 1982; Krowchuk et al, 1983). A systemic corticosteroid may be necessary if kerions are present. At least one month of therapy usually is required for clinical cure. Shampoos containing selenium sulfide, a sporicidal agent active against the causative organism of tinea capitis, are effective adjunctively in combination with oral griseofulvin.

Dermatophytic infections of the palms usually require two to three months of treatment; the fingernails usually respond within six months, although nine months may be necessary. Toenail infections seldom respond until growth of a normal nail occurs, which may take 15 months or longer, and reinfection develops frequently; therefore, some authorities do not recommend griseofulvin for toenail infections. Some forms of onychomycosis are almost completely resistant to therapy. Treatment of these infections with griseofulvin must be continued until infected keratinous structures have been eradicated as determined by clinical and laboratory examinations. In stubborn infections, concomitant treatment with topical antifungal and/or keratolytic agents in areas of hyperkeratosis may be helpful.

Ketoconazole is used in systemic fungal diseases and is currently being evaluated for severe infections of the scalp, beard, and nails when griseofulvin is contraindicated or the organism is resistant (see Chapter 76, Antifungal Agents for Systemic Mycoses).

ADVERSE REACTIONS, PRECAUTIONS, AND INTERACTIONS. The most common minor reaction is headache, which usually disappears in a few days, even with continued therapy. Other reactions include dysgeusia, dryness of the mouth, gastrointestinal disturbances (nausea, vomiting, diarrhea), arthralgia, peripheral neuritis, vertigo, and fever. Griseofulvin occasionally causes syncope, blurred vision, photosensitivity, insomnia, and rash. Rarely, it may cause serum sickness, angioedema, confusion, lapses of memory, and impaired judgment that may affect the performance of routine tasks. This compound also may produce estrogen-like effects in children. Patients sensitive to penicillin rarely may be sensitive to griseofulvin.

Serious reactions associated with the use of griseofulvin occur infrequently. Leukopenia is observed occasionally and granulocytopenia may develop after use of large doses and/or prolonged therapy. It may be advisable to perform blood counts occasionally during therapy.

Griseofulvin may cause hepatotoxicity and is contraindicated in patients with acute intermittent porphyria or a history of that condition, hepatocellular failure, and hypersensitivity to the drug.

Three cases of urticaria and fixed drug eruption have been reported (Feinstein et al, 1984).

The safe use of griseofulvin during pregnancy has not been established. Therefore, potential benefits must be weighed against the possible hazards if griseofulvin is considered for use in women of childbearing age.

Griseofulvin decreases the activity of coumarin-type anticoagulants (eg, warfarin) by metabolic enzyme induction, and dosage adjustments may be required. Conversely, barbiturates depress griseofulvin activity by decreasing its systemic absorption, and an increase in dosage of the latter may be required.

PHARMACOKINETICS. Griseofulvin is only administered orally. The rate of absorption and the total amount of drug absorbed are enhanced after a high-fat meal (Ginsburg et al, 1983).

During long-term administration, griseofulvin is deposited in the skin, hair, and nails and is actively secreted from eccrine sweat glands. The drug appears to move in and out of the stratum corneum quite rapidly and lesions begin to heal within a few days after treatment is initiated. The stratum corneum is cleared of drug two to three days after therapy is discontinued.

Griseofulvin is extensively metabolized by the liver. The half-life ranges from 24 to 36 hours; therefore, once-daily administration is usually adequate. However, administration every six hours is recommended to maintain effective serum concentrations and lessen side effects when large doses are required initially to control severe infections. Plasma levels can be detected for four days after therapy has been stopped.

DOSAGE AND PREPARATIONS. Griseofulvin was marketed originally in a macrocrystalline form that required the use of large doses to achieve and maintain effective blood levels. A microcrystalline form has now replaced the macrocrystalline preparations, and the same blood levels can be achieved with smaller doses.

An ultramicrocrystalline form produces the same blood levels as the microcrystalline form at a further one-third reduction in dosage (not one-half as originally claimed) (Straughn et al, 1980). However, there is no convincing evidence that further reducing the particle size confers any significant advantage. Therefore, there appears to be no practical therapeutic difference between these two forms. The dosage required to assure comparable blood levels of the ultramicrocrystalline form of griseofulvin are cited below.

Regardless of the form administered, griseofulvin should be taken with milk or other fat-containing foods to maximize absorption (Ginsburg et al, 1983).

MICROCRYSTALLINE FORM:

Oral: *Adults,* 500 mg daily in single or divided doses with meals for minor infections; 750 mg to 1 g daily in divided doses has been recommended for severe infections. *Children,* approximately 10 mg/kg daily in single or divided doses with meals. Divided dosage regimens usually are indicated only if the patient cannot tolerate a single daily dose or large initial doses are required. Because griseofulvin is absorbed over a relatively long period, once-daily administration maintains adequate blood levels.

    Generic. Capsules 250 mg.
    Fulvicin-U/F (Schering). Tablets 250 and 500 mg.
    Grifulvin V (Ortho). Suspension (pediatric) 125 mg/5 ml; tablets 250 and 500 mg.
    Grisactin (Ayerst). Capsules 125 and 250 mg; tablets 500 mg.

ULTRAMICROCRYSTALLINE FORM:

Oral: *Adults,* 330 mg daily in single or divided doses with meals is satisfactory in most patients with tinea corporis, tinea cruris, and tinea capitis. For fungal infections that are more difficult to eradicate, such as tinea pedis and tinea unguium, 660 mg in divided doses is recommended. Approximately 7.26 mg/kg/day is effective for most *children.* On this basis, the following dosages are suggested for administration in single or divided amounts: *Children weighing 16 to 27 kg,* 125 to 187.5 mg daily; *over 27 kg,* 187.5 to 375 mg daily; *2 years or younger,* dosage has not been established. Clinical experience with griseofulvin in children with tinea capitis indicates that a single daily dose is effective.

Clinical relapse will occur if the medication is discontinued before the infecting organism is eradicated.

    Fulvicin P/G (Schering). Tablets 125, 165, 250, and 330 mg.
    Grisactin Ultra (Ayerst). Tablets 125, 250, and 330 mg.
    Gris-PEG (Herbert). Tablets 125 and 250 mg.

HALOPROGIN

[Halotex]

USES. Haloprogin is a synthetic topical antifungal agent used to treat superficial dermatophytic (tinea) infections, including tinea versicolor. Its cure and relapse rates are similar to those of tolnaftate, but, unlike tolnaftate, haloprogin is effective in cutaneous candidal infections.

ADVERSE REACTIONS AND PRECAUTIONS. Adverse reactions include local irritation, burning sensation, and vesicle formation. Haloprogin may exacerbate pruritus, maceration,

and pre-existing lesions. If sensitization is noted, the drug should be discontinued and not used again. Contact with the eyes must be avoided.

DOSAGE AND PREPARATIONS.

Topical: The preparation is applied liberally to the affected area twice daily for two to four weeks. Interdigital lesions may require up to four weeks of therapy. If there is no improvement after four weeks, haloprogin should be discontinued and the diagnosis reconfirmed.

    Halotex (Westwood). Cream 1% in 15 and 30 g containers; solution 1% in 10 and 30 ml containers.

TOLNAFTATE

[Aftate, Tinactin, Zeasorb-AF]

This nonprescription drug is effective topically in the treatment of dermatophytic (tinea) fungal infections, including tinea versicolor. The powder and aerosol forms are also effective prophylactically against athlete's foot, but they should not be used to prevent jock itch and ringworm. Fungal infections of the scalp, nails, soles, and palms usually do not respond to topical antifungal agents. Tolnaftate is not effective in candidal or bacterial infections.

Alternating use of 10% salicylic acid ointment (as needed for keratolysis) with tolnaftate may improve the effectiveness of the latter in hyperkeratotic lesions. Topical haloprogin, clotrimazole, or miconazole is recommended for lesions refractory to tolnaftate.

Tolnaftate is well tolerated. Sensitization is rare, and irritation occurs infrequently.

DOSAGE AND PREPARATIONS.

Topical: One or two drops of solution or a small amount of cream or powder is rubbed into lesions twice daily for two to three weeks; treatment for four to six weeks may be required. The powder or powder aerosol may be used following the original treatment period to help maintain remission in patients susceptible to tinea.

    Aftate (Plough). Gel 1% in 15 g containers; powder 1% in 45 and 67.5 g containers; powder (aerosol) 1% in 105 and 150 g containers; liquid (aerosol) 1% in 120 ml containers; liquid (pump spray) 1% in 45 ml containers (all forms nonprescription).
    Tinactin (Schering). Cream 1% in 15 g containers; liquid (aerosol) 1% in 120 ml containers; powder 1% in 45 g containers; powder (aerosol) 1% in 120 g containers; solution 1% in 10 ml containers (all forms nonprescription).
    Zeasorb-AF (Stiefel). Powder 1% in 45 g containers.

COMPOUND UNDECYLENIC ACID

This nonprescription mixture of undecylenic acid and zinc undecylenate is effective topically in dermatophytic (tinea) infections except for tinea versicolor; it is not effective in candidal or bacterial infections (Landau, 1983).

The most extensive use of compound undecylenic acid has been for tinea pedis (athlete's foot). Its effectiveness in this condition compares favorably with that of tolnaftate.

Compound undecylenic acid is well tolerated, but it should be discontinued if irritation develops.

Under normal conditions of topical use, clinically significant quantities of this mixture are not absorbed from the skin.

DOSAGE AND PREPARATIONS.
Topical: The ointment or powder is applied once or twice daily to the involved area. A common practice is to apply powder or aerosol in the morning and an ointment or aerosol at night.

> **Generic.** Ointment containing undecylenic acid 5% and zinc undecylenate 20% (nonprescription).

> Available Trademark.
> **Desenex Ointment, Powder, Aerosol Powder, Solution, Foam, Soap** (Pharmacraft) (all forms nonprescription).

Imidazoles

CLOTRIMAZOLE

[Lotrimin, Gyne-Lotrimin, Mycelex, Mycelex-G]

ACTIONS AND USES. Clotrimazole is closely related chemically to miconazole (Sawyer et al, 1975). It affects the permeability of fungi by interfering with the biosynthesis of ergosterol, which causes disorganization of the plasma membrane (Beggs et al, 1981). A systemic preparation is not available in the United States.

Clotrimazole is useful when applied topically in dermatophytic (tinea) infections, including tinea versicolor; cutaneous candidiasis; and candidal infections of the mucous membranes and mucocutaneous junctions (eg, orocutaneous [perleche], oropharyngeal [thrush], perianal, intertriginous and vulvovaginal areas). Clinical cure for dermatophytic and candidal infections of the skin, mucous membranes, and mucocutaneous junctions usually requires two weeks to one month, depending on the site and extent of involvement.

Initial studies support the prophylactic use of the troche form in selected patients (eg, those receiving cytotoxic and immunosuppressant drugs) (Owens et al, 1984). This dosage form also may be adequate for mild to moderate involvement of the esophagus; however, systemic therapy with amphotericin B (with or without flucytosine) or oral ketoconazole may be necessary in patients with more severe infections (Mathieson and Dutta, 1983; Kodsi and Goldberg, 1983; Shectman et al, 1984).

In order to improve compliance and minimize relapses and recurrent infections, treatment of vulvovaginal candidiasis has been modified to reduce exposure time by utilizing the highest dose possible commensurate with acceptable side effects. Treatment regimens have been modified from seven days to three days to one day (single dose) and doses increased from 100 to 200 to 500 mg, respectively. All regimens appear to be equally effective; however, some physicians use the lower daily doses for three or seven days in pregnant women to limit peak blood concentrations.

A mixture of clotrimazole and betamethasone has been introduced in the United States. Data are limited, but in one controlled study, the combination was only slightly more effective than either of the components used alone in patients with tinea corporis and tinea cruris; however, the onset of effect was shortened appreciably (Katz et al, 1984).

ADVERSE REACTIONS AND PRECAUTIONS. Adverse effects after topical use of clotrimazole include erythema; stinging, blistering, and peeling of the skin; edema; pruritus; and urticaria.

Adverse reactions after use of the troche form include nausea and vomiting (incidence, about 5%). Reversible elevation of SGOT to abnormal levels occurs in 15% of patients receiving troches. Abdominal cramping and diarrhea have been reported. The manufacturer recommends periodic assessment of hepatic function, particularly in patients with pre-existing hepatic impairment. The safety and effectiveness of clotrimazole troches in children less than 3 years have not been established; therefore, use of this dosage form in these patients is not recommended.

Following vaginal application, mild vaginal burning, erythema, and irritation have occurred.

Pregnancy is not a contraindication to the topical cutaneous application of clotrimazole. Adequate studies on vulvovaginal infections during the first trimester of pregnancy are not available; however, use during the second and third trimesters has not been associated with ill effects in the neonate. Cutaneous and intravaginal preparations are classified in FDA Pregnancy Category B and the oral troche in FDA Pregnancy Category C.

Clotrimazole is embryotoxic in rats and mice when given in doses 100 times the adult human dose (in mg/kg), possibly secondary to maternal toxicity. The drug was not teratogenic in mice, rabbits, and rats when given in doses up to 200 times the human dose. There are no adequate, well-controlled reproductive studies in pregnant women.

Preparations of clotrimazole are not intended for ophthalmic use and should be used with caution around the eyes.

DOSAGE AND PREPARATIONS.
Topical: A sufficient amount of cream, solution, or lotion to cover the affected and surrounding area is applied twice daily morning and evening.

> **Lotrimin** (Schering), **Mycelex** (Miles). Cream 1% in 15, 30, 45 (**Lotrimin** only), and 90 g containers; solution 1% in 10 and 30 ml containers; and lotion 1% (**Lotrimin** only) in 30 ml containers.
> AVAILABLE MIXTURE.
> **Lotrisone** (Schering). Cream containing clotrimazole 1% and betamethasone dipropionate 0.05% in 15 and 45 g containers.

Intravaginal: One tablet is inserted into the vagina nightly for seven days or one applicatorful of cream is inserted into the vagina nightly for seven to 14 days.

For nonpregnant patients, an alternative, equally effective regimen is two tablets (200 mg) inserted into the vagina nightly for three days; studies also support the efficacy of a single 500-mg dose as a vaginal tablet (Hughes and Kriedman, 1984; Fleury et al, 1985).

Gyne-Lotrimin (Schering), *Mycelex-G* (Miles). Cream (vaginal) 1% in 45 and 90 g (*Mycelex-G* only) containers with applicator; tablets (vaginal) 100 and 500 mg (*Mycelex-G* only) with applicator.

Oral: One troche five times a day for 14 consecutive days; the troche must be dissolved slowly in the mouth.

Mycelex (Miles). Troche 10 mg.

ECONAZOLE NITRATE
[Spectazole]

ACTIONS AND USES. This imidazole affects the permeability of fungi by interfering with the biosynthesis of ergosterol, which causes disorganization of the plasma cell membrane (Beggs et al, 1981).

Econazole is available only for topical application in the treatment of tinea skin infections, including tinea versicolor and cutaneous candidiasis (Heel et al, 1978). Oral griseofulvin may be required in moderately severe tinea infections of the palms, soles, and nails. Econazole is not labeled for use in tinea capitis. Its final role in all tinea infections remains to be determined; limited comparative studies with other topical imidazoles suggest that it is equally effective.

ADVERSE REACTIONS AND PRECAUTIONS. Side effects in controlled studies are reported to be infrequent (3.3%) and minor (eg, pruritus, subjective burning and stinging, erythema). The incidence of sensitization is very low. Overdose of econazole has not been reported. No systemic toxicity has occurred following topical administration because of limited absorption.

PREGNANCY AND LACTATION. Econazole was not teratogenic when administered orally to mice, rabbits, or rats. Fetotoxic or embryotoxic effects were observed in mice, rabbits, and/or rats receiving oral doses 80 or 40 times the human dermal dose. Econazole should be used in the first trimester only when administration is considered essential (FDA Pregnancy Category C).

It is not known whether econazole is excreted in human milk. Oral administration to lactating rats resulted in excretion of econazole and/or metabolites in milk and these substances were found in nursing pups. Therefore, caution should be exercised when econazole is administered to nursing women.

PHARMACOKINETICS. Econazole is not used systemically, and clinically insignificant amounts (less than 1%) are absorbed after topical application to the skin.

DOSAGE AND PREPARATIONS.

Topical: The preparation is applied to affected areas twice daily morning and evening in patients with tinea pedis, tinea cruris, tinea corporis, and cutaneous candidiasis, and once daily in patients with tinea versicolor. Candidal infections and tinea cruris and corporis should be treated for two weeks and tinea pedis for one month to reduce the possibility of recurrence.

Spectazole (Ortho). Cream 1% in 15, 30, and 85 g containers.

KETOCONAZOLE
[Nizoral]

Ketoconazole is the only imidazole that is adequately absorbed orally. Because of the potential for adverse reactions following systemic administration, oral ketoconazole should be reserved for superficial cutaneous infections that do not respond to conventional topical drugs or to griseofulvin. A topical cream preparation of ketoconazole has been approved recently for use in superficial mycoses.

Ketoconazole plays a prominent role in the treatment of a number of systemic mycoses, and it is the drug of choice for chronic mucocutaneous candidiasis. See the evaluation in Chapter 76, Antifungal Agents for Systemic Mycoses, for a more complete discussion.

Nizoral (Janssen). Tablets 200 mg.
(Investigational use)

MICONAZOLE NITRATE
[Micatin, Monistat-Derm, Monistat 7, Monistat 3]

ACTIONS AND USES. Miconazole is a synthetic imidazole with broad in vitro antifungal activity. This drug affects fungal permeability by interfering with the biosynthesis of ergosterol to cause disorganization of the plasma membrane (Beggs et al, 1981).

Miconazole is effective topically in dermatophytic infections of the intertriginous and glabrous skin and in tinea versicolor. However, griseofulvin is preferred in moderate to severe dermatophytoses of the scalp, beard, palms, and fingernails. Miconazole also is useful in superficial cutaneous and vaginal candidal infections. Clinical evidence suggests that the course of treatment is usually shorter with miconazole cream than nystatin suppositories in vulvovaginal candidiasis. A few patients with persistent, recurrent vaginal infections may benefit from use of a nonabsorbable oral antifungal agent (eg, nystatin) in addition to vaginal antifungal therapy to eliminate a gastrointestinal source of infection.

ADVERSE REACTIONS AND PRECAUTIONS. Side effects after topical application consist of irritation, burning, or maceration. If these reactions appear to be caused by hypersensitivity or if undue discomfort occurs, the drug should be discontinued. Miconazole should be used cautiously around the eyes.

After vulvovaginal application of 100 mg/day for 14 days, burning, pruritus, or irritation occurred in 6% to 7% of patients in controlled studies; only 0.9% of the patients discontinued therapy. Doses of 200 mg/day caused burning, pruritus, or irritation in 2% of patients in controlled studies; urticaria and skin rash occurred in less than 0.5%. Only 0.3% of patients discontinued therapy.

Small amounts of miconazole are absorbed from the vagina; however, no adverse effects or complications attributable to the drug have been reported in infants of women treated for vulvovaginal candidiasis during pregnancy.

DOSAGE AND PREPARATIONS.
Topical: A sufficient amount of cream to cover the affected area is applied twice daily in the morning and evening. The lotion is most suitable for intertriginous areas; the cream should be applied sparingly to such areas. Two weeks of therapy are usually sufficient, but four weeks are recommended for infections of the soles. If no improvement is seen after one month of therapy, the diagnosis should be reconfirmed.

    Micatin (Advanced Care Products). Cream 2% in 15 and 30 g containers; powder (aerosol) 2% in 90 g containers; powder 2% in 45 g containers; liquid (aerosol) 2% in 105 g containers (nonprescription).

    Monistat-Derm (Ortho). Cream 2% in 15, 30, and 85 g containers; lotion 2% in 30 and 60 ml containers.

Intravaginal: One applicatorful of cream is inserted high in the vagina or one 100-mg suppository is inserted nightly for seven days; alternatively, to increase compliance, one 200-mg suppository may be inserted nightly for three days. In resistant cases, the course of therapy may be repeated after the diagnosis has been reconfirmed.

    Monistat 7 (Ortho). Cream 2% in 47 g containers with applicator; suppositories 100 mg with applicator.

    Monistat 3 (Ortho). Suppositories 200 mg with applicator.

Polyene Antibiotics

AMPHOTERICIN B
[Fungizone]

Although intravenous amphotericin B has a broad spectrum of activity in systemic mycoses, its topical application is limited to the treatment of cutaneous and some acute mucocutaneous candidal infections (eg, diaper rash, otomycosis, perleche, intertrigo); no vaginal preparation is available. Amphotericin B is not effective in dermatophytic (tinea) infections.

Topical amphotericin B is not well absorbed and no systemic effects have been observed. Local irritation (pruritus, burning, and erythema) is reported occasionally, most often after application on intertriginous areas.

DOSAGE AND PREPARATIONS.
Topical: Formulations are applied two to four times daily for an appropriate length of time, depending on the degree of involvement, its location, and the patient's response (see manufacturer's literature).

    Fungizone (Squibb). Cream and ointment 3% in 20 g containers; lotion 3% in 30 ml containers.

NYSTATIN
[Mycostatin, Nilstat, O-V Statin]

ACTIONS AND USES. Nystatin is an antifungal polyene antibiotic derived from *Streptomyces noursei*. This drug has no effect on the normal flora of the intestine and is not absorbed from the gastrointestinal tract. Its clinical use usually is limited to infections of the skin and mucous membranes of the mouth, esophagus, and vagina caused by all species of *Candida*. Nystatin is administered orally, vaginally, and topically but is too toxic for parenteral use.

Vaginal candidiasis responds well to topical nystatin, but the tablet form appears to be somewhat less effective than miconazole cream and a longer duration of therapy is required to effect a cure.

ADVERSE REACTIONS. Adverse reactions occur infrequently and are mild and transitory. Nausea, vomiting, and diarrhea may develop after oral administration. Irritation occurs rarely after topical application, but hypersensitivity has not been observed. Resistance to nystatin has not been reported clinically.

No adverse effects or complications have been attributed to nystatin in infants born to women treated with nystatin vaginal tablets during pregnancy.

DOSAGE AND PREPARATIONS.
Oral: *Adults* (tablets), 500,000 to 1,000,000 units three times daily. *Adults and children* (suspension), 400,000 to 600,000 units four times daily (one-half of dose in each side of mouth), held in the mouth for a time before swallowing; *infants,* 200,000 units four times daily; *premature and low-birth-weight infants,* 100,000 units four times daily. Treatment should be continued for at least 48 hours after disappearance of symptoms.

    Mycostatin (Squibb), **Nilstat** (Lederle), **Generic.** Drops (oral suspension) 100,000 units/ml; tablets (oral) 500,000 units.

Vaginal: 100,000 to 200,000 units daily for two weeks.

    Generic. Tablets (vaginal) 100,000 units.

    Mycostatin (Squibb), **Nilstat** (Lederle). Tablets (vaginal) 100,000 units with applicator.

    O-V Statin (Squibb). Oral/vaginal therapy pack containing 42 tablets (oral) 500,000 units and 14 tablets (vaginal) 100,000 units.

Topical: The ointment or cream is applied to lesions twice daily. The powder is preferred for moist lesions and is applied two or three times daily; however, caking may occur and result in local irritation. For use in the eye, see Chapter 73, Topical Anti-infective Agents: Otic and Ophthalmic Preparations.

Generic. Cream 100,000 units/g in 15 g containers.

Mycostatin (Squibb). Cream and ointment 100,000 units/g in 15 and 30 g containers; powder 100,000 units/g in 15 g containers.

Nilstat (Lederle). Cream 100,000 units/g in 15 and 240 g containers; ointment 100,000 units/g in 15 g containers.

ANTIVIRAL AGENTS FOR WARTS AND MOLLUSCUM CONTAGIOSUM

Certain DNA and RNA viruses primarily affect the skin (Millikan, 1982). DNA viruses commonly associated with skin disease include herpesviruses, poxviruses (eg, molluscum contagiosum), and papovaviruses (eg, human papilloma virus that causes a number of verrucous diseases [warts]). RNA viruses are exemplified by picornaviruses (enteroviruses) that include Coxsackie A and B viruses, which are responsible for hand, foot, and mouth disease, viral exanthemas and enanthemas (vesicular stomatitis), and togavirus (arborvirus) and paramyxovirus, which cause rubella and rubeola, respectively.

Vaccines to prevent rubella and rubeola are discussed in Chapter 62, Agents for Active and Passive Immunity; the treatment of herpes infections is discussed in Chapter 79, Antiviral Agents. The discussion on topical antiviral drug therapy in this section is limited to the treatment of warts and molluscum contagiosum.

More than 40 human papilloma virus subtypes have been identified and associated with the various forms of warts (Rees, 1984). Clinical forms include common (verruca vulgaris), digitate or filiform, flat, palmar, plantar, plantar mosaic, myrmecia (anthill), paronychial or periungual, anogenital (condyloma), oral, and laryngeal.

Common warts disappear spontaneously in about 50% of patients after one year; the same odds apply again in the following year. Intervention is indicated when warts are painful, subject to trauma or secondary infection, or cosmetically objectionable. Therapy that produces little or no scarring is preferred (Bunney, 1983; Anderson, 1985).

Drug Selection: The therapy selected depends on the type of wart, number of lesions, and anatomic location. Application of topical keratolytic agents, with periodic paring of lesions, is employed for most common warts. Keratolytic agents should be applied carefully and repeated to minimize destruction of normal tissue. The natural resolution of warts is presumed to depend upon the release of antigen systemically during the keratolytic process, which results in antibody formation and/or cell-mediated immunity (Rees, 1984). Salicyclic acid 5% to 17% in collodion is effective and well tolerated by most individuals. A salicylic acid 40% plaster also is available but is primarily used to remove plantar warts. A cure rate for common warts approximating 70% has been obtained with nightly applications of equal parts of salicylic acid 17% and lactic acid 17% (Bunney, 1983). Bichloroacetic acid (Kahlenberg solution) and trichloroacetic acid are effective keratolytic agents in concentrations of 30% to 50%, although salicylic acid is less destructive and is usually preferred.

The cure rate with cryotherapy is similar to that with salicylic acid and lactic acid. The recommended interval between treatments is two weeks and no more than three weeks; three treatments are sufficient for most patients. Electrodesiccation with curettage and surgical excision are less desirable because of the potential for scar formation.

Cantharidin [Cantharone] is most useful for periungual common warts and molluscum contagiosum. Podophyllin [Podoben] generally is preferred for condyloma acuminatum (moist or venereal warts), especially for multiple or large cauliflower-like lesions; however, it is much less effective in nonmoist areas (eg, penile shaft, proximal thighs).

In investigational studies, human leukocyte interferon appeared to be quite effective for condyloma when applied topically (Vesterinen et al, 1984), intralesionally (Geffen et al, 1984), or intramuscularly (Schonfeld et al, 1984). Results of initial trials in juvenile laryngeal papilloma (White, 1983) and the adult form (Bomholt, 1983) also appear promising.

CANTHARIDIN
[Cantharone]

Cantharidin produces intraepidermal vesiculation and resolves various types of warts caused by the human papilloma virus, especially the periungual variety, and the flat wart-like lesions (smooth, waxy, umbilicated papules) of molluscum contagiosum caused by the poxvirus. An occlusive bandage is applied after use of cantharidin and is removed in 24 hours. The blister that forms will break, crust, and fall off in about ten days.

Burning and stinging may be noted after topical application. A severe inflammatory response may occur in patients with molluscum contagiosum. Cantharidin is quite toxic if taken orally; it should not be prescribed for home use.

Cantharone (Seres). Liquid containing cantharidin 0.7% in a vehicle containing ether 35%, acetone, ethocel, and flexible collodion in 7.5 ml containers.

PODOPHYLLIN
[Podoben]

Podophyllin resin is an extract of *Podophyllum peltatum* (May apple). A 20% to 25% dispersion in compound benzoin tincture and alcohol is applied at weekly intervals principally to treat condyloma acuminatum. Occlusion enhances effectiveness. This preparation should be removed 4 to 12 hours after application.

Encouraging results have been obtained with the investigational agent, podophyllotoxin (an active ingredient of podophyllin resin) (von Krogh, 1983). Application of 0.25 ml of podophyllotoxin 0.5% to 1% twice daily for three days appears to be safer than traditional podophyllin therapy, even when self-administered under supervision in an experimental setting.

Podophyllin should be applied sparingly on extensive lesions because it can be absorbed and produce psychotoxic confusional states, severe peripheral neuropathy, adynamic ileus, renal damage, and leukopenia and thrombocytopenia; fatalities have been reported (Cassidy et al, 1982). Because podophyllin is a teratogen, its use during pregnancy is contraindicated (Karol et al, 1980). *Podophyllin should not be given to the patient for self-administration.*

> **Podoben** (Maurry). Podophyllin 25% in compound benzoin tincture 10% and isopropyl alcohol 72% in 5 ml containers.
>
> Available Mixture.
> **Cantharone Plus** (Seres). Liquid containing podophyllin 5%, cantharidin 1%, and salicylic acid 30% in octylphenylpolyethylene glycol 0.5%, cellosolve, ethocel, collodion, castor oil, and acetone in 7.5 ml containers.

SALICYLIC ACID

USES. Salicylic acid 3% to 6% in an ointment base is a keratolytic agent useful in thinning or removal of calluses. Concentrations of 5% to 17% in collodion are effective and well tolerated by most patients for the removal of common warts. Combinations of salicylic acid 10% to 20% and lactic acid 10% to 20% in flexible collodion also have been used (Bunney, 1983). Controlled studies are required to determine if lactic acid enhances the effect of salicylic acid. A concentration of 40% has been applied as a plaster, principally for removal of plantar warts; efficacy is variable.

ADVERSE REACTIONS AND PRECAUTIONS. This drug is absorbed readily and is excreted slowly in the urine. Thus, salicylic acid should not be applied over large areas, in high concentrations, or for prolonged periods. Caution must be exercised when a 40% plaster is used, particularly on the extremities, in diabetics, or in patients with peripheral vascular disease, since acute inflammation and ulceration may occur after excessive use. This acid is not effective in a zinc oxide paste (eg, Lassar's Plain Zinc Paste) because it forms zinc salicylate, which is pharmacologically inactive.

Ointments containing salicylic acid are odorless and do not stain the skin.

Salicylic acid is classified in FDA Pregnancy Category C.

DOSAGE AND PREPARATIONS. The collodion solution is applied to warts. After drying, an adhesive moleskin is applied to the affected area for one to three days. The softened necrotic tissue is pared with a scalpel blade or scissors. Applications and parings are repeated as necessary. Plantar warts generally require longer exposures and more frequent debridement.

> SALICYLIC ACID, U.S.P.:
> **Generic.** Powder.
> SALICYLIC ACID COLLODION, U.S.P.,
> SALICYLIC ACID PLASTER, U.S.P.:
> Numerous commercial products available. Selected concentrations (usually 5% to 17%) can be compounded by a pharmacist.
> AVAILABLE MIXTURES.
> **Hydrisalic** (Pedinol). Gel containing salicylic acid 6% in a propylene glycol, ethyl alcohol, and hydroxypropylcellulose vehicle in 30 g containers.
> **Keralyt** (Westwood). Gel containing salicylic acid 6% in a propylene glycol, alcohol 19.4%, and hydroxypropylcellulose vehicle in 30 g containers.
> **Duofilm** (Stiefel), **Salactic Film** (Pedinol), **Viranol** (American Dermal). Flexible collodion containing salicylic acid 16.7% and

lactic acid 16.7% in 10 ml (**Viranol** only) and 15 ml (**Duofilm** and **Salactic Film** only) containers.
> BENZOIC AND SALICYLIC ACIDS OINTMENT:
> Mixture available generically under the name Whitfield's Ointment in 30, 45, and 454 g containers.

ANTI-INFESTATION AGENTS

Organisms from the phylum, Arthropoda, that parasitize man belong to one of two main classes (ie, Arachnida, Insecta). The principal parasite of Arachnida that infests man is known by the trivial name itch mite and causes scabies. The principal parasites of the class Insecta that infest man are *Pediculus humanus* var capitis (head lice), *Pediculus humanus* var humanus (body lice), and *Phthirus pubis* (pubic lice, crabs) and cause pediculosis.

Scabies

Scabies occurs when the gravid female itch mite, *Sarcoptes scabiei* var hominis, invades the skin. Adult female mites are approximately 0.4 x 0.3 mm and attack cracks and folds of the skin. A 10 mm serpiginous burrow may be established in the horny layer of the epidermis in as little as 15 minutes and the mite remains in the burrow, laying one or two eggs daily for the last 14 days of her entire life span (about one month). The eggs hatch in about three to four days; the larvae migrate to the skin surface where they mature in 10 to 17 days.

TRANSMISSION. Skin-to-skin contact, usually prolonged, is necessary to transmit scabies, which is classified as a sexually transmitted disease. However, prolonged nonsexual contact probably accounts for most transmission, especially between children and adults and between patients and medical staff. Children sleeping with infested parents can acquire the disease. In crusted (Norwegian) scabies in immunocompromised patients, mite populations are prodigious, and the shedding of epidermal scales containing numerous mites causes rapid spread of the disease, even to individuals who are exposed briefly.

Scabies epidemics are alleged to occur in 25- to 30-year cycles, which are hypothesized to result from a form of "immunity" that develops during infestation. However, this immunity is not absolute and lasts only for several months after infestation (Orkin and Maibach, 1985). A recent reassessment of the evidence does not support the occurrence of cycles (Burkhart, 1983).

SIGNS AND SYMPTOMS. Pruritus occurs after scabies is fully developed and usually is accompanied by papular dermatitis. During severe infestations, induration, crusting, and even nodules may occur. Irritation and pruritus are caused by sensitization to acarine products. Scratching can lead to excoriation and secondary infection.

Burrows may not be visible or may not appear in the classic form. When burrows are apparent, they appear as wavy lines several millimeters long, usually surrounded by mild inflammation and erythema. In adults, burrows are observed most frequently on the sides and webs of fingers, the ulnar border of the hand, the volar aspects of the wrists, the points of the elbows, the axillary folds, the margins of the feet, the areolae of the nipples and intertriginous folds of the breasts in women, and the genitalia in men. In infants, small children, and bedridden individuals, scabietic eruptions are common on the head, neck, and buttocks, and the symptoms of secondary infection are more likely to obscure the characteristic lesion than in adults.

Crusted scabies is characterized by a psoriasiform dermatitis on the hands and feet associated with dystrophic nails. This rare form of scabies is highly contagious and is observed most often in mentally retarded patients in institutions who are unable to care for themselves and in physically or immunologically debilitated individuals. Crusted scabies differs so markedly from classic scabies that it often is not diagnosed until attending personnel begin to develop common scabies.

See Orkin and Maibach, 1985, for a detailed discussion of scabies.

DIAGNOSIS. Classic scabies often is diagnosed easily in adults, but diagnosis can be difficult in infants and children.

The pathognomonic lesion is the burrow produced by the gravid female. Secondary lesions include vesicles, pustules, excoriations, and crusts. Identification of the mite from direct skin scrapings or cutaneous biopsy ensures a definitive diagnosis, which is not always attainable, especially if the physician is inexperienced in searching for the parasite. Mineral oil or microscope immersion oil, which is more viscous and easier to use, is preferred by a few physicians to potassium hydroxide solution or water as a medium in which to examine skin scrapings (Hazelrigg, 1978), since mites that adhere to the oil remain alive and motile; dry scraping followed by contact with potassium hydroxide kills and fragments the mites. The contact with 10% potassium hydroxide should be brief.

Since scabietic lesions can mimic any pruritic skin disease, differential diagnosis must exclude such common conditions as atopic dermatitis, impetigo, ecthyma, seborrheic dermatitis, eczematous dermatitis, dermatitis herpetiformis, psoriasis, papular urticaria, pediculosis, and chickenpox.

MANAGEMENT. The first goal of treatment is to identify the source of the infestation and avoid or remove this source. Treatment of an infested individual also should include the simultaneous administration of a scabicide to the sexual partner(s) of the patient or other household members who have prolonged skin-to-skin contact with the patient (eg, a child who shares a bed with an infested parent or sibling). Such therapy may prevent the "ping-pong" passing of the disease from one individual to the other.

Disinfestation of Fomites: Away from the human body, the scabies mite survives in a moist environment for only one or two days. Fomites may play a significant role in the transmission of scabies (Burkhart, 1983). If disinfestation of fomites is necessary, intimate clothing and bedding used within the previous 48 hours may be machine washed and dried using the hot cycles of the washer and dryer. No other measures are necessary, except for crusted scabies.

Secondary Bacterial Infection: This is the most common complication of scabietic infestations. Scratching, particularly in individuals with poor personal hygiene, can lead to dermatoses that range from pustules to furunculosis. If the infecting organism is a beta-hemolytic *Streptococcus*, acute glomerulonephritis may develop. Appropriate topical antibacterial preparations may be effective in mild secondary infections, but systemic antibiotics occasionally are required for moderate to severe pyodermas.

Drug Application: Medication is curative only when correctly utilized. Claims by a patient that he has undergone scabicidal therapy at an earlier date should not lead a physician to a misdiagnosis. Often an individual may undertake self-medication, which ameliorates symptoms without curing the infestation. Moreover, during self-medication, the patient may apply the drug erratically or only on areas that exhibit definite pruritus, thereby allowing some infested areas to escape treatment.

Pruritus may persist for several weeks after treatment because of residual eggs and feces, which prompts patients to apply preparations more frequently and for longer periods than prescribed. Physicians should, therefore, give careful instructions on the use of scabicides and prescribe only the amount needed for a given course of therapy with *no refills*. If a preparation is used too often or for too long a period, it may cause dermatitis that is mistaken for persistence of the infestation which, in turn, is aggravated by further application of the drug. The patient should be instructed not to use topical preparations other than those prescribed.

Drug Selection: Crotamiton [Eurax] and lindane (gamma benzene hexachloride) [Kwell, Scabene] are the drugs of choice for treating scabies. There are no definitive data to prove that either drug is ovicidal. Two or more applications of crotamiton are recommended by the manufacturer, but only one application of lindane usually is necessary; therefore, lindane is preferred.

Sulfur ointment is useful, but it is messy, has a bad odor, and stains clothing. Nevertheless, sulfur may be a preferred agent for infants, young children, or pregnant women. Benzyl benzoate is effective in scabies but is rarely used in the United States. Monosulfiram [Tetmosol] is used in England as a substitute for benzyl benzoate, particularly in children, since benzyl benzoate often stings when applied to the skin. Monosulfiram is diluted with two to three parts of water before application. Adults using this drug must be warned to avoid alcohol immediately before and during therapy since monosulfiram is related to disulfiram [Antabuse].

An emulsion concentrate (NBIN) containing chlorophenothane 6%, benzyl benzoate 68%, benzocaine 12%, and polysorbate 80 14% is recommended by the World Health Organization as a relatively inexpensive scabicide that can be compounded from materials readily obtainable even in developing countries. The preparation requires a 1:15 dilution with water before application. This mixture is not available in the United States. Thiabendazole, given orally or applied topically as a 10% solution (Hernández-Pérez, 1976), also is used in other countries.

Pediculosis

Pediculosis in man is caused by three types of lice: *Phthirus pubis* (crab louse), which primarily infests the pubic skin and hair; *Pediculus humanus* (body louse), which inhabits clothing and infests the trunk and limbs only to feed; and *Pediculus capitis* (head louse), which affects the scalp.

Differences in the habits of crab, body, and head lice produce three distinct public health problems. The distinction is most evident in countries with high standards of hygiene, where regular laundering of clothing has almost eliminated body louse infestations. Today, people harboring body lice are mostly vagrants or those living in substandard housing with poor facilities for maintaining cleanliness; the worst cases often involve elderly, infirm, or mentally retarded individuals.

Head lice infestations are not restricted to any socioeconomic group and are prominent in some industrial areas. Children are affected more often than adults, and girls or young women are infested more commonly than boys or young men (Busvine, 1980). Good personal hygiene often does not preclude head louse infestation but may reduce its intensity.

The population affected by crab lice cannot be defined clearly, but they are likely to be sexually active or belong to a family with a promiscuous member.

Louse infestations per se generally are not dangerous or injurious to health. *P. capitis* has never been established as a primary vector for any disease. Body lice can transmit typhus, relapsing fever, and, rarely, trench fever. Louse-borne diseases now occur only in a few parts of the world, since they can spread only where there is a high proportion of infested individuals.

INCIDENCE. The frequency of head and crab louse infestations is increasing, but there is no evidence that body louse infestations are on the rise. Regular bathing and shampooing do not ensure freedom from crab or head lice. However, poor personal hygiene by those already infested may increase the possibility of secondary bacterial infection. Head louse infestations have increased without regard to race or socioeconomic barriers with the exception of American blacks, who are rarely infested with head lice; the reason for the decreased prevalence in blacks has not been explained.

Long hair or complex hairdos are of contributory importance only when they impede early detection of an infestation, when amounts of pediculicide are insufficient to saturate long hair, or when they make combing to eliminate the nits difficult.

TRANSMISSION. Crab lice are transferred from one individual to another by sexual contact. Children can acquire the disease from infested adults through close personal contact, such as sleeping with an infested parent.

Body lice are transmitted by contact with infested clothing or bedding, since the louse lives in garment seams and visits the body only to feed. Thus, the body louse can be removed from the host by removing infested clothing. The continued existence of the louse depends upon the continuous wearing of infested clothing for a major portion of each day.

Head lice move from the head of one host to that of another, and direct person-to-person spread of head lice is believed to be the predominant mode of transmission. Exchange of combs, headwear, or other wearing apparel also may play a role.

SIGNS AND SYMPTOMS. Pruritus with scratching, excoriation, and, sometimes, secondary bacterial infection are associated with louse infestations. Symptoms are caused by an allergic reaction to saliva deposited by the parasite into the skin. Lightly infested individuals are often asymptomatic.

DIAGNOSIS. Pediculosis pubis and capitis may be diagnosed by identifying the adult louse or, more commonly, eggs (nits) attached to the hair shaft initially at the hair-skin junction. Pediculosis pubis usually involves the pubic region but can spread to the trunk, legs, and axillae and rarely involves the margins of the eyebrows and eyelashes (mainly in children), scalp, and mustache. Pediculosis capitis generally is found on the scalp and is common in children; the occipital and postauricular regions are most commonly involved. In rare instances, the beard and other exceptionally hairy areas may harbor head lice.

Pediculosis corporis can be confirmed by the presence of lice or nits in the seams of clothing, usually where clothing comes in contact with the axillae, or at the beltline and collar. Except in heavily infested individuals, parasites may be almost absent from the body.

MANAGEMENT. Pediculosis capitis, pubis, and corporis are managed by disinfestation of fomites and proper application of agents that kill the lice and nits.

Disinfestation of Fomites: General decontamination procedures have been described for all three kinds of lice. Heat is lethal to lice and their eggs; therefore, personal articles can be disinfected by machine washing in hot water and/or drying using the hot cycle of the dryer. Eggs are killed after five minutes at 51.5 C (135 F) or 30 minutes at 49.5 C (117 F), and adult lice succumb to slightly lower temperatures. Combs and brushes can be disinfected by soaking for one hour in saponated cresol solution 2% or the equivalent (eg, Lysol, Pine-Sol) or heating in water to about 60 C for five to ten minutes. Clothing or bedding that cannot be washed may be dry cleaned or placed in a plastic bag and sealed for ten days (head lice and crab lice). Head lice die in about 48 hours without a blood meal and nits kept at room temperature for ten days do not hatch. Similarly, crab lice separated from the host die in less than 24 hours. Body lice may survive for four to ten days away from the host, and eggs may hatch up to 30 days after removal from the host. Shaving or cutting the hair is not necessary.

Cleaning of houses, wards, or other rooms inhabited by infested individuals should be limited to thorough vacuuming. Fumigation is not necessary, but may be a useful alternative procedure to decontaminate the clothing of individuals with body louse infestation. Several preparations containing pyrethroids (eg, R & C Spray III, Li-Ban Spray) are relatively safe, usually effective, and much easier to use than most fumigation procedures. If fumigation is necessary, clothing or bedding can be placed in an air-tight metal container or plastic bag and exposed to ethyl formate 2 ml/L (60 ml/ft^3) for one hour. Longer exposure times (five hours or more) achieve the same results with lower concentrations of ethyl formate (0.5 ml/L, 15 ml/ft^3). In either case, the cost is low. Clothing retains a slight odor of ethyl formate upon removal from the fumigating container, which soon disperses. Ethyl formate is no more flammable or toxic than benzene, and small quantities can be handled safely.

Drug Selection: The treatment for head and crab lice is somewhat similar, because these insects live directly on the patient; therapy for body lice is markedly different since these insects live and lay their eggs on clothing. Although the procedures differ, the contact insecticides used are similar.

Shampoos containing lindane and pyrethrins synergized with piperonyl butoxide are the drugs of choice for the treatment of head and pubic pediculosis (Rasmussen, 1983). Both agents appear to be equally effective. The recommended exposure is only four minutes for lindane shampoo and ten minutes for the pyrethrins. Little probability of significant absorption occurs for the pyrethrins; however, lindane may be difficult to wash off completely. Retreatment with lindane after seven days is seldom necessary, but the patient should be examined a week later to determine that no living lice are present. A single retreatment with pyrethrins is recommended seven days following initial therapy.

Another pyrethroid, permethrim [Nix], currently is being investigated.

Malathion lotion 0.5% [Prioderm] has been used widely in Europe to treat head and pubic lice but was withdrawn from the United States market in 1985. It has some ovicidal activity, is one of the least toxic organophosphorus insecticides, and is highly effective against both head and pubic lice; however, it requires an 8- to 12-hour exposure time to eliminate lice.

Petrolatum ophthalmic ointment is used to treat crab louse (*P. pubis*) infestation of the eyelashes. The ointment is applied thickly twice daily for eight days. An ophthalmic ointment containing physostigmine 0.25% also has been applied, but undesirable effects on vision, pupillary size, and accommodation have limited its usefulness.

Carbaryl [Sevin], a cholinesterase inhibitor insecticide, is used in England and some other countries as a pediculicide in the form of a shampoo. Although about 10% of an applied dose may be absorbed, carbaryl has low toxicity when applied topically. When poisoning does occur, the signs and symptoms may be indistinguishable from those caused by organophosphorus compounds (Murphy, 1980).

Chlorophenothane (DDT) was one of the first synthetic insecticides used against lice. However, body lice have become resistant in many countries, and head lice are resistant in some areas outside the United States. DDT is not ovicidal and furnishes no residual protection. Anxiety about environmental contamination with DDT has restricted its use, and it is no longer available in the United States.

Powder preparations are often useful in managing head lice in areas where houses are poorly heated and hot running water is not available. These conditions make wetting the hair unacceptable to patients, especially in the winter. Powders also have been found to be more convenient than lotions or shampoos in controlling head lice in jails and prisons where the daily admission and discharge rate is high. Under these circumstances, it is easier to shake on a powder than it is to ensure that a recalcitrant or inebriated person will apply a lotion or shampoo properly. Powders also control body lice when a change of clothes or laundry facilities is not readily available.

As with scabicides, patients tend to use pediculicides more frequently than necessary. To avoid toxicity and/or irritant dermatitis, pediculicides should not be applied more than twice a week.

Drug Evaluations

BENZYL BENZOATE

This agent has been widely used outside the United States to treat scabies but has been supplanted by crotamiton and lindane in this country.

Benzyl benzoate is relatively nontoxic but may irritate the skin and eyes. Increased pruritus and irritation (manifested by burning and stinging, particularly of the genitalia and scalp) are common. Contact with the eyes and urethral meatus should be avoided. There is no evidence that this drug is absorbed through the skin in amounts sufficient to cause systemic toxicity. Benzyl benzoate is converted to hippuric acid following ingestion, but systemic toxic symptoms have not been described in man. In animals, this agent has been reported to cause progressive incoordination, central nervous system excitation, convulsions, and death.

DOSAGE AND PREPARATIONS.
Topical: After thorough cleansing with soap and water for ten minutes, a preparation containing approximately 25% of the drug is applied to the entire body below the neck; after this application has dried, the medication may be reapplied and the residue washed off 24 hours later. Benzyl benzoate may be applied nightly or every other night for a total of three applications.
 Generic. Emulsion 50% in pt and gal containers (nonprescription).

CROTAMITON
[Eurax]

Crotamiton is effective in scabies. It is claimed to have antipruritic activity independent of its scabietic effects but this has been questioned (Smith et al, 1985). Two applications, 24 hours apart, are recommended by the manufacturer; a cleansing bath should be taken 48 hours after the second application. Occasionally, more than two applications are necessary to attain the same degree of effectiveness as one application of lindane; therefore, the latter is preferred.

Crotamiton rarely causes allergic contact dermatitis but occasionally produces irritant contact dermatitis and may be particularly irritating to denuded skin.

DOSAGE AND PREPARATIONS.

Topical: The preparation is massaged into the skin of the whole body, working from the chin down. When the head and face are involved (eg, infants), these areas also should be treated. Particular attention should be given to the body folds, hands, feet (including the soles), and intertriginous areas. Contact with the eyes, mouth, and urethral meatus should be avoided. Two or more applications at 24-hour intervals eradicate most scabietic infestations. A cleansing bath should be taken 48 hours following the last application. In resistant cases, treatment may be repeated one week later or an alternative drug used.

 Eurax (Westwood). Cream 10% in 60 g containers; lotion 10% in 60 and 474 ml containers.

LINDANE (Gamma Benzene Hexachloride)
[Kwell, Scabene]

USES. Lindane is a drug of choice for the treatment of scabies. Lindane shampoo also is highly effective for head and pubic lice, and it may have some ovicidal activity. Lice have become resistant in a few countries, but this is not as serious a problem in the United States.

ADVERSE REACTIONS AND PRECAUTIONS. The potential for serious toxicity is considerable if the preparation is misused; therefore, it is important that the patient or family be given adequate instructions in use of lindane (Rasmussen, 1981).

As usually formulated, lindane is irritating to the eyes and mucosa. Allergic contact dermatitis has not been documented, but irritant contact dermatitis has occurred when the drug was applied in excessive amounts, too frequently, or for extended periods. If irritation becomes evident, the drug should be washed off and not used again. Lindane is absorbed through intact skin and is toxic if absorbed in excessive amounts. Some authorities have expressed concern about the absorption of lindane cream or lotion after the recommended 8- to 12-hour exposure time for scabies, especially in children. This agent is excreted slowly in the urine (half-life, approximately 20 hours).

Lindane should be used with caution in pregnant women. It penetrates skin and has the potential for central nervous system toxicity. Studies indicate that the potential for toxic effects of topical lindane is greater in the young. Careful attention to recommended dosage is advised.

If accidental ingestion occurs, prompt gastric lavage eliminates much of the preparation. Oil-type laxatives should be avoided since they enhance absorption. Systemic toxicity is usually manifested as central nervous system stimulation progressing to convulsions; intravenous diazepam or barbiturates counteract this effect. Intravenous calcium gluconate also may be beneficial, but epinephrine should be avoided.

DOSAGE AND PREPARATIONS.
Topical: For scabies, *adults and children*, no more than 20 to 30 g of lotion or cream is applied to all parts of the body except the face. The eyes, eyelashes, and mucous membranes should be avoided. The medication is washed off thoroughly following overnight exposure (8 to 12 hours). It can be applied again after a seven-day interval, but usually only one treatment is required. When used in *infants,* the manufacturers' recommended dose should not be exceeded.

For head lice, *adults and children*, up to 30 ml of shampoo is massaged into the hair for four minutes. The hair is then thoroughly rinsed with warm water and towel dried. Treatment is repeated in one week. For pubic lice, *adults and children,* the shampoo is applied to the affected and adjacent hairy areas, particularly the pubic mons and perianal region, and is removed after four minutes; in hairy individuals, the thighs, trunk, and axillary regions also should be shampooed. When the hair is dry, any remaining nits or nit shells should be removed with a fine-toothed comb and tweezers. Retreatment in seven days is indicated only if gross signs of infestation (new nits, living lice) are present. The lotion or cream is less convenient than the shampoo for head and pubic lice, and a longer exposure time is recommended (8 to 12 hours). Lindane should not be used for *P. pubis* infestations of the eyelashes (see the discussion on Drug Selection in the section on Pediculosis).

For body lice, a thin layer of lotion or cream is applied to infested and adjacent hairy areas, left on for 8 to 12 hours, and removed by showering or bathing.

 Generic. Lotion and shampoo 1% in 60, 474, and 3,792 ml containers.
 Kwell (Reed & Carnrick). Cream 1% (for scabies) in 57 and 454 g containers; lotion 1% in 59 and 474 ml containers; shampoo 1% (for head and pubic lice) in 59 and 474 ml containers.
 Scabene (Stiefel). Lotion and shampoo 1% in 59 and 474 ml containers.

PYRETHRINS AND PIPERONYL BUTOXIDE
[A-200 Pyrinate, R & C Shampoo, RID]

Pyrethrins synergized with piperonyl butoxide are available without prescription in liquid form in concentrations ranging from 0.17% to 0.3%. These contact insecticides are alternative preparations of choice for the treatment of head and pubic lice.

Topical absorption from intact skin is poor. Toxicology studies in animals indicate that pyrethrins are among the safest insecticides available.

Impurities in poor quality extracts of pyrethrins may cause allergic dermatitis; persons sensitive to ragweed may be susceptible. Pharmaceutical formulations generally do not cross react in patch tests on humans sensitized to ragweed pollen, but caution is advised.

Because commercial formulations are irritating to the eyes and mucous membranes, they should not be used to treat *P. pubis* infestations of the eyelashes (see the discussion on Drug Selection in the section on Pediculosis).

DOSAGE AND PREPARATIONS.
Topical: Liquid preparations are applied to the hair, scalp, or other infested area until the hair is thoroughly wet. After ten minutes, the insecticide is removed by shampooing and rinsing with warm water. Remaining nits or nit shells should be

removed with a fine-toothed comb and tweezers. Treatment should be repeated in one week.

A-200 Pyrinate (Norcliff Thayer). Gel containing pyrethrins 0.33%, piperonyl butoxide 4%, and deodorized kerosene 5.33% in 30 g containers; liquid containing pyrethrins 0.17%, piperonyl butoxide 2%, and deodorized kerosene 5% in 60 and 120 ml containers (both forms nonprescription).

R & C Shampoo (Reed & Carnrick). Shampoo containing pyrethrins 0.3%, piperonyl butoxide 3%, petroleum distillate 1.2% in 60 and 120 ml containers (nonprescription).

RID (Pfipharmecs). Liquid containing pyrethrins 0.3%, piperonyl butoxide 3%, and petroleum distillate 2.4% in 60 and 120 ml containers (nonprescription).

SULFUR

This compound is applied topically as a 6% (range, 5% to 10%) ointment of precipitated sulfur in petrolatum to treat scabies. Only a few authorities consider sulfur to be a preferred scabicide for infants, young children, and pregnant women.

Sulfur ointment has staining properties and an unpleasant odor; rarely, it causes irritation and dermatitis if used frequently.

DOSAGE AND PREPARATIONS.

Topical: Following a cleansing scrub using tepid water and soap, the skin is dried and sulfur ointment is applied nightly for three nights. The patient may bathe each night prior to application of the drug or once, 24 hours after the last application.

No pharmaceutical dosage form is available; compounding is necessary for prescription. The usual formulation is a 6% ointment of precipitated sulfur in petrolatum.

ANTISEPTICS AND DISINFECTANTS

Antiseptics

These antimicrobial agents are applied topically to living tissues (usually intact skin, mucous membranes, or wounds) to destroy microorganisms or inhibit their reproduction or metabolic activities. Antiseptics are included in some formulations employed by health care personnel as surgical hand scrubs, as handwashes to reduce the risk of cross contamination, and for preoperative skin preparation. Antimicrobial soaps that contain antiseptics reduce skin bacteria for a deodorant effect.

Skin cleansers and protectants for the laity may contain antiseptics to minimize the potential for infection associated with minor cuts, abrasions, burns, or insect bites. However, such use is of limited value. These agents should be considered, at best, only adjuncts to adequate removal of dirt and organic matter by sudsing, emulsification, irrigation, and debridement techniques (Larson, 1985) and use of protective dressings that assure adequate drainage.

Although the use of antiseptics by health care personnel is effective, controversy exists as to which antiseptics are most effective and safe (Sebben, 1983; Rutala and Cole, 1984). The antiseptics most widely employed by health care personnel include ethyl and isopropyl alcohols; cationic surface-active agents (eg, benzalkonium); the biguanide, chlorhexidine; iodine compounds (ie, iodine solution, iodine tincture, povidone-iodine); and the phenolic compounds, triclosan, parachlorometaxylenol, and hexachlorophene. These antiseptics, except for hexachlorophene, are incorporated into OTC products. Also available are chlorine compounds (eg, sodium hypochlorite, oxychlorosene), hydrogen peroxide, mercurial compounds (eg, thimerosal), and phenolic compounds (eg, phenol, hexylresorcinol).

Silver nitrate is used prophylactically for ophthalmia neonatorum; silver sulfadiazine is used most often to treat burns. The phenolic compound, triclosan, and the carbanilide, triclocarban, are also used principally as components of antimicrobial soaps for deodorant purposes.

Disinfectants

These substances are used on inanimate objects to destroy microorganisms and prevent infection. Some disinfectants are used as antiseptics if they can be diluted sufficiently to avoid injuring living tissues while retaining antimicrobial activity. The principal disinfectants available are the aldehydes, formaldehyde and glutaral; elemental chlorine; and the phenolic compound, cresol.

Sterilization is the complete and total destruction of all microbial life, including vegetative bacteria, spores, fungi, and viruses. Ethylene oxide is the only chemical available that is approved for sterilization of objects that cannot be heated or sterilized by other physical methods (eg, radiation).

Drug Evaluations

ETHYL ALCOHOL

ISOPROPYL ALCOHOL

Alcohols are applied to reduce local bacterial flora prior to penetration with needles or other sharp instruments and as a preoperative wash. Their antiseptic action can be enhanced by prior mechanical cleansing of the skin with water and a detergent and gentle rubbing with sterile gauze during application.

Ethyl alcohol is widely used for skin antisepsis. Its bactericidal effects result from rapid coagulation of protein. The 70% aqueous solution is more effective in reducing the surface tension of bacterial cells than absolute alcohol; the latter precipitates protoplasm at the periphery of the cell and thus tends to retard penetration of the agent.

Isopropyl alcohol has slightly greater bactericidal activity than ethyl alcohol due to its greater depression of surface tension. It rapidly kills vegetative forms of most bacteria when used full strength or as a 70% aqueous solution.

Ethyl and isopropyl alcohol are used as cleansers, lubricants, and rubefacients for bedridden patients. Rubbing alcohol contains about 70% (by volume) ethyl alcohol. Alcohol is applied to cool the skin but it may irritate inflamed or denuded tissue, especially after repeated use. Application of an emollient after an alcohol rub alleviates the dry feeling.

Ethyl and isopropyl alcohol are potent virucidal agents (Klein and Deforest, 1983). Neither has reliable fungicidal or sporicidal activity in any concentration and they are not useful for sterilization of instruments.

Alcohols should not be used to disinfect wounds because they irritate tissues, resulting in painful burning and stinging, and they precipitate protein to form a coagulated mass in which bacteria may grow.

ETHYL ALCOHOL:
Alcohol, U.S.P., Diluted Alcohol, U.S.P., Rubbing Alcohol, N.F. (nonprescription).
ISOPROPYL ALCOHOL:
Isopropyl Alcohol, N.F. (nonprescription).

FORMALDEHYDE

GLUTARAL

Formaldehyde is a potent, volatile, wide-spectrum germicide that has been used as a vapor and as a solution in water (formalin). The vapor is irritating when inhaled or applied to the skin in the concentrations required for antisepsis. Therefore, formaldehyde is used principally as a disinfectant in concentrations of 2% to 8%. Formaldehyde has an anhidrotic action when applied to palms and soles but not axillae.

Glutaral (glutaraldehyde) is a potent dialdehyde with a wide range of antimicrobial activity; it is rapidly sporicidal and possesses tuberculocidal activity. A 2% aqueous solution buffered with sodium carbonate 0.3% to a pH of 7.5 to 8.5 disinfects and sterilizes surgical and endoscopic instruments and plastic and rubber apparatus used for respiratory therapy and anesthesia. Glutaral loses activity within two weeks after preparation because it tends to polymerize in alkaline solution, which is the optimum pH for germicidal activity. A stabilized alkaline solution with a longer use life is now available (Cidex-7) (Miner et al, 1977). The combination product, glutaral-phenate sterilizing solution [Sporicidin] appears to be more active and stable against spores than glutaral alone (Sebben, 1984).

Like formaldehyde, glutaral has an anhidrotic action when applied to palms and soles. It generally is not used on the axilla because of its irritant and sensitizing properties. Glutaral generally does not cross react with formaldehyde.

FORMALDEHYDE SOLUTION, U.S.P.:
Solution containing 37% by weight of formaldehyde with methanol added to prevent polymerization.
GLUTARAL:
Cidex Solution, Cidex-7 (Surgikos). Solution 2% (nonprescription).
AVAILABLE MIXTURE.
Sporicidin (Sporicidin Co) (nonprescription).

TRICLOCARBAN

This carbanilide is used as an antimicrobial in bar soap; it has antibacterial and antifungal actions. Currently, the concen-

tration is limited by the FDA to 1.5%, and use of triclocarban is currently restricted to inclusion in bar soaps; additional data on substantivity, absorption, distribution, blood levels, excretion, and safety are needed before final guidelines for use of triclocarban can be established.

Coast (Procter & Gamble), *Dial* (Armour-Dial), *Jergens Clear Complexion Bar* (Jergens), *Safeguard* (Procter & Gamble), *Zest* (Procter & Gamble) (all nonprescription).

ETHYLENE OXIDE

Ethylene oxide is readily diffusible, noncorrosive, and antimicrobial to all organisms at room temperature. This gaseous alkylating agent is widely used as an alternative to heat sterilization of drugs and medical devices. It reacts with chloride and water to produce two active germicides, 2-chloroethanol and ethylene glycol. Special sterilizing chambers are required because the gas must remain in contact with the objects for several hours. *Adequate airing* of sterilized materials is important to minimize skin irritation in nonsensitized individuals who come into contact with such materials. Ethylene oxide also is a pulmonary irritant when inhaled. It is too toxic to be applied topically as an antiseptic.

Ethylene oxide and 2-chloroethanol (but not ethylene glycol, an alkylating agent) are mutagenic in animals, and some concern exists about the current OSHA exposure limit for workers of 1 ppm over an eight-hour period.

HYDROGEN PEROXIDE

When hydrogen peroxide comes into contact with catalase, an enzyme found in blood and most tissues, it rapidly decomposes into oxygen and water in wounds and on mucous membranes. The liberated oxygen has little bactericidal effect except, possibly, on anaerobes, but it does loosen masses of infected detritus in wounds. Hydrogen peroxide has little effect on intact skin because the oxygen is released so slowly.

When diluted with one or more parts of water, hydrogen peroxide is sometimes employed as a mouthwash, but its use to treat stomatitis and gingivitis may irritate the tongue and buccal mucosa. The 3% solution often is instilled in the external ear to aid in removal of cerumen. It should never be instilled in closed body cavities or abscesses from which the gas has no free egress. Hemiplegia has followed its use to irrigate the pleural cavity; presumably this is caused by the passage of the gas into the vascular system, resulting in cerebral embolism.

Generic. Solution 3% (nonprescription).

CHLORHEXIDINE GLUCONATE
[Hibiclens, Hibistat]

Chlorhexidine is a chlorophenyl biguanide with a relatively broad spectrum of antimicrobial activity (Aly and Maibach, 1983; Goldblum et al, 1983; Sebben, 1983). At pH 5.0 to 8.0, it is most effective against gram-positive (10 mcg/ml) and gram-negative (50 mcg/ml) bacteria. Bacterial spores are prevented from germinating but are not killed except at elevated temperatures. High concentrations of serum proteins reduce the bacteriostatic and bactericidal effects of chlorhexidine. Its effectiveness is somewhat reduced by blood and other organic matter. Although high levels of surfactants also may reduce the bacteriostatic and bactericidal effects of chlorhexidine, this problem has been minimized by careful formulation.

Chlorhexidine is rapid acting, has considerable skin substantivity (residual adherence), has low potential for producing contact sensitivity and photosensitivity with long-term clinical use, and is poorly absorbed, even after many daily hand washings.

Hibiclens is used as an antiseptic wound and general skin cleanser, for preoperative preparation of the patient, as a surgical scrub, and as a handwash for health care personnel. It contains a 4% concentration in a sudsing base formulation. Hibistat is a germicidal hand rinse; the clear, colorless liquid contains 0.5% weight/weight chlorhexidine gluconate in 70% isopropyl alcohol with emollients.

> **Hibiclens Skin Cleanser, Hibistat Hand Rinse** (Stuart) (nonprescription).

MERCURIAL COMPOUNDS

Although organic mercurial compounds are less irritating and less toxic than inorganic compounds, they have only weak bacteriostatic activity and are less effective than ethyl alcohol. Serum and tissue proteins reduce antimicrobial activity and skin sensitization is common. Consequently, the antiseptic and disinfectant uses of mercurial compounds are limited, and only thimerosal is available.

To avoid systemic absorption of mercury, organic mercurials should not be used on large areas of denuded skin, and prolonged repeated applications in the mouths of infants should be avoided. Acute poisoning with suicidal intent damages gastrointestinal mucosa and can cause severe chemical nephrosis with albuminuria, oliguria, azotemia, and irreversible acute renal failure. Dimercaprol is an effective antidote if therapy is begun within four hours (see Chapter 80, Drugs Used in the Treatment of Poisoning).

> THIMEROSAL:
> (All forms nonprescription)
> **Generic.** Solution, swabs, tincture.
> **Mersol** (Century). Tincture.
> **Merthiolate** (Lilly). Aerosol, solution, tincture.

CATIONIC SURFACTANTS

Soaps are anionic and organic quaternary ammonium compounds are cationic surface-active agents. Both classes of detergents emulsify sebaceous material, which is then removed with dirt and microbes. The mild desquamating effect of the quaternary ammonium compounds aids in cleansing. Their antimicrobial properties are limited and solutions are prone to contamination; thus, their usefulness as antiseptics is often less than desired (Sebben, 1983). Nevertheless, these compounds are widely used as industrial and home detergents, emulsifiers, and sanitizers. Their antimicrobial action is ascribed to alteration of microbial membrane permeability.

BENZALKONIUM CHLORIDE
[Ionax, Zephiran]

This is the prototype of the organic quaternary ammonium compounds. It is active against gram-positive and gram-negative bacteria, some fungi (including yeasts), and certain protozoa (eg, *Trichomonas vaginalis*). Strains of *Pseudomonas aeruginosa* are more resistant and require longer exposure. Aqueous solutions are ineffective against *Mycobacterium tuberculosis, Clostridium,* and other spore-forming bacteria and viruses.

Benzalkonium chloride may be used preoperatively to diminish the number of organisms on intact skin and mucous membranes. It is applied to minor lacerations, wounds, and abrasions to limit infection. Organic material, soap, and other anionic substances inactivate benzalkonium chloride; therefore, soap should be rinsed off thoroughly with water and alcohol 70% before this agent is applied.

Concentrated solutions can produce corrosive skin lesions with deep necrosis and scarring. Properly diluted solutions are not ordinarily irritating or sensitizing; however, if they are used under occlusive dressings, casts, or packs, irritation may occur. Caution is advisable when irrigating body cavities with benzalkonium chloride, for systemic absorption may cause muscle weakness.

The following concentrations are recommended: For use on intact skin, minor wounds, and abrasions, 1:750 (tincture or aqueous solutions); for mucous membranes and broken or diseased skin, 1:2,000 to 1:5,000 (aqueous solution); for storage of instruments, 1:750 to 1:5,000 (aqueous solution). An antirust agent should be added to retard corrosion of metallic instruments. Solutions should be checked periodically for contamination by resistant bacteria and spores and replenished frequently to maintain effective bactericidal concentrations.

The quaternary ammonium compounds are adsorbed and inactivated by cotton fabrics, cellulose sponges, certain plastics (particularly polyvinyl chloride), or other porous materials. For this reason, these agents are of uncertain efficacy in cold sterilization of catheters, flexible endoscopes, or other instruments.

> **Generic.** Solution, concentrate (both forms nonprescription).
> **Ionax** (Owen). Foam aerosol, scrub paste (both forms nonprescription).
> **Zephiran** (Winthrop-Breon). Solution (aqueous), concentrate, tincture, tincture spray (all forms nonprescription).

METHYLBENZETHONIUM CHLORIDE
[Diaparene]

This cationic surfactant is effective against gram-positive and gram-negative organisms. It is commonly used as a rinse for diapers and for bed linen and underclothes of incontinent adults to prevent irritant contact dermatitis; articles should be free of soap to avoid inactivation of the antiseptic. Methylbenzethonium is applied topically as a dusting powder around genitalia, rectum, and thighs and in intertriginous areas to prevent and treat perianal dermatitis, miliaria rubra, and intertrigo. It seldom produces irritation.

Diaparene (Glenbrook). Powder, perianal cream, ointment (all forms nonprescription).

CHLORINE COMPOUNDS

CHLORINE

SODIUM HYPOCHLORITE SOLUTION

OXYCHLOROSENE
[Clorpactin XCB, Clorpactin WCS-90]

Chlorine is a potent germicidal agent used to disinfect inanimate objects, water supplies, and swimming pools. It is not recommended for disinfecting medical instruments because of its corrosive properties. The germicidal action is due to elemental chlorine and to the hypochlorous acid that forms in aqueous solution. This effect is decreased by organic matter and an alkaline pH.

Sodium hypochlorite solution is used to disinfect utensils. The undiluted solution contains approximately 5% sodium hypochlorite and is too irritating for use as an antiseptic except in root canal therapy. Sodium hypochlorite solution diluted (modified Dakin's solution) contains 0.5% sodium hypochlorite adjusted to a neutral pH with sodium bicarbonate. It once was widely used to treat suppurating wounds, but its solvent action delays clotting.

Sodium hypochlorite causes allergic contact dermatitis. Patch test concentrations are 1:100 and 1:1,000 freshly prepared in water.

The germicidal chlorophor, oxychlorosene, is a mixture of hypochlorous acid and alkylbenzene sulfonates. The sulfonates appear to enhance the germicidal activity of hypochlorous acid by causing its slow release. The sodium salt is used as a topical antiseptic for preoperative preparation of the skin and for wound irrigation in a concentration of 0.2% to 0.4%. Concentrations of 0.1% to 0.2% are useful for urologic and ophthalmologic irrigations or applications.

SODIUM HYPOCHLORITE SOLUTION, N.F.:
Available generically and as household bleach (nonprescription).
DILUTED SODIUM HYPOCHLORITE SOLUTION, N.F.
OXYCHLOROSENE:
Clorpactin XCB (Guardian). Powder 5 g (for solution) (nonprescription).
OXYCHLOROSENE SODIUM:
Clorpactin WCS-90 (Guardian). Powder 2 g (for solution) (nonprescription).

IODINE COMPOUNDS

Elemental iodine is a powerful antimicrobial agent; adequate concentrations and duration of exposure can destroy all known bacteria, fungi, viruses, protozoa, and yeasts. Bacterial resistance to iodine is unknown. Elemental iodine is poorly soluble in water or alcohol and saturates in both at about 0.03% (300 ppm). Soluble iodine is referred to as free iodine. Additional iodine can be made soluble only by conversion to triiodide ion with an iodide salt, such as the inclusion of sodium iodide in U.S.P. iodine solution and U.S.P. iodine tincture. This reaction is reversible when the concentration of elemental iodine falls below the saturation level. The potentially reversible inorganic triiodide ion plus free iodine are together referred to as "available iodine," whereas free and complexed elemental iodine (I_2) in organic iodophors (eg, povidone-iodine) are together referred to as "available iodine." However, it is only free iodine that appears to possess significant antimicrobial activity (Favero, 1982).

Free iodine is an avid collector of electrons to form iodide ion. Iodine captures electrons from many organic molecules, such as glucose, starches, glycols, lipids, amino acids, and proteins, which is the basis for its rapid antimicrobial action. Once iodine is converted to iodide ion, antimicrobial activity is lost. Iodine cannot penetrate tissue without undergoing rapid conversion to inactive iodide ion, ie, it is active only on tissue surface. Nevertheless, iodophors remain active in the presence of blood, pus, serum, mucosal secretions, other tissue fluids, and soap.

Iodine can be used to disinfect water when other methods are not available; three drops of tincture of iodine added to one quart of water kills bacteria and amebae within 15 minutes.

Hypersensitivity reactions may occur after application of any of these compounds. Iodine solutions occasionally are taken with suicidal intent. The caustic action of elemental iodine affects the gastrointestinal mucosa. Suspensions of starch or protein or solutions of sodium thiosulfate may be ingested as antidotes.

IODINE SOLUTION, U.S.P.

IODINE TINCTURE

Iodine solution U.S.P. contains approximately 2% iodine and 2.4% sodium iodide in water (2% available iodine and 0.03% free iodine). It is preferred for superficial lacerations to prevent microbial infections, since it is effective and nonirritating. (Iodine Solution should not be confused with Strong Iodine Solution, U.S.P. [Lugol's solution], which is used to treat thyroid disease.)

Iodine tincture is a 2% solution of elemental iodine with 2.4% sodium iodide in water and 44% to 50% alcohol (2% available iodine and 0.03% free iodine). It is preferred to the older 7% iodine tincture, which caused severe burns, and to iodine solution for the decontamination of intact skin prior to intravenous injection or obtaining blood for microbial culture studies. The concentration of alcohol in iodine tincture is irritating to wounds and does not contribute appreciably to the antibacterial action.

Iodine Solution, U.S.P. (nonprescription).
Iodine Tincture, U.S.P. (nonprescription).

Iodophors

Iodophors are complexes of iodine and organic compounds that release free iodine from a reservoir of available iodine gradually and in low concentration. In addition to their medical use as antiseptics, iodophors are extensively employed as general disinfectants for household, industrial, farming, and veterinary purposes. Medical use is limited to the nonsurfactant aqueous and alcohol soluble povidone-iodine (polyvinylpyrrolidine-iodine complex).

POVIDONE-IODINE

The iodine complexed with povidone has no antimicrobial activity until it is released as free iodine in solution. It has the same broad antimicrobial spectrum as iodine solution and iodine tincture (the standard undiluted 10% aqueous povidone-iodine solutions are formulated to contain 1% available iodine but only 0.0002% [2 ppm] free iodine).

Although diluting the standard 10% aqueous povidone-iodine solution with water 1:10 increases the liberation of elemental iodine four- to fivefold and increases in vitro activity, in vivo, the antimicrobial activity of diluted solutions may be inadequate because the reservoir of available iodine is insufficient (Berkelman et al, 1982). In any event, if diluted prior to intended use, solutions are less stable and deteriorate rapidly on standing. Antiseptic activity ceases when povidone-iodine in dressings or on the skin becomes dry.

Povidone-iodine preparations are used as handwashes for health care personnel; as surgical scrubs; to prepare skin prior to surgery, injection, or aspiration; to treat minor cuts and abrasions; to treat burns (see the section on Chemotherapeutic Agents for Burns); and as a disinfectant for urinary catheters and peritoneal dialysis equipment. Povidone-iodine [Betadine] may be used locally as a vaginal disinfectant in the treatment of trichomoniasis. Its topical vaginal application elevates serum iodine concentrations; therefore, this drug should not be used repeatedly during pregnancy to avoid goiter and hypothyroidism in the fetus and newborn (see also Chapter 77, Antiprotozoal Agents).

Povidone-iodine is less irritating and less toxic than aqueous and alcoholic solutions of elemental iodine (Rodeheaver et al, 1982); however, irritation occurs occasionally, especially with use of solutions containing detergents. Local hypersensitivity reactions are uncommon, but individuals with a history of iodine sensitization should not use this agent.

(All forms nonprescription)
Generic. Ointment, solution, surgical scrub, vaginal douche.
Aerosol Spray:
Betadine (Purdue-Frederick).
Mouthwash and Gargle:
Betadine (Purdue-Frederick), ***Isodine*** (Blair).
Ointment:
ACU-dyne (Acme United), ***Betadine*** (Purdue-Frederick), ***Efodine*** (Fougera), ***Pharmadine*** (Sherwood), ***Polydine*** (Century).
Skin Cleanser:
ACU-dyne (Acme United), ***Betadine Liquid, Foam*** (Purdue-Frederick), ***Pharmadine*** (Sherwood).
Solution:
ACU-dyne (Acme United), ***Betadine*** (Purdue-Frederick), ***Isodine*** (Blair), ***Pharmadine*** (Sherwood), ***Polydine*** (Century).
Surgical Scrub:
Betadine (Purdue-Frederick), ***Mallisol*** (Mallard), ***Pharmadine*** (Sherwood).

PHENOLIC COMPOUNDS

PHENOL

SAPONIFIED CRESOL SOLUTION

HEXYLRESORCINOL

PARACHLOROMETAXYLENOL

PARABENS

Phenol and substituted phenols vary greatly in their antiseptic and disinfectant efficacy and safety. Phenol is bacteriostatic in concentrations of 1:500 to 1:800 and bactericidal and fungicidal in concentrations of 1:50 to 1:100. It is not effective against spores. Phenol is seldom used as an antiseptic or disinfectant. Because it possesses local anesthetic activity and has an antipruritic effect at concentrations of 0.5% to 1.5%, its primary use is as a component of topical antipruritic formulations.

Under certain conditions, phenol damages skin, which increases the rate of penetration; therefore, it should be applied only on small areas of skin and occlusive dressings, bandages, or diapers should not be used. Phenol should never be used in pregnant women, in infants under 6 months, or for diaper rash. Phenolic disinfectants have produced epidemics of neonatal hyperbilirubinemia when used to clean bassinets and mattresses in poorly ventilated nurseries. Fatalities have been documented in infants. Since phenol has been implicated as a tumor promoter in concentrations above 5%, controlled studies are under way to determine the carcinogenic, mutagenic, and teratogenic activities of this agent.

Cresol is a mixture of the three methyl isomers of phenol saponified in linseed oil. It is as toxic as phenol but three times more potent as a bactericide. Because of its irritating effect on the skin, use of cresol is limited to disinfection. However, neither phenol nor cresol should be used to disinfect rubber, plastic, or fabrics that may adsorb the agent, because burns may result when these come into contact with the skin.

Hexylresorcinol is a more effective and less toxic bactericide than phenol. It is used in antiseptic mouthwashes and as a skin wound cleanser, but it may be irritating.

Parachlorometaxylenol 0.5% to 2% is a more effective bactericide than phenol. It is a component of handwashes used by health care personnel and OTC mixtures used for acne, seborrhea, and otic infections. More data on skin absorption are needed before its safety can be established definitely.

The short alkyl esters of *p*-hydroxybenzoic acid are known as the *parabens*. Although they are seldom used as antiseptics, methylparaben and its homologues often are included in topical and some parenteral preparations as preservatives. The parabens may sensitize the skin, but the incidence is low.

Phenol, U.S.P. (nonprescription).
Saponified Cresol Solution (Lysol) (nonprescription).
Hexylresorcinol, N.F. (nonprescription).
Parachlorometaxylenol, U.S.P.
Medicated Lotion Soap (Vestal) 0.5% (nonprescription).

HEXACHLOROPHENE
[pHisoHex, pHiso Scrub, Septisol]

This chlorinated bisphenol compound has strong bacteriostatic activity and is most effective against gram-positive bacteria, including staphylococci. It has little activity against most gram-negative bacteria or spores. Hexachlorophene is used for handwashing by hospital and healthcare personnel, as a surgical hand scrub, and for preoperative preparation of the skin.

Although single washings of the skin are no more effective than soap in reducing the number of bacteria, regularly repeated scrubs steadily decrease bacterial flora. Cleansing with alcohol or washing with soap removes the antibacterial residue.

ADVERSE REACTIONS AND PRECAUTIONS. Hexachlorophene may produce irritation, but hypersensitivity reactions are rare. Preparations may cause a burning sensation on the skin and in the eyes, and suds containing this agent should be rinsed promptly from the eyes with water.

Hexachlorophene is absorbed through intact skin and mucosal surfaces. Since amounts sufficient to produce neurotoxic effects may be absorbed, it should not be applied in compresses and special precautions should be taken to avoid extensive application to broken, denuded, or burned skin. Systemic absorption causes symptoms characteristic of cerebral irritability. Hexachlorophene should not be used routinely for prophylactic total body bathing, especially for infants. When it is applied to clean small areas of pyoderma in infants, the residue should be rinsed off thoroughly. The drug is available only on prescription.

Emulsion 3%:
pHisoHex (Winthrop-Breon) in 150, 472, and 3,792 ml containers.

Foam 0.23% with alcohol 46%:
Septisol (Vestal) in 180 and 600 ml containers.

Sponge 3%:
pHiso Scrub (Winthrop-Breon).

TRICLOSAN

This 5-chloro-2-(2,4-dichlorophenoxy) phenol is an antimicrobial ingredient of bar soaps at concentrations no greater than 1%. It is also present in antiseptic, wound cleanser, and wound protectant products. The FDA has reclassified triclosan from category II to category III B (safe and effective) for hand washes and surgical hand scrubs for health care personnel and III E (effective) for preoperative skin preparation. Products containing triclosan should not be used in infants under 6 months because the cumulative effects of cutaneous absorption have not been determined.

Liquid 0.25%:
Septi-Soft (Vestal) in 240, 948, and 3,792 ml containers.
Solution 0.25%:
Septisol (Vestal) in 240, 948, and 3,792 ml containers.
Antimicrobial soaps as **Lifebuoy, Phase III**; also with triclocarban as **Irish Spring** (nonprescription).

SILVER COMPOUNDS

Silver nitrate and silver sulfadiazine [Silvadene] are the only silver compounds widely used. Colloidal silver preparations (eg, mild silver protein [Argyrol S.S. 10%]) are less corrosive, but their disinfecting properties do not equal those of the silver salts because less of the active free silver ion is available; therefore, they are not recommended for such use.

Silver sulfadiazine is used in burn therapy and in the treatment of chronic pressure ulcers (Kucan et al, 1981). See the discussion on Chemotherapeutic Agents for Burns.

SILVER NITRATE

This silver salt is strongly bactericidal when applied topically in relatively low concentrations; most microorganisms are destroyed rapidly by a 1:1,000 solution and a 1:10,000 solution is bacteriostatic.

In many states, instillation of two drops of 1% solution into the conjunctival sac of newborn infants is required by law to prevent ophthalmia neonatorum. (See Chapter 73, Topical Anti-infective Agents: Otic and Ophthalmic Preparations.)

Since silver nitrate is an effective germicide and astringent, a 0.1% to 0.5% solution is used on wet dressings but may stain tissue black due to reduction of silver deposits upon exposure to sunlight. Occasionally, 0.01% to 0.03% solutions are applied to irrigate the urethra and bladder.

Aqueous solutions of 0.5% silver nitrate are sometimes applied as dressings on second- and third-degree burns to prevent infections caused by *Pseudomonas aeruginosa*, *Proteus*, or other gram-negative and gram-positive organisms. The most important adverse effect with such use is depletion of sodium and chloride caused by precipitation of insoluble silver chloride; this is particularly likely if silver nitrate is applied to extensive areas over prolonged periods. Small amounts of silver nitrate may be absorbed through the skin after prolonged use, resulting in argyria, a permanent bluish-black discoloration of the skin (only one case of argyria has been reported in association with burn therapy). Pain lasting for one-half to one hour after application of dressings is common with concentrations exceeding 0.5% and occasionally with lower concentrations.

A solid preparation in a pencil-form applicator (toughened silver nitrate) or a cotton pledget dipped in 10% silver nitrate solution is used to cauterize wounds, fissures, aphthae, and granulomatous tissue.

Generic. Solution (ophthalmic) 1%; ointment; toughened sticks; applicators (nonprescription).

Cited References

Aly R, Maibach HI: Comparative evaluation of chlorhexidine gluconate (Hibiclens) and povidone-iodine (E-Z Scrub) sponge/brushes for presurgical hand scrubbing. Curr Ther Res 34:740-745, 1983.

Aly R, Maibach HI: Pyodermas: Avoiding empiric approach: Part I. Pathophysiology and evaluations. Part II. Differential diagnosis and treatment. Fam Med Rep 2:17-24; 25-32, (Winter/Spring) 1984.

Anderson FE: Warts: Fact and fiction. *Drugs* 30:368-375, 1985.

Beggs WH, et al: Action of imidazole-containing antifungal drugs. *Life Sci* 28:111-118, 1981.

Beggs WH, Polman DM: Fungicidal and fungistatic actions of tioconazole. *Curr Ther Res* 38:778-784, 1985.

Berkelman RL, et al: Increased bactericidal activity of dilute preparations of povidone-iodine solutions. *J Clin Microbiol* 15:635-639, 1982.

Bomholt A: Interferon therapy for laryngeal papillomatosis in adults. *Arch Otolaryngol* 109:550-552, 1983.

Bradbeer CS, et al: Butoconazole and miconazole in treating vaginal candidiasis. *Genitourinary Med* 61:270-272, 1985.

Bunney MH: Wart treatments. *Semin Dermatol* 2:101-108, 1983.

Burkhart CG: Scabies: Epidemiologic reassessment. *Ann Intern Med* 98:498-503, 1983.

Busvine JR: *Insects and Hygiene*, ed 3. London, Methuen, 1980.

Cassidy DE, et al: Podophyllum toxicity: Report of fatal case and review of literature. *J Toxicol Clin Toxicol* 19:35-44, 1982.

Clissold SP, Heel RC: Tioconazole: Review of its antimicrobial activity and therapeutic use in superficial mycoses. *Drugs* 31:29-51, 1986.

Cullen SI, et al: Treatment of tinea versicolor with new antifungal agent, ciclopirox olamine cream 1%. *Clin Therapeut* 7:574-583, 1985.

Degreef H, Dooms-Goossens A: Patch testing with silver sulfadiazine cream. *Contact Dermatitis* 12:33-37, 1985.

Demling RH: Burns. *N Engl J Med* 313:1389-1398, 1985.

East MO (ed): Tioconazole: Review of clinical studies in dermatology. *Dermatologica* 166(suppl 1):1-33, (June) 1983.

Ezzedeen FW, et al: Percutaneous absorption and disposition of iodochlorhydroxyquin in dogs. *J Pharmaceut Sci* 73:1369-1372, 1984.

Favero MS: Iodine: Champagne in tin cup. *Infection Control* 3:30-32, 1982.

Feinstein A, et al: Urticaria and fixed drug eruption in patient treated with griseofulvin. *J Am Acad Dermatol* 10:915-917, 1984.

Fisher AA: Adverse reactions to bacitracin, polymyxin, and gentamicin sulfate. *Cutis* 32:510-513, 1983.

Fleury F, et al: Therapeutic results obtained in vaginal mycoses after single dose treatment with 500 mg clotrimazole vaginal tablets. *Am J Obstet Gynecol* 152(part 2):968-970, 1985.

Fox CL Jr: Topical therapy and development of silver sulfadiazine. *Surg Gynecol Obstet* 157:82-88, 1983.

Geffen JR, et al: Intralesional administration of large doses of human leukocyte interferon for treatment of condylomata acuminata. *J Infect Dis* 150:612-615, 1984.

Ginsburg CM, et al: Effect of feeding on bioavailability of griseofulvin in children. *J Pediatr* 102:309-311, 1983.

Goldblum SE, et al: Comparison of 4% chlorhexidine gluconate in detergent base (Hibiclens) and povidone-iodine (Betadine) for skin preparation of hemodialysis patients and personnel. *Am J Kidney Dis* 11:548-552, 1983.

Hazelrigg DE: Scraping for scabies. *Am Fam Physician* 17:129, (Jan) 1978.

Heel RC, et al: Econazole: Review of its antifungal activity and therapeutic efficacy. *Drugs* 16:177-201, 1978.

Hernández-Pérez E: Topically applied thiabendazole in treatment of scabies. *Arch Dermatol* 112:1400-1401, 1976.

Hughes D, Kriedman T: Treatment of vulvovaginal candidiasis with 500-mg vaginal tablet of clotrimazole. *Clin Ther* 6:662-668, 1984.

Jacoby F: Care of massive burn wound. *Crit Care Q* 44-53, (Dec) 1984.

Jue SG, et al: Ciclopirox olamine 1% cream: Preliminary review of its antimicrobial activity and therapeutic use. *Drugs* 29:330-341, 1985.

Katz HI, et al: SCH 370 (clotrimazole-betamethasone dipropionate) cream in patients with tinea cruris or tinea corporis. *Cutis* 34:183-187, 1984.

Karol MD, et al: Podophyllum: Suspected teratogenicity from topical application. *Clin Toxicol* 16:283-286, 1980.

Kligman AM, et al: Evaluation of ciclopirox olamine cream for the treatment of tinea pedis: Multicenter double-blind comparative studies. *Clin Ther* 7:409-417, 1985.

Kodsi BE, Goldberg PK: Therapeutic strategy for esophageal candidiasis. *Drug Ther* 13:199-213, (April) 1983.

Klein M, Deforest A: Principles of viral inactivation, in Block SS (ed): *Disinfection, Sterilization, and Preservation*, ed 3. Philadelphia, Lea & Febiger, 1983, 422-434.

Krowchuk DP, et al: Current status of identification and management of tinea capitis. *Pediatrics* 72:625-631, 1983.

Kucan JO, et al: Comparison of silver sulfidiazine, povidone-iodine, and physiological saline in treatment of chronic pressure ulcers. *J Am Geriatr Soc* 29:232-235, 1981.

Lacey RW: Evolution of microorganisms and antibiotic resistance. *Lancet* 2:1022-1025, 1984.

Lachapelle JM: Occupational allergic contact dermatitis to povidone-iodine. *Contact Dermatitis* 11:189-190, 1984.

Landau JW: Commentary: Undecylenic acid and fungous infections. *Arch Dermatol* 119:351-353, 1983.

Larson E: Handwashing and skin: Physiologic and bacteriologic aspects. *Infection Control* 6:14-23, 1985.

Laude TA, et al: Tinea capitis in Brooklyn. *Am J Dis Child* 136:1047-1050, 1982.

Leyden JJ, Kligman AM: Rationale for topical antibiotics. *Cutis* 22:515-528, 1978.

MacMillan BG: Infections following burn injury. *Surg Clin North Am* 60:186-196, 1980.

Mathieson R, Dutta SK: Candida esophagitis. *Digest Dis Sci* 28:365-370, 1983.

Meech RJ, et al: Pathogenic mechanisms in recurrent genital candidosis in women. *NZ Med J* 98:1-5, 1985.

Millikan LE: Viral skin infections: Challenges in differential diagnosis and therapy. *Postgrad Med* 72:195-207, (Oct) 1982.

Miner NA, et al: Antimicrobial and other properties of new stabilized alkaline glutaraldehyde disinfectant/sterilizer. *Am J Hosp Pharm* 34:376-382, 1977.

Moleski RJ: Burn wound: Topical therapy for infection control. *Drug Intell Clin Pharmacol* 12:28-35, 1978.

Molnar JA, Burke JF: Metabolic and nutritional management: Avoiding pitfalls. *Drug Ther (Hosp)* 9:45-54, (Oct) 1984.

Moylan JA: Outpatient treatment of burns. *Postgrad Med* 73:235-242, (March) 1983.

Murphy SD: Pesticides, in Doull J, et al (eds): *The Basic Science of Poisons*, ed 2. New York, Macmillan, 1980, 357-408.

Orkin M, Maibach HI (eds): *Cutaneous Infestations and Insect Bites*. New York, Marcel Dekker, 1985.

Owens NJ, et al: Prophylaxis of oral candidiasis with clotrimazole troches. *Arch Intern Med* 144:290-293, 1984.

Pegg SP: Role of drugs in management of burns. *Drugs* 24:256-260, 1982.

Rasmussen JE: Problem of lindane. *J Am Acad Dermatol* 5:507-516, 1981.

Rasmussen JE: Advances in treatment of head and pubic lice. *Drug Ther* 13:185-192, (Nov) 1983.

Rees RB: Treatment of warts. *Semin Dermatol* 3:130-135, 1984.

Rodeheaver G, et al: Bactericidal activity and toxicity of iodine-containing solutions in wounds. *Arch Surg* 117:181-186, 1982.

Rudolph AH: Surefire ways to treat fungal infections of skin, scalp, and nails. *Mod Med* 122-128, (Jan) 1985.

Rutala WA, Cole EC: Antiseptics and disinfectants: Safe and effective? (editorial). *Infection Control* 5:215-218, 1984.

Sakurai K, et al: Mode of action of 6-cyclohexyl-1-hydroxy-4-methyl-2(1H)-pyridone ethanolamine salt (Hoe 296). *Chemotherapy* 24:68-76, 1978.

Sawyer PR, et al: Clotrimazole: Review of its antifungal activity and therapeutic efficacy. *Drugs* 9:424-447, 1975.

Schonfeld A, et al: Intramuscular human interferon-β injections in treatment of condylomata acuminata. *Lancet* 1:1038-1042, 1984.

Sebben JE: Surgical antiseptics. *J Am Acad Dermatol* 9:759-765, 1983.

Sebben JE: Sterilization and care of surgical instruments and supplies. *J Am Acad Dermatol* 11:381-394, 1984.

Shectman LB, et al: Clotrimazole treatment of oral candidiasis in patients with neoplastic disease. *Am J Med* 76:91-94, 1984.

Smith EB, et al: Crotamiton lotion in pruritus. *Int Dermatol* 23:684-685, 1985.

Sobel JD: Management of recurrent vulvovaginal candidiasis with intermittent ketoconazole prophylaxis. *Obstet Gynecol* 65:435-440, 1985.

Stohs SJ, et al: Percutaneous absorption of iodochlorhydroxyquin in humans. *J Invest Dermatol* 82:195-198, 1984.

Straughn AB, et al: Bioavailability of microsize and ultramicrosize griseofulvin products in man. *J Pharmacokinet Biopharm* 8:347-362, 1980.

Tannenbaum L, et al: 1% sulconazole cream v 2% miconazole cream in treatment of tinea versicolor: Double-blind multicenter study. *Arch Dermatol* 120:216-219, 1984.

Vesterinen E, et al: Topical treatment of flat vaginal condyloma with human leukocyte interferon. *Obstet Gynecol* 64:535-538, 1984.

von Krogh G: Condylomata acuminata 1983. *Semin Dermatol* 2:109-129, 1983.

White EC: Interferon joins attack on severe laryngeal papilloma. *JAMA* 250:1815, 1983.

Witkowski JA, Parish LC: Bacterial skin infections: Management of common streptococcal and staphylococcal lesions. *Postgrad Med* 72:166-185, (Oct) 1982.

Wolfe RA, et al: Mortality differences and speed of wound closure among specialized burn care facilities. *JAMA* 250:763-766, 1983.

Zellner PR, Bugyi S: Povidone-iodine in treatment of burn patients. *J Hosp Infect* Suppl A:139-146, (Mar 6) 1985.

Antimycobacterial Agents

TUBERCULOSIS

Tuberculosis is caused by *Mycobacterium tuberculosis*, a bacillus that can remain dormant in the human host for years. The disease is typically acquired by inhalation of aerosols of sputum containing the tubercle bacilli. Acquired cellular immunity usually renders the bacilli quiescent and most infected individuals never develop disease. When active tuberculosis does develop, it can become progressive, is potentially fatal, and may be transmitted to susceptible individuals. About one-third of all cases are discovered in patients with febrile pulmonary disease, another one-third in those with unrelated complaints, and the final one-third in those undergoing medical examinations.

It has been estimated that more than 10 million people in the United States are infected with tubercle bacilli (*Morbid Mortal Week Rep,* [Sept 16] 1983). In 1983, 23,532 tuberculosis cases were reported to the Centers for Disease Control (CDC), which represented a decrease of 7.8% from the previous year. However, among 38 notifiable communicable diseases reported to the CDC in 1979, tuberculosis was the leading cause of death and exceeded the combined total for the other 37 diseases (*Morbid Mortal Week Rep,* 1984). For the years 1979 to 1982, the average number of deaths annually was nearly 2,000.

Tuberculosis is a major health problem in recent Asian, Haitian, and Hispanic immigrants. For Indochinese refugees who entered the United States in 1980, the incidence was 480/100,000 (Powell et al, 1983); in southern Florida, the prevalence of tuberculosis among recent immigrants from Haiti was reported to be 650/100,000 (Pitchenik et al, 1982). Many of these cases appeared to be due to organisms resistant to antituberculosis drugs, including isoniazid (Pitchenik et al, 1982; *Morbid Mortal Week Rep,* [Oct 14] 1983).

Nationally, there has been an annual overall decrease in the incidence of tuberculosis since 1968. However, from 1976 through 1981, the incidence among children up to 14 years remained stable, apparently because of the high rates of disease among refugee Indochinese and Hispanic children. Also, more children than adults have miliary or meningeal tuberculosis (Powell et al, 1984). Thus, physicians practicing in certain communities are more likely to see active cases, many of which are due to drug-resistant organisms.

In the United States, it is mandatory for physicians to report not only newly diagnosed tuberculosis, but also patients who prematurely discontinue therapy. Detailed records of therapy, including changes in regimen, all bacteriologic reports, and the results of drug susceptibility tests, must be kept.

PATHOGENESIS. Infection with the tubercle bacillus results in two major immunologic responses: acquired immunity and tuberculin hypersensitivity. These two responses play an important role in the development of tuberculosis. They appear to be separate and distinct, are of a cellular nature, and are mediated by T-lymphocytes; different populations of T-cells probably are involved. The occurrence of overt disease primarily depends on the interplay between these immunologic events.

Tuberculous infections may take one of two general paths, depending on whether there has been previous exposure to the tubercule bacillus. Individuals with no prior exposure to the tubercle bacillus or other related mycobacteria (eg, BCG vaccine, *M. kansasii, M. avium-intracellulare*) have not developed an immunologic reaction to the organism, and infection in such an individual is known as the *primary* infection. Individuals with previous exposure have reacted immunologically to the tubercle bacillus and probably have acquired cellular immunity and tuberculin hypersensitivity. Infection in such individuals is known as *reinfection* tuberculosis.

Primary Infection: The lung is usually the first organ involved, since infection is usually via the lower respiratory tract. The tubercle bacilli initially lodge within an alveolus where they are soon taken up by macrophages and neutrophils. The ingested bacilli multiply within phagocytes, for they are resistant to the cells' destructive action. Since there is little resistance to multiplication, bacilli disseminate from the original pulmonary site, largely through the lymphatic system; extensive involvement of the hilar lymph nodes follows. In addition, there is spillover from the lymphatic vessels to the bloodstream, causing infection in other parts of the lungs, especially the apices, and in other organs and tissues. Thus, tuberculosis may become generalized within a few days. Most of the disseminated bacilli are taken up by mononuclear cells in lymphoid organs where they continue to multiply.

Resolution of the process usually occurs within a few weeks due to the acquisition of cell-mediated immunity. Coincident with this resolution, tuberculin positivity develops and there is a marked increase in the ability of macrophages to inhibit multiplication of the tubercle bacilli (acquired cellular immunity). The development of acquired immunity is considered to be of major importance in control of the disease.

Most persons with primary infection exhibit no clinical or radiographic evidence of disease other than a positive tuberculin skin test. In 5% to 10% of cases, however, clinical and/or radiographic signs, such as a pneumonic infiltrate, hilar adenopathy, and fever, do appear. A pneumonic process near the pleura may lead to pleural effusion and enlarged lymph nodes may cause atelectasis. In a small percentage of cases, a poor host response may lead to bronchogenic and/or miliary spread of disease to remote sites, such as the liver, bone marrow, lymph nodes, and meninges.

Endogenous Reactivation: Although the acquisition of cell-mediated immunity leads to the resolution of the primary infection in most persons, they remain at risk of disease reactivation for life. Reactivation or post-primary (adult-type) tuberculosis can occur at any site seeded with bacilli at the time of the primary infection, but is most commonly seen in the upper lobes of the lungs, perhaps due to the relatively high oxygen tension there. Endogenous reactivation probably accounts for more than 90% of tuberculosis cases in the United States.

Necrosis is a conspicuous feature of reactivation tuberculosis and is due to tissue destruction following the allergic inflammatory reaction to tuberculin. The lesion is localized because cellular immunity limits bacterial multiplication and dissemination. However, the disease may spread to adjacent tissue. Erosion of an infected bronchus may lead to bronchogenic spread or, if a blood vessel is affected, to hematogenous spread of the bacilli. Macrophages and lymphocytes do not function or survive in necrotic areas and, therefore, the benefits of acquired cellular immunity are lost at these sites.

Reinfection Tuberculosis: This occurs when individuals who have previously been infected and have acquired cellular immunity and delayed hypersensitivity to tuberculin are infected again. Clinically, it is indistinguishable from reactivation tuberculosis. Reinfection tuberculosis is rare in the United States but is relatively common in developing countries.

Drug Selection

The objectives of antituberculous chemotherapy are to eliminate tubercle bacilli rapidly and to prevent relapse. Ideally, therapy would render the sputum negative by both smear and culture and would keep the sputum consistently negative thereafter. The goal is to make the patient noninfectious as rapidly as possible and to maintain the noninfectious state permanently. There is general agreement that an effective therapeutic regimen should produce a failure-relapse rate of less than 5%.

There are two main principles of therapy for tuberculosis: (1) Therapy must consist of two or more drugs to which the tubercle organisms are susceptible. (2) Treatment must continue for three to six months after the sputum becomes negative to sterilize the lesions and prevent relapse.

Tubercle bacilli are killed by antituberculosis drugs only during replication. *Mycobacterium tuberculosis* is an obligate aerobe and the frequency of multiplication, as well as the level of metabolic activity, varies with the concentration of oxygen. In addition, bacilli are affected by the pH of their environment. Three replicating populations of tubercle bacilli are hypothesized to exist in the host: (1) those in cavitary lesions; (2) those in closed caseous lesions; and (3) those existing within macrophages.

In cavities, the oxygen tension is fairly high, the medium is neutral or slightly alkaline, and multiplication is active. In closed caseous lesions, the oxygen tension is low, the medium is neutral, and replication is slow and intermittent. The intracellular milieu of macrophages is acidic and multiplication is relatively slow. There is evidence that the efficacy of antituberculous drugs differs among these various bacterial populations (see Table 1). In addition, the host may harbor bacilli that are not replicating, have a low level of metabolic activity, and are not affected by antituberculous drugs.

Isoniazid [Dow-Isoniazid, Nydrazid] and rifampin [Rifadin, Rimactane] are the most potent antituberculous drugs available; they are thought to be bactericidal for extracellular (including cavitary) bacteria, intracellular (macrophages) bacteria, and bacteria in closed caseous lesions. However, both rifampin and pyrazinamide appear to be more active than isoniazid against slowly or intermittently replicating bacilli in macrophages and closed caseous lesions.

Pyrazinamide, although not very active in vitro, is believed

TABLE 1.
ACTION OF DRUGS DEPENDING UPON THE METABOLIC ACTIVITY OF TUBERCLE BACILLI

| | | Metabolic activity of tubercle bacilli | |
| | | Slowly multiplying | |
Drug	Actively multiplying (usually extracellular)	At acid pH (intracellular)	At neutral pH (extracellular)
Streptomycin	+++	0	0
Isoniazid	++	+	±
Rifampin	++	+	+
Pyrazinamide	+ or ±	++	0
Ethambutol	±	±	0

NOTE: *Metabolic activity is expressed on a scale of 0 to +++ as follows: 0 = no activity; ± = bacteriostatic activity; and +, ++, and +++ = bactericidal activity of increasing intensity.*
Adapted from Dutt AK, Stead WW: Present chemotherapy for tuberculosis. J Infect Dis 146:698–704, 1982.

to be quite active against intracellular bacilli in the acidic environment of the macrophages. These are the bacilli that are likely to cause relapses. Pyrazinamide had been considered a second-line drug, but recently has been used as a first-line drug in combination with isoniazid and rifampin. Clinical studies suggest that pyrazinamide is most useful during the initial phase of therapy and, because of its action against intracellular bacilli, may play an important role in decreasing relapses.

Streptomycin is believed to be bactericidal only for the large, rapidly multiplying, extracellular population of tubercle bacilli in cavitary lesions.

Ethambutol [Myambutol] is considered to be bacteriostatic only. Its greatest value in multidrug regimens is its ability to prevent or delay the emergence of organisms resistant to the other drugs in the regimen.

An important consideration in drug selection is the likelihood that drug-resistant organisms are present. The incidence of resistant strains varies with different population groups. In certain developing countries, tuberculosis is common and the incidence of resistance to isoniazid and streptomycin has been increasing, especially in patients who contracted disease in the Far East, Africa, or Central and South America.

In a study on patients who acquired infection in Korea, the resistance rate to isoniazid and streptomycin was 33% and 22%, respectively; in non-Korean isolates, the rates were 6% and 5%, respectively (Carpenter et al, 1982). In South Texas, where the majority of the population is Mexican-American, the reported incidence of resistance to isoniazid is 16.4%, ethambutol 3.9%, rifampin 10.6%, and streptomycin 7.8% (Carpenter et al, 1983). In a 20-year prospective study of primary drug-resistant tuberculosis among children in the United States (principally black or Puerto Rican), the overall resistance rate was 15.8% to one or more antituberculous drugs (Steiner et al, 1983).

In the United States, the incidence of primary drug resistance, particularly to streptomycin and isoniazid, is much greater (1) among children from households in which a family member has received unsuccessful treatment for tuberculosis;

(2) in some large inner city areas; and (3) in the foreign-born, especially those who immigrated during the last two decades from areas with a high incidence of tuberculosis (eg, Southeast Asia, Africa, South America).

Mutants naturally resistant to two drugs are rare (frequency about 10^{-11} organisms) and, to avoid their growth, it is imperative that dual *bactericidal* drug therapy be used initially in active tuberculosis and be continued long enough to eliminate populations that multiply infrequently.

The choice of agents depends primarily upon whether the organism can be presumed to be susceptible to the major antituberculous drugs. If there is any possibility of previous treatment with an antituberculous drug or if infection with drug-resistant organisms is suspected, special consideration must be given to selection of the initial chemotherapeutic agents. If drugs were given previously, it is important to use two drugs that the patient has not received previously until results of sensitivity studies are available.

In addition to the use of multiple drugs, adequate doses must be administered for sufficient periods to effect a cure. Supervised drug administration or reliable patient compliance is essential for successful therapy. With optimal treatment, the rate of cure approaches 100%.

A number of highly effective and relatively safe multiple-drug regimens are utilized to individualize treatment of active disease. Expanded knowledge of pharmacokinetics and pharmacodynamics and the availability of bactericidal drugs have altered approaches to drug selection and treatment, especially with respect to dosage schedules and duration of therapy. Authorities agree that the best chance to bring about rapid and complete recovery is when the diagnosis is first made, when the organisms are multiplying rapidly, and before chronic, often irreversible, changes occur.

A single drug should never be added to an initial regimen that may be failing. In this situation (which occurs rarely if optimal treatment is prescribed initially), two effective agents not previously administered should be added. It may be best to substitute an entirely new regimen on the basis of dependable bacterial susceptibility studies. Such specialized studies are readily available through many state health departments or large independent laboratories.

Less commonly used antituberculous drugs include capreomycin [Capastat], kanamycin [Kantrex, Klebcil], aminosalicylic acid, ethionamide [Trecator-SC], and cycloserine [Seromycin]. All are generally considered to be bacteriostatic. These drugs are less effective, more toxic, or less acceptable to patients and are reserved for use when organisms exhibit multiple resistance to the bactericidal drugs or when the latter are not tolerated or are contraindicated. They are more commonly employed in the retreatment of tuberculosis. Aminosalicylic acid is undesirable because of the gastrointestinal distress it produces, especially in adults. However, this drug is well tolerated in children under 2 years and may be substituted for ethambutol in these young patients, for they cannot be monitored satisfactorily for retrobulbar neuritis.

PREVENTIVE THERAPY. Preventive therapy of tuberculosis has one of the following two goals: (1) to prevent infection in an individual with a negative Mantoux skin test in the absence of anergy but who has had intimate contact with an active case; (2) to prevent active disease in an individual who is infected but does not have overt disease (significant reaction to Mantoux skin test but chest x-ray does not demonstrate active disease; therefore, subclinical infection is presumed). In the former, the regimen is referred to as true chemoprophylaxis, and in the latter, the regimen is referred to as chemoprophylaxis of subclinical infection (see Table 2).

Single-drug therapy is limited to preventive therapy. Isoniazid is the only drug approved for this use; however, rifampin has been used when isoniazid is contraindicated or not tolerated (Farer, 1982) (see Table 2).

On the basis of studies by the Public Health Service, it formerly was recommended that any person with a positive Mantoux skin test be given a course of chemoprophylaxis with isoniazid alone for one year. As a result, isoniazid was utilized in thousands of individuals. After the true risk of isoniazid-induced hepatitis became apparent with time, the indications for preventive treatment were modified.

At present, the Centers for Disease Control and the American Thoracic Society recommend preventive chemotherapy for (1) all household contacts and other close associates of patients with active pulmonary tuberculosis; (2) persons with a

positive Mantoux skin test and an abnormal chest x-ray consistent with previous tuberculous disease, including those with a past history of tuberculosis and inadequate chemotherapy; (3) individuals whose Mantoux skin test reaction is known to have converted from not significant to significant during the previous two years; (4) infected individuals at special risk of developing active tuberculosis because of treatment with adrenal corticosteroids or immunosuppressive agents; and (5) patients with diseases that lower resistance to the tubercle bacillus (particularly leukemia, Hodgkin's disease, diabetes, silicosis, and the postgastrectomy state). In addition, preventive treatment is considered mandatory for all positive tuberculin reactors under 6 years of age and is still recommended for reactors under 35 years, with the exception of pregnant women.

Recommendations for isoniazid prophylaxis during pregnancy are somewhat controversial. In both rats and rabbits, isoniazid has an embryocidal effect; however, no adverse effects on the fetus were reported in clinical studies involving more than 1,400 pregnancies (Coleman and Slutkin, 1984). Therefore, it has been recommended that, since preventive therapy is elective, administration of isoniazid should be deferred until after delivery for reactors of unknown duration who do not have additional risk factors.

Among older reactors, the risk of developing active tuberculosis must be weighed against the risk of isoniazid-induced hepatitis (Leff and Geppert, 1979; Sbarbaro and Iseman, 1981). Age appears to be the major risk factor (see the evaluation on Isoniazid); however, discontinuation of isoniazid is uncommon.

The risk of isoniazid-induced hepatitis is less than the risk of developing tuberculosis for patients exposed to active cases or those who had recent skin test conversion. Therefore, isoniazid should not be withheld from such individuals (Stead, 1981). Patients under 25 years who develop signs and symptoms of hepatitis during isoniazid prophylaxis may discontinue therapy if the serum level of aspartate aminotransferase is increased threefold or more. The hepatic reaction has cleared promptly when such guidelines were followed.

The assumptions on which the American Thoracic Society and the Centers for Disease Control based their recommendations for asymptomatic individuals with a positive skin test, even those under 35 years, have been challenged recently

TABLE 2.
CURRENT REGIMENS FOR THERAPEUTIC MANAGEMENT OF TUBERCULOSIS

Indications	Regimens
PREVENTIVE THERAPY[1] *True Chemoprophylaxis* (negative tuberculin skin test in absence of anergy; known intimate contact with active case).	*Adults,* isoniazid (orally 4 to 5 mg/kg or 300 mg daily) plus pyridoxine[2] (orally 15 to 50 mg daily). *Children,* isoniazid (orally 10 mg/kg daily to maximum of 300 mg); pyridoxine rarely necessary in younger children. Skin test is repeated in 3 months. If negative and contact with active case is broken, discontinue therapy. If positive or contact with active case is unbroken, continue treatment for 12 months. If supervision is required, isoniazid 15 mg/kg (adults, 900 mg) can be given twice weekly.

(Continued on next page)

Indications	Regimens

PREVENTIVE THERAPY (continued)

Chemoprophylaxis of Subclinical Infection to prevent active disease (positive tuberculin skin test; no evidence of active disease on chest x-ray).

1. Age 35 or younger *or* over age 35 with additional risk factors (diabetes, silicosis, postgastrectomy state, lymphoma, leukemia, disease- or drug-induced immunosuppression, close contact with an active case, intense skin reaction, known conversion of skin test from negative to positive within two years, hemodialysis for chronic renal failure, presence of small apical fibrotic inactive lesions on the chest x-ray film in sputum-negative patients).

   Isoniazid and pyridoxine dosage regimen as above for 12 months.

2. All PPD converters regardless of age.

   Adults, rifampin (orally, 10 to 20 mg/kg or 600 mg daily); *children,* maximum of 600 mg daily. Therapy is continued for 12 months.[3]

ACTIVE TUBERCULOSIS

Conventional-Course Chemotherapy (12 months)

1. Severely immunosuppressed patients.

2. Patients with complicated tuberculosis (ie, extensive or extrapulmonary tuberculosis) or associated conditions (eg, diabetes mellitus, silicosis, the postgastrectomy state). Many workers feel that short-course chemotherapy for nine months is adequate for these patients and recommend its routine use.

3. No contraindications to the use of isoniazid, rifampin or ethambutol; otherwise, see text.

   Adults, initially, isoniazid 300 mg and rifampin 600 mg are given daily for 20 weeks; *children* receive isoniazid 10 mg/kg (maximum 300 mg) and rifampin 15 mg/kg (maximum 600 mg) daily, followed by isoniazid 300 mg daily and ethambutol 15 mg/kg daily until sputum cultures remain negative for one year.

   If evidence exists that the individual is likely to harbor an isoniazid-resistant organism (ie, recent immigrant or contact with a person who has recently immigrated from many parts of Africa, Asia or South America), some physicians also give ethambutol 15 to 25 mg/kg daily initially to preclude monotherapy if the strain proves to be resistant.

Short-Course Chemotherapy (9 months)

1. Patients with uncomplicated pulmonary tuberculosis.

2. No contraindications to the use of isoniazid or rifampin; otherwise, see text.

   Adults and children, isoniazid 300 mg and rifampin 600 mg are given daily for 9 months; children receive isoniazid 10 mg/kg (maximum 300 mg) and rifampin 15 mg/kg (maximum 600 mg) daily. Alternatively, after one month of daily therapy, biweekly administration of isoniazid 15 mg/kg (usually 900 mg) and rifampin 600 mg for adults or isoniazid 20 mg/kg and rifampin 15 mg/kg for children may be given under supervision when compliance cannot be assured. Sputums are examined every month until conversion occurs (usually three months) and therapy is continued for at least six months after conversion. Follow-up sputum examinations are recommended for one year to assure the absence of relapse.

   If evidence exists that the individual is likely to harbor an isoniazid-resistant organism (ie, recent immigrant or contact with a person who has recently immigrated from many parts of Africa, Asia or South America), ethambutol 25 mg/kg daily is given initially to preclude monotherapy if the strain proves to be resistant to isoniazid; otherwise, ethambutol is discontinued.

---

[1]*In pregnant women, preventive therapy should be delayed until after delivery.*
[2]*The need for pyridoxine when isoniazid is given in this dose range is not yet proven.*
[3]*The use of rifampin for preventive therapy in tuberculosis is not yet proven.*

(Taylor et al, 1981) but are still generally accepted (Farer, 1982).

Persons with fibrotic lesions consistent with pulmonary tuberculosis are at increased risk of developing the disease. Treatment with isoniazid for 24 or 52 weeks significantly reduced the incidence of tuberculosis in these patients who where followed for five years (Comstock, 1983).

Rifampin has been suggested as an alternative for prophylaxis in contacts of patients with isoniazid-resistant organisms; however, its efficacy has not been proved (Farer, 1982).

ACTIVE DISEASE TREATMENT. Historically, individuals with tuberculosis were isolated but, as understanding of the means of infection transmission and the efficacy of therapy improved, it became apparent that isolation was not beneficial either to those infected or to society. As a result, affected individuals are now treated as outpatients if they are compliant and able to manage their own care and medication. Hospitalization is required only occasionally, usually when signs and symptoms are severe, when unrelated illnesses are present, when public health considerations of infectiousness are important, or when the patient cannot ingest medications and provide self-care. Patients who are potentially noncompliant (eg, alcoholics) require careful monitoring if they are not institutionalized.

The actual time necessary to produce a cure depends upon the drug regimen used and the patient's response to therapy. However, most patients can be cured with a nine-month regimen of isoniazid and rifampin. Some physicians feel that standard (18 months) therapy is superior to any shorter course (Buechner, 1983).

Conventional-course Chemotherapy: If the conventional, longer course of chemotherapy is considered desirable, adults are given isoniazid 300 mg and rifampin 600 mg daily for 20 weeks; children are given isoniazid 10 mg/kg (maximum 300 mg) daily and rifampin 15 mg/kg (maximum 600 mg) daily, followed by isoniazid 300 mg daily and ethambutol 15 mg/kg daily until sputum cultures remain negative for one year. This regimen has provided definitive cures and the lowest relapse rates in most patients in whom the organisms were originally susceptible and medication was taken consistently (Long et al, 1979). If there is evidence of an isoniazid-resistant organism (recent immigrant or contact with such a person), some physicians also give ethambutol 15 to 25 mg/kg daily initially to preclude monotherapy. Other physicians routinely initiate treatment with a regimen of three drugs (isoniazid, rifampin, and ethambutol) until the results of sensitivity studies are known. If the organism is found to be sensitive to isoniazid and rifampin, ethambutol is discontinued (Buechner, 1980).

Short-course Chemotherapy: A nine-month course of chemotherapy with isoniazid and rifampin has been effective in adults and children with pulmonary tuberculosis (including cavitary disease) and extrapulmonary tuberculosis. The short-course regimen is not recommended for the severely immunosuppressed patient.

Following the determination of baseline data, including hematocrit, white blood cell and platelet count, blood urea nitrogen, serum glutamic oxaloacetic transaminase, and bilirubin levels, selected adults are given isoniazid 300 mg and rifampin 600 mg daily for nine months; children receive isoniazid 10 mg/kg (maximum 300 mg) and rifampin 15 mg/kg (maximum 600 mg) daily for nine months.

Some authorities recommend that a third drug (ethambutol, streptomycin, or pyrazinamide) be added to the regimen during the first two months of therapy. Ethambutol should be added if an isoniazid-resistant organism is suspected (contact with a recent immigrant from Africa, Asia, or South America). Other authorities recommend using four bactericidal drugs (streptomycin, isoniazid, rifampin, and pyrazinamide) until the

results of susceptibility tests are known (Dutt and Stead, 1982).

Alternatively, after four to eight weeks of daily therapy, biweekly administration of isoniazid 15 mg/kg (usually 900 mg) and rifampin 600 mg for adults or isoniazid 20 mg/kg and rifampin 15 mg/kg for children may be considered if compliance can be assured (clinic attendance, pill counts, urine tests, and/or sputum cultures). Sputums are examined every month until conversion occurs (usually within three months), and therapy is continued for at least six months after conversion. Follow-up sputum examinations are recommended for one year to assure the absence of relapse. This short-term isoniazid-rifampin regimen should be followed *only if the organisms are sensitive to both drugs*.

Although a nine-month course of isoniazid-rifampin therapy has proved quite successful, a six-month course employing these two drugs alone was inadequate (Snider et al, 1984). An intensive initial regimen utilizing four bactericidal drugs (streptomycin, isoniazid, rifampin, and pyrazinamide) for eight weeks, followed by isoniazid and rifampin for an additional four months is an acceptable alternative to the nine-month regimen provided therapy can be supervised adequately (Snider et al, 1981, 1982; Aquinas, 1982; Stead and Dutt, 1982; British Thoracic Association, 1982; Tuberculosis Research Centre, 1983).

A six-month regimen consisting of isoniazid, rifampin, ethambutol, and pyrazinamide daily for two months, followed by isoniazid and rifampin daily for four months is also effective for pulmonary tuberculosis and is an acceptable alternative regimen provided it is fully supervised (Algerian Working Group/British Medical Research Council, 1984). Following short-course chemotherapy of less than six months, unacceptably high relapse rates were reported in most studies.

Combined chemotherapy can be administered two or three times weekly with little or no loss of effect if the mean daily dose of each agent is not decreased significantly (except for rifampin, the daily dose of which is not increased when given two or three times weekly). Best results with short-course chemotherapy were achieved when intermittent therapy was preceded by daily treatment with usual doses of the same agents for one to three months.

Intermittent outpatient chemotherapy is most useful in areas with a high incidence of tuberculosis and limited facilities for treatment, as in developing countries. In the United States, intermittent administration is very useful in recalcitrant patients, alcoholics, and others who cannot adhere to a daily regimen. The drugs must be given under the close supervision of a nurse or other health professional who ascertains compliance.

Adrenal Corticosteroids: These drugs have a mixed effect in tuberculosis. Although they ameliorate the symptoms of the disease, they also inhibit cell-mediated immunity and thus may activate a latent infection (Kasik, 1979). It was thought that decreased immunity may allow dormant and semidormant bacilli to multiply and thus become more vulnerable to the bactericidal action of antituberculosis drugs. However, in one study, prednisone did not influence the speed of sputum conversion, the response to chemotherapy, or the rate of bacteriologic relapse (Tuberculosis Research Centre, 1983).

In fulminating pulmonary tuberculosis, steroids may be useful adjuncts to intensive chemotherapy. Comatose patients are given large doses of methylprednisolone sodium succinate [Solu-Medrol] or an equivalent agent until they are conscious. Therapy should begin with 80 to 120 mg daily; 30 to 40 mg is injected initially and the remainder is added to intravenous fluids. If the patient is conscious, 30 to 40 mg of an oral preparation (usually prednisone) is given daily for the first few days of treatment. Steroid therapy may be required until the disease is controlled but, to avoid complications, usually should be limited to four to six weeks.

To avoid a rebound phenomenon, the total daily dose should be decreased very gradually every three days over two to six weeks as soon as the patient shows definite signs of improvement; this usually is observed within one week after beginning treatment. Administration of a larger dose is resumed if symptoms or signs of widespread disease recur (eg, fever, anemia).

The efficacy of corticosteroids in any form of tuberculosis has never been proved in a well-controlled study; nevertheless, many uncontrolled studies have suggested their efficacy, especially in patients with meningitis, peritonitis, pericarditis, and fulminating pulmonary tuberculosis.

For preparations, see Chapter 61, Adrenal Corticosteroids in Nonendocrine Diseases.

ACTIVE DISEASE RETREATMENT. For various reasons, treatment is not always optimal and retreatment is sometimes necessary. A single new drug should not be added to the combination administered previously unless there is proof that the strains are still susceptible to these agents. Since it is usually necessary to resume treatment before new sensitivity studies are available, the regimen should be dictated by the patient's previous treatment, therapeutic response, results of earlier susceptibility studies, and need for intensive chemotherapy.

When effective combined chemotherapy is discontinued prematurely (eg, after one month), satisfactory results often can be achieved with the same regimen. If therapy is inadequate, relapses are often due to strains having the same drug sensitivity as the original isolates (Mehrotra et al, 1984; Hong Kong Chest Service/Tuberculosis Research Centre, 1984). If the patient has received a number of courses of chemotherapy or has taken drugs for several months, it is important to prescribe two new drugs that are likely to be effective as determined by the patient's record.

If resistance to isoniazid alone is suspected, some investigators recommend that streptomycin 1 g daily for five days a week and pyrazinamide 30 mg/kg daily be given in addition to isoniazid and rifampin for the first six to eight weeks of treatment or until results of susceptibility studies are available. If the organisms are susceptible to both isoniazid and rifampin, streptomycin and pyrazinamide are discontinued for the remainder of the nine-month period or six months after sputum conversion. If isoniazid resistance is documented, streptomycin, rifampin, and pyrazinamide are administered for the same period (Stead and Dutt, 1981, 1982).

For critically ill patients with a poorly documented chemotherapeutic history, rifampin, ethambutol, capreomycin, and one or two older agents least likely to have been prescribed previously (eg, ethionamide, pyrazinamide, cycloserine) should be given.

Adverse Reactions

Although most antituberculous agents are well tolerated, all have some potential toxicity (Girling, 1982). The most serious error made by physicians is failure to recognize true toxicity promptly. A more common error is failure to distinguish between drug reactions and adverse events produced by the plethora of signs and symptoms that are not related to chemotherapy. The physician who diagnoses drug toxicity erroneously may delete one drug after another from the regimen, sometimes making inappropriate substitutions. Loss of drug susceptibility and therapeutic failure may be the end result.

Hypersensitivity reactions occur most often between the third and eighth week of treatment. If a drug or group of drugs is tolerated well for at least four months, a full course of chemotherapy usually can be completed. The most common early signs and symptoms of hypersensitivity are fever, which increases over a period of several days; tachycardia; anorexia; and malaise. At this time, results of laboratory studies are usually within normal limits, but eosinophilia and other abnormalities are observed rarely. If the offending drug is discontinued promptly, the patient soon recovers. If not, the reaction becomes progressively worse and is often accompanied by cutaneous reactions, including exfoliative dermatitis; hepatitis; renal abnormalities; and, occasionally, acute blood dyscrasias. Severe reactions can be fatal.

Patients who develop hypersensitivity to one antituberculous drug may be at greater than usual risk of reacting to others. When such reactions occur, all chemotherapy should be discontinued unless the disease is life-threatening (in which case, drugs least likely to produce these reactions are continued, possibly in conjunction with corticosteroids if indicated). When the reaction has subsided, treatment should be resumed with one drug at a time, beginning with a test dose, then adding other drugs as rapidly as they can be tolerated until the patient is again receiving adequate chemotherapy. Desensitization to streptomycin and some other drugs may be successful. However, with the number of effective agents available, it is not advisable to risk continuing treatment with a drug that has caused a serious reaction (eg, hepatitis).

Many of the adverse reactions reported in the literature have been noted infrequently, sometimes only once and without verification. Also, in combined chemotherapy, toxicity ascribed to one drug may actually have been caused by another or by a drug-drug interaction. In the evaluations that follow, emphasis is placed on those adverse reactions that are well documented and occur more than rarely; however, significant rare reactions also are cited. Adverse reactions that have been reported but not verified are so designated.

Precautions

Many toxic effects of the antimycobacterial agents, particularly those related to dosage, can be avoided by taking into account the patient's age, weight, and general health. Renal status is especially important, since impaired function may lead to proportionately high serum concentrations with increased danger of toxicity.

Relatively small doses may be sufficient to produce therapeutic serum concentrations in elderly or unusually small adults. Some antimycobacterial agents are prescribed routinely on the basis of body weight and consideration should be given to this factor when prescribing all drugs, especially those administered to children.

Although most agents are metabolized in the liver, evidence of hepatic dysfunction is seldom a deterrent in selecting a regimen. Alcoholic patients tolerate the usual regimens well even when cirrhosis is present. Nevertheless, when a history of alcoholism, infectious hepatitis, jaundice, or other hepatic disease is present, it is advisable to obtain a complete profile of liver function before beginning treatment. In fact, in any new case in which the patient has not been under regular medical supervision, it is wise to obtain baseline studies of the renal, hepatic, and hematopoietic systems.

Since most or all treatment is now given on an outpatient basis, the patient should receive information on the potential toxicity of the drugs in the regimen. Patients also must be monitored at regular intervals throughout treatment; weekly interviews should be scheduled for the first month or two. Laboratory studies should be performed promptly if clinically indicated by symptoms suggestive of hepatitis.

Drug Evaluations

AMINOSALICYLIC ACID

AMINOSALICYLATE SODIUM
[Teebacin]

ACTIONS AND USES. Until ethambutol became available, aminosalicylic acid (para-aminosalicylic acid, P.A.S.) was widely used in combination chemotherapy to deter the emergence of streptomycin- and isoniazid-resistant strains of tubercle bacilli. The antimycobacterial effect of aminosalicylic acid alone is scarcely discernible. The mechanism of action is presumed to be related to its structural similarity to para-aminobenzoic acid, and therefore its selective inhibition of synthesis of this agent in *Mycobacterium tuberculosis*.

Aminosalicylic acid is now seldom included in initial treatment programs; instead it is used almost exclusively as a substitute for ethambutol in regimens for children under 2 years. (These patients cannot be tested for ocular toxicity when ethambutol is administered.) The inclusion of aminosalicylic acid in retreatment regimens may prevent bacterial resistance to more potent agents.

ADVERSE REACTIONS AND PRECAUTIONS. Patient acceptance and tolerance of aminosalicylic acid are poor in adults; children are less affected. Therapy must be discontinued in approximately 20% of patients (15% because of intolerable gastrointestinal disturbances, particularly nausea, vomiting, and diarrhea, and 4% because of hypersensitivity reactions that occasionally are very serious or even fatal). Furthermore, investigators have estimated that 20% to 50% of patients who appear to tolerate aminosalicylic acid do not take the required amount of medication consistently.

Data are insufficient to evaluate the safety of aminosalicylic acid during pregnancy or lactation.

PHARMACOKINETICS. Oral absorption is relatively rapid and complete; the volume of distribution is 0.23 L/kg. The compound is approximately 50% acetylated, and 80% of the drug and its metabolites are eliminated in the urine. Dosage adjustment is required in the presence of renal failure. The half-life is 0.5 to 1.5 hours.

DOSAGE AND PREPARATIONS. This drug is usually administered as the sodium salt. The usual total daily dose of 12 g provides approximately 1.28 g of sodium, an amount that may be contraindicated in some patients.

Oral: Adults, 150 to 200 mg/kg daily (maximum, 12 g) in two or three doses after meals. There is evidence that a single dose of 6 g may be equally effective when combined with isoniazid or other potent agents administered once daily. *Children,* 200 to 300 mg/kg daily in three or four divided doses after meals.

AMINOSALICYLIC ACID:
Generic (P.A.S., Para-Aminosalicylic Acid). Powder (bulk).
AMINOSALICYLATE SODIUM:
Generic (P.A.S. Sodium, Para-Aminosalicylate Sodium), Teebacin (CMC). Powder (bulk); tablets 500 mg and 1 g.

CAPREOMYCIN SULFATE
[Capastat Sulfate]

	R	
Capreomycin IA	OH	$C_{25}H_{44}N_{14}O_8$
Capreomycin IB	H	$C_{25}H_{44}N_{14}O_7$

ACTIONS AND USES. Capreomycin is a polypeptide antibiotic isolated from a species of *Streptomyces*. It is chemically and pharmacologically related to viomycin and has similar potential toxicity; bacterial susceptibility studies show that cross resistance between the two drugs is common.

Capreomycin has a marked suppressive effect against *Mycobacterium tuberculosis* and *M. bovis* in vitro and in vivo. Most strains of *M. kansasii* also are susceptible, but other atypical mycobacteria often are resistant. This agent usually is reserved for retreatment regimens when parenteral therapy is indicated; it is given by deep intramuscular injection.

Compared to kanamycin (an antibiotic derived from another species of *Streptomyces*), capreomycin is less toxic and has a somewhat greater bacteriostatic effect. Capreomycin approaches streptomycin in therapeutic efficacy and, since there is no cross resistance between the two, it is useful in patients with streptomycin-resistant strains of tubercle bacilli. Nevertheless, because of potential nephrotoxicity, capreomycin cannot be substituted routinely for streptomycin.

When capreomycin is used with other effective agents that are administered orally every day, its prolonged daily use is rarely necessary. After two to four weeks, it can be given two or three times a week to reduce the risk of permanent renal damage without appreciably affecting efficacy.

ADVERSE REACTIONS, PRECAUTIONS, AND INTERACTIONS. Extensive experimental and clinical studies have demonstrated that renal damage is the most consistent and significant toxic effect of capreomycin. This is manifested by elevated urea nitrogen levels, decreased creatinine clearance, albuminuria, and cylindruria. Fatal toxic nephritis was reported in one patient given both capreomycin and aminosalicylic acid for one month. However, capreomycin must be discontinued because of nephrotoxicity in fewer than 10% of patients, and renal abnormalities usually disappear with cessation of treatment. Hypokalemia is a significant but relatively uncommon side effect; blood potassium levels should be monitored.

Capreomycin is potentially toxic to the eighth cranial nerve. However, daily use for two to four months has caused vestibular toxicity only infrequently and auditory toxicity rarely.

Because of its potential toxicity for the kidneys and eighth cranial nerve, capreomycin is rarely prescribed for patients with renal disease and should not be administered with other nephrotoxic or ototoxic agents (eg, colistin, gentamicin). It is advisable to obtain pertinent baseline laboratory data before beginning treatment with capreomycin, and all patients should have a monthly clinical workup and a weekly complete blood count, urinalysis, and serum profile screening. There is no evidence that previous damage to the eighth nerve precludes treatment with capreomycin, but impaired renal function must be considered, particularly with respect to dosage and frequency of administration.

Eosinophilia often occurs during treatment and occasionally has been marked. Definite hypersensitivity reactions, manifested by fever and rash, apparently are uncommon and are not severe.

A partial neuromuscular block has been demonstrated after large intravenous doses of capreomycin. This adverse effect was enhanced by ether anesthesia and antagonized by neostigmine.

In teratogenic studies, a questionable rib abnormality was reported in rats only. Data in humans are insufficient to evaluate this drug's safety during pregnancy or lactation.

PHARMACOKINETICS. The oral bioavailability of capreomycin is negligible. Absorption after intramuscular administration is rapid and complete (one to two hours). Only an insignificant amount is metabolized, and the drug is eliminated unchanged in the urine. The elimination half-life has not been determined, but, in normal volunteers, about 50% of capreomycin was excreted in the urine in 12 hours.

DOSAGE AND PREPARATIONS. The drug should be dissolved in 2 ml of sodium chloride injection or sterile water for injection; two to three minutes should be allowed for complete dissolution.

Intramuscular (deep): Adults, 15 mg/kg (approximately 1 g) daily for two to four weeks, followed by 1 g two or three times weekly for 6 to 12 months or longer, if necessary. Most patients tolerate 1 g daily for two to four months and occasionally for as long as six months. A dose of 20 mg/kg/day should not be exceeded. Information is inadequate to establish a dosage for *children.*

Capastat Sulfate (Lilly). Powder (sterile) 1 g (equivalent to base) in 5 ml containers.

CYCLOSERINE
[Seromycin]

USES. Although cycloserine is derived from a species of *Streptomyces*, it is chemically unrelated to and therefore exhibits no cross resistance with the aminoglycosides or the peptides, capreomycin and viomycin. It is a structural analogue of D-alanine and inhibits mycobacterial cell wall synthesis. This bacteriostatic antibiotic is administered orally and has proved to be an effective antimycobacterial agent when tolerated.

Cycloserine is used primarily for retreatment of nonresponsive or noncompliant patients. Doses that provide serum concentrations higher than the minimal inhibitory concentrations in vitro must be used for retreatment; this is probably necessary for all antimycobacterial agents but is particularly important for agents used in retreatment regimens.

ADVERSE REACTIONS AND PRECAUTIONS. The limiting factor in the use of cycloserine is its central nervous system toxicity, including both neurologic and psychic disturbances. Neurologic reactions vary from muscular twitching to seizures. It has been suggested that these reactions may be prevented by administering large doses of pyridoxine concomitantly (at least 100 mg three times daily); however, this use of pyridoxine is still investigational. Epilepsy is considered a relative contraindication to use of cycloserine.

Psychic disturbances range from nervousness to frank psychotic episodes. These effects occasionally are related to excessive serum concentrations, especially if the total daily dose exceeds 500 mg, but more often they cannot be predicted or prevented. Patients with a history of mental illness often tolerate cycloserine unusually well, whereas apparently stable individuals may develop a psychotic reaction soon after initiation of treatment, sometimes before therapeutic serum levels are achieved. Psychotic episodes occur in nearly 10% of patients treated with cycloserine and require prompt cessation of treatment. These reactions are nearly always reversible within two weeks. Large doses of chlorpromazine may hasten recovery. Until the patient's condition returns to normal, he should be watched closely and security measures taken if necessary. Suicide has occurred occasionally during a drug-induced psychotic reaction.

Hypersensitivity reactions are rare. Cycloserine is contraindicated in patients with severe renal insufficiency.

Data in humans are insufficient to evaluate the safety of cycloserine during pregnancy or lactation. Safety and dosage have not been established for children.

DRUG INTERACTIONS. If possible, isoniazid or ethionamide should not be given with cycloserine because of potential additive central nervous system toxicity. Ingestion of alcohol is inadvisable while the patient is receiving cycloserine, although many alcoholics have experienced no difficulty (presumably during periods of abstinence). This drug is contraindicated in active alcoholics.

PHARMACOKINETICS. Precise bioavailability data are not available, but cycloserine appears to be completely and rapidly absorbed (time to peak effect is three to four hours). It is widely distributed throughout body fluids and tissues, including cerebrospinal fluid. One-third of an administered dose is metabolized to an unidentified substance, and the remainder is eliminated unchanged in the urine. Because the drug is highly concentrated in the urine, large doses are not required in urinary tract tuberculosis. The half-life is approximately 8 to 12 hours.

DOSAGE AND PREPARATIONS.
Oral: Initially, 250 mg twice daily at 12-hour intervals for the first two weeks. The dose may be increased by 250 mg every few days (if tolerated) until therapeutic serum levels are obtained. The usual dosage is 500 mg to a maximum of 1 g daily in divided doses. It may be possible to administer a smaller total dose once a day without loss of therapeutic effect when cycloserine is used with other agents that are also prescribed once a day. Blood levels should be monitored during therapy. Best results occur with trough serum concentrations of 25 to 30 mcg/ml. Serum levels in excess of 30 mcg/ml have been associated with toxicity and should be avoided. Blood used to determine serum drug concentrations should be drawn before the patient's first dose of the day.
   Seromycin (Lilly). Capsules 250 mg.

ETHAMBUTOL HYDROCHLORIDE
   [Myambutol]

$$CH_3CH_2 \overset{\overset{\displaystyle CH_2OH}{|}}{\underset{\underset{\displaystyle H}{|}}{C}} \overset{+}{NH_2}CH_2CH_2\overset{+}{NH_2} \overset{\overset{\displaystyle H}{|}}{\underset{\underset{\displaystyle CH_2OH}{|}}{C}} CH_2CH_3 \quad 2Cl^-$$

SPECTRUM AND ACTIONS. *Mycobacterium tuberculosis*, *M. bovis*, and most strains of *M. kansasii* are highly susceptible to ethambutol, and some nonphotochromogens (mycobacterial group III organisms) are susceptible to this drug in vitro.

Ethambutol inhibits the synthesis of cell metabolites, which inhibits cell metabolism and results in cell death. It is effective only against actively growing bacilli.

USES. This synthetic bacteriostatic compound is an orally administered adjunct to the bactericidal antimycobacterial agents, isoniazid and rifampin, in conventional tuberculous chemotherapy programs. It occasionally is used initially in short-course chemotherapy to preclude monotherapy when resistance to isoniazid or rifampin is suspected. Because of its relative lack of toxicity and good patient acceptance, ethambutol has supplanted aminosalicylic acid in chemotherapeutic regimens. In retreatment and cases of primary resistance, ethambutol is of great value when combined with other effective antimycobacterial agents.

ADVERSE REACTIONS AND PRECAUTIONS. The only significant adverse effect produced by ethambutol is dose-related ocular toxicity; with initial doses of 25 mg/kg daily for two months followed by 15 mg/kg daily, the incidence is 0.8%. The visual changes generally are reversible over a period of weeks or months but, rarely, recovery is delayed for one year or more or the effects are irreversible. Eye involvement is bilateral and consistent with retrobulbar neuritis (decreased visual acuity, loss of color discrimination, constriction of visual fields, and central and peripheral scotomata). Currently recommended doses produce ocular toxicity only rarely in patients with normal renal function. The drug should be used cautiously in patients with impaired renal function.

Regular ophthalmologic examinations are not necessary during treatment, but the patient should report any visual changes promptly and should be questioned about vision during each regularly scheduled visit. Symptoms often precede objective evidence of toxicity. If a patient complains of blurring or fading of vision, a complete ophthalmologic examination should be performed at once. Ethambutol should be discontinued immediately if symptoms persist or visual acuity decreases significantly.

A complete ophthalmologic examination is mandatory to establish a baseline before beginning treatment with ethambutol if the patient has cataracts or other ocular abnormalities that make changes in vision difficult to detect or evaluate. Pretreatment examinations are not indicated routinely, however, in patients with normal vision or simple errors of refraction corrected by glasses.

The incidence of hypersensitivity to ethambutol is very low (about 0.1%) and reactions tend to be mild.

Patients treated with ethambutol have included many pregnant women, most of whom were already receiving chemotherapy before conception. No teratogenic effects definitely attributable to ethambutol have been reported. Data in humans are insufficient to evaluate the safety of this drug during lactation.

No toxic effects have been observed in children receiving therapeutic doses of ethambutol, but, because of the difficulty of determining visual acuity in small children and because aminosalicylic acid is relatively well tolerated in this age group, few children have been treated with ethambutol. However, in severe disease, particularly disseminated tuberculosis caused by highly resistant strains of bacilli, young children have received ethambutol for up to five years without evidence of toxicity.

PHARMACOKINETICS. Ethambutol is absorbed rapidly from the gastrointestinal tract (time to peak effect, two to four hours; bioavailability, 77% $\pm$ 8%). Volume of distribution is 1.6 $\pm$ 2 L/kg. Protein binding is about 40%. Ethambutol is excreted mainly by the kidneys; only 10% is converted to inactive metabolites. Clearance is 8.6 $\pm$ 0.8 ml/min/kg, and the elimination half-life is 3.1 $\pm$ 0.4 hours. Ethambutol does not penetrate intact meninges but can be detected in presumably therapeutic concentrations in the cerebrospinal fluid of patients with tuberculous meningitis.

DOSAGE AND PREPARATIONS. Because no practicable method of determining serum concentrations exists, ethambutol must be prescribed on the basis of body weight. The dose must be calculated carefully and adjusted if there are appreciable changes in the patient's weight. However, in the interest of compliance, doses should be rounded off to the nearest whole tablet.

Oral: 15 to 25 mg/kg given in one dose each day. In one suggested regimen, 15 mg/kg is given throughout treatment. In another, 25 mg/kg is administered for two months, followed by 15 mg/kg thereafter for the duration of therapy. These amounts are both safe and effective in patients with normal renal function. When ethambutol is given in a multiple-drug regimen twice a week, the usual single dose is 50 mg/kg.

Myambutol (Lederle). Tablets 100 and 400 mg.

ETHIONAMIDE
[Trecator-SC]

ACTIONS AND USES. This bacteriostatic drug is the thioamide of isonicotinic acid and is related chemically to isoniazid. Ethionamide is about one-tenth as active as isoniazid. Like the latter drug, it is widely distributed in the body, including the cerebrospinal fluid. It is effective against human and bovine strains of mycobacteria and against *M. kansasii*.

The usefulness of ethionamide in tuberculosis is limited because many patients cannot tolerate therapeutic doses. In approximately one-third of patients, ethionamide must be discontinued or the dose reduced. Most patients tolerate one-half to two-thirds of the usual total daily dose, but the therapeutic efficacy of these amounts is uncertain, particularly since ethionamide is used in retreatment regimens, often in combination with drugs having marginal antimycobacterial activity.

ADVERSE REACTIONS AND PRECAUTIONS. Ethionamide almost invariably causes gastrointestinal disturbances, most frequently anorexia, nausea, and vomiting. These effects are thought to be caused by its central nervous system actions rather than direct gastric irritation. Their severity may limit the total dosage to 250 mg twice daily in 50% of patients.

Ethionamide is potentially toxic to the liver. Abnormal results of liver function studies are noted in 9% of patients, and jaundice occurs in 1% to 3%. However, recovery is usually rapid when ethionamide is discontinued.

Hypersensitivity reactions are infrequent. Like isoniazid, ethionamide may cause peripheral neuritis, particularly in susceptible patients. Mental depression and hypothyroidism have occasionally been attributed to treatment with this agent. Gynecomastia, impotence, and purpura have been reported rarely.

Seizures associated with cycloserine therapy may be aggravated by the concomitant use of ethionamide.

Teratogenic effects were produced in animals given doses higher than those used in man. Data in humans are insufficient to evaluate the safety of ethionamide during pregnancy or lactation.

PHARMACOKINETICS. Ethionamide is presumably well absorbed orally (time to peak effect is about three hours) and is widely distributed (including cerebrospinal fluid). It is almost entirely metabolized. The half-life has not been determined, but therapeutic concentrations are obtained on a 12-hour dosing schedule.

DOSAGE AND PREPARATIONS.

Oral: 0.5 to 1 g daily in one to three doses after meals. Variations in dose and timing of administration may be tried. Some patients tolerate the drug best when a single dose is given at bedtime, whereas others prefer a single dose after the evening meal. When the total amount can be tolerated in one dose, serum concentrations are higher and a therapeutic effect is more likely than when small doses are administered two or three times a day.

Trecator-SC (Wyeth). Tablets 250 mg.

ISONIAZID
[Dow-Isoniazid, Nydrazid]

ACTIONS AND USES. Isoniazid is bactericidal for both extracellular and intracellular bacteria and may act by interfering with cell wall mycolic acid biosynthesis. This synthetic compound probably remains the best single antimycobacterial agent with respect to efficacy, toxicity, cost, ease of administration, and patient acceptance. It may be administered alone for prophylaxis but is used in combination regimens for chemotherapy of disease.

ADVERSE REACTIONS AND PRECAUTIONS. The metabolism of isoniazid is characterized by increased excretion of pyridoxine, which may result in peripheral neuritis, particularly when large doses are prescribed. The incidence is about 10% when 8 to 10 mg/kg of isoniazid is given. Peripheral neuritis occasionally produces bizarre symptoms and, therefore, may not be recognized promptly. In adults, it may be treated with pyridoxine 50 to 100 mg orally; in severe cases, parenteral administration may be more effective. Since peripheral neuritis is not always completely reversible, some clinicians administer pyridoxine 15 to 50 mg daily routinely to patients receiving usual doses of isoniazid, especially those with diabetes mellitus, alcoholism, or malnutrition. Those receiving larger doses or individuals with pre-existing symptoms of peripheral neuritis should receive 100 to 300 mg of pyridoxine daily. Isoniazid-induced peripheral neuritis is rare in children; some authorities do not feel that the routine use of pyridoxine is justified in this age group.

Convulsions have occurred in less than 1% of patients treated with isoniazid, and this drug has been administered without difficulty to many individuals being treated for convulsive disorders. Since the action of phenytoin may be potentiated by isoniazid, particularly in slow isoniazid acetylators, the blood level of phenytoin should be monitored when the two drugs are given simultaneously and the dose of the anticonvulsant reduced if indicated.

Reversible psychotic episodes may be precipitated in a small percentage of patients treated with very large doses of isoniazid. Arthralgia or arthritis has been noted infrequently.

Optic neuropathy has been reported rarely, but a causal relationship has not been established. This is true of many other abnormalities listed in the labeling of isoniazid preparations. It is probable that some of the reactions reported, including vasculitis with antinuclear antibodies, may be manifestations of a hypersensitivity reaction simulating systemic lupus erythematosus.

Isoniazid can cause hepatic inflammation and necrosis that probably are not hypersensitivity reactions. The incidence of hepatitis increases with age; it is uncommon in individuals less than 35 years, increases to about 1% between the ages of 35 and 49, and may be almost 2.5% after age 50. The daily consumption of alcohol may increase the risk of isoniazid-related hepatitis.

Patients should be monitored periodically for signs or symptoms of hepatitis or other significant adverse reactions. It is well known that serum transaminase levels are elevated during the first few months of treatment in at least 10% of patients, and more specific evidence of liver dysfunction sometimes is noted. All values usually return to normal and are not an indication for discontinuing treatment without clinical evidence of hepatitis. However, some clinicians routinely monitor serum transaminase levels and discontinue isoniazid therapy when the transaminase levels exceed three times normal.

In reproductive studies on mammals, no isoniazid-related congenital anomalies were observed. The concentration of isoniazid in breast milk is 20% or slightly more than that in the maternal serum; therefore, both mother and infant should receive supplemental pyridoxine. The infant also should be monitored periodically for signs and symptoms of hepatotoxicity.

PHARMACOKINETICS. For maximum therapeutic effect and convenience, isoniazid should be administered orally. It can be given parenterally (using oral dosage levels) if oral administration is not practical. In critical cases, both routes may be used until clinical improvement occurs. The bioavailability of isoniazid is generally reported to be 90%; however, a significant first-pass effect may be present. Time to peak effect is one to two hours, and volume of distribution is 0.16 ± 0.11 L/kg. Protein binding is clinically insignificant.

Isoniazid is almost completely metabolized by enzymatic acetylation and hydroxylation. Because of genetic heterogeneity, about one-half of the population in the United States acetylate isoniazid rapidly (mean half-life, 1.1 ± 0.2 hours; clearance, 7 ml/min/kg) and the other half acetylate this drug slowly (mean half-life, 3 ± 0.8 hours; clearance, 2.5 ml/min/kg). This wide range of plasma concentrations has little relevance to either efficacy or safety, although toxic concentrations accumulate more rapidly in slow acetylators with impaired renal function.

DOSAGE AND PREPARATIONS.
Oral, Intramuscular: Adults, for chemoprophylaxis, 4 to 5 mg/kg daily or 300 mg daily is given orally in a single dose. For chemotherapy, this dose is given with other antimycobacterial agents. For disseminated tuberculosis (particularly tuberculous meningitis) and pulmonary disease caused by atypical mycobacteria, 10 to 20 mg/kg daily. In critical cases, 300 mg daily may be given parenterally when oral administration is not possible. When chemotherapy is given twice a week, isoniazid is often prescribed in a dose of 15 mg/kg (usually, 900 mg).

Infants and children, for active tuberculosis, 10 to 20 mg/kg daily, depending on severity of infection, in one or more doses; for preventive therapy, 10 mg/kg daily (maximum, 300 mg daily) in one dose.
Generic. Powder (bulk); tablets 50, 100, and 300 mg.
Dow-Isoniazid (Merrell Dow). Tablets 300 mg.
Nydrazid (Squibb). Tablets 100 mg; solution (for injection) 100 mg/ml in 10 ml containers.
The following dual pack containing isoniazid and rifampin may be convenient if patients are taking both drugs.
Rimactane/INH (CIBA). Dual pack containing 30 isoniazid 300-mg tablets and 60 rifampin 300-mg capsules.
Rifamate (Merrell Dow). Capsules containing isoniazid 150 mg and rifampin 300 mg.

PYRAZINAMIDE

ACTIONS AND USES. Pyrazinamide, an analogue of nicotinamide, is not water soluble and exhibits antimycobacterial activity in vitro only in an acid medium, which makes susceptibility studies very difficult. Sophisticated studies of host metabolism have not explained pyrazinamide's mode of action. This drug is bactericidal, especially for intracellular tubercle bacilli; this may explain its efficacy in murine tuberculosis, which is primarily an intracellular disease. When pyrazinamide is administered with other agents, it may contribute to the total antimycobacterial effect.

Pyrazinamide was once considered a second-line agent, and had been used in the United States primarily for retreatment and only when the disease was a greater threat than the drug's potential toxicity. However, it may have value in short-course primary regimens when resistance to isoniazid is suspected (Fox, 1979; Stead and Dutt, 1981, 1982). Thus, some clinicians administer pyrazinamide with isoniazid and rifampin until results of susceptibility studies are available to avoid monotherapy and/or parenteral therapy (see the Introduction).

ADVERSE REACTIONS AND PRECAUTIONS. Pyrazinamide can cause hepatotoxicity, which apparently is dose related. A dose of 3 g daily is effective adjunctively when given with isoniazid in the initial treatment of tuberculosis, but the incidence of hepatotoxicity in this regimen is approximately 14% and deaths have occurred rarely from acute yellow atrophy of the liver. Liver damage from pyrazinamide is rarely serious, however, and currently used doses (approximately 30 mg/kg/day) cause hepatotoxicity much less commonly, especially when pyrazinamide is discontinued after two months. Pretreatment laboratory studies should include a complete liver function profile. Measurements of serum transaminases are usually recommended every two to four weeks throughout treatment.

Pyrazinamide almost routinely causes hyperuricemia, which is usually asymptomatic; serum uric acid levels of 12 to 14 mg/dl are not uncommon. If symptoms of gout develop and continued treatment with pyrazinamide is necessary, the patient may be given a uricosuric agent (eg, allopurinol, probenecid). A complete blood count, urinalysis, and serum profile screening should be performed monthly.

Data in humans are insufficient to evaluate the safety of pyrazinamide during pregnancy or lactation.

PHARMACOKINETICS. Pyrazinamide is well absorbed orally (time to peak effect is about two hours) and is widely distributed. It is hydrolyzed and hydroxylated to the major excretory product, 5-hydroxyprazinoic acid, which is eliminated principally by glomerular filtration. The elimination half-life is 10 to 16 hours.

DOSAGE AND PREPARATIONS.
Oral: *Adults,* 20 to 35 mg/kg daily in one or more doses (maximum, 3 g daily); *children,* information is inadequate to establish dosage.
   Pyrazinamide (Lederle). Tablets 500 mg.

RIFAMPIN
[Rifadin, Rimactane]

SPECTRUM, ACTIONS, AND USES. This semisynthetic antibiotic represents the greatest contribution to the chemotherapy of tuberculosis since the introduction of isoniazid, but a drawback is its cost. In vitro and in vivo, rifampin has a marked bactericidal effect against extracellular and intracellular *Mycobacterium tuberculosis,* *M. bovis,* and nearly all strains of *M. kansasii.* Some strains of scotochromogens (mycobacterial group II) and a few strains of nonphotochromogens (mycobacterial group III) are inhibited by low concentrations of the drug. Rifampin is most active during cell multiplication, but it also appears to have some effect on resting cells. Electron microscopy has revealed changes in the cytoplasm and disappearance of ribosomes in tubercle bacilli exposed to rifampin, which are probably due to inhibition of the B subunit of DNA-dependent RNA polymerase. Mycobacterial resistance to rifampin can be reduced markedly by combination therapy with isoniazid, ethambutol, streptomycin, or other effective antimycobacterial agents administered in therapeutic doses; thus, it is always administered with one or more of these drugs in active treatment or retreatment regimens.

Rifampin alone is used investigationally for preventive therapy as an alternative to isoniazid in patients who cannot tolerate the latter drug (see the Introduction). Rifampin also is effective in the treatment of leprosy (see the section on Leprosy).

ADVERSE REACTIONS AND PRECAUTIONS. Most patients tolerate and accept rifampin well. Abdominal distress, aching in muscles and joints, and cramping in the legs occur occasionally, especially during the first few weeks of treatment. During this period, asymptomatic jaundice is noted rarely but usually subsides without interruption of therapy. The subsidence may be caused by the increased biliary excretion of rifampin due to enzyme induction that occurs during the first few weeks of use, which reduces the half-life by about 40%. Jaundice with laboratory evidence of obstructive liver dysfunction may develop and may be alleviated by reducing the dose of rifampin but, if symptoms and signs of hepatitis also occur, therapy should be discontinued. Since both rifampin and bile are excreted by hepatic cells, jaundice may be caused by the competitive displacement of bilirubin, which then enters the blood, chiefly in conjugated form. This is most likely to occur when liver function is impaired or when rifampin is combined with isoniazid and other potentially hepatotoxic agents.

The incidence of liver dysfunction, as determined by elevated serum transaminase levels and other abnormalities, varies from 4% to 35%. In a USPHS cooperative study, marked elevation of SGPT (more than 100 units/ml) occurred in 4.2% of patients treated with rifampin in combination with isoniazid or isoniazid and ethambutol, but jaundice was not observed in any patient. When rifampin is administered to patients with impaired liver function, they should be kept under close medical supervision; serum enzyme levels should be monitored in alcoholics and those with pre-existing liver disease for at least the first two or three months of treatment.

Pruritus with or without rash has been noted in less than 3% of patients. Rifampin and its metabolites impart a reddish orange color to urine, feces, saliva, sweat, and tears; there also is at least one report (Lyons, 1979) of discoloration of soft contact lenses in patients taking rifampin. Patients should be informed of these problems to prevent anxiety.

Intermittent treatment with rifampin and other agents has been employed for years without significant toxicity. However, a serious reaction, assumed to be immunologic in nature, has occurred in about 1% of patients who received large doses (900 to 1,200 mg) intermittently or in whom treatment was resumed after a lapse of days or weeks. The mechanism is unknown, but rifampin-dependent antibodies have been demonstrated in the serum of some patients. The reaction is characterized by a severe flu-like syndrome with dyspnea, sometimes accompanied by wheezing; purpura associated with thrombocytopenia; leukopenia; and, occasionally, a state similar to true anaphylaxis. Rarely, hemolysis, hemoglobinuria, hematuria, and renal insufficiency also occurred. Treatment with rifampin had to be discontinued in only 3% of the patients, and most were able to tolerate the drug when the dose was reduced or when daily treatment was substituted for intermittent therapy.

One well-documented case of myopathy induced by rifampin has been reported (Jenkins and Emerson, 1981).

Teratogenic effects have not been reported in man, even after inadvertent administration during the first trimester of pregnancy. However, data in humans are still insufficient to conclude that rifampin is safe for use during pregnancy or lactation.

DRUG INTERACTIONS. Rifampin has immunosuppressive properties that have no clinical significance in the treatment of tuberculosis but presumably could interfere with certain immunization procedures or immunosuppressive therapy. It has been reported that rifampin interferes with the effectiveness of digitoxin, oral contraceptives, corticosteroids, sulfonylureas, quinidine (Twum-Barina and Carruthers, 1981), oral hypoglycemics, ketoconazole, dapsone, disopyramide, warfarin, and methadone through the induction of hepatic cytochrome P-450 enzymes and alterations in absorption and hepatic uptake (Baciewicz and Self, 1984). Therefore, adjustments in dosages of these agents may be indicated. The bentonite excipients in some aminosalicylic acid preparations may interfere with the oral absorption of rifampin.

PHARMACOKINETICS. Although the oral bioavailability of rifampin is reported to be 90% to 95%, repeated administration causes enzyme induction that increases the clearance of plasma rifampin and increases biliary excretion of the major metabolite, 2,5-o-desacetyl-rifampicin. Food interferes with the rate and extent of absorption. Rifampin diffuses freely into body tissues and fluids, including cerebrospinal fluid. The drug also crosses the placenta. Currently recommended doses produce peak serum levels in one to two hours; levels above the minimal inhibitory concentration persist for at least six hours. The volume of distribution is 1.6 ± 0.2 L/kg.

Rifampin is metabolized by the liver and is excreted mainly in the bile, although as much as one-third of a dose is eliminated in the urine as parent drug (50%) and active metabolites; therefore, therapeutic concentrations appear in the urine.

The half-life of the parent molecule is 1.5 to 5 hours, and the major metabolite is active. Initially, the mean half-life is 2.3 to 5.1 hours but decreases after repeated administration over a two-week period to approximately two hours because of enzyme induction (Kenny and Strates, 1981).

DOSAGE AND PREPARATIONS.

Oral: *Adults,* 600 mg or 10 to 20 mg/kg daily; *children,* 10 to 20 mg/kg (maximum, 600 mg daily). The drug should be given in a single dose one hour before a meal (usually breakfast) or two hours afterward.

Rifadin (Merrell Dow). Capsules 150 and 300 mg.

Rimactane (CIBA). Capsules 300 mg.

The following dual pack containing isoniazid and rifampin may be convenient if patients are taking both drugs.

Rimactane/INH (CIBA). Dual pack containing 30 isoniazid 300-mg tablets and 60 rifampin 300-mg capsules.

Rifamate (Merrell Dow). Capsules containing isoniazid 150 mg and rifampin 300 mg.

Intravenous: A formulation of rifampin for intravenous use is currently under study. *Adults,* 300 mg twice daily has been employed for tuberculosis (Nilsson and Boman, 1981). Pharmacokinetic studies show that serum concentrations after intravenous administration (150 to 600 mg) were similar to those obtained after oral administration of the same dose.

(Investigational route)

STREPTOMYCIN SULFATE

ACTIONS AND USES. Streptomycin was the first chemotherapeutic agent of undeniable efficacy in the treatment of tuberculosis. It must be administered intramuscularly, which limits its usefulness in long-term therapy. Streptomycin is the most effective and least toxic of the parenterally administered antibiotics derived from *Streptomyces.* It is bactericidal, principally for extracellular (including cavitary) tubercle bacilli, probably through a direct action on the bacterial ribosome to inhibit protein synthesis.

The combination of intramuscular streptomycin and isoniazid, the only other highly effective agent approved for parenteral use, has an immediate, marked, suppressive effect on susceptible organisms and often has been lifesaving in critical situations.

Streptomycin is of greatest value in the early weeks or months of therapy. Possibly because it is administered parenterally and high serum concentrations are produced rapidly, this drug appears to enhance the effect of agents administered orally, even such effective agents as ethambutol and isoniazid.

Parenteral administration of streptomycin is valuable when oral medication is contraindicated or when gastrointestinal absorption is impaired. In some cases, it may be advisable to give streptomycin on an outpatient basis twice a week in combination with two oral agents prescribed daily. Streptomycin also is useful in intermittent therapy, and it is one of the few agents that is effective against nonphotochromogens (mycobacterial group III organisms) in vitro.

ADVERSE REACTIONS AND PRECAUTIONS. Most individuals tolerate streptomycin well. Occasionally, transient headache or malaise occurs soon after injection. Clinically unimportant facial paresthesia, particularly around the mouth, is noted in approximately 15% of patients and may be accompanied by a tingling sensation in the hands.

When administered correctly, streptomycin is rarely toxic. Hypersensitivity reactions occur occasionally during the early weeks of treatment but are less common than with aminosalicylic acid and usually are less serious than with aminosalicylic acid or isoniazid. Although streptomycin is related to a family of potentially nephrotoxic drugs, it has been given daily for up to six months with little or no evidence of renal toxicity.

Streptomycin has a selective neurotoxic effect upon the eighth cranial nerve when large doses are administered for long periods (see Chapter 70, Aminoglycosides), and some patients receiving a total dose of 10 to 12 g may develop eighth nerve damage; usually, however, damage to the eighth nerve occurs only rarely when this agent is prescribed correctly. If usual adult doses are administered daily to young children for two months or more, permanent loss of labyrinthine function is almost a certainty. Advanced age and renal impairment predispose to ototoxicity. Baseline and periodic audiograms and caloric tests of vestibular function are recommended, especially with prolonged therapy.

A few reports of anaphylactic and hematopoietic reactions, including eosinophilia, agranulocytosis, and aplastic anemia, have appeared in the literature.

Teratogenicity has not been documented; however, the drug should not be administered during the first trimester of pregnancy or in total doses exceeding 20 g during the last half of pregnancy to minimize the possibility of congenital deafness.

Minimal amounts of streptomycin pass into breast milk when therapeutic serum levels are achieved in the mother.

DRUG INTERACTIONS. Like other aminoglycosides, streptomycin may interact with neuromuscular blocking drugs to intensify neuromuscular blockade and with other ototoxic (eg, ethacrynic acid, furosemide) or nephrotoxic (eg, cephalosporins, polymyxin) drugs.

PHARMACOKINETICS. Oral bioavailability of streptomycin is less than 1%. The drug is rapidly (time to peak effect is 30 to 90 minutes) and well absorbed after intramuscular injection. There is inadequate penetration into cells, including the tubercle bacillus, and into cerebrospinal fluid, even when the meninges are inflamed. Volume of distribution is 0.25 L/kg. Metabolism is negligible, and the drug is almost entirely eliminated by glomerular filtration. The rate of clearance approximates two-thirds of the simultaneous creatinine clearance. The elimination half-life is two to three hours; however, a deep compartment may release tissue-bound streptomycin slowly over many days.

DOSAGE AND PREPARATIONS.
(Doses and strengths expressed in terms of the base)
Intramuscular: *Adults,* 20 mg/kg (maximum, rarely more than 1 g) once a day for two to three weeks. Thereafter, the frequency of administration usually can be decreased to 1 g every other day or three times weekly and then to 1 g twice a week; patients with normal renal function tolerate this regimen well for months. Alternatively, streptomycin has been given in a dose of 25 to 30 mg/kg when chemotherapy is given twice weekly. The dose should be reduced in elderly patients, children, small adults, and individuals with impaired renal function.

> **Generic.** Powder 1 and 5 g; solution 400 mg/ml in 2.5 and 12.5 ml containers and 500 mg/ml in 10 ml containers.

Mixture

To achieve maximum therapeutic efficacy and minimal toxicity, it is essential to consider such factors as age, body weight, and renal function in prescribing each agent in a chemotherapeutic regimen. Patient compliance is also essential to successful therapy of tuberculosis. When the following fixed combination of isoniazid and rifampin meets the criteria of maximum therapeutic efficacy and minimal toxicity, compliance may be enhanced (*Morbid Mortal Week Rep,* 1980; Moulding, 1980).

> **Rifamate** (Merrell Dow). Capsules containing isoniazid 150 mg and rifampin 300 mg.

ATYPICAL MYCOBACTERIAL INFECTIONS

Mycobacteria other than *M. tuberculosis* may cause disease in humans. On culture, these bacteria form colonies that are not typical of *M. tuberculosis*, hence the term "atypical mycobacteria." Runyon (1965) classified atypical mycobacteria into four large groups on the basis of pigment production or rapid growth in culture.

Atypical mycobacteria vary in their susceptibility to drugs; some are completely susceptible and others are markedly resistant. Some strains of *M. kansasii* may be as susceptible to chemotherapy as *M. tuberculosis*, whereas others are resistant.

M. kansasii is the most important pathogen of Runyon's Group I (photochromogens) and is often associated with pulmonary disease. It is usually susceptible in vitro to commonly used antituberculous drugs. A current recommendation for therapy is a combination of isoniazid, rifampin, and ethambutol for approximately two years with negative cultures for six months recommended prior to discontinuance of therapy (Bass and Hawkins, 1983). However, a 12-month course of treatment employing a regimen of rifampin, isoniazid, and streptomycin was reported to be sufficient for initial treatment of pulmonary disease (Ahn et al, 1983).

In difficult cases, five or six agents may be administered simultaneously, including those having less potency and greater potential toxicity than the primary antimycobacterial drugs. Surgical resection in conjunction with chemotherapy may be necessary in selected patients.

The only member of Group II (scotochromogens) of clinical significance is *M. scrofulaceum*, so named because it may cause cervical lymphadenitis in children. Chemotherapy is of little benefit in this condition, and surgical excision is the recommended treatment.

The only other group of atypical mycobacteria causing pulmonary disease with any frequency is the nonphotochromogens (mycobacterial Group III organisms), including *M. avium-intracellulare* complex. The latter causes lung disease most commonly in individuals with pre-existing pulmonary conditions. Extrapulmonary disease is uncommon except in immunocompromised hosts. It is often encountered in patients with the acquired immunodeficiency syndrome (AIDS). Unfortunately, many strains are resistant to most antituberculous drugs. Nevertheless, individualized multiple-drug regimens chosen on the basis of susceptibility tests are effective in 35% to 75% of patients.

No particular drug regimen can be recommended for the treatment of *M. avium-intracellulare* infections in AIDS patients, although in one study utilizing ansamycin, an investigational derivative of rifampin, and clofazimine [Lamprene], an investigational agent used in leprosy, results were promising (Murray et al, 1984). In nonimmunocompromised patients, the disease is limited anatomically and surgical resection may provide the best chance of cure.

Members of Group IV, including *M. fortuitum*, are highly resistant to all available antimycobacterial drugs. Fortunately, the organisms are ubiquitous saprophytes that rarely cause disease; however, both pulmonary and extrapulmonary disease have been reported. Treatment with large doses of broad spectrum antibiotics having in vitro activity against these organisms (erythromycin, doxycycline, amikacin, sulfamethizole) has appeared to be helpful in isolated cases.

LEPROSY

Incidence: It has been estimated that 12 million people worldwide have leprosy (Hansen's disease). The majority of these cases are in India, China, and Africa; India alone has about 3.2 million registered cases. There are approximately 4,000 cases in the United States; New York, California, Hawaii, Florida, Louisiana, and Texas have the largest number. Endemic foci exist in Texas, Louisiana, and Hawaii. The increased incidence of leprosy in this country appears to be attributable entirely to immigrants, particularly those from Mexico, the Philippines, and Southeast Asia. Fifty-two percent of all cases occur in individuals 20 to 40 years; in the United States, 40% of patients are Hispanic.

Provided that the disease is under therapeutic control, leprosy is no longer a reason to deny an immigrant entry into the United States. Therefore, although the possibility is still remote, the likelihood of a physician encountering a patient with leprosy is greater today than ever before because of the ease of intercontinental travel, the fact that servicemen have been stationed in countries where leprosy is endemic, and the steady influx of immigrants from endemic areas.

There is little reason to fear that leprosy will spread throughout the United States because patient infectivity drops off markedly with chemotherapy. In recent years, no spread attributable to imported cases has been reported.

Although other possibilities exist, the most widely held view is that leprosy is spread by bacilli from the upper respiratory tract of infected persons that enter through the respiratory tract of susceptible individuals. The chief source of infection is the untreated or poorly treated patient with multibacillary disease. The infectivity rate does not appear to be high, and it is believed that the incubation period varies from three to ten years. The clinical attack rate in close family contacts of multibacillary cases is 5% to 10%. Hospitalization is unnecessary and, since therapy rapidly renders the patient noninfectious, isolation is not required.

Types: There are two major polar types of leprosy: tuberculoid and lepromatous. Intermediate between the two is the borderline or dimorphous type. Indeterminate leprosy is an early form manifested by a hypopigmented macule. Without treatment, the condition may progress to tuberculoid or lepromatous leprosy. Worldwide, tuberculoid leprosy is the most common form; however, in the United States, 67% of cases reported in 1981 were of the lepromatous type.

The different forms of leprosy are thought to be due to differences in cell-mediated immunity to *M. leprae*. The relative degree of host resistance to *M. leprae* is greatest in tuberculoid and most indeterminate forms; in the lepromatous type, resistance is severely compromised.

The different clinical forms of leprosy have been classified into five different groups (Ridley and Jopling, 1966) by subdividing the borderline type into three subgroups: borderline-tuberculoid (BT), borderline-lepromatous (BL), and mid-borderline (BB) between the two. The characteristics of these forms are shown in Table 3.

Paucibacillary leprosy includes the indeterminate, tuberculoid (TT), and borderline-tuberculoid (BT) groups; multibacillary leprosy includes the lepromatous (LL), borderline-lepromatous (BL), and mid-borderline (BB) groups. This classification of leprosy is very useful for prognosis and for determining therapy and duration of treatment.

Drug Selection

Generally, leprosy is best managed by specialists who, in the United States, are usually associated with the National Hansen's Disease Center (NHDC) at Carville, Louisiana, or with various outpatient clinics associated with NHDC located in states where the disease is most prevalent. Indeed, the resources of these facilities are usually required to establish a diagnosis.

Biopsies will be examined, at no cost, at the National Hansen's Disease Center. The biopsy should be taken entirely from within the lesion and preserved in neutral formalin. Once the diagnosis has been established, the attending physician must report the case to the state health department whether he decides to treat the patient himself or refers the patient to NHDC facilities.

Current recommendations for the treatment of leprosy may be obtained the NHDC at Carville, Louisiana ([504] 642-7771). This institution and its clinics provide free care to any leprosy patient irrespective of nationality or citizenship. Outpatient

TABLE 3.
A CLINICAL CLASSIFICATION OF HANSEN'S DISEASE BASED ON THE RIDLEY-JOPLING CLASSIFICATION

Observation or Test	Type of HD			
	TT	BT	BB-BL	LL
Number of skin lesions	Single usually	Single or few	Several or many	Very many
Size of lesions	Variable	Variable	Variable	Small
Surface of lesions	Very dry, sometimes scaly	Dry	Shiny	Shiny
Hair growth in lesions	Absent	Moderately diminished	Slightly diminished	Not affected
Sensation in lesions (not face)	Completely lost	Moderate-marked loss	Slight-moderate loss	No loss
AFB in smears	Nil	Nil or scanty	Several-many	Very many
AFB in nasal scrapings or in nose-blows	Nil	Nil	Nil (scanty rarely)	Very many
Lepromin test	Strongly positive (+++)	Weakly positive (+ or ++)	Negative	Negative

From Jopling WH: Clinical classification of Hansen's disease. The Star, Carville, Louisiana, May-June 1983. Reprinted with permission.

AFB = acid-fast bacilli
TT = tuberculoid
BT = borderline-tuberculoid
BB-BL = mid-borderline and borderline-lepromatous
LL = lepromatous

leprosy clinics are located in Los Angeles, San Francisco, San Diego, Seattle, Boston, Staten Island, Miami, New Orleans, and Chicago.

Regimens: Chemotherapy is the mainstay in the treatment of leprosy. The broad objectives of chemotherapy are (1) to render the patient noninfectious; (2) to prevent further bacterial multiplication; and (3) to avoid or treat reactions.

Treatment of leprosy with sulfones was introduced in 1943. For many years, monotherapy with dapsone was the treatment of choice; in the early years, small initial doses were given and the amount was increased gradually to maintenance levels. In subsequent years, full dosage levels were used throughout treatment. The widespread use of dapsone has resulted in the emergence of resistant *M. leprae*. Primary and secondary resistance to dapsone has been increasing since it was first reported in 1964. In some countries, primary resistance has been reported to be as high as 40%. In the United States, the problem of primary resistance is not as great as that of secondary resistance. At the NHDC in Carville, Louisiana, secondary resistance has been as high as 10%.

An additional problem in leprosy chemotherapy has been the presence of "persisters." These viable, fully drug-susceptible *M. leprae* are able to survive for many years in the patient, despite the presence of bactericidal concentrations of an antileprosy drug. These persisters are dormant bacilli that escape the action of antileprosy drugs, and they may cause relapses after the cessation of chemotherapy. No single drug eliminates these persisting organisms.

The persistence of *M. leprae* and the development of primary and secondary resistance to dapsone have led to recommendations that multiple-drug therapy be used for the treatment of leprosy. It is hoped that combination drug regimens will prevent the development of resistant strains of *M. leprae* where they do not already exist and/or shorten the treatment period.

For patients infected with sulfone-sensitive *M. leprae*, the NHDC currently advises the following regimens: Patients with indeterminate, tuberculoid, and borderline tuberculoid leprosy should receive dapsone 100 mg daily plus rifampin 600 mg daily for six months, followed by dapsone alone, which is given for three years after tests are negative for those with indeterminate and tuberculoid forms and for five years for those with the borderline tuberculoid form. Negativity is defined as skin scrapings negative for bacilli (BI = O) for one year, a negative biopsy, and no clinical evidence of activity, such as progressive skin lesions, neuropathy, or leprosy reaction. Patients with mid-borderline, borderline lepromatous, and lepromatous forms should receive dapsone 100 mg daily with rifampin 600 mg daily for three years; this is followed by dapsone alone for ten years beyond negativity in those with the mid-borderline forms, and indefinitely for those with borderline-lepromatous and lepromatous forms. Clofazimine 50 to 100 mg daily may be given in addition to dapsone and rifampin for the first three years, particularly if drug sensitivity studies are not done prior to the initiation of therapy or the patient has relapsed.

Mid-borderline, borderline-lepromatous, and lepromatous patients infected with sulfone-resistant bacilli should receive 100 mg of clofazimine daily indefinitely, together with rifampin 600 mg daily for the first three years. Rifampin 600 mg daily with ethionamide 250 mg daily, both given indefinitely, may be substituted for the clofazimine regimen in those who refuse to take it because of the pigmentation produced. Ongoing trials may indicate that these treatment intervals can be shortened by using combination drug therapy, but until sufficient data are available, the NHDC continues to recommend this more conservative approach.

In reviewing the existing world situation, particularly that in underdeveloped countries where cost and compliance are significant factors, the World Health Organization Study Group on Chemotherapy for Leprosy (WHO, 1982) felt that the widespread prevalence of dapsone resistance precluded the recommendation of dapsone plus *one* additional drug for multibacillary leprosy, since this was likely to give rise to multiple drug resistance. It therefore recommended that two additional drugs be combined with dapsone, one of which is rifampin because of its great potency. The Study Group also felt that multidrug regimens should allow a shortened course of therapy, noting that long-term treatment (up to life-long) is not feasible in most third world countries. The proposed regimen (Table 4) was designed for the treatment of all patients with multibacillary leprosy, including those who are newly diagnosed and previously untreated, as well as those previously treated with dapsone monotherapy, regardless of therapeutic outcome.

The World Health Organization Study Group (WHO, 1982) also has recommended only four drugs for combined chemotherapy: dapsone, rifampin, clofazimine, and ethionamide. (When available, prothionamide may replace the latter, although it has no particular advantage.) Dapsone is inexpensive and nontoxic in recommended dosages and is weakly bactericidal against *M. leprae* in man. Although expensive, rifampin is rapidly bactericidal for *M. leprae*; toxic effects have not occurred after monthly administration, although adverse effects may be encountered when this drug is given at shorter intervals. Clofazimine, an investigational drug in the United States, is also expensive and its major adverse effect is skin pigmentation. It is weakly bactericidal against the leprosy bacillus. Ethionamide has less bactericidal activity than rifampin; it is an alternative to clofazimine when the latter is unacceptable.

The WHO Study Group recommended short-course chemotherapy with rifampin and dapsone for all patients with paucibacillary leprosy (see Table 4). The Study Group reasoned that, since the bacterial load in paucibacillary leprosy is much lower than that in the multibacillary type, the probability of encountering drug-resistant mutants is insignificant. Also, bacterial persisters are likely to be contained by cell-mediated immunity, which is adequate in these patients. Therefore, short-course chemotherapy is feasible, especially with the bactericidal drug, rifampin. Patients are not expected to harbor rifampin-resistant *M. leprae* bacilli. The regimen should not be interrupted if reversal reactions occur.

Neither the multibacillary or paucibacillary regimen recommended by the WHO Study Group has been evaluated fully in large numbers of patients over a prolonged period. Because of leprosy's long incubation period, it may be several years before definitive results are obtained.

Household Contacts: A household contact has been defined as "anyone who has lived with the patient for at least one month since the onset of his symptoms." It has been established that 20% to 45% of leprosy cases may be traced to household contacts. Family members are said be eight times more likely to develop lepromatous leprosy and four times more likely to develop tuberculoid leprosy (Hendrick and

TABLE 4.
WHO RECOMMENDED STANDARD REGIMENS FOR CHEMOTHERAPY OF LEPROSY[1]

PAUCIBACILLARY FORMS[2] (I, TT, BT)[3]
    Rifampin: 600 mg once a month for six months. Supervised.
    Dapsone: 100 mg (1 to 2 mg/kg) daily for six months. Self-administered.
    It is recommended that follow-up continue for a minimum of four years.

MULTIBACILLARY FORMS[2] (LL, BL, BB)[4]
    Rifampin: 600 mg once monthly for patients over 35 kg; 450 mg for those less than 35 kg. Supervised.
    Dapsone: 100 mg/day (1 to 2 mg/kg). Self-administered.
    Clofazimine[5]: 300 mg once monthly, supervised, and 50 mg daily, self-administered.
    Treatment Period: Minimum two years (preferably to smear negativity).

[1]*WHO Study Group on Chemotherapy of Leprosy for Control Programmes. Chemotherapy of leprosy for control programmes. World Health Organization Technical Report Series 675. WHO, Geneva, 1982.*
[2]*These regimens still have to be evaluated in a significantly large number of patients over a long-term period.*
[3]*I, indeterminate; TT, tuberculoid; BT, borderline-tuberculoid*
[4]*LL, lepromatous; BL, borderline-lepromatous; BB, mid-borderline*
[5]*When clofazimine is unacceptable, it may be replaced by ethionamide 250 to 375 mg (5 to 10 mg/kg) daily, self-administered.*

Wilkin, 1982). It is recommended that all family members be screened once a year for at least five years.

Leprosy Reactions: Reactions occur during the treatment of leprosy in up to 50% of patients. Two types of reactions are seen: Type 1 (reversal) reactions in the borderline and tuberculoid forms and Type 2 (erythema nodosum leprosum [ENL]) reactions in the lepromatous and, occasionally, borderline forms.

Type 1 reactions commonly occur during the first six months of treatment. Neuritis is the predominant symptom and may become severe and lead to sensorimotor loss. Skin lesions may become erythematous, edematous, and occasionally ulcerate. There may be edema of the face, hands, or feet. This type of reaction is generally considered to be a phenomenon of delayed hypersensitivity associated with an increase in the cell-mediated immune response to *M. leprae.*

Type 2 reactions are associated most commonly with lepromatous leprosy. They usually occur later in the course of treatment than type 1 reactions. Crops of erythematous nodules may appear anywhere on the skin, often accompanied by fever and malaise. Neuritis, orchitis, iridocyclitis, arthritis, proteinuria, and lymphadenopathy also may occur. In severe reactions, lesions may become vesicular or bullous and break down. Muscle paralysis is less common and severe than in type 1 reactions. Type 2 reactions are thought to be generalized immune complex-mediated reactions involving complement activation and deposition of immune complexes in tissues and resemble an Arthus reaction.

Patients with mild leprosy reactions may require no treatment or can be treated with analgesic doses of aspirin. Antimonials (stibophen [Fuadin] and antimony potassium tartrate) have been used but, because of their toxic effects and the availability of more effective drugs, it is highly questionable whether these agents should be given.

Severe leprosy reactions of either type respond to corticosteroids; prednisone 60 mg daily is usually sufficient for initial control, and the dose often can be reduced gradually to an alternate-day schedule if prolonged therapy is required. Corticosteroids should be used whenever neuritis causes a progressive neural deficit or a skin ulceration appears.

Thalidomide is the treatment of choice for type 2 reactions, and is available only for this investigational use in the United States. It is of no value in type 1 reactions. After an initial dose of up to 400 mg daily (adults), the amount often can be decreased over two weeks to a maintenance level of 100 mg daily. Periodic attempts should be made to discontinue the drug; the course can be repeated if symptoms recur. Except under unusual circumstances, thalidomide is contraindicated in women of child-bearing age who might conceive during therapy. Clofazimine 300 mg daily also may slowly control leprosy reactions of either type.

In general, chemotherapy should be continued despite the appearance of a leprosy reaction, for discontinuing or reducing the dose of dapsone or any other medication will not immediately ameliorate the reactive episode. Withdrawal of therapy may have been responsible, at least in part, for the appearance of sulfone-resistant strains of *M. leprae.*

At best, the treatment of leprosy or leprosy reactions is difficult and complex and should be undertaken only by specialists or in consultation with them. Assistance is available at all times from the experts at NHDC.

See the evaluations for adverse reactions and precautions.

Drug Evaluations

DAPSONE

USES. This sulfone continues to be a drug of choice for all patients infected with sulfone-sensitive *Mycobacterium leprae.* Dapsone is inexpensive and nontoxic in the usual dosage range. A dose of 100 mg/day produces peak serum levels that exceed the MIC by a factor of approximately 500 and has some bactericidal activity against the leprosy bacillus. Maximum dosage should be used from the start of therapy and continued during leprosy reactions.

Dapsone has been administered alone for the treatment of indeterminate and tuberculoid forms and has been suggested for prophylaxis of household contacts of borderline and lepromatous patients. However, the increasing incidence of sulfone-resistant organisms has precipitated a re-evaluation of dapsone monotherapy and it is now recommended that other antileprosy drugs (most commonly rifampin and clofazimine) be given with dapsone.

ADVERSE REACTIONS. Adverse reactions are usually mild and occur infrequently with the doses used to treat leprosy. Nausea, vomiting, headache, dizziness, and tachycardia are uncommon, and methemoglobinemia, leukopenia, and agranulocytosis are rare with therapeutic doses.

Many patients receiving 100 mg/day experience an increased rate of erythrocyte destruction; however, this is severe only in occasional patients with glucose-6-phosphate dehydrogenase (G6PD) deficiency.

Deaths from agranulocytosis, aplastic anemia, and other blood dyscrasias have been associated with dapsone. Complete blood counts should be performed frequently; weekly for the first month, monthly for six months, and semimonthly thereafter in conjunction with baseline and periodic liver function tests.

A hypersensitivity reaction, termed the "sulfone syndrome," also occurs rarely. It begins one to four weeks after administration (Tomecki and Catalano, 1981) and is characterized by fever, malaise, exfoliative dermatitis, jaundice with hepatic necrosis, lymphadenopathy, methemoglobinemia, and anemia. The condition improves if dapsone is withdrawn and corticosteroid therapy is given. Peripheral neuritis has been reported rarely after administration of large doses.

No teratogenic effect has been reported to date, although neonatal mortality may be higher than normal; careful observation of the neonate is recommended (Farb et al, 1982). This drug is classified in FDA Pregnancy Category A. Mild reversible hemolytic anemia transmitted through breast milk has been reported in one infant (Sanders et al, 1982).

PHARMACOKINETICS. Dapsone is slowly (time to peak effect

is one to three hours) but completely absorbed after oral administration. The drug is 50% bound to plasma protein. The plasma elimination half-life ranges from 10 to 50 hours with a mean of 28 hours. About 70% to 80% of a dose is excreted as N-glucuronide or N-sulfamate conjugates. Dapsone is acetylated in the liver, and enterohepatic circulation accounts for appreciable tissue levels of dapsone three weeks after therapy is terminated. Rifampin lowers dapsone levels seven- to tenfold by increasing plasma clearance.

DOSAGE AND PREPARATIONS.
Oral: Adults and children, 100 mg (1 to 2 mg/kg) daily. Dapsone is usually given with other antileprosy drugs, most commonly rifampin and clofazimine. It is advisable to screen the patient for G6PD deficiency prior to initiation of therapy. If deficiency is found, the drug should be given more cautiously, starting with 25 mg twice weekly. If the patient cannot tolerate the drug and severe hemolysis occurs, clofazimine should be used instead.
   Generic. Tablets 25 and 100 mg.

ETHIONAMIDE
   [Trecator-SC]

The use of this drug for the treatment of leprosy is investigational in the United States. Ethionamide has been shown to be bactericidal for *Mycobacterium leprae* in mice; in man, its bactericidal effect is intermediate between that of dapsone and rifampin. It is used as an alternative to clofazimine in the triple-drug regimen (dapsone, rifampin, clofazimine) recommended by the WHO Study Group (WHO, 1982) when the latter is not acceptable. Ethionamide also has been used in combination regimens for the treatment of both sulfone-sensitive and sulfone-resistant leprosy.

The major adverse effect of ethionamide in leprosy patients is hepatotoxicity, especially when this drug is given with rifampin.

DOSAGE AND PREPARATIONS.
Oral: Adults, for multibacillary leprosy, 250 to 375 mg daily in combination with other antileprosy drugs (dapsone, rifampin) for at least two years.
   Trecator-SC (Wyeth). Tablets 250 mg.
   (Investigational indication)

CLOFAZIMINE (B663)
   [Lamprene]

USES. This fat-soluble riminophenazine dye has been used for the treatment of leprosy since the early 1960's. It has a bactericidal effect between that of dapsone and rifampin and is the treatment of choice (given with rifampin) when sulfone-

resistant *Mycobacterium leprae* are present. Clofazimine also has a marked anti-inflammatory effect and is given to control leprosy reactions. Its use is investigational in the United States, however, and it may be obtained only through the National Hansen's Disease Center.

Although only one case of *M. leprae* resistant to clofazimine has been reported, most investigators believe that this drug, like dapsone, should be used only in combination regimens to treat patients with lepromatous and borderline leprosy.

ADVERSE REACTIONS. Clofazimine, a red-colored compound that is deposited in the tissues, may discolor the skin and conjunctivae. The skin first develops a reddish hue that may progress to mahogany brown, while the leprosy lesions become even more pigmented and appear mauve, slate gray, or black. The degree of pigmentation varies from patient to patient; generally, the larger the dose and the more advanced the disease, the more pronounced the pigmentation will be. The conjunctivae become varying shades of red-brown. In addition, a red tint may appear in the urine, sputum, and sweat. All of these effects clear slowly after therapy is discontinued.

Diminished sweating and tear production may be noted and photosensitivity reactions have been reported. The most serious adverse effect of clofazimine is on the small bowel. Nausea, vomiting, and diarrhea may occur but are uncommon if the dose is 100 mg or less daily. Larger doses sometimes produce abdominal pain and, because of extensive deposition of the drug in the wall of the small bowel, which may become edematous, symptoms suggesting bowel obstruction occasionally develop.

Infants may be pigmented at birth or after ingesting the drug in maternal milk.

PHARMACOKINETICS. Clofazimine is absorbed orally, accumulates, and is retained for a long period in the body. It is excreted very slowly because it is extremely hydrophobic. The elimination half-life is about 70 days in man (Feng et al, 1981).

DOSAGE AND PREPARATIONS.
Oral: Adults, 50 to 100 mg daily. The WHO Study Group (WHO, 1982) has recommended 300 mg once monthly, supervised, and 50 mg daily, self-administered, for treatment of multibacillary leprosy. Control of leprosy reactions may require 100 mg three times daily, but the dose must be reduced at once if symptoms of gastrointestinal toxicity develop.
   Lamprene (Geigy). Capsules 50 and 100 mg.
   (Investigational drug)

RIFAMPIN
   [Rifadin, Rimactane]

USES. Rifampin is effective in the treatment of leprosy, but this use is investigational in the United States. It is much more rapidly bactericidal for *Mycobacterium leprae* than the other currently used drugs.

Reports indicate that oral doses of 300 to 600 mg daily (adults) render bacilli noninfective for the mouse footpad and, therefore, presumably noninfectious for contacts more rapidly than dapsone or clofazimine (several days versus two to three months). However, in humans, the longer-term response, as measured by clearance of skin lesions and reduction in the number of bacilli in skin smears, is no better.

Some patients have taken rifampin alone for as long as 10 years without problems. On the other hand, resistant strains of *M. leprae* have appeared in three to four years in patients given rifampin monotherapy. For this reason, it is now recommended that rifampin be used only in combination drug regimens. Usually these utilize rifampin plus dapsone (plus clofazimine in some patients) for infections with sulfone-sensitive *M. leprae* and rifampin plus either clofazimine or ethionamide for infections with sulfone-resistant *M. leprae*.

ADVERSE REACTIONS. The adverse effects of rifampin in the treatment of leprosy are the same as those observed when the drug is used to treat tuberculosis (see the section on Tuberculosis).

DOSAGE AND PREPARATIONS.
Oral: Adults, the usual dose is 600 mg daily. The WHO Study Group has recommended 600 mg once monthly under supervision in a regimen consisting of rifampin, dapsone, and clofazimine (WHO, 1982).

Rifadin (Merrell Dow). Capsules 150 and 300 mg.
Rimactane (CIBA). Capsules 300 mg.
(Investigational indication)

Cited References

Follow-up on guidelines for short-course tuberculosis chemotherapy. *Morbid Mortal Week Rep* 29:183-189, 1980.

Tuberculosis: United States, 1982. *Morbid Mortal Week Rep* 32:478-480, (Sept 16) 1983.

Primary resistance to antituberculosis drugs: United States. *Morbid Mortal Week Rep* 32:521-523, (Oct 14) 1983.

Tuberculosis: United States, 1983. *Morbid Mortal Week Rep* 33:77-78, 1984.

Ahn CH, et al: Short-course chemotherapy for pulmonary disease caused by *Mycobacterium kansasii. Am Rev Respir Dis* 128:1048-1050, 1983.

Algerian Working Group/British Medical Research Council Cooperative Study: Controlled clinical trial comparing 6-month and 12-month regimen in treatment of pulmonary tuberculosis in the Algerian Sahara. *Am Rev Respir Dis* 129:921-928, 1984.

Aquinas M: Short-course therapy for tuberculosis. *Drugs* 24:118-132, 1982.

Baciewicz AM, Self TH: Rifampin drug interactions. *Arch Intern Med* 144:1667-1671, 1984.

Bass JB Jr, Hawkins EL: Treatment of disease caused by nontuberculous mycobacteria. *Arch Intern Med* 143:1439-1441, 1983.

British Thoracic Association: Controlled trial of 6 months chemotherapy in pulmonary tuberculosis: Second report. Results during 24 months after end of chemotherapy. *Am Rev Respir Dis* 126:460-462, 1982.

Buechner HA: Medical management of tuberculosis. *Ration Drug Ther* 14:1-7, (Oct) 1980.

Buechner HA: Short course chemotherapy for tuberculosis: Treatment of choice? *Compr Ther* 9:59-63, (May) 1983.

Carpenter JL, et al: Drug-resistant *Mycobacterium tuberculosis* in Korean isolates. *Am Rev Respir Dis* 126:1092-1095, 1982.

Carpenter JL, et al: Antituberculosis drug resistance in south Texas. *Am Rev Respir Dis* 128:1055-1058, 1983.

Coleman DL, Slutkin G: Chemoprophylaxis against tuberculosis. *West J Med* 140:106-110, 1984.

Comstock GW: New data on preventative treatment with isoniazid. *Ann Intern Med* 98:663-665, 1983.

Dutt AK, Stead WW: Modern treatment of tuberculosis. *Compr Ther* 8:19-28, (Sept) 1982.

Farb H, et al: Clofazimine in pregnancy complicated by leprosy. *Obstet Gynecol* 59:122-123, 1982.

Farer LS: Chemoprophylaxis. *Am Rev Respir Dis* 125:102-107, 1982.

Feng PCC, et al: Metabolism of clofazimine in leprosy patients. *Drug Metab Dispos* 9:521-524, 1981.

Fox W: Current status of short-course chemotherapy. *Tubercle* 60:177-190, 1979.

Girling DJ: Adverse effects of antituberculosis drugs. *Drugs* 23:56-74, 1982.

Hendrick SS, Wilkin JK: Leprosy. *Am Fam Physician* 26:161-166, 1982.

Hong Kong Chest Service/Tuberculosis Research Centre, Madras/British Medical Research Council: Controlled trial of 2-month, 3-month, and 12-month regimens of chemotherapy for sputum-smear-negative pulmonary tuberculosis: Results at 60 months. *Am Rev Respir Dis* 130:23-28, 1984.

Jenkins P, Emerson PA: Myopathy induced by rifampicin. *Br Med J* 283:105-106, 1981.

Kasik JE: Tuberculosis and other mycobacterial disease, in Conn HF (ed): *Current Therapy 1979.* Philadelphia, WB Saunders, 1979, 155-160.

Kenny MT, Strates B: Metabolism and pharmacokinetics of antibiotic rifampin. *Drug Metab Rev* 12:159-218, 1981.

Leff A, Geppert EF: Public health and preventive aspects of pulmonary tuberculosis: Infectiousness, epidemiology, risk factors, classification, and preventive therapy. *Arch Intern Med* 139:1405-1410, 1979.

Long MW, et al: U.S. Public Health Service Cooperative trial of three rifampin-isoniazid regimens in treatment of pulmonary tuberculosis. *Am Rev Respir Dis* 119:879-894, 1979.

Lyons RW: Orange contact lenses from rifampin. *N Engl J Med* 300:372-373, 1979.

Mehrotra ML, et al: Shortest possible acceptable effective chemotherapy in ambulatory patients with pulmonary tuberculosis. Part II. Results during the 24 months after the end of chemotherapy. *Am Rev Respir Dis* 129:1016-1017, 1984.

Moulding TS: Short course chemotherapy: Use of combination tablets of isoniazid and rifampin, (letter). *Am Rev Respir Dis* 122:170-171, 1980.

Murray JF, et al: Pulmonary complications of acquired immunodeficiency syndrome. *N Engl J Med* 310:1682-1688, 1984.

Nilsson BS, Boman G: Intravenous use of rifampicin. *Eur J Respir Dis* 62:212-214, 1981.

Pitchenik AE, et al: Prevalence of tuberculosis and drug resistance among Haitians. *N Engl J Med* 307:162-165, 1982.

Powell KE, et al: Tuberculosis among Indochinese refugees in the United States. *JAMA* 249:1455-1460, 1983.

Powell KE, et al: Recent trends in tuberculosis in children. *JAMA* 251:1289-1292, 1984.

Ridley DS, Jopling WH: Classification of leprosy according to immunity: Five-group system. *Int J Lepr* 34:255-273, 1966.

Runyon EH: Pathogenic mycobacteria. *Bibl Tuberc Med Thorac* 21:235-237, 1965.

Sanders SW, et al: Hemolytic anemia induced by dapsone transmitted through breast milk. *Ann Intern Med* 96:465-466, 1982.

Sbarbaro JA, Iseman MD: Prophylactic treatment of tuberculosis. *Compr Ther* 7:14-19, (June) 1981.

Snider D Jr, et al: Preliminary results of six-month regimens studied in the United States and Poland. *Chest* 80:727-729, 1981.

Snider DE, et al: Successful intermittent treatment of smear positive pulmonary tuberculosis in 6 months: Cooperative study in Poland. *Am Rev Respir Dis* 125:265-267, 1982.

Snider DE Jr, et al: Six-months isoniazid-rifampin therapy for pulmonary tuberculosis: Report of United States Public Health Service cooperative trial. *Am Rev Respir Dis* 129:573-579, 1984.

Stead WW: Isoniazid prophylaxis, (letter). *Ann Intern Med* 95:393, 1981.

Stead WW, Dutt AK: Modern treatment of tuberculosis. *Drug Ther* 11:85-99, (May) 1981.

Stead WW, Dutt AK: Chemotherapy for tuberculosis today. *Am Rev*

Respir Dis 125:94-101, 1982.

Steiner P, et al: Continuing study of primary drug-resistant tuberculosis among children observed at Kings County Hospital Medical Center between years 1961 and 1980. *Am Rev Respir Dis* 128:425-428, 1983.

Taylor WC, et al: Should young adults with positive tuberculin test take isoniazid? *Ann Intern Med* 94:808-813, 1981.

Tomecki KJ, Catalano CJ: Dapsone hypersensitivity: Sulfone syndrome revisited. *Arch Dermatol* 117:38-39, 1981.

Tuberculosis Research Centre: Study of chemotherapy regimens of 5 and 7 months' duration and role of corticosteroids in treatment of sputum-positive patients with pulmonary tuberculosis in South India. *Tubercle* 64:73-91, 1983.

Twum-Barina Y, Carruthers SG: Quinidine-rifampin interaction. *N Engl J Med* 304:1466-1469, 1981.

World Health Organization: *Chemotherapy of Leprosy for Control Programmes*. WHO Technical Report Series No. 675, Publication No. ISBN 92 4 120675 6, Geneva, Switzerland, 1982.

Other Selected References

Banner AS: Tuberculosis: Clinical aspects and diagnosis. *Arch Intern Med* 139:1387-1390, 1979.

Geppert EF, Leff A: Pathogenesis of pulmonary and miliary tuberculosis. *Arch Intern Med* 139:1381-1383, 1979.

Leff A, et al: Tuberculosis: Chemotherapeutic triumph but persistent socioeconomic problem. *Arch Intern Med* 139:1375-1377, 1979.

Youmans GP: *Tuberculosis*. Philadelphia, WB Saunders, 1979.

Antifungal Agents for Systemic Mycoses

76

INTRODUCTION

DRUG SELECTION

DRUG EVALUATIONS

Amphotericin B

Flucytosine

Ketoconazole

Miconazole Nitrate

Potassium Iodide

For therapeutic purposes, fungal infections (mycoses) may be classified as superficial, deep, and systemic. This chapter describes the antifungal agents used for deep mycoses (relatively localized to regions other than the skin or mucous membranes), systemic (disseminated) mycoses, and chronic mucocutaneous candidiasis. Agents used for superficial mycoses are discussed in Chapter 74, Topical Anti-infective Agents: Drug Used on Skin and Mucous Membranes.

Chronic mucocutaneous candidiasis is uncommon. The skin, scalp, nails, and mucous membranes are usually involved. Although topical antifungal therapy may be adequate for mild cases, systemic therapy is usually required in moderate to severe cases.

Organisms causing aspergillosis, blastomycosis, coccidioidomycosis, cryptococcosis, histoplasmosis, mucormycosis, and paracoccidioidomycosis usually enter the body by inhalation. The infection is generally limited to the lung (eg, pulmonary blastomycosis, histoplasmosis, coccidioidomycosis) or other airway passages (mucormycosis of the nose and sinuses). The fungus may spread hematogenously, usually to specific organs (eg, cutaneous blastomycosis, cryptococcal meningitis) or, in the case of mucormycosis, by direct extension to the orbits and/or brain. Disseminated candidiasis is thought to spread from a mucocutaneous site rather than from the lung. Organisms causing chromomycosis, mycetoma, and sporotrichosis usually enter the body through the skin and spread only to contiguous tissues; therefore, they are often referred to as subcutaneous mycoses. Sporotrichosis disseminates only rarely.

Blastomycosis, chromomycosis, coccidioidomycosis, histoplasmosis, mycetoma, paracoccidioidomycosis, and sporotrichosis develop in normal individuals. The organisms that cause aspergillosis, candidiasis, cryptococcosis, and mucormycosis often are termed *opportunistic* pathogens, because they usually affect immunocompromised or debilitated individuals. Blastomycosis, coccidioidomycosis, histoplasmosis, sporotrichosis, aspergillosis, candidiasis, and cryptococcosis are most common in the United States. See Table 1, Medically Important Deep and Systemic Mycoses, for information on causative organisms, synonyms, and geographic distribution.

DRUG SELECTION

Treatment: Systemic mycoses are often difficult to diagnose. Since most antifungal agents are not active against bacteria and it is not always possible to differentiate among bacterial, fungal, and mixed infections solely on the basis of signs and symptoms, the causative organism should be identified before initiating treatment. Serologic tests are helpful in the diagnosis and management of cryptococcosis, coccidioidomycosis, and paracoccidioidomycosis. Histologic or cultural proof usually is required for diagnosis of a deep mycosis (Penn et al, 1983). Correct diagnosis is especially important because some antifungal drugs have a considerable potential for adverse reactions.

Drugs for deep and systemic mycoses include amphotericin B [Fungizone] and miconazole [Monistat i.v.], which are administered intravenously, and flucytosine [Ancobon], potassium

TABLE 1.
MEDICALLY IMPORTANT DEEP AND SYSTEMIC MYCOSES

Infection [Alternative Names]	Organism	Geographic and Demographic Distribution
Aspergillosis	*Aspergillus* species (especially *A. fumigatus*)	Worldwide. Immunocompromised patients are most susceptible.
Blastomycosis [North American Blastomycosis]	*Blastomyces dermatitidis*	North America, endemic in southeastern and north central United States; occasionally in Africa.
Candidiasis [Moniliasis; Thrush; Candidosis]	*Candida albicans* *C. parapsilosis* *C. tropicalis*	Worldwide. Immunocompromised patients are most susceptible.
Chromomycosis [Chromoblastomycosis]	*Fonsecaea (Hormodendrum) pedrosoi* *F. (H.) compactum* *F. (H.) dermatitidis* *Phialophora verrucosa* *Cladosporium carrioni*	Subcutaneous fungal infection found worldwide. Most common in subtropical countries. Men age 30 to 50 years working in agricultural areas are most commonly infected.
Coccidioidomycosis [San Joaquin Fever; Valley Fever]	*Coccidioides immitis*	Endemic in California (San Joaquin Valley) and other dry regions of southwestern United States (Arizona, New Mexico, Texas, Nevada, and southern Utah), northern Mexico, Central and South America (especially northern Argentina and Paraguay). Severe disease most prevalent in men age 25 to 55 years.
Cryptococcosis [Torulosis]	*Cryptococcus neoformans*	Worldwide. Most commonly affects men age 40 to 60 years. Immunocompromised patients are most susceptible.
Histoplasmosis	*Histoplasma capsulatum*	Principally North America in the central United States, particularly the Mississippi Valley. An African variant of the organism also exists. The young and elderly are most susceptible to disseminated infection.
Mucormycosis [Zygomycosis; Phycomycosis]	*Rhizopus, Mucor, Rhizomucor, Cunninghamella,* and *Absidia* species (eg, *Rhizopus oryzae, Mucor pusillus*)	Worldwide. Immunocompromised and debilitated patients are most susceptible.
Paracoccidioidomycosis [South American Blastomycosis]	*Paracoccidioides brasiliensis*	South America and Central America (most common in Brazil), especially in male agricultural workers age 20 to 50 years.
Sporotrichosis	*Sporothrix schenkii*	Subcutaneous fungal infection found worldwide. Most common in Central and South America. Agricultural workers, especially horticulturists, are most often affected.

iodide, and ketoconazole [Nizoral], which are administered orally.

Amphotericin B is the drug of choice for most systemic mycoses. Most experts prefer a combination of amphotericin B and flucytosine for cryptococcal meningitis (Dismukes et al, 1984), disseminated cryptococcosis, and candidiasis (Bennett et al, 1979; Smego et al, 1984). Ketoconazole is effective in some patients with localized, nonlife-threatening, extrameningeal blastomycosis, histoplasmosis, and cryptococcosis; however, amphotericin B is preferred by most clinicians for cryptococcosis because ketoconazole has not prevented cryptococcal meningitis even during active therapy in some

patients. Data in man are too fragmentary to assess the role of two investigational, potent azoles, itraconazole (Van Cutsem et al, 1985) and fluconazole (Humphrey et al, 1985).

Flucytosine is sometimes used alone for chromomycosis, but it is not used alone in other fungal infections because resistance develops rapidly. Only smaller lesions of chromomycosis respond to flucytosine as initial therapy; larger lesions should be resected and flucytosine given (with or without amphotericin B) after resection. Ketoconazole is only marginally effective in chromomycosis.

Ketoconazole is the drug of choice for chronic mucocutaneous candidiasis and paracoccidioidomycosis; however, prolonged therapy is required to avoid relapses. Amphotericin B [Fungizone] is the alternative therapy for chronic mucocutaneous candidiasis. Although ketoconazole is an alternative drug for blastomycosis, coccidioidomycosis, and histoplasmosis, amphotericin B generally is preferred for severe infections. Miconazole is rarely used as an alternative to amphotericin B in coccidioidomycosis since ketoconazole became available.

Potassium iodide is used only for the cutaneous-lymphatic form of sporotrichosis and is the drug of choice. Although ketoconazole also is used (investigational), it is only marginally effective. Amphotericin B is the drug of choice for extracutaneous or disseminated sporotrichosis.

Hydroxystilbamidine is so much less effective than amphotericin B or ketoconazole for blastomycosis that it is considered obsolete, and it is not available in the United States.

See Table 2 for suggested therapy for systemic mycoses. For further information on deep and systemic mycoses and their differential diagnosis and treatment, see the references at the end of the chapter (Mandell et al, 1985; Hoeprich, 1983 A), as well as reviews of drug treatment (American Thoracic Society, 1979; Medoff and Kobayashi, 1980; *Med Lett Drugs Ther*, 1982; Graybill and Craven, 1983; Hermans and Keys, 1983).

Chemoprophylaxis: Studies have been conducted on antifungal chemoprophylaxis primarily for prevention of systemic candidiasis and aspergillosis in neutropenic cancer patients. No well-defined criteria or uniform regimens have been established because the data are limited. Therefore, chemoprophylaxis of fungal infections, most commonly utilizing oral amphotericin B (oral form not available in the United States), nystatin, or ketoconazole, is investigational (Meunier-Carpentier, 1984; Cohen, 1984). In mice, the antifungal effect of amphotericin B was antagonized by ketoconazole; this has not been confirmed clinically but may be a problem when amphotericin B is required following use of ketoconazole chemoprophylaxis (Schaffner and Frick, 1985).

TABLE 2.
ANTIFUNGAL THERAPY FOR DEEP AND SYSTEMIC MYCOSES

Infection	Recommended Therapy	Alternative Treatment	Comments
Aspergillosis			
Disseminated or Pulmonary (invasive)	Amphotericin B (intravenous)		Immunosuppressed patients have required up to 1 mg/kg/day.
Pulmonary (noninvasive)			Therapy usually is not required.
Blastomycosis			
Disseminated or Pulmonary (chronic)	Amphotericin B (intravenous)	Ketoconazole (oral)	Ketoconazole is often preferred in patients with nonlife-threatening extrameningeal disease.
Pulmonary (acute, self-limited)			This infection is usually self-limited and does not require therapy.
Candidiasis			
Disseminated	Amphotericin B (intravenous) with or without Flucytosine (oral)		The combination of flucytosine 150 mg/kg/day with reduced doses of amphotericin B (0.3 mg/kg/day) minimizes the adverse reactions caused by the larger dose of amphotericin B required when it is used alone.
Chronic Mucocutaneous	Ketoconazole (oral)	Amphotericin B (intravenous)	Ketoconazole is effective and safer than amphotericin B; however, either drug must be given for prolonged periods to avoid relapses and this is especially difficult with amphotericin B because of toxicity. A topical candicidal agent may be a useful adjunct.

(Continued on next page)

TABLE 2.
ANTIFUNGAL THERAPY FOR DEEP AND SYSTEMIC MYCOSES (continued)

Infection	Recommended Therapy	Alternative Treatment	Comments
Chromomycosis			
Subcutaneous	Flucytosine (oral) with or without Amphotericin B (intravenous)	Ketoconazole (oral)	Only small lesions are responsive to flucytosine alone; larger lesions are resected and flucytosine (with or without amphotericin B) is given after resection. Intralesional injection of amphotericin B is reported to be effective in some patients.
Coccidioidomycosis			
Meningeal	Amphotericin B (intrathecal)		Intrathecal administration is required.
Chronic or Disseminated (nonmeningeal)	Amphotericin B (intravenous)	Ketoconazole (oral)	Ketoconazole is not usually employed in patients with severe disseminated coccidioidomycosis except when amphotericin B is ineffective, but it is useful to suppress the chronic stage of disease.
Pulmonary (acute, self-limited)			This infection is usually self-limited and does not require therapy.
Cryptococcosis			
Disseminated or Meningeal	Flucytosine (oral) plus Amphotericin B (intravenous)	Amphotericin B (intravenous)	In these life-threatening clinical forms of the disease, most investigators use a combination of flucytosine 150 mg/kg/day with reduced doses of amphotericin B (0.3 mg/kg/day) to minimize the adverse reactions caused by the larger dose of amphotericin B required when it is used alone.
Localized (nonmeningeal)	Amphotericin B (intravenous)	Ketoconazole (oral)	Although ketoconazole is effective in some patients with less severe infections of the lung, bone, and skin, it has not prevented cryptococcal meningitis in some patients.
Histoplasmosis			
Disseminated or Chronic Cavitary	Amphotericin B (intravenous)	Ketoconazole (oral)	Ketoconazole is an alternative in less severe, nonlife-threatening disease.
Pulmonary (acute, self-limited)			Nonprogressive pulmonary infection is usually self-limited and does not require therapy.
Mucormycosis			
Disseminated	Amphotericin B (intravenous)		
Paracoccidioidomycosis			
Cutaneous-lymphatic and/or Visceral-lymphatic	Ketoconazole (oral)	Amphotericin B (intravenous) Sulfonamides (oral)	Amphotericin B is preferred in severe, life-threatening infections or when ketoconazole is ineffective.

(Continued on next page)

Infection	Recommended Therapy	Alternative Treatment	Comments
Sporotrichosis			
Disseminated or Extracutaneous	Amphotericin B (intravenous)		
Cutaneous-lymphatic	Potassium Iodide (oral)	Ketoconazole* (oral)	Limited studies suggest that ketoconazole is only marginally effective in some cases. Local heat may be beneficial adjunctively.

*Investigational use

Drug Evaluations

AMPHOTERICIN B
[Fungizone]

ACTIONS. Amphotericin B is a polyene antibiotic produced by *Streptomyces nodosus*. Low concentrations inhibit the growth of fungi, protozoa, and algae. Concentrations near the upper limits of tolerance in man are fungicidal to some strains. Although amphotericin B binds to sterols in fungal and mammalian membranes, it binds more avidly to ergosterol in fungal membranes than to cholesterol in mammalian membranes. Binding to ergosterol in fungal cell membranes alters selective permeability.

USES. The combination of amphotericin B and flucytosine often is the treatment of choice in disseminated candidiasis and cryptococcosis. Amphotericin B is an alternative to ketoconazole in nonlife-threatening blastomycosis, histoplasmosis, and paracoccidioidomycosis but is the drug of choice in life-threatening cases, in patients with meningitis, or when ketoconazole is ineffective (Dismukes et al, 1985). Amphotericin B is the drug of choice for mucormycosis, although this infection, as well as invasive aspergillosis and coccidioidomycosis, is less responsive. Amphotericin B is indicated in disseminated and extracutaneous sporotrichosis, but potassium iodide is preferred for the cutaneous-lymphatic form. The subcutaneous mycoses, mycetoma (Mahgoub, 1985) and chromomycosis, appear to be least affected by amphotericin B. Intralesional injection has been reported to be effective in some patients with chromomycosis. Immunosuppressed patients with deep or systemic mycoses are more resistant to therapy than normal individuals with the same mycosis (Bodey, 1984; Hawkins and Armstrong, 1985; Wheat et al, 1985).

In one controlled study, empiric use of intravenous amphotericin B was beneficial in febrile cancer patients with granulocytopenia who did not respond to optimal antibacterial agents; therefore, it is recommended to prevent fungal superinfections and to control clinically undetected fungal invasion in such patients (Pizzo et al, 1982).

Amphotericin B has some effect, although it is not the drug of choice, in mucocutaneous leishmaniasis caused by *Leishmania braziliensis* (see Chapter 77, Antiprotozoal Agents).

RESISTANCE. Susceptibility to amphotericin B varies widely among species but is fairly uniform within a given species. The minimal inhibitory concentration (MIC) varies with the method, and there is no standard technique. Whatever method has been used, the small variation in MIC encountered within a given species does not predict response to therapy in humans and has no clinical value.

ADVERSE REACTIONS AND PRECAUTIONS. Amphotericin B should be employed only in patients who are observed closely and who have a confirmed diagnosis of a progressive, potentially fatal mycosis caused by a susceptible fungus. Therapy must be continued for a sufficient period, usually two to four months. This drug causes potentially dangerous reactions in most patients. Nevertheless, a full course of therapy usually can be administered if the side effects are managed appropriately.

An acute febrile reaction is most prominent early in therapy; azotemia is the most important reaction later. A shaking chill is often the initial symptom of the typical febrile reaction, which begins precipitously about two hours after an infusion is started. Fever is maximal about one hour after onset and subsides within the next hour or two. Intravenous infusion of hydrocortisone sodium succinate 25 to 50 mg just prior to the infusion may decrease the intensity of known reactions in patients not already receiving corticosteroids. Hydrocortisone should not be given routinely, however, because its immunosuppressant action may worsen the course of the mycosis. Meperidine or an antihistamine given prior to the infusion has been advocated when reactions to previous infusions were not controlled by other measures. Pretreatment with aspirin or acetaminophen ameliorates mild reactions.

In the acute phase of the febrile reaction, symptoms of anaphylaxis (wheezing and hypoxemia) may develop, particularly in patients with obstructive lung disease or congestive heart failure, but true anaphylaxis with hypotension, urticaria, or edema of the mucous membranes is rare. An allergic skin rash also occurs rarely. Patients with severe angina pectoris may develop chest pain.

Transient, dose-dependent azotemia is observed in almost all patients. There is minimal permanent renal damage, but impairment may become permanent in patients with pre-existing renal disease or in those receiving a total dose of more than 3 g. In patients without prior renal disease, the usual daily dose of 0.4 to 0.6 mg/kg produces a serum creatinine level of 1.7 to 3.5 mg/dl and a blood urea nitrogen level of 25 to 50 mg/dl. More severe azotemia (creatinine level above 3 mg/dl) may require reduction of dosage, improved hydration, and avoidance or elimination of diuretics or other nephrotoxic drugs. Renal tubular acidosis, hypokalemia, or hyponatremia may require treatment. Renal function should be monitored daily if the serum creatinine level rises rapidly to 2 mg/dl or more, and serum electrolytes should be monitored at least twice weekly. Sodium depletion is reported to increase susceptibility to renal impairment (Daneshmend and Warnock, 1983; Heidemann et al, 1983); in the latter study, supplemental sodium loading (150 mEq/day) reversed renal impairment and allowed a full course of amphotericin B therapy.

The hematocrit often falls during therapy to a stable level between 20% and 30%. Transfusion ordinarily should be avoided. A slight decrease in leukocyte count and, rarely, thrombocytopenia may occur. Nausea, vomiting, anorexia, and weight loss are common.

Heparin 1,000 units (10 mg) is often added to infusions in an attempt to decrease phlebitis. As intravenous therapy continues, patients may experience less phlebitis and anorexia if a double dose on alternate days is substituted gradually.

Intrathecal injection may cause nausea and vomiting; urinary retention; pain in the back, legs, or abdomen; headache; radiculitis; paresis (usually transient); paresthesias; tinnitus and diminished hearing; vertigo; and, rarely, impaired vision that may progress to blindness.

In pregnant women or those of childbearing age, therapy should be limited to life-threatening infections. At least six pregnant patients have been treated successfully without obvious teratogenic effects.

PHARMACOKINETICS. Amphotericin B is inadequately absorbed orally. It is injected intravenously for systemic fungal infections and intrathecally for coccidioidal meningitis.

Amphotericin B is highly protein bound (90% to 95%). The large volume of distribution (4.0 ± 0.4 L/kg) probably reflects binding to cell membranes and has no clinical significance. This drug penetrates extravascular compartments poorly. An initial plasma half-life of about 24 hours is followed by a slower terminal elimination half-life of about 15 days (Daneshmend and Warnock, 1983). After therapy is discontinued, amphotericin B can be detected in the serum for seven to eight weeks because it is released slowly from tissue depots. Metabolic pathways are unknown. The concentration in the serum is similar to that in urine. The serum concentration is not elevated in patients with impaired or absent renal function. Neither hemodialysis nor peritoneal dialysis removes a significant amount of drug.

DOSAGE AND PREPARATIONS. Detailed instructions for storage, preparation, and administration should be followed closely, because this drug is unstable under unfavorable conditions (eg, exposure to heat, low pH). The powder should be refrigerated and suspensions used the same day. Since the preparation is a colloidal suspension, any membrane filter used should have a mean pore diameter of greater than 1 micron. Suspensions are prepared by adding 10 ml of water for injection to 50 mg of amphotericin B and shaking the vial until the contents are clear. The desired dose is then added to 5% dextrose injection. The pH of the suspension should be 4.2 or above. The dose should not be added to infusates that contain bacteriostatic agents (eg, benzyl alcohol), potassium chloride, sodium chloride and other electrolytes because they cause the drug to precipitate. Cloudy solutions may produce low serum levels and should be discarded.

Intravenous (infusion): Daily dosage must be individualized on the basis of the severity of the disease and tolerance of the patient.

The total daily dose is administered as an infusion that usually is given over two to four hours. The initial dose in adults and children should not exceed 0.25 mg/kg (an initial dose of 1 mg often is preferred to test for a possible anaphylactic reaction). The amount may be increased by 5 to 10 mg daily or every other day to a maintenance level of 0.4 to 0.6 mg/kg/day. The alternate-day regimen is satisfactory for most chronic mycoses and reduces the frequency of phlebitis and acute reactions. Some clinicians prefer to give 1 mg/kg/day initially for several days to severely ill and immunocompromised patients; however, continued administration of this dose usually causes formidable problems in management. It may be necessary to give up to 0.8 mg/kg/day for a prolonged period in acute invasive aspergillosis.

The total dose of 30 mg/kg (1 to 3 g) for a course of therapy usually can be administered over six to ten weeks, but several months may be necessary to achieve a cure. Shorter periods may produce an inadequate response and lead to relapse. Whenever administration is interrupted for longer than seven days, therapy should be resumed gradually according to the above schedule.

When given with flucytosine for disseminated candidiasis or cryptococcosis, the initial regimen is amphotericin B 0.3 mg/kg/day plus flucytosine 37.5 mg/kg at six-hour intervals in the absence of renal impairment. Usually six weeks of therapy are required. Some authorities decrease the daily maintenance dose of flucytosine to 25 mg/kg at six-hour intervals depending on the tolerance and response of the patient.

Intrathecal: The suspension for lumbar intrathecal injection may be diluted in 10% dextrose. The patient is placed in a 30° Trendelenburg position for 30 to 45 minutes immediately after the injection to allow downward flow of the hyperbaric solution. Hydrocortisone sodium succinate 10 to 15 mg may be added to the solution to decrease chemical arachnoiditis, although the extra volume necessitates use of enough dextrose to maintain a hyperbaric final concentration.

For injections in the lateral cerebral ventricle employing a cisternal Ommaya reservoir, the solution is diluted in 5% dextrose with or without hydrocortisone sodium succinate 10 to 15 mg. The initial dose is approximately 0.05 mg; subsequent doses are increased by 0.1 mg three times a week to a maintenance dose of 0.5 mg two or three times a week.

Fungizone (Squibb). Powder (lyophilized, sterile) 50 mg.

FLUCYTOSINE
[Ancobon]

ACTIONS AND USES. Flucytosine, a synthetic agent, is administered orally to treat subcutaneous chromomycosis. Smaller lesions respond to flucytosine alone but larger lesions must be resected before flucytosine is used. Amphotericin B may be given concomitantly when the response to flucytosine alone is inadequate or the disease is extensive.

Flucytosine is used with amphotericin B to treat deep or systemic infections caused by *Candida* or *Cryptococcus neoformans*, because resistance develops rapidly when flucytosine is given alone; 5% to 15% of pretreatment isolates of *Candida* are resistant. Combined use also permits reduction in the dose of amphotericin B (see Dosage and Preparations).

Flucytosine is metabolized to fluorouracil and fluorodeoxyuridine monophosphate. Fluorouracil is incorporated into fungal RNA and inhibits protein synthesis. Fluorodeoxyuridine monophosphate inhibits DNA synthesis.

ADVERSE REACTIONS AND PRECAUTIONS. Flucytosine is less toxic than amphotericin B, but it may cause rash, nausea, vomiting, or diarrhea. The diarrhea can become protracted if flucytosine is continued. Perforation of the bowel as a result of colonic ulcers has been reported (Kerkering, 1982).

The most common serious adverse reaction is leukopenia or thrombocytopenia, either of which can be fatal. These reactions are dose related, are more likely to develop when the serum level of flucytosine exceeds 100 mcg/ml, and are usually reversible on discontinuing the drug.

Since flucytosine causes no renal toxicity, it is safe in patients with impaired renal function when the dosage is modified. Patients with severe or rapidly developing azotemia are difficult to treat unless serum levels are monitored frequently. Special caution is advised when flucytosine is administered with amphotericin B, because the latter's potential for inducing renal impairment may interfere with the elimination of flucytosine (Kerkering, 1982).

Elevation of hepatic enzymes (SGOT, SGPT, alkaline phosphatase) is noted occasionally. Three cases of patchy hepatic cell necrosis have been reported (Kerkering, 1982).

Flucytosine must be administered with care to patients with bone marrow depression (eg, caused by certain hematologic diseases, radiation, or drugs). An allergic skin reaction occurs occasionally.

The safety of flucytosine during pregnancy has not been established. Therefore, the drug should be given to pregnant patients only when serious or life-threatening systemic fungal infections exist, and contraceptive measures should be considered in women of childbearing age.

PHARMACOKINETICS. More than 80% of a dose of flucytosine is absorbed from the gastrointestinal tract, and peak serum levels are achieved in two to four hours (Daneshmend and Warnock, 1983). The drug is widely distributed in body water; protein binding is negligible. The volume of distribution is 0.57 ± 0.02 L/kg. Levels in the cerebrospinal fluid and central nervous system are about 80% of those in the serum. About 63% to 84% of a dose is eliminated principally unchanged in the urine. Clearance is approximately 75% of creatinine clearance. The serum half-life is three to six hours.

DOSAGE AND PREPARATIONS.

Oral: Adults and children with normal renal function, usually 37.5 mg/kg at six-hour intervals. When given with amphotericin B to patients with normal renal function, the initial regimen is amphotericin B 0.3 mg/kg/day with flucytosine 37.5 mg/kg at six-hour intervals. Usually six weeks of therapy is required. Some authorities decrease the daily maintenance dose to 25 mg/kg at six-hour intervals depending on the tolerance and response of the patient.

Serum levels of flucytosine should be monitored and the dosage adjusted accordingly. The following guidelines are recommended for patients with renal impairment (Kerkering, 1982): For those with creatinine clearances of 20 to 40 ml/min, the dosing interval is doubled or the dose is halved; for those with creatinine clearances of 10 to 20 ml/min, the interval is quadrupled or the dose is reduced fourfold. Patients undergoing hemodialysis should receive 37.5 mg/kg after each hemodialysis, and those on continuous peritoneal dialysis should receive a single daily dose of 37.5 mg/kg.

The desired peak blood level, usually measured two hours after oral administration, is 50 to 100 mcg/ml. Blood levels over 100 mcg/ml are not recommended because adverse reactions are more common.

Ancobon (Roche). Capsules 250 and 500 mg.

KETOCONAZOLE
[Nizoral]

ACTIONS. Ketoconazole is an antifungal imidazole (Restrepo et al, 1980; Heel et al, 1982; Levine, 1982; Graybill, 1983; Hume and Kerkering, 1983; Smith and Henry, 1984; Van Tyle, 1984). Like other imidazoles (clotrimazole, econazole, and miconazole), ketoconazole inhibits the cytochrome system that causes the 14-demethylation of lanosterol, the precursor of ergosterol, and thus interferes with ergosterol synthesis. This effect alters the permeability of the fungal cell membrane (Petersen et al, 1980; Beggs et al, 1981; Smith and Henry,

1984). High concentrations are required to inhibit the biosynthesis of cholesterol in mammals. Since yeast forms of *Candida albicans* are more susceptible to phagocytosis by leukocytes than are pseudohyphae, an additional action of the drug in *Candida* may be inhibition of the transformation of yeast to hyphal forms (Smith and Henry, 1984).

Ketoconazole is most active during active fungal growth. The effect is fungistatic, since fungicidal concentrations are not achieved with usual therapeutic doses. Consequently, cures are uncommon and relapse rates are high if adequate therapy is not given for a sufficient length of time.

USES. *Candidiasis:* Ketoconazole is the drug of choice for chronic mucocutaneous candidiasis, but it must be given for prolonged periods to avoid relapse (Graybill et al, 1980; Petersen et al, 1980; Jorizzo, 1982). Patients with disseminated disease often respond poorly and its usefulness in this form remains controversial; amphotericin B alone or with flucytosine remains the therapy of choice.

Paracoccidioidomycosis: Because it is especially effective in this infection, ketoconazole is preferred in mild to moderate disease; amphotericin B is preferred in severe, life-threatening disease.

Blastomycosis and Histoplasmosis: Ketoconazole is usually effective against all clinical forms of blastomycosis and histoplasmosis at daily doses of 400 to 800 mg; therefore, it is an alternative drug to amphotericin B and may be preferred except in patients with severe involvement or meningitis.

Coccidioidomycosis: Ketoconazole has some effect in nonmeningeal coccidioidomycosis (Catanzaro et al, 1982; Ross et al, 1982), but amphotericin B is preferred, especially when involvement is severe. The use of large oral doses of ketoconazole (1.2 g/day) to improve penetration into cerebrospinal fluid in patients with coccidioidal meningitis is investigational (Craven et al, 1983).

Cryptococcosis: Ketoconazole has been effective in a limited number of patients with nonmeningeal cryptococcosis. Experience is too limited to permit a recommendation at this time.

Chromomycosis: Although oral flucytosine alone or with amphotericin B is the therapy of choice, ketoconazole may improve (but seldom cures) this mycosis.

Sporotrichosis (Investigational): Limited studies suggest that ketoconazole is only marginally effective in cutaneous-lymphatic sporotrichosis; potassium iodide is the drug of choice. Amphotericin B remains the drug of choice for disseminated sporotrichosis.

Miscellaneous: Patients with *aspergillosis* and *mucormycosis* seldom respond to ketoconazole; amphotericin B is the drug of choice. No agent is effective in *mycetoma* caused by *Eumycetoma*. Ketoconazole is reported to be effective in some patients with *pseudallescheriasis* (Galgiani et al, 1984).

Dermatophytic and Superficial Candidal Infections (Investigational): A topical cream preparation of ketoconazole has been approved recently for use in superficial mycoses; oral use of this drug in superficial mycoses is investigational. Because of ketoconazole's potential for adverse reactions, it should be reserved for superficial cutaneous fungal infections that do not respond to conventional topical antifungal agents

or an established orally effective agent (ie, griseofulvin). (See Chapter 74, Topical Anti-infective Agents: Drugs Used on Skin and Mucous Membranes.)

Prostatic Carcinoma (Investigational): Ketoconazole suppresses the gonadal synthesis of testosterone and the adrenal synthesis of related androgens (Santen et al, 1983; Pont et al, 1984); therefore, the drug is being investigated in patients with prostatic carcinoma who are resistant to conventional therapy.

Hyperadrenalism (Investigational): Because daily doses of 600 to 800 mg inhibit adrenal steroidogenesis and may displace glucocorticoid from binding sites, ketoconazole is being investigated in Cushing's disease, hyperadrenalism secondary to adrenal rest tumor (Contreras et al, 1985), and small-cell lung carcinoma producing corticotropin (Angeli and Frairia, 1985; Shepherd et al, 1985; Stevens, 1985).

RESISTANCE. Resistance has been encountered only rarely in normally susceptible species. Efficacy cannot be predicted on the basis of in vitro susceptibility tests.

ADVERSE REACTIONS AND PRECAUTIONS. Nausea is dose related and occurs in about 17% of patients receiving 400 mg daily; headache, pruritus, dysfunctional uterine bleeding, dizziness, abdominal pain, constipation, diarrhea, somnolence, and nervousness have been reported less frequently (Dismukes et al, 1985).

The drug elevates hepatic enzyme levels temporarily in 2% to 5% of patients but they remain asymptomatic. Abrupt onset of hepatic injury resembling viral hepatitis occurs in about 1 in 12,000 patients and appears to be idiosyncratic. Fatalities have been reported in a few individuals who developed hepatic necrosis (Smith and Henry, 1984). Appropriate periodic monitoring of liver function is recommended. If values of liver function tests rise significantly or other signs and symptoms suggest hepatocellular dysfunction, ketoconazole should be discontinued.

Gynecomastia, infertility, decreased libido, or oligospermia occur in some males. The effect is dose dependent and is most likely to develop when doses exceed 600 mg/day. Ketoconazole suppresses the activity of cytochrome P450. Since testosterone synthesis is dependent on that enzyme, gonadal testosterone and adrenal androgen synthesis are inhibited (Pont et al, 1984; Santen et al, 1983). Doses of 600 to 800 mg/day may inhibit adrenal steroidogenesis, and reversible hypoadrenalism has been observed rarely (Tucker et al, 1985).

Doses of 80 mg/kg/day have caused syndactyly and oligodactyly in the offspring of rats. Data are insufficient to evaluate safety in pregnant women; therefore, ketoconazole should not be used during pregnancy unless the potential benefit justifies the risk to the fetus (FDA Pregnancy Category C). The drug is present in breast milk.

DRUG INTERACTIONS. Ketoconazole is reported to increase cyclosporine blood concentrations resulting in nephrotoxicity and increasing the serum creatinine concentration. The mechanism of this interaction is unknown; however, ketoconazole is known to inhibit some subsets of cytochrome P450 drug metabolizing enzymes (Brown et al, 1985).

Ketoconazole increased the prothrombin time in a few patients receiving coumarin derivatives (Smith, 1984). Cimetidine and probably ranitidine markedly decrease ketoconazole blood concentrations.

Rifampin administered with ketoconazole decreased anticipated serum ketoconazole concentrations; when this drug is administered with ketoconazole, therapeutic concentrations of ketoconazole may not be obtainable (Engelhard et al, 1984).

PHARMACOKINETICS

Absorption: Approximately one to two hours after a single 200-mg dose, the serum concentration is 1.6 to 6.9 mcg/ml and can be maintained with a single daily dose. Metabolic enzyme induction probably does not occur.

Higher serum levels are achieved if the drug is given without food. The absence of hydrochloric acid will lead to poor absorption of ketoconazole; therefore, especially in the elderly, it is advisable to rule out achlorhydria before ketoconazole is given. Since bioavailability depends upon gastric acidity, antacids, anticholinergic agents, and H_2 blocking agents (eg, cimetidine, ranitidine) should be avoided. Antacids may not interfere with absorption if they are given no less than two hours after ketoconazole.

Metabolism: Extensive hepatic degradation by microsomal enzymes occurs, and little active drug is excreted in the bile. Only 2% to 4% of a dose is eliminated unchanged in the urine.

Distribution: Ketoconazole is 95% to 97% bound to plasma proteins, principally albumin. Concentrations in the cerebrospinal fluid are only 1% to 4% of those in the serum at usual therapeutic doses. Only negligible concentrations occur in the peritoneal fluid of patients undergoing peritoneal dialysis.

Elimination: An initial half-life of one to four hours is probably more meaningful than the beta terminal half-life of 6 to 10 hours in view of the low serum concentrations associated with the longer half-life (Daneshmend and Warnock, 1983).

DOSAGE AND PREPARATIONS. The most effective dose and duration of therapy must be determined in each individual.

Oral: Adults, the usual initial dose is 400 mg daily for deep or systemic infection, increased to 600 to 800 mg daily if necessary. The minimum duration of therapy is six months. The high incidence of relapse or failure in some deep mycoses, such as coccidioidomycosis, has led to use of larger doses (up to 1.6 g) and longer courses of treatment (Dismukes et al, 1983; Hoeprich, 1983 B; Goodpasture et al, 1985), but large doses are often poorly tolerated. Chronic mucocutaneous candidiasis requires continuous maintenance therapy.

Children over 2 years, 3.3 mg/kg once daily; for deep infections, at least 6.6 mg/kg once daily for a minimum of six months.

Nizoral (Janssen). Tablets 200 mg.

MICONAZOLE NITRATE

[Monistat i.v.]

ACTIONS. Miconazole is a synthetic antifungal agent of the imidazole group that includes clotrimazole, econazole, and ketoconazole (Heel et al, 1980; Stevens, 1982; Stranz, 1980). Its fungistatic actions are similar to those of ketoconazole; it inhibits ergosterol synthesis, which alters the permeability of the fungal cell membrane (Beggs et al, 1981). Other actions also have been described (Beggs, 1984; Stevens, 1982).

USES. Although miconazole is occasionally regarded as an alternative to amphotericin B in the treatment of disseminated coccidioidomycosis, ketoconazole is much preferred as the drug of second choice. Miconazole has been effective in coccidioidomycosis not responsive to amphotericin B (Stevens, 1983); controlled studies are needed to clarify the role of miconazole in this disease.

Although miconazole is active in vitro against the organisms causing blastomycosis and histoplasmosis, the clinical effect is too variable to recommend its use. Organisms causing aspergillosis and mucormycosis are naturally resistant; otherwise, resistance has not been observed.

Miconazole is widely used topically for dermatophytic and candidal infections (see Chapter 74, Topical Anti-infective Agents: Drugs Used on Skin and Mucous Membranes).

ADVERSE REACTIONS AND PRECAUTIONS. Thrombophlebitis, thrombocytosis, pruritus, nausea, and anorexia are most common. Thrombophlebitis is not relieved by in-line filters, corticosteroids, bicarbonate, or heparin infusion; miconazole itself or an additive probably is responsible. Rotation of the infusion site every 48 to 72 hours is recommended. Rash, hyponatremia (probably caused by inappropriate secretion of antidiuretic hormone [SIADH]), and anemia also occur frequently.

Tachypnea, tachycardia, and ventricular tachycardia can be minimized by giving the infusion over a period of 60 to 120 minutes in a volume of at least 200 ml. Elevation of plasma triglycerides and cholesterol is common, and is caused by the vehicle, polyethoxylated castor oil. Neurologic disturbances (acute toxic psychoses, hallucinations, confusion, hyperesthesia, and anxiety) occur occasionally. Anaphylaxis has been reported. Erythrocyte aggregation (rouleaux formation) is noted commonly in blood smears.

Miconazole, like ketoconazole, is a potent inhibitor of hepatic cytochrome P450 drug metabolizing enzymes. This action is reported to be responsible for the prolonged prothrombin time seen in occasional patients receiving both miconazole and phenytoin (Rolan et al, 1983).

Miconazole is not teratogenic in rats or rabbits; however, clinical data are insufficient to determine the drug's safety during pregnancy.

PHARMACOKINETICS. The oral bioavailability of miconazole is about 25%; however, no oral preparation is available. Serum concentrations peak at 7.5 to 10 mcg/ml after intravenous doses of 1 g. Because fungistatic concentrations are not attained in urine, the drug must be given by catheter into the bladder for urinary fungal infections.

Miconazole is present to a variable extent (approximately 3% of the serum concentration) in the cerebrospinal fluid; therefore, intrathecal administration has been tried in fungal meningitis because intravenous therapy appears to be ineffective.

Miconazole is extensively metabolized in the liver, principally to inactive metabolites. An initial half-life of 20 to 30 minutes is followed by an intermediate half-life of one hour. The terminal beta half-life is about 20 hours and is not influenced by renal impairment (Daneshmend and Warnock, 1983); however, the drug must be given every eight hours. Miconazole is 91% to 93% bound to serum protein.

DOSAGE AND PREPARATIONS.

Intravenous: Adults, the dosage range depends upon the mycosis: for paracoccidioidomycosis, 200 mg to 1.2 g/day; for coccidioidomycosis, 1.8 to 3.6 g/day. The daily dose is divided into two or three infusions containing the appropriate fractional dose diluted in 200 ml of 0.9% sodium chloride or 5% dextrose solution and is infused over a period of 60 to 120 minutes. Therapy generally should be continued until the patient has recovered or the lesions have stabilized (usually 2 to 20 weeks).

Children, the total daily dose is 20 to 40 mg/kg and no single infusion should exceed 15 mg/kg.

Monistat i.v. (Janssen). Solution (sterile) 10 mg/ml in 20 ml containers.

POTASSIUM IODIDE

Potassium iodide is the drug of choice for cutaneous-lymphatic sporotrichosis. Local heat may be tried adjunctively or in patients allergic to iodides. Amphotericin B is the drug of choice for the extracutaneous and disseminated forms of the disease.

If symptoms of toxicity (brassy taste, heartburn, nausea, rhinitis, coryza, salivation, lacrimation, sneezing, burning of mouth and throat, ocular irritation, sialadenitis, and pustular acne over the cape area of the chest) become incapacitating, the dosage may require reduction.

DOSAGE AND PREPARATIONS.

Oral: Initially, 1 ml of a saturated solution (1 g/ml) is given three times daily; the amount is increased by 1 ml daily, depending upon tolerance, to a maximal daily dose of 12 to 15 ml. Cure requires at least six to eight weeks, and therapy should be continued for a minimum of four weeks after the disappearance or stabilization of the lesions.

Generic. Solution (saturated) 1 g/ml.

Cited References

Drugs for treatment of systemic fungal infections. *Med Lett Drugs Ther* 24:36-38, 1982.

American Thoracic Society: Treatment of fungal diseases. *Am Rev Respir Dis* 120:1393-1397, 1979.

Angeli A, Frairia R: Ketoconazole therapy in Cushing's disease, (letter). *Lancet* 1:821-822, 1985.

Beggs WH: Growth phase in relation to ketoconazole and miconazole susceptibilities of Candida albicans. *Antimicrob Agents Chemother* 25:316-318, 1984.

Beggs WH, et al: Action of imidazole-containing antifungal drugs. *Life Sci* 28:111-118, 1981.

Bennett JE, et al: Comparison of amphotericin B alone and combined with flucytosine in treatment of cryptococcal meningitis. *N Engl J Med* 301:126-131, 1979.

Bodey GP: Candidiasis in cancer patients. *Am J Med* 77(4D):13-19, 1984.

Brown MW, et al: Effect of ketoconazole on hepatic oxidative drug metabolism. *Clin Pharmacol Ther* 37:290-297, 1985.

Catanzaro A, et al: Ketoconazole for treatment of disseminated coccidioidomycosis. *Ann Intern Med* 96:436-440, 1982.

Cohen J: Empirical therapy in neutropenic patients. *J Antimicrob Chemother* 13:409-411, 1984.

Contreras P, et al: Adrenal rest tumor of liver causing Cushing's syndrome: Treatment with ketoconazole preceding apparent surgical cure. *J Clin Endocrinol Metab* 60:21-28, 1985.

Craven PC, et al: High-dose ketoconazole for treatment of fungal infections of central nervous system. *Ann Intern Med* 98:160-167, 1983.

Daneshmend TK, Warnock DW: Clinical pharmacokinetics of systemic antifungal drugs. *Clin Pharmakokinet* 8:17-42, 1983.

Dismukes WE, et al: Treatment of systemic mycoses with ketoconazole: Emphasis on toxicity and clinical response in 52 patients. *Ann Intern Med* 98:13-20, 1983.

Dismukes WE, et al: Comparison of two different treatment regimens of flucytosine and amphotericin B in cryptococcal meningitis, (abstract). *Program and Abstracts of the 24th Interscience Conference on Antimicrobial Agents and Chemotherapy.* Washington, DC, Oct 8-10, 1984, 286.

Dismukes WE, et al: Treatment of blastomycosis and histoplasmosis with ketoconazole: Results of prospective randomized clinical trial. *Ann Intern Med* 103:861-872, 1985.

Engelhard D, et al: Interaction of ketoconazole with rifampin and isoniazid. *N Engl J Med* 311:1681-1683, 1984.

Galgiani JN, et al: *Pseudallescheria boydii* infections treated with ketoconazole. *Chest* 86:219-224, 1984.

Goodpasture HC, et al: Treatment of central nervous system fungal infection with ketoconazole. *Arch Intern Med* 145:879-880, 1985.

Graybill JR (ed): Symposium on new developments in therapy for the mycoses. *Am J Med* 74(1B):1-90, 1983.

Graybill JR, Craven PC: Antifungal agents used in systemic mycoses: Activity and therapeutic use. *Drugs* 25:41-62, 1983.

Graybill JR, et al: Ketoconazole treatment of chronic mucocutaneous candidiasis. *Arch Dermatol* 116:1137-1141, 1980.

Hawkins CC, Armstrong D: Opportunistic organisms in the immunocompromised. *Consultant* 25:93-127, (May) 1985.

Heel RC, et al: Miconazole: Preliminary review of therapeutic efficacy in systemic fungal infections. *Drugs* 19:7-30, 1980.

Heel RC, et al: Ketoconazole: Review of therapeutic efficacy in superficial and systemic fungal infections. *Drugs* 23:1-36, 1982.

Heidemann HT, et al: Amphotericin B nephrotoxicity in humans decreased by salt repletion. *Am J Med* 75:476-481, 1983.

Hermans PE, Keys TF: Antifungal agents used for deep-seated mycotic infections. *Mayo Clin Pract* 58:223-231, 1983.

Hoeprich PD (ed): *Infectious Diseases: A Modern Treatise of Infectious Processes*, ed 3. Philadelphia, JB Lippincott, 1983 A.

Hoeprich PD: Ketoconazole in systemic mycoses, (editorial). *Ann Intern Med* 98:105, 1983 B.

Hume AL, Kerkering TM: Ketoconazole. *Drug Intell Clin Pharm* 17:169-174, 1983.

Humphrey MJ, et al: Pharmacokinetic evaluation of UK-49,858, metabolically stable thiazole antifungal drug, in animals and humans. *Antimicrob Agents Chemother* 28:648-653, 1985.

Jorizzo JL: Chronic mucocutaneous candidosis: Update, (editorial). *Arch Dermatol* 118:963-965, 1982.

Kerkering TM: Present status of flucytosine therapy. *Drug Ther* 12:75-79, 1982.

Levine HB (ed): *Ketoconazole in the Management of Fungal Disease.* New York, ADIS Press, 1982.

Mahgoub ES: Mycetoma. *Semin Dermatol* 4:230-239, 1985.

Mandell GL, et al (eds): Mycoses, in: *Principles and Practice of Infectious Diseases*, ed 2. New York, John Wiley & Sons, 1985, 1434-1504.

Medoff G, Kobayashi GS: Strategies in treatment of systemic fungal infections. *N Engl J Med* 302:145-155, 1980.

Meunier-Carpentier F: Chemoprophylaxis of fungal infections. *Am J Med* 76:652-656, 1984.

Penn RL, et al: Invasive fungal infections: Use of serologic tests in diagnosis and management. *Arch Intern Med* 143:1215-1220, 1983.

Petersen EA, et al: Treatment of chronic mucocutaneous candidiasis with ketoconazole. *Ann Intern Med* 93:791-795, 1980.

Pizzo PA, et al: Empiric antibiotic and antifungal therapy for cancer patients with prolonged fever and granulocytopenia. *Am J Med* 72:101-110, 1982.

Pont A, et al: High-dose ketoconazole therapy and adrenal and testicular function in humans. *Arch Intern Med* 144:2150-2153, 1984.

Restrepo A, et al (eds): First international symposium on ketoconazole. *Rev Infect Dis* 2:519-699, (July-Aug) 1980.

Rolan PE, et al: Phenytoin intoxication during treatment with parenteral miconazole. *Br Med J* 287:1760, 1983.

Ross JB, et al: Ketoconazole for treatment of chronic pulmonary coccidioidomycosis. *Ann Intern Med* 96:440-443, 1982.

Santen RJ, et al: Site of action of low dose ketoconazole on androgen biosynthesis in men. *Clin Endocrinol Metab* 57:732-736, 1983.

Schaffner A, Frick PG: Effect of ketoconazole on amphotericin B in model of disseminated aspergillosis. *J Infect Dis* 151:902-910, 1985.

Shepherd FA, et al: Ketoconazole: Use in treatment of ectopic adrenocorticotropic hormone production and Cushing's syndrome in small-cell lung cancer. *Arch Intern Med* 145:863-864, 1985.

Smego RA Jr, et al: Combined therapy with amphotericin B and 5-fluorocytosine for *Candida meningitis*. *Rev Infect Dis* 6:791-801, 1984.

Smith AG: Potentiation of oral anticoagulants by ketoconazole. *Br Med J* 288:188-189, 1984.

Smith EB, Henry JC: Ketoconazole: Orally effective antifungal agent: Mechanism of action, pharmacology, clinical efficacy and adverse effects. *Pharmacotherapy* 4:199-204, 1984.

Stevens DA: Current perspectives on miconazole. *Drug Ther* 12:85-92, 1982.

Stevens DA: Miconazole in treatment of coccidioidomycosis. *Drugs* 26:347-354, 1983.

Stevens DA: Ketoconazole metamorphosis: Antimicrobial becomes endocrine drug, (editorial). *Arch Intern Med* 145:813-815, 1985.

Stranz MH: Miconazole. *Drug Intell Clin Pharm* 14:86-95, 1980.

Tucker WS Jr, et al: Reversible adrenal insufficiency induced by ketoconazole. *JAMA* 253:2413-2414, 1985.

Van Cutsem J, et al: Itraconazole, new triazole that is orally active in aspergillosis. *Antimicrob Agents Chemother* 26:527-534, 1985.

Van Tyle JH: Ketoconazole: Mechanism of action, spectrum of activity, pharmacokinetics, drug interactions, adverse reactions and therapeutic use. *Pharmacotherapy* 4:343-373, 1984.

Wheat LJ, et al: Histoplasmosis in acquired immune deficiency syndrome. *Am J Med* 78:203-210, 1985.

The advent of jet flight, the involvement of American military forces in many parts of the world, and the increased immigration of people into the United States from Africa, Asia, and South America have increased the probability that a physician in the United States will be asked to diagnose and treat a parasitic disease.

All four classes of protozoa include pathogenic organisms: The *Sarcodina* (eg, *Entamoeba histolytica*) cause amebic disease. The *Mastigophora* (flagellates) produce dientamebiasis, giardiasis (lambliasis), leishmaniasis, trichomoniasis, and trypanosomiasis. The *Ciliophora* (ciliates) include at least one organism, *Balantidium coli*, that produces disease (balantidiasis). The *Sporozoa* cause malaria, toxoplasmosis, pneumocystosis, and coccidiosis (isosporiasis and cryptosporidiosis).

Therapy for protozoal infections presents a number of difficulties not usually encountered in other infections or parasitic diseases and there are no effective immunization proce-

dures. Chemotherapy often is less than ideal, frequently is toxic, and almost always is too expensive for single-patient use in developing countries with limited resources. Programs of mass chemotherapy have had only limited success. More effective measures include control of the insect vector (when one exists), elimination of the reservoir of infection, and improvement of sanitation and living conditions. Unfortunately, the people at risk are spread over large, sometimes inaccessible areas and often cannot comply with instructions given by a physician or health worker. Moreover, they are frequently infected with several organisms, which makes diagnosis, therapy, and follow-up complex. Even when individual cures are effected, the patient returns to an environment where reinfection is almost a certainty.

Drugs noted as being available from the Centers for Disease Control may be obtained by contacting the Drug Service, Centers for Disease Control, 1600 Clifton Road, Bldg 6, Room

161, Atlanta, GA 30333. During regular business hours (8 AM to 4:30 PM), the telephone number is (404) 329-3670; the emergency number is (404) 329-2888.

AMEBIASIS

Infection with *Entamoeba histolytica* causes intermittent amebiasis in millions of people worldwide, including 2% to 5% of the population in the United States. The prevalence rate among homosexuals is 25% to 32% in this country, although invasive amebiasis does not appear to have increased proportionately.

Amebiasis is transmitted when mature cysts are ingested (Harries, 1982; McGowan, 1984) or introduced by colonic irrigation. Each cyst develops into eight trophozoites, usually in the ileocecal region of the intestine. A colony is established in the cecum and later extends throughout the colon.

Trophozoites penetrate the mucosa and cause ulceration of the intestinal wall that may simulate ulcerative colitis. Diarrhea and abdominal pain are common in those with invasive disease, although most individuals remain asymptomatic while transmitting amebae by passing mature cysts in formed stools. *E. histolytica* occasionally invades the liver, where it may cause abscesses. Amebic abscesses rarely occur in other organs.

Definitive diagnosis is based on finding the organism in fresh or preserved stool specimens; serologic tests may aid in screening for invasive disease. The indirect hemagglutinin test is highly specific and is most commonly used, especially in those with liver involvement or severe colonic disease. Enzyme-linked immunosorbent assay (ELISA) and fluorescent serum antibody test are less specific but very sensitive. Strains of *E. histolytica* vary in virulence. Some investigators speculate that virulence is due to elaboration of proteinase cytotoxins (Lushbaugh et al, 1984), release of serotonin (McGowan et al, 1983), and/or contact-dependent cytotoxicity (Ravdin and Guerrant, 1982); however, these are not completely reliable markers for assessing the severity of human disease.

Classification of Amebicides: Some drugs act upon amebae only within the lumen of the bowel, whereas others affect the parasite in the intestinal wall or other organs. A few drugs act at more than one site.

Diloxanide (investigational) and iodoquinol (diiodohydroxyquin) [Yodoxin] act in the intestinal lumen. These agents and the antibiotic, paromomycin [Humatin], are termed oral luminal or contact amebicides.

Emetine; its analogue, dehydroemetine [Mebadin], which is as effective as emetine and probably less toxic; and chloroquine [Aralen] are tissue amebicides. The emetines are given parenterally and affect amebae in the intestinal wall and liver. Chloroquine is given orally and acts principally in the liver. It is appreciably less effective than the emetines but also is less toxic. It is not indicated for intestinal infection. Chloroquine alone probably is inadequate for amebic abscess but can be combined with iodoquinol and the emetines.

Metronidazole [Flagyl, Protostat] has a relatively low toxic potential and is highly effective against amebae. Although it is effective in the colonic lumen, its actions are most pronounced in tissue because most of the compound is absorbed during passage through the small intestine. For this reason, metronidazole often is classified as a tissue amebicide, and a luminal amebicide, most commonly iodoquinol, must be given after its administration to eradicate organisms in the intestine and avoid relapse.

Tetracycline and oxytetracycline act indirectly in the intestinal lumen and wall by modifying the flora necessary for survival of amebae. These antibiotics are not effective alone in amebiasis but may be used as adjuncts. Paromomycin may be effective alone in asymptomatic cyst passers as a luminal amebicide or following use of metronidazole or the emetines.

Other nitroimidazoles (tinidazole, ornidazole, and secnidazole) related to metronidazole but with appreciably longer half-lives are being investigated for use in amebiasis (Rossignol et al, 1984). The luminal amebicide, quinfamide (a dichloroacetyl quinolol derivative), also is in clinical trial (Guevara et al, 1983).

Drug Selection: The choice of amebicide(s) depends principally upon the severity of disease and site of involvement (luminal or extraintestinal); other factors influencing drug selection are pregnancy (eg, avoidance of metronidazole and tetracycline), drug allergy, or tolerance. Adverse reactions, precautions, and/or interactions should be reviewed before drug selection is finalized.

Chronic, nondysenteric, asymptomatic amebiasis (cyst carrier state) is treated with a luminal amebicide. The drug of choice is iodoquinol; paromomycin and diloxanide (available only from the CDC) are suitable alternatives. Because the asymptomatic cyst passer is not treated in endemic areas and because metronidazole is less effective as a luminal amebicide than as a tissue amebicide, this agent is not generally recommended to treat asymptomatic amebiasis.

In intestinal amebiasis, *E. histolytica* are present in the intestinal lumen, on the mucosal surface of the bowel, and in the walls of the intestine. Metronidazole is a drug of choice in combination with iodoquinol for mild to moderate disease. If metronidazole is not tolerated or is contraindicated, a tetracycline or paromomycin may be given with iodoquinol.

For severe disease, emetine or dehydroemetine with iodoquinol is an alternative regimen to metronidazole with iodoquinol. A tetracycline plus iodoquinol may be useful when metronidazole or the emetines are not effective, not tolerated, or contraindicated.

Abscesses can be treated with metronidazole. A luminal amebicide, usually iodoquinol, also is indicated to eliminate the primary source of infection and prevent relapses. Alternative therapy consists of emetine or dehydroemetine and iodoquinol with or without chloroquine. Liver abscesses may require drainage depending on the size and response to therapy; closed aspiration is preferred when there is a palpable mass (especially when the left lobe impinges on the diaphragm with potential pericardial involvement), persistent local tenderness, or markedly raised hemidiaphragm (Basile et al, 1983; Thompson et al, 1985). Ultrasound or computerized axial tomography is useful to locate the abscesses. Liver abscesses sometimes rupture into the lungs, pleura, pericardium, or peritoneum.

These complications are treated by drainage and administration of the same regimen used for hepatic amebiasis.

Complications of intestinal amebiasis include ameboma (a tumor-like mass of granulomatous tissue in the intestinal wall) and stricture, peritonitis, or intussusception. These conditions are treated with metronidazole alone or with emetine or dehydroemetine, a luminal amebicide, and a tetracycline. Intussusception must be reduced surgically during therapy. Peritonitis is a serious complication. Ulcerative postdysenteric colitis may respond to maintenance of an adequate fluid and electrolyte balance, blood transfusion, and a high-calorie diet. Sulfasalazine [Azulfidine] has been administered, but its effectiveness is unpredictable.

Dosage recommendations appear in the evaluations and Table 1.

Adverse Reactions and Precautions: All amebicidal drugs may cause gastrointestinal disturbances (eg, anorexia, nausea and vomiting, epigastric burning and pain, increased gastrointestinal motility, diarrhea, constipation) and fungal superinfections with prolonged use. Diloxanide often produces excessive flatulence.

Iodoquinol is related to clioquinol (iodochlorhydroxyquin), which has caused subacute myelo-optic neuropathy (SMON). Although iodoquinol has not produced this phenomenon when recommended doses were used to treat intestinal amebiasis, the maximum recommended dose should not be exceeded. Iodoquinol is contraindicated in patients who cannot tolerate iodine, and it interferes with certain thyroid function tests; therefore, it is contraindicated in patients with thyroid disorders.

For a more detailed discussion of adverse reactions, precautions, and contraindications, see the evaluations.

BALANTIDIASIS

Balantidiasis is caused by the ciliate protozoan, *Balantidium coli*, which infects the terminal ileum and cecum of the large intestine. Pigs may be reservoirs of infection and people who handle these animals may become infected from ingestion of the cyst form. However, the disease also is transmitted by man. The incidence of human balantidiasis is low and many individuals are asymptomatic, although diarrhea and abdominal pain may occur. In severe infections, a dysenteric syndrome similar to that observed in amebiasis develops.

Balantidiasis is treated with tetracycline. Iodoquinol and metronidazole are being investigated for use in this infection.

COCCIDIOSIS

Cryptosporidiosis: *Cryptosporidium*, an intracellular coccidian parasite similar to *Isospora belli*, commonly produces mild, self-limited diarrhea of two to four weeks' duration and a mild flu-like state in immunocompetent persons (Wolfson et al, 1985); an asymptomatic carrier phase also occurs. In immunocompromised individuals, especially those with acquired immunodeficiency syndrome, severe chronic diarrhea characterized by watery (cholera-like) or frothy nonbloody stools develops. Nausea, weakness, low-grade fever, anorexia, and severe abdominal cramps also are present. Biliary (Pitlik et al, 1983) and respiratory (Forgacs et al, 1983) symptoms are noted in a small percentage of patients with severe infection. Definitive diagnosis is based on signs, symptoms, and identification of oocysts in stool specimens.

The organism produces a similar infection in many animals,

TABLE 1.
RECOMMENDED THERAPY FOR AMEBIASIS*

Type of Infection	Therapy of Choice	Alternate Therapy
Asymptomatic (cyst carrier state)	Iodoquinol[1]	Diloxanide Furoate[2] or Paromomycin[3]
Mild to moderate intestinal disease	Metronidazole[5] followed by Iodoquinol[1]	Paromomycin[3] or Tetracycline[4] followed by Iodoquinol[1]
Severe intestinal disease	Metronidazole[5] followed by Iodoquinol[1]	Dehydroemetine[6] or Emetine[7] followed by Iodoquinol[1]
Tissue abscess (usually hepatic)	Metronidazole[5] followed by Iodoquinol[1]	Dehydroemetine[6] or Emetine[7] followed by Iodoquinol[1] with or without Chloroquine Phosphate[8]

*Except for emetine and dehydroemetine, all drugs are given orally.

[1]Adults, 650 mg three times daily for 20 days. Children, 30 to 40 mg/kg/day in two or three doses for 20 days (maximum, 2 g/day).

[2]Adults, 500 mg three times daily for 20 days. Children, 20 mg/kg/day in three doses for 10 days.

[3]Adults and children, 25 to 35 mg/kg/day in three doses for 7 to 10 days.

[4]Adults, 250 to 500 mg four times daily for 10 days. Children, 10 mg/kg (maximum, 600 mg) four times daily for 10 days.

[5]Adults, 750 mg three times daily for 5 to 10 days. Children, 35 to 50 mg/kg/day in three doses for 10 days.

[6]Adults, 1 to 1.5 mg/kg/day (maximum, 90 mg/day) for five days. Children, no more than 1 to 1.5 mg/kg/day in two doses for five days.

[7]Adults, 1 mg/kg/day (maximum, 60 mg/day) for five days. Children, no more than 0.5 mg/kg twice daily for five days.

[8]Adults, 1 g (600 mg base) daily for two days, then 500 mg (300 mg base) daily for two to three weeks. Children, 10 mg (base)/kg/day for 21 days (maximum, 300 mg (base)/day).

but does not appear to be to species-specific (Angus, 1983). Spread of the disease may occur through contact with pets, farm animals, and certain wild animals. Like giardiasis, *Cryptosporidium* has caused diarrhea in day-care centers (*Morbid Mortal Week Rep*, [Oct 26] 1984; Taylor et al, 1985).

Supportive therapy is usually adequate in immunocompetent patients. Moderate to severe diarrhea in immunocompromised patients is very resistant to therapy, and many anti-infective agents are ineffective (Miller et al, 1983).

The investigational macrolide antibiotic, spiramycin, has an antimicrobial spectrum similar to that of erythromycin and clindamycin and has terminated or controlled diarrhea in some patients (Portnoy et al, 1984; *Morbid Mortal Week Rep*, [March 9] 1984).

Isosporiasis: This coccidiosis is caused by *Isospora belli*, a human intracellular parasite that is harbored in the gut after transmission by contact with contaminated human excreta. The infection usually resolves in two to four weeks without treatment. A subacute febrile syndrome, headache, anorexia, and gastrointestinal symptoms (nonbloody diarrhea, abdominal tenderness and distension) are characteristic.

Bismuth subsalicylate [Pepto-Bismol] has been somewhat effective in the symptomatic treatment of isosporiasis. Furazolidone [Furoxone], trimethoprim/sulfamethoxazole [Bactrim, Septra], and a combination of pyrimethamine and sulfadiazine have been used investigationally in persistent human infections.

DIENTAMEBIASIS

Dientamebiasis is caused by the parasite, *Dientamoeba fragilis*, which presently is classified as a flagellate (Millet et al, 1983). Many authorities believe it to cause chronic, mild, lower intestinal symptoms, including persistent diarrhea. No cyst form exists and the trophozoite is highly labile and easily overlooked unless stools are examined immediately or preserved for later examination. Dientamebiasis is often associated with enterobiasis; most investigators believe that the trophozoite is transmitted within the pinworm egg.

Tetracycline or iodoquinol is effective. The drugs may be given consecutively for persistent infections (Wolfe, 1982).

GIARDIASIS

The terms, giardiasis and lambliasis, refer to infection of the gastrointestinal tract by *Giardia lamblia*. The infection can be transmitted sexually, but contact with contaminated surfaces or water is most common. Man is the principal host and main source of infection. Recent evidence indicates that giardiasis also may be transmitted by wild animals (especially bears) and possibly dogs (Farthing and Keusch, 1982).

G. lamblia is the most common flagellate in the gastrointestinal tract of man worldwide and often infects individuals returning to the United States following foreign travel; young children are especially susceptible. Giardiasis has occurred in endemic form in the United States (prevalence rate, 2% to 10% in the general population and 6% to 18% in homosexu-

als); 20% to 50% of infected persons are asymptomatic. Day-care centers are a reservoir for infection (Pickering et al, 1984; Child Day Care Infectious Disease Study Group, 1985).

The motile trophozoite of *G. lamblia* attaches to the mucosa of the small intestine. Trophozoites occasionally are present in the bile ducts and gallbladder. Cysts, the usual infective stage, are passed in formed stools but trophozoites are passed by individuals with frank diarrhea.

Signs and Symptoms: Positive diagnosis requires identification of trophozoites or cysts in fresh or preserved stool specimens, or by biopsy of small intestine mucosa. A fluorescent antibody test may be useful in symptomatic patients with no other intestinal parasites (Wittner et al, 1983). Symptoms commonly include foul diarrhea (with or without episodes of constipation), abdominal distention, foul flatulence, foul belching, bloating, heartburn, nocturnal borborygmi, vomiting, colicky pain related to food ingestion, and profound malaise. Weight loss may be present. Lactose intolerance frequently accompanies giardiasis. Because vitamin A is poorly absorbed and steatorrhea may be present, the infection may resemble celiac syndrome or kwashiorkor. The pain associated with giardiasis may mimic that of appendicitis, cholelithiasis, ulcer, or hiatal hernia.

Chronic giardiasis may be more common than previously believed (Chester et al, 1985). Increased frequency of constipation and upper gastrointestinal complaints that persist for a mean duration of 3.3 years typify chronic compared to acute giardiasis (symptoms less than six months).

Environmental sanitation is essential to limit the spread of giardiasis, eg, personal hygiene, examination of household contacts. Guidelines are available for the prevention and management of outbreaks in day-care centers (Pickering et al, 1984; Child Day Care Infectious Disease Study Group, 1985).

Drug Selection: Quinacrine [Atabrine] is the drug of choice for severely affected adults who can tolerate it. Severe nausea and vomiting or other toxic effects may preclude its use.

Metronidazole is beginning to replace quinacrine in moderate giardiasis (investigational indication), because it has similar activity and usually is less toxic, especially in children. Other related nitroimidazoles (tinidazole, ornidazole, and secnidazole) have appreciably longer half-lives and are being investigated for giardiasis (Rossignol et al, 1984). Most experience has been accrued with tinidazole in the prophylaxis and treatment of anaerobic infections (Carmine et al, 1982). A single dose of tinidazole 1.5 or 2 g was as effective as two doses of metronidazole (Jokipii and Jokipii, 1982) and a single 2-g dose was more effective than a single 2.4-g dose of metronidazole (Speelman, 1985).

Furazolidone also is an effective antigiardial agent. Cure rates exceeding 90% with few relapses have been reported, but the drug has not been as widely used as quinacrine in the United States. Furazolidone is available as a suspension, and it is usually well tolerated by children; therefore, it is an alternative drug of choice in children. At least seven and preferably ten days of therapy are recommended (Murphy and Nelson, 1983).

Combined therapy with quinacrine and metronidazole should be considered in individuals who do not respond to repeated courses of single-drug therapy (Smith et al, 1982).

Because lactose intolerance often occurs, patients should be advised to avoid milk products during treatment and for several weeks afterward.

LEISHMANIASIS

This disease remains largely *tropical* and *subtropical* in distribution because it is transmitted by blood-sucking insect vectors indigenous to these areas (Chance, 1981; Pearson, 1984). The infection results from invasion of the reticuloendothelial cells by the intracellular amastigote form of *Leishmania*, which is transmitted to man by sandflies of the genus *Phlebotomus* (Old World) or *Lutzomyia* (New World) from a reservoir of organisms present in rodents or other small animals.

In man, visceral, mucocutaneous, or cutaneous infection ranges from mild and self-limiting to severe and fatal. Visceral leishmaniasis (kala-azar) is caused by *L. donovani*; it usually has a gradual onset and is characterized by fever, weight loss, hepatosplenomegaly with hepatic dysfunction, hypoalbuminemia, hypergammaglobulinemia, pancytopenia, hemorrhage, and lymphadenopathy. If untreated, it often is fatal. Mucocutaneous leishmaniasis (espundia) is caused by *L. braziliensis*. Several forms occur in South America. Marked disfiguration is due to progressive ulceration of mucous membranes in the mouth, palate, pharynx, and nose. Cutaneous leishmaniasis (oriental sore) is caused by *L. tropica* or *L. major* (Old World leishmaniasis) and *L. braziliensis*, *L. mexicana*, or *L. peruviana* (New World leishmaniasis) and occurs as far north as Texas (Nelson et al, 1985). A nodule develops at the point of the insect bite and may crust or ulcerate and is very slow to heal. *Leishmania* organisms usually can be identified in tissue samples or from cultures taken from the borders of the skin ulcerations.

Drug Selection: Few drugs are uniformly effective in leishmaniasis. The pentavalent antimonial compounds (eg, sodium stibogluconate [Pentostam], meglumine antimoniate) are used most commonly (Bell, 1981). The East African form of the disease is relatively resistant to the antimonials; Mediterranean, Indian, Chinese, and Brazilian forms are more susceptible. The diamidines (eg, pentamidine [Pentam 300], hydroxystilbamidine) and amphotericin B [Fungizone] may be suitable alternatives if the antimonial agents are not effective or cannot be tolerated (World Health Organization, 1984). Local application of heat has accelerated healing in oriental sore.

Rifampin [Rifadin, Rimactane], trimethoprim/sulfamethoxazole [Bactrim, Septra], and metronidazole have produced results in leishmaniasis, and it is unclear whether the beneficial effect is related solely to prevention or elimination of secondary infection (Nelson et al, 1985).

MALARIA

Worldwide, malaria is the most common cause of morbidity and mortality from infection (Wyler, 1983; Garnham, 1984). Diminution in spraying programs and emergence of insecticide-resistant strains of mosquitoes and drug-resistant strains of *Plasmodium falciparum* in many areas have resulted in resurgence of this disease. *P. falciparum* produces the highest mortality among all plasmodial species that affect man.

Almost all cases of malaria in the United States result from exposure abroad. The few indigenous cases are induced by accidental blood inoculation among drug addicts or transfusion of infected blood.

PARASITE LIFE CYCLE AND CLINICAL COURSE. The four species of *Plasmodium* that cause malaria in man are *P. falciparum*, *P. vivax*, *P. ovale*, and *P. malariae*. The human phase of the life cycle begins when an infected female anopheline mosquito bites the host and injects sporozoites from her salivary glands. The sporozoites enter the circulation and rapidly reach the liver where they invade cells, develop into primary tissue schizonts (the primary exoerythrocytic forms), and mature into tissue merozoites. This asymptomatic (prepatent) period lasts 8 to 21 days, depending on the species. This asexual multiplication is termed schizogony. At the end of the prepatent period, the merozoites of all species enter the blood stream, invade red cells, develop into trophozoites (blood schizonts), and begin the erythrocytic cycle of schizogony. The erythrocytic cycle ends when the infected red cells rupture, releasing parasites (that reinvade other red cells), pigments, and other products. The clinical attack of malaria (ie, chills, fever, profuse sweating) occurs at this time.

In individuals infected with *P. vivax* and presumably with *P. ovale*, dormant hepatic forms (hypnozoites) are released into the circulation at various times to cause clinical relapses (Krotoski, 1985). This does not occur with *P. falciparum* and *P. malariae*.

After several cycles, some erythrocytic parasites develop into gametocytes, the sexual forms of the organism. If the infected person is then bitten by a female anopheline mosquito and gametocytes enter the mosquito, the cycle from human host to vector is completed and the disease is perpetuated. The sexual stage of parasite reproduction occurs in the mosquito.

DIAGNOSIS. Definitive diagnosis of malaria is made on the basis of clinical history and the presence of parasites on thick or thin peripheral blood films. The classical cycles of malarial paroxysms take place when the maturation phase of erythrocytic parasites becomes synchronized, although this may not be observed until after several attacks have occurred. In falciparum malaria, cyclic fever may not occur at all.

CLASSIFICATION OF ANTIMALARIAL AGENTS. These agents are classified principally on the basis of their action against the plasmodial organism at different stages in its life cycle.

Clinical Cure: Drugs used to cure the clinical attack of malaria (drugs that eliminate the asexual forms of the parasite) are known as blood schizonticidal agents. These include chloroquine [Aralen], hydroxychloroquine [Plaquenil], pyrimethamine [Daraprim], pyrimethamine/sulfadoxine [Fansidar], quinine sulfate and dihydrochloride, and quinidine gluconate (investigational indication).

Individuals traveling to certain geographic areas may receive antimalarial drugs that are not available in the United States: Amodiaquine [Camoquin] is an alternative to chloroquine (see the evaluation). Chloroguanide (proguanil) is a short-acting blood schizonticide that acts as a dihydrofolate reductase inhibitor, but *P. falciparum* and *P. vivax* develop resistance quite rapidly. It is one of the safer antimalarial drugs, but because of its antifolate action, it is not recommended during pregnancy. The combination of pyrimethamine/dapsone [Maloprim] is less preferred than the combination of pyrimethamine/sulfadoxine, because dapsone may cause agranulocytosis.

The investigational agent, mefloquine, is a quinolinemethanol derivative of chloroquine and a long-acting blood schizonticide (Jiang et al, 1982; Li et al, 1984; Harinasuta et al, 1985). It is effective against most chloroquine-resistant strains of *P. falciparum*. Since a few strains of *P. falciparum* resistant to mefloquine have already been reported, it is likely that this drug will be used in combination with other antimalarial agents for prophylaxis (eg, mefloquine/pyrimethamine/sulfadoxine [Fansimef]) (Ellis and Chiodini, 1984). Another investigational agent, artemisinine (qinghaosu), is a novel sesquiterpene peroxide that acts rapidly as a blood schizonticide; it is effective in the treatment of chloroquine-resistant strains of *P. falciparum* (Klayman, 1985). Since the recrudescence rate is high, it also will probably be used only in combination with other antimalarial drugs for treatment.

Clinical Prophylaxis: Suppressive agents inhibit the erythrocytic stage of parasite development and thus prevent clinical attacks in what is known as clinical or field prophylaxis. All of the drugs used for clinical cure can be given for clinical prophylaxis. They are administered weekly one to two weeks before, during, and six to eight weeks after visiting a malarious area.

Radical Cure: In radical cure, all asexual blood forms and all residual exoerythrocytic forms are completely eliminated from the body. Radical cure may be difficult to confirm, however. In falciparum and malariae malaria, there are no persisting exoerythrocytic forms and elimination of blood forms achieves both clinical and radical cure. Radical cure of the other forms of malaria requires additional therapy to eliminate residual exoerythrocytic forms; the drug of choice is primaquine. Patients who have achieved radical cure may give blood for transfusion.

Untreated or inadequately treated patients who survive initial attacks become partially immune, especially those with *P. falciparum* infection. These individuals may experience recrudescences and can transmit malaria by blood transfusion. Immunity wanes over a few years and frequent re-exposure is required to maintain immunity. Immunity is suppressed by severe illness, surgery, pregnancy, or immunosuppressive drugs.

The natural duration of untreated nonlethal infection with *P. vivax*, *P. ovale*, and *P. falciparum* is one to four years, and patients are essentially cured after these intervals. Untreated *P. malariae* infections last for many years, although cure is just as readily achieved as with the other species.

Causal Prophylaxis: Causal prophylaxis implies elimination of exoerythrocytic parasites before they invade red cells. Primaquine is the only drug with such activity for all four human species of malaria. Proguanil and pyrimethamine are active against *P. falciparum* only.

MANAGEMENT. Patients with mild to moderate malaria require supportive therapy and chemotherapy. Bedrest, antipyretics (aspirin or related analgesics) and/or sponging with tepid water, and maintenance of adequate fluid and salt balance may be required during acute attacks.

Hypervolemia, increased capillary permeability, and hyponatremia are often associated with moderate to severe acute malaria and require cautious fluid replacement, including blood transfusion.

Falciparum infection in a nonimmune individual can be eliminated if appropriate antimalarial therapy is initiated before overwhelming parasitemia develops. Complications include hemolytic anemia, toxic encephalopathy with confusion or coma ("cerebral malaria"), hemoglobinuria with renal failure (blackwater fever), noncardiac pulmonary edema, or hypoglycemia (White et al, 1983 A) associated with marked hyperinsulinemia (especially during pregnancy and severe disease). Prompt ancillary measures to treat these complications may be useful (Peters and Hall, 1985); packed red cells, antipyretics, assisted ventilation, exchange transfusions, plasma volume expanders or low-molecular-weight dextran, diuresis with mannitol, or dialysis also may be necessary. Anticonvulsants may be required for seizures due to cerebral malaria. Dexamethasone is contraindicated in cerebral malaria.

DRUG SELECTION. ***Treatment:*** Drug selection for treatment of a clinical attack of malaria depends upon the area visited (ie, areas with or without known chloroquine-resistant falciparum malaria), the probability of persisting exoerythrocytic forms (ie, *P. vivax*, *P. ovale*), whether the patient is pregnant (Bruce-Chwatt, 1983), and the existence of drug allergy or intolerance. In addition, some antimalarial agents have different pharmacokinetic parameters (eg, loading dose requirement, long half-life) (White, 1985) and unique adverse reactions, precautions, and interactions that should be reviewed before drug selection is finalized.

Clinical cure of an acute attack of malaria caused by *P. vivax*, *P. ovale*, *P. malariae*, or chloroquine-sensitive strains of *P. falciparum* is readily accomplished with a three-day course of chloroquine phosphate. If oral administration is not feasible, chloroquine hydrochloride may be administered intravenously (except in children) until an oral preparation can be used. Alternatively, oral quinine sulfate can be given or, in severe attacks, quinine dihydrochloride or quinidine gluconate (investigational indication) can be administered by slow intravenous infusion. No additional treatment is usually required in patients infected with chloroquine-sensitive *P. falciparum* and *P. malariae* but, to prevent relapses and to achieve radical cure in *P. vivax* and *P. ovale* infections, a two-week course of primaquine may be given after consideration of the fact that primaquine causes hemolysis in G6PD-deficient individuals. See also Table 2, Drug Selection for Malaria.

Treatment of chloroquine-resistant falciparum malaria should be initiated with oral quinine sulfate, if possible, or by slow intravenous infusion of quinine dihydrochloride or quinidine gluconate (investigational indication) in severe cases. When oral medication can be tolerated, sulfadiazine and pyrimethamine or the combination of pyrimethamine/sulfadoxine [Fansidar] can be given with quinine sulfate. Pyrimethamine and dapsone, available in fixed combination

TABLE 2.
DRUG SELECTION FOR MALARIA

Type	Therapy of Choice	Alternate Therapy
TREATMENT		
Mild to Moderate Uncomplicated Infection (oral therapy)		
Plasmodium falciparum (chloroquine-sensitive) *P. vivax* *P. ovale* *P. malariae*	Chloroquine Phosphate Primaquine Phosphate[1]	Quinine Sulfate Hydroxychloroquine Sulfate Pyrimethamine Chloroguanide Hydrochloride[2]
P. falciparum (chloroquine-resistant)	Quinine Sulfate + Pyrimethamine/Sulfadoxine [Fansidar] or Pyrimethamine + Sulfadiazine	Quinine Sulfate + Tetracycline Pyrimethamine/Dapsone [Maloprim][2] Mefloquine[2,3] Artemisinine[2,3]
Severe or Complicated Infection (generally intravenous therapy)		
P. falciparum (chloroquine-sensitive) *P. vivax* *P. ovale* *P. malariae*	Quinine Dihydrochloride	Quinidine Gluconate[4] Chloroquine Hydrochloride (not generally recommended in children)
P. falciparum (chloroquine-resistant)	Quinine Dihydrochloride + Pyrimethamine/Sulfadoxine [Fansidar] or Pyrimethamine + Sulfadiazine	Quinine Dihydrochloride or Quinidine Gluconate[4] + Tetracycline (oral or IV)
PROPHYLAXIS		
P. falciparum (areas containing chloroquine-sensitive strains) *P. vivax* *P. ovale* *P. malariae*	Chloroquine Phosphate Primaquine Phosphate[1]	Hydroxychloroquine Sulfate Pyrimethamine Amodiaquine Hydrochloride[2,5] Chloroguanide Hydrochloride[2]
P. falciparum (areas containing chloroquine-resistant strains)	Chloroquine Phosphate Pyrimethamine/Sulfadoxine [Fansidar][5,6]	Doxycycline [4,5] Pyrimethamine Amodiaquine Hydrochloride[2,5] + Pyrimethamine/Sulfadoxine [Fansidar][5] Chloroguanide Hydrochloride[2] Pyrimethamine/Dapsone [Maloprim][2] Mefloquine[2,3] Artemisinine[2,3]

[1]*Following chloroquine or other therapy initially, a course of primaquine may be given to eradicate exoerythrocytic forms of* P. vivax *and* P. ovale, *especially if exposure was prolonged.*
[2]*Not available in United States*
[3]*Investigational drug*
[4]*Investigational indication*
[5]*See also Table 3.*
[6]*Should be given only if febrile illness develops.*

[Maloprim] only outside the United States also is substituted on occasion. Alternatively, tetracycline in combination with quinine or quinidine may be substituted for the sulfonamide/pyrimethamine combination (Reacher et al, 1981). These regimens are also effective against chloroquine-sensitive strains, but chloroquine alone is preferable. (See Table 2.)

Mixed infections occur occasionally, but only those that include *P. falciparum* are significant. Treatment of the clinical attack with chloroquine or a similar agent eliminates parasitemia with all sensitive species, but relapses of *P. vivax* and *P. ovale* malaria are likely unless primaquine is given. Hence, if a mixed infection is suspected, after treatment of the clinical attack, the patient should be observed for a prolonged period or given a course of primaquine.

TABLE 3.
MALARIA PROPHYLAXIS FOR GEOGRAPHIC AREAS
CONTAINING CHLOROQUINE-RESISTANT PLASMODIUM FALCIPARUM[1]

Geographic Area of Exposure	Recommendation
AFRICA (Rural and Urban) Angola, Burundi, Central African Republic, Comoros, Ethiopia, Gabon, Kenya, Madagascar, Malawi, Mozambique, Namibia, Rwanda, Sudan (Northern Province), Tanzania, Uganda, Zaire (NE), Zambia (NE)	A
OCEANIA (Rural and Urban) Papua New Guinea, Solomon Islands, Vanuatu	A
SOUTH AMERICA (Exposure in rural malarious areas during evening and nighttime hours) Bolivia, Brazil,[2] Colombia, Ecuador,[3] French Guiana, Panama (East of Canal Zone, including the San Blas Islands), Peru (Northern Provinces), Surinam, Venezuela	A
ASIA (Exposure in rural malarious areas during evening and nighttime hours) Burma, China (Hainan Island and Southern Provinces), Indonesia,[4] Kampuchea,[5] Laos,[6] Malaysia, Philippines (Luzon, Basilan, Mindoro, Palawan, Mindanao Islands, Sulu Archipelago), Thailand, Vietnam	A
INDIAN SUBCONTINENT (Rural and Urban) Bangladesh (North and East), India, Pakistan (Ralwapindi)	B

RECOMMENDATION A:

Short-term Stay (<3 weeks)

    Preferred: Chloroquine plus Fansidar (For adults, Fansidar is HELD as a single dose [3 tablets]
          for self-treatment of a febrile illness when medical care
          not readily available.) Use of protective clothing,
          insect repellants, insect sprays, net, and screens is recommended.

    Alternative: Doxycycline

Longer Term Stay (>3 weeks)

    Preferred: Cholroquine plus Fansidar (see precautions for long-term use of Fansidar.
          For adults, Fansidar is HELD as a single dose [3 tablets]
          for self-treatment of a febrile illness when medical care
          not readily available). Use of protective clothing,
          insect repellants, insect sprays, net, and screen is recommended.

    Alternative: Amodiaquine[7] plus Fansidar

RECOMMENDATION B:

Chloroquine alone for short- or long-term stay

[1]Adapted from Morbid Mortal Week Rep, *(April 12) 1985 and (Jan 17) 1986.*
[2]*Malaria risk exists in urban areas of interior Amazon River region.*
[3]*Malaria risk exists in urban areas of Esmeraldas, Manabi, El Oro, and Guayas Provinces (including city of Guayaquil).*
[4]*Malaria risk exists in urban areas of Timor and Kalimantan Provinces. Irian Jaya should be considered as Oceania.*
[5]*Malaria risk exists in most urban areas.*
[6]*Malaria risk exists in all urban areas except Vientiane.*
[7]*Recent experience reveals an unpredicted and unexplained rise in the frequency of agranulocytosis associated with the use of amodiaquine; 7 of the 23 reported cases resulted in death (Morbid Mortal Week Rep, (March 14) 1986). Consequently, The Centers for Disease Control has withdrawn its prior recommendation for the prophylactic use of amodiaquine as an alternative for chloroquine when longer term stays (> 3 weeks) are anticipated.*

Clinical Prophylaxis: Four levels of resistance to chloroquine by *P. falciparum* have been described (Weniger et al, 1982; Wernsdorfer, 1984): RO or S (no resistance—clearance of the organism from the blood in seven days without recrudescence); RI (mild resistance—clearance as described for RO, but with recrudescence not due to reinfection within 28 days); RII (moderate resistance)—parasitemia decreased within seven days, but complete clearance not achieved); RIII (complete resistance)—chloroquine has no effect on the parasitemia. For drug selection, RI, RII, and RIII are considered resistant to chloroquine.

Table 2 lists drugs recommended for clinical prophylaxis of all forms of malaria, including both chloroquine-sensitive and -resistant *P. falciparum* strains. For drug selection for clinical prophylaxis of chloroquine-resistant falciparum malaria based on the geographic area of exposure, see Table 3.

For more complete information, see the evaluations.

Travelers should be informed that any regimen of prophylaxis is not absolutely effective and instructed to consult a physician if any symptoms appear.

Recommendations for prophylaxis of malaria are revised periodically by the Centers for Disease Control and appear in *Morbidity and Mortality Weekly Report (MMWR).* A supplement is usually published in August as a monograph entitled, *Health Information for International Travel.* The supplement is available from the Center for Prevention Services, Division of Quarantine, International Health Information, Centers for Disease Control, Atlanta, GA 30333. The CDC can be contacted for current information at (404)329-3670 during the day or at (404)329-2888 for emergencies at night and on weekends.

ADVERSE REACTIONS AND PRECAUTIONS. Certain antimalarial drugs induce hemolytic anemia in individuals with glucose-6-phosphate dehydrogenase (G6PD) deficiency. This X-linked condition occurs principally in people from regions historically endemic for malaria, including those of Mediterranean, African, and Southeast Asian ancestry. The Caucasian and Oriental variants of G6PD deficiency usually precipitate more severe reactions than the African variant. Primaquine and sulfonamides cause hemolytic anemia in these patients, but chloroquine and related 4-aminoquinolines do not.

Chloroquine or another 4-aminoquinoline is best suited for use during pregnancy, since they have not caused teratogenic effects. Pyrimethamine probably should be avoided because anomalies in the offspring of animals given this drug have been encountered, although no cases have been documented in humans. Use of primaquine probably should be postponed until after delivery; therefore, a pregnant women with *P. vivax* or *P. ovale* malaria should be given chloroquine until primaquine can be administered.

The 4-aminoquinolines and pyrimethamine (alone or with a long-acting sulfonamide) are well tolerated by children. The combination of pyrimethamine/sulfamethoxazole should be avoided in individuals sensitive to sulfonamides, because erythema multiforme, Stevens-Johnson syndrome, and toxic epidermal necrolysis have been reported.

Because chloroquine tablets are extremely bitter, a syrup or elixir form of chloroquine or amodiaquine has been used in some areas. Alternatively, chloroquine tablets can be pulverized and mixed with chocolate syrup to make an acceptable preparation for children.

Death from poisoning has occurred in children after accidental ingestion of antimalarial agents.

PNEUMOCYSTOSIS

Pneumocystis pneumonia is caused by the sporozoan parasite, *Pneumocystis carinii*, which usually does not cause infection unless immune responses are impaired by disease, drugs, and/or protein-calorie malnutrition. Definitive diagnosis is made by identification of the organism (pleomorphic trophozoite or cyst) in lung biopsy material or bronchoalveolar lavage fluid, clinical signs and symptoms, and laboratory data (ie, blood gases, roentgenograms). Counterimmunoelectrophoresis for peripheral circulating antigen and diffusion capacity are not reliable.

Signs and Symptoms: Early symptoms are usually generalized and include frequent dry cough, dyspnea and/or tachypnea, chest discomfort, and marked pallor. The most common and consistent findings are cyanosis, particularly of the perioral region; rales; and hypoxemia.

In overt disease, a condition designated as interstitial plasma cell pneumonia, the lungs are infiltrated and lung tissue takes on a honeycomb appearance. Untreated interstitial plasma cell pneumonia is fatal in more than 50% of patients. Death is often sudden with few, if any, premonitory signs.

Drug Selection: In the last decade, trimethoprim/sulfamethoxazole has replaced pentamidine as the drug of choice for pneumocystosis because it is equally effective and less toxic (Small et al, 1985). However, a higher proportion of immunocompromised patients, particularly those with acquired immunodeficiency syndrome (AIDS), have more frequent and serious adverse reactions to this combination than immunocompetent patients (Jaffe et al, 1983; Kovacs et al, 1984). Consequently, in some studies, it was necessary to substitute pentamidine for trimethoprim/sulfamethoxazole in 20% to 30% of immunocompromised patients (Siegel et al, 1984. Pentamidine should not be substituted before day six, because patients often get worse before they improve. (See the evaluation in Chapter 71, Sulfonamides and Trimethoprim.) Although pentamidine may be effective when trimethoprim/sulfamethoxazole has failed, there is no evidence that a combination of the two preparations is more effective than either preparation alone.

Patients unresponsive to trimethoprim/sulfamethoxazole or pentamidine may benefit from the investigational drug, difluoromethylornithine (DFMO) (Sjoerdsma and Schechter, 1984; Golden et al, 1984). DFMO inhibits the key enzyme in polyamine biosynthesis, ornithine decarboxylase (Tierney et al, 1985). Initial results have been encouraging, and the drug also is being investigated in African trypanosomiasis and other protozoan diseases.

Trimethoprim/sulfamethoxazole has prevented pneumocystosis in leukemic children (Hughes, 1982). The criteria for patient selection remain unsettled because of the large number of factors that must be considered (Pifer, 1983) and because not all studies have shown that this combination is beneficial for prophylaxis.

TOXOPLASMOSIS

Toxoplasmosis is caused by the obligate intracellular parasite, *Toxoplasma gondii*. This protozoan is distributed worldwide and infects a wide variety of creatures ranging from poikilotherms to man. Felines are definitive hosts, harboring the enteric sexual cycle (oocysts are shed in the feces) and extraintestinal asexual forms. Other animals, including man, are intermediate hosts in which only the asexual forms develop (ie, the tachyzoites or proliferative forms, the bradyzoites or encysted forms). Many animals and man may harbor and pass the parasite without clear evidence of disease. The infection can be contracted by ingesting cysts, usually in inadequately cooked or raw meat. The infection also may be transmitted by blood, blood products, marrow, and organs used for transplantation.

Signs and Symptoms: The acquired form of disease varies from an asymptomatic condition to severe systemic disease that may progress to encephalitis and death. The latter is especially likely in immunocompromised patients.

Maternal toxoplasmosis occurs in 2 to 3/1,000 pregnancies; about one-third transmit the infection to the fetus. One of 500 to 13,000 live newborns have congenital toxoplasmosis (Fine and Arndt, 1985). The fetus is most susceptible during the third trimester, but manifestations are most severe when exposure occurs during the first trimester. Clinical manifestations are present at birth in only 10% to 20% of exposed fetuses, and only one-fourth of this group develop severe signs and symptoms. The eyes, brain, and other organs may be damaged severely. Congenital toxoplasmosis has a characteristic syndrome of hydrocephalus, hepatosplenomegaly with jaundice, mental retardation, and bilateral retinochoroiditis, occasionally with microcephaly and cerebral calcification. When involvement is complete, the congenital disease usually is fatal.

In immunocompetent adults, acquired infection often is subclinical and patients frequently are asymptomatic for years following the infection. The most common symptoms are retinochoroiditis, lymphadenopathy, fever, and nonpruritic, red, macular rash on the palms and soles. A mild to moderate mononucleosis-like syndrome (prolonged low-grade fever, malaise, and enlarged lymph nodes) associated with a negative heterophil antibody test may occur in adults with mild infection. The most serious consequence of disease is meningoencephalitis. Toxoplasmosis may mimic other diseases, including atypical pneumonia, and may cause myocarditis progressing to heart failure.

Diagnosis: The most reliable diagnostic test is the IgM enzyme-linked immunosorbent assay (ELISA). The IgM-IFA (immunofluorescent antibody) test is less reliable but more helpful than a single-determination Sabin-Feldman dye test (which measures IgG antibody) because of the high incidence of positive titers in the normal population. It is important to remember that the absence of specific IgM antibody and/or no elevation in IgG antibody titer to *T. gondii* does not exclude toxoplasmosis in the immunocompromised host (Bach and Armstrong, 1983; Horowitz et al, 1983; Luft et al, 1983; Alonso et al, 1984).

Drug Selection: The treatment of choice for toxoplasmosis is trisulfapyrimidines or sulfadiazine with pyrimethamine [Daraprim]. Folinic acid (leucovorin) should be given with pyrimethamine (a folic acid antagonist) but is not recommended if acute leukemia is associated with toxoplasmosis, because it may accelerate the leukemia (see the evaluation). The investigational agent, spiramycin, may be used when any of the above agents is contraindicated. Trimethoprim/sulfamethoxazole is ineffective. Therapy is continued for about five weeks; there is no evidence that longer therapy is effective.

If the eyes are involved, some clinicians add clindamycin to the regimen. A corticosteroid also is indicated for ocular involvement, but always should be administered with antiparasitic agents.

In pregnant patients, therapeutic abortion should be considered if infection occurs during the first trimester. Spiramycin is recommended for maternal toxoplasmosis during the second or third trimester.

TRICHOMONIASIS

Vaginal infections caused by *Trichomonas vaginalis* are common and occur most frequently during the reproductive years when estrogen levels are high. Infections often recur, which indicates that trichomonads may persist in extravaginal foci, particularly the urethra. *T. vaginalis* has been found in the urine rather than the vaginal mucus and may be present in the male urethra, the periurethral glands and ducts, and the rectum of both sexes.

Trichomonal vaginitis, urethritis, and prostatovesiculitis are classified as sexually transmitted diseases, but infections may be acquired from contaminated items (eg, toilet articles, toilet seats) as well.

Diagnosis: Diagnosis is established by microscopic examination of a hanging drop preparation containing fresh exudate from the vagina, semen, or prostatic fluid obtained by massage or examination of urinary sediment. Trichomonal flagella usually are identified easily in fresh preparations, but special stains are required to identify them in fixed smears. When symptoms suggest trichomoniasis (eg, wet inflamed vagina; "strawberry" cervix; a thin, yellow, slightly alkaline, frothy, malodorous discharge) but parasites cannot be identified, cultures should be used to confirm the diagnosis and are usually required to establish a positive diagnosis in men. When signs and symptoms disappear and results of microscopic examination of appropriate samples are negative, initial infection is presumed to be controlled, although cultures are mandatory to confirm cures in patients of either sex. Sexual partners should be examined and treated if necessary. Intercourse should be avoided until a cure is confirmed.

Drug Selection: Metronidazole [Flagyl, Protostat] is the drug of choice (Aubert and Sesta 1982; Robbie and Sweet, 1983). Other nitroimidazoles (tinidazole, ornidazole, secnidazole) are undergoing clinical trial in other countries (Rossignol et al, 1984).

The locally acting anti-infective preparation, povidone-iodine

[Betadine], may be useful. Restoration of the normal vaginal pH by periodic vinegar douching may eliminate mild infections. It has been claimed that the vaginal instillation of lactobacilli is beneficial in vaginitis of any etiology by reducing the vaginal pH. However, lactobacilli do not restore vaginal flora to normal or eradicate specific pathogens and, therefore, have limited value.

A number of combination products are available for local application in the treatment of trichomoniasis. There is little objective evidence of their efficacy, and none of these mixtures are as effective as metronidazole. Some preparations are recommended not only for trichomoniasis but also for other vaginal infections characterized as bacterial, candidal, mixed, or "nonspecific."

Sulfonamides are undesirable for topical application because of their sensitizing properties, and the estrogen present in some mixtures may not be appropriate for some women. The quinoline derivatives in some mixtures may be useful, but aminacrine is of doubtful value. Some preparations contain alleged debriding agents (eg, allantoin) but these drugs have little value. Detergents and surfactants may exert some cleansing effect and improve the action of other ingredients, but this synergism has not been proved. For these reasons, the following mixtures are not recommended for trichomoniasis; *AAS* (Rugby), *Aci Jel* (Ortho), *AVC* (Merrell Dow), *AVC/Dienestrol* (Merrell Dow), *Vagisec* (Schmid), *Vagisec Plus* (Schmid).

Adverse Reactions and Precautions: Hypersensitivity reactions are the principal adverse effects of local trichomonacides. Burning, pruritus, or staining may occur but rarely necessitate discontinuation of therapy. Topical vaginal application of povidone-iodine elevates serum iodine concentrations. This drug should not be used repeatedly during pregnancy to avoid goiter and hypothyroidism in the fetus and newborn (Vorherr et al, 1980).

The adverse reactions produced by metronidazole are discussed in the evaluation.

TRYPANOSOMIASIS

African Trypanosomiasis: Sleeping sickness is caused by the bite of a *Glossina* (tsetse fly) infected by *Trypanosoma*. Two clinical types of African sleeping sickness are caused by two subtypes of *Trypanosoma brucei*: West African or Gambian (*T. gambiense*) transmitted by riverine tsetse flies, and East African or Rhodesian (*T. rhodesiense*) transmitted by woodland tsetse flies (Foulkes, 1981; Cochran and Rosen, 1983). Both subtypes produce similar symptoms, but the onset and progression of disease are more rapid with *T. rhodesiense* infection. In the earlier stages of disease, the organism localizes in the lymphatic system and causes intermittent attacks of fever, lymphadenopathy, hepatosplenomegaly, dyspnea, and tachycardia (hemolymphatic stage). When the organisms reach the central nervous system, the chronic, so-called sleeping sickness state begins, characterized by headache, disturbances in coordination, mental dullness, and apathy. As the disease progresses, the patient sleeps constantly, becomes emaciated, and, if untreated, will die.

The hemolymphatic stage of Rhodesian trypanosomiasis is treated with pentamidine; the Gambian form is treated with suramin. Melarsoprol [Arsobal] is the drug of choice to eliminate organisms in the central nervous system in either form of the disease.

Difluoromethylornithine (DFMO) inhibits the key enzyme in polyamine biosynthesis, ornithine decarboxylase (Tierney et al, 1985), and is being investigated in the treatment of African trypanosomiasis (Sjoerdsma and Schechter, 1984). Early reports are very promising.

Pentamidine has been given prophylactically for the Gambian form, but most experts caution against this use.

South American Trypanosomiasis: South American trypanosomiasis (Chagas disease) is transmitted to man by fecal contamination from reduviid bugs infected with *T. cruzi*. These parasites have been found in reservoir hosts as far north as Maryland. *T. cruzi* is regarded as distinct from the organisms causing African trypanosomiasis and somewhat resembles *Leishmania*.

Chagas disease is often asymptomatic but, when present, symptoms vary from region to region. Early signs are local swelling (chagoma) with severe inflammation at the site of the bite. Allergic reactions include rash, fever, and edema of the eyelids and face.

Chronic disease may be asymptomatic or, in certain geographic locations, may produce organomegaly, particularly megaesophagus and megacolon. *T. cruzi* has affinity for cardiac parenchymal cells and also attacks nerve cells in the mesenteric plexus; in some acute infections, acute myocarditis and/or meningoencephalitis develop. Complications affecting the central nervous system, such as meningoencephalitis, are often fatal, especially in young children. The most common manifestation is cardiomyopathy that occurs many years after the initial infection. Chronic cardiopathies are the usual cause of death in long-standing Chagas disease.

Chagas disease is resistant to most forms of therapy. Primaquine may be effective against extracellular trypanosomes (trypomastigotes) in the blood but is ineffective against intracellular forms (amastigotes). Nifurtimox [Lampit, Bayer 2502] acts against both intracellular and extracellular parasites; however, gastrointestinal reactions and peripheral neuritis limit its usefulness. Benznidazole, an analogue of metronidazole, is effective but toxic effects (hypersensitive skin reactions and dose-dependent polyneuropathy) are common.

Drug Evaluations

AMODIAQUINE HYDROCHLORIDE

This 4-aminoquinoline derivative is effective for the prophylaxis and treatment of acute attacks (clinical cure) of malaria caused by *Plasmodium vivax*, *P. ovale*, *P. malariae*, and susceptible strains of *P. falciparum*. Limited evidence suggests that isolates of chloroquine-resistant *P. falciparum* are less resistant to amodiaquine, which clears parasitemia more rapidly (Watkins et al, 1984); however, it has not been established in long-term trials that clinical cure is achieved more frequently with amodiaquine (Phillips, 1984). This drug is not available in the United States.

ADVERSE REACTIONS AND PRECAUTIONS. Adverse reactions include nausea, vomiting, diarrhea, fatigue, lassitude, and vertigo. Most gastrointestinal reactions can be minimized by administering the drug with meals. Reversible pigmentation of the palate, nail beds, and skin may occur when weekly antimalarial doses are given for prolonged periods (five weeks to six years).

Agranulocytosis is the most serious adverse reaction reported for amodiaquine. An unpredicted, unexplained rise in the frequency of agranulocytosis occurred during 1985 and 1986 when amodiaquine was used for malaria prophylaxis and this has generated considerable concern (*Morbid Mortal Week Rep*, [March 14] 1986). Of 23 reported cases of agranulocytosis, 7 resulted in death. The anticipated advantage of more rapid clearance of parasitemia with amodiaquine than with chloroquine must now be weighed against this potentially fatal reaction. The Centers for Disease Control has withdrawn its recommendation for the prophylactic use of amodiaquine as an alternative to chloroquine when long-term exposure (more than 3 weeks) is anticipated.

PHARMACOKINETICS. Amodiaquine is a prodrug. It is rapidly absorbed and converted to the active metabolite, desethyl amodiaquine (DAM). As with other 4-aminoquinolines (eg, chloroquine), the DAM blood concentration declines slowly. Its disposition in the body is unknown, but, unlike chloroquine, amodiaquine is not concentrated in the red blood cells (Salako and Idowu, 1985).

DOSAGE AND PREPARATIONS. All doses are expressed in terms of the base.
Oral: For treatment of malaria, *adults,* 600 mg initially, followed by 400 mg at 6, 24, and 48 hours. *Children,* 10 mg/kg initially, followed by 5 mg/kg at 6, 24, and 48 hours.

For prophylaxis of malaria, *adults,* 400 mg; *children less than 1 year,* 50 mg; *2 to 4 years,* 50 to 100 mg; *5 to 8 years,* 150 to 200 mg; *9 to 12 years,* 300 mg. Adjustments within age groups should be based on weight. This dose is given once weekly on the same day of the week beginning one to two weeks before, during, and for six weeks after the last exposure in the endemic area. Primaquine may be given after completing this six-week course, particularly if exposure has been heavy and prolonged (see that evaluation).
(Not available in the United States)

CHLOROQUINE HYDROCHLORIDE
[Aralen]

CHLOROQUINE PHOSPHATE
[Aralen Phosphate]

USES. Chloroquine, a 4-aminoquinoline, is the drug of choice for prophylaxis and treatment of acute attacks (clinical cure) of malaria caused by *Plasmodium vivax*, *P. ovale*, *P. malariae*, and susceptible strains of *P. falciparum*. It also is a component of the combination, Aralen Phosphate with Primaquine Phosphate, which may be used for prophylaxis of all susceptible species. The combination has no advantage over the individual drugs used in sequence. (See the evaluation.)

Chloroquine is combined occasionally with emetine or dehydroemetine and iodoquinol for the treatment of hepatic amebiasis. It is ineffective alone.

Chloroquine can be administered orally, intramuscularly, or intravenously. The phosphate salt is given only orally; the hydrochloride salt is given parenterally when severe nausea or vomiting occurs, when drug absorption is questionable, or when the infection is particularly severe. Special caution is necessary when using the parenteral form in children. Oral administration should be substituted as soon as practicable.

ADVERSE REACTIONS. Most adverse effects of antimalarial doses of chloroquine are relatively mild, since the amounts used for clinical prophylaxis are small and the larger doses employed to treat acute attacks are given only for short periods. Adverse effects are dose related and include gastrointestinal discomfort with nausea and diarrhea, pruritus, rash, headache, and central nervous system stimulation. Most gastrointestinal reactions can be minimized by administering the drug with meals. Administration once weekly rarely causes renal damage.

Adverse reactions and precautions associated with chloroquine's use in amebiasis resemble those occurring with its use in malaria, except that daily administration for a longer period may increase the frequency of gastrointestinal disturbances. When chloroquine is given for prolonged periods as an anti-inflammatory agent, more severe reactions may occur, especially reversible interference with visual accommodation (see Chapter 59, Antiarthritic Drugs, for a discussion of ocular toxicity).

Rapid intravenous injection causes dizziness, nausea, visual disturbances, and a transient fall in blood pressure. Acute overdosage can cause acute circulatory failure, convulsions, respiratory and cardiac arrest, and death.

PHARMACOKINETICS. Absorption of chloroquine is essentially complete and rapid. Taking chloroquine with food may augment bioavailability. Plasma binding is approximately 50%. Although the plasma half-life is about 48 hours, the drug is retained in certain tissues (eg, lungs, kidney, liver, eyes) and is excreted in the urine months and even years after therapy is discontinued. About 30% of a dose is metabolized to monodes-ethylchloroquine and bisdesethylchloroquine.

Chloroquine is excreted chiefly by nonrenal pathways; however, the renal excretion of unchanged chloroquine is increased in alkaline urine. Patients with severely depressed renal function (glomerular filtration rate, less than 10 ml/minute) who require prolonged therapy should receive a reduced dose (50 to 100 mg daily).

DOSAGE AND PREPARATIONS. All doses are expressed in terms of the base.

CHLOROQUINE PHOSPHATE:

Oral: For treatment of amebiasis, *adults,* 600 mg daily for two days, followed by 300 mg daily for two to three weeks. *Children,* 10 mg/kg (maximum, 600 mg) daily for three weeks.

For treatment of a clinical attack of malaria, adults, 600 mg, followed by 300 mg in six hours and daily for the next two days. *Children,* 10 mg/kg initially, followed by 5 mg/kg in six hours and daily for the next two days. Chloroquine resistance should be considered if a good response is not noted in two or three days.

For prophylaxis of malaria, *adults,* 300 mg; *children,* 5 mg/kg. The dose is given once weekly on the same day of the week beginning one to two weeks before the individual enters the malarious area, during, and for six weeks after leaving the area. Primaquine may be added to the regimen immediately after the individual has left an endemic area, particularly if exposure has been heavy and prolonged (see that evaluation).

> *Generic.* Tablets 250 mg (equivalent to 150 mg of base).
> *Aralen Phosphate* (Winthrop-Breon). Tablets 500 mg (equivalent to 300 mg of base).

CHLOROQUINE HYDROCHLORIDE:

Intramuscular: For treatment of a clinical attack of malaria, *adults,* 3 mg/kg initially, repeated, if necessary, at intervals of six hours (maximum, 1 g in 24 hours). The usual dose is 200 to 250 mg every six hours for three days. An oral preparation should be substituted as soon as possible. This route should be used in *infants and children* only when absolutely necessary, because of its potential for local irritation and even necrosis. The suggested dose is 6.25 mg/kg initially, repeated, if necessary, in six hours. The total dose should not exceed 12.5 mg/kg in 24 hours.

Intravenous: For treatment of a clinical attack of malaria, *adults*, 200 mg or 3 mg/kg infused over a period of at least one hour while monitoring cardiovascular status to detect hypotension or arrhythmias, then 3 mg/kg every six hours (maximum, 1 g/day). *Children,* not recommended.

> *Aralen* (Winthrop-Breon). Solution 50 mg (equivalent to 40 mg of base)/ml in 5 ml containers.

DEHYDROEMETINE

EMETINE HYDROCHLORIDE

ACTIONS AND USES. These salts of an ipecac alkaloid have a direct amebicidal effect against trophozoites of *Entamoeba histolytica* in the intestinal lumen but are not active against cysts. Extraintestinal (tissue) forms of *E. histolytica* also are affected. These agents are used with iodoquinol for severe intestinal amebiasis and extraintestinal amebiasis (usually hepatic abscess). Chloroquine phosphate occasionally is added to this regimen. However, metronidazole and iodoquinol are preferred for all forms of symptomatic amebiasis.

Emetines inhibit polypeptide chain elongation, thereby blocking protein synthesis in eukaryotic but not prokaryotic cells. Therefore, protein synthesis is inhibited in parasitic and mammalian cells but not in bacteria.

The emetines usually are administered by subcutaneous or deep intramuscular injection. They are not given intravenously because severe toxic reactions may occur.

ADVERSE REACTIONS. Adverse reactions are common, especially when the emetines are used for a prolonged period. The incidence of toxicity is similar with both drugs, although dehydroemetine may be slightly less cardiotoxic than emetine. The drugs accumulate in the body, and untoward effects are more frequent with repeated courses.

Cardiovascular reactions are the most serious and include precordial pain, dyspnea, tachycardia, hypotension, gallop rhythm, cardiac dilatation, congestive failure, and death. Electrocardiographic changes are those of conduction delay and can be of long duration (average, six weeks); alterations include widening of the QRS complex, prolongation of the P-R and Q-T intervals, alteration of the S-T segment, and flattening or inversion of the T wave. If these changes are observed, the drug should be discontinued immediately. Injury to the myocardium and other organs may occur.

Nausea, vomiting, and diarrhea are sometimes seen, even when the drugs are administered parenterally, and may make it difficult to assess the response to therapy in amebic dysentery. Headache, skeletal muscle weakness, stiffness, pain and muscle weakness at the site of injection, as well as eczematous, urticarial, or purpuric lesions also have been observed.

PRECAUTIONS. Patients receiving the emetines should be hospitalized and remain in bed during treatment. An electrocardiogram should be performed before therapy is initiated and repeated daily; the heart rate and blood pressure also should be monitored. The emetines should not be used during pregnancy, in patients with heart or kidney disease, or in children unless other therapy is ineffective. These drugs must be used with caution in debilitated or elderly patients. If a ten-day course of therapy is not successful, six weeks to two months should elapse before a second course is started to prevent cumulative toxicity.

PHARMACOKINETICS. The emetines are concentrated in the liver, kidney, spleen, and lung, which may contribute to their efficacy in hepatic amebiasis. It is assumed that the kidney is the major route of excretion in man, but documentation for this is not adequate.

DOSAGE AND PREPARATIONS.
EMETINE HYDROCHLORIDE:
Intramuscular (deep), Subcutaneous: Adults, 1 mg/kg daily (maximum, 60 mg daily) in one dose (alternatively, two divided doses may be given if the patient cannot tolerate one dose) for five days (preferred) or up to ten days; symptoms often improve after three days and allow the substitution of other drugs (eg, metronidazole). The dose should be reduced by one-half in *underweight, elderly, or debilitated patients. Children,* no more than 1 mg/kg daily in two doses for not more than five days. Multiple injection sites should be used to avoid abscesses.
   Generic. Solution 65 mg/ml in 1 ml containers.

DEHYDROEMETINE:
Intramuscular (deep), Subcutaneous: Adults, 1 to 1.5 mg/kg (maximum, 90 mg) daily in one dose for up to five days; *children,* 1 to 1.5 mg/kg daily in two divided doses for five days (preferred) or for ten days if necessary.
   Drug available from the Drug Service, Centers for Disease Control, Atlanta, GA 30333.

DILOXANIDE FUROATE

USES. This amebicide is an alternative to iodoquinol in asymptomatic or mildly symptomatic cyst carriers but is available only through the Centers for Disease Control. Diloxanide is less effective in symptomatic patients with intestinal amebiasis who are passing trophozoites or in those with acute amebic dysentery; metronidazole and iodoquinol are preferred. Diloxanide is of no value in extraintestinal amebiasis. Its mechanism of action is unknown.

ADVERSE REACTIONS AND PRECAUTIONS. Diloxanide is relatively safe, and discontinuation of therapy because of adverse reactions is only rarely necessary. Excessive flatulence is the most common side effect. Infrequently reported adverse reactions include esophagitis, nausea, vomiting, diarrhea, abdominal cramps, vague tingling sensations, pruritus, urticaria, and albuminuria. Abnormal results of hematologic and blood chemistry tests have not been noted.

Since the safety of diloxanide during pregnancy has not been determined, this drug should not be given to pregnant women. Also, it should not be administered to children under 2 years.

PHARMACOKINETICS. Diloxanide is rapidly and significantly absorbed from the gastrointestinal tract after oral administration. The ester is largely hydrolyzed in the intestine, and only diloxanide appears in the systemic circulation. Time to peak effect is approximately one hour. The elimination half-life is approximately six hours, and the major portion of diloxanide appears in the urine as the glucuronide.

DOSAGE AND PREPARATIONS.
Oral: Adults, 500 mg three times daily for ten days. *Children 2 years or older,* 20 mg/kg daily in three divided doses for ten days. Treatment may be repeated if the initial course is unsuccessful.
   In the United States, this preparation is available from the Drug Service, Centers for Disease Control, Atlanta, GA 30333.

FURAZOLIDONE
   [Furoxone]

USES. This nitrofuran is effective in the treatment of giardiasis. Although cure rates in excess of 90% with few relapses have been reported, this drug has not been widely used for giardiasis in the United States, because quinacrine or metronidazole is preferred. However, the liquid formulation of furazolidone may be preferred in children.

In addition to its antigiardial activity, furazolidone is effective against a variety of gram-positive and gram-negative enteric organisms, including *Salmonella, Shigella, Escherichia coli,* staphylococci, and enterococci. It has been used to treat bacterial enteritis and dysentery and shigellosis and may be effective in cholera. Furazolidone acts by interfering with several bacterial enzyme systems; resistance is minimal.

Furazolidone has been used investigationally in the treatment of persistent isosporiasis.

ADVERSE REACTIONS AND DRUG INTERACTIONS. Furazolidone usually is well tolerated, but nausea and vomiting occur occasionally and vesicular morbilliform pruritic rash has been reported. It may cause acute hemolysis in people with G6PD deficiency, and rarely, agranulocytosis. Traces of drug and metabolic degradation products in the urine may tint the urine brown.

Furazolidone produces a disulfiram-type reaction in some patients after ingestion of alcohol. Administration of furazolidone markedly inhibits the activity of monoamine oxidase, and a hypertensive reaction may occur if the drug is given with adrenergic agents, tricyclic compounds, or foods containing significant amounts of tyramine.

Other nitrofurans are discussed in Chapter 72, Miscellaneous Antibacterial Agents.

DOSAGE AND PREPARATIONS.
Oral: Adults, 100 mg four times daily for seven days. *Children,*

5 mg/kg daily divided into four doses for seven days. Alternatively, 8 mg/kg divided into three equal doses with meals for at least seven and preferably ten days (Murphy and Nelson, 1983). The drug should not be given to *infants under 1 month.*
Furoxone (Norwich-Eaton). Liquid 50 mg/15 ml; tablets 100 mg.

HYDROXYCHLOROQUINE SULFATE
[Plaquenil Sulfate]

Hydroxychloroquine, a 4-aminoquinoline, can be used orally for both prophylaxis and clinical cure of malaria caused by *Plasmodium vivax, P. malariae, P. ovale,* and susceptible strains of *P. falciparum*; however, it has no therapeutic advantage over chloroquine and is seldom used for this indication. Hydroxychloroquine is more commonly used than chloroquine as an anti-inflammatory agent for arthritis (see Chapter 59, Antiarthritic Drugs).

Adverse reactions caused by hydroxychloroquine are the same as those for chloroquine (see that evaluation).

DOSAGE AND PREPARATIONS. All doses are expressed in terms of the base.
Oral: For treatment of malaria, *adults,* 620 mg initially, followed by 310 mg in six hours and daily for the next two days. *Children,* 10 mg/kg initially, followed by 5 mg/kg in six hours and daily for the next two days.

For prophylaxis of malaria, *adults,* 310 mg, and *children,* 5 mg/kg (maximum, 310 mg/week); the dose is given once weekly on the same day of the week beginning one to two weeks before the individual enters the malarious area, during, and for six weeks after leaving the area.
Plaquenil Sulfate (Winthrop-Breon). Tablets 200 mg (equivalent to 155 mg of base).

IODOQUINOL (Diiodohydroxyquin)
[Yodoxin]

USES. This organic iodine compound acts against amebae in the intestinal lumen and is the drug of choice in the treatment of asymptomatic intestinal amebiasis (cyst carrier state). Diloxanide is preferred by some authorities, but it is available only from the Centers for Disease Control. Iodoquinol alone is not effective in symptomatic or extraintestinal amebiasis, but it

is given to eliminate luminal organisms after a course of metronidazole (preferred regimen).

Iodoquinol is reported to be effective in some patients with *Dientamoeba fragilis* and *Balantidium coli* infections.

Less than 10% of an oral dose of iodoquinol is recovered in the urine, largely as glucuronides and ethanol sulfates.

ADVERSE REACTIONS AND PRECAUTIONS. Occasional adverse reactions include nausea, abdominal cramps, pruritus ani, rash, acne, and slight enlargement of the thyroid gland.

Iodoquinol has caused subacute myelo-optic neuropathy (SMON) when doses larger than those recommended for amebiasis were given for three weeks. SMON is characterized by muscle pain and weakness, usually below the T-12 vertebra; painful dysesthesias, especially of the limbs, often associated with significant alteration of gait; and, in some instances, optic atrophy and blindness. Although these symptoms regress following discontinuation of the drug, they are not always completely reversible. Children appear to be most susceptible. Iodoquinol has not produced SMON as often as clioquinol, which is no longer available for systemic use in the United States.

The safety of iodoquinol during pregnancy or lactation has not been established.

Iodoquinol is contraindicated in patients hypersensitive to iodine and interferes with the results of some thyroid function tests; therefore, it is relatively contraindicated in patients with thyroid disorders.

DOSAGE AND PREPARATIONS.
Oral: For amebiasis, dientamebiasis (investigational use), and balantidiasis (investigational use), *adults,* 650 mg three times daily after meals for three weeks; *children,* 30 to 40 mg/kg daily in two or three doses (maximum, 2 g daily) for no more than three weeks. If required, the course may be repeated after a two- or three-week interval.
Generic. Tablets 650 mg.
Yodoxin (Glenwood). Tablets 210 and 650 mg; powder 25 g.

MELARSOPROL (MEL-B)

USES. This trivalent arsenical compound is the drug of choice for meningoencephalitis associated with the late stages of Gambian or Rhodesian trypanosomiasis. Melarsoprol is somewhat effective in the earlier stages but, because of its potential to cause encephalopathy, is not used until later in the course of disease.

ADVERSE REACTIONS AND PRECAUTIONS. Melarsoprol is very toxic and many adverse effects are those of arsenic poisoning. Potentially fatal reactive encephalopathy develops in approximately 12% of patients. Other reactions include abdominal pain, vomiting, hypotension, albuminuria, peripheral neuropathy, arthralgia, angioedema, and rashes. A

Herxheimer-like reaction may follow the first dose of melarsoprol. Patients receiving this drug should be hospitalized and monitored closely.

The drug is given intravenously but is irritating to tissues and care must be taken to avoid extravasation.

Information on dosage and precautions are available from the Drug Service, Centers for Disease Control, Atlanta, GA 30333.

METRONIDAZOLE
[Flagyl, Protostat]

USES. This synthetic nitroimidazole compound is amebicidal for *Entamoeba histolytica* at both intestinal (luminal) and extraintestinal (tissue) sites, and currently is the preferred drug for amebiasis except in asymptomatic cyst carriers. Because most of an oral dose is absorbed, another luminal amebicide must be given (generally iodoquinol) to eradicate organisms in the intestine and avoid relapse. See also the section on Amebiasis.

Metronidazole is a highly effective alternative to quinacrine in giardiasis and is an alternative to tetracycline in balantidiasis (investigational indication).

Metronidazole is the drug of choice in the treatment of *Trichomonas vaginalis* infection in men and women (Aubert and Sesta, 1982; Robbie and Sweet, 1983). This drug is active in semen, urine, and extravaginal (eg, prostate, seminal vesicles, epididymis), as well as vaginal, foci. It is active against *Gardnerella vaginalis* vaginitis but is inactive against *Candida* species that cause vaginitis.

Metronidazole also is the drug of choice for many serious anaerobic bacterial infections (see Chapter 72, Miscellaneous Antibacterial Agents).

ADVERSE REACTIONS AND PRECAUTIONS. The incidence of adverse effects is low. The most common reaction is nausea; diarrhea occurs less often. Other untoward effects include unpleasant taste, furry tongue, glossitis, stomatitis, anorexia, epigastric distress, vomiting, abdominal cramps, constipation, dizziness, ataxia, headache, urticaria, vaginal and urethral discomfort, and, rarely, darkening of the urine. Rarely, seizures and reversible peripheral neuropathy have been reported.

Temporary decreases in total (particularly polymorphonuclear) leukocyte counts have been reported following metronidazole therapy. Therefore, total and differential white cell counts should be performed periodically if the drug is given for longer than seven days, especially in very young, very old, or debilitated patients or if a second course of therapy is necessary because of relapse or reinfection. Metronidazole should be used with caution in individuals with or prone to blood dyscrasias, since the parent nitroimidazole nucleus may depress bone marrow activity. Similarly, it should be used cautiously in individuals with pronounced central nervous system disorders.

DRUG INTERACTIONS. Metronidazole interferes with the oxidation of alcohol to carbon dioxide. Thus, when taken with alcoholic beverages, it may produce a disulfiram [Antabuse]-type reaction (abdominal distress, nausea, vomiting, and headache) caused by accumulation of acetaldehyde.

Metronidazole inhibits the metabolism of warfarin and related coumarin anticoagulants. The doses of these anticoagulants should be reduced accordingly to maintain the desired prothrombin time.

PREGNANCY AND LACTATION. Metronidazole is carcinogenic in mice and probably rats, but not in hamsters and other animal species tested. It has not been shown to be carcinogenic in man. Since amebiasis can be life-threatening and metronidazole is generally well tolerated, use of the drug is justified, particularly when alternative therapy may expose the patient to a greater risk of toxicity.

Although the drug readily crosses the placenta, no effects on the fetus have been reported when metronidazole was used to treat amebiasis and trichomoniasis during pregnancy. However, since it has mutagenic activity against certain bacteria at concentrations readily obtainable in body fluids following therapeutic doses, it is recommended that metronidazole not be used during the first trimester and be avoided throughout pregnancy if possible until additional data on hazards to the fetus become available (FDA Pregnancy Category B).

Metronidazole is excreted in breast milk, but no adverse effects have been observed in nursing infants; however, no long-term surveillance data are available.

PHARMACOKINETICS. Metronidazole is well absorbed following oral administration. The extent of absorption is not affected significantly by food, although the rate may be slowed. It is widely distributed and minimally bound to plasma proteins. Urinary excretion of unchanged drug is 20%; hydroxy and acid metabolites account for the remainder of excreted drug. The elimination half-life is approximately eight hours (Ralph, 1983). The drug may accumulate in the plasma in the presence of hepatic insufficiency.

DOSAGE AND PREPARATIONS.
Oral: For amebiasis, *adults,* 750 mg three times daily for five to ten days; *children,* 35 to 50 mg/kg daily in three divided doses for ten days.

For giardiasis (investigational indication), *adults,* 250 to 500 mg three times daily for five to seven days or 2 g daily in a single dose for three days; *children,* 5 mg/kg three times daily for five to seven days.

For balantidiasis (investigational indication), *adults,* 750 mg three times daily for five to ten days; *children,* 35 to 50 mg/kg/day divided into three doses for ten days.

For trichomoniasis, the dosage should be individualized to ensure compliance and minimize reinfection. *Women,* one-day treatment, 2 g as a single dose (preferred if tolerated by the patient) or in two equally divided doses; seven-day treatment, 250 mg three times daily for seven consecutive days. *Men,* treatment is the same as for women.

Flagyl (Searle), **Protostat** (Ortho), **Generic.** Tablets 250 and 500 mg.

Additional Trademarks.
Metryl (Lemmon), **Satric** (Savage), **SK-Metronidazole** (Smith Kline & French).

NIFURTIMOX

USES. This nitrofuran derivative is potentially curative in the acute stage of South American trypanosomiasis (Chagas disease), because it inhibits both the extracellular and intracellular forms of *Trypanosoma cruzi* and reduces parasitemia. However, nifurtimox must be taken for months, and gastric upset makes compliance difficult. The mechanism of action is unknown. Nifurtimox is more effective against Argentinean and Chilean strains of the parasite than against Brazilian strains.

ADVERSE REACTIONS. Adverse reactions are more common in adults (incidence, 40% to 70%) than in children. They usually consist of anorexia, nausea, vomiting, abdominal pain, excitement, vertigo, headache, myalgia, insomnia, and skin rashes. Peripheral neuritis and psychoses also may be seen.

PHARMACOKINETICS. After oral administration, nifurtimox is extensively metabolized; the metabolites are excreted primarily by the kidney.

Information on dosage and preparations is available from the Drug Service, Centers for Disease Control, Atlanta, GA 30333.

PAROMOMYCIN SULFATE
[Humatin]

Paromomycin is a luminal amebicide. This aminoglycoside is generally administered with iodoquinol as an alternative to metronidazole with iodoquinol in the treatment of mild to moderate intestinal amebiasis caused by *Entamoeba histolytica*. Paromomycin also is an alternative to iodoquinol in the asymptomatic carrier state.

For use of paromomycin in intestinal tapeworm infections, see Chapter 78, Anthelmintics.

ADVERSE REACTIONS AND PRECAUTIONS. Frequently reported adverse reactions include nausea, increased gastrointestinal motility, abdominal pain, and diarrhea. Rash, headache, vertigo, and vomiting occur occasionally. Patients should be observed for signs of superinfection.

Paromomycin is poorly absorbed from the intact gastrointes-

tinal tract, and most of a single dose is eliminated in the feces. Nevertheless, to avoid excessive absorption (which may cause ototoxicity and nephrotoxicity), the drug should be used with caution in patients with intestinal inflammation or ulcerations.

DOSAGE AND PREPARATIONS.
Oral: *Adults and children,* 25 to 35 mg/kg daily in three divided doses with meals for seven to ten days. The course may be repeated after a two-week interval.
Humatin (Parke-Davis). Capsules equivalent to 250 mg of base.

PENTAMIDINE ISETHIONATE
[Pentam 300]

USES. This diamidine is active in trypanosomiasis, leishmaniasis, and pneumocystosis (Sands et al, 1985; Drake et al, 1985). Its mechanism of action may be inhibition of kinetoplast DNA replication in parasites.

Pentamidine is the drug of choice in the treatment of early Gambian sleeping sickness caused by *Trypanosoma gambiense* when central nervous system involvement is not present. It is an alternative drug for Rhodesian sleeping sickness when suramin is contraindicated. Melarsoprol is the preferred agent for either form when the central nervous system is involved. Pentamidine is ineffective in South American trypanosomiasis (Chagas disease).

This drug is a suitable alternative in visceral leishmaniasis if the preferred antimonial agents are ineffective (eg, Sudanese kala-azar) or not tolerated.

Pentamidine is an alternative to trimethoprim/sulfamethoxazole in pneumonia caused by *Pneumocystis carinii*.

ADVERSE REACTIONS AND PRECAUTIONS. Pentamidine may cause pain at the site of intramuscular injection, followed by tissue necrosis and abscess formation. Other reactions include nausea, vomiting, hypotension, tachycardia, arrhythmias, and hypoglycemia. Severe hypoglycemia has been associated with islet cell necrosis and inappropriately high plasma concentrations of insulin; daily monitoring of blood glucose is recommended.

Many patients develop renal and hepatic dysfunction and leukopenia that is usually reversible when the drug is discontinued. Thrombocytopenia also has been reported. Confusion, hallucinations, anemia, fever, thrombocytopenia, hypocalcemia, and Stevens-Johnson syndrome also have occurred.

Animal reproduction studies have not been conducted. Pentamidine should be used during pregnancy only if diagnosis is definitive and the agent is clearly needed (FDA Pregnancy Category C).

PHARMACOKINETICS. Since pentamidine is poorly absorbed from the gastrointestinal tract, it must be administered parenterally. Elimination from the serum is rapid but that from the body is slow and accumulation in tissue occurs. Pentamidine appears in the urine for six to eight weeks after cessation of therapy. The major path of excretion is via the kidney (about 80%), and the dose should be adjusted in patients with renal dysfunction. If the glomerular filtration rate (GFR) is 10 to 50 ml/minute, the dosage interval should be 24 to 36 hours. If the GFR is less than 10 ml/minute, the dosage interval should be 48 hours.

DOSAGE AND PREPARATIONS.

Intravenous (preferred), Intramuscular: Fatalities due to arrhythmias and severe hypotension have occurred, even after a single dose; therefore, the dose should be infused over at least 60 minutes to avoid hypotension and the blood pressure should be carefully monitored until it is stable.

For Gambian trypanosomiasis, *adults and children,* 4 mg/kg/day for 10 days.

For Rhodesian trypanosomiasis, *adults and children,* 4 mg/kg as a single dose once every three to six months.

For leishmaniasis, *adults and children,* 4 mg/kg/day three times weekly for 5 to 25 weeks, depending upon the response.

For pneumocystosis, *adults and children,* 4 mg/kg/day for 14 days.

> *Pentam 300* (LyphoMed). Powder 300 mg.

POVIDONE-IODINE
[Betadine]

Clinical evidence indicates that this water-soluble complex of polyvinylpyrrolidone and iodine may be beneficial in vaginal infections caused by *Trichomonas vaginalis* when extravaginal sources of reinfection are not present. Metronidazole is preferred.

ADVERSE REACTIONS AND PRECAUTIONS. Although povidone-iodine does not produce the degree of local irritation associated with use of tincture of iodine, reactions may occur in patients allergic to iodine.

Topical vaginal application of povidone-iodine elevates serum concentrations of iodine. Euthyroid women showed no evidence of thyroid dysfunction (Safran and Braverman, 1982); however, this drug should not be used repeatedly as a vaginal disinfectant during pregnancy to avoid goiter and hypothyroidism in the fetus and newborn (Vorherr et al, 1980).

DOSAGE AND PREPARATIONS.

Topical (vaginal): After swabbing the cervix and vulvovaginal area with a povidone-iodine solution in the office, one applicatorful of the gel is inserted nightly, followed by use of the douche preparation the next morning. Daily applications of gel and douche should be continued for at least two weeks. Infections may resolve in 10 to 15 days, or therapy may be required for two or three menstrual cycles.

> *Generic.* Douche; gel; solution.
> *Betadine* (Purdue Frederick). Douche 10% in 15, 30, 180, and 240 ml containers; gel 10% in 18 and 90 g containers; solution 10% in 15, 30, and 240 ml containers.

PRIMAQUINE PHOSPHATE

USES. Primaquine is the most effective and least toxic of the available 8-aminoquinolines. It is used almost exclusively to provide radical cure of malaria caused by the exoerythrocytic forms of *Plasmodium vivax* or *P. ovale.* Because of its potential for hemolysis, most experts advise using primaquine for travelers after their return from malarious areas only when exposure to *P. vivax* and *P. ovale* was prolonged.

Although primaquine is effective against the erythrocytic forms of plasmodia, it is not used for clinical or causal prophylaxis because of its slow onset of action and short half-life.

Primaquine controls parasitemia in South American trypanosomiasis (Chagas disease), but is ineffective against intracellular parasites (nifurtimox is preferred).

ADVERSE REACTIONS AND PRECAUTIONS. The most serious adverse effect is intravascular hemolysis manifested as acute hemolytic anemia in patients with glucose-6-phosphate dehydrogenase (G6PD) deficiency. Rarely, primaquine also may induce hemolysis in individuals with other defects of the erythrocytic pentose phosphate pathway of glucose metabolism and certain hemoglobinopathies. In healthy individuals with G6PD deficiency, the severity of hemolysis varies directly with the dose and degree of deficiency. There are many molecular variations and degrees of G6PD deficiency found among all races. In individuals with the African variant, the hemolytic anemia induced by a standard course of primaquine therapy is relatively mild, self-limited, and often asymptomatic. In those with the Mediterranean variant, clinically evident hemolysis with the usual dosage schedule is likely. Thus, in patients whose ethnic origin indicates the possibility of G6PD deficiency, screening for this deficiency prior to administering primaquine is necessary. Monitoring of the hemogram, including reticulocyte counts and bilirubin, is recommended, especially during the first and second weeks of therapy. The urine should be examined as well.

Primaquine also may cause abdominal discomfort, nausea, headache, interference with visual accommodation, and pruritus. Methemoglobinemia is common but rarely necessitates interruption of therapy. Leukopenia and agranulocytosis occur rarely. Primaquine may exacerbate psoriasis.

Although it has not been established conclusively that primaquine causes teratogenic effects in man, the use of this agent probably should be postponed until after delivery.

PHARMACOKINETICS. Limited studies suggest that primaquine is rapidly and completely absorbed, extensively distributed (apparent volume of distribution is 243 ± 70 L), and converted principally to carboxyprimaquine. The drug is not subject to extensive first-pass metabolism. Clearance is 24 ±

7.4 L/hour (Mihaly et al, 1985). Less than 5% of the administered dose is found in the urine (White, 1985).

DOSAGE AND PREPARATIONS. All doses are expressed in terms of the base.

Oral: For treatment of malaria (radical cure) due to *P. vivax* and *P. ovale* or to prevent relapses in travelers after their return from malarious areas when exposure to *P. vivax* and *P. ovale* was prolonged, *adults,* 15 mg, and *children,* 0.3 mg/kg. This dose is given daily for 14 days, preferably *consecutively* with chloroquine or other therapy, which is given on the first three days of an acute attack.

The hemolytic effect of primaquine is lessened by the following equally effective alternative regimens. For those with the African variant of G6PD deficiency, 45 mg once weekly for eight weeks; for those with the Caucasian or Oriental variants, 30 mg once weekly for 15 weeks. There is risk in these regimens, however, and it may be preferable to treat each relapse with chloroquine.

No pediatric formulation of primaquine is available and it may be more convenient to use the combination tablet containing chloroquine and primaquine or to break the primaquine tablet into the approximate dose portion in children. (See the evaluation on Chloroquine/Primaquine Phosphates.)

    Generic (Winthrop-Breon). Tablets 26.3 mg (equivalent to 15 mg of base).

PYRIMETHAMINE
[Daraprim]

USES. This potent dihydrofolate reductase inhibitor is used for the prophylaxis and treatment of malaria caused by susceptible species of *Plasmodium*. Because parasites readily develop resistance to this drug, it is given principally with sulfonamides for suppression of chloroquine-resistant *P. falciparum*. Folic acid antagonists should almost always be given with sulfonamides, for their combined activity is many times greater than that of either drug alone. Furthermore, the number of strains resistant to either agent is thought to be greatly decreased with use of the combination.

In the treatment of an acute attack of malaria due to a chloroquine-resistant organism, the combination of pyrimethamine, a sulfonamide, and quinine is the regimen of choice. A product combining sulfadoxine with pyrimethamine [Fansidar] is available.

Pyrimethamine with sulfadiazine or trisulfapyrimidines is the treatment of choice for toxoplasmosis. The combination of pyrimethamine and sulfadiazine is used investigationally to treat persistent isosporiasis.

ADVERSE REACTIONS AND PRECAUTIONS. The hazards from small, suppressive, antimalarial doses of pyrimethamine are minimal. However, prolonged administration may produce toxicity. Symptoms mainly reflect interference with folic acid metabolism. The effects, therefore, are most evident in rapidly dividing cells. Because pyrimethamine has an antifolate action and is teratogenic in animals, it is not recommended during pregnancy unless the risk of malaria outweighs the potential adverse effects.

If hematologic abnormalities appear, administration should be stopped and leucovorin (folinic acid) 3 to 9 mg is given intramuscularly or 10 mg is given orally each day until the blood cell count returns to safe levels. Alternatively, concomitant administration of 3 to 9 mg of leucovorin or folic acid usually prevents anemia, thrombocytopenia, and leukopenia without affecting the antiprotozoal action of pyrimethamine.

DOSAGE AND PREPARATIONS.

Oral: For prophylaxis of malaria, the following doses are given once weekly on the same day of the week: *Adults and children over 10 years,* 25 mg; *children 2 years and under,* 6.25 to 12.5 mg; *3 to 10 years,* 12.5 to 25 mg. Since adequate blood levels are obtained within a few hours after ingestion, administration need not be started until the day before entering an endemic area and should be continued for six weeks after return. However, it is strongly recommended that pyrimethamine be given with a sulfonamide for prophylaxis and treatment of chloroquine-resistant strains of *P. falciparum* malaria (see the evaluation on Pyrimethamine/Sulfadoxine).

For toxoplasmosis, *adults,* initially, 50 to 100 mg daily for one to three days, followed by 25 mg/day for three to four weeks plus trisulfapyrimidines 2 to 6 g daily in four to six divided doses for three to four weeks. Sulfadiazine may be used instead of trisulfapyrimidines (initially, 2 to 4 g, followed by 1 g every four to six hours for three to four weeks). *Children,* 2 mg/kg/day for three days (maximum, 25 mg/day), then 1 mg/kg/day for four weeks. This should be given with 100 to 200 mg/kg/day of trisulfapyrimidines in four to six divided doses for three to four weeks. *Infants,* 2 mg/kg/day for three days, then 1 mg/kg/day every two to three days for four weeks.

    Daraprim (Burroughs Wellcome). Tablets 25 mg.

QUINACRINE HYDROCHLORIDE
[Atabrine Hydrochloride]

ACTIONS AND USES. Metronidazole and other nitroimidazole compounds are replacing quinacrine in the treatment of giardiasis, because they are more active and less toxic. However, quinacrine may be preferred for initial therapy in adults, especially those with severe infection. Children do not tolerate quinacrine well; therefore, metronidazole (investigational indication) or furazolidone is more commonly used.

Quinacrine is obsolete in the treatment of tapeworm infections and malaria.

ADVERSE REACTIONS AND PRECAUTIONS. Nausea and vomiting are the most common adverse effects of quinacrine. Prolonged administration stains the skin yellow and produces a deep yellow urine, which can be confused with hepatitis. Toxic psychosis has been reported in 1.5% to 2% of adults taking this drug (Wolfe, 1981). Transient dizziness also may occur. Aplastic anemia, exfoliative dermatitis, atypical lichen planus, and acute hepatic necrosis are rare.

Quinacrine should be used cautiously in patients over 60 years and in those with a history of psychosis. This drug should not be used in patients with psoriasis, because it may exacerbate this condition. Treatment of pregnant women should be postponed until after delivery because giardiasis generally is not life-threatening and quinacrine poses a hazard to the fetus.

PHARMACOKINETICS. Quinacrine is well absorbed from the intestinal tract. It is widely distributed in tissues where it accumulates and is liberated slowly. Quinacrine is excreted in the urine; significant amounts can be detected in the urine two months after therapy is discontinued.

DOSAGE AND PREPARATIONS.
Oral: For giardiasis, *adults*, 100 mg three times daily after meals for seven days. *Children* (not commonly used), 2 mg/kg three times daily after meals for seven days (maximum, 300 mg/day).

Atabrine Hydrochloride (Winthrop-Breon). Tablets 100 mg.

QUININE SULFATE

QUININE DIHYDROCHLORIDE

QUINIDINE GLUCONATE

Quinine, pyrimethamine, and a sulfonamide (eg, sulfadoxine, sulfadiazine, dapsone) constitute the regimen of choice to treat chloroquine-resistant strains of *Plasmodium falciparum*; tetracycline or clindamycin can be substituted for the pyrimethamine/sulfonamide combination if patients are resistant or sensitive to either component. Unless they are not tolerated or contraindicated, the safer and more rapid-acting 4-aminoquinolines should be used instead of quinine in malaria caused by other species or chloroquine-sensitive *P. falciparum*. Quinine is not used for prophylaxis of malaria because of toxicity or lack of compliance.

Quinine has been used in the treatment of nocturnal leg cramps and myotonia congenita, as an antipyretic-analgesic, to induce labor, and as a local anesthetic or sclerosing agent. More effective drugs are available for these uses, except nocturnal leg cramps. Quinine's oxytocic effect is observed only with larger than recommended doses.

Quinine can be administered orally (sulfate) or intravenously (dihydrochloride). The intravenous route is preferred in patients with severe attacks when absorption of quinine sulfate cannot be assured.

A parenteral preparation of quinine is available only from the Centers for Disease Control. Consequently, quinidine gluconate (investigational indication) has been substituted for quinine in emergencies when intravenous administration for falciparum malaria is required and quinine dihydrochloride is not available (White et al, 1981; Phillips et al, 1985). However, because quinidine may be cardiotoxic, the heart should be monitored carefully.

ADVERSE REACTIONS AND PRECAUTIONS. The usual antimalarial dose of quinine sulfate frequently causes mild to moderate cinchonism (tinnitus, headache, altered auditory acuity, blurred vision, nausea, diarrhea), but symptoms seldom necessitate cessation of treatment. Severe symptoms develop only rarely (except with overdosage), most often when plasma levels exceed 10 mg/dl. Asthma may be precipitated in susceptible individuals. Urticaria is the most frequent allergic reaction and pruritus may develop with or without rash. Signs of hematologic toxicity include acute hemolysis, hypoprothrombinemia, thrombocytopenic purpura, and agranulocytosis. The precise role played by quinine in precipitating blackwater fever is unknown.

Blindness or other visual disturbances occurred within 4 to 14 hours after an overdose in 6 of 48 patients; the effect is reversible in most patients, but long-term visual impairment can result (Dyson et al, 1985).

Intravenous administration of the dihydrochloride salt may produce hypotension and acute circulatory failure. Very dilute solutions should be injected slowly and oral administration of the sulfate salt should be substituted as soon as possible. Any adverse reactions associated with quinine sulfate also may occur with the dihydrochloride salt.

Quinine should be given with caution to patients who have atrial fibrillation and to those who manifest idiosyncrasy to it in the form of cutaneous angioedema or visual or auditory symptoms. This drug is contraindicated in the presence of optic neuritis and tinnitus.

Quinine sulfate is classified in FDA Pregnancy Category X.

PHARMACOKINETICS. Quinine is well absorbed orally. It is widely distributed and metabolized primarily in the liver. The metabolites are excreted via the kidney. The normal elimination half-life ranges from 5 to 16 hours.

DOSAGE AND PREPARATIONS. All doses are expressed in terms of the base. Dosage adjustment is required in those with renal failure and the following are general guidelines: Glomerular filtration rate more than 50 ml/minute, 8-hour interval; 10 to 50 ml/minute, 8- to 12-hour interval; less than 10 ml/minute, 24-hour interval.
QUININE SULFATE:

Oral: For treatment of chloroquine-sensitive malaria, *adults,* 650 mg (or 10 mg/kg) every eight hours for seven to ten days. *Children,* 25 mg/kg/day in divided doses every eight hours for seven to ten days.

For treatment of chloroquine-resistant *P. falciparum* malaria in *adults,* the above dose is given; in severe infection, a loading dose of 20 mg/kg should be administered (White et al, 1983 B). Pyrimethamine 25 mg twice daily is added for the first three days and sulfadiazine 500 mg four times daily for five days, or the fixed-dose combination of pyrimethamine and sulfadoxine [Fansidar] should be added to the regimen (two to three tablets daily for three days in adults). Alternatively, quinine may be given for three to five days and tetracycline administered. The dosage of tetracycline is 1 g daily in divided doses every six hours for seven to ten days.

For *children,* quinine 25 mg/kg/day is given in divided doses every eight hours for three days, pyrimethamine 0.5 to 1 mg/kg/day is given in divided doses every 12 hours for three days (with supplemental folic acid), and sulfadiazine 120 to 150 mg/kg/day (maximum, 2 g/day) is given in divided doses every six hours for five days or the fixed-dose combination of pyrimethamine and sulfadoxine [Fansidar] should be added to the regimen (see the evaluation).

 Generic. Capsules 130, 195, 300, and 325 mg; tablets 260 and 325 mg.

QUININE DIHYDROCHLORIDE:

Intravenous: For treatment of severe malaria, *adults,* 600 mg (or 10 mg/kg) in 300 ml of 0.9% sodium chloride injection infused over at least a one-hour or preferably a four-hour period. This dose is repeated in six to eight hours (maximum total daily dose, 1.8 g). Cardiovascular status should be monitored to detect hypotension or arrhythmias. Following clinical response, quinine sulfate should be given orally as soon as practicable. *Infants and children,* 12.5 mg/kg infused over at least one hour or preferably four hours; the dose is repeated in six to eight hours if the oral dose cannot be tolerated (maximum, 25 mg/kg/day).

If the infection is caused by chloroquine-resistant *P. falciparum,* pyrimethamine plus a sulfonamide or tetracycline, should be added as described above.

 The drug may be obtained from the Drug Service, Centers for Disease Control, Atlanta, GA 30333.

QUINIDINE GLUCONATE:

Intravenous: For treatment of severe malaria (investigational indication), *adults and children,* a loading dose of 15 mg/kg is dissolved in 250 ml of 5% dextrose injection and infused over four hours while monitoring for hypotension and widening of the QRS interval; if either symptom occurs, the rate should be decreased or the infusion discontinued. Subsequent doses of 7.5 mg/kg are administered every eight hours for seven days either as four-hour infusions or as an equivalent oral dose of quinine or quinidine when the patient's condition has improved sufficiently.

 Generic. Suspension 80 mg/ml (equivalent to 50 mg/ml base) in 10 ml containers.

SODIUM STIBOGLUCONATE

MEGLUMINE ANTIMONIATE

ACTIONS AND USES. The pentavalent antimonial, sodium stibogluconate, is a drug of choice in treating visceral leishmaniasis (kala-azar) and also acts against the cutaneous and mucocutaneous forms. The antimonial compounds inhibit various enzymes in *Leishmania* and may act on parasite ribosomes, but their exact mode of action has not been fully established.

Although not available in the United States, meglumine antimoniate also is a drug of choice in cutaneous and mucocutaneous leishmanial infections and has some effect on visceral leishmaniasis.

The East African form of the disease is relatively resistant to the antimonials; Mediterranean, Indian, Chinese, and Brazilian forms are more susceptible.

ADVERSE REACTIONS AND PRECAUTIONS. Although sodium stibogluconate is better tolerated than trivalent antimonials, adverse reactions can be severe. The most common and serious effect is cardiotoxicity, usually manifested as ECG abnormalities and, occasionally, as severe bradycardia. Vasodilation and shock also have been observed. Liver and kidney function may be impaired. Milder reactions include nausea, vomiting, rash, headache, syncope, dyspnea, facial edema, and abdominal pain. Pain in joints and muscles may occur toward the end of a therapeutic course.

Pentavalent antimonials are generally contraindicated in the presence of cardiac, hepatic, or renal disease; pneumonia; tuberculosis; pregnancy; or in infants under 18 months.

PHARMACOKINETICS. Oral pentavalent antimonial compounds are absorbed too slowly to be effective; indeterminate amounts are reduced to trivalent antimony in the liver. Elimination data are incomplete, but up to 90% of the dose may be excreted in the urine following injection (Rees et al, 1980).

DOSAGE AND PREPARATIONS.

Intramuscular, Intravenous: For leishmaniasis, *adults and children,* 10 mg/kg/day for six to ten days. For the cutaneous form, the course may be repeated. For Old World visceral leishmaniasis, 15 to 20 mg/kg/day (maximum, 850 mg/day). The minimum duration recommended is 20 days; up to 30 days are required in some patients (Anabwani et al, 1983).

 Preparations of sodium antimony gluconate (sodium stibogluconate) are available from the Drug Service, Centers for Disease Control, Atlanta, GA 30333.

SURAMIN
[Bayer 205]

ACTIONS AND USES. Suramin is trypanosomicidal and is the drug of choice for the treatment of early (hemolymphatic) Rhodesian sleeping sickness when the central nervous system is not involved. It is an alternative drug in early Gambian sleeping sickness (pentamidine is preferred). When the parasite is entrenched within the central nervous system, melarsoprol is the drug of choice for both forms of disease. Suramin appears to be selectively absorbed into trypanosomes, perhaps by pinocytosis, where it binds with enzymes, often in a reversible fashion. The exact mechanism of action has not been explained.

Suramin also is used to destroy adult worms in onchocerciasis (see Chapter 78, Anthelmintics).

ADVERSE REACTIONS AND PRECAUTIONS. Suramin should be administered only in a hospital under close medical supervision. Adverse effects affecting the central nervous system are common and include paresthesias, hyperesthesia of the palms and soles, peripheral neuropathy, and photophobia. Loss of consciousness and seizures occur in approximately 0.3% of patients. Pruritus and urticaria may develop quickly, even with therapeutic doses, and other types of rashes, including exfoliative dermatitis, may develop later. Suramin is nephrotoxic and causes proteinuria, hematuria, and cylindruria. Rarely, blood dyscrasias and hemolytic anemia have been reported. Occasionally, a shock-like reaction characterized by nausea, vomiting, hypotension, and unconsciousness occurs immediately after injection. A 100- to 200-mg test dose should be administered before the first full therapeutic injection is given. If a severe reaction does not occur, therapy can be initiated.

PHARMACOKINETICS. Suramin is not well absorbed orally. It is tightly bound to proteins and persists in the circulation for months. This drug is released slowly from plasma proteins and excreted by the kidney.

DOSAGE AND PREPARATIONS.
Intravenous: For trypanosomiasis, *adults,* following a test dose of 100 to 200 mg, 10 to 15 mg/kg is given on days 1, 3, 7, 14, and 21. *Children,* 20 mg/kg given on the same days as for adults. A fresh solution must be prepared before each injection.

Suramin is available from the Drug Service, Centers for Disease Control, Atlanta, GA 30333.

TETRACYCLINES

These broad spectrum antibiotics are partially active against amebae in the intestinal lumen and wall. They are indirectly amebicidal in that they modify the intestinal flora necessary for amebic viability. Tetracycline and oxytetracycline are the most effective members of this group. They may be used with other drugs to treat mild to moderate invasive intestinal amebiasis (see also section on Amebiasis). The tetracyclines also are used to treat balantidiasis, dientamebiasis, and chloroquine-resistant *P. falciparum* malaria (given with quinine). Doxycycline is an alternative drug in the prophylaxis of chloroquine-resistant *P. falciparum* malaria (see Table 3).

For adverse reactions, precautions, and other uses, see Chapter 69, Tetracyclines and Chloramphenicol.

DOSAGE AND PREPARATIONS.
OXYTETRACYCLINE, TETRACYCLINE:
Oral: Adults, for amebiasis, 250 to 500 mg four times daily for ten days; *children, over 8 years*, 10 mg/kg (maximum, 600 mg) four times daily for ten days; *under 8 years*, not recommended.

For dientamebiasis, 250 mg four times daily for seven to ten days. For treatment of chloroquine-resistant *P. falciparum* malaria, 1 g daily in divided doses every six hours for seven to ten days.
DOXYCYCLINE:
Oral: For prophylaxis of chloroquine-resistant *P. falciparum* malaria, *adults*, 100 mg/day during the exposure period; *children*, 2 mg/kg/day.

See Chapter 69 for preparations.

Mixtures

CHLOROQUINE/PRIMAQUINE PHOSPHATES
[Aralen Phosphate with Primaquine Phosphate]

This combination of chloroquine and primaquine is suitable and safe for the prophylaxis of malaria when used for at least six weeks after the individual has left a malarious area. It has been especially effective in the long-term prophylaxis of vivax malaria in military personnel but has never achieved widespread acceptance for civilian use.

This combination is also more easily tolerated by individuals susceptible to the adverse effects of primaquine. The same adverse effects and precautions apply to the combination as for either drug used alone. See the evaluations for details.

DOSAGE AND PREPARATIONS.
Oral: For prophylaxis of malaria, *adults and children over 45 kg,* one tablet weekly on the same day of each week, starting two weeks before entering the malarious area, during, and for six weeks after leaving. For younger children, a suspension of the tablets is made in chocolate syrup or fruit juice so that each 5 ml contains 40 mg of chloroquine base and 6 mg of primaquine base. The following amounts are then given once weekly on the same day of each week: *Children 5 to 7 kg,* 2.5 ml; *8 to 11 kg,* 5 ml; *12 to 15 kg,* 7.5 ml; *16 to 20 kg,* 10 ml; *21 to 24 kg,* 12.5 ml; and *25 to 45 kg,* one-half tablet. These doses should not be exceeded.

Aralen Phosphate with Primaquine Phosphate (Winthrop-Breon). Tablets containing chloroquine phosphate 500 mg (equivalent to 300 mg of base) and primaquine phosphate 79 mg (equivalent to 45 mg of base).

PYRIMETHAMINE/SULFADOXINE
[Fansidar]

ACTIONS AND USES. This combination contains pyrimethamine and sulfadoxine in a fixed ratio of 20:1, respectively. It is indicated for the treatment of malaria caused by susceptible strains of plasmodia and is the drug of choice for prophylaxis of chloroquine-resistant *P. falciparum* malaria in selected endemic areas (see Table 3). It is effective against most strains of chloroquine-resistant *P. falciparum*. *P. vivax* does not respond to this combination.

This mixture acts by sequential blockade of two consecutive steps in the formation of folinic acid from aminobenzoic acid (PABA) by the parasite. Sulfadoxine prevents the parasite from utilizing PABA to synthesize folic acid; pyrimethamine, a folic acid antagonist, inhibits the enzyme, dihydrofolate reductase, thereby preventing formation of tetrahydrofolic acid (folinic acid).

ADVERSE REACTIONS. The adverse effects of the mixture are those characteristic of the sulfonamides (see Chapter 71, Sulfonamides and Trimethoprim) and pyrimethamine (see the evaluation).

The combination should be avoided in patients who are sensitive to or cannot tolerate the sulfonamides, because erythema multiforme, Stevens-Johnson syndrome, and toxic epidermal necrolysis have been reported. The incidence of these reactions during prophylactic use by American travelers ranges from 1:18,000 to 1:26,000, and ten fatalities have been reported (*Morbid Mortal Week Rep*, [Jan 4] 1985). Recommendations for American travelers have been revised because of these findings (*Morbid Mortal Week Rep*, [April 12] 1985) (see Table 3). Other serious reactions include serum sickness, exfoliative dermatitis, urticaria, and hepatitis.

Because the most severe cutaneous reactions have been associated only with multiple doses of Fansidar, individuals with renal insufficiency or liver damage may be particularly susceptible. Therefore, prophylactic (repeated) use of Fansidar is contraindicated in patients with severe renal insufficiency, marked liver parenchymal damage, or blood dyscrasias.

Overdosage may result in acute intoxication manifested by anorexia, nausea, vomiting, and central nervous system stimulation, including convulsions. Megaloblastic anemia, leukopenia, thrombocytopenia, glossitis, and crystalluria also may develop.

PHARMACOKINETICS. Both drugs are absorbed orally and achieve peak plasma concentrations at about the same time (eg, 2.5 to 6 hours for sulfadoxine, 1.5 to 8 hours for pyrimethamine). Elimination half-life is about 100 to 200 hours for sulfadoxine and 50 to 100 hours for pyrimethamine; these drugs are excreted primarily by the kidney.

DOSAGE AND PREPARATIONS.
Oral: For treatment of an acute attack of chloroquine-resistant *P. falciparum* malaria, a single daily dose should be given according to the following schedule: *Adults,* two to three tablets; *children 9 to 14 years,* two tablets; *4 to 8 years,* one tablet; *under 4 years,* one-half tablet.

For prophylaxis of malaria (if pyrimethamine/sulfadoxine is to be given rather than HELD as a single dose for self-treatment), *adults,* one tablet weekly one to two weeks before, during, and for six weeks after last exposure in endemic areas; *children 9 to 14 years,* three-fourths tablet weekly; *4 to 8 years,* one-half tablet weekly; *1 to 3 years,* one-fourth tablet weekly; *6 to 11 months,* one-eighth tablet weekly (see also Table 3).

> **Fansidar** (Roche). Tablets containing sulfadoxine 500 mg and pyrimethamine 25 mg.

Cited References

Adverse reactions to Fansidar and updated recommendations for its use in prevention of malaria. *Morbid Mortal Week Rep* 33:713-714, (Jan 4) 1985.

Agranulocytosis associated with use of amodiaquine for malarial prophylaxis. *Morbid Mortal Week Rep* 35:165-166, (March 14) 1986.

Cryptosporidiosis among children attending day-care centers: Georgia, Pennsylvania, Michigan, California, New Mexico. *Morbid Mortal Week Rep* 33:599-601, (Oct 26) 1984.

Need for malaria prophylaxis by travelers to areas with chloroquine-resistant *Plasmodium falciparum*. *Morbid Mortal Week Rep* 35:21-27, (Jan 17) 1986.

Revised recommendations for preventing malaria in travelers to areas with chloroquine resistant *Plasmodium falciparum*. *Morbid Mortal Week Rep* 34:185-195, (April 12) 1985.

Update: Treatment of cryptosporidiosis in patients with acquired immunodeficiency syndrome (AIDS). *Morbid Mortal Week Rep* 33:117-119, (March 9) 1984.

Alonso R, et al: Cerebral toxoplasmosis in acquired immune deficiency syndrome. *Arch Neurol* 41:321-323, 1984.

Anabwani GM, et al: Comparison of two dosage schedules of sodium stibogluconate in treatment of visceral leishmaniasis in Kenya. *Lancet* 1:210-213, 1983.

Angus KW: Cryptosporidiosis in man, domestic animals and birds: Review. *J R Soc Med* 76:62-70, 1983.

Aubert JM, Sesta HJ: Treatment of vaginal trichomoniasis: Single, 2-gram dose of metronidazole as compared with seven-day course. *J Reprod Med* 27:743-745, 1982.

Bach MC, Armstrong RM: Acute toxoplasmic encephalitis in normal adult. *Arch Neurol* 40:596-597, 1983.

Basile JA, et al: Amebic liver abscess: Surgeon's role in management. *Am J Surg* 146:67-71, 1983.

Bell DR: *Lecture Notes on Tropical Medicine*. Oxford, Blackwell Scientific, 1981.

Bruce-Chwatt LJ: Malaria and pregnancy, (editorial). *Br Med J* 286:1457-1458, 1983.

Carmine AA, et al: Tinidazole in anaerobic infections: Review of its antibacterial activity, pharmacological properties, and therapeutic efficacy. *Drugs* 24:85-117, 1982.

Chance ML: Leishmaniasis. *Br Med J* 283:1245-1247, 1981.

Chester AC, et al: Giardiasis as chronic disease. *Digest Dis Sci* 30:215-218, 1985.

Child Day Care Infectious Disease Study Group: Considerations of infectious diseases in day care centers. *Pediatr Infect Dis* 4:124-136, 1985.

Cochran R, Rosen T: African trypanosomiasis in United States. *Arch Dermatol* 119:670-674, 1983.

Drake S, et al: Pentamidine isethionate in treatment of *Pneumocystis carinii* pneumonia. *Clin Pharm* 4:507-516, 1985.

Dyson EH, et al: Death and blindness due to overdose of quinine. *Br Med J* 291:31-33, 1985.

Ellis CJ, Chiodini PL: Treatment of falciparum malaria. *J Antimicrob Chemother* 13:311-313, 1984.

Farthing MJG, Keusch GT: Giardiasis: Wilderness disease. *Drug Ther* 12:115-126, 1982.

Fine J-D, Arndt KA: TORCH syndrome: Clinical review. *J Am Acad Dermatol* 12:697-706, 1985.

Forgacs P, et al: Intestinal and bronchial cryptosporidiosis in immuno-deficient homosexual man. *Ann Intern Med* 99:793-794, 1983.

Foulkes JR: Human trypanosomiasis in Africa. *Br Med J* 283:1172-1174, 1981.

Garnham PCC: Present state of malaria research: Historical survey. *Experientia* 40:1305-1309, 1984.

Golden JA, et al: Pneumocystis carinii pneumonia treated with α-difluoromethylornithine: Prospective study among patients with acquired immunodeficiency syndrome. *West J Med* 141:613-623, 1984.

Guevara L, et al: Study with quinfamide in treatment of chronic amebiasis in adults. *Clin Therapeut* 6:43-46, 1983.

Harinasuta T, et al: Trials of mefloquine in vivax and of mefloquine plus 'Fansidar' in falciparum malaria. *Lancet* 1:885-888, 1985.

Harries J: Amoebiasis: Review. *J R Soc Med* 75:190-197, 1982.

Horowitz SL, et al: CNS toxoplasmosis in acquired immunodeficiency syndrome. *Arch Neurol* 40:649-652, 1983.

Hughes WT: Trimethoprim-sulfamethoxazole therapy for *Pneumocystis carinii* pneumonitis in children. *Rev Infect Dis* 4:602-607, 1982.

Jaffe HS, et al: Complications of co-trimoxazole in treatment of AIDS-associated pneumocystis carinii pneumonia in homosexual men. *Lancet* 2:1109-1111, 1983.

Jiang JB, et al: Antimalarial activity of mefloquine and qinghaosu. *Lancet* 2:285-288, 1982.

Jokipii L, Jokipii AMM: Treatment of giardiasis: Comparative evaluation of ornidazole and tinidazole as single oral dose. *Gastroenterology* 83:399-404, 1982.

Klayman DL: Qinghaosu (artemisinin): Antimalarial drug from China. *Science* 228:1049-1055, 1985.

Kovacs JA, et al: *Pneumocystis carinii* pneumonia: Comparison between patients with acquired immunodeficiency syndrome and patients with other immunodeficiencies. *Ann Intern Med* 100:663-671, 1984.

Krotoski WA: Discovery of hypnozoite and new theory of malarial relapse. *Trans R Soc Trop Med Hyg* 79:1-11, 1985.

Li G, et al: Randomised comparative study of mefloquine, qinghaosu, and pyrimethamine-sulfadoxine in patients with falciparum malaria. *Lancet* 2:1360-1361, 1984.

Luft BJ, et al: Outbreak of central-nervous-system toxoplasmosis in Western Europe and North America. *Lancet* 2:781-784, 1983.

Lushbaugh WB, et al: Proteinase activities of *Entamoeba histolytica* cytotoxin. *Gastroenterology* 87:17-27, 1984.

McGowan K: How to find and treat amebiasis. *Drug Ther* 14:159-174, (May) 1984.

McGowan K, et al: *Entamoeba histolytica* causes intestinal secretion: Role of serotonin. *Science* 221:762-764, 1983.

Mihaly GW, et al: Pharmacokinetics of primaquine in man. I. Studies of absolute bioavailability and effects of dose size. *Br J Clin Pharmacol* 19:745-750, 1985.

Miller RA, et al: Life-threatening diarrhea caused by Cryptosporidium in child undergoing therapy for acute lymphocytic leukemia. *J Pediatr* 103:256-259, 1983.

Millet V, et al: *Dientamoeba fragilis*, protozoan parasite in adult members of semicommunal group. *Digest Dis Sci* 28:335-339, 1983.

Murphy TV, Nelson JD: Five versus ten days' therapy with furazolidone for giardiasis. *Am J Dis Child* 137:267-270, 1983.

Nelson DA, et al: Clinical aspects of cutaneous leishmaniasis acquired in Texas. *J Am Acad Dermatol* 12:985-992, 1985.

Pearson RD: Leishmaniasis: Pathologic spectrum. *Hosp Pract* 19:100E-100X, (May) 1984.

Peters W, Hall AP: Treatment of severe falciparum malaria. *Br Med J* 291:1146-1147, 1985.

Phillips RE: Management of *Plasmodium falciparum* malaria. *Med J Aust* 141:511-516, 1984.

Phillips RE, et al: Intravenous quinidine for treatment of severe falciparum malaria: Clinical and pharmacokinetic studies. *N Engl J Med* 312:1273-1278, 1985.

Pickering LK, et al: Occurrence of *Giardia lamblia* in children in day care centers. *J Pediatr* 104:522-526, 1984.

Pifer LL: *Pneumocystis carinii*: Diagnostic dilemma. *Pediatr Infect Dis* 2:177-183, 1983.

Pitlik SD, et al: Human cryptosporidiosis: Spectrum of disease; report of six cases and review of literature. *Arch Intern Med* 143:2269-2275, 1983.

Portnoy D, et al: Treatment of intestinal cryptosporidiosis with spiramycin. *Ann Intern Med* 101:202-204, 1984.

Ralph ED: Clinical pharmacokinetics of metronidazole. *Clin Pharmacokinet* 8:43-62, 1983.

Ravdin JI, Guerrant RL: Review of parasite cellular mechanisms involved in pathogenesis of amebiasis. *Rev Infect Dis* 4:1185-1207, 1982.

Reacher M, et al: Drug therapy for *Plasmodium falciparum* malaria resistant to pyrimethamine-sulfadoxine (Fansidar): Study of alternate regimens in Eastern Thailand, 1980. *Lancet* 2:1066-1069, 1981.

Rees PH, et al: Renal clearance of pentavalent antimony (sodium stibogluconate). *Lancet* 2:226-229, 1980.

Robbie MO, Sweet RL: Metronidazole use in obstetrics and gynecology: Review. *Am J Obstet Gynecol* 145:865-881, 1983.

Rossignol J-F, et al: Nitroimidazoles in treatment of trichomoniasis, giardiasis, and amebiasis. *Int J Clin Pharmacol Ther Toxicol* 22:63-72, 1984.

Safran M, Braverman LE: Effect of chronic douching with polyvinylpyrrolidone-iodine on iodine absorption and thyroid function. *Obstet Gynecol* 60:35-40, 1982.

Salako LA, Idowu OR: Failure to detect amodiaquine in blood after oral administration. *Br J Clin Pharmacol* 20:307-311, 1985.

Sands M, et al: Pentamidine: Review. *Rev Infect Dis* 7:625-634, 1985.

Siegel SE, et al: Treatment of *Pneumocystis carinii* pneumonitis: Comparative trial of sulfamethoxazole-trimethoprim v pentamidine in pediatric patients with cancer; report from Childrens Cancer Study Group. *Am J Dis Child* 138:1051-1054, 1984.

Sjoerdsma A, Schechter PJ: Chemotherapeutic implications of polyamine biosynthesis inhibition. *Clin Pharmacol Ther* 35:287-300, 1984.

Small CB, et al: Treatment of *Pneumocystis carinii* pneumonia in acquired immunodeficiency syndrome. *Arch Intern Med* 145:837-840, 1985.

Smith PD, et al: Chronic giardiasis: Studies on drug sensitivity, toxin production, and host immune response. *Gastroenterology* 83:797-803, 1982.

Speelman P: Single-dose tinidazole for treatment of giardiasis. *Antimicrob Agents Chemother* 27:227-229, 1985.

Taylor JP, et al: Cryptosporidiosis outbreak in day-care center. *Am J Dis Child* 139:1023-1025, 1985.

Thompson JE Jr, et al: Amebic liver abscess: Therapeutic approach. *Rev Infect Dis* 7:171-179, 1985.

Tierney DF, et al: Polyamines in clinical disorders. *West J Med* 142:63-73, 1985.

Vorherr H, et al: Vaginal absorption of povidone-iodine. *JAMA* 244:2628-2629, 1980.

Watkins WM, et al: Effectiveness of amodiaquine as treatment for chloroquine-resistant *Plasmodium falciparum* infections in Kenya. *Lancet* 1:357-359, 1984.

Weniger BG, et al: High-level chloroquine resistance of *Plasmodium falciparum* malaria acquired in Kenya. *N Engl J Med* 307:1560-1562, 1982.

Wernsdorfer WH: Drug resistant malaria. *Endeavour* 8:166-171, 1984.

White NJ: Clinical pharmacokinetics of antimalarial drugs. *Clin Pharmacokinet* 10:187-215, 1985.

White NJ, et al: Quinidine in falciparum malaria. *Lancet* 2:1069-1071, 1981.

White NJ, et al: Severe hypoglycemia and hyperinsulinemia in falciparum malaria. *N Engl J Med* 309:61-66, 1983 A.

White NJ, et al: Quinine loading dose in cerebral malaria. *Am J Trop Med Hyg* 32:1-5, 1983 B.

Wittner M, et al: Diagnosis of giardiasis by two methods: Immunofluorescence and enzyme-linked immunosorbent assay. *Arch Pathol Lab Med* 107:524-527, 1983.

Wolfe MS: Diagnosis and management of giardiasis. *IM* 2:63-67, (June) 1981.

Wolfe MS: Treatment of intestinal protozoan infections. *Med Clin North Am* 66:707-720, 1982.

Wolfson JS, et al: Cryptosporidiosis in immunocompetent patients. *N Engl J Med* 312:1278-1282, 1985.

World Health Organization: *The Leishmaniases*. Geneva, WHO, Technical Report Series 701, 1984.

Wyler DJ: Malaria: Resurgence, resistance, and research, parts 1 and 2. *N Engl J Med* 308:875-878, 934-940, 1983.

Other Selected References

Drugs for parasitic infections. *Med Lett Drugs Ther* 28:9-18, 1986.

Health Information for International Travel 1984. US Dept of Health and Human Services publication no (CDC)84-8280. Atlanta,

Centers for Disease Control, 1984.

Beck JW, Davies JE: *Medical Parasitology*, ed 3. St Louis, CV Mosby, 1981.

Brown HW, Neva FA: *Basic Clinical Parasitology*, ed 5. Norwalk, CT, Appleton-Century-Crofts, 1983.

James DH, Gilles HM: *Human Antiparasitic Drugs: Pharmacology and Usage*. New York, John Wiley & Sons, 1985.

Katz M, et al: *Parasitic Diseases*. New York, Springer-Verlag, 1982.

Most H: Treatment of parasitic infections of travelers and immigrants. *N Engl J Med* 310:298-304, 1984.

Wade A (ed): *Martindale: The Extra Pharmacopoeia*, ed 28. London, The Pharmaceutical Press, 1982, 86-109.

Anthelmintics

INTRODUCTION

NEMATODE INFECTIONS

  Intestinal Infections

    Ascariasis (Roundworm Infection)

    Enterobiasis (Pinworm Infection)

    Trichuriasis (Whipworm Infection)

    Strongyloidiasis (Threadworm Infection)

    Uncinariasis (Hookworm Infection)

  Tissue Infections

    Cutaneous Larva Migrans (Creeping Eruption)

    Visceral Larva Migrans (Toxocariasis)

    Trichinosis (Trichinelliasis, Pork Roundworm Infection)

    Filariasis (Onchocerciasis, Lymphatic Filariasis, Loiasis, Dipetalonemiasis, Ozzardi Filariasis)

    Dirofilariasis (Dracontiasis, Dracunculiasis, Guinea Worm Infection)

CESTODE INFECTIONS

  Intestinal Infections

    Taeniasis (Beef and Pork Tapeworm Infection)

    Diphyllobothriasis (Fish Tapeworm Infection)

    Hymenolepiasis (Dwarf Tapeworm Infection)

    Dipylidiasis (Dog Tapeworm Infection)

  Tissue Infections

    Cysticercosis

    Echinococciasis (Hydatid Disease)

TREMATODE INFECTIONS

  Schistosomiasis (Blood Fluke Infections)

  Clonorchiasis and Opisthorchiasis (Chinese or Oriental Liver Fluke Infection)

  Fascioliasis (Sheep Liver Fluke Infection)

  Paragonimiasis (Lung Fluke Infection)

  Fasciolopsiasis (Giant Intestinal Fluke Infection)

DRUG EVALUATIONS

Parasitic worm infections are a major cause of disease in many areas of the world. Helminthiasis is often associated with squalid living conditions, but poor sanitation is not an absolute prerequisite to infection.

With few exceptions (eg, *Strongyloides stercoralis, Hymenolepis nana*), helminths do not multiply in the human host. Individuals who harbor many helminths but are not re-exposed lose worms over time; therefore, anthelmintics are not essential to effect a cure for some parasites (eg, whipworm, hookworm). On the other hand, in countries with a relatively high standard of living where individualized therapy is available, patients should be treated for most helminthic infections diagnosed unless the side effects of treatment are potentially more dangerous or unpleasant than the infection. Individualized treatment is often impractical in developing countries because of the prohibitive costs of medication, limited medical facilities, and the great potential for reinfection. It is apparent, therefore, that control of helminthiasis involves more than application of chemotherapeutic measures. Equally important adjunctive techniques may include removal of patients from the infected environment or cleansing the environment of the parasite or vector. Similarly, knowledge of when to treat and what signs or symptoms precede complications is of considerable value to the physician.

Disease Classification: The helminths that commonly infect man belong to two phyla: (1) the Nemathelminthes, which includes the class, Nematoda (roundworms), and (2) the Platyhelminthes (flatworms), which encompasses the classes, Cestoda (tapeworms) and Trematoda (flukes). For disease classification and suggested drug therapy, see Table 1.

Therapy: Anthelmintics act locally on worms in the gastrointestinal tract or systemically on those that have migrated into body tissues. Most common intestinal parasites can be eliminated easily and safely with an appropriate anthelmintic. Tissue infections (eg, muscle, liver, lung) may be more difficult to treat, are often of longer duration, and occasionally require additional supportive procedures, including surgery, for cure. The efficacy of therapy may be difficult to evaluate in complex infections, such as schistosomiasis. Criteria for satisfactory progress include relief of signs and symptoms; absence of the parasite in blood, stool, or tissue; reduction of the fecal egg count; and correction of biochemical abnormalities.

The relative specificity of anthelmintic drugs usually necessitates accurate diagnosis, although this may be less essential with broader spectrum agents, such as mebendazole [Vermox], pyrantel [Antiminth], or praziquantel [Biltricide]. Parasites occasionally can be identified by gross examination of the stool, but more often an appropriate specimen (stool, blood,

TABLE 1.
CLASSIFICATION OF THE MAJOR HELMINTHS
AND DRUGS USED TO TREAT HELMINTHIASIS

Parasite	Disease Name(s)	Geographical Distribution	Usual Source and Route of Infection
NEMATODES (ROUNDWORMS)			
Intestinal Infections			
Ascaris lumbricoides Roundworm	Ascariasis	Cosmopolitan (more common in tropics)	Human feces to soil to food
Enterobius vermicularis Pinworm, Seatworm	Enterobiasis	Cosmopolitan (less common in tropics)	Anal contact. Fecal or soil contamination to food
Trichuris trichiura Whipworm	Trichuriasis	Cosmopolitan (more common in tropics)	Human feces to soil to food
Strongyloides stercoralis Threadworm	Strongyloidiasis Cochin-China Diarrhea	Tropics and subtropics (more common in tropics)	Human feces to soil to skin
Ancylostoma duodenale Old World, European, or Common Hookworm	Uncinariasis Ancylostomiasis Miner's Anemia	Tropics and subtropics (Europe, North Africa, Middle and Far East, South America)	Human feces to soil to skin or food
Necator americanus New World or American Hookworm	Uncinariasis Necatoriasis	Tropics and subtropics (Americas, Italy, tropical Africa, Asia)	Human feces to soil to skin
Tissue Infections			
Ancylostoma braziliense	Cutaneous Larva Migrans Creeping Eruption	Tropics and subtropics (Asia, Africa, Americas, Pacific)	Cat and dog feces to soil to skin
Toxocara canis *T. cati*	Visceral Larva Migrans Toxocariasis	Cosmopolitan (common in North America and Europe)	Cat and dog feces to soil to skin
Trichinella spiralis Pork Roundworm	Trichinelliasis Trichinosis	Cosmopolitan (more common in Northern Hemisphere than in tropics)	Meat as food (usually pork)
Onchocerca volvulus	River Blindness (Filariasis) Onchocerciasis	Africa, Yemen, Central and South America	Insect bite
Wuchereria bancrofti	Lymphatic or Bancroftian Filariasis Wuchereriasis	Asia, Africa, Pacific, South America	Insect bite

Vector or Intermediate Host	Stage(s) in Man	Site(s) of Involvement	Drug(s) of Choice	Alternative Drugs
None	Larvae and Adults	Small Intestine	Pyrantel Pamoate or Mebendazole	Piperazine
None	Larvae and Adults	Cecum, Ascending Colon, Ileum	Pyrantel Pamoate or Mebendazole	Pyrvinium Pamoate, Piperazine
None	Larvae and Adults	Cecum, Upper Colon, Rectum, Appendix	Mebendazole[1]	None
None	Larvae and Adults	Small Intestine	Thiabendazole[1]	Cambendazole[2]
None	Larvae and Adults	Small Intestine	Pyrantel Pamoate[3] or Mebendazole	Bephenium Tetrachloroethylene
None	Larvae and Adults	Small Intestine	Pyrantel Pamoate[3] or Mebendazole	Bephenium Tetrachloroethylene
Cats Dogs	Larvae only (in epidermis)	Skin	Thiabendazole (oral and topical)	None
Dogs Cats	Larvae Only	Liver, Lungs; occasionally kidney, brain, eye	Mebendazole[3] or Thiabendazole plus Corticosteroids[3,4] if symptoms are severe, especially if there is ocular involvement	Diethylcarbamazine Citrate
Swine (mainly)	Larvae and Adults	Small intestine	Thiabendazole plus Corticosteroids[4]	Mebendazole,[5] Pyrantel Pamoate (kills only adult worms)
Simulium (Black fly)	Larvae (microfilariae) migrate and Adults (macrofilariae) in skin	Lymphatics, Blood, Skin, Subcutaneous Tissue, Eye	Diethylcarbamazine Citrate or Ivermectin[2] followed by Suramin[3]	Flubendazole,[2] Mebendazole[3]
Culex, Aedes, and *Anopheles* mosquitoes	Larvae (microfilariae in blood) and Adults (macrofilariae)	Lymphatics, Blood,	Diethylcarbamazine Citrate	None

(Continued on next page)

Parasite	Disease Name(s)	Geographical Distribution	Usual Source and Route of Infection
Brugia malayi *B. timori*	Lymphatic Malayan, or Brug's Filariasis Brugiasis	Southeast Asia (Malaya, Borneo, India, Ceylon, tropical China)	Insect bite
Loa loa	Loiasis Eyeworm Disease of Africa Calabar Swelling Disease (Filariasis)	West and Central Africa (Rain Forest)	Insect bite
Dipetalonema perstans	Filariasis Dipetalonemiasis	West and Central Africa, South America	Insect bite
Mansonella ozzardi	Ozzardi Filariasis	South America, West Indies	Insect bite
Dracunculus medinensis Guinea Worm	Dirofilariasis Dracunculiasis Dracontiasis	Tropics (West Africa, Nile Valley, Middle East, India, West Indies, Guyana)	Ingesting infected water fleas

CESTODES (TAPEWORMS)
Intestinal Infections

Parasite	Disease Name(s)	Geographical Distribution	Usual Source and Route of Infection
Taenia saginata Beef Tapeworm	Taeniasis	Cosmopolitan (mainly Middle East, Kenya, Ethiopia, South America, Mexico, Russia)	Beef as food
Taenia solium Pork Tapeworm	Taeniasis	Cosmopolitan (common in Mexico, Central and South America)	Pork as food
Diphyllobothrium latum Fish Tapeworm	Diphyllobothriasis	Cosmopolitan (more common in temperate areas)	Freshwater crustacea to fish to man
Hymenolepis nana Dwarf Tapeworm	Hymenolepiasis	Cosmopolitan	Human feces to soil to food. Fecal contamination
Dipylidium canium Dog Tapeworm	Dipylidiasis	Cosmopolitan	Dog or cat fleas to mouth

Vector or Intermediate Host	Stage(s) in Man	Site(s) of Involvement	Drug(s) of Choice	Alternative Drugs
Mansonoides mosquito	Larvae (microfilariae in blood) and Adults (macrofilariae)	Lymphatics, Blood,	Diethylcarbamazine Citrate	None
Chrysops (fly)	Larvae (microfilariae in blood) and Adults (macrofilariae)	Lymphatics, Blood, Subcutaneous Tissue, Skin	Diethylcarbamazine Citrate	None
Culicoides (a small black midge)	Larvae (microfilariae in blood) and Adults (macrofilariae)	Lymphatics, Blood, Serous Cavities	Diethylcarbamazine Citrate	None
Culicoides	Larvae (microfilariae in blood) and Adults (macrofilariae)	Lymphatics, Blood, Visceral Adipose Tissue	Diethylcarbamazine Citrate (therapy rarely indicated)	None
Cyclops (water flea)	Larvae and Adults	Loose Connective Tissue and Skin	Niridazole[6]	Metronidazole[6]
Cattle	Adults	Small Intestine	Niclosamide or Praziquantel[3]	Paromomycin
Swine	Adults	Small Intestine	Niclosamide or Praziquantel[3]	Paromomycin
Freshwater crustacea to fish to man	Adults	Ileum	Niclosamide or Praziquantel[3]	Paromomycin
None	Larvae and Adults	Small Intestine	Praziquantel[3]	Niclosamide Paromomycin
Dog or Cat flea	Adult	Small Intestine	Niclosamide or Praziquantel[3]	Paromomycin

(Continued on next page)

TABLE 1 (continued)

Parasite	Disease Name(s)	Geographical Distribution	Usual Source and Route of Infection
Tissue Infections			
Cysticercus cellulosae Cysticercoid stage of *Taenia solium*	Cysticercosis Neurocysticercosis	Cosmopolitan (common in Mexico, Central and South America)	*T. solium* eggs in fecal-contaminated food or soil, carrier self-contamination, or reverse peristalsis
Echinococcus granulosis *E. multilocularis*	Hydatid Disease Alveolar Hydatid Disease Echinococciasis	Cosmopolitan (wherever the triad of man, sheep or cattle, and dog is common)	Canine feces to soil to food. Fecal contamination
TREMATODES (FLUKES)			
Schistosoma haematobium Blood Fluke	Urinary Bilharziasis	Iraq, Africa, Near East, Madagascar	Skin penetration from contaminated water
Schistosoma mansoni Blood Fluke	Intestinal Bilharziasis	Africa, West Indies, South America, Middle East	Skin penetration from contaminated water
Schistosoma japonicum *S. mekongi* Oriental Blood Fluke	Oriental or Chinese Bilharziasis	Japan, China, Philippines, Celebes	Skin penetration from contaminated water
Schistosoma intercalatum African Blood Fluke	African Schistosomiasis	Africa	Skin penetration from contaminated water
Clonorchis sinensis Chinese Liver Fluke *Opisthorchis viverrini* Liver Fluke	Clonorchiasis Opisthorchiasis	Far East, mainly Japan, Korea, China, Vietnam	Human and animal feces to water to snail to soil to fish as food
Fasciola hepatica Sheep Liver Fluke	Fascioliasis	Cosmopolitan (more common in Europe, Cuba, and Chile)	Sheep feces to water to snail to wild water-cress and other pasture food plants
Paragonimus westermani Lung Fluke	Paragonimiasis	Far East, Central and South America	Human sputum and feces to soil to snail to freshwater crabs used as food
Fasciolopsis buski Giant Intestinal Fluke	Fasciolopsiasis	China, India, Indonesia, Thailand, Malaya, Taiwan	Swine feces to soil to snail to water plants (eg, water chestnuts)

[1] Follow-up therapy with pyrantel pamoate may be indicated if multiple infection with Ascaris roundworms and pinworms also present.

[2] Investigational drug

[3] Investigational use

[4] Thiabendazole is nematocidal in conventional doses during the early larval migration; corticosteroids are useful to reduce the marked inflammatory response that usually occurs during that migration.

Vector or Intermediate Host	Stage(s) in Man	Site(s) of Involvement	Drug(s) of Choice	Alternative Drugs
Swine	Larvae	Any tissue, especially skeletal muscle, central nervous system, and eye	Praziquantel[3]	None
Sheep, Cattle, Man, Deer, Dogs	Larvae	Encysted in liver, lung, and other tissues	Surgery	Albendazole[2] Flubendazole[2] Mebendazole[3] given as adjunct to surgery
Freshwater snail	Larvae (penetrate the skin) and Adults	Veins of urinary bladder, other tissues	Praziquantel	Metrifonate
Freshwater snail	Larvae (penetrate the skin) and Adults	Veins of small and large intestine, other tissues	Praziquantel	Oxamniquine
Freshwater snail	Larvae (penetrate the skin) and Adults	Veins of small and large intestine, other tissues	Praziquantel	Niridazole[7] Antimony Potassium Tartrate[7]
Freshwater snail	Larvae (penetrate the skin) and Adults	Veins of small and large intestine, other tissues	Praziquantel	Niridazole[7]
Snail, Fish (other definitive hosts are cats, dogs, rats)	Larvae and Adults	Biliary Tract	Praziquantel[3]	None
Snails (sheep and cattle are definitive hosts)	Larvae and Adults	Biliary Tract	Praziquantel[3]	Bithionol[2]
Snails, Freshwater crabs	Larvae and Adults	Lung; Occasionally central nervous and gastrointestinal systems	Praziquantel[3]	Bithionol[2]
Snails, Freshwater plants	Adults	Small Intestine	Praziquantel[3]	Tetrachloroethylene[3]

[5]*Mebendazole, used in a higher dose and for a longer duration than conventional use for intestinal worms, has been shown to kill encysted larvae (Levin, 1983).*

[6]*Although niridazole and metronidazole are used in this disease, their beneficial effect appears to be unrelated to any antiparasitic action; they probably minimize the high risk of secondary skin infection and inflammation that accompany the primary lesion.*

[7]*Because of their limited effectiveness, niridazole and antimony potassium tartrate generally are not recommended for this use in the United States.*

urine, sputum, aspirate, or biopsy) must be submitted to a parasitology laboratory for definitive diagnosis.

When the initial course of therapy with the drug of choice has not effected a cure and alternative therapy is more hazardous, retreatment with the first drug should be undertaken before another anthelmintic is prescribed. In mixed infections, which are very common and often unrecognized, the effect of therapy on each of the species present must be considered.

For sources of anthelmintic drugs, see Table 2. Drugs available from the CDC may be obtained by contacting the Drug Service, Centers for Disease Control, 1600 Clifton Road, Bldg 6, Room 161, Atlanta, GA 30333. During regular business hours (8 AM to 4:30 PM), the telephone number is (404) 329-3670; the emergency number is (404) 329-2888.

NEMATODE INFECTIONS

Intestinal Infections

ASCARIASIS (ROUNDWORM INFECTION). Ascariasis is the most common helminthic disease worldwide. Approximately one-third of the world population (more than one billion people) is infected with this parasite. The incidence is greatest in tropical countries with low standards of hygiene, but infections also occur in temperate climates.

Infection usually follows ingestion of embryonated eggs on raw vegetables or soil (pica in children). Larvae hatch in the duodenum, penetrate the duodenal wall, and migrate in the venous and lymphatic systems through the liver and heart to the lungs; this process takes approximately four days. During the next ten days, the larvae molt twice in the lungs, penetrate the alveoli, ascend the pulmonary tree to the epiglottis, and are swallowed. Upon reaching the duodenum for the second time, larvae develop into adult worms, which produce eggs that are passed in the feces. The entire cycle takes 60 to 75 days; the adult lifespan is 6 to 18 months. Reinfection occurs commonly in endemic areas.

Most individuals are asymptomatic. Acute symptoms and signs during migration include fever, cough, and pulmonary infiltration. A clinical diagnosis usually cannot be made, although pneumonitis associated with eosinophilia and generalized allergic manifestations (Loeffler's syndrome) may be suggestive. The presence of eggs in a stool sample is definitive. Abdominal distress, epigastric pain, anorexia, nausea, and vomiting are likely to be associated with intestinal obstruction due to masses of worms.

Ascariasis always should be treated because serious complications may follow migration of adult worms into the pancreatic and bile ducts, gallbladder, or liver. Complete obstruction of the appendix or intestinal lumen may occur, and asphyxia or aspiration pneumonia may result from vomiting. Byproducts or breakdown products of worms may cause severe reactions in sensitized individuals.

Pyrantel [Antiminth] and mebendazole [Vermox] are drugs of choice in ascariasis; piperazine [Antepar] is a less effective alternative. Levamisole and bephenium hydroxynaphthoate also are effective, but are used principally in other parts of the world. (See the evaluation on levamisole in Chapter 63,

Immunomodulators.) When treating mixed infections that include ascariasis, agents that are ineffective for ascariasis should be avoided initially, because ascarids may be stimulated to migrate.

ENTEROBIASIS (PINWORM INFECTION). Enterobiasis occurs more often in temperate areas than in the tropics and is the most common parasitic disease in the United States. Although it is thought to be a childhood ailment, infection is not uncommon in adults. Because Enterobius eggs can survive for a few days away from the body, soiled clothing or bed linen, dirt under the fingernails, toys, and house dust may be sources of infection.

The disease is transmitted by ingestion of mature eggs; the usual route is anus to hand to mouth. First-stage larvae hatch in the duodenum, molt three times, and mature in two to five weeks. Adult worms inhabit the cecum and occupy part of the ascending colon and ileum in heavy infections. Following copulation, the male worm usually is passed in the feces. The female deposits eggs on the perianal and perineal skin. The diagnosis may be facilitated by the use of transparent adhesive tape to collect eggs from the perianal skin. Occasionally, larvae that hatch on the perianal skin may migrate back up the anus to produce reinfection that may persist for months. Adult worms live for about eight weeks.

Although most patients are asymptomatic, pruritus ani and vulvae may occur and may be severe enough to result in persistent scratching during the day and restlessness or insomnia at night. There may be eosinophilia of up to 12%, but it is seldom a useful diagnostic sign. Rare serious complications include intra-abdominal inflammation, appendicitis, peritoneal granulomas, and allergic urticaria. Migration of worms may cause vaginitis and, rarely, endometritis or salpingitis. Enterobiasis is often associated with dientamebiasis.

Because of the relative ubiquity of Enterobius vermicularis, it is important that good personal hygiene, including nail cleaning and careful hand washing following defecation or urination, be instituted with drug therapy to prevent reinfection.

Mebendazole and pyrantel pamoate are drugs of choice in pinworm infection. Piperazine and pyrvinium [Povan] are less preferred alternatives. All members of a family should be treated at least once. Since developing larvae and eggs may not be killed with a single dose, some physicians recommend a second dose in two weeks.

TRICHURIASIS (WHIPWORM INFECTION). Trichuriasis occurs worldwide, is most common in tropical climates, and often is found in immigrants and travelers returning from such areas. Almost one billion people harbor the Trichuris parasite. Infection is acquired by ingesting embryonated eggs, usually on raw vegetables. First-stage larvae hatch in the small intestine or colon and penetrate the mucosa where they develop for an additional week. Immature worms usually inhabit the cecum but also may be found in the upper colon, rectum, or appendix. In three to four months, the female begins to produce eggs. Adult worms often live for three years but can survive for ten years or longer. Since worms do not multiply in the human host, an existing infection can become heavier only by ingesting additional eggs.

Trichuriasis seldom produces discernible symptoms, although some individuals (especially children) with a heavy

TABLE 2.
ANTHELMINTIC DRUGS

| Generic Name | Source | | Principal Use(s) |
	U.S.	Foreign	
DRUGS OF CHOICE AND ALTERNATIVE DRUGS			
Albendazole[1]	Valbazen [Smith Kline & French]	United Kingdom [Smith Kline & French][2]	Echinococciasis
Bithionol[1, 2]	CDC (Bithin, Lorothidol)	Japan (Bitin)	Fasciolasis Paragonimiasis
Cambendazole[1, 2]	Equiben, Novazole [Merck Sharp & Dohme]	United Kingdom [Merck Sharp & Dohme]	Strongyloidiasis
Diethylcarbamazine Citrate[2]	CDC	Canada, United Kingdom, Australia, West Germany (Hetrazan [Lederle]); France (Notezine)	Filariasis Visceral Larva Migrans[3]
Flubendazole[1]	---	Belgium [Janssen]	Echinococciasis[3] Onchocerciasis
Ivermectin[1]	Eqvalan, Ivomec [Merck Sharp & Dohme]	United Kingdom (Ivomec [Merck Sharp & Dohme])	Onchocerciasis
Mebendazole	Vermox [Janssen]	Canada, United Kingdom, Australia, South Africa, West Germany (Vermox [Janssen])	Ascariasis Echinococciasis[3] Enterobiasis Onchocerciasis[3] Trichinosis[3] Trichuriasis Uncinariasis
Metrifonate[1]	CDC (Bilarcil)	West Germany (Bilarcil [Bayer])	Schistosomiasis (*S. haematobium*)
Niclosamide	Niclocide [Miles]	Canada, United Kingdom, Australia, South Africa, West Germany (Yomesan [Bayer]); Argentina (Sulqui)	Cestodiasis
Niridazole[1]	CDC (Ambilhar)	United Kingdom, South Africa (Ambilhar [CIBA]	Dirofilariasis Schistosomiasis (*S. japonicum*)
Oxamniquine	Vansil [Pfipharmecs]	South Africa (Vansil [Pfizer]); Brazil (Mansil [Pfizer])	Schistosomiasis (*S. mansoni*)
Paromomycin	Humatin [Parke-Davis]	Argentina (Gabbromicina [Montedison]); West Germany (Gabbromycin [Farmitalia])	Cestodiasis
Piperazine Citrate	Antepar [Burroughs Wellcome]	Switzerland (Helmizin, Wurmsirup [Siegfried]); France (Piperol Forte); Japan (Pipenin)	Ascariasis Enterobiasis Fasciolopsiasis[3]

(Continued on next page)

TABLE 2.
ANTHELMINTIC DRUGS (continued)

Generic Name	Source U.S.	Source Foreign	Principal Use(s)
DRUGS OF CHOICE AND ALTERNATIVE DRUGS (continued)			
Praziquantel	Biltricide [Miles]	West Germany (Biltricide [Bayer])	Cestodiasis[3] Clonorchiasis[3] Cysticercosis[3] Fascioliasis[3] Fasciolopsiasis[3] Opisthorchiasis[3] Paragonimiasis[3] Schistosomiasis
Pyrantel Pamoate	Antiminth [Pfipharmecs]	Canada, South Africa, Argentina, France (Combantrin [Pfizer]); West Germany (Helmex [Pfizer])	Ascariasis Enterobiasis Trichinosis[3] Uncinariasis[3]
Pyrvinium Pamoate	Povan [Parke-Davis]	Canada, Australia (Vanquin [Parke-Davis]); Argentina (Tru [Elea])	Enterobiasis
Suramin[1]	CDC (Fourneau 309, Bayer 205, Germanin, Moranyl, Belganyl, Naphuride, Antrypol, Naganol)	West Germany (Germanin [Bayer])	Onchocerciasis
Tetrachloroethylene[3]	Nema Worm Capsules [Parke-Davis][2]	---	Fasciolopsiasis
Thiabendazole	Mintezol [Merck Sharp & Dohme]	Canada, United Kingdom, Australia, South Africa (Mintezol [Merck Sharp & Dohme]); Argentina (Foldan)	Larva Migrans Strongyloidiasis Trichinosis[3]
SECONDARY AGENTS*			
Antimony Potassium Tartrate	---	United Kingdom	Schistosomiasis (S. haematobium, S. mansoni, S. japonicum)
Bephenium Hydroxy-naphthoate	---	United Kingdom, South Africa, West Germany (Alcopar [Burroughs Wellcome])	Ascariasis Uncinariasis
Hycanthone Mesylate	---	United Kingdom, South Africa (Etrenol [Winthrop])	Schistosomiasis (S. haematobium, S. mansoni)
Levamisole	---	United Kingdom (Ketrax [ICI]); Argentina (Meglum, Stimamizol); South Africa (Ergamisol)	Ascariasis
Stibocaptate	CDC (Astiban [Rochel])	United Kingdom (Astiban [Rochel])	Schistosomiasis (S. haematobium, S. japonicum, S. mansoni)

[1]Investigational drug in the U.S.
[2]Veterinary product
[3]Investigational indication in the U.S.
*These anthelmintics generally are less effective, have a limited spectrum of action, and/or possess a greater potential for serious adverse reactions. They have no role in therapy and are not available in the United States (except stibocaptate). Since availability and cost are important in the selection of drugs, they may be used in developing countries in certain endemic regions.

worm burden may develop diarrhea or dysentery. There may be eosinophilia of up to 15%, but it is seldom a useful diagnostic sign. When the worm load is extremely heavy, rectal prolapse may occur and expose a mucosa covered with small white worms. Anemia may be observed in malnourished or heavily infected children.

Patients with heavy infections must be treated. Mebendazole is the drug of choice.

STRONGYLOIDIASIS (THREADWORM INFECTION). Strongyloidiasis generally is restricted to tropical and subtropical areas. It is common in both southern Europe and the southern United States. Disease occurs when third-stage larvae penetrate the intact skin (usually on the feet or lower limbs), enter the cutaneous blood vessels, and are carried to the lungs. Larvae migrate to the alveoli, molt twice, and, as immature adults, ascend the bronchi and trachea and are swallowed. Upon reaching the small intestine, they burrow into the mucosa of the duodenum and jejunum. After about 17 days, the female begins to lay eggs, which hatch into first-stage larvae. These larvae are passed in the feces; if the feces are deposited on soil, the larvae feed on bacteria and molt twice, developing into the nonfeeding infectious third-stage larvae, which can survive for about two weeks under optimum conditions. They can be killed by drying, excessive moisture, or temperatures below 8 C.

Despite the potential severity of strongyloidiasis, the infection is usually asymptomatic. Mild infection is associated with abdominal pain and occasionally with intermittent diarrhea and eosinophilia. Rash, especially over the thighs and buttocks, and intense pruritus may occur for a few days after infiltration of the parasite, followed by mild chest pains and cough. Symptoms of moderate infection include diarrhea, duodenitis (resembling peptic ulcer), and eosinophilia. Pneumonia also has been observed. The manifestations of severe infection (hyperinfection syndrome or disseminated strongyloidiasis) include vomiting, acute abdominal pain, voluminous foul-smelling stools, malabsorption syndrome, dehydration, electrolyte imbalance, and secondary bacteremia. Edema and paralytic ileus may develop, and the mortality rate is high in certain patients (eg, immunocompromised host) (Davidson et al, 1984).

Strongyloidiasis should always be treated. If untreated, even in initially asymptomatic individuals, a cyclic autoinfection may develop in which larvae penetrate the colon or perianal mucosa, migrate through the systemic circulation, and re-enter the intestine. Such an infection may be maintained for many years and result in a massive worm burden. Severe autoinfection can be fatal, especially in patients receiving corticosteroids or other immunosuppressive drugs (Davidson et al, 1984). These agents should be discontinued if possible.

Thiabendazole [Mintezol] usually controls the infection. In serious infections that do not respond to thiabendazole or in patients who cannot tolerate this drug, a veterinary preparation, cambendazole, has been reported to be effective (Bicalho et al, 1983).

UNCINARIASIS (HOOKWORM INFECTION). The two major hookworm diseases that affect man, *ancylostomiasis* and *necatoriasis,* occur in the tropics and subtropics. Both are common in Africa, Asia, and South America and to a lesser extent in northern Australia, Japan, and Portugal. *Necator* also is found in the southern United States and West Indies and *Ancylostoma* in Italy and the North African littoral. Hookworm infection is most common in rural areas where there is high rainfall and shade, low standards of sanitation, and the inhabitants often go barefoot.

Infection occurs when third-stage larvae penetrate the skin or are swallowed (frequent with *Ancylostoma duodenale*). Larvae migrate by way of the lymphatics, venules, and the venous bloodstream via the heart to the lungs where they penetrate the alveoli, ascend the bronchi and trachea, and are swallowed. When larvae reach the small intestine, they attach themselves to the luminal walls by means of a buccal capsule where they suck blood. As tissue erodes and is digested, the worms move to new sites. Shallow ulcerations are created at the site of attachment and lead to blood loss. Blood also passes from the anus of the worm. The segmented egg is passed in the feces. If deposited on soil, the first-stage larvae hatch in 24 hours, feed on organic material or bacteria, and molt twice to form the third-stage, nonfeeding, filariform larvae. These larvae can survive for about four weeks in shaded, moist, sandy soil.

A process of arrested development has been described for *Ancylostoma* organisms in India. Larvae that invade the body during the latter part of the monsoon season may remain dormant until the following year when they develop into adults. Thus, an infection may be manifested many months after an individual has left the endemic area.

Nausea, vomiting, and abdominal pain may occur during acute infections. Chronic blood loss is characteristic of hookworm infections and individuals with marginal iron intake or inadequate iron stores (eg, malnourished children, some menstruating women) are especially prone to anemia. Patients with satisfactory iron intake may develop anemia if blood loss cannot be compensated by the normal erythropoietic mechanisms. Thus, symptoms and signs of progressive iron deficiency anemia may occur, and this condition must be corrected at the same time that anthelmintic therapy is begun. Additional symptoms include abdominal fullness, epigastric pain, and cough due to pneumonitis that occurs when large numbers of worms are migrating through the lungs. Local erythema and pruritus ("ground itch") may develop at the site of skin penetration.

The incidence of hookworm infection has decreased markedly in the United States (except for some areas in the South) and the species is almost universally *Necator*. Some cases are imported and the species usually is unknown at the time of treatment. Pyrantel (investigational use) and mebendazole are the drugs of choice for treating either variety of hookworm. Bephenium and tetrachloroethylene are effective, but they are used principally in other parts of the world. Individuals with light worm burdens are asymptomatic and may not require treatment in the absence of anemia.

Tissue Infections

CUTANEOUS LARVA MIGRANS (CREEPING ERUPTION). This skin infection most often is caused by *Ancylostoma braziliense*, a species of hookworm common in cats and dogs, but also may be caused by *Uncinaria stenocephala* or *A. caninum*. It occurs on the southeastern and gulf coasts of the United States and in many tropical and subtropical areas, including tropical South America, Africa, and the Malay peninsula.

Filariform larvae usually penetrate the skin of the feet, legs, and hands. Individuals often are infected by lying on beaches contaminated by dog and cat feces. The larvae migrate around in the skin at the rate of 1 to 2 cm daily for several months but usually do not visceralize in man. Rarely, some larvae reach the lungs and cause eosinophilia and patchy pulmonary infiltration. An allergic reaction to the worm causes intense pruritus ("ground itch") that leads to scratching, excoriation of the skin, and secondary infection. The appearance of the lesion left by the entrance of the larvae and the occurrence of an erythematous, serpiginous, intracutaneous tract or burrow usually are diagnostic.

Thiabendazole, used both systemically and topically, eradicates this parasite. In countries where infection is common, ethyl chloride spray is used with topical formulations containing bacitracin, polymyxin B, and neomycin (eg, Mycitracin, Neo-Polycin, Neosporin) to control associated bacterial skin infections.

VISCERAL LARVA MIGRANS (TOXOCARIASIS). This condition is due to the prolonged larval migration of animal nematodes in human tissue other than skin. It is caused by ascaris of the dog (*Toxocara canis*) or cat (*T. cati*) or by other nematodes (eg, *Toxascaris leonina*). Human infection occurs when eggs containing second-stage larvae are ingested in soil or on raw vegetables contaminated by dog or cat feces. Sand boxes in public playgrounds are a common source of infection in young children. After the larvae hatch in the intestine, they migrate by way of the bloodstream or peritoneal serosa to the lungs and liver. The larvae are very thin and sometimes pass through the sinusoids to the kidney, brain, or eyes.

Infections with smaller numbers of larvae may be asymptomatic; eosinophilia may be present. Moderate to severe infection is manifested by persistent hypereosinophilia, hepatomegaly, and pneumonitis, particularly in children. Visceral larva migrans usually is self-limiting (duration, 18 months). It is diagnosed on suspicion aroused by the eosinophilia and is confirmed by serologic examination.

Specific treatment usually is not required; when the infection is severe, mebendazole or thiabendazole (both investigational) and a corticosteroid have been reported to minimize inflammation. Diethylcarbamazine is an alternative drug.

TRICHINOSIS (TRICHINELLIASIS, PORK ROUNDWORM INFECTION). This infection occurs worldwide. Areas of high incidence include eastern Europe and parts of western Europe, especially Poland, Austria, Germany, and Yugoslavia, where raw pork products are popular. Cases also have been reported in the Arctic, South America, Asia, and East Africa. The incidence of infection in the United States has decreased markedly over the past few years, and infection is uncommon in Great Britain and France. Australia has no indigenous trichinelliasis.

The most common reservoir of infection for man is the domestic pig, but other carnivores may host *Trichinella spiralis*, including the wild boar, bear, fox, wildcat, weasel, martin, lynx, badger, and rat. Human infection typically is acquired when undercooked pork or pork products containing encysted larvae are ingested. The cyst wall is digested in the stomach, and first-stage larvae invade the mucosa of the duodenum where they molt four times. Fertilized females appear in the intestinal lumen in less than two days and begin to produce first-stage larvae that are deposited in the ileal mucosa. Adult females live for only a few weeks. The larvae are carried to skeletal muscle by the blood stream and lymphatics and become encysted in a collagenous capsule in about 17 days. Thus, three weeks are required before encysted larvae will appear in a press preparation or digested specimen of a muscle biopsy or the bentonite flocculation serologic test becomes strongly positive. Some encysted larvae live for years, while others die and are calcified within a few months.

Trichinosis may cause gastrointestinal upset, fever, myalgia, periorbital edema, sore throat, and eosinophilia (25% to 50%). The great majority of affected individuals recover following the use of aspirin and supportive therapy, but cysts remain in the muscles. A small percentage of patients develop life-threatening complications, such as congestive heart failure, meningitis, neuritis, or a Guillain-Barré-type syndrome.

Thiabendazole has some effect on the migrating larvae but has little effect on encapsulated forms. It kills adult female worms and may decrease worm load. Corticosteroids are useful during larval migration to reduce inflammation, but they may increase production of larvae. Mebendazole has been used investigationally in large doses for a prolonged period to kill encysted larvae (Levin, 1983). Pyrantel kills only adult forms.

FILARIASIS. These infections are transferred to man by insect bite. Filariasis is confined exclusively to the tropics and subtropics, because the insects that serve as vectors or reservoirs are found only in these areas. Microfilariae are ingested by certain insects while taking a blood meal from infected persons and are passed to noninfected individuals in the same fashion. Although the diseases caused by these tissue-invasive nematodes are of greatest concern in endemic areas, travelers returning from these areas rarely harbor parasites (*Loa loa* may be an exception).

Onchocerciasis (Onchocerca volvulus infection): This infection is rare in travelers returning from the tropics, because the areas where these infections are endemic (West and Central Africa, Central and South America) are not popular tourist areas, and prolonged exposures are required generally to produce infections. The disease is characterized by skin irritation occurring about one year after the infection is acquired, skin nodules, and corneal opacities. Macrofilariae (adults) are located in skin nodules and are relatively innocuous; however, the microfilariae (larvae) migrate to many tissues and cause severe symptoms and signs. Degenerating microfilariae can provoke a serious inflammatory response (Mazotti reaction), especially in the skin and eye. Blindness occurs only in individuals with large worm burdens who have lived in an endemic area for years.

Diethylcarbamazine followed by suramin is the most effective regimen of treatment for onchocerciasis (Edwards, 1984), but is not often used in the United States because of toxicity. Diethylcarbamazine is effective only against the microfilariae, while suramin kills the macrofilariae. Intermittent administration of diethylcarbamazine controls the signs and symptoms of disease (eg, when reinfection is chronic and parenteral suramin is not readily available, practical, or warranted because of its toxicity). Suramin has some microfilaricidal activity, but its use alone initially may produce a severe allergic reaction affecting the eye.

Suramin is relatively more toxic (substantial nephrotoxicity) than diethylcarbamazine and must be given intravenously. Diethylcarbamazine is well tolerated and safe, but allergic reactions (especially those causing ocular complications) may occur due to disintegration and redistribution of microfilariae (Mazzoti reaction). The concomitant use of corticosteroids to minimize this allergic response may decrease the effectiveness of diethylcarbamazine. Reduction of the dose of diethylcarbamazine during initial therapy appears to control this reaction more effectively.

The investigational use of mebendazole or flubendazole (preferred but not available in the United States) may be an acceptable alternative. These benzimidazoles affect adult worms much more than the larvae; therefore, fewer ocular complications have been observed. Ultimately, long-term suppression of microfilariae results from the embryocidal and macrofilaricidal activities of these drugs. Side effects have been minimal but flubendazole causes severe irritation at the site of injection (Dominguez-Vasquez et al, 1983).

Ivermectin, a potent oral agent, is being evaluated in onchocerciasis (Aziz et al, 1982; Campbell et al, 1983; *Lancet*, [Nov 3] 1984; Awadzi et al, 1984; Lariviere et al, 1985). This microfilaricidal drug appears to be superior to diethylcarbamazine, because fewer Mazzoti reactions occur (Greene et al, 1985). Although it acts slowly, a single oral dose is as effective as eight days of diethylcarbamazine. Like flubendazole, even microfilariae contained in the adult worm are killed; the drug has little or no effect on adult worms.

Lymphatic Filariasis (Wuchereriasis, Brugiasis): Wuchereriasis (caused by *Wuchereria bancrofti*) and brugiasis (caused by *Brugia malayi*) are serious diseases (WHO Expert Committee on Filariasis, 1984). It is unlikely that a visitor to an endemic area will become infected based on studies of the rates of infection among American servicemen stationed in the southwest Pacific during World War II and French soldiers in Indochina during the 1950's.

Individuals with light infections, even those who live in the tropics, may be asymptomatic. Heavier infections may produce (1) a syndrome described as "filarial fevers" or paroxysmal inflammatory filariasis (Weller and Arnow, 1983); and (2) lymphatic obstruction by macrofilariae that causes severe edema with hydrocele or elephantiasis.

The syndrome of tropical pulmonary eosinophilia may develop and is characterized by nocturnal paroxysmal cough, hypereosinophilia (3,000 to 50,000 cells/mm³), elevated sedimentation rate, radiologic evidence of diffuse miliary lesions or increased bronchovascular markings, high titers of filarial and IgE antibodies, and impaired (restrictive-type) pulmonary function. Hepatosplenomegaly and lymphadenopathy have been observed. Chronic pulmonary fibrosis results if the disease is untreated.

Paroxysmal inflammatory filariasis is characterized by chills and fever lasting two to ten days and associated with headache, nausea, vomiting, diaphoresis, constipation, urticarial

rash, lymphadenitis, and lymphangitis that develops in a retrograde fashion. These episodes occur in paroxysms and may last for many years.

Diethylcarbamazine has microfilaricidal activity. It also has sufficient macrofilaricidal activity against *W. bancrofti*, *B. malayi*, and *B. timori*, which cause lymphatic filariasis, to be curative when used alone in large doses for prolonged periods (WHO Expert Committee on Filariasis, 1984).

Loiasis, Dipetalonemiasis, Ozzardi Filariasis: Microfilariae of *Loa loa*, *Dipetalonema perstans*, or *Mansonella ozzardi* may be found in the blood of individuals who have lived in an endemic area for a significant period of time. Travelers to these areas usually are not affected except possibly for loiasis. Of the three infections, loiasis is the most important clinically. Localized painful swelling of the arms and legs develops 3 to 12 months following infection and often subsides in a few days. Similar swelling may be noted around the eyes when the adult worms are in the subcutaneous tissues around the eye. Neurologic disturbances are rare. Eosinophilia develops, especially after treatment.

Patients with dipetalonemiasis usually are asymptomatic, but fever, swelling, arthritis, hepatomegaly with abdominal pain, and hypereosinophilia may occur.

Mansonella worms are usually regarded as nonpathogenic, although fever, headache, lymphadenitis, and erythematous rashes have occurred. Cold extremities also have been reported, presumably caused by a filarial toxin.

Diethylcarbamazine is effective against *Loa loa* and *Dipetalonema perstans*; the drug is rarely needed for infections caused by *Mansonella ozzardi*.

Dirofilariasis (Dracontiasis, Dracunculiasis, Guinea Worm Infection): This disease is acquired by ingesting infected water fleas from contaminated shallow ponds or wells. The larvae penetrate the intestinal wall and mature in loose connective tissue, especially in the legs and feet. The male worm dies after copulation. The adult gravid female emerges, usually from the foot or leg through an ulceration that has formed, approximately one year after infection. A few weeks before the worm appears at the skin surface, patients often develop urticaria. If the condition is recognized before the worms burst through the skin and cause an inflammatory reaction, they can be extracted with a forceps. Intense, painful, inflammatory reactions, often with secondary bacterial infections and tetanus, may occur if the disease is untreated or treated improperly.

Although the benzimidazole, niridazole, and the nitroimidazole, metronidazole [Flagyl, Metryl], are used in this disease, their beneficial action appears unrelated to any antiparasitic effect; however, they minimize the high risk of secondary skin infection and inflammation (*Lancet*, 1983).

CESTODE INFECTIONS

Intestinal Infections

TAENIASIS (BEEF AND PORK TAPEWORM INFECTION). These tapeworm infections occur worldwide and result from ingestion of raw or undercooked meat containing live cysticerci; man is the only definitive host. The adult worm fastens itself to the intestinal wall by means of suckers, hooks, or grooves in the scolex (head) and develops a long strobilum (body) composed of segmental proglottids. Eggs pass out of the bowel, either free or in gravid segments, and, following ingestion by the appropriate intermediate host, hatch to form the larval stage. These larvae penetrate the intestinal mucosa and develop into encysted forms, thereby completing the cycle. Intermediate hosts for *Taenia saginata* are cattle, llamas, buffalo, and related species. *T. saginata* rarely produces symptoms; reports of abdominal discomfort, weight loss, and excessive hunger are not well documented. The usual intermediate hosts for *T. solium* are domestic swine and wild boars. Although the adult form of *T. solium* rarely causes signs and symptoms, cysticercosis is a danger (see below).

DIPHYLLOBOTHRIASIS (FISH TAPEWORM INFECTION). *Diphyllobothrium* infections are acquired by eating undercooked or raw fish containing a plerocercoid, which is the form infective to man. Once the adult worm develops, eggs are excreted in the feces. If deposited in water, a ciliated embryo hatches and may be eaten by a freshwater flea, which, in turn, is eaten by various freshwater fish. Most individuals harbor a single tapeworm and remain asymptomatic for years. Even infections with multiple tapeworms only occasionally cause minor complaints of abdominal discomfort, malaise, or weight loss. *D. latum* utilizes vitamin B_{12} and folic acid in unusually large quantities and may cause megaloblastic anemia, but this manifestation is not common. Therefore, infection, particularly with the larger species, often first becomes apparent when a segment (proglottid) is passed in the stool.

HYMENOLEPIASIS (DWARF TAPEWORM INFECTION). This disease is acquired by fecal contamination of the hands or food or from contact with contaminated soil. The definitive hosts are man, rats, and mice. No intermediate host is required. Eggs are immediately infective and enter the cells of intestinal villi. The intracellular egg develops into a cercocyst (an intermediate stage), from which the adult tapeworm hatches.

Hymenolepis nana is the most common tapeworm affecting man in this country. Infections involving large numbers of worms (up to 1,000) have been reported, particularly in mental hospitals or schools for young children where fecal-oral exposure is difficult to control. Anorexia, diarrhea, abdominal pain, headache, dizziness, and occasional seizures have been reported but are not well documented.

DIPYLIDIASIS (DOG TAPEWORM INFECTION). Unlike other intestinal tapeworms, *Dipylidium caninum* has an obligate intermediate host, the flea. More rarely, a louse or other arthropod may be the intermediate host. Fleas feed on eggs in proglottids passed by infected dogs or cats. The infection occurs primarily in children, who ingest fleas infected with the larval form (cysticercoid) of the organism. The adult worm develops in the small intestine in three to four weeks.

Patients often are asymptomatic but may complain of anorexia, abdominal pain, anal pruritus, weight loss, and irritability. Gravid segments (proglottids in short chains) may be observed in stool or on the perineum. These segments often are confused with pinworms (Hamrick et al, 1983).

Therapy: Tapeworms should be treated when diagnosed. The drug of choice for beef, pork, fish, and dog tapeworm infections is a single dose of niclosamide [Niclocide]. Praziquantel is also effective in all intestinal tapeworm infections (investigational use). It is the drug of choice for the dwarf tapeworm infection because a single dose kills both the cercocyst and adult worm compared to five days of treatment required for niclosamide. Unlike niclosamide, it is absorbed systemically but appears to be safe (Most, 1984; Pearson and Guerrant, 1983; Weniger and Schantz, 1984). Other drugs (eg, paromomycin) are not as effective or are potentially more toxic.

Tissue Infections

CYSTICERCOSIS. Man may be both the definitive and intermediate host of *Taenia solium* and *T. saginata*; however, cysticercosis due to *T. saginata* is extremely rare in man. *T. solium* can be acquired by ingestion of ova in contaminated food or soil. Autoinfection can occur. The mechanism is unclear. In any event, the larvae in the small intestine invade tissues, usually the brain, subcutaneous tissues, and skeletal muscles, to cause cysticercosis.

Light infections appear to be tolerated during migration, and only mild fever and slight muscular pain may be present. However, mortality is high in those with heavy infections. Encysted cysticerci in the muscles and subcutaneous tissues generally are well tolerated. Although severe symptoms occur with ocular, cardiac, and spinal involvement, they are most common with cerebral cysticercosis (neurocysticercosis). Symptoms of pressure or inflammatory reactions (eg, epilepsy, cerebral hypertension, blurred vision, iritis, iridocyclitis, retinal detachment) may be the first signs of involvement and may not occur until the encysted cysticerci die (three to five years).

Praziquantel is effective in some patients with neurocysticercosis (Pearson and Guerrant, 1983; Nash and Neva, 1984; Sotelo et al, 1984, 1985) and produces complete resolution of some cysts. Generally, a 14-day course of therapy is recommended. Adjunctive therapy with anticonvulsants, corticosteroids, or surgery for cerebral ventricular obstruction may be required.

ECHINOCOCCIASIS (HYDATID DISEASE). Only the larval form of this parasite develops in man, who is not the definitive host for either *Echinococcus granulosus* or *E. multilocularis*. Nevertheless, the infection may be serious because of formation of hydatid cysts. The disease is transmitted to man by ingestion of eggs excreted by infected canines (eg, dogs, wolves, foxes). Eggs may be picked up from the soil (pica in children) or while petting or skinning the animal and are transferred by licking the fingers. Hence, children are affected more often than adults. Cysts can take as long as 20 to 30 years to develop and usually are less than 10 cm in diameter but may grow much larger. They occur most often in the liver, except for a Canadian variant in which the lung is involved more frequently.

Hydatid disease is treated surgically. The role of mebendazole in the primary resolution of such cysts is unclear. It may be used to shrink cysts either preoperatively or in inoperable patients or to prevent secondary echinococciasis if spillage has occurred intraoperatively; however, these uses have not been established (Kune et al, 1983).

Albendazole, a benzimidazole related to mebendazole, has the same cestocidal and nematocidal actions (Prasad et al, 1985; Misra et al, 1985). Because it is much better absorbed systemically and attains higher concentration in the cystic fluid of hydatid disease, it is being investigated in this form of cestodiasis (Saimot et al, 1983; Morris et al, 1985). Nevertheless, considerably more data on the natural history of echinococciasis are required in addition to specific pharmacokinetic data on albendazole and comparison with flubendazole (investigational) before its definitive role in hydatid disease can be established (*Lancet*, [Sept 22] 1984; Schantz, 1985).

TREMATODE INFECTIONS

SCHISTOSOMIASIS (BLOOD FLUKE INFECTIONS). Freshwater snails are the intermediate hosts for these flukes, which produce infection by cercarial penetration of the skin. Transmission of the disease does not occur in the United States because the appropriate snails are not indigenous to this country. Swimmers' itch is sometimes seen in the United States. This irritation is caused by an animal schistosome that penetrates the skin but does not fully develop before it dies.

Acute Schistosomiasis: Dermatitis, which results from cercarial penetration of the skin, develops two to eight days after contracting the infection (Nash et al, 1982). Acute schistosomiasis (Katayama fever) may resemble serum sickness and follows the maturation of adult worms. Fever accompanied by cough, lymphadenopathy, anorexia, weight loss, malaise, angioedema, myalgia, urticaria, and eosinophilia may develop in two to eight weeks. Leukocytosis and elevated levels of alkaline phosphatase, IgG, IgE, and especially IgM are characteristic. Definitive diagnosis is based on identification of eggs in the feces five to six weeks after exposure. Stool sedimentation may be necessary because the eggs are so few in number. Signs and symptoms abate over three to four months without treatment even though the adult worms and eggs persist; the only therapy is supportive.

Chronic Schistosomiasis: The vasculature of the intestinal tract (intestinal polyposis), biliary system (hepatosplenomegaly), and, less commonly, the lungs may be sites of involvement in chronic schistosomiasis.

Chronic schistosomiasis produced by *Schistosoma mansoni, S. japonicum*, and *S. mekongi* affects the liver and is characterized by the gradual development of asymptomatic hepatosplenomegaly. Hepatic fibrosis (Symmer's fibrosis of the liver) and granulomata are typical pathologic findings. Variceal bleeding may be a late finding and is due to portal hypertension. Spinal cord disease (eg, transverse myelitis) is rare and appears to be caused by deposition of ova in spinal cord vessels. *S. japonicum* rarely invades the brain.

The urinary tract is most commonly involved in infection caused by *S. haematobium*. Painless hematuria, dysuria, and white cells in the urine are characteristic. Definitive diagnosis is based on identification of eggs in the urine. An association between bladder cancer and endemic schistosomiasis has been demonstrated, but the exact role of the schistosome remains elusive (Hicks, 1983).

Therapy: Active infection in acute and chronic schistosomiasis usually responds to chemotherapy. Praziquantel is the drug of choice in all forms (Nash et al, 1982; Pearson and Guerrant, 1983; Most, 1984; Weniger and Schantz, 1984). Oxamniquine [Vansil] is an alternative in *S. mansoni* infections and metrifonate in *S. haematobium* infection. The latter is well tolerated. Since antimony potassium tartrate and niridazole are only somewhat effective in *S. japonicum, S. mekongi*, and *S. intercalatum* infections and there is considerable concern about niridazole's potential carcinogenicity, their use for these organisms generally is not recommended in the United States. The hepatic fibrosis that occurs in chronic schistosomiasis cannot be reversed by drug therapy.

CLONORCHIASIS AND OPISTHORCHIASIS (CHINESE OR ORIENTAL LIVER FLUKE INFECTION). Infection sometimes occurs in patients who have traveled to the Far East and is common in the United States in Southeast Asian refugees. The disease is acquired by eating undercooked, raw, dried, or pickled freshwater fish. The larvae ascend the biliary tree from the duodenum and mature in the bile ducts. The disease is usually asymptomatic, but ascending cholangitis, biliary stones, and cholangiocarcinoma that cause malaise, epigastric pain, and tender hepatomegaly may develop. Eosinophilia is rare. The parasite may live for 40 years in man.

Praziquantel is effective and appears to be safe in the treatment of clonorchiasis and opisthorchiasis (Pearson and Guerrant, 1983; Most, 1984; Weniger and Schantz, 1984). Biliary obstruction may require surgery.

FASCIOLIASIS (SHEEP LIVER FLUKE INFECTION). This is the only indigenous fluke infection in the continental United States. The disease usually results from ingesting watercress and other aquatic plants collected from areas contaminated by animal excreta; a snail is required as an intermediate host.

Symptoms begin one to three months after acquiring the disease. Their severity depends upon the worm burden. The usual pattern is loss of appetite, slight fever, lassitude, and a dull ache in the hepatic area. The liver may be tender and enlarged. Urticaria also may be present and there may be a considerable eosinophilia.

Although experience is limited, praziquantel is effective (Pearson and Guerrant, 1983; Weniger and Schantz, 1984). Oral bithionol is a much less preferred alternative.

PARAGONIMIASIS (LUNG FLUKE INFECTION). *Paragonimus westermani*, which occurs in the Far East and Central and South America, is the most common etiologic agent of this disease in man. *P. kellicotti* appears to be limited to the Americas, but this organism and other species (eg, *P. skrjabini, P. heterotremus, P. africanus*) that are found in Africa, China, and other Far Eastern countries only infrequently infect man. Pulmonary symptoms, often with hemoptysis, are the primary manifestations of disease but gastrointestinal and central nervous system symptoms also may develop.

Currently available data suggest that praziquantel is effective and safer than the alternative drug, bithionol (Pearson and Guerrant, 1983; Most, 1984; Pachucki et al, 1984; Weniger and Schantz, 1984). Bithionol is not effective when the parasite is localized in the brain or spinal cord.

FASCIOLOPSIASIS (GIANT INTESTINAL FLUKE INFECTION). The giant intestinal fluke (*Fasciolopsis buski*) occurs primarily in Southeast Asia and is normally found in pigs. Eggs are passed in the feces and a snail acts as an intermediate host. Humans acquire the infection by eating raw vegetables grown in contaminated water (eg, water chestnuts).

Most infections are asymptomatic. Heavy infections may produce abdominal symptoms simulating peptic ulcer. Alternating diarrhea and constipation may be noted. Edema of the face and trunk sometimes occurs, especially in children. In its most severe form, intestinal stasis, ulceration, and complete bowel obstruction requiring surgical intervention have been reported.

Fasciolopsiasis is more responsive to therapy than some related infections. An early study demonstrated a 100% cure rate with praziquantel (Bunnag et al, 1983), which is the drug of choice if cost is not a limiting factor. Tetrachloroethylene is the preferred alternative but is available only as a veterinary product in the United States. Piperazine is less effective.

Drug Evaluations

DIETHYLCARBAMAZINE CITRATE

USES. Diethylcarbamazine destroys the microfilariae of *Wuchereria bancrofti, Brugia malayi, B. timori, Loa loa, Dipetalonema perstans*, and *Onchocerca volvulus*. Large doses given for prolonged periods kill or sterilize adult females of these species (except *Onchocerca*) and, therefore, usually are curative. The mechanism of action is unknown. The adults of *O. volvulus* must be removed surgically or treated with suramin sodium; otherwise, microfilariae generally reappear a few months after treatment with diethylcarbamazine (Edwards, 1984). The investigational microfilaricide, ivermectin, is at least as effective as diethylcarbamazine, does not cause allergic ocular complications because of its slow action, and does not cause migration of the microfilariae (see the Introduction).

Diethylcarbamazine has been used investigationally in visceral larva migrans.

ADVERSE REACTIONS. Adverse reactions directly attributable to diethylcarbamazine are usually mild and consist of headache, dizziness, weakness, nausea, and vomiting.

Allergic reactions caused by substances released when microfilariae are destroyed (Mazzoti reaction) are usually mild in patients with wuchereriasis but may be serious in those with onchocerciasis and loiasis. Effects include pedal edema that may be severe, intense pruritus, dermatitis, fever, colic, arthritis, and lymphadenitis. Ocular complications include punctate keratitis, uveitis, retinal pigment atrophy, and chorioretinitis. Tachycardia sometimes occurs. Allergic encephalopathy (reaction to dead microfilariae) is rare in patients treated for loiasis. These reactions usually subside within three to seven days, and doses larger than those that initiated the adverse effects may be administered without further problems.

PHARMACOKINETICS. Diethylcarbamazine is absorbed rapidly from the gastrointestinal tract. Peak blood concentrations are reached in approximately four hours. Renal excretion of unchanged compound and metabolites is complete 48 hours after a single dose.

DOSAGE AND PREPARATIONS. A gradual increase in dosage and/or the concomitant administration of antihistamines or corticosteroids is advisable to minimize allergic effects, particularly when there is ocular involvement with onchocerciasis. If reactions are severe, the dose should be reduced or treatment interrupted.

Oral: Adults, for infections caused by *Loa loa, W. bancrofti, B. malayi, B. timori,* and *D. perstans,* day 1: 50 mg; day 2, 50 mg three times; day 3, 100 mg three times; day 4 through day 21, 2 mg/kg three times a day. *Children,* day 1, 25 to 50 mg; day 2, 25 to 50 mg three times; day 3, 50 to 100 mg three times; day 4 through day 21, 2 mg/kg three times a day.

Because severe Mazzoti reactions are more likely when treating *O. volvulus* infections, the dosage schedule for either systemic or ocular onchocerciasis is: *Adults,* initially, 25 mg daily for three days, then 50 mg/day for five days, 100 mg/day for three days, and maintenance at 150 mg/day for two to three weeks. *Infants and small children,* 0.5 mg/kg three times daily (maximum, 25 mg daily) for three days, 1 mg/kg three times daily (maximum, 50 mg daily) for three or four days; 1.5 mg/kg three times daily (maximum, 100 mg daily) for three or four days, and maintenance at 2 mg/kg three times daily (maximum, 150 mg daily) for two to three weeks. An alternative maintenance dose for adults and children is 3 mg/kg three times daily for three weeks.

See the evaluation on Suramin Sodium for follow-up treatment of onchocerciasis. Some experts believe that *Loa loa* infections should be treated in the same manner as *O. volvulus* infections because of the potential for severe reactions.

Generic. Tablets 50, 200, and 400 mg. Available from the Drug Service, Centers for Disease Control. See the Introduction for address and telephone numbers.

MEBENDAZOLE
[Vermox]

USES. Mebendazole is a broad spectrum anthelmintic and is the drug of choice in trichuriasis (whipworm infection). Multiple doses have produced cure rates as high as 94% (particularly in children). Retreatment may be necessary in massive whipworm infections (more than 40,000 eggs/g of feces); the drug may decrease the fecal egg count by 70% to 99% even in refractory infections.

Mebendazole is a drug of choice for enterobiasis (pinworm infection) and both types of uncinariasis (hookworm infection) that commonly infect man. Single doses have produced cure rates of 90% to 100% in enterobiasis, and cure rates of approximately 95% have been reported after multiple doses were given to treat hookworm infection.

Mebendazole is an alternative drug in ascariasis but worms

have migrated to the mouths of a few children with heavy infections. Since a single dose of pyrantel is equally effective, this drug is preferred.

Because of its wide spectrum, mebendazole may be particularly useful in mixed infections. Large doses are being investigated in trichinosis (pork tissue roundworm), onchocerciasis, toxocariasis, and hydatid disease caused by *Echinococcus granulosus* (see the Introduction).

ADVERSE REACTIONS AND PRECAUTIONS. Occasional adverse effects include transient abdominal pain, diarrhea, fever, pruritus, and skin rash.

Reversible neutropenia may occur, especially when larger than usual doses are given to treat hydatid disease or trichinosis (Levin et al, 1983).

Mebendazole is reported to increase the secretion of insulin, which potentiates the action of exogenously administered insulin and oral hypoglycemic drugs (Caprio et al, 1984).

Teratogenic effects occurred in rats but not in dogs, sheep, or horses; nevertheless, this anthelmintic is contraindicated during pregnancy (FDA Pregnancy Category C).

PHARMACOKINETICS. Mebendazole has very low solubility and is poorly and variably but rapidly absorbed (less than 5% to 10%). Bioavailability is only 2.1% to 3.3% because of very high first-pass elimination (Dawson et al, 1985). Following a single oral dose of 10 mg/kg, peak plasma concentrations ranged from 17.5 to 500 ng/ml in 1.5 to 7.5 hours. The mean peak concentration after an initial dose (69.5 ng/ml) increased following chronic therapy (137.4 ng/ml) (Braithwaite et al, 1982). Systemic bioavailability is enhanced by concomitant ingestion of food. Three polar metabolites that undergo extensive enterohepatic recycling have been identified.

The elimination half-life of mebendazole has ranged from 2.8 to 9 hours; however, based upon studies in which the drug was given intravenously, these values may be more related to absorption rather than elimination half-life. The elimination half-life is prolonged in patients with impaired hepatic function. Unchanged mebendazole and its major metabolites are eliminated in the urine. Mebendazole is highly bound to plasma protein. Concentrations in tissue and hydatid cyst material from two patients ranged from 59.5 to 206.6 ng/g.

DOSAGE AND PREPARATIONS.
Oral: Adults and children, for most hookworm, roundworm, and whipworm infections, 100 mg morning and evening for three consecutive days; pinworm infections are usually cured by a single 100-mg dose. If cure is not achieved with initial therapy, a second course may be given two weeks later.

For trichinosis (investigational use), *adults,* 200 to 400 mg three times daily for three days, then 400 to 500 mg three times daily for ten days.

For hydatid disease (investigational use limited to patients with severe disease because of drug toxicity), 40 to 50 mg/kg/day in four divided doses for three to eight months to shrink cysts; the same dose can be given for three weeks postoperatively if there is spillage during surgery. The white count should be monitored frequently, especially during the first few weeks (Levin et al, 1983). A gradual increase in dosage may be indicated to determine individual tolerance. Some physicians recommend up to 200 mg/kg/day in four

divided doses to reach a blood concentration of 80 ng/ml, which appears to correlate well with drug efficacy.

Mebendazole has not been extensively investigated in *children under 2 years,* and the relative benefit:risk ratio must be considered when it is used in these patients.

Vermox (Janssen). Tablets (chewable) 100 mg.

METRIFONATE

$$(CH_3O)_2\overset{\overset{\displaystyle OH}{|}}{\underset{\underset{\displaystyle O}{||}}{P}}CHCCl_3$$

ACTIONS AND USES. Metrifonate, an organophosphorus cholinesterase inhibitor, acts by paralyzing worm musculature. It is slowly metabolized to dichlorvos in man.

Metrifonate is an alternative to praziquantel, the drug of choice, in *Schistosoma haematobium* infection of the urinary tract. The cure rate in this condition is 90% to 95%. Metrifonate has anticholinesterase activity; however, therapeutic doses are usually well tolerated.

ADVERSE REACTIONS AND PRECAUTIONS. Side effects usually are mild and transient and include abdominal discomfort, pain, diarrhea, vomiting, weakness, headache, dizziness, and vertigo. These effects probably are unrelated to effects on plasma cholinesterase. Plasma cholinesterase levels are depressed to approximately 5% of pretreatment values within six hours after the drug is administered and return to normal within four to six weeks. Therefore, metrifonate should be avoided when cholinesterase levels are already depressed (eg, in patients with genetic variants, severe liver disease, those living in areas where there is extensive use of organophosphorus insecticides). Furthermore, cholinesterase-inhibiting muscle relaxants should be avoided during surgery in any patient taking metrifonate unless assisted ventilation is used.

Mutagenicity and organ damage developed in animals after prolonged use of large doses of this drug. Toxicity from overdose is related to metrofinate's anticholinesterase action (see Chapter 80, Drugs Used in the Treatment of Poisoning).

DOSAGE AND PREPARATIONS.
Oral: 5 to 15 mg/kg every two weeks for three doses.
Available from the Drug Service, Centers for Disease Control (see the Introduction for address and telephone numbers). (Investigational drug)

NICLOSAMIDE
[Niclocide]

USES. Niclosamide is a drug of choice for intestinal tapeworm infections due to *Taenia saginata, T. solium, Diphyllobothrium latum,* and *Dipylidium caninum.* Interference with glucose uptake in the parasite is the proposed mechanism of action.

This anthelmintic can be given orally without intubation, and its use does not require hospitalization. Praziquantel is an alternative drug of choice for these infections, but it is preferred by some authorities for dwarf tapeworm (*H. nana*) infection, because a single-dose regimen is effective.

Concomitant use of a laxative is not necessary except in *T. solium* infections. Niclosamide may destroy *T. solium* segments during therapy, which release viable eggs; therefore, the laxative should be administered one to two hours after use of the anthelmintic to avoid cysticercosis.

ADVERSE REACTIONS AND PRECAUTIONS. Absorption is minimal and no serious adverse reactions have been reported. Up to 10% of patients may experience malaise, mild abdominal pain, and nausea on the day the drug is administered. Since tapeworm infections generally are not life-threatening, treatment of pregnant women should be postponed until after delivery.

DOSAGE AND PREPARATIONS. For intestinal tapeworm infections except *H. nana*, the patient should omit breakfast but may eat two hours after the last dose. *The tablets should be chewed thoroughly and swallowed with a little water.*
Oral: Adults, 2 g as a single dose. *Children weighing more than 34 kg (75 lb),* 1.5 g (three tablets) as a single dose; *11 to 34 kg (25 to 75 lb),* 1 g (two tablets) as a single dose.

For *H. nana* infections in *adults,* the drug should be administered daily for five successive days.
  Niclocide (Miles). Tablets (chewable) 500 mg.

NIRIDAZOLE
[Ambilhar]

USES. This investigational drug is only moderately effective against *Schistosoma japonicum, S. mekongi,* and *S. intercalatum.* It causes many adverse reactions; there is also concern about its carcinogenic potential, especially in immunocompromised patients. Therefore, niridazole is not recommended for infections due to these organisms in the United States; praziquantel is the drug of choice.

Niridazole is the drug of choice for dirofilariasis (dracontiasis, dracunculiasis). Its beneficial action appears to be unrelated to any antiparasitic effect. Rather, it minimizes secondary skin inflammation and infection that accompany the primary lesion of guinea worm infection.

ADVERSE REACTIONS. Children usually experience fewer untoward effects than adults. Gastrointestinal disturbances (eg, anorexia, abdominal cramping, vomiting, and diarrhea) are reversible upon discontinuation of the drug. Headache, dizziness, rashes, and, occasionally, electrocardiographic changes and neuropsychiatric disturbances (eg, insomnia, anxiety, confusion, hallucinations, seizures) also have been seen. Hemolytic anemia may occur in patients with G6PD deficiency.

Transient reduction in spermatogenesis has been reported experimentally, but additional studies are needed to determine the relevance of these effects on human spermatozoa.

PRECAUTIONS. The dose of niridazole should be reduced in patients with a history of liver disease, neuropsychiatric or convulsive disorders, decompensated heart disease, or renal insufficiency. If possible, niridazole should not be given with isoniazid to avoid additive hepatotoxic and neuropsychiatric actions.

Since experiments using body fluids of humans and mice have demonstrated that niridazole is mutagenic in small doses against certain bacteria, the drug should not be given to pregnant women. Additional studies are needed to ascertain its carcinogenicity.

PHARMACOKINETICS. Niridazole is absorbed from the gastrointestinal tract over 10 to 15 hours; peak plasma levels are attained after six hours. Considerable plasma binding occurs, and niridazole and its metabolites are uniformly distributed throughout tissues. It is metabolized extensively by the liver. The metabolites are excreted in the urine and feces, causing dark brown discoloration.

DOSAGE AND PREPARATIONS.
Oral: Adults and children, 25 mg/kg daily (maximum, 1.5 g) in two divided doses for five to ten days. For children, therapy is continued for 10 days in schistosomiasis and for 15 days in dirofilariasis.
  Ambilhar (CIBA). Available from the Drug Service, Centers for Disease Control (see the Introduction for address and telephone numbers).
  (Investigational drug)

OXAMNIQUINE
[Vansil]

USES. Oxamniquine, a tetrahydroquinoline derivative, has schistosomicidal activity and is an alternative to praziquantel in *Schistosoma mansoni* infections. This drug can be given orally as well as intramuscularly (the oral route is preferred) and the course of treatment is relatively short. In South America, especially Brazil, 100% cure rates have been reported following single doses. In Africa, the drug must be administered for several days to produce a 90% to 100% cure rate.

The mechanism of action is not established; however, muscular paralysis that impairs the adult worm's suckers is known to occur.

ADVERSE REACTIONS AND PRECAUTIONS. The most common side effects are dizziness and somnolence. Nausea, vomiting, fever, eosinophilia, transient pulmonary infiltration, liver function test abnormalities, electroencephalographic changes, hallucinations, and seizures also have been reported. Oxamniquine should not be given to patients with epilepsy, decompensated congestive heart failure, or renal failure.

Although there is no evidence of teratogenicity or carcinogenicity with oxamniquine, these problems have been reported with related compounds. Thus, this compound should be avoided in pregnant women (FDA Pregnancy Category C).

PHARMACOKINETICS. Oxamniquine is well absorbed after oral administration and time to peak plasma concentration is about three hours. Most of an administered dose is extensively metabolized in the liver, principally on a first-pass mechanism, and excreted in the urine. The elimination half-life of parent drug is 1 to 2.5 hours.

DOSAGE AND PREPARATIONS.

Oral: Adults (western hemisphere), 15 mg/kg as a single dose given after a meal or late in the day to minimize side effects; *(Africa)* 15 mg/kg twice daily for two days. *Children (western hemisphere),* 20 mg/kg in two equally divided doses two to eight hours apart; *(Africa)* 15 mg/kg twice daily for two days. *Intramuscular: (South America only)* 7.5 mg/kg as a single dose given after a meal or late in the day.

> *Vansil* (Pfipharmecs). Capsules 250 mg.

PIPERAZINE CITRATE
[Antepar]

USES. Piperazine is an alternative drug for the treatment of ascariasis and enterobiasis. Pyrantel or mebendazole are preferred for both infections. A single dose of piperazine cures approximately 70% of individuals with ascariasis. Two doses given on successive days increase the cure rate to between 90% and 100%. *Ascaris* worms are passed, paralyzed and alive, one to three days after treatment. A laxative is not needed to expel the worms from the gut.

In enterobiasis, the majority of worms are passed alive and active during the first four days of therapy. A seven-day course of treatment usually is needed for optimal effects.

Piperazine causes a reversible hyperpolarization-type of muscle paralysis in the helminths. It is readily absorbed from the gastrointestinal tract and most of an oral dose is excreted in the urine within 24 hours.

ADVERSE REACTIONS AND PRECAUTIONS. Therapeutic doses do not usually cause adverse effects, but nausea, vomiting, diarrhea, and allergic reactions may develop. With larger doses, as in inadvertent overdosage or when the drug accumulates in the presence of renal insufficiency, muscular incoordination or weakness, vertigo, dysphasia, confusion, and myoclonic contractions have been reported. These effects usually disappear when the drug is discontinued. Piperazine may induce or exacerbate epileptic seizures in predisposed patients. For these reasons, it is contraindicated in patients with renal or hepatic insufficiency or epilepsy.

No harmful effects on the fetus have been reported after use of piperazine in pregnant women.

DOSAGE AND PREPARATIONS. (Doses and strengths expressed in terms of the hexahydrate salt that is formed in solution from the citrate salt.)

Oral: For ascariasis, *adults and children,* 75 mg/kg (maximum, 3.5 g) once daily for two consecutive days. For enterobiasis, *adults and children,* 65 mg/kg (maximum, 2.5 g) once daily for seven consecutive days. The course should be repeated after a one-week interval. Fasting before treatment is not necessary.

> *Generic.* Syrup 500 mg/5 ml; tablets 250 and 500 mg.
> *Antepar* (Burroughs Wellcome). Tablets 500 mg.

PRAZIQUANTEL
[Biltricide]

ACTIONS. Praziquantel, a pyrazino-isoquinoline, has a broad spectrum of activity against trematodes (flukes) and cestodes (tapeworms). It causes loss of intracellular calcium resulting in paralysis and dislodgement of worms from sites of attachment. Bleb formation on the integument is followed by rupture and extensive vacuolization, which allows phagocytic attachment and lysis of the parasite.

USES. *Schistosomiasis (Blood Flukes):* Praziquantel is especially useful for all *Schistosoma* (blood flukes) that are pathogenic in man, ie, *S. mansoni, S. haematobium, S. japonicum, S. mekongi, S. intercalatum* (Nash et al, 1982; Pearson and Guerrant, 1983; Most, 1984; Weniger and Schantz, 1984). It is the drug of choice for infections caused by all of the above organisms. Alternative chemotherapy for *S. mansoni* (oxamniquine) and *S. haematobium* (metrifonate) are available if cost, availability, or other factors militate against use of praziquantel. Niridazole and antimony potassium tartrate are alternatives for *S. japonicum, S. mekongi,* and *S. intercalatum,* but they are seldom effective and are toxic.

Praziquantel is equally effective in both acute and chronic schistosomiasis. Hepatic fibrosis is not reversed by drug treatment; however, the pathogenic process usually can be halted and fecal egg counts markedly reduced or eliminated.

Clonorchiasis, Opisthorchiasis, Fascioliasis, Paragonimiasis, Fasciolopsiasis: Praziquantel is being investigated for use in these trematode infections. Very good cure rates have been documented for clonorchiasis, opisthorchiasis, and paragonimiasis (Pachucki et al, 1984), and in limited studies, for fascioliasis and fasciolopsiasis. Praziquantel is considered the drug of choice in infections caused by *Clonorchis* and *Opisthorchis* species (Chinese or Oriental liver flukes), and most authorities recommend that it replace bithionol as the drug of choice in paragonimiasis and fascioliasis. Results of limited studies show that praziquantel is probably more effective than tetrachloroethylene in the treatment of fasciolopsiasis (Bunnag et al, 1983).

Taeniasis, Diphyllobothriasis, Hymenolepiasis: Although most of this drug is systemically absorbed, praziquantel is as effective as niclosamide and appears to be quite safe in intestinal infections caused by *Taenia saginata, T. solium*, and *Diphyllobothrium latum*. A single dose of praziquantel seems to be as effective as niclosamide given for five days in dwarf tapeworm infection. Thus, praziquantel is the drug of choice in hymenolepiasis even though it is investigational for this use.

Cysticercosis: Praziquantel is effective in the treatment of cysticercosis (including neurocysticercosis) caused by *Taenia solium* (Nash and Neva, 1984; Sotelo et al, 1984). Results of early studies show that the drug produces partial or complete cyst resolution and is an effective addition to surgery, anticonvulsants, or corticosteroids in the management of this serious parasitic disease.

ADVERSE REACTIONS AND PRECAUTIONS. The following adverse reactions are much more likely to occur after use of larger doses. Dizziness, headache, malaise, abdominal pain, and nausea are relatively common but generally mild and transient. Lassitude, diarrhea, urticaria, pruritus, fever, sweating, pruritic rash, and mild to moderate increases in SGOT and SGPT levels occur less frequently, but also are usually transient and reversible. Vomiting also occurs.

Praziquantel is related chemically to sedative and antianxiety agents. Because drowsiness develops relatively frequently, the patient should be advised to use caution while driving or performing activities that require mental alertness until one day after the last dose is taken.

A syndrome consisting of headache, hyperthermia, seizures, intracranial hypertension, and/or arachnoiditis develops in almost all patients treated for neurocysticercosis with praziquantel. This syndrome is presumed to result from an inflammatory response to dead and dying organisms in cerebrospinal fluid and nervous tissue. Since destruction of parasites within the eye may cause irreparable lesions, the treatment of ocular cysticercosis should be undertaken only by experts.

No serious drug interactions have been reported.

Experience with acute praziquantel overdosage in humans is limited. The oral LD_{50} in animals ranges from 1 to 2.8 g/kg.

The safety of praziquantel in children under 4 years of age has not been established.

PREGNANCY AND LACTATION. Reproduction studies performed in rats and rabbits using up to 40 times the human dose revealed no evidence of impaired fertility or harm to the fetus. The abortion rate in rats increased when three times the single human therapeutic dose was given. There are no well-controlled studies in pregnant women. This drug should be used during pregnancy only if clearly needed (FDA Pregnancy Category B).

Praziquantel appears in human breast milk in concentrations about one-fourth those in maternal serum. Women should not nurse on the day praziquantel is given and for 72 hours thereafter.

PHARMACOKINETICS. About 80% of an oral dose is absorbed; however, extensive first-pass hepatic hydroxylation in the circulation markedly reduces the amount of unchanged praziquantel (Leopold et al, 1978). A single 50-mg oral dose in healthy adults produces peak serum concentrations of 1 mcg/ml in one to two hours. The anthelmintic activity of metabolites is unknown. Distribution in the tissues is not well documented, but the cerebrospinal fluid concentration is 10% to 20% of that in the serum (free and bound) and about 25% appears in human milk.

Metabolites of praziquantel are excreted principally (80%) in the urine; their half-lives are four to five hours. Praziquantel has a serum half-life of 0.8 to 1.5 hours.

DOSAGE AND PREPARATIONS. Since praziquantel has a bitter taste, the tablets should not be chewed before swallowing to avoid gagging and emesis.

Oral: For *Schistosoma japonicum* and *S. mekongi* infections, *adults and children over 4 years*, 60 mg/kg/day in three equal doses every four to six hours. For infections caused by *S. haematobium* and *S. mansoni*, 40 mg/kg in a single dose.

For fascioliasis, fasciolopsiasis, paragonimiasis, clonorchiasis, and opisthorchiasis (investigational uses), *adults and children over 4 years*, 75 mg/kg daily given in three equal doses every four to six hours. Treatment is for one day in fascioliasis and fasciolopsiasis, for one or two days in paragonimiasis, and for one to three days in clonorchiasis and opisthorchiasis; the course may be repeated for clonorchiasis or opisthorchiasis if required.

For taeniasis and diphyllobothriasis (investigational uses), *adults and children over 4 years*, 10 to 20 mg/kg in a single dose.

For hymenolepiasis (investigational use), *adults and children over 4 years*, 15 to 25 mg/kg in a single dose.

For cysticercosis (investigational use), *adults and children over 4 years*, 50 mg/kg/day in three equal doses every four to six hours for 14 days. Concomitant corticosteroid treatment (eg, dexamethasone 6 to 16 mg daily, prednisone 30 to 40 mg daily) is recommended in patients with cerebral involvement. Therapy may be repeated in three to six months if necessary.

Biltricide (Miles). Tablets 600 mg.

PYRANTEL PAMOATE
[Antiminth]

ACTIONS AND USES. Pyrantel is a drug of choice for ascariasis and enterobiasis; cure rates are 90% to 100% following a single dose. Most authorities consider it a drug of choice for uncinariasis (hookworm infections) (investigational use). Cure rates ranging from 48% to 93% for *Necator americanus* and 92% to 93% for *Ancylostoma duodenale* have been reported. This drug is ineffective in trichuriasis (whipworm) and strongyloidiasis (threadworm) infections. Pyrantel kills only the adult form of *Trichinella spiralis*; it has no effect on the larva encysted form.

Pyrantel acts as a depolarizing neuromuscular blocking agent that paralyzes the worms, which are then expelled from the body, usually without requiring a laxative.

ADVERSE REACTIONS AND PRECAUTIONS. Systemic adverse reactions include anorexia, nausea, headache, dizziness, drowsiness, and rash. Other untoward effects that probably result from local activity in the gut are abdominal pain, vomiting, and diarrhea. Transient elevation of the SGOT level may occur; therefore, pyrantel should be used with caution in patients with pre-existing liver dysfunction.

There has been little experience with the drug in children under 2 years, and its safety during pregnancy has not been determined.

PHARMACOKINETICS. Pyrantel is poorly and incompletely absorbed from the gastrointestinal tract; most of an oral dose is excreted unchanged in the feces and about 7% is excreted unchanged in the urine.

DOSAGE AND PREPARATIONS.
(Dosage expressed in terms of the base)
Oral: Adults and children, for ascariasis and enterobiasis, a single dose of 11 mg/kg (maximum, 1 g); for uncinariasis (investigational use), this dose is given for three consecutive days. Fasting before treatment is not necessary. Dosage may be repeated in one month if indicated.
   Antiminth (Pfipharmecs). Oral suspension 250 mg/5 ml (equivalent to base).

PYRVINIUM PAMOATE
[Povan]

USES. Pyrvinium pamoate is the salt of a cyanine dye. It is an alternative to pyrantel and mebendazole in enterobiasis (pinworm infection); a single oral dose produces cure rates of up to 96%. However, since reinfection is common, a second course of therapy should be given two or three weeks after the first; a cure cannot be assured until perianal swabs of cellophane tape are free of eggs for five to six weeks.

ADVERSE REACTIONS AND PRECAUTIONS. Pyrvinium is minimally absorbed from the gastrointestinal tract. Nausea, abdominal cramps, vomiting, and, rarely, photosensitivity occur. Patients should be told that the drug stains stools bright red and will stain clothing if vomited.

DOSAGE AND PREPARATIONS. (Dosage expressed in terms of the base)
Oral: For enterobiasis, *adults and children,* a single dose of 5 mg/kg, repeated in two or three weeks. The tablets should be swallowed immediately and not chewed.
   Povan (Parke-Davis). Tablets 50 mg (equivalent to base).

SURAMIN SODIUM

USES. Suramin, a complex derivative of urea, is used parenterally in the treatment of African trypanosomiasis (see Chapter 77, Antiprotozoal Agents). It also has been used investigationally with diethylcarbamazine to kill the adult *Onchocerca.* Multiple doses of suramin kill adult female *O. volvulus* within one or two months, but males remain alive longer. Microfilariae disappear over a period of several months. The mechanism of action of suramin is unknown.

ADVERSE REACTIONS AND PRECAUTIONS. The need for multiple doses and the potentially dangerous adverse reactions limit the usefulness of suramin; close medical supervision during treatment is essential.

Suramin may cause nausea, vomiting, colic, urticaria, severe local irritation on extravasation, and, in very sensitive persons, shock, syncope, acute circulatory failure, and seizures. Because suramin has some microfilaricidal activity, allergic reactions to proteins released by degenerating microfilariae (eg, pruritus, rash, fever, edema, burning and hyperesthesia of the soles, photophobia, iritis, lacrimation) occur but generally are less intense than with diethylcarbamazine. The drug may cause albuminuria, casts, hematuria, and, rarely, agranulocytosis or hemolytic anemia, exfoliative dermatitis, nephritis, and renal failure. It is contraindicated in patients with severe renal or ocular disease.

PHARMACOKINETICS. Suramin must be administered parenterally. It is extensively and tightly bound to plasma protein; low plasma concentrations persist for as long as three months after terminating administration.

DOSAGE AND PREPARATIONS.
Intravenous: A 10% solution in water for injection is used. For onchocerciasis (investigational use), *adults,* 100 mg initially to test tolerance, then 1 g weekly for five weeks. The total dose should not exceed 5.5 g, since larger doses may cause renal toxicity. *Children,* 100 mg initially to test tolerance, then 10 to 15 mg/kg weekly for five weeks. Severe local irritation results from extravasation. The drug may be administered intramuscularly if the intravenous route is impractical.
   Available from the Drug Service, Centers for Disease Control (see the Introduction for address and telephone numbers). (Investigational indication)

TETRACHLOROETHYLENE

$$Cl_2C = CCl_2$$

USES. Tetrachloroethylene was used extensively in hookworm infections, but more effective and less toxic agents are now available. However, it has been used investigationally as an alternative to praziquantel for fasciolopsiasis (intestinal giant fluke infection). It is available in the United States only as a veterinary preparation (eg, Nema Worm Capsules).

ADVERSE REACTIONS. Nausea, vomiting, dizziness, and inebriation occur occasionally. Syncope has been reported rarely. Tetrachloroethylene has been used safely in severely anemic patients.

PHARMACOKINETICS. Sufficient tetrachloroethylene may be absorbed from the gut to produce inebriation. If it is absorbed orally, tetrachloroethylene is excreted largely by the lungs.

DOSAGE AND PREPARATIONS.

Oral: Adults and children, 0.1 ml/kg (maximum, 5 ml). Only a low-bulk, low-fat meal should be eaten the evening before treatment, and alcohol must be avoided before and for 24 hours after use of tetrachloroethylene. Breakfast is omitted and the drug is given early in the morning; the patient should remain recumbent for the next four hours if possible. No laxative should be given, since this increases the toxic effects and decreases the effectiveness of the drug.

Available in the United States only in veterinary preparations (eg, **Nema Worm Capsules** [Parke-Davis]). These capsules contain pure tetrachloroethylene. Available sizes are 0.2, 0.5, 1, 2.5, and 5 ml.

THIABENDAZOLE

[Mintezol]

USES. Thiabendazole is the drug of choice in *Strongyloides stercoralis* (threadworm) infection; cure rates of almost 100% have been achieved. It may be lifesaving in disseminated strongyloidiasis (hyperinfection syndrome), which occurs primarily in immunocompromised patients. It also is the drug of choice for oral and topical therapy of cutaneous larva migrans caused by *Ancylostoma braziliense* and for oral therapy in visceral larva migrans due to *Toxocara canis* and *T. cati.*

In trichinosis, thiabendazole reduces the number of developing and migrating larvae of *Trichinella spiralis*; activity also has been demonstrated against adult female *T. spiralis* in the intestine. Thiabendazole is ineffective against encysted larvae.

Although this drug is useful in other nematode infections (ie, ascariasis, trichuriasis, uncinariasis, enterobiasis), safer and more effective drugs are available.

Thiabendazole is proposed to act by inhibiting the helminth-specific enzyme, fumarate reductase.

ADVERSE REACTIONS AND PRECAUTIONS. Common untoward effects are dizziness, drowsiness, giddiness, anorexia, nausea, and vomiting. Diarrhea, fever, epigastric distress, flushing, chills, angioedema, pruritus, lethargy, rash, and headache occur less frequently. Additional adverse reactions include tinnitus, conjunctival injection, blurred vision, hypotension, syncope, anaphylaxis, numbness, seizures, transient leukopenia, lymphadenopathy, enuresis, hyperglycemia, impaired liver function, jaundice, xanthopsia, crystalluria, hematuria, and collapse. A few cases of erythema multiforme and Stevens-Johnson syndrome have been reported. When used to treat ascariasis, live *Ascaris* sometimes appear in the mouth and nose.

Thiabendazole should be used cautiously in patients with impaired liver or kidney function. It may interfere with the metabolism of xanthine derivatives and increase the blood concentration of theophylline.

The safety of this drug during pregnancy and lactation has not been established (FDA Pregnancy Category C).

PHARMACOKINETICS. Thiabendazole is well absorbed after oral administration; time to peak concentration is about one hour. Much of the drug is metabolized to 5-hydroxythiabendazole, which is then conjugated to the glucuronide or sulfate. Most of the drug is excreted in the urine within 24 hours.

DOSAGE AND PREPARATIONS.

Oral: Adults and children, for strongyloidiasis, 25 mg/kg twice daily (maximum, 3 g/day) for two days. Therapy should be continued for at least five days in disseminated infections (hyperinfection syndrome), which occur primarily in immunocompromised patients.

For cutaneous larva migrans, topical therapy alone is preferred except when lesions are widespread. (A topical formulation is not available; however, the oral suspension can be applied directly in a 5- to 7.5-cm area over the end of the larval burrow or tunnel in the skin.) If oral therapy is required, 25 mg/kg is given twice daily (maximum, 3 g/day) for two to five days. If active lesions are still present two days after completion of therapy, a second course is recommended. Concomitant topical therapy also is recommended.

For visceral larva migrans, 25 mg/kg twice daily (maximum, 3 g/day) for five days. For trichinosis (investigational use), 25 mg/kg twice daily for five days. When the drug is used to treat trichinosis or visceral larva migrans involving the eye, concomitant administration of corticosteroids may be needed to minimize the severe inflammatory reaction to the dying larvae.

For ascariasis, uncinariasis, and trichuriasis, 25 mg/kg twice daily (maximum, 3 g/day) for two to four days.

Mintezol (Merck Sharp & Dohme). Suspension (oral) 500 mg/5 ml; tablets (chewable) 500 mg.

Cited References

After smallpox, guineaworm? (editorial). *Lancet* 1:161-162, 1983.

Albendazole: Worms and hydatid disease, (editorial). *Lancet* 2:675-676, (Sept 22) 1984.

Ivermectin in onchocerciasis, (editorial). *Lancet* 2:1021, (Nov 3) 1984.

Awadzi K, et al: Ivermectin in onchocerciasis, (letter). *Lancet* 2:921, 1984.

Aziz M, et al: Efficacy and tolerance of ivermectin in human onchocerciasis. *Lancet* 2:171-173, 1982.

Bicalho SA, et al: Cambendazole in treatment of human strongyloidiasis. *Eur J Clin Pharmacol* 32:1181-1183, 1983.

Braithwaite PA, et al: Clinical pharmacokinetics of high dose mebendazole in patients treated for cystic hydatid disease. *Eur J Clin Pharmacol* 22:161-169, 1982.

Bunnag D, et al: Field trial on treatment of fasciolopsiasis with praziquantel. *Southeast Asian J Trop Med Public Health* 14:216-219, 1983.

Campbell WC, et al: Ivermectin: Potent new antiparasitic agent. *Science* 221:823-828, 1983.

Caprio S, et al: Improvement of metabolic control in diabetic patients during mebendazole administration: Preliminary studies. *Diabetologia* 27:52-55, 1984.

Davidson RA, et al: Risk factors for strongyloidiasis: Case-control study. *Arch Intern Med* 144:321-324, 1984.

Dawson M, et al: Pharmacokinetics and bioavailability of tracer dose of [³H]-mebendazole in man. *Br J Clin Pharmacol* 19:79-86, 1985.

Dominguez-Vazquez A, et al: Comparison of flubendazole and diethyl-carbamazine in treatment of onchocerciasis. *Lancet* 1:139-142, 1983.

Edwards G: Recent advances in chemotherapy of onchocerciasis. *TIPS* 192-195, (May) 1984.

Greene BM, et al: Comparison of ivermectin and diethylcarbamazine in treatment of onchocerciasis. *N Engl J Med* 313:133-138, 1985.

Hamrick HJ, et al: Two cases of dipylidiasis (dog tapeworm infection) in children: Update on old problem. *Pediatrics* 72:114-117, 1983.

Hicks RM: Canopic worm: Role of bilharziasis in aetiology of human bladder cancer. *J R Soc Med* 76:16-22, 1983.

Kune GA, et al: Hydatid disease in Australia: Prevention, clinical presentation, and treatment. *Med J Aust* 2:385-388, 1983.

Lariviere M, et al: Double-blind study of ivermectin and diethylcarbamazine in African onchocerciasis patients with ocular involvement. *Lancet* 2:174-177, 1985.

Leopold G, et al: Clinical pharmacology in normal volunteers of praziquantel, new drug against schistosomes and cestodes: Example of complex study covering both tolerance and pharmacokinetics. *Eur J Clin Pharmacol* 14:281-291, 1978.

Levin ML: Treatment of trichinosis with mebendazole. *Am J Trop Med Hyg* 32:980-983, 1983.

Levin MH, et al: Severe, reversible neutropenia during high-dose mebendazole therapy for echinococcosis. *JAMA* 249:2929-2931, 1983.

Misra PK, et al: Albendazole in treatment of intestinal helminthiasis in children. *Curr Med Res Opin* 9:516-519, 1985.

Morris DL, et al: Albendazole: Objective evidence of response in human hydatid disease. *JAMA* 253:2053-2057, 1985.

Most H: Treatment of parasitic infections of travelers and immigrants. *N Engl J Med* 310:298-304, 1984.

Nash TE, Neva FA: Recent advances in diagnosis and treatment of cerebral cysticercosis. *N Engl J Med* 311:1492-1496, 1984.

Nash TE, et al: Schistosome infections in humans: Perspectives and recent findings. *Ann Intern Med* 97:740-754, 1982.

Pachucki CT, et al: American paragonimiasis treated with praziquantel. *N Engl J Med* 311:582-583, 1984.

Pearson RD, Guerrant RL: Praziquantel: Major advance in anthelmintic therapy. *Ann Intern Med* 99:195-198, 1983.

Prasad R, et al: Albendazole in treatment of intestinal helminthiasis in children. *Clin Therapeut* 7:164-168, 1985.

Saimot AG, et al: Albendazole as potential treatment for human hydatidosis. *Lancet* 2:652-656, 1983.

Schantz PM: Effective medical treatment for hydatid disease? (editorial). *JAMA* 253:2095-2097, 1985.

Sotelo J, et al: Therapy of parenchymal brain cysticercosis with praziquantel. *N Engl J Med* 310:1001-1007, 1984.

Sotelo J, et al: Praziquantel in treatment of neurocysticercosis: Long-term follow-up. *Neurology* 35:752-755, 1985.

Weller PF, Arnow PM: Paroxysmal inflammatory filariasis: Filarial fevers, (editorial). *Arch Intern Med* 143:1523-1524, 1983.

Weniger BG, Schantz PM: Praziquantel and refugee health. *JAMA* 251:2391-2392, 1984.

WHO Expert Committee on Filariasis: *Lymphatic Filariasis.* Geneva, World Health Organization, Technical Report Series 702, 1984.

Other Selected References

Drugs for parasitic infections. *Med Lett Drugs Ther* 28:9-18, 1986.

Health Information for International Travel 1984. US Dept of Health and Human Services, publication no (CDC)84-8280. Atlanta, Centers for Disease Control, 1984.

Beck JW, Davies JE: *Medical Parasitology,* ed 3. St Louis, CV Mosby, 1981.

Brown HW, Neva FA: *Basic Clinical Parasitology,* ed 5. Norwalk, CT, Appleton-Century-Crofts, 1983.

James DH, Gilles HM: *Human Antiparasitic Drugs: Pharmacology and Usage.* New York, John Wiley & Sons, 1985.

Katz M, et al: *Parasitic Diseases.* New York, Springer-Verlag, 1982.

Most H: Treatment of parasitic infections of travelers and immigrants. *N Engl J Med* 310:298-304, 1984.

Wade A (ed): *Martindale: The Extra Pharmacopoeia,* ed 28. London, The Pharmaceutical Press, 1982, 86-109.

Antiviral Agents

Compared to the remarkable progress made in the treatment of bacterial diseases in the past four decades, there have been few notable advances in the chemotherapy of viral diseases. Only a small number of useful antiviral agents is available for a limited number of infections. Much simpler organisms than bacteria, viruses are obligate intracellular parasites that utilize many biochemical mechanisms of the infected host cells. Therefore, it is more difficult to achieve selective antiviral activity because there are fewer virus-specific functions that may be interrupted by chemical agents. This also means that it is difficult to obtain antiviral activity without also affecting some aspect of normal host cell metabolism and thus causing toxic effects in uninfected host cells.

Earlier antiviral drugs, such as idoxuridine [Herplex, Stoxil] and cytarabine [Cytosar-U], have had limited clinical usefulness because of low therapeutic indices. An additional problem is that, by the time frank symptoms appear, several cycles of virus multiplication may have occurred. This is particularly true in acute infections, such as the common cold and influenza, in which rapid multiplication of the virus occurs prior to the development of clinical illness. Agents that inhibit virus replication may be ineffective unless given during the stage of significant virus multiplication. Therefore, antiviral agents must be given early during the course of infection or they must be given prophylactically (eg, in influenza).

As understanding of viral structures, enzymes, and replicative mechanisms has increased, it has become clear that there are macromolecules and functions unique to viruses. These include host cell surface receptors to which viruses attach or are adsorbed and viral-encoded enzymes (eg, herpesvirus-induced thymidine kinase). Exploitation of such functions has led to the development of the four antiviral drugs (amantadine [Symmetrel], vidarabine [Vira-A], acyclovir [Zovirax], and ribavirin [Virazole]) currently licensed for clinical use. Some promising investigational agents (eg, bromovinyldeoxyuridine [BVDU], dihydroxypropoxymethylguanine [DHPG], fluoroiodoaracytosine [FIAC], rimantadine) also exhibit selective antiviral activity. With increased understanding of the molecular biology of virus multiplication, additional virus-specific functions should

be discovered that will serve as targets for attack by future, highly effective antiviral drugs.

CLASSIFICATION AND BIOLOGY OF VIRUSES

Viruses are composed of a nucleic acid core surrounded by a protein-containing outer coat. The viral genome contains either ribonucleic acid (RNA) or deoxyribonucleic acid (DNA), but never both, and viruses are classified on this basis. Viruses can be subdivided further by characteristics such as morphology, whether the virus shell has an envelope, whether viral multiplication occurs in the nucleus or cytoplasm of the infected cell, and serologic type.

Selected RNA viruses that infect humans and the typical diseases that they cause are as follows (classification is initially by virus family) (Melnick, 1980):

> *Picornaviridae*—polioviruses (poliomyelitis), coxsackieviruses and echoviruses (aseptic meningitis), and rhinoviruses (common cold).
> *Reoviridae*—rotaviruses (diarrhea).
> *Togaviridae*—various mosquito-borne encephalitis viruses (encephalitis), yellow fever virus (yellow fever), and rubella virus (rubella).
> *Orthomyxoviridae*—influenza viruses (influenza).
> *Paramyxoviridae*—parainfluenza viruses (croup, pneumonia, bronchitis), mumps virus (mumps), measles virus (measles), and respiratory syncytial virus (bronchiolitis, pneumonia).
> *Rhabdoviridae*—rabies virus (rabies).
> *Coronaviridae*—coronaviruses (respiratory illnesses).
> *Bunyaviridae*—California encephalitis viruses (encephalitis).
> *Retroviridae*—human T-cell lymphotropic viruses (leukemia/lymphoma, acquired immunodeficiency syndrome).

Selected DNA viruses that infect humans and the typical diseases that they cause are as follows (classification is initially by virus family) (Melnick, 1980):

> *Papovaviridae*—papilloma viruses (warts, progressive multifocal leukoencephalopathy).

Adenoviridae—adenoviruses (acute respiratory diseases, keratitis).
Herpesviridae—herpes simplex types 1 and 2 ("cold" sores, keratitis, genital infections, encephalitis), varicella-zoster (chickenpox, shingles), cytomegalovirus (cytomegalic inclusion disease), and Epstein-Barr virus (infectious mononucleosis, association with Burkitt's lymphoma).
Chordopoxviridae—variola virus (smallpox).

Although the precise mechanisms of infection are often different and quite specific for individual viruses, the general cellular infective process proceeds along the following scheme: Initially, viruses adsorb onto the surface of a host cell by electrostatic interaction. For some viruses (eg, influenza virus, poliovirus), attachment to specific receptor sites has been demonstrated. It is likely that most viruses attach to virus-specific receptors, accounting for cell and tissue tropism. Viruses then penetrate the host cell membrane by pinocytosis and their nucleic acid is released by an uncoating process. Following uncoating, the replication, transcription, and translation of the viral genome occur. These events result in the production of sufficient quantities of viral nucleic acid and protein to form a new generation of virions (ie, complete infectious virus particles). In the classic cytolytic infection, the replicative mechanisms of the host cell are turned off and the host cell dies. Once the viral components have been manufactured, they are assembled and released as mature virions to begin the cycle again. The processes involved are numerous and complex and utilize not only cellular enzyme systems, but also viral enzymes produced for specialized functions.

Certain viruses (eg, adenoviruses, papovaviruses, retroviruses, herpesviruses) are capable of transforming cells into a malignant state. All or part of the viral genome is integrated into the host cell genome, thus creating a new cell type with features of a malignant cell. (For further information, see Klein, 1980, and Dulbecco and Ginsberg, 1980.)

Although some viral infections are chronic (eg, chronic mononucleosis, hepatitis B and non-A/non-B, warts, molluscum contagiosum), many of those seen clinically are acute. They may remain localized (eg, common cold, influenza) or disseminate via the bloodstream to other parts of the body (eg, chickenpox, smallpox). With the latter, symptoms may appear only after an incubation period when a secondary target organ becomes involved. Acute viral infections usually terminate when a sufficient immune response develops to the infecting virus; for some viruses, this immunity may persist for the entire lifetime of the host. However, recurrences of certain viral infections are common, because (1) the virus persists within the host in a latent state (eg, herpesviruses), (2) multiple viral serotypes exist that do not exhibit significant cross-immunity (eg, rhinoviruses), or (3) antigenic shift occurs (eg, influenza viruses).

NONDRUG TREATMENT OF VIRAL INFECTIONS

Since chemotherapeutic approaches are still limited, symptomatic and supportive treatment (eg, bed rest, analgesics, antipyretics) is the only management for many viral diseases, particularly acute respiratory infections.

IMMUNIZATION. Active immunization utilizing viral vaccines to stimulate the normal host defense mechanisms is the most effective means of controlling many viral diseases. Vaccination prevents measles, rubella, mumps, poliomyelitis, yellow fever, smallpox, and hepatitis B. Despite the problems of antigenic shifts, vaccination against influenza often provides short-term protection and is recommended annually for high-risk individuals (eg, patients with underlying diseases, the elderly). Unfortunately, vaccines have not been developed for all viruses and this would appear to be impractical in some cases. For example, the rhinoviruses have 100 known antigenically distinct serotypes. Also, with the possible exception of rabies vaccine, most vaccines do not prevent the spread of active infections within the host.

Passive immunization with human immune globulin or equine antiserum is another nondrug approach to combat viral infections. For example, hyperimmune globulins are very useful in the prophylaxis of varicella, rabies, and hepatitis B.

For detailed discussion of active and passive immunization, see Chapter 62.

INTERFERONS. Vaccines and available antiviral drugs possess narrow spectra. Consequently, their uses are limited to selected viral infections. Clinically effective, broad spectrum antiviral agents are generally unavailable. One of the attractive features of the investigational antiviral substances, interferons, is their broad spectrum.

Interferon is a general term applied to a family of glycoproteins produced by animal, including human, cells infected with viruses or stimulated by various other natural and synthetic substances. The current nomenclature for the three principal types of interferons appears below:

HUMAN INTERFERON NOMENCLATURE*

New Nomenclature	Old Nomenclature
IFN-α	Le (leukocyte), type I, pH 2 stable, foreign cell-induced, classical
IFN-β	F (fibroblast), Fi, type I, pH 2 stable
IFN-r	IIF (immune), type II, T, pH 2 labile, antigen-induced, mitogen-induced

*Prefix denotes animal of origin: For example, HuIFN = human; MuIFN = murine.
Adapted from Stiehm ER, et al: Interferon: Immunobiology and clinical significance. Ann Intern Med 96:80-93, 1982.

There are several interferon (IFN) subtypes. More than 20 IFN-α genes have been postulated, but not all have been clearly identified with a product. However, at least 14 distinct subtypes of IFN-α have been cloned using recombinant DNA techniques. Up to five IFN-β mRNAs have been identified, but only two gene products, IFN-β_1 and IFN-β_2, have been established. IFN-β_1 represents over 90% of the interferon produced by fibroblasts. Thus far, only one type of IFN-γ has been described. This interferon bears little homology to the IFN-α or IFN-β species but shares many of their biological functions. In humans, the main cluster of IFN-producing genes is on chromosome 9 (IFN-α and IFN-β_1). Chromosomes 2 and 5 have been associated with the production of IFN-β_2, $_5$, while chromosome 12 is associated with IFN-γ production.

Actions: Binding of interferon to the intact cell membrane is the first step in establishing its antiviral effect. IFN binds to specific cell surface receptors; IFN-γ appears to have a different receptor from either IFN-α or -β, which may explain the synergistic antiviral and antitumor effects sometimes observed when IFN-γ is given with either of the other two IFN species.

A prevalent view of interferon action (Preble and Friedman, 1983) is that, following binding, there is synthesis of new cellular RNAs and proteins, which mediate the antiviral effect. Chromosome 21 is required to develop the antiviral state in humans no matter which species of IFN is employed. At least three of the newly synthesized proteins in IFN-treated cells appear to be associated with the development of the antiviral state: (1) a 2'-5' oliogoadenylate (2-5A) synthetase, (2) a protein kinase, and (3) an endonuclease. The antiviral state is not fully expressed until these primed cells are infected with virus.

Double stranded RNA, which is produced during the replication of many viruses, activates 2-5A synthetase and protein kinase. The activated 2-5A synthetase catalyzes the polymerization of ATP into 2'-5' oligonucleotides that in turn activate endogenous cellular endoribonuclease, which degrades viral RNA. The activated protein kinase phosphorylates the alpha subunit of eukaryotic initiation factor 2 resulting in inhibition of viral protein synthesis. The combined effects of protein kinase and endonuclease in IFN-treated cells are thought to result in inhibition of virus protein synthesis and, hence, virus replication. However, it is not yet known how these enzymes discriminate between host and virus protein synthesis.

Although the foregoing postulate on IFN's mechanism of action explains its inhibition of virus replication, interferon does not appear to act by inhibiting virus-specific RNA or protein synthesis in other virus cell systems. For example, interferon appears to inhibit the final maturation of retroviruses in infected cells so that they are not released into the medium but instead accumulate on the cell surface. If interferon is removed, virus release proceeds normally. Other enzymes and proteins have been described in IFN-treated cells. For a detailed review of the actions of interferons, see Becker, 1984.

In addition to their antiviral effect, interferons have a number of other useful biological properties including inhibition of cell proliferation and enhancement of the cytotoxic activities of lymphocytes, the expression of cell surface antigens, and the phagocytic and tumoricidal activities of macrophages. These properties may play an important role in the in vivo antiviral and antitumor effects of the interferons.

Sources: Although interferons exhibit broad spectrum antiviral activity, they are relatively species-specific, usually having maximal activity only in cells from the same or closely related species. Until recently, the amount of human interferons available for clinical trials was limited and preparations were impure. To circumvent the early limited supply of exogenous human interferon, compounds that stimulate the endogenous production of interferon by host cells were investigated. Interferon inducers include certain microorganisms (eg, viruses, *Rickettsia*, *Mycoplasma*, coliform bacteria), microbial ex-

tracts, certain dyes (eg, methylene blue, acridine orange), tilorone, and synthetic polymers; however, none of these agents have been shown to be safe or effective in man.

Clinical investigations with exogenous human interferons have been performed and a number are still ongoing. Most of the early studies utilized semipurified interferon (HuIFN-α) from buffy-coat leukocytes stimulated with Sendai virus. A few studies employed fibroblast interferon from poly rI:rC-induced human fibroblasts grown in culture. The general consensus has been that these preparations have some antiviral effects in a number of infections. For example, leukocyte IFN administered prophylactically as a nasal spray reduced the incidence and severity of colds caused by rhinoviruses (Greenberg et al, 1982; Scott et al, 1982) and suppressed varicella in immunocompromised children with cancer (Arvin et al, 1982 A); when given prophylactically, leukocyte IFN significantly reduced the incidence of cytomegalovirus reactivation syndromes and opportunistic infections in renal transplant patients (Hirsch et al, 1983). However, in infants with congenital rubella, treatment only decreased pharyngeal virus excretion temporarily (Arvin et al, 1982 B). Leukocyte IFN used in combination with synthetic antiviral agents was effective in chronic hepatitis B infection (Smith et al, 1982), herpetic keratitis (Colin et al, 1983), and progressive cutaneous herpes simplex infection (Shalev et al, 1984).

As with leukocyte interferon from buffy coats, recombinant leukocyte interferon (rHuIFN-α_2) given prophylactically in the form of nasal spray or drops prevented infection and reduced the severity and frequency of illness and virus shedding in experimentally challenged subjects (Samo et al, 1983; Hayden and Gwaltney, 1983) and in patients naturally infected with rhinoviruses (Herzog et al, 1983; Farr et al, 1984). In two other studies, rHuIFN-α_2 self-administered for seven days by healthy individuals exposed to another family member with cold-like symptoms reduced the symptoms of respiratory illness in recipients by 39% to 41%. This beneficial effect was confined to rhinovirus infections. When rhinoviral colds alone were considered, the IFN prevented colds in 78% to 79% of patients. Also, IFN shortened the course of rhinovirus colds with 76% fewer symptom days (Douglas et al, 1986; Hayden et al, 1986). In addition, intranasal rHuIFN-α_2 was effective prophylactically in reducing the incidence of colds, severity of symptoms, and virus multiplication in experimental respiratory coronavirus infection (Higgins et al, 1983). Its administration to patients with chronic hepatitis B temporarily suppressed Dane particle-associated polymerase activity (Smith et al, 1983). However, when given therapeutically to marrow transplant patients with serious cytomegalovirus or adenovirus infection, no favorable effect was observed (Meyers et al, 1983).

No well controlled trials have been reported that demonstrate the antiviral efficacy of HuIFN-γ, although a pharmacokinetic study in cancer patients has been published (Gutterman et al, 1984).

Not only are the clinical antiviral activities of cell culture and recombinant interferon preparations similar, if not identical, but so are their adverse effects. Fever has occurred in most patients receiving interferons intramuscularly or intravenously. Headache and myalgia are common. Malaise and fatigue have been observed and become more pronounced with additional doses. Interferons produced reversible dose-related leukopenia and thrombocytopenia. Nausea and vomiting, erythema and pain at the site of intramuscular injection, and transient alopecia also have been observed.

In clinical studies employing rHuIFN-α_2 intranasally, nasal irritation with discharge of blood-tinged mucus, superficial erosions of the nasal mucosa, and transient leukopenia were reported (Hayden and Gwaltney, 1983; Samo et al, 1983; Farr et al, 1984; Douglas et al, 1986; Hayden et al, 1986).

In pharmacokinetic studies in humans who were given rHuIFN-α_2 intravenously, intramuscularly, and subcutaneously, the severity of adverse effects was related to the route of administration (Willis et al, 1984).

DRUG THERAPY FOR VIRAL INFECTIONS

Classification and Uses

Pyrimidine and Purine Antimetabolites: Many compounds considered to be potential antiviral drugs are antimetabolites that inhibit nucleic acid synthesis. The clinical usefulness of these pyrimidine and purine derivatives is related directly to their ability to selectively block viral, as opposed to host, nucleic acid synthesis. Particular emphasis has been placed on the development of such drugs to treat herpesvirus infections.

Cytarabine [Cytosar-U], a cytidine analogue used to treat acute myelogenous leukemia, was originally developed as an antiviral drug. This agent inhibits herpesvirus DNA synthesis but has a greater inhibitory effect on dividing host cells, causing severe bone marrow and gastrointestinal toxicity. Therefore, cytarabine is not used clinically as an antiviral drug.

Idoxuridine [Herplex, Stoxil] and trifluridine [Vioptic] are analogues of thymidine. When administered systemically, these substituted nucleosides are phosphorylated by both viral and cellular thymidine kinases to the active triphosphorylated derivatives, which inhibit viral and cellular DNA synthesis. The result is both antiviral activity and sufficient host cytotoxicity to prevent their systemic use for viral infections. The toxicity is not significant, however, when idoxuridine and trifluridine are applied topically to the eye to treat herpes simplex keratitis; most authorities consider trifluridine to be superior to idoxuridine (see Chapter 73, Topical Anti-infective Agents: Otic and Ophthalmic Preparations). In England and other countries, the topical application of idoxuridine dissolved in dimethyl sulfoxide (DMSO) has been reported to be effective in cutaneous herpes simplex and herpes zoster lesions. However, in a randomized, double-blind, controlled trial, 30% idoxuridine in DMSO had no effect on the clinical manifestations of initial or recurrent genital herpesvirus infections (Silvestri et al, 1982).

Vidarabine [Vira-A] and acyclovir [Zovirax] are purine nucleoside analogues with selective activity against herpesviruses. Vidarabine is phosphorylated by host kinases to the active 5'-triphosphate (ara-ATP). This triphosphate competitively inhibits DNA-dependent DNA polymerases of DNA viruses approximately 40 times more than those of host cells. In addition, vidarabine is incorporated into terminal positions of both cellular and herpesvirus DNA, thus inhibiting completion of DNA chains. Therefore, viral DNA synthesis is blocked at lower doses, resulting in a relatively selective antiviral effect. However, large doses of vidarabine are cytotoxic to dividing host cells because antiviral selectivity is not absolute.

Vidarabine, administered intravenously, is effective in biopsy-proven herpes simplex encephalitis (Whitley et al, 1977, 1981), neonatal herpes simplex infection (Whitley et al, 1980), and herpes zoster (Whitley et al, 1976) and varicella (Whitley et al, 1982 A) infections in immunocompromised patients. Vidarabine also is used topically to treat herpes simplex keratitis (see Chapter 73). It has limited use in mucocutaneous herpesvirus infections in immunocompromised hosts (Whitley et al, 1984). In chronic hepatitis B infection, vidarabine decreased Dane particle-associated polymerase activity temporarily but pretreatment levels were observed following cessation of therapy (Pollard et al, 1978; Bassendine et al, 1981; Hoofnagle et al, 1984). In two separate trials, cytomegalovirus (CMV) infections in bone marrow (Kraemer et al, 1978) or renal transplant (Marker et al, 1980) patients were not altered by vidarabine therapy. However, in one small study (Pollard et al, 1980) of progressive CMV retinitis, 20 mg/kg/day of vidarabine seemed to alter the course of the disease, although significant adverse effects were observed. The drug is not useful in genital herpesvirus or smallpox infections.

A major disadvantage of vidarabine is its poor solubility, which necessitates the use of large volumes of intravenous fluid and prolonged infusion times (see the evaluation). Another drawback is its deamination by adenosine deaminase to hypoxanthine arabinoside, which has much weaker antiviral activity. This has led to the search for derivatives resistant to deamination by this enzyme. Cyclaradine, a carbocyclic analogue, is as potent as vidarabine in vitro and is resistant to deamination by adenosine deaminase (Vince and Daluge, 1977). However, although cyclaradine is a promising compound (Vince et al, 1983), clinical trials have not yet been reported.

Acyclovir, a nucleoside analogue of guanosine, is probably the best example of an antimetabolite with selective antiviral activity. In infected cells, herpesvirus kinase (commonly called thymidine kinase, but perhaps more accurately referred to as a pyrimidine kinase) converts acyclovir to acyclovir monophosphate, a nucleotide analogue. In uninfected host cells (eg, Vero, HeLas), this phosphorylation is limited; depending upon the virus strain/host cell system employed, the rate is 30 to 120 times faster in extracts prepared from infected cells than in those from uninfected host cells. (Uninfected cells apparently contain an enzyme other than thymidine kinase, which phosphorylates acyclovir to a limited extent.) Following conversion to the monophosphate, the compound is further converted to the diphosphate by cellular guanylate kinase and finally to the triphosphate (acyclo-GTP) by a number of cellular enzymes. Once formed, acyclo-GTP may remain in the cell for a prolonged period.

The initial reaction in the phosphorylation sequence is critical, for the specificity of the viral enzyme is quite different from that of thymidine kinase from the uninfected cell. The herpesvirus thymidine kinase binds 200 times more strongly to acyclovir and phosphorylates it 3 million times faster than does host cell thymidine kinase.

Acyclo-GTP is a potent inhibitor of viral DNA polymerase and inhibits cellular alpha-DNA polymerase to a much lesser degree. Cellular beta-DNA polymerase is insensitive to the compound. Acyclo-GTP can be incorporated into growing chains of DNA by viral and, to a much lesser extent, cellular DNA polymerase. When this incorporation occurs, DNA chain growth is terminated, apparently because acyclovir does not have a 3'-hydroxyl group on which chain elongation can continue and the acyclo-GMP-terminated template binds and inactivates the viral DNA polymerase.

Acyclovir is available in intravenous, topical, and oral forms. Intravenous acyclovir has been shown to be effective in immunocompromised patients for the treatment of mucocutaneous herpes (Mitchell et al, 1981; Chou et al, 1981; Wade et al, 1982 A; Meyers et al, 1982) and for the treatment and prophylaxis of herpes simplex (Spector et al, 1982; Saral et al, 1981, 1983) and herpes zoster infections (Selby et al, 1979; Spector et al, 1982; Balfour et al, 1983; Serota et al, 1982; Meyers et al, 1984). In immunocompetent patients, intravenous acyclovir has been effective in primary genital herpes (Mindel et al, 1982; Corey et al, 1983) and·herpes zoster infections (Peterslund et al, 1981, 1984; Bean et al, 1982; Esmann et al, 1982).

A recent collaborative study that compared intravenous acyclovir and vidarabine in the treatment of herpes simplex encephalitis concluded that acyclovir was the treatment of choice. Mortality in the vidarabine and acyclovir groups was, respectively, 43% versus 13% at one month, 54% versus 19% at six months, and 54% versus 28% overall. In patients less than 30 years old, the mortality rate was 6% for those treated with acyclovir and 45% for those treated with vidarabine. Six months after therapy, 14% of those in the vidarabine group and 38% of those in the acyclovir group were functionally normal (Whitley et al, 1986).

Topical acyclovir has been efficacious in the treatment of mucocutaneous herpesvirus infections in immunocompromised patients (Spruance et al, 1982; Whitley et al, 1982 B) but has not been shown to be so in immunocompetent patients (Spruance et al, 1982, 1984). In the latter, topical administration has been useful for the management of primary, but not recurrent, genital herpes infections (Corey et al, 1982 A and B; Luby et al, 1984). Many studies support the efficacy of topical acyclovir in the treatment of herpes simplex keratitis, but this use is still investigational.

A number of clinical studies on oral acyclovir have been conducted. In immunocompromised patients, oral acyclovir suppressed symptomatic attacks of mucocutaneous and other herpes simplex virus infections (Straus et al, 1982, 1984 A), prevented herpes simplex virus reactivation after transplantation (Wade et al, 1984), and was credited with eliminating the dissemination of varicella-zoster virus in children (Novelli et al, 1984).

Oral and intravenous acyclovir were reported to be equally effective in reducing pain and accelerating the rate of healing in herpes zoster (Peterslund et al, 1984). However, results of other studies employing oral acyclovir in herpes zoster are inconclusive (McKendrick et al, 1984) and recommendations for its use in this disease must await analysis of ongoing trials.

In immunocompetent patients, oral acyclovir was effective in primary herpes genitalis (Nilsen et al, 1982; Bryson et al, 1983; Mertz et al, 1984) and was reported to reduce recurrences (Straus et al, 1984 B; Douglas et al, 1984; Mindel et al, 1984). In two multicenter crossover trials employing the oral form, efficacy in genital herpes simplex infections was suggested (Thin et al, 1985; Ruhnek-Forsbeck et al, 1985). However, further studies are needed to define the indications, dose, and duration of treatment of genital herpes with oral acyclovir.

Two derivatives of acyclovir have shown promise for the treatment of herpesvirus infections. One, 6-deoxyacyclovir (2-amino-9-((2-hydroxyethoxy)methyl)-9H-purine, A515U), is a prodrug that is well absorbed after oral administration. It is converted to acyclovir by xanthine oxidase and is also oxidized by aldehyde oxidase to metabolites. This drug and its metabolites are inactive in vitro against herpes simplex virus type 1. However, in laboratory animals and man, 6-deoxyacyclovir is extensively converted into the active metabolite, acyclovir. In clinical studies involving both patients with hematologic malignancies and healthy volunteers, oral 6-deoxyacyclovir was well tolerated and well absorbed; plasma concentrations of acyclovir were comparable to those achieved after intravenous administration of acyclovir and much higher than those obtained after oral administration of acyclovir (Krenitsky et al, 1984; Selby et al, 1984; Whiteman et al, 1984). These studies suggest that 6-deoxyacyclovir may be superior to the parent compound for oral administration. The greater absorption of the prodrug and the higher plasma levels of acyclovir obtained may be important in therapy against less sensitive viruses, such as varicella-zoster, and may decrease the likelihood of viral resistance. Since the drug is metabolized to its active form by xanthine oxidase, the simultaneous use of allopurinol, which inhibits this enzyme, must be avoided.

The acyclic nucleoside, 9-(1,3-dihydroxy-2-propoxymethyl) guanine (DHPG), is an analogue of acyclovir with considerably more activity against CMV. In vitro, it inhibited the replication of HSV-1 and -2, CMV, and EBV. DHPG is also active against both thymidine kinase- and DNA polymerase-altered mutants resistant to acyclovir. In mice, DHPG was more active than acyclovir against herpesvirus encephalitis and vaginitis. Like acyclovir, the activity of DHPG in herpesvirus-infected cells depends upon phosphorylation by virus-induced thymidine kinase. Also like acyclovir, DHPG monophosphate is further converted to the di- and triphosphate by cellular kinases. In cells infected by HSV-1 or -2, the triphosphate (DHPGTP) competitively inhibits the incorporation of GTP into virus DNA; DHPGTP is incorporated at internal and terminal sites of viral DNA, thus inhibiting DNA synthesis. The mode of action of DHPG against CMV and EBV is not known, but it has been suggested that these viruses may induce a cellular thymidine kinase or other kinase that carries on the obligatory initial phosphorylation of DHPG to the active monophosphate (Smee et al, 1983; Cheng et al, 1983; Mar et al, 1983; Frank et al, 1984).

DHPG is of clinical interest not only because of its greater potency and broader spectrum of activity against herpesviruses, but also because it is active against some mutants resistant to acyclovir. Trials of the drug in patients with CMV infection are in progress. In one preliminary study involving only two patients with CMV retinitis, intravenous DHPG was reported to heal retinal lesions and resolve viremia and viral shedding (Felsenstein et al, 1985). In three patients with AIDS, DHPG halted progressive hemorrhagic retinitis and symptomatic pneumonitis due to CMV. In these patients, the virus rapidly returned and lesions progressed when treatment was discontinued (Bach et al, 1985). In a second study on CMV infections in AIDS patients (seven with retinitis, one with only pneumonitis), intravenous DHPG produced substantial improvement in all eight patients. However, all surviving patients experienced clinical or virologic relapses within 30 days after ending therapy. Maintenance regimens consisting of two to five doses of 2.5 mg/kg weekly did not prevent relapses, either because of clinical reactivation or the development of leukopenia requiring cessation of therapy (Masur et al, 1986). However, it should be noted that AIDS patients are likely to experience recurrences of all infections. In one study on ten bone marrow transplant recipients with biopsy-proven CMV pneumonia treated with DHPG, viruria and viremia ceased after four days of treatment in all patients with initially positive urine or blood cultures. Also, CMV was eliminated from respiratory secretions after a median of eight days; however, only one patient survived the pneumonia (Shepp et al, 1985).

Ribavirin [Virazole], a recently approved drug, exhibits a broad antiviral spectrum that includes both RNA and DNA viruses. The mechanisms of its antiviral effect are poorly understood and probably are not the same for all viruses; however, its ability to alter nucleotide pools and the packaging of mRNA appears to be important. This process is not totally virus specific, but there is a certain selectivity in that infected cells produce more mRNA than noninfected cells. A major action is the inhibition by ribavirin-5′-monophosphate of inosine monophosphate dehydrogenase, an enzyme essential for DNA synthesis. This inhibition may have direct effects on the intracellular level of GMP; other nucleotide levels may be altered, but the mechanisms are presently unknown. The 5′-triphosphate of ribavirin inhibits the formation of the 5′-guanylation capping on the mRNA of vaccinia and Venezuelan equine encephalitis viruses. In addition, the triphosphate is a potent inhibitor of viral mRNA (guanine-7-) methyltransferase of vaccinia virus. The capacity of viral mRNA to support protein synthesis is markedly reduced by ribavirin; high concentrations of ribavirin also inhibit cellular protein synthesis. It has been suggested that ribavirin may inhibit influenza A RNA-dependent RNA polymerase.

Results of clinical trials employing oral ribavirin have suggested that this form is marginally effective in the prophylaxis of influenza A and B infections and, possibly, in the treatment of influenza A. Aerosolized ribavirin has been more effective in controlling influenza infections. In an early study on influenza A infections (Knight et al, 1981), fever and illness disappeared more rapidly and virus shedding was reduced in treated patients compared to controls; in a more recent study, the duration of fever was shorter and recovery was more rapid with use of ribavirin aerosol (Wilson et al, 1984). More rapid defervescence, resolution of clinical illness, and reduction of viral shedding in nasal secretions also were observed in patients with influenza B infections treated with aerosolized ribavirin (McClung et al, 1983).

Ribavirin has been reported to be effective by other routes in several other human viral infections, including measles, genital herpes infections, herpes zoster, and acute hepatitis types A and B (Fernandez, 1980; Uylangco et al, 1981; Bierman et al, 1981; Minkoff et al, 1980). When given intravenously or orally, it also has been reported to significantly reduce mortality in patients with Lassa fever (McCormick et al, 1986). In vitro, ribavirin inhibits the replication of HTLV-III, the retrovirus considered to be the etiologic agent of AIDS, and is in clinical trials in patients with AIDS.

Use of aerosolized ribavirin in adults and children with respiratory syncytial virus (RSV) infections reduced the severity of illness and virus shedding (Hall et al, 1983 A and B). Repeated courses eliminated simultaneous infection with both parainfluenza and RSV in an infant with severe combined immunodeficiency syndrome (McIntosh et al, 1984).

In a double-blind, placebo-controlled trial, aerosolized ribavirin was evaluated in RSV lower respiratory tract disease in 26 infants, including those with underlying cardiopulmonary disease. Treated infants improved significantly faster as measured by illness severity score, arterial blood gas values, and amount of virus shed from nasal washes. In addition, a generally good outcome was observed in 27 nonrandomized severely ill infants with congenital heart disease who were treated with ribavirin aerosol. (About one-third of infants with congenital heart disease may die from RSV infection.) No adverse effects were observed in any of the infants studied and no ribavirin-resistant RSV strains were isolated despite prolonged treatment in some infants (Hall et al, 1985). Aerosol therapy with ribavirin appears to have the advantage of producing very high pulmonary drug levels with little systemic absorption. In patients receiving eight or more hours of continuous therapy, the mean peak level in tracheal secretions may be 100 times greater than the minimum inhibitory concentration preventing the RSV replication in vitro (Connor et al, 1984).

As this book went to press, the Food and Drug Administration approved ribavirin aerosol for the treatment of selected hospitalized infants and young children with severe lower respiratory tract infections due to RSV. The manufacturer's package insert should be consulted for further information.

The investigational agent, bromovinyldeoxyuridine (BVDU), is a potent inhibitor of herpes simplex virus type 1 (HSV-1) and varicella-zoster virus (VZV). In vitro, it is somewhat more potent than acyclovir against HSV-1 and approximately 1,000 times more potent against VZV; however, it is about 50 times less potent than acyclovir against HSV-2. It is also effective against several herpesviruses infecting animals.

Like acyclovir, the selectivity of BVDU is based upon the phosphorylation of the parent compound by herpesvirus thymidine kinase, which restricts its action to virus-infected cells. When added to cells infected with HSV-1 and HSV-2, virus-encoded thymidine kinase rapidly converts the parent compound to the 5′-monophosphate form. In cells infected with

HSV-1, but not HSV-2, the monophosphate is further phosphorylated to the 5'-diphosphates and 5'-triphosphates. The triphosphate inhibits viral DNA polymerase much more than cellular DNA polymerases. In addition, the triphosphate is incorporated into viral DNA, which may also contribute to its antiviral activity. The difference in sensitivity of HSV-1 and HSV-2 to BVDU is thought to be due to the induction of a dTMP kinase by HSV-1 but not HSV-2. This kinase catalyzes the phosphorylation of BVDU monophosphate to the diphosphate. The triphosphate of BVDU inhibits HSV-1 and HSV-2 DNA polymerases equally; thus, the differential susceptibility of the two viruses is at the level of the dTMP kinase rather than at the DNA polymerase level.

In preliminary, uncontrolled, clinical trials, topical BVDU appeared to be effective in treating herpetic keratitis (Maudgal et al, 1981 A) and the oral form appeared to be beneficial in mucocutaneous herpes simplex and zoster infections in immunocompromised patients (de Clercq et al, 1980; Wildiers and de Clercq, 1984), VZV infections in leukemic children (Benoit et al, 1985), and ophthalmic zoster in the elderly (Maudgal et al, 1981 B). No adverse effects were reported in any of these studies. Controlled trials are required to assess efficacy more fully.

Fluoroiodoaracytosine (FIAC) is another potent selective inhibitor of herpesviruses. Like acyclovir and BVDU, its activity depends on phosphorylation by herpesvirus thymidine kinase. FIAC is phosphorylated 1,200 to 9,000 times better by the virus enzyme than by enzymes of normal host cells. The parent compound is converted rapidly to the triphosphate in infected cells, is selectively utilized by virus DNA polymerase, and is incorporated into viral DNA, resulting in the formation of very short chains. In vitro, FIAC has greater antiviral activity than acyclovir against HSV-1; it also is active against HSV-2, VZV, and CMV. Although it is highly active against the latter, its mechanism of action against this virus is not well understood. CMV does not produce its own thymidine kinase, but does increase the production of the cellular enzyme. In vitro, the therapeutic index of the drug has been calculated to be about 500.

An uncontrolled clinical trial with FIAC suggested that this agent was effective in the treatment of VZV infections in immunocompromised patients (Young et al, 1983). Clinical trials of this agent in CMV infections have not yet been reported.

Amantadine and Derivatives: Amantadine [Symmetrel] is a highly selective antiviral drug that inhibits the growth of known subtypes of influenza A viruses (H2N2 and H3N2). It has no clinical activity against influenza B viruses. Therefore, this drug is used prophylactically and therapeutically in infections caused by influenza type A virus only (see the evaluation). It is also widely used in parkinsonism (see Chapter 11, Drugs Used in Extrapyramidal Movement Disorders).

Although amantadine was the first antiviral agent to be approved in the United States, its mechanism of action is not yet completely understood. Influenza A viruses differ in their susceptibility to amantadine, and the drug may have different actions depending upon the concentration and virus strain. Early studies indicated that amantadine acted by preventing the penetration and/or uncoating of influenza A viruses. In more recent studies, low concentrations of the drug were shown to inhibit virus assembly by interacting with virus hemagglutinin; high concentrations appear to inhibit an early stage of the infection involving fusion between the virus envelope and the membrane of secondary lysosomes. Additional studies are needed to further clarify the mechanism(s) by which this drug inhibits susceptible virus strains.

There is general agreement that the efficacy of amantadine when used prophylactically in influenza A infections averages 70% to 80% (range, 0% to 100%), approximately the same as with influenza vaccines.

Rimantadine, an investigational analogue of amantadine, has a spectrum and mechanism of action similar to those of the parent drug. It does not appear to inhibit virus adsorption or penetration, but it may interfere with virus uncoating, possibly by inhibiting release of M protein from viral ribonucleoproteins. Workers in the Soviet Union, where rimantadine has been employed extensively, have suggested that the compound may act by inhibiting RNA-dependent RNA polymerase or the synthesis of virus-specific RNA. As with amantadine, additional studies are necessary to clarify the mechanism(s) of action.

Several clinical studies conducted in the United States demonstrated the prophylactic and therapeutic efficacy of rimantadine against influenza A infections (Dolin et al, 1982; Quarles et al, 1981; Van Voris et al, 1981). It has not been shown to have any effect on influenza B infections.

Most investigators agree that rimantadine causes fewer adverse effects than amantadine after use of identical dosages; higher plasma drug levels are obtained with amantadine, which could account for the higher incidence of adverse effects with this drug. In the elderly, however, serum levels were nearly three times higher than those in younger adults, possibly due to decreased renal function in older individuals; therefore, a reduction of dosage of amantadine may be necessary to reduce the incidence of adverse effects (Patriarca et al, 1984).

Miscellaneous Investigational Drugs: Many compounds are being evaluated for selective antiviral activity. The following have shown some potential for clinical use.

Inosiplex [Isoprinosine] (inosine pranobex, methisoprinol) is a mixture of three compounds: inosine, dimethylaminoisopropanol, and paracitamidobenzoic acid. It is being used in Europe to treat a number of viral diseases, including herpesvirus, rhinovirus, and influenza A infections and viral hepatitis, but results of clinical studies are equivocal (Chang and Heel, 1981). Inosiplex has been investigated in the United States for use in influenza, rhinovirus, herpes simplex, and herpes zoster infections with variable results. It was reported to be effective in the long-term treatment of subacute sclerosing panencephalitis, but this finding is controversial (Dyken et al, 1982; Durant et al, 1982; Haddah and Risk, 1980).

The mechanism of action of inosiplex is not known. It was postulated early that the drug modifies ribosomes so that binding of virus mRNA occurs but translation of the message is inhibited. Claims also have been made that inosiplex is an immune modulator, since the drug potentiates in vitro lymphocyte responses to mitogens. Finally, it has been suggested that inosiplex has a dual antiviral effect in that it supports lymphocyte functions by promoting cellular RNA synthesis and translational ability but suppresses viral RNA synthesis (Ohnishi et al, 1982). In humans, inosiplex is rapidly metabolized; the half-life is 50 minutes after oral administration and 3 minutes after intravenous injection.

Enviroxime is a benzimidazole derivative that is being evaluated for use against rhinoviruses, the primary causative organisms of the common cold. In vitro, it inhibits the replication of a wide range of rhinoviruses and also has antiviral effects against coxsackie-, echo-, and polioviruses. The proposed mechanism of action is interference with macromolecular synthesis in infected cells through inhibition of a viral RNA polymerase. In vitro studies have shown that enviroxime added to cell cultures a few hours after virus inoculation still significantly inhibits replication, thus suggesting a primary action during a late phase of replication. Some efficacy was observed against experimentally induced rhinovirus type 9 infection after combined oral and intranasal administration (Phillpotts et al, 1981), but more recent studies failed to demonstrate significant effects on artificially induced rhinovirus infections when the drug was administered only intranasally (Hayden and Gwaltney, 1982; Levandowski et al, 1982; Phillpotts et al, 1983).

Oral enviroxime is not well tolerated; adverse effects include nausea, vomiting, diarrhea, abdominal pain, and headache. However, the drug is well tolerated when given intranasally. Further studies are needed before the potential clinical usefulness of this compound can be determined.

Foscarnet sodium (trisodium phosphonoformate, PFA), a pyrophosphate analogue of phosphonoacetic acid (PAA), has potent in vitro and in vivo activity against herpesvirus. In laboratory animals, PAA produced liver degeneration, gingivitis, and severe dermal toxicity and accumulated in bone. Thus, it was considered too toxic for human use. PFA is considerably less toxic and no dermal effects have been observed. Both PAA and PFA inhibit the DNA polymerases of all human herpesviruses through similar mechanisms of action. These drugs are thought to act by blocking the pyrophosphate binding site, thus inhibiting the formation of the 3'-5'-phosphodiester bond between primer and substrate and preventing chain elongation. In addition to inhibiting herpesvirus DNA polymerase, PFA also inhibits influenza A RNA-dependent RNA polymerase and the reverse transcriptases of several animal retroviruses; cellular DNA polymerase α is approximately 80 times more resistant to this action than herpesvirus DNA polymerases. The antiviral spectrum of PFA in vitro includes herpes simplex virus types 1 and 2, varicella-zoster virus, cytomegalovirus, Epstein-Barr virus, African swine fever, HTLV-III, and various animal retroviruses (avian myeloblastosis, visna, and murine leukemia virus). PFA has also demonstrated activity against HTLV-III reverse transcriptase.

There have been few clinical trials with PFA. In one preliminary trial in patients with recurrent herpes labialis, topical application of a 3% cream significantly shortened the vesicular period and decreased the development of new vesicles (Wallin et al, 1980). PFA also is undergoing clinical trials in patients with AIDS. A drawback to the use of PFA is that, like PAA, it is deposited in bone; however, in mice, 50% of bound PFA is released within three weeks. Additional clinical trials are necessary to fully evaluate the therapeutic potential of this agent.

Resistance

As with other microorganisms, virus mutants may arise that are resistant to certain antiviral drugs.

In herpesviruses, two encoded enzymes, thymidine kinase (TK) and DNA polymerase, are intimately involved in the action of antiherpesvirus drugs in current use or being investigated (acyclovir, vidarabine, BVDU, FIAC, PFA). As might be expected, loss or reduction of thymidine kinase activity or subtle alterations in viral thymidine kinase or DNA polymerase markedly reduces the sensitivity of herpesviruses to these drugs. For example, five types of mutants have been isolated by passage of virus in cell cultures maintained in the presence of acyclovir: (1) mutants with absent or low production of TK, (2) mutants producing altered TK, (3) mutants with altered DNA polymerase, (4) mutants deficient in TK and with altered DNA polymerase, and (5) mutants with altered TK and DNA polymerase.

Acquired resistance in mutants isolated from cell cultures, animals, and man has been reported for idoxuridine, vidarabine, cytarabine, trifluorothymidine, acyclovir, BVDU, FIAC, PAA, and PFA. TK-defective mutants are inherently resistant to all drugs whose action is mediated through this enzyme; thus, TK- mutants have been described that are cross resistant to idoxuridine, cytarabine, acyclovir, and BVDU (Field et al, 1981). It is rather facile to isolate a TK-resistant mutant in cell culture; a single passage of virus in cells cultured in the presence of any of the TK-mediated drugs is sufficient to isolate TK-resistant viruses.

Resistance through alterations in herpesvirus DNA polymerase may lead to cross resistance. It was reported early that mutants resistant to PAA were always resistant to the analogue, PFA, and mutants resistant to PAA have been reported to be resistant to acyclovir and vice versa. The physical map limits of sequences within the HSV-1 DNA polymerase locus that contain mutations conferring resistance to BVDU have been defined. The region of resistance mutation for vidarabine is closely linked to that for PAA and acyclovir and overlaps with that for BVDU; however, the latter can be transferred separately (Crumpacker et al, 1982 A and B). Thus, cross resistance to the herpesvirus drugs, PAA, PFA, acyclovir, and vidarabine, due to an altered DNA polymerase can be expected, at least in vitro. The resistance of herpesvirus DNA polymerase to BVDU appears to be independent of its resistance to PAA, acyclovir, and vidarabine.

Fortunately, resistant herpesvirus mutants do not emerge often in humans or animals undergoing chemotherapy, even though they arise readily in drug-treated cell cultures. Attempts to isolate resistant viruses from experimentally infected animals treated with acyclovir have been generally unsuccessful. It is thought that conditions exist in vivo that limit the development of resistance. By far the most frequently isolated resistant mutants from infected cell cultures or patients are those that are defective in TK production. These TK- mutants appear to be present in clinical isolates both before and after therapy with acyclovir. TK-deficient mutants are less virulent than the wild strains and considerably less capable of establishing latency in experimental animals. A clinical isolate of an HSV mutant with resistance due to an altered TK has been reported. Clinical isolates of resistant mutants with an altered DNA polymerase have not yet been reported. As might be anticipated, resistant strains of herpesviruses have been encountered more frequently in immunocompromised patients receiving acyclovir. However, such isolates all have been TK-deficient mutants. Thus, at the moment, resistance is not a significant clinical problem with the antiherpesvirus drugs.

Herpesviruses also exhibit a different type of resistance that poses a major problem. Latent herpesviruses persist for prolonged periods in certain areas of the body (eg, neural cells of ganglia for herpes simplex and varicella-zoster viruses). This latent infection is punctuated by episodes of active viral replication and disease recurrence. Unfortunately, the currently available antiherpesvirus drugs must be given during active viral multiplication to be effective. None are active against latent virus and, therefore, active infections can be expected once treatment is stopped.

Compared to the antiherpesvirus drugs, resistance to the anti-influenza drugs, amantadine and rimantadine, appears to develop less frequently. Strains of influenza A resistant to amantadine have emerged following a single passage in cell cultures containing the compound. Resistant mutants of influenza A also have been isolated from infected mice treated with amantadine. Mutants with increased resistance to the drug were observed after a single passage; after six passages, most of the isolated strains were completely resistant to amantadine and rimantadine (Oxford et al, 1970). Amantadine- and rimantadine-resistant influenza strains have been isolated from patients in whom neither compound was used prophylactically (Heider et al, 1981).

The mechanism of resistance to amantadine has not been firmly established, but investigators reported that gene 7, which codes for the M (matrix) protein, seems to segregate with amantadine resistance (Lubeck et al, 1978; Hay et al, 1979; Scholtissek and Faulkner, 1979; Hamzawi et al, 1981). Unfortunately, little field work has been conducted in search of amantadine- or rimantadine-resistant influenza strains in persons treated with these agents or in their contacts; thus, it is not yet possible to gauge the clinical significance of resistant mutants. There is a possibility, however, that resistance could spread between influenza viruses by recombination and reassortment.

Drug Evaluations

ACYCLOVIR SODIUM (Parenteral)
[Zovirax]

ACTIONS. The antiviral spectrum of acyclovir is limited to

herpesviruses. In vitro, the order of decreasing susceptibility to its antiviral activity is HSV-1, HSV-2, varicella-zoster, cytomegalovirus. Epstein-Barr virus (EBV) also is sensitive. Acyclovir is 160 times more potent than vidarabine against herpes simplex type 1 in tissue culture experiments. The specific activation of acyclovir by herpesvirus thymidine kinase and the subsequent preferential inhibition of viral DNA polymerase by acyclo GTP provide the drug with a high degree of selective activity (see the Introduction). A 3,000-fold greater concentration of acyclovir is required to inhibit the growth of host cells than to inhibit viral replication.

The mechanism of action of acyclovir against CMV and EBV appears to be somewhat different than against herpes simplex or varicella-zoster viruses. Unlike the latter viruses, neither CMV nor EBV code for their own thymidine kinase. In cells infected by these viruses, acyclovir is poorly phosphorylated; however, once phosphorylated to the triphosphate, both CMV and EBV DNA polymerase are quite sensitive to the drug.

USES. A number of double-blind, placebo-controlled studies support the efficacy of acyclovir both systemically and topically in various herpesvirus infections (see also the following evaluation on topical acyclovir).

In immunocompromised patients with mucocutaneous herpes simplex infections, the median times to cessation of new lesion formation, lesion crusting, lesion healing, cessation of pain, and termination of viral shedding were shorter in patients in the acyclovir group than in those in the placebo group (Mitchell et al, 1981; Chou et al, 1981; Wade et al, 1982 B; Meyers et al, 1982).

Acyclovir also appears to be effective in other herpes simplex infections in immunocompromised patients. When intravenous acyclovir was given to herpes simplex virus-seropositive recipients of bone marrow transplants for 18 days beginning three days before transplantation, no patient developed lesions during the course of therapy (Saral et al, 1981). One-half of the treated patients developed mild herpes simplex infections after cessation of therapy, however, indicating that acyclovir cannot eradicate latent infection. Similarly, acyclovir prevented reactivation of HSV infections when given prophylactically to leukemic patients receiving timed sequential chemotherapy (Saral et al, 1983), but infection recurred in many patients after cessation of acyclovir when cancer chemotherapy was resumed.

The efficacy of acyclovir against herpes zoster infections in immunocompromised patients has been demonstrated in several clinical trials (Selby et al, 1979; Spector et al, 1982; Serota et al, 1982; Balfour et al, 1983; Meyers et al, 1984). In one trial, 40 marrow transplant patients were treated with acyclovir for VZV infections (Meyers et al, 1984) and a rapid antiviral effect was noted; the median times to cessation of virus positivity, new lesion formation, and total pustulation were shorter than those reported for vidarabine. In a prospective randomized trial, acyclovir and vidarabine given intravenously were compared in 22 severely compromised patients who presented within 72 hours of onset of VZV infection. Cutaneous dissemination of infection did not occur in any of the 10 evaluable patients treated with acyclovir; in comparison, 5 of the evaluable 10 recipients of vidarabine developed localized dermatomal disease. Acyclovir also was superior to vidarabine in shortening the period of virus shedding, new lesion formation, the median interval until the first decrease in pain, the pustulation and crusting of all lesions, and the complete healing of lesions and in reducing the incidence of fever. The authors concluded that acyclovir was the drug of choice for the treatment of varicella-zoster infection in immunocompromised patients (Shepp et al, 1986).

Studies also have demonstrated the effectiveness of acyclovir in immunocompetent patients with herpes zoster (Peterslund et al, 1981, 1984; Bean et al, 1982; Esmann et al, 1982). Reduction in pain and erythema, prevention of new lesion formation, and decrease in healing time were reported. Presently, use of this drug for prophylaxis of HSV infections and treatment of herpes encephalitis or herpes zoster infection is investigational.

In patients with normal immune systems, acyclovir has been effective in primary genital herpesvirus infections. When compared to placebo controls, patients receiving acyclovir showed more rapid healing, earlier cessation of pain and pruritus, and earlier termination of viral shedding (Corey et al, 1983; Mindel et al, 1982).

Results of clinical studies employing acyclovir to treat CMV disease in immunocompromised patients are equivocal. In one study, organ transplant patients with CMV disease were given acyclovir 500 mg/M^2 three times daily intravenously for seven days (Balfour et al, 1982). These patients experienced more rapid defervescence and clinical improvement than placebo controls. In a second study, however, marrow transplant patients with CMV pneumonia were given doses ranging from 400 to 1,200 mg/M^2 without favorable effect (Wade et al, 1982 B).

ADVERSE REACTIONS AND PRECAUTIONS. In general, intravenous acyclovir has not produced serious adverse effects. Elevations in blood urea nitrogen and creatinine concentrations have been reported and were more common when the drug was administered as an intravenous bolus. The elevations returned to normal after cessation of therapy and, in some cases, despite continued therapy. Decreasing the dose or increasing water intake reversed the effect. The proposed mechanism for this nephrotoxic action is crystallization of acyclovir in renal tubules, which was observed previously in animal studies. Therefore, it is recommended that acyclovir be administered by slow infusion over one hour. Caution should be exercised in dehydrated patients or those with impaired renal function.

Phlebitis at the injection site and delirium in two patients also have been reported. This drug is classified in FDA Pregnancy Category C.

PHARMACOKINETICS. Following intravenous administration, acyclovir exhibits dose-dependent pharmacokinetics in the range of 0.5 to 15 mg/kg. In adults, when 5 mg/kg was given in one-hour infusions every eight hours, mean steady-state peak and trough concentrations of 9.8 mcg/ml and 0.7 mcg/ml, respectively, were achieved.

Acyclovir is widely distributed in tissues and body fluids. Concentrations attained in the cerebrospinal fluid are approximately 50% of those in the plasma. Plasma protein binding is low (9% to 33%). The drug is excreted by glomerular filtration and tubular secretion, primarily in unchanged form. The half-life is about 2.5 hours in adults and children with normal renal function.

DOSAGE AND PREPARATIONS.
Intravenous: Acyclovir should be administered by intravenous infusion. Rapid or bolus intravenous, intramuscular, or subcutaneous injection must be avoided. Therapy should be initiated as early as possible following onset of symptoms. Dosage adjustments are necessary in patients with renal impairment (see the manufacturer's recommendations).

For mucosal and cutaneous herpes simplex infections in immunocompromised patients, *adults,* 5 mg/kg infused at a constant rate over a one-hour period every eight hours (15 mg/kg/day) for seven days; *children under 12 years,* 250 mg/M^2 infused at a constant rate over a one-hour period every eight hours (750 mg/M^2/day) for seven days.

For severe initial episodes of herpes genitalis in immunocompetent patients, the same dosages as above are administered for five days.

For herpes zoster infections in both immunocompetent and immunocompromised patients (investigational indication), *adults and children over 12 years*, 5 to 12 mg/kg over a one-hour period every eight hours for seven days.
   Zovirax (Burroughs Wellcome). Powder (sterile) equivalent to 500 mg base in 10 ml containers.

ACYCLOVIR (Topical)
[Zovirax Ointment 5%]

USES. A topical ointment containing acyclovir 5% in polyethylene glycol is used for the management of initial genital herpes infections. A double-blind, placebo-controlled study showed that the application of acyclovir ointment to lesions four or six times a day promoted healing, relieved pain and pruritus, and decreased the duration of viral shedding in patients with initial infections (Corey et al, 1982 A and B). In contrast, no clinical benefit was noted in patients with recurrent herpes genitalis, although some decrease in the duration of viral shedding was observed (Luby et al, 1984). Acyclovir does not eradicate latent herpesvirus and, therefore, does not prevent recurrences of active disease (see also the Introduction). Thus, the use of topical acyclovir in genital herpes is limited to active initial infections.

Topical acyclovir also has been used for limited, nonlife-threatening, mucocutaneous herpes simplex infections, mainly herpes labialis, in immunocompromised patients. The duration of viral shedding was reduced and the duration of pain was decreased slightly (Whitley et al, 1982 B). No evidence of clinical benefit has been observed in immunocompetent patients with herpes labialis, although some decrease in duration of viral shedding has been seen (Spruance et al, 1982, 1984).

A number of clinical trials have established the effectiveness of an ophthalmic ointment containing acyclovir 3% in the treatment of herpes simplex keratitis. However, this use is currently investigational.

ADVERSE REACTIONS AND PRECAUTIONS. The most common adverse effect is mild pain, including transient burning and stinging, at the site of application. Pruritus, rash, and vulvitis also have been reported. These adverse effects probably are caused by the application of ointment to tender and sensitive lesions, since placebo-treated patients also experienced these undesirable effects.

DOSAGE AND PREPARATIONS.

Topical: Sufficient ointment to cover all lesions should be applied every three hours six times a day for seven days. The dose/application depends upon the total lesion area but should approximate a one-half inch ribbon of ointment/4 in² of surface area. A finger cot or rubber glove should be used to prevent autoinoculation of other body sites and transmission of infection to other persons. Therapy should be initiated as early as possible following onset of signs and symptoms.

   Zovirax (Burroughs Wellcome). Ointment 5% (50 mg/g) in a polyethylene glycol base in 15 g containers.

ACYCLOVIR (Oral)
[Zovirax]

USES. Oral acyclovir is indicated for the treatment of initial episodes of genital herpes virus infections and management of recurrences in certain patients.

   Treatment of primary genital herpes infection with oral acyclovir 200 mg given five times daily for five to ten days significantly reduced viral shedding, time to crusting, duration of local pain, and severity of symptoms (Nilsen et al, 1982; Bryson et al, 1983; Mertz et al, 1984); however, treatment did not appear to influence recurrence rates.

   Oral acyclovir also has been beneficial in the treatment of recurrent genital herpes infections. In a multicenter trial involving 250 patients with recurrent genital herpes, oral acyclovir 200 mg given five times daily for five days reduced virus shedding and shortened the time to healing of lesions. The effects were more pronounced when patients self-initiated therapy early in the course of recurrences. However, therapy did not appear to affect the latent state, for there was no difference in times to the next recurrence between drug and placebo groups (Reichman et al, 1984). In a randomized, double-blind trial, acyclovir 200 mg four times daily for 12 weeks reduced the mean monthly recurrence rate and median time to first recurrence (Mindel et al, 1984). In other studies in which acyclovir was administered in two, three, or five daily doses over a four-month period, significantly fewer recurrences were reported in treated patients compared to placebo-controlled groups (Straus et al, 1984 B; Douglas et al, 1984). The efficacy of oral acyclovir in recurrent genital herpes infection has been confirmed in more recent studies (Ruhnek-Forsbeck et al, 1985; Shepp et al, 1985). In all these studies, however, recurrences followed cessation of therapy, although disease was less severe. In one study, the time to first recurrence was similar in both drug- and placebo-controlled groups (Straus et al 1984 B). In other studies, the median time to first recurrence was significantly shorter in the treated groups (Douglas et al, 1984; Mindel et al, 1984). This discrepancy may be due to differences in study design or patient populations.

   Long-term (four months) therapy does not appear to have any lasting effect on the natural history of the disease, for

recurrences return to pretreatment frequencies following cessation of therapy (Douglas et al, 1984). In addition, lesions in treated patients contained resistant virus, although in later recurrences the virus appeared to be drug-sensitive (Straus et al, 1984 B). Thus, studies to date suggest that oral acyclovir is useful for maintenance therapy rather than for cure of genital herpes, but no recommendations can be made regarding episodic versus continuous therapy until further studies are completed.

   In a number of clinical trials, oral acyclovir was reported to have significant efficacy against other herpesvirus infections in both immunocompromised and immunocompetent patients. Symptomatic attacks of mucocutaneous herpes simplex infections were suppressed in immunocompromised patients during the course (up to 65 days) of drug administration (Straus et al, 1982). In recurrent infections in immunodeficient patients, 200 mg five times daily for five days reduced virus shedding, alleviated signs and symptoms, and increased time to recurrence (Straus et al, 1984 A). In the clinical trials, however, recurrences always followed cessation of therapy. In the latter study, however, expected recurrences were suppressed by the administration of one capsule (200 mg) twice daily.

   In a prospective, randomized, double-blind, placebo-controlled trial, oral acyclovir was reported to be safe and effective in preventing herpesvirus reactivation after marrow transplantation when 400 mg five times daily was given from one week before to four weeks after transplantation (Wade et al, 1984).

   In an uncontrolled study, dissemination of varicella-zoster virus in immunocompromised children was prevented by oral acyclovir 400 mg five times daily for ten days (Novelli et al, 1984). In a double-blind, randomized trial in elderly patients with acute zoster infections, oral acyclovir 400 mg five times daily for five days was as effective as intravenous acyclovir in shortening the duration of pain and accelerating the healing rate (Peterslund et al, 1984). However, in a double-blind, placebo-controlled trial conducted in immunocompetent patients over 50 years with herpes zoster, the only statistically significant difference demonstrated by a similar regimen of oral acyclovir was a decrease in the days of new lesion formation within the affected dermatome after day zero (McKendrick et al, 1984). Further studies are required to unequivocally establish the usefulness of oral acyclovir for the treatment of zoster infections.

ADVERSE REACTIONS. Acyclovir is well tolerated when given orally. The most frequently reported reactions during short-term administration are nausea and/or vomiting (incidence 2.7%) and headache (0.6%); the most common reactions during long-term administration are headache (13.1%), diarrhea (8.8%), nausea and/or vomiting (8%), vertigo (3.6%), and arthralgia (3.6%). Acyclovir has not affected results of laboratory tests, except for one report of increased mean corpuscular volume of erythrocytes and mean corpuscular hemoglobin concentrations (Straus et al, 1984 A) and another report of elevated bilirubin levels (Douglas et al, 1984).

   Large doses of acyclovir decreased spermatogenesis in some animals and, in some acute studies, were reported to produce mutagenic effects. Because chromosome breaks may occur at high drug concentrations, acyclovir should not be used during pregnancy unless the potential benefits outweigh the risks to the fetus (FDA Pregnancy Category C). No adequate controlled studies have been done in pregnant women and it is not known whether the drug is secreted in human milk.

PHARMACOKINETICS. Acyclovir is slowly and variably absorbed; peak levels are achieved in one to four hours. Bioavailability is 15% to 30%. Depending upon the dose employed, peak plasma levels range from 0.3 to 2 mcg/ml. The half-life of oral acyclovir is 3.3 hours. After administration of 200 mg orally, levels of 0.19 mcg/ml and 0.8 mcg/ml, respectively, were attained in saliva and vaginal secretions. Ten to fifteen percent of the administered dose is excreted unchanged in the urine, and 15% to 25% is excreted unchanged in stools.

DOSAGE AND PREPARATIONS.

Oral: Adults, for initial episodes of genital herpes, 200 mg five times daily for ten days. For chronic suppressive therapy for recurrent disease, 200 mg three to five times daily for up to six months. For intermittent therapy for recurrent disease, 200 mg five times daily for five days. Therapy should begin at the earliest sign of recurrence. In patients with renal impairment (creatinine clearance $\leq$10 ml/min/1.73 M^2), the drug should be given every 12 hours.

Zovirax (Burroughs Wellcome). Capsules 200 mg.

AMANTADINE HYDROCHLORIDE
[Symmetrel]

ACTIONS AND USES. Amantadine has a narrow antiviral spectrum. All influenza A subtypes and some C strains are inhibited in vitro; influenza B strains are rarely sensitive. Strains of influenza A differ in sensitivity; in vitro inhibitory concentrations vary from 0.2 to 30 mcg/ml, depending upon the assay system employed. Sendai and rubella viruses also are sensitive to amantadine in vitro. Early studies suggested that amantadine acted by inhibiting viral penetration and/or uncoating, but more recent studies indicate that its inhibitory effect may involve interaction with the virion M (matrix) protein (see the Introduction).

Amantadine is useful in the prophylaxis and treatment of influenza A infections (National Institutes of Health Consensus Development Conference, 1980). Approximately 70% of recipients exposed to influenza A viruses are protected. Although early immunization is preferred, amantadine is recommended when vaccine is unavailable or contraindicated, particularly in children and adults at high risk because of underlying diseases, elderly patients in semiclosed institutional environments, and individuals with vital community functions (eg, policemen, firemen, hospital personnel). Since amantadine does not interfere with the immune response to influenza A vaccine, it can be administered concomitantly to provide interim protection or to augment the prophylactic effect in a previously vaccinated individual.

Amantadine also is effective in the treatment of active influenza A infection when administered within 48 hours after the onset of symptoms. This drug is of no clinical value in infections caused by influenza B or other myxoviruses.

ADVERSE REACTIONS AND PRECAUTIONS. Amantadine is well tolerated by most patients during short- and long-term use. Central nervous system side effects are most common and include difficulty in thinking, confusion, lightheadedness, hallucinations, anxiety, and insomnia. These symptoms are mild, usually occur shortly after therapy is started, are reversible on discontinuation of the drug, and often cease even when administration is continued. Activities requiring mental alertness (eg, driving) should be avoided until it is reasonable to assume that these symptoms will not occur. More severe adverse effects, such as mental depression and psychosis, are usually associated with doses exceeding 200 mg daily. Less common untoward effects include anorexia, nausea, vomiting, and orthostatic hypotension. Rarely, leukopenia and neutropenia are observed; other hematologic disorders have not been reported.

Livedo reticularis occasionally associated with ankle edema has occurred with use of amantadine in parkinsonism, particularly in women given the drug for a month or longer (see Chapter 11). This reaction has not been observed with the smaller doses used for influenza.

The manufacturer reports that congestive heart failure developed in a few patients receiving amantadine. The dose may require careful adjustment in patients with pre-existing congestive heart failure or peripheral edema.

Caution also must be exercised when amantadine is administered to patients with impaired renal function, liver disease, epilepsy, and psychosis or severe psychoneurosis not controlled by psychotropic agents.

In certain laboratory animals, large doses have been embryotoxic and teratogenic. Thus, amantadine should be used in pregnant women only after the risks to the fetus are weighed against the benefit to the patient (FDA Pregnancy Category C). Amantadine is excreted in milk and thus should not be given to nursing mothers.

DRUG INTERACTIONS. The peripheral and central adverse effects of anticholinergic drugs are increased by the concomitant use of amantadine. Acute psychotic reactions identical to those caused by atropine poisoning have occurred with combined therapy. Psychotic reactions also have developed occasionally in patients receiving amantadine and levodopa. If signs of central toxicity develop, the dose of anticholinergic drug or levodopa should be reduced while the patient is receiving amantadine.

PHARMACOKINETICS. Amantadine is absorbed rapidly and completely after oral administration; peak serum levels of approximately 0.3 mcg/ml are achieved two to four hours after administration of 2.5 mg/kg. The half-life in the serum averages 20 hours (range, 9 to 37 hours). When the usual adult dose of 100 mg is given every 12 hours, maximal tissue concentrations are reached in approximately 48 hours. Amantadine is not metabolized in humans, and about 90% of an administered dose is excreted unchanged in the urine. The drug crosses the blood-brain barrier and a cerebrospinal fluid concentration approximating 60% of that in the plasma may be attained. Because the drug may accumulate, the dose should be decreased or therapy discontinued in patients with impaired renal function.

DOSAGE AND PREPARATIONS.

Oral: For prophylaxis of influenza A infections, *adults,* 100 mg twice daily; *children 1 to 9 years,* 4.4 to 8.8 mg/kg daily in two or three equal doses (maximum, 150 mg daily); *9 to 12 years,* 100 mg twice daily.

Prophylactic administration should be started in anticipation of contact or as soon as possible after exposure to influenza A viruses. Amantadine should be given for at least ten days following a known exposure or throughout the risk period, which in most communities is four to six weeks. Dosage can be continued for up to 90 days in cases of possible repeated and unknown exposures. When used with inactivated influenza A vaccine (to provide interim protection until adequate antibody titers develop), amantadine is continued for two to three weeks after administration of vaccine.

For treatment of established influenza A, the same dosage used for prophylaxis should be administered within 48 hours after onset of illness and continued for four to five days.

Symmetrel (DuPont). Capsules 100 mg; syrup 50 mg/5 ml.

VIDARABINE
[Vira-A]

ACTIONS AND USES. Vidarabine is converted to ara-ATP, the active metabolite, which preferentially inhibits viral DNA polymerase (see the Introduction). In vitro, the drug is active against herpes simplex types 1 and 2, varicella-zoster, cytomegalovirus, and vaccinia viruses. Cytomegalovirus and vaccinia virus are most resistant. Vidarabine is inactive against adenoviruses. Among the RNA viruses, only rhabdoviruses (vesicular stomatitis and rabies viruses) and retroviruses (Rous sarcoma, Gross murine leukemia, and Rauscher murine leukemia viruses) are susceptible.

When administered by intravenous infusion, vidarabine is useful in the treatment of herpes simplex encephalitis. In a multicenter, double-blind, placebo-controlled study (Whitley et al, 1977), vidarabine 15 mg/kg/day for ten days decreased overall mortality from 70% to 28%, and reduced debilitating

neurologic sequelae in individuals who exhibited only lethargy when therapy was begun. Although vidarabine reduced mortality in semicomatose and comatose patients, it did not alter morbidity or prevent serious neurologic sequelae in these patients. The results of this trial were confirmed in a later study (Whitley et al, 1981).

Early and accurate diagnosis of herpes simplex encephalitis is essential to achieve maximum benefits. This disease should be suspected whenever there is a history of febrile encephalopathy, disordered mental state, reduced consciousness, and focal cerebral signs. Examination of the cerebrospinal fluid, electroencephalography, and a brain scan using computerized axial tomography may be helpful, but a brain biopsy is essential to confirm the diagnosis (see Whitley et al, 1982 C). Specimens are negative in over one-half of patients suspected of having this disease. Treating such patients with vidarabine not only subjects them to the adverse effects of the drug but, more importantly, may deprive them of effective therapy for other diseases.

A recent study has demonstrated that intravenous acyclovir is more effective than vidarabine for the treatment of herpes simplex encephalitis and is the drug of choice for this infection (Whitley et al, 1986). Thus, it has been suggested that vidarabine be restricted to patients who have not responded to acyclovir, those with acyclovir-resistant strains, or individuals who relapse after acyclovir therapy.

Intravenous vidarabine has been effective for other severe herpesvirus infections in double-blind, placebo-controlled, clinical trials. In neonatal herpes simplex infections, vidarabine decreased both mortality and morbidity (Whitley et al, 1980). Once again, however, efficacy was related inversely to the severity of the disease. In neonates who experienced only localized skin, eye, or mouth infections, vidarabine 15 mg/kg/day for ten days prevented severe ocular and neurologic sequelae. In more severely affected infants with central nervous system and disseminated disease, the drug reduced mortality from 74% to 38% and morbidity (at 1 year of age) in survivors from 89% to 71%. Although the number of patients was small, outcome was better in those with localized central nervous system disease than in those with disseminated disease. Vidarabine appears to slow the process of neurologic impairment but cannot reverse existing damage.

Vidarabine also is indicated to treat localized herpes zoster and chickenpox infections in immunocompromised adults and children, respectively. Results in patients with herpes zoster who received vidarabine within 72 hours after onset of symptoms were compared to those achieved in untreated controls; the former experienced faster rates of healing (ie, earlier cessation of new vesicle formation, shorter times to total pustulation and scabbing), decreased cutaneous dissemination and visceral complications, and reduced duration of postherpetic neuralgia (Whitley et al, 1976; Whitley et al, 1982 D). Efficacy was similar in immunocompromised children with chickenpox (Whitley et al, 1982 A). However, a more recent clinical trial compared intravenous vidarabine with acyclovir for the treatment of varicella-zoster infections in immunocompromised patients and concluded that acyclovir was preferred in these patients (Shepp et al, 1986).

Intravenous vidarabine has not been effective in cytomegalovirus or smallpox infections.

A topical ophthalmic preparation of vidarabine [Vira-A] is effective in herpes simplex keratitis (see Chapter 73, Topical Anti-infective Agents: Otic and Ophthalmic Preparations). However, vidarabine is not useful in herpes simplex labialis or genitalis.

ADVERSE REACTIONS AND PRECAUTIONS. When therapeutic doses are given intravenously, vidarabine causes minimal or no adverse effects in most patients. The most common side effects (incidence, 10% to 15%) are gastrointestinal disturbances (eg, anorexia, nausea, vomiting, diarrhea), which are usually mild. Central nervous system disturbances noted occasionally include tremors, dizziness, confusion, hallucinations, ataxia, and psychoses. Doses of 20 mg/kg/day or more cause more pronounced central nervous system effects; cytotoxic effects, leukopenia, and thrombocytopenia also become apparent.

Patients with impaired renal function (eg, renal transplant patients) excrete ara-Hx, the major metabolite of vidarabine, slowly and may require reduced doses to avoid accumulation and severe adverse reactions. Liver function and hematologic tests are recommended because elevated SGOT and bilirubin levels and/or decreased hemoglobin, hematocrit, and white blood cell counts occasionally have been associated with vidarabine therapy.

Supportive care may be required in patients who are susceptible to fluid overload or cerebral edema, which is a common consequence of herpes simplex encephalitis. Measures to combat increased intracranial pressure should be utilized; elevation of the head, administration of mannitol and/or glycerin, and hyperventilation to maintain a decreased arterial PCO_2 level are recommended.

Vidarabine is teratogenic in laboratory animals. Therefore, its use in pregnant women should be avoided if possible (FDA Pregnancy Category C).

DRUG INTERACTIONS. Increased neurotoxicity has been reported in patients receiving allopurinol with vidarabine. This is probably due to increased blood levels of ara-Hx resulting from inhibition of xanthine oxidase by allopurinol. A reduction in vidarabine dosage should be considered when these two drugs are given together.

PHARMACOKINETICS. Because of poor aqueous solubility, vidarabine must be administered in large volumes of fluid by continuous intravenous infusion over a 12- to 24-hour period. It is rapidly deaminated to arabinosylhypoxanthine (ara-Hx), which has much weaker antiviral activity. Peak plasma levels of ara-Hx and vidarabine range from 3 to 6 mcg/ml and 0.2 to 0.4 mcg/ml, respectively, after slow infusion of 10 mg/kg of vidarabine. These levels reflect the slow rate of infusion and lack of accumulation. The plasma half-life of ara-Hx is approximately four hours, and excretion is primarily via the kidneys. Approximately 60% of a daily dose is recovered in urine as ara-Hx; only 1% to 3% is parent drug. Ara-Hx levels in cerebrospinal fluid are about one-third those in plasma.

DOSAGE AND PREPARATIONS.
Intravenous: The solubility of vidarabine in intravenous solutions is limited; a maximum of 450 mg can be dissolved in 1 L of fluid. The drug should be administered by slow, continuous infusion over a 12- to 24-hour period. Rapid or bolus injection must be avoided.

Adults and children, for herpes simplex encephalitis, 15 mg/kg daily for ten days. For neonatal herpes simplex infection (investigational indication), the same dosage is employed. For varicella-zoster in immunocompromised patients, 10 mg/kg/day for five days (Whitley et al, 1981).

Vira-A (Parke-Davis). Suspension (sterile) 200 mg monohydrate (equivalent to 187.4 mg of base)/ml in 5 ml containers.

Cited References

Arvin AM, et al: Human leukocyte interferon for treatment of varicella in children with cancer. *N Engl J Med* 306:761-765, 1982 A.

Arvin AM, et al: Alpha interferon administration to infants with congenital rubella. *Antimicrob Agents Chemother* 21:259-261, 1982 B.

Bach MC, et al: 9-(1,3 dihydroxy-2-propoxymethyl) guanine for cytomegalovirus infections in patients with acquired immunodeficiency syndrome. *Ann Intern Med* 103:381-384, 1985.

Balfour HH Jr, et al: Acyclovir in immunocompromised patients with cytomegalovirus disease: Controlled trial at one institution. *Am J Med* 73(1A):241-248, 1982.

Balfour HH Jr, et al: Acyclovir halts progression of herpes zoster in immunocompromised patients. *N Engl J Med* 308:1448-1453, 1983.

Bassendine MF, et al: Adenine arabinoside therapy in HBsAG-positive chronic liver disease: Controlled study. *Gastroenterology* 80:1016-1022, 1981.

Bean B, et al: Acyclovir therapy for acute herpes zoster. *Lancet* 2:118-121, 1982.

Becker Y (ed): *Antiviral Drugs and Interferon: The Molecular Basis of Their Activity.* Boston, Martinus Nijhoff, 1984.

Benoit Y, et al: Oral BVDU treatment of varicella and zoster in children with cancer. *Eur J Pediatr* 143:198-202, 1985.

Bierman SM, et al: Clinical efficacy of ribavirin in treatment of genital herpes simplex virus infection. *Chemotherapy* 27:139-145, 1981.

Bryson YJ, et al: Treatment of first episodes of genital herpes simplex virus infection with oral acyclovir. *N Engl J Med* 308:916-921, 1983.

Chang T-W, Heel RC: Ribavirin and inosiplex: Review of their present status in viral diseases. *Drugs* 22:111-128, 1981.

Cheng Y-C, et al: Unique spectrum of activity of 9-[(1,3-dihydroxy-2-propoxy) methyl]-guanine against herpesviruses in vitro and its mode of action against herpes simplex virus type 1. *Proc Natl Acad Sci USA* 80:2767-2770, 1983.

Chou S, et al: Controlled clinical trial of intravenous acyclovir in heart-transplant patients with mucocutaneous herpes simplex infections. *Lancet* 1:1392-1394, 1981.

Colin J, et al: Combination therapy for dendritic keratitis with human leukocyte interferon and acyclovir. *Am J Ophthalmol* 95:346-348, 1983.

Connor JD, et al: Ribavirin pharmacokinetics in children and adults during therapeutic trials, in Smith RA, et al (eds): *Clinical Applications of Ribavirin.* Orlando, FL, Academic Press, 1984, 107-123.

Corey L, et al: Trial of topical acyclovir in genital herpes simplex virus infections. *N Engl J Med* 306:1313-1319, 1982 A.

Corey L, et al: Double-blind controlled trial of topical acyclovir in genital herpes simplex infection. *Am J Med* 73(1A):326-334, 1982 B.

Corey L, et al: Intravenous acyclovir for treatment of primary genital herpes. *Ann Intern Med* 98:914-921, 1983.

Crumpacker CS, et al: Resistance of herpes simplex virus to adenine arabinoside and E-5-(2-bromovinyl)-2'-deoxyuridine: Physical analysis. *J Infect Dis* 146:167-172, 1982 A.

Crumpacker CS, et al: Resistance to antiviral drugs of herpes simplex virus isolated from patient treated with acyclovir. *N Engl J Med* 306:343-346, 1982 B.

de Clercq E, et al: Oral (E)-5-(2-bromovinyl)-2'-deoxyuridine in severe herpes zoster. *Br Med J* 281:1178, 1980.

Dolin R, et al: Controlled trial of amantadine and rimantadine in prophylaxis of influenza A infections. *N Engl J Med* 307:580-584, 1982.

Douglas JM, et al: Double-blind study of oral acyclovir for suppression of recurrences of genital herpes simplex virus infection. *N Engl J Med* 310:1551-1556, 1984.

Douglas RM, et al: Prophylactic efficacy of intranasal alpha₂-interferon against rhinovirus infections in family setting. *N Engl J Med* 314:65-70, 1986.

Dulbecco R, Ginsberg HS: *Virology.* Hagerstown, MD, Harper & Row, 1980.

Durant RH, et al: Influence of inosiplex treatment on neurological disability of patients with subacute sclerosing panencephalitis. *J Pediatr* 101:288-293, 1982.

Dyken PR, et al: Long-term follow-up of subacute sclerosing panencephalitis patients treated with inosiplex. *Ann Neurol* 11:359-364, 1982.

Esmann V, et al: Therapy of acute herpes zoster with acyclovir in non-immunocompromised host. *Am J Med* 73(1A):320-325, 1982.

Farr BM, et al: Intranasal interferon-α2 for prevention of natural rhinovirus colds. *Antimicrob Agents Chemother* 26:31-34, 1984.

Felsenstein D, et al: Treatment of cytomegalovirus retinitis with 9-[2-hydroxy-1-(hydroxymethyl) ethoxymethyl] guanine. *Ann Intern Med* 103:377-380, 1985.

Fernandez H: Ribavirin: Summary of clinical trials—Herpes genitalis and measles, in Smith RA, Kirkpatrick W (eds): *Ribavirin: A Broad Spectrum Antiviral Agent.* New York, Academic Press, 1980, 215-230.

Field H, et al: Sensitivity of acyclovir-resistant mutants of herpes simplex virus to other antiviral drugs. *J Infect Dis* 143:281-285, 1981.

Frank KB, et al: Interaction of herpes simplex virus-induced DNA polymerase with 9- (1,3-dihydroxy-2-propoxymethyl) guanine triphosphate. *J Biol Chem* 259:1566-1569, 1984.

Greenberg SB, et al: Prophylactic effect of low doses of human leukocyte interferon against infection with rhinovirus. *J Infect Dis* 145:542-546, 1982.

Gutterman JU, et al: Pharmacokinetic study of partially pure γ-interferon in cancer patients. *Cancer Res* 44:4164-4170, 1984.

Haddah FS, Risk WS: Isoprinosine treatment in 18 patients with subacute sclerosing panencephalitis: Controlled study. *Ann Neurol* 7:185-188, 1980.

Hall CB, et al: Aerosolized ribavirin treatment of infants with respiratory syncytial viral infection: Randomized double-blind study. *N Engl J Med* 308:1443-1447, 1983 A.

Hall CB, et al: Ribavirin treatment of experimental respiratory syncytial viral infection: Controlled double-blind study in young adults. *JAMA* 249:2666-2670, 1983 B.

Hall CB, et al: Ribavirin treatment of respiratory syncytial virus infection in infants with underlying cardiopulmonary disease. *JAMA* 254:3047-3051, 1985.

Hamzawi M, et al: Amantadine-sensitivity of recombinant and parental influenza virus strains. *Med Microbiol Immunol* 169:259-268, 1981.

Hay AJ, et al: Matrix protein gene determines amantadine-sensitivity of influenza viruses. *J Gen Virol* 42:189-191, 1979.

Hayden FG, Gwaltney JM Jr: Prophylactic activity of intranasal enviroxime against experimentally induced rhinovirus type 39 infection. *Antimicrob Agents Chemother* 21:892-897, 1982.

Hayden FG, Gwaltney JM Jr: Intranasal interferon α2 for prevention of rhinovirus infection and illness. *J Infect Dis* 148:543-550, 1983.

Hayden FG, et al: Prevention of natural colds by contact prophylaxis with intranasal alpha₂-interferon. *N Engl J Med* 314:71-75, 1986.

Heider H, et al: Occurrence of amantadine- and rimantadine-resistant influenza A virus strains during 1980 epidemic. *Acta Virol* 25:395-400, 1981.

Herzog C, et al: Intranasal interferon for contact prophylaxis against common cold in families, (letter). *Lancet* 2:962, 1983.

Higgins PG, et al: Intranasal interferon as protection against experimental respiratory coronavirus infection in volunteers. *Antimicrob Agents Chemother* 24:713-715, 1983.

Hirsch MS, et al: Effects of interferon-alpha on cytomegalovirus reactivation syndromes in renal-transplant recipients. *N Engl J Med* 308:1489-1493, 1983.

Hoofnagle JH, et al: Randomized controlled trial of adenine arabinoside monophosphate for chronic type B hepatitis. *Gastroenterology* 86:150-157, 1984.

Klein G (ed): *Viral Oncology.* New York, Raven Press, 1980.

Knight V, et al: Ribavirin aerosol in influenza A infections, (abstract 876). *21st Interscience Conference on Antimicrobial Agents and Chemotherapy.* Chicago, Nov 4-6, 1981.

Kraemer KG, et al: Prophylactic adenine arabinoside following marrow transplantation. *Transplant Proc* 10:237-240, 1978.

Krenitsky TA, et al: 6-deoxyacyclovir: Xanthine oxidase-activated prodrug of acyclovir. *Proc Natl Acad Sci USA* 81:3209-3213, 1984.

Levandowski RA, et al: Topical enviroxime against rhinovirus infection. *Antimicrob Agents Chemother* 22:1004-1007, 1982.

Lubeck J, et al: Susceptibility of influenza A viruses to amantadine is influenced by gene coding for M protein. *J Virol* 28:710-716, 1978.

Luby JP, et al: Collaborative study of patient-initiated treatment of recurrent genital herpes with topical acyclovir or placebo. *J Infect Dis* 150:1-6, 1984.

Mar E-C, et al: Effect of 9-(1,3 dihydroxy-2-propoxymethyl) guanine on human cytomegalovirus replication in vitro. *Antimicrob Agents Chemother* 24:518-521, 1983.

Marker SC, et al: Trial of vidarabine for cytomegalovirus infection in renal transplant patients. *Arch Intern Med* 140:1441-1444, 1980.

Masur H, et al: Effect of 9-(1, 3-dihydroxy-2-propoxymethyl) guanine on serious cytomegalovirus disease in eight immunosuppressed homosexual men. *Ann Intern Med* 104:41-44, 1986.

Maudgal PC, et al: Efficacy of (E)-5-(2-bromovinyl)-2'-deoxyuridine in topical treatment of herpes simplex keratitis. *Albrecht Von Graefes Arch Klin Exp Ophthalmol* 216:261-268, 1981 A.

Maudgal PC, et al: Preliminary results of oral BVDU treatment of herpes zoster ophthalmicus. *Bull Soc Belg Ophthalmol* 193:49-56, 1981 B.

McClung HW, et al: Ribavirin aerosol treatment of influenza B virus infection. *JAMA* 249:2671-2674, 1983.

McCormick JB, et al: Lassa fever: Effective therapy with ribavirin. *N Engl J Med* 314:20-26, 1986.

McIntosh K, et al: Treatment of respiratory viral infection in immunodeficient infant with ribavirin aerosol. *Am J Dis Child* 138:305-308, 1984.

McKendrick MW, et al: Oral acyclovir in herpes zoster. *J Antimicrob Chemother* 14:661-665, 1984.

Melnick JL: Taxonomy of viruses, 1980. *Prog Med Virol* 26:214-232, 1980.

Mertz GJ, et al: Double-blind placebo-controlled trial of oral acyclovir in first-episode genital herpes simplex virus infection. *JAMA* 252:1147-1151, 1984.

Meyers JD, et al: Multicenter collaborative trial of intravenous acyclovir for treatment of mucocutaneous herpes simplex virus infection in immunocompromised host. *Am J Med* 73(1A):229-235, 1982.

Meyers JD, et al: Recombinant leukocyte A interferon for treatment of serious viral infections after marrow transplant: Phase I study. *J Infect Dis* 148:551-556, 1983.

Meyers JD, et al: Acyclovir treatment of varicella-zoster virus infection in compromised host. *Transplantation* 37:571-574, 1984.

Mindel A, et al: Intravenous acyclovir treatment for primary genital herpes. *Lancet* 1:697-700, 1982.

Mindel A, et al: Prophylactic oral acyclovir in recurrent genital herpes. *Lancet* 2:57-59, 1984.

Minkoff DI, et al: Clinical use of ribavirin and treatment of herpes zoster in otherwise normal adults, in Smith RA, Kirkpatrick W (eds): *Ribavirin: A Broad Spectrum Antiviral Agent.* New York, Academic Press, 1980, 185-199.

Mitchell CD, et al: Acyclovir therapy for mucocutaneous herpes simplex infections in immunocompromised patients. *Lancet* 1:1389- 1392, 1981.

National Institutes of Health Consensus Development Conference: Amantadine: Does it have role in prevention and treatment of influenza? *Ann Intern Med* 92:256-258, 1980.

Nilsen AE, et al: Efficacy of oral acyclovir in treatment of initial and recurrent genital herpes. *Lancet* 2:571-573, 1982.

Novelli VM, et al: Acyclovir administered perorally in immunocompromised children with varicella-zoster infections. *J Infect Dis* 149:478, 1984.

Ohnishi H, et al: Mechanism of host defense suppression induced by viral infection: Mode of action of inosiplex as antiviral agent. *Infect Immun* 38:243-250, 1982.

Oxford JS, et al: In vivo selection of influenza A2 strain resistant to amantadine. *Nature* 226:82-83, 1970.

Patriarca PA, et al: Safety of prolonged administration of rimantadine hydrochloride in prophylaxis of influenza A virus infections in nursing homes. *Antimicrob Agents Chemother* 26:101-103, 1984.

Peterslund NA, et al: Acyclovir in herpes zoster. *Lancet* 2:827-830, 1981.

Peterslund NA, et al: Oral and intravenous acyclovir are equally effective in herpes zoster. *J Antimicrob Chemother* 14:185-189, 1984.

Phillpotts RJ, et al: Activity of enviroxime against rhinovirus infection in man. *Lancet* 1:1342-1344, 1981.

Phillpotts RJ, et al: Therapeutic activity of enviroxime against rhinovirus infection in volunteers. *Antimicrob Agents Chemother* 23:671-675, 1983.

Pollard RB, et al: Effect of vidarabine on chronic hepatitis B virus infection. *JAMA* 239:1648-1650, 1978.

Pollard RB, et al: Cytomegalovirus retinitis in immunosuppressed hosts: I. Natural history and effects of treatment with adenine arabinoside. *Ann Intern Med* 93:655-664, 1980.

Preble OT, Friedman RM: Interferon-induced alterations in cells: Relevance to viral and nonviral diseases. *Laboratory Invest* 49:4-18, 1983.

Quarles JM, et al: Comparison of amantadine and rimantadine for prevention of type A (Russian) influenza. *Antiviral Res* 1:149-155, 1981.

Reichman RC, et al: Treatment of recurrent genital herpes simplex infections with oral acyclovir: Controlled trial. *JAMA* 251:2103-2107, 1984.

Ruhnek-Forsbeck M, et al: Treatment of recurrent genital herpes simplex infections with oral acyclovir. *J Antimicrob Chemother* 16:621-628, 1985.

Samo TC, et al: Efficacy and tolerance of intranasally applied recombinant leukocyte A interferon in normal volunteers. *J Infect Dis* 148:535-542, 1983.

Saral R, et al: Acyclovir prophylaxis of herpes simplex virus infections: Randomized, double-blind controlled trial in bone marrow transplant recipients. *N Engl J Med* 305:63-67, 1981.

Saral R, et al: Acyclovir prophylaxis against herpes simplex virus infection in patients with leukemia: Randomized, double-blind, placebo-controlled study. *Ann Intern Med* 99:773-776, 1983.

Scholtissek C, Faulkner GP: Amantadine-resistant and -sensitive influenza A strains and recombinants. *J Gen Virol* 44:807-815, 1979.

Scott GM, et al: Purified interferon as protection against rhinovirus infection. *Br Med J* 284:1822-1825, 1982.

Selby PJ, et al: Parenteral acyclovir therapy for herpesvirus infections in man. *Lancet* 2:1267-1270, 1979.

Selby P, et al: Amino (hydroxyethoxymethyl) purine: New well-absorbed prodrug of acyclovir. *Lancet* 2:1428-1430, 1984.

Serota FT, et al: Acyclovir treatment of herpes zoster infections: Use in children undergoing bone marrow transplantation. *JAMA* 247:2132-2135, 1982.

Shalev Y, et al: Progressive cutaneous herpes simplex infection in acute myeloblastic leukemia: Successful treatment with interferon and cytarabine. *Arch Dermatol* 120:922-926, 1984.

Shepp DH, et al: Activity of 9-[2-hydroxy-1-(hydroxymethyl) ethoxymethyl] guanine in treatment of cytomegalovirus pneumonia. *Ann Intern Med* 103:368-373, 1985.

Shepp DH, et al: Treatment of varicella-zoster virus infection in severely immunocompromised patients: Randomized comparison of acyclovir and vidarabine. *N Engl J Med* 314:208-212, 1986.

Silvestri DL, et al: Ineffectiveness of topical idoxuridine in dimethyl sulfoxide for therapy for genital herpes. *JAMA* 248:953-959, 1982.

Smee DF, et al: Anti-herpesvirus activity of acyclic nucleoside 9-(1,3-dihydroxy-2-propoxymethyl) guanine. *Antimicrob Agents Chemother* 23:676-682, 1983.

Smith CI, et al: Vidarabine monophosphate and human leukocyte interferon in chronic hepatitis B infection. *JAMA* 247:2261-2265, 1982.

Smith CI, et al: Acute Dane particle suppression with recombinant leukocyte A interferon in chronic hepatitis B virus infection. *J Infect Dis* 148:907-913, 1983.

Spector SA, et al: Treatment of herpes virus infections in immunocompromised patients with acyclovir by continuous intravenous infusion. *Am J Med* 73(1A):229-235, 1982.

Spruance SL, et al: Treatment of herpes simplex labialis with topical acyclovir in polyethylene glycol. *J Infect Dis* 146:85-90, 1982.

Spruance SL, et al: Early, patient-initiated treatment of herpes labialis with topical 10% acyclovir. *Antimicrob Agents Chemother* 25:553-555, 1984.

Straus SE, et al: Acyclovir for chronic mucocutaneous herpes simplex virus infection in immunosuppressed patients. *Ann Intern Med* 96:270-277, 1982.

Straus SE, et al: Oral acyclovir to suppress recurring herpes simplex virus infections in immunodeficient patients. *Ann Intern Med* 100:522-524, 1984 A.

Straus SE, et al: Suppression of frequently recurring genital herpes: Placebo-controlled double-blind trial of oral acyclovir. *N Engl J Med* 310:1545-1550, 1984 B.

Thin RN, et al: Recurrent genital herpes suppressed by oral acyclovir: Multicentre double blind trial. *J Antimicrob Chemother* 16:219-226, 1985.

Uylangco CV, et al: Double-blind placebo-controlled evaluation of ribavirin in treatment of acute measles. *Clin Therapeut* 3:389-396, 1981.

Van Voris LP, et al: Successful treatment of naturally occurring influenza A/USSR/77 147NI. *JAMA* 245:1128-1131, 1981.

Vince R, Daluge S: Carbocyclic arabinosyladenine: Adenosine deaminase resistant antiviral agent. *J Med Chem* 20:612-613, 1977.

Vince R, et al: Carbocyclic arabinofuranosyladenine (Cyclaradine): Efficacy against genital herpes in guinea pigs. *Science* 221:1405-1406, 1983.

Wade JC, et al: Intravenous acyclovir to treat mucocutaneous herpes simplex virus infection after marrow transplantation: Double-blind trial. *Ann Intern Med* 96:265-269, 1982 A.

Wade JC, et al: Treatment of cytomegalovirus pneumonia with high-dose acyclovir. *Am J Med* 73(1A):249-256, 1982 B.

Wade JC, et al: Oral acyclovir for prevention of herpes simplex virus reactivation after marrow transplantation. *Ann Intern Med* 100:823-828, 1984.

Wallin J, et al: Treatment of recurrent herpes labialis with trisodium phosphonoformate, in Nelson JD, Grassi C (eds): *Current Chemotherapy and Infectious Disease*. Washington, DC, American Society for Microbiology, 1980, 1361-1362.

Whiteman PD, et al: Tolerance and pharmacokinetics of A515U, acyclovir analogue, in health volunteers. *Proc BPS* 149P-150P, (Sept 11-14) 1984.

Whitley RJ, et al: Adenine arabinoside therapy of herpes zoster in immunosuppressed: NIAID Collaborative Antiviral Study. *N Engl J Med* 294:1193-1199, 1976.

Whitley RJ, et al: Adenine arabinoside therapy of biopsy-proved herpes simplex encephalitis: NIAID Collaborative Antiviral Study. *N Engl J Med* 297:289-294, 1977.

Whitley RJ, et al: Vidarabine therapy of neonatal herpes simplex infection. *Pediatrics* 66:495-501, 1980.

Whitley RJ, et al: Herpes simplex encephalitis: Vidarabine therapy and diagnostic problems. *N Engl J Med* 304:313-318, 1981.

Whitley R, et al: Vidarabine therapy of varicella in immunosuppressed patients. *J Pediatr* 101:125-131, 1982 A.

Whitley RJ, et al: Mucocutaneous herpes simplex virus infections in immunocompromised patients: Model for evaluation of topical antiviral agents. *Am J Med* 73(1A):236-240, 1982 B.

Whitley RJ, et al: Herpes simplex encephalitis: Clinical assessment. *JAMA* 247:317-320, 1982 C.

Whitley RJ, et al: Early vidarabine therapy to control complications of herpes zoster in immunosuppressed patients. *N Engl J Med* 307:971-975, 1982 D.

Whitley RJ, et al: Vidarabine therapy for mucocutaneous herpes simplex virus infections in immunocompromised host. *J Infect Dis* 149:1-8, 1984.

Whitley RJ, et al: Vidarabine versus acyclovir therapy in herpes simplex encephalitis. *N Engl J Med* 314:144-149, 1986.

Wildiers J, de Clercq E: Oral (E)-5-(2-bromovinyl)-2'-deoxyuridine treatment of severe herpes zoster in cancer patients. *Eur J Cancer Clin Oncol* 20:471-476, 1984.

Wills RJ, et al: Interferon kinetics and adverse reactions after intravenous, intramuscular, and subcutaneous injection. *Clin Pharmacol Ther* 35:722-727, 1984.

Wilson SZ, et al: Treatment of influenza A(H1N1) virus infection with ribavirin aerosol. *Antimicrob Agents Chemother* 26:200-203, 1984.

Young CW, et al: Phase I evaluation of 2'-fluoro-5-iodo-1-β-D-arabinofuranosylcytosine in immunosuppressed patients with herpesvirus infection. *Cancer Res* 43:5006-5009, 1983.

Other Selected References

Belshe RB (ed): *Textbook of Human Virology*. Littleton, MA, PSG Publishing Company, 1984.

Stuart-Harris CH, Oxford J (eds): *Problems of Antiviral Therapy*. New York, Academic Press, 1983.

Drugs Used in the Treatment of Poisoning

80

Principles of Therapy

There are four basic elements in the treatment of poisoning, and their sequence of initiation depends upon the circumstances.

Individual Assessment: An immediate evaluation of the putative intoxication must be made to determine if it is (1) life-threatening and already compromises vital functions, (2) poses a potential hazard, or (3) is harmless or essentially so. A poison control center, particularly a regional center, can provide information and advice on management. This is useful because early identification of the ingredients and their potential toxicity can save time and lessen the chance of complications. It is important to remember that hazard is associated not only with the potency of a poison, but also with the quantity ingested, the extent of exposure, and the presence of other ingredients, including solvents. See the references for information on the general management of poisoning.

Estimates of the dose, the time elapsed since exposure, and the physical status of the patient determine whether induced vomiting, gastric lavage, supportive care (particularly hydration), or specific therapy is required and the sequence of use. Care must be exercised when assessing the hazard, since the experience of poison control centers and emergency rooms has shown that approximately 50% of all histories taken in this situation are incorrect as to substance, quantity, and even actual exposure. Factors that may affect the patient's re-sponse to the poison (ie, age, presence of hereditary and other diseases, current drug therapy, allergy to drugs) also should be considered.

Blood and urine samples to determine a baseline for monitoring elimination of the toxin, glucose, electrolytes, and acid-base disturbances may aid in assessing therapy. Identification of the suspected toxin in the blood or urine is necessary occasionally to verify exposure. Quantitative determinations are needed for relatively few substances, eg, acetaminophen, salicylate, iron, lead, methyl alcohol, theophylline, lithium, digitalis glycosides; for some of these, two plasma samples obtained one or more hours apart, depending on half-life, may be required to determine if the concentration of the toxic substance is rising or falling before deciding whether specific therapy is needed or can be discontinued.

Supportive Care: Hypoventilation can be avoided by ensuring an adequate airway with suction, humidified oxygen, insertion of an airway, and mechanical ventilation as required. Anticonvulsants may be necessary if seizures interfere with ventilation. A reliable venous access with a venous catheter should be established in comatose patients. Volume depletion secondary to vomiting, diarrhea, and sweating must be corrected promptly with normal saline or Ringer's solution, particularly in young children. Hypotension severe enough to require correction, whether due to volume depletion or peripheral pooling, frequently necessitates monitoring of central venous or pulmonary wedge pressure to determine fluid needs.

1633

Any adult in coma of unknown etiology should receive at least 50 ml (25 g) of dextrose 50% intravenously immediately without waiting for the blood glucose determination to prevent brain damage from hypoglycemia. Thiamine 100 mg may be injected simultaneously if alcoholism is suspected. Many comatose adults may be given naloxone empirically (2.4 to 4 mg at five-minute intervals) when opioids are suspected of causing the coma. For children in coma of unknown etiology, dextrose 20% to 25% (0.5 g/kg) is administered over a five- to ten-minute period. This is particularly important in known or suspected intoxication from ethyl alcohol, a salicylate, or an oral hypoglycemic drug.

Termination of Exposure: Eliminating the poison from the gut, skin, or eyes before extensive absorption or damage can occur usually avoids the necessity for further therapeutic intervention. The elimination of some drugs may be increased by altering the pH of the urine (ion trapping). The excretion of basic drugs (eg, amphetamine, phencyclidine) is promoted by acidifying the urine and that of acidic drugs (eg, aspirin, phenobarbital) by making the urine more alkaline. Diuretics or cathartics generally do not increase clearance significantly.

Dialysis and hemoperfusion through charcoal may be useful for drugs that are not significantly protein bound (less of an obstacle in hemoperfusion than in hemodialysis) and have a low apparent volume of distribution (eg, alcohol, ethylene glycol). Otherwise, these procedures usually are reserved for patients whose renal function has been affected by the intoxication.

Specific Drug Therapy: It is estimated that specific drug therapy is required in no more than 2% of poisonings.

Agents and Procedures Used to Terminate Exposure to Poisons

TOPICAL EXPOSURE. Initially, contaminated clothing should be removed and all routes of exposure should be determined. When the eyes are involved, the lids should be retracted and the eyes flushed immediately with tap water poured from a container to avoid mechanical injury from a high-force stream. When giving instructions by telephone, adequate compliance may be achieved by specifying that flushing of the eyes be maintained for at least 15 minutes "by the clock." When the skin is affected, water and, if the poison and/or solvent is lipid soluble, tincture of green soap may aid in removing the poison. The hair should be shampooed if contaminated (eg, pesticide spray).

INGESTION. The stomach should be emptied after ingestion of most poisons (for exceptions, see Contraindications). An emetic should be administered or lavage performed unless the patient has experienced *significant* return of ingested material by spontaneous emesis (Goldfrank et al, 1986). Induced emesis is preferred to lavage in alert patients with an active gag reflex. Lavage is usually less efficient than induced vomiting, especially when plant material or large tablets or capsules have been swallowed. Induced emesis also may partially empty the upper small intestine.

Mechanically induced gagging is ineffective and hazardous. Hypertonic sodium chloride should not be used because toxic

amounts may be absorbed. Deaths from hypernatremia have occurred following its use as an emetic or irrigant for gastric lavage.

Emetics: Ipecac syrup is the emetic of first choice (Easom and Lovejoy, 1979). The amount of stomach contents removed by emesis varies widely, and activated charcoal may be indicated after vomiting has ceased. Effectiveness is increased by concomitant ingestion of water, but the amount should be limited to 300 ml in adults and 10 ml/kg in children to reduce pyloric emptying. Apomorphine is not recommended. It offers no advantage over syrup of ipecac, is less convenient to prepare for use, and may depress the central nervous system.

Lavage: If vomiting cannot be induced by emetics, gastric lavage with a large bore orogastric tube (adults, 36 to 42 French; children, 26 to 28 French) should be started, preferably within three hours after ingestion (see Contraindications). Lavage may be effective even six or more hours after ingestion, depending upon the rate of disintegration and dissolution of the formulation ingested, the formation of concretions or bezoars, and whether gastrointestinal transit time is prolonged by the poison.

To minimize the chances of aspiration, the patient should be placed on his left side with the face near the edge of the table and the legs elevated. In comatose patients, a cuffed endotracheal tube should be used. Stomach contents should be aspirated by suction before instilling the lavage solution. Tap water may be used as the lavage irrigant but 0.9% or 0.45% sodium chloride solution is preferred in young children, because even a 5% increase in body fluid volume of electrolyte-free water may cause dilutional hyponatremia. Lavage fluid should be at room temperature; cooled fluid may produce hypothermia. Lavage using small amounts of fluid (about 300 ml in adults and 10 ml/kg in small children) should be repeated until returns are clear and at least 2 liters of fluid in children and 5 liters in adults have been employed. Thereafter, activated charcoal should be instilled through the lavage tube and allowed to remain in the stomach.

Contraindications: Emetics are contraindicated in the presence of convulsions, shock, coma or imminent coma, altered sensorium, or inadequate gag reflex. They should not be used after ingestion of strongly caustic substances, such as strong alkalis (lye) or acids, since additional injury (eg, perforated esophagus with mediastinitis) may occur. Alkali ingestions should be diluted with water or milk and the patient should be examined for esophageal ulceration.

Emetics and lavage may be contraindicated after ingestion of the following high-viscosity aliphatic petroleum distillates: (1) mineral seal or signal oils present in furniture and oil-containing polishes, because they are most likely to cause severe aspiration pneumonitis; and (2) fuel, motor, cutting, mineral, suntan, and baby oils, which are nontoxic but may cause lipid pneumonia if aspirated.

Emesis is indicated on ingestion of 10 ml/kg or more of naphthas, gasoline, or kerosene; any quantity of turpentine or diesel oil; or a significant amount of a hydrocarbon containing benzene, a halogenated hydrocarbon, a pesticide, camphor, metals, pine wood distillate, or other particularly toxic ingredient.

Lavage with boluses of 300 to 500 ml of fluid initially,

especially on a full stomach, may force material through the pylorus where it cannot be recovered. Aspiration of vomitus into the bronchial tree is a potential hazard of both gastric lavage and drug-induced vomiting; however, in conscious patients, the hazard is less with use of emetics.

Drug Evaluations

AGENTS FOR GENERAL MANAGEMENT

Emetic

SYRUP OF IPECAC

ACTIONS AND USES. Ipecac alkaloids act locally on the gastric mucosa and centrally on the chemoreceptor trigger zone to induce vomiting. Vomiting occurs within 30 minutes in about 90% of patients (average time, less than 20 minutes). Emesis may be more effective if water is taken immediately after administration of the syrup. Although less desirable, clear carbonated beverages may be used. Milk should not be employed because it delays the onset of emesis. About 10% of patients will vomit again if fluids are ingested within two hours after the initial induction of emesis. Vomiting after this interval may be ascribed to the intoxicant rather than to ipecac.

Ipecac syrup is available without prescription in a maximum amount of 30 ml. Physicians often recommend that an ounce of the syrup be stored in the home when children become 1 year old so that it is readily available for immediate administration when a physician recommends its use by telephone.

ADVERSE REACTIONS AND PRECAUTIONS. Adverse effects caused by syrup of ipecac are not significant if the recommended dose is not exceeded. In children under 3 years, drowsiness may be anticipated in about 20% and diarrhea in about 25%. Less than 4% experience coughing or choking in association with emesis.

Activated charcoal should not be given concomitantly, because it adsorbs ipecac and may reduce the emetic effect; it should, however, be given after vomiting has subsided to reduce absorption of any poison remaining in the stomach and small bowel.

For contraindications, see the introduction.

DOSAGE AND PREPARATIONS.
Oral: Children over 1 year and adults, 15 or 30 ml (the lower dose usually is adequate), followed by one to two glasses of water depending on age; *infants 9 to 11 months,* 10 ml (two teaspoonsful), preceded or followed by 120 to 240 ml (one-half to one full glass) of water; *infants 6 to 8 months,* 5 ml (one teaspoonful). Accumulating evidence shows that a dose of 15 ml probably is both safe and effective in infants 8 to 12 months. In patients older than 1 year, doses may be repeated once after 30 minutes if vomiting has not occurred. If vomiting does not occur within 45 minutes after the first dose, gastric lavage may be indicated to remove the toxin.

The administration of syrup of ipecac to infants 6 to 8

months old should be conducted under medical supervision and not in the home.

Generic. Syrup in 15 and 30 ml containers (alcohol 1.5%) (nonprescription).

Adsorbent

ACTIVATED CHARCOAL

This adsorbent is a useful adjunct in the treatment of acute poisoning. It should be given as soon after ingestion of the poisonous substance as possible or after emesis has ceased if syrup of ipecac has been given, although effectiveness has been demonstrated even after several hours, particularly if bowel sounds are absent. If activated charcoal is being given repetitively, it may be started at any time and continued for days.

Although the efficacy of charcoal has not been determined for many drugs in vivo, it is known to reduce the gastrointestinal absorption of drugs that commonly cause poisoning, such as analgesics (salicylates, acetaminophen, propoxyphene), antianxiety agents, hypnotics, and tricyclic antidepressants. This agent does not affect the absorption of mineral acids, alkalis, and drugs that are insoluble in aqueous acidic solution; adsorption of ferrous sulfate is low. Cyanide is partially adsorbed but then released slowly in the intestine; however, the addition of activated charcoal to lavage fluid may be useful. Activated charcoal is less effective in poisoning caused by rapidly absorbed agents. Repeated doses may be effective for drugs that are absorbed slowly or recycled through the enterohepatic system or by gastric secretion. Since charcoal is mildly constipating, it should be combined with a cathartic (eg, magnesium citrate, sorbitol) when multiple doses are given; this does not affect its binding capacity. This also will speed elimination of the charcoal-toxin complex. Usually there appears to be little desorption of poison from charcoal during its passage through the gastrointestinal tract provided that the quantity of activated charcoal is large compared to the toxin (Neuvonen, 1982).

Activated charcoal in water is usually acceptable to children but its appearance may be unappetizing. If charcoal with water is refused, commercial preparations containing activated charcoal in 70% sorbitol can be used. This suspension has no gritty oral residue and its sweetness is attractive to children. This combination also has the advantage of inducing an exceptionally rapid intestinal transit time: In fasted subjects, the mean transit time of activated charcoal is about 25 hours; this is reduced to 1.1 hours with activated charcoal in sorbitol (Krenzelok, 1984). However, sorbitol limits the quantity of charcoal that can be administered, causes liquid stools (Mayersohn et al, 1977), and may evoke spontaneous emesis. Care should be exercised not to induce volume depletion in young children.

Charcoal adsorbs ipecac; thus, syrup of ipecac should be given before activated charcoal is used. Activated charcoal is then given after vomiting has subsided.

Charcoals from different sources vary in adsorption capacity. The most effective are those of small particle size (large total surface area) and low mineral content. Petroleum-based charcoals with a greater surface area than those now employed as gastric adsorbents are being investigated. The advantage of such a charcoal is that a smaller quantity is required. Charcoal PX-21 [SuperChar] was found to have about three times the adsorptive capacity of Norit A while retaining a similar adsorption rate (Cooney and Kane, 1980; Cooney, 1980).

DOSAGE AND PREPARATIONS.

Oral: Adults, 50 to 100 g, *children*, 25 to 50 g or 1 g/kg, administered with water orally or through the lavage tube after gastric lavage. Charcoal is not toxic and, therefore, there is no maximum dose limit. Doses can be repeated at two-hour intervals for poisons that undergo enterohepatic circulation (eg, glutethimide, digitoxin, theophylline, *Amanita phalloides* toxin) or are resecreted into the stomach (eg, phencyclidine, phenobarbital, tricyclic antidepressants).

Generic. Liquid; powder (nonprescription).

Available Trademarks.
Powder: *Acta-Char* (Gulf Bio-Systems), *CharcoalantiDote* (U.S. Products).
Powder in water: *Actidose-Aqua* (Paddock), *Liqui-Char* (Bowman), *Liquid-Antidose* (U.S. Products).
Powder in sorbitol: *Acta-Char Liquid* (Gulf Bio-Systems), *Actidose* (Paddock).
Powder (PX-21): *SuperChar* (Gulf Bio-Systems).
Liquid (PX-21) in sorbitol: *SuperChar Liquid* (Gulf Bio-Systems). (All forms nonprescription)

Agents Affecting Urinary Excretion

AMMONIUM CHLORIDE

This acidifying salt temporarily reduces urinary pH and can be given to impede the renal tubular reabsorption of organic bases and thus enhance their urinary excretion. However, significant enhancement of urinary excretion requires that the base have a pKa close to neutral, a small volume of distribution, and be appreciably eliminated via the kidney. Only a few organic bases (eg, amphetamines) have these properties. Routine acidification of the urine to treat overdose of an organic base is neither safe nor advisable. Ammonium chloride should not be used for forced diuresis to hasten excretion of poisons. Tolerance develops within two to three days.

ADVERSE REACTIONS AND PRECAUTIONS. Adequate doses frequently cause gastric irritation, nausea, and vomiting. Absorption also may be erratic, depending upon the toxic substance ingested. Ammonium chloride is relatively contraindicated in patients with impaired hepatic or renal function, because of the risk of ammonium toxicity, and in patients with convulsions or in prolonged coma (Penn et al, 1971) to avoid complications of an acid urine in myoglobinuria.

DOSAGE AND PREPARATIONS.

Oral: Adults, 1 to 2 g four or six times daily. *Children,* 75 mg/kg/day. Urinary pH should be monitored and the dosage adjusted accordingly. The development of tolerance to ammo-

nium chloride following three consecutive days of therapy will usually necessitate interruption of administration for three to four days.

Generic. Tablets (plain) 500 mg; tablets (enteric-coated) 500 mg and 1 g (nonprescription).

Intravenous Infusion: This route is required only rarely in the management of intoxications. The rate of infusion in adults usually should not exceed 0.4 mEq/min. Repeated determinations of serum bicarbonate are required.

Generic. Solution 2.14% (0.4 mEq/ml) in 500 ml containers and 26.75% (5 mEq/ml) in 20 ml containers for dilution in 0.9% sodium chloride injection.

SODIUM BICARBONATE

ACTIONS AND USES. Sodium bicarbonate is used to treat metabolic acidosis (see Chapter 46, Replenishers and Regulators of Water and Electrolytes). It alkalizes urine, which interferes with the renal tubular reabsorption of organic acids (eg, aspirin, phenobarbital) and enhances their excretion.

PRECAUTIONS. Excessive bicarbonate may alkalize the plasma and interfere with the passage of organic acids out of the brain, which prolongs central nervous system toxicity. Potassium depletion caused by aspirin poisoning also may be aggravated.

The maximum sodium tolerance is 250 mEq/M²/24 hours in healthy persons (1 g of sodium bicarbonate contains 11.9 mEq of sodium). Sodium bicarbonate must be used with caution in patients with congestive heart failure or liver disease. Patients with renal insufficiency given usual doses or those with normal renal function receiving prolonged therapy may experience systemic alkalosis manifested by irritability, neuromuscular excitability, and tetany.

DOSAGE AND PREPARATIONS.

Oral: Adults, 300 mg to 1.8 g one to four times daily, usually before meals and at bedtime. The urinary pH of each patient should be monitored and the dosage adjusted accordingly. The dosage should be based on the degree of metabolic acidosis, sodium overload, and potassium depletion. A persistent aciduria despite theoretically adequate doses of sodium bicarbonate suggests a need for the concurrent use of potassium chloride.

Generic. Powder; tablets 325 and 650 mg (nonprescription).

Intravenous: *Adults,* 2 to 5 mEq/kg, and *children,* 1 to 2 mEq/kg administered over a four- to eight-hour period; the specific amount depends upon the degree of metabolic acidosis.

Generic. Solution 4.2% (0.5 mEq/ml) in 10 ml containers, 5% (0.595 mEq/ml) in 500 ml containers, 7.5% (0.892 mEq/ml) and 8.4% (1 mEq/ml) in 10 and 50 ml containers.

AGENTS FOR SPECIFIC THERAPY

Metal Antagonists

Heavy metal poisoning continues to be a serious toxicologic problem. Metal ions enter the body following parenteral administration for medical use, through ingestion or inhalation, and, occasionally, through abraded or intact skin. The absorption and distribution of organic and inorganic metallic compounds usually are quite different.

Heavy metal ions react with two or more ligands of an organic compound through at least one coordinate covalent bond. The resulting product is either a stable heterocyclic compound, termed a chelate (claw), or a less stable, nonheterocyclic compound, referred to as a complex. Medically useful heavy metal antagonists are nonionic, water soluble, and chemically stable and they are eliminated in the urine and/or feces via bile. The electrophilic ligands of metal antagonists compete with electrophilic physiologic ligands for the free metal ion in vivo. The stability constant of a metal antagonist is an overall representation of affinity and dissociation. If the metal antagonist has a higher stability constant than the existing physiologic complex or chelate in vivo, the metal antagonist will gradually displace the bound metal. Because none of the metal antagonists are specific for only one metal cation, long-term use may cause trace element deficiencies. The intensity and type of deficiency depend upon the nature of the metal antagonist.

Heavy Metal Poisoning: Other than terminating exposure, the only successful approach to the treatment of acute heavy metal poisoning is inactivation of the metal ion by metal antagonists. The agents administered primarily for this purpose are edetate calcium disodium [Calcium Disodium Versenate] for lead; deferoxamine [Desferal] for iron; dimercaprol [BAL in Oil] for arsenic, inorganic mercury salts, or gold and, in conjunction with EDTA, for the initial management of lead encephalopathy (not for iron); and penicillamine [Cuprimine, Depen] for arsenic, copper, lead, gold, and mercury. Edetate disodium [Endrate, Sodium Versenate] has high affinity for calcium and is used in severe hypercalcemia. It should *not* be used to treat heavy metal poisoning. No specific therapy can be recommended for poisoning by cadmium or thallium.

Therapy is most effective when it is begun immediately after exposure to the heavy metal. If the time elapsed between ingestion of the toxic material and initiation of therapy is sufficient to allow incorporation of the metal into certain metal-avid binding sites in tissue and bone, prolonged therapy will be needed.

The severe adverse reactions produced by penicillamine and dimercaprol and the pain associated with the intramuscular administration of edetate calcium disodium and dimercaprol have stimulated searches for less toxic, orally effective agents to treat lead poisoning. An investigational drug, 2,3-dimercaptosuccinic acid, which is similar to dimercaprol chemically but is water soluble, may represent such an agent (Graziano et al, 1985). Clinically, it mobilizes and enhances the excretion of lead; experimentally, it is active against mercury and arsenic as well. The currently suggested dose of this drug for lead poisoning is 3 to 5 mg/kg orally at six-hour intervals.

Similarly, alternatives to penicillamine have been sought for removal of copper in Wilson's disease. Zinc sulfate, which increases the fecal elimination of copper, has been tried, but too little experience has accumulated to define its role in Wilson's disease (Hoogenraad et al, 1984; Caillie-Bertrand et

al, 1985). The chelating agent, triethylenetetramine (trien), was introduced for use in patients unable to tolerate penicillamine (Walshe, 1982) and was approved in late 1985 for this indication under Orphan Drug status as trientine hydrochloride [Cuprid].

Radioactive Isotope Poisoning: Because of the increasing use of radioactive isotopes in biomedical and industrial research, the possibility of accidental ingestion of a radioactive heavy metal is increasing. Poisoning with a conventional radioactive isotope, such as iron, can be treated with deferoxamine to hasten excretion. However, treatment is more difficult if a more exotic metal, such as uranium, radium, strontium, plutonium, or yttrium, is involved. Neither radium nor strontium can be removed from the body because their stability constants with various metal antagonists are about the same as those of calcium. However, their rate of excretion can be increased by infusion of calcium salts in conjunction with oral administration of ammonium chloride. The excretion of plutonium, thorium, uranium, yttrium, and some other radioactive isotopes can be increased considerably by chelation with edetate calcium disodium. Pentetic acid (trisodium zinc diethylenetriaminepentaacetate, DTPA), currently available only as an investigational drug in this country, hastens the excretion of lanthanum, yttrium, americium, scandium, and plutonium but not strontium, polonium, or uranium. The daily dose is 1 g (30 micromole/kg) administered intravenously over one hour.

Miscellaneous Indications: Some metal antagonists have been tried in conditions other than heavy metal poisoning or in diseases associated with heavy metal retention (eg, penicillamine in Wilson's disease, primary biliary cirrhosis, cystinuria, rheumatoid arthritis, chronic active hepatitis; deferoxamine in hemochromatosis). Metal antagonists are ineffective in porphyria, scleroderma, angina pectoris, nephrocalcinosis, calcified mitral stenosis, otosclerosis, atherosclerosis, and sarcoidosis.

Adverse Reactions and Precautions: Because of the wide variation in toxic manifestations, it is impossible to generalize about the adverse reactions and precautions of metal antagonists. Although serious toxic effects can occur, adverse reactions are rarely life-threatening, usually reversible, and generally less severe than the effects of heavy metal poisoning.

EDETATE CALCIUM DISODIUM
[Calcium Disodium Versenate]

ACTIONS AND USES. This drug is used primarily to treat lead poisoning (plumbism). The chelates formed are water soluble, not easily dissociated, and readily excreted by the kidneys. Edetate calcium disodium does not produce negative calcium balance. It is capable of binding and increasing the excretion of zinc, but these actions are thought to be clinically insignificant if therapy is limited to five days, followed by a two- to five-day drug-free interval to permit recovery from the zinc depletion.

Edetate calcium disodium is of questionable or unproved value in poisoning caused by cadmium, chromium, manganese, nickel, vanadium, and zinc. It is ineffective in poisoning caused by mercury, gold, or arsenic.

The optimal pH range for the combination of edetate calcium disodium with lead includes all physiologic values. When treating lead poisoning in *adults,* the drug is given intravenously for three to five days to allow continued chelation and excretion of the heavy metal as it is released from tissues into extracellular fluid. Peak excretion of chelated lead occurs within 24 to 48 hours.

Too rapid mobilization of lead results in deposition in lead-avid soft tissues at a rate faster than its urinary clearance, which may exacerbate toxicity. Thus, the preferred treatment for severe lead poisoning (blood lead concentration greater than 70 mcg/dl), especially lead encephalopathy in children, is combined therapy with edetate calcium disodium and dimercaprol. This combination increases the excretion of lead and is less toxic than either agent alone. The first dose of dimercaprol should *always* precede the first dose of edetate calcium disodium by at least four hours.

Penicillamine may be administered orally for follow-up therapy when necessary (see the evaluation). The concentration of lead in the blood should be kept below 25 mcg/dl and the erythrocyte protoporphyrin below 35 mcg/dl. Children who have received chelation therapy should have lead and protoporphyrin evaluations five to seven days after therapy and after one to four weeks. If the reduction is maintained, laboratory determinations may be scheduled at two- to four-week intervals for six months, then at three-month intervals until the child is 6 years old (Piomelli et al, 1984).

DIAGNOSIS OF POISONING. Guidelines established by the Centers for Disease Control for the diagnosis and treatment of lead poisoning have been reviewed (Centers for Disease Control, 1985; Piomelli et al, 1984). Toxicity is defined as a lead concentration exceeding 25 mcg/dl of whole blood with a blood erythrocyte protoporphyrin concentration greater than 35 mcg/dl.

When the concentration of lead is between 25 and 55 mcg/dl and derangement of heme synthesis is suspected (erythrocyte protoporphyrin whole blood concentration is greater than 35 mcg/dl in children), a mobilization test often is performed to determine the need for chelation therapy. Initially, edetate calcium disodium 500 mg/M^2 (to a maximum of 1 g) diluted in 250 ml/M^2 of dextrose 5% is infused intravenously over at least one hour. An eight-hour urine sample is collected. The concentration of lead in the urine (mcg/ml) is multiplied by the urine volume (ml) to obtain the total excretion of lead (mcg). This figure is divided by the quantity of edetate calcium disodium (mg) to obtain the "lead excretion ratio." Chelation therapy is recommended if the ratio is greater than 0.60 (see Table 1). The result of this test is valid only when renal function is normal

and lead-free glass or plastic ware is used during urine collection and analysis.

The mobilization test is omitted and appropriate chelation therapy given immediately to symptomatic patients or to those with lead concentrations greater than 55 mcg/dl of whole blood.

ADVERSE REACTIONS AND PRECAUTIONS. Pain at the site of intramuscular injection, transient bone marrow depression, hypotension, cheilosis, chills, fever, and histamine-like reactions (sneezing, nasal congestion, and lacrimation) occur. Occasionally, proteinuria, microscopic hematuria, and large epithelial cells in the urinary sediment are observed. The most serious reaction is acute necrosis of the proximal renal tubules.

Patients who are dehydrated from repeated vomiting should receive intravenous fluids before chelation to ensure an adequate urine flow; however, excessive fluid must be avoided in patients with encephalopathy.

Edetate calcium disodium should be used cautiously in reduced doses in patients with pre-existing mild renal disease, and it is contraindicated in patients who are or who become anuric or severely oliguric. If anuria develops during therapy, edetate calcium disodium should be discontinued immediately. Urinalysis and blood urea nitrogen, serum creatinine, calcium, and phosphorus levels should be measured before treatment is begun and on the third and fifth days of therapy.

Since steroids enhance the renal toxicity of edetate calcium disodium in animals, they should not be used to prevent or relieve the cerebral edema that may accompany lead encephalopathy. Repeated doses of mannitol are recommended for this purpose.

Some patients may develop hypercalcemia, since lead displaces calcium from the chelate. Edetate calcium disodium interferes with the duration of action of zinc insulin preparations by forming a chelate with zinc.

PHARMACOKINETICS. Edetate calcium disodium is not metabolized and is excreted within 24 hours exclusively by glomerular filtration. Therefore, adequate urine flow should be established before initiating therapy. This agent is eliminated from the plasma by first-order kinetics (half-life, 20 to 60 minutes). Excretion is unaffected by urinary pH.

Edetate calcium disodium is poorly absorbed from the gastrointestinal tract. Furthermore, the absorption of any lead present in the intestine may be increased, because the lead chelate formed is more soluble than the lead itself. After absorption, the chelate dissociates and releases free lead ions, which can produce toxic reactions. Thus, oral administration for prophylaxis may enhance lead absorption in workers exposed to this metal (an oral preparation is no longer marketed). The most effective way to prevent chronic exposure is to maintain proper industrial hygiene.

DOSAGE AND PREPARATIONS.
Intravenous Infusion: This is the preferred route of administration in adults. Since edetate calcium disodium is eliminated by the kidneys and renal function is related to body surface area, the dosage is calculated on this basis.

Adults, 1.5 g/M^2/day in two divided doses for three to five days. For mildly symptomatic adults or adults with whole blood

TABLE 1.
CHELATION THERAPY IN CHILDREN WITH LEAD TOXICITY

Condition	Management
Acute encephalopathy Blood lead concentration usually >100 mcg/dl	Dimercaprol 75 mg/M^2 is given by deep intramuscular injection every four hours. Four hours after the initial dose of dimercaprol, continuous intravenous infusion of edetate calcium disodium 1.5 g/M^2/24 hours is begun. The first course of combined therapy is of five days' duration. Therapy is discontinued for two days, then resumed for an additional five days if the blood lead concentration remains elevated. One or more additional courses are indicated, with five- to seven-day drug-free periods between, if the blood lead concentration is ≥50 mcg/dl within 48 hours after treatment has been stopped. The use of oral penicillamine follow-up treatment should be considered (see text).
Symptomatic intoxication without encephalopathy or **Asymptomatic with blood lead concentration >70 mcg/dl**	Dimercaprol 50 mg/M^2 is given by deep intramuscular injection every four hours. Four hours after the initial dose of dimercaprol, continuous intravenous infusion* of edetate calcium disodium 1 g/M^2/24 hours is begun. Combined therapy is continued for five days,** then as above.
Asymptomatic with blood lead concentration between 56–69 mcg/dl	Edetate calcium disodium* 1 g/M^2/day is given by continuous intravenous infusion for five days. Additional courses are indicated if the blood lead concentration rebounds.
Asymptomatic with blood lead concentration between 25–55 mcg/dl	A diagnostic mobilization test is performed with edetate calcium disodium as outlined in text.
If test ratio >0.70	Edetate calcium disodium* 1 g/M^2/day is given by continuous intravenous infusion for five days.
If test ratio 0.60–0.69 age <3 years	Edetate calcium disodium* 1 g/M^2/day is given by continuous intravenous infusion for three days.
age >3 years	No treatment.
If test ratio <0.60	No treatment.

* *Less desirably, edetate calcium disodium 175 mg/M^2 may be given every four hours by slow intravenous infusion over 15 to 20 minutes or by deep intramuscular injection at a site separate from dimercaprol.*

***After three days of therapy, if the blood lead concentration has fallen to ≤50 mcg/dl, dimercaprol may be discontinued, but edetate calcium disodium should be continued for the full five-day course.*

Adapted from Centers for Disease Control, 1985.

lead levels of 50 to 70 mcg/dl, the total daily dose may be reduced to 1 g/M^2. Each dose is diluted in 250 or 500 ml of sodium chloride injection or 5% dextrose injection and administered over six to eight hours. Therapy is then interrupted for at least two days (preferably two weeks) to allow redistribution of lead from inaccessible storage sites and a second course is then given if necessary. The maximum 24-hour dose in adults should not exceed 50 mg/kg (1.75 g/M^2), even in severe poisoning.

For *children,* intramuscular injection is preferred to avoid extravasation or excessive fluid load in encephalopathy. If the intravenous route is chosen, treatment courses and doses are the same as for adults with the following exceptions: The maximum 24-hour dose may be increased to 75 mg/kg in very severe poisoning, but the total amount of fluid administered per dose must be reduced as required and the concentration of edetate must not exceed 0.5% in the parenteral fluid. If intake volume must be decreased further, the drug should be given intramuscularly. Children may require more than two courses of therapy when mobilization of lead from labile skeletal stores approaches the critical blood level of 70 mcg/dl. Therapy should be continued intermittently until the blood lead concentration remains below 50 mcg/dl.

Intramuscular (deep): *Adults,* the dose and treatment schedule are the same as for intravenous use. The drug is administered as a 20% solution. Generally, procaine is added to a final concentration of 0.5% to minimize pain following injection.

Children, see Table 1.

Calcium Disodium Versenate (Riker). Solution (sterile) 100 mg/ml in 10 ml containers.

DEFEROXAMINE MESYLATE
[Desferal]

$$H_3\overset{+}{N}(CH_2)_5\underset{\underset{OH}{|}}{N}C(CH_2)_2CNH(CH_2)_5\underset{\underset{OH}{|}}{N}C(CH_2)_2CNH(CH_2)_5\underset{\underset{OH}{|}}{N}CCH_3 \quad CH_3SO_3^-$$

ACTIONS. Deferoxamine, a compound obtained from *Streptomyces pilosus*, is a potent and highly specific iron chelating agent. It readily complexes with ferric ion to form ferrioxamine, a stable, water-soluble chelate; it also has limited affinity for ferrous ion. In addition to combining with free ionic iron, deferoxamine can remove iron from ferritin and hemosiderin, except in bone marrow. It is much less effective against transferrin and does not remove iron from cytochromes, myoglobin, or hemoglobin. Deferoxamine 100 mg binds 8.5 mg of iron.

USES. Deferoxamine is used in severe, acute iron intoxication. Primary management should include gastric emptying and control of metabolic acidosis and hypovolemic shock. In adults, gastric lavage with sodium bicarbonate (4 ampuls diluted 1:4 with normal saline) or sodium phosphate (Fleet's Phospho-Soda diluted 1:4 in normal saline) solutions, which form nonabsorbable iron salts, may be helpful (Czajka et al, 1981). However, the repeated indiscriminate use of such a solution in children has caused complications, including hypernatremia, hyperphosphatemia, and hypocalcemia, with more potential risk than iron poisoning.

Deferoxamine also promotes iron excretion in secondary hemochromatosis (Weatherall et al, 1983). It usually is administered intramuscularly or by slow subcutaneous infusion in patients with chronic anemia and iron overload secondary to multiple blood transfusions. A negative net accumulation of iron may be demonstrated in some patients. These patients also should receive supplemental intravenous deferoxamine during blood transfusion (the drug should be given separately from the blood). No tolerance to deferoxamine was demonstrated over a period of two years. Total dose and duration of therapy must be individualized on the basis of an initial dose-response curve. The goal is to use the minimum amount of deferoxamine that prevents net iron accumulation.

Deferoxamine is less effective in primary hemochromatosis than phlebotomy (Young et al, 1979; Halliday and Bassett, 1980). However, deferoxamine is useful when venesection is contraindicated (eg, when the patient is hypoproteinemic or too anemic to tolerate blood loss).

Urinary excretion of the ferrioxamine complex accounts for two-thirds of the iron eliminated; the remainder is excreted in bile. The ferrioxamine complex has a characteristic reddish color; thus, the appearance of reddish brown urine after injection of deferoxamine is presumptive evidence of elevated serum iron levels and an indication for further therapy. However, the absence of this color *does not rule out* severe, acute iron poisoning.

DIAGNOSIS OF POISONING. Probably over 90% of cases of overdose do not require deferoxamine. However, in severe poisoning, the shorter the interval between the ingestion of iron and the administration of deferoxamine, the greater the probability of recovery without sequelae. The first phase (30 to 120 minutes) of acute iron intoxication includes signs and symptoms caused principally by gastrointestinal irritation and necrosis. Although infrequent, an asymptomatic phase may then ensue that can be misleading. Therefore, the patient must continue to be monitored closely, and deferoxamine may have to be administered to avoid or reduce the later phases of acidosis, hepatic failure, oliguria, pulmonary edema, and vasomotor collapse.

Severe poisoning requiring immediate chelation therapy may be correlated with serum iron concentrations greater than 500 mcg/dl. A serum concentration in excess of 1,000 mcg/dl is potentially lethal, and exchange transfusion should be considered in addition to chelation therapy. Samples should be obtained within four hours of ingestion because iron undergoes rapid redistribution into tissue.

While the serum iron concentration is being determined, an estimate of potential severity may be based on history and other findings. Iron in excess of total iron binding capacity indicates a serum iron greater than 300 mcg/dl and suggests initiation of chelation therapy. If diarrhea, vomiting, leukocytosis, or hyperglycemia is present or an abdominal radiograph is positive, the serum iron concentration probably exceeds 300 mcg/dl. If vomiting is absent or the patient remains asymptomatic for at least six hours after ingestion, the serum iron concentration is probably below this value (Lacouture et al, 1981).

The minimal toxic dose is 20 to 60 mg/kg elemental iron; the potentially lethal dose is 60 mg/kg elemental iron. The ingested dose (mg/kg) equals the number of tablets ingested multiplied by the milligrams of elemental iron per tablet divided by the child's weight (kg). To calculate milligrams of elemental iron in solid preparations of iron salts, see Table 2. A compilation of the elemental iron content in liquid formulations of iron salts and for multicomponent drug products is available (Krenzelok and Hoff, 1979). Although uncommon, toxicity has been reported following the ingestion of children's multivitamin preparations containing iron.

ADVERSE REACTIONS AND PRECAUTIONS. Deferoxamine generally is well tolerated. Rapid intravenous injection can cause hypotension, tachycardia, erythema, and urticaria. Some patients experience a local histamine-like reaction or induration following subcutaneous administration for chronic iron overload (hemochromatoses); this reaction is rare when the drug is given intramuscularly. Severe, transient pain at the site of injection may occur.

Patients receiving long-term therapy to treat chronic iron storage disease have experienced mild allergic-type dermatologic reactions (wheals, pruritus), diarrhea, dysuria, abdominal discomfort, leg cramps, tachycardia, and fever. Visual and auditory neurotoxicity can be produced, particularly with larger doses in younger patients, but usually is reversible when the dosage is reduced (Olivieri et al, 1986).

There are no absolute contraindications to the use of deferoxamine in acute iron intoxication or hemochromatosis. Since the drug and the ferrioxamine complex are excreted primarily by the kidneys, deferoxamine generally is contraindi-

TABLE 2.
ELEMENTAL IRON CONTENT
OF SOLID FERROUS SALT PREPARATIONS

Component	% Elemental Iron	To Obtain Approximate mg Elemental Iron Divide mg of Iron Salt by
Ferrous sulfate (anhydrous)	36.77	2.7
Ferrous sulfate monohydrate*	32.87	3
Ferrous sulfate heptahydrate**	20.01	5
Ferrous gluconate (anhydrous)	12.52	8
Ferrous gluconate dihydrate	11.58	8.6
Ferrous fumarate	32.87	3

*Synonym: Dried ferrous sulfate
**Synonym: Ferrous Sulfate, U.S.P.

cated in patients with severe renal disease or anuria. Exchange transfusion or hemodialysis may be required in patients with acute renal failure or life-threatening symptoms (especially shock) refractory to treatment or when the amount of iron is so large that maximum recommended doses of deferoxamine cannot be expected to complex with more than a fraction of the free iron available. Chelation therapy, except that for acute iron intoxication, should be withheld, if possible, during pregnancy.

PHARMACOKINETICS. Deferoxamine has an apparent volume of distribution of about 60% of body weight. It is metabolized rapidly by tissues and plasma. The half-life following intravenous administration is about one hour.

DOSAGE AND PREPARATIONS.

Acute Iron Poisoning:

Intravenous: This route is employed *only* for *adults and children* with signs of cardiovascular shock, a serum iron level greater than 500 mcg/dl, or free iron in the plasma. A dose of 10 mg/kg/hr is infused for four hours, followed by 5 mg/kg/hr for the next eight hours, then 2 to 5 mg/kg/hr until the serum iron level falls to 100 mcg/dl or less (Temple, 1981). (However, whether deferoxamine is given or not, in the absence of continuing absorption and/or an enormous overdose, serum iron will fall rapidly four to ten hours after ingestion.) Faster rates of administration or bolus injections may cause severe hypotension. The rate of infusion should never exceed 15 mg/kg/hr, and the total dose should not exceed 240 mg/kg/24 hr (6 g/24 hr).

Intramuscular: Deferoxamine should be prepared by adding 2 ml of sterile water for injection to each vial. This route is usually reserved for *adults and children* not in shock or in whom an intravenous site is not available. Initially, 1 g followed by 0.5 g at four-hour intervals for two doses. Subsequent doses of 0.5 g may be administered every 4 to 12 hours, as necessary. The total dose should not exceed 6 g/24 hr.

Chronic Iron Overload (Hemochromatoses):

Continuous subcutaneous or intravenous infusion is recommended for iron overload associated with hemochromatoses, because more iron is eliminated per unit dose of deferoxamine than with intramuscular bolus administration. The concomitant oral administration of ascorbic acid (0.5 to 1 g twice daily) may improve the chelating action of deferoxamine in hemochromatosis. Its use should be discontinued, however, if signs and symptoms of cardiac decompensation occur. Since there is considerable dose-response variation, the dosage and duration of therapy should be adjusted by monitoring the urinary excretion of iron.

Intramuscular, Intravenous: Adults, 0.5 to 1 g daily is administered intramuscularly. In addition, 2 g is administered by slow infusion (not to exceed 15 mg/kg/hr) over a 12-hour period with each unit of blood transfused. Deferoxamine can be administered at the same time as blood but must not be mixed in the same container.

Subcutaneous: Adults and children, 20 to 40 mg/kg/day is slowly infused by pump, usually in the anterior abdominal wall over a 12-hour period during the night.

Desferal (CIBA). Powder for solution (lyophilized, sterile) 500 mg.

DIMERCAPROL
[BAL in Oil]

$$\underset{\text{SH \quad SH}}{\overset{\text{CH}_2\text{CH}_2\text{CH}_2\text{OH}}{|\quad\quad|}}$$

ACTIONS AND USES. Dimercaprol antagonizes the toxic effects of arsenic, mercury, and gold by forming chelates or complexes. It is not useful in arsine (AsH_3) poisoning. Therapy is most effective when begun within one or two hours after ingestion. Retrospective clinical studies reveal that dimercaprol removes mercury when given within four hours after ingestion, but efficacy is reduced after six hours. Dimercaprol is used only in acute mercury poisoning.

Although this drug increases the urinary and fecal excretion of lead, edetate calcium disodium or penicillamine is preferred. However, for severe lead poisoning in *children* (lead encephalopathy), the combination of dimercaprol and edetate calcium disodium is preferred, since some studies suggest that this regimen hastens excretion of lead and reduces the incidence of brain damage. Dimercaprol may accelerate the excretion of copper in Wilson's disease (hepatolenticular degeneration), but penicillamine is the drug of choice.

Dimercaprol is not beneficial in antimony or bismuth poisoning and should *not* be used in iron, cadmium, or selenium poisoning because the complexes formed are more nephrotoxic than the metal alone.

This drug is not effective orally for systemic intoxications.

ADVERSE REACTIONS AND PRECAUTIONS. Adverse reactions are generally mild and transitory. In addition to pain at the site of injection sometimes associated with sterile abscesses, they include, in approximate order of frequency, nausea with occasional vomiting; headache; mild conjunctivitis, lacrimation, rhinorrhea, and salivation; burning sensation in the lips, mouth, and throat and feeling of constriction or pain in the throat, chest, or hands; tingling or burning paresthesias in the hands and penis; sweating; and abdominal pain (Klaassen, 1985). Many of these effects, as well as symptoms of serum sickness, are relieved by an antihistamine. Dimercaprol imparts an unpleasant odor to the breath. Drug-induced fever may persist throughout therapy in children.

Dimercaprol consistently causes moderate to marked increases in both systolic and diastolic blood pressure accompanied by tachycardia. It also may induce metabolic acidosis with elevated serum lactate levels. Continued use of large doses damages capillaries, resulting in loss of protein and fluid from the circulation. Dimercaprol may induce hemolysis in patients with glucose-6-phosphate dehydrogenase deficiency and should be utilized in such patients only in life-threatening situations.

Dimercaprol is contraindicated in patients with impaired liver function. It may be used for lead poisoning in patients with virtually complete renal impairment since both dimercaprol and its complex with lead can be excreted in the bile (Chisolm, 1968). However, dimercaprol is potentially nephrotoxic. If acute renal failure develops during therapy, dimercaprol should be continued with extreme caution, since toxic serum concentrations of dimercaprol may appear. Because the chelate rapidly dissociates in an acid medium, releasing the bound metal, *the urine should be kept alkaline.*

Dimercaprol forms a toxic complex with and should not be used in conjunction with medicinal iron. Severe iron deficiency anemia during dimercaprol therapy should be managed by blood transfusion.

PHARMACOKINETICS. Peak plasma concentrations of dimercaprol are obtained 30 to 60 minutes after intramuscular administration. About 50% of the drug is excreted in the bile; the remainder is metabolized rapidly. A single dose is eliminated completely in about four hours.

DOSAGE AND PREPARATIONS. *Dimercaprol in oil must never be given intravenously.* Doses in excess of 5 mg/kg should be avoided since vomiting, seizures, and coma may be induced.

Intramuscular: Adults and children, for mild arsenic or gold poisoning, 2.5 mg/kg four times daily for two days, two times on the third day, then once daily for ten days; for severe arsenic or gold poisoning, 3 mg/kg every four hours for two days, four times on the third day, then twice daily for ten days.

For acute mercury poisoning, 5 mg/kg initially, followed by 2.5 mg/kg one or two times daily for ten days. The suggested dosage based on body surface area is: for very severe poisoning, 750 mg/M^2/day in divided doses every four hours; for less severe poisoning, 500 mg/M^2/day in divided doses every four hours; for mild poisoning, 333 mg/M^2/day in divided doses every four to six hours. Dosage is adjusted as described above.

For dosage used in lead poisoning, see Table 1.

BAL in Oil (Hynson, Westcott & Dunning). Solution (sterile) 100 mg/ml in peanut oil in 3 ml containers.

PENICILLAMINE
[Cuprimine, Depen]

$$CH_3 - \underset{\underset{CH_3}{|}}{\overset{\overset{SH}{|}}{C}} - \underset{\underset{H}{|}}{\overset{\overset{NH_2}{|}}{C}} - \overset{\overset{O}{||}}{C}OH$$

ACTIONS. This sulfhydryl compound, an inactive degradation product of penicillin, is now manufactured synthetically to avoid contamination with trace amounts of penicillin. It combines with copper, iron, mercury, lead, gold, and arsenic to form soluble complexes that are readily excreted by the kidneys. Penicillamine itself is oxidized to a disulfide derivative and is also excreted by the kidneys.

USES. This orally effective agent is superior to other metal antagonists for chelating copper and is used primarily to remove excess copper in patients with Wilson's disease. Continuous penicillamine therapy promotes long-term survival in these patients; prophylactic administration is now recommended for individuals homozygous for Wilson's disease before symptoms develop.

Penicillamine chelates lead less effectively than edetate calcium disodium or dimercaprol but has the advantage of being effective orally. It is not the drug of choice for severe lead intoxication, although it may be given after initial therapy with edetate calcium disodium. Penicillamine is useful in asymptomatic patients with moderately elevated blood levels of lead. However, unless excessive oral lead exposure is terminated, absorption of lead may be enhanced by penicillamine.

Although dimercaprol is the standard therapy for arsenic poisoning, penicillamine is equally effective (Peterson and Rumack, 1977). It also may be substituted for dimercaprol in acute inorganic mercury poisoning.

ADVERSE REACTIONS AND PRECAUTIONS. Although the adverse reactions associated with short-term administration are generally acceptable, penicillamine can produce serious and even fatal reactions. Side effects, precautions, and contraindications for the use of penicillamine are described in detail in Chapter 31, Agents Used to Treat Urologic Disorders.

DOSAGE AND PREPARATIONS.

Oral: For Wilson's disease, *infants over 6 months and young children,* a single daily dose of 250 mg dissolved in fruit juice; *older children and adults,* initially, 125 or 250 mg daily, increased gradually over a four- to eight-week period as indicated by side effects and urinary copper excretion. The usual maintenance dose is 250 mg four times daily; however, if efficacy is not compromised, it is recommended that the total daily dose be limited to 500 to 750 mg to minimize untoward effects. Although these guidelines are helpful, dosage must be individualized and can be determined only by measuring the urinary excretion of copper. If the patient is on a low-copper diet and is using an oral cation exchange resin, negative copper balance will result if the urinary excretion of copper is 1 mg or more every 24 hours.

Penicillamine should be given on an empty stomach at least one hour before meals and at bedtime; the last dose should be given at least three hours after the evening meal. Patients also should be maintained on a low-copper diet.

For lead poisoning, *adults and children,* 600 mg/M^2 daily (see Table 1) until the concentration of lead remains below 50 mcg/dl of whole blood (usually four weeks to several months). Side effects can be minimized by initiating therapy with 25% of the calculated dose, increasing to 50% after one week and to the full dose after another week with monitoring for possible toxicity. A low-calcium diet augments lead sequestration.

For acute arsenic poisoning, *adults and children,* 100 mg/kg/day in four divided doses before meals to a maximum of 1 g/day for five days. After a drug-free interval of three to five days, therapy may be reinstituted if symptoms reappear. When the urinary excretion of arsenic falls below 50 mcg/24 hours, further chelation therapy is unnecessary (Peterson and Rumack, 1977).

For acute mercury poisoning, *adults,* 250 mg four times a day; *children,* 100 mg/kg/day for 3 to 10 days guided by the urinary excretion of mercury (Rumack and Peterson, 1980).

> **Cuprimine** (Merck Sharp & Dohme). Capsules 125 and 250 mg. If necessary, these capsules may be opened and the drug suspended in any liquid, except milk.
> **Depen** (Wallace). Tablets 250 mg.

TRIENTINE HYDROCHLORIDE
[Cuprid]

$$H_2NCH_2CH_2NHCH_2CH_2NHCH_2CH_2NH_2 \quad \cdot \, 2HCl$$

ACTIONS AND USES. Trientine is a chelating agent employed to remove excess copper in Wilson's disease. Until more experience accumulates, its use should be restricted to patients who cannot tolerate penicillamine. This drug is of no value in other conditions that respond to penicillamine, such as rheumatoid arthritis and cystinuria, and it is not useful in primary biliary cirrhosis (Epstein and Sherlock, 1980).

ADVERSE REACTIONS AND PRECAUTIONS. Trientine was approved under Orphan Drug status in late 1985. Therefore, the usual extensive preclinical and clinical studies required prior to marketing were not conducted. A limited number of patients (about 200 in the United States) require the agent. The only adverse response noted to date is iron deficiency, which can be corrected by supplementation. However, since iron and trientine inhibit each other's absorption, administration of these agents should be separated by at least two hours.

Trientine causes contact dermatitis and bronchitis and asthma have occurred after this drug was inhaled by chemical workers. The patient should be asked to report any occurrence of fever or skin lesions during the first month of therapy.

Trientine is classified in FDA Pregnancy Category C.

DOSAGE AND PREPARATIONS. Trientine should be given on an empty stomach at least one hour before or two hours after meals and at least one hour apart from any other drug, food, or milk. The capsules should be swallowed whole with water and not chewed.

Oral: Initially, 500 to 750 mg/day for *children* and 750 mg to 1.25 g/day for *adults* in two, three, or four divided doses. This may be increased to a maximum of 1.5 g/day in *children under 12 years* and to 2 g/day for *adults.* The daily dose is increased only if the clinical response is inadequate or the free serum copper concentration is persistently above 20 mcg/dl.

> **Cuprid** (Merck Sharp & Dohme). Capsules 250 mg.

Miscellaneous Specific Antidotes

NALOXONE HYDROCHLORIDE
[Narcan]

ACTIONS AND USES. Naloxone is the drug of choice to treat respiratory depression known or suspected to be caused by opioid overdose; it promptly increases the respiratory rate and volume. Since naloxone does not cause respiratory depression or affect that produced by barbiturates or other respiratory depressants, lack of response suggests that the depression is not the result of opioid overdose or that multiple-agent intoxication is involved.

Naloxone reverses the agonist effects of pentazocine [Talwin] and other mixed agonist-antagonists and terminates the psychotogenic and dysphoric effects sometimes caused by these drugs. It also terminates coma and convulsions associated with large doses of propoxyphene [Darvon] or meperidine [Demerol] in drug abusers (Martin, 1976) or after overdose in children (Lovejoy et al, 1974). In addition, naloxone counteracts other actions of the opioids, such as analgesia, cardiovascular and gastrointestinal effects, biliary duct spasm, pupillary response, release of antidiuretic hormone, and hyperglycemia.

Naloxone may be administered postoperatively to reverse severe respiratory depression caused by opioids. However, since it also decreases the analgesic and sedative effects of these drugs, the dose must be selected carefully. Too rapid reversal may cause nausea and vomiting or tachycardia and hypertension; these reactions may be due to catecholamine release, since they sometimes occur following administration of naloxone to opioid- and pain-free subjects (Azar et al, 1981). Pulmonary edema and disturbances of cardiac rhythm are extremely rare and have been reported only in critically ill patients receiving multiple doses.

Naloxone is effective in neonatal respiratory depression caused by large doses of morphine-like drugs administered to the mother during labor and delivery. The antagonist should be injected intravenously in the infant after delivery if postnatal respiratory depression is present. It should be kept in mind that, if the mother is dependent on morphine-like drugs, the infant is also dependent and may exhibit withdrawal symptoms after birth (hypertonia, sweating, continuous shrill cry, failure to feed). Because an antagonist will precipitate a withdrawal reaction in these infants, careful monitoring is essential after the desired effect is achieved.

The pupillography test using naloxone has been useful when employed by trained personnel to diagnose opioid addiction, but small doses must be administered cautiously to avoid precipitating a severe withdrawal syndrome in opioid-dependent individuals. Chemical methods that detect opioids in the urine are more sensitive and are preferable.

Naloxone has been given with various morphine-like analgesics in an attempt to prevent respiratory depression while retaining the analgesic effect, but there is little evidence to support the use of such combined therapy.

ADVERSE REACTIONS AND PRECAUTIONS. Naloxone may precipitate a withdrawal syndrome in opioid-dependent patients. Although the syndrome is relatively self-limited (15 to 60 minutes), naloxone should be administered in increments to dependent patients until respiratory depression is reversed.

This drug has been notably free from adverse reactions. Tolerance and psychic or physical dependence do not develop. Naloxone is not subject to the Controlled Substances Act.

PHARMACOKINETICS. The onset of action is rapid; an effect usually is noted within two minutes after intravenous injection and only slightly later after intramuscular, subcutaneous, sublingual, or endotracheal injection, but the intravenous route is preferred. The duration of action may be shorter than that of most opioids. The apparent volume of distribution is 2.77 ± 0.16 L/kg. The half-life is 48.6 ± 7.3 minutes in normal subjects and 29.9 ± 2.6 minutes when hepatic microsomal enzymes have been induced (eg, after use of barbiturates or prolonged intake of alcohol). *Thus, repeated doses may be necessary to treat respiratory depression.*

DOSAGE AND PREPARATIONS. *Naloxone is given to antagonize opioid-induced respiratory depression immediately after the establishment of a clear airway and adequate assistance of respiration.* Although the intravenous route is preferred, the same dosage is effective almost as rapidly following sublingual, endotracheal, intramuscular, or subcutaneous administration.

Intravenous: For respiratory depression caused by opioid overdosage, *adults and children,* 2 mg (five ampuls) as a bolus. Larger doses (as much as 20 times the usual quantity) may be required for poisoning with propoxyphene [Darvon] or pentazocine [Talwin] or massive overdoses of other analgesics. If a single dose of 2 mg fails to reverse symptoms in suspected narcotic overdosage, an additional 2 to 4 mg should be administered by bolus. Because of its short half-life, additional doses of naloxone may be required at 20- to 60-minute intervals, especially with overdose of long-acting opioids such as methadone. Alternatively, after a satisfactory response to the initial dose, approximately 60% of the amount necessary for reversal may be given hourly: Ten times the hourly dose is added to 1 L of dextrose 5% in water and infused at the rate of about 100 ml/hr, adjusted to maintain a satisfactory ventilatory response without evoking withdrawal symptoms (Goldfrank, 1986).

For postoperative respiratory depression caused by opioids, *adults,* 0.1 to 0.2 mg (1.5 mcg/kg) at two- to three-minute intervals until the desired effect is achieved. The drug also has been given by continuous infusion (3.66 mcg/kg/hr) to counteract respiratory depression induced by morphine anesthesia (Johnstone et al, 1974).

Intravenous, Intramuscular, Subcutaneous: To reverse opioid-induced respiratory depression in *newborn infants,* 0.01 mg/kg initially, repeated once in three to five minutes if

there is no response. The dose may be repeated in 30 to 90 minutes, depending upon the degree of depression.

Narcan (DuPont). Solution 0.4 mg/ml in 1 and 10 ml containers and 0.02 mg/ml in 2 ml containers (*Narcan Neonatal*) with methylparaben and propylparaben as preservatives.

NALTREXONE HYDROCHLORIDE
[Trexan]

ACTIONS AND USES. Naltrexone resembles naloxone in its ability to competitively antagonize opioid drugs. An oral dose suppresses the psychological and physical effects of opioids for 48 to 72 hours. The sole indication for naltrexone is maintenance of an opioid-free state in abusers. Unlike methadone, which also is used for this purpose, it has no agonist activity. Therefore, it is not a scheduled drug and may be prescribed by physicians outside of specialized clinics and drug abuse programs. Compliance is essential to efficacy; verification of regular naltrexone use and urinalysis are essential, and job counseling, psychotherapy, and physician and family support enhance compliance. Drug therapy to lessen anxiety, depression, or insomnia may be required during initial use of naltrexone.

ADVERSE REACTIONS AND PRECAUTIONS. Shortly after beginning therapy with naltrexone, minor disturbances, particularly nausea, loss of energy, mental depression, and dysphoria, may develop. These effects usually diminish in 30 to 60 days and also occur in normal volunteers. It has been speculated that this response may be ascribed to blockade of endogenous opioids (Hollister et al, 1981).

The most serious adverse reaction is dose-related hepatotoxicity. Since liver dysfunction is common in many drug abusers, it is recommended that serum transaminases be measured before initiating therapy, monthly during the first six months, and periodically thereafter. A threefold or greater increase in the transaminase level is an indication for discontinuation of the medication.

Antidiarrheal and antitussive preparations containing opioids are ineffective in patients treated with naltrexone. If pain relief is required, a nonsteroidal drug, regional anesthesia, or inhalational anesthetic, such as nitrous oxide, must be used. Patients given naltrexone should wear a bracelet or necklace indicating such use.

PHARMACOKINETICS. In the absence of food, absorption following oral administration of naltrexone is rapid and complete; a maximum concentration is attained in the plasma within one hour. However, there is extensive first-pass metabolism in the liver, and only about 5% of a dose reaches the systemic circulation. The variability in hepatic extraction among individuals probably accounts for the discrepancies reported in pharmacokinetic data.

The principal metabolite, 6-β-naltrexol, exhibits only weak antiopioid activity and, despite its longer elimination half-life, it is presumed that this metabolite does not contribute to the clinical effect of naltrexone. The volume of distribution of naltrexone at steady state is 16.1 ± 5.2 L/kg (Verebey et al, 1976). The clearance (total) is approximately 94 L/hr and the elimination half-life is approximately four hours (Meyer et al, 1984). There is no evidence that prolonged administration results in accumulation of naltrexone or its metabolites.

DOSAGE AND PREPARATIONS. Naltrexone should not be administered unless the patient has been opioid-free for seven to ten days as confirmed by chemical urinalysis and a naloxone challenge test.

Oral: To prevent readdiction in former opioid abusers, initially, 25 mg. If no signs of an opioid withdrawal syndrome become apparent within one hour, the remainder of the daily dose may be administered. Doses of 100 to 150 mg three times per week usually are employed. However, dose schedules may be tailored to the probable compliance of the patient, eg, 50 mg per day, 100 mg every other day, 150 mg every third day, 100 mg on Monday and Wednesday and 150 mg on Friday.

Trexan (DuPont). Tablets 50 mg.

Subcutaneous (Investigational): Because of notoriously poor compliance, studies are in progress utilizing a biodegradable bead containing naltrexone that would require subcutaneous implantation only once a month (Chiang et al, 1985).

ACETYLCYSTEINE
[Mucomyst]

$$HSCH_2CHCOH$$
$$\underset{\underset{O}{\overset{\|}{NHCCH_3}}}{|}$$

This mucolytic drug is used as an antidote for severe acetaminophen poisoning (Rumack et al, 1983) characterized by ingestion of more than 140 mg/kg or a plasma concentration indicating risk of hepatotoxicity (see the figure). Values obtained prior to four hours may give spuriously low concentrations due to incomplete absorption. Approximately two-thirds of patients fulfilling these criteria develop symptoms of hepatotoxicity and should benefit from therapy. Acetaminophen-induced hepatic damage is thought to be produced by a reactive intermediate of a minor metabolite that is normally inactivated by conjugation with glutathione. Overdosage occurs when 70% or more of glutathione is depleted. The sulfhydryl compound, acetylcysteine, is an effective antidote.

Because of the low incidence of side effects associated with acetylcysteine, therapy should be initiated immediately without waiting for plasma acetaminophen determinations. The decision to continue therapy may then be guided by the laboratory results. The incidence of hepatotoxicity is 100% when plasma acetaminophen concentrations exceed 300 mcg/ml.

Acetylcysteine is hydrolyzed rapidly to cysteine after cellular penetration. Adverse reactions are minor; transient elevation of blood pressure may occur but arrhythmias have not been documented.

DOSAGE AND PREPARATIONS.
Oral: After emptying the stomach by gastric lavage or induced emesis, a loading dose of 140 mg/kg is given as a 5% solution in iced water, grapefruit juice, or a cola beverage. Additional doses of 70 mg/kg then are administered at four-hour intervals for 17 doses; however, the optimum number has not been determined and this number may be unnecessarily large.

Acetylcysteine has an extremely disagreeable odor and taste. To improve patient compliance, the drug may be ingested through a straw inserted through a plastic cap on an opaque cup. If frequent vomiting interferes, the material may be instilled through an oroduodenal tube.

Mucomyst (Mead Johnson). Solution (sterile) 10% and 20% in 4, 10, and 30 ml containers.

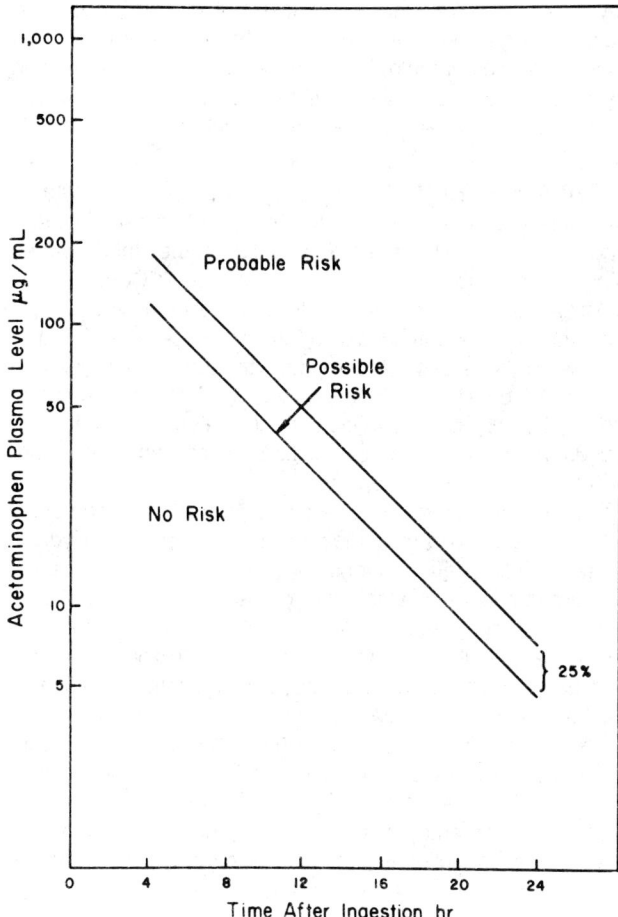

Plasma concentration of acetaminophen with time following a single acute ingestion to show probability of hepatotoxic risk.

Adapted from Rumack BH, et al. Arch Intern Med 141:380-385, 1981.

CYANIDE ANTIDOTE

ACTIONS AND USES. Cyanide ion combines principally with ferricytochrome oxidase to produce tissue hypoxia. A cyanide antidote kit is available and contains amyl nitrite for inhalation and sodium nitrite and sodium thiosulfate for intravenous injection. Nitrite ion converts hemoglobin to methemoglobin; the ferric ion formed competes with ferricytochrome oxidase for available cyanide ion. Cyanide ion is biotransformed to the relatively nontoxic thiocyanate ion by hepatic rhodanase and thiol-containing compounds normally present in the body. Sodium thiosulfate increases the biotransformation of cyanide to thiocyanate over thirtyfold (Sylvester et al, 1983).

Oxygen is an important adjunct in the treatment of cyanide poisoning. It permits the saturation of hemoglobin not converted to methemoglobin and may reactivate cyanide-depressed enzymatic processes, eg, carbohydrate metabolism (Way et al, 1984). No benefit is gained from hyperbaric oxygenation.

ADVERSE REACTIONS. Adverse reactions to recommended doses of cyanide antagonists in the cyanide antidote kit are seldom clinically significant in otherwise healthy individuals but may be clinically relevant in some situations (eg, prolonged sodium nitroprusside infusion in hypertensive patients). Large amounts of methemoglobin decrease the quantity of oxygen available for tissues, and nitrites also can produce cardiovascular instability, usually manifested as hypotension, especially during anesthesia.

ALTERNATIVE THERAPY. The use of the traditional cyanide antagonists is being re-evaluated in light of investigations in Europe using cobalt edetate and studies in the United States using hydroxocobalamin (Graham et al, 1977; Cottrell et al, 1978). Intravenous cobalt edetate 600 mg forms a relatively nontoxic complex with cyanide; another dose of 300 mg is administered if recovery is delayed. Although some physicians in England consider cobalt edetate to be the treatment of choice (the drug is not available in the United States), it often causes vomiting, and anaphylactic reactions and ventricular arrhythmias have been reported.

The vitamin, hydroxocobalamin [alphaRedisol], combines with cyanide ion to form cyanocobalamin (vitamin B_{12}). Hydroxocobalamin is given intravenously, but no commercial parenteral preparation is available that contains the amount of drug required to combat cyanide toxicity without administering excessive quantities of fluid. The role of hydroxocobalamin in cyanide poisoning is promising but investigational. No adverse reactions have been reported.

Results of animal experiments in which stroma-free methemoglobin solutions are injected intravenously have been promising (Ten Eyck et al, 1984). The advantages of administering exogenous methemoglobin over endogenous conversion are that the onset of action is immediate and the patient's oxygen-carrying capacity is not compromised.

DOSAGE AND PREPARATIONS.

Inhalation, Intravenous: Adults, oxygen therapy should be initiated and amyl nitrite inhaled from the crushable ampuls for 30 seconds of every minute until an intravenous route is established. Amyl nitrite then is discontinued and all of the sodium nitrite (300 mg) in the 10-ml ampul is administered intravenously. The 12.5 g of sodium thiosulfate contained in the 50-ml ampul is then administered intravenously. If symptoms persist, a second dose of sodium nitrite (one-half the amount of the first dose) should be given 30 minutes later. *Children,* oxygen therapy is initiated; 0.33 ml/kg of sodium nitrite solution is administered, followed immediately by 1.65 ml/kg of sodium thiosulfate solution.

If nitrite-induced methemoglobinemia becomes severe, whole blood may be given. *Under no circumstances* should methylene blue be used to treat the methemoglobinemia. This will cause release of cyanide ion and its use in these circumstances has resulted in fatalities (Arena, 1983).

Cyanide Antidote Package (Lilly). Each kit contains 12 crushable ampuls containing amyl nitrite 0.3 ml, two 10-ml containers of sodium nitrite 300 mg, two 50-ml containers of sodium thiosulfate 12.5 g, disposable syringes, stomach tube, and instructions. The expiration date on the kit must be observed.

PHYSOSTIGMINE SALICYLATE
[Antilirium]

ACTIONS AND USES. This tertiary amine alkaloid is an anticholinesterase. Its ability to penetrate the central nervous system is useful adjunctively in the treatment of severe central anticholinergic toxicity characterized by anxiety, disorientation, delirium, hyperactivity, hallucinations, illusions, impaired consciousness, and impaired memory. Physostigmine is less effective in antagonizing peripheral signs and symptoms (tachycardia; mydriasis; facial flushing; reduced sweating; hyperpyrexia; depressed bronchial, pharyngeal, nasal, and gastrointestinal secretions; decreased gastrointestinal and urinary tract motility).

This spectrum of anticholinergic toxicity is most characteristic of poisoning with atropine and scopolamine. Drugs with secondary anticholinergic activity include antihistamines, tricyclic antidepressants, certain antiemetics, some antiparkinson drugs (centrally acting anticholinergics), phenothiazines, and, to a lesser extent, butyrophenones. Physostigmine should *not* be used to treat overdosage with these drugs but may be useful as an adjunct to respiratory support if severe anticholinergic toxicity is suspected. It may aggravate some nonanticholinergic cardiac disturbances caused by the tricyclic antidepressants (eg, bradyarrhythmias, A-V conduction blocks).

Physostigmine should be reserved for serious situations, because it is potentially dangerous; *its routine use for the management of anticholinergic delirium is not recommended.* Treatment of acidosis with sodium bicarbonate and correction of inadequate minute volume usually are more appropriate. If the diagnosis of anticholinergic overdose is well documented, if supportive care has improved and stabilized vital signs, and if urine output is adequate, there may be little value in using physostigmine for arousal.

In some instances (ie, presence of convulsions, hypertension, supraventricular arrhythmias, severe hallucinations), documented anticholinergic toxicity may demand aggressive therapy, but mixed overdose of cocaine and a tricyclic antidepressant or overdose of a sympathomimetic agent must be ruled out first. Physostigmine may improve ventilation in marginal situations, thus avoiding the necessity for endotracheal intubation and mechanical ventilation, or improve the care of agitated, disoriented patients.

ADVERSE REACTIONS AND PRECAUTIONS. Hypersensitivity to physostigmine is uncommon. Slight to moderate bradycardia may occur; severe bradyarrhythmias are more likely to develop if physostigmine is given to overcome the effects of orphenadrine and tricyclic antidepressants. Severe hypotensive episodes are rare, although convulsions have been observed, particularly with too rapid administration. Excessive salivation, vomiting, urination, and defecation also may occur. The most dangerous sequela of vomiting may be aspiration, and adequate suction should always be available. In such instances, administration of atropine may be necessary. Such adverse reactions are less likely to occur when anticholinergic poisoning is established. In this instance, a return to more normal function occurs.

A dystonic extrapyramidal reaction should not be mistaken for central anticholinergic toxicity. The akinesia, akathisia, and dyskinesia of the former can be confused with the signs and symptoms of hyperactivity caused by the latter; however, there is little or no impairment of consciousness associated with dystonic extrapyramidal reactions. Physostigmine worsens the rigidity, tremor, and akinesia of parkinsonism and extrapyramidal dystonic reactions.

Because of its short duration of action, physostigmine gradually becomes ineffective over 30 to 60 minutes; therefore, continued observation of the patient is important.

Any cholinergic sign or symptom that is undesirable in a given clinical situation may be considered a relative contraindication (eg, precipitation of an asthmatic attack).

PHARMACOKINETICS. Physostigmine is almost completely hydrolyzed by the enzyme that it inhibits. It is relatively short acting (half-life, one to two hours). Renal impairment does not alter dosage.

DOSAGE AND PREPARATIONS.
Intravenous: Adults, 1 to 2 mg given slowly (1 mg/min). The dose may be repeated if life-threatening signs and symptoms recur. Frequent surveillance is essential to determine the appropriate dosage in any given individual. The response to a single dose seldom lasts longer than 30 to 60 minutes. Monitoring of blood pressure, heart rate, and autonomic nervous system function is required. *Children,* 0.5 mg given slowly. If toxic effects persist and no cholinergic effects are produced, the drug should be given at five-minute intervals to a maximum dose of 2 mg. The lowest total effective dose should be repeated if life-threatening signs and symptoms recur.

Antilirium (Forest). Solution 1 mg/ml in 1 and 2 ml containers.

PRALIDOXIME CHLORIDE
[Protopam Chloride]

ACTIONS AND USES. Pralidoxime (2-PAM) is a cholinesterase reactivator used primarily as an adjunct to atropine in the treatment of severe poisoning caused by pesticides that are organophosphate cholinesterase inhibitors.

In organophosphate poisoning, pralidoxime competes with the phosphorylated inhibited enzyme to form an oxime-phosphonate complex that liberates active cholinesterase. This occurs primarily at the neuromuscular junction in skeletal muscle and also at autonomic effector sites.

The relative specificity in its site of action determines the role of pralidoxime in anticholinesterase poisoning: It is used to reverse muscular paralysis, particularly that of the respiratory muscles. Atropine must be administered to treat symptoms originating at sites where pralidoxime is relatively ineffective, especially the respiratory center. Therefore, after securing the airway and providing respiratory assistance as required, atropine is given prior to pralidoxime to control convulsions, improve central respiratory function, and reduce bronchopulmonary secretions, hypersalivation, lacrimation, hyperhidrosis, nausea, vomiting, abdominal cramps, bradycardia, headache, lethargy, and drowsiness. One of the best indices for monitoring therapy is the amount of salivary secretion. Diazepam may be given cautiously if convulsions are not controlled by atropine. Only then should pralidoxime be administered.

If dermal exposure has occurred, clothing should be removed as soon as possible and the hair and skin washed thoroughly with soapy water or alcohol if required. Emergency room personnel should protect themselves from exposure.

Pralidoxime is most effective if administered immediately after poisoning. Generally, little is accomplished if the drug is given more than 36 hours after termination of exposure. When the poison has been ingested, however, exposure may continue for some time due to slow absorption from the lower bowel, and fatal relapses have been reported after initial improvement. Continued administration for several days may be useful in such patients. Close supervision is indicated for at least 48 to 72 hours.

Pralidoxime is not equally useful against all cholinesterase inhibitors. It has been most effective in poisoning caused by the organophosphate pesticide, parathion. Pralidoxime also has been effective in poisoning caused by the related agents, Mevinphos, Isoflurophate, Diazinon, Dursban, EPN, Guthion, methyl parathion, Phosdrin, Systox, and TEPP. (See the manufacturer's literature for additional substances.) Pralidoxime does *not* antagonize the effects of carbamate-type cholinesterase inhibitors (eg, neostigmine, pyridostigmine, ambenonium, which are used in the treatment of myasthenia gravis; the pesticides, Aldicarb, Baygon, Carbaryl [Sevin], Metalkamate, Oxyamyl).

DIAGNOSIS OF POISONING. Known exposure associated with compatible symptoms is enough evidence to initiate atropine therapy. If nicotinic effects persist, pralidoxime should be administered. Therapy should not await the results of laboratory tests; red blood cell, plasma cholinesterase, and, in parathion exposure, urinary paranitrophenol measurements help to confirm the diagnosis. Depression of the plasma cholinesterase level does not necessarily reflect nerve cholinesterase activity. The red blood cell cholinesterase concentration provides a more accurate index of intoxication; a level less than 50% of normal has been seen only with organophosphate ester poisoning. When pralidoxime is administered soon after the onset of poisoning, the red blood cell cholinesterase activity may be restored more rapidly than the plasma level. However, both plasma and red blood cell activities may remain depressed for a month or longer after intoxication; they also may be depressed in patients with subclinical chronic exposures. Therefore, exposure to anticholinesterase inhibitors, including organic phosphate pesticides, should be avoided for several weeks after poisoning.

ADVERSE REACTIONS AND PRECAUTIONS. Pralidoxime may cause dizziness, diplopia, impaired accommodation, headache, drowsiness, nausea, tachycardia, increased systolic and diastolic blood pressure, hyperventilation, and muscle weakness when given parenterally to individuals not exposed to anticholinesterase poisons. No significant toxic effects have been reported after prolonged oral administration.

The dose of pralidoxime should be reduced in patients with impaired renal function because blood levels are increased in these patients.

DOSAGE AND PREPARATIONS.
Intravenous: For severe poisoning (coma, cyanosis, respiratory depression) caused by organophosphate-containing substances, the following treatment program should be instituted: A patent airway is secured and, if necessary, artificial respiration with oxygen is begun. In *adults,* atropine 2 to 4 mg is given intravenously *after* adequate oxygenation is assured, and this dose is repeated at 5- to 10-minute intervals until secretions are inhibited or signs of atropine toxicity appear. For *children,* atropine 0.5 mg is given initially and repeated at 5- to 10-minute intervals until salivary secretions are inhibited. Some degree of atropinization should be maintained for at least 48 hours. *Adults,* after atropine, pralidoxime 1 g, preferably diluted in 100 ml of sodium chloride injection, is infused over a 30-minute period or injected at a rate not exceeding 200 mg/min. If the response is inadequate, this dose may be repeated in one hour. *Children* may be given 20 to 40 mg/kg using the same procedure. If infusion is not feasible, a 5% solution may be injected over a five-minute period.
Protopam Chloride (Ayerst). Powder (sterile) 1 g in 20 ml containers.
Oral: For mild poisoning (headache, blurred vision, mild muscarinic signs), exposure to the poison is terminated and atropine therapy is initiated. If necessary, 1 to 2 g of pralidoxime is given; this dose can be repeated in three hours. The patient should remain under the physician's supervision for at least 24 hours.
Protopam Chloride (Ayerst). Tablets 500 mg.

ETHANOL

ACTIONS AND USES. The toxicity of methanol (methyl or wood alcohol) and ethylene glycol (antifreeze) is caused by the metabolites of these compounds. Both are metabolized by the enzyme, alcohol dehydrogenase. Ethanol has a greater affinity for this enzyme and retards the rate of formation of toxic metabolites to a level at which they can be eliminated safely.

To avoid gastritis, an ethanol concentration no greater than 20% is recommended for oral use, but any blended whiskey can be substituted if necessary. Oral therapy is preferred to intravenous administration because of the large volumes that may be required. In comatose patients, ethanol can be administered by orogastric tube.

For intravenous administration, ethanol 10% in 5% dextrose in water solution is used (approximately 80 mg/ml of ethanol). Intravenous therapy obviates the concerns for absorption, concurrent drug administration (eg, activated charcoal), and airway management.

In adults, an oral or intravenous loading dose of 0.6 to 0.7 g/kg is given, followed by a maintenance dose of about 125 mg/kg/hr. Blood ethanol concentrations should be monitored and the maintenance dose adjusted to maintain a concentration between 100 and 150 mg/dl (Peterson, 1981). If rapid monitoring is not possible, the maintenance dose may be set arbitrarily at 125 to 150 mg/kg/hr.

The concurrent use of single-pass (not recirculating) hemodialysis markedly reduces morbidity in both methanol and ethylene glycol poisoning (Peterson et al, 1981 A). For methanol poisoning, hemodialysis should be instituted when blood methanol concentrations exceed 50 mg/dl or more than 35 ml has been ingested and, for ethylene glycol poisoning, when the volume of ethylene glycol ingested is greater than 100 ml. If hemodialysis is utilized, the ethanol maintenance dose must be increased to approximately 250 mg/kg/hr; however, because the specific amount depends on flow and extraction efficiency, the dose should be adjusted on the basis of serial blood alcohol determinations. An alternative is to add 95% ethanol to the dialysate to give a dialysate level of 100 mg/dl (Peterson et al, 1981 B); however this method is difficult to control and costly.

Because poisoning by these compounds also is associated with severe metabolic acidosis (formate and lactate), parenteral sodium bicarbonate must be administered if the serum bicarbonate concentration is below 15 mEq/L and the plasma pH is below 7.35 (see Chapter 46, Replenishers and Regulators of Water and Electrolytes).

ALTERNATIVE THERAPY. In methanol poisoning, acidosis and ocular damage result from accumulation of formic acid. A folate-dependent enzyme system is responsible for the oxidation of formic acid to carbon dioxide. Man and certain monkeys are relatively deficient in this system. In animals, the administration of the folate analogue, leucovorin calcium (citrovorum factor), increases the rate of metabolism of formic acid, which markedly reduces blood levels of the toxin (Noker et al, 1980). If the value of leucovorin calcium is substantiated in man, this drug would be extremely useful to treat methanol poisoning, particularly when hemodialysis is difficult (eg, in young children). Leucovorin calcium is essentially nontoxic (see Chapter 32, Agents Used to Treat Deficiency Anemias).

The alcohol dehydrogenase inhibitor, 4-methylpyrazole, is relatively nontoxic. Animal experiments suggest that this may be a satisfactory alternative to ethanol for use in methanol poisoning since monitoring of the serum concentration is not required and additive central nervous system depression does not occur (Blomstrand and Ingemansson, 1984).

References

General Management

Aronow R (ed): *Handbook of Common Poisonings in Children*, ed 2. Evanston, IL, American Academy of Pediatrics, 1983.

Doull J, et al (eds): *Toxicology: The Basic Science of Poisons*, ed 3. New York, Macmillan, in press.

Dreisbach RH: *Handbook of Poisoning*, ed 11. Los Altos, CA, Lange Medical Publications, 1983.

Gleason MN, et al: *Clinical Toxicology of Commercial Products*, ed 5. Baltimore, Williams & Wilkins, 1984.

Goldfrank LR, et al: *Toxicologic Emergencies,* ed 3. New York, Appleton-Century-Crofts, 1986.

Haddad LM, Winchester JF: *Clinical Management of Poisoning and Drug Overdose*. Philadelphia, WB Saunders, 1983.

Rumack BH, et al (eds): *POISINDEX:* An emergency poison management system. Denver, Micromedex, Inc (issued quarterly).

Adsorbent, Emetic, Urinary pH

Cooney DO: *Activated Charcoal: Antidotal and Other Medical Uses.* New York, Marcel Dekker, 1980.

Cooney DO, Kane RP: "Superactive" charcoal adsorbs drugs as fast as standard antidotal charcoal. *Clin Toxicol* 16:123-125, 1980.

Easom JM, Lovejoy FH Jr: Efficacy and safety of gastrointestinal decontamination in treatment of oral poisoning. *Pediatr Clin North Am* 26:827-836, 1979.

Krenzelok EP: Comparison of cathartics used with activated charcoal. *Vet Hum Toxicol* 26 (suppl 2):45, 1984.

Mayersohn M, et al: Evaluation of charcoal-sorbitol mixture as antidote for oral aspirin overdose. *Clin Toxicol* 11:561-567, 1977.

Neuvonen PJ: Clinical pharmacokinetics of oral activated charcoal in acute intoxications. *Clin Pharmacokinet* 7:465-489, 1982.

Penn AS, et al: Drugs, coma, and myoglobinuria. *Neurology* 21:453, 1971.

Metal Antagonists

Caillie-Bertrand MV, et al: Oral zinc sulfate for Wilson's disease. *Arch Dis Child* 60:656-659, 1985.

Catsch A, Harmuth-Hoene AE: Pharmacology and therapeutic applications of agents used in heavy metal poisoning, in Levine WG (ed): *International Encyclopedia of Pharmacology and Therapeutics, Section 70, Chelation of Heavy Metals.* Oxford, Pergamon Press, 1979, 107-224.

Centers for Disease Control: *Preventing Lead Poisoning in Young Children.* Atlanta, GA, Department of Health and Human Services, (Jan) 1985.

Chisolm JJ Jr: Use of chelating agents in treatment of acute and chronic lead intoxication in childhood. *J Pediatr* 73:1-38, 1968.

Czajka PA, et al: Iron poisoning: In vitro comparison of bicarbonate and phosphate lavage solutions. *J Pediatr* 98:491-494, 1981.

Epstein O, et al: Reduction of immune complexes and immunoglobulins induced by D-penicillamine in primary biliary cirrhosis. *N Engl J Med* 300:274-278, 1979.

Epstein O, Sherlock S: Triethylene triamine dihydrochloride toxicity in primary biliary cirrhosis. *Gastroenterology* 78:1442-1445, 1980.

Fleming CR, et al: Asymptomatic primary biliary cirrhosis: Presentation, histology, and results with D-penicillamine. *Mayo Clin Proc* 53:587-593, 1978.

Graziano JH, et al: 2,3-dimercaptosuccinic acid as antidote for lead intoxication. *Clin Pharmacol Ther* 37:431-438, 1985.

Halliday JW, Bassett ML: Treatment of iron storage disorders. *Drugs* 20:207-215, 1980.

Hoogenraad TU, et al: Effective treatment of Wilson's disease with oral sulfate: Two case reports. *Br Med J* 289:273-276, 1984.

Jain S, et al: Controlled trial of D-penicillamine therapy in primary biliary cirrhosis. *Lancet* 1:831-834, 1977.

Klaassen CD: Heavy metals and heavy-metal antagonists, in Gilman AG, et al (eds): *The Pharmacological Basis of Therapeutics*, ed 7. New York, Macmillan, 1985, 1605-1627.

Krenzelok EP, Hoff JV: Accidental childhood iron poisoning: Problem of marketing and labeling. *Pediatrics* 63:591-596, 1979.

Lacouture PG, et al: Emergency assessment of severity in iron overdose by clinical and laboratory methods. *J Pediatr* 99:89-91, 1981.

Olivieri NF, et al: Visual and auditory neurotoxicity in patients receiving subcutaneous deferoxamine infusions. *N Engl J Med* 314:869-873, 1986.

Peterson RG, Rumack BH: D-penicillamine therapy of acute arsenic poisoning. *J Pediatr* 91:661-666, 1977.

Piomelli S, et al: Management of childhood lead poisoning. *J Pediatr* 105:523-532, 1984.

Rumack BH, Peterson RG: Clinical toxicology, in Doull J, et al (eds): *Toxicology: The Basic Science of Poisons,* ed 2. New York, Macmillan, 1980, 677-698.

Temple AR: Management of acute iron poisoning. Poisoning Symposium. Denver, March 9-13, 1981.

Walshe JM: Treatment of Wilson's disease with trientine (triethylene tetramine) dihydrochloride. *Lancet* 1:643-647, 1982.

Weatherall DJ, et al: Iron loading in thalassemia: Five years with the pump, (editorial). *N Engl J Med* 308:456-458, 1983.

Young N, et al: Treatment of primary hemochromatosis with deferoxamine. *JAMA* 241:1152-1154, 1979.

Opioid Antagonists

Azar I, et al: Cardiovascular response following naloxone administration during enflurane anesthesia. *Anesth Analg* 60:237-238, 1981.

Chiang CN, et al: Clinical evaluation of naltrexone sustained-release preparation. *Drug Alcohol Depend* 16:1-8, 1985.

Goldfrank LR, et al: Dosing nomogram for continuous infusion intravenous naloxone. *Ann Emerg Med* 15:566-570, 1986.

Hollister LE, et al: Aversive effects of naltrexone in subjects not dependent on opiates. *Drug Alcohol Depend* 8:37-41, 1981.

Johnstone RE, et al: Reversal of morphine anesthesia with naloxone. *Anesthesiology* 41:361-367, 1974.

Lovejoy FH Jr, et al: Management of propoxyphene poisoning. *J Pediatr* 85:98-100, 1974.

Martin WR: Naloxone. *Ann Intern Med* 85:765-768, 1976.

Meyer MC, et al: Bioequivalence, dose-proportionality, and pharmacokinetics of naltrexone after oral administration. *J Clin Psychiatry* 45(9, Sec 2):15-19, 1984.

Verebey K, et al: Naltrexone: Disposition, metabolism and effects after acute and chronic dosing. *Clin Pharmacol Ther* 20:315-328, 1976.

Acetylcysteine

Rumack BH, et al: Acetaminophen overdosage: 662 cases with evaluation of oral acetylcysteine treatment. *Arch Intern Med* 141:380-385, 1981.

Rumack BH, et al: Acetaminophen, in Haddad LM, Winchester JF (eds): *Clinical Management of Poisoning and Drug Overdose.* Philadelphia, WB Saunders, 1983, 562-575.

Cyanide Antagonists

Arena JM: Cyanide, in Haddad LM, Winchester JF (eds): *Clinical Management of Poisoning and Drug Overdose*. Philadelphia, WB Saunders, 1983, 744-747.

Cottrell JE, et al: Prevention of nitroprusside-induced cyanide toxicity with hydroxocobalamin. *N Engl J Med* 298:809-811, 1978.

Graham DL, et al: Acute cyanide poisoning complicated by lactic acidosis and pulmonary edema. *Arch Intern Med* 137:1051-1055, 1977.

Sylvester DM, et al: Effects of thiosulfate on cyanide pharmacokinetics in dogs. *Toxicol Appl Pharmacol* 69:265-271, 1983.

Ten Eyck RP, et al: Stroma-free methemoglobin solution as antidote for cyanide poisoning: Preliminary study. *Clin Toxicol* 21:343-358, 1984.

Way JL, et al: Recent perspectives on toxicodynamic basis of cyanide antagonism. *Fund Appl Toxicol* 4:S231-S239, 1984.

Pralidoxime

Hayes WJ Jr: *Toxicology of Pesticides*. Baltimore, Williams & Wilkins, 1975, 410-416.

Murphy SD: Pesticides, in Doull J, et al (eds): *Toxicology: The Basic Science of Poisons*, ed 3. New York, Macmillan, in press.

Methanol and Ethylene Glycol Poisoning

Blomstrand R, Ingemansson SO: Studies on effect of 4-methylpyrazole on methanol poisoning using the monkey as animal model: With particular reference to ocular toxicity. *Drug Alcohol Depend* 13:343-355, 1984.

Noker PE, et al: Methanol toxicity: Treatment with folic acid and 5-formyl tetrahydrofolic acid. *Alcoholism: Clin Exp Res* 4:378-383, 1980.

Peterson CD: Oral ethanol doses in patients with methanol poisoning. *Am J Hosp Pharm* 38:1024-1027, 1981.

Peterson CD, et al: Ethylene glycol poisoning: Pharmacokinetics during therapy with ethanol and hemodialysis. *N Engl J Med* 304:21-23, 1981 A.

Peterson CD, et al: Ethanol for ethylene glycol poisoning. *N Engl J Med* 304:977-978, 1981 B.

Swartz RD, et al: Epidemic methanol poisoning: Clinical and biochemical analysis of recent episode. *Medicine (Baltimore)* 60:373-382, 1981.

Manufacturers

Abbott Laboratories, Abbott Park, North Chicago, Illinois 60064

Acme United Corporation, 100 Hicks Street, Bridgeport, Connecticut 06608

Adria Laboratories, Inc., P.O. Box 16529, Columbus, Ohio 43216

Aeroceuticals Health Care Products, 1175 Post Road East, Westport, Connecticut 06880

Akorn, Inc., 100 Akorn Drive, Abita Springs, Louisiana 70420

Alcon Laboratories, Inc., 6201 South Freeway, Fort Worth, Texas 76101

Allergan Pharmaceuticals, 2525 Dupont Drive, Irvine, California 92713

Aloe Creme Laboratories, Inc, 2313 N.W. 30th Place, Pompano Beach, Florida 33060

Alpha Therapeutic Corporation, 5555 Valley Boulevard, Los Angeles, California 90032

Alza Corporation, 950 Page Mill Road, Palo Alto, California 94303-0802

American Critical Care, Division of American Hospital Supply Corporation, 1600 Waukegan Road, McGaw Park, Illinois 60085

American Dermal Corporation, 12 Worlds Fair Drive, Somerset, New Jersey 08873

American McGaw, Division of American Hospital Supply Corporation, 2525 McGaw Avenue, Irvine, California 92714

American Optical Corporation, Soft Contact Lens Division, 55 New York Avenue, Farmingham, Massachusetts 01701

Anaquest, Inc., 2005 W. Beltline Road, Madison, Wisconsin 53713

Armour Pharmaceutical Company, 303 S. Broadway, Tarrytown, New York 10591

Armour-Dial, Inc., Armour Research Center, 1510l N. Scottsdale Road, Scottsdale, Arizona 85260

B. F. Ascher & Company, Inc., 15501 West 109th Street, Lenexa, Kansas 66219

Ascot Pharmaceuticals, Inc., 7701 North Austin Avenue, Skokie, Illinois 60077

Astra Pharmaceutical Products, Inc., 50 Otis Street, Westborough, Massachusetts 01581-4428

Ayerst Laboratories, Division of American Home Products Corporation, 685 Third Avenue, New York, New York 10017

Barnes-Hind, Inc., Division of Revlon Health Care Group, 895 Kifer Road, Sunnyvale, California 94086

Bayer AG, 5090 Leverkusen, West Germany

Beach Pharmaceuticals, Division of Beach Products, Inc., 5220 S. Manhattan Avenue, Tampa, Florida 33611

Beecham Laboratories, Division of Beecham, Inc., 501 Fifth Street, Bristol, Tennessee 37620

Beiersdorf, Inc., P.O. Box 5529, Norwalk, Connecticut 06856

Berlex Laboratories Inc., 300 Fairfield Road, Wayne, New Jersey 07470

Biocraft Laboratories, Inc., 92 Route 46, Elmwood Park, New Jersey 07407

Bio Products, Inc., 2820 Columbiana Road, Suite 210, Birmingham, Alabama 35216

BioSearch Medical Products, Inc., 35 Industrial Parkway, Somerville, New Jersey 08876

Blair Laboratories, Inc., Subsidiary of Purdue Frederick Company, 100 Connecticut Avenue, Norwalk, Connecticut 06856

Bock Pharmacal Company, P.O. Box 8519, St. Louis, Missouri 63126

Boehringer Ingelheim Ltd., 90 East Ridge, Ridgefield, Connecticut 06877

Bolar Pharmaceutical Company, 130 Lincoln Street, Copiague, New York 11726

Boots Co., Thane Road, Nottingham NG2 3AA, Great Britain

Boots Pharmaceuticals, Inc., 6540 Line Avenue, Shreveport, Louisiana 71106

Bowman Pharmaceutical, Inc., 119 Schroyer Avenue Northwest, Canton, Ohio 44702

Braintree Laboratories, Inc., P.O. Box 361, Braintree, Massachusetts 02184

Bristol Laboratories, Division of Bristol-Myers Company, P.O. Box 4755, Syracuse, New York 13221-4755

Bristol-Myers Oncology, Division of Bristol-Myers Company, P.O. Box 4755, Syracuse, New York 13221-4755

Bristol-Myers Products, Division of Bristol-Myers Company, 345 Park Avenue, New York, New York 10154

Britannia Pharmaceuticals, Ltd., Hamilton House, 87/89 Bell Street, Reigate, Surrey, RH2 7Y2, Great Britain

Burroughs Wellcome Company, 3030 Cornwallis Road, Research Triangle Park, North Carolina 27709

C & M Pharmacal, Inc., 1519 E. Eight Mile Road, Hazel Park, Michigan 48030

CMC-Consolidated Midland Corporation, 195 East Main Street, Brewster, New York 10509

Carnrick Laboratories, Inc., 65 Horse Hill Road, Cedar Knolls, New Jersey 07927

Caswell-Massey Company, Ltd., 111 Eighth Avenue, New York, New York 10011

Central Pharmaceuticals, Inc., 110-128 E. Third Street, Seymour, Indiana 47274

Century Pharmaceuticals, Inc., 10377 Hague Road, Indianapolis, Indiana 46256

Chesebrough-Ponds, Inc., 33 Benedict Place, Greenwich, Connecticut 06830

Ciba Pharmaceutical Company, Division of Ciba-Geigy Corporation, 556 Morris Avenue, Summit, New Jersey 07901

Colgate-Hoyt, Division of Colgate-Palmolive Company, 909 River Road, Piscataway, New Jersey 08854

Commerce Drug Company, Division of Del Laboratories, Inc., 565 Broad Hollow Road, Farmingdale, New Jersey 11735

Connaught Laboratories, Inc., Swiftwater, Pennsylvania 18370

CooperVision, Inc., Mountain View Division, 455 E. Middlefield Road, Mountain View, California 94039

Cutter, Biological Division of Miles Laboratories, Inc., 2200 Powell Street, Emeryville, California 94662

Davis & Geck, American Cyanamid Company, One Cyanamid Plaza, Wayne, New Jersey 07470

Dermalab Inc., 400 Country Club Drive, Bensenville, Illinois 60106

Dermik Laboratories, Inc., 500 Virginia Drive, Ft. Washington, Pennsylvania 19034

Dey Laboratories, Inc., 10246 Miller Road, Dallas, Texas 75238

Dista Products Company, Division of Eli Lilly and Company, Indianapolis, Indiana 46285

Doak Pharmacal Company, Inc., 700 Shames Drive, Westbury, New York 11590

Dorsey Laboratories, Division of Sandoz, Inc., P.O. Box 83288, Lincoln, Nebraska 68501

Du Pont Pharmaceuticals, Inc., Subsidiary of E.I. du Pont de Nemours & Company, Inc., Wilmington, Delaware 19898

Edlaw Preparations, Inc., 195 B Central Avenue, Farmingdale, New York 11735

Elder Pharmaceuticals, Inc., 3300 Hyland Avenue, Costa Mesa, California 92626

Elea Laboratories Saladillo 2452, 1440 Buenos Aires, Argentina

Elkins-Sinn, Inc., Subsidiary of A. H. Robins Company, 2 Esterbrook Lane, Cherry Hill, New Jersey 08034

Ex-Lax Pharmaceutical Company, Inc., Division of Sandoz, Inc., 605 Third Avenue, New York, New York 10158

Farmitalia Carb Erba GmbH, Merzhauser Strasse 112, Postfach 480, 7800 Freiburg, West Germany

Ferndale Laboratories, Inc., 780 W. Eight Mile Road, Ferndale, Michigan 48220

Fisons Corporation, Two Preston Court, Bedford, Massachusetts 01730

C. B. Fleet Company, Inc., 4615 Murray Place, Lynchburg, Virginia 24506

Fleming & Company, 1600 Fenpark Drive, Fenton, Missouri 63026

Flint Laboratories, Division of Travenol Laboratories, Inc., 1425 Lake Cook Road, Deerfield, Illinois 60015

Forest Pharmaceuticals, Inc., Subsidiary of Forest Laboratories, Inc., 2510 Metro Boulevard, Maryland Heights, Missouri 63043

E. Fougera & Company, Division of Altanta, Inc., 60 Baylis Road, Melville, New York 11747

Geigy Pharmaceuticals, Division of Ciba-Geigy Corporation, Ardsley, New York 10502

Genderm Corporation, 425 Huehl Road, Northbrook, Illinois 60062

Genentech, Inc., 460 Point San Bruno Boulevard, South San Francisco, California 94080

Gerber Products Company, 445 State Street, Fremont, Michigan 49412

Geriatric Pharmaceutical Corporation, 1249 North Franklin Place, Milwaukee, Wisconsin 53202

Gilbert Laboratories, 31 Fairmont Avenue, Chester, New Jersey 07930

Glaxo, Inc., 5 Moore Drive, Research Triangle Park, North Carolina 27709

Glenbrook Laboratories, Division of Sterling Drug Inc., 90 Park Avenue, New York, New York 10016

Glenwood Laboratories, Inc., 83 N. Summit Street, Tenafly, New Jersey 07670

Guardian Chemical Corporation, 230 Marcus Boulevard, Smithtown, New York 11787

Gulf Bio-Systems, Inc., 5310 Harvest Hill Road, Dallas, Texas 75230

W. E. Hauck, Inc., P.O. Box 1065, Roswell, Georgia 30075

Herbert Laboratories, 2525 Dupont Drive, Irvine, California 92715

Hermal Pharmaceutical Laboratories, Inc., Route 145, Oak Hill, New York 12460

Hoechst-Roussel Pharmaceuticals, Inc., Route 202-206 North, Somerville, New Jersey 08876

Holland-Rantos Company, Inc., 310 Enterprise Avenue, Trenton, New Jersey 08638

Hollister-Stier, Division of Miles Laboratories, Inc., 2535 N. Regal Street, Spokane, Washington 99207-3145

Hyland Therapeutics Division, Travenol Laboratories, Inc., 444 West Glenoaks Boulevard, Glendale, California 91202

Hynson, Westcott & Dunning, Inc., Charles & Chase Streets, Baltimore, Maryland 21201

Hyrex Pharmaceuticals, 3494 Democrat Road, Memphis, Tennessee 38118

ICI Pharmaceuticals, U.K. Imperial Chemical Industries Ltd., Pharmaceutical Division, Alderley Park, Macclesfield, Cheshire SK10 4TF, Great Britain

ICN Pharmaceuticals, Inc., 3300 Hyland Avenue, Costa Mesa California 92626

Immuno U.S., 1200 Parkdale Road, Rochester, Michigan 48063

Janssen Pharmaceutica, Inc., 40 Kingsbridge Road, Piscataway, New Jersey 08854

Jeffrey Martin, Inc., 410 Clermont Terrace, Union, New Jersey 07083

The Andrew Jergens Company, 2535 Spring Grove Avenue, Cincinnati, Ohio 45214

Johnson & Johnson Products, Inc., 501 George Street, New Brunswick, New Jersey 08903

KabiVitrum, Inc., 1131 Harbor Bay Parkway, Alameda, California 94501

Kay Pharmacal Company, Inc., P.O. Box 50375, 1312 N. Utica Avenue, Tulsa, Oklahoma 74150

Keene Pharmaceuticals, Inc., P.O. Box 7, Keene, Texas 76059

Key Pharmaceuticals, Inc., 4400 Biscayne Boulevard, Miami, Florida 33137

Knoll Pharmaceutical Company, 30 N. Jefferson Road, Whippany, New Jersey 07981

Kremers-Urban Company, see William H. Rorer., Inc.

Lactaid, Inc., 600 Fire Road, Pleasantville, New Jersey 08232

Lafayette Pharmacal, Inc., 4200 South Halen Street, Fort Worth, Texas 76109

Lakeside Pharmaceuticals, Division of Merrell Dow Pharmaceuticals, Inc., P.O. Box 429553, Cincinnati, Ohio 45242-9553

The Lannett Company, Inc., 9000 State Road, Philadelphia, Pennsylvania 79136

Laser, Inc., 2000 N. Main Street, Crown Point, Indiana 46307

Lederle Laboratories, Division of American Cyanamid Company, Pearl River, New York 10965

Leeming Division, Pfizer, Inc., 100 Jefferson Road, Parsippany, New Jersey 07054

Legere Pharmaceuticals, Inc., 7326 East Evans Road, Scottsdale, Arizona 85260

Lemmon Company, P.O. Box 630, Sellersville, Pennsylvania 18960

Lilly Research Laboratories, Division of Eli Lilly and Company, Indianapolis, Indiana 46285

Loma Linda Food Company, 11503 Pierce Street, Riverside, California 92515

Lyphomed, Inc., 2020 Ruby Street, Melrose Park, Illinois 60130

Mallard, Inc., 3021 Wabash Avenue, Detroit, Michigan 48216

Mallinckrodt, Inc., 675 McDonnell Boulevard, St. Louis, Missouri 63134

Marion Laboratories, Inc., P.O. Box 9627, Kansas City, Missouri 64134

Maurry Biological Co., Inc., 6109 South Western Avenue, Los Angeles, California 90047

Mayrand Inc., 4 Dundas Circle, Greensboro, North Carolina 27419

McNeil Consumer Products Company, McNeilab Inc., Fort Washington, Pennsylvania 19034

McNeil Pharmaceutical, McNeilab, Inc., Spring House, Pennsylvania 19477

Mead Johnson & Company, 2404 West Pennyslvania Street, Evansville, Indiana 47721

Medco Research, Inc., 8733 Beverly Boulevard, Los Angeles, California 90048

Med-Corp, Division of Life Medical Systems, Inc., 5310 Harvest Hill Road, Dallas, Texas 75230

Medical Market Specialties, Inc., P.O. Box 307, Cedar Grove, New Jersey 07009

Medicone Company, 225 Varick Street, New York, New York 10014

Menley & James Laboratories, A Smith Kline Beckman Company, P.O. Box 8082, Philadelphia, Pennsylvania 19101

The Mentholatum Company, 1360 Niagra Street, Buffalo, New York 14213

Merck Sharp & Dohme, Division of Merck & Co., Inc., West Point, Pennsylvania 19486

Merieux Institute, Inc., 7855 N.W. 12th Street, Suite 114, Miami, Florida 33126

Merrell Dow Pharmaceuticals, Inc., Subsidiary of The Dow Chemical Company, 2110 E. Galbraith Road, Cincinnati, Ohio 45215

Miles Pharmaceuticals, Division of Miles Laboratories, Inc., 400 Morgan Lane, West Haven, Connecticut 06516

Misemer Pharmaceutical, Inc., 4553 South Campbell, Springfield, Missouri 68507

Mission Pharmacal Company, P.O. Box 1676, San Antonio, Texas 78296

Montedison Farmaceutica, Arcos 2626, Buenos Aires, Argentina

Muro Pharmaceutical, Inc., 890 East Street, Tewksbury, Massachusetts 01876

Neutrogena Dermatologics, Division of Neutrogena Corporation, 5755 West 96th Street, Los Angeles, California 90045

Newport Pharmaceuticals International 897 W. 16th Street, Newport Beach, California 92660-0147

Norcliff Thayer, Inc., 303 South Broadway, Tarrytown, New York 10591

Nordisk-USA, 6500 Rock Spring Drive, Suite 304, Bethesda, Maryland 20817

Norwich Eaton Pharmaceuticals, Inc., P.O. Box 191, Norwich, New York 13815

Organon, Inc., 375 Mount Pleasant Avenue, West Orange, New Jersey 07052

Ortho Pharmaceutical Corporation, Route 202, Raritan, New Jersey 08869

Otis Clapp, l43 Albany Street, Cambridge, Massachusetts 02139

Owen Laboratories, 6201 South Freeway, P.O. Box 1959, Fort Worth, Texas 76101

Paddock Laboratories, Inc., 3101 Louisiana Avenue, North, Minneapolis, Minnesota 55427

Parke-Davis, Division of Warner-Lambert Company, 201 Tabor Road, Morris Plains, New Jersey 07950

Pedinol Pharmacal, Inc., 30 Banfi Plaza North, Farmingdale, New York 11735

Pennwalt Corporation, Pharmaceutical Division, 755 Jefferson Road, Rochester, New York 14623

Person & Covey, Inc., 616 Allen Avenue, Glendale, California 91201

The Pfeiffer Company, 43-45 North Washington Avenue, Wilkes Barre, Pennsylvania 18701

Pfipharmecs Division, Pfizer, Inc., 235 E. 42nd Street, New York, New York 10017

Pfizer, Inc., Laboratories Division, 235 E. 42nd Street, New York, New York 10017

Pharmacia, Inc., 800 Centennial Avenue, Piscataway, New Jersey 08854

Pharmacraft Division, Pennwalt Corporation, 755 Jefferson Road, Rochester, New York 14623

PharmFair, Inc., 110 Kennedy Drive, Houppauge, New York 11788

Plough, Inc., P.O. Box 377, Memphis, Tennessee 38151

Poythress Laboratories, Inc., 16 N. 22nd Street, Richmond, Virginia 23261

Proctor & Gamble Company, Cincinnati, Ohio 45201

The Purdue Frederick Company, 100 Connecticut Avenue, Norwalk, Connecticut 06856

Racei Laboratories, 330 South Kellogg, Building M, Goleta, California 93017

Rachelle Laboratories, Inc., Subsidiary of International Rectifier Corporation, 700 Henry Ford Avenue, Long Beach, California 90810

Reed & Carnrick, 1 New England Avenue, Piscataway, New Jersey 08854

Reid-Provident Laboratories, see Reid-Rowell, Inc.

Reid-Rowell, Inc., 640 Tenth Street N.W., Atlanta, Georgia 30318

Republic Drug Company, Inc., 175 Great Arrow, Buffalo, New York 14207

Requa Mfg. Co., Inc., 1 Seneca Place, Greenwich, Connecticut 06830

Research Industries Corporation, Pharmaceutical Division, 1847 West 2300 South, Salt Lake City, Utah 84119

Riker Laboratories, Inc., Subsidiary of 3M Company, 225-15-07 3M Center, St. Paul, Minnesota 55144

A. H. Robins Company, 1211 Sherwood Avenue, Richmond, Virginia 23220

Roche Laboratories, Division of Hoffmann-LaRoche, Inc., Nutley, New Jersey 07110

Roerig, Division of Pfizer Pharmaceuticals, 235 E. 42nd Street, New York, New York 10017

William H. Rorer, Inc., 500 Virginia Drive, Fort Washington, Pennsylvania 19034

Ross Laboratories, Division of Abbott Laboratories, 625 Cleveland Avenue, Columbus, Ohio 43216

Rowell Laboratories,Inc., see Reid-Rowell, Inc.

Roxane Laboratories, Inc., 330 Oak Street, Columbus, Ohio 43216

Rugby Laboratories, Inc., 20 Nassau Avenue, Rockville Centre, New York 11570

Rydelle Laboratories, Inc., 1525 Howe Street, Racine, Wisconsin 53403

Sandoz Pharmaceuticals, Division of Sandoz, Inc., 59 Route 10, East Hanover, New Jersey 07936

Sandoz Nutrition, Clinical Nutrition Division, 5320 West Twentythird Street, Minneapolis, Minnesota 55440

Sanofi Pharmaceuticals, Inc., 101 Park Avenue, New York, New York 10178

Savage Laboratories, Division of Altanta, Inc., 60 Baylis Road, Melville, New York 11747

Schein Pharmaceutical, Inc., 5 Harbor Park Drive, Port Washington, New York 11050

Schering Corporation, Galloping Hill Road, Kenilworth, New Jersey 07033

Schmid Products Company, Division of Schmid Laboratories, Inc., Route 46 West, Little Falls, New Jersey 07424

Sclavo, Inc., 5 Mansord Court, Wayne, New Jersey 07470

G. D. Searle & Company, 4901 Searle Parkway, Skokie, Illinois 60077

The Seatrace Company, P.O. Box 363, Gadsen, Alabama 35902

Seres Laboratories, Inc., 3331 Industrial Drive, Santa Rosa, California 95402

Serono Laboratories, Inc., 280 Pond Street, Randolph, Massachusetts 02368

Siegfried FBK, Mumphfer-Faehrster 68, Saeckingen/Baden, West Germany

Sherwood Laboratories, Inc., 160l East 361st Street, Willoughby, Ohio 44094

Sigma Tau, Inc., 723 North Beers Street, Holmdel, New Jersey 07733

Smith Laboratories, Inc., 2211 Sanders Road, Northbrook, Illinois 60062

Smith Kline & French Laboratories, 1900 Market Street, Philadelphia, Pennsylvania 19101

Spencer-Mead Inc., 270 W. Merrick Road, Valley Stream, New York 11582

E. R. Squibb & Sons, Inc., P.O. Box 4000, Princeton, New Jersey 08540

Squibb/Connaught, Inc., 330 Alexander Street, Princeton, New Jersey 08540

Squibb-Novo, Inc., 120 Alexander Street, Princeton, New Jersey 08540

Stiefel Laboratory, Inc., 2801 Ponce de Leon Boulevard, Coral Gables, Florida 33134

Stuart Pharmaceuticals, Division of ICI Americas, Inc., Wilmington, Delaware 19897

Surgikos, Inc., Division of Johnson & Johnson, P.O. Box 130, Arlington, Texas 76010

Syntex Laboratories, Inc., 3401 Hillview Avenue, Palo Alto, California 94303

Syosset Laboratories, 150 Eileen Way, Syosset, New York 11791

TAP Pharmaceuticals, 1400 Sheridan Road, North Chicago, Illinois 60064

3M Personal Care Products, 223-1N-08, St. Paul, Minnesota 55144

Travenol Laboratories, Inc., 1425 Lake Cook Road, Deerfield, Illinois 60015

Trimen Laboratories, Inc., 80 26th Street, Pittsburgh, Pennsylvania 15222

Ulmer Pharmacal, 2440 Fernbrook Lane, Plymouth, Minnesota 55441

The Upjohn Company, 7000 Portage Road, Kalamazoo, Michigan 49001

Upsher-Smith Laboratories, Inc., 14905 23rd Avenue North, Minneapolis, Minnesota 55441

U.S. Products, Inc., 12555 Biscayne Boulevard, North Maimi, Florida 33181

USV Laboratories, 303 S. Broadway, Tarrytown, New York 10591

The Vale Chemical Company, Inc., 1201 Liberty Street, Allentown, Pennsylvania 18102

Vestal Laboratories, 5075 Manchester Avenue, St. Louis, Missouri 63110

Vicks Health Care, Division of Richardson-Vicks Inc., 10 Westport Road, Wilton, Connecticut 06897

Vicks Pharmacy Products, Division of Richardson-Vicks, Inc., 10 Westport Road, Wilton, Connecticut 06897

VioBin Corporation, Subsidiary of A.H. Robins Company, 226 W. Livingston Street, Monticello, Illinois 61856

Vitaline Formulas, P.O. Box 6757, Incline Village, Nevada 89450

Vortech Pharmaceuticals, Ltd., P.O. Box 189, Dearborn, Michigan 48123

Wallace Laboratories, Division of Carter-Wallace, Inc., P.O. Box 1, Cranbury, New Jersey 08512

Warner/Lambert Company, 201 Tabor Road, Morris Plains, New Jersey 07950

Webcon Pharmaceuticals Division, Alcon Laboratories, Inc., 6201 South Freeway, Fort Worth, Texas 76101

West Chemical Products, Inc., 1855 S. Mt. Prospect Road, Des Plaines, Illinois 60618

Westwood Pharmaceuticals Inc., 100 Forest Avenue, Buffalo, New York 14213

Wharton Laboratories, Inc., 37-02 Forty-Eighth Avenue, Long Island City, New York 11101

Whitehall Laboratories, Division of American Home Products Corporation, 685 Third Avenue, New York, New York 10017

Willen Drug Company, 18 N. High Street, Baltimore, Maryland 21202

The J.B. Williams Company, Inc., 750 Walnut Avenue, Cranford, New Jersey 07016

Winthrop-Breon Laboratories, 90 Park Avenue, New York, New York 10016

Wyeth Laboratories, Division of American Home Products Corporation, P.O. Box 8299, Philadelphia, Pennsylvania 19101

W.F. Young, Inc., 111 Lyman Street, Springfield, Massachusetts 01103

Youngs Drug Products Corporation, 865 Centennial Avenue, Piscataway, New Jersey 08854